DAVIS'S DRUG GUIDE AT A GLANCE

BEERS REMS HIGH ALERT

meperidine (me-per-i-deen)
Demerol

Classification
Therapeutic: opioid analgesics
Pharmacologic: opioid agonists

Schedule II

Risk Evaluation and Mitigation Systems (REMS) Icon

The Beers Criteria for Potentially Inappropriate Medication Use in Older Adults

RED tab for High Alert medications

Icon for pharmacogenomic content

Life-threatening side effects in **RED**, CAPITALIZED letters

Drug-drug, drug-food, and drug-natural product interactions

Headings highlighting considerations for patient populations

- Geri—concerns for older adults
- OB and Lact—information for pregnant and breastfeeding patients
- Pedi—concerns for children
- Rep—considerations for patients of reproductive age

HIGH ALERT

warfarin (war-fa-rin)
Coumadin, Jantoven

Classification
Therapeutic: anticoagulants
Pharmacologic: coumarins

Indications
Prophylaxis and treatment of: Venous thrombosis, Pulmonary embolism, Atrial fibrillation with embolization. Management of myocardial infarction: Decreases risk of death, Decreases risk of subsequent MI, Decreases risk of future thromboembolic events. Prevention of thrombus formation and embolization after prosthetic valve placement.

Action
Interferes with hepatic synthesis of vitamin K-dependent clotting factors (II, VII, IX, and X). **Therapeutic Effects:** Prevention of thromboembolic events.

Pharmacokinetics
Absorption: Well absorbed from the GI tract after oral administration.
Distribution: Crosses the placenta but does not enter breast milk.
Protein Binding: 99%.
Metabolism and Excretion: Metabolized by the liver.
Half-life: 42 hr.

TIME/ACTION PROFILE (effects on coagulation tests)

ROUTE	ONSET	PEAK	DURATION
PO	36–72 hr	5–7 days†	2–5 days‡

†At a constant dose
‡After discontinuation

Contraindications/Precautions
Contraindicated in: Uncontrolled bleeding; Open wounds; Active ulcer disease; Recent brain, eye, or spinal cord injury or surgery; Severe liver or kidney disease; Uncontrolled hypertension; OB: Crosses placenta and may cause fatal hemorrhage in the fetus. May also cause congenital malformation.
Use Cautiously in: Malignancy; Patients with history of ulcer, liver disease, or acute kidney injury; History of poor compliance; Asian patients or those who carry the CYP2C9*2 allele and/or the CYP2C9*3 allele, or with the VKORC1 AA genotype (↑ risk of bleeding with standard dosing; lower initial doses should be considered); Geri: Due to greater than expected anticoagulant response, initiate and maintain at lower doses; Rep: Women of reproductive potential; Pedi: Has been used safely but may require more frequent PT/INR assessments.

Adverse Reactions/Side Effects
Derm: dermal necrosis. **GI:** cramps, nausea. **GU:** CALCIPHYLAXIS. **Hemat:** BLEEDING. **Misc:** fever.

Interactions
Drug-Drug: Androgens, capecitabine, cefotetan, chloramphenicol, clopidogrel, disulfiram, fluconazole, fluoroquinolones, itraconazole, metronidazole (including vaginal use), **thrombolytics, eptifibatide, tirofiban, sulfonamides, quinidine, quinine, NSAIDs, valproates,** and **aspirin** may ↑ the response to warfarin and ↑ the risk of bleeding. Chronic use of **acetaminophen** may ↑ the risk of bleeding. Chronic **alcohol** ingestion may ↓ action of warfarin; if chronic **alcohol** abuse results in significant liver damage, action of warfarin may be ↑ due to ↓ production of clotting factor. Acute **alcohol** ingestion may ↑ action of warfarin. **Barbiturates, carbamazepine, rifampin,** and **hormonal contraceptives containing estrogen** may ↓ the anticoagulant response to warfarin. **Many other drugs** may affect the activity of warfarin.
Drug-Natural Products: St. John's wort ↓ effect. ↑ bleeding risk with **anise, arnica, chamomile, clove, dong quai, fenugreek, feverfew, garlic, ginger, ginkgo, Panax ginseng, licorice,** and others.
Drug-Food: Ingestion of large quantities of **foods high in vitamin K content** (see list in Appendix K) may antagonize the anticoagulant effect of warfarin.

Route/Dosage
PO (Adults): 2–5 mg/day for 2–4 days; then adjust daily dose by results of INR. Initiate therapy with lower doses in geriatric or debilitated patients or in Asian patients or those with CYP2C9*2 and/or CYP2C9*3 alleles or VKORC1 AA genotype.
PO (Children >1 mo): *Initial loading dose*—0.2 mg/kg (maximum dose: 10 mg) for 2–4 days then adjust daily dose by results of INR, use 0.1 mg/kg if liver dysfunction is present. *Maintenance dose range*—0.05–0.34 mg/kg/day.

Availability (generic available)
Tablets: 1 mg, 2 mg, 2.5 mg, 3 mg, 4 mg, 5 mg, 6 mg, 7.5 mg, 10 mg. **Cost:** *Generic*—1 mg $10.83/100, 2 mg $10.83/100, 2.5 mg $10.83/100, 3 mg $10.83/100, 4 mg $10.83/100, 5 mg $8.52/100, 6 mg $10.64/100, 7.5 mg $10.83/100, 10 mg $10.83/100.

NURSING IMPLICATIONS

Assessment
- Assess for signs of bleeding and hemorrhage (bleeding gums; nosebleed; unusual bruising; tarry, black stools; hematuria; fall in hematocrit or BP; guaiac-positive stools, urine, or nasogastric aspirate).

= Canadian drug name. = Genetic implication. ~~Strikethrough~~ = Discontinued.
*CAPITALS indicates life-threatening; underlines indicate most frequent.

Clearly defined nursing responsibilities and priorities

NURSING IMPLICATIONS

Assessment

- Assess for signs of bleeding and hemorrhage (bleeding gums; nosebleed; unusual bruising; tarry, black stools; hematuria; fall in hematocrit or BP; guaiac-positive stools, urine, or nasogastric aspirate).
- Assess for evidence of additional or increased thrombosis. Symptoms depend on area of involvement.
- ***Lab Test Considerations:*** Monitor PT, INR and other clotting factors frequently during therapy; monitor more frequently in patients with renal impairment. Therapeutic PT ranges 1.3–1.5 times greater than control; however, the INR, a standardized system that provides a common basis for communicating and interpreting PT results, is usually referenced. Normal INR (not on anticoagulants) is 0.8–1.2. An INR of 2.5–3.5 is recommended for patients at very high risk of embolization (for example, patients with mitral valve replacement and ventricular hypertrophy). Lower levels are acceptable when risk is lower. Heparin may affect the PT/INR; draw blood for PT/INR in patients receiving both heparin and warfarin at least 5 hr after the IV bolus dose, 4 hr after cessation of IV infusion, or 24 hr after subcut heparin injection. Asian patients and those who carry the CYP2C9*2 allele and/or the CYP2C9*3 allele, or those with VKORC1 AA genotype may require more frequent monitoring and lower doses.
- Geri: Patients over 60 yr exhibit greater than expected PT/INR response. Monitor for side effects at lower therapeutic ranges.
- Pedi: Achieving and maintaining therapeutic PT/INR ranges may be more difficult in pediatric patients. Assess PT/INR levels more frequently.
- Monitor hepatic function and CBC before and periodically throughout therapy.
- Monitor stool and urine for occult blood before and periodically during therapy.
- ***Toxicity and Overdose:*** Withholding 1 or more doses of warfarin is usually sufficient if INR is excessively elevated or if minor bleeding occurs. If overdose occurs or anticoagulation needs to be immediately reversed, the antidote is vitamin K (phytonadione, Aquamephyton). Administration of whole blood or plasma also may be required in severe bleeding because of the delayed onset of vitamin K.

Implementation

- ***High Alert:*** Do not confuse Coumadin (warfarin) with Avandia (rosiglitazone) or Cardura (doxazosin). Do not confuse Jantoven (warfarin) with Janumet (sitagliptin/metformin) or Januvia (sitagliptin).
- Because of the large number of medications capable of significantly altering warfarin's effects, careful monitoring is recommended when new agents are started or other agents are discontinued. Interactive potential should be evaluated for all new medications (Rx, OTC, and herbal products).
- **PO:** Administer medication at same time each day. Medication requires 3–5 days to reach effective levels; usually begun while patient is still on heparin.
- Do not interchange brands; potencies may not be equivalent.

In-depth guidance for patient and family education

Patient/Family Teaching

- Instruct patient to take medication as directed. Take missed doses as soon as remembered that day; do not double doses. Inform health care professional of missed doses at time of checkup or lab tests. Inform patients that anticoagulant effect may persist for 2–5 days following discontinuation. Advise patient to read *Medication Guide* before starting therapy and with each Rx refill in case of changes.
- Review foods high in vitamin K (see Appendix K). Patient should have consistent limited intake of these foods, as vitamin K is the antidote for warfarin, and alternating intake of these foods will cause PT levels to fluctuate. Advise patient to avoid cranberry juice or products during therapy.
- Caution patient to avoid IM injections and activities leading to injury. Instruct patient to use a soft toothbrush, not to floss, and to shave with an electric razor during warfarin therapy. Advise patient that venipunctures and injection sites require application of pressure to prevent bleeding or hematoma formation.
- Advise patient to report any symptoms of unusual bleeding or bruising (bleeding gums; nosebleed; black, tarry stools; hematuria; excessive menstrual flow) and pain, color, or temperature change to any area of your body to health care professional immediately. Patients with a deficiency in protein C and/or S mediated anticoagulant response may be at greater risk for tissue necrosis.
- Instruct patient not to drink alcohol or take other Rx, OTC, or herbal products, especially those containing aspirin or NSAIDs, or to start or stop any new medications during warfarin therapy without advice of health care professional.
- Advise patient to notify health care professional if pregnancy is planned or suspected or if breast feeding.
- Instruct patient to carry identification describing medication regimen at all times and to inform all health care personnel caring for patient on anticoagulant therapy before lab tests, treatment, or surgery.
- Emphasize the importance of frequent lab tests to monitor coagulation factors.

More patient safety information than any other drug guide

Evaluation/Desired Outcomes

- Prolonged PT (1.3–2.0 times the control; may vary with indication) or INR of 2–4.5 without signs of hemorrhage.

= Canadian drug name. = Genetic implication. ~~Strikethrough~~ = Discontinued.
*CAPITALS indicates life-threatening; underlines indicate most frequent.

Find enhanced Canadian content throughout—in the monographs, appendices, and index.

STOP Med Errors

DAVIS'S DRUG GUIDE for NURSES®

SEVENTEENTH EDITION

April Hazard Vallerand, PhD, RN, FAAN
Director, PhD Program
Distinguished Professor
College of Nursing Alumni Endowed Professor
Wayne State University
College of Nursing
Detroit, Michigan

Cynthia A. Sanoski, BS, PharmD, BCPS, FCCP
Department Chair and Associate Professor
Thomas Jefferson University
Jefferson School of Pharmacy
Philadelphia, Pennsylvania

F.A. DAVIS
Philadelphia

F. A. Davis Company
1915 Arch Street
Philadelphia, PA 19103
www.fadavis.com

Printed in the United States of America

Last digit indicates print number 10 9 8 7 6 5 4 3 2 1
Editor-in-Chief, Nursing: Jean Rodenberger
Acquisitions Editor: Megan Klim
Content Project Manager: Amanda M. Minutola

NOTE: As new scientific information becomes available through basic and clinical research, recommended treatments and drug therapies undergo changes. The authors and publisher have done everything possible to make this book accurate, up to date, and in accord with accepted standards at the time of publication. However, the reader is advised always to check product information (package inserts) for changes and new information regarding dose and contraindications before administering any drug. Caution is especially urged when using new or infrequently ordered drugs.

Library of Congress Cataloging-in-Publication Data

Names: Vallerand, April Hazard, author. | Sanoski, Cynthia A., author.
Title: Davis's drug guide for nurses / April Hazard Vallerand, Cynthia A. Sanoski.
Other titles: Drug guide for nurses
Description: Seventeenth edition. | Philadelphia, PA : F.A. Davis Company, [2021] | Includes bibliographical references and index.
Identifiers: LCCN 2020000824 | ISBN 9781719640053 (hardback) | ISBN 9781719641135 (ebook)
Subjects: MESH: Pharmaceutical Preparations--administration & dosage | Drug Therapy--nursing | Pharmacology, Clinical--methods | Handbook | Nurses Instruction
Classification: LCC RM301.12 | NLM QV 735 | DDC 615.102/4613--dc23
LC record available at https://lccn.loc.gov/2020000824

DEDICATION

To my son, Ben, whose sensitivity and sense of humor make even the toughest day easier.
To my daughter, Katharine, whose dedication and passion in seeking her goals I admire.
Watching you both grow to become wonderful young adults gives me such pride and joy. Your support of my work inspires me. Thank you for sharing so much of your lives with me. I love you.

AHV

To my wonderful mother, Geraldine, who has provided her continual love, support, and wisdom as I continue to pursue all of my personal and professional goals.

CAS

ACKNOWLEDGMENTS

We offer our thanks to the students and nurses who have used our book for more than 30 years. We hope our book provides you with the current knowledge of pharmacotherapeutics you need to continue to give quality care in our rapidly changing health care environment.

April and Cindy

CONSULTANTS

Jamie Crawley, PhD, RN
Assistant Professor
University of Windsor
Faculty of Nursing
Windsor, ON, Canada

Wanda Edwards, PMHCNS-BC, NP
Instructor (Clinical)
Wayne State University
College of Nursing
Detroit, MI

Linda Felver, PhD, RN
Associate Professor
Oregon Health & Science University
School of Nursing
Portland, OR

Althea DuBose-Hayes, RD
Renal Dietitian
Greenfield Health System,
a division of Henry Ford Health System
Southfield, MI

Debbie Richmond, NP-C, ACRN
Wayne State University
Detroit, MI

Gladdi Tomlinson, RN, MSN
Professor of Nursing
Harrisburg Area Community College
Harrisburg, PA

Reviewers

Brandy Haley, PhD, RN
Dean of Nursing
University of Arkansas at Monticello
Monticello, Arkansas

Christina D. Brazier, MSN, BSN, RN
RN Instructor
West Georgia Technical College, School of Nursing
Waco, Georgia

Denise Dion, MSN-Ed, PCCN, CNE, RN
Director of Nursing
Central Arizona College
Coolidge, Arizona

Cinthia DosSantos Mesquita, MSN, RN
Nursing Instructor
Assabet Valley Regional Technical High School
Practical Nursing Program
Marlborough, Massachusetts

Becky L. Fields, PhD, RN
Nursing Program Director
Roane State Community College
Harriman, Tennessee

Concetta S. Fiorentino, DNP, RN, CNE, PCCN
Assistant Professor
Montgomery County Community College
Blue Bell, Pennsylvania

Joely T. Goodman, PhD, MSN, RN
Assistant Professor/Faculty Chair
Creighton University
Hastings, Nebraska

Dawn McLaughlin, MSN-MHA, RN
Associate Dean of Nursing
Rasmussen College
Ocala, Florida

Cynthia V. Olivas, DNP, RN
Interim Nursing Program Director
Doña Ana Community College
Las Cruces, New Mexico

Frenchy Savage, MSN, RN
Nursing Instructor
Dorsey Schools
Wayne, Michigan

Rachel Unger, RN, MSN
Staff Development, Quality Nurse, Instructor
Itasca Community College
Grand Rapids, Minnesota

Elizabeth Pettit, RN, MSN, CNE, CHSE
Assistant Nursing Professor
Pellissippi State Community College
Knoxville, Tennessee

Canadian Reviewers

Anan Ahmed, BSP, MSc, CDE
Pharmacist
University of Saskatchewan
Saskatoon, Saskatchewan

Duncan (Stewart) MacLennan, MN, PhD(c), NP
Assistant Teaching Professor and Nurse Practitioner
University of Alberta
Edmonton, Alberta

Kerry Mansell, BSP, PharmD, BA, MBA
Professor of Pharmacy
College of Pharmacy and Nutrition
University of Saskatchewan
Saskatoon, Saskatchewan

Wendy Neander, PhD (c), MN, BScN, BScv
Assistant Teaching Professor
School of Nursing
University of Victoria
Nanaimo, British Columbia

Jim Wohlgemuth, RN, MN, CTN-B
Instructor, Nursing Education & Health Studies
Grande Prairie Regional College
Grande Prairie, Alberta

CONTENTS

HOW TO USE *DAVIS'S DRUG GUIDE FOR NURSES*

Davis's Drug Guide for Nurses provides comprehensive, up-to-date drug information in well-organized, nursing-focused monographs. It also includes extensive supplemental material in 14 appendices, thoroughly addresses the issue of safe medication administration, and educates the reader about 50 different therapeutic classes of drugs. In this 17th edition, we have continued the tradition of focusing on safe medication administration by including **Medication Safety Tools** and even more information about health care's most vulnerable patients: children, the elderly, pregnant women, and breast feeding mothers. Look for more Pedi, Geri, OB, and Lactation headings throughout the monographs. We have also included a BEERS label at the top of applicable drug monographs for those medications listed in the Beers Criteria developed by the American Geriatrics Society. These medications are considered to be potentially inappropriate for use in older adults because they are associated with more risk than benefit in this patient population. In addition, we've included information relevant to Canadian students and nurses. You'll find an appendix comparing Canadian and U.S. pharmaceutical practices, more Canada-only combination drugs in the Combination Drugs appendix, and additional Canadian brand names in the drug monographs. To help you find this information quickly, we've also added a maple leaf icon (🍁) in the index next to each Canadian entry. We have added pharmacogenomic information throughout numerous monographs to guide the nurse in selecting and monitoring various drug therapies. To help you find this information quickly, we've added a double helix icon (🧬) to denote this information as it applies to specific drugs. Use this book to enhance your competence in implementing and evaluating medication therapies. The following sections describe the organization of *Davis's Drug Guide for Nurses* and explain how to quickly find the information you need.

Safe Medication Use Articles

"Medication Errors: Improving Practices and Patient Safety," "Detecting and Managing Adverse Drug Reactions," "Overview of Risk Evaluation and Mitigation Systems (REMS)," "Special Dosing Considerations," and "Educating Patients About Safe Medication Use" comprise the safe medication use articles and provide an overview of the medication safety issues that confront practitioners and patients. Leading off this series, the medication errors article familiarizes you with the systems issues and clinical situations repeatedly implicated in medication errors and suggests practical means to avoid them. It also teaches you about *high alert* medications, which have a greater potential to cause patient harm than other medications. "Detecting and Managing Adverse Drug Reactions" explains the different types of adverse reactions and provides guidance on how to detect and manage them. "Risk Evaluation and Mitigation Strategies (REMS)" explains strategies developed by the pharmaceutical industry and required by the Food and Drug Administration (FDA) to minimize adverse drug reactions from potentially dangerous drugs. We have highlighted the drugs that currently have approved REMS programs associated with their use by adding a REMS label at the top of applicable drug monographs. "Special Dosing Considerations" identifies the patient populations, such as neonates and patients with renal impairment, who require careful dose adjustments to ensure optimal therapeutic outcomes. "Educating Patients About Medication Use" reviews the most important teaching points for nurses to discuss with their patients and their families. In addition to these safety articles, other critical information is highlighted in red throughout the drug monographs. This allows the reader to quickly identify important information and to see how nursing practice, including assessment, implementation, and patient teaching, relates to it.

Classifications Profile

Medications in the same therapeutic class often share similar mechanisms of action, assessment guidelines, precautions, and interactions. The Classifications Profile provides summaries of the major therapeutic classifications used in *Davis's Drug Guide for Nurses*. It also provides patient teaching information common to all agents within the class and a list of drugs within each class.

Medication Safety Tools

Updated for this edition is a section with tables and charts that nurses can use for a quick but thorough reference to information that will help them avoid making medication errors. It includes lists of drugs that are associated with adverse reactions and falls in the elderly; proper dosing for pediatric intravenous medications; confused drug names; FDA-approved Tall Man letters and more.

Drug Monographs

Drug monographs are organized in the following manner:

High Alert Status: Some medications, such as chemotherapeutic agents, anticoagulants, and insulins, have a greater potential for harm than others. These medications have been identified by the *Institute for Safe Medication Practices* as **high alert drugs**. *Davis's Drug Guide for Nurses* includes a high alert tab in the upper right corner of the monograph header in appropriate medications to alert the nurse to the medication's risk. The term "high alert" is used in other parts of the monograph as well, to help the nurse administer these medications safely. See the article "Medication Errors: Improving Practices and Patient Safety" for a complete list of high alert medications in *Davis's Drug Guide for Nurses*. Refer to ISMP.org for all solutions, groups, and individual high alert drugs.

Generic/Brand Name: The generic name appears first, with a pronunciation key, followed by an alphabetical list of trade names. Canadian trade names are preceded by a maple leaf (🍁). Brand names that have been discontinued have a slash through them (~~Decadron~~). Common names, abbreviations, and selected foreign names are also included.

Classification: The therapeutic classification, which categorizes drugs by the disease state they are used to treat, appears first, followed by the pharmacologic classification, which is based on the drug's mechanism of action.

Controlled Substance Schedule: All drugs regulated by federal law are placed into one of five schedules, based on the drug's medicinal value, harmfulness, and potential for abuse or addiction. Schedule I drugs, the most dangerous and having no medicinal value, are not included in *Davis's Drug Guide for Nurses*. (See Appendix I for a description of the Schedule of Controlled Substances.)

Pregnancy Category: The FDA recently recommended discontinuation of the Pregnancy Category system (A, B, C, D, and X) since this categorization may not appropriately communicate the risk that a drug may have during pregnancy or breast feeding. Based on this guidance, the Pregnancy Categories have been removed from each of the drug monographs. These pregnancy letter categories have been replaced in drug prescribing information with a narrative summary that describes the potential risk of using the drug during pregnancy and breast feeding, as well as the potential impairment of fertility in women and men of reproductive potential. The drug monographs have been enhanced with this detailed information in these patient populations and highlighted by a *Rep* tag to call the user's attention to reproductive information.

Indications: Medications are approved by the FDA for specific disease states. This section identifies the diseases or conditions for which the drug is commonly used and includes significant unlabeled uses as well.

Action: This section contains a concise description of how the drug produces the desired therapeutic effect.

Pharmacokinetics: Pharmacokinetics refers to the way the body processes a medication by absorption, distribution, metabolism, and excretion. This section also includes information on the drug's half-life.

Absorption: Absorption describes the process that follows drug administration and its subsequent delivery to systemic circulation. If only a small fraction is absorbed following oral administration (diminished bioavailability), then the oral dose must be much greater than the parenteral dose.

Absorption into systemic circulation also follows other routes of administration such as topical, transdermal, intramuscular, subcutaneous, rectal, and ophthalmic routes. Drugs administered intravenously are 100% bioavailable.

Distribution: This section comments on the drug's distribution in body tissues and fluids. Distribution becomes important in choosing one drug over another, as in selecting an antibiotic that will penetrate the central nervous system to treat meningitis or in avoiding drugs that cross the placenta or concentrate in breast milk. Information on protein binding is included for drugs that are >95% bound to plasma proteins, which has implications for drug-drug interactions.

Metabolism and Excretion: Drugs are primarily eliminated from the body either by hepatic conversion to active or inactive compounds (metabolism or biotransformation) and subsequent excretion by the kidneys, or by renal elimination of unchanged drug. Therefore, drug metabolism and excretion information is important in determining dosage regimens and intervals for patients with impaired renal or hepatic function. The creatinine clearance (CCr) helps quantify renal function and guides dosage adjustments. Formulas to estimate CCr are included in Appendix F.

Half-Life: The half-life of a drug is the amount of time it takes for the drug concentration to decrease by 50% and roughly correlates with the drug's duration of action. Half-lives are given for drugs assuming the patient has normal renal or hepatic function. Conditions that alter the half-life are noted.

Time/Action Profile: The time/action profile table provides the drug's onset of action, peak effect, and duration of activity. This information can aid in planning administration schedules and allows the reader to appreciate differences in choosing one route over another.

Contraindications and Precautions: Situations in which drug use should be avoided are listed as contraindications. In general, most drugs are contraindicated in pregnancy or lactation, unless the potential benefits outweigh the possible risks to the mother or baby (e.g., anticonvulsants, antihypertensives, and antiretrovirals). Contraindications may be absolute (i.e., the drug in question should be avoided completely) or relative, in which certain clinical situations may allow cautious use of the drug. The precautions portion includes disease states or clinical situations in which drug use involves particular risks or in which dosage modification may be necessary. Extreme cautions are noted separately to draw attention to conditions under which use of the drug results in serious, potentially life-threatening consequences.

Adverse Reactions and Side Effects: Although it is not possible to include all reported reactions, major side effects for all drugs are included. Life-threatening adverse reactions or side effects are **CAPITALIZED**, and the most frequent side effects are <u>underlined</u>. Those underlined generally have an incidence of 10% or greater. Those not underlined occur in fewer than 10% but more than 1% of patients. Although life-threatening reactions may be rare (fewer than 1%), they are included because of their significance. The following abbreviations are used for body systems:

CNS: central nervous system
EENT: eye, ear, nose, and throat
Resp: respiratory
CV: cardiovascular
GI: gastrointestinal
GU: genitourinary
Derm: dermatologic
Endo: endocrinologic
F and E: fluid and electrolyte
Hemat: hematologic
Local: local
Metab: metabolic
MS: musculoskeletal
Neuro: neurologic
Misc: miscellaneous
Rep: reproductive

Interactions: Drug interactions are a significant risk for patients. As the number of medications a patient receives increases, so does the likelihood of drug-drug interactions. This section provides the most important drug-drug interactions and their physiological effects. Significant drug-food and drug-natural product interactions are also noted as are recommendations for avoiding or minimizing these interactions.

Route and Dosage: Routes of administration are grouped together and include recommended doses for adults, children, and other more specific age groups (such as geriatric patients). Dosage units are expressed in the terms in which they are usually prescribed. For example, penicillin G dosage is given in units rather than in milligrams. Dosing intervals also are provided in the manner in which they are frequently ordered. If a specific clinical situation (indication) requires a different dose or interval, this is listed separately for clarity. Specific dosing regimens for hepatic or renal impairment are also included.

Availability: This section lists the strengths and concentrations of available dose forms. Such information is useful in planning more convenient regimens (fewer tablets/capsules, less injection volume) and in determining whether certain dose forms are available (suppositories, oral concentrates, sustained- or extended-release forms). Flavors of oral liquids and chewable tablets have been included to improve compliance and adherence in pediatric patients. General availability and average wholesale prices of commonly prescribed drugs have also been added as an aid to nurses with prescriptive authority.

Nursing Implications: This section helps the nurse apply the nursing process to pharmacotherapeutics. The subsections provide a step-by-step guide to clinical assessment, implementation (drug administration), and evaluation of the outcomes of pharmacologic therapy.

Assessment: This section includes guidelines for assessing patient history and physical data before, during, and following drug therapy. Assessments specific to the drug's various indications are also included. The **Lab Test Considerations** section provides the nurse with information regarding which laboratory tests to monitor and how the results may be affected by the medication. It also includes dose modifications required for changes in lab values. **Toxicity and Overdose** alerts the nurse to therapeutic serum drug concentrations that must be monitored and signs and symptoms of toxicity. The antidote and treatment for toxicity or overdose of appropriate medications also are included.

Implementation: Guidelines specific for medication administration are discussed in this subsection. **High Alert** information, i.e., information that directly relates to preventing medication errors with inherently dangerous drugs, is included first if applicable. Sound-alike look-alike name confusion alerts are also included here. Other headings in this section provide data regarding routes of administration. **PO** describes when and how to administer the drug, whether tablets may be crushed or capsules opened, and when to administer the medication in relation to food. In addition, we have identified which opioids have *abuse deterrent* properties and describe the mechanism of these properties within the monograph. The **IV Administration** section includes specific information about administering the medication intravenously. This section has been thoroughly updated and contains a prominent IV Administration heading that introduces this section. Bold, red headings are included to highlight the recommended **diluents** and **concentrations**. These headings complement the **rate** heading and make this critical information easy to find. Several subsections comprise the IV Administration section. The first section, **IV Push**, which refers to administering medications from a syringe directly into a saline lock, Y-site of IV tubing, or a 3-way stopcock, provides details for reconstitution, concentration, dilution, and rate. **Rate** is also included for other methods of IV administration, intermittent or continuous infusion. **Intermittent Infusion** and **Continuous Infusion** specify standard dilution solutions and amounts, stability information, and rates. In addition, a quick reference for information about dilution amounts in neonates and infants, who are extremely sensitive to excess fluids, is contained in the new **Medication Safety Tools** section. **Y-Site Compatibility/Incompatibility** identifies medications compatible or incompatible with each drug when administered via Y-site injection or 3-way stopcock in IV tubing. Information for drugs not included in these lists is conflicting or unavailable. **Additive Compatibility/Incompatibility** identifies medications compatible or incompatible when admixed in solution. Compatibility of diluted medications administered through a Y-site for continuous or intermittent infusion is usually limited to 24 hours. **Solution Compatibility/Incompatibility** identifies compatible or incompatible solutions for dilution for administration purposes. Compatibility information is compiled from *Micromedex* and the manufacturer's package insert.

Patient/Family Teaching: This section includes information that should be taught to patients and/or families of patients. Side effects that should be reported, information on minimizing and managing side effects, details on administration, and follow-up requirements are presented. The nurse also should refer to the **Implementation** section for specific information to teach to the patient and family about taking the medication. **Home Care Issues** discusses aspects to be considered for medications taken in the home setting.

Evaluation: Outcome criteria for determination of the effectiveness of the medication are provided.

REFERENCES

1. Phillips LD, Gorski LA. *Manual of I.V. Therapeutics*. 6th Edition. F.A. Davis Company: Philadelphia, 2014.

EVIDENCE-BASED PRACTICE AND PHARMACOTHERAPEUTICS: Implications for Nurses

Note: The content below is an excerpt from an article written exclusively for the 12th edition of **Davis's Drug Guide for Nurses**. To access the full article, visit **DavisPlus**, F.A. Davis's online center for student and instructor ancillaries, at http://davisplus.fadavis.com.

The purpose of evidence-based practice is to improve the outcomes of treatment for patients. How pharmacologic agents affect patients is often the subject of research; such research is required by the Food and Drug Administration (FDA) before and after drug approval. Any medication can be the subject of an evidence-based clinical review article. But what does "evidence-based" mean and how does it relate to nursing?

According to Ingersoll, "Evidence-based nursing practice is the conscientious, explicit, and judicious use of theory-derived, research-based information in making decisions about care delivery to individuals or groups of patients and in consideration of individual needs and preferences" (2000, p. 152). Still subject to debate are questions about the sufficiency and quality of evidence. For example, what kind of evidence is needed? How much evidence is necessary to support, modify, or change clinical practice? And, were the studies reviewed of "good" quality and are their results valid?

In general, clinicians use **hierarchy of evidence** schemas to rank types of research reports from the most valuable and scientifically rigorous to the least useful. The hierarchy makes clear that some level of evidence about the effect of a particular treatment or condition exists, even if the evidence is considered weak. Figure 1 illustrates a hierarchy of evidence pyramid with widely accepted rankings: the most scientifically rigorous at the top, the least scientifically rigorous at the bottom. Practitioners and clinicians should look for the highest level of available evidence to answer their clinical questions. However, it is important that clinicians also apply the second fundamental principle of EBP, which is that evidence alone is not sufficient to make clinical decisions. Decision makers must always trade off the benefits and risks, and the costs associated with alternative treatment options, and by doing so, consider the patients' values and preferences.

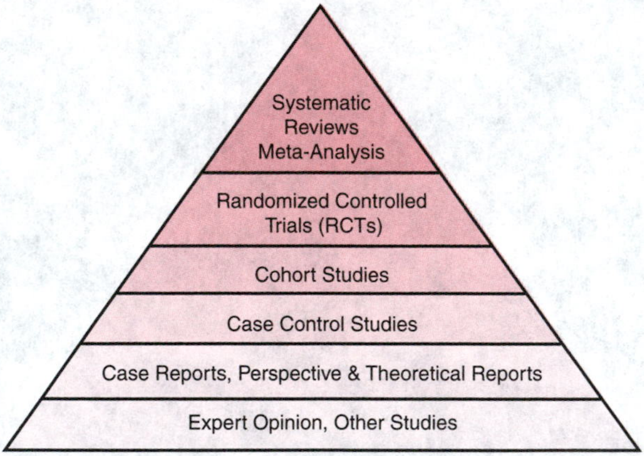

Figure 1: Hierarchy of Scientific Evidence Pyramid

Evidence-Based Practice and Its Importance in Pharmacology

Evidence-based practices in pharmacology generally are derived from well-designed randomized controlled trials (RCTs) or other experimental designs that investigate drugs' therapeutic and non-therapeutic effects. However, although FDA-approved pharmacologic agents have undergone rigorous testing through RCTs, nurses have the responsibility to evaluate the findings for the best scientific evidence available and to determine the most appropriate, safest, and efficacious drugs for their patients.

While numerous databases are available through Internet searches, two valuable and quickly accessible resources for evaluating the current highest level of pharmacologic evidence are 1) the Cochrane Database of Systematic Reviews and the Central Register of Controlled Trials and 2) the National Guidelines Clearinghouse (NGC), supported by the Agency for Healthcare Research and Quality (AHRQ). The Cochrane library and databases provide full text of high-quality, regularly updated systematic reviews, protocols, and clinical trials. The Web address is http://www.cochrane.org.

AHRQ's Evidence-Based Practice Centers (EPCs) provide evidence reports and technology assessments that can assist nurses in their efforts to provide the highest quality and safest pharmacologic health care available. The EPCs systematically review the relevant scientific literature, conduct additional analyses (when appropriate) prior to developing their reports and assessments, and provide guideline comparisons. The Web address is http://www.guideline.gov.

Evidence-based systematic reports and guidelines provide nurses with instantaneous access to the most current knowledge, enabling them to critically appraise the scientific evidence and its appropriateness to their patient population. This is especially important given the need for nurses to keep abreast of the rapidly changing pharmacologic agents in use. New drugs are approved each month, compelling nurses to know these drugs' intended uses, therapeutic effects, interactions, and adverse effects.

Evidence-based practice requires a shift from the traditional paradigm of clinical practice—grounded in intuition, clinical experience, and pathophysiologic rationale—to a paradigm in which nurses must combine clinical expertise, patient values and preferences, and clinical circumstances with the integration of the best scientific evidence in order to make conscientious, well-informed, research-based decisions that affect nursing patient care.

***

Linda S. Weglicki, PhD, RN, MSN
Health Scientist Administrator
Office of Extramural Programs
National Institute of Nursing Research
National Institutes of Health
Bethesda, Maryland

REFERENCES

1. DiCenso A, Guyatt G, Ciliska D. (2005). *Evidence-based nursing: A guide to clinical practice*. St. Louis, MO: Elsevier Mosby.
2. Guyatt G, Rennie D, Meade MO, Cook DJ. (2015). *Users' guide to the medical literature: Essentials of evidence-based clinical practice*. (3rd ed). New York, NY: McGraw Hill Education.
3. Ingersoll GL. Evidence-based nursing: What it is and what it isn't. *Nurs Outlook* 2000;48:151-2.

4. Institute of Medicine (IOM). (2001). *Crossing the quality chasm: A new health system for the 21st century*. Washington, DC: National Academy Press.
5. Leavitt SB. (2003). Evidence-based addiction medicine for practitioners: Evaluating and using research evidence in clinical practice. Addiction Treatment Forum, March. Retrieved May, 2007, from http://atforum.com/documents/EBAM_16_Pager.pdf
6. Melnyk BM, Fineout-Overholt E. (2015). *Evidence-based practice in nursing & healthcare: A guide to best practice*. (3rd ed). Philadelphia, PA: Wolters Kluwer Health.
7. Mick J. How to implement evidence-based nursing practice. *Nursing* 2017;47:36–43.
8. Polit DF, Beck CT. (2014). *Essentials of nursing research: Appraising evidence for nursing practice*. (8th ed). Philadelphia, PA: Wolters Kluwer Health.
9. Sackett D, Rosenberg W, Gray J, Haynes R, Richardson W. Evidence-based medicine: What it is and what it isn't. *BMJ* 1996;312:71-2.

PHARMACOGENOMICS

Introduction

Multiple variables influence the selection and optimization of drug therapy for each individual patient. Pharmacogenomics, the study of the influence of individual genetic variations on drug response in patients, may yield additional information to further enhance safe and effective medication use. Whereas the field originally focused on the effects of specific variants within individual genes on drug response (i.e., pharmacogenetics), efforts increasingly examine the role of multiple variants across the genome and their potential relationship to drug therapy outcomes.

As our understanding of pharmacogenomics and the biological relevance of specific genetic variants in individuals' drug metabolizing enzymes, drug transporter proteins, and drug target receptors to certain drug responses has increased, we have learned that multiple variations across the genome can contribute to significant and relatively predictable treatment outcomes. Virtually every therapeutic area involving medication use includes a drug for which documented genetic variability has the potential to affect drug response. Some of this information is included in the FDA-approved package insert prescribing information. For some agents, the suitability of a specific drug or the determination of an appropriate initial dose for an individual patient based on pharmacogenetic information has been incorporated into dosing algorithms and patient care. As such, it is essential that health care professionals can interpret and utilize this information to facilitate safer and more effective use of medications for individual patients.

Genetic Variation within the Human Genome

The human genome is comprised of approximately 3 billion nucleotide base pair sequences that encode for molecular DNA with, except for identical twins, each individual having his/her own unique human genome sequence. Four nucleotide bases (adenine, guanine, cytosine, and thymine) are responsible for constituting the sequence of each single strand of DNA. Variations in nucleotide sequences can occur, and contribute to alterations in the expression and activities of certain genes. The location of these variations within a DNA sequence on a particular chromosome can have a profound impact on the ultimate biological activity or characteristic of that gene or lead to little or unknown consequences.

Proteins are involved in most enzymatic, structural, and biologic functions associated with drug disposition and effects. The processes involved in DNA replication, RNA transcription, and translation to synthesized proteins are complex. Each of these processes is potentially susceptible to consequences of DNA sequence variations.

Genetic variations can take many forms, including single nucleotide base substitutions (e.g., a cytosine substituted for an adenine), insertions or deletions of a nucleotide base within a sequence, and deletions or extra copies of entire DNA sequences. Variations in DNA that occur at a frequency of greater than 1% in the population are called polymorphisms. The most common genetic variations in humans are referred to as single nucleotide polymorphisms (SNPs) and result from the substitution of one nucleotide base for another. The specific location of a SNP within a gene is important. As mentioned previously, genetic variations can be of unknown or no clinical consequence or they can lead to a truncated, dysfunctional, or complete lack of protein product that is associated with an alteration in drug response.

Clinical Significance of Genetic Polymorphisms

SNPs and other genetic variations influence drug response at different levels through alterations in the activities of enzymes or proteins involved in drug absorption, transport, metabolism, elimination, or at the drug target receptor (site of drug action). Clinically relevant polymorphisms have been identified for genes that encode for most of the common enzymes involved in drug metabolism. Most enzymes are localized intracellularly throughout a wide variety of tissues in the body, including the enterocytes that line the intestine and within hepatocytes. Variants that cause diminished or absent enzyme activity decrease drug metabolism processes. In this case, if the drug is metabolized to an inactive product, then the prolonged persistence of the parent drug in the body could result in excessive pharmacologic effects and potential toxicities may occur. If the drug requires enzymatic conversion to a pharmacologically active metabolite, drug response may be reduced or absent. In contrast, if the variation is due to extra copies of a gene that results in increased enzymatic activity, opposite effects on drug metabolism and response can occur.

Similar outcomes can be associated with polymorphisms in genes that encode for membrane transporter proteins that are responsible for drug transport into cells (influx), as well as proteins that participate in energy-dependent processes that export drugs out of cells (efflux transporters). Polymorphisms in drug transport proteins can influence drug response by altering drug gastrointestinal absorption, uptake and distribution in tissues, exposure to intracellular drug metabolizing enzymes, and elimination via the bile or urine. Finally, some genes that encode for certain drug receptors are highly polymorphic, resulting in attenuated or exaggerated drug responses. The number of polymorphic genes responsible for variations in drug response at drug receptors is relatively small compared to those associated with drug metabolizing enzymes or transport proteins; however, this area has undergone the least amount of study to date.

Incorporating Pharmacogenomic Information into Clinical Practice

Most drugs are initiated in individual patients based on knowledge about their safety and effectiveness within the general population. Information regarding patient characteristics (e.g., age, ethnicity, renal/hepatic function, concomitant disease, etc.) known to contribute to variability in drug response, when available, is considered at this time. Currently, there are more than 50 drugs with pharmacogenomic information included in the package insert. For selected agents, dosing recommendations based on an individual's genetic information (i.e., genotype) for specific drugs and drug classes are also considered. Genomic biomarkers can play an important role in identifying responders and non-responders, avoiding drug toxicity, and adjusting the dose of drugs to optimize their efficacy and safety. However, the typical strategy for most drug therapy is to monitor the patient's response to treatment and modify regimens as necessary. Patients who develop exaggerated pharmacologic responses or elicit no pharmacologic effect may be expressing a phenotype suggestive of altered drug disposition or target receptor effect that could be associated with an underlying genetic polymorphism. As we continue to learn more about these associations and can incorporate pharmacogenomic information into decisions regarding drug therapy for individual patients, the ultimate goal is to improve therapeutic outcomes by limiting drug exposure to patients that are most likely to derive no therapeutic benefit and/or experience toxic drug effects.

For example, some genetic variants are associated with hypersensitivity reactions to a specific drug. A prescriber who is contemplating initiating that drug for a patient may determine whether the patient possesses that variant in his or her DNA. If that specific variant is present, the prescriber might select an alternate agent, thereby avoiding a potentially life-threatening hypersensitivity reaction. In another example, patients who are determined to have a genetic variant that results in an inactive metabolizing enzyme would not be appropriate candidates for an analgesic drug that requires that enzyme to convert the drug to the active analgesia-producing form. On the other hand, if that metabolizing enzyme is responsible for conversion of an active parent drug to an inactive metabolite, the starting dose of the drug may be reduced or perhaps an alternate drug might be selected.

Several Clinical Laboratory Improvement Amendment (CLIA)-approved laboratories offer pharmacogenetic testing to identify relevant genetic polymorphisms that predict drug response and can be used to initiate appropriate drugs and dosing regimens for individual patients. Some of these tests, while recommended in drug prescribing information, are costly and may not be covered by insurance. Patients may not fully understand the utility of undergoing genetic testing and providing a specimen for DNA analysis, which is typically performed on a blood, saliva, buccal swab, or other tissue collection. On the other hand, patients who are engaged in their medical care may be familiar with the concept of "personalized medicine" and seek information about available tests to "individualize" their own drug therapy. Currently, four drugs are required to have pharmacogenetic testing performed before they are prescribed: cetuximab, trastuzumab, maraviroc, and dasatinib. Other drugs have labeling that include "test recommended" or "for information only." Health care professionals will need to be familiar with pharmacogenetic tests that are recommended for specific drug therapies, how to interpret the results of those tests, and how to incorporate pharmacogenetic data with other clinical information to optimize patient drug therapy and health care outcomes.

Pertinent Resources:

Cheek DJ, Bashore L, Brazeau DA. Pharmacogenomics and implications for nursing practice. *J Nurs Scolarsh* 2015;47:496–504.

Court MH. A pharmacogenomics primer. *J Clin Pharmacol* 2007;47:1087-1103.

Evans WE, McLeod HL. Pharmacogenomics – drug disposition, drug targets, and side effects. *N Engl J Med* 2003;348:538-49.

Evans WE, Relling MV. Moving towards individualized medicine with pharmacogenomics. *Nature* 2004;429:464-8.

NCBI Genetics Primer: http://www.ncbi.nlm.nih.gov/pmc/articles/PMC3860415/pdf/arcr-34-3-270.pdf

Roden DM, Altman RB, Benowitz NL, et al. Pharmacogenomics: challenges and opportunities. *Ann Intern Med* 2006;145:749-57.

Shin J, Kayser SR, Langaee TY. Pharmacogenetics: from discovery to patient care. *Am J Health-Syst Pharm* 2009;66:625-37.

Valdes R, Yin DT. Fundamentals of pharmacogenetics in personalized, precision medicine. *Clin Lab Med* 2016;36:447–59.

Weiss ST, McLeod HL, Flockhart DA, et al. Creating and evaluating genetic tests predictive of drug response. *Nat Rev Drug Disc* 2008;7:568-74.

Wilkinson GR. Drug metabolism and variability among patients in drug response. *N Engl J Med* 2005;352:2211-21.

MEDICATION ERRORS: Improving Practices and Patient Safety

It is widely acknowledged that medication errors result in thousands of adverse drug events, preventable reactions, and deaths per year. Nurses, physicians, pharmacists, patient safety organizations, the Food and Drug Administration, the pharmaceutical industry, Health Canada, and other parties share in the responsibility for determining how medication errors occur and designing strategies to reduce error.

One impediment to understanding the scope and nature of the problem has been the reactive "blaming, shaming, training" culture that singled out one individual as the cause of the error. Also historically, medication errors that did not result in patient harm—near-miss situations in which an error could have but didn't happen—or errors that did not result in serious harm were not reported. In contrast, serious errors often instigated a powerful punitive response in which one or a few persons were deemed to be at fault and, as a result, lost their jobs and sometimes their licenses.

In 1999, the Institute of Medicine (IOM) published *To Err Is Human: Building a Safer Health System*, which drew attention to the problem of medication errors. It pointed out that excellent health care providers do make medication errors, that many of the traditional processes involved in the medication-use system were error-prone, and that other factors, notably drug labeling and packaging, contributed to error. Furthermore, the IOM report, in conjunction with other groups such as the United States Pharmacopeia (USP) and the Institute for Safe Medication Practices (ISMP), called for the redesign of error-prone systems to include processes that anticipated the fallibility of humans working within the system. This initiative is helping shift the way the health care industry addresses medication errors from a single person/bad apple cause to a systems issue.

The National Coordinating Council for Medication Error Reporting and Prevention (NCC-MERP) developed the definition of a medication error that reflects this shift and captures the scope and breadth of the issue:

> "A medication error is any preventable event that may cause or lead to inappropriate medication use or patient harm while the medication is in the control of the health care professional, patient, or consumer. Such events may be related to professional practice, health care products, procedures, and systems, including prescribing; order communication; product labeling, packaging, and nomenclature; compounding; dispensing; distribution; administration; education; monitoring; and use."

Inherent in this definition's mention of related factors are the human factors that are part of the medication use system. For example, a nurse or pharmacist may automatically reach into the bin where dobutamine is usually kept, see "do" and "amine" but select dopamine instead of dobutamine. Working amidst distractions, working long hours or shorthanded, and working in a culture where perfection is expected and questioning is discouraged are other examples of the human factors and environmental conditions that contribute to error.

The goal for the design of any individual or hospital-wide medication use system is to determine where systems are likely to fail and to build in safeguards that minimize the potential for error. One way to begin that process is to become familiar with medications or practices that have historically been shown to be involved in serious errors.

High Alert Medications

Some medications, because of a narrow therapeutic range or inherent toxic nature, have a high risk of causing devastating injury or death if improperly ordered, prepared, stocked, dispensed, administered, or monitored. Although these medications may not be involved in more errors, they require special attention due to the potential for serious, possibly fatal consequences. These have been termed **high-alert medications**, to communicate the need for extra care and safeguards. Many of these drugs are used commonly in the general population or are used frequently in urgent clinical situations. The Joint Commission (TJC) monitors the use of frequently prescribed high-alert medications, which include insulin, opiates and narcotics, injectable potassium chloride (or phosphate) concentrate, intravenous anticoagulants (such as heparin), sodium chloride solutions above 0.9 percent, and others. See the High

Alert Drugs table in the **Medication Safety Tools** section, and Table 1 in this article for a complete list of the high alert meds found in *Davis's Drug Guide for Nurses*. (Visit the Institute for Safe Medication Practices at www.ismp.org for more information on high alert drugs.)

Causes of Medication Errors

Many contributing factors and discrete causes of error have been identified, including failed communication, poor drug distribution practices, dose miscalculations, drug packaging and drug-device related problems, incorrect drug administration, and lack of patient education.

Failed Communication: Failed communication covers many of the errors made in the ordering phase, and although ordering is performed by the prescriber, the nurse, the clerk, and the pharmacist who interpret that order are also involved in the communication process.

- ***Poorly handwritten or verbal orders.*** Handwriting is a major source of error and has led to inaccurate interpretations of the drug intended, the route of administration, the frequency, and dose. Telephone and verbal orders are likewise prone to misinterpretation.
- ***Drugs with similar-sounding or similar-looking names.*** Similar sounding names, or names that look similar when handwritten, are frequently confused. Amiodarone and amrinone (now renamed inamrinone to help prevent confusion), or Zebeta® and Diabeta® are two examples. The USP has identified over 700 "sound-alike, look-alike" drugs. Mix-ups are more likely when each drug has similar dose ranges and frequencies.

Several of the sound-alike/look-alike drugs were targeted for labeling intervention by the FDA, which requested manufacturers of 33 drugs with look-alike names to voluntarily revise the appearance of the established names. The revision visually differentiates the drug names by using "tall man" letters (capitals) to highlight distinguishing syllables (ex.: acetoHEXAMIDE versus acetaZOLAMIDE or buPROPrion versus busPIRone. See the TALL MAN Lettering table in the **Medication Safety Tools** section for the list of the pairs of drugs that are commonly confused, often with serious consequences.

- ***Misuse of zeroes in decimal numbers.*** Massive, ten-fold overdoses are traceable to not using a leading zero (.2 mg instead of 0.2 mg) or adding an unnecessary trailing zero (2.0 mg instead of 2 mg) in decimal expressions of dose. Similar overdosages are found in decimal expressions in which the decimal point is obscured by poor handwriting, stray marks, or lined orders sheets (e.g., reading 3.1 grams as 31 grams). Under-dosing also may occur by the same mechanism and prevent a desired, perhaps life-saving effect.
- ***Use of apothecary measures (grains, drams) or package units (amps, vials, tablets) instead of metric measures (grams, milligrams, milliequivalents).*** Apothecary measurements are poorly understood and their abbreviations are easily confused with other units of measurement. Use of such measures should be abandoned. Errors also occur when dosage units are used instead of metric weight. For example, orders for 2 tablets, 1 1/2 vials, or 2 ampules can result in overdose or underdose when the medications ordered come in various strengths.
- ***Misinterpreted abbreviations.*** Abbreviations can be misinterpreted or, when used in the dosage part of the order, can result in incorrect dosage of the correct medication. For example, lower or uppercase "U" for units has been read as a zero, making 10 u of insulin look like 100 units when handwritten. The Latin abbreviation "QOD" for every other day has been misinterpreted as QID (4 times per day). See Table 2 for a list of confusing abbreviations and safer alternatives.
- ***Ambiguous or incomplete orders.*** Orders that do not clearly specify dose, route, frequency, or indication do not communicate complete information and are open to misinterpretation.

Poor Distribution Practices: Poor distribution includes error-prone storing practices such as keeping similar-looking products next to each other. Dispensing multidose floor stock vials of potentially dangerous drugs instead of unit doses is also associated with error as is allowing non-pharmacists to dispense medications in the absence of the pharmacist.

Dose Miscalculations: Dose miscalculations are a prime source of medication error. Also, many medications need to be dose-adjusted for renal or hepatic impairment, age, height and weight, and body composition (i.e., correct for obesity). Complicated dosing formulas provide many opportunities to introduce error. Often vulnerable populations, such as premature infants, children, the elderly, and those with serious underlying illnesses, are at greatest risk.

Drug Packaging and Drug Delivery Systems: Similar packaging or poorly designed packaging encourages error. Drug companies may use the same design for different formulations, or fail to highlight information about concentration or strength. Lettering, type size, color, and packaging methods can either help or hinder drug identification.

Drug delivery systems include infusion pumps and rate controllers. Some models do not prevent free flow of medication, leading to sudden high dose infusion of potent and dangerous medications. The lack of safeguards preventing free flow and programming errors are among the problems encountered with infusion control devices.

Incorrect Drug Administration: Incorrect drug administration covers many problems. Misidentification of a patient, incorrect route of administration, missed doses, or improper drug preparation are types of errors that occur during the administration phase.

Lack of Patient Education: Safe medication use is enhanced in the hospital and the home when the patient is well informed. The knowledgeable patient can recognize when something has changed in his or her medication regimen and can question the health care provider. At the same time, many issues related to medication errors, such as ambiguous directions, unfamiliarity with a drug, and confusing packaging, affect the patient as well as the health care provider, underscoring the need for careful education. Patient education also enhances adherence, which is a factor in proper medication use.

Prevention Strategies

Since medication use systems are complex and involve many steps and people, they are error-prone. On an individual basis, nurses can help reduce the incidence of error by implementing the following strategies:

- Clarify any order that is not obviously and clearly legible. Ask the prescriber to print orders using block style letters.
- Do not accept orders with the abbreviation "u" or "IU" for units. Clarify the dosage and ask the prescriber to write out the word units.
- Clarify any abbreviated drug name or the abbreviated dosing frequencies q.d., QD, q.o.d., QOD, and q.i.d or QID. Suggest abandoning Latin abbreviations in favor of spelling out dosing frequency.
- Do not accept doses expressed in package units or volume instead of metric weight. Clarify any order written for number of ampules, vials, or tablets (e.g., calcium chloride, 1 ampule or epinephrine, 1 Bristojet).
- Decimal point errors can be hard to see. Suspect a missed decimal point and clarify any order if the dose requires more than 3 dosing units.
- If dose ordered requires use of multiple dosage units or very small fractions of a dose unit, review the dose, have another health care provider check the original order and recalculate formulas, and confirm the dose with the prescriber.
- If taking a verbal order, ask prescriber to spell out the drug name and dosage to avoid sound-alike confusion (e.g., hearing Cerebyx for Celebrex, or fifty for fifteen). Read back the order to the prescriber after you have written it in the chart. Confirm and document the indication to further enhance accurate communication.
- Clarify any order that does not include metric weight, dosing frequency, or route of administration.
- Check the nurse's/clerk's transcription against the original order. Make sure stray marks or initials do not obscure the original order.
- Do not start a patient on new medication by borrowing medications from another patient. This action bypasses the double check provided by the pharmacist's review of the order.
- Always check the patient's name band before administering medications. Verbally addressing a patient by name does not provide sufficient identification.
- Use the facility's standard drug administration times to reduce the chance of an omission error.
- Be sure to fully understand any drug administration device before using it. This includes infusion pumps, inhalers, and transdermal patches.

- Have a second practitioner independently check original order, dosage calculations, and infusion pump settings for high alert medications.
- Realize that the printing on packaging boxes, vials, ampoules, prefilled syringes, or any container in which a medication is stored can be misleading. Be sure to differentiate clearly the medication and the number of milligrams per milliliter versus the total number of milligrams contained within. Massive overdoses have been administered by assuming that the number of milligrams per ml is all that is contained within the vial or ampule. Read the label when obtaining the medication, before preparing or pouring the medication, and after preparing or pouring the medication.
- Educate patients about the medications they take. Provide verbal and written instructions and ask the patient to restate important points. Refer to Educating Patients about Safe Medication Use on page 29 for recommendations on what patients should understand about their medications.

As stated previously, errors are a result of problems within the medication use system and cannot be eliminated by the vigilance of any one group of health care providers. System redesign involves strong leadership from administration and all involved departments. Health care facilities should consider the following when addressing the issue of medication errors:

- Do not provide unit stock of critical, high alert medications. If eliminating these medications from floor stock is not feasible, consider reducing the number available and standardizing the concentrations or forms in which the medication is available.
- Create committees that address safety issues.
- Install a computer physician order entry (CPOE) system to help reduce prescribing orders. Link order entry to pertinent lab, allergy, and medication data.
- Implement bar code technology to ensure the right drug reaches the right patient.
- Develop policies that discourage error-prone prescribing practices such as inappropriate use of verbal orders, use of confusing dosing symbols, and use of abbreviations.
- Develop policies that encourage better communication of medication information such as requiring block-style printing of medications, including indication in prescription, and using both the trade and generic name in prescriptions.
- Ensure a reasonable workload for pharmacists and nurses, and provide a well-designed work area.
- Limit the availability of varying concentrations of high alert medications.
- Provide standard concentrations and infusion rate tables.
- Supply pharmacy and patient care areas with current reference material.
- Cultivate a culture that does not assign blame when medication errors occur but looks for root causes instead.
- Encourage staff to participate in the USP-ISMP-MERP error reporting program.

REFERENCES

1. Kohn LT, Corrigan JM, Donaldson MS (eds). *To Err Is Human: Building a Safer Health System.* National Academy Press, Washington, DC (1999).
2. National Coordinating Council for Medication Error Reporting and Prevention. http://www.nccmerp.org/about-medication-errors
3. Cohen MR. *Medication Errors.* American Pharmacists Association, Washington DC (2007).
4. Branowicki P, O'Neill JB, Dwyer JL, et al. Improving complex medication systems: an interdisciplinary approach. *J Nurs Adm* 2003;33:199-200.
5. Burke KG. Executive summary: the state of the science on safe medication administration symposium. *J Infus Nurs* 2005;28(2 Suppl):4-9.
6. ISMP. What's in a name? Ways to prevent dispensing errors linked to name confusion. *ISMP Medication Safety Alert!* 7(12) June 12, 2002. http://www.ismp.org/Newsletters/acutecare/archives/Jun02.asp
7. McPhillips HA, Stille CJ, Smith D, et al. Potential medication dosing errors in outpatient pediatrics. *J Pediatr* 2005;147:727-8.
8. Ofosu R, Jarrett P. Reducing nurse medicine administration errors. *Nurs Times* 2015;111:12–4.
9. Santell JP, Cousins DD, Medication errors related to product names. *Joint Commission J Qual Pt. Safety* 2005; 31:649-54.

Table 1: High Alert Medications in Davis's Drug Guide for Nurses

aldesleukin	erlotinib	mitoxantrone
alemtuzumab	esmolol	morphine
alitretinoin	etoposides	nalbuphine
amiodarone	fentanyl (buccal, transmucosal)	nateglinide
amphotericin B cholesteryl sulfate/ lipid complex/liposome	fentanyl (parenteral)	nesiritide
argatroban	fentanyl (transdermal)	nilotinib
arsenic trioxide	fludarabine	nitroprusside
asparaginase	fluorouracil	norepinephrine
azacitidine	fondaparinux	oxaliplatin
bendamustine	gefitinib	oxycodone compound
bevacizumab	gemcitabine	oxymorphone
bivalirudin	gemtuzumab ozogamicin	oxytocin
bleomycin	heparin	paclitaxel
bortezomib	heparins (low molecular weight)	pancuronium
buprenorphine	hydrocodone	panitumumab
busulfan	hydromorphone	pazopanib
butorphanol	hydroxyurea	pegaspargase
capecitabine	hypoglycemic agents, oral	pemetrexed
carboplatin	idarubicin	pentazocine
carmustine	ifosfamide	potassium phosphates
cetuximab	imatinib	potassium supplements
chloralhydrate	insulin mixtures	pramlintide
chlorambucil	insulins (intermediate-acting)	procarbazine
cisplatin	insulins (long-acting)	promethazine (IV)
cladribine	insulins (rapid-acting)	propofol
clofarabine	insulins (short-acting)	propranolol
codeine	irinotecan	repaglinide
colchicine (IV)	ixabepilone	rituximab
cyclophosphamide	labetalol	sodium chloride (hypertonic)
cytarabine	lapatinib	sunitinib
dacarbazine	lepirudin	temsirolimus
DAUNOrubicin hydrochloride	lidocaine	thalidomide
decitabine	magnesium sulfate (IV, parenteral)	thioguanine
digoxin	mechlorethamine	thrombolytic agents
DOBUTamine	melphalan	tirofiban
docetaxel	meperidine	topotecan
DOPamine	methadone	trastuzumab
DOXOrubicin hydrochloride	methotrexate	vinBLAStine
DOXOrubicin hydrochloride liposome	metoprolol	vinCRIStine
epinephrine	midazolam	vinorelbine
epirubicin	milrinone	warfarin
eptifibatide	mitomycin	

Table 2: Abbreviations and Symbols Associated with Medication Errors

Abbreviation/Symbol	Intended Meaning	Mistaken For	Recommendation
APAP	Acetaminophen	Not recognized as acetaminophen	Use full drug name
AZT	Zidovudine	Azathioprine	Use full drug name
CPZ	Compazine (prochlorperazine)	Thorazine (chlorpromazine)	Use full drug name
HCl	Hydrochloric acid	KCl (potassium chloride)	Use full drug name
HCT	Hydrocortisone	Hydrochlorothiazide	Use full drug name
HCTZ	Hydrochlorothiazide	Hydrocortisone	Use full drug name
IV Vanc	Intravenous vancomycin	Invanz (ertapenem)	Use full drug name
$MgSO_4$*	Magnesium sulfate	Morphine sulfate	Use full drug name
MS, MSO_4*	Morphine sulfate	Magnesium sulfate	Use full drug name
MTX	Methotrexate	Mitoxantrone	Use full drug name
"Nitro" drip	Nitroglycerin infusion	Nitroprusside infusion	Use full drug name

NoAC	Novel/new oral anticoagulant	No anticoagulant	Use full drug name
PCA	Procainamide	Patient controlled analgesia	Use full drug name
PTU	Propylthiouracil	Mercaptopurine	Use full drug name
T3	Tylenol with codeine no. 3	Liothyronine	Use full drug name
TAC	Triamcinolone	Tetracaine, Adrenalin, or Cocaine	Use full drug name
TNK	TNKase	tPA	Use full drug name
TPA or tPA	Tissue plasminogen activator (alteplase)	TNKase (tenecteplase)	Use full drug name
$ZnSO_4$	Zinc sulfate	Morphine sulfate	Use full drug name
μg	Microgram	Mg (milligram)	Use "mcg"
AD, AS, AU	Right ear, left ear, both ears	Right eye, left eye, both eyes	Spell out "right ear," "left ear," or "both ears"
BT	Bedtime	BID (twice daily)	Spell out "bedtime"
cc	cubic centimeters	u (units)	Use "ml"
D/C	Discharge or discontinue	One mistaken for the other	Spell out "discharge" or "discontinue"
HS or hs	Half strength or hour of sleep (at bedtime)	One mistaken for the other	Spell out "half strength" or "at bedtime"
IN	Intranasal	IM or IV	Spell out "intranasal" or use "NAS"
I.U.*	International Units	IV or 10	Spell out "units"
"Nitro" drip	Nitroglycerin infusion	Nitroprusside infusion	
OD, OS, OU	Right eye, left eye, both eyes	Right ear, left ear, both ears	Spell out "right eye," "left eye," or "both eyes"
o.d. or OD	Every day	Right eye	Spell out "daily"
q.d. or QD*	Every day	q.i.d. (4 times per day)	Spell out "daily"
qhs	Nightly at bedtime	qhr (every hour)	Spell out "at bedtime"
q.o.d. or QOD*	Every other day	q.i.d. (4 times per day) or qd (daily)	Spell out "every other day"
SC, SQ, sub q	Subcutaneously	SC mistaken as SL (sublingual); SQ as "5 every"; q in sub q as "every"	Use subcut or write out "subcutaneously"
SSRI	Sliding scale regular insulin	Selective serotonin reuptake inhibitor	Spell out "sliding scale insulin"
TIW	3 times a week	3 times a day or twice a week	Spell out "3 times weekly"
u or U*	units	0 (zero), 4 (four) or cc	Spell out "units"
/ (slash mark)	Per"	1 (numeral one)	Spell out "per"
+	Plus sign	"4" (numeral four)	Spell out "and"
Zero **after** a decimal point (e.g., 1.0 mg)*	1 mg	10 mg	DO NOT USE zero after a decimal point
No zero **before** a decimal point (e.g., .1 mg)*	.1 mg	1 mg	ALWAYS USE zero before a decimal point
@	At	2	Use "at"
>	Greater than	7 or <	Spell out "greater than"
<	Less than	L or >	Spell out "less than"
&	And	2	Use "and"
°	Hour	Zero (q 1° seen as q 10)	Use "hr," "h," or "hour"
Drug name and dose run together. Example: Inderal 40 mg	Inderal 40 mg	Inderal 140 mg	Leave space between drug name, dose, and unit of measure
Numerical dose and unit of measure run together. Example: 10 mg	10 mg	100 mg	Leave space between drug dose and unit of measure

*Appears on The Joint Commission's "Do Not Use" list of abbreviations.

Modified from ISMP's List of Error-Prone Abbreviations, Symbols, and Dose Designations, 2015.

DETECTING AND MANAGING ADVERSE DRUG REACTIONS

An *adverse drug reaction* (ADR) is any unexpected, undesired, or excessive response to a medication that results in:

- temporary or permanent serious harm or disability
- admission to a hospital, transfer to a higher level of care, or prolonged stay
- death.

Adverse drug reactions are distinguished from adverse drug events, in which causality is uncertain, and side effects, which may be bothersome to the patient and necessitate a change in therapy but are not considered serious. Although some ADRs are the result of medication errors, many are not.

Types of ADRs

The Food and Drug Administration (FDA) classifies ADRs into 2 broad categories: Type A and Type B. Type A reactions are predictable reactions based on the primary or secondary pharmacologic effect of the drug. Dose-related reactions and drug-drug interactions are examples of Type A reactions. Type B reactions are unpredictable, are not related to dose, and are not the result of the drug's primary or secondary pharmacologic effect. Idiosyncratic and hypersensitivity reactions are examples of Type B reactions.

Dose-Related Reactions (Toxic Reactions): In dose related reactions, the dose prescribed for the patient is excessive. Although a variety of mechanisms may interact, reasons for this type of reaction include:

- renal or hepatic impairment
- extremes in age (neonates and frail elderly)
- drug-drug or drug-food interactions
- underlying illness.

Dose-related reactions are often the result of preventable errors in prescribing in which physiologic factors such as age, renal impairment, and weight were not considered sufficiently, or in inadequate therapeutic monitoring. Medications with narrow therapeutic ranges (digoxin, aminoglycosides, antiepileptic drugs) and those that require careful monitoring or laboratory testing (anticoagulants, nephrotoxic drugs) are most frequently implicated in dose-related reactions. Dose-related reactions usually are managed successfully by temporarily discontinuing the drug and then reducing the dose or increasing the dosing interval. In some instances, the toxic effects need to be treated with another agent (e.g., Digibind for digoxin toxicity or Kayexalate for drug-induced hyperkalemia). Appropriately timed therapeutic drug level monitoring, review of new drugs added to an existing regimen that may affect the drug level, and frequent assessment of relevant laboratory values are critical to safe medical management and prevention of dose-related reactions.

Drug-Drug Interactions: Drug-drug interactions occur when the pharmacokinetic or pharmacodynamic properties of an individual drug affect another drug. Pharmacokinetics refers to the way the body processes a medication (absorption, distribution, metabolism, and elimination). In a drug-drug interaction, the pharmacokinetic properties of one drug can cause a change in drug concentration of another drug and an altered response. For example, one drug may block enzymes that metabolize a second drug. The concentration of the second drug is then increased and may become toxic or cause adverse reactions. Pharmacodynamic drug-drug interactions involve the known effects and side-effects of the drugs. For example, two drugs with similar therapeutic effects may act together in a synergistic way. The increased anticoagulant effects that occur when warfarin and aspirin are taken together, or the increased central nervous system (CNS) depression that results when two drugs with CNS depressant effects potentiate each other, are examples of pharmacodynamic drug-drug interactions. Certain classes of drugs are more likely to result in serious drug-drug interactions, and patients receiving these agents should be monitored carefully. The medication classes include anticoagulants, oral hypoglycemic agents, nonsteroidal anti-inflammatory agents, monoamine oxidase inhibitors, antihypertensives, antiepileptics, and antiretrovirals. In addition, specific drugs such as theophylline, cimetidine, lithium, and digoxin may result in serious ADRs.

Idiosyncratic Reactions: Idiosyncratic reactions occur without relation to dose and are unpredictable and sporadic. Reactions of this type may manifest in many different ways, including fever, blood dyscrasias, cardiovascular effects, or mental status changes. The time frame between the occurrence of a problem and initiation of therapy is sometimes the only clue linking drug to symptom. Some idiosyncratic reactions may be explained by genetic differences in drug-metabolizing enzymes.

Hypersensitivity Reactions: Hypersensitivity reactions are usually allergic responses. Manifestations of hypersensitivity reactions range from mild rashes, to nephritis, pneumonitis, hemolytic anemia, and anaphylaxis. Protein drugs (vaccines, enzymes) are frequently associated with hypersensitivity reactions. In most instances, antibody formation is involved in the process and therefore cross-sensitivity may occur. An example of this is hypersensitivity to penicillin and cross-sensitivity with other penicillins and/or cephalosporins. Documenting drugs to which the patient is allergic and the specific hypersensitivity reaction is very important. If the reaction to an agent is anaphylaxis the nurse should monitor the patient during administration of a cross-hypersensitive agent, especially during the initial dose, and ensure ready access to emergency resuscitative equipment.

Recognizing an ADR

Adverse drug reactions should be suspected whenever there is a negative change in a patient's condition, particularly when a new drug has been introduced. Strategies that can enhance recognition include knowing the side effect/adverse reaction profile of medications. Nurses should be familiar with a drug's most commonly encountered side effects and adverse reactions before administering it. (In *Davis's Drug Guide for Nurses*, most frequent adverse drug reactions are <u>underlined</u>, and life-threatening adverse reactions are CAPITALIZED and appear in second color in the **Adverse Reactions and Side Effects** section.) As always, monitoring the patient's response to a medication and ongoing assessment are key nursing actions. Learn to recognize patient findings that suggest an ADR has occurred. These include:

- rash
- change in respiratory rate, heart rate, blood pressure, or mental state
- seizure
- anaphylaxis
- diarrhea
- fever.

Any of these findings can suggest an ADR and should be reported and documented promptly so that appropriate interventions, including discontinuation of suspect medications, can occur. Prompt intervention can prevent a mild adverse reaction from escalating into a serious health problem. Other steps taken by the health care team when identifying and treating an ADR include:

1. Determining that the drug ordered was the drug given and intended.
2. Determining that the drug was given in the correct dosage by the correct route.
3. Establishing the chronology of events: time drug was taken and onset of symptoms.
4. Stopping the drug and monitoring patient status for improvement (dechallenge).
5. Restarting the drug, if appropriate, and monitoring closely for adverse reactions (rechallenge).

Prevention

Health care organizations have responded to consumer, regulator, and insurer pressures by developing programs that aim to eliminate preventable ADRs. In the inpatient setting, computer systems can display the patient's age, height, weight, and creatinine clearance or serum creatinine concentration and send an alert to the clinician if a prescribed dose is out of range for any of the displayed parameters. Allergy alerts and drug-drug interactions can be presented to the clinician at the time an order is entered.

In the outpatient setting, strategies that increase the patient's knowledge base and access to pharmacists and nurses may help prevent adverse reactions. Outpatient pharmacy computer systems that are linked within a chain of pharmacies may allow the pharmacist to view the patient's profile if the patient is filling a prescription in a pharmacy other than the usual one. Many pharmacy computers have dose limits and drug-drug reaction verification to assist pharmacists filling orders.

Such strategies are a valuable auxiliary to, but cannot replace, conscientious history taking, careful patient assessment, and ongoing monitoring. A thorough medication history including all prescription and nonprescription drugs, all side effects and adverse reactions encountered, allergies, and all pertinent physical data should be available to the prescriber. The prescriber is responsible for reviewing this data, along with current medications, laboratory values, and any other variable that affects drug response.

It is not expected that practitioners will remember all relevant information when prescribing. In fact, reliance on memory is error-fraught, and clinicians need to use available resources to verify drug interactions whenever adding a new drug to the regimen. Setting expectations that clinicians use evidence-based information rather than their memories when prescribing, dispensing, administering, or monitoring patients has the potential to reduce the incidence of preventable ADRs.

Reporting Adverse Drug Reactions in the U.S.:

Food and Drug Administration MedWatch Program: To monitor and assess the incidence of adverse reactions, the FDA sponsors MedWatch, a program that allows health care practitioners and consumers the opportunity to report serious adverse reactions or product defects encountered from medications, medical devices, special nutritional products, or other FDA-regulated items. The FDA considers serious those reactions that result in death, life-threatening illness or injury, hospitalization, disability, congenital anomaly, or those that require medical/surgical intervention.

In addition to reporting serious adverse reactions, health care providers should also report problems related to suspected contamination, questionable stability, defective components, or poor packaging/labeling. Reports should be submitted even if there is some uncertainty about the cause/effect relationship or if some details are missing. This reporting form may be accessed at https://www.fda.gov/safety/medwatch-fda-safety-information-and-adverse-event-reporting-program. Reports also may be faxed to the FDA (1-800-FDA-0178). Reactions to vaccines should be reported to the Vaccine Adverse Event Reporting System (VAERS; 1-800-822-7967). Nurses share with other health care providers an obligation to report adverse reactions to the MedWatch program so that all significant data can be analyzed for opportunities to improve patient care.

Reporting Adverse Drug Reactions in Canada:

The Marketed Health Products Directorate of Health Canada coordinates adverse reaction reporting activities, and analyzes reports submitted from regional centers in each province. MedEffect Canada encourages health professionals, patients and regulatory authorities to report adverse reactions as they occur, either by email, mail, or the Health Canada website. Health care professionals reporting adverse reactions are required to supply information regarding patient characteristics, details about the reaction(s), current treatment, and outcomes. Information identifying the patient or health care provider remains confidential.

Adverse reaction reports are analyzed to investigate any associations with the health product. Based on the outcome, regulatory bodies decide on a course of action, which may include performing additional post-marketing studies, re-assessment of the risk versus benefit of the product, packaging modification, addition of warnings in patient information leaflets, or issuing public alerts or market withdrawals. Updates regarding adverse reactions are published in the Health Product InfoWatch every month.

Access the following link for the Side Effect Reporting Form for consumers and health professionals: https://www.canada.ca/en/health-canada/services/drugs-health-products/medeffect-canada/adverse-reaction-reporting.html.

REFERENCES

1. Alhawassi TM, Krass I, Bajorek BV, Pont LG. A systematic review of the prevalence and risk factors for adverse drug reactions in the elderly in the acute care setting. *Clin Inter Aging* 2014;9:2079–86.
2. Bennett CL, Nebeker JR, Lyons EA, et al. The Research on Adverse Drug Events and Reports (RADAR) project. *JAMA.* 2005;293:2131-40.
3. Field TS, Gilman BH, Subramanian S, et al. The costs associated with adverse drug events among older adults in the ambulatory setting. *Med Care.* 2005;43:1171-6.
4. Petrone K, Katz P. Approaches to appropriate drug prescribing for the older adult. *Prim Care.* 2005; 32:755-75.
5. Pezalla E. Preventing adverse drug reactions in the general population. *Manag Care Interface.* 2005; 18:49-52.
6. Tache SV, Sonnichsen A, Ashcroft DM. Prevalence of adverse drug events in ambulatory care: a systematic review. *Ann Pharmacother* 2011;45:977–89.
7. Winterstein AG, Sauer BC, Hepler CD, Poole C. Identifying clinically significant preventable adverse drug events through a hospital's database of adverse drug reaction reports. *Am J Health-Syst Pharm* 2002;59:1742-9.
8. "Adverse Reaction Information." *MedEffect Canada.* October 2012. http://www.hc-sc.gc.ca/dhp-mps/medeff/advers-react-neg/index-eng.php#a5 (accessed 7 September 2017).

OVERVIEW OF RISK EVALUATION AND MITIGATION SYSTEMS (REMS)

Over the past several decades, the Food and Drug Administration (FDA) has employed a number of "risk management" programs designed to detect, evaluate, prevent, and mitigate drug adverse events for drugs with the potential for serious adverse drug reactions. Some of the risk management plans used by the FDA over the years have included the use of patient package inserts, medication guides, restricted access programs, and classification of drugs as controlled substances. These programs were acknowledged by the FDA as Risk Minimization Action Plans (RiskMAPS) in 2005. With these programs, the FDA only had the authority to mandate postmarketing commitments from drug manufacturers before the drug was approved; however, these requirements could not be enforced after the drug was approved.

The Food and Drug Administration Amendments Act of 2007 has given the FDA the authority to subject drugs to new risk identification and communication strategies in the postmarketing period. These new strategies, called Risk Evaluation and Mitigation Strategies (REMS), can be required for any drug or drug class that is associated with serious risks. The FDA can require a REMS if it believes that this program is necessary to ensure that the benefits outweigh the potential risks of the drug. The FDA can require a REMS either as part of the drug approval process or during the postmarketing period if new information becomes available regarding potentially harmful effects that are associated with the use of the drug.

Components of the REMS may include a medication guide, a patient package insert, and/or a communication plan. A REMS for New Drug Applications or Biologics License Applications requires a timetable for submission of assessment of the REMS. A variety of elements to ensure safe use of drugs can be required as part of the REMS if it is believed that a medication guide, patient package insert, or communication plan are not adequate to mitigate the serious risks associated with a particular drug. These elements may include the following:

- Health care providers who prescribe the drug are specifically trained and/or certified.
- Pharmacies, practitioners, or health care settings that dispense the drug are specifically trained and/or certified.
- The drug is dispensed to patients only in certain health care settings, such as hospitals.
- The drug is dispensed only to patients with evidence or other documentation of safe-use conditions, such as laboratory test results.
- Patients using the drug are subject to certain monitoring.
- Patients using the drug are enrolled in a registry.

The FDA maintains an updated list of these REMS programs at https://www.accessdata.fda.gov/scripts/cder/rems/index.cfm. A REMS tag has been added at the top of the monographs of drugs associated with these programs.

SPECIAL DOSING CONSIDERATIONS

For many patients the average dose range for a given drug can be toxic. The purpose of this section is to describe vulnerable patient populations for which special dosing considerations must be made to protect the patient and improve clinical outcomes.

The Pediatric Patient

Most drugs prescribed to children are not approved by the Food and Drug Administration (FDA) for use in pediatric populations. This does not mean it's wrong to prescribe these drugs to children, rather it means that the medications were not tested in children. The lack of pediatric drug information can result in patient harm or death, such as what occurred with the drug chloramphenicol. When given to very young children, chloramphenicol caused toxicity and multiple deaths. Referred to as "gray baby syndrome," this toxic reaction was eventually found to be dose dependent. The FDA now requires that new drugs that may be used in children include information for safe pediatric use.

The main reason for adjusting dosages in pediatric patients is body size, which is measured by body weight or body surface area (BSA). Weight-based pediatric drug dosages are expressed in number of milligrams per kilogram of body weight (mg/kg) while dosages calculated on BSA are expressed in number of milligrams per meter squared (mg/m^2). BSA is determined using a BSA nomogram or calculated by using formulas (Appendix F).

The neonate and the premature infant require additional adjustments secondary to immature function of body systems. For example, absorption may be incomplete or altered secondary to differences in gastric pH or motility. Distribution may be altered because of varying amounts of total body water, and metabolism and excretion can be delayed due to immature liver and kidney function. Furthermore, rapid weight changes and progressive maturation of hepatic and renal function require frequent monitoring and careful dosage adjustments. Gestational age, as well as weight, may be needed to properly dose some drugs in the neonate.

The Older Adult Patient

Absorption, distribution, metabolism, and excretion are altered in adults over 65 years of age, putting the older patient at risk for toxic reactions. Pharmacokinetic properties in older adults are affected by

- diminished gastrointestinal (GI) motility and blood flow, which delays absorption
- percentage of body fat, lean muscle mass, and total body water, which alters distribution
- decreased plasma proteins, especially in the malnourished patient, which alters distribution by allowing a larger proportion of free or unbound drug to circulate and exert effects
- diminshed hepatic function, which slows metabolism
- diminished renal function, which delays excretion.

Older adults should be prescribed the lowest possible effective dose at the initiation of therapy followed by careful titration of doses as needed. Just as importantly, they should be monitored very carefully for signs and symptoms of adverse drug reactions.

Another concern is that many older adult patients are prescribed multiple drugs and are at risk for polypharmacy. As the number of medications a patient takes increases, so does the risk for an adverse drug reaction. One drug may negate or potentiate the effects of another drug (drug-drug interaction). This situation is compounded by concurrent use of nonprescription drugs and natural products. In general, doses of most medications (especially digoxin, sedative/hypnotics, anticoagulants, nonsteroidal anti-inflammatory agents, antibiotics, and antihypertensives) should be decreased in the older adult population. The Beers List/Criteria, which appears in the *Medication Safety Tools* section, is a list of drugs to be used with caution in older adults, and is based on these concerns.

The Patient of Reproductive Age

Generally, pregnant women should avoid medications, except when absolutely necessary. Both the mother and the fetus must be considered. The placenta protects the fetus only from extremely large molecules. The fetus is particularly vulnerable during the first and the last trimesters of pregnancy. During the first trimester, vital organs are forming and ingestion of teratogenic drugs may lead to fetal malformation or miscarriage. Unfortunately, this is the time when a woman is least likely to know that she is pregnant. In the third trimester, drugs administered to the mother and transferred to the fetus may not be safely metabolized and excreted by the fetus. This is especially true of drugs administered near term. After the infant is delivered, he or she no longer has the placenta to help with drug excretion, and drugs administered before delivery may result in toxicity.

Of course, many conditions, such as asthma, diabetes, gastrointestinal disorders, and mental illness affect pregnant women and require long-term medication use. When the medications are used, whether over-the-counter or prescription, prescribing the lowest effective dose for the shortest period of time necessary is the rule.

The possibility of a medication altering sperm quality and quantity in a potential father also is an area of concern. Male patients should be informed of this risk when taking any medications known to have this potential.

Renal Impairment

The kidneys are the major organ of drug elimination. Failure to account for decreased renal function is a preventable source of adverse drug reactions. Renal function is measured by the creatinine clearance (CCr), which can be approximated in the absence of a 24-hour urine collection (Appendix F). In addition, dosages in the patients with renal impairment can be optimized by measuring blood levels of certain drugs (e.g., digoxin, aminoglycosides).

Patients with underlying renal impairment, premature infants with immature renal function, and older adults with an age-related decrease in renal function require careful dose adjustments. Renal function may fluctuate over time and should be re-assessed periodically.

Hepatic Impairment

The liver is the major organ of drug metabolism. It changes a drug from a relatively fat-soluble compound to a more water-soluble substance, which means that the drug can then be excreted by the kidneys. Liver function is not as easily quantified as renal function, and it therefore is difficult to predict the correct dosage for a patient with hepatic impairment based on laboratory tests.

A patient who is severely jaundiced or who has very low serum proteins (particularly albumin) can be expected to have some problems metabolizing drugs. In advanced liver disease, portal vascular congestion also impairs drug absorption. Examples of drugs that should be carefully dosed in patients with hepatic impairment include theophylline, diuretics, phenytoin, and sedatives. Some drugs (e.g., enalapril, carisoprodol) must be activated in the liver to exert their effect and are known as prodrugs. In patients with hepatic impairment, these drugs may not be converted to the active component, thereby resulting in decreased efficacy.

Heart Failure

Heart failure results in passive congestion of blood vessels in the gastrointestinal tract, which impairs drug absorption. Heart failure also slows drug delivery to the liver, delaying metabolism. Renal function is frequently compromised as well, adding to delayed elimination and prolonged drug action. Dosages of drugs metabolized mainly by the liver or excreted mainly by the kidneys should be decreased in patients with chronic heart failure.

Body Size

Drug dosing is often based on total body weight. However, some drugs selectively penetrate fatty tissues. If the drug does not penetrate fatty tissues (e.g., digoxin, gentamicin), dosages for the obese patient should be determined by ideal body weight or estimated lean body mass. Ideal body weight may be determined from tables of desirable weights or may be estimated using formulas for lean body mass when the patient's height and weight are known (Appendix F). If such adjustments are not made, considerable toxicity can result.

Body size is also a factor in patients who are grossly underweight. Older adults, chronic alcoholics, patients with acquired immune deficiency, and patients who are terminally ill from cancer or other debilitating illnesses need careful attention to dosing. Patients who have had a limb amputated also need to have this change in body size taken into account.

Drug Interactions

Use of multiple drugs, especially those known to interact with other drugs, may necessitate dosage adjustments. Drugs highly bound to plasma proteins, such as warfarin and phenytoin, may be displaced by other highly protein-bound drugs. When this phenomenon occurs, the drug that has been displaced exhibits an increase in its activity because the free or unbound drug is active.

Some drugs decrease the liver's ability to metabolize other drugs. Drugs capable of doing this include cimetidine and ketoconazole. Concurrently administered drugs that are also highly metabolized by the liver may need to be administered in decreased dosages. Other agents such as phenobarbital, other barbiturates, and rifampin are capable of stimulating the liver to metabolize drugs more rapidly, requiring larger doses to be administered. Concurrently administered drugs that are also highly metabolized by the liver may need to be administered in higher dosages.

Drugs that significantly alter urine pH can affect excretion of drugs for which the excretory process is pH dependent. Alkalinizing the urine will hasten the excretion of acidic drugs. An example of this is administering sodium bicarbonate in cases of aspirin overdose to promote the renal excretion of aspirin. Alkalinizing the urine will increase reabsorption of alkaline drugs, which prolongs and enhances drug action. Acidification of the urine will hasten the excretion of alkaline drugs. Acidification of the urine will also enhance reabsorption of acidic drugs, prolonging and enhancing drug action.

Some drugs compete for enzyme systems with other drugs. Allopurinol inhibits the enzyme involved in uric acid production, but it also inhibits metabolism (inactivation) of 6-mercaptopurine, greatly increasing its toxicity. The dosage of mercaptopurine needs to be significantly reduced when coadministered with allopurinol.

The same potential for interactions exists for some foods. Dietary calcium, found in high concentrations in dairy products, combines with tetracycline or fluoroquinolones and prevents their absorption. Foods high in pyridoxine (vitamin B_6) can negate the anti-Parkinsonian effect of levodopa. Grapefruit juice inhibits the enzyme that breaks down some drugs, and concurrent ingestion may significantly increase drug levels and the risk for toxicity.

Many commonly taken natural products interact with pharmaceutical drugs. St. John's wort, garlic, ephedra, and other natural products can interact with medications and cause known or unpredictable reactions.

Nurses and prescribers should consult drug references and remember that the average dosing range for drugs is intended for an average patient. However, every patient is an individual with specific drug-handling capabilities. Taking these special dosing considerations into account allows for an individualized drug regimen that promotes the desired therapeutic outcome and minimizes the risk of toxicity.

THE CYTOCHROME P450 SYSTEM: What Is It and Why Should I Care?[1]

Looking beyond the obvious takes time, energy, insight, and fortitude; yet this is what we are called to do. We are nurses—tireless care providers. Yet, when the subject of the liver's enzyme system, also called the cytochrome P450 system, is discussed, we feel the urge to run the other way . . . or better yet, to just ignore the conversation. Yet, can we do this as the tireless care provider? The answer to this question is clear and simple: no, we cannot. This is because numerous medications, nutrients, and herbal therapies are metabolized through the cytochrome P450 (CYP450) enzyme system. This system can be inhibited or induced by drugs, and once altered can be clinically significant in the development of drug-drug interactions that may cause unanticipated adverse reactions or therapeutic failures. This article will review the basic concepts of the CYP450 system and relate these concepts to clinically significant altered responses.

The CYP450 enzymes are essential for the production of numerous agents including cholesterol and steroids. Additionally, these enzymes are necessary for the detoxification of foreign chemicals and the metabolism of drugs. CYP450 enzymes are so named because they are bound to membranes within a cell (cyto) and contain a heme pigment (chrome and P) that absorbs light at a wavelength of 450 nm when exposed to carbon monoxide. There are more than 50 CYP450 enzymes, but the CYP1A2, CYP2C19, CYP2D6, CYP1A2, CYP3A4, and CYP3A5 enzymes are responsible for metabolizing 45% of drug metabolism. The CYP2D6 (20–30%), the CYP2C9 (10%), and the CYP2E1 and CYP1A2 (5%) complete this enzyme system.

Drugs that cause CYP450 drug interactions are referred to as either inhibitors or inducers. An inducing agent can increase the rate of another drug's metabolism by as much as two- to threefold that develops over a period of a week. When an inducing agent is prescribed with another medication, the dosage of the other medication may need to be adjusted since the rate of metabolism is increased and the effect of the medication reduced. This can lead to a therapeutic failure of the medication. Conversely, if a medication is taken with an agent that inhibits its metabolism, then the drug level can rise and possibly result in a harmful or adverse effect. Information regarding a drug's CYP450 metabolism and its potential for inhibition or induction can be found on the drug label and accessed through the U.S. Food and Drug Administration (FDA) or manufacturer's websites.

When we assess our patients and provide management modalities, these are implemented within a framework of the patient's heritage, race, and culture. This is also true in pharmacology as well (i.e., "pharmacogenetics"). This concept is important to examine since we know that there exists genetic variability, which may influence a patient's response to commonly prescribed drug classes. This genetic variability can be defined as polymorphism. Seven percent of Caucasians and 2–7% of African Americans are poor metabolizers of drugs dependent on CYP2D6, which metabolizes many beta blockers, antidepressants, and opioids. This is because the drug's metabolism via CYP450 enzymes exhibits genetic variability.

Recently, researchers have studied the genetic variability in metabolism among women who were prescribed tamoxifen and medications that inhibit the CYP2D6 enzyme. To review, tamoxifen is biotransformed to the potent antiestrogen, endoxifen, by this enzyme. CYP2D6 genetic variation (individuals considered extensive metabolizers versus poor metabolizers) and inhibitors of the enzyme markedly reduce endoxifen plasma concentrations in tamoxifen-treated patients.

The researchers concluded that CYP2D6 metabolism is an "independent predictor of breast cancer outcome in post-menopausal women receiving tamoxifen for early breast cancer. Determination of CYP2D6 genotype may be of value in selecting adjuvant hormonal therapy and it appears CYP2D6 inhibitors should be avoided in tamoxifen-treated women." Do oncology patients come to us with only their cancer and its treatment? No, they come with multifaceted dimensions and co-morbid conditions such as hypertension, dyslipidemia, depression, seizure disorders, etc. For example, several antidepressants (paroxetine [Paxil] and fluoxetine [Prozac]) are inhibitors of metabolism when given with drugs metabolized through the CYP2D6 enzyme, such as haloperidol (Haldol), metoprolol (Lopressor), and hydrocodone. Thus, the therapeutic response can be accentuated. Medications that inhibit the CYP3A4 enzyme, such as amiodarone and antifungals, can affect the therapeutic response of fentanyl, alprazolam (Xanax), and numerous statins; as a result, the effect of these drugs can be enhanced leading to potential toxic levels.

At times, these CYP450 inducers and inhibitors are commonly ingested items such as grapefruit juice and tobacco. In the case of grapefruit juice, there are numerous medications known to interact with grapefruit juice including statins, antiarrhythmic agents, immunosuppressive agents, and calcium channel blockers. Furthermore, the inhibition of the enzyme system seems to be dose dependent; thus, the more a patient drinks, the more the inhibition that occurs. Additionally, the effects can last for several days if grapefruit juice is consumed on a regular basis. Luckily, the effect of this is not seen with other citrus juices.

Hopefully, this brief review has opened the door to your inquisitive nature on how the liver's enzyme system is affected by numerous medications and why some patients experience clinically significant unanticipated adverse reactions or therapeutic failures.

CYP1A2

Substrates	Inhibitors	Inducers
alosetron, amitriptyline, clozapine, cyclobenzaprine, desipramine, diazepam, duloxetine, fluvoxamine, imipramine, mexiletine, mirtazapine, olanzapine, propranolol, ropinirole, theophylline, (R)-warfarin	cimetidine, ciprofloxacin, fluvoxamine, ketoconazole, lidocaine, mexiletine	carbamazepine, cigarette smoke, phenobarbital, rifampin

CYP2C9

Substrates	Inhibitors	Inducers
celecoxib, glimepiride, glipizide, losartan, montelukast, nateglinide, phenytoin, sulfamethoxazole, voriconazole, (S)-warfarin	amiodarone, efavirenz, fluconazole, fluvastatin, ketoconazole, sulfamethoxazole, zafirlukast	carbamazepine, phenobarbital, phenytoin, rifampin

CYP2C19

Substrates	Inhibitors	Inducers
citalopram, diazepam, escitalopram, esomeprazole, imipramine, lansoprazole, nelfinavir, omeprazole, pantoprazole, phenytoin, rabeprazole, voriconazole	efavirenz, esomeprazole, fluoxetine, fluvoxamine, lansoprazole, omeprazole, rabeprazole, sertraline, ticlopidine	carbamazepine, phenytoin, rifampin

CYP2D6

Substrates	Inhibitors	Inducers
amitriptyline, aripiprazole, atomoxetine, codeine, desipramine, dextromethorphan, duloxetine, flecainide, fluoxetine, haloperidol, imipramine, lidocaine, metoprolol, mexiletine, mirtazapine, nefazodone, nortriptyline, oxycodone, paroxetine, propafenone, propranolol, risperidone, ritonavir, tramadol, venlafaxine	amiodarone, cimetidine, clozapine, desipramine, duloxetine, fluoxetine, haloperidol, lidocaine, methadone, paroxetine, pimozide, quinidine, ritonavir, sertraline, ticlopidine	None

CYP3A Substrates	Inhibitors	Inducers
alprazolam, amiodarone, aprepitant, aripiprazole, atorvastatin, boceprevir, buspirone, calcium channel blockers, carbamazepine, cilostazol, citalopram, clarithromycin, clonazepam, cyclosporine, dapsone, diazepam, disopyramide, efavirenz, ergot derivatives, erlotinib, erythromycin, escitalopram, estrogens, fentanyl, gefitinib, glucocorticoids, imatinib, indinavir, irinotecan, itraconazole, ketoconazole, lansoprazole, lidocaine, losartan, lovastatin, methadone, midazolam, mirtazapine, montelukast, nateglinide, nefazodone, nelfinavir, nevirapine, ondansetronoxycodone, paclitaxel, pimozide, protease inhibitors, quetiapine, quinidine, repaglinide, rifabutin, sildenafil, simvastatin, sirolimus, sorafenib, sunitinib, tacrolimus, tadalafil, tamoxifen, telaprevir, theophylline, tiagabine, ticlopidine, vardenafil, (R)-warfarin, zolpidem, zonisamide	amiodarone, aprepitant, cimetidine, clarithromycin, cyclosporine, diltiazem, efavirenz, erythromycin, fluconazole, grapefruit juice, imatinib, indinavir, itraconazole, ketoconazole, metronidazole, nefazodone, nelfinavir, quinidine, ritonavir, saquinavir, sertraline, verapamil, voriconazole	carbamazepine, efavirenz, nevirapine, phenobarbital, phenytoin, rifabutin, rifampin, St. John's wort

REFERENCES

1. Arcangelo VP, Peterson AM, Wilbur V, Reinhold JA. (2017). Pharmacotherapeutics for Advanced Practice: A Practical Approach. (4th ed). Philadelphia: Wolters Kluwer.
2. Krau SD. Cytochrome p450, part 1: what nurses really need to know. *Nurs Clin North Am* 2013; 48:671–80.
3. Krau SD. Cytochrome p450, part 2: what nurses need to know about the cytochrome p450 family systems. *Nurs Clin North Am* 2013;48:681–96.
4. Krau SD. Cytochrome p450, part 3: drug interactions: essential concepts and considerations. *Nurs Clin North Am* 2013;48:697–706.
5. Lynch T, Price, A. The effect of P450 metabolism on drug response, interactions, and adverse effects. *Am Fam Physician* 2007;76:391–7.

EDUCATING PATIENTS ABOUT SAFE MEDICATION USE

Research has shown that patients need information about several medication-related topics, no matter what the medication. A well-informed patient and/or family can help prevent medication errors by hospital staff and is less likely to make medication errors at home. Adherence to the medication regimen is another goal achieved through patient education.

Before beginning any teaching, however, always assess the patient's current knowledge by asking if he or she is familiar with the medication, how it is taken at home, what precautions or follow-up care is required, and other questions specific to each drug. Based on the patient's current knowledge level and taking into consideration factors such as readiness to learn, environmental and social barriers to learning or adherence, and cultural factors, discuss the following:

1. **Generic and brand names of the medication.** Patients should know both the brand and generic names of each medication for two reasons. It helps them identify their medications when a generic equivalent is substituted for a brand name version, and it prevents patients or health care providers from making sound-alike confusion errors when giving or documenting a medication history. An example of this is saying Celebrex but meaning or hearing Cerebyx.

2. **Purpose of the medication.** Patients have a right to know what the therapeutic benefit of the medication will be but also should be told the consequences of not taking the prescribed medication. This may enhance adherence. For example, a patient may be more likely to take blood pressure medication if told lowering high blood pressure will prevent heart attack, kidney disease, or stroke, rather than saying only that it will lower blood pressure.

3. **Dosage and how to take the medication.** To derive benefit and avoid adverse reactions or other poor outcomes, the patient must know how much of the medication to take and when to take it. Refer to dosages in metric weight (i.e., milligram, gram) rather than dosage unit (tablet) or volume (1 teaspoon). The patient must also be informed of the best time to take the medication, for example, on an empty or a full stomach, before bedtime, or with or without other medications. If possible, help the patient fit the medication schedule into his or her own schedule, so that taking the medication is not difficult or forgotten.

4. **What to do if a dose is missed.** Always explain to patients what to do if a dose is missed. Patients have been reported to take a double dose of medications when a missed dose occurs, putting themselves at risk for side effects and adverse reactions.

5. **Duration of therapy.** It is not uncommon for patients to stop taking a medication when they feel better or to discontinue a medication when they cannot perceive a benefit. For very long term, even lifelong therapy, the patient may need to be reminded that the medication helps maintain the current level of wellness. Patients may need to be reminded to finish short-term courses of medications even though they frequently will feel much better before the prescription runs out. Some medications cannot be discontinued abruptly and patients should be warned to consult a health care professional before discontinuing such agents. Patients will need to know to refill prescriptions several days before running out or to take extra medication if traveling.

6. **Minor side effects and what to do if they occur.** Inform the patient that all medications have potential side effects. Explain the most common side effects associated with the medication and how to avoid or manage them if they occur. An informed patient is less likely to stop taking a medication because of a minor and potentially avoidable side effect.

7. **Serious side effects and what to do if they occur.** Inform the patient of the possibility of serious side effects. Describe signs and symptoms associated with serious side effects, and tell the

patient to immediately inform a physician or nurse should they occur. Tell the patient to call before the next dose of the medication is scheduled and to not assume that the medication is the source of the symptom and prematurely discontinue it.

8. **Medications to avoid.** Drug-drug interactions can dampen drug effects, enhance drug effects, or cause life-threatening adverse events such as cardiac dysrhythmias, hepatitis, renal failure, or internal bleeding. The patient and family need to know which other medications, including which over-the-counter medications, to avoid.

9. **Foods to avoid and other precautions.** Food-drug interactions are not uncommon and can have effects similar to drug-drug interactions. Excessive sun exposure resulting in severe dermal reactions is not uncommon and represents an environmental-drug interaction. Likewise, the patient should be informed of what activities to avoid, in case the medication affects alertness or coordination, for example.

10. **How to store the medication:** Medications must be stored properly to maintain potency. Most medications should not be stored in the bathroom medicine cabinet because of excess heat and humidity. In addition, thoughtful storage practices, such as separating two family members' medications, can prevent mix-ups and inadvertent accessibility by children (or pets). Review storage with patients and ask about current methods for storing medications.

11. **Follow-up care.** Anyone taking medication requires ongoing care to assess effectiveness and appropriateness of medications. Many medications require invasive and noninvasive testing to monitor blood levels; hematopoietic, hepatic, or renal function; or other effects on other body systems. Ongoing medical evaluation may result in dosage adjustments, change in medication, or discontinuation of medication.

12. **What not to take.** Inform patients not to take expired medications or someone else's medication. Warn them not to self-medicate with older, no-longer-used prescriptions even if the remaining supply is not expired. Tell patients to keep a current record of all medications taken and to ask health care providers if new medications are meant to replace a current medication.

As you teach, encourage the patient and the family to ask questions. Providing feedback about medication questions will increase their understanding and help you identify areas that need reinforcement. Also, ask patients to repeat what you have said and return to demonstrate application or administration techniques.

Stress the importance of concurrent therapies. Medications often are only a part of a recommended therapy. Review with the patient and family other measures that will enhance or maintain health. Always consider the cultural context in which health information is provided and plan accordingly. This might include obtaining a same-gender translator or adjusting dosing times to avoid conflict with traditional rituals.

Finally, provide written instructions in a simple and easy-to-read format. Keep in mind that most health care information is written at a 10th grade reading level, while many patients read at a 5th grade level. Tell patients to keep the written instructions, so that they can be reviewed at home, when stress levels are lower and practical difficulties in maintaining the medication plan are known.

● ANTI-ALZHEIMER'S AGENTS

PHARMACOLOGIC PROFILE

General Use
Management of Alzheimer's dementia.

General Action and Information
All agents act by ↑ the amount of acetylcholine in the CNS by inhibiting cholinesterase. No agents to date can slow the progression of Alzheimer's dementia. Current agents may temporarily improve cognitive function and therefore improve quality of life.

Contraindications
Hypersensitivity.

Precautions
Use cautiously in patients with a history of "sick sinus syndrome" or other supraventricular cardiac conduction abnormalities (may cause bradycardia). Cholinergic effects may result in adverse GI effects (nausea, vomiting, diarrhea, weight loss) and may also ↑ gastric acid secretion resulting in GI bleeding, especially during concurrent NSAID therapy. Other cholinergic effects may include urinary tract obstruction, seizures, or bronchospasm.

Interactions
Additive effects with other drugs having cholinergic properties. May exaggerate the effects of succinylcholine-type muscle relaxation during anesthesia. May ↓ therapeutic effects of anticholinergics.

NURSING IMPLICATIONS

Assessment
- Assess cognitive function (memory, attention, reasoning, language, ability to perform simple tasks) throughout therapy.
- Monitor nausea, vomiting, anorexia, and weight loss. Notify health care professional if these side effects occur.

Patient/Family Teaching
- Instruct patient and caregiver that medication should be taken as directed.
- Advise patient and caregiver to notify health care professional if nausea, vomiting, anorexia, and weight loss occur.

Evaluation/Desired Outcomes
- Temporary improvement in cognitive function (memory, attention, reasoning, language, ability to perform simple tasks) in patients with Alzheimer's disease.

CLASSIFICATIONS

• ANTIANEMICS

PHARMACOLOGIC PROFILE

General Use
Prevention and treatment of anemias.

General Action and Information
Iron (ferric carboxymaltose, ferric pyrophosphate citrate, ferrous fumarate, ferrous gluconate, ferrous sulfate, ferumoxytol, iron dextran, iron sucrose, polysaccharide-iron complex, sodium ferric gluconate complex) is required for production of hemoglobin, which is necessary for oxygen transport to cells. Cyanocobalamin and hydroxocobalamin (vitamin B_{12}) and folic acid are water-soluble vitamins that are required for red blood cell production. Darbepoetin, epoetin, and methoxy polyethylene glycol-epoetin beta stimulate production of red blood cells.

Contraindications
Undiagnosed anemias. Hemochromatosis, hemosiderosis, hemolytic anemia (Iron). Uncontrolled hypertension (darbepoetin, epoetin, and methoxy polyethylene glycol-epoetin beta).

Precautions
Use parenteral iron (ferric carboxymaltose, ferric pyrophosphate citrate, ferumoxytol, iron dextran, iron sucrose, sodium ferric gluconate complex) cautiously in patients with a history of allergy or hypersensitivity reactions.

Interactions
Oral iron can ↓ the absorption of tetracyclines, fluoroquinolones, or penicillamine. Vitamin E may impair the therapeutic response to iron. Phenytoin and other anticonvulsants may ↓ the absorption of folic acid. Darbepoetin and epoetin may ↑ the requirement for heparin during hemodialysis.

NURSING IMPLICATIONS

Assessment
- Assess patient's nutritional status and dietary history to determine possible causes for anemia and need for patient teaching.

Implementation
- Iron salts are available in combination with many vitamins and minerals (see Appendix B).

Patient/Family Teaching
- Encourage patients to comply with diet recommendations of health care professional. Explain that the best source of vitamins and minerals is a well-balanced diet with foods from the four basic food groups.
- Patients self-medicating with vitamin and mineral supplements should be cautioned not to exceed RDA. The effectiveness of mega doses for treatment of various medical conditions is unproven and may cause side effects.

Evaluation/Desired Outcomes
- Resolution of anemia.

• ANTIANGINALS

PHARMACOLOGIC PROFILE

General Use
Nitrates are used to treat and prevent attacks of angina. Only nitrates (sublingual, lingual spray, topical, or intravenous) may be used in the acute treatment of attacks of angina pectoris. Calcium channel blockers, beta blockers, and ranolazine are used prophylactically in long-term management of angina.

General Action and Information
Several different groups of medications are used in the treatment of angina pectoris. The nitrates (isosorbide dinitrate, isosorbide mononitrate, and nitroglycerin) are available as a translingual spray, sublingual tablets, sublingual powder, intravenous solution, transdermal patch, topical ointment, and sustained-release oral dosage forms. Nitrates dilate coronary arteries and cause systemic vasodilation (↓ preload). Calcium channel blockers dilate coronary arteries (some also slow heart rate). Beta blockers ↓ myocardial oxygen consumption via a ↓ in heart rate. Ranolazine ↓ myocardial oxygen consumption.

Contraindications
Hypersensitivity. Avoid use of beta blockers or calcium channel blockers in advanced heart block, cardiogenic shock, or decompensated HF.

Precautions
Beta blockers should be used cautiously in patients with diabetes mellitus, pulmonary disease, or hypothyroidism.

Interactions
Nitrates, calcium channel blockers, and beta blockers may cause hypotension with other antihypertensives or acute ingestion of alcohol. Verapamil, diltiazem, and beta blockers may have additive myocardial depressant effects when used with other agents that affect cardiac function. Verapamil, diltiazem, and ranolazine have a number of other significant drug-drug interactions.

NURSING IMPLICATIONS

Assessment
- Assess location, duration, intensity, and precipitating factors of patient's anginal pain.
- Monitor BP and pulse periodically throughout therapy.

Implementation
- Available in various dose forms. See specific drugs for information on administration.

Patient/Family Teaching
- Instruct patient on concurrent nitrate therapy and prophylactic antianginals to continue taking both medications as ordered and to use sublingual/translingual nitroglycerin as needed for anginal attacks.
- Advise patient to contact health care professional immediately if chest pain does not improve; worsens after therapy; is accompanied by diaphoresis or shortness of breath; or if severe, persistent headache occurs.
- Caution patient to make position changes slowly to minimize orthostatic hypotension.
- Advise patient to avoid concurrent use of alcohol with these medications.

Evaluation/Desired Outcomes

- Decrease in frequency and severity of anginal attacks.
- Increase in activity tolerance.

• ANTIANXIETY AGENTS

PHARMACOLOGIC PROFILE

General Use

Antianxiety agents are used in the management of various forms of anxiety, including generalized anxiety disorder (GAD). Some agents are more suitable for intermittent or short-term use (benzodiazepines) while others are more useful long-term (buspirone, doxepin, fluoxetine, paroxetine, sertraline, venlafaxine).

General Action and Information

Most agents cause generalized CNS depression. Benzodiazepines may produce tolerance with long-term use and have potential for psychological or physical dependence. These agents have NO analgesic properties.

Contraindications

Hypersensitivity. Should not be used in comatose patients or in those with pre-existing CNS depression. Should not be used in patients with uncontrolled severe pain. Avoid use during pregnancy or lactation.

Precautions

Use cautiously in patients with hepatic impairment, severe renal impairment, or severe underlying pulmonary disease (benzodiazepines only). Use with caution in patients who may be suicidal or who may have had previous drug addictions. Patients may be more sensitive to CNS depressant effects; dosage ↓ may be required.

Interactions

Mainly for benzodiazepines; additive CNS depression with alcohol, antihistamines, some antidepressants, opioid analgesics, or phenothiazines may occur. Most agents should not be used with MAO inhibitors.

NURSING IMPLICATIONS

Assessment

- Monitor BP, pulse, and respiratory status frequently throughout IV administration.
- Prolonged high-dose therapy may lead to psychological or physical dependence. Restrict the amount of drug available to patient, especially if patient is depressed, suicidal, or has a history of addiction.
- **Anxiety:** Assess degree of anxiety and level of sedation (ataxia, dizziness, slurred speech) before and periodically throughout therapy.

Implementation

- Patients changing to buspirone from other antianxiety agents should receive gradually ↓ doses. Buspirone will not prevent withdrawal symptoms.

Patient/Family Teaching

- May cause daytime drowsiness. Caution patient to avoid driving and other activities requiring alertness until response to medication is known.

- Advise patient to avoid the use of alcohol and other CNS depressants concurrently with these medications.
- Advise patient to inform health care professional if pregnancy is planned or suspected.

Evaluation/Desired Outcomes

- Decrease in anxiety level.

• ANTIARRHYTHMICS

PHARMACOLOGIC PROFILE

General Use

Suppression of cardiac arrhythmias.

General Action and Information

Correct cardiac arrhythmias by a variety of mechanisms, depending on the group used. The therapeutic goal is ↓ symptomatology and ↑ hemodynamic performance. Choice of agent depends on etiology of arrhythmia and individual patient characteristics. Treatable causes of arrhythmias should be corrected before therapy is initiated (e.g., electrolyte disturbances, other drugs). Antiarrhythmics are generally classified by their effects on cardiac conduction tissue (see the following table). Adenosine, atropine, and digoxin are also used as antiarrhythmics.

MECHANISM OF ACTION OF MAJOR ANTIARRHYTHMIC DRUGS

CLASS	DRUGS	MECHANISM
IA	quinidine, procainamide, disopyramide	Na channel blockers, ↑ APD and ERP, ↓ membrane responsiveness
IB	lidocaine, phenytoin, mexiletine	Na channel blockers, ↓ APD and ERP
IC	flecainide, propafenone	Profound slowing of conduction by blocking Na channels, markedly depress phase 0; propafenone also has beta-blocking properties
II	esmolol, propranolol, metoprolol	Beta-blockers; ↓ AV nodal conduction, ↓ automaticity
III	amiodarone, dofetilide, dronedarone, ibutilide, sotalol	K channel blockers; amiodarone and dronedarone also have Na channel, beta-receptor, and Ca-channel blocking properties; sotalol also has beta-blocking properties
IV	diltiazem, verapamil	Non-dihydropyridine Ca channel blockers; ↓ AV nodal conduction

APD = action-potential duration; AV = atrioventricular; Ca = calcium; ERP = effective refractory period; K = potassium; Na = sodium.

Contraindications

Differ greatly among various agents. See individual drugs.

Precautions

Differ greatly among agents used. Appropriate dosage adjustments should be made in elderly patients and those with renal or hepatic impairment, depending on agent chosen. Correctable causes (electrolyte abnormalities, drug toxicity) should be evaluated. See individual drugs.

Interactions

Differ greatly among agents used. See individual drugs.

CLASSIFICATIONS

NURSING IMPLICATIONS

Assessment

- Monitor ECG, pulse, and BP continuously throughout IV administration and periodically throughout oral administration.

Implementation

- Take apical pulse before administration of oral doses. Withhold dose and notify physician or other health care professional if heart rate is <50 bpm.

Patient/Family Teaching

- Instruct patient to take oral doses around the clock, as directed, even if feeling better.
- Instruct patient or family member on how to take pulse. Advise patient to report changes in pulse rate or rhythm to health care professional.
- Caution patient to avoid taking OTC medications without consulting health care professional.
- Advise patient to carry identification describing disease process and medication regimen at all times.
- Emphasize the importance of follow-up exams to monitor progress.

Evaluation/Desired Outcomes

- Resolution of cardiac arrhythmias without detrimental side effects.

• ANTIASTHMATICS

PHARMACOLOGIC PROFILE

General Use

Management of acute and chronic episodes of reversible bronchoconstriction. Goal of therapy is to treat acute attacks (short-term control) and to ↓ incidence and intensity of future attacks (long-term control). The choice of modalities depends on the continued requirement for short term control agents.

General Action and Information

Adrenergic bronchodilators and phosphodiesterase inhibitors both work by ↑ intracellular levels of cyclic-3', 5'-adenosine monophosphate (cAMP); adrenergics by ↑ production and phosphodiesterase inhibitors by ↓ breakdown. ↑ levels of cAMP produce bronchodilation. Corticosteroids act by ↓ airway inflammation. Anticholinergics (ipratropium) produce bronchodilation by ↓ intracellular levels of cyclic guanosine monophosphate (cGMP). Leukotriene receptor antagonists and mast cell stabilizers ↓ the release of substances that can contribute to bronchospasm.

Contraindications

Inhaled corticosteroids, long-acting adrenergic agents, and mast cell stabilizers should not be used during acute attacks of asthma.

Precautions

Adrenergic bronchodilators and anticholinergics should be used cautiously in patients with cardiovascular disease. Chronic use of systemic corticosteroids should be avoided in children or during pregnancy or lactation. Patients with diabetes may experience loss of glycemic control during corticosteroid therapy. Corticosteroids should never be abruptly discontinued.

Interactions
Adrenergic bronchodilators and phosphodiesterase inhibitors may have additive CNS and cardiovascular effects with other adrenergic agents. Cimetidine ↑ theophylline levels and the risk of toxicity. Corticosteroids may ↓ the effectiveness of antidiabetics. Corticosteroids may cause hypokalemia which may be additive with potassium-losing diuretics and may also ↑ the risk of digoxin toxicity.

NURSING IMPLICATIONS

Assessment
- Assess lung sounds and respiratory function prior to and periodically throughout therapy.
- Assess cardiovascular status of patients taking adrenergic bronchodilators or anticholinergics. Monitor for ECG changes and chest pain.

Implementation
- **Inhaln:** Shake inhaler well, and allow at least 1 min between inhalations of aerosol medication. Prime the inhaler before first use. Use of spacer recommended for children.

Patient/Family Teaching
- Instruct patient to take antiasthmatics as directed. Do not take more than prescribed or discontinue without discussing with health care professional.
- Advise patient to avoid smoking and other respiratory irritants.
- Instruct patient in correct use of metered-dose inhaler or other administration devices (see Appendix D).
- Advise patient to contact health care professional promptly if the usual dose of medication fails to produce the desired results, if symptoms worsen after treatment, or if toxic effects occur.
- Patients using inhalation medications and bronchodilators should be advised to use the bronchodilator first and allow 5 min to elapse before administering other medications, unless otherwise directed by health care professional.

Evaluation/Desired Outcomes
- Prevention of and reduction in symptoms of asthma.

• ANTICHOLINERGICS

PHARMACOLOGIC PROFILE

General Use
Atropine—Bradyarrhythmias. **Ipratropium**—bronchospasm (inhalation) and rhinorrhea (intranasal). **Scopolamine**—Nausea and vomiting related to motion sickness and vertigo. **Propantheline and glycopyrrolate**— ↓ gastric secretory activity and ↑ esophageal sphincter tone. Atropine and scopolamine are also used as ophthalmic mydriatics. **Benztropine and trihexyphenidyl**—Parkinson's disease. **Oxybutynin and tolterodine**—Overactive bladder.

General Action and Information
Competitively inhibit the action of acetylcholine. In addition, atropine, glycopyrrolate, propantheline, and scopolamine are antimuscarinic in that they inhibit the action of acetylcholine at sites innervated by postganglionic cholinergic nerves.

Contraindications

Hypersensitivity, narrow-angle glaucoma, severe hemorrhage, tachycardia (due to thyrotoxicosis or cardiac insufficiency), or myasthenia gravis.

Precautions

Geriatric and pediatric patients are more susceptible to adverse effects. Use cautiously in patients with urinary tract pathology; those at risk for GI obstruction; and those with chronic renal, hepatic, pulmonary, or cardiac disease.

Interactions

Additive anticholinergic effects (dry mouth, dry eyes, blurred vision, constipation) with other agents possessing anticholinergic activity, including antihistamines, antidepressants, quinidine, and disopyramide. May alter GI absorption of other drugs by inhibiting GI motility and ↑ transit time. Antacids may ↓ absorption of orally administered anticholinergics.

NURSING IMPLICATIONS

Assessment

- Assess vital signs and ECG frequently during IV drug therapy. Report any significant changes in heart rate or BP or increase in ventricular ectopy or angina promptly.
- Monitor intake and output ratios in elderly or surgical patients; may cause urinary retention.
- Assess patient regularly for abdominal distention and auscultate for bowel sounds. Constipation may become a problem. Increasing fluids and adding bulk to the diet may help alleviate constipation.

Implementation

- **PO:** Administer oral doses of glycopyrrolate, propantheline, or scopolamine 30 min before meals.
- Scopolamine transdermal patch should be applied at least 4 hr before travel.

Patient/Family Teaching

- Instruct patient that frequent rinses, sugarless gum or candy, and good oral hygiene may help relieve dry mouth.
- May cause drowsiness. Caution patient to avoid driving or other activities requiring alertness until response to medication is known.
- **Ophth:** Advise patients that ophthalmic preparations may temporarily blur vision and impair ability to judge distances. Dark glasses may be needed to protect eyes from bright light.

Evaluation/Desired Outcomes

- Increase in heart rate.
- Decrease in nausea and vomiting related to motion sickness or vertigo.
- Dryness of mouth.
- Dilation of pupils.
- Decrease in GI motility.
- Resolution of signs and symptoms of Parkinson's disease.
- Decreased urinary frequency, urgency, and urge incontinence.

• ANTICOAGULANTS

PHARMACOLOGIC PROFILE

General Use
Prevention and treatment of thromboembolic disorders including deep vein thrombosis, pulmonary embolism, and atrial fibrillation. Also used in the management of myocardial infarction (MI) sequentially or in combination with thrombolytics and/or antiplatelet agents.

General Action and Information
Anticoagulants are used to prevent clot extension and formation. They do not dissolve clots. The main types of anticoagulants in common use are parenteral heparins, oral warfarin, oral/parenteral direct thrombin inhibitors, and oral/parenteral factor Xa inhibitors. When initiating warfarin, unfractionated heparin or a low-molecular weight heparin is usually administered concomitantly initially since warfarin takes several days to produce therapeutic anticoagulation. Once a therapeutic anticoagulant effect is achieved with warfarin, the unfractionated heparin or low-molecular weight heparin will be discontinued. Unfractionated heparin (at lower doses), a low-molecular weight heparin (at lower doses), or fondaparinux are mostly used to prevent deep vein thrombosis after certain surgical procedures or situations in which prolonged bedrest increases the risk of thromboembolism. Argatroban is used to provide anticoagulation in patients who have developed thrombocytopenia during heparin therapy.

Contraindications
Underlying coagulation disorders, ulcer disease, malignancy, recent surgery, or active bleeding.

Precautions
Anticoagulation should be undertaken cautiously in any patient with a potential site for bleeding. Pregnant or lactating patients should not receive warfarin. Heparin does not cross the placenta. All anticoagulants should be used cautiously in patients receiving epidural analgesia.

Interactions
Warfarin is highly protein bound and may displace or be displaced by other highly protein-bound drugs. The resultant interactions depend on which drug is displaced. Bleeding may be potentiated by aspirin or large doses of penicillins or penicillin-like drugs, cefotetan, cefoperazone, valproic acid, or NSAIDs.

NURSING IMPLICATIONS

Assessment
- Assess patient taking anticoagulants for signs of bleeding and hemorrhage (bleeding gums; nosebleed; unusual bruising; tarry, black stools; hematuria; fall in hematocrit or BP; guaiac-positive stools; urine; or NG aspirate).
- Assess patient for evidence of additional or increased thrombosis. Symptoms will depend on area of involvement.
- **Lab Test Considerations:** Monitor prothrombin time (PT) or international normalized ratio (INR) with warfarin therapy, activated partial thromboplastin time (aPTT) with full-dose heparin therapy and hematocrit, and other clotting factors frequently during therapy.

- **Toxicity and Overdose:** If overdose occurs or anticoagulation needs to be immediately reversed, the antidote for heparins is protamine sulfate; for warfarin, the antidote is vitamin K (phytonadione); for dabigatran, the antidote is idarucizumab; for rivaroxaban and apixaban, the antidote is andexanet alfa. Administration of fresh frozen plasma or prothrombin complex concentrate may also be required in severe bleeding due to warfarin, the oral direct thrombin inhibitors, or the oral factor Xa inhibitors.

Implementation
- Inform all health care professionals caring for patient of anticoagulant therapy. Venipunctures and injection sites require application of pressure to prevent bleeding or hematoma formation.
- Use an infusion pump with continuous infusions to ensure accurate dosage.

Patient/Family Teaching
- Caution patient to avoid activities leading to injury, to use a soft toothbrush and electric razor, and to report any symptoms of unusual bleeding or bruising to health care professional immediately.
- Instruct patient not to take OTC medications, especially those containing aspirin, NSAIDs, or alcohol, without advice of health care professional.
- Review foods high in vitamin K (see Appendix K) with patients on warfarin. Patient should have consistent limited intake of these foods, as vitamin K is the antidote for warfarin and greatly alternating intake of these foods will cause the INR to fluctuate.
- Emphasize the importance of frequent lab tests to monitor the degree of anticoagulation with unfractionated heparin or warfarin.
- Instruct patient to carry identification describing medication regimen at all times and to inform all health care professionals caring for patient of anticoagulant therapy before laboratory tests, treatment, or surgery.

Evaluation/Desired Outcomes
- Prevention of undesired clotting and its sequelae without signs of hemorrhage. Prevention of stroke, MI, and death in patients at risk.

• ANTICONVULSANTS

PHARMACOLOGIC PROFILE

General Use
Anticonvulsants are used to ↓ the incidence and severity of seizures due to various etiologies. Some anticonvulsants are used parenterally in the immediate treatment of seizures. It is not uncommon for patients to require more than one anticonvulsant to control seizures on a long-term basis. Several anticonvulsants are evaluated with serum level monitoring. Several anticonvulsants also are used to treat neuropathic pain.

General Action and Information
Anticonvulsants include a variety of agents, all capable of depressing abnormal neuronal discharges in the CNS that may result in seizures. They may work by preventing the spread of seizure activity, depressing the motor cortex, raising seizure threshold, or altering levels of neurotransmitters, depending on the group. See individual drugs.

Contraindications
Previous hypersensitivity.

Precautions

Use cautiously in patients with severe hepatic or renal impairment; dose adjustment may be required. Choose agents carefully in pregnant and lactating women. Fetal hydantoin syndrome may occur in offspring of patients who receive phenytoin during pregnancy.

Interactions

Barbiturates stimulate the metabolism of other drugs that are metabolized by the liver, ↓ their effectiveness. Phenytoin is highly protein-bound and may displace or be displaced by other highly protein-bound drugs. Lamotrigine, tiagabine, and topiramate are capable of interacting with several other anticonvulsants. Many drugs are capable of lowering seizure threshold and may ↓ the effectiveness of anticonvulsants, including tricyclic antidepressants and phenothiazines. For more specific interactions, see individual drugs.

NURSING IMPLICATIONS

Assessment

- Assess location, duration, and characteristics of seizure activity.
- **Toxicity and Overdose:** Monitor serum drug levels routinely throughout anticonvulsant therapy, especially when adding or discontinuing other medications.

Implementation

- Administer anticonvulsants around the clock. Abrupt discontinuation may precipitate status epilepticus.
- Implement seizure precautions.

Patient/Family Teaching

- Instruct patient to take medication every day, exactly as directed.
- May cause drowsiness. Caution patient to avoid driving or other activities requiring alertness until response to medication is known. Do not resume driving until physician gives clearance based on control of seizures.
- Advise patient to avoid taking alcohol or other CNS depressants concurrently with these medications.
- Advise patient to carry identification describing disease process and medication regimen at all times.

Evaluation/Desired Outcomes

- Decrease or cessation of seizures without excessive sedation.
- Decreased neuropathic pain.

• ANTIDEPRESSANTS

PHARMACOLOGIC PROFILE

General Use

Used in the treatment of various forms of endogenous depression, often in conjunction with psychotherapy. Other uses include: Treatment of anxiety (doxepin, duloxetine, fluoxetine, paroxetine, sertraline, venlafaxine); Enuresis (imipramine); Chronic pain syndromes (amitriptyline, doxepin, duloxetine, imipramine, nortriptyline); Smoking cessation (bupropion); Bulimia (fluoxetine); Obsessive-compulsive disorder (fluoxetine, fluvoxamine, paroxetine, sertraline); Social anxiety disorder (paroxetine, sertraline, venlafaxine).

General Action and Information

Antidepressant activity is most likely due to preventing the reuptake of dopamine, norepinephrine, and serotonin by presynaptic neurons, resulting in accumulation of these neurotransmitters. The major classes of antidepressants are the tricyclic antidepressants, the selective serotonin reuptake inhibitors (SSRIs), and the serotonin/norepinephrine reuptake inhibitors (SNRIs). Most tricyclic agents possess significant anticholinergic and sedative properties, which explains many of their side effects (amitriptyline, amoxapine, desipramine, doxepin, imipramine, nortriptyline, trimipramine). The SSRIs are more likely to cause insomnia (citalopram, escitalopram, fluoxetine, fluvoxamine, paroxetine, sertraline, vortioxetine, vilazodone). The SNRIs include desvenlafaxine, duloxetine, levomilnacipran, milnacipran, and venlafaxine.

Contraindications

Hypersensitivity. Should not be used in narrow-angle glaucoma. Should not be used in pregnancy or lactation or immediately after MI.

Precautions

Use cautiously in older patients and those with pre-existing cardiovascular disease. Elderly men with prostatic enlargement may be more susceptible to urinary retention. Anticholinergic side effects of tricyclic antidepressants (dry eyes, dry mouth, blurred vision, and constipation) may require dosage modification or drug discontinuation. Dosage requires slow titration; onset of therapeutic response may be 2–4 wk. May ↓ seizure threshold, especially bupropion.

Interactions

Tricyclic antidepressants—May cause hypertension, tachycardia, and convulsions when used with MAO inhibitors. May prevent therapeutic response to some antihypertensives. Additive CNS depression with other CNS depressants. Sympathomimetic activity may be enhanced when used with other sympathomimetics. Additive anticholinergic effects with other drugs possessing anticholinergic properties. **MAO inhibitors**—Hypertensive crisis may occur with concurrent use of MAO inhibitors and amphetamines, methyldopa, levodopa, dopamine, epinephrine, norepinephrine, desipramine, imipramine, vasoconstrictors, or ingestion of tyramine-containing foods. Hypertension or hypotension, coma, convulsions, and death may occur with use of meperidine or other opioid analgesics and MAO inhibitors. Additive hypotension with antihypertensives or spinal anesthesia and MAO inhibitors. Additive hypoglycemia with insulin or oral hypoglycemic agents and MAO inhibitors. SSRIs, bupropion, or venlafaxine should not be used in combination with or within weeks of MAO inhibitors (see individual monographs). Risk of adverse reactions with MAO inhibitors may be ↑ by almotriptan, frovatriptan, rizatriptan, naratriptan, sumatriptan, or zolmitriptan.

NURSING IMPLICATIONS

Assessment

- Monitor mental status and affect. Assess for suicidal tendencies, especially during early therapy. Restrict amount of drug available to patient.
- **Toxicity and Overdose:** Concurrent ingestion of MAO inhibitors and tyramine-containing foods may lead to hypertensive crisis. Symptoms include chest pain, severe headache, nuchal rigidity, nausea and vomiting, photosensitivity, and enlarged pupils. Treatment includes IV phentolamine.

Implementation
- Administer drugs that are sedating at bedtime to avoid excessive drowsiness during waking hours, and administer drugs that cause insomnia in the morning.

Patient/Family Teaching
- Caution patient to avoid alcohol and other CNS depressants. Patients receiving MAO inhibitors should also avoid OTC drugs and foods or beverages containing tyramine (see Appendix K) during and for at least 2 wk after therapy has been discontinued, as they may precipitate a hypertensive crisis. A health care professional should be contacted immediately if symptoms of hypertensive crisis develop.
- Inform patient that dizziness or drowsiness may occur. Caution patient to avoid driving and other activities requiring alertness until response to the drug is known.
- Caution patient to make position changes slowly to minimize orthostatic hypotension.
- Advise patient to notify health care professional if dry mouth, urinary retention, or constipation occurs. Frequent rinses, good oral hygiene, and sugarless candy or gum may diminish dry mouth. An increase in fluid intake, fiber, and exercise may prevent constipation.
- Advise patient to notify health care professional of medication regimen and any herbal alternative therapies before treatment or surgery. MAO inhibitor therapy usually needs to be withdrawn at least 2 wk before use of anesthetic agents.
- Emphasize the importance of participation in psychotherapy and follow-up exams to evaluate progress.

Evaluation/Desired Outcomes
- Resolution of depression.
- Decrease in anxiety.
- Control of bedwetting in children over 6 yr of age.
- Management of chronic neurogenic pain.

• ANTIDIABETICS

PHARMACOLOGIC PROFILE

General Use
Insulin is used in the management of type 1 diabetes mellitus. It may also be used in type 2 diabetes mellitus when diet and/or oral medications fail to adequately control blood sugar. The choice of insulin preparation (rapid-acting, intermediate-acting, long-acting) depends on the degree of control desired, daily blood glucose fluctuations, and history of previous reactions. Oral agents non-insulin injectable agents are used primarily in type 2 diabetes mellitus. Oral agents are used when diet therapy alone fails to control blood glucose or symptoms or when patients are not amenable to using insulin or another injectable agent. Some oral agents may be used with insulin.

General Action and Information
Insulin, a hormone produced by the pancreas, lowers blood glucose by ↑ transport of glucose into cells and promotes the conversion of glucose to glycogen. It also promotes the conversion of amino acids to proteins in muscle, stimulates triglyceride formation, and inhibits the release of free fatty acids. Sulfonylureas, nateglinide, repaglinide, the dipeptidyl peptidase 4 (DPP-4) inhibitors (e.g. sitagliptin), and the glucagon-like peptide-1 (GLP-1) receptor agonists (e.g. exenatide) ↓ blood glucose by stimulating endogenous insulin se-

cretion by beta cells of the pancreas and by ↑ sensitivity to insulin at intracellular receptor sites. Intact pancreatic function is required. Acarbose and miglitol delay digestion of ingested carbohydrates, thus ↓ blood glucose, especially after meals. The thiazolidinediones (e.g. pioglitazone) and metformin ↑ insulin sensitivity. The sodium-glucose transporter 2 (SGLT2) inhibitors (e.g. empagliflozin) inhibit the reabsorption of glucose in the proximal renal tubule, thereby ↑ the excretion of glucose in the urine.

Contraindications

Insulin—Hypoglycemia. **Oral hypoglycemic agents**—Hypersensitivity (cross-sensitivity with other sulfonylureas and sulfonamides may exist). Hypoglycemia. Type 1 diabetes. Avoid use in patients with severe kidney, liver, thyroid, and other endocrine dysfunction. Should not be used in pregnancy or lactation. **DPP–4 inhibitors**—Type 1 diabetes. **GLP-1 agonists**—Personal or family history of medullary thyroid carcinoma. Multiple Endocrine Neoplasia syndrome type 2. **SGLT2 inhibitors**—Severe renal impairment.

Precautions

Insulin—Infection, stress, or changes in diet may alter requirements. **Oral hypoglycemic agents**—Use cautiously in geriatric patients. Dose ↓ may be necessary. Infection, stress, or changes in diet may alter requirements. Use sulfonylureas with caution in patients with a history of cardiovascular disease. Metformin may cause lactic acidosis. **DPP–4 inhibitors**—Use cautiously in patients with renal impairment, history of pancreatitis, or history of angioedema to another DPP-4 inhibitor. **GLP-1 agonists**—Use cautiously in patients with a history of pancreatitis or history of angioedema to another GLP-1 agonist. **SGLT2 inhibitors**—Use cautiously in patients with moderate renal impairment or history of pancreatitis. Hypovolemia, chronic kidney disease, HF, concurrent use of diuretics, NSAIDs, ACE inhibitors, or ARBs may ↑ risk of acute kidney injury. Previous amputation, peripheral vascular disease, neuropathy, or diabetic foot infection may ↑ risk of lower limb amputation.

Interactions

Insulin—Additive hypoglycemic effects with oral hypoglycemic agents. **Oral hypoglycemic agents**—Ingestion of alcohol may result in disulfiram-like reaction with some agents. Alcohol, corticosteroids, rifampin, glucagon, and thiazide and loop diuretics may ↓ effectiveness. Anabolic steroids, chloramphenicol, MAO inhibitors, most NSAIDs, salicylates, sulfonamides, and warfarin may ↑ hypoglycemic effect. Beta blockers may produce hypoglycemia and mask signs and symptoms of hypoglycemia. **DPP–4 inhibitors**—Use with insulin or sulfonylureas may ↑ hypoglycemic effect. **GLP-1 agonists**—Use with sulfonylureas may ↑ hypoglycemic effect. **SGLT2 inhibitors**—Use with insulin or sulfonylureas may ↑ hypoglycemic effect. NSAIDs, diuretics, ACE inhibitors, or ARBs may ↑ risk of acute kidney injury.

NURSING IMPLICATIONS

Assessment

- Observe patient for signs and symptoms of hypoglycemic reactions.
- Metformin, acarbose, miglitol, and the thiazolidinediones do not cause hypoglycemia when taken alone but may ↑ the hypoglycemic effect of other hypoglycemic agents.
- Patients who have been well controlled on metformin but develop illness or laboratory abnormalities should be assessed for ketoacidosis or lactic acidosis. Assess serum electrolytes, renal function, ketones, glucose, and, if indicated, blood pH and lactate and pyruvate levels. If either form of acidosis is present, discontinue metformin immediately and treat acidosis.

- **Lab Test Considerations:** Serum glucose and glycosylated hemoglobin should be monitored periodically throughout therapy to evaluate effectiveness of treatment.

Implementation

- Patients stabilized on a diabetic regimen who are exposed to stress, fever, trauma, infection, or surgery may require sliding scale insulin. Withhold oral hypoglycemic agents and reinstitute after resolution of acute illness.
- **Insulin:** Available in different types and strengths and from different species. Check type, species, source, dose, and expiration date with another licensed nurse. Do not interchange insulins without physician's order. Use only insulin syringes to draw up dose. Use only U100 syringes to draw up insulin lispro dose.

Patient/Family Teaching

- Explain to patient that medication controls hyperglycemia but does not cure diabetes. Therapy is long-term.
- Review signs of hypoglycemia and hyperglycemia with patient. If hypoglycemia occurs, advise patient to take a glass of orange juice or 2–3 tsp of sugar, honey, or corn syrup dissolved in water (glucose, not table sugar, if taking miglitol), and notify health care professional.
- Encourage patient to follow prescribed diet, medication, and exercise regimen to prevent hypoglycemic or hyperglycemic episodes.
- Instruct patient in proper testing of serum glucose and ketones.
- Advise patient to notify health care professional if nausea, vomiting, or fever develops; if unable to eat usual diet; or if blood glucose levels are not controlled.
- Advise patient to carry sugar or a form of glucose and identification describing medication regimen at all times.
- Insulin is the recommended method of controlling blood glucose during pregnancy. Counsel female patients to use a form of contraception other than oral contraceptives and to notify health care professional promptly if pregnancy is planned or suspected.
- **Insulin:** Instruct patient on proper technique for administration; include type of insulin, equipment (syringe and cartridge pens), storage, and syringe disposal. Discuss the importance of not changing brands of insulin or syringes, selection and rotation of injection sites, and compliance with therapeutic regimen.
- **Sulfonylureas:** Advise patient that concurrent use of alcohol may cause a disulfiram-like reaction (abdominal cramps, nausea, flushing, headache, and hypoglycemia).
- **Metformin:** Explain to patient the risk of lactic acidosis and the potential need for discontinuation of metformin therapy if a severe infection, dehydration, or severe or continuing diarrhea occurs or if medical tests or surgery is required.

Evaluation/Desired Outcomes

- Control of blood glucose levels without the appearance of hypoglycemic or hyperglycemic episodes.

• ANTIDIARRHEALS

PHARMACOLOGIC PROFILE

General Use

For the control and symptomatic relief of acute and chronic nonspecific diarrhea.

C L A S S I F I C A T I O N S

General Action and Information
Diphenoxylate/atropine, difenoxin/atropine, and loperamide slow intestinal motility and propulsion. Bismuth subsalicylate affects fluid content of the stool. Bismuth subsalicylate is also used as part of the management of peptic ulcer disease due to *Helicobacter pylori*. Polycarbophil acts as an antidiarrheal by taking on water within the bowel lumen to create a formed stool. Polycarbophil may also be used to treat constipation. Octreotide is used specifically for diarrhea associated with GI endocrine tumors.

Contraindications
Previous hypersensitivity. Severe abdominal pain of unknown cause, especially when associated with fever.

Precautions
Use cautiously in patients with severe liver disease or inflammatory bowel disease. Safety in pregnancy and lactation not established (diphenoxylate/atropine and loperamide). Octreotide may aggravate gallbladder disease.

Interactions
Polycarbophil ↓ the absorption of tetracycline. Octreotide may alter the response to insulin or oral hypoglycemic agents.

NURSING IMPLICATIONS

Assessment
- Assess the frequency and consistency of stools and bowel sounds before and throughout therapy.
- Assess patient's fluid and electrolyte status and skin turgor for dehydration.

Implementation
- Shake liquid preparations before administration.

Patient/Family Teaching
- Instruct patient to notify health care professional if diarrhea persists; or if fever, abdominal pain, or palpitations occur.

Evaluation/Desired Outcomes
- Decrease in diarrhea.

• ANTIEMETICS

PHARMACOLOGIC PROFILE

General Use
Phenothiazines, dolasetron, granisetron, metoclopramide, ondansetron, and palonosetron are used to manage nausea and vomiting of many causes, including surgery, anesthesia, and antineoplastic and radiation therapy. Aprepitant, fosaprepitant, netupitant, and rolapitant are used specifically with emetogenic chemotherapy. Dimenhydrinate, scopolamine, and meclizine are used almost exclusively to prevent motion sickness.

General Action and Information
Phenothiazines act on the chemoreceptor trigger zone to inhibit nausea and vomiting. Dimenhydrinate, scopolamine, and meclizine act as antiemetics mainly by diminishing mo-

tion sickness. Metoclopramide ↓ nausea and vomiting by its effects on gastric emptying. Dolasetron, granisetron, palonosetron, and ondansetron block the effects of serotonin at 5-HT_3 receptor sites. Aprepitant, fosaprepitant, netupitant, and rolapitant act as selective antagonists at substance P/neurokinin 1 receptors in the brain.

Contraindications
Previous hypersensitivity.

Precautions
Use phenothiazines cautiously in children who may have viral illnesses. Use dolasetron, granisetron, palonosetron, and ondansetron with caution in patients with QT interval prolongation. Choose agents carefully in pregnant patients (no agents are approved for safe use).

Interactions
Additive CNS depression with other CNS depressants including antidepressants, antihistamines, opioid analgesics, and sedative/hypnotics. Phenothiazines may produce hypotension when used with antihypertensives, nitrates, or acute ingestion of alcohol.

NURSING IMPLICATIONS
Assessment
- Assess nausea, vomiting, bowel sounds, and abdominal pain before and following administration.
- Monitor hydration status and intake and output. Patients with severe nausea and vomiting may require IV fluids in addition to antiemetics.

Implementation
- For prophylactic administration, follow directions for specific drugs so that peak effect corresponds to time of anticipated nausea.

Patient/Family Teaching
- Advise patient and family to use general measures to decrease nausea (begin with sips of liquids and small, nongreasy meals; provide oral hygiene; and remove noxious stimuli from environment).
- May cause drowsiness. Advise patient to call for assistance when ambulating and to avoid driving or other activities requiring alertness until response to medication is known.
- Advise patient to make position changes slowly to minimize orthostatic hypotension.

Evaluation/Desired Outcomes
- Prevention of, or decrease in, nausea and vomiting.

• ANTIFUNGALS

PHARMACOLOGIC PROFILE
General Use
Treatment of fungal infections. Infections of skin or mucous membranes may be treated with topical or vaginal preparations. Deep-seated or systemic infections require oral or parenteral therapy. Lipid-based formulations of amphotericin employ lipid encapsulation technology designed to ↓ nephrotoxicity.

General Action and Information
Kill (fungicidal) or stop growth of (fungistatic) susceptible fungi by affecting the permeability of the fungal cell membrane or protein synthesis within the fungal cell itself.

Contraindications
Previous hypersensitivity.

Precautions
Because most systemic antifungals may have adverse effects on bone marrow function, use cautiously in patients with depressed bone marrow reserve. Amphotericin B commonly causes renal impairment. Fluconazole requires dosage adjustment in the presence of renal impairment. Adverse reactions to fluconazole may be more severe in HIV-positive patients. The IV formulation of voriconazole should be avoided in patients with renal impairment.

Interactions
Differ greatly among various agents. See individual drugs.

NURSING IMPLICATIONS

Assessment
- Assess patient for signs of infection and assess involved areas of skin and mucous membranes before and throughout therapy. Increased skin irritation may indicate need to discontinue medication.

Implementation
- Available in various dosage forms. Refer to specific drugs for directions for administration.
- **Topical:** Consult physician or other health care professional for cleansing technique before applying medication. Wear gloves during application. Do not use occlusive dressings unless specified by physician or other health care professional.

Patient/Family Teaching
- Instruct patient on proper use of medication form.
- Instruct patient to continue medication as directed for full course of therapy, even if feeling better.
- Advise patient to report increased skin irritation or lack of therapeutic response to health care professional.

Evaluation/Desired Outcomes
- Resolution of signs and symptoms of infection. Length of time for complete resolution depends on organism and site of infection. Deep-seated fungal infections may require prolonged therapy (weeks–months). Recurrent fungal infections may be a sign of serious systemic illness.

• ANTIHISTAMINES

PHARMACOLOGIC PROFILE

General Use
Relief of symptoms associated with allergies, including rhinitis, urticaria, and angioedema, and as adjunctive therapy in anaphylactic reactions. Some antihistamines are used to treat

motion sickness (dimenhydrinate and meclizine), insomnia (diphenhydramine), Parkinson-like reactions (diphenhydramine), and other nonallergic conditions.

General Action and Information

Antihistamines block the effects of histamine at the H_1 receptor. They do not block histamine release, antibody production, or antigen-antibody reactions. Most antihistamines have anticholinergic properties and may cause constipation, dry eyes, dry mouth, and blurred vision. In addition, many antihistamines cause sedation. Some phenothiazines have strong antihistaminic properties (hydroxyzine and promethazine).

Contraindications

Hypersensitivity and angle-closure glaucoma. Should not be used in premature or newborn infants.

Precautions

Elderly patients may be more susceptible to adverse anticholinergic effects of antihistamines. Use cautiously in patients with pyloric obstruction, prostatic hypertrophy, hyperthyroidism, cardiovascular disease, or severe liver disease. Use cautiously in pregnancy and lactation.

Interactions

Additive sedation when used with other CNS depressants, including alcohol, antidepressants, opioid analgesics, and sedative/hypnotics. MAO inhibitors prolong and intensify the anticholinergic properties of antihistamines.

NURSING IMPLICATIONS

Assessment

- Assess allergy symptoms (rhinitis, conjunctivitis, hives) before and periodically throughout therapy.
- Monitor pulse and BP before initiating and throughout IV therapy.
- Assess lung sounds and character of bronchial secretions. Maintain fluid intake of 1500–2000 mL/day to decrease viscosity of secretions.
- **Nausea and Vomiting:** Assess degree of nausea and frequency and amount of emesis when administering for nausea and vomiting.
- **Anxiety:** Assess mental status, mood, and behavior when administering for anxiety.
- **Pruritus:** Observe the character, location, and size of affected area when administering for pruritic skin conditions.

Implementation

- When used for prophylaxis of motion sickness, administer at least 30 min and preferably 1–2 hr before exposure to conditions that may precipitate motion sickness.
- When administering concurrently with opioid analgesics (hydroxyzine, promethazine), supervise ambulation closely to prevent injury secondary to increased sedation.

Patient/Family Teaching

- Inform patient that drowsiness may occur. Avoid driving or other activities requiring alertness until response to drug is known.
- Caution patient to avoid using concurrent alcohol or CNS depressants.
- Advise patient that good oral hygiene, frequent rinsing of mouth with water, and sugarless gum or candy may help relieve dryness of mouth.
- Instruct patient to contact health care professional if symptoms persist.

Evaluation/Desired Outcomes
- Decrease in allergic symptoms.
- Prevention or decreased severity of nausea and vomiting.
- Relief of pruritus.
- Sedation when used as a hypnotic.

• ANTIHYPERTENSIVES

PHARMACOLOGIC PROFILE

General Use
Treatment of hypertension of many causes, most commonly essential hypertension. Parenteral products are used in the treatment of hypertensive emergencies. Oral treatment should be initiated as soon as possible and individualized to ensure adherence and compliance for long-term therapy. Therapy is initiated with agents having minimal side effects. When such therapy fails, more potent drugs with different side effects are added in an effort to control BP while causing minimal patient discomfort.

General Action and Information
As a group, the antihypertensives are used to lower BP to a normal level (<130–140 systolic and <80–90 mm Hg diastolic) or to the lowest level tolerated. The goal of antihypertensive therapy is prevention of end-organ damage. Antihypertensives are classified into groups according to their site of action. These include alpha-1 receptor antagonists, centrally-acting alpha-adrenergic agonists; beta blockers; vasodilators; ACE inhibitors; angiotensin II receptor blockers (ARBs); calcium channel blockers; renin inhibitors; and diuretics. Hypertensive emergencies may be managed with parenteral agents, such as nitroprusside, nicardipine, or beta blockers (e.g. esmolol, labetalol).

Contraindications
Hypersensitivity to individual agents.

Precautions
Choose agents carefully in pregnancy and during lactation. ACE inhibitors, ARBs, and aliskiren should be avoided during pregnancy. Centrally acting alpha-adrenergic agonists and beta blockers should be used only in patients who are compliant with their medications because abrupt discontinuation of these agents may result in rapid and excessive ↑ in BP (rebound phenomenon). Thiazide and loop diuretics may ↑ the risk of hyperglycemia. Vasodilators may cause tachycardia if used alone and are commonly used in combination with beta blockers. Some antihypertensives (e.g. hydralazine, minoxidil) cause sodium and water retention and are usually combined with a diuretic.

Interactions
Many drugs can negate the therapeutic effectiveness of antihypertensives, including NSAIDs, sympathomimetics, decongestants, appetite suppressants, SNRIs, and MAO inhibitors. Hypokalemia from diuretics may ↑ the risk of digoxin toxicity. Potassium supplements and potassium-sparing diuretics may cause hyperkalemia when used with ACE inhibitors, ARBs, or aliskiren.

NURSING IMPLICATIONS

Assessment

- Monitor BP and pulse frequently during dosage adjustment and periodically throughout therapy.
- Monitor intake and output ratios and daily weight with use of diuretics.
- Monitor frequency of prescription refills to determine compliance.

Implementation

- Many antihypertensives are available as combination products to enhance compliance (see Appendix B).

Patient/Family Teaching

- Instruct patient to continue taking medication, even if feeling well. Abrupt withdrawal may cause rebound hypertension. Medication controls, but does not cure, hypertension.
- Encourage patient to comply with additional interventions for hypertension (weight reduction, low-sodium diet, regular exercise, discontinuation of smoking, moderation of alcohol consumption, and stress management).
- Instruct patient and family on proper technique for monitoring BP. Advise them to check BP weekly and report significant changes.
- Caution patient to make position changes slowly to minimize orthostatic hypotension. Advise patient that exercise or hot weather may enhance hypotensive effects.
- Advise patient to consult health care professional before taking any OTC medications, especially cold remedies.
- Advise patient to inform health care professional of medication regimen before treatment or surgery.
- Patients taking ACE inhibitors, ARBs, or aliskiren should notify health care professional if pregnancy is planned or suspected.
- Emphasize the importance of follow-up exams to monitor progress.

Evaluation/Desired Outcomes

- Decrease in BP.

• ANTI-INFECTIVES

PHARMACOLOGIC PROFILE

General Use

Treatment and prophylaxis of various bacterial infections. See specific drugs for spectrum and indications. Some infections may require additional surgical intervention and supportive therapy.

General Action and Information

Kill (bactericidal) or inhibit the growth of (bacteriostatic) susceptible pathogenic bacteria. Not active against viruses or fungi. Anti-infectives are subdivided into categories depending on chemical similarities and antimicrobial spectrum.

Contraindications

Known hypersensitivity to individual agents. Cross-sensitivity among related agents may occur.

Precautions

Culture and susceptibility testing are desirable to optimize therapy. Dosage modification may be required in patients with hepatic or renal insufficiency. Use cautiously in pregnant and lactating women. Prolonged inappropriate use of broad spectrum anti-infective agents may lead to superinfection with fungi or resistant bacteria.

Interactions

Penicillins and aminoglycosides chemically inactivate each other and should not be physically admixed. Erythromycin and clarithromycin may ↓ hepatic metabolism of other drugs. Probenecid ↑ serum levels of penicillins and related compounds. Highly protein-bound anti-infectives such as sulfonamides may displace or be displaced by other highly bound drugs. See individual drugs. Extended-spectrum penicillins (piperacillin/tazobactam) and some cephalosporins (cefoperazone, cefotetan) may ↑ the risk of bleeding with anticoagulants, thrombolytic agents, antiplatelet agents, or NSAIDs. Fluoroquinolone absorption may be ↓ by antacids, bismuth subsalicylate, calcium, iron salts, sucralfate, and zinc salts.

NURSING IMPLICATIONS

Assessment

- Assess patient for signs and symptoms of infection prior to and throughout therapy.
- Determine previous hypersensitivities in patients receiving penicillins or cephalosporins.
- Obtain specimens for culture and sensitivity prior to initiating therapy. First dose may be given before receiving results.
- Monitor bowel function. Diarrhea, abdominal cramping, fever, and bloody stools should be reported to health care professional promptly as a sign of *Clostridium difficile*-associated diarrhea (CDAD).

Implementation

- Most anti-infectives should be administered around the clock to maintain therapeutic serum drug levels.

Patient/Family Teaching

- Instruct patient to continue taking medication around the clock until finished completely, even if feeling better.
- Advise patient to report the signs of superinfection (black, furry overgrowth on the tongue; vaginal itching or discharge; loose or foul-smelling stools) and allergy to health care professional.
- Instruct patient to notify health care professional if fever and diarrhea develop, especially if stool contains pus, blood, or mucus. Advise patient not to treat diarrhea without consulting health care professional.
- Instruct patient to notify health care professional if symptoms do not improve.

Evaluation/Desired Outcomes

- Resolution of the signs and symptoms of infection. Length of time for complete resolution depends on organism and site of infection.

• ANTINEOPLASTICS

PHARMACOLOGIC PROFILE

General Use

Used in the treatment of various solid tumors, lymphomas, and leukemias. Also used in some autoimmune disorders such as rheumatoid arthritis (cyclophosphamide, methotrexate). Often used in combinations to minimize individual toxicities and ↑ response. Chemotherapy may be combined with other treatment modalities such as surgery and radiation therapy. Dosages vary greatly, depending on extent of disease, other agents used, and patient's condition. Some agents (doxorubicin, irinotecan) are available in lipid-based formulations that have less toxicity with greater efficacy.

General Action and Information

Act by many different mechanisms (see the following table). Many affect DNA synthesis or function; others alter immune function or affect hormonal status of sensitive tumors. Action may not be limited to neoplastic cells.

MECHANISM OF ACTION OF SELECTED ANTINEOPLASTICS

MECHANISM OF ACTION	AGENT	EFFECTS ON CELL CYCLE
ALKYLATING AGENTS	busulfan	Cell cycle–nonspecific
Cause cross-linking of DNA	carboplatin	
	chlorambucil	
	cisplatin	
	cyclophosphamide	
	ifosfamide	
	melphalan	
	procarbazine	
	temozolamide	
ANTHRACYCLINES	daunorubicin	Cell cycle–nonspecific
Interfere with DNA and RNA synthesis	doxorubicin	
	epirubicin	
	idarubicin	
ANTITUMOR ANTIBIOTIC	bleomycin	Cell cycle–nonspecific (except bleomycin)
Interfere with DNA and RNA synthesis	mitomycin	
	mitoxantrone	
ANTIMETABOLITES	cytarabine	Cell cycle–specific, work mostly in S phase (DNA synthesis)
Take the place of normal proteins	fluorouracil	
	hydroxyurea	
	methotrexate	
ENZYMES	asparaginase	Cell-cycle phase–specific
Deplete asparagine	pegaspargase	
ENZYME INHIBITORS	irinotecan	Cell-cycle phase–specific
Inhibits topoisomerase	topotecan	
Inhibits kinase	imatinib	Unknown
HORMONAL AGENTS	bicalutamide	Unknown
Alter hormonal status in tumors that are sensitive	estramustine	
	flutamide	
	leuprolide	
	megestrol	
	nilutamide	
	tamoxifen	
	testosterone (androgens)	
	triptorelin	
HORMONAL AGENTS–AROMATASE INHIBITORS	anastrozole	Unknown

(continued) MECHANISM OF ACTION OF VARIOUS ANTINEOPLASTICS

MECHANISM OF ACTION	AGENT	EFFECTS ON CELL CYCLE
Inhibit enzyme responsible for activating estrogen	letrozole	
IMMUNE MODULATORS	aldesleukin alemtuzumab gemtuzumab toremifene trastuzumab	Unknown
PODOPHYLLOTOXIN DERIVATIVES Damages DNA before mitosis	etoposide	Cell-cycle phase–specific
TAXOIDS Interrupt interphase and mitosis	docetaxel paclitaxel	Cell-cycle phase–specific
VINCA ALKALOIDS Interfere with mitosis	vinblastine vincristine vinorelbine	Cell cycle–specific, work during M phase (mitosis)

Contraindications

Previous bone marrow depression or hypersensitivity. Contraindicated in pregnancy and lactation.

Precautions

Use cautiously in patients with active infections, ↓ bone marrow reserve, radiation therapy, or other debilitating illnesses. Use cautiously in patients with childbearing potential.

Interactions

Allopurinol ↓ metabolism of mercaptopurine. Toxicity from methotrexate may be ↑ by other nephrotoxic drugs or larger doses of aspirin or NSAIDs. Bone marrow depression is additive. See individual drugs.

NURSING IMPLICATIONS

Assessment

- Monitor for bone marrow depression. Assess for bleeding (bleeding gums, bruising, petechiae, guaiac stools, urine, and emesis) and avoid IM injections and rectal temperatures if platelet count is low. Apply pressure to venipuncture sites for 10 min. Assess for signs of infection during neutropenia. Anemia may occur. Monitor for ↑ fatigue, dyspnea, and orthostatic hypotension.
- Monitor intake and output ratios, appetite, and nutritional intake. Prophylactic antiemetics may be used. Adjusting diet as tolerated may help maintain fluid and electrolyte balance and nutritional status.
- Monitor IV site carefully and ensure patency. Discontinue infusion immediately if discomfort, erythema along vein, or infiltration occurs. Tissue ulceration and necrosis may result from infiltration.
- Monitor for symptoms of gout (↑ uric acid, joint pain, and edema). Encourage patient to drink at least 2 L of fluid each day. Allopurinol may be given to ↓ uric acid levels. Alkalinization of urine may be ordered to ↑ excretion of uric acid.

Implementation

- Solutions for injection should be prepared in a biologic cabinet. Wear gloves, gown, and mask while handling medication. Discard equipment in designated containers.
- Check dose carefully. Fatalities have resulted from dosing errors.

Patient/Family Teaching
- Caution patient to avoid crowds and persons with known infections. Health care professional should be informed immediately if symptoms of infection occur.
- Instruct patient to report unusual bleeding. Advise patient of thrombocytopenia precautions.
- These drugs may cause gonadal suppression; however, patient should still use birth control, as most antineoplastics are teratogenic. Advise patient to inform health care professional immediately if pregnancy is suspected.
- Discuss with patient the possibility of hair loss. Explore methods of coping.
- Instruct patient to inspect oral mucosa for erythema and ulceration. If ulceration occurs, advise patient to use sponge brush and to rinse mouth with water after eating and drinking. Topical agents may be used if mouth pain interferes with eating. Stomatitis pain may require treatment with opioid analgesics.
- Instruct patient not to receive any vaccinations without advice of health care professional. Antineoplastics may ↓ antibody response and ↑ risk of adverse reactions.
- Advise patient of need for medical follow-up and frequent lab tests.

Evaluation/Desired Outcomes
- Decrease in size and spread of tumor.
- Improvement in hematologic status in patients with leukemia.

• ANTIPARKINSON AGENTS

PHARMACOLOGIC PROFILE

General Use
Treatment of Parkinson's disease.

General Action and Information
Drugs used in the treatment of Parkinson's disease and other dyskinesias are aimed at restoring the natural balance of two major neurotransmitters in the CNS: acetylcholine and dopamine. The imbalance is a deficiency in dopamine that results in excessive cholinergic activity. Many of the drugs used are either anticholinergics (benztropine and trihexyphenidyl) or dopaminergic agonists (apomorphine, bromocriptine, levodopa/carbidopa, pramipexole, ropinirole, rotigotine). Entacapone and tolcapone inhibit the enzyme that breaks down levodopa, thereby enhancing its effects. Rasagiline and selegiline are MAO-B inhibitors that lead to ↑ concentrations of dopamine in the CNS.

Contraindications
Anticholinergics should be avoided in patients with angle-closure glaucoma.

Precautions
Use cautiously in patients with severe cardiac disease, pyloric obstruction, or prostatic enlargement.

Interactions
Pyridoxine, MAO inhibitors, benzodiazepines, phenytoin, phenothiazines, and haloperidol may antagonize the effects of levodopa. Agents that antagonize dopamine (phenothiazines, metoclopramide) may ↓ effectiveness of dopamine agonists.

NURSING IMPLICATIONS

Assessment
- Assess parkinsonian and extrapyramidal symptoms (akinesia, rigidity, tremors, pill rolling, mask facies, shuffling gait, muscle spasms, twisting motions, and drooling) before and throughout course of therapy. On-off phenomenon may cause symptoms to appear or improve suddenly.
- Monitor BP frequently during therapy. Instruct patient to remain supine during and for several hours after first dose of bromocriptine, as severe hypotension may occur.

Implementation
- In the carbidopa/levodopa combination, the number following the drug name represents the milligram of each respective drug.

Patient/Family Teaching
- May cause drowsiness or dizziness. Advise patient to avoid driving or other activities that require alertness until response to medication is known.
- Caution patient to make position changes slowly to minimize orthostatic hypotension.
- Instruct patient that frequent rinsing of mouth, good oral hygiene, and sugarless gum or candy may decrease dry mouth. Patient should notify health care professional if dryness persists (saliva substitutes may be used). Also notify the dentist if dryness interferes with use of dentures.
- Advise patient to confer with health care professional before taking OTC medications, especially cold remedies, or drinking alcoholic beverages. Patients receiving levodopa should avoid multivitamins. Vitamin B_6 (pyridoxine) may interfere with levodopa's action.
- Caution patient that decreased perspiration may occur. Overheating may occur during hot weather. Patients should remain indoors in an air-conditioned environment during hot weather.
- Advise patient to increase activity, bulk, and fluid in diet to minimize constipating effects of medication.
- Advise patient to notify health care professional if confusion, rash, urinary retention, severe constipation, visual changes, or worsening of parkinsonian symptoms occur.

Evaluation/Desired Outcomes
- Resolution of parkinsonian signs and symptoms
- Resolution of drug-induced extrapyramidal symptoms.

• ANTIPLATELET AGENTS

PHARMACOLOGIC PROFILE

General Use
Used to treat and prevent thromboembolic events such as stroke and MI.

General Action and Information
Inhibit platelet aggregation, prolong bleeding time, and are used to prevent MI or stroke (aspirin, clopidogrel, dipyridamole, ticlopidine, prasugrel, ticagrelor). Eptifibatide and tirofiban are used in the management of acute coronary syndromes. These agents are often used concurrently/sequentially with anticoagulants and thrombolytics.

Contraindications
Hypersensitivity, ulcer disease, active bleeding, and recent surgery.

Precautions
Use cautiously in patients at risk for bleeding (trauma, surgery). History of GI bleeding or ulcer disease. Safety not established in pregnancy, lactation, or children.

Interactions
Concurrent use with NSAIDs, heparin, thrombolytics, or warfarin, dabigatran, rivaroxaban, apixaban, edoxaban, or betrixaban may ↑ the risk of bleeding.

NURSING IMPLICATIONS

Assessment
- Assess patient for evidence of additional or ↑ thrombosis. Symptoms will depend on area of involvement.
- Assess patient taking antiplatelet agents for symptoms of stroke, peripheral arterial disease, or MI periodically throughout therapy.

Implementation
- Use an infusion pump with continuous infusions to ensure accurate dosage.

Patient/Family Teaching
- Instruct patient to notify health care professional immediately if any bleeding is noted.

Evaluation/Desired Outcomes
- Prevention of stroke, MI, and vascular death in patients at risk.

• ANTIPSYCHOTICS

PHARMACOLOGIC PROFILE

General Use
Treatment of acute and chronic psychoses, particularly when accompanied by ↑ psychomotor activity. Use of clozapine is limited to schizophrenia unresponsive to conventional therapy. Selected agents are also used as antihistamines or antiemetics. Chlorpromazine is also used in the treatment of intractable hiccups.

General Action and Information
Block dopamine receptors in the brain; also alter dopamine release and turnover. Peripheral effects include anticholinergic properties and alpha-adrenergic blockade. Typical antipsychotics include the phenothiazines and haloperidol. Atypical antipsychotics may have fewer adverse reactions compared to the typical antipsychotics and include aripiprazole, asenapine, brexpiprazole, cariprazine, clozapine, iloperidone, lurasidone, paliperidone, olanzapine, paliperidone, pimavanserin, quetiapine, risperidone, and ziprasidone. Phenothiazines differ in their ability to produce sedation (greatest with chlorpromazine and thioridazine), extrapyramidal reactions (greatest with prochlorperazine and trifluoperazine), and anticholinergic effects (greatest with chlorpromazine).

Contraindications
Hypersensitivity. Cross-sensitivity may exist among phenothiazines. Should not be used in angle-closure glaucoma. Should not be used in patients who have CNS depression.

CLASSIFICATIONS

Precautions

Safety in pregnancy and lactation not established. Use cautiously in patients with symptomatic cardiac disease. Avoid exposure to extremes in temperature. Use cautiously in severely ill or debilitated patients and patients with respiratory insufficiency, diabetes, prostatic hypertrophy, or intestinal obstruction. May ↓ seizure threshold. Clozapine may cause agranulocytosis. Most agents are capable of causing neuroleptic malignant syndrome. Should not be used routinely for anxiety or agitation not related to psychoses.

Interactions

Additive hypotension with acute ingestion of alcohol, antihypertensives, or nitrates. Antacids may ↓ absorption. Phenobarbital may ↑ metabolism and ↓ effectiveness. Additive CNS depression with other CNS depressants, including alcohol, antihistamines, antidepressants, opioid analgesics, or sedative/hypnotics. Lithium may ↓ blood levels and effectiveness of phenothiazines. May ↓ the therapeutic response to levodopa. May ↑ the risk of agranulocytosis with antithyroid agents.

NURSING IMPLICATIONS

Assessment

- Assess patient's mental status (orientation, mood, behavior) before and periodically throughout therapy.
- Monitor BP (sitting, standing, lying), pulse, and respiratory rate before and frequently during the period of dosage adjustment.
- Observe patient carefully when administering medication to ensure medication is actually taken and not hoarded.
- Monitor patient for onset of *akathisia*—restlessness or desire to keep moving—and extrapyramidal side effects; *parkinsonian effects*—difficulty speaking or swallowing, loss of balance control, pill rolling, mask-like face, shuffling gait, rigidity, tremors; and *dystonia*—muscle spasms, twisting motions, twitching, inability to move eyes, weakness of arms or legs—every 2 mo during therapy and 8–12 wk after therapy has been discontinued. Parkinsonian effects are more common in geriatric patients and dystonias are more common in younger patients. Notify health care professional if these symptoms occur, as ↓ in dosage or discontinuation of medication may be necessary. Trihexyphenidyl, benztropine, or diphenhydramine may be used to control these symptoms.
- Monitor for *tardive dyskinesia*—uncontrolled rhythmic movement of mouth, face, and extremities; lip smacking or puckering; puffing of cheeks; uncontrolled chewing; rapid or worm-like movements of tongue. Notify health care professional immediately if these symptoms occur; these side effects may be irreversible.
- Monitor for development of *neuroleptic malignant syndrome*—fever, respiratory distress, tachycardia, convulsions, diaphoresis, hypertension or hypotension, pallor, tiredness, severe muscle stiffness, loss of bladder control. Notify health care professional immediately if these symptoms occur.

Implementation

- Keep patient recumbent for at least 30 min following parenteral administration to minimize hypotensive effects.
- **PO:** Administer with **food**, **milk**, or a full glass of **water** to minimize gastric irritation.
- Dilute most concentrates in 120 mL of distilled or acidified tap water or **fruit juice** just before administration.

Patient/Family Teaching

- Advise patient to take medication exactly as directed and not to skip doses or double up on missed doses. Abrupt withdrawal may lead to gastritis, nausea, vomiting, dizziness, headache, tachycardia, and insomnia.
- Advise patient to make position changes slowly to minimize orthostatic hypotension.
- Medication may cause drowsiness. Caution patient to avoid driving or other activities requiring alertness until response to the medication is known.
- Caution patient to avoid taking alcohol or other CNS depressants concurrently with this medication.
- Advise patient to use sunscreen and protective clothing when exposed to the sun to prevent photosensitivity reactions. Extremes of temperature should also be avoided, as these drugs impair body temperature regulation.
- Advise patient that ↑ activity, bulk, and fluids in the diet helps minimize the constipating effects of this medication.
- Instruct patient to use frequent mouth rinses, good oral hygiene, and sugarless gum or candy to minimize dry mouth.
- Advise patient to notify health care professional of medication regimen before treatment or surgery.
- Emphasize the importance of routine follow-up exams and continued participation in psychotherapy as indicated.

Evaluation/Desired Outcomes

- Decrease in excitable, paranoic, or withdrawn behavior. Relief of nausea and vomiting. Relief of intractable hiccups.

• ANTIPYRETICS

PHARMACOLOGIC PROFILE

General Use

Used to lower fever of many causes (infection and inflammation).

General Action and Information

Antipyretics lower fever by affecting thermoregulation in the CNS and by inhibiting the action of prostaglandins peripherally. Many antipyretics affect platelet function; of these, aspirin has the most profound effect as compared with other salicylates or NSAIDs.

Contraindications

Avoid aspirin or NSAIDs in patients with bleeding disorders (risk of bleeding is less with other salicylates). Aspirin and other salicylates should be avoided in children and adolescents.

Precautions

Use aspirin or NSAIDs cautiously in patients with peptic ulcer disease. Avoid chronic use of large doses of acetaminophen.

Interactions

Large doses of aspirin may displace other highly protein-bound drugs. Additive GI irritation with aspirin and other NSAIDs or corticosteroids. Aspirin or NSAIDs may ↑ the risk of bleeding with other agents affecting hemostasis (anticoagulants, thrombolytic agents, antiplatelets, and antineoplastics).

NURSING IMPLICATIONS

Assessment

- Assess fever; note presence of associated symptoms (diaphoresis, tachycardia, and malaise).

Implementation

- Administration with food or antacids may minimize GI irritation.
- Available in oral and rectal dosage forms and in combination with other drugs.

Patient/Family Teaching

- Advise patient to consult health care professional if fever is not relieved by routine doses or if greater than 39.5°C (103°F) or lasts longer than 3 days.
- Centers for Disease Control and Prevention warns against giving aspirin to children or adolescents with varicella (chickenpox) or influenza-like or viral illnesses because of a possible association with Reye's syndrome.

Evaluation/Desired Outcomes

- Reduction of fever.

• ANTIRETROVIRALS

PHARMACOLOGIC PROFILE

General Use

The goal of antiretroviral therapy in the management of HIV infection is to improve CD4 cell counts and ↓ viral load. If accomplished, this generally results in slowed progression of the disease, improved quality of life, and ↓ opportunistic infections. Perinatal use of agents also prevents transmission of the virus to the fetus. Post-exposure and pre-exposure prophylaxis with certain antiretrovirals is also recommended.

General Action and Information

Because of the rapid emergence of resistance and toxicities of individual agents, HIV infection is almost always managed by a combination of agents. Selections and doses are based on individual toxicities, underlying organ system disease, concurrent drug therapy, and severity of illness.

Contraindications

Hypersensitivity. Because of highly varying toxicities among agents, see individual monographs for more specific information.

Precautions

Many agents require modification for renal impairment. Protease inhibitors may cause hyperglycemia and hyperlipidemia and should be used cautiously in patients with diabetes and patients at increased risk for cardiovascular disease. Hemophiliacs may also be at risk of bleeding when taking protease inhibitors. See individual monographs for specific information.

Interactions

There are many significant and potentially serious drug-drug interactions among the antiretrovirals. They are affected by drugs that alter metabolism; some agents themselves affect metabolism. See individual agents.

NURSING IMPLICATIONS

Assessment

- Assess patient for change in severity of symptoms of HIV and for symptoms of opportunistic infections throughout therapy.
- **Lab Test Considerations:** Monitor viral load and CD4 counts prior to and periodically during therapy.

Implementation

- Administer doses around the clock.

Patient/Family Teaching

- Instruct patient to take medication exactly as directed, around the clock, even if sleep is interrupted. Emphasize the importance of complying with therapy, not taking more than prescribed amount, and not discontinuing without consulting health care professional. Missed doses should be taken as soon as remembered unless almost time for next dose; patient should not double doses. Inform patient that long-term effects are unknown at this time.
- Instruct patient that antiretrovirals should not be shared with others.
- Inform patient that antiretroviral therapy does not cure HIV and does not ↓ the risk of transmission of HIV to others through sexual contact or blood contamination. Caution patient to use a condom during sexual contact and to avoid sharing needles or donating blood to prevent spreading the AIDS virus to others.
- Advise patient to avoid taking any Rx, OTC, or herbal products without consulting health care professional.
- Emphasize the importance of regular follow-up exams and blood counts to determine progress and to monitor for side effects.

Evaluation/Desired Outcomes

- Decrease in viral load and increase in CD4 counts in patients with HIV.

• ANTIRHEUMATICS

PHARMACOLOGIC PROFILE

General Use

Antirheumatics are used to manage symptoms of rheumatoid arthritis (pain, swelling) and in more severe cases to slow down joint destruction and preserve joint function. NSAIDs, aspirin, and other salicylates are used to manage symptoms such as pain and swelling, allowing continued motility and improved quality of life. Corticosteroids are reserved for more advanced swelling and discomfort, primarily because of their ↑ side effects, especially with chronic use. They can be used to control acute flares of disease. Neither NSAIDs nor corticosteroids prevent disease progression or joint destruction. Disease-modifying antirheumatics drugs (DMARDs) slow the progression of rheumatoid arthritis and delay joint destruction. DMARDs are reserved for severe cases because of their toxicity. Several months of therapy may be required before benefit is noted and maintained. Serious and frequent adverse reactions may require discontinuation of therapy, despite initial benefit.

General Action and Information

Both NSAIDs and corticosteroids have potent anti-inflammatory properties. DMARDs work by a variety of mechanisms. See individual agents, but most work by suppressing the autoimmune response thought to be responsible for joint destruction.

CLASSIFICATIONS

Contraindications
Hypersensitivity. Patients who are allergic to aspirin should not receive other NSAIDs. Corticosteroids should not be used in patients with active untreated infections.

Precautions
NSAIDs and corticosteroids should be used cautiously in patients with a history of GI bleeding. Corticosteroids should be used with caution in patients with diabetes. Many DMARDs have immunosuppressive properties and should be avoided in patients for whom immunosuppression poses a serious risk, including patients with active infections, underlying malignancy, and transplant recipients.

Interactions
NSAIDs may diminish the response to diuretics and other antihypertensives. Corticosteroids may augment hypokalemia from other medications and ↑ the risk of digoxin toxicity. DMARDs ↑ the risk of serious immunosuppression with other immunosuppressants. Live vaccines should not be given concurrently with DMARDs.

NURSING IMPLICATIONS

Assessment
- Assess patient monthly for pain, swelling, and range of motion.

Implementation
- Most agents require regular administration to obtain maximum effects.

Patient/Family Teaching
- Instruct patient to contact health care professional if no improvement is noticed within a few days.

Evaluation/Desired Outcomes
- Improvement in signs and symptoms of rheumatoid arthritis.

• ANTITUBERCULARS

PHARMACOLOGIC PROFILE

General Use
Used in the treatment and prevention of tuberculosis. Combinations are used in the treatment of active tuberculosis to rapidly ↓ the infectious state and delay or prevent the emergence of resistant strains. In selected situations, intermittent (twice weekly) regimens may be employed. Streptomycin is also used as an antitubercular. Rifampin is also used in the prevention of meningococcal meningitis and *Haemophilus influenzae* type B.

General Action and Information
Kill (tuberculocidal) or inhibit the growth of (tuberculostatic) mycobacteria responsible for causing tuberculosis. Combination therapy with two or more agents is required, unless used as prophylaxis (isoniazid alone).

Contraindications
Hypersensitivity. Severe liver disease.

Precautions
Use cautiously in patients with a history of liver disease or in elderly or debilitated patients. Ethambutol requires ophthalmologic follow-up. Safety in pregnancy and lactation not established, although selected agents have been used without adverse effects on the fetus. Compliance is required for optimal response.

Interactions
Isoniazid inhibits the metabolism of phenytoin. Rifampin significantly ↓ levels of many drugs.

NURSING IMPLICATIONS

Assessment
- Mycobacterial studies and susceptibility tests should be performed prior to and periodically throughout therapy to detect possible resistance.
- Assess lung sounds and character and amount of sputum periodically throughout therapy.

Implementation
- Most medications can be administered with food if GI irritation occurs.

Patient/Family Teaching
- Advise patient of the importance of continuing therapy even after symptoms have subsided.
- Emphasize the importance of regular follow-up exams to monitor progress and check for side effects.
- Inform patients taking rifampin that saliva, sputum, sweat, tears, urine, and feces may become red-orange to red-brown and that soft contact lenses may become permanently discolored.

Evaluation/Desired Outcomes
- Resolution of the signs and symptoms of tuberculosis. Negative sputum cultures.

• ANTIULCER AGENTS

PHARMACOLOGIC PROFILE

General Use
Treatment and prophylaxis of peptic ulcer and gastric hypersecretory conditions such as Zollinger-Ellison syndrome. Histamine H_2-receptor antagonists (blockers) and proton pump inhibitors are also used in the management of gastroesophageal reflux disease (GERD).

General Action and Information
Because a great majority of peptic ulcer disease may be traced to GI infection with the organism *Helicobacter pylori*, eradication of the organism ↓ symptomatology and recurrence. Anti-infectives with significant activity against the organism include amoxicillin, clarithromycin, metronidazole, and tetracycline. Bismuth also has anti-infective activity against *H. pylori*. *H. pylori* treatment regimens usually include: a proton pump inhibitor, and 2 anti-infectives with or without bismuth subsalicylate for 10–14 days. Other medications used in the management of gastric/duodenal ulcer disease are aimed at neutralizing

gastric acid (antacids), ↓ acid secretion (histamine H_2 antagonists, proton pump inhibitors, misoprostol), or protecting the ulcer surface from further damage (misoprostol, sucralfate). Histamine H_2-receptor antagonists competitively inhibit the action of histamine at the H_2 receptor, located primarily in gastric parietal cells, resulting in inhibition of gastric acid secretion. Misoprostol ↓ gastric acid secretion and ↑ production of protective mucus. Proton pump inhibitors prevent the transport of hydrogen ions into the gastric lumen.

Contraindications

Hypersensitivity. Pregnancy.

Precautions

Most histamine H_2 antagonists require dose reduction in renal impairment and in elderly patients. Magnesium-containing antacids should be used cautiously in patients with renal impairment. Misoprostol should be used cautiously in women of reproductive potential.

Interactions

Calcium- and magnesium-containing antacids ↓ the absorption of tetracycline and fluoroquinolones. Cimetidine inhibits the ability of the liver to metabolize several drugs, ↑ the risk of toxicity from warfarin, tricyclic antidepressants, theophylline, metoprolol, phenytoin, propranolol, and lidocaine. Omeprazole ↓ metabolism of phenytoin, diazepam, and warfarin. All agents that ↑ gastric pH will ↓ the absorption of itraconazole, ketoconazole, iron salts, erlotinib, nilotinib, atazanavir, nelfinavir, rilpivirine, and mycophenolate mofetil.

NURSING IMPLICATIONS

Assessment

- Assess patient routinely for epigastric or abdominal pain and frank or occult blood in the stool, emesis, or gastric aspirate.
- **Antacids:** Assess for heartburn and indigestion as well as the location, duration, character, and precipitating factors of gastric pain.
- **Histamine H_2 Antagonists:** Assess elderly and severely ill patients for confusion routinely. Notify health care professional promptly should this occur.
- **Misoprostol:** Assess women of reproductive potential for pregnancy. Medication is usually begun on 2nd or 3rd day of menstrual period following a negative serum pregnancy test within 2 wk of beginning therapy.

Implementation

- **Antacids:** Antacids cause premature dissolution and absorption of enteric-coated tablets and may interfere with absorption of other oral medications. Separate administration of antacids and other oral medications by at least 1 hr.
- Shake liquid preparations well before pouring. Follow administration with water to ensure passage to stomach. Liquid and powder dosage forms are considered to be more effective than chewable tablets.
- Chewable tablets must be chewed thoroughly before swallowing. Follow with half a glass of water.
- Administer 1 and 3 hr after meals and at bedtime for maximum antacid effect.
- **Misoprostol:** Administer with meals and at bedtime to reduce the severity of diarrhea.
- **Proton Pump Inhibitors:** Administer before meals, preferably in the morning. Capsules should be swallowed whole; do not open, crush, or chew.
- May be administered concurrently with antacids.

- **Sucralfate:** Administer on an empty stomach 1 hr before meals and at bedtime. Do not crush or chew tablets. Shake suspension well prior to administration. If nasogastric administration is required, consult pharmacist, as protein-binding properties of sucralfate have resulted in formation of a bezoar when administered with enteral feedings and other medications.

Patient/Family Teaching

- Instruct patient to take medication as directed for the full course of therapy, even if feeling better. If a dose is missed, it should be taken as soon as remembered but not if almost time for next dose. Do not double doses.
- Advise patient to avoid alcohol, products containing aspirin, NSAIDs, and foods that may cause an ↑ in GI irritation.
- Advise patient to report onset of black, tarry stools to health care professional promptly.
- Inform patient that cessation of smoking may help prevent the recurrence of duodenal ulcers.
- **Antacids:** Caution patient to consult health care professional before taking antacids for more than 2 wk or if problem is recurring. Advise patient to consult health care professional if relief is not obtained or if symptoms of gastric bleeding (black, tarry stools; coffee-ground emesis) occur.
- **Misoprostol:** Emphasize that sharing of this medication may be dangerous.
- Inform patient that misoprostol may cause spontaneous abortion. Women of reproductive potential must be informed of this effect through verbal and written information and must use contraception throughout therapy. If pregnancy is suspected, the woman should stop taking misoprostol and immediately notify her health care professional.
- **Sucralfate:** Advise patient to continue with course of therapy for 4–8 wk, even if feeling better, to ensure ulcer healing.
- Advise patient that an ↑ in fluid intake, dietary bulk, and exercise may prevent drug-induced constipation.

Evaluation/Desired Outcomes

- Decrease in GI pain and irritation. Prevention of gastric irritation and bleeding. Healing of duodenal ulcers can be seen by x-rays or endoscopy. Therapy with histamine H_2 antagonists is continued for at least 6 wk after initial episode. Decreased symptoms of GERD. Increase in the pH of gastric secretions (antacids). Prevention of gastric ulcers in patients receiving chronic NSAID therapy (misoprostol only).

• ANTIVIRALS

PHARMACOLOGIC PROFILE

General Use

Acyclovir, famciclovir, and valacyclovir are used in the management of herpes virus infections. Acyclovir and valacyclovir are also used in the management of chickenpox. Baloxavir, oseltamivir, peramivir, and zanamivir are used primarily in the prevention and/or treatment of influenza infection. Cidofovir, ganciclovir, valganciclovir, and foscarnet are used in the prevention and/or treatment of cytomegalovirus (CMV) infection. Penciclovir, famciclovir, valacyclovir, and docosanol are used in the treatment and prevention of orallfacial herpes simplex.

General Action and Information

Most agents inhibit viral replication.

Contraindications
Previous hypersensitivity.

Precautions
All except zanamivir require dose adjustment in renal impairment. Acyclovir may cause renal impairment. Acyclovir may cause CNS toxicity. Foscarnet ↑ risk of seizures.

Interactions
Acyclovir may have additive CNS and nephrotoxicity with drugs causing similar adverse reactions.

NURSING IMPLICATIONS

Assessment
- Assess patient for signs and symptoms of infection before and throughout therapy.
- **Ophth:** Assess eye lesions before and daily during therapy.
- **Topical:** Assess lesions before and daily during therapy.

Implementation
- Most systemic antiviral agents should be administered around the clock to maintain therapeutic serum drug levels.

Patient/Family Teaching
- Instruct patient to continue taking medication around the clock for full course of therapy, even if feeling better.
- Advise patient that antivirals do not prevent transmission to others. Precautions should be taken to prevent spread of virus.
- Instruct patient in correct technique for topical or ophthalmic preparations.
- Instruct patient to notify health care professional if symptoms do not improve.

Evaluation/Desired Outcomes
- Prevention or resolution of the signs and symptoms of viral infection. Length of time for complete resolution depends on organism and site of infection.

• BETA BLOCKERS

PHARMACOLOGIC PROFILE

General Use
Management of hypertension, angina pectoris, tachyarrhythmias, migraine headache (prophylaxis), MI, glaucoma (ophthalmic use), heart failure (HF) (bisoprolol, carvedilol, and sustained-release metoprolol only) and hyperthyroidism (management of symptoms only).

General Action and Information
Beta blockers compete with adrenergic (sympathetic) neurotransmitters (epinephrine and norepinephrine) for adrenergic receptor sites. Beta$_1$-adrenergic receptor sites are located chiefly in the heart where stimulation results in increased heart rate and myocardial contractility. Beta$_2$-adrenergic receptors are found mainly in bronchial and vascular smooth muscle and the uterus. Stimulation of beta$_2$-adrenergic receptors produces vasodilation, bronchodilation, and uterine relaxation. Beta blockers may be relatively selective for beta$_1$-adrenergic receptors (acebutolol, atenolol, betaxolol, bisoprolol, esmolol, and metoprolol) or nonselective (carvedilol, labetalol, nadolol, pindolol, propranolol, and timolol)

blocking both $beta_1$- and $beta_2$-adrenergic receptors. Carvedilol and labetalol have additional alpha-adrenergic blocking properties. Ophthalmic beta blockers ↓ production of aqueous humor.

Contraindications
Decompensated HF, acute bronchospasm, some forms of valvular heart disease, bradyarrhythmias, and heart block.

Precautions
Use cautiously in pregnant and lactating women (may cause fetal bradycardia and hypoglycemia). Use cautiously in any form of lung disease. Use with caution in patients with diabetes or severe liver disease. Beta blockers should not be abruptly discontinued in patients with cardiovascular disease.

Interactions
May cause additive myocardial depression and bradycardia when used with other agents having these effects (digoxin, diltiazem, verapamil, clonidine, and ivabradine). May antagonize the therapeutic effects of bronchodilators. May alter the requirements for insulin or hypoglycemic agents in patients with diabetes. Cimetidine may ↓ the metabolism and ↑ the effects of some beta blockers.

NURSING IMPLICATIONS

Assessment
- Monitor BP and pulse frequently during dosage adjustment and periodically throughout therapy.
- Monitor intake and output ratios and daily weight. Assess patient routinely for signs and symptoms of HF (dyspnea, rales/crackles, weight gain, peripheral edema, jugular venous distention).
- **Angina:** Assess frequency and severity of episodes of chest pain periodically throughout therapy.
- **Migraine Prophylaxis:** Assess frequency and severity of migraine headaches periodically throughout therapy.

Implementation
- Take apical pulse prior to administering. If heart rate is <50 bpm or if arrhythmias occur, hold medication and notify health care professional.

Patient/Family Teaching
- Instruct patient to continue taking medication, even if feeling well. Abrupt withdrawal may cause life-threatening arrhythmias, hypertension, or myocardial ischemia. Medication controls, but does not cure, hypertension.
- Encourage patient to comply with additional interventions for hypertension (weight reduction, low-sodium diet, regular exercise, smoking cessation, moderation of alcohol consumption, and stress management).
- Instruct patient and family on proper technique for monitoring BP. Advise them to check BP weekly and report significant changes to health care professional.
- Caution patient to make position changes slowly to minimize orthostatic hypotension. Advise patient that exercising or hot weather may enhance hypotensive effects.
- Advise patient to consult health care professional before taking any OTC medications or herbal/alternative therapies, especially cold remedies.

- Patients with diabetes should monitor blood glucose closely, especially if weakness, malaise, irritability, or fatigue occurs.
- Advise patient to advise health care professional of medication regimen prior to treatment or surgery.
- Advise patient to carry identification describing disease process and medication regimen at all times.
- Emphasize the importance of follow-up exams to monitor progress.
- **Ophth:** Instruct patient in correct technique for administration of ophthalmic preparations.

Evaluation/Desired Outcomes

- Decrease in BP.
- Decrease in frequency and severity of anginal attacks.
- Control of arrhythmias.
- Prevention of myocardial reinfarction.
- Prevention of migraine headaches.
- Decrease in tremors.
- Lowering of intraocular pressure.

• BONE RESORPTION INHIBITORS

PHARMACOLOGIC PROFILE

General Use

Bone resorption inhibitors are primarily used to treat and prevent osteoporosis in postmenopausal women. Other uses include treatment of osteoporosis due to other causes, including corticosteroid therapy, treatment of Paget's disease of the bone, and management of hypercalcemia.

General Action and Information

Bisphosphonates (alendronate, etidronate, ibandronate, pamidronate, risedronate, and zoledronic acid) inhibit resorption of bone by inhibiting hydroxyapatite crystal dissolution and osteoclast activity. Raloxifene binds to estrogen receptors, producing estrogen-like effects on bone including ↓ bone resorption and ↓ bone turnover.

Contraindications

Hypersensitivity. Bisphosphonates should not be used in patients with hypocalcemia. Raloxifene should not be used in women of reproductive potential or a history of thromboembolic disease.

Precautions

Use cautiously in patients with renal impairment; some agents should be avoided in moderate to severe renal impairment.

Interactions

Calcium supplements ↓ absorption of bisphosphonates. Aspirin may ↑ GI adverse reactions with bisphosphonates. Cholestyramine ↓ absorption of raloxifene (concurrent use is contraindicated).

NURSING IMPLICATIONS

Assessment

- Assess patients for low bone density before and periodically during therapy.
- Assess for symptoms of Paget's disease (bone pain, headache, decreased visual and auditory acuity, ↑ skull size).
- **Lab Test Considerations:** Monitor serum calcium in patients with osteoporosis. Monitor alkaline phosphatase in patients with Paget's disease.

Patient/Family Teaching

- Instruct patient to take medication exactly as directed.
- Encourage patient to participate in regular exercise and to modify behaviors that ↑ the risk of osteoporosis.

Evaluation/Desired Outcomes

- Prevention of, or decrease in, the progression of osteoporosis in postmenopausal women. Decrease in the progression of Paget's disease.

• BRONCHODILATORS

PHARMACOLOGIC PROFILE

General Use

Used in the treatment of reversible airway obstruction due to asthma or chronic obstructive pulmonary disease (COPD). Recommendations for management of asthma recommend that rapid-acting inhaled beta-agonist bronchodilators (not salmeterol, formoterol, arformoterol, indacaterol, olodaterol, or vilanterol) be reserved as acute relievers of bronchospasm; repeated or chronic use indicates the need for additional long-term control agents, including inhaled corticosteroids, mast cell stabilizers, long-acting bronchodilators (oral theophylline, beta$_2$-agonists, or anticholinergics), and leukotriene modifiers (montelukast, zafirlukast).

General Action and Information

Beta$_2$-adrenergic agonists (albuterol, arformoterol, epinephrine, formoterol, indacaterol, levalbuterol, metaproterenol, olodaterol, salmeterol, terbutaline, and vilanterol) produce bronchodilation by stimulating the production of cyclic adenosine monophosphate (cAMP). Onset of action allows use in management of acute attacks except for arformoterol, formoterol, indacaterol, olodaterol, salmeterol, and vilanterol, which have delayed onset. Phosphodiesterase inhibitors (aminophylline and theophylline) inhibit the breakdown of cAMP. Aclidinium, glycopyrrolate, ipratropium and tiotropium are anticholinergic compounds that produce bronchodilation by blocking the action of acetylcholine in the respiratory tract.

Contraindications

Hypersensitivity to agents or preservatives (bisulfites) used in their formulation. Avoid use in uncontrolled cardiac arrhythmias.

Precautions

Use cautiously in patients with diabetes, cardiovascular disease, or hyperthyroidism.

Interactions
Therapeutic effectiveness may be antagonized by concurrent use of beta blockers. Additive sympathomimetic effects with other adrenergic (sympathetic) drugs, including vasopressors and decongestants. Cardiovascular effects may be potentiated by antidepressants and MAO inhibitors.

NURSING IMPLICATIONS

Assessment
- Assess BP, pulse, respiration, lung sounds, and character of secretions before and throughout therapy.
- Patients with a history of cardiovascular problems should be monitored for ECG changes and chest pain.

Implementation
- Administer around the clock to maintain therapeutic plasma levels.

Patient/Family Teaching
- Emphasize the importance of taking only the prescribed dose at the prescribed time intervals.
- Encourage the patient to drink adequate liquids (2000 mL/day minimum) to ↓ the viscosity of the airway secretions.
- Advise patient to avoid OTC cough, cold, or breathing preparations without consulting health care professional and to minimize intake of xanthine-containing foods or beverages (colas, coffee, and chocolate), as these may ↑ side effects of theophylline.
- Caution patient to avoid smoking and other respiratory irritants.
- Instruct patient on proper use of metered-dose inhaler (see Appendix D).
- Advise patient to contact health care professional promptly if the usual dose of medication fails to produce the desired results, symptoms worsen after treatment, or toxic effects occur.
- Patients using other inhalation medications and bronchodilators should be advised to use bronchodilator first and allow 5 min to elapse before administering the other medication, unless otherwise directed by health care professional.

Evaluation/Desired Outcomes
- Decreased bronchospasm. Increased ease of breathing.

• CALCIUM CHANNEL BLOCKERS

PHARMACOLOGIC PROFILE

General Use
Used in the treatment of hypertension (amlodipine, diltiazem, felodipine, isradipine, nicardipine, nifedipine, nisoldipine, verapamil) or in the treatment and prophylaxis of angina pectoris or coronary artery spasm (amlodipine, diltiazem, felodipine, nicardipine, verapamil). Verapamil and diltiazem are also used as antiarrhythmics. Nimodipine is used to prevent neurologic damage due to certain types of cerebral vasospasm.

General Action and Information
Block calcium entry into cells of vascular smooth muscle and myocardium. Dilate coronary arteries in both normal and ischemic myocardium and inhibit coronary artery spasm.

Diltiazem and verapamil also ↓ AV nodal conduction. Nimodipine has a relatively selective effect on cerebral blood vessels.

Contraindications

Hypersensitivity. Contraindicated in bradycardia, 2nd- or 3rd-degree heart block, or decompensated HF (all except for amlodipine and felodipine).

Precautions

Safety in pregnancy and lactation not established. Use cautiously in patients with liver disease or uncontrolled arrhythmias.

Interactions

May cause additive bradycardia when used with other agents having these effects (beta blockers, digoxin, clonidine, and ivabradine). Effectiveness may be ↓ by phenobarbital or phenytoin and ↑ by propranolol or cimetidine. Verapamil and diltiazem may ↑ serum digoxin levels and cause toxicity.

NURSING IMPLICATIONS

Assessment

- Monitor BP and pulse frequently during dosage adjustment and periodically throughout therapy.
- Monitor intake and output ratios and daily weight. Assess patient routinely for signs and symptoms of HF (dyspnea, rales/crackles, weight gain, peripheral edema, jugular venous distention).
- **Angina:** Assess frequency and severity of episodes of chest pain periodically throughout therapy.
- **Arrhythmias:** ECG should be monitored continuously during IV therapy and periodically during long-term therapy with verapamil or diltiazem.
- **Cerebral Vasospasm:** Assess patient's neurological status (level of consciousness, movement) before and periodically during therapy with nimodipine.

Implementation

- May be administered without regard to meals.
- Do not open, crush, or chew sustained-release capsules.

Patient/Family Teaching

- Instruct patient to continue taking medication, even if feeling well.
- Caution patient to make position changes slowly to minimize orthostatic hypotension. Advise patient that exercising or hot weather may enhance hypotensive effects.
- Instruct patient on the importance of maintaining good dental hygiene and seeing dentist frequently for teeth cleaning to prevent tenderness, bleeding, and gingival hyperplasia (gum enlargement).
- Advise patient to consult health care professional before taking any OTC medications or herbal/alternative therapies, especially cold remedies.
- Advise patient to advise health care professional of medication regimen prior to treatment or surgery.
- Advise patient to carry identification describing disease process and medication regimen at all times.
- Emphasize the importance of follow-up exams to monitor progress.
- **Angina:** Instruct patients on concurrent nitrate therapy to continue taking both medications as directed and using SL nitroglycerin as needed for anginal attacks. Advise patient

to contact health care professional if chest pain worsens or does not improve after therapy, or is accompanied by diaphoresis or shortness of breath, or if severe, persistent headache occurs. Caution patient to discuss exercise precautions with health care professional prior to exertion.

- **Hypertension:** Encourage patient to comply with additional interventions for hypertension (weight reduction, low-sodium diet, regular exercise, smoking cessation, moderation of alcohol consumption, and stress management). Medication controls, but does not cure, hypertension.
- Instruct patient and family on proper technique for monitoring BP. Advise them to check BP weekly and report significant changes to health care professional.

Evaluation/Desired Outcomes

- Decrease in BP.
- Decrease in frequency and severity of anginal attacks.
- Decrease need for nitrate therapy.
- Increase in activity tolerance and sense of well-being.
- Suppression and prevention of supraventricular tachyarrhythmias.
- Improvement in neurological deficits due to vasospasm following subarachnoid hemorrhage.

• CENTRAL NERVOUS SYSTEM STIMULANTS

PHARMACOLOGIC PROFILE

General Use

Used in the treatment of narcolepsy and as adjunctive treatment in the management of attention deficit hyperactivity disorder (ADHD).

General Action and Information

Produce CNS stimulation by ↑ levels of neurotransmitters in the CNS. Produce CNS and respiratory stimulation, dilated pupils, ↑ motor activity and mental alertness, and a diminished sense of fatigue. In children with ADHD, these agents ↓ restlessness and ↑ attention span.

Contraindications

Hypersensitivity. Should not be used in pregnant or lactating women. Should not be used in hyperexcitable states. Avoid using in patients with psychotic personalities or suicidal/homicidal tendencies. Contraindicated in glaucoma and severe cardiovascular disease.

Precautions

Use cautiously in patients with a history of cardiovascular disease, hypertension, diabetes mellitus, or in elderly or debilitated patients. Continual use may result in psychological dependence or addiction.

Interactions

Additive sympathomimetic (adrenergic) effects. Use with MAO inhibitors can result in hypertensive crises. Alkalinizing the urine (sodium bicarbonate, acetazolamide) ↓ excretion and enhances effects of amphetamines. Acidification of the urine (ammonium chloride, large doses of ascorbic acid) ↓ effect of amphetamines. Phenothiazines may also ↓ effects. Methylphenidate may ↓ the metabolism and ↑ effects of other drugs (warfarin, anticonvulsants, tricyclic antidepressants).

NURSING IMPLICATIONS

Assessment

- Monitor BP, pulse, and respiration before administering and periodically during therapy.
- Monitor weight biweekly and inform health care professional of significant weight loss.
- Monitor height periodically in children; inform health care professional if growth inhibition occurs.
- May produce false sense of euphoria and well-being. Provide frequent rest periods and observe patient for rebound depression after the effects of the medication have worn off.
- **ADHD:** Assess attention span, impulse control, and interactions with others in children. Therapy may be interrupted at intervals to determine if symptoms are sufficient to warrant continued therapy.
- **Narcolepsy:** Observe and document frequency of episodes.

Patient/Family Teaching

- Instruct patient not to alter dose without consulting health care professional. These medications have high dependence and abuse potential. Abrupt cessation with high doses may cause extreme fatigue and mental depression.
- Advise patient to avoid intake of large amounts of caffeine.
- Advise patient that many of these medications have known abuse potential. Caution patient to protect the medications from theft, and never give them to anyone other than the individual for whom it was prescribed. Store the medications out of sight and reach of children, and in a location not accessible by others.
- Medication may impair judgment. Caution patient to avoid driving or other activities requiring judgment until response to medication is known.
- Inform patient that periodic holidays from the drug may be used to assess progress and decrease dependence.

Evaluation/Desired Outcomes

- Decreased frequency of narcoleptic episodes.
- Improved attention span and social interactions.

• CORTICOSTEROIDS

PHARMACOLOGIC PROFILE

General Use

Used in replacement doses (20 mg of hydrocortisone or equivalent) systemically to treat adrenocortical insufficiency. Larger doses are usually used for their anti-inflammatory, immunosuppressive, or antineoplastic activity. Used adjunctively in many other situations, including autoimmune diseases. Topical corticosteroids are used in a variety of inflammatory and allergic conditions. Inhaled corticosteroids are used in the chronic management of reversible airway disease (asthma); intranasal and ophthalmic corticosteroids are used in the management of chronic allergic and inflammatory conditions.

General Action and Information

Produce profound and varied metabolic effects, in addition to modifying the normal immune response and suppressing inflammation. Available in a variety of dosage forms, including oral, injectable, topical, ophthalmic, intranasal, and inhalation. Prolonged used of large amounts of topical, ophthalmic, intranasal, or inhaled agent may result in systemic absorption and/or adrenal suppression.

Contraindications

Serious infections (except for certain forms of meningitis). Do not administer live vaccines to patients on larger doses.

Precautions

Prolonged treatment will result in adrenal suppression. Do not discontinue abruptly. Additional doses may be needed during stress (surgery and infection). Safety in pregnancy and lactation not established. Long-term use in children will result in ↓ growth. May mask signs of infection. Use lowest dose possible for shortest time possible. Alternate-day therapy is preferable during long-term treatment.

Interactions

Additive hypokalemia with amphotericin B and potassium-losing diuretics. Hypokalemia may ↑ the risk of digoxin toxicity. May ↑ requirements for insulin or oral hypoglycemic agents. Phenytoin, phenobarbital, and rifampin stimulate metabolism and may ↓ effectiveness. Oral contraceptives may block metabolism. Cholestyramine and colestipol may ↓ absorption.

NURSING IMPLICATIONS

Assessment

- These drugs are indicated for many conditions. Assess involved systems prior to and periodically throughout course of therapy.
- Assess patient for signs of adrenal insufficiency (hypotension, weight loss, weakness, nausea, vomiting, anorexia, lethargy, confusion, restlessness) prior to and periodically throughout course of therapy.
- Children should have periodic evaluations of growth during chronic therapy.

Implementation

- If dose is ordered daily or every other day, administer in the morning to coincide with the body's normal secretion of cortisol.
- **PO:** Administer with meals to minimize gastric irritation.

Patient/Family Teaching

- Emphasize need to take medication exactly as directed. Review symptoms of adrenal insufficiency that may occur when stopping the medication and that may be life-threatening.
- Encourage patients on long-term therapy to eat a diet high in protein, calcium, and potassium and low in sodium and carbohydrates.
- These drugs cause immunosuppression and may mask symptoms of infection. Instruct patient to avoid people with known contagious illnesses and to report possible infections. Advise patient to consult health care professional before receiving any vaccinations.
- Discuss possible effects on body image. Explore coping mechanisms.
- Advise patient to carry identification in the event of an emergency in which patient cannot relate medical history.

Evaluation/Desired Outcomes
- Suppression of the inflammatory and immune responses in autoimmune disorders, allergic reactions, and organ transplants.
- Replacement therapy in adrenal insufficiency.
- Resolution of skin inflammation, pruritus, or other dermatologic conditions.

• DIURETICS
PHARMACOLOGIC PROFILE
General Use
Thiazide diuretics and loop diuretics are used alone or in combination in the treatment of hypertension or edema due to HF or other causes. Potassium-sparing diuretics have weak diuretic and antihypertensive properties and are used mainly to conserve potassium in patients receiving thiazide or loop diuretics. Osmotic diuretics are often used in the management of cerebral edema.

General Action and Information
Enhance the selective excretion of various electrolytes and water by affecting renal mechanisms for tubular secretion and reabsorption. Groups commonly used are thiazide diuretics and thiazide-like diuretics (chlorothiazide, chlorthalidone, hydrochlorothiazide, indapamide, and metolazone), loop diuretics (bumetanide, furosemide, and torsemide), potassium-sparing diuretics (amiloride, spironolactone, and triamterene), and osmotic diuretics (mannitol). Mechanisms vary, depending on agent.

Contraindications
Hypersensitivity. Thiazide and loop diuretics may exhibit cross-sensitivity with other sulfonamides.

Precautions
Use with caution in patients with renal or hepatic disease. Safety in pregnancy and lactation not established.

Interactions
Additive hypokalemia with corticosteroids, amphotericin B, and piperacillin/tazobactam. Hypokalemia may ↑ the risk of digoxin toxicity. Potassium-losing diuretics ↓ lithium excretion and may cause toxicity. Additive hypotension with other antihypertensives or nitrates. Potassium-sparing diuretics may cause hyperkalemia when used with potassium supplements, ACE inhibitors, angiotensin II receptor antagonists, and aliskiren.

NURSING IMPLICATIONS
Assessment
- Assess fluid status throughout therapy. Monitor daily weight, intake and output ratios, amount and location of edema, lung sounds, skin turgor, and mucous membranes.
- Assess patient for anorexia, muscle weakness, numbness, tingling, paresthesia, confusion, and excessive thirst. Notify health care professional promptly if these signs of electrolyte imbalance occur.
- **Hypertension:** Monitor BP and pulse before and during administration. Monitor frequency of prescription refills to determine compliance in patients treated for hypertension.

- **Increased Intracranial Pressure:** Monitor neurologic status and intracranial pressure readings in patients receiving osmotic diuretics to decrease cerebral edema.
- **Increased Intraocular Pressure:** Monitor for persistent or increased eye pain or decreased visual acuity.
- **Lab Test Considerations:** Monitor electrolytes (especially potassium), blood glucose, BUN, and serum uric acid levels before and periodically throughout course of therapy.
- Thiazide and loop diuretics may cause ↑ serum cholesterol, low-density lipoprotein (LDL) cholesterol, and triglyceride concentrations.

Implementation

- Administer oral diuretics in the morning to prevent disruption of sleep cycle.
- Many diuretics are available in combination with other antihypertensives or potassium-sparing diuretics.

Patient/Family Teaching

- Instruct patient to take medication exactly as directed. Advise patients on antihypertensive regimen to continue taking medication, even if feeling better. Medication controls, but does not cure, hypertension.
- Caution patient to make position changes slowly to minimize orthostatic hypotension. Caution patient that the use of alcohol, exercise during hot weather, or standing for long periods during therapy may enhance orthostatic hypotension.
- Instruct patient to consult health care professional regarding dietary potassium guidelines.
- Instruct patient to monitor weight weekly and report significant changes.
- Caution patient to use sunscreen and protective clothing to prevent photosensitivity reactions.
- Advise patient to consult health care professional before taking OTC medication concurrently with this therapy.
- Instruct patient to notify health care professional of medication regimen before treatment or surgery.
- Advise patient to contact health care professional immediately if muscle weakness, cramps, nausea, dizziness, or numbness or tingling of extremities occurs.
- Emphasize the importance of routine follow-up.
- **Hypertension:** Reinforce the need to continue additional therapies for hypertension (weight loss, regular exercise, restricted sodium intake, stress reduction, moderation of alcohol consumption, and cessation of smoking).
- Instruct patients with hypertension in the correct technique for monitoring weekly BP.

Evaluation/Desired Outcomes

- Decreased BP.
- Increased urine output.
- Decreased edema.
- Reduced intracranial pressure.
- Prevention of hypokalemia in patients taking diuretics.
- Treatment of hyperaldosteronism.

• HORMONES

PHARMACOLOGIC PROFILE

General Use

Used in the treatment of deficiency states including diabetes mellitus (insulin), diabetes insipidus (desmopressin), hypothyroidism (thyroid hormones), and menopause (estrogens or estrogens/progestins). Estrogenic and progestational hormones are used as contraceptive agents in various combinations and sequences. Hormones may be used to treat hormonally sensitive tumors (androgens, estrogens) and in other selected situations. See individual drugs.

General Action and Information

Natural or synthetic substances that have a specific effect on target tissue. Differ greatly in their effects, depending on individual agent and function of target tissue.

Contraindications

Differ greatly among individual agents; see individual entries.

Precautions

Differ greatly among individual agents; see individual entries.

Interactions

Differ greatly among individual agents; see individual entries.

NURSING IMPLICATIONS

Assessment

- Monitor patient for symptoms of hormonal excess or insufficiency.
- **Sex Hormones:** BP and hepatic function tests should be monitored periodically throughout therapy.

Implementation

- **Sex Hormones:** During hospitalization, continue to administer according to schedule followed prior to hospitalization.

Patient/Family Teaching

- Explain dose schedule (and withdrawal bleeding with female sex hormones).
- Emphasize the importance of follow-up exams to monitor effectiveness of therapy and to ensure proper development of children and early detection of possible side effects.
- **Female Sex Hormones:** Advise patient to report signs and symptoms of fluid retention, thromboembolic disorders, mental depression, or hepatic dysfunction to health care professional.

Evaluation/Desired Outcomes

- Resolution of clinical symptoms of hormone imbalance including menopause symptoms and contraception.
- Correction of fluid and electrolyte imbalances.
- Control of the spread of advanced metastatic breast or prostate cancer.
- Slowed progression of postmenopausal osteoporosis.

• IMMUNOSUPPRESSANTS

PHARMACOLOGIC PROFILE

General Use
Azathioprine, basiliximab, cyclosporine, everolimus, mycophenolate, sirolimus, and tacrolimus are used with corticosteroids in the prevention of transplantation rejection reactions. Muromonab-CD3 is used to manage rejection reactions not controlled by other agents. Azathioprine, cyclosporine, cyclophosphamide, and methotrexate are used in the management of selected autoimmune diseases (nephrotic syndrome of childhood and severe rheumatoid arthritis).

General Action and Information
Inhibit cell-mediated immune responses by different mechanisms. In addition to azathioprine and cyclosporine, which are used primarily for their immunomodulating properties, cyclophosphamide and methotrexate are used to suppress the immune responses in certain disease states (nephrotic syndrome of childhood and severe rheumatoid arthritis). Muromonab-CD3 is a recombinant immunoglobulin antibody that alters T-cell function. Basiliximab is a monoclonal antibody.

Contraindications
Hypersensitivity to drug or vehicle.

Precautions
Use cautiously in patients with infections. Safety in pregnancy and lactation not established.

Interactions
Allopurinol inhibits the metabolism of azathioprine. Drugs that alter liver-metabolizing processes may change the effect of cyclosporine, tacrolimus, or sirolimus. The risk of toxicity with methotrexate may be ↑ by other nephrotoxic drugs, large doses of aspirin, or NSAIDs. Muromonab-CD3 has additive immunosuppressive properties; concurrent immunosuppressive doses should be ↓ or eliminated.

NURSING IMPLICATIONS

Assessment
- Monitor for infection (vital signs, sputum, urine, stool, WBC). Notify physician or other health care professional immediately if symptoms occur.
- **Organ Transplant:** Assess for symptoms of organ rejection throughout therapy.
- **Lab Test Consideration:** Monitor CBC and differential throughout therapy.

Implementation
- Protect transplant patients from staff and visitors who may carry infection.
- Maintain protective isolation as indicated.

Patient/Family Teaching
- Reinforce the need for lifelong therapy to prevent transplant rejection. Review symptoms of rejection for transplanted organ and stress the need for patient to notify health care professional immediately if they occur.
- Advise patient to avoid contact with contagious persons. Patients should not receive vaccinations without first consulting with health care professional.
- Emphasize the importance of follow-up exams and lab tests.

Evaluation/Desired Outcomes

- Prevention or reversal of rejection of organ transplants or decrease in symptoms of autoimmune disorders.

• LAXATIVES

PHARMACOLOGIC PROFILE

General Use

Used to treat or prevent constipation or to prepare the bowel for radiologic or endoscopic procedures.

General Action and Information

Induce one or more bowel movements per day. Groups include stimulants (bisacodyl, sennosides), saline laxatives (magnesium salts and phosphates), stool softeners (docusate), bulk-forming agents (polycarbophil and psyllium), and osmotic cathartics (lactulose, polyethylene glycol/electrolyte). ↑ fluid intake, exercising, and adding more dietary fiber are also useful in the management of chronic constipation.

Contraindications

Hypersensitivity. Contraindicated in persistent abdominal pain, nausea, or vomiting of unknown cause, especially if accompanied by fever or other signs of an acute abdomen.

Precautions

Excessive or prolonged use may lead to dependence. Should not be used in children unless advised by a physician or other health care professional.

Interactions

Theoretically may ↓ the absorption of other orally administered drugs by ↓ transit time.

NURSING IMPLICATIONS

Assessment

- Assess patient for abdominal distention, presence of bowel sounds, and usual pattern of bowel function.
- Assess color, consistency, and amount of stool produced.

Implementation

- May be administered at bedtime for morning results.
- Taking oral doses on an empty stomach will usually produce more rapid results.
- Do not crush or chew enteric-coated tablets. Take with a full glass of water or juice.
- Stool softeners and bulk laxatives may take several days for results.

Patient/Family Teaching

- Advise patients, other than those with spinal cord injuries, that laxatives should be used only for short-term therapy. Long-term therapy may cause electrolyte imbalance and dependence.
- Advise patient to ↑ fluid intake to a minimum of 1500–2000 mL/day during therapy to prevent dehydration.
- Encourage patients to use other forms of bowel regulation: ↑ bulk in the diet, ↑ fluid intake, and ↑ mobility. Normal bowel habits are individualized and may vary from 3 times/day to 3 times/wk.

- Instruct patients with cardiac disease to avoid straining during bowel movements (Valsalva maneuver).
- Advise patient that laxatives should not be used when constipation is accompanied by abdominal pain, fever, nausea, or vomiting.

Evaluation/Desired Outcomes

- A soft, formed bowel movement.
- Evacuation of the colon.

• LIPID-LOWERING AGENTS

PHARMACOLOGIC PROFILE

General Use

Used as a part of a total plan including diet and exercise to $\downarrow$ blood lipids in an effort to $\downarrow$ the morbidity and mortality of atherosclerotic cardiovascular disease and its sequelae.

General Action and Information

HMG-CoA reductase inhibitors (atorvastatin, fluvastatin, lovastatin, pitavastatin, pravastatin, rosuvastatin, simvastatin) inhibit an enzyme involved in cholesterol synthesis. The PCSK9 inhibitors (alirocumab, evolocumab) facilitate clearing of LDL from the blood. Bile acid sequestrants (cholestyramine, colestipol, colesevelam) bind cholesterol in the GI tract. Ezetimibe inhibits the absorption of cholesterol in the small intestine. Fenofibrate, gemfibrozil, and niacin act by other mechanisms (see individual monographs).

Contraindications

Hypersensitivity. HMG-CoA reductase inhibitors are contraindicated in pregnancy.

Precautions

Safety of other drugs in pregnancy, lactation, and children not established. See individual drugs. Dietary therapy should be given a 2–3 mo trial before drug therapy is initiated.

Interactions

Bile acid sequestrants (cholestyramine and colestipol) may bind lipid-soluble vitamins (A, D, E, and K) and other concurrently administered drugs in the GI tract. The risk of myopathy from HMG-CoA reductase inhibitors is $\uparrow$ by niacin, erythromycin, gemfibrozil, and cyclosporine.

NURSING IMPLICATIONS

Assessment

- Obtain a diet history, especially in regard to **fat** and alcohol consumption.
- **Lab Test Considerations:** Serum cholesterol, LDL, HDL, and triglyceride levels should be evaluated before initiating and periodically throughout therapy. Medication should be discontinued if paradoxical increase in cholesterol level occurs.
- Liver function tests should be assessed before and periodically throughout therapy with HMG Co-A reductase inhibitors, niacin, and fibric acid derivatives. May cause an $\uparrow$ in levels.

Implementation

- See specific medications to determine timing of doses in relation to meals.

Patient/Family Teaching

- Advise patient that these medications should be used in conjunction with diet restrictions (**fat**, **cholesterol**, **carbohydrates**, and alcohol), exercise, and cessation of smoking.

Evaluation/Desired Outcomes

- Decreased serum cholesterol, triglyceride, and LDL levels and improved HDL levels.

• MINERALS/ELECTROLYTES/pH MODIFIERS

PHARMACOLOGIC PROFILE

General Use

Prevention and treatment of deficiencies or excesses of electrolytes and maintenance of optimal acid/base balance for homeostasis. Acidifiers and alkalinizers are also used to promote urinary excretion of substances that accumulate in certain disease states (kidney stones, uric acid).

General Action and Information

Electrolytes and minerals are necessary for many body processes. Maintenance of electrolyte levels within normal limits is required for many physiological processes such as cardiac, nerve, and muscle function; bone growth and stability; and a number of other activities. Minerals and electrolytes may also serve as catalysts in many enzymatic reactions. Acid/base balance allows for normal transfer of substances at the cellular and intracellular level.

Contraindications

Contraindicated in situations in which replacement would cause excess or when risk factors for retention are present.

Precautions

Use cautiously in disease states in which electrolyte imbalances are common such as significant hepatic or renal disease, adrenal or pituitary disorders.

Interactions

Depend on individual agents. Alkalinizers and acidifiers can alter the excretion of drugs for which elimination is pH dependent. See specific entries.

NURSING IMPLICATIONS

Assessment

- Observe patient carefully for evidence of electrolyte excess or insufficiency. Monitor lab values before and periodically throughout therapy.

Implementation

- **Potassium Chloride:** Do not administer potassium chloride undiluted.

Patient/Family Teaching

- Review diet modifications with patients with chronic electrolyte disturbances.

Evaluation/Desired Outcomes

- Return to normal serum electrolyte concentrations and resolution of clinical symptoms of electrolyte imbalance.
- Changes in pH or composition of urine, which prevent formation of renal calculi.

• NATURAL/HERBAL PRODUCTS

PHARMACOLOGIC PROFILE

General Use
These remedies are used for a wide variety of conditions. Prescriptions are not required and consumers have the choice of many products.

General Action and Information
Use of these agents is based on historical and sometimes anecdotal evidence. The FDA has little control over these agents, so currently there is little standardization among products.

Contraindications
Hypersensitivity. Most products are plant extracts that may contain a variety of impurities.

Precautions
Elderly, pediatric, and pregnant or lactating patients should be aware that these agents carry many of the same risks as prescription medications. Patients with serious chronic medical conditions should consult their health care professional before use.

Interactions
These agents have the ability to interact with prescription medications and may prevent or augment a desired therapeutic outcome. St. John's wort and kava-kava have the greatest risk for serious interactions.

NURSING IMPLICATIONS

Assessment
- Assess the condition for which the patient is taking the product.

Implementation
- **PO:** Administer with food if product associated with gastric irritation.

Patient/Family Teaching
- Discuss with patient the reason for using the product. Encourage patient to choose products with USP label, if possible, to guarantee content and purity of medication.
- Inform patient of known side effects and interactions with other medications.

Evaluation/Desired Outcomes
- Improvement in condition for which medication was taken.

• NONOPIOID ANALGESICS

PHARMACOLOGIC PROFILE

General Use
Used to control mild to moderate pain and/or fever. Phenazopyridine is used only to treat urinary tract pain, and capsaicin is used topically for a variety of painful syndromes.

General Action and Information
Most nonopioid analgesics inhibit prostaglandin synthesis peripherally for analgesic effect and centrally for antipyretic effect.

Contraindications
Hypersensitivity and cross-sensitivity among NSAIDs may occur.

Precautions
Use cautiously in patients with severe hepatic or renal disease, chronic alcohol use/abuse, or malnutrition.

Interactions
Long-term use of acetaminophen with NSAIDs may ↑ the risk of adverse renal effects. Prolonged high-dose acetaminophen may ↑ the risk of bleeding with warfarin. Hepatotoxicity may be additive with other hepatotoxic agents, including alcohol. NSAIDs ↑ the risk of bleeding with warfarin, thrombolytic agents, antiplatelet agents, some cephalosporins, and valproate (effect is greatest with aspirin). NSAIDs may also ↓ the effectiveness of diuretics and antihypertensives.

NURSING IMPLICATIONS

Assessment
- Patients who have asthma, allergies, and nasal polyps or who are allergic to tartrazine are at an ↑ risk for developing hypersensitivity reactions.
- **Pain:** Assess pain and limitation of movement; note type, location, and intensity prior to and at the peak (see Time/Action Profile) following administration.
- **Fever:** Assess fever and note associated signs (diaphoresis, tachycardia, malaise, chills).
- **Lab Test Considerations:** Hepatic, hematologic, and renal function should be evaluated periodically throughout prolonged high-dose therapy. Aspirin and most NSAIDs prolong bleeding time due to suppressed platelet aggregation and, in large doses, may cause prolonged prothrombin time. Monitor hematocrit periodically in prolonged high-dose therapy to assess for GI blood loss.

Implementation
- **PO:** Administer salicylates and NSAIDs after meals or with food to minimize gastric irritation.

Patient/Family Teaching
- Instruct patient to take salicylates and NSAIDs with a full glass of water and to remain in an upright position for 15–30 min after administration.
- Adults should not take acetaminophen longer than 10 days and children not longer than 5 days unless directed by health care professional. Short-term doses of acetaminophen with salicylates or NSAIDs should not exceed the recommended daily dose of either drug alone.
- Caution patient to avoid concurrent use of alcohol with this medication to minimize possible gastric irritation; 3 or more glasses of alcohol per day may ↑ the risk of GI bleeding with salicylates or NSAIDs. Caution patient to avoid taking acetaminophen, salicylates, or NSAIDs concurrently for more than a few days, unless directed by health care professional to prevent analgesic nephropathy.
- Advise patients on long-term therapy to inform health care professional of medication regimen prior to surgery. Aspirin, salicylates, and NSAIDs may need to be withheld prior to surgery.

Evaluation/Desired Outcomes
- Relief of mild to moderate discomfort.
- Reduction of fever.

CLASSIFICATIONS

• NONSTEROIDAL ANTI-INFLAMMATORY AGENTS

PHARMACOLOGIC PROFILE

General Use
NSAIDs are used to control mild to moderate pain, fever, and various inflammatory conditions, such as rheumatoid arthritis and osteoarthritis. Ophthalmic NSAIDs are used to ↓ postoperative ocular inflammation, to inhibit perioperative miosis, and to ↓ inflammation due to allergies.

General Action and Information
NSAIDs have analgesic, antipyretic, and anti-inflammatory properties. Analgesic and anti-inflammatory effects are due to inhibition of prostaglandin synthesis. Antipyretic action is due to vasodilation and inhibition of prostaglandin synthesis in the CNS. COX-2 inhibitors (celecoxib) may cause less GI bleeding.

Contraindications
Hypersensitivity to aspirin is a contraindication for the whole group of NSAIDs. Cross-sensitivity may occur.

Precautions
Use cautiously in patients with a history of bleeding disorders, GI bleeding, and severe hepatic, renal, or cardiovascular disease. Safe use in pregnancy is not established and, in general, should be avoided during the second half of pregnancy.

Interactions
NSAIDs prolong bleeding time and potentiate the effect of warfarin, thrombolytic agents, some cephalosporins, antiplatelet agents, and valproates. Prolonged use with aspirin may result in ↑ GI side effects and ↓ effectiveness. NSAIDs may also ↓ response to diuretics or antihypertensive therapy. COX-2 inhibitors do not negate the cardioprotective effect of low-dose aspirin.

NURSING IMPLICATIONS

Assessment
- Patients who have asthma, allergies, and nasal polyps or who are allergic to tartrazine are at an ↑ risk for developing hypersensitivity reactions.
- **Pain:** Assess pain and limitation of movement; note type, location, and intensity prior to and at the peak (see Time/Action Profile) following administration.
- **Fever:** Assess fever and note associated signs (diaphoresis, tachycardia, malaise, chills).
- **Lab Test Considerations:** Most NSAIDs prolong bleeding time due to suppressed platelet aggregation and, in large doses, may cause prolonged PT. Monitor periodically in prolonged high-dose therapy to assess for GI blood loss.

Implementation
- **PO:** Administer NSAIDs after meals or with food to minimize gastric irritation.

Patient/Family Teaching
- Instruct patient to take NSAIDs with a full glass of water and to remain in an upright position for 15–30 min after administration.
- Caution patient to avoid concurrent use of alcohol with this medication to minimize possible gastric irritation; 3 or more glasses of alcohol per day may ↑ the risk of GI bleeding with salicylates or NSAIDs. Caution patient to avoid taking acetaminophen, salicy-

lates, or NSAIDs concurrently for more than a few days, unless directed by health care professional to prevent analgesic nephropathy.

- Advise patient on long-term therapy to inform health care professional of medication regimen prior to surgery. NSAIDs may need to be withheld prior to surgery.

Evaluation/Desired Outcomes

- Relief of mild to moderate discomfort
- Reduction of fever.

• OPIOID ANALGESICS

PHARMACOLOGIC PROFILE

General Use

Management of moderate to severe pain. Fentanyl is also used as a general anesthetic adjunct.

General Action and Information

Opioids bind to opiate receptors in the CNS, where they act as agonists of endogenously occurring opioid peptides (eukephalins and endorphins). The result is alteration to the perception of and response to pain.

Contraindications

Hypersensitivity to individual agents.

Precautions

Use cautiously in patients with undiagnosed abdominal pain, head trauma or pathology, liver disease, or history of addiction to opioids. Use smaller doses initially in the elderly and those with respiratory diseases. Prolonged use may result in tolerance and the need for larger doses to relieve pain. Psychological or physical dependence may occur.

Interactions

↑ the CNS depressant properties of other drugs, including alcohol, antihistamines, antidepressants, sedative/hypnotics, phenothiazines, and MAO inhibitors. Use of partial-antagonist opioid analgesics (buprenorphine, butorphanol, and nalbuphine) may precipitate opioid withdrawal in physically dependent patients. Use with MAO inhibitors or procarbazine may result in severe paradoxical reactions (especially with meperidine). Nalbuphine may ↓ the analgesic effects of other concurrently administered opioid analgesics.

NURSING IMPLICATIONS

Assessment

- Assess type, location, and intensity of pain prior to and at peak following administration. When titrating opioid doses, ↑ of 25–50% should be administered until there is either a 50% ↓ in the patient's pain rating on a numerical or visual analogue scale or the patient reports satisfactory pain relief. A repeat dose can be safely administered at the time of the peak if previous dose is ineffective and side effects are minimal. Patients requiring higher doses of opioid agonist-antagonists should be converted to an opioid agonist.
- Opioid agonist-antagonists are not recommended for prolonged use or as first-line therapy for acute or cancer pain.
- An equianalgesic chart (see Appendix J) should be used when changing routes or when changing from one opioid to another.

- Assess BP, pulse, and respirations before and periodically during administration. If respiratory rate is <10/min, assess level of sedation. Physical stimulation may be sufficient to prevent significant hypoventilation. Dose may need to be ↓ by 25–50%. Initial drowsiness will diminish with continued use.
- Assess prior analgesic history. Antagonistic properties of agonist-antagonists may induce withdrawal symptoms (vomiting, restlessness, abdominal cramps, and ↑ BP and temperature) in patients physically dependent on opioids.
- Prolonged use may lead to physical and psychological dependence and tolerance. This should not prevent patient from receiving adequate analgesia. Most patients who receive opioid analgesics for pain do not develop psychological dependence. Progressively higher doses may be required to relieve pain with chronic therapy.
- Assess bowel function routinely. Prevention of constipation should be instituted with ↑ intake of fluids and bulk, stool softeners, and laxatives to minimize constipating effects. Stimulant laxatives should be administered routinely if opioid use exceeds 2–3 days, unless contraindicated.
- Monitor intake and output ratios. If significant discrepancies occur, assess for urinary retention and inform physician or other health care professional.
- **Toxicity and Overdose:** If an opioid antagonist is required to reverse respiratory depression or coma, naloxone is the antidote. Dilute the 0.4-mg ampule of naloxone in 10 mL of 0.9% NaCl and administer 0.5 mL (0.02 mg) by IV push every 2 min. For children and patients weighing <40 kg, dilute 0.1 mg of naloxone in 10 mL of 0.9% NaCl for a concentration of 10 mcg/mL and administer 0.5 mcg/kg every 1–2 min. Naloxone may also be administered intranasally to reverse opioid-induced respiratory depression or coma. Administer 1 spray (2 mg or 4 mg) in one nostril; may repeat dose every 2–3 min (with each subsequent dose being administered in alternate nostril). Titrate dose to avoid withdrawal, seizures, and severe pain.

Implementation

- Do not confuse morphine with hydromorphone or meperidine; errors have resulted in fatalities.
- Explain therapeutic value of medication before administration to enhance the analgesic effect.
- Regularly administered doses may be more effective than prn ("as needed") administration. Analgesic is more effective if given before pain becomes severe.
- Coadministration with nonopioid analgesics may have additive analgesic effects and may permit lower doses.
- Medication should be discontinued gradually after long-term use to prevent withdrawal symptoms.

Patient/Family Teaching

- Instruct patient on how and when to ask for pain medication.
- Advise patient that opioid analgesics have known abuse potential. Advise the patient to protect these medications from theft, and never give them to anyone other than the individual for whom it was prescribed. Store out of sight and reach of children, and in a location not accessible by others.
- Medication may cause drowsiness or dizziness. Caution patient to call for assistance when ambulating or smoking and to avoid driving or other activities requiring alertness until response to medication is known.
- Advise patient to make position changes slowly to minimize orthostatic hypotension.

- Caution patient to avoid concurrent use of alcohol or other CNS depressants with this medication.
- Encourage patient to turn, cough, and breathe deeply every 2 hr to prevent atelectasis.

Evaluation/Desired Outcomes

- Decreased severity of pain without a significant alteration in level of consciousness or respiratory status.

• SEDATIVE/HYPNOTICS

PHARMACOLOGIC PROFILE

General Use

Sedatives are used to provide sedation, usually prior to procedures. Hypnotics are used to manage insomnia. Selected agents are useful as anticonvulsants (clorazepate, diazepam, phenobarbital), skeletal muscle relaxants (diazepam), adjuncts in the management of alcohol withdrawal syndrome (chlordiazepoxide, diazepam, oxazepam), adjuncts in general anesthesia (droperidol), or as amnestics (midazolam, diazepam).

General Action and Information

Cause generalized CNS depression. May produce tolerance with chronic use and have potential for psychological or physical dependence. These agents have NO analgesic properties.

Contraindications

Hypersensitivity. Should not be used in comatose patients or in those with pre-existing CNS depression. Should not be used in patients with uncontrolled severe pain. Avoid use during pregnancy or lactation.

Precautions

Use cautiously in patients with hepatic impairment, severe renal impairment, or severe underlying pulmonary disease. Use with caution in patients who may be suicidal or who may have had previous drug addictions. Hypnotic use should be short-term. Geriatric patients may be more sensitive to CNS depressant effects; dosage ↓ may be required.

Interactions

Additive CNS depression with alcohol, antihistamines, some antidepressants, opioid analgesics, or phenothiazines. Barbiturates induce hepatic drug-metabolizing enzymes and can ↓ the effectiveness of drugs metabolized by the liver, including oral contraceptives. Should not be used with MAO inhibitors.

NURSING IMPLICATIONS

Assessment

- Monitor BP, pulse, and respiratory status frequently throughout IV administration. Prolonged high-dose therapy may lead to psychological or physical dependence. Restrict the amount of drug available to patient, especially if patient is depressed, suicidal, or has a history of addiction.
- **Insomnia:** Assess sleep patterns before and periodically throughout course of therapy.
- **Seizures:** Observe and record intensity, duration, and characteristics of seizure activity. Institute seizure precautions.

- **Muscle Spasms:** Assess muscle spasms, associated pain, and limitation of movement before and throughout therapy.
- **Alcohol Withdrawal:** Assess patient experiencing alcohol withdrawal for tremors, agitation, delirium, and hallucinations. Protect patient from injury.

Implementation

- Supervise ambulation and transfer of patients following administration of hypnotic doses. Remove cigarettes. Side rails should be raised and call bell within reach at all times. Keep bed in low position.

Patient/Family Teaching

- Discuss the importance of preparing the environment for sleep (dark room, quiet, avoidance of nicotine and caffeine). If less effective after a few weeks, consult health care professional; do not ↑ dose. Gradual withdrawal may be required to prevent reactions following prolonged therapy.
- May cause daytime drowsiness. Caution patient to avoid driving and other activities requiring alertness until response to medication is known.
- Advise patient to avoid the use of alcohol and other CNS depressants concurrently with these medications.
- Advise patient to inform health care professional if pregnancy is planned or suspected.

Evaluation/Desired Outcomes

- Improvement in sleep patterns.
- Control of seizures.
- Decrease in muscle spasms.
- Decreased tremulousness.
- More rational ideation when used for alcohol withdrawal.

• SKELETAL MUSCLE RELAXANTS

PHARMACOLOGIC PROFILE

General Use

Two major uses are spasticity associated with spinal cord diseases or lesions (baclofen and dantrolene) or adjunctive therapy in the symptomatic relief of acute painful musculoskeletal conditions (carisoprodol, chlorzoxazone, cyclobenzaprine, diazepam, and methocarbamol). IV dantrolene is also used to treat and prevent malignant hyperthermia.

General Action and Information

Act either centrally (baclofen, carisoprodol, cyclobenzaprine, metaxolone, and methocarbamol) or directly (dantrolene).

Contraindications

Baclofen and oral dantrolene should not be used in patients in whom spasticity is used to maintain posture and balance.

Precautions

Safety in pregnancy and lactation not established. Use cautiously in patients with a history of previous liver disease.

Interactions
Additive CNS depression with other CNS depressants, including alcohol, antihistamines, antidepressants, opioid analgesics, and sedative/hypnotics.

NURSING IMPLICATIONS

Assessment
- Assess patient for pain, muscle stiffness, and range of motion before and periodically throughout therapy.

Implementation
- Provide safety measures as indicated. Supervise ambulation and transfer of patients.

Patient/Family Teaching
- Encourage patient to comply with additional therapies prescribed for muscle spasm (rest, physical therapy, heat).
- Medication may cause drowsiness. Caution patient to avoid driving or other activities requiring alertness until response to drug is known.
- Advise patient to avoid concurrent use of alcohol or other CNS depressants with these medications.

Evaluation/Desired Outcomes
- Decreased musculoskeletal pain
- Decreased muscle spasticity
- Increased range of motion
- Prevention or decrease in temperature and skeletal rigidity in malignant hyperthermia.

• THROMBOLYTICS

PHARMACOLOGIC PROFILE

General Use
Acute management of ST-segment-elevation MI. Alteplase is also used in the management of acute pulmonary embolism and acute ischemic stroke.

General Action and Information
Converts plasminogen to plasmin, which then degrades fibrin in clots. Alteplase, reteplase, and tenecteplase directly activate plasminogen. Results in lysis of blood clots.

Contraindications
Hypersensitivity. Active internal bleeding, history of cerebrovascular accident, recent CNS trauma or surgery, neoplasm, or arteriovenous malformation, severe uncontrolled hypertension, and known bleeding tendencies.

Precautions
Recent (within 10 days) major surgery, trauma, GI or GU bleeding. Severe hepatic or renal disease. Subacute bacterial endocarditis or acute pericarditis. Use cautiously in geriatric patients. Safety not established in pregnancy, lactation, or children.

Interactions
Concurrent use with antiplatelet agents, NSAIDs, warfarin, dabigatran, rivaroxaban, apixaban, edoxaban, betrixaban, or heparins may ↑ the risk of bleeding, although these agents

are frequently used together or in sequence. Risk of bleeding may also be ↑ by concurrent use with cefotetan, cefoperazone, and valproic acid.

NURSING IMPLICATIONS

Assessment

- Begin therapy as soon as possible after the onset of symptoms.
- Monitor vital signs, including temperature, continuously for coronary thrombosis and at least every 4 hr during therapy for other indications. Do not use lower extremities to monitor BP.
- Assess patient carefully for bleeding every 15 min during the 1st hr of therapy, every 15–30 min during the next 8 hr, and at least every 4 hr for the duration of therapy. Frank bleeding may occur from sites of invasive procedures or from body orifices. Internal bleeding may also occur (↓ neurologic status; abdominal pain with coffee-ground emesis or black, tarry stools; hematuria; joint pain). If uncontrolled bleeding occurs, stop medication and notify physician immediately.
- Assess neurologic status throughout therapy.
- Altered sensorium or neurologic changes may be indicative of intracranial bleeding.
- **Coronary Thrombosis:** Monitor ECG continuously. Notify physician if significant arrhythmias occur. IV lidocaine or procainamide may be ordered prophylactically. Cardiac enzymes should be monitored. Coronary angiography may be ordered following therapy to monitor effectiveness of therapy.
- Monitor heart sounds and breath sounds frequently. Inform physician if signs of HF occur (rales/crackles, dyspnea, S3 heart sound, jugular venous distention).
- **Pulmonary Embolism:** Monitor pulse, BP, hemodynamics, and respiratory status (rate, degree of dyspnea, arterial blood gases).
- **Cannula/Catheter Occlusion:** Monitor ability to aspirate blood as indicator of patency. Ensure that patient exhales and holds breath when connecting and disconnecting IV syringe to prevent air embolism.
- **Acute Ischemic Stroke:** Assess neurologic status. Determine time of onset of stroke symptoms. Alteplase must be administered within 3–4.5 hr of onset (within 3 hr in patients >80 years, those taking oral anticoagulants, those with a baseline National Institutes of Health Stroke Scale score >25, or those with both a history of stroke and diabetes).
- **Lab Test Considerations:** Hematocrit, hemoglobin, platelet count, fibrin/fibrin degradation product (FDP/fdp) titer, fibrinogen concentration, prothrombin time, thrombin time, and activated partial thromboplastin time may be evaluated prior to and frequently throughout therapy. Bleeding time may be assessed prior to therapy if patient has received platelet aggregation inhibitors. Obtain type and cross match and have blood available at all times in case of hemorrhage. Stools should be tested for occult blood loss and urine for hematuria periodically during therapy.
- **Toxicity and Overdose:** If local bleeding occurs, apply pressure to site. If severe or internal bleeding occurs, discontinue infusion. Clotting factors and/or blood volume may be restored through infusions of whole blood, packed RBCs, fresh frozen plasma, or cryoprecipitate. Do not administer dextran, as it has antiplatelet activity. Aminocaproic acid may be used as an antidote.

Implementation

- This medication should be used only in settings in which hematologic function and clinical response can be adequately monitored.

- Starting two IV lines prior to therapy is recommended: one for the thrombolytic agent, the other for any additional infusions.
- Avoid invasive procedures, such as IM injections or arterial punctures, with this therapy. If such procedures must be performed, apply pressure to all arterial and venous puncture sites for at least 30 min. Avoid venipunctures at noncompressible sites (jugular vein, subclavian site).
- Systemic anticoagulation with heparin is usually begun several hours after the completion of thrombolytic therapy.
- Acetaminophen may be ordered to control fever.

Patient/Family Teaching
- Explain purpose of medication and the need for close monitoring to patient and family. Instruct patient to report hypersensitivity reactions (rash, dyspnea) and bleeding or bruising.
- Explain need for bedrest and minimal handling during therapy to avoid injury. Avoid all unnecessary procedures such as shaving and vigorous tooth brushing.

Evaluation/Desired Outcomes
- Lysis of thrombi and restoration of blood flow
- Prevention of neurologic sequelae in acute ischemic stroke
- Cannula or catheter patency.

• VACCINES/IMMUNIZING AGENTS

PHARMACOLOGIC PROFILE

General Use
Immune globulins provide passive immunization to infectious diseases by providing antibodies. Immunization with vaccines and toxoids containing bacterial or viral antigenic material results in endogenous production of antibodies.

General Action and Information
Immunity from immune globulins is rapid, but short-lived (up to 3 months). Active immunization with vaccine or toxoids produces prolonged immunity (years).

Contraindications
Hypersensitivity to product, preservatives, or other additives. Some products contain thimerisol, neomycin, and/or **egg protein**.

Precautions
Severe bleeding problems (IM injections).

Interactions
↓ antibody response to vaccine/toxoids and ↑ risk of adverse reactions in patients receiving concurrent antineoplastic, immunosuppressive, or radiation therapy.

NURSING IMPLICATIONS

Assessment
- Assess previous immunization history and history of hypersensitivity.

CLASSIFICATIONS

Implementation
- Measles, mumps, and rubella vaccine, trivalent oral polio virus vaccine, and diphtheria toxoid, tetanus toxoid, and pertussis vaccine may be given concurrently.
- Administer each immunization by appropriate route.

Patient/Family Teaching
- Inform patient/parent of potential and reportable side effects of immunization. Health care professional should be notified if patient develops fever over 39.4°C (103°F); difficulty breathing; hives; itching; swelling of the eyes, face, or inside of nose; sudden severe tiredness or weakness; or convulsions occur.
- Review next scheduled immunization with parent. Emphasize the importance of keeping a record of immunizations and dates given.

Evaluation/Desired Outcomes
- Prevention of diseases through active immunity.

• VASCULAR HEADACHE SUPPRESSANTS

PHARMACOLOGIC PROFILE

General Use
Used for acute treatment of vascular headaches (migraine, cluster headaches, migraine variants). Other agents such as some beta blockers and some calcium channel blockers are used for suppression of frequently occurring vascular headaches.

General Action and Information
Ergot derivatives (ergotamine, dihydroergotamine) directly stimulate alpha-adrenergic and serotonergic receptors, producing vascular smooth muscle vasoconstriction. Almotriptan, eletriptan, frovatriptan, naratriptan, rizatriptan, sumatriptan, and zolmitriptan produce vasoconstriction by acting as serotonin ($5\text{-}HT_1$) agonists.

Contraindications
Avoid using these agents in patients with ischemic cardiovascular disease.

Precautions
Use cautiously in patients who have a history of, or at risk for, cardiovascular disease.

Interactions
Avoid concurrent use of ergot derivative agents with serotonin agonist agents; see also individual agents.

NURSING IMPLICATIONS

Assessment
- Assess pain location, intensity, duration, and associated symptoms (photophobia, phonophobia, nausea, vomiting) during migraine attack and frequency of attacks.

Implementation
- Medication should be administered at the first sign of a headache.

Patient/Family Teaching

- Inform patient that medication should be used only during a migraine attack. It is meant to be used for relief of migraine attacks but not to prevent or reduce the number of attacks.
- Advise patient that lying down in a darkened room following medication administration may further help relieve headache.
- May cause dizziness or drowsiness. Caution patient to avoid driving or other activities requiring alertness until response to medication is known.
- Advise patient to avoid alcohol, which aggravates headaches.

Evaluation/Desired Outcomes

- Relief of migraine attack.

• VITAMINS

PHARMACOLOGIC PROFILE

General Use

Used in the prevention and treatment of vitamin deficiencies and as supplements in various metabolic disorders.

General Action and Information

Serve as components of enzyme systems that catalyze numerous varied metabolic reactions. Necessary for homeostasis. Water-soluble vitamins (B-vitamins and vitamin C) rarely cause toxicity. Fat-soluble vitamins (vitamins D and E) may accumulate and cause toxicity.

Contraindications

Hypersensitivity to additives, preservatives, or colorants.

Precautions

Dose should be adjusted to avoid toxicity, especially for fat-soluble vitamins.

Interactions

Pyridoxine in large amounts may interfere with the effectiveness of levodopa. Cholestyramine, colestipol, and mineral oil ↓ absorption of fat-soluble vitamins.

NURSING IMPLICATIONS

Assessment

- Assess patient for signs of vitamin deficiency before and periodically throughout therapy.
- Assess nutritional status through 24-hr diet recall. Determine frequency of consumption of vitamin-rich foods.

Implementation

- Because of infrequency of single vitamin deficiencies, combinations are commonly administered.

Patient/Family Teaching

- Encourage patients to comply with diet recommendations of physician or other health care professional. Explain that the best source of vitamins is a well-balanced diet with foods from the four basic food groups.

- Patients self-medicating with vitamin supplements should be cautioned not to exceed RDAs. The effectiveness of megadoses for treatment of various medical conditions is unproved and may cause side effects and toxicity.

Evaluation/Desired Outcomes

- Prevention of, or decrease in, the symptoms of vitamin deficiencies.

• WEIGHT CONTROL AGENTS

PHARMACOLOGIC PROFILE

General Use

These agents are used in the management of exogenous obesity as part of a regimen including a reduced-calorie diet. They are especially useful in the presence of other risk factors including hypertension, diabetes, or dyslipidemias.

General Action and Information

Phentermine is an anorexiant designed to ↓ appetite via its action in the CNS. Orlistat is a lipase inhibitor that ↓ absorption of dietary fat.

Contraindications

None of these agents should be used during pregnancy or lactation. Phentermine should not be used in patients with severe hepatic or renal disease, uncontrolled hypertension, known HF, or cardiovascular disease. Orlistat should not be used in patients with chronic malabsorption.

Precautions

Phentermine should be used cautiously in patients with a history of seizures, or angle-closure glaucoma and in geriatric patients.

Interactions

Phentermine may have additive, adverse effects with CNS stimulants, some vascular headache suppressants, MAO inhibitors, and some opioids (concurrent use should be avoided). Orlistat ↓ absorption of some fat-soluble vitamins and beta-carotene.

NURSING IMPLICATIONS

Assessment

- Monitor weight and dietary intake prior to and periodically during therapy. Adjust concurrent medications (antihypertensives, antidiabetics, lipid-lowering agents) as needed.

Implementation

Patient/Family Teaching

- Advise patient that regular physical activity, approved by healthcare professional, should be used in conjunction with medication and diet.

Evaluation/Desired Outcomes

- Slow, consistent weight loss when combined with a reduced-calorie diet.

abacavir/dolutegravir/lamivudine

(ah-**back**-ah-veer/doe-loo-**teg**-ra-vir/la-**mi**-vyoo-deen)

Triumeq

Classification

Therapeutic: antiretrovirals (combination)

Pharmacologic: integrase strand transfer inhibitors (INSTI) (dolutegravir), nucleoside reverse transcriptase inhibitors (abacavir, lamivudine)

Indications

Treatment of HIV-1 infection.

Action

Abacavir—Converted inside cells to carbovir triphosphate, its active metabolite. Carbovir triphosphate inhibits the activity of HIV-1 reverse transcriptase, which in turn terminates viral DNA growth. *Dolutegravir*—Inhibits HIV-1 integrase, which is required for viral replication. *Lamivudine*—After intracellular conversion to its active form (lamivudine-5-triphosphate), inhibits viral DNA synthesis by inhibiting the enzyme reverse transcriptase. **Therapeutic Effects:** Evidence of decreased viral replication and reduced viral load with slowed progression of HIV and its sequelae.

Pharmacokinetics

Abacavir

Absorption: Rapidly and extensively (83%) absorbed.

Distribution: Distributes into extravascular space and readily distributes into erythrocytes.

Metabolism and Excretion: Mostly metabolized by the liver; 1.2% excreted unchanged in urine.

Half-life: 1.5 hr.

Dolutegravir

Absorption: Absorption follows oral administration; bioavailability is unknown.

Distribution: Enters CSF.

Protein Binding: >98.9%.

Metabolism and Excretion: Metabolized primarily by the UGT1A1 enzyme system with some metabolism by CYP3A4. 53% excreted unchanged in feces. Metabolites are renally excreted, minimal renal elimination of unchanged drug. Poor metabolizers of dolutegravir have ↑ levels and ↓ clearance.

Half-life: 14 hr.

Lamivudine

Absorption: Well absorbed after oral administration (86% in adults, 66% in infants and children).

Distribution: Distributes into the extravascular space. Some penetration into CSF; remainder of distribution unknown.

Metabolism and Excretion: Mostly excreted unchanged in urine; <5% metabolized by the liver.

Half-life: *Adults*—3.7 hr; *children*—2 hr.

TIME/ACTION PROFILE (blood levels)

ROUTE	ONSET	PEAK	DURATION
PO	unknown	unknown	24 hr

Contraindications/Precautions

Contraindicated in: Hypersensitivity to any component (especially abacavir, rechallenge may be fatal); Resistance to any component; Presence of HLA-B*5701 allele; Concurrent use of dofetilide; Concurrent administration of lamivudine or abacavir alone or in other combination antiretroviral dose forms; Moderate to severe liver impairment; CCr <50 mL/min; Lactation: Breast feeding not recommended for HIV-infected patients.

Use Cautiously in: Underlying hepatitis B or C (may worsen liver function); Patients with HIV-1/HCV coinfection receiving interferon alfa with/without ribavirin (may be at risk for hepatic decompensation, dose alteration or discontinuation of interferon and/or ribavirin may be necessary); Mild hepatic impairment (if dose ↓ of abacavir is necessary, combination should be given as individual components); Women and obesity (↑ risk of lactic acidosis and severe hepatomegaly with steatosis); Underlying cardiovascular disease, including history of hypertension, hyperlipidema, smoking history, or diabetes mellitus; OB: Use only if potential benefit justifies potential risk to the fetus; Pedi: Children <40 kg (safety and effectiveness not established).

Adverse Reactions/Side Effects

Abacavir/dolutegravir/lamivudine.

CNS: fatigue, headache, insomnia. **CV:** MYOCARDIAL INFARCTION. **F and E:** LACTIC ACIDOSIS. **GI:** HEPATOMEGALY (WITH STEATOSIS), HEPATOTOXICITY (↑ WITH HEPATITIS B OR C), exacerbation of Hepatitis B. **Misc:** HYPERSENSITIVITY REACTIONS, immune reconstitution syndrome.

Interactions

Drug-Drug: Abacavir: Alcohol ↑ blood levels. May ↑ **methadone** metabolism in some patients; slight ↑ in **methadone** dosing may be needed. **Dolutegravir:** May ↑ blood levels and toxicity from **dofetilide**; concurrent use contraindicated. Blood levels and effectiveness are ↓ by **etravirine** (should not be used concurrently without atazanavir/ritonavir, darunavir/ritonavir or lopinavir/ritonavir). Blood levels and effectiveness are ↓ by **efavirenz, fosamprenavir/ritonavir, tipranavir/ritonavir, carbamazepine**, and **rifampin**; ↑ dosage of dolutegravir recommended. Blood levels and effectiveness may be ↓ by **nevirapine**; avoid concurrent use.

May ↑ blood levels and toxicity from **metformin**; do not exceed metformin dose of 1000 mg/day. Blood levels and effectiveness may be ↓ by other **metabolic inducers** including **oxcarbazepine**, **phenobarbital**, and **phenytoin**; avoid concurrent use. Absorption and effectiveness may be ↓ by cation-containing **antacids**, **buffered medications**, oral **calcium supplements**, oral **iron supplements**, **laxatives**, or **sucralfate**; dolutegravir should be taken 2 hr before or 6 hr after; may also take dolutegravir and calcium or iron supplements with food. **Lamivudine: Trimethoprim/sulfamethoxazole** ↑ levels (dose alteration may be necessary in renal impairment). ↑ risk of pancreatitis with concurrent use of other **drugs causing pancreatitis**. ↑ risk of neuropathy with concurrent use of other **drugs causing neuropathy**. Combination therapy with **tenofovir** and **abacavir** may lead to virologic nonresponse; avoid use. **Sorbitol** may ↓ levels; avoid concurrent use.

Drug-Natural Products: Levels and effectiveness may be ↓ **St. John's wort**; avoid concurrent use.

Route/Dosage

PO (Adults and Children ≥40 kg): One tablet (abacavir 600 mg/dolutegravir 50 mg/lamivudine 300 mg) once daily; *Concurrent efavirenz, fosamprenavir/ritonavir, tipranavir/ritonavir, carbamazepine, or rifampin*—additional 50–mg dose of dolutegravir is required separated by 12 hr.

Availability

Tablets: abacavir 600 mg/dolutegravir 50 mg/lamivudine 300 mg.

NURSING IMPLICATIONS

Assessment

- Assess patient for change in severity of HIV symptoms and for symptoms of opportunistic infections throughout therapy.
- Assess for signs of hypersensitivity reactions (fever; rash; gastrointestinal—nausea, vomiting, diarrhea, abdominal pain; constitutional—malaise, fatigue, achiness; respiratory—dyspnea, cough, pharyngitis). May also cause elevated liver function tests, increased creatine phosphokinase or serum creatinine, and lymphopenia. Patients who carry the HLA-B*5701 allele are at high risk for hypersensitivity reaction. Discontinue promptly if hypersensitivity reaction is suspected. Regardless of HLA-B*5701 status, permanently discontinue if hypersensitivity cannot be ruled out, even when other diagnoses are possible. Following a hypersensitivity reaction, never restart abacavir-containing products. More severe symptoms may occur within hr and may include life-threatening hypotension and death. Symptoms usually resolve upon discontinuation.
- May cause lactic acidosis and severe hepatomegaly with steatosis. Monitor patient for signs (↑ serum lactate levels, ↑ liver enzymes, liver enlargement on palpation). Therapy should be suspended if clinical or laboratory signs occur.
- Assess patient, especially pediatric patients, for signs of pancreatitis (nausea, vomiting, abdominal pain) periodically during therapy. May require discontinuation of therapy.
- Monitor patient for signs and symptoms of peripheral neuropathy (tingling, burning, numbness, or pain in hands or feet); may be difficult to differentiate from peripheral neuropathy of severe HIV disease. May require discontinuation of therapy.
- ***Lab Test Considerations:*** Obtain a negative pregnancy test prior to starting therapy.
- Monitor viral load and CD4 cell count regularly during therapy.
- Screen for HLA-B*5701 allele prior to initiation of therapy to decrease risk of hypersensitivity reaction. Screening is also recommended prior to reinitiation of abacavir in patients of unknown HLA-B*5701 status who have previously tolerated abacavir.
- Monitor liver function periodically. May cause ↑ levels of AST, ALT, and alkaline phosphatase, which usually resolve after interruption of therapy. Patients with concurrent Hepatitis B or C should be followed for at least several mo after stopping therapy. Lactic acidosis may occur with hepatic toxicity, causing hepatic steatosis; may be fatal, especially in women.
- May cause ↑ serum glucose, lipase, and triglyceride levels.

Implementation

- **PO:** Administer without regard to food.
- Take *Triumeq* 2 hr before or 6 hr after antacids, laxatives, other medications containing aluminum, magnesium, sucralfate, or buffering agents, calcium, or iron. Supplements containing calcium or iron can be taken with *Triumeq* if taken with food.

Patient/Family Teaching

- Emphasize the importance of taking *Triumeq* as directed. Must always be used in combination with other antiretroviral drugs. Do not take more than prescribed amount, and do not stop taking without consulting health care professional. Take missed doses as soon as remembered unless almost time for next dose; do not double doses. Advise patient to read the *Medication Guide* prior to starting therapy and with each Rx refill in case of changes.
- Instruct patient not to share medication with others.
- Inform patient that medication does not cure AIDS or prevent associated or opportunistic infections. Medication does not reduce the risk of transmission of HIV to others through sexual contact or blood contamination. Caution patient to use a condom, and avoid sharing needles or donating blood to prevent spreading the AIDS virus to others. Advise patient that the long-term effects of medication are unknown at this time.
- Advise patient of potential for hypersensitivity reactions that may result in death. Instruct patient to dis-

continue medication and notify health care professional immediately if symptoms of hypersensitivity or signs of Immune Reconstitution Syndrome (signs and symptoms of inflammation from previous infections) occur. A warning card summarizing symptoms of hypersensitivity is provided with each prescription; instruct patient to carry card at all times.

- Instruct patient to notify health care professional immediately if symptoms of lactic acidosis (tiredness or weakness, unusual muscle pain, trouble breathing, stomach pain with nausea and vomiting, cold especially in arms or legs, dizziness, fast or irregular heartbeat) or if signs of hepatotoxicity (yellow skin or whites of eyes, dark urine, light-colored stools, lack of appetite for several days or longer, nausea, abdominal pain) occur. These symptoms may occur more frequently in patients that are female, obese, or have been taking medications for a long time.
- Instruct patient to notify health care professional promptly if signs of peripheral neuropathy or pancreatitis occur.
- Advise patient to avoid sugarless gum or candy due to sorbitol content; may ↓ medication effectiveness.
- Inform patient that redistribution and accumulation of body fat may occur, causing central obesity, dorsocervical fat enlargement (buffalo hump), peripheral wasting, breast enlargement, and cushingoid appearance. The cause and long-term effects are not known.
- Advise patient to notify health care professional of all Rx or OTC medications, vitamins, or herbal products being taken and to consult with health care professional before taking other medications, especially methadone, St. John's wort, and other antiretrovirals.
- Rep: Advise female patient of reproductive potential to use effective contraception and to avoid breast feeding during therapy. Notify health care professional if pregnancy is planned or suspected. Switch to another antiviral regimen during 1st trimester. May consider *Triumeq* during 2nd and 3rd trimesters of pregnancy if expected benefit justifies potential risk to pregnant woman and fetus. Pregnant patients should be encouraged to enroll in the Antiretroviral Pregnancy Registry by calling 1-800-258-4263.
- Emphasize the importance of regular follow-up exams and blood counts to determine progress and monitor for side effects.

Evaluation/Desired Outcomes

- Delayed progression of AIDS, and decreased opportunistic infections in patients with HIV.
- Decrease in viral load and increase in CD4 cell counts.

⧖ abemaciclib

(a-bem-a-**sye**-klib)

Verzenio

Classification

Therapeutic: antineoplastics

Pharmacologic: kinase inhibitors

Indications

⧖ Advanced or metastatic hormone receptor (HR)-positive, human epidermal growth factor 2 (HER2)-negative breast cancer in women with disease progression following endocrine therapy (in combination with fulvestrant). ⧖ Advanced or metastatic HR-positive, HER2-negative breast cancer in women with disease progression following endocrine therapy and prior chemotherapy in the metastatic setting (as monotherapy). HR-positive, HER2-negative advanced or metastatic breast cancer in postmenopausal women (in combination with an aromatase inhibitor).

Action

Inhibits kinases (cyclin-dependent kinases 4 and 6) that are part of the signaling pathway for cell proliferation. **Therapeutic Effects:** Improved survival and decreased spread of breast cancer.

Pharmacokinetics

Absorption: 45% absorbed following oral administration.

Distribution: Extensively distributed to tissues.

Protein Binding: 96%.

Metabolism and Excretion: Primarily metabolized in the liver by CYP3A4 to several active metabolites; 81% excreted in feces, 3% in urine.

Half-life: 18.3 hr.

TIME/ACTION PROFILE (blood levels)

ROUTE	ONSET	PEAK	DURATION
PO	unknown	8 hr	24 hr

Contraindications/Precautions

Contraindicated in: OB: Pregnancy (may cause fetal harm); Lactation: Avoid breast feeding.

Use Cautiously in: Severe renal impairment (CCr <30 mL/min); Severe hepatic impairment (↓ dose); Rep: Women of reproductive potential; Pedi: Safety and effectiveness not established.

Adverse Reactions/Side Effects

CNS: dizziness, fatigue, headache. **CV:** VENOUS THROMBOEMBOLISM, peripheral edema. **Derm:** alopecia, pruritus, rash. **GI:** HEPATOTOXICITY, abdominal pain, ↓ appetite, constipation, diarrhea, dry mouth, dysgeusia, ↑ liver enzymes, nausea, stomatitis, vomiting. **GU:** ↑ serum creatinine, ↓ fertility (males). **Hemat:** ANEMIA, LEUKOPENIA, NEUTROPENIA, THROMBOCY-

TOPENIA. **Metab:** ↓ weight. **MS:** arthralgia. **Resp:** cough. **Misc:** INFECTION, fever.

Interactions

Drug-Drug: Strong CYP3A inhibitors, including **itraconazole** or **ketoconazole** may ↑ abemaciclib levels and risk of toxicity; avoid concurrent use with ketoconazole; ↓ abemaciclib dose when using other strong CYP3A4 inhibitors (resume original dose after 3–5 half-lives of offending drug have passed following discontinuation). **Strong CYP3A inducers**, including **rifampin** may ↓ abemaciclib levels and its effectiveness; avoid concurrent use.

Route/Dosage

PO (Adults): *With fulvestrant or an aromatase inhibitor*—150 mg twice daily; continue until disease progression or unacceptable toxicity. *As monotherapy*—200 mg twice daily; continue until disease progression or unacceptable toxicity. *Concurrent use of strong CYP3A inhibitor (other then ketoconazole)*—100 mg twice daily (with fulvestrant or as monotherapy); if dose already at 100 mg twice daily due to adverse reactions, ↓ dose to 50 mg twice daily; continue until disease progression or unacceptable toxicity.

Hepatic Impairment

PO (Adults): *Severe hepatic impairment (Child-Pugh C)*—With fulvestrant: 150 mg once daily; continue until disease progression or unacceptable toxicity. *As monotherapy*—200 mg once daily; continue until disease progression or unacceptable toxicity. *Concurrent use of strong CYP3A inhibitor (other then ketoconazole)*—100 mg once daily (with fulvestrant or as monotherapy); if dose already at 100 mg once daily due to adverse reactions, ↓ dose to 50 mg once daily; continue until disease progression or unacceptable toxicity.

Availability

Tablets: 50 mg, 100 mg, 150 mg, 200 mg.

NURSING IMPLICATIONS

Assessment

- Monitor for diarrhea, may result in dehydration and infection. *Grade 1:* no dose modification required. *Grade 2:* If resolves in 24 hrs to ≤Grade 1, suspend therapy until resolution. No dose reduction required. *Grade 2 that persists or recurs after resuming same dose despite maximum supportive measures:* Hold dose until diarrhea resolves to ≤Grade 1. Resume at next lower dose. *Grade 3 or 4 diarrhea or diarrhea that requires hospitalization,* withhold abemaciclib until resolves to ≤Grade 1, then resume at next lower dose.
- Monitor for signs and symptoms of venous thrombosis and pulmonary embolism and treat as needed.
- ***Lab Test Considerations:*** Verify negative pregnancy test before starting therapy.
- Monitor CBC before starting, every 2 wk for first 2 mo, monthly for next 2 mo, and as clinically indicated. *Grade 1 or 2 neutropenia:* No dose reduction required. *Grade 3:* Hold dose until resolves to ≤Grade 2. *Grade 3 recurrent or Grade 4:* Hold therapy until resolved to ≤Grade 2. Resume at next lower dose.
- Monitor ALT, AST, and serum bilirubin prior to starting therapy, every 2 wk for first 2 mo, monthly for next 2 mo, and as clinically indicated. *If Grade 1 (>upper limit of normal [ULN] to 3 times ULN), Grade 2 (>3.0 to 5.0 times ULN, without ↑ in total bilirubin >2 times ULN):* no dose reduction required. *If persistent or recurrent Grade 2, or Grade 3 (>5.0–20.0 x ULN), without ↑ in total bilirubin above 2 x ULN:* Withhold therapy until toxicity resolves to baseline or Grade 1. Resume at next lower dose. *If elevation in AST and/or ALT >3 x ULN with total bilirubin >2 x ULN, in the absence of cholestasis or Grade 4 (>20.0 x ULN):* discontinue therapy.
- May cause ↑ serum creatinine without glomerular function being affected. Monitor BUN, cystatin C, or calculated glomerular filtration rate to determine impaired renal function.

Implementation

- **PO:** Administer twice daily, at the same times each day, without regard to food. Swallow tablets whole; do not crush, break, or chew.

Patient/Family Teaching

- Instruct patient to take abemaciclib at the same times each day as directed. If patient vomits or misses a dose, omit dose and take next dose as scheduled. Do not ingest tablets that are broken, cracked, or not intact. Advise patient to read *Patient Information* before starting therapy and with each Rx refill in case of changes.
- Advise patient that at first sign of diarrhea, start antidiarrheal therapy (loperamide), increase oral fluids, and notify health care professional.
- Advise patient to notify health care professional if signs and symptoms of infection (fever, chills), liver problems (feeling very tired, pain on upper right side of abdomen, loss of appetite, unusual bleeding or bruising), or venous thromboembolism (pain or swelling in arms or legs, shortness of breath, chest pain, rapid breathing, rapid heart rate) occurs.
- Instruct patient to notify health care professional of all Rx or OTC medications, vitamins, or herbal products being taken and to consult with health care professional before taking other medications.
- Rep: May be teratogenic. Advise female patient to use effective contraception and avoid breast feeding during and for at least 3 wk after last dose of therapy. Inform male patient may impair fertility.

Evaluation/Desired Outcomes

- Decrease in the spread of breast cancer.

abiraterone (a-bi-ra-te-rone)

Yonsa, Zytiga

Classification

Therapeutic: antineoplastics

Pharmacologic: enzyme inhibitors

Indications

Zytiga: Treatment of metastatic castration-resistant prostate cancer (in combination with prednisone). **Zytiga:** Treatment of metastatic high-risk castration-sensitive prostate cancer (in combination with prednisone). **Yonsa:** Treatment of metastatic castration-resistant prostate cancer (in combination with methylprednisolone).

Action

Inhibits the enzyme 17α-hydroxylase/C17,20–lyase (CYP17), which is required for androgen production. May also result in increased mineralocortocoid production. **Therapeutic Effects:** Decreased androgen production with decreased spread of androgen-sensitive prostate cancer.

Pharmacokinetics

Absorption: Hydrolyzed to its active compound following oral administration.

Distribution: Unknown.

Protein Binding: >99%.

Metabolism and Excretion: Metabolized by esterases to inactive compounds; eliminated primarily in feces as unchanged drug and metabolites; 5% excreted in urine.

Half-life: 12 hr.

TIME/ACTION PROFILE (blood level)

ROUTE	ONSET	PEAK	DURATION
PO	unknown	2 hr	12 hr

Contraindications/Precautions

Contraindicated in: Severe hepatic impairment; Concurrent use of radium Ra 223 dichloride (↑ risk of fractures); OB: Pregnancy (may cause fetal harm); Lactation: Avoid breast feeding.

Use Cautiously in: HF, recent MI, other cardiovascular disease, ventricular arrhythmias; Electrolyte abnormalities or hypertension (correct/treat prior to initiation); Pre-existing liver disease (dose modification required for Child-Pugh Class B); Stress, infection, trauma, acute disease process (may result in adrenocortical insufficiency requiring additional corticosteroids); Rep: Women of reproductive potential and men with female partners of reproductive potential; Pedi: Safety not established.

Adverse Reactions/Side Effects

Noted for combination treatment with prednisone.

CV: TORSADES DE POINTES (in presence of hypokalemia), hypertension, arrhythmia, edema, QT interval prolongation (in presence of hypokalemia). **Derm:** hot flush. **Endo:** adrenocortical insufficiency (due to concurrent corticosteroid). **F and E:** hypokalemia. **GI:** HEPATOTOXICITY, diarrhea, dyspepsia. **GU:** ↓ fertility, nocturia, urinary frequency. **MS:** fracture, joint pain/discomfort. **Resp:** cough.

Interactions

Drug-Drug: Acts as an inhibitor of the CYP2D6 and CYP2C8 enzyme system; avoid concurrent use with agents that are substrates of CYP2D6, especially those with narrow therapeutic indices, including **thioridazine** and **dextromethorphan** (CYP2D6 substrates) as well as **pioglitazone** (CYP2C8 substrate); if concurrent use is necessary, dose ↓ of substrate may be required. Concurrent use of **strong CYP3A4 inducers**, including **carbamazepine**, **phenobarbital**, **phenytoin**, **rifabutin**, **rifapentine**, or **rifampin** may ↓ levels and effectiveness; avoid concurrent use.

Route/Dosage

Zytiga

PO (Adults): 1000 mg once daily; *Concurrent use of strong CYP3A4 inducer*—1000 mg twice daily.

Hepatic Impairment

PO (Adults): *Child-Pugh Class B*—250 mg once daily.

Yonsa

PO (Adults): 500 mg once daily; *Concurrent use of strong CYP3A4 inducer*—500 mg twice daily.

Hepatic Impairment

PO (Adults): *Child-Pugh Class B*—125 mg once daily.

Availability (generic available)

Tablets (Zytiga): 250 mg, 500 mg. **Tablets (Yonsa):** 125 mg.

NURSING IMPLICATIONS

Assessment

- Monitor BP and assess for fluid retention at least monthly. Control hypertension during therapy.
- Monitor for signs and symptoms of adrenocortical insufficiency (hypotension, weight loss, weakness, nausea, vomiting, anorexia, lethargy, confusion, restlessness), especially in patients under stress or who are withdrawn from or have decreased prednisone dose. Symptoms may be masked by abiraterone.
- ***Lab Test Considerations:*** Monitor AST, ALT, and bilirubin prior to starting therapy, every 2 wk for 3

mo, and monthly thereafter. Administer reduced dose to patients with baseline moderate hepatic impairment and monitor AST, ALT, and bilirubin prior to starting therapy, every wk for first mo, every 2 wk for 2 mo, and monthly thereafter. If clinical signs of hepatic toxicity occur, measure serum bilirubin, AST, and ALT promptly; monitor frequently if ↑ levels. If AST and/or ALT ↑ >5 times upper limit of normal or bilirubin ↑ >3 times upper limit of normal in patients with baseline moderate hepatic impairment, interrupt abiraterone. Following return of liver function to baseline or AST and ALT ↑>2.5 times upper limit of normal or bilirubin ↑ >1.5 times upper limit of normal may restart at a reduced dose of 750 mg once daily. Monitor serum transaminases and bilirubin every 2 wk for 3 mo and monthly thereafter. If hepatotoxicity recurs, may restart at 500 mg once daily following return to baseline or AST and ALT ↑ >2.5 times upper limit of normal or bilirubin ↑ >1.5 times upper limit of normal. If hepatotoxicity recurs at 500 mg dose, discontinue therapy. If concurrent ↑ ALT >3 times upper limit of normal and total bilirubin ↑>2 times upper limit of normal without biliary obstruction or other causes, permanently discontinue therapy.

- Monitor serum potassium and sodium at least monthly during therapy. May cause hypokalemia; control during therapy.
- May cause ↑ triglycerides and ↓ phosphorous.

Implementation

- Control hypertension and correct hypokalemia prior to starting therapy.
- **PO:** *For castration-resistant prostate cancer:* Administer once daily with twice daily prednisone on an empty stomach at least 1 hr before or 2 hrs after meals; food increases absorption and adverse reactions. Swallow tablets whole with water; do not crush, break, or chew. *For castration-sensitive prostate cancer:* Administer once daily with once daily prednisone on an empty stomach at least 1 hr before or 2 hrs after meals; food increases absorption. Swallow tablets whole with water; do not crush, break, or chew.
- Patients should also receive a gonadotropin-releasing hormone analog concurrently or should have had bilateral orchiectomy.

Patient/Family Teaching

- Instruct patient to take medications as directed and not to stop abiraterone, prednisone or gonadotropin-releasing hormone analog without consulting health care professional. If a dose is missed, take the following day. If more than 1 dose is missed, consult health care professional. Do not share medication with others, even if they have the same symptoms; may be dangerous.
- Advise patient to notify health care professional if signs and symptoms of high blood pressure, low potassium, and fluid retention (dizziness, fast heartbeats, feel faint or lightheaded, headache, confusion, muscle weakness, pain in legs, swelling in legs or feet), adrenal insufficiency, or hepatotoxicity (yellowing of skin and eyes, dark urine, pain in upper right quadrant, severe nausea or vomiting, difficulty concentrating, disorientation, confusion) occur or of side effects that are bothersome or persistent.
- Advise parents to notify health care professional of all Rx or OTC medications, vitamins, or herbal products being taken and to consult with health care professional before taking other medications.
- Rep: Male patients should use a condom and another form of contraception during sex with a women of reproductive potential during and for 3 wk after therapy. Pregnant women and women of reproductive potential should not touch tablets without wearing gloves. May impair reproductive function and fertility in males of reproductive potential.
- Explain need for continued follow-up exams and lab tests to assess possible side effects.

Evaluation/Desired Outcomes

- Decreased spread of androgen-sensitive prostate cancer.

acetaminophen (oral, rectal)

(a-seet-a-**min**-oh-fen)

✱Abenol, Acephen, ✱Acet, ✱Children Feverhalt, ✱Fortolin, Infant's Feverall, ✱Pediaphen, ✱Pediatrix, ✱Taminol, ✱Tempra, Tylenol

acetaminophen (intravenous)

Ofirmev

Classification

Therapeutic: antipyretics, nonopioid analgesics

Indications

PO, Rect: Treatment of: Mild pain, Fever. **IV:** Treatment of: Mild to moderate pain, Moderate to severe pain with opioid analgesics, Fever.

Action

Inhibits synthesis of prostaglandins that may serve as mediators of pain and fever, primarily in the CNS. Has no significant anti-inflammatory properties or GI toxicity. **Therapeutic Effects:** Analgesia. Antipyresis.

Pharmacokinetics

Absorption: Well absorbed following oral administration. Rectal absorption is variable. Intravenous administration results in complete bioavailability.

Distribution: Widely distributed. Crosses the placenta; enters breast milk in low concentrations.

Metabolism and Excretion: 85–95% metabolized by the liver (CYP2E1 enzyme system). Metabolites may be toxic in overdose situation. Metabolites excreted by the kidneys.

Half-life: Neonates: 7 hr; Infants and Children: 3–4 hr; Adults: 1–3 hr.

TIME/ACTION PROFILE (analgesia and antipyresis)

ROUTE	ONSET	PEAK	DURATION
PO	0.5–1 hr	1–3 hr	3–8 hr†
Rect	0.5–1 hr	1–3 hr	3–4 hr
IV‡	within 30 min	30 min	4–6 hr

†Depends on dose.

‡Antipyretic effects.

Contraindications/Precautions

Contraindicated in: Previous hypersensitivity; Products containing alcohol, aspartame, saccharin, sugar, or tartrazine (FDC yellow dye #5) should be avoided in patients who have hypersensitivity or intolerance to these compounds; Severe hepatic impairment/ active liver disease.

Use Cautiously in: Hepatic disease/renal disease (lower chronic doses recommended); Alcoholism, chronic malnutrition, severe hypovolemia or severe renal impairment (CCr <30 mL/min, ↑ dosing interval and ↓ daily dose may be necessary); Chronic alcohol use/abuse; Malnutrition; OB: Use in pregnancy only if clearly needed (for IV); Lactation: Use cautiously (for IV).

Adverse Reactions/Side Effects

CNS: agitation (↑ in children) (IV), anxiety (IV), headache (IV), fatigue (IV), insomnia (IV). **CV:** hypertension (IV), hypotension (IV). **Derm:** ACUTE GENERALIZED EXANTHEMATOUS PUSTULOSIS, STEVENS-JOHNSON SYNDROME, TOXIC EPIDERMAL NECROLYSIS, rash, urticaria. **F and E:** hypokalemia (IV). **GI:** HEPATOTOXICITY (↑ DOSES), constipation (↑ in children) (IV), ↑ liver enzymes, nausea (IV), vomiting (IV). **GU:** renal failure (high doses/chronic use). **Hemat:** neutropenia, pancytopenia. **MS:** muscle spasms (IV), trismus (IV). **Resp:** atelectasis (↑ in children) (IV), dyspnea (IV).

Interactions

Drug-Drug: Chronic high-dose acetaminophen (>2 g/day) may ↑ risk of bleeding with **warfarin** (INR should not exceed 4). Hepatotoxicity is additive with other **hepatotoxic substances**, including **alcohol**. Concurrent use of **isoniazid**, **rifampin**, **rifabutin**, **phenytoin**, **barbiturates**, and **carbamazepine** may ↑ the risk of acetaminophen-induced liver damage (limit self-medication); these agents will also ↓ therapeutic effects of acetaminophen. Concurrent use of **NSAIDs** may ↑ the risk of adverse renal effects (avoid chronic concurrent use). **Propranolol** ↓ metabolism and may ↑ effects. May ↓ effects of **lamotrigine** and **zidovudine**.

Route/Dosage

Children ≤12 yr should not receive >5 PO or rectal doses/24 hr without notifying physician or other health care professional. No dose adjustment needed when converting between IV and PO acetaminophen in adults and children ≥50 kg.

PO (Adults and Children >12 yr): 325–650 mg every 6 hr or 1 g 3–4 times daily or 1300 mg every 8 hr (not to exceed 3 g or 2 g/24 hr in patients with hepatic/ renal impairment).

PO (Children 1–12 yr): 10–15 mg/kg/dose every 6 hr as needed (not to exceed 5 doses/24 hr).

PO (Infants): 10–15 mg/kg/dose every 6 hr as needed (not to exceed 5 doses/24 hr).

PO (Neonates): 10–15 mg/kg/dose every 6–8 hr as needed.

IV (Adults and Children ≥13 yr and ≥50 kg): 1000 mg every 6 hr or 650 mg every 4 hr (not to exceed 1000 mg/dose, 4 g/day [by all routes], and less than 4 hr dosing interval).

IV (Adults and Children ≥13 yr and <50 kg): 15 mg/kg every 6 hr or 12.5 mg/kg every 4 hr (not to exceed 15 mg/kg/dose [up to 750 mg/dose], 75 mg/kg/ day [up to 3750 mg/day] [by all routes], and less than 4 hr dosing interval).

IV (Children 2–12 yr): 15 mg/kg every 6 hr or 12.5 mg/kg every 4 hr (not to exceed 15 mg/kg/dose [up to 750 mg/dose], 75 mg/kg/day [up to 3750 mg/day] [by all routes], and less than 4 hr dosing interval).

IV (Infants 29 days-2 yr): 15 mg/kg every 6 hr (not to exceed 60 mg/kg/day [by all routes]).

IV (Neonates Birth–28 days): 12.5 mg/kg every 6 hr (not to exceed 50 mg/kg [by all routes]).

Rect (Adults and Children >12 yr): 325–650 mg every 4–6 hr as needed or 1 g 3–4 times/day (not to exceed 4 g/24 hr).

Rect (Children 1–12 yr): 10–20 mg/kg/dose every 4–6 hr as needed.

Rect (Infants): 10–20 mg/kg/dose every 4–6 hr as needed.

Rect (Neonates): 10–15 mg/kg/dose every 6–8 hr as needed.

Availability (generic available)

Chewable tablets (fruit, bubblegum, or grape flavor): 80 mg^OTC, 160 mg^OTC. **Tablets:** 160 mg^OTC, 325 mg^OTC. **Caplets:** 325 mg^OTC. **Solution (berry, fruit, and grape flavor):** 100 mg/mL^OTC. **Liquid (mint):** 160 mg/5 mL^OTC. **Elixir (grape and cherry flavor):** 160 mg/5 mL^OTC. **Drops:** 160 mg/ 5 mL ^OTC. **Suspension:** ✱100 mg/mL^OTC, ✱160 mg/5 mL^OTC. **Syrup:** 160 mg/5 mL^OTC. **Suppositories:** 80 mg^OTC, 120 mg^OTC, 325 mg^OTC. **Solution for intravenous infusion:** 1000 mg/100 mL in 100-mL vials. ***In combination with:*** many other medications. See Appendix B.

NURSING IMPLICATIONS

Assessment

- Assess overall health status and alcohol usage before administering acetaminophen. Patients who are malnourished or chronically abuse alcohol are at higher risk of developing hepatotoxicity with chronic use of usual doses of this drug.
- Assess amount, frequency, and type of drugs taken in patients self-medicating, especially with OTC drugs. Prolonged use of acetaminophen increases risk of adverse hepatic and renal effects. For short-term use, combined doses of acetaminophen and salicylates should not exceed the recommended dose of either drug given alone. Do not exceed maximum daily dose of acetaminophen when considering all routes of administration and all combination products containing acetaminophen.
- Assess for rash periodically during therapy. May cause Stevens-Johnson syndrome. Discontinue therapy if rash (reddening of skin, blisters, and detachment of upper surface of skin peeling) or if accompanied with fever, general malaise, fatigue, muscle or joint aches, blisters, oral lesions, conjunctivitis, hepatitis, and/or eosinophilia.
- **Pain:** Assess type, location, and intensity prior to and 30–60 min following administration.
- **Fever:** Assess fever; note presence of associated signs (diaphoresis, tachycardia, and malaise).
- ***Lab Test Considerations:*** Evaluate hepatic, hematologic, and renal function periodically during prolonged, high-dose therapy.
- May alter results of blood glucose monitoring. May cause falsely ↓ values when measured with glucose oxidase/peroxidase method, but probably not with hexokinase/G6PD method. May also cause falsely ↑ values with certain instruments; see manufacturer's instruction manual.
- Increased serum bilirubin, LDH, AST, ALT, and prothrombin time may indicate hepatotoxicity.
- ***Toxicity and Overdose:*** If overdose occurs, **acetylcysteine** (Acetadote) is the antidote.

Implementation

- Do not confuse Tylenol with Tylenol PM. Do not confuse acetaminophen with acetazolamide.
- To prevent fatal medication errors ensure dose in milligrams (mg) and milliliters (mL) is not confused; dosing is based on weight for patients under 50 kg; program infusion pump for accuracy; and total daily dose of acetaminophen from all sources does not exceed maximum daily limits.
- When combined with opioids do not exceed the maximum recommended daily dose of acetaminophen.
- **PO:** Administer with a full glass of water.
- May be taken with food or on an empty stomach.

IV Administration

- **Intermittent Infusion:** *For 1000 mg dose*, insert vented IV set through septum of 100 mL vial; may be administered without further dilution. *For doses <1000 mg*, withdraw appropriate dose from vial place in a separate empty, sterile container for IV infusion. Place small volume pediatric doses up to 60 mL in a syringe and administer via syringe pump. Solution is clear and colorless; do not administer solutions that are discolored or contain particulate matter. Administer within 6 hrs of breaking vial seal. ***Rate:*** Infuse over 15 min. Monitor end of infusion in order to prevent air embolism, especially if acetaminophen is primary infusion.
- **Y-Site Compatibility:** buprenorphine, butorphanol, cefoxitin, ceftriaxone, clindamycin, D5W, dexamethasone, dexmedetomidine, D10W, D5/LR, D5/0.9% NaCl, diphenhydramine, dolasetron, droperidol, esmolol, fentanyl, gentamicin, granisetron, heparin, hydrocortisone, hydromorphone, ketorolac, LR, lidocaine, lorazepam, mannitol, meperidine, methylprednisolone, metoclopramide, midazolam, morphine, nalbuphine, 0.9% NaCl, ondansetron, oxytocin, piperacillin/tazobactam, potassium chloride, prochlorperazine, ranitidine, sufentanil, vancomycin.
- **Y-Site Incompatibility:** acyclovir, chlorpromazine, diazepam, metronidazole.
- **Additive Incompatibility:** Do not mix with other medications.

Patient/Family Teaching

- Advise patient to take medication exactly as directed and not to take more than the recommended amount. Chronic excessive use of >4 g/day (2 g in chronic alcoholics) may lead to hepatotoxicity, renal, or cardiac damage. Adults should not take acetaminophen longer than 10 days and children not longer than 5 days unless directed by health care professional. Short-term doses of acetaminophen with salicylates or NSAIDs should not exceed recommended daily dose of either drug alone.
- Advise patient to avoid alcohol (3 or more glasses per day increase the risk of liver damage) if taking more than an occasional 1–2 doses and to avoid taking concurrently with salicylates or NSAIDs for more than a few days, unless directed by health care professional.
- Advise patient to discontinue acetaminophen and notify health care professional if rash occurs.
- Inform patients with diabetes that acetaminophen may alter results of blood glucose monitoring. Advise patient to notify health care professional if changes are noted.
- Caution patient to check labels on all OTC products. Advise patients to avoid taking more than one product containing acetaminophen at a time to prevent toxicity.
- Advise patient to consult health care professional if discomfort or fever is not relieved by routine doses of this drug or if fever is greater than 39.5°C (103°F) or lasts longer than 3 days.

- Pedi: Advise parents or caregivers to check concentrations of liquid preparations. All OTC single ingredient acetaminophen liquid products now come in a single concentration of 160 mg/5 mL. Errors have resulted in serious liver damage. Have parents or caregivers determine the correct formulation and dose for their child (based on the child's age/weight), and demonstrate how to measure it using an appropriate measuring device.

Evaluation/Desired Outcomes

- Relief of mild to moderate pain.
- Reduction of fever.

acetylcysteine

(a-se-teel-**sis**-teen)
Acetadote, Cetylev

Classification
Therapeutic: antidotes (for acetaminophen toxicity), mucolytic

Indications

PO, IV: Antidote for the management of potentially hepatotoxic overdose of acetaminophen. **Inhaln:** Mucolytic in the management of conditions associated with thick viscid mucous secretions. **Unlabeled Use: PO:** Prevention of radiocontrast-induced renal dysfunction.

Action

PO, IV: Decreases the buildup of a hepatotoxic metabolite in acetaminophen overdosage. **Inhaln:** Degrades mucus, allowing easier mobilization and expectoration. **Therapeutic Effects: PO:** Prevention or lessening of liver damage following acetaminophen overdose. **Inhaln:** Lowers the viscosity of mucus.

Pharmacokinetics

Absorption: Absorbed from the GI tract following oral administration. Action is local following inhalation; remainder may be absorbed from pulmonary epithelium. IV administration results in complete bioavailability.
Distribution: Crosses the placenta; 0.47 L/kg.
Protein Binding: 83% bound to plasma proteins.
Metabolism and Excretion: Partially metabolized by the liver, 22% excreted renally.
Half-life: *Adults*—5.6 hr (↑ in hepatic impairment) *newborns*—11 hr.

TIME/ACTION PROFILE

ROUTE	ONSET	PEAK	DURATION
PO (antidote)	unknown	30–60 min	4 hr
IV (antidote)	unknown	unknown	unknown
Inhaln (mucolytic)	1 min	5–10 min	short

Contraindications/Precautions

Contraindicated in: Hypersensitivity.
Use Cautiously in: Severe respiratory insufficiency, asthma, or history of bronchospasm; History of GI bleeding (oral only); OB, Lactation: Safety not established.

Adverse Reactions/Side Effects

CNS: drowsiness. **CV:** vasodilation, tachycardia, hypotension. **EENT:** rhinorrhea. **Resp:** bronchospasm, bronchial/tracheal irritation, chest tightness, ↑ secretions. **GI:** nausea, vomiting, stomatitis. **Derm:** rash, clamminess, pruritus, urticaria. **Misc:** allergic reactions (primarily with IV), including ANAPHYLAXIS, ANGIOEDEMA, chills, fever.

Interactions

Drug-Drug: Activated charcoal may adsorb orally administered acetylcysteine and ↓ its effectiveness as an antidote.

Route/Dosage

Acetaminophen Overdose

PO (Adults and Children): 140 mg/kg initially, followed by 70 mg/kg every 4 hr for 17 additional doses.
IV (Adults and Children): *Loading dose*—150 mg/kg (maximum: 15 g) over 60 min initially followed by *First maintenance dose*—50 mg/kg (maximum: 5 g) over 4 hr, then *second maintenance dose*—100 mg/kg (maximum: 10 g) over 16 hr.

Mucolytic

Inhaln (Adults and Children 1–12 yrs): *Nebulization via face mask*—3–5 mL of 20% solution or 6–10 mL of the 10% solution 3–4 times daily; *nebulization via tent or croupette*—volume of 10–20% solution required to maintain heavy mist; *direct instillation*—1–2 mL of 10–20% solution every 1–4 hr; *intratracheal instillation via tracheostomy*—1–2 mL of 10–20% solution every 1–4 hr (up to 2–5 mL of 20% solution via tracheal catheter into particular segments of the bronchopulmonary tree).
Inhaln (Infants): *Nebulization*—1–2 mL of 20% solution or 2–4 mL of 10% solution 3–4 times daily.

Prevention of Radiocontrast-Induced Renal Dysfunction

PO (Adults): 600 mg twice daily for 2 days, beginning the day before the procedure.

Availability (generic available)

Effervescent tablets (lemon-mint flavor): 500 mg, 2.5 g. **Solution for inhalation:** 10% (100 mg/mL), 20% (200 mg/mL). **Solution for injection:** 20% (200 mg/mL).

NURSING IMPLICATIONS

Assessment

- **Antidote in Acetaminophen Overdose:** Assess type, amount, and time of acetaminophen ingestion. Assess plasma acetaminophen levels. Initial levels are drawn at least 4 hr after ingestion of acetaminophen. Plasma level determinations may be difficult to interpret following ingestion of extended-release preparations. Do not wait for results to administer dose.
- *IV:* Assess for anaphylaxis. Erythema and flushing are common, usually occurring 30–60 min after initiating infusion, and may resolve with continued administration. If rash, hypotension, wheezing, or dyspnea occur, initiate treatment for anaphylaxis (antihistamine and epinephrine). Interrupt acetylcysteine infusion until symptoms resolve and restart carefully. If anaphylaxis recurs, discontinue acetylcysteine and use alternative form of treatment.
- Assess patient for nausea, vomiting, and urticaria. Notify health care professional if these occur.
- **Mucolytic:** Assess respiratory function (lung sounds, dyspnea) and color, amount, and consistency of secretions before and immediately following treatment to determine effectiveness of therapy.
- ***Lab Test Considerations:*** Monitor AST, ALT, and bilirubin levels along with prothrombin time every 24 hr for 96 hr in patients with plasma acetaminophen levels indicating potential hepatotoxicity.
- Monitor cardiac and renal function (creatinine, BUN), serum glucose, and electrolytes. Maintain fluid and electrolyte balance; correct hypoglycemia.

Implementation

- After opening, solution for inhalation may turn light purple; does not alter potency. Refrigerate open vials and discard after 96 hr.
- Drug reacts with rubber and metals (iron, nickel, copper); avoid contact.
- **PO:** Dissolve effervescent tablets in 100 mL of water for a 50 mg/mL solution for patient weighing 1–19 kg, in 150 mL for patients weighing 20–59 kg, and in 300 mL for patients weighing 60 kg or more within 2 hrs of administration. May be administered by duodenal tube if patient is unable to swallow. If patient vomits loading dose or maintenance doses within 1 hr of administration, readminister dose.
- **Acetaminophen Overdose**—Empty stomach contents by inducing emesis or lavage prior to administration.

IV Administration

- **Intermittent Infusion:** Most effective if administered within 8 hr of acetaminophen ingestion. ***Diluent:*** Dilute in D5W. ***Concentration:*** **For loading dose:** *For patients 5–20 kg:* Dilute 150 mg in 3 mL/kg of diluent. *For patients 21–40 kg:* Dilute 150 mg/kg in 100 mL. *For patients 41–100 kg:* Dilute 150 mg/kg in 200 mL. **For Second Dose:** *For patients 5–20 kg:* Dilute 50 mg/kg in 7 mL/kg of diluent. *For patients 21–40 kg:* Dilute 50 mg/kg in 250 mL of diluent. *For patients 41–100 kg:* Dilute 50 mg/kg in 500 mL. **For Third Dose:** *For patients 5–20 kg:* Dilute 100 mg/kg in 14 mL/kg of diluent. *For patients 21–40 kg:* 100 mg/kg diluted in 500 mL of diluent. *For patients 41–100 kg:* Dilute 100 mg/kg in 1000 mL. Adjust fluid volume for patients requiring fluid restriction. Vials are single-use. Discard after using. Reconstituted solution is stable for 24 hr at room temperature. ***Rate:*** Administer **Loading Dose** over 1 hr.
- Administer **For Second Dose:** over 4 hr.
- Administer **For Third Dose:** over 16 hr.
- **Y-Site Compatibility:** heparin, naloxone, tigecycline, vancomycin.
- **Y-Site Incompatibility:** cefepime, ceftazidime.
- **Inhaln: Mucolytic**—Encourage adequate fluid intake (2000–3000 mL/day) to decrease viscosity of secretions.
- For nebulization, the 20% solution may be diluted with 0.9% NaCl for injection or inhalation or sterile water for injection or inhalation. May use 10% solution undiluted. May be administered by nebulization, or 1–2 mL may be instilled directly into airway. During administration, when 25% of medication remains in nebulizer, dilute with equal amount of 0.9% NaCl or sterile water.
- An increased volume of liquefied bronchial secretions may occur following administration. Have suction equipment available for patients unable to effectively clear airways.
- If bronchospasm occurs during treatment, discontinue and consult health care professional regarding possible addition of bronchodilator to therapy. Patients with asthma or hyperactive airway disease should be given a bronchodilator prior to acetylcysteine to prevent bronchospasm.
- Rinse patient's mouth and wash face following treatment, as drug leaves a sticky residue.

Patient/Family Teaching

- **Acetaminophen Overdose:** Explain purpose of medication to patient.
- **Inhaln:** Instruct patient to clear airway by coughing deeply before taking aerosol treatment.
- Inform patient that unpleasant odor of this drug becomes less noticeable as treatment progresses and medicine dissipates.

Evaluation/Desired Outcomes

- Decreased acetaminophen levels.
- No further increase in hepatic damage during acetaminophen overdose therapy.
- Decreased dyspnea and clearing of lung sounds when used as a mucolytic.
- Prevention of radiocontrast-induced renal dysfunction.

aclidinium/formoterol
(a-kli-**din**-ee-um/for-**moh**-te-rol)
Duaklir Genuair, Duaklir Pressair

Classification
Therapeutic: bronchodilators
Pharmacologic: anticholinergics, adrenergics

Indications
Maintenance treatment of COPD.

Action
Aclidinium—Acts as an anticholinergic by inhibiting the M_3 receptor in bronchial smooth muscle. *Formoterol*—$Beta_2$-adrenergic agonist that stimulates adenyl cyclase, resulting in accumulation of cyclic adenosine monophosphate and subsequent bronchodilation.
Therapeutic Effects: Improved airflow and ↓ exacerbations in COPD.

Pharmacokinetics
Absorption: *Aclidinium*—6% systemically absorbed following inhalation; *Formoterol*—majority of inhaled drug is swallowed and absorbed.
Distribution: Unknown.
Metabolism and Excretion: *Aclidinium*—Rapidly hydrolyzed; metabolites are not pharmacologically active. Metabolites are eliminated in urine (54–65%) and feces (20–33%); <1% excreted unchanged in urine. *Formoterol*—Mostly metabolized by the liver; 10–18% excreted unchanged in urine.
Half-life: *Aclidinium*—12 hr. *Formoterol*—10 hr.

TIME/ACTION PROFILE (bronchodilation)

ROUTE	ONSET	PEAK	DURATION
Inhalation	1 hr	2–4 hr	12 hr

Contraindications/Precautions
Contraindicated in: Hypersensitivity; Severe hypersensitivity to milk proteins; Asthma; Acutely deteriorating COPD or acute respiratory symptoms.
Use Cautiously in: Narrow-angle glaucoma; Prostatic hyperplasia or bladder neck obstruction; Severe hypersensitivity to milk proteins; History of hypersensitivity to atropine (cross-sensitivity may occur); Cardiovascular disease (including angina, hypertension, and arrhythmias); Diabetes; Seizure disorders; Glaucoma; Hyperthyroidism; Pheochromocytoma; Excessive use (may lead to tolerance and paradoxical bronchospasm); OB: Use only if potential maternal benefit justifies potential fetal risk; may inhibit contractions during labor; Lactation: Use while breast feeding only if potential maternal benefit justifies potential risk to infant; Pedi: Safety and effectiveness not established.

Adverse Reactions/Side Effects
CNS: dizziness, headache, insomnia, nervousness. **CV:** angina, arrhythmias, hypertension, hypotension, palpitations, tachycardia. **EENT:** worsening of narrow-angle glaucoma. **F and E:** hypokalemia. **GI:** dry mouth, nausea. **GU:** urinary retention. **Metab:** hyperglycemia. **MS:** arthralgia, muscle cramps. **Neuro:** tremor. **Resp:** PARADOXICAL BRONCHOSPASM, cough. **Misc:** HYPERSENSITIVITY REACTIONS (including anaphylaxis and angioedema).

Interactions
Drug-Drug: Concurrent use with **MAO inhibitors**, **tricyclic antidepressants**, or other **QT interval prolonging agents** may results in serious arrhythmias; use concurrently only with extreme caution. ↑ risk of hypokalemia with **theophylline**, **corticosteroids**, **loop diuretics**, and **thiazide diuretics**. **Beta blockers** may ↓ therapeutic effects. ↑ adrenergic effects may occur with concurrent use of **adrenergics**. May ↑ risk of anticholinergic effects with other **anticholingerics**.

Route/Dosage
Inhaln (Adults): One inhalation (aclidinium 400 mcg/formoterol 12 mcg) twice daily.

Availability
Powder for inhalation (contains lactose): aclidinium 400 mcg/formoterol 12 mcg/actuation.

NURSING IMPLICATIONS
Assessment
- Assess lung sounds, pulse, and BP before administration and during peak of medication. Note amount, color, and character of sputum produced. Closely monitor patients on higher dose for adverse effects.
- Monitor pulmonary function tests before initiating and periodically during therapy to determine effectiveness.
- Observe for paradoxical bronchospasm (wheezing, dyspnea, tightness in chest) and hypersensitivity reaction (rash; urticaria; swelling of the face, lips, or eyelids). If condition occurs, withhold medication and notify health care professional immediately.
- Monitor ECG periodically during therapy. May cause prolonged QTc interval.
- Monitor patient for signs of hypersensitivity reactions (difficulties in breathing or swallowing, swelling of tongue, lips and face), urticaria, or skin rash during therapy. Discontinue therapy and consider alternative if reaction occurs.
- ***Lab Test Considerations:*** May cause ↑ serum glucose and decreased serum potassium.

Implementation
- **Inhaln:** Administer as 1 inhalation twice daily, morning and evening. Inhaler is breath-activated.

Patient/Family Teaching

- Instruct patient to use medication as directed. Do not discontinue therapy without discussing with health care professional, even if feeling better. If a dose is missed skip dose and take next dose at regularly scheduled time. Do not double doses. Use a rapid-acting bronchodilator if symptoms occur before next dose is due. Caution patient not to use more than 1 time a day; may cause adverse effects, paradoxical bronchospasm, or loss of effectiveness of medication. Instruct patient to review *Patient Information* before starting therapy and with each Rx refill in case of changes.
- Caution patient not to use medication to treat acute symptoms. A rapid-acting inhaled beta-adrenergic bronchodilator should be used for relief of acute asthma attacks. Notify health care professional immediately if symptoms get worse or more inhalations than usual are needed from rescue inhaler.
- Instruct patient to contact health care professional immediately if shortness of breath is not relieved by medication or nausea, vomiting, shakiness, headache, fast or irregular heartbeat, sleeplessness, or signs and symptoms of narrow angle glaucoma (eye pain or discomfort, blurred vision, visual halos or colored images, red eyes) or urinary retention (difficulty passing urine, painful urination) occur.
- Advise patient to consult health care professional before taking any Rx, OTC, or herbal products or alcohol concurrently with this therapy. Caution patient also to avoid smoking and other respiratory irritants.
- Advise patient to notify health care professional if pregnancy is planned or suspected, or if breast feeding.

Evaluation/Desired Outcomes

- Bronchodilation with decreased airflow obstruction.

acyclovir (ay-**sye**-kloe-veer)

Sitavig, Zovirax

Classification
Therapeutic: antivirals
Pharmacologic: purine analogues

Indications

PO: Treatment of: Recurrent genital herpes infections. Localized cutaneous herpes zoster infections (shingles) and chickenpox (varicella). **Buccal:** Recurrent herpes labialis (cold sores) in nonimmunosuppressed patients. **IV:** Treatment of: Severe initial episodes of genital herpes in nonimmunosuppressed patients. Mucosal or cutaneous herpes simplex infections or herpes zoster infections (shingles) in immunosuppressed patients. Herpes simplex encephalitis. Neonatal herpes simplex infections. **Topical:** *Cream*—Recurrent herpes labialis (cold sores). *Ointment*—Treatment of limited non–life-threatening herpes simplex infections in immunocompromised patients (systemic treatment is preferred).

Action

Interferes with viral DNA synthesis. **Therapeutic Effects:** Inhibition of viral replication, decreased viral shedding, and reduced time for healing of lesions.

Pharmacokinetics

Absorption: Despite poor absorption (15–30%), therapeutic blood levels are achieved.
Distribution: Widely distributed. CSF concentrations are 50% of plasma. Crosses placenta; enters breast milk.
Protein Binding: <30%.
Metabolism and Excretion: >90% eliminated unchanged by kidneys; remainder metabolized by liver.
Half-life: Neonates: 4 hr; Children 1–12 yr: 2–3 hr; Adults: 2–3.5 hr (↑ in renal failure).

TIME/ACTION PROFILE (antiviral blood levels)

ROUTE	ONSET	PEAK	DURATION
PO	unknown	1.5–2.5 hr	4 hr
IV	prompt	end of infusion	8 hr

Contraindications/Precautions

Contraindicated in: Hypersensitivity to acyclovir or valacyclovir; Hypersensitivity to milk protein concentrate (buccal only).
Use Cautiously in: Pre-existing serious neurologic, hepatic, pulmonary, or fluid and electrolyte abnormalities; Renal impairment (dose alteration recommended if CCr <50 mL/min); Geri: Due to age related ↓ in renal function; Obese patients (dose should be based on ideal body weight); Patients with hypoxia; OB, Lactation: Safety not established.

Adverse Reactions/Side Effects

CNS: SEIZURES, dizziness, headache, hallucinations, trembling. **Derm:** STEVENS-JOHNSON SYNDROME, acne, hives, rash, unusual sweating. **Endo:** changes in menstrual cycle. **GI:** diarrhea, nausea, vomiting, ↑ liver enzymes, hyperbilirubinemia, abdominal pain, anorexia. **GU:** RENAL FAILURE, crystalluria, hematuria, renal pain. **Hemat:** THROMBOTIC THROMBOCYTOPENIC PURPURA/HEMOLYTIC UREMIC SYNDROME (high doses in immunosuppressed patients). **Local:** pain, phlebitis, local irritation. **MS:** joint pain. **Misc:** polydipsia.

Interactions

Drug-Drug: Probenecid and **theophylline** may ↑ levels and the risk of toxicity. **Valproic acid** or **phenytoin** may ↓ levels and effectiveness. Concurrent use of other **nephrotoxic drugs** may ↑ risk nephrotoxicity. **Zidovudine** and intrathecal **methotrexate** may ↑ risk of CNS side effects.

Route/Dosage

Initial Genital Herpes

PO (Adults and Children): 200 mg every 4 hr while awake (5 times/day) for 7–10 days or 400 mg every 8

hr for 7–10 days; maximum dose in children: 80 mg/kg/day in 3–5 divided doses.
IV (Adults and Children ≥12 yr): 5 mg/kg every 8 hr for 5 days.

Chronic Suppressive Therapy for Recurrent Genital Herpes

PO (Adults and Children): 400 mg twice daily or 200 mg 3–5 times/day for up to 12 mo. Maximum dose in children: 80 mg/kg/day in 2–5 divided doses.

Intermittent Therapy for Recurrent Genital Herpes

PO (Adults and Children): 200 mg every 4 hr while awake (5 times/day) or 400 mg every 8 hr or 800 mg every 12 hr for 5 days, start at first sign of symptoms. Maximum dose in children: 80 mg/kg/day in 2–5 divided doses.

Acute Treatment of Herpes Zoster in Immunosuppressed Patients

PO (Adults): 800 mg every 4 hr while awake (5 times/day) for 7–10 days. *Prophylaxis*—400 mg 5 times/day.
PO (Children): 250–600 mg/m²/dose 4–5 times/day.

Herpes Zoster in Immunocompetent Patients

PO (Adults and Children): 4000 mg/day in 5 divided doses for 5–7 days, maximum dose in children: 80 mg/kg/day in 5 divided doses.

Chickenpox

PO (Adults and Children): 20 mg/kg (not to exceed 800 mg/dose) 4 times daily for 5 days. Start within 24 hr of rash onset.

Mucosal and Cutaneous Herpes Simplex Infections in Immunosuppressed Patients

IV (Adults and Children >12 yr): 5 mg/kg every 8 hr for 7 days.
IV (Children 3 mo–12 yr): 10 mg/kg every 8 hr for 7 days.
Topical (Adults): 0.5 in. ribbon of 5% *ointment* for every 4-square-in. area every 3 hr (6 times/day) for 7 days.

Herpes Simplex Encephalitis

IV (Adults and Children ≥12 yr): 10 mg/kg every 8 hr for 10 days.
IV (Children 3 mo–12 yr): 20 mg/kg every 8 hr for 10 days.
IV (Children birth–3 mo): 20 mg/kg every 8 hr for 14–21 days.
IV (Neonates, premature): 10 mg/kg every 12 hr for 14–21 days.

Neonatal Herpes Simplex Infections

IV (Children post-menstrual age of ≥34 wk): 20 mg/kg every 8 hr for 21 days.
IV (Children post-menstrual age of <34 wk): 20 mg/kg every 12 hr for 21 days.

Varicella Zoster Infections in Immunosuppressed Patients

IV (Adults and Children ≥12 yr): 10 mg/kg every 8 hr for 7 days.
IV (Children <12 yr): 20 mg/kg every 8 hr for 7 days.

Renal Impairment

PO, IV (Adults and Children >3 mo): *CCr 25.1–50 mL/min/1.73 m²*—Normal dose every 12 hr; *CCr 10.1–25 mL/min/1.73 m²*—Normal dose every 24 hr; *CCr ≤10 mL/min/1.73 m²*—50% of dose every 24 hr.

Herpes Labialis

Topical (Adults and Children >12 yr): Apply 5 times/day for 4 days; start at first symptoms.
Buccal (Adults): Apply one 50–mg buccal tablet to the upper gum region within 1 hr of onset of prodromal symptoms (but before appearance of any lesions).

Availability (generic available)

Capsules: 200 mg. **Cost:** *Generic*—$97.70/100. **Tablets:** 400 mg, 800 mg. **Cost:** *Generic*—400 mg $6.99/30, 800 mg $17.91/30. **Buccal tablets:** 50 mg. **Oral suspension (banana flavor):** 200 mg/5 mL. **Cost:** *Generic*—$137.70/473 mL. **Solution for injection (requires dilution):** 50 mg/mL. **Cream:** 5%. **Cost:** $565.24/5 g. **Ointment:** 5%. **Cost:** *Generic*—$797.59/30 g. ***In combination with:*** hydrocortisone (Xerese). See Appendix B.

NURSING IMPLICATIONS

Assessment

- Assess lesions before and daily during therapy.
- Monitor frequency of recurrences.
- Monitor neurologic status in patients with herpes encephalitis.
- ***Lab Test Considerations:*** Monitor BUN, serum creatinine, and CCr before and during therapy. ↑ BUN and serum creatinine levels or ↓ CCr may indicate renal failure.

Implementation

- Do not confuse Zovirax with Doribax, Zyvox, or Zostrix.
- Start acyclovir treatment as soon as possible after herpes simplex symptoms appear and within 24 hr of a herpes zoster outbreak.
- **PO:** Acyclovir may be administered with food or on an empty stomach, with a full glass of water.

- Shake oral suspension well before administration.
- **Buccal:** Apply tablet with a dry finger to upper gum just above canine immediately after taking out of blister. Hold in place with pressure on lip for 30 sec to ensure adhesion. May be more comfortable to apply rounded side of tablet to gum surface. Apply on same side as herpes labialis symptoms within 1 hr of onset of symptoms, before appearance of herpes labialis lesions. Once applied, stays in position and dissolves slowly during day; do not crush, suck, chew, or swallow. May eat and drink while tablet is in place; avoid interfering with adhesion of tablet (chewing gum, touching, or pressing tablet after placement, wearing upper denture, brushing teeth). If the teeth need to be cleaned while tablet is in place, rinse mouth gently. Drink plenty of liquids to prevent dry mouth.

IV Administration

- **IV:** Maintain adequate hydration (2000–3000 mL/day), especially during first 2 hr after IV infusion, to prevent crystalluria.
- Observe infusion site for phlebitis. Rotate infusion site to prevent phlebitis.
- Do not administer acyclovir injectable topically, IM, subcut, PO, or in the eye.
- **Intermittent Infusion:** Reconstitute 500-mg or 1-g vial with 10 mL or 20 mL, respectively, of sterile water for injection. Do not reconstitute with bacteriostatic water with benzyl alcohol or parabens. Shake well to dissolve completely. ***Diluent:*** Dilute in at least 100 mL of D5W, 0.9% NaCl, dextrose/saline combinations or LR. ***Concentration:*** 7 mg/mL. Patients requiring fluid restriction: 10 mg/mL. ***Rate:*** Administer via infusion pump over 1 hr to minimize renal tubular damage.
- Use reconstituted solution within 12 hr. Once diluted for infusion, the solution should be used within 24 hr. Refrigeration results in precipitation, which dissolves at room temperature.
- **Y-Site Compatibility:** alemtuzumab, alfentanil, allopurinol, amikacin, aminophylline, amphotericin B lipid complex, amphotericin B liposome, ampicillin, anidulafungin, argatroban, arsenic trioxide, atracurium, azithromycin, bivalirudin, bleomycin, bumetanide, buprenorphine, busulfan, butorphanol, calcium chloride, calcium gluconate, carboplatin, carmustine, cefazolin, cefotaxime, cefoxitin, ceftaroline, ceftazidime, ceftriaxone, cefuroxime, chloramphenicol, cisplatin, clindamycin, cyclophosphamide, cytarabine, dactinomycin, dantrolene, dexamethasone, dexmedetomidine, digoxin, dimenhydrinate, diphenhydramine, docetaxel, doxorubicin liposome, doxycycline, enalaprilat, ephedrine, ertapenem, erythromycin lactobionate, etoposide, etoposide phosphate, famotidine, fentanyl, filgrastim, fluconazole, fluorouracil, fosphenytoin, furosemide, glycopyrrolate, heparin, hetastarch, hydrocortisone, hydromorphone, ifosfamide, imipenem/cilastatin, insulin, isoproterenol, leucovorin calcium, linezolid, lorazepam, magnesium sulfate, mannitol, melphalan, methohexital, methotrexate, methylprednisolone, metoprolol, metronidazole, milrinone, mitoxantrone, multivitamins, nafcillin, naloxone, nitroglycerin, octreotide, oxacillin, oxytocin, paclitaxel, pamidronate, pancuronium, pantoprazole, pemetrexed, penicillin G potassium, pentobarbital, perphenazine, phenobarbital, potassium acetate, potassium chloride, propofol, propranolol, ranitidine, remifentanil, rituximab, rocuronium, sodium acetate, sodium bicarbonate, succinylcholine, sufentanil, theophylline, thiopental, thiotepa, tigecycline, tirofiban, tobramycin, trastuzumab, trimethoprim/sulfamethoxazole, vancomycin, vasopressin, vinblastine, vincristine, voriconazole, zidovudine, zoledronic acid.
- **Y-Site Incompatibility:** acetaminophen, amifostine, amphotericin B deoxycholate, ampicillin/sulbactam, aztreonam, cefepime, chlorpromazine, ciprofloxacin, dacarbazine, daptomycin, daunorubicin, dexrazoxane, diazepam, dobutamine, dopamine, doxorubicin hydrochloride, epinephrine, epirubicin, eptifibatide, esmolol, fenoldopam, fludarabine, foscarnet, gemcitabine, haloperidol, hydralazine, hydroxyzine, idarubicin, irinotecan, ketamine, ketorolac, labetalol, levofloxacin, lidocaine, mesna, midazolam, mitomycin, mycophenolate, nicardipine, nitroprusside, ondansetron, palonosetron, pentamidine, phenylephrine, phenytoin, piperacillin/tazobactam, potassium phosphates, procainamide, prochlorperazine, promethazine, quinupristin/dalfopristin, sargramostim, sodium phosphates, streptozocin, tacrolimus, vecuronium, verapamil, vinorelbine.
- **Topical:** Apply to skin lesions only; do not use in the eye.

Patient/Family Teaching

- Instruct patient to take medication as directed for the full course of therapy. Take missed doses as soon as possible but not just before next dose is due; do not double doses. Acyclovir should not be used more frequently or longer than prescribed.
- Advise patients that the additional use of OTC creams, lotions, and ointments may delay healing and may cause spreading of lesions.
- Inform patient that acyclovir is not a cure; the virus lies dormant in the ganglia. Acyclovir will not prevent the spread of infection to others.
- Advise patient that condoms should be used during sexual contact and to avoid sexual contact while lesions are present.
- Instruct patient to consult health care professional if symptoms are not relieved after 7 days of topical therapy or if oral acyclovir does not decrease the frequency and severity of recurrences. Immunocompromised patients may require a longer time, usually 2 wk, for crusting over of lesions.

- Instruct women with genital herpes to have yearly Papanicolaou smears because they may be more likely to develop cervical cancer.
- **Topical:** Instruct patient to apply ointment in sufficient quantity to cover all lesions every 3 hr, 6 times/day for 7 days. 0.5-in. ribbon of ointment covers approximately 4 square in. Use a finger cot or glove when applying to prevent inoculation of other areas or spread to other people. Keep affected areas clean and dry. Loose-fitting clothing should be worn to prevent irritation.
- Avoid drug contact in or around eyes. Report any unexplained eye symptoms to health care professional immediately; ocular herpetic infection can lead to blindness.
- **Buccal:** Instruct patient on correct application and use of buccal tablet. If buccal tablet does not adhere or falls off within first 6 hrs, reposition immediately with same tablet. If tablet cannot be repositioned, apply new tablet. If swallowed within first 6 hrs, advise patient to drink a glass of water and apply a new tablet. Do not reapply if tablet falls out after 6 hrs.

Evaluation/Desired Outcomes

- Crusting over and healing of skin lesions.
- Decrease in frequency and severity of recurrences.
- Acceleration of complete healing and cessation of pain in herpes zoster.
- Decrease in intensity of chickenpox.

adalimumab (a-da-li-mu-mab)

Amjevita, Cyltezo, ✤Hadlima, Humira

Classification

Therapeutic: antirheumatics

Pharmacologic: DMARDs, monoclonal antibodies

Indications

Amjevita, Cyltezo, and Humira: Treatment of the following conditions: Moderately to severely active rheumatoid arthritis (may be used alone or with methotrexate or other non-biologic DMARDs), Psoriatic arthritis (may be used alone or with other non-biologic DMARDs), Active ankylosing spondylitis, Moderately to severely active Crohn's disease in patients who have responded inadequately to conventional therapy, Moderately to severely active ulcerative colitis in patients who have responded inadequately to immunosuppressants such as corticosteroids, azathioprine, or 6–mercaptopurine, Moderate to severely active polyarticular juvenile idiopathic arthritis (as monotherapy or with methotrexate), Moderate to severe chronic plaque psoriasis in patients who are candidates for systemic therapy or phototherapy and when other systemic therapies are deemed inappropriate. **Humira only:** Treatment of the following conditions: Moderate to severe hidradenitis suppurativa, Non-infectious intermediate, posterior and panuveitis.

Action

Neutralizes and prevents the action of tumor necrosis factor (TNF), resulting in anti-inflammatory and antiproliferative activity. **Therapeutic Effects:** Decreased pain and swelling with decreased rate of joint destruction in patients with rheumatoid arthritis, psoriatic arthritis, juvenile idiopathic arthritis, and ankylosing spondylitis. Reduced signs and symptoms and maintenance of clinical remission of Crohn's disease. Induction and maintenance of clinical remission of ulcerative colitis. Reduced severity of plaques. Reduced number of abscesses and inflammatory nodules. Decreased progression of uveitis.

Pharmacokinetics

Absorption: 64% absorbed after subcut administration.

Distribution: Synovial fluid concentrations are 31–96% of serum.

Metabolism and Excretion: Unknown.

Half-life: 14 days (range 10–20 days).

TIME/ACTION PROFILE (improvement)

ROUTE	ONSET	PEAK	DURATION
Subcut	8–26 wk	131 hr*	2 wk†

*Blood level.

†Following discontinuation.

Contraindications/Precautions

Contraindicated in: Hypersensitivity; Concurrent use of anakinra or abatacept; Active infection (including localized).

Use Cautiously in: History of chronic or recurrent infection or underlying illness/treatment predisposing to infection; History of exposure to tuberculosis; History of opportunistic infection; Patients residing, or who have resided, where tuberculosis, histoplasmosis, coccidioidomycoses, or blastomycosis is endemic; Preexisting or recent-onset CNS demyelinating disorders; History of lymphoma; OB: Use during pregnancy only if material benefit outweighs potential fetal risk; Lactation: Use while breast feeding only if maternal benefit outweighs risk to infant; Pedi: Children <2 yr (safety not established); ↑ risk of lymphoma (including hepatosplenic T-cell lymphoma [HSTCL] in patients with Crohn's disease or ulcerative colitis), leukemia, and other malignancies; Geri: ↑ risk of infection/malignancy.

Adverse Reactions/Side Effects

CNS: <u>headache</u>, Guillain-Barre syndrome, multiple sclerosis. **CV:** hypertension. **Derm:** <u>rash</u>, psoriasis. **EENT:** optic neuritis. **GI:** abdominal pain, nausea.

GU: hematuria. **Hemat:** neutropenia, thrombocytopenia. **Local:** injection site reactions. **Metab:** hyperlipidemia. **MS:** back pain. **Misc:** HYPERSENSITIVITY REACTIONS (including anaphylaxis and angioedema), INFECTION (including reactivation tuberculosis and other opportunistic infections due to bacterial, invasive fungal, viral, mycobacterial, and parasitic pathogens), MALIGNANCY (including lymphoma, HSTCL, leukemia, and skin cancer), fever.

Interactions

Drug-Drug: Concurrent use with **anakinra**, **abatacept**, or other **TNF blocking agents** ↑ risk of serious infections and is contraindicated. Concurrent use with **azathioprine** and/or **methotrexate** may ↑ risk of HSTCL. **Live vaccinations** should not be given concurrently. Risks and benefits should be considered before using live vaccinations in an infant exposed to adalimumab therapy *in utero*.

Route/Dosage

Rheumatoid Arthritis, Ankylosing Spondylitis, and Psoriatic Arthritis

Subcut (Adults): 40 mg every other wk; patients not receiving concurrent methotrexate may receive additional benefit by ↑ dose to 40 mg once weekly.

Crohn's Disease

Subcut (Adults): 160 mg initially on Day 1 (given in one day or over two consecutive days), followed by 80 mg 2 wk later on Day 15. Two wk later (Day 29), begin maintenance dose of 40 mg every other wk. Aminosalicylates, corticosteroids, and/or immunomodulatory agents (e.g. azathioprine, 6–mercaptopurine, methotrexate) may be continued during therapy.
Subcut (Children ≥6 yr and ≥40 kg): *Humira only*—160 mg initially on Day 1 (given in one day or over two consecutive days), followed by 80 mg 2 wk later on Day 15. Two wk later (Day 29), begin maintenance dose of 40 mg every other wk. Aminosalicylates, corticosteroids, and/or immunomodulatory agents (e.g. azathioprine, 6–mercaptopurine, methotrexate) may be continued during therapy.
Subcut (Children ≥6 yr and 17–<40 kg): *Humira only*—80 mg initially on Day 1, followed by 40 mg 2 wk later on Day 15. Two wk later (Day 29), begin maintenance dose of 20 mg every other wk. Aminosalicylates, corticosteroids, and/or immunomodulatory agents (e.g. azathioprine, 6–mercaptopurine, methotrexate) may be continued during therapy.

Ulcerative Colitis

Subcut (Adults): 160 mg initially on Day 1 (given in one day or over two consecutive days), followed by 80 mg 2 wk later on Day 15. Two wk later (Day 29), begin maintenance dose of 40 mg every other wk. Aminosalicylates, corticosteroids, and/or immunomodulatory agents (e.g. azathioprine, 6–mercaptopurine, methotrexate) may be continued during therapy. Should be continued only if patients have evidence of clinical remission by wk 8 of therapy.

Juvenile Idiopathic Arthritis

Subcut (Children 2–17 yr (Humira); 4–17 yr (Amjevita and Cyltezo): *10–<15 kg (Humira only)*—10 mg every other wk; *15–<30 kg (Humira and Amjevita only)*—20 mg every other wk; *≥30 kg*—40 mg every other wk.

Plaque Psoriasis

Subcut (Adults): 80 mg initially, then in 1 wk, begin regimen of 40 mg every other wk.

Uveitis

Subcut (Adults): 80 mg initially, then in 1 wk, begin regimen of 40 mg every other wk.
Subcut (Children ≥2 yr and ≥30 kg): 40 mg every other wk.
Subcut (Children ≥2 yr and 15–<30 kg): 20 mg every other wk.
Subcut (Children ≥2 yr and 10–<15 kg): 10 mg every other wk.

Hidradenitis Suppurativa

Subcut (Adults and Children ≥12 yr and ≥60 kg): 160 mg initially (given in one day or over two consecutive days), followed by 80 mg 2 wk later on Day 15. Two wk later (Day 29), begin maintenance dose of 40 mg every wk.
Subcut (Children ≥12 yr and 30–59 kg): 80 mg initially on Day 1, followed by 40 mg 1 wk later on Day 8. Two wk later (Day 22), begin maintenance dose of 40 mg every other wk.

Availability

Solution for injection (prefilled syringes): 10 mg/0.1 mL, 10 mg/0.2 mL, 20 mg/0.2 mL, 20 mg/0.4 mL, 40 mg/0.4 mL, 40 mg/0.8 mL, 80 mg/0.8 mL. **Solution for injection (vials):** 40 mg/0.8 mL. **Solution for injection (prefilled pens):** 40 mg/0.4 mL, 40 mg/0.8 mL, 80 mg/0.8 mL.

NURSING IMPLICATIONS

Assessment

- Assess for signs of infection (fever, dyspnea, flu-like symptoms, frequent or painful urination, redness or swelling at the site of a wound), including tuberculosis and Hepatitis B virus (HBV), prior to and periodically during therapy. Adalimumab is contraindicated in patients with active infection. New infections should be monitored closely; most common are upper respiratory tract infections, bronchitis, and urinary tract infections. Infections may be fatal, especially in patients taking immunosuppressive therapy.
- Monitor for injection site reactions (redness and/or itching, rash, hemorrhage, bruising, pain, or swelling). Rash will usually disappear within a few days. Application of a towel soaked in cold water may relieve pain or swelling.

- Assess patient for latex allergy. Needle cover of syringe contains latex and should not be handled by persons sensitive to latex.
- Monitor patient for signs of anaphylaxis (urticaria, dyspnea, facial edema) following injection. Medications (antihistamines, corticosteroids, epinephrine) and equipment should be readily available in the event of a severe reaction. Discontinue adalimumab immediately if anaphylaxis or other severe allergic reaction occurs.
- Assess patient for latent tuberculosis with a tuberculin skin test prior to initiation of therapy. Treatment of latent tuberculosis should be started before therapy with adalimumab.
- Assess for signs and symptoms of systemic fungal infections (fever, malaise, weight loss, sweats, cough, dyspnea, pulmonary infiltrates, serious systemic illness with or without concomitant shock). Ascertain if patient lives in or has traveled to areas of endemic mycoses. Consider empiric antifungal treatment for patients at risk of histoplasmosis and other invasive fungal infections until pathogens are identified. Consult with an infectious diseases specialist. Consider stopping adalimumab until infection has been diagnosed and adequately treated.
- **Arthritis:** Assess pain and range of motion before and periodically during therapy.
- **Crohn's Disease or Ulcerative Colitis:** Monitor frequency and consistency of bowel movements periodically during therapy.
- **Plaque Psoriasis:** Assess skin lesions periodically during therapy.
- **Hidradenitis Suppurativa:** Monitor skin lesions (abscesses, inflammatory nodules, draining fistulas) during therapy.
- **Uveitis:** Monitor signs and symptoms of uveitis (red eye with or without pain, photosensitivity, blurry vision, seeing "floaters" all of a sudden) during therapy.
- ***Lab Test Considerations:*** May cause agranulocytosis, granulocytopenia, leukopenia, pancytopenia, and polycythemia.
- Monitor CBC with differential periodically during therapy. May cause leukopenia, neutropenia, thrombocytopenia, and pancytopenia. Discontinue adalimumab if symptoms of blood dyscrasias (persistent fever) occur.
- Monitor for HBV blood tests before starting during, and for several mo after therapy is completed.

Implementation

- Administer a tuberculin skin test prior to administration of adalimumab. Patients with active latent TB should be treated for TB prior to therapy.
- Immunizations should be current prior to initiating therapy. Patients on adalimumab may receive concurrent vaccinations, except for live vaccines.
- Administer initial injection under supervision of a health care professional.
- Vial is for institutional use only. With training, patient may use pen and prefilled syringes at home.
- Do not administer solutions that are discolored or contain particulate matter. Discard unused solution.
- Other DMARDs should be continued during adalimumab therapy.
- **Subcut:** Solution may be left at room temperature for 15–30 min before injecting. Administer at a 45° angle in upper thighs or abdomen, avoiding the 2 inches around the navel. Put pressure on injection site for 10 sec, do not rub. Rotate injection sites; avoid areas that are tender, bruised, hard, or red. If multiple injections required per dose, administer in separate sites. Refrigerate prefilled syringes and pens.

Patient/Family Teaching

- Instruct patient on the correct technique for administering adalimumab. Review *Medication Guide*, preparation of dose, administration sites and technique, and disposal of equipment into a puncture-resistant container.
- Advise patient to use calendar stickers provided by manufacturer to assist in remembering when dose is due. If a dose is missed, instruct patient to administer as soon as possible, then take next dose according to regular schedule. If more than prescribed dose is taken, caution patient to consult health care professional or the HUMIRA Patient Resource Center at 1-800-4HUMIRA (448-6472).
- Caution patient to notify health care professional immediately if signs of infection, HBV (muscle aches, clay-colored bowel movements, feeling very tired, fever, dark urine, chills, skin or eyes look yellow, stomach discomfort, little or no appetite, skin rash, vomiting), severe rash, swollen face, or difficulty breathing occurs or if nervous system problems (numbness or tingling, problems vision, weakness in arms or legs, dizziness) occur while taking adalimumab.
- Advise patient to notify health care professional of all Rx or OTC medications, vitamins, or herbal products being taken and to consult with health care professional before taking other medications.
- Instruct patient to notify health care professional of medication regimen prior to treatment or surgery.
- Advise patient to avoid live vaccines during therapy.
- Rep: Advise female patients to notify health care professional if pregnancy is planned or suspected or if breast feeding. Encourage patient to contact the pregnancy registry by calling 1-877-311-8972 if pregnant.
- **Pen:** Clean area for injection with alcohol swab. Hold pen with gray cap pointing up. Check solution

through window; if discolored, cloudy, or contains flakes, discard solution. Turn pen over and point cap down to make sure solution reaches fill line; if not, do not use and contact pharmacist. Remove gray cap exposing the needle and the plum cap exposing the button; removing the plum cap activates the pen. Pinch skin and place pen, with window visible, against skin at a 90° angle and press button until a click is heard. Hold pen in place until all solution is injected (10 sec) and yellow marker is visible in window and has stopped moving. Continue to pinch skin throughout injection. Remove needle and press with a gauze pad or cotton ball for 10 sec. Do not rub injection site. Dispose of pen into a puncture-resistant container.

Evaluation/Desired Outcomes

- Decreased pain and swelling with decreased rate of joint destruction in patients with rheumatoid arthritis.
- Decreased signs and symptoms, slowed progression of joint destruction, and improved physical function in patients with psoriatic arthritis.
- Reduced signs and symptoms of ankylosing spondylitis.
- Decreased signs and symptoms, and maintenance of remission, in patients with Crohn's disease or ulcerative colitis.
- Reduced pain and swelling in patients moderate to severe polyarticular juvenile idiopathic arthritis in children 2 yr of age and older.
- Reduced severity of plaques in patients with severe chronic plaque psoriasis.
- Improvement in skin lesions in patients with hidradenitis suppurativa.
- Decreased progression of uveitis.

adenosine (a-den-oh-seen)

Adenocard, Adenoscan

Classification
Therapeutic: antiarrhythmics

Indications

Conversion of paroxysmal supraventricular tachycardia (PSVT) to normal sinus rhythm when vagal maneuvers are unsuccessful. As a diagnostic agent (with noninvasive techniques) to assess myocardial perfusion defects occurring as a consequence of coronary artery disease.

Action

Restores normal sinus rhythm by interrupting re-entrant pathways in the AV node. Slows conduction time through the AV node. Also produces coronary artery vasodilation. **Therapeutic Effects:** Restoration of normal sinus rhythm.

Pharmacokinetics

Absorption: Following IV administration, absorption is complete.

Distribution: Taken up by erythrocytes and vascular endothelium.

Metabolism and Excretion: Rapidly converted to inosine and adenosine monophosphate.

Half-life: <10 sec.

TIME/ACTION PROFILE (antiarrhythmic effect)

ROUTE	ONSET	PEAK	DURATION
IV	immediate	unknown	1–2 min

Contraindications/Precautions

Contraindicated in: Hypersensitivity; 2nd- or 3rd-degree AV block or sick sinus syndrome, unless a functional artificial pacemaker is present; Myocardial ischemia/infarction (only Adenoscan).

Use Cautiously in: Patients with a history of asthma (may induce bronchospasm); Unstable angina; OB, Lactation: Safety not established.

Adverse Reactions/Side Effects

CNS: SEIZURES (only with Adenoscan), STROKE (only with Adenoscan), apprehension, dizziness, headache, head pressure, lightheadedness. **EENT:** blurred vision, throat tightness. **Resp:** shortness of breath, chest pressure, hyperventilation. **CV:** MI, VENTRICULAR TACHYCARDIA, facial flushing, transient arrhythmias, chest pain, hypotension, palpitations. **GI:** metallic taste, nausea. **Derm:** burning sensation, facial flushing, sweating. **MS:** neck and back pain. **Neuro:** numbness, tingling. **Misc:** HYPERSENSITIVITY REACTIONS, heaviness in arms, pressure sensation in groin.

Interactions

Drug-Drug: Carbamazepine may ↑ risk of progressive heart block. **Dipyridamole** ↑ effects of adenosine (dose ↓ of adenosine recommended). Effects of adenosine ↓ by **theophylline** or **caffeine** (↑ doses of adenosine may be required). Concurrent use with **digoxin** may ↑ risk of ventricular fibrillation.

Route/Dosage

IV (Adults and Children >50 kg): *Antiarrhythmic (Adenocard)*—6 mg by rapid IV bolus; if no results, repeat 1–2 min later as 12-mg rapid bolus. This dose may be repeated (single dose not to exceed 12 mg). *Diagnostic use (Adenoscan)*—140 mcg/kg/min for 6 min (0.84 mg/kg total).

IV (Children <50 kg): *Antiarrhythmic*—0.05–0.1 mg/kg as a rapid bolus, may repeat in 1–2 min; if response is inadequate, may increase by 0.05–0.1 mg/kg until sinus rhythm is established or maximum dose of 0.3 mg/kg is used.

Availability (generic available)

Injection: 3 mg/mL in 2–mL vial (Adenocard), 3 mg/mL in 20–mL and 30-mL vials (Adenoscan).

NURSING IMPLICATIONS

Assessment

- Monitor heart rate frequently (every 15–30 sec) and ECG continuously during therapy. A short, transient period of 1st-, 2nd-, or 3rd-degree heart block or asystole may occur following injection; usually resolves quickly due to short duration of adenosine. Once conversion to normal sinus rhythm is achieved, transient arrhythmias (premature ventricular contractions, atrial premature contractions, sinus tachycardia, sinus bradycardia, skipped beats, AV nodal block) may occur, but generally last a few sec.
- Monitor BP during therapy.
- Assess respiratory status (breath sounds, rate) following administration. Patients with history of asthma may experience bronchospasm.

Implementation

IV Administration

- **IV:** Crystals may occur if adenosine is refrigerated. Warm to room temperature to dissolve crystals. Solution must be clear before use. Do not administer solutions that are discolored or contain particulate matter. Discard unused portions.
- **IV Push:** ***Diluent:*** Administer undiluted. ***Concentration:*** 3 mg/mL. ***Rate:*** Administer over 1–2 sec via peripheral IV as proximal as possible to trunk. Slow administration may cause increased heart rate in response to vasodilation. Follow each dose with 20 mL rapid saline flush to ensure injection reaches systemic circulation.
- **Intermittent Infusion (for use in diagnostic testing):** ***Diluent:*** Administer 30-mL vial undiluted. ***Concentration:*** 3 mg/mL. ***Rate:*** Administer at a rate of 140 mcg/kg/min over 6 min for a total dose of 0.84 mg/kg. Thallium-201 should be injected as close to the venous access as possible at the midpoint (after 3 min) of the infusion.

Patient/Family Teaching

- Caution patient to change positions slowly to minimize orthostatic hypotension. Doses >12 mg decrease BP by decreasing peripheral vascular resistance.
- Instruct patient to report facial flushing, shortness of breath, or dizziness.
- Advise patient to avoid products containing methylxanthines (caffeinated coffee, tea, carbonated drinks or drugs such as aminophylline or theophylline) prior to myocardial perfusion imaging study.

Evaluation/Desired Outcomes

- Conversion of supraventricular tachycardia to normal sinus rhythm.
- Diagnosis of myocardial perfusion defects.

ado-trastuzumab

(ado tras-**too**-zoo-mab)
Kadcyla

Classification
Therapeutic: antineoplastics
Pharmacologic: drug-antibody conjugates

Indications

Treatment of HER2-positive metastatic breast cancer in patients previously treated with trastuzumab and a taxane who have either received prior therapy for metastatic disease or developed disease recurrence during or within 6 mo of completing adjuvant therapy. Adjuvant treatment of HER2–positive early breast cancer in patients who have residual invasive disease after neoadjuvant taxane and trastuzumab-based therapy.

Action

A HER2-targeted antibody and microtubule inhibitor conjugate. Trastuzumab, the antibody, attaches to receptors and is taken into the cell, where the microtubule inhibitor, DM1, causes cell cycle arrest and death.
Therapeutic Effects: Decreased spread of metastatic breast cancer, with improved progression-free survival.

Pharmacokinetics

Absorption: IV administration results in complete bioavailability.
Distribution: Unknown.
Metabolism and Excretion: DM1 is metabolized by CYP3A4/5.
Half-life: 4 days.

TIME/ACTION PROFILE (comparative improvement in progression-free survival)

ROUTE	ONSET	PEAK	DURATION
IV	4–6 mo	10–12 mo	2 yr

Contraindications/Precautions

Contraindicated in: Interstitial lung disease or pneumonitis; Concurrent use of strong CYP3A4 inhibitors; OB: Pregnancy (may cause fetal harm); Lactation: Lactation.
Use Cautiously in: Underlying cardiovascular or pulmonary disease, including dyspnea at rest; Rep: Women of reproductive potential and men with female partners of reproductive potential should use effective contraception; Pedi: Safety and effectiveness not established.

Adverse Reactions/Side Effects

CNS: fatigue, headache, dizziness, insomnia, weakness. **CV:** HF, hypertension, peripheral edema. **Derm:** pruritus, rash. **EENT:** blurred vision, conjunctivitis, dry eyes, ↑ lacrimation. **F and E:** hypokalemia. **GI:** HEPATOTOXICITY, constipation, ↑ liver enzymes, nausea, altered taste, diarrhea, dry mouth, dyspepsia, stomatitis, vomiting. **GU:** ↓ fertility. **Hemat:** HEMORRHAGE, THROMBOCYTOPENIA, anemia, neutropenia. **MS:** musculoskeletal pain, arthralgia, myalgia. **Neuro:** peripheral neuropathy. **Resp:** INTERSTITIAL LUNG DISEASE, cough. **Misc:** HYPERSENSITIVITY REACTIONS, chills, infusion-related reactions, fever.

Interactions

Drug-Drug: Strong CYP3A4 inhibitors, including **atazanavir, clarithromycin, indinavir, itraconazole, ketoconazole, nefazodone, nelfinavir, ritonavir, saquinavir**, and **voriconazole** may ↑ levels and risk of toxicity; avoid concurrent use. Concurrent use of **anticoagulants**, or **antiplatelet agents**, especially during the first cycle, may ↑ risk of bleeding.

Route/Dosage

Should not be used interchangeably with trastuzumab.

Metastatic Breast Cancer

IV (Adults): 3.6 mg/kg every 3 wk until disease progression or unacceptable toxicity.

Early Breast Cancer

IV (Adults): 3.6 mg/kg every 3 wk (21–day cycle) for a total of 14 cycles unless there is disease progression or unacceptable toxicity.

Availability

Lyophilized powder for injection (requires reconstitution and dilution): 100 mg/vial, 160 mg/vial.

NURSING IMPLICATIONS

Assessment

- Evaluate left ventricular function in all patients prior to and every 3 mo during therapy. **For patients with metastatic disease:** *If symptomatic HF:* discontinue ado-trastuzumab. *If left ventricular ejection fraction (LVEF) <40%:* Hold dose. Repeat LVEF assessment within 3 wk. If LVEF <40% is confirmed, discontinue therapy. *If LVEF 40% to ≤45% and decrease is ≥10% points from baseline:* Hold dose. Repeat LVEF within 3 wk. If LVEF has not recovered to within 10% points from baseline, discontinue therapy. *If LVEF 40% to ≤45% and decrease is <10% points from baseline:* Continue therapy with ado-trastuzumab. Repeat LVEF within 3 wk. *If LVEF >45%:* Continue therapy. Discontinue therapy if symptomatic heart failure occurs. **For patients with early breast cancer:** *If LVEF <45%:* Hold dose. Repeat LVEF within 3 wk. If LVEF < 45% confirmed, discontinue therapy. *If LVEF 45% to < 50% and decrease is ≥ 10% points from baseline:* Hold dose. Repeat LVEF within 3 wk. *If the LVEF < 50% and not recovered to < 10% points from baseline, discontinue therapy. If LVEF 45% to < 50% and decrease is < 10% points from baseline:* Continue therapy. Repeat LVEF within 3 wk. *If LVEF ≥ 50%:* Continue therapy. *If symptomatic heart failure, Grade 3-4 left ventricular systolic dysfunction or Grade 3-4 heart failure, or Grade 2 heart failure accompanied by LVEF < 45%:* Discontinue therapy.
- Monitor infusion site closely for infiltration and extravasation closely. Within 24 hrs erythema, tenderness, skin irritation, pain, or swelling at infusion site is seen if extravasation occurs.
- Assess for signs and symptoms of infusion reactions (fever, chills, flushing, dyspnea, hypotension, wheezing, bronchospasm, tachycardia). Slow or interrupt therapy if symptoms are severe. Observe closely during first infusion. Permanently discontinue for life-threatening reactions.
- Monitor neurologic status before and during treatment. Assess for paresthesia (numbness, tingling, pain, burning sensation), loss of deep tendon reflexes (Achilles reflex is usually first involved), weakness (wrist drop or footdrop, gait disturbances), cranial nerve palsies (jaw pain, hoarseness, ptosis, visual changes), arthralgia, myalgia, muscle spasm, autonomic dysfunction (ileus, difficulty voiding, orthostatic hypotension, impaired sweating), and CNS dysfunction (decreased level of consciousness, agitation, hallucinations). Temporarily discontinue therapy in patients with Grade 3 or 4 peripheral neuropathy (severe symptoms; limiting self-care activities of daily living (ADL)) until resolution to ≤ Grade 2 (moderate symptoms; limiting instrumental ADL) neuropathy.
- Monitor for signs and symptoms of pulmonary toxicity (dyspnea, cough, fatigue, pulmonary infiltrates). Permanently discontinue therapy if interstitial lung disease or pneumonitis develops.
- Monitor for hemorrhage (central nervous system, respiratory, gastrointestinal hemorrhage) during therapy, especially in patients receiving anticoagulants, antiplatelet therapy, or who have thrombocytopenia.
- ***Lab Test Considerations:*** HER2 protein overexpression is used to determine whether treatment with ado-trastuzumab is indicated. HER2 protein overexpression should be determined by labs with proficiency in specific technology used. Information on approved tests is available at http://www.fda.gov/CompanionDiagnostics.
- Verify negative pregnancy status before starting therapy.
- Monitor serum transaminases and bilirubin prior to starting therapy and before each dose. **For patients with metastatic disease:** *If AST/ALT is Grade 2 (>2.5 to ≤5× upper limit of normal (ULN)):* Treat at same dose. *If AST/ALT is Grade 3 (>5 to ≤20× ULN):* Do not administer ado-trastuzumab until AST/

ALT recovers to Grade ≤2, and then reduce 1 dose level. *If AST/ALT is Grade 4 (>20× ULN):* Permanently discontinue ado-trastuzumab. *If serum bilirubin is Grade 2 (>1.5 to ≤3× ULN):* Hold dose until bilirubin recovers to Grade ≤1, then treat at same dose level. *If bilirubin is Grade 3 (>3 to ≤10× ULN):* Hold dose until bilirubin recovers to Grade ≤1, then reduce 1 dose level. *If bilirubin is Grade 4 (>10× ULN):* Permanently discontinue ado-trastuzumab. Permanently discontinue ado-trastuzumab in patients with AST/ALT >3× ULN and concomitant total bilirubin >2× ULN. **For patients with early breast cancer:** *If ALT Grade 2-3 (> 3.0 to ≤ 20 x ULN on day of scheduled treatment):* Hold dose until ALT recovers to Grade ≤1, then reduce one dose level. *If ALT Grade 4 (> 20 x ULN at any time):* Permanently discontinue therapy. *If AST Grade 2 (> 3.0 to ≤ 5 x ULN on day of scheduled treatment):* Hold dose until AST recovers to Grade ≤1, then treat with same dose. *If AST Grade 3 (> 5 to ≤ 20 x ULN on day of scheduled treatment):* Hold dose until AST recovers to Grade ≤1, then reduce one dose level. *If AST Grade 4 (> 20 x ULN at any time):* Permanently discontinue therapy. *If total bilirubin >1.0 to ≤ 2.0 x ULN on day of scheduled treatment:* Hold dose until total bilirubin ≤ 1.0× ULN, then reduce one dose level. *If total bilirubin >2 x ULN at any time:* Permanently discontinue therapy.

- Monitor platelet count prior to starting therapy and before each dose. Nadir of thrombocytopenia occurs by Day 8 and generally improves to Grade 0 or 1 by next scheduled dose. **For patients with metastatic disease:** *If thrombocytopenia is Grade 3 (platelets 25,000/mm³ to <50,000/mm³:* Hold dose until platelet count recovers to ≤Grade 1 (≥75,000/mm³), then treat at same dose level. *If thrombocytopenia is Grade 4 (platelets <25,000/mm₃):* Hold dose until platelet count recovers to ≤Grade 1, then reduce 1 dose level. **For patients with early breast cancer:** If Grade 2-3 on day of scheduled treatment (25,000 to < 75,000/mm³): Hold dose until platelet count recovers to Grade ≤1 (≥ 75,000/mm³), then treat at the same dose level. If 2 delays required due to thrombocytopenia, reduce dose by one level. *If Grade 4 at any time < 25,000/mm³:* Hold dose until platelet count recovers to Grade ≤1 (≥ 75,000/mm³), then reduce one dose level.
- May cause ↓ hemoglobin, neutrophils, and serum potassium.

Implementation

- ***High Alert:*** Do not confuse ado-trastuzumab (Kadcyla) with trastuzumab (Herceptin). Double check names. Trade name of administered product should be clearly recorded in patient file to improve traceability.
- ***High Alert:*** Fatalities have occurred with chemotherapeutic agents. Before administering, clarify all ambiguous orders; double check single, daily, and course-of-therapy dose limits; have second practitioner independently double check original order, dose calculations and infusion pump settings.
- Solution should be prepared in a biologic cabinet. Wear gloves, gown, and mask while handling medication. Discard IV equipment in specially designated containers.

IV Administration

- **Intermittent Infusion:** Reconstitute by slowly injecting 5 or 8 mL of sterile water for injection into 100 or 160 mg vial of ado-trastuzumab respectively, for a solution of 20 mg/mL. Swirl gently until dissolved; do not shake. Solution is clear, colorless to pale brown, and slightly opalescent; do not administer solutions that are discolored or contain particulate matter. Use reconstituted vials immediately or store in refrigerator up to 4 hr; then discard. Do not freeze. Calculate amount of solution needed. ***Diluent:*** Withdraw from vial and add to infusion bag containing 250 mL of 0.9% NaCl; do not use dextrose solutions. Gently invert bag to mix without foaming. Use diluted solution immediately; may be stored in refrigerator up to 24 hrs prior to use, then discard; do not freeze or shake. Administer every 3 wk (21–day cycle); if cycle is delayed, administer as soon as possible. Do not wait until next planned cycle; maintain 3-wk interval between doses. ***Rate:*** Infuse through a 0.2 or 0.22 micron in-line non-protein adsorptive polyethersulfone (PES) filter. Do not administer as IV push or bolus. *First infusion:* Infuse over 90 min; observe for infusion related reaction. *Subsequent infusions:* Infuse over 30 min if prior infusions were well tolerated. Observe patient during infusion and for at least 90 min after infusion.
- Management of increased serum transaminases, hyperbilirubinemia, left ventricular dysfunction, thrombocytopenia, pulmonary toxicity, or peripheral neuropathy may require temporary interruption, dose reduction, or discontinuation.
- Dose reduction schedule is: *Starting dose*—3.6 mg/kg; *First dose reduction*—3 mg/kg; *Second dose reduction*—2.4 mg/kg; *Requirement for further dose reduction*—discontinue therapy.
- **Y-Site Incompatibility:** Do not mix or administer with other medications.

Patient/Family Teaching

- Explain purpose of medication to patient. If a dose is missed administer as soon as possible; do not wait until next scheduled dose. Adjust schedule to maintain 3 wk interval between doses.

- Inform patient of potential liver injury and HF. Advise patient to notify health care professional immediately if signs and symptoms of liver injury (nausea, vomiting, abdominal pain, jaundice, dark urine, pruritus, anorexia) or HF (new onset or worsening shortness of breath, cough, swelling of ankles/legs, palpitations, weight gain of >5 lbs in 24 hrs, dizziness, loss of consciousness) occur.
- Advise patient to notify health care professional if signs of peripheral neuropathy (burning, numbness, pain in hands and feet/legs) occur.
- Rep: Ado-trastuzumab can cause fetal harm. Advise male and female patients to use a highly effective method (IUD, hormonal contraceptive, tubal ligation, partner's vasectomy) of contraception during and for at least 4 mo after last dose. Instruct patient to notify health care professional promptly if pregnancy is suspected and to avoid breast feeding for at least 7 mo after last dose. Encourage women who have been exposed to ado-trastuzumab either directly or through seminal fluid, to immediately report exposure to Genentech Adverse Event Line at 1-888-835-2555. May impair fertility in male and female patients.

Evaluation/Desired Outcomes

- Decreased spread of metastatic breast cancer.

afatinib (a-fa-ti-nib)

Gilotrif, Giotrif

Classification

Therapeutic: antineoplastics

Pharmacologic: kinase inhibitors

Indications

First-line treatment of metastatic non-small cell lung cancer (NSCLC) where the tumor has non-resistant epidermal growth factor receptor (EGFR) mutations detectable by an FDA-approved test. Treatment of metastatic squamous NSCLC progressing after platinum chemotherapy.

Action

Inhibits tyrosine kinases which results in slowed proliferation of specific tumor cell lines. **Therapeutic Effects:** Decreased spread of NSCLC.

Pharmacokinetics

Absorption: Well absorbed (92%) following oral administration; absorption is decreased by high fat meal.

Distribution: Unknown.

Metabolism and Excretion: Metabolites occur partly as protein-bound products. Excretion is primarily fecal (85%) as parent drug; 4% excreted in urine.

Half-life: 37 hr.

TIME/ACTION PROFILE (improved progression-free survival)

ROUTE	ONSET	PEAK	DURATION
PO	3 mo	12 mo	20 mo

Contraindications/Precautions

Contraindicated in: Tumors with resistant EGFR mutations; Lactation: Discontinue drug or discontinue breast feeding; OB: May cause fetal harm.

Use Cautiously in: Severe renal impairment (↓ dose); Severe hepatic impairment (dose adjustment may be necessary); Asian ethnicity (may be ↑ susceptible to interstitial lung disease); Rep: Women of reproductive potential; Pedi: Safety and effectiveness not established.

Adverse Reactions/Side Effects

Derm: STEVENS-JOHNSON SYNDROME, TOXIC EPIDERMAL NECROLYSIS, cutaneous reactions (including bullous/blistering/exfoliating reactions, acneiform eruptions and palmar-plantar erythrodysesthesia), dry skin, paronychia, pruritus, rash. **EENT:** conjunctivitis, epistaxis, keratitis, rhinorrhea. **GI:** HEPATOTOXICITY, PANCREATITIS, diarrhea, ↓ appetite, ↓ weight, nausea, stomatitis, vomiting. **F and E:** hypokalemia. **Resp:** INTERSTITIAL LUNG DISEASE. **Misc:** fever.

Interactions

Drug-Drug: Concurrent use of **P-gp inhibitors** including **amiodarone**, **cyclosporine**, **erythromycin**, **itraconazole**, **ketoconazole**, **quinidine ritonavir**, **saquinavir**, **tacrolimus**, or **verapamil** ↑ blood levels and the risk of toxicity; dosage adjustment may be necessary (ritonavir may be given concurrently or 6 hr after). Concurrent use of **P-gp inducers** including **carbamazepine**, **phenobarbital**, **phenytoin**, or **rifampin** ↓ blood levels and may ↓ effectiveness; dosage adjustment may be necessary.

Route/Dosage

PO (Adults): 40 mg once daily; *concurrent use of P-gp inhibitors*—↓ dose by 10 mg/day if necessary; *concurrent use of P-gp inducers*—↑ dose by 10 mg/day if necessary. Continue until disease progression or occurrence of unacceptable toxicity.

Renal Impairment

PO (Adults): *eGFR 15–29 mL/min*—30 mg once daily.

Availability

Tablets: 20 mg, 30 mg, 40 mg.

NURSING IMPLICATIONS

Assessment

- Monitor for diarrhea; occurs frequently. Provide patient with an antidiarrheal agent (loperamide) at the onset of diarrhea and until diarrhea ceases for 12 hrs. If diarrhea is severe and lasts more than 48 hr despite use of antidiarrheal agent (Grade 2 or higher), withhold afatinib until diarrhea resolves to Grade 1 or less, then resume with reduced dose of 10 mg/day.

- Assess for cutaneous reactions (bullous, blistering, exfoliative lesions; rash, erythema, acneiform rash) periodically during therapy. Discontinue afatinib if life-threatening lesions or prolonged Grade 2 cutaneous lesions lasting ≥7 days, intolerable Grade 2, or Grade 3 cutaneous reactions occur. Withhold afatinib until reaction resolves to Grade 1 or less and resume at 10 mg/day.
- Monitor for signs and symptoms of interstitial lung disease (lung infiltration, pneumonitis, acute respiratory distress syndrome, allergic alveolitis); 🧬 may occur more commonly in patients of Asian ethnicity. Withhold afatinib if symptoms occur; discontinue if interstitial lung disease is confirmed.
- ***Lab Test Considerations:*** Monitor liver function tests periodically during therapy. If severe decline in liver function occurs, discontinue afatinib. May cause ↑ AST and ALT.
- May cause hypokalemia.

Implementation

- **PO:** Administer once daily on an empty stomach, at least 1 hr before or 2 hrs after meals.

Patient/Family Teaching

- Instruct patient to take afatinib as directed. Take missed dose as soon as remembered unless within 12 hrs of next dose, then omit and take next dose at scheduled time; do not double doses.
- Caution patient to notify health care professional if signs and symptoms of keratitis (acute or worsening eye inflammation, lacrimation, light sensitivity, blurred vision, eye pain, and/or red eye) occur. Withhold if symptoms occur; if ulcerative keratitis is confirmed, discontinue afatinib. Advise patient that use of contact lenses is also a risk factor.
- Advise patient to wear sunscreen and protective clothing during therapy to minimize risk of skin disorders.
- Inform patient that diarrhea occurs in most patients and may cause dehydration and renal impairment. Notify health care professional if diarrhea is severe or persistent, if new or worsening lung symptoms (difficulty breathing, shortness of breath, cough, fever), symptoms of liver problems (yellow skin or whites of eyes, dark brown urine, pain on right side of abdomen, unusual bleeding or bruising, lethargy) or if symptoms of left ventricular dysfunction (shortness of breath, exercise intolerance, cough, fatigue, swelling or ankles or feet, palpitations, sudden weight gain) occur.
- Advise patient to notify health care professional of all Rx or OTC medications, vitamins, or herbal products being taken and to consult with health care professional before taking other medications.
- Rep: Advise female patients to use highly effective contraception during and for at least 2 wk after last dose and to avoid breast feeding. If pregnancy occurs, instruct patient to notify health care professional immediately.

Evaluation/Desired Outcomes

- Decreased spread of non-small cell lung cancer.

albuterol (al-byoo-ter-ole)

Accuneb, 🍁Airomir, Proair HFA, Proair Respiclick, Proventil HFA, 🍁Salbutamol, Ventolin HFA, 🍁Ventolin Diskus, 🍁Ventolin Nebules, VoSpire ER

Classification

Therapeutic: bronchodilators

Pharmacologic: adrenergics

Indications

Treatment or prevention of bronchospasm in asthma or chronic obstructive pulmonary disease (COPD). **Inhaln:** Prevention of exercise-induced bronchospasm. **PO:** Used as a long-term control agent in patients with chronic/persistent bronchospasm.

Action

Binds to $beta_2$-adrenergic receptors in airway smooth muscle, leading to activation of adenyl cyclase and increased levels of cyclic-3′, 5′-adenosine monophosphate (cAMP). Increases in cAMP activate kinases, which inhibit the phosphorylation of myosin and decrease intracellular calcium. Decreased intracellular calcium relaxes smooth muscle airways. Relaxation of airway smooth muscle with subsequent bronchodilation. Relatively selective for $beta_2$ (pulmonary) receptors. **Therapeutic Effects:** Bronchodilation.

Pharmacokinetics

Absorption: Well absorbed after oral administration but rapidly undergoes extensive metabolism.

Distribution: Small amounts appear in breast milk.

Metabolism and Excretion: Extensively metabolized by the liver and other tissues.

Half-life: Oral 2.7–5 hr; Inhalation: 3.8 hr.

TIME/ACTION PROFILE (bronchodilation)

ROUTE	ONSET	PEAK	DURATION
PO	15–30 min	2–3 hr	4–6 hr or more
PO–ER	30 min	2–3 hr	12 hr
Inhaln	5–15 min	60–90 min	3–6 hr

Contraindications/Precautions

Contraindicated in: Hypersensitivity to adrenergic amines.

Use Cautiously in: Cardiac disease; Hypertension; Hyperthyroidism; Diabetes; Glaucoma; Seizure disorders; Excess inhaler use may lead to tolerance and paradoxical bronchospasm; OB, Lactation, Pedi: Safety not established for pregnant women near term, breast-feeding women, and children <2 yr; Geri: ↑ risk of adverse reactions; may require dose ↓.

Adverse Reactions/Side Effects

CNS: nervousness, restlessness, tremor, headache, insomnia (Pedi: occurs more frequently in young children than adults), hyperactivity in children. **Resp:** PARADOXICAL BRONCHOSPASM (excessive use of inhalers). **CV:** chest pain, palpitations, angina, arrhythmias, hypertension. **GI:** nausea, vomiting. **Endo:** hyperglycemia. **F and E:** hypokalemia. **Neuro:** tremor.

Interactions

Drug-Drug: Concurrent use with other **adrenergic agents** will have ↑ adrenergic side effects. Use with **MAO inhibitors** may lead to hypertensive crisis. **Beta blockers** may negate therapeutic effect. May ↓ serum **digoxin** levels. Cardiovascular effects are potentiated in patients receiving **tricyclic antidepressants**. Risk of hypokalemia ↑ concurrent use of **potassium-losing diuretics**. Hypokalemia ↑ the risk of **digoxin** toxicity.

Drug-Natural Products: Use with caffeine-containing herbs (**cola nut**, **guarana**, **tea**, **coffee**) ↑ stimulant effect.

Route/Dosage

PO (Adults and Children ≥12 yr): 2–4 mg 3–4 times daily (not to exceed 32 mg/day) or 4–8 mg of extended-release tablets twice daily.

PO (Geriatric Patients): Initial dose should not exceed 2 mg 3–4 times daily, may be ↑ carefully (up to 32 mg/day).

PO (Children 6–12 yr): 2 mg 3–4 times daily or 0.3–0.6 mg/kg/day as extended-release tablets divided twice daily; may be carefully ↑ as needed (not to exceed 8 mg/day).

PO (Children 2–6 yr): 0.1 mg/kg 3 times daily (not to exceed 2 mg 3 times daily initially); may be carefully ↑ to 0.2 mg/kg 3 times daily (not to exceed 4 mg 3 times daily).

Inhaln (Adults and Children ≥4 yr): *Via metered-dose inhaler or dry powder inhaler*—2 inhalations every 4–6 hr (some patients may respond to 1 inhalation) or 2 inhalations 15 min before exercise; *NIH Guidelines for acute asthma exacerbation: Children*—4–8 puffs every 20 min for 3 doses then every 1–4 hr; *Adults*—4–8 puffs every 20 min for up to 4 hr then every 1–4 hr as needed.

Inhaln (Adults and Children >12 yr): *NIH Guidelines for acute asthma exacerbation via nebulization or IPPB*—2.5–5 mg every 20 min for 3 doses then 2.5–10 mg every 1–4 hr as needed; *Continuous nebulization*—10–15 mg/hr.

Inhaln (Children 2–12 yr): *NIH Guidelines for acute asthma exacerbation via nebulization or IPPB*—0.15 mg/kg/dose (minimum dose 2.5 mg) every 20 min for 3 doses then 0.15–0.3 mg/kg (not to exceed 10 mg) every 1–4 hr as needed *or* 1.25 mg 3–4 times daily for children 10–15 kg *or* 2.5 mg 3–4 times daily for children >15 kg; *Continuous nebulization*—0.5–3 mg/kg/hr.

Inhaln (Neonates): 1.25 mg/dose every 8 hr via nebulization or 1–2 puffs via MDI into the ventilator circuit every 6 hrs.

Availability (generic available)

Tablets: 2 mg, 4 mg. **Cost:** *Generic*—4 mg $565.87/100. **Extended-release tablets:** 4 mg, 8 mg. **Oral syrup (strawberry-flavored):** 2 mg/5 mL. **Metered-dose aerosol:** 90 mcg/inhalation in 6.7-g, 8-g, 8.5-g, and 18-g canisters (200 metered inhalations), 🍁100 mcg/spray. **Cost:** *Proair HFA*—$52.53/8.5-g canister; *Proventil HFA*—$62.62/6.7-g canister; *Ventolin HFA*—$19.08/8-g canister. **Inhalation solution:** 0.63 mg/3 mL (0.021%), 1.25 mg/3 mL (0.042%), 2.5 mg/3 mL (0.083%), 🍁1 mg/mL, 🍁2 mg/mL, 5 mg/mL (0.5%). **Cost:** *Generic*—2.5 mg/3 mL $40.82/90 mL, 5 mg/mL $51.02/60 mL. **Powder for inhalation (Proair Respiclick):** 90 mcg/inhalation (200 metered inhalations). **Powder for inhalation (Ventolin Diskus):** 🍁200 mcg. ***In combination with:*** ipratropium (Combivent). See Appendix B.

NURSING IMPLICATIONS

Assessment

- Assess lung sounds, pulse, and BP before administration and during peak of medication. Note amount, color, and character of sputum produced.
- Monitor pulmonary function tests before initiating therapy and periodically during therapy.
- Observe for paradoxical bronchospasm (wheezing). If condition occurs, withhold medication and notify health care professional immediately.
- ***Lab Test Considerations:*** May cause transient ↓ in serum potassium concentrations with nebulization or higher-than-recommended doses.

Implementation

- **PO:** Administer oral medication with meals to minimize gastric irritation.
- Extended-release tablets should be swallowed whole; do not break, crush, or chew.
- **Inhaln:** Shake inhaler well, and allow at least 1 min between inhalations of aerosol medication. Prime the inhaler before first use by releasing 4 test sprays into the air away from the face. *Proair Respiclick* does not require priming. Pedi: Use spacer for children <8 yr of age.
- For nebulization or IPPB, the 0.5-, 0.83-, 1-, and 2-mg/mL solutions do not require dilution before ad-

ministration. The 5 mg/mL (0.5%) solution must be diluted with 1–2.5 mL of 0.9% NaCl for inhalation. Diluted solutions are stable for 24 hr at room temperature or 48 hr if refrigerated.

- For nebulizer, compressed air or oxygen flow should be 6–10 L/min; a single treatment of 3 mL lasts about 10 min.
- IPPB usually lasts 5–20 min.

Patient/Family Teaching

- Instruct patient to take albuterol as directed. If on a scheduled dosing regimen, take missed dose as soon as remembered, spacing remaining doses at regular intervals. Do not double doses or increase the dose or frequency of doses. Caution patient not to exceed recommended dose; may cause adverse effects, paradoxical bronchospasm (more likely with first dose from new canister), or loss of effectiveness of medication.
- Instruct patient to contact health care professional immediately if shortness of breath is not relieved by medication or is accompanied by diaphoresis, dizziness, palpitations, or chest pain.
- Instruct patient to prime unit with 4 sprays before using and to discard canister after 200 sprays. Actuators should not be changed among products.
- Inform patient that these products contain hydrofluoroalkane (HFA) and the propellant and are described as non-CFC or CFC-free (contain no chlorofluorocarbons).
- Instruct patient to notify health care professional of all Rx or OTC medications, vitamins, or herbal products being taken and to consult health care professional before taking any OTC medications or alcoholic beverages concurrently with this therapy. Caution patient also to avoid smoking and other respiratory irritants.
- Inform patient that albuterol may cause an unusual or bad taste.
- **Inhaln:** Instruct patient in the proper use of the metered-dose inhaler or nebulizer (see Appendix D).
- Advise patients to use albuterol first if using other inhalation medications and allow 5 min to elapse before administering other inhalant medications unless otherwise directed.
- Advise patient to rinse mouth with water after each inhalation dose to minimize dry mouth and clean the mouthpiece with water at least once a wk.
- Instruct patient to notify health care professional if there is no response to the usual dose or if contents of one canister are used in less than 2 wk. Asthma and treatment regimen should be re-evaluated and corticosteroids should be considered. Need for increased use to treat symptoms indicates decrease in asthma control and need to re-evaluate patient's therapy.

Evaluation/Desired Outcomes

- Prevention or relief of bronchospasm.

---

alclometasone, See CORTICOSTEROIDS (TOPICAL/LOCAL).

---

alectinib (al-ekti-nib)

Alecensa, Alecensaro

Classification
Therapeutic: antineoplastics
Pharmacologic: kinase inhibitors

Indications

Patients with metastatic non-small cell lung cancer (NSCLC) that is positive for anaplastic lymphoma kinase (ALK).

Action

Inhibits tyrosine kinase receptors targeting anaplastic lymphoma kinase (ALK) and RET. **Therapeutic Effects:** Decreased spread of NSCLC.

Pharmacokinetics

Absorption: 37% absorbed following oral administration; high-fat, high-calorie meals ↑ absorption.
Distribution: Extensively distributed to tissues.
Protein Binding: 99%.
Metabolism and Excretion: Mostly metabolized by the liver (CYP3A4 enzyme system) to its active metabolite, M4 (also metabolized by CYP3A4). 84% excreted in feces unchanged; minimal excretion in urine.
Half-life: 33 hr (alectinib); 31 hr (M4 active metabolite).

TIME/ACTION PROFILE (blood levels)

ROUTE	ONSET	PEAK	DURATION
PO	unknown	4 hr	unknown

Contraindications/Precautions

Contraindicated in: OB: Pregnancy (may cause fetal harm); Lactation: Lactation.
Use Cautiously in: Severe renal impairment (CCr <30 mL/min); Moderate or severe hepatic impairment; Rep: Women of reproductive potential; Pedi: Safety and effectiveness not established.

Adverse Reactions/Side Effects

CNS: fatigue, headache. **CV:** bradycardia, edema. **Derm:** photosensitivity, rash. **EENT:** blurred vision, diplopia. **Endo:** hyperglycemia. **F and E:** hypocalcemia, hypokalemia, hyponatremia, hypophosphatemia. **GI:** HEPATOTOXICITY, constipation, diarrhea, hyperbilirubinemia, nausea, vomiting. **GU:** ↑ serum creatinine. **Hemat:** HEMORRHAGE, anemia, lymphopenia. **Metab:** ↑ weight. **MS:** back pain, ↑ creatine kinase, myalgia. **Resp:** INTERSTITIAL LUNG DISEASE, PULMONARY EMBOLISM, cough, dyspnea.

Interactions

Drug-Drug: None reported.

Route/Dosage

PO (Adults): 600 mg twice daily with food.

Availability

Capsules: 150 mg.

NURSING IMPLICATIONS

Assessment

- Monitor for signs and symptoms of interstitial lung disease/pneumonitis (worsening of respiratory symptoms, dyspnea, cough, fever). Withhold therapy if symptoms occur and permanently discontinue if no other potential causes are identified.
- Monitor heart rate and BP regularly during therapy. *If symptomatic bradycardia occurs*, withhold therapy until asymptomatic or heart rate ≥60 bpm. If concomitant medication identified as contributing and is discontinued, or its dose adjusted, resume alectinib at previous dose upon recovery to asymptomatic bradycardia or to heart rate ≥60 bpm. If no contributing medication identified, or if contributing medications are not discontinued or dose modified, resume alectinib at reduced dose upon recovery to asymptomatic bradycardia or to heart rate of ≥60 bpm. *If life-threatening bradycardia occurs*, permanently discontinue alectinib if no contributing medication is identified. If contributing medication is identified and discontinued, or its dose is adjusted, resume alectinib at reduced dose upon recovery to asymptomatic bradycardia or to heart rate of ≥60 bpm, with frequent monitoring as clinically indicated. Permanently discontinue alectinib in case of recurrence.
- Assess for myalgia periodically during therapy.
- ***Lab Test Considerations:*** Dose reduction schedule: 1st dose reduction—450 mg twice daily, 2nd dose reduction 300 mg twice daily. Discontinue if unable to tolerate 300 mg twice daily.
- Monitor liver function tests every 2 wk during first 3 mo of therapy, and then monthly and as clinically indicated during treatment. *If ALT or AST ↑ >5 times upper limit of normal (ULN) with total bilirubin ≤2 times ULN*, temporarily withhold until recovery to baseline or ≤3 times ULN, then resume at reduced dose. *If ALT or AST ↑ >3 times ULN with total bilirubin ↑ >2 times ULN in absence of cholestasis or hemolysis*, permanently discontinue alectinib. *If total bilirubin ↑ >3 times ULN*, temporarily withhold until recovery to baseline or to ≤1.5 times ULN, then resume at reduced dose.
- Assess CK every 2 wk during 1st mo of therapy and in patients reporting unexplained muscle pain, tenderness, or weakness. *If ↑ CK >5 times ULN*, temporarily withhold until recovery to baseline or ≤2.5 times ULN, then resume at same dose. *If ↑ CK >10 times ULN or 2nd occurrence of ↑ CK >5 times ULN*, temporarily withhold until recovery to baseline or ≤2.5 times ULN, then resume at reduced dose.
- Monitor serum creatinine periodically during therapy. *If Grade 3 renal impairment occurs*, hold doses until serum creatinine ≤ 1.5 times ULN, then resume at reduced dose. *If Grade 4 renal impairment occurs*, discontinue alectinib permanently.
- May cause hyperglycemia, hypocalcemia, hypokalemia, hypophosphatemia, and hyponatremia.
- May cause anemia and lymphopenia.

Implementation

- **PO:** Administer twice daily with food. Swallow capsules whole, do not open or dissolve capsule contents.

Patient/Family Teaching

- Instruct patient to take alectinib as directed. If a dose is missed or vomiting occurs after taking, omit dose and take next dose at scheduled time.
- Advise patient to use sunscreen and lip balm (SPF ≥50) and to wear protective clothing to prevent photosensitivity reaction.
- Advise patient to notify health care professional if signs and symptoms of liver problems (feeling tired, itchy skin, feeling less hungry than usual, nausea or vomiting, yellowing of skin or whites of eyes, pain on right side of stomach, dark urine, bleeding or bruising more easily than normal), respiratory problems (trouble breathing, shortness of breath, cough, fever), bradycardia (dizziness, lightheadedness, syncope), or myalgia (unexplained muscle pain, tenderness, or weakness) occur.
- Instruct patient to notify health care professional of all Rx or OTC medications, vitamins, or herbal products being taken and consult health care professional before taking any new medications.
- Rep: May cause teratogenic effects. Advise both male and female patients to use effective contraception during and for at least 1 wk following therapy. Advise female patients to avoid breast feeding during and for at least 1 wk following therapy.

Evaluation/Desired Outcomes

- Decreased spread of NSCLC.

alendronate (a-len-drone-ate)

Binosto, Fosamax

Classification

Therapeutic: bone resorption inhibitors
Pharmacologic: biphosphonates

Indications

Treatment and prevention of postmenopausal osteoporosis. Treatment of osteoporosis in men. Treatment of Paget's disease of the bone. Treatment of corticosteroid-induced osteoporosis in patients (men and women) who are receiving ≥7.5 mg of prednisone/day (or equivalent) with evidence of decreased bone mineral density.

Action
Inhibits resorption of bone by inhibiting osteoclast activity. **Therapeutic Effects:** Reversal of the progression of osteoporosis with decreased fractures. Decreased progression of Paget's disease.

Pharmacokinetics
Absorption: Poorly absorbed (0.6–0.8%) after oral administration.
Distribution: Transiently distributes to soft tissue, then distributes to bone.
Metabolism and Excretion: Excreted in urine.
Half-life: 10 yr (reflects release of drug from skeleton).

TIME/ACTION PROFILE (inhibition of bone resorption)

ROUTE	ONSET	PEAK	DURATION
PO	1 mo	3–6 mo	3 wk–7 mo†

†After discontinuation of alendronate.

Contraindications/Precautions
Contraindicated in: Abnormalities of the esophagus which delay esophageal emptying (i.e. strictures, achalasia); Inability to stand/sit upright for at least 30 min; Renal impairment (CCr <35 mL/min); OB: Pregnancy (may cause fetal harm).
Use Cautiously in: History of upper GI disorders; Pre-existing hypocalcemia or vitamin D deficiency; Invasive dental procedures, cancer, receiving chemotherapy, corticosteroids, or angiogenesis inhibitors, poor oral hygiene, periodontal disease, dental disease, anemia, coagulopathy, infection, or poorly-fitting dentures (may ↑ risk of jaw osteonecrosis); Lactation: Use while breast feeding only if potential maternal benefit justifies potential risk to infant; Pedi: Safety and effectiveness not established.

Adverse Reactions/Side Effects
CNS: headache. **CV:** atrial fibrillation. **Derm:** erythema, photosensitivity, rash. **EENT:** blurred vision, conjunctivitis, eye pain/inflammation. **GI:** abdominal distention, abdominal pain, acid regurgitation, constipation, diarrhea, dyspepsia, dysphagia, esophageal cancer, esophageal ulcer, esophagitis, flatulence, gastritis, nausea, taste perversion, vomiting. **MS:** musculoskeletal pain, femur fractures, osteonecrosis (primarily of jaw). **Resp:** asthma exacerbation.

Interactions
Drug-Drug: Calcium supplements, **antacids**, and **levothyroxine** may ↓ the absorption of alendronate. Doses >10 mg/day ↑ risk of adverse GI events when used with **NSAIDs**. IV **ranitidine** ↑ blood levels.
Drug-Food: Food significantly ↓ absorption. **Caffeine (coffee, tea, cola)**, **mineral water**, and **orange juice** also ↓ absorption.

Route/Dosage
PO (Adults): *Treatment of osteoporosis*—10 mg once daily or 70 mg once weekly. *Prevention of osteoporosis*—5 mg once daily or 35 mg once weekly. *Paget's disease*—40 mg once daily for 6 mo. Retreatment may be considered for patients who relapse. *Treatment of corticosteroid-induced osteoporosis in men and premenopausal women*—5 mg once daily. *Treatment of corticosteroid-induced osteoporosis in postmenopausal women not receiving estrogen*—10 mg once daily.

Availability (generic available)
Effervescent tablets (strawberry flavor): 70 mg. **Cost:** $168.00/4. **Oral solution (raspberry flavor):** 70 mg/75 mL. **Cost:** *Generic*—$23.44/75 mL. **Tablets:** 5 mg, 10 mg, 35 mg, 40 mg, 70 mg. **Cost:** *Generic*—10 mg $20.94/100, 35 mg $6.99/4, 70 mg $8.22/4. ***In combination with:*** Cholecalciferol (Fosamax plus D) See Appendix B.

NURSING IMPLICATIONS

Assessment
- **Osteoporosis:** Assess patients for low bone mass before and periodically during therapy.
- **Paget's Disease:** Assess for symptoms of Paget's disease (bone pain, headache, decreased visual and auditory acuity, increased skull size).
- ***Lab Test Considerations:*** *Osteoporosis:* Assess serum calcium before and periodically during therapy. Hypocalcemia and vitamin D deficiency should be treated before initiating alendronate therapy. May cause mild, transient ↑ of calcium and phosphate.
- **Paget's Disease:** Monitor alkaline phosphatase before and periodically during therapy. Alendronate is indicated for patients with alkaline phosphatase twice the upper limit of normal.

Implementation
- **PO:** Administer first thing in the morning with 6–8 oz plain water 30 min before other medications, beverages, or food. Oral solution should be followed by at least 2 oz of water. Swallow tablets whole; do not crush, break, or chew.
- For *effervescent tablets* dissolve 1 tablet in half a glass (4 oz) of plain room temperature water (not mineral water or flavored water). Wait at least 5 min after the effervescence stops, stir the solution for approximately 10 sec and drink contents.

Patient/Family Teaching
- Instruct patient on the importance of taking exactly as directed, first thing in the morning, 30 min before other medications, beverages, or food. Waiting longer than 30 min will improve absorption. Alendronate should be taken with 6–8 oz plain water

(mineral water, orange juice, coffee, and other beverages decrease absorption). If a dose is missed, skip dose and resume the next morning; do not double doses or take later in the day. If a weekly dose is missed, take the morning after remembered and resume the following wk on the chosen day. Do not take 2 tablets on the same day. Do not discontinue without consulting health care professional.

- Caution patient to remain upright for 30 min following dose to facilitate passage to stomach and minimize risk of esophageal irritation. Advise patient to discontinue alendronate and notify health care provider if pain or difficulty swallowing, retrosternal pain, or new/worsening heartburn occur.
- Advise patient to eat a balanced diet and consult health care professional about the need for supplemental calcium and vitamin D.
- Encourage patient to participate in regular exercise and to modify behaviors that increase the risk of osteoporosis (stop smoking, reduce alcohol consumption).
- Advise patient to inform health care professional of alendronate therapy prior to dental surgery.
- Caution patient to use sunscreen and protective clothing to prevent photosensitivity reactions.
- Advise patient to notify health care professional if blurred vision, eye pain, or inflammation occur.
- Advise female patient to notify health care professional if pregnancy is planned or suspected or if breast feeding.

Evaluation/Desired Outcomes

- Prevention of or decrease in the progression of osteoporosis in postmenopausal women. Reassess need for medication periodically. Consider discontinuation of alendronate after 3–5 yr in patients with low-risk of fractures. If discontinued, reassess fracture risk periodically.
- Treatment of osteoporosis in men.
- Decrease in the progression of Paget's disease.
- Treatment of corticosteroid-induced osteoporosis.

alfuzosin (al-fyoo-zo-sin)

Uroxatral, ✱Xatral

Classification

Therapeutic: urinary tract antispasmodics

Pharmacologic: peripherally acting antiadrenergics

Indications

Management of symptomatic benign prostatic hyperplasia (BPH).

Action

Selectively blocks $alpha_1$-adrenergic receptors in the lower urinary tract to relax smooth muscle in the bladder neck and prostate. **Therapeutic Effects:** Increased urine flow and decreased symptoms of BPH.

Pharmacokinetics

Absorption: 49% absorbed following oral administration; food enhances absorption.

Distribution: Unknown.

Metabolism and Excretion: Mostly metabolized by the liver (CYP3A4 enzyme system); 11% excreted unchanged in urine.

Half-life: 10 hr.

TIME/ACTION PROFILE

ROUTE	ONSET	PEAK	DURATION
PO-ER	within hr	8 hr	24 hr

Contraindications/Precautions

Contraindicated in: Hypersensitivity; Moderate to severe hepatic impairment; Potent inhibitors of the CYP3A4 enzyme system; Concurrent use of other alpha-adrenergic blocking agents; Severe renal impairment; Pedi: Children.

Use Cautiously in: Congenital or acquired QTc prolongation or concurrent use of other drugs known to prolong QTc; Mild hepatic impairment; Symptomatic hypotension; Concurrent use of antihypertensive agents, phosphodiesterase type 5 inhibitors, or nitrates (↑ risk of postural hypotension); Previous hypotensive episode with other medications; Geri: Consider age-related changes in body mass and cardiac, renal, and hepatic function when prescribing.

Adverse Reactions/Side Effects

CNS: dizziness, fatigue, headache. **EENT:** intraoperative floppy iris syndrome. **Derm:** TOXIC EPIDERMAL NECROLYSIS. **Resp:** bronchitis, sinusitis, pharyngitis. **CV:** postural hypotension. **GI:** abdominal pain, constipation, dyspepsia, nausea. **GU:** erectile dysfunction, priapism. **Hemat:** thrombocytopenia.

Interactions

Drug-Drug: Ketoconazole, **itraconazole**, and **ritonavir** ↓ metabolism and significantly ↑ levels and effects (concurrent use contraindicated). Levels are ↑ by **cimetidine**, **atenolol**, and **diltiazem**. May ↑ levels and effects of **atenolol** and **diltiazem** (monitor BP and heart rate). ↑ risk of hypotension with **antihypertensives**, **nitrates**, **phosphodiesterase type 5 inhibitors** (including **sildenafil**, **tadalafil**, and **vardenafil**) and acute ingestion of **alcohol**.

Route/Dosage

PO (Adults): 10 mg once daily.

Availability (generic available)

Extended-release tablets: 10 mg.

NURSING IMPLICATIONS

Assessment

- Assess for symptoms of benign prostatic hyperplasia (urinary hesitancy, feeling of incomplete bladder emptying, interruption of urinary stream, impairment of size and force of urinary stream, terminal urinary dribbling, straining to start flow, dysuria, urgency) before and periodically during therapy.

- Assess for orthostatic reaction and syncope. Monitor BP (lying and standing) and pulse frequently during initial dose adjustment and periodically thereafter. May occur within a few hr after initial doses and occasionally thereafter.
- Rule out prostatic carcinoma before therapy; symptoms are similar.

Implementation

- **PO:** Administer with food at the same meal each day. Tablets must be swallowed whole; do not crush, break, or chew.

Patient/Family Teaching

- Instruct patient to take medication with the same meal each day. Take missed doses as soon as remembered. If not remembered until next day, omit; do not double doses.
- May cause dizziness or drowsiness. Advise patient to avoid driving or other activities requiring alertness until response to the medication is known.
- Caution patient to avoid sudden changes in position to decrease orthostatic hypotension.
- Advise patient to consult health care professional before taking any cough, cold, or allergy remedies.
- Instruct patient to notify health care professional of medication regimen before any surgery, especially cataract surgery.
- Advise patient to notify health care professional if priapism, angina, frequent dizziness, rash, or fainting occurs.
- Emphasize the importance of follow-up exams to evaluate effectiveness of medication.
- Geri: Assess risk for falls; implement fall prevention program and instruct patient and family in preventing falls at home.

Evaluation/Desired Outcomes

- Decreased symptoms of benign prostatic hyperplasia.

alirocumab (a-li-**roe**-kyoo-mab)

Praluent

Classification

Therapeutic: lipid-lowering agents

Pharmacologic: proprotein convertase subtilisin kexin type 9 (PCSK9) inhibitor antibodies

Indications

Lowering of low density lipoprotein cholesterol (LDL-C) as an adjunct to diet, as monotherapy or in combination with other lipid-lowering therapies (e.g. statin, ezetimibe) in patients with primary hyperlipidemia. Reduction in risk of MI, stroke, and unstable angina requiring hospitalization in patients with established cardiovascular disease.

Action

A human monoclonal immunoglobulin (IgG1) produced in genetically engineered Chinese hamster ovary cells that binds to PCSK9 inhibiting its binding to the low density lipoprotein receptor (LDLR) resulting in ↑ number of LDLRs available to clear LDL from blood. **Therapeutic Effects:** ↓ LDL-C. Reduction in risk of MI, stroke, and unstable angina requiring hospitalization.

Pharmacokinetics

Absorption: Well absorbed (85%) following subcut administration.

Distribution: Mostly distributed in the circulatory system; crosses the placenta.

Metabolism and Excretion: Eliminated by binding to PCSK9 and by proteolytic degradation.

Half-life: 17–20 days.

TIME/ACTION PROFILE (effect circulating unbound PCSK9)

ROUTE	ONSET	PEAK	DURATION
subcut	rapid	4–8 hr	2 wk

Contraindications/Precautions

Contraindicated in: History of serious hypersensitivity to alirocumab.

Use Cautiously in: Severe renal/hepatic impairment; OB: Crosses the placenta, consider fetal risks; Lactation: Consider benefits of breast feeding against possible risk to infant; Pedi: Safety and effectiveness not established; Geri: Elderly patients may be more sensitive to drug effects.

Adverse Reactions/Side Effects

CNS: confusion. **Local:** injection site reactions. **Misc:** serious allergic reactions (including vasculitis).

Interactions

Drug-Drug: None noted.

Route/Dosage

Subcut (Adults): 75 mg every 2 wk; if desired LDL-C has not been achieved, may ↑ dose to 150 mg every 2 wk. If less frequent dosing desired, may initiate therapy with 300 mg every 4 wk; if desired LDL-C has not been achieved, may adjust dose to 150 mg every 2 wk. *Patients undergoing apheresis*—150 mg every 2 wk.

Availability

Solution for injection (prefilled pens or prefilled syringes): 75 mg/mL, 150 mg/mL.

NURSING IMPLICATIONS

Assessment

- Obtain a diet history, especially with regard to fat consumption.

- Monitor for signs and symptoms of hypersensitivity reactions (pruritus, rash, urticaria, hypersensitivity vasculitis and hypersensitivity reactions requiring hospitalization) during therapy. If severe symptoms occur, discontinue alirocumab.
- ***Lab Test Considerations:*** Assess LDL-C levels within 4–8 wk of initiating or titrating alirocumab for patients taking every 2 wk or just before next dose for patients taking every 4 wk, to assess response and adjust dose, if needed.

Implementation

- **Subcut:** Allow solution to warm to room temperature for 30–40 min before injecting. May be kept at room temperature for up to 30 days. Solution is clear and colorless to pale yellow; do not administer solutions that are cloudy or contain particulate matter. Do not shake. Inject into thigh, abdomen, or upper arm. Rotate sites with each injection. Do not inject into areas with skin disease or injury (sunburns, rashes, inflammation, skin infections). Do not reuse prefilled pen or syringe. Do not administer other injectable drugs at same site. Store in refrigerator; keep in original container, protect from light. Do not freeze.
- Administer 300 mg dose as two 150 mg injections in 2 different sites.

Patient/Family Teaching

- Instruct patient in correct technique for self-injection, care and disposal of equipment. Administer missed doses within 7 days, then resume original schedule. If not administered within 7 days, wait until next dose on original schedule. Advise patient to read *Patient Information* before starting therapy and with each Rx refill in case of changes.
- Advise patient that this medication should be used in conjunction with diet restrictions (fat, cholesterol, carbohydrates, alcohol), exercise, and cessation of smoking.
- Instruct patient to notify health care professional of all Rx or OTC medications, vitamins, or herbal products being taken and to consult health care professional before taking any other Rx, OTC, or herbal products.
- Advise patient to notify health care professional of medication regimen prior to treatment or surgery.
- Rep: Advise patient to notify health care professional if pregnancy is planned or suspected or if breast feeding. Encourage pregnant women to enroll in the pregnancy exposure registry that monitors pregnancy outcomes in women exposed to alirocumab during pregnancy by calling 1-877-311-8972 or go to https://mothertobaby.org/ongoing-study/praluent/ to enroll in or to obtain information about registry.

Evaluation/Desired Outcomes

- ↓ LDL-C levels.

allopurinol (al-oh-**pure**-i-nole)

Aloprim, Lopurin, Zyloprim

Classification

Therapeutic: antigout agents, antihyperuricemics

Pharmacologic: xanthine oxidase inhibitors

Indications

PO: Prevention of attack of gouty arthritis and nephropathy. **PO, IV:** Treatment of secondary hyperuricemia, which may occur during treatment of tumors or leukemias.

Action

Inhibits the production of uric acid by inhibiting the action of xanthine oxidase. **Therapeutic Effects:** Lowering of serum uric acid levels.

Pharmacokinetics

Absorption: Well absorbed (80%) following oral administration.

Distribution: Widely distributed in tissue and breast milk.

Protein Binding: <1%.

Metabolism and Excretion: Metabolized to oxypurinol, an active compound with a long half-life. 12% excreted unchanged, 76% excreted as oxypurinol.

Half-life: 1–3 hr (oxypurinol 18–30 hr).

TIME/ACTION PROFILE (hypouricemic effect)

ROUTE	ONSET	PEAK	DURATION
PO, IV	1–2 days	1–2 wk	1–3 wk†

†Duration after discontinuation of allopurinol.

Contraindications/Precautions

Contraindicated in: Hypersensitivity.

Use Cautiously in: Acute attacks of gout; Renal insufficiency (dose ↓ required if CCr <20 mL/min); Dehydration (adequate hydration necessary); OB, Lactation: Rarely used; Geri: Begin at lower end of dosage range.

Adverse Reactions/Side Effects

CNS: drowsiness. **CV:** hypotension, flushing, hypertension, bradycardia, and heart failure (reported with IV administration). **Derm:** <u>rash (discontinue drug at first sign of rash)</u>, urticaria. **GI:** diarrhea, hepatitis, nausea, vomiting. **GU:** renal failure, hematuria. **Hemat:** bone marrow depression. **Misc:** hypersensitivity reactions.

Interactions

Drug-Drug: Use with **mercaptopurine** and **azathioprine** ↑ bone marrow depressant properties—doses of these drugs should be ↓. Use with **ampicillin** or **amoxicillin** ↑ risk of rash. Use with **oral hypoglycemic agents** and **warfarin** ↑ effects of these drugs.

Use with **thiazide diuretics** or **ACE inhibitors** ↑ risk of hypersensitivity reactions. Large doses of allopurinol may ↑ risk of **theophylline** toxicity. May ↑ **cyclosporine** levels.

Route/Dosage

Management of Gout

PO (Adults and Children >10 yr): *Initially*—100 mg/day; ↑ at weekly intervals based on serum uric acid (not to exceed 800 mg/day). Doses >300 mg/day should be given in divided doses; *Maintenance dose*—100–200 mg 2–3 times daily. Doses of ≤300 mg may be given as a single daily dose.

Management of Secondary Hyperuricemia

PO (Adults and Children >10 yr): 600–800 mg/day in 2–3 divided doses starting 1–2 days before chemotherapy or radiation.

PO (Children 6–10 yr): 10 mg/kg/day in 2–3 divided doses (maximum 800 mg/day) or 300 mg daily in 2–3 divided doses.

PO (Children <6 yr): 10 mg/kg/day in 2–3 divided doses (maximum 800 mg/day) or 150 mg daily in 3 divided doses.

IV (Adults and Children >10 yr): 200–400 mg/m²/day (up to 600 mg/day) as a single daily dose or in divided doses every 8–24 hr.

IV (Children <10 yr): 200 mg/m²/day initially as a single daily dose or in divided doses every 8–24 hr (maximum dose 600 mg/day).

Renal Impairment

(Adults and Children): *CCr 10–50 mL/min*—↓ dose to 50% of recommended; *CCr <10 mL/min*—↓ dosage to 30% of recommended.

Availability (generic available)

Powder for injection: 500 mg/vial. **Tablets:** 100 mg, ✤200 mg, 300 mg. **Cost:** *Generic*—100 mg $10.83/100, 300 mg $10.83/100.

NURSING IMPLICATIONS

Assessment

- Monitor intake and output ratios. Decreased kidney function can cause drug accumulation and toxic effects. Ensure that patient maintains adequate fluid intake (minimum 2500–3000 mL/day) to minimize risk of kidney stone formation.
- Assess patient for rash or more severe hypersensitivity reactions. Discontinue allopurinol immediately if rash occurs. Therapy should be discontinued permanently if reaction is severe. Therapy may be reinstated after a mild reaction has subsided, at a lower dose (50 mg/day with very gradual titration). If skin rash recurs, discontinue permanently.
- **Gout:** Monitor for joint pain and swelling. Addition of colchicine or NSAIDs may be necessary for acute attacks. Prophylactic doses of colchicine or an NSAID should be administered concurrently during first 3–6 mo of therapy because of an increased frequency of acute attacks of gouty arthritis during early therapy.
- ***Lab Test Considerations:*** Serum and urine uric acid levels usually begin to ↓ 2–3 days after initiation of oral therapy.
- Monitor blood glucose in patients receiving oral hypoglycemic agents. May cause hypoglycemia.
- Monitor hematologic, renal, and liver function tests before and periodically during therapy, especially during the first few mo. May cause ↑ serum alkaline phosphatase, bilirubin, AST, and ALT levels. ↓ CBC and platelets may indicate bone marrow depression. ↑ BUN, serum creatinine, and CCr may indicate nephrotoxicity. These are usually reversed with discontinuation of therapy.

Implementation

- Do not confuse Zyloprim with zolpidem.
- **PO:** May be administered after milk or meals to minimize gastric irritation; give with plenty of fluid. May be crushed and given with fluid or mixed with food for patients who have difficulty swallowing.

IV Administration

- **Intermittent Infusion:** Reconstitute each 500 mg vial with 25 mL of sterile water for injection. Solution should be clear and almost colorless with only slight opalescence. ***Diluent:*** Dilute to desired concentration with 0.9% NaCl or D5W. Administer within 10 hr of reconstitution; do not refrigerate. Do not administer solutions that are discolored or contain particulate matter. ***Concentration:*** Not >6 m g/mL. ***Rate:*** Infusion should be initiated 24–48 hr before start of chemotherapy known to cause tumor cell lysis. Rate of infusion depends on volume of infusate (100–300 mg doses may be infused over 30 min). May be administered as a single infusion or equally divided infusions at 6-, 8-, or 12-hr intervals.
- **Y-Site Compatibility:** acyclovir, aminophylline, amphotericin B lipid complex, anidulafungin, argatroban, aztreonam, bivalirudin, bleomycin, bumetanide, buprenorphine, butorphanol, calcium gluconate, carboplatin, caspofungin, cefazolin, cefotetan, ceftazidime, ceftriaxone, cefuroxime, cisplatin, cyclophosphamide, dactinomycin, dexamethasone sodium phosphate, dexmedetomidine, docetaxel, doxorubicin liposome, enalaprilat, etoposide, famotidine, fenoldopam, filgrastim, fluconazole, fludarabine, fluorouracil, fosphenytoin, furosemide, ganciclovir, gemcitabine, granisetron, heparin, hetastarch, hydrocortisone, hydromorphone, ifosfamide,

leucovorin calcium, linezolid, lorazepam, mannitol, mesna, methotrexate, milrinone, mitoxantrone, morphine, octreotide, oxytocin, paclitaxel, pamidronate, pantoprazole, pemetrexed, piperacillin/tazobactam, potassium chloride, ranitidine, sodium acetate, thiotepa, tigecycline, tirofiban, trimethoprim/sulfamethoxazole, vancomycin, vasopressin, vinblastine, vincristine, voriconazole, zidovudine, zoledronic acid.

- **Y-Site Incompatibility:** alemtuzumab, amikacin, amiodarone, carmustine, cefotaxime, chlorpromazine, clindamycin, cytarabine, dacarbazine, daptomycin, daunorubicin, dexrazoxane, diltiazem, diphenhydramine, doxorubicin, doxycycline, droperidol, epirubicin, ertapenem, etoposide phosphate, floxuridine, foscarnet, gentamicin, haloperidol, hydroxyzine, idarubicin, imipenem/cilastatin, irinotecan, meperidine, methylprednisolone sodium succinate, metoprolol, minocycline, mitomycin, moxifloxacin, mycophenolate, nalbuphine, ondansetron, palonosetron, pancuronium, potassium acetate, prochlorperazine, promethazine, sodium bicarbonate, streptozocin, tacrolimus, tobramycin, topotecan, vecuronium, vinorelbine.

Patient/Family Teaching

- Instruct patient to take allopurinol as directed. Take missed doses as soon as remembered. If dosing schedule is once daily, do not take if remembered the next day. If dosing schedule is more than once a day, take up to 300 mg for next dose.
- Instruct patient to continue taking allopurinol along with an NSAID or colchicine during an acute attack of gout. Allopurinol helps prevent, but does not relieve, acute gout attacks.
- Alkaline diet may be ordered. Urinary acidification with large doses of vitamin C or other acids may increase kidney stone formation (see Appendix K). Advise patient of need for increased fluid intake.
- May occasionally cause drowsiness. Caution patient to avoid driving or other activities requiring alertness until response to drug is known.
- Instruct patient to report skin rash, blood in urine, or influenza symptoms (chills, fever, muscle aches and pains, nausea, or vomiting) to health care professional immediately; skin rash may indicate hypersensitivity.
- Advise patient that large amounts of alcohol increase uric acid concentrations and may decrease the effectiveness of allopurinol.
- Emphasize the importance of follow-up exams to monitor effectiveness and side effects.

Evaluation/Desired Outcomes

- Decreased serum and urinary uric acid levels. May take 2–6 wk to observe clinical improvement in patients treated for gout.

almotriptan (al-moe-**trip**-tan)

~~Axert~~

Classification

Therapeutic: vascular headache suppressants

Pharmacologic: 5-HT_1 agonists

Indications

Acute treatment of migraine headache (for adolescents, migraines should be ≥4 hr in duration).

Action

Acts as an agonist at specific 5-HT_1 receptor sites in intracranial blood vessels and sensory trigeminal nerves. **Therapeutic Effects:** Cranial vessel vasoconstriction with associated decrease in release of neuropeptides and resultant decrease in migraine headache.

Pharmacokinetics

Absorption: Well absorbed following oral administration (70%).

Distribution: Unknown.

Metabolism and Excretion: 40% excreted unchanged in urine; 27% metabolized by monoamine oxidase-A (MAO-A); 12% metabolized by CYP3A4 and CYP2D6; 13% excreted in feces as unchanged and metabolized drug.

Half-life: 3–4 hr.

TIME/ACTION PROFILE (Blood levels)

ROUTE	ONSET	PEAK	DURATION
PO	unknown	1–3 hr	unknown

Contraindications/Precautions

Contraindicated in: Hypersensitivity; Ischemic cardiovascular, cerebrovascular, or peripheral vascular syndromes (including ischemic bowel disease); History of significant cardiovascular disease; Uncontrolled hypertension; Should not be used within 24 hr of other 5-HT_1 agonists or ergot-type compounds (dihydroergotamine); Basilar or hemiplegic migraine; Concurrent MAO-A inhibitor therapy or within 2 wk of discontinuing MAO-A inhibitor therapy.

Use Cautiously in: Cardiovascular risk factors (hypertension, hypercholesterolemia, cigarette smoking, obesity, diabetes, strong family history, menopausal women or men >40 yr); use only if cardiovascular status has been evaluated and determined to be safe and first dose is administered under supervision; Impaired hepatic or renal function; Hypersensitivity to sulfonamides (cross-sensitivity may occur); OB, Lactation: Safety not established; Pedi: Children <12 yr (safety and effectiveness not established).

Adverse Reactions/Side Effects

CNS: drowsiness, headache. **CV:** CORONARY ARTERY VASOSPASM, MI, VENTRICULAR ARRHYTHMIAS, myocardial ischemia. **GI:** dry mouth, nausea. **Neuro:** paresthesia.

A

Interactions

Drug-Drug: Concurrent use with **MAO-A inhibitors** ↑ blood levels and the risk of adverse reactions (concurrent use or use within 2 wk or MAO inhibitor is contraindicated). Concurrent use with other **5-HT$_1$ agonists** or **ergot-type compounds (dihydroergotamine)** may result in additive vasoactive properties (avoid use within 24 hr of each other). ↑ serotonin levels and serotonin syndrome may occur when used concurrently with **SSRI and SNRI antidepressants**. Blood levels and effects may be ↑ by **ketoconazole**, **itraconazole**, **ritonavir**, and **erythromycin** (inhibitors of CYP3A4 enzymes).

Route/Dosage

PO (Adults and Children ≥12 yr): 6.25–12.5 mg initially, may repeat in 2 hr; not to exceed 2 doses per 24-hr period.

Hepatic/Renal Impairment

PO (Adults): 6.25 mg initially, may repeat in 2 hr; not to exceed 2 doses per 24-hr period.

Availability (generic available)

Tablets: 6.25 mg, 12.5 mg.

NURSING IMPLICATIONS

Assessment

- Assess pain location, character, intensity, and duration and associated symptoms (photophobia, phonophobia, nausea, vomiting) during migraine attack.
- Assess for serotonin syndrome (mental changes [agitation, hallucinations, coma], autonomic instability [tachycardia, labile BP, hyperthermia], neuromuscular aberrations [hyperreflexia, incoordination], and/or GI symptoms [nausea, vomiting, diarrhea]), especially in patients taking other serotonergic drugs (SSRIs, SNRIs).

Implementation

- **PO:** Tablets should be swallowed whole with liquid.

Patient/Family Teaching

- Inform patient that almotriptan should only be used during a migraine attack. It is meant to be used for relief of migraine attacks but not to prevent or reduce the number of attacks.
- Instruct patient to administer almotriptan as soon as symptoms of a migraine attack appear, but it may be administered any time during an attack. If migraine symptoms return, a 2nd dose may be used. Allow at least 2 hr between doses, and do not use more than 2 doses in any 24-hr period.
- If first dose does not relieve headache, additional almotriptan doses are not likely to be effective; notify health care professional.
- Caution patient not to take almotriptan within 24 hr of another vascular headache suppressant.
- Advise patient that lying down in a darkened room following almotriptan administration may further help relieve headache.
- Advise patient that overuse (use more than 10 days/month) may lead to exacerbation of headache (migraine-like daily headaches, or as a marked increase in frequency of migraine attacks). May require gradual withdrawal of almotriptan and treatment of symptoms (transient worsening of headache).
- **Advise patient to notify health care professional prior to next dose of almotriptan if pain or tightness in the chest occurs during use. If pain is severe or does not subside, notify health care professional immediately. If feelings of tingling, heat, flushing, heaviness, pressure, drowsiness, dizziness, tiredness, or sickness develop discuss with health care professional at next visit.**
- May cause dizziness or drowsiness. Caution patient to avoid driving or other activities requiring alertness until response to medication is known.
- Advise patient to avoid alcohol, which aggravates headaches, during almotriptan use.
- Advise patient to notify health care professional of all Rx or OTC medications, vitamins, or herbal products being taken and to consult with health care professional before taking other medications.
- Advise patient to notify health care professional immediately if signs or symptoms of serotonin syndrome occur.
- Advise females of reproductive potential to notify health care professional if pregnancy is planned or suspected, or if breast feeding.

Evaluation/Desired Outcomes

- Relief of migraine attack.

alogliptin (al-oh-glip-tin)

Nesina

Classification

Therapeutic: antidiabetics

Pharmacologic: dipeptidyl peptidase-4 (DDP-4) inhibitors

Indications

Adjunct to diet and exercise to improve glycemic control in type 2 diabetes mellitus.

Action

Acts as a competitive inhibitor of dipeptidyl peptidase-4 (DPP-4) which slows the inactivation of incretin hormones, thereby increasing their concentrations and reducing fasting and postprandial glucose concentrations. **Therapeutic Effects:** Improved control of blood glucose.

Pharmacokinetics

Absorption: Completely absorbed following oral administration (100%).

Distribution: Well distributed into tissues.

Metabolism and Excretion: Not extensively metabolized, 76% excreted unchanged in urine.

Half-life: 21 hr.

TIME/ACTION PROFILE (inhibition of DPP-4)

ROUTE	ONSET	PEAK†	DURATION
PO	unknown	1–2 hr	24 hr

†Multiple dosing.

Contraindications/Precautions

Contraindicated in: Type 1 diabetes; Diabetic ketoacidosis; Previous severe hypersensitivity reactions.

Use Cautiously in: Hepatic impairment; Renal impairment (dose ↓ required if CCr <60 mL/min); HF or renal impairment (↑ risk for worsening HF); OB: Use only if potential maternal benefit justifies potential fetal risk; Lactation: Use while breast feeding only if potential maternal benefit justifies potential risk to infant; Pedi: Safety and effectiveness not established; Geri: May have ↑ sensitivity to effects.

Adverse Reactions/Side Effects

CNS: headache. **CV:** HF. **Derm:** STEVENS-JOHNSON SYNDROME, bullous pemphigoid. **GI:** HEPATOTOXICITY, PANCREATITIS, ↑ liver enzymes. **MS:** RHABDOMYOLYSIS, arthralgia. **Misc:** HYPERSENSITIVITY REACTIONS (including anaphylaxis or angioedema).

Interactions

Drug-Drug: ↑ risk of hypoglycemia with **sulfonylureas** and **insulin**; dose adjustments may be necessary.

Route/Dosage

PO (Adults): 25 mg once daily.

Renal Impairment

PO (Adults): *CCr 30–59 mL/min*—12.5 mg once daily; *CCr 15–29 mL/min*—6.25 mg once daily; *CCr <15 mL/min or requiring hemodialysis*—6.25 mg once daily.

Availability

Tablets: 6.25 mg, 12.5 mg, 25 mg. ***In combination with:*** metformin (Kazano), pioglitazone (Oseni).

NURSING IMPLICATIONS

Assessment

- Observe for signs and symptoms of hypoglycemic reactions (abdominal pain, sweating, hunger, weakness, dizziness, headache, tremor, tachycardia, anxiety).
- Monitor for signs of pancreatitis (nausea, vomiting, anorexia, persistent severe abdominal pain, sometimes radiating to the back) during therapy. If pancreatitis occurs, discontinue alogliptin and monitor serum and urine amylase, amylase/CCr ratio, electrolytes, serum calcium, glucose, and lipase.
- Assess for signs and symptoms of HF (increasing shortness of breath, rapid increase in weight, swelling of feet) periodically during therapy.
- Assess for rash periodically during therapy. May cause Stevens-Johnson syndrome. Discontinue therapy if severe or if accompanied with fever, general malaise, fatigue, muscle or joint aches, blisters, oral lesions, conjunctivitis, hepatitis, and/or eosinophilia.
- ***Lab Test Considerations:*** Monitor hemoglobin A1C prior to and periodically during therapy.
- Monitor liver function tests prior to starting and periodically during therapy. Interrupt therapy and determine cause if significant ↑ in enzymes or abnormal tests persist or worsen. Do not restart therapy without explanation for abnormalities.
- Monitor renal function prior to and periodically during therapy.

Implementation

- Patients stabilized on a diabetic regimen who are exposed to stress, fever, trauma, infection, or surgery may require administration of insulin.
- **PO:** May be administered without regard to food.

Patient/Family Teaching

- Instruct patient to take alogliptin as directed. Take missed doses as soon as remembered, unless it is almost time for next dose; do not double doses. Advise patient to read *Medication Guide* before starting and with each Rx refill in case of changes.
- Explain to patient that alogliptin helps control hyperglycemia but does not cure diabetes. Therapy is usually long term.
- Instruct patient not to share this medication with others, even if they have the same symptoms; it may harm them.
- Encourage patient to follow prescribed diet, medication, and exercise regimen to prevent hyperglycemic or hypoglycemic episodes.
- Review signs of hypoglycemia and hyperglycemia with patient. If hypoglycemia occurs, advise patient to take a glass of orange juice or 2–3 tsp of sugar, honey, or corn syrup dissolved in water, and notify health care professional.
- Instruct patient in proper testing of blood glucose and urine ketones. These tests should be monitored closely during periods of stress or illness and health care professional notified if significant changes occur.
- Advise patient to stop taking alogliptin and notify health care professional promptly if symptoms of hypersensitivity reactions (rash; hives; swelling of face, lips, tongue, and throat; difficulty in breathing or swallowing), liver dysfunction (fatigue, nausea, vomiting, anorexia, right upper abdominal discomfort, dark urine, yellowing of skin or whites of eyes), HF, or pancreatitis occur.

- Advise patient to notify health care professional of all Rx or OTC medications, vitamins, or herbal products being taken and to consult with health care professional before taking other medications.
- Instruct patient to notify health care professional if severe joint pain occurs.
- Advise patient to notify health care professional if pregnancy is planned or suspected or if breast feeding.

Evaluation/Desired Outcomes

- Improved hemoglobin A1C, fasting plasma glucose and 2-hr post-prandial glucose levels.

alpelisib (al-pe-lisib)

Piqray

Classification
Therapeutic: antineoplastics
Pharmacologic: kinase inhibitors

Indications

Treatment of postmenopausal women and men with hormone receptor (HR)-positive, human epidermal growth factor receptor 2 (HER2)-negative, PIK3CA-mutated, advanced or metastatic breast cancer (in combination with fulvestrant).

Action

Acts as an inhibitor of phosphatidylinositol 3–kinase (PI3K). Mutations in the gene encoding the catalytic α-subunit of PI3K (PI3KCA) lead to activation of PI3Kα and Akt-signaling, cellular transformation, and tumor generation. Alpelisib inhibits phosphorylation of PI3K downstream targets (including Akt) and demonstrated activity in cell lines harboring a PIK3CA mutation.
Therapeutic Effects: Decreased progression of breast cancer.

Pharmacokinetics

Absorption: Well absorbed following oral administration.
Distribution: Widely distributed to tissues.
Metabolism and Excretion: Primarily metabolized via hydrolysis; also metabolized to a lesser extent by CYP3A4. Excreted in feces (36% as unchanged drug; 32% as metabolites) and urine (2% as unchanged drug; 7% as metabolites).
Half-life: 8–9 hr.

TIME/ACTION PROFILE (plasma concentrations)

ROUTE	ONSET	PEAK	DURATION
PO	unknown	2–4 hr	24 hr

Contraindications/Precautions

Contraindicated in: History of serious hypersensitivity reactions including anaphylaxis, Steven-Johnson syndrome, or erythema multiforme; History of Stevens-Johnson syndrome, erythema multiforme, or toxic epidermal necrolysis; Concurrent use of strong inducers or substrates of CYP3A; OB: Pregnancy (may cause fetal harm); Lactation: Lactation.
Use Cautiously in: Diabetes; Severe renal impairment (CCr ≤30 mL/min); Rep: Women of reproductive potential and men with female partners of reproductive potential; Pedi: Safety and effectiveness not established; Geri: May be more sensitive to drug effects.

Adverse Reactions/Side Effects

CNS: fatigue, headache, insomnia. **CV:** peripheral edema. **Derm:** ERYTHEMA MULTIFORME, STEVENS-JOHNSON SYNDROME, alopecia, dry skin, pruritus, rash. **Endo:** KETOACIDOSIS, hyperglycemia, hypoglycemia. **F and E:** hypocalcemia, hypokalemia. **GI:** DIARRHEA, abdominal pain, ↓ appetite, ↑ lipase, ↑ liver enzymes, metallic taste, nausea, stomatitis, vomiting. **GU:** acute kidney injury, ↓ fertility. **Hemat:** anemia, lymphocytopenia, thrombocytopenia. **Metab:** ↓ weight, hypertriglyceridemia, hypoalbuminemia, hypomagnesemia. **Resp:** PNEUMONITIS, cough. **Misc:** HYPERSENSITIVITY REACTIONS (including anaphylaxis), INFECTION, fever.

Interactions

Drug-Drug: Strong CYP3A4 inducers may ↓ levels and effectiveness; avoid concurrent use. **BCRP inhibitors** may ↑ levels and risk of toxicity; avoid concurrent use. May ↓ levels of **CYP2C9 substrates**, including **warfarin**.

Route/Dosage

PO (Adults): 300 mg once daily until disease progression or unacceptable toxicity.

Availability

Tablets: 50 mg, 150 mg, 200 mg.

NURSING IMPLICATIONS

Assessment

- Monitor for signs and symptoms of hypersensitivity reactions (dyspnea, flushing, rash, fever, tachycardia) during therapy. If symptoms occur, permanently discontinue alpelisib.
- Assess for skin reactions (prodrome of fever, flu-like symptoms, mucosal lesions, progressive skin rash) during therapy. *If rash is Grade 1 (< 10% body surface area (BSA) with active skin toxicity);* No dose adjustment needed. Initiate topical corticosteroid treatment. Consider adding oral antihistamine to manage symptoms. *If Grade 2 (10-30% BSA with active skin toxicity);* No dose adjustment necessary. Initiate or intensify topical corticosteroid and oral antihistamines. Consider low dose systemic corticosteroid treatment. *If Grade 3 (severe rash not responsive to medical management and >30%*

BSA with active skin toxicity): Hold alpelisib. Initiate or intensify topical/systemic corticosteroid and oral antihistamines. Once ≤ Grade 1, resume alpelisib at same dose level for first occurrence of rash, or at next lower dose level if second occurrence. *If Grade 4 (severe bullous, blistering or exfoliating skin conditions and any % BSA associated with extensive superinfection, with IV antibiotics indicated; life-threatening):* Permanently discontinue alpelisib.

- Monitor for signs and symptoms of pneumonitis (hypoxia, cough, dyspnea, interstitial infiltrates) during therapy. If pneumonitis is confirmed, discontinue alpelisib permanently.
- Monitor for signs and symptoms of diarrhea during therapy. *If Grade 1 diarrhea occurs,* do not adjust alpelisib dose. Start antidiarrheal therapy and monitor symptoms. *If Grade 2 diarrhea occurs,* start or intensify antidiarrheal therapy and monitor symptoms. Hold alpelisib until recovery to Grade ≤1, then resume at same dose. *If Grade 3 or 4 diarrhea occurs,* start or intensify antidiarrheal therapy and monitor symptoms. Hold alpelisib until recovery to Grade ≤1, then resume at the next lower dose.
- ***Lab Test Considerations:*** Obtain a negative pregnancy test before starting therapy.
- Information on FDA approved tests for the detection of PIK3CA mutations in breast cancer is available at: http://www.fda.gov/CompanionDiagnostics.
- May cause hyperglycemia. Before starting alpelisib therapy, test fasting blood glucose (FBG) and HbA1c; optimize blood glucose. After starting therapy, monitor blood glucose at least weekly for first 2 wk, then at least once every 4 wk, and as indicated. Monitor HbA1c every 3 mo and as indicated. *If Grade 1 FBG >upper limit of normal (ULN)-160 mg/dL or >ULN-8.9 mmol/L:* No dose adjustment needed. Initiate or intensify anti-diabetic treatment. *If Grade 2 FBG >160-250 mg/dL or >8.9-13.9 mmol/L:* No dose adjustment needed. Initiate or further intensify anti-diabetic therapy. If FBG does not decrease to ≤ 160 mg/dL or 8.9 mmol/L within 21 days, reduce alpelisib dose by 1 dose level and follow FBG value recommendations. *If Grade 3 >250-500 mg/dL or >13.9-27.8 mmol/L:* Hold alpelisib. Initiate or intensify oral anti-diabetic therapy and consider additional anti-diabetic agents for 1-2 days until hyperglycemia improves. Administer intravenous hydration and consider added intervention for electrolyte/ketoacidosis/hyperosmolar disturbances). If FBG decreases to ≤160 mg/dL or 8.9 mmol/L within 3 to 5 days under appropriate anti-diabetic therapy, resume alpelisib at 1 lower dose level. If FBG does not decrease to ≤160 mg/dL or 8.9 mmol/L within 3 to 5 days under appropriate anti-diabetic therapy, consult with a specialist in the treatment of hyperglycemia. If FBG does not decrease to ≤160 mg/dL or 8.9 mmol/L within 21 days following appropriate anti-diabetic therapy, permanently discontinue alpelisib. *If Grade 4 >500 m g/dL or ≥27.8 mmol/L:* Hold alpelisib. Initiate or intensify appropriate anti-diabetic therapy (administer intravenous hydration and consider appropriate intervention for electrolyte/ketoacidosis/hyperosmolar disturbances), re-check FBG within 24 hrs and as indicated. If FBG decreases to ≤500 mg/dL or 27.8 mmol/L, follow FBG recommendations for Grade 3. If FBG is confirmed at >500 m g/dL or 27.8 mmol/L, discontinue alpelisib permanently.

Implementation

- When starting at 300 mg once daily, two 150 mg tablets, dose adjustments for adverse reactions include *First-dose reduction:* 250 mg once daily, one 200 mg tablet and one 50 mg tablet. *Second-dose reduction:* 200 mg tablet once daily.
- **PO:** Administer with food once daily at same time of day. Swallow tablets whole, do not crush, break, or chew.
- When administered with fulvestrant, fulvestrant 500 mg is usually given on Days 1, 15, and 29, and once monthly thereafter.

Patient/Family Teaching

- Instruct patient to take alpelisib as directed. Take missed doses with food within 9 hrs of time usually taken. If >9 hrs, omit dose and take next dose next day at usual time. If patient vomits after dose, skip dose and take next dose next day. Advise patient to read *Patient Information* before starting and with each Rx refill in case of changes.
- Advise patients to notify health care professional of the signs and symptoms of hypersensitivity reactions, skin reaction, hyperglycemia (e.g., excessive thirst, urinating more often than usual or higher amount of urine than usual, or increased appetite with weight loss), and lung problems occur. Advise patients to immediately report new or worsening respiratory symptoms.
- If diarrhea occurs, advise patient to start antidiarrheal treatment, increase oral fluids, and notify health care professional.
- Advise patient to notify health care professional of all Rx or OTC medications, vitamins, or herbal products being taken and to consult health care professional before taking any new medications.
- Rep: May be teratogenic. Advise females of reproductive potential and males with female partners of reproductive potential to use effective contraception during and for 1 wk after last dose. Advise patient to avoid breast feeding during and for 1 wk after last dose. May impair fertility in male and female patients.

Evaluation/Desired Outcomes

- Decreased progression of breast cancer.

BEERS

ALPRAZolam (al-pray-zoe-lam)

Xanax, Xanax XR

Classification
Therapeutic: antianxiety agents
Pharmacologic: benzodiazepines

Schedule IV

Indications

Generalized anxiety disorder (GAD). Panic disorder. Anxiety associated with depression. **Unlabeled Use:** Management of symptoms of premenstrual syndrome (PMS) and premenstrual dysphoric disorder. Insomnia, irritable bowel syndrome (IBS), and other somatic symptoms associated with anxiety. Used as an adjunct with acute mania, acute psychosis.

Action

Acts at many levels in the CNS to produce anxiolytic effect. May produce CNS depression. Effects may be mediated by GABA, an inhibitory neurotransmitter. **Therapeutic Effects:** Relief of anxiety.

Pharmacokinetics

Absorption: Well absorbed (90%) from the GI tract; absorption is slower with extended-release tablets.
Distribution: Widely distributed, crosses blood-brain barrier. Probably crosses the placenta and enters breast milk. Accumulation is minimal.
Metabolism and Excretion: Metabolized by the liver (CYP3A4 enzyme system) to an active compound that is subsequently rapidly metabolized.
Half-life: 12–15 hr.

TIME/ACTION PROFILE (sedation)

ROUTE	ONSET	PEAK	DURATION
PO	1–2 hr	1–2 hr	up to 24 hr

Contraindications/Precautions

Contraindicated in: Hypersensitivity; Cross-sensitivity with other benzodiazepines may exist; Pre-existing CNS depression; Severe uncontrolled pain; Angle-closure glaucoma; Obstructive sleep apnea or pulmonary disease; Concurrent use with itraconazole or ketoconazole; OB, Lactation: Use in pregnancy or lactation may cause CNS depression, flaccidity, feeding difficulties, and seizures in infant.
Use Cautiously in: Renal impairment (↓ dose required); Hepatic impairment (↓ dose required); Concurrent use with nefazodone, fluvoxamine, cimetidine, fluoxetine, hormonal contraceptives, diltiazem, isoniazid, erythromycin, clarithromycin, or grapefruit juice (↓ dose may be necessary); History of suicide attempt or alcohol/drug dependence, debilitated patients (↓ dose required); Geri: Appears on Beers list. Elderly patients have ↑ sensitivity to benzodiazepines; associated with ↑ risk of falls and excessive CNS effects (↓ dose required); Pedi: Safety and effectiveness not established.

Adverse Reactions/Side Effects

CNS: <u>dizziness</u>, <u>drowsiness</u>, <u>lethargy</u>, confusion, depression, hangover, headache, paradoxical excitation. **EENT:** blurred vision. **GI:** constipation, diarrhea, nausea, vomiting, weight gain. **Derm:** rash. **Misc:** physical dependence, psychological dependence, tolerance.

Interactions

Drug-Drug: Use with **opioids** or other **CNS depressants**, including other **benzodiazepines**, **nonbenzodiazepine sedative/hypnotics**, **anxiolytics**, **general anesthetics**, **muscle relaxants**, **antipsychotics**, and **alcohol** may cause profound sedation, respiratory depression, coma, and death; reserve concurrent use for when alternative treatment options are inadequate. **Hormonal contraceptives**, **disulfiram**, **fluoxetine**, **isoniazid**, **metoprolol**, **propranolol**, **valproic acid**, **CYP3A4 inhibitors** (**erythromycin**, **ketoconazole**, **itraconazole**, **fluvoxamine**, **cimetidine**, **nefazodone**) ↑ levels and effects; dose adjustments may be necessary; concurrent use with ketoconazole and itraconazole contraindicated. May ↓ efficacy of **levodopa**. **CYP3A4 inducers** (**rifampin**, **carbamazepine**, or **barbiturates**) ↓ levels and effects. Sedative effects may be ↓ by **theophylline**. **Cigarette smoking** ↓ levels and effects.
Drug-Natural Products: **Kava-kava**, **valerian**, or **chamomile** can ↑ CNS depression.
Drug-Food: Concurrent ingestion of **grapefruit juice** ↑ levels and effects.

Route/Dosage

Anxiety

PO (Adults): 0.25–0.5 mg 2–3 times daily (not to exceed 4 mg/day).
PO (Geriatric Patients): Begin with 0.25 mg 2–3 times daily.

Panic Attacks

PO (Adults): 0.5 mg 3 times daily; may be ↑ by 1 mg or less every 3–4 days as needed (not to exceed 10 mg/day). *Extended-release tablets*—0.5–1 mg once daily in the morning, may be ↑ every 3–4 days by not more than 1 mg/day; up to 10 mg/day (usual range 3–6 mg/day).

Availability (generic available)

Tablets: 0.25 mg, 0.5 mg, 1 mg, 2 mg. **Cost:** *Generic*—0.25 mg $10.59/100, 0.5 mg $5.25/100, 1 mg $10.41/100, 2 mg $15.13/100. **Extended-release tablets:** 0.5 mg, 1 mg, 2 mg, 3 mg. **Cost:** *Generic*—1 mg $54.05/180, 2 mg $86.76/180, 3 mg $319.38/60. **Orally disintegrating tablets (orange-flavor):** 0.25 mg, 0.5 mg, 1 mg, 2 mg. **Cost:** *Generic*—0.25 mg $151.73/100, 0.5 mg $189.04/100, 1 mg $252.22/100, 2 mg $428.86/100. **Oral solution (concentrate):** 1 mg/mL. **Cost:** *Generic*—$81.10/30 mL.

NURSING IMPLICATIONS

Assessment

- Assess degree and manifestations of anxiety and mental status (orientation, mood, behavior) prior to and periodically during therapy.
- Assess patient for drowsiness, light-headedness, and dizziness. These symptoms usually disappear as therapy progresses. Dose should be reduced if these symptoms persist.
- Geri: Assess CNS effects and risk of falls. Institute falls prevention strategies.
- Prolonged high-dose therapy may lead to psychological or physical dependence. Risk is greater in patients taking >4 mg/day. Restrict the amount of drug available to patient. Assess regularly for continued need for treatment.
- ***Lab Test Considerations:*** Monitor CBC and liver and renal function periodically during long-term therapy. May cause ↓ hematocrit and neutropenia.
- ***Toxicity and Overdose:*** Flumazenil is the antidote for alprazolam toxicity or overdose. (Flumazenil may induce seizures in patients with a history of seizures disorder or who are taking tricyclic antidepressants).

Implementation

- Do not confuse Xanax (alprazolam) with Zantac (ranitidine), Fanapt (iloperidone), or Tenex (guanfacine).
- Do not confuse alprazolam with clonazepam or lorazepam.
- If early morning anxiety or anxiety between doses occurs, same total daily dose should be divided into more frequent intervals.
- **PO:** May be administered with food if GI upset occurs. Administer greatest dose at bedtime to avoid daytime sedation.
- Tablets may be crushed and taken with food or fluids if patient has difficulty swallowing. Do not crush, break, or chew extended-release tablets.
- Taper by 0.5 mg every 3 days to prevent withdrawal. Some patients may require longer tapering period (months).
- For *orally disintegrating tablets:* Remove tablet from bottle with dry hands just prior to taking medication. Place tablet on tongue. Tablet will dissolve with saliva; may also be taken with water. Remove cotton from bottle and reseal tightly to prevent moisture from entering bottle. If only ½ tablet taken, discard unused portion immediately; may not remain stable.

Patient/Family Teaching

- Instruct patient to take medication as directed; do not skip or double up on missed doses. If a dose is missed, take within 1 hr; otherwise, skip the dose and return to regular schedule. If medication is less effective after a few wk, check with health care professional; do not increase dose. Abrupt withdrawal may cause sweating, vomiting, muscle cramps, tremors, and seizures.
- Advise patient to not take more than prescribed or share medication with anyone.
- May cause drowsiness or dizziness. Caution patient to avoid driving and other activities requiring alertness until response to the medication is known. Geri: Instruct patient and family how to reduce falls risk at home.
- Advise patient to avoid drinking grapefruit juice during therapy.
- Advise patient to avoid the use of alcohol or other CNS depressants concurrently with alprazolam. Instruct patient to consult health care professional before taking Rx, OTC, or herbal products concurrently with this medication.
- Inform patient that benzodiazepines are usually prescribed for short-term use and do not cure underlying problems.

Evaluation/Desired Outcomes

- Decreased sense of anxiety without CNS side effects.
- Decreased frequency and severity of panic attacks.
- Decreased symptoms of premenstrual syndrome.

alteplase, See THROMBOLYTIC AGENTS.

amcinonide, See CORTICOSTEROIDS (TOPICAL/LOCAL).

amifostine (a-mi-fos-teen)

Ethyol

Classification

Therapeutic: cytoprotective agents

Indications

Reduces renal toxicity from cisplatin. Reduces the incidence of moderate to severe xerostomia from postoperative radiation for head and neck cancer in which the radiation port includes a large portion of the parotid glands.

Action

Converted by alkaline phosphatase in tissue to a free thiol compound that binds and detoxifies damaging metabolites of cisplatin and reactive oxygen species generated by radiation. **Therapeutic Effects:** Decreased renal damage from cisplatin. Decreased severity of xerostomia following radiation for head and neck cancer.

Pharmacokinetics

Absorption: IV administration results in complete bioavailability.
Distribution: Unknown.
Metabolism and Excretion: Rapidly cleared from plasma; converted to cytoprotective compounds by alkaline phosphatase in tissues.
Half-life: 8 min.

TIME/ACTION PROFILE

ROUTE	ONSET	PEAK	DURATION
IV	unknown	unknown	unknown

Contraindications/Precautions

Contraindicated in: Hypersensitivity to aminothiol compounds; Hypotension or dehydration; Concurrent antineoplastic therapy for other tumors (especially malignancies of germ cell origin); OB: Pregnancy (may cause fetal harm); Lactation: Lactation.
Use Cautiously in: Cardiovascular disease (↑ risk of adverse reactions); Pedi: Safety and effectiveness not established; Geri: ↑ risk of adverse reactions.

Adverse Reactions/Side Effects

CNS: dizziness, somnolence. **CV:** hypotension. **EENT:** blurred vision, diplopia, sneezing. **Derm:** DRUG REACTION WITH EOSINOPHILIA AND SYSTEMIC SYMPTOMS (DRESS), ERYTHEMA MULTIFORME, EXFOLIATIVE DERMATITIS, STEVENS-JOHNSON SYNDROME, TOXIC EPIDERMAL NECROLYSIS, TOXODERMA, flushing. **F and E:** hypocalcemia. **GI:** hiccups, nausea, vomiting. **Misc:** ANAPHYLAXIS, chills, injection site reactions.

Interactions

Drug-Drug: Concurrent use of **antihypertensives** ↑ risk of hypotension.

Route/Dosage

Reduction of Renal Damage with Cisplatin

IV (Adults): 910 mg/m² once daily, within 30 min before chemotherapy; if full dose is poorly tolerated, subsequent doses should be ↓ to 740 mg/m².

Reduction of Xerostomia from Radiation

IV (Adults): 200 mg/m² once daily starting 15–30 min before standard fraction radiation therapy.

Availability (generic available)

Powder for injection: 500 mg/vial.

NURSING IMPLICATIONS

Assessment

- Monitor BP before and every 5 min during infusion. Discontinue antihypertensives 24 hr prior to treatment. If significant hypotension requiring interruption of therapy occurs, place patient in Trendelenburg position and administer an infusion of 0.9% NaCl using a separate IV line. If BP returns to normal in 5 min and patient is asymptomatic, infusion may be resumed so that full dose may be given.
- Assess fluid status before administration. Correct dehydration before instituting therapy. Nausea and vomiting are frequent and may be severe. Administer prophylactic antiemetics including dexamethasone 20 mg IV and a serotonin-antagonist antiemetic (dolasetron, granisetron, ondansetron, palonosetron) before and during infusion. Monitor fluid status closely.
- Observe patient for signs and symptoms of anaphylaxis (rash, pruritus, laryngeal edema, wheezing). Discontinue the drug and notify physician or other health care professional immediately if these problems occur. Keep epinephrine, an antihistamine, and resuscitation equipment close by in case of an anaphylactic reaction.
- Monitor patient for skin reactions before, during, and after amifostine administration; reactions may be delayed by several wk after initiation of therapy. Permanently discontinue amifostine in patients who experience serious or severe cutaneous reactions or cutaneous reactions associated with fever or other symptoms of unknown cause. Withhold therapy and obtain dermatologic consultation and biopsy for cutaneous reactions or mucosal lesions of unknown cause appearing outside of injection site or radiation port, and for erythematous, edematous, or bullous lesions on the palms of the hand or soles of the feet.
- Monitor for signs and symptoms of DRESS (fever, rash, lymphadenopathy, and/or facial swelling, associated with involvement of other organ systems (hepatitis, nephritis, hematologic abnormalities, myocarditis, myositis) during therapy. May resemble an acute viral infection. Eosinophilia is often present. Discontinue therapy if signs occur.
- **Xerostomia:** Assess patient for dry mouth and mouth sores periodically during therapy.
- ***Lab Test Considerations:*** Monitor serum calcium concentrations before and periodically during therapy. May cause hypocalcemia. Calcium supplements may be necessary.

Implementation

IV Administration

- **Intermittent Infusion:** ***Diluent:*** Reconstitute with 9.7 mL of sterile 0.9% NaCl. Dilute further with 0.9% NaCl. Do not administer solutions that are discolored or contain particulate matter. Solution is stable for 5 hr at room temperature or 24 hr if refrigerated. ***Concentration:*** Adults: dilute dose to a final volume of 50 mL; Children: 5–40 mg/mL. ***Rate:*** *For renal toxicity:* Administer over 15 min within 30 min before chemotherapy administration. Longer infusion times are not as well tolerated. *For xerostomia:* Administer over 3 min starting 15–30 min prior to radiation therapy.

- **Y-Site Compatibility:** alemtuzumab, amikacin, aminophylline, amphotericin B liposome, ampicillin, ampicillin/sulbactam, anidulafungin, argatroban, aztreonam, bivalirudin, bleomycin, bumetanide, buprenorphine, butorphanol, calcium gluconate, carboplatin, carmustine, caspofungin, cefazolin, cefotaxime, cefotetan, cefoxitin, ceftazidime, ceftriaxone, cefuroxime, ciprofloxacin, clindamycin, cyclophosphamide, cytarabine, dacarbazine, dactinomycin, daptomycin, daunorubicin, dexamethasone, dexmedetomidine, dexrazoxane, diltiazem, diphenhydramine, dobutamine, docetaxel, docetaxel, dolasetron, dopamine, doxorubicin, doxycycline, droperidol, enalaprilat, epirubicin, ertapenem, etoposide, etoposide phosphate, famotidine, fenoldopam, floxuridine, fluconazole, fludarabine, fluorouracil, foscarnet, fosphenytoin, furosemide, gemcitabine, gentamicin, granisetron, haloperidol, heparin, hetastarch, hydrocortisone, hydromorphone, idarubicin, ifosfamide, imipenem/cilastatin, irinotecan, leucovorin, levofloxacin, linezolid, lorazepam, magnesium sulfate, mannitol, meperidine, mesna, methotrexate, methylprednisolone, metoclopramide, metronidazole, milrinone, mitomycin, morphine, moxifloxacin, nalbuphine, octreotide, ondansetron, oxaliplatin, paclitaxel, palonosetron, pamidronate, pancuronium, pantoprazole, pemetrexed, piperacillin/tazobactam, potassium acetate, potassium chloride, promethazine, ranitidine, rituximab, sodium acetate, sodium bicarbonate, streptozocin, tacrolimus, thiotepa, tigecycline, tirofiban, tobramycin, trastuzumab, trimethoprim/sulfamethoxazole, vancomycin, vasopressin, vecuronium, vinblastine, vincristine, vinorelbine, voriconazole, zidovudine, zoledronic acid.
- **Y-Site Incompatibility:** acyclovir, amiodarone, amphotericin B deoxycholate, amphotericin B lipid complex, chlorpromazine, cisplatin, ganciclovir, hydroxyzine, minocycline, mycophenolate, prochlorperazine, quinupristin/dalfopristin, topotecan.

Patient/Family Teaching

- Explain the purpose of amifostine infusion to patient.
- Inform patient that amifostine may cause hypotension, nausea, vomiting, flushing, chills, dizziness, somnolence, hiccups, and sneezing.
- Advise patient to notify health care professional if skin reactions, or signs and symptoms of anaphylaxis or DRESS occur.

Evaluation/Desired Outcomes

- Prevention of renal toxicity associated with repeated administration of cisplatin in patients with ovarian cancer.
- Decreased severity of xerostomia from radiation treatment of head and neck cancer.

amikacin, See AMINOGLYCOSIDES.

aMILoride, See DIURETICS (POTASSIUM-SPARING).

aminocaproic acid

(a-mee-noe-ka-**pro**-ik **a**-sid)

Amicar

Classification

Therapeutic: hemostatic agents

Pharmacologic: fibrinolysis inhibitors

Indications

Management of acute, life-threatening hemorrhage due to systemic hyperfibrinolysis or urinary fibrinolysis. **Unlabeled Use:** Prevention of recurrent subarachnoid hemorrhage. Prevention of bleeding following oral surgery in hemophiliacs. Management of severe hemorrhage caused by thrombolytic agents.

Action

Inhibits activation of plasminogen. **Therapeutic Effects:** Inhibition of fibrinolysis. Stabilization of clot formation.

Pharmacokinetics

Absorption: Rapidly absorbed following oral administration.

Distribution: Widely distributed.

Metabolism and Excretion: Mostly eliminated unchanged by the kidneys.

Half-life: Unknown.

TIME/ACTION PROFILE (peak blood levels)

ROUTE	ONSET	PEAK	DURATION
PO	unknown	2 hr	N/A
IV	unknown	2 hr	N/A

Contraindications/Precautions

Contraindicated in: Active intravascular clotting.

Use Cautiously in: Upper urinary tract bleeding; Cardiac, renal, or liver disease (dosage reduction may be required); Disseminated intravascular coagulation (should be used concurrently with heparin); OB, Lactation: Safety not established; Pedi: Do not use products containing benzyl alcohol with neonates.

Adverse Reactions/Side Effects

CNS: dizziness, malaise. **CV:** arrhythmias, hypotension (IV only). **EENT:** nasal stuffiness, tinnitus. **GI:** anorexia, bloating, cramping, diarrhea, nausea. **GU:** diuresis, renal failure. **MS:** myopathy.

Interactions

Drug-Drug: Concurrent use with **estrogens, conjugated** may result in a hypercoagulable state. Concurrent use with **clotting factors** may ↑ risk of thromboses.

Route/Dosage

Acute Bleeding Syndromes due to Elevated Fibrinolytic Activity

PO (Adults): 5 g 1st hr, followed by 1–1.25 g every hr for 8 hr or until hemorrhage is controlled; or 6 g over 24 hr after prostate surgery (not >30 g/day).
IV (Adults): 4–5 g over 1st hr, followed by 1 g/hr for 8 hr or until hemorrhage is controlled; or 6 g over 24 hr after prostate surgery (not >30 g/day).
PO, IV (Children): 100 mg/kg or 3 g/m^2 over 1st hr, followed by continuous infusion of 33.3 mg/kg/hr; or 1 g/m^2/hr (total dose not >18 g/m^2/24 hr).

Subarachnoid Hemorrhage

PO (Adults): *To follow IV*—3 g every 2 hr (36 g/day). If no surgery is performed, continue for 21 days after bleeding stops, then ↓ to 2 g every 2 hr (24 g/day) for 3 days, then 1 g every 2 hr (12 g/day) for 3 days.
IV (Adults): 36 g/day for 10 days followed by PO.

Prevention of Bleeding Following Oral Surgery in Hemophiliacs

PO (Adults): 75 mg/kg (up to 6 g) immediately after procedure, then every 6 hr for 7–10 days; syrup may also be used as an oral rinse of 1.25 g (5 mL) 4 times a day for 7–10 days.
IV, PO (Children): *Also for epistaxis*—50–100 mg/kg/dose administered IV every 6 hr for 2–3 days starting 4 hr before the procedure. After completion of IV therapy, aminocaproic acid should be given as 50–100 mg/kg/dose orally every 6 hr for 5–7 days.

Availability (generic available)

Tablets: 500 mg, 1000 mg. **Oral syrup (raspberry flavor):** 1.25 g/5 mL. **Solution for injection:** 250 mg/mL.

NURSING IMPLICATIONS

Assessment

- Monitor BP, pulse, and respiratory status as indicated by severity of bleeding.
- Monitor for overt bleeding every 15–30 min during acute bleed and periodically during therapy.
- Monitor neurologic status (pupils, level of consciousness, motor activity) in patients with subarachnoid hemorrhage.
- Monitor intake and output ratios frequently; notify health care professional if significant discrepancies occur.
- Assess for thromboembolic complications (especially in patients with history). Notify health care professional of positive Homans' sign, leg pain and edema, hemoptysis, dyspnea, or chest pain.
- ***Lab Test Considerations:*** Monitor platelet count and clotting factors prior to and periodically throughout therapy in patients with systemic fibrinolysis.
- ↑ CPK, AST, and serum aldolase may indicate myopathy.
- May ↑ serum potassium.

Implementation

- **PO:** Syrup may be used as an oral rinse, swished for 30 sec 4 times/day for 7–10 days for the control of bleeding during dental and oral surgery in hemophilic patients. Small amounts may be swallowed, except during 1st and 2nd trimesters of pregnancy. Syrup may be applied with an applicator in children or unconscious patients.

IV Administration

- **IV:** Stabilize IV catheter to minimize thrombophlebitis. Monitor site closely.
- **Intermittent Infusion:** ***Diluent:*** Do not administer undiluted. Dilute initial 4–5 g dose in 250 mL of sterile water for injection, 0.9% NaCl, D5W, or LR. Do not dilute with sterile water in patients with subarachnoid hemorrhage. ***Concentration:*** 20 mg/mL. ***Rate:*** Single doses: Administer over 1 hr. Rapid infusion rate may cause hypotension, bradycardia, or other arrhythmias.
- **Continuous Infusion:** Administer IV solution using infusion pump to ensure accurate dose. Administer via slow IV infusion.
- ***Rate:*** Initial dose may be followed by a continuous infusion of 1–1.25 g/hr in adults or 33.3 mg/kg/hr in children.
- **Y-Site Compatibility:** alemtuzumab, alfentanil, amikacin, aminophylline, amphotericin B deoxycholate, amphotericin B lipid complex, amphotericin B liposome, ampicillin, ampicillin/sulbactam, anidulafungin, argatroban, arsenic trioxide, atracurium, azithromycin, aztreonam, bivalirudin, bleomycin, bumetanide, buprenorphine, butorphanol, calcium chloride, calcium gluconate, carboplatin, carmustine, cefazolin, cefepime, cefotaxime, cefotetan, cefoxitin, ceftazidime, ceftriaxone, cefuroxime, cisatracurium, clindamycin, cyclophosphamide, cyclosporine, cytarabine, dacarbazine, daptomycin, dexamethasone, dexmedetomidine, digoxin, dilti-

azem, diphenhydramine, dobutamine, docetaxel, dopamine, droperidol, enalaprilat, ephedrine, epinephrine, epirubicin, ertapenem, erythromycin, esmolol, etoposide, etoposide phosphate, famotidine, fenoldopam, fentanyl, fluconazole, fludarabine, foscarnet, fosphenytoin, furosemide, gemcitabine, gentamicin, granisetron, haloperidol, heparin, hetastarch, hydrocortisone, hydromorphone, idarubicin, ifosfamide, imipenem/cilastatin, irinotecan, isoproterenol, ketorolac, labetalol, leucovorin calcium, levofloxacin, levorphanol, lidocaine, linezolid, lorazepam, magnesium sulfate, mannitol, meperidine, meropenem, mesna, methohexital, methylprednisolone, metoclopramide, metoprolol, metronidazole, milrinone, mitoxantrone, morphine, nalbuphine, naloxone, nitroglycerin, nitroprusside, octreotide, ondansetron, oxaliplatin, oxytocin, palonosetron, pamidronate, pancuronium, pantoprazole, pamidronate, pancuronium, pantoprazole, pemetrexed, pentamidine, pentobarbital, phenobarbital, phenylephrine, piperacillin/tazobactam, potassium acetate, potassium chloride, potassium phosphates, procainamide, promethazine, propranolol, ranitidine, remifentanil, rocuronium, sargramostim, sodium bicarbonate, sodium phosphates, succinylcholine, sufentanil, tacrolimus, theophylline, thiotepa, tigecycline, tirofiban, tobramycin, trimethoprim/sulfamethoxazole, vancomycin, vasopressin, vecuronium, verapamil, vincristine, voriconazole, zidovudine, zoledronic acid.

- **Y-Site Incompatibility:** acyclovir, amiodarone, caspofungin, chlorpromazine, ciprofloxacin, diazepam, doxycycline, filgrastim, ganciclovir, midazolam, mycophenolate, nicardipine, phenytoin, prochlorperazine, quinupristin/dalfopristin, thiopental.
- **Additive Incompatibility:** Do not admix with other medications.

Patient/Family Teaching

- Instruct patient to notify the nurse immediately if bleeding recurs or if thromboembolic symptoms develop.
- **IV:** Caution patient to make position changes slowly to avoid orthostatic hypotension.

Evaluation/Desired Outcomes

- Cessation of bleeding.
- Prevention of rebleeding in subarachnoid hemorrhage without occurrence of undesired clotting.

AMINOGLYCOSIDES

amikacin (am-i-**kay**-sin)
~~Amikin~~, Arikayce

gentamicin† (jen-ta-**mye**-sin)
~~Garamycin~~

neomycin (neo-oh-**mye**-sin)

streptomycin (strep-toe-**mye**-sin)

tobramycin† (toe-bra-**mye**-sin)
Bethkis, Kitabis Pak, TOBI, TOBI Podhaler

Classification
Therapeutic: anti-infectives
Pharmacologic: aminoglycosides

†See Appendix C for ophthalmic use

Indications

Amikacin, gentamicin, and tobramycin: Treatment of serious gram-negative bacterial infections and infections caused by staphylococci when penicillins or other less toxic drugs are contraindicated. **Streptomycin:** In combination with other agents in the management of active tuberculosis. **Neomycin:** Used orally to prepare the GI tract for surgery, to decrease the number of ammonia-producing bacteria in the gut as part of the management of hepatic encephalopathy, and to treat diarrhea caused by *Escherichia coli*. **Amikacin by inhalation:** Treatment of *Mycobacterium avium* complex (MAC) lung disease in patients who have limited or no other treatment options and who do not achieve negative sputum cultures after ≥6 consecutive mo of a multidrug treatment regimen (in combination with other antibacterial drugs). **Tobramycin by inhalation:** Management of *Pseudomonas aeruginosa* in cystic fibrosis patients. **Gentamicin, streptomycin:** In combination with other agents in the management of serious enterococcal infections. **Gentamicin IV:** Prevention of infective endocarditis. **Gentamicin (topical):** Treatment of localized infections caused by susceptible organisms. **Unlabeled Use:** Amikacin: In combination with other agents in the management of *Mycobacterium avium* complex infections.

Action

Inhibits protein synthesis in bacteria at level of 30S ribosome. **Therapeutic Effects:** Bactericidal action. **Spectrum:** Most aminoglycosides notable for activity against: *P. aeruginosa*, *Klebsiella pneumoniae*, *E. coli*, *Proteus*, *Serratia*, *Acinetobacter*, *Staphylococcus aureus*. In treatment of enterococcal infections, synergy with a penicillin is required. Streptomycin and amikacin also active against *Mycobacterium*.

Pharmacokinetics

Absorption: Well absorbed after IM administration. IV administration results in complete bioavailability. Some absorption follows administration by other routes. Minimal systemic absorption with neomycin (may accumulate in patients with renal failure).
Distribution: Widely distributed throughout extracellular fluid; cross the placenta; small amounts enter breast milk. Poor penetration into CSF (↑ when meninges are inflamed).
Metabolism and Excretion: Excretion is >90% renal.
Half-life: 2–4 hr (↑ in renal impairment).

TIME/ACTION PROFILE (blood levels*)

ROUTE	ONSET	PEAK	DURATION
PO (neomycin)	rapid	1–4 hr	N/A
IM	rapid	30–90 min	6–24 hr
IV	rapid	15–30 min†	6–24 hr

*All parenterally administered aminoglycosides.

†Postdistribution peak occurs 30 min after the end of a 30-min infusion and 15 min after the end of a 1-hr infusion.

Contraindications/Precautions

Contraindicated in: Hypersensitivity to aminoglycosides; Most parenteral products contain bisulfites and should be avoided in patients with known intolerance; Intestinal obstruction (neomycin only); OB: Avoid use of tobramycin, streptomycin, and inhaled amikacin during pregnancy (may cause fetal nephrotoxicity or deafness); Pedi: Products containing benzyl alcohol should be avoided in neonates.

Use Cautiously in: Renal impairment (dose adjustments necessary; blood level monitoring useful in preventing ototoxicity and nephrotoxicity); Hearing impairment; Neuromuscular diseases such as myasthenia gravis; Obese patients (dose should be based on ideal body weight); COPD or asthma (amikacin inhalation may worsen condition); Lactation: Safety not established; Pedi: Neonates have ↑ risk of neuromuscular blockade; difficulty in assessing auditory and vestibular function and immature renal function; safety and effectiveness of amikacin inhalation not established in children; Geri: Difficulty in assessing auditory and vestibular function and age-related renal impairment.

Adverse Reactions/Side Effects

CNS: ataxia, headache (amikacin inhalation only), anxiety (amikacin inhalation only), vertigo. **Derm:** rash (amikacin inhalation only). **EENT:** ototoxicity (vestibular and cochlear), voice alteration (amikacin inhalation only), epistaxis (amikacin inhalation only), oral candidiasis (amikacin inhalation only). **F and E:** hypomagnesemia. **GI:** diarrhea (amikacin inhalation only), nausea (amikacin inhalation only), diarrhea (neomycin only), dry mouth (amikacin inhalation only), metallic taste (amikacin inhalation only), nausea (neomycin only), vomiting (amikacin inhalation and neomycin only). **GU:** nephrotoxicity. **Metab:** ↓ weight (amikacin inhalation only). **MS:** muscle paralysis (high parenteral doses). **Neuro:** ↑ neuromuscular blockade. **Resp:** bronchospasm (amikacin inhalation only), cough (amikacin inhalation only), hemoptysis (amikacin inhalation only), apnea, bronchospasm (tobramycin inhalation only), hypersensitivity pneumonitis (amikacin inhalation only), wheezing (tobramycin inhalation only). **Misc:** hypersensitivity reactions.

Interactions

Drug-Drug: Inactivated by **penicillins** and **cephalosporins** when coadministered to patients with renal insufficiency. Possible respiratory paralysis after **inhalation anesthetics** or **neuromuscular blocking agents**. ↑ incidence of ototoxicity with **loop diuretics** or **mannitol (IV)**. ↑ incidence of nephrotoxicity with other **nephrotoxic drugs**. Neomycin may ↑ anticoagulant effects of **warfarin**. Neomycin may ↓ absorption of **digoxin** and **methotrexate**.

Route/Dosage

Amikacin

IM, IV (Adults and Children): 5 mg/kg every 8 hr or 7.5 mg/kg every 12 hr (not to exceed 1.5 g/day). *Mycobacterium avium complex*—7.5–15 mg/kg/day divided every 12–24 hr.

IM, IV (Neonates): *Loading dose*—10 mg/kg; *Maintenance dose*—7.5 mg/kg every 12 hr.

Inhaln (Adults): 590 mg once daily.

Renal Impairment

IM, IV (Adults): *Loading dose*—7.5 mg/kg, further dosing based on blood level monitoring and renal function assessment.

Gentamicin

Many regimens are used; most involve dosing adjusted on the basis of blood level monitoring and assessment of renal function.

IM, IV (Adults): 1–2 mg/kg every 8 hr (up to 6 mg/kg/day in 3 divided doses); *Once-daily dosing (unlabeled)*—4–7 mg/kg every 24 hr.

IM, IV (Children >5 yr): 2–2.5 mg/kg/dose every 8 hr; *Once daily*—5–7.5 mg/kg/dose every 24 hr; *Cystic fibrosis*—2.5–3.3 mg/kg/dose every 6–8 hr; *Hemodialysis*—1.25–1.75 mg/kg/dose postdialysis.

IM, IV (Children 1 mo–5 yr): 2.5 mg/kg/dose every 8 hr; *Once daily*—5–7.5 mg/kg/dose every 24 hr; *Cystic fibrosis*—2.5–3.3 mg/kg/dose every 6–8 hr; *Hemodialysis*—1.25–1.75 mg/kg/dose postdialysis.

IM, IV (Neonates full term and/or >1 wk): *Weight <1200 g*—2.5 mg/kg/dose every 18–24 hr; *Weight 1200–2000 g*—2.5 mg/kg/dose every 8–12 hr; *Weight >2000 g*—2.5 mg/kg/dose every 8 hr; *ECMO*—2.5 mg/kg/dose every 18 hr, subsequent doses based on serum concentrations; *Once daily*—3.5–5 mg/kg/dose every 24 hr.

IM, IV (Neonates premature and/or ≤1 wk): *Weight <1000 g*—3.5 mg/kg/dose every 24 hr; *Weight 1000–1200 g*—2.5 mg/kg/dose every 18–24 hr; *Weight >1200 g*—2.5 mg/kg/dose every 12 hr; *Once daily*—3.5–4 mg/kg/dose every 24 hr.

IT (Adults): 4–8 mg/day.

IT (Infants >3 mo and Children): 1–2 mg/day.

IT (Neonates): 1 mg/day.

Topical (Adults and Children >1 mo): Apply cream or ointment 3–4 times daily.

Renal Impairment

IM, IV (Adults): Initial dose of 2 mg/kg. Subsequent doses/intervals based on blood level monitoring and renal function assessment.

Neomycin

PO (Adults): *Preoperative intestinal antisepsis*—1 g every hr for 4 doses, then 1 g every 4 hr for 5 doses *or* 1 g at 1 PM, 2 PM, and 11 PM on day before surgery; *Hepatic encephalopathy*—1–3 g every 6 hr for 5–6 days; may be followed by 4 g/day chronically.

PO (Children): *Preoperative intestinal antisepsis*—15 mg/kg every 4 hr for 2 days *or* 25 mg/kg at 1 PM, 2 PM, and 11 PM on day before surgery; *Hepatic encephalopathy*—12.5–25 mg/kg every 6 hr for 5–6 days (maximum dose = 12 g/day).

Streptomycin

IM (Adults): *Tuberculosis*—1 g/day initially, ↓ to 1 g 2–3 times weekly; *Other infections*—250 mg–1 g every 6 hr *or* 500 mg–2 g every12 hr.

IM (Children): *Tuberculosis*—20 mg/kg/day (not to exceed 1 g/day); *Other infections*—5–10 mg/kg every 6 hr *or* 10–20 mg/kg every 12 hr.

Renal Impairment

IM (Adults): 1 g initially, further dosing determined by blood level monitoring and assessment of renal function.

Tobramycin

IM, IV (Adults): 1–2 mg/kg every 8 hr *or* 4–6.6 mg/kg/day every 24 hr.

IM, IV (Adults): 3–6 mg/kg/day in 3 divided doses, or 4–6.6 mg/kg once daily.

IM, IV (Children >5 yr): 6–7.5 mg/kg/day divided every 8 hr, up to 13 mg/kg/day divided every 6–8 hr in cystic fibrosis patients (dosing interval may vary from every 6 hr–every 24 hr, depending on clinical situation).

IM, IV (Children 1 mo–5 yr): 7.5 mg/kg/day divided every 8 hr, up to 13 mg/kg/day divided every 6–8 hr in cystic fibrosis.

IM, IV (Neonates): *Preterm <1000 g*—3.5 mg/kg/dose every 24 hr; *0–4 weeks, <1200 g*—2.5 mg/kg/dose every 18 hr; *Postnatal age <7 days*—2.5 mg/kg/dose every 12 hr; *Postnatal age ≥8 days, 1200–2000 g*—2.5 mg/kg/dose every 8–12 hr; *Postnatal age ≥8 days, >2000 g*—2.5 mg/kg/dose every 8 hr.

Inhaln (Adults and Children ≥6 yr): *Nebulizer solution*—300 mg twice daily for 28 days, then off for 28 days, then repeat cycle; *Powder for inhalation*—Inhale contents of four 28-mg capsules twice daily for 28 days, then off for 28 days, then repeat cycle.

Renal Impairment

IM, IV (Adults): 1 mg/kg initially, further dosing determined by blood level monitoring and assessment of renal function.

Availability

Amikacin (generic available)

Solution for injection (requires dilution): 250 mg/mL. **Suspension for oral inhalation:** 590 mg/8.4 mL.

Gentamicin (generic available)

Premixed infusion: 60 mg/50 mL, 80 mg/50 mL, 80 mg/100 mL, 100 mg/50 mL, 100 mg/100 mL, 120 mg/100 mL. **Solution for injection (requires dilution):** 10 mg/mL, 40 mg/mL. **Topical cream:** 0.1%. **Topical ointment:** 0.1%.

Neomycin (generic available)

Tablets: 500 mg. ***In combination with:*** other topical antibiotics or anti-inflammatory agents for skin, ear, and eye infections. See Appendix B.

Streptomycin (generic available)

Lyophilized powder for injection (requires reconstitution): 1 g/vial.

Tobramycin (generic available)

Lyophilized powder for injection (requires reconstitution and dilution): 1200 mg/vial. **Nebulizer solution (Bethkis):** 300 mg/4 mL. **Nebulizer solution (TOBI, Kitabis Pak):** 300 mg/5 mL. **Powder for inhalation (TOBI Podhaler):** 28 mg/capsule. **Solution for injection (requires dilution):** 10 mg/mL, 40 mg/mL.

NURSING IMPLICATIONS

Assessment

- Assess for infection (vital signs, wound appearance, sputum, urine, stool, WBC) at beginning of and throughout therapy.
- Obtain specimens for culture and sensitivity before initiating therapy. First dose may be given before receiving results.
- Evaluate eighth cranial nerve function by audiometry before and throughout therapy. Hearing loss is usually in high-frequency range. Prompt recognition and intervention are essential in preventing permanent damage. Monitor for vestibular dysfunction (vertigo, ataxia, nausea, vomiting). Eighth cranial nerve dysfunction is associated with persistently elevated peak aminoglycoside levels. Discontinue aminoglycosides if tinnitus or subjective hearing loss occurs.
- Monitor intake and output and daily weight to assess hydration status and renal function.
- Assess for signs of superinfection (fever, upper respiratory infection, vaginal itching or discharge, increasing malaise, diarrhea).
- **Hepatic Encephalopathy:** Monitor neurologic status. Before administering oral medication, assess patient's ability to swallow.
- ***Lab Test Considerations:*** Monitor renal function by urinalysis, specific gravity, BUN, creatinine, and CCr before and during therapy.

- May cause ↑ BUN, AST, ALT, serum alkaline phosphatase, bilirubin, creatinine, and LDH concentrations.
- May cause ↓ serum calcium, magnesium, potassium, and sodium concentrations (streptomycin and tobramycin).
- ***Toxicity and Overdose:*** Monitor blood levels periodically during oral, IM, and IV therapy; not needed for inhalation therapy. Timing of blood levels is important in interpreting results. Draw blood for peak levels 1 hr after IM injection and 30 min after a 30-min IV infusion is completed. Draw trough levels just before next dose. Peak level for **amikacin** is 20–30 mcg/mL; trough level should be <10 mcg/mL. Peak level for **gentamicin** and **tobramycin** should not exceed 10 mcg/mL; trough level should not exceed 2 mcg/mL. Peak level for **streptomycin** should not exceed 25 mcg/mL.

Implementation

- Keep patient well hydrated (1500–2000 mL/day) during therapy.
- **Preoperative Bowel Prep:** Neomycin is usually used in conjunction with erythromycin, a low-residue diet, and a cathartic or enema.
- **PO:** Neomycin may be administered without regard to meals.
- **IM:** IM administration should be deep into a well-developed muscle. Alternate injection sites.
- **IV:** If aminoglycosides and penicillins or cephalosporins must be administered concurrently, administer in separate sites, at least 1 hr apart.

Amikacin

IV Administration

- **Intermittent Infusion: *Diluent:*** Dilute with D5W, D10W, 0.9% NaCl, dextrose/saline combinations, or LR. Solution may be pale yellow without decreased potency. Stable for 24 hr at room temperature. ***Concentration:*** 10 mg/mL. ***Rate:*** Infuse over 30–60 min for adults and children and over 1–2 hr in infants.
- **Y-Site Compatibility:** acyclovir, aldesleukin, alemtuzumab, alfentanil, amifostine, aminophylline, amiodarone, amsacrine, anidulafungin, arsenic trioxide, ascorbic acid, atracurium, atropine, aztreonam, benztropine, bivalirudin, bleomycin, bumetanide, buprenorphine, butorphanol, calcium chloride, calcium gluconate, cangrelor, carboplatin, carmustine, caspofungin, cefazolin, cefepime, cefotaxime, cefotetan, cefoxitin, ceftaroline, ceftazidime, ceftriaxone, cefuroxime, chloramphenicol, chlorpromazine, cisatracurium, cisplatin, clindamycin, codeine, cyanocobalamin, cyclophosphamide, cyclosporine, cytarabine, dactinomycin, daptomycin, daunorubicin, dexamethasone, dexmedetomidine, digoxin, diltiazem, diphenhydramine, dobutamine, docetaxel, dopamine, doxacurium, doxorubicin hydrochloride, doxycycline, enalaprilat, ephedrine, epinephrine, epirubicin, epoetin alfa, eftifibatide, ertapenem, erythromycin, esmolol, etoposide, etoposide phosphate, famotidine, fentanyl, filgrastim, fluconazole, fludarabine, fluorouracil, foscarnet, fosphenytoin, furosemide, gemcitabine, gentamicin, glycopyrrolate, granisetron, hydrocortisone, hydromorphone, idarubicin, ifosfamide, imipenem/cilastatin, irinotecan, isoproterenol, ketamine, ketorolac, labetalol, leucovorin calcium, levofloxacin, lidocaine, linezolid, lorazepam, magnesium sulfate, mannitol, melphalan, meperidine, mesna, metaraminol, methotrexate, methyldopate, methylprednisolone, metoclopramide, metoprolol, midazolam, milrinone, mitoxantrone, morphine, multivitamins, mycophenolate, nafcillin, nalbuphine, naloxone, nicardipine, nitroglycerin, nitroprusside, norepinephrine, octreotide, ondansetron, oxaliplatin, oxytocin, paclitaxel, palonosetron, pamidronate, pancuronium, pemetrexed, papaverine, penicillin G, perphenazine, phenobarbital, phentolamine, phenylephrine, phytonadione, piperacillin/tazobactam, posaconazole, potassium acetate, potassium chloride, procainamide, prochlorperazine, promethazine, propranolol, protamine, pyridoxime, quinupristin/dalfopristin, ranitidine, remifentanil, rituximab, rocuronium, sargramostim, sodium acetate, sodium bicarbonate, streptokinase, succinylcholine, sufentanil, tacrolimus, theophylline, thiamine, thiotepa, tigecycline, tirofiban, tobramycin, tolazoline, topotecan, vancomycin, vasopressin, vecuronium, verapamil, vinblastine, vincristine, vinorelbine , voriconazole, warfarin, zidovudine, zoledronic acid.
- **Y-Site Incompatibility:** allopurinol, amphotericin B colloidal, amphotericin B lipid complex, amphotericin B liposome, azathioprine, dacarbazine, dantrolene, diazepam, diazoxide, folic acid, ganciclovir, heparin, hetastarch, indomethacin, mitomycin, pentamidine, pentobarbital, phenytoin, propofol, trastuzumab, trimethoprim/sulfamethoxazole.
- **Inhaln:** If using a bronchodilator or with known hyperreactive airway disease, chronic obstructive pulmonary disease, asthma, or bronchospasm, pre-treat with short-acting selective beta-2 agonists.
- Allow to come to room temperature before administering with *Lamira Nebulizer System* only. Shake vial well for 10–15 sec. until contents appear uniform and well mixed. Flip up plastic top of vial and pull down on metal ring to open. Remove metal ring and rubber stopper carefully. Pour contents of vial into medication reservoir of the nebulizer handset.

Gentamicin

IV Administration

- **Intermittent Infusion:** ***Diluent:*** Dilute each dose with D5W, 0.9% NaCl, or LR. Do not use solutions that are discolored or that contain a precipitate. ***Concentration:*** 10 mg/mL. ***Rate:*** Infuse slowly over 30 min–2 hr.
- **Y-Site Compatibility:** aldesleukin, alemtuzumab, alfentanil, alprostadil, amifostine, amikacin, aminophylline, amiodarone, amsacrine, anidulafungin, argatroban, ascorbic acid, atropine, aztreonam, benztropine, bivalirudin, bleomycin, bumetanide, buprenorphine, butorphanol, calcium chloride, calcium gluconate, carboplatin, carmustine, caspofungin, chlorpromazine, ciprofloxacin, cisatracurium, cisplatin, clindamycin, cyanocobalamin, cyclophosphamide, cyclosporine, cytarabine, dactinomycin, daptomycin, dexmedetomidine, dexrazoxane, digoxin, diltiazem, dimenhydrinate, diphenhydramine, dobutamine, docetaxel, dolasetron, dopamine, doxapram, doxorubicin, doxorubicin liposome, doxycycline, enalaprilat, ephedrine, epinephrine, epirubicin, epoetin alfa, eptifibatide, ertapenem, erythromycin, esmolol, etoposide, etoposide phosphate, famotidine, fenoldopam, fentanyl, fluconazole, fludarabine, fluorouracil, foscarnet, fosphenytoin, gemcitabine, glycopyrrolate, granisetron, hydromorphone, ifosfamide, imipenem/cilastatin, irinotecan, isoproterenol, ketamine, ketorolac, labetalol, leucovorin, levofloxacin, lidocaine, linezolid, lorazepam, magnesium sulfate, mannitol, melphalan, meperidine, meropenem, mesna, methylprednisolone, metoclopramide, metoprolol, metronidazole, midazolam, milrinone, mitoxantrone, morphine, multivitamins, mycophenolate, nalbuphine, naloxone, nicardipine, nitroglycerin, nitroprusside, norepinephrine, octreotide, ondansetron, oxaliplatin, oxytocin, paclitaxel, palonosetron, pamidronate, pancuronium, papaverine, phenobarbital, phentolamine, phenylephrine, phytonadione, posaconazole, potassium acetate, potassium chloride, procainamide, prochlorperazine, promethazine, propranolol, protamine, pyridoxine, ranitidine, remifentanil, rituximab, rocuronium, sargramostim, sodium acetate, sodium bicarbonate, streptokinase, succinylcholine, sufentanil, tacrolimus, telavancin, theophylline, thiamine, thiotepa, tigecycline, tirofiban, tobramycin, topotecan, trastuzumab, vancomycin, vasopressin, vecuronium, verapamil, vinblastine, vincristine, vinorelbine, vitamin B complex with C, voriconazole, zidovudine, zoledronic acid.
- **Y-Site Incompatibility:** allopurinol, amphotericin B colloidal, amphotericin B lipid complex, amphotericin B liposome, azathioprine, cangrelor, cefotetan, dacarbazine, dantrolene, diazepam, diazoxide, folic acid, ganciclovir, idarubicin, indomethacin, methotrexate, pemetrexed, pentamidine, pentobarbital, phenytoin, propofol, trimethoprim/sulfamethoxazole, warfarin.

Tobramycin

IV Administration

- **Intermittent Infusion:** ***Diluent:*** Dilute each dose of tobramycin in 50–100 mL of D5W, D10W, D5/0.9% NaCl, 0.9% NaCl, Ringer's or lactated Ringer's solution. ***Concentration:*** not >10 m g/mL. Pediatric doses may be diluted in proportionately smaller amounts. Stable for 24 hr at room temperature, 96 hr if refrigerated. ***Rate:*** Infuse slowly over 30–60 min in both adult and pediatric patients.
- **Y-Site Compatibility:** acyclovir, aldesleukin, alemtuzumab, alfentanil, alprostadil, alteplase, amifostine, aminophylline, amiodarone, anidulafungin, argatroban, ascorbic acid, atropine, aztreonam, benztropine, bivalirudin, bleomycin, bumetanide, buprenorphine, butorphanol, calcium chloride, calcium gluconate, carboplatin, carmustine, caspofungin, chloramphenicol, chlorpromazine, ciprofloxacin, cisatracurium, cisplatin, clindamycin, cyanocobalamin, cyclophosphamide, cyclosporine, cytarabine, dactinomycin, daptomycin, daunorubicin, dexmedetomidine, dexrazoxane, digoxin, diltiazem, dimenhydrinate, diphenhydramine, dobutamine, docetaxel, dolasetron, dopamine, doxorubicin, doxorubicin liposomal, doxycycline, enalaprilat, ephedrine, epinephrine, epirubicin, epoetin alfa, ertapenem, esmolol, etoposide, etoposide phosphate, famotidine, fenoldopam, fentanyl, filgrastim, fluconazole, fludarabine, fluorouracil, foscarnet, furosemide, gemcitabine, gentamicin, glycopyrrolate, granisetron, hydromorphone, idarubicin, ifosfamide, imipenem/cilastatin, irinotecan, isoproterenol, ketamine, ketorolac, labetalol, leucovorin, levofloxacin, lidocaine, linezolid, lorazepam, magnesium sulfate, mannitol, melphalan, meperidine, mesna, methotrexate, methylprednisolone, metoclopramide, metoprolol, metronidazole, midazolam, milrinone, mitomycin, mitoxantrone, morphine, multivitamins, mycophenolate, nalbuphine, naloxone, nicardipine, nitroglycerin, nitroprusside, norepinephrine, octreotide, ondansetron, oxaliplatin, oxytocin, paclitaxel, palonosetron, pamidronate, pancuronium, papaverine, phenobarbital, phentolamine, phenylephrine, phytonadione, potassium acetate, potassium chloride, procainamide, prochlorperazine, promethazine, propranolol, protamine, pyridoxine, quinupristin/dalfopristin, ranitidine, remifentanil, rituximab, rocuronium, sodium acetate, sodium bicarbonate, succinylcholine, sufentanil, tacrolimus, telavancin, theophylline, thiamine, thiotepa, tigecycline, tirofiban, topotecan, trastuzumab, vancomycin, vasopressin, vecuronium, verapamil, vinblastine, vincristine, vinorelbine, voriconazole, zidovudine, zoledronic acid.
- **Y-Site Incompatibility:** allopurinol, amphotericin B colloidal, amphotericin B lipid complex, ampho-

tericin B liposome, azathioprine, cangrelor, cefazolin, cefotetan, ceftriaxone, dacarbazine, dantrolene, dexamethasone, diazepam, diazoxide, folic acid, ganciclovir, hetastarch, indomethacin, oxacillin, pemetrexed, pentamidine, pentobarbital, phenytoin, piperacillin/tazobactam, propofol, sargramostim, trimethoprim/sulfamethoxazole.

- **Topical:** Cleanse skin before application. Wear gloves during application.
- **Inhaln:** Do not mix *TOBI* with dornase alpha in nebulizer.
- *TOBI Podhaler* capsules are not for oral use. Store capsules in blister until immediately before use. Use new Podhaler device provided with each weekly packet. Check to see capsule is empty after inhaling. If powder remains in capsule, repeat inhalation until capsule is empty.

Patient/Family Teaching

- Instruct patient to report signs of hypersensitivity, tinnitus, vertigo, hearing loss, rash, dizziness, or difficulty urinating.
- Advise patient of the importance of drinking plenty of liquids.
- Teach patients with a history of rheumatic heart disease or valve replacement the importance of using antimicrobial prophylaxis before invasive medical or dental procedures.
- Advise female patient to notify health care professional if pregnancy is planned or suspected or if breast feeding. May cause irreversible deafness in babies.
- **PO:** Instruct patient to take neomycin as directed for full course of therapy. Take missed doses as soon as possible if not almost time for next dose; do not take double doses.
- Caution patient that neomycin may cause nausea, vomiting, or diarrhea.
- **Topical:** Instruct patient to wash affected skin gently and pat dry. Apply a thin film of ointment. Apply occlusive dressing only if directed by health care professional. Patient should assess skin and inform health care professional if skin irritation develops or infection worsens.
- **Inhaln: Amikacin**: Advise patient to omit missed doses and administer next dose next day; do not double doses. Instruct patient to read *Medication Guide* before starting and with each Rx refill in case of changes.
- Advise patient to notify health care professional if signs and symptoms of allergic inflammation of lungs (fever, wheezing, coughing, shortness of breath, fast breathing), hemoptysis (coughing up blood), bronchospasm (shortness of breath, difficult or labored breathing, wheezing, coughing, chest tightness) or worsening of COPD occur. **Tobramycin**: Instruct patient to take inhalation twice daily as close to 12 hr apart as possible; not <6 hr apart. Solution is colorless to pale yellow and may darken with age without effecting quality. Administer over 15 min period using a hand-held PARI LC PLUS reusable nebulizer with a *PARI VIOS (for Bethkis) or DeVibiss Pulmo Aide (for TOBI)* compressor. Instruct patient on multiple therapies to take others first and use *tobramycin* last. Tobramycin-induced bronchospasm may be reduced if tobramycin is administered after bronchodilators. Instruct patient to sit or stand upright during inhalation and breathe normally through mouthpiece of nebulizer. Nose clips may help patient breath through mouth. Store at room temperature for up to 28 days. Advise patient to disinfect the nebulizer parts (except tubing) by boiling them in water for a full 10 min every other treatment day.
- Instruct patient in correct technique for use of *TOBI Podhaler*. Wipe mouthpiece with clean, dry cloth after use; do not wash with water.

Evaluation/Desired Outcomes

- Resolution of the signs and symptoms of infection. If no response is seen within 3–5 days, new cultures should be taken.
- Prevention of infection in intestinal surgery (neomycin).
- Improved neurologic status in hepatic encephalopathy (neomycin).
- Endocarditis prophylaxis (gentamicin).

BEERS HIGH ALERT

amiodarone

(am-ee-**oh**-da-rone)

Nexterone, Pacerone

Classification

Therapeutic: antiarrhythmics (class III)

Indications

Life-threatening ventricular arrhythmias unresponsive to less toxic agents. **Unlabeled Use: PO:** Management of supraventricular tachyarrhythmias. **IV:** As part of the Advanced Cardiac Life Support (ACLS) and Pediatric Advanced Life Support (PALS) guidelines for the management of ventricular fibrillation (VF)/pulseless ventricular tachycardia (VT) after cardiopulmonary resuscitation and defibrillation have failed; also for other life-threatening tachyarrhythmias.

Action

Prolongs action potential and refractory period. Inhibits adrenergic stimulation. Slows the sinus rate, increases PR and QT intervals, and decreases peripheral vascular resistance (vasodilation). **Therapeutic Effects:** Suppression of arrhythmias.

Pharmacokinetics

Absorption: Slowly and variably absorbed from the GI tract (35–65%). IV administration results in complete bioavailability.
Distribution: Distributed to and accumulates slowly in body tissues. Reaches high levels in fat, muscle, liver, lungs, and spleen. Crosses the placenta and enters breast milk.
Protein Binding: 96% bound to plasma proteins.
Metabolism and Excretion: Metabolized by the liver, excreted into bile. Minimal renal excretion. One metabolite has antiarrhythmic activity.
Half-life: 13–107 days.

TIME/ACTION PROFILE (suppression of ventricular arrhythmias)

ROUTE	ONSET	PEAK	DURATION
PO	2–3 days (up to 2–3 mo)	3–7 hr	wk–mos
IV	2 hr	3–7 hr	unknown

Contraindications/Precautions

Contraindicated in: Patients with cardiogenic shock; Severe sinus node dysfunction; 2nd- and 3rd-degree AV block; Bradycardia (has caused syncope unless a pacemaker is in place); Hypersensitivity to amiodarone or iodine; OB: May cause fetal harm (cardiac, thyroid, neurodevelopmental, neurological, and growth adverse effects); Lactation: Enters breast milk and can cause harm to the neonate; avoid breast feeding; Pedi: Safety not established; products containing benzyl alcohol should not be used in neonates.
Use Cautiously in: History of HF; Thyroid disorders; Corneal refractive laser surgery; Severe pulmonary or liver disease; Geri: Initiate therapy at the low end of the dosing range due to ↓ hepatic, renal, or cardiac function; comorbid disease; or other drug therapy.

Adverse Reactions/Side Effects

CNS: confusional states, disorientation, hallucinations, dizziness, fatigue, malaise, headache, insomnia. **EENT:** corneal microdeposits, abnormal sense of smell, dry eyes, optic neuritis, optic neuropathy, photophobia. **Resp:** ADULT RESPIRATORY DISTRESS SYNDROME (ARDS), PULMONARY FIBROSIS, PULMONARY TOXICITY. **CV:** HF, WORSENING OF ARRHYTHMIAS, QT INTERVAL PROLONGATION, bradycardia, hypotension. **GI:** anorexia, constipation, nausea, vomiting, abdominal pain, abnormal sense of taste, ↑ liver enzymes. **GU:** ↓ libido, epididymitis. **Derm:** TOXIC EPIDERMAL NECROLYSIS (rare), photosensitivity, blue discoloration. **Endo:** hypothyroidism, hyperthyroidism. **Neuro:** ataxia, involuntary movement, paresthesia, peripheral neuropathy, poor coordination, tremor.

Interactions

Drug-Drug: ↑ risk of QT prolongation with **fluoroquinolones**, **macrolides**, and **azole antifungals** (undertake concurrent use with caution). ↑ levels of **digoxin** (↓ dose of digoxin by 50%). ↑ levels of **class I antiarrhythmics** (**quinidine**, **mexiletine**, **lidocaine**, or **flecainide**—↓ doses of other drugs by 30–50%). ↑ levels of **cyclosporine**, **dextromethorphan**, **methotrexate**, **phenytoin**, **carvedilol**, and **theophylline**. **Phenytoin** ↓ amiodarone levels. ↑ activity of **warfarin** (↓ dose of warfarin by 33–50%). ↑ risk of bradyarrhythmias, sinus arrest, or AV heart block with **beta blockers**, **verapamil**, **diltiazem**, **digoxin**, **ivabradine**, or **clonidine**. ↑ risk of bradycardia when used with **ledipasvir/sofosbuvir** or with **sofosbuvir** with **simeprevir**. **Cholestyramine** may ↓ amiodarone levels. **Cimetidine** and **ritonavir** ↑ amiodarone levels. Risk of myocardial depression is ↑ by **volatile anesthetics**. ↑ risk of myopathy with **lovastatin** and **simvastatin** (do not exceed 40 mg/day of lovastatin or 20 mg/day of simvastatin).
Drug-Natural Products: **St. John's wort** induces enzymes that metabolize amiodarone; may ↓ levels and effectiveness. Avoid concurrent use.
Drug-Food: **Grapefruit juice** inhibits enzymes in the GI tract that metabolize amiodarone resulting in ↑ levels and risk of toxicity; avoid concurrent use.

Route/Dosage

Ventricular Arrhythmias

PO (Adults): 800–1600 mg/day in 1–2 doses for 1–3 wk, then 600–800 mg/day in 1–2 doses for 1 mo, then 400 mg/day maintenance dose.
PO (Children): 10 mg/kg/day (800 mg/1.72 m^2/day) for 10 days or until response or adverse reaction occurs, then 5 mg/kg/day (400 mg/1.72 m^2/day) for several wk, then ↓ to 2.5 mg/kg/day (200 mg/1.72 m^2/day) or lowest effective maintenance dose.
IV (Adults): 150 mg over 10 min, followed by 360 mg over the next 6 hr and then 540 mg over the next 18 hr. Continue infusion at 0.5 mg/min until oral therapy is initiated. If arrhythmia recurs, a small loading infusion of 150 mg over 10 min should be given; in addition, the rate of the maintenance infusion may be ↑. *Conversion to initial oral therapy*—If duration of IV infusion was <1 wk, oral dose should be 800–1600 mg/day; if IV infusion was 1–3 wk, oral dose should be 600–800 mg/day; if IV infusion was >3 wk, oral dose should be 400 mg/day. *ACLS guidelines for pulseless VF/VT*—300 mg IV push, may repeat once after 3–5 min with 150 mg IV push (maximum cumulative dose 2.2 g/24 hr; unlabeled).
IV: Intraosseous (Children and infants): *PALS guidelines for pulseless VF/VT*—5 mg/kg as a bolus; *Perfusion tachycardia*—5 mg/kg loading dose over 20–60 min (maximum of 15 mg/kg/day; unlabeled).

Supraventricular Tachycardia

PO (Adults): 600–800 mg/day for 1 wk or until desired response occurs or side effects develop, then ↓ to 400 mg/day for 3 wk, then maintenance dose of 200–400 mg/day.

PO (Children): 10 mg/kg/day (800 mg/1.72 m^2/day) for 10 days or until response or side effects occur, then 5 mg/kg/day (400 mg/1.72 m^2/day) for several wk, then ↓ to 2.5 mg/kg/day (200 mg/1.72 m^2/day) or lowest effective maintenance dose.

Availability (generic available)

Tablets: 100 mg, 200 mg, 400 mg. **Injection:** 50 mg/mL. **Premixed infusion (Nexterone):** 150 mg/100 mL D5W (does not contain polysorbate 80 or benzyl alcohol), 360 mg/200 mL D5W (does not contain polysorbate 80 or benzyl alcohol).

NURSING IMPLICATIONS

Assessment

- Monitor ECG continuously during IV therapy or initiation of oral therapy. Monitor heart rate and rhythm throughout therapy; PR prolongation, slight QRS widening, T-wave amplitude reduction with T-wave widening and bifurcation, and U waves may occur. QT prolongation may be associated with worsening of arrhythmias; monitor closely during IV therapy. Report bradycardia or increase in arrhythmias promptly; patients receiving IV therapy may require slowing rate, discontinuing infusion, or inserting a temporary pacemaker.
- Assess pacing and defibrillation threshold in patients with pacemakers and implanted defibrillators at beginning and periodically during therapy.
- Assess for signs of pulmonary toxicity (rales/crackles, decreased breath sounds, pleuritic friction rub, fatigue, dyspnea, cough, wheezing, pleuritic pain, fever, hemoptysis, hypoxia). Chest x-ray and pulmonary function tests are recommended before therapy. Monitor chest x-ray every 3–6 mo during therapy to detect diffuse interstitial changes or alveolar infiltrates. Bronchoscopy or gallium radionuclide scan may also be used for diagnosis. Usually reversible after withdrawal, but fatalities have occurred.
- **IV:** Assess for signs and symptoms of ARDS throughout therapy. Report dyspnea, tachypnea, or rales/crackles promptly. Bilateral, diffuse pulmonary infiltrates are seen on chest x-ray.
- Monitor BP frequently. Hypotension usually occurs during first several hrs of therapy and is related to rate of infusion. If hypotension occurs, slow rate.
- **PO:** Assess for neurotoxicity (ataxia, proximal muscle weakness, tingling or numbness in fingers or toes, uncontrolled movements, tremors); common during initial therapy, but may occur within 1 wk to several mo of initiation of therapy and may persist for more than 1 yr after withdrawal. Dose reduction is recommended. Assist patient during ambulation to prevent falls.
- Ophthalmic exams should be performed before and regularly during therapy and whenever visual changes (photophobia, halos around lights, decreased acuity) occur. May cause permanent loss of vision.
- Assess for signs of thyroid dysfunction, especially during initial therapy. Lethargy; weight gain; edema of the hands, feet, and periorbital region; and cool, pale skin suggest hypothyroidism and may require decrease in dose or discontinuation of therapy and thyroid supplementation. Tachycardia; weight loss; nervousness; sensitivity to heat; insomnia; and warm, flushed, moist skin suggest hyperthyroidism and may require discontinuation of therapy and treatment with antithyroid agents.
- ***Lab Test Considerations:*** Monitor liver and thyroid functions before and every 6 mo during therapy. Drug effects persist long after discontinuation. Thyroid function abnormalities are common, but clinical thyroid dysfunction is uncommon.
- Monitor AST, ALT, and alkaline phosphatase at regular intervals during therapy, especially in patients receiving high maintenance dose. If liver function studies are 3 times normal or double in patients with elevated baseline levels or if hepatomegaly occurs, dose should be reduced.
- May cause asymptomatic ↑ in ANA titer concentrations.
- Monitor serum potassium, calcium, and magnesium prior to starting and periodically during therapy. Hypokalemia, hypocalcemia, and/or hypomagnesemia may ↓ effectiveness or cause additional arrhythmias; correct levels before beginning therapy. Monitor closely when converting from IV to oral therapy, especially in geriatric patients.

Implementation

- ***High Alert:*** IV vasoactive medications are inherently dangerous; fatalities have occurred from medication errors involving amiodarone. Before administering, have second practitioner check original order, dose calculations, and infusion pump settings. Patients should be hospitalized and monitored closely during IV therapy and initiation of oral therapy. IV therapy should be administered only by clinicians experienced in treating life-threatening arrhythmias.
- Do not confuse amiodarone with amantadine.
- **PO:** May be administered with meals and in divided doses if GI intolerance occurs or if daily dose exceeds 1000 mg.

IV Administration

- **IV:** Administer via volumetric pump; drop size may be reduced, causing altered dosing with drop counter infusion sets.
- Administer through an in-line filter.
- Infusions exceeding 2 hr must be administered in glass or polyolefin bottles to prevent adsorption.

However, polyvinyl chloride (PVC) tubing must be used during administration because concentrations and infusion rate recommendations have been based on PVC tubing.

- **IV Push:** ***Diluent:*** Administer undiluted. May also be diluted in 20–30 mL of D5W or 0.9% NaCl. ***Concentration:*** 50 mg/mL. ***Rate:*** Administer IV push.
- **Intermittent Infusion:** ***Diluent:*** Dilute 150 mg of amiodarone in 100 mL of D5W. Infusion stable for 2 hr in PVC bag, or use pre-mixed bags. ***Concentration:*** 1.5 mg/mL. ***Rate:*** Infuse over 10 min. Do not administer IV push.
- **Continuous Infusion:** ***Diluent:*** Dilute 900 mg (18 mL) of amiodarone in 500 mL of D5W. Infusion stable for 24 hr in glass or polyolefin bottle. ***Concentration:*** 1.8 mg/mL. Concentration may range from 1–6 mg/mL (concentrations >2 mg/mL must be administered via central venous catheter). ***Rate:*** Infuse at a rate of 1 mg/min for the first 6 hr, then decrease infusion rate to 0.5 mg/min and continue until oral therapy initiated.
- **Y-Site Compatibility:** alemtuzumab, alfentanil, amikacin, amphotericin B lipid complex, anidulafungin, atracurium, atropine, bleomycin, buprenorphine, busulfan, butorphanol, calcium chloride, cangrelor, carboplatin, carmustine, caspofungin, cefepime, ceftaroline, chlorpromazine, ciprofloxacin, cisatracurium, cisplatin, clindamycin, cyclophosphamide, cyclosporine, dacarbazine, dactinomycin, daptomycin, daunorubicin, dexmedetomidine, dexrazoxane, diltiazem, diphenhydramine, docetaxel, dolasetron, dopamine, doxacurium, doxycycline, droperidol, enalaprilat, ephedrine, epinephrine, erythromycin lactobionate, esmolol, etoposide, etoposide phosphate, famotidine, fenoldopam, fluconazole, gemcitabine, gentamicin, glycopyrrolate, granisetron, hydralazine, hydromorphone, idarubicin, ifosfamide, irinotecan, isoproterenol, ketamine, labetalol, lidocaine, linezolid, lorazepam, mannitol, meperidine, mesna, metoclopramide, metoprolol, metronidazole, midazolam, milrinone, mitoxantrone, morphine, moxifloxacin, mycophenolate, nafcillin, nalbuphine, naloxone, nicardipine, nitroglycerin, octreotide, ondansetron, oxaliplatin, palonosetron, pancuronium, pemetrexed, penicillin G potassium, pentamidine, phentolamine, phenylephrine, procainamide, prochlorperazine, promethazine, propranolol, quinupristin/dalfopristin, remifentanil, rifampin, rocuronium, streptozocin, succinylcholine, sufentanil, tacrolimus, theophylline, tirofiban, tobramycin, topotecan, vancomycin, vasopressin, vecuronium, vinblastine, vincristine, vinorelbine, voriconazole, zidovudine, zoledronic acid.
- **Y-Site Incompatibility:** acyclovir, allopurinol, amifostine, aminocaproic acid, aminophylline, ampicillin, ampicillin/sulbactam, azithromycin, bivalirudin, cefotaxime, cefotetan, ceftazidime, chloramphenicol, cytarabine, dantrolene, dexamethasone, diazepam, digoxin, doxorubicin, ertapenem, fludarabine, fluorouracil, foscarnet, fosphenytoin, ganciclovir, heparin, hydrocortisone, imipenem-cilastatin, ketorolac, leucovorin, levofloxacin, melphalan, meropenem, methotrexate, micafungin, mitomycin, paclitaxel, pentobarbital, phenobarbital, phenytoin, piperacillin/tazobactam, potassium acetate, potassium phosphates, ranitidine, sodium acetate, sodium bicarbonate, sodium phosphates, thiopental, thiotepa, tigecycline, trimethoprim/sulfamethoxazole, verapamil.

Patient/Family Teaching

- Instruct patient to take amiodarone as directed. If a dose is missed, do not take at all. Consult health care professional if more than two doses are missed. Advise patient to read the *Medication Guide* prior to first dose and with each Rx refill in case of changes.
- Advise patient to avoid drinking grapefruit juice during therapy.
- Inform patient that side effects may not appear until several days, weeks, or yr after initiation of therapy and may persist for several mo after withdrawal.
- Teach patients to monitor pulse daily and report abnormalities.
- Advise patients that photosensitivity reactions may occur through window glass, thin clothing, and sunscreens. Protective clothing and sunblock are recommended during and for 4 mo after therapy. If photosensitivity occurs, dose reduction may be useful.
- Inform patients that bluish discoloration of the face, neck, and arms is a possible side effect of this drug after prolonged use. This is usually reversible and will fade over several mo. Notify health care professional if this occurs.
- Instruct male patients to notify health care professional if signs of epididymitis (pain and swelling in scrotum) occur. May require reduction in dose.
- Advise patient to notify health care professional of all Rx or OTC medications, vitamins, or herbal products being taken and to consult with health care professional before taking other medications, especially St. John's wort.
- Instruct patient to notify health care professional of medication regimen before treatment or surgery.
- Advise patient to notify health care professional if signs and symptoms of thyroid dysfunction occur.
- Advise female patient to notify health care professional if pregnancy is planned or suspected and to avoid breast feeding during therapy.
- Emphasize the importance of follow-up exams, including chest x-ray and pulmonary function tests every 3–6 mo and ophthalmic exams after 6 mo of therapy, and then annually.

Evaluation/Desired Outcomes

- Cessation of life-threatening ventricular arrhythmias. Adverse effects may take up to 4 mo to resolve.

BEERS

amitriptyline

(a-mee-**trip**-ti-leen)

Elavil, Levate

Classification

Therapeutic: antidepressants

Pharmacologic: tricyclic antidepressants

Indications

Depression. **Unlabeled Use:** Anxiety, insomnia, treatment-resistant depression. Chronic pain syndromes (i.e., fibromyalgia, neuropathic pain/chronic pain, headache, low back pain).

Action

Potentiates the effect of serotonin and norepinephrine in the CNS. Has significant anticholinergic properties. **Therapeutic Effects:** Antidepressant action.

Pharmacokinetics

Absorption: Well absorbed from the GI tract.

Distribution: Widely distributed.

Protein Binding: 95% bound to plasma proteins.

Metabolism and Excretion: Extensively metabolized by the liver. Some metabolites have antidepressant activity. Undergoes enterohepatic recirculation and secretion into gastric juices. Probably crosses the placenta and enters breast milk.

Half-life: 10–50 hr.

TIME/ACTION PROFILE (antidepressant effect)

ROUTE	ONSET	PEAK	DURATION
PO	2–3 wk (up to 30 days)	2–6 wk	days–wk

Contraindications/Precautions

Contraindicated in: Angle-closure glaucoma; Known history of QTc interval prolongation, recent MI, or heart failure.

Use Cautiously in: May ↑ risk of suicide attempt/ideation especially during dose early treatment or dose adjustment; risk may be greater in children or adolescents; Patients with pre-existing cardiovascular disease; Prostatic hyperplasia (↑ risk of urinary retention); History of seizures (threshold may be ↓); OB: Use only if clearly needed and maternal benefits outweigh risk to fetus; Lactation: May cause sedation in infant; Pedi: Children <12 yr (safety not established); Geri: Appears on Beers list. ↑ risk of adverse reactions including falls secondary to sedative and anticholinergic effects.

Adverse Reactions/Side Effects

CNS: SUICIDAL THOUGHTS, lethargy, sedation. **EENT:** blurred vision, dry eyes, dry mouth. **CV:** ARRHYTHMIAS, TORSADE DE POINTES, hypotension, ECG changes, QT interval prolongation. **GI:** constipation, hepatitis, paralytic ileus, ↑ appetite, weight gain. **GU:** urinary retention, ↓ libido. **Derm:** photosensitivity. **Endo:** changes in blood glucose, gynecomastia. **Hemat:** blood dyscrasias.

Interactions

Drug-Drug: Amitriptyline is metabolized in the liver by the cytochrome P450 2D6 enzyme, and its action may be affected by drugs that compete for metabolism by this enzyme, including other **antidepressants**, **phenothiazines**, **carbamazepine**, **class 1C antiarrhythmics** including **propafenone**, and **flecainide**; when these drugs are used concurrently with amitriptyline, dosage ↓ of one or the other or both may be necessary. Concurrent use of other drugs that inhibit the activity of the enzyme, including **cimetidine**, **quinidine**, **amiodarone**, and **ritonavir**, may result in ↑ effects of amitriptyline. May cause hypotension, tachycardia, and potentially fatal reactions when used with **MAO inhibitors** (avoid concurrent use—discontinue 2 wk before starting amitriptyline). Concurrent use with **SSRI antidepressants** may result in ↑ toxicity and should be avoided (**fluoxetine** should be stopped 5 wk before starting amitriptyline). Concurrent use with **clonidine** may result in hypertensive crisis and should be avoided. Concurrent use with **levodopa** may result in delayed or ↓ absorption of levodopa or hypertension. Blood levels and effects may be ↓ by **rifampin**, **rifapentine**, and **rifabutin**. Concurrent use with **moxifloxacin** ↑ risk of adverse cardiovascular reactions. ↑ CNS depression with other **CNS depressants** including **alcohol**, **antihistamines**, **clonidine**, **opioids**, and **sedative/hypnotics**. **Barbiturates** may alter blood levels and effects. **Adrenergic** and **anticholinergic** side effects may be ↑ with other agents having **anticholinergic** properties. **Phenothiazines** or **oral contraceptives** ↑ levels and may cause toxicity. **Nicotine** may ↑ metabolism and alter effects.

Drug-Natural Products: St. John's wort may ↓ serum concentrations and efficacy. Concomitant use of **kava-kava**, **valerian**, or **chamomile** can ↑ CNS depression. ↑ anticholinergic effects with **jimson weed** and **scopolia**.

Route/Dosage

PO (Adults): 75 mg/day in divided doses; may be ↑ up to 150 mg/day *or* 50–100 mg at bedtime, may ↑ by 25–50 mg up to 150 mg (in hospitalized patients, may initiate with 100 mg/day, and ↑ total daily dose up to 300 mg).

PO (Geriatric Patients): 10–25 mg at bedtime; may ↑ by 10–25 mg weekly if tolerated (usual dose range = 25–150 mg/day).

Availability (generic available)

Tablets: 10 mg, 25 mg, 50 mg, 75 mg, 100 mg, 150 mg. **Cost:** *Generic*—25 mg $9.33/100, 75 mg $9.83/100.

NURSING IMPLICATIONS

Assessment

- Obtain weight and BMI initially and periodically during treatment.
- Assess fasting glucose and cholesterol levels in overweight/obese individuals.
- Monitor BP and pulse before and during initial therapy. Notify health care professional of decreases in BP (10–20 mm Hg) or sudden increase in pulse rate. Patients taking high doses or with a history of cardiovascular disease should have ECG monitored before and periodically during therapy.
- **Depression:** Monitor mental status (orientation, mood behavior) frequently. Assess for suicidal tendencies, especially during early therapy. Restrict amount of drug available to patient.
- Assess for suicidal tendencies, especially during early therapy. Restrict amount of drug available to patient. Risk may be increased in children, adolescents, and adults ≤24 yrs. After starting therapy, children, adolescents, and young adults should be seen by health care professional at least weekly for 4 wk, every 3 wk for next 4 wk, and on advice of health care professional thereafter.
- **Pain:** Assess intensity, quality, and location of pain periodically during therapy. May require several wk for effects to be seen. Use pain scale to monitor effectiveness of medication. Assess for sexual dysfunction (decreased libido; erectile dysfunction). Geri: Geriatric patients started on amitriptyline may be at an increased risk for falls; start with low dose and monitor closely. Assess for anticholinergic effects (weakness and sedation).
- ***Lab Test Considerations:*** Assess leukocyte and differential blood counts, liver function, and serum glucose before and periodically during therapy. May cause an ↑ serum bilirubin and alkaline phosphatase. May cause bone marrow depression. Serum glucose may be ↑ or ↓.

Implementation

- Dose increases should be made at bedtime because of sedation. Dose titration is a slow process; may take wk to mo. May give entire dose at bedtime. Sedative effect may be apparent before antidepressant effect is noted. May require tapering to avoid withdrawal effects.
- **PO:** Administer medication with or immediately after a meal to minimize gastric upset. Tablet may be crushed and given with food or fluids.

Patient/Family Teaching

- Instruct patient to take medication as directed. If a dose is missed, take as soon as possible unless almost time for next dose; if regimen is a single dose at bedtime, do not take in the morning because of side effects. Advise patient that drug effects may not be noticed for at least 2 wk. Abrupt discontinuation may cause nausea, vomiting, diarrhea, headache, trouble sleeping with vivid dreams, and irritability.
- May cause drowsiness and blurred vision. Caution patient to avoid driving and other activities requiring alertness until response to drug is known.
- Orthostatic hypotension, sedation, and confusion are common during early therapy, especially in geriatric patients. Protect patient from falls and advise patient to make position changes slowly. Institute fall precautions. Advise patient to make position changes slowly. Refer as appropriate for nutrition/weight management and medical management.
- Advise patient to avoid alcohol or other CNS depressant drugs during and for 3–7 days after therapy has been discontinued.
- Advise patient, family and caregivers to look for suicidality, especially during early therapy or dose changes. Notify health care professional immediately if thoughts about suicide or dying, attempts to commit suicide, new or worse depression or anxiety, agitation or restlessness, panic attacks, insomnia, new or worse irritability, aggressiveness, acting on dangerous impulses, mania, or other changes in mood or behavior occur.
- Instruct patient to notify health care professional if urinary retention, dry mouth, or constipation persists. Sugarless candy or gum may diminish dry mouth, and an increase in fluid intake or bulk may prevent constipation. If symptoms persist, dose reduction or discontinuation may be necessary. Consult health care professional if dry mouth persists for >2 wk.
- Caution patient to use sunscreen and protective clothing to prevent photosensitivity reactions. Alert patient that medication may turn urine blue-green in color.
- Inform patient of need to monitor dietary intake. Increase in appetite may lead to undesired weight gain.
- Advise patient to notify health care professional of medication regimen before treatment or surgery. Medication should be discontinued as long as possible before surgery.
- Advise patient to notify health care professional if pregnancy is planned or suspected or if breast feeding.
- Therapy for depression is usually prolonged and should be continued for at least 3 mo to prevent relapse. Emphasize the importance of follow-up exams to monitor effectiveness, side effects, and improved coping skills. Advise patient and family that treatment is not a cure and symptoms can recur after discontinuation of medication.

Evaluation/Desired Outcomes

- Increased sense of well-being.
- Renewed interest in surroundings.

- Increased appetite.
- Improved energy level.
- Improved sleep.
- Decrease in chronic pain symptoms.
- Full therapeutic effects may be seen 2–6 wk after initiating therapy.

amLODIPine (am-loe-di-peen)

Norvasc

Classification

Therapeutic: antihypertensives

Pharmacologic: calcium channel blockers

Indications

Alone or with other agents in the management of hypertension, angina pectoris, and vasospastic (Prinzmetal's) angina.

Action

Inhibits the transport of calcium into myocardial and vascular smooth muscle cells, resulting in inhibition of excitation-contraction coupling and subsequent contraction. **Therapeutic Effects:** Systemic vasodilation resulting in decreased BP. Coronary vasodilation resulting in decreased frequency and severity of attacks of angina.

Pharmacokinetics

Absorption: Well absorbed after oral administration (64–90%).

Distribution: Probably crosses the placenta.

Protein Binding: 95–98%.

Metabolism and Excretion: Mostly metabolized by the liver.

Half-life: 30–50 hr (↑ in geriatric patients and patients with hepatic impairment).

TIME/ACTION PROFILE (cardiovascular effects)

ROUTE	ONSET	PEAK	DURATION
PO	unknown	6–9	24 hr

Contraindications/Precautions

Contraindicated in: Hypersensitivity; Systolic BP <90 mm Hg.

Use Cautiously in: Severe hepatic impairment (dose reduction recommended); Aortic stenosis; History of HF; OB, Lactation, Pedi: Children <6 yr (safety not established); Geri: Dose reduction recommended; ↑ risk of hypotension.

Adverse Reactions/Side Effects

CNS: dizziness, fatigue. **CV:** peripheral edema, angina, bradycardia, hypotension, palpitations. **Derm:** flushing. **GI:** gingival hyperplasia, nausea.

Interactions

Drug-Drug: Strong CYP3A4 inhibitors, including **ketoconazole, itraconazole, clarithromycin**, and **ritonavir** may ↑ levels. Additive hypotension may occur when used concurrently with **fentanyl**, other **antihypertensives, nitrates**, acute ingestion of **alcohol**, or **quinidine**. Antihypertensive effects may be ↓ by concurrent use of **nonsteroidal anti-inflammatory agents**. May ↑ risk of neurotoxicity with **lithium**. ↑ risk of myopathy with **simvastatin** (do not exceed 20 mg/day of simvastatin). May ↑ **cyclosporine** and **tacrolimus** levels.

Route/Dosage

PO (Adults): 5–10 mg once daily; *antihypertensive in fragile or small patients or patients already receiving other antihypertensives*—initiate at 2.5 mg/day, ↑ as required/tolerated (up to 10 mg/day) as an antihypertensive therapy with 2.5 mg/day in patients with hepatic insufficiency.

PO (Geriatric Patients): *Antihypertensive*—Initiate therapy at 2.5 mg/day, ↑ as required/tolerated (up to 10 mg/day); *antianginal*—initiate therapy at 5 mg/day, ↑ as required/tolerated (up to 10 mg/day).

PO (Children 6–17 yr): 2.5–5 mg once daily.

Hepatic Impairment

PO (Adults): *Antihypertensive*—Initiate therapy at 2.5 mg/day, ↑ as required/tolerated (up to 10 mg/day); *antianginal*—initiate therapy at 5 mg/day, ↑ as required/tolerated (up to 10 mg/day).

Availability (generic available)

Tablets: 2.5 mg, 5 mg, 10 mg. **Cost:** *Generic*—2.5 mg $11.35/100, 5 mg $12.86/100, 10 mg $8.42/100. ***In combination with:*** aliskiren/hydrochlorothiazide (Amturnide), atorvastatin (Caduet), benazepril (Lotrel), celecoxib (Consensi), olmesartan (Azor), olmesartan/hydrochlorothiazide (Tribenzor), perindopril (Prestalia), telmisartan (Twynsta), valsartan (Exforge), and valsartan/hydrochlorothiazide (Exforge HCT). See Appendix B.

NURSING IMPLICATIONS

Assessment

- Monitor BP and pulse before therapy, during dose titration, and periodically during therapy. Monitor ECG periodically during prolonged therapy.
- Monitor intake and output ratios and daily weight. Assess for signs of HF (peripheral edema, rales/crackles, dyspnea, weight gain, jugular venous distention).
- Monitor frequency of prescription refills to determine adherence.
- **Angina:** Assess location, duration, intensity, and precipitating factors of patient's anginal pain.

- ***Lab Test Considerations:*** Total serum calcium concentrations are not affected by calcium channel blockers.

Implementation

- Do not confuse amlodipine with amiloride.
- **PO:** May be administered without regard to meals.

Patient/Family Teaching

- Advise patient to take medication as directed, even if feeling well. Take missed doses as soon as possible within 12 hrs of missed dose. If >12 hrs since missed dose, skip dose and take next dose at scheduled time; do not double doses. May need to be discontinued gradually.
- Instruct patient on correct technique for monitoring pulse. Instruct patient to contact health care professional if heart rate is <50 bpm.
- Caution patient to change positions slowly to minimize orthostatic hypotension.
- May cause drowsiness or dizziness. Advise patient to avoid driving or other activities requiring alertness until response to the medication is known.
- Instruct patient on importance of maintaining good dental hygiene and seeing dentist frequently for teeth cleaning to prevent tenderness, bleeding, and gingival hyperplasia (gum enlargement).
- Instruct patient to notify health care professional of all Rx or OTC medications, vitamins, or herbal products being taken, to avoid alcohol, and to consult health care professional before taking any new medications, especially cold preparations.
- Advise patient to notify health care professional if irregular heartbeats, dyspnea, swelling of hands and feet, pronounced dizziness, nausea, constipation, or hypotension occurs or if headache is severe or persistent.
- Caution patient to wear protective clothing and use sunscreen to prevent photosensitivity reactions.
- Advise patient to inform health care professional of medication regimen before treatment or surgery.
- Instruct female patient to notify health care professional if pregnancy is planned or suspected or if breast feeding.
- **Angina:** Instruct patient on concurrent nitrate or beta-blocker therapy to continue taking both medications as directed and to use SL nitroglycerin as needed for anginal attacks.
- Advise patient to contact health care professional if chest pain does not improve or worsens after therapy, if it occurs with diaphoresis, if shortness of breath occurs, or if severe, persistent headache occurs.
- Caution patient to discuss exercise restrictions with health care professional before exertion.
- **Hypertension:** Encourage patient to comply with other interventions for hypertension (weight reduction, low-sodium diet, smoking cessation, moderation of alcohol consumption, regular exercise, and stress management). Medication controls but does not cure hypertension.
- Instruct patient and family in proper technique for monitoring BP. Advise patient to take BP weekly and to report significant changes to health care professional.

Evaluation/Desired Outcomes

- Decrease in BP.
- Decrease in frequency and severity of anginal attacks.
- Decrease in need for nitrate therapy.
- Increase in activity tolerance and sense of well-being.

amoxicillin (a-mox-i-**sill**-in)

~~Amoxil~~, ~~Trimox~~

Classification

Therapeutic: anti-infectives, antiulcer agents

Pharmacologic: aminopenicillins

Indications

Treatment of: Skin and skin structure infections, Otitis media, Sinusitis, Respiratory infections, Genitourinary infections. Endocarditis prophylaxis. Postexposure inhalational anthrax prophylaxis. Management of ulcer disease due to *Helicobacter pylori*. **Unlabeled Use:** Lyme disease in children <8 yr.

Action

Binds to bacterial cell wall, causing cell death. **Therapeutic Effects:** Bactericidal action; spectrum is broader than penicillins. **Spectrum:** Active against: Streptococci, Pneumococci, Enterococci, *Haemophilus influenzae*, *Escherichia coli*, *Proteus mirabilis*, *Neisseria meningitidis*, *N. gonorrhoeae*, *Shigella*, *Chlamydia trachomatis*, *Salmonella*, *Borrelia burgdorferi*, *H. pylori*.

Pharmacokinetics

Absorption: Well absorbed from duodenum (75–90%). More resistant to acid inactivation than other penicillins.

Distribution: Diffuses readily into most body tissues and fluids. CSF penetration increased when meninges are inflamed. Crosses placenta; enters breast milk in small amounts.

Metabolism and Excretion: 70% excreted unchanged in the urine; 30% metabolized by the liver.

Half-life: Neonates: 3.7 hr; Infants and Children: 1–2 hr; Adults: 0.7–1.4 hr.

TIME/ACTION PROFILE (blood levels)

ROUTE	ONSET	PEAK	DURATION
PO	30 min	1–2 hr	8–12 hr

Contraindications/Precautions

Contraindicated in: Hypersensitivity to penicillins (cross-sensitivity exists to cephalosporins and other beta-lactams).

Use Cautiously in: Severe renal impairment (↓ dose if CCr <30 mL/min); Infectious mononucleosis, acute lymphocytic leukemia, or cytomegalovirus infection (↑ risk of rash); OB, Lactation: Has been used safely.

Adverse Reactions/Side Effects

CNS: SEIZURES (high doses). **Derm:** rash, urticaria. **GI:** CLOSTRIDIUM DIFFICILE-ASSOCIATED DIARRHEA (CDAD), diarrhea, nausea, vomiting, ↑ liver enzymes. **Hemat:** blood dyscrasias. **Misc:** HYPERSENSITIVITY REACTIONS (including anaphylaxis), SERUM SICKNESS, superinfection.

Interactions

Drug-Drug: Probenecid ↓ renal excretion and ↑ blood levels of amoxicillin—therapy may be combined for this purpose. May ↑ effect of **warfarin**. May ↓ effectiveness of **oral contraceptives**. **Allopurinol** may ↑ frequency of rash.

Route/Dosage

Most Infections

PO (Adults): 250–500 mg every 8 hr *or* 500–875 mg every 12 hr (not to exceed 2–3 g/day).
PO (Children >3 mo): 25–50 mg/kg/day in divided doses every 8 hr *or* 25–50 mg/kg/day in divided doses every 12 hr; *Acute otitis media due to highly resistant strains of S. pneumoniae*—80–90 mg/kg/day in divided doses every 12 hr; *Postexposure inhalational anthrax prophylaxis*—<40 kg: 45 mg/kg/day in divided doses every 8 hr; >40 kg: 500 mg every 8 hr.
PO (Infants ≤3 mo and neonates): 20–30 mg/kg/day in divided doses every 12 hr.

H. Pylori

PO (Adults): *Triple therapy*—1000 mg amoxicillin twice daily with lansoprazole 30 mg twice daily and clarithromycin 500 mg twice daily for 14 days *or* 1000 mg amoxicillin twice daily with omeprazole 20 mg twice daily and clarithromycin 500 mg twice daily for 14 days *or* amoxicillin 1000 mg twice daily with esomeprazole 40 mg daily and clarithromycin 500 mg twice daily for 10 days. *Dual therapy*—1000 mg amoxicillin three times daily with lansoprazole 30 mg three times daily for 14 days.

Endocarditis Prophylaxis

PO (Adults): 2 g 1 hr prior to procedure.
PO (Children): 50 mg/kg 1 hr prior to procedure (not to exceed adult dose).

Gonorrhea

PO (Adults and Children ≥40 kg): Single 3 g dose.
PO (Children >2 yr and <40 kg): 50 mg/kg with probenecid 25 mg/kg as a single dose.

Renal Impairment

PO (Adults): *CCr 10–30 mL/min*—250–500 mg every 12 hr; *CCr <10 mL/min*—250–500 mg every 24 hr.

Availability (generic available)

Capsules: 250 mg, 500 mg. **Cost:** *Generic*—250 mg $5.90/30, 500 mg $5.90/30. **Chewable tablets (cherry, banana, peppermint flavors):** 125 mg, 250 mg. **Cost:** *Generic*—250 mg $15.89/30. **Powder for oral suspension (strawberry [125 mg/5 mL] and bubblegum [200 mg/5 mL, 250 mg/5 mL, 400 mg/5 mL] flavors):** 125 mg/5 mL, 200 mg/5 mL, 250 mg/5 mL, 400 mg/5 mL. **Cost:** *Generic*—125 mg/5 mL $4.11/150 mL, 200 mg/5 mL $6.84/75 mL, 250 mg/5 mL $6.09/100 mL, 400 mg/5 mL $7.33/75 mL. **Tablets:** 500 mg, 875 mg. **Cost:** *Generic*—875 mg $9.53/30. ***In combination with:*** clarithromycin and lansoprazole in a compliance package (Prevpac). See Appendix B.

NURSING IMPLICATIONS

Assessment

- Assess for infection (vital signs; appearance of wound, sputum, urine, and stool; WBC) at beginning of and throughout therapy.
- Obtain a history before initiating therapy to determine previous use of and reactions to penicillins or cephalosporins. Persons with a negative history of penicillin sensitivity may still have an allergic response.
- Observe for signs and symptoms of anaphylaxis (rash, pruritus, laryngeal edema, wheezing). Notify health care professional immediately if these occur.
- Obtain specimens for culture and sensitivity prior to therapy. First dose may be given before receiving results.
- Monitor bowel function. Diarrhea, abdominal cramping, fever, and bloody stools should be reported to health care professional promptly as a sign of Clostridium difficile-associated diarrhea (CDAD). May begin up to several wk following cessation of therapy.
- ***Lab Test Considerations:*** May cause ↑ serum alkaline phosphatase, LDH, AST, and ALT concentrations.
- May cause false-positive direct Coombs' test result.

Implementation

- **PO:** Administer around the clock. May be given without regard to meals or with meals to decrease GI side effects. Capsule contents may be emptied and swallowed with liquids. Extended-release tablets should be swallowed whole; do not crush, break, or chew. Chewable tablets should be crushed or chewed before swallowing with liquids.

- Shake oral suspension before administering. Suspension may be given straight or mixed in formula, milk, fruit juice, water, or ginger ale. Administer immediately after mixing. Discard refrigerated reconstituted suspension after 10 days.

Patient/Family Teaching

- Instruct patients to take medication around the clock and to finish the drug completely as directed, even if feeling better. Advise patients that sharing of this medication may be dangerous.
- Pedi: Teach parents or caregivers to calculate and measure doses accurately. Reinforce importance of using measuring device supplied by pharmacy or with product, not household items.
- Advise patient to report the signs of superinfection (furry overgrowth on the tongue, vaginal itching or discharge, loose or foul-smelling stools) and allergy.
- Instruct patient to notify health care professional immediately if diarrhea, abdominal cramping, fever, or bloody stools occur and not to treat with antidiarrheals without consulting health care professional.
- Instruct the patient to notify health care professional if symptoms do not improve.
- Teach patients with a history of rheumatic heart disease or valve replacement the importance of using antimicrobial prophylaxis before invasive medical or dental procedures.
- Instruct female patients taking oral contraceptives to use an alternate or additional nonhormonal method of contraception during therapy with amoxicillin and until next menstrual period.

Evaluation/Desired Outcomes

- Resolution of the signs and symptoms of infection. Length of time for complete resolution depends on the organism and site of infection.
- Endocarditis prophylaxis.
- Eradication of *H. pylori* with resolution of ulcer symptoms.
- Prevention of inhalational anthrax (postexposure).

amoxicillin/clavulanate

(a-mox-i-**sill**-in/klav-yoo-**lan**-ate)
Augmentin, Augmentin ES, Augmentin XR, ✱Clavulin

Classification
Therapeutic: anti-infectives
Pharmacologic: aminopenicillins/beta lactamase inhibitors

Indications

Treatment of a variety of infections including: Skin and skin structure infections, Otitis media, Sinusitis, Respiratory tract infections, Genitourinary tract infections.

Action

Binds to bacterial cell wall, causing cell death; spectrum of amoxicillin is broader than penicillin. Clavulanate resists action of beta-lactamase, an enzyme produced by bacteria that is capable of inactivating some penicillins. **Therapeutic Effects:** Bactericidal action against susceptible bacteria. **Spectrum:** Active against: Streptococci, Pneumococci, Enterococci, *Haemophilus influenzae*, *Escherichia coli*, *Proteus mirabilis*, *Neisseria meningitidis*, *N. gonorrhoeae*, *Staphylococcus aureus*, *Klebsiella pneumoniae*, *Shigella*, *Salmonella*, *Moraxella catarrhalis*.

Pharmacokinetics

Absorption: Well absorbed from the duodenum (75–90%). More resistant to acid inactivation than other penicillins.
Distribution: Diffuses readily into most body tissues and fluids. Does not readily enter brain/CSF; CSF penetration is ↑ in the presence of inflamed meninges. Crosses the placenta and enters breast milk in small amounts.
Metabolism and Excretion: 70% excreted unchanged in the urine; 30% metabolized by the liver.
Half-life: 1–1.3 hr.

TIME/ACTION PROFILE (peak blood levels)

ROUTE	ONSET	PEAK	DURATION
PO	30 min	1–2 hr	8–12 hr

Contraindications/Precautions

Contraindicated in: Hypersensitivity to penicillins or clavulanate; Suspension and chewable tablets contain aspartame and should be avoided in phenylketonurics; History of amoxicillin/clavulanate-associated cholestatic jaundice.
Use Cautiously in: Severe renal insufficiency (dose ↓ necessary); Infectious mononucleosis (↑ risk of rash); Hepatic impairment (dose cautiously, monitor liver function).

Adverse Reactions/Side Effects

CNS: SEIZURES (high doses). **GI:** CLOSTRIDIUM DIFFICILE-ASSOCIATED DIARRHEA (CDAD), diarrhea, hepatic dysfunction, nausea, vomiting. **GU:** vaginal candidiasis. **Derm:** rash, urticaria. **Hemat:** blood dyscrasias. **Misc:** allergic reactions including ANAPHYLAXIS and SERUM SICKNESS, superinfection.

Interactions

Drug-Drug: Probenecid ↓ renal excretion and ↑ blood levels of amoxicillin—therapy may be combined for this purpose. May ↑ the effect of **warfarin**. Concurrent **allopurinol** therapy ↑ risk of rash. May ↓ the effectiveness of **hormonal contraceptives**.
Drug-Food: Clavulanate absorption is ↓ by a **high fat** meal.

Route/Dosage

Most Infections (Dosing based on amoxicillin component)

PO (Adults and Children >40 kg): 250 mg every 8 hr or 500 mg every 12 hr.

Serious Infections and Respiratory Tract Infections

PO (Adults and Children >40 kg): 875 mg every 12 hr *or* 500 mg every 8 hr; *Acute bacterial sinusitis*—2000 mg every 12 hr for 10 days as extended release (XR) product; *Community-acquired pneumonia*—2000 mg every 12 hr for 7–10 days as extended release (XR) product.

Recurrent/persistent acute otitis media due to Multidrug-resistant *Streptococcus pneumonia, H. influenzae,* or *M. catarrhalis*

PO (Children <40 kg): 80–90 mg/kg/day in divided doses every 12 hr for 10 days (as ES formulation only).

Renal Impairment

PO (Adults): *CCr 10–30 mL/min*—250–500 mg every 12 hr (do not use 875 mg tablet); *CCr <10 mL/min*—250–500 mg every 24 hr.

Otitis Media, Sinusitis, Lower Respiratory Tract Infections, Serious Infections

PO (Children ≥3 mo): *200 mg/5 mL or 400 mg/5 mL suspension*—45 mg/kg/day divided every 12 hr; *125 mg/5 mL or 250 mg/5 mL suspension*—40 mg/kg/day divided every 8 hr.

Less Serious Infections

PO (Children ≥3 mo): *200 mg/5 mL or 400 mg/5 mL suspension*—25 mg/kg/day divided every 12 hr *or* 20 mg/kg/day divided every 8 hr (as 125 mg/5 mL or 250 mg/5 mL suspension).

PO (Children <3 mo): 15 mg/kg every 12 hr (125 mg/mL suspension recommended).

Availability (generic available)

Tablets: 250 mg amoxicillin with 125 mg clavulanate, 500 mg amoxicillin with 125 mg clavulanate, 875 mg amoxicillin with 125 mg clavulanate. **Cost:** *Generic*—500 mg $18.98/20, 875 mg $23.46/30. **Chewable tablets (cherry-banana flavor):** 200 mg amoxicillin with 28.5 mg clavulanate, 400 mg amoxicillin with 57 mg clavulanate. **Cost:** *Generic*—200 mg $36.17/20, 400 mg $68.93/20. **Extended-release tablets (scored):** 1000 mg amoxicillin with 62.5 mg clavulanate. **Cost:** *Generic*—$108.62/28. **Powder for oral suspension (125 mg/5 mL is banana flavor; 200 mg/5mL is fruit flavor; 250 mg/5 mL is orange flavor; 400 mg/5 mL is fruit flavor; 600 mg/5 mL is orange or strawberry-creme flavor):** 125 mg amoxicillin with 31.25 mg clavulanate/5 mL, 200 mg amoxicillin with 28.5 mg clavulanate/5 mL, 250 mg amoxicillin with 62.5 mg clavulanate/5 mL, 400 mg amoxicillin with 57 mg clavulanate/5 mL, 600 mg amoxicillin with 42.9 mg clavulanate/5 mL (ES formulation). **Cost:** *Generic*—200 mg $36.17/100 mL, 250 mg $86.43/100 mL, 400 mg $68.93/100 mL, 600 mg $83.03/125 mL.

NURSING IMPLICATIONS

Assessment

- Assess for infection (vital signs; appearance of wound, sputum, urine, and stool; WBC) at beginning of and throughout therapy.
- Obtain a history before initiating therapy to determine previous use of and reactions to penicillins or cephalosporins. Persons with a negative history of penicillin sensitivity may still have an allergic response.
- Observe for signs and symptoms of anaphylaxis (rash, pruritus, laryngeal edema, wheezing). Notify health care professional immediately if these occur.
- Obtain specimens for culture and sensitivity prior to therapy. First dose may be given before receiving results.
- Monitor bowel function. Diarrhea, abdominal cramping, fever, and bloody stools should be reported to health care professional promptly as a sign of Clostridium difficile-associated diarrhea (CDAD). May begin up to several wk following cessation of therapy.
- ***Lab Test Considerations:*** May cause ↑ serum alkaline phosphatase, LDH, AST, and ALT concentrations. Elderly men and patients receiving prolonged treatment are at ↑ risk for hepatic dysfunction.
- May cause false-positive direct Coombs' test result.

Implementation

- **PO:** Administer around the clock. Administer at the start of a meal to enhance absorption and to decrease GI side effects. Do not administer with high fat meals; clavulanate absorption is decreased. XR tablet is scored and can be broken for ease of administration. Capsule contents may be emptied and swallowed with liquids. Chewable tablets should be crushed or chewed before swallowing with liquids. Shake oral suspension before administering. Refrigerated reconstituted suspension should be discarded after 10 days.
- Two 250-mg tablets are not bioequivalent to one 500-mg tablet; 250-mg tablets and 250-mg chewable tablets are also not interchangeable. Two 500-mg tablets are not interchangeable with one 1000-mg XR tablet; amounts of clavulanic acid and durations of action are different. Augmentin ES 600 (600 mg/5 mL) does not contain the same amount of clavulanic acid as any of the other Augmentin suspensions. Suspensions are not interchangeable.
- Pedi: Do not administer 250-mg chewable tablets to children <40 kg due to clavulanate content. Children <3 mo should receive the 125-mg/5 mL oral solution.

Patient/Family Teaching

- Instruct patients to take medication around the clock and to finish the drug completely as directed, even if feeling better. Advise patients that sharing of this medication may be dangerous.
- Pedi: Teach parents or caregivers to calculate and measure doses accurately. Reinforce importance of using measuring device supplied by pharmacy or with product, not household items.
- Advise patient to report the signs of superinfection (furry overgrowth on the tongue, vaginal itching or discharge, loose or foul-smelling stools) and allergy.
- Instruct patient to notify health care professional immediately if diarrhea, abdominal cramping, fever, or bloody stools occur and not to treat with antidiarrheals without consulting health care professionals.
- Instruct the patient to notify health care professional if symptoms do not improve or if nausea or diarrhea persists when drug is administered with food.
- Instruct female patients taking oral contraceptives to use an alternate or additional method of contraception during therapy and until next menstrual period; may decrease effectiveness of hormonal contraceptives.

Evaluation/Desired Outcomes

- Resolution of the signs and symptoms of infection. Length of time for complete resolution depends on the organism and site of infection.

amphetamine mixtures

(am-**fet**-a-meen)

~~Adderall~~, Adderall XR, Mydayis

Classification

Therapeutic: central nervous system stimulants

Schedule II

Indications

ADHD. Narcolepsy.

Action

Causes release of norepinephrine from nerve endings. Pharmacologic effects are: CNS and respiratory stimulation, Vasoconstriction, Mydriasis (pupillary dilation). **Therapeutic Effects:** Increased motor activity, mental alertness, and decreased fatigue in narcoleptic patients. Increased attention span in ADHD.

Pharmacokinetics

Absorption: Well absorbed after oral administration.
Distribution: Widely distributed in body tissues, with high concentrations in the brain and CSF. Crosses placenta and enters breast milk.
Metabolism and Excretion: Some metabolism by the liver. Urinary excretion is pH-dependent. Alkaline urine promotes reabsorption and prolongs action.
Half-life: Children 6–12 yrs: 9–11 hr; Adults: 10–13 hr (depends on urine pH).

TIME/ACTION PROFILE (CNS stimulation)

ROUTE	ONSET	PEAK	DURATION
PO	tablet: 0.5–1 hr	tablet: 3 hr capsule: 7 hr	4–6 hr

Contraindications/Precautions

Contraindicated in: Hypersensitivity; Hyperexcitable states including hyperthyroidism; Psychotic personalities; Concurrent use or use within 14 days of MAO inhibitors or MAO-like drugs (linezolid or methylene blue); Suicidal or homicidal tendencies; Chemical dependence; Glaucoma; Structural cardiac abnormalities (may ↑ the risk of sudden death); End-stage renal disease; OB: Potentially embryotoxic.
Use Cautiously in: Cardiovascular disease (sudden death has occurred in children with structural cardiac abnormalities or other serious heart problems); History of substance use disorder (misuse may result in serious cardiovascular events/sudden death); Hypertension; Diabetes mellitus; Tourette's syndrome (may exacerbate tics); Severe renal impairment (↓ dose); Geri: Geriatric or debilitated patients may be more susceptible to side effects.

Adverse Reactions/Side Effects

CNS: <u>hyperactivity</u>, <u>insomnia</u>, <u>restlessness</u>, <u>tremor</u>, aggression, anger, behavioral disturbances, dizziness, hallucinations, headache, mania, irritability, skin picking, talkativeness, thought disorder, tics. **CV:** SUDDEN DEATH, <u>palpitations</u>, <u>tachycardia</u>, cardiomyopathy (increased with prolonged use, high doses), hypertension, hypotension, peripheral vasculopathy. **Derm:** alopecia, urticaria. **Endo:** growth inhibition (with long term use in children). **EENT:** blurred vision, mydriasis. **GI:** <u>anorexia</u>, constipation, cramps, diarrhea, dry mouth, metallic taste, nausea, vomiting. **GU:** erectile dysfunction, <u>libido changes</u>, priapism. **MS:** RHABDOMYOLYSIS. **Neuro:** paresthesia. **Misc:** HYPERSENSITIVITY REACTIONS (including anaphylaxis and angioedema), psychological dependence.

Interactions

Drug-Drug: Concurrent use with **MAO inhibitors** or **MAO-inhibitor-like drugs**, such as **linezolid** or **methylene blue** may result in serious, potentially fatal reactions; wait at least 14 days following discontinuation of MAO inhibitor before initiation of amphetamine mixtures. Drugs that affect serotonergic neurotransmitter systems, including **MAO inhibitors**, **tricyclic antidepressants**, **SSRIs**, **SNRIs**, **fentanyl**, **buspirone**, **tramadol**, **lithium**, and **triptans** ↑ risk of serotonin syndrome. ↑ adrenergic effects with other **adrenergics** or **thyroid preparations**. **Drugs that alkalinize urine** (**sodium bicarbonate**, **acetazolamide**) ↓ excretion, ↑ effects. **Drugs that acidify urine** (large doses of **ascorbic acid**) ↑ excretion, ↓ effects. ↑ risk of hypertension and bradycardia with **beta blockers**. ↑ risk of arrhythmias with **digoxin**. **Tricyclic antidepressants** may ↑ effect of amphetamine but may ↑ risk of arrhythmias, hypertension, or hyperpyrexia. **Proton pump inhibitors** may ↑ effects.

Drug-Natural Products: Use with **St. John's wort** may ↑ risk of serotonin syndrome.

Drug-Food: Foods that alkalinize the urine (fruit juices) can ↑ effect of amphetamine.

Route/Dosage

Dose is expressed in total amphetamine content (amphetamine + dextroamphetamine).

ADHD

PO (Adults): *Immediate-release tablets*—5 mg 1–2 times daily; may ↑ daily dose in 5–mg increments at weekly intervals; usual dose range = 5–40 mg/day in 1–3 divided doses. *Extended-release capsules (Adderall XR)*—20 mg once daily; *Extended-release capsules (Mydayis)*—12.5–25 mg once daily in the morning upon awakening; may ↑ daily dose in 12.5–mg increments at weekly intervals. (maximum dose = 50 mg/day).

PO (Children ≥13 yr): *Immediate-release tablets*—5 mg 1–2 times daily; may ↑ daily dose in 5–mg increments at weekly intervals; usual dose range = 5–40 mg/day in 1–3 divided doses. *Extended-release capsules (Adderall XR)*—10 mg once daily in the morning; may ↑ to 20 mg once daily in the morning after 1 wk; *Extended-release capsules (Mydayis)*—12.5 mg once daily in the morning upon awakening; may ↑ daily dose in 12.5–mg increments at weekly intervals (maximum dose = 25 mg/day).

PO (Children 6–12 yr): *Immediate-release tablets*—5 mg 1–2 times daily; may ↑ daily dose in 5–mg increments at weekly intervals; usual dose range = 5–40 mg/day in 1–3 divided doses. *Extended-release capsules (Adderall XR)*—5–10 mg once daily in the morning; may ↑ daily dose in 5–10–mg increments at weekly intervals (maximum dose = 30 mg/day).

PO (Children 3–5 yr): *Immediate-release tablets*—2.5 mg once daily in the morning; may ↑ daily dose in 2.5–mg increments at weekly intervals; usual dose range = 2.5–40 mg/day in 1–3 divided doses.

Renal Impairment

PO (Adults): *GFR 15–29 mL/min/1.73 m²*—Extended-release capsules (Adderall XR)—15 mg once daily in the morning; Extended–release capsules (Mydayis)—12.5 mg once daily in the morning upon awakening; may ↑ daily dose in 12.5–mg increments at weekly intervals (maximum dose = 25 mg/day).

Renal Impairment

(Children ≥13 yr): *GFR 15–29 mL/min/1.73 m²*—Extended–release capsules (Mydayis)—12.5 mg once daily in the morning upon awakening (maximum dose = 12.5 mg/day).

Renal Impairment

(Children ≥6 yr): *GFR 15–29 mL/min/1.73 m²*—Extended–release capsules (Adderall XR)—5 mg once daily in the morning (maximum dose = 20 mg/day in children 6–12 yrs).

Narcolepsy

PO (Adults and Children ≥13 yr): *Immediate-release tablets*—10 mg once daily in the morning; may ↑ daily dose in 10–mg increments at weekly intervals; usual dosage range = 5–60 mg/day in 1–3 divided doses.

PO (Children 6–12 yr): *Immediate-release tablets*—5 mg once daily; may ↑ daily dose in 5–mg increments at weekly intervals; usual dose range = 5–60 mg/day in 1–3 divided doses.

Availability (generic available)

Amount is expressed in total amphetamine content (amphetamine + dextroamphetamine).

Tablets: 5 mg, 7.5 mg, 10 mg, 12.5 mg, 15 mg, 20 mg, 30 mg. **Cost:** *Generic*—All strengths $171.40/100. **Extended-release capsules (Adderall XR):** 5 mg, 10 mg, 15 mg, 20 mg, 25 mg, 30 mg. **Cost:** *Generic*—All strengths $613.15/100. **Extended-release capsules (Mydayis):** 12.5 mg, 25 mg, 37.5 mg, 50 mg.

NURSING IMPLICATIONS

Assessment

- Monitor BP, pulse, and respiration before and periodically during therapy. Obtain a history (including assessment of family history of sudden death or ventricular arrhythmia), physical exam to assess for cardiac disease, and further evaluation (ECG and echocardiogram), if indicated. If exertional chest pain, unexplained syncope, or other cardiac symptoms occur, evaluate promptly.
- May produce a false sense of euphoria and well-being. Provide frequent rest periods and observe patient for rebound depression after the effects of the medication have worn off.
- Monitor closely for behavior change during therapy.
- Assess for risk of abuse prior to starting therapy. Monitor during therapy. Has high dependence and abuse potential. Tolerance to medication occurs rapidly; do not increase dose.
- Assess infants born to mothers taking amphetamines for symptoms of withdrawal (feeding difficulties, irritability, agitation, excessive drowsiness).

- **ADHD:** Monitor weight biweekly and height periodically and inform health care professional of significant loss.
- Assess child's attention span, impulse control, and interactions with others. Therapy may be interrupted at intervals to determine whether symptoms are sufficient to continue therapy.
- **Narcolepsy:** Observe and document frequency of narcoleptic episodes.
- ***Lab Test Considerations:*** May interfere with urinary steroid determinations.
- May cause ↑ plasma corticosteroid concentrations; greatest in evening.

Implementation

- **PO:** Administer in the morning to prevent insomnia. May be taken without regard to food. Individualize dose to therapeutic needs and response of patient. Use the lowest effective dose.
- May be taken without regard to food. Administer short acting doses 4–6 hrs apart.
- Extended-release capsules may be swallowed whole or opened and sprinkled on applesauce; swallow contents without chewing. Applesauce should be swallowed immediately; do not store. Do not divide contents of capsule; entire contents of capsule should be taken.
- **ADHD:** Pedi: When symptoms are controlled, dose reduction or interruption of therapy may be possible during summer mo or may be given on each of the 5 school days, with medication-free weekends and holidays.

Patient/Family Teaching

- Instruct patient to take medication once in the early morning as directed. With extended release capsule, avoid afternoon doses to prevent insomnia. Omit missed doses and resume schedule next day. Do not double doses. Advise patient and parents to read the *Medication Guide* prior to starting therapy and with each Rx refill in case of changes. Instruct patient not to alter dose without consulting health care professional. Abrupt cessation of high doses may cause extreme fatigue and mental depression.
- Advise patient that amphetamine mixtures are drugs with known abuse potential. Protect them from theft, and never give to anyone other than the individual for whom they were prescribed.
- Caution patients to inform health care professional if they have ever abused or been dependent on alcohol or drugs, or if they are now abusing or dependent on alcohol or drugs.
- Inform patient that the effects of drug-induced dry mouth can be minimized by rinsing frequently with water or chewing sugarless gum or candies.
- Advise patient to limit caffeine intake.
- May impair judgment. Advise patient to use caution when driving or during other activities requiring alertness until response to medication is known.
- Advise patient to notify health care professional of all Rx or OTC medications, vitamins, or herbal products being taken and to consult with health care professional before taking other medications, especially St. John's wort.
- Inform patient that periodic holidays from the drug may be used to assess progress and decrease dependence. Pedi: Children should be given a drug-free holiday each yr to reassess symptoms and treatment. Doses will change as children age due to pharmacokinetic changes such as slower hepatic metabolism.
- Advise patient and/or parents to notify health care professional of behavioral changes (new or worse behavior and thought problems, bipolar illness, or aggressive behavior or hostility; new psychotic symptoms such as hearing voices, believing things that are not true, are suspicious, or new manic symptoms).
- Advise patient to notify health care professional if symptoms of heart problems (chest pain, shortness of breath, fainting), nervousness, restlessness, insomnia, dizziness, anorexia, or dry mouth becomes severe. Pedi: If reduced appetite and weight loss occur, advise parents to provide high calorie meals when drug levels are low (at breakfast and or bedtime).
- Inform patients of risk of peripheral vasculopathy. Instruct patients to notify health care professional of any new numbness; pain; skin color change from pale, to blue, to red; or coolness or sensitivity to temperature in fingers or toes, and call if unexplained wounds appear on fingers or toes.
- Advise patient to notify health care professional of all Rx or OTC medications, vitamins, or herbal products being taken and to consult with health care professional before taking other medications.
- Rep: Advise patient to notify health care professional if pregnancy is planned or suspected, and to avoid breast feeding. May cause birth complications. Enroll women exposed to amphetamine mixtures during pregnancy by calling the National Pregnancy Registry for Psychostimulants at 1-866-961-2388 or online at https://womensmentalhealth.org/clinical-and-research-programs/pregnancyregistry/other-medications/. Monitor infants born to mothers taking amphetamines for symptoms of withdrawal (feeding difficulties, irritability, agitation, excessive drowsiness).
- Emphasize the importance of routine follow-up exams to monitor progress.
- **Home Care Issues:** Advise parents to notify school nurse of medication regimen.

Evaluation/Desired Outcomes

- Improved attention span.
- Decrease in narcoleptic symptoms.

A

HIGH ALERT

AMPHOTERICIN B
(am-foe-**ter**-i-sin bee)

amphotericin B deoxycholate
✱Fungizone

amphotericin B lipid complex
Abelcet

amphotericin B liposome
AmBisome

Classification
Therapeutic: antifungals

Indications
IV: Treatment of progressive, potentially fatal fungal infections. The lipid complex, and liposome formulations should be considered for patients who are intolerant (e.g., renal dysfunction) or refractory to amphotericin B dexycholate. **Amphotericin B liposome:** Management of suspected fungal infections in febrile neutropenic patients: Treatment of visceral leishmaniasis, Treatment of cryptococcal meningitis in HIV patients.

Action
Binds to fungal cell membrane, allowing leakage of cellular contents. Toxicity (especially acute infusion reactions and nephrotoxicity) is less with lipid formulations. **Therapeutic Effects:** Can be fungistatic or fungicidal (depends on concentration achieved and susceptibility of organism). **Spectrum:** Active against: Aspergillosis, Blastomycosis, Candidiasis, Coccidioidomycosis, Cryptococcosis, Histoplasmosis, Leishmaniasis (liposomal formulation only), Mucormycosis.

Pharmacokinetics
Absorption: IV administration results in complete bioavailability.

Distribution: Extensively distributed to body tissues and fluids. Poor penetration into CSF.

Metabolism and Excretion: Elimination is very prolonged. Detectable in urine up to 7 wk after discontinuation.

Half-life: Biphasic—initial phase, 24–48 hr; terminal phase, 15 days. *Cholesteryl sulfate*—28 hr. *Lipid complex*—174 hr. *Liposomal*—100–153 hr.

TIME/ACTION PROFILE (blood levels)

ROUTE	ONSET	PEAK	DURATION
IV	rapid	end of infusion	24 hr

Contraindications/Precautions
Contraindicated in: Hypersensitivity; Lactation: Potential for distribution into breast milk and toxicity in infant; discontinue nursing.

Use Cautiously in: Renal impairment or electrolyte abnormalities; Patients receiving concurrent leukocyte transfusions (↑ risk of pulmonary toxicity); OB: Has been used safely.

Adverse Reactions/Side Effects
CNS: anxiety, confusion, headache, insomnia. **Resp:** dyspnea, hypoxia, wheezing. **CV:** chest pain, hypotension, tachycardia, edema, hypertension. **GI:** diarrhea, hyperbilirubinemia, ↑ liver enzymes, nausea, vomiting, abdominal pain. **GU:** nephrotoxicity, hematuria. **F and E:** hyperglycemia, hypocalcemia, hypokalemia, hypomagnesemia. **Hemat:** anemia, leukopenia, thrombocytopenia. **Derm:** pruritus, rashes. **Local:** phlebitis. **MS:** arthralgia, myalgia. **Misc:** HYPERSENSITIVITY REACTIONS, chills, fever, acute infusion reactions.

Interactions
Drug-Drug: ↑ risk of nephrotoxicity, bronchospasm, and hypotension with **antineoplastics**. Concurrent use with **corticosteroids** ↑ risk of hypokalemia. Concurrent use with **zidovudine** may ↑ the risk of myelotoxicity and nephrotoxicity. Concurrent use with **flucytosine** ↑ antifungal activity but may ↑ the risk of toxicity from flucytosine. Combined use with **azole antifungals** may induce fungal resistance. ↑ risk of nephrotoxicity with other **nephrotoxic agents** such as **aminoglycosides**, **cyclosporine**, or **tacrolimus**. Hypokalemia from amphotericin ↑ the risk of **digoxin** toxicity. Hypokalemia may enhance the curariform effects of **neuromuscular blocking agents**.

Route/Dosage
Specific dosage and duration of therapy depend on nature of infection being treated.

Amphotericin Deoxycholate
IV (Adults): Give test dose of 1 mg. If test dose tolerated, initiate therapy with 0.25 mg/kg/day (doses up to 1.5 mg/kg/day may be used, depending on type of infection) (alternate-day dosing may also be used); *Bladder irrigation*—Instill 50 mcg/mL solution into bladder daily for 5–10 days.

IV (Infants and Children): Give test dose of 0.1 mg/kg (maximum dose 1 mg) or may administer initial dose of 0.25–1 mg/kg/day over 6 hr (without test dose) (some infections may require 1.5 mg/kg/day; alternate-day dosing may be used).

IT (Adults): 25–300 mcg every 48–72 hr, ↑ to 500 mcg–1 mg as tolerated (maximum total dose = 15 mg).

IT (Children): 25–100 mcg every 48–72 hr; ↑ to 500 mcg as tolerated.

Amphotericin B Lipid Complex (Abelcet)

IV (Adults and Children): 2.5–5 mg/kg every 24 hr (no test dose needed).

Amphotericin B Liposome (AmBisome)

IV (Adults and Children): *Empiric therapy*—3 mg/kg every 24 hr; *Documented infections*—3–5 mg/kg every 24 hr; *Visceral leishmaniasis (immunocompetent patients)*—3 mg/kg every 24 hr on days 1–5, then 3 mg/kg every 24 hr on days 14 and 21; *Visceral leishmaniasis (immunosuppressed patients)*—4 mg/kg every 24 hr on days 1–5, then 4 mg/kg every 24 hr on days 10, 17, 24, 31, and 38; *Cryptococcal meningitis in HIV patients*—6 mg/kg every 24 hr.

Availability (generic available)

Amphotericin Deoxycholate

Powder for injection: 50 mg/vial.

Amphotericin B Lipid Complex

Suspension for injection: 5 mg/mL.

Amphotericin B Liposome

Powder for injection: 50 mg/vial.

NURSING IMPLICATIONS

Assessment

- Monitor patient closely during test dose and the first 1–2 hr of each dose for fever, chills, headache, anorexia, nausea, or vomiting. Premedicating with antipyretics, corticosteroids, antihistamines, meperidine, and antiemetics may decrease these reactions. Febrile reaction usually subsides within 4 hr after the infusion is completed.
- Assess injection site frequently for thrombophlebitis or leakage. Drug is very irritating to tissues.
- Monitor vital signs every 15 min during test dose and every 30 min for 2–4 hr after administration. Meperidine and dantrolene have been used to prevent and treat rigors. Assess respiratory status (lung sounds, dyspnea) daily. If respiratory distress occurs, discontinue infusion immediately; anaphylaxis may occur. Equipment for cardiopulmonary resuscitation should be readily available.
- Monitor intake and output and weigh daily. Adequate hydration (2000–3000 mL/day) and maintaining sodium balance may minimize nephrotoxicity.
- ***Lab Test Considerations:*** Monitor CBC, BUN and serum creatinine, and potassium and magnesium levels daily. If BUN and serum creatinine ↑ significantly, may need to discontinue or consider switching to lipid complex, or liposomal formulation.

Implementation

- Do not confuse amphotericin deoxycholate with amphotericin B lipid complex (Abelcet), or amphotericin B liposome (AmBisome); they are not interchangeable.
- This drug should be administered IV only to hospitalized patients or those under close supervision. Diagnosis should be confirmed before administration.

Amphotericin B Deoxycholate

IV Administration

- **Test dose:** Reconstitute 50-mg vial with 10 mL of sterile water for injection to achieve a concentration of 5 mg/mL. Reconstituted vial stable for 24 hr at room temperature or 1 wk if refrigerated. ***Diluent:*** Further dilute with 500 mL of D5W. May be diluted in 250 mL of D5W if being administered via a central venous catheter. Protect infusion from light. Infusion stable for 24 hr at room temperature or 2 days if refrigerated. To obtain test dose, withdraw 1 mg (10 mL) from 500 mL infusion and further dilute with D5W to a total volume of 20 mL. ***Concentration:*** 0.05 mg/mL. ***Rate:*** Infuse over 10–30 min to determine patient tolerance. Pedi: Infuse over 30–60 min.
- **Intermittent Infusion:** ***Diluent:*** Reconstitute and dilute 50-mg vial as per the directions above. ***Concentration:*** Final concentration of infusion should not exceed 0.1 mg/mL for peripheral infusion or 0.25 mg/mL for central line administration. ***Rate:*** Infuse slowly over 4–6 hr.
- **Y-Site Compatibility:** aldesleukin, aminocaproic acid, argatroban, carmustine, dactinomycin, diltiazem, etoposide, hydromorphone, ifosfamide, lorazepam, octreotide, oxaliplatin, tacrolimus, thiotepa, zidovudine, zoledronic acid.
- **Y-Site Incompatibility:** acyclovir, alemtuzumab, alfentanil, allopurinol, amifostine, amikacin, ampicillin, ampicillin/sulbactam, anidulafungin, atropine, azithromycin, aztreonam, benztropine, bivalirudin, bleomycin, bumetanide, butorphanol, calcium chloride, calcium gluconate, cangrelor, carboplatin, caspofungin, cefepime, cefotetan, ceftaroline, chloramphenicol, chlorpromazine, cisplatin, clindamycin, cyanocobalamin, cyclophosphamide, cytarabine, dacarbazine, dantrolene, daptomycin, daunorubicin, dexamethasone, dexmedetomidine, dexrazoxane, diazepam, digoxin, diphenhydramine, dobutamine, docetaxel, dolasetron, dopamine, doxorubicin, doxorubicin liposome, doxycycline, ephedrine, epinephrine, epirubicin, epoetin alfa, eptifibatide, ertapenem, erythromycin, esmolol, etoposide phosphate, famotidine, fenoldopam, filgrastim, fluconazole, fludarabine, fluorouracil, foscarnet, fosphenytoin, ganciclovir, gemcitabine, gentamicin, glycopyrrolate, granisetron, haloperidol, hetastarch, hydralazine, hydrocortisone, hydroxyzine, idarubicin, irinotecan, isoproterenol, ketorolac, labetalol, leucovorin, levofloxacin, lidocaine, linezolid, melphalan, meperidine, meropenem, mesna, methotrexate, methylprednisolone, metoclopramide, metoprolol, metronidazole, midazolam, milrinone, mitomycin, mitoxantrone, morphine, mycophenolate, nafcillin, nalbuphine, nicardipine, nitroprus-

A

side, norepinephrine, ondansetron, oxacillin, paclitaxel, palonosetron, pamidronate, pancuronium, pantoprazole, papaverine, pemetrexed, penicillin G, pentamidine, phenylephrine, phenytoin, piperacillin/tazobactam, potassium acetate, potassium chloride, prochlorperazine, promethazine, propofol, propranolol, protamine, pyridoxine, quinupristin/dalfopristin, rituximab, rocuronium, sodium acetate, sodium bicarbonate, succinylcholine, telavancin, thiamine, tigecycline, tirofiban, tobramycin, topotecan, trastuzumab, trimethoprim/sulfamethoxazole, vancomycin, vasopressin, vecuronium, verapamil, vinblastine, vincristine, vinorelbine, voriconazole.

- **Solution Incompatibility:** LR injection, saline solutions.

Amphotericin B Lipid Complex

IV Administration

- **Intermittent Infusion:** ***Diluent:*** Shake vial gently until yellow sediment at bottom has dissolved. Withdraw dose from required number of vials with 18-gauge needle. Replace needle from syringe filled with amphotericin B lipid complex with 5-micron filter needle. Each filter needle may be used to filter the contents of no more than 4 vials. Insert filter needle of syringe into IV bag of D5W and empty contents of syringe into bag. Protect from light. Infusion is stable for 6 hr at room temperature or 48 hr if refrigerated. ***Concentration:*** Final concentration of infusion should be 1 mg/mL; a concentration of 2 mg/mL can be used for pediatric patients or patients who cannot tolerate large volumes of fluid. ***Rate:*** Do not use an in-line filter. Infuse at a rate of 2.5 mg/kg/hr via infusion pump. If infusion exceeds 2 hr, mix contents by shaking infusion bag every 2 hr. If administering through an existing line, flush line with D5W before infusion or use a separate line.
- **Y-Site Compatibility:** acyclovir, allopurinol, aminocaproic acid, aminophylline, amiodarone, anidulafungin, argatroban, azithromycin, aztreonam, bumetanide, buprenorphine, busulfan, butorphanol, carboplatin, carmustine, cefazolin, cefepime, cefotaxime, cefotetan, cefoxitin, ceftazidime, ceftriaxone, cefuroxime, chloramphenicol, chlorpromazine, cisatracurium, clindamycin, cyclophosphamide, cyclosporine, cytatabine, dactimomycin, dexamethasone, digoxin, diphenhydramine, docetaxel, doxorubicin liposome, enalaprilat, ephedrine, epinephrine, eptifibatide, ertapenem, etoposide, famotidine, fentanyl, fludarabine, fluorouracil, fosphenytoin, furosemide, ganciclovir, granisetron, heparin, hydrocortisone, hydromorphone, ifosfamide, insulin, ketorolac, lidocaine, linezolid, lorazepam, mannitol, melphalan, meperidine, methotrexate, methylprednisolone, metoclopramide, mitomycin, nafcillin, nitroglycerin, nitroprusside, octreotide, oxaliplatin, paclitaxel, pamidronate, pantoprazole, pemetrexed, pentobarbital, phenobarbital, piperacillin/tazobactam, procainamide, ranitidine, succinylcholine, sufentanil, tacrolimus, telavancin, theophylline, thiopental, thiotepa, verapamil, vinblastine, vincristine, zidovudine, zoledronic acid.
- **Y-Site Incompatibility:** alemtuzumab, alfentanil, amifostine, amikacin, ampicillin, ampicillin/sulbactam, bivalirudin, bleomycin, calcium chloride, calcium gluconate, caspofungin, ciprofloxacin, cisplatin, dacarbazine, dantrolene, daptomycin, daunorubicin, dexmedetomidine, dexrazoxane, diazepam, diltiazem, dobutamine, dolasetron, dopamine, doxorubicin, doxycycline, droperidol, epirubicin, erythromycin, esmolol, etoposide phosphate, fenoldopam, fluconazole, foscarnet, gemcitabine, gentamicin, glycopyrrolate, haloperidol, hydralazine, hydroxyzine, idarubicin, imipenem/cilastatin, irinotecan, isoproterenol, labetalol, leucovorin, levofloxacin, magnesium sulfate, meropenem, mesna, metoprolol, metronidazole, midazolam, milrinone, mitoxantrone, morphine, moxifloxacin, mycophenolate, nalbuphine, naloxone, nicardipine, norepinephrine, ondansetron, pancuronium, pentamidine, phenylephrine, phenytoin, potassium acetate, potassium phosphates, prochlorperazine, promethazine, propranolol, quinupristin/dalfopristin, remifentanil, rocuronium, sodium acetate, sodium bicarbonate, sodium phosphates, streptozocin, tirofiban, tobramycin, topotecan, trimethoprim/sulfamethoxazole, vancomycin, vasopressin, vecuronium, vinorelbine, voriconazole.
- **Solution Incompatibility:** saline solutions.

Amphotericin B Liposome

IV Administration

- **Intermittent Infusion:** ***Diluent:*** Reconstitute each 50–mg vial with 12 mL of sterile water for injection to achieve concentration of 4 mg/mL. Immediately shake vial vigorously for at least 30 sec until all particulate matter is completely dispersed. Reconstituted vials are stable for 24 hr if refrigerated. Withdraw appropriate volume for dilution into a syringe. Attach the 5-micron filter to the syringe and inject syringe contents into an appropriate volume of D5W. Infusion should be administered within 6 hr of dilution. ***Concentration:*** Final concentration of infusion should be 1–2 mg/mL; a lower concentration (0.2–0.5 mg/mL) may be used for infants and small children. ***Rate:*** Infuse over 2 hr. Infusion time may be shortened to 1 hr if patient tolerates infusion without any adverse reactions. If discomfort occurs during infusion, duration of infusion may be increased. May be administered through an in-line filter with pore diameter of at least 1 micron.

If administering through an existing line, flush line with D5W before infusion or use a separate line.

- **Y-Site Compatibility:** acyclovir, amifostine, aminocaproic acid, aminophylline, anidulafungin, argatroban, atropine, azithromycin, bivalirudin, bumetanide, buprenorphine, busulfan, butorphanol, carboplatin, carmustine, cefazolin, cefoxitin, ceftriaxone, cefuroxime, clindamycin, cyclophosphamide, cytarabine, dactinomycin, daptomycin, dexamethasone, dexmedetomidine, diphenhydramine, doxorubicin liposomal, enalaprilat, ephedrine, epinephrine, eptifibatide, ertapenem, esmolol, etoposide, famotidine, fenoldopam, fentanyl, fludarabine, fluorouracil, foscarnet, fosphenytoin, furosemide, granisetron, haloperidol, heparin, hydrocortisone, hydromorphone, ifosfamide, isoproterenol, ketorolac, lidocaine, linezolid, mesna, methotrexate, methylprednisolone, metoprolol, milrinone, mitomycin, nitroglycerin, nitroprusside, octreotide, oxaliplatin, oxytocin, palonosetron, pamidronate, pancuronium, pantoprazole, pemetrexed, pentobarbital, phenobarbital, phenylephrine, piperacillin/tazobactam, potassium acetate, potassium chloride, procainamide, ranitidine, sufentanil, tacrolimus, theophylline, thiopental, thiotepa, tigecycline, trimethoprim/sulfamethoxazole, vasopressin, vincristine, voriconazole, zidovudine, zoledronic acid.
- **Y-Site Incompatibility:** alemtuzumab, alfentanil, amikacin, ampicillin, ampicillin/sulbactam, aztreonam, bleomycin, calcium chloride, calcium gluconate, caspofungin, cefepime, cefotaxime, cefotetan, ceftazidime, chlorpromazine, ciprofloxacin, cisplatin, cyclosporine, dacarbazine, daunorubicin, dexrazoxane, diazepam, digoxin, diltiazem, dobutamine, docetaxel, dolasetron, dopamine, doxorubicin, doxycycline, droperidol, epirubicin, erythromycin, etoposide phosphate, gemcitabine, gentamicin, hetastarch, hydroxyzine, idarubicin, imipenem/cilastatin, irinotecan, labetalol, leucovorin, levofloxacin, lorazepam, magnesium sulfate, mannitol, meperidine, meropenem, metoclopramide, metronidazole, midazolam, mitoxantrone, morphine, mycophenolate, nalbuphine, naloxone, nicardipine, ondansetron, paclitaxel, pentamidine, phenytoin, potassium phosphates, prochlorperazine, promethazine, propranolol, quinupristin/dalfopristin, sodium bicarbonate, sodium phosphates, telavancin, tobramycin, vancomycin, vecuronium, verapamil, vinblastine, vinorelbine.
- **Solution Incompatibility:** Do not dilute or admix with saline solutions, other medications, or solutions containing a bacteriostatic agent.

Patient/Family Teaching

- Explain need for long duration of IV therapy.
- **IV:** Inform patient of potential side effects and discomfort at IV site. Advise patient to notify health care professional if side effects occur.
- **Home Care Issue:** Instruct family or caregiver on dilution, rate, and administration of drug and proper care of IV equipment.

Evaluation/Desired Outcomes

- Resolution of signs and symptoms of infection. Several wk to mo of therapy may be required to prevent relapse.

ampicillin/sulbactam

(am-pi-**sil**-in/sul-**bak**-tam)

Unasyn

Classification

Therapeutic: anti-infectives

Pharmacologic: aminopenicillins/beta lactamase inhibitors

Indications

Treatment of the following infections: Skin and skin structure infections, soft-tissue infections, Otitis media, Intra-abdominal infections, Sinusitis, Respiratory infections, Genitourinary infections, Meningitis, Septicemia.

Action

Binds to bacterial cell wall, resulting in cell death; spectrum is broader than that of penicillin. Addition of sulbactam increases resistance to beta-lactamases, enzymes produced by bacteria that may inactivate ampicillin. **Therapeutic Effects:** Bactericidal action. **Spectrum:** Active against: Streptococci, Pneumococci, Enterococci, *Haemophilus influenzae*, *Escherichia coli*, *Proteus mirabilis*, *Neisseria meningitidis*, *N. gonorrhoeae*, *Shigella*, *Salmonella*, *Bacteroides fragilis*, *Moraxella catarrhalis*. Use should be reserved for infections caused by beta-lactamase–producing strains.

Pharmacokinetics

Absorption: Well absorbed from IM sites.

Distribution: Ampicillin diffuses readily into bile, blister and tissue fluids. Poor CSF penetration unless meninges are inflamed. Crosses the placenta; enters breast milk in small amounts.

Metabolism and Excretion: Ampicillin is variably metabolized by the liver (12–50%). Renal excretion is also variable. Sulbactam is eliminated unchanged in urine.

Protein Binding: *Ampicillin*—28%; *sulbactam*—38%.

Half-life: *Ampicillin*—1–1.8 hr; *sulbactam*—1–1.3 hr.

TIME/ACTION PROFILE (blood levels)

ROUTE	ONSET	PEAK	DURATION
IM	rapid	1 hr	6–8 hr
IV	immediate	end of infusion	6–8 hr

A

Contraindications/Precautions

Contraindicated in: Hypersensitivity to penicillins or sulbactam; History of cholestatic jaundice or hepatic dysfunction with ampicillin/sulbactam.

Use Cautiously in: Severe renal insufficiency (dosage ↓ required if CCr <30 mL/min); Epstein-Barr virus infection, acute lymphocytic leukemia, or cytomegalovirus infection (↑ risk of rash).

Adverse Reactions/Side Effects

CNS: SEIZURES (high doses). **GI:** HEPATOTOXICITY, CLOSTRIDIUM DIFFICILE-ASSOCIATED DIARRHEA (CDAD), diarrhea, cholestasis, nausea, vomiting. **Derm:** ERYTHEMA MULTIFORME, STEVENS-JOHNSON SYNDROME, TOXIC EPIDERMAL NECROLYSIS, acute generalized exanthematous pustulosis, rash, urticaria. **Hemat:** blood dyscrasias. **Local:** pain at IM site, pain at IV site. **Misc:** allergic reactions including ANAPHYLAXIS and SERUM SICKNESS, phlebitis, superinfection, ↑ liver enzymes.

Interactions

Drug-Drug: Probenecid ↓ renal excretion and ↑ levels of ampicillin—therapy may be combined for this purpose. May potentiate the effect of **warfarin**. Concurrent **allopurinol** therapy (↑ risk of rash). May ↓ levels and effectiveness of **hormonal contraceptives**.

Route/Dosage

Dosage based on ampicillin component.

IM, IV (Adults and Children ≥40 kg): 1–2 g ampicillin every 6–8 hr (not to exceed 12 g ampicillin/day).

IM, IV (Children ≥1 yr): 100–200 mg ampicillin/kg/day divided every 6 hr; *Meningitis*—200–400 mg ampicillin/kg/day divided every 6 hr; maximum dose: 8 g ampicillin/day.

IM, IV (Infants >1 mo): 100–150 mg ampicillin/kg/day divided every 6 hr.

Renal Impairment

IM, IV (Adults , Children, and Infants): *CCr 15–29 mL/min*—Administer every 12 hr; *CCr 5–14*—Administer every 24 hr.

Availability (generic available)

Powder for injection: 1.5 g/vial (1 g ampicillin with 500 mg sulbactam), 3 g/vial (2 g ampicillin with 1 g sulbactam), 15 g/vial (10 g ampicillin with 5 g sulbactam).

NURSING IMPLICATIONS

Assessment

- Assess patient for infection (vital signs, wound appearance, sputum, urine, stool, and WBCs) at beginning and throughout therapy.
- Obtain a history before initiating therapy to determine previous use of, and reactions to, penicillins or cephalosporins. Persons with a negative history of penicillin sensitivity may still have an allergic response.
- Obtain specimens for culture and sensitivity before therapy. First dose may be given before receiving results.
- Observe patient for signs and symptoms of anaphylaxis (rash, pruritus, laryngeal edema, wheezing). Discontinue the drug and notify the physician or other health care professional immediately if these occur. Keep epinephrine, an antihistamine, and resuscitation equipment close by in the event of an anaphylactic reaction.
- Monitor bowel function. Diarrhea, abdominal cramping, fever, and bloody stools should be reported to health care professional promptly as a sign of CDAD. May begin up to several mo following cessation of therapy.
- Monitor for rash, may lead to severe skin reactions.
- ***Lab Test Considerations:*** Monitor hepatic function periodically during therapy. May cause ↑ AST, ALT, LDH, bilirubin, alkaline phosphatase, BUN, and creatinine.
- May cause ↓ hemoglobin, hematocrit, RBC, WBC, neutrophils, and lymphocytes.
- May cause transient ↓ estradiol, total conjugated estriol, estriol-glucuronide, or conjugated estrone in pregnant women.
- May cause a false-positive Coombs' test result.

Implementation

- **IM:** Reconstitute for IM use by adding 3.2 mL of sterile water or 0.5% or 2% lidocaine HCl to the 1.5-g vial or 6.4 mL to the 3-g vial. Administer within 1 hr of preparation, deep IM into well-developed muscle.

IV Administration

- **IV Push:** ***Diluent:*** Reconstitute 1.5-g vial with 3.2 mL of sterile water for injection and the 3-g vial with 6.4 mL. ***Concentration:*** 375 mg ampicillin/sulbactam per mL. ***Rate:*** Administer over at least 10–15 min within 1 hr of reconstitution. More rapid administration may cause seizures.
- **Intermittent Infusion:** Reconstitute vials as per directions above. ***Diluent:*** Further dilute in 50–100 mL of 0.9% NaCl, D5W, D5/0.45% NaCl, or LR. Stability of solution varies from 2–8 hr at room temperature or 3–72 hr if refrigerated, depending on concentration and diluent. ***Concentration:*** Final concentration of infusion should be 3–45 mg of ampicillin/sulbactam per mL. ***Rate:*** Infuse over 15–30 min.
- **Y-Site Compatibility:** alemtuzumab, amifostine, aminocaproic acid, anidulafungin, argatroban, azithromycin, bivalirudin, bleomycin, cangrelor, carboplatin, carmustine, cefepime, cisplatin, cyclophosphamide, cytarabine, dactinomycin, daptomycin, dexmedetomidine, dexrazoxane, docetaxel,

doxorubicin liposomal, eptifibatide, etoposide, etoposide phosphate, fenoldopam, filgrastim, fludarabine, fluorouracil, foscarnet, fosphenytoin, gemcitabine, granisetron, hydromorphone, ifosfamide, irinotecan, leucovorin, levofloxacin, linezolid, mesna, methotrexate, metronidazole, milrinone, mitomycin, octreotide, oxaliplatin, paclitaxel, palonosetron, pamidronate, pancuronium, pantoprazole, pemetrexed, potassium acetate, remifentanil, rituximab, rocuronium, sodium acetate, televancin, thiotepa, tigecycline, tirofiban, trastuzumab, vecuronium, vinblastine, vincristine, voriconazole, zoledronic acid.

- **Y-Site Incompatibility:** acyclovir, amiodarone, amphotericin B deoxycholate, amphotericin B lipid complex, amphotericin B liposome, azathioprine, caspofungin, chlorpromazine, ciprofloxacin, dacarbazine, dantrolene, daunorubicin, diazepam, diazoxide, dobutamine, dolasetron, doxorubicin, doxycycline, epirubicin, ganciclovir, haloperidol, hydralazine, hydrocortisone, hydroxyzine, idarubicin, lansoprazole, lorazepam, methylprednisolone, midazolam, mitoxantrone, mycophenolate, nicardipine, ondansetron, papaverine, pentamidine, phenytoin, prochlorperazine, promethazine, protamine, quinupristin/dalfopristin, sargramostim, topotecan, tranexamic acid, trimethoprim/sulfamethoxazole, verapamil, vinorelbine, If aminoglycosides and penicillins must be given concurrently, administer in separate sites at least 1 hr apart.

Patient/Family Teaching

- Advise patient to report rash, signs of superinfection (furry overgrowth on the tongue, vaginal itching or discharge, loose or foul-smelling stools) and allergy.
- Caution patient to notify health care professional if fever and diarrhea occur, especially if stool contains blood, pus, or mucus. Advise patient not to treat diarrhea without consulting health care professional. May occur up to several wk after discontinuation of medication.
- Rep: Advise patients taking oral contraceptives to use an alternative or additional nonhormonal method of contraception while taking ampicillin/sulbactam and until next menstrual period.
- Instruct the patient to notify health care professional if symptoms do not improve.

Evaluation/Desired Outcomes

- Resolution of signs and symptoms of infection. Length of time for complete resolution depends on the organism and site of infection.

anastrozole (a-nass-troe-zole)

Arimidex

Classification

Therapeutic: antineoplastics

Pharmacologic: aromatase inhibitors

Indications

Adjuvant treatment of postmenopausal hormone receptor-positive early breast cancer. Initial therapy in women with postmenopausal hormone receptor-positive or hormone receptor unknown, locally advanced, or metastatic breast cancer. Advanced postmenopausal breast cancer in women with disease progression despite tamoxifen therapy.

Action

Inhibits the enzyme aromatase, which is partially responsible for conversion of precursors to estrogen. **Therapeutic Effects:** Lowers levels of circulating estrogen, which may halt progression of estrogen-sensitive breast cancer.

Pharmacokinetics

Absorption: 83–85% absorbed following oral administration.

Distribution: Unknown.

Metabolism and Excretion: 85% metabolized by the liver; 11% excreted renally.

Half-life: 50 hr.

TIME/ACTION PROFILE (lowering of serum estradiol)

ROUTE	ONSET	PEAK	DURATION
PO	within 24 hr	14 days	6 days†

†Following cessation of therapy.

Contraindications/Precautions

Contraindicated in: OB: Pregnancy (may cause fetal harm); Lactation: Lactation.

Use Cautiously in: Ischemic heart disease; Rep: Women of reproductive potential; Pedi: Safety not established.

Adverse Reactions/Side Effects

CNS: headache, weakness, dizziness. **CV:** MYOCARDIAL INFARCTION, angina, peripheral edema. **Derm:** rash, sweating. **EENT:** pharyngitis. **F and E:** hypercalcemia. **GI:** nausea, abdominal pain, anorexia, constipation, diarrhea, dry mouth, vomiting. **GU:** ↓ fertility (females), pelvic pain, vaginal bleeding, vaginal dryness. **Metab:** hypercholesterolemia, weight gain. **MS:** back pain, arthritis, bone pain, carpal tunnel syndrome, fracture, myalgia. **Neuro:** paresthesia. **Resp:** cough, dyspnea. **Misc:** allergic reactions including ANGIOEDEMA, URTICARIA, ANAPHYLAXIS, hot flashes, pain.

Interactions

Drug-Drug: None significant.

Route/Dosage

PO (Adults): 1 mg once daily.

Availability (generic available)

Tablets: 1 mg.

NURSING IMPLICATIONS

Assessment

- Assess patient for pain and other side effects periodically during therapy.
- ***Lab Test Considerations:*** Obtain a negative pregnancy test before starting therapy.
- May cause ↑ GGT, AST, ALT, alkaline phosphatase, total cholesterol, and LDL cholesterol levels.

Implementation

- **PO:** Take medication consistently with regard to food.

Patient/Family Teaching

- Instruct patient to take medication as directed. Take missed doses as soon as remembered unless it is almost time for next dose. Do not double doses. Advise patient to read the *Patient Information* leaflet before starting and with each Rx refill; changes may occur.
- Inform patient of potential for adverse reactions, and advise patient to notify health care professional immediately if allergic reactions (swelling of the face, lips, tongue, and/or throat, difficulty in swallowing and/or breathing), liver problems (general feeling of not being well, yellowing of skin or whites of eyes, pain on the right side of abdomen), skin reactions (lesions, ulcers, or blisters), or chest pain occurs.
- Advise patient that vaginal bleeding may occur during first few wk after changing over from other hormonal therapy. Continued bleeding should be evaluated.
- Teach patient to report increase in pain so treatment can be initiated.
- Rep: May be teratogenic. Advise female patients of reproductive potential to use effective contraception during and for at least 3 wk after last dose of therapy, to avoid breast feeding for at least 2 wk after last dose, and to notify health care professional immediately if pregnancy is planned or suspected. May impair female fertility.

Evaluation/Desired Outcomes

- Slowing of disease progression in women with advanced breast cancer.

🧬 ANGIOTENSIN-CONVERTING ENZYME (ACE) INHIBITORS

benazepril (ben-**aye**-ze-pril)
Lotensin

captopril (**kap**-toe-pril)
~~Capoten~~

enalapril/enalaprilat
(e-**nal**-a-pril/e-**nal**-a-pril-at)
Epaned, Vasotec, 🍁Vasotec IV

fosinopril (foe-**sin**-oh-pril)
~~Monopril~~

lisinopril (lyse-**in**-oh-pril)
Prinivil, Qbrelis, Zestril

moexipril (moe-**eks**-i-pril)
~~Univasc~~

perindopril (pe-**rin**-do-pril)
~~Aceon~~, 🍁Coversyl

quinapril (**kwin**-a-pril)
Accupril

ramipril (ra-**mi**-pril)
Altace

trandolapril (tran-**doe**-la-pril)
🍁Mavik

Classification
Therapeutic: antihypertensives
Pharmacologic: ACE inhibitors

Indications

Alone or with other agents in the management of hypertension. **Captopril, enalapril, fosinopril, lisinopril, quinapril, ramipril, trandolapril:** Management of HF. **Captopril, lisinopril, ramipril, trandolapril:** Reduction of risk of death or development of HF following MI. **Enalapril:** Slowed progression of left ventricular dysfunction into overt heart failure. **Ramipril:** Reduction of the risk of MI, stroke, and death from cardiovascular disease in patients at risk (>55 yr old with a history of CAD, stroke, peripheral vascular disease, or diabetes with another cardiovascular risk factor). **Captopril:** ↓ progression of diabetic nephropathy. **Perindopril:** Reduction of risk of death from cardiovascular causes or nonfatal MI in patients with stable CAD.

Action

ACE inhibitors block the conversion of angiotensin I to the vasoconstrictor angiotensin II. ACE inhibitors also prevent the degradation of bradykinin and other vasodilatory prostaglandins. ACE inhibitors also ↑ plasma renin levels and ↓ aldosterone levels. Net result is systemic vasodilation. **Therapeutic Effects:** Lowering of BP in hypertensive patients. Improved symptoms in patients with HF (selected agents only). ↓ development of overt heart failure (enalapril only). Improved survival and ↓ development of overt HF after MI (selected agents only). ↓ risk of death from cardiovascular causes or MI in patients with stable CAD (perindopril only). ↓ risk of MI, stroke or death from cardiovascular causes in high-risk patients (ramipril only). ↓ progression of diabetic nephropathy (captopril only).

Pharmacokinetics

Absorption: *Benazepril*—37% absorbed after oral administration. *Captopril*—60–75% absorbed after oral administration (↓ by food). *Enalapril*—55–75% absorbed after oral administration. *Enalaprilat*—IV administration results in complete bioavailability. *Fosinopril*—36% absorbed after oral administration. *Lisinopril*—25% absorbed after oral administration (much variability). *Moexipril*—13% bioavailability as moexiprilat after oral administration (↓ by food). *Perindopril*—25% bioavailability as perindoprilat after oral administration. *Quinapril*—60% absorbed after oral administration (high-fat meal may ↓ absorption). *Ramipril*—50–60% absorbed after oral administration. *Trandolapril*—70% bioavailability as trandolapril at after oral administration.

Distribution: All ACE inhibitors cross the placenta. *Benazepril, captopril, enalapril, fosinopril, quinapril*, and *trandolapril*—Enter breast milk. *Lisinopril*—Minimal penetration of CNS. *Ramipril*—Probably does not enter breast milk. *Trandolapril*—Enters breast milk.

Protein Binding: *Benazepril*—95%, *Fosinopril*—99.4%, *Moexipril*—90%, *Quinapril*—97%.

Metabolism and Excretion: *Benazepril*—Converted by the liver to benazeprilat, the active metabolite. 20% excreted by kidneys; 11–12% nonrenal (biliary elimination). *Captopril*—50% metabolized by the liver to inactive compounds, 50% excreted unchanged by the kidneys. *Enalapril, enalaprilat*—Enalapril is converted by the liver to enalaprilat, the active metabolite; primarily eliminated by the kidneys. *Fosinopril*—Converted by the liver and GI mucosa to fosinoprilat, the active metabolite—50% excreted in urine, 50% in feces. *Lisinopril*—100% eliminated by the kidneys. *Moexipril*—Converted by liver and GI mucosa to moexiprilat, the active metabolite; 13% excreted in urine, 53% in feces. *Perindopril*—Converted by the liver to perindoprilat, the active metabolite; primarily excreted in urine. *Quinapril*—Converted by the liver, GI mucosa, and tissue to quinaprilat, the active metabolite: 96% eliminated by the kidneys. *Ramipril*—Converted by the liver to ramiprilat, the active metabolite; 60% excreted in urine, 40% in feces. *Trandolapril*—Converted by the liver to trandolaprilat, the active metabolite; 33% excreted in urine, 66% in feces.

Half-life: *Benazeprilat*—10–11 hr. *Captopril*—2 hr (↑ in renal impairment). *Enalapril*—2 hr (↑ in renal impairment). *Enalaprilat*—35–38 hr (↑ in renal impairment). *Fosinoprilat*—12 hr. *Lisinopril*—12 hr (↑ in renal impairment). *Moexiprilat*—2–9 hr (↑ in renal impairment). *Perindoprilat*—3–10 hr (↑ in renal impairment). *Quinaprilat*—3 hr (↑ in renal impairment). *Ramiprilat*—13–17 hr (↑ in renal impairment). *Trandolaprilat*—22.5 hr (↑ in renal impairment).

TIME/ACTION PROFILE (effect on BP—single dose†)

ROUTE	ONSET	PEAK	DURATION
Benazepril	within 1 hr	2–4 hr	24 hr
Captopril	15–60 min	60–90 min	6–12 hr
Enalapril PO	1 hr	4–8 hr	12–24 hr
Enalapril IV	15 min	1–4 hr	4–6 hr
Fosinopril	within 1 hr	2–6 hr	24 hr
Lisinopril	1 hr	6 hr	24 hr
Moexipril	within 1 hr	3–6 hr	up to 24 hr
Perindoprilat	within 1–2 hr	3–7 hr	up to 24 hr
Quinapril	within 1 hr	2–4 hr	up to 24 hr
Ramipril	within 1–2 hr	3–6 hr	24 hr
Trandolapril	within 1–2 hr	4–10 hr	up to 24 hr

†Full effects may not be noted for several wks.

Contraindications/Precautions

Contraindicated in: Hypersensitivity; History of angioedema with previous use of ACE inhibitors (also in absence of previous use of ACE inhibitors for benazepril); Concurrent use with aliskiren in patients with diabetes or moderate-to-severe renal impairment (CCr <60 mL/min); Concurrent use with sacubitril/valsartan; must be a 36–hr wash-out period after switching to/from sacubitril/valsartan; OB: Pregnancy (may cause fetal harm); Lactation: Lactation.

Use Cautiously in: Renal impairment, hepatic impairment, hypovolemia, hyponatremia, concurrent diuretic therapy; Black patients with hypertension (monotherapy less effective, may require additional therapy; ↑ risk of angioedema); Rep: Women of reproductive potential; Surgery/anesthesia (hypotension may be exaggerated); Pedi: Safety not established for most agents; benazepril, fosinopril, and lisinopril may be used in children ≥6 yr (captopril and enalapril may be used in children of all ages); Geri: Initial dose ↓ recommended for most agents due to age-related ↓ in renal function.

Exercise Extreme Caution in: Family history of angioedema.

Adverse Reactions/Side Effects

CNS: dizziness, drowsiness, fatigue, headache, insomnia, vertigo, weakness. **CV:** hypotension, chest pain, edema, tachycardia. **Derm:** flushing, pruritus, rashes. **Endo:** hyperuricemia. **F and E:** hyperkalemia. **GI:** taste disturbances, abdominal pain, anorexia, constipation, diarrhea, nausea, vomiting. **GU:** erectile dysfunction, proteinuria, renal dysfunction, renal failure. **Hemat:** AGRANULOCYTOSIS, neutropenia (captopril only). **MS:** back pain, muscle cramps, myalgia. **Resp:** cough, dyspnea. **Misc:** ANGIOEDEMA, fever.

Interactions

Drug-Drug: Concurrent use with **sacubitril** ↑ risk of angioedema; concurrent use contraindicated; do not administer within 36 hr of switching to/from **sacubitril/valsartan**. Excessive hypotension may occur with concurrent use of **diuretics** and other **anti-**

hypertensives. ↑ risk of hyperkalemia with concurrent use of **potassium supplements**, **potassium-sparing diuretics**, or **potassium-containing salt substitutes**. ↑ risk of hyperkalemia, renal dysfunction, hypotension, and syncope with concurrent use of **angiotensin II receptor blockers** or **aliskiren**; avoid concurrent use with aliskiren in patients with diabetes or CCr <60 mL/min; avoid concurrent use with angiotensin II receptor blockers. **NSAIDs** and selective **COX-2 inhibitors** may blunt the antihypertensive effect and ↑ the risk of renal dysfunction. Absorption of fosinopril may be ↓ by **antacids** (separate administration by 1–2 hr). ↑ levels and may ↑ risk of **lithium** toxicity. Quinapril may ↓ absorption of **tetracycline**, **doxycycline**, and **fluoroquinolones** (because of magnesium in tablets). ↑ risk of angioedema with **temsirolimus**, **sirolimus**, or **everolimus**.
Drug-Food: Food significantly ↓ absorption of captopril and moexipril (administer drugs 1 hr before meals).

Route/Dosage

Benazepril

🧬 **PO (Adults):** 10 mg once daily, ↑ gradually to maintenance dose of 20–40 mg/day in 1–2 divided doses (begin with 5 mg/day in patients receiving diuretics).
PO (Children ≥6 yr): 0.2 mg/kg once daily; may be titrated up to 0.6 mg/kg/day (or 40 mg/day).

Renal Impairment

PO (Adults): *CCr <30 mL/min*—Initiate therapy with 5 mg once daily.

Renal Impairment

PO (Children ≥6 yr): *CCr <30 mL/min*—Contraindicated.

Captopril

PO (Adults): *Hypertension*—12.5–25 mg 2–3 times daily, may be ↑ at 1–2 wk intervals up to 150 mg 3 times daily (begin with 6.25–12.5 mg 2–3 times daily in patients receiving diuretics) (maximum dose = 450 mg/day); *HF*—25 mg 3 times daily (6.25–12.5 mg 3 times daily in patients who have been vigorously diuresed); titrated up to target dose of 50 mg 3 times daily; *Post-MI*—6.25-mg test dose, followed by 12.5 mg 3 times daily, may be ↑ up to 50 mg 3 times daily; *Diabetic nephropathy*—25 mg 3 times daily.
PO (Children): *HF*—0.3 mg/kg–0.5 mg/kg/dose 3 times daily, titrate up to a maximum of 6 mg/kg/day in 2–4 divided doses; *Older Children*—6.25–12.5 mg/dose every 12–24 hr, titrate up to a maximum of 6 mg/kg/day in 2–4 divided doses.
PO (Infants): *HF*—0.15–0.3 mg/kg/dose, titrate up to a maximum of 6 mg/kg/day in 1–4 divided doses.
PO (Neonates): *HF*—0.05–0.1 mg/kg/dose every 8–24 hr, may ↑ as needed up to 0.5 mg/kg every 6–24 hr; *Premature neonates*—0.01 mg/kg/dose every 8–12 hr.

Renal Impairment

PO (Adults): *CCr 10–50 mL/min*—Administer 75% of dose; *CCr <10 mL/min*—Administer 50% of dose.

Enalapril/Enalaprilat

PO (Adults): *Hypertension*—2.5–5 mg once daily, ↑ as required up to 40 mg/day in 1–2 divided doses (initiate therapy at 2.5 mg once daily in patients receiving diuretics); *HF*—2.5 mg 1–2 times daily, titrated up to target dose of 10 mg twice daily; begin with 2.5 mg once daily in patients with hyponatremia (serum sodium <130 mEq/L); *Asymptomatic left ventricular dysfunction*—2.5 mg twice daily, titrated up to a target dose of 10 mg twice daily.
PO (Children >1 mo): *Hypertension*—0.08 mg/kg once daily; may be slowly titrated up to a maximum of 0.58 mg/kg/day.
IV (Adults): *Hypertension*—0.625–1.25 mg (0.625 mg if receiving diuretics) every 6 hr; can be titrated up to 5 mg every 6 hr.
IV (Children >1 mo): *Hypertension*—5–10 mcg/kg/dose given every 8–24 hr.

Renal Impairment

PO, IV (Adults): *Hypertension CCr 10–50 mL/min*—Administer 75% of dose; *CCr <10 mL/min*—Administer 50% of dose.

Renal Impairment

PO, IV (Children >1 mo): *CCr <30 mL/min*—Contraindicated.

Fosinopril

PO (Adults): *Hypertension*—10 mg once daily, may be ↑ as required up to 80 mg/day. *HF*—10 mg once daily (5 mg once daily in patients who have been vigorously diuresed), may be ↑ over several wk up to 40 mg/day.
PO (Children ≥6 yr and >50 kg): *Hypertension*—5–10 mg once daily.

Lisinopril

PO (Adults): *Hypertension*—10 mg once daily, can be ↑ up to 20–40 mg/day (initiate therapy at 5 mg/day in patients receiving diuretics); *HF*—5 mg once daily; may be titrated every 2 wk up to 40 mg/day; begin with 2.5 mg once daily in patients with hyponatremia (serum sodium <130 mEq/L); *Post-MI*—5 mg once daily for 2 days, then 10 mg daily.
PO (Children ≥6 yr): *Hypertension*—0.07 mg/kg once daily (up to 5 mg/day), may be titrated every 1–2 wk up to 0.6 mg/kg/day (or 40 mg/day).

Renal Impairment

PO (Adults): *CCr 10–30 mL/min*—Begin with 5 mg once daily; may be slowly titrated up to 40 mg/day; *CCr*

<10 ml/min—Begin with 2.5 mg once daily; may be slowly titrated up to 40 mg/day.

Renal Impairment

(Children ≥6 yr): *CCr <30 mL/min*—Contraindicated.

Moexipril

PO (Adults): 7.5 mg once daily, may be ↑ up to 30 mg/day in 1–2 divided doses (begin with 3.75 mg/day in patients receiving diuretics).

Renal Impairment

PO (Adults): *CCr ≤40 mL/min*—Initiate therapy at 3.75 mg once daily, may be titrated upward carefully to 15 mg/day.

Perindopril

PO (Adults): *Hypertension*—4 mg once daily, may be slowly titrated up to 16 mg/day in 1–2 divided doses (should not exceed 8 mg/day in elderly patients) (begin with 2–4 mg/day in 1–2 divided doses in patients receiving diuretics); *Stable CAD*—4 mg once daily for 2 wk, may be ↑, if tolerated, to 8 mg once daily; for elderly patients, begin with 2 mg once daily for 1 wk (may be ↑, if tolerated, to 4 mg once daily for 1 wk, then, ↑ as tolerated to 8 mg once daily).

Renal Impairment

PO (Adults): *CCr 30–60 mL/min*—2 mg/day initially, may be slowly titrated up to 8 mg/day in 1–2 divided doses.

Quinapril

PO (Adults): *Hypertension*—10–20 mg once daily initially, may be titrated every 2 wk up to 80 mg/day in 1–2 divided doses (initiate therapy at 5 mg/day in patients receiving diuretics); *HF*—5 mg twice daily initially, may be titrated at weekly intervals up to 20 mg twice daily.

Renal Impairment

PO (Adults): *CCr >60 mL/min*—Initiate therapy at 10 mg/day; *CCr 30–60 mL/min*—Initiate therapy at 5 mg/day; *CCr 10–30 mL/min*—Initiate therapy at 2.5 mg/day.

Ramipril

PO (Adults): *Hypertension*—2.5 mg once daily, may be ↑ slowly up to 20 mg/day in 1–2 divided doses (initiate therapy at 1.25 mg/day in patients receiving diuretics). *HF post-MI*—1.25–2.5 mg twice daily initially, may be ↑ slowly up to 5 mg twice daily. *Reduction in risk of MI, stroke, and death from cardiovascular causes*—2.5 mg once daily for 1 wk, then 5 mg once daily for 3 wk, then ↑ as tolerated to 10 mg once daily (can also be given in 2 divided doses).

Renal Impairment

PO (Adults): *CCr <40 mL/min*—Initiate therapy at 1.25 mg once daily, may be slowly titrated up to 5 mg/day in 1–2 divided doses.

Trandolapril

PO (Adults): *Hypertension*—1 mg once daily (2 mg once daily in black patients); *HF post-MI*—Initiate therapy at 1 mg once daily, titrate up to 4 mg once daily if possible.

Renal Impairment

PO (Adults): *CCr <30 mL/min*—Initiate therapy at 0.5 mg once daily, may be slowly titrated upward (maximum dose = 4 mg/day).

Hepatic Impairment

PO (Adults): Initiate therapy at 0.5 mg once daily, may be slowly titrated upward (maximum dose = 4 mg/day).

Availability

Benazepril (generic available)

Tablets: 5 mg, 10 mg, 20 mg, 40 mg. **Cost:** *Generic*—All strengths $10.83/100. ***In combination with:*** amlodipine (Lotrel) and hydrochlorothiazide (Lotensin HCT). See Appendix B.

Captopril (generic available)

Tablets: 12.5 mg, 25 mg, 50 mg, 100 mg. **Cost:** *Generic*—12.5 mg $77.18/100, 25 mg $83.44/100, 50 mg $143.08/100, 100 mg $190.54/100. ***In combination with:*** hydrochlorothiazide (Capozide). See Appendix B.

Enalapril (generic available)

Oral solution (mixed berry flavor): 1 mg/mL. **Tablets:** 2.5 mg, 5 mg, 10 mg, 20 mg. **Cost:** *Generic*—2.5 mg $88.33/100, 5 mg $106.37/100, 10 mg $117.81/100, 20 mg $167.64/100. ***In combination with:*** hydrochlorothiazide (Vaseretic). See Appendix B.

Enalaprilat (generic available)

Solution for injection: 1.25 mg/mL.

Fosinopril (generic available)

Tablets: 10 mg, 20 mg, 40 mg. **Cost:** *Generic*—All strengths $107.08/90. ***In combination with:*** hydrochlorothiazide. See Appendix B.

Lisinopril (generic available)

Oral solution: 1 mg/mL. **Tablets:** 2.5 mg, 5 mg, 10 mg, 20 mg, 30 mg, 40 mg. **Cost:** *Generic*—2.5 mg $9.63/100, 5 mg $10.83/100, 10 mg $6.99/100, 20 mg $9.14/100, 30 mg $10.83/100, 40 mg $7.41/100. ***In combination with:*** hydrochlorothiazide (Prinzide, Zestoretic). See Appendix B.

Moexipril (generic available)

Tablets: 7.5 mg, 15 mg. **Cost:** *Generic*—7.5 mg $138.92/100, 15 mg $145.54/100. ***In combination with:*** hydrochlorothiazide (Uniretic).

Perindopril (generic available)

Tablets: 2 mg, 4 mg, 8 mg. **Cost:** *Generic*—2 mg $189.77/100, 4 mg $221.27/100, 8 mg $268.76/100. ***In combination with:*** amlodipine (Prestalia). See Appendix B.

A

Quinapril (generic available)

Tablets: 5 mg, 10 mg, 20 mg, 40 mg. **Cost:** *Generic*—5 mg $27.20/100, 10 mg $39.19/100, 20 mg $21.04/100, 40 mg $27.50/100. ***In combination with:*** hydrochlorothiazide (Accuretic, Quinaretic). See Appendix B.

Ramipril (generic available)

Capsules: 1.25 mg, 2.5 mg, 5 mg, 10 mg. **Cost:** *Generic*—1.25 mg $153.01/100, 2.5 mg $180.61/100, 5 mg $189.49/100, 10 mg $221.72/100.

Trandolapril (generic available)

Tablets: 1 mg, 2 mg, 4 mg. **Cost:** *Generic*—All strengths $123.93/100. ***In combination with:*** verapamil (Tarka). See Appendix B.

NURSING IMPLICATIONS

Assessment

- **Hypertension:** Monitor BP and pulse frequently during initial dose adjustment and periodically during therapy. Notify health care professional of significant changes.
- Monitor frequency of prescription refills to determine adherence.
- Assess patient for signs of angioedema (swelling of face, extremities, eyes, lips, tongue, difficulty in swallowing or breathing); may occur at any time during therapy. Discontinue medication and provide supportive care.
- **HF:** Monitor weight and assess patient routinely for resolution of fluid overload (peripheral edema, rales/crackles, dyspnea, weight gain, jugular venous distention).
- ***Lab Test Considerations:*** Monitor BUN, creatinine, and electrolyte levels periodically. Serum potassium, BUN and creatinine may be ↑, whereas sodium levels may be ↓. If ↑ BUN or serum creatinine concentrations occur, dose reduction or withdrawal may be required.
- Monitor CBC periodically during therapy. Certain drugs may rarely cause slight ↓ in hemoglobin and hematocrit, leukopenia, and eosinophilia.
- May cause ↑ AST, ALT, alkaline phosphatase, serum bilirubin, uric acid, and glucose.
- Assess urine protein prior to and periodically during therapy for up to 1 yr in patients with renal impairment or those receiving >150 m g/day of captopril. If excessive or ↑ proteinuria occurs, re-evaluate ACE inhibitor therapy.
- *Captopril:* May cause positive ANA titer.
- *Captopril:* May cause false-positive test results for urine acetone.
- *Captopril:* Monitor CBC with differential prior to initiation of therapy, every 2 wk for first 3 mo, and periodically for up to 1 yr in patients at risk for neutropenia (patients with renal impairment or collagen-vascular disease) or at first sign of infection. Discontinue therapy if neutrophil count is <1000/mm³.

Implementation

- Do not confuse Accupril with Aciphex. Do not confuse benazepril with Benadryl. Do not confuse captopril with carvedilol. Do not confuse Zestril with Zegerid, Zetia, or Zyprexa.
- Correct volume depletion, if possible, before initiation of therapy.
- **PO:** Precipitous drop in BP during first 1–3 hr after first dose may require volume expansion with normal saline but is not usually considered an indication for stopping therapy. Discontinuing diuretic therapy or cautiously increasing salt intake 2–3 days before initiation may ↓ risk of hypotension. Monitor closely for at least 1 hr after BP has stabilized. Resume diuretics if BP is not controlled.

Benazepril

- **PO:** For patients with difficulty swallowing tablets, pharmacist may compound oral suspension; stable for 30 days if refrigerated. Shake suspension before each use.

Captopril

- **PO:** Administer 1 hr before or 2 hr after meals. May be crushed if patient has difficulty swallowing. Tablets may have a sulfurous odor.
- An oral solution may be prepared by crushing a 25-mg tablet and dissolving it in 25–100 mL of water. Shake for at least 5 min and administer within 30 min.

Enalapril

- **PO:** For patients with difficulty swallowing tablets, oral solution is available ready to use. Shake solution before each use. Solution is stable at controlled room temperature for 60 days.

Enalaprilat

IV Administration

- **IV Push:** ***Diluent:*** May be administered undiluted. ***Concentration:*** 1.25 mg/mL. ***Rate:*** Administer over at least 5 min.
- **Intermittent Infusion:** ***Diluent:*** Dilute in up to 50 mL of D5W, 0.9% NaCl, D5/0.9% NaCl, or D5/LR. Diluted solution is stable for 24 hr. ***Rate:*** Administer as a slow infusion over at least 5 min.
- **Y-Site Compatibility:** acyclovir, alemtuzumab, alfentanil, allopurinol, amifostine, amikacin, aminocaproic acid, aminophylline, amiodarone, amphotericin B lipid complex, amphotericin B liposome, anidulafungin, argatroban, ascorbic acid, atropine, azathioprine, azithromycin, aztreonam, benztropine,

bivalirudin, bleomycin, bumetanide, buprenorphine, butorphanol, calcium chloride, calcium gluconate, cangrelor, carboplatin, carmustine, cefazolin, cefotaxime, cefotetan, cefoxitin, ceftaroline, ceftazidime, ceftriaxone, cefuroxime, chloramphenicol, chlorpromazine, cisatracurium, cisplatin, cladribine, clindamycin, cyanocobalamin, cyclophosphamide, cyclosporine, cytarabine, dacarbazine, dactinomycin, daptomycin, daunorubicin, dexamethasone, dexmedetomidine, dexrazoxane, digoxin, diltiazem, diphenhydramine, dobutamine, docetaxel, dolasetron, dopamine, doxorubicin, doxorubicin liposomal, doxycycline, ephedrine, epinephrine, epirubicin, epoetin, eptifibatide, ertapenem, erythromycin, esmolol, etoposide, etoposide phosphate, famotidine, fenoldopam, fentanyl, filgrastim, fluconazole, fludarabine, fluorouracil, folic acid, foscarnet, fosphenytoin, furosemide, ganciclovir, gemcitabine, gentamicin, glycopyrrolate, granisetron, heparin, hetastarch, hydrocortisone, hydromorphone, idarubicin, ifosfamide, imipenem/cilastatin, indomethacin, insulin, irinotecan, isoproterenol, ketorolac, labetalol, leucovorin, levofloxacin, lidocaine, linezolid, lorazepam, magnesium sulfate, mannitol, melphalan, meperidine, meropenem, mesna, methotrexate, methylprednisolone, metoclopramide, metoprolol, metronidazole, midazolam, milrinone, mitomycin, mitoxantrone, morphine, moxifloxacin, multivitamins, mycophenolate, nafcillin, nalbuphine, naloxone, nicardipine, nitroglycerin, nitroprusside, norepinephrine, octreotide, ondansetron, oxacillin, oxaliplatin, oxytocin, paclitaxel, palonosetron, pamidronate, pancuronium, papaverine, pemetrexed, penicillin G, pentamidine, pentobarbital, phenobarbital, phentolamine, phenylephrine, phytonadione, piperacillin/tazobactam, potassium acetate, potassium chloride, potassium phosphates, procainamide, prochlorperazine, promethazine, propofol, propranolol, protamine, pyridoxine, quinupristin/dalfopristin, ranitidine, remifentanil, rituximab, rocuronium, sodium acetate, sodium bicarbonate, succinylcholine, sufentanil, tacrolimus, tetracycline, theophylline, thiamine, thiotepa, tigecycline, tirofiban, tobramycin, topotecan, trastuzumab, vancomycin, vasopressin, vecuronium, verapamil, vinblastine, vincristine, vinorelbine, voriconazole, zoledronic acid.

- **Y-Site Incompatibility:** amphotericin B colloidal, caspofungin, cefepime, dantrolene, diazepam, diazoxide, phenytoin.

Lisinopril

- **PO:** Oral solution is clear to slightly opalescent. Administer without dilution.

Moexipril

- **PO:** Administer moexipril on an empty stomach, 1 hr before a meal.

Ramipril

- **PO:** Capsules may be opened and sprinkled on applesauce, or dissolved in 4 oz water or apple juice for patients with difficulty swallowing. Effectiveness is same as capsule. Prepared mixtures can be stored for up to 24 hr at room temperature or up to 48 hr if refrigerated.

Trandolapril

- **PO:** May be taken with or without food.

Patient/Family Teaching

- Instruct patient to take medication as directed at the same time each day, even if feeling well. Take missed doses as soon as possible but not if almost time for next dose. Do not double doses. Warn patient not to discontinue ACE inhibitor therapy unless directed by health care professional.
- Caution patient to avoid salt substitutes or foods containing high levels of potassium or sodium unless directed by health care professional (see Appendix K).
- Caution patient to change positions slowly to minimize hypotension. Use of alcohol, standing for long periods, exercising, and hot weather may ↑ orthostatic hypotension.Instruct patient to notify health care professional of all Rx or OTC medications, vitamins, or herbal products being taken and consult health care professional before taking any new medications, especially cough, cold, or allergy remedies.
- May cause dizziness. Caution patient to avoid driving and other activities requiring alertness until response to medication is known.
- Advise patient to inform health care professional of medication regimen prior to treatment or surgery.
- Advise patient that medication may cause impairment of taste that generally resolves within 8–12 wk, even with continued therapy.
- Instruct patient to notify health care professional immediately if rash; mouth sores; sore throat; fever; swelling of hands or feet; irregular heart beat; chest pain; dry cough; hoarseness; swelling of face, eyes, lips, or tongue; difficulty swallowing or breathing occur; or if taste impairment or skin rash persists. Persistent dry cough may occur and may not subside until medication is discontinued. Consult health care professional if cough becomes bothersome. Also notify health care professional if nausea, vomiting, or diarrhea occurs and continues.
- Advise diabetic patients to monitor blood glucose closely, especially during first mo of therapy; may cause hypoglycemia.
- Advise women of childbearing age to use contraception and notify health care professional if pregnancy is planned or suspected. If pregnancy is detected, discontinue medication as soon as possible. May be teratogenic.
- Emphasize the importance of follow-up examinations to monitor progress.
- **Hypertension:** Encourage patient to comply with additional interventions for hypertension (weight re-

A

duction, low sodium diet, discontinuation of smoking, moderation of alcohol consumption, regular exercise, and stress management). Medication controls but does not cure hypertension.

- Instruct patient and family on correct technique for monitoring BP. Advise them to check BP at least weekly and to report significant changes to health care professional.

Evaluation/Desired Outcomes

- Decrease in BP without appearance of excessive side effects.
- Decrease in signs and symptoms of HF (some drugs may also improve survival).
- Decrease in development of overt HF (enalapril).
- Reduction of risk of death or development of HF following MI.
- Reduction of risk of death from cardiovascular causes and MI in patients with stable CAD (perindopril).
- Reduction of risk of MI, stroke, or death from cardiovascular causes in patients at high-risk for these events (ramipril).
- Decrease in progression of diabetic nephropathy (captopril).

ANGIOTENSIN II RECEPTOR ANTAGONISTS

azilsartan (a-zill-**sar**-tan)
Edarbi

candesartan (can-de-**sar**-tan)
Atacand

eprosartan (ep-roe-**sar**-tan)
Teveten

irbesartan (ir-be-**sar**-tan)
Avapro

losartan (loe-**sar**-tan)
Cozaar

olmesartan (ole-me-**sar**-tan)
Benicar, Olmetec

telmisartan (tel-mi-**sar**-tan)
Micardis

valsartan (val-**sar**-tan)
Diovan

Classification
Therapeutic: antihypertensives
Pharmacologic: angiotensin II receptor antagonists

Indications

Alone or with other agents in the management of hypertension. Treatment of diabetic nephropathy in patients with type 2 diabetes and hypertension (irbesartan and losartan only). Management of HF (New York Heart Association class II-IV) in patients who cannot tolerate ACE inhibitors (candesartan and valsartan only) or in combination with an ACE inhibitor and beta-blocker (candesartan only). Prevention of stroke in patients with hypertension and left ventricular hypertrophy (losartan only). Reduction of risk of death from cardiovascular causes in patients with left ventricular systolic dysfunction after MI (valsartan only). Reduction of risk of myocardial infarction, stroke, or cardiovascular death in patients ≥55 yr who are at high risk for cardiovascular events and are unable to take ACE inhibitors (telmisartan only).

Action

Blocks vasoconstrictor and aldosterone-producing effects of angiotensin II at receptor sites, including vascular smooth muscle and the adrenal glands. **Therapeutic Effects:** Lowering of BP. Slowed progression of diabetic nephropathy (irbesartan and losartan only). Reduced cardiovascular death and hospitalizations due to HF in patients with HF (candesartan and valsartan only). Decreased risk of cardiovascular death in patients with left ventricular systolic dysfunction who are post-MI (valsartan only). Decreased risk of stroke in patients with hypertension and left ventricular hypertrophy (effect may be less in black patients) (losartan only).

Pharmacokinetics

Absorption: *Azilsartan*— Azilsartan medoxomil is converted to azilsartan, the active component. 60% absorbed; *Candesartan*—Candesartan cilexetil is converted to candesartan, the active component; 15% bioavailability of candesartan; *Eprosartan*—13% absorbed after oral administration; *Irbesartan*—60–80% absorbed after oral administration; *Losartan*—well absorbed, with extensive first-pass hepatic metabolism, resulting in 33% bioavailability; *Olmesartan*—Olmesartan medoxomil is converted to olmesartan, the active component; 26% bioavailability of olmesartan; *Telmisartan*—42–58% absorbed following oral administration (bioavailability ↑ in patients with hepatic impairment); *Valsartan*—10–35% absorbed following oral administration.
Distribution: All angiotensin receptor blockers (ARBs) cross the placenta; *Candesartan*—enters breast milk.
Protein Binding: All ARBs are >90% protein-bound.
Metabolism and Excretion: *Azilsartan*—50% metabolized by the liver, primarily by the CYP2C9 enzyme system. 55% eliminated in feces, 42% in urine (15% as unchanged drug); *Candesartan*—Minor metabolism by the liver; 33% excreted in urine, 67% in fe-

ces (via bile); *Eprosartan*—Excreted primarily unchanged in feces via biliary excretion; *Irbesartan*—Some hepatic metabolism; 20% excreted in urine, 80% in feces; *Losartan*—Undergoes extensive first-pass hepatic metabolism; 14% is converted to an active metabolite. 4% excreted unchanged in urine; 6% excreted in urine as active metabolite; some biliary elimination; *Olmesartan*—30–50% excreted unchanged in urine, remainder eliminated in feces via bile; *Telmisartan*—Excreted mostly unchanged in feces via biliary excretion; *Valsartan*—Minor metabolism by the liver; 13% excreted in urine, 83% in feces.

Half-life: *Azilsartan*—11 hr; *Candesartan*—9 hr; *Eprosartan*—20 hr; *Irbesartan*—11–15 hr; *Losartan*—2 hr (6–9 hr for metabolite); *Olmesartan*—13 hr; *Telmisartan*—24 hr; *Valsartan*—6 hr.

TIME/ACTION PROFILE (antihypertensive effect with chronic dosing)

DRUG	ONSET	PEAK	DURATION
Azilsartan	within 2 hr	18 hr	24 hr
Candesartan	2–4 hr	4 wk	24 hr
Eprosartan	1–2 hr	2–3 wk	12–24 hr
Irbesartan	within 2 hr	2 wk	24 hr
Losartan	6 hr	3–6 wk	24 hr
Olmesartan	within 1 wk	2 wk	24 hr
Telmisartan	within 3 hr	4 wk	24 hr
Valsartan	within 2 hr	4 wk	24 hr

Contraindications/Precautions

Contraindicated in: Hypersensitivity; Concurrent use with aliskiren in patients with diabetes or moderate-to-severe renal impairment (CCr <60 mL/min); Severe hepatic impairment (candesartan); OB: Can cause injury or death of fetus—if pregnancy occurs, discontinue immediately; Lactation: Discontinue drug or use formula.

Use Cautiously in: HF (may result in azotemia, oliguria, acute renal failure and/or death); Volume- or salt-depleted patients or patients receiving high doses of diuretics (correct deficits before initiating therapy or initiate at lower doses); Black patients (may not be effective); Impaired renal function due to primary renal disease or HF (may worsen renal function); Obstructive biliary disorders (telmisartan) or hepatic impairment (losartan, or telmisartan); Women of childbearing potential; Pedi: Safety not established in children <18 yr (<6 yr for losartan, olmesartan, and valsartan).

Adverse Reactions/Side Effects

CNS: dizziness, anxiety, depression, fatigue, headache, insomnia, weakness. **CV:** hypotension, chest pain, edema, tachycardia. **Derm:** rashes. **EENT:** nasal congestion, pharyngitis, rhinitis, sinusitis. **GI:** abdominal pain, diarrhea, drug-induced hepatitis, dyspepsia, nausea, vomiting. **GU:** impaired renal function. **F and E:** hyperkalemia. **MS:** arthralgia, back pain, myalgia. **Misc:** ANGIOEDEMA.

Interactions

Drug-Drug: NSAIDs and selective **COX-2 inhibitors** may blunt the antihypertensive effect and ↑ the risk of renal dysfunction. ↑ antihypertensive effects with other **antihypertensives** and **diuretics**. Telmisartan may ↑ serum **digoxin** levels. Concurrent use of **potassium-sparing diuretics**, **potassium-containing salt substitutes**, or **potassium supplements** may ↑ risk of hyperkalemia. ↑ risk of hyperkalemia, renal dysfunction, hypotension, and syncope with concurrent use of **ACE inhibitors** or **aliskiren**; avoid concurrent use with aliskiren in patients with diabetes or CCr <60 mL/min; avoid concurrent use with ACE inhibitors. Candesartan, valsartan, and irbesartan may ↑ **lithium** levels. Irbesartan and losartan may ↑ effects of **amiodarone**, **fluoxetine**, **glimepiride**, **glipizide**, **phenytoin**, **rosiglitazone**, and **warfarin**. **Rifampin** may ↓ effects of losartan. ↑ risk of renal dysfunction when telmisartan used with **ramipril** (concurrent use not recommended). **Colesevelam** may ↓ olmesartan levels; administer olmesartan ≥4 hr before colesevelam.

Route/Dosage

Azilsartan

PO (Adults): 80 mg once daily, initial dose may be ↓ to 40 mg once daily if high doses of diuretics are used concurrently.

Candesartan

PO (Adults): *Hypertension*—16 mg once daily; may be ↑ up to 32 mg/day in 1–2 divided doses (begin therapy at a lower dose in patients who are receiving diuretics or are volume depleted). *HF*—4 mg once daily initially, dose may be doubled at 2 wk intervals up to target dose of 32 mg once daily.

PO (Children 6–16 yr and >50 kg): 8–16 mg/day (in 1–2 divided doses); may be ↑ up to 32 mg/day (in 1–2 divided doses).

PO (Children 6–16 yr and <50 kg): 4–8 mg/day (in 1–2 divided doses); may be ↑ up to 16 mg/day (in 1–2 divided doses).

PO (Children 1–5 yr): 0.20 mg/kg/day (in 1–2 divided doses); may be ↑ up to 0.4 mg/kg/day (in 1–2 divided doses).

Hepatic Impairment

PO (Adults): *Moderate hepatic impairment*—Initiate at 8 mg once daily.

Eprosartan

PO (Adults): 600 mg once daily; may be ↑ to 800 mg/day (in 1–2 divided doses) (usual range 400–800 mg/day).

Renal Impairment

PO (Adults): *CCr <60 mL/min*—Do not exceed 600 mg/day.

Irbesartan

PO (Adults): *Hypertension*—150 mg once daily; may be ↑ to 300 mg once daily. Initiate therapy at 75 mg once daily in patients who are receiving diuretics or are volume depleted. *Type 2 diabetic nephropathy*—300 mg once daily.

Losartan

PO (Adults): *Hypertension*—50 mg once daily initially (range 25–100 mg/day as a single daily dose or 2 divided doses) (initiate therapy at 25 mg once daily in patients who are receiving diuretics or are volume depleted). *Prevention of stroke in patients with hypertension and left ventricular hypertrophy*—50 mg once daily initially; hydrochlorothiazide 12.5 mg once daily should be added and/or dose of losartan ↑ to 100 mg once daily followed by an ↑ in hydrochlorothiazide to 25 mg once daily based on BP response. *Type 2 diabetic nephropathy*—50 mg once daily, may ↑ to 100 mg once daily depending on BP response.

Hepatic Impairment

PO (Adults): 25 mg once daily initially; may be ↑ as tolerated.
PO (Children >6 yr): *Hypertension*—0.7 mg/kg once daily (up to 50 mg/day), may be titrated up to 1.4 mg/kg/day (or 100 mg/day).

Renal Impairment

PO (Children >6 yr): *CCr <30 mL/min*—Contraindicated.

Olmesartan

PO (Adults): 20 mg once daily; may be ↑ up to 40 mg once daily (patients who are receiving diuretics or are volume-depleted should be started on lower doses).
PO (Children 6–16 yr): *≥35 kg*—20 mg once daily; may be ↑ after 2 wk up to 40 mg once daily; *20–34.9 kg*—10 mg once daily; may be ↑ after 2 wk up to 20 mg once daily.

Telmisartan

PO (Adults): *Hypertension*—40 mg once daily (volume-depleted patients should start with 20 mg once daily); may be titrated up to 80 mg/day; *Cardiovascular risk reduction*—80 mg once daily.

Valsartan

PO (Adults): *Hypertension*—80 mg or 160 mg once daily initially in patients who are not volume-depleted; may be ↑ to 320 mg once daily; *HF*—40 mg twice daily, may be titrated up to target dose of 160 mg twice daily as tolerated; *Post-MI*—20 mg twice daily (may be initiated ≥ 12 hr after MI); dose may be titrated up to target dose of 160 mg twice daily, as tolerated.
PO (Children 6–16 yr): *Hypertension*—1.3 mg/kg once daily (maximum dose = 40 mg/day); may be ↑ up to 2.7 mg/kg once daily (maximum dose = 160 mg/day).

Availability

Azilsartan

Tablets: 40 mg, 80 mg. **Cost:** All strengths $113.23/30. ***In combination with:*** chlorthalidone (Edarbyclor); see Appendix B.

Candesartan (generic available)

Tablets: 4 mg, 8 mg, 16 mg, 32 mg. **Cost:** *Generic*—4 mg $99.16/30, 8 mg $99.16/30, 16 mg $285.56/30, 32 mg $386.60/30. ***In combination with:*** hydrochlorothiazide (Atacand HCT); see Appendix B.

Eprosartan (generic available)

Tablets: 400 mg, 600 mg. **Cost:** *Generic*—600 mg $102.78/30. ***In combination with:*** hydrochlorothiazide (Teveten HCT); see Appendix B.

Irbesartan (generic available)

Tablets: 75 mg, 150 mg, 300 mg. **Cost:** *Generic*—75 mg $10.44/90, 150 mg $279.97/90, 300 mg $31.13/90. ***In combination with:*** hydrochlorothiazide (Avalide); see Appendix B.

Losartan (generic available)

Tablets: 25 mg, 50 mg, 100 mg. **Cost:** *Generic*—25 mg $151.43/90, 50 mg $67.88/30, 100 mg $277.36/90. ***In combination with:*** hydrochlorothiazide (Hyzaar); see Appendix B.

Olmesartan (generic available)

Tablets: 5 mg, 20 mg, 40 mg. **Cost:** 5 mg $288.15/90, 20 mg $358.41/90, 40 mg $543.45/100. ***In combination with:*** hydrochlorothiazide (Benicar HCT); amlodipine (Azor); see Appendix B.

Telmisartan (generic available)

Tablets: 20 mg, 40 mg, 80 mg. **Cost:** 20 mg $445.33/90, 40 mg $441.19/90, 80 mg $441.19/90. ***In combination with:*** hydrochlorothiazide (Micardis HCT); amlodipine (Twynsta); see Appendix B).

Valsartan (generic available)

Tablets: 40 mg, 80 mg, 160 mg, 320 mg. **Cost:** 40 mg $330.05/90, 80 mg $428.25/90, 160 mg $469.86/90, 320 mg $581.92/90. ***In combination with:*** amlodipine (Exforge); hydrochlorothiazide (Diovan HCT); amlodipine and hydrochlorothiazide (Exforge HCT); see Appendix B.

NURSING IMPLICATIONS

Assessment

- Assess BP (lying, sitting, standing) and pulse periodically during therapy. Notify health care professional of significant changes.
- Monitor frequency of prescription refills to determine adherence.
- Assess patient for signs of angioedema (dyspnea, facial swelling). May rarely cause angioedema.

- **HF:** Monitor daily weight and assess patient routinely for resolution of fluid overload (peripheral edema, rales/crackles, dyspnea, weight gain, jugular venous distention).
- ***Lab Test Considerations:*** Monitor renal function and electrolyte levels periodically. Serum potassium, BUN, and serum creatinine may be ↑.
- May cause ↑ AST, ALT, and serum bilirubin (candesartan and olmesartan only).
- May cause ↑ uric acid, slight ↓ in hemoglobin and hematocrit, neutropenia, and thrombocytopenia.

Implementation

- Do not confuse Benicar with Mevacor. Do not confuse Diovan with Zyban.
- Correct volume depletion, if possible, prior to initiation of therapy.
- **PO:** May be administered without regard to meals.

Losartan

- **PO:** For patients with difficulty swallowing tablets, pharmacist can compound oral suspension; stable for 4 wk if refrigerated. Shake suspension before each use.

Patient/Family Teaching

- Emphasize the importance of continuing to take as directed, even if feeling well. Take missed doses as soon as remembered if not almost time for next dose; do not double doses. Instruct patient to take medication at the same time each day. Warn patient not to discontinue therapy unless directed by health care professional.
- Caution patient to avoid salt substitutes containing potassium or food containing high levels of potassium or sodium unless directed by health care professional. See Appendix K.
- Caution patient to avoid sudden changes in position to decrease orthostatic hypotension. Use of alcohol, standing for long periods, exercising, and hot weather may increase orthostatic hypotension.
- May cause dizziness. Caution patient to avoid driving or other activities requiring alertness until response to medication is known.
- Instruct patient to notify health care professional of all Rx or OTC medications, vitamins, or herbal products being taken and consult health care professional before taking any new medications, especially NSAIDs and cough, cold, or allergy remedies.
- Instruct patient to notify health care professional of medication regimen prior to treatment or surgery.
- Instruct patient to notify health care professional immediately if swelling of face, eyes, lips, or tongue occurs, or if difficulty swallowing or breathing occurs.
- Advise women with reproductive potential to use contraception and notify health care professional if pregnancy is suspected or planned, or if breast feeding. If pregnancy is detected, discontinue medication as soon as possible.
- Emphasize the importance of follow-up exams to evaluate effectiveness of medication.
- **Hypertension:** Encourage patient to comply with additional interventions for hypertension (weight reduction, low-sodium diet, discontinuation of smoking, moderation of alcohol consumption, regular exercise, stress management). Medication controls but dose not cure hypertension.
- Instruct patient and family on proper technique for monitoring BP. Advise them to check BP at least weekly and to report significant changes.

Evaluation/Desired Outcomes

- Decrease in BP without appearance of excessive side effects.
- Slowed progression of diabetic nephropathy (irbesartan, losartan).
- Decreased cardiovascular death and HF-related hospitalizations in patients with HF (candesartan).
- Decreased hospitalizations in patients with HF (valsartan).
- Decreased risk of cardiovascular death in patients with left ventricular systolic dysfunction after MI (valsartan).
- Reduced risk of stroke in patients with hypertension and left ventricular hypertrophy (losartan).
- Reduction of risk of myocardial infarction, stroke, or cardiovascular death (telmisartan).

anidulafungin

(a-**ni**-du-la-fun-gin)

Eraxis

Classification

Therapeutic: antifungals

Pharmacologic: echinocandins

Indications

Candidemia and other serious candidal infections including intra-abdominal abscess, peritonitis. Esophageal candidiasis.

Action

Inhibits the synthesis of fungal cell wall. **Therapeutic Effects:** Death of susceptible fungi. **Spectrum:** Active against *Candida albicans*, *C. glabrata*, *C. parapsilosis*, and *C. tropicalis*.

Pharmacokinetics

Absorption: IV administration results in complete bioavailability.

Distribution: Crosses the placenta.

Metabolism and Excretion: Undergoes chemical degradation without hepatic metabolism; <1% excreted in urine.

Half-life: 40–50 hr.

TIME/ACTION PROFILE (blood levels)

ROUTE	ONSET	PEAK	DURATION
IV	rapid	end of infusion	24 hr

Contraindications/Precautions

Contraindicated in: Hypersensitivity.

Use Cautiously in: Underlying liver disease (may worsen); OB, Lactation: Pregnancy or lactation; Pedi: Safety not established.

Adverse Reactions/Side Effects

Resp: bronchospasm, dyspnea. **CV:** hypotension. **GI:** diarrhea, ↑ liver enzymes. **Derm:** flushing, rash, urticaria. **F and E:** hypokalemia. **Misc:** ANAPHYLAXIS, infusion reaction.

Interactions

Drug-Drug: None noted.

Route/Dosage

IV (Adults): *Esophageal candidiasis*—100 mg loading dose on day 1, then 50 mg daily. *Candidemia and other candidal infections*—200 mg loading dose on day 1, then 100 mg daily.

Availability

Lyophilized powder for IV use (requires reconstitution): 50 mg/vial.

NURSING IMPLICATIONS

Assessment

- Assess infected area and monitor cultures before and periodically during therapy.
- Specimens for culture should be taken before instituting therapy. Therapy may be started before results are obtained.
- Monitor for signs and symptoms of anaphylaxis (rash, urticaria, flushing, pruritus, bronchospasm, dyspnea, hypotension); usually related to histamine release. To decrease risk, do not exceed a rate of infusion of 1.1 mg/min.
- ***Lab Test Considerations:*** May cause ↑ ALT, AST, alkaline phosphatase, and hepatic enzymes.
- May cause hypokalemia.
- May cause neutropenia and leukopenia.

Implementation

IV Administration

- **Intermittent Infusion:** Reconstitute each 50 mg vial with 15 mL or the 100 mg vial with 30 mL of sterile water for injection for a concentration of 3.33 mg/mL. May be stored in refrigerator for up to 1 hr. ***Diluent:*** Further dilute within 24 hr by transferring contents of reconstituted vial into IV bag of D5W or 0.9% NaCl. For the 50 mg dose, dilute with 85 mL for an infusion volume of 100 mL. For the 100 mg dose, dilute with 170 mL for an infusion volume of 200 mL. For the 200 mg dose, dilute with 340 mL for a total infusion volume of 400 mL. ***Concentration:*** Final concentration should not exceed 0.5 mg/mL. Do not administer solutions that are discolored or contain particulate matter. Store reconstituted solution in refrigerator; do not freeze. Administer within 24 hr. ***Rate:*** Administer at a rate not to exceed 1.1 mg/min (1.4 mL/min or 84 mL/hr).
- **Y-Site Compatibility:** acyclovir, alemtuzumab, alfentanil, allopurinol, amifostine, amikacin, aminophylline, amiodarone, amphotericin B lipid complex, amphotericin B liposome, ampicillin, ampicillin/sulbactam, argatroban, aresnic trioxide, atracurium, azithromycin, aztreonam, bivalirudin, bleomycin, bumetanide, buprenorphine, bulsulfan, butorphanol, calcium chloride, calcium gluconate, carboplatin, carmustine, caspofungin, cefazolin, cefepime, cefotaxime, cefotetan, cefoxitin, ceftazidime, ceftriaxone, cefuroxime, chloramphenicol, ciprofloxacin, cisatracurium, cisplatin, clindamycin, cyclophosphamide, cyclosporine, cytarabine, dacarbazine, dactinomycin, daunorubicin hydrochloride, dexamethasone, dexmedetomidine, digoxin, diltiazem, diphenhydramine, dobutamine, docetaxel, dolasetron, dopamine, doxacurium, doxorubicin hydrochloride, doxorubicin liposome, doxycycline, droperidol, enalaprilat, ephedrine, epinephrine, epirubicin, eptifibatide, erythromycin, esmolol, etoposide, etoposide phosphate, famotidine, fenoldopam, fentanyl, fluconazole, fludarabine, fluorouracil, foscarnet, fosphenytoin, furosemide, ganciclovir, gemcitabine, gentamicin, glycopyrrolate, granisetron, haloperidol, heparin, hydralazine, hydrocortisone, hydromorphone, idarubicin, ifosfamide, imipenem/cilastatin, insulin, irinotecan, isoproterenol, ketorolac, labetalol, leucovorin, levofloxacin, linezolid, lorazepam, mannitol, melphalan, meperidine, meropenem, mesna, metaraminol, methotrexate, methyldopate, methylprednisolone, metoclopramide, metoprolol, metronidazole, midazolam, milrinone, mitomycin, mitoxantrone, morphine, mycophenolate, nafcillin, naloxone, nicardipine, nitroglycerin, nitroprusside, norepinephrine, octreotide, ondansetron, oxaliplatin, oxytocin, paclitaxel, palonosetron, pamidronate, pancuronium, pantoprazole, pentamidine, pentobarbital, phenobarbital, phentolamine, phenylephrine, piperacillin/tazobactam, potassium acetate, potassium chloride, procainamide, prochlorperazine, promethazine, propranolol, quinupristin/dalfopristin, ranitidine, remifentanil, rocuronium, sodium acetate, streptozocin, succinylcholine, sufentanil, tacrolimus, theophylline, thiopental, thiotepa, tirofiban, tobramycin, topotecan, trimethoprim/sulfamethoxazole, vancomycin, vasopressin, vecuronium, verapamil, vinblastine, vincristine, vinorelbine, voriconazole, zidovudine, zoledronic acid.
- **Y-Site Incompatibility:** amphotericin B deoxycholate, dantrolene, diazepam, ertapenem, magnesium sulfate, nalbuphine, pemetrexed, phenytoin, potas-

sium phosphates, sodium bicarbonate, sodium phosphates.

Patient/Family Teaching
- Explain purpose of medication to patient.
- Instruct patient to notify health care professional if signs and symptoms of anaphylaxis occur or if diarrhea becomes pronounced.

Evaluation/Desired Outcomes
- Resolution of clinical and laboratory indications of fungal infections. Duration of therapy should be based on the patients clinical response. Therapy should be continued for at least 14 days after the last positive culture. For esophageal candidiasis, treatment should continue for at least 7 days following resolution of symptoms.

ANTIFUNGALS (TOPICAL)

butenafine (byoo-**ten**-a-feen)
Lotrimin Ultra, Mentax

ciclopirox (sye-kloe-**peer**-ox)
Loprox, Penlac, ✱Stieprox

clotrimazole (kloe-**trye**-ma-zole)
✱Canesten, ✱Clotrimaderm, Lotrimin AF, Mycelex, ✱Neo-Zol

econazole (ee-**kon**-a-zole)
Ecoza

ketoconazole
(kee-toe-**koe**-na-zole)
Extina, ✱Ketoderm, Nizoral, Nizoral A-D, Xolegel

luliconazole (loo-li-**kon**-a-zole)
Luzu

miconazole (mye-**kon**-a-zole)
Fungoid, Lotrimin AF, Micatin, ✱Micozole, Zeasorb-AF

naftifine (**naff**-ti-feen)
Naftin

nystatin (nye-**stat**-in)
~~Mycostatin~~, ✱Nyaderm, Nystop

oxiconazole (ox-i-**kon**-a-zole)
Oxistat

sulconazole (sul-**kon**-a-zole)
Exelderm

terbinafine (ter-**bin**-a-feen)
✱Lamisil, Lamisil AT

tolnaftate (tol-**naff**-tate)
✱Canesten, ✱EZ Clear, ✱Flexitol, ✱Fungicure, ✱Fungifoam, Lamisil AF, Podactin, ✱Proclearz, Tinactin

Classification
Therapeutic: antifungals (topical)

Indications
Treatment of a variety of cutaneous fungal infections, including cutaneous candidiasis, tinea pedis (athlete's foot), tinea cruris (jock itch), tinea corporis (ringworm), tinea versicolor, seborrheic dermatitis, dandruff, and onychomycosis of fingernails and toes.

Action
Butenafine, nystatin, clotrimazole, econazole, ketoconazole, luliconazole, miconazole, naftifine, oxiconazole, sulconazole, and terbinafine affect the synthesis of the fungal cell wall, allowing leakage of cellular contents. Tolnaftate distorts the hyphae and stunts mycelial growth in fungi. Ciclopirox inhibits the transport of essential elements in the fungal cell, disrupting the synthesis of DNA, RNA, and protein. **Therapeutic Effects:** Decrease in symptoms of fungal infection.

Pharmacokinetics
Absorption: Absorption through intact skin is minimal.
Distribution: Distribution after topical administration is primarily local.
Metabolism and Excretion: Metabolism and excretion not known following local application.
Half-life: *Butenafine*—35 hr; *Ciclopirox*—5.5 hr (gel); *Terbinafine*—21 hr.

TIME/ACTION PROFILE (resolution of symptoms/lesions†)

ROUTE	ONSET	PEAK	DURATION
Butenafine	unknown	up to 4 wk	unknown
Luliconazole	unknown	3–4 wk	unknown
Tolnaftate	24–72 hr	unknown	unknown

† Only the drugs with known information included in this table.

Contraindications/Precautions
Contraindicated in: Hypersensitivity to active ingredients, additives, preservatives, or bases; Some products contain alcohol or bisulfites and should be avoided in patients with known intolerance.
Use Cautiously in: Nail and scalp infections (may require additional systemic therapy); OB, Lactation: Safety not established.

Adverse Reactions/Side Effects
Local: burning, itching, local hypersensitivity reactions, redness, stinging.

Interactions
Drug-Drug: Econazole may ↑ levels of and risk of bleeding from **warfarin**.

Route/Dosage

Butenafine

Topical (Adults and Children >12 yr): Apply once daily for 2 wk for tinea corporis, tinea cruris, or tinea versicolor. Apply once daily for 4 wk or once daily for 7 days for tinea pedis.

Ciclopirox

Topical (Adults and Children >10 yr): *Cream/lotion*—Apply twice daily for 2–4 wk; *Topical solution (nail lacquer)*—Apply to nails at bedtime or 8 hr prior to bathing for up to 48 wk. Each daily application should be made over the previous coat and then removed with alcohol every 7 days; *Gel*—Apply twice daily for 4 wk; *Shampoo*—5–10 mL applied to scalp, lather and leave on for 3 min, rinse; repeat twice weekly for 4 wk (at least 3 days between applications).

Clotrimazole

Topical (Adults and Children >3 yr): Apply twice daily for 1–4 wk.

Econazole

Topical (Adults and Children): Apply once daily for tinea pedis (for 4 wk), tinea cruris (for 2 wk), tinea corporis (for 2 wk), or tinea versicolor (for 2 wk). Apply twice daily for cutaneous candidiasis (for 2 wk).

Ketoconazole

Topical (Adults): Apply cream once daily for cutaneous candidiasis (for 2 wk), tinea corporis (for 2 wk), tinea cruris (for 2 wk), tinea pedis (for 6 wk), or tinea versicolor (for 2 wk). Apply cream twice daily for seborrheic dermatitis (for 4 wk). For dandruff, use shampoo twice weekly (wait 3–4 days between treatments) for 4 wk, then intermittently.

Luliconazole

Topical (Adults and Children ≥12 yr): *Interdigital tinea pedis*—Apply to affected and surrounding areas once daily for 2 wk; *Tinea cruris*—Apply to affected and surrounding areas once daily for 1 wk.
Topical (Adults and Children ≥2 yr): *Tinea corporis*—Apply to affected and surrounding areas once daily for 1 wk.
Topical (Adults): *Interdigital tinea pedis*—Apply to affected and surrounding areas once daily for 2 wk; *Tinea cruris and tinea corporis*—Apply to affected and surrounding areas once daily for 1 wk.

Miconazole

Topical (Adults and Children >2 yr): Apply twice daily. Treat tinea cruris for 2 wk and tinea pedis or tinea corporis for 4 wk.

Naftifine

Topical (Adults): *Interdigital tinea pedis*—Apply cream or gel once daily for 2 wk; *Tinea cruris or tinea corporis*—apply cream once daily for 2 wk.
Topical (Children ≥12 yr): *Interdigital tinea pedis*—Apply cream or gel once daily for 2 wk.
Topical (Children ≥2 yr): *Tinea corporis*—Apply cream once daily for 2 wk.

Nystatin

Topical (Adults and Children): Apply 2–3 times daily until healing is complete.

Oxiconazole

Topical (Adults and Children): Apply cream or lotion 1–2 times daily for tinea pedis (for 4 wk), tinea corporis (for 2 wk), or tinea cruris (for 2 wk). Apply cream once daily for tinea versicolor (for 2 wk).

Sulconazole

Topical (Adults): Apply 1–2 times daily (twice daily for tinea pedis). Treat tinea corporis, tinea cruris, or tinea versicolor for 3 wk, and tinea pedis for 4 wk.

Terbinafine

Topical (Adults): Apply twice daily for tinea pedis (for 1 wk) or daily for tinea cruris or tinea corporis for 1 wk.

Tolnaftate

Topical (Adults): Apply twice daily for tinea cruris (for 2 wk), tinea pedis (for 4 wk), or tinea corporis (for 4 wk).

Availability

Butenafine (generic available)

Cream: 1%$^{Rx, OTC}$.

Ciclopirox (generic available)

Cream: 0.77%. **Gel:** 0.77%. **Lotion:** 🍁 1%. **Nail lacquer:** 8%. **Shampoo:** 1%, 🍁 1.5%. **Suspension:** 0.77%.

Clotrimazole (generic available)

Cream: 1%^{OTC}. **Solution:** 1%^{OTC}. ***In combination with:*** betamethasone (Lotrisone). See Appendix B.

Econazole (generic available)

Cream: 1%. **Foam:** 1%.

Ketoconazole (generic available)

Cream: 2%. **Foam:** 2%. **Gel:** 2%. **Shampoo:** 1%^{OTC}, 2%.

Luliconazole

Cream: 1%.

Miconazole (generic available)

Cream: 2%$^{Rx, OTC}$. **Ointment:** 2%^{OTC}. **Powder:** 2%^{OTC}. **Solution:** 2%^{OTC}. **Spray liquid:** 2%^{OTC}. **Spray pow-

der: 2%^{OTC}. **Tincture:** 2%^{OTC}. ***In combination with:*** zinc oxide (Vusion). See Appendix B.

Naftifine
Cream: 1%, 2%. **Gel:** 1%, 2%.

Nystatin (generic available)
Cream: 100,000 units/g$^{Rx, OTC}$. **Ointment:** 100,000 units/g$^{Rx, OTC}$. **Powder:** 100,000 units/g$^{Rx, OTC}$. ***In combination with:*** triamcinolone. See Appendix B.

Oxiconazole (generic available)
Cream: 1%. **Lotion:** 1%.

Sulconazole
Cream: 1%. **Solution:** 1%.

Terbinafine (generic available)
Cream: 1%^{OTC}. **Gel:** 1%^{OTC}. **Spray liquid:** 1%^{OTC}.

Tolnaftate (generic available)
Cream: 1%^{OTC}. **Powder:** 1%^{OTC}. **Solution:** 1%^{OTC}. **Spray liquid:** 1%^{OTC}. **Spray powder:** 1%^{OTC}.

NURSING IMPLICATIONS

Assessment
- Inspect involved areas of skin and mucous membranes before and frequently during therapy. Increased skin irritation may indicate need to discontinue medication.

Implementation
- Consult health care professional for proper cleansing technique before applying medication.
- Choice of vehicle is based on use. Ointments, creams, and liquids are used as primary therapy. Lotion is usually preferred in intertriginous areas; if cream is used, apply sparingly to avoid maceration. Powders are usually used as adjunctive therapy but may be used as primary therapy for mild conditions (especially for moist lesions).
- **Topical:** Apply small amount to cover affected area completely. Avoid use of occlusive wrappings or dressings unless directed by health care professional.
- **Nail lacquer:** Avoid contact with skin other than skin immediately surrounding treated nail. Avoid contact with eyes or mucous membranes. Removal of unattached, infected nail, as frequently as monthly, by health care professional is needed with use of this medication. Up to 48 wk of daily application and professional removal may be required to achieve clear or almost clear nail. 6 mo of treatment may be required before results are noticed.
- **Ciclopirox or Ketoconazole shampoo:** Moisten hair and scalp thoroughly with water. Apply sufficient shampoo to produce enough lather to wash scalp and hair and gently massage it over the entire scalp area for approximately 1 min. Rinse hair thoroughly with warm water. Repeat process, leaving shampoo on hair for an additional 3 min. After the 2nd shampoo, rinse and dry hair with towel or warm air flow. Shampoo twice a wk for 4 wk with at least 3 days between each shampooing and then intermittently as needed to maintain control.
- **Ketoconazole foam:** Hold container upright and dispense foam into cap of can or other smooth surface; dispensing directly on to hand is not recommended as the foam begins to melt immediately on contact with warm skin. Pick up small amounts with fingertips and gently massage into affected areas until absorbed. Move hair to allow direct application to skin.

Patient/Family Teaching
- Instruct patient to apply medication as directed for full course of therapy, even if feeling better. Emphasize the importance of avoiding the eyes.
- Caution patient that some products may stain fabric, skin, or hair. Check label information. Fabrics stained from cream or lotion can usually be cleaned by hand washing with soap and warm water; stains from ointments can usually be removed with standard cleaning fluids.
- Patients with athlete's foot should be taught to wear well-fitting, ventilated shoes, to wash affected areas thoroughly, and to change shoes and socks at least once a day.
- Advise patient to report increased skin irritation or lack of response to therapy to health care professional.
- **Nail lacquer:** File away loose nail and trim nails every 7 days after solution is removed with alcohol. Do not use nail polish on treated nails. Inform health care professional if patient has diabetes mellitus before using.

Evaluation/Desired Outcomes
- Decrease in skin irritation and resolution of infection. Early relief of symptoms may be seen in 2–3 days. For *Candida,* tinea cruris, and tinea corporis, 2 wk are needed, and for tinea pedis, therapeutic response may take 3–4 wk. Recurrent fungal infections may be a sign of systemic illness.

ANTIFUNGALS (VAGINAL)

butoconazole (byoo-toe-**kon**-a-zole)
Gynezole-1, Mycelex-3

clotrimazole (kloe-**trye**-ma-zole)
Canesten, Clotrimaderm, Gyne-Lotrimin-3, Mycelex-7

miconazole (mye-**kon**-a-zole)
Monistat-1, Monistat-3, Monistat-7, Vagistat-3

terconazole (ter-**kon**-a-zole)
Terazol-3, Terazol-7

tioconazole (tye-oh-**kon**-a-zole)
1-Day, Monistat-1Day, Vagistat-1

Classification
Therapeutic: antifungals (vaginal)

Indications
Treatment of vulvovaginal candidiasis.

Action
Affects the permeability of the fungal cell wall, allowing leakage of cellular contents. Not active against bacteria. **Therapeutic Effects:** Inhibited growth and death of susceptible *Candida*, with decrease in accompanying symptoms of vulvovaginitis (vaginal burning, itching, discharge).

Pharmacokinetics
Absorption: Absorption through intact skin is minimal.
Distribution: Unknown. Action is primarily local.
Metabolism and Excretion: Negligible with local application.
Half-life: Not applicable.

TIME/ACTION PROFILE

ROUTE	ONSET	PEAK	DURATION
All agents	rapid	unknown	24 hr

Contraindications/Precautions
Contraindicated in: Hypersensitivity to active ingredients, additives, or preservatives; OB: Safety not established; Lactation: Safety not established.
Use Cautiously in: None noted.

Adverse Reactions/Side Effects
Derm: *terconazole*—TOXIC EPIDERMAL NECROLYSIS. **GU:** itching, pelvic pain, vulvovaginal burning. **Misc:** *terconazole*—ANAPHYLAXIS.

Interactions
Drug-Drug: Concurrent use of vaginal miconazole with **warfarin** ↑ risk of bleeding/bruising (appropriate monitoring recommended).

Route/Dosage

Butoconazole
Vag (Adults and Children ≥12 yr): 1 applicatorful (5 g) at bedtime for 3 days (Mycelex-3) *or* one applicatorful single dose (Gynezole-1).

Clotrimazole
Vag (Adults and Children >12 yr): *Vaginal tablets*—100 mg at bedtime for 7 nights (preferred regimen for pregnancy) *or* 200 mg at bedtime for 3 nights. *Vaginal cream*—1 applicatorful (5 g) of 1% cream at bedtime for 7 days *or* 1 applicatorful (5 g) of 2% cream at bedtime for 3 days.

Miconazole
Vag (Adults and Children ≥12 yr): *Vaginal suppositories*—one 100-mg suppository at bedtime for 7 days *or* one 200-mg suppository at bedtime for 3 days *or* one 1200-mg suppository as a single dose. *Vaginal cream*—1 applicatorful of 2% cream at bedtime for 7 days *or* 1 applicatorful of 4% cream at bedtime for 3 days. *Combination packages*—contain a cream or suppositories as well as an external vaginal cream (may be used twice daily for up to 7 days, as needed, for symptomatic management of itching).

Terconazole
Vag (Adults): *Vaginal cream*—1 applicatorful (5 g) of 0.4% cream at bedtime for 7 days *or* 1 applicatorful (5 g) of 0.8% cream at bedtime for 3 days. *Vaginal suppositories*—1 suppository (80 mg) at bedtime for 3 days.

Tioconazole
Vag (Adults and Children ≥12 yr): 1 applicatorful (4.6 g) at bedtime as a single dose.

Availability

Butoconazole
Vaginal cream: 2%^Rx, OTC^.

Clotrimazole (generic available)
Vaginal tablets: 100 mg^OTC^, 200 mg^OTC^. **Vaginal cream:** 1%^OTC^, 2%^OTC^.

Miconazole (generic available)
Vaginal cream: 2%^OTC^, 4%^OTC^. **Vaginal suppositories:** 100 mg^OTC^, 200 mg^Rx, OTC^. ***In combination with:*** combination package of three 200-mg suppositories and 2% external cream^OTC^; one 1200-mg suppository and 2% external cream^OTC^; 4% vaginal cream and 2% external cream^OTC^; seven 100-mg suppositories and 2% external cream^OTC^; 2% vaginal cream and 2% external cream^OTC^.

Terconazole (generic available)
Vaginal cream: 0.4%, 0.8%. **Vaginal suppositories:** 80 mg.

Tioconazole
Vaginal ointment: 6.5%^OTC^.

NURSING IMPLICATIONS

Assessment
- Inspect involved areas of skin and mucous membranes before and frequently during therapy. Increased skin irritation may indicate need to discontinue medication.

Implementation
- Consult health care professional for proper cleansing technique before applying medication.

- **Vag:** Applicators are supplied for vaginal administration.

Patient/Family Teaching

- Instruct patient to apply medication as directed for full course of therapy, even if feeling better. Therapy should be continued during menstrual period.
- Instruct patient on proper use of vaginal applicator. Medication should be inserted high into the vagina at bedtime. Instruct patient to remain recumbent for at least 30 min after insertion. Advise use of sanitary napkins to prevent staining of clothing or bedding.
- Advise patient to avoid using tampons while using this product.
- Advise patient to consult health care professional regarding intercourse during therapy. Vaginal medication may cause minor skin irritation in sexual partner. Advise patient to refrain from sexual contact during therapy or have male partner wear a condom. Some products may weaken latex contraceptive devices. Another method of contraception should be used during treatment.
- Advise patient to report to health care professional increased skin irritation or lack of response to therapy. A second course may be necessary if symptoms persist.
- Instruct patient to stop using medication and notify health care professional if rash or signs and symptoms of anaphylaxis (wheezing, rash, hives, shortness of breath) occur.
- Advise patient to dispose of applicator after each use (except for terconazole).

Evaluation/Desired Outcomes

- Decrease in skin irritation and vaginal discomfort. Therapeutic response is usually seen after 1 wk. Diagnosis should be reconfirmed with smears or cultures before a second course of therapy to rule out other pathogens associated with vulvovaginitis. Recurrent vaginal infections may be a sign of systemic illness.

apixaban (a-pix-a-ban)

Eliquis

Classification
Therapeutic: anticoagulants
Pharmacologic: factor Xa inhibitors

Indications

Decreases risk of stroke/systemic embolism associated with nonvalvular atrial fibrillation. Prevention of deep vein thrombosis that may lead to pulmonary embolism following knee or hip replacement surgery. Treatment of and reduction in risk of recurrence of deep vein thrombosis (DVT) or pulmonary embolism (PE).

Action

Acts as a selective, reversible site inhibitor of factor Xa, inhibiting both free and bound factor. Does not affect platelet aggregation directly, but does inhibit thrombin-induced platelet aggregation. Decreases thrombin generation and thrombus development. **Therapeutic Effects:** Treatment and prevention of thromboembolic events.

Pharmacokinetics

Absorption: 50% absorbed following oral administration.
Distribution: Unknown.
Metabolism and Excretion: 25% metabolized (mostly by CYP3A4) and excreted in urine and feces. Biliary and direct intestinal excretion account for fecal elimination.
Half-life: 6 hr (12 hr after repeated dosing due to prolonged absorption).

TIME/ACTION PROFILE (effect on hemostasis)

ROUTE	ONSET	PEAK	DURATION
PO	unknown	3–4 hr†	24 hr

†Blood levels.

Contraindications/Precautions

Contraindicated in: Previous severe hypersensitivity reactions; Active pathological bleeding; Severe hepatic impairment; Not recommended for use in patients with prosthetic heart valves; Concurrent use of strong dual inducers of CYP3A4 and P-gp; PE with hemodynamic instability or requiring thrombolysis or pulmonary embolectomy; Lactation: Lactation.
Use Cautiously in: Neuroaxial spinal anesthesia or spinal puncture, especially if concurrent with an indwelling epidural catheter, drugs affecting hemostasis, history of traumatic/repeated spinal puncture or spinal deformity (↑ risk of spinal hematoma); Discontinuation ↑ risk of thromboses; Surgery; Renal impairment (dose ↓ may be required; Moderate hepatic impairment (↑ risk of bleeding); Concurrent use of strong dual inhibitors of CYP3A4 and P-gp systems (dose ↓ required); OB: Use during pregnancy only if potential benefit outweighs possible risks to mother and fetus; Pedi: Safety and effectiveness not established.

Adverse Reactions/Side Effects

Hemat: BLEEDING. **Misc:** hypersensitivity reactions including ANAPHYLAXIS.

Interactions

Drug-Drug: ↑ risk of bleeding with other **anticoagulants**, **aspirin**, **clopidogrel**, **ticagrelor**, **prasugrel**, **fibrinolytics**, **NSAIDs**, **SNRIs**, or **SSRIs**. Concurrent use of strong inhibitors of both the CYP3A4 and P-gp enzyme systems (including **itraconazole**, **ketoconazole**, and **ritonavir**) ↑ levels and bleeding risk; may need to ↓ apixaban dose or avoid concurrent use. Inducers of the CYP3A4 enzyme system and the P-gp system including **carbamazepine**, **phenytoin**, **rifampin** will ↓ levels and may ↑ risk of thromboses; avoid concomitant use.

Drug-Natural Products: Concurrent use **St. John's wort**, a strong dual inducer of the CYP3A4 and P-gp enzyme systems can ↓ levels and ↑ risk of thromboses and should be avoided.

Route/Dosage

Reduction in Risk of Stroke/Systemic Embolism in Nonvalvular Atrial Fibrillation

PO (Adults): 5 mg twice daily; *Any 2 of the following: age ≥80 yr, weight ≤60 kg, serum creatinine ≥1.5 mg/dL*—2.5 mg twice daily; *Concurrent use of strong inhibitors of both CYP3A4 and P-gp*—2.5 mg twice daily; if patient already taking 2.5 mg twice daily, avoid concomitant use.

Renal Impairment

PO (Adults): *HD*—5 mg twice daily; *HD and either age ≥80 yr or weight ≤60 kg*—2.5 mg twice daily.

Prevention of Deep Vein Thrombosis Following Knee or Hip Replacement Surgery

PO (Adults): 2.5 mg twice daily, initiated 12–24 hr post-operatively (when hemostasis is achieved) continued for 35 days after hip replacement or 12 days after knee replacement; *Concurrent use of strong inhibitors of both CYP3A4 and P-gp*—Avoid concomitant use.

Treatment of DVT or PE

PO (Adults): 10 mg twice daily for 7 days, then 5 mg twice daily; *Concurrent use of strong inhibitors of both CYP3A4 and P-gp*—2.5 mg twice daily.

Reduction in Risk of Recurrence of DVT or PE

PO (Adults): 2.5 mg twice daily after ≥6 mo of treatment of DVT or PE; *Concurrent use of strong inhibitors of both CYP3A4 and P-gp*—Avoid concomitant use.

Availability

Tablets: 2.5 mg, 5 mg.

NURSING IMPLICATIONS

Assessment

- Assess patient for symptoms of stroke, DVT, PE, bleeding, or peripheral vascular disease periodically during therapy.
- ***Toxicity and Overdose:*** Antidote is andexanet alfa. Effects persist for at least 24 hrs after last dose. Oral activated charcoal decreases apixaban absorption, lowering plasma concentrations. Other agents and hemodialysis do not have a significant effect.

Implementation

- When *converting from warfarin*, discontinue warfarin and start apixaban when INR is <2.0.
- When *converting from apixaban to warfarin*, apixaban affects INR, so INR measurements may not be useful for determining appropriate dose of warfarin. If continuous anticoagulation is necessary, discontinue apixaban and begin both a parenteral anticoagulant and warfarin at time of next dose of apixaban, discontinue parenteral anticoagulant when INR reaches acceptable range.
- When *switching between apixaban and anticoagulants other than warfarin*, discontinue one being taken and begin the other at the next scheduled dose.
- *For surgery*, discontinue apixaban at least 48 hrs before invasive or surgical procedures with a moderate or high risk of unacceptable or clinically significant bleeding or at least 24 hrs prior to procedures with a low risk of bleeding or where the bleeding would be non-critical in location and easily controlled.
- **PO:** Administer twice daily without regard to food.
- For patients who cannot swallow tablet, 5 mg and 2.5 mg tablets can be crushed, suspended in water, D5W, or apple juice, or mixed with applesauce and administered immediately orally. May also be suspended in 60 mL of water or D5W and promptly administered through a nasogastric tube.

Patient/Family Teaching

- Instruct patient to take apixaban as directed. Take missed doses as soon as remembered on the same day and resume twice daily administration; do not double doses. Do not discontinue without consulting health care professional; may increase risk of having a stroke, DVT, or PE. If temporarily discontinued, restart as soon as possible. Store apixaban at room temperature. Advise patient to read *Medication Guide* before beginning therapy and with each Rx refill in case of changes.
- Inform patient that they may bruise and bleed more easily or longer than usual. Advise patient to notify health care professional immediately if signs of bleeding (unusual bruising, pink or brown urine, red or black, tarry stools, coughing up blood, vomiting blood, pain or swelling in a joint, headache, dizziness, weakness, recurring nose bleeds, unusual bleeding from gums, heavier than normal menstrual bleeding, dyspepsia, abdominal pain, epigastric pain) occurs or if injury occurs, especially head injury.
- Caution patient to notify health care professional if skin rash or signs of severe allergic reaction (chest pain or tightness, swelling of face or tongue, trouble breathing or wheezing, feeling dizzy or faint) occur.
- Advise patient to notify health care professional of medication regimen prior to treatment or surgery.
- Instruct patient to notify health care professional of all Rx or OTC medications, vitamins, or herbal prod-

ucts being taken and consult health care professional before taking any new medications, especially St. John's wort. Risk of bleeding is increased with aspirin, NSAIDs, warfarin, heparin, SSRIs or SNRIs.

- Inform patient having had neuraxial anesthesia or spinal puncture to watch for signs and symptoms of spinal or epidural hematomas (numbness or weakness of legs, bowel or bladder dysfunction). Notify health care professional immediately if symptoms occur.
- Advise female patient to notify health care professional if pregnancy is planned or suspected or if breast feeding.

Evaluation/Desired Outcomes

- Reduction in the risk and treatment of stroke and systemic embolism.

aprepitant (oral)

(a-**prep**-i-tant)

Emend

aprepitant (injection)

(a-**prep**-i-tant)

Cinvanti

fosaprepitant (injection)

(fos-a-**prep**-i-tant)

Emend

Classification

Therapeutic: antiemetics

Pharmacologic: neurokinin antagonists

Indications

PO, IV: Prevention of: Acute and delayed nausea and vomiting associated with initial and repeat courses of highly emetogenic chemotherapy, Nausea and vomiting associated with initial and repeat courses of moderately emetogenic chemotherapy.

Action

Acts as a selective antagonist at substance P/neurokinin 1 (NK_1) receptors in the brain. **Therapeutic Effects:** Decreased nausea and vomiting associated with chemotherapy. Augments the antiemetic effects of dexamethasone and 5-HT_3 antagonists.

Pharmacokinetics

Absorption: 60–65% absorbed following oral administration. Following IV administration, fosaprepitant is rapidly converted to aprepitant, the active component. IV administration results in complete bioavailability.

Distribution: Crosses the blood brain barrier; remainder of distribution unknown.

Protein Binding: 95–99%.

Metabolism and Excretion: Mostly metabolized by the liver (CYP3A4 enzyme system); not renally excreted.

Half-life: *Aprepitant*—9–13 hr.

TIME/ACTION PROFILE (antiemetic effect)

ROUTE	ONSET	PEAK	DURATION
PO	1 hr	4 hr*	24 hr
IV	rapid	end of infusion*	24 hr

*Blood level.

Contraindications/Precautions

Contraindicated in: Hypersensitivity; Concurrent use with pimozide (risk of life-threatening adverse cardiovascular reactions); Lactation: May cause unwanted effects in nursing infants.

Use Cautiously in: Concurrent use with any CYP3A4 substrates; Concurrent use with strong or moderate CYP3A4 inhibitors; Concurrent use with strong CYP3A4 inducers; OB: Use only if clearly needed; Pedi: Children <6 mo (IV) and <6 mo (PO) (safety and effectiveness not established).

Adverse Reactions/Side Effects

CNS: headache. **CV:** dizziness, fatigue, weakness. **Derm:** STEVENS-JOHNSON SYNDROME. **GI:** diarrhea. **Misc:** HYPERSENSITIVITY REACTIONS (including anaphylaxis), hiccups, infusion reactions (fosaprepitant IV only).

Interactions

Drug-Drug: May ↑ levels of **CYP3A4 substrates**, including **docetaxel**, **paclitaxel**, **etoposide**, **irinotecan**, **ifosfamide**, **imatinib**, **vinorelbine**, **vinblastine**, **vincristine**, **midazolam**, **triazolam**, and **alprazolam**; concurrent use should be undertaken with caution. **Moderate or strong CYP3A4 inhibitors**, including **ketoconazole**, **itraconazole**, **nefazodone**, **clarithromycin**, **ritonavir**, **nelfinavir**, and **diltiazem**) may ↑ levels and risk of adverse reactions. **Strong CYP3A4 inducers**, including **rifampin**, **carbamazepine**, and **phenytoin** may ↓ levels and effects. ↑ levels and effects of **dexamethasone** (regimen reflects a 50% dose ↓); a similar effect occurs with **methylprednisolone** (↓ IV dose by 25%, ↓ PO dose by 50% when used concurrently). May ↓ the effects of **warfarin** (carefully monitor INR for 2 wk), **oral contraceptives** (use alternate method), and **phenytoin**.

Route/Dosage

Prevention of Nausea and Vomiting Associated with Highly Emetogenic Chemotherapy

PO (Adults): *Capsules or suspension*—125 mg given 1 hr prior to chemotherapy (Day 1) (with dexamethasone 12 mg PO given 30 min prior to chemotherapy and a 5-HT_3 antagonist given prior to chemotherapy), then 80 mg once daily for 2 days (Days 2 and 3) (with dexamethasone 8 mg once daily for 3 days [Days 2–4]).

IV (Adults): *Fosaprepitant*—150 mg given 30 min prior to chemotherapy on Day 1 (with dexamethasone 12 mg PO given 30 min prior to chemotherapy and a 5-HT_3 antagonist prior to chemotherapy). Continue dexamethasone on Days 2–4 (8 mg PO on Day 2, 8 mg twice daily on Days 3 and 4); *Aprepitant*—130 mg given 30 min prior to chemotherapy on Day 1 (with dexamethasone 12 mg PO given 30 min prior to chemotherapy and a 5-HT_3 antagonist prior to chemotherapy). Continue dexamethasone on Days 2–4 (8 mg PO on Day 2, 8 mg twice daily on Days 3 and 4).
PO (Children ≥12 yr): *Capsules*—125 mg given 1 hr prior to chemotherapy (Day 1) (with PO dexamethasone at 50% of recommended dose given 30 min prior to chemotherapy and a 5-HT_3 antagonist given prior to chemotherapy), then 80 mg once daily for 2 days (Days 2 and 3) (with PO dexamethasone at 50% of recommended dose once daily for 3 days [Days 2–4]).
PO (Children 6 mo–<12 yr and >6 kg): *Suspension*—3 mg/kg (max dose = 125 mg) given 1 hr prior to chemotherapy (Day 1) (with PO dexamethasone at 50% of recommended dose given 30 min prior to chemotherapy and a 5-HT_3 antagonist given prior to chemotherapy), then 2 mg/kg (max dose = 80 mg) once daily for 2 days (Days 2 and 3) (with PO dexamethasone at 50% of recommended dose once daily for 3 days [Days 2–4]).
IV (Children 12–17 yr and ≥6 kg): *Single-day chemotherapy regimen*—150 mg given 30 min prior to chemotherapy on Day 1 (with PO dexamethasone at 50% of recommended dose given 30 min prior to chemotherapy and a 5-HT_3 antagonist given prior to chemotherapy). Continue dexamethasone on Day 2; *Multi-day chemotherapy regimen*—115 mg given 30 min prior to chemotherapy on Day 1 (with PO dexamethasone at 50% of recommended dose given 30 min prior to chemotherapy and a 5-HT_3 antagonist given prior to chemotherapy), then 80 mg PO once daily (capsules) for 2 days (Days 2 and 3) (with PO dexamethasone at 50% of recommended dose once daily for 2 days [Days 2 and 3].
IV (Children 2–<12 yr and ≥6 kg): *Single-day chemotherapy regimen*—4 mg/kg (max dose = 150 mg) given 30 min prior to chemotherapy on Day 1 (with PO dexamethasone at 50% of recommended dose given 30 min prior to chemotherapy and a 5-HT_3 antagonist given prior to chemotherapy). Continue dexamethasone on Day 2; *Multi-day chemotherapy regimen*—3 mg/kg (max dose = 115 mg) given 30 min prior to chemotherapy on Day 1 (with PO dexamethasone at 50% of recommended dose given 30 min prior to chemotherapy and a 5-HT_3 antagonist given prior to chemotherapy), then 2 mg/kg (max dose = 80 mg) (oral suspension) PO once daily for 2 days (Days 2 and 3) (with PO dexamethasone at 50% of recommended dose once daily for 2 days [Days 2 and 3].
IV (Children 6 mo-<2 yr and ≥6 kg): *Single-day chemotherapy regimen*—5 mg/kg (max dose = 150 mg) given 30 min prior to chemotherapy on Day 1 (with PO dexamethasone at 50% of recommended dose given 30 min prior to chemotherapy and a 5-HT_3 antagonist given prior to chemotherapy). Continue dexamethasone on Day 2; *Multi-day chemotherapy regimen*—3 mg/kg (max dose = 115 mg) given 30 min prior to chemotherapy on Day 1 (with PO dexamethasone at 50% of recommended dose given 30 min prior to chemotherapy and a 5-HT_3 antagonist given prior to chemotherapy), then 2 mg/kg (max dose = 80 mg) (oral suspension) PO once daily for 2 days (Days 2 and 3) (with PO dexamethasone at 50% of recommended dose once daily for 2 days [Days 2 and 3].

Prevention of Nausea and Vomiting Associated with Moderately Emetogenic Chemotherapy

PO (Adults): *Capsules or suspension*—125 mg given 1 hr prior to chemotherapy (Day 1) (with dexamethasone 12 mg PO given 30 min prior to chemotherapy and a 5-HT_3 antagonist), then 80 mg once daily for 2 days (Days 2 and 3).
IV (Adults): *Fosaprepitant*—150 mg given 30 min prior to chemotherapy on Day 1 (with dexamethasone 12 mg PO given 30 min prior to chemotherapy and a 5-HT_3 antagonist prior to chemotherapy); *Aprepitant*—100 mg given 30 min prior to chemotherapy on Day 1 (with dexamethasone 12 mg PO given 30 min prior to chemotherapy and a 5-HT_3 antagonist prior to chemotherapy). Continue aprepitant 80 mg PO on Days 2 and 3.
PO (Children ≥12 yr): *Capsules*—125 mg given 1 hr prior to chemotherapy (Day 1) (with PO dexamethasone at 50% of recommended dose given 30 min prior to chemotherapy and a 5-HT_3 antagonist), then 80 mg once daily for 2 days (Days 2 and 3).
PO (Children 6 mo–<12 yr and >6 kg): *Suspension*—3 mg/kg (max dose = 125 mg) given 1 hr prior to chemotherapy (Day 1) (with PO dexamethasone at 50% of recommended dose given 30 min prior to chemotherapy and a 5-HT_3 antagonist given prior to chemotherapy), then 2 mg/kg (max dose = 80 mg) once daily for 2 days (Days 2 and 3) (with PO dexamethasone at 50% of recommended dose once daily for 3 days [Days 2–4]).
IV (Children 12–17 yr and ≥6 kg): *Single-day chemotherapy regimen*—150 mg given 30 min prior to chemotherapy on Day 1 (with PO dexamethasone at 50% of recommended dose given 30 min prior to chemotherapy and a 5-HT_3 antagonist given prior to chemotherapy). Continue dexamethasone on Day 2; *Multi-day chemotherapy regimen*—115 mg given 30 min prior to chemotherapy on Day 1 (with PO dexamethasone at 50% of recommended dose given 30 min

prior to chemotherapy and a 5-HT_3 antagonist given prior to chemotherapy), then 80 mg PO once daily (capsules) for 2 days (Days 2 and 3) (with PO dexamethasone at 50% of recommended dose once daily for 2 days [Days 2 and 3].

IV (Children 2–<12 yr and ≥6 kg): *Single–day chemotherapy regimen*—4 mg/kg (max dose = 150 mg) given 30 min prior to chemotherapy on Day 1 (with PO dexamethasone at 50% of recommended dose given 30 min prior to chemotherapy and a 5-HT_3 antagonist given prior to chemotherapy). Continue dexamethasone on Day 2; *Multi–day chemotherapy regimen*—3 mg/kg (max dose = 115 mg) given 30 min prior to chemotherapy on Day 1 (with PO dexamethasone at 50% of recommended dose given 30 min prior to chemotherapy and a 5-HT_3 antagonist given prior to chemotherapy), then 2 mg/kg (max dose = 80 mg) (oral suspension) PO once daily for 2 days (Days 2 and 3) (with PO dexamethasone at 50% of recommended dose once daily for 2 days [Days 2 and 3].

IV (Children 6 mo-<2 yr and ≥6 kg): *Single–day chemotherapy regimen*—5 mg/kg (max dose = 150 mg) given 30 min prior to chemotherapy on Day 1 (with PO dexamethasone at 50% of recommended dose given 30 min prior to chemotherapy and a 5-HT_3 antagonist given prior to chemotherapy). Continue dexamethasone on Day 2; *Multi–day chemotherapy regimen*—3 mg/kg (max dose = 115 mg) given 30 min prior to chemotherapy on Day 1 (with PO dexamethasone at 50% of recommended dose given 30 min prior to chemotherapy and a 5-HT_3 antagonist given prior to chemotherapy), then 2 mg/kg (max dose = 80 mg) (oral suspension) PO once daily for 2 days (Days 2 and 3) (with PO dexamethasone at 50% of recommended dose once daily for 2 days [Days 2 and 3].

Availability (generic available)

Capsules: 40 mg, 80 mg, 125 mg. **Emulsion for injection (aprepitant):** 7.2 mg/mL. **Lyophilized powder for injection (fosaprepitant) (requires reconstitution and dilution):** 150 mg/vial. **Powder for oral suspension (requires reconstitution):** 125 mg/pouch.

NURSING IMPLICATIONS

Assessment

- Assess nausea, vomiting, appetite, bowel sounds, and abdominal pain prior to and following administration.
- Monitor hydration, nutritional status, and intake and output. Patients with severe nausea and vomiting may require IV fluids in addition to antiemetics.
- Assess for rash periodically during therapy. May cause Stevens-Johnson syndrome. Discontinue therapy if severe rash or if accompanied with fever, general malaise, fatigue, muscle or joint aches, blisters, skin peeling, sores, oral lesions, conjunctivitis, hepatitis, and/or eosinophilia.
- Monitor for signs and symptoms of infusion site reaction (erythema, edema, pain, thrombophlebitis). Treat symptomatically. Avoid infusion into small veins or through a butterfly catheter.
- Monitor for signs and symptoms of hypersensitivity reactions (flushing, erythema, dyspnea, hypotension, syncope) periodically during therapy. If symptoms occur, discontinue therapy and treat symptoms; do not reinitiate therapy if symptoms occur with first use.
- ***Lab Test Considerations:*** Monitor clotting status closely during the 2 wk period, especially at 7–10 days, following aprepitant therapy in patients on chronic warfarin therapy.
- May cause mild, transient ↑ in alkaline phosphatase, AST, ALT, and BUN.
- May cause proteinuria, erythrocyturia, leukocyturia, hyperglycemia, hyponatremia, and ↑ leukocytes.
- May cause ↓ hemoglobin and WBC.

Implementation

- For chemotherapy, aprepitant/fosaprepitant is given as part of a regimen that includes a corticosteroid and a 5-HT_3 antagonist (see Route/Dosage).
- **PO:** Administer daily for 3 days. *Day 1*—administer 1 hr prior to chemotherapy. *Days 2 and 3*—administer once in the morning. May be administered without regard to food. Swallow capsules whole; do not open, crush, or chew.
- Oral suspension may be used for pediatric patients or those with difficulty swallowing. Refrigerate suspension; may be stored at room temperature for up to 3 hrs before use. To administer, take cap off, place dispenser in patient's mouth along inner cheek. Dispense slowly. Discard after 72 hrs.

IV Administration

aprepitant

- **IV Push:** ***Diluent:*** 0.9% NaCl or D5W. *For Highly-Emetogenic Chemotherapy:* Using 130 mL of diluent, withdraw 18 mg aprepitant from vial and add to bag for 148 mL. *For Moderately-Emetogenic Chemotherapy:* Using 100 mL of diluent, withdraw 14 mL aprepitant from vial and add to bag for 114 mL. Mix by gently inverting bag 4–5 times. Solution is an opaque, off-white emulsion. Do not administer solutions that are discolored or contain particulate matter. May be stored at room temperature for 6 hrs if mixed with 0.9% NaCl or 12 hrs if mixed with D5W or in refrigerator for up to 72 hrs. ***Rate:*** Inject over 2 min. Flush line with 0.9% NaCl before and after injection.
- **Solution Incompatibility:** Incompatible with solutions containing divalent cations (calcium, magnesium) including LR and Hartmann's solution.

fosaprepitant

- **Intermittent Infusion:** Inject 5 mL of 0.9% NaCl for Injection into vial. Swirl gently; avoid shaking or jetting saline into vial. ***Diluent:*** Prepare an infusion bag of 145 mL 0.9% NaCl. Withdraw entire volume from vial, and transfer to infusion bag for a total volume of 150 mL. ***Concentration:*** 1 mg/mL. Gently invert bag 2–3 times. Solution is stable for 24 hr at room temperature. Inspect solution for particulate matter. Do not administer solutions that are discolored or contain particulate matter. Solution is stable for 24 hr at room temperature. ***Rate:*** Infuse over 20–30 min, 30 min prior to chemotherapy.

- **Y-Site Compatibility:** dexamethasone, granisetron, methylprednisolone, ondansetron, palonosetron.
- **Solution Incompatibility:** Incompatible with solutions containing divalent cations (calcium, magnesium) including LR.

Patient/Family Teaching

- Instruct patient to take aprepitant as directed. Direct patient to read the *Patient Package Insert* before starting therapy and each time Rx renewed in case of changes.
- Instruct patient to notify health care professional if nausea and vomiting occur prior to administration.
- Advise patient to notify health care professional immediately if symptoms of hypersensitivity reaction (hives, rash, itching, redness of the face/skin, difficulty in breathing or swallowing) occur.
- Instruct patient to notify health care professional of all Rx or OTC medications, vitamins, or herbal products being taken and consult health care professional before taking any new medications.
- Advise patient and family to use general measures to decrease nausea (begin with sips of liquids and small, non-greasy meals; provide oral hygiene; remove noxious stimuli from environment).
- Rep: Caution patient that aprepitant and fosaprepitant may decrease effectiveness of oral contraceptives. Advise patient to use alternate nonhormonal methods of contraception during and for 1 mo following treatment. Advise patient to notify health care professional if pregnancy is planned or suspected or if breast feeding.

Evaluation/Desired Outcomes

- Decreased nausea and vomiting associated with chemotherapy.
- Augmentation of antiemetic effects of dexamethasone and 5-HT_3 antagonists.

HIGH ALERT

argatroban (ar-gat-tro-ban)

Classification
Therapeutic: anticoagulants
Pharmacologic: thrombin inhibitors

Indications

Prophylaxis or treatment of thrombosis in patients with heparin-induced thrombocytopenia. As an anticoagulant in patients with or at risk for heparin-induced thrombocytopenia who are undergoing percutaneous coronary intervention (PCI).

Action

Inhibits thrombin by binding to its receptor sites. Inhibition of thrombin prevents activation of factors V, VIII, and XII; the conversion of fibrinogen to fibrin; platelet adhesion and aggregation. **Therapeutic Effects:** Decreased thrombus formation and extension with decreased sequelae of thrombosis (emboli, postphlebitic syndromes).

Pharmacokinetics

Absorption: IV administration results in complete bioavailability.
Distribution: Unknown.
Metabolism and Excretion: Mostly metabolized by the liver; excreted primarily in feces via biliary excretion. 16% excreted unchanged in urine, 14% excreted unchanged in feces.
Half-life: 39–51 min (↑ in hepatic impairment).

TIME/ACTION PROFILE (anticoagulant effect)

ROUTE	ONSET	PEAK	DURATION
IV	immediate	1–3 hr	2–4 hr

Contraindications/Precautions

Contraindicated in: Major bleeding; Hypersensitivity.
Use Cautiously in: Hepatic impairment (↓ initial infusion rate recommended); OB: Use only if potential maternal benefit justifies potential fetal risk; Lactation: Use while breast feeding only if potential maternal benefit justifies potential risk to infant; Pedi: Safety and effectiveness not established.

Adverse Reactions/Side Effects

CV: hypotension. **GI:** diarrhea, nausea, vomiting. **Hemat:** BLEEDING. **Misc:** HYPERSENSITIVITY REACTIONS (including anaphylaxis), fever.

Interactions

Drug-Drug: Risk of bleeding may be ↑ by concurrent use of **antiplatelet agents, thrombolytic agents,** or **other anticoagulants**.
Drug-Natural Products: ↑ bleeding risk with **anise, arnica, chamomile, clove, feverfew, garlic, ginger, ginkgo, Panax ginseng,** and others.

Route/Dosage

IV (Adults): 2 mcg/kg/min as a continuous infusion; adjust infusion rate on the basis of activated partial thromboplastin time (aPTT). *Patients undergoing PCI*—350 mcg/kg bolus followed by infusion at 25 mcg/kg/min, activated clotting time (ACT) should be assessed 5–10 min later. If ACT is 300–450 sec, procedure may be started. If ACT <300 sec, give additional bolus of 150 mcg/kg and ↑ infusion rate to 30 mcg/kg/min. If ACT is >450 sec infusion rate should be ↓ to 15 mcg/kg/min and ACT rechecked after 5–10 min. If thrombotic complications occur or ACT drops to <300 sec, an additional bolus of 150 mcg/kg may be given and the infusion rate ↑ to 40 mcg/kg/min followed by ACT monitoring. If anticoagulation is required after surgery, lower infusion rates should be used.

Hepatic Impairment

IV (Adults): 0.5 mcg/kg/min as a continuous infusion; adjust infusion rate on the basis of aPTT.

Availability (generic available)

Premixed infusion: 50 mg/50 mL, 125 mg/125 mL, 250 mg/250 mL. **Solution for injection:** 100 mg/mL.

NURSING IMPLICATIONS

Assessment

- Monitor vital signs periodically during therapy. Unexplained decreases in BP may indicate hemorrhage. Assess patient for bleeding. Minimize arterial and venous punctures, IM injections, and use of urinary catheters, nasotracheal intubation, and nasogastric tubes. Avoid noncompressible sites for IV access. Monitor for blood in urine, lower back pain, pain or burning on urination. If bleeding cannot be controlled with pressure, decrease dose or discontinue argatroban immediately.
- Monitor for signs of anaphylaxis (rash, coughing, dyspnea) throughout therapy.
- ***Lab Test Considerations:*** Monitor aPTT prior to initiation of continuous infusion, 2 hrs after initiation of therapy, and periodically during therapy to confirm aPTT is within desired therapeutic range.
- For patients undergoing PCI, monitor ACT as described in Route and Dose section.
- Assess hemoglobin, hematocrit, and platelet count prior to, and periodically during, argatroban therapy. May cause ↓ hemoglobin and hematocrit. Unexplained ↓ hematocrit may indicate hemorrhage.
- Use of argatroban concurrently with multiple doses of warfarin will result in more prolonged prothrombin time and international normalized ratio (INR) (although there is not an ↑ in vitamin K-dependent factor X_a activity) than when warfarin is used alone. Monitor INR daily during concomitant therapy. Repeat INR 4–6 hr after argatroban is discontinued. If repeat value is below desired therapeutic value for warfarin alone, restart argatroban therapy and continue until desired therapeutic range for warfarin alone is reached. To obtain the INR for warfarin alone when dose of argatroban is >2 mcg/kg/min, temporarily reduce argatroban dose to 2 mcg/kg/min; INR for combined therapy may then be obtained 4–6 hr after argatroban dose was reduced.
- ***Toxicity and Overdose:*** There is no specific antidote for argatroban. If overdose occurs, discontinue argatroban. Anticoagulation parameters usually return to baseline within 2–4 hr after discontinuation.

Implementation

- Do not confuse argatroban with Aggrastat (tirofiban).
- All parenteral anticoagulants should be discontinued before argatroban therapy is initiated. Oral anticoagulation may be initiated with maintenance dose of warfarin; do not administer loading dose. Discontinue argatroban therapy when INR for combined therapy is >4.

IV Administration

- **IV:** Do not administer solutions that are cloudy or contain particulate matter. Discard unused portion.
- **IV Push:** ***Diluent:*** Bolus dose of 350 mcg/kg should be given prior to continuous infusion in patients undergoing PCI. For Diluent information, see Continuous Infusion section below. ***Rate:*** Administer bolus over 3–5 min.
- **Continuous Infusion:** ***Diluent:*** Dilute each 100 mg/mL in 0.9% NaCl, D5W, or LR. ***Concentration:*** 1 mg/mL. Mix by repeated inversion for 1 min. Diluted solution is slightly viscous, clear, and colorless to pale yellow; may show a slight haziness that disappears upon mixing; solution must be clear before use. Solution is stable at controlled room temperature and ambient light for 24 hrs, or for 96 hrs at controlled room temperature or refrigerated and protected from light; do not expose to direct sunlight. Pre-mixed solutions are clear and colorless. Store at room temperature, do not refrigerate or freeze. ***Rate:*** Based on patient's weight (See Route/Dosage section). Dose adjustment may be made 2 hr after starting infusion or changing dose until steady-state aPTT is 1.5–3 times the initial baseline value (not to exceed 100 sec).
- **Y-Site Compatibility:** acyclovir, alemtuzumab, alfentanil, allopurinol, amifostine, amikacin, aminocaproic acid, aminophylline, amiodarone, amphotericin B deoxycholate, amphotericin B lipid complex, amphotericin B liposome, ampicillin, ampicillin/sulbactam, anidulafungin, arsenic trioxide, atracurium, atropine, azithromycin, aztreonam, bivalirudin, bleomycin, bumetanide, buprenorphine, busulfan, butorphanol, calcium acetate, calcium chloride, calcium gluconate, carboplatin, carmustine, caspofungin, cefazolin, cefotaxime, cefotetan, cefoxitin, ceftazidime, ceftriaxone, cefuroxime, chloramphenicol, chlorpromazine, ciprofloxacin, cisatracurium, cisplatin, clindamycin, cyclophosphamide, cyclosporine, cytarabine, dacarbazine, dactinomycin, dantrolene, daptomycin, daunorubicin, dexamethasone, dexmedetomidine, dexrazoxane, digoxin, diltiazem, diphenhydramine, dobutamine, docetaxel, dopamine, doxorubicin, doxorubicin liposomal, doxycycline, droperidol, enalaprilat, ephedrine, epinephrine, epirubicin, eptifibatide, ertapenem, erythromycin, esmolol, etoposide, etoposide phos-

A

phate, famotidine, fenoldopam, fentanyl, fluconazole, fludarabine, fluorouracil, foscarnet, fosphenytoin, furosemide, ganciclovir, gemcitabine, gentamicin, glycopyrrolate, granisetron, haloperidol, heparin, hydralazine, hydrocortisone, hydromorphone, ibutilide, idarubicin, ifosfamide, imipenem/cilastatin, insulin, irinotecan, isoproterenol, ketorolac, labetalol, leucovorin, levofloxacin, lidocaine, linezolid, lorazepam, magnesium sulfate, mannitol, melphalan, meperidine, meropenem, mesna, methotrexate, methylprednisolone, metoclopramide, metoprolol, midazolam, milrinone, mitomycin, mitoxantrone, morphine, moxifloxacin, mycophenolate, nafcillin, nalbuphine, naloxone, nicardipine, nitroglycerin, nitroprusside, norepinephrine, octreotide, ondansetron, oxaliplatin, oxytocin, paclitaxel, palonosetron, pamidronate, pancuronium, pantoprazole, pentamidine, pentobarbital, phenobarbital, phentolamine, phenylephrine, phenytoin, piperacillin/tazobactam, potassium acetate, potassium chloride, potassium phosphates, procainamide, prochlorperazine, promethazine, propranolol, quinupristin/dalfopristin, ranitidine, remifentanil, rocuronium, sodium acetate, sodium bicarbonate, sodium phosphates, streptozocin, succinylcholine, sufentanil, tacrolimus, theophylline, thiopental, thiotepa, tigecycline, tirofiban, tobramycin, topotecan, trimethoprim/sulfamethoxazole, vancomycin, vasopressin, vecuronium, verapamil, vinblastine, vincristine, vinorelbine, voriconazole, zidovudine, zoledronic acid.

- **Y-Site Incompatibility:** cefepime, dantrolene, diazepam, phenytoin.

Patient/Family Teaching

- Inform patient of the purpose of argatroban.
- Advise patient to avoid other products known to affect bleeding.
- Instruct patient to notify health care professional immediately if any bleeding or signs and symptoms of allergic reaction is noted.

Evaluation/Desired Outcomes

- Decreased thrombus formation and extension.
- Decreased sequelae of thrombosis (emboli, postphlebitic syndromes).

BEERS

ARIPiprazole (a-ri-pip-ra-zole)

Abilify, Abilify Maintena, Aristada, Aristada Initio

Classification

Therapeutic: antipsychotics, mood stabilizers

Pharmacologic: serotonin-dopamine activity modulators (SDAM)

Indications

Schizophrenia (Abilify, Abilify Maintena, and Aristada). Acute treatment of manic and mixed episodes associated with bipolar I disorder (as monotherapy or with lithium or valproate) (Abilify only). Maintenance treatment of bipolar I disorder (as monotherapy) (Abilify Maintena). Adjunctive treatment of depression (Abilify only). Agitation associated with schizophrenia or bipolar disorder (Abilify only). Irritability associated with autistic disorder (Abilify only). Tourette's disorder (Abilify only).

Action

Psychotropic activity may be due to agonist activity at dopamine D_2 and serotonin 5-HT_{1A} receptors and antagonist activity at the 5-HT_{2A} receptor. Also has $alpha_1$ adrenergic blocking activity. **Therapeutic Effects:** Decreased manifestations of schizophrenia. Decreased mania in bipolar patients. Decreased symptoms of depression. Decreased agitation associated with schizophrenia or bipolar disorder. Decreased emotional and behavioral symptoms of irritability. Decreased incidence of tics.

Pharmacokinetics

Absorption: Well absorbed (87%) following oral administration; 100% following IM injection.

Distribution: Extensive extravascular distribution.

Protein Binding: >99%.

Metabolism and Excretion: Mostly metabolized by the liver (CYP3A4 and CYP2D6 isoenzymes); the CYP2D6 enzyme system exhibits genetic polymorphism; ~7% of population may be poor metabolizers (PMs) and may have significantly ↑ aripiprazole concentrations and an ↑ risk of adverse effects (↓ dose by 50% in PMs); one metabolite (dehydro-aripiprazole) has antipsychotic activity. 18% excreted unchanged in feces; <1% excreted unchanged in urine.

Half-life: *Aripiprazole*—75 hr; *dehydro-aripiprazole—94 hr*; ER injectable suspension: 30–46 days (Abilify Maintena); 29–35 days (Aristada).

TIME/ACTION PROFILE (antipsychotic effect)

ROUTE	ONSET	PEAK	DURATION
PO	unknown	2 wk	unknown
ER-IM	unknown	unknown	unknown

Contraindications/Precautions

Contraindicated in: Hypersensitivity; CYP2D6 PMs or concurrent use of strong CYP3A4 inhibitors, strong CYP2D6 inhibitors, or strong CYP3A4 inducers (Aristada Initio only); Lactation: Excreted in breast milk; discontinue drug or bottle feed.

Use Cautiously in: Known cardiovascular or cerebrovascular disease; Conditions which cause hypotension (dehydration, treatment with antihypertensives or diuretics); Diabetes (may ↑ risk of hyperglycemia); Seizure disorders; Patients at risk for aspiration pneumonia or falls; Concurrent ketoconazole or other potential CYP3A4 inhibitors (↓ aripiprazole dose by 50%); Concurrent quinidine, fluoxetine, paroxetine, or other potential CYP2D6 inhibitors; Concurrent carbamazepine or other potential CYP3A4 inducers; OB: Neonates at ↑ risk for extrapyramidal symptoms and withdrawal after delivery when exposed during the 3rd trimester; use only if maternal benefit outweighs risk to fetus; Pedi: May ↑ risk of suicide attempt/ideation especially during dose early treatment or dose adjustment; risk may be greater in children, adolescents, and young adults taking antidepressants (safety in children/adolescents not established); Geri: ↑ risk of mortality in elderly patients treated for psychosis related to dementia/neurocognitive disorders.

Adverse Reactions/Side Effects

CNS: SUICIDAL THOUGHTS, drowsiness, extrapyramidal reactions, akathisia, confusion, depression, fatigue, hostility, impaired cognitive function, impulse control disorders (eating/binge eating, gambling, sexual, shopping), insomnia, lightheadedness, manic reactions, nervousness, restlessness, sedation, seizures, tardive dyskinesia. **CV:** bradycardia, chest pain, edema, hypertension, orthostatic hypotension, tachycardia. **Derm:** dry skin, ecchymosis, skin ulcer, sweating. **EENT:** blurred vision, conjunctivitis, ear pain. **GI:** constipation, anorexia, ↑ salivation, nausea, vomiting, weight gain, weight loss. **GU:** urinary incontinence. **Hemat:** AGRANULOCYTOSIS, anemia, leukopenia, neutropenia. **Metab:** dyslipidemia, hyperglycemia. **MS:** muscle cramps, neck pain. **Neuro:** tremor, abnormal gait. **Resp:** dyspnea. **Misc:** HYPERSENSITIVITY REACTIONS, NEUROLEPTIC MALIGNANT SYNDROME, ↓ heat regulation, injection site reactions.

Interactions

Drug-Drug: **Ketoconazole**, **clarithromycin**, or other **strong CYP3A4 inhibitors** ↓ metabolism and ↑ effects (↓ aripiprazole dose by 50%). **Quinidine**, **fluoxetine**, **paroxetine**, or **other strong CYP2D6 inhibitors** ↓ metabolism and ↑ effects (↓ aripiprazole dose by at least 50%). Concurrent **carbamazepine** or **other potential CYP3A4 inducers** ↑ metabolism and ↓ effects (double aripiprazole dose).

Route/Dosage

If used concurrently with combination of strong, moderate, or weak CYP3A4 and CYP2D6 inhibitors, ↓ oral aripiprazole dose by 75%. Aripiprazole dose should be ↓ by 75% in CYP2D6 PMs who are concomitantly receiving a strong CYP3A4 inhibitor. Do NOT substitute Aristada Initio for Aristada.

Schizophrenia

PO (Adults): 10 or 15 mg once daily; doses up to 30 mg/day have been used; increments in dosing should not be made before 2 wk at a given dose.

PO (Children 13–17 yr): 2 mg once daily; ↑ to 5 mg once daily after 2 days, and then to target dose of 10 mg once daily after another 2 days; may further ↑ dose in 5-mg increments if needed (max: 30 mg/day).

IM (Adults): *Abilify Maintena*—400 mg every mo; after 1st injection, continue treatment with oral aripiprazole (10–20 mg/day) for 14 days; if no adverse reactions to 400 mg/mo dose, may ↓ dose to 300 mg every mo. *CYP2D6 PMs*—↓ dose to 300 mg monthly; *CYP2D6 PMs concomitantly receiving strong CYP3A4 inhibitor*—↓ dose to 200 mg monthly; *Concomitant therapy with strong CYP2D6 or CYP3A4 inhibitor*—↓ dose to 300 mg monthly (if originally receiving 400 mg monthly) or 200 mg monthly (if originally receiving 300 mg monthly); *Concomitant therapy with strong CYP2D6 and CYP3A4 inhibitor*—↓ dose to 200 mg monthly (if originally receiving 400 mg monthly) or 160 mg monthly (if originally receiving 300 mg monthly); *Concomitant therapy with CYP3A4 inducer*—Avoid use.

IM (Adults): *Aristada with Aristada Initio*—administer 675–mg injection of Aristada Initio with first injection of Aristada (dose is based on total daily dose of oral aripiprazole; if patient receiving 10 mg/day of oral aripiprazole, administer 441 mg every mo; if patient receiving 15 mg/day of oral aripiprazole, administer 662 mg every mo, 882 mg every 6 wk, or 1064 mg every 2 mo; if patient receiving ≥20 mg/day of oral aripiprazole, administer 882 mg every mo) (initial Aristada dose can be given on same day as or within 10 days of Aristada Initio) AND one dose of oral aripiprazole 30 mg; *Aristada without Aristada Initio*—Dose is based on total daily dose of oral aripiprazole; if patient receiving 10 mg/day of oral aripiprazole, administer 441 mg every mo; if patient receiving 15 mg/day of oral aripiprazole, administer 662 mg every mo, 882 mg every 6 wk, or 1064 mg every 2 mo; if patient receiving ≥20 mg/day of oral aripiprazole, administer 882 mg every mo; after 1st injection; continue treatment with oral aripiprazole for 21 days; *Concomitant therapy with strong CYP2D6 or CYP3A4 inhibitor for >2 wk*—↓ dose of Aristada to 441 mg monthly (if originally receiving 662 mg monthly) or 662 mg monthly (if originally receiving 882 mg monthly); no dose adjustment necessary if originally receiving 441 mg monthly; avoid use of Aristada Initio; *CYP2D6 PMs concomitantly receiving strong CYP3A4 inhibitor for >2 wk*—↓ dose of Aristada to 441 mg monthly (if originally receiving 662 mg or 882 mg monthly); no dose adjustment necessary if originally receiving 441 mg monthly; avoid use of Aristada Initio; *Concomitant therapy with strong CYP2D6 and CYP3A4 inhibitor*—avoid use of Aristada in patients requiring 662 mg or 882 mg monthly dose; no dose adjustment of Aristada necessary if originally receiving 441 mg monthly; avoid use of Aristada Initio; *Concomitant therapy with CYP3A4 inducer*—↑ dose of Aristada to 662 mg monthly (if originally receiving 441 mg monthly); no dose adjustment if Aristada necessary if originally receiving 662 mg or 882 mg monthly; avoid use of Aristada Initio.

Acute Manic or Mixed Episodes Associated with Bipolar I Disorder

PO (Adults): 15 mg once daily as monotherapy or 10–15 mg once daily with lithium or valproate; target dose is 15 mg once daily; may ↑ to 30 mg once daily, if needed.

PO (Children 10–17 yr): 2 mg once daily; ↑ to 5 mg once daily after 2 days, and then to target dose of 10 mg once daily after another 2 days; may further ↑ dose in 5-mg increments if needed (max: 30 mg/day).

Maintenance Treatment of Bipolar I Disorder

IM (Adults): 400 mg every mo; after 1st injection, continue treatment with oral aripiprazole (10–20 mg/day) for 14 days; if no adverse reactions to 400 mg/mo dose, may ↓ dose to 300 mg every mo. *CYP2D6 PMs*—↓ dose to 300 mg monthly; *CYP2D6 PMs concomitantly receiving strong CYP3A4 inhibitor*—↓ dose to 200 mg monthly; *Concomitant therapy with strong CYP2D6 or CYP3A4 inhibitor*—↓ dose to 300 mg monthly (if originally receiving 400 mg monthly) or 200 mg monthly (if originally receiving 300 mg monthly); *Concomitant therapy with strong CYP2D6 and CYP3A4 inhibitor*—↓ dose to 200 mg monthly (if originally receiving 400 mg monthly) or 160 mg monthly (if originally receiving 300 mg monthly); *Concomitant therapy with CYP3A4 inducer*—Avoid use.

Depression

PO (Adults): 2–5 mg once daily, may titrate upward at 1-wk intervals to 5–10 mg once daily (max: 15 mg/day).

Irritability Associated with Autistic Disorder

PO (Children 6–17 yr): 2 mg once daily; ↑ to 5 mg once daily after at least 1 wk; may further ↑ dose in 5-mg increments if needed at ≥1-wk intervals (max: 15 mg/day).

Tourette's Disorder

PO (Children 6–18 yr and ≥50 kg): 2 mg once daily; ↑ to target dose of 5 mg once daily after 2 days; may further ↑ dose if needed at ≥1-wk intervals (max: 10 mg/day).

PO (Children 6–18 yr and <50 kg): 2 mg once daily; ↑ to 5 mg once daily after 2 days, and then to target dose of 10 mg once daily after 5 days; may further ↑ dose in 5-mg increments if needed at ≥1-wk intervals (max: 20 mg/day).

Availability (generic available)

Tablets: 2 mg, 5 mg, 10 mg, 15 mg, 20 mg, 30 mg. **Cost:** 2 mg $2,208.52/90, 5 mg $2,208.52/90, 10 mg $2,208.52/90, 15 mg $2,208.52/90, 20 mg $3,107.38/90, 30 mg $3,107.38/90. **Orally disintegrating tablets (vanilla flavor):** 10 mg, 15 mg. **Cost:** All strengths $955.82/30. **Extended-release injectable suspension (Abilify Maintena) :** 300 mg/vial or prefilled syringe, 400 mg/vial or prefilled syringe. **Extended-release injectable suspension (Aristada) (in prefilled syringes):** 441 mg/1.6 mL, 662 mg/2.4 mL, 882 mg/3.2 mL, 1064 mg/3.9 mL. **Extended-release injectable suspension (Aristada Initio) (in prefilled syringes):** 675 mg/2.4 mL. **Oral solution (orange cream):** 1 mg/mL.

NURSING IMPLICATIONS

Assessment

- Assess mental status (orientation, mood, behavior) before and periodically during therapy. Assess for suicidal tendencies, especially during early therapy for depression. Restrict amount of drug available to patient. Risk may be increased in children, adolescents, and adults ≤24 yrs.
- Assess weight and BMI initially and throughout therapy. Compare weight of children and adolescents with that expected during normal growth.
- Monitor BP (sitting, standing, lying), pulse, and respiratory rate before and periodically during therapy.
- Observe patient carefully when administering medication to ensure that medication is actually taken and not hoarded or cheeked.
- Monitor patient for onset of akathisia (restlessness or desire to keep moving) and extrapyramidal side effects (*parkinsonian*—difficulty speaking or swallowing, loss of balance control, pill rolling of hands, masklike face, shuffling gait, rigidity, tremors; and *dystonic*—muscle spasms, twisting motions, twitching, inability to move eyes, weakness of arms or legs) periodically throughout therapy. Report these symptoms.
- Monitor for tardive dyskinesia (uncontrolled rhythmic movement of mouth, face, and extremities; lip smacking or puckering; puffing of cheeks; uncontrolled chewing; rapid or worm-like movements of tongue). Notify health care professional immediately if these symptoms occur, as these side effects may be irreversible.
- Monitor for development of neuroleptic malignant syndrome (fever, muscle rigidity, altered mental status, respiratory distress, tachycardia, seizures, diaphoresis, hypertension or hypotension, pallor, tiredness, loss of bladder control). Notify health care professional immediately if these symptoms occur.
- Assess for falls risk. Drowsiness, orthostatic hypotension, and motor and sensory instability increase risk. Institute prevention if indicated.
- ***Lab Test Considerations:*** May cause ↑ creatinine phosphokinase.

- Monitor CBC frequently during initial mo of therapy in patients with pre-existing or history of low WBC. May cause leukopenia, neutropenia, or agranulocytosis. Discontinue therapy if this occurs.
- Monitor blood glucose and cholesterol levels prior to starting and periodically during therapy.

Implementation

- Do not confuse aripiprazole with rabeprazole.
- *Aristada Initio* is only used as a one-time dose to initiate *Aristada* therapy or if doses of *Aristada* are missed. Administer missed doses as soon as possible, may supplement next *Aristada* injection with *Aristada Initio.* **If last Aristada injection 441 mg** *and time since last injection ≤6 wk,* do not supplement; *if >6 wk and ≤ 7 wk since last dose,* supplement with single dose of *Aristada Initio*; *if >7 wk since last dose,* re-initiate with a single dose of *Aristada Initio* and a single dose of oral aripiprazole 30 mg. **If last Aristada injection 662 mg or 882 mg** *and time since last injection ≤8 wk,* do not supplement; *if >8 wk and ≤12 wk since last dose,* supplement with single dose of *Aristada Initio*; *if ≥12 wk since last dose,* re-initiate with a single dose of *Aristada Initio* and a single dose of oral aripiprazole 30 mg. **If last Aristada injection 1064 mg** *and time since last injection ≤10 wk,* do not supplement; *if >8 wk and ≤12 wk since last dose,* supplement with single dose of *Aristada Initio*; *if ≥12 wk since last dose,* re-initiate with a single dose of *Aristada Initio* and a single dose of oral aripiprazole 30 mg.
- **PO:** Administer once daily without regard to meals.
- *Orally disintegrating tablets:* Do not open blister until ready to administer. For single tablet removal, open package and peel back foil on blister to expose tablet. Do not push tablet through foil; may damage tablet. Immediately upon opening blister, using dry hands, remove tablet and place entire orally disintegrating tablet on tongue. Tablet disintegration occurs rapidly in saliva. Take tablet without liquid; but if needed, it can be taken with liquid. Do not attempt to split tablet.
- **Extended-Release IM:** *Abilify Maintena* is available in vials or dual chamber prefilled syringes. *For vials,* reconstitute 300 mg dose with 1.5 mL and 400 mg dose with 1.9 mL of sterile water for injection; discard extra sterile water. Withdraw air to equalize pressure in vial. Shake vial vigorously for 30 sec until suspension is uniform; suspension is opaque and milky white. If injection is not given immediately, shake vial vigorously to resuspend prior to injection. Do not store suspension in syringe. Determine volume needed for dose: from 400 mg vial: 400 mg = 2 mL, 300 mg = 1.5 mL, 200 mg = 1.0, and 160 mg = 0.8 mL. From 300 mg vial: 300 mg = 1.5 mL, 200 mg = 1 mL, and 160 mg = 0.8 mL. *For prefilled syringes,* push plunger rod slightly to engage threads. Rotate plunger rod until rod stops rotating to release diluent; middle stopper will be at indicator line. Vertically shake syringe vigorously for 20 sec until drug is uniformly milky-white. *For deltoid site,* use 23 gauge needle, 1 inch in length for non-obese patients and 22 gauge 1.5 inch for obese patients. *For gluteal site,* use 22 gauge needle, 1.5 inches in length for non-obese patients and 22 gauge, 2 inch for obese patients. Inject deep into deltoid or gluteal site; do not massage. Continue oral dosing of aripiprazole for 2 wk after first dose of *Abilify Maintena*.
- If 2nd or 3rd doses of *Abilify Maintena* are missed and >4 wk and <5 wk since last injection, administer injection as soon as possible. If >5 wk since last injection, restart concomitant oral aripiprazole for 14 days with next administered injection. If fourth or subsequent doses are missed and >4 wk and <6 wk since last injection, administer injection as soon as possible. If >6 wk since last injection, restart concomitant oral aripiprazole for 14 days with next administered injection.
- *Aristada* comes in a kit with several needle sizes. Tap syringe at least 10 times to dislodge settled material and shake syringe vigorously for at least 30 sec to ensure suspension is uniform. Shake again if syringe not used within 15 min. Select needle and injection site. Deltoid may be used for 441 mg dose only. May use gluteal site for all doses. Remove air from syringe. Inject entire contents rapidly and continuously over <10 sec.

Patient/Family Teaching

- Advise patient to take medication as directed and not to skip doses or double up on missed doses. Take missed doses as soon as remembered unless almost time for the next dose. Emphasize importance of maintaining regular scheduled injections when taking *Abilify Maintena or Aristada.*
- Inform patient of possibility of extrapyramidal symptoms and tardive dyskinesia. Instruct patient to report these symptoms immediately.
- Advise patient to make position changes slowly to minimize orthostatic hypotension.
- Medication may cause drowsiness and lightheadedness. Caution patient to avoid driving or other activities requiring alertness until response to medication is known.
- Advise patient and family to notify health care professional if thoughts about suicide or dying, attempts to commit suicide; new or worse depression; new or worse anxiety; feeling very agitated or restless; panic attacks; trouble sleeping; new or worse irritability; acting aggressive; being angry or violent; acting on dangerous impulses; an extreme increase in activity and talking; other unusual changes in behavior or mood or if signs and symptoms of high blood sugar (feel very thirsty, urinating more than usual, feel very hungry, feel weak or tired, nausea, confusion, breath smells fruity) occur.

- Inform patient that aripiprazole may cause weight gain. Advise patient to monitor weight periodically. Notify health care professional of significant weight gain.
- Instruct patient to notify health care professional of all Rx or OTC medications, vitamins, or herbal products being taken and to consult health care professional before taking any new medications. Caution patient to avoid taking alcohol or other CNS depressants concurrently with this medication.
- Advise patient that extremes in temperature should be avoided, because this drug impairs body temperature regulation.
- Advise patient to notify health care professional if new or increased eating/binge eating, gambling, sexual, shopping, or other impulse control disorders occur.
- Advise patient to notify health care professional of medication regimen prior to treatment or surgery.
- Advise female patients to notify health care professional if pregnancy is planned or suspected and to avoid breast feeding during therapy. Encourage pregnant patients to enroll in registry by contacting National Pregnancy Registry for Atypical Antipsychotics at 1-866-961-2388 or visit http://womensmentalhealth.org/clinical-and-research-programs/pregnancyregistry/.
- Emphasize the importance of routine follow-up exams and continued participation in psychotherapy as indicated.

Evaluation/Desired Outcomes

- Decrease in excitable, paranoid, or withdrawn behavior.
- Decrease incidence of mood swings in patients with bipolar disorders.
- Increased sense of well-being in patients with depression.
- Decreased agitation associated with schizophrenia or bipolar disorder.
- Decreased emotional and behavioral symptoms of irritability.
- Decrease in tics.

BEERS

asenapine (a-sen-a-peen)

Saphris

Classification

Therapeutic: antipsychotics, mood stabilizers

Pharmacologic: dibenzo-oxepino pyrroles

Indications

Schizophrenia. Acute treatment of manic/mixed episodes associated with bipolar I disorder (as monotherapy or with lithium or valproate). Maintenance treatment of manic/mixed episodes associated with bipolar I disorder (as monotherapy).

Action

May act through combined antagonism of dopaminergic (D_2) and 5-HT_{2A} receptors. **Therapeutic Effects:** Decreased symptoms of acute schizophrenia and mania/mixed episodes of bipolar I disorder.

Pharmacokinetics

Absorption: 35% absorbed following SL administration.

Distribution: Rapidly distributed throughout the body. Vd is approximately 20–25 L/kg; 95% bound to plasma proteins.

Metabolism and Excretion: Highly metabolized; primarily by CYP1A2 and UGTA14 enzyme systems 50% excreted in urine, 40% in feces, primarily as metabolites.

Half-life: 24 hr.

TIME/ACTION PROFILE (antipsychotic effect)

ROUTE	ONSET	PEAK	DURATION
SL	unknown	0.5–1.5 hr†	12–24 hr

†Blood levels.

Contraindications/Precautions

Contraindicated in: Hypersensitivity; Dementia-related psychoses; Severe hepatic impairment; Lactation: Avoid use.

Use Cautiously in: History of cardiac arrhythmias, congenital QT prolongation, electrolyte abnormalities (especially hypomagnesemia or hypokalemia; correct prior to use) or concurrent use of medications known to prolong the QTc interval (may ↑ risk of life-threatening arrhythmias); History of seizures or conditions/medications known to ↓ seizure threshold; History of leukopenia/neutropenia; Strenuous exercise, exposure to extreme heat, concurrent medications with anticholinergic activity, or risk of dehydration; History of suicide attempt; Dehydration, hypovolemia, concurrent use of antihypertensive medications, history of myocardial infarction/ischemic heart disease/HF/conduction abnormalities/cerebrovascular disease (↑ risk of hypotension); Patients at risk for falls; Geri: ↑ risk of adverse reactions; consider age-related ↓ in hepatic function, cardiovascular status, and concurrent medications; ↑ risk of mortality and stroke/TIA in elderly patients treated for dementia-related psychosis; OB: Neonates at ↑ risk for extrapyramidal symptoms and withdrawal after delivery when exposed during the 3rd trimester; use only if benefit outweighs risk to fetus; Pedi: Children <10 yr (safety and effectiveness not established).

Adverse Reactions/Side Effects

CNS: NEUROLEPTIC MALIGNANT SYNDROME, SEIZURES, SUICIDAL THOUGHTS, akathisia, dizziness, drowsiness, extrapyramidal symptoms, anxiety, fatigue, syncope, tardive dyskinesia. **CV:** QT INTERVAL PROLONGATION, bradycardia, orthostatic hypotension, tachycardia. **GI:** oral hypoesthesia, dry mouth, dyspepsia, dysphagia, oral blisters, oral inflammation, oral peeling/sloughing, oral ulcers. **Endo:** dyslipidemia, hyperglycemia, hyperprolactinemia. **Hemat:** AGRANULOCYTOSIS, leukopenia, neutropenia. **Metab:** weight gain, ↑ appetite. **Misc:** HYPERSENSITIVITY REACTIONS (including anaphylaxis, angioedema, hypotension, tachycardia, swollen tongue, dyspnea, wheezing, and rash).

Interactions

Drug-Drug: Concurrent use of **QTc interval prolonging drugs** including **Class 1A antiarrhythmics** such as **quinidine** and **procainamide** or **Class 3 antiarrhythmics** including **amiodarone** and **sotalol** or other **antipsychotics** including **ziprasidone**, **chlorpromazine** or **thioridazine** or certain **antibiotics** such as **moxifloxacin**; may ↑ risk of torsade de pointes and/or sudden death; avoid concurrent use. **Fluvoxamine**, a strong inhibitor of CYP1A2, ↑ levels and risk of toxicity; use cautiously. Similar effects may occur with **paroxetine**, a CYP2D6 substrate and inhibitor. Drugs having similar properties (**substrates/inhibitors of CYP2D6**) should also be used cautiously with asenapine. ↑ risk of CNS depression with other **CNS depressants** including **antihistamines**, some **antidepressants**, **sedative/hypnotics**, and **alcohol**.

Route/Dosage

Schizophrenia

SL (Adults): 5 mg twice daily; may ↑ to 10 mg twice daily after 1 wk.

Acute Manic/Mixed Episodes Associated with Bipolar I Disorder

SL (Adults): *Monotherapy*—10 mg twice daily; may ↓ to 5 mg twice daily if tolerated poorly; continue on the dose that caused stabilization as maintenance therapy; *Adjunctive therapy with lithium or valproate*—5 mg twice daily; may ↑ to 10 mg twice daily.
SL (Children 10–17 yr): *Monotherapy*—2.5 mg twice daily; may ↑ to 5 mg twice daily after 3 days; may ↑ to 10 mg twice daily after another 3 days.

Availability

Sublingual tablets (black cherry flavor): 2.5 mg, 5 mg, 10 mg.

NURSING IMPLICATIONS

Assessment

- Assess mental status (orientation, mood, behavior) before and periodically during therapy. Assess for suicidal tendencies. Restrict amount of drug available to patient. Risk may be increased in children, adolescents, and adults ≤24 yrs.
- Assess weight and BMI initially and throughout therapy.
- Monitor BP (sitting, standing, lying) and pulse before and periodically during therapy.
- Observe patient carefully when administering medication to ensure that medication is actually taken and not hoarded or cheeked.
- Monitor patient for onset of akathisia (restlessness or desire to keep moving) and extrapyramidal side effects (*parkinsonian*—difficulty speaking or swallowing, loss of balance control, pill rolling of hands, masklike face, shuffling gait, rigidity, tremors; and *dystonic*—muscle spasms, twisting motions, twitching, inability to move eyes, weakness of arms or legs) periodically throughout therapy. Report these symptoms.
- Monitor for tardive dyskinesia (uncontrolled rhythmic movement of mouth, face, and extremities; lip smacking or puckering; puffing of cheeks; uncontrolled chewing; rapid or worm-like movements of tongue). Notify health care professional immediately if these symptoms occur, as these side effects may be irreversible.
- Monitor for development of neuroleptic malignant syndrome (fever, muscle rigidity, altered mental status, respiratory distress, tachycardia, seizures, diaphoresis, hypertension or hypotension, pallor, tiredness, loss of bladder control). Discontinue asenapine and notify health care professional immediately if these symptoms occur.
- Monitor for symptoms related to hyperprolactinemia (menstrual abnormalities, galactorrhea, sexual dysfunction).
- Assess for falls risk. Drowsiness, orthostatic hypotension, and motor and sensory instability increase risk. Institute prevention if indicated.
- Assess patient for signs and symptoms of hypersensitivity reactions, including anaphylaxis, angioedema, hypotension, tachycardia, swollen tongue, dyspnea, wheezing, and rash.
- ***Lab Test Considerations:*** Obtain fasting blood glucose, lipid profile, and cholesterol levels initially and periodically during therapy.
- Monitor CBC frequently during initial mo of therapy in patients with pre-existing or history of low WBC. May cause leukopenia, neutropenia, or agranulocytosis. Monitor patients with neutropenia for fever or other symptoms of infection and treat promptly. Discontinue therapy if ANC <1000/mm^3 occurs.
- May cause transient ↑ in serum ALT.

Implementation

- **SL:** Open packet immediately before use by firmly pressing thumb button and pulling out tablet pack. Do not push tablet through or cut or tear tablet pack. Peel back colored tab and gently remove tablet. Place tablet under tongue and allow to dissolve completely; dissolves in saliva within sec. Do not split, crush, chew, or swallow tablets. Avoid eating or drinking for 10 min after administration. Slide tablet pack back into case until it clicks.

Patient/Family Teaching

- Advise patient to take medication as directed and not to skip doses or double up on missed doses. Take missed doses as soon as remembered unless almost time for the next dose.
- Inform patient of possibility of extrapyramidal symptoms and tardive dyskinesia. Instruct patient to report these symptoms immediately.
- Advise patient to make position changes slowly to minimize orthostatic hypotension. Protect from falls.
- Medication may cause drowsiness and dizziness. Caution patient to avoid driving or other activities requiring alertness until response to medication is known.
- Advise patient and family to notify health care professional if thoughts about suicide or dying, attempts to commit suicide; new or worse depression; new or worse anxiety; feeling very agitated or restless; panic attacks; trouble sleeping; new or worse irritability; acting aggressive; being angry or violent; acting on dangerous impulses; an extreme increase in activity and talking; other unusual changes in behavior or mood or if signs and symptoms of hypersensitivity reactions (difficulty breathing, itching, swelling of the face, tongue or throat, feeling lightheaded) occur.
- Inform patient that oral ulcers, blisters, peeling/sloughing, and inflammation may occur at application site. Advise patient to notify health care professional if these occur, may require discontinuation. Inform patient that numbness or tingling of mouth or throat may occur shortly after administration of asenapine; usually resolves within 1 hr.
- Instruct patient to notify health care professional of all Rx or OTC medications, vitamins, or herbal products being taken, to avoid alcohol, and to consult health care professional before taking any new medications and to avoid taking alcohol or other CNS depressants concurrently with this medication.
- Advise patient that extremes in temperature should be avoided, because this drug impairs body temperature regulation.
- Advise patient to notify health care professional of medication regimen prior to treatment or surgery.
- Advise female patients to notify health care professional if pregnancy is planned or suspected and to avoid breast feeding during therapy. Encourage pregnant patients to enroll in registry by contacting National Pregnancy Registry for Atypical Antipsychotics at 1-866-961-2388 or visit http://womensmentalhealth.org/clinical-and-research-programs/pregnancyregistry/.
- Emphasize the importance of routine follow-up exams and continued participation in psychotherapy as indicated.

Evaluation/Desired Outcomes

- Decrease in excitable, paranoic, or withdrawn behavior.
- Decrease incidence of mood swings in patients with bipolar disorders.
- Decreased agitation associated with schizophrenia or bipolar disorder.

BEERS

aspirin (as-pir-in)

Acuprin, ✱Asaphen, Aspergum, Aspir-Low, Aspirtab, Bayer Aspirin, Bayer Timed-Release Arthritic Pain Formula, Easprin, Ecotrin, 8-Hour Bayer Timed-Release, Empirin, ✱Entrophen, Halfprin, Healthprin, ✱Lowprin, Norwich Aspirin, ✱Novasen, ✱Rivasa, Sloprin, St. Joseph Adult Chewable Aspirin, Therapy Bayer, Vazalore, ZORprin

Classification

Therapeutic: antipyretics, nonopioid analgesics

Pharmacologic: salicylates

Indications

Inflammatory disorders including: Rheumatoid arthritis, Osteoarthritis. Mild to moderate pain. Fever. Prophylaxis of transient ischemic attacks and MI. **Unlabeled Use:** Adjunctive treatment of Kawasaki disease.

Action

Produce analgesia and reduce inflammation and fever by inhibiting the production of prostaglandins. Decreases platelet aggregation. **Therapeutic Effects:** Analgesia. Reduction of inflammation. Reduction of fever. Decreased incidence of transient ischemic attacks and MI.

Pharmacokinetics

Absorption: Well absorbed from the upper small intestine; absorption from enteric-coated preparations may be unreliable; rectal absorption is slow and variable.

Distribution: Rapidly and widely distributed; crosses the placenta and enters breast milk.

Metabolism and Excretion: Extensively metabolized by the liver; inactive metabolites excreted by the kidneys. Amount excreted unchanged by the kidneys depends on urine pH; as pH increases, amount excreted unchanged increases from 2–3% up to 80%.

Half-life: 2–3 hr for low doses; up to 15–30 hr with larger doses because of saturation of liver metabolism.

TIME/ACTION PROFILE (analgesia/fever reduction)

ROUTE	ONSET	PEAK	DURATION
PO	5–30 min	1–3 hr	3–6 hr

Contraindications/Precautions

Contraindicated in: Hypersensitivity to aspirin or other salicylates; Cross-sensitivity with other NSAIDs may exist (less with nonaspirin salicylates); Bleeding disorders or thrombocytopenia; Pedi: May increase risk of Reye's syndrome in children or adolescents with viral infections.

Use Cautiously in: History of GI bleeding or ulcer disease; Chronic alcohol use/abuse; Severe hepatic or renal disease; OB: Salicylates may have adverse effects on fetus and mother and should be avoided during pregnancy, especially during the 3rd trimester; Lactation: Safety not established; Geri: ↑ risk of adverse reactions especially GI bleeding; more sensitive to toxic levels.

Adverse Reactions/Side Effects

Derm: rash, urticaria. **EENT:** tinnitus. **GI:** GI BLEEDING, dyspepsia, epigastric distress, nausea, abdominal pain, anorexia, hepatotoxicity, vomiting. **Hemat:** anemia, hemolysis. **Misc:** HYPERSENSITIVITY REACTIONS (including anaphylaxis and laryngeal edema).

Interactions

Drug-Drug: May ↑ the risk of bleeding with **warfarin**, **heparin**, **heparin-like agents**, **thrombolytic agents**, **dipyridamole**, **clopidogrel**, **tirofiban**, or **eptifibatide**, although these agents are frequently used safely in combination and in sequence. **Ibuprofen:** may negate the cardioprotective antiplatelet effects of low-dose aspirin. May ↑ risk of bleeding with **cefotetan** and **valproic acid**. May ↑ activity of **penicillins**, **phenytoin**, **methotrexate**, **valproic acid**, **oral hypoglycemic agents**, and **sulfonamides**. **Urinary acidification** ↑ reabsorption and may ↑ serum salicylate levels. **Alkalinization of the urine** or the ingestion of large amounts of **antacids** ↑ excretion and ↓ serum salicylate levels. May blunt the therapeutic response to **diuretics** and **ACE inhibitors**. ↑ risk of GI irritation with **NSAIDs**.

Drug-Natural Products: ↑ anticoagulant effect and bleeding risk with **arnica**, **chamomile**, **clove**, **feverfew**, **garlic**, **ginger**, **ginkgo**, **Panax ginseng**, and others.

Drug-Food: Foods capable of acidifying the urine (see Appendix K) may ↑ serum salicylate levels.

Route/Dosage

Pain/Fever

PO, Rect (Adults): 325–1000 mg every 4–6 hr (not to exceed 4 g/day). *Extended-release tablets*—650 mg every 8 hr or 800 mg every 12 hr.

PO, Rect (Children 2–11 yr): 10–15 mg/kg/dose every 4–6 hr; maximum dose: 4 g/day.

Inflammation

PO (Adults): 2.4 g/day initially; ↑ to maintenance dose of 3.6–5.4 g/day in divided doses (up to 7.8 g/day for acute rheumatic fever).

PO (Children): 60–100 mg/kg/day in divided doses (up to 130 mg/kg/day for acute rheumatic fever).

Prevention of Transient Ischemic Attacks

PO (Adults): 50–325 mg once daily.

Prevention of Myocardial Infarction/Antiplatelet Effects

PO (Adults): 80–325 mg once daily. *Suspected acute MI*—160 mg as soon as MI is suspected.

PO (Children): 3–10 mg/kg/day given once daily (round dose to a convenient amount).

Kawasaki Disease

PO (Children): 80–100 mg/kg/day in 4 divided doses until fever resolves; may be followed by maintenance dose of 3–5 mg/kg/day as a single dose for up to 8 wk.

Availability (generic available)

Capsules: 325 mg[OTC]. **Tablets:** 81 mg[OTC], 162.5 mg[OTC], 325 mg[OTC], 500 mg[OTC], 650 mg[OTC], 🍁975 mg[OTC]. **Chewable tablets:** 🍁80 mg[OTC], 81 mg[OTC]. **Chewing gum:** 227 mg[OTC]. **Dispersible tablets:** 325 mg[OTC], 500 mg[OTC]. **Enteric-coated (delayed-release) tablets:** 80 mg[OTC], 165 mg[OTC], 🍁300 mg[OTC], 325 mg[OTC], 500 mg[OTC], 🍁600 mg[OTC], 650 mg[OTC], 975 mg[OTC]. **Extended-release tablets:** 🍁325 mg[OTC], 650 mg[OTC], 800 mg. **Delayed-release capsules:** 🍁325 mg[OTC], 🍁500 mg[OTC]. **Suppositories:** 60 mg[OTC], 120 mg[OTC], 125 mg[OTC], 130 mg[OTC], 🍁150 mg[OTC], 🍁160 mg[OTC], 195 mg[OTC], 200 mg[OTC], 300 mg[OTC], 🍁320 mg[OTC], 325 mg[OTC], 600 mg[OTC], 🍁640 mg[OTC], 650 mg[OTC], 1.2 g[OTC]. ***In combination with:*** antihistamines, decongestants, cough suppressants[OTC], and opioids. See Appendix B.

NURSING IMPLICATIONS

Assessment

- Patients who have asthma, allergies, and nasal polyps or who are allergic to tartrazine are at an increased risk for developing hypersensitivity reactions.
- **Pain:** Assess pain and limitation of movement; note type, location, and intensity before and at the peak (see Time/Action Profile) after administration.
- **Fever:** Assess fever and note associated signs (diaphoresis, tachycardia, malaise, chills).
- ***Lab Test Considerations:*** Monitor hepatic function before antirheumatic therapy and if symptoms of hepatotoxicity occur; more likely in patients, especially children, with rheumatic fever, systemic lupus erythematosus, juvenile arthritis, or pre-existing hepatic disease. May cause ↑ serum AST, ALT, and alkaline phosphatase, especially when plasma concentrations exceed 25 mg/100 mL. May return to

normal despite continued use or dose reduction. If severe abnormalities or active liver disease occurs, discontinue and use with caution in future.

- Monitor serum salicylate levels periodically with prolonged high-dose therapy to determine dose, safety, and efficacy, especially in children with Kawasaki disease.
- May alter results of serum uric acid, urine vanillylmandelic acid (VMA), protirelin-induced thyroid-stimulating hormone (TSH), urine hydroxyindoleacetic acid (5-HIAA) determinations, and radionuclide thyroid imaging.
- Prolongs bleeding time for 4–7 days and, in large doses, may cause prolonged prothrombin time. Monitor hematocrit periodically in prolonged high-dose therapy to assess for GI blood loss.
- ***Toxicity and Overdose:*** Monitor for the onset of tinnitus, headache, hyperventilation, agitation, mental confusion, lethargy, diarrhea, and sweating. If these symptoms appear, withhold medication and notify health care professional immediately.

Implementation

- Use lowest effective dose for shortest period of time.
- **PO:** Administer after meals or with food or an antacid to minimize gastric irritation. Food slows but does not alter the total amount absorbed.
- Do not crush or chew enteric-coated tablets. Do not take antacids within 1–2 hr of enteric-coated tablets. Chewable tablets may be chewed, dissolved in liquid, or swallowed whole. Some extended-release tablets may be broken or crumbled but must not be ground up before swallowing. See manufacturer's prescribing information for individual products.

Patient/Family Teaching

- Instruct patient to take salicylates with a full glass of water and to remain in an upright position for 15–30 min after administration.
- Advise patient to report tinnitus; unusual bleeding of gums; bruising; black, tarry stools; or fever lasting longer than 3 days.
- Caution patient to avoid concurrent use of alcohol with this medication to minimize possible gastric irritation; 3 or more glasses of alcohol per day may increase risk of GI bleeding. Caution patient to avoid taking concurrently with acetaminophen or NSAIDs for more than a few days, unless directed by health care professional to prevent analgesic nephropathy.
- Instruct patients on a sodium-restricted diet to avoid effervescent tablets or buffered-aspirin preparations.
- Tablets with an acetic (vinegar-like) odor should be discarded.
- Advise patients on long-term therapy to inform health care professional of medication regimen before surgery. Aspirin may need to be withheld for 1 wk before surgery.
- Pedi: Centers for Disease Control and Prevention warns against giving aspirin to children or adolescents with varicella (chickenpox) or influenza-like or viral illnesses because of a possible association with Reye's syndrome.
- **Transient Ischemic Attacks or MI:** Advise patients receiving aspirin prophylactically to take only prescribed dose. Increasing dose has not been found to provide additional benefits.

Evaluation/Desired Outcomes

- Relief of mild to moderate discomfort.
- Increased ease of joint movement. May take 2–3 wk for maximum effectiveness.
- Reduction of fever.
- Prevention of transient ischemic attacks.
- Prevention of MI.

aspirin, See SALICYLATES.

atenolol (a-ten-oh-lole)

Tenormin

Classification

Therapeutic: antianginals, antihypertensives

Pharmacologic: beta blockers

Indications

Management of hypertension. Management of angina pectoris. Prevention of MI.

Action

Blocks stimulation of $beta_1$ (myocardial)-adrenergic receptors. Does not usually affect $beta_2$ (pulmonary, vascular, uterine)-receptor sites. **Therapeutic Effects:** Decreased BP and heart rate. Decreased frequency of attacks of angina pectoris. Prevention of MI.

Pharmacokinetics

Absorption: 50–60% absorbed after oral administration.

Distribution: Minimal penetration of CNS. Crosses the placenta and enters breast milk.

Metabolism and Excretion: 40–50% excreted unchanged by the kidneys; remainder excreted in feces as unabsorbed drug.

Half-life: 6–9 hr.

TIME/ACTION PROFILE (cardiovascular effects)

ROUTE	ONSET	PEAK	DURATION
PO	1 hr	2–4 hr	24 hr

Contraindications/Precautions

Contraindicated in: Uncompensated HF; Pulmonary edema; Cardiogenic shock; Bradycardia or heart block.

Use Cautiously in: Renal impairment (dosage ↓ recommended if CCr ≤35 mL/min); Hepatic impairment; Geri: ↑ sensitivity to beta blockers; initial dose ↓ recommended; Pulmonary disease (including asthma; beta selectivity may be lost at higher doses); Diabetes mellitus (may mask signs of hypoglycemia); Thyrotoxicosis (may mask symptoms); Patients with a history of severe allergic reactions (intensity of reactions may be ↑); OB: Crosses the placenta and may cause fetal/neonatal bradycardia, hypotension, hypoglycemia, or respiratory depression; Lactation, Pedi: Safety not established.

Adverse Reactions/Side Effects

CNS: fatigue, weakness, anxiety, depression, dizziness, drowsiness, insomnia, memory loss, mental status changes, nervousness, nightmares. **EENT:** blurred vision, stuffy nose. **Resp:** bronchospasm, wheezing. **CV:** BRADYCARDIA, HF, PULMONARY EDEMA, hypotension, peripheral vasoconstriction. **GI:** constipation, diarrhea, ↑ liver enzymes, nausea, vomiting. **GU:** erectile dysfunction, ↓ libido, urinary frequency. **Derm:** rashes. **Endo:** hyperglycemia, hypoglycemia. **MS:** arthralgia, back pain, joint pain. **Misc:** drug-induced lupus syndrome.

Interactions

Drug-Drug: General anesthesia, **IV phenytoin**, and **verapamil** may cause additive myocardial depression. Additive bradycardia may occur with **digoxin**. Additive hypotension may occur with other **antihypertensives**, acute ingestion of **alcohol**, or **nitrates**. Concurrent use with **amphetamine**, **cocaine**, **ephedrine**, **epinephrine**, **norepinephrine**, **phenylephrine**, or **pseudoephedrine** may result in unopposed alpha-adrenergic stimulation (excessive hypertension, bradycardia). Concurrent **thyroid** administration may ↓ effectiveness. May alter the effectiveness of **insulins** or **oral hypoglycemic agents** (dosage adjustments may be necessary). May ↓ the effectiveness of **theophylline**. May ↓ the beneficial beta$_1$-cardiovascular effects of **dopamine** or **dobutamine**. Use cautiously within 14 days of **MAO inhibitor** therapy (may result in hypertension).

Route/Dosage

PO (Adults): *Antianginal*—50 mg once daily; may be ↑ after 1 wk to 100 mg/day (up to 200 mg/day). *Antihypertensive*—25–50 mg once daily; may be ↑ after 2 wk to 50–100 mg once daily. *MI*—50 mg, then 50 mg 12 hr later, then 100 mg/day as a single dose or in 2 divided doses for 6–9 days or until hospital discharge.

Renal Impairment

PO (Adults): *CCr 15–35 mL/min*—dosage should not exceed 50 mg/day; *CCr <15 mL/min*—dosage should not exceed 50 mg every other day.

Availability (generic available)

Tablets: 25 mg, 50 mg, 100 mg. **Cost:** *Generic*—All strengths $10.83/100. ***In combination with:*** chlorthalidone (Tenoretic). See Appendix B.

NURSING IMPLICATIONS

Assessment

- Monitor BP, ECG, and pulse frequently during dose adjustment period and periodically throughout therapy.
- Monitor intake and output ratios and daily weights. Assess routinely for HF (dyspnea, rales/crackles, weight gain, peripheral edema, jugular venous distention).
- Monitor frequency of prescription refills to determine adherence.
- **Angina:** Assess frequency and characteristics of angina periodically during therapy.
- ***Lab Test Considerations:*** May cause ↑ BUN, serum lipoprotein, potassium, triglyceride, and uric acid levels.
- May cause ↑ ANA titers.
- May cause ↑ in blood glucose levels.
- ***Toxicity and Overdose:*** Monitor patients receiving beta blockers for signs of overdose (bradycardia, severe dizziness or fainting, severe drowsiness, dyspnea, bluish fingernails or palms, seizures). Notify health care professional immediately if these signs occur.

Implementation

- **PO:** Take apical pulse before administering drug. If <50 bpm or if arrhythmia occurs, withhold medication and notify health care professional.

Patient/Family Teaching

- Instruct patient to take atenolol as directed at the same time each day, even if feeling well; do not skip or double up on missed doses. Take missed doses as soon as possible up to 8 hr before next dose. Abrupt withdrawal may cause life-threatening arrhythmias, hypertension, or myocardial ischemia.
- Advise patient to make sure enough medication is available for weekends, holidays, and vacations. A written prescription may be kept in wallet in case of emergency.
- Teach patient and family how to check pulse and BP. Instruct them to check pulse daily and BP biweekly and to report significant changes.
- May cause drowsiness or dizziness. Caution patients to avoid driving or other activities that require alertness until response to the drug is known.
- Advise patients to change positions slowly to minimize orthostatic hypotension.
- Caution patient that atenolol may increase sensitivity to cold.
- Instruct patient to notify health care professional of all Rx or OTC medications, vitamins, or herbal products being taken, to avoid alcohol, and to consult health care professional before taking any new medications, especially cold preparations.
- Patients with diabetes should closely monitor blood glucose, especially if weakness, malaise, irritability, or fatigue occurs. Medication does not block sweating as a sign of hypoglycemia.

- Advise patient to notify health care professional if slow pulse, difficulty breathing, wheezing, cold hands and feet, dizziness, light-headedness, confusion, depression, rash, fever, sore throat, unusual bleeding, or bruising occurs.
- Instruct patient to inform health care professional of medication regimen before treatment or surgery.
- Advise female patient to notify health care professional if pregnancy is planned or suspected, or if breast feeding.
- Advise patient to carry identification describing disease process and medication regimen at all times.
- **Hypertension:** Reinforce the need to continue additional therapies for hypertension (weight loss, sodium restriction, stress reduction, regular exercise, moderation of alcohol consumption, and smoking cessation). Medication controls but does not cure hypertension.

Evaluation/Desired Outcomes

- Decrease in BP.
- Reduction in frequency of angina.
- Increase in activity tolerance.
- Prevention of MI.

atezolizumab

(a-te-zoe-**liz**-ue-mab)

Tecentriq

Classification

Therapeutic: antineoplastics

Pharmacologic: monoclonal antibodies, programmed death ligand 1 (PD-L1) inhibitors

Indications

Locally advanced or metastatic urothelial carcinoma in patients who are not eligible for cisplatin-containing chemotherapy and whose tumors express PD-L1, or are not eligible for any platinum-containing chemotherapy regardless of the level of PD-L1 tumor expression, or have disease progression during or following any platinum-containing chemotherapy, or have disease progression within 12 mo of neoadjuvant or adjuvant chemotherapy. Metastatic non-small cell lung cancer (NSCLC) in patients who have disease progression during or following platinum-containing chemotherapy. Patients with epidermal growth factor receptor (EGFR) or anaplastic lymphoma kinase (ALK) genomic tumor aberrations should have disease progression on FDA-approved therapy for these aberrations prior to receiving atezolizumab. Metastatic non-squamous, non-small cell lung cancer (NSq NSCLC) as first-line therapy in patients who have no EGFR or ALK genomic tumor aberrations (in combination with bevacizumab, paclitaxel, and carboplatin). Unresectable, locally advanced or metastatic triple-negative breast cancer in patients whose tumors express PD-L1 (in combination with paclitaxel protein-bound). Extensive-stage small cell lung cancer (SCLC) as first-line therapy (in combination with carboplatin and etoposide).

Action

Binds to programmed death ligand 1 (PD-L1) to prevent its interaction with the programmed cell death-1 (PD-1) and B7.1 (or CD80) receptors, which activates the anti-tumor immune response. **Therapeutic Effects:** Decreased spread of urothelial carcinoma. Decreased spread of NSCLC, SCLC, and triple-negative breast cancer with increased survival.

Pharmacokinetics

Absorption: IV administration results in complete bioavailability.

Distribution: Minimally distributed to tissues.

Metabolism and Excretion: Unknown.

Half-life: 27 days.

TIME/ACTION PROFILE (blood levels)

ROUTE	ONSET	PEAK	DURATION
IV	unknown	unknown	unknown

Contraindications/Precautions

Contraindicated in: OB: Pregnancy (may cause fetal harm); Lactation: Lactation.

Use Cautiously in: Rep: Women of reproductive potential; Pedi: Safety and effectiveness not established.

Adverse Reactions/Side Effects

CNS: ENCEPHALITIS, MENINGITIS. **CV:** peripheral edema, myocarditis. **Derm:** pruritus, rash. **Endo:** hypothyroidism, adrenal insufficiency, hyperglycemia, hyperthyroidism, hypophysitis, type 1 diabetes mellitus. **F and E:** hyponatremia, dehydration. **GI:** COLITIS/DIARRHEA, HEPATOTOXICITY, PANCREATITIS, constipation, ↓ appetite, nausea, vomiting, abdominal pain, ↑ liver enzymes. **GU:** hematuria, acute kidney injury, ↓ fertility (females), ↑ serum creatinine, urinary obstruction. **Hemat:** lymphopenia, anemia. **Metab:** hypoalbuminemia. **MS:** arthralgia, ↑ alkaline phosphatase. **Neuro:** GUILLAIN-BARRE SYNDROME, MYASTHENIA GRAVIS. **Resp:** INTERSTITIAL LUNG DISEASE, cough, dyspnea. **Misc:** INFECTIONS (including herpes encephalitis and tuberculosis), INFUSION-RELATED REACTIONS, fatigue, fever.

Interactions

Drug-Drug: None known.

Route/Dosage

Urothelial Carcinoma or Previously Treated NSCLC

IV (Adults): 840 mg every 2 wk *or* 1200 mg every 3 wk *or* 1680 mg every 4 wk until disease progression or unacceptable toxicity.

NSq NSCLC

IV (Adults): 1200 mg every 3 wk (followed by bevacizumab, paclitaxel, and carboplatin) for a maximum of 4–6 cycles, then 1200 mg every 3 wk (followed by bevacizumab) until disease progression or unacceptable toxicity; if bevacizumab is discontinued after the 4–6 cycles of combination chemotherapy, continue with atezolizumab (as monotherapy) at a dose of 840 mg every 2 wk *or*1200 mg every 3 wk *or*1680 mg every 4 wk until disease progression or unacceptable toxicity.

SCLC

IV (Adults): 1200 mg every 3 wk (followed by carboplatin and etoposide) for 4 cycles, then continue with atezolizumab (as monotherapy) at a dose of 840 mg every 2 wk *or*1200 mg every 3 wk *or*1680 mg every 4 wk until disease progression or unacceptable toxicity.

Triple-Negative Breast Cancer

IV (Adults): 840 mg on Days 1 and 15 of each 28–day cycle (with paclitaxel protein-bound being administered on Days 1, 8, 15 of each 28–day cycle) until disease progression or unacceptable toxicity.

Availability

Solution for injection (requires dilution): 60 mg/mL.

NURSING IMPLICATIONS

Assessment

- Monitor for signs and symptoms of pneumonitis (new or worsening cough, dyspnea, chest pain) during therapy. Monitor with x-rays as needed. *For ≥Grade 2 pneumonitis,* administer corticosteroids at a dose of 1–2 mg/kg/day prednisolone equivalents followed by a taper. *For Grade 3 or 4 pneumonitis,* permanently discontinue atezolizumab.
- Monitor for signs and symptoms of hepatitis (jaundice, severe nausea or vomiting, pain on right side of abdomen, lethargy, dark urine, unusual bleeding or bruising, anorexia) periodically during therapy.
- Monitor for signs and symptoms of diarrhea or colitis (blood in stools, dark tarry stools, abdominal pain or tenderness) periodically during therapy. *For Grade 2 or 3,* hold atezolizumab until Grade 1 or resolved and corticosteroid dose ≤prednisone 10 mg per day (or equivalent). *For Grade 4,* permanently discontinue atezolizumab.
- Monitor for signs and symptoms of adrenal insufficiency (extreme tiredness, dizziness or fainting, frequent urination, nausea or vomiting, changes in mood or behavior, ↓ sex drive, irritability, forgetfulness), hypophysitis (unusual headaches, persistent headaches, vision problems), hyperthyroidism, and Type 1 diabetes periodically during therapy. *If Grades 2, 3, or 4 occur,* hold dose until Grade 1 or resolved and clinically stable on hormone replacement therapy.
- Monitor for signs and symptoms of meningitis or encephalitis (fever, confusion, changes in mood or behavior, extreme sensitivity to light, neck stiffness) during therapy. If symptoms occur, permanently discontinue atezolizumab. Administer 1–2 mg/kg/day methylprednisolone or equivalent. Convert to oral prednisone 60 mg/day or equivalent once improved. When symptoms improve to ≤Grade 1, taper steroids over ≥1 mo.
- Monitor for signs and symptoms of motor or sensory neuropathy (severe muscle weakness, numbness or tingling in hands or feet) periodically during therapy. For any grade of myasthenic syndrome/myasthenia gravis or Guillaine-Barre syndrome, permanently discontinue atezolizumab. Institute treatment as needed. Consider systemic corticosteroids at a dose of 1–2 mg/kg/day prednisone.
- Monitor for signs and symptoms of pancreatitis (abdominal pain) during therapy. *If Grade 2 or 3 pancreatitis,* withhold atezolizumab. Treat with methylprednisolone IV 1–2 mg/kg/day or equivalent. Once symptoms improve, follow with 1–2 mg/kg/day of oral prednisone or equivalent. Resume atezolizumab if symptoms of pancreatitis resolved and corticosteroid reduced to ≤10 mg/day oral prednisone or equivalent. *For Grade 4 or recurrent pancreatitis,* permanently discontinue atezolizumab.
- Monitor for signs and symptoms of infection (fever, cough, frequent urination, flu-like symptoms, painful urination) periodically during therapy. Treat suspected or confirmed infections with antibiotics. *For ≥Grade 3 or 4 infections,* withhold atezolizumab until Grade 1 or resolved.
- Monitor for signs and symptoms of infusion-related reactions (chills or shaking, itching or rash, flushing, dyspnea, wheezing, dizziness, fever, feeling faint, back or neck pain, facial swelling) during therapy. *For Grade 1 or 2,* interrupt or slow infusion. *For Grade 3 or 4 infusion reactions,* permanently discontinue atezolizumab.
- ***Lab Test Considerations:*** Obtain a negative pregnancy test before starting therapy.
- Determine PD-L1 expression in locally advanced or metastatic urothelial carcinoma or triple-negative breast cancer via tests at http://www.fda.gov/CompanionDiagnostics. Information on FDA-approved tests for the determination of PD-L1.
- Monitor AST, ALT, and serum bilirubin prior to and periodically during therapy. *If AST or ALT >3 and up to 8 times upper limit of normal (ULN) or total bilirubin >1.5 and up to 3 times ULN* hold dose until Grade 1 or resolved and corticosteroid dose ≤prednisone 10 mg per day (or equivalent). *If AST or ALT >8 times ULN or total bilirubin >3 times ULN,* permanently discontinue atezolizumab.
- Monitor thyroid function prior to and periodically during therapy. *If asymptomatic,* continue therapy. *For symptomatic hypothyroidism (extreme tiredness, weight gain, constipation, feeling cold, hair loss, deepening voice),* withhold atezolizumab and begin thyroid replacement therapy as needed with-

out corticosteroids. *For symptomatic hyperthyroidism (hunger, irritability, mood swings, weight loss),* hold atezolizumab until Grade 1 or resolved and clinically stable on hormone replacement therapy. Resume therapy when symptoms of hyper— or hypothyroidism are controlled and thyroid function is improving.

- Monitor blood glucose periodically during therapy. For type 1 diabetes, begin treatment with insulin. For ≥Grade 2, 3, or 4 hyperglycemia (fasting glucose >250–500 mg/dL), hold atezolizumab until Grade 1 or resolved and control is achieved on insulin replacement therapy.
- Monitor serum amylase or lipase in patients with symptoms of pancreatitis. If serum amylase or lipase levels ≥Grade 3 (>2x upper limit of normal), withhold atezolizumab. Treat with methylprednisolone IV 1–2 mg/kg/day or equivalent. Once symptoms improve, follow with 1–2 mg/kg/day of oral prednisone or equivalent. Resume atezolizumab if symptoms of pancreatitis resolved and corticosteroid ↓ to ≤10 mg/day oral prednisone or equivalent.
- May cause lymphopenia, hyponatremia, anemia, ↑ alkaline phosphatase, ↑creatinine, and hypoalbuminemia.

Implementation

IV Administration

- **Intermittent Infusion:** ***Diluent:*** Dilute 20 mL of atezolizumab in 250 mL of 0.9% NaCl in a polyvinyl chloride, polyethylene, or polyolefin infusion bag.Gently invert to dilute; do not shake. Solution is clear and colorless to slightly yellow. Do not administer solutions that are discolored or contain particulate matter. Administer immediately once prepared or store for ≤6 hrs at room temperature (including infusion time) or ≤24 hrs if refrigerated. Do not freeze.
- Administer atezolizumab before chemotherapy or other antineoplastic drugs when given on same day. ***Rate:*** Administer over 60 min with or without a sterile, non-pyrogenic, low-protein binding in-line filter (0.2–0.22 micron); do not administer via IV push or bolus. If first infusion is tolerated, subsequent infusions may be infused over 30 min.
- **Y-Site Incompatibility:** Do not administer other drugs through same IV line.

Patient/Family Teaching

- Advise patient to notify health care professional immediately if symptoms of pneumonitis, hepatitis, colitis, endocrine problems, meningitis, nervous system problems, ocular inflammatory toxicity (blurry or double vision, eye pain or redness), pancreatitis, infection, infusion-related reactions, or rash occur.
- Advise patient to notify health care professional of all Rx or OTC medications, vitamins, or herbal products being taken and to consult with health care professional before taking other medications.
- Rep: May be teratogenic. Advise females to use effective contraception during and for ≥5 mo after last dose. Inform females atezolizumab may impair fertility. Advise patient to avoid breast feeding during and for ≥5 mo after last dose.

Evaluation/Desired Outcomes

- Decreased spread of urothelial carcinoma.
- Decreased spread of NSCLC, SCLC, and triple-negative breast cancer with increased survival.

⧖ atomoxetine
(a-to-**mox**-e-teen)
Strattera

Classification
Therapeutic: agents for attention deficit disorder
Pharmacologic: selective norepinephrine reuptake inhibitors

Indications

Attention-Deficit/Hyperactivity Disorder (ADHD).

Action

Selectively inhibits the presynaptic transporter of norepinephrine. **Therapeutic Effects:** Increased attention span.

Pharmacokinetics

Absorption: Well absorbed following oral administration.
Distribution: Unknown.
Protein Binding: 98%.
Metabolism and Excretion: Mostly metabolized by the liver (CYP2D6 enzyme pathway). ⧖ A small percentage of the population are poor metabolizers and will have higher blood levels with ↑ effects.
Half-life: 5 hr.

TIME/ACTION PROFILE

ROUTE	ONSET	PEAK	DURATION
PO	unknown	1–2 hr	12–24 hr

Contraindications/Precautions

Contraindicated in: Hypersensitivity; Concurrent or within 2 wk therapy with MAO inhibitors; Angle-closure glaucoma; Pheochromocytoma; Hypertension, tachycardia, cardiovascular, or cerebrovascular disease.
Use Cautiously in: Pre-existing psychiatric illness; Pedi: May ↑ risk of suicide attempt/ideation especially during dose early treatment or dose adjustment; risk may be greater in children or adolescents; Concurrent albuterol or vasopressors (↑ risk of adverse cardiovas-

cular reactions); OB: Use only if benefits outweigh risks to fetus; Lactation, Pedi: Safety not established.

Adverse Reactions/Side Effects

CNS: SUICIDAL THOUGHTS, dizziness, fatigue, mood swings, behavioral disturbances, hallucinations, hostility, mania, thought disorder; *Adults*, insomnia. **CV:** hypertension, orthostatic hypotension, QT interval prolongation, syncope, tachycardia. **GI:** HEPATOTOXICITY, dyspepsia, nausea, vomiting; *Adults*, dry mouth, constipation. **Derm:** ↑ sweating, rash, urticaria. **GU:** *Adults*—dysmenorrhea, ejaculatory problems, erectile dysfunction, libido changes, priapism, urinary hesitation, urinary retention. **Metab:** ↓ appetite, weight/growth loss. **MS:** RHABDOMYOLYSIS. **Neuro:** *Adults*—paresthesia. **Misc:** allergic reactions including ANGIONEUROTIC EDEMA and ANAPHYLAXIS.

Interactions

Drug-Drug: Concurrent use with **MAO inhibitors** may result in serious, potentially fatal reactions (do not use within 2 wk of each other). ↑ risk of cardiovascular effects with **albuterol** or **vasopressors** (use cautiously). **Drugs which inhibit the CYP2D6 enzyme pathway** (**quinidine**, **fluoxetine**, **paroxetine**) will ↑ blood levels and effects, dose ↓ recommended.

Route/Dosage

PO (Children and Adolescents <70 kg): 0.5 mg/kg/day initially, may be ↑ every 3 days to a daily target dose of 1.2 mg/kg, given as a single dose in the morning or evenly divided doses in the morning and late afternoon/early evening (not to exceed 1.4 mg/kg/day or 100 mg/day whichever is less). *If taking concurrent CYP2D6 inhibitor (quinidine, fluoxetine, paroxetine)*—0.5 mg/kg/day initially, may ↑ if needed to 1.2 mg/kg/day after 4 wk.

PO (Adults, Adolescents, and Children >70 kg): 40 mg/day initially, may be ↑ every 3 days to a daily target dose of 80 mg/day given as a single dose in the morning or evenly divided doses in the morning and late afternoon/early evening; may be further ↑ after 2–4 wk up to 100 mg/day. *If taking concurrent CYP2D6 inhibitor (quinidine, fluoxetine, paroxetine)*—40 mg/day initially, may ↑ if needed to 80 mg/day after 4 wk.

Hepatic Impairment

PO (Adults and Children): *Moderate hepatic impairment (Child-Pugh Class B)*—↓ initial and target dose by 50%; *Severe hepatic impairment (Child-Pugh Class C)*—↓ initial and target dose to 25% of normal.

Availability (generic available)

Capsules: 10 mg, 18 mg, 25 mg, 40 mg, 60 mg, 80 mg, 100 mg.

NURSING IMPLICATIONS

Assessment

- Assess attention span, impulse control, and interactions with others.
- Monitor BP and pulse periodically during therapy. Obtain a history (including assessment of family history of sudden death or ventricular arrhythmia), physical exam to assess for cardiac disease, and further evaluation (ECG and echocardiogram), if indicated. If exertional chest pain, unexplained syncope, or other cardiac symptoms occur, evaluate promptly.
- Monitor growth, body height, and weight in children.
- Assess for signs of liver injury (pruritus, dark urine, jaundice, right upper quadrant tenderness, unexplained "flu-like" symptoms) during therapy. Monitor liver function tests at first sign of liver injury. Discontinue and do not restart atomoxetine in patients with jaundice or laboratory evidence of liver injury.
- Monitor closely for notable changes in behavior that could indicate the emergence or worsening of suicidal thoughts or behavior or depression.

Implementation

- Do not confuse atomoxetine with atorvastatin.
- **PO:** Administer without regard to food. Capsules should be swallowed whole; do not open, crush, or chew. Doses may be discontinued without tapering.

Patient/Family Teaching

- Instruct patient to take medication as directed. Take missed doses as soon as possible, but should not take more than the total daily amount in any 24-hr period. Advise patient and parents to read the *Medication Guide* prior to starting therapy and with each Rx refill.
- Inform patient that sharing this medication may be dangerous.
- Advise patient and family to notify health care professional if thoughts about suicide or dying, attempts to commit suicide; new or worse depression; new or worse anxiety; feeling very agitated or restless; panic attacks; trouble sleeping; new or worse irritability; acting aggressive or hostile; being angry or violent; acting on dangerous impulses; an extreme increase in activity and talking; other unusual changes in behavior or mood occur or if signs and symptoms of severe liver injury (pruritus, dark urine, jaundice, right upper quadrant tenderness, or unexplained "flu-like" symptoms) occur.
- Instruct patient to notify health care professional of all Rx or OTC medications, vitamins, or herbal products being taken and consult health care professional before taking any new medications.
- May cause dizziness. Caution patient to avoid driving or other activities requiring alertness until response to medication is known.
- Advise female patients to notify health care professional if pregnancy is planned or suspected or if they are breast feeding.

Evaluation/Desired Outcomes

- Improved attention span and social interactions in ADHD.

atorvastatin, See HMG-CoA REDUCTASE INHIBITORS (statins).

atovaquone (a-toe-va-kwone)

Mepron

Classification

Therapeutic: anti-infectives

Indications

Treatment of mild to moderate *Pneumocystis jirovecii* pneumonia (PJP) in patients who are unable to tolerate trimethoprim/sulfamethoxazole. Prophylaxis of *PJP*.

Action

Inhibits the action of enzymes necessary to nucleic acid and ATP synthesis. **Therapeutic Effects:** Active against *P. jirovecii*.

Pharmacokinetics

Absorption: Absorption is poor but is increased by food, particularly fat.

Distribution: Enters CSF in very low concentrations (<1% of plasma levels).

Protein Binding: >99.9%.

Metabolism and Excretion: Undergoes enterohepatic recycling; elimination occurs in feces.

Half-life: 2.2–2.9 days.

TIME/ACTION PROFILE (blood levels)

ROUTE	ONSET	PEAK	DURATION
PO	unknown	1–8 hr; 24–96 hr†	12 hr

†Two peaks are due to enterohepatic recycling.

Contraindications/Precautions

Contraindicated in: Hypersensitivity; Lactation: Avoid breast feeding in patients infected with HIV.

Use Cautiously in: ↓ hepatic, renal, or cardiac function (dose modification may be necessary); GI disorders (absorption may be limited); OB: Use only if potential maternal benefit justifies potential fetal risk; Pedi: Safety not established.

Adverse Reactions/Side Effects

CNS: headache, insomnia. **Derm:** rash. **GI:** diarrhea, nausea, vomiting. **Resp:** cough. **Misc:** fever.

Interactions

Drug-Drug: Rifampin or **rifabutin** may ↓ levels and efficacy; concurrent use not recommended. **Tetracycline** may ↓ levels and efficacy; use caution when using concurrently. **Metoclopramide** may ↓ levels and efficacy; use only if no other alternative available. May ↓ **indinavir** levels and efficacy; use caution when using concurrently.

Drug-Food: Food ↑ absorption.

Route/Dosage

Treatment

PO (Adults): 750 mg twice daily for 21 days.

PO (Children): 40 mg/kg/day (unlabeled).

Prevention

PO (Adults and Adolescents 13–16 yr): 1500 mg once daily.

Availability (generic available)

Suspension: 750 mg/5 mL. ***In combination with:*** proguanil (Malarone). See Appendix B.

NURSING IMPLICATIONS

Assessment

- Assess patient for signs of infection (vital signs, lung sounds, sputum, WBCs) at beginning of and throughout therapy.
- Obtain specimens prior to initiating therapy. First dose may be given before receiving results.
- ***Lab Test Considerations:*** Monitor hematologic and hepatic functions. May cause mild, transient anemia and neutropenia. May also cause ↑ serum amylase, AST, ALT, and alkaline phosphatase.
- Monitor electrolytes. May cause hyponatremia.

Implementation

- **PO:** Administer with food twice daily for 21 days for treatment and once daily for prevention.
- Shake suspension gently prior to administration.

Patient/Family Teaching

- Instruct patient to take atovaquone as directed around the clock for full course of therapy, even if feeling better. Emphasize the importance of taking atovaquone with food, especially foods high in fat; taking without food may decrease plasma concentrations and effectiveness.
- Advise patient to notify health care professional if rash occurs.
- Advise female patient to notify health care professional if pregnancy is planned or suspected and to avoid breast feeding.

Evaluation/Desired Outcomes

- Resolution of the signs and symptoms of infection.

BEERS

atropine† (at-ro-peen)

Atro-Pen

Classification

Therapeutic: antiarrhythmics

Pharmacologic: anticholinergics, antimuscarinics

†See Appendix C for ophthalmic use

Indications

IM: Given preoperatively to decrease oral and respiratory secretions. **IV:** Treatment of sinus bradycardia and heart block. **IV:** Reversal of adverse muscarinic effects of anticholinesterase agents (neostigmine, physostigmine, or pyridostigmine). **IM, IV:** Treatment of anticholinesterase (organophosphate pesticide) poisoning. **Inhaln:** Treatment of exercise-induced bronchospasm.

Action

Inhibits the action of acetylcholine at postganglionic sites located in: Smooth muscle, Secretory glands, CNS (antimuscarinic activity). Low doses decrease: Sweating, Salivation, Respiratory secretions. Intermediate doses result in: Mydriasis (pupillary dilation), Cycloplegia (loss of visual accommodation), Increased heart rate. GI and GU tract motility are decreased at larger doses. **Therapeutic Effects:** Increased heart rate. Decreased GI and respiratory secretions. Reversal of muscarinic effects. May have a spasmolytic action on the biliary and genitourinary tracts.

Pharmacokinetics

Absorption: Well absorbed following subcut or IM administration.

Distribution: Readily crosses the blood-brain barrier. Crosses the placenta and enters breast milk.

Metabolism and Excretion: Mostly metabolized by the liver; 30–50% excreted unchanged by the kidneys.

Half-life: Children <2 yr: 4–10 hr; Children >2 yr: 1.5–3.5 hr; Adults: 4–5 hr.

TIME/ACTION PROFILE (inhibition of salivation)

ROUTE	ONSET	PEAK	DURATION
IM, subcut	rapid	15–50 min	4–6 hr
IV	immediate	2–4 min	4–6 hr

Contraindications/Precautions

Contraindicated in: Hypersensitivity; Angle-closure glaucoma; Acute hemorrhage; Tachycardia secondary to cardiac insufficiency or thyrotoxicosis; Obstructive disease of the GI tract.

Use Cautiously in: Intra-abdominal infections; Prostatic hyperplasia; Chronic renal, hepatic, pulmonary, or cardiac disease; OB, Lactation: Safety not established; IV administration may produce fetal tachycardia; Pedi: Infants with Down syndrome have increased sensitivity to cardiac effects and mydriasis. Children may have increased susceptibility to adverse reactions. Exercise care when prescribing to children with spastic paralysis or brain damage; Geri: Increased susceptibility to adverse reactions.

Adverse Reactions/Side Effects

CNS: drowsiness, confusion, hyperpyrexia. **EENT:** blurred vision, cycloplegia, photophobia, dry eyes, mydriasis. **CV:** tachycardia, palpitations, arrhythmias. **GI:** dry mouth, constipation, impaired GI motility. **GU:** urinary hesitancy, retention, impotency. **Resp:** tachypnea, pulmonary edema. **Misc:** flushing, decreased sweating.

Interactions

Drug-Drug: ↑ anticholinergic effects with other **anticholinergics**, including **antihistamines**, **tricyclic antidepressants**, **quinidine**, and **disopyramide**. Anticholinergics may alter the absorption of other **orally administered drugs** by slowing motility of the GI tract. **Antacids** ↓ absorption of **anticholinergics**. May ↑ GI mucosal lesions in patients taking oral **potassium chloride** tablets. May alter response to **beta-blockers**.

Route/Dosage

Preanesthesia (To Decrease Salivation/Secretions)

IM, IV, Subcut (Adults): 0.4–0.6 mg 30–60 min pre-op.

IM, IV, Subcut (Children >5 kg): 0.01–0.02 mg/kg/dose 30–60 min preop to a maximum of 0.4 mg/dose; minimum: 0.1 mg/dose.

IM, IV, Subcut (Children <5 kg): 0.02 mg/kg/dose 30–60 min preop then every 4–6 hr as needed.

Bradycardia

IV (Adults): 0.5–1 mg; may repeat as needed every 5 min, not to exceed a total of 2 mg (every 3–5 min in Advanced Cardiac Life Support guidelines) or 0.04 mg/kg (total vagolytic dose).

IV (Children): 0.02 mg/kg (maximum single dose is 0.5 mg in children and 1 mg in adolescents); may repeat every 5 min up to a total dose of 1 mg in children (2 mg in adolescents).

Endotracheal (Children): use the IV dose and dilute before administration.

Reversal of Adverse Muscarinic Effects of Anticholinesterases

IV (Adults): 0.6–12 mg for each 0.5–2.5 mg of neostigmine methylsulfate or 10–20 mg of pyridostigmine bromide concurrently with anticholinesterase.

Organophosphate Poisoning

IM (Adults): 2 mg initially, then 2 mg every 10 min as needed up to 3 times total.

IV (Adults): 1–2 mg/dose every 10–20 min until atropinic effects observed then every 1–4 hr for 24 hr; up to 50 mg in first 24 hr and 2 g over several days may be given in severe intoxication.

IM (Children >10 yr >90 lbs): 2 mg.

IM (Children 4–10 yr 40–90 lbs): 1 mg.

IM (Children 6 mo–4 yr 15–40 lbs): 0.5 mg.

IV (Children): 0.02–0.05 mg/kg every 10–20 min until atropinic effects observed then every 1–4 hr for 24 hr.

Bronchospasm

Inhaln (Adults): 0.025–0.05 mg/kg/dose every 4–6 hr as needed; maximum 2.5 mg/dose.

Inhaln (Children): 0.03–0.05 mg/kg/dose 3–4 times/day; maximum 2.5 mg/dose.

Availability (generic available)

Injection: 0.05 mg/mL, 0.1 mg/mL, 0.4 mg/mL, 1 mg/mL, 0.5 mg/0.7 mL Auto-injector, 1 mg/0.7 mL Auto-injector, 2 mg/0.7 mL Auto-injector.

NURSING IMPLICATIONS

Assessment

- Assess vital signs and ECG tracings frequently during IV drug therapy. Report any significant changes in heart rate or BP, or increased ventricular ectopy or angina to health care professional promptly.
- Monitor intake and output ratios in elderly or surgical patients because atropine may cause urinary retention.
- Assess patients routinely for abdominal distention and auscultate for bowel sounds. If constipation becomes a problem, increasing fluids and adding bulk to the diet may help alleviate constipation.
- ***Toxicity and Overdose:*** If overdose occurs, physostigmine is the antidote.

Implementation

- **IM:** Intense flushing of the face and trunk may occur 15–20 min following IM administration. In children, this response is called "atropine flush" and is not harmful.

IV Administration

- **IV Push:** ***Diluent:*** Administer undiluted. ***Rate:*** Administer over 1 min; more rapid administration may be used during cardiac resuscitation (follow with 20 mL saline flush). Slow administration (over >1 min) may cause a paradoxical bradycardia (usually resolved in approximately 2 min).
- **Y-Site Compatibility:** alfentanyl, amikacin, aminophylline, amiodarone, argatroban, ascorbic acid, azathioprine, aztreonam, benztropine, bivalirudin, bumetanide, buprenorphine, butorphanol, calcium chloride, calcium gluconate, cefazolin, cefotaxime, cefotetan, cefoxitin, ceftazidime, ceftriaxone, cefuroxime, chloramphenicol, chlorpromazine, clindamycin, cyanocobalamin, cyclosporine, dexamethasone, dexmedetomidine, digoxin, diphenhydramine, dobutamine, dopamine, doxycycline, enalaprilat, ephedrine, epinephrine, epoetin alfa, eptifibatide, erythromycin, esmolol, etomidate, famotidine, fenoldopam, fentanyl, fluconazole, folic acid, furosemide, ganciclovir, gentamicin, glycopyrrolate, heparin, hydrocortisone sodium succinate, hydromorphone, imipenem/cilastatin, indomethacin, insulin, isoproterenol, ketamine, ketorolac, labetalol, lidocaine, magnesium sulfate, mannitol, meperidine, meropenem, methadone, methyldopate, methylprednisolone, metoclopramide, metoprolol, midazolam, morphine, multivitamins, nafcillin, nalbuphine, naloxone, nitroglycerin, nitroprusside, norepinephrine, ondansetron, oxacillin, oxytocin, palonosetron, papaverine, penicillin G, pentamidine, pentobarbital, phenobarbital, phentolamine, phenylephrine, phytonadione, potassium chloride, procainamide, prochlorperazine, promethazine, propranolol, protamine, pyridoxime, ranitidine, sodium bicarbonate, streptokinase, succinylcholine, sufentanil, theophylline, thiamine, tirofiban, tobramycin, tolazoline, vancomycin, vasopressin, verapamil, vitamin B complex with C.
- **Y-Site Incompatibility:** amphotericin B deoxycholate, dantrolene, diazepam, diazoxide, pantoprazole, phenytoin, trimethoprim/sulfamethoxazole, thiopental.
- **Endotracheal:** Dilute with 5–10 mL of 0.9% NaCl.
- ***Rate:*** Inject directly into the endotracheal tube followed by several positive pressure ventilations.

Patient/Family Teaching

- May cause drowsiness. Caution patients to avoid driving or other activities requiring alertness until response to medication is known.
- Instruct patient that oral rinses, sugarless gum or candy, and frequent oral hygiene may help relieve dry mouth.
- Caution patients that atropine impairs heat regulation. Strenuous activity in a hot environment may cause heat stroke. Advise patient to notify health care professional of all Rx or OTC medications, vitamins, or herbal products being taken and to consult with health care professional before taking other medications.
- Pedi: Instruct parents or caregivers that medication may cause fever and to notify health care professional before administering to a febrile child.
- Geri: Inform male patients with benign prostatic hyperplasia that atropine may cause urinary hesitancy and retention. Changes in urinary stream should be reported to health care professional.

Evaluation/Desired Outcomes

- Increase in heart rate.
- Dryness of mouth.
- Reversal of muscarinic effects.

avanafil (av-an-a-fil)

Stendra

Classification

Therapeutic: erectile dysfunction agents

Pharmacologic: phosphodiesterase type 5 inhibitors

Indications

Treatment of erectile dysfunction.

Action

Enhances effects of nitric oxide released during sexual stimulation. Nitric oxide activates guanylate cyclase, which produces ↑ levels of cyclic guanosine monophosphate (cGMP). cGMP produces smooth muscle relaxation of the corpus cavernosum, which promotes ↑ blood flow and subsequent erection. Inhibits the enzyme phosphodiesterase type 5 (PDE5), PDE5 inactivates cGMP. **Therapeutic Effects:** Enhanced blood flow to the corpus cavernosum and erection sufficient to allow sexual intercourse. Requires sexual stimulation.

Pharmacokinetics

Absorption: Rapidly absorbed following oral administration.

Distribution: Minimal amounts enter semen.

Protein Binding: 99%.

Metabolism and Excretion: Mostly metabolized by the liver (primarily by the CYP3A4 enzyme system), metabolites excreted in feces (62%) and urine (21%). One metabolite had inhibitory activity on PDE5.

Half-life: 5 hr.

TIME/ACTION PROFILE (effect on BP)

ROUTE	ONSET	PEAK	DURATION
PO	within 1 hr	1–2 hr	unknown

Contraindications/Precautions

Contraindicated in: Hypersensitivity; Concurrent use of nitrates or riociguat; Severe renal or hepatic impairment; Concurrent use of strong CYP3A4 inhibitors; Serious underlying cardiovascular disease (including history of MI, stroke, or serious arrhythmia within 6 mo), cardiac failure, or coronary artery disease with unstable angina, angina with sexual intercourse; History of HF, coronary artery disease, uncontrolled hypertension (BP >170/110 mm Hg) or hypotension (BP <90/50 mm Hg), dehydration, autonomic dysfunction, or severe left ventricular outflow obstruction; Hereditary degenerative retinal disorders; Women.

Use Cautiously in: Serious underlying cardiovascular disease or conditions in which sexual activity is not advised; History of sudden severe vision loss or non-arteritic ischemic optic neuropathy (NAION); may ↑ risk of recurrence; Low cup to disk ratio, age >50 yr, diabetes, hypertension, coronary artery disease, hyperlipidemia, or smoking (↑ risk of NAION); Alpha adrenergic blockers (patients should be on stable dose of alpha blockers before treatment, initiate with 50 mg dose); Anatomic penile deformity (angulation, cavernosal fibrosis, Peyronie disease); Conditions associated with priapism (sickle cell anemia, multiple myeloma, leukemia); Concurrent use of moderate CYP3A4 inhibitors (initiate with 50 mg dose); History of hearing loss; Bleeding disorders or peptic ulceration; Geri: Elderly may be more sensitive to drug effects; Pedi: Safety not established.

Adverse Reactions/Side Effects

CNS: headache, dizziness. **EENT:** nasal congestion, nasopharyngitis, sudden hearing/vision loss. **GU:** priapism. **Derm:** flushing. **MS:** back pain.

Interactions

Drug-Drug: Concurrent use of **nitrates** may cause serious, life-threatening hypotension and is contraindicated. Concurrent use of **riociguat** may result in severe hypotension; concurrent use contraindicated. Blood levels and effects may be ↑ by **CYP3A4 inhibitors**, concurrent use of **strong CYP3A4 inhibitors** including **atazanavir**, **clarithromycin**, **indinavir**, **itraconazole**, **ketoconazole**, **nefazodone**, **nelfinavir**, and **saquinavir** is contraindicated. A similar but lesser effect is expected with **moderate CYP3A4 inhibitors** including **erythromycin**, **aprepitant**, **diltiazem**, **fluconazole**, **fosamprenavir**, **ritonavir**, and **verapamil**; initial dose should not exceed 50 mg/24 hr. ↑ risk of hypotension with **alpha-adrenergic blockers**, **antihypertensives**, and **alcohol** (more than 3 units); dosage adjustments may be necessary.

Route/Dosage

PO (Adults): 100 mg 15 min prior to sexual activity, not to exceed once daily (range 50–200 mg, use lowest effective dose); *Concurrent alpha-blockers or moderate CYP3A4 inhibitors*—50 mg, not to exceed once daily.

Availability

Tablets: 50 mg, 100 mg, 200 mg.

NURSING IMPLICATIONS

Assessment

- Determine erectile dysfunction before administration. Avanafil has no effect in the absence of sexual stimulation.

Implementation

- **PO:** Administer dose as needed for erectile dysfunction at least 15 min prior to sexual activity.
- May be administered without regard to food.

Patient/Family Teaching

- Instruct patient to take avanafil as needed for ED at least 15 min before sexual activity and not more than once per day. Inform patient that sexual stimulation is required for an erection to occur after taking avanafil.
- Advise patient that avanafil is not indicated for use in women.
- Caution patient not to take avanafil concurrently with alpha adrenergic blockers (unless on a stable dose) or nitrates. If chest pain occurs after taking avanafil, instruct patient to seek immediate medical attention.
- Advise patient to avoid excess alcohol intake (≥3 units) in combination with avanafil; may increase risk of orthostatic hypotension, increased heart rate, decreased standing BP, dizziness, headache.

- Instruct patient to notify health care professional promptly if erection lasts longer than 4 hr, if they are not satisfied with their sexual performance, develop unwanted side effects or if they experience sudden or decreased vision loss in one or both eyes or loss or decrease in hearing, ringing in the ears, or dizziness.
- Advise patient to notify health care professional of all Rx or OTC medications, vitamins, or herbal products being taken and to consult with health care professional before taking other medications that may interact with avanafil.
- Inform patient that avanafil offers no protection against sexually transmitted diseases. Counsel patient that protection against sexually transmitted diseases and HIV infection should be considered.

Evaluation/Desired Outcomes

- Male erection sufficient to allow intercourse.

azaTHIOprine

(ay-za-**thye**-oh-preen)

Azasan, Imuran

Classification

Therapeutic: immunosuppressants

Pharmacologic: purine antagonists

Indications

Prevention of renal transplant rejection (with corticosteroids, local radiation, or other cytotoxic agents). Treatment of severe, active, erosive rheumatoid arthritis unresponsive to more conventional therapy. **Unlabeled Use:** Management of Crohn's disease or ulcerative colitis.

Action

Antagonizes purine metabolism with subsequent inhibition of DNA and RNA synthesis. **Therapeutic Effects:** Suppression of cell-mediated immunity and altered antibody formation.

Pharmacokinetics

Absorption: Readily absorbed after oral administration.

Distribution: Crosses the placenta. Enters breast milk in low concentrations.

Metabolism and Excretion: Metabolized to 6–mercaptopurine, which is further metabolized (one route is by thiopurine methyltransferase [TPMT] to form an inactive metabolite; nucleotide diphosphatase [NUDT15] is also involved in inactivation process). Minimal renal excretion of unchanged drug.

Half-life: 3 hr.

TIME/ACTION PROFILE

ROUTE	ONSET	PEAK	DURATION
PO (anti-inflammatory)	6–8 wk	12 wk	unknown

Contraindications/Precautions

Contraindicated in: Hypersensitivity; Concurrent use of mycophenolate; OB: Has been shown to cause fetal harm; Lactation: Appears in breast milk.

Use Cautiously in: Infection; Malignancies; ↓ bone marrow reserve; Previous or concurrent radiation therapy; Other chronic debilitating illnesses; Severe renal impairment/oliguria (↑ sensitivity); TPMT or NUDT15 enzyme deficiency (alternative therapy or substantial dose ↓ are required to avoid hematologic adverse events); Rep: Women of reproductive potential; Pedi: ↑ risk of hepatosplenic T-cell lymphoma [HSTCL] in patients with inflammatory bowel disease.

Adverse Reactions/Side Effects

CNS: PROGRESSIVE MULTIFOCAL LEUKOENCEPHALOPATHY. **Derm:** alopecia, rash. **EENT:** retinopathy. **GI:** anorexia, hepatotoxicity, nausea, vomiting, diarrhea, mucositis, pancreatitis. **Hemat:** anemia, leukopenia, pancytopenia, thrombocytopenia. **MS:** arthralgia. **Resp:** pulmonary edema. **Misc:** MALIGNANCY (including post-transplant lymphoma, HSTCL, and skin cancer), SERUM SICKNESS, chills, fever, Raynaud's phenomenon, retinopathy.

Interactions

Drug-Drug: Febuxostat inhibits the metabolism of azathioprine, increasing toxicity; concurrent use not recommended. Additive myelosuppression with **antineoplastics**, **cyclosporine**, and **myelosuppressive agents**. **Allopurinol** inhibits the metabolism of azathioprine, increasing toxicity. Dose of azathioprine should be ↓ to 25–33% of the usual dose when used with allopurinol. May ↓ antibody response to **live-virus vaccines** and ↑ the risk of adverse reactions.

Drug-Natural Products: Concomitant use with **echinacea** and **melatonin** may interfere with immunosuppression.

Route/Dosage

Renal Allograft Rejection Prevention

PO (Adults and Children): 3–5 mg/kg/day initially; maintenance dose 1–3 mg/kg/day.

Rheumatoid Arthritis

PO (Adults and Children): 1 mg/kg/day for 6–8 wk, ↑ by 0.5 mg/kg/day every 4 wk until response or up to 2.5 mg/kg/day, then ↓ by 0.5 mg/kg/day every 4–8 wk to minimal effective dose.

Inflammatory Bowel Disease (Crohn's Disease or Ulcerative Colitis) (unlabeled use)

PO (Adults and Children): 50 mg once daily; may ↑ by 25 mg/day every 1–2 wk as tolerated to target dose of 2–3 mg/kg/day.

Availability (generic available)

Tablets: 50 mg, 75 mg, 100 mg.

NURSING IMPLICATIONS

Assessment

- Assess for infection (vital signs, sputum, urine, stool, WBC) during therapy.
- Monitor intake and output and daily weight. Decreased urine output may lead to toxicity with this medication.
- **Rheumatoid Arthritis:** Assess range of motion; degree of swelling, pain, and strength in affected joints; and ability to perform activities of daily living before and periodically during therapy.
- ***Lab Test Considerations:*** Monitor renal, hepatic, and hematologic functions before beginning therapy, weekly during the 1st mo, bimonthly for the next 2–3 mo, and monthly thereafter.
- Leukocyte count of <3000 or platelet count of <100,000/mm^3 may necessitate a reduction in dose or temporary discontinuation.
- ↓ in hemoglobin may indicate bone marrow suppression.
- Hepatotoxicity may be manifested by ↑ alkaline phosphatase, bilirubin, AST, ALT, and amylase concentrations. Usually occurs within 6 mo of transplant, rarely with rheumatoid arthritis, and is reversible on discontinuation of azathioprine.
- May ↓ serum and urine uric acid and plasma albumin.

Implementation

- Do not confuse azathioprine with azacitidine.
- Protect transplant patients from staff members and visitors who may carry infection. Maintain protective isolation as indicated.
- **PO:** May be administered with or after meals or in divided doses to minimize nausea.

Patient/Family Teaching

- Instruct patient to take azathioprine as directed. If a dose is missed on a once-daily regimen, omit dose; if on several-times-a-day dosing, take as soon as possible or double next dose. Consult health care professional if more than 1 dose is missed or if vomiting occurs shortly after dose is taken. Do not discontinue without consulting health care professional.
- Advise patient to report unusual tiredness or weakness; cough or hoarseness; fever or chills; lower back or side pain; painful or difficult urination; severe diarrhea; black, tarry stools; blood in urine; or transplant rejection to health care professional immediately.
- Reinforce the need for lifelong therapy to prevent transplant rejection.
- Inform patient of increased risk of malignancy.
- Instruct patient to notify health care professional of all Rx or OTC medications, vitamins, or herbal products being taken and consult health care professional before taking any new medications or receiving any vaccinations while taking this medication.
- Advise patient to avoid contact with persons with contagious diseases and persons who have recently taken oral poliovirus vaccine or other live viruses.
- Rep: This drug may have teratogenic properties. Advise patient to use contraception during and for at least 4 mo after therapy is completed and to avoid breast feeding during therapy.
- Emphasize the importance of follow-up exams and lab tests.
- **Rheumatoid Arthritis:** Concurrent therapy with salicylates, NSAIDs, or corticosteroids may be necessary. Patient should continue physical therapy and adequate rest. Explain that joint damage will not be reversed; goal is to slow or stop disease process.

Evaluation/Desired Outcomes

- Prevention of transplant rejection.
- Decreased stiffness, pain, and swelling in affected joints in 6–8 wk in rheumatoid arthritis. Therapy is discontinued if no improvement in 12 wk.

azilsartan, See ANGIOTENSIN II RECEPTOR ANTAGONISTS.

azithromycin

(aye-**zith**-roe-mye-sin)

Zithromax, ~~Zmax~~

Classification

Therapeutic: agents for atypical mycobacterium, anti-infectives

Pharmacologic: macrolides

Indications

Treatment of the following infections due to susceptible organisms: Upper respiratory tract infections, including streptococcal pharyngitis, acute bacterial exacerbations of chronic bronchitis and tonsillitis, Lower respiratory tract infections, including bronchitis and pneumonia, Acute otitis media, Skin and skin structure infections, Nongonococcal urethritis, cervicitis, gonorrhea, and chancroid. Prevention of disseminated *Mycobacterium avium* complex (MAC) infection in patients with advanced HIV infection. **Unlabeled Use:** Prevention of bacterial endocarditis. Treatment of cystic fibrosis lung disease. Treatment and post-exposure prophylaxis of pertussis in infants.

Action

Inhibits protein synthesis at the level of the 50S bacterial ribosome. **Therapeutic Effects:** Bacteriostatic action against susceptible bacteria. **Spectrum:** Active against the following gram-positive aerobic bacteria: *Staphylococcus aureus*, *Streptococcus pneumoniae*, *S. pyogenes* (group A strep). Active against these gram-negative aerobic bacteria: *Haemophilus influenzae*, *Moraxella catarrhalis*, *Neisseria gonorrhoeae*. Also active against: *Bordetella pertussis*, *Mycoplasma*, *Legionella*, *Chlamydia pneumoniae*, *Ureaplasma urealyticum*, *Borrelia burgdorferi*, *M. avium*. Not active against methicillin-resistant *S. aureus*.

Pharmacokinetics

Absorption: Rapidly absorbed (40%) after oral administration. IV administration results in complete bioavailability.

Distribution: Widely distributed to body tissues and fluids. Intracellular and tissue levels exceed those in serum; low CSF levels.

Protein Binding: 7–51%.

Metabolism and Excretion: Mostly excreted unchanged in bile; 4.5% excreted unchanged in urine.

Half-life: 11–14 hr after single dose; 2–4 days after several doses.

TIME/ACTION PROFILE (serum)

ROUTE	ONSET	PEAK	DURATION
PO	rapid	2.5–3.2 hr	24 hr
IV	rapid	end of infusion	24 hr

Contraindications/Precautions

Contraindicated in: Hypersensitivity to azithromycin, erythromycin, or other macrolide anti-infectives; History of cholestatic jaundice or hepatic dysfunction with prior use of azithromycin; QT interval prolongation, hypokalemia, hypomagnesemia, or bradycardia; Concurrent use of quinidine, procainamide, dofetilide, amiodarone, or sotalol.

Use Cautiously in: Severe hepatic impairment (dose adjustment may be required); Severe renal impairment (CCr <10 mL/min); Myasthenia gravis (may worsen symptoms); Geri: May have ↑ risk of QT interval prolongation; OB: Use only if potential maternal benefit justifies potential fetal risk; Lactation: Use during breast feeding only if potential maternal benefit justifies potential risk to infant; Pedi: Neonates (↑ risk of infantile hypertrophic pyloric stenosis at up to 42 days of life).

Adverse Reactions/Side Effects

CNS: dizziness, seizures, drowsiness, fatigue, headache. **CV:** TORSADES DE POINTES, chest pain, hypotension, palpitations, QT interval prolongation. **Derm:** ACUTE GENERALIZED EXANTHEMATOUS PUSTULOSIS, DRUG REACTION WITH EOSINOPHILIA AND SYSTEMIC SYMPTOMS (DRESS), STEVENS-JOHNSON SYNDROME, TOXIC EPIDERMAL NECROLYSIS, photosensitivity, rash. **EENT:** ototoxicity. **F and E:** hyperkalemia. **GI:** HEPATOTOXICITY, CLOSTRIDIUM DIFFICILE-ASSOCIATED DIARRHEA (CDAD), abdominal pain, diarrhea, nausea, cholestatic jaundice, ↑ liver enzymes, dyspepsia, flatulence, melena, oral candidiasis, pyloric stenosis. **GU:** nephritis, vaginitis. **Hemat:** anemia, leukopenia, thrombocytopenia. **Misc:** HYPERSENSITIVITY REACTIONS (including anaphylaxis and angioedema).

Interactions

Drug-Drug: **Quinidine**, **procainamide**, **dofetilide**, **sotalol**, and **amiodarone** may ↑ risk of QT interval prolongation; concurrent use should be avoided. **Aluminum-** and **magnesium-containing antacids** ↓ peak levels. **Nelfinavir** ↑ levels (monitor carefully); azithromycin also ↓ nelfinavir levels. **Efavirenz** ↑ levels. May ↑ the effects and risk of toxicity of **warfarin** and **zidovudine**. Other macrolide anti-infectives have been known to ↑ levels and effects of **digoxin**, **theophylline**, **ergotamine**, **dihydroergotamine**, **triazolam**, **carbamazepine**, **cyclosporine**, **tacrolimus**, and **phenytoin**; careful monitoring of concurrent use is recommended.

Route/Dosage

Most Respiratory and Skin Infections

PO (Adults): 500 mg on 1st day, then 250 mg/day for 4 more days (total dose of 1.5 g); *Acute bacterial sinusitis*— 500 mg once daily for 3 days.

PO (Children ≥ 6 mo): *Pneumonia/Pertussis*— 10 mg/kg (not to exceed 500 mg/dose) on 1st day, then 5 mg/kg once daily (not to exceed 250 mg/dose) for 4 more days. *Pharyngitis/tonsilitis*— 12 mg/kg once daily for 5 days (not to exceed 500 mg/dose); *Acute bacterial sinusitis*— 10 mg/kg once daily for 3 days.

PO (Neonates): *Pertussis, treatment and post-exposure prophylaxis*— 10 mg/kg once daily for 5 days.

Otitis Media

PO (Children ≥6 mo): 30 mg/kg single dose (not to exceed 1500 mg/dose) *or* 10 mg/kg once daily (not to exceed 500 mg/dose) for 3 days *or* 10 mg/kg (not to exceed 500 mg/dose) on 1st day, then 5 mg/kg once daily (not to exceed 250 mg/dose) for 4 more days.

Acute Bacterial Exacerbations of Chronic Bronchitis

PO (Adults): 500 mg on 1st day, then 250 mg once daily for 4 more days (total dose of 1.5 g) *or* 500 mg once daily for 3 days.

Community-Acquired Pneumonia

IV, PO (Adults): *More severe*— 500 mg IV every 24 hr for at least 2 doses, then 500 mg PO every 24 hr for a

🍁 = Canadian drug name. ⚕ = Genetic implication. ~~Strikethrough~~ = Discontinued.
*CAPITALS indicates life-threatening; underlines indicate most frequent.

total of 7–10 days; *Less severe*—500 mg PO, then 250 mg/day PO for 4 more days.

PO (Children >6 mo): 10 mg/kg on 1st day, then 5 mg/kg once daily for 4 more days.

Pelvic Inflammatory Disease

IV, PO (Adults): 500 mg IV every 24 hr for 1–2 days, then 250 mg PO every 24 hr for a total of 7 days.

Endocarditis Prophylaxis

PO (Adults): 500 mg 1 hr before procedure.

PO (Children): 15 mg/kg 1 hr before procedure.

Nongonococcal Urethritis, Cervicitis, Chancroid, Chlamydia

PO (Adults): Single 1-g dose.

PO (Children): *Chancroid:* Single 20-mg/kg dose (not to exceed 1000 mg/dose). *Urethritis or cervicitis:* Single 10-mg/kg dose (not >1000 mg/dose).

Gonorrhea

PO (Adults): Single 2-g dose.

Prevention of Disseminated MAC Infection

PO (Adults): 1.2 g once weekly (alone or with rifabutin).

PO (Children): 5 mg/kg once daily (not >250 mg/dose) or 20 mg/kg (not >1200 mg/dose) once weekly (alone or with rifabutin).

Cystic Fibrosis

PO (Children ≥6 yrs, ≥40 kg): 500 mg every Monday, Wednesday, and Friday.

PO (Children ≥6 yrs, 25 kg to <40 kg): 250 mg every Monday, Wednesday, and Friday.

Availability (generic available)

Powder for injection (requires reconstitution and dilution): 500 mg/vial. **Powder for oral suspension (cherry and banana flavor) (requires reconstitution):** 1 g/pkt. **Cost:** *Generic*—$72.45/3 pkts. **Powder for oral suspension (cherry, creme de vanilla, and banana flavor) (requires reconstitution):** 100 mg/5 mL, 200 mg/5 mL. **Cost:** *Generic*—100 mg/5 mL $34.88/15 mL, 200 mg/5 mL $34.88/22.5 mL. **Tablets:** 250 mg, 500 mg, 600 mg. **Cost:** *Generic*—250 mg $8.82/6, 500 mg $10.03/3, 600 mg $104.62/30.

NURSING IMPLICATIONS

Assessment

- Assess patient for infection (vital signs; appearance of wound, sputum, urine, and stool; WBC) at beginning of and throughout therapy.
- Obtain specimens for culture and sensitivity before initiating therapy. First dose may be given before receiving results.
- Observe for signs and symptoms of anaphylaxis (rash, pruritus, laryngeal edema, wheezing). Notify health care professional immediately if these occur.
- Assess patient for skin rash frequently during therapy. Discontinue azithromycin at first sign of rash; may be life-threatening. Stevens-Johnson syndrome or toxic epidermal necrolysis may develop. Treat symptomatically; may recur once treatment is stopped.
- ***Lab Test Considerations:*** May cause ↑ serum bilirubin, AST, ALT, LDH, and alkaline phosphatase concentrations.
- May cause ↑ creatine phosphokinase, potassium, prothrombin time, BUN, serum creatinine, and blood glucose concentrations.
- May occasionally cause ↓ WBC and platelet count.

Implementation

- **PO:** Administer 1 hr before or 2 hr after meals.
- For administration of single 1-g packet, thoroughly mix entire contents of packet with 2 oz (60 mL) of water. Drink entire contents immediately; add an additional 2 oz of water, mix and drink to assure complete consumption of dose. Do not use the single packet to administer doses other than 1000 mg of azithromycin. Pedi: 1-g packet is not for pediatric use.

IV Administration

- **Intermittent Infusion:** ***Diluent:*** Reconstitute each 500-mg vial with 4.8 mL of sterile water for injection to achieve a concentration of 100 mg/mL. Reconstituted solution is stable for 24 hr at room temperature. Further dilute the 500-mg dose in 250 mL or 500 mL of 0.9% NaCl, 0.45% NaCl, D5W, LR, D5/0.45% NaCl, or D5/LR. Infusion is stable for 24 hr at room temperature or for 7 days if refrigerated. ***Concentration:*** Final concentration of infusion is 1–2 mg/mL. ***Rate:*** Administer the 1-mg/mL solution over 3 hr or the 2-mg/mL solution over 1 hr. Do not administer as a bolus.
- **Y-Site Compatibility:** acyclovir, alemtuzumab, alfentanil, aminocaproic acid, aminophylline, amphotericin B lipid complex, amphotericin B liposome, ampicillin, ampicillin/sulbactam, anidulafungin, argatroban, arsenic trioxide, atracurium, bivalirudin, bleomycin, bumetanide, buprenorphine, butorphanol, calcium chloride, calcium gluconate, cangrelor, carboplatin, carmustine, cefazolin, cefepime, cefotetan, cefoxitin, ceftaroline, ceftazidime, cisatracurium, cisplatin, cyclophosphamide, cyclosporine, cytarabine, dacarbazine, daptomycin, daunorubicin, dexamethasone, dexmedetomidine, dexrazoxane, digoxin, diltiazem, diphenhydramine, dobutamine, docetaxel, dopamine, doxorubicin liposome, doxycycline, droperidol, enalaprilat, ephedrine, epinephrine, eptifibatide, ertapenem, esmolol, etoposide, etoposide phosphate, fenoldopam, fluconazole, fluorouracil, foscarnet, fosphenytoin, ganciclovir, gemcitabine, granisetron, haloperidol, heparin, hetastarch, hydrocortisone, hydromorphone, idarubicin, ifosfamide, irinotecan, isoproterenol, labetalol, leucovorin, lidocaine, linezolid, lorazepam,

magnesium sulfate, mannitol, meperidine, meropenem, mesna, methohexital, methotrexate, methylprednisolone, metoclopramide, milrinone, nalbuphine, naloxone, nitroglycerin, nitroprusside, octreotide, ondansetron, oxaliplatin, oxytocin, paclitaxel, palonosetron, pamidronate, pancuronium, pantoprazole, pemetrexed, pentobarbital, phenobarbital, phenylephrine, potassium acetate, potassium phosphates, procainamide, prochlorperazine, promethazine, propranolol, ranitidine, remifentanil, rocuronium, sodium acetate, sodium bicarbonate, sodium phosphates, succinylcholine, sufentanil, tacrolimus, telavancin, thiotepa, tigecycline, tirofiban, trimethoprim/sulfamethoxazole, vancomycin, vasopressin, vecuronium, verapamil, vincristine, voriconazole, zidovudine, zoledronic acid.

- **Y-Site Incompatibility:** amiodarone, amphotericin B deoxycholate, chlorpromazine, diazepam, doxorubicin, epirubicin, midazolam, mitoxantrone, mycophenolate, nicardipine, pentamidine, phenytoin, quinupristin/dalfopristin, thiopental.

Patient/Family Teaching

- Instruct patients to take medication as directed and to finish the drug completely, even if they are feeling better. Take missed doses as soon as possible unless almost time for next dose; do not double doses. Advise patients that sharing of this medication may be dangerous.
- Instruct patient not to take azithromycin with food or antacids.
- May cause drowsiness and dizziness. Caution patient to avoid driving or other activities requiring alertness until response to medication is known.
- Advise patient to use sunscreen and protective clothing to prevent photosensitivity reactions.
- Advise patient to report symptoms of chest pain, palpitations, yellowing of skin or eyes, or signs of superinfection (black, furry overgrowth on the tongue; vaginal itching or discharge; loose or foul-smelling stools) or rash.
- Instruct patient to notify health care professional if fever and diarrhea develop, especially if stool contains blood, pus, or mucus. Advise patient not to treat diarrhea without advice of health care professional.
- Advise patients being treated for nongonococcal urethritis or cervicitis that sexual partners should also be treated.
- Instruct parents, caregivers, or patient to notify health care professional if symptoms do not improve.
- Rep: Advise female patient of reproductive potential to notify health care professional if pregnancy is planned or suspected or if breast feeding. Advise women to monitor breast-fed infant for diarrhea, vomiting, or rash.

Evaluation/Desired Outcomes

- Resolution of the signs and symptoms of infection. Length of time for complete resolution depends on the organism and site of infection.

aztreonam (az-**tree**-oh-nam)

Azactam, Cayston

Classification

Therapeutic: anti-infectives

Pharmacologic: monobactams

Indications

Treatment of serious gram-negative infections including: Septicemia, Skin and skin structure infections, Intra-abdominal infections, Gynecologic infections, Respiratory tract infections, Urinary tract infections. Useful for treatment of multi-resistant strains of some bacteria including aerobic gram-negative pathogens. **Inhaln:** To improve respiratory symptoms in cystic fibrosis (CF) patients with *Pseudomonas aeruginosa.*

Action

Binds to the bacterial cell wall membrane, causing cell death. **Therapeutic Effects:** Bactericidal action against susceptible bacteria. **Spectrum:** Displays significant activity against gram-negative aerobic organisms only: *Escherichia coli*, *Serratia*, *Klebsiella oxytoca or pneumoniae*, *Citrobacter*, *Proteus mirabilis*, *Pseudomonas aeruginosa*, *Enterobacter*, *Haemophilus influenzae*. Not active against: *Staphylococcus aureus*, *Enterococcus*, *Bacteroides fragilis*, *Streptococci*.

Pharmacokinetics

Absorption: Well absorbed following IM administration. Low absorption follows administration by inhalation.

Distribution: Widely distributed. Crosses the placenta and enters breast milk in low concentrations. High concentrations achieved in sputum with inhalation.

Protein Binding: 56%.

Metabolism and Excretion: 60–70% excreted unchanged by the kidneys. 10% of inhaled dose excreted unchanged in urine. Small amounts metabolized by the liver.

Half-life: Adults: 1.5–2 hr; Children: 1.7 hr; Neonates: 2.4–9 hr(↑ in renal impairment).

TIME/ACTION PROFILE (blood levels)

ROUTE	ONSET	PEAK	DURATION
IM	rapid	60 min	6–8 hr
IV	rapid	end of infusion	6–8 hr
Inhaln	rapid	unknown	Several hr

Contraindications/Precautions

Contraindicated in: Hypersensitivity.

Use Cautiously in: Renal impairment (dosage ↓ required if CCr 30 mL/min or less); Cross-sensitivity with penicillins or cephalosporins may occur rarely. Has been used safely in patients with a history of penicillin or cephalosporin allergy; Patients with FEV_1 <25% or >75% predicted, or patients colonized with *Burkholderia cepacia* (safety and effectiveness not established); OB, Lactation: Safety not established; Pedi: Children <7 yr (inhalation) (safety and effectiveness not established); Geri: Consider age-related ↓ in renal function.

Adverse Reactions/Side Effects

CNS: SEIZURES. **EENT:** nasal congestion (inhalation), nasopharyngeal pain (inhalation). **CV:** chest discomfort (inhalation). **GI:** CLOSTRIDIUM DIFFICILE-ASSOCIATED DIARRHEA (CDAD), abdominal pain (inhalation), altered taste, diarrhea, nausea, vomiting. **Resp:** cough (inhalation), wheezing (inhalation), bronchospasm (inhalation). **Derm:** rash. **Local:** pain at IM site, phlebitis at IV site. **Misc:** allergic reactions including ANAPHYLAXIS, fever (inhalation), superinfection.

Interactions

Drug-Drug: Serum levels may be ↑ by **furosemide** or **probenecid**.

Route/Dosage

IM, IV (Adults): *Moderately severe infections*—1–2 g every 8–12 hr; *severe or life-threatening infections (including those due to Pseudomonas aeruginosa)*—2 g every 6–8 hr; *urinary tract infections*—0.5–1 g every 8–12 hr.

IV (Children 1 mo–16 yr): *Mild to moderate infections*—30 mg/kg every 8 hr; *moderate to severe infections*—30 mg/kg every 6–8 hr; *cystic fibrosis*—50 mg/kg every 6–8 hr.

IV (Neonates >2 kg): 30 mg/kg every 6–8 hr.

IV (Neonates ≤2 kg): 30 mg/kg every 8–12 hr.

Inhaln (Adults and Children >7 yr): 75 mg three times daily for 28 days.

Renal Impairment

IV (Adults): *CCr 10–30 mL/min*—1–2 g initially, then 50% of usual dosage at usual interval; *CCr <10 mL/min*—500 mg–2 g initially, then 25% of usual dosage at usual interval (⅛ of initial dose should also be given after each hemodialysis session).

Availability (generic available)

Injection: 500 mg/vial, 1 g/vial, 2 g/vial. **Premixed containers:** 1 g/50 mL, 2 g/50 mL. **Lyphilized powder for use with diluent provided in Altera Nebulizer System only (Cayston):** 75 mg/vial with 1 mL ampule of diluent (0.17% sodium chloride).

NURSING IMPLICATIONS

Assessment

- Assess for infection (vital signs; wound appearance, sputum, urine, and stool; WBC) at beginning of and throughout therapy.
- Obtain a history before initiating therapy to determine previous use of and reactions to penicillins and cephalosporins. Patients allergic to these drugs may exhibit hypersensitivity reactions to aztreonam. However, aztreonam can often be used in these patients.
- Obtain specimens for culture and sensitivity before initiating therapy. First dose may be given before receiving results.
- Assess respiratory status prior to and following inhalation therapy.
- Observe for signs and symptoms of anaphylaxis (rash, pruritus, laryngeal edema, wheezing). Notify the health care professional immediately if these occur.
- Monitor bowel function. Report diarrhea, abdominal cramping, fever, and bloody stools to health care professional promptly as a sign of Clostridium difficile-associated diarrhea (CDAD). May begin up to several wk following cessation of therapy.
- ***Lab Test Considerations:*** May cause ↑ in AST, ALT, alkaline phosphatase, LDH, and serum creatinine. May cause ↑ prothrombin and partial thromboplastin times, and positive Coombs' test.

Implementation

- After adding diluent to vial, shake immediately and vigorously. Not for multidose use; discard unused solution. IV route is recommended if single dose >1 g or for severe or life-threatening infection.
- **IM:** Use 15-mL vial and dilute each gram of aztreonam with at least 3 mL of 0.9% NaCl, or sterile or bacteriostatic water for injection. Stable at room temperature for 48 hr or 7 days if refrigerated.
- Administer into large, well-developed muscle.

IV Administration

- **IV Push:** Reconstitute 15 mL vial with 6–10 mL of sterile water for injection. ***Rate:*** Administer slowly over 3–5 min by direct injection or into tubing of a compatible solution.
- **Intermittent Infusion:** Reconstitute 15 mL vial with 3 mL of sterile water for injection. ***Diluent:*** Dilute further with 0.9% NaCl, Ringer's or LR, D5W, D10W, D5/0.9% NaCl, D5/0.45% NaCl, D5/0.2% NaCl, D5/LR, or sodium lactate. ***Concentration:*** Do not exceed 50 mg/mL. Solution is stable for 48 hr at room temperature and 7 days if refrigerated. Solutions range from colorless to light, straw yellow or may develop a pink tint upon standing; this does not affect potency. ***Rate:*** Infuse over 20–60 min.
- **Y-Site Compatibility:** alemtuzumab, alfentanil, allopurinol, amifostine, amikacin, aminophylline, amphotericin B lipid complex, anidulafungin, argatroban, ascorbic acid, atracurium, atropine,

benztropine, bivalirudin, bleomycin, bumetanide, buprenorphine, butorphanol, calcium chloride, calcium gluconate, carboplatin, carmustine, caspofungin, cefazolin, cefepime, cefotaxime, cefotetan, cefoxitin, ceftazidime, ceftriaxone, cefuroxime, chloramphenicol, ciprofloxacin, cisatracurium, cisplatin, clindamycin, cyanocobalamin, cyclophosphamide, cyclosporine, cytarabine, dacarbazine, dactinomycin, daptomycin, dexamethasone sodium phosphate, dexmedetomidine, digoxin, diltiazem, dobutamine, docetaxel, dopamine, doxacurium, doxorubicin hydrochloride, doxorubicin liposome, doxycycline, droperidol, enalaprilat, ephedrine, epinephrine, epirubicin, epoetin alfa, eptifibatide, ertapenem, esmolol, etoposide, etoposide phosphate, famotidine, fenoldopam, fentanyl, filgrastim, floxuridine, fluconazole, fludarabine, fluorouracil, folic acid, foscarnet, furosemide, gemcitabine, gentamicin, glycopyrrolate, granisetron, heparin, hetastarch, hydrocortisone, hydromorphone, idarubicin, ifosfamide, insulin, irinotecan, isoproterenol, ketorolac, labetalol, leucovorin, levofloxacin, lidocaine, linezolid, magnesium sulfate, mannitol, melphalan, meperidine, mesna, metaraminol, methotrexate, methoxamine, methyldopate, methylprednisolone sodium succinate, metoclopramide, metoprolol, midazolam, milrinone, morphine, multivitamins, nafcillin, nalbuphine, naloxone, nicardipine, nitroglycerin, nitroprusside, norepinephrine, octreotide, ondansetron, oxacillin, oxaliplatin, oxytocin, paclitaxel, palonosetron, pamidronate, pancuronium, pemetrexed, penicillin G, phenobarbital, phentolamine, phenylephrine, phytonadione, piperacillin/tazobactam, potassium acetate, potassium chloride, procainamide, propofol, propranolol, protamine, pyridoxime, ranitidine, remifentanil, rituximab, rocuronium, sargramostim, sodium acetate, sodium bicarbonate, streptokinase, succinylcholine, sufentanil, tacrolimus, theophylline, thiamine, thiotepa, tigecycline, tirofiban, tobramycin, tolazoline, trimetaphan, vasopressin, vecuronium, verapamil, vinblastine, vincristine, vinorelbine, voriconazole, zidovudine, zoledronic acid.

- **Y-Site Incompatibility:** acyclovir, amphotericin B cholesteryl, amphotericin B deoxycholate, amphotericin B liposome, amsacrine, azathioprine, azithromycin, chlorpromazine, dantrolene, daunorubicin hydrochloride, diazepam, diazoxide, erythromycin, ganciclovir, indomethacin, lorazepam, metronidazole, mitomycin, mitoxantrone, mycophenolate, pantoprazole, papaverine, pentamidine, pentobarbital, phenytoin, prochlorperazine, streptozocin, trastuzumab.
- **Inhaln:** Open glass aztreonam vial by removing metal ring and pulling tab, and removing gray rubber stopper. Twist tip of diluent ampule and squeeze contents into glass aztreonam vial. Replace rubber stopper and swirl gently until contents are completely dissolved. Administer immediately after reconstitution using *Altera Nebulizer System*. Pour reconstituted solution into handset of nebulizer. Turn unit on. Place mouthpiece into mouth and breathe normally only through mouth. Administration takes 2–3 min. Do not use other nebulizers or mix with other medications. Do not administer IV or IM. Refrigerate azotreonam and diluent; may be stored at room temperature for up to 28 days. Protect from light.
- Administer short-acting bronchodilator between 15 min and 4 hr or long-acting bronchodilator between 30 min and 12 hr prior to treatment. If taking multiple inhaled therapies, administer in the following order: bronchodilator, mucolytic, and lastly, aztreonam.

Patient/Family Teaching

- Advise patient to report the signs of superinfection (furry overgrowth on the tongue, vaginal itching or discharge, loose or foul-smelling stools) and allergy.
- Instruct patient to notify health care professional if fever and diarrhea develop, especially if stool contains blood, pus, or mucus. Advise patient not to treat diarrhea without consulting health care professional.
- Advise patient to notify health care professional if new or worsening symptoms or signs of anaphylaxis occur.
- **Inhaln:** Instruct patient to use aztreonam as directed for the full 28–day course, even if feeling better. If a dose is missed, take all 3 daily doses, as long as doses are at least 4 hrs apart. Skipping doses or not completing full course of therapy may decrease effectiveness and increase likelihood of bacterial resistance not treatable in the future. Inform patient of the importance of using a bronchodilator prior to treatment and in use and cleaning of nebulizer.

Evaluation/Desired Outcomes

- Resolution of signs and symptoms of infection. Length of time for complete resolution depends on the organism and site of infection.
- Improvement in respiratory symptoms in patients with cystic fibrosis.

baclofen (bak-loe-fen)

Gablofen, Lioresal, Ozobax

Classification

Therapeutic: antispasticity agents, skeletal muscle relaxants (centrally acting)

Indications

PO: Treatment of reversible spasticity due to multiple sclerosis or spinal cord lesions. **IT:** Treatment of severe spasticity of cerebral or spinal origin (should be reserved for patients who do not respond or are intolerant to oral baclofen) (should wait at least one yr in patients with traumatic brain injury before considering therapy). **Unlabeled Use:** Management of pain in trigeminal neuralgia.

Action

Inhibits reflexes at the spinal level. **Therapeutic Effects:** Decreased muscle spasticity; bowel and bladder function may also be improved.

Pharmacokinetics

Absorption: Well absorbed after oral administration.

Distribution: Widely distributed; crosses the placenta.

Protein Binding: 30%.

Metabolism and Excretion: 70–80% eliminated unchanged by the kidneys.

Half-life: 2.5–4 hr.

TIME/ACTION PROFILE (effects on spasticity)

ROUTE	ONSET	PEAK	DURATION
PO	hr–wk	unknown	unknown
IT	0.5–1 hr	4 hr	4–8 hr

Contraindications/Precautions

Contraindicated in: Hypersensitivity.

Use Cautiously in: Patients in whom spasticity maintains posture and balance; Patients with epilepsy (may ↓ seizure threshold); Renal impairment (↓ dose may be required); OB, Lactation: Safety not established; Pedi: Children <4 yr (intrathecal) (safety not established); Geri: ↑ risk of CNS side effects.

Adverse Reactions/Side Effects

CNS: SEIZURES (IT), dizziness, drowsiness, fatigue, weakness, confusion, depression, headache, insomnia. **CV:** edema, hypotension. **Derm:** pruritus, rash. **EENT:** nasal congestion, tinnitus. **GI:** nausea, constipation. **GU:** frequency. **Metab:** hyperglycemia, ↑ weight. **Neuro:** ataxia. **Misc:** hypersensitivity reactions, sweating.

Interactions

Drug-Drug: ↑ CNS depression with other **CNS depressants** including **alcohol**, **antihistamines**, **opioid analgesics**, and **sedative/hypnotics**. Use with **MAO inhibitors** may lead to ↑ CNS depression or hypotension.

Drug-Natural Products: Concomitant use of **kava-kava**, **valerian**, or **chamomile** can ↑ CNS depression.

Route/Dosage

PO (Adults): 5 mg 3 times daily. May increase every 3 days by 5 mg/dose up to 80 mg/day (some patients may have a better response to 4 divided doses).

PO (Children ≥8 yr): 30–40 mg daily divided every 8 hr; titrate to a maximum of 120 mg/day.

PO (Children 2–7 yr): 20–30 mg daily divided every 8 hr; titrate to a maximum of 60 mg/day.

PO (Children <2 yr): 10–20 mg daily divided every 8 hr; titrate to a maximum of 40 mg/day.

IT (Adults): 100–800 mcg/day infusion; dose is determined by response during screening phase.

IT (Children ≥4 yr): 25–1200 mcg/day infusion (average 275 mcg/day); dose is determined by response during screening phase.

Availability (generic available)

Oral solution (grape flavor): 1 mg/mL. **Solution for intrathecal injection:** 50 mcg/mL, 500 mcg/mL, 1000 mcg/mL, 2000 mcg/mL. **Tablets:** 5 mg, 10 mg, 20 mg. **Cost:** *Generic*— 10 mg $10.83/100, 20 mg $11.04/100.

NURSING IMPLICATIONS

Assessment

- Assess muscle spasticity before and periodically during therapy.
- Observe patient for drowsiness, dizziness, or ataxia. May be alleviated by a change in dose.
- **IT:** Monitor patient closely during test dose and titration. Resuscitative equipment should be immediately available for life-threatening or intolerable side effects.
- ***Lab Test Considerations:*** May cause ↑ in serum glucose, alkaline phosphatase, AST, and ALT levels.

Implementation

- **PO:** Administer with milk or food to minimize gastric irritation.
- **IT:** For *screening phase,* dilute for a concentration of 50 mcg/mL with sterile preservative-free NaCl for injection. Test dose should be administered over at least 1 min. Observe patient for a significant decrease in muscle tone or frequency or severity of spasm. If response is inadequate, 2 additional test doses, each 24 hr apart, 75 mcg/1.5 mL and 100 mcg/2 mL respectively, may be administered. Patients with an inadequate response should not receive chronic IT therapy. Avoid use of prefilled syringes for filling reservoir of pump; prefilled syringes are not sterile.

- Dose titration for implantable IT pumps is based on patient response. If no substantive response after dose increase, check pump function and catheter patency.

Patient/Family Teaching

- Instruct patient to take baclofen as directed. Take a missed dose within 1 hr; do not double doses. Caution patient to avoid abrupt withdrawal of this medication; may precipitate an acute withdrawal reaction (hallucinations, increased spasticity, seizures, mental changes, restlessness). Discontinue baclofen gradually over 2 wk or more.
- May cause dizziness and drowsiness. Advise patient to avoid driving or other activities requiring alertness until response to drug is known.
- Instruct patient to change positions slowly to minimize orthostatic hypotension.
- Advise patient to avoid concurrent use of alcohol or other CNS depressants while taking this medication.
- Instruct patient to notify health care professional if frequent urge to urinate or painful urination, constipation, nausea, headache, insomnia, tinnitus, depression, or confusion persists.
- Advise patient to report signs and symptoms of hypersensitivity (rash, itching) promptly.
- Rep: Advise female patient of reproductive potential to notify health care professional if pregnancy is planned or suspected or if breast feeding. Inform patient that use during pregnancy may cause withdrawal symptoms (increased muscle tone, tremor, jitteriness, seizures) in infants starting hrs to days after delivery.
- **IT:** Caution patient and caregiver not to discontinue IT therapy abruptly. May result in fever, mental status changes, exaggerated rebound spasticity, and muscle rigidity. Advise patient not to miss scheduled refill appointments and to notify health care professional promptly if signs of withdrawal occur.

Evaluation/Desired Outcomes

- Decrease in muscle spasticity and associated musculoskeletal pain with an increased ability to perform activities of daily living.
- Decreased pain in patients with trigeminal neuralgia. May take wk to obtain optimal effect.

baloxavir (ba-**lox**-**a**-veer)

Xofluza

Classification
Therapeutic: antivirals
Pharmacologic: endonuclease inhibitors

Indications

Treatment of acute uncomplicated influenza in patients who have been symptomatic for ≤48 hr.

Action

Inhibits the endonuclease activity of the polymerase acidic protein in the viral RNA polymerase complex that is required for viral gene transcription, thereby resulting in inhibition of influenza virus replication. **Therapeutic Effects:** Reduced duration of flu-related symptoms.

Pharmacokinetics

Absorption: Administered as a prodrug (baloxavir marboxil) which is rapidly absorbed from the GI tract and converted by the liver to the active form, baloxavir.
Distribution: Extensively distributed to tissues.
Protein Binding: 93–94%.
Metabolism and Excretion: Rapidly metabolized by the liver by UGT1A3 to baloxavir, the active metabolite. Primarily excreted in feces (80%); 15% excreted in urine (3% as active metabolite).
Half-life: 79 hr.

TIME/ACTION PROFILE (plasma concentrations)

ROUTE	ONSET	PEAK	DURATION
PO	unknown	4 hr	unknown

Contraindications/Precautions

Contraindicated in: Hypersensitivity.
Use Cautiously in: OB: Use during pregnancy only if potential maternal benefit justifies potential fetal risk; Lactation: Use while breast feeding only if potential maternal benefit justifies potential risk to infant; Pedi: Children <12 yr or <40 kg (safety and effectiveness not established).

Adverse Reactions/Side Effects

CNS: headache. **EENT:** nasopharyngitis. **GI:** diarrhea, nausea.

Interactions

Drug-Drug: Medications containing divalent or trivalent cations, including **calcium**, **iron**, **magnesium**, **selenium**, or **zinc** may ↓ absorption of baloxavir; avoid concurrent use. May ↓ the therapeutic effect of the **live attenuated influenza vaccine**.
Drug-Food: **Calcium** in foods or **dairy products** may ↓ absorption of baloxavir; avoid concurrent administration.

Route/Dosage

PO (Adults and Children ≥12 yr and ≥80 kg): 80 mg as a single dose.
PO (Adults and Children ≥12 yr and 40–<80 kg): 40 mg as a single dose.

Availability

Tablets: 20 mg, 40 mg.

NURSING IMPLICATIONS

Assessment

- Monitor influenza symptoms (sudden onset of fever, cough, headache, fatigue, muscular weakness, sore throat). Additional supportive treatment may be indicated to treat symptoms.

- Monitor for signs and symptoms of hypersensitivity reactions (anaphylaxis, angioedema, urticaria, erythema multiforme) following therapy.

Implementation

- **PO:** Administer 2 tablets without regard to food within 48 hr of onset of symptoms. Avoid taking dairy products, calcium-fortified beverages, polyvalent cation-containing laxatives, antacids or oral supplements (calcium, iron, magnesium, selenium, or zinc) at same time.

Patient/Family Teaching

- Instruct patient to take baloxavir as directed. Advise patient to read *Patient Information* before taking baloxavir.
- Advise patient to notify health care professional immediately if signs and symptoms of hypersensitivity reactions (rash, hives, difficulty breathing, swelling of lips, face, and throat) occur.
- Advise patient to consult health care professional before receiving a live attenuated influenza vaccine after taking baloxavir.
- Advise patient that baloxavir is not a substitute for a flu shot. Patients should receive annual flu shot according to immunization guidelines.
- Advise patient to notify health care professional of all Rx or OTC medications, vitamins, or herbal products being taken and to consult health care professional before taking any new medications.
- Advise females of reproductive potential to notify health care professional if pregnancy is planned or suspected, or if breast feeding.

Evaluation/Desired Outcomes

- Reduced duration or prevention of flu-related symptoms.

baricitinib (bar-i-**sye**-ti-nib)

Olumiant

Classification

Therapeutic: antirheumatics

Pharmacologic: kinase inhibitors

Indications

Moderately to severely active rheumatoid arthritis (RA) in patients who have had an inadequate response/intolerance to ≥1 tumor necrosis factor inhibitor therapies (as monotherapy or in combination with methotrexate or other nonbiologic disease-modifying antirheumatic drugs [DMARDs]) (not to be used with other Janus kinase [JAK] inhibitors, biologic DMARDs or potent immunosuppressants including azathioprine and cyclosporine).

Action

Acts as a JAK inhibitor which prevents the activation of signal transducers and activators of transcription resulting in a reduction in immunoglobulins and C-reactive protein. **Therapeutic Effects:** Improvement in clinical and symptomatic parameters of RA.

Pharmacokinetics

Absorption: Well absorbed following oral administration (80%).

Distribution: Widely distributed into tissues.

Metabolism and Excretion: Metabolized by the liver by CYP3A4; primarily excreted in the urine (69% as unchanged drug); 15% excreted in feces as unchanged drug.

Half-life: 12 hr.

TIME/ACTION PROFILE (clinical improvement)

ROUTE	ONSET	PEAK	DURATION
PO	1 wk	3 mo	unknown

Contraindications/Precautions

Contraindicated in: Active infection; Moderate-to-severe renal impairment (CCr <60 mL/min); Severe hepatic impairment; Increased risk for thrombosis; Absolute lymphocyte count <500 cells/mm^3, absolute neutrophil count (ANC) <1000 cells/mm^3, or hemoglobin levels <8 g/dL; Lactation: Lactation.

Use Cautiously in: Active malignancy (other than non-melanoma skin cancer); Diverticulitis (↑ risk of GI perforation); OB: Use during pregnancy only if potential maternal benefit justifies potential fetal risk; Pedi: Safety and effectiveness not established; Geri: Infection risk may be ↑.

Adverse Reactions/Side Effects

CV: ARTERIAL THROMBOSIS, DEEP VEIN THROMBOSIS. **GI:** GI PERFORATION, ↑ liver enzymes, nausea. **GU:** ↑ serum creatinine. **Hemat:** anemia, lymphopenia, neutropenia, thrombocytosis. **Metab:** ↑ lipids. **MS:** ↑ creatine kinase. **Resp:** PULMONARY EMBOLISM. **Misc:** INFECTION (including tuberculosis, bacterial, invasive fungal infections, viral, and other infections due to opportunistic pathogens), MALIGNANCY.

Interactions

Drug-Drug: Probenecid may ↑ levels and risk of toxicity; avoid concurrent use.

Route/Dosage

PO (Adults): 2 mg once daily.

Availability

Film-coated tablets: 2 mg.

NURSING IMPLICATIONS

Assessment

- Assess pain and range of motion before and periodically during therapy.
- Assess for signs of infection (fever, dyspnea, flu-like symptoms, frequent or painful urination, redness or swelling at the site of a wound), including tuberculosis and hepatitis B virus (HBV), prior to and periodically during therapy. Baricitinib is contraindicated in patients with active infection. New infections should be monitored closely; most common are upper respiratory tract infections, bronchitis, and urinary tract infections. Infections may be fatal, especially in patients taking immunosuppressive therapy.
- Assess patient for latent tuberculosis with a tuberculin skin test prior to initiation of therapy. Treatment of latent tuberculosis should be started before therapy with baricitinib.
- ***Lab Test Considerations:*** May cause neutropenia. Monitor ANC at baseline and periodically during therapy. *If ANC ≥1000 cells/mm³*, maintain dose. *If ANC <1000 cells/mm³*, hold baricitinib until ANC ≥1000 cells/mm³.
- May cause lymphopenia. Monitor absolute lymphocyte count (ALC) at baseline and periodically during therapy. *If ALC ≥500 cells/mm³*, maintain dose. *If ALC <500 cells/mm³*, hold baricitinib until ALC ≥500 cells/mm³. Do not start therapy if ALC <500 cells/mm³.
- May cause anemia. Monitor hemoglobin at baseline and periodically during therapy. *If hemoglobin ≥8 g/dL*, maintain dose. *If hemoglobin <8 g/dL*, hold baricitinib until hemoglobin ≥8 g/dL. Do not start therapy if hemoglobin <8 g/dL.
- Monitor liver enzymes at baseline and periodically during therapy. If elevations in AST or ALT and liver injury is suspected, hold baricitinib until cause determined.
- May cause elevations in serum lipids. Monitor total cholesterol, low-density lipoprotein (LDL) cholesterol, and high-density lipoprotein (HDL) cholesterol 12 wk after starting therapy.

Implementation

- Administer a tuberculin skin test prior to administration of baricitinib. Patients with active latent TB should be treated for TB prior to therapy.
- Immunizations should be current prior to initiating therapy. Patients on baricitinib may receive concurrent vaccinations, except for live vaccines.
- **PO:** Administer once daily without regard to food.

Patient/Family Teaching

- Instruct patient to take baricitinib as directed. Advise patient to read *Medication Guide* before starting therapy and with each Rx refill in case of changes.
- Advise patient to notify health care professional if signs and symptoms of infections (fever; sweating; chills; muscle aches; cough; shortness of breath; blood in your phlegm; weight loss; warm, red, or painful skin or sores on body; diarrhea or stomach pain; burning during urination or urinating more often than normal, feeling tired) blood clots in legs (swelling, pain or tenderness in leg, sudden unexplained chest pain, shortness of breath), stomach problems (fever, stomach-area pain that does not go away, change in bowel habits) occur.
- Advise patient to notify health care professional of all Rx or OTC medications, vitamins, or herbal products being taken and to consult with health care professional before taking other medications.
- Inform patients that baricitinib may increase risk of certain cancers. Instruct patients to notify health care professional if they have ever had any type of cancer.
- Advise patient to avoid live vaccines during therapy.
- Advise patient to notify health care professional if pregnancy is planned or suspected, or if breast feeding.

Evaluation/Desired Outcomes

- Decreased pain and swelling with decreased rate of joint destruction in patients with rheumatoid arthritis.

basiliximab (ba-sil-ix-i-mab)
Simulect

Classification
Therapeutic: immunosuppressants
Pharmacologic: monoclonal antibodies

Indications

Prevention of acute organ rejection in patients undergoing renal transplantation; used with corticosteroids and cyclosporine.

Action

Binds to and blocks specific interleukin-2 (IL-2) receptor sites on activated T lymphocytes. **Therapeutic Effects:** Prevention of acute organ rejection following renal transplantation.

Pharmacokinetics

Absorption: IV administration results in complete bioavailability.

Distribution: Unknown.

Metabolism and Excretion: Unknown.

Half-life: 7.2 days.

TIME/ACTION PROFILE (effect on immune function)

ROUTE	ONSET	PEAK	DURATION
IV	2 hr	unknown	36 days

Contraindications/Precautions

Contraindicated in: Hypersensitivity; OB: May affect fetal developing immune system; Lactation: May enter breast milk.

B

Use Cautiously in: Women with childbearing potential; Geri: Due to greater incidence of infection.

Adverse Reactions/Side Effects

Noted for patients receiving corticosteroids and cyclosporine in addition to basiliximab.
CNS: dizziness, headache, insomnia, weakness.
EENT: abnormal vision, cataracts. **Resp:** coughing.
CV: HEART FAILURE, edema, hypertension, angina, arrhythmias, hypotension. **GI:** abdominal pain, constipation, diarrhea, dyspepsia, moniliasis, nausea, vomiting, GI bleeding, gingival hyperplasia, stomatitis. **Derm:** acne, wound complications, hypertrichosis, pruritus.
Endo: hyperglycemia, hypoglycemia. **F and E:** acidosis, hypercholesterolemia, hyperkalemia, hyperuricemia, hypocalcemia, hypokalemia, hypophosphatemia. **Hemat:** bleeding, coagulation abnormalities.
MS: back pain, leg pain. **Neuro:** tremor, neuropathy, paresthesia. **Misc:** hypersensitivity reactions including ANAPHYLAXIS, infection, weight gain, chills.

Interactions

Drug-Drug: Immunosuppression may be ↑ with other **immunosuppressants**.
Drug-Natural Products: Concommitant use with **echinacea** and **melatonin** may interfere with immunosuppression.

Route/Dosage

IV (Adults and Children ≥35 kg): 20 mg given 2 hr before transplantation; repeated 4 days after transplantation. Second dose should be withheld if complications or graft loss occurs.
IV (Children <35 kg): 10 mg given 2 hr before transplantation; repeated 4 days after transplantation. Second dose should be withheld if complication or graft loss occurs.

Availability

Powder for reconstitution: 20 mg/vial, 10 mg/vial.

NURSING IMPLICATIONS

Assessment

- Monitor for signs of anaphylactic or hypersensitivity reactions (hypotension, tachycardia, cardiac failure, dyspnea, wheezing, bronchospasm, pulmonary edema, respiratory failure, urticaria, rash, pruritus, sneezing) at each dose. Onset of symptoms is usually within 24 hr. Resuscitation equipment and medications for treatment of severe hypersensitivity should be readily available. If a severe hypersensitivity reaction occurs, basiliximab therapy should be permanently discontinued. Patients who have previously received basiliximab should only receive subsequent therapy with extreme caution.
- Monitor for infection (fever, chills, rash, sore throat, purulent discharge, dysuria). Notify physician immediately if these symptoms occur; may necessitate discontinuation of therapy.
- ***Lab Test Considerations:*** May cause ↑ or ↓ hemoglobin, hematocrit, serum glucose, potassium, and calcium concentrations.
- May cause ↑ serum cholesterol levels.
- May cause ↑ BUN, serum creatinine, and uric acid concentrations.
- May cause ↓ serum magnesium, phosphate, and platelet levels.

Implementation

IV Administration

- Basiliximab is usually administered concurrently with cyclosporine and corticosteroids.
- Reconstitute with 2.5 mL or 5 mL of sterile water for injection for the 10 mg or 20 mg vial, respectively. Shake gently to dissolve powder.
- **IV Push:** ***Diluent:*** May be administered undiluted. Bolus administration may be associated with nausea, vomiting, and local reactions (pain). ***Concentration:*** 4 mg/mL. ***Rate:*** Administer over 20–30 min via peripheral or central line.
- **Intermittent Infusion:** ***Diluent:*** Dilute further with 25–50 mL of 0.9% NaCl or D5W. Gently invert bag to mix; do not shake, to avoid foaming. Solution is clear to opalescent and colorless; do not administer solutions that are discolored or contain particulate matter. Discard unused portion. Administer within 4 hr or may be refrigerated for up to 24 hr. Discard after 24 hr. ***Concentration:*** 0.08–0.16 mg/mL. ***Rate:*** Administer over 20–30 min via peripheral or central line.
- **Additive Incompatibility:** Do not admix; do not administer in IV line containing other medications.

Patient/Family Teaching

- Explain purpose of medication to patient. Explain that patient will need to resume lifelong therapy with other immunosuppressive drugs after completion of basiliximab course.
- May cause dizziness. Caution patient to avoid driving or other activities requiring alertness until response is known.
- Instruct patient to continue to avoid crowds and persons with known infections, because basiliximab also suppresses the immune system.

Evaluation/Desired Outcomes

- Prevention of acute organ rejection in patients receiving renal transplantation.

becaplermin (be-kap-lerm-in)

Regranex

Classification

Therapeutic: wound/ulcer/decubiti healing agent

Pharmacologic: platelet-derived growth factors

Indications

Treatment of lower extremity diabetic neuropathic ulcers extending to subcut tissue or beyond and having adequate blood supply.

Action

Promotes chemotaxis of cells involved in wound repair and enhances formation of granulation tissue. **Therapeutic Effects:** Improved healing.

Pharmacokinetics

Absorption: Minimal absorption (<3%).

Distribution: Action is primarily local.

Metabolism and Excretion: Unknown.

Half-life: Unknown.

TIME/ACTION PROFILE (improvement in ulcer healing)

ROUTE	ONSET	PEAK	DURATION
Topical	within 10 wk	unknown	unknown

Contraindications/Precautions

Contraindicated in: Known hypersensitivity to becaplermin or parabens; Known neoplasm at site of application; Wounds that close by primary intention.

Use Cautiously in: Known malignancy; OB, Lactation, Pedi: Safety not established.

Adverse Reactions/Side Effects

Derm: erythematous rash at application site. **Misc:** MALIGNANCY.

Interactions

Drug-Drug: None known.

Route/Dosage

Topical (Adults): Length of gel *in inches* from 15- or 7.5-g tube = length × width of ulcer area × 0.6; from the 2-g tube = length × width of ulcer area × 1.3. Length of gel *in centimeters* from 15- or 7.5-g tube = length × width of ulcer area ÷ 4; from the 2-g tube = length × width of ulcer area ÷ 2; for 12 hr each day.

Availability

Gel: 0.01%.

NURSING IMPLICATIONS

Assessment

- Assess size, color, drainage, and skin surrounding wound at weekly or biweekly intervals. Amount of gel to be applied is recalculated based on wound size.

Implementation

- **Topical:** Calculated amount is applied as a thin layer (1/16-in. thick) and covered with a moist saline dressing for 12 hr; dressing is removed, ulcer rinsed and redressed with moist dressing without becaplermin for rest of day. Process is repeated daily.
- Store gel in refrigerator; do not freeze. Do not use beyond expiration date on crimped end of tube.

Patient/Family Teaching

- Instruct patient on proper technique for application. Wash hands before applying gel and use cotton swab or tongue depressor to aid in application. Tip of tube should not come in contact with ulcer or any other surface; recap tightly after each use. Squeeze calculated amount of gel onto a clean, firm, nonabsorbable surface (wax paper). Spread gel with swab or tongue depressor over the ulcer surface in an even layer to the thickness of a dime. Cover with a saline-moistened gauze dressing.
- Do not apply more than calculated amount; has not been shown to be beneficial. If a dose is missed, apply as soon as remembered. If not remembered until next day, skip dose and return to regular dosing schedule. Do not double doses.
- After 12 hr, rinse ulcer gently with saline or water to remove residual gel and cover with saline-moistened gauze.
- Emphasize the importance of strict wound care and non–weight-bearing program.

Evaluation/Desired Outcomes

- Improved healing of ulcers. If the ulcer does not decrease in size by 30% within 10 wk or if complete healing has not occurred within 20 wk, continuation of therapy should be reassessed.

beclomethasone, See CORTICOSTEROIDS (INHALATION) and CORTICOSTEROIDS (NASAL).

belatacept (be-lat-a-sept)

Nulojix

Classification

Therapeutic: immunosuppressants

Pharmacologic: fusion proteins

Indications

Prevention of organ rejection following kidney transplant in adult patients; in combination with basiliximab induction, mycophenolate, and corticosteroids.

Action

Binds to CD80 and CD86 sites, thereby blocking T-cell costimulation; result is inhibition of T-lymphocyte proliferation and cytokine production. **Therapeutic**

Effects: Prolonged graft survival with decreased production of anti-donor antibodies following kidney transplantation.

Pharmacokinetics

Absorption: IV administration results in complete bioavailability.
Distribution: Unknown.
Metabolism and Excretion: Unknown.
Half-life: 9.8 days.

TIME/ACTION PROFILE

ROUTE	ONSET	PEAK	DURATION
IV	unknown	end of infusion	up to 4 wk

Contraindications/Precautions

Contraindicated in: Epstein-Barr virus (EBV) seronegativity or unknown EBV serostatus; Liver transplantation; Lactation: Avoid breast feeding.
Use Cautiously in: Cytomegalovirus (CMV) infection/T-cell depleting therapy (↑ risk of post-transplant lymphoproliferative disorder [PTLD]), CMV prophylaxis recommended for 3 mo following transplant; Change in body weight >10% (dose adjustment recommended); Unknown tuberculosis status (latent infection should be treated prior to use); Evidence of polyoma virus-associated nephropathy (PVAN), ↓ immunosuppression may be necessary; OB: Use only if potential benefit to mother outweighs potential risk to fetus; Pedi: Safety and effectiveness not established.

Adverse Reactions/Side Effects

CNS: PROGRESSIVE MULTIFOCAL LEUKOENCEPHALOPATHY (PML), headache. **Resp:** cough. **CV:** hypertension, peripheral edema. **GI:** constipation, diarrhea, nausea, vomiting. **GU:** proteinuria. **Endo:** new-onset diabetes mellitus. **F and E:** hyperkalemia, hypokalemia. **Hemat:** anemia, leukopenia. **Misc:** POST-TRANSPLANT LYMPHOPROLIFERATIVE DISORDER (PTLD), ↑ RISK OF MALIGNANCY, SERIOUS INFECTIONS, fever, graft dysfunction, infusion reactions.

Interactions

Drug-Drug: May ↓ antibody response to and ↑ risk of adverse reactions from **live virus vaccines**; avoid use during treatment. May ↑ levels and toxicity of **mycophenolate mofetil**; ↓ dose of mycophenolate mofetil. Concurrent use with **antithymocyte globulin** may ↑ risk of venous thrombosis of renal allograft; separate administration by 12 hr.

Route/Dosage

Prescribed dose must be evenly divisible by 12.5 to ensure accurate preparation.
IV (Adults): *Initial phase*—10 mg/kg on day of transplant/prior to implantation, day 5 (96 hr after day 1 dose), and at end of wk 2, 4, 8, and 12 following transplantation; *Maintenance phase*—10 mg/kg at end of wk 16 and then every 4 wk (±3 days).

Availability

Lyophilized powder for injection (requires reconstitution): 250 mg/vial.

NURSING IMPLICATIONS

Assessment

- Assess for symptoms of organ rejection throughout therapy.
- Assess for signs of progressive multifocal leukoencephalopathy (hemiparesis, apathy, confusion, cognitive deficiencies, and ataxia) periodically during therapy.
- Monitor for signs and symptoms of infection (fever, dyspnea) periodically during therapy.
- Assess for signs and symptoms of post-transplant lymphoproliferative disorder (changes in mood or usual behavior, confusion, problems thinking, loss of memory, changes in walking or talking, decreased strength or weakness on one side of the body, changes in vision) during and for at least 36 mo post-transplant.
- Monitor for infusion reactions (hypotension, hypertension) during therapy.
- ***Lab Test Considerations:*** May cause hyperkalemia, hypokalemia, hypophosphatemia, hyperglycemia, hypocalcemia, hypercholesterolemia, hypomagnesemia, and hyperuricemia.

Implementation

- Pre-medication is not required.
- Cortisone doses should be consistent with clinical trials experience. Cortisone doses were tapered to between 10–20 mg/day by first 6 wk after transplant, then remained at 10 mg (5–10 mg) per day for first 6 mo after transplant.
- Treat patient for latent tuberculosis prior to therapy.
- Prophylaxis for *Pneumocystis jiroveci* is recommended after transplant.

IV Administration

- **Intermittent Infusion:** Calculate number of vials required for total infusion dose. Reconstitute contents of each vial with 10.5 mL of 0.9% NaCl or D5W using the silicone-free disposable syringe provided and an 18–21 gauge needle for a concentration of 25 mg/mL. Direct stream of diluent to wall of vial. Rotate and invert vial gently; do not shake to avoid foaming. Solution is clear to slightly opalescent and colorless to pale yellow; do not use if opaque particles, discoloration, or other particles are present. Calculate total volume needed for infusion dose. ***Diluent:*** Dilute further with 0.9% NaCl or D5W if reconstituted with sterile water for injection, 0.9%

NaCl if reconstituted with 0.9% NaCl, or with D5W if reconstituted with D5W. ***Concentration:*** 2 mg/mL. Withdraw amount of diluent from infusion container equal to volume of infusion dose. Using same silicone-free disposable syringe used for reconstitution, withdraw required amount of belatacept solution from vial, inject into infusion container, and rotate gently to mix. Typical infusion volume is 100 mL, but may range from 50–250 mL. Transfer from vial to infusion container immediately; infusion must be completed within 24 hr of reconstitution. May be refrigerated and protected from light for 24 hr. Do not administer solutions that are discolored or contain particulate matter. Discard unused solution in vials. ***Rate:*** Infuse over 30 min using a non-pyrogenic, low-protein-binding filter with 0.2–1.2 micron pore size.

- **Y-Site Incompatibility:** Do not mix or infuse in same line with other agents.

Patient/Family Teaching

- Reinforce the need for lifelong therapy to prevent transplant rejection. Review symptoms of rejection for the transplanted organ, and stress need to notify health care professional immediately if signs of rejection or infection occur.
- Advise patient to avoid contact with persons with contagious diseases.
- Inform patient of the increased risk of skin cancer and other malignancies. Advise patient to use sunscreen with a high protection factor and wear protective clothing to decrease risk of skin cancer.
- Advise patient to notify health care professional of all Rx or OTC medications, vitamins, or herbal products being taken and to consult with health care professional before taking other medications.
- Advise patient to notify health care professional immediately if signs or symptoms of infection, post-transplant lymphoproliferative disorder or progressive multifocal leukoencephalopathy occur.
- Advise patients to avoid live vaccines during therapy.
- Rep: Advise female patients to notify health care professional if pregnancy is planned or suspected or if breast feeding. Encourage patients who become pregnant or whose partners have received belatacept to register with the National Transplant Pregnancy Registry (NTPR) by calling 1-877-955-6877.
- Emphasize the importance of routine follow-up laboratory tests.

Evaluation/Desired Outcomes

- Prevention of rejection of transplanted kidneys.

belimumab (be-li-moo-mab)

Benlysta

Classification

Therapeutic: immunosuppressants

Pharmacologic: monoclonal antibodies

Indications

Active autoantibody-positive systemic lupus erythematosus (SLE) in patients currently receiving standard therapy.

Action

A monoclonal antibody produced by recombinant DNA technique that specifically binds.to B-lymphocyte stimulator protein (BLyS), thereby inactivating it. **Therapeutic Effects:** ↓ survival of B cells, including autoreactive ones and ↓ differentiation into immunoglobulin-producing plasma cells. Result is ↓ disease activity with lessened damage/improvement in mucocutaneous, musculoskeletal, and immunologic manifestations of SLE.

Pharmacokinetics

Absorption: 74% absorbed after subcut administration; IV administration results in complete bioavailability.

Distribution: Unknown.

Metabolism and Excretion: Unknown.

Half-life: 19.4 days.

TIME/ACTION PROFILE (reduction in activated B cells)

ROUTE	ONSET	PEAK	DURATION
IV or subcut	8 wk	unknown	52 wk†

†With continuous treatment.

Contraindications/Precautions

Contraindicated in: Hypersensitivity; Concurrent use of other biologicals or cyclophosphamide; Concurrent use of live vaccines; Receiving therapy for chronic infection.

Use Cautiously in: Infections (consider temporary withdrawal for acute infections, treat aggressively); Previous history of depression or suicidal ideation (may worsen); OB, Lactation: Use only if potential maternal benefit outweighs potential fetal risk; Rep: Women of reproductive potential; Pedi: Children <5 yr (safety and effectiveness not established); Geri: May be more sensitive to drug effects, consider age-related changes in renal, hepatic and cardiac function, concurrent drug therapy, and chronic disease states.

Adverse Reactions/Side Effects

CNS: PROGRESSIVE MULTIFOCAL LEUKOENCEPHALOPATHY (PML), SUICIDAL IDEATION/BEHAVIOR, depression, insomnia, migraine, anxiety, fatigue. **Derm:** rash. **GI:** nausea, diarrhea. **GU:** cystitis. **Hemat:** leukopenia. **MS:** extremity pain, myalgia. **Misc:** ANAPHYLAXIS, INFECTION, infusion reactions, fever, facial edema.

Interactions

Drug-Drug: ↑ risk of adverse reactions and ↓ immune response to **live vaccines**; should not be given concurrently.

Route/Dosage

IV (Adults and Children ≥5 yr): 10 mg/kg every 2 wk for 3 doses, then 10 mg/kg every 4 wk.
Subcut (Adults): 200 mg once weekly; if transitioning from IV therapy, give first subcut dose 1–4 wk after last IV dose.

Availability

Lyophilized powder for injection (requires reconstitution and dilution): 120 mg/vial, 400 mg/vial. **Solution for injection (prefilled syringes and autoinjectors):** 200 mg/mL.

NURSING IMPLICATIONS

Assessment

- Monitor patient for signs of anaphylaxis (hypotension, angioedema, urticaria, rash, pruritus, wheezing, dyspnea, facial edema) during and following injection. Medications (antihistamines, corticosteroids, epinephrine) and equipment should be readily available in the event of a severe reaction. Discontinue belimumab immediately if anaphylaxis or other severe allergic reaction occurs.
- Monitor for infusion reactions (headache, nausea, skin reactions, bradycardia, myalgia, headache, rash, urticaria, hypotension). There is insufficient evidence to determine whether premedication diminishes frequency or severity. Infusion rate may be slowed or interrupted if an infusion reaction occurs.
- Assess for signs of infection (fever, dyspnea, flu-like symptoms, frequent or painful urination, redness or swelling at the site of a wound), including tuberculosis, prior to injection. Belimumab is contraindicated in patients with active infection. New infections should be monitored closely; most common are upper respiratory tract infections, bronchitis, and urinary tract infections. Signs and symptoms of inflammation may be lessened due to suppression from belimumab. Infections may be fatal, especially in patients taking immunosuppressive therapy. If patient develops a serious infection, consider discontinuing belimumab until infection is controlled.
- Assess mental status and mood changes. Inform health care professional if patient demonstrates significant ↑ in depressed mood, anxiety, nervousness, or insomnia.
- Assess for signs of progressive multifocal leukoencephalopathy (hemiparesis, apathy, confusion, cognitive deficiencies, and ataxia) periodically during therapy.

Implementation

- Consider premedication for prophylaxis against infusion reactions and hypersensitivity reactions.
- **Subcut:** Allow autoinjector or prefilled syringe to sit at room temperature for 30 min prior to injection; do not use other methods of warming. Solution is clear to opalescent and colorless to pale yellow. Do not inject solutions that are discolored or contain particulate matter. Administer first injection under supervision of health care professional into abdomen or thigh. Rotate injection sites each wk. Avoid areas of tenderness, bruising, redness, or hardness. Refrigerate autoinjectors and prefilled syringes prior to use; do not freeze or shake. Avoid exposure to heat. May be stored at room temperature if protected from sunlight for up to 12 hrs.

IV Administration

- **Intermittent Infusion:** Remove belimumab from refrigerator and allow to stand 10–15 min to reach room temperature. Using a 21–25 gauge needle, reconstitute 120 mg vial with 1.5 mL and 400 mg vial with 4.8 mL of sterile water for injection by directing stream toward side of vial to minimize foaming. Swirl gently for 60 sec. Allow vial to sit at room temperature during reconstitution, swirling gently for 60 sec every 5 min until powder is dissolved. Do not shake. Reconstitution usually takes 10–15 min, but may take up to 30 min. Protect from sunlight. Solution is opalescent and colorless to pale yellow and without particles. Small bubbles are expected and acceptable. ***Concentration:*** 80 mg/mL. ***Diluent:*** 0.9% NaCl, 0.45% NaCl or LR. Remove volume of patient's dose from a 250 mL infusion bag and discard. Replace with required amount of reconstituted solution. Gently invert bag to mix. Do not administer solutions that are discolored or contain particulate matter. Discard unused solution in vial. If not used immediately, refrigerate and protect from light. Solution is stable for 8 hrs. ***Rate:*** Infuse over 1 hr; may slow or interrupt rate if patient develops an infusion reaction.
- **Y-Site Incompatibility:** Do not administer with dextrose solutions or other solutions or medications.

Patient/Family Teaching

- Instruct patient in correct technique for subcut injection. Inject on the same day each wk. Inject missed doses as soon as remembered, then resume on usual day or start a new weekly schedule from the day missed dose was administered. Do not inject 2 doses on same day. Advise patient to read *Medication Guide* prior to each treatment session in case of changes.
- Caution patient to notify health care professional immediately if signs of infection (fever, sweating, chills, muscle aches, cough, shortness of breath, blood in phlegm, weight loss, warm, red or painful skin or sores, diarrhea or stomach pain, burning on urination, urinary frequency, feeling tired), progressive multifocal leukoencephalopathy, severe rash, swollen face, or difficulty breathing occurs while taking.

- Advise patient, family, and caregivers to look for depression and suicidality, especially during early therapy or dose changes. Notify health care professional immediately if thoughts about suicide or dying, attempts to commit suicide; new or worse depression or anxiety; agitation or restlessness; panic attacks; insomnia; new or worse irritability; aggressiveness; acting on dangerous impulses, mania, or other changes in mood or behavior, or if symptoms of serotonin syndrome occur.
- Caution patient to avoid receiving live vaccines for 30 days before and during belimumab therapy.
- Instruct patient to notify health care professional of all Rx or OTC medications, vitamins, or herbal products being taken and consult health care professional before taking any new medications.
- Rep: Advise women of childbearing potential to use adequate contraception during and for at least 4 mo after final treatment and to notify health care professional if breast feeding. Encourage pregnant patients to enroll in registry by calling 1-877-681-6296.

Evaluation/Desired Outcomes

- Improvement in mucocutaneous, musculoskeletal, and immunologic disease activity in patients with SLE.

benazepril, **See ANGIOTENSIN-CONVERTING ENZYME (ACE) INHIBITORS.**

benralizumab

(ben-ra-**liz**-ue-mab)

Fasenra

Classification

Therapeutic: antiasthmatics

Pharmacologic: monoclonal antibodies, interleukin antagonists

Indications

Add-on maintenance treatment of severe asthma that is of an eosinophilic phenotype.

Action

Interleukin-5 (IL-5) antagonist that inhibits binding of IL-5 to the surface of the eosinophil, which reduces the production and survival of eosinophils. **Therapeutic Effects:** Decreased incidence of asthma exacerbations. Reduction in use of maintenance oral corticosteroid therapy.

Pharmacokinetics

Absorption: 58% absorbed following subcut administration.

Distribution: Minimally distributed to tissues.

Metabolism and Excretion: Degraded by proteolytic enzymes located throughout the body.

Half-life: 15 days.

TIME/ACTION PROFILE (blood levels)

ROUTE	ONSET	PEAK	DURATION
Subcut	unknown	unknown	unknown

Contraindications/Precautions

Contraindicated in: Hypersensitivity; Acute bronchospasm or status asthmaticus.

Use Cautiously in: Pre-existing helminth infections; OB: Use only if potential maternal benefit outweighs potential fetal risk; Lactation: Use only if potential maternal benefit outweighs potential risk to child; Pedi: Children <12 yr (safety and effectiveness not established).

Adverse Reactions/Side Effects

CNS: headache. **EENT:** pharyngitis. **Misc:** HYPERSENSITIVITY REACTIONS (including anaphylaxis, angioedema, urticaria, and rash), fever, injection site reactions.

Interactions

Drug-Drug: None known.

Route/Dosage

Subcut (Adults and Children ≥12 yr): 30 mg every 4 wk for first three doses, then 30 mg every 8 wk thereafter.

Availability

Solution for subcut injection (prefilled syringe): 30 mg/mL.

NURSING IMPLICATIONS

Assessment

- Assess lung sounds, pulse, and BP periodically during therapy. Note amount, color, and character of sputum produced.
- Monitor for signs and symptoms of hypersensitivity reactions (rash, pruritus, hives, swelling of face and neck, dyspnea, fainting, dizziness, feeling lightheaded) periodically during therapy; usually occur within hrs, but may occur days after injection. Discontinue medication if reaction occurs.

Implementation

- **Subcut:** Administer every 4 wk for the 1st three doses and every 8 wk thereafter in upper arm, thigh or abdomen. Store in refrigerator; protect from light. Do not freeze or shake. Leave carton at room temperature for 30 min before administration. Solution is clear to opalescent, colorless to slightly yellow; may contain a few translucent or white to off-white particles. Do not administer if liquid is cloudy, discolored, or contains large particles or foreign particulate matter. Do not expel the air bubble prior to administration. Pinch skin to inject medication.

Patient/Family Teaching

- Instruct patient to have medication administered by health care professional as scheduled.
- Advise patient that benralizumab should not be used to treat an acute asthma attack. Patient should con-

tinue asthma medications, including corticosteroids, unless otherwise instructed by health care professional.

- Advise patient to stop using medication and notify health care professional immediately if signs and symptoms of hypersensitivity reactions occur.
- Instruct patient to notify health care professional of all Rx or OTC medications, vitamins, or herbal products being taken and to consult health care professional before taking any OTC medications or alcoholic beverages concurrently with this therapy. Caution patient also to avoid smoking and other respiratory irritants.
- Instruct patient whose systemic corticosteroids have been recently reduced or withdrawn to carry a warning card indicating the need for supplemental systemic corticosteroids in the event of stress or severe asthma attack unresponsive to bronchodilators.
- Advise patient to have helminth infections treated before starting benralizumab therapy.
- Advise female patients to notify health care professional if pregnancy is planned or suspected or if breast feeding.

Evaluation/Desired Outcomes

- Decreased incidence of asthma exacerbations. Reduction in use of maintenance oral corticosteroid therapy.

benzathine penicillin G, **See PENICILLINS.**

BEERS

benztropine (benz-troe-peen)

Cogentin

Classification

Therapeutic: antiparkinson agents

Pharmacologic: anticholinergics

Indications

Adjunctive treatment of all forms of Parkinson's disease, including drug-induced extrapyramidal effects and acute dystonic reactions.

Action

Blocks cholinergic activity in the CNS, which is partially responsible for the symptoms of Parkinson's disease. Restores the natural balance of neurotransmitters in the CNS. **Therapeutic Effects:** Reduction of rigidity and tremors.

Pharmacokinetics

Absorption: Well absorbed following PO and IM administration.

Distribution: Unknown.

Metabolism and Excretion: Unknown.

Half-life: Unknown.

TIME/ACTION PROFILE (antidyskinetic activity)

ROUTE	ONSET	PEAK	DURATION
PO	1–2 hr	several days	24 hr
IM, IV	within min	unknown	24 hr

Contraindications/Precautions

Contraindicated in: Hypersensitivity; Children <3 yr; Angle-closure glaucoma; Tardive dyskinesia.

Use Cautiously in: Prostatic hyperplasia; Seizure disorders; Cardiac arrhythmias; OB, Lactation: Safety not established; Geri: ↑ risk of adverse reactions.

Adverse Reactions/Side Effects

CNS: confusion, depression, dizziness, hallucinations, headache, sedation, weakness. **EENT:** blurred vision, dry eyes, mydriasis. **CV:** arrhythmias, hypotension, palpitations, tachycardia. **GI:** constipation, dry mouth, ileus, nausea. **GU:** hesitancy, urinary retention. **Misc:** decreased sweating.

Interactions

Drug-Drug: Additive anticholinergic effects with **drugs sharing anticholinergic properties**, such as **antihistamines, phenothiazines, quinidine, disopyramide**, and **tricyclic antidepressants**. Counteracts the cholinergic effects of **bethanechol**. **Antacids** and **antidiarrheals** may ↓ absorption.

Drug-Natural Products: ↑ anticholinergic effect with **angel's trumpet, jimson weed**, and **scopolia**.

Route/Dosage

Parkinsonism

PO (Adults): 1–2 mg/day in 1–2 divided doses (range 0.5–6 mg/day).

Acute Dystonic Reactions

IM, IV (Adults): 1–2 mg, then 1–2 mg PO twice daily.

Drug-Induced Extrapyramidal Reactions

PO, IM, IV (Adults): 1–4 mg given once or twice daily (1–2 mg 2–3 times daily may also be used PO).

Availability (generic available)

Tablets: 0.5 mg, 1 mg, 2 mg. **Cost:** *Generic*—0.5 mg $26.07/100, 1 mg $25.74/100, 2 mg $51.86/100. **Injection:** 1 mg/mL.

NURSING IMPLICATIONS

Assessment

- Assess parkinsonian and extrapyramidal symptoms (restlessness or desire to keep moving, rigidity, tremors, pill rolling, masklike face, shuffling gait, muscle spasms, twisting motions, difficulty speaking or swallowing, loss of balance control) before and throughout therapy.

- Assess bowel function daily. Monitor for constipation, abdominal pain, distention, or absence of bowel sounds.
- Monitor intake and output ratios and assess patient for urinary retention (dysuria, distended abdomen, infrequent voiding of small amounts, overflow incontinence).
- Patients with mental illness are at risk of developing exaggerated symptoms of their disorder during early therapy with benztropine. Withhold drug and notify physician or other health care professional if significant behavioral changes occur.
- **IM/IV:** Monitor pulse and BP closely and maintain bedrest for 1 hr after administration. Advise patients to change positions slowly to minimize orthostatic hypotension.

Implementation

- **PO:** Administer with food or immediately after meals to minimize gastric irritation. May be crushed and administered with food if patient has difficulty swallowing.
- **IM:** Parenteral route is used only for dystonic reactions.

IV Administration

- **IV Push:** IV route is rarely used because onset is same as with IM route. ***Rate:*** Administer at a rate of 1 mg over 1 min.
- **Y-Site Compatibility:** alfentanil, amikacin, aminophylline, ascorbic acid, atracurium, atropine, azathioprine, aztreonam, bumetanide, buprenorphine, butorphanol, calcium chloride, calcium gluconate, cefazolin, cefotaxime, cefotetan, cefoxitin, ceftazidime, ceftriaxone, cefuroxime, chlorpromazine, clindamycin, cyanocobalamin, cyclosporine, dexamethasone, digoxin, diphenhydramine, dobutamine, dopamine, doxycycline, enalaprilat, ephedrine, epinephrine, epoetin alfa, erythromycin, esmolol, famotidine, fentanyl, fluconazole, folic acid, gentamicin, glycopyrrolate, heparin, hydrocortisone, imipenem/cilastatin, insulin, isoproterenol, ketorolac, labetalol, lidocaine, magnesium sulfate, mannitol, meperidine, metaraminol, methyldopate, methylprednisolone, metoclopramide, metoprolol, midazolam, morphine, multivitamins, nafcillin, nalbuphine, naloxone, nitroglycerin, nitroprusside, norepinephrine, ondansetron, oxacillin, oxytocin, papaverine, penicillin G, pentamidine, phenobarbital, phentolamine, phenylephrine, phytonadione, potassium chloride, procainamide, prochlorperazine, promethazine, propranolol, protamine, pyridoxime, ranitidine, sodium bicarbonate, streptokinase, succinylcholine, sufentanil, tacrolimus, theophylline, thiamine, tobramycin, tolazoline, vancomycin, vasopressin, verapamil.
- **Y-Site Incompatibility:** amphotericin B deoxycholate, chloramphenicol, dantrolene, diazepam, diazoxide, furosemide, ganciclovir, indomethacin, pentobarbital, phenytoin, sulfamethoxazole/trimethoprim.

Patient/Family Teaching

- Encourage patient to take benztropine as directed. Take missed doses as soon as possible, up to 2 hr before the next dose. Taper gradually when discontinuing or a withdrawal reaction may occur (anxiety, tachycardia, insomnia, return of parkinsonian or extrapyramidal symptoms).
- May cause drowsiness or dizziness. Advise patient to avoid driving or other activities that require alertness until response to the drug is known.
- Instruct patient that frequent rinsing of mouth, good oral hygiene, and sugarless gum or candy may decrease dry mouth. Patient should notify health care professional if dryness persists (saliva substitutes may be used). Also, notify the dentist if dryness interferes with use of dentures.
- Caution patient to change positions slowly to minimize orthostatic hypotension.
- Instruct patient to notify health care professional if difficulty with urination, constipation, abdominal discomfort, rapid or pounding heartbeat, confusion, eye pain, or rash occurs.
- Advise patient to confer with health care professional before taking OTC medications, especially cold remedies, or drinking alcoholic beverages.
- Caution patient that this medication decreases perspiration. Overheating may occur during hot weather. Patient should notify health care professional if unable to remain indoors in an air-conditioned environment during hot weather.
- Advise patient to avoid taking antacids or antidiarrheals within 1–2 hr of this medication.
- Emphasize the importance of routine follow-up exams.

Evaluation/Desired Outcomes

- Decrease in tremors and rigidity and an improvement in gait and balance. Therapeutic effects are usually seen 2–3 days after the initiation of therapy.

betamethasone, See CORTICOSTEROIDS (SYSTEMIC) and CORTICOSTEROIDS (TOPICAL/LOCAL).

betrixaban (be-**trix**-a-ban)

Bevyxxa

Classification

Therapeutic: anticoagulants
Pharmacologic: factor Xa inhibitors

Indications
Prevention of venous thromboembolism in patients hospitalized for an acute medical illness who are at increased risk for thromboembolic events.

Action
Selective inhibitor of factor Xa. Decreases thrombin generation and thrombus development. Does not inhibit platelet aggregation. **Therapeutic Effects:** Prevention of deep vein thrombosis and pulmonary embolism.

Pharmacokinetics
Absorption: 34% absorbed following oral administration. Bioavailability ↓ by food.
Distribution: Widely distributed.
Metabolism and Excretion: Undergoes minimal metabolism. Primarily excreted unchanged in the feces; 18% excreted unchanged in urine.
Half-life: 19–27 hr.

TIME/ACTION PROFILE (anticoagulant effect)

ROUTE	ONSET	PEAK	DURATION
PO	unknown	3–4 hr	24 hr

Contraindications/Precautions
Contraindicated in: Hypersensitivity; Active bleeding; Prosthetic heart valve; Moderate or severe hepatic impairment.
Use Cautiously in: Neuraxial anesthesia/spinal puncture (↑ risk of spinal/epidural hematoma and potential paralysis); Severe renal impairment (dose ↓ required for CCr 15–29 mL/min); OB: Use only if potential maternal benefit justifies potential fetal risk; Lactation: Use while breast feeding only if potential maternal benefit justifies potential risk to infant; Pedi: Safety and effectiveness not established.

Adverse Reactions/Side Effects
F and E: hypokalemia. **GI:** constipation. **Hemat:** BLEEDING.

Interactions
Drug-Drug: ↑ risk of bleeding with other **anticoagulants**, **aspirin**, **clopidogrel**, **ticagrelor**, **prasugrel**, **fibrinolytics**, **NSAIDs**, **SNRIs**, or **SSRIs**. **P-gp inhibitors**, including **amiodarone**, **azithromycin**, **clarithromycin**, **ketoconazole** (oral), or **verapamil** may ↑ levels and risk of bleeding; ↓ betrixaban dose. **P-glycoprotein inducers**, including **carbamazepine**, **phenytoin**, or **rifampin** may ↓ levels and efficacy; avoid concurrent use.

Route/Dosage
PO (Adults): 160 mg on Day 1, then 80 mg once daily starting on Day 2 for a total duration of 35–42 days; *Concurrent use of P-gp inhibitor*—80 mg on Day 1, then 40 mg once daily starting on Day 2 for a total duration of 35–42 days.

Renal Impairment
(Adults): *CCr 15–29 mL/min*—80 mg on Day 1, then 40 mg once daily starting on Day 2 for a total duration of 35–42 days.

Availability
Capsules: 40 mg, 80 mg.

NURSING IMPLICATIONS

Assessment
- Monitor for bleeding. Discontinue betrixaban if active pathological bleeding occurs. Concomitant drugs (aspirin, other antiplatelet agents, other antithrombotic agents, fibrinolytic therapy, chronic use of NSAIDs) may increase risk of bleeding. Anticoagulant effects of betrixaban persist for about 72 hr after last dose; there is no established way to reverse anticoagulant effects. Anticoagulant effects cannot be reliably monitored with standard laboratory tests. No reversal agent is available; protamine sulfate, vitamin K, and tranexamic acid do not reverse anticoagulant activity. Effects of hemodialysis are unknown.
- Monitor frequently for signs and symptoms of neurological impairment (numbness or weakness of legs, bowel, or bladder dysfunction, back pain, tingling, muscle weakness); if noted, urgent treatment is required. Intrathecal or epidural catheters should not be removed earlier than 72 hr after last dose of betrixaban. Next dose of betrixaban should be given >5 hr after removal of catheter.

Implementation
- **PO:** Administer once daily with food.

Patient/Family Teaching
- Instruct patient to take betrixaban as directed. Take missed doses as soon as remembered on same day. Return to regular schedule next day. Do not double doses in one day. Do not discontinue without consulting health care professional; stopping may increase risk of stroke.
- Caution patient that they may bleed more easily, longer, or bruise more easily during therapy. Advise patient to notify health care professional immediately if bleeding or a fall, especially with head injury, occurs.
- Advise patient to notify health care professional of all Rx or OTC medications, vitamins, or herbal products being taken and to consult with health care professional before taking other medications, especially other aspirin or NSAIDs.
- Advise patient to notify health care professional of therapy before surgery, medical, or dental procedures are scheduled.

- Advise female patient to notify health care professional if pregnancy is planned or suspected or if breast feeding.

Evaluation/Desired Outcomes

- Prevention of deep vein thrombosis and pulmonary embolism.

bevacizumab

(be-va-**siz**-uh-mab)
Avastin, Mvasi, Zirabev

Classification
Therapeutic: antineoplastics
Pharmacologic: monoclonal antibodies

Indications

Avastin, Mvasi, and Zirabev: Treatment of the following conditions: Metastatic colorectal cancer (in combination with IV 5–fluorouracil-based chemotherapy as first-line or second-line therapy). Metastatic colorectal cancer in patients who have progressed on a first-line regimen containing bevacizumab (in combination with fluoropyrimidine-irinotecan- or fluoropyrimidine-oxaliplatin-based chemotherapy), First-line treatment of patients with unresectable, locally advanced, recurrent or metastatic non-squamous, non-small cell lung cancer (in combination with carboplatin and paclitaxel), Recurrent glioblastoma (as monotherapy), Metastatic renal cell carcinoma (in combination with interferon alfa), Persistent, recurrent, or metastatic cervical cancer (in combination with paclitaxel and cisplatin or paclitaxel and topotecan), **Avastin only:** Treatment of the following conditions: Platinum-resistant recurrent epithelial ovarian, fallopian tube, or primary peritoneal cancer (in combination with paclitaxel, pegylated liposomal doxorubicin, or topotecan), Platinum-sensitive recurrent epithelial ovarian, fallopian tube, or primary peritoneal cancer (in combination with carboplatin and paclitaxel or carboplatin and gemcitabine followed by bevacizumab as a single agent), Stage III or IV epithelial ovarian, fallopian tube, or primary peritoneal cancer following initial surgical resection (in combination with carboplatin and paclitaxel followed by bevacizumab as a single agent).

Action

A monoclonal antibody that binds to vascular endothelial growth factor (VEGF), preventing its attachment to binding sites on vascular endothelium, thereby inhibiting growth of new blood vessels (angiogenesis). **Therapeutic Effects:** Decreased metastatic disease progression and microvascular growth.

Pharmacokinetics

Absorption: IV administration results in complete bioavailability.
Distribution: Unknown.
Metabolism and Excretion: Unknown.
Half-life: 20 days (range 11–50 days).

TIME/ACTION PROFILE

ROUTE	ONSET	PEAK	DURATION
IV	rapid	end of infusion	14 days

Contraindications/Precautions

Contraindicated in: Hypersensitivity; Recent hemoptysis or other serious recent bleeding episode; First 28 days after major surgery; OB: Pregnancy (can cause fetal harm); Lactation: Discontinue nursing during treatment and, due to long half-life, for several wk following treatment.
Use Cautiously in: Cardiovascular disease; Diabetes (↑ risk of arterial thromboembolic events); Previous use of anthracyclines (↑ risk of HF); Rep: Women of reproductive potential; Pedi: Safety not established (cases of non-mandibular osteonecrosis reported); Geri: ↑ risk of serious adverse reactions including arterial thromboembolic events.

Adverse Reactions/Side Effects

CNS: POSTERIOR REVERSIBLE ENCEPHALOPATHY SYNDROME (PRES). **CV:** HF, THROMBOEMBOLIC EVENTS, hypertension, hypotension. **Derm:** NECROTIZING FASCIITIS. **GI:** GI PERFORATION. **GU:** ↑ serum creatinine, nephrotic syndrome, ovarian failure, proteinuria. **Hemat:** BLEEDING. **Resp:** HEMOPTYSIS, non-gastrointestinal fistulas, nasal septum perforation. **Misc:** WOUND DEHISCENCE, impaired wound healing, infusion reactions.

Interactions

Drug-Drug: ↑ blood levels of SN 38 (the active metabolite of **irinotecan**); significance is not known. ↑ risk of microangiopathic hemolytic anemia when used with **sunitinib**; concurrent use should be avoided.

Route/Dosage

Colorectal Cancer

IV (Adults): 5 mg/kg every 14 days when given with bolus-IFL chemotherapy regimen *or* 10 mg/kg every 14 days when given with FOLFOX4 chemotherapy regimen *or*5 mg/kg every 14 days or 7.5 mg/kg every 21 days when given with a fluoropyrimidine-irinotecan or fluoropyrimidine-oxaliplatin based chemotherapy regimen.

Lung Cancer

IV (Adults): 15 mg/kg every 3 wk when given with carboplatin and paclitaxel.

Glioblastoma

IV (Adults): 10 mg/kg every 14 days.

Renal Cell Carcinoma

IV (Adults): 10 mg/kg every 14 days when given with interferon alfa.

B

Cervical Cancer

IV (Adults): 15 mg/kg every 3 wk when given with paclitaxel and cisplatin or paclitaxel and topotecan.

Platinum-Resistant Epithelial Ovarian, Fallopian Tube, or Primary Peritoneal Cancer

IV (Adults): 10 mg/kg every 2 wk when given with paclitaxel, pegylated liposomal doxorubicin, or topotecan (weekly) *or* 15 mg/kg every 3 wk when given with topotecan (every 3 wk).

Platinum-Sensitive Epithelial Ovarian, Fallopian Tube, or Primary Peritoneal Cancer

IV (Adults): 15 mg/kg every 3 wk when given with carboplatin and paclitaxel for 6–8 cycles, followed by 15 mg/kg every 3 wk as a single agent *or* 15 mg/kg every 3 wk when given with carboplatin and gemcitabine for 6–10 cycles, followed by 15 mg/kg every 3 wk as a single agent.

Stage III or IV Epithelial Ovarian, Fallopian Tube, or Primary Peritoneal Cancer Following Surgical Resection

IV (Adults): 15 mg/kg every 3 wk when given with carboplatin and paclitaxel for up to 6 cycles, followed by 15 mg/kg every 3 wk as a single agent for a total up to 22 cycles or until disease progression, whichever occurs earlier .

Availability

Solution for injection (requires dilution): 25 mg/mL.

NURSING IMPLICATIONS

Assessment

- Assess for signs of GI perforation (abdominal pain associated with constipation, fever, nausea, and vomiting), fistula formation, and wound dehiscence during therapy; discontinue therapy if this occurs.
- Assess for signs of hemorrhage (epistaxis, hemoptysis, bleeding) and thromboembolic events (stroke, MI, deep vein thrombosis, pulmonary embolus) during therapy; may require discontinuation. Do not administer to patients with recent history of hemoptysis of ≥1/2 teaspoon (2.5 mL) of red blood.
- Monitor BP every 2–3 wk during therapy. Temporarily suspend therapy during severe hypertension not controlled with medical management; permanently discontinue if hypertensive crisis occurs.
- Assess for infusion reactions (stridor, wheezing, hypertension, oxygen desaturation, chest pain, headache, rigors, diaphoresis) during therapy. If clinically significant reaction occurs, hold therapy until resolved and resume at decreased rate. Stop therapy if severe reaction occurs.
- Assess for signs of HF (dyspnea, peripheral edema, rales/crackles, jugular venous distension) during therapy. Discontinue therapy if symptoms occur.
- Monitor for signs of PRES (headache, seizure, lethargy, confusion, blindness). Hypertension may or may not be present. May occur within 16 hr to 1 yr of initiation of therapy. Treat hypertension if present and discontinue bevacizumab therapy. Symptoms usually resolve within days.
- Monitor wound healing. If wound healing complications requiring medical intervention or necrotizing fasciitis occur, discontinue therapy.
- ***Lab Test Considerations:*** Monitor serial urinalysis for proteinuria during therapy. Patients with a 2+ or greater urine dipstick require further testing with a 24-hr urine collection. Suspend therapy for ≥2 grams of proteinuria/24 hr and resume when proteinuria is <2 g/24 hr. Discontinue therapy in patients with nephrotic syndrome.
- May cause leukopenia, thrombocytopenia, hypokalemia, and hyperbilirubinemia.
- May cause ↑ serum creatinine.

Implementation

- Avoid administration for at least 28 days following major surgery; surgical incision should be fully healed due to potential for impaired wound healing.

IV Administration

- **Intermittent Infusion:** ***Diluent:*** Dilute prescribed dose in 100 mL of 0.9% NaCl. Do not shake. Discard unused portions. Solution is colorless to pale yellow; do not administer solution that is discolored or contains particulate matter. Stable if refrigerated for up to 8 hr. ***Rate:*** Administer initial dose over 90 min. If well tolerated, second infusion may be administered over 60 min. If well tolerated, all subsequent infusions may be administered over 30 min. **Do not administer as an IV push or bolus.**
- **Additive Incompatibility:** Do not mix or administer with dextrose solutions.

Patient/Family Teaching

- Inform patient of purpose of medication.
- Advise patient of the need for monitoring BP periodically during therapy; notify health care professional if BP is elevated.
- Advise patient to report any signs of bleeding, unusual bleeding, high fever, rigors, sudden onset of worsening neurological function, or persistent or severe abdominal pain, severe constipation, or vomiting immediately to health care professional.
- Inform patient of increased risk of wound healing complications and arterial thromboembolic events.
- Rep: Bevacizumab is teratogenic. Advise female patients to use effective contraception during and for 6 mo after last dose and to avoid breast feeding. Inform female patient of reproductive potential of risk

of ovarian failure that may lead to sterility following therapy.

Evaluation/Desired Outcomes

- Decreased metastatic disease progression and microvascular growth.

bezlotoxumab

(bez-loe-**tox**-ue-mab)

Zinplava

Classification

Therapeutic: antidiarrheals

Pharmacologic: monoclonal antibodies

Indications

Reduction in recurrence of *Clostridium difficile* infection (CDI) in patients who are receiving antibacterial drug treatment of CDI and are at a high risk for CDI recurrence.

Action

Binds to *Clostridium difficile* toxin B and neutralizes its effects. **Therapeutic Effects:** Reduced CDI recurrence.

Pharmacokinetics

Absorption: IV administration results in complete bioavailability.

Distribution: Minimally distributed to tissues.

Metabolism and Excretion: Eliminated primarily through catabolism.

Half-life: 19 days.

TIME/ACTION PROFILE (blood levels)

ROUTE	ONSET	PEAK	DURATION
IV	unknown	unknown	unknown

Contraindications/Precautions

Contraindicated in: None.

Use Cautiously in: Heart failure; OB, Lactation: Safety not established; Pedi: Safety and effectiveness not established.

Adverse Reactions/Side Effects

CV: HF. **CNS:** headache. **GI:** nausea. **Misc:** infusion reactions, fever.

Interactions

Drug-Drug: None known.

Route/Dosage

IV (Adults): 10 mg/kg as a single dose.

Availability

Solution for injection (requires dilution): 25 mg/mL.

NURSING IMPLICATIONS

Assessment

- Assess for signs and symptoms of CDI prior to and following therapy.

Implementation

- Not for treatment of CDI; must be used with antibacterial agents.

IV Administration

- **Intermittent Infusion:** ***Diluent:*** Withdraw volume from bezlotoxumab vial based on patient weight and transfer to IV bag of 0.9% NaCl or D5W. Invert gently to mix; do not shake. Solution is clear to moderately opalescent, colorless to pale yellow; do not administer solutions that are discolored or contain particulate matter. ***Concentration:*** 1 mg/mL to 10 mg/mL. Store in refrigerator for up to 24 hrs or at room temperature protected from light for up to 16 hrs prior to preparation; do not freeze. ***Rate:*** Infuse over 60 min using a sterile, non-pyrogenic, low-protein binding 0.205 micron in-line or add-on filter. Do not administer as IV push or bolus. May be infused via central line or peripheral catheter.
- **Y-Site Incompatibility:** Do not administer other drugs simultaneously through same infusion line.

Patient/Family Teaching

- Inform patient that bezlotoxumab does not replace antibacterial treatment for their CDI infection. Antibacterial medications must be continued as directed.
- Rep: Advise female patient to notify health care professional if pregnancy is planned or suspected or if breast feeding.

Evaluation/Desired Outcomes

- Decrease in recurrence of CDI.

bicalutamide

(bye-ka-**loot**-a-mide)

Casodex

Classification

Therapeutic: antineoplastics

Pharmacologic: antiandrogens

Indications

Treatment of metastatic prostate carcinoma in conjunction with luteinizing hormone–releasing hormone (LHRH) analogs (goserelin, leuprolide).

Action

Antagonizes the effects of androgen at the cellular level. **Therapeutic Effects:** Decreased spread of prostate carcinoma.

Pharmacokinetics

Absorption: Well absorbed after oral administration.

Distribution: Unknown.

Protein Binding: 96%.

Metabolism and Excretion: Mostly metabolized by the liver.

Half-life: 5.8 days.

TIME/ACTION PROFILE (blood levels)

ROUTE	ONSET	PEAK	DURATION
PO	unknown	31.3 hr	unknown

Contraindications/Precautions

Contraindicated in: Hypersensitivity; Women.

Use Cautiously in: Moderate to severe liver impairment; Rep: Men with female partners of reproductive potential; Pedi: Safety not established.

Adverse Reactions/Side Effects

CNS: weakness, dizziness, headache, insomnia. **CV:** chest pain, hypertension, peripheral edema. **Derm:** alopecia, photosensitivity, rash, sweating. **Endo:** breast pain, gynecomastia. **GI:** HEPATOTOXICITY, constipation, diarrhea, nausea, abdominal pain, ↑ liver enzymes, vomiting. **GU:** erectile dysfunction, ↓ fertility, hematuria, incontinence, nocturia, urinary tract infections. **Hemat:** anemia. **Metab:** hyperglycemia, weight loss. **MS:** back pain, pelvic pain, bone pain. **Neuro:** paresthesia. **Resp:** dyspnea. **Misc:** generalized pain, hot flashes, flu-like syndrome, infection.

Interactions

Drug-Drug: May ↑ the effect of **warfarin**.

Route/Dosage

PO (Adults): 50 mg once daily (must be given concurrently with LHRH analog).

Availability (generic available)

Tablets: 50 mg.

NURSING IMPLICATIONS

Assessment

- Assess patient for adverse GI effects. Diarrhea is the most common cause of discontinuation of therapy.
- ***Lab Test Considerations:*** Monitor serum prostate-specific antigen (PSA) periodically to determine response to therapy. If levels rise, assess patient for disease progression. May require periodic LHRH analogue administration without bicalutamide.
- Monitor serum transaminases before, regularly during first 4 mo of therapy, and periodically during therapy. May cause ↑ serum alkaline phosphatase, AST, ALT, and bilirubin concentrations. If patient is jaundiced or if transaminases ↑>2 times normal, discontinue bicalutamide; levels usually return to normal after discontinuation.
- May cause ↑ BUN and serum creatinine, and ↓ hemoglobin and WBCs.
- May cause ↓ glucose tolerance in males taking LHRH agonists concurrently; monitor blood glucose in patients receiving bicalutamide in combination with LHRH agonists.
- Monitor PT/INR closely in patients taking warfarin. May lead to severe bleeding.

Implementation

- Start treatment with bicalutamide at the same time as LHRH analogue.
- **PO:** May be administered in the morning or evening, without regard to food.

Patient/Family Teaching

- Instruct patient to take bicalutamide along with the LHRH analog as directed at the same time each day. If a dose is missed, omit and take the next dose at regular time; do not double doses. Do not discontinue without consulting health care professional. Advise patient to read *Patient Information* prior to starting and with each Rx refill in case of changes.
- May cause dizziness. Caution patient to avoid driving or other activities requiring alertness until response to medication is known.
- Advise patient to stop taking bicalutamide and notify health care professional immediately of symptoms of liver dysfunction (nausea, vomiting, abdominal pain, fatigue, anorexia, "flu-like" symptoms, dark urine, jaundice, or right upper quadrant tenderness) or interstitial lung disease (trouble breathing with or without a cough or fever).
- Advise patient to notify health care professional of all Rx or OTC medications, vitamins, or herbal products being taken and to consult health care professional before taking any new medications.
- Instruct patient to report severe or persistent diarrhea.
- Discuss with patient the possibility of hair loss, breast enlargement and breast pain. Explore methods of coping.
- Advise patient to use sunscreen, avoid sunlight or sunlamps and tanning beds, and wear protective clothing to prevent photosensitivity reactions.
- Rep: Advise female and male patients to use effective contraception during and for 130 days after last dose of therapy. Female patients should avoid breast feeding during therapy. Advise male patients bicalutamide may impair fertility.
- Emphasize the importance of regular follow-up exams and blood tests to determine progress; monitor for side effects.

Evaluation/Desired Outcomes

- Decreased spread of prostate carcinoma.

bictegravir/emtricitabine/tenofovir alafenamide

(bik-**teg**-ra-vir/em-trye-**sye**-ta-been/ten-**of**-oh-veer al-a-**fen**-a-mide)

Biktarvy

Classification
Therapeutic: antiretrovirals
Pharmacologic: nucleoside reverse transcriptase inhibitors, integrase strand transfer inhibitors (INSTI)

Indications
Management of HIV infection in patients who have no antiretroviral treatment history or in those on a stable antiretroviral regimen with HIV-1 RNA <50 copies/mL for ≥3 mo and no history of treatment failure or no known substitutions associated with resistance to the individual components of the medication (to replace their current antiretroviral regimen).

Action
Bictegravir—Inhibits HIV-1 integrase, which is required for viral replication; *Emtricitabine*—Phosphorylated intracellularly where it inhibits HIV reverse transcriptase, resulting in viral DNA chain termination; *Tenofovir*—Phosphorylated intracellularly where it inhibits HIV reverse transcriptase resulting in disruption of DNA synthesis. **Therapeutic Effects:** Slowed progression of HIV infection and decreased occurrence of sequelae.

Pharmacokinetics
Absorption: *Bictegravir*—Extent of absorption following oral administration unknown; *Emtricitabine*—Well absorbed (93%) following oral administration; *Tenofovir*—Tenofovir alafenamide is a prodrug, which is hydrolyzed into tenofovir, the active component; absorption enhanced by high-fat meals.
Distribution: *Bictegravir, emtricitabine, and tenofovir*—Unknown.
Protein Binding: *Bictegravir*—>99%.
Metabolism and Excretion: *Bictegravir*—Primarily metabolized by the CYP3A4 isoenzyme and UGT1A1 in the liver; 60% excreted in feces, 35% excreted in urine; *Emtricitabine*—Undergoes some metabolism, 70% excreted in urine, 14% excreted in feces; *Tenofovir*—Tenofovir is phosphorylated to tenofovir diphosphate (active metabolite); 32% excreted in feces, <1% excreted in urine.
Half-life: *Bictegravir*—17.3 hr; *Emtricitabine*—10.4 hr; *Tenofovir alafenamide*—0.51 hr; *Tenofovir diphosphate*—150–180 hr.

TIME/ACTION PROFILE (plasma concentrations)

ROUTE	ONSET	PEAK	DURATION
bictegravir PO	unknown	2–4 hr	24 hr
emtricitabine PO	unknown	1.5–2 hr	24 hr
tenofovir PO	unknown	0.5–2 hr	24 hr

Contraindications/Precautions
Contraindicated in: Concurrent use of dofetilide or rifampin; Severe renal impairment; Severe hepatic impairment; Lactation: Breast feeding not recommended in patients with HIV.
Use Cautiously in: Hepatitis B co-infection; History of suicidal ideation or depression (↑ risk of suicidal thoughts); Renal impairment or receiving nephrotoxic medications (↑ risk of renal impairment); OB: Use during pregnancy only if potential benefit justifies potential fetal risk; Pedi: Children weighing <25 kg (safety and effectiveness not established).

Adverse Reactions/Side Effects
CNS: abnormal dreams, dizziness, fatigue, headache, insomnia. **GI:** LACTIC ACIDOSIS/HEPATOMEGALY WITH STEATOSIS, diarrhea, ↑ amylase, ↑ liver enzymes, nausea. **GU:** renal impairment. **Hemat:** neutropenia. **Metab:** hyperlipidemia. **MS:** ↑ creatine kinase. **Misc:** ACUTE EXACERBATION OF HEPATITIS B, immune reconstitution syndrome.

Interactions
Drug-Drug: Bictegravir may ↑ **dofetilide** levels and the risk of torsades de pointes; concurrent use contraindicated. **Rifampin** may ↓ bictegravir levels and its effectiveness; concurrent use contraindicated. Medications that compete for active tubular secretion, including **acyclovir**, **cidofovir**, **ganciclovir**, **valacyclovir**, **valganciclovir**, or **aminoglycosides** may ↑ emtricitabine and tenofovir levels and toxicity. Nephrotoxic agents, including **NSAIDs** ↑ risk of nephrotoxicity with tenofovir; avoid concurrent use. **Carbamazepine**, **oxcarbazepine**, **phenobarbital**, **phenytoin**, **rifabutin**, and **rifapentine** may ↓ bictegravir and tenofovir levels and their effectiveness; avoid concurrent use. Administration with **antacids**, containing **magnesium** or **aluminum** ↓ absorption of bictegravir; take ≥2 hr before or ≥6 hr after magnesium- or aluminum-containing antacids. Administration with supplements or antacids containing **calcium** or **iron**↓ absorption of bictegravir; take at the same time as calcium or iron supplements with food (and not on an empty stomach). May ↑ **metformin** levels.
Drug-Natural Products: St. John's wort may ↓ bictegravir and tenofovir levels and their effectiveness; avoid concurrent use.

Route/Dosage
PO (Adults and Children ≥25 kg): 1 tablet once daily.

Availability
Tablets: bictegravir 50 mg/emtricitabine 200 mg/tenofovir alafenamide 25 mg.

NURSING IMPLICATIONS
Assessment
- Assess patient for change in severity of HIV symptoms and for symptoms of opportunistic infections during therapy.
- May cause lactic acidosis and severe hepatomegaly with steatosis. Monitor patient for signs (increased

serum lactate levels, elevated liver enzymes, liver enlargement on palpation). Therapy should be suspended if clinical or laboratory signs occur.

- ***Lab Test Considerations:*** Monitor viral load and CD4 cell count regularly during therapy.
- Test patients for chronic hepatitis B virus (HBV) before initiating therapy. Medication is not indicated for treatment of HBV. Exacerbations of HBV have occurred upon discontinuation of therapy.
- Assess serum creatinine, estimated CCr, urine glucose and urine protein during therapy. Also monitor serum phosphorous in patients with chronic kidney disease. Discontinue therapy in patients who develop clinically significant ↓ renal function or evidence of Fanconi syndrome.
- Monitor liver function tests in patients co-infected with HIV and HBV who discontinue *Biktarvy*. May cause an exacerbation of hepatitis B. May cause ↑ AST, ALT, bilirubin, creatine kinase, serum amylase, serum lipase, and triglycerides.
- May cause ↓ neutrophil count.
- May cause ↑ LDL cholesterol.

Implementation

- **PO:** Administer once daily without regard for food.
- Administer medication at least 2 hr before or 6 hr after antacids containing aluminum or magnesium. Medication may be taken with food at same time as supplements or antacids containing iron or calcium.

Patient/Family Teaching

- Emphasize the importance of taking medication as directed. Do not take more than prescribed amount and do not stop taking without consulting health care professional. Take missed doses as soon as remembered, but not if almost time for next dose; do not double doses. Advise patient to read *Patient Information* before starting therapy and with each Rx refill in case of changes.
- Instruct patient that medication should not be shared with others.
- Inform patient that medication does not cure AIDS or prevent associated or opportunistic infections. Therapy does not reduce the risk of transmission of HIV to others through sexual contact or blood contamination. Caution patient to use a condom and to avoid sharing needles or donating blood to prevent spreading the AIDS virus to others.
- Instruct patient to notify health care professional immediately if symptoms of lactic acidosis (tiredness or weakness, unusual muscle pain, trouble breathing, stomach pain with nausea and vomiting, cold especially in arms or legs, dizziness, fast or irregular heartbeat) or if signs of hepatotoxicity (yellow skin or whites of eyes, dark urine, light colored stools, lack of appetite for several days or longer, nausea, abdominal pain) occur.
- Instruct patient to notify health care professional of all Rx or OTC medications, vitamins, or herbal products being taken and consult health care professional before taking any new medications, especially St. John's wort.
- Advise patient to notify health care professional if signs and symptoms of immune reconstitution syndrome (signs and symptoms of an infection) occur.
- Rep: Advise patient taking oral contraceptives to use a nonhormonal method of birth control during therapy. If pregnancy is suspected notify health care professional promptly. Encourage pregnant women to enroll in the Antiretroviral Pregnancy Registry by calling 1-800-258-4263. Advise female patient to avoid breast feeding during therapy.
- Emphasize the importance of regular follow-up exams and blood counts to determine progress and monitor for side effects.

Evaluation/Desired Outcomes

- Delayed progression of AIDS and decreased opportunistic infections in patients with HIV.
- Decrease in viral load and increase in CD4 cell counts.

binimetinib (bin-i-me-ti-nib)

Mektovi

Classification
Therapeutic: antineoplastics
Pharmacologic: kinase inhibitors

Indications

Treatment of metastatic/unresectable melanoma with the BRAF V600E or V600K mutation (in combination with encorafenib).

Action

Inhibits the activity of mitogen-activated extracellular kinase (MEK) 1 and 2 which are enzymes that normally promote cellular proliferation. **Therapeutic Effects:** Decreased progression of melanoma.

Pharmacokinetics

Absorption: At least 50% absorbed following oral administration.
Distribution: Extensively distributed to tissues.
Protein Binding: 97%.
Metabolism and Excretion: Mostly metabolized by the liver via glucuronidation. 62% excreted in feces (32% as unchanged drug); 31% excreted in urine (6.5% as unchanged drug).
Half-life: 3.5 hr.

TIME/ACTION PROFILE (blood levels)

ROUTE	ONSET	PEAK	DURATION
PO	unknown	1.6 hr	unknown

Contraindications/Precautions

Contraindicated in: OB: Pregnancy (may cause fetal harm); Lactation: Lactation.

Use Cautiously in: Left ventricular ejection fraction <50%; History of retinal vein occlusion; Uncontrolled glaucoma or history of hypercoagulability (↑ risk of retinal vein occlusion); Moderate or severe hepatic impairment (↓ dose); Rep: Women of reproductive potential; Pedi: Safety and effectiveness not established.

Adverse Reactions/Side Effects

CNS: dizziness, fatigue. **CV:** CARDIOMYOPATHY, DEEP VENOUS THROMBOSIS, hypertension, peripheral edema. **Derm:** rash. **EENT:** retinopathy, visual impairment, macular edema, retinal detachment, retinal vein occlusion, uveitis. **F and E:** hyponatremia. **GI:** HEPATOTOXICITY, abdominal pain, constipation, diarrhea, ↑ liver enzymes, nausea, vomiting, colitis. **GU:** ↑ serum creatinine. **Hemat:** HEMORRHAGE, anemia, leukopenia, lymphopenia, neutropenia. **MS:** RHABDOMYOLYSIS, ↑ creatine kinase. **Resp:** INTERSTITIAL LUNG DISEASE, PULMONARY EMBOLISM. **Misc:** fever.

Interactions

Drug-Drug: None reported.

Route/Dosage

PO (Adults): 45 mg twice daily; continue until disease progression or unacceptable toxicity.

Hepatic Impairment

PO (Adults): *Moderate or severe hepatic impairment*—30 mg twice daily; continue until disease progression or unacceptable toxicity.

Availability

Tablets: 15 mg.

NURSING IMPLICATIONS

Assessment

- Monitor cardiac function (LVEF) by ECG or multigated acquisition (MUGA) scan before starting therapy with binimetinib, one mo after initiation of therapy, and then at 2- to 3-mo intervals during therapy. *If asymptomatic, absolute decrease in LVEF of greater than 10% from baseline that is also below lower limit of normal (LLN) occurs,* hold binimetinib for up to 4 wk and evaluate LVEF every 2 wk. Resume binimetinib at reduced dose if present: LVEF is at or above LLN and absolute decrease from baseline is 10% or less and patient is asymptomatic. If LVEF does not recover within 4 wk, permanently discontinue binimetinib. *If symptomatic HF occurs with absolute decrease in LVEF >20% from baseline that is also below LLN,* discontinue binimetinib permanently.
- Monitor for signs and symptoms of venous thromboembolism (shortness of breath, chest pain, arm or leg swelling, cool or pale arm or leg) during therapy. *If uncomplicated deep vein thrombosis (DVT) or pulmonary embolus (PE) occurs,* hold binimetinib. If improves to Grade 0-1, resume at reduced dose. If not improved, permanently discontinue. *If life-threatening PE occurs,* permanently discontinue binimetinib.
- Assess for visual symptoms at each visit. Perform regular ophthalmologic exams. Monitor for signs and symptoms of ocular toxicities (blurred vision, loss of vision, other vision changes, see color dots, halo around objects), swelling, redness, photophobia, eye pain). *If symptomatic retinopathy/retinal pigment epithelial detachments occur,* hold binimetinib for up to 10 days. If improves and becomes asymptomatic, resume at same dose. If not improved, resume at a lower dose or permanently discontinue. *If any grade retinal vein occlusion (RVO) occurs,* permanently discontinue binimetinib. *If Grade 1-3 uveitis occurs,* if Grade 1 or 2 does not respond to specific ocular therapy, or for Grade 3 uveitis, withhold binimetinib for up to 6 wk. If improved, resume at same or reduced dose. If not improved, permanently discontinue binimetinib. *If Grade 4 uveitis occurs,* permanently discontinue therapy.
- Monitor for signs and symptoms of interstitial lung disease or pneumonitis (cough, dyspnea, hypoxia, pleural effusion, infiltrates) during therapy. *If Grade 2 occurs,* hold binimetinib for up to 4 wk. If improved to Grade 0-1, resume at reduced dose. If not resolved within 4 wk, permanently discontinue binimetinib. *If Grade 3 or 4 occurs,* discontinue binimetinib permanently.
- Assess for bleeding (headaches, dizziness, feeling weak, coughing up blood or blood clots, vomiting blood or vomit looks like "coffee grounds", red or black stools that look like tar) during therapy. *If recurrent Grade 2 or first occurrence of Grade 3 occurs,* hold binimetinib for up to 4 wk. If improves to Grade 0-1 or to pretreatment/baseline levels, resume at reduced dose. If no improvement, permanently discontinue binimetinib. *If first occurrence of Grade 4 hemorrhagic event occurs,* permanently discontinue binimetinib, or hold for up to 4 wk. If improves to Grade 0-1 or to pretreatment/baseline levels, then resume at reduced dose. If no improvement, permanently discontinue. *If recurrent Grade 3 hemorrhagic event occurs,* consider discontinuing binimetinib permanently. *If recurrent Grade 4 hemorrhagic event occurs,* permanently discontinue therapy.
- ***Lab Test Considerations:*** Obtain a negative pregnancy test prior to starting therapy.
- Information on FDA-approved tests for the detection of BRAF V600 mutations in melanoma is available at: http://www.fda.gov/CompanionDiagnostics.

B

- Monitor liver function tests before starting therapy, monthly during therapy, and as indicated. *If Grade 2 AST or ALT increased,* continue dose. If no improvement within 2 wk, hold binimetinib until improved to Grade 0-1 or to pretreatment/baseline levels and resume at same dose. *If Grade 3 or 4 AST or increased ALT occurs,* consider permanently discontinuing binimetinib.
- May cause rhabdomyolysis. Monitor CPK and creatinine levels prior to starting therapy, periodically during therapy, and as indicated. *If Grade 4 asymptomatic CPK elevation or any Grade CPK elevation with symptoms or with renal impairment occurs,* hold dose for up to 4 wk. If improved to Grade 0-1 resume at reduced dose. If not resolved within 4 wk, permanently discontinue binimetinib.

Implementation

- Dose adjustments for adverse reactions include: First dose reduction, 30 mg twice daily. If patient unable to tolerate 30 mg twice daily, discontinue binimetinib.
- **PO:** Administer twice daily, about 12 hr apart, without regard to food. Usually taken with encorafenib.

Patient/Family Teaching

- Instruct patient to take medication as directed. Take missed doses as soon as remembered, but not closer than 6 hr to next dose. If patient vomits after dose, omit and take next dose when scheduled.
- Advise patient to notify health care professional promptly if signs and symptoms of HF, venous thromboembolism (sudden onset of difficulty breathing, leg pain, swelling), changes in vision, interstitial lung disease (new or worsening cough or dyspnea), hepatotoxicity (jaundice, dark urine, nausea, vomiting, loss of appetite, fatigue, bruising, bleeding), rhabdomyolysis (unusual or new onset weakness, myalgia, darkened urine), or hemorrhage occur.
- Rep: Advise females of reproductive potential to use effective contraception during and for at least 30 days after last dose and to avoid breast feeding for 3 days after last dose. Advise patient to notify health care professional if pregnancy is planned or suspected.

Evaluation/Desired Outcomes

- Decreased progression of melanoma.

bisacodyl (bis-a-**koe**-dill)

Bisac-Evac, ♣Bisacolax, Biscolax, ♣Carter's Little Pills, ♣Codulax, Correctol, Dacodyl, Doxidan, Dulcolax, Ex-Lax Ultra, Femilax, Fleet Laxative, ♣Soflax-Ex

Classification
Therapeutic: laxatives
Pharmacologic: stimulant laxatives

Indications

Treatment of constipation. Evacuation of the bowel before radiologic studies or surgery. Part of a bowel regimen in spinal cord injury patients.

Action

Stimulates peristalsis. Alters fluid and electrolyte transport, producing fluid accumulation in the colon. **Therapeutic Effects:** Evacuation of the colon.

Pharmacokinetics

Absorption: Variable absorption follows oral administration; rectal absorption is minimal; action is local in the colon.

Distribution: Small amounts of metabolites excreted in breast milk.

Metabolism and Excretion: Small amounts absorbed are metabolized by the liver.

Half-life: Unknown.

TIME/ACTION PROFILE (evacuation of bowel)

ROUTE	ONSET	PEAK	DURATION
PO	6–12 hr	unknown	unknown
Rectal	15–60 min	unknown	unknown

Contraindications/Precautions

Contraindicated in: Hypersensitivity; Abdominal pain; Obstruction; Nausea or vomiting (especially with fever or other signs of an acute abdomen).

Use Cautiously in: Severe cardiovascular disease; Anal or rectal fissures; Excess or prolonged use (may result in dependence); OB, Lactation: May be used during pregnancy and lactation.

Adverse Reactions/Side Effects

GI: abdominal cramps, nausea, diarrhea, rectal burning. **F and E:** hypokalemia (with chronic use). **MS:** muscle weakness (with chronic use). **Misc:** protein-losing enteropathy, tetany (with chronic use).

Interactions

Drug-Drug: Antacids, histamine H_2-receptor antagonists, and **gastric acid–pump inhibitors** may remove enteric coating of tablets resulting in gastric irritation/dyspepsia. May ↓ the absorption of other **orally administered drugs** because of ↑ motility and ↓ transit time.

Drug-Food: Milk may remove enteric coating of tablets, resulting in gastric irritation/dyspepsia.

Route/Dosage

PO (Adults and Children ≥12 yr): 5–15 mg/day (up to 30 mg/day) as a single dose.

PO (Children 3–11 yr): 5–10 mg/day (0.3 mg/kg) as a single dose.

Rect (Adults and Children ≥12 yr): 10 mg/day single dose.

Rect (Children 2–11 yr): 5–10 mg/day single dose.
Rect (Children <2 yr): 5 mg/day single dose.

Availability (generic available)

Enteric-coated tablets: 5 mg[OTC]. **Enteric coated and delayed release:** 5 mg[OTC]. **Suppositories:** 10 mg[OTC]. **Rectal solution:** 10 mg/30 mL[OTC]. ***In combination with:*** In Bowel Preparation kits with Magnesium citrate (Evac-Q-Kwik[OTC], EZ-EM Prep Kit[OTC], LiquiPrep Bowel Evacuant[OTC], Tridate Bowel Cleansing Kit[OTC]), Phosphate/biphosphate (Fleet Prep Kit. No. 1[OTC], Fleet Prep Kit No. 2[OTC], Fleet Prep Kit No. 3[OTC]), sennosides (X-Prep Bowel Evacuant Kit #1[OTC]), sennosides, magnesium citrate, magnesium sulfate (X-Prep Bowel Evacuant Kit #2[OTC]). See Appendix B.

NURSING IMPLICATIONS

Assessment

- Assess patient for abdominal distention, presence of bowel sounds, and usual pattern of bowel function.
- Assess color, consistency, and amount of stool produced.

Implementation

- Do not confuse Dulcolax (bisacodyl) with Dulcolax (docusate sodium).
- May be administered at bedtime for morning results.
- **PO:** Taking on an empty stomach will produce more rapid results.
- Do not crush or chew enteric-coated tablets. Take with a full glass of water or juice.
- Do not administer oral doses within 1 hr of milk or antacids; this may lead to premature dissolution of tablet and gastric or duodenal irritation.
- **Rect:** Suppository or enema can be given at the time a bowel movement is desired. Lubricate suppositories with water or water-soluble lubricant before insertion. Encourage patient to retain the suppository or enema 15–30 min before expelling.

Patient/Family Teaching

- Advise patients, other than those with spinal cord injuries, that laxatives should be used only for short-term therapy. Prolonged therapy may cause electrolyte imbalance and dependence.
- Advise patient to increase fluid intake to at least 1500–2000 mL/day during therapy to prevent dehydration.
- Encourage patients to use other forms of bowel regulation (increasing bulk in the diet, increasing fluid intake, or increasing mobility). Normal bowel habits may vary from 3 times/day to 3 times/wk.
- Instruct patients with cardiac disease to avoid straining during bowel movements (Valsalva maneuver).
- Advise patient that bisacodyl should not be used when constipation is accompanied by abdominal pain, fever, nausea, or vomiting.

Evaluation/Desired Outcomes

- Soft, formed bowel movement when used for constipation.
- Evacuation of colon before surgery or radiologic studies, or for patients with spinal cord injuries.

bisoprolol (bis-oh-proe-lol)

~~Zebeta~~

Classification
Therapeutic: antihypertensives
Pharmacologic: beta blockers

Indications

Management of hypertension.

Action

Blocks stimulation of $beta_1$ (myocardial)-adrenergic receptors. Does not usually affect $beta_2$ (pulmonary, vascular, uterine)-receptor sites. **Therapeutic Effects:** Decreased BP and heart rate.

Pharmacokinetics

Absorption: Well absorbed after oral administration, but 20% undergoes first-pass hepatic metabolism.
Distribution: Unknown.
Metabolism and Excretion: 50% excreted unchanged by the kidneys; remainder renally excreted as metabolites; 2% excreted in feces.
Half-life: 9–12 hr.

TIME/ACTION PROFILE (antihypertensive effect)

ROUTE	ONSET	PEAK	DURATION
PO	unknown	1–4 hr	24 hr

Contraindications/Precautions

Contraindicated in: Uncompensated HF; Pulmonary edema; Cardiogenic shock; Bradycardia or heart block.
Use Cautiously in: Renal impairment (dosage ↓ recommended); Hepatic impairment (dosage ↓ recommended); Pulmonary disease (including asthma; $beta_1$ selectivity may be lost at higher doses); avoid use if possible; Diabetes mellitus (may mask signs of hypoglycemia); Thyrotoxicosis (may mask symptoms); Patients with a history of severe allergic reactions (intensity of reactions may be ↑); OB, Lactation, Pedi: Safety not established; crosses the placenta and may cause fetal/neonatal bradycardia, hypotension, hypoglycemia, or respiratory depression; Geri: ↑ sensitivity to beta blockers; initial dosage ↓ recommended.

Adverse Reactions/Side Effects

CNS: <u>fatigue</u>, <u>weakness</u>, anxiety, depression, dizziness, drowsiness, insomnia, memory loss, mental status changes, nervousness, nightmares. **EENT:** blurred vision, stuffy nose. **Resp:** bronchospasm, wheezing. **CV:** BRADYCARDIA, HF, PULMONARY EDEMA, hypotension, peripheral vasoconstriction. **GI:** constipation, diarrhea, ↑ liver function tests, nausea, vomiting. **GU:** erectile dysfunction, ↓ libido, urinary frequency. **Derm:** rash. **Endo:** hyperglycemia, hypoglycemia. **MS:** arthralgia, back pain, joint pain. **Misc:** drug-induced lupus syndrome.

Interactions

Drug-Drug: General anesthetics, **IV phenytoin**, and **verapamil** may cause additive myocardial depression. Additive bradycardia may occur with **digoxin**, **diltiazem**, **verapamil**, or **clonidine**. Additive hypotension may occur with other **antihypertensives**, acute ingestion of **alcohol**, or **nitrates**. Concurrent use with **amphetamine**, **cocaine**, **ephedrine**, **epinephrine**, **norepinephrine**, **phenylephrine**, or **pseudoephedrine** may result in unopposed alpha-adrenergic stimulation (excessive hypertension, bradycardia). Concurrent thyroid preparation administration may ↓ effectiveness. May alter the effectiveness of **insulins** or **oral hypoglycemic agents** (dose adjustments may be necessary). May ↓ the effectiveness of **theophylline**. May ↓ the beta$_1$-cardiovascular effects of **dopamine** or **dobutamine**. Use cautiously within 14 days of **MAO inhibitor** therapy (may result in hypertension).

Route/Dosage

PO (Adults): 5 mg once daily, may be ↑ to 10 mg once daily (range 2.5–20 mg/day).

Renal Impairment

Hepatic Impairment

PO (Adults): *CCr <40 mL/min*— Initiate therapy with 2.5 mg/day, titrate cautiously.

Availability (generic available)

Tablets: 5 mg, 10 mg. ***In combination with:*** hydrochlorothiazide (Ziac). See Appendix B.

NURSING IMPLICATIONS

Assessment

- Monitor BP, ECG, and pulse frequently during dosage adjustment period and periodically throughout therapy.
- Monitor intake and output ratios and daily weights. Assess routinely for signs and symptoms of HF (dyspnea, rales/crackles, weight gain, peripheral edema, jugular venous distention).
- Monitor frequency of prescription refills to determine adherence.
- ***Lab Test Considerations:*** May cause increased BUN, serum lipoprotein, potassium, triglyceride, and uric acid levels.
- May cause increased ANA titers.
- May cause increase in blood glucose levels.

Implementation

- **PO:** Take apical pulse before administering. If <50 bpm or if arrhythmia occurs, withhold medication and notify physician or other health care professional.
- May be administered without regard to meals.

Patient/Family Teaching

- Instruct patient to take medication exactly as directed, at the same time each day, even if feeling well; do not skip or double up on missed doses. If a dose is missed, it should be taken as soon as possible up to 4 hr before next dose. Abrupt withdrawal may precipitate life-threatening arrhythmias, hypertension, or myocardial ischemia.
- Teach patient and family how to check pulse and BP. Instruct them to check pulse daily and BP biweekly and to report significant changes to health care professional.
- May cause drowsiness. Caution patients to avoid driving or other activities that require alertness until response to the drug is known.
- Advise patients to change positions slowly to minimize orthostatic hypotension.
- Caution patient that this medication may increase sensitivity to cold.
- Instruct patient to notify health care professional of all Rx or OTC medications, vitamins, or herbal products being taken and to consult health care professional before taking any Rx, OTC, or herbal products, especially cold preparations, concurrently with this medication. Patients on antihypertensive therapy should also avoid excessive amounts of coffee, tea, and cola.
- Diabetics should closely monitor blood glucose, especially if weakness, malaise, irritability, or fatigue occurs. Medication does not block dizziness or sweating as signs of hypoglycemia.
- Advise patient to notify health care professional if slow pulse, difficulty breathing, wheezing, cold hands and feet, dizziness, light-headedness, confusion, depression, rash, fever, sore throat, unusual bleeding, or bruising occurs.
- Instruct patient to inform health care professional of medication regimen before treatment or surgery.
- Advise patient to carry identification describing disease process and medication regimen at all times.
- **Hypertension:** Reinforce the need to continue additional therapies for hypertension (weight loss, sodium restriction, stress reduction, regular exercise, moderation of alcohol consumption, and smoking cessation). Medication controls but does not cure hypertension.

Evaluation/Desired Outcomes

- Decrease in BP.

HIGH ALERT

bivalirudin (bi-val-i-roo-din)

Angiomax

Classification

Therapeutic: anticoagulants

Pharmacologic: thrombin inhibitors

Indications

Used in conjunction with aspirin in patients with unstable angina who are undergoing percutaneous transluminal angioplasty (PTCA). Used in conjunction with aspirin in patients with or at risk of heparin-induced thrombocytopenia (HIT) or heparin-induced thrombocytopenia and thrombosis syndrome (HITTS) who are undergoing percutaneous coronary intervention (PCI). Used in conjunction with aspirin and with provisional glycoprotein IIb/IIIa inhibitor therapy in patients who are undergoing PCI.

Action

Specifically and reversibly inhibits thrombin by binding to its receptor sites. Inhibition of thrombin prevents activation of factors V, VIII, and XII; the conversion of fibrinogen to fibrin; platelet adhesion and aggregation. **Therapeutic Effects:** Decreased acute ischemic complications in patients with unstable angina (death, MI, or the urgent need for revascularization procedures).

Pharmacokinetics

Absorption: IV administration results in complete bioavailability.

Distribution: Unknown.

Metabolism and Excretion: Cleared from plasma by a combination of renal mechanisms and proteolytic breakdown.

Half-life: 25 min (↑ in renal impairment).

TIME/ACTION PROFILE (anticoagulant effect)

ROUTE	ONSET	PEAK	DURATION
IV	immediate	unknown	1–2 hr

Contraindications/Precautions

Contraindicated in: Active major bleeding; Hypersensitivity.

Use Cautiously in: Any disease state associated with an ↑ risk of bleeding; Heparin-induced thrombocytopenia or heparin-induced thrombocytopenia-thrombosis syndrome; Patients with unstable angina not undergoing PTCA; Patients with other acute coronary syndromes; Concurrent use with other platelet aggregation inhibitors (safety not established); Renal impairment (↓ infusion rate if CCr <30 mL/min); OB: Safety not established; Lactation: Use while breast feeding only if benefit to patient outweighs potential risk to infant; Pedi: Safety and effectiveness not established.

Adverse Reactions/Side Effects

CNS: headache, anxiety, insomnia, nervousness. **CV:** ACUTE STENT THROMBOSIS (especially in patients with ST-segment elevation mi undergoing PCI), hypotension, bradycardia, hypertension. **GI:** nausea, abdominal pain, dyspepsia, vomiting. **Hemat:** BLEEDING. **Local:** injection site pain. **MS:** back pain. **Misc:** pain, fever, pelvic pain.

Interactions

Drug-Drug: Risk of bleeding may be ↑ by concurrent use of **heparin**, **low molecular weight heparins**, **clopidogrel**, **thrombolytics**, or any other **drugs that inhibit coagulation**.

Drug-Natural Products: ↑ risk of bleeding with **arnica**, **chamomile**, **clove**, **dong quai**, **feverfew**, **garlic**, **ginger**, **gingko**, **Panax ginseng**, and others.

Route/Dosage

IV (Adults): 0.75 mg/kg as a bolus injection, followed by an infusion at a rate of 1.75 mg/kg/hr for the duration of the PCI/PTCA procedure. For patients without HIT/HITTS, an activated clotting time (ACT) should be performed 5 min after bolus dose and an additional bolus dose of 0.3 mg/kg may be administered if needed. Continuation of the infusion (at a rate of 1.75 mg/kg/hr) for up to 4 hr post-procedure is optional (should be considered in patients with ST-segment elevation MI). If needed, the infusion may be continued beyond this initial 4 hr at a rate of 0.2 mg/kg/hr for up to 20 hr. Therapy should be initiated prior to the procedure and given in conjunction with aspirin.

Renal Impairment

IV (Adults): No ↓ in the bolus dose is needed in any patient with renal impairment. *GFR 10–29 mL/min*—↓ infusion rate to 1 mg/kg/hr; *Dialysis-dependent patients (off dialysis)*—↓ infusion rate to 0.25 mg/kg/hr. ACT should be monitored in all patients with renal impairment.

Availability (generic available)

Lyophilized powder for injection (requires reconstitution and dilution): 250 mg/vial. **Premixed infusion:** 250 mg/50 mL 0.9% NaCl, 500 mg/100 mL 0.9% NaCl.

NURSING IMPLICATIONS

Assessment

- Assess for bleeding. Most common is oozing from the arterial access site for cardiac catheterization. Minimize use of arterial and venous punctures, IM injections, and use of urinary catheters, nasotracheal intubation, and nasogastric tubes. Avoid noncompressible sites for IV access. If bleeding cannot be controlled with pressure, discontinue bivalirudin immediately.
- Monitor vital signs. May cause bradycardia, hypertension, or hypotension. An unexplained decrease in BP may indicate hemorrhage.
- Monitor patients with STEMI undergoing primary PCI with bivalirudin for acute stent thrombosis for at least 24 hrs in a facility capable of managing ischemic complications.

B

- ***Lab Test Considerations:*** Assess hemoglobin, hematocrit, and platelet count prior to bivalirudin therapy and periodically during therapy. May cause ↓ hemoglobin and hematocrit. An unexplained ↓ in hematocrit may indicate hemorrhage.
- Bivalirudin interferes with INR measurements; INR may not be useful in determining appropriate dose of warfarin.
- Monitor ACT periodically in patients with renal dysfunction.

Implementation

- Administer IV just prior to PTCA, in conjunction with aspirin 300 mg to 325 mg/day. Do not administer IM.

IV Administration

- **IV Push:** (for bolus dose) Reconstitute each 250-mg vial with 5 mL of sterile water for injection. Reconstituted vials are stable for 24 hr if refrigerated. ***Diluent:*** Further dilute in 50 mL of D5W or 0.9% NaCl. Withdraw bolus dose out of bag. Infusion is stable for 24 hr at room temperature. ***Concentration:*** Final concentration of infusion is 5 mg/mL. ***Rate:*** Administer as a bolus injection.
- **Intermittent Infusion:** Reconstitute each 250-mg vial as per the above directions. ***Diluent:*** Further dilute in 50 mL of D5W or 0.9% NaCl. If infusion is to be continued after 4 hr (at a rate of 0.2 mg/kg/hr), reconstituted vial should be diluted in 500 mL of D5W or 0.9% NaCl. Infusion is stable for 24 hr at room temperature. ***Concentration:*** 5 mg/mL (for infusion rate of 1.75 mg/kg/hr); 0.5 mg/mL (for infusion rate of 0.2 mg/kg/hr). ***Rate:*** Based on patient's weight (see Route/Dosage section).
- **Y-Site Compatibility:** acyclovir, alfentanil, allopurinol, amifostine, amikacin, aminocaproic acid, aminophylline, amphotericin B liposome, ampicillin, ampicillin-sulbactam, anidulafungin, argatroban, arsenic trioxide, atropine, azithromycin, aztreonam, bleomycin, bumetanide, buprenorphine, busulfan, butorphanol, calcium chloride, calcium gluconate, cangrelor, carboplatin, carmustine, cefazolin, cefepime, cefotaxime, cefotetan, cefoxitin, ceftazidime, ceftriaxone, cefuroxime, chloramphenicol, ciprofloxacin, cisatracurium, cisplatin, clindamycin, cyclophosphamide, cyclosporine, cytarabine, dacarbazine, dactinomycin, daptomycin, daunorubicin, dexamethasone, dexmedetomidine, dexrazoxane, digoxin, diltiazem, diphenhydramine, docetaxel, dopamine, doxorubicin, doxorubicin liposomal, doxycycline, droperidol, enalaprilat, ephedrine, epinephrine, epirubicin, epoprostenol, eptifibatide, ertapenem, erythromycin, esmolol, etoposide, etoposide phosphate, fenoldopam, fentanyl, fluconazole, fludarabine, fluorouracil, foscarnet, fosphenytoin, furosemide, ganciclovir, gemcitabine, gentamicin, glycopyrrolate, granisetron, heparin, hydralazine, hydrocortisone, hydromorphone, idarubicin, ifosfamide, imipenem/cilastatin, insulin, irinotecan, isoproterenol, ketorolac, leucovorin, levofloxacin, lidocaine, linezolid, magnesium sulfate, mannitol, melphalan, meperidine, meropenem, mesna, methotrexate, methylprednisolone, metoclopramide, metoprolol, metronidazole, midazolam, milrinone, mitomycin, mitoxantrone, morphine, moxifloxacin, mycophenolate, nafcillin, nalbuphine, naloxone, nicardipine, nitroglycerin, nitroprusside, norepinephrine, octreotide, ondansetron, oxaliplatin, oxytocin, paclitaxel, palonosetron, pamidronate, pancuronium, pemetrexed, pentobarbital, phenobarbital, phenylephrine, piperacillin-tazobactam, potassium acetate, potassium chloride, potassium phosphates, procainamide, propranolol, ranitidine, remifentanil, rocuronium, sodium acetate, sodium bicarbonate, sodium phosphates, streptozocin, succinylcholine, sufentanil, tacrolimus, theophylline, thiopental, thiotepa, tigecycline, tirofiban, tobramycin, topotecan, trimethoprim/sulfamethoxazole, vasopressin, vecuronium, verapamil, vinblastine, vincristine, vinorelbine, voriconazole, warfarin, zidovudine, zoledronic acid.
- **Y-Site Incompatibility:** alteplase, amiodarone, amphotericin B deoxycholate, amphotericin B lipid complex, caspofungin, chlorpromazine, dantrolene, diazepam, dobutamine, pentamidine, phenytoin, prochlorperazine, quinupristin/dalfopristin, reteplase, streptokinase, vancomycin.

Patient/Family Teaching

- Inform patient of the purpose of bivalirudin.
- Instruct patient to notify health care professional immediately if any bleeding or bruising is noted.
- Instruct patient to notify health care professional of all Rx or OTC medications, vitamins, or herbal products being taken and consult health care professional before taking any new medications.
- Advise female patients of reproductive potential to notify health care professional if pregnancy is planned or suspected or of breast feeding.

Evaluation/Desired Outcomes

- Decreased acute ischemic complications in patients with unstable angina (death, MI, or the urgent need for revascularization procedures).

HIGH ALERT

bleomycin (blee-oh-**mye**-sin)

Blenoxane

Classification

Therapeutic: antineoplastics
Pharmacologic: antitumor antibiotics

Indications
Treatment of: Lymphomas, Squamous cell carcinoma, Testicular embryonal cell carcinoma, Choriocarcinoma, Teratocarcinoma. Intrapleural administration to prevent the reaccumulation of malignant effusions.

Action
Inhibits DNA and RNA synthesis. **Therapeutic Effects:** Death of rapidly replicating cells, particularly malignant ones.

Pharmacokinetics
Absorption: Well absorbed from IM and subcut sites. Absorption follows intrapleural and intraperitoneal administration.

Distribution: Widely distributed, concentrates in skin, lungs, peritoneum, kidneys, and lymphatics.

Metabolism and Excretion: 60–70% excreted unchanged by the kidneys.

Half-life: 2 hr (↑ in renal impairment).

TIME/ACTION PROFILE (tumor response)

ROUTE	ONSET	PEAK	DURATION
IV, IM, Subcut	2–3 wk	unknown	unknown

Contraindications/Precautions
Contraindicated in: Hypersensitivity; OB, Lactation: Potential for fetal, infant harm.

Use Cautiously in: Renal impairment (dose ↓ required if CCr <35 mL/min); Pulmonary impairment; Nonmalignant chronic debilitating illness; Patients with childbearing potential; Geri: ↑ risk of pulmonary toxicity and reduction in renal function.

Adverse Reactions/Side Effects
CNS: aggressive behavior, disorientation, weakness. **Resp:** PULMONARY FIBROSIS, pneumonitis. **CV:** hypotension, peripheral vasoconstriction. **GI:** anorexia, nausea, stomatitis, vomiting. **Derm:** hyperpigmentation, mucocutaneous toxicity, alopecia, erythema, rashes, urticaria, vesiculation. **Hemat:** anemia, leukopenia, thrombocytopenia. **Local:** pain at tumor site, phlebitis at IV site. **Metab:** weight loss. **Misc:** ANAPHYLACTOID REACTIONS, chills, fever.

Interactions
Drug-Drug: Hematologic toxicity ↑ with concurrent use of **radiation therapy** and other **antineoplastics**. Concurrent use with **cisplatin** ↓ elimination of bleomycin and may ↑ toxicity. ↑ risk of pulmonary toxicity with other **antineoplastics** or thoracic **radiation therapy**. **General anesthesia** ↑ the risk of pulmonary toxicity. ↑ risk of Raynaud's phenomenon when used with **vinblastine**.

Route/Dosage
Lymphoma patients should receive initial test doses of 2 units or less for the first 2 doses.

IV, IM, Subcut (Adults and Children): 0.25–0.5 unit/kg (10–20 units/m^2) weekly or twice weekly initially. If favorable response, lower maintenance doses given (1 unit/day or 5 units/wk IM or IV). May also be given as continuous IV infusion at 0.25 unit/kg or 15 units/m^2/day for 4–5 days.

Intrapleural (Adults): 15–20 units instilled for 4 hr, then removed.

Availability (generic available)
Injection: 15 units/vial, 30 units/vial.

NURSING IMPLICATIONS
Assessment
- Monitor vital signs before and frequently during therapy.
- Assess for fever and chills. May occur 3–6 hr after administration and last 4–12 hr.
- Monitor for anaphylactic (fever, chills, hypotension, wheezing) and idiosyncratic (confusion, hypotension, fever, chills, wheezing) reactions. Keep resuscitation equipment and medications on hand. Lymphoma patients are at particular risk for idiosyncratic reactions that may occur immediately or several hrs after therapy, usually after the 1st or 2nd dose.
- Assess respiratory status for dyspnea and rales/crackles. Monitor chest x-ray before and periodically during therapy. Pulmonary toxicity occurs primarily in geriatric patients (age 70 or older) who have received 400 or more units or at lower doses in patients who received other antineoplastics or thoracic radiation. May occur 4–10 wk after therapy. Discontinue and do not resume bleomycin if pulmonary toxicity occurs.
- Assess nausea, vomiting, and appetite. Weigh weekly. Modify diet as tolerated. Antiemetics may be given before administration.
- ***Lab Test Considerations:*** Monitor CBC before and periodically during therapy. May cause thrombocytopenia and leukopenia (nadir occurs in 12 days and usually returns to pretreatment levels by day 17).
- Monitor baseline and periodic renal and hepatic function.

Implementation
- ***High Alert:*** Fatalities have occurred with chemotherapeutic agents. Before administering, clarify all ambiguous orders; double-check single, daily, and course-of-therapy dose limits; have second practitioner independently double-check original order and dose calculations.
- Prepare solution in a biologic cabinet. Wear gloves, gown, and mask while handling medication. Discard equipment in specially designated containers.
- Lymphoma patients should receive a 1- or 2-unit test dose 2–4 hr before initiation of therapy. Monitor closely for anaphylactic reaction. May not detect reactors.

- Premedication with acetaminophen, corticosteroids, and diphenhydramine may reduce drug fever and risk of anaphylaxis.
- Reconstituted solution is stable for 24 hr at room temperature and for 14 days if refrigerated.
- **IM Subcut:** Reconstitute vial with 1–5 mL of sterile water for injection, 0.9% NaCl, or bacteriostatic water for injection. Do not reconstitute with diluents containing benzyl alcohol when used for neonates.

IV Administration

- **Intermittent Infusion:** Prepare IV doses by diluting 15-unit vial with at least 5 mL of 0.9% NaCl. ***Diluent:*** Further dilute dose in 50 to 1000 mL of D5W or 0.9% NaCl. ***Rate:*** Administer slowly over 10 min.
- **Y-Site Compatibility:** allopurinol, amifostine, aminocaproic acid, aminophylline, amiodarone, anidulafungin, atracurium, aztreonam, bivalirudin, bumetanide, busulfan, calcium chloride, calcium gluconate, carboplatin, carmustine, caspofungin, cefepime, chlorpromazine, cimetidine, cisatracurium, cisplatin, codeine, cyclophosphamide, cyclosporine, cytarabine, dacarbazine, dactinomycin, daptomycin, daunorubicin, dexamethasone, dexmedetomidine, dexrazoxane, digoxin, diltiazem, diphenhydramine, dobutamine, docetaxel, dopamine, doxacurium, doxorubicin, doxorubicin liposome, droperidol, enalaprilat, epinephrine, epirubicin, ertapenem, esmolol, etoposide, etoposide phosphate, famotidine, fenoldopam, filgrastim, fludarabine, fluorouracil, fosphenytoin, furosemide, gemcitabine, glycopyrrolate, granisetron, haloperidol, heparin, hetastarch, hydralazine, hydrocortisone, idarubicin, ifosfamide, insulin, isoproterenol, ketorolac, labetalol, leucovorin calcium, levofloxacin, lidocaine, magnesium sulfate, mannitol, melphalan, meperidine, mesna, metaraminol, methotrexate, methyldopate, methylprednisolone, metoclopramide, metoprolol, milrinone, mitomycin, mitoxantrone, naloxone, nicardipine, nitroglycerin, norepinephrine, octreotide, ondansetron, oxaliplatin, paclitaxel, palonosetron, pancuronium, pantoprazole, pemetrexed, phentolamine, phenylephrine, piperacillin/tazobactam, potassium chloride, potassium phosphates, procainamide, quinupristin/dalfopristin, rituximab, sargramostim, sodium acetate, thiotepa, tirofiban, trastuzumab, vinblastine, vincristine, vinorelbine, voriconazole.
- **Y-Site Incompatibility:** amphotericin B liposome, dantrolene, phenytoin, tigecycline.
- **Intrapleural:** Dissolve 60 units in 50–100 mL of 0.9% NaCl.
- May be administered through thoracotomy tube. Position patient as directed.

Patient/Family Teaching

- Instruct patient to notify health care professional if fever, chills, wheezing, faintness, diaphoresis, shortness of breath, prolonged nausea and vomiting, or mouth sores occur.
- Encourage patient not to smoke because this may worsen pulmonary toxicity.
- Explain to the patient that skin toxicity may manifest itself as skin sensitivity, hyperpigmentation (especially at skin folds and points of skin irritation), and skin rashes and thickening.
- Instruct patient to inspect oral mucosa for erythema and ulceration. If ulceration occurs, advise patient to use sponge brush and rinse mouth with water after eating and drinking. Opioid analgesics may be required if pain interferes with eating.
- Discuss with patient the possibility of hair loss. Explore coping strategies.
- Advise patient of the need for contraception during therapy.
- Instruct patient not to receive any vaccinations without advice of health care professional.
- Emphasize need for periodic lab tests to monitor for side effects.

Evaluation/Desired Outcomes

- Decrease in tumor size without evidence of hypersensitivity or pulmonary toxicity.

bortezomib (bor-tez-o-mib)

Velcade

Classification

Therapeutic: antineoplastics

Pharmacologic: proteasome inhibitors

Indications

Multiple myeloma (as initial therapy or after progression); with melphalan and prednisone. Mantle cell lymphoma.

Action

Inhibits proteasome, a regulator of intracellular protein catabolism, resulting in disruption of various intracellular processes. Cytotoxic to a variety of cancerous cells. **Therapeutic Effects:** Death of rapidly replicating cells, particularly malignant ones.

Pharmacokinetics

Absorption: IV administration results in complete bioavailability.

Distribution: Unknown.

Metabolism and Excretion: Mostly metabolized by the liver (P450 enzymes); excretion is unknown.

Half-life: 9–15 hr.

TIME/ACTION PROFILE

ROUTE	ONSET	PEAK	DURATION
IV	unknown	38 days*	unknown

*Median time to response based on clinical parameters.

Contraindications/Precautions

Contraindicated in: Hypersensitivity to bortezomib, boron, or mannitol; Intrathecal administration (may cause death); OB: Pregnancy (may cause fetal harm); Lactation: Lactation.

Use Cautiously in: Moderate to severe hepatic impairment (may ↑ levels, risk of toxicity); History of or risk factors for HF; Rep: Women of reproductive potential and men with female partners of reproductive potential; Pedi: Safety not established.

Adverse Reactions/Side Effects

CNS: PROGRESSIVE MULTIFOCAL LEUKOENCEPHALOPATHY (PML), POSTERIOR REVERSIBLE ENCEPHALOPATHY SYNDROME (PRES), fatigue, malaise, weakness, dizziness, syncope. **CV:** hypotension, HF. **Derm:** STEVENS-JOHNSON SYNDROME, TOXIC EPIDERMAL NECROLYSIS. **EENT:** blurred vision, diplopia. **GI:** LIVER FAILURE, anorexia, constipation, diarrhea, nausea, vomiting. **Hemat:** THROMBOTIC THROMBOCYTOPENIC PURPURA/HEMOLYTIC UREMIC SYNDROME, BLEEDING, anemia, neutropenia, thrombocytopenia. **Neuro:** peripheral neuropathy. **Resp:** pneumonia. **Misc:** fever, tumor lysis syndrome.

Interactions

Drug-Drug: Concurrent neurotoxic medications including **amiodarone**, some **antivirals**, **nitrofurantoin**, **isoniazid**, or **HMG-CoA reductase inhibitors** may ↑ risk of peripheral neuropathy.

Route/Dosage

Previously Untreated Multiple Myeloma

IV, Subcut (Adults): 1.3 mg/m² twice weekly for Cycles 1–4 (days 1, 4, 8, 11, 22, 25, 29, and 32; no treatment during cycle 3), then once weekly for Cycles 5–9 (days 1, 8, 22, and 29; no treatment during Cycle 7); further cycles/doses depend on response and toxicity.

Previously Untreated Mantle Cell Lymphoma

IV, Subcut (Adults): 1.3 mg/m² twice weekly on days 1, 4, 8, and 11, followed by a 10–day rest (days 12–21); repeat for 5 additional cycles; further cycles/doses depend on response and toxicity.

Relapsed Multiple Myeloma and Mantle Cell Lymphoma

IV, Subcut (Adults): 1.3 mg/m² twice weekly for 2 wk (days 1, 4, 8, and 11), followed by a 10-day rest; further cycles/doses depend on response and toxicity. Patients with multiple myeloma who have previously responded to bortezomib therapy and who have relapsed ≥6 mo after prior bortezomib therapy can be started on their last tolerated dose; dose should be given twice weekly (days 1, 4, 8, and 11) every 3 wk for a maximum of 8 cycles.

Hepatic Impairment

IV (Adults): *Moderate or severe hepatic impairment*—0.7 mg/m² per injection for the first cycle, then may ↑ to 1 mg/m² per injection or ↓ further to 0.5 mg/m² per injection, based on tolerability.

Availability

Lyophilized powder for injection (requires reconstitution): 3.5 mg/vial.

NURSING IMPLICATIONS

Assessment

- Monitor vital signs frequently during therapy. May cause fever and orthostatic hypotension requiring adjustment of antihypertensives, hydration, or administration of mineralocorticoids.
- Monitor for GI adverse effects. May require antidiarrheals, antiemetics, and fluid and electrolyte replacement to prevent dehydration. Weigh weekly; modify diet as tolerated.
- Monitor for signs and symptoms of tumor lysis syndrome (tachypnea, tachycardia, hypotension, pulmonary edema). Patients with high tumor burden prior to treatment are at increased risk.
- Monitor for signs of PRES (headache, seizure, lethargy, confusion, blindness). Hypertension may or may not be present. May occur within 16 hr to 1 yr of initiation of therapy. Treat hypertension if present and discontinue bortezomib therapy. Symptoms usually resolve within days.
- Assess for any new signs or symptoms that may be suggestive of PML, an opportunistic infection of the brain caused by the JC virus, that leads to death or severe disability; withhold dose and notify health care professional promptly. PML symptoms may begin gradually but usually worsen rapidly. Symptoms vary depending on which part of brain is infected (mental function declines rapidly and progressively, causing dementia; speaking becomes increasingly difficult; partial blindness; difficulty walking; rarely, headaches and seizures occur). Diagnosis is usually made via gadolinium-enhanced MRI and CSF analysis. Risk of PML increases with the number of infusions. Withhold bortezomib at first sign of PML.
- Monitor for signs and symptoms of thrombotic angiopathy (thrombocytopenia, microangiopathic hemolytic anemia, acute kidney injury). Discontinue therapy immediately if clinical or lab symptoms occur.
- ***Lab Test Considerations:*** Obtain a negative pregnancy test before starting therapy.
- Monitor CBC frequently during therapy. Assess platelet count before each dose. Dose modifications for hematologic toxicity are made based on indication and concurrent drug therapy; see manufacturer's recommendations. The nadir of thrombocytopenia is day 11 and recovery is usually by next cycle. Occurs more commonly in cycles 1 and 2, but may occur throughout therapy. May require discontinuation of therapy.
- Monitor blood glucose levels closely in patients taking oral hypoglycemic agents; may require adjustment of antidiabetic agent dose.

Implementation

- Should be administered under the supervision of a physician experienced in the use of antineoplastic therapy.
- Solution should be prepared in a biologic cabinet. Wear gloves, gown, and mask while handling medication. Discard IV equipment in specially designated containers.

IV Administration

- **Subcut:** Reconstitute each vial with 1.4 mL of 0.9% NaCl. ***Concentration:*** 2.5 mg/mL. Solution should be clear and colorless; do not administer solutions that are discolored or contain particulate matter. May inject into thigh or abdomen; rotate injection sites. Inject into sites at least 1 inch from other sites and avoid tender, bruised, erythematous, or indurated sites. If local injection site reactions occur, may inject a less concentrated (1 mg/mL) solution.
- **IV Push:** Reconstitute each vial with 3.5 mL of 0.9% NaCl. Solution should be clear and colorless; do not administer solutions that are discolored or contain particulate matter. ***Concentration:*** 1 mg/mL. Administer reconstituted solution within 8 hr at room temperature; 3 of the 8 hr may be stored in a syringe. ***Rate:*** Administer as a 3–5 sec bolus injection twice weekly for 2 wk followed by a 10-day rest period. At least 72 hr should elapse between consecutive doses.
- *If peripheral neuropathy is Grade 1 (paresthesia or loss of reflexes without pain or loss of function)* continue prescribed dose. *If paresthesia is Grade 1 with pain or Grade 2 (interfering with function but not with daily activities)* reduce dose to 1.0 mg/m². *If peripheral neuropathy is Grade 2 with pain or Grade 3 (interfering with activities of daily living)* withhold dose until toxicity resolves, then re-initiate with a reduced dose of 0.7 mg/m² and decrease frequency to once/wk. *If peripheral neuropathy is Grade 4 (permanent sensory loss that interferes with daily function)* discontinue bortezomib.

Patient/Family Teaching

- Caution the patient that dehydration may occur with vomiting or diarrhea. Advise patient to maintain fluid intake and to notify health care professional if dizziness or fainting occurs.
- Instruct patient to contact health care professional if they experience new or worsening signs of peripheral neuropathy (tingling, numbness, pain, burning feeling in the feet or hands, weakness in the arms or legs), PML (progressive weakness on one side of the body or clumsiness of limbs, disturbance of vision; changes in thinking, memory, and orientation leading to confusion and personality changes), or if symptoms of dehydration (dizziness, fainting) due to vomiting or diarrhea; rash; shortness of breath; cough; swelling of feet, ankles, or legs; bleeding, infection, convulsions; persistent headache; reduced eyesight; increase in BP or blurred vision occur.
- May cause dizziness and blurred vision. Caution patient to avoid driving or other activities requiring alertness until response to medication is known.
- Advise patient to notify health care professional of all Rx or OTC medications, vitamins, or herbal products being taken and consult health care professional before taking Rx, OTC, or herbal products, especially St. John's wort.
- Advise diabetic patients taking oral hypoglycemic agents to monitor blood glucose frequently and notify health care professional of changes in blood sugar.
- Rep: Advise female patient of reproductive potential to use effective contraception during and for 7 mo after last dose and to avoid breast feeding during therapy and for 2 mo after therapy. Advise male patient with female partner of reproductive potential to use effective contraception for 4 mo after last dose of bortezomib. Patient should notify health care professional immediately if pregnancy is suspected. May impair fertility for male and female patients.

Evaluation/Desired Outcomes

- Decrease in serum and urine myeloma protein.
- Decrease in size and spread of malignancy.

brentuximab

(bren-**tux**-i-mab)

Adcetris

Classification

Therapeutic: antineoplastics

Pharmacologic: drug-antibody conjugates

Indications

Classical Hodgkin lymphoma (cHL) in patients who have failed autologous hematopoietic stem cell transplant (auto-HSCT) or who have failed ≥2 prior multi-agent chemotherapies and are not candidates for auto-HSCT. cHL in patients who are at high risk of relapse or progression as post-auto-HSCT consolidation. Previously untreated stage III or IV cHL (in combination with doxorubicin, vinblastine, and dacarbazine). Systemic anaplastic large cell lymphoma after failure of ≥1 multi-agent chemotherapy regimen. Primary cutaneous anaplastic large cell lymphoma or CD30-expressing mycosis fungoides in patients who have received prior systemic therapy. Previously untreated systemic anaplastic large cell lymphoma or other CD30–expressing peripheral T-cell lymphoma (in combination with cyclophosphamide, doxorubicin, and prednisone).

Action

An antibody-drug conjugate (ADC) made up three parts: an antibody specific for human CD30 (cAC10, a cell membrane protein of the tumor necrosis factor receptor), a microtubule disrupting agent monomethyl auristatin (MMAE), and a protease-cleavable linker that attaches MMAE covalently to cAC10. The combination disrupts the intracellular microtubule network causing cell-cycle arrest and apoptotic cellular death. **Therapeutic Effects:** Decreased spread of lymphoma.

Pharmacokinetics

Absorption: IV administration results in complete bioavailability.
Distribution: Unknown.
Metabolism and Excretion: Small amounts of MMAE that are released are metabolized by the liver and eliminated mostly by the kidneys.
Half-life: *ADC*—4–6 days.

TIME/ACTION PROFILE (blood levels)

ROUTE	ONSET	PEAK	DURATION
IV (ADC)	unknown	end of infusion	3 wk
IV (MMAE)	unknown	1–3 days	3 wk

Contraindications/Precautions

Contraindicated in: Concurrent use of bleomycin (↑ risk of pulmonary toxicity); Severe renal impairment (CCr <30 mL/min); Moderate or severe hepatic impairment; OB: May cause fetal harm; avoid pregnancy; Lactation: Breast feeding should be avoided.
Use Cautiously in: Preexisting GI involvement (↑ risk of GI perforation); Rep: Women of reproductive potential and males with female partners of reproductive potential; Pedi: Safety and effectiveness not established.

Adverse Reactions/Side Effects

CNS: PROGRESSIVE MULTIFOCAL LEUKOENCEPHALOPATHY (PML), anxiety, dizziness, fatigue, headache, insomnia. **CV:** peripheral edema. **Derm:** STEVENS-JOHNSON SYNDROME, TOXIC EPIDERMAL NECROLYSIS, alopecia, night sweats, pruritus, rash, dry skin. **GI:** BOWEL OBSTRUCTION, ENTEROCOLITIS, GI HEMORRHAGE, GI PERFORATION, GI ULCER, ILEUS, HEPATOTOXICITY, NEUTROPENIC COLITIS, PANCREATITIS, abdominal pain, constipation, ↓ appetite, diarrhea, nausea, vomiting, ulcer. **GU:** ↓ fertility. **Hemat:** NEUTROPENIA, THROMBOCYTOPENIA, anemia. **Metab:** weight loss. **MS:** arthralgia, back pain, extremity pain, myalgia, muscle spasm. **Neuro:** peripheral neuropathy. **Resp:** ACUTE RESPIRATORY DISTRESS SYNDROME, INTERSTITIAL LUNG DISEASE, cough, dyspnea, oropharyngeal pain. **Misc:** INFUSION REACTIONS (including anaphylaxis), TUMOR LYSIS SYNDROME, fever, lymphadenopathy, chills.

Interactions

Drug-Drug: MMAE is both a substrate and inhibitor of the CYP3A4/5 enzyme system. **Bleomycin** may ↑ risk of pulmonary toxicity; concurrent use contraindicated. **Strong CYP3A4 inhibitors**, including **ketoconazole** may ↑ levels and risk of adverse reactions. **Strong CYP3A4 inducers**, including **rifampin**, may ↓ levels and effectiveness.

Route/Dosage

Relapsed cHL or Relapsed Systemic Anaplastic Large Cell Lymphoma

IV (Adults): 1.8 mg/kg (max dose = 180 mg) every 3 wk until disease progression or unacceptable toxicity.

Renal Impairment

IV (Adults): *CCr <30 mL/min*—Avoid use.

Hepatic Impairment

IV (Adults): *Mild (Child-Pugh A)*—1.2 mg/kg (max dose = 120 mg) every 3 wk until disease progression or unacceptable toxicity; *Moderate (Child-Pugh B) or severe (Child-Pugh C)*—Avoid use.

cHL Consolidation

IV (Adults): 1.8 mg/kg (max dose = 180 mg) every 3 wk until a maximum of 16 cycles completed, disease progression, or unacceptable toxicity. Initiate therapy within 4–6 wk post-auto-HSCT or upon recovery of auto-HSCT.

Renal Impairment

IV (Adults): *CCr <30 mL/min*—Avoid use.

Hepatic Impairment

IV (Adults): *Mild (Child-Pugh A)*—1.2 mg/kg (max dose = 120 mg) every 3 wk until a maximum of 16 cycles completed, disease progression or unacceptable toxicity; *Moderate (Child-Pugh B) or severe (Child-Pugh C)*—Avoid use.

Previously Untreated Stage III or IV cHL

IV (Adults): 1.2 mg/kg (max dose = 120 mg) every 2 wk until a maximum of 12 doses completed, disease progression or unacceptable toxicity.

Renal Impairment

IV (Adults): *CCr <30 mL/min*—Avoid use.

Hepatic Impairment

IV (Adults): *Mild (Child-Pugh A)*—0.9 mg/kg (max dose = 90 mg) every 2 wk until a maximum of 12 doses completed, disease progression or unacceptable toxicity; *Moderate (Child-Pugh B) or severe (Child-Pugh C)*—Avoid use.

Relapsed Primary Cutaneous Anaplastic Large Cell Lymphoma or CD-30 Expressing Mycosis Fungoides

IV (Adults): 1.8 mg/kg (max dose = 180 mg) every 3 wk until a maximum of 16 cycles completed, disease progression, or unacceptable toxicity.

Renal Impairment

IV (Adults): *CCr <30 mL/min*—Avoid use.

B

Hepatic Impairment

IV (Adults): *Mild (Child-Pugh A)*—1.2 mg/kg (max dose = 120 mg) every 3 wk until a maximum of 16 cycles completed, disease progression, or unacceptable toxicity; *Moderate (Child-Pugh B) or severe (Child-Pugh C)*—Avoid use.

Previously Untreated Systemic Anaplastic Large Cell Lymphoma or Other CD-30 Expressing Peripheral T-Cell Lymphomas

IV (Adults): 1.8 mg/kg (max dose = 180 mg) every 3 wk with each cycle of chemotherapy for 6–8 doses.

Renal Impairment

IV (Adults): *CCr <30 mL/min*—Avoid use.

Hepatic Impairment

IV (Adults): *Mild (Child-Pugh A)*—1.2 mg/kg (max dose = 120 mg) every 3 wk with each cycle of chemotherapy for 6–8 doses; *Moderate (Child-Pugh B) or severe (Child-Pugh C)*—Avoid use.

Availability

Lyophilized powder for injection (requires reconstitution and dilution): 50 mg/vial.

NURSING IMPLICATIONS

Assessment

- Monitor for signs and symptoms of peripheral neuropathy (hypoesthesia, hyperesthesia, paresthesia, discomfort, burning, neuropathic pain, weakness). *For new or worsening neuropathy Grade 2 or 3,* delay next dose until neuropathy improves to Grade 1 or baseline, then restart at 1.2 mg/kg. *If Grade 4 peripheral neuropathy occurs,* discontinue therapy.
- Monitor temperature periodically during therapy, especially if neutropenic.
- Assess for signs and symptoms of infusion-related reaction, including anaphylaxis (rash, pruritus, dyspnea, swelling of face and neck). If anaphylaxis occurs, discontinue infusion immediately; do not restart. Treat other infusion-related reactions by stopping and treating symptoms. Premedicate patient prior to subsequent infusions with acetaminophen, an antihistamine, and a corticosteroid.
- Monitor for tumor lysis syndrome due to rapid reduction in tumor volume (acute renal failure, hyperkalemia, hypocalcemia, hyperuricemia, or hypophosphatemia). Risks are higher in patients with greater tumor burden and rapidly proliferating tumors; may be fatal. Correct electrolyte abnormalities, monitor renal function and fluid balance, and administer supportive care, including dialysis, as indicated.
- Assess for skin rash frequently during therapy. Discontinue at first sign of rash; may be life-threatening. Stevens-Johnson syndrome may develop. Treat symptomatically; may recur once treatment is stopped.
- Assess for any new signs or symptoms that may be suggestive of PML, an opportunistic infection of the brain caused by the JC virus, that leads to death or severe disability; withhold dose and notify health care professional promptly. PML symptoms may begin gradually but usually worsen rapidly. Symptoms vary depending on which part of brain is infected (mental function declines rapidly and progressively, causing dementia; speaking becomes increasingly difficult; partial blindness; difficulty walking; rarely, headaches and seizures occur). Diagnosis is usually made via gadolinium-enhanced MRI and CSF analysis. Risk of PML increases with the number of infusions. Withhold brentuximab at first sign of PML.
- Monitor for signs and symptoms of pulmonary toxicity (cough, dyspnea) during therapy. If new or worsening pulmonary symptoms occur, hold brentuximab during assessment and until symptoms improve.
- Monitor for severe abdominal pain during therapy; may cause pancreatitis.
- ***Lab Test Considerations:*** Verify negative pregnancy status prior to starting therapy.
- Monitor CBC prior to each dose and more frequently in patients with Grade 3 or 4 neutropenia. Prolonged (≥1 wk) severe neutropenia may occur. Hold dose of brentuximab for Grade 3 or 4 neutropenia until resolution to baseline or Grade 2 or lower. Consider growth factor support for subsequent cycles for patients who developed Grade 3 or 4 neutropenia. Discontinue brentuximab or reduce dose to 1.2 mg/kg in patients with recurrent Grade 4 neutropenia despite use of growth factors.
- Monitor liver enzymes and bilirubin periodically during therapy. Signs of new, worsening, or recurrent hepatotoxicity may require decrease in dose, or interruption or discontinuation of therapy.

Implementation

IV Administration

- Premedicate patients with previously untreated Stage III or IV cHL who are treated with brentuximab in combination with chemotherapy with G-CSF beginning with Cycle 1.
- **Intermittent Infusion:** Calculate dose and number of brentuximab vials needed. Calculate for 100 kg for patients weighing >100 kg. Reconstitute each 50 mg vial with 10.5 mL of sterile water for injection for a concentration of 5 mg/mL. Direct stream to side of vial. Swirl gently; do not shake. Solution should be clear to slightly opalescent, and colorless. Do not administer solutions that are discolored or contain a precipitate. Withdraw volume of brentuxi-

mab dose from infusion bag of at least 100 mL. ***Diluent:*** 0.9% NaCl, D5W, or LR. ***Concentration:*** 0.4 — 1.8 mg/mL. Invert bag gently to mix. Dilute immediately into infusion bag or store solution in refrigerator; use within 24 hrs of reconstitution. Do not freeze. ***Rate:*** Infuse over 30 min. Do not administer as IV push or bolus.

- **Y-Site Incompatibility:** Do not administer with other products.

Patient/Family Teaching

- Instruct patient to notify health care professional of any numbness or tingling of hands or feet or any muscle weakness.
- Advise patient to notify health care professional immediately if signs and symptoms of infection (fever of ≥100.5°F, chills, cough, pain on urination), hepatotoxicity (fatigue, anorexia, right upper abdominal discomfort, dark urine, jaundice), PML (changes in mood or usual behavior, confusion, thinking problems, loss of memory, changes in vision, speech, or walking, decreased strength or weakness on one side of body), pulmonary toxicity, GI complications or pancreatitis (abdominal pain, nausea, vomiting, diarrhea, rash), or infusion reactions (fever, chills, rash, breathing problems within 24 hr of infusion) occur.
- Rep: Caution female and male patients with a partner with reproductive potential to use effective contraception during therapy and for at least 6 mo after last dose and to avoid breast feeding during therapy. If pregnancy is suspected, notify health care professional promptly. Inform male patients therapy may impair fertility.

Evaluation/Desired Outcomes

- Decreased spread of lymphoma.

REMS

brexanolone (brex-an-oh-lone)

Zulresso

Classification

Therapeutic: antidepressants

Pharmacologic: corticosteroids, gamma aminobutyric acid (GABA) enhancers

Schedule IV

Indications

Postpartum depression.

Action

Although not fully understood, thought to be related to positive allosteric modulation of GABA-A receptors. **Therapeutic Effects:** Reduction in depressive symptoms.

Pharmacokinetics

Absorption: IV administration results in complete absorption.

Distribution: Extensively distributed to tissues.

Metabolism and Excretion: Extensively metabolized via keto-reduction, glucuronidation, and sulfation to inactive metabolites. Primarily excreted in feces (47%) and urine (42%) as metabolites.

Half-life: 9 hr.

TIME/ACTION PROFILE (reduction in depressive symptoms)

ROUTE	ONSET	PEAK	DURATION
IV	1–2 hr	60–72 hr	At least 30 days

Contraindications/Precautions

Contraindicated in: End-stage renal disease (CCr <15 mL/min) (↑ accumulation of solubilizing agent).

Use Cautiously in: OB: Safety not established; Lactation: Enters breast milk; use while breast feeding only if potential maternal benefit justifies potential risk to infant; Pedi: May ↑ risk of suicide thoughts/behaviors.

Adverse Reactions/Side Effects

CNS: SUICIDAL THOUGHTS/BEHAVIORS, dizziness, presyncope, sedation, vertigo, altered consciousness, loss of consciousness. **CV:** tachycardia. **Derm:** flushing. **GI:** dry mouth, diarrhea, dyspepsia, oropharyngeal pain.

Interactions

Drug-Drug: Use with **benzodiazepines** or other **CNS depressants**, including **opioids**, **non-benzodiazepine sedative/hypnotics**, **anxiolytics**, **muscle relaxants**, and **alcohol** may cause profound sedation, loss of consciousness, and/or respiratory depression; avoid concurrent use, if possible.

Route/Dosage

IV (Adults): 30 mcg/kg/hr for 4 hr, then ↑ to 60 mcg/kg/hr for 20 hr, then ↑ to 90 mcg/kg/hr for 28 hr, then ↓ to 60 mcg/kg/hr for 4 hr, then ↓ to 30 mcg/kg/hr for 4 hr, then discontinue. Total duration of infusion = 60 hr.

Availability

Solution for injection (requires dilution): 5 mg/mL.

NURSING IMPLICATIONS

Assessment

- Monitor for hypoxia using continuous pulse oximetry equipped with alarm. Assess for excessive sedation every 2 hrs during planned, non-sleep periods. Stop infusion immediately if signs or symptoms of excessive sedation occur. Time to full recovery from loss or altered state of consciousness ranges from 15–60 min after infusion is stopped. Infusion may be resumed at same or lower dose after symptoms resolve. If hypoxia occurs, immediately stop infusion and do not resume.
- Assess for suicidal tendencies, especially during early therapy. Risk may be increased in adults ≤24 yr. Consider changing therapeutic regimen, including discontinuing brexanolone, in patients whose depression becomes worse or who experience emergent suicidal thoughts and behaviors.

B

Implementation

- Start brexanolone therapy early enough during the day to allow for recognition of excessive sedation.
- Brexanolone is only available through a restricted Risk Evaluation and Mitigation Strategy (REMS) called the Zulresso REMS due to potential harm from excessive sedation or sudden loss of consciousness. Healthcare facilities must enroll to ensure medication is only given to patients enrolled in program. Pharmacies must be certified with the program. Patients must be enrolled before receiving brexanolone.
- **Continuous Infusion:** Prepare 5 infusion bags for 60 hr period, more if patient weighs ≥90 kg. For each bag, prepare and store in polyolefin, non-DEHP, nonlatex bag, only. Dilute in infusion bag immediately after initial puncture of vial. Withdraw 20 mL of brexanolone from vial and place in infusion bag. ***Diluent:*** Dilute with 40 mL of sterile water for injection, and further dilute with 40 mL of 0.9% NaCl 100 mL volume. ***Concentration:*** 1 mg/mL. Immediately place infusion bag in refrigerator until use. Solution is clear and colorless; do not administer solutions that are discolored or contain particulate matter. Solution is stable for up to 96 hrs if refrigerated. Diluted solution is stable for 12 hr at room temperature. Each 60 hr infusion requires at least 5 bags. Discard bag after 12 hrs of infusion. ***Rate:*** Using a programmable peristaltic infusion pump to ensure accurate delivery. See Route and Dosage for rate. Use a dedicated line; do not mix with other medications in bag or line. Prime infusion line with admixture before inserting into pump and connecting to venous catheter. Use a PVC, non-DEHP, nonlatex infusion set. Do not use in-line filter infusion sets.

Patient/Family Teaching

- Explain purpose of medication to patient and family and requirements of Zulresso REMS program. Advise patient to read *Medication Guide* before starting brexanolone.
- Advise patient to notify health care professional if excessive sedation occurs during infusion. Patients must not be the primary caregiver of dependents and must be accompanied during interactions with their child(ren).
- Caution patient to avoid driving and activities requiring alertness until response from medication is known.
- Instruct patient to notify health care professional of all Rx or OTC medications, vitamins, or herbal products being taken and consult health care professional before taking any new medications. Advise patient to avoid taking other CNS depressants or alcohol.
- Rep: Advise females of reproductive potential to notify health care professional if they could possibly be pregnant prior to therapy. Advise pregnant women and females of reproductive potential of the potential risk to a fetus. Encourage patient to enroll in the registry that monitors pregnancy outcomes in women exposed to antidepressants during pregnancy. To register patients, healthcare professionals call the National Pregnancy Registry for Antidepressants at 1-844-405-6185 or online at https://womensmentalhealth.org/clinical-and-researchprograms/pregnancyregistry/antidepressants/.

Evaluation/Desired Outcomes

- Decreased symptoms of postpartum depression.

BEERS

brexpiprazole

(brex-**pip**-ra-zole)

Rexulti

Classification

Therapeutic: none assigned, antipsychotics, antidepressants

Pharmacologic: serotonin-dopamine activity modulators (SDAM)

Indications

Treatment of schizophrenia. Adjunctive treatment of major depressive disorder.

Action

Psychotropic activity may be due to partial agonist activity at dopamine D_2 and serotonin 5-HT_{1A} receptors and antagonist activity at the 5-HT_{2A} receptor. **Therapeutic Effects:** Decreased manifestations of schizophrenia including excitable, paranoic, or withdrawn behavior. Improvement in symptoms of depression with increased sense of wellbeing.

Pharmacokinetics

Absorption: Well absorbed (95%) following oral administration.

Distribution: Displays extravascular distribution.

Protein Binding: >99%.

Metabolism and Excretion: Metabolized by CYP3A4 and CYP2D6; 25% excreted in urine (<1% unchanged), 46% in feces (14% unchanged).

Half-life: 91 hr.

TIME/ACTION PROFILE (improvement in symptoms)

ROUTE	ONSET	PEAK	DURATION
PO (schizophrenia)	within 1–2 wk	4–6 wk	unknown
PO (depression)	within 1 wk	5 wk	unknown

Contraindications/Precautions

Contraindicated in: Hypersensitivity.

Use Cautiously in: History of seizures, concurrent use of medications that may ↓ seizure threshold; Pre-existing cardiovascular disease, dehydration, hypotension, concurrent antihypertensives, diuretics, electrolyte imbalance (↑ risk of orthostatic hypotension, correct deficits before treatment); Pre-existing low WBC (may ↑ risk of leukopenia/neutropenia; History of diabetes, metabolic syndrome or dyslipidemia (may exacerbate); Patients <24 yr (may ↑ suicidal ideation/behaviors, monitor carefully); Patients at risk for falls; Poor CYP2D6 metabolizers (PM), dose ↓ required; Geri: Elderly patients with dementia-induced psychoses (↑ risk of serious adverse cardiovascular reactions and death), consider age, concurrent medical conditions and medications, renal/hepatic/cardiac function; OB: Safety not established; use during third trimester may result in extrapyramidal/withdrawal symptoms in infant; Lactation: Consider health benefits against risk of adverse effects in infant; Pedi: Safety and effectiveness not established (may ↑ suicidal ideation/behaviors).

Adverse Reactions/Side Effects

CNS: SEIZURES, abnormal dreams, dizziness, drowsiness, headache, restlessness, urges (eating, gambling, sexual, shopping). **EENT:** blurred vision. **CV:** cerebrovascular adverse reactions (↑ in elderly patients with dementia-related psychoses), orthostatic hypotension/syncope. **GI:** abdominal pain, constipation, diarrhea, dry mouth, dysphagia, excess salivation, flatulence. **Hemat:** agranulocytosis, leukopenia, neutropenia. **Metab:** ↑ appetite, ↑ weight, hyperglycemia/diabetes, dyslipidemia. **Neuro:** akathisia, dystonia, extrapyramidal symptoms, tardive dyskinesia, tremor. **Misc:** NEUROLEPTIC MALIGNANT SYNDROME, allergic reactions including ANAPHYLAXIS, body temperature dysregulation.

Interactions

Drug-Drug: Concurrent use with strong CYP3A4 inhibitors including **clarithromycin**, **itraconazole** or **ketoconazole** ↑ blood levels, effects and risk of adverse reactions; ↓ dose of brexpiprazole required. Concurrent use with strong CYP2D6 inhibitors including **fluoxetine**, **paroxetine**, or **quinidine** ↑ blood levels, effects and risk of adverse reactions; ↓ dose of brexpiprazole required. Combined use of **strong or moderate CYP3A4 inhibitors with strong or moderate CYP2D6 inhibitors** in addition to brexpiprazole including the following combinations **itraconazole + quinidine**, **fluconazole + paroxetine**, **itraconazole + duloxetine** or **fluconazole + duloxetine** ↑ blood levels, effects and risk of toxicity; ↓ dose of brexpiprazole required. Concurrent use of **strong inducers of CYP3A4** including **rifampin** ↓ blood levels and effectiveness; ↑ dose of brexpiprazole required. Concurrent use of **antihypertensives** or **diuretics** (↑ risk of hypotension). Concurrent use of **medications that may ↓ seizure threshold** (↑ risk of seizures).

Drug-Natural Products: Concurrent use of **St. John's wort** ↓ blood levels and effectiveness; ↑ dose of brexpiprazole required.

Route/Dosage

PO (Adults): *Schizophrenia*—1 mg once daily for the 1st 4 days (Days 1–4), then ↑ to 2 mg once daily for the next 3 days (Days 5–8), then ↑ to 4 mg once daily on Day 8 (not to exceed 4 mg once daily); *Major depressive disorder*—0.5 or 1 mg once daily initially, may be ↑ to 2 mg once daily (not to exceed 3 mg once daily); *Known CYP2D6 poor metabolizers*—use 50% of the usual dose. *Concurrent use of strong CYP2D6 inhibitors (schizophrenia only) or CYP3A4 inhibitors*—use 50% of the usual dose; *Concurrent use of strong/moderate CYP2D6 inhibitors AND strong/moderate CYP3A4 inhibitors*—use 25% of the usual dose; *Known CYP2D6 poor metabolizer taking concurrent strong/moderate CYP3A4 inhibitors*—use 25% of the usual dose; *Concurrent use of strong CYP3A4 inducers*—double usual dose over 1–2 wk; titrate by clinical response.

Hepatic Impairment

PO (Adults): *Moderate to severe hepatic impairment [Child-Pugh score ≥7]*—maximum daily dose should not exceed 3 mg for schizophrenia or 2 mg for major depressive disorder.

Renal Impairment

PO (Adults): *Moderate/severe/end-stage renal impairment [CCr <60 mL/min]*—maximum daily dose should not exceed 3 mg for schizophrenia or 2 mg for major depressive disorder.

Availability

Tablets: 0.25 mg, 0.5 mg, 1 mg, 2 mg, 3 mg, 4 mg.

NURSING IMPLICATIONS

Assessment

- Assess mental status (orientation, mood, behavior) before and periodically during therapy. Assess for suicidal tendencies, especially during early therapy for depression. Restrict amount of drug available to patient. Risk may be increased in children, adolescents, and adults ≤24 yrs.
- Assess weight and BMI initially and throughout therapy.
- Obtain fasting blood glucose and cholesterol levels initially and periodically during therapy.
- Monitor BP (sitting, standing, lying), pulse, and respiratory rate before and periodically during therapy.
- Observe patient carefully when administering medication to ensure that medication is actually taken and not hoarded or cheeked.
- Monitor patient for onset of akathisia (restlessness or desire to keep moving) and extrapyramidal side effects (*parkinsonian*—difficulty speaking or swallowing, loss of balance control, pill rolling of hands, masklike face, shuffling gait, rigidity, tremors; and

B

dystonic—muscle spasms, twisting motions, twitching, inability to move eyes, weakness of arms or legs) periodically throughout therapy. Report these symptoms.

- Monitor for tardive dyskinesia (uncontrolled rhythmic movement of mouth, face, and extremities; lip smacking or puckering; puffing of cheeks; uncontrolled chewing; rapid or worm-like movements of tongue). Notify health care professional immediately if these symptoms occur, as these side effects may be irreversible.
- Monitor for development of neuroleptic malignant syndrome (fever, muscle rigidity, altered mental status, respiratory distress, tachycardia, seizures, diaphoresis, hypertension or hypotension, pallor, tiredness, loss of bladder control). Notify health care professional immediately if these symptoms occur.
- Assess for falls risk. Drowsiness, orthostatic hypotension, and motor and sensory instability increase risk. Institute prevention if indicated.
- ***Lab Test Considerations:*** Monitor CBC frequently during initial mo of therapy in patients with pre-existing or history of low WBC. May cause leukopenia, neutropenia, or agranulocytosis. Discontinue therapy if severe neutropenia (ANC <1000 mm^3 occurs).
- Monitor blood glucose and cholesterol levels initially and periodically during therapy.

Implementation

- **PO:** Administer once daily without regard to meals.

Patient/Family Teaching

- Advise patient to take medication as directed and not to skip doses or double up on missed doses. Take missed doses as soon as remembered unless almost time for the next dose. Do not stop taking brexpiprazole without consulting health care professional. Advise patient to read *Medication Guide* before starting and with each Rx refill in case of changes.
- Inform patient of possibility of extrapyramidal symptoms and tardive dyskinesia. Instruct patient to report these symptoms immediately.
- Advise patient to make position changes slowly to minimize orthostatic hypotension. Protect from falls.
- Medication may cause drowsiness and lightheadedness. Caution patient to avoid driving or other activities requiring alertness until response to medication is known.
- Advise patient and family to notify health care professional if thoughts about suicide or dying, attempts to commit suicide; new or worse depression; new or worse anxiety; feeling very agitated or restless; panic attacks; trouble sleeping; new or worse irritability; acting aggressive; being angry or violent; acting on dangerous impulses; an extreme increase in activity and talking; other unusual changes in behavior or mood occur.
- Inform patient that brexipiprazole may cause weight gain. Advise patient to monitor weight periodically. Notify health care professional of significant weight gain.
- Instruct patient to notify health care professional of all Rx or OTC medications, vitamins, or herbal products being taken and to consult health care professional before taking any new medications. Caution patient to avoid taking alcohol or other CNS depressants concurrently with this medication.
- Advise patient that extremes in temperature should be avoided, because this drug impairs body temperature regulation.
- Advise patient to notify health care professional if new or increased eating/binge eating, gambling, sexual, shopping, or other impulse control disorders occur.
- Advise patient to notify health care professional of medication regimen prior to treatment or surgery.
- Advise female patients to notify health care professional if pregnancy is planned or suspected and to avoid breast feeding during therapy. Encourage pregnant patients to enroll in registry by contacting National Pregnancy Registry for Atypical Antipsychotics at 1-866-961-2388 or visit http://womensmentalhealth.org/clinical-and-research-programs/pregnancyregistry/.
- Emphasize the importance of routine follow-up exams and continued participation in psychotherapy as indicated.

Evaluation/Desired Outcomes

- Decrease in excitable, paranoic, or withdrawn behavior.
- Increased sense of wellbeing in patients with depression.

brigatinib (bri-**ga**-ti-nib)

Alunbrig

Classification

Therapeutic: antineoplastics

Pharmacologic: kinase inhibitors

Indications

Metastatic non-small cell lung cancer (NSCLC) that is positive for anaplastic lymphoma kinase (ALK) in patients who have progressed on or intolerant to crizotinib.

Action

Inhibits receptor tyrosine kinases including anaplastic lymphoma kinase (ALK), insulin-like growth factor—1 receptor (IGF-1R), ROS1, and FMS-like tyrosine kinase-3 (FLT-3). **Therapeutic Effects:** Decreased spread of lung cancer.

Pharmacokinetics

Absorption: Well absorbed following oral administration. Bioavailability reduced by high fat meals.
Distribution: Extensively distributed to tissues.
Metabolism and Excretion: Mostly metabolized by the liver (CYP2C8 and CYP3A4 isoenzymes); also induces CYP3A. 27% excreted in feces unchanged, 22% eliminated unchanged in urine.
Half-life: 25 hr.

TIME/ACTION PROFILE (blood levels)

ROUTE	ONSET	PEAK	DURATION
PO	unknown	1–4 hr	unknown

Contraindications/Precautions

Contraindicated in: Concurrent use of moderate or strong inhibitors/inducers of the CYP3A enzyme system; OB: May cause fetal harm; Lactation: Avoid breast feeding.
Use Cautiously in: Diabetes; Severe renal or hepatic impairment; Rep: Women of reproductive potential and men with female sexual partners of reproductive potential; Pedi: Safety and effectiveness not established.

Adverse Reactions/Side Effects

CNS: headache, insomnia. **CV:** BRADYCARDIA, HYPERTENSION. **Derm:** rash. **EENT:** blurred vision, ↓ visual acuity, diplopia, cataracts, macular edema. **Endo:** hyperglycemia. **F and E:** hypophosphatemia. **GI:** abdominal pain, constipation, ↓ appetite, diarrhea, ↑ amylase, ↑ lipase, ↑ liver enzymes, nausea, vomiting. **Hemat:** anemia, ↑ activated partial thromboplastin time, lymphopenia. **MS:** arthralgia, back pain, ↑ creatine phosphokinase, muscle spasms, myalgia. **Neuro:** peripheral neuropathy. **Resp:** INTERSTITIAL LUNG DISEASE/PNEUMONITIS, cough, dyspnea, hypoxia, pneumonia. **Misc:** fatigue, fever.

Interactions

Drug-Drug: Strong or moderate CYP3A inhibitors, including **clarithromycin**, **cobicistat**, **conivaptan**, **indinavir**, **itraconazole**, **ketoconazole**, **lopinavir**, **nefazodone**, **nelfinavir**, **posaconazole**, **ritonavir**, **saquinavir**, and **voriconazole** may ↑ levels; concurrent use should be avoided; if concurrent therapy must be used, ↓ brigatinib dose. **Strong CYP3A inducers**, including **carbamazepine**, **phenytoin**, and **rifampin** may ↓ levels and effectiveness; concurrent use should be avoided; if concurrent therapy with moderate CYP3A inducer must be used, ↓ brigatinib dose. May ↓ levels of **CYP3A substrates**, including **hormonal contraceptives**. **Beta-blockers**, **verapamil**, **diltiazem**, **digoxin**, and **clonidine** may ↑ risk of bradycardia; avoid concurrent use, if possible.
Drug-Natural Products: Concurrent use of **St. John's wort** may ↓ levels and effectiveness and should be avoided.
Drug-Food: Grapefruit or **grapefruit juice** may ↑ levels and should be avoided.

Route/Dosage

PO (Adults): 90 mg once daily for 7 days, then 180 mg once daily. Continue until disease progression or unacceptable toxicity. *Concurrent use of strong CYP3A inhibitor*—If previously taking 180 mg once daily, ↓ dose to 90 mg once daily; if previously taking 90 mg once daily, ↓ dose to 60 mg once daily; *Concurrent use of moderate CYP3A inhibitor*—If previously taking 180 mg once daily, ↓ dose to 120 mg once daily; if previously taking 120 mg once daily, ↓ dose to 90 mg once daily; if previously taking 90 mg once daily, ↓ dose to 60 mg once daily; *Concurrent use of moderate CYP3A inducer*—↑ daily dose in 30–mg increments after 7 days of treatment with the dose used prior to initiation of moderate CYP3A inducer; dose may be ↑ up to a maximum of twice the dose that was tolerated prior to initiating the moderate CYP3A inducer.

Renal Impairment

PO (Adults): *Severe renal impairment (CCr 15–29 mL/min)*—If previously taking 180 mg once daily, ↓ dose to 90 mg once daily; if previously taking 90 mg once daily, ↓ dose to 60 mg once daily.

Hepatic Impairment

PO (Adults): *Severe hepatic impairment (Child–Pugh C)*—If previously taking 180 mg once daily, ↓ dose to 120 mg once daily; if previously taking 120 mg once daily, ↓ dose to 90 mg once daily; if previously taking 90 mg once daily, ↓ dose to 60 mg once daily.

Availability

Film-coated tablets: 30 mg, 90 mg, 180 mg.

NURSING IMPLICATIONS

Assessment

- Assess respiratory function (lung sounds, dyspnea, oxygen saturation) periodically during therapy.
- Monitor for signs and symptoms of interstitial lung disease (ILD) or pneumonitis (difficulty breathing, shortness or breath, cough with or without mucus, fever) periodically during therapy. **Grade 1:** *If new pulmonary symptoms occur during first 7 days of therapy,* hold brigatinib until recovery to baseline, then resume at same dose; do not escalate to 180 mg if ILD/pneumonitis is suspected. *If new pulmonary symptoms occur after first 7 days of therapy,* hold brigatinib until recovery to baseline, then resume at same dose. *If ILD/pneumonitis recurs,* permanently discontinue brigatinib. **Grade 2:** *If new pulmonary symptoms occur during first 7 days of therapy,* hold brigatinib until recovery to baseline, then resume at same dose; do not escalate to 180 mg if ILD/pneumonitis is suspected. *If new pulmonary*

symptoms occur after first 7 days of therapy, hold brigatinib until recovery to baseline. If ILD/pneumonitis is suspected, resume at next lower dose; if not, resume at same dose. *If ILD/pneumonitis recurs,* permanently discontinue brigatinib. **Grade 3 or 4:** Permanently discontinue brigatinib for ILD/pneumonitis.

- Monitor BP prior to therapy, after 2 wk, and monthly during therapy. Control BP prior to therapy. Monitor blood pressure after 2 wk and at least monthly during therapy. *If Grade 3 hypertension (SBP ≥160 mmHg or DBP ≥100 mmHg) occurs,* hold brigatinib until hypertension ≤Grade 1 (SBP <140 mmHg and DBP <90 mmHg), then resume brigatinib at next lower dose. *If recurrence of Grade 3:* withhold therapy until recovery to ≤Grade 1, and resume at next lower dose or permanently discontinue treatment. *If Grade 4 hypertension (life-threatening consequences, urgent intervention indicated) occurs,* hold brigatinib until ≤Grade 1, and resume at next lower dose or permanently discontinue. *Grade 4 recurrence:* permanently discontinue brigatinib.
- Monitor for bradycardia (HR <60 bpm) periodically during therapy, especially if concurrent medications decrease HR. *If symptomatic bradycardia (dizziness, lightheadedness, fainting) occurs,* hold brigatinib until asymptomatic bradycardia or resting heart rate of ≥60 bpm. *If concomitant medication known to cause bradycardia is identified and discontinued or dose reduced,* resume at same dose once asymptomatic or resting heart rate of ≥60 bpm. *If no concomitant medication known to cause bradycardia, or if contributing concomitant medications are not discontinued or dose reduced,* resume brigatinib at next lower dose upon recovery to asymptomatic bradycardia or to resting heart rate of ≥60 bpm. *If bradycardia with life-threatening consequences or urgent intervention needed,* permanently discontinue brigatinib if no contributing concomitant medication is identified. *If contributing concomitant medication is identified and discontinued or dose reduced,* resume therapy at next lower dose when recovered to asymptomatic bradycardia or to a resting heart rate of ≥60 bpm, with frequent monitoring. *Grade 4 recurrence:* permanently discontinue therapy.
- Monitor for visual changes (blurred vision, diplopia, reduced visual acuity) periodically during therapy. *If Grade 2 or 3 visual disturbance occurs,* hold doses until recovery to Grade 1 or baseline, then resume at next lower dose. *If Grade 4 visual disturbance occurs,* discontinue brigatinib permanently.
- ***Lab Test Considerations:*** Obtain a negative pregnancy before starting therapy.
- Monitor CPK levels periodically during therapy. *If Grade 3 CPK ↑ (>5.0 × upper limit of normal [ULN]) occurs,* hold therapy until ≤Grade 1 (≤2.5 × ULN) or to baseline, then resume at same dose. *If Grade 4 CPK ↑ (>10.0 × ULN) or recurrence of Grade 3 ↑ occurs,* hold brigatinib until ≤Grade 1 (≤2.5 × ULN) or to baseline, then resume therapy at next lower dose.
- Monitor serum lipase and amylase periodically during therapy. *If Grade 3 lipase or amylase ↑ (>2.0 × ULN) occurs,* hold brigatinib until ≤Grade 1 (≤1.5 × ULN) or baseline, then resume brigatinib at same dose. *If Grade 4 lipase or amylase ↑ (>5.0 × ULN) or recurrence of Grade 3 ↑ occurs,* hold brigatinib until ≤Grade 1 (≤ 1.5 × ULN) or baseline, then resume therapy at next lower dose.
- Monitor fasting serum glucose prior to starting and periodically during therapy. May cause new or worsening hyperglycemia. Use antihyperglycemic medications as needed. If adequate hyperglycemic control cannot be achieved with medical management, hold brigatinib until adequate hyperglycemic control is achieved and consider reducing dose or discontinue brigatinib.

Implementation

- **PO:** Administer daily without regard to food. Swallow tablets whole; do not crush, break, or chew. If therapy is interrupted for 14 days or longer, other than adverse reactions, resume therapy at 90 mg once daily for 7 days before increasing to previously tolerated dose.

Patient/Family Teaching

- Instruct patient to take brigatinib as directed. If patient vomits or misses a dose, omit dose and take next dose as scheduled. Do not double doses. Advise patient to read *Patient Information* before starting therapy and with each Rx refill in case of changes.
- Advise patient to avoid eating grapefruit or drinking grapefruit juice during therapy.
- Advise patient to notify health care professional if signs and symptoms of lung problems (cough, chest pain, fever), hypertension (headaches, dizziness, blurred vision, chest pain, shortness of breath), bradycardia (dizziness, lightheadedness, feeling faint), visual changes (double vision, seeing flashes of light, blurry vision, light hurting eyes, new or increased floaters), symptoms of pancreatitis (upper abdominal pain, weight loss, nausea), new or worsening symptoms of myalgia (unexplained muscle pain, tenderness, or weakness), or hyperglycemia (feeling very thirsty, needing to urinate more than usual, feeling very hungry, nausea, feeling weak or tired, feeling confused) occur, may require dose reduction or discontinuation.
- Instruct patient to notify health care professional of all Rx or OTC medications, vitamins, or herbal products being taken and consult health care profes-

sional before taking any new medications, especially St. John's wort.

- Rep: May be teratogenic. Advise female patient of reproductive potential to use effective non-hormonal contraception during and for at least 4 mo after final dose. Advise males with female partners of reproductive potential to use effective contraception during and for at least 3 mo after last dose of brigatinib. Advise patient to avoid breast feeding during and for 1 wk after last dose. Inform male patient that brigatinib may reduce fertility.

Evaluation/Desired Outcomes

- Decreased spread in lung cancer.

brivaracetam

(briv-a-**ra**-se-tam)

Briviact, Brivlera

Classification

Therapeutic: anticonvulsants

Indications

Partial-onset seizures (as monotherapy or adjunctive therapy).

Action

Displays a high and selective affinity for synaptic vesicle protein 2A (SV2A) in the brain, which may contribute to its anticonvulsant effect. **Therapeutic Effects:** Decreased incidence of seizures.

Pharmacokinetics

Absorption: Rapidly and completely absorbed following oral administration.

Distribution: Widely distributed to tissues.

Metabolism and Excretion: Hepatic and extrahepatic amidase-mediated hydrolysis of the amide moiety to form carboxylic acid metabolite (primary route) and hydroxylation primarily by CYP2C19 to form the hydroxy metabolite (secondary route) (all metabolites inactive). The CYP2C19 enzyme system exhibits genetic polymorphism; poor metabolizers may have significantly ↑ brivaracetam concentrations and an ↑ risk of adverse effects. >95% excreted by the kidneys (<10% excreted unchanged).

Half-life: 9 hr.

TIME/ACTION PROFILE (blood levels)

ROUTE	ONSET	PEAK	DURATION
PO	unknown	1–4hr†	unknown

†1 hr in fasting state; 4 hr with high-fat meal.

Contraindications/Precautions

Contraindicated in: Hypersensitivity; End-stage renal disease; Lactation: Discontinue brivaracetam or discontinue breast feeding.

Use Cautiously in: All patients (may ↑ risk of suicidal thoughts/behaviors); Patients who are known or suspected to be poor CYP2C19 metabolizers (may require dose ↓); Hepatic impairment (dose ↓ recommended); OB: Use only if potential maternal benefit justifies potential fetal risk; Pedi: Children <4 yr (safety and effectiveness not established); Geri: ↓ renal and hepatic function (dose ↓ may be necessary).

Adverse Reactions/Side Effects

CNS: SUICIDAL THOUGHTS/BEHAVIOR, aggression, agitation, anger, apathy, belligerence, anxiety, depression, dizziness, drowsiness, hallucinations, irritability, mood swings, paranoia, psychosis, restlessness, tearfulness, euphoria, fatigue. **EENT:** nystagmus. **GI:** constipation, dysgeusia, nausea, vomiting. **Hemat:** leukopenia. **Neuro:** ataxia, balance disorder, coordination difficulties, vertigo. **Local:** infusion site pain. **Misc:** HYPERSENSITIVITY REACTIONS (including bronchospasm and angioedema).

Interactions

Drug-Drug: CYP2C19 inducers including rifampin may ↓ levels and effectiveness; ↑ dose of brivaracetam by up to 100%. Concurrent use with **carbamazepine** may ↑ levels of carbamazepine-epoxide (active metabolite); consider ↓ dose of carbamazepine if tolerability issues occur. May ↑ levels of **phenytoin**.

Route/Dosage

PO, IV (Adults and Children ≥16 yrs): 50 mg twice daily; may be titrated down to 25 mg twice daily or up to 100 mg twice daily based on tolerability and effectiveness.

PO (Children 4–<16 yr and ≥50 kg): 25–50 mg twice daily; may be titrated up to 100 mg twice daily based on tolerability and effectiveness.

PO (Children 4–<16 yr and 20–<50 kg): 0.5-1 mg/kg twice daily; may be titrated up to 2 mg/kg twice daily based on tolerability and effectiveness.

PO (Children 4–<16 yr and 11–<20 kg): 0.5-1.25 mg/kg twice daily; may be titrated up to 2.5 mg/kg twice daily based on tolerability and effectiveness.

Hepatic Impairment

PO, IV (Adults and Children ≥16 yr): 25 mg twice daily; titrate based on tolerability and effectiveness (max dose = 75 mg twice daily).

Hepatic Impairment

PO (Children ≥4 yr and ≥50 kg): 25 mg twice daily; titrate based on tolerability and effectiveness (max dose = 75 mg twice daily).

Hepatic Impairment

PO (Children ≥4 yr and 20–<50 kg): 0.5 mg/kg twice daily; titrate based on tolerability and effectiveness (max dose = 1.5 mg/kg twice daily).

Hepatic Impairment

PO (Children ≥4 yr and 11–<20 kg): 0.5 mg/kg twice daily; titrate based on tolerability and effectiveness (max dose = 2 mg/kg twice daily).

Availability
Oral solution (raspberry-flavored): 10 mg/mL. **Solution for injection:** 10 mg/mL. **Tablets:** 10 mg, 25 mg, 50 mg, 75 mg, 100 mg.

NURSING IMPLICATIONS
Assessment
- Assess mental status (orientation, mood, behavior) before and periodically during therapy. Monitor closely for notable changes in behavior that could indicate the emergence or worsening of suicidal thoughts or behavior or depression.
- Monitor for signs and symptoms of bronchospasm (wheezing, dyspnea) and angioedema (rash, pruritus, perioral swelling) during therapy. If signs of hypersensitivity occur discontinue brivaracetam.
- ***Lab Test Considerations:*** May cause ↓ WBC and neutrophil counts.

Implementation
- Initiate therapy with oral or IV administration. IV administration may be used when oral dose is not feasible; administer at same dose and frequency as oral doses.
- **PO:** Administer twice daily without regard to food. Swallow tablets whole with liquid; do not crush or chew.
- Use a calibrated measuring device for accuracy with oral solution. Dilution is not necessary, May be administered via nasogastric or gastrostomy tube. Oral solution is stable for 5 mo after opening.

IV Administration
- **Intermittent Infusion:** ***Diluent:*** May be administered undiluted or diluted with 0.9% NaCl, LR, or D5W. Solution is clear and colorless; do not administer solutions that are discolored or contain particulate matter. Solution is stable for up to 4 hr at room temperature; may be stored in polyvinyl chloride bags. ***Rate:*** Administer over 2–15 min.

Patient/Family Teaching
- Instruct patient to take brivaracetam as directed. ↓ dose gradually; do not stop abruptly to minimize risk of ↑ seizure frequency and status epilepticus. Advise patient to read *Medication Guide* prior to therapy and with each Rx refill in case of changes.
- May cause drowsiness, fatigue, dizziness, and balance problems. Caution patient to avoid driving or other activities requiring alertness until response to medication is known. Do not resume driving until physician gives clearance based on control of seizure disorder.
- Advise patient and family to notify health care professional if behavioral changes, thoughts about suicide or dying, attempts to commit suicide; new or worse depression; new or worse anxiety; feeling very agitated or restless; panic attacks; trouble sleeping; new or worse irritability; acting aggressive; being angry or violent; acting on dangerous impulses; an extreme increase in activity and talking, other unusual changes in behavior or mood occur.
- Advise patient to notify health care professional of all Rx or OTC medications, vitamins, or herbal products being taken and to consult with health care professional before taking other medications.
- Rep: Advise female patients to notify health care professional if pregnancy is planned or suspected or if breast feeding. Encourage patients who become pregnant to enroll in the North American Antiepileptic Drug (NAAED) Pregnancy Registry by calling 1-888-233-2334 or on the web at www.aedpregnancyregistry.org. Enrollment must be done by patients themselves.

Evaluation/Desired Outcomes
- Decreased incidence of partial-onset seizures.

REMS

brodalumab (broe-**dal**-ue-mab)
Siliq

Classification
Therapeutic: antipsoriatics
Pharmacologic: interleukin antagonists

Indications
Moderate-to-severe plaque psoriasis in patients who are candidates for systemic therapy or phototherapy and have failed to respond or have lost response to other systemic therapies.

Action
A monoclonal antibody that acts as an antagonist of interleukin (IL)–17RA by selectively binding to it and preventing its interaction with numerous interleukin cytokines. Antagonism prevents production of inflammatory cytokines and chemokines. **Therapeutic Effects:** Decreased plaque formation and spread.

Pharmacokinetics
Absorption: 55% absorbed following subcut administration.
Distribution: Minimally distributed to tissues.
Metabolism and Excretion: Primarily eliminated by being catabolized into small peptides and amino acids.
Half-life: Unknown.

TIME/ACTION PROFILE (blood levels)

ROUTE	ONSET	PEAK	DURATION
Subcut	unknown	3 days	unknown

Contraindications/Precautions

Contraindicated in: Crohn's disease (may worsen disease); Active tuberculosis.

Use Cautiously in: History of suicidality or depression; Chronic infection or history of recurrent infection; OB, Lactation: Safety not established; Pedi: Safety and effectiveness not established.

Adverse Reactions/Side Effects

CNS: SUICIDAL THOUGHTS/BEHAVIORS, headache.
EENT: oropharyngeal pain. **GI:** Crohn's disease, diarrhea, nausea. **Hemat:** neutropenia. **MS:** arthralgia, myalgia. **Misc:** INFECTIONS (including reactivation tuberculosis), fatigue, injection site reactions.

Interactions

Drug-Drug: May ↓ antibody response to **live-virus vaccine** and ↑ risk of adverse reactions (do not administer concurrently). May affect activity of CYP450 enzymes and may alter the effectiveness/toxicity of drugs that are substrates of CYP450 (including **warfarin** and **cyclosporine**); close monitoring is recommended and necessary dose modifications undertaken.

Route/Dosage

Subcut (Adults): 210 mg at Wk 0, 1, and 2 then 210 mg every 2 wk; consider discontinuing therapy if adequate response not achieved after 12–16 wk of therapy.

Availability

Solution for subcutaneous injection (prefilled syringes): 210 mg/1.5 mL.

NURSING IMPLICATIONS

Assessment

- Assess skin lesions prior to and periodically during therapy.
- Assess for tuberculosis (TB) infection prior to starting therapy. Begin treatment for latent TB prior to brodalumab administration; do not administer to patients with active TB infection.
- Assess for new or worsening symptoms of depression, anxiety, other mood disorders, or suicidality. Refer to mental health professional as appropriate. Re-evaluate risks and benefits of brodalumab if depression occurs.
- Monitor for signs and symptoms of infection (fever, sweats, chills, muscle aches, cough, dyspnea, sore throat or difficulty swallowing, warm, red or painful skin or sores, diarrhea or stomach pain, burning or frequency of urination) during therapy. If serious infection develops or is not responding to therapy, monitor patient closely and discontinue brodalumab until infection resolves.

Implementation

- Available only through restricted program called Siliq REMS due to suicide risks. Providers must be certified, patients must sign a Patient-Provider Agreement form, and pharmacies must be certified and only dispense to patients authorized to receive brodalumab. Further information and a list of qualified pharmacies can be found at www.SILIQREMS.com or by calling 855-511-6135.
- **Subcut:** Allow prefilled syringe to reach room temperature for approximately 30 min before injecting. Do not warm any other way. Solution is clear to slightly opalescent, colorless to slightly yellow. A few translucent to white, amorphous proteinaceous particles may be present; do not administer if solution is cloudy or discolored. Inject full dose (1.5 mL) into thigh, abdomen, or upper arm. Pinch skin and inject at a 45° or 90° angle. Do not rub injection site. Do not inject in skin areas that are tender, bruised, red, hard, thick, scaly, or affected by psoriasis. Store in refrigerator or at room temperature for up to 14 days; do not return to refrigerator after room temperature. Protect from light. Do not freeze.

Patient/Family Teaching

- Advise patient to administer injection as directed, according to schedule. Health care professional should supervise first self-injection. Instruct patient to inject full dose, and to use proper technique for syringe and needle disposal. Inform patient that they must enroll in SILIQ REMS program and to carry SILIQ Patient Wallet Card at all times and share with other health care professionals. Card describes symptoms which, if experienced, should prompt patient to seek immediate medical evaluation. Provide patient with telephone number and website for pharmacies participating in SILIQ REMS program.
- Caution patient to avoid live vaccines during therapy.
- May cause depression or suicide. Instruct patients and caregivers to monitor for emergence of suicidal thoughts and behaviors. Notify health care professional immediately if suicidal thoughts, new or worsening depression, anxiety, changes in behavior or mood, thoughts of suicide, dying, or hurting self, or acting on dangerous impulses occur. Instruct patient to carry wallet card and to call the national Suicide Prevention Lifeline at 1-800-273-8255 if they experience suicidal thoughts.
- Instruct patient to notify health care professional if signs and symptoms of infection occur.
- Instruct patient to notify health care professional of all Rx or OTC medications, vitamins, or herbal products being taken and consult health care professional before taking any new medications.
- Rep: Advise female patient to notify health care professional if pregnancy is planned or suspected or if breast feeding.

Evaluation/Desired Outcomes

- Decrease in plaque formation and spread of plaque psoriasis. Consider discontinuing if adequate response not achieved after 12–16 wk. Treatment beyond 16 wk in patients without an adequate response is not likely to result in greater success.

budesonide, See CORTICOSTEROIDS (INHALATION), CORTICOSTEROIDS (NASAL), and CORTICOSTEROIDS (SYSTEMIC).

bumetanide (byoo-**met**-a-nide)

~~Bumex~~, ✱ Burinex

Classification
Therapeutic: diuretics
Pharmacologic: loop diuretics

Indications

Edema due to heart failure, hepatic disease, or renal impairment. **Unlabeled Use:** Reversal of oliguria in preterm neonates.

Action

Inhibits the reabsorption of sodium and chloride from the loop of Henle and distal renal tubule. Increases renal excretion of water, sodium chloride, magnesium, potassium, and calcium. Effectiveness persists in impaired renal function. **Therapeutic Effects:** Diuresis and subsequent mobilization of excess fluid (edema, pleural effusions).

Pharmacokinetics

Absorption: Well absorbed after oral or IM administration.
Distribution: Widely distributed.
Protein Binding: 72–96%.
Metabolism and Excretion: Partially metabolized by liver; 50% eliminated unchanged by kidneys and 20% excreted in feces.
Half-life: 60–90 min (6 hr in neonates).

TIME/ACTION PROFILE (diuretic effect)

ROUTE	ONSET	PEAK	DURATION
PO	30–60 min	1–2 hr	4–6 hr
IM	30–60 min	1–2 hr	4–6 hr
IV	2–3 min	15–45 min	2–3 hr

Contraindications/Precautions

Contraindicated in: Hypersensitivity; Cross-sensitivity with thiazides and sulfonamides may occur; Hepatic coma or anuria.
Use Cautiously in: Severe liver disease (may precipitate hepatic coma; concurrent use with potassium-sparing diuretics may be necessary); Electrolyte depletion; Diabetes mellitus; Increasing azotemia; Lactation, Pedi: Safety not established; bumetanide is a potent displacer of bilirubin and should be used cautiously in critically ill or jaundiced neonates because of risk of kernicterus. Injection contains benzyl alcohol, which may cause gasping syndrome in neonates; Geri: May have ↑ risk of side effects, especially hypotension and electrolyte imbalance, at usual doses.

Adverse Reactions/Side Effects

CNS: dizziness, encephalopathy, headache. **EENT:** hearing loss, tinnitus. **CV:** hypotension. **GI:** diarrhea, dry mouth, nausea, vomiting. **GU:** ↑ BUN, excessive urination. **Derm:** STEVENS-JOHNSON SYNDROME, TOXIC EPIDERMAL NECROLYSIS, photosensitivity, pruritis, rash. **Endo:** hyperglycemia, hyperuricemia. **F and E:** dehydration, hypocalcemia, hypochloremia, hypokalemia, hypomagnesemia, hyponatremia, hypovolemia, metabolic alkalosis. **MS:** arthralgia, muscle cramps, myalgia.

Interactions

Drug-Drug: ↑ risk of hypotension with **antihypertensives**, **nitrates**, or acute ingestion of **alcohol**. ↑ risk of hypokalemia with other **diuretics**, **amphotericin B**, **stimulant laxatives**, and **corticosteroids**. Hypokalemia may ↑ risk of **digoxin** toxicity. ↓ **lithium** excretion, may cause **lithium** toxicity. ↑ risk of ototoxicity with **aminoglycosides**. **NSAIDS** ↓ effects of bumetanide.

Route/Dosage

PO (Adults): 0.5–2 mg/day given in 1–2 doses; titrate to desired response (maximum daily dose = 10 mg/day).
PO (Infants and Children): 0.015–0.1 mg/kg/dose every 6–24 hrs (maximum: 10 mg/day).
PO (Neonates): 0.01–0.05 mg/kg/dose every 12–24 in term neonates or every 24–48 hrs in preterm neonates.
IM, IV (Adults): 0.5–1 mg/dose, may repeat every 2–3 hr as needed (up to 10 mg/day).
IM, IV (Infants and Children): 0.015–0.1 mg/kg/dose every 6–24 hrs (maximum: 10 mg/day).
IM, IV (Neonates): 0.01–0.05 mg/kg/dose every 12–24 in term neonates or every 24–48 hrs in preterm neonates.

Availability (generic available)

Tablets: 0.5 mg, 1 mg, 2 mg, ✱ 5 mg. **Cost:** *Generic*—0.5 mg $30.20/100, 1 mg $44.52/100, 2 mg $75.18/100. **Injection:** 0.25 mg/mL.

NURSING IMPLICATIONS

Assessment

- Assess fluid status during therapy. Monitor daily weight, intake and output ratios, amount and location of edema, lung sounds, skin turgor, and mucous membranes. Notify health care professional if thirst, dry mouth, lethargy, weakness, hypotension, or oliguria occurs.

✱ = Canadian drug name. ⧖ = Genetic implication. ~~Strikethrough~~ = Discontinued.
*CAPITALS indicates life-threatening; underlines indicate most frequent.

- Monitor BP and pulse before and during administration. Monitor frequency of prescription refills to determine compliance.
- Assess patients receiving digoxin for anorexia, nausea, vomiting, muscle cramps, paresthesia, and confusion; ↑ risk of digoxin toxicity due to potassium-depleting effect of diuretic. Potassium supplements or potassium-sparing diuretics may be used concurrently to prevent hypokalemia.
- Assess patient for tinnitus and hearing loss. Audiometry is recommended for patients receiving prolonged high-dose IV therapy. Hearing loss is most common after rapid or high-dose IV administration in patients with decreased renal function or those taking other ototoxic drugs.
- Assess for allergy to sulfonamides.
- Assess patient for skin rash frequently during therapy. Discontinue bumetanide at first sign of rash; may be life-threatening. Stevens-Johnson syndrome or toxic epidermal necrolysis may develop. Treat symptomatically; may recur once treatment is stopped.
- Geri: Diuretic use is associated with increased risk for falls in older adults. Assess falls risk and implement fall prevention strategies.
- ***Lab Test Considerations:*** Monitor electrolytes, renal and hepatic function, serum glucose, and uric acid levels before and periodically during therapy. May cause ↓ serum sodium, potassium, calcium, and magnesium concentrations. May also cause ↑ BUN, serum glucose, creatinine, and uric acid levels.

Implementation

- If administering twice daily, give last dose no later than 5 PM to minimize disruption of sleep cycle.
- IV is preferred over IM for parenteral administration.
- **PO:** May be taken with food to minimize gastric irritation.

IV Administration

- **IV Push:** ***Diluent:*** Administer undiluted. ***Concentration:*** 0.25 mg/mL. ***Rate:*** Administer slowly over 1–2 min.
- **Continuous Infusion:** ***Diluent:*** May dilute in D5W or 0.9% NaCl. May also administer as undiluted drug. Protect from light. ***Concentration:*** Not to exceed 0.25 mg/mL. ***Rate:*** Infuse over 5 min. May be administered over 12 hr for patients with renal impairment.
- **Y-Site Compatibility:** acyclovir, alfentanil, allopurinol, amifostine, amikacin, aminocaproic acid, aminophylline, amiodarone, amphotericin B lipid complex, amphotericin B liposome, anidulafungin, argatroban, ascorbic acid, atropine, azithromycin, aztreonam, benztropine, bivalirudin, bleomycin, buprenorphine, butorphanol, calcium chloride, calcium gluconate, carboplatin, carmustine, caspofungin, cefazolin, cefepime, cefotaxime, cefoxitin, ceftaroline, ceftazidime, ceftriaxone, cefuroxime, chloramphenicol, cisatracurium, cisplatin, cladribine, clindamycin, cyanocobalamin, cyclophosphamide, cyclosporine, cytarabine, dactinomycin, daptomycin, dexamethasone, dexmedetomidine, dexrazoxane, digoxin, diltiazem, diphenhydramine, dobutamine, docetaxel, dopamine, doxorubicin, doxorubicin liposomal, doxycycline, enalaprilat, ephedrine, epinephrine, epirubicin, epoetin alfa, eptifibatide, ertapenem, erythromycin, esmolol, etoposide, etoposide phosphate, famotidine, fentanyl, filgrastim, fluconazole, fludarabine, fluorouracil, folic acid, furosemide, gemcitabine, gentamicin, glycopyrrolate, granisetron, heparin, hetastarch, hydrocortisone sodium succinate, hydromorphone, idarubicin, ifosfamide, imipenem/cilastatin, indomethacin, insulin, irinotecan, isoproterenol, ketorolac, labetalol, leucovorin calcium, levofloxacin, lidocaine, linezolid, lorazepam, magnesium sulfate, mannitol, melphalan, meperidine, methotrexate, methyldopate, methylprednisolone sodium succinate, metoclopramide, metoprolol, metronidazole, micafungin, milrinone, mitoxantrone, morphine, moxifloxacin, multivitamins, mycophenolate, nafcillin, nalbuphine, naloxone, nitroglycerin, nitroprusside, norepinephrine, octreotide, ondansetron, oxacillin, oxaliplatin, oxytocin, paclitaxcel, palonosetron, pamidronate, pancuronium, pantoprazole, pemetrexed, penicillin G, pentobarbital, phenobarbital, phentolamine, phenylephrine, phytonadione, piperacillin/tazobactam, potassium acetate, potassium chloride, procainamide, promethazine, propofol, propranolol, protamine, pyridoxime, ranitidine, remifentanil, rifampin, rituximab, rocuronium, sodium acetate, sodium bicarbonate, streptokinase, succinylcholine, sufentanil, tacrolimus, theophylline, thiamine, thiotepa, tigecycline, tirofiban, tobramycin, tolazoline, trastuzumab, vancomycin, vasopressin, vecuronium, verapamil, vinblastine, vincristine, vinorelbine, voriconazole, zoledronic acid.
- **Y-Site Incompatibility:** alemtuzumab, amphotericin B deoxycholate, azathioprine, chlorpromazine, dantrolene, diazepam, diazoxide, fenoldopam, ganciclovir, haloperidol, papaverine, pentamidine, phenytoin, quinupristin/dalfopristin, trimethoprim/sulfamethoxazole.

Patient/Family Teaching

- Instruct patient to take bumetanide as directed. Take missed doses as soon as possible; do not double doses.
- Caution patient to change positions slowly to minimize orthostatic hypotension. Caution patient that drinking alcohol, exercising during hot weather, or standing for long periods may enhance orthostatic hypotension.
- Instruct patient to consult health care professional regarding a diet high in potassium. See Appendix K.
- Advise patient to contact health care professional of gain more than 3 lbs in one day.

- Instruct patient to notify health care professional of all Rx or OTC medications, vitamins, or herbal products being taken and to consult health care professional before taking any OTC medications concurrently with this therapy.
- Instruct patient to notify health care professional of medication regimen before treatment or surgery.
- Caution patient to use sunscreen and protective clothing to prevent photosensitivity reactions.
- Advise patient to contact health care professional immediately if rash, muscle weakness, cramps, nausea, dizziness, numbness, or tingling of extremities occurs.
- Advise patients with diabetes to monitor blood glucose closely; may cause increased levels.
- Emphasize the importance of routine follow-up examinations.
- Geri: Caution older patients or their caregivers about increased risk for falls. Suggest strategies for fall prevention.

Evaluation/Desired Outcomes

- Decrease in edema.
- Decrease in abdominal girth and weight.
- Increase in urinary output.

bupivacaine, See EPIDURAL LOCAL ANESTHETICS.

REMS HIGH ALERT

buprenorphine

(byoo-pre-**nor**-feen)

Belbuca, Buprenex, Butrans, Probuphine, Sublocade, ~~Subutex~~

Classification

Therapeutic: opioid analgesics

Pharmacologic: opioid agonists/antagonists

Schedule III

Indications

IM, IV: Management of moderate to severe acute pain. **Buccal, Transdermal:** Pain that is severe enough to require daily, around-the-clock long-term opioid treatment and for which alternative treatment options (e.g. non-opioid analgesics or immediate-release opioids) are inadequate. **SL:** Treatment of opioid dependence (preferred for induction only); suppresses withdrawal symptoms in opioid detoxification. **Subdermal:** Maintenance treatment of opioid dependence in patients who have achieved and sustained prolonged (≥3 mo) clinical stability on low-to-moderate doses of a transmucosal buprenorphine-containing product (≤8 mg/day). **Subcut:** Treatment of opioid dependence in patients who have initiated treatment with a transmucosal buprenorphine-containing product (8–24 mg/day) for ≥7 days.

Action

Binds to opiate receptors in the CNS. Alters the perception of and response to painful stimuli while producing generalized CNS depression. Has partial antagonist properties that may result in opioid withdrawal in physically dependent patients when used as an analgesic.

Therapeutic Effects: IM, IV, Transdermal: Decreased severity of pain. **SL:** Suppression of withdrawal symptoms during detoxification and maintenance from heroin or other opioids. Produces a relatively mild withdrawal compared to other agents. **Subdermal:** Continued cessation of opioid use. **Subcut:** Continued cessation of opioid use.

Pharmacokinetics

Absorption: Well absorbed after IM and SL use; 46–65% absorbed with buccal use; 15% of transdermal dose absorbed through skin; IV administration results in complete bioavailability.

Distribution: Crosses the placenta; enters breast milk. CNS concentration is 15–25% of plasma.

Protein Binding: 96%.

Metabolism and Excretion: Mostly metabolized by the liver mostly via the CYP3A4 enzyme system; one metabolite is active; 70% excreted in feces; 27% excreted in urine.

Half-life: 2–3 hr (IV); 27 hr (buccal); 26 hr (transdermal); 37 hr (SL); 24–48 hr (subdermal); 43–60 days (subcut).

TIME/ACTION PROFILE (analgesia)

ROUTE	ONSET	PEAK	DURATION
IM	15 min	60 min	6 hr†
IV	rapid	less than 60 min	6 hr†
SL	unknown	unknown	unknown
Transdermal	unknown	unknown	7 days
Buccal	unknown	unknown	unknown
Subdermal	unknown	unknown	unknown
Subcut	unknown	unknown	unknown

†4–5 hr in children.

Contraindications/Precautions

Contraindicated in: Hypersensitivity; Significant respiratory depression (transdermal, buccal); Acute or severe bronchial asthma (transdermal, buccal); Paralytic ileus (transdermal, buccal); Acute, mild, intermittent, or postoperative pain (transdermal); Long QT syndrome; Concurrent use of class I or III antiarrhythmics; Lactation: Enters breast milk; avoid use or discontinue nursing.

Use Cautiously in: ↑ intracranial pressure; Compromised respiratory function including COPD, cor pulmonale, diminished respiratory reserve, hypoxia, hypercapnia or respiratory depression of other causes; Severe renal impairment; Moderate or severe hepatic impairment (dose ↓ needed for severe impairment); Hypothyroidism; Seizure disorders; Adrenal insufficiency; Alcoholism; Biliary tract disease; Acute pancreatitis; Debilitated patients (dose ↓ required); Oral mucositis (dose ↓ required) (buccal); Undiagnosed abdominal pain; Hypokalemia, hypomagnesemia, unstable atrial fibrillation, symptomatic bradycardia, unstable HF, or myocardial ischemia; Prostatic hyperplasia; OB: Safety not established; prolonged use of buccal, transdermal, subdermal, or SL buprenorphine during pregnancy can result in neonatal opioid withdrawal syndrome; Pedi: Safety and effectiveness not established in children (SL and transdermal) or children <2 yr (parenteral); Geri: ↑ risk of respiratory depression (dose ↓ required).

Adverse Reactions/Side Effects

CNS: confusion, dysphoria, hallucinations, sedation, dizziness, euphoria, floating feeling, headache, unusual dreams. **CV:** hypertension, hypotension, palpitations, QT interval prolongation. **Derm:** sweating, clammy feeling, erythema, pruritus, rash. **EENT:** blurred vision, diplopia, miosis (high doses). **Endo:** adrenal insufficiency. **GI:** HEPATOTOXICITY, nausea, constipation, dry mouth, ileus, vomiting. **GU:** urinary retention. **Resp:** RESPIRATORY DEPRESSION. **Misc:** HYPERSENSITIVITY REACTIONS (including anaphylaxis, angioedema, and bronchospasm), injection site reactions, physical dependence, psychological dependence, tolerance.

Interactions

Drug-Drug: Concurrent use with **class Ia antiarrhythmics**, **class III antiarrhythmics**, or other **QT interval prolonging medications** may ↑ risk of QT interval prolongation; avoid concurrent use. Use with **benzodiazepines** or other **CNS depressants** including other **opioids**, **non-benzodiazepine sedative/hypnotics**, **anxiolytics**, **general anesthetics**, **muscle relaxants**, **antipsychotics**, and **alcohol** may cause profound sedation, respiratory depression, coma, and death; reserve concurrent use for when alternative treatment options are inadequate. Use with extreme caution in patients receiving **MAO inhibitors** (↑ CNS and respiratory depression and hypotension—↓ buprenorphine dose by 50%; may need to ↓ **MAO inhibitor** dose; do not use transdermal formulation within 14 days of **MAO inhibitor**). May ↓ effectiveness of other **opioid analgesics**. Inhibitors of the CYP3A4 enzyme system including **itraconazole**, **ketoconazole**, **erythromycin**, **ritonavir**, **indinavir**, **saquinavir**, **atazanavir**, or **fosamprenavir** may ↑ blood levels and effects; may need to ↓ buprenorphine dose. Inducers of the CYP3A4 enzyme system including **carbamazepine**, **rifampin**, or **phenytoin** may ↓ blood levels and effects; buprenorphine dose modification may be necessary during concurrent use. Concurrent abuse of buprenorphine and **benzodiazepines** may result in coma and death. Drugs that affect serotonergic neurotransmitter systems, including **tricyclic antidepressants**, **SSRIs**, **SNRIs**, **MAO inhibitors**, **TCAs**, **tramadol**, **trazodone**, **mirtazapine**, **5–HT$_3$ receptor antagonists**, **linezolid**, **methylene blue**, and **triptans** ↑ risk of serotonin syndrome.

Drug-Natural Products: Concomitant use of **kava-kava**, **valerian**, **chamomile**, or **hops** can ↑ CNS depression.

Route/Dosage

Analgesia

IM, IV (Adults): 0.3 mg every 4–6 hr as needed. May repeat initial dose after 30 min (up to 0.3 mg every 4 hr or 0.6 mg every 6 hr); 0.6-mg doses should be given only IM.

IM, IV (Children 2–12 yr): 2–6 mcg (0.002–0.006 mg)/kg every 4–6 hr.

Transdermal (Adults): *Opioid-naïve*—Transdermal system delivering 5–20 mcg/hr applied every 7 days. Initiate with 5 mcg/hr system; each dose titration may occur after 72 hr; do not exceed dose of 20 mcg/hr (due to ↑ risk of QT interval prolongation); *Previously taking <30 mg/day of morphine or equivalent*—Initiate with 5 mcg/hr system; each dose titration may occur after 72 hr; do not exceed dose of 20 mcg/hr (due to ↑ risk of QT interval prolongation); apply patch every 7 days; *Previously taking 30–80 mg/day of morphine or equivalent*—Initiate with 10 mcg/hr system; each dose titration may occur after 72 hr; do not exceed dose of 20 mcg/hr (due to ↑ risk of QT interval prolongation); apply patch every 7 days; *Previously taking >80 mg/day of morphine or equivalent*—Consider use of alternate analgesic.

Buccal (Adults): *Opioid-naïve*—Initiate therapy with 75 mcg once daily or every 12 hr for ≥4 days, then ↑ dose to 150 mcg every 12 hr; may then titrate dose in increments of 150 mcg every 12 hr no more frequently than every 4 days; do not exceed dose of 450 mcg every 12 hr (based on clinical studies); *Previously taking <30 mg/day of morphine or equivalent*—Initiate therapy with 75 mcg once daily or every 12 hr for ≥4 days, then ↑ dose to 150 mcg every 12 hr; may then titrate dose in increments of 150 mcg every 12 hr no more frequently than every 4 days; do not exceed dose of 900 mcg every 12 hr (due to ↑ risk of QT interval prolongation); *Previously taking 30–89 mg/day of morphine or equivalent*—Initiate therapy with 150 mcg every 12 hr for ≥4 days; may then titrate dose in increments of 150 mcg every 12 hr no more frequently than every 4 days; do not exceed dose of 900 mcg every 12 hr (due to ↑ risk of QT interval prolongation); *Previously taking 90–160 mg/day of morphine or equivalent*—Initiate therapy with 300 mcg every 12 hr for ≥4 days; may then titrate dose in increments of 150 mcg every 12 hr no more frequently than every 4 days; do not exceed dose of 900 mcg every 12 hr (due to ↑ risk of QT interval prolongation); *Previously taking >160 mg/day of morphine or equivalent*—Consider use of alternate analgesic; *Patients with oral mucositis*—↓ initial dose by 50% then titrate dose in increments of 75 mcg every 12 hr no more frequently than every 4 days.

Hepatic Impairment

Transdermal (Adults): *Mild to moderate hepatic impairment*—Initiate with 5 mcg/hr system.

Hepatic Impairment

Buccal (Adults): *Severe hepatic impairment*—↓ initial dose by 50% then titrate dose in increments of 75 mcg every 12 hr no more frequently than every 4 days.

Treatment of Opioid Dependence

SL (Adults): *Induction*—8 mg once daily on Day 1, then 16 mg once daily on Day 2–4; *Maintenance*—Patients should preferably be transitioned to buprenorphine/naloxone; if patient cannot tolerate naloxone, then can use buprenorphine (usual dosage range = 4–24 mg/day); recommended target dose = 16 mg/day; dose can be ↑ or ↓ by 2–4 mg, as needed to prevent signs/symptoms of opioid withdrawal.
Subcut (Adults): 300 mg once monthly for 2 mo, then 100 mg once monthly; may ↑ maintenance dose to 300 mg once monthly if patient reports illicit opioid use or has positive urine drug screen for illicit opioid use.
Subdermal (Adults): Insert 4 implants in inner side of upper arm and then remove at end of 6 mo.

Hepatic Impairment

SL (Adults): *Severe hepatic impairment*—↓ initial dose and adjustment dose by 50%.

Availability (generic available)

Extended-release solution for injection (prefilled syringes) (Sublocade): 100 mg/0.5 mL, 300 mg/1.5 mL. **Sublingual tablets:** 2 mg, 8 mg. **Solution for injection (Buprenex):** 300 mcg (0.3 mg)/mL. **Transdermal system (Butrans):** 5 mcg/hr, 7.5 mcg/hr, 10 mcg/hr, 15 mcg/hr, 20 mcg/hr. **Buccal film (Belbuca):** 75 mcg, 150 mcg, 300 mcg, 450 mcg, 600 mcg, 750 mcg, 900 mcg. **Implant:** 74.2 mg/implant. ***In combination with:*** naloxone (Bunavail, Suboxone, Zubsolv). See Appendix B.

NURSING IMPLICATIONS

Assessment

- Monitor for signs and symptoms of adrenal insufficiency (nausea, vomiting, anorexia, fatigue, weakness, dizziness, and low blood pressure) during therapy. If adrenal insufficiency is suspected, confirm with diagnostic testing. If confirmed, treat with physiologic doses of replacement corticosteroids. Wean patient off opioid to allow adrenal recovery and continue corticosteroids until adrenal function recovers. Other opioids may be tried.
- **Pain:** Assess type, location, and intensity of pain before and 1 hr after IM and 5 min (peak) after IV administration. When titrating opioid doses, increases of 25–50% should be administered until there is either a 50% reduction in the patient's pain rating on a numerical or visual analogue scale or the patient reports satisfactory pain relief. A repeat dose can be safely administered at the time of the peak if previous dose is ineffective and side effects are minimal. Single doses of 600 mcg (0.6 mg) should be administered IM. Patients requiring doses higher than 600 mcg (0.6 mg) should be converted to an opioid agonist. Buprenorphine is not recommended for prolonged use (except buccal or transdermal) or as first-line therapy for acute or cancer pain. SL and subdermal formulations should not be used to relieve pain.
- An equianalgesic chart (see Appendix J) should be used when changing routes or when changing from one opioid to another.
- Assess level of consciousness, BP, pulse, and respirations before and periodically during administration, especially within first 24–72 hrs of buccal therapy. If respiratory rate is <10/min, assess level of sedation. Dose may need to be decreased by 25–50%. Buprenorphine 0.3–0.4 mg has approximately equal analgesic and respiratory depressant effects to morphine 10 mg.
- Assess previous analgesic history. Antagonistic properties may induce withdrawal symptoms (vomiting, restlessness, abdominal cramps, increased BP and temperature) in patients who are physically dependent on opioid agonists. Symptoms may occur up to 15 days after discontinuation and persist for 1–2 wk.
- Buprenorphine has a lower potential for dependence than other opioids; however, prolonged use may lead to physical and psychological dependence and tolerance. This should not prevent patient from receiving adequate analgesia. Most patients receiving buprenorphine for pain rarely develop psychological dependence. If tolerance develops, changing to an opioid agonist may be required to relieve pain.
- Assess bowel function routinely. Prevent constipation with increased intake of fluids and bulk, and laxatives to minimize constipating effects. Administer stimulant laxatives routinely if opioid use exceeds 2–3 days, unless contraindicated. Consider drugs for opioid-induced constipation.
- **Transdermal:** Assess risk for opioid addiction, abuse, or misuse prior to administration. Monitor for respiratory depression, especially during initiation or following dose increase; serious, life-threat-

ening, or fatal respiratory depression may occur. Misuse or abuse of *Butrans* by chewing, swallowing, snorting or injecting buprenorphine extracted from transdermal system will result in the uncontrolled delivery of buprenorphine and risk of overdose and death.

- Maintain frequent contact during periods of changing analgesic requirements, including initial titration, between the prescriber, other members of the healthcare team, the patient, and the caregiver/family.
- **Treatment of Opioid Dependence:** Assess patient for signs and symptoms of opioid withdrawal before and during therapy.
- Examine *Probuphine* insertion site 1 wk after insertion for infection, wound healing, and implant extrusion. Patients should be seen at least monthly for counseling and psychological support.
- ***Lab Test Considerations:*** May cause ↑ serum amylase and lipase levels.
- Monitor liver function tests prior to and periodically during opioid dependence therapy.
- ***Toxicity and Overdose:*** If an opioid antagonist is required to reverse respiratory depression or coma, naloxone (Narcan) is the antidote. Dilute the 0.4-mg ampule of naloxone in 10 mL of 0.9% NaCl and administer 0.5 mL (0.02 mg) by IV push every 2 min. For children and patients weighing <40 kg, dilute 0.1 mg of naloxone in 10 mL of 0.9% NaCl for a concentration of 10 mcg/mL and administer 0.5 mcg/kg every 1–2 min. Titrate dose to avoid withdrawal, seizures, and severe pain. Naloxone may not completely reverse respiratory depressant effects of buprenorphine; may require mechanical ventilation, oxygen, IV fluids, and vasopressors.

Implementation

- Do not confuse buprenorphine with hydromorphone.
- **Pain:** Explain therapeutic value of medication before administration to enhance the analgesic effect.
- Regularly administered doses may be more effective than prn administration. Analgesic is more effective if given before pain becomes severe.
- Coadministration with nonopioid analgesics has additive effects and may permit lower opioid doses.
- FDA strongly encourages health care professionals to complete a REMS-compliant education program that includes all the elements of the FDA Education *Blueprint for Health Care Providers Involved in the Management or Support of Patients with Pain,* available at www.fda.gov/OpioidAnalgesicREMSBlueprint. Information on programs can be found at 1-800-503-0784 or www.opioidanalgesicrems.com.
- **Buccal:** Have patient wet inside of cheek with tongue or rinse mouth with water. Apply film immediately after removal from package. Place yellow side of film against inside of cheek. Hold film in place with dry fingers for 5 sec, then leave in place on inside of cheek until fully dissolved. If chewed or swallowed, may result in lower peak concentrations and lower bioavailability. Do not administer if package seal if broken or film is cut, damaged, or changed. Avoid applying to areas of mouth with sores or lesions. To dispose of unused film, remove from foil package, drop into toilet and flush.
- **IM:** Administer IM injections deep into well-developed muscle. Rotate sites of injections.

IV Administration

- **IV Push:** May give IV undiluted. ***High Alert:*** Administer slowly. Rapid administration may cause respiratory depression, hypotension, and cardiac arrest. ***Rate:*** Give over at least 2 min.
- **Y-Site Compatibility:** acetaminophen, acyclovir, alfentanil, allopurinol, amifostine, amikacin, aminocaproic acid, amiodarone, amphotericin B lipid complex, amphotericin B liposome, anidulafungin, argatroban, arsenic trioxide, ascorbic acid, atracurium, atropine, azithromycin, aztreonam, benztropine, bivalirudin, bleomycin, bumetanide, butorphanol, calcium chloride, calcium gluconate, carboplatin, carmustine, cefazolin, cefepime, cefotaxime, cefotetan, cefoxitin, ceftazidime, ceftriaxone, cefuroxime, chloramphenicol, chlorpromazine, cisatracurium, cisplatin, cladribine, clindamycin, cyanocobalamin, cyclophosphamide, cyclosporine, cytarabine, dactinomycin, daptomycin, daunorubicin, dexamethasone, dexmedetomidine, dexrazoxane, digoxin, diltiazem, diphenhydramine, dobutamine, docetaxel, dolasetron, dopamine, doxorubicin, doxycycline, enalaprilat, ephedrine, epinephrine, epirubicin, epoetin alfa, eptifibatide, ertapenem, erythromycin, esmolol, etoposide, etoposide phosphate, famotidine, fenoldopam, fentanyl, filgrastim, fluconazole, fludarabine, foscarnet, fosphenytoin, gemcitabine, gentamicin, glycopyrrolate, granisetron, heparin, hetastarch, hydrocortisone, idarubicin, ifosfamide, imipenem/cilastatin, insulin, irinotecan, isoproterenol, ketorolac, labetalol, leucovorin calcium, levofloxacin, lidocaine, linezolid, lorazepam, magnesium sulfate, mannitol, melphalan, meperidine, mesna, methotrexate, methylprednisolone, metoclopramide, metoprolol, metronidazole, midazolam, milrinone, mitomycin, mitoxantrone, morphine, multivitamins, mycophenolate, nafcillin, nalbuphine, naloxone, nicardipine, nitroglycerin, nitroprusside, norepinephrine, octreotide, ondansetron, oxacillin, oxaliplatin, oxytocin, paclitaxel, palonosetron, pamidronate, pancuronium, papaverine, pemetrexed, penicillin G, pentamidine, phentolamine, phenylephrine, phytonadione, piperacillin/tazobactam, potassium acetate, potassium chloride, procainamide, prochlorperazine, promethazine, propofol, propranolol, protamine, pyridoxine, quinupristin/dalfopristin, ranitidine, remifentanil, rituximab, rocuronium, sodium acetate, streptokinase,

succinylcholine, sufentanil, tacrolimus, theophylline, thiamine, thiotepa, tigecycline, tirofiban, tobramycin, topotecan, trastuzumab, vancomycin, vasopressin, vecuronium, verapamil, vinblastine, vincristine, vinorelbine, voriconazole, zoledronic acid.

- **Y-Site Incompatibility:** alemtuzumab, aminophylline, ampicillin, azathioprine, dantrolene, diazepam, diazoxide, doxorubicin liposomal, fluorouracil, gemtuzumab, indomethacin, pantoprazole, pentobarbital, phenobarbital, phenytoin, sodium bicarbonate, trimethoprim/sulfamethoxazole.
- **Transdermal:** Buprenorphine may cause withdrawal in patients who are already taking opioids. For conversion from other opioids to buprenorphine transdermal, taper current around-the-clock opioids for up to 7 days to no more than 30 mg of morphine or equivalent per day before beginning treatment with buprenorphine transdermal. May use short-acting analgesics as needed until analgesic efficacy with buprenorphine transdermal is attained. Buprenorphine transdermal may not provide adequate analgesia for patients requiring greater than 80 mg/day oral morphine equivalents.
- Apply system to flat, hairless, nonirritated, and nonirradiated site on the upper outer arm, upper chest, upper back or the side of the chest. If skin preparation is necessary, use clear water and clip, do not shave, hair. Allow skin to dry completely before application. Apply immediately after removing from package. Do not alter the system (i.e., cut) in any way before application. Remove liner from adhesive layer and press firmly in place with palm of hand for 30 sec, especially around the edges, to make sure contact is complete. Remove used system and fold so that adhesive edges are together. Flush system down toilet immediately on removal or follow the institutional policy. Apply new system to a different site. After removal, wait a minimum of 3 wk before applying to the same site. If patch falls off during 7-day dosing interval, dispose of patch and place a new patch on at a different site.
- May be titrated no less than every 72 hrs. Dose adjustments in 5 mcg/hr, 7.5 mcg/hr, or 10 mcg/hr increments may be used by using no more than two patches.
- To discontinue, taper dose gradually to prevent signs and symptoms of withdrawal; consider introduction of immediate-release opioid medication.
- **Treatment of Opioid Dependence:** Must be prescribed by health care professional with special training.
- **SL:** Induction is usually started with buprenorphine SL over 3–4 days. Initial dose should be administered at least 4 hr after last opioid dose and preferably when early signs of opioid withdrawal appear. Once patient is on a stable dose, maintenance therapy with buprenorphine/naloxone (Suboxone) is preferred for continued, unsupervised treatment.
- Administer sublingually. Usually takes 2–10 min for tablets to dissolve. If more than one tablet is prescribed, place multiple tablets under the tongue or 2 at a time until all tablets are dissolved. Do not chew or swallow; decreases amount of medication absorbed. Not used for analgesia; may cause death in opioid naïve patients.
- **Subcut:** *Sublocade* is for patients who have initiated treatment with a transmucosal buprenorphine product followed by dose adjustment for at least 7 days. Prepare and administer only by health care professional. Use syringe and needle provided by manufacturer. Remove from refrigerator at least 15 min before injection to allow to reach room temperature. Do not open foil pouch until patient has arrived. Discard if left at room temperature for >7 days. Do not administer solutions that are discolored or contain particulate matter. Pinch injection site and administer into abdomen; do not rub. May cause a lump that will decrease over several wk. Do not administer IV or IM. If discontinued, withdrawal effects will be delayed (2–5 mo) due to long half-life. Monitor patients discontinuing for withdrawal signs and symptoms. May use transmucosal buprenorphine to treat withdrawal.
- **Subdermal:** Patient must meet selection criteria before insertion: Prolonged stability on transmucosal buprenorphine dose of ≤8 mg/day without supplementation for ≥3 mo. Rx for supplemental buprenorphine should not be provided. If additional doses are required assess patient promptly. Amount of buprenorphine may not be adequate for stable maintenance. Alternate products may be required.
- Follow package insert instructions for insertion of *Probuphine*. Inserts must be removed after 6 mo. A new implant may be inserted into contralateral arm for a second 6 mo period. No additional implants are allowed. If a second implant is not inserted, maintain patient on previous dose of transmucosal buprenorphine.
- *Probuphine* implants are only available through the Probuphine REMS Program at www.probuphinerems.com or by calling 1–844–859–6341. Due to risk of complications of migration, protrusion and expulsion, and nerve damage associated with the insertion and removal of implant, health care professionals must be certified by enrolling and completing live training with demonstrated competency, patients must be monitored to make sure implants are removed by a certified health care professional, and implants are available to certified prescribers through a restricted distribution program.

Patient/Family Teaching

- Instruct patient on risk of addiction, abuse, and misuse, which could lead to death. Discuss safe use, risks, and proper storage and disposal of opioid analgesics with patients and caregivers with each Rx. The Patient Counseling Guide (PCG) is available at www.fda.gov/OpioidAnalgesicREMSPCG. Advise patient not to share buprenorphine with others and to protect from theft or misuse.
- Medication may cause drowsiness or dizziness. Advise patient to call for assistance when ambulating and to avoid driving or other activities requiring alertness until response to medication is known, especially within 24–48 hrs after subdermal implant insertion.
- Advise patient to avoid concurrent use of alcohol or other CNS depressants.
- Instruct patient to notify health care professional of all Rx or OTC medications, vitamins, or herbal products being taken and to consult health care professional before taking any Rx, OTC, or herbal products, especially CNS depressants.
- Rep: Advise patient to notify health care professional if pregnancy is planned or suspected, or if breast feeding. Inform patient of potential for neonatal opioid withdrawal syndrome with prolonged use during pregnancy.
- **Pain:** Instruct patient on how and when to ask for pain medication.
- Encourage patients on bedrest to turn, cough, and deep-breathe every 2 hr to prevent atelectasis.
- Instruct patient to change positions slowly to minimize orthostatic hypotension.
- Advise patient that good oral hygiene, frequent mouth rinses, and sugarless gum or candy may decrease dry mouth.
- **Buccal:** Instruct patient on proper technique of buccal film and to avoid eating or drinking until film dissolves. Apply at same time each day. Avoid touching or moving buccal film with tongue or fingers. Do not stop using buprenorphine without consulting health care professional. Advise patient to read *Instructions for Use* prior to starting therapy and with each Rx refill in case of changes.
- Advise patient to notify health care professional if the dose does not control pain.
- **Transdermal:** Instruct patient in correct method for application, removal, storage, and disposal of transdermal system. Wear patches for 7 days. May be worn while bathing, showering, or swimming. Do not discontinue or change dose without consulting health care professional. Instruct patient to read the *Medication Guide* prior to starting and with each Rx refill.
- Advise patients and caregivers/family members of the potential side effects. Instruct patient to notify health care professional if pain is not controlled or if bothersome side effects occur. Contact immediately if difficulty or changes in breathing, unusual deep "sighing" breathing, slow or shallow breathing, new or unusual snoring, slow heartbeat, severe sleepiness, cold, clammy skin, feeling faint, dizzy, confused, or cannot think, walk, or talk normally, or if swelling or blistering around patch occurs.
- Advise patient that fever, electric blankets, heating pads, saunas, hot tubs, and heated water beds increase release of buprenorphine from patch.
- Advise patient referred for MRI test to discuss patch with referring health care professional and MRI facility to determine if removal of patch is necessary prior to test and for directions for replacing patch.
- **Opioid Dependence:** Explain techniques for use to patient.
- Caution patient that buprenorphine may be a target for people who abuse drugs; store medications in a safe place to protect them from theft. Selling or giving this medication to others is against the law.
- Caution patient that injection of *Suboxone* can lead to severe withdrawal symptoms.
- Advise patient if admitted to the emergency department to inform treating health care professional and emergency room staff of physical dependence on opioids and of treatment regimen.
- Advise patient to notify health care professional promptly if faintness, dizziness, confusion, slowed breathing, skin or whites of eyes turn yellow, urine turns dark, light-colored stools, decreased appetite, nausea, or abdominal pain occur.
- **SL:** Instruct patient in correct use of medication; directions for use must be followed exactly. Medication must be used regularly, not occasionally. Take missed doses as soon as remembered; if almost time for next dose, skip missed dose and return to regular dosing schedule. Do not take 2 doses at once unless directed by health care professional. Do not discontinue use without consulting health care professional; abrupt discontinuation may cause withdrawal symptoms. If medication is discontinued, flush unused tablets down the toilet if a drug take-back option is not readily available. **Subcut:** Inform patient *Sublocade* is only available through a restricted program, *Sublocade* REMS program. *Sublocade* can only be dispensed to directly to a health care provider. **Subdermal:** Advise patient to notify health care professional if bleeding, signs and symptoms of infection (excessive or worsening itching, pain, irritation, redness, or swelling), weakness or numbness in arm after the insertion or removal procedure, shortness of breath) occur.

Evaluation/Desired Outcomes

- Decrease in severity of pain without a significant alteration in level of consciousness or respiratory status.
- Suppression of withdrawal symptoms during detoxification and maintenance from heroin or other opioids.

B

buPROPion (byoo-proe-pee-on)

Aplenzin, Forfivo XL, ~~Wellbutrin~~, Wellbutrin SR, Wellbutrin XL, ~~Zyban~~

Classification

Therapeutic: antidepressants, smoking deterrents

Pharmacologic: aminoketones

Indications

Treatment of depression (with psychotherapy). Depression with seasonal affective disorder. Smoking cessation. **Unlabeled Use:** Treatment of ADHD (adults). To increase sexual desire in women.

Action

Decreases neuronal reuptake of dopamine in the CNS. Diminished neuronal uptake of serotonin and norepinephrine (less than tricyclic antidepressants). **Therapeutic Effects:** Diminished depression. Decreased craving for cigarettes.

Pharmacokinetics

Absorption: Although well absorbed, rapidly and extensively metabolized by the liver.

Distribution: Unknown.

Metabolism and Excretion: Extensively metabolized by the liver into 3 active metabolites (CYP2B6 involved in formation of one of the active metabolites).

Half-life: 14 hr (active metabolites may have longer half-lives).

TIME/ACTION PROFILE (antidepressant effect)

ROUTE	ONSET	PEAK	DURATION
PO	1–3 wk	unknown	unknown

Contraindications/Precautions

Contraindicated in: Hypersensitivity; Concurrent use of MAO inhibitors or MAO-like drugs (linezolid or methylene blue); Concurrent use of ritonavir; Seizure disorders; Arteriovenous malformation, severe head injury, CNS tumor, CNS infection, severe stroke, anorexia nervosa, bulimia, or abrupt discontinuation of alcohol, benzodiazepines, barbiturates, or antiepileptic drugs (↑ risk of seizures); Lactation: Potential for serious adverse reactions in nursing infants.

Use Cautiously in: Renal/hepatic impairment (↓ dose recommended) (Forfivo XL not recommended in patients with renal or hepatic impairment); Recent history of MI; History of suicide attempt; Unstable cardiovascular status; May ↑ risk of suicide attempt/ideation especially during early treatment or dose adjustment; this risk appears to be greater in adolescents or children; Psychiatric illness; Angle-closure glaucoma; OB: Use during pregnancy only if maternal benefit outweighs potential risk to fetus; Geri: ↑ risk of drug accumulation; ↑ sensitivity to effects.

Exercise Extreme Caution in: Severe hepatic cirrhosis (↓ dose required); Pedi: ↑ risk of suicidal thinking and behavior. Observe carefully, especially at initiation of therapy and during ↑ or ↓ in dose.

Adverse Reactions/Side Effects

CNS: HOMICIDAL THOUGHTS/BEHAVIOR, SEIZURES, SUICIDAL THOUGHTS/BEHAVIOR, agitation, headache, aggression, anxiety, delusions, depression, hallucinations, hostility, insomnia, mania, panic, paranoia, psychoses. **CV:** hypertension. **Derm:** photosensitivity. **Endo:** hyperglycemia, hypoglycemia, syndrome of inappropriate ADH secretion. **GI:** dry mouth, nausea, vomiting, change in appetite, weight gain, weight loss. **Neuro:** tremor.

Interactions

Drug-Drug: Concurrent use with **MAO-inhibitors** may ↑ risk of hypertensive reactions; concurrent use contraindicated; at least 14 days should elapse between discontinuation of MAO inhibitor and initiation of bupropion (or visa versa). Concurrent use with **MAO-inhibitor like drugs**, such as **linezolid** or **methylene blue** may ↑ risk of hypertensive reactions; concurrent use contraindicated; do not start therapy in patients receiving **linezolid** or **methylene blue**; if **linezolid** or **methylene blue** need to be started in a patient receiving bupropion, immediately discontinue bupropion and monitor for 2 wk or until 24 hr after last dose of linezolid or methylene blue, whichever comes first (may resume bupropion therapy 24 hr after last dose of linezolid or methylene blue). ↑ risk of adverse reactions when used with **amantadine** or **levodopa**. ↑ risk of seizures with **phenothiazines**, **antidepressants**, **theophylline**, **corticosteroids**, **OTC stimulants/anorectics**, or cessation of **alcohol** or **benzodiazepines** (avoid or minimize alcohol use). **Ritonavir**, **lopinavir/ritonavir**, and **efavirenz** may ↓ levels; may need to ↑ bupropion dose. May ↑ **citalopram** levels. **Carbamazepine** may ↓ blood levels and effectiveness. Concurrent use with **nicotine** replacement may cause hypertension. ↑ risk of bleeding with **warfarin**. Bupropion and one of its metabolites inhibit the CYP2D6 enzyme system and may ↑ levels and risk of toxicity from **antidepressants** (SSRIs and tricyclic), **haloperidol**, **risperidone**, **thioridazine**, **beta blockers**, **flecainide**, and **propafenone**. May ↓ levels and efficacy of **tamoxifen**. May ↓ the efficacy of **tamoxifen**. May ↓ **digoxin** levels.

Route/Dosage

Depression

PO (Adults): *Immediate-release*—100 mg twice daily initially; after 3 days may ↑ to 100 mg 3 times daily; after at least 4 wk of therapy, may ↑ up to 450 mg/day in divided doses (not to exceed 150 mg/dose; wait at least 6 hr between doses at the 300 mg/day dose or at least 4 hr between doses at the 450-mg/day dose). *12–hr sustained-release*—150 mg once daily in the morning; after 3 days, may ↑ to 150 mg twice daily with at least 8 hr between doses; after at least 4 wk of therapy, may ↑ to a maximum daily dose of 400 mg given as 200 mg twice daily. *24–hr extended-release (Wellbutrin XL)*—150 mg once daily in the morning, may be ↑ after 4 days to 300 mg once daily; some patients may require up to 450 mg/day as a single daily dose. *24–hr extended-release (Aplenzin)*—174 mg once daily in the morning, may be ↑ after 4 days to 348 mg once daily; some patients may require up to 522 mg/day as a single daily dose. *24–hr extended-release (Forfivo XL)*—450 mg once daily (should NOT be used as initial therapy; it should only be used in patients who have been receiving 300 mg/day of another bupropion formulation for at least 2 wk and require titration up to 450 mg/day or in those patients receiving 450 mg/day of another bupropion formulation).

Hepatic Impairment

PO (Adults): *Moderate-to-severe hepatic impairment (Aplenzin)*—Max dose: 174 mg every other day.

Seasonal Affective Disorder

PO (Adults): *24–hr extended-release (Wellbutrin XL)*—150 mg/day in the morning; if dose is well tolerated, ↑ to 300 mg/day in one wk. Doses should be tapered to 150 mg/day for 2 wk before discontinuing; *24–hr extended-release (Aplenzin)*—174 mg once daily in the morning, may be ↑ after 7 days to 348 mg once daily.

Hepatic Impairment

PO (Adults): *Moderate-to-severe hepatic impairment (Aplenzin)*—Max dose: 174 mg every other day.

Smoking cessation

PO (Adults): *12–hr sustained release*—150 mg once daily for 3 days, then 150 mg twice daily for 7–12 wk (doses should be at least 8 hr apart).

Availability (generic available)

Immediate-release tablets: 75 mg, 100 mg. **Cost:** *Generic*—75 mg $79.43/100, 100 mg $106.01/100. **12–Hour sustained-release tablets:** 100 mg, 150 mg, 200 mg. **Cost:** *Generic*—100 mg $51.12/180, 150 mg $59.60/180, 200 mg $52.33/180. **24–Hour extended-release tablets (Wellbutrin XL):** 150 mg, 300 mg. **Cost:** *Generic*—150 mg $74.84/90, 300 mg $63.94/90. **24–Hour extended-release tablets (Aplenzin):** 174 mg, 348 mg, 522 mg. **Cost:** 174 mg $359.09/30, 348 mg $473.36/30, 522 mg $1,077.23/30. **24–Hour extended-release tablets (Forfivo XL):** 450 mg. **Cost:** $176.40/30.

NURSING IMPLICATIONS

Assessment

- Assess mental status and mood changes in all patients, especially during initial few mo of therapy and during dose changes. Risk may be increased in children, adolescents, and adults ≤24 yrs. Inform health care professional if patient demonstrates significant increase in signs of depression (depressed mood, loss of interest in usual activities, significant change in weight and/or appetite, insomnia or hypersomnia, psychomotor agitation or retardation, increased fatigue, feelings of guilt or worthlessness, slowed thinking or impaired concentration, suicide attempt or suicidal/homicidal ideation). If so, restrict amount of drug available to patient.
- ***Lab Test Considerations:*** Monitor hepatic and renal function closely in patients with kidney or liver impairment to prevent ↑ serum and tissue bupropion concentrations.
- May cause false-positive urine test for amphetamines.

Implementation

- Do not confuse bupropion with buspirone. Do not confuse *Wellbutrin SR* with *Wellbutrin XL*. Do not administer bupropion (*Wellbutrin products*) with Zyban, which contain the same ingredients.
- Administer doses in equally spaced time increments during the day to minimize the risk of seizures. Risk of seizures increases fourfold in doses greater than 450 mg per day.
- May be initially administered concurrently with sedatives to minimize agitation. This is not usually required after the 1st wk of therapy.
- Insomnia may be decreased by avoiding bedtime doses. May require treatment during 1st wk of therapy.
- Nicotine patches, gum, inhalers, and spray may be used concurrently with bupropion.
- When converting from other brands of bupropion to *Aplenzin* 522 mg/day *Aplenzin* is equivalent to 450 mg/day bupropion HCl, 348 mg/day *Aplenzin* is equivalent to 300 mg/day bupropion HCl, and 174 mg/day *Aplenzin* is equivalent to 150 mg/day bupropion HCl.
- **PO:** Swallow sustained-release or extended-release tablets whole; do not break, crush, or chew.
- May be administered with food to lessen GI irritation.
- **Seasonal Affective Disorder:** Begin administration in autumn prior to the onset of depressive symptoms. Continue therapy through winter and begin to taper and discontinue in early spring.

Patient/Family Teaching

- Instruct patient to take bupropion as directed at the same time each day. Missed doses should be omitted. Do not double doses or take more than prescribed. May require 4 wk or longer for full effects.

Do not discontinue without consulting health care professional. May require gradual reduction before discontinuation. Advise patient to read *Medication Guide* before starting and with each Rx refill in case of changes.

- May impair judgment or motor and cognitive skills. Caution patient to avoid driving and other activities requiring alertness until response to medication is known.
- Advise patient, family, and caregivers to look for suicidality, especially during early therapy or dose changes. Notify health care professional immediately if thoughts about suicide or dying, attempts to commit suicide, new or worse depression or anxiety, agitation or restlessness, panic attacks, insomnia, new or worse irritability, aggressiveness, acting on dangerous impulses, mania, or other changes in mood or behavior occur.
- Instruct patient to notify health care professional of all Rx or OTC medications, vitamins, or herbal products being taken, to avoid alcohol during therapy and to consult with health care professional before taking other medications with bupropion, such as *Zyban*.
- Inform patient that frequent mouth rinses, good oral hygiene, and sugarless gum or candy may minimize dry mouth. If dry mouth persists for more than 2 wk, consult health care professional regarding use of saliva substitute.
- Instruct patient to notify health care professional of all Rx or OTC medications, vitamins, or herbal products being taken and consult health care professional before taking any new medications.
- Advise patient to notify health care professional if rash or other troublesome side effects occur.
- Inform patient that unused shell of XL tablets may appear in stool; this is normal.
- Advise patient to use sunscreen and protective clothing to prevent photosensitivity reactions.
- Advise patient to notify health care professional of medication regimen before treatment or surgery.
- Instruct female patients to inform health care professional if pregnancy is planned or suspected or if breast feeding or planning to breast feed.
- Emphasize the importance of follow-up exams to monitor progress. Encourage patient participation in psychotherapy.
- **Smoking Cessation:** Smoking should be stopped during the 2nd wk of therapy to allow for the onset of bupropion and to maximize the chances of quitting.
- Advise patient to stop taking bupropion and contact a health care professional immediately if agitation, depressed mood, and any changes in behavior that are not typical of nicotine withdrawal, or if suicidal thoughts or behavior occur.

Evaluation/Desired Outcomes

- Increased sense of well-being.
- Renewed interest in surroundings. Acute episodes of depression may require several mo of treatment.
- Cessation of smoking.

bupropion/naltrexone

(byoo-**proe**-pee-on nal-**trex**-one)
Contrave

Classification
Therapeutic: weight control agents
Pharmacologic: aminoketones, opioid antagonists

Indications

Adjunct to calorie-reduced diet and increased physical activity for chronic weight management in obese patients (BMI ≥30 kg/m^2) or overweight patients (BMI ≥27 kg/m^2) with at least one other comorbidity (hypertension, type 2 diabetes, or dyslipidemia).

Action

Bupropion—an antidepressant that acts as a weak inhibitor of neuronal reuptake of dopamine and norepinephrine. *Naltrexone*—acts as an opioid antagonist. In combination they affect two different brain areas involved in food intake: the hypothalamic appetite regulatory center and mesolimbic dopamine circuit reward system. **Therapeutic Effects:** Decreased appetite with associated weight loss.

Pharmacokinetics

Bupropion

Absorption: Well absorbed but rapidly metabolized by the liver. Absorption is enhanced by a high-fat meal.

Distribution: Parent drug and metabolites enter breast milk.

Metabolism and Excretion: Extensively metabolized; three metabolites are pharmacologically active. Excretion is mostly renal as metabolites, minimal renal excretion of unchanged drug.

Half-life: 21 hr (longer for some metabolites).

Naltrexone

Absorption: Well absorbed orally, undergoes extensive first pass hepatic metabolism resulting in 5–40% bioavailability. Absorption is enhanced by a high-fat meal.

Distribution: Parent drug and metabolites enter breast milk.

Metabolism and Excretion: Metabolized to 6–beta-naltrexol. Both parent drug and metabolite are pharmacologically active. Excretion is mostly renal as metabolite, less than 2% as unchanged drug.

Half-life: *naltrexone*—5 hr; *6–beta-naltrexol*—13 hr.

TIME/ACTION PROFILE (weight loss)

ROUTE	ONSET	PEAK	DURATION
PO	within 4 wk	6 mos	unknown

Contraindications/Precautions

Contraindicated in: Known hypersensitivity to bupropion or naltrexone; Uncontrolled hypertension; End-stage renal disease; Seizure disorders; Anorexia or bulimia; During withdrawal from or discontinuation of alcohol, benzodiazepines, barbiturates or antiepileptics; Chronic opioid/opiate agonist or partial agonist use or acute opiate withdrawal; During/within 14 days of MAOIs; Concurrent use of CYP2B6 inducers; Concurrent use of other bupropion-containing medications; OB: Pregnancy (may cause fetal harm); Lactation: Discontinue bupropion/naltrexone or discontinue breast feeding; Pedi: Not recommended for use in children.

Use Cautiously in: History of suicidal behavior/ideation; History of seizure risk (avoid administration with a high-fat meal, adhere to recommended dose); History of cardiac/cerebrovascular disease; History of angle-closure glaucoma; Diabetes mellitus (weight loss may result in hypoglycemia if treatment is not adjusted); Concurrent use of drugs that ↓ seizure threshold; Moderate to severe renal impairment (use lower dose); Hepatic impairment (use lower dose); Geri: Elderly may be ↑ sensitive to adverse CNS reactions and ↓ renal elimination; Concurrent ingestion of alcohol (avoid or reduce consumption).

Adverse Reactions/Side Effects

CNS: HOMICIDAL THOUGHTS/BEHAVIOR, SEIZURES, SUICIDAL THOUGHTS/BEHAVIOR, headache, aggression, agitation, anxiety, delusions, depression, dizziness, hallucinations, hostility, insomnia, mania, panic, paranoia, psychosis. **CV:** hypertension, tachycardia. **EENT:** angle-closure glaucoma (bupropion), tinnitus. **GI:** nausea, constipation, vomiting, abdominal pain, diarrhea, dry mouth, dysgeusia, hepatotoxicity (naltrexone). **Derm:** hot flush, sweating. **Neuro:** tremor. **Misc:** allergic reactions including ANAPHYLAXIS/ANAPHYLACTOID REACTIONS.

Interactions

Drug-Drug: Concurrent or use within 14 days with **MAOIs** ↑ risk of hypertensive reactions. Bupropion inhibits the CYP2D6 enzyme system and can ↑ blood levels and risk of adverse reactions from **antidepressants** including **SSRIs** and many **tricyclic antidepressants**, **antipsychotics** including **haloperidol**, **risperidone**, and **thioridazine**, **beta-blockers** including **metoprolol**, and **Type 1C antiarrhythmics** including **flecanide** and **propafenone**. Dose adjustments may be necessary. Blood levels and effectiveness may be ↓ by **CYP2B6 inducers** including **carbamazepine**, **efavirenz**, **ritonavir**, **lopinavir**, **phenobarbital**, and **phenytoin**; concurrent use should be avoided. Blood levels and risk of toxicity of bupropion may be ↑ by **CYP2B6 inhibitors** including **clopidogrel** (dose should not exceed one tablet twice daily). Concurrent use of **drugs that ↓ seizure threshold** may ↑ risk of seizures. **Dopaminergic drugs** including **amantadine** and **levodopa** may ↑ risk of CNS toxicity. Concurrent use with **opioids** may ↑ risk of overdose. Concurrent ingestion of **alcohol** may ↑ risk of neuropsychiatric reactions (reduce consumption or avoid). May ↓ renal excretion of and ↑ blood levels/risk of toxicity from **amantadine**, **amiloride**, **cimetidine**, **dopamine**, **famotidine**, **memantine**, **metformin**, **pindolol**, **procainamide**, **ranitidine**, **varenicline**, and **oxaliplatin** (careful monitoring is recommended). May ↑ sensitivity to **opioids**.

Route/Dosage

PO (Adults): *Wk 1*—one tablet in the morning; *wk 2*—one tablet in the morning and one tablet in the evening; *wk 3*—two tablets in the morning and one tablet in the evening; *wk 4 and onward*—two tablets in the morning and two tablets in the evening; *concurrent use of CYP2B6 inhibitors*—dose should not exceed one tablet twice daily.

Renal Impairment

PO (Adults): *Moderate to severe renal impairment*—dose should not exceed one tablet in the morning and one tablet in the evening.

Hepatic Impairment

PO (Adults): Dose should not exceed one tablet in the morning.

Availability

Extended-release tablets: 90 mg bupropion/8 mg naltrexone.

NURSING IMPLICATIONS

Assessment

- Monitor for weight loss and adjust concurrent medications (antihypertensives, antidiabetics, lipid-lowering agents) as needed.
- Assess mental status and mood changes, especially during initial few mo of therapy. Risk may be increased in children, adolescents, and adults ≤24 yrs. Inform health care professional if patient demonstrates significant increase in signs of depression (depressed mood, loss of interest in usual activities, insomnia or hypersomnia, psychomotor agitation or retardation, increased fatigue, feelings of guilt or worthlessness, slowed thinking or impaired concentration, irritability, hostility, suicide or homicide attempt or suicidal ideation). Restrict amount of drug available to patient.
- Monitor BP and heart rate periodically during therapy, especially in patient with hypertension.
- Monitor for signs and symptoms of anaphylactic reactions (pruritus, urticaria, hives, angioedema, dyspnea). Discontinue therapy and treat symptomatically.

- ***Lab Test Considerations:*** Monitor blood glucose prior to and during therapy in patients with type 2 diabetes; may cause hypoglycemia.
- May cause false-positive urine test for amphetamines.

Implementation

- **PO:** Administer in the morning and evening according to dose escalation schedule. Swallow tablets whole; do not break, crush, or chew.
- Do not administer with a high-fat meal; may increase risk of seizures.

Patient/Family Teaching

- Instruct patient to take medication as directed, following the dose escalation schedule. If a dose is missed, omit and wait until next scheduled dose; do not double doses. Advise patient to read *Medication Guide* before starting therapy and with each Rx refill in case of changes.
- Instruct patient to adhere to a reduced-calorie diet and increased physical activity.
- Advise patient, family, and caregivers to look for suicidality, especially during early therapy. Notify health care professional immediately if thoughts about suicide, homicide, or dying, attempts to commit suicide, new or worse depression or anxiety, agitation or restlessness, panic attacks, insomnia, new or worse irritability, aggressiveness, hostility, acting on dangerous impulses, mania, or other changes in mood or behavior occur.
- Advise patient to notify health care professional if signs and symptoms of liver damage (stomach pain lasting more than a few days, dark urine, yellowing of skin and whites of eyes, tiredness) occurs.
- Advise patients they may be more sensitive to opioids, even at lower doses, during therapy. Patients physically dependant on opioid analgesics should wait at least 7–10 days without opioids, or 2 wk without methadone, before beginning bupropion/naltrexone.
- Advise patient to notify health care professional of all Rx or OTC medications, vitamins, or herbal products being taken and to consult with health care professional before taking other medications and to minimize or avoid alcohol during therapy.
- Instruct female patients to inform health care professional if pregnancy is planned or suspected and to avoid breast feeding during therapy.

Evaluation/Desired Outcomes

- Decreased appetite with associated weight loss. Evaluate therapy after 12 wk at maintenance dose. If patient has not lost 5% of baseline body weight discontinue medication; clinically meaningful weight loss is unlikely.

busPIRone (byoo-**spye**-rone)

~~BuSpar~~

Classification
Therapeutic: antianxiety agents

Indications

Management of anxiety.

Action

Binds to serotonin and dopamine receptors in the brain. Increases norepinephrine metabolism in the brain. **Therapeutic Effects:** Relief of anxiety.

Pharmacokinetics

Absorption: Rapidly absorbed.
Distribution: Unknown.
Protein Binding: 95% bound to plasma proteins.
Metabolism and Excretion: Extensively metabolized by the liver (CYP3A4 enzyme system); 20–40% excreted in feces.
Half-life: 2–3 hr.

TIME/ACTION PROFILE (relief of anxiety)

ROUTE	ONSET	PEAK	DURATION
PO	7–10 days	3–4 wk	unknown

Contraindications/Precautions

Contraindicated in: Hypersensitivity; Severe hepatic or renal impairment; Concurrent use of MAO inhibitors; Ingestion of large amounts of grapefruit juice.
Use Cautiously in: Patients receiving other antianxiety agents (other agents should be slowly withdrawn to prevent withdrawal or rebound phenomenon); Patients receiving other psychotropics; Lactation, OB, Pedi: Safety not established.

Adverse Reactions/Side Effects

CNS: dizziness, drowsiness, excitement, fatigue, headache, insomnia, nervousness, weakness, personality changes. **EENT:** blurred vision, nasal congestion, sore throat, tinnitus, altered taste or smell, conjunctivitis. **Resp:** chest congestion, hyperventilation, shortness of breath. **CV:** chest pain, palpitations, tachycardia, hypertension, hypotension, syncope. **GI:** nausea, abdominal pain, constipation, diarrhea, dry mouth, vomiting. **GU:** changes in libido, dysuria, urinary frequency, urinary hesitancy. **Derm:** rashes, alopecia, blisters, dry skin, easy bruising, edema, flushing, pruritus. **Endo:** irregular menses. **MS:** myalgia. **Neuro:** incoordination, numbness, paresthesia, tremor. **Misc:** clamminess, sweating, fever.

Interactions

Drug-Drug: Use with **MAO inhibitors** may result in hypertension and is not recommended. **Erythromycin**,

nefazodone, **ketoconazole**, **itraconazole**, **ritonavir**, and other **inhibitors of CYP3A4** ↑ blood levels and effects of buspirone; dose reduction is recommended (↓ to 2.5 mg twice daily with erythromycin; ↓ to 2.5 mg once daily with nefazodone). **Rifampin**, **dexamethasone**, **phenytoin**, **phenobarbital**, **carbamazepine**, and other **inducers of CYP3A4** ↓ blood levels and effects of buspirone; dose adjustment may be necessary. Avoid concurrent use with **alcohol**.
Drug-Natural Products: Concomitant use of **kava-kava**, **valerian**, or **chamomile** can ↑ CNS depression.
Drug-Food: Grapefruit juice ↑ serum levels and effect; ingestion of large amounts of grapefruit juice is not recommended.

Route/Dosage

PO (Adults): 7.5 mg twice daily; ↑ by 5 mg/day every 2–4 days as needed (not to exceed 60 mg/day). Usual dose is 20–30 mg/day (in 2 divided doses).

Availability (generic available)

Tablets: 5 mg, 7.5 mg, 10 mg, 15 mg, 30 mg. **Cost:** *Generic*—5 mg $77.12/100, 7.5 mg $109.08/100, 10 mg $134.50/100, 15 mg $201.92/100, 30 mg $218.10/100.

NURSING IMPLICATIONS

Assessment

- Assess degree and manifestations of anxiety before and periodically during therapy.
- Buspirone does not appear to cause physical or psychological dependence or tolerance. However, patients with a history of substance use disorder should be assessed for tolerance or impaired control. Restrict amount of drug available to these patients.

Implementation

- Do not confuse buspirone with bupropion.
- Patients changing from other antianxiety agents should receive gradually decreasing doses. Buspirone will not prevent withdrawal symptoms.
- **PO:** May be administered with food to minimize gastric irritation. Food slows but does not alter extent of absorption.

Patient/Family Teaching

- Instruct patient to take buspirone exactly as directed. Take missed doses as soon as possible if not just before next dose; do not double doses. Do not take more than amount prescribed.
- May cause dizziness or drowsiness. Caution patient to avoid driving or other activities requiring alertness until response to the medication is known.
- Advise patient to avoid concurrent use of alcohol or other CNS depressants.
- Instruct patient to notify health care professional of all Rx or OTC medications, vitamins, or herbal products being taken and to consult health care professional before taking any Rx, OTC, or herbal products.
- Instruct patient to notify health care professional if any chronic abnormal movements occur (dystonia, motor restlessness, involuntary movements of facial or cervical muscles) or if pregnancy is suspected.
- Emphasize the importance of follow-up exams to determine effectiveness of medication.

Evaluation/Desired Outcomes

- Increase in sense of well-being.
- Decrease in subjective feelings of anxiety. Some improvement may be seen in 7–10 days. Optimal results take 3–4 wk of therapy. Buspirone is usually used for short-term therapy (3–4 wk). If prescribed for long-term therapy, efficacy should be periodically assessed.

HIGH ALERT

busulfan (byoo-**sul**-fan)

Busulfex, Myleran

Classification
Therapeutic: antineoplastics
Pharmacologic: alkylating agents

Indications

PO: Treatment of chronic myelogenous leukemia (CML) and bone marrow disorders. **IV:** With cyclophosphamide as a conditioning regimen before allogenic hematopoietic progenitor cell transplantation for CML.

Action

Disrupts nucleic acid function and protein synthesis (cell-cycle phase–nonspecific). **Therapeutic Effects:** Death of rapidly growing cells, especially malignant ones.

Pharmacokinetics

Absorption: Rapidly absorbed from the GI tract.
Distribution: Unknown.
Metabolism and Excretion: Extensively metabolized by the liver.
Half-life: 2.5 hr.

TIME/ACTION PROFILE (effects on blood counts)

ROUTE	ONSET	PEAK	DURATION
PO	1–2 wk	weeks	up to 1 mo†
IV	unknown	unknown	13 days‡

†Complete recovery may take up to 20 mo.
‡After administration of last dose.

Contraindications/Precautions

Contraindicated in: Hypersensitivity; Failure to respond to previous courses; OB: Pregnancy (may cause fetal harm); Lactation: Lactation.
Use Cautiously in: Active infections; ↓ bone marrow reserve; Obese patients (base dose on ideal body

B

weight); Other chronic debilitating diseases; Rep: Women of reproductive potential and men with female partners of reproductive potential; Geri: Begin therapy at lower end of dose range due to ↑ frequency of impaired cardiac, hepatic, or renal function.

Adverse Reactions/Side Effects

Incidence and severity of adverse reactions and side effects are increased with IV use.

CNS: *IV*—SEIZURES, CEREBRAL HEMORRHAGE/COMA, anxiety, confusion, depression, dizziness, headache, encephalopathy, mental status changes, weakness. **CV:** *PO*—CARDIAC TAMPONADE (WITH HIGH-DOSE CYCLOPHOSPHAMIDE); *IV*, chest pain, hypotension, tachycardia, thrombosis, arrhythmias, atrial fibrillation, cardiomegaly, ECG changes, edema, heart block, heart failure, hypertension, pericardial effusion, ventricular extrasystoles. **Derm:** *PO*—itching, rash, acne, alopecia, erythema nodosum, exfoliative dermatitis, hyperpigmentation. **EENT:** *PO*—cataracts; *IV*, epistaxis, pharyngitis, ear disorders. **Endo:** *PO and IV*—hyperuricemia; *IV*, hyperglycemia; *PO*, sterility, gynecomastia. **F and E:** hypokalemia, hypomagnesemia, hypophosphatemia. **GI:** *PO*—drug-induced hepatitis, nausea, vomiting; *IV*, abdominal enlargement, anorexia, constipation, diarrhea, dry mouth, hematemesis, nausea, rectal discomfort, vomiting, abdominal pain, dyspepsia, hepatic veno-occlusive disease (↑ in allogenic transplantation), hepatomegaly, pancreatitis, stomatitis. **GU:** oliguria, dysuria, hematuria, ↓ fertility. **Hemat:** BONE MARROW DEPRESSION. **Local:** inflammation/pain at injection site. **MS:** arthralgia, myalgia, back pain. **Resp:** *PO*—PULMONARY FIBROSIS; *IV*, alveolar hemorrhage, asthma, atelectasis, cough, hemoptysis, hypoxia, pleural effusion, pneumonia, rhinitis, sinusitis. **Misc:** allergic reactions, chills, fever, infection.

Interactions

Drug-Drug: Concurrent or previous (within 72 hr) use of **acetaminophen** may ↓ elimination and ↑ toxicity. Concurrent use with high-dose **cyclophosphamide** in patients with thalassemia may result in cardiac tamponade. **Itraconazole**, **metronidazole**, or **deferasirox** may ↑ levels and risk of toxicity. **Phenytoin** may ↓ levels and effectiveness. Long-term continuous therapy with **thioguanine** may ↑ risk of hepatic toxicity. ↑ bone marrow suppression with other **antineoplastics** or **radiation therapy**. May ↓ the antibody response to and ↑ risk of adverse reactions from **live-virus vaccines**.

Route/Dosage

Many other regimens are used. See current protocols for up-to-date dosage.

PO (Adults): *Induction*—1.8 mg/m^2/day or 60 mcg (0.06 mg)/kg/day until WBCs <15,000/mm^3. Usual dose is 4–8 mg/day (range 1–12 mg/day). *Maintenance*—1–3 mg/day.

PO (Children): 0.06–0.12 mg/kg/day or 1.8–4.6 mg/m^2/day initially. Titrate dose to maintain WBC of approximately 20,000/mm^3.

IV (Adults): 0.8 mg/kg every 6 hr (dose based on ideal body weight or actual weight, whichever is less; in obese patients, dosage should be based on adjusted ideal body weight) for 4 days (total of 16 doses); given in combination with cyclophosphamide.

Availability (generic available)

Tablets: 2 mg. **Solution for injection:** 6 mg/mL.

NURSING IMPLICATIONS

Assessment

- ***High Alert:*** Monitor for bone marrow depression. Assess for bleeding (bleeding gums, bruising, petechiae, guaiac stools, urine, emesis) and avoid IM injections and taking rectal temperatures. Apply pressure to venipuncture sites for at least 10 min. Assess for signs of infection (fever, chills, sore throat, cough, hoarseness, lower back or side pain, difficult or painful urination) during neutropenia. Anemia may occur. Monitor for increased fatigue, dyspnea, and orthostatic hypotension. Notify health care professional if these symptoms occur.
- Monitor intake and output ratios and daily weights. Report significant changes in totals.
- Monitor for symptoms of gout (increased uric acid, joint pain, lower back or side pain, swelling of feet or lower legs). Encourage patient to drink at least 2 L of fluid each day. Allopurinol may be given to decrease uric acid levels. Alkalinization of urine may be ordered to increase excretion of uric acid.
- Assess for pulmonary fibrosis (fever, cough, shortness of breath) periodically during and after therapy. Discontinue therapy at the first sign of pulmonary fibrosis. Usually occurs 8 mo–10 yr (average 4 yr) after initiation of therapy.
- **IV:** Premedicate patient with phenytoin before IV administration to minimize the risk of seizures.
- Administer antiemetics before IV administration and on a fixed schedule during IV administration.
- ***Lab Test Considerations:*** Monitor CBC with differential and platelet count before and weekly during therapy. The nadir of leukopenia occurs within 10–15 days and the nadir of WBC at 11–30 days. Recovery usually occurs within 12–20 wk. Notify health care professional if WBC is <15,000/mm^3 or if a precipitous drop occurs. Institute thrombocytopenia precautions if platelet count is <150,000/mm^3. Bone marrow depression may be severe and progressive, with recovery taking 1 mo–2 yr after discontinuation of therapy.
- Monitor serum ALT, bilirubin, alkaline phosphatase, and uric acid before and periodically during therapy. May cause ↑ uric acid levels.

- May cause false-positive cytology results of breast, bladder, cervix, and lung tissues.

Implementation

- ***High Alert:*** Fatalities have occurred with chemotherapeutic agents. Before administering, clarify all ambiguous orders; double check single, daily, and course-of-therapy dose limits; have second practitioner independently double check original order, calculations, and infusion pump settings.
- ***High Alert:*** Do not confuse Myleran with Alkeran or Leukeran.
- **PO:** Administer at the same time each day. Administer on an empty stomach to decrease nausea and vomiting.

IV Administration

- **IV:** Prepare solution in a biologic cabinet. Wear gloves, gown, and mask while handling IV medication. Discard IV equipment in specially designated containers.
- **Intermittent Infusion:** ***Diluent:*** Dilute with 10 times the volume of busulfan using 0.9% NaCl or D5W. ***Concentration:*** ≥0.5 mg/mL. When drawing busulfan from vial, use needle with 5-micron nylon filter provided, remove calculated volume from vial, remove needle and filter, replace needle and inject busulfan into diluent. Do not use polycarbonate syringes with busulfan. Only use filters provided with busulfan. Always add busulfan to diluent, not diluent to busulfan. Solution diluted with 0.9% NaCl or D5W is stable for 8 hr at room temperature and solution diluted with 0.9% NaCl is stable for 12 hr if refrigerated. Administration must be completed during this time. Solution is clear and colorless; do not administer solutions that are discolored or contain a precipitate. ***Rate:*** Administer via central venous catheter over 2 hr every 6 hr for 4 days for a total of 16 doses. Use infusion pump to administer entire dose over 2 hr.
- **Y-Site Compatibility:** acyclovir, amiodarone, amphotericin B lipid complex, amphotericin B liposome, anidulafungin, argatroban, arsenic trioxide, bivalirudin, bleomycin, caspofungin, dacarbazine, daptomycin, dexmedetomidine, dexrazoxane, diltiazem, docetaxel, dolasetron, ertapenem, fenoldopam, foscarnet, fosphenytoin, granisetron, hetastarch, hydromorphone, leucovorin calcium, levofloxacin, linezolid, lorazepam, meperidine, metronidazole, milrinone, moxifloxacin, octreotide, ondansetron, paclitaxel, palonosetron, pancuronium, piperacillin/tazobactam, potassium acetate, quinupristin/dalfopristin, rituximab, sodium acetate, tacrolimus, tigecycline, tirofiban, trastuzumab, vasopressin, vinblastine, zoledronic acid.
- **Y-Site Incompatibility:** idarubicin, thiotepa, vecuronium, voriconazole.

Patient/Family Teaching

- Instruct patient to take medication as directed, at the same time each day, even if nausea and vomiting are a problem. Consult health care professional if vomiting occurs shortly after dose is taken. If a dose is missed, do not take at all; do not double doses.
- Advise patient to notify health care professional if fever; sore throat; signs of infection; lower back or side pain; difficult or painful urination; sores in the mouth or on the lips; chills; dyspnea; persistent cough; bleeding gums; bruising; petechiae; or blood in urine, stool, or emesis occurs. Instruct patient to use soft toothbrush and electric razor. Caution patient not to drink alcoholic beverages or take products containing aspirin or NSAIDs.
- Caution patient to avoid crowds and persons with known infections. Health care professional should be informed immediately if symptoms of infection occur.
- Discuss with patient the possibility of hair loss. Explore methods of coping.
- Instruct patient not to receive any vaccinations without advice of health care professional.
- Advise patient to notify health care professional if unusual bleeding; bruising; or flank, stomach, or joint pain occurs. Advise patients on long-term therapy to notify health care professional immediately if cough, shortness of breath, and fever occur or if darkening of skin, diarrhea, dizziness, fatigue, anorexia, confusion, or nausea and vomiting become pronounced.
- Inform patient of increased risk of a second malignancy with busulfan.
- Rep: Advise female patients of reproductive potential to use effective contraception during and for 6 mo after last dose and to avoid breast feeding during therapy. Advise men with female partners of reproductive potential to use effective contraception during and for 3 mo after last dose of therapy. Women need to use contraception even if amenorrhea occurs. May impair fertility in male and female patients.

Evaluation/Desired Outcomes

- Decrease in leukocyte count to within normal limits.
- Decreased night sweats.
- Increase in appetite.
- Increased sense of well-being. Therapy is resumed when leukocyte count reaches 50,000/mm³.

---

butenafine, **See ANTIFUNGALS (TOPICAL).**

---

butoconazole, **See ANTIFUNGALS (VAGINAL).**

HIGH ALERT

cabazitaxel (ka-ba-zi-tax-el)

Jevtana

Classification
Therapeutic: antineoplastics
Pharmacologic: taxoids

Indications

Hormone-refractory metastatic prostate cancer previously treated with a regimen including docetaxel (used in combination with prednisone).

Action

Binds to intracellular tubulin and promotes its assembly into microtubules while inhibiting disassembly. Result is inhibition of mitosis and interphase. **Therapeutic Effects:** Death of rapidly replicating cells, particularly malignant ones, with ↓ spread of metastatic prostate cancer.

Pharmacokinetics

Absorption: IV administration results in complete bioavailability.
Distribution: Equally distributed between blood and plasma.
Metabolism and Excretion: Extensively (>95%) metabolized by the liver, 80–90% by CYP3A4/5 enzyme system. Metabolites are excreted in urine and feces. Minimal renal excretion.
Half-life: *Terminal elimination*—95 hr.

TIME/ACTION PROFILE (blood levels)

ROUTE	ONSET	PEAK	DURATION
IV	rapid	end of infusion	unknown

Contraindications/Precautions

Contraindicated in: Severe hypersensitivity to cabazitaxel or polysorbate 80; Neutrophil count ≤1,500/mm^3; Hepatic impairment (total bilirubin ≥3x upper limit of normal [ULN]); Concurrent use of strong CYP3A4 inhibitors or inducers; OB: Avoid use during pregnancy (may cause fetal harm); Lactation: Avoid breast feeding.
Use Cautiously in: Concurrent use of moderate CYP3A4 inhibitors; Patients with neutropenia or a history of pelvic radiation, adhesions, ulceration, or GI bleeding (↑ risk of GI and urinary adverse reactions); Concomitant use of steroids, NSAIDs, or antithrombotics (↑ risk of GI adverse reactions); Severe renal impairment (CCr <30 mL/min) or end-stage renal disease; Hemoglobin <10 g/dL; Lung disease (↑ risk of pulmonary toxicity); Mild or moderate hepatic impairment (dose ↓ required); Rep: Women of reproductive potential; Geri: ↑ risk of adverse reactions (especially neutropenia and febrile neutropenia); Pedi: Safety and effectiveness not established.

Adverse Reactions/Side Effects

CNS: weakness, fatigue. **Resp:** ACUTE RESPIRATORY DISTRESS SYNDROME, INTERSTITIAL LUNG DISEASE, dyspnea. **CV:** arrhythmias, hypotension. **GI:** DIARRHEA, ENTEROCOLITIS, GI BLEED, GI PERFORATION, ILEUS, abdominal pain, abnormal taste, anorexia, constipation, nausea, vomiting, dyspepsia. **GU:** RENAL FAILURE, hematuria, cystitis. **Derm:** alopecia. **F and E:** electrolyte imbalance. **Hemat:** NEUTROPENIA, THROMBOCYTOPENIA, anemia, leukopenia, thrombocytopenia. **MS:** arthralgia, back pain, muscle spasms. **Neuro:** peripheral neuropathy. **Misc:** allergic reactions including ANAPHYLAXIS, fever.

Interactions

Drug-Drug: **Strong CYP3A inhibitors** including **ketoconazole**, **itraconazole**, **clarithromycin**, **atazanavir**, **indinavir**, **nefazodone**, **nelfinavir**, **ritonavir**, **saquinavir**, and **voriconazole** ↑ levels and risk of toxicity; concomitant use contraindicated. **Strong CYP3A inducers** including **phenytoin**, **carbamazepine**, **rifampin**, **rifabutin**, **rifapentin**, and **phenobarbital** may ↓ levels and effectiveness; concomitant use contraindicated.
Drug-Natural Products: **St. John's wort** may ↓ levels and effectiveness; concomitant use contraindicated.

Route/Dosage

PO (Adults): 20 mg/m^2 every 3 wk (with prednisone 10 mg PO daily). A dose of 25 mg/m^2 may be considered in select patients.

Hepatic Impairment

PO (Adults): *Mild hepatic impairment (total bilirubin >1x to ≤1.5x ULN or AST >1.5x ULN)*—20 mg/m^2 every 3 wk (with prednisone 10 mg PO daily); *Moderate hepatic impairment (total bilirubin >1.5x to ≤3x ULN)*—15 mg/m^2 every 3 wk (with prednisone 10 mg PO daily); *Severe hepatic impairment (total bilirubin >3x ULN)*—Contraindicated.

Availability

Viscous solution for injection (requires two dilutions prior to IV administration): 40 mg/mL (contains polysorbate 80) comes with diluent (5.7 mL of 13% [w/w] ethanol in water for injection).

NURSING IMPLICATIONS

Assessment

- Assess for hypersensitivity reactions (generalized rash/erythema, hypotension, bronchospasm, swelling of face). May occur within min following initiation of infusion. If severe reactions occur, discontinue infusion immediately and provide supportive therapy.
- Assess for signs and symptoms of GI toxicity (abdominal pain and tenderness, fever, persistent constipation, nausea, vomiting, severe diarrhea); may

result in death due to electrolyte imbalance. Premedication is recommended. Treat with rehydration, antidiarrheal, or antiemetic therapy as needed. If Grade ≥3 diarrhea or persisting diarrhea occurs despite appropriate medication, fluid and electrolyte replacement, delay treatment until improvement or resolution, then reduce dose to 20 mg/mL.

- Assess for signs and symptoms of peripheral neuropathy (pain, burning, numbness in hands, feet, or legs) during therapy. *If Grade 2 occurs,* withhold until improvement or resolution, then reduce dose to 20 mg/mL. *If ≥Grade 3 occurs,* discontinue therapy.
- Monitor for signs and symptoms of respiratory compromise (trouble breathing, dyspnea, chest pain, cough, fever) during therapy. Interrupt therapy if new or worsening symptoms occur. Consider discontinuation.
- ***Lab Test Considerations:*** Monitor CBC weekly during cycle 1 and before each treatment cycle thereafter. Do not administer if neutrophils ≤1500/mm³. If prolonged grade 3 neutropenia (>1 wk) despite appropriate medication including filgrastim, delay treatment until neutrophil count is >1500 mm³, then reduce dose to 20 mg/m². Use filgrastim for secondary prophylaxis. Risk is ↑ in elderly patients.
- If febrile neutropenia occurs, delay therapy until improvement or resolution and neutrophil count is >1500/mm³, then reduce dose to 20 mg/m². Use filgrastim for primary or secondary prophylaxis.
- Discontinue cabazitaxel if prolonged Grade 3 neutropenia, febrile neutropenia, or Grade 3 diarrhea occur at the 20 mg/m² dose.
- May cause hematuria.
- May cause Grade 3–4 ↑ AST, ↑ ALT, and ↑ bilirubin.

Implementation

- ***High Alert:*** Fatalities have occurred with chemotherapeutic agents. Before administering, clarify all ambiguous orders; double check single, daily, and course-of-therapy dose limits; have second practitioner independently double check original order and dose calculations.
- Prepare solution in a biologic cabinet. Wear gloves, gown, and mask while handling medication. Discard equipment in specially designated containers. If solution comes in contact with skin or mucosa, wash with soap and water immediately.
- Premedicate at least 30 min before each dose with antihistamine (diphenhydramine 25 mg or equivalent), corticosteroid (dexamethasone 8 mg or equivalent), and H_2 antagonist (ranitidine 50 mg or equivalent). Antiemetic prophylaxis, PO or IV, is recommended.

IV Administration

- **First Dilution: *Diluent:*** Mix vial with entire contents of supplied diluent. Direct needle to inside wall of vial and inject slowly to avoid foaming. Mix gently by repeated inversions for at least 45 sec; do not shake. Let stand for a few min to allow foam to dissipate. ***Concentration:*** 10 mg/mL. **Second Dilution: *Diluent:*** Withdraw recommended dose from cabazitaxel solution and dilute further into a sterile 250 mL PVC-free container of 0.9% NaCl or D5W. If dose >65 mg is required, use a larger volume of infusion vehicle so concentration does not exceed 0.26 mg/mL. Gently invert container to mix. ***Concentration:*** 0.10–0.26 mg/mL. Stable for 8 hr (including 1 hr infusion) at room temperature or 24 hr if refrigerated. May crystallize over time. Do not use if crystallized, discolored, or contains particulate matter; discard. ***Rate:*** Infuse over 1 hr at room temperature through a 0.22 micrometer nominal pore size filter.
- **Y-Site Incompatibility:** Do not mix with other medication.

Patient/Family Teaching

- Instruct patient to take oral prednisone as prescribed and to notify health care professional if a dose is missed or not taken in time.
- Advise patient to notify health care professional immediately if signs or symptoms of hypersensitivity reactions; fever; sore throat; signs of infection; lower back or side pain; difficult or painful urination; sores on the mouth or on the lips; bleeding gums; bruising; petechiae; blood in urine, stool, or emesis; unusual swelling, shortness of breath, trouble breathing, chest pain, cough, or fever occur. Caution patient to avoid crowds and persons with known infections. Instruct patient to use soft toothbrush and electric razor and to avoid falls. Patient should also be cautioned not to drink alcoholic beverages or to take products containing aspirin or NSAIDs; may precipitate GI hemorrhage.
- Instruct patient to notify health care professional of all Rx or OTC medications, vitamins, or herbal products being taken and consult health care professional before taking any new medications, especially St. John's wort.
- May cause dizziness. Caution patient to avoid driving or other activities requiring alertness until response to medication is known.
- Instruct patient not to receive any vaccinations without advice of health care professional.
- Rep: Advise female patients of the need for contraception and to avoid breast feeding during therapy. Advise male patients with female partners of reproductive potential to use effective contraception during and for at least 3 mo after last dose of cabazitaxel. May impair fertility in males of reproductive potential.
- Emphasize need for periodic lab tests to monitor for side effects. Advise patient to monitor temperature frequently.

Evaluation/Desired Outcomes

- ↓ in size and spread of metastatic prostate cancer.

calcitriol, See VITAMIN D COMPOUNDS.

HIGH ALERT

CALCIUM SALTS

calcium acetate (25% Ca or 12.6 mEq/g)
(**kal**-see-um **ass**-e-tate)
PhosLo, Phoslyra

calcium carbonate (40% Ca or 20 mEq/g)
(**kal**-see-um **kar**-bo-nate)
Calci-Chew, Caltrate, Maalox , Oysco, Titralac, Tums, Tums E-X

calcium chloride (27% Ca or 13.6 mEq/g)
(**kal**-see-um **kloh**-ride)
❖Calciject

calcium citrate (21% Ca or 12 mEq/g) (**kal**-see-um **si**-trate)
Cal-Citrate 250

calcium gluconate (9% Ca or 4.5 mEq/g)
(**kal**-see-um **gloo**-koh-nate)

calcium lactate (13% Ca or 6.5 mEq/g) (**kal**-see-um **lak**-tate)
Cal-Lac

tricalcium phosphate (39% Ca or 19.5 mEq/g)
(tri-**kal**-see-um **foss**-fate)
Posture

Classification
Therapeutic: mineral and electrolyte replacements/supplements
Pharmacologic: antacids

Indications
PO, IV: Treatment and prevention of hypocalcemia. **PO:** Adjunct in the prevention of postmenopausal osteoporosis. **IV:** Emergency treatment of hyperkalemia and hypermagnesemia and adjunct in cardiac arrest or calcium channel blocking agent toxicity (calcium chloride, calcium gluconate). **Calcium carbonate:** May be used as an antacid. **Calcium acetate:** Control of hyperphosphatemia in end-stage renal disease.

Action
Essential for nervous, muscular, and skeletal systems. Maintain cell membrane and capillary permeability. Act as an activator in the transmission of nerve impulses and contraction of cardiac, skeletal, and smooth muscle. Essential for bone formation and blood coagulation. Binds to dietary phosphate to form an insoluble calcium phosphate complex, which is excreted in the feces, resulting in decreased serum phosphorus concentrations (calcium acetate). **Therapeutic Effects:** Replacement of calcium in deficiency states. Control of hyperphosphatemia in end-stage renal disease without promoting aluminum absorption (calcium acetate).

Pharmacokinetics
Absorption: Absorption from the GI tract requires vitamin D. IV administration results in complete bioavailability.
Distribution: Readily enters extracellular fluid. Crosses the placenta and enters breast milk.
Metabolism and Excretion: Excreted mostly in the feces; 20% eliminated by the kidneys.
Half-life: Unknown.

TIME/ACTION PROFILE (effects on serum calcium)

ROUTE	ONSET	PEAK	DURATION
PO	unknown	unknown	unknown
IV	immediate	immediate	0.5–2 hr

Contraindications/Precautions
Contraindicated in: Hypercalcemia; Renal calculi; Ventricular fibrillation; Concurrent use of calcium supplements (calcium acetate).
Use Cautiously in: Patients receiving digoxin; Severe respiratory insufficiency; Renal impairment; Cardiac disease; OB: Hypercalcemia may ↑ risk of maternal and fetal complications; Lactation: Breast feeding not expected to harm infant provided that serum calcium levels monitored.

Adverse Reactions/Side Effects
CNS: syncope (IV only), tingling. **CV:** CARDIAC ARREST (IV only), arrhythmias, bradycardia. **F and E:** hypercalcemia. **GI:** constipation, diarrhea (oral solution only), nausea, vomiting. **GU:** calculi, hypercalciuria. **Local:** phlebitis (IV only).

Interactions
Drug-Drug: Hypercalcemia ↑ the risk of **digoxin** toxicity. Chronic use with **antacids** in renal insufficiency may lead to milk-alkali syndrome. **Calcium supplements**, including calcium-containing antacids, may ↑ risk of hypercalcemia; avoid concurrent use. Ingestion by mouth ↓ the absorption of orally administered **phenytoin** and **iron salts**; take 1 hr before or 3

hr after oral calcium supplements. Excessive amounts may ↓ the effects of **calcium channel blockers**. Calcium acetate may ↓ absorption of orally administered **tetracyclines**; take ≥1 hr before calcium acetate. Calcium acetate may ↓ absorption of orally administered **fluoroquinolones**; take ≥2 hr before or 6 hr after calcium acetate. Calcium acetate may ↓ absorption of orally administered **levothyroxine**; take ≥4 hr before or 4 hr after calcium acetate. ↓ absorption of **etidronate** and **risedronate** (do not take within 2 hr of calcium supplements). Concurrent use with **diuretics (thiazide)** may result in hypercalcemia. May ↓ the ability of **sodium polystyrene sulfonate** to decrease serum potassium.
Drug-Food: Cereals, **spinach**, or **rhubarb** may ↓ the absorption of calcium supplements.

Route/Dosage

Doses are expressed in mg, g, or mEq of calcium.
PO (Adults): *Prevention of hypocalcemia, treatment of depletion, osteoporosis*—1–2 g/day. *Antacid*—0.5–1.5 g as needed (calcium carbonate only). *Hyperphosphatemia in end-stage renal disease (calcium acetate only)*—1334 mg with each meal, may ↑ gradually (in absence of hypercalcemia) to achieve target serum phosphate levels (usual dose = 2001–2668 mg with each meal).
PO (Children): *Supplementation*—45–65 mg/kg/day.
PO (Infants): *Neonatal hypocalcemia*—50–150 mg/kg (not to exceed 1 g).
IV (Adults): *Emergency treatment of hypocalcemia, cardiac standstill*—7–14 mEq. *Hypocalcemic tetany*—4.5–16 mEq; repeat until symptoms are controlled. *Hyperkalemia with cardiac toxicity*—2.25–14 mEq; may repeat in 1–2 min. *Hypermagnesemia*—7 mEq.
IV (Children): *Emergency treatment of hypocalcemia*—1–7 mEq. *Hypocalcemic tetany*—0.5–0.7 mEq/kg 3–4 times daily.
IV (Infants): *Emergency treatment of hypocalcemia*—<1 mEq. *Hypocalcemic tetany*—2.4 mEq/kg/day in divided doses.

Availability (generic available)

Calcium Acetate

Gelcaps: 667 mg (169 mg elemental Ca). **Oral solution:** 667 mg (169 mg elemental Ca)/5 mL. **Tablets:** 667 mg (169 mg elemental Ca).

Calcium Carbonate

Chewable tablets: 420 mg (168 mg Ca)^OTC, 500 mg (200 mg Ca)^OTC, 750 mg (300 mg Ca)^OTC, 1 g (400 mg Ca)^OTC, 1.25 g (500 mg Ca)^OTC. **Oral suspension:** 1.25 g (500 mg Ca)/5 mL^OTC. **Powder:** 6.5 g (2400 mg Ca)/packet^OTC. **Tablets:** 600 mg (240 mg Ca)^OTC, 650 mg (260 mg Ca)^OTC, 1.25 g (500 mg Ca)^OTC, 1.5 g (600 mg Ca)^OTC.

Calcium Chloride

Solution for injection: 10% (1.36 mEq/mL).

Calcium Citrate

Tablets: 250 mg^OTC.

Calcium Gluconate

Premixed infusion (in sodium chloride): 1 g/50 mL (4.65 mEq/50 mL), 2 g/100 mL (9.3 mEq/100 mL). **Solution for injection:** 10% (0.45 mEq/mL). **Tablets:** 500 mg (45 mg Ca)^OTC.

Calcium Lactate

Tablets: 500 mg^OTC, 650 mg (84.5 mg Ca)^OTC.

Tricalcium Phosphate

Tablets: 600 mg (234 mg Ca)^OTC.

NURSING IMPLICATIONS

Assessment

- **Calcium Supplement/Replacement:** Observe patient closely for symptoms of hypocalcemia (paresthesia, muscle twitching, laryngospasm, colic, cardiac arrhythmias, Chvostek's or Trousseau's sign). Notify health care professional if these occur. Protect symptomatic patients by elevating and padding siderails and keeping bed in low position.
- Monitor BP, pulse, and ECG frequently throughout parenteral therapy. May cause vasodilation with resulting hypotension, bradycardia, arrhythmias, and cardiac arrest. Transient increases in BP may occur during IV administration, especially in geriatric patients or in patients with hypertension.
- Assess IV site for patency. Extravasation may cause cellulitis, necrosis, and sloughing.
- Monitor patient on digoxin for signs of toxicity.
- **Antacid:** When used as an antacid, assess for heartburn, indigestion, and abdominal pain. Inspect abdomen; auscultate bowel sounds.
- ***Lab Test Considerations:*** Monitor serum calcium or ionized calcium, chloride, sodium, potassium, magnesium, albumin, and parathyroid hormone (PTH) concentrations before and periodically during therapy for treatment of hypocalcemia.
- *For patients with hyperphosphatemia*: Monitor serum calcium twice weekly during adjustment phase. If serum calcium level is >12 mg/dL, discontinue therapy and start hemodialysis as needed; lower dose or temporarily stop therapy for calcium level between 10.5 and 11.9 mg/dL.
- May cause ↓ serum phosphate concentrations with excessive and prolonged use. When used to treat hyperphosphatemia in renal failure patients, monitor phosphate levels.
- ***Toxicity and Overdose:*** Assess patient for nausea, vomiting, anorexia, thirst, severe constipation, paralytic ileus, and bradycardia. Contact health care professional immediately if these signs of hypercalcemia occur.

Implementation

- ***High Alert:*** Errors with IV calcium gluconate and chloride have occurred secondary to confusion over which salt is ordered. Clarify incomplete orders. Confusion has occurred with milligram doses of calcium chloride and calcium gluconate, which are not equal. Chloride and gluconate forms are routinely available on most hospital crash carts; specify form of calcium desired.

- Do not confuse Os-Cal (calcium carbonate) with Asacol (mesalamine).
- In arrest situations, the use of calcium chloride is now limited to patients with hyperkalemia, hypocalcemia, and calcium channel blocker toxicity.
- **PO:** Administer calcium carbonate or phosphate 1–1.5 hr after meals and at bedtime. Chewable tablets should be well chewed before swallowing. Dissolve effervescent tablets in glass of water. Follow oral doses with a full glass of water, except when using calcium carbonate as a phosphate binder in renal dialysis. Administer on an empty stomach before meals to optimize effectiveness in patients with hyperphosphatemia.
- **IM:** IM administration of calcium salts can cause severe necrosis and tissue sloughing. Do not administer IM.

IV Administration

- **IV:** IV solution should be warmed to body temperature and given through a small-bore needle in a large vein to minimize phlebitis. Do not administer through a scalp vein. May cause cutaneous burning sensation, peripheral vasodilation, and drop in BP. Patient should remain recumbent for 30–60 min after IV administration.
- If infiltration occurs, discontinue IV. May be treated with application of heat, elevation, and local infiltration of normal saline, 1% procaine HCl, or hyaluronidase.
- ***High Alert:*** Administer slowly. High concentrations may cause cardiac arrest. Rapid administration may cause tingling, sensation of warmth, and a metallic taste. Halt infusion if these symptoms occur, and resume infusion at a slower rate when they subside.
- Do not administer solutions that are not clear or that contain a precipitate.

Calcium Chloride

IV Administration

- **IV Push:** May be administered undiluted by IV push.
- **Intermittent/Continuous Infusion:** May be diluted with D5W, D10W, 0.9% NaCl, D5/0.25% NaCl, D5/0.45% NaCl, D5/0.9% NaCl, or D5/LR.
- ***Rate:*** Maximum rate for adults is 0.7–1.4 mEq/min (0.5–1 mL of 10% solution); for children, 0.5 mL/min.
- **Y-Site Compatibility:** acyclovir, alemtuzumab, alfentanil, amikacin, aminocaproic acid, aminophylline, amiodarone, anidulafungin, argatroban, ascorbic acid, atropine, azithromycin, aztreonam, benztropine, bivalirudin, bleomycin, bumetanide, buprenorphine, butorphanol, calcium gluconate, carboplatin, carmustine, caspofungin, cefotaxime, cefotetan, cefoxitin, ceftaroline, chloramphenicol, chlorpromazine, cisplatin, clindamycin, cyanocobalamin, cyclophosphamide, cyclosporine, cytarabine, dacarbazine, dactinomycin, daptomycin, dexmedetomidine, dexrazoxane, digoxin, diltiazem, diphenhydramine, dobutamine, docetaxel, dopamine, doxorubicin, doxycycline, enalaprilat, ephedrine, epinephrine, epirubicin, epoetin alfa, eptifibatide, ertapenem, erythromycin, esmolol, etoposide, etoposide phosphate, famotidine, fenoldopam, fentanyl, fluconazole, fludarabine, furosemide, ganciclovir, gemcitabine, gentamicin, glycopyrrolate, granisetron, heparin, hetastarch, hydromorphone, idarubicin, ifosfamide, insulin, irinotecan, isoproterenol, labetalol, leucovorin, lidocaine, linezolid, lorazepam, mannitol, meperidine, mesna, methotrexate, metoclopramide, metoprolol, metronidazole, micafungin, midazolam, milrinone, mitomycin, mitoxantrone, morphine, moxifloxacin, multivitamin, mycophenolate, nafcillin, nalbuphine, naloxone, nicardipine, nitroglycerin, nitroprusside, norepinephrine, octreotide, ondansetron, oxaliplatin, oxytocin, paclitaxel, palonosetron, pancuronium, papaverine, penicillin G, pentobarbital, phenobarbital, phenylephrine, phytonadione, piperacillin/tazobactam, potassium acetate, potassium chloride, procainamide, promethazine, propranolol, protamine, pyridoxine, ranitidine, rocuronium, streptokinase, succinylcholine, sufentanil, tacrolimus, theophylline, thiamine, thiotepa, tigecycline, tirofiban, tobramycin, topotecan, vancomycin, vasopressin, vecuronium, verapamil, vinblastine, vincristine, vinorelbine, voriconazole.
- **Y-Site Incompatibility:** amphotericin B colloidal, amphotericin B lipid complex, amphotericin B liposome, azathioprine, cefazolin, ceftazidime, ceftriaxone, cefuroxime, dantrolene, diazepam, diazoxide, doxorubicin liposomal, fluorouracil, folic acid, foscarnet, fosphenytoin, haloperidol, indomethacin, ketorolac, magnesium sulfate, methylprednisolone, pantoprazole, pemetrexed, phenytoin, potassium phosphates, prochlorperazine, propofol, quinupristin/dalfopristin, sodium bicarbonate, sodium phosphates, trimethoprim/sulfamethoxazole.

Calcium Gluconate

IV Administration

- **IV Push:** Administer slowly by IV push. ***Rate:*** Maximum administration rate for adults is 1.5–2 mL/min.
- **Continuous Infusion:** May be further diluted in 1000 mL of D5W, D10W, D20W, D5/0.9% NaCl, 0.9% NaCl, D5/LR, or LR.
- ***Rate:*** Administer at a rate not to exceed 200 mg/min over 12–24 hr.

- **Y-Site Compatibility:** acyclovir, aldesleukin, alemtuzumab, alfentanil, allopurinol, amifostine, amikacin, aminocaproic acid, aminophylline, anidulafungin, argatroban, arsenic trioxide, ascorbic acid, azathioprine, azithromycin, aztreonam, benztropine, bivalirudin, bleomycin, bumatanide, buprenorphine, butorphanol, calcium chloride, carboplatin, carmustine, caspofungin, cefazolin, cefepime, cefotaxime, cefotetan, ceftaroline, ceftazidime, ceftolozane/tazobactam, cefuroxime, chloramphenicol, chlorpromazine, ciprofloxacin, cisatracurium, cisplatin, cladribine, clindamycin, cyanocobalamin, cyclophosphamide, cyclosporine, cytarabine, dacarbazine, dactinomycin, daptomycin, daunorubicin, dexmedetomidine, dexrazoxane, digoxin, diltiazem, diphenhydramine, dobutamine, docetaxel, dolasetron, dopamine, doxacurium, doxapram, doxorubicin, doxorubicin liposomal, doxycycline, enalaprilat, epinephrine, epirubicin, epoetin alfa, eptifibatide, ertepenem, erythromycin, esmolol, etoposide, etoposide phosphate, famotidine, fenoldopam, fentanyl, filgrastim, fludarabine, fluorouracil, folic acid, furosemide, ganciclovir, gemcitabine, gentamicin, glycopyrrolate, granisetron, heparin, hetastarch, hydromorphone, idarubicin, ifosfomide, insulin regular, irinotecan, isuvuconazonium, isoproterenol, ketamine, labetalol, leucovorin calcium, levofloxacin, lidocaine, linezolid, lorazepam, magnesium sulfate, mannitol, melphalan, meperidine, meropenem/vaborbactam, mesna, metaraminol, methohexital, methotrexate, methyldopate, metoclopramide, metoprolol, micafungin, midazolam, milrinone, mitomycin, mitoxantrone, morphine, moxifloxacin, multivitamins, nafcillin, nalbuphine, naloxone, nicardipine, nitroglycerin, nitroprusside, norepinephrine, octreotide, ondansetron, oritavancin, oxaliplatin, oxytocin, paclitaxel, palonosetron, pancuronium, papaverine, penicillin G, pentamidine, pentobarbital, phenobarbital, phentolamine, phenylephrine, phytonadione, piperacillin/tazobactam, plazomicin, potassium acetate, potassium chloride, procainamide, prochlorperazine, promethazine, propofol, propranolol, protamine, pyridoxime, ranitidine, remifentanil, rituximab, rocuronium, sargramostim, sodium acetate, streptokinase, succinylcholine, sufentanil, tacrolimus, telavancin, theophylline, thiamine, thiotepa, tigecycline, tirofiban, tobramycin, tolazoline, traztuzumab, vancomycin, vasopressin, vecuronium, verapamil, vinblastine, vincristine, vinorelbine, vitamin B complex with C, voriconazole.
- **Y-Site Incompatibility:** amphotericin B deoxycholate, amphotericin B lipid complex, amphotericin B liposome, cangrelor, ceftriaxone, dantrolene, diazepam, diazoxide, foscarnet, fosphenytoin, gemtuzumab, indomethacin, methylprednisolone, minocycline, mycophenolate, oxacillin, pemetrexed, phenytoin, potassium phosphates, quinypristin/dalfopristin, sodium bicarbonate, sodium phosphates, tedizolid, topotecan, trimethoprim/sulfamethoxazole.

Patient/Family Teaching

- Instruct patient not to take enteric-coated tablets within 1 hr of calcium carbonate; this will result in premature dissolution of the tablets.
- Do not administer concurrently with foods containing large amounts of oxalic acid (spinach, rhubarb), phytic acid (brans, cereals), or phosphorus (milk or dairy products). Administration with milk products may lead to milk-alkali syndrome (nausea, vomiting, confusion, headache). Do not take within 1–2 hr of other medications if possible.
- Instruct patients on a regular schedule to take missed doses as soon as possible, then go back to regular schedule.
- Advise patient that calcium carbonate may cause constipation. Review methods of preventing constipation (increasing bulk in diet, increasing fluid intake, increasing mobility) and using laxatives. Severe constipation may indicate toxicity.
- Advise patient to avoid excessive use of tobacco or beverages containing alcohol or caffeine.
- Advise patient to notify health care professional if pregnancy is planned or suspected, or if breast feeding. Monitor infants born to mothers with hypocalcemia for signs of hypocalcemia or hypercalcemia (neuromuscular irritability, apnea, cyanosis, and cardiac rhythm disorders).
- **Calcium Supplement:** Encourage patients to maintain a diet adequate in vitamin D (see Appendix K).
- **Osteoporosis:** Advise patients that exercise has been found to arrest and reverse bone loss. Patient should discuss any exercise limitations with health care professional before beginning program.
- **Hyperphosphatemia:** Advise patient to notify health care professional promptly if signs and symptoms of hypercalcemia (constipation, anorexia, nausea, vomiting, confusion, stupor) occur.
- Advise patient to avoid taking calcium-containing supplements, including calcium-based antacids, during therapy.

Evaluation/Desired Outcomes

- Increase in serum calcium levels.
- Decrease in the signs and symptoms of hypocalcemia.
- Resolution of indigestion.
- Control of hyperphosphatemia in patients with renal failure (calcium acetate only).

canagliflozin

(kan-a-gli-**floe**-zin)

Invokana

Classification

Therapeutic: antidiabetics

Pharmacologic: sodium-glucose co-transporter 2 (SGLT2) inhibitors

Indications

Adjunct to diet and exercise in the management of type 2 diabetes mellitus. To reduce the risk of major adverse cardiovascular events in patients with type 2 diabetes mellitus and established cardiovascular disease.

Action

Inhibits proximal renal tubular sodium-glucose co-transporter 2 (SGLT2), which determines reabsorption of glucose from the tubular lumen. Inhibits reabsorption of glucose, lowers renal threshold for glucose, and increases excretion of glucose in urine. **Therapeutic Effects:** Improved glycemic control. Reduction in risk of cardiovascular death, nonfatal MI, and nonfatal stroke.

Pharmacokinetics

Absorption: Well absorbed (65%) following oral administration.
Distribution: Extensive tissue distribution.
Protein Binding: 99%.
Metabolism and Excretion: Mostly metabolized by UDP-glucuronyl transferases (UGT) to inactive metabolites, minimal metabolism by CYP3A4 (7%). 50% excreted in feces as parent drug and metabolites, 33% as metabolites in urine, <1% excreted in urine as unchanged drug.
Half-life: 10.6 hr.

TIME/ACTION PROFILE (effects on A1C)

ROUTE	ONSET	PEAK	DURATION
PO	unknown	unknown	24 hr

Contraindications/Precautions

Contraindicated in: Hypersensitivity; Severe renal impairment (eGFR <45 mL/min/1.73 m^2), end-stage renal disease or on dialysis; Type 1 diabetes; Severe hepatic impairment; Lactation: Avoid use, discontinue breast feeding or discontinue canagliflozin.
Use Cautiously in: eGFR <60 mL/min/1.73 m^2 (monitor frequently) (↑ risk of adverse reactions related to ↓ intravascular volume); History of pancreatitis, pancreatic surgery, reduced caloric intake due to illness or surgery, or alcohol abuse (↑ risk of ketoacidosis); Hypovolemia, chronic kidney disease, HF, or concurrent use of diuretics, NSAIDs, ACE inhibitors, or ARBs (↑ risk of acute kidney injury); Previous amputation, peripheral vascular disease, neuropathy, or diabetic foot infection (↑ risk of lower limb amputation); Geri: ↑ risk of adverse reactions related to ↓ intravascular volume; Hypotension (correct prior to treatment, especially if eGFR 30–60 mL/min, age >75 yr, or concurrent use of loop diuretics, ACE inhibitors, or ARBs; OB: Use during pregnancy only if potential maternal benefit justifies potential fetal risk; Pedi: Safety and effectiveness not established.

Adverse Reactions/Side Effects

CV: hypotension. **Endo:** hypoglycemia (↑ with other medications). **F and E:** KETOACIDOSIS, hypermagnesemia, hyperphosphatemia, thirst. **GI:** abdominal pain, constipation, nausea. **GU:** NECROTIZING FASCIITIS OF PERINEUM (FOURNIER'S GANGRENE), UROSEPSIS, female mycotic infections, acute kidney injury, glucosuria, male mycotic infections, ↓ renal function, urinary tract infection (including pyelonephritis), ↑ urination, vulvovaginal pruritus. **Metab:** hyperlipidemia. **MS:** bone fractures, lower limb amputation. **Misc:** HYPERSENSITIVITY REACTIONS (including anaphylaxis or angioedema).

Interactions

Drug-Drug: Blood levels are ↓ by **UGT inducers** including **phenobarbital**, **phenytoin**, **rifampin**, and **ritonavir**; ↑ dose may be required. ↑ risk of hypoglycemia with **insulin** or **insulin secretagogues**; dose adjustments may be required. May ↑ blood levels and effects of **digoxin**; levels should be monitored. ↑ risk of hyperkalemia with **potassium-sparing diuretics** or **medications that interfere with the renin-angiotensin-aldosterone system**. Concurrent use with **NSAIDs**, **diuretics**, **ACE inhibitors**, or **angiotensin receptor blockers** may ↑ risk of acute kidney injury.

Route/Dosage

PO (Adults): *eGFR ≥ 60 mL/min/1.73 m^2*— 100 mg once daily initially, may be ↑ to 300 mg once daily; *Concurrent use of UGT inducers (phenobarbital, phenytoin, rifampin, ritonavir)*—if maintenance dose is 100 mg daily, may require ↑ to 300 mg daily.

Renal Impairment

PO (Adults): *eGFR 45–60 mL/min/1.73 m^2*— 100 mg once daily.

Availability

Tablets: 100 mg, 300 mg. ***In combination with:*** metformin (Invokamet); metformin XR (Invokamet XR). See Appendix B.

NURSING IMPLICATIONS

Assessment

- Observe patient for signs and symptoms of hypoglycemic reactions (abdominal pain, sweating, hunger, weakness, dizziness, headache, tremor, tachycardia, anxiety).
- Monitor for signs and symptoms of volume depletion (dizziness, feeling faint, weakness, orthostatic hypotension) after initiating therapy.
- Monitor for infection, new pain, tenderness, erythema, swelling, sores, or ulcers involving lower limbs, with fever or malaise; discontinue canagliflozin if these occur.
- ***Lab Test Considerations:*** Monitor hemoglobin A1C prior to and periodically during therapy.

- May cause ↑ uric acid levels.
- Monitor renal function prior to and periodically during therapy, especially in patients with eGFR <60 mL/min/1.73 m^2. May ↑ serum creatinine and ↓ eGFR.
- May cause ↑ serum potassium, magnesium, and phosphate levels. Monitor electrolytes periodically during therapy.
- May cause ↑ LDL-C. Monitor serum lipid levels periodically during therapy.
- Causes positive test for urine glucose.
- Monitor for ketoacidosis, especially during prolonged fasting for illness or surgery. May require temporary discontinuation of therapy.

Implementation

- Patients stabilized on a diabetic regimen who are exposed to stress, fever, trauma, infection, or surgery may require administration of insulin.
- Correct volume depletion prior to beginning therapy with canagliflozin.
- **PO:** Administer before the first meal of the day.

Patient/Family Teaching

- Instruct patient to take canagliflozin as directed. Take missed doses as soon as remembered, unless it is almost time for next dose; do not double doses. Advise patient to read the *Medication Guide* before starting and with each Rx refill in case of changes.
- Explain to patient that canagliflozin helps control hyperglycemia but does not cure diabetes. Therapy is usually long term.
- Instruct patient not to share this medication with others, even if they have the same symptoms; it may harm them.
- Encourage patient to follow prescribed diet, medication, and exercise regimen to prevent hyperglycemic or hypoglycemic episodes.
- Review signs of hypoglycemia and hyperglycemia with patient. If hypoglycemia occurs, advise patient to take a glass of orange juice or 2–3 tsp of sugar, honey, or corn syrup dissolved in water, and notify health care professional.
- Instruct patient in proper testing of blood glucose and urine ketones, especially during periods of stress or illness. Inform patient that canagliflozin will cause a positive test result when testing for urine glucose. Notify health care professional if significant changes occur.
- Advise patient to notify health care professional if new pain or tenderness, sores or ulcers, or infections involving the leg or foot occur and to immediately seek care if pain or tenderness, redness, or swelling of the genitals or area from the genitals back to the rectum, along with a fever above 100.4°F or malaise occur.
- Inform patient that canagliflozin may cause yeast infections. Women may have signs and symptoms of a vaginal yeast infection (vaginal odor, white or yellow vaginal discharge [may be lumpy or look like cottage cheese], vaginal itching). Men may have signs and symptoms of a yeast infection of the penis (redness, itching, or swelling of penis; rash on penis; foul smelling discharge from penis; pain in skin around penis). Advise patient to notify health care professional if yeast infection occurs.
- Advise patient to notify health care professional promptly if rash; hives; or swelling of face, lips, or throat occur.
- Inform patient of increased risk for urinary tract infections, hypotension, and bone fractures and discuss factors that may increase risk.
- Advise patient to notify health care professional of all Rx or OTC medications, vitamins, or herbal products being taken and to consult with health care professional before taking other medications, especially other oral hypoglycemic medications.
- Advise patient to notify health care professional if pregnancy is planned or suspected and to avoid breast feeding during therapy.

Evaluation/Desired Outcomes

- Improved hemoglobin A1C and glycemic control in adults with Type II diabetes.
- Reduction in risk of cardiovascular death, nonfatal MI, and nonfatal stroke.

candesartan, See ANGIOTENSIN II RECEPTOR ANTAGONISTS.

cangrelor (kan-**grel**-or)

Kengreal

Classification

Therapeutic: antiplatelet agents

Pharmacologic: platelet aggregation inhibitors

Indications

Adjunct to percutaneous coronary intervention (PCI) to ↓ risk of periprocedural MI, repeat coronary revascularization or stent thrombosis in patients not currently receiving a $P2Y_{12}$ platelet inhibitor and are not receiving a glycoprotein IIb/IIIa inhibitor.

Action

Inhibits platelet aggregation by reversibly interacting with platelet $P2Y_{12}$ADP-receptors, preventing signal transduction and platelet activation. **Therapeutic Effects:** ↓ risk of periprocedural MI, repeat coronary revascularization or stent thrombosis associated with PCI.

Pharmacokinetics

Absorption: IV administration results in complete bioavailability.

Distribution: Unk.

Protein Binding: 97–98%.

Metabolism and Excretion: Metabolized rapidly in the blood stream; metabolites do not have antiplatelet activity. 58% excreted by kidneys, 35% in feces.
Half-life: 3–6 min.

TIME/ACTION PROFILE (antiplatelet effect)

ROUTE	ONSET	PEAK	DURATION
IV	rapid	2 min	1 hr†

† following discontinuation.

Contraindications/Precautions

Contraindicated in: Hypersensitivity; Significant severe bleeding.
Use Cautiously in: CCr <30 mL/min (↑ risk of further decline in renal function); OB: Consider potential maternal benefits and fetal risks; Pedi: Safe and effective use in children has not been established.

Adverse Reactions/Side Effects

Resp: dyspnea. **Hemat:** bleeding. **Misc:** allergic reactions including ANAPHYLAXIS.

Interactions

Drug-Drug: Concurrent use of other **$P2Y_{12}$ inhibitors** including **clopidogrel**, **prasugrel**, or **tigagrelor**↑ risk of bleeding. Blocks antiplatelet effects of concurrently administered **clopidogrel** or **prasugrel**.

Route/Dosage

IV (Adults): 30 mcg/kg bolus prior to PCI, then 4 mcg/kg/min infusion for 2 hr or duration of procedure, whichever is longer; should be followed by initiation of an oral $P2Y_{12}$ platelet inhibitor.

Availability

Lyophilized powder for IV injection (requires reconstitution): 50 mg/vial.

NURSING IMPLICATIONS

Assessment

- Monitor for signs and symptoms of bleeding during and following infusion.
- Monitor for signs and symptoms of hypersensitivity reaction (bronchospasm, angioedema, stridor) during therapy. Discontinue therapy and treat symptomatically.

Implementation

- **IV Push:** Reconstitute each 50 mg vial with 5 mL of sterile water for injection. Swirl gently until dissolved; avoid vigorous mixing. Allow foam to settle. Solution is clear and colorless to pale yellow; do not administer solutions that are discolored or contain particulate matter. ***Diluent:*** Withdraw reconstituted solution and add to 250 mL of 0.9% NaCl or D5W. Dilute immediately. Stable for 12 hrs if diluted with D5W or 24 hrs if diluted with 0.9% NaCl at room temperature. Discard unused portion. ***Concentration:*** 200 mcg/mL. Patients >100 kg will require at least 2 bags. ***Rate:*** Administer rapidly over <1 min from diluted bag via IV push or pump. Ensure bolus completely administered before beginning infusion.
- **Intermittent Infusion:** Start infusion immediately after administration of bolus. ***Rate:*** 4 mcg/kg/min for at least 2 hrs or duration of PCI, whichever is longer.
- **Y-Site Incompatibility:** Infusion requires a dedicated line.
- To maintain platelet inhibition, administer either ticagrelor 180 mg PO at any time during or immediately after discontinuation, or prasugrel 60 mg PO or clopidogrel 600 mg PO immediately after discontinuation of infusion; do not administer prasugrel or clopidogrel prior to discontinuation of infusion.

Patient/Family Teaching

- Caution patient to notify health care professional if bleeding occurs.
- Advise female patient to notify health care professional if pregnancy is suspected or if breast feeding.

Evaluation/Desired Outcomes

- ↓ risk of periprocedural MI, repeat coronary revascularization or stent thrombosis associated with PCI.

cannabidiol (kan-a-bidye-ol)

Epidiolex

Classification
Therapeutic: anticonvulsants
Pharmacologic: cannabinoids

Schedule V

Indications

Seizures associated with Lennox-Gastaut syndrome or Dravet syndrome.

Action

Cannabidiol is a cannabinoid that naturally occurs in the *Cannabis sativa* plant. Mechanism of anticonvulsant effect unknown; does not work by interacting with cannabinoid receptors. **Therapeutic Effects:** Reduction in frequency of atonic, tonic, clonic, and tonic-clonic seizures.

Pharmacokinetics

Absorption: Extent of absorption unknown. High fat/high calorie meals increase extent of absorption.
Distribution: Extensively distributed to tissues.
Protein Binding: >94%.
Metabolism and Excretion: Primarily metabolized in the liver by the CYP2C9 and CYP3A4 isoenzymes to an active metabolite (7-OH-CBD). Primarily excreted in feces.
Half-life: 56–61 hr.

TIME/ACTION PROFILE (plasma concentrations)

ROUTE	ONSET	PEAK	DURATION
PO	unknown	2.5–5 hr	unknown

Contraindications/Precautions

Contraindicated in: Hypersensitivity to cannabidiol or sesame oil.

Use Cautiously in: Concurrent use of valproic acid or clobazam; Concurrent use of sedatives, hypnotics, or other psychoactive drugs (↑ risk of adverse effects); Elevated liver enzymes (at baseline); Moderate to severe hepatic impairment; OB: Use only if the potential benefit justifies the potential risk to the fetus; Lactation: Use only if the potential benefit justifies the potential risk to the infant; Geri: Choose dose carefully, considering concurrent disease states, drug therapy, and age-related ↓ in hepatic and renal function; Pedi: Children <2 yr (safety and effectiveness not established).

Adverse Reactions/Side Effects

CNS: SUICIDAL THOUGHTS/BEHAVIORS, drowsiness, fatigue, insomnia, aggressive behavior, agitation. **Derm:** rash. **EENT:** dry mouth. **GI:** HEPATOTOXICITY, ↓ appetite, diarrhea, ↑ liver enzymes, abdominal pain, ↓ weight. **GU:** ↑ serum creatinine. **Hemat:** anemia. **Neuro:** ataxia. **Misc:** hypersensitivity reactions (angioedema, pruritus), infection, physical dependence, psychological dependence (high doses or prolonged therapy).

Interactions

Drug-Drug: Concurrent use of **valproic acid** or **clobazam** ↑ risk of hepatotoxicity. **Moderate or strong CYP2C9 or CYP3A4 inhibitors** may ↑ levels and risk of toxicity; consider ↓ cannabidiol dose. **Strong CYP2C9 or CYP3A4 inducers** may ↓ levels and effectiveness; consider ↑ cannabidiol dose. May ↑ levels and risk of toxicity of **CYP2C8, CYP2C9, or CYP2C19 substrates**; consider ↓ dose of CYP2C8, CYP2C9, or CYP2C19 substrate. May ↑ or ↓ levels of **CYP1A2 or CYP2B6 substrates**; consider ↓ dose of CYP1A2 or CYP2B6 substrate. Additive CNS depression with **alcohol**, **antihistamines**, **barbiturates**, **benzodiazepines**, **muscle relaxants**, **opioid analgesics**, **tricyclic antidepressants**, and **sedative/hypnotics**.

Route/Dosage

PO (Adults and Children ≥2 yr): 2.5 mg/kg twice daily; can ↑ dose to 5 mg/kg twice daily in 1 wk. If further reduction in seizure frequency needed, may continue to ↑ dose on weekly basis (every other day if more rapid titration warranted) in increments of 2.5 mg/kg twice daily (max dose = 10 mg/kg twice daily).

Hepatic Impairment

PO (Adults and Children ≥2 yr): *Moderate hepatic impairment (Child–Pugh B)*—1.25 mg/kg twice daily; can ↑ dose to 2.5 mg/kg twice daily in 1 wk. If further reduction in seizure frequency needed, may continue to ↑ dose on weekly basis (every other day if more rapid titration warranted) in increments of 1.25 mg/kg twice daily (max dose = 5 mg/kg twice daily); *Severe hepatic impairment (Child–Pugh C)*—0.5 mg/kg twice daily; can ↑ dose to 1 mg/kg twice daily in 1 wk. If further reduction in seizure frequency needed, may continue to ↑ dose on weekly basis (every other day if more rapid titration warranted) in increments of 0.5 mg/kg twice daily (max dose = 2 mg/kg twice daily).

Availability

Oral solution (strawberry flavor): 100 mg/mL.

NURSING IMPLICATIONS

Assessment

- Assess location, duration, and characteristics of seizure activity. Institute seizure precautions.
- Monitor closely for notable changes in behavior that could indicate the emergence or worsening of suicidal thoughts or behavior or depression.
- Monitor for signs and symptom of hepatotoxicity (unexplained nausea, vomiting, right upper quadrant abdominal pain, fatigue, anorexia, jaundice and/or dark urine). If signs and symptoms occur, promptly measure serum transaminases and total bilirubin and interrupt or discontinue treatment with cannabidiol.
- Monitor for signs and symptoms of hypersensitivity reactions (pruritus, erythema, and angioedema) during therapy. Discontinue cannabidiol if symptoms occur.
- ***Lab Test Considerations:*** Obtain serum transaminases (ALT, AST) and total bilirubin levels before starting therapy. Elevations usually respond to decreased dose or discontinuation of therapy. Monitor levels at 1, 3, and 6 mo after starting therapy, within 1 mo following dose changes, and as needed thereafter. Discontinue cannabidiol if transaminase levels >3 times upper limit of normal (ULN) and bilirubin levels >2 times ULN. Also discontinue therapy if transaminase persistently >5 times ULN.

Implementation

- **PO:** Administer orally twice daily. Use calibrated measuring device included with cannabidiol to ensure accurate dosing. Solution is strawberry flavored clear, colorless to yellow. Store at room temperature; do not refrigerate or freeze. Discard 12 wk after bottle is first opened.

Patient/Family Teaching

- Instruct patient to take cannabidiol as directed. Advise patient not to stop cannabidiol without consulting health care professional; must be gradually discontinued to prevent seizures. Advise patient to read the *Medication Guide* before starting therapy and with each Rx refill in case of changes.
- May cause drowsiness. Caution patient to avoid driving or other activities requiring alertness until re-

sponse to medication is known. Tell patient not to resume driving until health care professional gives clearance based on control of seizure disorder.

- Advise patient to notify health care professional promptly if signs and symptoms of hepatotoxicity occur.
- Instruct patient to notify health care professional of all Rx or OTC medications, vitamins, or herbal products being taken and consult health care professional before taking any new medications.
- Inform patients and families of risk of suicidal thoughts and behavior and advise that behavioral changes, emergency or worsening signs and symptoms of depression, unusual changes in mood, or emergence of suicidal thoughts, behavior, or thoughts of self-harm should be reported to health care professional immediately.
- Inform patients of potential for positive cannabis drug screens.
- Rep: Advise female patients to notify health care professional if pregnancy is planned or suspected or if breast feeding. Encourage patients who become pregnant to enroll in the North American Antiepileptic Drug (NAAED) Pregnancy Registry by calling 1-888-233-2334 or on the web at www.aedpregnancyregistry.org. Enrollment must be done by patients themselves.

Evaluation/Desired Outcomes

- Decreased frequency and intensity of seizure activity.

HIGH ALERT

capecitabine

(ka-pe-**site**-a-been)

Xeloda

Classification

Therapeutic: antineoplastics

Pharmacologic: antimetabolites

Indications

Metastatic colorectal cancer. Adjuvant treatment for Dukes' C colon cancer following primary resection. Metastatic breast cancer that has worsened despite prior therapy with anthracycline (daunorubicin, doxorubicin, idarubicin) (to be used in combination with docetaxel). Metastatic breast cancer that is resistant to both paclitaxel and an anthracycline (daunorubicin, doxorubicin, idarubicin) or is resistant to paclitaxel and further anthracycline therapy is contraindicated.

Action

Converted in tissue to 5-fluorouracil, which inhibits DNA and RNA synthesis by preventing thymidine production. The enzyme responsible for the final step in the conversion to 5-fluorouracil may be found in higher concentrations in some tumors. **Therapeutic Effects:** Death of rapidly replicating cells, particularly malignant ones.

Pharmacokinetics

Absorption: Well absorbed after oral administration.

Distribution: Unknown.

Metabolism and Excretion: Metabolized mostly in tissue and by the liver to 5-fluorouracil; 5-fluorouracil is metabolized by dihydropyrimidine dehydrogenase to a less toxic compound; inactive metabolites are excreted primarily in urine.

Half-life: 45 min.

TIME/ACTION PROFILE (blood levels)

ROUTE	ONSET	PEAK	DURATION
PO	unknown†	1.5 hr (2 hr for 5-FU)‡	unknown

†Onset of antineoplastic effect is 6 wk.

‡Peak 5-FU levels occur at 2 hr.

Contraindications/Precautions

Contraindicated in: Hypersensitivity to capecitabine or 5-fluorouracil; Severe renal impairment (CCr <30 mL/min); OB: Pregnancy (may cause fetal harm); Lactation: Potential for serious adverse effects in nursing infants.

Use Cautiously in: Dihydropyrimidine dehydrogenase deficiency (patients at ↑ risk of 5-fluorouracil toxicity); Mild-moderate renal impairment (↓ starting dose to 75% in patients with CCr 30–50 mL/min); Hepatic impairment; Coronary artery disease; Rep: Women of reproductive potential and men with female partners of reproductive potential; Pedi: Safety not established; Geri: ↑ risk of severe diarrhea in patients ≥80 yr.

Adverse Reactions/Side Effects

CNS: fatigue, headache, dizziness, insomnia. **CV:** edema, chest pain. **Derm:** STEVENS-JOHNSON SYNDROME, TOXIC EPIDERMAL NECROLYSIS, dermatitis, hand-and-foot syndrome, nail disorder, alopecia, erythema, rashes. **EENT:** eye irritation, epistaxis, rhinorrhea. **F and E:** dehydration. **GI:** DIARRHEA, NECROTIZING ENTEROCOLITIS, abdominal pain, anorexia, constipation, dysgeusia, hyperbilirubinemia, nausea, stomatitis, vomiting, dyspepsia, xerostomia. **GU:** acute renal failure, ↓ fertility. **Hemat:** anemia, leukopenia, thrombocytopenia. **MS:** arthralgia, myalgia. **Neuro:** peripheral neuropathy. **Resp:** cough, dyspnea. **Misc:** fever.

Interactions

Drug-Drug: May ↑ risk of bleeding with **warfarin**; monitor PT/INR frequently. Toxicity ↑ by concurrent **leucovorin**. **Antacids** may ↑ absorption. May ↑ levels and risk of toxicity from **phenytoin** (may need to ↓ phenytoin dose). ↑ incidence of acute renal failure with other **nephrotoxic drugs**. **Allopurinol** may ↓ levels

of capecitabine's active metabolite and its overall effectiveness; avoid concurrent use.
Drug-Food: Food ↑ absorption, although capecitabine should be given within 30 min after a meal.

Route/Dosage

PO (Adults): 1250 mg/m² twice daily for 14 days, followed by 7-day rest period; given in 3-wk cycles.

Renal Impairment

PO (Adults): *CCr 30–50 mL/min*—↓ initial dose to 75% of usual.

Availability (generic available)

Tablets: 150 mg, 500 mg.

NURSING IMPLICATIONS

Assessment

- Assess for signs of infection (fever, chills, sore throat, cough, hoarseness, pain in lower back or side, difficult or painful urination). Assess for bleeding (bleeding gums; bruising; petechiae; and guaiac-test stools, urine, and emesis). Avoid IM injections and taking rectal temperatures. Apply pressure to venipuncture sites for 10 min. Anemia may occur. Monitor for increased fatigue, dyspnea, and orthostatic hypotension.
- Assess mucous membranes, number and consistency of stools, and frequency of vomiting. Notify health care professional if symptoms of toxicity (stomatitis, uncontrollable vomiting, diarrhea, fever) occur; drug may need to be discontinued or dose decreased. Patients with severe diarrhea should be monitored carefully, administered antidiarrheal agents (loperamide) and given fluid and electrolyte replacements if they become dehydrated. Grade 2 diarrhea (4–6 stools/day or nocturnal stools), Grade 3 (7–9 stools/day or incontinence and malabsorption), Grade 4 (≥10 stools/day or grossly bloody diarrhea or need for parenteral support). If grade 2, 3, or 4 diarrhea occurs, immediately stop therapy until diarrhea resolves or decreases in intensity to Grade 1. Grade 3 or 4 diarrhea usually lasts 5 days.
- Assess patient for mucocutaneous and dermatologic toxicity (Stevens-Johnson syndrome, toxic epidermal necrolysis, hand-and-foot syndrome). Grade 1 (numbness, dysesthesia/paresthesia, tingling, painless swelling or erythema of hands and/or feet and/or discomfort which does not disrupt normal activities). Grade 2 (painful erythema and swelling of hands and/or feet and/or discomfort affecting the patient's activities of daily living). Grade 3 (moist desquamation, ulceration, blistering or severe pain of hands and/or feet and/or severe discomfort causing patient to be unable to work or perform activities of daily living). Persistent or severe hand-and-foot syndrome of Grade 2 and above can lead to loss of fingerprints, affecting patient identification. *If Grade 2 or 3 occurs,* interrupt therapy until Grade 1. Decrease doses following Grade 3.
- ***Lab Test Considerations:*** Monitor hepatic (serum alkaline phosphatase, AST, ALT, and bilirubin), renal, and hematologic (hematocrit, hemoglobin, leukocyte, platelet count) function before and periodically during therapy. May cause leukopenia, anemia, and thrombocytopenia. Leukopenia may require discontinuation of therapy. Therapy should be interrupted if serum bilirubin ↑ to 1.5 times normal or greater; may be reinstituted after bilirubin returns to normal.
- Monitor PT or INR frequently in patients receiving warfarin and capecitabine to adjust warfarin dose. May cause ↑ bleeding within a few days to several mo of initiation of therapy to 1 mo following discontinuation of therapy. Risk is greater in patients over 60 yr.

Implementation

- ***High Alert:*** Fatalities have occurred with chemotherapeutic agents. Before administering, clarify all ambiguous orders; double-check single, daily, and course-of-therapy dose limits; have second practitioner independently double-check original order and dose calculations. Do not confuse Xeloda (capecitabine) with Xenical (orlistat).
- Dose modifications are based on degree of toxicity encountered. Once a dose has been reduced because of toxicity, it should not be increased at a later time. See manufacturer's recommendations.
- **PO:** Administer every 12 hr for 2 wk, followed by a 1-wk rest period. Swallow tablets whole; do not crush or cut. Tablets should be taken with water within 30 min after a meal.

Patient/Family Teaching

- Instruct patient to take medication every 12 hr with water within 30 min after a meal. Missed doses should be omitted; continue regular schedule. Do not double dose. Advise patient to read *Patient Package Insert* before starting and with each Rx refill in case of changes.
- Inform patient of the most common side effects. Instruct patient to notify health care provider immediately if any of the following occur: diarrhea (>4 bowel movements in a day or any diarrhea at night), vomiting (more than once in 24 hr), nausea (loss of appetite and significant decrease in daily food intake), stomatitis (pain, redness, swelling, or sore in mouth), hand-and-foot syndrome (pain, swelling, or redness of hands and/or feet), skin reactions (rash, blisters, peeling of skin), fever, or infection (temperature of ≥100.5° F or other signs of infection).
- Instruct patient to notify health care professional if he or she is taking folic acid.
- Instruct patient to notify health care professional if fever; chills; sore throat; signs of infection; yellowing of skin or eyes; abdominal pain; joint or flank pain; swelling of feet or legs; bleeding gums; bruising; petechiae; or blood in urine, stool, or emesis occurs. Caution patient to avoid crowds and persons with known infections. Instruct patient to use soft toothbrush and electric razor. Patients should be cau-

tioned not to drink alcoholic beverages or take products containing aspirin or NSAIDs.
- Advise patient to rinse mouth with clear water after eating and drinking and to avoid flossing to minimize stomatitis. Viscous lidocaine may be used if mouth pain interferes with eating. Stomatitis pain may require treatment with opioid analgesics.
- Advise patient to notify health care professional of all Rx or OTC medications, vitamins, or herbal products being taken and to consult with health care professional before taking other medications.
- Rep: Advise female patient to use effective contraception during and for at least 6 mo after last dose. Advise male patients with female partners of reproductive potential to use effective contraception for at least 3 mo after last dose. Avoid breast feeding for 2 wk after last dose. May impair fertility of female and male patients of reproductive potential.
- Emphasize the importance of routine follow-up lab tests to monitor progress and to check for side effects.

Evaluation/Desired Outcomes
- Tumor regression.

capsaicin (kap-say-sin)
Capzasin-HP, Capzasin-P, DiabetAid Pain and Tingling Relief, Qutenza, Zostrix, Zostrix-HP

Classification
Therapeutic: nonopioid analgesics (topical)

Indications
Temporary management of pain due to rheumatoid arthritis and osteoarthritis. Treatment of pain associated with postherpetic neuralgia (topical and transdermal) or diabetic neuropathy. **Unlabeled Use:** Treatment of postmastectomy pain syndrome. Treatment of complex regional pain syndrome.

Action
Topical: May deplete and prevent the reaccumulation of a chemical (substance P) responsible for transmitting painful impulses from peripheral sites to the CNS. **Transdermal**: Initially stimulates the transient receptor potential vanilloid 1 (TRPV1) receptors on nociceptive nerve fibers in the skin; this is followed by pain relief thought to be due to a reduction in TRPV1–expressing nociceptive nerve endings. **Therapeutic Effects:** Relief of discomfort associated with painful peripheral syndromes.

Pharmacokinetics
Absorption: Unknown.
Distribution: Unknown.
Metabolism and Excretion: Unknown.
Half-life: Unknown.

TIME/ACTION PROFILE

ROUTE	ONSET	PEAK	DURATION
topical	1–2 wk	2–4 wk†	unknown
transdermal	unknown	unknown	unknown

†May take up to 6 wk for head and neck neuralgias.

Contraindications/Precautions
Contraindicated in: Hypersensitivity to capsaicin or hot peppers; Not for use near eyes or on open or broken skin.
Use Cautiously in: OB, Lactation: Safety not established; Pedi: Safety not established in children <18 yr (transdermal) or <2 yr (topical).

Adverse Reactions/Side Effects
CV: *Patch*—↑ BP. **Derm:** pain (after application of patch), transient burning. **Resp:** cough.

Interactions
Drug-Drug: None significant.

Route/Dosage
Topical (Adults and Children ≥2 yr): Apply to affected areas 3–4 times daily.
Transdermal (Adults): Apply up to 4 patches for 60 min (single use); may be repeated every 3 mo, as needed based on pain (should not be used more frequently than every 3 mo).

Availability (generic available)
Cream: 0.1%^{OTC}, 0.025%^{OTC}, 0.035%^{OTC}, 0.075%^{OTC}. **Gel:** 0.025%^{OTC}. **Lotion:** 0.025%^{OTC}. **Topical liquid:** 0.15%^{OTC}. **Transdermal patch:** 0.0225%/patch, 0.025%/patch, 0.03%/patch, 0.035%/patch, 0.05%/patch, 8% (179 mg)/patch. ***In combination with:*** methylsalicylate (Ziks^{OTC}). See Appendix B.

NURSING IMPLICATIONS
Assessment
- Assess pain intensity and location before and periodically throughout therapy.
- **Transdermal:** Monitor BP periodically during application.

Implementation
- Do not confuse Zostrix (capsaicin) with Zovirax (acyclovir).
- **Topical:** Apply to affected area not more than 3–4 times daily. Avoid getting medication into eyes or on broken or irritated skin. Do not bandage tightly.
- Topical lidocaine may be applied during the first 1–2 wk of treatment to reduce initial discomfort.
- **Transdermal:** Identify treatment area (painful area including areas of hypersensitivity and allodynia) and mark on the skin. If needed, clip hair (do not shave) in and around treatment area to promote

patch adherence. Cut patch to size and shape of treatment area. Gently wash area with mild soap and water and dry thoroughly. Apply topical anesthetic to the entire treatment area and surrounding 1–2 cm and keep the local anesthetic in place until skin is anesthetized prior to the application of patch. Remove the topical anesthetic with a dry wipe. Gently wash treatment area with mild soap and water and dry. Use only nitrile gloves when handling capsaicin and cleaning capsaicin residue from skin; latex gloves do not provide adequate protection. Apply patch to dry, intact skin. Apply patch within 2 hr of opening pouch. Tear pouch open along the three dashed lines and remove patch. Inspect patch and identify the outer surface backing layer with the printing on one side and the capsaicin-containing adhesive on the other side. Adhesive side of the patch is covered by a clear, unprinted, diagonally cut release liner. Cut patch before removing protective release liner. Peel a small section of the release liner back and place adhesive side of patch on treatment area. While slowly peeling back release liner from under patch with one hand, use other hand to smooth the patch down on to skin. Once patch is applied, leave in place for 60 min. To ensure patch maintains contact with treatment area, a dressing, such as rolled gauze, may be used. Instruct the patient not to touch the patch or treatment area.

- Even following use of a local anesthetic prior to administration of capsaicin, patients may experience substantial procedural pain. Prepare to treat acute pain during and following application with local cooling (such as an ice pack) and/or appropriate analgesic medication (opioids).
- Remove patches by gently and slowly rolling inward. After removal, generously apply *Cleansing Gel* to treatment area and leave on for at least 1 min. Remove *Cleansing Gel* with a dry wipe and gently wash area with mild soap and water and dry thoroughly. Aerosolization of capsaicin can occur upon rapid removal of patches. Remove patches gently and slowly by rolling adhesive side inward. If irritation of eyes or airways occurs, remove affected individual from the vicinity. Flush eyes and mucous membranes with cool water. Inhalation of airborne capsaicin can result in coughing or sneezing. Provide supportive care if shortness of breath develops. If skin not intended to be treated comes in contact with capsaicin, apply *Cleansing Gel* for 1 min and wipe off with dry gauze. After *Cleansing Gel* has been wiped off, wash area with soap and water.

Patient/Family Teaching

- **Topical:** Instruct patient on the correct method for application of capsaicin. Rub cream into affected area well so that little or no cream is left on the surface. Gloves should be worn during application or hands should be washed immediately after application. If application is to hands for arthritis, do not wash hands for at least 30 min after application.
- Advise patient to apply missed doses as soon as possible unless almost time for next dose. Pain relief lasts only as long as capsaicin is used regularly.
- Advise patient that transient burning may occur with application, especially if applied fewer than 3–4 times daily. Burning usually disappears after the first few days but may continue for 2–4 wk or longer. Burning is increased by heat, sweating, bathing in warm water, humidity, and clothing. Burning usually decreases in frequency and intensity the longer capsaicin is used. Decreasing number of daily doses will not lessen burning but may decrease amount of pain relief and may prolong period of burning.
- Caution patient to flush area with water if capsaicin gets into eyes and to wash with warm, but not hot, soapy water if capsaicin gets on other sensitive areas of the body.
- Instruct patient with herpes zoster (shingles) not to apply capsaicin cream until lesions have healed completely.
- Advise patient to discontinue use and notify health care professional if pain persists longer than 1 mo, worsens, or if signs of infection are present.
- **Transdermal:** Inform patient that treated area may be sensitive for a few days to heat (e.g., hot showers or baths, direct sunlight, vigorous exercise).
- Advise patient that exposure of skin to capsaicin may result in transient erythema and burning sensation. Instruct patients not to touch patch and if they accidentally touch patch it may burn and/or sting.
- Instruct patient to notify health care professional immediately if irritation of eyes or airways occurs, or if any of the side effects become severe.
- If opioids are used to treat pain from patch, caution patient that opioids may cause drowsiness and to avoid driving or other activities requiring alertness until response to medication is known.
- May cause transient increases in BP. Instruct patients to inform health care professional if they have experienced any recent cardiovascular event.
- Instruct patients to notify health care professional if pregnancy is planned or suspected or if breast feeding.

Evaluation/Desired Outcomes

- Decrease in discomfort associated with:
- Postherpetic neuropathy.
- Diabetic neuropathy.
- Rheumatoid arthritis.
- Osteoarthritis. Pain relief usually begins within 1–2 wk with arthritis, 2–4 wk with neuralgias, and 4–6 wk with neuralgias of the head and neck.

captopril, See ANGIOTENSIN-CONVERTING ENZYME (ACE) INHIBITORS.

carBAMazepine
(kar-ba-**maz**-e-peen)
Carbatrol, Carnexiv, Epitol, Equetro, Mazepine, TEGretol, TEGretol CR, TEGretol XR, Teril

Classification
Therapeutic: anticonvulsants, mood stabilizers

Indications
IV, PO: Treatment of tonic-clonic, mixed, and complex-partial seizures. **PO:** Management of pain in trigeminal neuralgia. **Equetro only:** Acute manic or mixed episodes associated with bipolar I disorder. **Unlabeled Use:** Other forms of neurogenic pain.

Action
Decreases synaptic transmission in the CNS by affecting sodium channels in neurons. **Therapeutic Effects:** Prevention of seizures. Relief of pain in trigeminal neuralgia. Decreased mania.

Pharmacokinetics
Absorption: Oral absorption is slow but complete. Suspension produces earlier, higher peak, and lower trough levels. IV administration results in complete bioavailability.
Distribution: Widely distributed. Crosses the blood-brain barrier. Crosses the placenta rapidly and enters breast milk in high concentrations.
Protein Binding: *Carbamazepine*—75–90%; *epoxide*—50%.
Metabolism and Excretion: Extensively metabolized in the liver by cytochrome P450 3A4 to active epoxide metabolite; epoxide metabolite has anticonvulsant and antineuralgic activity.
Half-life: *Carbamazapine*—single dose—25–65 hr, chronic dosing—*Children*—8–14 hr; *Adults*—12–17 hr; *epoxide*—34±9 hr.

TIME/ACTION PROFILE (anticonvulsant activity)

ROUTE	ONSET	PEAK	DURATION
PO	up to 1 mo†	4–5 hr‡	6–12 hr
PO-ER	up to 1 mo†	2–3–12 hr‡	12 hr
IV	unknown	unknown	unknown

†Onset of antineuralgic activity is 8–72 hr.
‡Listed for tablets; peak level occurs 1.5 hr after a chronic dose of suspension.

Contraindications/Precautions
Contraindicated in: Hypersensitivity to carbamazepine or tricyclic antidepressants; Bone marrow suppression; Concomitant use or use within 14 days of MAO inhibitors; Concurrent use of nefazodone or NNRTIs that are CYP3A4 substrates; Moderate-to-severe renal impairment (IV only); OB: Use only if potential benefits outweigh risks to the fetus; additional vitamin K during last wk of pregnancy has been recommended; Lactation: Discontinue drug or bottle feed.
Use Cautiously in: All patients (may ↑ risk of suicidal thoughts/behaviors); Cardiac or hepatic disease; Renal failure (dosing adjustment required for CCr <10 mL/min); Mild renal impairment (IV only); ↑ intraocular pressure; Geri: Older men with prostatic hyperplasia may be at ↑ risk for acute urinary retention or difficulty initiating stream; Pedi: Safety and effectiveness of IV formulation not established.
Exercise Extreme Caution in: Patients positive for HLA-B*1502 or HLA-A*3101 alleles (unless benefits clearly outweigh the risks) (↑ risk of serious skin reactions).

Adverse Reactions/Side Effects
CNS: SUICIDAL THOUGHTS, ataxia, drowsiness, fatigue, psychosis, sedation, vertigo. **EENT:** blurred vision, corneal opacities, nystagmus. **Resp:** pneumonitis. **CV:** HF, edema, heart block, hypertension, hypotension, syncope. **GI:** HEPATOTOXICITY, PANCREATITIS, ↑ liver enzymes, weight gain. **GU:** hesitancy, renal impairment (IV only), urinary retention. **Derm:** DRUG REACTION WITH EOSINOPHILIA AND SYSTEMIC SYMPTOMS (DRESS), STEVENS-JOHNSON SYNDROME, TOXIC EPIDERMAL NECROLYSIS, nail shedding, photosensitivity, rash, urticaria. **F and E:** syndrome of inappropriate antidiuretic hormone (SIADH), hyponatremia. **Hemat:** AGRANULOCYTOSIS, APLASTIC ANEMIA, THROMBOCYTOPENIA, eosinophilia, leukopenia, lymphadenopathy. **Misc:** chills, fever.

Interactions
Drug-Drug: May significantly ↓ levels of **nefazodone** or **NNRTIs** that are CYP3A4 substrates; concurrent use contraindicated. Concurrent or recent (within 2 wk) use of **MAO inhibitors** may result in hyperpyrexia, hypertension, seizures, and death; use contraindicated. May ↓ levels/effectiveness of **acetaminophen**, **alprazolam**, **aprepitant**, **buprenorphine**, **bupropion**, **calcium channel blockers**, **citalopram**, **clonazepam**, **corticosteroids**, **cyclosporine**, **doxycycline**, **estrogen-containing contraceptives**, **everolimus**, **haloperidol**, **imatinib**, **itraconazole**, **lamotrigine**, **levothyroxine**, **methadone**. **midazolam**, **olanzapine**, **paliperidone**, **phenytoin**, **protease inhibitors**, **risperidone**, **sertraline**, **sirolimus**, **tacrolimus**, **tadalafil**, **theophylline**, **tiagabine**, **topiramate**, **tramadol**, **trazodone**, **tricyclic antidepressants**, **valproic acid**, **warfarin**, **ziprasidone**, and **zonisamide**. May ↓ **aripiprazole** levels; double the aripiprazole dose. May ↓ **temsirolimus** and **lapatinib** levels; avoid concurrent use. **Aprepitant**, **cimetidine**, **ciprofloxacin**, **clarithromycin**, **danazol**, **dantrolene**, **diltiazem**, **erythromycin**, **fluconazole**, **fluoxetine**, **fluvoxamine**, **isoni-**

C

azid, **itraconazole**, **ketoconazole**, **loratadine**, **olanzapine**, **omeprazole**, **oxybutynin**, **protease inhibitors**, **trazodone**, **voriconazole**, and **verapamil** may ↑ carbamazepine levels; may ↑ risk of toxicity. Enzyme inducers such as **rifampin**, **phenobarbital**, and **phenytoin** may ↓ levels. May ↑ risk of hepatotoxicity from **isoniazid**. May ↑ risk of CNS toxicity from **lithium**. May ↓ effects of **nondepolarizing neuromuscular blocking agents**. May ↑ risk of toxicity from **cyclophosphamide**.

Drug-Food: Grapefruit juice ↑ serum levels and oral bioavailability by 40% and therefore may ↑ effects.

Route/Dosage

IV route should only be used when oral administration is not possible. When converting from immediate-release to extended-release formulation, administer same total daily dose (in 2 divided doses).

Seizures

PO (Adults and Children >12 yr): 200 mg twice daily (immediate-release [IR] tablets and extended-release [ER] tablets/capsules) or 100 mg 4 times daily (suspension); ↑ by up to 200 mg/day in divided doses (every 12 hr for ER tablets; every 6–8 hr for IR tablets and suspension) every 7 days until therapeutic levels are achieved (usual range = 600–1200 mg/day); not to exceed 1000 mg/day in children 12–15 yrs old or 1200 mg/day in children 15–18 yrs old or 1600 mg/day in adults.

PO (Children 6–12 yr): 100 mg twice daily (IR tablets or ER tablets/capsules) or 50 mg 4 times daily (suspension). ↑ by up to 100 mg/day in divided doses (every 12 hr for ER tablets; every 6–8 hr for IR tablets and suspension) every 7 days until therapeutic levels are achieved (usual range = 400–800 mg/day); not to exceed 1000 mg/day.

PO (Children <6 yr): 10–20 mg/kg/day in 2–3 divided doses (IR tablets) or in 4 divided doses (suspension); may be ↑ at weekly intervals until optimal response and therapeutic levels are achieved; not to exceed 35 mg/kg/day.

IV (Adults): Total daily dose = 70% of total daily oral carbamazepine dose. Divide total daily dose into 4 separate doses administered every 6 hr. Should not be used for >7 days.

Trigeminal Neuralgia

PO (Adults): 100 mg twice daily (IR or ER tablets), 200 mg once daily (ER capsules), or 50 mg 4 times daily (suspension); ↑ by up to 200 mg/day in divided doses (every 12 hr for IR tablets or ER tablets/capsules; every 6 hr for suspension) as needed until pain is relieved (usual range = 400–800 mg/day); not to exceed 1200 mg/day.

Acute Manic or Mixed Episodes Associated with Bipolar I Disorder

PO (Adults): *Equetro*—200 mg twice daily; ↑ by 200 mg/day until optimal response is achieved; not to exceed 1600 mg/day.

Availability (generic available)

Tablets: 200 mg. **Cost:** *Generic*—$7.18/100. **Chewable tablets:** 100 mg, 200 mg. **Cost:** *Generic*—$23.11/100. **Extended-release capsules (Carbatrol, Equetro):** 100 mg, 200 mg, 300 mg. **Cost:** *Generic*—All strengths $214.48/60. **Extended-release tablets (Tegretol XR):** 100 mg, 200 mg, 400 mg. **Cost:** *Generic*—200 mg $113.31/100, 400 mg $224.76/100. **Oral suspension (citrus/vanilla flavor):** 100 mg/5 mL. **Cost:** *Generic*—$74.77/450 mL. **Solution for injection (requires dilution):** 10 mg/mL.

NURSING IMPLICATIONS

Assessment

- Monitor closely for changes in behavior that could indicate the emergence or worsening of suicidal thoughts or behavior or depression.
- Monitor for changes in skin condition in early therapy. Stevens-Johnson syndrome and toxic epidermal necrolysis are significantly more common in patients with a particular human leukocyte antigen (HLA) allele, HLA-B*1502 (occurs almost exclusively in patients with Asian ancestry, including South Asian Indians). Screen patients of Asian ancestry for the HLA-B*1502 allele before starting treatment with carbamazepine. If positive, carbamazepine should not be started unless the expected benefit outweighs increased risk of serious skin reactions. Patients who have been taking carbamazepine for more than a few mo without developing skin reactions are at low risk of these events ever developing.
- Monitor for signs and symptoms of DRESS syndrome (fever, rash, and/or lymphadenopathy with organ system involvement, [hepatitis, nephritis, hematologic abnormalities, myocarditis, myositis]) resembling an acute viral infection with eosinophilia. Discontinue carbamazepine if other cause not determined.
- **Seizures:** Assess frequency, location, duration, and characteristics of seizure activity.
- **Trigeminal Neuralgia:** Assess for facial pain (location, intensity, duration). Ask patient to identify stimuli that may precipitate facial pain (hot or cold foods, bedclothes, touching face).
- **Bipolar Disorder:** Assess mental status (mood, orientation, behavior) and cognitive abilities before and periodically during therapy.
- ***Lab Test Considerations:*** Monitor CBC, including platelet count, reticulocyte count, and serum iron, at baseline, weekly during the first 2 mo, and yearly thereafter for evidence of potentially fatal blood cell abnormalities. Discontinue therapy if bone marrow depression occurs.
- Perform genetic testing for the HLA-B*1502 allele in patients of Asian ancestry prior to beginning therapy.
- Perform liver function tests, urinalysis, electrolytes, serum creatinine, and BUN at baseline and routinely

performed. May cause ↑ AST, ALT, serum alkaline phosphatase, bilirubin, BUN, urine protein, and urine glucose levels.

- Monitor serum ionized calcium levels every 6 mo or if seizure frequency increases. Thyroid function tests and ionized serum calcium concentrations may be ↓; hypocalcemia ↓ seizure threshold.
- Monitor ECG and serum electrolytes before and periodically during therapy. May cause hyponatremia.
- May occasionally cause ↑ serum cholesterol, high-density lipoprotein, and triglyceride concentrations.
- May cause false-negative pregnancy test results with tests that determine human chorionic gonadotropin.
- ***Toxicity and Overdose:*** Serum blood levels should be routinely monitored during therapy. Therapeutic levels range from 4–12 mcg/mL.

Implementation

- Do not confuse carbamazepine with oxcarbazepine. Do not confuse Tegretol with Tegretol XR.
- Implement seizure precautions as indicated.
- **PO:** Administer medication with food to minimize gastric irritation. May take at bedtime to reduce daytime sedation. Tablets may be crushed if patient has difficulty swallowing. Do not crush or chew extended-release tablets. Extended-release capsules may be opened and the contents sprinkled on applesauce or other similar foods.
- Do not administer suspension simultaneously with other liquid medications or diluents; mixture produces an orange rubbery mass.

IV Administration

- Return to previous oral dose as soon as possible.
- **Intermittent Infusion:** Dilute dose in 100 mL of 0.9% NaCl, LR, or D5W and mix gently. Solution is stable for 4 hrs at room temperature or 24 hrs if refrigerated. Do not infuse solutions that are discolored, cloudy, or contain particulate matter. ***Rate:*** Infuse over 30 min.

Patient/Family Teaching

- Instruct patient to take carbamazepine around the clock, as directed. Take missed doses as soon as possible but not just before next dose; do not double doses. Notify health care professional if more than one dose is missed. Discontinue gradually to prevent seizures. Instruct patient to read the *Medication Guide* before starting and with each Rx refill in case of changes.
- Advise patient to avoid grapefruit and grapefruit juice during therapy.
- Advise patient to notify health care professional of all Rx or OTC medications, vitamins, or herbal products being taken and to consult with health care professional before taking other medications.
- May cause dizziness or drowsiness. Advise patients to avoid driving or other activities requiring alertness until response to medication is known.
- Instruct patient to report behavioral changes, skin rash, fever, sore throat, mouth ulcers, easy bruising, petechiae, unusual bleeding, abdominal pain, chills, rash, pale stools, dark urine, or jaundice to health care professional immediately. Advise patient and family to notify health care professional if thoughts about suicide or dying, attempts to commit suicide; new or worse depression; new or worse anxiety; feeling very agitated or restless; panic attacks; trouble sleeping; new or worse irritability; acting aggressive; being angry or violent; acting on dangerous impulses; an extreme increase in activity and talking, other unusual changes in behavior or mood occur.
- Inform patient that coating of *Tegretol XR* is not absorbed, but is excreted in feces and may be visible in stool.
- Advise patient not to take alcohol or other CNS depressants concurrently with this medication.
- Caution patients to use sunscreen and protective clothing to prevent photosensitivity reactions.
- Inform patient that frequent mouth rinses, good oral hygiene, and sugarless gum or candy may help reduce dry mouth. Saliva substitute may be used. Consult dentist if dry mouth persists >2 wk.
- Instruct patient to notify health care professional of medication regimen before treatment or surgery.
- Rep: Advise female patients to use a nonhormonal form of contraception while taking carbamazepine, to avoid breast feeding, and to notify health care professional if pregnancy is planned or suspected or if breast feeding. Encourage patients who become pregnant to enroll in the North American Antiepileptic Drug (NAAED) Pregnancy Registry by calling 1-888-233-2334 or on the web at www.aedpregnancyregistry.org. Enrollment must be done by patients themselves.
- Emphasize the importance of follow-up lab tests and eye exams to monitor for side effects.
- **Seizures:** Advise patients to carry identification describing disease and medication regimen at all times.

Evaluation/Desired Outcomes

- Absence or reduction of seizure activity.
- Decrease in trigeminal neuralgia pain. Patients with trigeminal neuralgia who are pain-free should be reevaluated every 3 mo to determine minimum effective dose.
- Decreased mania and depressive symptoms in bipolar I disorder.

carbidopa/levodopa

(**kar**-bi-doe-pa/**lee**-voe-doe-pa)

Duopa, Duodopa, Rytary, Sinemet, Sinemet CR

Classification

Therapeutic: antiparkinson agents

Pharmacologic: dopamine agonists

Indications

Parkinson's disease. Not useful for drug-induced extrapyramidal reactions.

Action

Levodopa is converted to dopamine in the CNS, where it serves as a neurotransmitter. Carbidopa, a decarboxylase inhibitor, prevents peripheral destruction of levodopa. **Therapeutic Effects:** Relief of tremor and rigidity in Parkinson's syndrome.

Pharmacokinetics

Absorption: Well absorbed following oral administration.

Distribution: Widely distributed. *Levodopa*—enters the CNS in small concentrations. *Carbidopa*—does not cross the blood-brain barrier but does cross the placenta. Both enter breast milk.

Metabolism and Excretion: *Levodopa*—mostly metabolized by the GI tract and liver. *Carbidopa*—30% excreted unchanged by the kidneys.

Half-life: *Levodopa*—1 hr; *carbidopa*—1–2 hr.

TIME/ACTION PROFILE (antiparkinson effects)

ROUTE	ONSET	PEAK	DURATION
Carbidopa	unknown	unknown	5–24 hr
Levodopa	10–15 min	unknown	5–24 hr or more
Carbidopa/levodopa sustained release	unknown	2 hr	12 hr

Contraindications/Precautions

Contraindicated in: Hypersensitivity; Angle-closure glaucoma; Nonselective MAO inhibitor therapy; Malignant melanoma; Undiagnosed skin lesions; Some products contain tartrazine, phenylalanine, or aspartame and should be avoided in patients with known hypersensitivity.

Use Cautiously in: History of cardiac, psychiatric, or ulcer disease; OB, Pedi: Safety not established; Lactation: May ↓ serum prolactin; levodopa enters breast milk.

Adverse Reactions/Side Effects

CNS: depression, involuntary movements, anxiety, confusion, dizziness, drowsiness, hallucinations, memory loss, psychiatric problems, sudden sleep onset, urges (gambling, sexual). **CV:** orthostatic hypotension. **EENT:** blurred vision, mydriasis. **GI:** GI HEMORRHAGE (enteral suspension), GI ISCHEMIA (enteral suspension), GI OBSTRUCTION (enteral suspension), GI PERFORATION (enteral suspension), HEPATOTOXICITY, INTUSSUSCEPTION (enteral suspension), PANCREATITIS (enteral suspension), PERITONITIS (enteral suspension), constipation, nausea, vomiting, anorexia, bezoar (enteral suspension), dry mouth. **Derm:** melanoma. **Hemat:** hemolytic anemia, leukopenia. **MS:** dyskinesias. **Neuro:** neuropathy. **Misc:** MELANOMA, darkening of urine or sweat.

Interactions

Drug-Drug: Use with **nonselective MAO inhibitors** may result in hypertensive reactions; concurrent use contraindicated (MAO inhibitor must be discontinued ≥2 wk before initiating carbidopa/levodopa). ↑ risk of arrhythmias with **inhalation hydrocarbon anesthetics** (especially **halothane**; if possible discontinue 6–8 hr before anesthesia). **Phenothiazines**, **haloperidol**, **papaverine**, and **phenytoin** may ↓ effect of levodopa. Large doses of **pyridoxine** may ↓ beneficial effects of levodopa. Concurrent use with **methyldopa** may alter the effectiveness of levodopa and ↑ risk of CNS side effects. ↑ hypotension may result with concurrent **antihypertensives**. **Anticholinergics** may ↓ absorption of levodopa. ↑ risk of adverse reactions with **selegiline** or **cocaine**.

Drug-Natural Products: Kava-kava may ↓ levodopa effectiveness.

Drug-Food: Ingestion of foods containing large amounts of **pyridoxine** may ↓ effect of levodopa.

Route/Dosage

Carbidopa/Levodopa

PO (Adults): 25 mg carbidopa/100 mg levodopa 3 times daily; may be ↑ every 1–2 days until desired effect is achieved (max = 8 tablets of 25 mg carbidopa/100 mg levodopa/day).

Enteral (Adults): Patients must be converted to and be on stable dose of PO immediate-release carbidopa/levodopa tablets before initiation of enteral suspension therapy. *Morning dose for Day 1 (mL) (to be administered over 10–30 min)* = (Amount of levodopa (in mg) in first dose of immediate-release carbidopa/levodopa taken by patient on previous day * 0.8)/20; *Continuous dose for Day 1 (mL) (to be administered over 16 hr)* = Determine amount of levodopa (in mg) patient received from immediate-release carbidopa/levodopa doses throughout 16 waking hrs of previous day (do not include doses of immediate-release carbidopa/levodopa taken at night when calculating the levodopa amount). Then, subtract amount of first levodopa dose (in mg) taken by patient on previous day. Divide result by 20 to obtain the # of mL to be administered over 16 hr. Do not exceed dose of 2000 mg. At end of daily 16-hr infusion, patients will disconnect the pump from feeding tube and take their night-time dose of oral immediate-release carbidopa/levodopa tablets.

Total daily dose can be titrated after Day 1 based on patient response and tolerability.

Carbidopa/Levodopa Extended-Release (doses of all other dosage forms of carbidopa/levodopa and Rytary are not interchangeable)

PO (Adults): *Patients not currently receiving levodopa (Sinemet CR)*—50 mg carbidopa/200 mg levodopa twice daily (minimum of 6 hr apart) initially. *Patients not currently receiving levodopa (Rytary)*—23.75 mg carbidopa/95 mg levodopa 3 times daily x 3 days, then 36.25 mg carbidopa/145 mg levodopa 3 times daily. May continue to ↑ dose as needed (max dose = 97.5 mg carbidopa/390 mg levodopa 3 times daily). May also ↑ frequency of administration up to 5 times daily (max dose = 612.5 mg carbidopa/2450 mg levodopa/day). *Conversion from immediate-release (IR) carbidopa/levodopa to Sinemet CR*—initiate therapy with at least 10% more levodopa content/day (may need up to 30% more) given at 4–8 hr intervals while awake. Allow 3 days between dosage changes; some patients may require larger doses and shorter dosing intervals. *Conversion from IR carbidopa/levodopa to Rytary*—If taking 400–549 mg/day of IR levodopa, give 3 capsules of Rytary 23.75 mg carbidopa/95 mg levodopa 3 times daily. If taking 550–749 mg/day of IR levodopa, give 4 capsules of Rytary 23.75 mg carbidopa/95 mg levodopa 3 times daily. If taking 750–949 mg/day of IR levodopa, give 3 capsules of Rytary 36.25 mg carbidopa/145 mg levodopa 3 times daily. If taking 950–1249 mg/day of IR levodopa, give 3 capsules of Rytary 48.75 mg carbidopa/195 mg levodopa 3 times daily. If taking ≥1250 mg/day of IR levodopa, give 4 capsules of Rytary 48.75 mg carbidopa/195 mg levodopa 3 times daily or 3 capsules of Rytary 61.25 mg carbidopa/245 mg levodopa 3 times daily; may then titrate as needed (max daily dose = 612.5 mg carbidopa/2450 mg levodopa).

Availability (generic available)

Tablets: 10 mg carbidopa/100 mg levodopa, 25 mg carbidopa/100 mg levodopa, 25 mg carbidopa/250 mg levodopa. **Cost:** *Generic*—10 mg/100 mg $25.28/100, 25 mg/100 mg $28.91/100, 25 mg/250 mg $19.22/100. **Orally disintegrating tablets (mint):** 10 mg carbidopa/100 mg levodopa, 25 mg carbidopa/100 mg levodopa, 25 mg carbidopa/250 mg levodopa. **Cost:** *Generic*—10 mg/100 mg $121.48/100, 25 mg/100 mg $137.18/100, 25 mg/250 mg $174.76/100. **Extended-release tablets (Sinemet CR):** 25 mg carbidopa/100 mg levodopa, 50 mg carbidopa/200 mg levodopa. **Cost:** *Generic*—25 mg/100 mg $93.90/100, 50 mg/200 mg $180.50/100. **Extended-release capsules (Rytary):** 23.75 mg carbidopa/95 mg levodopa, 36.25 mg carbidopa/145 mg levodopa, 48.75 mg carbidopa/195 mg levodopa, 61.25 mg carbidopa/245 mg levodopa. **Enteral suspension (Duopa):** 4.63 mg carbidopa/20 mg levodopa/mL in 100–mL single-use cassettes, 🍁 5 mg carbidopa/20 mg levodopa/mL in 100–mL single-use cassettes. ***In combination with:*** entacapone (Stalevo); see Appendix B.

NURSING IMPLICATIONS

Assessment

- Assess parkinsonian symptoms (akinesia, rigidity, tremors, pill rolling, shuffling gait, mask-like face, twisting motions, and drooling) during therapy. "On-off phenomenon" may cause symptoms to appear or improve suddenly.
- Assess BP and pulse frequently during period of dose adjustment.
- **Duopa:** Monitor for signs and symptoms of GI complications (abdominal pain, prolonged constipation, nausea, vomiting, fever, melanotic stool) during therapy.
- ***Lab Test Considerations:*** May cause false-positive test results in Coombs' test.
- May cause ↑ serum glucose. Dipstick for urine ketones may reveal false-positive results.
- Monitor hepatic and renal function and CBC periodically in patients on long-term therapy. May cause ↑ AST, ALT, bilirubin, alkaline phosphatase, LDH, and serum protein-bound iodine concentrations.
- May cause ↓ hemoglobin, ↓ hematocrit, agranulocytosis, hemolytic and nonhemolytic anemia, thrombocytopenia, leukopenia, and ↑ WBC.
- ***Toxicity and Overdose:*** Assess for signs of toxicity (involuntary muscle twitching, facial grimacing, spasmodic eye winking, exaggerated protrusion of tongue, behavioral changes). Consult health care professional if symptoms occur.

Implementation

- Do not confuse Sinemet with Janumet.
- In the carbidopa/levodopa combination, the number following the drug name represents the milligrams of each respective drug.
- In preoperative patients or patients who are NPO, confer with health care professional about continuing medication administration using oral disintegrating tablets.
- **PO:** Administer on a regular schedule. Hospitalized patients should be continued on same schedule as at home. Administer while awake, not around the clock to improve sleep and prevent side effects.
- Controlled-release tablets may be administered as whole or half tablets, but they should not be crushed or chewed.
- For *orally disintegrating tablets,* just prior to administration remove tablet from bottle with dry hands. Immediately place tablet on top of tongue.

Tablet will dissolve in sec, then swallow with saliva. Administration with liquid is not necessary.

- *For enteral administration,* administer *DUOPA* into the jejunum through a percutaneous endoscopic gastrostomy with jejunal tube (PEG-J) with CADD-Legacy 1400 portable infusion pump. Take suspension out of refrigerator 20 min prior to use; must be at room temperature for use. Administer over 16 hrs. If extra dose is needed, set function at 1 mL (20 mg of levodopa) when starting; may be adjusted in 0.2 mL increments. Limit to 1 extra dose every 2 hrs. Frequent extra doses may cause or worsen dyskinesias. Discontinue gradually; do not stop abruptly.
- *For extended-release capsules,* administer without regard to food. Swallow capsules whole; do not chew, divide, or crush. For patients with difficulty swallowing, open capsule and sprinkle entire contents on 1–2 tablespoons of applesauce; consume immediately. Do not store mixture for future use. Inform patients that first dose of day may be taken 1–2 hrs before eating, as a high fat, high calorie meal may delay the absorption of levodopa and onset of action by 2–3 hrs. Discontinue gradually; do not stop abruptly. When adjusting dose of extended-release capsules, keep dose of other Parkinson's medications stable; dose may need to be increased in patients taking COMT inhibitor. Extended-release capsules may be administered 3–5 times daily if more frequent dosing is needed and tolerated.

Patient/Family Teaching

- Instruct patient to take medication at regular intervals as directed. Do not change dose regimen or take additional antiparkinson drugs, including more carbidopa/levodopa, without consulting health care professional. Take missed doses as soon as remembered, unless next scheduled dose is within 2 hr; do not double doses.
- Explain that gastric irritation may be decreased by eating food shortly after taking medications but that high-protein meals may impair levodopa's effects. Dividing daily protein intake among all the meals may help ensure adequate protein intake and drug effectiveness. Do not drastically alter diet during carbidopa/levodopa therapy without consulting health care professional.
- May cause sudden onset of sleep, drowsiness, or dizziness. Advise patient to avoid driving and other activities that require alertness until response to drug is known.
- Caution patient to change positions slowly to minimize orthostatic hypotension. Health care professional should be notified if orthostatic hypotension occurs.
- Instruct patient that frequent rinsing of mouth, good oral hygiene, and sugarless gum or candy may decrease dry mouth.
- Caution patient to monitor skin lesions for any changes. Health care professional should be notified promptly because carbidopa/levodopa may activate malignant melanoma.
- Advise patient to notify health care professional of all Rx or OTC medications, vitamins, or herbal products being taken and to consult with health care professional before taking other medications, especially cold remedies. Large amounts of vitamin B_6 (pyridoxine) and iron may interfere with the action of levodopa.
- Inform patient that harmless darkening of saliva, urine, or sweat may occur.
- Advise patient to notify health care professional if signs and symptoms of GI complications, palpitations, urinary retention, involuntary movements, behavioral changes, severe nausea and vomiting, new skin lesions, or new or increased gambling, sexual, or other intense urges occur. Dose reduction may be required.
- Inform patient that sometimes a "wearing-off" effect may occur at end of dosing interval. Notify health care professional if this poses a problem to lifestyle.
- Advise female patients to notify health care professional if pregnancy is planned or suspected or if breast feeding.

Evaluation/Desired Outcomes

- Resolution of parkinsonian signs and symptoms. Therapeutic effects usually become evident after 2–3 wk of therapy but may require up to 6 mo. Patients who take this medication for several yr may experience a decrease in the effectiveness of this drug.

carbonyl iron, See IRON SUPPLEMENTS.

HIGH ALERT

CARBOplatin (kar-boe-**pla**-tin)

~~Paraplatin~~

Classification
Therapeutic: antineoplastics
Pharmacologic: alkylating agents

Indications

Advanced ovarian carcinoma (with other agents). Palliative treatment of ovarian carcinoma unresponsive to other modalities.

Action

Inhibits DNA synthesis by producing cross-linking of parent DNA strands (cell-cycle phase–nonspecific). **Therapeutic Effects:** Death of rapidly replicating cells, particularly malignant ones.

Pharmacokinetics

Absorption: IV administration results in complete bioavailability.
Distribution: Unknown.

Protein Binding: Platinum is irreversibly bound to plasma proteins.
Metabolism and Excretion: Excreted mostly by the kidneys.
Half-life: *Carboplatin*—2.6–5.9 hr (increased in renal impairment); *platinum*—5 days.

TIME/ACTION PROFILE (effects on blood counts)

ROUTE	ONSET	PEAK	DURATION
IV	unknown	21 days	28 days

Contraindications/Precautions

Contraindicated in: Hypersensitivity to carboplatin, cisplatin, or mannitol; OB, Lactation: Pregnancy or lactation.
Use Cautiously in: Hearing loss; Electrolyte abnormalities; Renal impairment (dose ↓ recommended if CCr <60 mL/min); Active infections; Diminished bone marrow reserve (dose ↓ recommended); Other chronic debilitating illnesses; Geri: ↑ risk of thrombocytopenia, consider renal function in dose determination; Patients with childbearing potential; Pedi: Safety not established.

Adverse Reactions/Side Effects

CNS: weakness. **EENT:** ototoxicity. **GI:** abdominal pain, nausea, vomiting, constipation, diarrhea, hepatitis, stomatitis. **GU:** gonadal suppression, nephrotoxicity. **Derm:** alopecia, rash. **F and E:** hypocalcemia, hypokalemia, hypomagnesemia, hyponatremia. **Hemat:** ANEMIA, LEUKOPENIA, THROMBOCYTOPENIA. **Metab:** hyperuricemia. **Neuro:** peripheral neuropathy. **Misc:** hypersensitivity reactions including ANAPHYLACTIC-LIKE REACTIONS.

Interactions

Drug-Drug: ↑ nephrotoxicity and ototoxicity with other **nephrotoxic** and **ototoxic drugs (aminoglycosides, loop diuretics)**. ↑ bone marrow depression with other **bone marrow–depressing drugs** or **radiation therapy**. May ↓ antibody response to **live-virus vaccines** and ↑ risk of adverse reactions.

Route/Dosage

Other dosing formulas are used.
IV (Adults): *Initial treatment*—300 mg/m² with cyclophosphamide at 4-wk intervals. *Treatment of refractory tumors*—360 mg/m² as a single dose; may be repeated at 4-wk intervals, depending on response.

Renal Impairment

IV (Adults): *CCr 41–59 mL/min*—initial dose 250 mg/m²; *CCr 16–40 mL/min*—initial dose 200 mg/m².

Availability (generic available)

Solution for injection: 10 mg/mL.

NURSING IMPLICATIONS

Assessment

- Assess for nausea and vomiting; often occur 6–12 hr after therapy (1–4 hr for aqueous solution) and may persist for 24 hr. Prophylactic antiemetics may be used. Adjust diet as tolerated to maintain fluid and electrolyte balance and ensure adequate nutritional intake. May require discontinuation of therapy.
- Monitor for bone marrow depression. Assess for bleeding (bleeding gums, bruising, petechiae, guaiac stools, urine, and emesis) and avoid IM injections and rectal temperatures if platelet count is low. Apply pressure to venipuncture sites for 10 min. Assess for signs of infection during neutropenia. Anemia may occur and may be cumulative; transfusions are frequently required. Monitor for increased fatigue, dyspnea, and orthostatic hypotension.
- Monitor for signs of anaphylaxis (rash, urticaria, pruritus, facial swelling, wheezing, tachycardia, hypotension). Discontinue medication immediately and notify physician if these occur. Epinephrine and resuscitation equipment should be readily available.
- Audiometry is recommended before initiation of therapy and subsequent doses. Ototoxicity manifests as tinnitus and unilateral or bilateral hearing loss in high frequencies and becomes more frequent and severe with repeated doses. Ototoxicity is more pronounced in children.
- ***Lab Test Considerations:*** Monitor CBC, differential, and clotting studies before and weekly during therapy. The nadirs of thrombocytopenia and leukopenia occur after 21 days and recover by 30 days after a dose. Nadir of granulocyte counts usually occurs after 21–28 days and recovers by day 35. Withhold subsequent doses until neutrophil count is >2000/mm³ and platelet count is >100,000/mm³.
- Monitor renal function and serum electrolytes before initiation of therapy and before each course of carboplatin.
- Monitor hepatic function before and periodically during therapy. May cause ↑ serum bilirubin, alkaline phosphatase, and AST concentrations.

Implementation

- ***High Alert:*** Fatalities have occurred with chemotherapeutic agents. Before administering, clarify all ambiguous orders; double-check single, daily, and course-of-therapy dose limits; have second practitioner independently double-check original order, calculations, and infusion pump settings.
- ***High Alert:*** Do not confuse carboplatin with cisplatin.
- ***High Alert:*** Carboplatin should be administered in a monitored setting under the supervision of a physician experienced in cancer chemotherapy.

IV Administration

- Solution should be prepared in a biologic cabinet. Wear gloves, gown, and mask while handling medication. Discard equipment in specially designated containers.
- Do not use aluminum needles or equipment during preparation or administration; aluminum reacts with the drug.
- **Intermittent Infusion:** ***Concentration:*** 0.5 mg/mL. Stable for 8 hr at room temperature. ***Rate:*** Infuse over 15–60 min.
- **Y-Site Compatibility:** acyclovir, alemtuzumab, alfentanil, allopurinol, amifostine, amikacin, aminocaproic acid, aminophylline, amiodarone, amphotericin B deoxycholate, amphotericin B lipid complex, amphotericin B liposome, ampicillin, ampicillin/sulbactam, anidulafungin, argatroban, atracurium, azithromycin, aztreonam, bivalirudin, bleomycin, bumetanide, buprenorphine, butorphanol, calcium chloride, calcium gluconate, caspofungin, cefazolin, cefepime, cefotaxime, cefotetan, cefoxitin, ceftazidime, ceftriaxone, cefuroxime, ciprofloxacin, cisatracurium, cisplatin, cladribine, clindamycin, cyclophosphamide, cyclosporine, cytarabine, dacarbazine, daptomycin, dexamethasone, dexmedetomidine, dexrazoxane, digoxin, diltiazem, diphenhydramine, docetaxel, dolasetron, dopamine, doxacurium, doxorubicin hydrochloride, doxycycline, droperidol, enalaprilat, ephedrine, ertapenem, erythromycin, esmolol, etoposide, etoposide phosphate, famotidine, fenoldopam, fentanyl, filgrastim, fluconazole, fludarabine, fluorouracil, foscarnet, fosphenytoin, furosemide, ganciclovir, gemcitabine, gentamicin, glycopyrrolate, granisetron, haloperidol, heparin, hetastarch, hydrocortisone, hydromorphone, idarubicin, ifosfamide, imipenem/cilastatin, insulin, isoproterenol, ketorolac, labetalol, levofloxacin, lidocaine, linezolid, lorazepam, magnesium sulfate, mannitol, melphalan, meperidine, meropenem, mesna, metaraminol, methotrexate, methyldopate, methylprednisolone, metoclopramide, metoprolol, metronidazole, micafungin, midazolam, milrinone, mitomycin, mitoxantrone, morphine, moxifloxacin, nafcillin, nalbuphine, naloxone, nicardipine, nitroglycerine, nitroprusside, norepinephrine, octreotide, ondansetron, oxaliplatin, paclitaxel, palonosetron, pamidronate, pancuronium, pantoprazole, pemetrexed, pentamidine, pentobarbital, phenobarbital, phenylephrine, piperacillin/tazobactam, potassium acetate, potassium chloride, potassium phosphates, prochlorperazine, promethazine, propofol, propranolol, quinupristin/dalfopristin, ranitidine, remifentanil, rituximab, rocuronium, sargramostim, sodium acetate, sodium bicarbonate, sodium phosphates, succinylcholine, sufentanil, tacrolimus, theophylline, thiotepa, tigecycline, tirofiban, tobramycin, trastuzumab, trimethoprim/sulfamethoxazole, vancomycin, vecuronium, verapamil, vinblastine, vincristine, vinorelbine, voriconazole, zidovudine, zoledronic acid.
- **Y-Site Incompatibility:** amphotericin B deoxycholate, chlorpromazine, diazepam, leucovorin calcium, phenytoin, procainamide, thiopental.

Patient/Family Teaching

- Instruct patient to notify health care professional promptly if fever; chills; sore throat; signs of infection; lower back or side pain; difficult or painful urination; bleeding gums; bruising; pinpoint red spots on skin; blood in stools, urine, or emesis; increased fatigue, dyspnea, or orthostatic hypotension occurs.
- Caution patient to avoid crowds and persons with known infections. Instruct patient to use soft toothbrush and electric razor and to avoid falls. Caution patients not to drink alcoholic beverages or take medication containing aspirin or NSAIDs because they may precipitate gastric bleeding.
- Instruct patient to promptly report any numbness or tingling in extremities or face, decreased coordination, difficulty with hearing or ringing in the ears, unusual swelling, or weight gain to health care professional.
- Instruct patient not to receive any vaccinations without advice of health care professional and to avoid contact with persons who have received oral polio vaccine within the past several mo.
- Advise patient of the need for contraception (if patient is not infertile as a result of surgical or radiation therapy).
- Instruct patient to inspect oral mucosa for erythema and ulceration. If ulceration occurs, advise patient to notify health care professional, rinse mouth with water after eating, and use sponge brush. Mouth pain may require treatment with opioids.
- Discuss with patient the possibility of hair loss. Explore methods of coping.
- Emphasize the need for periodic lab tests to monitor for side effects.

Evaluation/Desired Outcomes

- Decrease in size or spread of ovarian carcinoma.

BEERS

cariprazine (kar-**ip**-ra-zeen)

Vraylar

Classification

Therapeutic: antipsychotics

Indications

Schizophrenia. Acute treatment of mania/mixed episodes associated with bipolar I disorder. Depressive episodes associated with bipolar I disorder.

Action

Acts as a partial agonist at dopamine D_2 receptors in the CNS and serotonin $5-HT_{1A}$; also acts an antagonist at $5-HT_{2A}$ receptors. **Therapeutic Effects:** Decreased incidence and severity of symptoms of schizophrenia. Decreased occurrence and severity of mania associated with bipolar 1 disorder.

Pharmacokinetics

Absorption: Well absorbed following oral administration.

Distribution: Unknown.

Protein Binding: 91–97%.

Metabolism and Excretion: Two metabolites, desmethyl cariprazine (DCAR) and didesmethyl cariprazine (DDCAR), have antipsychotic activity. Metabolism occurs mostly via the CYP3A4 enzyme system, with further metabolism resulting in inactive metabolites; 21% excreted urine, 1.2% as unchanged drug.

Half-life: Cariprazine—2–4 days; *DDCAR*—1–3 wk.

TIME/ACTION PROFILE (improvement in symptoms)

ROUTE	ONSET	PEAK	DURATION
PO (schizophrenia)	within 1–2 wk	4–6 wk	2 wk†
PO (mania due to bipolar 1 disorder)	within 5–7 days	2–3 wk	2 wk†

†Blood levels of drug and active metabolites following discontinuation.

Contraindications/Precautions

Contraindicated in: Hypersensitivity.

Use Cautiously in: Known cerebrovascular/cardiovascular disease, dehydration, concurrent use of diuretics/antihypertensives or syncope (↑ risk of orthostatic hypotension); Pre-existing ↓ WBC or ANC or history of drug-induced leukopenia/neutropenia; At risk of aspiration or falls; OB: Neonates exposed in the third trimester may experience extrapyramidal symptoms/withdrawal; Lactation: Use while breast feeding only if potential maternal benefit justifies potential risk to infant; Pedi: Safety and effectiveness not established; may ↑ risk of suicide attempt/ideation in children or adolescents; Geri: Elderly patients with dementia-related psychosis (↑ risk of adverse cardiovascular effects and death), consider age-related ↓ in renal/hepatic/cardiovascular function, concurrent disease states and medications (↓ initial dose recommended).

Adverse Reactions/Side Effects

CNS: SUICIDAL THOUGHTS/BEHAVIORS, drowsiness, headache, agitation, dizziness, fatigue, insomnia, restlessness. **CV:** hypertension, orthostatic hypotension, tachycardia. **Derm:** STEVENS-JOHNSON SYNDROME, rash. **EENT:** blurred vision. **GI:** dyspepsia, nausea, ↓ appetite, constipation, diarrhea, dry mouth, dysphagia (↑ aspiration risk), ↑ liver enzymes, vomiting. **Hemat:** AGRANULOCYTOSIS, leukopenia, neutropenia. **Metab:** dyslipidemia, hyperglycemia/diabetes mellitus, weight gain. **MS:** arthralgia, back pain, extremity pain. **Neuro:** akathisia, extrapyramidal symptoms, tardive dyskinesia. **Resp:** cough. **Misc:** NEUROLEPTIC MALIGNANT SYNDROME, body temperature dysregulation.

Interactions

Drug-Drug: Levels, effects and risk of toxicity ↑ by concurrent use of **strong CYP3A4 inhibitors** including **itraconazole** and **ketoconazole**; concurrent use not recommended. Levels and effectiveness may be ↓ by concurrent use of **strong CYP3A4 inducers** including **carbamazepine** and **rifampin**; concurrent use not recommended. Concurrent use of **diuretics** or **antihypertensives** may ↑ risk of orthostatic hypotension/syncope.

Route/Dosage

Schizophrenia or Acute Treatment of Mania/Mixed Episodes Associated with Bipolar I Disorder

PO (Adults): 1.5 mg once daily; may ↑ to 3 mg once daily on Day 2; further dosage adjustments can be made in increments of 1.5 mg or 3 mg depending on response/tolerability (max dose = 6 mg once daily). *Initiation of strong CYP3A4 inhibitor while on stable dose of cariprazine*—↓ dose by 50%; *Initiation of cariprazine while on stable dose of strong CYP3A4 inhibitor*—1.5 mg once daily on Day 1 and 3 (no dose on Day 2), then 1.5 mg once daily starting on Day 4; may titrate depending on response/tolerance up to max dose of 3 mg once daily.

Depressive Episodes Associated with Bipolar I Disorder

PO (Adults): 1.5 mg once daily; may ↑ to 3 mg once daily on Day 15 depending on response/tolerability (max dose = 3 mg once daily); *Initiation of strong CYP3A4 inhibitor while on stable dose of cariprazine*—↓ dose by 50%; *Initiation of cariprazine while on stable dose of strong CYP3A4 inhibitor*—1.5 mg once daily on Day 1 and 3 (no dose on Day 2), then 1.5 mg once daily starting on Day 4; may titrate depending on response/tolerance up to max dose of 3 mg once daily.

Availability

Capsules: 1.5 mg, 3 mg, 4.5 mg, 6 mg.

NURSING IMPLICATIONS

Assessment

- Assess mental status (orientation, mood, behavior) before and periodically during therapy. Monitor for worsening depression and emergence of suicidal thoughts and behaviors.
- Assess weight and BMI at baseline and frequently during therapy.

- Monitor BP (sitting, standing, lying), pulse, and respiratory rate before and periodically during therapy.
- Observe patient carefully when administering medication to ensure that medication is actually taken and not hoarded or cheeked.
- Monitor for adverse reactions and patient response for several wk after starting therapy and after each dose increase. Due to long action, may not occur for several wks. Consider reducing dose or discontinuing drug if severe adverse reactions occur.
- Monitor patient for onset of akathisia (restlessness or desire to keep moving) and extrapyramidal side effects (*parkinsonian*—difficulty speaking or swallowing, loss of balance control, pill rolling of hands, masklike face, shuffling gait, rigidity, tremors; and *dystonic*—muscle spasms, twisting motions, twitching, inability to move eyes, weakness of arms or legs) periodically throughout therapy. Report these symptoms.
- Monitor for tardive dyskinesia (uncontrolled rhythmic movement of mouth, face, and extremities; lip smacking or puckering; puffing of cheeks; uncontrolled chewing; rapid or worm-like movements of tongue). Notify health care professional immediately if these symptoms occur, as these side effects may be irreversible.
- Monitor for development of neuroleptic malignant syndrome (fever, muscle rigidity, altered mental status, respiratory distress, tachycardia, seizures, diaphoresis, hypertension or hypotension, pallor, tiredness, loss of bladder control). Notify health care professional immediately if these symptoms occur.
- Assess for skin reactions (rash, toxic skin reactions, bullous exanthema).
- Assess for falls risk. Drowsiness, orthostatic hypotension, and motor and sensory instability increase risk. Institute prevention if indicated.
- ***Lab Test Considerations:*** Monitor CBC frequently during therapy in patients with pre-existing or history of low WBC. May cause leukopenia, neutropenia, or agranulocytosis. Discontinue therapy if severe neutropenia (ANC $<1000\ mm^3$) occurs.
- Monitor fasting blood glucose and lipid profile before, soon after starting, and periodically during therapy.

Implementation

- **PO:** Administer once daily without regard to meals.

Patient/Family Teaching

- Advise patient to take medication as directed and not to skip doses or double up on missed doses. Take missed doses as soon as remembered unless almost time for the next dose. Do not stop taking cariprazine without consulting health care professional.
- Inform patient of possibility of extrapyramidal symptoms and tardive dyskinesia. Instruct patient to report these symptoms immediately.
- Advise patient to make position changes slowly to minimize orthostatic hypotension. Protect from falls.
- Medication may cause drowsiness. Caution patient to avoid driving or other activities requiring alertness until response to medication is known.
- Advise patient and family to notify health care professional of new or worse depression; new or worse anxiety; feeling very agitated or restless; panic attacks; trouble sleeping; new or worse irritability; acting aggressive; being angry or violent; acting on dangerous impulses; an extreme increase in activity and talking; other unusual changes in behavior or mood; or rash occur.
- Inform patient that cariprazine may cause weight gain. Advise patient to monitor weight periodically. Notify health care professional of significant weight gain.
- Instruct patient to notify health care professional of all Rx or OTC medications, vitamins, or herbal products being taken and to consult health care professional before taking any new medications. Caution patient to avoid taking alcohol or other CNS depressants concurrently with this medication.
- Advise patient that extremes in temperature should be avoided, because this drug impairs body temperature regulation.
- Advise patient to notify health care professional of medication regimen prior to treatment or surgery.
- Rep: Advise female patients to notify health care professional if pregnancy is planned or suspected and to avoid breast feeding during therapy. Encourage pregnant patients to enroll in registry by contacting National Pregnancy Registry for Atypical Antipsychotics at 1-866-961-2388 or visit http://womensmentalhealth.org/clinical-and-research-programs/pregnancyregistry/. Monitor neonates of women pregnant while taking cariprazine for extrapyramidal and/or withdrawal symptoms and manage symptoms appropriately.

Evaluation/Desired Outcomes

- Decrease in excitable, paranoid, or withdrawn behavior.
- Decreased occurrence and severity of mania associated with bipolar 1 disorder.

carvedilol (kar-**ve**-di-lole)

Coreg, Coreg CR

Classification

Therapeutic: antihypertensives

Pharmacologic: beta blockers

Indications

Hypertension. HF (ischemic or cardiomyopathic) with digoxin, diuretics, and ACE inhibitors. Left ventricular dysfunction after myocardial infarction.

Action

Blocks stimulation of $beta_1$ (myocardial) and $beta_2$ (pulmonary, vascular, and uterine)-adrenergic receptor sites. Also has alpha$_1$ blocking activity, which may result in orthostatic hypotension. **Therapeutic Effects:** Decreased heart rate and BP. Improved cardiac output, slowing of the progression of HF and decreased risk of death.

Pharmacokinetics

Absorption: Well absorbed but rapidly undergoes extensive first-pass hepatic metabolism, resulting in 25–35% bioavailability. Food slows absorption.
Distribution: Unknown.
Protein Binding: 98%.
Metabolism and Excretion: Extensively metabolized (primarily by CYP2D6 and CYP2C9; the CYP2D6 enzyme system exhibits genetic polymorphism); ~7% of population may be poor metabolizers and may have significantly ↑ carvedilol concentrations and an ↑ risk of adverse effects); excreted in feces via bile, <2% excreted unchanged in urine.
Half-life: 7–10 hr.

TIME/ACTION PROFILE (cardiovascular effects)

ROUTE	ONSET	PEAK	DURATION
PO	within 1 hr	1–2 hr	12 hr
PO-CR	unknown	5 hr	24 hr

Contraindications/Precautions

Contraindicated in: History of serious hypersensitivity reaction (Stevens-Johnson syndrome, angioedema, anaphylaxis); Pulmonary edema; Cardiogenic shock; Bradycardia, heart block or sick sinus syndrome (unless a pacemaker is in place); Decompensated HF requiring IV inotropic agents (wean before starting carvedilol); Severe hepatic impairment; Asthma or other bronchospastic disorders.
Use Cautiously in: HF (condition may deteriorate during initial therapy); Diabetes mellitus (may mask signs of hypoglycemia); Thyrotoxicosis (may mask symptoms); Peripheral vascular disease; History of severe allergic reactions (intensity of reactions may be ↑); Patients undergoing cataract surgery (↑ risk of intraoperative floppy iris syndrome); OB: Crosses placenta and may cause fetal/neonatal bradycardia, hypotension, hypoglycemia, or respiratory depression; Lactation: Use while breast feeding only if potential maternal benefit justifies potential risk to infant; Pedi: Safety and effectiveness not established; Geri: ↑ sensitivity to beta blockers; initial dose ↓ recommended.

Adverse Reactions/Side Effects

CNS: dizziness, fatigue, weakness, anxiety, depression, drowsiness, insomnia, memory loss, mental status changes, nervousness, nightmares. **CV:** BRADYCARDIA, HF, PULMONARY EDEMA. **Derm:** STEVENS-JOHNSON SYNDROME, TOXIC EPIDERMAL NECROLYSIS, itching, rashes, urticaria. **EENT:** blurred vision, dry eyes, intraoperative floppy iris syndrome, nasal stuffiness. **Endo:** hyperglycemia, hypoglycemia. **GI:** diarrhea, constipation, nausea. **GU:** erectile dysfunction, ↓ libido. **MS:** arthralgia, back pain, muscle cramps. **Neuro:** paresthesia. **Resp:** bronchospasm, wheezing. **Misc:** HYPERSENSITIVITY REACTIONS (including anaphylaxis and angioedema), drug-induced lupus syndrome.

Interactions

Drug-Drug: General anesthetics, IV phenytoin, diltiazem, and **verapamil** may cause ↑ myocardial depression. ↑ risk of bradycardia with **digoxin**. **Amiodarone** or **fluconazole** may ↑ levels. ↑ hypotension may occur with other **antihypertensives**, acute ingestion of **alcohol**, or **nitrates**. Concurrent use with **clonidine** ↑ hypotension and bradycardia. May ↑ withdrawal phenomenon from **clonidine** (discontinue carvedilol first). Concurrent administration of **thyroid preparations** may ↓ effectiveness. May alter the effectiveness of **insulins** or **oral hypoglycemic agents** (dose adjustments may be necessary). May ↓ effectiveness of **theophylline**. May ↓ beneficial beta$_1$-cardiovascular effects of **dopamine** or **dobutamine**. Use cautiously within 14 days of **MAO inhibitor** therapy (may result in hypotension/bradycardia). **Cimetidine** may ↑ toxicity from carvedilol. Concurrent **NSAIDs** may ↓ antihypertensive action. Effectiveness may be ↓ by **rifampin**. May ↑ serum **digoxin** levels. May ↑ blood levels of **cyclosporine** (monitor blood levels).

Route/Dosage

PO (Adults): *Hypertension*—6.25 mg twice daily, may be ↑ every 7–14 days up to 25 mg twice daily *or extended-release*—20 mg once daily, dose may be doubled every 7–14 days up to 80 mg once daily; *HF*—3.125 mg twice daily for 2 wk; may be ↑ to 6.25 mg twice daily. Dose may be doubled every 2 wk as tolerated (not to exceed 25 mg twice daily in patients <85 kg or 50 mg twice daily in patients >85 kg) *or extended-release*—10 mg once daily, dose may be doubled every 2 wk as tolerated up to 80 mg once daily; *Left ventricular dysfunction after MI*—6.25 mg twice daily, ↑ after 3–10 days to 12.5 twice daily then to target dose of 25 mg twice daily; some patients may require lower initial doses and slower titration *or extended-release*—20 mg once daily, dose may be doubled every 3–10 days up to 80 mg once daily.

Availability (generic available)

Extended-release capsules: 10 mg, 20 mg, 40 mg, 80 mg. **Cost:** all strengths $175.36/30. **Tablets:** 3.125 mg, 6.25 mg, 12.5 mg, 25 mg. **Cost:** *Generic*—All strengths $7.18/100.

NURSING IMPLICATIONS

Assessment

- Monitor BP and pulse frequently during dose adjustment period and periodically during therapy. Assess for orthostatic hypotension when assisting patient up from supine position. If heart rate decreases below 55 beats/min, decrease dose.

- Monitor intake and output ratios and daily weight. Assess patient routinely for evidence of fluid overload (peripheral edema, dyspnea, rales/crackles, fatigue, weight gain, jugular venous distention). Patients may experience worsening of symptoms during initiation of therapy for HF.
- **Hypertension:** Check frequency of refills to determine adherence.
- ***Lab Test Considerations:*** May cause ↑ BUN, serum lipoprotein, potassium, triglyceride, and uric acid levels.
- May cause ↑ ANA titers.
- May cause ↑ in blood glucose levels.
- ***Toxicity and Overdose:*** Monitor patients receiving beta blockers for signs of overdose (bradycardia, severe dizziness or fainting, severe drowsiness, dyspnea, bluish fingernails or palms, seizures). Notify health care professional immediately if these signs occur.

Implementation

- Do not confuse carvedilol with captopril.
- Discontinuation of concurrent clonidine should be gradual, with carvedilol discontinued first over 1–2 wk with limitation of physical activity; then, after several days, discontinue clonidine.
- **PO:** Take apical pulse before administering. If <50 bpm or if arrhythmia occurs, withhold medication and notify health care professional.
- Administer with food to minimize orthostatic hypotension.
- Administer extended-release capsules in the morning. Swallow whole; do not crush or chew. Extended-release capsules may be opened and sprinkled on cold applesauce and taken immediately; do not store mixture.
- To convert from immediate-release to extended-release product, doses of 3.125 mg twice daily can be converted to 10 mg daily; doses of 6.25 mg twice daily can be converted to 20 mg daily; doses of 12.5 mg twice daily can be converted to 40 mg daily; and doses of 25 mg twice daily can be converted to 80 mg daily.

Patient/Family Teaching

- Instruct patient to take medication as directed, at the same time each day, even if feeling well. Do not skip or double up on missed doses. Take missed doses as soon as possible up to 4 hr before next dose. Abrupt withdrawal may precipitate life-threatening arrhythmias, hypertension, or myocardial ischemia. Discontinue carvedilol slowly over 1–2 wk. Advise patient to read *Patient Information* before starting therapy and with each Rx refill in case of changes.
- Advise patient to make sure enough medication is available for weekends, holidays, and vacations. A written prescription may be kept in wallet in case of emergency.
- Teach patient and family how to check pulse and BP. Instruct them to check pulse daily and BP biweekly. Advise patient to hold dose and contact health care professional if pulse is <50 bpm or BP changes significantly.
- May cause drowsiness or dizziness. Caution patients to avoid driving or other activities that require alertness until response to the drug is known.
- Advise patient to change positions slowly to minimize orthostatic hypotension, especially during initiation of therapy or when dose is increased.
- Caution patient that this medication may increase sensitivity to cold.
- Instruct patient to notify health care professional of all Rx or OTC medications, vitamins, or herbal products being taken and to consult health care professional before taking other Rx, OTC, or herbal products, especially cold preparations, concurrently with this medication.
- Advise patients with diabetes to closely monitor blood glucose, especially if weakness, malaise, irritability, or fatigue occurs. Medication may mask some signs of hypoglycemia, but dizziness and sweating may still occur.
- Advise patient to notify health care professional if slow pulse, difficulty breathing, wheezing, cold hands and feet, dizziness, confusion, depression, rash, fever, sore throat, unusual bleeding, or bruising occurs.
- Instruct patient to inform health care professional of medication regimen before treatment or surgery.
- Advise females of reproductive potential to notify health care professional if pregnancy is planned or suspected, or if breast feeding. If carvedilol is taken during third trimester, monitor newborn for symptoms of hypotension, bradycardia, hypoglycemia, and respiratory depression and manage accordingly.
- Advise patient to carry identification describing disease process and medication regimen at all times.
- **Hypertension:** Reinforce the need to continue additional therapies for hypertension (weight loss, sodium restriction, stress reduction, regular exercise, moderation of alcohol consumption, and smoking cessation). Medication controls but does not cure hypertension.

Evaluation/Desired Outcomes

- Decrease in BP without appearance of detrimental side effects.
- Decrease in severity of HF.

caspofungin (kas-po-**fun**-gin)

Cancidas

Classification

Therapeutic: antifungals (systemic)
Pharmacologic: echinocandins

C

Indications
Invasive aspergillosis refractory to, or intolerant of, other therapies. Candidemia and associated serious infections (intra-abdominal abscesses, peritonitis, pleural space infections). Esophageal candidiasis. Suspected fungal infections in febrile neutropenic patients.

Action
Inhibits the synthesis of β (1, 3)-D-glucan, a necessary component of the fungal cell wall. **Therapeutic Effects:** Death of susceptible fungi.

Pharmacokinetics
Absorption: IV administration results in complete bioavailability.
Distribution: Widely distributed to tissues.
Protein Binding: 97%.
Metabolism and Excretion: Slowly and extensively metabolized; <1.5% excreted unchanged in urine.
Half-life: Polyphasic: *β phase*—9–11 hr; *γ phase*—40–50 hr.

TIME/ACTION PROFILE

ROUTE	ONSET	PEAK	DURATION
IV	unknown	end of infusion	24 hr

Contraindications/Precautions
Contraindicated in: Hypersensitivity; Concurrent use with cyclosporine; OB: Pregnancy (may cause fetal harm).
Use Cautiously in: Moderate hepatic impairment (↓ maintenance dose recommended); Lactation: Use while breast feeding only if potential maternal benefit justifies potential risk to infant.

Adverse Reactions/Side Effects
CNS: headache, chills. **Derm:** STEVENS-JOHNSON SYNDROME, TOXIC EPIDERMAL NECROLYSIS, flushing, pruritus, rash. **GI:** diarrhea, ↑ liver enzymes, nausea, vomiting. **GU:** ↑ serum creatinine. **Local:** venous irritation at injection site. **Resp:** bronchospasm. **Misc:** HYPERSENSITIVITY REACTIONS (including anaphylaxis and angioedema), fever.

Interactions
Drug-Drug: Concurrent use with **cyclosporine** is not recommended due to ↑ risk of hepatic toxicity. May ↓ blood levels and effects of **tacrolimus**. Blood levels and effectiveness may be ↓ by **rifampin**; maintenance dose should be ↑ to 70 mg (in patients with normal liver function). Blood levels and effectiveness also may be ↓ by **efavirenz**, **nelfinavir**, **nevirapine**, **phenytoin**, **dexamethasone**, or **carbamazepine**; an ↑ in the maintenance dose to 70 mg should be considered in patients who are not clinically responding.

Route/Dosage
IV (Adults): 70 mg initially followed by 50 mg once daily; duration determined by clinical situation and response; *Esophageal candidiasis*—50 mg once daily; duration determined by clinical situation and response.
IV (Children ≥3 mo): 70 mg/m² (max: 70 mg) initially followed by 50 mg/m² once daily (max: 70 mg/day); duration determined by clinical situation and response.
IV (Infants 1 to <3 mo and Neonates): 25 mg/m²/dose once daily.

Hepatic Impairment
IV (Adults): *Moderate hepatic impairment*—70 mg initially followed by 35 mg once daily; duration determined by clinical situation and response.

Availability (generic available)
Powder for injection (requires reconstitution and dilution): 50 mg/vial, 70 mg/vial.

NURSING IMPLICATIONS

Assessment
- Assess patient for signs and symptoms of fungal infections prior to and periodically during therapy.
- Assess for skin rash frequently during therapy. Discontinue at first sign of rash; may be life-threatening. Stevens-Johnson syndrome may develop. Treat symptomatically; may recur once treatment is stopped.
- Monitor patient for signs of anaphylaxis (rash, dyspnea, stridor, facial swelling, angioedema, pruritus, sensation of warmth, bronchospasm) during therapy.
- ***Lab Test Considerations:*** May cause ↑ serum alkaline phosphatase, serum creatinine, AST, ALT, eosinophils, and urine protein and RBCs. May also cause ↓ serum potassium, hemoglobin, hematocrit, and WBCs.

Implementation
IV Administration
- **Intermittent Infusion:** Allow refrigerated vial to reach room temperature. *For 70-mg or 50-mg dose*—Reconstitute vials with 10.8 mL of 0.9% NaCl, sterile water for injection, bacteriostatic water for injection with methylparaben and propylparaben, or bacteriostatic water for injection with 0.9% benzyl alcohol. Use preservative-free diluents for neonates. Do not dilute with dextrose solutions. Reconstituted solution is stable for 1 hr at room temperature. ***Diluent:*** Withdraw 10 mL from vial and add to 250 mL of 0.9% NaCl, 0.45% NaCl, 0.225% NaCl, or LR. The 50-mg dose also can be diluted in 100 mL when volume restriction is necessary. Infusion is stable for 24 hr at room temperature or 48 hr if refrigerated. *For 35-mg dose*—Reconstitute a 50-mg

or 70-mg vial as per the directions above. Remove the volume of drug equal to the calculated loading dose or calculated maintenance dose based on a concentration of 7 mg/mL (if reconstituted from the 70-mg vial) or a concentration of 5 mg/mL (if reconstituted from the 50-mg vial). White cake should dissolve completely. Mix gently until a clear solution is obtained. Do not use a solution that is cloudy, discolored, or contains precipitates. ***Concentration:*** 0.14–0.47 mg/mL. ***Rate:*** Infuse over 1 hr.

- **Y-Site Compatibility:** alemtuzumab, alfentanil, allopurinol, amifostine, amikacin, aminophylline, amiodarone, anidulafungin, argatroban, arsenic trioxide, atracurium, aztreonam, bleomycin, bumetanide, busulfan, butorphanol, calcium acetate, calcium chloride, calcium gluconate, carboplatin, carmustine, chlorpromazine, ciprofloxacin, cisatracurium, cisplatin, cyclophosphamide, cyclosporine, dacarbazine, dactinomycin, daptomycin, daunorubicin, dexmedetomidine, dexrazoxane, diltiazem, diphenhydramine, dobutamine, docetaxel, dolasetron, dopamine, doxorubicin, doxorubicin liposome, doxycycline, droperidol, epinephrine, epirubicin, erythromycin, esmolol, etoposide, etoposide phosphate, famotidine, fenoldopam, fentanyl, fluconazole, fludarabine, ganciclovir, gemcitabine, gentamicin, glycopyrrolate, granisetron, haloperidol, hydrocortisone sodium succinate, hydromorphone, idarubicin, ifosfamide, imipenem/cilastatin, insulin, irinotecan, isoproterenol, labetalol, leucovorin, levofloxacin, linezolid, magnesium sulfate, mannitol, melphalan, meperidine, meropenem, mesna, methyldopate, metoclopramide, metoprolol, midazolam, milrinone, mitomycin, mitoxantrone, morphine, moxifloxacin, mycophenolate, nalbuphine, naloxone, nicardipine, nitroglycerin, norepinephrine, octreotide, ondansetron, oxaliplatin, oxytocin, paclitaxel, palonosetron, pentamidine, phentolamine, phenylephrine, posaconazole, potassium acetate, potassium chloride, procainamide, prochlorperazine, promethazine, propranolol, quinupristin/dalfopristin, remifentanil, rocuronium, streptozocin, succinylcholine, sufentanil, tacrolimus, telavancin, theophylline, thiopental, thiotepa, tigecycline, tirofiban, tobramycin, topotecan, vancomycin, vasopressin, vecuronium, verapamil, vinblastine, vincristine, vinorelbine, voriconazole, zidovudine, zoledronic acid.
- **Y-Site Incompatibility:** aminocaproic acid, amphotericin B lipid complex, amphotericin B liposome, ampicillin, ampicillin/sulbactam, bivalirudin, blinatumomab, cefazolin, cefepime, cefotaxime, cefotetan, cefoxitin, ceftaroline, ceftazidime, ceftriaxone, cefuroxime, chloramphenicol, clindamycin, dantrolene, dexamethasone, diazepam, digoxin, enalaprilat, ephedrine, ertapenem, fluorouracil, foscarnet, fosphenytoin, furosemide, heparin, ketorolac, lidocaine, methotrexate, methylprednisolone, nafcillin, nitroprusside, pamidronate, pancuronium, pemetrexed, pentobarbital, phenobarbital, phenytoin, piperacillin/tazobactam, potassium phosphates, ranitidine, sodium acetate, sodium bicarbonate, sodium phosphates, trimethoprim/sulfamethoxazole.
- **Solution Incompatibility:** Solutions containing dextrose.

Patient/Family Teaching

- Explain the purpose of caspofungin to patient and family.
- Advise patient to notify health care professional immediately if symptoms of allergic reactions (rash, facial swelling, pruritus, sensation of warmth, difficulty breathing) occur.
- Advise female patient to notify health care professional if pregnancy is planned or suspected or if breast feeding.

Evaluation/Desired Outcomes

- Decrease in signs and symptoms of fungal infections. Duration of therapy is determined based on severity of underlying disease, recovery from immunosuppression, and clinical response.

cefaclor, See CEPHALOSPORINS—SECOND GENERATION.

cefadroxil, See CEPHALOSPORINS—FIRST GENERATION.

ceFAZolin, See CEPHALOSPORINS—FIRST GENERATION.

cefdinir, See CEPHALOSPORINS—THIRD GENERATION.

cefditoren, See CEPHALOSPORINS—THIRD GENERATION.

cefepime (seff-e-peem)

Maxipime

Classification

Therapeutic: anti-infectives

Pharmacologic: fourth-generation cephalosporins

Indications

Treatment of the following infections caused by susceptible organisms: Uncomplicated skin and skin structure infections, Bone and joint infections, Uncomplicated and complicated urinary tract infections, Respiratory tract infections, Complicated intra-abdominal infections (with metronidazole), Septicemia. Empiric treatment of febrile neutropenic patients.

Action

Binds to the bacterial cell wall membrane, causing cell death. **Therapeutic Effects:** Bactericidal action against susceptible bacteria. **Spectrum:** Similar to that of second- and third-generation cephalosporins, but activity against staphylococci is less, whereas activity against gram-negative pathogens is greater, even for organisms resistant to first-, second-, and third-generation agents. Notable is increased action against: *Enterobacter, Haemophilus influenzae* (including β-lactamase-producing strains), *Escherichia coli, Klebsiella pneumoniae, Neisseria, Proteus, Providencia, Pseudomonas aeruginosa, Serratia, Moraxella catarrhalis* (including β-lactamase-producing strains). Not active against methicillin-resistant staphylococci or enterococci.

Pharmacokinetics

Absorption: Well absorbed after IM administration; IV administration results in complete bioavailability.
Distribution: Widely distributed. Crosses the placenta; enters breast milk in low concentrations. Some CSF penetration.
Protein Binding: 20%.
Metabolism and Excretion: 85% excreted unchanged in urine.
Half-life: *Adults*—2 hr (↑ in renal impairment); *Children 2 mo–6 yr*—1.7–1.9 hr.

TIME/ACTION PROFILE

ROUTE	ONSET	PEAK	DURATION
IM	rapid	1–2 hr	12 hr
IV	rapid	end of infusion	12 hr

Contraindications/Precautions

Contraindicated in: Hypersensitivity to cephalosporins; Serious hypersensitivity to penicillins.
Use Cautiously in: Renal impairment (↓ dosing/↑ dosing interval recommended if CCr ≤60 mL/min); History of GI disease, especially colitis; Patients with hepatic dysfunction or poor nutritional status (may be at ↑ risk of bleeding); Geriatric patients (dose adjustment due to age-related ↓ in renal function may be necessary); OB, Lactation: Pregnancy and lactation (safety not established).

Adverse Reactions/Side Effects

CNS: ENCEPHALOPATHY, SEIZURES (↑ risk in renal impairment), aphasia, headache. **GI:** CLOSTRIDIUM DIFFICILE-ASSOCIATED DIARRHEA (CDAD), diarrhea, nausea, vomiting. **Derm:** rashes, pruritis, urticaria. **Hemat:** bleeding, eosinophilia, hemolytic anemia, neutropenia, thrombocytopenia. **Local:** pain at IM site, phlebitis at IV site. **Misc:** allergic reactions including ANAPHYLAXIS, superinfection, fever.

Interactions

Drug-Drug: Probenecid ↓ excretion and ↑ blood levels. Concurrent use of **loop diuretics** or **aminoglycosides** may ↑ risk of nephrotoxicity.

Route/Dosage

IM (Adults): *Mild-to-moderate uncomplicated or complicated urinary tract infections due to Escherichia coli*—0.5–1 g every 12 hr.
IV (Adults): *Moderate-to-severe pneumonia*—1–2 g every 12 hr. *Mild-to-moderate uncomplicated or complicated urinary tract infections*—0.5–1 g every 12 hr. *Severe uncomplicated or complicated urinary tract infections, moderate-to-severe uncomplicated skin and skin structure infections, complicated intra-abdominal infections*—2 g every 12 hr. *Empiric treatment of febrile neutropenia*—2 g every 8 hr.
IV (Children 1 mo–16 yr): *Uncomplicated and complicated urinary tract infections, uncomplicated skin and skin structure infections, pneumonia*—50 mg/kg every 12 hr (not to exceed 2 g/dose). *Febrile neutropenia*—50 mg/kg every 8 hr (not to exceed 2 g/dose).
IV (Neonates postnatal age ≥14 days): 50 mg/kg every 12 hr.
IV (Neonates postnatal age <14 days): 30 mg/kg every 12 hr; consider 50 mg/kg every 12 hr for *Pseudomonas* infections.

Renal Impairment

IM, IV (Adults): (See Manufacturer's specific recommendations) *CCr 30–60 mL/min*—0.5–1 g every 24 hr or 2 g every 12–24 hr; *CCr 11–29 mL/min*—0.5–2 g every 24 hr; *CCr <11 mL/min*—250 mg–1 g every 24 hr.

Availability (generic available)

Powder for injection: 500 mg, 1 g, 2 g. **Premixed containers:** 1 g/50 mL D5W, 2 g/100 mL D5W.

NURSING IMPLICATIONS

Assessment

- Assess patient for infection (vital signs; appearance of wound, sputum, urine, and stool; WBC) at beginning of and throughout therapy.
- Before initiating therapy, obtain a history to determine previous use of and reactions to penicillins or cephalosporins. Persons with a negative history of penicillin sensitivity may still have an allergic response.
- Obtain specimens for culture and sensitivity before initiating therapy. First dose may be given before receiving results.

- Observe patient for signs and symptoms of anaphylaxis (rash, pruritus, laryngeal edema, wheezing). Discontinue the drug and notify health care professional immediately if these symptoms occur. Keep epinephrine, an antihistamine, and resuscitation equipment close by in the event of an anaphylactic reaction.
- Monitor bowel function. Diarrhea, abdominal cramping, fever, and bloody stools should be reported to health care professional promptly as a sign of Clostridium difficile-associated diarrhea (CDAD). May begin up to several wk following cessation of therapy.
- ***Lab Test Considerations:*** May cause positive results for Coombs' test in patients receiving high doses or in neonates whose mothers were given cephalosporins before delivery.
- May cause ↑ serum AST, ALT, bilirubin, BUN, and creatinine.
- May rarely cause leukopenia, neutropenia, thrombocytopenia, and eosinophilia.

Implementation

- **IM:** Reconstitute IM doses with sterile or bacteriostatic water for injection, 0.9% NaCl, or D5W. May be diluted with lidocaine to minimize injection discomfort.
- Inject deep into a well-developed muscle mass; massage well.
- IM route should only be used for treatment of mild-to-moderate uncomplicated or complicated urinary tract infections due to *Escherichia coli*.

IV Administration

- **IV:** Monitor injection site frequently for phlebitis (pain, redness, swelling). Change sites every 48–72 hr to prevent phlebitis.
- If aminoglycosides are administered concurrently, administer in separate sites, if possible, at least 1 hr apart. If second site is unavailable, flush lines between medications.
- **Intermittent Infusion:** Reconstitute with 5 mL sterile water, 0.9% NaCl, or D5W for the 500-mg vial, or 10 mL for the 1-g or 2-g vials. ***Diluent:*** Dilute further in 50–100 mL of D5W, 0.9% NaCl, D10W, D5/0.9% NaCl, or D5/LR. ***Concentration:*** Maximum 40 mg/mL.
- Solution is stable for 24 hr at room temperature and 7 days if refrigerated. ***Rate:*** Administer over 20–30 min.
- **Y-Site Compatibility:** amikacin, amiodarone, amphotericin B lipid complex, ampicillin-sulbactam, anidulafungin, azithromycin, aztreonam, bivalirudin, bleomycin, bumetanide, buprenorphine, butorphanol, calcium gluconate, carboplatin, carmustine, cyclophosphamide, cytarabine, dactinomycin, daptomycin, dexamethasone sodium phosphate, dexmedetomidine, docetaxel, doxorubicin liposome, eptifibatide, fenoldopam, fluconazole, fludarabine, fluorouracil, foscarnet, fosphenytoin, furosemide, gentamicin, granisetron, hetastarch, hydrocortisone sodium phosphate, hydrocortisone sodium succinate, hydromorphone, imipenem-cilastatin, insulin, ketamine, leucovorin, levofloxacin, linezolid, lorazepam, melphalan, mesna, methotrexate, methylprednisolone sodium succinate, metronidazole, milrinone, octreotide, oxytocin, paclitaxel, palonosetron, pamidronate, pancuronium, piperacillin-tazobactam, potassium acetate, ranitidine, remifentanil, rocuronium, sargramostim, sodium acetate, sodium bicarbonate, sufentanil, telavancin, thiotepa, tigecycline, tirofiban, tobramycin, trimethoprim/sulfamethoxazole, vasopressin, zidovudine, zoledronic acid.
- **Y-Site Incompatibility:** acetylcysteine, acyclovir, alemtuzumab, amphotericin B cholesteryl, amphotericin B deoxycholate, amphotericin B liposome, argatroban, caspofungin, chlorpromazine, ciprofloxacin, cisplatin, dacarbazine, daunorubicin, dexrazoxane, diazepam, diltiazem, diphenhydramine, dolasetron, doxorubicin hydrochloride, droperidol, enalaprilat, epirubicin, erythromycin, etoposide, etoposide phosphate, famotidine, filgrastim, floxuridine, ganciclovir, gemcitabine, haloperidol, idarubicin, ifosfamide, irinotecan, magnesium sulfate, mannitol, meperidine, metoclopramide, midazolam, mitomycin, mitoxantrone, nalbuphine, ondansetron, oxaliplatin, pantoprazole, pemetrexed, phenytoin, prochlorperazine, promethazine, quinupristin/dalfopristin, streptozocin, tacrolimus, theophylline, vecuronium, vinblastine, vincristine, vinorelbine, voriconazole.

Patient/Family Teaching

- Advise patient to report signs of superinfection (furry overgrowth on the tongue, vaginal itching or discharge, loose or foul-smelling stools) and allergy.
- Instruct patient to notify health care professional if fever and diarrhea develop, especially if stool contains blood, pus, or mucus. Advise patient not to treat diarrhea without consulting health care professional.

Evaluation/Desired Outcomes

- Resolution of the signs and symptoms of infection. Length of time for complete resolution depends on the organism and site of infection.

cefixime, See CEPHALOSPORINS—THIRD GENERATION.

cefotaxime, See CEPHALOSPORINS—THIRD GENERATION.

cefoTEtan, See CEPHALOSPORINS—SECOND GENERATION.

cefOXitin, See CEPHALOSPORINS—SECOND GENERATION.

cefpodoxime, See CEPHALOSPORINS—THIRD GENERATION.

cefprozil, See CEPHALOSPORINS—SECOND GENERATION.

ceftaroline (sef-tar-oh-leen)

Teflaro

Classification

Therapeutic: anti-infectives

Pharmacologic: cephalosporin derivatives

Indications

Acute bacterial skin/skin structure infections. Community-acquired pneumonia.

Action

Binds to bacterial cell wall membrane, causing cell death. **Therapeutic Effects:** Bactericidal action against susceptible bacteria. **Spectrum:** *Treatment of skin/skin structure infections*—Active against *Staphylococcus aureus* (including methicillin-susceptible and -resistant strains), *Streptococcus pyogenes*, *Streptococcus agalactiae*, *Escherichia coli*, *Klebsiella pneumoniae*, and *Klebsiella oxytoca*; *Treatment of community acquired pneumonia*—*Streptococcus pneumoniae* (including pneumonia with bacteremia), *Staphylococcus aureus* (methicillin-susceptible strains only), *Haemophilus influenzae*, *Klebsiella pneumoniae*, *Klebsiella oxytoca*, and *Escherichia coli*.

Pharmacokinetics

Absorption: IV administration results in complete bioavailability of parent drug.
Distribution: Unknown.
Metabolism and Excretion: Ceftaroline fosamil is rapidly converted by plasma phosphatases to ceftaroline, the active metabolite; 88% excreted in urine, 6% in feces.
Half-life: 2.6 hr (after multiple doses).

TIME/ACTION PROFILE (blood levels)

ROUTE	ONSET	PEAK	DURATION
IV	rapid	end of infusion	12 hr

Contraindications/Precautions

Contraindicated in: Known serious hypersensitivity to cephalosporins.

Use Cautiously in: Known hypersensitivity to other beta-lactams; Renal impairment (dosage ↓ required for CCr ≤50 mL/min in adults); OB: Use only if potential maternal benefit justifies potential fetal risk; Lactation: Use while breast feeding only if potential maternal benefit justifies potential risk to infant; Pedi: Neonates <34 wk (gestational age) or <12 days (postnatal age) (acute bacterial skin/skin structure infections) and infants <2 mo (community-acquired pneumonia) (safety and effectiveness not established); Geri: Dose adjustment may be necessary for age-related ↓ in renal function.

Adverse Reactions/Side Effects

Derm: rash. **GI:** CLOSTRIDIUM DIFFICILE-ASSOCIATED DIARRHEA (CDAD), diarrhea, nausea. **Hemat:** hemolytic anemia. **Local:** phlebitis at injection site. **Misc:** HYPERSENSITIVITY REACTIONS (including anaphylaxis).

Interactions

Drug-Drug: None noted.

Route/Dosage

Acute Bacterial Skin/Skin Structure Infections

IV (Adults): 600 mg every 12 hr for 5–14 days.
IV (Children 2–17 yr and >33 kg): 400 mg every 8 hr for 5–14 days *or* 600 mg every 12 hr for 5–14 days.
IV (Children 2–17 yr and ≤33 kg): 12 mg/kg every 8 hr for 5–14 days.
IV (Children 2 mo–<2 yr): 8 mg/kg every 8 hr for 5–14 days.
IV (Neonates 0–<2 mo): 6 mg/kg every 8 hr for 5–14 days.

Renal Impairment

IV (Adults): *CCr >30 to ≤50 mL/min*—400 mg every 12 hr; *CCr ≥15 to ≤30 mL/min*—300 mg every 12 hr; *CCr <15 mL/min including hemodialysis*—200 mg every 12 hr.

Community-Acquired Pneumonia

IV (Adults): 600 mg every 12 hr for 5–7 days.
IV (Children 2–17 yr and >33 kg): 400 mg every 8 hr for 5–14 days *or* 600 mg every 12 hr for 5–14 days.
IV (Children 2–17 yr and ≤33 kg): 12 mg/kg every 8 hr for 5–14 days.
IV (Children 2 mo–<2 yr): 8 mg/kg every 8 hr for 5–14 days.

Renal Impairment

IV (Adults): *CCr >30 to ≤50 mL/min*—400 mg every 12 hr; *CCr ≥15 to ≤30 mL/min*—300 mg every 12 hr; *CCr <15 mL/min including hemodialysis*—200 mg every 12 hr.

Availability

Powder for injection (requires reconstitution and dilution): 400 mg/vial, 600 mg/vial.

NURSING IMPLICATIONS

Assessment

- Assess for infection (vital signs; appearance of wound, sputum, urine, and stool; WBC) at beginning of and throughout therapy.
- Before initiating therapy, obtain a history to determine previous use of and reactions to penicillins, cephalosporins, or carbapenems. Persons with a negative history of sensitivity may still have an allergic response.
- Obtain specimens for culture and sensitivity before initiating therapy. First dose may be given before receiving results.
- Observe patient for signs and symptoms of anaphylaxis (rash, pruritus, laryngeal edema, wheezing). Discontinue the drug and notify health care professional immediately if these symptoms occur. Keep epinephrine, an antihistamine, and resuscitation equipment close by in the event of an anaphylactic reaction.
- Monitor bowel function. Diarrhea, abdominal cramping, fever, and bloody stools should be reported to health care professional promptly as a sign of Clostridium difficile-associated diarrhea (CDAD). May begin up to several mo following cessation of therapy.
- ***Lab Test Considerations:*** May cause seroconversion from a negative to a positive direct Coombs' test. If anemia develops during or after therapy, perform a direct Coombs' test. If drug-induced hemolytic anemia is suspected, discontinue ceftaroline and provide supportive care.

Implementation

IV Administration

- **Intermittent Infusion:** Reconstitute with 20 mL of sterile water for injection, 0.9% NaCl, D5W, or LR. ***Diluent:*** Dilute further with 50–250 mL of same diluent unless reconstituted with sterile water for injection, then use 0.9% NaCl, D5W, D2.5W, 0.45% NaCl, or LR. Mix gently to dissolve. Solution is clear to light or dark yellow; do not administer solutions that are discolored or contain particulate matter. Solution is stable for 6 hr at room temperature or 24 hr if refrigerated. ***Rate:*** Infuse over 5–60 min.
- **Y-Site Compatibility:** acyclovir, amikacin, aminophylline, amiodarone, azithromycin, bumetanide, calcium chloride, calcium gluconate, ciprofloxacin, cisatracurium, clindamycin, cyclosporine, dexamethasone, digoxin, diltiazem, diphenhydramine, dopamine, enalaprilat, esomeprazole, famotidine, fentanyl, fluconazole, furosemide, gentamicin, granisetron, haloperidol, heparin, hydrocortisone, hydromorphone, insulin regular, insulin lispro, levofloxacin, lidocaine, lorazepam, mannitol, meperidine, methylprednisolone, metoclopramide, metoprolol, midazolam, milrinone, morphine, moxifloxacin, multivitamins, norepinephrine, ondansetron, pantoprazole, potassium chloride, promethazine, propofol, ranitidine, remifentanil, sodium bicarbonate, tobramycin, trimethoprim/sulfamethoxazole, vasopressin, voriconazole.
- **Y-Site Incompatibility:** caspofungin, diazepam, filgrastim, labetalol, potassium phosphates, sodium phosphates.

Patient/Family Teaching

- Explain the purpose of ceftaroline to patient. Emphasize the importance of completing therapy, even if feeling better.
- Instruct patient to notify health care professional if fever and diarrhea develop, especially if stool contains blood, pus, or mucus. Advise patient not to treat diarrhea without consulting health care professional.

Evaluation/Desired Outcomes

- Resolution of the signs and symptoms of infection. Length of time for complete resolution depends on the organism and site of infection.

cefTAZidime, See CEPHALOSPORINS—THIRD GENERATION.

ceftazidime/avibactam

(sef-**tay**-zi-deem/tay-zoe-**bak**-tam)
Avycaz

Classification
Therapeutic: anti-infectives
Pharmacologic: third-generation cephalosporins, beta lactamase inhibitors

Indications

Complicated intra-abdominal infections (in combination with metronidazole). Complicated urinary tract infections (including pyelonephritis). Hospital-acquired and ventilator-associated bacterial pneumonia.

Action

Ceftazidime—Binds to the bacterial cell wall membrane, causing cell death. *Avibactam*—Inhibits beta-lactamase, an enzyme that destroys penicillins and cephalosporins. **Therapeutic Effects:** Death of susceptible bacteria with resolution of infection. **Spectrum:** Active against *Escherichia coli*, *Klebsiella pneumoniae*, *Proteus mirabilis*, *Haemophilus influenzae*, *Enterobacter cloacae*, *Klebsiella oxytoca*, *Pseudomonas aeruginosa*, *Citrobacter freundii*, and *Serratia marcescens*.

Pharmacokinetics

Absorption: IV administration results in complete bioavailability.

Distribution: *Ceftazidime*—Widely distributed, enters breast milk in low concentrations; *avibactam*—widely distributed.

Metabolism and Excretion: *ceftazidime*—minimally metabolized, 80–90% excreted unchanged in urine; *avibactam*—minimally metabolized, mainly excreted unchanged in urine.

Half-life: *Ceftazidime*—2.8–3.3 hr (↑ in renal impairment); *avibactam*—2.2–2.7 hr.

TIME/ACTION PROFILE (blood levels)

ROUTE	ONSET	PEAK	DURATION
IV	rapid	end of infusion	8 hr (↑ in renal impairment)

Contraindications/Precautions

Contraindicated in: Known hypersensitivity to ceftazidime, other cephalosporins or avibactam-containing products; cross-sensitivity with other penicillins, carbapenems, and cephalosporins may occur.

Use Cautiously in: CCr 30–50 mL/min (efficacy may be ↓, monitor renal function frequently and adjust dose if necessary); OB: Use only if potential material benefit justifies potential fetal risk; Lactation: Use cautiously in breast-feeding women; Pedi: Safety and effectiveness not established in children <3 mo (complicated intra-abdominal infections and complicated urinary tract infections) and <18 yr (hospital-acquired and ventilator-associated bacterial pneumonia); Geri: Consider age-related impairment of renal function.

Adverse Reactions/Side Effects

CNS: SEIZURES (↑ in renal impairment), anxiety, dizziness, headache. **F and E:** hypokalemia. **GI:** CLOSTRIDIUM DIFFICILE-ASSOCIATED DIARRHEA (CDAD), diarrhea, nausea, vomiting. **Hemat:** eosinophilia, thrombocytopenia. **Misc:** HYPERSENSITIVITY REACTIONS (including anaphylaxis and serious skin reactions).

Interactions

Drug-Drug: Probenecid may ↓ renal excretion of avibactam; concurrent administration is not recommended.

Route/Dosage

Complicated Intra-abdominal Infections and Complicated Urinary Tract Infections

IV (Adults): 2.5 g (2 g ceftazidime/0.5 g avibactam) every 8 hr. Duration of therapy = 5–14 days (complicated intra-abdominal infections); 7–14 days (complicated urinary tract infections).

IV (Children ≥2 yr): 62.5 mg/kg (50 mg/kg ceftazidime/12.5 mg/kg avibactam) (max dose = 2.5 g [2 g ceftazidime/0.5 g avibactam]) every 8 hr. Duration of therapy = 5–14 days (complicated intra-abdominal infections); 7–14 days (complicated urinary tract infections).

IV (Children 6 mo–<2 yr): 62.5 mg/kg (50 mg/kg ceftazidime/12.5 mg/kg avibactam) every 8 hr. Duration of therapy = 5–14 days (complicated intra-abdominal infections); 7–14 days (complicated urinary tract infections).

IV (Children 3 mo–<6 mo): 50 mg/kg (40 mg/kg ceftazidime/10 mg/kg avibactam) every 8 hr. Duration of therapy = 5–14 days (complicated intra-abdominal infections); 7–14 days (complicated urinary tract infections).

Renal Impairment

IV (Adults): *CCr 31–50 mL/min*—1.25 g (1 g ceftazidime/0.25 g avibactam) every 8 hr; *CCr 16–30 mL/min*—0.94 g (0.75 g ceftazidime/0.19 g avibactam) every 12 hr; *CCr 6–15 mL/min*—0.94 g (0.75 g ceftazidime/0.19 g avibactam) every 24 hr; *CCr ≤5 mL/min*—0.94 g (0.75 g ceftazidime/0.19 g avibactam) every 48 hr: *Hemodialysis*—Administer dose after hemodialysis on hemodialysis days.

Renal Impairment

IV (Children ≥2 yr): *CCr 31–50 mL/min*—31.25 mg/kg (25 mg/kg ceftazidime/6.25 mg/kg avibactam) (max dose = 1.25 g [1 g ceftazidime/0.25 g avibactam]) every 8 hr; *CCr 16–30 mL/min*—23.75 mg/kg (19 mg/kg ceftazidime/4.75 mg/kg avibactam) (max dose = 0.94 g [0.75 g ceftazidime/0.19 g avibactam]) every 12 hr; *CCr 6–15 mL/min*—23.75 mg/kg (19 mg/kg ceftazidime/4.75 mg/kg avibactam) (max dose = 0.94 g [0.75 g ceftazidime/0.19 g avibactam]) every 24 hr; *CCr ≤5 mL/min*—23.75 mg/kg (19 mg/kg ceftazidime/4.75 mg/kg avibactam) (max dose = 0.94 g [0.75 g ceftazidime/0.19 g avibactam]) every 48 hr; *Hemodialysis*—Administer dose after hemodialysis or on hemodialysis days.

Hospital-acquired and Ventilator-associated Bacterial Pneumonia

IV (Adults): 2.5 g (2 g ceftazidime/0.5 g avibactam) every 8 hr. Duration of therapy = 5–14 days (complicated intra-abdominal infections); 7–14 days (complicated urinary tract infections).

Renal Impairment

IV (Adults): *CCr 31–50 mL/min*—1.25 g (1 g ceftazidime/0.25 g avibactam) every 8 hr; *CCr 16–30 mL/min*—0.94 g (0.75 g ceftazidime/0.19 g avibactam) every 12 hr; *CCr 6–15 mL/min*—0.94 g (0.75 g ceftazidime/0.19 g avibactam) every 24 hr; *CCr ≤5 mL/min*—0.94 g (0.75 g ceftazidime/0.19 g avibactam) every 48 hr: *Hemodialysis*—Administer dose after hemodialysis on hemodialysis days.

Availability

Powder for injection (requires reconstitution and dilution): ceftazidime 2 g/avibactam 0.5 g/vial.

NURSING IMPLICATIONS

Assessment

- Assess for infection (vital signs; appearance of wound, sputum, urine, and stool; WBC) at beginning of and throughout therapy.
- Before initiating therapy, obtain a history to determine previous use of and reactions to penicillins,

C

cephalosporins or carbapenems. Persons with a negative history of sensitivity may still have an allergic response.

- Obtain specimens for culture and sensitivity before initiating therapy. First dose may be given before receiving results.
- Observe patient for signs and symptoms of anaphylaxis (rash, pruritus, laryngeal edema, wheezing). Discontinue the drug and notify health care professional immediately if these symptoms occur. Keep epinephrine, an antihistamine, and resuscitation equipment close by in the event of an anaphylactic reaction.
- Monitor bowel function. Diarrhea, abdominal cramping, fever, and bloody stools should be reported to health care professional promptly as a sign of CDAD. May begin up to several mo following cessation of therapy.
- Monitor for signs and symptoms of encephalopathy (disturbance of consciousness including confusion, hallucinations, stupor, coma), myoclonus, and seizures during and following therapy. May require immediate treatment, dose adjustment, or discontinuation of therapy.
- ***Lab Test Considerations:*** May cause seroconversion from a negative to a positive direct Coombs' test. If anemia develops during or after therapy, perform a direct Coombs' test.
- May cause a false-positive reaction for glucose in urine with certain methods; use enzymatic glucose oxidase reactions.

Implementation

IV Administration

- **Intermittent Infusion:** Reconstitute with 10 mL of sterile water for injection. 0.9% NaCl, D5W, D5/0.9% NaCl, D5/0.45% NaCl, D2.5/0.9% NaCl, D2.5/0.45% NaCl, or LR. Mix gently. ***Diluent:*** Use same diluent used for reconstitution for a volume between 50 mL and 250 mL. ***Concentration:*** 40 and 10 mg/mL of ceftazidime and avibactam, respectively to 8 and 2 mg/mL of ceftazidime and avibactam, respectively. Solution ranges from clear to light yellow; do not administer solutions that are discolored or contain particulate matter. Solution is stable for 12 hrs at room temperature or 24 hrs if refrigerated. ***Rate:*** Infuse over 2 hrs.
- **Y-Site Compatibility:** daptomycin, dexmedetomidine, dopamine, ertapenem, furosemide, gentamicin, heparin, imipenem/cilastatin, linezolid, magnesium sulfate, meropenem, norepinephrine, phenylephrine, potassium chloride, potassium phosphates, sodium bicarbonate, tobramycin, vasopressin, vecuronium.

Patient/Family Teaching

- Explain the purpose of ceftazidime/avibactam to patient.
- Instruct patient to notify health care professional if fever and diarrhea develop, especially if stool contains blood, pus, or mucus. Advise patient not to treat diarrhea without consulting health care professional.
- Advise patient to notify health care professional immediately if signs and symptoms of allergic reactions or nervous system reactions occur.
- Advise female patient to notify health care professional if pregnancy is planned or suspected or if breast feeding.

Evaluation/Desired Outcomes

- Resolution of the signs and symptoms of infection. Length of time for complete resolution depends on the organism and site of infection.

ceftolozane/tazobactam
(sef-**tol**-o-zane/taz-oh-**bak**-tam)
Zerbaxa

Classification
Therapeutic: anti-infectives
Pharmacologic: cephalosporin derivatives, beta lactamase inhibitors

Indications

Complicated intra-abdominal infections (cIAI) (in combination with metronidazole). Complicated urinary tract infections (cUTI) (including pyelonephritis). Hospital-acquired bacterial pneumonia (HABP) and ventilator-associated bacterial pneumonia (VABP).

Action

Ceftolozane: binds to bacterial cell wall membrane, causing cell death. Spectrum is extended compared with other penicillins. Tazobactam: Inhibits beta-lactamase, an enzyme that can destroy penicillins. **Therapeutic Effects:** Death of susceptible bacteria. **Spectrum:** Active against *Bacteroides fragilis, Enterobacter cloacae, Escherichia coli, Haemophilus influenzae, Klebsiella oxytoca, Klebsiella pneumoniae, Proteus mirabilis, Pseudomonas aeruginosa, Serratia marcesens, Streptococcus anginosus, Streptococcus constellatus*, and *Streptococcus salivarius*.

Pharmacokinetics

Absorption: IV administration results in complete bioavailability.

Distribution: Unknown.

Metabolism and Excretion: *Ceftolozane*—minimal metabolism, excreted almost entirely (>95%) unchanged in urine; *tazobactam*—80% excreted unchanged in urine, some metabolized to an inactive M1 metabolite which is excreted unchanged in urine.

Half-life: *Ceftolozane*—2.8 hr; *tazobactam*—0.9 hr.

TIME/ACTION PROFILE

ROUTE	ONSET	PEAK	DURATION
IV	rapid	end of infusion	8 hr

Contraindications/Precautions

Contraindicated in: Known serious hypersensitivity to ceftolozane/tazbactam, piperacillin/tazobactam or other beta-lactams.

Use Cautiously in: CCr 30–<50 mL/min (effectiveness may be ↓); CCr <50 mL/min (dose adjustment recommended); OB: Use during pregnancy only if potential benefit outweighs potential risks; Lactation: Use cautiously if breast feeding; Pedi: Safety and effectiveness not established.

Adverse Reactions/Side Effects

CNS: anxiety, dizziness, headache, insomnia. **CV:** atrial fibrillation, hypotension. **Derm:** rash. **F and E:** hypokalemia. **GI:** abdominal pain, constipation, diarrhea, CLOSTRIDIUM DIFFICILE-ASSOCIATED DIARRHEA (CDAD), nausea, vomiting. **Hemat:** anemia, thrombocytosis. **Misc:** HYPERSENSITIVITY REACTIONS (including anaphylaxis).

Interactions

Drug-Drug: None reported.

Route/Dosage

cIAI or cUTI

IV (Adults): 1.5 g (1 g ceftolozane/0.5 g tazobactam) every 8 hr for 4–14 days for cIAI or 7 days for cUTI.

Renal Impairment

(Adults): *CCr 30–50 mL/min*—750 mg (500 mg ceftolozane/250 mg tazobactam) every 8 hr; *CCr 15–29 mL/min*—375 mg (250 mg ceftolozane/125 mg tazobactam) every 8 hr; *End-stage renal disease on hemodialysis*—Single loading dose of 750 mg (500 mg ceftolozane/250 mg tazobactam), then 150 mg (100 mg ceftolozane/50 mg tazobactam) every 8 hr (on dialysis days administer as soon as possible after dialysis).

HABP or VABP

IV (Adults): 3 g (2 g ceftolozane/1 g tazobactam) every 8 hr for 8–14 days.

Renal Impairment

(Adults): *CCr 30–50 mL/min*—1.5 g (1 g ceftolozane/0.5 g tazobactam) every 8 hr; *CCr 15–29 mL/min*—750 mg (500 mg ceftolozane/250 mg tazobactam) every 8 hr; *End-stage renal disease on hemodialysis*—Single loading dose of 2.25 g (1.5 g ceftolozane/0.75 g tazobactam), then 450 mg (300 mg ceftolozane/150 mg tazobactam) every 8 hr (on dialysis days administer as soon as possible after dialysis).

Availability

Powder for injection (requires reconstitution and dilution): 1 g ceftolozane/0.5 g tazobactam/vial.

NURSING IMPLICATIONS

Assessment

- Assess for infection (vital signs; appearance of wound, sputum, urine, and stool; WBC) at beginning of and throughout therapy.
- Before initiating therapy, obtain a history to determine previous use of and reactions to penicillins, cephalosporins, or other beta-lactams. Persons with a negative history of sensitivity may still have an allergic response.
- Obtain specimens for culture and sensitivity before initiating therapy. First dose may be given before receiving results.
- Observe patient for signs and symptoms of anaphylaxis (rash, pruritus, laryngeal edema, wheezing). Discontinue the drug and notify health care professional immediately if these symptoms occur. Keep epinephrine, an antihistamine, and resuscitation equipment close by in the event of an anaphylactic reaction.
- Monitor bowel function. Diarrhea, abdominal cramping, fever, and bloody stools should be reported to health care professional promptly as a sign of (CDAD). May begin up to several mo following cessation of therapy.
- ***Lab Test Considerations:*** Monitor creatinine clearance at least daily in patients with changing renal function and adjust dose accordingly.

Implementation

IV Administration

- **Intermittent Infusion:** Reconstitute with 10 mL of sterile water for injection or 0.9% NaCl for injection; shake gently to dissolve for final volume of 11.4 mL. ***Diluent:*** Withdraw 11.4 mL for 1.5 g (1.0 g/0.5 g dose, 5.7 mL for 750 mg (500 mg/250 mg) dose, 2.9 mL for 375 mg (250 mg/125 mg) dose, or 1.2 mL for 150 mg (100 mg/50 mg) dose and add to 100 mL of 0.9% NaCl or D5W. Solution is clear, colorless to slightly yellow; do not administer solutions that are discolored or contain particulate matter. Solution is stable for 24 hr at room temperature or 7 days if refrigerated; do not freeze. ***Rate:*** Infuse over 1 hr.
- **Y-Site Compatibility:** amikacin, amiodarone, ampicillin/sulbactam, anidulafungin, azithromycin, bumetanide, calcium chloride, calcium gluconate, cefazolin, cefepime, ceftaroline, ceftazidime, ceftriaxone, cefuroxime, ciprofloxacin, cisatracurium, daptomycin, dexamethasone, dexmedetomidine, digoxin, diltiazem, diphenhydramine, dobutamine, dopamine, doxycycline, ephedrine, epinephrine, eptifibatide, ertapenem, esmolol, esomeprazole, famotidine, fentanyl, filgrastim, fosphenytoin, furosemide, gentamicin, heparin, hydrocortisone, hydromorphone, insulin regular, labetalol, levofloxa-

cin, lidocaine, linezolid, lorazepam, magnesium sulfate, mannitol, meperidine, meropenem, mesna, metoclopramide, micafungin, midazolam, milrinone, morphine, mycophenolate, naloxone, nicardipine, nitroglycerin, nitroprusside, norepinephrine, octreotide, ondansetron, pantoprazole, penicillin G, phenylephrine, piperacillin/tazobactam, potassium chloride, potassium phosphates, ranitidine, rocuronium, sodium bicarbonate, sodium phosphates, tacrolimus, tigecycline, tobramycin, vancomycin, vasopressin, vecuronium.

- **Y-Site Incompatibility:** albumin human, amphotericin B lipid complex, amphotericin B liposome, caspofungin, cyclosporine, phenytoin, propofol.
- **Additive Incompatibility:** Do not mix with other drugs or solutions.

Patient/Family Teaching

- Explain the purpose of ceftolozane/tazobactam to patient.
- Instruct patient to notify health care professional if fever and diarrhea develop, especially if stool contains blood, pus, or mucus. Advise patient not to treat diarrhea without consulting health care professional.
- Advise female patient to notify health care professional if pregnancy is planned or suspected or if breast feeding.

Evaluation/Desired Outcomes

- Resolution of the signs and symptoms of infection. Length of time for complete resolution depends on the organism and site of infection.

cefTRIAXone, See CEPHALOSPORINS—THIRD GENERATION.

cefuroxime, See CEPHALOSPORINS—SECOND GENERATION.

celecoxib (sel-e-**kox**-ib)

CeleBREX

Classification

Therapeutic: antirheumatics, nonsteroidal anti-inflammatory agents

Pharmacologic: COX-2 inhibitors

Indications

Relief of signs and symptoms of osteoarthritis, rheumatoid arthritis, ankylosing spondylitis, and juvenile rheumatoid arthritis. Management of acute pain including primary dysmenorrhea.

Action

Inhibits the enzyme COX-2. This enzyme is required for the synthesis of prostaglandins. Has analgesic, anti-inflammatory, and antipyretic properties. **Therapeutic Effects:** Decreased pain and inflammation caused by arthritis or spondylitis. Decreased pain.

Pharmacokinetics

Absorption: Bioavailability unknown.

Distribution: 97% bound to plasma proteins; extensive tissue distribution.

Metabolism and Excretion: Mostly metabolized by the hepatic CYP2C9 isoenzyme; the CYP2C9 enzyme system exhibits genetic polymorphism; poor metabolizers may have significantly ↑ celecoxib concentrations and an ↑ risk of adverse effects; <3% excreted unchanged in urine and feces.

Half-life: 11 hr.

TIME/ACTION PROFILE (pain reduction)

ROUTE	ONSET	PEAK	DURATION
PO	24–48 hr	unknown	12–24 hr†

†After discontinuation.

Contraindications/Precautions

Contraindicated in: Hypersensitivity; Cross-sensitivity may exist with other NSAIDs, including aspirin; History of allergic-type reactions to sulfonamides; History of asthma, urticaria, or allergic-type reactions to aspirin or other NSAIDs, including the aspirin triad (asthma, nasal polyps, and severe hypersensitivity reactions to aspirin); Advanced renal disease; Severe hepatic dysfunction; Coronary artery bypass graft (CABG) surgery; OB: Should not be used in late pregnancy (may cause premature closure of the ductus arteriosus).

Use Cautiously in: Cardiovascular disease or risk factors for cardiovascular disease (may ↑ risk of serious cardiovascular thrombotic events, myocardial infarction, and stroke, especially with prolonged use or use of higher doses); avoid use in patients with recent MI or HF; Pre-existing renal disease, heart failure, liver dysfunction, concurrent diuretic, or ACE inhibitor therapy (↑ risk of renal impairment); Long duration of NSAID use, smoking, alcohol use, advanced liver disease, coagulopathy, and poor general health (↑ risk of GI bleeding); Hypertension or fluid retention; Renal impairment (may precipitate acute renal failure); Serious dehydration (correct deficits before administering); Patients who are known or suspected to be poor CYP2C9 metabolizers (↓ initial dose by 50%); Pre-existing asthma; Pedi: Safety not established in children <2 yr or for longer than 6 mo; Geri: ↑ risk of GI bleeding; Lactation: Lactation.

Exercise Extreme Caution in: History of peptic ulcer disease or GI bleeding.

Adverse Reactions/Side Effects

CNS: dizziness, headache, insomnia. **CV:** HF, MYOCARDIAL INFARCTION, STROKE, THROMBOSIS, edema, hypertension. **Derm:** EXFOLIATIVE DERMATITIS, STEVENS-JOHNSON SYNDROME, TOXIC EPIDERMAL NECROLYSIS, rash.

F and E: hyperkalemia. **GI:** GI BLEEDING, abdominal pain, diarrhea, dyspepsia, flatulence, nausea.

Interactions

Drug-Drug: CYP2C9 inhibitors may ↑ levels. May ↓ effectiveness of **ACE inhibitors**, **thiazide diuretics**, and **furosemide**. **Fluconazole** ↑ levels (use lowest recommended dosage). ↑ risk of GI bleeding with **anticoagulants**, **aspirin**, **clopidogrel**, **ticagrelor**, **prasugrel**, **corticosteroids**, **fibrinolytics**, **SNRIs**, or **SSRIs**. May ↑ serum **lithium** levels. Does not inhibit the cardioprotective effect of low-dose **aspirin**.

Route/Dosage

PO (Adults): *Osteoarthritis*—200 mg once daily *or* 100 mg twice daily. *Rheumatoid arthritis*—100–200 mg twice daily. *Ankylosing spondylitis*—200 mg once daily *or* 100 mg twice daily; may ↑ dose after 6 wk to 400 mg daily. *Acute pain, including dysmenorrhea*—400 mg initially, then a 200-mg dose if needed on the first day; then 200 mg twice daily as needed.

Hepatic Impairment

PO (Adults): *Moderate hepatic impairment (Child-Pugh Class B)*—↓ dose by 50%.
PO (Children ≥2 yr, ≥10 kg–≤25 kg): *Juvenile rheumatoid arthritis*—50 mg twice daily.
PO (Children ≥2 yr, ≥25 kg): *Juvenile rheumatoid arthritis*—100 mg twice daily.

Availability (generic available)

Capsules: 50 mg, 100 mg, 200 mg, 400 mg. **Cost:** 100 mg $387.18/100, 200 mg $621.67/100, 400 mg $1,576.25/180. ***In combination with:*** amlodipine (Consensi). See Appendix B.

NURSING IMPLICATIONS

Assessment

- Assess range of motion, degree of swelling, and pain in affected joints before and periodically throughout therapy.
- Assess patient for allergy to sulfonamides, aspirin, or NSAIDs. Patients with these allergies should not receive celecoxib.
- Assess patient for skin rash frequently during therapy. Discontinue at first sign of rash; may be life-threatening. Stevens-Johnson syndrome may develop. Treat symptomatically; may recur once treatment is stopped.
- ***Lab Test Considerations:*** May cause ↑ AST and ALT levels.
- May cause hypophosphatemia, hyperkalemia, and ↑ BUN.

Implementation

- Do not confuse Celebrex (celecoxib) with Celexa (citalopram) or Cerebyx (fosphenytoin).
- **PO:** May be administered without regard to meals. Capsules may be opened and sprinkled on applesauce and ingested immediately with water. Mixture may be stored in the refrigerator for up to 6 hr.

Patient/Family Teaching

- Instruct patient to take celecoxib exactly as directed. Do not take more than prescribed dose. Increasing doses does not appear to increase effectiveness. Use lowest effective dose for shortest period of time. Advise patient to read *Medication Guide* before starting therapy and with each Rx refill in case of changes.
- Advise patient to notify health care professional promptly if signs or symptoms of GI toxicity (abdominal pain, black stools), cardiovascular effects (chest pain, shortness of breath, weakness, slurring of speech), skin rash, unexplained weight gain, or edema occurs. Patients should discontinue celecoxib and notify health care professional if signs and symptoms of hepatotoxicity (nausea, fatigue, lethargy, pruritus, jaundice, upper right quadrant tenderness, flu-like symptoms) occur.
- May cause hypertension. Instruct patient in correct technique for monitoring BP and to notify health care professional if significant changes occur.
- Rep: Advise patient to notify health care professional if pregnancy is planned or suspected or if breast feeding. Avoid celecoxib after 30 wk of gestation.

Evaluation/Desired Outcomes

- Reduction in joint pain in patients with osteoarthritis.
- Reduction in joint tenderness, pain, and joint swelling in patients with rheumatoid arthritis and juvenile rheumatoid arthritis.
- Decreased pain.
- Decreased pain with dysmenorrhea.

cephalexin, See CEPHALOSPORINS—FIRST GENERATION.

CEPHALOSPORINS—FIRST GENERATION

cefadroxil (sef-a-**drox**-ill)
~~Duricef~~

ceFAZolin (sef-**a**-zoe-lin)
~~Ancef~~

cephalexin (sef-a-**lex**-in)
Keflex

Classification
Therapeutic: anti-infectives
Pharmacologic: first-generation cephalosporins

Indications

Treatment of the following infections caused by susceptible organisms: Skin and skin structure infections (including burn wounds), Pneumonia, Urinary tract infections, Bone and joint infections, Septicemia. Not suitable for the treatment of meningitis. **Cefadroxil:** Pharyngitis and/or tonsillitis. **Cefazolin:** Perioperative prophylaxis, biliary tract infections, genital infections, bacterial endocarditis prophylaxis for dental and upper respiratory tract procedures. **Cephalexin:** Otitis media.

Action

Bind to bacterial cell wall membrane, causing cell death. **Therapeutic Effects:** Bactericidal action against susceptible bacteria. **Spectrum:** Active against many gram-positive cocci including: *Streptococcus pneumoniae*, Group A beta-hemolytic streptococci, Penicillinase-producing staphylococci. Not active against: Methicillin-resistant staphylococci, *Bacteroides fragilis*, *Enterococcus*. Active against some gram-negative rods including: *Klebsiella pneumoniae*, *Proteus mirabilis*, *Escherichia coli*.

Pharmacokinetics

Absorption: *Cefadroxil* and *cephalexin* are well absorbed following oral administration. *Cefazolin* is well absorbed following IM administration.
Distribution: Widely distributed. Cefazolin penetrates bone and synovial fluid well. All cross the placenta and enter breast milk in low concentrations. Minimal CSF penetration.
Metabolism and Excretion: Excreted almost entirely unchanged by the kidneys.
Half-life: *Cefadroxil*—60–120 min; *cefazolin*—90–150 min; *cephalexin*—50–80 min (all are ↑ in renal impairment).

TIME/ACTION PROFILE (blood levels)

ROUTE	ONSET	PEAK	DURATION
Cefadroxil PO	rapid	1.5–2 hr	12–24 hr
Cefazolin IM	rapid	0.5–2 hr	6–12 hr
Cefazolin IV	rapid	5 min	6–12 hr
Cephalexin PO	rapid	1 hr	6–12 hr

Contraindications/Precautions

Contraindicated in: Hypersensitivity to cephalosporins; Serious hypersensitivity to penicillins.
Use Cautiously in: Renal impairment (dosage ↓ and/or ↑ dosing interval recommended for: *cefadroxil* and *cephalexin*, if CCr ≤50 mL/min, and *cefazolin*, if CCr <30 mL/min; History of GI disease, especially colitis; Geri: Dose adjustment due to age-related ↓ in renal function may be necessary; OB, Lactation: Half-life is shorter and blood levels lower during pregnancy; have been used safely.

Adverse Reactions/Side Effects

CNS: SEIZURES (high doses). **GI:** CLOSTRIDIUM DIFFICILE-ASSOCIATED DIARRHEA (CDAD), diarrhea, nausea, vomiting, cramps. **Derm:** STEVENS-JOHNSON SYNDROME, rashes, pruritis, urticaria. **Hemat:** agranulocytosis, eosinophilia, hemolytic anemia, neutropenia, thrombocytopenia. **Local:** pain at IM site, phlebitis at IV site. **Misc:** allergic reactions including ANAPHYLAXIS and SERUM SICKNESS, superinfection.

Interactions

Drug-Drug: Probenecid ↓ excretion and ↑ blood levels of renally excreted cephalosporins. Concurrent use of **loop diuretics** or **aminoglycosides** may ↑ risk of renal toxicity.

Route/Dosage

Cefadroxil

PO (Adults): *Pharyngitis and tonsillitis*—500 mg every 12 hr or 1 g every 24 hr for 10 days. *Skin and soft-tissue infections*—500 mg every 12 hr or 1 g every 24 hr. *Urinary tract infections*—500 mg–1 g every 12 hr or 1–2 g every 24 hr.
PO (Children): *Pharyngitis, tonsillitis, or impetigo*—15 mg/kg every 12 hr or 30 mg/kg every 24 hr for 10 days. *Skin and soft-tissue infections*—15 mg/kg every 12 hr. *Urinary tract infections*—15 mg/kg every 12 hr.

Renal Impairment

PO (Adults): *CCr 25–50 mL/min*—500 mg every 12 hr; *CCr 10–25 mL/min*—500 mg every 24 hr; *CCr <10 mL/min*—500 mg every 36 hr.

Cefazolin

IM, IV (Adults): *Moderate to severe infections*—500 mg–2 g every 6–8 hr (maximum 12 g/day). *Mild infections with gram-positive cocci*—250–500 mg every 8 hr. *Uncomplicated urinary tract infections*—1 g every 12 hr. *Pneumococcal pneumonia*—500 mg every 12 hr. *Infective endocarditis or septicemia*—1–1.5 g every 6 hr. *Perioperative prophylaxis*—1 g given 30–60 min prior to incision. Additional 500 mg–1 g should be given for surgeries ≥2 hr. 500 mg–1 g should then be given for all surgeries every 6–8 hr for 24 hr postoperatively.
IM, IV (Children and Infants >1 mo): 16.7–33.3 mg/kg every 8 hr (maximum 6 g/day); *Bacterial endocarditis prophylaxis in penicillin-allergic patients:* 25 mg/kg 30 min prior to procedure (maximum dose = 1 g).
IM, IV (Neonates ≤7 days): 40 mg/kg/day divided every 12 hr.
IM, IV (Neonates >7 days and ≤2 kg): 40 mg/kg/day divided every 12 hr.
IM, IV (Neonates >7 days and >2 k g): 60 mg/kg/day divided every 8 hr.

Renal Impairment

IM, IV (Adults): *CCr 10–30 mL/min*—Administer every 12 hr; *CCr ≤10 mL/min*—Administer every 24 hr.

C

Cephalexin

PO (Adults): *Most infections*—250–500 mg every 6 hr. *Uncomplicated cystitis, skin and soft-tissue infections, streptococcal pharyngitis*—500 mg every 12 hr.
PO (Children): *Most infections*—25–50 mg/kg/day divided every 6–8 hr (can be administered every 12 hr in skin/skin structure infections or streptococcal pharyngitis). *Otitis media*—18.75–25 mg/kg every 6 hr (maximum = 4 g/day).

Renal Impairment

PO (Adults): *CCr 10–50 mL/min*—500 mg every 8–12 hr; *CCr <10 mL/min*—250–500 mg every 12–24 hr.

Availability

Cefadroxil (generic available)

Capsules: 500 mg. **Tablets:** 1 g. **Oral suspension (orange-pineapple flavor):** 250 mg/5 mL, 500 mg/5 mL.

Cefazolin (generic available)

Powder for injection: 500 mg/vial, 1 g/vial, 10 g/vial, 20 g/vial. **Premixed containers:** 1 g/50 mL D5W, 2 g/50 mL D5W.

Cephalexin (generic available)

Capsules: 250 mg, 500 mg, 750 mg. **Tablets:** 250 mg, 500 mg. **Oral suspension:** 125 mg/5 mL, 250 mg/5 mL.

NURSING IMPLICATIONS

Assessment

- Assess for infection (vital signs; appearance of wound, sputum, urine, and stool; WBC) at beginning and during therapy.
- Before initiating therapy, obtain a history to determine previous use of and reactions to penicillins or cephalosporins. Persons with a negative history of penicillin sensitivity may still have an allergic response.
- Obtain specimens for culture and sensitivity before initiating therapy. First dose may be given before receiving results.
- Observe patient for signs and symptoms of anaphylaxis (rash, pruritus, laryngeal edema, wheezing). Discontinue drug and notify health care professional immediately if these problems occur. Keep epinephrine, an antihistamine, and resuscitation equipment close by in case of an anaphylactic reaction.
- Monitor bowel function. Diarrhea, abdominal cramping, fever, and bloody stools should be reported to health care professional promptly as a sign of Clostridium difficile-associated diarrhea (CDAD). May begin up to several wk following cessation of therapy.
- Assess patient for skin rash frequently during therapy. Discontinue cephalosporins at first sign of rash; may be life-threatening. Stevens-Johnson syndrome or toxic epidermal necrolysis may develop. Treat symptomatically; may recur once treatment is stopped.
- ***Lab Test Considerations:*** May cause positive results for Coombs' test in patients receiving high doses or in neonates whose mothers were given cephalosporins before delivery.
- May cause ↑ serum AST, ALT, alkaline phosphatase, bilirubin, LDH, BUN, creatinine.
- May rarely cause leukopenia, neutropenia, agranulocytosis, thrombocytopenia, or eosinophilia.

Implementation

- Do not confuse cefazolin with cefotetan, cefoxitin, ceftazidime, or ceftriaxone. Do not confuse Keflex with Keppra.
- **PO:** Administer around the clock. May be administered on full or empty stomach. Administration with food may minimize GI irritation. Shake oral suspension well before administering. Use calibrated measuring device with liquid preparations. Refrigerate oral suspensions.

Cefazolin

- **IM:** Reconstitute IM doses with 2 mL or 2.5 mL of sterile water for injection to achieve a final concentration of 225–330 mg/mL.
- Inject deep into a well-developed muscle mass; massage well.

IV Administration

- **IV:** Monitor site frequently for thrombophlebitis (pain, redness, swelling). Change sites every 48–72 hr to prevent phlebitis.
- Do not use solutions that are cloudy or contain a precipitate.
- If aminoglycosides are administered concurrently, administer in separate sites, if possible, at least 1 hr apart. If second site is unavailable, flush line between medications.
- **IV Push:** ***Diluent:*** 0.9% NaCl, D5W, D10W, dextrose/saline combinations, D5/LR. ***Concentration:*** 100 mg/mL. May use up to 138 mg/mL in fluid-restricted patients. ***Rate:*** May administer over 3–5 min.
- **Intermittent Infusion:** ***Diluent:*** Reconstituted 500-mg or 1-g solution may be diluted in 50–100 mL of 0.9% NaCl, D5W, D10W, dextrose/saline combinations, D5/LR. Solution is stable for 24 hr at room temperature and 10 days if refrigerated. ***Concentration:*** 20 mg/mL. ***Rate:*** Administer over 10–60 min.
- **Y-Site Compatibility:** acyclovir, alfentanil, allopurinol, alprostadil, amifostine, aminocaproic acid, aminophylline, amphotericin B lipid complex, amphotericin B liposome, anidulafungin, argatroban, ascorbic acid, atracurium, atropine, azithromycin, aztreonam, benztropine, bivalirudin, bleomycin, bumetanide, buprenorphine, butorphanol, calcium gluconate, carboplatin, carmustine, cefotetan, cefoxitin, ceftazidime, ceftriaxone, cefuroxime, chloram-

pheniocol, cisplatin, clindamycin, cyanocobalamin, cyclophosphamide, cyclosporine, cytarabine, dactinomycin, daptomycin, dexamethasone, dexmedetomidine, digoxin, diltiazem, docetaxel, doxacurium, doxapram, doxorubicin liposome, enalaprilat, ephedrine, epinephrine, epirubicin, epoetin alfa, eptifibatide, esmolol, etoposide, etoposide phosphate, fenoldopam, fentanyl, filgrastim, fluconazole, fludarabine, fluorouracil, folic acid, foscarnet, furosemide, gemcitabine, glycopyrrolate, granisetron, heparin, hydrocortisone, ifosfamide, imipenem/cilastatin, indomethacin, insulin, irinotecan, isoproterenol, ketamine, ketorolac, leucovorin, lidocaine, linezolid, lorazepam, mannitol, melphalan, meperidine, metaraminol, methotrexate, methyldopate, methylprednisolone, metoclopramide, metoprolol, metronidazole, midazolam, milrinone, morphine, multivitamins, nafcillin, nalbuphine, naloxone, nicardipine, nitroglycerin, nitroprusside, norepinephrine, octreotide, ondansetron, oxacillin, oxaliplatin, oxytocin, paclitaxel, palonosetron, pamidronate, pancuronium, penicillin G, perphenazine, phenobarbital, phenylephrine, phytonadione, potassium acetate, potassium chloride, procainamide, propofol, propranolol, ranitidine, remifentanil, rituximab, sargramostim, sodium acetate, sodium bicarbonate, streptokinase, succinylcholine, sufentanil, tacrolimus, theophylline, thiamine, thiotepa, tigecycline, tirofiban, tolazoline, trastuzumab, vasopressin, vecuronium, verapamil, vinblastine, vincristine, vitamin B complex with C, voriconazole, warfarin, zoledronic acid.

- **Y-Site Incompatibility:** alemtuzumab, amphotericin B cholesteryl, azathioprine, calcium chloride, caspofungin, cefotaxime, chlorpromazine, dantrolene, diazepam, diazoxide, diphenhydramine, dobutamine, dolasetron, dopamine, doxorubicin hydrochloride, doxycycline, erythromycin, ganciclovir, haloperidol, hydralazine, hydroxyzine, idarubicin, levofloxacin, mitoxantrone, mycophenolate, papaverine, pemetrexed, pentamidine, pentobarbital, phentolamine, phenytoin, prochlorperazine, promethazine, protamine, pyridoxime, quinupristin/dalfopristin, sodium citrate, tobramycin, trimethoprim/sulfamethoxazole, vinorelbine.

Patient/Family Teaching

- Instruct patient to take medication around the clock at evenly spaced times and to finish the medication completely as directed, even if feeling better. Take missed doses as soon as possible unless almost time for next dose; do not double doses. Instruct parents or caregivers to use calibrated measuring device with liquid preparations. Advise patient that sharing this medication may be dangerous.
- Advise patient to report signs of superinfection (furry overgrowth on the tongue, vaginal itching or discharge, loose or foul-smelling stools) and allergy.
- Instruct patient to notify health care professional if rash, or fever and diarrhea develop, especially if diarrhea contains blood, mucus, or pus. Advise patient not to treat diarrhea without consulting health care professional.

Evaluation/Desired Outcomes

- Resolution of signs and symptoms of infection. Length of time for complete resolution depends on the organism and site of infection.
- Decreased incidence of infection when used for prophylaxis.

CEPHALOSPORINS—SECOND GENERATION

cefaclor (**sef**-a-klor)

cefoTEtan (sef-oh-**tee**-tan)
Cefotan

cefOXitin (se-**fox**-i-tin)
Mefoxin

cefprozil (sef-**proe**-zil)

cefuroxime (se-fyoor-**ox**-eem)
~~Ceftin~~, Zinacef

Classification
Therapeutic: anti-infectives
Pharmacologic: second-generation cephalosporins

Indications

Treatment of the following infections caused by susceptible organisms: Respiratory tract infections, Skin and skin structure infections, Bone and joint infections (not cefaclor or cefprozil), Urinary tract infections (not cefprozil). **Cefotetan and cefoxitin:** Intra-abdominal and gynecologic infections. **Cefuroxime:** Meningitis, gynecologic infections, and Lyme disease. **Cefaclor, cefprozil, cefuroxime:** Otitis media. **Cefoxitin and cefuroxime:** Septicemia. **Cefotetan, cefoxitin, cefuroxime:** Perioperative prophylaxis.

Action

Bind to bacterial cell wall membrane, causing cell death. **Therapeutic Effects:** Bactericidal action against susceptible bacteria. **Spectrum:** Similar to that of first-generation cephalosporins but have ↑ activity against several other gram-negative pathogens including: *Haemophilus influenzae*, *Escherichia coli*, *Klebsiella pneumoniae*, *Morganella morganii*, *Neisseria gonorrhoeae* (including penicillinase-producing strains), *Proteus*, *Providencia*, *Serratia marcescens*, *Moraxella catarrhalis*. Not active against methicillin-resistant staphylococci or enterococci. **Cefuroxime:** Active against *Borrelia burgdorferi*. **Cefotetan and cefoxitin:** Active against *Bacteroides fragilis*.

Pharmacokinetics

Absorption: *Cefotetan*, *cefoxitin*, and *cefuroxime*—well absorbed following IM administration. *Cef-*

aclor, cefprozil, and *cefuroxime*—well absorbed following oral administration.
Distribution: Widely distributed. Penetration into CSF is poor, but adequate for cefuroxime (IV) to be used in treating meningitis. All cross the placenta and enter breast milk in low concentrations.
Metabolism and Excretion: Excreted primarily unchanged by the kidneys.
Half-life: *Cefaclor*—30–60 min; *cefotetan*—3–4.6 hr; *cefoxitin*—40–60 min; *cefprozil*—90 min; *cefuroxime*—60–120 min (all are ↑ in renal impairment).

TIME/ACTION PROFILE

ROUTE	ONSET	PEAK	DURATION
Cefaclor PO	rapid	30–60 min	6–12 hr
Cefaclor PO-CD	unknown	unknown	12 hr
Cefotetan IM	rapid	1–3 hr	12 hr
Cefotetan IV	rapid	end of infusion	12 hr
Cefoxitin IM	rapid	30 min	4–8 hr
Cefoxitin IV	rapid	end of infusion	4–8 hr
Cefprozil PO	unknown	1–2 hr	12–24 hr
Cefuroxime PO	unknown	2–3 hr	8–12 hr
Cefuroxime IM	rapid	15–60 min	6–12 hr
Cefuroxime IV	rapid	end of infusion	6–12 hr

Contraindications/Precautions
Contraindicated in: Hypersensitivity to cephalosporins; Serious hypersensitivity to penicillins.
Use Cautiously in: Renal impairment (↓ dose/↑ dosing interval recommended for: *cefotetan* if CCr ≤30 mL/min, *cefoxitin* if CCr ≤50 mL/min, *cefprozil* if CCr <30 mL/min, *cefuroxime* if CCr <30 mL/min); Patients with hepatic dysfunction, poor nutritional state, or cancer may be at ↑ risk for bleeding; History of GI disease, especially colitis; *Cefprozil (oral suspension)* contains aspartame and should be avoided in patients with phenylketonuria; Geri: Dose adjustment due to age-related ↓ in renal function may be necessary; may also be at ↑ risk for bleeding with *cefotetan* or *cefoxitin*; OB, Lactation: Have been used safely.

Adverse Reactions/Side Effects
CNS: SEIZURES (high doses). **Derm:** rash, urticaria. **GI:** CLOSTRIDIUM DIFFICILE-ASSOCIATED DIARRHEA (CDAD), diarrhea, cramps, nausea, vomiting. **Hemat:** agranulocytosis, bleeding (↑ with cefotetan and cefoxitin), eosinophilia, hemolytic anemia, neutropenia, thrombocytopenia. **Local:** pain at IM site, phlebitis at IV site. **Misc:** HYPERSENSITIVITY REACTIONS (including anaphylaxis and serum sickness), superinfection.

Interactions
Drug-Drug: Probenecid ↓ excretion and ↑ blood levels. If **alcohol** is ingested within 48–72 hr of cefotetan, a disulfiram-like reaction may occur. Cefotetan may ↑ risk of bleeding with **anticoagulants**, **antiplatelet agents**, **thrombolytics**, and **NSAIDs**. **Antacids** ↓ absorption of cefaclor. Concurrent use of **aminoglycosides** or **loop diuretics** may ↑ risk of nephrotoxicity.

Route/Dosage
Cefaclor
PO (Adults): 250–500 mg every 8 hr or 375–500 mg every 12 hr as extended-release tablets.
PO (Children >1 mo): 6.7–13.4 mg/kg every 8 hr or 10–20 mg/kg every 12 hr (up to 1 g/day).

Cefotetan
IM, IV (Adults): *Most infections*—1–2 g every 12 hr. *Severe/life-threatening infections*—2–3 g every 12 hr. *Urinary tract infections*—500 mg–2 g every 12 hr *or* 1–2 g every 24 hr. *Perioperative prophylaxis*—1–2 g 30–60 min before initial incision (one-time dose).

Renal Impairment
IM, IV (Adults): *CCr 10–30 mL/min*—Usual adult dose every 24 hr *or* ½ usual adult dose every 12 hr; *CCr <10 mL/min*—Usual adult dose every 48 hr *or* ¼ usual adult dose every 12 hr.

Cefoxitin
IM, IV (Adults): *Most infections*—1 g every 6–8 hr. *Severe infections*—1 g every 4 hr *or* 2 g every 6–8 hr. *Life-threatening infections*—2 g every 4 hr *or* 3 g every 6 hr. *Perioperative prophylaxis*—2 g 30–60 min before initial incision, then 2 g every 6 hr for up to 24 hr.
IM, IV (Children and Infants >3 mo): *Most infections*—13.3–26.7 mg/kg every 4 hr *or* 20–40 mg/kg every 6 hr. *Perioperative prophylaxis*—30–40 mg/kg within 60 min of initial incision, then 30–40 mg/kg every 6 hr for up to 24 hr.

Renal Impairment
IM, IV (Adults): *CCr 30–50 mL/min*—1–2 g every 8–12 hr; *CCr 10–29 mL/min*—1–2 g every 12–24 hr; *CCr 5–9 mL/min*—0.5–1 g every 12–24 hr; *CCr <5 mL/min*—0.5–1 g every 24–48 hr.

Cefprozil
PO (Adults): *Most infections*—250–500 mg every 12 hr *or* 500 mg every 24 hr.
PO (Children 6 mo–12 yr): *Otitis media*—15 mg/kg every 12 hr. *Acute sinusitis*—7.5–15 mg/kg every 12 hr (higher dose should be used for moderate-to-severe infections).

PO (Children 2–12 yr): *Pharyngitis/tonsillitis*—7.5 mg/kg every 12 hr. *Skin/skin structure infections*—20 mg/kg every 24 hr.

Renal Impairment

PO (Adults and Children ≥6 mo): *CCr <30 mL/min*—½ of usual dose at normal dosing interval.

Cefuroxime

PO (Adults and Children >12 yr): *Pharyngitis/tonsillitis, maxillary sinusitis, uncomplicated UTIs*—250 mg every 12 hr. *Bronchitis, uncomplicated skin/skin structure infections*—250–500 mg every 12 hr. *Gonorrhea*—1 g (single dose). *Lyme disease*—500 mg every 12 hr for 20 days.
PO (Children 3 mo–12 yr): *Otitis media, acute bacterial maxillary sinusitis, impetigo*—250 mg every 12 hr.
IM, IV (Adults): *Uncomplicated urinary tract infections, skin/skin structure infections, disseminated gonococcal infections, uncomplicated pneumonia*—750 mg every 8 hr. *Bone/joint infections, severe or complicated infections*—1.5 g every 8 hr. *Life-threatening infections*—1.5 g every 6 hr. *Meningitis*—3 g every 8 hr. *Perioperative prophylaxis*—1.5 g IV 30–60 min before initial incision; 750 mg IM/IV every 8 hr can be given when procedure prolonged. *Prophylaxis during open-heart surgery*—1.5 g IV at induction of anesthesia and then every 12 hr for 3 additional doses. *Gonorrhea*—1.5 g IM (750 mg in two sites) with 1 g probenecid PO.
IM, IV (Children and Infants >3 mo): *Most infections*—12.5–25 mg/kg every 6 hr *or* 16.7–33.3 mg/kg every 8 hr (max dose = 6 g/day). *Bone and joint infections*—50 mg/kg every 8 hr (max dose = 6 g/day). *Bacterial meningitis*—50–60 mg/kg every 6 hr *or* 66.7–80 mg/kg every 8 hr.

Renal Impairment

IM, IV (Adults): *CCr 10–29 mL/min*—Give standard dose every 24 hr; *CCr <10 mL/min (no hemodialysis)*—Give standard dose every 48 hr; *Hemodialysis*—Give an additional dose at end of each dialysis session.

Availability

Cefaclor (generic available)

Capsules: 250 mg, 500 mg. **Extended-release tablets:** 375 mg, 500 mg. **Oral suspension (strawberry):** 125 mg/5 mL, 187 mg/5 mL, 250 mg/5 mL, 375 mg/5 mL.

Cefotetan (generic available)

Powder for injection (requires reconstitution and dilution): 1 g/vial, 2 g/vial, 10 g/vial. **Premixed infusion:** 1 g/50 mL, 2 g/50 mL.

Cefoxitin (generic available)

Powder for injection (requires reconstitution and dilution): 1 g/vial, 2 g/vial, 10 g/vial. **Premixed infusion:** 1 g/50 mL D5W, 2 g/50 mL D5W.

Cefprozil (generic available)

Oral suspension (bubblegum flavor): 125 mg/5 mL, 250 mg/5 mL. **Tablets:** 250 mg, 500 mg.

Cefuroxime (generic available)

Powder for injection (requires reconstitution and dilution): 750 mg/vial, 1.5 g/vial, 7.5 g/vial. **Premixed infusion:** 750 mg/50 mL, 1.5 g/50 mL. **Tablets:** 250 mg, 500 mg.

NURSING IMPLICATIONS

Assessment

- Assess for infection (vital signs; appearance of wound, sputum, urine, and stool; WBC) at beginning and during therapy.
- Before initiating therapy, obtain a history to determine previous use of and reactions to penicillins or cephalosporins. Persons with a negative history of penicillin sensitivity may still have an allergic response.
- Obtain specimens for culture and sensitivity before initiating therapy. First dose may be given before receiving results.
- Observe patient for signs and symptoms of anaphylaxis (rash, pruritus, laryngeal edema, wheezing). Discontinue the drug immediately if these symptoms occur. Keep epinephrine, an antihistamine, and resuscitation equipment close by in the event of an anaphylactic reaction.
- Monitor bowel function. Diarrhea, abdominal cramping, fever, and bloody stools should be reported to health care professional promptly as a sign of Clostridium difficile-associated diarrhea (CDAD). May begin up to several wk following cessation of therapy.
- ***Lab Test Considerations:*** May cause positive results for Coombs' test in patients receiving high doses or in neonates whose mothers were given cephalosporins before delivery.
- *Cefotetan*—monitor prothrombin time and assess patient for bleeding (guaiac stools; check for hematuria, bleeding gums, ecchymosis) daily in high-risk patients; may cause hypoprothrombinemia.
- May cause ↑ serum AST, ALT, alkaline phosphatase, bilirubin, LDH, BUN, and serum creatinine.
- *Cefoxitin* may cause falsely ↑ test results for serum and urine creatinine; do not obtain serum samples within 2 hr of administration.
- May rarely cause leukopenia, neutropenia, agranulocytosis, thrombocytopenia, and eosinophilia.

Implementation

- Do not confuse cefotetan with cefazolin, cefoxitin, ceftazidime, or ceftriaxone.
- **PO:** Administer around the clock. May be administered on full or empty stomach. Administration with food may minimize GI irritation. Shake oral suspension well before administering.
- Administer cefaclor extended-release tablets with food; do not crush, break, or chew.

- Do not administer *cefaclor* within 1 hr of antacids.
- *Cefuroxime* tablets should be swallowed whole, not crushed; crushed tablets have a strong, persistent bitter taste. Tablets may be taken without regard to meals.
- **IM:** Reconstitute IM doses with sterile or bacteriostatic water for injection or 0.9% NaCl for injection. May be diluted with lidocaine to minimize injection discomfort.
- Inject deep into a well-developed muscle mass; massage well.

IV Administration

- **IV:** Change sites every 48–72 hr to prevent phlebitis. Monitor site frequently for thrombophlebitis (pain, redness, swelling).
- If aminoglycosides are administered concurrently, administer in separate sites if possible, at least 1 hr apart. If second site is unavailable, flush line between medications.
- **IV Push:** Dilute each cephalosporin in at least 1 g/10 mL. Do not use preparations containing benzyl alcohol for neonates. ***Rate:*** Administer slowly over 3–5 min.

Cefotetan

- **Intermittent Infusion: *Diluent:*** Reconstituted solution may be further diluted in 50–100 mL of D5W or 0.9% NaCl. Solution may be colorless or yellow. Solution is stable for 24 hr at room temperature or 96 hr if refrigerated. ***Concentration:*** 10–40 mg/mL. ***Rate:*** Administer over 20–30 min.
- **Y-Site Compatibility:** acyclovir, alfentanil, allopurinol, amifostine, aminocaproic acid, aminophylline, amphotericin B lipid complex, anidulafungin, argatroban, ascorbic acid, atropine, azithromycin, aztreonam, benztropine, bivalirudin, bleomycin, bumetanide, buprenorphine, butorphanol, calcium chloride, calcium gluconate, carboplatin, carmustine, cefazolin, cefotaxime, cefoxitin, ceftriaxone, cefuroxime, chloramphenicol, cisplatin, clindamycin, cyanocobalamin, cyclophosphamide, cyclosporine, cytarabine, dacarbazine, dactinomycin, daptomycin, dexamethasone, dexmedetomidine, dexrazoxane, digoxin, diltiazem, docetaxel, dopamine, doxorubicin liposomal, enalaprilat, ephedrine, epinephrine, epoetin alfa, eptifibatide, etoposide, etoposide phosphate, fenoldopam, fentanyl, filgrastim, fluconazole, fludarabine, fluorouracil, folic acid, foscarnet, fosphenytoin, furosemide, gemcitabine, glycopyrrolate, granisetron, heparin, hetastarch, hydrocortisone, hydromorphone, ifosfamide, imipenem/cilastatin, irinotecan, isoproterenol, ketorolac, leucovorin, levofloxacin, lidocaine, linezolid, lorazepam, magnesium sulfate, mannitol, melphalan, methotrexate, methylprednisolone, metoclopramide, metoprolol, metronidazole, milrinone, mitoxantrone, morphine, multivitamins, nafcillin, nalbuphine, naloxone, nitroglycerin, nitroprusside, norepinephrine, octreotide, oxacillin, oxaliplatin, oxytocin, paclitaxel, palonosetron, pamidronate, pancuronium, penicillin G, phenylephrine, phytonadione, potassium acetate, potassium chloride, procainamide, propofol, propranolol, pyridoxine, ranitidine, remifentanil, rituximab, rocuronium, sargramostim, sodium acetate, streptokinase, succinylcholine, sufentanil, tacrolimus, theophylline, thiamine, thiotepa, tigecycline, tirofiban, topotecan, vasopressin, vecuronium, verapamil, vinblastine, vincristine, voriconazole, zoledronic acid.
- **Y-Site Incompatibility:** alemtuzumab, amiodarone, amphotericin B colloidal, amphotericin B liposome, azathioprine, caspofungin, chlorpromazine, dantrolene, daunorubicin hydrochloride, diazepam, diphenhydramine, dobutamine, dolasetron, doxorubicin hydrochloride, doxycycline, epirubicin, erythromycin, esmolol, ganciclovir, gentamicin, haloperidol, hydralazine, hydroxyzine, idarubicin, indomethacin, labetalol, minocycline, mitomycin, mycophenolate, pantoprazole, papaverine, pemetrexed, pentamidine, pentobarbital, phenobarbital, phentolamine, phenytoin, prochlorperazine, promethazine, protamine, quinupristin/dalfopristin, sodium bicarbonate, tobramycin, trastuzumab, trimethoprim/sulfamethoxazole, vinorelbine.

Cefoxitin

- **Intermittent Infusion: *Diluent:*** Reconstituted solution may be further diluted in 50–100 mL of D5W, D10W, 0.9% NaCl, dextrose/saline combinations, D5/LR, Ringer's or LR. Stable for 24 hr at room temperature and 1 wk if refrigerated. Darkening of powder does not alter potency. ***Concentration:*** 40 mg/mL. ***Rate:*** Administer over 30–60 min.
- **Continuous Infusion:** May be diluted in 500–1000 mL for continuous infusion.
- **Y-Site Compatibility:** acetaminophen, acyclovir, alfentanil, amifostine, aminocaproic acid, aminophylline, amphotericin B lipid complex, amphotericin B liposome, anidulafungin, argatroban, ascorbic acid, atropine, azithromycin, aztreonam, benztropine, bivalirudin, bleomycin, bumetanide, buprenorphine, butorphanol, calcium chloride, calcium gluconate, cangrelor, carboplatin, carmustine, cefazolin, cefotaxime, cefotetan, ceftazidime, ceftriaxone, cefuroxime, chloramphenicol, cisplatin, clindamycin, cyanocobalamin, cyclophosphamide, cyclosporine, cytarabine, dacarbazine, dactinomycin, daptomycin, dexamethasone, dexmedetomidine, dexrazoxane, digoxin, diltiazem, docetaxel, dopamine, doxorubicin liposome, enalaprilat, ephedrine, epinephrine, epoetin alfa, eptifibatide, esmolol, etoposide, etoposide phosphate, fentanyl, fluconazole,

fludarabine, fluorouracil, folic acid, foscarnet, fosphenytoin, furosemide, gemcitabine, glycopyrrolate, granisetron, heparin, hydrocortisone, hydromorphone, ifosfamide, imipenem/cilastatin, indomethacin, irinotecan, isoproterenol, ketorolac, leucovorin, lidocaine, linezolid, lorazepam, magnesium sulfate, mannitol, meperidine, mesna, methotrexate, metoclopramide, metoprolol, metronidazole, midazolam, milrinone, mitomycin, morphine, multivitamins, nafcillin, nalbuphine, naloxone, nitroglycerin, nitroprusside, norepinephrine, octreotide, ondansetron, oxacillin, oxaliplatin, oxytocin, paclitaxel, palonosetron, pamidronate, pantoprazole, penicillin G, phenylephrine, phytonadione, potassium acetate, potassium chloride, procainamide, propofol, propranolol, pyridoxine, ranitidine, remifentanil, rituximab, rocuronium, sodium acetate, streptokinase, succinylcholine, sufentanil, tacrolimus, theophylline, thiamine, thiotepa, tigecycline, tirofiban, topotecan, vasopressin, vecuronium, verapamil, vinblastine, vincristine, voriconazole, zoledronic acid.

- **Y-Site Incompatibility:** alemtuzumab, azathioprine, caspofungin, chlorpromazine, dantrolene, daunorubicin, diazepam, diazoxide, diphenhydramine, dobutamine, dolasetron, doxorubicin hydrochloride, doxycycline, epirubicin, erythromycin, fenoldopam, filgrastim, ganciclovir, haloperidol, hydralazine, hydroxyzine, idarubicin, insulin, labetalol, levofloxacin, methylprednisolone, minocycline, mitoxantrone, mycophenolate, papaverine, pemetrexed, pentamidine, pentobarbital, phenobarbital, phentolamine, phenytoin, prochlorperazine, promethazine, protamine, quinupristin/dalfopristin, sodium bicarbonate, trastuzumab, trimethoprim/sulfamethoxazole, vinorelbine.

Cefuroxime

- **IV Push:** Reconstitute 750 mg vial with 8.3 mL, 1.5 g vial with 16 mL, and 7.5 g vial with 77 mL of sterile water for injection, respectively. Do not use preparations containing benzyl alcohol for neonates. ***Rate:*** Administer slowly over 3–5 min.
- **Intermittent Infusion:** ***Diluent:*** Dilute further in 50–100 mL of 0.9% NaCl, D5W, or 0.45% NaCl. Stable for 24 hr at room temperature and 7 days if refrigerated. ***Concentration:*** 10–40 mg/mL. ***Rate:*** Administer over 15–60 min.
- **Continuous Infusion:** May also be diluted in 500–1000 mL 0.9% NaCl, D5W, D10W, D5/0.9% NaCl, D5/.45 NaCl, or 1/6 M Sodium Lactate Injection for continuous infusion.
- **Y-Site Compatibility:** acyclovir, alfentanil, allopurinol, amifostine, aminocaproic acid, aminophylline, amphotericin B lipid complex, amphotericin B liposome, anidulafungin, argatroban, arsenic trioxide, ascorbic acid, atracurium, atropine, aztreonam, benztropine, bivalirudin, bleomycin, bumetanide, buprenorphine, butorphanol, calcium gluconate, cangrelor, carboplatin, carmustine, cefazolin, cefotaxime, cefotetan, cefoxitin, ceftazidime, ceftolozane/tazobactam, ceftriaxone, chloramphenicol, cisplatin, clindamycin, cyclophosphamide, cyanocobalamin, cyclophosphamide, cyclosporine, cytarabine, dacarbazine, dactinomycin, daptomycin, dexmedetomidine, dexrazoxane, digoxin, diltiazem, docetaxel, dopamine, doxorubicin liposomal, enalaprilat, ephedrine, epinephrine, epoetin alfa, eptifibatide, erythromycin, esmolol, etoposide, etoposide phosphate, famotidine, fenoldopam, fentanyl, fludarabine, fluorouracil, folic acid, foscarnet, fosphenytoin, furosemide, gemcitabine, gemtuzumab, glycopyrrolate, granisetron, heparin, hetastarch, hydrocortisone, hydromorphone, ifosfamide, imipenem/cilastatin, indomethacin, insulin, regular, irinotecan, isoproterenol, ketamine, ketorolac, leucovorin calcium, levofloxacin, lidocaine, linezolid, lorazepam, mannitol, melphalan, meperidine, meropenem/vaborbactam, mesna, metaraminol, methotrexate, methyldopate, methylprednisolone, metoclopramide, metoprolol, milrinone, morphine, multivitamins, nafcillin, nalbuphine, naloxone, nitroglycerin, nitroprusside, norepinephrine, octreotide, ondansetron, oxacillin, oxaliplatin, oxytocin, paclitaxel, palonosetron, pamidronate, pancuronium, pemetrexed, penicillin G, perphenazine, phenylephrine, phytonadione, potassium acetate, potassium chloride, procainamide, propofol, propranolol, pyridoxine, ranitidine, remifentanil, rituximab, rocuronium, sargramostim, sodium acetate, streptokinase, succinylcholine, sufentanil, tacrolimus, tedizolid, theophylline, thiamine, thiotepa, tigecycline, tirofiban, topotecan, trastuzumab, vasopressin, vecuronium, verapamil, vinblastine, vincristine, voriconazole, zoledronic acid.
- **Y-Site Incompatibility:** alemtuzumab, azathioprine, calcium chloride, caspofungin, chlorpromazine, dantrolene, daunorubicin, daunorubicin, dexamethasone, diazepam, diphenhydramine, dobutamine, dolasetron, doxorubicin hydrochloride, doxycycline, epirubicin, filgrastim, ganciclovir, haloperidol, hydralazine, hydroxyzine, idarubicin, isavuconazonium, labetalol, magnesium sulfate, midazolam, minocycline, mitomycin, mitoxantrone, mycophenolate, nicardipine, papaverine, pentamidine, penatzocine, pentobarbital, phenobarbital, phentolamine, phenytoin, prochlorperazine, promethazine, protamine, quinupristin/dalfopristin, sodium bicarbonate, trimethoprim/sulfamethoxazole, vinorelbine.

Patient/Family Teaching

- Instruct patient to take medication around the clock at evenly spaced times and to finish the medication completely, even if feeling better. Take missed doses as soon as possible unless almost time for next dose; do not double doses. Use calibrated measuring device with liquid preparations. Advise patient that sharing of this medication may be dangerous.

- Advise patient to report signs of superinfection (furry overgrowth on the tongue, vaginal itching or discharge, loose or foul-smelling stools) and allergy.
- Caution patients that concurrent use of alcohol with *cefotetan* may cause a disulfiram-like reaction (abdominal cramps, nausea, vomiting, headache, hypotension, palpitations, dyspnea, tachycardia, sweating, flushing). Alcohol and alcohol-containing medications should be avoided during and for several days after therapy.
- Instruct patient to notify health care professional if fever and diarrhea develop, especially if stool contains blood, pus, or mucus. Advise patient not to treat diarrhea without consulting health care professional.
- Advise females of reproductive potential to notify health care professional if pregnancy is planned or suspected, or if breast feeding.

Evaluation/Desired Outcomes

- Resolution of signs and symptoms of infection. Length of time for complete resolution depends on the organism and site of infection.
- Decreased incidence of infection when used for prophylaxis.

CEPHALOSPORINS—THIRD GENERATION

cefdinir (**sef**-di-nir)
~~Omnicef~~

cefditoren (sef-dye-**tor**-en)
Spectracef

cefixime (sef-**ik**-seem)
Suprax

cefotaxime (sef-oh-**taks**-eem)
~~Claforan~~

cefpodoxime (sef-poe-**dox**-eem)
~~Vantin~~

cefTAZidime (sef-**tay**-zi-deem)
Fortaz, Tazicef

cefTRIAXone (sef-try-**ax**-one)
~~Rocephin~~

Classification
Therapeutic: anti-infectives
Pharmacologic: third-generation cephalosporins

Indications

Treatment of the following infections caused by susceptible organisms: Skin and skin structure infections (not cefixime), Urinary and gynecologic infections (not cefdinir or cefditoren), Respiratory tract infections (not cefdinir or cefditoren). **Cefotaxime, ceftazidime, ceftriaxone:** Meningitis and bone/joint infections. **Cefotaxime, ceftazidime, ceftriaxone:** Intra-abdominal infections and septicemia. **Cefdinir, cefixime, cefpodoxime, ceftriaxone:** Otitis media. **Cefotaxime, ceftriaxone:** Perioperative prophylaxis. **Ceftazidime:** Febrile neutropenia. **Cefotaxime, ceftriaxone:** Lyme disease.

Action

Bind to the bacterial cell wall membrane, causing cell death. **Therapeutic Effects:** Bactericidal action against susceptible bacteria. **Spectrum:** Similar to that of second-generation cephalosporins, but activity against staphylococci is less, whereas activity against gram-negative pathogens is greater, even for organisms resistant to first- and second-generation agents. Notable is increased action against: *Enterobacter, Haemophilus influenzae, Escherichia coli, Klebsiella pneumoniae, Neisseria gonorrhoeae, Citrobacter, Morganella, Proteus, Providencia, Serratia, Moraxella catarrhalis, Borrelia burgdorferi*. Some agents have activity against *N. meningitidis* (cefotaxime, ceftazidime, ceftriaxone). Some agents have enhanced activity against *Pseudomonas aeruginosa* (ceftazidime). Not active against methicillin-resistant staphylococci or enterococci. Some agents have activity against anaerobes, including *Bacteroides fragilis* (cefotaxime, ceftriaxone).

Pharmacokinetics

Absorption: *Cefotaxime, ceftazidime,* and *ceftriaxone* are well absorbed after IM administration. *Cefixime* 40–50% absorbed after oral administration (oral suspension); *cefdinir* 16–25% absorbed after oral administration. *Cefditoren pivoxil* and *cefpodoxime proxetil* are prodrugs that are converted to their active components in GI tract during absorption (*cefditoren*—14% absorbed [↑ by high-fat meal] *cefpodoxime*—50% absorbed).

Distribution: Widely distributed. Cross the placenta; enter breast milk in low concentrations. CSF penetration better than with first- and second-generation agents.

Protein Binding: *Ceftriaxone* ≥90%.

Metabolism and Excretion: *Cefdinir, ceftazidime,* and *cefditoren*—>85% excreted in urine. *Cefpodoxime*—30% excreted in urine. *Ceftriaxone* and *cefotaxime*—partly metabolized and partly excreted in the urine. *Cefixime*—50% excreted unchanged in urine, ≥10% in bile.

Half-life: *Cefdinir*—1.7 hr; *cefditoren*—1.6 hr; *cefixime*—3–4 hr; *cefotaxime*—1–1.5 hr; *cefpodoxime*—2–3 hr; *ceftazidime*—2 hr; *ceftriaxone*—6–9 hr (all except *ceftriaxone* are ↑ in renal impairment).

TIME/ACTION PROFILE

ROUTE	ONSET	PEAK	DURATION
Cefdinir PO	rapid	2–4 hr	12–24 hr
Cefditoren PO	rapid	1.5–3 hr	12 hr
Cefixime PO	rapid	2–6 hr	24 hr
Cefotaxime IM	rapid	0.5 hr	4–12 hr
Cefotaxime IV	rapid	end of infusion	4–12 hr
Cefpodoxime PO	unknown	2–3 hr	12 hr
Ceftazidime IM	rapid	1 hr	6–12 hr
Ceftazidime IV	rapid	end of infusion	6–12 hr
Ceftriaxone IM	rapid	1–2 hr	12–24 hr
Ceftriaxone IV	rapid	end of infusion	12–24 hr

Contraindications/Precautions

Contraindicated in: Hypersensitivity to cephalosporins; Serious hypersensitivity to penicillins; Pedi: Premature neonates up to a postmenstrual age of 41 wk (ceftriaxone only); Pedi: Hyperbilirubinemic neonates (may lead to bilirubin encephalopathy); Pedi: Neonates ≤28 days requiring calcium-containing IV solutions (↑ risk of precipitation formation); Carnitine deficiency or inborn errors of metabolism (cefditoren only); Hypersensitivity to milk protein (ceftidoren only; contains sodium caseinate).

Use Cautiously in: Renal impairment (↓ dosing/↑ dosing interval recommended for: *cefdinir* if CCr <30 mL/min, *cefixime* if CCr ≤60 mL/min, *cefotaxime* if CCr <20 mL/min, *cefpodoxime* if CCr <30 mL/min, *ceftazidime* if CCr ≤50 mL/min, *cefditoren* if CCr <50 mL/min); Combined severe hepatic and renal impairment (dose ↓/↑ dosing interval recommended for *ceftriaxone*); Diabetes (*cefdinir* suspension contain sucrose); Phenylketonuria (*cefixime* chewable tablets contain aspartame); History of GI disease, especially colitis; OB, Lactation: Have been used safely; Pedi: ↑ risk of urolithiasis and acute renal failure (ceftriaxone only); Geri: Dose adjustment due to age-related ↓ in renal function may be necessary.

Adverse Reactions/Side Effects

CNS: SEIZURES (high doses), headache. **Derm:** STEVENS-JOHNSON SYNDROME, rash, urticaria. **GI:** *Clostridium difficile*-ASSOCIATED DIARRHEA, diarrhea, nausea, vomiting, cholelithiasis (ceftriaxone), cramps, pancreatitis (ceftriaxone). **GU:** acute renal failure (ceftriaxone), hematuria, urolithiasis (ceftriaxone), vaginal moniliasis. **Hemat:** agranulocytosis, bleeding, eosinophilia, hemolytic anemia, lymphocytosis, neutropenia, thrombocytopenia, thrombocytosis. **Local:** pain at IM site, phlebitis at IV site. **Misc:** HYPERSENSITIVITY REACTIONS (including anaphylaxis and serum sickness), superinfection.

Interactions

Drug-Drug: Probenecid ↓ excretion and ↑ serum levels (cefdinir, cefditoren, cefixime, cefotaxime, cefpodoxime, ceftriaxone). Concurrent use of **loop diuretics, aminoglycosides**, or **NSAIDs** may ↑ risk of nephrotoxicity. **Antacids** ↓ absorption of cefdinir, cefditoren, and cefpodoxime. **Iron supplements** ↓ absorption of cefdinir. **H_2-receptor antagonists** ↓ absorption of cefditoren and cefpodoxime. Cefixime may ↑ **carbamazepine** levels. Ceftriaxone should not be administered concomitantly with any calcium-containing solutions. Ceftriaxone may ↑ risk of bleeding with **warfarin**.

Route/Dosage

Cefdinir

PO (Adults ≥13 yr): 300 mg every 12 hr *or* 600 mg every 24 hr (use every 12 hr dosing only for community-acquired pneumonia or skin and skin structure infections).

PO (Children 6 mo–12 yr): 7 mg/kg every 12 hr (use only for skin/skin structure infections) *or* 14 mg/kg every 24 hr; dose should not exceed 600 mg/day.

Renal Impairment

PO (Adults and Children ≥13 yr): *CCr <30 mL/min*—300 mg every 24 hr.

Renal Impairment

PO (Children 6 mo–12 yr): *CCr <30 mL/min*—7 mg/kg every 24 hr.

Cefditoren

PO (Adults and Children ≥12 yr): *Pharyngitis/tonsillitis, skin/skin structure infections*—200 mg twice daily; *Acute bacterial exacerbation of chronic bronchitis or community acquired pneumonia*—400 mg twice daily.

Renal Impairment

PO (Adults): *CCr 30–49 mL/min*—dose should not exceed 200 mg twice daily; *CCr <30 mL/min*—dose should not exceed 200 mg once daily.

Cefixime

PO (Adults and Children >12 yr or >50 kg): *Most infections*—400 mg once daily; *Gonorrhea*—400 mg single dose.

PO (Children): 8 mg/kg once daily *or* 4 mg/kg every 12 h.

Renal Impairment

PO (Adults): *CCr 21–60 mL/min*—75% of standard dose once daily; *CCr ≤20 mL/min*—50% of standard dose once daily.

Cefotaxime

IM, IV (Adults and Children >12 yr): *Most uncomplicated infections*—1 g every 12 hr. *Moderate or severe infections*—1–2 g every 6–8 hr. *Life-threatening infections*—2 g every 4 hr (maximum dose = 12

g/day). *Gonococcal urethritis/cervicitis or rectal gonorrhea in females*—500 mg IM (single dose). *Rectal gonorrhea in males*—1 g IM (single dose). *Perioperative prophylaxis*—1 g 30–90 min before initial incision (one-time dose).
IM, IV (Children 1 mo–12 yr): *<50 kg*—100–200 mg/kg/day divided every 6–8 hr. *Meningitis*—200 mg/kg/day divided every 6 hr. *Invasive pneumococcal meningitis*—225–300 mg/kg/day divided every 6–8 hr. *≥50 kg*—see adult dosing.
IV (Neonates 1–4 wk): 50 mg/kg every 6–8 hr.
IV (Neonates ≤1 wk): 50 mg/kg every 8–12 hr.

Renal Impairment
(Adults): *CCr <20 mL/min*—↓ dose by 50%.

Cefpodoxime
PO (Adults): *Most infections*—200 mg every 12 hr. *Skin and skin structure infections*—400 mg every 12 hr. *Urinary tract infections/pharyngitis*—100 mg every 12 hr. *Gonorrhea*—200 mg single dose.
PO (Children 2 mo–12 yr): *Pharyngitis/tonsillitis/otitis media/acute maxillary sinusitis*—5 mg/kg every 12 hr (not to exceed 200 mg/dose).

Renal Impairment
PO (Adults): *CCr <30 mL/min*—↑ dosing interval to every 24 hr.

Ceftazidime
IM, IV (Adults and Children ≥12 yr): *Pneumonia and skin/skin structure infections*—500 mg–1 g every 8 hr. *Bone and joint infections*—2 g every 12 hr. *Severe and life-threatening infections*—2 g every 8 hr. *Complicated urinary tract infections*—500 mg every 8–12 hr. *Uncomplicated urinary tract infections*—250 mg every 12 hr. *Cystic fibrosis lung infection caused by* P. aeruginosa—30–50 mg/kg every 8 hr (maximum dose = 6 g/day).
IM, IV (Children 1 mo–12 yr): 33.3–50 mg/kg every 8 hr (maximum dose = 6 g/day).
IM, IV (Neonates ≤4 wk): 50 mg/kg every 8–12 hr.

Renal Impairment
IM, IV (Adults): *CCr 31–50 mL/min*—1 g every 12 hr; *CCr 16–30 mL/min*—1 g every 24 hr; *CCr 6–15 mL/min*—500 mg every 24 hr; *CCr <5 mL/min*—500 mg every 48 hr.

Ceftriaxone
IM, IV (Adults): *Most infections*—1–2 g every 12–24 hr. *Gonorrhea*—250 mg IM (single dose). *Meningitis*—2 g every 12 hr. *Perioperative prophylaxis*—1 g 30–120 min before initial incision (single dose).
IM, IV (Children): *Most infections*—25–37.5 mg/kg every 12 hr *or* 50–75 mg/kg every 24 hr; dose should not exceed 2 g/day. *Meningitis*—100 mg/kg every 24 hr *or* 50 mg/kg every 12 hr; dose should not exceed 4 g/day. *Acute otitis media*—50 mg/kg IM single dose; dose should not exceed 1 g. *Uncomplicated gonorrhea*—125 mg IM (single dose).

Availability

Cefdinir (generic available)
Capsules: 300 mg. **Oral suspension (strawberry):** 125 mg/5 mL, 250 mg/5 mL. **Cost:** *Generic*—125 mg/5 mL $51.00/60 mL, 250 mg/5 mL $99.48/60 mL.

Cefditoren (generic available)
Tablets: 200 mg, 400 mg. **Cost:** *Generic*—All strengths $294.81/20.

Cefixime (generic available)
Capsules: 400 mg. **Chewable tablets (contain aspartame):** 100 mg, 150 mg, 200 mg. **Cost:** 100 mg $170.77/10, 200 mg $341.51/10. **Oral suspension (strawberry):** 100 mg/5 mL, 200 mg/5 mL, 500 mg/5 mL. **Cost:** 100 mg/5 mL $170.77/50 mL, 200 mg/5 mL $341.55/50 mL, 500 mg/5 mL $170.77/10 mL. **Tablets:** 400 mg. **Cost:** $1008.49/50.

Cefotaxime (generic available)
Powder for injection (requires reconstitution and dilution): 500 mg/vial, 1 g/vial, 2 g/vial, 10 g/vial.

Cefpodoxime (generic available)
Oral suspension (lemon creme): 50 mg/5 mL, 100 mg/5 mL. **Cost:** *Generic*—50 mg/5 mL $35.28/50 mL, 100 mg/5 mL $86.17/50 mL. **Tablets:** 100 mg, 200 mg. **Cost:** *Generic*—100 mg $134.74/20, 200 mg $169.14/20.

Ceftazidime (generic available)
Powder for injection (requires reconstitution and dilution): 500 mg/vial, 1 g/vial, 2 g/vial, 6 g/vial. **Premixed infusion:** 1 g/50 mL, 2 g/50 mL.

Ceftriaxone (generic available)
Powder for injection (requires reconstitution and dilution): 250 mg/vial, 500 mg/vial, 1 g/vial, 2 g/vial, 10 g/vial, 100 g/vial. **Premixed infusion:** 1 g/50 mL, 2 g/50 mL.

NURSING IMPLICATIONS

Assessment
- Assess for infection (vital signs; appearance of wound, sputum, urine, and stool; WBC) at beginning of and throughout therapy.
- Before initiating therapy, obtain a history to determine previous use of and reactions to penicillins or cephalosporins. Persons with a negative history of penicillin sensitivity may still have an allergic response.
- Obtain specimens for culture and sensitivity before initiating therapy. First dose may be given before receiving results.

- Observe for signs and symptoms of anaphylaxis (rash, pruritus, laryngeal edema, wheezing). Discontinue drug and notify health care professional immediately if these symptoms occur. Keep epinephrine, an antihistamine, and resuscitation equipment close by in the event of an anaphylactic reaction.
- Monitor bowel function. Diarrhea, abdominal cramping, fever, and bloody stools should be reported to health care professional promptly as a sign of Clostridium difficile-associated diarrhea (CDAD). May begin up to several wk following cessation of therapy.
- Assess patient for skin rash frequently during therapy. Discontinue at first sign of rash; may be life-threatening. Stevens-Johnson syndrome may develop. Treat symptomatically; may recur once treatment is stopped.
- Pedi: Assess newborns for jaundice and hyperbilirubinemia before making decision to use ceftriaxone (should not be used in jaundiced or hyperbilirubinemic neonates).
- ***Lab Test Considerations:*** May cause positive results for Coombs' test in patients receiving high doses or in neonates whose mothers were given cephalosporins before delivery.
- Monitor prothrombin time and assess patient for bleeding (guaiac stools; check for hematuria, bleeding gums, ecchymosis) daily in patients receiving *cefditoren*, as this agent may cause hypoprothrombinemia.
- May cause ↑ serum AST, ALT, alkaline phosphatase, bilirubin, LDH, BUN, and serum creatinine.
- May rarely cause leukopenia, neutropenia, agranulocytosis, thrombocytopenia, eosinophilia, lymphocytosis, and thrombocytosis.

Implementation

- Do not confuse ceftazidime with cefazolin, cefoxitin, cefotetan, or ceftriaxone.
- Cefditoren is not recommended for prolonged use since other piralate-containing compounds have caused clinical manifestations of carnitine deficiency when used over a period of mo.
- **PO:** Administer around the clock. May be administered on full or empty stomach. Administration with food may minimize GI irritation. Shake oral suspension well before administering. Administer *cefditoren* with meals to enhance absorption. Administer *cefpodoxime tablets* with meals to enhance absorption (suspension may be administered without regard to meals.
- *Cefixime oral suspension* should be used to treat otitis media (results in higher peak concentrations than tablets).
- Do not administer *cefdinir* or *cefpodoxime* within 2 hr before or after an antacid. Do not administer *cefpodoxime* within 2 hr before or after an H_2 receptor antagonist. Do not administer *cefdinir* within 2 hr before or after iron supplements. Do not administer *cefditoren* concomitantly with antacids.
- **IM:** Reconstitute IM doses with sterile or bacteriostatic water for injection or 0.9% NaCl for injection. May be diluted with lidocaine to minimize injection discomfort. Do not administer lidocaine-containing ceftriaxone IV.
- Inject deep into a well-developed muscle mass; massage well.

IV Administration

- **IV:** Monitor injection site frequently for phlebitis (pain, redness, swelling). Change sites every 48–72 hr to prevent phlebitis.
- If aminoglycosides are administered concurrently, administer in separate sites, if possible, at least 1 hr apart. If second site is unavailable, flush lines between medications.
- **IV Push:** Dilute cephalosporins in at least 1 g/10 mL. Avoid IV push administration of *ceftriaxone*. Do not use preparations containing benzyl alcohol for neonates. ***Rate:*** Administer slowly over 3–5 min.

Cefotaxime

- **Intermittent Infusion:** ***Diluent:*** Reconstituted solution may be further diluted in D5W, D10W, lactated Ringer's solution, D5/0.25% NaCl, D5/0.45% NaCl, D5/0.9% NaCl, or 0.9% NaCl. ***Concentration:*** 20–60 mg/mL. Solution may appear light yellow to amber. Solution is stable for 24 hr at room temperature and 5 days if refrigerated. ***Rate:*** Administer over 20–30 min.
- **Y-Site Compatibility:** acyclovir, alfentanil, alprostadil, amifostine, amikacin, aminocaproic acid, aminophylline, amphotericin B lipid complex, anidulafungin, argatroban, arsenic trioxide, ascorbic acid, atracurium, atropine, aztreonam, benztropine, bivalirudin, bleomycin, bumetanide, buprenorphine, butorphanol, calcium chloride, calcium gluconate, cangrelor, carboplatin, carmustine, cefotetan, cefoxitin, ceftriaxone, cefuroxime, cisplatin, clindamycin, cyanocobalamin, cyclophosphamide, cyclosporine, cytarabine, dactinomycin, daptomycin, dexamethasone, dexmedetomidine, dexrazoxane, digoxin, diltiazem, dimenhydrinate, docetaxel, dopamine, doxorubicin liposomal, doxycycline, enalaprilat, ephedrine, epinephrine, epirubicin, epoetin alfa, eptifibatide, erythromycin, esmolol, etoposide, etoposide phosphate, famotidine, fenoldopam, fentanyl, fludarabine, fluorouracil, folic acid, foscarnet, fosphenytoin, furosemide, glycopyrrolate, granisetron, heparin, hetastarch, hydrocortisone, hydromorphone, ifosfamide, imipenem/cilastatin, indomethacin, insulin, isoproterenol, ketamine, ketorolac, leucovorin, lidocaine, linezolid, lorazepam, magnesium sulfate, mannitol, melphalan, meperidine, mesna, methotrexate, methyldopate, metoclopramide, metoprolol, midazolam, milrinone, morphine, multivitamins, nafcillin, nalbuphine, naloxone, nicardipine, nitroglycerin, nitroprusside, norepinephrine, octreotide, ondansetron, oxacillin, oxaliplatin, oxytocin, paclitaxel, palonosetron, pamidronate, pancu-

ronium, penicillin G, perphenazine, phenylephrine, phytonadione, potassium acetate, potassium chloride, procainamide, propofol, propranolol, pyridoxine, ranitidine, remifentanil, rituximab, rocuronium, sargramostim, sodium acetate, streptokinase, succinylcholine, sufentanil, tacrolimus, theophylline, thiamine, thiotepa, tigecycline, tirofiban, tobramycin, tolazoline, topotecan, vasopressin, verapamil, vinblastine, vinorelbine, voriconazole, zoledronic acid.

- **Y-Site Incompatibility:** alemtuzumab, allopurinol, amiodarone, amphotericin B liposome, azathioprine, caspofungin, cefazolin, ceftazidime, chloramphenicol, chlorpromazine, dacarbazine, dantrolene, daunorubicin, diazepam, diphenhydramine, dobutamine, dolasetron, doxorubicin, filgrastim, ganciclovir, gemcitabine, haloperidol, hydralazine, hydroxyzine, idarubicin, irinotecan, labetalol, methylprednisolone, minocycline, mitomycin, mitoxantrone, mycophenolate, pantoprazole, papaverine, pemetrexed, pentamidine, pentobarbital, phenobarbital, phenytoin, prochlorperazine, promethazine, protamine, quinupristin/dalfopristin, sodium bicarbonate, trastuzumab, trimethoprim/sulfamethoxazole, vecuronium.

Ceftazidime

- **Intermittent Infusion:** ***Diluent:*** Reconstituted solution may be further diluted in at least 1 g/10 mL of 0.9% NaCl, D5W, D10W, dextrose/saline combinations, or LR. Dilution causes CO_2 to form inside vial, resulting in positive pressure; vial may require venting after dissolution to preserve sterility of vial. Not required with L-arginine formulation (Ceftaz). Solution may appear yellow to amber; darkening does not alter potency. Solution is stable for 18 hr at room temperature and 7 days if refrigerated. ***Concentration:*** 40 mg/mL. ***Rate:*** Administer over 15–30 min.
- **Y-Site Compatibility:** acyclovir, alfentanil, allopurinol, amifostine, aminocaproic acid, aminophylline, amphotericin B lipid complex, anakinra, anidulafungin, argatroban, atropine, aztreonam, benztropine, bivalirudin, bleomycin, bumetanide, buprenorphine, butorphanol, calcium gluconate, cangrelor, carboplatin, carmustine, cefazolin, cefotetan, cefoxitin, ceftriaxone, cefuroxime, ciprofloxacin, cisplatin, clindamycin, cyanocobalamin, cyclophosphamide, cyclosporine, cytarabine, dacarbazine, dactinomycin, daptomycin, dexamethasone, dexmedetomidine, dexrazoxane, digoxin, diltiazem, dimenhydrinate, docetaxel, dopamine, enalaprilat, ephedrine, epinephrine, epoetin alfa, eptifibatide, esmolol, etoposide, etoposide phosphate, famotidine, fenoldopam, fentanyl, filgrastim, fludarabine, fluorouracil, folic acid, foscarnet, fosphenytoin, furosemide, gemcitabine, glycopyrrolate, granisetron, heparin, hetastarch, hydrocortisone, hydromorphone, ibuprofen, ifosfamide, imipenem/cilastatin, indomethacin, insulin, irinotecan, isoproterenol, ketamine, ketorolac, labetalol, leucovorin calcium, levofloxacin, lidocaine, linezolid, lorazepam, magnesium sulfate, mannitol, melphalan, meperidine, mesna, methotrexate, methylprednisolone, metoclopramide, metoprolol, metronidazole, milrinone, mitomycin, morphine, multivitamins, nafcillin, nalbuphine, naloxone, nitroglycerin, norepinephrine, octreotide, oxacillin, oxaliplatin, oxytocin, paclitaxel, palonosetron, pamidronate, pancuronium, penicillin G, phenobarbital, phentolamine, phenylephrine, phytonadione, potassium acetate, potassium chloride, procainamide, propranolol, pyridoxine, ranitidine, remifentanil, rituximab, rocuronium, sodium acetate, sodium bicarbonate, streptokinase, succinylcholine, sufentanil, tacrolimus, telavancin, thiotepa, tigecycline, tirofiban, trastuzumab, vasopressin, vecuronium, vinblastine, vincristine, vinorelbine, voriconazole, zidovudine, zoledronic acid.
- **Y-Site Incompatibility:** acetylcysteine, alemtuzumab, amiodarone, amphotericin B liposome, ascorbic acid, azathioprine, calcium chloride, caspofungin, cefotaxime, chloramphenicol, chlorpromazine, dantrolene, daunorubicin, diazepam, diazoxide, diphenhydramine, doxorubicin, doxorubicin liposome, doxycycline, epirubicin, ganciclovir, haloperidol, hydralazine, hydroxyzine, idarubicin, midazolam, mitoxantrone, mycophenolate, nitroprusside, papaverine, pemetrexed, pentamidine, phenytoin, prochlorperazine, promethazine, protamine, quinupristin/dalfopristin, thiamine, topotecan, trimethoprim/sulfamethoxazole, verapamil, warfarin.

Ceftriaxone

- **Intermittent Infusion:** Reconstitute each 250-mg vial with 2.4 mL, each 500-mg vial with 4.8 mL, each 1-g vial with 9.6 mL, and each 2-g vial with 19.2 mL of sterile water for injection, 0.9% NaCl, or D5W for a concentration of 100 mg/mL. ***Diluent:*** Solution should be further diluted in 50–100 mL of 0.9% NaCl, D5W, D10W, D5/0.45% NaCl, or D5/0.9% NaCl. Solution may appear light yellow to amber. Solution is stable for 3 days at room temperature. ***Concentration:*** 40 mg/mL. ***Rate:*** Infuse over 30 min.
- **Y-Site Compatibility:** acetaminophen, acyclovir, alfentanil, allopurinol, amifostine, aminocaproic acid, aminophylline, amphotericin B lipid complex, amphotericin B liposome, anidulafungin, argatroban, atropine, aztreonam, benztropine, bivalirudin, bumetanide, buprenorphine, butorphanol, cangrelor, carboplatin, carmustine, cefazolin, cefotaxime, cefotetan, cefoxitin, ceftazidime, cefuroxime, cisatracurium, cisplatin, cyanocobalamin, cyclophosphamide, cyclosporine, cytarabine, dactinomycin, dap-

tomycin, dexamethasone, dexmedetomidine, dexrazoxane, digoxin, diltiazem, docetaxel, dopamine, doxorubicin liposome, doxycycline, enalaprilat, ephedrine, epinephrine, epoetin alfa, eptifibatide, erythromycin, esmolol, etoposide, etoposide phosphate, fenoldopam, fentanyl, fludarabine, fluorouracil, folic acid, foscarnet, fosphenytoin, furosemide, gemcitabine, glycopyrrolate, granisetron, heparin, hydrocortisone, hydromorphone, ifosfamide, indomethacin, insulin, isoproterenol, ketorolac, levofloxacin, lidocaine, linezolid, lorazepam, mannitol, melphalan, meperidine, mesna, methotrexate, methylprednisolone, metoclopramide, metoprolol, metronidazole, midazolam, milrinone, morphine, multivitamins, nafcillin, nalbuphine, naloxone, nicardipine, nitroglycerin, nitroprusside, norepinephrine, octreotide, oxacillin, oxaliplatin, oxytocin, paclitaxel, palonosetron, pamidronate, pantoprazole, pemetrexed, penicillin G, phenobarbital, phentolamine, phenylephrine, phytonadione, potassium acetate, potassium chloride, procainamide, propranolol, pyridoxine, ranitidine, remifentanil, rituxumab, rocuronium, sargramostim, sodium acetate, sodium bicarbonate, succinylcholine, sufentanil, tacrolimus, telavancin, theophylline, thiamine, thiotepa, tigecycline, tirofiban, topotecan, trastuzumab, vasopressin, vecuronium, verapamil, vinblastine, vincristine, voriconazole, warfarin, zidovudine, zoledronic acid.

- **Y-Site Incompatibility:** alemtuzumab, ascorbic acid, azathioprine, calcium chloride, calcium gluconate, caspofungin, chloramphenicol, chlorpromazine, clindamycin, dacarbazine, dantrolene, daunorubicin, diazepam, diazoxide, diphenhydramine, dobutamine, doxorubicin, epirubicin, filgrastim, ganciclovir, haloperidol, hetastarch, hydralazine, hydroxyzine, idarubicin, imipenem/cilastatin, irinotecan, labetalol, leucovorin, mitoxantrone, mycophenolate, papaverine, pentamidine, pentobarbital, phenytoin, prochlorperazine, promethazine, protamine, quinupristin/dalfopristin, tobramycin, trimethoprim/sulfamethoxazole, vinorelbine. Calcium-containing solutions, including parenteral nutrition, should not be mixed or co-administered, even via different infusion lines at different sites in patients <28 days old. In older patients, flush line thoroughly between infusions.

Patient/Family Teaching

- Instruct patient to take medication around the clock and to finish the medication completely, even if feeling better. Take missed doses as soon as possible unless almost time for next dose; do not double doses. Advise patient that sharing of this medication may be dangerous.
- Pedi: Instruct parents or caregivers to use calibrated measuring device with liquid preparations.
- Advise patient to report signs of superinfection (furry overgrowth on the tongue, vaginal itching or discharge, loose or foul-smelling stools) and allergy.
- Instruct patient to notify health care professional if rash, fever and diarrhea develop, especially if stool contains blood, pus, or mucus. Advise patient not to treat diarrhea without consulting health care professional.
- Advise females of reproductive potential to notify health care professional if pregnancy is planned or suspected, or if breast feeding.

Evaluation/Desired Outcomes

- Resolution of the signs and symptoms of infection. Length of time for complete resolution depends on the organism and site of infection.
- Decreased incidence of infection when used for prophylaxis.

ceritinib (se-ri-ti-nib)

Zykadia

Classification

Therapeutic: antineoplastics

Pharmacologic: kinase inhibitors

Indications

Anaplastic lymphoma kinase (ALK)-positive, metastatic non-small cell lung cancer (NSCLC).

Action

Acts as a tyrosine kinase inhibitor, inhibiting anaplastic lymphoma kinase as well as other kinases, resulting in decreased growth of certain malignant cell lines.

Therapeutic Effects: Slowed progression of metastatic NSCLC.

Pharmacokinetics

Absorption: Absorption follows oral administration; food significantly ↑ absorption and may ↑ risk of adverse reactions.

Distribution: Slight preference to distribute from plasma into red blood cells.

Metabolism and Excretion: Metabolized in the liver (mostly by CYP3A) and is a substrate of P-glycoprotein (P-gp); 68% eliminated unchanged in feces, 1.3% in urine.

Half-life: 41 hr.

TIME/ACTION PROFILE (clinical response)

ROUTE	ONSET	PEAK	DURATION
PO	unknown	4–6 hr (blood level)	7.1–7.4 mos

Contraindications/Precautions

Contraindicated in: OB: Pregnancy (may cause fetal harm); Lactation: Lactation; Congenital long QT syndrome.

Use Cautiously in: Moderate to severe hepatic impairment/severe renal impairment (CCr <30 mL/min); HF, bradycardia, electrolyte abnormalities, or concurrent use of QT prolonging medications; Concurrent use of strong CYP3A4 inhibitors; Rep: Women of reproductive potential and men with female partners of reproductive potential; Pedi: Safety and effectiveness not established.

Adverse Reactions/Side Effects

CNS: fatigue. **CV:** BRADYCARDIA, TORSADE DE POINTES, QT interval prolongation. **Derm:** rash. **Endo:** hyperglycemia. **F and E:** hypophosphatemia. **GI:** HEPATOTOXICITY, PANCREATITIS, abdominal pain, ↓ appetite, constipation, diarrhea, esophagitis/reflux/dysphagia, ↑ lipase, ↑ liver enzymes, nausea, vomiting. **GU:** ↑ creatinine. **Hemat:** anemia. **Resp:** INTERSTITIAL LUNG DISEASE/PNEUMONITIS.

Interactions

Drug-Drug: Concurrent use of strong **CYP3A inhibitors** including **ketoconazole**, and **nefazodone** ↑ levels and the risk of toxicities; avoid concurrent use; if unavoidable, ↓ ceritinib dose. Strong **CYP3A inducers** including **carbamazepine**, **phenytoin**, and **rifampin** may ↓ levels and effectiveness; avoid concurrent use. May ↑ levels and the risk of toxicity of CYP3A4 and CYP2C9 substrates, including **alfentanil**, **cyclosporine**, **dihydroergotamine**, **ergotamine**, **fentanyl**, **phenytoin**, **pimozide**, **quinidine**, **sirolimus**, **tacrolimus**, and **warfarin**; dose of these medications may need to be ↓. **Beta-blockers**, **diltiazem**, **verapamil**, **digoxin**, and **clonidine** may ↑ risk of bradycardia; avoid concurrent use, if possible. Concurrent use of **QT interval prolonging medications** may ↑ risk of QT interval prolongation and torsade de pointes.

Drug-Food: **Grapefruit/grapefruit juice** ↑ levels and the risk of toxicity; concurrent ingestion should be avoided. **St. John's wort** ↓ levels and effectiveness; concurrent use should be avoided.

Route/Dosage

PO (Adults): 450 mg once daily; continue until disease progression or unacceptable toxicity; *Concurrent use of strong CYP3A inhibitors*—↓ dose by ⅓, rounded to the nearest 150-mg strength.

Hepatic Impairment

PO (Adults): *Severe hepatic impairment*—↓ dose by ⅓, rounded to the nearest 150-mg strength.

Availability

Tablets: 150 mg.

NURSING IMPLICATIONS

Assessment

- Assess for signs and symptoms of interstitial lung disease or pneumonitis (trouble breathing, shortness of breath, fever, cough with or without mucus, chest pain). If these symptoms occur, discontinue therapy permanently.
- Monitor ECG periodically during therapy. *If QTc interval is >500 msec on at least 2 separate ECGs,* hold ceritinib until QTc interval <481 msec or recovery to baseline if QTc ≥481 msec, then resume ceritinib with a 150 mg dose reduction. *If QTc interval prolongation occurs in combination with torsades de pointes or polymorphic ventricular tachycardia or signs and symptoms of serious arrhythmia,* discontinue ceritinib permanently.
- *If symptomatic bradycardia that is not life-threatening occurs,* hold ceritinib until recovery to asymptomatic bradycardia or a heart rate ≥ 60 bpm, evaluate concurrent medications causing bradycardia, and adjust dose of ceritinib. *If clinically significant bradycardia requiring intervention or life-threatening bradycardia in patients taking concurrent medication known to cause bradycardia or a medication known to cause hypotension occurs,* hold ceritinib until recovery to asymptomatic bradycardia or a heart rate ≥60 bpm. *If concurrent medication can be adjusted or discontinued,* resume ceritinib with a 150 mg dose reduction and frequent monitoring. *If life-threatening bradycardia occurs in patients not taking medications known to cause bradycardia or hypotension,* discontinue ceritinib permanently.
- Assess for nausea, vomiting, diarrhea. If severe or intolerable nausea, vomiting, or diarrhea continue despite optimal antiemetic or antidiarrheal therapy, hold ceritinib until improved; then resume with a 150 mg dose reduction.
- ***Lab Test Considerations:*** Test patient for ALK positivity in tumor specimens through an FDA approved test prior to starting therapy.
- Monitor liver function tests at least monthly. *If ALT or AST >5 times the upper limit of normal (ULN) and total bilirubin is ≤2 x ULN,* hold ceritinib until recovery to baseline or ≤3 x ULN, then resume ceritinib with a 150 mg dose reduction. *If ALT or AST >3 x ULN and total bilirubin is >2 x ULN in the absence of cholestasis or hemolysis,* permanently discontinue ceritinib.
- Monitor fasting blood glucose prior to and periodically during therapy. *If persistent hyperglycemia >250 m g/dL despite anti-hyperglycemic therapy,* hold ceritinib until hyperglycemia is adequately controlled, then resume with a 150 mg dose reduction. *If adequate hyperglycemic control cannot be achieved,* discontinue therapy.
- May cause ↓ hemoglobin and serum phosphate; ↑ creatinine.
- Monitor serum lipase and amylase prior to and periodically during therapy. May cause ↑ serum lipase and amylase. *If ↑ lipase or amylase >2 x upper ULN,* hold ceritinib and monitor serum lipase and

amylase. *When recovery to <1.5 x ULN,* resume with 150 mg dose reduction.

Implementation

- **PO:** Administer on an empty stomach, at least 1 hr before or 2 hr after meals.

Patient/Family Teaching

- Instruct patient to take ceritinib as directed. Take missed doses as soon as remembered unless within 12 hrs of next dose. If vomiting occurs, do not administer additional dose, continue with next scheduled dose. Instruct patient to read *Patient Information* prior to starting therapy and with each Rx refill in case of changes.
- Inform patient to avoid consuming grapefruit and grapefruit juice during therapy.
- Advise patient to notify health care professional if nausea, vomiting, and diarrhea is severe or persistent; if signs and symptoms of hepatotoxicity (feeling tired, itchy skin, skin or whites of eyes turn yellow, nausea and vomiting, decreased appetite, pain on right side of stomach, dark or brown, tea-colored urine, bleed or bruise easily); pneumonitis; QTc interval prolongation or bradycardia (new chest pain, changes in heartbeat, palpitations, dizziness, fainting, or changes in or use of a new heart or BP medication); hyperglycemia (increased thirst, increased hunger, headaches, trouble thinking or concentration, urinating often, blurred vision, tiredness, breath smells like fruit), or pancreatitis (upper abdominal pain that may spread to the back and get worse with eating) occur.
- Rep: Advise female patient of reproductive potential to use effective contraceptives during and for at least 6 mo following completion of therapy, to notify health care provider if pregnancy is planned or suspected, and to avoid breast feeding during and for at least 2 wk after end of therapy. Advise males with female partners of reproductive potential to use condoms during therapy and for 3 mo following completion of therapy.

Evaluation/Desired Outcomes

- Slowed progression of metastatic NSCLC.

certolizumab

(ser-toe-**liz**-u-mab)

Cimzia

Classification

Therapeutic: gastrointestinal anti-inflammatories, antirheumatics

Pharmacologic: tumor necrosis factor blockers, DMARDs, monoclonal antibodies

Indications

Moderately-to-severely active Crohn's disease when response to conventional therapy has been inadequate. Moderately-to-severely active rheumatoid arthritis. Active psoriatic arthritis. Active ankylosing spondylitis. Moderate-to-severe plaque psoriasis in patients who are not candidates for systemic therapy or phototherapy. Active non-radiographic axial spondyloarthritis with objective signs of inflammation.

Action

Neutralizes tumor necrosis factor (TNF), a prime mediator of inflammation; pegylation provides a long duration of action. **Therapeutic Effects:** Decreased signs/symptoms of Crohn's disease. Decreased pain and swelling, decreased rate of joint destruction and improved physical function in rheumatoid arthritis. Decreased joint swelling and pain in psoriatic arthritis. Decreased spinal pain and inflammation in ankylosing spondylitis. Reduced severity of plaques. Decreased pain and swelling, reduced C-reactive protein levels, and improved physical function in axial spondyloarthritis.

Pharmacokinetics

Absorption: 80% absorbed following SC administration.

Distribution: Unknown.

Metabolism and Excretion: Unknown.

Half-life: 14 days.

TIME/ACTION PROFILE (blood levels)

ROUTE	ONSET	PEAK	DURATION
Subcut	unknown	50–120 hr	2–4 wk

Contraindications/Precautions

Contraindicated in: Hypersensitivity; Active infection (including localized); Concurrent use of anakinra.

Use Cautiously in: History of chronic or recurrent infection or underlying illness/treatment predisposing to infection; History of exposure to tuberculosis; History of opportunistic infection; Patients residing, or who have resided, where tuberculosis, histoplasmosis, coccidioidomycoses, or blastomycosis is endemic; History of demyelinating disorders (may exacerbate); History of heart failure; Geri: May ↑ risk of infections; OB: Use in pregnancy only if clearly needed; Lactation: Breast feed only if potential benefits justify potential risk to fetus; Pedi: Safety not established; ↑ risk of lymphoma (including hepatosplenic T-cell lymphoma [HSTCL] in patients with Crohn's disease), leukemia, and other malignancies.

Adverse Reactions/Side Effects

Derm: psoriasis, skin reactions (rarely severe). **Hemat:** hematologic reactions. **MS:** arthralgia. **Misc:** HYPERSENSITIVITY REACTIONS (including anaphylaxis, angioedema, serum sickness, and urticaria), INFECTIONS (including reactivation tuberculosis, hepatitis B reactivation, and other opportunistic infections due to bacterial, invasive fungal, viral, mycobacterial, and parasitic pathogens), MALIGNANCY (including lymphoma, HSTCL, leukemia, and skin cancer), lupus-like syndrome.

Interactions

Drug-Drug: Concurrent use with **anakinra** ↑ risk of serious infections (contraindicated). Concurrent use with **azathioprine** and/or **methotrexate** may ↑ risk of HSTCL. May ↓ antibody response to or ↑ risk of adverse reactions to **live vaccines** (contraindicated).

Route/Dosage

Crohn's Disease

Subcut (Adults): 400 mg (given as two 200–mg injections) initially, repeat 2 and 4 wk later; may be followed by maintenance dose of 400 mg (given as two 200–mg injections) every 4 wk.

Rheumatoid Arthritis or Psoriatic Arthritis

Subcut (Adults): 400 mg (given as two 200–mg injections) initially, repeat 2 and 4 wk later; then maintenance dose of 200 mg every 2 wk (400 mg [given as two 200–mg injections] every 4 wk may be used alternatively).

Ankylosing Spondylitis or Non-Radiographic Axial Spondyloarthritis

Subcut (Adults): 400 mg (given as two 200–mg injections) initially, repeat 2 and 4 wk later; then maintenance dose of 200 mg every 2 wk or 400 mg (given as two 200–mg injections) every 4 wk.

Plaque Psoriasis

Subcut (Adults): 400 mg (given as two 200–mg injections) every 2 wk; *Patients ≤90 kg*—may consider giving 400 mg (given as two 200–mg injections) initially, then repeat 2 and 4 wk later; then maintenance dose of 200 mg every 2 wk.

Availability

Lyophilized powder for injection (requires reconstitution): 200 mg/vial. **Solution for injection (prefilled syringes):** 200 mg/mL.

NURSING IMPLICATIONS

Assessment

- **Crohn's Disease:** Assess abdominal pain and frequency, quantity, and consistency of stools at beginning and during therapy.
- **Arthritis/Ankylosing Spondylitis:** Assess pain and range of motion before and periodically during therapy.
- Assess for signs of infection (fever, sore throat, dyspnea, WBC) prior to and during therapy. Monitor all patients for active TB (persistent cough, wasting, weight loss, low grade fever) during therapy, even if initial test was negative. Do not begin certolizumab during an active infection, including chronic or localized infections. If infection develops, monitor closely and discontinue certolizumab if infection becomes serious.
- Evaluate patients at risk for hepatitis B virus (HBV) infection for prior evidence of HBV infection before initiating therapy. Monitor carriers of HBV closely for clinical and lab signs of active HBV infection during and for several mo following discontinuation of therapy. If HBV reactivation occurs, discontinue certolizumab and initiate antiviral therapy.
- Monitor for signs of hypersensitivity reactions (angioedema, dyspnea, hypotension, rash, serum sickness, urticaria). If reactions occur, discontinue certolizumab and treat symptomatically.
- Assess for signs and symptoms of systemic fungal infections (fever, malaise, weight loss, sweats, cough, dyspnea, pulmonary infiltrates, serious systemic illness with or without concomitant shock). Ascertain if patient lives in or has traveled to areas of endemic mycoses. Consider empiric antifungal treatment for patients at risk of histoplasmosis and other invasive fungal infections until the pathogens are identified. Consult with an infectious diseases specialist. Consider stopping certolizumab until the infection has been diagnosed and adequately treated.
- ***Lab Test Considerations:*** May cause anemia, leukopenia, pancytopenia, and thrombocytopenia.
- Monitor CBC with differential periodically during therapy. May cause leukopenia, neutropenia, thrombocytopenia, and pancytopenia. Discontinue certolizumab if symptoms of blood dyscrasias (persistent fever) occur.
- May cause ↑ liver enzymes.
- May cause erroneously ↑ aPTT.

Implementation

- Perform test for latent TB. If positive for latent TB, active TB in whom an adequate course of treatment cannot be confirmed, and for patients with a negative test for TB who have risk factors for tuberculosis infection, begin treatment for TB prior to starting certolizumab therapy. Monitor for TB throughout therapy, even if latent TB test is negative.
- Allow vial to sit at room temperature for 30 min prior to reconstituting; do not use other warming methods. Reconstitute vial by adding 1 mL of sterile water for injection, using a 20-gauge needle, for a concentration of 200 mg/mL. Gently swirl so all powder comes into contact with sterile water; do not shake. Leave vial undisturbed for as long as 30 min to fully reconstitute. Solution is clear and colorless to pale yellow; do not administer solutions that are cloudy, discolored or contain particulate matter. Do not leave reconstituted solution at room temperature for >2 hr prior to injection. May be refrigerated for up to 24 hr prior to injection; do not freeze.
- **Subcut:** Allow solution to sit at room temperature for 30 min prior to injection; do not use other warming methods. Give 400-mg dose as two injec-

tions of 200 mg each. Using a new 20-gauge needle for each vial, withdraw reconstituted solution into 2 separate syringes each containing 1 mL (200 mg/mL) of certolizumab. Switch each 20-gauge needle to a 23-gauge needle and inject the full contents of each syringe subcut into separate sides of the abdomen or thigh. Avoid areas of skin tenderness, bruising, redness or hardness, or scars or stretch marks.
- Assess for latex allergies. Needle shield inside the removable cap of prefilled syringes contains a derivative of natural rubber latex.

Patient/Family Teaching

- Advise patient of potential benefits and risks of certolizumab. Instruct patient in correct technique for injection, and care and disposal of equipment. Advise patient to read the *Medication Guide* prior to starting therapy.
- Inform patient of risk of infection. Advise patient to notify health care professional if symptoms of infection (fever, cough, flu-like symptoms, or open cuts or sores), including TB or reactivation of HBV infection, occur.
- Counsel patient about possible risk of lymphoma and other malignancies while receiving certolizumab.
- Advise patient to notify health care professional if signs of hypersensitivity reactions (rash, swollen face, difficulty breathing), or new or worsening medical conditions such as heart or neurological disease or autoimmune disorders occur and to report signs of bone marrow depression (bruising, bleeding, or persistent fever).
- Advise patient to notify health care professional of all Rx or OTC medications, vitamins, or herbal products being taken and to consult with health care professional before taking other medications.
- Rep: Advise patient to notify health care professional if pregnancy is planned or suspected or if breast feeding. Encourage women who become pregnant to enroll in the MotherToBaby Pregnancy Studies conducted by the Organization of Teratology Information Specialists (OTIS). The OTIS AutoImmune Diseases Study at 1-877-311-8972 or visit http://mothertobaby.org/pregnancy-studies/.

Evaluation/Desired Outcomes

- Decrease in signs and symptoms of Crohn's disease.
- Decreased pain and swelling with decreased rate of joint destruction in patients with rheumatoid arthritis.
- Decreased joint swelling and pain in psoriatic arthritis.
- Decreased spinal pain and inflammation in ankylosing spondylitis.
- Reduced severity of plaques.
- Decreased pain and swelling, reduced C-reactive protein levels, and improved physical function in axial spondyloarthritis.

cetirizine (se-ti-ra-zeen)

✤ Aller Relief, ✤ Reactine, ✤ Rhinaris Relief, ZyrTEC

Classification

Therapeutic: allergy, cold, and cough remedies, antihistamines

Pharmacologic: piperazines (peripherally selective)

Indications

Relief of allergic symptoms caused by histamine release including: Seasonal and perennial allergic rhinitis, Chronic urticaria.

Action

Antagonizes the effects of histamine at H_1-receptor sites; does not bind to or inactivate histamine. Anticholinergic effects are minimal and sedation is dose related. **Therapeutic Effects:** Decreased symptoms of histamine excess (sneezing, rhinorrhea, ocular tearing and redness, pruritus).

Pharmacokinetics

Absorption: Well absorbed following oral administration.

Distribution: Unknown.

Protein Binding: 93%.

Metabolism and Excretion: Excreted primarily unchanged by the kidneys.

Half-life: 7.4–9 hr (↓ in children to 6.2 hr, ↑ in renal impairment up to 19–21 hr).

TIME/ACTION PROFILE (antihistaminic effects)

ROUTE	ONSET	PEAK	DURATION
PO	30 min	4–8 hr	24 hr

Contraindications/Precautions

Contraindicated in: Hypersensitivity to cetirizine, hydroxyzine or any component; Lactation: Excreted in breast milk; not recommended for use.

Use Cautiously in: Patients with hepatic or renal impairment (dose ↓ recommended if CCr ≤31 mL/min or hepatic function is impaired); OB, Pedi: Safety not established for pregnant women or children <6 mo; Geri: Initiate at lower doses.

Adverse Reactions/Side Effects

CNS: dizziness, drowsiness (significant with doses >10 mg/day), fatigue. **Derm:** acute generalized exanthematous pustulosis. **EENT:** pharyngitis. **GI:** dry mouth.

Interactions

Drug-Drug: Additive CNS depression may occur with **alcohol**, **opioid analgesics**, or **sedative/hypnotics**. **Theophylline** may ↓ clearance and ↑ toxicity.

Route/Dosage

PO (Adults and children ≥6 yr): 5–10 mg given once or divided twice daily.

PO (Children 2–5 yr): 2.5 mg once daily initially, may be ↑ to 5 mg once daily or 2.5 mg every 12 hr.
PO (Children 1–2 yr): 2.5 mg once daily; may be ↑ to 2.5 mg every 12 hr.
PO (Children 6–12 mo): 2.5 once daily.

Hepatic/Renal Impairment

PO (Adults and Children ≥12 yr): *CCr ≤31 mL/min, hepatic impairment or hemodialysis*—5 mg once daily.

Hepatic/Renal Impairment

PO (Children 6–11 yr): start therapy at <2.5 mg/day.

Hepatic/Renal Impairment

PO (Children <6 yr): use not recommended.

Availability (generic available)

Tablets: 5 mg[OTC], 10 mg[OTC]. **Capsules:** 5 mg[OTC], 10 mg[OTC]. **Chewable tablets (grape):** 5 mg[OTC], 10 mg[OTC]. **Orally disintegrating tablets:** 10 mg. **Syrup (banana-grape and bubblegum flavors):** 1 mg/mL[OTC]. ***In combination with:*** pseudoephedrine (Zyrtec-D 12 hr) (See Appendix B).

NURSING IMPLICATIONS

Assessment

- Assess allergy symptoms (rhinitis, conjunctivitis, hives) before and periodically during therapy.
- Assess lung sounds and character of bronchial secretions. Maintain fluid intake of 1500–2000 mL/day to decrease viscosity of secretions.
- ***Lab Test Considerations:*** May cause false-negative result in allergy skin testing.

Implementation

- Do not confuse cetirizine with sertraline or stavudine. Do not confuse Zyrtec (cetirizine) with Zerit (Stavudine), Lipitor (atorvastatin), Zantac (ranitidine), Zocor (simvastatin), Zyprexa (olanzapine), Zyrtec-D (cetirizine/pseudoephedrine), Zyrtec Itchy Eye Drops (ketotifen fumarate).
- **PO:** Administer once daily without regard to food.

Patient/Family Teaching

- Instruct patient to take medication as directed.
- May cause dizziness and drowsiness. Caution patient to avoid driving or other activities requiring alertness until response to medication is known.
- Advise patient to avoid taking alcohol or other CNS depressants concurrently with this drug.
- Advise patient that good oral hygiene, frequent rinsing of mouth with water, and sugarless gum or candy may minimize dry mouth. Patient should notify dentist if dry mouth persists >2 wk.
- Instruct patient to contact health care professional if rash or dizziness occurs or if symptoms persist.

Evaluation/Desired Outcomes

- Decrease in allergic symptoms.

cetuximab (se-**tux**-i-mab)

Erbitux

Classification
Therapeutic: antineoplastics
Pharmacologic: monoclonal antibodies

Indications

Locally or regionally advanced squamous cell carcinoma of the head and neck with radiation. Recurrent or metastatic squamous cell carcinoma of the head and neck progressing after platinum-based therapy. Recurrent or metastatic squamous cell carcinoma of the head and neck in combination with platinum-based therapy with 5-fluorouracil. *K-ras* wild-type, epidermal growth factor receptor (EGFR)-expressing metastatic colorectal cancer in patients who have not responded to irinotecan and oxaliplatin or are intolerant to irinotecan. In combination with irinotecan in patients with *K-ras* wild-type, EGFR-expressing metastatic colorectal cancer who have not responded to irinotecan alone. First-line treatment of *K-ras* wild-type, EGFR-expressing metastatic colorectal cancer in combination with irinotecan, 5-fluorouracil, and leucovorin (FOLFIRI).

Action

Binds specifically to EGFR, thereby preventing the binding of endogenous epidermal growth factor (EGF). This prevents cell growth and differentiation processes. Combination with irinotecan enhances antitumor effects of irinotecan. **Therapeutic Effects:** Decreased tumor growth and spread.

Pharmacokinetics

Absorption: IV administration results in complete bioavailability.
Distribution: Unknown.
Metabolism and Excretion: Unknown.
Half-life: 97–114 hr.

TIME/ACTION PROFILE

ROUTE	ONSET	PEAK	DURATION
IV	unknown	unknown	unknown

Contraindications/Precautions

Contraindicated in: Hypersensitivity to cetuximab or murine (mouse) proteins; *RAS*-mutant metastatic colorectal cancer or unknown *RAS* mutation status (↑ mortality and tumor progression); OB: Pregnancy (may cause fetal harm); Lactation: Lactation.

Use Cautiously in: Exposure to sunlight (may exacerbate dermatologic toxicity); Rep: Women of reproductive potential; Pedi: Safety not established.

Adverse Reactions/Side Effects

Most adverse reactions reflect combination therapy with irinotecan.

CNS: malaise, depression, headache, insomnia. **CV:** CARDIOPULMONARY ARREST, PULMONARY EMBOLISM, SUDDEN CARDIAC DEATH. **Derm:** STEVENS-JOHNSON SYNDROME, TOXIC EPIDERMAL NECROLYSIS, acneform dermatitis, hypertrichosis, nail disorder, pruritus, skin desquamation, skin infection. **EENT:** conjunctivitis, ulcerative keratitis. **F and E:** dehydration, hypomagnesemia, peripheral edema. **GI:** abdominal pain, constipation, diarrhea, nausea, vomiting, anorexia, stomatitis. **GU:** ↓ fertility (females), renal failure. **Hemat:** anemia, leukopenia. **MS:** back pain. **Metab:** ↓ weight. **Resp:** cough, dyspnea, interstitial lung disease. **Misc:** INFUSION REACTIONS, fever, desquamation of mucosal epithelium.

Interactions

Drug-Drug: None reported.

Route/Dosage

Head & Neck Cancer with Radiation or in Combination with Platinum-Based Therapy with 5-Fluorouracil

IV (Adults): 400 mg/m² administered 1 wk prior to initiation of radiation therapy or on the day of initiation of platinum-based therapy with 5-fluorouracil (complete infusion 1 hr to prior to starting platinum-based therapy with 5-fluorouracil), followed by weekly maintenance doses of 250 mg/m² for the duration of radiation therapy or until disease progression or unacceptable toxicity with platinum-based therapy with 5-fluorouracil (complete infusion 1 hr prior to radiation therapy or platinum-based therapy with 5-fluorouracil). Dose modification recommended for dermatologic toxicity.

Head and Neck Cancer Monotherapy

IV (Adults): 400 mg/m² initial loading dose, followed by weekly maintenance doses of 250 mg/m² until disease progression or unacceptable toxicity; dose modification recommended for dermatologic toxicity.

Colorectal Cancer

IV (Adults): 400 mg/m² initial loading dose, followed by weekly maintenance doses of 250 mg/m² until disease progression or unacceptable toxicity; dose modification recommended for dermatologic toxicity.

Availability

Solution for injection: 2 mg/mL.

NURSING IMPLICATIONS

Assessment

- Assess for infusion reaction (rapid onset of airway obstruction [bronchospasm, stridor, hoarseness], urticaria, hypotension, loss of consciousness, myocardial infarction, cardiopulmonary arrest) for at least 1 hr following infusion. Longer observation periods may be required for those who experience infusion reactions. Most reactions occur during first dose, but may also occur in later doses. For severe reactions, immediately stop infusion and discontinue cetuximab permanently. Epinephrine, corticosteroids, IV antihistamines, bronchodilators, and oxygen should be available for reactions. Mild to moderate reactions (chills, fever, dyspnea) may be managed by slowing rate of infusion and administration of antihistamines. *If infusion reaction is Grade 1 or 2,* reduce infusion rate by 50%. *If infusion reaction is Grade 3 or 4,* discontinue immediately and permanently.
- Assess for acute onset or worsening of pulmonary symptoms. Delay infusion 1–2 wk; if condition improves, continue at dose that was being administered at the time of occurrence. If no improvement in 2 wk or interstitial lung disease (ILD) is confirmed, discontinue cetuximab and treat appropriately.
- Assess for dermatologic toxicities (acneform rash, skin drying and fissuring, inflammatory and infectious sequelae [blepharitis, cheilitis, cellulitis, cyst]). Treat symptomatically. Acneform rash usually occurs within initial 2 wk of therapy and resolves following cessation, but may continue up to 28 days following therapy. *For 1st occurrence of acneform rash,* delay infusion 1–2 wk; if improvement, continue at 250 mg/m², if no improvement, discontinue cetuximab. *For 2nd occurrence,* delay infusion 1–2 wk; if improvement, reduce dose to 200 mg/m², if no improvement, discontinue cetuximab. *For 3rd occurrence,* delay infusion 1–2 wk; if improvement, reduce dose to 150 mg/m², if no improvement, discontinue cetuximab. *For 4th occurrence,* discontinue cetuximab.
- ***Lab Test Considerations:*** Obtain a negative pregnancy test before starting therapy.
- Determine Ras mutation and EGFR-expression status using FDA-approved tests prior to initiating treatment. Only patients whose tumors are K-Ras wild-type should receive cetuximab.
- May cause anemia and leukopenia.
- Monitor serum electrolytes, especially serum magnesium, potassium, and calcium, closely during and periodically for at least 8 wk following infusion. May cause hypomagnesemia, hypocalcemia, and hypokalemia; may occur from days to mo after initiation of therapy. May require electrolyte replacement. May lead to cardiopulmonary arrest and sudden death.

Implementation

- Premedicate with histamine$_1$ antagonist (diphenhydramine 50 mg) 30–60 min prior to first dose; base subsequent administration on presence and severity of infusion reactions.

IV Administration

- Administer through a low protein binding 0.22-micrometer in-line filter placed as proximal to patient as possible. Solution should be clear and colorless and may contain a small amount of white amorphous cetuximab particles. Do not shake or dilute.

- Can be administered via infusion pump or syringe pump. Cetuximab should be piggybacked to the patient's infusion line.
- Observe patient for 1 hr following infusion.
- **Intermittent Infusion:** *For administration via infusion pump:* Draw up volume of a vial using vented spike needle or other transfer device. Transfer to a sterile evacuated container or bag. Repeat with new needle for each vial until calculated volume is in container. Affix infusion line and prime with cetuximab before starting infusion.
- *For administration via syringe pump:* Draw up volume of a vial using sterile syringe attached to an appropriate vented spike needle. Place syringe into syringe driver of a syringe pump and set rate. Connect infusion line and prime with cetuximab. Use a new needle and filter for each vial. ***Diluent:*** Do not dilute. ***Concentration:*** 2 mg/mL. ***Rate:*** Administer over 2 hr at a rate not to exceed 10 mg/min. Use 0.9% NaCl to flush line at end of infusion.
- Cetuximab infusion must be completed 1 hr prior to FOLFIRI (irinotecan, 5-fluorouracil, leucovorin) regimen. May infuse subsequent weekly infusions over 1 hr.

Patient/Family Teaching

- Explain purpose of cetuximab and potential side effects to patient.
- Advise patient to notify health care professional if dermatologic changes (itchy, dry, scaly, or cracking skin, and inflammation, infection or swelling at base of nails or loss of the nails), conjunctivitis, blepharitis, or decreased vision, and signs and symptoms of pulmonary toxicity (new or worsening cough, chest pain, shortness of breath), infusion reactions (fever, chills, or breathing problems) promptly. Risk for infusion reactions in patients who have had a tick bite or red meat allergy.
- Caution patient to wear sunscreen and hats and limit sun exposure during therapy during and for 2 mo following last dose of cetuximab.
- Rep: Advise females of reproductive potential and male patients with female partners of reproductive potential to use effective contraception during and for 2 mo after last dose of therapy and to avoid breast feeding during and for 2 mo following therapy.

Evaluation/Desired Outcomes

- Decreased tumor growth and spread.

chlorothiazide, See DIURETICS (THIAZIDE).

chlorthalidone (thiazide-like), See DIURETICS (THIAZIDE).

cholecalciferol, See VITAMIN D COMPOUNDS.

choline and magnesium salicylates, See SALICYLATES.

ciclesonide, See CORTICOSTEROIDS (NASAL).

ciclopirox, See ANTIFUNGALS (TOPICAL).

cilostazol (sil-os-tah-zol)

~~Pletal~~

Classification

Therapeutic: antiplatelet agents

Pharmacologic: platelet aggregation inhibitors

Indications

Reduction of the symptoms of intermittent claudication as measured by increased walking distance.

Action

Inhibits the enzyme cyclic adenosine monophosphate (cAMP) phosphodiesterase III (PDE III), which results in increased cAMP in platelets and blood vessels, producing inhibition of platelet aggregation and vasodilation. **Therapeutic Effects:** Reduced symptoms of intermittent claudication with improved walking distance.

Pharmacokinetics

Absorption: Slowly absorbed after oral administration.

Distribution: Unknown.

Protein Binding: 95–98% bound to plasma proteins; one active metabolite is 97.4% bound, the other is 66% bound.

Metabolism and Excretion: Extensively metabolized by the liver, two metabolites have platelet aggregation inhibitory activity; metabolites are mostly excreted by the kidneys.

Half-life: *Cilostazol and its active metabolites*—11–13 hr.

TIME/ACTION PROFILE (symptom reduction)

ROUTE	ONSET	PEAK	DURATION
PO	2–4 wk	up to 12 wk	unknown

Contraindications/Precautions

Contraindicated in: Hypersensitivity; HF; OB: Potential for congenital defects, stillbirth, and low birth weight; Lactation: Potential risk to nursing infants; discontinue or bottle feed.

Use Cautiously in: Pedi: Safety not established.

Adverse Reactions/Side Effects

CNS: headache, dizziness. **CV:** hypotension, left ventricular outflow obstruction, palpitations, tachycardia. **GI:** diarrhea.

Interactions

Drug-Drug: Concurrent administration of **ketoconazole**, **itraconazole**, **erythromycin**, **diltiazem**, **fluconazole**, **miconazole**, **fluvoxamine**, **fluoxetine**, **nefazodone**, **sertraline**, or **omeprazole** ↓ metabolism and ↑ levels and activity of cilostazol (use lower doses). Concurrent use with **aspirin** has additive effects on platelet function.

Drug-Food: **Grapefruit juice** inhibits metabolism and ↑ effects; concurrent use should be avoided.

Route/Dosage

PO (Adults): 100 mg twice daily (50 mg twice daily if receiving inhibitors of cilostazol metabolism).

Availability (generic available)

Tablets: 50 mg, 100 mg.

NURSING IMPLICATIONS

Assessment

- Assess patient for intermittent claudication before and periodically during therapy.
- ***Lab Test Considerations:*** May occasionally cause anemia, hyperlipemia, hyperuricemia, and albuminuria. May prolong bleeding time.

Implementation

- **PO:** Administer on an empty stomach, 1 hr before or 2 hr after meals.

Patient/Family Teaching

- Instruct patient to take cilostazol on an empty stomach, exactly as directed.
- Advise patient to avoid grapefruit juice during therapy.
- May cause dizziness. Caution patient to avoid driving or other activities requiring alertness until response to medication is known.
- Advise patient to avoid smoking; nicotine constricts blood vessels.

Evaluation/Desired Outcomes

- Relief from cramping in calf muscles, buttocks, thighs, and feet during exercise.
- Improvement in walking endurance. Therapeutic effects may be seen in 2–4 wk.

cimetidine, See HISTAMINE H_2 ANTAGONISTS.

cinacalcet (sin-a-**kal**-set)

Sensipar

Classification

Therapeutic: hypocalcemics

Pharmacologic: calcimimetic agents

Indications

Secondary hyperparathyroidism in patients with chronic kidney disease (CKD) on dialysis. Hypercalcemia caused by parathyroid carcinoma. Severe hypercalcemia in patients with primary hyperparathyroidism who are unable to undergo parathyroidectomy.

Action

Increases sensitivity of calcium-sensing receptors located on the surface of chief cells of parathyroid gland to levels of extracellular calcium. This decreases parathyroid hormone production with resultant decrease in serum calcium. **Therapeutic Effects:** Decreased bone turnover and fibrosis. Decreased serum calcium.

Pharmacokinetics

Absorption: Well absorbed following oral administration, absorption is enhanced by food and further enhanced by a high fat meal.

Distribution: Unknown.

Protein Binding: 93–97%.

Metabolism and Excretion: Highly metabolized by CYP3A4, CYP2D6, and CYP1A2 enzyme systems; 80% excreted in urine as metabolites, 15% in feces.

Half-life: 30–40 hr.

TIME/ACTION PROFILE (effect on PTH levels)

ROUTE	ONSET	PEAK	DURATION
PO	rapid	2–6 hr	6–12 hr

Contraindications/Precautions

Contraindicated in: Hypersensitivity; Hypocalcemia.

Use Cautiously in: History of seizure disorder (↑ risk of seizures with hypocalcemia); Chronic kidney disease patients who are not being dialyzed (↑ risk of hypocalcemia); Intact parathyroid hormone (iPTH) level <150 pg/mL (dose ↓ or discontinuation may be warranted); Moderate or severe hepatic impairment; Congenital long QT syndrome, QT interval prolongation, family history of long QT syndrome or sudden cardiac death, or concurrent use of QT interval prolonging medications; OB: Safety not established; Lactation: Use while breast feeding only if potential maternal benefit justifies potential risk to infant; Pedi: Safety not established.

Adverse Reactions/Side Effects

CNS: seizures. **CV:** ARRHYTHMIA, TORSADE DE POINTES, HF exacerbation, hypotension, QT interval prolongation. **F and E:** HYPOCALCEMIA. **GI:** nausea, vomiting. **Metab:** adynamic bone disease.

Interactions

Drug-Drug: Concurrent use of **QT interval prolonging medications** may ↑ risk of QT interval prolongation and/or torsade de pointes, especially in patients with hypocalcemia. Inhibits CYP2D6 and may ↑ levels of **flecainide**, **vinblastine**, **thioridazine**, **metoprolol**, **carvedilol**, and most **tricyclic antidepressants**; dose adjustments may be necessary. **Strong CYP3A4 inhibitors** including **ketoconazole**, **itraconazole**, and **erythromycin** may ↑ levels and risk of toxicity; monitoring and dose adjustment may be necessary.

Route/Dosage

PO (Adults): *Secondary hyperparathyroidism in CKD patients on dialysis*—30 mg once daily; may ↑ dose every 2–4 wk (dose range 30–180 mg once daily) based on iPTH levels; *Parathyroid carcinoma or primary hyperparathyroidism*—30 mg twice daily; may titrate every 2–4 wk up to 90 mg 3–4 times daily based on serum calcium levels.

Availability

Tablets: 30 mg, 60 mg, 90 mg.

NURSING IMPLICATIONS

Assessment

- Monitor for signs and symptoms of hypocalcemia (paresthesias, myalgias, cramping, tetany, convulsions) during therapy. If calcium levels decrease to below normal, serum calcium may be increased by adjusting dose (see Lab Test Considerations) and providing supplemental serum calcium, initiating or increasing dose of calcium-based phosphate binder or vitamin D.
- Monitor ECG for prolonged QT interval periodically during therapy.
- ***Lab Test Considerations:*** Monitor serum calcium and phosphorus levels within 1 wk after initiation of therapy or dose adjustment and monthly for patients with hyperparathyroidism or every 2 mo for patients with parathyroid carcinoma once maintenance dose has been established, especially in patients with a history of seizure disorder. Therapy should not be initiated in patients with serum calcium less than the lower limit of normal (8.4 mg/dL).
- If serum calcium ↓ below 8.4 mg/dL but remains above 7.5 mg/dL, or if symptoms of hypocalcemia occur, use calcium-containing phosphate binders and/or vitamin D sterols to ↑ serum calcium. If serum calcium ↓ below 7.5 mg/dL, or if symptoms of hypocalcemia persist and the dose of vitamin D cannot be ↑, withhold administration of cinacalcet until serum calcium levels reach 8.0 mg/dL, and/or symptoms of hypocalcemia resolve. Re-initiate therapy using next lowest dose of cinacalcet.
- Monitor serum iPTH levels 1 to 4 wk after initiation of therapy or dose adjustment, and every 1 to 3 mo after maintenance dose has been established. If iPTH levels ↓ below 150–300 pg/mL, reduce dose or discontinue cinacalcet. Assess iPTH levels no earlier than 12 hr after dose.
- Monitor liver function tests in patients with moderate to severe hepatic impairment during therapy.

Implementation

- Cinacalcet may be used alone or in combination with vitamin D and/or phosphate binders.
- **PO:** Administer with food or shortly after a meal. Take tablets whole, do not crush, break or chew.

Patient/Family Teaching

- Instruct patient to take cinacalcet as directed.
- Advise patient to report signs and symptoms of hypocalcemia, GI bleeding (black tarry stools, abdominal pain), nausea and vomiting to health care professional promptly.
- Advise females of reproductive potential to notify health care professional if pregnancy is planned or suspected, or if breast feeding.
- Emphasize the importance of follow-up lab tests to monitor safely and efficacy.

Evaluation/Desired Outcomes

- Decreased serum calcium levels.

HIGH ALERT

CISplatin (sis-**pla**-tin)

~~Platinol~~

Classification

Therapeutic: antineoplastics

Pharmacologic: alkylating agents

Indications

Metastatic testicular and ovarian carcinoma. Advanced bladder cancer. Head and neck cancer. Cervical cancer. Lung cancer. Other tumors.

Action

Inhibits DNA synthesis by producing cross-linking of parent DNA strands (cell-cycle phase–nonspecific). **Therapeutic Effects:** Death of rapidly replicating cells, particularly malignant ones.

Pharmacokinetics

Absorption: IV administration results in complete bioavailability.

Distribution: Widely distributed; accumulates for months; enters breast milk.

Metabolism and Excretion: Excreted mainly by the kidneys.

Half-life: 30–100 hr.

TIME/ACTION PROFILE (effects on blood counts)

ROUTE	ONSET	PEAK	DURATION
IV	unknown	18–23 days	39 days

Contraindications/Precautions

Contraindicated in: Hypersensitivity; OB, Lactation: Pregnancy or lactation.

Use Cautiously in: Hearing loss; Renal impairment (dosage ↓ recommended); HF; Electrolyte abnormalities; Active infections; Bone marrow depression; Geri: ↑ risk of nephrotoxicity and peripheral neuropathy; Rep: Women of reproductive potential.

Adverse Reactions/Side Effects

CNS: REVERSIBLE POSTERIOR LEUKOENCEPHALOPATHY SYNDROME (RPLS), SEIZURES, malaise, weakness. **EENT:** ototoxicity, tinnitus. **GI:** HEPATOTOXICITY, nausea, vomiting, diarrhea. **GU:** nephrotoxicity, sterility. **Derm:** alopecia. **F and E:** hypocalcemia, hypokalemia, hypomagnesemia. **Hemat:** LEUKOPENIA, THROMBOCYTOPENIA, anemia. **Local:** phlebitis at IV site. **Metab:** hyperuricemia. **Neuro:** peripheral neuropathy. **Misc:** anaphylactoid reactions.

Interactions

Drug-Drug: ↑ risk of nephrotoxicity and ototoxicity with other **nephrotoxic** and **ototoxic drugs (aminoglycosides, loop diuretics)**. ↑ risk of hypokalemia and hypomagnesemia with **loop diuretics** and **amphotericin B**. May ↓ **phenytoin** levels. ↑ bone marrow depression with other **antineoplastics** or **radiation therapy**. May ↓ antibody response to **live-virus vaccines** and ↑ adverse reactions.

Route/Dosage

Other regimens are used.

IV (Adults): *Metastatic testicular tumors*—20 mg/m² daily for 5 days repeated every 3–4 wk. *Metastatic ovarian cancer*—75–100 mg/m², repeat every 4 wk in combination with cyclophosphamide *or* 100 mg/m² every 3 wk if used as a single agent. *Advanced bladder cancer*—50–70 mg/m² every 3–4 wk as a single agent.

Availability (generic available)

Injection: 1 mg/mL.

NURSING IMPLICATIONS

Assessment

- Monitor vital signs frequently during administration. Report significant changes.
- Monitor intake and output and specific gravity frequently during therapy. To reduce risk of nephrotoxicity, maintain urinary output of at least 100 mL/hr for 4 hr before initiating and for at least 24 hr after administration.
- Encourage patient to drink 2000–3000 mL/day of water to promote excretion of uric acid. Allopurinol and alkalinization of urine may be used to help prevent uric acid nephropathy.
- Assess patency of IV site frequently during therapy. Cisplatin may cause severe irritation and necrosis of tissue if extravasation occurs. If a large amount of highly concentrated cisplatin solution extravasates, mix 4 mL of 10% sodium thiosulfate with 6 mL of sterile water or 1.6 mL of 25% sodium thiosulfate with 8.4 mL of sterile water and inject 1–4 mL (1 mL for each mL extravasated) through existing line or cannula. Inject subcut if needle has been removed. Sodium thiosulfate inactivates cisplatin.
- Severe and protracted nausea and vomiting usually occur 1–4 hr after a dose; vomiting may last for 24 hr. Administer parenteral antiemetic agents 30–45 min before therapy and routinely around the clock for the next 24 hr. Monitor amount of emesis and notify health care professional if emesis exceeds guidelines to prevent dehydration. Nausea and anorexia may persist for up to 1 wk.
- Monitor for bone marrow depression. Assess for bleeding (bleeding gums, bruising, petechiae, stools, urine, and emesis) and avoid IM injections and taking rectal temperatures if platelet count is low. Apply pressure to venipuncture sites for 10 min. Assess for signs of infection during neutropenia. Anemia may occur. Monitor for increased fatigue, dyspnea, and orthostatic hypotension.
- Monitor for signs of anaphylaxis (facial edema, wheezing, dizziness, fainting, tachycardia, hypotension). Discontinue medication immediately and report symptoms. Epinephrine and resuscitation equipment should be readily available.
- Medication may cause ototoxicity and neurotoxicity. Assess patient frequently for dizziness, tinnitus, hearing loss, loss of coordination, loss of taste, or numbness and tingling of extremities; may be irreversible. Notify health care professional promptly if these occur. Audiometry should be performed before initiation of therapy and before subsequent doses. Hearing loss is more frequent with children and usually occurs first with high frequencies and may be unilateral or bilateral.
- Monitor for inadvertent cisplatin overdose. Doses >100 m g/m²/cycle once every 3–4 wk are rarely used. Differentiate daily doses from total dose/cycle. Symptoms of high cumulative doses include muscle cramps (localized, painful involuntary skeletal muscle contractions of sudden onset and short duration) and are usually associated with advanced stages of peripheral neuropathy.
- Monitor for signs of RPLS (headache, seizure, lethargy, confusion, blindness). Hypertension may or may not be present. May occur within 16 hr to 1 yr

of initiation of therapy. Treat hypertension if present and discontinue cisplatin therapy. Symptoms usually resolve within days.

- ***Lab Test Considerations:*** Monitor CBC with differential and platelet count before and routinely throughout therapy. The nadir of leukopenia, thrombocytopenia, and anemia occurs within 18–23 days and recovery 39 days after a dose. Withhold further doses until WBC is >4000/mm³ and platelet count is >100,000/mm³.
- Monitor BUN, serum creatinine, and CCr before initiation of therapy and before each course of cisplatin to detect nephrotoxicity. May cause ↑ BUN and creatinine and ↓ calcium, magnesium, phosphate, sodium, and potassium levels that usually occur 2nd wk after a dose. Do not administer additional doses until BUN is <25 mg/dL and serum creatinine is <1.5 mg/dL. May cause ↑ uric acid level, which usually peaks 3–5 days after a dose.
- May cause transiently ↑ serum bilirubin and AST concentrations.
- May cause positive Coombs' test result.

Implementation

- ***High Alert:*** Fatalities have occurred with chemotherapeutic agents. Before administering, clarify all ambiguous orders; double-check single, daily, and course-of-therapy dose limits; have second practitioner independently double-check original order, calculations, and infusion pump settings.
- Do not confuse cisplatin with carboplatin. To prevent confusion, orders should include generic and brand names. Administer under supervision of a physician experienced in use of cancer chemotherapeutic agents.
- Solution should be prepared in a biologic cabinet. Wear gloves, gown, and mask while handling medication. If powder or solution comes in contact with skin or mucosa, wash thoroughly with soap and water. Discard equipment in specially designated containers.
- Hydrate patient with at least 1–2 L of IV fluid 8–12 hr before initiating therapy with cisplatin. Amifostine may be administered to minimize nephrotoxicity.
- Do not use aluminum needles or equipment during preparation or administration. Aluminum reacts with this drug, forms a black or brown precipitate, and renders the drug ineffective.
- Unopened vials of powder and constituted solution must not be refrigerated.

IV Administration

- **Intermittent Infusion:** Solution should be clear and colorless; discard if turbid or if it contains precipitates.
- ***Diluent:*** Dilution in 2 L of 5% dextrose in 0.3% or 0.45% NaCl containing 37.5 g of mannitol is recommended. ***Concentration:*** Keep under 0.5 mg/mL to prevent tissue necrosis. ***Rate:*** Variable. Administer over 6–8 hr. Maximum rate 1 mg/min.
- **Continuous Infusion:** Has been administered as continuous infusion over 24 hr to 5 days with resultant decrease in nausea and vomiting. ***High Alert:*** Clarify dose to ensure cumulative dose is not confused with daily dose; errors may be fatal.
- **Y-Site Compatibility:** acyclovir, alfentanil, allopurinol, amikacin, aminophylline, amiodarone, ampicillin, ampicillin/sulbactam, anidulafungin, argatroban, azithromycin, aztreonam, bivalirudin, bleomycin, bumetanide, buprenorphine, butorphanol, calcium chloride, calcium gluconate, carmustine, caspofungin, cefazolin, cefotaxime, cefotetan, ceftazidime, ceftriaxone, cefuroxime, chlorpromazine, ciprofloxacin, cisatracurium, cladribine, clindamycin, cyclophosphamide, cyclosporine, cytarabine, dactinomycin, daptomycin, daunorubicin hydrochloride, dexamethasone, dexmedetomidine, dexrazoxane, digoxin, diltiazem, diphenhydramine, dobutamine, docetaxel, dolasetron, dopamine, doxacurium, doxorubicin, doxorubicin liposome, doxycycline, droperidol, enalaprilat, ephedrine, epinephrine, epirubicin, ertapenem, erythromycin, esmolol, etoposide, etoposide phosphate, famotidine, fenoldopam, fentanyl, filgrastim, fluconazole, fludarabine, fluorouracil, foscarnet, fosphenytoin, furosemide, ganciclovir, gemcitabine, gentamicin, glycopyrrolate, granisetron, haloperidol, heparin, hetastarch, hydrocortisone, hydromorphone, idarubicin, ifosfamide, imipenem/cilastatin, indomethacin, irinotecan, isoproterenol, ketorolac, labetalol, leucovorin calcium, levofloxacin, levorphanol, lidocaine, linezolid, lorazepam, magnesium sulfate, mannitol, melphalan, meperidine, meropenem, methotrexate, methylprednisolone, metoclopramide, metoprolol, metronidazole, midazolam, milrinone, mitomycin, mitoxantrone, moxifloxacin, nafcillin, naloxone, nicardipine, nitroglycerin, nitroprusside, norepinephrine, octreotide, ondansetron, oxaliplatin, paclitaxel, palonosetron, pamidronate, pancuronium, pemetrexed, pentamidine, pentobarbital, phenobarbital, phenylephrine, phenytoin, potassium acetate, potassium chloride, potassium phosphates, procainamide, prochlorperazine, promethazine, propofol, propranolol, quinupristin/dalfopristin, ranitidine, remifentanil, rituximab, sargramostim, sodium acetate, sodium bicarbonate, sodium phosphates, succinylcholine, sufentanil, tacrolimus, theophylline, thiopental, tigecycline, tirofiban, tobramycin, topotecan, trastuzumab, vancomycin, vasopressin, vecuronium, verapamil, vinblastine, vincristine, vinorelbine, voriconazole, zidovudine, zoledronic acid.
- **Y-Site Incompatibility:** amifostine, amphotericin B deoxycholate, amphotericin B lipid complex, amphotericin B liposome, cefepime, dantrolene, diaze-

pam, insulin, pantoprazole, piperacillin/tazobactam, thiotepa.

Patient/Family Teaching

- Instruct patient to report pain at injection site immediately.
- Instruct patient to notify health care professional promptly if fever; chills; cough; hoarseness; sore throat; signs of infection; lower back or side pain; painful or difficult urination; bleeding gums; bruising; petechiae; blood in stools, urine, or emesis; increased fatigue; dyspnea; or orthostatic hypotension occurs. Caution patient to avoid crowds and persons with known infections. Instruct patient to use soft toothbrush and electric razor and to avoid falls. Caution patient not to drink alcoholic beverages or take medication containing aspirin or NSAIDs; may precipitate gastric bleeding.
- Instruct patient to report promptly any numbness or tingling in extremities or face, difficulty with hearing or tinnitus, unusual swelling, or joint pain.
- Instruct patient not to receive any vaccinations without advice of health care professional.
- Advise patient of the need for contraception, although cisplatin may cause infertility.
- Emphasize the need for periodic lab tests to monitor for side effects.

Evaluation/Desired Outcomes

- Decrease in size or spread of malignancies. Therapy should not be administered more frequently than every 3–4 wk, and only if lab values are within acceptable parameters and patient is not exhibiting signs of ototoxicity or other serious adverse effects.

citalopram (si-tal-oh-pram)

CeleXA

Classification
Therapeutic: antidepressants
Pharmacologic: selective serotonin reuptake inhibitors (SSRIs)

Indications

Depression. **Unlabeled Use:** Premenstrual dysphoric disorder (PMDD). Obsessive-compulsive disorder (OCD). Panic disorder. Generalized anxiety disorder (GAD). Post-traumatic stress disorder (PTSD). Social anxiety disorder (social phobia).

Action

Selectively inhibits the reuptake of serotonin in the CNS. **Therapeutic Effects:** Antidepressant action.

Pharmacokinetics

Absorption: 80% absorbed after oral administration.
Distribution: Enters breast milk.
Metabolism and Excretion: Mostly metabolized by the liver (10% by CYP3A4 and 2C19 enzymes); excreted unchanged in urine.
Half-life: 35 hr.

TIME/ACTION PROFILE (antidepressant effect)

ROUTE	ONSET	PEAK	DURATION
PO	1–4 wk	unknown	unknown

Contraindications/Precautions

Contraindicated in: Hypersensitivity; Concurrent use of MAO inhibitors or MAO-like drugs (linezolid or methylene blue); Concurrent use of pimozide; Congenital long QT syndrome, bradycardia, hypokalemia, hypomagnesemia, recent myocardial infarction, decompensated heart failure (↑ risk of QT interval prolongation); Concurrent use of QT interval prolonging drugs.
Use Cautiously in: History of mania; History of suicide attempt/ideation (↑ risk during early therapy and during dose adjustment); History of seizure disorder; Illnesses or conditions that are likely to result in altered metabolism or hemodynamic responses; Severe renal or hepatic impairment (maximum dose of 20 mg/day in patients with hepatic impairment); Poor metabolizers of CYP2C19 (↑ risk of QT interval prolongation) (maximum dose of 20 mg/day); Concurrent use of CYP2C19 inhibitors (↑ risk of QT interval prolongation) (maximum dose of 20 mg/day); Angle-closure glaucoma; OB: Use during third trimester may result in neonatal serotonin syndrome requiring prolonged hospitalization, respiratory and nutritional support; Lactation: Present in breast milk and may result in lethargy with ↓ feeding in infants; weigh risk/benefits; Pedi: May ↑ risk of suicide attempt/ideation especially during early treatment or dose adjustment in children/adolescents (unlabeled for pediatric use); Geri: ↓ doses recommended (maximum dose of 20 mg/day in patients >60 yr).

Adverse Reactions/Side Effects

CNS: NEUROLEPTIC MALIGNANT SYNDROME, SUICIDAL THOUGHTS, apathy, confusion, drowsiness, insomnia, weakness, agitation, amnesia, anxiety, ↓ libido, dizziness, fatigue, impaired concentration, ↑ depression, migraine headache. **EENT:** abnormal accommodation. **Resp:** cough. **CV:** TORSADE DE POINTES, postural hypotension, QT interval prolongation, tachycardia. **GI:** abdominal pain, anorexia, diarrhea, dry mouth, dyspepsia, flatulence, ↑ saliva, nausea, altered taste, ↑ appetite, vomiting. **GU:** amenorrhea, dysmenorrhea, ejaculatory delay, erectile dysfunction, polyuria. **Derm:** sweating, photosensitivity, pruritus, rash. **Metab:** weight loss, weight gain. **F and E:** hyponatremia. **MS:** arthralgia, myalgia. **Neuro:** tremor, paresthesia. **Misc:** SEROTONIN SYNDROME, fever, yawning.

Interactions

Drug-Drug: May cause serious, potentially fatal reactions when used with **MAO inhibitors**; concurrent use contraindicated; allow at least 14 days between citalopram and **MAO inhibitors**. Concurrent use with **MAO-inhibitor like drugs**, such as **linezolid** or **methylene blue**, may ↑ risk of serotonin syndrome;

concurrent use contraindicated; do not start therapy in patients receiving **linezolid** or **methylene blue**; if **linezolid** or **methylene blue** need to be started in a patient receiving citalopram, immediately discontinue citalopram and monitor for signs/symptoms of serotonin syndrome for 2 wk or until 24 hr after last dose of linezolid or methylene blue, whichever comes first (may resume citalopram therapy 24 hr after last dose of linezolid or methylene blue). Concurrent use with **pimozide** may result in prolongation of the QTc interval and is contraindicated. **QT interval prolonging drugs** may ↑ the risk of QT interval prolongation and torsade de pointes (concurrent use should be avoided). **CYP2C19 inhibitors**, including **cimetidine** may ↑ levels and the risk of toxicity (maximum dose = 20 mg/day). Drugs that affect serotonergic neurotransmitter systems, including **tricyclic antidepressants**, **SNRIs**, **fentanyl**, **buspirone**, **tramadol**, **amphetamines**, and **triptans** ↑ risk of serotonin syndrome. Use cautiously with other **centrally acting drugs** (including **alcohol**, **antihistamines**, **opioid analgesics**, and **sedative/hypnotics**; concurrent use with **alcohol** is not recommended). Serotonergic effects may be ↑ by **lithium** (concurrent use should be carefully monitored). **Ketoconazole**, **itraconazole**, **erythromycin**, and **omeprazole** may ↑ levels. **Carbamazepine** may ↓ blood levels. May ↑ levels of **metoprolol**. Use cautiously with **tricyclic antidepressants** due to unpredictable effects on serotonin and norepinephrine reuptake. ↑ risk of bleeding with **aspirin**, **NSAIDs**, **clopidogrel**, or **warfarin**.

Drug-Natural Products: ↑ risk of serotonergic side effects including serotonin syndrome with **St. John's wort** and **SAMe**.

Route/Dosage

PO (Adults): 20 mg once daily initially, may be ↑ in 1 wk to 40 mg/day (maximum dose); *Poor metabolizer of CYP2C19 or concurrent use of CYP2C19 inhibitor*—Do not exceed dose of 20 mg/day.

PO (Geriatric Patients): 20 mg once daily initially (do not exceed dose of 20 mg/day in patients >60 yr).

Hepatic Impairment

PO (Adults): 20 mg once daily (do not exceed dose of 20 mg/day).

Availability (generic available)

Tablets: 10 mg, 20 mg, 40 mg. **Cost:** *Generic*—10 mg $7.11/100, 20 mg $9.73/100, 40 mg $10.83/100. **Oral solution (peppermint flavor):** 10 mg/5 mL. **Cost:** *Generic*—10 mg/5 mL $117.50/240 mL.

NURSING IMPLICATIONS

Assessment

- Monitor mood changes during therapy.
- Assess for suicidal tendencies, especially during early therapy and dose changes. Restrict amount of drug available to patient. Risk may be increased in children, adolescents, and adults ≤24 yr. After starting therapy, children, adolescents, and young adults should be seen by health care professional at least weekly for 4 wk, every 3 wk for the next 4 wk, and on advice of health care professional thereafter.
- Assess for sexual dysfunction (erectile dysfunction; decreased libido).
- Assess for serotonin syndrome (mental changes [agitation, hallucinations, coma], autonomic instability [tachycardia, labile BP, hyperthermia], neuromuscular aberrations [hyperreflexia, incoordination], and/or GI symptoms [nausea, vomiting, diarrhea]), especially in patients taking other serotonergic drugs (SSRIs, SNRIs, triptans).
- ***Lab Test Considerations:*** Monitor electrolytes (potassium and magnesium) in patients at risk for electrolyte imbalances prior to and periodically during therapy.

Implementation

- Do not confuse with Celebrex (celecoxib), Cerebyx (fosphenytoin), or Zyprexa (olanzapine).
- **PO:** Administer as a single dose in the morning or evening without regard to food.

Patient/Family Teaching

- Instruct patient to take citalopram as directed. Take missed doses as soon as remembered unless almost time for next dose; do not double doses. Do not stop abruptly; may cause anxiety, irritability, high or low mood, feeling restless or changes in sleep habits, headache, sweating, nausea, dizziness, electric shock-like sensations, shaking, and confusion. Advise patient to read the *Medication Guide* prior to starting therapy and with each refill in case of changes.
- May cause drowsiness, dizziness, impaired concentration, and blurred vision. Caution patient to avoid driving and other activities requiring alertness until response to the drug is known.
- Instruct patient to notify health care professional of all Rx or OTC medications, vitamins, or herbal products being taken and to consult health care professional before taking any other Rx, OTC, or herbal products, especially alcohol or other CNS depressants and St. John's wort.
- Caution patient to change positions slowly to minimize dizziness.
- Advise patient, family, and caregivers to look for suicidality, especially during early therapy or dose changes. Notify health care professional immediately if thoughts about suicide or dying, attempts to commit suicide, new or worse depression or anxiety, agitation or restlessness, panic attacks, insomnia, new or worse irritability, aggressiveness, acting on dangerous impulses, mania, or other changes in mood or behavior or if symptoms of serotonin syndrome occur.

- Advise patient to use sunscreen and wear protective clothing to prevent photosensitivity reactions.
- Inform patient that frequent mouth rinses, good oral hygiene, and sugarless gum or candy may minimize dry mouth. If dry mouth persists for more than 2 wk, consult health care professional regarding use of saliva substitute.
- Instruct female patients to inform health care professional if pregnancy is planned or suspected, or if breast feeding. If used during pregnancy should be tapered during third trimester to avoid neonatal serotonin syndrome.
- Emphasize the importance of follow-up exams to monitor progress.

Evaluation/Desired Outcomes

- Increased sense of well-being.
- Renewed interest in surroundings. May require 1–4 wk of therapy to obtain antidepressant effects.

clarithromycin

(kla-**rith**-roe-mye-sin)

~~Biaxin~~, Biaxin XL

Classification

Therapeutic: agents for atypical mycobacterium, anti-infectives, antiulcer agents

Pharmacologic: macrolides

Indications

Respiratory tract infections including streptococcal pharyngitis, sinusitis, bronchitis, and pneumonia. Treatment (with ethambutol) and prevention of disseminated *Mycobacterium avium* complex (MAC). Treatment of following pediatric infections: Otitis media, Sinusitis, Pharyngitis, Skin/skin structure infections. Part of a combination regimen for ulcer disease due to *Helicobacter pylori*. Endocarditis prophylaxis.

Action

Inhibits protein synthesis at the level of the 50S bacterial ribosome. **Therapeutic Effects:** Bacteriostatic action. **Spectrum:** Active against these gram-positive aerobic bacteria: *Staphylococcus aureus*, *S. pneumoniae*, *S. pyogenes* (group A strep). Active against these gram-negative aerobic bacteria: *Haemophilus influenzae*, *Moraxella catarrhalis*. Also active against: *Mycoplasma*, *Legionella*, *H. pylori*, *M. avium*.

Pharmacokinetics

Absorption: Rapidly absorbed (50%) after oral administration.

Distribution: Widely distributed; tissue levels may exceed those in serum.

Protein Binding: 65–70%.

Metabolism and Excretion: 10–15% converted by the liver to 14-hydroxyclarithromycin, which has anti-infective activity; 20–30% excreted unchanged in urine. Metabolized by and also inhibits the CYP3A enzyme system.

Half-life: Dose-dependent and prolonged with renal dysfunction *250-mg dose*—3–4 hr; *500-mg dose*—5–7 hr.

TIME/ACTION PROFILE (serum levels)

ROUTE	ONSET	PEAK	DURATION
PO	unknown	2 hr	12 hr
PO-XL	unknown	4 hr	24 hr

Contraindications/Precautions

Contraindicated in: Hypersensitivity to clarithromycin, erythromycin, or other macrolide anti-infectives; History of cholestatic jaundice or hepatic dysfunction with clarithromycin; Concurrent use of pimozide, ergotamine, dihydroergotamine, lovastatin, simvastatin, disopyramide, quinidine, procainamide, dofetilide, amiodarone, or sotalol; Concurrent use of colchicine in patients with hepatic or renal impairment; QT interval prolongation, hypokalemia, hypomagnesemia, or bradycardia; OB: Pregnancy (may cause fetal harm); avoid use unless no alternatives are available.

Use Cautiously in: Coronary artery disease (may ↑ risk of mortality); Severe liver or renal impairment (dose adjustment required if CCr <30 mL/min); Myasthenia gravis; Lactation: Use during breast feeding only if benefit to patient outweighs potential risk to infant; Pedi: Children <6 mo (safety and effectiveness not established); Geri: May have ↑ risk of QT interval prolongation.

Adverse Reactions/Side Effects

CNS: headache. **CV:** TORSADES DE POINTES, QT interval prolongation. **Derm:** ACUTE GENERALIZED EXANTHEMATOUS PUSTULOSIS, DRUG RASH WITH EOSINOPHILIA AND SYSTEMIC SYMPTOMS (DRESS), STEVENS-JOHNSON SYNDROME, TOXIC EPIDERMAL NECROLYSIS, pruritus, rash. **GI:** HEPATOTOXICITY, CLOSTRIDIUM DIFFICILE-ASSOCIATED DIARRHEA (CDAD), abdominal pain/discomfort, abnormal taste, diarrhea, dyspepsia, nausea. **Misc:** HYPERSENSITIVITY REACTIONS (including anaphylaxis and angioedema).

Interactions

Drug-Drug: Clarithromycin is an inhibitor of the CYP3A enzyme system. Concurrent use with other agents metabolized by this system can ↑ levels and risk of toxicity. May prolong the QT interval and ↑ risk of arrhythmias with **pimozide**; concurrent use contraindicated. May ↑ levels of **ergotamine** and **dihydroergotamine** and risk for acute ergot toxicity; concurrent use contraindicated. **Disopyramide**, **quinidine**, **procainamide**, **dofetilide**, **sotalol**, and **amiodarone** may ↑ risk of QT interval prolongation; concurrent use should be avoided. ↑ risk of rhabdomyolysis with **lovastatin** and **simvastatin**; concurrent use contraindicated. May ↑ serum levels and the risk of toxicity from **carbamazepine**, some **benzodiazepines (midazolam, triazolam, alprazolam)**, **cyclosporine**, **disopyramide**, **quinidine**, **ergot alkaloids**, **felodipine**, **omeprazole**, **tacrolimus**, **digoxin**, **quetiapine**, or **theophylline**. May ↑ levels and effects of **omepra-**

zole. **Ritonavir** ↑ blood levels (↓ clarithromycin dose in patients with CCr <60 mL/min). ↑ levels and risk of myopathy from **atorvastatin** and **pravastatin**; use lowest dose of these agents; do not exceed atorvastatin dose of 20 mg/day or pravastatin dose of 40 mg/day. May ↑ or ↓ effects of **zidovudine**. Blood levels are ↑ by **delavirdine** and **fluconazole**. Blood levels may be ↓ by **rifampin**, **rifabutin**, **efavirenz**, and **nevirapine**. May ↑ levels and risk of toxicity from **colchicine**; ↓ colchicine dose in patients with normal renal and hepatic function; concurrent use is contraindicated in patients with renal or hepatic impairment. May ↑ **calcium channel blocker** levels and the risk for hypotension, bradycardia, and lactic acidosis. Concomitant use with **calcium channel blockers** metabolized by CYP3A4, including **verapamil**, **diltiazem**, **amlodipine**, and **nifedipine** may ↑ the risk of acute kidney injury, especially in patients older than 65 yr. May ↑ **warfarin** levels and the risk for bleeding. May ↑ blood levels and effects of **sildenafil**, **tadalafil**, and **vardenafil**; concurrent use not recommended. May ↑ levels of **tolterodine**. Concurrent use with **atazanavir** may ↑ clarithromycin and atazanavir levels; ↓ clarithromycin dose by 50%. Concurrent use with **itraconazole** may ↑ clarithromycin and itraconazole levels. Concurrent use with **saquinavir** may ↑ clarithromycin and saquinavir levels.

Route/Dosage

PO (Adults): *Pharyngitis/tonsillitis*— 250 mg every 12 hr for 10 days; *Acute maxillary sinusitis*— 500 mg every 12 hr for 14 days or 1000 mg once daily for 14 days as XL tablets; *Acute exacerbation of chronic bronchitis*— 250–500 mg every 12 hr for 7–14 days or 1000 mg once daily for 7 days as XL tablets; *Community-acquired pneumonia*— 250 mg every 12 hr for 7–14 days or 1000 mg once daily for 7 days as XL tablets; *Skin/skin structure infections*— 250 mg every 12 hr for 7–14 days; *H. pylori*— 500 mg 2–3 times daily with a proton pump inhibitor (lansoprazole or omeprazole) or ranitidine with or without amoxicillin for 10–14 days; *Endocarditis prophylaxis*— 500 mg 1 hr before procedure; *MAC prophylaxis/treatment*— 500 mg twice daily, for active infection another antimycobacterial is required.

PO (Children ≥6 mo): *Most infections*— 15 mg/kg/day divided every 12 hr for 7–14 days (up to 500 mg/dose for MAC). *Endocarditis prophylaxis*— 15 mg/kg 1 hr before procedure.

Renal Impairment

PO (Adults): *CCr <30 mL/min*— 250 mg 1–2 times daily, a 500-mg initial dose may be used.

PO (Children): *CCr <30 mL/min*— ↓ dose by 50% or double dosing interval.

Availability (generic available)

Tablets: 250 mg, 500 mg. **Extended-release tablets:** 500 mg. **Oral suspension (fruit punch and vanilla flavors):** 125 mg/5 mL, 250 mg/5 mL. ***In combination with:*** amoxicillin and lansoprazole as part of a compliance package (Prevpac); See Appendix B.

NURSING IMPLICATIONS

Assessment

- Assess patient for infection (vital signs; appearance of wound, sputum, urine, and stool; WBC) at beginning of and during therapy.
- Obtain specimens for culture and sensitivity before initiating therapy. First dose may be given before receiving results.
- Monitor bowel function. Diarrhea, abdominal cramping, fever, and bloody stools should be reported to health care professional promptly as a sign of Clostridium difficile-associated diarrhea (CDAD). May begin up to several wk after cessation of therapy.
- Assess patient for skin rash frequently during therapy. Discontinue clarithromycin at first sign of rash; may be life-threatening. Stevens-Johnson syndrome may develop. Treat symptomatically; may recur once treatment is stopped.
- **Ulcers:** Assess patient for epigastric or abdominal pain and frank or occult blood in the stool, emesis, or gastric aspirate.
- ***Lab Test Considerations:*** May rarely cause ↑ serum AST, ALT, total bilirubin, and alkaline phosphatase concentrations.
- May occasionally cause ↑ BUN.

Implementation

- **PO:** Administer around the clock, without regard to meals; may be administered with milk. Food slows but does not decrease the extent of absorption.
- Administer XL tablets with food or milk. Swallow whole; do not crush, break, or chew.
- Shake suspension well before administration. Store suspension at room temperature; do not refrigerate.
- Do not administer within 4 hr of zidovudine.

Patient/Family Teaching

- Instruct patient to take medication around the clock and to finish the drug completely as directed, even if feeling better. Take missed doses as soon as possible, unless almost time for next dose. Do not double doses. Advise patient that sharing of this medication may be dangerous.
- May cause dizziness, vertigo, confusion and disorientation. Caution patient to avoid driving and other activities requiring alertness until response to medication is known.
- Advise patient to report the signs of superinfection (black, furry overgrowth on the tongue; vaginal itching or discharge; loose or foul-smelling stools).
- Instruct patient to notify health care professional if rash, or fever and diarrhea develop, especially if

stool contains blood, pus, or mucus. Advise patient not to treat diarrhea without consulting health care professional.

- Caution patients taking zidovudine that clarithromycin and zidovudine must be taken at least 4 hr apart.
- Advise patient to notify health care professional of all Rx or OTC medications, vitamins, or herbal products being taken and to consult with health care professional before taking other medications.
- Rep: May cause fetal harm. Advise patient to notify health care professional immediately if pregnancy is planned or suspected or if breast feeding.
- Instruct the patient to notify health care professional if symptoms do not improve within a few days.

Evaluation/Desired Outcomes

- Resolution of the signs and symptoms of infection. Length of time for complete resolution depends on the organism and site of infection.
- Treatment of ulcers.
- Endocarditis prophylaxis.

clindamycin (klin-da-**mye**-sin)

Cleocin, Cleocin T, Clinda-Derm, ✱Clinda-T, Clindagel, Clindesse, Clindets, ✱Dalacin C, ✱Dalacin T, Evoclin

Classification

Therapeutic: anti-infectives

Indications

PO, IM, IV: Treatment of: Skin and skin structure infections, Respiratory tract infections, Septicemia, Intra-abdominal infections, Gynecologic infections, Osteomyelitis, Endocarditis prophylaxis. **Topical:** Severe acne. **Vag:** Bacterial vaginosis. **Unlabeled Use: PO, IM, IV:** Treatment of *Pneumocystis jiroveci* pneumonia, CNS toxoplasmosis, and babesiosis.

Action

Inhibits protein synthesis in susceptible bacteria at the level of the 50S ribosome. **Therapeutic Effects:** Bactericidal or bacteriostatic, depending on susceptibility and concentration. **Spectrum:** Active against most gram-positive aerobic cocci, including: Staphylococci, *Streptococcus pneumoniae*, other streptococci, but not enterococci. Has good activity against those anaerobic bacteria that cause bacterial vaginosis, including *Bacteroides fragilis*, *Gardnerella vaginalis*, *Mobiluncus* spp., *Mycoplasma hominis*, and *Corynebacterium*. Also active against *Pneumocystis jirovecii*, *Propionibacterium acnes*, and *Toxoplasma gondii*.

Pharmacokinetics

Absorption: Well absorbed following PO/IM administration. Minimal absorption following topical/vaginal use.

Distribution: Widely distributed. Does not significantly cross blood-brain barrier. Crosses the placenta; enters breast milk.

Protein Binding: 94%.

Metabolism and Excretion: Mostly metabolized by the liver (by CYP3A4).

Half-life: Neonates: 3.6–8.7 hr; Infants up to 1 yr: 3 hr; Children and adults: 2–3 hr.

TIME/ACTION PROFILE (blood levels)

ROUTE	ONSET	PEAK	DURATION
PO	rapid	60 min	6–8 hr
IM	rapid	1–3 hr	6–8 hr
IV	rapid	end of infusion	6–8 hr

Contraindications/Precautions

Contraindicated in: Hypersensitivity; Regional enteritis or ulcerative colitis (topical foam); Previous *Clostridium difficile*—associated diarrhea; Severe liver impairment; Diarrhea; Known alcohol intolerance (topical solution, suspension).

Use Cautiously in: OB: Safety not established for topical administration; systemic administration during 2nd and 3rd trimesters not associated with ↑ risk of congenital abnormalities; approved for vaginal use in 3rd trimester of pregnancy; injection contains benzyl alcohol which can cross placenta; Lactation: Appears in breast milk (when given PO or IV) and exposes infant to drug and its side effects; not known whether appears in breast milk after vaginal or topical administration; Pedi: Injection contains benzyl alcohol which can cause gasping syndrome in infants and neonates.

Adverse Reactions/Side Effects

CNS: dizziness, headache, vertigo. **CV:** arrhythmias, hypotension. **Derm:** DRUG REACTION WITH EOSINOPHILIA AND SYSTEMIC SYMPTOMS (DRESS), ERYTHEMA MULTIFORME, STEVENS-JOHNSON SYNDROME, TOXIC EPIDERMAL NECROLYSIS, rash, urticaria. **GI:** CLOSTRIDIUM DIFFICILE ASSOCIATED DIARRHEA, diarrhea, bitter or metallic taste, nausea, vomiting. **Local:** local irritation (topical products), phlebitis at IV site. **Misc:** HYPERSENSITIVITY REACTIONS (including anaphylaxis).

Interactions

Drug-Drug: May enhance the neuromuscular blocking action of other **neuromuscular blocking agents**. **CYP3A4 inhibitors** may ↑ levels. **CYP3A4 inducers**, including **rifampin** may ↓ levels and lead to therapeutic failure. **Topical:** Concurrent use with **irritants**, **abrasives**, or **desquamating agents** may result in additive irritation.

Route/Dosage

PO (Adults): *Most infections*—150–450 mg every 6 hr. *Pneumocystis jiroveci pneumonia*—1200–1800 mg/day in divided doses with 15–30 mg primaquine/day (unlabeled). *CNS toxoplasmosis*—1200–2400 mg/day in divided doses with pyrimethamine 50–100 mg/day (unlabeled); *Bacterial endocarditis prophylaxis*—600 mg 1 hr before procedure.

PO (Children >1 mo): 10–30 mg/kg/day divided every 6–8 hr; maximum dose 1.8 g/day. *Bacterial en-*

docarditis prophylaxis—20 mg/kg 1 hr before procedure.
IM, IV (Adults): *Most infections*—300–600 mg every 6–8 hr *or* 900 mg every 8 hr (up to 4.8 g/day IV has been used; single IM doses of >600 mg are not recommended). *Pneumocystis jiroveci pneumonia*—2400–2700 mg/day in divided doses with primaquine (unlabeled). *Toxoplasmosis*—1200–4800 mg/day in divided doses with pyrimethamine. *Bacterial endocarditis prophylaxis*—600 mg 30 min before procedure.
IM, IV (Children >1 mo): 25–40 mg/kg/day divided every 6–8 hr; maximum dose: 4.8 g/day. *Bacterial endocarditis prophylaxis*—20 mg/kg 30 min before procedure; maximum dose: 600 mg.
IM, IV (Infants <1 mo and <2 kg): 5 mg/kg every 8–12 hr; *≥2 kg*—20–30 mg/kg/day divided every 6–8 hr.
Vag (Adults and Adolescents): *Cleocin, Clindamax*—1 applicatorful (5 g) at bedtime for 3 or 7 days (7 days in pregnant patients); *Clindesse*—one applicatorful (5 g) single dose; *or* 1 suppository (100 mg) at bedtime for 3 nights.
Topical (Adults and Adolescents): *Solution*—1% solution/suspension applied twice daily (range 1–4 times daily). *Foam, gel*—1% foam or gel applied once daily.

Availability (generic available)

Capsules: 75 mg, 150 mg, 300 mg. **Oral suspension:** 75 mg/5 mL. **Solution for injection:** 150 mg/mL. **Premixed infusion (in 0.9% NaCl):** 300 mg/50 mL, 600 mg/50 mL, 900 mg/50 mL. **Topical:** 1% lotion, gel, foam, solution, suspension, single-use applicators. **Vaginal cream:** 2%. **Vaginal suppositories (ovules):** 100 mg. ***In combination with:*** benzoyl peroxide (Acanya, BenzaClin, Onexton), tretinoin (Veltin, Ziana); (see Appendix B).

NURSING IMPLICATIONS

Assessment

- Assess for infection (vital signs; appearance of wound, sputum, urine, and stool; WBC) at beginning of and during therapy.
- Obtain specimens for culture and sensitivity prior to initiating therapy. First dose may be given before receiving results.
- Monitor bowel elimination. Report diarrhea, abdominal cramping, fever, and bloody stools to health care professional promptly as a sign of Clostridium difficile-associated diarrhea (CDAD). May begin up to several wk following the cessation of therapy.
- Assess patient for hypersensitivity (skin rash, urticaria).
- ***Lab Test Considerations:*** Monitor CBC; may cause transient ↓ in leukocytes, eosinophils, and platelets.
- May cause ↑ alkaline phosphatase, bilirubin, CPK, AST, and ALT concentrations.

Implementation

- Do not confuse Clindesse with Clindets.
- **PO:** Administer with a full glass of water. May be given with or without meals. Shake liquid preparations well. Do not refrigerate. Stable for 14 days at room temperature.
- **IM:** Inject undiluted. Do not administer >600 m g in a single IM injection.

IV Administration

- **Intermittent Infusion:** ***Diluent:*** Vials must be diluted before use. Dilute a dose of 300 mg or 600 mg in 50 mL and a dose of 900 mg or 1200 mg in 100 mL. Compatible diluents include D5W, 0.9% NaCl, D5/0.9% NaCl, D5/0.45% NaCl, or LR. Admixed solution stable for 16 days at room temperature. Premixed infusion is already diluted and ready to use. ***Concentration:*** Not to exceed 18 mg/mL. ***Rate:*** Infuse over 10–60 min. Not to exceed 30 mg/min. Hypotension and cardiopulmonary arrest have been reported following rapid IV administration.
- **Y-Site Compatibility:** acetaminophen, acyclovir, alemtuzumab, alfentanil, amifostine, amikacin, aminocaproic acid, aminophylline, amiodarone, amphotericin B lipid complex, amphotericin B liposome, anakinra, anidulafungin, argatroban, arsenic trioxide, ascorbic acid, atropine, aztreonam, benztropine, bivalirudin, bleomycin, bumetanide, buprenorphine, butorphanol, calcium chloride, calcium gluconate, cangrelor, carboplatin, carmustine, cefazolin, cefotaxime, cefotetan, cefoxitin, ceftaroline, ceftazidime, cefuroxime, chloramphenicol, cisatracurium, cisplatin, cyanocobalamin, cyclophosphamide, cyclosporine, cytarabine, dacarbazine, dactinomycin, daptomycin, dexamethasone, dexmedetomidine, dexrazoxane, digoxin, diltiazem, diphenhydramine, dobutamine, docetaxel, dolasetron, dopamine, doxorubicin, doxorubicin liposomal, doxycycline, enalaprilat, ephedrine, epinephrine, epirubicin, epoetin alfa, eptifibatide, esmolol, etoposide, etoposide phosphate, famotidine, fenoldopam, fentanyl, fludarabine, fluorouracil, folic acid, foscarnet, fosphenytoin, furosemide, gemcitabine, gentamicin, glycopyrrolate, granisetron, heparin, hetastarch, hydrocortisone, hydromorphone, ifosfamide, imipenem/cilastatin, indomethacin, insulin regular, irinotecan, isoproterenol, ketamine, ketorolac, leucovorin, levofloxacin, lidocaine, linezolid, lorazepam, magnesium sulfate, mannitol, melphalan, meperidine, mesna, methotrexate, methyldopate, methylprednisolone, metoclopramide, metoprolol, milrinone, morphine, multivitamins, nafcillin, nalbuphine, naloxone, nitroglycerin, nitroprusside, norepinephrine, octreotide, ondansetron, oxacillin, ox-

aliplatin, oxytocin, paclitaxel, palonosetron, pamidronate, pancuronium, pemetrexed, penicillin G, phenobarbital, phenylephrine, phytonadione, piperacillin/tazobactam, potassium acetate, potassium chloride, procainamide, propofol, propranolol, protamine, pyridoxine, ranitidine, remifentanil, rituximab, rocuronium, sargramostim, sodium acetate, sodium bicarbonate, succinylcholine, sufentanil, tacrolimus, theophylline, thiamine, thiotepa, tigecycline, tirofiban, tobramycin, vancomycin, vasopressin, vecuronium, verapamil, vinblastine, vincristine, vinorelbine, vitamin B complex with C, voriconazole, zidovudine, zoledronic acid.

- **Y-Site Incompatibility:** allopurinol, azathioprine, caspofungin, ceftriaxone, chlorpromazine, dantrolene, daunorubicin, diazepam, filgrastim, ganciclovir, haloperidol, hydroxyzine, idarubicin, minocycline, mitomycin, mitoxantrone, mycophenolate, papaverine, pentamidine, pentobarbital, phentolamine, phenytoin, prochlorperazine, promethazine, quinupristin/dalfopristin, topotecan, trastuzumab, trimethoprim/sulfamethoxazole.
- **Vag:** Applicators are supplied for vaginal administration. When treating bacterial vaginosis, concurrent treatment of male partner is not usually necessary.
- **Topical:** Contact with eyes, mucous membranes, and open cuts should be avoided during topical application. If accidental contact occurs, rinse with copious amounts of cool water.
- Wash affected areas with warm water and soap, rinse, and pat dry prior to application. Apply to entire affected area.

Patient/Family Teaching

- Instruct patient to take medication around the clock at evenly spaced times and to finish completely as directed, even if feeling better. Take missed doses as soon as possible unless almost time for next dose. Do not double doses. Advise patient that sharing of this medication may be dangerous.
- Instruct patient to notify health care professional immediately if diarrhea, abdominal cramping, fever, or bloody stools occur and not to treat with antidiarrheals without consulting health care professional.
- Advise patient to report signs of superinfection (furry overgrowth on the tongue, vaginal or anal itching or discharge).
- Notify health care professional if no improvement within a few days.
- Patients with a history of rheumatic heart disease or valve replacement need to be taught the importance of antimicrobial prophylaxis before invasive medical or dental procedures.
- Rep: Advise female patient of reproductive potential to notify health care professional if pregnancy is planned or suspected or if breast feeding. Use with caution during 1st trimester. If breast feeding, alternate drugs are preferred. If breast feeding continued, monitor infant for diarrhea, thrush, and diaper rash.
- **IV:** Inform patient that bitter or metallic taste occurring with IV administration is not clinically significant.
- **Vag:** Instruct patient on proper use of vaginal applicator. Insert high into vagina at bedtime. Instruct patient to remain recumbent for at least 30 min following insertion. Advise patient to use sanitary napkin to prevent staining of clothing or bedding. Continue therapy during menstrual period.
- Advise patient to refrain from vaginal sexual intercourse during treatment.
- Caution patient that mineral oil in clindamycin cream may weaken latex or rubber contraceptive devices. Such products should not be used within 72 hr of vaginal cream.
- **Topical:** Caution patient applying topical clindamycin that solution is flammable (vehicle is isopropyl alcohol). Avoid application while smoking or near heat or flame.
- Advise patient to notify health care professional if excessive drying of skin occurs.
- Advise patient to wait 30 min after washing or shaving area before applying.

Evaluation/Desired Outcomes

- Resolution of the signs and symptoms of infection. Length of time for complete resolution depends on the organism and site of infection.
- Endocarditis prophylaxis.
- Improvement in acne vulgaris lesions. Improvement should be seen in 6 wk but may take 8–12 wk for maximum benefit.

clobetasol, See CORTICOSTEROIDS (TOPICAL/LOCAL).

clocortolone, See CORTICOSTEROIDS (TOPICAL/LOCAL).

BEERS

clonazePAM (kloe-**na**-ze-pam)

KlonoPIN, Rivotril

Classification

Therapeutic: anticonvulsants

Pharmacologic: benzodiazepines

Schedule IV

Indications

Treatment of Lennox-Gastaut, akinetic, or myoclonic seizures. Panic disorder with or without agoraphobia. **Unlabeled Use:** Uncontrolled leg movements during sleep. Neuralgias. Infantile spasms. Sedation. Adjunct management of acute mania, acute psychosis, or insomnia.

Action

Anticonvulsant effects may be due to presynaptic inhibition. Produces sedative effects in the CNS, probably by stimulating inhibitory GABA receptors. **Therapeutic Effects:** Prevention of seizures. Decreased manifestations of panic disorder.

Pharmacokinetics

Absorption: Well absorbed from the GI tract.
Distribution: Probably crosses the blood-brain barrier and the placenta.
Protein Binding: 85%.
Metabolism and Excretion: Mostly metabolized by the liver.
Half-life: 18–50 hr.

TIME/ACTION PROFILE (anticonvulsant activity)

ROUTE	ONSET	PEAK	DURATION
PO	20–60 min	1–2 hr	6–12 hr

Contraindications/Precautions

Contraindicated in: Hypersensitivity to clonazepam or other benzodiazepines; Severe hepatic impairment; OB: Pregnancy (may cause fetal harm); Lactation: Lactation.

Use Cautiously in: All patients (may ↑ risk of suicidal thoughts/behaviors); Angle-closure glaucoma; Obstructive sleep apnea; Chronic respiratory disease; History of porphyria; Pedi: Children <18 yr (panic disorder) (safety and effectiveness not established); Geri: May experience excessive sedation at usual doses; ↓ dose recommended.

Adverse Reactions/Side Effects

CNS: SUICIDAL THOUGHTS, behavioral changes, drowsiness, fatigue, slurred speech, ataxia, sedation, abnormal eye movements, diplopia, nystagmus. **CV:** palpitations. **Derm:** rash. **GI:** constipation, diarrhea, hepatitis, weight gain. **GU:** dysuria, nocturia, urinary retention. **Hemat:** anemia, eosinophilia, leukopenia, thrombocytopenia. **Neuro:** ataxia, hypotonia. **Resp:** ↑ secretions. **Misc:** fever, physical dependence, psychological dependence, tolerance.

Interactions

Drug-Drug: Use with **opioids** or other **CNS depressants**, including other **benzodiazepines**, **nonbenzodiazepine sedative/hypnotics**, **anxiolytics**, **general anesthetics**, **muscle relaxants**, **antipsychotics**, and **alcohol** may cause profound sedation, respiratory depression, coma, and death; reserve concurrent use for when alternative treatment options are inadequate. **Cimetidine**, **hormonal contraceptives**, **disulfiram**, **fluoxetine**, **isoniazid**, **ketoconazole**, **metoprolol**, **propranolol**, or **valproic acid** may ↓ metabolism and ↑ toxicity of clonazepam. May ↓ efficacy of **levodopa**. **Rifampin** or **barbiturates** may ↑ metabolism and ↓ effectiveness. Sedative effects may be ↓ by **theophylline**. May ↑ serum **phenytoin** levels. **Phenytoin** may ↓ levels.

Drug-Natural Products: Concomitant use of **kava-kava**, **valerian**, or **chamomile** can ↑ CNS depression.

Route/Dosage

PO (Adults): 0.5 mg 3 times daily; may ↑ by 0.5–1 mg every 3 days. Total daily maintenance dose not to exceed 20 mg. *Panic disorder*—0.125 mg twice daily; ↑ after 3 days toward target dose of 1 mg/day (some patients may require up to 4 mg/day).

PO (Children ≤10 yr or ≤30 kg): Initial daily dose 0.01–0.03 mg/kg/day (not to exceed 0.05 mg/kg/day) given in 2–3 equally divided doses; ↑ by no more than 0.25–0.5 mg every 3 days until therapeutic blood levels are reached (not to exceed 0.2 mg/kg/day).

Availability (generic available)

Tablets: ✱ 0.25 mg, 0.5 mg, 1 mg, 2 mg. **Cost:** *Generic*—0.5 mg $11.77/100, 1 mg $11.25/100, 2 mg $15.59/100. **Orally disintegrating tablets:** 0.125 mg, 0.25 mg, 0.5 mg, 1 mg, 2 mg. **Cost:** *Generic*—0.125 mg $77.93/60, 0.25 mg $77.93/60, 0.5 mg $77.80/60, 1 mg $88.91/60, 2 mg $123.19/60.

NURSING IMPLICATIONS

Assessment

- Observe and record intensity, duration, and location of seizure activity.
- Assess degree and manifestations of anxiety and mental status (orientation, mood, behavior) prior to and periodically during therapy.
- Assess need for continued treatment regularly.
- Assess patient for drowsiness, unsteadiness, and clumsiness. These symptoms are dose related and most severe during initial therapy; may decrease in severity or disappear with continued or long-term therapy.
- Monitor closely for notable changes in behavior that could indicate the emergence or worsening of suicidal thoughts or behavior or depression.
- ***Lab Test Considerations:*** Patients on prolonged therapy should have CBC and liver function test results evaluated periodically. May cause an ↑ in serum bilirubin, AST, and ALT.
- May cause ↓ thyroidal uptake of ^{123}I, and ^{131}I.
- ***Toxicity and Overdose:*** Therapeutic serum concentrations are 20–80 mg/mL. Flumazenil antagonizes clonazepam toxicity or overdose (may induce seizures in patients with history of seizure disorder or who are on tricyclic antidepressants).

Implementation

- Do not confuse clonazepam with alprazolam, clonidine, clozapine, clobazam, or lorazepam. Do not confuse Klonopin with clonidine.
- Institute seizure precautions for patients on initial therapy or undergoing dose manipulations.
- **PO:** Administer with food to minimize gastric irritation. Tablets may be crushed if patient has difficulty swallowing. Administer largest dose at bedtime to avoid daytime sedation. Taper by 0.25 mg every 3 days to decrease signs and symptoms of withdrawal. Some patients may require longer taper period (months).
- Orally disintegrating tablets should be left in the package until use. Remove from the blister pouch. Do not push tablet through the blister; peel open the blister pack with dry hands and place tablet on tongue. Tablet will dissolve rapidly and be swallowed with saliva. No liquid is needed to take the orally disintegrating tablet.

Patient/Family Teaching

- Instruct patient to take medication exactly as directed. Take missed doses within 1 hr or omit; do not double doses. Abrupt withdrawal of clonazepam may cause status epilepticus, tremors, nausea, vomiting, and abdominal and muscle cramps. Instruct patient to read the *Medication Guide* before starting and with each Rx refill, changes may occur.
- Advise patient that clonazepam is usually prescribed for short-term use and does not cure underlying problems.
- Advise patient to not share medication with others.
- May cause drowsiness or dizziness. Advise patient to avoid driving or other activities requiring alertness until response to drug is known.
- Instruct patient to notify health care professional of all Rx or OTC medications, vitamins, or herbal products being taken and to consult health care professional before taking any other Rx, OTC, or herbal products. Caution patient to avoid taking alcohol or other CNS depressants concurrently with this medication.
- Advise patient to notify health care professional of medication regimen prior to treatment or surgery.
- Instruct patient and family to notify health care professional of unusual tiredness, bleeding, sore throat, fever, clay-colored stools, yellowing of skin, or behavioral changes. Advise patient and family to notify health care professional if thoughts about suicide or dying, attempts to commit suicide; new or worse depression; new or worse anxiety; feeling very agitated or restless; panic attacks; trouble sleeping; new or worse irritability; acting aggressive; being angry or violent; acting on dangerous impulses; an extreme increase in activity and talking; other unusual changes in behavior or mood occur.
- Advise female patients to notify health care professional if pregnancy is planned or suspected or if breast feeding. Encourage pregnant patients to enroll in North American Antiepileptic Drug (NAAED) Pregnancy Registry to collect information about safety of antiepileptic drugs during pregnancy. To enroll, patients can call 1-888-233-2334.
- Patient on anticonvulsant therapy should carry identification at all times describing disease process and medication regimen.
- Emphasize the importance of follow-up exams to determine effectiveness of the medication.

Evaluation/Desired Outcomes

- Decrease or cessation of seizure activity without undue sedation. Dose adjustments may be required after several mo of therapy.
- Decrease in frequency and severity of panic attacks.
- Relief of leg movements during sleep.
- Decrease in pain from neuralgia.

BEERS

cloNIDine (klon-i-deen)

Catapres, Catapres-TTS, Duraclon, Kapvay

Classification

Therapeutic: antihypertensives
Pharmacologic: adrenergics (centrally acting)

Indications

PO, Transdermal: Mild to moderate hypertension. **PO:** Attention-deficit hyperactivity disorder (ADHD) (as monotherapy or as adjunctive to stimulants) (Kapvay only). **Epidural:** Management of cancer pain unresponsive to opioids alone. **Unlabeled Use:** Management of opioid withdrawal. Adjunctive treatment of neuropathic pain.

Action

Stimulates alpha-adrenergic receptors in the CNS, which results in decreased sympathetic outflow inhibiting cardioacceleration and vasoconstriction centers. Prevents pain signal transmission to the CNS by stimulating alpha-adrenergic receptors in the spinal cord. **Therapeutic Effects:** Decreased BP. Decreased pain. Improvement in ADHD symptoms.

Pharmacokinetics

Absorption: Well absorbed from the GI tract and skin. Enters systemic circulation following epidural use. Some absorption follows sublingual administration.
Distribution: Widely distributed; enters CNS. Crosses the placenta readily; enters breast milk in high concentrations.
Metabolism and Excretion: Mostly metabolized by the liver; 40–60% eliminated unchanged in urine.
Half-life: *Neonates*—44–72 hr; *Children*—8–12 hr; *Adults: Plasma*—12–16 hr (↑ in renal impairment); *CNS*—1.3 hr.

TIME/ACTION PROFILE (PO, TD = antihypertensive effect; epidural = analgesia)

ROUTE	ONSET	PEAK	DURATION
PO	30–60 min	1–3 hr	8–12 hr
Transdermal	2–3 days	unknown	7 days†
Epidural	unknown	unknown	unknown

†8 hr following removal of patch.

Contraindications/Precautions

Contraindicated in: Hypersensitivity; *Epidural*—injection site infection, anticoagulant therapy, or bleeding problems.

Use Cautiously in: Serious cardiac or cerebrovascular disease; Renal insufficiency; Pedi: Safety and efficacy not established for ADHD in children <6 yr; evaluation for cardiac disease should precede initiation of therapy for ADHD in children; Geri: Appear on Beers list due to ↑ risk of orthostatic hypotension and adverse CNS effects in geriatric patients (↓ dose recommended); OB, Lactation: Safety not established.

Adverse Reactions/Side Effects

CNS: drowsiness, depression, dizziness, hallucinations, nervousness, nightmares. **EENT:** dry eyes. **CV:** AV block, bradycardia, hypotension (↑ with epidural), palpitations. **GI:** dry mouth, constipation, nausea, vomiting. **GU:** erectile dysfunction. **Derm:** rash, sweating. **F and E:** sodium retention. **Metab:** weight gain. **Neuro:** paresthesia. **Misc:** withdrawal phenomenon.

Interactions

Drug-Drug: Additive sedation with **CNS depressants**, including **alcohol**, **antihistamines**, **opioid analgesics**, and **sedative/hypnotics**. Additive hypotension with other **antihypertensives** and **nitrates**. Additive bradycardia with **beta blockers**, **diltiazem**, **verapamil**, or **digoxin**. **MAO inhibitors**, **amphetamines**, or **tricyclic antidepressants** may ↓ antihypertensive effect. Withdrawal phenomenon may be ↑ by discontinuation of **beta blockers**. Epidural clonidine prolongs the effects of epidurally administered **local anesthetics**. May ↓ effectiveness of **levodopa**.

Route/Dosage

PO (Adults and Adolescents ≥12 yr): *Hypertension (immediate-release)*—100 mcg (0.1 mg) twice daily, ↑ by 100–200 mcg (0.1–0.2 mg)/day every 2–4 days; usual maintenance dose is 200–600 mcg (0.2–0.6 mg)/day in 2–3 divided doses (up to 2.4 mg/day). *Urgent treatment of hypertension (immediate-release)*—200 mcg (0.2 mg) loading dose, then 100 mcg (0.1 mg) every hr until BP is controlled or 800 mcg (0.8 mg) total has been administered; follow with maintenance dosing; *Opioid withdrawal (immediate-release)*—300 mcg (0.3 mg)–1.2 mg/day, may be ↓ by 50%/day for 3 days, then discontinued or ↓ by 100–200 mcg (0.1–0.2 mg)/day.

PO (Geriatric Patients): *Hypertension (immediate–release)*—100 mcg (0.1 mg) at bedtime initially, ↑ as needed.

PO (Children): *Hypertension (immediate-release)*—Initial 5–10 mcg/kg/day divided into 2 or 3 doses, then ↑ gradually to 5–25 mcg/kg/day in divided doses every 6 hr; maximum dose: 0.9 mg/day. *ADHD (Kapvay-extended release) (children >6 yr)*—0.1 mg once daily at bedtime; after 1 wk, ↑ dose to 0.1 mg in AM and at bedtime; after 1 wk, ↑ dose to 0.1 mg in AM and 0.2 mg at bedtime; after 1 wk, ↑ dose to 0.2 mg in AM and at bedtime (max dose = 0.4 mg/day). *ADHD (Immediate release) (children >6 yr, <45 kg)*—0.05 mg once daily at bedtime; then ↑ every 3–7 days to 0.05 mg twice daily; then 0.05 mg 3 times daily; then 0.05 mg 4 times daily. *Neuropathic pain (immediate-release)*—2 mcg/kg/dose every 4–6 hr then ↑ gradually over days up to 4 mcg/kg/dose every 4–6 hr.

PO (Neonates): *Neonatal abstinence syndrome*—0.5–1 mcg/kg/dose every 4–6 hr. Once stabilized taper by 0.25 mcg/kg/dose every 6 hr.

Transdermal (Adults): *Hypertension*—Transdermal system delivering 100–300 mcg (0.1–0.3 mg)/24 hr applied every 7 days. Initiate with 100 mcg (0.1 mg)/24 hr system; dosage increments may be made every 1–2 wk when system is changed.

Transdermal (Children): Once stable oral dose is reached, children may be switched to a transdermal system equivalent closest to the total daily oral dose.

Epidural (Adults): 30 mcg/hr initially; titrated according to need.

Epidural (Children): 0.5 mcg/kg/hr initially; titrated according to need up to 2 mcg/kg/hr.

Availability (generic available)

Tablets: 🍁 25 mcg (0.025 mg), 100 mcg (0.1 mg), 200 mcg (0.2 mg), 300 mcg (0.3 mg). **Cost:** *Generic*—0.1 mg $6.80/100, 0.2 mg $6.99/100, 0.3 mg $6.99/100. **Extended-release tablets (Kapvay):** 0.1 mg. **Cost:** All strengths $366.60/60. **Transdermal systems:** Catapres-TTS 1, releases 0.1 mg/24 hr, Catapres-TTS 2, releases 0.2 mg/24 hr, Catapres-TTS 3, releases 0.3 mg/24 hr. **Cost:** *Generic*—0.1 mg/24 hr $132.49/4 patches, 0.2 mg/24 hr $223.06/4 patches, 0.3 mg/24 hr $309.44/4 patches. **Solution for epidural injection (Duraclon):** 100 mcg/mL, 500 mcg/mL.

NURSING IMPLICATIONS

Assessment

- **Hypertension:** Monitor intake and output ratios and daily weight, and assess for edema daily, especially at beginning of therapy.
- Monitor BP and pulse prior to starting, frequently during initial dose adjustment and dose increases and periodically throughout therapy. Titrate slowly in patients with cardiac conditions or those taking other sympatholytic drugs. Report significant changes.

- **Pain:** Assess location, character, and intensity of pain prior to, frequently during first few days, and routinely throughout administration.
- Monitor for fever as potential sign of catheter infection.
- **Opioid Withdrawal:** Monitor patient for signs and symptoms of opioid withdrawal (tachycardia, fever, runny nose, diarrhea, sweating, nausea, vomiting, irritability, stomach cramps, shivering, unusually large pupils, weakness, difficulty sleeping, gooseflesh).
- **ADHD:** Assess attention span, impulse control, and interactions with others.
- ***Lab Test Considerations:*** May cause transient ↑ in blood glucose levels.
- May cause ↓ urinary catecholamine and vanillylmandelic acid (VMA) concentrations; these may ↑ on abrupt withdrawal.
- May cause weakly positive Coombs' test result.

Implementation

- Do not confuse clonidine with clonazepam (Klonopin) or clozapine.
- Do not substitute between clonidine products on a mg-per-mg basis, because of differing pharmacokinetic profiles.
- In the perioperative setting, continue clonidine up to 4 hr prior to surgery and resume as soon as possible thereafter. Do not interrupt *transdermal clonidine* during surgery. Monitor BP carefully.
- **PO:** Administer last dose of the day at bedtime. May be taken without regard for food.
- Swallow extended-release tablets whole; do not crush, break, or chew.
- **Transdermal:** Transdermal system should be applied once every 7 days. May be applied to any hairless site; avoid cuts or calluses. Absorption is greater when placed on chest or upper arm and decreased when placed on thigh. Rotate sites. Wash area with soap and water; dry thoroughly before application. Apply firm pressure over patch to ensure contact with skin, especially around edges. Remove old system and discard. System includes a protective adhesive overlay to be applied over medication patch to ensure adhesion, should medication patch loosen.
- **Epidural:** Dilute 500 mcg/mL with 0.9% NaCl for a concentration of 100 mcg/mL. Do not administer solutions that are discolored or contain a precipitate. Discard unused portion.

Patient/Family Teaching

- Instruct patient to take clonidine at the same time each day, even if feeling well. Take missed dose as soon as remembered. If dose of extended-release product is missed, omit dose and take next dose as scheduled. Do not take more than the prescribed daily dose in any 24 hr. If more than 1 oral dose in a row is missed or if transdermal system is late in being changed by 3 or more days, consult health care professional. All routes of clonidine should be gradually discontinued over 2–4 days to prevent rebound hypertension.
- Advise patient to make sure enough medication is available for weekends, holidays, and vacations. A written prescription may be kept in wallet in case of emergency.
- May cause drowsiness, which usually diminishes with continued use. Advise patient to avoid driving or other activities requiring alertness until response to medication is known.
- Caution patient to avoid sudden changes in position to decrease orthostatic hypotension. Use of alcohol, standing for long periods, exercising, and hot weather may increase orthostatic hypotension.
- If dry mouth occurs, frequent mouth rinses, good oral hygiene, and sugarless gum or candy may decrease effect. If dry mouth continues for more than 2 wk, consult health care professional.
- Caution patients with contact lenses that clonidine may cause dryness of eyes.
- Caution patient to avoid concurrent use of alcohol or other CNS depressants with this medication.
- Instruct patient to notify health care professional of all Rx or OTC medications, vitamins, or herbal products being taken and to consult health care professional before taking any other Rx, OTC, or herbal products, especially cough, cold, or allergy remedies.
- Advise patient to notify health care professional of medication regimen prior to treatment or surgery.
- Advise patient to notify health care professional if itching or redness of skin (with transdermal patch), mental depression, swelling of feet and lower legs, paleness or cold feeling in fingertips or toes, or vivid dreams or nightmares occur. May require discontinuation of therapy, especially with depression.
- **Hypertension:** Encourage patient to comply with additional interventions for hypertension (weight reduction, low-sodium diet, discontinuation of smoking, moderation of alcohol consumption, regular exercise, and stress management). Medication helps control but does not cure hypertension.
- Instruct patient and family on proper technique for BP monitoring. Advise them to check BP at least weekly and report significant changes.
- **Transdermal:** Instruct patient on proper application of transdermal system. Do not cut or trim unit. Transdermal system can remain in place during bathing or swimming.
- Advise patient referred for MRI test to discuss patch with referring health care professional and MRI facility to determine if removal of patch is necessary prior to test and for directions for replacing patch.
- Pedi: Advise parents to notify school nurse of medication regimen.

Evaluation/Desired Outcomes

- Decrease in BP.
- Decrease in severity of pain.
- Decrease in the signs and symptoms of opioid withdrawal.
- Improved attention span and social interactions in ADHD.

C

clopidogrel (kloh-pid-oh-grel)
Plavix

Classification
Therapeutic: antiplatelet agents
Pharmacologic: platelet aggregation inhibitors

Indications
Acute coronary syndrome (ST-segment elevation MI, non-ST-segment elevation MI, or unstable angina). Patients with established peripheral arterial disease, recent MI, or recent stroke.

Action
Inhibits platelet aggregation by irreversibly inhibiting the binding of ATP to platelet receptors. **Therapeutic Effects:** Reduction in risk of MI and stroke.

Pharmacokinetics
Absorption: Well absorbed following oral administration; rapidly metabolized to an active antiplatelet compound. Parent drug has no antiplatelet activity.
Distribution: Unknown.
Protein Binding: *Clopidogrel*—98%; *active metabolite*—94%.
Metabolism and Excretion: Rapidly and extensively converted by the liver (CYP2C19) to its active metabolite, which is then eliminated 50% in urine and 45% in feces; 2% of Whites, 4% of Blacks, and 14% of Asians have CYP2C19 genotype that results in reduced metabolism of clopidogrel (poor metabolizers) into its active metabolite (may result in ↓ antiplatelet effects).
Half-life: 6 hr (active metabolite 30 min).

TIME/ACTION PROFILE (effects on platelet function)

ROUTE	ONSET	PEAK	DURATION
PO	within 24 hr	3–7 days	5 days†

†Following discontinuation.

Contraindications/Precautions
Contraindicated in: Hypersensitivity to clopidogrel or prasugrel; Pathologic bleeding (peptic ulcer, intracranial hemorrhage); Concurrent use of omeprazole or esomeprazole; CYP2C19 poor metabolizers; Lactation: Lactation.
Use Cautiously in: Patients at risk for bleeding (trauma, surgery, or other pathologic conditions); History of GI bleeding/ulcer disease; Severe hepatic impairment; Hypersensitivity to another thienopyridine (prasugrel); OB: Use only if clearly indicated; Pedi: Safety and effectiveness not established.

Adverse Reactions/Side Effects
Incidence of adverse reactions similar to that of aspirin. **CNS:** depression, dizziness, fatigue, headache. **CV:** chest pain, edema, hypertension. **Derm:** ACUTE GENERALIZED EXANTHEMATOUS PUSTULOSIS, DRUG RASH WITH EOSINOPHILIA AND SYSTEMIC SYMPTOMS, STEVENS-JOHNSON SYNDROME, TOXIC EPIDERMAL NECROLYSIS, pruritus, purpura, rash. **EENT:** epistaxis. **GI:** GI BLEEDING, abdominal pain, diarrhea, dyspepsia, gastritis. **Hemat:** BLEEDING, NEUTROPENIA, THROMBOTIC THROMBOCYTOPENIC PURPURA. **Metab:** hypercholesterolemia. **MS:** arthralgia, back pain. **Resp:** cough, dyspnea, eosinophilic pneumonia. **Misc:** HYPERSENSITIVITY REACTIONS (including anaphylaxis), fever.

Interactions
Drug-Drug: Concurrent **eptifibatide, tirofiban, aspirin, NSAIDs, heparin, LMWHs, thrombolytic agents, SSRIs, SNRIs, prasugrel,** or **warfarin** may ↑ risk of bleeding. May ↓ metabolism and ↑ effects of **phenytoin, repaglinide, tamoxifen, torsemide, fluvastatin,** and many **NSAIDs**; avoid concurrent use with **repaglinide**. Concurrent use with the CYP2C19 inhibitors, **omeprazole,** or **esomeprazole** may ↓ antiplatelet effects; avoid concurrent use; may consider using **H_2 antagonist** or another **proton pump inhibitor** (e.g., **dexlansoprazole, lansoprazole,** or **pantoprazole**). **Opioids** may ↓ absorption of clopidogrel and its active metabolite and ↓ antiplatelet effects; consider using parenteral antiplatelet in patients with acute coronary syndrome if concurrent use of opioids needed.
Drug-Natural Products: ↑ bleeding risk with **anise, arnica, chamomile, clove, fenugreek, feverfew, garlic, ginger, ginkgo, Panax ginseng,** and others.

Route/Dosage
Recent MI, Stroke, or Peripheral Arterial Disease
PO (Adults): 75 mg once daily.

Acute Coronary Syndrome
PO (Adults): 300 mg initially, then 75 mg once daily; aspirin 75–325 mg once daily should be given concurrently.

Availability (generic available)
Tablets: 75 mg, 300 mg. **Cost:** *Generic*—75 mg $23.46/90.

NURSING IMPLICATIONS
Assessment
- Assess patient for symptoms of stroke, peripheral vascular disease, or MI periodically during therapy.
- Monitor patient for signs of thrombotic thrombocytic purpura (thrombocytopenia, microangiopathic

hemolytic anemia, neurologic findings, renal dysfunction, fever). May rarely occur, even after short exposure (<2 wk). Requires prompt treatment.

- ***Lab Test Considerations:*** Monitor bleeding time during therapy. Prolonged bleeding time, which is time- and dose-dependent, is expected.
- Monitor CBC with differential and platelet count periodically during therapy. Neutropenia and thrombocytopenia may rarely occur.
- May cause ↑ serum bilirubin, hepatic enzymes, total cholesterol, nonprotein nitrogen (NPN), and uric acid concentrations.

Implementation

- Do not confuse Plavix (clopidogrel) with Paxil (paroxetine) or Pradaxa (dabigatran).
- Discontinue clopidogrel 5–7 days before planned surgical procedures. If clopidogrel must be temporarily discontinued, restart as soon as possible. Premature discontinuation of therapy may increase risk of cardiovascular events.
- **PO:** Administer once daily without regard to food.

Patient/Family Teaching

- Instruct patient to take medication exactly as directed. Take missed doses as soon as possible unless almost time for next dose; do not double doses. Do not discontinue clopidogrel without consulting health care professional; may increase risk of cardiovascular events. Advise patient to read the *Medication Guide* before starting clopidogrel and with each Rx refill in case of changes.
- Advise patient to notify health care professional promptly if signs and symptoms of bleeding (unexpected bleeding or bleeding that lasts a long time; blood in urine [pink, red or brown urine], red or black stools [looks like tar], bruises without known cause or get larger; cough up blood or blood clots; vomit blood or vomit looks like coffee grounds); fever, weakness, chills, sore throat, rash, unusual bleeding or bruising, extreme skin paleness, purple skin patches, yellowing of skin or eyes, or neurological changes occur.
- Advise patient to notify health care professional of medication regimen prior to treatment or surgery.
- Caution patient to avoid taking omeprazole or esomeprazole during therapy. Consult health care professional for other options.
- Instruct patient to notify health care professional of all Rx or OTC medications, vitamins, or herbal products being taken and to consult health care professional before taking any other Rx, OTC, or herbal products, especially those containing aspirin or NSAIDs or proton pump inhibitors.
- Advise female patient to notify health care professional if pregnancy is planned or suspected, or if breast feeding.

Evaluation/Desired Outcomes

- Prevention of stroke, MI, and vascular death in patients at risk.

clotrimazole, See ANTIFUNGALS (TOPICAL) and ANTIFUNGALS (VAGINAL).

BEERS REMS

cloZAPine (kloe-za-peen)

Clozaril, ~~FazaClo~~, Versacloz

Classification
Therapeutic: antipsychotics

Indications

Schizophrenia unresponsive to or intolerant of standard therapy with other antipsychotics (treatment refractory). To reduce recurrent suicidal behavior in schizophrenic patients.

Action

Binds to dopamine receptors in the CNS. Also has anticholinergic and alpha-adrenergic blocking activity. Produces fewer extrapyramidal reactions and less tardive dyskinesia than standard antipsychotics but carries high risk of hematologic abnormalities. **Therapeutic Effects:** Diminished schizophrenic behavior. Diminished suicidal behavior.

Pharmacokinetics

Absorption: Well absorbed after oral administration.
Distribution: Rapid and extensive distribution; crosses blood-brain barrier and placenta.
Protein Binding: 95%.
Metabolism and Excretion: Mostly metabolized on first pass through the liver (by CYP1A2, CYP2D6, and CYP3A4 isoenzymes); (the CYP2D6 enzyme system exhibits genetic polymorphism; ~7% of population may be poor metabolizers and may have significantly ↑ clozapine concentrations and an ↑ risk of adverse effects).
Half-life: 8–12 hr.

TIME/ACTION PROFILE (antipsychotic effect)

ROUTE	ONSET	PEAK	DURATION
PO	unknown	wk	4–12 hr

Contraindications/Precautions

Contraindicated in: Hypersensitivity; Bone marrow depression; Severe CNS depression/coma; Uncontrolled epilepsy; Clozapine-induced agranulocytosis or severe granulocytopenia; Lactation: Lactation.
Use Cautiously in: Long QT syndrome; Risk factors for QT interval prolongation or ventricular arrhythmias (i.e., recent myocardial infarction, heart failure, arrhythmias); Concurrent use of CYP1A2, CYP2D6, or CYP3A4 inhibitors or QT-interval prolonging drugs; Hypokalemia or hypomagenesemia; Prostatic enlargement; Angle-closure glaucoma; Malnourished or dehydrated patients, patients with cardiovascular, cerebrovascular, hepatic, or renal disease, or patients

on antihypertensives (use lower initial dose, titrate more slowly); Risk factors for stroke (↑ risk of stroke in patients with dementia); Diabetes; Seizure disorder; Patients at risk for falls; OB: Neonates at ↑ risk for extrapyramidal symptoms and withdrawal after delivery when exposed during the 3rd trimester; use only if potential maternal benefit justifies potential fetal risk; Pedi: Children <16 yr (safety and effectiveness not established); Geri: ↑ risk of mortality in elderly patients treated for dementia-related psychosis.

Adverse Reactions/Side Effects

CNS: NEUROLEPTIC MALIGNANT SYNDROME, SEIZURES, dizziness, sedation. **CV:** CARDIAC ARREST, DEEP VEIN THROMBOSIS, HF, MITRAL VALVE INCOMPETENCE, MYOCARDITIS, TORSADE DE POINTES, VENTRICULAR ARRHYTHMIAS, hypotension, tachycardia, bradycardia, ECG changes, hypertension, syncope, QT interval prolongation. **Derm:** rash, sweating. **EENT:** visual disturbances. **GI:** HEPATOTOXICITY, constipation, abdominal discomfort, dry mouth, ↑ salivation, nausea, vomiting, weight gain. **GU:** nocturnal enuresis. **Endo:** hyperglycemia, hyperlipidemia, weight gain. **Hemat:** AGRANULOCYTOSIS, LEUKOPENIA. **Neuro:** extrapyramidal reactions. **Resp:** PULMONARY EMBOLISM. **Misc:** fever.

Interactions

Drug-Drug: ↑ anticholinergic effects with other **agents having anticholinergic properties**, including **antihistamines**, **quinidine**, **disopyramide**, and **antidepressants**. Concurrent use with strong **CYP1A2 inhibitors**, including **fluvoxamine** or **ciprofloxacin** may ↑ levels; ↓ clozapine dose to ⅓ of the original dose during concurrent use. Concurrent use with moderate or weak **CYP1A2 inhibitors**, including **oral contraceptives** or **caffeine** may ↑ levels; consider ↓ clozapine dose. Concurrent use with **CYP2D6 inhibitors** or **CYP3A4 inhibitors**, including **cimetidine**, **escitalopram**, **erythromycin**, **paroxetine**, **bupropion**, **fluoxetine**, **quinidine**, **duloxetine**, **terbinafine**, or **sertraline** may ↑ levels; consider ↓ clozapine dose. Concurrent use with **CYP1A2 inducers** or **CYP3A4 inducers**, including **nicotine**, **carbamazepine**, **phenytoin**, or **rifampin** may ↓ levels; concurrent use with strong CYP3A4 inducers not recommended. ↑ CNS depression with **alcohol**, **antidepressants**, **antihistamines**, **opioid analgesics**, or **sedative/hypnotics**. ↑ hypotension with **nitrates**, acute ingestion of **alcohol**, or **antihypertensives**. ↑ risk of bone marrow suppression with **antineoplastics** or **radiation therapy**. Use with **lithium** ↑ risk of adverse CNS reactions, including seizures. ↑ risk of QT interval prolongation with other **agents causing QT interval prolongation**.

Drug-Natural Products: Caffeine-containing herbs (**cola nut**, **tea**, **coffee**) may ↑ serum levels and side effects. **St. John's wort** may ↓ blood levels and efficacy.

Route/Dosage

PO (Adults): 12.5 mg 1–2 times daily initially; ↑ by 25–50 mg/day over a period of 2 wk up to target dose of 300–450 mg/day. May then be ↑ by up to 100 mg/day once or twice weekly (not to exceed 900 mg/day). Treatment should be continued for at least 2 yr in patients with suicidal behavior.

Availability (generic available)

Orally disintegrating tablets (mint): 12.5 mg, 25 mg, 100 mg, 150 mg, 200 mg. **Oral suspension :** 50 mg/mL. **Tablets:** 25 mg, 100 mg.

NURSING IMPLICATIONS

Assessment

- Monitor patient's mental status (orientation, mood, behavior) before and periodically during therapy. Titrate slowly and monitor closely; may cause orthostatic hypotension, bradycardia, syncope, and cardiac arrest.
- Monitor BP (sitting, standing, lying) and pulse rate before and frequently during initial dose titration.
- Assess weight and BMI initially and periodically during therapy. Refer as appropriate for nutritional/weight management and medical management.
- Observe patient carefully when administering medication to ensure that medication is actually taken and not hoarded or cheeked.
- Monitor for signs of myocarditis (unexplained fatigue, dyspnea, tachypnea, fever, chest pain, palpitations, other signs and symptoms of heart failure, ECG changes, such as ST-T wave abnormalities, arrhythmias, or tachycardia during first mo of therapy). If these occur, clozapine should be discontinued and not restarted.
- Monitor patient for onset of akathisia (restlessness or desire to keep moving) and extrapyramidal side effects (*parkinsonian*—difficulty speaking or swallowing, loss of balance control, pill-rolling motion of hands, mask-like face, shuffling gait, rigidity, tremors and dystonic muscle spasms, twisting motions, twitching, inability to move eyes, weakness of arms or legs) every 2 mo during therapy and 8–12 wk after therapy has been discontinued. Notify health care professional if these symptoms occur; reduction in dose or discontinuation of medication may be necessary. Trihexyphenidyl or benzotropine may be used to control these symptoms.
- Monitor for possible tardive dyskinesia (uncontrolled rhythmic movement of mouth, face, and extremities; lip smacking or puckering; puffing of cheeks; uncontrolled chewing; rapid or worm-like movements of tongue). Report these symptoms immediately; may be irreversible.
- Monitor frequency and consistency of bowel movements. Increasing bulk and fluids in the diet may help to minimize constipation.

- Clozapine lowers the seizure threshold. Institute seizure precautions for patients with history of seizure disorder.
- Transient fevers may occur, especially during first 3 wk of therapy. Fever is usually self-limiting but may require discontinuation of medication. Also, monitor for development of neuroleptic malignant syndrome (fever, respiratory distress, tachycardia, seizures, diaphoresis, hypertension or hypotension, pallor, tiredness). Notify health care professional immediately if these symptoms occur.
- Assess respiratory status during therapy. If deep-vein thrombosis, acute dyspnea, chest pain, or other respiratory signs and symptoms occur, consider pulmonary embolism.
- Assess for falls risk. Drowsiness, orthostatic hypotension, and motor and sensory instability increase risk. Institute prevention if indicated.
- Monitor for signs and symptoms of hepatotoxicity (fatigue, malaise, anorexia, nausea, jaundice, hyperbilirubinemia, coagulopathy, hepatic encephalopathy). May require permanent discontinuation if combined with elevated transaminases.
- ***Lab Test Considerations:*** Monitor WBC, absolute neutrophil count (ANC), and differential count before initiation of therapy. ANC must be ≥1500/mm^3 for the general population and ≥1000/mm^3 for patients with documented Benign Ethnic Neutropenia (BEN) for patient to begin therapy. Monitor ANC weekly for the first 6 mo, then biweekly for the second 6 mo, then, if maintained within acceptable parameters, monthly after 12 mo. *If mild neutropenia (ANC 1000–1499/mm^3) occurs,* continue therapy and monitor ANC 3 times/wk until ANC ≥1500/mm^3. Once ANC ≥1500/mm^3, return to patient's last ANC monitoring interval. *If moderate neutropenia (ANC 500–999/mm^3) occurs,* recommend hematology consultation. Interrupt therapy for suspected clozapine-induced neutropenia. Resume therapy once ANC ≥1000/mm^3. Monitor ANC daily until ANC ≥1000/mm^3 then 3 times/wk until ANC ≥1500/mm^3. Once ANC ≥1500/mm^3, check ANC weekly for 4 wk, then return to patient's last ANC monitoring interval. *If severe neutropenia (<500/mm^3) occurs,* recommend hematology consultation. Interrupt therapy for suspected clozapine-induced neutropenia. Do not rechallenge unless benefit outweighs risk. Monitor ANC daily until ANC ≥1000/mm^3, then 3 times/wk until ANC ≥1500/mm^3. If patient rechallenged, resume therapy as a new patient using normal monitoring once ANC ≥1500/mm^3. For patients with **Benign Ethnic Neutropenia (BEN)**, obtain at least 2 baseline ANC levels before starting therapy. Monitor ANC weekly for the first 6 mo, then biweekly for the second 6 mo, then, if maintained within acceptable parameters, monthly after 12 mo. *If neutropenia (ANC 500–999/mm^3) occurs,* recommend hematology consultation and continue therapy. Monitor ANC 3 times/wk until ANC ≥1000/mm^3 or at patient's known baseline. Once ANC ≥1000/mm^3, check ANC weekly for 4 wk, then return to patient's last ANC monitoring interval. *If severe neutropenia (<500/mm^3) occurs,* recommend hematology consultation. Interrupt therapy for suspected clozapine-induced neutropenia. Do not rechallenge. Monitor ANC daily until ANC ≥500/mm^3, then 3 times/wk until ANC ≥patient's baseline. If patient rechallenged, resume therapy as a new patient using normal monitoring once ANC ≥1000/mm^3 or at patient's baseline.
- Assess fasting blood glucose and cholesterol levels initially and throughout therapy.
- Monitor liver function tests periodically during therapy or if clinical signs of hepatotoxicity occur.
- ***Toxicity and Overdose:*** Overdose is treated with activated charcoal and supportive therapy. Monitor patient for several days because of risk of delayed effects.
- Avoid use of epinephrine and its derivatives when treating hypotension, and avoid quinidine and procainamide when treating arrhythmias.

Implementation

- Do not confuse clozapine with clonazepam or clonidine. Do not confuse Clozaril with Colazal.
- Because of the risk of severe neutropenia, clozapine is only available through restricted program called *Clozapine REMS Program*. Health care professionals must be trained and certified to prescribe clozapine. Patients must be enrolled in the program and comply with ANC testing and monitoring requirements. Pharmacies dispensing clozapine must be trained and certified with program and must dispense only to patients eligible to receive clozapine.
- **PO:** Administer capsules with food or milk to decrease gastric irritation.
- Leave oral disintegrating tablet in blister until time of use. Do not push tablet through foil. Just before use, peel foil and gently remove disintegrating tablet. Immediately place tablet in mouth and allow to disintegrate and swallow with saliva. If ½ tablet dose used, destroy other half of tablet.
- Oral solution may be taken without regard to food. Shake bottle for suspension for 10 sec prior to withdrawing. Use oral syringes and oral adaptor provided for accurate dosing. Do not store dose in syringe; wash between doses.

Patient/Family Teaching

- Instruct patient to take medication as directed. If clozapine is stopped for >2 days, do not restart medication, notify health care professional for new dosing instructions. Patients on long-term therapy may need to discontinue gradually over 1–2 wk.
- Explain purpose and procedures for *Clozapine REMS Program* to patient.
- Inform patient of possibility of extrapyramidal symptoms. Instruct patient to report these symptoms immediately.

- Inform patient that cigarette smoking can decrease clozapine levels. Risk for relapse increases if patient begins or increases smoking.
- Advise patient to change positions slowly to minimize orthostatic hypotension. Protect from falls.
- May cause seizures and drowsiness. Caution patient to avoid driving or other activities requiring alertness while taking clozapine.
- Instruct patient to notify health care professional of all Rx or OTC medications, vitamins, or herbal products being taken and to consult health care professional before taking any other medications. Caution patient to avoid concurrent use of alcohol and other CNS depressants.
- Instruct patient to use frequent mouth rinses, good oral hygiene, and sugarless gum or candy to minimize dry mouth.
- Advise patient to notify health care professional of medication regimen before treatment or surgery.
- Instruct patient to notify health care professional promptly if unexplained fatigue, dyspnea, tachypnea, chest pain, palpitations, sore throat, fever, lethargy, weakness, malaise, or flu-like symptoms occur.
- Rep: Advise female patients to notify health care professional if pregnancy is planned or suspected, or if breast feeding. Consider early screening for gestational diabetes if used during preganacy. Neonates exposed to antipsychotic drugs during third trimester are at risk for extrapyramidal and/or withdrawal symptoms following delivery. Monitor neonates for symptoms of agitation, hypertonia, hypotonia, tremor, somnolence, respiratory distress, and feeding difficulties. May require NICU.
- Advise patient of need for continued medical follow-up for psychotherapy, eye exams, and laboratory tests.

Evaluation/Desired Outcomes

- Decreased positive symptoms (delusions, hallucinations) of schizophrenia.
- Decrease in negative symptoms (social withdrawal, flat, blunt affect) of schizophrenia.

cobimetinib

(koe-bi-**me**-ti-nib)
Cotellic

Classification
Therapeutic: antineoplastics
Pharmacologic: kinase inhibitors

Indications

Treatment of metastatic/unresectable melanoma with the BRAF V600E or V600K mutation (in combination with vemurafenib).

Action

Inhibits the activity of mitogen-activated extracellular kinase (MEK) 1 and 2 which are enzymes that normally promote cellular proliferation. **Therapeutic Effects:** Decreased progression of melanoma.

Pharmacokinetics

Absorption: 46% absorbed following oral administration.
Distribution: Extensively distributed to tissues.
Protein Binding: 95%.
Metabolism and Excretion: Mostly metabolized by the liver (via CYP3A4 enzyme system and glucuronidation). 6.6% excreted in feces unchanged; 20% excreted in urine (mostly as metabolites).
Half-life: 44 hr.

TIME/ACTION PROFILE (blood levels)

ROUTE	ONSET	PEAK	DURATION
PO	unknown	2.4 hr	unknown

Contraindications/Precautions

Contraindicated in: Concurrent use of strong or moderate CYP3A4 inhibitors or inducers; OB: May cause fetal harm; Lactation: Breast feeding should be avoided during treatment and for 2 wk after therapy.
Use Cautiously in: Left ventricular ejection fraction <50%; Severe renal impairment (CCr <30 mL/min); Rep: Women of childbearing potential (use effective contraception); Pedi: Safety and effectiveness not established.

Adverse Reactions/Side Effects

CV: CARDIOMYOPATHY, hypertension. **Derm:** alopecia, erythema, photosensitivity, rash. **EENT:** retinopathy. **F and E:** hyperkalemia, hypocalcemia, hypokalemia, hyponatremia, hypophosphatemia. **GI:** HEPATOTOXICITY, diarrhea, hypoalbuminemia, nausea, stomatitis, vomiting. **GU:** ↑ serum creatinine, ↓ fertility. **Hemat:** HEMORRHAGE, anemia, lymphopenia, thrombocytopenia. **MS:** ↑ creatine kinase, RHABDOMYOLYSIS. **Misc:** MALIGNANCY, fever.

Interactions

Drug-Drug: Strong or moderate CYP3A4 inhibitors, including **itraconazole**, may ↑ levels; avoid concurrent use. Strong or moderate CYP3A4 inducers, including **carbamazepine**, **efavirenz**, **phenytoin**, and **rifampin** may ↓ levels; avoid concurrent use.
Drug-Natural Products: St. John's wort may ↓ levels; avoid concurrent use.

Route/Dosage

PO (Adults): 60 mg once daily for days 1–21 of each 28–day cycle; continue until disease progression or unacceptable toxicity; *Concurrent short-term use of moderate CYP3A4 inhibitor*—20 mg once daily; resume 60 mg once daily once 3A4 inhibitor discontinued (avoid use of strong or moderate CYP3A4 inhibitor if patient already taking reduced dose of 20–40 mg once daily).

Availability

Tablets: 20 mg.

NURSING IMPLICATIONS

Assessment

- Assess skin prior to starting therapy and every 2 mo during and for 6 mo following therapy for new lesions. If new lesions appear evaluate and remove as needed. If Grade 2 (intolerable), Grade 3 or 4 rash or other skin reactions occur, withhold or reduce dose.
- Monitor for bleeding and hemorrhage periodically during therapy. *If Grade 3 hemorrhage occurs,* withhold therapy for up to 4 wk. If improved to Grade 0 or 1, resume at next lower dose. If not improved within 4 wk, permanently discontinue. *If Grade 4 hemorrhage occurs,* permanently discontinue therapy.
- Monitor left ventricular ejection fraction (LVEF) prior to initiation, 1 mo after initiation, and every 3 mo until discontinuation. *If asymptomatic, absolute ↓ LVEF from baseline of >10% and <institutional lower limit of normal (LLN),* withhold therapy for 2 wk; repeat LVEF. *Resume at next lower dose if all of following are present:* LVEF is ≥LLN and absolute ↓ from baseline LVEF ≤10%. *Discontinue permanently if any of following are present:* LVEF is <LLN or absolute ↓ from baseline LVEF >10%. *If symptomatic LVEF ↓ from baseline,* withhold therapy for up to 4 wk, repeat LVEF. *Resume at next lower dose if all of following are present:* symptoms resolve and LVEF is ≥LLN and absolute ↓ from baseline LVEF is ≤10%. *Discontinue permanently if any of following are present:* symptoms persist, or LVEF <LLN, or absolute ↓ from baseline LVEF >10%. If restarting cobimetinib after a dose reduction or interruption, evaluate LVEF at approximately 2 wk, 4 wk, 10 wk, and 16 wk, and as clinically indicated.
- Perform ophthalmological evaluations periodically during therapy and if patient reports new or worsening visual disturbances. *If serious retinopathy occurs,* withhold therapy for up to 4 wk. If signs and symptoms improve, resume at next lower dose. If not improved or symptoms recur at lower dose within 4 wk, permanently discontinue. *If retinal vein occlusion occurs,* permanently discontinue therapy.
- Assess for photosensitivity during therapy. *If Grade 2 (intolerable), Grade 3 or Grade 4 photosensitivity occurs,* withhold therapy up to 4 wk. If improved to Grade 0 or 1, resume at next lower dose. If not improved within 4 wk, permanently discontinue.
- ***Lab Test Considerations:*** May cause ↑ AST, ALT, alkaline phosphatase, and GGT. Monitor liver function tests before initiation and monthly during therapy, and as clinically indicated. *For 1st occurrence of Grade 4 hepatotoxicity,* withhold therapy up to 4 wk. If improved to Grade 0 or 1, resume at next lower dose. If not improved to Grade 0 or 1 within 4 wk, permanently discontinue. *If Grade 4 hepatotoxicity recurs,* discontinue therapy permanently.
- Obtain CPK and serum creatinine levels at baseline and periodically during therapy. If Grade 4 CPK ↑ or any CPK ↑ and myalgia occur, withhold therapy up to 4 wk. If improved to Grade 3 or lower, resume at next lower dose level. If not improved within 4 wk, permanently discontinue.
- May cause hypophosphatemia, hyponatremia, hypoalbuminemia, hypokalemia, hyperkalemia, and hypocalcemia.
- May cause anemia, lymphopenia, and thrombocytopenia.

Implementation

- **PO:** Administer three 20-mg tablets once daily without regard to food.

Patient/Family Teaching

- Instruct patient to take cobimetinib as directed. If dose is missed or vomiting occurs after dose, do not repeat, take next dose as scheduled.
- Advise patient to notify health care professional immediately if skin changes (new wart, skin sore that bleeds or does not heal, change in size or color of mole, signs and symptoms of bleeding (blood in urine, red or black stools, unusual or excessive vaginal bleeding, bleeding of gums, abdominal pain, headache, dizziness, feeling weak), cardiomyopathy (persistent coughing or wheezing, tiredness, shortness of breath, increased heart rate, swelling of ankles and feet), eye problems (blurred vision, halos, distorted vision, other vision changes, partly missing vision), liver injury (yellowing of skin or white of eyes, feeling tired or weak, dark or brown [tea color] urine, loss of appetite, nausea or vomiting), rhabdomyolysis (muscle aches, dark, reddish urine, muscle spasms, weakness), or rash occur.
- Advise patient to avoid sun exposure, wear protective clothing and use a broad-spectrum UVA/UVB sunscreen and lip balm (SPF ≥30) when outdoors. May require dose reduction or discontinuation.
- Advise patient to notify health care professional of all Rx or OTC medications, vitamins, or herbal products being taken and to consult with health care professional before taking other medications, especially St. John's wort.
- Rep: May be teratogenic. Advise patient use effective contraception and avoid breast feeding during and for at least 2 wk following therapy. May reduce fertility in females and males of reproductive potential.

Evaluation/Desired Outcomes

- Decrease in progression of melanoma.

C

REMS HIGH ALERT

codeine (koe-deen)

Classification

Therapeutic: allergy, cold, and cough remedies, antitussives, opioid analgesics

Pharmacologic: opioid agonists

Schedule II, III, IV, V (depends on content)

Indications

Management of mild to moderate pain. Antitussive (in smaller doses). **Unlabeled Use:** Management of diarrhea.

Action

Binds to opiate receptors in the CNS. Alters the perception of and response to painful stimuli while producing generalized CNS depression. Decreases cough reflex. Decreases GI motility. **Therapeutic Effects:** Decreased severity of pain. Suppression of the cough reflex. Relief of diarrhea.

Pharmacokinetics

Absorption: 50% absorbed from the GI tract.

Distribution: Widely distributed. Crosses the placenta; enters breast milk.

Protein Binding: 7%.

Metabolism and Excretion: Mostly metabolized by the liver (primarily via CYP2D6); 10% converted to morphine; the CYP2D6 enzyme system exhibits genetic polymorphism (some patients [1–10% Whites, 3% African Americans, 16–28% North Africans/Ethiopians/Arabs] may be ultra-rapid metabolizers and may have ↑ morphine concentrations and an ↑ risk of adverse effects); 5–15% excreted unchanged in urine.

Half-life: 2.5–4 hr.

TIME/ACTION PROFILE (analgesia)

ROUTE	ONSET	PEAK	DURATION
PO	30–45 min	60–120 min	4 hr

Contraindications/Precautions

Contraindicated in: Hypersensitivity; Significant respiratory depression; Acute or severe bronchial asthma (in unmonitored setting or in absence of resuscitative equipment); Known or suspected GI obstruction (including paralytic ileus); Concurrent use of MAO inhibitors (or use within the past 14 days); Ultra-rapid CYP2D6 metabolizers of codeine; Lactation: Avoid use in breast feeding (↑ risk of drowsiness and respiratory depression in infant); Pedi: Children <12 yr, children <18 yr following tonsillectomy and/or adenoidectomy, and children 12–18 yr who are postoperative, have obstructive sleep apnea, obesity, or severe pulmonary disease, neuromuscular disease; or are taking other medications that cause respiratory depression (↑ risk of respiratory depression and death).

Use Cautiously in: Head trauma; ↑ intracranial pressure; Severe renal, hepatic, or pulmonary disease; Hypothyroidism; Adrenal insufficiency; Alcoholism; Prostatic hyperplasia; Undiagnosed abdominal pain; Geri: Geriatric or debilitated patients (dose ↓ required; more susceptible to CNS depression, constipation); OB: Has been used during labor; respiratory depression may occur in the newborn.

Adverse Reactions/Side Effects

CNS: confusion, sedation, dysphoria, euphoria, floating feeling, hallucinations, headache, unusual dreams. **CV:** hypotension, bradycardia. **Derm:** flushing, sweating. **EENT:** blurred vision, diplopia, miosis. **GI:** constipation, nausea, vomiting. **GU:** urinary retention. **Resp:** respiratory depression. **Misc:** physical dependence, psychological dependence, tolerance.

Interactions

Drug-Drug: MAO inhibitors ↑ risk of adverse reactions; concurrent use or use within previous 14 days contraindicated. Additive CNS depression with **alcohol**, **antidepressants**, **antihistamines**, **benzodiazepines**, and **sedative/hypnotics**. **CYP3A4 inhibitors**, including **erythromycin**, **clarithromycin**, **ketoconazole**, **itraconazole**, and **protease inhibitors** may ↑ levels and risk of respiratory depression. **CYP3A4 inducers** may ↓ levels. **CYP2D6 inhibitors**, including **amiodarone** and **quinidine** may ↓ analgesic effects. Administration of **partial antagonists (buprenorphine**, **butorphanol**, or **nalbuphine)** may precipitate opioid withdrawal in physically dependent patients. **Nalbuphine** may ↓ analgesia.

Drug-Natural Products: Concomitant use of **kava-kava**, **valerian**, **skullcap**, **chamomile**, or **hops** can ↑ CNS depression.

Route/Dosage

PO (Adults): *Analgesic*—15–60 mg every 4 hr as needed (not to exceed 360 mg/day). *Antitussive*—10–20 mg every 4–6 hr as needed (not to exceed 120 mg/day). *Antidiarrheal*—30 mg up to 4 times daily.

Renal Impairment

(Adults): *CCr 10–50 mL/min*—Administer 75% of the dose; *CCr <10 mL/min*—Administer 50% of the dose.

Availability (generic available)

Tablets: 15 mg, 30 mg, 60 mg. **Oral solution:** ✱10 mg/5 mL, ✱25 mg/5 mL. ***In combination with:*** antihistamines, decongestants, antipyretics, caffeine, butalbital, and nonopioid analgesics. See Appendix B.

NURSING IMPLICATIONS

Assessment

- Assess BP, pulse, and respirations before and periodically during administration. If respiratory rate is <10/min, assess level of sedation. Physical stimulation may be sufficient to prevent significant hypoventilation. Dose may need to be decreased by 25–50%. Initial drowsiness will diminish with continued use.
- Assess bowel function routinely. Prevention of constipation should be instituted with increased intake of fluids, bulk, and laxatives to minimize constipating effects. Stimulant laxatives should be administered routinely if opioid use exceeds 2–3 days, unless contraindicated. Consider drugs for opioid induced constipation.
- **Pain:** Assess type, location, and intensity of pain before and 1 hr (peak) after administration. When titrating opioid doses, increases of 25–50% should be administered until there is either a 50% reduction in the patient's pain rating on a numerical or visual analogue scale or the patient reports satisfactory pain relief. A repeat dose can be safely administered at the time of the peak if previous dose is ineffective and side effects are minimal.
- An equianalgesic chart (see Appendix J) should be used when changing routes or when changing from one opioid to another.
- Prolonged use may lead to physical and psychological dependence and tolerance. This should not prevent patient from receiving adequate analgesia. Most patients who receive codeine for pain do not develop psychological dependence. If progressively higher doses are required, consider conversion to a stronger opioid.
- Assess risk for opioid addiction, abuse, or misuse prior to administration.
- **Cough:** Assess cough and lung sounds during antitussive use.
- ***Lab Test Considerations:*** May cause ↑ plasma amylase and lipase concentrations.
- ***Toxicity and Overdose:*** If an opioid antagonist is required to reverse respiratory depression or coma, naloxone (Narcan) is the antidote. Dilute the 0.4-mg ampule of naloxone in 10 mL of 0.9% NaCl and administer 0.5 mL (0.02 mg) by IV push every 2 min. For children and patients weighing <40 kg, dilute 0.1 mg of naloxone in 10 mL of 0.9% NaCl for a concentration of 10 mcg/mL and administer 0.5 mcg/kg every 2 min. Titrate dose to avoid withdrawal, seizures, and severe pain.

Implementation

- ***High Alert:*** Accidental overdosage of opioid analgesics has resulted in fatalities. Before administering, clarify all ambiguous orders.
- Explain therapeutic value of medication before administration to enhance the analgesic effect.
- Regularly administered doses may be more effective than prn administration. Analgesic is more effective if given before pain becomes severe.
- Coadministration with nonopioid analgesics may have additive analgesic effects and permit lower doses.
- FDA strongly encourages health care professionals to complete a REMS-compliant education program that includes all the elements of the FDA Education *Blueprint for Health Care Providers Involved in the Management or Support of Patients with Pain,* available at www.fda.gov/OpioidAnalgesicREMSBlueprint. Information on programs can be found at 1-800-503-0784 or www.opioidanalgesicrems.com.
- Medications should be discontinued gradually after long-term use to prevent withdrawal symptoms.
- When combined with nonopioid analgesics (aspirin, acetaminophen) #2 = 15 mg, #3 = 30 mg, #4 = 60 mg codeine. Codeine as an individual drug is a Schedule II substance. In combination with other drugs, tablet form is Schedule III, and elixir or cough suppressant is Schedule V (see Appendix I).
- **PO:** Oral doses may be administered with food or milk to minimize GI irritation.

Patient/Family Teaching

- Instruct patient on how and when to ask for and take pain medication.
- Advise patient that codeine is a drug with known abuse potential. Protect it from theft, and never give to anyone other than the individual for whom it was prescribed.
- Instruct patient on risk of addiction, abuse, and misuse, which could lead to death. Discuss safe use, risks, and proper storage and disposal of opioid analgesics with patients and caregivers with each Rx. The Patient Counseling Guide (PCG) is available at www.fda.gov/OpioidAnalgesicREMSPCG. Advise patient not to share codeine with others and to protect from theft or misuse.
- May cause drowsiness or dizziness. Advise patient to call for assistance when ambulating or smoking. Caution ambulatory patient to avoid driving or other activities requiring alertness until response to medication is known.
- Advise patient to change positions slowly to minimize orthostatic hypotension.
- Caution patient to avoid concurrent use of alcohol or other CNS depressants with this medication.
- Encourage patient to turn, cough, and breathe deeply every 2 hr to prevent atelectasis.
- Advise patient that good oral hygiene, frequent mouth rinses, and sugarless gum or candy may decrease dry mouth.
- Rep: Advise patient to notify health care professional if pregnancy is planned or suspected, or if breast feeding. Inform patient of potential for neonatal opioid withdrawal syndrome with prolonged use during pregnancy. Monitor neonate for signs and

symptoms of withdrawal symptoms (irritability, hyperactivity and abnormal sleep pattern, high pitched cry, tremor, vomiting, diarrhea, and/or failure to gain weight); usually occur the first days after birth.

Evaluation/Desired Outcomes

- Decrease in severity of pain without a significant alteration in level of consciousness or respiratory status.
- Suppression of cough.
- Control of diarrhea.

HIGH ALERT

colchicine (kol-chi-seen)

Colcrys, Gloperba, Mitigare

Classification

Therapeutic: antigout agents

Indications

Prophylaxis and treatment of acute attacks of gouty arthritis (oral solution is only for prophylaxis). Familial Mediterranean fever.

Action

Interferes with the functions of WBCs in initiating and perpetuating the inflammatory response to monosodium urate crystals. **Therapeutic Effects:** Decreased pain and inflammation in acute attacks of gout. Reduced number of attacks of gout and familial Mediterranean fever.

Pharmacokinetics

Absorption: 45% absorbed from the GI tract, then re-enters GI tract from biliary secretions, when more absorption may occur.
Distribution: Concentrates in WBCs.
Metabolism and Excretion: Partially metabolized by the liver by CYP3A4; also a substrate for P-glycoprotein. Secreted in bile back into GI tract; eliminated in the feces. 40–65% excreted in the urine as unchanged drug.
Half-life: 27–31 hr.

TIME/ACTION PROFILE (anti-inflammatory activity)

ROUTE	ONSET	PEAK	DURATION
PO	12 hr	24–72 hr	unknown

Contraindications/Precautions

Contraindicated in: Hypersensitivity; Use of P-glycoprotein inhibitors or strong CYP3A4 inhibitors in patients with renal or hepatic impairment; Renal and hepatic impairment.
Use Cautiously in: Renal impairment (dose ↓ suggested if CCr <80 mL/min); OB, Lactation, Pedi: Safety not established for gout; Geri: Elderly or debilitated patients (toxicity may be cumulative).

Adverse Reactions/Side Effects

Derm: alopecia. **GI:** diarrhea, nausea, vomiting, abdominal pain. **Hemat:** AGRANULOCYTOSIS, APLASTIC ANEMIA, leukopenia, thrombocytopenia. **Neuro:** peripheral neuritis.

Interactions

Drug-Drug: Concurrent use of strong **CYP3A4 inhibitors**, including **atazanavir**, **clarithromycin**, **darunavir/ritonavir**, **indinavir**, **itraconazole**, **ketoconazole**, **lopinavir/ritonavir**, **nefazodone**, **nelfinavir**, **ritonavir**, **saquinavir**, or **tipranavir/ritonavir**, may ↑ levels and risk of toxicity; ↓ colchicine dose in patients with normal renal or hepatic function; concurrent use in patients with renal or hepatic impairment is contraindicated. Concurrent use of **P-glycoprotein inhibitors**, including **cyclosporine** or **ranolazine** may ↑ levels and risk of toxicity; ↓ colchicine dose in patients with normal renal or hepatic function; concurrent use in patients with renal or hepatic impairment is contraindicated. Moderate **CYP3A4 inhibitors**, including **aprepitant**, **diltiazem**, **erythromycin**, **fluconazole**, **fosamprenavir**, or **verapamil** may ↑ levels and risk of toxicity; ↓ colchicine dose. Additive bone marrow depression may occur with **bone marrow depressants** or **radiation therapy**. ↑ risk of rhabdomyolysis with **HMG-CoA reductase inhibitors**, **gemfibrozil**, **fenofibrate**, or **digoxin**. Additive adverse GI effects with **NSAIDs**. May cause reversible malabsorption of **vitamin B_{12}**.
Drug-Food: **Grapefruit juice** may ↑ levels and risk of toxicity; ↓ colchicine dose.

Route/Dosage

Treatment of Acute Gout Attacks

PO (Adults): 1.2 mg initially, then 0.6 mg 1 hr later (maximum dose of 1.8 mg in 1 hr); *Concomitant use of strong CYP3A4 inhibitors in patients with normal renal and hepatic function (atazanavir, clarithromycin, darunavir/ritonavir, indinavir, itraconazole, ketoconazole, lopinavir/ritonavir, nefazodone, nelfinavir, ritonavir, saquinavir, tipranavir/ritonavir)*—0.6 mg × 1 dose, then 0.3 mg 1 hr later (do not repeat treatment course for ≥3 days); *Concomitant use of moderate CYP3A4 inhibitors (aprepitant, diltiazem, erythromycin, fluconazole, fosamprenavir, grapefruit juice, verapamil)*—1.2 mg × 1 dose (do not repeat for ≥3 days); *Concomitant use of P-glycoprotein inhibitors (cyclosporine, ranolazine) in patients with normal renal and hepatic function*—0.6 mg × 1 dose (do not repeat for ≥3 days).

Renal Impairment

PO (Adults): *CCr <30 mL/min*—1.2 mg initially, then 0.6 mg 1 hr later; do not repeat treatment course for ≥2 wk; *Dialysis*—0.6 mg × 1 dose; do not repeat treatment course for ≥2 wk.

Prevention of Acute Gout Attacks

PO (Adults): 0.6 mg once or twice daily; *Concomitant use of strong CYP3A4 inhibitors (atazanavir, clarithromycin, darunavir/ritonavir, indinavir, itraconazole, ketoconazole, lopinavir/ritonavir, nefazodone, nelfinavir, ritonavir, saquinavir, tipranavir/ritonavir) or P-glycoprotein inhibitors (cyclosporine, ranolazine) in patients with normal renal and hepatic function*—if original dose was 0.6 mg twice daily, ↓ to 0.3 mg once daily; if original dose was 0.6 mg once daily, ↓ to 0.3 mg every other day; *Concomitant use of moderate CYP3A4 inhibitors (aprepitant, diltiazem, erythromycin, fluconazole, fosamprenavir, grapefruit juice, verapamil)*—if original dose was 0.6 mg twice daily, ↓ to 0.3 mg twice daily or 0.6 mg once daily; if original dose was 0.6 mg once daily, ↓ to 0.3 mg once daily.

Renal Impairment

PO (Adults): *CCr <30 mL/min*—0.3 mg once daily; *Dialysis*—0.3 mg twice weekly.

Familial Mediterranean Fever

PO (Adults and Children >12 yr): 1.2–2.4 mg/day (in 1–2 divided doses); may ↑ or ↓ dose in 0.3-mg/day increments based on safety and efficacy; *Concomitant use of strong CYP3A4 inhibitors (atazanavir, clarithromycin, darunavir/ritonavir, indinavir, itraconazole, ketoconazole, lopinavir/ritonavir, nefazodone, nelfinavir, ritonavir, saquinavir, tipranavir/ritonavir) or P-glycoprotein inhibitors (cyclosporine, ranolazine) in patients with normal renal and hepatic function*—Do not exceed 0.6 mg/day (may be given as 0.3 mg twice daily); *Concomitant use of moderate CYP3A4 inhibitors (aprepitant, diltiazem, erythromycin, fluconazole, fosamprenavir, grapefruit juice, verapamil)*—Do not exceed 1.2 mg/day (may be given as 0.6 mg twice daily).

PO (Children 6–12 yr): 0.9–1.8 mg/day (in 1–2 divided doses).

PO (Children 4–6 yr): 0.3–1.8 mg/day (in 1–2 divided doses).

Renal Impairment

PO (Adults): *CCr 30–50 mL/min*—dose ↓ may be necessary; *CCr <30 mL/min or dialysis*—0.3 mg/day.

Availability (generic available)

Capsules: 0.6 mg. **Oral solution (cherry flavor):** 0.6 mg/5 mL. **Tablets:** 0.6 mg, 🍁1 mg. ***In combination with:*** probenecid (Col-Probenecid). See Appendix B.

NURSING IMPLICATIONS

Assessment

- Monitor intake and output ratios. Fluids should be encouraged to promote a urinary output of at least 2000 mL/day.
- **Gout:** Assess involved joints for pain, mobility, and edema throughout therapy. During initiation of therapy, monitor for drug response every 1–2 hr.
- **Familial Mediterranean fever:** Assess for signs and symptoms of familial Mediterranean fever (abdominal pain, chest pain, fever, chills, recurrent joint pain, red and swollen skin lesions) periodically during therapy.
- ***Lab Test Considerations:*** In patients receiving prolonged therapy, monitor baseline and periodic CBC; report significant ↓ in values. May cause ↓ platelet count, leukopenia, aplastic anemia, and agranulocytosis.
- May cause ↑ in AST and alkaline phosphatase.
- May cause false-positive results for urine hemoglobin.
- May interfere with results of urinary 17-hydroxycorticosteroid concentrations.
- ***Toxicity and Overdose: High Alert:*** Assess patient for toxicity (muscle pain or weakness, tingling or numbness in fingers or toes; pale or gray color to lips, tongue, or palms of hands; severe diarrhea or vomiting; unusual bleeding, bruising, sore throat, fatigue, malaise, or weakness or tiredness). If these symptoms occur, discontinue colchicine and treat symptomatically. Opioids may be needed to treat diarrhea.

Implementation

- Do not confuse colchicine with Cortrosyn.
- Intermittent therapy with 3 days between courses may be used to decrease risk of toxicity.
- **PO:** Administer without regard to meals.
- Use an accurate measuring device for solution; a teaspoon is not accurate. Solution is slightly hazy, red liquid with a cherry odor.

Patient/Family Teaching

- Instruct patient to take colchicine as directed. Review medication administration schedule. Take missed doses as soon as remembered unless almost time for next dose. Do not double doses.
- Instruct patients taking prophylactic doses not to increase to therapeutic doses during an acute attack to prevent toxicity. An NSAID or corticosteroid, preferably via intrasynovial injection, should be used to treat acute attacks.
- Advise patient to avoid grapefruit and grapefruit juice during therapy; may increase risk of toxicity.
- Advise patient to follow recommendations of health care professional regarding weight loss, diet, and alcohol consumption.
- Instruct patient to report muscle pain or weakness, tingling or numbness in fingers or toes; pale or gray color to lips, tongue, or palms of hands; severe diarrhea or vomiting; unusual bleeding, bruising, sore throat, fatigue, malaise, or weakness or tiredness promptly. Hold colchicine if symptoms of toxicity occur.
- Instruct patient to notify health care professional of all Rx or OTC medications, vitamins, or herbal products being taken and to notify health care professional before taking any other Rx, OTC, or herbal products.
- Surgery may precipitate an acute attack of gout. Advise patient to confer with health care professional

regarding dose 3 days before surgical or dental procedures.

- Rep: Advise female patient to notify health care professional if pregnancy is planned or suspected or if breast feeding. Inform males with female partners of reproductive potential that colchicine may cause infertility that reverses when colchicine is stopped.

Evaluation/Desired Outcomes

- Decrease in pain and swelling in affected joints within 12 hr.
- Relief of symptoms within 24–48 hr.
- Prevention of acute gout attacks.
- Reduced number of attacks of familial Mediterranean fever.

colesevelam (koe-le-**sev**-e-lam)

Lodalis, Welchol

Classification
Therapeutic: lipid-lowering agents
Pharmacologic: bile acid sequestrants

Indications

Adjunctive therapy to diet and exercise for the reduction of LDL cholesterol in patients with primary hypercholesterolemia; may be used alone or in combination with statins. Adjunctive therapy to diet and exercise for the reduction of LDL cholesterol in children 10–17 yr with heterozygous familial hypercholesterolemia if diet therapy fails (LDL cholesterol remains ≥190 mg/dL or remains ≥160 mg/dL [with family history of premature cardiovascular disease or ≥2 risk factors for cardiovascular disease]); may be used alone or in combination with statin. Adjunctive therapy to diet and exercise to improve glycemic control in patients with type 2 diabetes.

Action

Binds bile acids in the GI tract. Results in increased clearance of cholesterol. Mechanism for lowering blood glucose unknown. **Therapeutic Effects:** Decreased cholesterol and blood glucose.

Pharmacokinetics

Absorption: Not absorbed; action is primarily local in the GI tract.
Distribution: Unknown.
Metabolism and Excretion: Unknown.
Half-life: Unknown.

TIME/ACTION PROFILE (cholesterol-lowering effect)

ROUTE	ONSET	PEAK	DURATION
PO	24–48 hr	2 wk	unknown

Contraindications/Precautions

Contraindicated in: Hypersensitivity; Bowel obstruction; Triglycerides >500 m g/dL; History of pancreatitis due to hypertriglyceridemia.
Use Cautiously in: Triglycerides >300 m g/dL; Dysphagia, swallowing disorders, severe GI motility disorders, or major GI tract surgery; Phenylketonuria (oral suspension packets contain phenylalanine); OB: Safety not established; not systemically absorbed; use during pregnancy not expected to result in fetal exposure; Lactation: Not systemically absorbed; not expected to be present in breast milk; Pedi: Children <10 yr (safety not established).

Adverse Reactions/Side Effects

GI: constipation, dyspepsia.

Interactions

Drug-Drug: May ↓ absorption of **glyburide**, **glimepiride**, **glipizide**, **levothyroxine**, **olmesartan**, **phenytoin**, **cyclosporine**, **warfarin**, and **estrogen-containing oral contraceptives** (give ≥4 hr before colesevelam). May ↑ levels of **metformin extended-release**.

Route/Dosage

Hyperlipidemia

PO (Adults and Children 10–17 yr): 6 tablets once daily *or* 3 tablets twice daily *or* one 3.75–g packet once daily *or* one 3.75–g chewable bar once daily.

Type 2 Diabetes

PO (Adults): 6 tablets once daily *or* 3 tablets twice daily *or* one 3.75–g packet once daily *or* one 3.75–g chewable bar once daily.

Availability (generic available)

Chewable bars (chocolate, strawberry, and caramel flavors): 3.75 g/bar. **Tablets:** 625 mg. **Granules for oral suspension:** 3.75 g/packet (contains 27 mg phenylalanine).

NURSING IMPLICATIONS

Assessment

- **Hypercholesterolemia:** Obtain a diet history, especially in regard to fat consumption.
- **Type 2 Diabetes:** Observe patient for signs and symptoms of hypoglycemic reactions (sweating, hunger, weakness, dizziness, tremor, tachycardia, anxiety).
- ***Lab Test Considerations:*** Monitor serum total cholesterol, LDL, and triglyceride levels before initiating, 4–6 wk after starting, and periodically during therapy. May cause hypertriglyceridemia.
- Monitor serum glucose and glycosylated hemoglobin periodically during therapy in patients with diabetes.

Implementation

- Patients stabilized on a diabetic regimen who are exposed to stress, fever, trauma, infection, or surgery may require administration of insulin.
- **PO:** Administer once or twice daily with meals. Colesevelam should be taken with a liquid. For oral suspension, empty the entire contents of one packet into a glass or cup. Add 1 cup (8 oz) of water, fruit juice, or a diet soft drink; do not take in dry form to avoid esophageal distress.
- Administer chewable bar with a meal. Chewable bars contain approximately 80 calories per bar.

Patient/Family Teaching

- Instruct patient to take medication as directed; do not skip doses or double up on missed doses.
- Instruct patient to notify health care professional of all Rx or OTC medications, vitamins, or herbal products being taken and consult health care professional before taking other Rx, OTC, or herbal products.
- Advise patients taking oral vitamin supplementation or oral contraceptives to take their vitamins at least 4 hr prior to colesevelam, especially those taking warfarin. Colesevelam may decrease absorption of fat-soluble vitamins A, D, E, and K.
- Instruct patient to consume a diet that promotes bowel regularity. Patients should be instructed to promptly discontinue colesevelam and notify health care professional if severe abdominal pain or severe constipation or symptoms of acute pancreatitis (severe abdominal pain with or without nausea and vomiting) occur.
- Rep: Insulin is the recommended method of controlling blood sugar during pregnancy. Counsel female patients that colesevelam may reduce efficacy of oral contraceptives. Advise females of reproductive potential to take oral contraceptives at least 4 hrs prior to taking colesevelam or use a form of contraception other than oral contraceptives and to notify health care professional promptly if pregnancy is planned or suspected.
- **Hypercholesterolemia:** Advise patient that this medication should be used in conjunction with diet restrictions (fat, cholesterol, carbohydrates, alcohol), exercise, and cessation of smoking.
- **Diabetes:** Explain to patient that this medication controls hyperglycemia but does not cure diabetes. Therapy is long term.
- Review signs of hypoglycemia and hyperglycemia with patient. If hypoglycemia occurs, advise patient to drink a glass of orange juice or ingest 2–3 tsp of sugar, honey, or corn syrup dissolved in water or an appropriate number of glucose tablets and notify health care professional.
- Encourage patient to follow prescribed diet, medication, and exercise regimen to prevent hypoglycemic or hyperglycemic episodes.
- Instruct patient in proper testing of serum glucose and ketones. These tests should be closely monitored during periods of stress or illness and health care professional notified if significant changes occur.
- Advise patient to carry a form of sugar (sugar packets, candy) and identification describing disease process and medication regimen at all times.

Evaluation/Desired Outcomes

- Decrease in serum total cholesterol, LDL cholesterol, apolipoprotein, and blood glucose levels.
- Control of blood glucose levels without the appearance of hypoglycemic or hyperglycemic episodes.

conivaptan (con-i-**vap**-tan)

Vaprisol

Classification
Therapeutic: electrolyte modifiers
Pharmacologic: vasopressin antagonists

Indications

To increase serum sodium in hospitalized patients with euvolemic or hypervolemic hyponatremia.

Action

Antagonizes vasopressin at V_2 receptor sites in renal collecting ducts, resulting in excretion of free water. **Therapeutic Effects:** Increased serum sodium concentrations. Improved fluid status.

Pharmacokinetics

Absorption: IV administration results in complete bioavailability.
Distribution: Unknown.
Protein Binding: 99% protein bound.
Metabolism and Excretion: Metabolized solely by the CYP3A4 enzyme system. 83% excreted in feces as metabolites, 12% in urine (as metabolites).
Half-life: 5 hr.

TIME/ACTION PROFILE

ROUTE	ONSET	PEAK	DURATION
IV	unknown	12 hr	end of infusion

Contraindications/Precautions

Contraindicated in: Hypersensitivity; Hypovolemic hyponatremia; Concurrent use of ketonconazole, itraconazole, clarithromycin, ritonavir, or indinavir; Lactation: Avoid breast feeding.
Use Cautiously in: Moderate or severe hepatic impairment (↓ dose recommended); Severe renal impairment (not recommended if CCr <30 mL/min); OB: Safety not established; Pedi: Safety and effectiveness not established.

Adverse Reactions/Side Effects

CNS: headache, confusion, insomnia. **CV:** hypertension, hypotension. **GI:** diarrhea. **GU:** ↓ fertility (females), polyuria. **F and E:** dehydration, hypokalemia, hypomagnesemia, hyponatremia. **Local:** infusion reactions. **Misc:** fever, thirst.

C

Interactions

Drug-Drug: Blood levels and effects are ↑ by **ketoconazole, itraconazole, clarithromycin, ritonavir,** or **indinavir**; concurrent use is contraindicated. ↑ blood levels and may ↑ effects of **midazolam, simvastatin, lovastatin, amlodipine**, and **other drugs metabolized by CYP3A4**; careful monitoring recommended. May ↑ **digoxin** levels.

Route/Dosage

IV (Adults): 20 mg loading dose initially, followed by 20 mg/day as a continuous infusion for 2–4 days. May titrate conivaptan up to 40 mg/day as a continuous infusion if serum sodium is not rising at desired rate. Total duration of therapy should not exceed 4 days.

Hepatic Impairment

(Adults): *Moderate or severe hepatic impairment*—10 mg loading dose initially, followed by 10 mg/day as a continuous infusion for 2–4 days; may titrate up to 20 mg/day as a continuous infusion if serum sodium is not rising at desired rate.

Availability

Premixed infusion: 20 mg/100 mL D5W.

NURSING IMPLICATIONS

Assessment

- Monitor injection site during administration. Frequently causes erythema, pain, swelling and phlebitis. May require discontinuation of therapy.
- Monitor vital signs frequently during therapy. Discontinue therapy if patient becomes hypovolemic and hypotensive. Therapy may be resumed at a reduced dose once patient is euvolemic and no longer hypotensive, if patient remains hyponatremic.
- Assess neurologic status during administration. Overly rapid rise in serum sodium may cause neurologic sequelae.
- ***Lab Test Considerations:*** Monitor serum sodium concentration frequently during therapy. If serum sodium rises at an undesirably rapid rate (>12 mEq/L/24 hr), discontinue administration of conivaptan. If serum sodium continues to rise, do not resume therapy. If hyponatremia persists or recurs (after discontinuation for rapid rise of serum sodium) and patient has no evidence of neurologic sequelae from rapid increase, conivaptan may be resumed at a reduced dose.
- May cause hyperglycemia, hypoglycemia, hypokalemia, hypomagnesemia, and hyponatremia.

Implementation

IV Administration

- Administer IV through large veins and rotate infusion site every 24 hr to minimize risk of vascular irritation.

Loading Dose

- **Intermittent Infusion:** ***Diluent:*** Premixed containers require no further dilution. ***Concentration:*** 0.2 mg/mL. ***Rate:*** Administer over 30 min.

Continuous Infusion

- **Continuous Infusion:** ***Diluent:*** Premixed containers require no further dilution. ***Concentration:*** 0.2 mg/mL. ***Rate:*** Administer continuous infusion at a rate of 20 mg/24 hr. If patient requires 40 mg/24 hr continuous infusion, infuse 20 mg over 12 hr, followed by 20 mg over 12 hr.
- **Additive Incompatibility:** Do not admix with LR, furosemide, or combine with any other product in the same IV line or bag.

Patient/Family Teaching

- Explain purpose of medication to patient.
- Instruct patient to notify health care professional if pain or redness occurs at infusion site.

Evaluation/Desired Outcomes

- Restoration of normal fluid and electrolyte balance.

CONTRACEPTIVES, HORMONAL

MONOPHASIC ORAL CONTRACEPTIVES

ethinyl estradiol/desogestrel
(**eth**-in-il es-tra-**dye**-ole/dess-oh-**jess**-trel)
Apri-28, ~~Desogen-28~~, Emoquette, Enskyce, Isibloom, Kalliga, Reclipsen, Solia

ethinyl estradiol/drospirenone
(**eth**-in-il es-tra-**dye**-ole/droe-**spy**-re-nown)
Beyaz, Gianvi, Kemeya, Kyra, Lo-Zumandimine, Loryna, Nikki, Ocella, Safyral, Syeda, Tydemy, ~~Vestura~~, Yaela, Yasmin, Yaz, Zarah, Zumandimine

ethinyl estradiol/ethynodiol
(**eth**-in-il es-tra-**dye**-ole/e-thye-noe-**dye**-ole)
Kelnor, Lo-Malmorede, Malmorede, Zovia 1/35–28, Zovia 1/50–28

ethinyl estradiol/levonorgestrel
(**eth**-in-il es-tra-**dye**-ole/lee-voe-nor-**jess**-trel)
Afirmelle, Altavera, Aubra, Aviane-28, Ayuna, Balcoltra, Cerinta, Chateal, Fal-

mina, Kurvelo, Lessina-28, Levora-28, Lutera, Marlissa, Orsythia, Portia-28, Sronyx, Vienva

ethinyl estradiol/norethindrone
(**eth**-in-il es-tra-**dye**-ole/nor-eth-**in**-drone)
Alyacen 1/35, Aurovela Fe 1.5/30, Balziva-28, Blisovi Fe 1.5/30, Blisovi 24 Fe, Briellyn, Cyclafem 0.5/35, Cyclafem 1/35, Cyonanz, Dasetta 1/35, Femcon Fe, Generess Fe, Gildagia, Gildess 1/20, Gildess Fe 1/20, Gildess 1.5/30, Gildess Fe 1.5/30, Hailey 1.5/30, Hailey Fe 1/20, Hailey Fe 1.5/30, Jinteli, Junel 1/20, Junel 1.5/30, Junel Fe 1/20, Junel Fe 1.5/30, Kaitlib Fe, Larin 1/20, Larin 1.5/30, Larin Fe 1/20, Larin Fe 1.5/30, Loestrin 21 1/20, Loestrin 21 1.5/30, Loestrin Fe 1/20, Loestrin Fe 1.5/30, Mibelas 24 Fe, Microgestin 1/20, Microgestin 1.5/30, Microgestin Fe 1/20, Microgestin Fe 1.5/30, Necon 0.5/35, Necon 1/35, Nexesta Fe, Norinyl 1/35, Norminest Fe, Nortrel 0.5/35, Nortrel 1/35, Nylia 1/35, Ortho-Novum 1/35, Philith, Pirmella 1/35, Taytulla, Vyfemla, Wera, Wymzya Fe, Zenchent, Zenchent Fe

ethinyl estradiol/norgestimate
(**eth**-in-il es-tra-**dye**-ole/nor-**jes**-ti-mate)
Estarylla, Mono-Linyah, Mili, Mononessa, Ortho-Cyclen-28, Previfem, Sprintec

ethinyl estradiol/norgestrel
(**eth**-in-il es-tra-**dye**-ole/nor-**jess**-trel)
Cryselle, Elinest, Low-Ogestrel–28, Ogestrel–28

mestranol/norethindrone
(**mes**-tre-nole/nor-eth-**in**-drone)
Necon 1/50, ~~Norinyl 1/50~~

BIPHASIC ORAL CONTRACEPTIVES

ethinyl estradiol/desogestrel
(**eth**-in-il es-tra-**dye**-ole/dess-oh-**jess**-trel)
Azurette, Bekyree, Kariva, Kimidess, Pimtrea, Viorele, Volnea

ethinyl estradiol/norethindrone
(**eth**-in-il es-tra-**dye**-ole/nor-eth-**in**-drone)
Lo Loestrin Fe, Necon 10/11

TRIPHASIC ORAL CONTRACEPTIVES

ethinyl estradiol/desogestrel
(**eth**-in-il es-tra-**dye**-ole/dess-oh-**jess**-trel)
Caziant, Cyclessa, Velivet

ethinyl estradiol/levonorgestrel
(**eth**-in-il ess-tra-**dye**-ole/lee-voe-nor-**jess**-trel)
Elifemme, Enpresse-28, Levonest, Trivora–28

ethinyl estradiol/norethindrone
(**eth**-in-il es-tra-**dye**-ole/nor-eth-**in**-drone)
Alyacen 7/7/7, Aranelle, Cyclafem 7/7/7, Dasetta 7/7/7, Estrostep Fe, Leena, Necon 7/7/7, Nortrel 7/7/7, Nylia 7/7/7, Ortho-Novum 7/7/7–28, Pirmella 7/7/7, Tilia Fe, Tri-Legest-21, Tri-Legest Fe, Tri-Norinyl-28

ethinyl estradiol/norgestimate
(**eth**-in-il es-tra-**dye**-ole/nor-**jess**-ti-mate)
Ortho Tri-Cyclen-28, Ortho Tri-Cyclen Lo, Tri-Estarylla, Tri-Linyah, Tri-Lo-Estarylla, Tri-Lo-Mili, Tri-Previfem, Tri-Sprintec, TriNessa

FOURPHASIC ORAL CONTRACEPTIVES

estradiol valerate/dienogest
(es-tra-**dye**-ole **val**-er-ate/dye-**en**-oh-jest)
Natazia

EXTENDED-CYCLE ORAL CONTRACEPTIVE

ethinyl estradiol/levonorgestrel
(**eth**-in-il ess-tra-**dye**-ole/lee-voe-nor-**jess**-trel)
Amethia, Amethia Lo, Amethyst, Ashlyna, Camrese, Camrese Lo, Daysee, Iclevia, Introvale, Jaimiess, Jolessa, LoSeasonique, Quartette, Quasense, Seasonale, Seasonique, Setlakin, Simpesse, Sylevia

C

PROGESTIN-ONLY ORAL CONTRACEPTIVES

norethindrone (nor-eth-**in**-drone)
Camila, Errin, Jencycla, Jolivette, Micronor, Nora-BE

drospirenone
Slynd

CONTRACEPTIVE IMPLANT

etonogestrel (e-toe-no-**jess**-trel)
Nexplanon

EMERGENCY CONTRACEPTIVE

levonorgestrel
(**lee**-voe-nor-**jess**-trel)
Fallback Solo, Plan B One-Step

ulipristal (u-li-**priss**-tal)
Ella, Logilia

INJECTABLE CONTRACEPTIVE

medroxyprogesterone
(me-**drox**-ee-proe-**jess**-te-rone)
Depo-Provera, Depo-subQ Provera 104

INTRAUTERINE CONTRACEPTIVE

levonorgestrel
(**lee**-voe-nor-**jess**-trel)
Kyleena, Liletta, Mirena, Skyla

VAGINAL RING CONTRACEPTIVE

ethinyl estradiol/etonogestrel
(**eth**-in-il ess-tra-**dye**-ole/e-toe-noe-**jess**-trel)
NuvaRing

TRANSDERMAL CONTRACEPTIVE

ethinyl estradiol/norelgestromin
(**eth**-in-il ess-tra-**dye**-ole/nor-el-**jess**-troe-min)
Xulane

Classification
Therapeutic: contraceptive hormones

Indications

Prevention of pregnancy. Regulation of menstrual cycle. Emergency contraception (some products). Treatment of heavy menstrual bleeding in women who choose to use intrauterine contraception as their method of contraception (Mirena). Treatment of heavy menstrual bleeding in women who choose to use an oral contraceptive as their method of contraception (Natazia). Treatment of premenstrual dysphoric disorder (Beyaz, Yaz, Yasmin). Management of acne in women >14 yr who desire contraception, have no health problems, and have failed topical treatment. Increase folate levels in women who desire oral contraception to reduce the risk of neural tube defects in a pregnancy that occurs while taking or shortly after discontinuing the product.

Action

Monophasic Oral Contraceptives: Provide a fixed dosage of estrogen/progestin over a 21-day cycle. Ovulation is inhibited by suppression of follicle-stimulating hormone (FSH) and luteinizing hormone (LH). May alter cervical mucus and the endometrial environment, preventing penetration by sperm and implantation of the egg. **Biphasic Oral Contraceptives:** Ovulation is inhibited by suppression of FSH and LH. May alter cervical mucus and the endometrial environment, preventing penetration by sperm and implantation of the egg. In addition, smaller dose of progestin in phase 1 allows for proliferation of endometrium. Larger amount in phase 2 allows for adequate secretory development. **Triphasic Oral Contraceptives:** Ovulation is inhibited by suppression of FSH and LH. May alter cervical mucus and the endometrial environment, preventing penetration by sperm and implantation of the egg. Varying doses of estrogen/progestin may more closely mimic natural hormonal fluctuations. **Fourphasic Oral Contraceptives:** Ovulation is inhibited by suppression of FSH and LH. May alter cervical mucus and the endometrial environment, preventing penetration by sperm and implantation of the egg. Doses of estrogen decrease while doses of progestin increase over the 28-day cycle. **Extended-cycle:** Provides continuous estrogen/progestin for 84 days (365 days for Lybrel), then off for 7 days (low-dose estrogen-only tablet taken during these 7 days with LoSeasonique and Seasonique), resulting in 4 menstrual periods/yr (no periods/yr for Lybrel). **Progressive Estrogen:** Contains constant amount of progestin with 3 progressive doses of estrogen. **Progestin-Only Contraceptives/Contraceptive Implant/Intrauterine Levonorgestrel/Medroxyprogesterone Injection:** Mechanism not clearly known. May alter cervical mucus and the endometrial environment, preventing penetration by sperm and implantation of the egg. Ovulation may also be suppressed. **Emergency Contraceptive Pills (ECPs):** Inhibit ovulation/fertilization; may also alter tubal transport of sperm/egg and prevent implantation. **Vaginal Ring, Transdermal Patch:** Inhibits ovulation, decreases sperm entry into uterus, decreases likelihood of implantation. **Anti-acne effect:** Combination of estrogen/progestin may increase sex hormone binding globulin (SHBG) resulting in decreased unbound testosterone, which may be a cause of acne. **Therapeutic Effects:** Prevention of pregnancy. Decreased severity of acne. Decrease in menstrual blood loss. Decrease in premenstrual disphoric disorder. Decrease in vasomotor symptoms or symptoms of vulvar and vaginal atrophy due to menopause. Increase in folate levels and prevention of neural tube defects.

Pharmacokinetics

Absorption: *Ethinyl estradiol*—rapidly absorbed; *Norethindrone*—65% absorbed; *Desogestrel and levonorgestrel*—100% absorbed; *Dienogest*—91% absorbed. Others are well absorbed after oral administration. Slowly absorbed from implant, subcutaneous or IM injection. Some absorption follows intrauterine implantation.

Distribution: Unknown.

Protein Binding: *Ethinyl estradiol*—97–98%; *Drospirenone*—97%; *Dienogest*—90%; *Ulipristal*—>94%.

Metabolism and Excretion: *Ethinyl estradiol and norethindrone*—undergo extensive first-pass hepatic metabolism. *Mestranol*—is rapidly converted to ethinyl estradol. *Desogestrel*—is rapidly metabolized to 3-keto-desogestrel, the active metabolite. Most agents are metabolized by the liver.

Half-life: *Ethinyl estradiol*—6–20 hr; *Levonorgestrel*—45 hr; *Norethindrone*—5–14 hr; *Desogestrel (metabolite)*—38 ± 20 hr; *Drospirenone*—30 hr; *Norgestimate (metabolite)*—12–20 hr; *Dienogest*—11 hr; *others*—unknown; *Ulipristal*—32 hr.

TIME/ACTION PROFILE (prevention of pregnancy)

ROUTE	ONSET	PEAK	DURATION
PO	1 mo	1 mo	1 mo†
Implant	1 mo	1 mo	5 yr
Intrauterine system	1 mo	1 mo	5 yr
IM	1 mo	1 mo	3 mo
Subcut	unknown	1 wk	3 mo

†Only during mo of taking contraceptive.

Contraindications/Precautions

Contraindicated in: Hypersensitivity; History of cigarette smoking and age >35 yr (↑ risk of cardiovascular or thromboembolic phenomenon); History of thromboembolic disease (e.g., DVT, PE, MI, stroke); Protein C, protein S, or antithrombin deficiency or other thrombophilic disorder; Cerebrovascular disease; Coronary artery disease; Valvular heart disease or thrombogenic heart rhythms; Major surgery with extended periods of immobility; Diabetes with vascular disease; Headache with focal neurological symptoms or migraine headaches with aura; Women >35 yr with migraine headaches; Uncontrolled hypertension; Breast cancer or any other estrogen- or progestin-sensitive cancer; Abnormal genital bleeding; Liver disease or liver tumors; Hypersensitivity to parabens (injectable only); Concurrent use of combinations containing ombitasvir/paritaprevir/ritonavir (with or without dasubavir) (↑ risk of liver enzyme elevations); *Drosperinone-containing products only*—Renal impairment, liver disease, or adrenal insufficiency (↑ risk of hyperkalemia); *Intrauterine levonorgestrel only*—Intrauterine anomaly, postpartum endometriosis, multiple sexual partners, pelvic inflammatory disease, liver disease, genital actinomycosis, immunosuppression, IV drug abuse, untreated genitourinary infection, history of ectopic pregnancy; OB: Pregnancy; Lactation: Avoid use; ↑ risk of uterine rupture with intrauterine levonorgestrel.

Use Cautiously in: Presence of other cardiovascular risk factors (obesity, hyperglycemia, hypertension); History or family history of hypertriglyceridemia (↑ risk of pancreatitis); Diabetes mellitus, bleeding disorders, concurrent anticoagulant therapy or headaches; Hereditary angioedema; Pedi: Avoid use before menarche.

Adverse Reactions/Side Effects

CNS: depression, headache. **CV:** THROMBOEMBOLISM, edema, hypertension, Raynaud's phenomenon, thrombophlebitis. **Derm:** melasma, rash. **EENT:** contact lens intolerance, optic neuritis, retinal thrombosis. **Endo:** hyperglycemia. **F and E:** *Drosperinone-containing products only*—hyperkalemia. **GI:** PANCREATITIS, abdominal cramps, bloating, cholestatic jaundice, gallbladder disease, liver tumors, nausea, vomiting. **GU:** amenorrhea, breakthrough bleeding, dysmenorrhea, spotting, *Intrauterine levonorgestrel only*—uterine imbedment/uterine rupture. **MS:** *Injectable medroxyprogesterone only*—bone loss. **Misc:** HYPERSENSITIVITY REACTIONS (including anaphylaxis and angioedema), weight change.

Interactions

Drug-Drug: Oral contraceptive efficacy may be ↓ by **penicillins**, **chloramphenicol**, **barbiturates**, chronic **alcohol** use, **carbamazepine**, **oxcarbazepine**, **bosentan**, **felbamate**, systemic **corticosteroids**, **phenytoin**, **topiramate**, **primidone**, **modafinil**, **rifampin**, **rifabutin**, **nelfinavir**, **ritonavir**, **darunavir/ritonavir**, **fosamprenavir/ritonavir**, **lopinavir/ritonavir**, **tipranavir/ritonavir**, **nevirapine**, **efavirenz**, **colesevelam**, or **tetracyclines**. **CYP3A4 inducers**, including **barbiturates**, **bosentan**, **carbamazepine**, **oxcarbazepine**, **phenytoin**, **topiramate**, **felbamate**, **rifampin** may ↓ effectiveness of ulipristal; avoid concomitant use. May ↑ effects/risk of toxicity of some **benzodiazepines**, **beta blockers**, **corticosteroids**, **cyclosporine**, **tizanidine**, **theophylline**, and **voriconazole**. ↑ risk of hepatotoxicity with **dantrolene** (estrogen only). **Indinavir**, **atazanavir/ritonavir**, **etravirine**, **itraconazole**, **ketoconazole**, **fluconazole**, **voriconazole**, **rosuvastatin**, and **atorvastatin** may ↑ effects/risk of toxicity. **Smoking** ↑ risk of thromboembolic phenomena (estrogen only). May ↓ levels of **acetaminophen**,

temazepam, **lamotrigine**, **lorazepam**, **oxazepam**, or **morphine**. Concurrent use of combinations containing **ombitasvir/paritaprevir/ritonavir** with ethinyl estradiol-containing products may ↑ risk of elevated liver enzymes; avoid concurrent use. *Drosperinone-containing products only*—concurrent use with **NSAIDs**, **potassium-sparing diuretics**, **potassium supplements**, **ACE inhibitors**, **aldosterone receptor antagonists**, or **angiotensin II receptor antagonists** may result in hyperkalemia. *Drosperinone-containing products only*—concurrent use with strong **CYP3A4 inhibitors**, including **ketoconazole**, **itraconazole**, **voriconazole**, **protease inhibitors**, or **clarithromycin** may ↑ risk of hyperkalemia; consider monitoring K+ concentrations. Ulipristal may ↑ levels of **P-glycoprotein substrates**, including **dabigatran** and **digoxin**.

Drug-Natural Products: Concomitant use with **St. John's wort** may ↓ contraceptive efficacy and cause breakthrough bleeding and irregular menses.

Drug-Food: **Grapefruit juice** may ↑ effects/risk of toxicity.

Route/Dosage

Monophasic Oral Contraceptives

PO (Adults): On 21-day regimen, take first tablet on first Sunday after menses begins (take on Sunday if menses begins on Sunday) for 21 days, then skip 7 days and begin again. Regimen may also be started on first day of menses, continue for 21 days, then skip 7 days and begin again. Some regimens contain 7 placebo tablets, so that 1 tablet is taken every day for 28 days.

Biphasic Oral Contraceptives

PO (Adults): Given in 2 phases. First phase is 10 days of smaller amount of progestin. Second phase is larger amount of progestin. Amount of estrogen remains constant for same length of time (total of 21 days), then skip 7 days and begin again. Some regimens contain 7 placebo tablets for 28-day regimen.

Triphasic Oral Contraceptives

PO (Adults): Progestin amount varies throughout 21-day cycle. Estrogen component stays the same or may vary. Some regimens contain 7 placebo tablets for 28-day regimen.

Fourphasic Oral Contraceptives

PO (Adults): Given in 4 phases. First phase contains higher amount of estrogen and no progestin. Second and third phases contains lower amount of estrogen, and increasing amounts of progestin. Fourth phase contains low dose of estrogen only. Also contains 2 placebo tablets to complete 28-day regimen.

Extended-Cycle Contraceptive

PO (Adults): *Daysee, LoSeasonique, Quartette, Seasonale and Seasonique*. Start taking first active pill on first Sunday after menses begins (if first day is Sunday, begin then), continue for 84 days of active pill, followed by 7 days of placebo tablets (low-dose estrogen tablets for Daysee, LoSeasonique, Quartette, and Seasonique), then resume 84/7 cycle again. For *Lybrel*, begin taking the first pill during the first day of the menstrual cycle and start the next pack the day after the previous pack ends.

Progestin-Only Oral Contraceptives

PO (Adults): Start on first day of menses. Taken daily and continuously.

Progressive Estrogen Oral Contraceptives

PO (Adults): Estrogen amount increases every 7 days throughout 21-day cycle. Progestin component stays the same. Some regimens contain 7 placebo tablets for 28-day regimen.

Emergency Contraceptive

PO (Adults and Adolescents): *Plan B*—1 tablet within 72 hr of unprotected intercourse followed by 1 more tablet 12 hr later; *Lo/Ovral*—4 white tablets within 72 hr of unprotected intercourse followed by 4 more white tablets 12 hr later; *Levlen*—4 light orange tablets within 72 hr of unprotected intercourse followed by 4 more light orange tablets 12 hr later; *Tri-Levlen*—4 yellow tablets within 72 hr of unprotected intercourse followed by 4 more yellow tablets 12 hr later; *Ulipristal*—1 tablet as soon as possible within 120 hr (5 days) after unprotected intercourse or known/suspected contraceptive failure.

Injectable Contraceptive

medroxyprogesterone (Depo-Provera)

IM (Adults): 150 mg within first 5 days of menses or within 5 days postpartum, if not breast feeding. If breast feeding, give 6 wk postpartum; repeat every 3 mo.

medroxyprogesterone (Depo-Sub Q Provera 104)

Subcut (Adults): 104 mg within first 5 days of menses or within 5 days postpartum, if not breast feeding. If breast feeding, give 6 wk postpartum; repeat every 12–14 wk.

Intrauterine Contraceptive

Intrauterine (Adults): Insert one device into uterine cavity within 7 days of menses or immediately after 1st trimester abortion. Skyla should be removed or replaced after 3 yr. Kyleena, Liletta, and Mirena should be removed or replaced after 5 yr.

Vaginal Ring Contraceptive

Vag (Adults): One ring inserted on or prior to day 5 of menstrual cycle. Ring is left in place for 3 wk, then removed for 1 wk, then a new ring is inserted.

Transdermal Patch

Transdermal (Adults): Patch is applied on day 1 of menstrual cycle (or convenient day in first wk), changed weekly thereafter for 3 wk. Wk 4 is patch-free. Cycle is then repeated.

Acne

PO (Adults): *Ortho Tri-Cyclen*—Take daily for 21 days, off for 7 days.

Availability

Combination Estrogen/Progestin Oral Contraceptives (generic available)

Oral contraceptive tablets: Usually in monthly packs with enough (21) active tablets to complete a 28-day cycle. Some contain 7 inert tablets to complete the cycle with or without supplemental iron, Beyaz and Safyral —contain 0.451 mg of levomefolate calcium/tablet.

Extended-Cycle Contraceptive

Tablets: *LoSeasonique*—active tablets containing 0.02 mg ethinyl estradiol, 0.1 mg levonorgestrel, and 7 tablets containing 0.01 mg ethinyl estradiol; *Quartette*—42 tablets containing 0.02 mg ethinyl estradiol and 0.15 mg levonorgestrel, 21 tablets containing 0.025 mg ethinyl estradiol and 0.15 mg levonorgestrel, 21 tablets containing 0.03 mg ethinyl estradiol and 0.15 mg levonorgestrel, and 7 tablets containing 0.01 mg ethinyl estradiol; *Seasonale*—84 active tablets containing 0.03 mg ethinyl estradiol and 0.15 mg levonorgestrel and 7 inactive tablets; *Daysee and Seasonique*—active tablets containing 0.03 mg ethinyl estradiol, 0.15 mg levonorgestrel, and 7 tablets containing 0.01 mg ethinyl estradiol; *Lybrel*—28 active tablets containing 0.09 mg levonorgestrel and 0.02 mg ethinyl estradiol.

Levonorgestrel (generic available)

Emergency contraceptives: 2 tablets containing 0.75 mg levonorgestrel (Plan B). **Intrauterine system (Kyleena):** contains 19.5 mg levonorgestrel (releases 9 mcg/day). **Intrauterine system (Liletta):** contains 52 mg levonorgestrel (releases 14.7 mcg/day). **Intrauterine system (Mirena):** contains 52 mg levonorgestrel (releases 20 mcg/day). **Intrauterine system (Skyla):** contains 13.5 mg levonorgestrel (releases 14 mcg/day).

Etonorgestrel

Implant: Rod contains 68 mg etonogestrel.

Ulipristal

Tablets: 30 mg.

Medroxyprogesterone (generic available)

Injectable IM: 150 mg/mL. **Injectable Subcutaneous:** 104 mg/0.65 mL (in pre-filled syringes).

Vaginal Ring Contraceptive

Ring: delivers 0.015 mg ethinyl estradiol and 0.120 mg etonogestrel/day.

Transdermal Patch

Patch (Xulane): contains 0.53 mg ethinyl estradiol and 4.86 mg of norelgestromin; releases 35 mcg ethinyl estradiol/150 mcg norelgestromin per 24 hr.

NURSING IMPLICATIONS

Assessment

- Assess BP before and periodically during therapy.
- Exclude the possibility of pregnancy on the basis or history and/or physical exam or a pregnancy test before administering emergency contraceptives.
- **Acne:** Assess skin lesion before and periodically during therapy.
- **Menopausal Symptoms:** Assess vasomotor symptoms or symptoms of vulvar and vaginal atrophy due to menopause prior to and periodically during therapy.
- ***Lab Test Considerations:*** Monitor hepatic function periodically during therapy.
- *Estrogens only*—May cause ↑ serum glucose, sodium, triglyceride, VHDL, total cholesterol, prothrombin, and factors VII, VIII, IX, and X levels. May cause ↓ LDL and antithrombin III levels.
- May cause false interpretations of thyroid function tests.
- *Progestins only*—May cause ↑ LDL concentrations. May cause ↓ serum alkaline phosphatase and HDL concentrations.
- *Drosperidone-containing contraceptives* —monitor serum potassium during first treatment cycle in women on long-term treatment with strong CYP3A4 inhibitors; may ↑ serum potassium concentration.

Implementation

- Do not confuse Ortho Tri-Cyclen with Ortho Tri-Cyclen Lo. Do not confuse Yasmin with Yaz.
- **PO:** Oral doses may be administered with or immediately after food to reduce nausea. Chewable tablets may be swallowed whole or chewed; if chewed follow with 8 oz of liquid.
- For extended-cycle tablets, *Jolessa, Quasense, Seasonale, Seasonique,* or *LoSeasonique*—take active tablets for 84 days and followed by the placebo tablets for 7 days; for *Lybrel*—Take 1 pill each day for 28 days, then start the next set of pills daily for the next 28 days.
- For *Emergency Contraception:* Tablets are taken as soon as possible and within 72 hr after unprotected intercourse. Two doses are taken 12 hr apart. Emergency contraception products are available without a prescription to all women of child-bearing age.
- *Ulipristal:* Administer 1 tablet as soon as possible within 120 hr (5 days) after unprotected intercourse or a known or suspected contraceptive failure. May be taken without regard to food. If vomiting occurs

within 3 hr of dose, may repeat. May be taken at any time during the menstrual cycle. Ulipristal may be less effective in women with a body mass index >30 kg/m^2.

- **Subcut:** Shake vigorously before use to form a uniform suspension. Inject slowly (over 5–7 sec) at a 45° angle into fatty area of anterior thigh or abdomen every 12 to 14 wk. If more than 14 wk elapse between injections, rule out pregnancy prior to administration. Do not rub area after injection.
- When switching from other hormonal contraceptives, administer within dosing period (7 days after taking last active pill, removing patch or ring, or within the dosing period for IM injection).
- **IM:** Shake vial vigorously just before use to ensure uniform suspension. Administer deep IM into gluteal or deltoid muscle. If period between injections is >14 wk, determine that patient is not pregnant before administering the drug.
- Injectable medroxyprogesterone may lead to bone loss, especially in women younger than 21 yr. Injectable medroxyprogesterone should be used for >2 yr only if other methods of contraception are inadequate. If used long term, women should use supplemental calcium and vitamin D, and monitor bone mineral density.
- **Intrauterine system:** Health care providers are advised to become thoroughly familiar with the insertion instructions before attempting insertion. Following insertion counsel patient on what to expect following insertion. Give patient *Follow-up Reminder Card* provided with product. Discuss expected bleeding patterns during the first mo of use. Prescribe analgesics, if indicated. Patients should be reexamined and evaluated 4 to 12 wk after insertion and once a yr thereafter, or more frequently if clinically indicated.

Patient/Family Teaching

- Instruct patient to take oral medication as directed at the same time each day. Pills should be taken in proper sequence and kept in the original container. Advise patient not to skip pills even if not having sex very often. Advise patient to read *Patient Guide* before starting and with each Rx refill in case of changes.
- *If single daily dose is missed:* Take as soon as remembered; if not until next day, take 2 tablets and continue on regular dosing schedule. *If 2 days in a row are missed:* Take 2 tablets a day for the next 2 days and continue on regular dosing schedule, using a 2nd method of birth control for the remaining cycle. *If 3 days in a row are missed:* Discontinue medication and use another form of birth control until period begins or pregnancy is ruled out; then begin a new cycle of tablets. *For 28-day dosing schedule:* If schedule is followed for first 21 days and 1 dose is missed of the last 7 tablets, it is important to take the 1st tablet of next month's cycle on the regularly scheduled day. Advise patient taking *Natazia* to follow *Patient Guide* for what to do if a pill is missed.
- Advise patient taking *Jolessa, Quasense, Seasonale, Sesonique,* or *LoSeasonique extended-cycle tablets* that withdrawal bleeding should occur during the 7 days following discontinuation of the active tablets. If withdrawal bleeding does not occur, notify health care professional. Advise patient taking *Lybrel* that no withdrawal bleeding should occur.
- For initial use of *Jolessa, Quasense, Seasonale, Seasonique,* or *LoSeasonique extended cycle tablets*, caution patient to use a nonhormonal method of contraception until she has taken the first 7 days of active tablets. Each 91-day cycle should start on the same day of the wk. If started later than the proper day or 2 or more days are missed, a 2nd nonhormonal method of contraception should be used until she has taken the pink tablet for 7 days. Transient spotting or bleeding may occur. If bleeding is persistent or prolonged, notify health care professional.
- Advise patient taking extended cycle tablets that spotting or light bleeding may occur, especially during first 3 mo. Continue medication; notify health care professional if bleeding lasts >70 k days.
- Advise patient of the need to use another form of contraception for the first 3 wk when beginning to use *oral contraceptives*.
- Instruct patient to notify health care professional of all Rx or OTC medications, vitamins, or herbal products being taken and consult health care professional before taking any new medications.
- Advise patient that a 2nd method of birth control should also be used during each cycle in which any of the following are used: *Oral contraceptives*—ampicillin, corticosteroids, antiretroviral protease inhibitors, barbiturates, carbamazepine, chloramphenicol, dihydroergotamine, corticosteroids (systemic), mineral oil, oral neomycin, oxcarbazapine, penicillin V, phenylbutazone, primidone, rifampin, sulfonamides, tetracyclines, topiramate, bosentan, or valproic acid.
- Explain dose schedule and maintenance routine. Discontinuing medication suddenly may cause withdrawal bleeding.
- If nausea becomes a problem, advise patient that eating solid food often provides relief. If nausea persists or vomiting or diarrhea occur, use a nonhormonal method of contraception and notify health care professional.
- Advise patient to report signs and symptoms of fluid retention (swelling of ankles and feet, weight gain), thromboembolic disorders (pain, swelling, tenderness in extremities, headache, chest pain, blurred vision), mental depression, hepatic dysfunction (yel-

lowed skin or eyes, pruritus, dark urine, light-colored stools), or abnormal vaginal bleeding. Women with a strong family history of breast cancer, fibrocystic breast disease, abnormal mammograms, or cervical dysplasia should be monitored for breast cancer at least yearly. Risk of thromboembolism is highest in 1st yr of use and increased when a combination hormonal contraceptive is restarted after a break in use of at least 4 wk.

- Instruct patient to stop taking medication and notify health care professional if pregnancy is suspected.
- Caution patient that cigarette smoking during estrogen therapy may increase risk of serious side effects, especially for women over age 35.
- Caution patients to use sunscreen and protective clothing to prevent increased pigmentation.
- Caution patient that hormonal contraceptives do not protect against HIV or other sexually transmitted diseases.
- Advise patient to notify health care professional of medication regimen before treatment or surgery.
- Emphasize the importance of routine follow-up physical exams including BP; breast, abdomen, and pelvic examinations; and Papanicolaou smears every 6–12 mo.
- **Emergency Contraception:** Instruct patient to take emergency contraceptive as directed. Advise patient that they should not take emergency contraceptives if they know or suspect they are pregnant; emergency contraceptives are not for use to end an existing pregnancy. Advise patient to contact health care professional if they vomit within 3 hr after taking ulipristal.
- Inform patient that *ulipristal* may reduce the effectiveness of hormonal contraceptives. Advise patient to use a non-hormonal contraceptive during that menstrual cycle. Advise patient to wait at least 5 days after taking *ulipristal* to resume taking hormonal contraceptives.
- Advise patient to notify health care professional and consider the possibility of pregnancy if their period is delayed by more than 1 wk beyond the expected date after taking *ulipristal*.
- Inform patient that emergency contraceptives are not to be used as a routine form of contraception or to be used repeatedly within the same menstrual cycle.
- Advise patient to notify health care professional if severe lower abdominal pain occurs 3–5 wk after taking *ulipristal* to be evaluated for an ectopic pregnancy.
- Advise female patients to avoid breast feeding if taking *ulipristal*.
- **IM Subcut:** Advise patient to maintain adequate amounts of dietary calcium and vitamin D to help prevent bone loss.
- **Transdermal:** Instruct patient on application of patch. First patch should be applied within 24 hr of menstrual period. If applied after Day 1 of menstrual period, a nonhormonal method of contraception should be used for the next 7 days. Day of application becomes *Patch Change Day*. Patches are worn for 1 wk and changed on the same day of each wk for 3 wk. Wk 4 is patch-free. Withdrawal bleeding is expected during this time.
- Apply patch to clean, dry, intact, healthy skin on buttock, abdomen, upper outer arm, or upper torso in a place where it won't be rubbed by tight clothing. Do not place on skin that is red, irritated, or cut, and do not place on breasts. Do not apply make-up, creams, lotions, powders, or other topical products to area of patch application.
- To apply patch open foil pouch by tearing along edge using fingers. Peel pouch apart and open flat. Grasp a corner of the patch firmly and remove gently from foil pouch. Use fingernail to lift one corner of the patch and peel patch **and** the plastic liner off the foil liner. Do not remove clear liner as patch is removed. Peel away half of the clear liner without touching sticky surface. Apply the sticky surface and remove the rest of the liner. Press down firmly with palm of hand for 10 sec; make sure the edges stick well.
- On *Patch Change Day* remove patch and apply new one immediately. Used patch still contains some active hormones; fold in half so it sticks to itself and throw away. Apply new patches to a new spot to prevent skin irritation; may be applied in same anatomic area.
- Following patch-free wk, apply a new patch on *Patch Change Day*, the day after Day 28, no matter when the menstrual cycle begins.
- If patch becomes partially or completely detached for less than 1 day, reapply patch or apply new patch. If patch is detached for more than 1 day, apply a new patch immediately and use a nonhormonal form of contraception for the next 7 days. Cycle will now start over with a new *Patch Change Day*. If patch is no longer sticky, apply a new patch; do not use tape or wraps to keep patch in place.
- If patch is not changed on *Patch Change Day* in the first wk of the cycle, apply new patch immediately upon remembering and use a nonhormonal method of contraception for next 7 days. If patch change is missed for 1 or 2 days during Wk 2 or 3, apply new patch immediately and apply next patch on usual *Patch Change Day*. No backup contraception is needed. If patch change is missed for more than 2 days during Wk 2 or 3, stop the cycle and start a new 4-wk contraceptive cycle by applying new patch immediately and using a nonhormonal method of contraception for the next 7 days. If patch is not removed on *Patch Change Day* in Wk 4, remove as soon as remembered and start next cycle on usual *Patch Change Day*. No additional contraception is needed.
- Advise patient referred for MRI test to discuss patch with referring health care professional and MRI facility to determine if removal of patch is necessary prior to test and for directions for replacing patch.

- **NuvaRing:** *If a hormonal contraceptive was not used in the past mo*, insert *NuvaRing* between Days 1 and 5 of the menstrual cycle (Day 1 = first day of menstrual period), even if bleeding has not finished. Use a nonhormonal method of birth control other than a diaphragm during the first 7 days of ring use. *If switching from a combination estrogen/progesterone oral contraceptive*, insert *NuvaRing* any time during first 7 days after last tablet and no later than the day a new pill cycle would have started. No extra birth control is needed. *If switching from a mini-pill*, start using *NuvaRing* on any day of the mo; do not skip days between last pill and first day of *NuvaRing* use. *If switching from an implant*, start using *NuvaRing* on same day implant is removed. *If switching from an injectable contraceptive*, start using *NuvaRing* on the day when next injection is due. *If switching from a progestin-containing IUD*, start using *NuvaRing* on the same day as IUD is removed. A nonhormonal method of contraception, other than the diaphragm, should be used for the first 7 days of *NuvaRing* use when switching from the mini-pill, implant, injectable contraceptive, or IUD.
- *NuvaRing* comes in a reclosable foil pouch. Instruct patient to wash hands, then remove *NuvaRing* from pouch; keep pouch for ring disposal. Using a position of comfort (lying down, squatting, or standing with one leg up), hold *NuvaRing* between thumb and index finger and press opposite sides of the ring together. Gently push folded ring into vagina. Exact position is not important for function of *NuvaRing*. Most women do not feel *NuvaRing* once it is in place. If discomfort is felt, *NuvaRing* may not be inserted far enough into vagina; use finger to push further into vagina. *There is no danger of NuvaRing being pushed in too far or getting lost*. Once inserted, leave *NuvaRing* in place for 3 wk.
- Remove ring 3 wk after insertion on same day and time of insertion. Remove by hooking finger under forward rim or by holding ring between index and middle finger and pulling out. Place ring in foil pouch and dispose; do not throw in toilet. Menstrual period will usually start 2–3 days after ring is removed and may not have finished before next ring is inserted. To continue contraceptive protection, new ring must be inserted 1 wk after last one was removed, even if menstrual period has not stopped.
- If *NuvaRing* slips out of vagina and has been out less than 3 hr, contraceptive protection is still in place. *NuvaRing* can be rinsed in cool to tepid water and should be reinserted as soon as possible. If ring is lost, insert a new ring and continue same schedule as lost ring. If *NuvaRing* has been out of vagina for more than 3 hr, a nonhormonal method of contraception, other than a diaphragm, should be used for the next 7 days.
- *If NuvaRing has been left in for an extra wk or less (4 wk total or less)*, remove and insert a new ring after a 1-wk ring-free break. If *NuvaRing* has been left in place for more than 4 wk, woman should check to be sure she is not pregnant. A nonhormonal method of contraception, other than a diaphragm, must be used for the next 7 days.
- Advise patient to avoid using other female barrier contraceptives (diaphragm, cervical cap, female condom) with Nuvaring.
- **Intrauterine system:** Advise patient to notify health care professional if pelvic pain or pain during sex, unusual vaginal discharge or genital sores, unexplained fever, exposure to sexually transmitted infections, very severe or migraine headaches, yellowing of skin or whites of the eyes, very severe vaginal bleeding or bleeding that lasts a long time occurs, if a menstrual period is missed, or if *Mirena's* threads cannot be felt.

Evaluation/Desired Outcomes

- Prevention of pregnancy.
- Regulation of the menstrual cycle.
- Decrease in menstrual blood loss.
- Decrease in acne.
- Decrease in symptoms of premenstrual dysphoric disorder.
- Decrease in vasomotor symptoms or symptoms of vulvar and vaginal atrophy due to menopause.

CORTICOSTEROIDS (INHALATION)

beclomethasone
(be-kloe-**meth**-a-sone)
🍁QVAR, QVAR Redihaler

budesonide (byoo-**dess**-oh-nide)
Pulmicort Flexhaler,
🍁Pulmicort Nebuamp, Pulmicort Respules, 🍁Pulmicort Turbuhaler

fluticasone (floo-**ti**-ka-sone)
Armonair Respiclick, Arnuity Ellipta, Flovent Diskus, Flovent HFA

mometasone (mo-**met**-a-sone)
Asmanex HFA, Asmanex Twisthaler

Classification
Therapeutic: antiasthmatics, anti-inflammatories (steroidal)
Pharmacologic: corticosteroids (inhalation)

Indications

Maintenance treatment of asthma as prophylactic therapy. May decrease the need for or eliminate use of systemic corticosteroids in patients with asthma.

Action

Potent, locally acting anti-inflammatory and immune modifier. **Therapeutic Effects:** Decreased frequency and severity of asthma attacks. Improves asthma symptoms.

Pharmacokinetics

Absorption: *Beclomethasone*—20%; *budesonide*—6–13% (Flexhaler), 6% (Respules); *fluticasone*—<7% (aerosol), 8–14% (powder); *mometasone*—<1%. Action is primarily local after inhalation.
Distribution: 10–25% is deposited in airways if a spacer device is not used. All cross the placenta and enter breast milk in small amounts.
Metabolism and Excretion: *Beclomethasone*—after inhalation, beclomethasone dipropionate is converted to beclomethasone monopropionate, an active metabolite that adds to its potency, primarily excreted in feces (<10% excreted in urine; *Budesonide, fluticasone, mometasone*—metabolized by the liver (primarily by CYP3A4) after absorption from lungs; *Budesonide*—60% excreted in urine, 40% in feces; *fluticasone*—primarily excreted in feces (<5% excreted in urine); *mometasone*—75% excreted in feces.
Half-life: *Beclomethasone*—2.8 hr; *budesonide*—2–3.6 hr; *fluticasone*—7.8 hr (propionate); 24 hr (furoate); *mometasone*—5 hr.

TIME/ACTION PROFILE (improvement in symptoms)

ROUTE	ONSET	PEAK	DURATION
Inhalation	within 24 hr‡	1–4 wk†	unknown

†Improvement in pulmonary function; ↓ airway responsiveness may take longer.
‡2–8 days for budesonide respule.

Contraindications/Precautions

Contraindicated in: Some products contain alcohol or lactose and should be avoided in patients with known hypersensitivity or intolerance; Acute attack of asthma/status asthmaticus.
Use Cautiously in: Active untreated infections; Diabetes or glaucoma; Underlying immunosuppression (due to disease or concurrent therapy); Systemic corticosteroid therapy (should not be abruptly discontinued when inhalation therapy is started; additional corticosteroids needed in stress or trauma); Hepatic impairment (fluticasone); OB, Lactation: Safety not established; Pedi: Prolonged or high-dose therapy may lead to complications.

Adverse Reactions/Side Effects

CNS: headache, agitation, depression, dizziness, fatigue, insomnia, restlessness. **EENT:** dysphonia, hoarseness, cataracts, glaucoma, nasal congestion, pharyngitis, sinusitis. **Endo:** adrenal suppression (↑ dose, long-term therapy only), ↓ growth (children), ↓ bone mineral density. **GI:** diarrhea, dry mouth, dyspepsia, esophageal candidiasis, taste disturbances, nausea. **MS:** back pain. **Resp:** bronchospasm, cough, wheezing. **Misc:** CHURG-STRAUSS SYNDROME, HYPERSENSITIVITY REACTIONS (including anaphylaxis, laryngeal edema, urticaria, and bronchospasm).

Interactions

Drug-Drug: Strong **CYP3A4 inhibitors**, including **ritonavir**, **atazanavir**, **clarithromycin**, **conivaptan**, **indinavir**, **itraconazole**, **ketoconazole**, **lopinavir**, **nefazodone**, **nelfinavir**, **saquinavir**, and **voriconazole** ↓ metabolism and ↑ levels of budesonide, mometasone, and fluticasone; concurrent use with fluticasone not recommended.

Route/Dosage

Beclomethasone

Inhaln (Adults and Children ≥12 yr): *No prior treatment with inhaled corticosteroid*—40–80 mcg twice daily (max dose = 320 mcg twice daily); *Prior treatment with inhaled corticosteroid*—40–320 mcg twice daily (starting dose should be based on dose of previous inhaled corticosteroid and disease severity) (max dose = 320 mcg twice daily).
Inhaln (Children 4–11 yr): *No prior treatment with inhaled corticosteroid*—40 mcg twice daily (max = 80 mcg twice daily); *Prior treatment with inhaled corticosteroid*—40 mcg twice daily (max = 80 mcg twice daily).

Budesonide (Pulmicort Flexhaler)

Inhaln (Adults): 180–360 mcg twice daily (not to exceed 720 mcg twice daily).
Inhaln (Children ≥6 yr): 180–360 mcg twice daily (not to exceed 360 mcg twice daily).

Budesonide (Pulmicort Respules)

Inhaln (Children 1–8 yr): *Previously on bronchodilators alone*—0.5 mg once daily or 0.25 mg twice daily (not to exceed 0.5 mg/day); *Previously on other inhaled corticosteroids*—0.5 mg once daily or 0.25 mg twice daily (not to exceed 1 mg/day); *Previously on oral corticosteroids*—1 mg once daily or 0.5 mg twice daily (not to exceed 1 mg/day).

Fluticasone (Aerosol Inhaler)

Inhaln (Adults and Children ≥12 yr): *Previously on bronchodilators alone*—88 mcg twice daily initially, may be ↑ up to 440 mcg twice daily; *Previously on other inhaled corticosteroids*—88–220 mcg twice daily initially, may be ↑ up to 440 mcg twice daily; *Previously on oral corticosteroids*—440 mcg twice daily initially, may be ↑ up to 880 mcg twice daily.
Inhaln (Children 4–11 yr): 88 mcg twice daily (not to exceed 88 mcg twice daily).

Fluticasone (Dry Powder Inhaler)

Inhaln (Adults and Children ≥12 yr): *No prior treatment with inhaled corticosteroid*—Propionate (Flovent Diskus): 100 mcg twice daily initially, may ↑

dose in 2 wk if not adequately responding (max dose = 1,000 mcg twice daily); Propionate (Armonair Respiclick): 55 mcg twice daily initially, may ↑ dose in 2 wk if not adequately responding (max dose = 232 mcg twice daily); Furoate: 100 mcg once daily, may ↑ dose in 2 wk to 200 mcg once daily if not adequately responding (max dose = 200 mcg once daily); *Prior treatment with inhaled corticosteroid*—Propionate (Armonair Respiclick): 55–232 mcg twice daily (starting dose should be based on dose of previous inhaled corticosteroid and disease severity) (max dose = 232 mcg twice daily); Furoate: 100–200 mcg once daily (max dose = 200 mcg once daily).

Inhaln (Children 5–11 yr): Furoate: 50 mcg once daily.

Inhaln (Children 4–11 yr): *No prior treatment with inhaled corticosteroid*—Propionate (Flovent Diskus): 50 mcg twice daily initially, may ↑ dose in 2 wk to 100 mcg twice daily if not adequately responding (max dose = 100 mcg twice daily).

Mometasone (Aerosol Inhaler)

Inhaln (Adults and Children ≥12 yr): *Previously on medium-dose inhaled corticosteroids*—Two 100–mcg inhalations twice daily; *Previously on high-dose inhaled corticosteroids or oral corticosteroids*—Two 200–mcg inhalations twice daily (not to exceed 800 mcg/day).

Mometasone (Dry Powder Inhaler)

Inhaln (Adults and Children ≥12 yr): *Previously on bronchodilators or other inhaled corticosteroids*—220 mcg once daily in evening, up to 440 mcg/day as a single dose or 2 divided doses; *Previously on oral corticosteroids*—440 mcg twice daily (not to exceed 880 mcg/day).

Inhaln (Children 4–11 yr): 110 mcg once daily in evening (not to exceed 110 mcg/day).

Availability

Beclomethasone

Inhalation aerosol: 40 mcg/metered inhalation in 10.6-g canister (delivers 120 metered inhalations), 🍁 50 mcg/metered inhalation in 6.5-g canister (delivers 100 metered inhalations) and 12.4-g canister (delivers 200 metered inhalations), 80 mcg/metered inhalation in 10.6-g canister (delivers 120 metered inhalations), 🍁 100 mcg/metered inhalation in 6.5-g canister (delivers 100 metered inhalations) and 12.4-g canister (delivers 200 metered inhalations). **Cost:** 40 mcg/metered inhalation $130.16/inhaler, 80 mcg/metered inhalation $173.67/inhaler.

Budesonide (generic available)

Inhalation powder (Flexhaler): 90 mcg/metered inhalation (delivers 60 metered inhalations), 180 mcg/metered inhalation (delivers 120 metered inhalations). **Cost:** 90 mcg/metered inhalation $143.87/inhaler, 180 mcg/metered inhalation $192.65/inhaler. **Inhalation powder (Turbuhaler):** 🍁 100 mcg/metered inhalation (delivers 200 metered inhalations), 🍁 200 mcg/metered inhalation (delivers 200 metered inhalations), 🍁 400 mcg/metered inhalation (delivers 200 metered inhalations). **Inhalation suspension (Respules):** 0.25 mg/2 mL in single-dose ampules (5 ampules/envelope), 0.5 mg/2 mL in single-dose ampules (5 ampules/envelope), 1 mg/2 mL in single-dose ampules (5 ampules/envelope). ***In combination with:*** formoterol (Symbicort). See Appendix B.

Fluticasone

Inhalation aerosol (propionate) (Flovent-HFA): 44 mcg/metered inhalation in 10.6-g canisters (delivers 120 metered inhalations), 🍁 50 mcg/metered inhalation in 13-g canisters (delivers 120 metered inhalations), 110 mcg/metered inhalation in 12-g canisters (delivers 120 metered inhalations), 🍁 125 mcg/metered inhalation in 7.5-g canisters (delivers 60 metered inhalations) and 13-g canisters (delivers 120 metered inhalations, 220 mcg/metered inhalation in 12-g canisters (delivers 120 metered inhalations), 🍁 250 mcg/metered inhalation in 7.5-g canisters (delivers 60 metered inhalations) and 13-g canisters (delivers 120 metered inhalations. **Cost:** 44 mcg/inhalation $137.82/inhaler, 110 mcg/inhalation $181.43/inhaler, 220 mcg/inhalation $278.14/inhaler. **Powder for inhalation (propionate) (Flovent Diskus):** 50 mcg/blister, 100 mcg/blister, 250 mcg/blister, 🍁 500 mcg/blister. **Cost:** 50 mcg $144.47/60 blisters, 250 mcg $134.71/28 blisters. **Powder for inhalation (propionate) (Armonair Respiclick):** 55 mcg/metered inhalation (delivers 60 metered inhalations), 113 mcg/metered inhalation (delivers 60 metered inhalations), 232 mcg/metered inhalation (delivers 60 metered inhalations). **Powder for inhalation (furoate) (Arnuity Ellipta):** 50 mcg/blister, 100 mcg/blister, 200 mcg/blister. ***In combination with:*** salmeterol (Advair Diskus, Advair HFA, AirDuo RespiClick, Wixhela Inhub); vilanterol (Breo Ellipta); umeclidinium and vilanterol (Trelegy Ellipta). See Appendix B.

Mometasone

Inhalation aerosol (Asmanex HFA): 100 mcg/metered inhalation in 13-g canisters (120 metered inhalations), 200 mcg/metered inhalation in 13-g canisters (120 metered inhalations). **Powder for inhalation (Asmanex Twisthaler):** 🍁 100 mcg/metered inhalation (30 metered inhalations), 110 mcg (delivers 100 mcg/metered inhalation; in packages of 7 and 30 inhalation units), 🍁 200 mcg/metered inhalation (60 metered inhalations), 220 mcg (delivers 200 mcg/metered inhalation; in packages of 14, 30, 60, and 120 inhalation units), 🍁 400 mcg/metered inhalation (30 and 60 metered inhalations). **Cost:** 110 mcg $88.75/7 inhalation units, 110 mcg $157.90/30 inhalation units, 220 mcg $88.75/14 inhalation units, 220 mcg $170.47/30 inhalation units, 220 mcg $200.32/60 inhalation units, 220 mcg $287.09/120 inhalation units.

NURSING IMPLICATIONS

Assessment

- Monitor respiratory status and lung sounds. Assess pulmonary function tests periodically during and for several mo after a transfer from systemic to inhalation corticosteroids.
- Assess patients changing from systemic corticosteroids to inhalation corticosteroids for signs of adrenal insufficiency (anorexia, nausea, weakness, fatigue, hypotension, hypoglycemia) during initial therapy and periods of stress. If these signs appear, notify health care professional immediately; condition may be life-threatening.
- Monitor for withdrawal symptoms (joint or muscular pain, lassitude, depression) during withdrawal from oral corticosteroids.
- Monitor growth rate in children receiving chronic therapy; use lowest possible dose.
- May cause decreased bone mineral density during prolonged therapy. Monitor patients with increased risk (prolonged immobilization, family history of osteoporosis, postmenopausal status, tobacco use, advanced age, poor nutrition, chronic use of drugs that can reduce bone mass [anticonvulsants, oral corticosteroids]) for fractures.
- Monitor for signs and symptoms of hypersensitivity reactions (rash, pruritis, swelling of face and neck, dyspnea) periodically during therapy.
- ***Lab Test Considerations:*** Periodic adrenal function tests may be ordered to assess degree of hypothalamic-pituitary-adrenal (HPA) axis suppression in chronic therapy. Children and patients using higher than recommended doses are at highest risk for HPA suppression.
- May cause ↑ serum and urine glucose concentrations if significant absorption occurs.

Implementation

- Do not confuse Flovent with Flonase.
- After desired clinical effect has been obtained, attempts should be made to decrease dose to lowest amount required to control symptoms. Gradually decrease dose every 2–4 wk as long as desired effect is maintained. If symptoms return, dose may briefly return to starting dose.
- **Inhaln:** Allow at least 1 min between inhalations.

Patient/Family Teaching

- Advise patient to take medication as directed. Take missed doses as soon as remembered unless almost time for next dose. Instruct patient to read the *Patient Information and Instructions for Use* before using and with each Rx refill, in case of new information. Advise patient not to discontinue medication without consulting health care professional; gradual decrease is required.
- Advise patients using inhalation corticosteroids and bronchodilator to use bronchodilator first and to allow 5 min to elapse before administering the corticosteroid, unless otherwise directed by health care professional.
- Advise patient that inhalation corticosteroids should not be used to treat an acute asthma attack but should be continued even if other inhalation agents are used.
- Patients using inhalation corticosteroids to control asthma may require systemic corticosteroids for acute attacks. Advise patient to use regular peak flow monitoring to determine respiratory status.
- Caution patient to avoid smoking, known allergens, and other respiratory irritants.
- Advise patient to notify health care professional if sore throat or sore mouth occurs.
- Advise patient to stop using medication and notify health care professional immediately if signs and symptoms of hypersensitivity reactions occur.
- Advise female patients to notify health care professional if pregnancy is planned or suspected or if breast feeding.
- Instruct patient whose systemic corticosteroids have been recently reduced or withdrawn to carry a warning card indicating the need for supplemental systemic corticosteroids in the event of stress or severe asthma attack unresponsive to bronchodilators.
- Advise patient to have regular eye exams. May increase risk for eye problems (glaucoma, cataracts, blurred vision).
- **Metered-Dose Inhaler:** Instruct patient in proper use of metered-dose inhaler. Most inhalers require priming before first use. Shake inhaler well. Exhale completely, and then close lips firmly around mouthpiece. While breathing in deeply and slowly, press down on canister. Hold breath for as long as possible to ensure deep instillation of medication. Remove inhaler from mouth and breathe out gently. Allow 1–2 min between inhalations. Rinse mouth with water or mouthwash after each use to minimize fungal infections, dry mouth, and hoarseness. Clean mouthpiece weekly with clean, dry tissue or cloth. Do not place in water (see Appendix D).
- **Pulmicort Flexhaler:** Advise patient to follow instructions supplied. Before first-time use, prime unit by turning cover and lifting off; hold upright with mouthpiece up and twist brown grip fully to right, then fully to left until it clicks. To administer dose, hold upright, twist brown grip fully to right, then fully to left until it clicks. Turn head away from inhaler and exhale (do not blow into inhaler). Do not shake inhaler. Place mouthpiece between lips and inhale deeply and forcefully. Remove inhaler from mouth and exhale (do not exhale into mouthpiece). Repeat procedure if 2nd dose required. Replace cover; rinse mouth with water (do not swallow).

C

- **Pulmicort Respules:** Administer with a jet nebulizer connected to adequate air flow, equipped with a mouthpiece or face mask. Adjust face mask to avoid exposing eyes to nebulized medication. Wash face after use of face mask. Ultrasonic nebulizers are not adequate for administration and not recommended. Store respules upright, away from heat and protected from light. Do not refrigerate or freeze. Respules are stable for 2 wk at room temperature after opening aluminum foil envelope. Open respules must be used promptly. Unused respules should be returned to aluminum foil envelope.
- **Flovent Diskus/Arnuity Ellipta:** Do not use with a spacer. Exhale completely and then close lips firmly around mouthpiece. While breathing in deeply and slowly, press down on canister. Hold breath for as long as possible to ensure deep instillation of medication. Remove inhaler from mouth and breathe out gently. Allow 1–2 min between inhalations. After inhalation, rinse mouth with water and spit out (see Appendix D). Never wash the mouthpiece or any part of the Diskus inhaler. Discard Diskus inhaler device (Flovent Diskus) 6 wk (50-mcg strength) or 2 mo (100-mcg and 250-mcg strengths) or blister tray (Arnuity Ellipta) 6 wk after removal from protective foil overwrap pouch or after all blisters have been used (whichever comes first).
- **Asmanex Twisthaler:** Advise patient to remove cap while device is in upright position. To administer dose, exhale fully, then place mouthpiece between lips and inhale deeply and forcefully. Remove device from mouth and hold breath for 10 sec before exhaling (do not exhale into mouthpiece). Wipe the mouthpiece dry, if necessary, and replace the cap on the device. Rinse mouth with water. Advise patient to discard twisthaler 45 days from opening or when dose counter reads "00," whichever comes first.

Evaluation/Desired Outcomes

- Decreased frequency and severity of asthma attacks.
- Improvement in symptoms of asthma.

CORTICOSTEROIDS (NASAL)

beclomethasone
(be-kloe-**meth**-a-sone)
Beconase AQ, QNASL, ✱~~Rivanase AQ~~

budesonide (byoo-**dess**-oh-nide)
Rhinocort Allergy, Rhinocort Aqua, ✱Rhinocort Turbuhaler

ciclesonide (sye-**kles**-oh-nide)
Omnaris, Zetonna

flunisolide (floo-**niss**-oh-lide)
~~Nasalide~~

fluticasone (floo-**ti**-ka-sone)
✱Avamys, Flonase Allergy Relief, Flonase Sensimist, Xhance

mometasone (moe-**met**-a-sone)
✱Mosaspray, Nasonex

triamcinolone
(trye-am-**sin**-oh-lone)
Nasacort Allergy 24 HR, ✱Nasacort AQ

Classification
Therapeutic: anti-inflammatories (steroidal)
Pharmacologic: corticosteroids (nasal)

Indications

Seasonal or perennial allergic rhinitis. Nonallergic rhinitis (fluticasone). Treatment of nasal polyps.

Action

Potent, locally acting anti-inflammatory and immune modifier. **Therapeutic Effects:** ↓ in symptoms of allergic or nonallergic rhinitis. ↓ in symptoms of nasal polyps.

Pharmacokinetics

Absorption: *Beclomethasone*—27–44% absorbed; *budesonide*—34% absorbed; *flunisolide*—50% absorbed; *ciclesonide, fluticasone, mometasone*—negligible absorption. Action of all agents is primarily local following nasal use.
Distribution: All agents cross the placenta and enter breast milk in small amounts.
Metabolism and Excretion: Following absorption from nasal mucosa, corticosteroids are rapidly and extensively metabolized by the liver.
Half-life: *Beclomethasone*—2.7 hr; *budesonide*—2–3 hr; *ciclesonide*—unknown; *flunisolide*—1–2 hr; *fluticasone*—7.8 hr; *mometasone*—5.8 hr; *triamcinolone*—3–5.4 hr.

TIME/ACTION PROFILE (improvement in symptoms)

ROUTE	ONSET	PEAK	DURATION
Beclomethasone	1–3 days	up to 2 wk	unknown
Budesonide	1–2 days	2 wk	unknown
Ciclesonide	1–2 days	2–5 wk	unknown
Flunisolide	few days	up to 3 wk	unknown
Fluticasone	few days	unknown	unknown
Mometasone	within 2 days	1–2 wk	unknown
Triamcinolone	few days	3–4 days	unknown

Contraindications/Precautions

Contraindicated in: Some products contain alcohol, propylene, or polyethylene glycol and should be avoided in patients with known hypersensitivity or intolerance.

Use Cautiously in: Active untreated infections; Diabetes or glaucoma; Underlying immunosuppression (due to disease or concurrent therapy); Systemic corticosteroid therapy (should not be abruptly discontinued when intranasal therapy is started); History of ↑ intraocular pressure, glaucoma, or cataracts; Recent nasal trauma, septal ulcers, or surgery (wound healing may be impaired by nasal corticosteroids); OB, Lactation, Pedi: Pregnancy, lactation, or children <12 yr (beclomethasone [QNASL]), <6 yr (beclomethasone [Beconase AQ], budesonide, ciclesonide, flunisolide) <4 yr (fluticasone [Flonase Allergy Relief]) or <2 yr (fluticasone [Flonase Sensimist], mometasone, triamcinolone) (safety not established; prolonged or high-dose therapy may lead to complications).

Adverse Reactions/Side Effects

CNS: dizziness, headache. **Derm:** rash (fluticasone), urticaria (fluticasone). **EENT:** blurred vision, cataracts, epistaxis, glaucoma, ↑ intraocular pressure, nasal burning, nasal congestion, nasal irritation, nasal perforation, nasal ulceration, pharyngitis, rhinorrhea, sneezing, tearing eyes. **Endo:** adrenal suppression (high-dose, long-term therapy only), growth suppression (children). **GI:** dry mouth, esophageal candidiasis, nausea, vomiting. **Resp:** bronchospasm, cough. **Misc:** HYPERSENSITIVITY REACTIONS (including anaphylaxis and angioedema).

Interactions

Drug-Drug: Strong CYP3A4 inhibitors, including **atazanavir**, **clarithromycin**, **cobicistat**, **indinavir**, **itraconazole**, **ketoconazole**, **nefazodone**, **nelfinavir**, **ritonavir**, and **saquinavir** may ↑ levels of budesonide, ciclesonide, fluticasone, and mometason and ↑ the risk of adverse reactions.

Route/Dosage

Beclomethasone

Intranasal (Adults and Children ≥12 yr): *Beconase AQ*—1–2 sprays in each nostril twice daily (not to exceed 2 metered sprays in each nostril twice daily); *QNASL*—2 sprays in each nostril once daily.

Intranasal (Children 6–12 yr): 1–2 sprays in each nostril twice daily; once adequate control achieved, ↓ dose to 1 spray in each nostril twice daily.

Budesonide

Intranasal (Adults and Children ≥12 yr): 1 spray in each nostril once daily (not to exceed 4 sprays in each nostril once daily). For OTC use, administer 2 sprays in each nostril once daily; once symptoms improve, ↓ to 1 spray in each nostril once daily.

Intranasal (Children 6–11 yr): 1 spray in each nostril once daily (not to exceed 2 sprays in each nostril once daily).

Ciclesonide

Intranasal (Adults and Children ≥12 yr): *Omnaris (for perennial allergic rhinitis only)*—2 sprays in each nostril once daily (not to exceed 2 sprays in each nostril/day); *Zetonna*—1 spray in each nostril once daily (not to exceed 1 spray in each nostril/day).

Intranasal (Adults and Children ≥6 yr): *Omnaris (for seasonal allergic rhinitis only)*—2 sprays in each nostril once daily (not to exceed 2 sprays in each nostril/day).

Flunisolide

Intranasal (Adults and Children >14 yr): 2 sprays in each nostril twice daily, may be ↑ to 2 sprays in each nostril 3 times daily if greater effect needed after 4–7 days (not to exceed 8 sprays in each nostril/day).

Intranasal (Children 6–14 yr): 1 spray in each nostril 3 times daily or 2 sprays in each nostril twice daily (not to exceed 4 sprays in each nostril/day).

Fluticasone

Intranasal (Adults): *Fluticasone Rx*—2 sprays in each nostril once daily or 1 spray in each nostril twice daily (not to exceed 2 sprays in each nostril/day); after several days, attempt to ↓ dose to 1 spray in each nostril once daily.

Intranasal (Adults and Children ≥12 yr): *Flonase Sensimist (OTC) and Flonase Allergy Relief (OTC)*—2 sprays in each nostril once daily; after 1 wk, may adjust to 1–2 sprays in each nostril once daily; discuss with health care professional if need to continue longer than 6 mo.

Intranasal (Children 4–11 yr): *Flonase Allergy Relief (OTC)*—1 spray in each nostril once daily; discuss with health care professional if need to continue longer than 2 mo.

Intranasal (Children ≥4 yr): *Fluticasone Rx*—1 spray in each nostril once daily; may ↑ to 2 sprays in each nostril once daily if no response; once symptoms controlled, attempt to ↓ dose to 1 spray in each nostril once daily.

Intranasal (Children 2–11 yrs): *Flonase Sensimist (OTC)*—1 spray in each nostril once daily; discuss with health care professional if need to continue longer than 2 mo.

Mometasone

Intranasal (Adults and Children >12 yr): *Treatment of seasonal and perennial allergic rhinitis*—2 sprays in each nostril once daily (not to exceed 2 sprays in each nostril once daily).

Intranasal (Adults): *Nasal polyps*—2 sprays in each nostril twice daily (not to exceed 2 sprays in each nostril twice daily).

Intranasal (Children 2–11 yr): *Treatment of seasonal and perennial allergic rhinitis*—1 spray in each nostril once daily.

Triamcinolone

Intranasal (Adults and Children ≥12 yr): 2 sprays in each nostril once daily; not to be used in children for longer than 2 mo.
Intranasal (Children 6–11 yr): 1 spray in each nostril once daily (not to exceed 2 sprays in each nostril/day); not to be used for longer than 2 mo.
Intranasal (Children 2–5 yr): 1 spray in each nostril once dailyl not to be used for longer than 2 mo.

Availability

Beclomethasone

Nasal spray (Beconase AQ): 42 mcg/metered spray in 25-g bottles (delivers 180 metered sprays). **Cost:** $173.37/bottle. **Nasal spray (QNASL):** 40 mcg/metered spray in 4.9-g bottles (delivers 60 metered sprays), 80 mcg/metered spray in 8.7-g bottles (delivers 120 metered sprays). **Cost:** $139.94/bottle.

Budesonide (generic available)

Nasal spray (Rhinocort Allergy): 32 mcg/metered spray in 5-mL bottle (delivers 60 metered sprays)^OTC^, and 8.43-mL bottle (delivers 120 metered sprays)^OTC^. **Nasal spray (Rhinocort Aqua):** 32 mcg/metered spray in 8.6-g canister (delivers 120 metered sprays), 5-mL bottle (delivers 60 metered sprays)^OTC^, and 8.43-mL bottle (delivers 120 metered sprays)^OTC^, 🍁64 mcg/metered spray (delivers 120 metered sprays). **Cost:** $153.97/bottle. **Nasal spray (Rhinocort Turbuhaler):** 🍁100 mcg/metered spray (delivers 200 metered sprays).

Ciclesonide

Nasal spray (Omnaris): 50 mcg/metered spray in 12.5-g bottle (delivers 120 metered sprays). **Cost:** $152.07/bottle. **Nasal spray (Zetonna):** 37 mcg/actuation in 6.1-g bottle (delivers 60 metered sprays). **Cost:** $159.43/bottle.

Flunisolide (generic available)

Nasal solution: 25 mcg/metered spray in 25-mL bottle (delivers 200 metered sprays). **Cost:** *Generic*—$44.56/bottle.

Fluticasone (generic available)

Nasal spray : 50 mcg/metered spray in 16-g bottle (delivers 120 metered sprays). **Cost:** *Generic*—$19.52/bottle. **Nasal spray (Flonase Allergy Relief):** 50 mcg/metered spray in 9.9-mL bottle (delivers 60 metered sprays)^OTC^. **Nasal spray (Flonase Sensimist):** 27.5 mcg/spray in 9.9-mL bottle (delivers 60 metered sprays). **Nasal spray (Avamys):** 🍁27.5 mcg/spray in 4.5-g bottle (delivers 30 metered sprays) and 10-g bottle (delivers 120 metered sprays). **Nasal spray (Xhance):** 93 mcg/spray in 16-mL bottle (delivers 120 metered sprays). ***In combination with:*** azelastine (Dymista); see Appendix B.

Mometasone (generic available)

Nasal spray (scent-free): 50 mcg/metered spray in 17-g bottle (delivers 120 metered sprays). **Cost:** $162.27/bottle.

Triamcinolone (generic available)

Nasal spray: 55 mcg/metered spray in 6.7-mL bottle (delivers 30 metered sprays)^OTC^, 10.8-mL bottle (delivers 60 metered sprays) ^OTC^ and 16.9-mL bottle (delivers 120 metered sprays) ^OTC^. **Cost:** *Generic*—$86.05/bottle.

NURSING IMPLICATIONS

Assessment

- Monitor degree of nasal stuffiness, amount and color of nasal discharge, and frequency of sneezing.
- Monitor for signs of adverse effects on nasal mucosa (nasal discomfort, epistaxis, nasal ulceration, *Candida albicans* infection, nasal septal perforation, impaired wound healing) periodically during therapy. Avoid use in patients with recent nasal ulcers, nasal surgery, or nasal trauma.
- Patients on long-term therapy should have periodic otolaryngologic examinations to monitor nasal mucosa and passages for infection or ulceration.
- Monitor growth rate in children receiving chronic therapy; use lowest possible dose.
- ***Lab Test Considerations:*** Periodic adrenal function tests may be ordered to assess degree of hypothalamic-pituitary-adrenal (HPA) axis suppression in chronic therapy. Children and patients using higher than recommended doses are at highest risk for HPA suppression.

Implementation

- Do not confuse Flonase with Flovent.
- After desired clinical effect is obtained, decrease dose to lowest effective amount. Gradually decrease dose every 2–4 wk as long as desired effect is maintained. If symptoms return, dose may briefly return to starting dose.
- **Intranasal:** Patients also using a nasal decongestant should be given decongestant 5–15 min before corticosteroid nasal spray. If patient is unable to breathe freely through nasal passages, instruct patient to blow nose gently in advance of medication administration.

Patient/Family Teaching

- Advise patient to take medication as directed. Take missed doses as soon as remembered unless almost time for next dose.
- Caution patient not to exceed maximal daily dose of nasal spray.
- Instruct patient in correct technique for administering nasal spray (see Appendix D). Most nasal sprays include directions with pictures. Instruct patient to

read patient information sheet prior to use. Most nasal sprays require priming prior to first use or use after 7 days. Shake well before use. Warn patient that temporary nasal stinging may occur.

- Instruct patient to gently blow nose to clear nostrils prior to administering dose.
- Instruct patient to stop medication and notify health care professional immediately if signs of anaphylaxis (rash, hives, difficulty breathing, swollen lips or throat) or if changes in vision occur.
- Instruct patient to notify health care professional of all Rx or OTC medications, vitamins, or herbal products being taken and consult health care professional before taking other Rx, OTC, or herbal products.
- Advise female patients to notify health care professional if pregnancy is planned or suspected or if breast feeding.
- Instruct patient to notify health care professional if symptoms do not improve within 1 mo, if symptoms worsen, or if sneezing or nasal irritation occurs.

Evaluation/Desired Outcomes

- Resolution of nasal stuffiness, discharge, and sneezing in seasonal or perennial allergic rhinitis or nonallergic rhinitis.
- Reduction in symptoms of nasal polyps.

CORTICOSTEROIDS (SYSTEMIC)

short-acting corticosteroids

cortisone (**kor**-ti-sone)

hydrocortisone
(hye-droe-**kor**-ti-sone)
Cortef, Cortenema, Solu-CORTEF

intermediate-acting corticosteroids

methylPREDNISolone
(meth-ill-pred-**niss**-oh-lone)
Depo-Medrol, Medrol, Solu-MEDROL

prednisoLONE
(pred-**niss**-oh-lone)
~~Orapred~~, Orapred ODT, Pediapred, Prelone

predniSONE (**pred**-ni-sone)
Rayos, ✱Winipred

triamcinolone
(trye-am-**sin**-oh-lone)
Aristospan, Kenalog, Zilretta

long-acting corticosteroids

betamethasone
(bay-ta-**meth**-a-sone)
✱Betaject, Celestone Soluspan, ~~Celestone~~

budesonide (byoo-**dess**-oh-nide)
✱Cortiment, Entocort EC, Uceris

dexamethasone
(dex-a-**meth**-a-sone)
Decadron

Classification
Therapeutic: antiasthmatics, corticosteroids
Pharmacologic: corticosteroids (systemic)

Indications

Cortisone, hydrocortisone: Management of adrenocortical insufficiency. **Betamethasone, dexamethasone, hydrocortisone, prednisolone, prednisone, methylprednisolone, triamcinolone:** Used systemically and locally in a wide variety of chronic diseases including: Inflammatory, Allergic, Hematologic, Neoplastic, Autoimmune disorders. **Methylprednisolone, prednisone:** With other immunosuppressants in the prevention of organ rejection in transplantation surgery. Asthma. **Dexamethasone:** Management of cerebral edema: Diagnostic agent in adrenal disorders. **Budesonide (Entocort EC):** Treatment of mild to moderate Crohn's disease involving ileum and/or ascending colon. **Budesonide (Entocort EC):** Maintenance of clinical remission for up to 3 mo of mild to moderate Crohn's disease involving ileum and/or ascending colon. **Budesonide (Uceris):** Induction of remission of active, mild to moderate ulcerative colitis. **Unlabeled Use:** Short-term administration to high-risk mothers before delivery to prevent respiratory distress syndrome in the newborn (betamethasone, dexamethasone). Adjunctive therapy of hypercalcemia (prednisone, prednisolone, methylprednisolone). Management of acute spinal cord injury (methylprednisolone). Adjunctive management of nausea and vomiting from chemotherapy (dexamethasone, prednisone, prednisolone, methylprednisolone). Management of croup (dexamethasone). Treatment of airway edema prior to extubation (dexamethasone). Facilitation of ventilator weaning in neonates with bronchopulmonary dysplasia (dexamethasone).

Action

In pharmacologic doses, all agents suppress inflammation and the normal immune response. All agents have numerous intense metabolic effects (see Adverse Reactions/Side Effects). Suppress adrenal function at chronic doses of *betamethasone*—0.6 mg/day; *cortisone, hydrocortisone*—20 mg/day; *dexamethasone*—0.75 mg/day; *methylprednisolone, triamcinolone*—4 mg/day; *prednisone/prednisolone*—5 mg/

day. **Cortisone, hydrocortisone:** Replace endogenous cortisol in deficiency states. **Cortisone, hydrocortisone:** Have potent mineralocorticoid (sodium-retaining) activity. **Prednisolone, prednisone:** Have minimal mineralocorticoid activity. **Betamethasone, dexamethasone, methylprednisolone, triamcinolone:** Have negligible mineralocorticoid activity. **Budesonide:** Local anti-inflammatory activity in the lumen of the GI tract. **Therapeutic Effects:** Suppression of inflammation and modification of the normal immune response. Replacement therapy in adrenal insufficiency. **Budesonide:** Improvement in symptoms/sequelae of Crohn's disease and induction of remission of ulcerative colitis.

Pharmacokinetics

Absorption: Well absorbed after oral administration (except budesonide). Sodium phosphate and sodium succinate salts are rapidly absorbed after IM administration. Acetate and acetonide salts are slowly but completely absorbed after IM administration. Absorption from local sites (intra-articular, intralesional) is slow but complete. Bioavailability of budesonide is 9–21%.
Distribution: All are widely distributed, cross the placenta, and probably enter breast milk.
Metabolism and Excretion: All are metabolized mostly by the liver to inactive metabolites. *Cortisone* is converted by the liver to hydrocortisone. *Prednisone* is converted by the liver to prednisolone, which is then metabolized by the liver.
Half-life: *Betamethasone*—3–5 hr (plasma), 36–54 hr (tissue). *Budesonide*—2.0–3.6 hr. *Cortisone*—0.5 hr (plasma), 8–12 hr (tissue). *Dexamethasone*—3–4.5 hr (plasma), 36–54 hr (tissue). *Hydrocortisone*—1.5–2 hr (plasma), 8–12 hr (tissue). *Methylprednisolone*—>3.5 hr (plasma), 18–36 hr (tissue). *Prednisolone*—2.1–3.5 hr (plasma), 18–36 hr (tissue). *Prednisone*—3.4–3.8 hr (plasma), 18–36 hr (tissue). *Triamcinolone*—2–5 hr (plasma), 18–36 hr (tissue).

TIME/ACTION PROFILE (anti-inflammatory activity)

ROUTE	ONSET	PEAK	DURATION
Betamethasone IM (acetate/ sodium phosphate)	1–3 hr	unknown	1 wk
Budesonide PO	unknown	unknown	unknown
Cortisone PO	rapid	2 hr	1.25–1.5 days
Dexamethasone PO	unknown	1–3 hr	2.75 days
Dexamethasone IM, IV (sodium phosphate)	rapid	unknown	2.75 days
Hydrocortisone PO	unknown	1–2 hr	1.25–1.5 days
Hydrocortisone IM (sodium succinate)	rapid	1 hr	variable
Hydrocortisone IV (sodium succinate)	rapid	unknown	unknown
Methylprednisolone PO	unknown	1–2 hr	1.25–1.5 days
Methylprednisolone IM (acetate)	6–48 hr	4–8 days	1–4 wk
Methylprednisolone IM, IV (sodium succinate)	rapid	unknown	unknown
Prednisolone PO	unknown	1–2 hr	1.25–1.5 days
Prednisone PO	unknown	1–2 hr	1.25–1.5 days
Triamcinolone IM (acetonide)	24–48 hr	unknown	1–6 wk
Triamcinolone Intralesional (hexacetonide)	slow	unknown	4 days–4 wk

Contraindications/Precautions

Contraindicated in: Active untreated infections (may be used in patients being treated for some forms of meningitis); Lactation: Avoid chronic use; Known alcohol, bisulfite, cow's milk, or tartrazine hypersensitivity or intolerance (some products contain these and should be avoided in susceptible patients); Administration of live virus vaccines.
Use Cautiously in: Chronic treatment (will lead to adrenal suppression; use lowest possible dose for shortest period of time); Hypothyroidism; Immunosuppression; Cirrhosis; Stress (surgery, infections); supplemental doses may be needed; Potential infections may mask signs (fever, inflammation); Traumatic brain injury (high doses may be associated with ↑ mortality); OB: Safety not established; Pedi: Children (chronic use will result in ↓ growth; use lowest possible dose for shortest period of time); Pedi: Neonates (avoid use of benzyl alcohol containing injectable preparations; use preservative-free formulations).

Adverse Reactions/Side Effects

Adverse reactions/side effects are much more common with high-dose/long-term therapy.
CNS: depression, euphoria, headache, ↑ intracranial pressure (children only), personality changes, psychoses, restlessness. **CV:** hypertension. **Derm:** acne, ↓ wound healing, ecchymoses, fragility, hirsutism, petechiae. **EENT:** cataracts, ↑ intraocular pressure. **Endo:** PHEOCHROMOCYTOMA, adrenal suppression, hyperglycemia. **F and E:** fluid retention (long-term high

doses), hypokalemia, hypokalemic alkalosis. **GI:** PEPTIC ULCERATION, anorexia, nausea, vomiting. **Hemat:** THROMBOEMBOLISM, leukocytosis, thrombophlebitis. **Metab:** weight gain. **MS:** muscle wasting, osteoporosis, avascular necrosis of joints, muscle pain. **Misc:** cushingoid appearance (moon face, buffalo hump), ↑ susceptibility to infection.

Interactions

Drug-Drug: ↑ risk of hypokalemia with **thiazide** and **loop diuretics**, or **amphotericin B**. Hypokalemia may ↑ risk of **digoxin** toxicity. May increase requirement for **insulin** or **oral hypoglycemic agents**. **Phenytoin**, **phenobarbital**, and **rifampin** ↑ metabolism; may ↓ effectiveness. **Hormonal contraceptives** may ↓ metabolism. ↑ risk of adverse GI effects with **NSAIDs** (including aspirin). At chronic doses that suppress adrenal function, may ↓ antibody response to and ↑ risk of adverse reactions from **live-virus vaccines**. May ↑ serum concentrations of **cyclosporine** and **tacrolimus**. May ↑ risk of tendon rupture from **fluoroquinolones**. **Antacids** ↓ absorption of prednisone and dexamethasone. **CYP3A4 inhibitors**, including **clarithromycin**, **cobicistat**, **itraconazole**, **ketoconazole**, or **ritonavir** may ↑ levels and the risk of toxicity. May ↓ **isoniazid** levels and effectiveness. May antagonize the effects of **anticholinergic agents** in myasthenia gravis.
Drug-Food: **Grapefruit juice** ↑ serum levels and effects of budesonide (avoid concurrent use).

Route/Dosage

Betamethasone

IM (Adults): 0.5–9 mg as betamethasone sodium phosphate/acetate suspension. *Prevention of respiratory distress syndrome in newborn*—12 mg daily for 2–3 days before delivery (unlabeled).
IM (Children): *Adrenocortical insufficiency*—17.5 mcg/kg/day (500 mcg/m²/day) in 3 divided doses every 3rd day or 5.8–8.75 mcg/kg (166–250 mcg/m²)/day as a single dose.

Budesonide

PO (Adults): *Active Crohn's disease (Entocort EC)*—9 mg once daily in the morning for ≤8 wk; may repeat 8-wk course for recurring episodes. *Maintenance of remission of Crohn's disease (Entocort EC)*—6 mg once daily for up to 3 mo; once symptoms are controlled, taper to complete cessation; *Induction of remission of ulcerative colitis (Uceris)*—9 mg once daily for up to 8 wk; once symptoms are controlled, taper to complete cessation.
PO (Children 8–17 yr and >25 kg): *Active Crohn's disease (Entocort EC)*—9 mg once daily in the morning for up to 8 wk, then 6 mg once daily in the morning for 2 wk.

Hepatic Impairment

(Adults): *Moderate hepatic impairment (Child-Pugh Class B)*—3 mg once daily in the morning.

Cortisone

PO (Adults): 25–300 mg/day in divided doses every 12–24 hr.
PO (Children): *Adrenocortical insufficiency*—0.7 mg/kg/day (20–25 mg/m²/day) in divided doses every 8 hr. *Other uses*—2.5–10 mg/kg/day (75–300 mg/m²/day) in divided doses every 6–8 hr.

Dexamethasone

PO, IM, IV (Adults): *Anti-inflammatory*—0.75–9 mg daily in divided doses every 6–12 hr. *Airway edema or extubation*—0.5–2 mg/kg/day divided every 6 hr; begin 24 hr prior to extubation and continue for 24 hr post-extubation. *Cerebral edema*—10 mg IV, then 4 mg IM or IV every 6 hr until maximal response achieved, then switch to PO regimen and taper over 5–7 days.
PO, IM, IV (Children): *Airway edema or extubation*—0.5–2 mg/kg/day divided every 6 hr; begin 24 hr prior to extubation and continue for 24 hr post-extubation. *Anti-inflammatory*—0.08–0.3 mg/kg/day or 2.5–10 mg/m²/day divided every 6–12 hr. *Physiologic replacement*—0.03–0.15 mg/kg/day or 0.6–0.75 mg/m²/day divided every 6–12 hr.
PO (Adults): *Suppression test*—1 mg at 11 PM or 0.5 mg every 6 hr for 48 hr.
IV (Children): *Chemotherapy-induced emesis*—5–20 mg given 15–30 min before treatment; *Cerebral edema*—Loading dose 1–2 mg/kg followed by 1–1.5 mg/kg/day divided every 4–6 hr for 5 days (not to exceed 16 mg/day); then taper over 1–6 wk; *Bacterial meningitis*—0.6 mg/kg/day divided every 6 hr for 4 days (start at time of first antibiotic dose).
IV, PO (Adults): *Chemotherapy-induced emesis*—10–20 mg given 15–30 min before each treatment or 10 mg every 12 hr on each treatment day; *Delayed nausea/vomiting*—4–10 mg PO 1–2 times/day for 2–4 days *or* 8 mg PO every 12 hr for 2 days, then 4 mg PO every 12 hr for 2 days *or* 20 mg PO 1 hr before chemotherapy, then 10 mg PO every 12 hr after chemotherapy, then 8 mg PO every 12 hr for 2 days, then 4 mg PO every 12 hr for 2 days.
IS (Adults): 0.4–6 mg/day.

Hydrocortisone

PO (Adults): 20–240 mg/day in 1–4 divided doses.
PO (Children): *Adrenocortical insufficiency*—0.56 mg/kg/day (15–20 mg/m²/day) as a single dose or in divided doses. *Other uses*—2–8 mg/kg/day (60–240 mg/m²/day) as a single dose or in divided doses.
IM, IV (Adults): 100–500 mg every 2–6 hr (range 100–8000 mg/day).
IM, IV (Children): *Adrenocortical insufficiency*—0.186–0.28 mg/kg/day (10–12 mg/m²/day) in 3 divided doses. *Other uses*—0.666–4 mg/kg (20–120 mg/m²) every 12–24 hr.

Rect (Adults): *Retention enema*—100 mg nightly for 21 days or until remission occurs.

Methylprednisolone

PO (Adults): *Multiple sclerosis*—160 mg/day for 7 days, then 64 mg every other day for 1 mo. *Other uses*—2–60 mg/day as a single dose or in 2–4 divided doses. *Asthma exacerbations*—120–180 mg/day in divided doses 3–4 times/day for 48 hr, then 60–80 mg/day in 2 divided doses.
PO (Children): *Anti-inflammatory/Immunosuppressive*—0.5–1.7 mg/kg/day (5–25 mg/m²/day) in divided doses every 6–12 hr. *Asthma exacerbations*—1 mg/kg every 6 hr for 48 hr, then 1–2 mg/kg/day (maximum: 60 mg/day) divided twice daily.
IM, IV (Adults): *Most uses: methylprednisolone sodium succinate*—40–250 mg every 4–6 hr. *High-dose "pulse" therapy: methylprednisolone sodium succinate*—30 mg/kg IV every 4–6 hr for up to 72 hr. *Status asthmaticus: methylprednisolone sodium succinate*—2 mg/kg IV, then 0.5–1 mg/kg IV every 6 hr for up to 5 days. *Multiple sclerosis: methylprednisolone sodium succinate*—160 mg/day for 7 days, then 64 mg every other day for 1 mo. *Adjunctive therapy of P. jiroveci pneumonia in AIDS patients: methylprednisolone sodium succinate*—30 mg twice daily for 5 days, then 30 mg once daily for 5 days, then 15 mg once daily for 10 days. *Acute spinal cord injury: methylprednisolone sodium succinate*—30 mg/kg IV over 15 min initially, followed in 45 min with a continuous infusion of 5.4 mg/kg/hr for 23 hr (unlabeled).
IM, IV (Children): *Anti-inflammatory/Immunosuppressive*—0.5–1.7 mg/kg/day (5–25 mg/m²/day) in divided doses every 6–12 hr. *Acute spinal cord injury: methylprednisolone sodium succinate*—30 mg/kg IV over 15 min initially, followed in 45 min with a continuous infusion of 5.4 mg/kg/hr for 23 hr (unlabeled). *Status asthmaticus*—2 mg/kg IV, then 0.5–1 mg/kg IV every 6 hr. *Lupus nephritis*—30 mg/kg IV every other day for 6 doses.
IM (Adults): *Methylprednisolone acetate*—40–120 mg daily, weekly, or every 2 wk.

Prednisolone

PO (Adults): *Most uses*—5–60 mg/day as a single dose or in divided doses. *Multiple sclerosis*—200 mg/day for 7 days, then 80 mg every other day for 1 mo. *Asthma exacerbations*—120–180 mg/day in divided doses 3–4 times/day for 48 hr, then 60–80 mg/day in 2 divided doses.
PO (Children): *Anti-inflammatory/Immunosuppressive*—0.1–2 mg/kg/day in 1–4 divided doses; *Nephrotic syndrome*—2 mg/kg/day (60 mg/m²/day) in 1–3 divided doses daily (maximum dose: 80 mg/day) until urine is protein-free for 4–6 wk, followed by 2 mg/kg/dose (40 mg/m²/dose) every other day in the morning; gradually taper off over 4–6 wk; *Asthma exacerbations*—1 mg/kg every 6 hr for 48 hr, then 1–2 mg/kg/day (maximum: 60 mg/day) divided twice daily.

Prednisone

PO (Adults): *Most uses*—5–60 mg/day as a single dose or in divided doses. *Multiple sclerosis*—200 mg/day for 1 wk, then 80 mg every other day for 1 mo. *Adjunctive therapy of P. jiroveci pneumonia in AIDS patients*—40 mg twice daily for 5 days, then 40 mg once daily for 5 days, then 20 mg once daily for 10 days.
PO (Children): *Nephrotic syndrome*—2 mg/kg/day initially given in 1–3 divided doses (maximum 80 mg/day) until urine is protein-free for 4–6 wk. Maintenance dose of 2 mg/kg/day every other day in the morning, gradually taper off after 4–6 wk. *Asthma exacerbation*—1 mg/kg every 6 hr for 48 hr, then 1–2 mg/kg/day (maximum 60 mg/day) in divided doses twice daily.

Triamcinolone

IM (Adults): *Triamcinolone acetonide*—40–80 mg every 4 wk.
Intra-articular (Adults): *Triamcinolone hexacetonide*—2–20 mg every 3–4 wk (dose depends on size of joint to be injected, amount of inflammation, and amount of fluid present); *Triamcinolone acetonide*—32 mg as a single dose into the knee joint.
IM (Children): *Triamcinolone acetonide*—40 mg every 4 wk or 30–200 mcg/kg (1–6.25 mg/m²) every 1–7 days.

Availability

Betamethasone (generic available)

Suspension for injection (sodium phosphate and acetate): 6 mg (total)/mL.

Budesonide (generic available)

Extended-release capsules (Entocort EC): 3 mg. **Cost:** *Generic*—$397.88/30. **Extended-release tablets (Uceris):** 9 mg. **Cost:** $1,482.00/30.

Cortisone (generic available)

Tablets: 25 mg. **Cost:** *Generic*—$108.00/100.

Dexamethasone (generic available)

Elixir (raspberry flavor): 0.5 mg/5 mL. **Cost:** *Generic*—$63.68/237 mL. **Oral solution (cherry flavor):** 0.5 mg/5 mL, 1 mg/mL. **Cost:** *Generic*—0.5 mg/5 mL $63.69/240 mL, 1 mg/mL $23.74/30 mL. **Solution for injection (sodium phosphate):** 4 mg/mL, 10 mg/mL. **Tablets:** 0.5 mg, 0.75 mg, 1 mg, 1.5 mg, 2 mg, 4 mg, 6 mg. **Cost:** *Generic*—0.5 mg $20.76/100, 0.75 mg $36.39/100, 1 mg $35.00/100, 1.5 mg $27.14/100, 2 mg $68.54/100, 4 mg $64.25/100, 6 mg $107.07/100.

Hydrocortisone (generic available)

Enema: 100 mg/60 mL. **Cost:** *Generic*—$48.80/480 mL. **Powder for injection (sodium succinate):** 100 mg/vial, 250 mg/vial, 500 mg/vial, 1 g. **Tablets:** 5 mg, 10 mg, 20 mg. **Cost:** *Generic*—5 mg $16.95/50, 10 mg $57.30/100, 20 mg $78.81/100.

Methylprednisolone (generic available)

Powder for injection (sodium succinate): 40 mg/vial, 125 mg/vial, 500 mg/vial, 1 g/vial, 2 g/vial. **Suspension for injection (acetate):** 20 mg/mL, 40 mg/mL, 80 mg/mL. **Tablets:** 2 mg, 4 mg, 8 mg, 16 mg, 32 mg. **Cost:** *Generic*—4 mg $142.93/100, 8 mg $50.26/25, 16 mg $155.29/50, 32 mg $115.62/25.

Prednisolone (generic available)

Oral solution: 5 mg/5 mL, 10 mg/5 mL, 15 mg/5 mL, 20 mg/5 mL, 25 mg/5 mL. **Cost:** *Generic*—5 mg/5 mL $98.09/120 mL, 15 mg/5 mL $25.80/237 mL, 25 mg/5 mL $186.00/237 mL. **Orally disintegrating tablets (grape flavor):** 10 mg, 15 mg, 30 mg. **Cost:** 10 mg $394.84/48, 15 mg $593.71/48, 30 mg $846.02/48.

Prednisone (generic available)

Delayed-release tablets: 1 mg, 2 mg, 5 mg. **Oral solution:** 5 mg/5 mL, 5 mg/mL. **Cost:** *Generic*—1 mg/mL $24.45/120 mL, 5 mg/mL $42.32/30 mL. **Tablets:** 1 mg, 2.5 mg, 5 mg, 10 mg, 20 mg, 50 mg. **Cost:** *Generic*—1 mg $11.04/30, 2.5 mg $7.41/30, 5 mg $8.32/30, 10 mg $10.84/30, 50 mg $13.77/30.

Triamcinolone (generic available)

Extended-release suspension for intra-articular injection (acetonide) (requires reconstitution) (Zilretta): 32 mg/vial. **Suspension for intra-articular injection (hexacetonide):** 5 mg/mL, 20 mg/mL. **Suspension for intramuscular injection (acetonide):** 10 mg/mL, 40 mg/mL, 80 mg/mL.

NURSING IMPLICATIONS

Assessment

- These drugs are indicated for many conditions. Assess involved systems before and periodically during therapy.
- Assess for signs of adrenal insufficiency (hypotension, weight loss, weakness, nausea, vomiting, anorexia, lethargy, confusion, restlessness) before and periodically during therapy.
- Monitor intake and output ratios and daily weights. Observe patient for peripheral edema, steady weight gain, rales/crackles, or dyspnea. Notify health care professional if these occur.
- Children should have periodic evaluations of growth; may slow growth.
- **Cerebral Edema:** Assess for changes in level of consciousness and headache during therapy.
- **Budesonide:** Assess signs of Crohn's disease and ulcerative colitis (diarrhea, crampy abdominal pain, fever, bleeding from rectum) during therapy. Monitor frequency and consistency of bowel movements periodically during therapy.
- **Rect:** Assess symptoms of ulcerative colitis (diarrhea, bleeding, weight loss, anorexia, fever, leukocytosis) periodically during therapy.
- ***Lab Test Considerations:*** Monitor serum electrolytes and glucose. May cause hyperglycemia, especially in persons with diabetes. May cause hypokalemia. Patients on prolonged therapy should routinely have CBC, serum electrolytes, and serum and urine glucose evaluated. May ↓ WBCs. May ↓ serum potassium and calcium and ↑ serum sodium concentrations.
- Guaiac-test stools. Promptly report presence of guaiac-positive stools.
- May ↑ serum cholesterol and lipid values. May ↓ uptake of thyroid ^{123}I or ^{131}I.
- Suppress reactions to allergy skin tests.
- Periodic adrenal function tests may be ordered to assess degree of hypothalamic-pituitary-adrenal axis suppression in systemic and chronic topical therapy.
- **Dexamethasone Suppression Test: :** To diagnose Cushing's syndrome: Obtain baseline cortisol level; administer dexamethasone at 11 PM and obtain cortisol levels at 8 AM the next day. Normal response is a ↓ cortisol level.
- Alternative method: Obtain baseline 24-hr urine for 17-hydroxycorticosteroid (OHCS) concentrations, then begin 48-hr administration of dexamethasone. Second 24-hr urine for 17-OHCS is obtained after 24 hr of dexamethasone.

Implementation

- Do not confuse prednisone with prednisolone. Do not confuse Solu-Cortef with Solu-Medrol.
- If dose is ordered daily or every other day, administer in the morning to coincide with the body's normal secretion of cortisol.
- Periods of stress, such as surgery, may require supplemental systemic corticosteroids.
- Patients with mild to moderate Crohn's disease may be switched from oral prednisolone without adrenal insufficiency by gradually decreasing prednisolone doses and adding budesonide.
- **PO:** Administer with meals to minimize GI irritation.
- Tablets may be crushed and administered with food or fluids for patients with difficulty swallowing. Capsules and extended-release tablets should be swallowed whole; do not open, crush, break, or chew. *Entocort EC* (budesonide) capsules can be opened and contents sprinkled on to 1 tbsp of applesauce for patients unable to swallow capsule. Applesauce must not be hot and must be soft enough to swallow without chewing. Mix granules with applesauce and consume entire contents within 30 min of mixing. Do not chew or crush the granules. Do not save the applesauce and granules for future use. Follow with a glass (8 oz) of cool water to ensure complete swallowing of granules.
- Use calibrated measuring device to ensure accurate dose of liquid forms.

C

- For orally disintegrating tablets (ODT), remove tablet from blister just prior to dosing. Peel blister pack open, and place tablet on tongue; may be swallowed whole or allowed to dissolve in mouth, with or without water. Tablets are friable; do not cut, split, or break.
- Avoid consumption of grapefruit juice during therapy with budesonide or methylprednisolone.
- **IM Subcut:** Shake suspension well before drawing up. IM doses should not be administered when rapid effect is desirable. Do not dilute with other solution or admix. Do not administer suspensions IV.

Dexamethasone

IV Administration

- **IV Push:** ***Diluent:*** May be given undiluted. ***Concentration:*** 4–10 mg/mL. ***Rate:*** Administer over 1–4 min if dose is <10 mg.
- **Intermittent Infusion:** ***Diluent:*** High-dose therapy should be added to D5W or 0.9% NaCl solution. Solution should be clear and colorless to light yellow; use diluted solution within 24 hr. ***Concentration:*** Up to 10 mg/mL. ***Rate:*** Administer infusions over 15–30 min.
- **Y-Site Compatibility:** acetaminophen, acyclovir, alfentanil, allopurinol, amifostine, amikacin, aminocaproic acid, aminophylline, amphotericin B lipid complex, amphotericin B liposome, amsacrine, anidulafungin, argatroban, arsenic trioxide, ascorbic acid, atracurium, atropine, azithromycin, aztreonam, benztropine, bivalirudin, bleomycin, bumetanide, buprenorphine, butorphanol, cangrelor, carboplatin, carmustine, cefazolin, cefepime, cefotaxime, cefotetan, cefoxitin, ceftaroline, ceftazidime, ceftolozane/tazobactam, ceftriaxone, chloramphenicol, cisatracurium, cisplatin, cladribine, clindamycin, cyanocobalamin, cyclophosphamide, cyclosporine, cytarabine, dacarbazine, dactinomycin, daptomycin, dexmedetomidine, digoxin, diltiazem, dimenhydrinate, docetaxel, dopamine, doxorubicin, doxorubicin liposomal, enalaprilat, ephedrine, epinephrine, epoetin alfa, eptifibatide, ertapenem, etoposide, etoposide phosphate, famotidine, fentanyl, filgrastim, fluconazole, fludarabine, fluorouracil, folic acid, fosaprepitant, foscarnet, fosphenytoin, furosemide, ganciclovir, gemcitabine, glycopyrrolate, granisetron, heparin, hetastarch, hydrocortisone, hydromorphone, ifosfamide, imipenem/cilastatin, indomethacin, insulin, regular, irinotecan, isavuconazonium, isoproterenol, ketorolac, leucovorin calcium, levofloxacin, lidocaine, linezolid, lorazepam, mannitol, melphalan, meropenem, meropenem/vaborbactam, mesna, methohexital, methyldopate, methylprednisolone, metoclopramide, metoprolol, metronidazole, miconazole, milrinone, mitomycin, morphine, moxifloxacin, multivitamin, nafcillin, nalbuphine, naloxone, nitroglycerin, nitroprusside, norepinephrine, octreotide, ondansetron, oxaliplatin, oxytocin, paclitaxel, palonosetron, pamidronate, pancuronium, pemetrexed, penicillin G, pentobarbital, phenobarbital, phenylephrine, phytonadione, piperacillin/tazobactam, plazomicin, potassium acetate, potassium chloride, procainamide, prochlorperazine, propofol, propranolol, pyridoxine, ranitidine, remifentanil, rituximab, sargramostim, sodium acetate, sodium bicarbonate, streptokinase, succinylcholine, sufentanil, tacrolimus, tedizolid, telavancin, theophylline, thiamine, thiotepa, tigecycline, tirofiban, trastuzumab, vancomycin, vasopressin, vecuronium, verapamil, vinblastine, vincristine, vinorelbine, vitamin B complex with C, voriconazole, zidovudine, zoledronic acid.
- **Y-Site Incompatibility:** alemtuzumab, amiodarone, blinatumomab, caspofungin, cefuroxime, ciprofloxacin, dacarbazine, dantrolene, daunorubicin, diazepam, diphenhydramine, dobutamine, doxycycline, epirubicin, esmolol, fenoldopam, gemtuzumab, haloperidol, hydroxyzine, idarubicin, labetalol, magnesium sulfate, midazolam, minocycline, mitoxantrone, mycophenolate, nicardipine, pantoprazole, papaverine, pentamidine, phenytoin, prochlorperazine, protamine, quinupristin/dalfopristin, tobramycin, topotecan, trimethoprim/sulfamethoxazole.

Hydrocortisone

IV Administration

- **IV Push:** ***Diluent:*** Reconstitute with provided solution (i.e., Act-O-Vials) or 2 mL of bacteriostatic water or saline for injection. ***Concentration:*** 50 mg/mL. ***Rate:*** Administer each 100 mg over at least 30 sec. Doses 500 mg and larger should be infused over at least 10 min.
- **Intermittent/Continuous Infusion:** ***Diluent:*** May be added to 50–1000 mL of D5W, 0.9% NaCl, or D5/0.9% NaCl. Diluted solutions should be used within 24 hr. ***Concentration:*** 1–5 mg/mL. Concentrations of up to 60 mg/mL have been used in fluid restricted adults. ***Rate:*** Administer over 20–30 min or at prescribed rate.
- **Hydrocortisone sodium succinate: Y-Site Compatibility:** acetaminophen, acyclovir, alemtuzumab, alfentanil, allopurinol, amifostine, amikacin, aminophylline, amphotericin B lipid complex, amphotericin B liposome, amsacrine, anidulafungin, argatroban, ascorbic acid, atracurium, atropine, azithromycin, aztreonam, benztropine, bivalirudin, bleomycin, bumetanide, buprenorphine, butorphanol, cangrelor, carboplatin, carmustine, caspofungin, cefazolin, cefepime, cefotaxime, cefotetan, cefoxitin, ceftaroline, ceftazidime, ceftriaxone, cefuroxime, chloramphenicol, chlorpromazine, cisatra-

curium, cisplatin, cladribine, clindamycin, cyanocobalamin, cyclophosphamide, cyclosporine, cytarabine, dactinomycin, daptomycin, dexamethasone, dexmedetomidine, dexrazoxane, digoxin, docetaxel, dopamine, doxacurium, doxorubicin hydrochloride, doxorubicin liposome, droperidol, enalaprilat, ephedrine, epinephrine, epirubicin, epoetin alfa, eptifibatide, ertapenem, erythromycin, estrogens, conjugated, etoposide, famotidine, fenoldopam, fentanyl, filgrastim, fluconazole, fludarabine, fluorouracil, folic acid, foscarnet, fosphenytoin, furosemide, gemcitabine, glycopyrrolate, granisetron, heparin, hetastarch, hydromorphone, ifosfamide, imipemem/cilastatin, indomethacin, insulin, irinotecan, isoproterenol, ketamine, ketorolac, leucovorin calcium, levofloxacin, lidocaine, linezolid, lorazepam, mannitol, melphalan, metaraminol, methotrexate, methoxamine, methyldopate, methylergonovine, metoclopramide, metoprolol, metronidazole, milrinone, mitoxantrone, morphine, moxifloxacin, multivitamins, nafcillin, naloxone, neostigmine, nitroglycerin, nitroprusside, norepinephrine, octreotide, ondansetron, oxacillin, oxaliplatin, oxytocin, paclitaxel, palonosetron, pamidronate, pancuronium, pantoprazole, pemetrexed, penicillin G, pentobarbital, phenobarbital, phentolamine, phenylephrine, phytonadione, piperacillin/tazobactam, potassium acetate, potassium chloride, procainamide, prochlorperazine, propofol, propranolol, pyridostigmine, ranitidine, remifentanil, rituximab, scopolamine, sodium acetate, sodium bicarbonate, streptokinase, succinylcholine, sufentanil, tacrolimus, telavancin, theophylline, thiotepa, tigecycline, tirofiban, topotecan, trastuzumab, vasopressin, vecuronium, verapamil, vinblastine, vincristine, vinorelbine, voriconazole, zoledronic acid.

- **Y-Site Incompatibility:** amiodarone, amphotericin B colloidal, ampicillin/sulbactam, azathioprine, ciprofloxacin, dantrolene, diazepam, diazoxide, dobutamine, dolasetron, doxycycline, ganciclovir, haloperidol, idarubicin, labetalol, midazolam, mycophenolate, nalbuphine, pentamidine, phenytoin, protamine, pyridoxime, quinupristin/dalfopristin, rocuronium, sargramostim, thiamine, trimethoprim/sulfamethoxazole.

Methylprednisolone sodium succinate

IV Administration

- **IV Push:** ***Diluent:*** Reconstitute with provided solution (Act-O-Vials, Univials) or 2 mL of bacteriostatic water (with benzyl alcohol) for injection. Use preservative-free diluent for use in neonates. Acetate injection is not for IV use. ***Concentration:*** Maximum concentration 125 mg/mL. ***Rate:*** Low dose (<1.8 mg/kg or <125 mg/dose): May be administered IV push over 1 to several min. Moderate dose (2 mg/kg or 250 mg/dose): give over 15–30 min. High dose (15 mg/kg or 500 mg/dose): give over 30 min. Doses 15 mg/kg or 1 g give over 1 hr.
- **Intermittent/Continuous Infusion:** ***Diluent:*** May be diluted further in D5W, 0.9% NaCl, or D5/0.9% NaCl and administered as intermittent or continuous infusion at the prescribed rate. ***Concentration:*** Maximum 2.5 mg/mL. Solution may form a haze upon dilution.
- **Y-Site Compatibility:** acetaminophen, acyclovir, alfentanil, alprostadil, amifostine, amikacin, aminophylline, amphotericin B lipid complex, amphotericin B liposome, anidulafungin, argatroban, ascorbic acid, atracurium, atropine, azithromycin, aztreonam, benztropine, bivalirudin, bleomycin, bumetanide, buprenorphine, butorphanol, cangrelor, carboplatin, carmustine, cefazolin, cefepime, cefotetan, ceftaroline, ceftazidime, ceftriaxone, cefuroxime, chloramphenicol, chlorpromazine, cisplatin, cladribine, clindamycin, cyanocobalamin, cyclophosphamide, cyclosporine, cytarabine, dactinomycin, daptomycin, dexamethasone, dexmedetomidine, digoxin, dobutamine, dopamine, doxacurium, doxorubicin liposome, enalaprilat, ephedrine, epinephrine, epoetin alfa, eptifibatide, ertapenem, erythromycin, etoposide, fentanyl, fluconazole, fludarabine, fluorouracil, folic acid, fosaprepitant, furosemide, gentamicin, glycopyrrolate, granisetron, hetastarch, hydromorphone, ifosfamide, imipenem/cilastatin, insulin, isoproterenol, ketorolac, labetalol, levofloxacin, linezolid, lorazepam, mannitol, melphalan, metaraminol, methotrexate, methoxamine, methyldopate, metoclopramide, metoprolol, metronidazole, milrinone, morphine, moxifloxacin, multivitamin, nafcillin, naloxone, nitroglycerin, nitroprusside, norepinephrine, octreotide, oxaliplatin, oxytocin, pamidronate, pancuronium, pemetrexed, penicillin G, pentobarbital, phenobarbital, phenylephrine, piperacillin/tazobactam, potassium acetate, procainamide, prochlorperazine, propranolol, ranitidine, remifentanil, rituximab, sodium acetate, sodium bicarbonate, streptokinase, succinylcholine, sufentanil, tacrolimus, theophylline, thiotepa, tirofiban, tobramycin, tolazoline, topotecan, trastuzumab, vasopressin, verapamil, vincristine, voriconazole, zoledronic acid.
- **Y-Site Incompatibility:** alemtuzumab, allopurinol, amphotericin B colloidal, ampicillin/sulbactam, amsacrine, calcium chloride, calcium gluconate, caspofungin, cefotaxime, cefoxitin, ciprofloxacin, dacarbazine, dantrolene, daunorubicin, dexrazoxane, diazepam, diazoxide, diphenhydramine, docetaxel, dolasetron, doxycycline, epirubicin, etoposide phosphate, fenoldopam, filgrastim, foscarnet, ganciclovir, gemcitabine, haloperidol, hydralazine, idarubicin, irinotecan, magnesium sulfate, mitoxantrone, mycophenolate, nalbuphine, paclitaxel, palonosetron, pantoprazole, papaverine, pentamidine, phenytoin, promethazine, propofol, protamine, pyridoxime, quinupristin/dalfopristin, rocuronium, sargramos-

tim, thiamine, trimethoprim/sulfamethoxazole, vancomycin, vecuronium, vinorelbine.

Patient/Family Teaching

- Instruct patient on correct technique of medication administration. Advise patient to take medication as directed. Take missed doses as soon as remembered unless almost time for next dose. Do not double doses. Stopping the medication suddenly may result in adrenal insufficiency (anorexia, nausea, weakness, fatigue, dyspnea, hypotension, hypoglycemia). If these signs appear, notify health care professional immediately. This can be life threatening. Advise patient to read *Patient Information* before starting and with each Rx refill in case of changes.
- Advise patient to avoid consumption of grapefruit juice during therapy with *budesonide* or *methylprednisolone*; may increase blood levels.
- Corticosteroids cause immunosuppression and may mask symptoms of infection. Instruct patient to avoid people with known contagious illnesses and to report possible infections immediately.
- *Prelone* syrup should not be refrigerated, *Pediapred* solution may be refrigerated, *Orapred* solution should be refrigerated.
- Caution patient to avoid vaccinations without first consulting health care professional.
- Review side effects with patient. Instruct patient to inform health care professional promptly if severe abdominal pain or tarry stools occur. Patient should also report unusual swelling, weight gain, tiredness, bone pain, bruising, nonhealing sores, visual disturbances, or behavior changes.Advise patient to notify health care professional if signs and symptoms of hypercorticism (acne, thicker or more hair on body and face; bruise easily; fatty pad or hump between shoulders (buffalo hump); rounding of face (moon face); pink or purple stretch marks on skin of abdomen, thighs, breasts and arms; ankle swelling), adrenal suppression (tiredness, weakness, nausea and vomiting, low blood pressure), worsening of allergies (eczema, rhinitis), and infection (fever, chills, pain, feeling tired, aches, nausea and vomiting). May worsen existing tuberculosis, fungal, bacterial, viral, or parasitic infections, or ocular herpes simplex.
- Instruct patient to notify health care professional of all Rx or OTC medications, vitamins, or herbal products being taken and to consult health care professional before taking any Rx, OTC, or herbal products.
- Instruct patient to notify health care professional immediately if exposed to chicken pox or measles.
- Advise patient to notify health care professional of medication regimen before treatment or surgery.
- Discuss possible effects on body image. Explore coping mechanisms.
- Instruct patient to inform health care professional if symptoms of underlying disease return or worsen.
- Advise patient to carry identification describing disease process and medication regimen in the event of emergency in which patient cannot relate medical history.
- Explain need for continued medical follow-up to assess effectiveness and possible side effects of medication. Periodic lab tests and eye exams may be needed.
- **Long-term Therapy:** Encourage patient to eat a diet high in protein, calcium, and potassium, and low in sodium and carbohydrates (see Appendix K). Alcohol should be avoided during therapy; may ↑ risk of GI irritation.
- If rectal dose used 21 days, decrease to every other night for 2–3 wk to decrease gradually.

Evaluation/Desired Outcomes

- Decrease in presenting symptoms with minimal systemic side effects.
- Suppression of the inflammatory and immune responses in autoimmune disorders, allergic reactions, and neoplasms.
- Management of symptoms in adrenal insufficiency.
- Improvement of symptoms/sequelae of Crohn's disease and ulcerative colitis (decreased frequency of liquid stools, decreased abdominal complaints, improved sense of well being).
- Improvement in symptoms of ulcerative colitis. Clinical symptoms usually improve in 3–5 days. Mucosal appearance may require 2–3 mo to improve.
- Induction of remission of ulcerative colitis.

CORTICOSTEROIDS (TOPICAL/ LOCAL)

alclometasone
(al-kloe-**met**-a-sone)
~~Aclovate~~

amcinonide (am-**sin**-oh-nide)

betamethasone
(bay-ta-**meth**-a-sone)
✱Betaderm, Beta-Val, ✱Beteflam, ✱Celestoderm V, ✱Celestoderm V/2, Dermabet, Diprolene, Diprolene AF, ✱Diprosone, Luxiq, ✱Rivasone, ✱Rolene, ✱Rosone, Sernivo, ✱Valisone, Valnac

clobetasol (kloe-**bay**-ta-sol)
Clobex, ✱Dermovate, Impoyz, Olux, Olux-E, ~~Temovate~~, ~~Temovate E~~

clocortolone (kloe-**kore**-toe-lone)
Cloderm

desonide (**des**-oh-nide)
Desonate, DesOwen, ✱ Tridesilon, Verdeso

desoximetasone
(dess-ox-i-**met**-a-sone)
✱ Desoxi, Topicort

diflorasone (dye-**flor**-a-sone)

fluocinolone (floo-oh-**sin**-oh-lone)
Capex, Derma-Smoothe/FS,
✱ Fluoderm, Synalar

fluocinonide (floo-oh-**sin**-oh-nide)
✱ Lidemol, ✱ Lidex, ✱ Lyderm,
✱ Tiamol, ✱ Topactin, Vanos

flurandrenolide
(flure-an-**dren**-oh-lide)
Cordran, Cordran SP

fluticasone (floo-**ti**-ka-sone)
Cutivate

halcinonide (hal-**sin**-oh-nide)
Halog

halobetasol (hal-oh-**bay**-ta-sol)
Bryhali, Ultravate

hydrocortisone
(hye-droe-**kor**-ti-sone)
Ala-Cort, Ala-Scalp, Anusol HC,
✱ Barriere-HC, Cortaid, Cortifoam,
✱ Cortoderm, ✱ Emo-Cort, ✱ Hyderm,
✱ Hydroval, Locoid, Pandel,
✱ Prevex HC, ✱ Sarna HC, Texacort

mometasone (moe-**met**-a-sone)
✱ Elocom, ~~Elocon~~

prednicarbate (pred-ni-**kar**-bate)
Dermatop

triamcinolone
(trye-am-**sin**-oh-lone)
✱ Aristocort C, ✱ Aristocort R, Kenalog, ✱ Triaderm, Triderm

Classification
Therapeutic: anti-inflammatories (steroidal)
Pharmacologic: corticosteroids (topical)

Indications
Moderate to severe plaque psoriasis. Inflammation and pruritus associated with corticosteroid-responsive dermatoses.

Action
Suppress normal immune response and inflammation. **Therapeutic Effects:** Suppression of dermatologic inflammation and immune processes. Clearing of plaques.

Pharmacokinetics
Absorption: Minimal. Prolonged use on large surface areas, application of large amounts, or use of occlusive dressings may ↑ systemic absorption.
Distribution: Remain primarily at site of action.
Metabolism and Excretion: Usually metabolized in skin; some have been modified to resist local metabolism and have a prolonged local effect.
Half-life: *Betamethasone*—3–5 hr (plasma), 36–54 hr (tissue). *Dexamethasone*—3–4.5 hr (plasma), 36–54 hr (tissue). *Hydrocortisone*—1.5–2 hr (plasma), 8–12 hr (tissue). *Triamcinolone*—2–>5 hr (plasma), 18–36 hr (tissue).

TIME/ACTION PROFILE (response depends on condition being treated)

ROUTE	ONSET	PEAK	DURATION
Topical	min–hr	hr–days	hr–days

Contraindications/Precautions
Contraindicated in: Hypersensitivity or known intolerance to corticosteroids or components of vehicles (ointment or cream base, preservative, alcohol); Untreated bacterial or viral infections.
Use Cautiously in: Hepatic impairment; Diabetes mellitus, cataracts, glaucoma, or tuberculosis (use of large amounts of high-potency agents may worsen condition); Patients with pre-existing skin atrophy; OB, Lactation: Chronic use at high dosages may result in adrenal suppression in mother and growth suppression in children; Pedi: Children may be more susceptible to adrenal and growth suppression. Clobetasol not recommended for children <18 yr (cream, lotion, shampoo, spray) or <12 yr (foam, gel, ointment, solution); desoximetasone not recommended for children <10 yr (cream, ointment, gel) or <18 yr (spray).

Adverse Reactions/Side Effects
Derm: allergic contact dermatitis, atrophy, burning, dryness, edema, folliculitis, hypersensitivity reactions, hypertrichosis, hypopigmentation, irritation, maceration, miliaria, perioral dermatitis, secondary infection, striae. **EENT:** cataracts, glaucoma. **Misc:** adrenal suppression (↑ dose, long-term therapy).

Interactions
Drug-Drug: None significant.

Route/Dosage
Topical (Adults and Children): 1–4 times daily (depends on product, preparation, and condition being treated).
Rect (Adults): hydrocortisone *Aerosol foam*—90 mg 1–2 times/day for 2–3 wk; then adjusted.

C

Availability

Alclometasone (generic available)

Cream: 0.05%. **Cost:** *Generic*—$97.51/45 g. **Ointment:** 0.05%. **Cost:** *Generic*—$50.47/15 g.

Amcinonide (generic available)

Cream: 0.1%. **Cost:** *Generic*—$38.88/30 g. **Lotion:** 0.1%. **Cost:** *Generic*—$325.73/60 mL. **Ointment:** 0.1%. **Cost:** *Generic*—$388.80/60 g.

Betamethasone (generic available)

Aerosol foam: 0.12%. **Cost:** *Generic*—$236.90/50 g. **Cream:** 0.05%, 0.1%. **Cost:** *Generic*—0.05% $39.51/15 g, 0.1% $24.17/15 g. **Gel:** 0.05%. **Cost:** *Generic*—$61.48/15 g. **Lotion:** 0.05%, 0.1%. **Cost:** *Generic*—0.05% $66.87/60 mL, 0.1% $78.09/60 mL. **Ointment:** 0.05%, 0.1%. **Cost:** *Generic*—0.05% $43.22/15 g, 0.1% $20.34/15 g. **Spray:** 0.05%. ***In combination with:*** calcipotriene (Enstilar, Taclonex), clotrimazole (Lotrisone); see Appendix B.

Clobetasol (generic available)

Cream: 0.025%, 0.05%. **Cost:** *Generic*—$24.94/30 g. **Foam:** 0.05%. **Cost:** *Generic*—$551.63/100 g. **Gel:** 0.05%. **Cost:** *Generic*—$47.87/30 g. **Lotion:** 0.05%. **Cost:** *Generic*—$288.96/59 mL. **Ointment:** 0.05%. **Cost:** *Generic*—$22.96/30 g. **Scalp solution:** 0.05%. **Cost:** *Generic*—$21.31/25 mL. **Shampoo:** 0.05%. **Cost:** *Generic*—$385.29/118 mL. **Spray:** 0.05%. **Cost:** $335.22/59 mL.

Clocortolone

Cream: 0.1%. **Cost:** $183.74/30 g.

Desonide (generic available)

Cream: 0.05%. **Cost:** *Generic*—$88.27/15 g. **Foam:** 0.05%. **Cost:** $630.00/100 g. **Gel:** 0.05%. **Cost:** $449.16/60 g. **Lotion:** 0.05%. **Cost:** *Generic*—$274.42/59 mL. **Ointment:** 0.05%. **Cost:** *Generic*—$70.30/15 g.

Desoximetasone (generic available)

Cream: 0.05%, 0.25%. **Cost:** *Generic*—0.05% $195.09/100 g, 0.25% $197.03/60 g. **Gel:** 0.05%. **Cost:** *Generic*—$87.57/15 g. **Ointment:** 0.25%. **Cost:** *Generic*—$279.97/60 g. **Spray:** 0.25%. **Cost:** $502.50/100 mL.

Diflorasone (generic available)

Cream: 0.05%. **Cost:** *Generic*—$169.23/30 g. **Ointment:** 0.05%. **Cost:** *Generic*—$179.53/30 g.

Fluocinolone (generic available)

Cream: 0.01%, 0.025%. **Cost:** *Generic*—0.01% $44.57/15 g, 0.025% $33.93/15 g. **Oil:** 0.01%. **Cost:** *Generic*—$197.90/20 mL. **Ointment:** 0.025%. **Cost:** *Generic*—$33.93/15 g. **Shampoo:** 0.01%. **Cost:** $416.76/120 mL. **Solution:** 0.01%. **Cost:** *Generic*—$178.80/60 mL. ***In combination with:*** hydroquinone and tretinoin (Tri-Luma). See Appendix B.

Fluocinonide (generic available)

Cream: 0.05%, 0.1%. **Cost:** *Generic*—0.05% $22.32/30 g; *Vanos (0.1%)*—$965.89/60 g. **Gel:** 0.05%. **Cost:** *Generic*—$67.10/60 g. **Ointment:** 0.05%. **Cost:** *Generic*—$55.76/60 g. **Solution:** 0.05%. **Cost:** *Generic*—$100.99/60 mL.

Flurandrenolide (generic available)

Cream: 0.025%, 0.05%. **Cost:** 0.05% $204.60/30 g. **Lotion:** 0.05%. **Cost:** $394.68/60 mL. **Ointment:** 0.05%. **Tape:** 4 mcg/cm². **Cost:** $214.96/1 unit.

Fluticasone (generic available)

Cream: 0.05%. **Cost:** *Generic*—$34.37/30 g. **Lotion:** 0.05%. **Cost:** *Generic*—$389.95/60 mL. **Ointment:** 0.005%. **Cost:** *Generic*—$34.30/30 g.

Halcinonide

Cream: 0.1%. **Cost:** $226.55/60 g. **Ointment:** 0.1%. **Cost:** $133.22/30 g.

Halobetasol (generic available)

Cream: 0.05%. **Cost:** *Generic*—$193.26/50 g. **Foam:** 0.05%. **Lotion:** 0.05%, 0.1%. **Ointment:** 0.05%. **Cost:** *Generic*—$88.67/15 g.

Hydrocortisone (generic available)

Cream: 0.1%, 0.2%, 0.5%Rx, OTC, 1%Rx, OTC, 2.5%. **Gel:** 1%Rx, OTC. **Lotion:** 1%Rx, OTC, 2.5%. **Ointment:** 0.1%, 0.2%, 0.5%Rx, OTC, 1%Rx, OTC, 2.5%. **Rectal cream:** 1%, 2.5%. **Solution:** 0.1%, 1%, 2.5%. ***In combination with:*** acetic acid, antifungals, anti-infectives, antihistamines, urea, and benzoyl peroxide in various otic and topical preparations. See Appendix B.

Mometasone (generic available)

Cream: 0.1%. **Cost:** *Generic*—$15.59/15 g. **Ointment:** 0.1%. **Cost:** *Generic*—$28.10/15 g. **Lotion:** 🍁 0.1%. **Cost:** $58.20/30 mL. **Solution:** 0.1%.

Prednicarbate (generic available)

Cream: 0.1%. **Cost:** *Generic*—$23.08/15 g. **Ointment:** 0.1%. **Cost:** *Generic*—$30.00/15 g.

Triamcinolone (generic available)

Cream: 0.025%, 0.1%, 0.5%. **Cost:** *Generic*—0.025% $4.45/15 g, 0.1% $5.57/15 g, 0.5% $10.11/15 g. **Lotion:** 0.025%, 0.1%. **Cost:** *Generic*—0.025% $37.79/60 mL, 0.1% $90.00/60 mL. **Ointment:** 0.025%, 0.1%, 0.5%. **Cost:** *Generic*—0.025% $10.11/80 g, 0.1% $5.58/15 g, 0.5% $10.10/15 g. **Spray:** 0.147 mg/g. ***In combination with:*** acetic acid, antifungals, anti-infectives, antihistamines, urea, and benzoyl peroxide in various otic and topical preparations. See Appendix B.

NURSING IMPLICATIONS

Assessment

- Assess affected skin before and daily during therapy. Note degree of inflammation, pruritus, and/or plaques. Notify health care professional if symptoms of infection (increased pain, erythema, purulent exudate) develop.

- ***Lab Test Considerations:*** Adrenal function tests may be ordered to assess degree of hypothalamic-pituitary-adrenal (HPA) axis suppression in long-term topical therapy. Children and patients with dose applied to a large area, using an occlusive dressing, or using high-potency products are at highest risk for HPA suppression.
- May cause ↑ serum and urine glucose concentrations if significant absorption occurs.

Implementation

- Choice of vehicle depends on site and type of lesion. Ointments are more occlusive and preferred for dry, scaly lesions. Creams should be used on oozing or intertriginous areas, where the occlusive action of ointments might cause folliculitis or maceration. Creams may be preferred for esthetic reasons even though they may dry skin more than ointments. Gels, aerosols, lotions, and solutions are useful in hairy areas.
- **Topical:** Apply *ointments, creams,* or *gels* sparingly as a thin film to clean, slightly moist skin. Wear gloves. Apply occlusive dressing only if specified by health care professional.
- Apply *lotion, solution,* or *gel* to hair by parting hair and applying a small amount to affected area. Rub in gently. Protect area from washing, clothing, or rubbing until medication has dried. Hair may be washed as usual but not right after applying medication.
- Use *aerosols* by shaking well and spraying on affected area, holding container 3–6 in. away. Spray for about 2 sec to cover an area the size of a hand. Do not inhale. If spraying near face, cover eyes.
- Shake *Sernivo spray* before using. Spray affected area and rub in gently. Discontinue if control not achieved or after 4 wk of use.

Patient/Family Teaching

- Instruct patient on correct technique of medication administration. Emphasize importance of avoiding the eyes. Apply missed doses as soon as remembered unless almost time for the next dose.
- Caution patient to use only as directed. Avoid using cosmetics, bandages, dressings, or other skin products over the treated area unless directed by health care professional.
- Advise parents of pediatric patients not to apply tight-fitting diapers or plastic pants on a child treated in the diaper area; these garments work as an occlusive dressing and may cause more of the drug to be absorbed.
- Advise patient to consult health care professional before using medicine for condition other than indicated.
- Caution women that medication should not be used extensively, in large amounts, or for protracted periods if they are pregnant or planning to become pregnant. Advise female patients of reproductive potential to notify health care professional if pregnancy is planned or suspected, or if breast feeding.
- Instruct patient to inform health care professional if symptoms of underlying disease return or worsen or if symptoms of infection develop.
- **Fluticasone:** Advise patient to avoid excessive natural or artificial exposure (tanning booth, sun lamp) to areas where lotion is applied.

Evaluation/Desired Outcomes

- Resolution of skin inflammation, pruritus, or other dermatologic conditions.
- Clearing of plaques in plaque psoriasis.

cortisone, See CORTICOSTEROIDS (SYSTEMIC).

crisaborole (kris-a-**bor**-ole)

Eucrisa

Classification

Therapeutic: anti-inflammatories

Pharmacologic: phosphodiesterase type 4 inhibitors

Indications

Mild to moderate atopic dermatitis.

Action

Inhibits phosphodiesterase 4 (PDE-4) resulting in ↑ intracellular cyclic adenosine monophosphate levels.

Therapeutic Effects: Decreased severity of atopic dermatitis.

Pharmacokinetics

Absorption: Minimal systemic absorption through intact skin.

Distribution: Local distribution after topical administration.

Protein Binding: 97%.

Metabolism and Excretion: Metabolized through liver into inactive metabolites; metabolites excreted in urine.

Half-life: Unknown.

TIME/ACTION PROFILE (improvement in symptoms)

ROUTE	ONSET	PEAK	DURATION
Topical	8 days	Unknown	Unknown

Contraindications/Precautions

Contraindicated in: Hypersensitivity.

Use Cautiously in: OB, Lactation: Safety not established; Pedi: Safety not established in children <2 yrs.

Adverse Reactions/Side Effects

Derm: burning, stinging. **Misc:** hypersensitivity reactions.

Interactions

Drug-Drug: None known.

Route/Dosage

Topical (Adults and Children ≥2 yrs): Apply a thin layer to affected areas twice daily.

Availability

Ointment: 2%.

NURSING IMPLICATIONS

Assessment

- Assess skin lesions periodically during therapy.

Implementation

- **Topical:** Apply a thin layer to affected areas twice daily. Do not apply to ophthalmic, oral or vaginal areas. Wash hands after applying ointment.

Patient/Family Teaching

- Instruct patient or parent to apply as directed. For topical use only.
- Advise patient or parent to discontinue therapy and notify health care professional if signs and symptoms of hypersensitivity (pruritus, swelling, erythema) at application site or a distant site occur.
- Instruct patient to notify health care professional of all Rx or OTC medications, vitamins, or herbal products being taken and consult health care professional before taking any new medications.
- Rep: Advise female patient to notify health care professional if pregnancy is planned or suspected or if breast feeding.

Evaluation/Desired Outcomes

- Decreased severity of atopic dermatitis.

crizotinib (kriz-oh-ti-nib)

Xalkori

Classification

Therapeutic: antineoplastics

Pharmacologic: kinase Inhibitors

Indications

Metastatic non-small cell lung cancer (NSCLC) that is positive for anaplastic lymphoma kinase (ALK) or ROS1.

Action

Inhibits receptor tyrosine kinases including anaplastic lymphoma kinase (ALK), Hepatocyte Growth Factor Receptor (HGFR, c-Met), ROS1, and Recepteur d'Origine Nantais (RON). **Therapeutic Effects:** Decreased spread of lung cancer and improved survival.

Pharmacokinetics

Absorption: 43% absorbed following oral administration.

Distribution: Extensively distributed to tissues.

Metabolism and Excretion: Mostly metabolized by the liver (CYP3A4/5 enzyme system), also acts as a inhibitor of CYP3A. 53% excreted in feces unchanged, 2.3% eliminated unchanged in urine.

Half-life: 42 hr.

TIME/ACTION PROFILE (blood levels)

ROUTE	ONSET	PEAK	DURATION
PO	unknown	4–6 hr	unknown

Contraindications/Precautions

Contraindicated in: Concurrent use of strong CYP3A inhibitors or inducers; Congenital long QT syndrome; OB: May cause fetal harm; Lactation: Breast feeding should be avoided.

Use Cautiously in: Heart failure, bradyarrhythmias, electrolyte abnormalities, concurrent medications that prolong QT interval (↑ risk of arrhythmias); Asian patients (↑ blood levels); Moderate or severe hepatic impairment (↓ dose); Severe renal impairment; Rep: Women of reproductive potential and men with female sexual partners of reproductive potential; Pedi: Safety and effectiveness not established.

Adverse Reactions/Side Effects

CNS: fatigue, headache, insomnia. **CV:** QT INTERVAL PROLONGATION, bradycardia, edema, chest pain. **Derm:** rash. **EENT:** visual disturbances. **Endo:** ↓ testosterone. **GI:** HEPATOTOXICITY, constipation, diarrhea, nausea, vomiting, abdominal pain, dysgeusia, esophagitis, ↓ appetite, stomatitis. **GU:** ↓ fertility, renal impairment. **Neuro:** neuropathy. **Resp:** PNEUMONITIS. **Misc:** fever.

Interactions

Drug-Drug: **Strong CYP3A inhibitors** including **atazanavir**, **clarithromycin**, **indinavir**, **itraconazole**, **ketoconazole**, **nefazodone**, **nelfinavir**, **ritonavir**, **saquinavir**, and **voriconazole** may ↑ levels; concurrent use should be avoided. **Strong CYP3A inducers** including **carbamazepine**, **phenobarbital**, **phenytoin**, **rifabutin**, and **rifampin** may ↓ levels and effectiveness; concurrent use should be avoided. May ↑ levels of **alfentanil**, **cyclosporine**, **dihydroergotamine**, **ergotamine**, **fentanyl**, **pimozide**, **quinidine**, **sirolimus**, and **tacrolimus**; avoid concurrent use. **Beta-blockers**, **verapamil**, **diltiazem**, **digoxin**, and **clonidine** may ↑ risk of bradycardia; avoid concurrent use, if possible.

Drug-Natural Products: Concurrent use of **St. John's wort** may ↓ levels and effectiveness and should be avoided.

Drug-Food: **Grapefruit** or **grapefruit juice** may ↑ levels and should be avoided.

Route/Dosage

PO (Adults): 250 mg twice daily until disease progression or unacceptable toxicity.

Renal Impairment

PO (Adults): *CCr <30 mL/min (not on dialysis)*—250 mg once daily.

Hepatic Impairment

PO (Adults): *Moderate hepatic impairment (AST and total bilirubin >1.5x and ≤3x ULN)*—200 mg twice daily; *Severe hepatic impairment (AST and total bilirubin >3x ULN)*—250 mg once daily.

Availability

Capsules: 200 mg, 250 mg.

NURSING IMPLICATIONS

Assessment

- Assess respiratory function (lung sounds, dyspnea, oxygen saturation) periodically during therapy.
- Monitor for signs and symptoms of pneumonitis (difficulty breathing, shortness or breath, cough with or without mucus, fever) periodically during therapy. *If any Grade of pneumonitis occurs,* permanently discontinue.
- Assess for signs and symptoms of neuropathy (burning, dysesthesia, hyperesthesia, hypoesthesia, neuralgia, paresthesia, peripheral neuropathy sensory and motor) periodically during therapy. Usually Grade 1.
- Monitor ECG periodically during therapy in patients with HF, bradyarrhythmias, electrolyte imbalances, or taking medications that may prolong QT interval. *If QTc >500 ms on at least 2 separate ECGs,* hold until recovery to baseline or to a QTc <481 ms, then resume at next lower dose. *If QTc >500 ms or ≥60 ms change from baseline with torsade de pointes or polymorphic ventricular tachycardia or signs/symptoms of serious arrhythmia,* permanently discontinue. *If symptomatic bradycardia occurs,* hold dose until heart rate return to ≥60 bpm. Evaluate concomitant medications, if contributing medication is identified and dose reduced or discontinued, return to previous dose of crizotinib once heart rate is ≥60 bpm and/or bradycardia is asymptomatic. If no contributing medication is identified or dose modifications are not made, resume crizotinib at a reduced dose once heart rate ≥60 bpm and/or bradycardia is asymptomatic. *If bradycardia is life-threatening and no contributing medication identified,* discontinue crizotinib. If contributing medication is identified and dose is reduced or discontinued, reduce crizotinib dose to 250 mg once daily with frequent monitoring once heart rate ≥60 bpm and/or bradycardia is asymptomatic.
- Monitor vision during therapy. If visual loss (Grade 4 Ocular Disorder) occurs, discontinue crizotinib during evaluation of severe vision loss. Perform an ophthalmological evaluation consisting of best corrected visual acuity, retinal photographs, visual fields, optical coherence tomography (OCT) and other evaluations as appropriate for new onset of severe visual loss.
- ***Lab Test Considerations:*** Test patient for ALK or ROS1 positivity in tumor specimens through an FDA approved test http://www.fda.gov/companiondiagnostics prior to starting therapy.
- Obtain a negative pregnancy test prior to starting therapy.
- Monitor CBC with differential monthly and as clinically indicated; more frequently if Grade 3 or 4 toxicities occur. *If Grade 3 hematologic toxicity occurs,* hold dose until recovery to Grade ≤2, then resume same dose schedule. *If Grade 4 hematologic toxicity occurs,* hold until recovery to Grade ≤2, then resume at next lower dose. May also cause Grade 3 or 4 neutropenia, thrombocytopenia, and lymphopenia.
- Monitor liver function tests every 2 wk during first 2 mo, then monthly and as clinically indicated; more frequently if Grade 2, 3, 4 abnormalities occur. *If ALT or AST ↑ >5 x upper limit of normal (ULN) with total bilirubin ≤ 1.5 times ULN,* hold crizotinib until recovery to baseline or ≤ 3 x ULN, then resume at next lower dose. *If ALT or AST ↑ >3 x ULN with concurrent total bilirubin ↑ >1.5 x ULN (in the absence of cholestasis or hemolysis),* permanently discontinue crizotinib. *If Grade 3 or 4 AST or ALT ↑ with Grade ≤1 total bilirubin occurs,* hold until recovery to Grade ≤1 or baseline, then resume at 200 mg twice daily.

Implementation

- **PO:** Administer twice daily without regard to food. Swallow capsules whole, do not crush, dissolve, or open.

Patient/Family Teaching

- Instruct patient to take crizotinib as directed; do not change dose or stop taking without consulting health care professional. If vomiting occurs, do not take extra dose, just take next dose at regular scheduled time. Take missed doses as soon as remembered unless <6 hr until next dose. If <6 hr to next dose, skip dose and return to regular schedule; do not double doses. Advise patient to read the *Patient Information leaflet* before starting and with each Rx refill in case of changes.
- Advise patient to avoid eating grapefruit or drinking grapefruit juice during therapy.
- Caution patient that dizziness and visual disorders may occur. Advise patient to avoid driving or other activities requiring alertness until response to medication is known. Visual disturbances generally start within 2 wk of therapy. Instruct patient to notify health care professional if flashes of light, blurry vision, light sensitivity, or new or worse vitreous floaters occur; ophthalmological evaluation should be considered.

- Advise patient to notify health care professional immediately if signs and symptoms of liver problems (weakness, fatigue, anorexia, nausea, vomiting, abdominal pain (especially RUQ abdominal pain), jaundice, dark urine, generalized pruritus, bleeding); lung problems (trouble breathing or shortness of breath, cough with or without mucous, fever); or heart problems (dizziness or fainting, abnormal heartbeats) occur.
- Inform patient that nausea, diarrhea, vomiting, and constipation are common side effects and usually occur during first few days of therapy. Standard antiemetic, antidiarrheal, and laxative medications are usually effective.
- Instruct patient to notify health care professional of all Rx or OTC medications, vitamins, or herbal products being taken and consult health care professional before taking any new medications, especially St. John's wort.
- Rep: Instruct women of reproductive potential to use effective contraception during and for at least 45 days following discontinuation of therapy and to avoid breast feeding during therapy. Because of potential for genotoxicity, advise males with female partners of reproductive potential to use condoms during treatment and for at least 90 days after final dose. May cause reduced fertility in females and males of reproductive potential; may be irreversible.

Evaluation/Desired Outcomes

- Decrease spread of non-small cell lung cancer.

cyanocobalamin, See VITAMIN B_{12} PREPARATIONS.

BEERS

cyclobenzaprine

(sye-kloe-**ben**-za-preen)

Amrix, ~~Flexeril~~

Classification

Therapeutic: skeletal muscle relaxants (centrally acting)

Indications

Management of acute painful musculoskeletal conditions associated with muscle spasm. **Unlabeled Use:** Management of fibromyalgia.

Action

Reduces tonic somatic muscle activity at the level of the brainstem. Structurally similar to tricyclic antidepressants. **Therapeutic Effects:** Reduction in muscle spasm and hyperactivity without loss of function.

Pharmacokinetics

Absorption: Well absorbed from the GI tract.
Distribution: Unknown.
Protein Binding: 93%.
Metabolism and Excretion: Mostly metabolized by the liver.
Half-life: 1–3 days.

TIME/ACTION PROFILE (skeletal muscle relaxation)

ROUTE	ONSET	PEAK†	DURATION
PO	within 1 hr	3–8 hr	12–24 hr
Extended release	unknown	unknown	24 hr

†Full effects may not occur for 1–2 wk.

Contraindications/Precautions

Contraindicated in: Hypersensitivity; Should not be used within 14 days of MAO inhibitor therapy; Immediate period after MI; Severe or symptomatic cardiovascular disease; Cardiac conduction disturbances; Hyperthyroidism.
Use Cautiously in: Cardiovascular disease; OB: Use only if potential maternal benefit justifies potential fetal risk; Lactation: Use while breast feeding only if potential maternal benefit justifies potential risk to infant; Pedi: Children <15 yr (safety and effectiveness not established); Geri: Appears on Beers list. Poorly tolerated due to anticholinergic effects.

Adverse Reactions/Side Effects

CNS: dizziness, drowsiness, confusion, fatigue, headache, nervousness. **CV:** arrhythmias. **EENT:** dry mouth, blurred vision. **GI:** constipation, dyspepsia, nausea, unpleasant taste. **GU:** urinary retention.

Interactions

Drug-Drug: Additive CNS depression with other **CNS depressants**, including **alcohol**, **antihistamines**, **opioid analgesics**, and **sedative/hypnotics**. Additive anticholinergic effects with **drugs possessing anticholinergic properties**, including **antihistamines**, **antidepressants**, **atropine**, **disopyramide**, **haloperidol**, and **phenothiazines**. Avoid use within 14 days of **MAO inhibitors** (hyperpyretic crisis, seizures, and death may occur). Drugs that affect serotonergic neurotransmitter systems, including **tricyclic antidepressants**, **SSRIs**, **SNRIs**, **fentanyl**, **buspirone**, **tramadol**, and **triptans** ↑ risk of serotonin syndrome.
Drug-Natural Products: Concomitant use of **kava-kava**, **valerian**, **chamomile**, or **hops** can ↑ CNS depression.

Route/Dosage

PO (Adults and Children ≥15 yo): *Acute painful musculoskeletal conditions*—Immediate-release: 10

mg 3 times daily (range 20–40 mg/day in 2–4 divided doses; not to exceed 60 mg/day); Extended-release: 15–30 mg once daily. *Fibromyalgia*—5–40 mg at bedtime (unlabeled).

Availability (generic available)

Extended-release capsules (Amrix): 15 mg, 30 mg. **Cost:** All strengths $1,437.60/60. **Tablets:** 5 mg, 7.5 mg, 10 mg. **Cost:** *Generic*—5 mg $9.43/100, 10 mg $8.32/100.

NURSING IMPLICATIONS

Assessment

- Assess patient for pain, muscle stiffness, and range of motion before and periodically throughout therapy.
- Geri: Assess geriatric patients for anticholinergic effects (sedation and weakness).
- Assess for serotonin syndrome (mental changes [agitation, hallucinations, coma], autonomic instability [tachycardia, labile BP, hyperthermia], neuromuscular aberrations [hyperreflexia, incoordination], and/or GI symptoms [nausea, vomiting, diarrhea]), especially in patients taking other serotonergic drugs (SSRIs, SNRIs, triptans).

Implementation

- **PO:** May be administered with meals to minimize gastric irritation.
- Swallow extended-release capsules whole; do not open, crush, or chew. Capsules may be opened and contents sprinkled onto applesauce; swallow immediately without chewing. Rinse mouth to make sure contents have been swallowed.

Patient/Family Teaching

- Instruct patient to take medication as directed, at the same time each day; do not take more than the prescribed amount. Take missed doses within 1 hr of time ordered; otherwise, return to normal dose schedule. Do not double doses. Do not stop abruptly, may cause nausea, headache, and malaise; discontinue gradually.
- Medication may cause drowsiness, dizziness, and blurred vision. Caution patient to avoid driving or other activities requiring alertness until response to drug is known.
- Advise patient to avoid concurrent use of alcohol or other CNS depressants with this medication.
- If constipation becomes a problem, advise patient that increasing fluid intake and bulk in diet and stool softeners may alleviate this condition.
- Instruct patient to notify health care professional of all Rx or OTC medications, vitamins, or herbal products being taken and to consult health care professional before taking any other Rx, OTC, or herbal products.
- Advise patient to notify health care professional if symptoms of urinary retention (distended abdomen, feeling of fullness, overflow incontinence, voiding small amounts) occur.
- Instruct patient to notify health care professional immediately if signs and symptoms of serotonin syndrome, irregular or abnormal heartbeats, fast heartbeat, or allergic reaction (difficulty breathing, hives, swelling of face or tongue, itching) occur.
- Inform patient that good oral hygiene, frequent mouth rinses, and sugarless gum or candy may help relieve dry mouth.
- Advise female of reproductive potential to notify health care professional if pregnancy is planned or suspected or if breast feeding.

Evaluation/Desired Outcomes

- Relief of muscular spasm in acute skeletal muscle conditions. Maximum effects may not be evident for 1–2 wk. Use is usually limited to 2–3 wk; however, has been effective for at least 12 wk in the management of fibromyalgia.

HIGH ALERT

cyclophosphamide

(sye-kloe-**fos**-fa-mide)

~~Cytoxan~~, Procytox

Classification

Therapeutic: antineoplastics, immunosuppressants

Pharmacologic: alkylating agents

Indications

Alone or with other modalities in the management of: Hodgkin's disease, Malignant lymphomas, Multiple myeloma, Leukemias, Mycosis fungoides, Neuroblastoma, Ovarian carcinoma, Breast carcinoma, and a variety of other tumors. Minimal change nephrotic syndrome in children. **Unlabeled Use:** Severe active rheumatoid arthritis or granulomatosis with polyangiitis.

Action

Interferes with DNA replication and RNA transcription, ultimately disrupting protein synthesis (cell-cycle phase–nonspecific). **Therapeutic Effects:** Death of rapidly replicating cells, particularly malignant ones. Also has immunosuppressant action in smaller doses.

Pharmacokinetics

Absorption: Inactive parent drug is well absorbed from the GI tract. Converted to active drug by the liver.

Distribution: Widely distributed. Limited penetration of the blood-brain barrier. Crosses the placenta; enters breast milk.

Metabolism and Excretion: Converted to active drug by the liver; 30% eliminated unchanged by the kidneys.

Half-life: 4–6.5 hr.

TIME/ACTION PROFILE (effects on blood counts)

ROUTE	ONSET	PEAK	DURATION
PO, IV	7 days	7–15 days	21 days

Contraindications/Precautions

Contraindicated in: Hypersensitivity; OB: Pregnancy (may cause fetal harm); Lactation: Lactation.

Use Cautiously in: Active infections; Bone marrow depression; Other chronic debilitating illnesses; Rep: Women of reproductive potential.

Adverse Reactions/Side Effects

CV: MYOCARDIAL FIBROSIS, hypotension. **Derm:** alopecia. **Endo:** gonadal suppression, syndrome of inappropriate antidiuretic hormone (SIADH). **GI:** anorexia, nausea, vomiting. **GU:** HEMORRHAGIC CYSTITIS, hematuria, ↓ fertility. **Hemat:** LEUKOPENIA, thrombocytopenia, anemia. **Metab:** hyperuricemia. **Resp:** PULMONARY FIBROSIS. **Misc:** secondary neoplasms.

Interactions

Drug-Drug: Phenobarbital or **rifampin** may ↑ toxicity of cyclophosphamide. Concurrent **allopurinol** or **thiazide diuretics** may exaggerate bone marrow depression. May prolong neuromuscular blockade from **succinylcholine**. Cardiotoxicity may be additive with other **cardiotoxic agents** (e.g., **cytarabine**, **daunorubicin**, **doxorubicin**). May ↓ serum **digoxin** levels. Additive bone marrow depression with other **antineoplastics** or **radiation therapy**. May potentiate the effects of **warfarin**. May ↓ antibody response to **live-virus vaccines** and ↑ risk of adverse reactions. Prolongs the effects of **cocaine**.

Route/Dosage

Many regimens are used.

PO (Adults): 1–5 mg/kg/day.

PO (Children): *Induction*—2–8 mg/kg/day (60–250 mg/m²/day) in divided doses for 6 days or longer. *Maintenance*—2–5 mg/kg (50–150 mg/m²/day) twice weekly.

IV (Adults): 40–50 mg/kg in divided doses over 2–5 days *or* 10–15 mg/kg every 7–10 days *or* 3–5 mg/kg twice weekly *or* 1.5–3 mg/kg/day. Other regimens may use larger doses.

IV (Children): *Induction*—2–8 mg/kg/day (60–250 mg/m²/day) in divided doses for 6 days or longer. Total dose for 7 days may be given as a single weekly dose. *Maintenance*—10–15 mg/kg every 7–10 days or 30 mg/kg every 3–4 wk.

Availability (generic available)

Capsules: 25 mg, 50 mg. **Lyophilized powder for injection (requires reconstitution):** 🍁200 mg/vial, 500 mg/vial, 1 g/vial, 2 g/vial.

NURSING IMPLICATIONS

Assessment

- Monitor BP, pulse, respiratory rate, and temperature frequently during administration. Report significant changes.
- Monitor urinary output frequently during therapy. To reduce the risk of hemorrhagic cystitis and to promote excretion of uric acid, fluid intake should be at least 3000 mL/day for adults and 1000–2000 mL/day for children. May be administered with mesna. Alkalinization of the urine may be used to help prevent uric acid nephropathy.
- Monitor for bone marrow depression. Assess for bleeding (bleeding gums, bruising, petechiae, guaiac stools, urine, and emesis) and avoid IM injections and taking rectal temperatures if platelet count is low. Apply pressure to venipuncture sites for 10 min. Assess for signs of infection during neutropenia. Anemia may occur. Monitor for increased fatigue, dyspnea, and orthostatic hypotension.
- Assess nausea, vomiting, and appetite. Weigh weekly. Antiemetics may be given 30 min before administration of medication to minimize GI effects. Anorexia and weight loss can be minimized by feeding frequent light meals.
- Assess cardiac and respiratory status for dyspnea, rales/crackles, cough, weight gain, edema. Pulmonary toxicity may occur after prolonged therapy. Cardiotoxicity may occur early in therapy and is characterized by symptoms of HF.
- ***Lab Test Considerations:*** Monitor CBC with differential and platelet count before and periodically during therapy. The nadir of leukopenia occurs in 7–12 days (recovery in 17–21 days). Leukocytes should be maintained at 2500–4000/mm³. May also cause thrombocytopenia (nadir 10–15 days), and rarely causes anemia.
- Monitor BUN, creatinine, and uric acid before and frequently during therapy to detect nephrotoxicity.
- Monitor ALT, AST, LDH, and serum bilirubin before and frequently during therapy to detect hepatotoxicity.
- Urinalysis should be evaluated before initiating therapy and frequently during therapy to detect hematuria or change in specific gravity indicative of SIADH.
- May suppress positive reactions to skin tests for *Candida*, mumps, *Trichophyton*, and tuberculin purified-protein derivative (PPD). May also produce false-positive results in Papanicolaou smears.

Implementation

- ***High Alert:*** Fatalities have occurred with chemotherapeutic agents. Before administering, clarify all ambiguous orders; double-check single, daily, and course-of-therapy dose limits; have second practitioner independently double-check original order, calculations, and infusion pump settings.

- Do not confuse cyclophosphamide with cyclosporine.
- **PO:** Administer in the morning. Swallow tablets whole; do not crush, break, or chew.

IV Administration

- **IV:** Solution should be prepared in a biologic cabinet. Wear gloves, gown, and mask while handling medication. If powder or solution comes in contact with skin or mucosa, wash thoroughly with soap and water. Discard equipment in specially designated containers.
- **IV Push:** Reconstitute each 100 mg with 5 mL of 0.9% NaCl. Swirl gently to dissolve. Do not reconstitute with sterile water for injection; results in a hypotonic solution not suitable for IV push. ***Concentration:*** 20 mg/mL. Administer reconstituted solution undiluted. ***Rate:*** Inject very slowly.
- **Intermittent Infusion:** Reconstitute each 100 mg with 5 mL of 0.9% NaCl or sterile water for injection. Swirl gently to dissolve. Use solution reconstituted with sterile water for injection immediately; solution reconstituted with 0.9% NaCl may be stored at room temperature for 24 hr or if refrigerated for 6 days. Do not administer solutions that contain clear or yellow viscous liquid. ***Diluent:*** May be further diluted in up to 250 mL of D5W, D5/0.9% NaCl, or 0.45% NaCl. ***Concentration:*** minimum 2 mg/mL. ***Rate:*** Infuse very slowly. May reduce rate-dependent adverse reactions (facial swelling, headache, nasal congestion, scalp burning).
- **Y-Site Compatibility:** acyclovir, alemtuzumab, alfentanil, allopurinol, amifostine, amikacin, aminocaproic acid, aminophylline, amiodarone, amphotericin B lipid complex, amphotericin B liposome, ampicillin/sulbactam, anidulafungin, argatroban, arsenic trioxide, atracurium, azithromycin, aztreonam, bivalirudin, bleomycin, bumetanide, buprenorphine, butorphanol, calcium chloride, calcium gluconate, carboplatin, carmustine, caspofungin, cefazolin, cefepime, cefotaxime, cefotetan, cefoxitin, ceftazidime, ceftriaxone, cefuroxime, chloramphenicol, chlorpromazine, ciprofloxacin, cisatracurium, cisplatin, cladribine, clindamycin, cyclosporine, cytarabine, dacarbazine, dactinomycin, daptomycin, daunorubicin hydrochloride, dexamethasone, dexmedetomidine, dexrazoxane, digoxin, diltiazem, diphenhydramine, dobutamine, docetaxel, dolasetron, dopamine, doxorubicin, doxorubicin liposome, doxycycline, droperidol, enalaprilat, ephedrine, epinephrine, epirubicin, ertapenem, erythromycin, esmolol, etoposide, etoposide phosphate, famotidine, fenoldopam, fentanyl, filgrastim, fluconazole, fludarabine, fluorouracil, foscarnet, fosphenytoin, furosemide, ganciclovir, gemcitabine, gentamicin, granisetron, haloperidol, heparin, hetastarch, hydralazine, hydrocortisone, hydromorphone, idarubicin, imipenem/cilastatin, insulin regular, irinotecan, isoproterenol, ketorolac, labetalol, leucovorin calcium, levofloxacin, lidocaine, linezolid, lorazepam, magnesium sulfate, mannitol, melphalan, meperidine, meropenem, mesna, methotrexate, methylprednisolone, metoclopramide, metoprolol, metronidazole, midazolam, milrinone, mitomycin, mitoxantrone, morphine, moxifloxacin, nafcillin, nalbuphine, naloxone, nicardipine, nitroglycerin, nitroprusside, norepinephrine, octreotide, ondansetron, oxacillin, oxaliplatin, oxytocin, paclitaxel, palonosetron, pamidronate, pancuronium, pantoprazole, pemetrexed, penicillin G, pentamidine, pentobarbital, phenobarbital, phentolamine, phenylephrine, piperacillin/tazobactam, potassium acetate, potassium chloride, potassium phosphates, procainamide, prochlorperazine, promethazine, propofol, propranolol, quinupristin/dalfopristin, ranitidine, remifentanil, rituximab, rocuronium, sargramostim, sodium acetate, sodium bicarbonate, sodium phosphates, succinylcholine, sufentanil, tacrolimus, theophylline, thiopental, thiotepa, tigecycline, tirofiban, tobramycin, topotecan, trastuzumab, trimethoprim/sulfamethoxazole, vancomycin, vasopressin, vecuronium, verapamil, vinblastine, vincristine, vinorelbine, voriconazole, zidovudine, zoledronic acid.
- **Y-Site Incompatibility:** amphotericin B deoxycholate, diazepam, phenytoin.

Patient/Family Teaching

- Instruct patient to take dose in early morning. Emphasize need for adequate fluid intake for 72 hr after therapy. Patient should void frequently to decrease bladder irritation from metabolites excreted by the kidneys. Report hematuria immediately. If a dose is missed, contact health care professional. Advise caregivers to use gloves when handling capsules. If capsule opens, wash hands thoroughly.
- Instruct patient to notify health care professional promptly if fever; sore throat; signs of infection; lower back or side pain; difficult or painful urination; sores in the mouth or on the lips; yellow discoloration of skin or eyes; bleeding gums; bruising; petechiae; blood in urine, stool, or emesis; unusual swelling of ankles or legs; joint pain; shortness of breath; cough, palpitations, weight gain of more than 5 lb in 24 hr, dizziness, loss of consciousness or confusion occurs. Caution patient to avoid crowds and persons with known infections. Instruct patient to use soft toothbrush and electric razor and to avoid falls. Patient should also be cautioned not to drink alcoholic beverages or to take products containing aspirin or NSAIDs; may precipitate GI hemorrhage.
- Discuss with patient the possibility of hair loss. Explore methods of coping. May also cause darkening of skin and fingernails.
- Instruct patient not to receive any vaccinations without advice of health care professional.

- Rep: Advise patient that this medication may cause sterility and menstrual irregularities or cessation of menses. This drug is also teratogenic; females should use highly effective contraceptive measures for up to 1 yr after completion and men should continue to wear condoms for at least 4 mo after completion of therapy.

Evaluation/Desired Outcomes

- Decrease in size or spread of malignant tumors.
- Improvement of hematologic status in patients with leukemia. Maintenance therapy is instituted if leukocyte count remains between 2500 and 4000/mm^3 and if patient does not demonstrate serious side effects.
- Management of minimal change nephrotic syndrome in children.

cycloSPORINE†

(sye-kloe-spor-een)

Gengraf, Neoral, SandIMMUNE

Classification

Therapeutic: immunosuppressants, antirheumatics (DMARD)

Pharmacologic: polypeptides (cyclic)

†See Appendix C for ophthalmic use

Indications

PO, IV: Prevention and treatment of rejection in renal, cardiac, and hepatic transplantation (with corticosteroids). **PO:** Treatment of severe active rheumatoid arthritis (Neoral only). Treatment of severe recalcitrant psoriasis in adult nonimmunocompromised patients (Neoral only). **Unlabeled Use:** Management of recalcitrant ulcerative colitis. Treatment of steroid-resistant nephrotic syndrome. Treatment of severe steroid-resistant autoimmune disease. Prevention and treatment of graft vs. host disease in bone marrow transplant patients.

Action

Inhibits normal immune responses (cellular and humoral) by inhibiting interleukin-2, a factor necessary for initiation of T-cell activity. **Therapeutic Effects:** Prevention of rejection reactions. Slowed progression of rheumatoid arthritis or psoriasis.

Pharmacokinetics

Absorption: Erratically absorbed (range 10–60%) after oral administration, with significant first-pass metabolism by the liver. Microemulsion (Neoral) has better bioavailability.

Distribution: Widely distributed, mainly into extracellular fluid and blood cells. Crosses the placenta; enters breast milk.

Protein Binding: 90–98%.

Metabolism and Excretion: Extensively metabolized by the liver by CYP3A4 (first pass); excreted in bile, small amounts excreted unchanged in urine.

Half-life: Children—7 hr; adults—19 hr.

TIME/ACTION PROFILE (blood levels)

ROUTE	ONSET	PEAK	DURATION
PO	unknown†	2–6 hr	unknown
IV	unknown	end of infusion	unknown

†Onset of action in rheumatoid arthritis is 4–8 wk and may last 4 wk after discontinuation; for psoriasis, onset is 2–6 wk and lasts 6 wk following discontinuation.

Contraindications/Precautions

Contraindicated in: Hypersensitivity to cyclosporine or polyoxyethylated castor oil (vehicle for IV form); Disulfiram therapy or known alcohol intolerance (IV and oral liquid dose forms contain alcohol); Patients with psoriasis receiving immunosuppressants or radiation; Renal impairment (in patients with rheumatoid arthritis or psoriasis); Uncontrolled hypertension; OB, Lactation: Should not be given unless benefits outweigh risks.

Use Cautiously in: Severe hepatic impairment (dose ↓ recommended); Renal impairment (frequent dose changes may be necessary); Active infection; Pedi: Larger or more frequent doses may be required.

Adverse Reactions/Side Effects

CNS: POSTERIOR REVERSIBLE ENCEPHALOPATHY SYNDROME, PROGRESSIVE MULTIFOCAL LEUKOENCEPHALOPATHY, SEIZURES, tremor, confusion, flushing, headache, psychiatric problems. **CV:** hypertension. **Derm:** hirsutism, acne, psoriasis. **F and E:** hyperkalemia, hypomagnesemia. **GI:** HEPATOTOXICITY, diarrhea, nausea, vomiting, abdominal discomfort, anorexia, pancreatitis. **GU:** nephrotoxicity. **Hemat:** anemia, leukopenia, thrombocytopenia. **Metab:** hyperlipidemia, hyperuricemia. **Neuro:** hyperesthesia, paresthesia. **MS:** lower extremity pain. **Misc:** MALIGNANCY, gingival hyperplasia, hypersensitivity reactions, infection (including activation of latent viral infections such as BK virus-associated nephropathy).

Interactions

Drug-Drug: Azithromycin, clarithromycin, allopurinol, amiodarone, bromocriptine, colchicine, danazol, digoxin, diltiazem, erythromycin, fluconazole, fluoroquinolones, imatinib, itraconazole, ketoconazole, voriconazole, metoclopramide, methylprednisolone, nefazodone, nicardipine, protease inhibitors, quinupristin/dalfopristin, verapamil, or **hormonal contraceptives** may ↑ serum levels and risk of toxicity. ↑ immunosuppression with other **immunosuppressants** (cyclophosphamide, azathioprine, corticosteroids). **Carbamazepine**, **nafcillin**, **octreotide**, **orlistat**, **oxcarbazepine**, **phenobarbital**, **phenytoin**, **rifampin**, **rifabutin**, or **terbinafine** may ↓ levels and effect. **Bosentan** may significantly ↓ levels; avoid concurrent use. ↑ risk of hyperkalemia with **potassium-sparing diuretics**, **potassium supplements**, or **ACE inhibitors**. May ↑ levels and risk of toxicity of **aliskiren**, **bosentan**, **colchicine**, **digoxin**, **etoposide**, **HMG-CoA reductase inhibitors**, **methotrexate**, **nifedipine**, **repaglinide**, and **sirolimus**. May ↑ levels and risk of toxicity of **ambrisentan**; do not titrate dose of ambrisentan up to maximum daily dose. May ↑ levels of and risk of bleeding with **dabigatran**; avoid concurrent use. May ↓ antibody response to **live-virus vaccines** and ↑ risk of adverse reactions; avoid concurrent use. Concurrent use with **tacrolimus** should be avoided. ↑ risk of renal impairment with **ciprofloxacin**, **aminoglycosides**, **vancomycin**, **trimethoprim/sulfamethoxazole**, **melphalan**, **amphotericin B**, **ketoconazole**, **colchicine**, **NSAIDS**, **cimetidine**, **ranitidine**, or **fibric acid derivatives**.

Drug-Natural Products: Concomitant use with **echinacea** and **melatonin** may interfere with immunosuppression. Use with **St. John's wort** may cause ↓ serum levels and organ rejection for transplant patients.

Drug-Food: Concurrent ingestion of **grapefruit or grapefruit juice** may ↑ serum levels and should be avoided. **Food** ↓ absorption of microemulsion products (Neoral).

Route/Dosage

Doses are adjusted on the basis of serum level monitoring.

Prevention of Transplant Rejection (Sandimmune)

PO (Adults and Children): 14–18 mg/kg/dose 4–12 hr before transplant then 5–15 mg/kg/day divided every 12–24 hr postoperatively, taper by 5% weekly to maintenance dose of 3–10 mg/kg/day.

IV (Adults and Children): 5–6 mg/kg/dose 4–12 hr before transplant, then 2–10 mg/kg/day in divided doses every 8–24 hr; change to PO as soon as possible.

Prevention of Transplant Rejection (Neoral)

PO (Adults and Children): 4–12 mg/kg/day divided every 12 hr (dose varies depending on organ transplanted).

Rheumatoid Arthritis (Neoral only)

PO (Adults and Children): 2.5 mg/kg/day given in 2 divided doses; may ↑ by 0.5–0.75 mg/kg/day after 8 and 12 wk, up to 4 mg/kg/day. ↓ dose by 25–50% if adverse reactions occur.

Severe Psoriasis (Neoral only)

PO (Adults): 2.5 mg/kg/day given in 2 divided doses, for at least 4 wk; then may ↑ by 0.5 mg/kg/day every 2 wk, up to 4 mg/kg/day. ↓ dose by 25–50% if adverse reactions occur.

Autoimmune Diseases (Neoral only)

PO (Adults and Children): 1–3 mg/kg/day.

Availability (generic available)

Microemulsion soft gelatin capsules (Gengraf, Neoral): 25 mg, 50 mg, 100 mg. **Microemulsion oral solution (Gengraf, Neoral):** 100 mg/mL. **Soft gelatin capsules (Sandimmune):** 25 mg, 100 mg. **Oral solution (Sandimmune):** 100 mg/mL. **Solution for injection (Sandimmune):** 50 mg/mL.

NURSING IMPLICATIONS

Assessment

- Monitor serum creatinine level, intake and output ratios, daily weight, and BP during therapy. Report significant changes.
- Assess for any new signs or symptoms that may be suggestive of progressive multifocal leukoencephalopathy (PML), an opportunistic infection of the brain caused by the Jakob Cruzfeldt (JC) virus, that may be fatal; withhold dose and notify health care professional promptly. PML symptoms may begin gradually (hemiparesis, apathy, confusion, cognitive deficiencies, and ataxia) and may include deteriorating renal function and renal graft loss.
- Monitor for signs and symptoms of posterior reversible encephalopathy syndrome (PRES) (impaired consciousness, convulsions, visual disturbances including blindness, loss of motor function, movement disorders and psychiatric disturbances, papilloedema, visual impairment). Usually reversible with discontinuation of cyclosporine. Occurs more often in patients with liver transplant than kidney transplant.
- **Prevention of Transplant Rejection:** Assess for symptoms of organ rejection throughout therapy.
- **IV:** Monitor patient for signs and symptoms of hypersensitivity (wheezing, dyspnea, flushing of face or neck) continuously during at least the first 30 min of each treatment and frequently thereafter. Oxygen, epinephrine, and equipment for treatment of anaphylaxis should be available with each IV dose.
- **Arthritis:** Assess pain and limitation of movement prior to and during administration.
- Prior to initiating therapy, perform a physical exam including BP on 2 occasions to determine baseline. Monitor BP every 2 wk during initial 3 mo, then monthly if stable. If hypertension occurs, dose should be reduced.
- **Psoriasis:** Assess skin lesions prior to and during therapy.
- ***Lab Test Considerations:*** Measure serum creatinine, BUN, CBC, magnesium, potassium, uric acid, and lipids at baseline, every 2 wk during initial ther-

apy, and then monthly if stable. Nephrotoxicity may occur; report significant increases.

- May cause hepatotoxicity; monitor for ↑ AST, ALT, alkaline phosphatase, amylase, and bilirubin.
- May cause ↑ serum potassium and uric acid levels and ↓ serum magnesium levels.
- Serum lipid levels may be ↑.
- ***Toxicity and Overdose:*** Evaluate serum cyclosporine levels periodically during therapy. Dose may be adjusted daily, in response to levels, during initiation of therapy. Guidelines for desired serum levels will vary among institutions.

Implementation

- Do not confuse cyclosporine with cyclophosphamide or cycloserine. Do not confuse Sandimmune (cyclosporine) with Sandostatin (octreotide).
- Given with other immunosuppressive agents. Protect transplant patients from staff and visitors who may carry infection. Maintain protective isolation as indicated.
- Microemulsion products (Neoral) and other products (Sandimmune) are not interchangeable.
- **PO:** Draw up oral solution in the pipette provided with the medication. Mix oral solution with milk, chocolate milk, apple juice, or orange juice, preferably at room temperature. Stir well and drink at once. Use a glass container and rinse with more diluent to ensure that total dose is taken. Administer oral doses with meals. Wipe pipette dry; do not wash after use.

IV Administration

- **Intermittent Infusion:** ***Diluent:*** Dilute each 1 mL (50 mg) of IV concentrate immediately before use with 20–100 mL of D5W or 0.9% NaCl for injection. Solution is stable for 24 hr in D5W. In 0.9% NaCl, it is stable for 6 hr in a polyvinylchloride container and 12 hr in a glass container at room temperature. ***Concentration:*** 2.5 mg/mL. ***Rate:*** Infuse slowly over 2–6 hr via infusion pump.
- **Continuous Infusion:** May be administered over 24 hr.
- **Y-Site Compatibility:** alemtuzumab, alfentanil, amikacin, aminocaproic acid, aminophylline, amiodarone, amphotericin B lipid complex, anidulafungin, argatroban, ascorbic acid, atropine, azithromycin, aztreonam, benztropine, bivalirudin, bleomycin, bumetanide, buprenorphine, butorphanol, calcium chloride, calcium gluconate, carboplatin, carmustine, caspofungin, cefazolin, cefotaxime, cefotetan, cefoxitin, ceftaroline, ceftazidime, ceftriaxone, cefuroxime, chloramphenicol, chlorpromazine, cisplatin, clindamycin, cyclophosphamide, cytarabine, dacarbazine, dactinomycin, daptomycin, daunorubicin hydrochloride, dexamethasone, dexmedetomidine, dexrazoxane, digoxin, diltiazem, diphenhydramine, dobutamine, docetaxel, dolasetron, dopamine, doxorubicin hydrochloride, doxorubicin liposomal, doxycycline, enalaprilat, ephedrine, epinephrine, epirubicin, epoetin alfa, ertapenem, erythromycin, esmolol, etoposide, etoposide phosphate, famotidine, fenoldopam, fentanyl, fluconazole, fludarabine, fluorouracil, folic acid, foscarnet, fosphenytoin, furosemide, ganciclovir, gemcitabine, gentamicin, glycopyrrolate, granisetron, heparin, hetastarch, hydrocortisone, hydromorphone, ifosfamide, imipenem/cilastatin, indomethacin, irinotecan, isoproterenol, ketorolac, labetalol, leucovorin calcium, levofloxacin, lidocaine, linezolid, lorazepam, mannitol, meperidine, meropenem, methotrexate, methylprednisolone, metoclopramide, metoprolol, metronidazole, micafungin, midazolam, milrinone, mitoxantrone, morphine, moxifloxacin, multivitamins, nafcillin, nicardipine, nitroglycerin, nitroprusside, norepinephrine, octreotide, ondansetron, oxacillin, oxaliplatin, oxytocin, paclitaxel, palonosetron, pamidronate, pancuronium, papaverine, pemetrexed, penicillin G, pentamidine, phentolamine, phenylephrine, phytonadione, piperacillin/tazobactam, potassium acetate, potassium chloride, procainamide, prochlorperazine, promethazine, propofol, propranolol, protamine, pyridoxine, quinupristin/dalfopristin, ranitidine, sargramostim, sodium acetate, sodium bicarbonate, streptokinase, succinylcholine, sufentanil, tacrolimus, theophylline, thiamine, thiotepa, tigecycline, tirofiban, tobramycin, tolazoline, topotecan, vancomycin, vasopressin, vecuronium, verapamil, vinblastine, vincristine, vinorelbine, zoledronic acid.
- **Y-Site Incompatibility:** amphotericin B liposome, cyanocobalamin, dantrolene, diazepam, idarubicin, nalbuphine, pentobarbital, phenobarbital, phenytoin, rituximab, trastuzumab, trimethoprim/sulfamethoxazole, voriconazole.

Patient/Family Teaching

- Instruct patient to take medication at the same time each day with meals, as directed. Take missed doses as soon as remembered within 12 hr. Do not skip doses or double up on missed doses. Do not discontinue medication without advice of health care professional.
- Reinforce the need for lifelong therapy to prevent transplant rejection. Review symptoms of rejection for transplanted organ, and stress need to notify health care professional immediately if they occur.
- Instruct patients and/or parents to notify health care professional if diarrhea develops; decreases absorption of cyclosporine and can result in rejection.
- Instruct patient to avoid grapefruit and grapefruit juice to prevent interaction with cyclosporine.
- Advise patient of common side effects (nephrotoxicity, ↑ BP, hand tremors, increased facial and body

hair, gingival hyperplasia). Advise patients that if hair growth is excessive, depilatories or waxing can be used.

- Teach patient the correct method for monitoring BP. Instruct patient to notify health care professional of significant changes in BP or if hematuria, increased frequency, cloudy urine, decreased urine output, fever, sore throat, tiredness, or unusual bruising occurs.
- Instruct patient on proper oral hygiene. Meticulous oral hygiene and dental examinations for teeth cleaning and plaque control every 3 mo will help decrease gingival inflammation and hyperplasia.
- Instruct patient to notify health care professional of all Rx or OTC medications, vitamins, or herbal products being taken and consult health care professional before taking other Rx, OTC, or herbal products or receiving any vaccinations while taking this medication.
- Advise patient to notify health care professional if pregnancy is planned or suspected, or if breast feeding.
- Emphasize the importance of follow-up exams and lab tests.

Evaluation/Desired Outcomes

- Prevention of rejection of transplanted tissues.
- Decrease in severity of pain in patients with rheumatoid arthritis.
- Increased ease of joint movement in patients with rheumatoid arthritis.
- Decrease in progression of psoriasis.

HIGH ALERT

cytarabine (sye-**tare**-a-been)

cytosine arabinoside, Cytosar, ~~Cytosar-U~~

Classification
Therapeutic: antineoplastics
Pharmacologic: antimetabolites

Indications

IV: Used mainly in combination chemotherapeutic regimens for the treatment of leukemias and non-Hodgkin's lymphomas. **IT:** Prophylaxis and treatment of meningeal leukemia.

Action

Inhibits DNA synthesis by inhibiting DNA polymerase (cell-cycle S-phase–specific). **Therapeutic Effects:** Death of rapidly replicating cells, particularly malignant ones.

Pharmacokinetics

Absorption: Absorption occurs from subcut sites, but blood levels are lower than with IV administration; IT administration results in negligible systemic exposure.

Distribution: Widely distributed; IV- and subcut-administered cytarabine crosses the blood-brain barrier but not in sufficient quantities. Crosses the placenta.

Metabolism and Excretion: Metabolized mostly by the liver; <10% excreted unchanged by the kidneys. Metabolism to inactive drug in the CSF is negligible because the enzyme that metabolizes it is present in very low concentrations in the CSF.

Half-life: *IV, subcut*—1–3 hr; *IT*—100–236 hr.

TIME/ACTION PROFILE (IV, subcut—effects on WBCs; IT—levels in CSF)

ROUTE	ONSET	PEAK	DURATION
Subcut, IV (1st phase)	24 hr	7–9 days	12 days
Subcut, IV (2nd phase)	15–24 days	15–24 days	25–34 days
IT	rapid	5 hr	14–28 days

Contraindications/Precautions

Contraindicated in: Hypersensitivity; OB, Lactation: Pregnancy or lactation; Active meningeal infection (IT only).

Use Cautiously in: Active infections; ↓ bone marrow reserve; Renal/hepatic impairment; Other chronic debilitating illnesses; Rep: Women of reproductive potential.

Adverse Reactions/Side Effects

CNS: CNS dysfunction (high dose), confusion, drowsiness, headache. **EENT:** corneal toxicity (high dose), hemorrhagic conjunctivitis (high dose), visual disturbances (including blindness). **Resp:** PULMONARY EDEMA (high dose). **CV:** edema. **GI:** HEPATOTOXICITY, nausea, vomiting, severe GI ulceration (high dose), stomatitis. **GU:** urinary incontinence. **Derm:** alopecia, rash. **Endo:** sterility. **Hemat:** *(less with IT use)*—anemia, leukopenia, thrombocytopenia. **Metab:** hyperuricemia. **Neuro:** *Intrathecal only*—CHEMICAL ARACHNOIDITIS, abnormal gait. **Misc:** cytarabine syndrome, fever.

Interactions

Drug-Drug: ↑ bone marrow depression with other **antineoplastics** or **radiation therapy**. ↑ risk of cardiomyopathy when used in high-dose regimens with **cyclophosphamide**. May ↓ antibody response to **live-virus vaccines** and ↑ risk of adverse reactions. May ↓ absorption of **digoxin** tablets. May ↓ the efficacy of **gentamicin** when used to treat *Klebsiella pneumoniae* infections. Recent treatment with **asparaginase** may ↑ risk of pancreatitis. ↑ neurotoxicity with concurrently administered **IT antineoplastics** (IT only).

Route/Dosage

Dose regimens vary widely.

IV (Adults): *Induction dose*—200 mg/m²/day for 5 days every 2 wk as a single agent *or* 2–6 mg/kg/day

(100–200 mg/m²/day) as a single daily dose *or* in 2–3 divided doses for 5–10 days or until remission occurs as part of combination chemotherapy. *Maintenance*—70–200 mg/m²/day for 2–5 days monthly. *Refractory leukemias/lymphomas*—3 g/m² every 12 hr for up to 12 doses.
Subcut (Adults): *Maintenance*—1–1.5 mg/kg every 1–4 wk.
IT (Adults): Usual dose = 30 mg/m² every 4 days; range = 5–75 mg/m² once daily for 4 days or every 4 days until CNS findings normalize, followed by one additional treatment.

Availability (generic available)

Powder for injection: 100 mg, 500 mg, 1 g, 2 g. **Solution for injection:** 20 mg/mL, 100 mg/mL. ***In combination with:*** daunorubicin (Vyxeos). See Appendix B.

NURSING IMPLICATIONS

Assessment

- Monitor for bone marrow depression. Assess for bleeding (bleeding gums, bruising, petechiae, guaiac stools, urine, and emesis) and avoid IM injections and taking rectal temperatures if platelet count is low. Apply pressure to venipuncture sites for 10 min. Assess for signs of infection during neutropenia. Anemia may occur. Monitor for increased fatigue, dyspnea, and orthostatic hypotension.
- Monitor intake and output ratios and daily weights. Report significant changes in totals.
- Monitor for symptoms of gout (increased uric acid, joint pain, edema). Encourage patient to drink at least 2 L of fluid each day. Allopurinol may decrease uric acid levels. Alkalinization of urine may increase excretion of uric acid.
- Assess nutritional status. Nausea and vomiting may occur within 1 hr of administration, especially if IV dose is administered rapidly, less severe if medication is infused slowly. Administering an antiemetic prior to and periodically throughout therapy and adjusting diet as tolerated may help maintain fluid and electrolyte balance and nutritional status.
- Monitor patient for development of *cytarabine* or *ara-C syndrome* (fever, myalgia, bone pain, chest pain, maculopapular rash, conjunctivitis, malaise), which usually occurs 6–12 hr following administration. Corticosteroids may be used for treatment or prevention. If patient responds to corticosteroids, continue cytarabine and corticosteroids.
- Assess patient for respiratory distress and pulmonary edema. Occurs with high doses rarely; may be fatal.
- Monitor patient for signs of anaphylaxis (rash, dyspnea, swelling). Epinephrine, corticosteroids, and resuscitation equipment should be readily available.
- **IT:** CSF flow should be evaluated prior to IT therapy. Administer directly into CSF via an intraventricular reservoir or by direct injection into the lumbar sac slowly over 1–5 min. Following administration by lumbar puncture, patient should lie flat for 1 hr.

  Chemical arachnoiditis (nausea, vomiting, headache, fever, back pain, CSF pleocytosis and neck rigidity, neck pain, or meningism) is an expected side effect of IT cytarabine. Incidence and severity of symptoms may be decreased with coadministration of dexamethasone. 4 mg bid, PO or IV, for 5 days beginning on day of injection.
- Monitor patients receiving IT therapy continuously for the development of neurotoxicity (myelopathy, personality changes, dysarthria, ataxia, confusion, somnolence, coma). If neurotoxicity develops, decrease amount of subsequent doses and discontinue if neurotoxicity persists. Risk may be increased if cytarabine is administered intrathecally and IV within a few days.
- ***Lab Test Considerations:*** Monitor CBC with differential and platelet count prior to and frequently during therapy. Leukocyte counts begin to drop within 24 hr of administration. The initial nadir occurs in 7–9 days. After a small ↑ in the count, the second, deeper nadir occurs 15–24 days after administration. Platelet counts begin to ↓ 5 days after a dose, with a nadir at 12–15 days. Leukocyte and platelet counts usually begin to ↑ 10 days after the nadirs. Therapy is usually withdrawn if leukocyte count is <1000/mm³ or platelet count is <50,000/mm³. Bone marrow aspirations are recommended every 2 wk until remission occurs.
- Monitor renal (BUN and serum creatinine) and hepatic function (AST, ALT, bilirubin, alkaline phosphatase, and LDH) prior to and routinely during therapy.
- May cause ↑ uric acid concentrations.

Implementation

- ***High Alert:*** Fatalities have occurred with chemotherapeutic agents. Before administering, clarify all ambiguous orders; double-check single, daily, and course-of-therapy dose limits; have second practitioner independently double-check original order, calculations, and infusion pump settings.
- ***High Alert:*** Do not confuse high-dose and regular therapy. Fatalities have occurred with high-dose therapy.
- Solution should be prepared in a biologic cabinet. Wear gloves, gown, and mask while handling IV medication. Discard IV equipment in specially designated containers.
- May be given subcut, direct IV, intermittent IV, continuous IV, or IT.
- **IV Subcut:** Reconstitute 100-mg vials with 5 mL of bacteriostatic water for injection with benzyl alcohol

0.9% for a concentration of 20 mg/mL. Reconstitute 500-mg vials with 10 mL for a concentration of 50 mg/mL, 1-g vials with 10 mL, and 2-g vials with 20 mL for a concentration of 100 mg/mL. Reconstituted solution is stable for 48 hr. Do not administer a cloudy or hazy solution.

IV Administration

- **IV Push:** ***Diluent:*** Administer undiluted. ***Concentration:*** 100 mg/mL. ***Rate:*** Administer each 100 mg over 1–3 min.
- **Intermittent Infusion:** ***Diluent:*** May be further diluted in 0.9% NaCl, D5W, D10W, D5/0.9% NaCl, Ringer's solution, LR, or D5/LR. ***Concentration:*** Dilute doses in 100 mL of diluent. ***Rate:*** Infuse over 15–30 min.
- **Continuous Infusion:** Rate and concentration for IV infusion are ordered individually.
- **Y-Site Compatibility:** acyclovir, alemtuzumab, alfentanil, amifostine, amikacin, aminocaproic acid, aminophylline, amphotericin B lipid complex, amphotericin B liposome, ampicillin, ampicillin/sulbactam, anidulafungin, argatroban, azithromycin, aztreonam, bivalirudin, bleomycin, bumetanide, buprenorphine, butorphanol, calcium chloride, calcium gluconate, carboplatin, carmustine, cefazolin, cefepime, cefotaxime, cefotetan, cefoxitin, ceftazidime, ceftriaxone, cefuroxime, chlorpromazine, ciprofloxacin, cisatracurium, cisplatin, cladribine, clindamycin, cyclophosphamide, cyclosporine, dacarbazine, daunorubicin, dexamethasone, dexmedetomidine, dexrazoxane, digoxin, diltiazem, diphenhydramine, dobutamine, docetaxel, dopamine, doxorubicin, doxorubicin liposome, doxycycline, droperidol, enalaprilat, ephedrine, epinephrine, ertapenem, erythromycin, esmolol, etoposide, etoposide phosphate, famotidine, fenoldopam, fentanyl, filgrastim, fluconazole, fludarabine, foscarnet, fosphenytoin, furosemide, gemcitabine, gentamicin, granisetron, haloperidol, heparin, hydrocortisone, hydromorphone, idarubicin, ifosfamide, imipenem/cilastatin, insulin, irinotecan, isoproterenol, ketorolac, labetalol, leucovorin, levofloxacin, levorphanol, lidocaine, linezolid, lorazepam, magnesium sulfate, mannitol, melphalan, meperidine, meropenem, mesna, methohexital, methotrexate, methylprednisolone, metoclopramide, metoprolol, metronidazole, midazolam, milrinone, mitoxantrone, morphine, moxifloxacin, nalbuphine, naloxone, nicardipine, nitroglycerin, nitroprusside, norepinephrine, octreotide, ondansetron, oxaliplatin, paclitaxel, palonosetron, pamidronate, pancuronium, pantoprazole, pemetrexed, pentamidine, pentobarbital, phenobarbital, phenylephrine, piperacillin/tazobactam, potassium acetate, potassium chloride, potassium phosphate, procainamide, prochlorperazine, promethazine, propofol, propranolol, quinupristin/dalfopristin, ranitidine, remifentanil, rituximab, rocuronium, sargramostim, sodium acetate, sodium bicarbonate, sodium phosphate, succinylcholine, sufentanil, tacrolimus, theophylline, thiopental, thiotepa, tigecycline, tirofiban, tobramycin, trastuzumab, trimethoprim/sulfamethoxazole, vancomycin, vasopressin, vecuronium, verapamil, vincristine, vinorelbine, voriconazole, zidovudine, zoledronic acid.
- **Y-Site Incompatibility:** allopurinol, amiodarone, amphotericin B deoxycholate, daptomycin, diazepam, ganciclovir, phenytoin.
- **IT: Reconstitute IT doses with preservative-free 0.9% NaCl or autologous spinal fluid. Use immediately to prevent bacterial contamination. Instruct patient to lie flat for 1 hr following IT injection. Monitor for immediate toxic reactions.**

Patient/Family Teaching

- Caution patient to avoid crowds and persons with known infections. Report symptoms of infection (fever, chills, cough, hoarseness, sore throat, lower back or side pain, painful or difficult urination) immediately.
- Instruct patient to report unusual bleeding. Advise patient of thrombocytopenia precautions (use soft toothbrush and electric razor, avoid falls, do not drink alcoholic beverages or take medication containing aspirin or NSAIDs; may precipitate gastric bleeding).
- Instruct patient to inspect oral mucosa for redness and ulceration. If mouth sores occur, advise patient to use sponge brush and rinse mouth with water after eating and drinking. Stomatitis may require treatment with opioid analgesics.
- Instruct patient not to receive any vaccinations without advice of health care professional.
- Rep: Advise patient that this medication may have teratogenic effects. Contraception should be used during therapy and for at least 4 mo after therapy is concluded.
- Emphasize the need for periodic lab tests to monitor for side effects.
- **IT:** Inform patient about the expected side effects (headache, nausea, vomiting, fever) and about early signs of neurotoxicity. Instruct patient to notify health care professional if these signs occur.

Evaluation/Desired Outcomes

- Improvement of hematopoietic values in leukemias.
- Decrease in size and spread of the tumor in non-Hodgkin's lymphomas. Therapy is continued every 2 wk until patient is in complete remission or thrombocyte count or leukocyte count falls below acceptable levels.
- Treatment of lymphomatous meningitis.

D

dabigatran (da-bi-**gat**-ran)

Pradaxa

Classification

Therapeutic: anticoagulants

Pharmacologic: thrombin inhibitors

Indications

To reduce the risk of stroke/systemic embolization associated with nonvalvular atrial fibrillation. Treatment of deep vein thrombosis or pulmonary embolism in patients who have been treated with parenteral anticoagulant for 5–10 days. To reduce the risk of recurrence of deep vein thrombosis or pulmonary embolism in patients who have been previously treated. Prevention of deep vein thrombosis and pulmonary embolism following hip replacement surgery.

Action

Acts as a direct inhibitor of thrombin. **Therapeutic Effects:** Lowered risk of thrombotic sequelae (stroke and systemic embolization) of nonvalvular atrial fibrillation.

Pharmacokinetics

Absorption: 3–7% absorbed following oral administration.

Distribution: Unknown.

Metabolism and Excretion: Of the amount absorbed, mostly excreted by kidneys (80%); 86% of ingested dose is eliminated in feces due to poor bioavailability.

Half-life: 12–17 hr.

TIME/ACTION PROFILE (effects on coagulation)

ROUTE	ONSET	PEAK	DURATION
PO	within hrs	unknown	2 days†

†Following discontinuation, 3–5 days in renal impairment.

Contraindications/Precautions

Contraindicated in: Hypersensitivity; Active pathological bleeding; Concurrent use of P-glycoprotein (P-gp) inducers; Prosthetic heart valves (mechanical or bioprosthetic); OB: Use not recommended in pregnancy; Lactation: Lactation.

Use Cautiously in: Neuroaxial spinal anesthesia or spinal puncture, especially if concurrent with an indwelling epidural catheter, drugs affecting hemostasis, history of traumatic/repeated spinal puncture or spinal deformity (↑ risk of spinal hematoma); Concurrent medications/pre-existing conditions that ↑ bleeding risk (other anticoagulants, antiplatelet agents, fibrinolytics, heparins, chronic NSAID use, labor and delivery); Renal impairment; Surgical procedures (discontinue 1–2 days prior if CCr ≥50 mL/min or 3–4 days prior if CCr <50 mL/min; Pedi: Safety and effectiveness not established; Geri: ↑ risk of bleeding.

Adverse Reactions/Side Effects

GI: abdominal pain, diarrhea, dyspepsia, gastritis, esophageal ulceration, nausea. **Hemat:** BLEEDING, thrombocytopenia. **Misc:** HYPERSENSITIVITY REACTIONS (including anaphylaxis and angioedema).

Interactions

Drug-Drug: Concurrent use of other **anticoagulants**, **antiplatelet agents**, **fibrinolytics**, **heparins**, **prasugrel**, **clopidogrel**, or chronic use of **NSAIDs** ↑ risk of bleeding. Concurrent use of **P-gp inducers** including **rifampin** ↓ levels and effectiveness; avoid concurrent use. **P-gp inhibitors**, including **dronedarone**, **ketoconazole (systemic)**, **verapamil**, **quinidine**, and **ticagrelor** may ↑ levels and the risk of bleeding; concomitant use should be avoided in patients with CCr 15–30 mL/min.

Route/Dosage

Reduction in Risk of Stroke/Systemic Embolism in Nonvalvular Atrial Fibrillation

PO (Adults): 150 mg twice daily.

Renal Impairment

PO (Adults): *CCr 30–50 mL/min and taking dronedarone or systemic ketoconazole*—75 mg twice daily; *CCr <30 mL/min and taking P-gp inhibitor*—Avoid concomitant use; *CCr 15–30 mL/min*—75 mg twice daily; *CCr <15 mL/min or on dialysis*—Not recommended.

Treatment of and Reduction in Risk of Recurrence of Deep Vein Thrombosis or Pulmonary Embolism

PO (Adults): 150 mg twice daily.

Renal Impairment

PO (Adults): *CCr <50 mL/min and taking P-gp inhibitor*—Avoid concomitant use; *CCr <30 mL/min or on dialysis*—Not recommended.

Prevention of Deep Vein Thrombosis and Pulmonary Embolism Following Hip Replacement Surgery

PO (Adults): 110 mg taken 1–4 hr after surgery and once hemostasis achieved, then 220 mg once daily for 28–35 days; if unable to start on day of surgery, once hemostasis achieved, start with 220 mg once daily.

Renal Impairment

PO (Adults): *CCr ≤30 mL/min or on dialysis*—Not recommended; *CCr <50 mL/min and taking P-gp inhibitor*—Avoid concomitant use.

Availability
Capsules: 75 mg, 110 mg, 150 mg.

NURSING IMPLICATIONS
Assessment
- Assess for symptoms of stroke or peripheral vascular disease periodically during therapy.
- Assess for symptoms of bleeding and blood loss; may be fatal. If reversal of anticoagulant effect is required, may use idarucizumab.
- ***Lab Test Considerations:*** Use aPTT or ECT, not INR, to assess anticoagulant activity, if needed.
- Monitor renal function prior to and periodically during therapy. Patients with renal impairment may require dose reduction or discontinuation.

Implementation
- Do not confuse dabigatran with vigabatrin. Do not confuse Pradaxa (dabigatran) with Plavix (clopidogrel).
- When *converting from warfarin*, discontinue warfarin and start dabigatran when INR is <2.0.
- When *converting from dabigatran to warfarin*, adjust starting time based on creatinine clearance. For *CCr >50 mL/min*, start warfarin 3 days before discontinuing dabigatran. For *CCr 31–50 mL/min*, start warfarin 2 days before discontinuing dabigatran. For *CCr 15–30 mL/min*, start warfarin 1 day before discontinuing dabigatran. For *CCr <15 mL/min*, no recommendations can be made. INR will better reflect warfarin's effect after dabigatran has been stopped for at least 2 days.
- When *converting from parenteral anticoagulants*, start dabigatran up to 2 hr before next dose of parenteral drug is due or at time of discontinuation of parenteral therapy.
- When *converting from dabigatran to parenteral anticoagulants*, wait 12 hrs (CCr ≥30 mL/min) or 24 hr (CCr <30 mL/min) after last dose of dabigatran before initiating parenteral anticoagulant therapy.
- *For surgery*, discontinue dabigatran 1–2 days (CCr ≥50 mL/min) or 3–5 days (CCr <50 mL/min) before invasive or surgical procedures; consider longer times for major surgery, spinal puncture, or placement of a spinal or epidural catheter. If surgery cannot be delayed, bleeding risk is ↑. Assess bleeding risk with ecarin clotting time (ECT) or a PTT if ECT is not available.
- **PO:** Administer twice daily with a full glass of water without regard to food. Swallow capsule whole; do not open, crush, or chew; may result in increased exposure.
- If dabigatran is discontinued, consider starting another anticoagulant; discontinuation of dabigatran increases risk of thromboembolic events.

Patient/Family Teaching
- Instruct patient to take dabigatran as directed. Take missed doses as soon as remembered within 6 hr. If <6 hr until next dose, skip dose and take next dose when scheduled; do not double doses. Do not discontinue without consulting health care professional. If temporarily discontinued, restart as soon as possible. Store dabigatran at room temperature. After opening bottle, use within 4 mo; discard unused dabigatran after 4 mo. Advise patient to read *Medication Guide* before starting therapy and with each Rx refill in case of changes.
- Inform patient that they may bleed more easily or longer than usual. Advise patient to notify health care professional immediately if signs of bleeding (unusual bruising; pink or brown urine; red or black, tarry stools; coughing up blood; vomiting blood; pain or swelling in a joint; headache; dizziness; weakness; recurring nose bleeds; unusual bleeding from gums; heavier than normal menstrual bleeding; dyspepsia; abdominal pain; epigastric pain) occur.
- Advise patient to notify health care professional of medication regimen prior to treatment or surgery.
- Instruct patient to notify health care professional of all Rx or OTC medications, vitamins, or herbal products being taken and consult health care professional before taking any new medications.
- Advise female patient to notify health care professional if pregnancy is planned or suspected or if breast feeding.

Evaluation/Desired Outcomes
- Reduction in the risk of stroke and systemic embolism.

dabrafenib (da-**braf**-e-nib)
Tafinlar

Classification
Therapeutic: antineoplastics
Pharmacologic: kinase inhibitors

Indications
Metastatic/unresectable melanoma in patients with the BRAF V600E mutation. Metastatic/unresectable melanoma in patients with the BRAF V600E or V600K mutation (in combination with trametinib). Adjuvant treatment of melanoma in patients with the BRAF V600E or V600K mutation and lymph node involvement following complete resection (in combination with trametinib). Metastatic non-small-cell lung cancer (NSCLC) in patients with the BRAF V600E mutation (in combination with trametinib). Locally advanced or metastatic anaplastic thyroid cancer (ATC) in patients with the BRAF V600E mutation and no satisfactory locoregional treatment options (in combination with trametinib).

Action
Inhibits kinase, an enzyme that promotes cell proliferation. **Therapeutic Effects:** Decreased spread/progression of melanoma, NSCLC, and ATC.

Pharmacokinetics

Absorption: Well absorbed (95%) following oral administration.

Distribution: Unknown.

Protein Binding: 99.7%.

Metabolism and Excretion: Mostly metabolized by CYP 2C8 and CYP3A4 enzyme systems; two metabolites (hydroxy-dabrafenib and desmethyl-1–dabrafenib) have antineoplastic activity. Excreted as metabolites in feces (72%) and urine (23%).

Half-life: *Dabrafenib*—8 hr; *hydroxy-dabrafenib*—10 hr, *desmethyl-1–dabrafenib*—21–22 hr.

TIME/ACTION PROFILE (progression-free survival)

ROUTE	ONSET	PEAK	DURATION
PO	within 1 mo	1–2 mo	8 mo

Contraindications/Precautions

Contraindicated in: OB: Pregnancy (may cause fetal harm); Lactation: Lactation; Concurrent use of CYP 3A4/CYP2C8 inhibitors or inducers (may significantly alter levels and effects).

Use Cautiously in: BRAF Wild-type melanoma (may ↑ proliferation); History of glucose-6–phosphate dehydrogenase deficiency (may cause hemolytic anemia); Moderate to severe hepatic impairment (blood levels may be ↑); Moderate to severe renal impairment; OB: Patients with reproductive potential (hormonal contraceptives may be less effective, additional methods required); Pedi: Safety and effectiveness not established.

Adverse Reactions/Side Effects

CNS: headache, fatigue. **CV:** HF, THROMBOEMBOLISM. **Derm:** alopecia, hyperkeratosis, palmar-plantar erythrodysesthesia, papilloma, cutaneous squamous cell carcinoma. **EENT:** iritis, retinal detachment, uveitis. **Endo:** hyperglycemia. **F and E:** hypophosphatemia, hyponatremia. **GI:** constipation, pancreatitis. **Hemat:** BLEEDING. **MS:** arthralgia, back pain, myalgia. **Resp:** cough, nasopharyngitis. **Misc:** MALIGNANCY, fever including serious febrile reactions, ↑ alkaline phosphatase, chills, tumor promotion.

Interactions

Drug-Drug: Concurrent use of strong inhibitors of CYP3A4 or CYP2C8, including **ketoconazole**, **nefazodone**, **clarithromycin**, and **gemfibrozil** ↑ levels and the risk of toxicity and should be avoided. Careful monitoring for toxicity is required. Concurrent use of **strong inducers of CYP3A4 or CYP2C8** including **carbamazepine**, **phenobarbital**, **phenytoin**, and **rifampin** ↓ levels and may ↓ effectiveness. Careful monitoring for decreased results is required. **Drugs that ↑ gastric pH** including **antacids**, **H_2–receptor antagonists** and **proton pump inhibitors** may ↓ levels and effectiveness. May ↓ effectiveness of other **CYP3A4 substrates** and **CYP2C9 substrates**, including **midazolam**, **warfarin**, **dexamethasone**, and **hormonal contraceptives**.

Drug-Natural Products: St. John's wort ↓ levels and may ↓ effectiveness; concurrent use should be avoided.

Route/Dosage

PO (Adults): 150 mg twice daily, continued until disease progression or unacceptable toxicity.

Availability

Capsules: 50 mg, 75 mg.

NURSING IMPLICATIONS

Assessment

- Perform skin examinations prior to starting therapy and every 2 mo during and for 6 mo after completion of therapy. *If intolerable Grade 2 skin toxicity, Grade 3 or Grade 4 occurs,* hold dabrafenib for up to 3 wk. If improved, resume at a lower dose. If not improved, permanently discontinue.
- Monitor temperature. *If fever is 101.3°F to 104°F,* hold dabrafenib until fever resolves, then resume at same dose. *If fever is >104°F or complicated by rigors, hypotension, dehydration, or renal failure,* hold until fever resolves, then resume at a reduced dose. *For first reduction,* decrease dose to 100 mg twice daily. *For second dose reduction,* decrease dose to 75 mg twice daily. *For third dose reduction,* decrease dose to 50 mg twice daily. *If unable to tolerate 50 mg twice daily,* discontinue dabrafenib.
- Monitor for signs and symptoms of ocular toxicities (blurred vision, loss of vision, other vision changes, see color dots, halo around objects), swelling, redness, photophobia, eye pain). May require steroid and mydriatic ophthalmic drops. *If iritis occurs,* do not modify dabrafenib dose. If severe uveitis or mild to moderate uveitis that does not respond to ocular therapy, hold dabrafenib for up to 6 wk. If improved to Grade 0–1, resume at same or lower dose. If not improved, permanently discontinue therapy.
- Monitor cardiac function (LVEF) by ECG or multigated acquisition (MUGA) scan before starting therapy with dabrafenib with trametinib, one mo after initiation of therapy, and then at 2- to 3-mo intervals during therapy. *If symptomatic HF occurs with absolute decrease in LVEF >20% from baseline that is below LLN,* hold dabrafenib until improved to institutional LLN and absolute decrease to ≤10% compared to baseline, then resume at same dose.
- Monitor for signs and symptoms of venous thromboembolism (shortness of breath, chest pain, arm or leg swelling, cool or pale arm or leg) during therapy. *If uncomplicated deep vein thrombosis*

(DVT) or pulmonary embolus (PE) occurs, do not modify dabrafenib dose. Withhold trametinib for up to 3 wk. If improved to Grade 0-1, resume at lower dose. If not improved, permanently discontinue. *If life-threatening PE occurs,* permanently discontinue dabrafenib and trametinib.

- Monitor for signs and symptoms of interstitial lung disease or pneumonitis (cough, dyspnea, hypoxia, pleural effusion, infiltrates) during therapy. If signs and symptoms occur, do not modify dabrafenib dose; permanently discontinue trametinib.
- Assess for bleeding (headaches, dizziness, feeling weak, coughing up blood or blood clots, vomiting blood or vomit looks like "coffee grounds," red or black stools that look like tar) during therapy. *If Grade 3 hemorrhagic event occurs,* withhold dabrafenib and trametinib for up to 3 wk, if improved resume at lower level. *If Grade 4 hemorrhagic event occurs,* permanently discontinue dabrafenib and trametinib.
- ***Lab Test Considerations:*** Obtain a negative pregnancy test prior to starting therapy.
- Information on FDA-approved tests for the detection of BRAF V600 mutations in melanoma is available at: http://www.fda.gov/CompanionDiagnostics.
- May cause hyperglycemia requiring increase in dose of or initiation of insulin or oral hypoglycemic agents. Monitor serum glucose levels in patients with pre-existing diabetes or hyperglycemia.
- May cause hypophosphatemia, ↑ alkaline phosphatase, and hyponatremia.
- Monitor for hemolytic anemia in patients with glucose-6–phosphate dehydrogenase (G6PD) deficiency.

Implementation

- Evidence of BRAF V600E or V600K mutation status must be confirmed prior to starting therapy with dabrafenib.
- **PO:** Administer twice daily about 12 hrs apart. Administer on an empty stomach at least 1 hr before or 2 hrs after a meal. Swallow capsules whole; do not open, crush, break, or chew.
- When administered with trametinib, administer once-daily dose of trametinib at same time each day with either morning or evening dose of dabrafenib.

Patient/Family Teaching

- Instruct patient to take dabrafenib as directed at least 1 hr before or 2 hrs after meals. Take missed doses as soon as remembered unless within 6 hrs of next dose, then skip missed dose and take regularly scheduled dose. Advise patient to read *Medication Guide* before starting therapy and with each Rx refill in case of changes.
- Inform patient that dabrafenib increases risk of developing new cutaneous malignancies. Notify health care professional immediately if new lesions (wart, skin sore or reddish bump that bleeds or does not heal) or changes in size or color of existing moles or lesions occur.
- Advise patient to notify health care professional of all Rx or OTC medications, vitamins, or herbal products being taken and to consult with health care professional before taking other medications, especially St. John's wort.
- Inform patient of potential side effects. Advise patient to notify health care professional if fever, signs and symptoms of hyperglycemia (increased thirst, urinating more often than normal, breath smells like fruit), or eye problems, bleeding, thromboembolism, heart failure (heart pounding or racing, shortness of breath, swelling of ankles and feet, feeling lightheaded) occur.
- Rep: Advise females of reproductive potential and males (including those who have had vasectomies) with female partner of reproductive potential to use a highly effective form of contraception during and for at least 2 wk after last dose of dabrafenib. Use a non-hormonal form of contraception; dabrafenib may decrease effectiveness of hormonal contraceptives. Advise patient to notify health care professional if pregnancy is suspected and to avoid breast feeding during and for 2 wk after last dose. Advise patients to seek counseling on fertility and family planning prior to beginning therapy; may permanently impair fertility in females and males.

Evaluation/Desired Outcomes

- Decrease in progression of malignant melanoma, NSCLC, and ATC.

HIGH ALERT

dacarbazine (da-**kar**-ba-zeen)

DTIC, DTIC-Dome

Classification

Therapeutic: antineoplastics

Pharmacologic: alkylating agents

Indications

Treatment of metastatic malignant melanoma (single agent). Treatment of Hodgkin's disease as second-line therapy (with other agents).

Action

Disrupts DNA and RNA synthesis (cell-cycle phase–nonspecific). **Therapeutic Effects:** Death of rapidly growing tissue cells, especially malignant ones.

Pharmacokinetics

Absorption: IV administration results in complete bioavailability.

Distribution: Large volume of distribution; probably concentrates in liver; some CNS penetration.

Metabolism and Excretion: 50% metabolized by the liver, 50% excreted unchanged by the kidneys.

Half-life: 5 hr (↑ in renal and hepatic dysfunction).

TIME/ACTION PROFILE (effects on blood counts)

ROUTE	ONSET	PEAK	DURATION
IV (WBCs)	16–20 days	21–25 days	3–5 days
IV (platelets)	unknown	16 days	3–5 days

Contraindications/Precautions

Contraindicated in: Hypersensitivity; OB, Lactation: Pregnancy or lactation.

Use Cautiously in: Active infections; Bone marrow depression; Pedi: Children (safety not established); Renal dysfunction; Hepatic dysfunction.

Adverse Reactions/Side Effects

GI: HEPATIC NECROSIS, anorexia, nausea, vomiting, diarrhea, hepatic vein thrombosis. **Derm:** alopecia, facial flushing, photosensitivity, rash. **Endo:** gonadal suppression. **Hemat:** anemia, leukopenia, thrombocytopenia. **Local:** pain at IV site, phlebitis at IV site, tissue necrosis. **MS:** myalgia. **Neuro:** facial paresthesia. **Misc:** ANAPHYLAXIS, fever, flu-like syndrome, malaise.

Interactions

Drug-Drug: Additive bone marrow depression with other **antineoplastics**. **Carbamazepine**, **phenobarbital**, and **rifampin** may ↑ metabolism and decrease effectiveness. Blood levels may be ↑ with **amiodarone**, **ciprofloxacin**, **fluvoxamine**, **ketoconazole**, **ofloxacin**, **isoniazid**, or **miconazole**. May ↓ antibody response to **live-virus vaccines** and ↑ risk of adverse reactions.

Route/Dosage

Other regimens are used.

IV (Adults): *Malignant melanoma*—2–4.5 mg/kg/day for 10 days administered every 4 wk *or* 250 mg/m²/day for 5 days administered every 3 wk. *Hodgkin's disease*—150 mg/m²/day for 5 days (in combination with other agents) administered every 4 wk *or* 375 mg/m² (in combination with other agents) administered every 15 days.

Availability

Powder for injection: 200 mg.

NURSING IMPLICATIONS

Assessment

- Monitor vital signs prior to and frequently during therapy.
- Monitor for bone marrow depression. Assess for bleeding (bleeding gums, bruising, petechiae, guaiac stools, urine, and emesis) and avoid IM injections and rectal temperatures if platelet count is low. Apply pressure to venipuncture sites for 10 min. Assess for signs of infection during neutropenia. Anemia may occur. Monitor for increased fatigue, dyspnea, and orthostatic hypotension.
- Monitor IV site closely. Dacarbazine is an irritant. Instruct patient to notify health care professional immediately if discomfort at IV site occurs. Discontinue IV immediately if infiltration occurs. Applications of hot packs may relieve pain, burning sensation, and irritation at injection site.
- Monitor intake and output, appetite, and nutritional intake. Assess for nausea and vomiting, which may be severe and last 1–12 hr. Administration of an antiemetic prior to and periodically during therapy, restricting oral intake for 4–6 hr prior to administration, and adjusting diet as tolerated may help maintain fluid and electrolyte balance and nutritional status. Nausea usually decreases on subsequent doses.
- ***Lab Test Considerations:*** Monitor CBC and differential prior to and periodically throughout therapy. The nadir of thrombocytopenia occurs in 16 days. The nadir of leukopenia occurs in 3–4 wk. Recovery begins in 5 days. Withhold dose and notify physician if platelet count is <100,000/mm³ or leukocyte count is <4000/mm³.
- Monitor for increased AST, ALT, BUN, and serum creatinine. May cause hepatic necrosis.

Implementation

- ***High Alert:*** Fatalities have occurred with chemotherapeutic agents. Before administering, clarify all ambiguous orders; double-check single, daily, and course-of-therapy dose limits; have second practitioner independently double-check original order, calculations, and infusion pump settings.

IV Administration

- Prepare solution in a biologic cabinet. Wear gloves, gown, and mask while handling medication. Discard equipment in designated containers.
- Reconstitute each 200-mg vial with 19.7 mL of sterile water for injection. Solution is colorless or clear yellow. Do not use solution that has turned pink. ***Concentration:*** 10 mg/mL. Solution is stable for 8 hr at room temperature and for 72 hr if refrigerated.
- **Intermittent Infusion:** ***Diluent:*** Further dilute with up to 250 mL of D5W or 0.9% NaCl. Stable for 24 hr if refrigerated or 8 hr at room temperature. ***Rate:*** Administer over 30–60 min.
- **Y-Site Compatibility:** amifostine, aztreonam, bivalirudin, caspofungin, daptomycin, dexmedetomidine, docetaxel, doxorubicin liposome, ertapenem, etoposide phosphate, fenoldopam, filgrastim, fludarabine, granisetron, hetastarch, levofloxacin, melphalan, octreotide, ondansetron, oxaliplatin, paclitaxel, palonosetron, quinupristin/dalfopristin, sargramostim, thiotepa, tigecycline, tirofiban, vinorelbine, voriconazole.
- **Y-Site Incompatibility:** allopurinol, amphotericin B liposome, cefepime, pantoprazole, pemetrexed, piperacillin/tazobactam.

Patient/Family Teaching

- Instruct patient to notify health care professional if fever; chills; sore throat; signs of infection; bleeding gums; bruising; petechiae; abdominal pain; yellowing of eyes; or blood in urine, stool, or emesis occurs. Caution patient to avoid crowds and persons with known infections. Instruct patient to use soft toothbrush and electric razor. Patients should be cautioned not to drink alcoholic beverages or take products containing aspirin or NSAIDs; may increase GI irritation.
- May cause photosensitivity. Instruct patient to avoid sunlight or wear protective clothing and use sunscreen for 2 days after therapy.
- Instruct patient to inform health care professional if flu-like syndrome occurs. Symptoms include fever, myalgia, and general malaise. May occur after several courses of therapy. Usually occurs 1 wk after administration. May persist for 1–3 wk. Acetaminophen may be used for relief of symptoms.
- Discuss with patient the possibility of hair loss. Explore coping strategies.
- Advise patient of the need for a nonhormonal method of contraception.
- Instruct patient not to receive any vaccinations without advice of health care professional.

Evaluation/Desired Outcomes

- Decrease in size and spread of malignant melanoma or Hodgkin's lymphoma.

dalbavancin (dal-ba-**van**-sin)

Dalvance

Classification

Therapeutic: anti-infectives

Pharmacologic: lipoglycopeptides

Indications

Treatment of skin/skin structure infections due to susceptible bacteria.

Action

Binds to bacterial cell wall resulting in cell death. **Therapeutic Effects:** Bactericidal action against susceptible bacteria with resolution of infection. **Spectrum:** Active against *Staphylococcus aureus* (including methicillin-susceptible and resistant strains), *Streptococcus agalactiae*, *Streptococcus anginosus* (including *S. anginosus*, *S. intermidius*, and *S. constellatus*) and *Streptococcus pyogenes*.

Pharmacokinetics

Absorption: IV administration results in complete bioavailability.

Distribution: Penetrates tissues and fluids.

Metabolism and Excretion: 33% eliminated unchanged in urine, 12% eliminated as inactive metabolite, 20% excreted in feces.

Half-life: 346 hr.

TIME/ACTION PROFILE (blood levels)

ROUTE	ONSET	PEAK	DURATION
IV	unknown	end of infusion	1 wk

Contraindications/Precautions

Contraindicated in: Hypersensitivity.

Use Cautiously in: Renal impairment (dose adjustment required for CCr <30 mL/min; Moderate to severe hepatic impairment; Geri: Consider age-related decrease in renal function; OB: Use during pregnancy only if potential benefit justifies potential risk to the fetus; Lactation: Use cautiously if breast feeding; Pedi: Safe and effective use in children has not been established.

Adverse Reactions/Side Effects

CNS: headache. **Derm:** pruritus, rash. **GI:** CLOSTRIDIUM DIFFICILE-ASSOCIATED DIARRHEA (CDAD), ↑ liver enzymes, nausea. **Misc:** HYPERSENSITIVITY REACTIONS (including anaphylaxis), infusion reactions (including Red-Man Syndrome).

Interactions

Drug-Drug: None noted.

Route/Dosage

IV (Adults): 1500 mg once *or* 1000 mg followed 1 wk later by 500 mg.

Renal Impairment

IV (Adults): *CCr <30 mL/min*—1125 mg once *or* 750 mg followed 1 wk later by 375 mg.

Availability

Lyophylized powder for injection (requires reconstitution and dilution): 500 mg/vial.

NURSING IMPLICATIONS

Assessment

- Assess for infection (vital signs; appearance of wound, sputum, urine, and stool; WBC) at beginning of and during therapy.
- Obtain specimens for culture and sensitivity prior to therapy. First dose may be given before receiving results.
- Monitor bowel function. Diarrhea, abdominal cramping, fever, and bloody stools should be reported to health care professional promptly as a sign of Clostridium difficile-associated diarrhea (CDAD). May begin up to 2 mo following cessation of therapy.
- Monitor for infusion reactions (Red-man syndrome—flushing of upper body, urticaria, pruritus, rash, back pain). May resolve with stopping or slowing infusion.
- ***Lab Test Considerations:*** Monitor hepatic function tests. May cause ↑ ALT, AST, and bilirubin.

Implementation

IV Administration

- **Intermittent Infusion:** Reconstitute with 25 mL of sterile water or D5W in each 500 mg vial. Alternate gentle swirling and inverting to avoid foaming, until completely dissolved. Do not shake. Reconstituted vial contains a clear colorless to yellow solution. Do not administer solutions that are discolored or contain particulate matter. Transfer reconstituted solution into D5W. ***Concentration:*** 1 mg/mL to 5 mg/mL. Discard unused solution. May be refrigerated or kept at room temperature; do not freeze. Infuse within 48 hr of reconstitution. Do not administer solutions containing particulate matter. ***Rate:*** Infuse over 30 min.
- **Y-Site Incompatibility:** Do not infuse with other medications or electrolytes. Saline solutions may cause precipitation. Flush line before and after infusion with D5W.

Patient/Family Teaching

- Instruct patient to notify health care professional if signs and symptoms of hypersensitivity reactions (rash, hives, dyspnea, facial swelling) occur.
- Instruct patient to notify health care professional immediately if diarrhea, abdominal cramping, fever, or bloody stools occur and not to treat with antidiarrheals without consulting health care professionals.
- Advise patient to notify health care professional of all Rx or OTC medications, vitamins, or herbal products being taken and to consult with health care professional before taking other medications.
- Advise female patients to use effective contraception during therapy and to notify health care professional if pregnancy is suspected or if breast feeding.
- Instruct the patient to notify health care professional if symptoms do not improve.

Evaluation/Desired Outcomes

- Resolution of the signs and symptoms of infection. Length of time for complete resolution depends on the organism and site of infection.

dalfampridine

(dal-**fam**-pri-deen)

Ampyra, ♣Fampyra

Classification

Therapeutic: anti-multiple sclerosis agents

Pharmacologic: potassium channel blockers

Indications

Treatment of multiple sclerosis, to improve walking speed.

Action

Acts as a potassium channel blocker, which may increase conduction of action potentials. **Therapeutic Effects:** Increased walking speed in patients with multiple sclerosis.

Pharmacokinetics

Absorption: Rapidly and completely absorbed (96%).

Distribution: Unknown.

Metabolism and Excretion: 96% eliminated in urine, 0.5% in feces.

Half-life: 5.2–6.5 hr.

TIME/ACTION PROFILE (improvement in walking speed)

ROUTE	ONSET	PEAK	DURATION
PO	unknown	3–4 hr	24 hr

Contraindications/Precautions

Contraindicated in: Hypersensitivity; History of seizures; Moderate/severe renal impairment (CCr ≤50 mL/min) (↑ risk of seizures); Lactation: Avoid use.

Use Cautiously in: Mild renal impairment (CCr 51–80 mL/min) (↑ risk of seizures); Geri: Consider age-related ↓ in renal function; OB: Use only if potential benefit justifies potential risk to fetus; Pedi: Safety and effectiveness not established.

Adverse Reactions/Side Effects

CNS: SEIZURES, dizziness, headache, insomnia, weakness. **EENT:** nasopharyngitis, pharyngolaryngeal pain. **GI:** constipation, dyspepsia, nausea. **GU:** urinary tract infection. **MS:** back pain. **Neuro:** balance disorder, multiple sclerosis relapse, paresthesia. **Misc:** ANAPHYLAXIS.

Interactions

Drug-Drug: Cimetidine may ↑ levels and ↑ risk of seizures.

Route/Dosage

PO (Adults): 10 mg twice daily.

Availability (generic available)

Extended-release tablets: 10 mg.

NURSING IMPLICATIONS

Assessment

- Assess walking speed in patients with multiple sclerosis prior to and periodically during therapy.
- Monitor for seizures during therapy, risk increases with increased dose. If seizure occurs, discontinue therapy.
- Monitor for signs and symptoms of anaphylaxis (dyspnea, wheezing, urticaria, angioedema of the throat or tongue) during therapy.

- ***Lab Test Considerations:*** Monitor CCr prior to and at least yearly during therapy; renal impairment may require dose reduction or discontinuation.

Implementation

- Administer tablets twice daily approximately 12 hr apart without regard to food. Swallow tablets whole; do not break, crush, chew, or dissolve.

Patient/Family Teaching

- Instruct patient to take dalfampridine as directed, with approximately 12 hrs between tablets. If a dose is missed, omit and take next scheduled dose on time; do not double doses. May increase risk of seizures. Advise patient to read *Medication Guide* prior to beginning therapy and with each Rx refill; new information may be available.
- Instruct patient to notify health care professional of all Rx or OTC medications, vitamins, or herbal products being taken and consult health care professional before taking any new medications.
- If a seizure or signs or symptoms of anaphylaxis occur, advise patient to notify health care professional immediately, to discontinue dalfampridine and do not restart medication.
- Advise female patient to notify health care professional if pregnancy is planned or suspected or if breast feeding.

Evaluation/Desired Outcomes

- Improved walking and increased walking speed in patients with multiple sclerosis.

dalteparin, See HEPARINS (LOW MOLECULAR WEIGHT).

dantrolene (dan-troe-leen)

Dantrium, Ryanodex

Classification

Therapeutic: skeletal muscle relaxants (direct acting)

Indications

PO: Treatment of spasticity associated with: Spinal cord injury, stroke, cerebral palsy, multiple sclerosis. Prophylaxis of malignant hyperthermia. **IV:** Emergency treatment of malignant hyperthermia. Prevention of malignant hyperthermia in patients at high risk. **Unlabeled Use:** Management of neuroleptic malignant syndrome.

Action

Acts directly on skeletal muscle, causing relaxation by decreasing calcium release from sarcoplasmic reticulum in muscle cells. Prevents intense catabolic process associated with malignant hyperthermia. **Therapeutic Effects:** Reduction of muscle spasticity. Treatment and prevention of malignant hyperthermia.

Pharmacokinetics

Absorption: 35% absorbed after oral administration. IV administration results in complete bioavailability.

Distribution: Unknown.

Metabolism and Excretion: Almost entirely metabolized by the liver.

Half-life: 8.7–11.4 hr.

TIME/ACTION PROFILE (effects on spasticity)

ROUTE	ONSET	PEAK	DURATION
PO	1 wk	unknown	6–12 hr
IV	rapid	rapid	unknown

Contraindications/Precautions

Contraindicated in: No contraindications to IV form in treatment of malignant hyperthermia; Lactation: Lactation; Situations in which spasticity is used to maintain posture or balance.

Use Cautiously in: Cardiac, pulmonary, or previous liver disease; Women and patients >35 yr (↑ risk of hepatotoxicity); Geri: Use lowest possible dose (may have ↑ risk of hepatotoxicity); OB: Use only if benefit outweighs potential risk to fetus.

Adverse Reactions/Side Effects

CNS: drowsiness, muscle weakness, confusion, dizziness, headache, insomnia, malaise, nervousness. **EENT:** excessive lacrimation, visual disturbances. **Resp:** dyspnea, pleural effusions, respiratory depression. **CV:** changes in BP, heart failure, tachycardia. **GI:** HEPATOTOXICITY, diarrhea, anorexia, cramps, dysphagia, GI bleeding, nausea, vomiting. **GU:** crystalluria, dysuria, frequency, erectile dysfunction, incontinence, nocturia. **Derm:** flushing, pruritus, sweating, urticaria. **Hemat:** anemia, aplastic anemia, eosinophilia, leukopenia, thrombocytopenia. **Local:** irritation at IV site, phlebitis. **MS:** myalgia. **Misc:** ANAPHYLAXIS, chills, drooling, fever.

Interactions

Drug-Drug: Calcium channel blockers may ↑ risk of cardiovsacular collapse; avoid concomitant use. Additive CNS depression with **CNS depressants**, including **alcohol**, **antihistamines**, **opioid analgesics**, **sedative/hypnotics**, and parenteral **magnesium sulfate**. ↑ risk of hepatotoxicity with other **hepatotoxic agents** or **estrogens**. ↑ risk of arrhythmias with **verapamil**. ↑ neuromuscular blocking effects of **vecuronium**.

Drug-Natural Products: Concomitant use of **kava-kava**, **valerian**, **chamomile**, or **hops** can ↑ CNS depression.

Route/Dosage

PO (Adults): *Spasticity*—25 mg once daily for 7 days, then 25 mg 2 times daily for 7 days, then 50 mg 3 times daily for 7 days, then 100 mg 3 times daily; may ↑ to 100 mg 4 times daily, if needed. *Prevention of*

malignant hyperthermia—4–8 mg/kg/day in 3–4 divided doses for 1–2 days before procedure, last dose 3–4 hr preop. *Posthyperthermic crisis follow-up*—4–8 mg/kg/day in 3–4 divided doses for 1–3 days after IV treatment.
PO (Children >5 yr): *Spasticity*—0.5 mg/kg once daily for 7 days, then 0.5 mg/kg 3 times daily for 7 days, then 1 mg/kg 3 times daily for 7 days, then 2 mg/kg 3 times daily (not to exceed 400 mg/day). *Prevention of malignant hyperthermia*—4–8 mg/kg/day in 3–4 divided doses for 1–2 days before procedure, last dose 3–4 hr preop. *Posthyperthermic crisis follow-up*—4–8 mg/kg/day in 3–4 divided doses for 1–3 days after IV treatment.
IV (Adults and Children): *Treatment of malignant hyperthermia*—at least 1 mg/kg, continued until symptoms ↓ or a cumulative dose of 10 mg/kg has been given. If symptoms reappear, dose may be repeated. *Prevention of malignant hyperthermia*—2.5 mg/kg given 75 min before surgery.

Availability (generic available)

Capsules: 25 mg, 50 mg, 100 mg. **Powder for injection:** 20 mg/vial, 250 mg/vial.

NURSING IMPLICATIONS

Assessment

- Assess bowel function periodically. Persistent diarrhea may warrant discontinuation of therapy.
- **Muscle Spasticity:** Assess neuromuscular status and muscle spasticity before initiating and periodically during therapy to determine response.
- **Malignant Hyperthermia:** Assess previous anesthesia history of all surgical patients. Also assess for family history of reactions to anesthesia (malignant hyperthermia or perioperative death).
- Monitor ECG, vital signs, electrolytes, and urine output continuously when administering IV for malignant hyperthermia.
- Monitor patient for difficulty swallowing and choking during meals on the day of administration.
- ***Lab Test Considerations:*** Monitor liver function frequently during therapy. Liver function abnormalities (↑ AST, ALT, alkaline phosphatase, bilirubin, GGTP) may require discontinuation of therapy.
- Evaluate renal function and CBC before and periodically during therapy in patients receiving prolonged therapy.

Implementation

- **PO:** If gastric irritation becomes a problem, may be administered with food. Oral suspensions may be made by opening capsules and adding them to fruit juices or other liquids. Drink immediately after mixing.
- Oral dose for spasticity should be divided into 4 doses/day.
- Oral dose is not indicated for neuroleptic malignant syndrome.

IV Administration

- Reconstitute each 20 mg of **Dantrium** with 60 mL of sterile water for injection (without a bacteriostatic agent). Shake until solution is clear. Solution must be used within 6 hr. Protect diluted solution from direct light.
- Reconstitute **Ryanodex** by adding 5 mL of sterile water for injection; do not reconstitute with other solutions. Shake vial to ensure uniform orange suspension. Do not administer solutions that are discolored or contain particulate matter. Solution is stable for 6 hrs at room temperature.

Treatment of Malignant Hyperthermia

- **IV Push:** Administer reconstituted solution without further dilution. ***Rate:*** Administer each single dose by rapid continuous IV push through Y-tubing. Follow immediately with subsequent doses as indicated. Medication is very irritating to tissues; observe infusion site frequently to avoid extravasation.

Prevention of Malignant Hyperthermia

- **IV Push:** Rates of products for prevention differ. ***Rate:*** Inject **Ryanodex** over at least 1 min starting 75 min before surgery into catheter with free flowing 0.9% NaCl or D5W or into a patent indwelling catheter, flush before and after injection.
- **Intermittent Infusion:** Reconstitute required number of **Dantrium** vials as above and transfer to a larger volume sterile plastic bag (do not use glass bottles). ***Rate:*** Administer over 1 hr beginning 75 min before anesthesia.
- **Y-Site Compatibility:** acyclovir, paclitaxel, palonosetron.
- **Y-Site Incompatibility:** alemtuzumab, alfentanil, amikacin, aminophylline, amphotericin B deoxycholate, amphotericin B lipid complex, ampicillin, ampicillin/sulbactam, anidulafungin, argatroban, arsenic trioxide, ascorbic acid, asparaginase, atropine, azathioprine, aztreonam, benztropine, bivalirudin, bleomycin, bumetanide, buprenorphine, butorphanol, calcium chloride, calcium gluconate, carmustine, caspofungin, cefotaxime, cefotetan, cefoxitin, ceftazidime, ceftriaxone, cefuroxime, chloramphenicol, chlorpromazine, cisplatin, clindamycin, cyanocobalamin, cyclosporine, dactinomycin, daptomycin, dexamethasone, diazepam, diazoxide, digoxin, diltiazem, diphenhydramine, dobutamine, docetaxel, dopamine, doxorubicin liposome, doxycycline, enalaprilat, ephedrine, epinephrine, epoetin alfa, ertapenem, erythromycin, esmolol, etoposide, etoposide phosphate, famotidine, fenoldopam, fentanyl, fluconazole, fludarabine, folic acid, foscarnet, fosphenytoin, furosemide, ganciclo-

vir, gemcitabine, gentamicin, glycopyrrolate, granisetron, haloperidol, heparin, hetastarch, hydralazine, hydrocortisone, hydromorphone, hydroxyzine, idarubicin, imipenem/cilastatin, indomethacin, insulin, irinotecan, isoproterenol, ketorolac, labetalol, leucovorin, lidocaine, linezolid, lorazepam, magnesium sulfate, mannitol, meperidine, mesna, metaraminol, methyldopate, methylprednisolone, metoclopramide, metoprolol, metronidazole, midazolam, milrinone, mitoxantrone, morphine, moxifloxacin, multivitamins, mycophenolate, nafcillin, nalbuphine, naloxone, nitroglycerin, nitroprusside, norepinephrine, octreotide, ondansetron, oxacillin, oxaliplatin, oxytocin, pamidronate, pancuronium, pantoprazole, papaverine, pemetrexed, penicillin G, pentamidine, pentobarbital, phenobarbital, phenylephrine, phenytoin, phytonadione, piperacillin/tazobactam, potassium acetate, potassium chloride, procainamide, prochlorperazine, promethazine, propranolol, protamine, pyridoxime, ranitidine, sodium acetate, sodium bicarbonate, streptokinase, succinylcholine, sufentanil, tacrolimus, theophylline, thiamine, thiotepa, tigecycline, tirofiban, tobramycin, tolazoline, topotecan, trimethoprim/sulfamethoxazole, vancomycin, vasopressin, vecuronium, verapamil, vinblastine, vinorelbine, voriconazole, zoledronic acid.

Patient/Family Teaching

- Advise patient not to take more medication than the amount prescribed, to minimize risk of hepatotoxicity and other side effects. If a dose is missed, do not take unless remembered within 1 hr. Do not double doses.
- May cause dizziness, drowsiness, visual disturbances, and muscle weakness. Advise patient to avoid driving and other activities requiring alertness until response to drug is known. After IV dose for surgery, patients may experience decreased grip strength, leg weakness, light-headedness, and difficulty swallowing for up to 48 hr. Caution patients to avoid activities requiring alertness and to use caution when walking down stairs and eating during this period.
- Advise patient to avoid taking alcohol or other CNS depressants concurrently with this medication.
- Instruct patient to notify health care professional if rash; itching; yellow eyes or skin; dark urine; or clay-colored, bloody, or black, tarry stools occur or if nausea, weakness, malaise, fatigue, or diarrhea persists. May require discontinuation of therapy.
- Advise patient to wear sunscreen and protective clothing to prevent photosensitivity reactions.
- Emphasize the importance of follow-up exams to check progress in long-term therapy and blood tests to monitor for side effects.
- **Malignant Hyperthermia:** Patients with malignant hyperthemia should carry identification describing disease process at all times.

Evaluation/Desired Outcomes

- Relief of muscle spasm in musculoskeletal conditions. One wk or more may be required to see improvement; if there is no observed improvement in 45 days, the medication is usually discontinued.
- Prevention of or decrease in temperature and skeletal rigidity in malignant hyperthermia.

DAPTOmycin (dap-to-**mye**-sin)
Cubicin, Cubicin RF

Classification
Therapeutic: anti-infectives
Pharmacologic: cyclic lipopeptide antibacterial agents

Indications

Complicated skin and skin structure infections caused by Gram-positive bacteria. *Staphylococcus aureus* bacteremia, including right-sided infective endocarditis caused by methicillin-susceptible and methicillin-resistant strains (in adults). *Staphylococcus aureus* bacteremia (in pediatric patients).

Action

Causes rapid depolarization of membrane potential following binding to bacterial membrane; this results in inhibition of protein, DNA, and RNA synthesis. **Therapeutic Effects:** Death of bacteria with resolution of infection. **Spectrum:** Active against *Staphylococcus aureus* (including methicillin-resistant strains), *Streptococcus pyogenes*, *Streptococcus agalactiae*, some *Streptococcus dysgalactiae*, and *Enterococcus faecalis* (vancomycin-susceptible strains).

Pharmacokinetics

Absorption: IV administration results in complete bioavailability.
Distribution: Unknown.
Protein Binding: 92%.
Metabolism and Excretion: Metabolism not known; mostly excreted by kidneys.
Half-life: 8.1 hr.

TIME/ACTION PROFILE

ROUTE	ONSET	PEAK	DURATION
IV	rapid	end of infusion	24 hr

Contraindications/Precautions

Contraindicated in: Hypersensitivity.
Use Cautiously in: CCr <30 mL/min (dose ↓ required); Moderate-to-severe renal impairment (may have ↓ clinical response); Geri: May have ↓ clinical response with ↑ risk of adverse reactions; OB: Use only if clearly needed; Lactation: Lactation; Pedi: Children <1 yr (↑ risk of muscular, neuromuscular, and CNS effects; avoid use).

Adverse Reactions/Side Effects

CNS: dizziness. **CV:** hypertension, hypotension. **Derm:** DRUG RASH WITH EOSINOPHILIA AND SYSTEMIC SYMPTOMS (DRESS), pruritus, rash. **GI:** CLOSTRIDIUM DIFFICILE-ASSOCIATED DIARRHEA (CDAD), constipation, diarrhea, nausea, vomiting, ↑ liver enzymes. **GU:** renal failure. **Hemat:** anemia. **Local:** injection site reactions. **MS:** ↑ creatine kinase. **Resp:** EOSINOPHILIC PNEUMONIA, dyspnea. **Misc:** ANGIOEDEMA, fever.

Interactions

Drug-Drug: Tobramycin ↑ blood levels. Concurrent **HMG-CoA reductase inhibitors** may ↑ the risk of myopathy.

Route/Dosage

Complicated Skin/Skin Structure Infections

IV (Adults): 4 mg/kg every 24 hr for 7–14 days.
IV (Children 12–17 yr): 5 mg/kg every 24 hr for up to 14 days.
IV (Children 7–11 yr): 7 mg/kg every 24 hr for up to 14 days.
IV (Children 2–6 yr): 9 mg/kg every 24 hr for up to 14 days.
IV (Children 1–<2 yr): 10 mg/kg every 24 hr for up to 14 days.

Renal Impairment

IV (Adults): *CCr <30 mL/min*—4 mg/kg every 48 hr for 7–14 days; *Hemodialysis and CAPD*—4 mg/kg every 48 hr for 7–14 days with dose administered after hemodialysis on hemodialysis days.

Staphylococcus aureus Bacteremia/Right-Sided Infective Endocarditis

IV (Adults): 6 mg/kg every 24 hr for 2–6 wk.

Renal Impairment

IV (Adults): *CCr <30 mL/min*—6 mg/kg every 48 hr for 2–6 wk; *Hemodialysis and CAPD*—6 mg/kg every 48 hr for 2–6 wk with dose administered after hemodialysis on hemodialysis days.

Staphylococcus aureus Bacteremia

IV (Children 12–17 yr): 7 mg/kg every 24 hr for up to 42 days.
IV (Children 7–11 yr): 9 mg/kg every 24 hr for up to 42 days.
IV (Children 1–6 yr): 12 mg/kg every 24 hr for up to 42 days.

Availability (generic available)

Lyophilized powder for injection (requires reconstitution): 350 mg/vial, 500 mg/vial.

NURSING IMPLICATIONS

Assessment

- Assess for infection (vital signs; appearance of wound, sputum, urine, and stool; WBC) at beginning of and throughout therapy.
- Monitor bowel function. Diarrhea, abdominal cramping, fever, and bloody stools should be reported to health care professional promptly as a sign of Clostridium difficile-associated diarrhea (CDAD). May begin up to several wk following cessation of therapy.
- Monitor for signs and symptoms of eosinophilic pneumonia (new onset or worsening fever, dyspnea, difficulty breathing, new infiltrates on chest imaging studies). Discontinue daptomycin if symptoms occur.
- Monitor for signs and symptoms of DRESS (fever, rash, lymphadenopathy, and/or facial swelling, associated with involvement of other organ systems (hepatitis, nephritis, hematologic abnormalities, myocarditis, myositis) during therapy. May resemble an acute viral infection. Eosinophilia is often present. Discontinue therapy if signs occur.
- Monitor for development of muscle pain or weakness, particularly of distal extremities. Discontinue daptomycin in patients with unexplained signs and symptoms of myopathy in conjunction with CPK elevation >1000 units/L, or in patients without reported symptoms who have marked elevations in CPK >2000 units/L. Consider temporarily suspending agents associated with rhabdomyolysis (HMG-CoA reductase inhibitors) in patients receiving daptomycin.
- ***Lab Test Considerations:*** Monitor CPK weekly, more frequently in patients with unexplained ↑. Discontinue daptomycin if CPK >1000 units/L and signs and symptoms of myopathy occur. In patients with renal insufficiency, monitor both renal function and CPK more frequently.
- May cause false prolongation of PT and ↑ INR.

Implementation

- Do not confuse daptomycin with dactinomycin. Do not confuse Cubicin with Cubicin RF.

IV Administration

Cubicin

- **IV Push:** Reconstitute 500-mg vial with 10 mL of 0.9% NaCl inserted toward wall of vial. Rotate vial gently to wet powder. Allow to stand for 10 min undisturbed. Swirl vial gently to completely reconstitute solution. Reconstituted vials are stable for 12 hr at room temperature or 48 hr if refrigerated. ***Concentration:*** 50 mg/mL. ***Rate:*** Administer over 2 min (for adults only).

- **Intermittent Infusion:** *Adults:* ***Diluent:*** Dilute further in 50 mL of 0.9% NaCl. Solution is stable for 12 hr at room temperature or 48 hr if refrigerated. Do not administer solutions that are cloudy or contain a precipitate. ***Rate:*** Infuse over 30 min. Do not infuse daptomycin with ReadyMED elastomeric infusion pumps due to incompatibility.
- **Intermittent Infusion:** *Children 1–6 yrs:* ***Diluent:*** Dilute further into a 25 mL IV infusion bag of 0.9% NaCl. ***Rate:*** Infuse over 60 min at a rate of 0.42 mL/min.
- **Intermittent Infusion:** *Children 7–17 yrs:* ***Diluent:*** Dilute further into a 50 mL IV infusion bag of 0.9% NaCl. ***Rate:*** Infuse over 30 min at a rate of 1.67 mL/min.

Cubicin RF

- **IV Push:** Reconstitute with 10 mL of sterile water for injection or bacteriostatic water for injection through center of rubber stopper into vial. Use a beveled sterile transfer needle that is 21 gauge or smaller, pointing transfer needle toward the wall of the vial. Rotate or swirl vial to mix. ***Concentration:*** 50 mg/mL. Do not use saline solutions to reconstitute. Remove reconstituted solution from vial using a beveled sterile needle that is 21 gauge or smaller. Solution is stable for 1 day at room temperature or 3 days if refrigerated. Do not administer solutions that are cloudy or contain particulate matter. ***Rate:*** Inject over 2 min (for adults only).
- **Intermittent Infusion:** *Adults:* ***Diluent:*** Dilute further into a 50 mL IV infusion bag of 0.9% NaCl. If reconstituted with sterile water, solution is stable for 19 hrs at room temperature or 3 days if refrigerated. If reconstituted with bacteriostatic water, solution is stable for 2 days at room temperature or 5 days if refrigerated. ***Rate:*** Infuse over 30 min.
- **Intermittent Infusion:** *Children 1–6 yrs:* ***Diluent:*** Dilute further into a 25 mL IV infusion bag of 0.9% NaCl. ***Rate:*** Infuse over 60 min at a rate of 0.42 mL/min.
- **Intermittent Infusion:** *Children 7–17 yrs:* ***Diluent:*** Dilute further into a 50 mL IV infusion bag of 0.9% NaCl. ***Rate:*** Infuse over 30 min at a rate of 1.67 mL/min.
- **Y-Site Compatibility:** alfentanil, amifostine, amikacin, aminocaproic acid, aminophylline, amiodarone, amphotericin B liposome, ampicillin, ampicillin/sulbactam, argatroban, arsenic trioxide, azithromycin, aztreonam, bivalirudin, bleomycin, bumetanide, buprenorphine, busulfan, butorphanol, calcium chloride, calcium gluconate, cangrelor, carboplatin, carmustine, caspofungin, cefazolin, cefepime, cefotaxime, cefotetan, cefoxitin, ceftazidime, ceftriaxone, cefuroxime, chloramphenicol, chlorpromazine, ciprofloxacin, cisatracurium, cisplatin, clindamycin, cyclophosphamide, cyclosporine, dacarbazine, dactinomycin, daunorubicin, dexamethasone sodium phosphate, dexmedetomidine, dexrazoxane, digoxin, diltiazem, diphenhydramine, dobutamine, docetaxel, dopamine, doxorubicin, doxorubicin liposome, doxycycline, droperidol, enalaprilat, ephedrine, epinephrine, epirubicin, eptifibatide, ertapenem, erythromycin, esmolol, etoposide, etoposide phosphate, famotidine, fenoldopam, fentanyl, fluconazole, fludarabine, fluorouracil, foscarnet, fosphenytoin, furosemide, ganciclovir, gentamicin, glycopyrrolate, granisetron, haloperidol, heparin, hydralazine, hydrocortisone sodium succinate, hydromorphone, idarubicin, ifosfamide, insulin, irinotecan, isoproterenol, ketorolac, labetalol, leucovorin, levofloxacin, lidocaine, linezolid, lorazepam, magnesium sulfate, mannitol, melphalan, meperidine, meropenem, mesna, methylprednisolone sodium succinate, metoclopramide, metoprolol, midazolam, milrinone, mitoxantrone, morphine, moxifloxacin, mycophenolate, nafcillin, nalbuphine, naloxone, nicardipine, nitroprusside, norepinephrine, octreotide, ondansetron, oxaliplatin, oxytocin, paclitaxel, palonosetron, pamidronate, pancuronium, pemetrexed, pentamidine, phenobarbital, phentolamine, phenylephrine, piperacillin/tazobactam, potassium acetate, potassium chloride, potassium phosphate, procainamide, prochlorperazine, promethazine, propranolol, quinupristin/dalfopristin, ranitidine, rocuronium, sodium acetate, sodium bicarbonate, sodium phosphate, succinylcholine, tacrolimus, theophylline, thiotepa, tigecycline, tirofiban, tobramycin, topotecan, trimethoprim/sulfamethoxazole, vasopressin, vecuronium, verapamil, vinblastine, vincristine, vinorelbine, voriconazole, zidovudine, zoledronic acid.
- **Y-Site Incompatibility:** acyclovir, alemtuzumab, allopurinol, amphotericin B deoxycholate, amphotericin B lipid complex, cytarabine, dantrolene, gemcitabine, imipenem/cilastatin, methotrexate, metronidazole, mitomycin, nitroglycerin, pantoprazole, pentobarbital, phenytoin, remifentanil, streptozocin, sufentanil, thiopental, vancomycin.

Patient/Family Teaching

- Inform patient of purpose of daptomycin.
- Instruct patient to notify health care professional if fever and diarrhea develop, especially if stool contains blood, pus, or mucus. Advise patient not to treat diarrhea without consulting health care professional.
- May cause dizziness. Caution patient to avoid driving or other activities requiring alertness until response to medication is known.
- Advise patient to notify health care professional immediately if signs and symptoms of eosinophilic pneumonia occur.
- Advise females of reproductive potential to notify health care professional if pregnancy is planned or suspected, or if breast feeding.

Evaluation/Desired Outcomes

- Resolution of the signs and symptoms of infection. Length of time for complete resolution depends on the organism and site of infection.

darbepoetin (dar-be-**poh**-e-tin)
Aranesp

Classification
Therapeutic: antianemics
Pharmacologic: hormones (rDNA), erythropoiesis stimulating agents (ESA)

Indications

Anemia associated with chronic kidney disease (CKD). Chemotherapy-induced anemia in patients with non-myeloid malignancies when there is ≥2 additional mo of planned chemotherapy.

Action

Stimulates erythropoiesis (production of red blood cells). **Therapeutic Effects:** Maintains and may elevate red blood cell counts, decreasing the need for transfusions.

Pharmacokinetics

Absorption: 30–50% following subcut administration; IV administration results in complete bioavailability.
Distribution: Confined to the intravascular space.
Metabolism and Excretion: Unknown.
Half-life: *Subcut*—49 hr; *IV*—21 hr.

TIME/ACTION PROFILE (↑ in RBCs)

ROUTE	ONSET	PEAK	DURATION
IV, Subcut	2–6 wk	unknown	unknown

Contraindications/Precautions

Contraindicated in: Hypersensitivity; Uncontrolled hypertension; Patients with cancer receiving hormonal agents, biologic products, or radiotherapy, unless also receiving concomitant myelosuppressive chemotherapy; Patients receiving chemotherapy when anticipated outcome is cure; Patients with cancer receiving myelosuppressive chemotherapy in whom the anemia can be managed by transfusion; Patients who require immediate correction of anemia when RBC transfusions can be used instead.
Use Cautiously in: Cardiovascular disease or stroke; Underlying hematologic diseases, including hemolytic anemia, sickle-cell anemia, thalassemia and porphyria (safety not established); OB, Lactation: Safety not established.

Adverse Reactions/Side Effects

CNS: SEIZURES, dizziness, fatigue, headache, weakness. **CV:** HF, MI, STROKE, THROMBOEMBOLIC EVENTS (especially with hemoglobin >11 g/dL), edema, hypertension, hypotension, chest pain. **Derm:** ERYTHEMA MULTIFORME, STEVENS-JOHNSON SYNDROME, TOXIC EPIDERMAL NECROLYSIS, pruritus. **GI:** abdominal pain, nausea, diarrhea, vomiting, constipation. **Hemat:** pure red cell aplasia. **MS:** myalgia, arthralgia, back pain, limb pain. **Resp:** cough, dyspnea, bronchitis. **Misc:** ALLERGIC REACTIONS (including anaphylaxis and angioedema), ↑ MORTALITY AND ↑ TUMOR GROWTH (WITH HEMOGLOBIN ≥12 G/DL), fever, sepsis.

Interactions

Drug-Drug: None reported.

Route/Dosage

Anemia due to Chronic Kidney Disease

(Do not initiate if hemoglobin ≥10 g/dL; should only consider initiating therapy in patients not on dialysis if rate of hemoglobin decline indicates likelihood of requiring a red blood cell transfusion and a goal is to reduce the risk of alloimmunization and/or red blood cell transfusion risks).

IV, Subcut (Adults): *Starting treatment with darbepoetin (no previous epoetin)*—0.45 mcg/kg once weekly or 0.75 mcg/kg every 2 wk (for patients on dialysis); 0.45 mcg/kg every 4 wk (for patients not on dialysis); use lowest dose sufficient to ↓ the need for red blood cell transfusions (do not exceed hemoglobin of 10 g/dL [patients not on dialysis] or 11 g/dL [patients on dialysis]); if Hgb ↑ by >1.0 g/dL in 2 wk, ↓ dose by 25%; if Hgb ↑ by <1.0 g/dL after 4 wk of therapy (with adequate iron stores), ↑ dose by 25%; do not ↑ dose more frequently than every 4 wk. *Conversion from epoetin to darbepoetin*—weekly epoetin dose <2500 units = 6.25 mcg/wk darbepoetin, weekly epoetin dose 2500–4999 units = 12.5 mcg/wk darbepoetin, weekly epoetin dose 5000–10,999 units = 25 mcg/wk darbepoetin, weekly epoetin dose 11,000–17,999 units = 40 mcg/wk darbepoetin, weekly epoetin dose 18,000–33,999 units = 60 mcg/wk darbepoetin, weekly epoetin dose 34,000–89,999 units = 100 mcg/wk darbepoetin, weekly epoetin dose >90,000 units = 200 mcg/wk darbepoetin.

IV, Subcut (Children): *Starting treatment with darbepoetin (no previous epoetin)*—0.45 mcg/kg once weekly (may also start with 0.75 mcg/kg every 2 wk in patients not on dialysis); use lowest dose sufficient to ↓ the need for red blood cell transfusions (do not exceed hemoglobin of 12 g/dL; if Hgb ↑ by >1.0 g/dL in 2 wk, ↓ dose by 25%; if Hgb ↑ by <1.0 g/dL after 4 wk of therapy (with adequate iron stores), ↑ dose by 25%; do not ↑ dose more frequently than every 4 wk.

Anemia due to Chemotherapy

(Use only for chemotherapy-related anemia and discontinue when chemotherapy course is completed; do not initiate if hemoglobin ≥10 g/dL.).

Subcut (Adults): 2.25 mcg/kg weekly or 500 mcg every 3 wk; target Hgb should not exceed 12 g/dL. If Hgb ↑ by >1.0 g/dL in 2 wk or or reaches a level needed to avoid red blood cell transfusions, ↓ dose by 40%; if Hgb ↑ by <1.0 g/dL after 6 wk of therapy, ↑ dose to 4.5 mcg/kg weekly.

Availability

Solution for injection (single-dose vials): 25 mcg/1 mL, 40 mcg/1 mL, 60 mcg/1 mL, 100 mcg/1 mL, 200 mcg/1 mL, 300 mcg/1 mL. **Solution for injection (prefilled syringes):** 10 mcg/0.4 mL, 25 mcg/0.42 mL, 40 mcg/0.4 mL, 60 mcg/0.3 mL, 100 mcg/0.5 mL, 150 mcg/0.3 mL, 200 mcg/0.4 mL, 300 mcg/0.6 mL, 500 mcg/1 mL.

NURSING IMPLICATIONS

Assessment

- Monitor BP before and during therapy. Inform health care professional if severe hypertension is present or if BP begins to increase. Additional antihypertensive therapy may be required during initiation of therapy.
- Monitor response for symptoms of anemia (fatigue, dyspnea, pallor).
- Monitor dialysis shunts (thrill and bruit) and status of artificial kidney during hemodialysis. May need to increase heparin dose to prevent clotting. Monitor patients with underlying vascular disease for impaired circulation.
- Monitor for allergic reactions (rash, utricaria). Discontinue darbepoetin if signs of anaphylaxis (dyspnea, laryngeal swelling) occur.
- Assess patient for skin rash frequently during therapy. Discontinue darbepoetin at first sign of rash; may be life-threatening. Stevens-Johnson syndrome or toxic epidermal necrolysis may develop. Treat symptomatically; may recur once treatment is stopped.
- **Lab Test Considerations:** May cause ↑ in WBCs and platelets. May ↓ bleeding times.
- Monitor serum ferritin, transferrin, and iron levels prior to and during therapy to assess need for concurrent iron therapy. Administer supplemental iron therapy if transferrin saturation <20% or serum ferritin is <100 mcg/mL.
- Monitor hemoglobin weekly until the hemoglobin level is stable and sufficient to minimize the need for RBC transfusion after starting therapy and after each dose adjustment.
- Monitor hemoglobin before and weekly during initial therapy, for 4 wk after a change in dose, and regularly after target range has been reached and maintenance dose is determined. Monitor other hematopoietic parameters (CBC with differential and platelet count) before and periodically during therapy. *If hemoglobin ↑ of more than 1.0 g/dL in any 2-wk period or hemoglobin reaches a level needed to avoid RBC transfusion,* ↓ dose by 40%. *If hemoglobin exceeds a level needed to avoid RBC transfusion,* withhold dose until hemoglobin approaches level where RBC transfusions may be required and reinitiate at a dose 40% below the previous dose. *If hemoglobin ↑ by less than 1 g/dL and remains below 10 g/dL after 6 wk of therapy,* ↑ dose to 4.5 mcg/kg/wk (if on weekly therapy) or do not adjust dose (if on every 3 wk schedule). *If there is no response as measured by hemoglobin levels or if RBC transfusions are still required after 8 wk of therapy,* following completion of a chemotherapy course, discontinue darbepoetin. Hemoglobin >11 g/dL increases the likelihood of life-threatening cardiovascular complications, cardiac arrest, neurologic events (seizures, stroke), hypertensive reactions, HF, vascular thrombosis/ischemia/infarction, acute MI, and fluid overload/edema.
- If ↑ in hemoglobin is less than 1 g/dL over 4 wk and iron stores are adequate, dose may be ↑ by 25% of previous dose. Use the lowest dose possible to avoid transfusions.
- Monitor renal function studies and electrolytes closely; resulting increased sense of well-being may lead to decreased compliance with other therapies for renal failure.
- **Anemia of Chronic Kidney Disease:** Monitor hemoglobin at least weekly until stable, then at least monthly. Do not increase dose more frequently than once every 4 wk. Decreases in dose can be made more frequently. Avoid frequent dose adjustments. *If hemoglobin ↑ >1 g/dL in a 2-wk period,* ↓ dose by 25% or more. *If hemoglobin ↑ by <1 g/dL over 4 wk (and iron stores are adequate),* ↑ dose by 25%. *If no response after 12 wk of escalation,* further dose ↑ is unlikely to improve response and may increase risks. Use lowest dose that will maintain Hgb level sufficient to reduce need for transfusions.
- **Adults with Anemia of Chronic Kidney Disease on Dialysis**: Start darbepoetin when hemoglobin >10 g/dL. If hemoglobin ≥11 g/dL, reduce or hold dose. **Adults with Anemia of Chronic Kidney Disease not on Dialysis**: Start darbepoetin only when hemoglobin <10 g/dL AND rate of hemoglobin decline indicates likelihood of requiring a RBC transfusion AND reducing risk of alloimmunization and/or other RBC transfusion-related risks is a goal. If hemoglobin level >10 g/dL, reduce or hold dose, and use lowest darbepoetin dose sufficient to reduce need for RBC transfusions. **Children with Anemia of Chronic Kidney Disease**: Start epoetin only when hemoglobin <10 g/dL. If hemoglobin level >12 g/dL, reduce or hold dose. Monitor renal function studies and electrolytes closely; resulting increased sense of well-being may lead to decreased compliance with other therapies for renal failure. Increases in BUN, serum creatinine, uric acid, phosphorus, and potassium may occur.

Implementation

- Transfusions are still required for severe symptomatic anemia. Supplemental iron should be initiated with darbepoetin and continued during therapy. Correct deficiencies of folic acid or vitamin B_{12} prior to therapy.
- Institute seizure precautions in patients who experience greater than a 1.0 g/dL increase in hemoglobin in a 2-wk period or exhibit any change in neurologic status.
- *For conversion from epoetin alfa to darbepoetin,* if epoetin was administered 2–3 times/wk administer darbepoetin once a wk. If patient was receiving epoetin once/wk, darbepoetin may be administered once every 2 wk. Route of administration should remain consistent.
- Dose adjustments should not be more frequent than once/mo.
- Do not shake vial; inactivation of medication may occur. Do not administer vials containing solution that is discolored or contains particulate matter. Discard vial immediately after withdrawing dose. Do not pool unused portions.
- **Subcut:** This route is often used for patients not requiring dialysis.

IV Administration

- **IV Push:** Administer undiluted. ***Rate:*** May be administered as direct injection or bolus over 1–3 min into IV tubing or via venous line at end of dialysis session.
- **Y-Site Incompatibility:** Do not administer in conjunction with other drugs or solutions.

Patient/Family Teaching

- Instruct patient to read the *Medication Guide* prior to beginning therapy and with each Rx refill in case of changes. Inform patients of risks and benefits of darbepoetin.
- Discuss ways of preventing self-injury in patients at risk for seizures. Driving and activities requiring continuous alertness should be avoided.
- Advise patient to stop darbopoetin and notify health care professional immediately if severe skin reactions (skin rash with itching, blisters, skin sores, peeling, areas of skin coming off) or signs and symptoms of serious allergic reactions (rash, itching, shortness of breath, wheezing, dizziness and fainting due to drop in blood pressure, swelling around mouth or eyes, fast pulse, sweating) occur.
- Inform patient that use of darbepoetin may result in shortened overall survival and/or ↓ time to tumor progression. May also cause MI or stroke. Advise patient to notify health care professional immediately if chest pain; trouble breathing or shortness of breath; pain in legs, with or without swelling; a cool or pale arm or leg; sudden confusion, trouble speaking, or trouble understanding others' speech; sudden numbness or weakness in face, arm, or leg, especially on one side of body; sudden trouble seeing; sudden trouble walking, dizziness, loss of balance or coordination; loss of consciousness (fainting); or hemodialysis vascular access stops working.
- Advise patient to notify health care professional of darbopoetin prior to surgery.
- Advise patient to notify health care professional if pregnancy is planned or suspected or if breast feeding.
- **Anemia of Chronic Kidney Disease**: Stress importance of compliance with dietary restrictions, medications, and dialysis. Foods high in iron and low in potassium include liver, pork, veal, beef, mustard and turnip greens, peas, eggs, broccoli, kale, blackberries, strawberries, apple juice, watermelon, oatmeal, and enriched bread. Darbepoetin will result in increased sense of well-being, but it does not cure underlying disease.
- **Home Care Issues:** Home dialysis patients determined to be able to safely and effectively administer darbepoetin should be taught proper dose, administration technique with syringe, auto-injector or IV use, and disposal of equipment. *Information for Patients and Caregivers* should be provided to patient along with medication.

Evaluation/Desired Outcomes

- Increase in hemoglobin not to exceed 11 g/dL with improvement in symptoms of anemia in patients with chronic renal failure or with chemotherapy-induced anemia.

darifenacin (dar-i-**fen**-a-sin)

Enablex

Classification

Therapeutic: urinary tract antispasmodics

Pharmacologic: anticholinergics

Indications

Overactive bladder with symptoms (urge incontinence, urgency, frequency).

Action

Acts as a muscarinic (cholinergic) receptor antagonist; antagonizes bladder smooth muscle contraction. **Therapeutic Effects:** Decreased symptoms of overactive bladder.

Pharmacokinetics

Absorption: 15–19% absorbed.

Distribution: Unknown.

Protein Binding: 98%.

Metabolism and Excretion: Extensively metabolized by the CYP2D6 enzyme system in most individuals;

poor metabolizers (7% of Caucasians, 2% of African Americans) have less CYP2D6 activity with less metabolism occurring. Some metabolism via CYP3A4 enzyme system. 60% excreted renally as metabolites, 40% in feces as metabolites.
Half-life: 13–19 hr.

TIME/ACTION PROFILE

ROUTE	ONSET	PEAK	DURATION
PO	unknown	7 hr	24 hr

Contraindications/Precautions

Contraindicated in: Hypersensitivity; Urinary retention; Gastric retention; Uncontrolled angle-closure glaucoma; Severe hepatic impairment.
Use Cautiously in: Concurrent use of CYP3A4 inhibitors (use lower dose/clinical monitoring may be necessary); Moderate hepatic impairment (lower dose recommended); Bladder outflow obstruction; GI obstructive disorders, ↓ GI motility, severe constipation or ulcerative colitis; Myasthenia gravis; Angle-closure glaucoma; OB: Use only if potential maternal benefit justifies potential fetal risk; Lactation, Pedi: Safety not established.

Adverse Reactions/Side Effects

CNS: confusion, dizziness, drowsiness, hallucinations, headache. **EENT:** blurred vision. **GI:** constipation, dry mouth, dyspepsia, nausea. **Metab:** heat intolerance. **Misc:** ANGIOEDEMA.

Interactions

Drug-Drug: Strong CYP3A4 inhibitors, including **ketoconazole**, **itraconazole**, **ritonavir**, **nelfinavir**, **clarithromycin**, and **nefazodone** may ↑ levels and risk of toxicity; daily dose should not exceed 7.5 mg. Concurrent use of **moderate CYP3A4 inhibitors**, especially those with narrow therapeutic indices, including **flecainide**, **thioridazine**, and **tricyclic antidepressants**, should be undertaken with caution.

Route/Dosage

PO (Adults): 7.5 mg once daily, may ↑ after 2 wk to 15 mg once daily.

Availability

Extended-release tablets: 7.5 mg, 15 mg. **Cost:** All strengths $599.48/90.

NURSING IMPLICATIONS

Assessment

- Monitor voiding pattern and assess symptoms of overactive bladder (urinary urgency, urinary incontinence, urinary frequency) to and periodically during therapy.

Implementation

- Do not confuse Enablex (darifenacin) with Effexor XR (venlafaxine).
- **PO:** Administer once daily without regard to food. Extended-release tablets must be swallowed whole; do not break, crush, or chew.

Patient/Family Teaching

- Instruct patient to take darifenacin as directed. If a dose is missed, skip dose and take next day; do not take 2 doses in same day. Advise patient to read the *Patient Information* before starting therapy and with each Rx refill in case of changes.
- Do not share darifenacin with others; may be dangerous.
- Inform patient of potential anticholinergic side effects (constipation, urinary retention, blurred vision, heat prostration in a hot environment).
- May cause dizziness, drowsiness, confusion, and blurred vision. Caution patient to avoid driving and other activities that require alertness until response to medication is known.
- Instruct patient to notify health care professional of all Rx or OTC medications, vitamins, or herbal products being taken and consult health care professional before taking any new medications.
- Advise female patient to notify health care professional if pregnancy is planned or suspected or if breast feeding.

Evaluation/Desired Outcomes

- Decrease in symptoms of overactive bladder (urge urinary incontinence, urgency, frequency).

darunavir (da-ru-na-veer)

Prezista

Classification
Therapeutic: antiretrovirals
Pharmacologic: protease inhibitors

Indications

HIV infection (must be used with ritonavir and with other antiretrovirals).

Action

Inhibits HIV-1 protease, selectively inhibiting the cleavage of HIV-encoded specific polyproteins in infected cells. This prevents the formation of mature virus particles. **Therapeutic Effects:** Increased CD4 cell counts and decreased viral load with subsequent slowed progression of HIV infection and its sequelae.

Pharmacokinetics

Absorption: *Without ritonavir*—37% absorbed following oral administration; *with ritonavir*—82%. Food ↑ absorption by 30%.
Distribution: Unknown.
Protein Binding: 95% bound to plasma proteins.
Metabolism and Excretion: Extensively metabolized by CYP3A enzyme system. 41% eliminated unchanged in feces, 8% in urine.
Half-life: 15 hr.

TIME/ACTION PROFILE

ROUTE	ONSET	PEAK	DURATION
PO	unknown	2.5–4 hr	12 hr

Contraindications/Precautions

Contraindicated in: Concurrent use of alfuzosin, dronedarone, colchicine (in renal/hepatic impairment), elbasvir/grazoprevir, ergot derivatives, ivabradine, lomitapide, lovastatin, lurasidone, midazolam (PO), naloxegol, pimozide, ranolazine, rifampin, sildenafil (Revatio), simvastatin, triazolam, or St. John's wort; Lactation: Avoid breast feeding (HIV may be transmitted in human milk).

Use Cautiously in: Hepatic impairment; Sulfa allergy; OB: May be used during pregnancy (if benefits of use generally outweigh fetal risk); Pedi: Children <3 yr (safety and efficacy not established); Geri: Consider age-related impairment in hepatic function, concurrent chronic disease states and drug therapy.

Adverse Reactions/Side Effects

Based on concurrent use with ritonavir.

Derm: DRUG RASH WITH EOSINOPHILIA AND SYSTEMIC SYMPTOMS (DRESS), STEVENS-JOHNSON SYNDROME, TOXIC EPIDERMAL NECROLYSIS, rash, acute generalized exanthematous pustulosis. **Endo:** Graves' disease, hyperglycemia. **GI:** HEPATOTOXICITY, autoimmune hepatitis, constipation, diarrhea, nausea, vomiting. **Metab:** body fat redistribution. **MS:** polymyositis. **Neuro:** Guillan-Barré syndrome. **Misc:** immune reconstitution syndrome.

Interactions

Drug-Drug: Darunavir and ritonavir are both inhibitors of CYP3A, CYP2D6, and P-gp and are metabolized by CYP3A. Multiple drug-drug interactions can be expected with drugs that share, inhibit, or induce these pathways. Consult product information for more specific details. May ↑ levels and risk of toxicity from **alfuzosin, dronedarone, elbasvir/grazoprevir, ergot derivatives (dihydroergotamine, ergotamine, methylergonovine), ivabradine, lomitapide, lovastatin, lurasidone, midazolam (oral), pimozide, ranolazine, sildenafil (Revatio), simvastatin,** and **triazolam**; concurrent use contraindicated. May ↑ **naloxegol** levels which can precipitate opioid withdrawal symptoms; concurrent use contraindicated. May ↑ **colchicine** levels and cause serious/life-threatening reactions; ↓ dose of colchicine; concurrent use contraindicated in patients with renal or hepatic impairment. **Rifampin** ↑ metabolism and may ↓ antiretroviral effectiveness, concurrent use is contraindicated. Concurrent use with **indinavir** may ↑ darunavir and indinavir levels. ↑ levels and risk of myopathy from **atorvastatin, rosuvastatin,** or **pravastatin**; use lowest dose of these agents; do not exceed atorvastatin dose of 20 mg/day. Concurrent use with **efavirenz** results in ↓ darunavir levels and ↑ efavirenz levels; use combination cautiously. **Lopinavir/ritonavir** may ↓ levels; concurrent use not recommended. **Saquinavir** may ↓ levels; concurrent use not recommended. May ↑ **maraviroc** levels; ↓ maraviroc dose to 150 mg twice daily. May ↑ levels of **lidocaine, quinidine, disopyramide, mexiletine, propafenone, flecainide,** and **amiodarone**; use cautiously and with available blood level monitoring. ↑ **digoxin** levels; blood level monitoring recommended. May ↑ **carbamazepine** levels; blood level monitoring recommended. May ↓ **phenytoin** or **phenobarbital** levels; blood level monitoring recommended. May ↑ **clonazepam** levels. May ↓ levels of **warfarin**; monitor INR. May ↑ levels of **trazodone, amitriptyline, desipramine, imipramine,** and **nortriptyline**; use cautiously and ↓ dose if necessary. May ↑ levels of **clarithromycin**; ↓ dose of clarithromycin if CCr ≤60 mL/min. May ↑ levels of **ketoconazole, isavuconazole,** and **itraconazole**; do not exceed itraconazole or ketoconazole dose >200 mg/day. **Ketoconazole, isavuconazole, itraconazole,** and **posaconazole** may ↑ levels. May ↓ levels of **voriconazole**; concurrent use not recommended. Concurrent use with **rifabutin** ↑ rifabutin levels and ↑ darunavir levels (may be due to ritonavir); ↓ rifabutin dose to 150 mg every other day. **Rifapentin** may ↓ levels; concurrent use not recommended. May ↑ levels of **beta-blockers**; may need to ↓ dose. May ↑ levels of **amlodipine, diltiazem, felodipine, nifedipine, nicardipine,** or **verapamil**; monitor clinical response carefully. **Dexamethasone** may ↓ levels/effects; consider use of alternative corticosteroid, such as beclomethasone or prednisolone. May ↑ levels of systemic, inhaled, nasal, or ophthalmic **corticosteroids (betamethasone, budesonide, ciclesonide, dexamethasone, fluticasone, methylprednisolone, mometasone,** or **triamcinolone**; consider alternative corticosteroid such as beclomethasone, prednisone, or prednisolone. May ↑ levels of **cyclosporine, tacrolimus,** or **sirolimus**; blood level monitoring recommended. May ↑ levels of **everolimus**; concurrent use not recommended. May ↑ levels of **irinotecan**; discontinue darunavir/ritonavir ≥1 wk before starting irinotecan therapy. May ↓ levels of **methadone**; may need to ↑ dose. May ↑ **risperidone** and **thioridazine** levels; may need to ↓ dose. May ↑ levels of **sildenafil, vardenafil, tadalafil,** or **avanafil**; single dose should not exceed the following (sildenafil 25 mg in 48 hr; vardenafil 2.5 mg in 72 hr; tadalafil 10 mg in 72 hr); concurrent use with avanafil not recommended. May ↓ levels of **sertraline** and **paroxetine**; adjust dose by clinical response. May ↓ levels and contraceptive efficacy of some combined **hormonal contraceptives** and **progestin-only contraceptives** (alternative methods of nonhormonal contraception recommended). May ↑ risk of hyperkalemia when used with **drospirenone**. May ↑ levels of **salmeterol**; concurrent use not recommended. May ↑ **bosentan** levels; initiate bosentan at 62.5 mg once daily or every other day once patient receiving darunavir for ≥10 days; if patient already receiving bosentan, discontinue bosentan ≥36 hr before initiation of darunavir and then restart bosentan ≥10 days later at 62.5 mg once daily or every other day. May ↑ **tadalafil (Adcirca)** levels; initiate tadalafil (Adcirca) at 20 mg once daily once patient receiving darunavir for ≥1 wk; if patient already receiving tadalafil (Adcirca), discontinue tadalafil (Adcirca) ≥24 hr before initiation of darunavir and then restart tadalafil (Adcirca) ≥7 days later at 20 mg once daily. May ↑ **lumefantrine** levels and risk of QT interval prolongation. May ↑ **quetiapine** levels; consider alternative antipsychotic therapy; if not possible, ↓ quetiapine dose to ⅙ of current dose. May ↑ levels of and risk of bleeding with **apixaban**, **dabigatran**, and **rivaroxaban**; concurrent use not recommended. May ↑ **dasatinib** and **nilotinib** levels; may need to ↓ dose or ↑ dosing interval of dasatinib and nilotinib. May ↑ **vinblastine** and **vincristine** levels; may need to temporarily hold darunavir-ritonavir or initiate another antiretroviral regimen. May ↑ levels of **buspirone**, **diazepam**, **estazolam**, **midazolam (IV)**, and **zolpidem**; ↓ dose of sedative. May ↓ **omeprazole** levels; consider ↑ omeprazole dose (not to exceed 40 mg/day). May ↑ levels of **glecaprevir/pibrentasvir**; concurrent use not recommended. May ↑ **ticagrelor** levels; concurrent use not recommended. May ↑ **fesoterodine** and **solifenacin** levels; should not exceed fesoterdine dose of 4 mg once daily or solifenacin dose of 5 mg once daily.

Drug-Natural Products: **St. John's wort** ↑ metabolism and may ↓ antiretroviral effectiveness; concurrent use contraindicated.

Route/Dosage

Genotypic testing of the baseline virus is recommended prior to initiating treatment in therapy-experienced patients. This testing is performed to screen for darunavir resistance associated substitutions, which may be helpful in determining whether the HIV virus will be susceptible to darunavir.

PO (Adults): *Therapy-naive*—800 mg once daily with ritonavir 100 mg once daily; *Therapy-experienced (with no darunavir resistance associated substitution)*—800 mg once daily with ritonavir 100 mg once daily; *Therapy-experienced (with ≥1 darunavir resistance associated substitution or if genotypic testing not performed)*—600 mg twice daily with ritonavir 100 mg twice daily; *Pregnancy*—600 mg twice daily with ritonavir 100 mg twice daily; if patient taking 800 mg once daily with ritonavir 100 mg once daily before pregnancy, may continue with this regimen if they are virologically suppressed (HIV-1 RNA <50 copies/mL), and if switch to twice daily regimen may compromise tolerability or compliance.

PO (Oral suspension or tablets) (Children 3–17 yr and ≥40 kg): *Therapy-naive*—800 mg once daily with ritonavir 100 mg once daily; *Therapy-experienced (with no darunavir resistance associated substitution)*—800 mg once daily with ritonavir 100 mg once daily; *Therapy-experienced (with ≥1 darunavir resistance associated substitution or if genotypic testing not performed)*—600 mg twice daily with ritonavir 100 mg twice daily.

PO (Oral suspension or tablets) (Children 3–17 yr and 30–39.9 kg): *Therapy-naive*—675 mg once daily with ritonavir 100 mg once daily; *Therapy-experienced (with no darunavir resistance associated substitution)*—675 mg once daily with ritonavir 100 mg once daily; *Therapy-experienced (with ≥1 darunavir resistance associated substitution or if genotypic testing not performed)*—450 mg twice daily with ritonavir 60 mg twice daily.

PO (Oral suspension or tablets) (Children 3–17 yr and 15–29.9 kg): *Therapy-naive*—600 mg once daily with ritonavir 100 mg once daily; *Therapy-experienced (with no darunavir resistance associated substitution)*—600 mg once daily with ritonavir 100 mg once daily; *Therapy-experienced (with ≥1 darunavir resistance associated substitution or if genotypic testing not performed)*—375 mg twice daily with ritonavir 48 mg twice daily.

PO (Oral suspension only) (Children 3–17 yr and 14–14.9 kg): *Therapy-naive*—490 mg once daily with ritonavir 96 mg once daily; *Therapy-experienced (with no darunavir resistance associated substitution)*—490 mg once daily with ritonavir 96 mg once daily; *Therapy-experienced (with ≥1 darunavir resistance associated substitution or if genotypic testing not performed)*—280 mg twice daily with ritonavir 48 mg twice daily.

PO (Oral suspension only) (Children 3–17 yr and 13–13.9 kg): *Therapy-naive*—455 mg once daily with ritonavir 80 mg once daily; *Therapy-experienced (with no darunavir resistance associated substitution)*—455 mg once daily with ritonavir 80 mg once daily; *Therapy-experienced (with ≥1 darunavir resistance associated substitution or if genotypic testing not performed)*—260 mg twice daily with ritonavir 40 mg twice daily.

PO (Oral suspension only) (Children 3–17 yr and 12–12.9 kg): *Therapy-naive*—420 mg once daily with ritonavir 80 mg once daily; *Therapy-experienced (with no darunavir resistance associated substitution)*—420 mg once daily with ritonavir 80 mg once daily; *Therapy-experienced (with ≥1 darunavir resistance associated substitution or if genotypic testing not performed)*—240 mg twice daily with ritonavir 40 mg twice daily.

PO (Oral suspension only) (Children 3–17 yr and 11–11.9 kg): *Therapy-naive*—385 mg once daily with ritonavir 64 mg once daily; *Therapy-experienced (with no darunavir resistance associated substitution)*—385 mg once daily with ritonavir 64 mg

once daily; *Therapy-experienced (with ≥1 darunavir resistance associated substitution or if genotypic testing not performed)*—220 mg twice daily with ritonavir 32 mg twice daily.
PO (Oral suspension only) (Children 3–17 yr and 10–10.9 kg): *Therapy-naive*—350 mg once daily with ritonavir 64 mg once daily; *Therapy-experienced (with no darunavir resistance associated substitution)*—350 mg once daily with ritonavir 64 mg once daily; *Therapy-experienced (with ≥1 darunavir resistance associated substitution or if genotypic testing not performed)*—200 mg twice daily with ritonavir 32 mg twice daily.

Availability (generic available)

Oral suspension: 100 mg/mL. **Tablets:** 75 mg, 150 mg, 600 mg, 800 mg. ***In combination with:*** cobicistat (Prezcobix); cobicistat, emtricitabine, tenofovir alafenamide (Symtuza). See Appendix B.

NURSING IMPLICATIONS

Assessment

- Assess patient for change in severity of HIV symptoms and for symptoms of opportunistic infections during therapy.
- Assess for allergy to sulfonamides.
- Monitor patient for development of rash; usually maculopapular and self-limited. May cause Stevens-Johnson syndrome or toxic epidermal necrolysis. Discontinue therapy if severe or if accompanied with fever, general malaise, fatigue, muscle or joint aches, blisters, oral lesions, conjunctivitis, hepatitis, and/or eosinophilia.
- Monitor for signs and symptoms of DRESS (fever, rash, lymphadenopathy, and/or facial swelling, associated with involvement of other organ systems (hepatitis, nephritis, hematologic abnormalities, myocarditis, myositis) during therapy. May resemble an acute viral infection. Eosinophilia is often present. Discontinue therapy if signs occur.
- ***Lab Test Considerations:*** Obtain HIV genotypic testing for antiretroviral treatment experienced patients prior to starting therapy.
- Monitor viral load and CD4 counts regularly during therapy.
- May cause ↑ serum AST, ALT, GGT, total bilirubin, alkaline phosphatase, pancreatic amylase, pancreatic lipase, triglycerides, total cholesterol, and uric acid concentrations. Monitor hepatic function prior to and periodically during therapy. Hepatotoxicity may require interruption or discontinuation of therapy.

Implementation

- **PO:** Must be administered with a meal or light snack along with ritonavir 100 mg to be effective. The type of food is not important. Tablets should be swallowed whole with water or milk; do not chew.
- Administer oral suspension 8 mL dose and two 4-mL doses using syringe provided along with ritonavir and food.

Patient/Family Teaching

- Emphasize the importance of taking darunavir with ritonavir exactly as directed, at evenly spaced times throughout day. Do not take more than prescribed amount and do not stop taking without consulting health care professional. If a dose of darunavir or ritonavir is missed by more than 6 hr, wait and take next dose at regularly scheduled time. If missed by less than 6 hr, take darunavir and ritonavir immediately and then take next dose at regularly scheduled time. If a dose is skipped, do not double doses. Advise patient to read the *Patient Information* sheet before starting therapy and with each Rx renewal in case changes have been made.
- Instruct patient that darunavir should not be shared with others.
- Instruct patient to notify health care professional of all Rx or OTC medications, vitamins, or herbal products being taken and consult health care professional before taking any new medications, especially St. John's wort.
- Inform patient that darunavir does not cure AIDS or prevent associated or opportunistic infections. Darunavir does not reduce the risk of transmission of HIV to others through sexual contact or blood contamination. Caution patient to use a condom during sexual contact and to avoid sharing needles or donating blood to prevent spreading the AIDS virus to others. Advise patient that the long-term effects of darunavir are unknown at this time.
- Inform patient that darunavir may cause hyperglycemia, hepatotoxicity, and severe skin reactions. Advise patient to notify health care professional promptly if signs of hyperglycemia (increased thirst or hunger; unexplained weight loss; increased urination; fatigue; or dry, itchy skin), hepatotoxicity (unexplained fatigue, anorexia, nausea, jaundice, abdominal pain, or dark urine), DRESS, or rash occur.
- Advise patient to notify health care professional if signs and symptoms of immune reconstitution syndrome (signs and symptoms of an infection) occur.
- Inform patient that redistribution and accumulation of body fat may occur, causing central obesity, dorsocervical fat enlargement (buffalo hump), peripheral wasting, breast enlargement, and cushingoid appearance. The cause and long-term effects are not known.
- Rep: Instruct females using hormonal contraceptives to use an alternative nonhormonal method of con-

traception. Advise patient to notify health care professional if pregnancy is planned or suspected and to avoid breast feeding. If pregnant patient is exposed to darunavir, register patient in *Antiretroviral Pregnancy Registry* by calling 1-800-258-4263.
- Emphasize the importance of regular follow-up exams and blood counts to determine progress and monitor for side effects.

Evaluation/Desired Outcomes
- Delayed progression of AIDS and decreased opportunistic infections in patients with HIV.
- Decrease in viral load and improvement in CD4 cell counts.

darunavir/cobicistat/emtricitabine/tenofovir alafenamide
(da-**roo**-na-veer/koe-**bik**-i-stat/em-tri-**si**-ti-been/te-**noe**-fo-veer al-a-**fen**-a-mide)
Symtuza

Classification
Therapeutic: antiretrovirals, pharmacoenhancers
Pharmacologic: protease inhibitors, enzyme inhibitors, nucleoside reverse transcriptase inhibitors

Indications
HIV-1 infection in patients who have no prior antiretroviral treatment history or who are virologically suppressed (HIV-1 RNA less than 50 copies/mL) on a stable antiretroviral regimen for ≥6 mo and have no known substitutions associated with resistance to darunavir or tenofovir.

Action
Darunavir—Inhibits HIV-1 protease, selectively inhibiting the cleavage of HIV-encoded specific polyproteins in infected cells. This prevents the formation of mature virus particles. *Cobicistat*—Strongly inhibits CYP3A enzymes, enhancing systemic exposure to darunavir. *Emtricitabine*—Phosphorylated intracellularly where it inhibits HIV reverse transcriptase, resulting in viral DNA chain termination. *Tenofovir alafenamide*—Phosphorylated intracellularly where it inhibits HIV reverse transcriptase resulting in disruption of DNA synthesis. **Therapeutic Effects:** Increased CD4 cell counts and decreased viral load with subsequent slowed progression of HIV infection and its sequelae.

Pharmacokinetics
Darunavir
Absorption: Food enhances oral absorption.
Distribution: Unknown.
Protein Binding: 95%.
Metabolism and Excretion: Extensively metabolized by CYP3A; 41% excreted unchanged in feces, 8% in urine.
Half-life: 9.4 hr.
Cobicistat
Absorption: Absorption follows oral administration.
Distribution: Unknown.
Protein Binding: 97–98%.
Metabolism and Excretion: Metabolized by CYP3A and to a small extent by CYP2D6; 86.2% excreted in feces, 8.2% in urine.
Half-life: 3.2 hr.
Emtricitabine
Absorption: 93% absorbed following oral administration.
Distribution: Unknown.
Metabolism and Excretion: Not significantly metabolized; 86% excreted in urine, 14% in feces.
Half-life: 7.5 hr.
Tenofovir Alafenamide
Absorption: Tenofovir alafenamide is a prodrug, which is hydrolyzed into tenofovir, the active component; absorption enhanced by high-fat meals.
Distribution: Unknown.
Metabolism and Excretion: Tenofovir is phosphorylated to tenofovir diphosphate (active metabolite); 32% excreted in feces, <1% in urine.
Half-life: 0.5 hr.

TIME/ACTION PROFILE (plasma concentrations)

ROUTE	ONSET	PEAK	DURATION
darunavir	unknown	3 hr	24 hr
cobicistat	unknown	3 hr	24 hr
emtricitabine PO	rapid	1.5 hr	24 hr
tenofovir PO	unknown	0.5 hr	24 hr

Contraindications/Precautions
Contraindicated in: Concurrent use of alfuzosin, carbamazepine, dronedarone, colchicine (in renal/hepatic impairment), elbasvir/grazoprevir, ergot derivatives, ivabradine, lomitapide, lovastatin, lurasidone, midazolam (PO), naloxegol, phenobarbital, phenytoin, pimozide, ranolazine, rifampin, sildenafil (Revatio), simvastatin, triazolam, or St. John's wort; Severe renal impairment (CCr <30 mL/min); Severe hepatic impairment (Child-Pugh Class C); OB: Pregnancy (significantly lower concentrations of darunavir and cobicistat during 2nd and 3rd trimesters); Lactation: HIV may be transmitted in human milk, breast feeding is not recommended.
Use Cautiously in: Hepatitis B or C infection or hepatic impairment; Sulfonamide allergy; Hemophilia (↑ risk of bleeding); Pedi: Safety and effectiveness not established; Geri: Consider age-related impairment in hepatic function, concurrent chronic disease states and drug therapy.

Adverse Reactions/Side Effects

CNS: fatigue, headache. **Derm:** ACUTE GENERALIZED EXANTHEMATOUS PUSTULOSIS, DRUG REACTION WITH EOSINOPHILIA AND SYSTEMIC SYMPTOMS (DRESS), STEVENS-JOHNSON SYNDROME, TOXIC EPIDERMAL NECROLYSIS, rash. **Endo:** Graves' disease, hyperglycemia. **GI:** ACUTE EXACERBATION OF HEPATITIS B, HEPATOTOXICITY, LACTIC ACIDOSIS/HEPATOMEGALY WITH STEATOSIS, abdominal pain, autoimmune hepatitis, diarrhea, flatulence, nausea. **GU:** renal impairment. **Metab:** hyperlipidemia. **MS:** polymyositis. **Neuro:** Guillan-Barré syndrome. **Misc:** immune reconstitution syndrome, redistribution of body fat.

Interactions

Drug-Drug: ↑ levels and risk of toxicity from **alfuzosin, dronedarone, elbasvir/grazoprevir, ergot derivatives (dihydroergotamine, ergotamine, methylergonovine), ivabradine, lomitapide, lovastatin, lurasidone, midazolam (oral), pimozide, ranolazine, sildenafil (Revatio), simvastatin,** and **triazolam**; concurrent use contraindicated. May ↑ **naloxegol** levels which can precipitate opioid withdrawal symptoms; concurrent use contraindicated. **Strong CYP3A4 inducers**, including **carbamazepine, phenobarbital, phenytoin,** and **rifampin** may ↓ cobicistat, darunavir, and tenofovir levels and their effectiveness; concurrent use contraindicated. ↑ levels/risk of adverse reactions with **colchicine**; concurrent use in patients with renal/hepatic impairment contraindicated; for others ↓ dose (*for gout flare*—0.6 mg followed by 0.3 mg one hr later, may repeat no sooner than 3 days, *for prophylaxis of gout flare*—if dose was originally 0.6 mg twice daily, ↓ to 0.3 mg once daily, if original regimen was 0.6 mg once daily, ↓ to 0.3 mg every other day, *for treatment of familial Mediterranean fever*—dose should not exceed 0.6 mg once daily or 0.3 mg twice daily). **Clarithromycin** and **erythromycin** may ↑ levels of darunavir and cobicistat; consider alternative anti-infectives. ↑ levels/risk of toxicity with **dasatinib**, **nilotinib**, **vinblastine**, and **vincristine**; careful monitoring for toxicity and dose adjustments recommended. May ↑ bleeding risk with **apixaban** and **rivaroxaban**; may need to adjust apixaban dose; avoid concurrent use with rivaroxaban. Effect on **warfarin** is not known; monitor INR. **Oxcarbazepine** and **eslicarbazepine** may ↓ cobicistat and tenofovir levels and their effectiveness; consider alternative anticonvulsant or antiretroviral therapy. May ↑ levels of **clonazepam**; careful anticonvulsant monitoring recommended. May ↑ levels/effects of **tricyclic antidepressants** and **trazodone**; careful dosing of antidepressants recommended (effect on **SSRIs** is unknown). May ↑ levels of **ketoconazole**, **isavuconazonium**, and **itraconazole**; effect on **voriconazole** unknown; concurrent use with voriconazole not recommended. Effects are unknown with **artemether/lumefantrine**; monitor for ↓ antimalarial activity or QT prolongation. ↑ levels/effects/risk of adverse reaction including neutropenia and uveitis with **rifabutin**; lower rifabutin dose to 150 mg every other day. **Rifapentine** ↓ darunavir and tenofovir levels; concurrent use not recommended. May ↑ levels/effects of **neuroleptics that are metabolized by CYP3A or CYP2D6**, including **perphenazine**, **risperidone**, and **thioridazine**; ↓ dose of neuroleptic may be necessary. May ↑ levels of **quetiapine**; if taking quetiapine when initiating therapy, consider alternative antiretroviral therapy or ↓ quetiapine dose to ⅙ of the original dose and monitor for adverse effects. ↑ levels/effects of **beta-blockers metabolized by CYP2D6**, including **metoprolol**, **carvedilol**, and **timolol**; clinical monitoring recommended. ↑ levels/effects of **calcium channel blockers metabolized by CYP3A**, including **amlodipine**, **diltiazem**, **felodipine**, **nifedipine**, or **verapamil**; careful monitoring recommended. ↑ level and risk of toxicity with **antiarrhythmics** including **amiodarone**, **disopyramide**, **flecainide**, **mexiletine**, **propafenone**, and **quindine**; careful monitoring and titration is recommended. May ↑ levels and risk of toxicity with **digoxin**; closely monitor digoxin levels and adjust dose as needed. **Dexamethasone** may ↓ levels of cobicistat and darunavir; consider use of alternative corticosteroid, such as prednisone or prednisolone. May ↑ levels of systemic, inhaled, nasal, or ophthalmic **corticosteroids (betamethasone**, **budesonide**, **ciclesonide**, **dexamethasone**, **fluticasone**, **methylprednisolone**, **mometasone**, or **triamcinolone**; consider alternative corticosteroid such as beclomethasone, prednisone, or prednisolone. Concurrent use with **bosentan** may result in ↑ levels/toxicity of bosentan and ↓ levels darunavir and cobicistat; dose alteration is required (*initiating bosentan in patients already receiving darunavir/cobicistat/emtricitabine/tenofovir alafenamide for ≥10 days*—bosentan 62.5 mg daily or every other day, depending on tolerance; *initiating darunavir/cobicistat/emtricitabine/tenofovir alafenamide in patient already receiving bosentan* —discontinue bosentan for 10 days, resume bosentan at 62.5 mg daily or every other day, depending on tolerance). May ↑ levels of **glecaprevir/pibrentasvir**; concurrent use not recommended. Nephrotoxic agents, including **NSAIDs**, ↑ risk of nephrotoxicity; avoid concurrent use. May ↓ levels and contraceptive efficacy of some combined **hormonal contraceptives**; additional or alternative methods of nonhormonal contraception recommended. May ↑ risk of hyperkalemia when used with **drospirenone**. ↑ levels and risk of toxicity from **immunosuppressants metabolized by CYP3A**, including **cyclosporine**, **everolimus**, **sirolimus**, and **tacrolimus**; therapeutic monitoring recommended. May ↑ levels of **irinotecan**;

D

discontinue darunavir/cobicistat/emtricitabine/tenofovir alafenamide ≥1 wk before starting irinotecan therapy. ↑ levels of **salmeterol** and may ↑ risk of serious adverse cardiovascular events; concurrent use is not recommended. ↑ levels and risk of myopathy from **atorvastatin**, **fluvastatin**, **pitavastatin**, **pravastatin**, or **rosuvastatin**; use lowest dose of these agents; do not exceed atorvastatin or rosuvastatin dose of 20 mg/day. May ↑ levels/risk of respiratory depression with opioids, including **buprenorphine**, **buprenorphine/naloxone**, **fentanyl**, **oxycodone**, and **tramadol**; carefully monitor for **opioid** effects, dose adjustment of opioid may be necessary. May ↑ levels and risk of adverse cardiovascular, ophthalmic, and genitourinary effects of **PDE-5 inhibitors**, including **avanafil**, **sildenafil**, **tadalafil**, and **vardenafil**; **avanafil** use is not recommended, *sildenafil* —use for pulmonary hypertension is contraindicated, when used for erectile dysfunction single dose should not exceed 25 mg/48 hr, *tadalafil* —for pulmonary hypertension-initiating tadalafil in patients receiving darunavir/cobicistat/emtricitabine/tenofovir alafenamide for ≥7 days—20 mg once daily initially, may be titrated to 40 mg once daily, initiating darunavir/cobicistat/emtricitabine/tenofovir alafenamide in patients receiving tadalafil—discontinue tadalafil 24 hr prior to initiating therapy, after 7 days reinstitute tadalafil at 20 mg once daily, may be ↑ to 40 mg once daily; for erectile dysfunction single dose should not exceed 10 mg/72 hr; *vardenafil*—for erectile dysfunction single dose should not exceed 2.5 mg/72 hr. May ↑ levels and risk of bleeding with **ticagrelor**; concurrent use not recommended. ↑ levels/ effects and risk of excess sedation/respiratory depression from some **sedative/hypnotics metabolized by CYP3A** including **buspirone**, **diazepam**, and **parenteral midazolam**; concurrent with **other sedative/hypnotics metabolized by CYP3A** should be undertaken with caution; dose ↓ may be necessary. May ↑ **fesoterodine** and **solifenacin** levels; should not exceed fesoterodine dose of 4 mg once daily or solifenacin dose of 5 mg once daily.

Drug-Natural Products: **St. John's wort** may ↓ cobicstat, darunavir, and tenofovir levels and their effectiveness; concurrent use contraindicated.

Route/Dosage

PO (Adults): One tablet (darunavir 800 mg/cobicistat 150 mg/emtricitabine 200 mg/tenofovir alafenamide 10 mg) once daily.

Availability

Tablets: darunavir 800 mg/cobicistat 150 mg/emtricitabine 200 mg/tenofovir alafenamide 10 mg.

NURSING IMPLICATIONS

Assessment

- Assess patient for change in severity of HIV symptoms and for symptoms of opportunistic infections during therapy.
- Assess for allergy to sulfonamides.
- Monitor for development of rash. May cause Stevens-Johnson syndrome or toxic epidermal necrolysis. Discontinue therapy if severe or if accompanied with fever, general malaise, fatigue, muscle or joint aches, blisters, oral lesions, conjunctivitis, hepatitis, and/or eosinophilia.
- ***Lab Test Considerations:*** Monitor viral load and CD4 count before and routinely during therapy to determine response.
- Assess for hepatitis B virus (HBV). *Symtuza* is not approved for administration in patients with HIV and HBV. If therapy is discontinued, may cause severe exacerbation of hepatitis B. Monitor liver function in co-infected patients for several mo after stopping therapy.
- Monitor liver function tests prior to, during, and following therapy. May cause ↑ LDL cholesterol, total cholesterol, and triglyceride concentrations. Lactic acidosis may occur with hepatic toxicity causing hepatic steatosis; may be fatal, especially in women. Discontinue therapy if symptoms occur.
- Calculate serum creatinine, CCr, urine glucose, and urine protein prior to and periodically during therapy and when clinically indicated. In patients with chronic kidney disease, assess serum creatinine, creatinine clearance, serum phosphorus, urine glucose, and urine protein prior to and periodically during therapy. May cause hypophosphatemia in patients with renal impairment.
- May cause hyperglycemia and glycosuria.

Implementation

- **PO:** Administer once daily with food. For patients who are unable to swallow the whole tablet, may be split into two pieces using a tablet-cutter, and consume entire dose immediately after splitting.

Patient/Family Teaching

- Instruct patient on the importance of taking medication as directed, even if feeling better. Do not take more than prescribed amount and do not stop taking without consulting health care professional. Discontinuing therapy may lead to severe exacerbations. Take missed doses as soon as remembered unless almost time for next dose; do not double doses. Advise patient to read *Patient Information* prior to starting therapy and with each Rx refill in case of changes. Caution patient not to share or trade *Symtuza* with others.
- Inform patient of importance of hepatitis B testing before starting antiretroviral therapy.
- Inform patient that *Symtuza* does not cure AIDS and does not reduce the risk of transmission of HIV to others through sexual contact or blood contamination. Caution patient to use a condom and avoid sharing needles or donating blood to prevent spreading HIV to others.
- Advise patient to notify health care professional immediately if symptoms of lactic acidosis (nausea,

vomiting, unusual or unexpected stomach discomfort, unusual muscle pain, difficulty breathing, feeling cold, especially in arms and legs, dizziness, fast or irregular heartbeat, and weakness or tiredness), liver problems (yellow skin or whites of eyes, dark urine, light colored stools, loss of appetite, nausea, stomach pain), or signs of immune reconstitution syndrome (signs and symptoms of an infection or inflammation) occur.

- Instruct patient to notify health care professional of all Rx or OTC medications, vitamins, or herbal products being taken and consult health care professional before taking any new medications, especially St. John's wort.
- Inform patient that redistribution and accumulation of body fat may occur, causing central obesity, dorsocervical fat enlargement (buffalo hump), peripheral wasting, breast enlargement, and cushingoid appearance. The cause and long-term effects are not known.
- Rep: Advise patient to notify health care professional if pregnancy is planned or suspected. Encourage pregnant women to enroll in the Antiretroviral Pregnancy Registry by calling 1-800-258-4263. Advise female patient that pregnancy is not recommended during *Symtuza*™ and avoid breast feeding during therapy.
- Emphasize the importance of regular follow-up exams and blood counts to determine progress and monitor for side effects.

Evaluation/Desired Outcomes

- Slowed progression of HIV infection and decreased occurrence of sequelae.

HIGH ALERT

DAUNOrubicin hydrochloride

(daw-noe-**roo**-bi-sin **hye**-dro-**klor**-ide)

✦Cerubidine

Classification

Therapeutic: antineoplastics
Pharmacologic: anthracyclines

Indications

In combination with other antineoplastics in the treatment of leukemias.

Action

Forms a complex with DNA, which subsequently inhibits DNA and RNA synthesis (cell-cycle phase-nonspecific). **Therapeutic Effects:** Death of rapidly replicating cells, particularly malignant ones. Also has immunosuppressive properties.

Pharmacokinetics

Absorption: Administered IV only, resulting in complete bioavailability.
Distribution: Widely distributed. Crosses the placenta.
Metabolism and Excretion: Extensively metabolized by the liver. Converted partially to a compound that also has antineoplastic activity (daunorubicinol); 40% eliminated by biliary excretion.
Half-life: *Daunorubicin* —18.5 hr. *Daunorubicinol*—26.7 hr.

TIME/ACTION PROFILE (effects on blood counts)

ROUTE	ONSET	PEAK	DURATION
IV	7–10 days	10–14 days	21 days

Contraindications/Precautions

Contraindicated in: Hypersensitivity to daunorubicin or any other components in the formulation; Symptomatic HF/arrhythmias; OB: Pregnancy (may cause fetal harm); Lactation: Lactation.
Use Cautiously in: Active infections or decreased bone marrow reserve; May reactivate skin lesions produced by previous radiation therapy; Hepatic or renal impairment (dosage ↓ recommended if serum creatinine >3 mg/dL or serum bilirubin >1.2 m g/dL); Patients who have received previous anthracycline therapy or who have underlying cardiovascular disease (↑ risk of cardiotoxicity); Rep: Women of reproductive potential; Geri: Geriatric patients or patients with other chronic debilitating illnesses (dose ↓ recommended for patients ≥60 yr).

Adverse Reactions/Side Effects

CV: CARDIOTOXICITY, arrhythmias. **Derm:** alopecia. **EENT:** rhinitis, abnormal vision, sinusitis. **GI:** nausea, vomiting, esophagitis, hepatoxicity, stomatitis. **GU:** red urine, gonadal suppression. **Hemat:** anemia, leukopenia, thrombocytopenia. **Local:** phlebitis at IV site. **Metab:** hyperuricemia. **Misc:** chills, fever.

Interactions

Drug-Drug: Additive myelosuppression with other **antineoplastics**. May ↓ antibody response to **live-virus vaccines** and ↑ risk of adverse reactions. **Cyclophosphamide** and **trastuzumab** ↑ risk of cardiotoxicity; avoid use of daunorubicin for up to 7 mo after discontinuing trastuzumab. May ↑ risk of hepatotoxicity with other **hepatotoxic agents**.

Route/Dosage

Other dose regimens are used. In adults, cumulative dose should not exceed 550 mg/m² (450 mg/m² if previous chest radiation).

IV (Adults <60 yr): 45 mg/m²/day for 3 days in first course, then for 2 days of second course (as part of combination regimen).
IV (Adults ≥60 yr): 30 mg/m²/day for 3 days in first course, then for 2 days of second course (as part of combination regimen).
IV (Children >2 yr): 25 mg/m² once weekly (as part of combination regimen). In children <2 yr or BSA <0.5 m², dose should be determined on a mg/kg basis.

Availability (generic available)

Powder for injection (requires reconstitution and dilution): 🍁20 mg/vial. **Solution for injection (requires dilution):** 5 mg/mL.

NURSING IMPLICATIONS

Assessment

- Monitor vital signs before and frequently during therapy.
- Monitor for bone marrow depression. Assess for bleeding (bleeding gums; bruising; petechiae; guaiac stools, urine, and emesis) and avoid IM injections and taking rectal temperatures if platelet count is low. Apply pressure to venipuncture sites for 10 min. Assess for signs of infection during neutropenia. Anemia may occur. Monitor for increased fatigue, dyspnea, and orthostatic hypotension.
- Assess IV site frequently for inflammation or infiltration. Instruct patient to notify nurse immediately if pain or irritation at injection site occurs. If extravasation occurs, infusion must be stopped and restarted in another vein to avoid damage to subcut tissue. Notify health care professional immediately. Daunorubicin is a vesicant. Standard treatments include local injections of steroids and application of ice compresses.
- Monitor intake and output, appetite, and nutritional intake. Assess for nausea and vomiting, which, although mild, may persist for 24–48 hr. Administration of an antiemetic before and periodically during therapy and adjusting diet as tolerated may help maintain fluid and electrolyte balance and nutritional status. Encourage fluid intake of 2000–3000 mL/day. Allopurinol and alkalinization of the urine may be used to help prevent urate stone formation.
- Assess for evidence of cardiotoxicity, which manifests as HF (peripheral edema, dyspnea, rales/crackles, weight gain, jugular venous distention) and usually occurs 1–6 mo after initiation of therapy. Obtain chest x ray, echocardiography, ECGs, and radionuclide angiography determination of ejection fraction before each course of therapy and periodically during therapy. A 30% decrease in QRS voltage and decrease in systolic ejection fraction are early signs of cardiotoxicity. Patients who receive total cumulative doses >550/mm², who have a history of cardiac disease, or who have received mediastinal radiation are at greater risk of developing cardiotoxicity. May be irreversible and fatal, but usually responds to early treatment.
- ***Lab Test Considerations:*** Monitor uric acid levels periodically during therapy.
- Monitor CBC and differential before and frequently during therapy. The leukocyte count nadir occurs 10–14 days after administration. Recovery usually occurs within 21 days after administration of daunorubicin.
- Monitor AST, ALT, LDH, and serum bilirubin prior to each course of therapy. May cause transiently ↑ serum alkaline phosphatase, bilirubin, and AST concentrations.
- Monitor renal function before each course of therapy.

Implementation

- ***High Alert:*** Fatalities have occurred with chemotherapeutic agents. Before administering, clarify all ambiguous orders; double-check single, daily, and course-of-therapy dose limits; have second practitioner independently double-check original order, calculations, and infusion pump settings.
- Do not confuse daunorubicin hydrochloride with doxorubicin, or idarubicin. To prevent confusion, orders should include generic and brand name.

IV Administration

- Solution should be prepared in a biologic cabinet. Wear gloves, gown, and mask while handling IV medication. Discard IV equipment in specially designated containers.
- **IV:** Reconstitute each 20 mg with 4 mL of sterile water for injection for a concentration of 5 mg/mL. Shake gently to dissolve. Reconstituted medication is stable for 24 hr at room temperature, 48 hr if refrigerated. Protect from sunlight.
- Do not use aluminum needles when reconstituting or injecting daunorubicin, as aluminum darkens the solution.
- **IV Push:** ***Diluent:*** Dilute further in 10–15 mL of 0.9% NaCl. Administer IV push through Y-site into free-flowing infusion of 0.9% NaCl or D5W. ***Rate:*** Administer over at least 2–3 min. Rapid administration rate may cause facial flushing or erythema along the vein.
- **Intermittent Infusion:** ***Diluent:*** May also be diluted in 50–100 mL of 0.9% NaCl. ***Rate:*** Administer 50 mL over 10–15 min or 100 mL over 30–45 min.
- **Y-Site Compatibility:** alemtuzumab, alfentanil, amifostine, amikacin, amiodarone, anidulafungin, argatroban, arsenic trioxide, atracurium, bivalirudin, bleomycin, bumetanide, buprenorphine, butorphanol, calcium chloride, calcium gluconate, carboplatin, carmustine, caspofungin, chlorpromazine, ciprofloxacin, cisatracurium, cisplatin, cyclophosphamide, cyclosporine, cytarabine, dacarbazine, dactinomycin, daptomycin, dexmedetomidine, dexrazoxane, digoxin, diltiazem, diphenhydramine, dobutamine, docetaxel, dolasetron, dopamine,

doxycycline, droperidol, enalaprilat, ephedrine, epinephrine, erythromycin, esmolol, etoposide, etoposide phosphate, famotidine, fenoldopam, fentanyl, filgrastim, fluconazole, gemcitabine, gentamicin, glycopyrrolate, granisetron, haloperidol, hetastarch, hydralazine, hydrocortisone, hydromorphone, idarubicin, imipenem/cilastatin, insulin regular, irinotecan, isoproterenol, labetalol, leucovorin calcium, lidocaine, linezolid, lorazepam, magnesium sulfate, mannitol, melphalan, meperidine, meropenem, metaraminol, methotrexate, methyldopate, metoclopramide, metoprolol, metronidazole, midazolam, milrinone, mitomycin, morphine, moxifloxacin, nalbuphine, naloxone, nitroglycerin, norepinephrine, octreotide, ondansetron, oxaliplatin, paclitaxel, palonosetron, pancuronium, pentamindine, phentolamine, phenylephrine, potassium acetate, potassium choride, potassium phosphates, procainamide, prochlorperazine, promethazine, propranolol, quinupristin/dalfopristin, ranitidine, remifentanil, rituximab, sodium acetate, sodium bicarbonate, sodium phosphates, streptozocin, succinylcholine, sufentanil, tacrolimus, theophylline, thiotepa, tigecycline, tobramycin, tolazoline, topotecan, trastuzumab, vancomycin, vecuronium, verapamil, vinblastine, vincristine, vinorelbine, voriconazole, zidovudine, zoledronic acid.

- **Y-Site Incompatibility:** acyclovir, allopurinol, aminophylline, amphotericin B lipid complex, amphotericin B liposome, ampicillin, ampicillin/sulbactam, aztreonam, cefazolin, cefepime, cefotaxime, cefotetan, cefoxitin, ceftazidime, ceftriaxone, cefuroxime, chloramphenicol, clindamycin, dantrolene, dexamethasone, diazepam, ertapenem, fludarabine, foscarnet, fosphenytoin, furosemide, ganciclovir, heparin, indomethacin, ketorolac, levofloxacin, methohexital, methylprednisolone, mitoxantrone, nafcillin, nitroprusside, pantoprazole, pemetrexed, pentobarbital, phenobarbital, phenytoin, piperacillin/tazobactam, thiopental, trimethoprim/sulfamethoxazole.
- **Additive Incompatibility:** Manufacturer does not recommend admixing daunorubicin hydrochloride.

Patient/Family Teaching

- Instruct patient to notify health care professional if fever; chills; sore throat; signs of infection; bleeding gums; bruising; petechiae; or blood in urine, stool, or emesis occurs. Caution patient to avoid crowds and persons with known infections. Instruct patient to use soft toothbrush and electric razor. Patient should be cautioned not to drink alcoholic beverages or take products containing aspirin or NSAIDs.
- Instruct patient to inspect oral mucosa for erythema and ulceration. If ulceration occurs, advise patient to use sponge brush and rinse mouth with water after eating and drinking. Stomatitis pain may require management with opioid analgesics. Period of highest risk is 3–7 days after administration of dose.
- Instruct patient to notify health care professional immediately if irregular heartbeat, shortness of breath, or swelling of lower extremities occurs.
- Discuss with patient possibility of hair loss. Explore methods of coping. Regrowth of hair usually begins within 5 wk after discontinuing therapy.
- Inform patient that medication may turn urine reddish color for 1–2 days after administration.
- Instruct patient not to receive any vaccinations without advice of health care professional.
- Rep: Inform patient that this medication may have teratogenic effects. Advise females of reproductive potential and males with a partner of reproductive potential to use effective contraception during therapy and for at least 4 mo after last dose and to avoid breast feeding during therapy. Inform patient that daunorubicin may cause irreversible gonadal suppression.
- Emphasize the need for periodic lab tests to monitor for side effects.

Evaluation/Desired Outcomes

- Improvement of hematologic status in patients with leukemia.

deferoxamine

(de-fer-**ox**-a-meen)

Desferal

Classification

Therapeutic: antidotes

Pharmacologic: heavy metal antagonists

Indications

Acute toxic iron ingestion. Secondary iron overload syndromes associated with multiple transfusion therapy.

Action

Chelates unbound iron, forming a water-soluble complex (ferrioxamine) in plasma that is easily excreted by the kidneys. **Therapeutic Effects:** Removal of excess iron. Also chelates aluminum.

Pharmacokinetics

Absorption: Poorly absorbed after oral administration. Well absorbed after IM administration and subcut administration.

Distribution: Appears to be widely distributed.

Metabolism and Excretion: Metabolized by tissues and plasma enzymes. Unchanged drug and chelated form excreted by the kidneys; 33% of iron removed is eliminated in the feces via biliary excretion.

Half-life: 1 hr.

TIME/ACTION PROFILE (effects on hematologic parameters)

ROUTE	ONSET	PEAK	DURATION
IV	rapid	unknown	unknown
IM	unknown	unknown	unknown
Subcut	unknown	unknown	unknown

Contraindications/Precautions

Contraindicated in: Severe renal disease; Anuria; OB: Rep: Early pregnancy or childbearing potential (however, may be used safely in pregnant patients with moderate-to-severe acute iron intoxication).
Use Cautiously in: Pedi: Children <3 yr (safety not established).

Adverse Reactions/Side Effects

EENT: blurred vision, cataracts, ototoxicity. **CV:** hypotension, tachycardia. **GI:** abdominal pain, diarrhea. **GU:** red urine. **Derm:** erythema, flushing, urticaria. **Local:** induration at injection site, pain at injection site. **MS:** leg cramps. **Misc:** allergic reactions, fever, shock after rapid IV administration.

Interactions

Drug-Drug: Ascorbic acid may ↑ effectiveness of deferoxamine but may also ↑ cardiac iron toxicity.

Route/Dosage

Acute Iron Ingestion

IM, IV (Adults and Children ≥3 yr): 1 g, then 500 mg every 4 hr for 2 doses. Additional doses of 500 mg every 4–12 hr may be needed (not to exceed 6 g/24 hr).

Chronic Iron Overload

IM, IV (Adults and Children ≥3 yr): 500 mg–1 g daily IM; additional doses of 2 g should be given IV for each unit of blood transfused (not to exceed 1 g/day in absence of transfusions; 6 g/day if patient receives transfusions).
Subcut (Adults and Children ≥3 yr): 1–2 g/day (20–40 mg/kg/day) infused over 8–24 hr.

Availability (generic available)

Powder for injection: 500 mg/vial, 2 g/vial.

NURSING IMPLICATIONS

Assessment

- In acute poisoning, assess time, amount, and type of iron preparation ingested.
- Monitor signs of iron toxicity: early acute (abdominal pain, bloody diarrhea, emesis), late acute (decreased level of consciousness, shock, metabolic acidosis).
- Monitor vital signs closely, especially during IV administration. Report hypotension, erythema, urticaria, or signs of allergic reaction. Keep epinephrine, an antihistamine, and resuscitation equipment close by in the event of an anaphylactic reaction.
- May cause oculotoxicity or ototoxicity. Report decreased visual acuity or hearing loss. Audiovisual exams should be performed every 3 mo in patients with chronic iron overload.
- Monitor intake and output and urine color. Inform health care professional if patient is anuric. Chelated iron is excreted primarily by the kidneys; urine may turn red.
- ***Lab Test Considerations:*** Monitor serum iron, total iron binding capacity (TIBC), ferritin levels, and urinary iron excretion before and periodically during therapy.
- Monitor liver function studies to assess damage from iron poisoning.

Implementation

- IM route is preferred in acute iron intoxication unless patient is in shock.
- Reconstitute 500-mg vial with 2 mL and 2-g vial with 8 mL of sterile water for injection for a concentration of 213 mg/mL. Dissolve powder completely before administration. Solution is yellow and is stable for 1 wk after reconstitution if protected from light. Discard unused portion.
- Used in conjunction with induction of emesis or gastric aspiration and lavage with sodium bicarbonate, and supportive measures for shock and metabolic acidosis in acute poisoning.
- **IM:** Administer deep IM and massage well. Rotate sites. IM administration may cause transient severe pain.
- **Subcut:** Reconstitute 500-mg vial with 5 mL and 2-g vial with 20 mL of sterile water for injection. ***Concentration:*** 95 mg/mL. Subcut route used to treat chronically elevated iron therapy is administered into abdominal subcut tissue via infusion pump for 8–24 hr per treatment.

IV Administration

- **IV:** Reconstitute 500-mg vial with 5 mL and 2-g vial with 20 mL of sterile water for injection. ***Concentration:*** 95 mg/mL. ***Diluent:*** D5W, 0.9% NaCl, 0.45% NaCl, or LR. Dissolve powder completely before administration. Solution is clear and colorless to slightly yellow. Administer within 3 hr of reconstitution; 24 hr if prepared under laminar flow hood. Discard unused portion. ***Rate:*** Maximum infusion rate is 15 mg/kg/hr for first 1000 mg. May be followed by 500 mg infused over 4 hr at a slower rate not to exceed 125 mg/hr. Rapid infusion rate may cause hypotension, erythema, urticaria, wheezing, convulsions, tachycardia, or shock.
- May be administered at the same time as blood transfusion in persons with chronically elevated serum iron levels. Use separate site for administration.

Patient/Family Teaching

- Reinforce need to keep iron preparations, all medications, and hazardous substances out of the reach of children.
- Reassure patient that red coloration of urine is expected and reflects excretion of excess iron.

- May cause dizziness or impairment of vision or hearing. Caution patient to avoid driving or other activities requiring alertness until response from medication is known.
- Advise patient not to take vitamin C preparations without consulting health care professional, because tissue toxicity may increase.
- Encourage patients requiring chronic therapy to keep follow-up appointments for lab tests. Eye and hearing exams may be monitored every 3 mo.

Evaluation/Desired Outcomes

- Return of serum iron concentrations to a normal level (50–150 mcg/100 mL).

degarelix (deg-a-rel-ix)

Firmagon

Classification
Therapeutic: antineoplastics
Pharmacologic: GnRH antagonist

Indications

Management of advanced prostate cancer.

Action

Reversibly brings to GnRH receptors in the pituitary gland, causing a decrease in the release of gonadotropins and testosterone. **Therapeutic Effects:** Decreased spread of prostate cancer.

Pharmacokinetics

Absorption: Well absorbed from depot following water.
Distribution: .
Metabolism and Excretion: 70–80% undergoes hepatic metabolism and biliary excretion, most metabolites excreted in feces; 20–30% excreted unchanged in urine.
Half-life: 53 days.

TIME/ACTION PROFILE (decrease in testosterone levels)

ROUTE	ONSET	PEAK	DURATION
SC	within 1 wk	2 wk	1 mo

Contraindications/Precautions

Contraindicated in: Previous hypersensitivity; OB: Pregnancy (may cause fetal harm) or child-bearing women; Lactation: Not recommended for use in women.
Use Cautiously in: Severe hepatic/renal impairment; Previous history of cardiovascular disease including congenital long QT syndrome, electrolyte abnormalities, HF, concurrent use of class IA or class III antiarrhythmics (may ↑ the risk of QT prolongation); Geri: May be more sensitive to drug effects; Pedi: Safety and effectiveness not established.

Adverse Reactions/Side Effects

CNS: dizziness, headache, insomnia, weakness. **CV:** QT INTERVAL PROLONGATION. **GI:** ↑ liver enzymes, diarrhea, nausea. **GU:** erectile dysfunction, testicular atrophy. **Endo:** gynecomastia, pituitary gonadal suppression. **Local:** injection site reactions. **Metab:** hot flashes, weight gain, ↓ bone density. **Misc:** hypersensitivity reactions including ANAPHYLAXIS, ANGIOEDEMA, AND URTICARIA, fever, sweating.

Interactions

Drug-Drug: Concurrent use with **class IA antiarrhythmics**, including **procainamide** and **quinidine** or **class III antiarrhythmics** including **amiodarone** or **sotalol** may ↑ risk of QT prolongation and serious arrhythmias.

Route/Dosage

Subcut (Adults): 240 mg initially (given as two injections of 120 mg each), followed by maintenance dose of 80 mg every 28 days.

Availability

Powder for subcutaneous injection (requires reconstitution): 80 mg/vial, 120 mg/vial.

NURSING IMPLICATIONS

Assessment

- Assess patient for hot flashes and other side effects.
- Monitor for signs and symptoms of hypersensitivity reactions (rash, wheezing, shortness of breath). Treat symptomatically and discontinue degarelix if symptoms occur.
- Monitor ECG periodically during therapy, especially in patients with congenital long QT syndrome, HF, frequent electrolyte abnormalities, and in patients taking drugs known to prolong QT interval.
- ***Lab Test Considerations:*** Measure serum prostate-specific antigen (PSA) periodically to determine effect. If PSA ↑, measure serum testosterone concentrations.
- May affect pituitary gonadotropic or gonadal functions.
- Monitor electrolyte levels periodically during therapy; correct abnormalities.

Implementation

- **Subcut:** Reconstitute each 120-mg vial with 3 mL and each 80-mg vial with 4.2 mL sterile water using 21 gauge, 2-inch reconstitution needle. Keep vial upright and swirl very gently until liquid is clear, without undissolved powder or particles. If powder adheres to vial over the liquid surface, vial can be tilted slightly to dissolve powder. Avoid shaking to prevent foam; ring of small air bubbles on surface of liquid is acceptable. Tilt vial slightly, keeping needle in lowest part of vial and withdraw 3 mL for 120-mg dose or 4 mL for 80-mg dose. Exchange reconstitution needle for 27 gauge, 1¼-inch administration needle. Remove air bubbles. Grasp abdominal skin and insert needle deeply at angle not <45°. Inject in an area free of pressure from belts, waistbands, or other types of clothing. Administer immediately after reconstitution. If administering 240-mg loading dose, repeat 120-mg injection for the 2nd dose.

Patient/Family Teaching

- Explain purpose of medication to patient. Instruct patient to notify health care professional if an injection is missed. Advise patient to read *Patient Labeling* before starting and with each Rx refill in case of changes.
- Inform patient of possible side effects (hot flashes, flushing, increased weight, decreased sex drive, erectile dysfunction). Advise patient that redness, swelling, and itching at injection site is usually mild, self-limiting, and decreases within 3 days.
- Instruct patient to notify health care professional of all Rx or OTC medications, vitamins, or herbal products being taken and consult health care professional before taking any new medications.
- Advise female patient that women who are pregnant or who plan to become pregnant or breast feed should not take degarelix.

Evaluation/Desired Outcomes

- Decrease in the spread of prostate cancer.

REMS

denosumab (de-**no**-su-mab)

Prolia, Xgeva

Classification

Therapeutic: bone resorption inhibitors

Pharmacologic: monoclonal antibodies

Indications

Prolia. Treatment of osteoporosis in postmenopausal women who are at high risk for fracture or those who have failed/are intolerant of conventional osteoporosis therapy. To increase bone mass in men with osteoporosis who are at high risk for fracture or those who have failed/are intolerant of conventional osteoporosis therapy. Treatment of glucocorticoid-induced osteoporosis in men and women at high risk for fracture who are initiating or continuing systemic glucocorticoids at a daily dosage of ≥7.5 mg of prednisone and are expected to remain on glucocorticoids for ≥6 mo. To increase bone mass in men receiving androgen deprivation therapy for nonmetastatic prostate cancer who are at high risk for fracture. To increase bone mass in women receiving adjuvant aromatase inhibitor therapy for breast cancer who are at high risk for fracture. **Xgeva**. Prevention of skeletal-related events in patients with multiple myeloma and in patients with bone metastases from solid tumors. Giant cell tumor of bone that is unresectable or where surgical resection is likely to result in severe morbidity. Treatment of hypercalcemia of malignancy that is refractory to bisphosphonate therapy.

Action

A monoclonal antibody that binds specifically to the human receptor activator of nuclear factor kappa-B-ligand (RANKL), which is required for formation, function, and survival of osteoclasts. Binding inhibits osteoclast formation, function, and survival. **Therapeutic Effects:** ↓ bone resorption with ↓ occurrence of fractures (vertebral, nonvertebral, hip) or other skeletal-related events (e.g., radiation therapy to bone, surgery to bone, spinal cord compression). ↑ bone mass.

Pharmacokinetics

Absorption: Well absorbed following subcutaneous administration.

Distribution: Unknown.

Metabolism and Excretion: Unknown.

Half-life: 25.4 days.

TIME/ACTION PROFILE (effects on bone resorption)

ROUTE	ONSET	PEAK	DURATION
Subcut	1 mo	unknown†	12 mo‡

†Maximum ↓ in serum calcium occurs at 10 days.
‡Following discontinuation.

Contraindications/Precautions

Contraindicated in: Hypersensitivity; Hypocalcemia (correct before administering); adequate supplemental calcium and vitamin D required; OB: Pregnancy (may cause fetal harm); Lactation: Lactation (↓ mammary gland development and lactation).

Use Cautiously in: Conditions associated with hypocalcemia including hypoparathyroidism, previous thyroid/parathyroid surgery, malabsorption syndromes, history of small intestinal excision, inadequate/no calcium supplementation, renal impairment/hemodialysis (CCr <30 mL/min and/or on dialysis); monitoring of calcium levels and calcium and vitamin D intake recommended; Invasive dental procedures, cancer, receiving chemotherapy, corticosteroids, or angiogenesis inhibitors, poor oral hygiene, diabetes. gingival infections, periodontal disease, dental disease, anemia, coagulopathy, infection, or poorly-fitting dentures (may ↑ risk of jaw osteonecrosis); History of osteoporosis or prior fractures (↑ risk of multiple vertebral fractures upon drug discontinuation); Concurrent use of immunosuppressants or diseases resulting in immunosuppression (↑ risk of infection); Rep: Women of reproductive potential; Pedi: Safety and effectiveness not established; Geri: May be more sensitive to drug effects.

Adverse Reactions/Side Effects

CNS: headache. **Derm:** dermatitis, eczema, rashes. **F and E:** hypocalcemia, hypophosphatemia, hypercalcemia. **GI:** PANCREATITIS, diarrhea, nausea. **GU:** cystitis. **Metab:** hypercholesterolemia. **MS:** back pain, extremity pain, musculoskeletal pain, atypical femoral fracture, osteonecrosis of the jaw, suppression of bone turnover. **Resp:** dyspnea, cough. **Misc:** HYPERSENSITIVITY REACTIONS (including anaphylaxis), infection.

Interactions

Drug-Drug: Concurrent use of **immunosuppressants** ↑ risk of infection. Concurrent use of **calcimimetic drugs** may ↑ risk of hypocalcemia.

Route/Dosage

Prolia

Subcut (Adults): 60 mg every 6 mo.

Xgeva

Subcut (Adults): *Multiple myeloma or bone metastasis from solid tumors*— 120 mg every 4 wk; *Giant cell tumor of bone*— 120 mg every 4 wk, with additional doses of 120 mg given on Days 8 and 15 of first mo of therapy; *Hypercalcemia of malignancy*— 120 mg every 4 wk, with additional doses of 120 mg given on Days 8 and 15 of first mo of therapy.

Availability

Solution for injection (Prolia) (prefilled syringe): 60 mg/mL. **Solution for injection (Xgeva):** 120 mg/1.7 mL.

NURSING IMPLICATIONS

Assessment

- Assess patients via bone density study for low bone mass before and periodically during therapy.
- Perform a routine oral exam prior to initiation of therapy. Dental exam with appropriate preventative dentistry should be considered prior to therapy. Patients with history of tooth extraction, poor oral hygiene, gingival infections, diabetes, or use of a dental appliance or those taking immunosuppressive therapy, angiogenesis inhibitors, or systemic corticosteroids are at greater risk for osteonecrosis of the jaw.
- Monitor for signs and symptoms of hypersensitivity reactions (hypotension, dyspnea, upper airway edema, lip swelling, rash, pruritus, urticaria). Treat symptomatically and discontinue medication if symptoms occur.
- ***Lab Test Considerations:*** Verify negative pregnancy status of patient before starting therapy.
- Assess serum calcium, phosphorous, and magnesium levels before and periodically during therapy, especially during first wks of therapy. Correct hypocalcemia and vitamin D deficiency before starting therapy. May cause mild, transient ↑ of calcium and phosphate. Supplement with calcium, magnesium, and vitamin D as needed.
- May cause hypercalcemia within the yr following discontinuation. Monitor for signs and symptoms of hypercalcemia, assess serum calcium periodically, reevaluate the patient's calcium and vitamin D supplementation requirements and manage as clinically.
- May cause anemia.
- May cause hypercholesterolemia.

Implementation

- Grey needle cap on single-use prefilled *Prolia* syringe should not be handled by people sensitive to latex.
- **Subcut:** Remove from refrigerator and bring to room temperature by standing in original container for 15–30 min prior to administration; do not warm in any other way. Do not shake. Administer using a 27–gauge needle in the upper arm, upper thigh, or abdomen. Solution is clear and colorless to pale yellow, and may contain trace amounts of translucent to white proteinaceous particles. Do not use if solution is discolored or contains many particles. Manually activate the green safety guard *after* the injection is given, not before.
- Patients should receive calcium 1000 mg and 400 IU vitamin D daily.

Patient/Family Teaching

- Explain the purpose of denosumab to patient. If a dose is missed, administer injection as soon as possible.
- Advise patient once treatment is stopped there may be an increased risk of having broken bones in the spine, especially in patients who have had a fracture or who have had osteoporosis. Advise patients not to interrupt therapy without their health care professional advice.
- Advise patient to eat a balanced diet and consult health care professional about the need for supplemental calcium and vitamin D (see Appendix K).
- Advise patient to notify health care professional immediately if signs of hypersensitivity, hypocalcemia (spasms, twitches, or cramps in muscles; numbness or tingling in fingers, toes, or around mouth), infection (fever, chills, skin that is red, swollen, hot, or tender to touch; severe abdominal pain, frequent or urgent need to urinate or burning during urination), or skin reactions (redness, itching, rash, dry or leathery feeling, blisters that ooze or become crusty, peeling), or osteonecrosis of the jaw (pain, numbness, swelling of or drainage from the jaw, mouth, or teeth) occur.
- Encourage patient to participate in regular exercise and to modify behaviors that ↑ the risk of osteoporosis (stop smoking, reduce alcohol consumption).

- Advise patient to take good care of teeth and gums (brush and floss regularly) and to inform health care professional of therapy prior to dental surgery.
- Inform patient of increased risk of fractures upon discontinuation. If denosumab is discontinued, consider another bone resorption inhibitor.
- Rep: Instruct female of reproductive potential to use highly effective contraception during and for at least 5 mo after therapy is completed. Advise patient to notify health care professional if pregnancy is planned or suspected or if breast feeding.

Evaluation/Desired Outcomes

- Reversal of the progression of osteoporosis with ↓ fractures and other sequelae.
- ↑ bone mass.
- Decreased growth of giant cell tumors.
- Reduction in hypercalcemia of malignancy that is refractory to bisphosphonate therapy.

BEERS

desipramine

(dess-**ip**-ra-meen)

Norpramin

Classification

Therapeutic: antidepressants

Pharmacologic: tricyclic antidepressants

Indications

Depression. **Unlabeled Use:** Chronic pain syndromes. Anxiety. Insomnia.

Action

Potentiates the effect of serotonin and norepinephrine in the CNS. Has significant anticholinergic properties. **Therapeutic Effects:** Antidepressant action (may develop only over several wk).

Pharmacokinetics

Absorption: Well absorbed from the GI tract.

Distribution: Widely distributed.

Protein Binding: 90–92%.

Metabolism and Excretion: Mostly metabolized by the liver (CYP2D6 isoenzyme); one metabolite is pharmacologically active (2-hydroxydesipramine); the CYP2D6 enzyme system exhibits genetic polymorphism; ~7% of population may be poor metabolizers (PMs) and may have significantly ↑ desipramine concentrations and an ↑ risk of adverse effects. Small amounts enter breast milk.

Half-life: 12–27 hr.

TIME/ACTION PROFILE (antidepressant effect)

ROUTE	ONSET	PEAK	DURATION
PO	2–3 wk	2–6 wk	days–wk

Contraindications/Precautions

Contraindicated in: Angle-closure glaucoma; Recent MI, heart failure, known history of QTc prolongation.

Use Cautiously in: Patients with pre-existing cardiovascular disease; Family history of sudden death, cardiac arrhythmias, or conduction disturbances; Prostatic hyperplasia (↑ susceptibility to urinary retention); History of seizures (threshold may be ↓; seizures may precede the development of cardiac arrhythmias or death); May ↑ risk of suicide attempt/ideation especially during early treatment or dose adjustment; risk may be greater in children or adolescents; OB: Use during pregnancy only if potential maternal benefit outweighs risk to fetus; Lactation: Use during breast feeding only if potential maternal benefit outweighs risk to infant; Pedi: Children <12 yr (safety not established); Geri: ↑ sensitivity to effects.

Adverse Reactions/Side Effects

CNS: drowsiness, fatigue. **CV:** ARRHYTHMIAS, hypotension, ECG changes. **Derm:** photosensitivity. **EENT:** blurred vision, dry eyes, dry mouth. **Endo:** changes in blood glucose, gynecomastia. **GI:** constipation, drug-induced hepatitis, paralytic ileus, ↑ appetite, weight gain. **GU:** urinary retention, ↓ libido. **Hemat:** blood dyscrasias.

Interactions

Drug-Drug: Desipramine is metabolized in the liver by the cytochrome P450 2D6 enzyme and its action may be affected by drugs which compete for metabolism by or alter the activity of this enzyme including other **antidepressants**, **phenothiazines**, **carbamazepine**, **class 1C antiarrthythmics** (**propafenone** or **flecainide**); when used concurrently dose ↓ of one or the other or both may be necessary. Concurrent use of other drugs that inhibit the activity of the enzyme, including **cimetidine**, **quinidine**, **amiodarone**, and **ritonavir**, may result in ↑ effects. May cause hypotension, tachycardia, and potentially fatal reactions when used with **MAO inhibitors** (avoid concurrent use—discontinue 2 wk prior to). Concurrent use with **SSRI antidepressants** may result in ↑ toxicity and should be avoided (fluoxetine should be stopped 5 wk before). Concurrent use with **clonidine** may result in hypertensive crisis and should be avoided. **Phenytoin** may ↓ levels and effectiveness; ↑ doses of desipramine may be required to treat depression. Concurrent use with **levodopa** may result in delayed/↓ absorption of levodopa or hypertension. Blood levels and effects may be ↓ by **rifampin**, **carbamazepine**, and **barbiturates**. Concurrent use with **moxifloxacin** ↑ risk of adverse cardiovascular reactions. ↑ CNS depression with other **CNS depressants** including **alcohol**, **antihistamines**, **clonidine**, **opioid analgesics**, and **sedative/hypnotics**. **Barbiturates** may alter blood levels and effects. **Adrenergic** and **anticholinergic** side effects may be ↑ with other **agents having these properties**.

Hormonal contraceptives ↑ levels and may cause toxicity. **Cigarette smoking** may ↑ metabolism and alter effects.
Drug-Natural Products: Concomitant use of **kava-kava, valerian,** or **chamomile** can ↑ CNS depression. ↑ anticholinergic effects with **jimson weed** and **scopolia**.

Route/Dosage

PO (Adults): 100–200 mg/day as a single dose or in divided doses (up to 300 mg/day).
PO (Geriatric Patients): 25–50 mg/day in divided doses (up to 150 mg/day).
PO (Children >12 yr): 25–50 mg/day in divided doses, may ↑ as needed up to 100 mg/day.
PO (Children 6–12 yr): 10–30 mg/day (1–5 mg/kg/day) in divided doses.

Availability (generic available)

Tablets: 10 mg, 25 mg, 50 mg, 75 mg, 100 mg, 150 mg.

NURSING IMPLICATIONS

Assessment

- Obtain weight and BMI initially and periodically throughout therapy.
- Assess fasting blood glucose and cholesterol levels for overweight/obese individuals.
- Refer as appropriate for nutrition/weight management and medical management.
- Monitor BP and pulse prior to and during initial therapy. Notify health care professional of decreases in BP (10–20 mm Hg) or sudden increase in pulse rate. Monitor ECG prior to and periodically during therapy in patients taking high doses or with a history of cardiovascular disease.
- **Depression:** Monitor mental status (orientation, mood, behavior) frequently. Assess for suicidal tendencies, especially during early therapy. Restrict amount of drug available to patient.
- Assess mental status and mood changes, especially during initial few mo of therapy and during dose changes. Risk may be increased in children, adolescents, and adults ≤24 yrs. Inform health care professional if patient demonstrates significant increase in signs of depression (depressed mood, loss of interest in usual activities, significant change in weight and/or appetite, insomnia or hypersomnia, psychomotor agitation or retardation, increased fatigue, feelings of guilt or worthlessness, slowed thinking or impaired concentration, suicide attempt or suicidal ideation). Restrict amount of drug available to patient.
- **Pain:** Assess intensity, quality, and location of pain periodically during therapy.
- ***Lab Test Considerations:*** Assess leukocyte and differential blood counts, liver function, and serum glucose periodically. May cause an ↑ serum bilirubin and alkaline phosphatase. May cause bone marrow depression. Serum glucose may be ↑ or ↓.
- Serum levels may be monitored in patients who fail to respond to usual therapeutic dose.

Implementation

- Do not confuse despiramine with disopyramide.
- Begin dose increases at bedtime due to sedation. Dose titration is a slow process; may take wk to mo. May give entire dose at bedtime.
- Taper to avoid withdrawal effects. Reduce dose by half for 3 days then reduce again by half for 3 days, then discontinue.
- **PO:** Administer medication with or immediately after a meal to minimize gastric upset. Tablet may be crushed and given with food or fluids.

Patient/Family Teaching

- Instruct patient to take medication as directed. Take missed doses as soon as possible unless almost time for next dose; if regimen is a single dose at bedtime, do not take in the morning because of side effects. Advise patient that drug effects may not be noticed for at least 2 wk. Abrupt discontinuation may cause nausea; vomiting; diarrhea; headache; trouble sleeping, with vivid dreams; and irritability. Instruct patient to read the *Medication Guide* prior to starting and with each Rx refill in case of changes.
- May cause drowsiness and blurred vision. Caution patient to avoid driving and other activities requiring alertness until response to drug is known.
- Orthostatic hypotension, sedation, and confusion are common during early therapy, especially in the elderly. Protect patient from falls. Institute fall precautions. Advise patient to make position changes slowly.
- Advise patient to avoid alcohol or other CNS depressant drugs during and for 3–7 days after therapy has been discontinued.
- Advise patient, family, and caregivers to look for suicidality, especially during early therapy or dose changes. Notify health care professional immediately if thoughts about suicide or dying, attempts to commit suicide, new or worse depression or anxiety, agitation or restlessness, panic attacks, insomnia, new or worse irritability, aggressiveness, acting on dangerous impulses, mania, or other changes in mood or behavior occur.
- Instruct patient to notify health care professional if urinary retention, dry mouth, or constipation persists. Sugarless candy or gum may diminish dry mouth, and an increase in fluids or bulk may prevent constipation. If symptoms persist, dose reduction or discontinuation may be necessary. Consult health care professional if dry mouth persists for more than 2 wk.

- Caution patient to use sunscreen and protective clothing to prevent photosensitivity reactions.
- Inform patient of need to monitor dietary intake. Increase in appetite may lead to undesired weight gain.
- Alert patient that medication may turn urine blue-green in color.
- Advise patient to notify health care professional of medication regimen prior to treatment or surgery.
- Advise female patients to notify health care professional if pregnancy is planned or suspected or if breast feeding. Enroll pregnant patients in National Pregnancy Registry for Antidepressants at 1-844-405-6185 or http://womensmentalhealth.org/clinical-and-researchprograms/pregnancyregistry/antidepressants to monitor pregnancy outcomes in women exposed to antidepressants.
- Therapy for depression is usually prolonged. Emphasize the importance of follow-up exams to monitor effectiveness and side effects and to improve coping skills.

Evaluation/Desired Outcomes

- Increased sense of well-being.
- Renewed interest in surroundings.
- Increased appetite.
- Improved energy level.
- Improved sleep.
- Decrease in chronic pain symptoms.
- Full therapeutic effects may be seen 2–6 wk after initiating therapy.

BEERS

desmopressin

(des-moe-**press**-in)

DDAVP, DDAVP Melt, DDAVP Rhinal Tube, DDAVP Rhinyle, Nocdurna, Octostim, Stimate

Classification

Therapeutic: hormones

Pharmacologic: antidiuretic hormones

Indications

PO, SL, Subcut, IV, Intranasal: Treatment of central diabetes insipidus caused by a deficiency of vasopressin. **IV, Intranasal:** Controls bleeding in certain types of hemophilia and von Willebrand's disease. **Intranasal, SL:** Nocturia due to nocturnal polyuria in patients who awaken ≥2 times per night to void (Nocdurna only). **PO, SL:** Primary nocturnal enuresis.

Action

An analogue of naturally occurring vasopressin (antidiuretic hormone). Primary action is enhanced reabsorption of water in the kidneys. **Therapeutic Effects:** Prevention of nocturnal enuresis. Maintenance of appropriate body water content in diabetes insipidus. Control of bleeding in certain types of hemophilia or von Willebrand's disease. Reduction in number of episodes of nocturia.

Pharmacokinetics

Absorption: <1% absorbed following oral or SL administration; nasal solution 10–20% absorbed; nasal spray 3–4% absorbed.

Distribution: Distribution not fully known. Enters breast milk.

Metabolism and Excretion: Primarily excreted in urine.

Half-life: *PO*—1.5–2.5 hr; *SL*—2.8 hr; *IV*—75 min (↑ in renal impairment); *Intranasal*—1.8–3.5 hr.

TIME/ACTION PROFILE (PO, intranasal = antidiuretic effect; IV = effect on factor VIII activity)

ROUTE	ONSET	PEAK	DURATION
PO	1 hr	4–7 hr	unknown
SL	unknown	unknown	unknown
Intranasal	1 hr	1–5 hr	8–20 hr
IV	within min	15–30 min	3 hr†

†4–24 hr in mild hemophilia A.

Contraindications/Precautions

Contraindicated in: Hypersensitivity; Hypersensitivity to chlorobutanol; Patients with severe type I, type IIB, or platelet-type (pseudo) von Willebrand's disease, hemophilia A with factor VIII levels <5% or hemophilia B; Renal impairment (CCr <50 mL/min); Current or a history of hyponatremia; Polydipsia (Nocdurna only); Concurrent use with loop diuretics or systemic/inhaled glucocorticoids (Nocdurna only); Known or suspected syndrome of inappropriate antidiuretic hormone secretion (Nocdurna only); Conditions that can lead to electrolyte or fluid imbalances, including gastroenteritis, salt-wasting nephropathies, or infection (Nocdurna only); HF (NYHA class II-IV) (Nocdurna only); Uncontrolled hypertension (Nocdurna only).

Use Cautiously in: Angina pectoris; Hypertension; Patients at risk for hyponatremia; Patients at risk for ↑ intracranial hypertension (Nocdurna only); Urinary retention (Nocdurna only); Women (↑ risk of hyponatremia; require ↓ dose) (Nocdurna only); Patients who require use of other intranasal medications; Geri: ↑ risk of hyponatremia; OB, Lactation: Safety not established; Nocdurna not recommended for treatment of nocturia in pregnancy; Pedi: Safety and effectiveness not established (Nocdurna only).

Adverse Reactions/Side Effects

CNS: SEIZURES, dizziness, drowsiness, headache, listlessness. **CV:** edema, hypertension, hypotension, tachycardia (large IV doses only). **Derm:** flushing. **EENT:** *intranasal*—epistaxis, nasal congestion, nasal discomfort, rhinitis, sneezing. **F and E:** HYPONATREMIA, fluid retention. **GI:** dry mouth, mild abdominal cramps, nausea. **GU:** vulval pain. **Local:** phlebitis at IV site. **MS:** back pain. **Resp:** dyspnea.

Interactions

Drug-Drug: Loop diuretics, systemic glucocorticoids, or **inhaled glucocorticoids** ↑ risk of severe hyponatremia; concurrent use with Nocdurna contraindicated. **Carbamazepine**, **chlorpromazine**, **lamotrigine**, **NSAIDs**, **opioids**, **SSRIs**, **sulfonylureas**, **TCAs**, or **thiazide diuretics** may ↑ risk of fluid retention and hyponatremia. **Demeclocycline**, **lithium**, or **norepinephrine** may diminish the antidiuretic response to desmopressin. Large doses may enhance the effects of **vasopressors**.

Route/Dosage

Primary Nocturnal Enuresis

PO (Adults and Children ≥6 yr): 0.2 mg at bedtime; may be titrated up to 0.6 mg at bedtime to achieve desired response.
SL (Adults and Children): 120 mcg 1 hr before bedtime; may be titrated up to 360 mcg at bedtime to achieve desired response.

Diabetes Insipidus

PO (Adults and Children): 0.05 mg twice daily; adjusted as needed (usual range: 0.1–1.2 mg/day for adults or 0.1–0.8 mg/day for children in 2–3 divided doses).
SL (Adults and Children): 60 mcg 3 times daily; adjusted as needed (usual range: 120–720 mcg/day in 2–3 divided doses).
Intranasal (Adults and Children ≥12 yr): *DDAVP*—5–40 mcg (0.0.05–0.4 mL) in 1–3 divided doses.
Intranasal (Children 3 mo–12 yr): *DDAVP*—5–30 mcg (0.05–0.3 mL) in 1–2 divided doses.
Subcut, IV (Adults and Children ≥12 yr): 2–4 mcg/day in 2 divided doses.
Subcut, IV (Children <12 yr): 0.1–1 mcg/day in 1–2 divided doses.

Hemophilia A/von Willebrand's Disease

Intranasal (Adults and Children >50 kg): *Stimate*—1 spray (150 mcg) in each nostril.
Intranasal (Adults and Children ≤50 kg): *Stimate*—1 spray (150 mcg) in one nostril.
IV (Adults and Children >3 mo): 0.3 mcg/kg, repeated as needed.

Nocturia

SL (Adults): *Women*—27.7 mcg 1 hr before bedtime; 25 mcg at bedtime (Canadian dose); *Men*—55.3 mcg 1 hr before bedtime; 50 mcg at bedtime (Canadian dose).

Availability (generic available)

Nasal spray (DDAVP): 10 mcg/spray in 5–mL bottle (contains 50 sprays). **Nasal spray (Stimate):** 150 mcg/spray in 2.5–mL bottle (contains 25 sprays). **Nasal solution (DDAVP Rhinal Tube):** 2.5-mL bottle with applicator tubes (10 mcg/mL). **Solution for injection:** 4 mcg/mL. **Sublingual tablet (Nocdurna):** ✱ 25 mcg, 27.7 mcg, ✱ 50 mcg, 55.3 mcg, ✱ 60 mcg, ✱ 120 mcg, ✱ 240 mcg. **Tablets:** 0.1 mg, 0.2 mg.

D

NURSING IMPLICATIONS

Assessment

- Chronic intranasal use may cause tolerance or if administered more frequently than every 24–48 hr IV tachyphylaxis (short-term tolerance) may develop.
- **Nocturnal Enuresis:** Monitor frequency of enuresis during therapy. Use cautiously in patients at risk for water intoxication with hyponatremia.
- Do not use intranasal form for nocturnal enuresis.
- **Nocturia**: Assess for possible causes of nocturia, including excessive fluid intake before bedtime, and address other treatable causes of nocturia.
- **Diabetes Insipidus:** Monitor urine and plasma osmolality and urine volume frequently. Assess patient for symptoms of dehydration (excessive thirst, dry skin and mucous membranes, tachycardia, poor skin turgor). Weigh patient daily and assess for edema.
- **Hemophilia:** Monitor plasma factor VIII coagulant, factor VIII antigen, and ristocetin cofactor. May also assess activated partial thromboplastin time (aPTT) for hemophilia A and skin bleeding time for von Willebrand's disease. Assess patient for signs of bleeding.
- Monitor BP and pulse during IV infusion.
- Monitor intake and output and adjust fluid intake (especially in children and elderly) to avoid overhydration in patients receiving desmopressin for hemophilia.
- ***Lab Test Considerations:*** Begin *Nocdurna* with a normal serum sodium level. Assess serum sodium concentration is normal before starting or resuming *Nocdurna*, within 1 wk, 1 mo after starting and periodically during therapy. Patients ≥65 yrs and older and patients at ↑ risk of hyponatremia may require more frequent monitoring. May need to hold or discontinue therapy if hyponatremia occurs.
- *Nocdurna:* Obtain a 24-hr urine collection to confirm diagnosis of nocturnal polyuria before starting therapy.
- ***Toxicity and Overdose:*** Signs and symptoms of water intoxication include confusion, drowsiness, headache, weight gain, difficulty urinating, seizures, and coma.
- Treatment of overdose includes decreasing dose and, if symptoms are severe, administration of furosemide.

Implementation

- Do not confuse desmopressin with vasopressin.
- IV desmopressin has 10 times the antidiuretic effect of intranasal desmopressin.
- **PO:** Begin oral doses 12 hr after last intranasal dose. Monitor response closely.
- **Diabetes Insipidus:** Parenteral dose for antidiuretic effect is administered IV push or subcut.
- **Hemophilia:** Parenteral dose for control of bleeding is administered via IV infusion. If used preoperatively, administer 30 min prior to procedure.
- **SL:** Administer 1 hr before bedtime. Place tablet under tongue until dissolved completely. *Nocdurna:* Limit fluid intake for at least 1 hr before until 8 hrs after administration. Use without fluid reduction may lead to fluid retention and hyponatremia.

IV Administration

- **IV Push:** (for diabetes insipidus) ***Diluent:*** Administer undiluted. ***Concentration:*** 4 mcg/mL. ***Rate:*** Administer over 1 min.
- **Intermittent Infusion (for hemophilia and von Willebrand's disease):** ***Diluent:*** Dilute each dose in 50 mL of 0.9% NaCl for adults and children >10 kg and in 10 mL in children weighing <10 kg. ***Concentration:*** maximum 0.5 mcg/mL. ***Rate:*** Infuse slowly over 15–30 min.
- **Y-Site Compatibility:** naloxone.
- **Intranasal:** If intranasal dose is used preoperatively, administer 2 hr before procedure.

Patient/Family Teaching

- Advise patient to notify health care professional if bleeding is not controlled or if headache, dyspnea, heartburn, nausea, abdominal cramps, vulval pain, or severe nasal congestion or irritation occurs.
- Caution patient to avoid concurrent use of alcohol with this medication.
- **Diabetes Insipidus:** Instruct patient on intranasal administration. Medication is supplied with a flexible calibrated catheter (rhinyle). Draw solution into rhinyle. Insert one end of tube into nostril, blow on the other end to deposit solution deep into nasal cavity. An air-filled syringe may be attached to the plastic catheter for children, infants, or obtunded patients. Tube should be rinsed under water after each use.
- If nasal spray is used, prime pump prior to first use by pressing down 4 times. Caution patient that nasal spray should not be used beyond the labeled number of sprays; subsequent sprays may not deliver accurate dose. Do not attempt to transfer remaining solution to another bottle.
- Instruct patient to take missed doses as soon as remembered but not if it is almost time for the next dose. Do not double doses.
- Advise patient that rhinitis or upper respiratory infection may decrease effectiveness of this therapy. If increased urine output occurs, patient should contact health care professional for dosage adjustment.
- Patients with diabetes insipidus should carry identification at all times describing disease process and medication regimen.
- **Nocturia:** Instruct patient to place tablet under tongue 1 hr before bedtime and empty bladder immediately before bedtime.
- Advise patient to limit fluid intake before bedtime and to avoid caffeine and alcohol before bedtime.
- Advise patient to notify health care professional immediately if signs and symptoms of hyponatremia (headache, feeling restless, drowsiness, muscle cramps, nausea or vomiting, fatigue, dizziness, change in mental condition [hallucinations, confusion, decreased awareness or alertness] occur.
- Instruct patient to notify health care professional if fever, infection, or diarrhea occurs. May need to hold medication.
- Instruct patient to notify health care professional of all Rx or OTC medications, vitamins, or herbal products being taken and to consult with health care professional before taking other medications.
- Advise female of reproductive potential to notify health care professional if pregnancy is planned or suspected or if breast feeding.

Evaluation/Desired Outcomes

- Decreased frequency of nocturnal enuresis.
- Decrease in urine volume.
- Relief of polydipsia.
- Increased urine osmolality.
- Control of bleeding in hemophilia.
- Reduced frequency of episodes of nocturia.

desonide, See CORTICOSTEROIDS (TOPICAL/LOCAL).

desoximetasone, See CORTICOSTEROIDS (TOPICAL/LOCAL).

desvenlafaxine

(des-ven-la-**fax**-een)

~~Khedezla~~, Pristiq

Classification

Therapeutic: antidepressants

Pharmacologic: selective serotonin/norepinephrine reuptake inhibitors

Indications

Major depressive disorder.

Action

Inhibits serotonin and norepinephrine reuptake in the CNS. **Therapeutic Effects:** Decrease in depressive symptomatology, with fewer relapses/recurrences.

D

Pharmacokinetics

Absorption: 80% absorbed following oral administration.
Distribution: Enters breast milk.
Metabolism and Excretion: 55% metabolized by the liver, 45% excreted unchanged in urine.
Half-life: 10 hr.

TIME/ACTION PROFILE (blood levels)

ROUTE	ONSET	PEAK	DURATION
PO	unknown	7.5 hr	24 hr

Contraindications/Precautions

Contraindicated in: Hypersensitivity to venlafaxine or desvenlafaxine; Concurrent use of MAO inhibitors or MAO-like drugs (linezolid or methylene blue); Should not be used concurrently with venlafaxine.
Use Cautiously in: Untreated cerebrovascular or cardiovascular disease, including untreated hypertension (control BP before initiating therapy); Bipolar disorder (may activate mania/hypomania); Renal impairment (consider modifications, dose should not exceed 50 mg/day, especially in moderate to severe renal impairment); History of seizures or neurologic impairment; Hepatic impairment (dose should not exceed 100 mg/day); Angle-closure glaucoma; OB, Lactation: Use only if maternal benefit outweighs fetal/infant risk; Pedi: ↑ risk of suicidal thinking and behavior (suicidality) in children and adolescents with major depressive disorder and other psychiatric disorders. Observe closely for suicidality and behavior changes; Geri: Consider age-related ↓ in renal function, ↓ body mass, concurrent disease states, and medications.

Adverse Reactions/Side Effects

CNS: NEUROLEPTIC MALIGNANT SYNDROME, SEIZURES, SUICIDAL THOUGHTS, anxiety, dizziness, drowsiness, insomnia, headache, teeth grinding, vertigo. **CV:** hypertension. **Derm:** ERYTHEMA MULTIFORME, STEVENS-JOHNSON SYNDROME, TOXIC EPIDERMAL NECROLYSIS, sweating. **EENT:** ↑ intraocular pressure, mydriasis. **F and E:** hyponatremia. **GI:** PANCREATITIS, ↓ appetite, constipation, nausea. **GU:** male sexual dysfunction. **Hemat:** ↑ risk of bleeding. **Metab:** hypercholesterolema, hyperlipidemia. **Resp:** eosinophilic pneumonia, interstitial lung disease. **Misc:** SEROTONIN SYNDROME.

Interactions

Drug-Drug: Concurrent use with **MAO inhibitors** may result in serious, potentially fatal reactions (wait at least 2 wk after stopping MAO inhibitor before initiating desvenlafaxine; wait at least 1 wk after stopping desvenlafaxine before starting an MAO inhibitor). Concurrent use with **MAO-inhibitor like drugs**, such as **linezolid** or **methylene blue** may ↑ risk of serotonin syndrome; concurrent use contraindicated; do not start therapy in patients receiving **linezolid** or **methylene blue**; if **linezolid** or **methylene blue** need to be started in a patient receiving desvenlafaxine, immediately discontinue desvenlafaxine and monitor for signs/symptoms of serotonin syndrome for 2 wk or until 24 hr after last dose of linezolid or methylene blue, whichever comes first (may resume desvenlafaxine therapy 24 hr after last dose of linezolid or methylene blue). ↑ risk of bleeding with **NSAIDs**, **aspirin**, **warfarin**, or **clopidogrel**. Use cautiously with other **CNS-active drugs**, including **alcohol** or **sedative/hypnotics**; effects of combination are unknown. Drugs that affect serotonergic neurotransmitter systems, including **tricyclic antidepressants**, **SNRIs**, **fentanyl**, **buspirone**, **tramadol**, **amphetamines**, and **triptans** ↑ risk of serotonin syndrome. **Ketoconazole** may ↑ the effects of desvenlafaxine. May ↑ levels of CYP2D6 substrates, including **desipramine**, **atomoxetine**, **dextromethorphan**, **metoprolol**, **nebivolol**, **perphenazine**, and **tolterodine**; if using desvenlafaxine at dose of 400 mg/day, ↓ dose of CYP2D6 substrate by 50%.

Route/Dosage

PO (Adults): 50 mg once daily (range = 50–400 mg/day).

Renal Impairment

PO (Adults): *CCr 30–50 mL/min*—50 mg once daily; *CCr <30 mL/min*—50 mg every other day or 25 mg once daily.

Hepatic Impairment

PO (Adults): *Moderate-to-severe hepatic impairment*—50 mg once daily (not to exceed 100 mg/day).

Availability (generic available)

Extended-release tablets: 25 mg, 50 mg, 100 mg. **Cost:** *Generic*—All strengths $174.14/30.

NURSING IMPLICATIONS

Assessment

- Assess mental status and mood changes, especially during initial few mo of therapy and during dose changes. Inform health care professional if patient demonstrates significant increase in signs of depression (depressed mood, loss of interest in usual activities, significant change in weight and/or appetite, insomnia or hypersomnia, psychomotor agitation or retardation, increased fatigue, feelings of guilt or worthlessness, slowed thinking or impaired concentration, suicide attempt or suicidal ideation).
- Assess suicidal tendencies, especially in early therapy. Restrict amount of drug available to patient. Risk may be increased in children, adolescents, and adults ≤24 yr.

- Monitor BP before and periodically during therapy. Sustained hypertension may be dose related; decrease dose or discontinue therapy if this occurs.
- Monitor appetite and nutritional intake; weigh weekly. Report continued weight loss. Adjust diet as tolerated to support nutritional status.
- Assess for serotonin syndrome (mental changes [agitation, hallucinations, coma], autonomic instability [tachycardia, labile BP, hyperthermia], neuromuscular aberrations [hyperreflexia, incoordination], and/or GI symptoms [nausea, vomiting, diarrhea]), especially in patients taking other serotonergic drugs (SSRIs, SNRIs, triptans).
- Assess patient for skin rash frequently during therapy. Discontinue at first sign of rash; may be life-threatening. Stevens-Johnson syndrome may develop. Treat symptomatically; may recur once treatment is stopped.
- ***Lab Test Considerations:*** May cause ↑ fasting serum total cholesterol, LDL, cholesterol, and triglycerides.
- May cause transient proteinuria, not usually associated with ↑ BUN or serum creatinine.
- May cause hyponatremia.
- May cause false-positive immunoassay screening tests for phencyclidine (PCP) and amphetamine.

Implementation

- Do not confuse Pristiq (desvenlafaxine) with Prilosec (omeprazole).
- **PO:** Administer at the same time each day, with or without food. Swallow tablets whole; do not crush, break, chew, or dissolve.

Patient/Family Teaching

- Instruct patient to take medication exactly as directed at the same time each day. Take missed doses as soon as possible unless almost time for next dose. Do not double doses or discontinue abruptly; gradually decrease before discontinuation to prevent dizziness, nausea, headache, irritability, insomnia, diarrhea, anxiety, fatigue, abnormal dreams, and hyperhidrosis.
- Advise patient, family, and caregivers to look for suicidality, especially during early therapy or dose changes. Notify health care professional immediately if thoughts about suicide or dying, attempts to commit suicide, new or worse depression or anxiety, agitation or restlessness, panic attacks, insomnia, new or worse irritability, aggressiveness, acting on dangerous impulses, mania, or other changes in mood or behavior or if symptoms of serotonin syndrome occur.
- May cause drowsiness or dizziness. Caution patient to avoid driving or other activities requiring alertness until response to the drug is known.
- Caution patient to avoid taking alcohol or other CNS-depressant drugs during therapy and of increased risk of bleeding with concomitant use of NSAIDs, aspirin, or other drugs that affect coagulation. Instruct patient to notify health care professional of all Rx or OTC medications, vitamins, or herbal products being taken, especially St. John's wort, and to consult health care professional before taking other Rx, OTC, or herbal products.
- Instruct patient to notify health care professional if signs of allergy (rash, hives, swelling, difficulty breathing) occur.
- Inform patient that remains of tablet may pass into stool, but medication has already been absorbed.
- Instruct female patients to inform health care professional if pregnancy is planned or suspected and to avoid breast feeding.
- Emphasize the importance of follow-up exams to monitor progress.

Evaluation/Desired Outcomes

- Increased sense of well-being.
- Renewed interest in surroundings. Need for therapy should be periodically reassessed. Therapy is usually continued for several mo.

dexamethasone, See CORTICOSTEROIDS (SYSTEMIC).

BEERS

dexlansoprazole

(dex-lan-**soe**-pra-zole)

Dexilant

Classification

Therapeutic: antiulcer agents

Pharmacologic: proton-pump inhibitors

Indications

Healing of erosive esophagitis (EE). Maintenance of healed EE and relief of heartburn. Treatment of heartburn from nonerosive gastroesophageal reflux disease (GERD).

Action

Binds to an enzyme in the presence of acidic gastric pH, preventing the final transport of hydrogen ions into the gastric lumen. **Therapeutic Effects:** Diminished accumulation of acid in the gastric lumen, with lessened acid reflux.

Pharmacokinetics

Absorption: Well absorbed following oral administration.

Distribution: Unknown.

Protein Binding: 96–99%.

Metabolism and Excretion: Extensively metabolized by the liver (CYP2C19 and CYP3A4 enzyme systems are involved); the CYP2C19 enzyme system exhibits genetic polymorphism; 15–20% of Asian patients and 3–5% of Caucasian and Black patients may be poor metabolizers and may have significantly ↑ dexlan-

soprazole concentrations and an ↑ risk of adverse effects); no active metabolites. No renal elimination.
Half-life: 1–2 hr.

TIME/ACTION PROFILE (blood levels)

ROUTE	ONSET	PEAK*	DURATION
PO	unknown	1–2 hr (1st); 4–5 hr (2nd)	24 hr

*Reflects effects of delayed release capsule.

Contraindications/Precautions

Contraindicated in: Hypersensitivity; Severe hepatic impairment; Concurrent use of rilpivirine; Lactation: Lactation.

Use Cautiously in: Moderate hepatic impairment (daily dose should not exceed 30 mg); Patients using high doses for >1 yr (↑ risk of hip, wrist, or spine fractures and fundic gland polyps); Patients using therapy for >3 yr (↑ risk of vitamin B_{12} deficiency); Pedi: Children <12 yr (safety and effectiveness not established).

Adverse Reactions/Side Effects

Derm: cutaneous lupus erythematosus. **F and E:** hypomagnesemia (especially if treatment duration ≥3 mo). **GI:** CLOSTRIDIUM DIFFICILE-ASSOCIATED DIARRHEA (CDAD), abdominal pain, diarrhea, flatulence, fundic gland polyps, nausea, vomiting. **GU:** acute interstitial nephritis. **Hemat:** vitamin B_{12} deficiency. **MS:** bone fracture. **Misc:** HYPERSENSITIVITY REACTIONS (including anaphylaxis), systemic lupus erythematosus.

Interactions

Drug-Drug: May ↓ absorption of drugs requiring acid pH, including **ketoconazole**, **itraconazole**, **atazanavir**, **nelfinavir**, **rilpivirine**, **ampicillin esters**, **iron salts**, **erlotinib**, and **mycophenolate mofetil**; concurrent use with **rilpivirine** contraindicated; avoid concurrent use with **atazanavir** and **nelfinavir**. May ↑ levels of **digoxin**, **methotrexate**, and **tacrolimus**. May ↑ effect of **warfarin**. Hypomagnesemia ↑ risk of **digoxin** toxicity.

Route/Dosage

PO (Adults and Children ≥12 yr): *Healing of EE*—60 mg once daily for up to 8 wk; *Maintenance of healed EE*—30 mg once daily for up to 6 mo (adults) and up to 16 wk (12–17 yr old); *GERD*—30 mg once daily for 4 wk.

Hepatic Impairment

PO (Adults): *Moderate hepatic impairment*—daily dose should not exceed 30 mg.

Availability (generic available)

Delayed-release capsules: 30 mg, 60 mg.

NURSING IMPLICATIONS

Assessment

- Assess patient routinely for epigastric or abdominal pain and for frank or occult blood in stool, emesis, or gastric aspirate.
- Monitor bowel elimination. Diarrhea, abdominal cramping, fever, and bloody stools should be reported to health care professional promptly as a sign of Clostridium difficile-associated diarrhea (CDAD).
- ***Lab Test Considerations:*** May cause abnormal liver function tests, including ↑ AST, ALT, and ↑ or ↓ serum bilirubin.
- May cause ↑ serum creatinine and BUN, ↑ blood glucose, and ↑ serum potassium, and ↓ serum magnesium levels.
- May cause ↓ platelet levels.
- May also cause ↑ gastrin and total protein levels.
- Monitor INR and prothrombin time in patients taking warfarin.

Implementation

- Do not confuse Dexilant (dexlansoprazole) with duloxetine.
- **PO:** May be administered without regard to food. Swallow capsules whole or may be opened and sprinkled on 1 tbsp of applesauce and swallowed immediately, without crushing or chewing, for patients with difficulty swallowing.
- Capsules may be opened and granules emptied into 20 mL water. Withdraw entire mixture into syringe; swirl gently to mix. Administer mixture into mouth or NG tube immediately; do not save for later. Rinse syringe with 10 mL of water twice to ensure all medication administered.
- Administer for shortest time possible.

Patient/Family Teaching

- Instruct patient to take medication as directed for the full course of therapy, even if feeling better. Take missed doses as soon as remembered.
- Advise patient to avoid alcohol, products containing aspirin or NSAIDs, and foods that may cause an increase in GI irritation.
- Advise patient to report onset of black, tarry stools; diarrhea; or abdominal pain to health care professional promptly, especially if accompanied by fever or bloody stools. Do not treat with antidiarrheals without consulting health care professional.
- Advise patient to notify health care professional if signs and symptoms of hypomagnesemia (seizures, dizziness, abnormal or fast heartbeat, jitteriness, jerking movements or shaking [tremors], muscle weakness, spasms of the hands and feet, cramps or muscle aches, spasm of the voice box) occur.
- Instruct patient to notify health care professional of all Rx or OTC medications, vitamins, or herbal prod-

ucts being taken and to consult with health care professional before taking other medications.
- Advise female patients to notify health care professional if pregnancy is planned or suspected or if breast feeding.

Evaluation/Desired Outcomes
- Decrease in abdominal pain, heartburn, gastric irritation, and bleeding in patients with GERD; may require up to 4 wk of therapy.
- Healing in patients with erosive esophagitis; may require up to 8 wk of therapy for healing and 6 mo of therapy for maintenance.

dexmedetomidine
(dex-me-de-**to**-mi-deen)
Precedex

Classification
Therapeutic: sedative/hypnotics

Indications
Sedation of initially intubated and mechanically ventilated patients during treatment in an intensive care setting; should not be used for >24 hr. Sedation of non-intubated patients before and/or during surgical and other procedures.

Action
Acts as a relatively selective alpha-adrenergic agonist with sedative properties. **Therapeutic Effects:** Sedation.

Pharmacokinetics
Absorption: IV administration results in complete bioavailability.
Distribution: Unknown.
Protein Binding: 94%.
Metabolism and Excretion: Mostly metabolized by the liver, some metabolism by P450 enzyme system. Metabolites are mostly excreted in urine.
Half-life: 2 hr.

TIME/ACTION PROFILE (sedation)

ROUTE	ONSET	PEAK	DURATION
IV	rapid	unknown	unknown

Contraindications/Precautions
Contraindicated in: Hypersensitivity.
Use Cautiously in: Hepatic impairment (lower doses may be required); Advanced heart block; Severe left ventricular dysfunction; OB, Lactation, Pedi: Safety not established; Geri: ↑ risk of bradycardia and hypotension (consider dose ↓).

Adverse Reactions/Side Effects
CV: BRADYCARDIA, SINUS ARREST, hypotension, transient hypertension. **GI:** dry mouth, nausea, vomiting. **Hemat:** anemia. **Resp:** hypoxia. **Misc:** fever.

Interactions
Drug-Drug: Sedation is enhanced by **anesthetics**, other **sedative/hypnotics**, and **opioid analgesics**.
Drug-Natural Products: Concomitant use of **kava-kava, valerian, skullcap, chamomile,** or **hops** can ↑ CNS depression.

Route/Dosage
ICU Sedation
IV (Adults): *Loading infusion*—1 mcg/kg over 10 min followed by *maintenance infusion* of 0.2–0.7 mcg/kg/hr for maximum of 24 hr; rate is adjusted to achieve desired level of sedation.
IV (Children): *Loading infusion*—0.5–1 mcg/kg followed by *maintenance infusion* of 0.2–1 mcg/kg/hr. Children <1 yr may require higher end of infusion rate.

Procedural Sedation
IV (Adults): *Loading infusion*—1 mcg/kg (0.5 mcg/kg for ophthalmic surgery or patients >65 yr) over 10 min followed by *maintenance infusion* of 0.6 mcg/kg/hr; rate is adjusted to achieve desired level of sedation (usual range 0.2–1 mcg/kg/hr) (maintenance infusion of 0.7 mcg/kg/hr recommended for fiberoptic intubation until endotracheal tube secured).

Availability (generic available)
Solution for injection (requires further dilution): 100 mcg/mL. **Premixed infusion (in 0.9% NaCl):** 80 mcg/20 mL, 200 mcg/50 mL, 400 mcg/100 mL.

NURSING IMPLICATIONS
Assessment
- Assess level of sedation throughout therapy. Dose is adjusted based on level of sedation.
- Monitor ECG and BP continuously throughout therapy. May cause hypotension, bradycardia, and sinus arrest.
- ***Toxicity and Overdose:*** Atropine IV may be used to modify the vagal tone.

Implementation
- Do not confuse dexmedetomidine with dexamethasone.
- Dexmedetomidine should be administered only in intensive care settings with continuous monitoring.
- A loading dose may not be required when converting patient from another sedative.

IV Administration
- **Continuous Infusion:** ***Diluent:*** To prepare infusion, withdraw 2 mL of dexmedetomidine and add to 48 mL of 0.9 NaCl for a total of 50 mL. ***Concentration:*** 4 mcg/mL. Shake gently. Solution should be clear; do not administer solutions that are discolored or contain particulate matter. Ampules and vials are for single use only. ***Rate:*** Administer *loading infusion* over 10 min, followed by *maintenance*

infusion of 0.2–0.7 mcg/kg/hr for ICU sedation and 0.2–1.0 mcg/kg/hr for procedural sedation. Adjust dose to achieve desired level of sedation. Administer via infusion pump to ensure accurate rate.

- **Y-Site Compatibility:** 20% mannitol, acyclovir, alemtuzumab, alfentanil, allopurinol, amifostine, amikacin, aminophylline, amiodarone, amphotericin B liposome, ampicillin, ampicillin/sulbactam, anidulafungin, argatroban, asparaginase, atropine, azithromycin, aztreonam, bivalirudin, bleomycin, bumetanide, buprenorphine, busulfan, butorphanol, calcium chloride, calcium gluconate, carboplatin, carmustine, caspofungin, cefazolin, cefepime, cefotaxime, cefotetan, cefoxitin, ceftazidime, ceftriaxone, cefuroxime, chlorpromazine, ciprofloxacin, cisatracurium, cisplatin, clindamycin, cyclophosphamide, cyclosporine, cytarabine, dacarbazine, dactinomycin, daptomycin, daunorubicin hydrochloride, dexamethasone, dexrazoxane, digoxin, diltiazem, diphenhydramine, dobutamine, docetaxel, dolasetron, dopamine, doxacurium, doxorubicin hydrochloride, doxycycline, droperidol, enalaprilat, ephedrine, epinephrine, ertapenem, erythromycin, esmolol, etomidate, etoposide, etoposide phosphate, famotidine, fenoldopam, fentanyl, fluconazole, fludarabine, fluorouracil, foscarnet, fosphenytoin, furosemide, ganciclovir, gemcitabine, gentamicin, glycopyrrolate, granisetron, haloperidol, heparin, hydrocortisone, hydromorphone, idarubicin, ifosfamide, imipenem/cilastatin, insulin, isoproterenol, ketorolac, labetalol, leucovorin, levofloxacin, levorphanol, lidocaine, linezolid, lorazepam, magnesium sulfate, mannitol, meperidine, meropenem, mesna, methohexital, methotrexate, methylprednisolone, metoclopramide, metoprolol, metronidazole, midazolam, milrinone, mitomycin, mitoxantrone, morphine, moxifloxacin, mycophenolate, nalbuphine, naloxone, nicardipine, nitroglycerin, nitroprusside, norepinephrine, octreotide, ondansetron, oxaliplatin, oxytocin, paclitaxel, palonosetron, pamidronate, pancuronium, pemetrexed, pentamidine, pentobarbital, phenobarbital, phenylephrine, piperacillin/tazobactam, plasma substitute, potassium acetate, potassium chloride, potassium phosphate, prochlorperazine, promethazine, propofol, propranolol, quinapristin/dalfopristin, ranitidine, remifentanil, rocuronium, sodium acetate, sodium bicarbonate, sodium phosphates, succinylcholine, sufentanil, tacrolimus, theophylline, thiopental, thiotepa, tigecycline, tirofiban, tobramycin, topotecan, trimethoprim/sulfamethoxazole, vancomycin, vasopressin, vecuronium, verapamil, vinblastine, vincristine, vinorelbine, voriconazole, zidovudine, zoledronic acid.
- **Y-Site Incompatibility:** amphotericin B deoxycholate, amphotericin B lipid complex, blood, diazepam, irinotecan, pantoprazole, plasma, phenytoin.

Patient/Family Teaching

- Explain to patient and family the purpose of the medication.

Evaluation/Desired Outcomes

- Sedation for up to 24 hr.

dexrazoxane (dex-ra-**zox**-ane)

Totect, Zinecard

Classification

Therapeutic: cardioprotective agents

Indications

Reducing incidence and severity of cardiomyopathy from doxorubicin in women with metastatic breast cancer who have already received a cumulative dose of doxorubicin >300 m g/m². Treatment of extravasation resulting from IV anthracycline chemotherapy.

Action

Acts as an intracellular chelating agent. **Therapeutic Effects:** Diminishes the cardiotoxic effects of doxorubicin. Decreased damage from extravasation of anthracyclines.

Pharmacokinetics

Absorption: IV administration results in complete bioavailability.

Distribution: Unknown.

Metabolism and Excretion: Some metabolism occurs; 42% eliminated in urine.

Half-life: 2.1–2.5 hr.

TIME/ACTION PROFILE (cardioprotective effect)

ROUTE	ONSET	PEAK	DURATION
IV	rapid	unknown	unknown

Contraindications/Precautions

Contraindicated in: Any other type of chemotherapy except other anthracyclines (doxorubicin-like agents); Hepatic impairment; OB: Pregnancy (may cause fetal harm); Lactation: Lactation.

Use Cautiously in: CCr <40 mL/min (↓ dose); Rep: Women of reproductive potential and men with female partners of reproductive potential; Pedi: Safety and effectiveness not established.

Adverse Reactions/Side Effects

GU: ↓ fertility (males). **Hemat:** NEUTROPENIA, leukopenia, thrombocytopenia. **Local:** pain at injection site. **Misc:** HYPERSENSITIVITY REACTIONS (including anaphylaxis and angioedema), MALIGNANCY.

Interactions

Drug-Drug: Myelosuppression may be ↑ by **antineoplastics** or **radiation therapy**. Antitumor effects of concurrent combination chemotherapy with **fluorouracil** and **cyclophosphamide** may be ↓ by dexrazoxane.

Route/Dosage

Cardioprotective

IV (Adults): 10 mg of dexrazoxane/1 mg doxorubicin.

Renal Impairment

IV (Adults): ↓ dose by 50%.

Extravasation Protection

IV (Adults): 1000 mg/m² (maximum 2000 mg) given on days 1 and 2, and followed by a dose of 500 mg/m² (maximum 1000 mg) on day 3.

Renal Impairment

IV (Adults): *CCr <40 mL/min*—↓ dose by 50%.

Availability (generic available)

Lyophilized powder for injection (Zinecard): 250 mg/vial, 500 mg/vial. **Lyophilized powder for injection (Totect):** 500 mg/vial.

NURSING IMPLICATIONS

Assessment

- **Cardioprotective:** Assess extent of cardiomyopathy (cardiomegaly on x ray, basilar rales, S gallop, dyspnea, decline in left ventricular ejection fraction) prior to and periodically during therapy.
- **Extravasation protection:** Assess site of extravasation for pain, burning, swelling, and redness.
- ***Lab Test Considerations:*** Obtain a negative pregnancy test before starting therapy.
- Monitor CBC and platelet count frequently during therapy. Thrombocytopenia, leukopenia, neutropenia, and granulocytopenia from chemotherapy may be more severe at nadir with dexrazoxane therapy.
- Monitor liver function tests periodically during therapy. May cause reversible ↑ of liver enzymes.

Implementation

IV Administration

- Solution should be prepared in a biologic cabinet. Wear gloves, gown, and mask while handling IV medication. Discard IV equipment in specially designated containers.
- Do not administer solutions that are discolored or contain particulate matter. Reconstituted solution and diluted solution are stable in an IV bag for 6 hr at room temperature or if refrigerated. Discard unused solutions.
- **Extravasation Protection:** Administer as soon as possible within 6 hr of extravasation. Remove cooling procedures, such as ice packs, at least 15 min before administration to allow sufficient blood flow to area of extravasation.
- *Totect*: **Intermittent Infusion:** Reconstitute *Totect* with 50 mL sterile water for injection. May also reconstitute with sodium lactate injection by adding 1.67 mL of 5 mEq/mL sodium lactate injection to 50 mL sterile water for injection to make 50 mL of 0.167M sodium lactate injection solution. ***Concentration:*** 10 mg/mL . ***Diluent:*** Withdraw dose volume within 30 min of reconstitution and inject into 1000 mL bag of LR or if reconstituted with sodium lactate, inject into 1000 mL 0.9% NaCl. Solution is stable for 4 hrs at room temperature or 12 hrs if refrigerated. ***Rate:*** Infuse over 1–2 hr in a large caliber vein.
- **Cardioprotective:** Doxorubicin should be administered within 30 min following dexrazoxane administration.
- *Zinecard*: **Intermittent Infusion:** Reconstitute *Zinecard* with 25 mL sterile water for injection for 250 mg vial or 50 mL for 500 mg vial. ***Concentration:*** 10 mg/mL. ***Diluent:*** Dilute reconstituted solution further in LR. ***Concentration:*** 1.3–5 mg/mL. Solution is stable for 1 hr at room temperature or 4 hrs if refrigerated. ***Rate:*** Infuse over 15 min. Administer doxorubicin within 30 min of completion of *Zinecard* infusion.
- **Additive Incompatibility:** Do not mix with other medications.
- **Y-Site Compatibility:** alemtuzumab, alfentanil, amifostine, amikacin, amiodarone, ampicillin, ampicillin/sulbactam, anidulafungin, argatroban, arsenic trioxide, atracurium, azithromycin, aztreonam, bivalirudin, bleomycin, bumetanide, buprenorphine, busulfan, butorphanol, calcium chloride, calcium gluconate, carboplatin, carmustine, caspofungin, cefazolin, cefotaxime, cefotetan, cefoxitin, ceftazidime, ceftriaxone, cefuroxime, chloramphenicol, chlorpromazine, ciprofloxacin, cisatracurium, cisplatin, clindamycin, cyclophosphamide, cyclosporine, cytarabine, dactinomycin, daptomycin, daunorubicin, dexmedetomidine, digoxin, diltiazem, diphenhydramine, docetaxel, dolasetron, dopamine, doxacurium, doxorubicin, doxorubicin liposomal, doxycycline, droperidol, enalaprilat, ephedrine, epinephrine, epirubicin, eptifibatide, ertapenem, erythromycin, esmolol, etoposide, etoposide phosphate, famotidine, fenoldopam, fentanyl, fluconazole, fludarabine, fluorouracil, foscarnet, fosphenytoin, gemcitabine, gentamycin, glycopyrrolate, granisetron, haloperidol, heparin, hetastarch, hydralazine, hydrocortisone, hydromorphone, idarubicin, ifosfamide, imipenem/cilastatin, insulin, regular, irinotecan, isoproterenol, ketorolac, leucovorin calcium, levofloxacin, lidocaine, linezolid, lorazepam, magnesium sulfate, mannitol, melphalan, meperidine, meropenem, mesna, metaraminol, methyldopate, metoclopramide, metoprolol, midazolam, milrinone, mitoxantrone, morphine, moxifloxacin, myco-

phenolate, nalbuphine, naloxone, nicardipine, nitroglycerin, nitroprusside, norepinephrine, octreotide, ondansetron, oxaliplatin, paclitaxel, palonosetron, pamidronate, pancuronium, pemetrexed, pentamidine, phenobarbital, phentolamine, phenylephrine, piperacillin/tazobactam, polmyxin B, potassium acetate, potassium chloride, potassium phosphates, procainamide, prochlorperazine, promethazine, propranolol, quinupristin/dalfopristin, ranitidine, remifentanil, rituximab, rocuronium, sodium acetate, sodium bicarbonate, streptozocin, succinylcholine, sufentanil, tacrolimus, theophylline, thiotepa, tigecycline, tirofiban, tobramycin, topotecan, vancomycin, vasopressin, vecuronium, verapamil, vinblastine, vincristine, vinorelbine, voriconazole, zoledronic acid.

Patient/Family Teaching

- Explain the purpose of the medication to the patient.
- Emphasize the need for continued monitoring of cardiac function.
- Rep: Dexrazoxane may be teratogenic. Advise females of reproductive potential to use highly effective contraception during and for 6 mo after last dose of dexrazoxane and to avoid breast feeding during and for 2 wk after last dose. Advise males with female partners of reproductive poential to use highly effective contreption during and for 3 mo after last dose. Advise patient to notify health care professional immediately if pregnancy is suspected. May impair fertility in males.

Evaluation/Desired Outcomes

- Reduction of incidence and severity of cardiomyopathy associated with doxorubicin administration in women with metastatic breast cancer.
- Decrease in late sequalae (site pain, fibrosis, atrophy, and local sensory disturbance) following extravasation of anthracycline chemotherapeutic agents.

dextromethorphan

(dex-troe-meth-**or**-fan)

✱Balminil DM, ✱Benylin DM, ✱Bronchophan Forte DM, ✱Buckley's DM, ✱Cough Syrup DM, Creo-Terpin, Creomulsion Adult Formula, Creomulsion for Children, Delsym, ✱Delsym DM, ✱DM Children's Cough Syrup, ✱DM Cough Syrup, ✱Dry Cough Syrup, Father John's, Hold DM, ✱Koffex DM, ✱Neocitran Thin Strips Cough, Pediacare Children's Long-Acting Cough, Robafin Cough, Robitussin Children's Cough Long-Acting, Robitussin Cough Long-Acting, Robitussin CoughGels Long-Acting, Robitussin Lingering Cold Long-Acting CoughGels, Scot-Tussin Diabetes, ✱Sedatuss DM, ✱Sucrets Cough Control, ✱Sucrets DM, ✱Triaminic DM, ✱Triaminic Long-Acting Cough, Triaminic Thin Strips Children's Long-Acting Cough, Triaminic Children's Cough Long-Acting, Vicks 44 Cough Relief, ✱Vicks Custom Care Dry Cough, Vicks DayQuil Cough, Vicks Nature Fusion Cough

Classification

Therapeutic: allergy, cold, and cough remedies, antitussives

Indications

Symptomatic relief of coughs caused by minor viral upper respiratory tract infections or inhaled irritants. Most effective for chronic nonproductive cough. A common ingredient in nonprescription cough and cold preparations.

Action

Suppresses the cough reflex by a direct effect on the cough center in the medulla. Related to opioids structurally but has no analgesic properties. **Therapeutic Effects:** Relief of irritating nonproductive cough.

Pharmacokinetics

Absorption: Rapidly absorbed from the GI tract. Extended-release product is slowly absorbed.

Distribution: Unknown. Probably crosses the placenta and enters breast milk.

Metabolism and Excretion: Metabolized to dextrorphan, an active metabolite. Dextromethorphan and dextrorphan are renally excreted.

Half-life: Unknown.

TIME/ACTION PROFILE (cough suppression)

ROUTE	ONSET	PEAK	DURATION
PO	15–30 min	unknown	3–6 hr†
PO-ER	unknown	unknown	9–12 hr

†Up to 8 hr for gelcaps.

Contraindications/Precautions

Contraindicated in: Hypersensitivity; Patients taking MAO inhibitors or SSRIs; Should not be used for chronic productive coughs; Some products contain alcohol and should be avoided in patients with known intolerance.

Use Cautiously in: Cough that lasts more than 1 wk or is accompanied by fever, rash, or headache—health care professional should be consulted; History of drug abuse or drug-seeking behavior (capsules have been abused resulting in deaths); Diabetes (some products contain sucrose); OB: Pregnancy (has been used safely); Lactation: Lactation; Pedi: Children <4 yr (OTC cough and cold products containing this medication should be avoided).

Adverse Reactions/Side Effects

CNS: *high dose*—dizziness, sedation. **GI:** nausea.

Interactions

Drug-Drug: Use with **MAO inhibitors** may result in serotonin syndrome (nausea, confusion, changes in BP); concurrent use should be avoided. ↑ CNS depression with **antihistamines**, **alcohol**, **antidepressants**, **sedative/hypnotics**, or **opioids**. **Amiodarone**, **fluoxetine**, or **quinidine** may ↑ blood levels and adverse reactions from dextromethorphan.

Route/Dosage

PO (Adults and Children >12 yr): 10–20 mg every 4 hr *or* 30 mg every 6–8 hr *or* 60 mg of extended-release preparation bid (not to exceed 120 mg/day).
PO (Children 6–12 yr): 5–10 mg every 4 hr *or* 15 mg every 6–8 hr *or* 30 mg of extended-release preparation every 12 hr (not to exceed 60 mg/day).
PO (Children 4–6 yr): 2.5–5 mg every 4 hr *or* 7.5 mg every 6–8 hr *or* 15 mg of extended-release preparation every 12 hr (not to exceed 30 mg/day).

Availability (generic available)

Gelcaps: 30 mg[OTC]. **Lozenges (cherry):** 2.5 mg[OTC], 5 mg[OTC]. **Liquid (cherry, grape):** 3.5 mg/5 mL[OTC], 5 mg/5 mL, 7.5 mg/5 mL[OTC], 15 mg/5 mL[OTC], 30 mg/5 mL[OTC]. **Syrup (cherry, cherry bubblegum):** 7.5 mg/5 mL[OTC], 15 mg/15 mL[OTC], 10 mg/5 mL[OTC]. **Extended-release suspension (orange):** 30 mg/5 mL[OTC]. **Drops (Grape):** 7.5 mg/0.8 mL[OTC], 7.5 mg/1 mL[OTC]. **Orally-disintegrating strips (cherry, grape):** 7.5 mg[OTC], 15 mg[OTC]. ***In combination with:*** antihistamines, decongestants, and expectorants in cough and cold preparations[OTC], quinidine sulfate (Nuedexta). See Appendix B.

NURSING IMPLICATIONS

Assessment

- Assess frequency and nature of cough, lung sounds, and amount and type of sputum produced. Unless contraindicated, maintain fluid intake of 1500–2000 mL to decrease viscosity of bronchial secretions.

Implementation

- Dextromethorphan 15–30 mg is equivalent in cough suppression to codeine 8–15 mg.
- **PO:** Do not give fluids immediately after administering to prevent dilution of vehicle. Shake oral suspension well before administration.

Patient/Family Teaching

- Instruct patient to cough effectively: Sit upright and take several deep breaths before attempting to cough.
- Advise patient to minimize cough by avoiding irritants, such as cigarette smoke, fumes, and dust. Humidification of environmental air, frequent sips of water, and sugarless hard candy may also decrease the frequency of dry, irritating cough.
- Caution patient to avoid taking more than the recommended dose or taking alcohol or other CNS depressants concurrently with this medication; fatalities have occurred. Caution parents to avoid OTC cough and cold products while breast feeding or to children <4 yrs.
- May occasionally cause dizziness. Caution patient to avoid driving or other activities requiring alertness until response to the medication is known.
- Advise patient that any cough lasting over 1 wk or accompanied by fever, chest pain, persistent headache, or skin rash warrants medical attention.

Evaluation/Desired Outcomes

- Decrease in frequency and intensity of cough without eliminating patient's cough reflex.

BEERS

diazePAM (dye-**az**-e-pam)

Diastat, Valium

Classification

Therapeutic: antianxiety agents, anticonvulsants, sedative/hypnotics, skeletal muscle relaxants (centrally acting)
Pharmacologic: benzodiazepines

Schedule IV

Indications

Adjunct in the management of: Anxiety Disorder, Athetosis, Anxiety relief prior to cardioversion (injection), Stiffman Syndrome, Preoperative sedation, Conscious sedation (provides light anesthesia and anterograde amnesia). Treatment of status epilepticus/uncontrolled seizures (injection). Skeletal muscle relaxant. Management of the symptoms of alcohol withdrawal. **Unlabeled Use:** Anxiety associated with acute myocardial infarction, insomnia.

Action

Depresses the CNS, probably by potentiating GABA, an inhibitory neurotransmitter. Produces skeletal muscle relaxation by inhibiting spinal polysynaptic afferent pathways. Has anticonvulsant properties due to enhanced presynaptic inhibition. **Therapeutic Effects:** Relief of anxiety. Sedation. Amnesia. Skeletal muscle relaxation. Decreased seizure activity.

Pharmacokinetics

Absorption: Rapidly absorbed from the GI tract. Absorption from IM sites may be slow and unpredictable. Well absorbed (90%) from rectal mucosa.

Distribution: Widely distributed. Crosses the blood-brain barrier. Crosses the placenta; enters breast milk.

Metabolism and Excretion: Highly metabolized by the hepatic P450 enzymes (CYP2C19 and CYP3A4); the CYP2C19 enzyme system exhibits genetic polymorphism; 15–20% of Asian patients and 3–5% of Caucasian and Black patients may be poor metabolizers and may have significantly ↑ diazepam concentrations and an ↑ risk of adverse effects. Some products of metabolism are active as CNS depressants.

Half-life: Neonates: 50–95 hr; Infants 1 mo–2 yr: 40–50 hr; Children 2–12 yr: 15–21 hr; Children 12–16 yr: 18–20 hr; Adults: 20–50 hr (up to 100 hr for metabolites).

TIME/ACTION PROFILE (sedation)

ROUTE	ONSET	PEAK	DURATION
PO	30–60 min	1–2 hr	up to 24 hr
IM	within 20 min	0.5–1.5 hr	unknown
IV	1–5 min	15–30 min	15–60 min†
Rectal	2–10 min	1–2 hr	4–12 hr

†In status epilepticus, anticonvulsant duration is 15–20 min.

Contraindications/Precautions

Contraindicated in: Hypersensitivity; Cross-sensitivity with other benzodiazepines may occur; Comatose patients; Myasthenia gravis; Severe pulmonary impairment; Sleep apnea; Severe hepatic dysfunction; Pre-existing CNS depression; Uncontrolled severe pain; Angle-closure glaucoma; Some products contain alcohol, propylene glycol, or tartrazine and should be avoided in patients with known hypersensitivity or intolerance; OB: ↑ risk of congenital malformations; Pedi: Children <6 mo (for oral; safety not established); Lactation: Recommend to discontinue drug or bottle-feed.

Use Cautiously in: Severe renal impairment; History of suicide attempt or drug dependence; Debilitated patients (dose ↓ required); Patients with low albumin; Pedi: Metabolites can accumulate in neonates. Injection contains benzyl alcohol which can cause potentially fatal gasping syndrome in neonates; Geri: Long-acting benzodiazepines cause prolonged sedation in the elderly. Appears on *Beers list* and is associated with ↑ risk of falls (↓ dose required or consider short-acting benzodiazepine).

Adverse Reactions/Side Effects

CNS: dizziness, drowsiness, lethargy, depression, hangover, ataxia, slurred speech, headache, paradoxical excitation. **EENT:** blurred vision. **Resp:** RESPIRATORY DEPRESSION. **CV:** hypotension (IV only). **GI:** constipation, diarrhea (may be caused by propylene glycol content in oral solution), nausea, vomiting, weight gain. **Derm:** rashes. **Local:** pain (IM), phlebitis (IV), venous thrombosis. **Misc:** physical dependence, psychological dependence, tolerance.

Interactions

Drug-Drug: Use with **opioids** or other **CNS depressants**, including other **benzodiazepines, nonbenzodiazepine sedative/hypnotics, anxiolytics, general anesthetics, muscle relaxants, antipsychotics**, and **alcohol** may cause profound sedation, respiratory depression, coma, and death; reserve concurrent use for when alternative treatment options are inadequate. **Cimetidine, hormonal contraceptives, disulfiram, fluoxetine, isoniazid, ketoconazole, metoprolol, propranolol,** or **valproic acid** may ↓ the metabolism of diazepam, enhancing its actions. May ↓ the efficacy of **levodopa**. **Rifampin** or **barbiturates** may ↑ the metabolism and ↓ effectiveness of diazepam. Sedative effects may be ↓ by **theophylline**. Concurrent use of **ritonavir** is not recommended.

Drug-Natural Products: Concomitant use of **kava-kava, valerian,** or **chamomile** can ↑ CNS depression.

Route/Dosage

Antianxiety

PO (Adults): 2–10 mg 2–4 times daily.

IM, IV (Adults): 2–10 mg, may repeat in 3–4 hr as needed.

PO (Children >6 mo): 1–2.5 mg 3–4 times daily.

IM, IV (Children >1 mo): 0.04–0.3 mg/kg/dose every 2–4 hr to a maximum of 0.6 mg/kg within an 8 hr period if necessary.

Precardioversion

IV (Adults): 5–15 mg 5–10 min precardioversion.

Pre-endoscopy

IV (Adults): 2.5–20 mg.

IM (Adults): 5–10 mg 30 min pre-endoscopy.

Pediatric Conscious Sedation for Procedures

PO (Children >6 mo): 0.2–0.3 mg/kg (not to exceed 10 mg/dose) 45–60 min prior to procedure.

Status Epilepticus/Acute Seizure Activity

IV (Adults): 5–10 mg, may repeat every 10–15 min to a total of 30 mg, may repeat regimen again in 2–4 hr (IM route may be used if IV route unavailable); larger doses may be required.

IM, IV (Children ≥5 yr): 0.05–0.3 mg/kg/dose given over 3–5 min every 15–30 min to a total dose of 10 mg, repeat every 2–4 hr.

IM, IV (Children 1 mo–5 yr): 0.05–0.3 mg/kg/dose given over 3–5 min every 15–30 min to maximum dose of 5 mg, repeat in 2–4 hr if needed.
IV (Neonates): 0.1–0.3 mg/kg/dose given over 3–5 min every 15–30 min to maximum dose of 2 mg.
Rect (Adults and Children >12 yr): 0.2 mg/kg; may repeat 4–12 hr later.
Rect (Children 6–11 yr): 0.3 mg/kg; may repeat 4–12 hr later.
Rect (Children 2–5 yr): 0.5 mg/kg; may repeat 4–12 hr later.

Febrile Seizure Prophylaxis

PO (Children >1 mo): 1 mg/kg/day divided every 8 hr at first sign of fever and continue for 24 hr after fever is gone.

Skeletal Muscle Relaxation

PO (Adults): 2–10 mg 3–4 times daily.
PO (Geriatric Patients or Debilitated Patients): 2–2.5 mg 1–2 times daily initially.
PO (Children >6 mo): 1–2.5 mg 3–4 times daily.
IM, IV (Adults): 5–10 mg; may repeat in 2–4 hr (larger doses may be required for tetanus).
IM, IV (Geriatric Patients or Debilitated Patients): 2–5 mg; may repeat in 2–4 hr (larger doses may be required for tetanus).
IM, IV (Children ≥5 yr): *Tetanus*—5–10 mg every 3–4 hr.
IM, IV (Children >1 mo): *Tetanus*—1–2 mg every 3–4 hr.

Alcohol Withdrawal

PO (Adults): 10 mg 3–4 times in first 24 hr, ↓ to 5 mg 3–4 times daily.
IM, IV (Adults): 10 mg initially, then 5–10 mg in 3–4 hr as needed; larger or more frequent doses have been used.

Psychoneurotic Reactions

IM, IV (Adults): 2–10 mg, may be repeated in 3–4 hr.

Availability (generic available)

Tablets: 2 mg, 5 mg, 10 mg. **Cost:** *Generic*—2 mg \$7.51/100, 5 mg \$10.74/100, 10 mg \$10.84/100. **Oral solution:** 1 mg/mL, 5 mg/mL (Intensol). **Cost:** *Generic*—1 mg/mL \$2.44/5 mL, 5 mg/mL \$33.98/30 mL. **Injection:** 5 mg/mL (contains 10% alcohol and 40% propylene glycol). **Rectal gel delivery system:** 2.5 mg, 10 mg, 20 mg.

NURSING IMPLICATIONS

Assessment

- Monitor BP, pulse, and respiratory rate prior to and periodically throughout therapy and frequently during IV therapy.
- Assess IV site frequently during administration; diazepam may cause phlebitis and venous thrombosis.
- Prolonged high-dose therapy may lead to psychological or physical dependence. Restrict amount of drug available to patient. Observe depressed patients closely for suicidal tendencies.
- Conduct regular assessment of continued need for treatment.
- Geri: Assess risk of falls and institute fall prevention strategies.
- **Anxiety:** Assess mental status (orientation, mood, behavior) and degree of anxiety.
- Assess level of sedation (ataxia, dizziness, slurred speech) prior to and periodically throughout therapy.
- **Seizures:** Observe and record intensity, duration, and location of seizure activity. The initial-dose of diazepam offers seizure control for 15–20 min after administration. Institute seizure precautions.
- **Muscle Spasms:** Assess muscle spasm, associated pain, and limitation of movement prior to and during therapy.
- **Alcohol Withdrawal:** Assess patient experiencing alcohol withdrawal for tremors, agitation, delirium, and hallucinations. Protect patient from injury.
- ***Lab Test Considerations:*** Evaluate hepatic and renal function and CBC periodically during prolonged therapy. May cause ↑ transaminases and alkaline phosphatase.
- ***Toxicity and Overdose:*** Flumazenil is an adjunct in the management of toxicity or overdose. (Flumazenil may induce seizures in patients with a history of seizures disorder or who are on tricyclic antidepressants.)

Implementation

- Do not confuse diazepam with diltiazem.
- Patient should be kept on bedrest and observed for at least 3 hr following parenteral administration.
- If opioid analgesics are used concurrently with parenteral diazepam, decrease opioid dose by ⅓ and titrate dose to effect.
- Use lowest effective dose. Taper by 2 mg every 3 days to decrease withdrawal symptoms. Some patients may require longer taper periods (mo).
- **PO:** Tablets may be crushed and taken with food or water if patient has difficulty swallowing.
- Mix Intensol preparation with liquid or semisolid food such as water, juices, soda, applesauce, or pudding. Administer entire amount immediately. Do not store.
- **IM:** IM injections are painful and erratically absorbed. If IM route is used, inject deeply into deltoid muscle for maximum absorption.

IV Administration

- **IV:** Resuscitation equipment should be available when diazepam is administered IV.
- **IV Push:** ***Diluent:*** For IV administration do not dilute or mix with any other drug. If IV push is not feasible, administer IV push into tubing as close to insertion site as possible. Continuous infusion is not recommended due to precipitation in IV fluids and

absorption of diazepam into infusion bags and tubing. Injection may cause burning and venous irritation; avoid small veins. ***Concentration:*** 5 mg/mL. ***Rate:*** Administer slowly at a rate of 5 mg/min in adults. Infants and children should receive 1–2 mg/min. Rapid injection may cause apnea, hypotension, bradycardia, or cardiac arrest.

- **Y-Site Compatibility:** docetaxel, methadone, piperacillin/tazobactam.
- **Y-Site Incompatibility:** acetaminophen, acyclovir, alemtuzumab, alfentanil, amikacin, aminocaproic acid, aminophylline, amphotericin B cholesteryl, amphotericin B deoxycholate, amphotericin B lipid complex, amphotericin B liposome, ampicillin, ampicillin/sulbactam, anidulafungin, argatroban, ascorbic acid, atracurium, atropine, azathioprine, aztreonam, azithromycin, benztropine, bivalirudin, bleomycin, bumetanide, buprenorphine, butorphanol, calcium chloride, calcium gluconate, carboplatin, carmustine, caspofungin, cefazolin, cefepime, cefotaxime, cefotetan, cefoxitin, ceftaroline, ceftazidime, ceftriaxone, cefuroxime, chloramphenicol, chlorpromazine, cisplatin, clindamycin, cyanocobalamin, cyclophosphamide, cyclosporine, cytarabine, dactinomycin, dantrolene, dexamethasone, dexmedetomidine, dexrazoxane, diazoxide, digoxin, diltiazem, diphenhydramine, dopamine, doxacurium, doxorubicin, doxorubicin liposomal, doxycycline, enalaprilat, ephedrine, epinephrine, epirubicin, epoetin alfa, eptifibatide, ertapenem, erythromycin, esmolol, etoposide, etoposide phosphate, famotidine, fenoldopam, fluconazole, fludarabine, fluorouracil, folic acid, foscarnet, furosemide, ganciclovir, gemcitabine, gentamicin, glycopyrrolate, granisetron, haloperidol, heparin, hetastarch, hydralazine, hydrocortisone, hydroxycobalamin, hydroxyzine, idarubicin, ifosfamide, imipenem/cilastatin, indomethacin, insulin, irinotecan, isoproterenol, ketorolac, labetalol, leucovorin calcium, levofloxacin, lidocaine, linezolid, magnesium chloride, mannitol, meperidine, meropenem, metaraminol, methotrexate, methoxamine, methyldopate, methylprednisolone, metoclopramide, metoprolol, metronidazole, midazolam, milrinone, mitoxantrone, multivitamin, mycophenolate, nalbuphine, naloxone, nitroglycerin, nitroprusside, norepinephrine, octreotide, oxacillin, oxaliplatin, oxytocin, paclitaxel, palonosetron, pancuronium, pantoprazole, papaverine, pemetrexed, penicillin G, pentamidine, pentobarbital, phenobarbital, phentolamine, phenylephrine, phenytoin, phytonadione, potassium acetate, potassium chloride, procainamide, prochlorperazine, promethazine, propofol, propranolol, protamine, pyridoxime, quinupristin/dalfopristin, ranitidine, rocuronium, sodium acetate, sodium bicarbonate, streptokinase, succinylcholine, tacrolimus, theophylline, thiamine, thiotepa, tigecycline, tirofiban, tobramycin, tolazoline, trimethoprim/sulfamethoxazole, vancomycin, vasopressin, vecuronium, verapamil, vinblastine, vincristine, vinorelbine, vitamin B complex with C, voriconazole, zoledronic acid.
- **Rect:** Do not repeat *Diastat* rectal dose more than 5 times/mo or 1 episode every 5 days. Round dose up to next available dose unit.
- Diazepam injection has been used for rectal administration. Instill via catheter or cannula fitted to the syringe or directly from a 1-mL syringe inserted 4–5 cm into the rectum. A dilution of diazepam injection with propylene glycol containing 1 mg/mL has also been used.
- Do not dilute with other solutions, IV fluids, or medications.

Patient/Family Teaching

- Instruct patient to take medication as directed and not to take more than prescribed or increase dose if less effective after a few wk without checking with health care professional. Review package insert for Diastat rectal gel with patient/caregiver prior to administration. Abrupt withdrawal of diazepam may cause insomnia, unusual irritability or nervousness, and seizures. Advise patient that sharing of this medication may be dangerous.
- Medication may cause drowsiness, clumsiness, or unsteadiness. Advise patient to avoid driving or other activities requiring alertness until response to medication is known. Geri: Advise geriatric patients of increased risk for CNS effects and potential for falls.
- Caution patient to avoid taking alcohol or other CNS depressants concurrently with this medication.
- Advise patient to notify health care professional if pregnancy is planned or suspected or if breast feeding.
- Emphasize the importance of follow-up examinations to determine effectiveness of the medication.
- **Seizures:** Patients on anticonvulsant therapy should carry identification describing disease process and medication regimen at all times.

Evaluation/Desired Outcomes

- Decrease in anxiety level. Full therapeutic antianxiety effects occur after 1–2 wk of therapy.
- Decreased recall of surgical or diagnostic procedures.
- Control of seizures.
- Decrease in muscle spasms.
- Decreased tremulousness and more rational ideation when used for alcohol withdrawal.

D

BEERS

DICLOFENAC† (dye-kloe-fen-ak)

diclofenac (oral)
Zorvolex

diclofenac potassium (oral)
Cambia, ~~Cataflam~~, Zipsor

diclofenac sodium (oral)
✱Voltaren, ✱Voltaren SR, ~~Voltaren XR~~

diclofenac sodium (rectal suppository)
✱Voltaren

diclofenac sodium (topical gel)
Solaraze, Voltaren

diclofenac sodium (topical solution)
Pennsaid

diclofenac epolamine (transdermal patch)
Flector

Classification
Therapeutic: nonopioid analgesics, nonsteroidal anti-inflammatory agents

†For ophthalmic use see Appendix C

Indications

PO: Management of inflammatory disorders including: Rheumatoid arthritis, Osteoarthritis, Ankylosing spondylitis. Primary dysmenorrhea. Relief of mild to moderate pain. Acute treatment of migraines (powder for oral solution). **Topical:** Management of: Actinic keratoses (Solaraze), Osteoarthritis (Voltaren Gel, Pennsaid [for knees]). **Transdermal:** Acute pain due to minor strains, sprains, and contusions.

Action

Inhibits prostaglandin synthesis. **Therapeutic Effects:** Suppression of pain and inflammation. Relief of acute migraine attacks. **Topical (Solaraze):** Clearance of actinic keratosis lesions.

Pharmacokinetics

Absorption: Undergoes first-pass metabolism by liver which results in 50% bioavailability. Oral diclofenac sodium is a delayed-release dose form. Diclofenac potassium is an immediate-release dose form. 6–10% of topical gel is systemically absorbed.
Distribution: Crosses the placenta.
Protein Binding: >99%.
Metabolism and Excretion: Metabolized by the liver (primarily by CYP2C9) to several metabolites; 65% excreted in urine, 35% in bile.
Half-life: 2 hr.

TIME/ACTION PROFILE

ROUTE	ONSET	PEAK	DURATION
PO (inflammation)	few days–1 wk	≥2 wk	unknown
PO (pain)	30 min	unknown	up to 8 hr
Top (gel and patch)	unknown	10–20 hr	unknown
Top (solution)	unknown	unknown	unknown

Contraindications/Precautions

Contraindicated in: Hypersensitivity to diclofenac or other components of formulation; Cross-sensitivity may occur with other NSAIDs including aspirin; Active GI bleeding/ulcer disease; Coronary artery bypass graft (CABG) surgery; Exudative dermatitis, eczema, infectious lesions, burns, or wounds.
Use Cautiously in: Severe renal/hepatic impairment; Cardiovascular disease or risk factors for cardiovascular disease (may ↑ risk of serious cardiovascular thrombotic events, myocardial infarction, and stroke, especially with prolonged use or use of higher doses); avoid use in patients with recent MI or HF; HF or edema; History of porphyria; History of peptic ulcer disease and/or GI bleeding; Bleeding tendency or concurrent anticoagulant therapy; OB, Lactation: Not recommended for use during 2nd half of pregnancy; Pedi: Safety and effectiveness only established for transdermal patch in children ≥6 yr;; Geri: Dose ↓ recommended; more susceptible to adverse effects, including GI bleeding.

Adverse Reactions/Side Effects

CNS: dizziness, headache. **CV:** HF, MYOCARDIAL INFARCTION, STROKE, edema, hypertension. **Derm:** EXFOLIATIVE DERMATITIS, STEVENS-JOHNSON SYNDROME, TOXIC EPIDERMAL NECROLYSIS, pruritus, rashes, eczema, photosensitivity. **EENT:** tinnitus. **F and E:** hyperkalemia. **GI:** GI BLEEDING, HEPATOTOXICITY, abdominal pain, constipation, diarrhea, dyspepsia, flatulence, heartburn, ↑ liver enzymes, nausea, vomiting. **GU:** acute renal failure, hematuria. **Hemat:** anemia, prolonged bleeding time. **Local:** *Topical only*—contact dermatitis, dry skin, exfoliation. **Misc:** HYPERSENSITIVITY REACTIONS (including anaphylaxis).

Interactions

Primarily noted for oral administration.

Drug-Drug: ↑ adverse GI effects with **aspirin**, other **NSAIDs**, or **corticosteroids**. May ↓ effectiveness of **diuretics** or **antihypertensives**. May ↑ levels/risk of toxicity from **cyclosporine**, **lithium**, or **methotrexate**. ↑ risk of bleeding with **anticoagulants**, **aspirin**, **clopidogrel**, **ticagrelor**, **prasugrel**, **corticosteroids**, **fibrinolytics**, **SNRIs**, or **SSRIs**. **CYP2C9 inhibitors**, including **voriconazole** may ↑ levels/risk of toxicity. **CYP2C9 inducers**, including **rifampin**, may

↓ levels/effectiveness. Concurrent use of oral **NSAIDs** during topical diclofenac therapy should be minimized.

Drug-Natural Products: ↑ bleeding risk with **arnica**, **chamomile**, **clove**, **dong quai**, **feverfew**, **garlic**, **ginger**, **ginkgo**, ***Panax ginseng***, and others.

Route/Dosage

Different formulations of oral diclofenac (diclofenac capsules, diclofenac sodium enteric-coated tablets, diclofenac sodium extended-release tablets, and diclofenac potassium immediate-release tablets) are not bioequivalent and should not be substituted on a mg-to-mg basis.

Diclofenac

PO (Adults): *Acute pain*—18–35 mg 3 times daily; *Osteoarthritis*—35 mg 3 times daily.

Hepatic Impairment

PO (Adults): Do not exceed dose of 18 mg 3 times daily.

Diclofenac Potassium

PO (Adults): *Analgesic/antidysmenorrheal (Cataflam)*—100 mg initially, then 50 mg 3 times daily as needed; *Analgesic (Zipsor)*—25 mg 4 times daily; *Rheumatoid arthritis (Cataflam)*—50 mg 3–4 times daily; *Osteoarthritis (Cataflam)*—50 mg 2–3 times daily; *Osteoarthritis (Cambia)*—one packet (50 mg) given as a single dose.

Diclofenac Sodium

PO (Adults): *Rheumatoid arthritis (delayed-release [enteric-coated] tablets)*—50 mg 3–4 times daily *or* 75 mg twice daily (usual maintenance dose 25 mg 3 times daily). *Rheumatoid arthritis (extended-release tablets)*—100 mg once daily; if unsatisfactory response, dose may be ↑ to 100 mg twice daily. *Osteoarthritis (delayed-release [enteric-coated] tablets)*—50 mg 2–3 times daily *or* 75 mg twice daily. *Osteoarthritis (extended-release tablets)*—100 mg once daily. *Ankylosing spondylitis (delayed-release [enteric-coated] tablets)*—25 mg 4 times daily, with an additional 25 mg given at bedtime, if necessary.

Topical (Adults): *Solaraze*—Apply to lesions twice daily for 60–90 days; *Voltaren gel*—Lower extremities (knees, ankles, feet): Apply 4 g to affected area 4 times daily (maximum of 16 g per joint/day); Upper extremities (elbows, wrists, hands): Apply 2 g to affected area 4 times daily (maximum of 8 g per joint/day). Maximum total body dose should not exceed 32 g/day; *Pennsaid*—Apply 40 drops to affected knee(s) 4 times daily.

Rect (Adults): Insert 50 mg or 100 mg as single dose to substitute for final oral daily dose (max combined dose [rectal and oral]: 100 mg/day).

Diclofenac Epolamine

Transdermal (Adults and Children ≥6 yr): *Flector*—Apply 1 patch to most painful area twice daily.

Availability (generic available)

Diclofenac capsules (Zorvolex): 18 mg, 35 mg. **Diclofenac epolamine transdermal patch (Flector):** 180 mg/patch. **Cost:** $239.70/30. **Diclofenac potassium immediate-release tablets (Cataflam):** 50 mg. **Cost:** *Generic*—$156.55/100. **Diclofenac potassium liquid-filled capsules (Zipsor):** 25 mg. **Cost:** $478.80/100. **Diclofenac potassium powder for oral solution (Cambia):** 50 mg/packet. **Cost:** $29.04/1 pkt. **Diclofenac sodium delayed-release (enteric-coated) tablets:** 25 mg, 50 mg, 75 mg. **Cost:** *Generic*—25 mg $142.18/100, 50 mg $147.23/100, 75 mg $177.39/100. **Diclofenac sodium extended-release tablets:** 🍁75 mg, 100 mg. **Cost:** *Generic*—100 mg $281.42/100. **Diclofenac sodium gel:** 1% (Voltaren gel), 3% (Solaraze). **Cost:** 1% $46.48/100 g, 3% $931.92/100 g. **Diclofenac sodium rectal suppository:** 🍁50 mg, 🍁100 mg. **Diclofenac sodium topical solution:** 1.5%. **Cost:** $289.67/150 mL. ***In combination with:*** misoprostol (Arthrotec). See Appendix B.

NURSING IMPLICATIONS

Assessment

- Patients who have asthma, aspirin-induced allergy, and nasal polyps are at ↑ risk for developing hypersensitivity reactions.
- Monitor BP closely during initiation of treatment and periodically during therapy in patients with hypertension.
- Assess patient for skin rash frequently during therapy. Discontinue at first sign of rash; may be life-threatening. Stevens-Johnson syndrome may develop. Treat symptomatically; may recur once treatment is stopped.
- **Pain:** Assess pain and limitation of movement; note type, location, and intensity before and 30–60 min after administration.
- **Arthritis:** Assess arthritic pain (note type, location, intensity) and limitation of movement before and periodically during therapy.
- **Actinic Keratosis:** Assess lesions prior to and periodically during therapy.
- ***Lab Test Considerations:*** Diclofenac has minimal effect on bleeding time and platelet aggregation.
- May cause ↓ in hemoglobin and hematocrit.
- Monitor CBC and liver function tests within 4–8 wk of initiating diclofenac and periodically during therapy. May cause ↑ serum alkaline phosphatase, LDH, AST, and ALT concentrations.
- Monitor BUN and serum creatinine periodically during therapy. May cause ↑ BUN and serum creatinine.

Implementation

- Administration in higher than recommended doses does not provide increased effectiveness but may cause increased side effects. Use lowest effective dose for shortest period of time.
- **PO:** Take with food or milk to minimize gastric irritation. May take first 1–2 doses on an empty stomach for more rapid onset. Do not crush or chew enteric-coated or extended-release tablets.
- **Dysmenorrhea:** Administer as soon as possible after the onset of menses. Prophylactic treatment has not been shown to be effective.
- **Topical: Gel** should be applied to intact skin; do not use on open wounds. An adequate amount of gel should be applied to cover the entire lesion.
- **Topical:** Dispense **solution** 10 drops at a time either directly onto knee or first into the hand and then onto knee. Spread solution evenly around front, back, and sides of the knee. Repeat until 40 drops have been applied and knee is completely covered with solution.
- **Transdermal:** Apply patch to the most painful area twice a day. Do not apply to nonintact or damaged skin resulting from any etiology (exudative dermatitis, eczema, infected lesion, burns, wounds). Avoid contact with eyes; wash hands after applying, handling, or removing patch.

Patient/Family Teaching

- Instruct patient to take diclofenac as directed and not take more than recommended. Advise patient that overuse (use more than 10 days/mo) may lead to exacerbation of headache (migraine-like daily headaches, or as a marked increase in frequency of migraine attacks). May require gradual withdrawal of diclofenac and treatment of symptoms (transient worsening of headache).
- Caution patient to avoid concurrent use of alcohol, aspirin, acetaminophen, other NSAIDs, or other OTC medications without consulting health care professional.
- Instruct patient to notify health care professional of medication regimen before treatment or surgery.
- May cause serious side effects: CV (MI or stroke), GI (ulcers, bleeding), skin (exfoliative dermatitis, Stevens-Johnson Syndrome, toxic epidermal necrolysis), and hypersensitivity (anaphylaxis). May occur without warning symptoms. Advise patient to stop medication and notify health care professional immediately if symptoms of CV side effects (chest pain, shortness of breath, weakness, slurring of speech), GI side effects (epigastric pain, dyspepsia, melena, hematemesis), skin side effects (skin rash, blisters, fever, itching), or hypersensitivity reactions (difficulty breathing or swelling of face or throat) occur. Inform patient that risk for heart attack or stroke that can lead to death increases with longer use of NSAID medications and in people who have heart disease and that risk of ulcer increases with concurrent use of corticosteroids and anticoagulants, longer use, smoking, drinking alcohol, older age, and having poor health.
- Advise patient to notify health care professional promptly if unexplained weight gain, swelling of arms and legs or hands and feet, nausea, fatigue, lethargy, rash, pruritus, yellowing of skin or eyes, itching, stomach pain, vomiting blood, bloody or tarry stools, or flu-like symptoms occur.
- Instruct patient to notify health care professional of all Rx or OTC medications, vitamins, or herbal products being taken and to consult with health care professional before taking other medications.
- Instruct female patients to inform health care professional if they plan or suspect pregnancy. Caution female patient to avoid use of diclofenac in last trimester of pregnancy and to notify health care professional if breast feeding.
- **PO:** Instruct patient to take diclofenac with a full glass of water and to remain in an upright position for 15–30 min after administration. Take missed doses as soon as possible within 1–2 hr if taking once or twice a day or unless almost time for next dose if taking more than twice a day. Do not double doses.
- May cause drowsiness or dizziness. Caution patient to avoid driving or other activities requiring alertness until response to medication is known.
- Caution patient to wear sunscreen and protective clothing to prevent photosensitivity reactions.
- **Topical:** Advise patient to minimize use of concurrent NSAIDs during topical therapy. Instruct patient to read *Medication Guide* before starting therapy and with each Rx refill in case changes have been made.
- *Pennsaid:* Instruct patient to avoid touching treated knee and allowing another person to touch knee until completely dry. Cover knee with clothing until completely dry. Avoid covering lesion with occlusive dressing or tight clothing, and avoid applying sunscreen, insect repellent, lotion, moisturizer, or cosmetics to the affected area. Do not use heating pads, sunlamps, and tanning beds. Protect treated knee from sunlight; wear protective clothes when in sunlight. Avoid showers or baths for at least 30 min after application.
- *Solaraze:* Advise patient that it may take up to 1 mo for complete healing of the lesion to occur.
- **Transdermal:** Instruct patient on correct application procedure for patch. Apply patch to most painful area. Change patch every 12 hr. Remove patch if irritation occurs. Fold used patches so adhesive sticks to itself and discard where children and pets cannot get them. Encourage patient to read the *NSAID Medication Guide* that accompanies the prescription.
- Instruct patients if patch begins to peel off to tape the edges. Do not wear patch during bathing or shower-

ing. Bathing should take place between scheduled patch removal and application.

- Advise patient referred for MRI test to discuss patch with referring health care professional and MRI facility to determine if removal of patch is necessary prior to test and for directions for replacing patch.

Evaluation/Desired Outcomes

- Decrease in severity of mild-to-moderate pain.
- Increased ease of joint movement. Patients who do not respond to one NSAID may respond to another. May require 2 wk or more for maximum effects.
- Decrease in or healing of lesions in actinic keratosis. Optimal effect may not be seen until 30 days after discontinuation of therapy. Lesions that do not heal should be re-evaluated.

dicloxacillin, See PENICILLINS, PENICILLINASE RESISTANT.

diflorasone, See CORTICOSTEROIDS (TOPICAL/LOCAL).

BEERS HIGH ALERT

digoxin (di-jox-in)

Lanoxin, Toloxin

Classification

Therapeutic: antiarrhythmics, inotropics

Pharmacologic: digitalis glycosides

Indications

Heart failure. Atrial fibrillation and atrial flutter (slows ventricular rate). Paroxysmal atrial tachycardia.

Action

Increases the force of myocardial contraction. Prolongs refractory period of the AV node. Decreases conduction through the SA and AV nodes. **Therapeutic Effects:** Increased cardiac output (positive inotropic effect) and slowing of the heart rate (negative chronotropic effect).

Pharmacokinetics

Absorption: 60–80% absorbed after oral administration of tablets; 70–85% absorbed after administration of elixir; 80% absorbed from IM sites (IM route not recommended due to pain/irritation).

Distribution: Widely distributed; crosses placenta and enters breast milk.

Metabolism and Excretion: Excreted almost entirely unchanged by the kidneys.

Half-life: 36–48 hr (↑ in renal impairment).

TIME/ACTION PROFILE (antiarrhythmic or inotropic effects, provided that a loading dose has been given)

ROUTE	ONSET	PEAK	DURATION
Digoxin–PO	30–120 min	2–8 hr	2–4 days†
Digoxin–IM	30 min	4–6 hr	2–4 days†
Digoxin–IV	5–30 min	1–4 hr	2–4 days†

†Duration listed is that for normal renal function; in impaired renal function, duration will be longer.

Contraindications/Precautions

Contraindicated in: Hypersensitivity; Uncontrolled ventricular arrhythmias; AV block (in absence of pacemaker); Idiopathic hypertrophic subaortic stenosis; Constrictive pericarditis; Known alcohol intolerance (elixir only).

Use Cautiously in: Hypokalemia (↑ risk of digoxin toxicity); Hypercalcemia (↑ risk of toxicity, especially with mild hypokalemia); Hypomagnesemia (↑ risk of digoxin toxicity); Diuretic use (may cause electrolyte abnormalities including hypokalemia and hypomagnesemia); Hypothyroidism; Myocardial infarction; Renal impairment (dose ↓ required); Obesity (base dose on ideal body weight); OB: Monitor neonates for signs/symptoms of digoxin toxicity; monitor levels in mother during pregnancy as levels may fluctuate during pregnancy and post-partum periods; may lead to ↑ risk of arrhythmias during labor and delivery; Lactation: Similar concentrations in serum and breast milk result in subtherapeutic levels in infant, use with caution; Geri: Very sensitive to toxic effects; dose adjustments required for age-related ↓ in renal function and body weight.

Adverse Reactions/Side Effects

CNS: fatigue, headache, weakness. **CV:** ARRHYTHMIAS, bradycardia, ECG changes, AV block, SA block. **EENT:** blurred vision, yellow or green vision. **GI:** anorexia, nausea, vomiting, diarrhea. **Hemat:** thrombocytopenia. **Metab:** electrolyte imbalances with acute digoxin toxicity.

Interactions

Drug-Drug: **Thiazide** and **loop diuretics**, **piperacillin/tazobactam**, **amphotericin B**, **corticosteroids**, and excessive use of **laxatives** may cause hypokalemia which may ↑ risk of toxicity. **Quinidine** and **ritonavir** may ↑ levels and lead to toxicity; ↓ digoxin dose by 30–50%. **Amiodarone** may ↑ levels and lead to toxicity; ↓ digoxin dose by 50%. **Cyclosporine**, **itraconazole**, **mirabegron**, **propafenone**, **quinine**, **spironolactone**, and **verapamil** may ↑ levels and lead to toxicity; serum level monitoring/dose ↓ may be required. Levels may be ↓ by some **antineoplastics** (**bleomycin**, **carmustine**, **cyclophosphamide**, **cytarabine**, **doxorubicin**, **methotrexate**, **procarba-**

zine, vincristine), **activated charcoal, cholestyramine, colestipol, metoclopramide, penicillamine, rifampin**, or **sulfasalazine**. In a small percentage (10%) of patients gut bacteria metabolize digoxin to inactive compounds; **macrolide anti-infectives (erythromycin, azithromycin, clarithromycin)** and **tetracyclines**, by killing these bacteria, will cause ↑ levels and toxicity; dose may need to be ↓ for up to 9 wk. Additive bradycardia may occur with **beta blockers, diltiazem, verapamil, clonidine, ivabradine**, and other **antiarrhythmics (quinidine, disopyramide)**. Concurrent use of **sympathomimetics** may ↑ risk of arrhythmias. **Thyroid hormones** may ↓ therapeutic effects.

Drug-Natural Products: Licorice and stimulant natural products (**aloe**) may ↑ risk of potassium depletion. **St. John's wort** may ↓ levels and effect.

Drug-Food: Concurrent ingestion of a **high-fiber meal** may ↓ absorption. Administer digoxin 1 hr before or 2 hrs after such a meal.

Route/Dosage

For rapid effect, a larger initial loading/digitalizing dose should be given in several divided doses over 12–24 hr. Maintenance doses are determined for digoxin by renal function. All dosing must be evaluated by individual response. In general, doses required for atrial arrhythmias are higher than those for inotropic effect.

IV, IM (Adults): *Digitalizing dose*—0.5–1 mg given as 50% of the dose initially and one quarter of the initial dose in each of 2 subsequent doses at 6–12 hr intervals.

IV, IM (Children >10 yr): *Digitalizing dose*—8–12 mcg/kg given as 50% of the dose initially and one quarter of the initial dose in each of 2 subsequent doses at 6–12 hr intervals.

IV, IM (Children 5–10 yr): *Digitalizing dose*—15–30 mcg/kg given as 50% of the dose initially and one quarter of the initial dose in each of 2 subsequent doses at 6–12 hr intervals.

IV, IM (Children 2–5 yr): *Digitalizing dose*—25–35 mcg/kg given as 50% of the dose initially and one quarter of the initial dose in each of 2 subsequent doses at 6–12 hr intervals.

IV, IM (Children 1–24 mo): *Digitalizing dose*—30–50 mcg/kg given as 50% of the dose initially and one quarter of the initial dose in each of 2 subsequent doses at 6–12 hr intervals.

IV, IM (Infants–full term): 20–30 mcg/kg given as 50% of the dose initially and one quarter of the initial dose in each of 2 subsequent doses at 6–12 hr intervals.

IV, IM (Infants–premature): *Digitalizing dose*—15–25 mcg/kg given as 50% of the dose initially and one quarter of the initial dose in each of 2 subsequent doses at 6–12 hr intervals.

PO (Adults): *Digitalizing dose*—0.75–1.5 mg given as 50% of the dose initially and one quarter of the initial dose in each of 2 subsequent doses at 6–12 hr intervals. *Maintenance dose*—0.125–0.5 mg/day depending on patient's lean body weight, renal function, and serum level.

PO (Geriatric Patients): Initial daily dose should not exceed 0.125 mg.

PO (Children >10 yr): *Digitalizing dose*—10–15 mcg/kg given as 50% of the dose initially and one quarter of the initial dose in each of 2 subsequent doses at 6–12 hr intervals. *Maintenance dose*—2.5–5 mcg/kg given daily as a single dose.

PO (Children 5–10 yr): *Digitalizing dose*—20–35 mcg/kg given as 50% of the dose initially and one quarter of the initial dose in each of 2 subsequent doses at 6–12 hr intervals. *Maintenance dose*—5–10 mcg/kg given daily in 2 divided doses.

PO (Children 2–5 yr): *Digitalizing dose*—30–40 mcg/kg given as 50% of the dose initially and one quarter of the initial dose in each of 2 subsequent doses at 6–12 hr intervals. *Maintenance dose*—7.5–10 mcg/kg given daily in 2 divided doses.

PO (Children 1–24 mo): *Digitalizing dose*—35–60 mcg/kg given as 50% of the dose initially and one quarter of the initial dose in each of 2 subsequent doses at 6–12 hr intervals. *Maintenance dose*—10–15 mcg/kg given daily in 2 divided doses.

PO (Infants–full term): *Digitalizing dose*—25–35 mcg/kg given as 50% of the dose initially and one quarter of the initial dose in each of 2 subsequent doses at 6–12 hr intervals. *Maintenance dose*—6–10 mcg/kg given daily in 2 divided doses.

PO (Infants–premature): *Digitalizing dose*—20–30 mcg/kg given as 50% of the dose initially and one quarter of the initial dose in each of 2 subsequent doses at 6–12 hr intervals. *Maintenance dose*—5–7.5 mcg/kg given daily in 2 divided doses.

Availability (generic available)

Elixir (lime flavor): 0.05 mg/mL. **Cost:** *Generic*—$42.10/60 mL. **Solution for injection:** 0.25 mg/mL. **Solution for injection (pediatric):** 0.1 mg/mL. **Tablets:** 0.0625 mg, 0.125 mg, 0.25 mg. **Cost:** *Generic*—All strengths $27.75/10.

NURSING IMPLICATIONS

Assessment

- Monitor apical pulse for 1 full min before administering. Withhold dose and notify health care professional if pulse rate is <60 bpm in an adult, <70 bpm in a child, or <90 bpm in an infant. Notify health care professional promptly of any significant changes in rate, rhythm, or quality of pulse.
- Pedi: Heart rate varies in children depending on age, ask health care professional to specify at what heart rates digoxin should be withheld.
- Monitor BP periodically in patients receiving IV digoxin.
- Monitor ECG during IV administration and 6 hr after each dose. Notify health care professional if bradycardia or new arrhythmias occur.

- Observe IV site for redness or infiltration; extravasation can lead to tissue irritation and sloughing.
- Monitor intake and output ratios and daily weights. Assess for peripheral edema, and auscultate lungs for rales/crackles throughout therapy.
- Before administering initial loading dose, determine whether patient has taken any digoxin in the preceding 2–3 wk.
- ***Lab Test Considerations:*** Evaluate serum electrolyte levels (especially potassium, magnesium, and calcium) and renal and hepatic function periodically during therapy. Notify health care professional before giving dose if patient is hypokalemic. Hypokalemia, hypomagnesemia, or hypercalcemia may make the patient more susceptible to digitalis toxicity. Pedi: Neonates may have falsely elevated serum digoxin concentrations due to a naturally occurring substance chemically similar to digoxin.
- ***Toxicity and Overdose:*** Therapeutic serum digoxin levels range from 0.5–2 ng/mL. Serum levels may be drawn 6–8 hr after a dose is administered; usually drawn immediately before the next dose. Geri: Older adults are at increased risk for toxic effects of digoxin (on Beers list) due to age-related decreased renal clearance; may exist even when serum creatinine levels are normal. Digoxin requirements in older adult may change and a formerly therapeutic dose can become toxic.
- Observe for signs and symptoms of toxicity. *In adults and older children,* first symptoms of toxicity usually include abdominal pain, anorexia, nausea, vomiting, visual disturbances, bradycardia, and other arrhythmias. *In infants and small children,* first signs of overdose are usually cardiac arrhythmias. If these appear, withhold drug and notify health care professional immediately.
- If signs of toxicity occur and are not severe, discontinuation of digoxin may be all that is required.
- Correct electrolyte abnormalities, thyroid dysfunction, and concomitant medications. Administer potassium to maintain serum potassium between 4.0 and 5.5 mmol/L. Monitor ECG for evidence of potassium toxicity (peaked T waves).
- Treatment of life-threatening arrhythmias may include administration of digoxin immune Fab *(Digibind)*, which binds to the digitalis glycoside molecule in the blood and is excreted by the kidneys.

Implementation

- Do not confuse Lanoxin (digoxin) with levothyroxine or naloxone.
- ***High Alert:*** Digoxin has a narrow therapeutic range. Medication errors associated with digoxin include miscalculation of pediatric doses and insufficient monitoring of digoxin levels. Have second practitioner independently check original order and dose calculations.
- For rapid digitalization, initial dose is higher than maintenance dose; 50% of total digitalizing dose is given initially. Administer remainder of dose in 25% increments at 4–8 hr intervals.
- When changing from parenteral to oral dose forms, dose adjustments may be necessary because of pharmacokinetic variations in percentage of digoxin absorbed: 100 mcg (0.1 mg) digoxin injection = 125 mcg (0.125 mg) tablet or 125 mcg (0.125 mg) of elixir.
- **PO:** Administer oral preparations consistently with regard to meals. Tablets can be crushed and administered with food or fluids if patient has difficulty swallowing. Use calibrated measuring device for elixir; calibrated dropper is not accurate for doses of less than 0.2 mL or 10 mcg.
- **IM:** Administer deep into gluteal muscle and massage well to reduce painful local reactions. Do not administer more than 2 mL of digoxin in each IM site. IM administration is not generally recommended.

IV Administration

- **IV Push:** ***Diluent:*** May be administered undiluted. May also dilute 1 mL of digoxin in 4 mL of sterile water for injection, D5W, or 0.9% NaCl. Less diluent will cause precipitation. Use diluted solution immediately. ***Rate:*** Administer over at least 5 min.
- **Y-Site Compatibility:** acyclovir, alemtuzumab, alfentanil, amikacin, aminocaproic acid, aminophylline, amphotericin B lipid complex, anidulafungin, argatroban, arsenic trioxide, ascorbic acid, atracurium, atropine, azathioprine, azithromycin, aztreonam, benztropine, bivalirudin, bleomycin, bumetanide, buprenorphine, butorphanol, calcium chloride, calcium gluconate, cangrelor, carboplatin, carmustine, cefazolin, cefotaxime, cefotetan, cefoxitin, ceftaroline, ceftazidime, ceftriaxone, cefuroxime, chloramphenicol, chlorpromazine, ciprofloxacin, cisatracurium, cisplatin, clindamycin, cyanocobalamin, cyclophosphamide, cyclosporine, cytarabine, dacarbazine, dactinomycin, daptomycin, daunorubicin, dexamethasone, dexmedetomidine, dexrazoxane, diltiazem, dimenhydrinate, diphenhydramine, dobutamine, docetaxel, dolasetron, dopamine, doxorubicin liposome, doxycycline, enalaprilat, ephedrine, epinephrine, epirubicin, epoetin alfa, eptifibatide, ertapenem, erythromycin, esmolol, etoposide, etoposide phosphate, famotidine, fenoldopam, fentanyl, fludarabine, fluorouracil, folic acid, fosfomycin, fosphenytoin, furosemide, ganciclovir, gemcitabine, gentamicin, glycopyrrolate, granisetron, heparin, hetastarch, hydrocortisone sodium succinate, hydromorphone, ifosfamide, imipenem/cilastatin, indomethacin, irinotecan, isoproterenol, ketamine, ketorolac, labetalol, leucovorin calcium, levofloxacin, lidocaine, linezolid, lorazepam, mag-

nesium sulfate, mannitol, meperidine, meropenem, mesna, methohexital, methotrexate, methylprednisolone sodium succinate, metoclopramide, metoprolol, midazolam, milrinone, mitomycin, morphine, moxifloxacin, multivitamins, mycophenolate, nafcillin, nalbuphine, naloxone, nicardipine, nitroglycerin, nitroprusside, norepinephrine, octreotide, ondansetron, oxacillin, oxaliplatin, oxytocin, palonosetron, pamidronate, pancuronium, pantoprazole, papaverine, pemetrexed, penicillin G, pentobarbital, phenobarbital, phentolamine, phenylephrine, phytonadione, piperacillin/tazobactam, potassium acetate, potassium chloride, procainamide, prochlorperazine, promethazine, propranolol, protamine, pyridoxine, ranitidine, remifentanil, rituximab, rocuronium, sodium acetate, sodium bicarbonate, streptomycin, succinylcholine, sufentanil, tacrolimus, theophylline, thiamine, thiotepa, tigecycline, tirofiban, tobramycin, trastuzumab, vancomycin, vasopressin, vecuronium, verapamil, vinblastine, vincristine, vinorelbine, vitamin B complex with C, voriconazole, zoledronic acid.

- **Y-Site Incompatibility:** amiodarone, amphotericin B deoxycholate, amphotericin B liposome, caspofungin, dantrolene, diazepam, diazoxide, doxorubicin, foscarnet, idarubicin, minocycline, mitoxantrone, paclitaxel, pentamidine, phenytoin, propofol, quinupristin/dalfopristin, telavancin, topotecan, trimethoprim/sulfamethoxazole.

Patient/Family Teaching

- Instruct patient to take medication as directed, at same time each day. Teach parents or caregivers of infants and children how to accurately measure medication. Take missed doses within 12 hr of scheduled dose or omit. Do not double doses. Consult health care professional if doses for 2 or more days are missed. Do not discontinue medication without consulting health care professional.
- Teach patient to take pulse and to contact health care professional before taking medication if pulse rate is <60 or >100.
- Pedi: Teach parents or caregivers that changes in heart rate, especially bradycardia, are among the first signs of digoxin toxicity in infants and children. Instruct parents or caregivers in apical heart rate assessment and ask them to notify health care professional if heart rate is outside of range set by health care professional before administering the next scheduled dose.
- Review signs and symptoms of digitalis toxicity with patient and family. Advise patient to notify health care professional immediately if these or symptoms of HF occur. Inform patient that these symptoms may be mistaken for those of colds or flu.
- Instruct patient to keep digoxin tablets in their original container and not to mix in pill boxes with other medications; may look similar to and may be mistaken for other medications.
- Advise patient that sharing of this medication can be dangerous.
- Instruct patient to notify health care professional of all Rx or OTC medications, vitamins, or herbal products being taken and to consult health care professional before taking other Rx, OTC, or herbal products, especially St. John's wort. Advise patient to avoid taking antacids or antidiarrheals within 2 hr of digoxin.
- Advise patient to notify health care professional of this medication regimen before treatment.
- Patients taking digoxin should carry identification describing disease process and medication regimen at all times.
- Geri: Review fall prevention strategies with older adults and their families.
- Advise female patient to notify health care professional if pregnancy is planned or suspected, may increase risk for low birth weight or preterm birth. Monitor neonates for signs and symptoms of digoxin toxicity (vomiting, cardiac arrhythmias).
- Emphasize the importance of routine follow-up exams to determine effectiveness and to monitor for toxicity.

Evaluation/Desired Outcomes

- Decrease in severity of HF.
- Increase in cardiac output.
- Decrease in ventricular response in atrial tachyarrhythmias.
- Termination of paroxysmal atrial tachycardia.

dilTIAZem (dil-tye-a-zem)

Cardizem, Cardizem CD, Cardizem LA, Cartia XT, Taztia XT, Tiazac, ✱Tiazac XC

Classification

Therapeutic: antianginals, antiarrhythmics (class IV), antihypertensives
Pharmacologic: calcium channel blockers

Indications

Hypertension. Angina pectoris and vasospastic (Prinzmetal's) angina. Supraventricular tachyarrhythmias and rapid ventricular rates in atrial flutter or fibrillation.

Action

Inhibits transport of calcium into myocardial and vascular smooth muscle cells, resulting in inhibition of excitation-contraction coupling and subsequent contraction. **Therapeutic Effects:** Systemic vasodilation resulting in decreased BP. Coronary vasodilation resulting in decreased frequency and severity of attacks of angina. Reduction of ventricular rate in atrial fibrillation or flutter.

Pharmacokinetics

Absorption: Well absorbed, but rapidly metabolized after oral administration.

Distribution: Unknown.
Protein Binding: 70–80%.
Metabolism and Excretion: Mostly metabolized by the liver (CYP3A4 enzyme system).
Half-life: 3.5–9 hr.

TIME/ACTION PROFILE

ROUTE	ONSET	PEAK	DURATION
PO	30 min	2–3 hr	6–8 hr
PO–CD, LA, XT	unknown	14 days†	up to 24 hr
IV	2–5 min	2–4 hr	unknown

†Maximum antihypertensive effect with chronic therapy.

Contraindications/Precautions

Contraindicated in: Hypersensitivity; Sick sinus syndrome; 2nd- or 3rd-degree AV block (unless an artificial pacemaker is in place); Systolic BP <90 mm Hg; Recent MI or pulmonary congestion; Concurrent use of rifampin.
Use Cautiously in: Severe hepatic impairment (↓ dose recommended); Geri: ↓ dose; slower IV infusion rate recommended; ↑ risk of hypotension; consider age-related decrease in body mass, ↓ hepatic/renal/cardiac function, concurrent drug therapy, and other disease states); Severe renal impairment; Serious ventricular arrhythmias or HF; OB, Lactation, Pedi: Safety not established.

Adverse Reactions/Side Effects

CNS: abnormal dreams, anxiety, confusion, dizziness, drowsiness, headache, nervousness, psychiatric disturbances, weakness. **EENT:** blurred vision, disturbed equilibrium, epistaxis, tinnitus. **Resp:** cough, dyspnea. **CV:** ARRHYTHMIAS, HF, peripheral edema, bradycardia, chest pain, hypotension, palpitations, syncope, tachycardia. **GI:** ↑ liver enzymes, anorexia, constipation, diarrhea, dry mouth, dysgeusia, dyspepsia, nausea, vomiting. **GU:** dysuria, nocturia, polyuria, sexual dysfunction, urinary frequency. **Derm:** STEVENS-JOHNSON SYNDROME, dermatitis, erythema multiforme, flushing, sweating, photosensitivity, pruritus/urticaria, rash. **Endo:** gynecomastia, hyperglycemia. **Hemat:** anemia, leukopenia, thrombocytopenia. **Metab:** weight gain. **MS:** joint stiffness, muscle cramps. **Neuro:** paresthesia, tremor. **Misc:** gingival hyperplasia.

Interactions

Drug-Drug: ↑ hypotension may occur when used with **fentanyl**, other **antihypertensives**, **nitrates**, acute ingestion of **alcohol**, or **quinidine**. Antihypertensive effects may be ↓ by **NSAIDs**. May ↑ **digoxin** levels. May ↑ levels of and risk of myopathy from **simvastatin** and **lovastatin**. Concurrent use with **beta blockers**, **clonidine**, **digoxin**, **disopyramide**, **ivabradine**, or **phenytoin** may result in bradycardia, conduction defects, or HF; avoid concurrent use with ivabradine. **Phenobarbital** and **phenytoin** may ↑ metabolism and ↓ effectiveness. May ↓ metabolism of and ↑ risk of toxicity from **cyclosporine**, **quinidine**, or **carbamazepine**. **Cimetidine** and **ranitidine** ↑ levels and effects. May ↑ or ↓ the effects of **lithium** or **theophylline**.
Drug-Food: Grapefruit juice ↑ levels and effect.

Route/Dosage

PO (Adults): 30–120 mg 3–4 times daily or 180–240 mg once daily as CD or XR capsules or LA tablets (up to 360 mg/day); *Concurrent simvastatin therapy*—Diltiazem dose should not exceed 240 mg/day and simvastatin dose should not exceed 10 mg/day.
IV (Adults): 0.25 mg/kg; may repeat in 15 min with a dose of 0.35 mg/kg. May follow with continuous infusion at 10 mg/hr (range 5–15 mg/hr) for up to 24 hr.

Availability (generic available)

Tablets: 30 mg, 60 mg, 90 mg, 120 mg. **Cost:** *Generic*—30 mg $10.44/100, 60 mg $22.25/100, 90 mg $26.89/100. **Extended-release capsules (Cardizem CD, Tiazac, Cartia XT, Taztia XT):** 120 mg, 180 mg, 240 mg, 300 mg, 360 mg, 420 mg. **Cost:** *Generic*—180 mg $58.19/100, 240 mg $63.54/100, 420 mg $171.49/100. **Extended-release tablets (Cardizem LA):** 120 mg, 180 mg, 240 mg, 300 mg, 360 mg, 420 mg. **Solution for injection:** 5 mg/mL.

NURSING IMPLICATIONS

Assessment

- Monitor BP and pulse prior to therapy, during dose titration, and periodically during therapy. Monitor ECG periodically during prolonged therapy. May cause prolonged PR interval.
- Monitor intake and output ratios and daily weight. Assess for signs of HF (peripheral edema, rales/crackles, dyspnea, weight gain, jugular venous distention).
- Monitor frequency of prescription refills to determine adherence.
- Patients receiving digoxin concurrently with calcium channel blockers should have routine serum digoxin levels checked and be monitored for signs and symptoms of digoxin toxicity.
- Assess for rash periodically during therapy. May cause Stevens-Johnson syndrome. Discontinue therapy if severe or if accompanied with fever, general malaise, fatigue, muscle or joint aches, blisters, oral lesions, conjunctivitis, hepatitis and/or eosinophilia.
- **Angina:** Assess location, duration, intensity, and precipitating factors of patient's anginal pain.
- **Arrhythmias:** Monitor ECG continuously during administration. Report bradycardia or prolonged hypotension promptly. Emergency equipment and

medication should be available. Monitor BP and pulse before and frequently during administration.

- ***Lab Test Considerations:*** Total serum calcium concentrations are not affected by calcium channel blockers.
- Monitor serum potassium periodically. Hypokalemia ↑ the risk of arrhythmias and should be corrected.
- Monitor renal and hepatic functions periodically during long-term therapy. May cause ↑ in hepatic enzymes after several days of therapy, which return to normal on discontinuation of therapy.

Implementation

- Do not confuse Cardizem (diltiazem) with Cardene (nicardipine). Do not confuse Tiazac (diltiazem) with Ziac (bisoprolol/hydrochlorothiazide). Do not confuse diltiazem with diazepam.
- **PO:** May be administered without regard to meals. May be administered with meals if GI irritation becomes a problem.
- Do not open, crush, break, or chew extended-release tablets. Empty tablets that appear in stool are not significant.

IV Administration

- **IV Push: *Diluent:*** Administer bolus dose undiluted. ***Concentration:*** 5 mg/mL. ***Rate:*** Administer over 2 min.
- **Continuous Infusion: *Diluent:*** Dilute 125 mg in 100 mL, 250 mg in 250 mL, or 250 mg in 500 mL of 0.9% NaCl, D5W, or D5/0.45% NaCl. Infusion is stable for 24 hr at room temperature or if refrigerated. ***Concentration:*** 125 mg/125 mL (1 mg/mL), 250 mg/300 mL (0.83 mg/mL), 250 mg/550 mL (0.45 mg/mL). ***Rate:*** See Route/Dosage section. Titrate to patient's heart rate and BP response.
- **Y-Site Compatibility:** albumin, alemtuzumab, alfentanil, amifostine, amikacin, aminocaproic acid, amiodarone, amphotericin B deoxycholate, anidulafungin, argatroban, atracurium, azithromycin, aztreonam, bivalirudin, bleomycin, bumetanide, buprenorphine, busulfan, butorphanol, calcium chloride, calcium gluconate, cangrelor, carboplatin, carmustine, caspofungin, cefazolin, cefotaxime, cefotetan, cefoxitin, ceftaroline, ceftazidime, ceftriaxone, cefuroxime, chlorpromazine, ciprofloxacin, cisatracurium, cisplatin, clindamycin, cyclophosphamide, cyclosporine, cytarabine, dacarbazine, dactinomycin, daptomycin, daunorubicin, dexamethasone, dexmedetomidine, dexrazoxane, digoxin, diphenhydramine, dobutamine, docetaxel, dolasetron, dopamine, doxorubicin, doxycycline, droperidol, enalaprilat, ephedrine, epinephrine, epirubicin, eptifibatide, ertapenem, erythromycin, esmolol, etoposide, etoposide phosphate, famotidine, fenoldopam, fentanyl, fluconazole, fludarabine, foscarnet, fosphenytoin, gemcitabine, gentamicin, glycopyrrolate, granisetron, haloperidol, hetastarch, hydralazine, hydromorphone, idarubicin, ifosfamide, imipenem/cilastatin, irinotecan, isoproterenol, labetalol, leucovorin calcium, levofloxacin, lidocaine, linezolid, lorazepam, magnesium sulfate, mannitol, melphalan, meperidine, meropenem, metoclopramide, metoprolol, metronidazole, midazolam, milrinone, mitoxantrone, morphine, moxifloxacin, multivitamins, mycophenolate, nalbuphine, naloxone, nicardipine, nitroglycerin, nitroprusside, norepinephrine, octreotide, ondansetron, oxacillin, oxaliplatin, oxytocin, paclitaxel, palonosetron, pamidronate, pancuronium, pemetrexed, penicillin G potassium, pentamidine, phentolamine, phenylephrine, potassium acetate, potassium chloride, potassium phosphates, prochlorperazine, promethazine, propranolol, quinupristin/dalfopristin, ranitidine, remifentanil, rocuronium, sodium acetate, streptozocin, succinylcholine, sufentanil, tacrolimus, telavancin, theophylline, thiotepa, tigecycline, tirofiban, tobramycin, topotecan, trimethoprim/sulfamethoxazole, vancomycin, vasopressin, vecuronium, verapamil, vinblastine, vincristine, vinorelbine, voriconazole, zidovudine, zoledronic acid.
- **Y-Site Incompatibility:** allopurinol, amphotericin B lipid complex, amphotericin B liposome, cefepime, chloramphenicol, dantrolene, diazepam, doxorubicin liposomal, fluorouracil, furosemide, ganciclovir, ketorolac, methotrexate, micafungin, mitomycin, pantoprazole, pentobarbital, phenobarbital, phenytoin, piperacillin/tazobactam, rifampin, thiopental.

Patient/Family Teaching

- Advise patient to take medication as directed at the same time each day, even if feeling well. Take missed doses as soon as possible unless almost time for next dose; do not double doses. May need to be discontinued gradually.
- Advise patient to avoid large amounts (6–8 glasses of grapefruit juice/day) during therapy.
- Instruct patient on correct technique for monitoring pulse. Instruct patient to contact health care professional if heart rate is <50 bpm.
- Caution patient to change positions slowly to minimize orthostatic hypotension.
- May cause drowsiness or dizziness. Advise patient to avoid driving or other activities requiring alertness until response to the medication is known.
- Instruct patient on importance of maintaining good dental hygiene and seeing dentist frequently for teeth cleaning to prevent tenderness, bleeding, and gingival hyperplasia (gum enlargement).
- Instruct patient to notify health care professional of all Rx or OTC medications, vitamins, or herbal products being taken and to avoid concurrent use of alcohol or OTC medications and herbal products, especially NSAIDs and cold preparations, without consulting health care professional.
- Advise patient to notify health care professional if rash, irregular heartbeats, dyspnea, swelling of hands and feet, pronounced dizziness, nausea, con-

stipation, or hypotension occurs or if headache is severe or persistent.

- Caution patient to wear protective clothing and use sunscreen to prevent photosensitivity reactions.
- Advise female patient to notify health care professional if pregnancy is planned or suspected or if breast feeding.
- **Angina:** Instruct patient on concurrent nitrate or beta-blocker therapy to continue taking both medications as directed and to use SL nitroglycerin as needed for anginal attacks.
- Advise patient to contact health care professional if chest pain does not improve, worsens after therapy, or occurs with diaphoresis; if shortness of breath occurs; or if severe, persistent headache occurs.
- Caution patient to discuss exercise restrictions with health care professional before exertion.
- **Hypertension:** Encourage patient to comply with other interventions for hypertension (weight reduction, low-sodium diet, smoking cessation, moderation of alcohol consumption, regular exercise, and stress management). Medication controls but does not cure hypertension.
- Instruct patient and family in proper technique for monitoring BP. Advise patient to take BP weekly and to report significant changes to health care professional.

Evaluation/Desired Outcomes

- Decrease in BP.
- Decrease in frequency and severity of anginal attacks.
- Decrease in need for nitrate therapy.
- Increase in activity tolerance and sense of well-being.
- Suppression and prevention of tachyarrhythmias.

dimethyl fumarate

(dye-**meth**-il **fue**-ma-rate)

Tecfidera

Classification

Therapeutic: anti-multiple sclerosis agents

Indications

Relapsing forms of multiple sclerosis, including clinically isolated syndrome, relapsing-remitting disease, and active secondary progressive disease.

Action

Activates nuclear factor (Nrf2) pathway involved in cellular response to oxidative stress. **Therapeutic Effects:** Decreased incidence/severity of relapse with decreased progression of lesions and disability.

Pharmacokinetics

Absorption: Following oral administration rapidly converted to active metabolite monomethyl fumarate (MMF) by enzymes in GI tract, blood, and tissue.

Distribution: Unknown.

Metabolism and Excretion: MMF is metabolized by the tricarboxylic acid (TCA) cycle. 60% eliminated via exhalation of CO_2. Minor amounts eliminated by renal (16%) and fecal (1%) routes, trace amounts in urine.

Half-life: *MMF*—1 hr.

TIME/ACTION PROFILE (effects on disability)

ROUTE	ONSET	PEAK	DURATION
PO	24 wk	60 wk	Unknown

Contraindications/Precautions

Contraindicated in: Hypersensitivity.

Use Cautiously in: Serious infections (treatment may be withheld); OB: Use only if potential maternal benefit justifies potential fetal risk; Lactation: Use cautiously if breast feeding; Pedi: Safety and effectiveness not established.

Adverse Reactions/Side Effects

CNS: PROGRESSIVE MULTIFOCAL LEUKOENCEPHALOPATHY (PML). **Derm:** flushing, erythema, pruritus, rash. **GI:** HEPATOTOXICITY, abdominal pain, diarrhea, nausea, dyspepsia, ↑ liver enzymes, vomiting. **Hemat:** lymphopenia. **Misc:** HYPERSENSITIVITY REACTIONS (including anaphylaxis and angioedema).

Interactions

Drug-Drug: None noted.

Route/Dosage

PO (Adults): 120 mg twice daily for one wk, then 240 mg twice daily.

Availability

Extended-release capsules: 120 mg, 240 mg.

NURSING IMPLICATIONS

Assessment

- Monitor for signs and symptoms of infections (fever, sore throat). Consider withholding medication until serious infections are resolved.
- Monitor for signs and symptoms of PML (progressive weakness on one side of body or clumsiness of limbs, disturbance of vision, changes in thinking, memory, and orientation causing confusion and personality changes). Symptoms are diverse, progress over days to weeks. Withhold medication and obtain diagnostic evaluation.
- ***Lab Test Considerations:*** Monitor CBC with lymphocyte count before initiating therapy, after 6 mo, and every 6–12 mo thereafter. If lymphocyte count

is <0.5 × 10^9/L for >6 mo, may interrupt therapy. Consider withholding therapy for patients with serious infections.

- Obtain serum aminotransferase, alkaline phosphatase, and total bilirubin levels prior to starting therapy and as clinically indicated. May cause ↑ hepatic transaminases. Discontinue therapy if clinically significant liver injury is suspected.
- May cause transient ↑ mean eosinophil count during first 2 mo of therapy.

Implementation

- **PO:** Administer 120 mg twice daily for 7 days then increase to maintenance dose of 240 mg twice daily without regard to food. For patients with difficulty tolerating maintenance dose, may temporarily decrease to 120 mg twice daily; resume maintenance dose within 4 wk. Swallow capsules whole; do not open, crush, chew, or sprinkle on food. Discard any unused capsules 90 days after opening.

Patient/Family Teaching

- Instruct patient to take dimethyl fumarate as directed. Advise patient to read *Patient Information* before starting therapy and with each Rx refill in case of changes.
- Caution patient not to share medication with others, even if they have the same symptoms; may be dangerous.
- May cause flushing (warmth, redness, itching, and/or burning sensation). Usually begins after starting and resolves over time. Administration of dimethyl fumarate with food or administration of non-enteric coated aspirin (up to a dose of 325 mg) 30 min prior to dimethyl fumarate dosing may decrease incidence or severity of flushing.
- Advise patient to notify health care professional promptly if signs and symptoms of PML (new or worsening weakness; trouble using their arms or legs; or changes to thinking, eyesight, strength or balance) or hypersensitivity reactions (difficulty breathing, urticaria, swelling of throat and tongue) occur.
- Advise patient to notify health care professional of all Rx or OTC medications, vitamins, or herbal products being taken and to consult with health care professional before taking other medications.
- Rep: Advise female patient to notify health care professional if pregnancy is planned or suspected, or if breast feeding. Patients who become pregnant should be encouraged to join the pregnancy registry by calling 1-866-810-1462 or visiting www.tecfiderapregnancyregistry.com.

Evaluation/Desired Outcomes

- Decreased incidence/severity of relapse of multiple sclerosis.

dinoprostone

(dye-noe-**prost**-one)

Cervidil, Prepidil, Prostin E

Classification

Therapeutic: cervical ripening agent

Pharmacologic: oxytocics, prostaglandins

Indications

Endocervical Gel and Vaginal Insert: Used to "ripen" the cervix in pregnancy at or near term when induction of labor is indicated. **Vaginal Suppository:** Used for the following indications: Induction of midtrimester abortion, Management of missed abortion up to 28 wk, Management of nonmetastatic gestational trophoblastic disease (benign hydatidiform mole).

Action

Produces contractions similar to those occurring during labor at term by stimulating the myometrium (oxytocic effect). Initiates softening, effacement, and dilation of the cervix ("ripening"). Also stimulates GI smooth muscle. **Therapeutic Effects:** Initiation of labor. Expulsion of fetus.

Pharmacokinetics

Absorption: Rapidly absorbed.

Distribution: Unknown. Action is mostly local.

Metabolism and Excretion: Metabolized by enzymes in lung, kidneys, spleen, and liver tissue.

Half-life: Unknown.

TIME/ACTION PROFILE

ROUTE	ONSET	PEAK	DURATION
Cervical ripening (gel)	rapid	30–45 min	unknown
Cervical ripening (insert)	rapid	unknown	12 hr
Abortion time (suppository)	10 min	12–24 hr	2–3 hr

Contraindications/Precautions

Contraindicated in: Hypersensitivity to prostaglandins or additives in the gel or suppository; The gel/insert should be avoided in situations in which prolonged uterine contractions should be avoided, including: Previous cesarean section or uterine surgery; Cephalopelvic disproportion; Traumatic delivery or difficult labor; Multiparity (≥6 term pregnancies); Hyperactive or hypertonic uterus; Fetal distress (if delivery is not imminent); Unexplained vaginal bleeding; Placenta previa; Vasa previa; Active herpes genitalis; Obstetric emergency requiring surgical intervention; Situations in which vaginal delivery is contraindicated; Presence of acute pelvic inflammatory disease or ruptured membranes; Concurrent oxytocic therapy (wait for 30 min after removing insert before using oxytocin).

Use Cautiously in: Uterine scarring; Asthma; Hypotension; Cardiac disease; Adrenal disorders; Anemia; Jaundice; Diabetes mellitus; Epilepsy; Glaucoma; Pulmonary, renal, or hepatic disease; Multiparity (up to 5 previous term pregnancies); Women >30 yr, those with complications during pregnancy, and those with a gestational age >40 wk (↑ risk of disseminated intravascular coagulation).

Adverse Reactions/Side Effects

Endocervical Gel, Vaginal Insert.

GU: uterine contractile abnormalities, warm feeling in vagina. **MS:** back pain. **Misc:** AMNIOTIC FLUID EMBOLISM, fever.

Suppository

CNS: headache, drowsiness, syncope. **CV:** hypotension, hypertension. **GI:** diarrhea, nausea, vomiting. **GU:** UTERINE RUPTURE, urinary tract infection, uterine hyperstimulation, vaginal/uterine pain. **Resp:** cough, dyspnea, wheezing. **Misc:** HYPERSENSITIVITY REACTIONS (including anaphylaxis), chills, fever.

Interactions

Drug-Drug: Augments the effects of other **oxytocics**.

Route/Dosage

Cervical Ripening

Vag (Adults , Cervical): *Endocervical gel*—0.5 mg; if response is unfavorable, may repeat in 6 hr (not to exceed 1.5 mg/24 hr). *Vaginal insert*—one 10-mg insert.

Abortifacient

Vag (Adults): One 20-mg suppository, repeat every 3–5 hr (not to exceed 240 mg total or longer than 48 hr).

Availability

Endocervical gel (Prepidil): 0.5 mg dinoprostone in 3 g of gel vehicle in a prefilled syringe with catheters. **Vaginal insert (Cervidil):** 10 mg. **Vaginal suppository (Prostin E Vaginal):** 20 mg.

NURSING IMPLICATIONS

Assessment

- **Abortifacient:** Monitor frequency, duration, and force of contractions and uterine resting tone. Opioid analgesics may be administered for uterine pain.
- Monitor temperature, pulse, and BP periodically during therapy. Dinoprostone-induced fever (elevation >1.1°C or 2°F) usually occurs within 15–45 min after insertion of suppository. This returns to normal 2–6 hr after discontinuation or removal of suppository from vagina.
- Auscultate breath sounds. Wheezing and sensation of chest tightness may indicate hypersensitivity reaction.
- Assess for nausea, vomiting, and diarrhea in patients receiving suppository. Vomiting and diarrhea occur frequently. Patient should be premedicated with antiemetic and antidiarrheal.
- Monitor amount and type of vaginal discharge. Notify health care professional immediately if symptoms of hemorrhage (increased bleeding, hypotension, pallor, tachycardia) occur.
- **Cervical Ripening:** Monitor uterine activity, fetal status, and dilation and effacement of cervix continuously throughout therapy. Assess for hypertonus, sustained uterine contractility, and fetal distress. Insert should be removed at the onset of active labor.

Implementation

- **Abortifacient:** Warm the suppository to room temperature just before use. Store suppositories in freezer.
- Wear gloves when handling unwrapped suppository to prevent absorption through skin. Insert high into vagina.
- Patient should remain supine for 10 min after insertion of suppository; then she may be ambulatory.
- **Vaginal Insert:** Place vaginal insert transversely in the posterior vaginal fornix immediately after removing from foil package. Warming of insert and sterile conditions are not required. Use vaginal insert only with a retrieval system. Use minimal amount of water-soluble lubricant during insertion; avoid excess because it may hamper release of dinoprostone from insert. Patient should remain supine for 2 hr after insertion, then may ambulate. Store vaginal inserts in freezer.
- Vaginal insert delivers dinoprostone 0.3 mg/hr over 12 hr. Remove insert at the onset of active labor, before amniotomy, or after 12 hr.
- Oxytocin should not be used during or <30 min after removal of insert.
- **Endocervical Gel:** Determine degree of effacement before insertion of the endocervical catheter. Do not administer above the level of the internal os. Use a 20-mm endocervical catheter if no effacement is present and a 10-mm catheter if the cervix is 50% effaced.
- Use caution to prevent contact of dinoprostone gel with skin. Wash hands thoroughly with soap and water after administration.
- Bring gel to room temperature just before administration. Do not force warming with external sources (water bath, microwave). Remove peel-off seal from end of syringe; then remove the protective end cap and insert end cap into plunger stopper assembly in barrel of syringe. Aseptically remove catheter from package. Firmly attach catheter hub to syringe tip; click is evidence of attachment. Fill catheter with sterile gel by pushing plunger to expel air from cath-

eter before administration to patient. Gel is stable for 24 mo if refrigerated.

- Patient should be in dorsal position with cervix visualized using a speculum. Introduce gel with catheter into cervical canal using sterile technique. Administer gel by gentle expulsion from syringe and then remove catheter. Do not attempt to administer small amount of gel remaining in syringe. Use syringe for only 1 patient; discard syringe, catheter, and unused package contents after using.
- Patient should remain supine for 15–30 min after administration to minimize leakage from cervical canal.
- Oxytocin may be administered 6–12 hr after desired response from dinoprostone gel. If no cervical/uterine response to initial dose of dinoprostone is obtained, repeat dose may be administered in 6 hr.

Patient/Family Teaching

- Explain purpose of medication and vaginal exams.
- **Abortifacient:** Instruct patient to notify health care professional immediately if fever and chills, foul-smelling vaginal discharge, lower abdominal pain, or increased bleeding occurs.
- Provide emotional support throughout therapy.
- **Cervical Ripening:** Inform patient that she may experience a warm feeling in her vagina during administration.
- Advise patient to notify health care professional if contractions become prolonged.

Evaluation/Desired Outcomes

- Complete abortion. Continuous administration for more than 2 days is not usually recommended.
- Cervical ripening and induction of labor.

BEERS

diphenhydrAMINE (oral, parenteral)

(dye-fen-**hye**-dra-meen)

✱Aller-Aide, ✱Allerdryl, ✱Allergy Formula, AllerMax, ✱Allernix, Banophen, Benadryl Dye-Free Alergy, Benadryl Allergy, Benadryl, ✱Benylin, ✱Calmex, Compoz, Compoz Nighttime Sleep Aid, ✱Dimetane Allergy, Diphen AF, Diphen Cough, ✱Diphenhist, ✱Dormex, ✱Dormiphen, Genahist, 40 Winks, Hyrexin-50, ✱Insomnal, Maximum Strength Nytol, Maximum Strength Sleepinal, Midol PM, Miles Nervine, ✱Nadryl, Nighttime Sleep Aid, Nytol, Scot-Tussin Allergy DM, Siladril, Silphen, Sleep-Eze 3, Sleepwell 2-night, Sominex, Snooze Fast, Sominex, Tusstat, Twilite, Unisom Nighttime Sleep-Aid

Classification

Therapeutic: allergy, cold, and cough remedies, antihistamines, antitussives

Indications

Relief of allergic symptoms caused by histamine release including: Anaphylaxis, Seasonal and perennial allergic rhinitis, Allergic dermatoses. Parkinson's disease and dystonic reactions from medications. Mild nighttime sedation. Prevention of motion sickness. Antitussive (syrup only).

Action

Antagonizes the effects of histamine at H_1-receptor sites; does not bind to or inactivate histamine. Significant CNS depressant and anticholinergic properties. **Therapeutic Effects:** Decreased symptoms of histamine excess (sneezing, rhinorrhea, nasal and ocular pruritus, ocular tearing and redness, urticaria). Relief of acute dystonic reactions. Prevention of motion sickness. Suppression of cough.

Pharmacokinetics

Absorption: Well absorbed after oral or IM administration but 40–60% of an oral dose reaches systemic circulation due to first-pass metabolism.

Distribution: Widely distributed. Crosses the placenta; enters breast milk.

Metabolism and Excretion: 95% metabolized by the liver.

Half-life: 2.4–7 hr.

TIME/ACTION PROFILE (antihistaminic effects)

ROUTE	ONSET	PEAK	DURATION
PO	15–60 min	2–4 hr	4–8 hr
IM	20–30 min	2–4 hr	4–8 hr
IV	rapid	unknown	4–8 hr

Contraindications/Precautions

Contraindicated in: Hypersensitivity; Acute attacks of asthma; Lactation: Lactation; Known alcohol intolerance (some liquid products).

Use Cautiously in: Severe liver disease; Angle-closure glaucoma; Seizure disorders; Prostatic hyperplasia; Peptic ulcer; May cause paradoxical excitation in young children; Hyperthyroidism; OB: Safety not established; Geri: Appears on *Beers list*. Geriatric patients are more susceptible to adverse drug reactions and anticholinergic effects (delirium, acute confusion, dizziness, dry mouth, blurred vision, urinary retention, constipation, tachycardia); dose ↓ or nonanticholinergic antihistamine recommended.

Adverse Reactions/Side Effects

CNS: <u>drowsiness</u>, dizziness, headache, paradoxical excitation (increased in children). **EENT:** blurred vision, tinnitus. **CV:** hypotension, palpitations. **GI:** anorexia, dry mouth, constipation, nausea. **GU:** dysuria, frequency, urinary retention. **Derm:** photosensitivity. **Resp:** chest tightness, thickened bronchial secretions, wheezing. **Local:** pain at IM site.

Interactions

Drug-Drug: ↑ risk of CNS depression with other **antihistamines**, **alcohol**, **opioid analgesics**, and **sedative/hypnotics**. ↑ anticholinergic effects with **tricyclic antidepressants**, **quinidine**, or **disopyramide**. **MAO inhibitors** intensify and prolong the anticholinergic effects of antihistamines.

Drug-Natural Products: Concomitant use of **kava-kava**, **valerian**, or **chamomile** can ↑ CNS depression.

Route/Dosage

PO (Adults and Children >12 yr): *Antihistaminic/antiemetic/antivertiginic*—25–50 mg every 4–6 hr, not to exceed 300 mg/day. *Antitussive*—25 mg every 4 hr as needed, not to exceed 150 mg/day. *Antidyskinetic*—25–50 mg every 4 hr (not to exceed 400 mg/day). *Sedative/hypnotic*—50 mg 20–30 min before bedtime.

PO (Children 6–12 yr): *Antihistaminic/antiemetic/antivertiginic*—12.5–25 mg every 4–6 hr (not to exceed 150 mg/day). *Antidyskinetic*—1–1.5 mg/kg every 6–8 hr as needed (not to exceed 300 mg/day). *Antitussive*—12.5 mg every 4 hr (not to exceed 75 mg/day). *Sedative/hypnotic*—1 mg/kg/dose 20–30 min before bedtime (not to exceed 50 mg).

PO (Children 2–6 yr): *Antihistaminic/antiemetic/antivertiginic*—6.25–12.5 mg every 4–6 hr (not to exceed 37.5 mg/day). *Antidyskinetic*—1–1.5 mg/kg every 4–6 hr as needed (not to exceed 300 mg/day). *Antitussive*—6.25 mg every 4 hr (not to exceed 37.5 mg/24 hr). *Sedative/hypnotic*—1 mg/kg/dose 20–30 min before bedtime (not to exceed 50 mg).

IM, IV (Adults): 25–50 mg every 4 hr as needed (may need up to 100-mg dose, not to exceed 400 mg/day).

IM, IV (Children): 1.25 mg/kg (37.5 mg/m²) 4 times daily (not to exceed 300 mg/day).

Topical (Adults and Children ≥2 yr): Apply to affected area up to 3–4 times daily.

Availability (generic available)

Capsules: 25 mg^Rx, OTC^, 50 mg^Rx, OTC^. **Tablets:** 🍁 12.5 mg^Rx, OTC^, 25 mg^Rx, OTC^, 50 mg^Rx, OTC^. **Chewable tablets (grape flavor):** 25 mg^Rx, OTC^. **Orally disintegrating strips (cherry and grape flavor):** 12.5 mg^Rx, OTC^, 25 mg^OTC^. **Orally disintegrating tablets:** 12.5 mg^OTC^, 25 mg^OTC^, 50 mg^Rx, OTC^. **Elixir (cherry and other flavors):** 12.5 mg/5 mL^Rx, OTC^. **Syrup (cherry and raspberry flavor):** 🍁 6.25 mg/5 mL^Rx, OTC^, 12.5 mg/5 mL^Rx, OTC^. **Cream:** 1%^Rx, OTC^, 2%^Rx, OTC^. **Topical gel:** 2%^OTC^. **Topical spray:** 2%^OTC^. **Topical stick:** 2%^OTC^. **Injection:** 50 mg/mL. ***In combination with:*** analgesics, decongestants, and expectorants, in OTC pain, sleep, cough, and cold preparations. See Appendix B.

NURSING IMPLICATIONS

Assessment

- Diphenhydramine has multiple uses. Determine why the medication was ordered and assess symptoms that apply to the individual patient. Geri: Appears in the *Beers list.* May cause sedation and confusion due to increased sensitivity to anticholinergic effects. Monitor carefully, assess for confusion, delirium, other anticholinergic side effects and fall risk. Institute measures to prevent falls.
- **Prevention and Treatment of Anaphylaxis:** Assess for urticaria and for patency of airway.
- **Allergic Rhinitis:** Assess degree of nasal stuffiness, rhinorrhea, and sneezing.
- **Parkinsonism and Extrapyramidal Reactions:** Assess movement disorder before and after administration.
- **Insomnia:** Assess sleep patterns.
- **Motion Sickness:** Assess nausea, vomiting, bowel sounds, and abdominal pain.
- **Cough Suppressant:** Assess frequency and nature of cough, lung sounds, and amount and type of sputum produced. Unless contraindicated, maintain fluid intake of 1500–2000 mL daily to decrease viscosity of bronchial secretions.
- **Pruritus:** Assess degree of itching, skin rash, and inflammation.
- ***Lab Test Considerations:*** May ↓ skin response to allergy tests. Discontinue 4 days before skin testing.

Implementation

- Do not confuse Benadryl with benazepril. Do not confuse diphenhydramine with dimenhydrinate.
- When used for insomnia, administer 20 min before bedtime and schedule activities to minimize interruption of sleep.
- When used for prophylaxis of motion sickness, administer at least 30 min and preferably 1–2 hr before exposure to conditions that may precipitate motion sickness.
- **PO:** Administer with meals or milk to minimize GI irritation. Capsule may be emptied and contents taken with water or food.
- Orally disintegrating tablets and strips should be left in the package until use. Remove from the blister pouch. Do not push tablet through the blister; peel open the blister pack with dry hands and place tablet on tongue. Tablet will dissolve rapidly and be swallowed with saliva. No liquid is needed to take the orally disintegrating tablet.
- **IM:** Administer 50 mg/mL into well-developed muscle. Avoid subcut injections.

IV Administration

- **IV Push:** ***Diluent:*** May be further diluted in 0.9% NaCl, 0.45% NaCl, D5W, D10W, dextrose/saline combinations, Ringer's solution, LR, and dextrose/Ringer's combinations. ***Concentration:*** 25 mg/mL. ***Rate:*** Infuse at a rate not to exceed 25 mg/min.
- **Y-Site Compatibility:** acetaminophen, aldesleukin, alemtuzumab, alfentanil, amifostine, amikacin, aminocaproic acid, amiodarone, amphotericin B lipid complex, amphotericin B liposome, amsacrine, anidulafungin, argatroban, ascorbic acid, atracurium, atropine, azithromycin, benztropine, bivalirudin, bleomycin, bumetanide, buprenorphine, butorphanol, calcium chloride, calcium gluconate, carboplatin, carmustine, caspofungin, ceftaroline, chlorpromazine, ciprofloxacin, cisatracurium, cisplatin, cladribine, clindamycin, cyanocobalamin, cyclophosphamide, cyclosporine, cytarabine, dacarbazine, dactinomycin, daptomycin, daunorubicin hydrochloride, dexmedetomidine, dexrazoxane, digoxin, diltiazem, dobutamine, docetaxel, dolasetron, dopamine, doxorubicin, doxorubicin liposome, doxycycline, enalaprilat, ephedrine, epinephrine, epirubicin, epoetin alfa, eptifibatide, ertapenem, erythromycin, esmolol, etoposide, etoposide phosphate, famotidine, fenoldopam, fentanyl, filgrastim, fluconazole, fludarabine, folic acid, fosphenytoin, gemcitabine, gentamicin, glycopyrrolate, granisetron, hetastarch, hydromorphone, idarubicin, ifosfamide, imipenem/cilastatin, irinotecan, isoproterenol, ketamine, labetalol, leucovorin calcium, levofloxacin, lidocaine, linezolid, lorazepam, magnesium sulfate, mannitol, melphalan, meperidine, meropenem, metaraminol, methotrexate, methyldopate, metoclopramide, metoprolol, metronidazole, midazolam, mitomycin, mitoxantrone, morphine, moxifloxacin, multiple vitamins, mycophenolate, nalbuphine, naloxone, nicardipine, nitroglycerin, norepinephrine, octreotide, ondansetron, oxaliplatin, oxytocin, paclitaxel, palonosetron, pamidronate, papaverine, pemetrexed, penicillin G, pentamidine, phentolamine, phenylephrine, phytonadione, piperacillin/tazobactam, potassium acetate, potassium chloride, procainamide, prochlorperazine, promethazine, propofol, propranolol, protamine, pyridoxime, quinipristin/dalfopristin, ranitidine, remifentanil, rituximab, rocuronium, sargramostim, sodium acetate, streptokinase, succinylcholine, sufentanil, tacrolimus, theophylline, thiamine, thiotepa, tigecycline, tirofiban, tobramycin, tolazoline, topotecan, trastuzumab, vancomycin, vasopressin, vecuronium, verapamil, vinblastine, vincristine, vinorelbine, vitamin B complex with C, voriconazole, zoledronic acid.
- **Y-Site Incompatibility:** allopurinol, aminophylline, amphotericin B deoxycholate, ampicillin, azathioprine, cefazolin, cefepime, cefotaxime, cefotetan, cefoxitin, ceftazidime, ceftriaxone, cefuroxime, chloramphenicol, dantrolene, dexamethasone, diazepam, diazoxide, fluorouracil, foscarnet, furosemide, ganciclovir, indomethacin, insulin, ketorolac, methylprednisolone, milrinone, nitroprusside, oxacillin, pantoprazole, pentobarbital, phenobarbital, phenytoin, sodium bicarbonate, trimethoprim/sulfamethoxazole.
- **Topical:** Apply a thin coat and rub gently until absorbed. Only for topical use; avoid ingestion.

Patient/Family Teaching

- Instruct patient to take medication as directed; do not exceed recommended amount. Caution patient not to use oral OTC diphenhydramine products with any other product containing diphenhydramine, including products used topically.
- May cause drowsiness. Caution patient to avoid driving or other activities requiring alertness until response to drug is known.
- May cause dry mouth. Inform patient that frequent oral rinses, good oral hygiene, and sugarless gum or candy may minimize this effect. Notify health care professional if dry mouth persists for more than 2 wk.
- Teach sleep hygiene techniques (dark room, quiet, bedtime ritual, limit daytime napping, avoidance of nicotine and caffeine) to patients taking diphenhydramine to aid sleep.
- Advise patient to use sunscreen and protective clothing to prevent photosensitivity reactions.
- Caution patient to avoid use of alcohol and other CNS depressants concurrently with this medication.
- Pedi: Can cause excitation in children. Caution parents or caregivers about proper dose calculation; overdose, especially in infants and children, can cause hallucinations, seizures, or death. Caution parents to avoid OTC cough and cold products while breast feeding or to children $<$4 yr.
- Geri: Instruct older adults to avoid OTC products that contain diphenhydramine due to increased sensitivity to anticholinergic effects and potential for adverse reactions related to these effects.
- Advise patients taking diphenhydramine in OTC preparations to notify health care professional if symptoms worsen or persist for more than 7 days.

Evaluation/Desired Outcomes

- Prevention of, or decreased urticaria in, anaphylaxis or other allergic reactions.
- Decreased dyskinesia in parkinsonism and extrapyramidal reactions.
- Sedation when used as a sedative/hypnotic.
- Prevention of or decrease in nausea and vomiting caused by motion sickness.
- Decrease in frequency and intensity of cough without eliminating cough reflex.

DIURETICS (POTASSIUM-SPARING)

aMILoride (a-**mill**-oh-ride)
✤Midamor

spironolactone (speer-oh-no-**lak**-tone)
Aldactone

triamterene (trye-**am**-ter-een)
Dyrenium

Classification
Therapeutic: diuretics
Pharmacologic: potassium-sparing diuretics

Indications

Counteract potassium loss caused by other diuretics. Used with other agents (thiazides) to treat edema or hypertension. Primary hyperaldosteronism (spironolactone only). **Unlabeled Use: Spironolactone:** Management of HF (low doses).

Action

Inhibition of sodium reabsorption in the kidney while saving potassium and hydrogen ions (spironolactone achieves this effect by antagonizing aldosterone receptors). **Therapeutic Effects:** Weak diuretic and antihypertensive response when compared with other diuretics. Conservation of potassium.

Pharmacokinetics

Absorption: *Amiloride*—30–90% absorbed; *spironolactone*—>90% absorbed; *triamterene*—30–70% absorbed.

Distribution: *Amiloride* and *triamterene*—widely distributed; all cross the placenta and enter breast milk.

Protein Binding: *Spironolactone* >90%.

Metabolism and Excretion: *Amiloride*—50% eliminated unchanged in urine, 40% excreted in the feces; *spironolactone*—converted by the liver to its active diuretic compound (canrenone); *triamterene*—80% metabolized by the liver, some excretion of unchanged drug.

Half-life: *Amiloride*—6–9 hr; *spironolactone*—78–84 min (spironolactone); 13–24 hr (canrenone); *triamterene*—1.7–2.5 hr.

TIME/ACTION PROFILE (diuretic effect)

ROUTE	ONSET	PEAK	DURATION
Amiloride	2 hr†	6–10 hr†	24 hr†
Spironolactone	unknown	2–3 days‡	2–3 days‡
Triamterene	2–4 hr†	1–several days‡	7–9 hr†

†Single dose.
‡Multiple doses.

Contraindications/Precautions

Contraindicated in: Hypersensitivity; Hyperkalemia; Anuria; Acute renal insufficiency; Significant renal dysfunction (CCr ≤30 mL/min or SCr >2.5 m g/dL).

Use Cautiously in: Hepatic dysfunction; Geri: Presence of age-related renal dysfunction may lead to ↑ risk of hyperkalemia; Diabetes (↑ risk of hyperkalemia); History of gout or kidney stones (triamterene only); Concurrent use of potassium supplements or potassium-containing salt substitutes; OB, Lactation, Pedi: Safety not established.

Adverse Reactions/Side Effects

CNS: dizziness; *spironolactone only*, clumsiness, headache. **CV:** arrhythmias. **GI:** *amiloride*—constipation, nausea, vomiting. **GU:** *spironolactone*—erectile dysfunction; *triamterene*—, nephrolithiasis. **Derm:** STEVENS-JOHNSON SYNDROME, TOXIC EPIDERMAL NECROLYSIS; *triamterene*—photosensitivity. **Endo:** *spironolactone*—breast tenderness, gynecomastia, irregular menses, voice deepening. **F and E:** <u>hyperkalemia</u>, hyponatremia. **Hemat:** *spironolactone*—agranulocytosis; *triamterene*—hemolytic anemia, thrombocytopenia. **MS:** muscle cramps. **Misc:** allergic reactions.

Interactions

Drug-Drug: ↑ hypotension with acute ingestion of **alcohol**, other **antihypertensives**, or **nitrates**. Use with **ACE inhibitors**, **angiotensin II receptor antagonists**, **NSAIDS**, **potassium supplements**, **cyclosporine**, or **tacrolimus** ↑ risk of hyperkalemia. May ↑ levels/risk of toxicity from **lithium**. Effectiveness may be ↓ by **NSAIDs**. Spironolactone may ↑ effects of **digoxin**.

Route/Dosage

Amiloride

PO (Adults): *HTN*—5–10 mg/day (up to 20 mg).
PO (Children 1–17 yr): 0.4–0.625 mg/kg/day (maximum = 20 mg/day) (unlabeled use).

Spironolactone

PO (Adults): *Edema*—25–200 mg/day in 1–2 divided doses. *HTN*—50–100 mg/day in 1–2 divided doses. *Diuretic-induced hypokalemia*—25–100 mg/day in 1–2 divided doses. *Diagnosis of primary hyperaldosteronism*—100–400 mg/day in 1–2 divided doses. *HF*—12.5–25 mg/day (unlabeled use).
PO (Children 1–17 yr): *Diuretic, HTN*—1 mg/kg/day in 1–2 divided doses (should not exceed 3.3 mg/kg/day or 100 mg/day) (unlabeled use). *Diagnosis of primary hyperaldosteronism*—125–375 mg/m^2/day in 1–2 divided doses (unlabeled use).
PO (Neonates): 1–3 mg/kg/day in 1–2 divided doses.

Triamterene

PO (Adults): *HTN*—100 mg twice daily (not to exceed 300 mg/day; lower doses in combination products).

PO (Children): *HTN*—1–2 mg/kg/day in 2 divided doses; should not exceed 4 mg/kg/day or 300 mg/day.

Availability

Amiloride (generic available)

Tablets: 5 mg. **Cost:** *Generic*—$59.00/100.

Spironolactone (generic available)

Tablets: 25 mg, 50 mg, 100 mg. **Cost:** *Generic*—25 mg $10.83/100, 50 mg $23.97/100, 100 mg $24.87/100. ***In combination with:*** hydrochlorothiazide (Aldactazide). See Appendix B.

Triamterene

Capsules: 50 mg, 100 mg. **Cost:** 50 mg $404.14/100, 100 mg $372.44/100. ***In combination with:*** hydrochlorothiazide (Dyazide, Maxzide). See Appendix B.

NURSING IMPLICATIONS

Assessment

- Monitor intake and output ratios and daily weight during therapy.
- If medication is given as an adjunct to antihypertensive therapy, monitor BP before administering.
- Assess patient frequently for development of hyperkalemia (fatigue, muscle weakness, paresthesia, confusion, dyspnea, ECG changes, cardiac arrhythmias). Patients who have diabetes mellitus or kidney disease and geriatric patients are at increased risk of developing these symptoms.
- Periodic ECGs are recommended in patients receiving prolonged therapy.
- Assess patient for skin rash frequently during therapy. Discontinue diuretic at first sign of rash; may be life-threatening. Stevens-Johnson syndrome or toxic epidermal necrolysis may develop. Treat symptomatically; may recur once treatment is stopped.
- ***Lab Test Considerations:*** Serum potassium levels should be evaluated before and routinely during therapy. Withhold drug and notify health care professional if patient becomes hyperkalemic.
- Monitor BUN, serum creatinine, and electrolytes before and periodically during therapy. May cause ↑ serum magnesium, BUN, creatinine, potassium, and urinary calcium excretion levels. May also cause ↓ sodium levels.
- Discontinue potassium-sparing diuretics 3 days before a glucose tolerance test because of risk of severe hyperkalemia.
- *Spironolactone* may cause false ↑ of plasma cortisol concentrations. Spironolactone should be withdrawn 4–7 days before test.
- Monitor platelet count and total and differential leukocyte count periodically during therapy in patients taking *triamterene*.

Implementation

- Do not confuse amiloride with amlodipine.
- **PO:** Administer in AM to avoid interrupting sleep pattern.
- Administer with food or milk to minimize gastric irritation and to increase bioavailability.
- *Triamterene* capsules may be opened and contents mixed with food or fluids for patients with difficulty swallowing.

Patient/Family Teaching

- Emphasize the importance of continuing to take this medication, even if feeling well. Instruct patient to take medication at the same time each day. Take missed doses as soon as remembered unless almost time for next dose. Do not double doses.
- Caution patient to avoid salt substitutes and foods that contain high levels of potassium or sodium unless prescribed by health care professional.
- May cause dizziness. Caution patient to avoid driving or other activities requiring alertness until response to medication is known.
- Instruct patient to notify health care professional of all Rx or OTC medications, vitamins, or herbal products being taken and to consult health care professional before taking any OTC medications concurrently with this therapy, especially OTC decongestants, cough or cold preparations, or appetite suppressants due to potential for increased BP.
- Advise patients taking *triamterene* to use sunscreen and protective clothing to prevent photosensitivity reactions.
- Instruct patient to notify health care professional of medication regimen before treatment or surgery.
- Advise patient to notify health care professional if rash, muscle weakness or cramps; fatigue; or severe nausea, vomiting, or diarrhea occurs.
- Emphasize the need for follow-up exams to monitor progress.
- **Hypertension:** Reinforce need to continue additional therapies for hypertension (weight loss, restricted sodium intake, stress reduction, moderation of alcohol intake, regular exercise, and cessation of smoking). Medication helps control but does not cure hypertension.
- Teach patient and family the correct technique for checking BP weekly.

Evaluation/Desired Outcomes

- Increase in diuresis and decrease in edema while maintaining serum potassium level in an acceptable range.
- Decrease in BP.
- Prevention of hypokalemia in patients taking diuretics.
- Treatment of hyperaldosteronism.

D

DIURETICS (THIAZIDE)

chlorothiazide
(klor-oh-**thye**-a-zide)
Diuril

chlorthalidone (thiazide–like)
(klor-**thal**-i-doan)
~~Thalitone~~

hydroCHLOROthiazide
(hye-droe-klor-oh-**thye**-a-zide)
Microzide, Oretic, ✱Urozide

Classification
Therapeutic: antihypertensives, diuretics
Pharmacologic: thiazide diuretics

Indications
Management of mild to moderate hypertension. Treatment of edema associated with: HF, Renal dysfunction, Cirrhosis, Glucocorticoid therapy, Estrogen therapy.

Action
Increases excretion of sodium and water by inhibiting sodium reabsorption in the distal tubule. Promotes excretion of chloride, potassium, magnesium, and bicarbonate. May produce arteriolar dilation. **Therapeutic Effects:** Lowering of BP in hypertensive patients and diuresis with mobilization of edema.

Pharmacokinetics
Absorption: All are rapidly absorbed after oral administration.
Distribution: All cross the placenta and enter breast milk.
Metabolism and Excretion: All are excreted mainly unchanged by the kidneys.
Half-life: *Chlorothiazide*—1–2 hr; *chlorthalidone*—35–50 hr; *hydrochlorothiazide*—6–15 hr.

TIME/ACTION PROFILE (diuretic effect)

ROUTE	ONSET	PEAK	DURATION
Chlorothiazide PO	2 hr	4 hr	6–12 hr
Chlorothiazide IV	15 min	30 min	2 hr
Chlorthalidone	2 hr	2 hr	48–72 hr
Hydrochlorothiazide†	2 hr	3–6 hr	6–12 hr

†Onset of antihypertensive effect is 3–4 days and does not become maximal for 7–14 days of dosing.

Contraindications/Precautions
Contraindicated in: Hypersensitivity (cross-sensitivity with other thiazides or sulfonamides may exist); Some products contain tartrazine and should be avoided in patients with known intolerance; Anuria; Lactation: Lactation.
Use Cautiously in: Renal or hepatic impairment; OB: Pregnancy (jaundice or thrombocytopenia may be seen in the newborn).

Adverse Reactions/Side Effects
CNS: dizziness, drowsiness, lethargy, weakness. **CV:** hypotension. **EENT:** acute angle-closure glaucoma (hydrochlorothiazide), acute myopia (hydrochlorothiazide). **GI:** anorexia, cramping, hepatitis, nausea, pancreatitis, vomiting. **Derm:** STEVENS-JOHNSON SYNDROME, photosensitivity, rash. **Endo:** hyperglycemia. **F and E:** hypokalemia, dehydration, hypercalcemia, hypochloremic alkalosis, hypomagnesemia, hyponatremia, hypophosphatemia, hypovolemia. **Hemat:** thrombocytopenia. **Metab:** hypercholesterolemia, hyperuricemia. **MS:** muscle cramps.

Interactions
Drug-Drug: Additive hypotension with other **antihypertensives**, acute ingestion of **alcohol**, or **nitrates**. Additive hypokalemia with **corticosteroids**, **amphotericin B**, or **piperacillin/tazobactam**. May ↑ **lithium** levels. **Cholestyramine** or **colestipol** ↓ absorption. Hypokalemia ↑ risk of **digoxin** toxicity. **NSAIDs** may ↓ effectiveness.

Route/Dosage
When used as a diuretic in adults, generally given daily, but may be given every other day or 2–3 days/wk.

Chlorothiazide
PO (Adults): 125 mg–2 g/day in 1–2 divided doses.
PO (Children >6 mos): 20 mg/kg/day in 1–2 divided doses (maximum dose = 1 g/day).
PO (Neonates ≤6 mo): 10–20 mg/kg every 12 hr (maximum dose = 375 mg/day).
IV (Adults): 500 mg–1 g/day in 1–2 divided doses.
IV (Children >6 mos): 4 mg/kg/day in 1–2 divided doses (maximum dose = 20 mg/kg/day) (unlabeled use).
IV (Neonates ≤6 mo): 1–4 mg/kg every 12 hr (maximum dose = 20 mg/kg/day) (unlabeled use).

Chlorthalidone
PO (Adults): 12.5–100 mg once daily (daily doses above 25 mg are associated with greater likelihood of electrolyte abnormalities).

Hydrochlorothiazide
PO (Adults): 12.5–100 mg/day in 1–2 divided doses (up to 200 mg/day); not to exceed 50 mg/day for hypertension; daily doses above 25 mg are associated with greater likelihood of electrolyte abnormalities.
PO (Children >6 mo): 1–3 mg/kg/day in 2 divided doses (not to exceed 37.5 mg/day).

PO (Children <6 mo): 1–3 mg/kg/day in 2 divided doses.

Availability

Chlorothiazide (generic available)

Tablets: 250 mg, 500 mg. **Cost:** *Generic*—250 mg $13.08/100, 500 mg $25.25/100. **Oral suspension:** 250 mg/5 mL. **Cost:** *Generic*— $63.36/237 mL. **Powder for injection:** 500 mg/vial.

Chlorthalidone (generic available)

Tablets: 25 mg, 50 mg. **Cost:** *Generic*—25 mg $55.17/100, 50 mg $68.04/100, 100 mg $101.25/100. ***In combination with:*** atenolol (Tenoretic), clonidine (Clorpres). See Appendix B.

Hydrochlorothiazide (generic available)

Tablets: 12.5 mg, 25 mg, 50 mg. **Cost:** *Generic*—12.5 mg $82.43/100, 25 mg $8.48/100, 50 mg $16.45/100. **Capsules:** 12.5 mg. ***In combination with:*** numerous antihypertensive agents. See Appendix B.

NURSING IMPLICATIONS

Assessment

- Monitor BP, intake, output, and daily weight and assess feet, legs, and sacral area for edema daily.
- Assess patient, especially if taking digoxin, for anorexia, nausea, vomiting, muscle cramps, paresthesia, and confusion. Notify health care professional if these signs of electrolyte imbalance occur. Patients taking digoxin are at risk of digoxin toxicity because of the potassium-depleting effect of the diuretic.
- If hypokalemia occurs, consideration may be given to potassium supplements or ↓ dose of diuretic.
- Assess patient for allergy to sulfonamides. Assess patient for skin rash frequently during therapy. Discontinue diuretic at first sign of rash; may be life-threatening. Stevens-Johnson syndrome may develop. Treat symptomatically; may recur once treatment is stopped.
- **Hypertension:** Monitor BP before and periodically during therapy.
- Monitor frequency of prescription refills to determine compliance.
- ***Lab Test Considerations:*** Monitor electrolytes (especially potassium), blood glucose, BUN, serum creatinine, and uric acid levels before and periodically throughout therapy.
- May cause ↑ in serum and urine glucose in diabetic patients.
- May cause ↑ in serum bilirubin, calcium, creatinine, and uric acid, and ↓ in serum magnesium, potassium, sodium, and urinary calcium concentrations.
- May cause ↑ serum cholesterol, low-density lipoprotein, and triglyceride concentrations.

Implementation

- Do not confuse hydrochlorothiazide with hydroxyzine or hydralazine.
- Administer in the morning to prevent disruption of sleep cycle.
- Intermittent dose schedule may be used for continued control of edema.
- **PO:** May give with food or milk to minimize GI irritation. Tablets may be crushed and mixed with fluid to facilitate swallowing.

IV Administration

- **Intermittent Infusion:** Reconstitute chlorothiazide with at least 18 mL of sterile water for injection. Shake to dissolve. Stable for 24 hr at room temperature. ***Diluent:*** May be given undiluted or may be diluted further with D5W or 0.9% NaCl. ***Concentration:*** Up to 28 mg/mL. ***Rate:*** If administered undiluted may give by IV push over 3–5 min. If diluted, may run over 30 min.
- **Y-Site Compatibility:** alprostadil, aminophylline, atropine, calcium chloride, calcium gluconate, chloramphenicol, cyclophosphamide, dexamethasone, digoxin, epinephrine, erythromycin, furosemide, gentamicin, heparin, hydrocortisone sodium succinate, isoproterenol, lidocaine, methohexital, methyldopate, norepinephrine, oxytocin, penicillin G, phenobarbital, phentolamine, potassium chloride, procainamide, propranolol, succinylcholine.
- **Y-Site Incompatibility:** chlorpromazine, hydralazine, prochlorperazine, promethazine.

Patient/Family Teaching

- Instruct patient to take this medication at the same time each day. Take missed dose as soon as remembered but not just before next dose is due. Do not double doses.
- Instruct patient to monitor weight biweekly and notify health care professional of significant changes.
- Caution patient to change positions slowly to minimize orthostatic hypotension. This may be potentiated by alcohol.
- Advise patient to use sunscreen and protective clothing to prevent photosensitivity reactions.
- Instruct patient to discuss dietary potassium requirements with health care professional (see Appendix K).
- Instruct patient to notify health care professional of medication regimen before treatment or surgery.
- Advise patient to report rash, muscle weakness, cramps, nausea, vomiting, diarrhea, or dizziness to health care professional.
- Emphasize the importance of routine follow-up exams.
- **Hypertension:** Advise patients to continue taking the medication even if feeling better. Medication controls but does not cure hypertension.
- Encourage patient to comply with additional interventions for hypertension (weight reduction, low-sodium diet, regular exercise, smoking cessation, moderation of alcohol consumption, and stress management).

- Instruct patient and family in correct technique for monitoring weekly BP.
- Instruct patient to notify health care professional of all Rx or OTC medications, vitamins, or herbal products being taken and to consult health care professional before taking other Rx, OTC, or herbal products, especially cough or cold preparations.

Evaluation/Desired Outcomes

- Decrease in BP.
- Increase in urine output.
- Decrease in edema.

divalproex sodium, **See VALPROATES.**

HIGH ALERT

DOBUTamine

(doe-**byoo**-ta-meen)

~~Dobutrex~~

Classification

Therapeutic: inotropics

Pharmacologic: adrenergics

Indications

Short-term (<48 hr) management of heart failure caused by depressed contractility from organic heart disease or surgical procedures.

Action

Stimulates $beta_1$ (myocardial)-adrenergic receptors with relatively minor effect on heart rate or peripheral blood vessels. **Therapeutic Effects:** Increased cardiac output without significantly increased heart rate.

Pharmacokinetics

Absorption: Administered by IV infusion only, resulting in complete bioavailability.
Distribution: Unknown.
Metabolism and Excretion: Metabolized by the liver and other tissues.
Half-life: 2 min.

TIME/ACTION PROFILE (inotropic effects)

ROUTE	ONSET	PEAK	DURATION
IV	1–2 min	10 min	brief (min)

Contraindications/Precautions

Contraindicated in: Hypersensitivity to dobutamine or bisulfites; Idiopathic hypertrophic subaortic stenosis.
Use Cautiously in: History of hypertension (↑ risk of exaggerated pressor response); MI; Atrial fibrillation (pretreatment with digoxin recommended); History of ventricular atopic activity (may be exacerbated); Hypovolemia (correct before administration); OB: Safety not established.

Adverse Reactions/Side Effects

CNS: headache. **CV:** <u>hypertension</u>, <u>increased heart rate</u>, <u>premature ventricular contractions</u>, angina pectoris, arrhythmias, hypotension, palpitations. **GI:** nausea, vomiting. **Local:** phlebitis. **Resp:** shortness of breath. **Misc:** hypersensitivity reactions, nonanginal chest pain.

Interactions

Drug-Drug: Use with **nitroprusside**; may have a synergistic effect on ↑ cardiac output. **Beta blockers** may negate the effect of dobutamine. ↑ risk of arrhythmias or hypertension with some **anesthetics** (**cyclopropane, halothane**), **MAO inhibitors, oxytocics**, or **tricyclic antidepressants**.

Route/Dosage

IV (Adults and Children): 2.5–15 mcg/kg/min; titrate to response (max dose = 40 mcg/kg/min).
IV (Neonates): 2–15 mcg/kg/min.

Availability (generic available)

Solution for injection (requires dilution): 12.5 mg/mL. **Premixed infusion:** 250 mg/250 mL, 500 mg/250 mL, 1000 mg/250 mL.

NURSING IMPLICATIONS

Assessment

- Monitor BP, heart rate, ECG, pulmonary capillary wedge pressure (PCWP), cardiac output, CVP, and urinary output continuously during the administration. Report significant changes in vital signs or arrhythmias. Consult physician for parameters for pulse, BP, or ECG changes for adjusting dose or discontinuing medication.
- Palpate peripheral pulses and assess appearance of extremities routinely during dobutamine administration. Notify health care professional if quality of pulse deteriorates or if extremities become cold or mottled.
- ***Lab Test Considerations:*** Monitor potassium concentrations during therapy; may cause hypokalemia.
- Monitor electrolytes, BUN, creatinine, and prothrombin time weekly during prolonged therapy.
- ***Toxicity and Overdose:*** If overdose occurs, reduction or discontinuation of therapy is the only treatment necessary because of the short duration of dobutamine.

Implementation

- ***High Alert:*** IV vasoactive medications are potentially dangerous. Have second practitioner independently check original order, dose calculations, and infusion pump settings. Do not confuse dobutamine with dopamine. If available as floor stock, store in separate areas.

- Correct hypovolemia with volume expanders before initiating dobutamine therapy.
- Administer into a large vein and assess administration site frequently. Extravasation may cause pain and inflammation.

IV Administration

- **Continuous Infusion:** ***Diluent:*** Vials must be diluted before use. Dilute 250–1000 mg in 250–500 mL of D5W, 0.9% NaCl, 0.45% NaCl, D5/0.45% NaCl, D5/0.9% NaCl, or LR. Admixed infusions stable for 48 hr at room temperature and 7 days if refrigerated. Premixed infusions are already diluted and ready to use. ***Concentration:*** 0.25–5 mg/mL. ***Rate:*** Based on patient's weight (see Route/Dosage section). Administer via infusion pump to ensure precise amount delivered. Titrate to patient response (heart rate, presence of ectopic activity, BP, urine output, CVP, PCWP, cardiac index). Dose should be titrated so heart rate does not increase by >10% of baseline.
- **Y-Site Compatibility:** alemtuzumab, alfentanil, alprostadil, amifostine, amikacin, aminocaproic acid, anidulafungin, argatroban, arsenic trioxide, ascorbic acid, atracurium, atropine, azithromycin, aztreonam, benztropine, bleomycin, bumetanide, buprenorphine, butorphanol, calcium chloride, calcium gluconate, cangrelor, carboplatin, caspofungin, chlorpromazine, ciprofloxacin, cisatracurium, cisplatin, cladribine, clindamycin, cyanocobalamin, cyclophosphamide, cyclosporine, cytarabine, dactinomycin, daptomycin, daunorubicin, dexmedetomidine, digoxin, diltiazem, diphenhydramine, docetaxel, dolasetron, dopamine, doxorubicin, doxorubicin liposome, doxycycline, enalaprilat, ephedrine, epinephrine, epirubicin, epoetin alfa, eptifibatide, erythromycin, esmolol, etoposide phosphate, famotidine, fenoldopam, fentanyl, fluconazole, fludarabine, fosfomycin, gemcitabine, gentamicin, glycopyrrolate, granisetron, hetastarch, hydromorphone, idarubicin, ifosfamide, irinotecan, isoproterenol, ketamine, labetalol, leucovorin calcium, levofloxacin, lidocaine, linezolid, lorazepam, magnesium sulfate, mannitol, meperidine, mesna, methyldopate, methylprednisolone sodium succinate, metoclopramide, metoprolol, milrinone, mitoxantrone, morphine, moxifloxacin, multivitamins, mycophenolate, nafcillin, nalbuphine, naloxone, nicardipine, nitroglycerin, norepinephrine, octreotide, ondansetron, oxaliplatin, oxytocin, paclitaxel, palonosetron, pamidronate, pancuronium, papaverine, pentamidine, phentolamine, phenylephrine, posaconazole, potassium acetate, potassium chloride, procainamide, prochlorperazine, promethazine, propranolol, protamine, pyridoxime, ranitidine, remifentanil, rituximab, rocuronium, sodium acetate, streptokinase, succinylcholine, sufentanil, tacrolimus, televancin, theophylline, thiamine, thiotepa, tigecycline, tirofiban, tobramycin, tolazoline, topotecan, trastuzumab, vancomycin, vasopressin, vecuronium, verapamil, voriconazole, zidovudine, zoledronic acid.
- **Y-Site Incompatibility:** acyclovir, alteplase, aminophylline, amphotericin B deoxycholate, amphotericin B lipid complex, amphotericin B liposome, ampicillin, ampicillin/sulbactam, azathioprine, bivalirudin, carmustine, cefazolin, cefotaxime, cefotetan, cefoxitin, ceftriaxone, cefuroxime, chloramphenicol, dacarbazine, dantrolene, dexamethasone, dexrazoxane, diazoxide, ertapenem, fluorouracil, folic acid, foscarnet, fosphenytoin, ganciclovir, hydrocortisone sodium succinate, hydroxycobalamin, ibuprofen, indomethacin, ketorolac, methotrexate, micafungin, mitomycin, oxacillin, pantoprazole, pemetrexed, penicillin G, pentobarbital, phenobarbital, phenytoin, piperacillin/tazobactam, sodium bicarbonate, thiopental, trimethoprim/sulfamethoxazole, warfarin.

Patient/Family Teaching

- Explain to patient the dobutamine and the need for frequent monitoring.
- Advise patient to inform nurse immediately if chest pain; dyspnea; or numbness, tingling, or burning of extremities occurs.
- Instruct patient to notify nurse immediately of pain or discomfort at the site of administration.
- **Home Care Issues:** Instruct caregiver on proper care of IV equipment.
- Instruct caregiver to report signs of worsening HF (shortness of breath, orthopnea, decreased exercise tolerance), abdominal pain, and nausea or vomiting to health care professional promptly.

Evaluation/Desired Outcomes

- Increase in cardiac output.
- Improved hemodynamic parameters.
- Increased urine output.

HIGH ALERT

DOCEtaxel (doe-se-**tax**-el)

Taxotere

Classification

Therapeutic: antineoplastics

Pharmacologic: taxoids

Indications

Breast cancer (locally advanced/metastatic breast cancer or with doxorubicin and cyclophosphamide as adjuvant treatment of operable node-positive disease). Non–small-cell lung cancer (locally advanced/metastatic) after failure on platinum regimen or with cisplatin as initial therapy. Metastatic castration-resistant prostate cancer (with prednisone). Squamous cell carcinoma of the head and neck (locally advanced) with cisplatin and fluorouracil. Gastric adenocarcinoma (advanced) with cisplatin and fluorouracil as initial therapy.

Action

Interferes with normal cellular microtubule function required for interphase and mitosis. **Therapeutic Effects:** Death of rapidly replicating cells, particularly malignant ones.

Pharmacokinetics

Absorption: IV administration results in complete bioavailability.
Distribution: Unknown.
Metabolism and Excretion: Extensively metabolized by the liver; metabolites undergo fecal elimination.
Half-life: 11.1 hr.

TIME/ACTION PROFILE (effect on blood counts)

ROUTE	ONSET	PEAK	DURATION
IV	rapid	5–9 days	7 days

Contraindications/Precautions

Contraindicated in: Hypersensitivity to docetaxel, paclitaxel or medications formulated with polysorbate 80; Known alcohol intolerance; Neutrophil count $<1500/mm^3$; Liver impairment (serum bilirubin >upper limit of normal, ALT and/or AST >1.5 times upper limit of normal, with alkaline phosphatase >2.5 times upper limit of normal); OB: Pregnancy (may cause fetal harm); Lactation: Lactation.
Use Cautiously in: Rep: Women of reproductive potential and men with female partners of reproductive potential; Pedi: Efficacy not established.

Adverse Reactions/Side Effects

CNS: fatigue, weakness, alcohol intoxication. **CV:** ASCITES, CARDIAC TAMPONADE, PERICARDIAL EFFUSION, PULMONARY EDEMA, peripheral edema. **Derm:** alopecia, edema, rash, dermatitis, desquamation, erythema, nail disorders. **EENT:** cystoid macular edema. **GI:** ENTEROCOLITIS, NEUTROPENIC COLITIS, diarrhea, nausea, stomatitis, vomiting. **GU:** amenorrhea, ↓ fertility (males). **Hemat:** anemia, leukopenia, thrombocytopenia. **Local:** injection site reactions. **MS:** myalgia, arthralgia. **Neuro:** neurosensory deficits, peripheral neuropathy. **Resp:** ACUTE RESPIRATORY DISTRESS SYNDROME, INTERSTITIAL LUNG DISEASE, PULMONARY FIBROSIS, bronchospasm, dyspnea. **Misc:** HYPERSENSITIVITY REACTIONS (including anaphylaxis), MALIGNANCY (including leukemias, myelodysplastic syndrome, non-Hodgkin's lymphoma, and renal cancer).

Interactions

Drug-Drug: ↑ bone marrow depression may occur with other **antineoplastics** or **radiation therapy**. Strong inhibitors of CYP3A4, including **atazanavir**, **clarithromycin**, **indinavir**, **itraconazole**, **ketoconazole**, **nefazodone**, **nelfinavir**, **ritonavir**, **saquinavir**, or **voriconazole** ↑ levels and the risk of toxicity; avoid concomitant use (if need to use, ↓ docetaxel dose by 50%).

Route/Dosage

IV (Adults): *Breast cancer*—60–100 mg/m² every 3 wk; *Breast cancer adjuvant therapy*—75 mg/m² every 3 wk for 6 cycles (with doxorubicin and cyclophosphamide); *Non–small-cell lung cancer*—75 mg/m² every 3 wk (alone or with platinum); *Prostate cancer*—75 mg/m² every 3 wk (with oral prednisone); *Squamous cell head and neck cancer*—75 mg/m² every 3 wk for 3–4 cycles (with cisplatin and fluorouracil); *Gastric adenocarcinoma*—75 mg/m² every 3 wk (with cisplatin and fluorouracil).

Availability (generic available)

Solution for injection (concentrate): 10 mg/mL (dose of 100 mg/m² contains 0.15 g/m² of ethanol), 20 mg/mL (dose of 100 mg/m² contains 1.975 g/m² of ethanol).

NURSING IMPLICATIONS

Assessment

- Monitor vital signs before and after administration.
- Assess infusion site for patency. Docetaxel is not a vesicant. If extravasation occurs, discontinue docetaxel immediately and aspirate the IV needle. Apply cold compresses to the site for 24 hr.
- Monitor for signs and symptoms of hypersensitivity reactions (bronchospasm, hypotension, erythema) continuously during infusion; most common after first and second doses of docetaxel. Treat mild to moderate reactions symptomatically and slow or stop infusion until reaction subsides. Discontinue therapy if severe reactions occur. Do not readminister docetaxel to patients with previous severe reactions. Severe edema may also occur. Weigh patients before each treatment. Fluid accumulation may result in edema, ascites, and pleural or pericardial effusions. Pretreatment with corticosteroids is recommended to minimize edema and hypersensitivity reactions. PO furosemide may be used to treat edema. For hormone-refractory metastatic prostate cancer (given with prednisone), premedicate with dexamethasone.
- Monitor for bone marrow depression. Assess for bleeding (bleeding gums, bruising, petechiae; guaiac stools, urine, and emesis) and avoid IM injections and taking rectal temperatures if platelet count is low. Apply pressure to venipuncture sites for 10 min. Assess for signs of infection during neutropenia. Anemia may occur. Monitor for increased fatigue, dyspnea, and orthostatic hypotension.

- Assess for rash. May occur on feet or hands but may also occur on arms, face, or thorax, usually with pruritus. Rash usually occurs within 1 wk after infusion and resolves before next infusion.
- Assess for development of neurosensory deficit (paresthesia, dysesthesia, pain, burning). May also cause weakness. Pyridoxine may be used to minimize symptoms. Severe symptoms may require dose reduction or discontinuation.
- Assess for arthralgia and myalgia, which are usually relieved by nonopioid analgesics but may be severe enough to require treatment with opioid analgesics.
- Assess for diarrhea and stomatitis. If Grade 3 or 4, reduce dose.
- ***Lab Test Considerations:*** Obtain a negative pregnancy test before starting therapy.
- Monitor CBC and differential before each treatment. Frequently causes neutropenia (<2000 neutrophils/mm^3); may require dose adjustment. If neutrophil count <1500/mm^3, hold dose. Neutropenia is reversible and not cumulative. The nadir is 8 days, with a duration of 7 days. May also cause thrombocytopenia and anemia.
- Monitor liver function studies (AST, ALT, alkaline phosphatase, bilirubin) before each cycle. If AST/ALT >2.5 to ≤5 times upper limit of normal (ULN) and alkaline phosphatase ≤2.5 times ULN, or AST/ALT >1.5 to ≤5 x upper limit of normal and alkaline phosphatase >2.5 to ≤5 x ULN, reduce dose by 20%. If AST/ALT >5 x upper limit of normal and/or alkaline phosphatase >5 times ULN, discontinue therapy.

Implementation

- ***High Alert:*** Fatalities have occurred with chemotherapeutic agents. Before administering, clarify all ambiguous orders; double-check single, daily, and course-of-therapy dose limits; have second practitioner independently double-check original order, calculations, and infusion pump settings.
- ***High Alert:*** Do not confuse Taxotere (docetaxel) with Taxol (paclitaxel).
- Premedicate with dexamethasone 8 mg twice daily for 3 days starting 1 day before docetaxel infusion to reduce incidence and severity of fluid retention and hypersensitivity reactions. Premedicate patients with hormone-refractory metastatic prostate cancer with PO dexamethasone 8 mg, at 12 hr, 3 hr and 1 hr before docetaxel infusion.
- Solution should be prepared in a biologic cabinet. Wear gloves, gown, and mask while handling medication. If powder or solution comes in contact with skin or mucosa, wash thoroughly with soap and water. Discard equipment in specially designated containers.

IV Administration

- **Intermittent Infusion:** *For injection concentrate:* Before dilution, allow vials to stand at room temperature for 5 min. Solution is pale yellow to brownish yellow. *For powder for injection:* Allow number of vials required for dose to stand at room temperature for 5 min. Reconstitute with diluent provided, 1 mL for 20-mg vial or 4 mL for 80-mg vial. Shake vial to dissolve. Solution should be clear; do not administer solutions that are discolored or contain a precipitate. Allow solution to stand for a few min for air bubbles to dissipate. May be refrigerated for up to 8 hrs. ***Concentration:*** 20 mg/0.8 mL for 20-mg vial; 24 mg/mL for 80-mg vial. ***Diluent:*** Withdraw required amount and inject into 250-mL bag of 0.9% NaCl or D5W. If a dose >200 mg is required, use a larger volume diluent so that concentration of 0.74 mg/mL is not exceeded. Rotate gently to mix. Do not administer solutions that are cloudy or contain a precipitate. Diluted solution must be infused within 6 hrs. ***Concentration:*** 0.3 mg/mL to 0.74 mg/mL. ***Rate:*** Administer over 1 hr.
- **Y-Site Compatibility:** acyclovir, alfentanil, allopurinol, amifostine, amikacin, aminocaproic acid, aminophylline, amiodarone, amphotericin B lipid complex, ampicillin, ampicillin/sulbactam, anidulafungin, argatroban, atracurium, azithromycin, aztreonam, bivalirudin, bleomycin, bumetanide, buprenorphine, busulfan, butorphanol, calcium chloride, calcium gluconate, carboplatin, carmustine, caspofungin, cefazolin, cefepime, cefotaxime, cefotetan, cefoxitin, ceftazidime, ceftriaxone, cefuroxime, chlorpromazine, ciprofloxacin, cisatracurium, cisplatin, clindamycin, cyclophosphamide, cyclosporine, cytarabine, dacarbazine, dactinomycin, daptomycin, daunorubicin, dexamethasone, dexmedetomidine, dexrazoxane, diazepam, digoxin, diltiazem, diphenhydramine, dobutamine, dolasetron, dopamine, doxorubicin, doxycycline, droperidol, enalaprilat, ephedrine, epinephrine, epirubicin, ertapenem, erythromycin, esmolol, etoposide, etoposide phosphate, famotidine, fenoldopam, fentanyl, fluconazole, fludarabine, fluorouracil, foscarnet, fosphenytoin, furosemide, ganciclovir, gemcitabine, gentamicin, glycopyrrolate, granisetron, haloperidol, heparin, hetastarch, hydralazine, hydrocortisone, hydromorphone, ifosfamide, imipenem/cilastatin, insulin regular, irinotecan, isoproterenol, ketorolac, labetalol, leucovorin, levofloxacin, lidocaine, linezolid, lorazepam, magnesium sulfate, mannitol, meperidine, meropenem, mesna, methotrexate, methyldopate, metoclopramide, metoprolol, metronidazole, midazolam, milrinone, mitoxantrone, morphine, moxifloxacin, nafcillin, naloxone, nicardipine, nitroglycerin, nitroprusside, norepinephrine, octreotide, ondansetron, oxaliplatin, palonosetron, pamidronate, pancuronium, pantoprazole, pemetrexed, pentamidine, pentobarbital, phenobarbital, phenylephrine, piperacillin/tazobactam, potassium acetate, potassium chloride, potassium phosphates, procainamide, prochlorperazine, promethazine, propranolol, quinupristin/dalfopristin, ranitidine, remifentanil, rituximab, rocuronium,

sodium acetate, sodium bicarbonate, sodium phosphates, succinylcholine, sufentanil, tacrolimus, theophylline, thiotepa, tigecycline, tirofiban, tobramycin, trastuzumab, trimethoprim/sulfamethoxazole, vancomycin, vasopressin, vecuronium, verapamil, vinblastine, vincristine, vinorelbine, voriconazole, zidovudine, zoledronic acid.

- **Y-Site Incompatibility:** amphotericin B liposome, dantrolene, doxorubicin liposome, idarubicin, methylprednisolone, mitomycin, nalbuphine, phenytoin.

Patient/Family Teaching

- Instruct patient to report symptoms of hypersensitivity reactions (trouble breathing; sudden swelling of face, lips, tongue, throat; trouble swallowing; hives; rash; redness all over body) immediately to health care professional immediately.
- Advise patient to notify health care professional if fever >101°F; chills; sore throat; signs of infection; bleeding gums; bruising; petechiae; or blood in urine, stool, or emesis occur. Caution patient to avoid crowds and persons with known infections. Instruct patient to use soft toothbrush and electric razor.
- Patient should be cautioned to avoid alcohol and products containing aspirin or NSAIDs.
- Fatigue is a frequent side effect of docetaxel. Advise patient that frequent rest periods and pacing of activities may minimize fatigue.
- Instruct patient to notify health care professional if signs of fluid retention (peripheral edema in the lower extremities, weight gain, dyspnea), colitis (abdominal pain or tenderness, diarrhea, with or without fever). yellow skin, weakness, paresthesia, gait disturbances, swelling of the feet, or joint or muscle aches occur.
- Alcohol content of docetaxel may impair CNS. Caution patient to avoid driving or other activities requiring alertness until response to medication is known.
- Instruct patient to inspect oral mucosa for redness and ulceration. If mouth sores occur, advise patient to use sponge brush and rinse mouth with water after eating and drinking.
- Instruct patient to notify health care professional of all Rx or OTC medications, vitamins, or herbal products being taken and consult health care professional before taking any new medications.
- Advise patient to notify health care professional if changes in vision occur. Obtain a prompt and comprehensive ophthalmologic examination. May require discontinuation of docetaxel and use of a non-taxane cancer therapy.
- Discuss with patient the possibility of hair loss. Complete hair loss usually begins after 1 or 2 treatments and is reversible after discontinuation of therapy. Explore coping strategies.
- Instruct patient not to receive any vaccinations without advice of health care professional.
- Rep: Advise females of reproductive potential to use effective contraception during and for 6 mo after last dose of therapy and to avoid breast feeding during and for 1 wk after last dose. Advise men with female partners of reproductive potential to use effective contraception during and for 3 mo after last dose of therapy. May impair fertility in male patients,.
- Emphasize the need for periodic lab tests to monitor for side effects.

Evaluation/Desired Outcomes

- Decrease in size or spread of malignancy in women with advanced breast cancer.
- Decrease in size or spread of malignancy in locally advanced or metastatic non–small-cell lung cancer, squamous cell carcinoma of the head and neck, and gastric adenocarcinoma.
- Decreased size or spread of advanced metastatic hormone-refractory prostate cancer.

DOCUSATE (dok-yoo-sate)

docusate calcium
Kao-Tin, Kaopectate Stool Softener

docusate sodium
Colace, Correctol, Diocto, Docu-Soft, Docusoft S, DOK, ✱Dosolax, DSS, Dulcolax, Dulcolax Stool Softener, Enemeez, Fleet Pedialax, Fleet Sof-Lax, Phillips Liquid-Gels, ✱Selax, Silace, ✱Soflax

Classification
Therapeutic: laxatives
Pharmacologic: stool softeners

Indications

PO: Prevention of constipation (in patients who should avoid straining, such as after MI or rectal surgery).
Rect: Used as enema to soften fecal impaction.

Action

Promotes incorporation of water into stool, resulting in softer fecal mass. May also promote electrolyte and water secretion into the colon. **Therapeutic Effects:** Softening and passage of stool.

Pharmacokinetics

Absorption: Small amounts may be absorbed from the small intestine after oral administration. Absorption from the rectum is not known.
Distribution: Unknown.

Metabolism and Excretion: Amounts absorbed after oral administration are eliminated in bile.
Half-life: Unknown.

TIME/ACTION PROFILE (softening of stool)

ROUTE	ONSET	PEAK	DURATION
PO	12–72 hr	unknown	unknown
Rectal	2–15 min	unknown	unknown

Contraindications/Precautions

Contraindicated in: Hypersensitivity; Abdominal pain, nausea, or vomiting, especially when associated with fever or other signs of an acute abdomen.
Use Cautiously in: Excessive or prolonged use may lead to dependence; Should not be used if prompt results are desired; OB, Lactation: Has been used safely.

Adverse Reactions/Side Effects

EENT: throat irritation. **GI:** mild cramps, diarrhea. **Derm:** rashes.

Interactions

Drug-Drug: None significant.

Route/Dosage

Docusate Calcium

PO (Adults): 240 mg once daily.

Docusate Sodium

PO (Adults and Children >12 yr): 50–400 mg in 1–4 divided doses.
PO (Children 6–12 yr): 40–150 mg in 1–4 divided doses.
PO (Children 3–6 yr): 20–60 mg in 1–4 divided doses.
PO (Children <3 yr): 10–40 mg in 1–4 divided doses.
PO (Infants): 5 mg/kg/day in 1–4 divided doses.
Rect (Adults): 50–100 mg or 1 unit containing 283 mg docusate sodium, soft soap, and glycerin.

Availability (generic available)

Docusate Calcium

Capsules: 240 mg^{OTC}.

Docusate Sodium (generic available)

Tablets: 100 mg^{OTC}. **Capsules:** 50 mg^{OTC}, 100 mg^{OTC}, 250 mg^{OTC}. **Syrup:** 20 mg/5 mL^{OTC}. **Liquid:** 50 mg/5 mL^{OTC}. **Enema:** 283 mg/5 mL^{OTC}. ***In combination with:*** stimulant laxatives^{OTC}. See Appendix B.

NURSING IMPLICATIONS

Assessment

- Assess for abdominal distention, presence of bowel sounds, and usual pattern of bowel function.
- Assess color, consistency, and amount of stool produced.

Implementation

- Do not confuse Colace with Cozaar. Do not confuse Dulcolax (docusate sodium) with Dulcolax (bisacodyl). Do not confuse Kaopectate Stool Softener (docusate calcium) with Kaopectate (bismuth subsalicylate).
- This medication does not stimulate intestinal peristalsis; stimulant laxative may be required for constipation.
- **PO:** Administer with a full glass of water or juice. May be administered on an empty stomach for more rapid results.
- Oral solution may be diluted in milk, infant formula, or fruit juice to decrease bitter taste.
- Do not administer within 2 hr of other laxatives, especially mineral oil. May cause increased absorption.
- **Rect:** Administer as a retention or flushing enema.

Patient/Family Teaching

- Advise patients that laxatives should be used only for short-term therapy. Long-term therapy may cause electrolyte imbalance and dependence.
- Encourage patients to use other forms of bowel regulation, such as increasing bulk in the diet, increasing fluid intake (6–8 full glasses/day), and increasing mobility. Normal bowel habits are variable and may vary from 3 times/day to 3 times/wk.
- Instruct patients with cardiac disease to avoid straining during bowel movements (Valsalva maneuver).
- Advise patient not to use laxatives when abdominal pain, nausea, vomiting, or fever is present.
- Advise patient not to take docusate within 2 hr of other laxatives.

Evaluation/Desired Outcomes

- A soft, formed bowel movement, usually within 24–48 hr. Therapy may take 3–5 days for results. Rectal dose forms produce results within 2–15 min.

dofetilide (doe-fet-il-ide)

Tikosyn

Classification
Therapeutic: antiarrhythmics (class III)

Indications

Maintenance of normal sinus rhythm (delay in time to recurrence of atrial fibrillation/atrial flutter [AF/AFl]) in patients with AF/AFl lasting more than one wk, and who have been converted to normal sinus rhythm. Conversion of AF and AFl to normal sinus rhythm.

Action

Blocks cardiac ion channels responsible for transport of potassium. Increases monophasic action potential duration. Increases effective refractory period. **Therapeutic Effects:** Prevention of recurrent AF/AFl. Conversion of AF/AFl to normal sinus rhythm.

Pharmacokinetics

Absorption: Well absorbed (>90%) following oral administration.

Distribution: Unknown.
Metabolism and Excretion: 80% excreted by kidneys via cationic renal secretion, mostly as unchanged drug; 20% excreted as inactive metabolites; some metabolism in the liver via cytochrome P450 system (CYP3A4 isoenzyme).
Half-life: 10 hr.

TIME/ACTION PROFILE (blood levels)

ROUTE	ONSET	PEAK	DURATION
PO	within hrs	2–3 hr†	12–24 hr

†Steady state levels are achieved after 2–3 days.

Contraindications/Precautions

Contraindicated in: Hypersensitivity; Congenital or acquired prolonged QT syndromes; Baseline QT interval or QTc of >440 msec (500 msec in patients with ventricular conduction abnormalities); CCr <20 mL/min; Concurrent use of verapamil, cimetidine, dolutegravir, ketoconazole, itraconazole, trimethoprim, megestrol, prochlorperazine, hydrochlorothiazide, or other QT-interval prolonging drugs; Lactation: Lactation.
Use Cautiously in: Underlying electrolyte abnormalities (↑ risk of serious arrhythmias; correct prior to administration); CCr 20–60 mL/min (dose ↓ recommended); Severe hepatic impairment; OB: Use only when potential maternal benefit justifies potential fetal risk; Pedi: Safety not established.

Adverse Reactions/Side Effects

CNS: dizziness, headache. **CV:** VENTRICULAR ARRHYTHMIAS (including torsade de pointes), chest pain, QT interval prolongation.

Interactions

Drug-Drug: **Hydrochlorothiazide**, **verapamil**, **cimetidine**, **ketoconazole**, **itraconazole**, **trimethoprim**, **megestrol**, **dolutegravir**, and **prochlorperazine** ↑ dofetilide levels and the risk of QT interval prolongation with arrhythmias; concurrent use is contraindicated. **QT interval prolonging drugs** may ↑ the risk of QT interval prolongation with arrhythmias; concurrent use contraindicated. **Amiloride**, **metformin**, and **triamterene** may also ↑ dofetilide levels; use with caution. Inhibitors of the cytochrome P450 system (CYP450 3A4 isoenzyme) including **macrolide anti-infectives**, **azole antifungals**, **protease inhibitor antiretrovirals**, **SSRI antidepressants**, **amiodarone**, **diltiazem**, **nefazodone**, **quinine**, and **zafirlukast** may also ↑ blood levels and the risk of arrhythmias and concurrent use should be undertaken with caution. Should not be used concurrently with other **class I or III antiarrhythmics** due to ↑ risk of arrhythmias. Hypokalemia or hypomagnesemia from **potassium-depleting diuretics** ↑ the risk of arrhythmias; correct abnormalities prior to administration. Concurrent use of **digoxin** may ↑ the risk of arrhythmias.
Drug-Food: **Grapefruit juice** may ↑ levels; avoid concurrent use.

Route/Dosage

Dosing should be adjusted according to renal function and assessment of QT interval.
PO (Adults): *Starting dose*—500 mcg twice daily; *maintenance dose*—250 mcg twice daily (not to exceed 500 mcg twice daily).

Renal Impairment

PO (Adults): *CCr 40–60 mL/min Starting dose*—250 mcg twice daily; *maintenance dose*—125 mcg twice daily; *CCr 20–40 mL/min Starting dose*—125 mcg twice daily; *maintenance dose*—125 mcg once daily.

Availability (generic available)

Capsules: 125 mcg, 250 mcg, 500 mcg.

NURSING IMPLICATIONS

Assessment

- Monitor ECG, pulse, and BP continuously during initiation of therapy and for at least 3 days or a minimum of 12 hrs after electrical or pharmacological conversion to normal sinus rhythm, whichever is greater, then periodically during therapy. Evaluate QTc (or QT interval if heart rate <60 bpm) prior to initiation of therapy and every 3 mo during therapy. If QTc exceeds 440 msec (500 msec in patients with ventricular conduction abnormalities), discontinue dofetilide and monitor patient until QTc returns to baseline.
- Within 2–3 hrs after first dose, determine QTc or QT (if heart rate is less than 60 beats per min). If QTc or QT >15% compared to baseline or if QTc or QT >500 msec (550 msec in patients with ventricular conduction abnormalities), adjust doses as follows: *if initial dose was 500 mcg twice daily,* change to 250 mcg twice daily; *if initial dose was 250 mcg twice daily,* administer 125 mcg twice daily; *if initial dose was 125 mcg twice daily,* give 125 mcg once a day. Determine QTc or QT within 2–3 hrs after each subsequent dose for hospital doses 2–5. No further down titration is recommended. Discontinue dofetilide if at any time after 2nd dose is given QTc or QT is >500 msec (550 msec in patients with ventricular conduction abnormalities).
- Assess the patient's medication history including OTC, Rx, and natural/herbal products, with emphasis on those that interact with dofetilide (see Interactions).

- ***Lab Test Considerations:*** Calculate creatinine clearance prior to administration to determine dose and every 3 mo during therapy.
- Correct hypokalemia before starting therapy. Maintain serum potassium in normal range during dofetilide therapy.

Implementation

- Dofetilide must be initiated or reinitiated and monitored for at least 3 days in a setting that provides continuous ECG monitoring and has personnel trained in the management of serious ventricular arrhythmias. Due to the potential for life-threatening ventricular arrhythmias, dofetilide is usually used for patients with highly symptomatic AF/AFl.
- Patients with AF should be anticoagulated according to usual protocol prior to electrical or pharmacological cardioversion.
- Make sure patient has an adequate supply of dofetilide prior to discharge to prevent interruption of therapy.
- Patients should not be discharged from the hospital within 12 hr of electrical or pharmacological conversion to normal sinus rhythm.
- **PO:** Administer at the same time each day without regard to food.

Patient/Family Teaching

- Instruct patient to take medication as directed, even if feeling well. If a dose is missed, skip dose; do not double next dose. Take next dose at usual time.
- Advise patient to avoid grapefruit juice during therapy; may increase drug levels.
- Advise patient to read *Medication Guide* prior to starting therapy and each Rx refill in case of changes. Emphasize need for adherence with therapy, potential for drug interactions, and need for periodic monitoring to minimize the risk of serious arrhythmias.
- Instruct patient or family member on how to take pulse. Advise patient to report changes in pulse rate or rhythm to health care professional.
- May cause dizziness. Caution patient to avoid driving or other activities requiring alertness until response to medication is known.
- Advise patient to inform health care professional of medication regimen prior to treatment or surgery.
- Instruct patient to notify health care professional of all Rx or OTC medications, vitamins, or herbal products being taken and to consult health care professional before taking other Rx, OTC, or herbal products.
- Advise patient to consult health care professional immediately if they faint, become dizzy, or have fast heartbeats. If health care professional is unavailable, instruct patient to go to nearest hospital emergency department, take remaining dofetilide capsules to hospital, and show them to health care professional. If symptoms associated with altered electrolyte balance such as excessive or prolonged diarrhea, sweating, or vomiting or loss of appetite or thirst occur, notify health care professional immediately.
- Advise female patient to notify health care professional if pregnancy is planned or suspected and to avoid breast feeding during therapy.
- Emphasize the importance of routine follow-up exams to monitor progress.

Evaluation/Desired Outcomes

- Prevention of recurrent AF/AFl.
- Conversion of AF/AFl to normal sinus rhythm.
- If patients do not convert to normal sinus rhythm within 24 hr of initiation of therapy, electrical conversion should be considered.

dolasetron (dol-a-se-tron)

Anzemet

Classification

Therapeutic: antiemetics

Pharmacologic: 5-HT_3 antagonists

Indications

PO: Prevention of nausea and vomiting associated with emetogenic chemotherapy.

Action

Blocks the effects of serotonin at receptor sites (selective antagonist) located in vagal nerve terminals and in the chemoreceptor trigger zone in the CNS. **Therapeutic Effects:** Decreased incidence and severity of nausea/vomiting associated with emetogenic chemotherapy or surgery.

Pharmacokinetics

Absorption: Well absorbed but rapidly metabolized to hydrodolasetron, the active metabolite.

Distribution: Unknown.

Metabolism and Excretion: 61% of hydrodolasetron is excreted unchanged by the kidneys.

Half-life: *Hydrodolasetron*—8.1 hr (shorter in children).

TIME/ACTION PROFILE (antiemetic effect)

ROUTE	ONSET	PEAK	DURATION
PO	unknown	1–2 hr	up to 24 hr

Contraindications/Precautions

Contraindicated in: Hypersensitivity; Congenital long QT syndrome; Complete heart block (unless pacemaker present).

Use Cautiously in: Patients with risk factors for cardiac conduction abnormalities (underlying structural heart disease, sick sinus syndrome, atrial fibrillation and slow ventricular rate, myocardial ischemia, concurrent beta-blocker, verapamil, diltiazem, or antiarrhythmic therapy); Hypokalemia, hypomagnesemia, concurrent therapy with diuretics, or history of cumulative high-dose anthracycline therapy; Geri: ↑ risk for cardiac conduction abnormalities; OB, Lactation: Safety not established.

Adverse Reactions/Side Effects

CNS: headache (increased in cancer patients), dizziness, fatigue, syncope. **CV:** CARDIAC ARREST, TORSADE DE POINTES, VENTRICULAR ARRHYTHMIAS, bradycardia, heart block, hypertension, hypotension, PR interval prolongation, QRS interval prolongation, QT interval prolongation, tachycardia. **GI:** diarrhea, dyspepsia. **GU:** oliguria. **Derm:** pruritus. **Misc:** SEROTONIN SYNDROME, chills, fever, pain.

Interactions

Drug-Drug: Concurrent **diuretic** or **antiarrhythmic** therapy or cumulative **high-dose anthracycline therapy** may ↑ risk of conduction abnormalities. Blood levels and effects of hydrodolasteron are ↑ by **atenolol** and **cimetidine**. Blood levels and effects of hydrodolasetron are ↓ by **rifampin**. ↑ risk of QT interval prolongation with other **agents causing QT interval prolongation**. Drugs that affect serotonergic neurotransmitter systems, including **SSRIs**, **SNRIs**, **tricyclic antidepressants**, **MAOIs**, **fentanyl**, **lithium**, **buspirone**, **tramadol**, **methylene blue**, and **triptans** ↑ risk of serotonin syndrome.

Route/Dosage

Prevention of Chemotherapy-Induced Nausea/Vomiting

PO (Adults): 100 mg given within 1 hr before chemotherapy.
PO (Children 2–16 yr): 1.8 mg/kg given within 1 hr before chemotherapy (not to exceed 100 mg).

Availability

Tablets: 50 mg, 100 mg.

NURSING IMPLICATIONS

Assessment

- Assess patient for nausea, vomiting, abdominal distention, and bowel sounds before and after administration.
- Monitor ECG in patients with HF, bradycardia, underlying heart disease, renal impairment, and elderly patients.
- ***Lab Test Considerations:*** Monitor serum potassium and magnesium prior to and periodically during therapy.

Implementation

- **PO:** Administer within 1 hr before chemotherapy.

Patient/Family Teaching

- Explain purpose of dolasetron to patient.
- Advise patient to notify health care professional if nausea or vomiting occurs.
- Advise patient to notify health care professional if symptoms of abnormal heart rate or rhythm (racing heart beat, shortness of breath, dizziness, fainting) occur.

Evaluation/Desired Outcomes

- Prevention of nausea and vomiting associated with emetogenic cancer chemotherapy.

🧬 dolutegravir
(doe-loo-**teg**-ra-vir)
Tivicay

Classification
Therapeutic: antiretrovirals
Pharmacologic: integrase strand transfer inhibitors (INSTI)

Indications

Treatment of HIV-1 infection (in combination with other antiretrovirals). Treatment of HIV-1 infection in patients to replace the current antiretroviral regimen in those who are virologically suppressed (HIV-1 RNA <50 copies/mL) on a stable antiretroviral regimen for ≥6 mo with no history of treatment failure or known substitutions associated with resistance to either dolutegravir or rilpivirine (in combination with rilpivirine).

Action

Inhibits HIV-1 integrase, which is required for viral replication. **Therapeutic Effects:** Evidence of decreased viral replication and reduced viral load with slowed progression of HIV and its sequelae.

Pharmacokinetics

Absorption: Absorption follows oral administration; bioavailability is unknown.
Distribution: Enters CSF.
Protein Binding: >98.9%.
Metabolism and Excretion: Metabobolized primarily by the UGT1A1 enzyme system with some metabolism by CYP3A4. 53% excreted unchanged in feces. Metabolites are renally excreted, minimal renal elimination of unchanged drug. 🧬 Poor metabolizers of dolutegravir have ↑ levels and ↓ clearance.
Half-life: 14 hr.

TIME/ACTION PROFILE (blood levels)

ROUTE	ONSET	PEAK	DURATION
PO	unknown	2–3 hr	12–24 hr†

†Depends on concurrent use of metabolic inducers.

Contraindications/Precautions

Contraindicated in: Concurrent use of dofetilide; Severe hepatic impairment; OB: Avoid use through first trimester of pregnancy (may ↑ risk of neural tube defects); Lactation: Breast feeding not recommended in HIV-infected patients.

Use Cautiously in: Underlying hepatic disease, including hepatitis B or C (↑ risk fo hepatotoxicity); Severe renal impairment; Geri: Consider age-related ↓ in cardiac, renal and hepatic function, chronic disease states and concurrent medications; Rep: Women of reproductive potential; Pedi: Children <30 kg or INSTI-experienced with resistance documented to other INSTIs (raltegravir) (safety and effectiveness not established).

Adverse Reactions/Side Effects

CNS: headache, insomnia, fatigue. **Derm:** pruritus. **GI:** HEPATOTOXICITY (↑ WITH HEPATITIS B OR C). **GU:** renal impairment. **MS:** myositis. **Misc:** hypersensitivity reactions (including rash, constitutional symptoms, and liver injury), immune reconstitution syndrome.

Interactions

Drug-Drug: May ↑ blood levels and toxicity from **dofetilide**; concurrent use contraindicated. Blood levels and effectiveness are ↓ by **etravirine** (should not be used concurrently without atazanavir/ritonavir, darunavir/ritonavir or lopinavir/ritonavir). Blood levels and effectiveness are ↓ by **efavirenz**, **fosamprenavir/ritonavir**, **tipranavir/ritonavir**, **carbamazepine**, and **rifampin**; ↑ dose of dolutegravir recommended. Blood levels and effectiveness may be ↓ by **nevirapine**; avoid concurrent use. May ↑ blood levels and toxicity from **metformin**; do not exceed metformin dose of 1000 mg/day. Blood levels and effectiveness may be ↓ by **oxcarbazepine**, **phenobarbital**, **phenytoin**; avoid concurrent use. Absorption and effectiveness may be ↓ by cation-containing **antacids**, **buffered medications**, **calcium supplements** (oral), **iron supplements** (oral), **laxatives**, or **sucralfate**; dolutegravir should be taken 2 hr before or 6 hr after; may also take dolutegravir and calcium or iron supplements with food.

Drug-Natural Products: Blood levels and effectiveness may be ↓ by **St. John's wort**; avoid concurrent use.

Route/Dosage

PO (Adults): *Treatment-naïve or treatment-experienced INSTI-naïve patients or virologically suppressed (HIV RNA <50 copies/mL) patients switching to dolutegravir plus rilpivirine*—50 mg once daily; *Treatment-naïve or treatment-experienced INSTI-naïve patients currently receiving efavirenz, fosamprenavir/ritonavir, tipranavir/ritonavir, carbamazepine, or rifampin*—50 mg twice daily; *INSTI-experienced with certain INSTI-associated resistance substitutions or clinically suspected INSTI resistance (consider other combinations that do not include metabolic inducers)*—50 mg twice daily.

PO (Children ≥40 kg): *Treatment-naïve or treatment-experienced INSTI-naïve patients*—50 mg once daily; *Treatment-naïve or treatment-experienced INSTI-naïve patients currently receiving efavirenz, fosamprenavir/ritonavir, tipranvir/ritonavir, carbamazepine, or rifampin*—50 mg twice daily.

PO (Children 30–39 kg): *Treatment-naïve or treatment-experienced INSTI-naïve patients*—35 mg once daily; *Treatment-naïve or treatment-experienced INSTI-naïve patients currently receiving efavirenz, fosamprenavir/ritonavir, tipranvir/ritonavir, carbamazepine, or rifampin*—35 mg twice daily.

Availability

Tablets: 10 mg, 25 mg, 50 mg. ***In combination with:*** abacavir and lamivudine (Triumeq); lamivudine (Dovato); rilpivirine (Juluca). See Appendix B.

NURSING IMPLICATIONS

Assessment

- Assess patient for change in severity of HIV symptoms and for symptoms of opportunistic infections during therapy.
- Monitor for signs and symptoms of hypersensitivity reactions (rash, fever, malaise, fatigue, muscle or joint aches, blisters or peeling of skin, oral blisters or lesions, conjunctivitis, facial edema, hepatitis, eosinophilia, angioedema, difficulty breathing). Discontinue therapy and do not restart.
- ***Lab Test Considerations:*** Monitor viral load and CD4 counts regularly during therapy.
- Obtain a negative pregnancy test before starting therapy.
- May cause ↓ ANC, hemoglobin, total neutrophils, and platelet counts.
- Monitor liver function periodically during therapy. May cause ↑ serum glucose, lipase, AST, ALT, total bilirubin, creatine kinase concentrations.

Implementation

- **PO:** May be administered without regard to food.
- Administer 2 hrs before or 6 hrs after calcium and iron supplements.

Patient/Family Teaching

- Emphasize the importance of taking dolutegravir as directed. Do not take more than prescribed amount and do not stop taking without consulting health care professional. Take missed doses as soon as remembered unless within 4 hr of next dose; then skip dose. Do not double doses. Advise patient to read *Patient Information* before starting therapy and with each Rx renewal in case of changes.
- Instruct patient that dolutegravir should not be shared with others.
- Instruct patient to notify health care professional of all Rx or OTC medications, vitamins, or herbal products being taken and consult health care professional before taking any new medications, especially St. John's wort.
- Inform patient that dolutegravir does not cure AIDS or prevent associated or opportunistic infections. Dolutegravir does not reduce the risk of transmission of HIV to others through sexual contact or

blood contamination. Caution patient to use a condom during sexual contact and to avoid sharing needles or donating blood to prevent spreading the AIDS virus to others. Advise patient that the long-term effects of dolutegravir are unknown at this time.
- Advise patient to notify health care professional if signs and symptoms of hypersensitivity occur.
- Advise patient to notify health care professional if signs and symptoms of immune reconstitution syndrome (signs and symptoms of an infection) occur.
- Rep: Advise patients to notify health care professional if pregnancy is planned or suspected. Avoid breast feeding during therapy. Pregnant patients should be encouraged to enroll in the Antiretroviral Pregnancy Registry by calling 1-800-258-4263.
- Emphasize the importance of regular follow-up exams and blood counts to determine progress and monitor for side effects.

Evaluation/Desired Outcomes
- Delayed progression of AIDS and decreased opportunistic infections in patients with HIV.
- Decrease in viral load and improvement in CD4 cell counts.

dolutegravir/rilpivirine
(doe-loo-**teg**-ra-vir/ril-pi-**vir**-een)
Juluca

Classification
Therapeutic: antiretrovirals
Pharmacologic: integrase strand transfer inhibitors (INSTI), non-nucleoside reverse transcriptase inhibitors

Indications
Treatment of HIV-1 infection in patients who are virologically suppressed (HIV-1 RNA < 50 copies/mL) on a stable antiretroviral regimen for ≥6 mo with no history of treatment failure and no known resistance to dolutegravir or rilpivirine.

Action
Dolutegravir—inhibits HIV-1 integrase, which is required for viral replication. *Rilpivirine*—inhibits HIV-replication by non-competitively inhibiting HIV reverse transcriptase. **Therapeutic Effects:** Increased CD4 cell counts and decreased viral load with subsequent slowed progression of HIV infection and its sequelae.

Pharmacokinetics
Dolutegravir
Absorption: Absorption follows oral administration; bioavailability is unknown.
Distribution: Enters CSF.
Protein Binding: >98.9%.
Metabolism and Excretion: Metabolized primarily by the UGT1A1 enzyme system with some metabolism by CYP3A4. 53% excreted unchanged in feces. Metabolites are renally excreted; minimal renal elimination of unchanged drug.
Half-life: 14 hr.
Rilpivirine
Absorption: Well absorbed following oral administration.
Distribution: Unknown.
Protein Binding: 99.7%.
Metabolism and Excretion: Mostly metabolized by the liver via CYP3A; 25% excreted in feces unchanged, <1% excreted unchanged in urine.
Half-life: 50 hr.

TIME/ACTION PROFILE (blood levels)

ROUTE	ONSET	PEAK	DURATION
Dolutegravir (PO)	unknown	2–3 hr	12–24 hr†
Rilpivirine (PO)	unknown	4–5 hr	24 hr

†Depends on concurrent use of metabolic inducers.

Contraindications/Precautions
Contraindicated in: Hypersensitivity; Concurrent use of carbamazepine, dexamethasone, dofetilide, oxcarbazepine, phenobarbital, phenytoin, proton pump inhibitors, rifampin, rifapentine, and St. John's wort; OB: Avoid use through first trimester of pregnancy (may ↑ risk of neural tube defects); Lactation: Breast feeding not recommended in patients with HIV.
Use Cautiously in: Underlying hepatic disease, including hepatitis B or C (↑ risk for hepatotoxicity); Severe renal impairment; History of depression or suicide attempt; Rep: Women of reproductive potential; Geri: Consider age-related ↓ in cardiac, renal and hepatic function, chronic disease states and concurrent medications; Pedi: Safety and effectiveness not established.

Adverse Reactions/Side Effects
CNS: SUICIDAL THOUGHTS, depression, headache, dizziness. **CV:** QTc interval prolongation. **Derm:** DRUG REACTION WITH EOSINOPHILIA AND SYSTEMIC SYMPTOMS (DRESS), pruritus, rash. **Endo:** hyperglycemia. **GI:** HEPATOTOXICITY, ↑ lipase. **GU:** ↑ serum creatinine. **MS:** ↓ bone mineral density. **Misc:** hypersensitivity reactions (including rash, constitutional symptoms, and liver injury), fatigue, immune reconstitution syndrome.

Interactions
Drug-Drug: May ↑ levels and risk of toxicity of **dofetilide**; concurrent use contraindicated. **CYP3A inducers**, including **carbamazepine**, **dexamethasone** (more than a single dose), **oxcarbazepine**, **phenobarbital**, **phenytoin**, **rifampin**, or **rifapen-**

tine may ↓ levels and effectiveness and promote virologic resistance; concurrent use contraindicated. By causing an ↑ in gastric pH, **proton pump inhibitors** ↓ rilpivirine levels and effectiveness and may promote virologic resistance; concurrent use contraindicated. May ↑ blood levels and toxicity from **metformin**; do not exceed metformin dose of 1000 mg/day. Cation-containing products, including **calcium supplements** (oral), **iron supplements** (oral), **laxatives**, **buffered medications**, or **sucralfate** may ↓ dolutegravir levels and effectiveness; give 4 hr before or 6 hr after products containing polyvalent cations. Concurrent use with **antacids** may ↓ rilpivirine levels and effectiveness; administer ≥4 hr before or ≥6 hr after antacids. Concurrent use with **H_2 receptor antagonists** may ↓ rilpivirine levels and effectiveness; administer ≥4 hr before or ≥12 hr after H_2 receptor antagonist. **Rifabutin** may ↓ rilpivirine levels; give additional rilipivirine 25–mg tablet once daily with a meal during concurrent use. **Clarithromycin** or **erythromycin** may ↑ rilpivirine levels; consider azithromycin. Concurrent use with **QT interval prolonging drugs** may ↑ risk of torsade de pointes. May ↓ **methadone** levels; monitor clinical effects.

Drug-Natural Products: St. John's wort may ↓ levels and effectiveness and promote virologic resistance; concurrent use contraindicated.

Route/Dosage

PO (Adults): One tablet once daily.

Availability

Tablets: dolutegravir 50 mg/rilpivirine 25 mg.

NURSING IMPLICATIONS

Assessment

- Assess for change in severity of HIV symptoms and for symptoms of opportunistic infections during therapy.
- Monitor for signs and symptoms of DRESS (fever, rash, lymphadenopathy, and/or facial swelling, associated with involvement of other organ systems (hepatitis, nephritis, hematologic abnormalities, myocarditis, myositis) during therapy. May resemble an acute viral infection. Eosinophilia is often present. Discontinue therapy if signs occur.
- Assess mental status (orientation, mood, behavior) before and periodically during therapy. Monitor closely for notable changes in behavior that could indicate the emergence or worsening of suicidal thoughts or behavior or depression.
- Monitor for signs and symptoms of hypersensitivity reactions (rash, fever, malaise, fatigue, muscle or joint aches, blisters or peeling of skin, oral blisters or lesions, conjunctivitis, facial edema, hepatitis, eosinophilia, angioedema, difficulty breathing). Discontinue therapy and do not restart.
- Assess mental status (orientation, mood, behavior) before and periodically during therapy. Monitor closely for notable changes in behavior that could indicate the emergence or worsening of suicidal thoughts or behavior or depression.
- ***Lab Test Considerations:*** Monitor viral load and CD4 counts regularly during therapy.
- Perform a pregnancy test prior to starting therapy.
- Monitor liver function tests before and periodically during therapy, especially in patients with underlying liver disease or marked ↑ transaminase. May cause ↑ AST, ALT, and total bilirubin.

Implementation

- **PO:** Administer one daily with a meal.
- Administer dolutegravir/rilpivirine ≥4 hr before or ≥6 hr after antacids and ≥4 hr before or ≥12 hrs after H_2 receptor antagonists.

Patient/Family Teaching

- Emphasize the importance of taking dolutegravir/rilpivirine as directed. Do not take more than prescribed amount and do not stop taking without consulting health care professional. Take missed doses as soon as remembered unless with a meal. Do not double doses. Advise patient to read *Patient Information* before starting therapy and with each Rx renewal in case of changes.
- Inform patient that dolutegravir/rilpivirine does not cure HIV or prevent associated or opportunistic infections. Dolutegravir/rilpivirine does not reduce the risk of transmission of HIV to others through sexual contact or blood contamination. Caution patient to use a condom during sexual contact and to avoid sharing needles or donating blood to prevent spreading the HIV virus to others. Advise patient that the long-term effects of dolutegravir/rilpivirine are unknown at this time.
- Advise patient to notify health care professional if signs and symptoms of skin rash and allergic reactions and hepatotoxicity (skin or white of eyes turns yellow/jaundice, dark urine, light-colored stools, nausea or vomiting, loss of appetite, pain, aching, or tenderness on the right side of stomach).
- Inform patients and families of risk of suicidal thoughts and behavior and advise that behavioral changes, emergent or worsening signs and symptoms of depression, unusual changes in mood, or emergence of suicidal thoughts, behavior, or thoughts of self-harm should be reported to health care professional immediately.
- Immune reconstitution syndrome may trigger opportunistic infections or autoimmune disorders. Notify health care professional if symptoms (signs and symptoms of an infection) occur.
- Advise patient to notify health care professional of all Rx or OTC medications, vitamins, or herbal products being taken and to consult with health care professional before taking other medications, especially St. John's wort.
- Rep: Advise patients to use effective contraception, especially during conception and the 1st trimester

and to notify health care professional if pregnancy is planned or suspected. Advise patient to avoid breast feeding during therapy. Encourage women who become pregnant during therapy to enroll in Antiviral Pregnancy Registry by calling 1-800-258-4263.

Evaluation/Desired Outcomes

- Delayed progression of AIDS and decreased opportunistic infections in patients with HIV.

donepezil (doe-nep-i-zill)

Aricept, ~~Aricept ODT~~

Classification

Therapeutic: anti-Alzheimer's agents

Pharmacologic: cholinergics (cholinesterase inhibitors)

Indications

Mild, moderate, or severe dementia/neurocognitive disorder associated with Alzheimer's disease.

Action

Inhibits acetylcholinesterase thus improving cholinergic function by making more acetylcholine available. **Therapeutic Effects:** May temporarily lessen some of the dementia associated with Alzheimer's disease. Enhances cognition. Does not cure the disease.

Pharmacokinetics

Absorption: Well absorbed after oral administration.

Distribution: Unknown.

Protein Binding: 96%.

Metabolism and Excretion: Partially metabolized by the liver (CYP2D6 and CYP3A4 enyzmes) and partially excreted by kidneys (17% unchanged). Two metabolites are pharmacologically active.

Half-life: 70 hr.

TIME/ACTION PROFILE (improvement in symptoms)

ROUTE	ONSET	PEAK	DURATION
PO	unknown	several wk	6 wk†

†Return to baseline after discontinuation.

Contraindications/Precautions

Contraindicated in: Hypersensitivity to donepezil or piperidine derivatives.

Use Cautiously in: Underlying cardiac disease, especially sick sinus syndrome or supraventricular conduction defects; History of ulcer disease or currently taking NSAIDs; History of seizures; History of asthma or obstructive pulmonary disease; OB: Safety not established; Lactation: Use during breast feeding only if benefit to patient outweighs potential risk to infant; Pedi: Safety and effectiveness not established.

Adverse Reactions/Side Effects

CNS: headache, abnormal dreams, depression, dizziness, drowsiness, fatigue, insomnia, syncope, sedation (unusual). **CV:** atrial fibrillation, hypertension, hypotension, vasodilation. **Derm:** ecchymoses. **GI:** diarrhea, nausea, anorexia, vomiting, weight gain (unusual). **GU:** frequent urination. **Metab:** hot flashes, weight loss. **MS:** arthritis, muscle cramps.

Interactions

Drug-Drug: Exaggerates muscle relaxation from **succinylcholine**. Interferes with the action of **anticholinergics**. ↑ cholinergic effects of **bethanechol**. May ↑ risk of GI bleeding from **NSAIDs**. **Quinidine** and **ketoconazole** ↓ metabolism of donepezil. **Rifampin**, **carbamazepine**, **dexamethasone**, **phenobarbital**, and **phenytoin** induce the enzymes that metabolize donepezil and may ↓ its effects.

Drug-Natural Products: Jimson weed and **scopolia** may antagonize cholinergic effects.

Route/Dosage

Mild to Moderate Alzheimer's Disease

PO (Adults): 5 mg once daily; may ↑ to 10 mg once daily after 4–6 wk (dose should not exceed 5 mg/day in frail, elderly females).

Severe Alzheimer's Disease

PO (Adults): 5 mg once daily; may ↑ to 10 mg once daily after 4–6 wk; after 3 mo, may then ↑ to 23 mg once daily.

Availability (generic available)

Orally disintegrating tablets: 5 mg, 10 mg. **Cost:** *Generic*—All strengths $233.62/30. **Tablets:** 5 mg, 10 mg, 23 mg. **Cost:** *Aricept*—23 mg $1,059.91/90; *Generic*—All strengths $23.97/90. ***In combination with:*** memantine (Namzaric). See Appendix B.

NURSING IMPLICATIONS

Assessment

- Assess cognitive function (memory, attention, reasoning, language, ability to perform simple tasks) periodically during therapy.
- Monitor heart rate periodically during therapy. May cause bradycardia.

Implementation

- Do not confuse Aricept with Aciphex or Azilect.
- **PO:** Administer in the evening just before going to bed. May be taken without regard to food.
- *Oral disintegrating tablets* should be allowed to dissolve on tongue; follow with water.
- Swallow *23 mg tablet* whole. Do not split, crush, or chew; may increase rate of absorption.

Patient/Family Teaching

- Emphasize the importance of taking donepezil daily, as directed. Missed doses should be skipped and regular schedule returned to the following day. Do not take more than prescribed; higher doses do not increase effects but may increase side effects.
- Inform patient/family that it may take weeks before improvement in baseline behavior is observed.
- Caution patient and caregiver that donepezil may cause dizziness. Advise patient to avoid driving and other activities requiring alertness until response to medication is known.
- Advise patient and caregiver to notify health care professional if nausea, vomiting, diarrhea, or changes in color of stool occur or if new symptoms occur or previously noted symptoms increase in severity.
- Instruct patient to notify health care professional of all Rx or OTC medications, vitamins, or herbal products being taken and to consult health care professional before taking other Rx, OTC, or herbal products.
- Advise patient and caregiver to notify health care professional of medication regimen before treatment or surgery.
- Advise females of reproductive potential to notify health care professional if pregnancy is planned or suspected or if breast feeding.
- Emphasize the importance of follow-up exams to monitor progress.

Evaluation/Desired Outcomes

- Improvement in cognitive function (memory, attention, reasoning, language, ability to perform simple tasks) in patients with Alzheimer's disease.

HIGH ALERT

DOPamine (dope-a-meen)

Intropin, Revimine

Classification

Therapeutic: inotropics, vasopressors
Pharmacologic: adrenergics

Indications

Adjunct to standard measures to improve: BP, Cardiac output, Urine output in treatment of shock unresponsive to fluid replacement. Increase renal perfusion (low doses).

Action

Small doses (0.5–3 mcg/kg/min) stimulate dopaminergic receptors, producing renal vasodilation. Larger doses (2–10 mcg/kg/min) stimulate dopaminergic and $beta_1$-adrenergic receptors, producing cardiac stimulation and renal vasodilation. Doses greater than 10 mcg/kg/min stimulate alpha-adrenergic receptors and may cause renal vasoconstriction. **Therapeutic Effects:** Increased cardiac output, increased BP, and improved renal blood flow.

Pharmacokinetics

Absorption: Administered IV only, resulting in complete bioavailability.
Distribution: Widely distributed but does not cross the blood-brain barrier.
Metabolism and Excretion: Metabolized in liver, kidneys, and plasma.
Half-life: 2 min.

TIME/ACTION PROFILE (hemodynamic effects)

ROUTE	ONSET	PEAK	DURATION
IV	1–2 min	up to 10 min	<10 min

Contraindications/Precautions

Contraindicated in: Tachyarrhythmias; Pheochromocytoma; Hypersensitivity to bisulfites (some products).
Use Cautiously in: Hypovolemia; Myocardial infarction; Occlusive vascular diseases; Geri: Older patients may be more susceptible to adverse effects; OB: Pregnancy and lactation (safety not established).

Adverse Reactions/Side Effects

CNS: headache. **EENT:** mydriasis (high dose). **Resp:** dyspnea. **CV:** arrhythmias, hypotension, angina, ECG change, palpitations, vasoconstriction. **GI:** nausea, vomiting. **Derm:** piloerection. **Local:** irritation at IV site.

Interactions

Drug-Drug: Use with **MAO inhibitors, ergot alkaloids (ergotamine), doxapram**, or some **antidepressants** results in severe hypertension. Use with IV **phenytoin** may cause hypotension and bradycardia. Use with **general anesthetics** may result in arrhythmias. **Beta blockers** may antagonize cardiac effects.

Route/Dosage

IV (Adults): *Dopaminergic (renal vasodilation) effects*—1–5 mcg/kg/min. *Beta-adrenergic (cardiac stimulation) effects*—5–15 mcg/kg/min. *Alpha-adrenergic (increased peripheral vascular resistance) effects*—>15 mcg/kg/min; infusion rate may be increased as needed.
IV (Children and Infants): 1–20 mcg/kg/min, depending on desired response (1–5 mcg/kg/min has been used to improve renal blood flow).
IV (Neonates): 1–20 mcg/kg/min.

Availability (generic available)

Injection for dilution: 40 mg/mL, 80 mg/mL, 160 mg/mL. **Premixed injection:** 200 mg/250 mL, 400 mg/250 mL, 800 mg/250 mL, 800 mg/500 mL.

NURSING IMPLICATIONS

Assessment

- Monitor BP, heart rate, pulse pressure, ECG, pulmonary capillary wedge pressure (PCWP), cardiac output, CVP, and urinary output continuously during administration. Report significant changes in vital signs or arrhythmias. Consult physician for parameters for pulse, BP, or ECG changes for adjusting dose or discontinuing medication.

- Monitor urine output frequently throughout administration. Report decreases in urine output promptly.
- Palpate peripheral pulses and assess appearance of extremities routinely during dopamine administration. Notify physician if quality of pulse deteriorates or if extremities become cold or mottled.
- If hypotension occurs, administration rate should be increased. If hypotension continues, more potent vasoconstrictors (norepinephrine) may be administered.
- ***Toxicity and Overdose:*** If excessive hypertension occurs, rate of infusion should be decreased or temporarily discontinued until BP is decreased.

Implementation

- ***High Alert:*** IV vasoactive medications are potentially dangerous. Have second practitioner independently check original order, dose calculations, and infusion pump settings. Do not confuse dopamine with dobutamine. If both are available as floor stock, store in separate areas.
- Correct hypovolemia with volume expanders before initiating dopamine therapy.
- Extravasation may cause severe irritation, necrosis, and sloughing of tissue. Administer into a large vein and assess administration site frequently. If extravasation occurs, affected area should be infiltrated liberally with 10–15 mL of 0.9% NaCl containing 5–10 mg of phentolamine. For pediatric patients, use 1 mL of phentolamine dilution to infiltrate (do not exceed 5 mg total). Infiltration within 12 hr of extravasation produces immediate hyperemic changes.

IV Administration

- **Continuous Infusion: *Diluent:*** Dopamine vials must be diluted before use. Dilute 200–800 mg of dopamine in 250–500 mL of 0.9% NaCl, D5W, D5/LR, D5/0.45% NaCl, D5/0.9% NaCl, or LR. Admixed solution is stable for 24 hr. Discard solutions that are cloudy, discolored, or contain a precipitate. Premixed infusions are already diluted and ready to use. ***Concentration:*** 0.8–3.2 mg/mL. ***Rate:*** Based on patient's weight (see Route/Dosage section). Infusion must be administered via infusion pump to ensure precise amount delivered. Titrate to response (BP, heart rate, urine output, peripheral perfusion, presence of ectopic activity, cardiac index). Decrease rate gradually when discontinuing to prevent marked decreases in BP.
- **Y-Site Compatibility:** amifostine, amikacin, aminophylline, amiodarone, anidulafungin, argatroban, atracurium, atropine, aztreonam, bivalirudin, bumetanide, calcium chloride, calcium gluconate, caspofungin, cefotaxime, cefoxitin, ceftazidime, ceftriaxone, cefuroxime, cimetidine, ciprofloxacin, cisatracurium, cladribine, clindamycin, cyclosporine, daptomycin, dexamethasone sodium phosphate, dexmedetomidine, digoxin, diltiazem, diphenhydramine, dobutamine, docetaxel, doxorubicin liposome, doxycycline, droperidol, enalaprilat, epinephrine, ertapenem, erythromycin, esmolol, etoposide phosphate, famotidine, fenoldopam, fentanyl, fluconazole, foscarnet, gemcitabine, gentamicin, granisetron, haloperidol, heparin, hydrocortisone sodium succinate, hydromorphone, imipenem/cilastatin, isoproterenol, ketorolac, labetalol, levofloxacin, lidocaine, linezolid, lorazepam, magnesium sulfate, meperidine, methylprednisolone sodium succinate, metoclopramide, metoprolol, metronidazole, micafungin, midazolam, milrinone, morphine, nafcillin, nicardipine, nitroglycerin, nitroprusside, norepinephrine, ondansetron, oxaliplatin, palonosetron, pancuronium, pantoprazole, pemetrexed, penicillin G potassium, phenylephrine, phytonadione, piperacillin/tazobactam, potassium chloride, procainamide, prochlorperazine, promethazine, propofol, propranolol, protamine, ranitidine, remifentanil, sargramostim, streptokinase, tacrolimus, theophylline, thiotepa, tigecycline, tirofiban, tobramycin, tolazoline, vancomycin, vasopressin, vecuronium, verapamil, vitamin B complex with C, voriconazole, warfarin, zidovudine.
- **Y-Site Incompatibility:** acyclovir, alteplase, amphotericin B cholesteryl sulfate, ampicillin, cefazolin, chloramphenicol, diazepam, ganciclovir, indomethacin, insulin, lansoprazole, phenytoin, thiopental, trimethoprim/sulfamethoxazole.

Patient/Family Teaching

- Explain to patient the rationale for instituting this medication and the need for frequent monitoring.
- Advise patient to inform nurse immediately if chest pain; dyspnea; numbness, tingling, or burning of extremities occurs.
- Instruct patient to inform nurse immediately of pain or discomfort at the site of administration.

Evaluation/Desired Outcomes

- Increase in BP.
- Increase in peripheral circulation.
- Increase in urine output.

doravirine/lamivudine/tenofovir disoproxil fumarate

(**dor**-a-**vir**-een/la-**mi**-vyoo-deen/te-**noe**-fo-veer dye-soe-**prox**-il **fue**-ma-rate)

Delstrigo

Classification

Therapeutic: antiretrovirals

Pharmacologic: non-nucleoside reverse transcriptase inhibitors, nucleoside reverse transcriptase inhibitors

Indications

HIV-1 infection in patients with no prior antiretroviral treatment history. To replace the current antiretroviral regimen in patients with HIV-1 infection who are virologically suppressed (HIV-1 RNA <50 copies/mL), receiving a stable antiretroviral regimen with no history of treatment failure, and have no known substitutions associated with resistance to doravirine, lamivudine, or tenofovir disoproxil fumarate.

Action

Doravirine—Binds to the enzyme reverse transcriptase, which results in disrupted viral DNA synthesis. *Lamivudine*—After intracellular conversion to its active form (lamivudine-5-triphosphate), inhibits viral DNA synthesis by inhibiting the enzyme HIV reverse transcriptase. *Tenofovir disoproxil fumarate*—Phosphorylated intracellularly where it inhibits HIV reverse transcriptase resulting in disruption of DNA synthesis.

Therapeutic Effects: Evidence of decreased viral replication and reduced viral load with slowed progression of HIV and its sequelae.

Pharmacokinetics

Doravirine

Absorption: 64% absorbed following oral administration.

Distribution: Extensively distributed to tissues.

Metabolism and Excretion: Primarily metabolized in the liver by CYP3A enzymes. Primarily excreted in feces (as metabolites), 6% unchanged in urine.

Half-life: 15 hr.

Lamivudine

Absorption: 86% absorbed after oral administration.

Distribution: Extensively distributed to tissues.

Metabolism and Excretion: 71% excreted unchanged in urine by glomerular filtration and active tubular secretion.

Half-life: 5–7 hr.

Tenofovir

Absorption: 25% absorbed after oral administration.

Distribution: Extensively distributed to tissues.

Metabolism and Excretion: 70–80% excreted unchanged in urine by glomerular filtration and active tubular secretion.

Half-life: 17 hr.

TIME/ACTION PROFILE (plasma concentrations)

ROUTE	ONSET	PEAK	DURATION
doravirine (PO)	unknown	2 hr	24 hr
lamivudine (PO)	unknown	unknown	24 hr
tenofovir (PO)	unknown	1 hr	24 hr

Contraindications/Precautions

Contraindicated in: Previous hypersensitivity reaction to lamivudine; Concurrent use of carbamazepine, enzalutamide, mitotane, oxcarbazepine, phenobarbital, phenytoin, rifampin, rifapentine, and St. John's wort; Concurrent or recent use of nephrotoxic medications; CCr <50 mL/min; Lactation: Breast feeding not recommended in women infected with HIV.

Use Cautiously in: Coinfection with hepatitis B virus (HBV) (hepatitis may recur after discontinuation of lamivudine and ↑ risk of lamivudine-resistant HBV); Severe hepatic impairment (Child-Pugh Class C); OB: Safety of doravirine not established; Pedi: Safety and effectiveness not established; Geri: Consider age-related ↓ in organ function and body mass, concurrent disease states and medications.

Adverse Reactions/Side Effects

CNS: abnormal dreams, dizziness, insomnia, sedation. **Derm:** rash. **Endo:** Graves' disease. **GI:** HEPATOTOXICITY (↑ with hepatitis B or C), autoimmune hepatitis, diarrhea, hyperbilirubinemia, ↑ lipase, ↑ liver enzymes, nausea. **GU:** ACUTE RENAL FAILURE/FANCONI SYNDROME, ↑ serum creatinine. **MS:** arthralgia, ↓ bone mineral density, ↑ creatine kinase, muscle weakness, myalgia, osteomalacia, polymyositis. **Neuro:** Guillan-Barré syndrome. **Misc:** immune reconstitution syndrome.

Interactions

Drug-Drug: **Strong CYP3A inducers**, including **carbamazepine**, **enzalutamide**, **mitotane**, **oxcarbazepine**, **phenobarbital**, **phenytoin**, **rifampin**, and **rifapentine** may significantly ↓ levels and effectiveness of doravirine; concurrent use contraindicated; should discontinue these medications for ≥4 wk before initiating doravirine/lamivudine/tenofovir disoproxil fumarate therapy. **Rifabutin** may ↓ levels and effectiveness of doravirine; take one doravirine 100–mg tablet 12 hr after doravirine/lamivudine/tenofovir disoproxil fumarate dose. Nephrotoxic drugs, including **acyclovir**, **aminoglycosides**, **cidofovir**, **ganciclovir**, **NSAIDs**, **valacyclovir**, or **valganciclovir** may ↑ risk of nephrotoxicity; avoid recent or concurrent use. **Ledipasvir/sofosbuvir** and **sofosbuvir/velpatasvir** may ↑ tenofovir levels and risk of toxicity; closely monitor. Medications containing **sorbitol** may ↓ lamivudine levels; avoid concurrent use.

Drug-Natural Products: St. John's wort may significantly ↓ levels and effectiveness of doravirine; concurrent use contraindicated; should discontinue this medication for ≥4 wk before initiating doravirine therapy.

Route/Dosage

PO (Adults): One tablet (doravirine 100 mg/lamivudine 300 mg/tenofovir disoproxil fumarate 300 mg) once daily.

Availability

Tablets: doravirine 100 mg/lamivudine 300 mg/tenofovir disoproxil fumarate 300 mg.

NURSING IMPLICATIONS

Assessment

- Assess for change in severity of HIV symptoms and for symptoms of opportunistic infections during therapy.
- Assess bone mineral density (BMD) in patients with HIV who have a history of pathologic bone fracture or other risk factors for osteoporosis or bone loss. Consider supplementation with calcium and vitamin D.
- ***Lab Test Considerations:*** Monitor viral load and CD4 cell count regularly during therapy.
- Assess for hepatitis B virus (HBV). *Delstrigo™* is not approved for administration in patients with HIV and HBV. If therapy is discontinued, may cause severe exacerbation of hepatitis B. Monitor liver function in co-infected patients for several mo after stopping therapy.
- Monitor liver function tests before and periodically during therapy, especially in patients with underlying liver disease or marked ↑ transaminases. May cause ↑ serum creatinine, AST, ALT, total bilirubin, total cholesterol, LDL, and triglycerides. May cause lactic acidosis and severe hepatomegaly with steatosis. These events are more likely to occur if patients are female, obese, or receiving nucleoside analogue medications for extended periods of time. Monitor patient for signs (increased serum lactate levels, elevated liver enzymes, liver enlargement on palpation). Therapy should be suspended if clinical or laboratory signs occur.
- Assess serum creatinine, creatinine clearance, urine glucose, and urine protein before starting and periodically during therapy. Also assess serum phosphorous in patients with chronic kidney disease. Patients taking nephrotoxic agents, including NSAIDs, are at increased risk for renal impairment.

Implementation

- Administer once daily without regard to meals.

Patient/Family Teaching

- Instruct patient on the importance of taking medication as directed, even if feeling better. Do not take more than prescribed amount and do not stop taking without consulting health care professional. Discontinuing therapy may lead to severe exacerbations. Take missed doses as soon as remembered unless almost time for next dose; do not double doses. Advise patient to read *Patient Information* prior to starting therapy and with each Rx refill in case of changes. Caution patient not to share or trade *Delstrigo™* with others.
- Inform patient of importance of hepatitis B testing before starting antiretroviral therapy.
- Inform patient that *Delstrigo™* does not cure AIDS and does not reduce the risk of transmission of HIV to others through sexual contact or blood contamination. Caution patient to use a condom and avoid sharing needles or donating blood to prevent spreading HIV to others.
- Advise patient to notify health care professional if bone pain (bone pain that does not go away or worsening bone pain; pain in arms, legs, hands or feet; broken bones, muscle pain or weakness). May be symptoms of a bone or kidney problem.
- Advise patient to notify health care professional if signs and symptoms of immune reconstitution syndrome (signs and symptoms of an infection) occur.
- Instruct patient to notify health care professional of all Rx or OTC medications, vitamins, or herbal products being taken and consult health care professional before taking any new medications, especially St. John's wort.
- Rep: Advise patient to notify health care professional if pregnancy is planned or suspected. Encourage pregnant women to enroll in the Antiretroviral Pregnancy Registry by calling 1-800-258-4263. Advise female patient that pregnancy is not recommended during *Delstrigo™* and avoid breast feeding during therapy.
- Emphasize the importance of regular follow-up exams and blood counts to determine progress and monitor for side effects.

Evaluation/Desired Outcomes

- Delayed progression of AIDS and decreased opportunistic infections in patients with HIV.
- Decrease in viral load and increase in CD4 cell counts.

BEERS

doxazosin (dox-ay-zoe-sin)

Cardura, Cardura XL

Classification

Therapeutic: antihypertensives

Pharmacologic: peripherally acting antiadrenergics

Indications

Hypertension (alone or with other agents) (immediate-release only). Symptomatic benign prostatic hyperplasia (BPH).

Action

Dilates both arteries and veins by blocking postsynaptic alpha$_1$-adrenergic receptors. **Therapeutic Effects:** Lowering of BP. Increased urine flow and decreased symptoms of BPH.

Pharmacokinetics

Absorption: Well absorbed following oral administration.

Distribution: Probably enters breast milk; rest of distribution unknown.

Protein Binding: 98–99%.

Metabolism and Excretion: Extensively metabolized by the liver.

Half-life: 22 hr.

TIME/ACTION PROFILE

ROUTE	ONSET	PEAK	DURATION
PO†	1–2 hr	2–6 hr	24 hr
PO-XL‡	5 wk	unknown	unknown

†Antihypertensive effect.

‡Improved urinary flow and BPH symptoms.

Contraindications/Precautions

Contraindicated in: Hypersensitivity.

Use Cautiously in: Hepatic dysfunction; Gastrointestinal narrowing (XL only); Geri: Appears on Beers list. Geriatric patients are at ↑ risk for hypotension; OB, Lactation, Pedi: Safety not established; Patients undergoing cataract surgery (↑ risk of intraoperative floppy iris syndrome).

Adverse Reactions/Side Effects

CNS: dizziness, headache, depression, drowsiness, fatigue, nervousness, weakness. **EENT:** abnormal vision, blurred vision, conjunctivitis, epistaxis, intraoperative floppy iris syndrome. **Resp:** dyspnea. **CV:** first-dose orthostatic hypotension, arrhythmias, chest pain, edema, palpitations. **GI:** abdominal discomfort, constipation, diarrhea, dry mouth, flatulence, nausea, vomiting. **GU:** ↓ libido, priapism, sexual dysfunction. **Derm:** flushing, rash, urticaria. **MS:** arthralgia, arthritis, gout, myalgia.

Interactions

Drug-Drug: ↑ risk of hypotension with **sildenafil**, **tadalafil**, **vardenafil**, other **antihypertensives**, **nitrates**, or acute ingestion of **alcohol**. **NSAIDs**, **sympathomimetics**, or **estrogens** may ↓ effects of antihypertensive therapy.

Route/Dosage

Hypertension

PO (Adults): —1 mg once daily, may be gradually ↑ at 2-wk intervals to 2–16 mg/day; incidence of postural hypotension greatly ↑ at doses >4 mg/day. *BPH*—1 mg once daily, may be gradually increased to 8 mg/day.

Benign Prostatic Hyperplasia

PO (Adults): *Immediate release*—1 mg once daily, may be ↑ every 1–2 wk up to 8 mg/day; *Extended release*—4 mg once daily (with breakfast), may be ↑ in 3–4 wk to 8 mg/day.

Availability (generic available)

Tablets: 1 mg, 2 mg, 4 mg, 8 mg. **Cost:** *Generic*—1 mg $60.00/100, 2 mg $79.89/100, 4 mg $85.34/100, 8 mg $60.41/100. **Extended-release tablets:** 4 mg, 8 mg. **Cost:** 4 mg $84.62/30, 8 mg $88.90/30.

NURSING IMPLICATIONS

Assessment

- Monitor BP and pulse 2–6 hr after first dose, with each increase in dose, and periodically during therapy. Report significant changes.
- Assess for first-dose orthostatic hypotension and syncope. Incidence may be dose related. Observe patient closely during this period and take precautions to prevent injury.
- Monitor intake and output ratios and daily weight, and assess for edema daily, especially at beginning of therapy. Report weight gain or edema.
- **BPH:** Assess patient for symptoms of prostatic hyperplasia (urinary hesitancy, feeling of incomplete bladder emptying, interruption of urinary stream, impairment of size and force of urinary stream, terminal urinary dribbling, straining to start flow, dysuria, urgency) prior to and periodically during therapy.

Implementation

- Do not confuse Cardura with Coumadin.
- **PO:** Administer daily dose at bedtime.
- XL tablets should be swallowed whole; do not break, crush, or chew.
- **Hypertension:** May be administered concurrently with a diuretic or other antihypertensive.

Patient/Family Teaching

- Emphasize the importance of continuing to take this medication, even if feeling well. Instruct patient to take medication at the same time each day. Take missed doses as soon as remembered unless almost time for next dose. Do not double doses.

- May cause drowsiness or dizziness. Advise patient to avoid driving or other activities requiring alertness until response to medication is known.
- Caution patient to change positions slowly to decrease orthostatic hypotension. May cause syncopal episodes, especially within first 24 hr of therapy, with dose increase, and with resumption of therapy after interruption.
- Instruct patient to notify health care professional of all Rx or OTC medications, vitamins, or herbal products being taken and to avoid concurrent use of alcohol or OTC medications and herbal products, especially cold preparations, without consulting health care professional, especially cough, cold, or allergy remedies.
- Advise male patient to notify health care professional if priapism or erection of longer than 4 hr occurs; may lead to permanent impotence if not treated.
- Advise female patient to notify health care professional if pregnancy is planned or suspected or if breast feeding.
- Emphasize the importance of follow-up visits to determine effectiveness of therapy.
- **Hypertension:** Instruct patient and family on proper technique for BP monitoring. Advise them to check BP at least weekly and report significant changes.
- Encourage patient to comply with additional interventions for hypertension (weight reduction, low-sodium diet, smoking cessation, moderation of alcohol consumption, regular exercise, and stress management).

Evaluation/Desired Outcomes

- Decrease in BP without appearance of side effects.
- Decrease in urinary symptoms of BPH.

doxercalciferol, See VITAMIN D COMPOUNDS.

HIGH ALERT

DOXOrubicin

(dox-oh-**roo**-bi-sin)

✤Adriamycin PFS, ✤Myocet

Classification

Therapeutic: antineoplastics

Pharmacologic: anthracyclines

Indications

Alone or with other modalities in the treatment of various solid tumors including: Breast, Ovarian, Bladder, Bronchogenic carcinoma, Malignant lymphomas and leukemias.

Action

Inhibits DNA and RNA synthesis by forming a complex with DNA; action is cell-cycle S-phase–specific. Also has immunosuppressive properties. **Therapeutic Effects:** Death of rapidly replicating cells, particularly malignant ones.

Pharmacokinetics

Absorption: Administered IV only, resulting in complete bioavailability.

Distribution: Widely distributed; does not cross the blood-brain barrier; extensively bound to tissues.

Metabolism and Excretion: Mostly metabolized by the liver (primarily by CYP2D6 and CYP3A4). Converted by liver to an active compound. Excreted predominantly in the bile, 50% as unchanged drug. Less than 5% eliminated unchanged in the urine.

Half-life: 16.7 hr.

TIME/ACTION PROFILE (effect on blood counts)

ROUTE	ONSET	PEAK	DURATION
IV	10 days	14 days	21–24 days

Contraindications/Precautions

Contraindicated in: Hypersensitivity; OB: Pregnancy (may cause fetal harm); Lactation: Lactation.

Use Cautiously in: History of cardiac disease or high cumulative doses of anthracyclines; Depressed bone marrow reserve; Hepatic impairment (↓ dose if serum bilirubin >1.2 m g/dL); Pedi, Geri: Children, geriatric patients, mediastinal radiation, concurrent cyclophosphamide (↑ risk of cardiotoxicity); Rep: Women of reproductive potential;.

Adverse Reactions/Side Effects

CV: CARDIOMYOPATHY, ECG changes. **Derm:** alopecia, photosensitivity. **Endo:** sterility, prepubertal growth failure with temporary gonadal impairment (children only). **GI:** diarrhea, esophagitis, nausea, stomatitis, vomiting. **GU:** red urine. **Hemat:** anemia, leukopenia, thrombocytopenia. **Local:** phlebitis at IV site, tissue necrosis. **Metab:** hyperuricemia. **Resp:** recall pneumonitis. **Misc:** hypersensitivity reactions.

Interactions

Drug-Drug: CYP2D6 inhibitors, **CYP3A4 inhibitors**, and **P-glycoprotein inhibitors** may ↑ risk of toxicity; avoid concurrent use. **CYP2D6 inducers**, **CYP3A4 inducers**, and **P-glycoprotein inducers** may ↓ effect and ↑ risk of therapeutic failure; avoid concurrent use. ↑ bone marrow depression with other **antineoplastics** or **radiation therapy**. Pediatric patients who have received concurrent doxorubicin and **dactinomycin** have an ↑ risk of recall pneumonitis at variable times following local radiation therapy. May ↑

skin reactions at previous **radiation therapy** sites. If **paclitaxel** is administered first, clearance of doxorubicin is ↓ and the incidence and severity of neutropenia and stomatitis are ↑ (problem is diminished if doxorubicin is administered first). Hematologic toxicity is ↑ and prolonged by concurrent use of **cyclosporine**; risk of coma and seizures is also ↑. Incidence and severity of neutropenia and thrombocytopenia are ↑ by concurrent **progesterone**. **Phenobarbital** may ↑ clearance and decrease effects of doxorubicin. Doxorubicin may ↓ metabolism and ↑ effects of **phenytoin**. **Streptozocin** may ↑ the half-life of doxorubicin (dosage ↓ of doxorubicin recommended). May ↑ risk of hemorrhagic cystitis from **cyclophosphamide**. May ↑ risk of hepatotoxicity from **mercaptopurine**. Cardiac toxicity may be ↑ by **radiation therapy** or **cyclophosphamide**. ↑ risk of cardiac toxicity with **trastuzumab**; avoid use of doxorubicin for up to 7 mo after discontinuing trastuzumab. If **dexrazoxane** is administered at initiation of doxorubicin-containing regimens, may ↑ risk of therapeutic failure and tumor progression. May ↓ antibody response to **live-virus vaccines** and ↑ risk of adverse reactions.

Route/Dosage

Other regimens are used.

IV (Adults): 60–75 mg/m² daily, repeat every 21 days; or 25–30 mg/m² daily for 2–3 days, repeat every 3–4 wk or 20 mg/m²/wk. Total cumulative dose should not exceed 550 mg/m² without monitoring of cardiac function or 400 mg/m² in patients with previous chest radiation or other cardiotoxic chemotherapy.

IV (Children): 30 mg/m²/day for 3 days every 4 wk.

Hepatic Impairment

IV (Adults): *Serum bilirubin 1.2–3 mg/dL*—↓ dose by 50%; *Serum bilirubin 3.1–5 mg/dL*—↓ dose by 75%.

Availability (generic available)

Powder for injection (requires reconstitution and dilution): 10 mg/vial, 20 mg/vial, 50 mg/vial, 🍁 150 mg/vial. **Solution for injection (requires dilution):** 2 mg/mL.

NURSING IMPLICATIONS

Assessment

- Monitor BP, pulse, respiratory rate, and temperature frequently during administration. Report significant changes.
- Monitor for bone marrow depression. Assess for bleeding (bleeding gums, bruising, petechiae, guaiac stools, urine, and emesis) and avoid IM injections and taking rectal temperatures if platelet count is low. Apply pressure to venipuncture sites for 10 min. Assess for signs of infection during neutropenia. Anemia may occur. Monitor for increased fatigue, dyspnea, and orthostatic hypotension.
- Monitor intake and output ratios, and report occurrence of significant discrepancies. Encourage fluid intake of 2000–3000 mL/day. Allopurinol and alkalinization of the urine may be used to decrease serum uric acid levels and to help prevent urate stone formation.
- Severe and protracted nausea and vomiting may occur as early as 1 hr after therapy and may last 24 hr. Administer parenteral antiemetics 30–45 min prior to therapy and routinely around the clock for the next 24 hr as indicated. Monitor amount of emesis and notify health care professional if emesis exceeds guidelines to prevent dehydration.
- Monitor for development of signs of cardiac toxicity, which may be either acute and transient (ST segment depression, flattened T wave, sinus tachycardia, and extrasystoles) or late onset (usually occurs 1–6 mo after initiation of therapy) and characterized by intractable HF (peripheral edema, dyspnea, rales/crackles, weight gain). Chest x ray, echocardiography, ECGs, and radionuclide angiography may be ordered prior to and periodically during therapy. Cardiotoxicity is more prevalent in children younger than 2 yr and geriatric patients. Dexrazoxane may be used to prevent cardiotoxicity in patients receiving cumulative doses of >300 m g/m².
- Assess injection site frequently for redness, irritation, or inflammation during and for up to 2 hr after completion of infusion. Doxorubicin is a vesicant but may infiltrate painlessly even if blood returns on aspiration of infusion needle. Severe tissue damage may occur if doxorubicin extravasates. If extravasation occurs, stop infusion immediately, restart, and complete dose in another vein. Local infiltration of antidote is not recommended. If extravasation is suspected, intermittent application of ice to site for 15 min. 4 times daily for 3 days may be useful. Because of the progressive nature of extravasation reactions, close observation and plastic surgery consultation are recommended. Blistering, ulceration, and/or persistent pain are indications for wide excision surgery, followed by split-thickness skin grafting. May use dexrazoxane to treat extravasation. Administer first infusion of dexrazoxane as soon as possible within 6 hr of extravasation. Remove ice packs for at least 15 min prior to and during dexrazoxane administration. Recommended dose of dexrazoxane for day 1 is 1000 mg/m² (up to 2000 mg); the dose for day 2 is 1000 mg/m² (up to 2000 mg); the dose for day 3 is 500 mg/m² (up to 1000 mg). Dexrazoxane is administered as an IV infusion over 1–2 hr. If swelling, redness, and/or pain persists beyond 48 hr, immediate consultation for possible debridement is indicated.
- Assess oral mucosa frequently for development of stomatitis. Increased dosing interval and/or decreasing dose is recommended if lesions are painful or interfere with nutrition.
- ***Lab Test Considerations:*** Monitor CBC and differential prior to and periodically during therapy. WBC nadir occurs 10–14 days after administration,

and recovery usually occurs by the 21st day. Thrombocytopenia and anemia may also occur. Increased dosing interval and/or decreased dose is recommended if ANC is <1000 cells/mm^3 and/or platelet count is <50,000 cells/mm^3.
- Monitor renal (BUN and creatinine) and hepatic (AST, ALT, LDH, and serum bilirubin) function prior to and periodically during therapy. Dose reduction is required for bilirubin >1.2 m g/dL or serum creatinine >3 m g/dL.
- May cause ↑ serum and urine uric acid concentrations.

Implementation

- ***High Alert:*** Fatalities have occurred with incorrect administration of chemotherapeutic agents. Before administering, clarify all ambiguous orders; double-check single, daily, and course-of-therapy dose limits; have second practitioner independently double-check original order, calculations, and infusion pump settings.
- ***High Alert:*** Do not confuse doxorubicin hydrochloride with doxorubicin liposomal (Doxil) or with daunorubicin hydrochloride or with idarubicin. Clarify orders that do not include both generic and brand names.
- Solution should be prepared in a biologic cabinet. Wear gloves, gown, and mask while handling medication. Discard IV equipment in specially designated containers.
- Aluminum needles may be used to administer doxorubicin but should not be used during storage, because prolonged contact results in discoloration of solution and formation of a dark precipitate. Solution is red.

IV Administration

- **IV Push:** ***Diluent:*** Dilute each 10 mg with 5 mL of 0.9% NaCl (nonbacteriostatic) for injection. Shake to dissolve completely. Do not add to IV solution. Reconstituted medication is stable for 24 hr at room temperature and 48 hr if refrigerated. Protect from sunlight. ***Concentration:*** 2 mg/mL. ***Rate:*** Administer each dose over 3–5 min through Y-site of a free-flowing infusion of 0.9% NaCl or D5W. Facial flushing and erythema along involved vein frequently occur when administration is too rapid.
- **Intermittent Infusion:** Has also been mixed in 100–250 mL of 0.9% NaCl. ***Rate:*** Infuse over 30–60 min.
- **Y-Site Compatibility:** alemtuzumab, alfentanil, amifostine, amikacin, anidulafungin, argatroban, arsenic trioxide, aztreonam, bivalirudin, bleomycin, bumetanide, buprenorphine, butorphanol, calcium chloride, calcium gluconate, carboplatin, carmustine, caspofungin, chlorpromazine, ciprofloxacin, cisplatin, cladribine, clindamycin, cyclophosphamide, cyclosporine, cytarabine, dacarbazine, dactinomycin, daptomycin, dexamethasone, dexmedetomidine, dexrazoxane, diltiazem, diphenhydramine, dobutamine, docetaxel, dolasetron, dopamine, doxycycline, droperidol, enalaprilat, ephedrine, epinephrine, erythromycin, esmolol, etoposide, etoposide phosphate, famotidine, fenoldopam, fentanyl, filgrastim, fluconazole, fludarabine, gemcitabine, gentamicin, granisetron, haloperidol, hetastarch, hydrocortisone, hydromorphone, ifosfamide, imipenem/cilastatin, irinotecan, isoproterenol, ketorolac, labetalol, leucovorin calcium, levorphanol, lidocaine, linezolid, lorazepam, mannitol, melphalan, meperidine, mesna, methotrexate, metoclopramide, metoprolol, midazolam, milrinone, mitomycin, morphine, moxifloxacin, nalbuphine, naloxone, nicardipine, nitroglycerin, nitroprusside, octreotide, ondansetron, oxaliplatin, paclitaxel, palonosetron, pamidronate, pancuronium, phenylephrine, potassium acetate, potassium chloride, procainamide, prochlorperazine, promethazine, propranolol, quinupristin/dalfopristin, ranitidine, sargramostim, sodium acetate, sufentanil, tacrolimus, theophylline, thiotepa, tigecycline, tirofiban, tobramycin, topotecan, trastuzumab, vancomycin, vasopressin, vecuronium, verapamil, vinblastine, vincristine, vinorelbine, zidovudine, zoledronic acid.
- **Y-Site Incompatibility:** acyclovir, allopurinol, aminophylline, amiodarone, amphotericin B deoxycholate, amphotericin B lipid complex, amphotericin B liposome, ampicillin, ampicillin/sulbactam, azithromycin, cefazolin, cefepime, cefotaxime, cefotetan, cefoxitin, ceftazidime, ceftriaxone, cefuroxime, diazepam, digoxin, ertapenem, foscarnet, fosphenytoin, ganciclovir, magnesium sulfate, meropenem, methohexital, minocycline, pantoprazole, pemetrexed, pentamidine, pentobarbital, phenobarbital, phenytoin, piperacillin/tazobactam, potassium phosphates, propofol, rituximab, sodium phosphates, thiopental, trimethoprim/sufamethoxazole, voriconazole.

Patient/Family Teaching

- Instruct patient to notify health care professional promptly if fever; sore throat; signs of infection; bleeding gums; bruising; petechiae; blood in stools, urine, or emesis; increased fatigue; dyspnea; or orthostatic hypotension occurs. Caution patient to avoid crowds and persons with known infections. Instruct patient to use soft toothbrush and electric razor and to avoid falls. Caution patient not to drink alcoholic beverages or take medication containing aspirin or NSAIDs, because these may precipitate gastric bleeding.
- Instruct patient to report pain at injection site immediately.

- Instruct patient to inspect oral mucosa for erythema and ulceration. If ulceration occurs, advise patient to use sponge brush, rinse mouth with water after eating and drinking, and confer with health care professional if mouth pain interferes with eating. Pain may require treatment with opioid analgesics. The risk of developing stomatitis is greatest 5–10 days after a dose; usual duration is 3–7 days.
- Instruct patient to notify health care professional immediately if irregular heartbeat, shortness of breath, swelling of lower extremities, or skin irritation (swelling, pain, or redness of feet or hands) occurs.
- Discuss the possibility of hair loss with patient. Explore methods of coping. Regrowth usually occurs 2–3 mo after discontinuation of therapy.
- Instruct patient not to receive any vaccinations without advice of health care professional.
- Inform patient that medication may cause urine to appear red for 1–2 days.
- Instruct patient to notify health care professional if skin irritation occurs at site of previous radiation therapy.
- Advise family and/or caregivers to take precautions (i.e., latex gloves) in handling body fluids for at least 5 days post-treatment.
- Instruct patient to notify health care professional of all Rx or OTC medications, vitamins, or herbal products being taken and to consult health care professional before taking other Rx, OTC, or herbal products.
- Inform patient that doxorubicin may increase risk of developing secondary cancers.
- Rep: May have teratogenic effects. Advise females of reproductive potential and males with female partners of reproductive potential to use effective contraception during and for at least 4 mo after therapy is concluded and avoid breast feeding during therapy. Inform patient before initiating therapy that this medication may cause irreversible gonadal suppression, or irreversible amenorrhea or early menopause.
- Emphasize the need for periodic lab tests to monitor for side effects.

Evaluation/Desired Outcomes

- Decrease in size or spread of malignancies in solid tumors.
- Improvement of hematologic status in leukemias.

HIGH ALERT

DOXOrubicin, liposomal

(dox-oh-**roo**-bi-sin **lye**-poe-sohm-al)

Caelyx, Doxil

Classification

Therapeutic: antineoplastics

Pharmacologic: anthracyclines

Indications

AIDS-related Kaposi's sarcoma (KS) in patients who cannot tolerate or fail conventional therapy. Ovarian cancer that has progressed or recurred after platinum-based chemotherapy. Multiple myeloma with bortezomib in patients who have not previously received bortezomib and have received at least one prior therapy.

Action

Inhibits DNA and RNA synthesis by forming a complex with DNA; action is cell-cycle S-phase–specific. Also has immunosuppressive properties. Encapsulation in a liposome increases uptake by tumors, prolongs action, and may decrease some toxicity. **Therapeutic Effects:** Death of rapidly replicating cells, particularly malignant ones.

Pharmacokinetics

Absorption: Administered IV only, resulting in complete bioavailability.

Distribution: Widely distributed; does not cross the blood-brain barrier; extensively bound to tissues (↑ concentrations delivered to KS lesions due to liposomal carrier).

Metabolism and Excretion: Mostly metabolized by the liver with conversion to an active compound. Excreted mostly in bile, 50% as unchanged drug. <5% eliminated unchanged in the urine.

Half-life: 55 hr.

TIME/ACTION PROFILE (effect on blood counts)

ROUTE	ONSET	PEAK	DURATION
IV	10 days	14 days	21–24 days

Contraindications/Precautions

Contraindicated in: Hypersensitivity; OB: Pregnancy (may cause fetal harm); Lactation: Lactation.

Use Cautiously in: Pre-existing cardiac disease or ↑ cumulative doses of anthracyclines; Depressed bone marrow reserve; Hepatic impairment (dose ↓ required if serum bilirubin >1.2 m g/dL); Rep: Women of reproductive potential; Geri, Pedi: Children, geriatric patients, prior mediastinal radiation, concurrent cyclophosphamide (↑ risk of cardiotoxicity).

Adverse Reactions/Side Effects

CNS: weakness. **CV:** CARDIOMYOPATHY. **Derm:** hand-foot syndrome, alopecia. **GI:** nausea, diarrhea, ↑ alkaline phosphatase, moniliasis, ORAL MALIGNANCY, stomatitis, vomiting. **Hemat:** anemia, leukopenia, thrombocytopenia. **Local:** injection site reactions. **Misc:** ANAPHYLACTOID ALLERGIC REACTIONS, acute infusion-related reactions, fever.

Interactions

Drug-Drug: ↑ bone marrow depression with other **antineoplastics** or **radiation therapy**. Pediatric patients who have received concurrent doxorubicin and **dactinomycin** have ↑ risk of recall pneumonitis following local radiation therapy. May ↑ skin reactions at previous **radiation therapy** sites. If **paclitaxel** is administered first, clearance of doxorubicin is ↓ and incidence and severity of neutropenia and stomatitis are ↑ (problem is less if doxorubicin is administered first). Hematologic toxicity is ↑ by concurrent use of **cyclosporine**; risk of coma and seizures is also ↑. Incidence and severity of neutropenia and thrombocytopenia are ↑ by concurrent **progesterone**. **Phenobarbital** may ↑ clearance and ↓ effects of doxorubicin. Doxorubicin may ↓ metabolism and ↑ effects of **phenytoin**. **Streptozocin** may ↑ the half-life of doxorubicin (dose reduction of doxorubicin recommended). May ↑ risk of hemorrhagic cystitis from **cyclophosphamide** or hepatitis from **mercaptopurine**. Cardiac toxicity may be ↑ by **radiation therapy** or **cyclophosphamide**. May ↓ antibody response to **live-virus vaccines** and ↑ risk of adverse reactions.

Route/Dosage

AIDS-Related KS

IV (Adults): 20 mg/m² every 3 wk until disease progression or unacceptable toxicity.

Ovarian Cancer

IV (Adults): 50 mg/m² every 4 wk until disease progression or unacceptable toxicity.

Multiple Myeloma

IV (Adults): 30 mg/m² on day 4 (after bortezomib) of each 21–day cycle for 8 cycles or until disease progression or unacceptable toxicity.

Availability (generic available)

Liposomal dispersion for injection (requires dilution): 2 mg/mL.

NURSING IMPLICATIONS

Assessment

- Monitor BP, pulse, respiratory rate, and temperature frequently during administration. Report significant changes.
- Monitor for acute infusion-related reactions consisting of flushing, shortness of breath, facial swelling, headache, chills, chest pain, back pain, chest or throat tightness, fever, tachycardia, pruritus, rash, cyanosis, syncope, bronchospasm, asthma, apnea, and hypotension. Reactions usually resolve over 1 day and are usually limited to first dose. Slowing infusion rate may minimize this reaction. Reaction is thought to be due to liposome.
- Observe for signs and symptoms of anaphylaxis (rash, pruritus, laryngeal edema, wheezing). Discontinue doxorubicin liposome and notify health care professional immediately if these problems occur. Keep epinephrine, an antihistamine, and resuscitation equipment close by in case of an anaphylactic reaction.
- Monitor for bone marrow depression. Assess for bleeding (bleeding gums, bruising, petechiae, guaiac stools, urine, and emesis) and avoid IM injections and taking rectal temperatures if platelet count is low. Apply pressure to venipuncture sites for 10 min. Assess for signs of infection during neutropenia. Anemia may occur. Monitor for increased fatigue, dyspnea, and orthostatic hypotension.
- Monitor intake and output ratios, and report occurrence of significant discrepancies. Encourage fluid intake of 2000–3000 mL/day. Allopurinol and alkalinization of the urine may be used to decrease serum uric acid levels and to help prevent urate stone formation.
- Severe and protracted nausea and vomiting may occur as early as 1 hr after therapy and may last 24 hr. Administer parenteral antiemetics 30–45 min prior to therapy and routinely around the clock for the next 24 hr as indicated. Monitor amount of emesis and notify health care professional if emesis exceeds guidelines to prevent dehydration.
- Assess left ventricular cardiac function (MUGA or echocardiogram) prior to initiation of therapy, during treatment to detect acute changes, and after treatment to detect delayed cardiotoxicity. Monitor for development of signs of cardiac toxicity, which may be either acute and transient (ST segment depression, flattened T wave, sinus tachycardia, and extrasystoles) or late onset (usually occurs 1–6 mo after initiation of therapy) and characterized by intractable HF (peripheral edema, dyspnea, rales/crackles, weight gain); occurs more frequently in patients receiving a cumulative dose of ≥550 mg/m². Cardiotoxicity is more prevalent in children younger than 2 yr and geriatric patients. Dexrazoxane may be used to prevent cardiotoxicity in patients receiving cumulative doses of >300 m g/m².
- Assess injection site frequently for redness, irritation, or inflammation. Doxorubicin liposome is an irritant but may infiltrate painlessly even if blood returns on aspiration of infusion needle. Severe tissue damage may occur if doxorubicin liposome extravasates. If extravasation occurs, stop infusion immediately, restart, and complete dose in another vein. If possible, withdraw 3–5 mL of blood to remove doxorubicin liposome. Apply ice to site for 15 min 4 times daily for 3 days. Local infiltration of antidote is not recommended. Delineate the infiltrated area on patient's skin with a felt-tip marker. Elevate for 48 hr above heart level using a sling or stockinette dressing with an observation window cut in the dressing. Avoid pressure or friction. Do not rub the area. Observe for signs of increased erythema, pain, or skin necrosis. If increased symptoms occur, consult a

plastic surgeon. After 48 hr, encourage patient to use extremity normally to promote full range of motion.

- Assess oral mucosa frequently for development of stomatitis. Increased dosing interval and/or decreased dose is recommended if lesions are painful or interfere with nutrition. *For Grade 1: Painless ulcers, erythema, or mild soreness,* If no previous Grade 3 or 4 toxicity: no dose adjustment. If previous Grade 3 or 4 toxicity: delay up to 2 wk then ↓ dose by 25%. *For Grade 2: Painful erythema, edema, or ulcers, but can eat,* Delay dosing up to 2 wk or until resolved to Grade 0-1. Discontinue therapy if no resolution after 2 wk. If resolved to Grade 0-1 within 2 wk: if no previous Grade 3 or 4 stomatitis: resume therapy at previous dose. If previous Grade 3 or 4 toxicity: ↓ dose by 25%. *For Grade 3: Painful erythema, edema, or ulcers, and cannot eat,* Delay dosing up to 2 wk or until resolved to Grade 0-1. ↓ dose by 25% and return to original dose interval. If no resolution after 2 wk, discontinue therapy. *For Grade 4: Requires parenteral or enteral support,* Delay dosing up to 2 wk or until resolved to Grade 0-1. ↓ dose by 25% and return to original dose interval. If no resolution after 2 wk, discontinue therapy.
- Continue to assess oral mucosa regularly during and for at least 6 yr for ulceration or any discomfort; may indicate secondary oral cancer.
- Monitor for skin toxicity with prolonged use; hand-foot syndrome (HFS) usually occurs after 6 wk of treatment and consists of swelling, pain, and erythema of the hands and feet. This may progress to desquamation but usually regresses after 2 wk. In severe cases, modification and delay of future doses of doxorubicin liposome may be necessary. *For Grade 1: Mild erythema, swelling, or desquamation not interfering with daily activities,* if no previous Grade 3 or 4 HFS: no dose adjustment. If previous Grade 3 or 4 HFS: delay dose up to 2 wk, then ↓ dose by 25%. *For Grade 2: Erythema, desquamation, or swelling interfering with, but not precluding normal physical activities; small blisters or ulcerations less than 2 cm in diameter,* delay dosing up to 2 wk or until resolved to Grade 0-1. Discontinue therapy if no resolution after 2 wk. If resolved to Grade 0-1 within 2 wk: if no previous Grade 3 or 4 HFS: continue treatment at previous dose. If previous Grade 3 or 4 toxicity: ↓ dose by 25%. *For Grade 3: Blistering, ulceration, or swelling interfering with walking or normal daily activities; cannot wear regular clothing,* Delay dosing up to 2 wk or until resolved to Grade 0-1, then ↓ dose by 25%. Discontinue therapy if no resolution after 2 wk. *For Grade 4: Diffuse or local process causing infectious complications, or a bed ridden state or hospitalization,* Delay dosing up to 2 wk or until resolved to Grade 0-1, then ↓ dose by 25%. Discontinue therapy if no resolution after 2 wk.
- ***Lab Test Considerations:*** Obtain negative pregnancy test before starting therapy.
- Monitor CBC and differential prior to and periodically during therapy. The WBC nadir occurs 10–14 days after administration, and recovery usually occurs by the 21st day. Thrombocytopenia and anemia may also occur. ↑ dosing interval and/or ↓ dose is recommended if ANC is <1000 cells/mm³ and/or platelet count is <50,000 cells/mm³. *If ANC 1500–1900 cells/mm³ and platelets 75,000–150,000 cells/mm³ (Grade 1)*, resume treatment with no dose reduction. *If ANC 1000–<1500 cells/mm³ and platelets 50,000–<75,000 cells/mm³ (Grade 2),* wait until ANC >1500 and platelets >75,000; then redose with no dose reduction. *If ANC 500–999 cells/mm³ and platelets 25,000–<50,000 cells/mm³ (Grade 3),* wait until ANC >1500 and platelets >75,000; then redose with no dose reduction. *If ANC <500 and platelets <25,000 cells/mm³ (Grade 4),* wait until ANC >1500 and platelets >75,000, then redose at 25% dose reduction or continue full dose with prophylactic granulocyte growth factor.
- **Recommended modifications of doxorubicin liposomal when administered with bortezomib.** *If fever ≥38°C and ANC <1,000/mm³,* withhold dose for this cycle if before Day 4; ↓ dose by 25%, if after Day 4 of previous cycle. *If on any day of drug administration after Day 1 of each cycle: Platelet count <25,000/mm³ or Hemoglobin <8 g/dL or ANC <500/mm³,* withhold dose for this cycle if before Day 4; ↓ dose by 25%, if after Day 4 of previous cycle AND if bortezomib is reduced for hematologic toxicity. *If Grade 3 or 4 non-hematologic drug related toxicity,* do not dose until recovered to Grade <2, then ↓ dose by 25%.
- Monitor renal (BUN and creatinine) and hepatic (AST, ALT, LDH, and serum bilirubin) function prior to and periodically during therapy. Dose reduction is required for bilirubin >1.2 m g/dL or serum creatinine >3 m g/dL.
- May cause ↑ serum and urine uric acid concentrations.

Implementation

- ***High Alert:*** Fatalities have occurred with incorrect administration of chemotherapeutic agents. Before administering, clarify all ambiguous orders; double-check single, daily, and course-of-therapy dose limits; have second practitioner independently double-check original order, calculations, and infusion pump settings.
- ***High Alert:*** Do not confuse doxorubicin liposomal (Doxil) with doxorubicin hydrochloride or with daunorubicin hydrochloride. Do not confuse Doxil (doxorubicin liposomal) with Paxil (paroxetine). Clarify orders that do not include both generic and brand names.

- Prepare solution in a biologic cabinet. Wear gloves, gown, and mask while handling medication. Discard IV equipment in specially designated containers.
- Aluminum needles may be used to administer doxorubicin but should not be used during storage, because prolonged contact results in discoloration of solution and formation of a dark precipitate. Solution is red.
- Do not increase dose if reduction is made due to toxicity.

IV Administration

- **Intermittent Infusion:** ***Diluent:*** Dilute dose, up to 90 mg, in 250 mL and doses >90 mg in 500 mL of D5W. Do not dilute with other diluents or diluents containing a bacteriostatic agent. Solution is not clear, but a translucent red liposomal dispersion. Do not use in-line filters. Refrigerate diluted solutions and administer within 24 hr of dilution. ***Rate:*** Initial rate of infusion should be 1 mg/min to minimize risk of infusion reactions. If no reactions occur, increase rate to complete administration within 1 hr. Do not administer as a bolus or undiluted solution. Rapid infusion may increase infusion-related reactions.
- **Y-Site Compatibility:** acyclovir, alfentanil, allopurinol, amifostine, amikacin, aminocaproic acid, aminophylline, amphotericin B lipid complex, amphotericin B liposomal, ampicillin, ampicillin/sulbactam, anidulafungin, argatroban, azithromycin, aztreonam, bivalirudin, bleomycin, bumetanide, butorphanol, calcium gluconate, carboplatin, caspofungin, cefazolin, cefepime, cefotaxime, cefotetan, cefoxitin, ceftriaxone, cefuroxime, chloramphenicol, chlorpromazine, ciprofloxacin, cisatracurium, cisplatin, clindamycin, cyclophosphamide, cyclosporine, cytarabine, dacarbazine, daptomycin, dexamethasone sodium phosphate, dexmedetomidine, dexrazoxane, digoxin, diphenhydramine, dobutamine, dopamine, droperidol, enalaprilat, ephedrine, epinephrine, eptifibatide, ertapenem, erythromycin, esmolol, etoposide, etoposide phosphate, famotidine, fenoldopam, fentanyl, fluconazole, fluorouracil, foscarnet, fosphenytoin, furosemide, ganciclovir, gentamicin, glycopyrrolate, granisetron, haloperidol, heparin, hydrocortisone sodium succinate, hydromorphone, ifosfamide, imipenem/cilastatin, insulin regular, irinotecan, isoproterenol, ketorolac, labetalol, leucovorin, levofloxacin, lidocaine, linezolid, lorazepam, magnesium sulfate, meropenem, mesna, methotrexate, methyldopate, methylprednisolone, metoprolol, midazolam, milrinone, moxifloxacin, mycophenolate, nafcillin, nalbuphine, naloxone, nicardipine, nitroglycerin, nitroprusside, norepinephrine, octreotide, ondansetron, oxaliplatin, palonosetron, pamidronate, pancuronium, pantoprazole, pemetrexed, pentamidine, pentobarbital, phenobarbital, phentolamine, phenylephrine, potassium acetate, potassium chloride, potassium phosphates, procainamide, prochlorperazine, propranolol, quinupristin/dalfopristin, ranitidine, remifentanil, rituximab, rocuronium, sodium acetate, sodium phosphates, succinylcholine, sufentanil, tacrolimus, thiopental, tigecycline, tirofiban, tobramycin, topotecan, trastuzumab, trimethoprim/sulfamethoxazole, vancomycin, vasopressin, vecuronium, verapamil, vinblastine, vincristine, vinorelbine, voriconazole, zidovudine, zoledronic acid.
- **Y-Site Incompatibility:** amiodarone, amphotericin B deoxycholate, buprenorphine, calcium chloride, ceftazidime, dantrolene, diazepam, diltiazem, docetaxel, dolasetron, gemcitabine, hydralazine, hydroxyzine, mannitol, metoclopramide, mitoxantrone, morphine, paclitaxel, phenytoin, piperacillin/tazobactam, promethazine, sodium bicarbonate, theophylline.

Patient/Family Teaching

- Instruct patient to notify health care professional promptly if fever; sore throat; signs of infection; bleeding gums; bruising; petechiae; blood in stools, urine, or emesis; increased fatigue; dyspnea; or orthostatic hypotension occurs. Caution patient to avoid crowds and persons with known infections. Instruct patient to use soft toothbrush and electric razor and to avoid falls. Caution patient not to drink alcoholic beverages or take medication containing aspirin or NSAIDs; may precipitate gastric bleeding.
- Instruct patient to report pain at injection site immediately.
- Instruct patient to inspect oral mucosa for erythema and ulceration. If ulceration occurs, advise patient to use sponge brush, rinse mouth with water after eating and drinking, and confer with health care professional if mouth pain interferes with eating. Pain may require treatment with opioid analgesics. The risk of developing stomatitis is greatest 5–10 days after a dose; the usual duration is 3–7 days.
- Instruct patient to notify health care professional immediately if irregular heartbeat, shortness of breath, swelling of lower extremities, or skin irritation (swelling, pain, or redness of feet or hands) occurs.
- Discuss the possibility of hair loss with patient. Explore methods of coping. Regrowth usually occurs 2–3 mo after discontinuation of therapy.
- Instruct patient not to receive any vaccinations without advice of health care professional.
- Inform patient that medication may cause urine to appear red for 1–2 days.
- Instruct patient to notify health care professional if skin irritation occurs at site of previous radiation therapy.
- Advise family and/or caregivers to take precautions (i.e., latex gloves) in handling body fluids for at least 5 days post-treatment.

- Rep: May have teratogenic effects. Advise females of reproductive potential and males with female partners of reproductive potential to use effective contraception during and for at least 6 mo after last dose of therapy. Inform patient before initiating therapy that this medication may cause irreversible gonadal suppression. In females, may cause infertility, amenorrhea, and premature menopause. In men, may result in oligospermia, azoospermia, and permanent loss of fertility. Some sperm counts have returned to normal several yr after therapy ended. Advise female patient to avoid breast feeding during therapy.
- Emphasize the need for periodic lab tests to monitor for side effects.

Evaluation/Desired Outcomes

- Decrease in size or spread of malignancies.
- Arrested progression of KS in patients with HIV infection.

doxycycline, See TETRACYCLINES.

doxylamine/pyridoxine
(dox-**il**-a-meen peer-ih-**dox**-een)
Bonjesta, Diclegis, Diclectin

Classification
Therapeutic: antiemetics
Pharmacologic: antihistamines, vitamin B6 analogues

Indications
Treatment of nausea and vomiting during pregnancy that has not responded to conservative management.

Action
Combination of an antihistamine and a vitamin B_6 analog. Mechanism not known. **Therapeutic Effects:** Decreased nausea and vomiting associated with pregnancy.

Pharmacokinetics
Absorption: Well absorbed following oral administration. Food delays/↓ absorption.
Distribution: Doxylamine probably enters breast milk.
Metabolism and Excretion: Doxylamine is mostly metabolized by the liver, inactive metabolites are renally excreted. Pyridoxine is a pro-drug, converted to its active metabolite by the liver.
Half-life: *Doxylamine*—12.5 hr; *pyridoxine*—0.4–0.5 hr.

TIME/ACTION PROFILE (anti-emetic effect)

ROUTE	ONSET	PEAK	DURATION
PO	unknown	unknown	8–24 hr

Contraindications/Precautions
Contraindicated in: Hypersensitivity to doxylamine or pyridoxine; Concurrent use of MAOIs; Lactation: Doxylamine probably enters breast milk and may cause irritability, excitement, or sedation in infants; breast feeding should be avoided.
Use Cautiously in: Asthma; ↑ intraocular pressure or narrow angle glaucoma; Stenosing peptic ulcer or pyloroduodenal obstruction; Urinary bladder-neck obstruction; Pedi: Safety and effectiveness not established.

Adverse Reactions/Side Effects
CNS: drowsiness.

Interactions
Drug-Drug: ↑ risk of CNS depression with other **CNS depressants** including **alcohol**, other **antihistamines**, **opioid analgesics**, and **sedative/hypnotics**. Concurrent use of **MAOIs** ↑ intensity/duration of adverse CNS (anticholinergic) reactions.

Route/Dosage

Delayed-Release Tablets
PO (Adults): *Day 1*—2 tablets (doxylamine 10 mg/pyridoxine 10 mg) at bedtime; if symptoms are controlled continue this regimen; *Day 2, if symptoms persist into afternoon on day 2*—2 tablets at bedtime on day 2 and then 1 tablet in the morning on day 3 and 2 tablets in the evening; if symptoms are controlled, continue this regimen; *Day 4, if symptoms persist*—1 tablet in the morning, 1 tablet mid-afternoon and 2 tablets at bedtime (not to exceed four tablets daily).

Extended-Release Tablets
PO (Adults): *Day 1*—1 tablet (doxylamine 20 mg/pyridoxine 20 mg) at bedtime; if symptoms are controlled, continue this regimen; *Day 2, if symptoms persist on day 2*—1 tablet in AM and 1 tablet at bedtime on day 2; if symptoms are controlled, continue this regimen (not to exceed two tablets daily).

Availability (generic available)
Delayed-release tablets (Diclegis): doxylamine 10 mg/pyridoxine 10 mg. **Extended-release tablets (Bonjesta):** doxylamine 20 mg/pyridoxine 20 mg.

NURSING IMPLICATIONS

Assessment
- Assess for frequency and amount of emesis daily during therapy. Reassess need for medication as pregnancy progresses.
- Monitor hydration status to prevent dehydration.
- ***Lab Test Considerations:*** May cause false positive urine screening tests for methadone, opiates, and PCP.

Implementation
- **PO:** Administer on an empty stomach with a full glass of water; food delays onset of medication. Swallow tablets whole; do not crush, break, or chew.

Patient/Family Teaching

- Instruct patient to take as directed. Do not take more than prescribed amount.
- May cause drowsiness. Caution patient to avoid driving and other activities requiring alertness until response to medication is known.
- Advise patient to avoid alcohol and CNS depressants, including sedatives, tranquilizers, antihistamines, opioids, and some cough and cold medications with doxylamine pyridoxine.
- Instruct patient to notify health care professional of all Rx or OTC medications, vitamins, or herbal products being taken and consult health care professional before taking any new medications.
- Advise female patient to avoid breast feeding during therapy.

Evaluation/Desired Outcomes

- Decrease in frequency of nausea and vomiting during pregnancy.

BEERS

dronedarone (droe-**ned**-a-rone)

Multaq

Classification

Therapeutic: antiarrhythmics

Pharmacologic: benzofurans

Indications

Reduces the risk of hospitalization for atrial fibrillation (AF) in patients in sinus rhythm with a history of paroxysmal or persistent AF.

Action

Has several antiarrhythmic properties; prolongs PR and QTc intervals. **Therapeutic Effects:** Suppression of AF/AFL.

Pharmacokinetics

Absorption: Poor bioavailability (4%) due to extensive first-pass hepatic metabolism (4%); food ↑ bioavailability (15%).

Distribution: Unknown.

Protein Binding: >98%.

Metabolism and Excretion: Undergoes extensive first-pass hepatic metabolism; mostly by the CYP3A enzyme system. 6% excreted in urine as metabolites, 84% was excreted in feces as metabolites. Minimal elimination as unchanged drug.

Half-life: 13–19 hr.

TIME/ACTION PROFILE (antiarrhythmic effect)

ROUTE	ONSET	PEAK	DURATION
PO	unknown†	3–6 hr‡	12 hr

†Steady state blood levels are attained at 4–8 days.
‡Peak levels after individual doses.

Contraindications/Precautions

Contraindicated in: Class IV heart failure or Class II–III heart failure with recent decompensation requiring hospitalization; Permanent AF; Second- or third-degree atrioventricular (AV) block or sick sinus syndrome (unless a pacemaker is present); Heart rate <50 bpm; Concurrent use of strong CYP3A inhibitors or drugs/herbal products that prolong the QT interval; liver or lung toxicity related to previous amiodarone use; QTc interval ≥500 msec; PR interval >280 msec; Concurrent use of Class I or III antiarrhythmics including amiodarone, flecainide, propafenone, quinidine, disopyramide, dofetilide, and sotalol; must be discontinued prior to treatment; Severe hepatic impairment; OB: May cause fetal harm; Lactation: Avoid use.

Use Cautiously in: New/worsening heart failure; Hypokalemia or hypomagnesemia (may ↑ risk of arrhythmias); Mild or moderate hepatic impairment; Rep: Women of reproductive potential (use effective contraception); Pedi: Safety and effectiveness not established.

Adverse Reactions/Side Effects

CNS: <u>weakness</u>. **CV:** HF, QTc prolongation. **GI:** <u>HEPATOTOXICITY</u>, <u>abdominal pain</u>, <u>diarrhea</u>, nausea, taste abnormality, <u>vomiting</u>. **Resp:** PNEUMONITIS, PULMONARY FIBROSIS. **GU:** ACUTE RENAL FAILURE, renal impairment. **Derm:** photosensitivity. **Misc:** ANGIOEDEMA.

Interactions

Drug-Drug: Dronedarone is metabolized by CYP3A and is a moderate inhibitor of CYP3A and CYP2D6 enzyme systems; interactions may occur with other drugs that are substrates for or are metabolized by these systems. Dronedarone also inhibits P-gp, which can result in ↑ absorption of certain drugs. Concurrent use of **strong CYP3A inhibitors** including **ketoconazole**, **itraconazole**, **voriconazole**, **cyclosporine**, **clarithromycin**, **nefazodone**, and **ritonavir** or **drugs that prolong the QT interval** including **phenothiazine antipsychotics**, **tricyclic antidepressants**, and other **Class I and III antiarrhythmics** ↑ risk of serious adverse cardiovascular reactions; concurrent use contraindicated. Concurrent use of CYP3A4 inducers including **rifampin**, **phenobarbital**, **carbamazepine**, or **phenytoin** ↓ blood levels and effectiveness and should be avoided. ↑ **digoxin** levels and the risk of toxicity (discontinue or ↓ dose of digoxin by 50% before treatment and monitor carefully). May ↑ **dabigatran** and **warfarin** levels and the risk of bleeding. Avoid concurrent use of other **antiarrhythmics**, including **amiodarone**, **flecainide**, **propafenone**, **quinidine**, **disopyramide**, **dofetilide**, and **sotalol** due to ↑ risk of adverse cardiovascular reactions; discontinue prior to dronedarone therapy (concurrent use is contraindicated). Concurrent use of **diltiazem**, **verapamil**, **digoxin**, or **beta-blockers** ↑ risk of

bradycardia (initiate at lower dose and ↑ only after ECG evaluation). May also ↑ levels and effects of **tricyclic antidepressants**, and **selective serotonin reuptake inhibitors (SSRIs)**. May ↑ levels and risk of toxicity of some **HMG-CoA reductase inhibitors (statins)**; do not exceed simvastatin dose of 10 mg/day. Concurrent use with **CYP 3A substrates** including **sirolimus** and **tacrolimus** may ↑ risk of serious adverse reactions; monitor and adjust dosage carefully.
Drug-Natural Products: St. John's wort ↓ blood levels and may ↓ effectiveness; avoid concurrent use.
Drug-Food: Grapefruit juice may ↑ levels and the risk of toxicity; avoid concurrent ingestion.

Route/Dosage
PO (Adults): 400 mg twice daily.

Availability
Tablets: 400 mg.

NURSING IMPLICATIONS

Assessment
- Assess for signs and symptoms of atrial fibrillation or atrial flutter (palpitations, abnormal ECG) periodically during therapy. If atrial fibrillation occurs, cardiovert or discontinue dronedarone; increases risk of stroke, hospitalization for HF, and death.
- Monitor ECG periodically and at least every 3 mo during therapy. If QTc ≥500 ms or PR interval >280 ms, discontinue therapy.
- Assess for signs and symptoms of hepatic injury (anorexia, nausea, vomiting, fever, malaise, fatigue, right upper quadrant pain, jaundice, dark urine, or itching) during therapy. If hepatic injury is suspected, discontinue therapy and test serum enzymes (AST, ALT), alkaline phosphatase, and serum bilirubin to determine liver injury. If liver injury occurs, begin treatment. Do not restart therapy without another explanation for liver injury.
- Assess for signs of pulmonary toxicity (dyspnea, nonproductive cough) periodically during therapy. If pulmonary toxicity occurs, discontinue therapy.
- ***Lab Test Considerations:*** Monitor serum hepatic enzymes periodically, especially during first 6 mo of therapy.
- Monitor serum potassium and magnesium levels during therapy and maintain within normal range. May cause hypokalemia and hypomagnesemia.
- Monitor serum creatinine levels periodically during therapy. Serum creatinine levels ↑ by about 0.1 mg/dL following initiation of therapy with a rapid onset and plateau after 7 days; reversible with discontinuation. If ↑ and plateau occurs, use increased value as new baseline.

Implementation
- Patient should be on concurrent antithrombotic therapy.
- **PO:** Administer twice daily with morning and evening meals.

Patient/Family Teaching
- Instruct patient to take dronedarone as directed. Do not stop taking dronedarone, even if feeling better, without consulting health care professional. If a dose is missed, omit and take next dose at regularly scheduled time; do not double dose. Advise patient to read *Medication Guide* before starting therapy and with each Rx refill in case of changes.
- Advise patient to avoid grapefruit juice during therapy; may increase drug levels.
- Advise patient to notify health care professional if signs and symptoms of HF (weight gain, dependent edema, increasing shortness of breath), hepatic injury, or pulmonary toxicity occur.
- Instruct patient to notify health care professional of all Rx or OTC medications, vitamins, or herbal products being taken and to consult with health care professional before taking other medications, especially St. John's wort.
- May be teratogenic. Caution female patients of reproductive potential to use effective contraception during therapy and to notify health care professional if pregnancy is planned or suspected or if breast feeding.

Evaluation/Desired Outcomes
- Reduction in hospitalization of patients with paroxysmal or persistent atrial fibrillation or atrial flutter.

dulaglutide (doo-la-**gloo**-tide)
Trulicity

Classification
Therapeutic: antidiabetics
Pharmacologic: glucagon-like peptide-1 (GLP-1) receptor agonists

Indications
Adjunct treatment to diet and exercise in the management of adults with type 2 diabetes mellitus; not recommended as first line therapy, as a substitute for insulin, in patients with type 1 diabetes, or for ketoacidosis.

Action
Acts as an acylated human Glucagon-Like Peptide-1 (GLP-1, an incretin) receptor agonist; increases intracellular cyclic AMP (cAMP) leading to insulin release when glucose is elevated, which then subsides as blood glucose decreases toward euglycemia. Also decreases glucagon secretion and delays gastric emptying. **Therapeutic Effects:** Improved glycemic control.

Pharmacokinetics
Absorption: *0.75 mg dose*—65% absorbed following subcutaneous administration; *1.5 mg dose*—47% absorbed following subcutaneous administration.
Distribution: Unknown.
Metabolism and Excretion: Degraded by protein catabolic processes.

Half-life: 5 days.

TIME/ACTION PROFILE (↓ in HbA_{1c})

ROUTE	ONSET	PEAK	DURATION
subcut	within 4 wk	13 wk	unknown

Contraindications/Precautions

Contraindicated in: Hypersensitivity; Personal or family history of medullary thyroid carcinoma; Multiple Endocrine Neoplasia syndrome type 2; History of pancreatitis; Type 1 diabetes; Diabetic ketoacidosis; Severe gastrointestinal disease (including severe gastroparesis).

Use Cautiously in: History of angioedema or anaphylaxis to another GLP-1 receptor agonist; Hepatic/renal impairment; OB: Use only if potential maternal benefit justifies potential fetal risk; Lactation: Use only if potential maternal benefit justifies potential risk to infant; Pedi: Safety and effectiveness not established.

Adverse Reactions/Side Effects

CNS: fatigue. **Derm:** pruritus, rash. **Endo:** THYROID C-CELL TUMORS. **GI:** PANCREATITIS, abdominal pain, nausea, vomiting, constipation, ↓ appetite, diarrhea, dyspepsia. **GU:** acute renal failure. **Local:** injection site reactions. **Misc:** HYPERSENSITIVITY REACTIONS including anaphylaxis and angioedema.

Interactions

Drug-Drug: Concurrent use with **insulin** or **agents that increase insulin secretion** including **sulfonylureas** may ↑ the risk of serious hypoglycemia, use cautiously and consider dose ↓ of insulin or agents increasing insulin secretion. May alter absorption of concomitantly administered **oral medications** due to delayed gastric emptying.

Route/Dosage

Subcut (Adults): 0.75 mg once weekly; may ↑ to 1.5 mg once weekly to obtain glycemic control.

Availability

Solution for injection (prefilled pens): 0.75 mg/0.5 mL, 1.5 mg/0.5 mL.

NURSING IMPLICATIONS

Assessment

- Observe patient taking concurrent insulin for signs and symptoms of hypoglycemic reactions (sweating, hunger, weakness, dizziness, tremor, tachycardia, anxiety, headache, blurred vision, slurred speech, irritability).
- If thyroid nodules or elevated serum calcitonin are noted, patient should be referred to an endocrinologist.
- Monitor for pancreatitis (persistent severe abdominal pain, sometimes radiating to the back, with or without vomiting). If pancreatitis is suspected, discontinue dulaglutide; if confirmed, do not restart dulaglutide.
- ***Lab Test Considerations:*** Monitor serum HbA_{1c} periodically during therapy to evaluate effectiveness.
- May ↑ lipase and pancreatic amylase.

Implementation

- Do not confuse Trulicity (dulaglutide) with Toujeo (insulin glargine), Tradjenta (linagliptin), or Tresiba (insulin degludec).
- Patients stabilized on a diabetic regimen who are exposed to stress, fever, trauma, infection, or surgery may require administration of insulin.
- **Subcut:** Administer once weekly at any time of the day, without regard to food. Day of wk may be changed as long as at least 72 hr before next dose. Inject into abdomen, thigh, or upper arm. Solution should be clear and colorless; do not administer solutions that are discolored or contain particulate matter.

Patient/Family Teaching

- Instruct patient on use of pen and to take dulaglutide as directed. Follow manufacturer's instructions for pen use. Pen should never be shared between patients, even if needle is changed. Store pen in refrigerator; do not freeze. After initial use, pen may be stored at room temperature up to 14 days. Advise patient to read the *Patient Medication Guide* before starting dulaglutide and with each Rx refill in case of changes.
- Take missed dose as soon as remembered as long as 3 days (72 hr) until next scheduled dose. If less than 3 days until next scheduled dose, skip and take next scheduled dose.
- Inform patient that nausea is the most common side effect, but usually decreases over time.
- Advise patient taking insulin and dulaglutide to never mix insulin and dulaglutide together. Give as 2 separate injections. Both injections may be given in the same body area, but should not be given right next to each other.
- Explain to patient that this medication controls hyperglycemia but does not cure diabetes. Therapy is long-term.
- Review signs of hypoglycemia and hyperglycemia with patient. If hypoglycemia occurs, advise patient to take a glass of orange juice or 2–3 tsp of sugar, honey, or corn syrup dissolved in water and notify health care professional.
- Encourage patient to follow prescribed diet, medication, and exercise regimen to prevent hypoglycemic or hyperglycemic episodes.
- Instruct patient in proper testing of serum glucose and ketones. These tests should be closely monitored during periods of stress or illness, and health

care professional should be notified if significant changes occur.

- Advise patient to notify health care professional of all Rx or OTC medications, vitamins, or herbal products being taken and consult health care professional before taking any new medications.
- Advise patient to notify discontinue dulaglutide and health care professional immediately if signs of pancreatitis (nausea, vomiting, abdominal pain) or hypersensitivity (swelling of face, lips, tongue or throat, problems breathing or swallowing, severe rash or itching, fainting or feeling dizzy, very rapid heartbeat) occur.
- Inform patient of risk of benign and malignant thyroid C-cell tumors. Advise patient to notify health care professional if symptoms of thyroid tumors (lump in neck, hoarseness, trouble swallowing, shortness of breath) or if signs of allergic reaction (swelling of face, lips, tongue, or throat; fainting or feeling dizzy; very rapid heartbeat; problems breathing or swallowing; severe rash or itching) occur.
- Advise patient to inform health care professional of medication regimen before treatment or surgery.
- Advise patient to carry a form of sugar (sugar packets, candy) and identification describing disease process and medication regimen at all times.
- Insulin is the preferred method of controlling blood glucose during pregnancy. Counsel female patients to notify health care professional if pregnancy is planned or suspected or if breast feeding.
- Emphasize the importance of routine follow-up exams.

Evaluation/Desired Outcomes

- Improved glycemic control.

DULoxetine (do-lox-e-teen)

Cymbalta, Drizalma Sprinkle

Classification

Therapeutic: antidepressants

Pharmacologic: selective serotonin/norepinephrine reuptake inhibitors

Indications

Cymbalta and Drizalma Sprinkle: Treatment of the following conditions: Major depressive disorder, Diabetic peripheral neuropathic pain, Generalized anxiety disorder, Chronic musculoskeletal pain (including chronic lower back pain and chronic pain from osteoarthritis). **Cymbalta only:** Fibromyalgia.

Action

Inhibits serotonin and norepinephrine reuptake in the CNS. Both antidepressant and pain inhibition are centrally mediated. **Therapeutic Effects:** Decreased depressive symptomatology. Decreased neuropathic pain. Decreased symptoms of anxiety. Decreased pain.

Pharmacokinetics

Absorption: Well absorbed following oral administration.

Distribution: Unknown.

Protein Binding: Highly (> 90%) protein-bound.

Metabolism and Excretion: Mostly metabolized, primarily by the CYP2D6 and CYP1A2 enzyme pathways; the CYP2D6 enzyme system exhibits genetic polymorphism; ~7% of population may be poor metabolizers (PMs) and may have significantly ↑ duloxetine concentrations and an ↑ risk of adverse effects.

Half-life: 12 hr.

TIME/ACTION PROFILE (blood levels)

ROUTE	ONSET	PEAK	DURATION
PO	unknown	6 hr	12 hr

Contraindications/Precautions

Contraindicated in: Hypersensitivity; Concurrent use of MAO inhibitors or MAO-like drugs (linezolid or methylene blue); Severe renal impairment (CCr <30 mL/min); Hepatic impairment or substantial alcohol use (↑ risk of hepatitis).

Use Cautiously in: History of suicide attempt or ideation; History of mania (may activate mania/hypomania); Concurrent use of other centrally acting drugs (↑ risk of adverse reactions); History of seizure disorder; Diabetes (may worsen glycemic control); Angle-closure glaucoma; OB: Use during 3rd trimester may result in neonatal serotonin syndrome requiring prolonged hospitalization, respiratory and nutritional support; Lactation: Use while breast feeding only if potential maternal benefit justifies potential risk to infant; Pedi: May ↑ risk of suicide attempt/ideation especially during dose early treatment or dose adjustment; risk may be greater in children or adolescents; Geri: ↑ risk of orthostatic hypotension and falls.

Adverse Reactions/Side Effects

CNS: NEUROLEPTIC MALIGNANT SYNDROME, SEIZURES, SUICIDAL THOUGHTS, fatigue, drowsiness, insomnia, activation of mania, dizziness, fainting, falls, nightmares. **CV:** ↑ BP, orthostatic hypotension. **Derm:** ERYTHEMA MULTIFORME, STEVENS-JOHNSON SYNDROME, ↑ sweating, pruritus, rash. **EENT:** blurred vision, ↑ intraocular pressure. **F and E:** hyponatremia. **GI:** HEPATOTOXICITY, PANCREATITIS, ↓ appetite, constipation, dry mouth, nausea, diarrhea, ↑ liver enzymes, gastritis, vomiting. **GU:** dysuria, abnormal orgasm, erectile dysfunction, ↓ libido, urinary retention. **Neuro:** tremor. **Misc:** SEROTONIN SYNDROME.

Interactions

Drug-Drug: Concurrent use with **MAO inhibitors** may result in serious potentially fatal reactions (Do not use within 14 days of discontinuing MAOI. Wait at least 5 days after stopping duloxetine to start MAOI). Concurrent use with **MAO-inhibitor-like drugs**, such as **linezolid** or **methylene blue** may ↑ risk of serotonin syndrome; concurrent use contraindicated; do not start therapy in patients receiving **linezolid** or **methylene blue**; if **linezolid** or **methylene blue** need to be started in a patient receiving duloxetine, immediately discontinue duloxetine and monitor for signs/symptoms of serotonin syndrome for 5 days or until 24 hr after last dose of linezolid or methylene blue, whichever comes first (may resume duloxetine therapy 24 hr after last dose of linezolid or methylene blue). ↑ risk of hepatotoxicity with alcohol use disorder/**alcohol** abuse. Drugs that affect serotonergic neurotransmitter systems, including **tricyclic antidepressants**, **SSRIs**, **fentanyl**, **buspirone**, **tramadol**, **amphetamines**, and **triptans** ↑ risk of serotonin syndrome. **Strong CYP1A2 inhibitors**, including **cimetidine**, **ciprofloxacin**, and **fluvoxamine**, may ↑ levels; avoid concurrent use. **Drugs that inhibit CYP2D6**, including **paroxetine**, **fluoxetine**, and **quinidine** ↑ levels of duloxetine and may increase the risk of adverse reactions. Duloxetine also inhibits CYP2D6 and may ↑ levels of drugs metabolized by CYP2D6, including **tricyclic antidepressants**, **phenothiazines**, and **class Ic antiarrhythmics** (**propafenone** and **flecainide**); concurrent use should be undertaken with caution. ↑ risk of serious arrhythmias with **thioridazine**; avoid concurrent use. ↑ risk of bleeding with **aspirin**, **NSAIDs**, or **warfarin**.

Drug-Natural Products: Use with **St. John's wort** ↑ serotonin syndrome.

Route/Dosage

Major Depressive Disorder

PO (Adults): 40–60 mg/day (as 20 mg or 30 mg twice daily or as 60 mg once daily) as initial therapy, then 60 mg once daily as maintenance therapy.

Generalized Anxiety Disorder

PO (Adults ≥65 yr): 30 mg once daily for 2 wk; may then consider ↑ to 60 mg once daily, then may ↑ by 30 mg once daily to maintenance dose of 60–120 mg once daily.

PO (Adults <65 yr): 30–60 mg once daily as initial therapy (if initiated on 30 mg once daily, should titrate to 60 mg once daily after 1 wk), then may ↑ by 30 mg once daily to maintenance dose of 60–120 mg once daily.

PO (Children 7–17 yr): 30 mg once daily for 2 wk; may then consider ↑ to 60 mg once daily; recommended maintenance dose = 30–60 mg once daily (not to exceed 120 mg once daily).

Diabetic Peripheral Neuropathic Pain

PO (Adults): 60 mg once daily.

Fibromyalgia

PO (Adults): 30 mg once daily for 1 wk, then ↑ to 60 mg once daily.

Chronic Musculoskeletal Pain

PO (Adults): 60 mg once daily (may also be started on 30 mg once daily and ↑ to 60 mg once daily after 1 wk).

Availability (generic available)

Delayed-release capsules: 20 mg, 30 mg, 40 mg, 60 mg. **Cost:** 20 mg $437.15/60, 30 mg $473.58/60, 60 mg $478.64/60. **Delayed-release sprinkle capsules:** 20 mg, 30 mg, 40 mg, 60 mg.

NURSING IMPLICATIONS

Assessment

- Monitor BP before and periodically during therapy. Sustained hypertension may be dose related; decrease dose or discontinue therapy if this occurs.
- Monitor appetite and nutritional intake. Weigh weekly. Report continued weight loss. Adjust diet as tolerated to support nutritional status.
- Assess for sexual dysfunction (erectile dysfunction; decreased libido) periodically during therapy.
- Monitor closely for notable changes in behavior that could indicate the emergence or worsening of suicidal thoughts or behavior or depression, especially in early therapy or during dose changes. Risk may be increased in children, adolescents, and adults ≤24 yr. Restrict amount of drug available to patient.
- Assess for serotonin syndrome (mental changes [agitation, hallucinations, coma], autonomic instability [tachycardia, labile BP, hyperthermia], neuromuscular aberrations [hyperreflexia, incoordination], and/or GI symptoms [nausea, vomiting, diarrhea]), especially in patients taking other serotonergic drugs (SSRIs, SNRIs, triptans).
- Assess for rash periodically during therapy. May cause Stevens-Johnson syndrome. Discontinue therapy if severe or if accompanied with fever, general malaise, fatigue, muscle or joint aches, blisters, oral lesions, conjunctivitis, hepatitis and/or eosinophilia.
- **Depression or Anxiety:** Assess mental status (orientation, mood, and behavior). Inform health care professional if patient demonstrates significant increase in anxiety, nervousness, or insomnia.
- **Pain or Fibromyalgia:** Assess intensity, quality, and location of pain periodically during therapy. May require several wk for effects to be seen.
- ***Lab Test Considerations:*** May cause ↑ ALT, AST, bilirubin, CPK, and alkaline phosphatase.
- May cause hyponatremia.
- Monitor blood sugar and hemoglobin A1c. May cause slight ↑ in blood glucose.

Implementation

- Do not confuse duloxetine with fluoxetine, paroxetine, or Dexilant (dexlansoprazole). Do not confuse Cymbalta (duloxetine) with Symbyax (olanzapine/fluoxetine).

- **PO:** May be administered without regard to meals. Capsules should be swallowed whole. Do not crush, chew, or open and sprinkle contents on food or liquids; may affect enteric coating.
- *Drizalma Sprinkle:* May be administered without regard to meals. Swallow sprinkle whole; do not chew or crush capsule. Capsule can be opened and contents sprinkled over applesauce. Swallowed along with a small amount (tablespoonful) of applesauce immediately; do not store for later use.
- *Drizalma Sprinkle:* May be administered via NG tube. Open capsule and add contents to an all plastic catheter tip syringe; add 50 mL of water. Gently shake syringe for 10 sec. Promptly deliver through a 12 French or larger nasogastric tube. Ensure no pellets are left in syringe. Rinse with additional water (about 15 mL) if needed.

Patient/Family Teaching

- Instruct patient to take duloxetine as directed at the same time each day. Take missed doses as soon as possible unless time for next dose. Do not stop abruptly; may cause dizziness, headache, nausea, diarrhea, paresthesia, irritability, vomiting, insomnia, anxiety, hyperhidrosis, and fatigue; must be decreased gradually. Advise patient to read *Medication Guide* before starting therapy and with each Rx refill in case of changes.
- Encourage patient and family to be alert for emergence of anxiety, agitation, panic attacks, insomnia, irritability, hostility, impulsivity, akathisia, hypomania, mania, worsening of depression and suicidal ideation, especially during early antidepressant therapy. If these symptoms occur, notify health care professional.
- May cause drowsiness. Caution patient to avoid driving or other activities requiring alertness until response to medication is known.
- Advise patient to make position changes slowly to minimize orthostatic hypotension and falls, especially in elderly patients and those taking antihypertensive medications.
- Instruct patient to notify health care professional of all Rx or OTC medications, vitamins, or herbal products being taken and to consult with health care professional before taking other medications.
- Instruct patient to notify health care professional if signs of serotonin syndrome (mental status changes: agitation, hallucinations, coma); autonomic instability (tachycardia, labile BP, hyperthermia); neuromuscular aberrations (hyperreflexia, incoordination); and/or gastrointestinal symptoms (nausea, vomiting, diarrhea); liver damage (pruritus, dark urine, jaundice, right upper quadrant tenderness, unexplained "flu-like" symptoms) or rash occur.
- Advise patient to avoid taking alcohol during duloxetine therapy.
- Rep: Instruct patient to notify health care professional if pregnancy is planned or suspected or if breast feeding. Encourage patients exposed to duloxetine during pregnancy to enroll in the National Pregnancy Registry for Antidepressants at 1-844-405-6185 or visiting online at https://womensmentalhealth.org/clinical-and-research-programs/pregnancyregistry/antidepressants/.

Evaluation/Desired Outcomes

- Increased sense of well-being.
- Renewed interest in surroundings. Need for therapy should be periodically reassessed. Patients may notice improvement within 1–4 wk, but should be advised to continue therapy as directed. Therapy is usually continued for several mo.
- Decrease in neuropathic pain associated with diabetic peripheral neuropathy.
- Decrease in chronic musculoskeletal pain and pain and soreness associated with fibromyalgia.
- Decrease in anxiety.

dupilumab (doo-**pil**-ue-mab)

Dupixent

Classification

Therapeutic: anti-inflammatories, antiasthmatics

Pharmacologic: interleukin antagonists

Indications

Moderate-to-severe atopic dermatitis not controlled by other prescription therapies or when these therapies cannot be used (with or without topical corticosteroids). Add-on maintenance treatment of moderate-to-severe asthma that is of an eosinophilic phenotype or that is dependent on oral corticosteroids. Add-on maintenance treatment of inadequately controlled chronic rhinosinusitis with nasal polyposis.

Action

Monoclonal antibody that inhibits interleukin-4 (IL-4) and IL-13, which inhibits cytokine-induced inflammatory responses. Mechanism in asthma not fully established. **Therapeutic Effects:** Decreased severity of atopic dermatitis. Decreased incidence of asthma exacerbations. Reduction in nasal polyps and nasal congestion.

Pharmacokinetics

Absorption: 61–64% absorbed following subcut administration.

Distribution: Minimally distributed to tissues.

Metabolism and Excretion: Degraded by proteolytic enzymes located throughout the body.

Half-life: Unknown.

TIME/ACTION PROFILE (plasma concentrations)

ROUTE	ONSET	PEAK	DURATION
Subcut	unknown	1 wk	unknown

Contraindications/Precautions

Contraindicated in: Hypersensitivity; Acute bronchospasm or status asthmaticus.

Use Cautiously in: Pre-existing helminth infections; OB: Use only if potential maternal benefit outweighs potential fetal risk; Lactation: Use only if potential maternal benefit outweighs potential risk to child; Pedi: Children <12 yr (safety and effectiveness not established).

Adverse Reactions/Side Effects

CV: vasculitis. **EENT:** conjunctivitis, keratitis. **Hemat:** eosinophilia. **Resp:** eosinophilic pneumonia. **Misc:** HYPERSENSITIVITY REACTIONS (including anaphylaxis, rash, erythema nodosum, and serum sickness), injection site reactions.

Interactions

Drug-Drug: Avoid use of **live vaccines**.

Route/Dosage

Atopic Dermatitis

Subcut (Adults and Children ≥12 yr and ≥60 kg): 600 mg (given as two 300–mg injections) initially, then 300 mg in 2 wk, then 300 mg every 2 wk.

Subcut (Children ≥12 yr and <60 kg): 400 mg (given as two 200–mg injections) initially, then 200 mg in 2 wk, then 200 mg every 2 wk.

Asthma

Subcut (Adults and Children ≥12 yr): 400 mg (given as two 200–mg injections) initially, then 200 mg in 2 wk, then 200 mg every 2 wk *or* 600 mg (given as two 300–mg injections) initially, then 300 mg in 2 wk, then 300 mg every 2 wk. *Patients with oral corticosteroid-dependent asthma or concomitant moderate-to-severe atopic dermatitis*—600 mg (given as two 300–mg injections) initially, then 300 mg in 2 wk, then 300 mg every 2 wk.

Chronic Rhinosinusitis with Nasal Polyposis

Subcut (Adults): 300 mg every 2 wk.

Availability

Solution for injection (prefilled syringes): 300 mg/2 mL, 200 mg/1.14 mL.

NURSING IMPLICATIONS

Assessment

- Monitor for signs and symptoms of hypersensitivity reactions (rash, urticaria, erythema nodosum, serum sickness) during therapy. If severe reaction occurs, treat symptomatically and discontinue dupilumab.
- Monitor for signs and symptoms of conjunctivitis and keratitis (eye redness or irritation) periodically during therapy.
- Monitor lung sounds periodically during therapy.
- Monitor for signs and symptoms of rhinosinusitis periodically during therapy.

Implementation

- **Subcut:** Dose must be divided into two injections for 400 mg and 600 mg doses. Administer at different sites. Thigh and abdomen may be used if patient administers dose. May also use upper arm if administered by caregiver. Rotate site with each injection; do not inject in skin that is tender, damaged, bruised, or scarred. Allow solution to reach room temperature (45 min for 300 mg dose, 30 min for 200 mg dose) before injecting. Solution is clear to slightly opalescent, colorless to pale yellow; do not administer solutions that are cloudy, discolored, or contain particulate matter.

Patient/Family Teaching

- Instruct patient and caregiver in correct injection technique and disposal of equipment. Administer missed dose as soon as remembered if within 7 days, then resume original schedule. If longer than 7 days, skip dose and resume with next scheduled dose.
- Inform patient that dupilumab is not used for acute asthma symptoms or exacerbations. Instruct patient to notify health care professional if asthma symptoms remain uncontrolled or worsen after starting dupilumab therapy.
- Instruct patient to notify health care professional of all Rx or OTC medications, vitamins, or herbal products being taken and to consult health care professional before taking other Rx, OTC, or herbal products.
- Advise patient to avoid live vaccines during therapy.
- Advise patient to have helminth infections treated before starting dupilumab therapy.
- Advise females of reproductive potential to notify health care professional if pregnancy is planned or suspected or if breast feeding.

Evaluation/Desired Outcomes

- Decreased severity of atopic dermatitis.
- Decreased incidence of asthma exacerbations.
- Reduction in symptoms of chronic rhinosinusitis with nasal polyposis.

dutasteride (doo-tas-te-ride)

Avodart

Classification

Therapeutic: benign prostatic hyperplasia (BPH) agents

Pharmacologic: androgen inhibitors

Indications

Management of the symptoms of benign prostatic hyperplasia (BPH) in men with an enlarged prostate gland (alone or with tamsulosin).

Action

Inhibits the enzyme 5-alpha-reductase, which is responsible for converting testosterone to its potent metabolite 5-alpha-dihydrotestosterone in the prostate gland and other tissues. 5-Alpha-dihydrotestosterone is partly responsible for prostatic hyperplasia. **Therapeutic Effects:** Reduced prostate size with associated decrease in urinary symptoms.

Pharmacokinetics

Absorption: Well absorbed (60%) following oral administration; also absorbed through skin.
Distribution: 11.5% of serum concentration partitions into semen.
Protein Binding: 99% bound to albumin; 96.6% bound to alpha-1 glycoprotein.
Metabolism and Excretion: Mostly metabolized by the liver via the CYP3A4 metabolic pathway; metabolites are excreted in feces.
Half-life: 5 wk.

TIME/ACTION PROFILE (reduction in dihydrotestosterone levels†)

ROUTE	ONSET	PEAK	DURATION
PO	unknown	1–2 wk	unknown

†Symptoms may only improve over 3–12 mo.

Contraindications/Precautions

Contraindicated in: Hypersensitivity; Cross-sensitivity with other 5-alpha-reductase inhibitors may occur; Women; Pedi: Children.
Use Cautiously in: Hepatic impairment.

Adverse Reactions/Side Effects

CNS: depressed mood. **GU:** PROSTATE CANCER (high-grade), ↓ libido, ejaculation disorders, erectile dysfunction, testicular pain, testicular swelling. **Endo:** gynecomastia. **Derm:** rash, urticaria. **Misc:** ALLERGIC REACTIONS, ANGIOEDEMA.

Interactions

Drug-Drug: Blood levels and effects may be ↑ by **ritonavir**, **ketoconazole**, **verapamil**, **diltiazem**, **cimetidine**, **ciprofloxacin**, or other **CYP3A4 enzyme inhibitors**.

Route/Dosage

PO (Adults): 0.5 mg once daily (with or without tamsulosin).

Availability (generic available)

Soft gelatin capsules: 0.5 mg. ***In combination with:*** tamsulosin (Jalyn); see Appendix B.

NURSING IMPLICATIONS

Assessment

- Assess patient for symptoms of prostatic hyperplasia (urinary hesitancy, feeling of incomplete bladder emptying, interruption of urinary stream, impairment of size and force of urinary stream, terminal urinary dribbling, straining to start flow, dysuria, urgency) before and periodically during therapy.
- Digital rectal examinations should be performed before and periodically during therapy for BPH.
- ***Lab Test Considerations:*** Serum prostate-specific antigen (PSA) concentrations, used to screen for prostate cancer, decrease by about 20% within the 1st mo of therapy and stabilize at about 50% of the pretreatment level within 6 mo. New baseline PSA concentrations should be established at 3 and 6 mo of therapy and evaluated periodically during therapy. Any increase in PSA during dutaseride therapy may be a sign of prostate cancer and should be evaluated, even those within normal limits. Isolated PSA values from men taking dutaseride for 3 mo or more should be doubled for comparison in untreated men.

Implementation

- **PO:** Administer once daily with or without meals. Do not break, crush, or chew capsule.

Patient/Family Teaching

- Instruct patient to take dutasteride at the same time each day as directed, even if symptoms improve or are unchanged. Take missed doses as soon as remembered later in the day or omit dose. Do not make up by taking double doses the next day.
- Caution patient that sharing of dutasteride may be dangerous.
- Inform patient that the volume of ejaculate may be decreased during therapy but that this will not interfere with normal sexual function.
- Advise patient to avoid donating blood for at least 6 mo after last dose of dutasteride to prevent a pregnant female from receiving dutasteride through a blood transfusion.
- Inform patient of potential increase risk in high-grade prostate cancer.
- Caution patient that dutasteride poses a potential risk to a male fetus. Women who are pregnant or may become pregnant should avoid exposure to semen of a partner taking dutasteride and should not handle dutasteride because of the potential for absorption.
- Emphasize the importance of periodic follow-up exams to determine whether a clinical response has occurred.

Evaluation/Desired Outcomes

- Decrease in urinary symptoms of BPH.

econazole, See ANTIFUNGALS (TOPICAL).

edaravone (e-dar-a-vone)

Radicava

Classification

Therapeutic: agents for amyotrophic lateral sclerosis

Indications

Amyotrophic lateral sclerosis (ALS).

Action

Unknown. **Therapeutic Effects:** Improved functional ability.

Pharmacokinetics

Absorption: IV administration results in complete bioavailability.

Distribution: Unknown.

Protein Binding: 92%.

Metabolism and Excretion: Metabolized via sulfation and glucuronidation into inactive metabolites. Primarily eliminated in urine (1% as unchanged drug).

Half-life: 4.5–6 hr.

TIME/ACTION PROFILE (blood levels)

ROUTE	ONSET	PEAK	DURATION
PO	unknown	1 hr	unknown

Contraindications/Precautions

Contraindicated in: Hypersensitivity; Sulfite allergy.

Use Cautiously in: OB: Safety not established; Lactation: Consider benefits of breast feeding against possible risk to infant; Pedi: Safety and effectiveness not established.

Adverse Reactions/Side Effects

CNS: headache. **Derm:** contusion, dermatitis, eczema, fungal infection (tinea). **GU:** glycosuria. **Neuro:** gait abnormality. **Misc:** HYPERSENSITIVITY REACTIONS (including anaphylaxis).

Interactions

Drug-Drug: None known.

Route/Dosage

IV (Adults): 60 mg once daily for 14 day, followed by a drug-free period of 14 days. Each subsequent cycle should consist of 60 mg once daily for 10 days out of 14 days, followed by a drug-free period of 14 days.

Availability

Premixed infusion: 30 mg/100 mL.

NURSING IMPLICATIONS

Assessment

- Assess respiratory and functional status prior to and periodically during therapy.
- Monitor for signs and symptoms of hypersensitivity reactions or sulfite allergic reactions (redness, wheals, erythema multiforme, urticaria, decreased blood pressure, dyspnea) with each infusion. If reaction occurs, discontinue therapy and treat with standard care.

Implementation

- **Intermittent Infusion:** Do not use if oxygen indicator has turned blue or purple before opening package. Use within 24 hrs of opening overwrap. Solution is clear and colorless; do not administer solutions that are discolored or contain particulate matter. ***Rate:*** Infuse as 2 consecutive infusion bags over 60 min at 1 mg/min.
- **Y-Site Incompatibility:** Do not mix with other medications.

Patient/Family Teaching

- Explain purpose of medication to patient.
- Instruct patient to notify health care professional immediately if signs and symptoms of hypersensitivity or allergic reactions occur.
- Advise patient to notify health care professional if pregnancy is planned or suspected or if breast feeding.

Evaluation/Desired Outcomes

- Improved functional ability.

edoxaban (e-dox-a-ban)

🍁Lixiana, Savaysa

Classification

Therapeutic: anticoagulants

Pharmacologic: factor Xa inhibitors

Indications

Reduction of stroke/systemic embolization (SE) risk associated with nonvalvular atrial fibrillation (NVAF).

Action

Selective inhibitor of factor Xa. Does not inhibit platelet aggregation directly, but does inhibit thrombin-induced platelet aggregation. Decreases thrombin generation and thrombus development. **Therapeutic Effects:** Decreased thrombotic events associated with atrial fibrillation including stroke and systemic embolization. Treatment of deep vein thrombosis (DVT) and pulmonary embolism (PE) after 5–10 days of parenteral anticoagulant.

Pharmacokinetics

Absorption: 62% absorbed following oral administration.
Distribution: Unknown.
Metabolism and Excretion: Minimal metabolism, one metabolite is pharmacologically active. Excreted mostly unchanged in urine.
Half-life: 10–14 hr.

TIME/ACTION PROFILE (anticoagulant effect)

ROUTE	ONSET	PEAK	DURATION
PO	unknown	1–2 hr	24 hr

Contraindications/Precautions

Contraindicated in: Active bleeding; CCr >95 mL/min (↓ effectiveness); Concurrent use of other anticoagulants or rifampin; Presence of mechanical heart valves or severe mitral stenosis; Moderate to severe hepatic impairment; Lactation: Avoid breast feeding.
Use Cautiously in: Elective/planned invasive/surgical procedures (discontinue at least 24 hr prior to ↓ risk of bleeding); Premature discontinuation (↑ risk of ischemic events); Neuroaxial anesthesia/spinal puncture (↑ risk of spinal/epidural hematoma and potential paralysis); Renal impairment (dose reduction required for CCr 15–50 mL/min); Deteriorating or improving renal function (may require dose change); Body weight ≤60 kg (requires lower dose); OB: Use during pregnancy only if potential benefit outweighs potential risk to fetus; Pedi: Safe and effective use in children has not been established.

Adverse Reactions/Side Effects

GI: abnormal liver function tests. **Hemat:** BLEEDING, anemia.

Interactions

Drug-Drug: ↑ risk of bleeding with other **anticoagulants, aspirin, clopidogrel, ticagrelor, prasugrel, fibrinolytics, NSAIDs, SNRIs,** or **SSRIs**. Rifampin may ↓ blood levels and effectiveness and is contraindicated. Concurrent use of **P-gp inhibitors** including **azithromycin, clarithromcyin, erythromycin, itraconazole** (oral), **ketoconazole** (oral), **quinidine**, or **verapamil** ↑ blood levels and the risk of bleeding (lower dose required).

Route/Dosage

Treatment of NVAF

PO (Adults): 60 mg once daily.

Renal Impairment

PO (Adults): *CCr 15–50 mL/min*—30 mg once daily.

Treatment of DVT/PE

PO (Adults >60 kg): 60 mg once daily.
PO (Adults ≤60 kg or certain concurrent P-gp inhibitors): 30 mg once daily.

Renal Impairment

PO (Adults CCr 15–50 mL/min): 30 mg once daily.

Availability

Tablets: 15 mg, 30 mg, 60 mg.

NURSING IMPLICATIONS

Assessment

- Monitor for bleeding. Discontinue edoxaban if active pathological bleeding occurs. Concomitant drugs (aspirin, other antiplatelet agents, other antithrombotic agents, fibrinolytic therapy, chronic use of NSAIDs) may increase risk of bleeding. Anticoagulant effects of edoxaban persist for about 24 hr after last dose; there is no established way to reverse anticoagulant effects. Anticoagulant effects cannot be reliably monitored with standard laboratory tests. No reversal agent is available; protamine sulfate, vitamin K, and tranexamic acid do not reverse anticoagulant activity. May consider prothrombin complex concentrates (PCC), or other procoagulant reversal agents such as activated prothrombin complex concentrate (APCC) or recombinant factor VIIa (r-FVIIa). If PCC is used, monitoring anticoagulation effect of edoxaban using clotting test (PT, INR, or aPTT) or anti-FXa activity is not useful. Hemodialysis does not significantly contribute to edoxaban clearance.
- Monitor frequently for signs and symptoms of neurological impairment (numbness or weakness of legs, bowel, or bladder dysfunction, back pain, tingling, muscle weakness); if noted, urgent treatment is required. Intrathecal or epidural catheters should not be removed earlier than 12 hr after last dose of edoxaban. Next dose of edoxaban should not be given less than 2 hr after removal of catheter.
- ***Lab Test Considerations:*** Assess creatinine clearance (CCr) using Cockcroft-Gault equation CCr = (140 − age) × (weight in kg) × (0.85 if female)/(72 × creatinine in mg/dL) before starting therapy.

Implementation

- Discontinue edoxaban at least 24 hr prior to invasive or surgical procedures; may increase risk of bleeding. Edoxaban may be restarted as soon as adequate hemostasis is established; time to onset of pharmacodynamic effect is 1–2 hr.
- **PO:** Tablets may be crushed and mixed with 2–3 oz of water and immediately administered by mouth or through a gastric tube. May also mix with applesauce and administered immediately.
- *If transitioning from warfarin or other vitamin K antagonists to edoxaban,* discontinue warfarin and start edoxaban when INR ≤2.5. *If transitioning from oral anticoagulants other than warfarin or other Vitamin K antagonists to edoxaban,* discontinue current oral anticoagulant and start edoxaban at time of next scheduled dose of other oral antico-

agulant. *If transitioning from low molecular weight heparin (LMWH) to edoxaban,* discontinue LMWH and start edoxaban at time of next scheduled administration of LMWH. *If transitioning from unfractionated heparin to edoxaban,* discontinue infusion and start edoxaban 4 hr later.

- *If transitioning from edoxaban to warfarin,* Oral Option: For patients taking 60 mg of edoxaban, reduce dose to 30 mg and begin warfarin concomitantly. For patients taking 30 mg edoxaban, reduce dose to 15 mg and begin warfarin concomitantly. Measure INR at least weekly and just prior to daily dose of edoxaban to minimize influence of edoxaban on INR measurements. Once stable INR ≥2.0 achieved, discontinue edoxaban and continue warfarin. Parenteral Option: Discontinue edoxaban and administer a parenteral anticoagulant and warfarin at time of next scheduled edoxaban dose. Once stable INR ≥2.0 achieved, discontinue parenteral anticoagulant and continue warfarin. *If transitioning from edoxaban to non-Vitamin-K Dependant Oral anticoagulant,* discontinue edoxaban and start other oral anticoagulant at time of next dose of edoxaban. *If transitioning from edoxaban to parenteral anticoagulant,* discontinue edoxaban and start parenteral anticoagulant at time of next dose of edoxaban.

Patient/Family Teaching

- Instruct patient to take edoxaban as directed. Take missed doses as soon as remembered on same day. Return to regular schedule next day. Do not double doses in one day. Do not discontinue without consulting health care professional; stopping may increase risk of stroke.
- Caution patient that they may bleed more easily, longer, or bruise more easily during therapy. Advise patient to notify health care professional immediately if bleeding or a fall, especially with head injury, occurs.
- Advise patient to notify health care professional of all Rx or OTC medications, vitamins, or herbal products being taken and to consult with health care professional before taking other medications, especially other aspirin or NSAIDs.
- Advise patient to notify health care professional of therapy before surgery, medical, or dental procedures are scheduled.
- Advise female patient to notify health care professional if pregnancy is planned or suspected. Avoid breast feeding during therapy.

Evaluation/Desired Outcomes

- Decreased thrombotic events (stroke and systemic embolization) associated with atrial fibrillation.
- Treatment of deep vein thrombosis (DVT) and pulmonary embolism (PE).

elagolix (el-a-**goe**-lix)

Orilissa

Classification
Therapeutic: analgesics
Pharmacologic: GnRH antagonist

E

Indications

Moderate to severe pain associated with endometriosis.

Action

Competitively binds to and inhibits gonadotropin-releasing hormone (GnRH) receptors in the pituitary gland, causing a decrease in the release of estradiol and progesterone by the ovaries. **Therapeutic Effects:** Reduction in dysmenorrhea and non-menstrual pelvic pain.

Pharmacokinetics

Absorption: Rapidly absorbed.
Distribution: Unknown.
Metabolism and Excretion: Primarily metabolized in the liver via CYP3A enzymes; some metabolism by CYP2D6, CYP2C8, and UGT. 90% of dose excreted in feces, <3% in urine.
Half-life: 4–6 hr.

TIME/ACTION PROFILE (plasma concentrations)

ROUTE	ONSET	PEAK	DURATION
PO	unknown	1 hr	24 hr

Contraindications/Precautions

Contraindicated in: Osteoporosis (may ↑ risk of bone loss); Severe hepatic impairment; Concurrent use of strong organic anion transporting polypeptide (OATP) 1B1 inhibitors; OB: Pregnancy (may ↑ risk of early pregnancy loss).
Use Cautiously in: History of low-trauma fracture or other risk factors for osteoporosis; History of suicidal thoughts/behaviors or depression; Moderate hepatic impairment (use lower dose); Lactation: Use while breast feeding only if potential maternal benefit justifies potential risk to infant; Rep: Women of reproductive potential; Pedi: Safety and effectiveness not established.

Adverse Reactions/Side Effects

CNS: SUICIDAL THOUGHTS/BEHAVIOR, headache, anxiety, depression, dizziness, insomnia, mood swings. **Derm:** rash. **Endo:** hot flushes, night sweats. **GI:** nausea, abdominal pain, constipation, diarrhea, ↑ liver enzymes. **GU:** ↓ libido, menstrual irregularities. **Metab:** dyslipidemia, ↑ weight. **MS:** arthralgia, ↓ bone density.

Interactions

Drug-Drug: Strong OATP1B1 inhibitors, including **cyclosporine** and **gemfibrozil** may significantly

↑ levels; concurrent use contraindicated. **Estrogen-containing contraceptives** may ↓ effectiveness; impact of **progestin-containing contraceptives** on effectiveness unknown; recommended to use non-hormonal contraceptives. May ↓ levels of **CYP3A substrates**, including **midazolam**. May ↑ levels of **CYP2C19 substrates**, including **omeprazole**; consider ↓ omeprazole dose when using higher doses (>40 mg/day). May ↑ levels of **P-glycoprotein substrates**, including **digoxin**; closely monitor digoxin levels. **Strong CYP3A inhibitors** may ↑ levels; limit concurrent use with elagolix 200 mg twice daily to ≤1 mo; limit concurrent use with elagolix 150 mg once daily to ≤6 mo. **CYP3A inducers**, including **rifampin** may ↓ levels; concurrent use with elagolix 200 mg twice daily not recommended; limit concurrent use with elagolix 150 mg once daily to ≤6 mo. May ↓ **rosuvastatin** levels; consider ↑ rosuvastatin dose.

Route/Dosage

PO (Adults): *No dyspareunia*—150 mg once daily for max duration of 24 mo; *Coexisting dyspareunia*—200 mg twice daily for max duration of 6 mo.

Hepatic Impairment

PO (Adults): *Moderate hepatic impairment (Child-Pugh Class B)*—150 mg once daily for max duration of 6 mo.

Availability

Tablets: 150 mg, 200 mg.

NURSING IMPLICATIONS

Assessment

- Assess bone mineral density in patients with a history of a low-trauma fracture or other risk factors for osteoporosis or bone loss. Vitamin D and calcium supplements may be considered.
- Assess for depression and mood changes during therapy. Refer patients with new or worsening depression, anxiety or other mood changes, suicidal ideation and behavior to a mental health professional. Consider benefits and risks of continuing elagolix.
- ***Lab Test Considerations:*** Obtain a negative pregnancy test before starting therapy. Use lowest effective dose for limited duration to minimize bone loss.
- Monitor liver function tests periodically during therapy. May cause ↑ AST and ALT.
- May cause ↑ lipid levels during first 2 mo of therapy, then usually remains stable.

Implementation

- **PO:** Administer at the same time each day without regard to food.

Patient/Family Teaching

- Instruct patient to take elagolix as directed. Take missed doses as soon as remembered if same day as missed dose, then return to regular dosing schedule; do not double doses. Advise patient to read *Medication Guide* before starting and with each Rx refill in case of changes.
- Inform patient that elagolix may change menstrual periods (irregular bleeding or spotting, a decrease in menstrual bleeding, no bleeding at all), and make it hard to know if you are pregnant. Watch for other signs of pregnancy (breast tenderness, weight gain, nausea).
- Advise patient and family to notify health care professional if signs and symptoms of mood or behavior changes (thoughts about suicide or dying, try to commit suicide, new or worse depression, new or worse anxiety, other unusual changes in behavior or mood) or liver problems (yellowing of skin or whites of eyes, dark amber-colored urine, feeling tired, nausea and vomiting, generalized swelling, right upper abdomen pain, bruising easily) occur.
- Advise patient to notify health care professional of all Rx or OTC medications, vitamins, or herbal products being taken and to consult with health care professional before taking other medications, especially birth control pills.
- Rep: Advise females of reproductive potential to use effective nonhormonal contraception during and for 1 wk after last dose. Hormonal contraceptives may decrease effectiveness of elagolix. to notify health care professional if pregnancy is planned or suspected, or if breast feeding. Encourage patient to enroll in pregnancy registry to monitor outcomes of women who become pregnant while taking elagolix by calling 1-833-782-7241. Discontinue elagolix if pregnancy occurs.

Evaluation/Desired Outcomes

- Reduction in dysmenorrhea and non-menstrual pelvic pain.

elbasvir/grazoprevir

(**elb**-as-vir/graz-**oh**-pre-vir)

Zepatier

Classification

Therapeutic: antivirals

Pharmacologic: NS5A inhibitors, protease inhibitors

Indications

Chronic hepatitis C virus (HCV) genotypes 1 or 4 infection (with or without ribavirin).

Action

Elbasvir—inhibits the HCV NS5A protein, resulting in inhibition of viral replication; *Grazoprevir*—inhibits the HCV NS3/4A protease, resulting in inhibition of viral replication. **Therapeutic Effects:** Decreased levels of HCV with sustained virologic response and lessened sequelae of chronic HCV infection.

Pharmacokinetics

Elbasvir

Absorption: Well absorbed following oral administration.

Distribution: Extensively distributed to tissues.

Protein Binding: >99.9%.

Metabolism and Excretion: Partially metabolized by CYP3A4. >90% excreted in feces and <1% eliminated in urine.

Half-life: 24 hr.

Grazoprevir

Absorption: Well absorbed following oral administration.

Distribution: Extensively distributed to tissues.

Protein Binding: >98.8%.

Metabolism and Excretion: Partially metabolized by CYP3A4. >90% excreted in feces and <1% eliminated in urine.

Half-life: 31 hr.

TIME/ACTION PROFILE (blood levels)

ROUTE	ONSET	PEAK	DURATION
elbasvir (PO)	unknown	3 hr	24 hr
grazoprevir (PO)	unknown	2 hr	24 hr

Contraindications/Precautions

Contraindicated in: Moderate or severe hepatic impairment (Child-Pugh B or C); Concurrent use of organic anion transporting polypeptides 1B1/3 (OATP1B1/3) inhibitors, strong CYP3A inducers, or efavirenz; Situations when ribavirin is contraindicated (when ribavirin required); OB: Pregnant women or men whose partners are pregnant (when ribavirin is required; ribavirin may cause fetal harm); Lactation: Discontinue elbasvir/grazoprevir or discontinue breast feeding (when ribavirin required).

Use Cautiously in: Patients who are female or of Asian ancestry (↑ risk of liver enzyme elevation); Patients awaiting liver transplantation or liver transplant recipients (safety and effectiveness not established); Receiving immunosuppressant or chemotherapy medications (↑ risk of hepatitis B virus reactivation); OB: Safety not established (when ribavirin not required); Lactation: Weigh benefits of breast feeding against possible adverse effects (when ribavirin not required); Geri: ↑ risk of liver enzyme elevation in elderly patients; Pedi: Safety and effectiveness not established.

Adverse Reactions/Side Effects

CNS: headache, insomnia. **GI:** abdominal pain, diarrhea, ↑ liver enzymes, nausea. **Misc:** ANGIOEDEMA, fatigue, hepatitis B virus reactivation.

Interactions

Drug-Drug: **OATP1B1/3 inhibitors**, including **atazanavir**, **cyclosporine**, **darunavir**, **lopinavir**, **saquinavir**, or **tipranavir** may ↑ levels/toxicity of grazoprevir; concurrent use contraindicated. **Strong CYP3A inducers**, including **phenytoin**, **carbamazepine**, or **rifampin** may ↓ levels/effectiveness of elbasvir and grazoprevir; concurrent use contraindicated. **Efavirenz** may ↓ levels/effectiveness of elbasvir and grazoprevir; concurrent use contraindicated. **Moderate CYP3A inducers**, including **nafcillin**, **bosentan**, **etravirine**, and **modafanil** may ↓ levels/effectiveness of elbasvir and grazoprevir; concurrent use not recommended. **Strong CYP3A inhibitors**, including **ketoconazole** and **cobicistat-containing regimens** may ↑ levels/toxicity of elbasvir and grazoprevir; concurrent use not recommended. May ↑ levels/toxicity of **tacrolimus**; frequent monitoring of tacrolimus whole blood concentrations recommended. May ↑ levels/toxicity of **atorvastatin**, **fluvastatin**, **lovastatin**, **rosuvastatin**, and **simvastatin**; rosuvastatin dose should not exceed 10 mg/day; atorvastatin dose should not exceed 20 mg/day; use lowest possible dose of fluvastatin, lovastatin, and simvastatin and monitor closely for myopathy. May cause fluctuations in INR when used with **warfarin**; closely monitor INR.

Drug-Natural Products: **St. John's wort** may ↓ levels/effectiveness of elbasvir and grazoprevir; concurrent use contraindicated.

Route/Dosage

Patients with HCV genotype 1a infection should be tested for the presence of virus with NS5A resistance-associated polymorphisms prior to initiation of therapy to determine the most appropriate dosage regimen and duration of therapy

PO (Adults): *Genotype 1a: Treatment-naïve or Peg-interferon/ribavirin-experienced without baseline NS5A polymorphisms*— 1 tablet once daily for 12 wk; *Genotype 1a: Treatment-naïve or Peg-interferon/ribavirin-experienced with baseline NS5A polymorphisms*— 1 tablet once daily for 16 wk in combination with ribavirin; *Genotype 1b: Treatment-naïve or Peg-interferon/ribavirin-experienced*— 1 tablet once daily for 12 wk; *Genotype 1a or 1b: Peg-interferon/ribavirin/ HCV NS3/4A protease inhibitor-experienced*— 1 tablet once daily for 12 wk in combination with ribavirin; *Genotype 4: Treatment-naïve*— 1 tablet once daily for 12 wk; *Genotype 4: Peg-interferon/ribavirin-experienced*— 1 tablet once daily for 16 wk in combination with ribavirin.

Availability

Tablets: elbasvir 50 mg/grazoprevir 100 mg.

NURSING IMPLICATIONS

Assessment

- Monitor for signs and symptoms of hepatitis B reactivation or hepatitis (jaundice, dark urine, light colored stools, fatigue, weakness, loss of appetite, nausea, vomiting, stomach pain) during therapy.
- ***Lab Test Considerations:*** Measure hepatitis B surface antigen (HBsAg) and hepatitis core antibody (anti-HBc) in all patients before starting hepatitis C virus therapy. May cause hepatitis B virus reactivation. Monitor for clinical and laboratory signs of hepatitis flare (↑ AST, ALT, bilirubin, liver failure, death) or HBV reactivation (rapid ↑ in serum HBV DNA level) during HCV treatment and post-treatment follow-up.
- Test all patients for current or prior hepatitis B virus (HBV) infection by measuring hepatitis B surface antigen (HBsAg) and hepatitis B core antibody (anti-HBc) before starting therapy. Monitor for HBV reactivation during and following therapy. Test patient with HCV genotype 1a infection for presence of virus with NS5A resistance-associated polymorphisms prior to starting therapy with Zepatier™ to determine dose regimen and duration.
- Monitor liver function tests (AST, ALT, bilirubin, alkaline phosphatase) prior to, at treatment wk 8, at treatment wk 12 if patient receiving 16 wk therapy, and as clinically indicated during therapy. If persistently ALT ↑ >10 times upper limit of normal, consider discontinuing elbasvir/grazoprevir. Discontinue therapy if ↑ ALT and signs and symptoms of liver inflammation or ↑ conjugated bilirubin, alkaline phosphatase, or INR.

Implementation

- **PO:** Administer one tablet daily without regard to food.

Patient/Family Teaching

- Instruct patient to take *Zepatier™* as directed. Keep tablet in blister pack until ready to take dose. Do not skip or miss doses, or stop medication without consulting health care professional. Advise patient to read *Patient Information* before starting and with each Rx refill in case of changes.
- Advise patient to notify health care professional promptly if signs and symptoms of liver inflammation (fatigue, weakness, lack of appetite, nausea and vomiting, jaundice, discolored feces) occur.
- Advise patient to notify health care professional if they have a history of HBV. May cause reactivation.
- Instruct patient to notify health care professional of all Rx or OTC medications, vitamins, or herbal products being taken and consult health care professional before taking any new medications, especially St. John's wort.
- Rep: Advise all patients to notify health care professional if pregnancy is planned or suspected or if breast feeding. Advise male and female patients who take *Zepatier™* with ribavirin to use effective contraception during and for 6 mo after therapy is completed. Notify health care professional immediately if pregnancy is suspected.

Evaluation/Desired Outcomes

- Decreased levels of HCV with sustained virologic response and lessened sequelae of chronic HCV infection.

elvitegravir/cobicistat/emtricitabine/tenofovir alafenamide

(el-vi-**teg**-ra-vir/koe-**bik**-i-stat/em-trye-**sye**-ta-been/ten-**of**-oh-vir al-a-**fen**-a-mide)

Genvoya

Classification

Therapeutic: antiretrovirals

Pharmacologic: integrase strand transfer inhibitors (INSTI), enzyme inhibitors, nucleoside reverse transcriptase inhibitors

Indications

Management of HIV infection in treatment-naïve adults. Management of HIV infection in patients with HIV-1 RNA <50 copies/mL (to replace their current antiretroviral regimen) who are on a stable antiretroviral regimen for ≥6 mo, have no history of treatment failure, and have no known substitutions associated with resistance to the individual medications in the combination product.

Action

Elvitegravir—An integrase strand transfer inhibitor that inhibits an enzyme necessary for viral replication. *Cobicistat*—A pharmacokinetic enhancer (inhibits CYP3A and CYP2D6) that increases systemic exposure to elvitegravir. *Emtricitabine*—Phosphorylated intracellularly where it inhibits HIV reverse transcriptase, resulting in viral DNA chain termination. *Tenofovir alafenamide*—Phosphorylated intracellularly where it inhibits HIV reverse transcriptase resulting in disruption of DNA synthesis. When compared to tenofovir disoproxil fumarate, tenofovir alafenamide is associated with fewer episodes of renal impairment and reductions in bone mineral density. **Therapeutic Effects:** Slowed progression of HIV infection and decreased occurrence of sequelae.

Pharmacokinetics

elvitegravir

Absorption: Absorption follows oral administration.
Distribution: Unknown.
Protein Binding: 98–99%.
Metabolism and Excretion: Metabolized by CYP3A; 94.5% eliminated in feces, 6.7% in urine.
Half-life: 12.9 hr.

cobicistat
Absorption: Absorption follows oral administration.
Distribution: Unknown.
Protein Binding: 97–98%.
Metabolism and Excretion: Metabolized by CYP3A and to a small extent by CYP2D6; 86.2% eliminated in feces, 8.2% in urine.
Half-life: 3.5 hr.
emtricitabine
Absorption: Rapidly and extensively absorbed; 93% bioavailable.
Distribution: Unknown.
Metabolism and Excretion: Some metabolism; 86% eliminated in urine, 14% in feces.
Half-life: 10 hr.
tenofovir alafenamide
Absorption: Tenofovir alafenamide is a prodrug, which is hydrolyzed into tenofovir, the active component; absorption enhanced by high-fat meals.
Distribution: Unknown.
Metabolism and Excretion: Tenofovir is phosphorylated to tenofovir diphosphate (active metabolite); 32% excreted in feces, <1% in urine.
Half-life: 0.51 hr.

TIME/ACTION PROFILE (blood levels)

ROUTE	ONSET	PEAK	DURATION
elvitegravir PO	unknown	4 hr	24 hr
cobicistat PO	unknown	3 hr	24 hr
emtricitabine PO	rapid	1–2 hr	24 hr
tenofovir alafenamide PO	unknown	0.5 hr	24 hr

Contraindications/Precautions

Contraindicated in: Severe hepatic impairment; Concurrent use of alfuzosin, carbamazepine, ergot derivatives, lomitapide, lovastatin, lurasidone, phenobarbital, phenytoin, pimozide, rifampin, sildenafil (Revatio), simvastatin, triazolam, or St. John's wort; Severe renal impairment (CCr <30 mL/min AND not receiving chronic hemodialysis); Severe hepatic impairment; OB: Not recommended in pregnancy (significantly lower concentrations of elvitegravir and cobicistat); Lactation: HIV-infected women should not breast feed due to risk of viral transmission.
Use Cautiously in: Female patients or obese patients (may be at ↑ risk for lactic acidosis/hepatic steatosis); Chronic hepatitis B virus infection (may exacerbate following discontinuation); Concurrent use of nephrotoxic drugs (↑ risk of renal impairment); Geri: Elderly may be more sensitive to drug effects; consider age-related ↓ in renal, hepatic, and cardiovascular function; concurrent disease states and medications; Pedi: Children <25 kg (safety and effectiveness not established).
Exercise Extreme Caution in: Hepatitis B (may cause severe acute exacerbation).

Adverse Reactions/Side Effects

CNS: headache. **F and E:** hypophosphatemia. **GI:** LACTIC ACIDOSIS/HEPATOMEGALY WITH STEATOSIS, POST-TREATMENT ACUTE EXACERBATION OF HEPATITIS B, nausea, diarrhea. **GU:** proteinuria, renal impairment. **Metab:** ↑ lipids. **Misc:** fatigue, immune reconstitution syndrome.

Interactions

Drug-Drug: May alter blood levels and effects of other drugs metabolized by the CYP3A or CYP2D6 enzyme systems. Other drugs that induce the CYP3A system can alter blood levels and effects. Concurrent administration of other drugs that depend mainly on CYP3A for metabolism and whose blood levels, when ↑, are associated with serious/life-threatening adverse reactions including **alfuzosin**, **dihydroergotamine**, **ergotamine**, **lomitapide**, **lovastatin**, **lurasidone**, **methylergonovine**, **pimozide**, **sildenafil** (when used for pulmonary hypertension), **simvastatin**, and **triazolam**; concurrent use contraindicated. **Carbamazepine**, **phenobarbital**, **phenytoin**, or **rifampin** may significantly ↓ levels/effectiveness of cobicistat and elvitegravir and ↑ risk of resistance; concurrent use contraindicated. Nephrotoxic agents, including **NSAIDs** and **aminoglycosides** may ↑ risk of nephrotoxicity; avoid concurrent use. Drugs that induce CYP3A will ↓ levels/effectiveness of elvitegravir, cobicistat, and tenofovir alafenamide. Drugs that inhibit CYP3A will ↑ levels/toxicity of cobicistat. **Acyclovir**, **cidofovir**, **ganciclovir**, **valacyclovir**, and **valganciclovir** may ↓ renal elimination and ↑ levels/toxicity of emtricitabine and tenofovir alafenamide. **Antacids**, including **aluminum hydroxide** and **magnesium hydroxide**, may ↓ levels/effectiveness of elvitegravir; separate administration by ≥2 hr. May ↑ levels/toxicity of **amiodarone**, **digoxin**, **disopyramide**, **flecainide**, **lidocaine**, **mexiletine**, **propafenone** and **quinidine**; careful monitoring recommended. May alter effects of **warfarin**; careful monitoring of INR recommended. Concurrent use with **clarithromycin** may ↑ levels/toxicity of clarithromycin and/or cobicistat (for patients with CCr 50–60 mL/min, ↓ dose of clarithromycin by 50%). May ↑ levels/toxicity of **ethosuximide**; clinical monitoring recommended. **Oxcarbamazepine** may ↓ levels/effectiveness of cobicistat, elvitegravir, and tenofovir alafenamide; consider using alternative anticonvulsant. May ↑ levels/toxicity of **SSRIs** (except sertraline), **tricyclic antidepressants**, and **trazodone**; careful titration and monitoring recommended. Concurrent use with **itraconazole**, **ketoconazole**, or **voriconazole**

may ↑ levels/toxicity of itraconazole, ketoconazole, voriconazole, elvitegravir, and cobicistat; (max dose of ketoconazole or itraconazole = 300 mg/day; assess risk vs. benefit before using voriconazole). May ↑ levels/toxicity of **colchicine**; concurrent use contraindicated in renal or hepatic impairment; *Dosing adjustment for gout flares*—0.6 mg, then 0.3 mg 1 hr later, do not repeat for ≥3 days; *Dosing adjustment for gout flare prophylaxis*—0.3 mg once daily if original regimen was 0.6 mg twice daily, 0.3 mg every other day if original regimen was 0.6 mg once daily; *Dosing adjustment for treatment of familial Mediterranean fever*—not to exceed 0.6 mg daily, may be given as 0.3 mg twice daily. **Rifabutin** or **rifapentine** may ↓ levels/effectiveness of cobicistat, elvitegravir, and tenofovir alafenamide and may foster resistance; concurrent use not recommended. May ↑ levels/toxicity of **beta blockers**; careful monitoring recommended; ↓ dose of beta blocker if necessary. May ↑ levels/toxicity of **calcium channel blockers** including **amlodipine**, **diltiazem**, **felodipine**, **nicardipine**, **nifedipine**, and **verapamil**; careful monitoring recommended. Concurrent use of **corticosteroids that induce CYP3A**, including **budesonide**, **dexamethasone**, **methylprednisolone**, or inhaled **betamethasone**, **ciclesonide**, **fluticasone**, **mometasone**, and **triamcinolone**, may ↓ levels/effectiveness and ↑ risk of resistance to elvitegravir (consider use of other corticosteroids, such as beclomethasone, prednisolone, or prednisone). Concurrent use of **corticosteroids that are metabolized by CYP3A** including **budesonide**, **dexamethasone**, **methylprednisolone**, or inhaled **betamethasone**, **ciclesonide**, **fluticasone**, **mometasone**, and **triamcinolone** may ↑ risk of Cushing's disease and adrenal suppression (consider use of other corticosteroids, such as beclomethasone, prednisolone, or prednisone). May ↑ levels/toxicity of **bosentan**; initiate bosentan at 62.5 mg once daily or every other day if already receiving elvitegravir/cobicistat/emtricitabine/tenofovir alafenamide for ≥10 days; if already receiving bosentan, discontinue bosentan ≥36 hr prior to starting elvitegravir/cobicistat/emtricitabine/tenofovir alafenamide; after 10 days, bosentan may be restarted at 62.5 mg once daily or every other day. May ↑ levels/toxicity of **atorvastatin**; initiate atorvastatin at lowest dose titrate cautiously; do not exceed dose of 20 mg/day. May ↑ levels/toxicity of **norgestimate** and ↓ levels of **ethinyl estradiol**; due to unpredictable effects, nonhormonal contraceptive methods should be considered. ↑ risk of hyperkalemia with contraceptives containing **drospirenone**; closely monitor serum potassium concentrations. May ↑ levels/toxicity of **immunosuppressants**, including **cyclosporine**, **sirolimus**, and **tacrolimus**; careful monitoring recommended. **Cyclosporine** may ↑ levels/toxicity of cobicistat and elvitegravir; careful monitoring recommended. May ↑ levels/toxicity of **buprenorphine** and ↓ levels of **naloxone**; carefully monitor for sedation and altered cognitive effects. May ↑ levels of **fentanyl**, and **tramadol**; monitor for respiratory depression; consider ↓ tramadol dose. May ↑ levels of and risk of adverse cardiovascular effects with **salmeterol**, concurrent use not recommended. ↑ levels/toxicity of **neuroleptics**, including **perphenazine**, **risperidone**, and **thioridazine**; may need to ↓ dose of neuroleptic. May ↑ levels of **quetiapine**; if taking quetiapine when initiating therapy, consider alternative antiretroviral therapy or ↓ quetiapine dose to ⅙ of the original dose and monitor for adverse effects. May ↑ levels/toxicity of **PDE5 inhibitors**, including **sildenafil**, **tadalafil**, and **vardenafil**; *Dosing adjustment for pulmonary hypertension*—sildenafil is contraindicated; in patients who have received elvitegravir/cobicistat/emtricitabine/tenofovir alafenamide for ≥7 days, start tadalafil at 20 mg once daily and carefully titrate if tolerating to 40 mg once daily; in patients already receiving tadalafil, discontinue tadalafil for ≥24 hr before initiating elvitegravir/cobicistat/emtricitabine/tenofovir alafenamide; after ≥1 wk, resume tadalafil at 20 mg once daily and titrate if tolerating to 40 mg once daily; *Dosing adjustment for erectile dysfunction*—sildenafil dose should not exceed 25 mg in 48 hr, vardenafil dose should not exceed 2.5 mg in 72 hr, and tadalafil dose should not exceed 10 mg in 72 hr. ↑ levels/toxicity of **sedative/hypnotics**, including **midazolam** (parenteral), **diazepam**, **buspirone**, and **zolpidem**; consider dose ↓ of parenteral midazolam; clinical monitoring and dose ↓, if necessary, is recommended for other sedative/hypnotics. May ↑ bleeding risk with **rivaroxaban**; avoid concurrent use. May ↑ bleeding risk with **apixaban**; if taking apixaban 5–10 mg twice daily, ↓ apixaban dose by 50%; if taking apixaban 2.5 mg twice daily, avoid concurrent use. May ↑ bleeding risk with **betrixaban**; ↓ betrixaban dose by 50%. May ↑ bleeding risk with **dabigatran**; may need to avoid concurrent use if patient has moderate or severe renal impairment (depends on dabigatran indication). May ↑ bleeding risk with **edoxaban**; ↓ edoxaban dose by 50% when used for VTE treatment in patients with moderate or severe renal impairment.

Drug-Natural Products: **St. John's wort** may significantly ↓ levels/effectiveness of cobicistat and elvitegravir and ↑ risk of resistance; concurrent use contraindicated.

Route/Dosage

PO (Adults and Children ≥25 kg): 1 tablet once daily.

Renal Impairment

PO (Adults): *CCr <15 mL/min AND receiving chronic hemodialysis*—1 tablet once daily (give after dialysis on dialysis days).

Availability

Tablets: elvitegravir 150 mg/cobicistat 150 mg/emtricitabine 200 mg/tenofovir alafenamide 10 mg.

NURSING IMPLICATIONS

Assessment

- Assess patient for change in severity of HIV symptoms and for symptoms of opportunistic infections during therapy.
- ***Lab Test Considerations:*** Monitor viral load and CD4 count before and routinely during therapy to determine response.
- Assess for hepatitis B virus (HBV). *Genvoya* is not approved for administration in patients with HIV and HBV. If therapy is discontinued, may cause severe exacerbation of hepatitis B. Monitor liver function in co-infected patients for several mo after stopping therapy.
- Monitor liver function tests prior to, during and following therapy. May cause ↑ LDL cholesterol, total cholesterol, and triglyceride concentrations. Lactic acidosis may occur with hepatic toxicity causing hepatic steatosis; may be fatal, especially in women. Discontinue therapy if symptoms occur.
- Calculate serum creatinine, CCr, urine glucose, and urine protein prior to and periodically during therapy and when clinically indicated. In patients with chronic kidney disease, assess serum creatinine, creatinine clearance, serum phosphorus, urine glucose, and urine protein prior to and periodically during therapy. May cause hypophosphatemia in patients with renal impairment.
- May cause hyperglycemia and glycosuria.

Implementation

- Do not confuse elvitegravir, cobicistat, emtricitabine, and tenofovir alafenamide with elvitegravir, cobicistat, emtricitabine, and tenofovir disoproxil fumarate.
- **PO:** Administer once daily with food.
- Administer antacids at least 2 hr before or after medication.

Patient/Family Teaching

- Instruct patient on the importance of taking medication as directed, even if feeling better. Do not take more than prescribed amount and do not stop taking without consulting health care professional. Discontinuing therapy may lead to severe exacerbations. Take missed doses as soon as remembered unless almost time for next dose; do not double doses. Advise patient to read *Patient Information* prior to starting therapy and with each Rx refill in case of changes. Caution patient not to share or trade *Genvoya*™ with others.
- Inform patient of importance of hepatitis B testing before starting antiretroviral therapy.
- Advise patients if antacids containing aluminum, magnesium hydroxide, or calcium carbonate, take at least 2 hrs before or after *Genvoya*™.
- Instruct patient to notify health care professional of all Rx or OTC medications, vitamins, or herbal products being taken and consult health care professional before taking any new medications, especially St. John's wort.
- Advise patient to notify health care professional immediately if symptoms of lactic acidosis (nausea, vomiting, unusual or unexpected stomach discomfort, unusual muscle pain, difficulty breathing, feeling cold, especially in arms and legs, dizziness, fast or irregular heartbeat, and weakness or tiredness) liver problems (yellow skin or whites of eyes, dark urine, light colored stools, loss of appetite, nausea, stomach pain) or signs of Immune Reconstitution Syndrome (signs and symptoms of an infection or inflammation) occur.
- Inform patient that *Genvoya* does not cure AIDS and does not reduce the risk of transmission of HIV to others through sexual contact or blood contamination. Caution patient to use a condom and avoid sharing needles or donating blood to prevent spreading HIV to others.
- Rep: Advise patient to notify health care professional if pregnancy is planned or suspected. Encourage pregnant women to enroll in the Antiretroviral Pregnancy Registry by calling 1-800-258-4263. Advise female patient to avoid breast feeding during therapy.
- Emphasize the importance of regular follow-up exams and blood counts to determine progress and monitor for side effects.

Evaluation/Desired Outcomes

- Slowed progression of HIV infection and decreased occurrence of sequelae.

empagliflozin

(em-pag-gli-**floe**-zin)
Jardiance

Classification
Therapeutic: antidiabetics
Pharmacologic: sodium-glucose co-transporter 2 (SGLT2) inhibitors

Indications

Adjunct to diet and exercise in the management of type 2 diabetes. To reduce risk of cardiovascular death in patients with type 2 diabetes and established cardiovascular disease.

Action

Inhibits proximal renal tubular sodium-glucose co-transporter 2 (SGLT2) which determines reabsorption of glucose from the tubular lumen. Inhibits reabsorption of glucose, lowers renal threshold for glucose and increases excretion of glucose in urine. **Therapeutic Effects:** Improved glycemic control. Reduced death due to cardiovascular causes.

Pharmacokinetics

Absorption: Well absorbed following oral administration.

Distribution: Enters red blood cells, remainder of distribution unknown.

Metabolism and Excretion: Minimally metabolized; excreted in feces (41.2% mostly as unchanged drug) and urine (54.4% half as unchanged drug, half as metabolites).

Half-life: 12.4 hr.

TIME/ACTION PROFILE (↓ in A1c)

ROUTE	ONSET	PEAK	DURATION
PO	within 6 wk	12 wk	unknown

Contraindications/Precautions

Contraindicated in: Hypersensitivity; Severe renal impairment (eGFR <30 mL/min/1.73 m^2/end-stage renal disease/dialysis); Type 1 diabetes; Diabetic ketoacidosis; Lactation: Avoid use, discontinue breast feeding or discontinue empagliflozin.

Use Cautiously in: Moderate renal impairment (eGFR 30–<45 mL/min/1.73 m^2); use not recommended; Hypotension (correct prior to treatment, especially in renal impairment, age >65 yr, or concurrent use of loop diuretics, ACE inhibitors, or ARBs; History of bladder cancer; History of pancreatitis, pancreatic surgery, reduced caloric intake due to illness or surgery, or alcohol abuse (↑ risk of ketoacidosis); Hypovolemia, chronic kidney disease, HF (↑ risk of acute kidney injury); OB: Use only if potential maternal benefit justifies potential fetal risk; Pedi: Safety and effectiveness not established; Geri: ↑ risk of adverse reactions related to ↓ intravascular volume.

Adverse Reactions/Side Effects

CV: hypotension, volume depletion. **Endo:** hypoglycemia (↑ with other medications). **F and E:** KETOACIDOSIS, hyperphosphatemia. **GU:** NECROTIZING FASCIITIS OF PERINEUM (FOURNIER'S GANGRENE), UROSEPSIS, acute kidney injury, genital mycotic infections, ↑ urination, urinary tract infection (including pyelonephritis), renal impairment. **Metab:** hyperlipidemia. **Misc:** HYPERSENSITIVITY REACTIONS (including angioedema).

Interactions

Drug-Drug: ↑ risk of hypotension with **antihypertensives** or **diuretics**. ↑ risk of hypoglycemia with other **antidiabetics** (dose adjustments may be required). ↑ risk of acute kidney injury with **diuretics**, **ACE inhibitors**, **angiotensin receptor blockers**, or **NSAIDs**.

Route/Dosage

PO (Adults): 10 mg once daily, may be ↑ to 25 mg once daily.

Availability

Tablets: 10 mg, 25 mg. ***In combination with:*** linagliptin (Glyxambi); metformin (Synjardy); metformin XR (Synjardy XR). See Appendix B.

NURSING IMPLICATIONS

Assessment

- Observe patient for signs and symptoms of hypoglycemic reactions (sweating, hunger, weakness, dizziness, confusion, headache, tremor, tachycardia, irritability, drowsiness).
- Monitor for signs and symptoms of volume depletion (dizziness, feeling faint, weakness, orthostatic hypotension) after initiating therapy, especially in elderly patients and patients with renal impairment, low systolic BP, or on diuretics.
- Monitor for signs and symptoms of urinary tract infection during therapy. Treat promptly.
- Monitor for infection, new pain, tenderness, erythema, swelling, sores, or ulcers involving lower limbs, with fever or malaise; discontinue empagliflozin if these occur.
- Assess for ketoacidosis in patients presenting with signs and symptoms of dehydration and metabolic acidosis (nausea, vomiting, abdominal pain, malaise, shortness of breath), regardless of blood glucose level. Discontinue empagliflozin and treat promptly (insulin, fluid and caloric replacement) if suspected. Consider risk factors for ketoacidosis (pancreatic insulin deficiency, caloric restriction, alcohol abuse) before starting empagliflozin.
- ***Lab Test Considerations:*** Monitor hemoglobin A1C prior to and periodically during therapy.
- May ↑ serum creatinine and ↓ eGFR. Monitor renal function prior to starting and periodically during therapy. Do not begin therapy if eGFR <45 mL/min/1.73 m^2. Discontinue therapy if eGFR is persistently <45 mL/min/1.73 m^2.
- May cause ↑ serum phosphate levels. Monitor electrolytes periodically during therapy.
- May cause ↑ LDL-C. Monitor serum lipid levels periodically during therapy.
- May cause ↑ hematocrit.
- Monitor for ketoacidosis, especially during prolonged fasting for illness or surgery. May require temporary discontinuation of therapy.

Implementation

- Patients stabilized on a diabetic regimen who are exposed to stress, fever, trauma, infection, or surgery may require administration of insulin.
- Correct volume depletion prior to beginning therapy with empagliflozin.
- **PO:** Administer once daily in the morning with or without food.

Patient/Family Teaching

- Instruct patient to take empagliflozin as directed. Take missed doses as soon as remembered, unless it is almost time for next dose; do not double doses. Advise patient to read the *Medication Guide* before starting and with each Rx refill in case of changes.
- Explain to patient that empagliflozin helps control hyperglycemia but does not cure diabetes. Therapy is usually long term.

- Instruct patient not to share this medication with others, even if they have the same symptoms; it may harm them.
- Encourage patient to follow prescribed diet, medication, and exercise regimen to prevent hyperglycemic or hypoglycemic episodes.
- Review signs of hypoglycemia and hyperglycemia with patient. If hypoglycemia occurs, advise patient to take a glass of orange juice or 2–3 tsp of sugar, honey, or corn syrup dissolved in water, and notify health care professional.
- Instruct patient in proper testing of serum glucose and ketones, especially during periods of stress or illness. Inform patient that empagliflozin will cause a positive test result when testing for urine glucose. Notify health care professional if significant changes occur.
- Advise patient to notify health care professional if new pain or tenderness, sores or ulcers, or infections involving the leg or foot occur and to immediately seek care if pain or tenderness, redness, or swelling of the genitals or area from the genitals back to the rectum, along with a fever above 100.4°F or malaise occur.
- Advise patient to notify health care professional if signs and symptoms of hypotension occur and to maintain adequate hydration as dehydration may increase risk of hypotension.
- Inform patient that empagliflozin may cause mycotic (yeast) infections. Women may have signs and symptoms of a vaginal yeast infection (vaginal odor, white or yellow vaginal discharge [may be lumpy or look like cottage cheese], vaginal itching). Men may have signs and symptoms of a yeast infection of the penis (redness, itching or swelling of penis; rash on penis; foul smelling discharge from penis; pain in skin around penis). Advise patient to notify health care professional if yeast infection occurs.
- Advise patient to notify health care professional if signs and symptoms of urinary tract infection (burning feeling when passing urine, cloudy urine, pain in pelvis or back) occur.
- Advise patient to notify health care professional of all Rx or OTC medications, vitamins, or herbal products being taken and to consult with health care professional before taking other medications, especially other oral hypoglycemic medications.
- Advise patient to notify health care professional promptly if signs and symptoms of hypersensitivity reactions (rash; raised red patches on skin; swelling of face, lips, tongue, throat; difficulty breathing or swallowing) occur.
- Advise patient to notify health care professional if pregnancy is planned or suspected and to avoid breast feeding during therapy.
- Encourage patient to follow up with routine lab tests for blood glucose and renal function.

Evaluation/Desired Outcomes

- Improved hemoglobin A1C and glycemic control in adults with Type 2 diabetes.

E

emtricitabine

(em-tri-**si**-ti-been)

Emtriva

Classification

Therapeutic: antiretrovirals

Pharmacologic: nucleoside reverse transcriptase inhibitors

Indications

HIV infection (with other antiretrovirals).

Action

Phosphorylated intracellularly where it inhibits HIV reverse transcriptase, resulting in viral DNA chain termination. **Therapeutic Effects:** Slowed progression of HIV infection and decreased occurrence of sequelae. Increases CD4 cell counts and decreases viral load.

Pharmacokinetics

Absorption: Rapidly and extensively absorbed; 93% bioavailable.

Distribution: Unknown.

Metabolism and Excretion: Some metabolism, 86% renally excreted, 14% fecal excretion.

Half-life: 10 hr.

TIME/ACTION PROFILE (blood levels†)

ROUTE	ONSET	PEAK	DURATION
PO	rapid	1–2 hr	24 hr

†Normal renal function.

Contraindications/Precautions

Contraindicated in: Hypersensitivity; Lactation: Breast feeding not recommended in HIV-infected patients.

Use Cautiously in: Hepatitis B co-infection (may exacerbate following discontinuation); Renal impairment; OB: Use during pregnancy only if benefit to patient outweighs potential risk to fetus; Geri: May be at ↑ risk for adverse effects.

Adverse Reactions/Side Effects

CNS: dizziness, headache, insomnia, weakness, depression, nightmares. **Derm:** rash, skin discoloration. **F and E:** LACTIC ACIDOSIS. **GI:** abdominal pain, diarrhea, nausea, SEVERE HEPATOMEGALY WITH STEATOSIS, dyspepsia, vomiting. **MS:** arthralgia, myalgia. **Neuro:** neuropathy, paresthesia. **Resp:** cough, rhinitis. **Misc:** immune reconstitution syndrome.

Interactions

Drug-Drug: None noted.

Route/Dosage

PO (Adults ≥18 yr): 200 mg once daily.

Renal Impairment

PO (Adults ≥18 yr): *CCr 30–49 mL/min*—200 mg every 48 hr; *CCr 15–29 mL/min*—200 mg every 72 hr; *CCr <15 mL/min*—200 mg every 96 hr.

Availability (generic available)

Capsules: 200 mg. **Oral solution (cotton candy flavor):** 10 mg/mL. ***In combination with:*** efavirenz and tenofovir (Atripla); tenofovir (Truvada); rilpivirine and tenofovir (Complera); elvitegravir, cobicistat, and tenofovir disoproxil fumarate (Stribild); cobicistat, darunavir, and tenofovir alafenamide (Symtuza). See Appendix B.

NURSING IMPLICATIONS

Assessment

- Assess patient for change in severity of HIV symptoms and for symptoms of opportunistic infections during therapy.
- May cause lactic acidosis and severe hepatomegaly with steatosis. These events are more likely to occur if patients are female, obese, or receiving nucleoside analogue medications for extended periods of time. Monitor patient for signs (increased serum lactate levels, elevated liver enzymes, liver enlargement on palpation). Therapy should be suspended if clinical or laboratory signs occur.
- ***Lab Test Considerations:*** Monitor viral load and CD4 cell count regularly during therapy.
- Test patients for chronic hepatitis B virus (HBV) before initiating therapy. Emtricitabine is not indicated for treatment of HBV. If therapy is discontinued, may cause severe exacerbation of hepatitis B. Monitor liver function in co-infected patients for several mo after stopping therapy.
- May cause ↑ AST, ALT, bilirubin, creatine kinase, serum amylase, serum lipase, and triglycerides. May cause ↑ or ↓ serum glucose. May cause ↓ neutrophil count.

Implementation

- **PO:** May be administered with or without food.

Patient/Family Teaching

- Emphasize the importance of taking emtricitabine as directed. It must always be used in combination with other antiretroviral drugs. Do not take more than prescribed amount and do not stop taking without consulting health care professional. Take missed doses as soon as remembered, but not if almost time for next dose; do not double doses. Advise patient to read *Patient Information* before starting therapy and with each Rx refill in case of changes.
- Instruct patient that emtricitabine should not be shared with others.
- Inform patient that emtricitabine does not cure AIDS or prevent associated or opportunistic infections. Emtricitabine does not reduce the risk of transmission of HIV to others through sexual contact or blood contamination. Caution patient to use a condom and to avoid sharing needles or donating blood to prevent spreading the AIDS virus to others. Advise patient that the long-term effects of emtricitabine are unknown at this time.
- Instruct patient to notify health care professional of all Rx or OTC medications, vitamins, or herbal products being taken and consult health care professional before taking any new medications.
- Instruct patient to notify health care professional immediately if symptoms of lactic acidosis (tiredness or weakness, unusual muscle pain, trouble breathing, stomach pain with nausea and vomiting, cold especially in arms or legs, dizziness, fast or irregular heartbeat) or if signs of hepatotoxicity (yellow skin or whites of eyes, dark urine, light colored stools, lack of appetite for several days or longer, nausea, abdominal pain) occur. These symptoms may occur more frequently in patients that are female, obese, or have been taking medications like emtricitabine for a long time.
- Advise patient to notify health care professional if signs and symptoms of Immune Reconstitution Syndrome (signs and symptoms of an infection) occur.
- Rep: Advise patient to notify health care professional if pregnancy is planned or suspected. Encourage pregnant women to enroll in the Antiretroviral Pregnancy Registry by calling 1-800-258-4263. Advise female patient to avoid breast feeding during therapy.
- Emphasize the importance of regular follow-up exams and blood counts to determine progress and monitor for side effects.

Evaluation/Desired Outcomes

- Delayed progression of AIDS and decreased opportunistic infections in patients with HIV.
- Decrease in viral load and increase in CD4 cell counts.

emtricitabine/rilpivirine/tenofovir alafenamide

(em-tri-**sye**-ti-been/**ril**-pi-vir-een/te-**noe**-fo-veer al-a-**fen**-a-mide)

Odefsey

Classification

Therapeutic: antiretrovirals

Pharmacologic: nucleoside reverse transcriptase inhibitors, non-nucleoside reverse transcriptase inhibitors

Indications

Management of HIV infection in treatment-naïve patients with HIV-1 RNA <100,000 copies/mL at the start of therapy (for use as a complete regimen). Management of HIV infection in patients on a stable antiretroviral regimen with HIV-1 RNA <50 copies/mL for ≥6 mo and have no history of treatment failure or no known substitutions associated with resistance to the individual components of the medication (to replace their current antiretroviral regimen).

Action

Emtricitabine—Phosphorylated intracellularly where it inhibits HIV reverse transcriptase, resulting in viral DNA chain termination. *Rilpivirine*—Inhibits HIV-replication by noncompetitively inhibiting HIV reverse transcriptase. *Tenofovir*—Phosphorylated intracellularly where it inhibits HIV reverse transcriptase resulting in disruption of DNA synthesis. **Therapeutic Effects:** Slowed progression of HIV infection and decreased occurrence of sequelae.

Pharmacokinetics

emtricitabine

Absorption: Rapidly and extensively absorbed; 93% bioavailable.

Distribution: Unknown.

Metabolism and Excretion: Some metabolism, 86% renally excreted, 14% fecal excretion.

Half-life: 10 hr.

rilpivirine

Absorption: Well absorbed following oral administration.

Distribution: Unknown.

Protein Binding: 99.7%.

Metabolism and Excretion: Primarily metabolized by the liver via CYP3A; 25% excreted in feces unchanged, <1% excreted unchanged in urine.

Half-life: 50 hr.

tenofovir alafenamide

Absorption: Tenofovir alafenamide is a prodrug, which is hydrolyzed into tenofovir, the active component; absorption enhanced by high-fat meals.

Distribution: Unknown.

Metabolism and Excretion: Tenofovir is phosphorylated to tenofovir diphosphate (active metabolite); 32% excreted in feces, <1% in urine.

Half-life: 0.51 hr.

TIME/ACTION PROFILE (blood levels)

ROUTE	ONSET	PEAK	DURATION
emtricitabine PO	rapid	1–2 hr	24 hr
rilpivirine PO	unknown	4–5 hr	24 hr
tenofovir PO	unknown	1 hr	24 hr

Contraindications/Precautions

Contraindicated in: Concurrent use of carbamazepine, oxcarbazepine, phenobarbital, phenytoin, rifampin, rifapentine, proton pump inhibitors, dexamethasone (>1 dose), or St. John's wort; Severe renal impairment (CCr <30 mL/min); Lactation: HIV-infected patients should not breast feed.

Use Cautiously in: History of suicidal ideation or depression; HIV-1 RNA >100,000 copies/mL (↑ risk of virologic failure); Hepatitis B or C infection or hepatic impairment; Renal impairment or receiving nephrotoxic medications (↑ risk of renal impairment); Severe hepatic impairment; OB: Use during pregnancy only if potential benefit justifies potential fetal risk (monitor viral load closely); Pedi: Children <12 yr (safety and effectiveness not established).

E

Adverse Reactions/Side Effects

CNS: SUICIDAL ATTEMPTS/THOUGHTS, depression, headache, sleep disturbances. **CV:** QT INTERVAL PROLONGATION. **Derm:** DRUG REACTION WITH EOSINOPHILIA AND SYSTEMIC SYMPTOMS (DRESS). **GI:** ACUTE EXACERBATION OF HEPATITIS B, HEPATOTOXICITY, LACTIC ACIDOSIS/HEPATOMEGALY WITH STEATOSIS. **GU:** renal impairment. **Metab:** hyperlipidemia. **Misc:** immune reconstitution syndrome.

Interactions

Drug-Drug: Strong CYP3A4 inducers, including **carbamazepine**, **oxcarbazepine**, **phenobarbital**, **phenytoin**, **dexamethasone** (more than a single dose), **rifampin**, and **rifapentine** may ↓ rilpivirine levels and its effectiveness; concurrent use contraindicated. **Proton pump inhibitors** including **esomeprazole**, **lansoprazole**, **omeprazole**, **pantoprazole**, and **rabeprazole** ↑ gastric pH and may ↓ rilpivirine levels and its effectiveness; concurrent use contraindicated. Concurrent use of **QT interval prolonging medications** may ↑ risk of torsades de pointes. Medications that compete for active tubular secretion, including **acyclovir**, **cidofovir**, **ganciclovir**, **valacyclovir**, **valganciclovir**, or **aminoglycosides** may ↑ emtricitabine and tenofovir levels and toxicity; avoid if possible. **Antacids** including **aluminum hydroxide**, **magnesium hydroxide**, and **calcium carbonate** ↑ gastric pH and may ↓ rilpivirine levels; administer antacid ≥2 hr before or ≥4 hr after. Blood levels and effectiveness may be ↓ by **H_2-antagonists** including **cimetidine**, **famotidine**, **nizatidine**, and **ranitidine**↑ gastric pH and may ↓ rilpivirine levels; administer H_2-antagonist ≥12 hr before or ≥4 hr after. Nephrotoxic agents, including **NSAIDs** ↑ risk of nephrotoxicity; avoid concurrent use. **Rifabutin** may ↓ rilpivirine and tenofovir alafenamide levels and their effectiveness; concurrent use not recommended. **Fluconazole**, **itraconazole**, **ketoconazole**, **posaconazole**, and **voriconazole** may ↑ rilpivirine and tenofovir alafenamide levels and risk of toxicity. May ↓ **ketoconazole** levels. May alter requirements for **methadone** maintenance. **Clarithromycin** or **ery-**

thromycin may ↑ rilpivirine levels and risk of toxicity; consider azithromycin as an alternative. **Ledipasvir/sofosbuvir**, **sofosbuvir/velpatasvir**, and **sofosbuvir/velpatasvir/voxilaprevir** may ↑ tenofovir levels.
Drug-Natural Products: **St. John's wort** may ↓ rilpivirine levels and its effectiveness; concurrent use contraindicated.

Route/Dosage

PO (Adults and Children ≥12 yr and ≥35 kg): 1 tablet once daily.

Availability

Tablets: emtricitabine 200 mg/rilpivirine 25 mg/ tenofovir alafenamide 25 mg.

NURSING IMPLICATIONS

Assessment

- Assess for change in severity of HIV symptoms and for symptoms of opportunistic infections during therapy.
- Monitor for signs and symptoms of DRESS (fever; rash with fever, blisters, mucosal involvement, eye inflammation (conjunctivitis); lymphadenopathy, and/or facial swelling, associated with involvement of other organ systems (hepatitis, nephritis, hematologic abnormalities, myocarditis, myositis) during therapy. May resemble an acute viral infection. Eosinophilia is often present. Discontinue therapy if signs occur.
- Assess mental status (orientation, mood, behavior) before and periodically during therapy. Monitor closely for notable changes in behavior that could indicate the emergence or worsening of suicidal thoughts or behavior or depression.
- ***Lab Test Considerations:*** Monitor viral load and CD4 cell count regularly during therapy.
- Assess for hepatitis B virus (HBV). *Odefsey* is not approved for administration in patients with HIV and HBV. If therapy is discontinued, may cause severe exacerbation of hepatitis B. Monitor liver function in co-infected patients for several mo after stopping therapy.
- Monitor liver function tests before and periodically during therapy, especially in patients with underlying liver disease or marked ↑ transaminase. May cause ↑ serum creatinine, AST, ALT, total bilirubin, total cholesterol, LDL, and triglycerides. May cause lactic acidosis and severe hepatomegaly with steatosis. These events are more likely to occur if patients are female, obese, or receiving nucleoside analogue medications for extended periods of time. Monitor patient for signs (increased serum lactate levels, elevated liver enzymes, liver enlargement on palpation). Therapy should be suspended if clinical or laboratory signs occur.
- Assess serum creatinine, creatinine clearance, urine glucose, and urine protein before starting and periodically during therapy. Also assess serum phosphorous in patients with chronic kidney disease. Patients taking nephrotoxic agents, including NSAIDs are at increased risk for renal impairment.

Implementation

- **PO:** Administer once daily with a meal.

Patient/Family Teaching

- Instruct patient to take medication as directed. Avoid missing doses, may result in development of resistance. Do not stop taking *Odefsey* without consulting health care professional. Advise patient to read *Patient Information* before starting and with each Rx refill in case of changes.
- Instruct patient that *Odefsey* should not be shared with others.
- Advise patient to notify health care professional immediately if symptoms of lactic acidosis (nausea, vomiting, unusual or unexpected stomach discomfort, and weakness), hypersensitivity (swelling of face, eyes, lips, mouth, tongue or throat; difficulty swallowing shortness of breath), severe liver problems (yellow skin or white part of eyes, dark "tea-colored" urine, light-colored stools, loss of appetite, nausea, stomach-area pain), or DRESS occur.
- Inform patients and families of risk of suicidal thoughts and behavior and advise that behavioral changes, emergency or worsening signs and symptoms of depression, unusual changes in mood, or emergence of suicidal thoughts, behavior, or thoughts of self-harm should be reported to health care professional immediately.
- Immune reconstitution syndrome may trigger opportunistic infections or autoimmune disorders. Notify health care professional if symptoms occur.
- Advise patient to notify health care professional of all Rx or OTC medications, vitamins, or herbal products being taken and to consult with health care professional before taking other medications, especially St. John's wort.
- **Rep:** Advise patients to notify health care professional if pregnancy is planned or suspected. Advise patient to avoid breast feeding during *Odefsey* therapy. Encourage women who become pregnant during *Odefsey* therapy to enroll in Antiviral Pregnancy Registry by calling 1-800-258-4263.

Evaluation/Desired Outcomes

- Delayed progression of AIDS and decreased opportunistic infections in patients with HIV.
- Decrease in viral load and increase in CD4 cell counts.

enalapril/enalaprilat, See ANGIOTENSIN-CONVERTING ENZYME (ACE) INHIBITORS.

encorafenib

(en-koe-**raf**-e-nib)

Braftovi

Classification

Therapeutic: antineoplastics

Pharmacologic: kinase inhibitors

Indications

Treatment of metastatic or unresectable melanoma in patients with the BRAF V600E or V600K mutation (in combination with binimetinib).

Action

Kinase inhibitor that targets BRAF V600E, a mutated enzyme that promotes tumor cell proliferation. **Therapeutic Effects:** Improvement in progression-free survival and overall survival in patients with melanoma.

Pharmacokinetics

Absorption: Well absorbed (86%) following oral administration.

Distribution: Extensively distributed to tissues.

Metabolism and Excretion: Mostly metabolized by CYP3A4 and CYP2C19 enzyme systems. Primarily excreted as metabolites in feces (42%) and urine (45%).

Half-life: 3.5 hr.

TIME/ACTION PROFILE (plasma concentrations)

ROUTE	ONSET	PEAK	DURATION
PO	unknown	2 hr	24 hr

Contraindications/Precautions

Contraindicated in: Wild-type BRAF melanoma (may ↑ proliferation); Long QT syndrome, bradyarrhythmias, severe or decompensated HF, hypokalemia, or hypomagnesemia (↑ risk of QT interval prolongation); Concurrent use of QT-interval prolonging medications; Baseline QTc interval >500 msec; Concurrent use of strong or moderate CYP3A4 inhibitors or inducers (may significantly alter levels and effects); OB: Pregnancy (may cause fetal harm); Lactation: Lactation.

Use Cautiously in: Moderate or severe hepatic impairment; Severe renal impairment; Rep: Women of reproductive potential; Pedi: Safety and effectiveness not established.

Adverse Reactions/Side Effects

CNS: INTRACRANIAL HEMORRHAGE, dizziness, headache, fatigue, facial paralysis. **CV:** QT interval prolongation. **Derm:** BASAL CELL CARCINOMA, CUTANEOUS SQUAMOUS CELL CARCINOMA, alopecia, dry skin, hyperkeratosis, pruritus, rash, nodule formation. **EENT:** uveitis. **Endo:** hyperglycemia. **F and E:** hypermagnesemia, hyponatremia. **GU:** ↑ serum creatinine, ↓ fertility (males). **GI:** GI HEMORRHAGE, PANCREATITIS, abdominal pain, constipation, ↑ liver enzymes, nausea, vomiting. **Hemat:** BLEEDING, anemia, leukopenia, lymphopenia, neutropenia. **MS:** arthralgia, myalgia. **Neuro:** peripheral neuropathy. **Misc:** HYPERSENSITIVITY REACTIONS, MALIGNANCY, fever.

Interactions

Drug-Drug: QT interval prolonging drugs may ↑ the risk of QT interval prolongation and torsades de pointes; avoid concurrent use. **Strong or moderate CYP3A4 inhibitors**, including **diltiazem** and **posaconazole** may ↑ levels and risk of toxicity; avoid concurrent use, if possible (if must use concurrently, ↓ encorafenib dose). **Strong or moderate CYP3A4 inducers** may ↓ levels and effectiveness; avoid concurrent use. May ↓ effectiveness of **hormonal contraceptives**; use non-hormonal method of contraception.

Drug-Natural Products: St. John's wort may ↓ levels and effectiveness; avoid concurrent use.

Drug-Food: Grapefruit juice may ↑ levels and risk of toxicity; avoid concurrent use.

Route/Dosage

PO (Adults): 450 mg once daily until disease progression or unacceptable toxicity. *Concurrent use of moderate CYP3A4 inhibitor*—225 mg once daily (if planned dose 450 mg once daily); 150 mg once daily (if planned dose 300 mg once daily); 75 mg once daily (if planned dose 150 mg once daily); *Concurrent use of strong CYP3A4 inhibitor*—150 mg once daily (if planned dose 450 mg once daily); 75 mg once daily (if planned dose 300 mg once daily or 150 mg once daily).

Availability

Capsules: 75 mg.

NURSING IMPLICATIONS

Assessment

- Assess skin for lesions prior to starting, every 2 months during, and for up to 6 months following discontinuation of therapy. Manage suspicious skin lesions with excision and dermatopathologic evaluation. *For Grade 2 lesion,* if no improvement in 2 wk, hold encorafenib until Grade 0-1. Resume at same dose. *For Grade 3,* hold encorafenib until Grade 0-1. Resume at same dose if first occurrence or reduce dose if recurrent. *For Grade 4,* discontinue encorafenib permanently.
- Monitor for Non-Cutaneous RAS Mutation-positive Malignancies. Permanently discontinue encorafenib if these malignancies occur.
- Monitor for signs and symptoms of hemorrhage (bleeding GI, rectal, anal, hemorrhoidal) periodically during therapy. *If Grade 2 or 1st occurrence of Grade 3:* Withhold encorafenib up to 4 wk. If im-

proves to Grade 0-1 or to pretreatment level, resume at reduced dose. If no improvement, permanently discontinue encorafenib. *If 1st occurrence of Grade 4:* Discontinue encorafenib permanently or withhold up to 4 wk. If improves to Grade 0-1 or to pretreatment level, resume at reduced dose. If no improvement, permanently discontinue encorafenib. *If recurrent Grade 3:* Consider permanently discontinuing encorafenib. *If recurrent Grade 4:* permanently discontinue encorafenib.

- Monitor ECG in patients who already have or are at risk of QTc prolongation, including patients with known long QT syndromes, clinically significant bradyarrhythmias, severe or uncontrolled heart failure and those taking other medications leading to QT prolongation. *If QTcF >500 ms and ≤60 ms increase from baseline,* hold encorafenib until QTcF ≤500 ms. Resume at reduced dose. If occurs more than once, permanently discontinue encorafenib. *If QTcF >500 ms and >60 ms increase from baseline,* discontinue encorafenib permanently.
- Assess for signs and symptoms of uveitis (visual changes, eye pain) during therapy. Perform ophthalmologic exam regularly and for new or worsening visual disturbances; follow new or persistent ophthalmologic findings. *If Grade 1 or 2 does not respond to ocular therapy, or for Grade 3 uveitis,* withhold encorafenib for up to 6 wk. If improved, resume at same or reduced dose. If not improved, permanently discontinue encorafenib. *If Grade 4 uveitis occurs,* permanently discontinue encorafenib.
- ***Lab Test Considerations:*** Verify negative pregnancy status of females of reproductive potential prior to starting therapy.
- Monitor serum electrolytes periodically during therapy. Correct hypokalemia and hypomagnesemia prior to and during therapy. May also cause hyponatremia and hyperglycemia.
- May cause anemia, leukopenia, lymphopenia, and neutropenia.
- Monitor liver function periodically during therapy. May cause ↑ serum creatinine, GGT, AST, ALT, and alkaline phosphatase. *If Grade 2 AST or ALT ↑:* continue encorafenib dose. If no improvement within 4 wk, hold encorafenib until Grade 0-1 or to baseline levels, then resume at same dose. If no improvement, permanently discontinue encorafenib. *If Grade 3 AST or ALT ↑:* Consider permanently discontinuing encorafenib. *If Grade 4 AST or ALT ↑:* Permanently discontinue encorefenib.

Implementation

- Confirm the presence of a BRAF V600E or V600K mutation in tumor specimens prior to initiating therapy. Information on FDA-approved tests for the detection of BRAF V600E and V600K mutations in melanoma is available at http://www.fda.gov/CompanionDiagnostics.
- **Reduced dose recommendations**: *First dose reduction:* 300 mg (four 75 mg capsules) orally once daily. *Second dose reduction:* 225 mg (three 75 mg capsules) orally once daily. *Subsequent modification:* Permanently discontinue if unable to tolerate encorafenib 225 mg (three 75 mg capsules) once daily.
- **PO:** Administer once daily without regard to food in combination with binimetinib. If binimetinib is held, reduce encorafenib to maximum dose of 300 mg once daily until binimetinib is resumed. Store in original, tightly capped bottle at room temperature; do not remove desiccant, protect from moisture.

Patient/Family Teaching

- Instruct patient to take encorafenib with binimetinib as directed. Take missed dose within 12 hr of missed dose; do not take dose within 12 hr of next dose. Advise patient to read *Medication Guide* before starting therapy and with each Rx refill in case of changes.
- Inform patient that grapefruit products may increase amount of encorafenib in the body. Avoid grapefruit and grapefruit juice during therapy.
- Inform patient that encorafenib increases risk of developing new cutaneous malignancies. Notify health care professional immediately if new lesions (wart, skin sore or reddish bump that bleeds or does not heal) or changes in size or color of existing moles or lesions occur.
- Advise patient to notify health care professional immediately if signs and symptoms of bleeding (headaches, dizziness, weakness, coughing up blood or blood clots, vomiting blood or vomit looks like "coffee grounds", red or black stools that look like tar); liver dysfunction (yellow skin or whites of eyes; feeling tired; urine turns dark or brown; nausea or vomiting; loss of appetite; pain on right side of stomach); changes heart rhythm (feeling faint, lightheaded, dizzy, heart beating irregularly or fast); or eye problems (blurred vision, loss of vision, other vision changes, seeing colored dots, seeing halos or blurred outline around objects, eye pain, swelling, redness) occur.
- Advise patient to notify health care professional of all Rx or OTC medications, vitamins, or herbal products being taken and to consult with health care professional before taking other medications, especially St. John's wort.
- Rep: Advise female patient to use a highly effective form of contraception and avoid breast feeding during and for at least 2 wk after last dose of encorafenib. Use a non-hormonal form of contraception; encorafenib may decrease effectiveness of hormonal contraceptives. Advise patient to notify health care professional if pregnancy is suspected and to avoid breast feeding during and for at least 2 wk after last dose. Advise patients to seek counseling on fertility and family planning prior to beginning therapy; may impair fertility in males.

- Inform patient that regular assessments of skin and assessments for signs and symptoms of other malignancies must be done every 2 mo during and for up to 6 mo after therapy. Advise patient to notify health care professional immediately if any changes in skin occur.

Evaluation/Desired Outcomes

- Decreased spread of melanoma.

enoxaparin, See HEPARINS (LOW MOLECULAR WEIGHT).

entacapone (en-**tak**-a-pone)

Comtan

Classification

Therapeutic: antiparkinson agents

Pharmacologic: catechol-*O*-methyltransferase inhibitors

Indications

With levodopa/carbidopa to treat idiopathic Parkinson's disease when signs and symptoms of end-of-dose "wearing-off" (so-called fluctuating patients) occur.

Action

Acts as a selective and reversible inhibitor of the enzyme catechol *O*-methyltransferase (COMT). Inhibition of this enzyme prevents the breakdown of levodopa, increasing availability to the CNS. **Therapeutic Effects:** Prolongs duration of response to levodopa with end-of-dose motor fluctuations. Decreased signs and symptoms of Parkinson's disease.

Pharmacokinetics

Absorption: 35% absorbed following oral administration; absorption is rapid.

Distribution: Unknown.

Protein Binding: 98%.

Metabolism and Excretion: Minimal amounts excreted unchanged; highly metabolized followed by biliary excretion.

Half-life: *Initial phase*—0.4–0.7 hr; *second phase*—2.4 hr.

TIME/ACTION PROFILE (inhibition of COMT)

ROUTE	ONSET	PEAK	DURATION
PO	unknown	unknown	up to 8 hr

Contraindications/Precautions

Contraindicated in: Hypersensitivity; Concurrent nonselective MAO inhibitor therapy; Psychotic disorder.

Use Cautiously in: Hepatic impairment; Concurrent use of drugs that are metabolized by COMT; OB, Lactation: Safety not established; Pedi: No identified use in children.

Adverse Reactions/Side Effects

CNS: NEUROLEPTIC MALIGNANT SYNDROME, agitation, aggressive behavior, confusion, delirium, disorientation, dizziness, hallucinations, paranoid ideation, syncope, urges (gambling, sexual). **Resp:** pulmonary infiltrates, pleural effusion, pleural thickening. **CV:** hypotension. **Derm:** melanoma. **GI:** abdominal pain, colitis, diarrhea, nausea (during initiation), retroperitoneal fibrosis. **GU:** brownish-orange discoloration of urine. **MS:** RHABDOMYOLYSIS, dyskinesia. **Neuro:** dyskinesia.

Interactions

Drug-Drug: Concurrent use with selective **MAO inhibitors** is not recommended; both agents inhibit the metabolic pathways of catecholamines. Concurrent use of drugs that are metabolized by COMT such as **isoproterenol**, **epinephrine**, **norepinephrine**, **dopamine**, **dobutamine**, and **methyldopa** may ↑ risk of tachycardia, ↑ BP, and arrhythmias. **Probenecid**, **cholestyramine**, **erythromycin**, **rifampin**, **ampicillin**, and **chloramphenicol** may interfere with biliary elimination of entacapone; use concurrently with caution.

Route/Dosage

PO (Adults): 200 mg with each dose of levodopa/carbidopa up to a maximum of 8 times daily.

Availability (generic available)

Tablets: 200 mg. ***In combination with:*** levodopa/carbidopa (Stalevo), see Appendix B.

NURSING IMPLICATIONS

Assessment

- Assess parkinsonian and extrapyramidal symptoms (restlessness or desire to keep moving, rigidity, tremors, pill rolling, mask-like face, shuffling gait, muscle spasms, twisting motions, difficulty speaking or swallowing, loss of balance control) prior to and during therapy. Dyskinesia may increase with therapy.
- Monitor patient for development of diarrhea. Usually occurs within 4 to 12 wk of start of therapy, but may occur as early as the first wk and as late as mo after initiation of therapy.
- Monitor patient for signs and symptoms of neuroleptic malignant syndrome (elevated temperature, muscular rigidity, altered consciousness, elevated CPK). Symptoms have been associated with rapid dose reduction or withdrawal of other dopaminergic drugs. Withdrawal should be gradual.

Implementation

- **PO:** Always administer entacapone with levodopa/carbidopa. Entacapone has no antiparkinsonism effects of its own.

Patient/Family Teaching

- Encourage patient to take entacapone as directed. Take missed doses as soon as possible, up to 2 hr before the next dose. Taper gradually when discontinuing or a withdrawal reaction may occur.
- May cause dizziness or hallucinations. Advise patient to avoid driving or other activities that require alertness until response to the drug is known.
- Inform patient that nausea may occur, especially at initiation of therapy and diarrhea. Advise patient with diarrhea to drink fluids to maintain adequate hydration and monitor for weight loss. If diarrhea is prolonged, may resolve with discontinuation. Therapy may cause change in urine color to brownish orange.
- Caution patient to change positions slowly to minimize orthostatic hypotension.
- Advise patient to notify health care professional if suspicious or unusual skin changes, agitation, aggression, delirium, hallucinations, or new or increased gambling, sexual, or other intense urges occur.
- Instruct patient to notify health care professional if pregnancy is planned or suspected, or if breast feeding.
- Emphasize the importance of routine follow-up exams.

Evaluation/Desired Outcomes

- Decreased signs and symptoms of Parkinson's disease.

entecavir (en-tek-aveer)

Baraclude

Classification

Therapeutic: antivirals

Pharmacologic: nucleoside analogues

Indications

Chronic hepatitis B infection with evidence of active viral replication and either persistent elevations in AST or ALT or histologically active disease.

Action

Phosphorylated intracellularly to active form which acts as an analogue of guanosine, interfering with viral DNA synthesis. **Therapeutic Effects:** Decreased hepatic damage due to chronic hepatitis B infection.

Pharmacokinetics

Absorption: Well absorbed following oral administration.

Distribution: Extensive tissue distribution.

Metabolism and Excretion: 62–73% excreted unchanged by kidneys.

Half-life: Plasma—128–149 hr; intracellular—15 hr.

TIME/ACTION PROFILE (blood levels)

ROUTE	ONSET	PEAK	DURATION
PO	rapid	0.5–1 hr	24 hr

Contraindications/Precautions

Contraindicated in: Hypersensitivity.

Use Cautiously in: Renal impairment (dose ↓ recommended if CCr <50 mL/min; Liver transplant recipients (careful monitoring of renal function recommended); Patients coinfected with HIV (unless receiving highly active antiretroviral therapy; at ↑ risk for resistance); OB: Safety not established; Lactation: Use during breast feeding only if benefit to patient outweighs potential risk to infant; Pedi: Children <2 yr (safety and effectiveness not established); Geri: ↑ risk of toxicity due to age-related ↓ in renal function.

Adverse Reactions/Side Effects

CNS: dizziness, fatigue, headache. **Derm:** alopecia, rash. **F and E:** LACTIC ACIDOSIS. **GI:** HEPATOMEGALY (WITH STEATOSIS), dyspepsia, nausea.

Interactions

Drug-Drug: Concurrent use of drugs which may impair renal function may ↑ blood levels and risk of toxicity.

Route/Dosage

PO (Adults and Children >16 yr): *Compensated liver disease*—0.5 mg once daily (1 mg once daily if history of lamivudine resistance); *Decompensated liver disease*—1 mg once daily.

Renal Impairment

PO (Adults and Children >16 yr): *CCr 30–<50 mL/min*—0.25 mg once daily or 0.5 mg every 48 hr (0.5 mg once daily or 1 mg every 48 hr if history of lamivudine resistance) *CCr 10–<30 mL/min*—0.15 mg once daily or 0.5 mg every 72 hr (0.3 mg once daily or 1 mg every 72 hr if history of lamivudine resistance); *CCr <10 mL/min*—0.05 mg once daily or 0.5 mg every 7 days (0.1 mg once daily or 1 mg every 7 days if history of lamivudine resistance).

PO (Children 2–<16 yr and >30 kg): 0.5 mg once daily (1 mg once daily if history of lamivudine resistance).

PO (Children 2–<16 yr and >26–30 kg): 0.45 mg once daily (0.9 mg once daily if history of lamivudine resistance).

PO (Children 2–<16 yr and >23–26 kg): 0.4 mg once daily (0.8 mg once daily if history of lamivudine resistance).

PO (Children 2–<16 yr and >20–23 kg): 0.35 mg once daily (0.7 mg once daily if history of lamivudine resistance).

PO (Children 2–<16 yr and >17–20 kg): 0.3 mg once daily (0.6 mg once daily if history of lamivudine resistance).

PO (Children 2–<16 yr and >14–17 kg): 0.25 mg once daily (0.5 mg once daily if history of lamivudine resistance).
PO (Children 2–<16 yr and >11–14 kg): 0.2 mg once daily (0.4 mg once daily if history of lamivudine resistance).
PO (Children 2–<16 yr and 10–11 kg): 0.15 mg once daily (0.3 mg once daily if history of lamivudine resistance).

Availability (generic available)
Oral solution (orange flavor): 0.05 mg/mL. **Tablets:** 0.5 mg, 1 mg.

NURSING IMPLICATIONS
Assessment
- Monitor signs of hepatitis (jaundice, fatigue, anorexia, pruritus) during and for several mo following discontinuation of therapy. Exacerbations may occur when therapy is discontinued.
- May cause lactic acidosis and severe hepatomegaly with steatosis. Monitor patient for signs (↑ serum lactate levels, elevated liver enzymes, liver enlargement on palpation). Suspend therapy if clinical or laboratory signs occur.
- ***Lab Test Considerations:*** Monitor liver function closely during and for several mo following discontinuation of therapy. May cause ↑ AST, ALT, bilirubin, amylase, lipase, creatinine, and serum glucose. May cause ↓ serum albumin.

Implementation
- **PO:** Administer on an empty stomach at least 2 hr before or after a meal. Use oral solution for dose <0.5 mg and children up to 30 kg. Children >30 kg can use oral solution or tablet. Oral solution is ready to use; do not dilute or mix with water or any other liquid. Hold spoon in a vertical position and fill gradually to mark corresponding to prescribed dose. Rinse dosing spoon with water after each daily dose. Store in outer carton at room temperature. After opening, solution can be used until expiration date on bottle.

Patient/Family Teaching
- Instruct patient to take entecavir as directed. Advise patient to read the *Patient Information* with each refill and to take entecavir as directed. Take missed doses as soon as possible unless almost time for next dose. Do not run out of entecavir; get more when supply runs low. Do not double doses. Emphasize the importance of compliance with full course of therapy, not taking more than the prescribed amount, and not discontinuing without consulting health care professional. Inform patient that hepatitis exacerbation may occur upon discontinuation of therapy. Caution patient not to share medication with others.
- Inform patient that entecavir does not cure HBV disease, but may lower the amount of HBV in the body, lower the ability of HBV to multiply and infect new liver cells, and may improve the condition of the liver. Entecavir does not reduce the risk of transmission of HBV to others through sexual contact or blood contamination. Caution patient to use a condom during sexual contact and avoid sharing needles or donating blood to prevent spreading HBV to others.
- Advise patient to notify health care professional promptly if signs of lactic acidosis (weakness or tiredness; unusual muscle pain; trouble breathing; stomach pain with nausea and vomiting; feeling cold, especially in arms or legs; dizziness, fast or irregular heartbeat) or hepatotoxicity (jaundice, dark urine, light-colored bowel movements, anorexia, nausea, lower stomach pain) occur.
- May cause dizziness. Caution patient to avoid driving or other activities requiring alertness until response to medication is known.
- Instruct patient to notify health care professional of all Rx or OTC medications, vitamins, or herbal products being taken and to consult with health care professional before taking other medications.
- Discuss the possibility of hair loss with patient. Explore methods of coping.
- Rep: Advise patient to notify health care professional if pregnancy is planned or suspected. Encourage pregnant women to enroll in the Antiretroviral Pregnancy Registry by calling 1-800-258-4263. Advise female patient to avoid breast feeding during therapy.
- Emphasize the importance of regular follow-up exams and blood tests to determine progress and monitor for side effects.

Evaluation/Desired Outcomes
- Decreased hepatic damage due to chronic hepatitis B infection.

enzalutamide
(en-za-**loo**-ta-mide)
Xtandi

Classification
Therapeutic: antineoplastics
Pharmacologic: androgen receptor inhibitors

Indications
Management of castration-resistant prostate cancer.

Action
Acts as an androgen receptor inhibitor, preventing the binding of androgen; also inhibits androgen nuclear translocation and DNA interaction. Decreases prolif-

eration and induces cell death of prostate cancer cells. **Therapeutic Effects:** Decreased growth and spread of prostate cancer.

Pharmacokinetics

Absorption: Well absorbed following oral administration.

Distribution: Unknown.

Protein Binding: *Enzalutamide*—97–98%; *N-desmethylenzalutamide*—95%.

Metabolism and Excretion: Extensively metabolized by the liver (CYP2C8 and CYP3A4 enzyme systems); one metabolite (N-desmethylenzalutamide) has antineoplastic activity. Metabolites are primarily renally excreted, only minimal amounts as unchanged drug.

Half-life: *Enzalutamide*—5.8 days; *N-desmethylenzalutamide*—7.8–8.6 days.

TIME/ACTION PROFILE (improved survival)

ROUTE	ONSET	PEAK	DURATION
PO	3 mo	unknown	unknown

Contraindications/Precautions

Contraindicated in: OB: Rep: Pregnancy (may cause fetal harm) or women of reproductive potential.

Use Cautiously in: History of seizures, underlying brain pathology, cerebrovascular accident, transient ischemic attack (within 12 mo), brain metastases or brain arteriovenous malformation (may ↑ risk of seizures); Rep: Men with female partners of reproductive potential; Geri: May be more sensitive to drug effects; Pedi: Safety and effectiveness not established.

Adverse Reactions/Side Effects

CNS: POSTERIOR REVERSIBLE ENCEPHALOPATHY SYNDROME (PRES), SEIZURES, SPINAL CORD COMPRESSION/CAUDA EQUINA SYNDROME, headache, weakness, anxiety, dizziness, hallucinations, insomnia, mental impairment disorders. **CV:** peripheral edema, hypertension, ischemic heart disease. **Derm:** hot flush, dry skin, pruritus. **EENT:** epistaxis. **GI:** diarrhea. **GU:** hematuria, urinary frequency. **MS:** arthralgia, musculoskeletal pain, fracture, muscular stiffness, muscular weakness. **Neuro:** hypoesthesia, paresthesia. **Misc:** HYPERSENSITIVITY REACTIONS, falls.

Interactions

Drug-Drug: Strong CYP2C8 inhibitors, including **gemfibrozil**, may ↑ levels and risk of toxicity; avoid concurrent use (if concurrent administration necessary, ↓ enzalutamide dose). **Strong CYP3A4 inducers**, including **carbamazepine**, **phenobarbital**, **phenytoin**, **rifabutin**, **rifampin**, and **rifapentine** may ↓ levels and response; avoid concurrent use (if concurrent administration necessary, ↑ enzalutamide dose). May ↓ levels of **CYP3A4, CYP2C9, and CYP2C19 substrates** that have narrow therapeutic indexes including **cyclosporine**, **fentanyl**, **phenytoin**, **sirolimus**, **tacrolimus**, and **warfarin**; avoid concurrent use. **Drugs that ↓ seizure threshold** may ↑ risk of seizures.

Drug-Natural Products: St. John's wort may ↓ levels and response; avoid concurrent use (if concurrent administration necessary, ↑ enzalutamide dose).

Route/Dosage

Patients taking enzalutamide should also receive gonadotropin-releasing hormone (GnRH) analog concurrently or should have had bilateral orchiectomy.

PO (Adults): 160 mg (four 40-mg capsules) once daily; if ≥Grade 3 toxicity or intolerable adverse reactions occur, discontinue for 1 wk and resume at the same or lower dose (80 or 120 mg). *Concurrent use of strong CYP2C8 inhibitors*—80 mg once daily; *Concurrent use of strong CYP3A4 inducers*—240 mg once daily.

Availability

Capsules: 40 mg.

NURSING IMPLICATIONS

Assessment

- Monitor for seizures. Implement seizure precautions. If a seizure occurs during therapy, permanently discontinue enzalutamide therapy.
- Monitor for signs and symptoms of PRES (seizure, headache, lethargy, confusion, blindness, other visual and neurological disturbances, hypertension) during therapy. Diagnosis is made with MRI. Discontinue enzalutamide in patients who develop PRES.
- Monitor for signs and symptoms of hypersensitivity reactions (swelling of face, tongue, lips or throat; dyspnea). Discontinue enzalutamide if serious hypersensitivity reactions occur.
- Monitor for signs and symptoms of ischemic heart disease (chest pain, fainting, dyspnea). Permanently discontinue enzalutamide if Grade 3 or 4 ischemic heart disease symptoms occur.
- Assess risk of falls and fractures periodically during therapy.
- ***Lab Test Considerations:*** May cause hematuria.

Implementation

- **PO:** Administer 4 capsules once daily without regard to food. Swallow capsules whole; do not open, dissolve, or chew.
- If ≥Grade 3 toxicity or intolerable side effects occur, hold dose for 1 wk or until symptoms improve to <Grade 2, then resume at same or reduced dose (120 mg or 80 mg).

Patient/Family Teaching

- Instruct patient to take enzalutamide as directed at the same time each day. Take missed doses as soon as remembered within the same day. If a whole day is missed, omit dose and take next day's scheduled dose; do not double doses. Advise patient not to interrupt, modify dose, or stop taking enzalutamide without consulting health care professional. Advise patient to read *Patient Information* before starting therapy and with each Rx refill in case of changes.

- May cause seizures, dizziness, mental impairment, paresthesia, hypoesthesia, falls, and hallucinations. Caution patient to avoid driving and other activities requiring alertness until response to medication is known. Notify health care professional immediately if loss of consciousness, seizure, chest pain, or signs and symptoms of PRES or hypersensitivity reactions occur.
- Inform patient of common side effects associated with enzalutamide: asthenia/fatigue, back pain, diarrhea, arthralgia, hot flush, peripheral edema, musculoskeletal pain, headache, upper and lower respiratory infection, muscular weakness, dizziness, insomnia, spinal cord compression, cauda equina syndrome, hematuria, paresthesia, anxiety, and hypertension. Notify health care professional if falls or problems thinking clearly, or if side effects are bothersome.
- Instruct patient to notify health care professional of all Rx or OTC medications, vitamins, or herbal products being taken and to consult health care professional before taking other Rx, OTC, or herbal products.
- Rep: Caution patients that enzalutamide is teratogenic and may cause loss of pregnancy. Advise patient to avoid pregnancy and breast feeding during and for 3 mo following completion of therapy. Instruct females of reproductive potential to avoid handling enzalutamide tablets. Advise males with female partners of reproductive potential to use a condom and effective contraception during and for 3 mo after last dose. May impair fertility in males.

Evaluation/Desired Outcomes

- Decreased growth and spread of prostate cancer.

HIGH ALERT

EPINEPHrine (ep-i-nef-rin)

Adrenaclick, Adrenalin, ✱Allerject, ✱Anapen, ✱Anapen Junior, ~~AsthmaNefrin~~, Auvi-Q, EpiPen, Primatene Mist, ✱S-2 (racepinephrine), Symjepi, ~~Twin-Ject~~

Classification

Therapeutic: antiasthmatics, bronchodilators, vasopressors

Pharmacologic: adrenergics

See Appendix C for ophthalmic use

Indications

Subcut, IM, IV: Severe allergic reactions. **IV:** Hypotension associated with septic shock. **Inhaln:** Upper airway obstruction and croup (racemic epinephrine). Temporary relief of mild symptoms of intermittent asthma (over-the-counter). **Local/Spinal:** Adjunct in the localization/prolongation of anesthesia. **Unlabeled Use:** IV, Intracardiac, Intratracheal, Intraosseous (part of advanced cardiac life support [ACLS] and pediatric advanced life support [PALS] guidelines): Cardiac arrest. **Subcut, IM:** Reversible airway disease due to asthma or COPD.

Action

Results in the accumulation of cyclic adenosine monophosphate (cAMP) at beta-adrenergic receptors. Affects both $beta_1$ (cardiac)-adrenergic receptors and $beta_2$ (pulmonary)-adrenergic receptor sites. Produces bronchodilation. Also has alpha-adrenergic agonist properties, which result in vasoconstriction. Inhibits the release of mediators of immediate hypersensitivity reactions from mast cells. **Therapeutic Effects:** Bronchodilation. Maintenance of heart rate and BP. Localization/prolongation of local/spinal anesthetic.

Pharmacokinetics

Absorption: IV administration results in complete bioavailability; well absorbed following subcut administration; some absorption may occur following repeated inhalation of large doses.

Distribution: Does not cross the blood-brain barrier; crosses the placenta and enters breast milk.

Metabolism and Excretion: Action is rapidly terminated by metabolism and uptake by nerve endings.

Half-life: Unknown.

TIME/ACTION PROFILE (bronchodilation)

ROUTE	ONSET	PEAK	DURATION
Inhaln	1 min	unknown	1–3 hr
Subcut	5–10 min	20 min	<1–4 hr
IM	6–12 min	unknown	<1–4 hr
IV	rapid	20 min	20–30 min

Contraindications/Precautions

Contraindicated in: Hypersensitivity to adrenergic amines; Some products may contain bisulfites and should be avoided in patients with known hypersensitivity or intolerance.

Use Cautiously in: Cardiac disease (angina, tachycardia, MI); Hypertension; Hyperthyroidism; Parkinson's disease; Pheochromocytoma; Diabetes; Cerebral arteriosclerosis; Glaucoma (except for ophthalmic use); Excessive use may lead to tolerance and paradoxical bronchospasm (inhaler); OB: Use only if potential maternal benefit outweighs potential risks to fetus; Lactation: High intravenous doses of epinephrine might ↓ milk production or letdown. Low-dose epidural, topical, inhaled, or ophthalmic epinephrine are unlikely to interfere with breast feeding (NIH); Pedi: Children <12

E

yr (over-the-counter product only); Geri: More susceptible to adverse reactions; may require ↓ dose.

Adverse Reactions/Side Effects

CNS: nervousness, restlessness, tremor, headache, insomnia. **CV:** angina, arrhythmias, hypertension, tachycardia. **Derm:** skin and soft tissue infections (including necrotizing fasciitis and myonecrosis). **Endo:** hyperglycemia. **GI:** nausea, vomiting. **GU:** renal impairment. **Resp:** PARADOXICAL BRONCHOSPASM (EXCESSIVE USE OF INHALERS), pulmonary edema.

Interactions

Drug-Drug: Concurrent use with other **adrenergic agents** will have additive adrenergic side effects. Use with **MAO inhibitors** may lead to hypertensive crisis. **Beta blockers** may negate therapeutic effect. **Tricyclic antidepressants** enhance pressor response to epinephrine.
Drug-Natural Products: Use with caffeine-containing herbs (**cola nut, guarana, mate, tea, coffee**) ↑ stimulant effect.

Route/Dosage

Subcut, IM (Adults and Children ≥30 kg): *Severe anaphylaxis*—0.3–0.5 mg (single dose not to exceed 0.5 mg); may repeat every 10–15 min as needed.
Subcut (Children <30 kg): *Severe anaphylaxis*—0.01 mg/kg (not to exceed 0.3 mg/dose); may repeat every 10–15 min as needed; *Auvi-Q or Symjepi (15–30 kg)*—0.15 mg; may repeat if anaphylactic symptoms persist; *Auvi-Q (7.5–15 kg)*—0.1 mg; may repeat if anaphylactic symptoms persist.
IV (Adults): *Severe anaphylaxis*—0.1–0.25 mg every 5–15 min; may be followed by 1–4 mcg/min continuous infusion; *Cardiopulmonary resuscitation (ACLS guidelines)*—1 mg every 3–5 min; *Bradycardia (ACLS guidelines)*—2–10 mcg/min continuous infusion; *Hypotension associated with septic shock*—0.05–2 mcg/kg/min continuous infusion; titrate every 10–15 min by 0.05–0.2 mcg/kg/min to achieve desired mean arterial pressure.
IV (Children): *Severe anaphylaxis*—0.1 mg (less in younger children); may be followed by 0.1 mcg/kg/min continuous infusion (may be ↑ up to 1.5 mcg/kg/min); *Symptomatic bradycardia/pulseless arrest (PALS guidelines)*—0.01 mg/kg, may be repeated every 3–5 min, higher doses (up to 0.1–0.2 mg/kg) may be considered; may also be given by the intraosseous route. May also be given by the endotracheal route in doses of 0.1–0.2 mg/kg diluted to a volume of 3–5 mL with normal saline followed by several positive pressure ventilations.
Inhaln (Adults): *Inhalation solution*—1 inhalation of 1% solution; may be repeated after 1–2 min; additional doses may be given every 3 hr; *Racepinephrine*—Via hand nebulizer, 2–3 inhalations of 2.25% solution; may repeat in 5 min with 2–3 more inhalations, up to 4–6 times daily.
Inhaln (Children >1 mo): 0.25–0.5 mL of 2.25% racemic epinephrine solution diluted in 3 mL normal saline.
Inhaln (Adults and Children ≥12 yr): *Over-the-counter inhaler*—1–2 inhalations every 4 hr as needed (max = 8 inhalations/day).
IV, Intratracheal (Neonates): 0.01–0.03 mg/kg every 3–5 min as needed.
Intracardiac (Adults): 0.3–0.5 mg.
Endotracheal (Adults): *Cardiopulmonary resuscitation (ACLS guidelines)*—2–2.5 mg.
Topical (Adults and Children ≥6 yr): *Nasal decongestant*—Apply 1% solution as drops, spray, or with a swab.
Intraspinal (Adults and Children): 0.2–0.4 mL of 1:1000 solution.
With Local Anesthetics (Adults and Children): Use 1:200,000 solution with local anesthetic.

Availability (generic available)

Inhalation aerosol: 0.125 mg/inhalation (160 metered inhalations)[OTC]. **Inhalation solution (racepinephrine):** 2.25%. **Intranasal solution:** 1 mg/mL (1:1000). **Solution for injection:** 1 mg/mL (1:1000). **Solution for injection (autoinjectors) (Adrenaclick, Auvi-Q, EpiPen):** 0.1 mg/0.1 mL (1:1000), 0.15 mg/0.15 mL (1:1000), 0.15 mg/0.3 mL (1:2000), 0.3 mg/0.3 mL (1:1000). **Solution for injection (prefilled syringes):** 0.1 mg/mL (1:10,000), 0.15 mg/0.3 mL (1:2000), 0.3 mg/0.3 mL (1:1000).

NURSING IMPLICATIONS

Assessment

- Monitor IV infusion site for extravasation (cold, hard, pallid appearance). If blanching occurs, may change infusion site to allow effects of local vasoconstriction to subside. If extravasation occurs, infiltrate area liberally with 10 mL to 15 mL of 0.9% NaCl with 5 mg to 10 mg of phentolamine using a syringe with a fine needle within 12 hrs of extravasation. Local hyperemic changes are immediate.
- **Bronchodilator:** Assess lung sounds, respiratory pattern, pulse, and BP before administration and during peak of medication. Note amount, color, and character of sputum produced, and notify health care professional of abnormal findings.
- Monitor pulmonary function tests before and periodically during therapy.
- Observe for paradoxical bronchospasm (wheezing). If condition occurs, withhold medication and notify health care professional immediately.
- Observe patient for drug tolerance and rebound bronchospasm. Patients requiring more than 3 inhalation treatments in 24 hr should be under close supervision. If minimal or no relief is seen after 3–5 inhalation treatments within 6–12 hr, further treatment with aerosol alone is not recommended.
- Assess for hypersensitivity reaction (rash; urticaria; swelling of the face, lips, or eyelids). If condition oc-

curs, withhold medication and notify health care professional immediately.

- **Vasopressor:** Monitor BP, pulse, ECG, and respiratory rate frequently during IV administration. Continuous ECG, hemodynamic parameters, and urine output should be monitored continuously during IV administration.
- Monitor for chest pain, arrhythmias, heart rate >110 bpm, and hypertension. Consult health care professional for parameters of pulse, BP, and ECG changes for adjusting dose or discontinuing medication.
- **Shock:** Assess volume status. Correct hypovolemia prior to administering epinephrine IV.
- **Nasal Decongestant:** Assess patient for nasal and sinus congestion prior to and periodically during therapy.
- ***Lab Test Considerations:*** May cause transient ↓ in serum potassium concentrations with nebulization or at higher than recommended doses.
- May cause an ↑ in blood glucose and serum lactic acid concentrations.
- ***Toxicity and Overdose:*** Symptoms of overdose include persistent agitation, chest pain or discomfort, decreased BP, dizziness, hyperglycemia, hypokalemia, seizures, tachyarrhythmias, persistent trembling, and vomiting.
- Treatment includes discontinuing adrenergic bronchodilator and other beta-adrenergic agonists and symptomatic, supportive therapy. Cardioselective beta blockers are used cautiously because they may induce bronchospasm.

Implementation

- Do not confuse epinephrine with ephedrine.
- ***High Alert:*** Patient harm or fatalities have occurred from medication errors with epinephrine. Epinephrine is available in various concentrations, strengths, and percentages and used for different purposes. Packaging labels may be confused or products incorrectly diluted. Dilutions should be prepared by a pharmacist. IV doses should be expressed in milligrams not ampules, concentration, or volume. Prior to administration, have second practitioner independently check original order, dose calculations, concentration, route of administration, and infusion pump settings.
- Medication should be administered promptly at the onset of bronchospasm.
- Use a tuberculin syringe with a 26-gauge ½-in. needle for subcut injection to ensure that correct amount of medication is administered.
- Tolerance may develop with prolonged or excessive use. Effectiveness may be restored by discontinuing for a few days and then readministering.
- Do not use solutions that are pinkish or brownish or that contain a precipitate.
- For anaphylactic shock, volume replacement should be administered concurrently with epinephrine. Antihistamines and corticosteroids may be used in conjunction with epinephrine.
- **IM Subcut:** Administer into anterolateral thigh, through clothing if necessary for anaphylaxis. Hold child's leg firmly to limit movement during injection to prevent lacerations, bent needles, and broken/embedded needles. Avoid injecting into gluteal muscle; may not be effective for anaphylaxis and may cause infection. Medication can cause irritation of tissue. Rotate injection sites to prevent tissue necrosis. Massage injection sites well after administration to enhance absorption and to decrease local vasoconstriction. Avoid IM administration in gluteal muscle.

IV Administration

- **IV Push:** ***Diluent:*** The 1:10,000 solution can be administered undiluted. Dilute 1 mg (1 mL) of a 1:1000 solution in 9 mL of 0.9% NaCl to prepare a 1:10,000 solution. ***Concentration:*** 0.1 mg/mL (1:10,000). ***Rate:*** Administer each 1 mg (10 mL) of a 1:10,000 solution over at least 1 min; more rapid administration may be used during cardiac resuscitation. Follow each dose with 20 mL IV saline flush.
- **Continuous Infusion:** ***Diluent:*** Dilute 1 mg (1 mL) of a 1:1000 solution in 250 mL of D5W or 0.9% NaCl. Protect from light. Infusion stable for 24 hr. ***Concentration:*** 4 mcg/mL. ***Rate:*** See Route/Dosage section. Titrate to response (BP, heart rate, respiratory rate).
- **Y-Site Compatibility:** meropenem/vaborbactam, plazomicin.
- **Inhaln:** When using epinephrine inhalation solution, 10 drops of 1% base solution should be placed in the reservoir of the nebulizer.
- The 2.25% inhalation solution of racepinephrine must be diluted for use in the combination nebulizer/respirator.
- Allow 1–2 min to elapse between inhalations of epinephrine inhalation solution to make certain the second inhalation is necessary.
- When epinephrine is used concurrently with corticosteroid or ipratropium inhalations, administer bronchodilator first and other medications 5 min apart to prevent toxicity from inhaled fluorocarbon propellants.
- **Endotracheal:** Epinephrine can be injected directly into the bronchial tree via the endotracheal tube if the patient has been intubated. Perform 5 rapid insufflations; forcefully administer 10 mL containing 2–2.5 mg epinephrine (1 mg/mL) directly into tube; follow with 5 quick insufflations.

Patient/Family Teaching

- Instruct patient to take medication exactly as directed. If on a scheduled dosing regimen, take a missed dose as soon as possible; space remaining doses at regular intervals. Do not double doses. Caution patient not to exceed recommended dose; may cause adverse effects, paradoxical bronchospasm, or loss of effectiveness of medication.

- Instruct patient to contact health care professional immediately if shortness of breath is not relieved by medication or is accompanied by diaphoresis, dizziness, palpitations, or chest pain.
- Advise patient to consult health care professional before taking any OTC medications or alcoholic beverages concurrently with this therapy. Caution patient also to avoid smoking and other respiratory irritants.
- **Inhaln:** Review correct administration technique (aerosolization, IPPB) with patient.
- Do not spray inhaler near eyes.
- Advise patients to use bronchodilator first if using other inhalation medications, and allow 5 min to elapse before administering other inhalant medications, unless otherwise directed.
- Advise patient to rinse mouth with water after each inhalation dose to minimize dry mouth.
- Advise patient to maintain adequate fluid intake (2000–3000 mL/day) to help liquefy tenacious secretions.
- Advise patient to consult health care professional if respiratory symptoms are not relieved or worsen after treatment or if chest pain, headache, severe dizziness, palpitations, nervousness, or weakness occurs.
- Advise patient to notify health care professional if pregnancy is planned or suspected or if breast feeding.
- **Autoinjector:** Instruct patients using auto-injector for anaphylactic reactions to remove gray safety cap, placing black tip on thigh at right angle to leg. Press hard into thigh until auto-injector functions, hold in place for 10 sec, remove, and discard properly. Massage injected area for 10 sec. Pedi: Teach parents or caregivers signs and symptoms of anaphylaxis, how to use auto-injector safely, and to get the child to a hospital as soon as possible. Instruct parents or caregivers to teach child how to manage his or her allergy, how to self-inject, and what to do in an emergency. For children too young to self-inject and who will be separated from parent, tell parents to always discuss allergy and use of auto-injector with responsible adult.

Evaluation/Desired Outcomes

- Prevention or relief of bronchospasm.
- Increase in ease of breathing.
- Prevention of bronchospasm or reduction of frequency of acute asthma attacks in patients with chronic asthma.
- Prevention of exercise-induced asthma.
- Reversal of signs and symptoms of anaphylaxis.
- Increase in cardiac rate and output, when used in cardiac resuscitation.
- Increase in BP, when used as a vasopressor.
- Localization of local anesthetic.
- Decrease in sinus and nasal congestion.

HIGH ALERT

epiRUBicin (ep-i-roo-bi-sin)

Ellence, ✱Pharmorubicin PFS

Classification
Therapeutic: antineoplastics
Pharmacologic: anthracyclines

Indications

A component of adjuvant therapy for evidence of axillary tumor involvement following resection of primary breast cancer.

Action

Inhibits DNA and RNA synthesis by forming a complex with DNA. **Therapeutic Effects:** Death of rapidly replicating cells, particularly malignant ones.

Pharmacokinetics

Absorption: IV administration results in complete bioavailability.
Distribution: Rapidly and widely distributed; concentrates in RBCs.
Metabolism and Excretion: Extensively and rapidly metabolized by the liver and other tissues.
Half-life: 35 hr.

TIME/ACTION PROFILE (effect on WBCs)

ROUTE	ONSET	PEAK	DURATION
IV	unknown	10–14 days	21 days

Contraindications/Precautions

Contraindicated in: Hypersensitivity to epirubicin, other anthracyclines, or related compounds; Baseline neutrophil count <1500 cells/mm^3; HF; Recent MI; Severe arrhythmias; Previous treatment with anthracyclines up to the maximum cumulative dose; Severe hepatic impairment; Concurrent cimetidine therapy; OB: May cause fetal harm (avoid use during 1st trimester); Lactation: Lactation.
Use Cautiously in: Cardiovascular disease, prior or concomitant radiation therapy to mediastinal or pericardial area, previous therapy with anthracyclines, or concomitant use of cardiotoxic drugs (↑ risk of cardiotoxicity); Severe renal impairment (serum creatinine >5 mg/dL); consider ↓ dose; Hepatic impairment (dose ↓ recommended for bilirubin >1.2 mg/dL or AST >2.2–4 times upper limit of normal); Depressed bone marrow reserve; OB: Use during 2nd or 3rd trimester only if potential maternal benefit justifies potential fetal risk; Rep: Women of reproductive potential and men with female partners of reproductive potential; Pedi: Safety and effectiveness not established; ↑ risk of acute cardiotoxicity and chronic HF; Geri: ↑ risk of toxicity in females ≥70 yr.

Adverse Reactions/Side Effects

CNS: lethargy. **CV:** HF (dose-related), bradycardia, heart block, thromboembolism, ventricular tachycardia. **Derm:** alopecia, flushing, itching, photosensitivity, radiation-recall reaction, rash, skin/nail hyperpigmentation. **Endo:** gonadal suppression. **GI:** nausea, vomiting, anorexia, diarrhea, mucositis. **GU:** amenorrhea, ↓ fertility, ↓ sperm production. **Hemat:** LEUKOPENIA, anemia, thrombocytopenia, treatment-related leukemia/myelodysplastic syndromes. **Local:** injection site reactions, phlebitis at IV site, tissue necrosis. **Metab:** hot flashes, hyperuricemia. **Misc:** ANAPHYLAXIS, INFECTION.

Interactions

Drug-Drug: Cimetidine ↑ blood levels and risk of serious toxicity; avoid concurrent use. Additive hematologic and gastrointestinal toxicity with other **antineoplastics** or **radiation therapy**. Use with other cardiotoxic drugs may ↑ risk of cardiotoxicity; avoid concurrent use. May ↓ antibody response to **live-virus vaccines** and ↑ risk of adverse reactions. **Trastuzumab** may ↑ risk of cardiotoxicity; avoid use of epirubicin for up to 7 mo after discontinuing trastuzumab.

Route/Dosage

IV (Adults): 100–120 mg/m² repeated in 3–4 wk cycles (total dose may be given on Day 1 or split and given in equally divided doses on Day 1 and Day 8 of each cycle) (combination regimens may employ concurrent 5-fluorouracil and cyclophosphamide).

Hepatic Impairment

IV (Adults): *Bilirubin 1.2–3 mg/dL or AST 2–4x ULN*—use 50% of recommended starting dose; *Bilirubin >3 m g/dL or AST >4x ULN*—use 25% of recommended starting dose.

Availability (generic available)

Solution for injection: 2 mg/mL.

NURSING IMPLICATIONS

Assessment

- Monitor for bone marrow depression. Assess for bleeding (bleeding gums, bruising, petechiae, guaiac stools, urine, and emesis) and avoid IM injections and taking rectal temperatures if platelet count is low. Apply pressure to venipuncture sites for 10 min. Assess for signs of infection during neutropenia. Anemia may occur. Monitor for increased fatigue, dyspnea, and orthostatic hypotension.
- Severe nausea and vomiting may occur. Administer parenteral antiemetic agents 30–45 min prior to therapy and routinely around the clock for next 24 hr as indicated. Monitor amount of emesis and notify health care professional if emesis exceeds guidelines to prevent dehydration.
- Measure cardiac function, using ECG and a multigated radionuclide angiography (MUGA) scan or an ECHO, prior to therapy. Perform repeated evaluations of left ventricular ejection fraction during therapy. Monitor for development of signs of cardiac toxicity, which may occur early (ST-T wave changes, sinus tachycardia, and extrasystoles) or late (may occur mo to yr after termination of therapy). Delayed cardiac toxicity is characterized by cardiomyopathy, tachycardia, peripheral edema, dyspnea, rales/crackles, weight gain, hepatomegaly, ascites, pleural effusion. Toxicity is usually dependent on cumulative dose.
- Assess injection site frequently for redness, irritation, or inflammation. Burning or stinging during infusion may indicate infiltration and infusion should be discontinued and restarted in another vein. Epirubicin is a vesicant but may infiltrate painlessly even if blood returns on aspiration of infusion needle. Severe tissue damage may occur if epirubicin extravasates. If extravasation occurs, stop infusion immediately, restart, and complete dose in another vein.
- Assess oral mucosa frequently for development of stomatitis (pain, burning, erythema, ulcerations, bleeding, infection). Increased dosing interval and/or decreased dosing is recommended if lesions are painful or interfere with nutrition.
- ***Lab Test Considerations:*** Obtain negative pregnancy test before starting therapy.
- Monitor CBC and differential before and during each cycle of therapy. Epirubicin should not be administered to patients with a baseline neutrophil count <1500 cells/mm³. The WBC nadir occurs 10–14 days after administration, and recovery usually occurs by the 21st day. Severe thrombocytopenia and anemia may also occur.
- Monitor renal (BUN and creatinine) and hepatic (AST, ALT, LDH, and serum bilirubin) function prior to and periodically during therapy. Dose reduction is required for bilirubin >1.2 m g/dL, AST 2–4 times the upper limit of normal, or serum creatinine >5 m g/dL.

Implementation

- ***High Alert:*** Fatalities have occurred with incorrect administration of chemotherapeutic agents. Before administering, clarify ambiguous orders; double-check single, daily, and course-of-therapy dose limits; have second practitioner independently double-check original order, calculations and infusion pump settings. Epirubicin should be administered only under the supervision of a physician experienced in the use of cancer chemotherapeutic agents.
- ***High Alert:*** Do not confuse epirubicin with eribulin.
- Prepare solution in a biologic cabinet. Wear gloves, gown, and mask while handling medication. Discard IV equipment in specially designated containers.
- Administer prophylactic anti-infective therapy with trimethoprim/sulfamethoxazole or a fluoroquino-

lone and antiemetic therapy prior to administration of epirubicin.

- Do not administer subcut or IM.

IV Administration

- **Intermittent Infusion:** ***Diluent:*** Administer undiluted. Solution is clear red. Use epirubicin within 24 hr of penetration of rubber stopper. Discard unused solution. ***Concentration:*** 2 mg/mL. ***Rate:*** Administer initial dose of 100–120 mg/m² over 15–20 min through free-flowing infusion of 0.9% NaCl or D5W. Lower doses may be infused for shorter periods, but not less than over 3 min. Do not administer via IV push. Facial flushing and erythema along involved vein frequently occur when administration is too rapid. Venous sclerosis may result from injection into a small vein or repeated injections into the same vein. Avoid veins over joints or in extremities with compromised venous or lymphatic drainage.
- **Y-Site Compatibility:** alemtuzumab, alfentanil, amifostine, amikacin, aminocaproic acid, anidulafungin, argatroban, arsenic trioxide, atracurium, aztreonam, bivalirudin, bleomycin, bumetanide, buprenorphine, butorphanol, calcium chloride, calcium gluconate, carboplatin, caspofungin, cefazolin, cefotaxime, chlorpromazine, ciprofloxacin, cisatracurium, cisplatin, clindamycin, cyclophosphamide, cyclosporine, dacarbazine, daptomycin, dexrazoxane, digoxin, diltiazem, diphenhydramine, dobutamine, docetaxel, dolasetron, dopamine, doxacurium, doxacycline, droperidol, enalaprilat, ephedrine, epinephrine, erythromycin, etoposide, etoposide phosphate, famotidine, fenoldopam, fentanyl, fluconazole, gemcitabine, gentamicin, granisetron, haloperidol, hetastarch, hydrocortisone, hydromorphone, ifosfamide, imipenem cilastatin, insulin, regular, isoproterenol, labetalol, levofloxacin, lidocaine, linezolid, lorazepam, mannitol, meperidine, mesna, methotrexate, metoclopramide, metoprolol, metronidazole, midazolam, milrinone, mitomycin, morphine, moxifloxacin, nalbuphine, naloxone, nicardipine, nitroglycerin, nitroprusside, norepinephrine, octreotide, ondansetron, oxaliplatin, paclitaxel, palonosetron, pamidronate, pancuronium, pentamidine, phenylephrine, potassium acetate, potassium chloride, procainamide, prochlorperazine, promethazine, propranolol, quinapristin/dalfopristin, ranitidine, remifentanil, rocuronium, sodium acetate, succinylcholine, sufentanil, tacrolimus, theophylline, thiotepa, tirofiban, tobramycin, vancomycin, vasopressin, vecuronium, verapamil, vinblastine, vincristine, vinorelbine, voriconazole, zidovudine, zoledronic acid.
- **Y-Site Incompatibility:** acyclovir, allopurinol, aminophylline, amphotericin B deoxycholate, amphotericin B lipid complex, amphotericin B liposome, ampicillin, ampicillin/sulbactam, azithromycin, cefepime, cefotetan, cefoxitin, ceftazidime, ceftriaxone, cefuroxime, dexamethasone, diazepam, ertapenem, fluorouracil, foscarnet, fosphenytoin, furosemide, ganciclovir, heparin, hydrocortisone, ketorolac, leucovorin calcium, magnesium sulfate, meropenem, methohexital, methylprednisolone, nafcillin, pantoprazole, pemetrexed, pentobarbital, phenobarbital, phenytoin, piperacillin/tazobactam, potassium phosphates, sodium bicarbonate, sodium phosphates, thiopental, tigecycline, trimethoprim/sulfamethoxazole.

Patient/Family Teaching

- Instruct patient to notify health care professional promptly if fever; sore throat; signs of infection; bleeding gums; bruising; petechiae; blood in stools, urine, or emesis; increased fatigue; dyspnea; or orthostatic hypotension occurs. Caution patient to avoid crowds and persons with known infections. Instruct patient to use soft toothbrush and electric razor and to avoid falls. Patient should be cautioned not to drink alcoholic beverages or take medication containing aspirin or NSAIDs, because these may precipitate gastric bleeding.
- Instruct patient to report pain at injection site immediately.
- Instruct patient to inspect oral mucosa for erythema and ulceration. If ulceration occurs, advise patient to use sponge brush, rinse mouth with water after eating and drinking, and confer with health care professional if mouth pain interferes with eating. Pain may require treatment with opioid analgesics. Patients usually recover by the third wk of therapy.
- Instruct patient to notify health care professional of all Rx or OTC medications, vitamins, or herbal products being taken and to avoid concurrent use of alcohol or OTC medications and herbal products, especially cold preparations, without consulting health care professional, especially cimetidine.
- Instruct patient to notify health care professional immediately if vomiting, dehydration, fever, evidence of infection, symptoms of HF, or pain at injection site occurs. Patients should be informed of the risk of irreversible cardiac damage and treatment-related leukemia.
- Discuss the possibility of hair loss with patient. Explore methods of coping. Regrowth usually occurs 2–3 mo after discontinuation of therapy.
- Instruct patient not to receive any vaccinations without advice of health care professional.
- Inform patient that medication may cause urine to appear red for 1–2 days.
- Instruct patient to notify health care professional if skin irritation occurs at site of previous radiation therapy. May cause hyperpigmentation of the skin and nails. Advise patient to use sunscreen and protective clothing to prevent photosensitivity reactions.
- Rep: May have teratogenic effects. Advise females of reproductive potential to use effective contraception during and for 6 mo after last dose of therapy and to avoid breast feeding for at least 7 days after last dose

of epirubicin. Advise males with female partners of reproductive potential to use effective contraception during and for 3 mo after last dose of therapy and to use condoms during and for at least 7 days after last dose of epirubicin. Inform females and males that epirubicin may cause permanent loss of fertility.
- Emphasize the need for periodic lab tests to monitor for side effects.

Evaluation/Desired Outcomes
- Decrease in size or spread of malignancies in patients with axillary node tumor involvement following resection of primary breast cancer.

eplerenone (e-ple-re-none)
Inspra

Classification
Therapeutic: antihypertensives
Pharmacologic: aldosterone antagonists

Indications
Hypertension (alone, or with other agents). LV systolic dysfunction and evidence of HF post-MI.

Action
Blocks the effects of aldosterone by attaching to mineralocorticoid receptors. **Therapeutic Effects:** Lowering of BP. Improves survival in patients with evidence of HF post-MI.

Pharmacokinetics
Absorption: Well absorbed following oral administration.
Distribution: Unknown.
Metabolism and Excretion: Mostly metabolized by the liver (CYP3A enzyme system); <5% excreted unchanged by the kidneys.
Half-life: 4–6 hr.

TIME/ACTION PROFILE (antihypertensive effect)

ROUTE	ONSET	PEAK	DURATION
PO	unknown	4 wk	unknown

Contraindications/Precautions
Contraindicated in: Serum potassium >5.5 mEq/L; Type 2 diabetes with microalbuminuria (for patients with HTN; ↑ risk of hyperkalemia); Serum creatinine >2 mg/dL in males or >1.8 mg/dL in females (for patients with HTN); CCr ≤30 mL/min (for all patients); CCr <50 mL/min (for patients with HTN); Concurrent use of potassium supplements or potassium-sparing diuretics (for patients with HTN); Concurrent use of strong inhibitors of the CYP3A4 enzyme system (ketoconazole, itraconazole, nefazodone, clarithromycin, ritonavir, or nelfinavir); Lactation: Lactation.

Use Cautiously in: Moderate hepatic impairment; OB: Use only if potential maternal benefit justifies potential fetal risk; Pedi: Safety and effectiveness not established; Geri: ↑ risk of hyperkalemia due to age-related ↓ in renal function.

Adverse Reactions/Side Effects
CNS: dizziness, fatigue. **Endo:** abnormal vaginal bleeding, gynecomastia. **F and E:** HYPERKALEMIA. **GI:** abnormal liver function tests, abdominal pain, diarrhea. **GU:** albuminuria. **Metab:** hypercholesterolemia, hypertriglyceridemia. **Misc:** flu-like symptoms.

Interactions
Drug-Drug: Concurrent use of strong CYP3A inhibitors, including **ketoconazole**, **itraconazole**, **nefazodone**, **clarithromycin**, **ritonavir**, or **nelfinavir** significantly ↑ effects of eplerenone; concurrent use contraindicated. Concurrent use of moderate CYP3A inhibitors, including **erythromycin**, **saquinavir**, **fluconazole**, or **verapamil** may ↑ levels; ↓ dose of eplerenone. **NSAIDs** may ↓ antihypertensive effects. Concurrent use of **ACE inhibitors** or **Angiotensin II receptor blockers** may ↑ risk of hyperkalemia.

Route/Dosage
Hypertension
PO (Adults): 50 mg once daily initially; may be ↑ to 50 mg twice daily; *Patients receiving concurrent moderate CYP3A4 inhibitors (erythromycin, saquinavir, verapamil, fluconazole)*—25 mg once daily initially; may be ↑ to 25 mg twice daily.

HF Post-MI
PO (Adults): 25 mg daily once initially; ↑ in 4 wk to 50 mg once daily; *Patients receiving concurrent moderate CYP3A4 inhibitors (erythromycin, saquinavir, verapamil, fluconazole)*—Do not exceed 25 mg once daily.

Availability (generic available)
Tablets: 25 mg, 50 mg.

NURSING IMPLICATIONS
Assessment
- Monitor BP periodically during therapy.
- Monitor prescription refills to determine adherence.
- ***Lab Test Considerations:*** May cause hyperkalemia. Monitor serum potassium levels prior to starting therapy, within the first wk, at 1 mo following start of therapy or dose adjustment, and periodically thereafter. Monitor serum potassium and serum creatinine in 3–7 days in patients who start taking a moderate CYP3A4 inhibitor.
- May cause ↓ serum sodium and ↑ serum triglyceride, cholesterol, ALT, GGT, creatinine, and uric acid levels.

Implementation

- Do not confuse Inspra (eplerenone) with Spiriva (tiotropium).
- **PO:** Administer once daily. May be increased to twice daily if response is inadequate.

Patient/Family Teaching

- Instruct patient to take medication as directed at the same time each day, even if feeling well.
- Encourage patient to comply with additional interventions for hypertension (weight reduction, discontinuation of smoking, moderation of alcohol consumption, regular exercise, stress management). Medication controls, but does not cure, hypertension.
- Instruct patient and family on correct technique for monitoring BP. Advise them to monitor BP at least weekly, and notify health care professional of significant changes.
- Inform patient not to use potassium supplements, salt substitutes containing potassium, or other Rx, OTC, or herbal products without consulting health care professional.
- May cause dizziness. Caution patient to avoid driving or other activities requiring alertness until response to medication is known.
- Advise patient to notify health care professional if dizziness, diarrhea, vomiting, rapid or irregular heartbeat, lower extremity edema, or difficulty breathing occur.
- Advise patient to inform health care professional of treatment regimen prior to treatment or surgery.
- Advise patient to notify health care professional if pregnancy is planned or suspected. Advise patient to avoid breast feeding during therapy.
- Emphasize the importance of follow-up exams to check serum potassium.

Evaluation/Desired Outcomes

- Decrease in BP without appearance of side effects.
- Improvement in survival in patients with evidence of HF post-MI.

epoetin (e-poe-e-tin)

Epogen, ✱Eprex, Procrit, Retacrit

Classification
Therapeutic: antianemics
Pharmacologic: hormones, erythropoiesis stimulating agents (ESA)

Indications

Anemia associated with chronic kidney disease (CKD). Anemia secondary to zidovudine (AZT) therapy in HIV-infected patients. Anemia from chemotherapy in patients with nonmyeloid malignancies when there is ≥2 additional mo of planned chemotherapy. Reduction of need for allogeneic red blood cell transfusions in patients undergoing elective, noncardiac, nonvascular surgery.

Action

Stimulates erythropoiesis (production of red blood cells). **Therapeutic Effects:** Maintains and may elevate RBCs, decreasing the need for transfusions.

Pharmacokinetics

Absorption: Well absorbed after subcut administration.

Distribution: Unknown.

Metabolism and Excretion: Unknown.

Half-life: *Children and Adults*—4–13 hr; *Neonates*—11–17 hr.

TIME/ACTION PROFILE (increase in RBCs)

ROUTE	ONSET†	PEAK	DURATION
IV, Subcut	7–10 days	within 2 mo	2 wk‡

†Increase in reticulocytes.
‡After discontinuation.

Contraindications/Precautions

Contraindicated in: Hypersensitivity to albumin or mammalian cell-derived products; Uncontrolled hypertension; Patients with erythropoietin levels >200 mUnits/mL; Patients with cancer receiving hormonal agents, biologic products, or radiotherapy, unless also receiving concomitant myelosuppressive chemotherapy; Patients receiving chemotherapy when anticipated outcome is cure; Patients with cancer receiving myelosuppressive chemotherapy in whom the anemia can be managed by transfusion; Patients who require immediate correction of anemia when RBC transfusions can be used instead; Patients scheduled for surgery who are willing to donate autologous blood; Patients undergoing cardiac or vascular surgery; OB, Lactation: Multidose vials should not be used as they contain benzyl alcohol and may cause fatal gasping syndrome in fetus in-utero and breast-fed infants; Pedi: Neutropenia in newborns; multidose vials should not be used as they contain benzyl alcohol, which can cause potentially fatal gasping syndrome in neonates and infants.

Use Cautiously in: History of seizures or stroke; Cardiovascular disease; History of porphyria; OB: Evidence of fetal harm in animal studies—use only if potential benefit outweighs potential risk to fetus; OB, Lactation: Little published information, however, erythropoetin alfa is a normal constituent of breast milk.

Adverse Reactions/Side Effects

CNS: SEIZURES, headache. **CV:** HF, MI, STROKE, THROMBOEMBOLIC EVENTS (especially with hemoglobin >11 g/dL), hypertension. **Derm:** ERYTHEMA MULTIFORME, STEVENS-JOHNSON SYNDROME, TOXIC EPIDERMAL NECROLYSIS, transient rashes. **Endo:** restored fertility, resumption of menses. **Misc:** ↑ MORTALITY AND ↑ TUMOR GROWTH (with hemoglobin >12 g/dL).

Interactions

Drug-Drug: May ↑ requirement for **heparin** anticoagulation during hemodialysis.

Route/Dosage

Anemia of CKD

(Do not initiate if hemoglobin ≥10 g/dL).

Subcut, IV (Adults): 50–100 units/kg 3 times weekly initially; use lowest dose sufficient to ↓ the need for red blood cell transfusions (do not exceed hemoglobin of 11 g/dL [patients on dialysis] or 10 g/dL [patients not on dialysis]); if Hgb ↑ by >1.0 g/dL in 2 wk, ↓ dose by 25%; if Hgb ↑ by <1.0 g/dL after 4 wk of therapy (with adequate iron stores), ↑ dose by 25%; do not ↑ dose more frequently than every 4 wk.

Subcut, IV (Children 1 mo–16 yr): 50 units/kg 3 times weekly initially; use lowest dose sufficient to ↓ the need for red blood cell transfusions (do not exceed hemoglobin of 12 g/dL; if Hgb ↑ by >1.0 g/dL in 2 wk, ↓ dose by 25%; if Hgb ↑ by <1.0 g/dL after 4 wk of therapy (with adequate iron stores), ↑ dose by 25%; do not ↑ dose more frequently than every 4 wk.

Anemia Secondary to AZT Therapy

Subcut, IV (Adults): 100 units/kg 3 times weekly for 8 wk; if inadequate response, may ↑ by 50–100 units/kg every 4–8 wk (max: 300 units/kg 3 times weekly).

Subcut, IV (Children 8 mo–17 yr): 50–400 units/kg 2–3 times weekly.

Anemia from Chemotherapy

(Use only for chemotherapy-related anemia and discontinue when chemotherapy course is completed; do not initiate if hemoglobin ≥10 g/dL).

Subcut (Adults): 150 units/kg 3 times weekly or 40,000 units weekly; adjust dose to maintain lowest hemoglobin level sufficient to avoid blood transfusions (do not exceed hemoglobin of 12 g/dL); if Hgb ↑ by >1.0 g/dL in 2 wk or reaches a level needed to avoid red blood cell transfusions, ↓ dose by 25%; if Hgb ↑ by <1.0 g/dL (and remains <10 g/dL) after initial 4 wk of therapy (with adequate iron stores), ↑ dose to 300 units/kg 3 times weekly or 60,000 units weekly.

IV (Children 5–18 yr): 600 units/kg weekly; adjust dose to maintain lowest hemoglobin level sufficient to avoid blood transfusions (do not exceed hemoglobin of 12 g/dL); if Hgb ↑ by >1.0 g/dL in 2 wk or reaches a level needed to avoid red blood cell transfusions, ↓ dose by 25%; if Hgb ↑ by <1.0 g/dL (and remains <10 g/dL) after initial 4 wk of therapy (with adequate iron stores), ↑ dose to 900 units/kg (maximum = 60,000 units) weekly.

Surgery

Subcut (Adults): 300 units/kg/day for 10 days before surgery, day of surgery, and 4 days after *or* 600 units/kg 21, 14, and 7 days before surgery and on day of surgery.

Availability

Solution for injection: 2,000 units/mL, 3,000 units/mL, 4,000 units/mL, 10,000 units/mL, 20,000 units/mL, 40,000 units/mL. **Solution for injection (prefilled syringes):** ✱ 1,000 units/0.5 mL, ✱ 2,000 units/0.5 mL, ✱ 3,000 units/0.3 mL, ✱ 4,000 units/0.4 mL, ✱ 5,000 units/0.5 mL, ✱ 6000 units/0.6 mL, ✱ 8,000 units/0.8 mL, ✱ 10,000 units/1 mL, ✱ 20,000 units/0.5 mL, ✱ 30,000 units/0.75 mL, ✱ 40,000 units/1 mL.

NURSING IMPLICATIONS

Assessment

- Monitor BP before and during therapy. Inform health care professional if severe hypertension is present or if BP begins to increase. Additional antihypertensive therapy may be required during initiation of therapy.
- Monitor for symptoms of anemia (fatigue, dyspnea, pallor).
- Monitor dialysis shunts (thrill and bruit) and status of artificial kidney during hemodialysis. Heparin dose may need to be increased to prevent clotting. Monitor patients with underlying vascular disease for impaired circulation.
- ***Lab Test Considerations:*** May cause ↑ in WBCs and platelets. May ↓ bleeding times.
- Monitor serum ferritin, transferrin, and iron levels to assess need for concurrent iron therapy. Administer supplemental iron therapy when serum ferritin <100 mcg/L or when serum transferrin saturation <20%.
- Monitor hemoglobin weekly until the hemoglobin level is stable and sufficient to minimize the need for RBC transfusion after starting therapy and after each dose adjustment.
- **Anemia of Chronic Kidney Disease:** Monitor hemoglobin at least weekly until stable, then at least monthly. Do not increase dose more frequently than once every 4 wk. Decreases in dose can be made more frequently. Avoid frequent dose adjustments. *If hemoglobin ↑ >1 g/dL in a 2-wk period,* ↓ dose by 25% or more. *If hemoglobin ↑ by <1 g/dL over 4 wk (and iron stores are adequate),* ↑ dose by 25%. If no response after 12 wk of escalation, further dose ↑ is unlikely to improve response and may increase risks. Use lowest dose that will maintain Hgb level sufficient to reduce need for transfusions.
- **Adults with Anemia of Chronic Kidney Disease on Dialysis:** Start epoetin when hemoglobin >10 g/dL. If hemoglobin ≥11 g/dL, reduce or hold dose.
- **Adults with Anemia of Chronic Kidney Disease not on Dialysis:** Start epoetin only when hemoglobin <10 g/dL AND rate of hemoglobin decline indicates likelihood of requiring a RBC transfusion AND reducing risk of alloimmunization and/or other RBC transfusion-related risks is a goal. If hemoglobin level >10 g/dL, reduce or hold dose, and use lowest epoetin dose sufficient to reduce need for RBC transfusions.

- **Children with Anemia of Chronic Kidney Disease:** Start epoetin only when hemoglobin <10 g/dL. If hemoglobin level >12 g/dL, reduce or hold dose.
- Monitor renal function studies and electrolytes closely; resulting increased sense of well-being may lead to decreased compliance with other therapies for renal failure. Increases in BUN, creatinine, uric acid, phosphorus, and potassium may occur.
- **Anemia Secondary to Zidovudine Therapy:** Before initiating therapy, determine serum erythropoietin level before transfusion. Patients receiving zidovudine with endogenous serum erythropoietin levels >500 mUnits/mL may not respond to therapy. *If hemoglobin does not ↑ after 8 wk of therapy,* ↑ dose by 50–100 units/kg at 4–8 wk intervals until hemoglobin reaches level needed to avoid RBC transfusions or 300 units/kg. *If hemoglobin ≥12 g/dL,* hold dose until hemoglobin drops to <11 g/dL, then ↓ dose by 25%. *If ↑ in hemoglobin is not achieved at a dose of 300 Units/kg for 8 wk,* discontinue therapy.
- **Anemia from Chemotherapy:** Start epoetin only if hemoglobin ≥10 g/dL and there is an additional 2 mo of planned chemotherapy. Patients with lower baseline serum erythropoietin levels may respond more rapidly; not recommended if levels >200 mUnits/mL. *If hemoglobin ↑ by >1.0 g/dL in any 2-wk period or hemoglobin reaches level needed to avoid RBC transfusion,* ↓ dose by 25%. *If hemoglobin ↑ <1 g/dL after 4 wk in absence of RBC transfusion) and remains <10 g/dL,* ↑ dose to 300 units/kg three times per wk in adults or 60,000 units weekly (adults) or 900 units/kg (max: 60,000 units) in children. *If no response in hemoglobin levels or if RBC transfusions are still required after 8 wk of therapy,* discontinue epoetin.
- **Surgery:** Implement prophylaxis of deep venous thrombosis during therapy.

Implementation

IV Administration

- Transfusions are still required for severe symptomatic anemia. Supplemental iron should be initiated with epoetin and continued throughout therapy.
- Institute seizure precautions in patients who experience greater than a 4-point increase in hematocrit in a 2-wk period or exhibit any change in neurologic status. Risk of seizures is greatest during the first 90 days of therapy.
- Do not shake vial; inactivation of medication may occur. Solution is clear and colorless; do not administer solutions that are discolored, cloudy, or contain a precipitate. Discard vial immediately after withdrawing dose from single-use 1-mL vial. Refrigerate multidose 2-mL vial; stable for 21 days after initial entry.
- **Subcut:** This route is often used for patients not requiring dialysis.
- May be admixed in syringe immediately before administration with 0.9% NaCl with benzyl alcohol 0.9% in a 1:1 ratio to prevent injection site discomfort.
- **IV Push:** ***Diluent:*** Administer undiluted or dilute with an equal amount of 0.9% NaCl. ***Concentration:*** 1000–40,000 units/mL. ***Rate:*** May be administered as direct injection or bolus over 1–3 min into IV tubing or via venous line at end of dialysis session.
- **Y-Site Compatibility:** alfentanil, amikacin, aminophylline, ascorbic acid, atracurium, atropine, azathioprine, aztreonam, benztropine, bumetanide, buprenorphine, butorphanol, calcium chloride, calcium gluconate, cefazolin, cefotaxime, cefotetan, cefoxitin, ceftazidime, ceftriaxone, cefuroxime, chloramphenicol, clindamycin, cyanocobalamin, cyclosporine, dexamethasone, digoxin, diphenhydramine, dobutamine, dopamine, doxycycline, enalaprilat, ephedrine, epinephrine, erythromycin, esmolol, famotidine, fentanyl, fluconazole, folic acid, furosemide, ganciclovir, gentamicin, glycopyrrolate, heparin, hydrocortisone, imipenem-cilastatin, indomethacin, insulin, regular, isoproterenol, ketorolac, labetalol, lidocaine, magnesium sulfate, mannitol, meperidine, methyldopate, methylprednisolone, metoclopramide, metoprolol, morphine, multivitamins, nafcillin, nalbuphine, naloxone, nitroglycerin, nitroprusside, norepinephrine, ondansetron, oxacillin, oxytocin, penicillin G, pentobarbital, phenobarbital, phentolamine, phenylephrine, phytonadione, potassium chloride, procainamide, promethazine, propranolol, protamine, pyridoxine, ranitidine, sodium bicarbonate, streptokinase, succinylcholine, sufentanil, theophylline, tobramycin, vasopressin, verapamil.
- **Y-Site Incompatibility:** amphotericin B deoxycholate, chlorpromazine, dantrolene, diazepam, haloperidol, midazolam, minocycline, pentamidine, phenytoin, prochlorperazine, trimethoprim/sulfamethoxazole, vancomycin.

Patient/Family Teaching

- Advise patient to read the *Medication Guide* prior to initiating therapy and with each Rx refill in case of changes. Patient must sign the patient-health care provider acknowledgment form before each course of therapy.
- Explain rationale for concurrent iron therapy (increased red blood cell production requires iron).
- Discuss ways of preventing self-injury in patients at risk for seizures. Driving and activities requiring continuous alertness should be avoided.
- Inform patient that use of epoetin may result in shortened overall survival and/or ↓ time to tumor progression.
- Advise patient to notify health care professional immediately if signs and symptoms of blood clots (chest pain, trouble breathing or shortness of breath; pain in the legs, with or without swelling; a cool or pale arm or leg; sudden confusion; trouble speaking or trouble understanding others' speech; sudden numbness or weakness in the face, arm, or

leg, especially on one side of the body; sudden trouble seeing; sudden trouble walking, dizziness, loss of balance or coordination; loss of consciousness or fainting; hemodialysis vascular access stops working), allergic reactions (rash, itching, shortness of breath, wheezing, dizziness and fainting, swelling around mouth or eyes, fast pulse, sweating), skin reactions (blisters, skin sores, peeling, or areas of skin coming off) occur.

- Advise patient to inform health care professional of medication prior to treatment or surgery.
- Rep: Discuss possible return of menses and fertility with health care professional. Advise female patients of reproductive potential to notify health care professional if pregnancy is planned or suspected or if breast feeding.
- **Anemia of Chronic Renal Failure:** Stress importance of compliance with dietary restrictions, medications, and dialysis. Foods high in iron and low in potassium include liver, pork, veal, beef, mustard and turnip greens, peas, eggs, broccoli, kale, blackberries, strawberries, apple juice, watermelon, oatmeal, and enriched bread. Epoetin will result in increased sense of well-being, but it does not cure underlying disease.
- **Home Care Issues:** Home dialysis patients determined to be able to safely and effectively administer epoetin should be taught proper dosage, administration technique, and disposal of equipment. *Information for Home Dialysis Patients* should be provided to patient along with medication.

Evaluation/Desired Outcomes

- Increase in hematocrit to 30–36% with improvement in symptoms of anemia in patients with chronic renal failure.
- Increase in hematocrit in anemia secondary to zidovudine therapy.
- Increase in hematocrit in patients with anemia resulting from chemotherapy.
- Reduction of need for transfusions after surgery.

eprosartan, See ANGIOTENSIN II RECEPTOR ANTAGONISTS.

HIGH ALERT

eptifibatide (ep-ti-**fib**-a-tide)

Integrilin

Classification

Therapeutic: antiplatelet agents
Pharmacologic: glycoprotein IIb/IIIa inhibitors

Indications

Acute coronary syndrome (unstable angina/non-Q-wave MI), including patients who will be managed medically and those who will undergo percutaneous coronary intervention (PCI) that may consist of percutaneous transluminal angioplasty (PCTA) or atherectomy. Treatment of patients undergoing PCI. Usually used concurrently with aspirin and heparin.

Action

Decreases platelet aggregation by reversibly antagonizing the binding of fibrinogen to the glycoprotein IIb/IIIa binding site on platelet surfaces. **Therapeutic Effects:** Inhibition of platelet aggregation resulting in decreased incidence of new MI, death, or refractory ischemia, reducing the need for repeat urgent cardiac intervention.

Pharmacokinetics

Absorption: IV administration results in complete bioavailability.
Distribution: Unknown.
Metabolism and Excretion: 50% excreted by the kidneys.
Half-life: 2.5 hr.

TIME/ACTION PROFILE (effects on platelet function)

ROUTE	ONSET	PEAK	DURATION
IV	immediate	following bolus	brief†

†Inhibition is reversible following cessation of infusion.

Contraindications/Precautions

Contraindicated in: Hypersensitivity; Active internal bleeding or history of bleeding within previous 30 days; Severe uncontrolled hypertension (systolic BP >200 mm Hg and/or diastolic BP >110 mm Hg); Major surgical procedure within 6 wk; History of hemorrhagic stroke or other stroke within 30 days; Concurrent use of other glycoprotein IIb/IIIa receptor antagonists; Platelet count <100,000/mm³; Severe renal insufficiency (serum creatinine ≥4 mg/dL) or dependency on renal dialysis.
Use Cautiously in: Geri: ↑ risk of bleeding; Renal insufficiency (↓ infusion rate if CCr <50 mL/min); OB, Pedi: Pregnancy, lactation, or children (safety not established; use in pregnancy only if clearly needed).

Adverse Reactions/Side Effects

Noted for patients receiving heparin and aspirin in addition to eptifibatide.
CV: hypotension. **Hemat:** BLEEDING (including GI and intracranial bleeding, hematuria, and hematomas), thrombocytopenia.

Interactions

Drug-Drug: ↑ risk of bleeding with other drugs that affect hemostasis (**heparins**, **warfarin**, **NSAIDs**, **thrombolytic agents**, **dipyridamole**, **clopidogrel**, some **cephalosporins**, **valproates**).

Drug-Natural Products: ↑ bleeding risk with **arnica**, **chamomile**, **clove**, **dong quai**, **feverfew**, **garlic**, **ginger**, **ginkgo**, and ***Panax ginseng***.

Route/Dosage

Acute Coronary Syndrome

IV (Adults ≤121 kg): 180 mcg/kg as a bolus dose, followed by 2 mcg/kg/min until hospital discharge or surgical intervention (up to 72 hr).

Percutaneous Coronary Intervention

IV (Adults): 180 mcg/kg as a bolus dose, immediately before PCI, followed by 2 mcg/kg/min infusion; a 2nd bolus of 180 mcg/kg is given 10 min after 1st bolus; infusion should continue for 18–24 or hospital discharge (minimum of 12 hr).

Renal Impairment

(Adults CCr <50 mL/min): 180 mcg/kg bolus followed by 1 mcg/kg/min infusion; 2nd bolus of 180 mcg/kg is given 10 min after first bolus for patients undergoing PCI.

Availability (generic available)

Solution for injection: 20 mg/10 mL, 75 mg/100 mL, 200 mg/100 mL.

NURSING IMPLICATIONS

Assessment

- Assess for bleeding. Most common sites are arterial access site for cardiac catheterization or GI or GU tract. Arterial and venous punctures, IM injections, and use of urinary catheters, nasotracheal intubation, and NG tubes should be minimized. Noncompressible sites for IV access should be avoided. If bleeding cannot be controlled with pressure, discontinue eptifibatide and heparin immediately.
- ***Lab Test Considerations:*** Prior to eptifibatide therapy, assess hemoglobin or hematocrit, platelet count, serum creatinine, and PT/aPTT. Activated clotting time (ACT) should also be measured in patients undergoing PCI.
- Maintain the aPTT between 50 and 70 sec unless PCI is to be performed. Maintain ACT between 300 and 350 sec during PCI.
- Arterial sheath should not be removed unless aPTT <45 sec.
- If platelet count decreases to <100,000 and is confirmed, eptifibatide and heparin should be discontinued and condition monitored and treated.

Implementation

- ***High Alert:*** Accidental overdose of antiplatelet medications has resulted in patient harm or death from internal hemorrhage or intracranial bleeding. Have second practitioner independently check original order, dose calculations, and infusion pump settings.
- Most patients receive heparin and aspirin concurrently with eptifibatide.
- After PCI, femoral artery sheath may be removed during eptifibatide treatment only after heparin has been discontinued and its effects mostly reversed.
- Do not administer solutions that are discolored or contain particulate matter. Discard unused portion.

IV Administration

- **IV Push:** ***High Alert: Diluent:*** Withdraw appropriate loading dose from bolus vial (20 mg/10-mL vial) into a syringe. Administer undiluted. ***Concentration:*** 2 mg/mL. ***Rate:*** Administer over 1–2 min.
- **Continuous Infusion:** ***Diluent:*** Administer undiluted directly from the 100-mL vial via an infusion pump. ***Concentration:*** 0.75 mg/mL or 2 mg/mL (depends on vial used). ***Rate:*** Based on patient's weight (see Route/Dosage section).
- **Y-Site Compatibility:** alemtuzumab, alfentanil, alteplase, amikacin, amiodarone, amphotericin B lipid complex, amphotericin B liposome, ampicillin, ampicillin/sulbactam, anidulafungin, argatroban, atracurium, atropine, azithromycin, aztreonam, bivalirudin, bumetanide, buprenorphine, butorphanol, calcium chloride, calcium gluconate, cangrelor, cefepime, cefotaxime, cefotetan, ceftazidime, ceftriaxone, cefuroxime, ciprofloxacin, cisatracurium, clindamycin, cyclosporine, daptomycin, dexamethasone, dexrazoxane, digoxin, diltiazem, diphenhydramine, dobutamine, dolasetron, dopamine, doxorubicin liposomal, doxycycline, droperidol, enalaprilat, ephedrine, epinephrine, ertapenem, erythromycin, esmolol, famotidine, fentanil, fluconazole, foscarnet, fosphenytoin, ganciclovir, gentamicin, granisetron, haloperidol, heparin, hydrocortisone, hydromorphone, imipenem/cilastatin, isoproterenol, ketorolac, labetalol, leucovorin, levofloxacin, lidocaine, linezolid, lorazepam, magnesium sulfate, mannitol, meperidine, meropenem, methylprednisolone, metoclopramide, metoprolol, micafungin, midazolam, milrinone, morphine, nalbuphine, naloxone, nicardipine, nitroglycerin, nitroprusside, octreotide, ondansetron, oxytocin, palonosetron, pancuronium, pemetrexed, pentobarbital, phenobarbital, phenylephrine, piperacillin/tazobactam, potassium acetate, potassium chloride, potassium phosphates, procainamide, prochlorperazine, promethazine, propranolol, ranitidine, remifentanil, rocuronium, sodium bicarbonate, sodium phosphates, succinylcholine, sufentanil, theophylline, tigecycline, tirofiban, tobramycin, vancomycin, vecuronium, verapamil, zidovudine, zoledronic acid.
- **Y-Site Incompatibility:** acyclovir, amphotericin B deoxycholate, chlorpromazine, diazepam, furosemide, methohexital, mycophenolate, pentamidine, phenytoin, thiopental.

Patient/Family Teaching
- Inform patient of the purpose of eptifibatide.
- Instruct patient to notify health care professional immediately if any bleeding is noted.

Evaluation/Desired Outcomes
- Inhibition of platelet aggregation, resulting in decreased incidence of new MI, death, or refractory ischemia with the need for repeat urgent cardiac intervention.

erenumab (e-ren-ue-mab)
Aimovig

Classification
Therapeutic: vascular headache suppressants
Pharmacologic: monoclonal antibodies, calcitonin gene-related peptide receptor antagonists

Indications
Migraine prevention.

Action
Monoclonal antibody that binds to the calcitonin gene-related peptide (CGRP) receptor, which reduces the neuroinflammatory and vasodilatory effects of CGRP.
Therapeutic Effects: Reduction in frequency of migraines.

Pharmacokinetics
Absorption: Well absorbed (82%) following subcutaneous administration.
Distribution: Some tissue distribution.
Metabolism and Excretion: *Low concentrations*—Eliminated through saturable binding to CGRP receptor; *High concentrations*—Eliminated through non-specific, non-saturable proteolytic pathway.
Half-life: 28 days.

TIME/ACTION PROFILE (plasma concentrations)

ROUTE	ONSET	PEAK	DURATION
Subcut	unknown	6 days	1 mo

Contraindications/Precautions
Contraindicated in: Hypersensitivity.
Use Cautiously in: Geri: Choose dose carefully, considering concurrent disease states, drug therapy, and age-related ↓ in hepatic and renal function; OB: Safety and effectiveness not established; Lactation: Use only if potential maternal benefit justifies potential risk to infant; Pedi: Safety and effectiveness not established.

Adverse Reactions/Side Effects
GI: constipation. **Local:** injection site reactions. **MS:** muscle spasm. **Misc:** HYPERSENSITIVITY REACTIONS (including anaphylaxis and angioedema).

Interactions
Drug-Drug: None known.

Route/Dosage
Subcut (Adults): 70 mg once monthly; may ↑ dose, if needed, to 140 mg once monthly.

Availability
Solution for injection (prefilled syringes and autoinjectors): 70 mg/mL, 140 mg/mL.

NURSING IMPLICATIONS

Assessment
- Assess frequency and intensity of migraines.
- Assess for latex allergy. Needle shield within white or orange cap of prefilled autoinjector and gray needle cap of prefilled syringe contain dry natural rubber (a derivative of latex), may cause allergic reactions in individuals sensitive to latex.
- Monitor for signs and symptoms of hypersensitivity reactions (rash, angioedema, anaphylaxis); usually occur within hrs of injection but >1 wk after injection. If reaction is severe, discontinue erenumab and treat as needed.

Implementation
- **Subcut:** Prior to use allow vial to sit at room temperature for at least 30 min, protect from direct sunlight. Do no use other methods to warm solution (hot water or microwave). Do not shake. Solution is clear to opalescent, colorless to light yellow; do not administer solutions that are discolored, cloudy, or contain particulate matter. Store in refrigerator in original carton to protect from light; do not freeze. May be stored up to 7 days at room temperature.
- Inject entire contents into abdomen, thigh, or upper arm. Do not inject into areas where the skin is tender, bruised, red, or hard.

Patient/Family Teaching
- Instruct patient to take as directed. Administer missed doses as soon as possible and schedule next dose 1 mo from last dose administered. Educate patient and/or caregiver on correct technique for injection and disposal of equipment. Advise patient to read Patient Information before starting therapy and with each Rx refill in case of changes.
- Instruct patient to notify health care professional immediately if signs and symptoms of hypersensitivity reaction (swelling of face, mouth, tongue or throat, trouble breathing, rash) occur.
- Advise patient to notify health care professional if severe constipation occurs; may cause serious complications.

- Advise patient to notify health care professional of all Rx or OTC medications, vitamins, or herbal products being taken and to consult with health care professional before taking other medications.
- Advise female patients to notify health care professional if pregnancy is planned or suspected or if breast feeding.

Evaluation/Desired Outcomes

- Decrease in frequency and intensity of migraines.

ergocalciferol, See VITAMIN D COMPOUNDS.

erlotinib (er-lo-ti-nib)

Tarceva

Classification

Therapeutic: antineoplastics

Pharmacologic: enzyme inhibitors

Indications

Treatment of metastatic non–small-cell lung cancer (NSCLC) that has epidermal growth factor exon 19 deletions or exon 21 substitution mutations in patients who are receiving first-line, maintenance or second or greater line treatment after progression following ≥1 previous chemotherapy regimen. First-line therapy for locally advanced, surgically unresectable, or metastatic pancreatic cancer (with gemcitabine).

Action

Inhibits the enzyme tyrosine kinase, which is associated with human epidermal growth factor receptor (EGFR); blocks growth stimulation signals in cancer cells. **Therapeutic Effects:** Decreased spread of lung or pancreatic cancer with increased survival.

Pharmacokinetics

Absorption: 60% absorbed; bioavailability ↑ to 100% with food.

Distribution: Unknown.

Protein Binding: 93% protein bound.

Metabolism and Excretion: Mostly metabolized by the liver (CYP3A4 enzyme system).

Half-life: 36 hr.

TIME/ACTION PROFILE (blood levels)

ROUTE	ONSET	PEAK	DURATION
Oral	unknown	4 hr	24 hr

Contraindications/Precautions

Contraindicated in: OB: Pregnancy (may cause fetal harm); Lactation: Lactation.

Use Cautiously in: Hepatic impairment; Previous chemotherapy/radiation, pre-existing lung disease, metastatic lung disease (may ↑ risk of interstitial lung disease); Rep: Women of reproductive potential; Pedi: Safety and effectiveness not established.

Adverse Reactions/Side Effects

CNS: CEREBROVASCULAR ACCIDENT (pancreatic cancer patients), fatigue. **CV:** MYOCARDIAL INFARCTION/ISCHEMIA (pancreatic cancer patients). **Derm:** BULLOUS AND EXFOLIATIVE SKIN DISORDERS, rash, dry skin, pruritus. **EENT:** abnormal eyelash growth, conjunctivitis, corneal perforation, corneal ulceration, keratitis, ↓ tear production. **GI:** HEPATOTOXICITY, GI PERFORATION, diarrhea, abdominal pain, anorexia, nausea, stomatitis, vomiting, ↑ liver enzymes. **GU:** RENAL FAILURE. **Hemat:** microangiopathic hemolytic anemia with thrombocytopenia (pancreatic cancer patients). **Resp:** INTERSTITIAL LUNG DISEASE, dyspnea, cough.

Interactions

Drug-Drug: Strong CYP3A4 inhibitors, including **atazanavir**, **clarithromycin**, **indinavir**, **itraconazole**, **ketoconazole**, **nefazodone**, **nelfinavir**, **ritonavir**, **saquinavir**, or **voriconazole** ↑ levels and the risk of toxicity; consider alternative therapy or ↓ erlotinib dose. **Strong CYP3A4 inducers**, including **rifampin**, **rifabutin**, **rifapentine**, **phenytoin**, **carbamazepine**, or **phenobarbital** ↓ levels and may ↓ response; consider alternative therapy or ↑ erlotinib dose. **CYP1A2 inhibitors**, including **ciprofloxacin**, may ↑ levels and the risk of toxicity; consider ↓ erlotinib dose if used with CYP3A4 inhibitor. **Smoking** may ↓ levels and may ↓ response; avoid smoking during therapy or consider ↑ erlotinib dose if smoking continues. **Moderate CYP1A2 inducers**, including **teriflunomide**, **rifampin**, or **phenytoin**; avoid concurrent use or ↑ erlotinib dose. May ↓ **midazolam** levels. May ↑ risk of bleeding with **warfarin**. ↓ levels with **proton pump inhibitors**, **H_2 blockers**, and **antacids**; avoid concurrent use with **proton pump inhibitors**; take 10 hr after **H_2 antagonist** and ≥2 hr before next dose of **H_2 antagonist**; separate from **antacid** by several hrs.

Drug-Natural Products: St. John's wort may ↓ levels and may ↓ response; alternative therapy or ↑ dose should be considered.

Drug-Food: Grapefruit juice or **grapefruit**, a strong CYP3A4 inhibitor, ↑ levels and the risk of toxicity; consider dose ↓.

Route/Dosage

PO (Adults): *NSCLC*—150 mg once daily; *Pancreatic cancer*—100 mg once daily. *Concurrent use of strong CYP3A4 inhibitor or concurrent use of CYP3A4 and CYP1A2 inhibitor (e.g., ciprofloxacin)*—Consider ↓ dose in 50 mg increments (avoid concomitant use, if possible); *Concurrent use of strong CYP3A4 inducer*—consider ↑ dose by 50 mg every 2 wk (max dose = 450 mg/day) (avoid concomitant use, if possible); *Concurrent cigarette smoking or concurrent use of moderate CYP1A2 inducer*—↑ dose by 50 mg every 2 wk (max dose = 300 mg/day);

immediately ↓ dose to recommended initial dose for indication upon smoking cessation.

Availability (generic available)

Tablets: 25 mg, 100 mg, 150 mg.

NURSING IMPLICATIONS

Assessment

- Assess respiratory status prior to and periodically during therapy. If dyspnea, cough, or fever occur, discontinue erlotinib, assess for interstitial lung disease, and institute treatment as needed.
- Assess for diarrhea. Usually responds to loperamide but may require dose reduction or discontinuation of therapy if unresponsive to therapy or patient becomes dehydrated.
- Assess skin throughout therapy. If bullous, blistering, and exfoliative skin conditions, including Stevens-Johnson syndrome/toxic epidermal necrolysis, occur, interrupt or discontinue treatment. Skin rash may require treatment with corticosteroids or anti-infectives with anti-inflammatory properties; acne treatments may aggravate dry skin and erythema.
- Assess eyes periodically during therapy. Discontinue erlotinib if corneal ulceration occurs. Withhold erlotinib if Grade 3 or 4 keratitis, or Grade 2 lasting >2 wk, or if acute or worsening eye pain or disorders occur.
- Assess for GI pain. Patients receiving concomitant antiangiogenic agents, corticosteroids, NSAIDs, and/or taxane-based chemotherapy, or who have prior history of peptic ulceration or diverticular disease, are at increased risk for GI perforation. Permanently discontinue erlotinib in patients who develop gastrointestinal perforation.
- ***Lab Test Considerations:*** Test patients for epidermal growth factor receptor (EGFR) exon 19 deletions or exon 21 (L858R) substitution mutations in plasma or tumor specimens prior to starting therapy; presence is required for therapy.
- Monitor liver function tests (AST, ALT, bilirubin, alkaline phosphatase) periodically during therapy. Consider dose reduction or discontinuation of therapy if severe changes in liver function (doubling or tripling of transaminase levels in *patients with pre-existing hepatic impairment* or total bilirubin ≥3 times upper limit of normal and/or transaminases ≥5 times upper limit of normal in *patients without pre-existing hepatic impairment*) occur.
- Monitor renal function and electrolytes in patients at risk for dehydration. Withhold therapy if dehydration or Grade 3 or 4 renal toxicity occurs.
- Monitor INR regularly in patients taking warfarin. May cause ↑ INR.

Implementation

- Do not confuse Tarceva (erlotinib) with Tresiba (insulin degludec).
- **PO:** Administer at least 1 hr before or 2 hr after food.

Patient/Family Teaching

- Instruct patient to take erlotinib as directed.
- Advise patient to notify health care professional if severe or persistent diarrhea, nausea, anorexia, vomiting, onset or worsening of skin rash, unexplained dyspnea or cough, eye irritation, or signs and symptoms of a cerebrovascular accident (sudden weakness; paralysis [an inability to move] or numbness of the face, arms, or legs, especially on one side of the body; confusion; trouble speaking or understanding speech; trouble seeing in one or both eyes; problems breathing; dizziness, trouble walking, loss of balance or coordination, unexplained falls; loss of consciousness; sudden and severe headache) occur.
- Instruct patient to avoid proton pump inhibitors and if antacids are necessary, separate antacids and erlotinib dose by several hrs. If therapy with H_2 antagonists is required, take erlotinib 10 hrs after H_2 antagonist and at least 2 hrs before next dose of H_2 antagonist.
- Advise patient to notify health care professional of all Rx or OTC medications, vitamins, or herbal products being taken and consult health care professional before taking any new medications.
- Advise patient to wear sunscreen and protective clothing to decrease skin reactions.
- Instruct patient to discontinue smoking during therapy; smoking decreases blood levels of erlotinib.
- Rep: Caution patient to use highly effective contraceptive during and for at least 1 mo after completion of therapy and to avoid breast feeding during and for at least 2 wk following last dose. Advise female patients to notify health care professional if pregnancy is planned or suspected.

Evaluation/Desired Outcomes

- Decrease in spread of non–small-cell lung or pancreatic cancer with increased survival.

ertapenem (er-ta-**pen**-em)

INVanz

Classification
Therapeutic: anti-infectives
Pharmacologic: carbapenems

Indications

Moderate to severe: complicated intra-abdominal infections, complicated skin and skin structure infections, community acquired pneumonia, complicated urinary tract infections (including pyelonephritis), acute pelvic infections including postpartum endomyometritis, septic abortion, and postsurgical gynecologic infections.

Prophylaxis of surgical site infection following elective colorectal surgery.

Action

Binds to bacterial cell wall, resulting in cell death. Ertapenem resists the actions of many enzymes that degrade most other penicillins and penicillin-like anti-infectives. **Therapeutic Effects:** Bactericidal action against susceptible bacteria. **Spectrum:** Active against the following aerobic gram-positive organisms: *Staphylococcus aureus* (methicillin-susceptible strains only), *Staphylococcus epidermidis*, *Streptococcus agalactiae*, *S. pneumoniae* (penicillin-susceptible strains only), and *S. pyogenes*. Also active against the following gram-negative aerobic organisms: *Escherichia coli*, *Haemophilus influenzae* (beta-lactamase negative strains), *Klebsiella pneumonia*, *Moraxella catarrhalis*, and *Providencia rettgeri*. Addition anaerobic spectrum includes *Bacteroides fragilis*, *B. distasonis*, *B. ovatus*, *B. thetaiotamicron*, *B. uniformis*, *B. vulgatis*, *Clostridium clostrioforme*, *Eubacterium lentum*, *Peptostreptococcus*, *Porphyromonas asaccharolytica*, and *Prevotella bivia*.

Pharmacokinetics

Absorption: 90% after IM administration; IV administration results in complete bioavailability.
Distribution: Enters breast milk.
Metabolism and Excretion: Mostly excreted by the kidneys.
Half-life: 1.8 hr (↑ in renal impairment).

TIME/ACTION PROFILE (blood levels)

ROUTE	ONSET	PEAK	DURATION
IM	rapid	2 hr	24 hr
IV	rapid	end of infusion	24 hr

Contraindications/Precautions

Contraindicated in: Hypersensitivity; Cross-sensitivity may occur with penicillins, cephalosporins, and other carbapenems; Hypersensitivity to lidocaine (may be used as a diluent for IM administration).
Use Cautiously in: History of multiple hypersensitivity reactions; Seizure disorders; Renal impairment; OB: Safety not established; Lactation: Use during breast feeding only if benefit to patient outweighs potential risk to infant; Pedi: Safety and effectiveness not established; Geri: ↑ sensitivity due to age-related ↓ in renal function.

Adverse Reactions/Side Effects

CNS: SEIZURES, headache. **Derm:** ACUTE GENERALIZED EXANTHEMATOUS PUSTULOSIS. **GI:** CLOSTRIDIUM DIFFICILE-ASSOCIATED DIARRHEA (CDAD), diarrhea, nausea, vomiting. **GU:** vaginitis. **Local:** phlebitis at IV site, pain at IM site. **Misc:** HYPERSENSITIVITY REACTIONS (including anaphylaxis).

Interactions

Drug-Drug: Probenecid ↓ excretion and ↑ levels. May ↓ serum **valproate** levels (↑ risk of seizures).

Route/Dosage

IV, IM (Adults and Children ≥13 yrs): 1 g once daily for up to 14 days (IV) or 7 days (IM).
IV, IM (Children 3 mo–12 yrs): 15 mg/kg twice daily (not to exceed 1 g/day) for up to 14 days (IV) or 7 days (IM).

Renal Impairment

IM, IV (Adults): *CCr ≤30 mL/min/1.73 m²*—500 mg once daily.

Availability (generic available)

Powder for injection (requires reconstitution): 1 g/vial.

NURSING IMPLICATIONS

Assessment

- Assess for infection (vital signs; appearance of wound, sputum, urine, and stool; WBC) at beginning of and during therapy.
- Obtain a history before initiating therapy to determine previous use of and reactions to penicillins, cephalosporins, or carbapenems. Persons with a negative history of penicillin sensitivity may still have an allergic response.
- Obtain specimens for culture and sensitivity before initiating therapy. First dose may be given before receiving results.
- Observe patient for signs and symptoms of anaphylaxis (rash, pruritus, laryngeal edema, wheezing). Discontinue the drug and notify the physician immediately if these occur. Have epinephrine, an antihistamine, and resuscitative equipment close by in the event of an anaphylactic reaction.
- Monitor bowel function. Diarrhea, abdominal cramping, fever, and bloody stools should be reported to health care professional promptly as a sign of Clostridium difficile-associated diarrhea (CDAD). May begin up to several wk following cessation of therapy.
- ***Lab Test Considerations:*** May cause ↑ AST, ALT, serum alkaline phosphatase levels.
- May cause ↑ platelet and eosinophil counts.

Implementation

- **IM:** Reconstitute 1-g vial with 3.2 mL of 1% lidocaine without epinephrine. Shake well to form solution. Immediately withdraw contents and inject deep into large muscle mass. Use reconstituted solution within 1 hr.

IV Administration

- **Intermittent Infusion: *Diluent:*** Reconstitute 1-g vial with 10 mL of sterile water for injection or 0.9% NaCl using a 21–gauge or smaller diameter needle and shake well. *For adults and pediatric patients 13 yrs and older:* further dilute in 50 mL of 0.9% NaCl. *For pediatric patients 3 mo to 12 yr:* immediately withdraw a volume equal to 15 mg/kg (not to exceed 1 g/day) and dilute in 0.9% NaCl to a final concentration of 20 mg/mL or less. Administer within 6 hr of reconstitution. ***Rate:*** Infuse over 30 min.

- **Y-Site Compatibility:** acyclovir, alfentanil, amifostine, amikacin, aminocaproic acid, aminophylline, amphotericin B lipid complex, amphotericin B liposome, argatroban, arsenic trioxide, atracurium, azithromycin, aztreonam, bivalirudin, bleomycin, bumetanide, buprenorphine, busulfan, butorphanol, calcium chloride, calcium gluconate, cangrelor, carboplatin, carmustine, chloramphenicol, cisatracurium, cyclophosphamide, cyclosporine, cytarabine, dacarbazine, dactinomycin, daptomycin, dexamethasone, dexmedetomidine, dexrazoxane, digoxin, diltiazem, diphenhydramine, docetaxel, dolasetron, dopamine, doxacurium, doxorubicin liposome, doxycycline, enalaprilat, ephedrine, epinephrine, eptifibatide, erythromycin, esmolol, etoposide phosphate, famotidine, fenoldopam, fluconazole, fludarabine, fluorouracil, foscarnet, fosfomycin, fosphenytoin, furosemide, ganciclovir, gemcitabine, gentamicin, glycopyrrolate, granisetron, haloperidol, heparin, hydrocortisone, hydromorphone, ifosfamide, insulin, regular, irinotecan, isoproterenol, ketorolac, labetalol, leucovorin calcium, levofloxacin, lidocaine, linezolid, lorazepam, magnesium sulfate, mannitol, melphalan, meperidine, meropenem/vaborbactam, mesna, methotrexate, methyldopate, methylprednisolone, metoclopramide, metronidazole, milrinone, mitomycin, morphine, moxifloxacin, nalbuphine, naloxone, nitroglycerin, nitroprusside, norepinephrine, octreotide, oxaliplatin, oxytocin, paclitaxel, pamidronate, pancuronium, pantoprazole, pemetrexed, pentobarbital, phenobarbital, phentolamine, phenylephrine, potassium acetate, potassium chloride, potassium phosphates, procainamide, propranolol, ranitidine, remifentanil, rocuronium, sodium acetate, sodium bicarbonate, sodium phosphates, streptozocin, succinylcholine, sufentanil, tacrolimus, telavancin, theophylline, thiotepa, tigecycline, tirofiban, tobramycin, trimethoprim/sulfamethoxazole, vancomycin, vasopressin, vecuronium, vinblastine, vincristine, vinorelbine, voriconazole, zidovudine, zoledronic acid.
- **Y-Site Incompatibility:** alemtuzumab, allopurinol, amiodarone, anidulafungin, caspofungin, chlorpromazine, dantrolene, daunorubicin hydrochloride, diazepam, dobutamine, doxorubicin hydrochloride, droperidol, epirubicin, hydralazine, hydroxyzine, idarubicin, isavuconazonium, midazolam, minocycline, mitoxantrone, nicardipine, ondansetron, pentamidine, phenytoin, prochlorperazine, promethazine, quinupristin/dalfopristin, thiopental, topotecan, verapamil.

Patient/Family Teaching

- Advise patient to report the signs of superinfection (black, furry overgrowth on the tongue; vaginal itching or discharge; loose or foul-smelling stools) and allergy.
- Caution patient to notify health care professional if fever and diarrhea occur, especially if stool contains blood, pus, or mucus. Advise patient not to treat diarrhea without consulting health care professional. May occur up to several wk after discontinuation of medication. Consult health care professional before treating with antidiarrheals.

Evaluation/Desired Outcomes

- Resolution of the signs and symptoms of infection. Length of time for complete resolution depends on the organism and site of infection.

E

ERYTHROMYCIN†
(eh-rith-roe-**mye**-sin)

erythromycin base
~~E-Mycin~~, ✱Eryc, Ery-Tab, ~~PCE~~

erythromycin ethylsuccinate
E.E.S, EryPed

erythromycin lactobionate
Erythrocin

erythromycin stearate
Erythrocin Stearate, ✱Erythro-S

erythromycin (topical)
Erygel

Classification
Therapeutic: anti-infectives
Pharmacologic: macrolides
†See Appendix C for ophthalmic use

Indications

IV, PO: Infections caused by susceptible organisms including: Upper and lower respiratory tract infections, Otitis media (with sulfonamides), Skin and skin structure infections, Pertussis, Diphtheria, Erythrasma, Intestinal amebiasis, Pelvic inflammatory disease, Nongonococcal urethritis, Syphilis, Legionnaires' disease, Rheumatic fever. Useful when penicillin is the most appropriate drug but cannot be used because of hypersensitivity, including: Streptococcal infections, Treatment of syphilis or gonorrhea. **Topical:** Treatment of acne.

Action

Suppresses protein synthesis at the level of the 50S bacterial ribosome. **Therapeutic Effects:** Bacteriostatic action against susceptible bacteria. **Spectrum:**

Active against many gram-positive cocci, including: Streptococci, Staphylococci. Gram-positive bacilli, including: *Clostridium*, *Corynebacterium*. Several gram-negative pathogens, notably: *Neisseria*, *Legionella pneumophila*. *Mycoplasma* and *Chlamydia* are also usually susceptible.

Pharmacokinetics

Absorption: Variable absorption from the duodenum after oral administration (dependent on salt form). Absorption of enteric-coated products is delayed. Minimal absorption may follow topical or ophthalmic use.

Distribution: Widely distributed. Minimal CNS penetration. Crosses placenta; enters breast milk.

Protein Binding: 70–80%.

Metabolism and Excretion: Partially metabolized by the liver, excreted mainly unchanged in the bile; small amounts excreted unchanged in the urine.

Half-life: Neonates: 2.1 hr; Adults: 1.4–2 hr.

TIME/ACTION PROFILE (blood levels)

ROUTE	ONSET	PEAK	DURATION
PO	1 hr	1–4 hr	6–12 hr
IV	rapid	end of infusion	6–12 hr

Contraindications/Precautions

Contraindicated in: Hypersensitivity; Concurrent use of dihydroergotamine, ergotamine, lovastatin, pimozide, or simvastatin; Long QT syndrome; Hypokalemia; Hypomagnesemia; Heart rate <50 bpm; Known alcohol intolerance (most topicals); Tartrazine sensitivity (some products contain tartrazine—FDC yellow dye #5); Products containing benzyl alcohol should be avoided in neonates.

Use Cautiously in: Liver/renal disease; OB: May be used in pregnancy to treat chlamydial infections or syphilis; Myasthenia gravis (may worsen symptoms); Geri: ↑ risk of ototoxicity if parenteral dose >4 g/day, ↑ risk of QTc interval prolongation.

Adverse Reactions/Side Effects

CNS: seizures (rare). **CV:** TORSADES DE POINTES, VENTRICULAR ARRHYTHMIAS, QT interval prolongation. **Derm:** rash. **EENT:** ototoxicity. **GI:** CLOSTRIDIUM DIFFICILE-ASSOCIATED DIARRHEA (CDAD), nausea, vomiting, abdominal pain, cramping, diarrhea, hepatitis, infantile hypertrophic pyloric stenosis, pancreatitis (rare). **GU:** interstitial nephritis. **Local:** phlebitis at IV site. **Misc:** HYPERSENSITIVITY REACTIONS (including anaphylaxis).

Interactions

Drug-Drug: Concurrent use with **pimozide** may ↑ levels and the risk for serious arrhythmias (concurrent use contraindicated); similar effects may occur with **diltiazem**, **verapamil**, **ketoconazole**, **itraconazole**, **nefazodone**, and **protease inhibitors**; avoid concurrent use. May ↑ levels of **ergotamine** and **dihydroergotamine** and risk for acute ergot toxicity; concurrent use contraindicated. Concurrent use with **lovastatin** or **simvastatin** may ↑ risk of rhabdomyolysis. Concurrent use with **amiodarone**, **dofetilide**, or **sotalol** may ↑ risk of torsades de pointe; avoid concurrent use. May ↑ **verapamil** levels and the risk for hypotension, bradycardia, and lactic acidosis. ↑ blood levels and effects of **sildenafil**, **tadalafil**, and **vardenafil**; use lower doses. Concurrent **rifabutin** or **rifampin** may ↓ effect of erythromycin and ↑ risk of adverse GI reactions. ↑ levels and risk of toxicity from **alfentanil**, **alprazolam**, **bromocriptine**, **carbamazepine**, **cyclosporine**, **cilostazol**, **diazepam**, **disopyramide**, **ergot alkaloids**, **felodipine**, **methylprednisolone**, **midazolam**, **quinidine**, **rifabutin**, **tacrolimus**, **triazolam**, or **vinblastine**. May ↑ levels of **lovastatin** and **simvastatin** and ↑ the risk of myopathy/rhabdomyolysis. May ↑ serum **digoxin** levels. **Theophylline** may ↓ blood levels. May ↑ **colchicine** levels and the risk for toxicity; use lower starting and maximum dose of colchicine. May ↑ **theophylline** levels and the risk for toxicity; ↓ theophylline dose. May ↑ **warfarin** levels and the risk for bleeding.

Route/Dosage

250 mg of erythromycin base or stearate = 400 mg of erythromycin ethylsuccinate.

Most Infections

PO (Adults): *Base, stearate*—250 mg every 6 hr, *or* 333 mg every 8 hr, *or* 500 mg every 12 hr. *Ethylsuccinate*—400 mg every 6 hr *or* 800 mg every 12 hr.

PO (Children >1 mo): *Base and ethylsuccinate*—30–50 mg/kg/day divided every 6–8 hr (max = 2 g/day as base or 3.2 g/day as ethylsuccinate). *Stearate*—30–50 mg/kg/day divided every 6 hr (max = 2 g/day).

PO (Neonates): *Ethylsuccinate*—20–50 mg/kg/day divided every 6–12 hr.

IV (Adults): 250–500 mg (up to 1 g) every 6 hr.

IV (Children >1 mo): 15–50 mg/kg/day divided every 6 hr (max = 4 g/day).

Acne

Topical (Adults and Children >12 yr): 2% gel, solution, or pledgets twice daily.

Availability (generic available)

Erythromycin Base

Delayed-release capsules: 250 mg, 333 mg. **Delayed—release tablets:** 250 mg, 333 mg, 500 mg.

Erythromycin Ethylsuccinate

Oral suspension (fruit, cherry, orange, or banana flavor): 200 mg/5 mL, 400 mg/5 mL. **Tablets:** 400 mg.

Erythromycin Lactobionate

Powder for injection (requires reconstitution and dilution): 500 mg/vial, 1 g.

Erythromycin Stearate

Film-coated tablets: 250 mg.

Erythromycin Topical Preparations

Gel: 2%. **Pledgets:** 2%. **Solution:** 2%. ***In combination with:*** benzoyl peroxide (Benzamycin). See Appendix B.

NURSING IMPLICATIONS

Assessment

- Assess for infection (vital signs; appearance of wound, sputum, urine, and stool; WBC) at beginning of and during therapy.
- Obtain specimens for culture and sensitivity before initiating therapy. First dose may be given before receiving results.
- Monitor bowel function. Diarrhea, abdominal cramping, fever, and bloody stools should be reported to health care professional promptly as a sign of Clostridium difficile-associated diarrhea (CDAD). May begin up to several wk following cessation of therapy.
- ***Lab Test Considerations:*** Monitor liver function tests periodically on patients receiving high-dose, long-term therapy.
- May cause ↑ serum bilirubin, AST, ALT, and alkaline phosphatase concentrations.
- May cause false ↑ of urinary catecholamines.

Implementation

- **PO:** Administer around the clock. *Erythromycin film-coated tablets (base and stearate)* are absorbed better on an empty stomach, at least 1 hr before or 2 hr after meals; may be taken with food if GI irritation occurs. *Enteric-coated erythromycin (base)* may be taken without regard to meals. *Erythromycin ethylsuccinate* is best absorbed when taken with meals. Take each dose with a full glass of water.
- Use calibrated measuring device for liquid preparations. Shake well before using.
- Do not crush or chew delayed-release capsules or tablets; swallow whole. *Erythromycin base delayed-release capsules* may be opened and sprinkled on applesauce, jelly, or ice cream immediately before ingestion. Entire contents of the capsule should be taken.

IV Administration

- **IV:** Add 10 mL of sterile water for injection without preservatives to 250- or 500-mg vials and 20 mL to 1-g vial. Solution is stable for 7 days after reconstitution if refrigerated.
- **Intermittent Infusion:** ***Diluent:*** Dilute in 0.9% NaCl or D5W. ***Concentration:*** 1–5 mg/mL. ***Rate:*** Administer slowly over 20–60 min to avoid phlebitis. Assess for pain along vein; slow rate if pain occurs; apply ice and notify health care professional if unable to relieve pain.
- **Continuous Infusion:** May also be administered as an infusion over 4 hr. ***Diluent:*** 0.9% NaCl, D5W, or LR. ***Concentration:*** 1 g/L.

Erythromycin Lactobionate

- **Y-Site Compatibility:** acyclovir, alemtuzumab, alfentanil, amikacin, aminocaproic acid, aminophylline, amiodarone, anidulafungin, argatroban, atropine, azathioprine, benztropine, bivalirudin, bleomycin, bumetanide, buprenorphine, butorphanol, calcium chloride, calcium gluconate, cangrelor, carboplatin, carmustine, caspofungin, cefotaxime, ceftriaxone, cefuroxime, chlorpromazine, cisplatin, cyanocobalamin, cyclophosphamide, cyclosporine, cytarabine, dacarbazine, dactinomycin, daptomycin, daunorubicin hydrochloride, dexmedetomidine, dexrazoxane, digoxin, diltiazem, diphenhydramine, dobutamine, docetaxel, dolasetron, dopamine, doxorubicin, doxorubicin liposomal, enalaprilat, ephedrine, epinephrine, epirubicin, epoetin alfa, eptifibatide, ertapenem, esmolol, etoposide, etoposide phosphate, famotidine, fenoldopam, fentanyl, fluconazole, fludarabine, fluorouracil, folic acid, foscarnet, fosphenytoin, gemcitabine, gentamicin, glycopyrrolate, granisetron, hetastarch, hydrocortisone, hydromorphone, idarubicin, ifosfamide, imipenem/cilastatin, insulin, irinotecan, isoproterenol, labetalol, leucovorin, levofloxacin, lidocaine, lorazepam, mannitol, meperidine, mesna, methotrexate, methyldopate, methylprednisolone, metoclopramide, metoprolol, metronidazole, midazolam, milrinone, mitoxantrone, morphine, multivitamins, mycophenolate, nafcillin, nalbuphine, naloxone, nicardipine, nitroglycerin, norepinephrine, octreotide, ondansetron, oxacillin, oxaliplatin, oxytocin, paclitaxel, palonosetron, pamidronate, pancuronium, papaverine, pentamidine, perphenazine, phenylephrine, phytonadione, piperacillin/tazobactam, potassium acetate, potassium chloride, procainamide, prochlorperazine, promethazine, propranolol, protamine, pyridoxine, ranitidine, sodium acetate, sodium bicarbonate, streptokinase, succinylcholine, sufentanil, tacrolimus, theophylline, thiamine, thiotepa, tigecycline, tirofiban, tobramycin, topotecan, vancomycin, vasopressin, vecuronium, verapamil, vinblastine, vincristine, vinorelbine, vitamin B complex with C, voriconazole, zidovudine, zoledronic acid.
- **Y-Site Incompatibility:** amphotericin B colloidal, amphotericin B lipid complex, amphotericin B liposome, ascorbic acid, aztreonam, cefazolin, cefepime, cefotetan, cefoxitin, dantrolene, diazepam, diazoxide, doxycycline, furosemide, ganciclovir, indomethacin, ketorolac, metaraminol, nitroprusside, pemetrexed, pentobarbital, phenytoin, trimethoprim/sulfamethoxazole.
- **Topical:** Cleanse area before application. Wear gloves during application.

Patient/Family Teaching

- Instruct patient to take medication around the clock and to finish the drug completely as directed, even if feeling better. Take missed doses as soon as remembered, with remaining doses evenly spaced throughout day. Advise patient that sharing of this medication may be dangerous.
- May cause nausea, vomiting, diarrhea, or stomach cramps; notify health care professional if these effects persist or if severe abdominal pain, yellow discoloration of the skin or eyes, darkened urine, pale stools, or unusual tiredness develops. May cause infantile hypertrophic pyloric stenosis in infants; notify health care professional if vomiting and irritability occur.
- Caution patient to notify health care professional if fever and diarrhea occur, especially if stool contains blood, pus, or mucus. Advise patient not to treat diarrhea without consulting health care professional. May occur up to several wk after discontinuation of medication.
- Advise patient to report signs of superinfection (black, furry overgrowth on the tongue; vaginal itching or discharge; loose or foul-smelling stools).
- Advise females of reproductive potential to notify health care professional if pregnancy is planned or suspected, or if breast feeding.
- Instruct patient to notify health care professional if symptoms do not improve.

Evaluation/Desired Outcomes

- Resolution of the signs and symptoms of infection. Length of time for complete resolution depends on the organism and site of infection.
- Improvement of acne lesions.

escitalopram

(ess-sit-**al**-o-pram)

✱Cipralex, Lexapro

Classification

Therapeutic: antidepressants

Pharmacologic: selective serotonin reuptake inhibitors (SSRIs)

Indications

Major depressive disorder. Generalized anxiety disorder (GAD). **Unlabeled Use:** Panic disorder. Obsessive-compulsive disorder (OCD). Post-traumatic stress disorder (PTSD). Social anxiety disorder (social phobia). Premenstrual dysphoric disorder (PMDD).

Action

Selectively inhibits the reuptake of serotonin in the CNS. **Therapeutic Effects:** Antidepressant action.

Pharmacokinetics

Absorption: 80% absorbed following oral administration.

Distribution: Enters breast milk.

Metabolism and Excretion: Mostly metabolized by the liver (primarily CYP3A4 and CYP2C19 isoenzymes); 7% excreted unchanged by kidneys.

Half-life: ↑ in elderly and patients with hepatic impairment.

TIME/ACTION PROFILE (antidepressant effect)

ROUTE	ONSET	PEAK	DURATION
PO	within 1–4 wk	unknown	unknown

Contraindications/Precautions

Contraindicated in: Hypersensitivity; Concurrent pimozide; Concurrent use of MAO inhibitors or MAO-like drugs (linezolid or methylene blue); Concurrent use of citalopram; Angle-closure glaucoma.

Use Cautiously in: History of mania (may activate mania/hypomania); History of seizures; Patients at risk for suicide; Hepatic impairment (dose ↓ recommended); Severe renal impairment; OB: Neonates exposed to SSRIs in the 3rd trimester may develop drug discontinuation syndrome manifested by respiratory distress, feeding difficulty, and irritability; Lactation: Use while breast feeding only if potential maternal benefit justifies potential risk to infant; Pedi: May ↑ risk of suicide attempt/ideation especially during early treatment or dose adjustment; safety not established in children <12 yr; Geri: ↓ doses recommended due to ↓ drug clearance in older patients.

Adverse Reactions/Side Effects

CNS: NEUROLEPTIC MALIGNANT SYNDROME, SUICIDAL THOUGHTS, insomnia, dizziness, drowsiness, fatigue. **Derm:** sweating. **Endo:** syndrome on inappropriate secretion of antidiuretic hormone (SIADH). **F and E:** hyponatremia. **GI:** diarrhea, nausea, abdominal pain, constipation, dry mouth, indigestion. **GU:** anorgasmia, ↓ libido, ejaculatory delay, erectile dysfunction. **Metab:** ↑ appetite. **Misc:** SEROTONIN SYNDROME.

Interactions

Drug-Drug: May cause serious, potentially fatal reactions when used with **MAO inhibitors**; allow at least 14 days between escitalopram and **MAO inhibitors**. Concurrent use with **MAO-inhibitor-like drugs**, such as **linezolid** or **methylene blue** may ↑ risk of serotonin syndrome; concurrent use contraindicated; do not start therapy in patients receiving **linezolid** or **methylene blue**; if **linezolid** or **methylene blue** need to be started in a patient receiving escitalopram, immediately discontinue escitalopram and monitor for signs/symptoms of serotonin syndrome for 2 wk or until 24 hr after last dose of linezolid or methylene blue, whichever comes first (may resume escitalopram therapy 24 hr after last dose of linezolid or methylene blue). Concurrent use with **pimozide** may result in prolongation of the QTc interval and is contraindicated. Use cautiously with other **centrally acting drugs** (including **alcohol, antihistamines, opioid analgesics**, and **sedative/hypnotics**; concurrent use with **alcohol**

is not recommended). Drugs that affect serotonergic neurotransmitter systems, including **tricyclic antidepressants, SNRIs, fentanyl, buspirone, tramadol, amphetamines**, and **triptans** ↑ risk of serotonin syndrome. **Cimetidine** may ↑ levels. Serotonergic effects may be ↑ by **lithium** (concurrent use should be carefully monitored). **Carbamazepine** may ↓ levels. May ↑ levels of **metoprolol**. Use cautiously with **tricyclic antidepressants** due to unpredictable effects on serotonin and norepinephrine reuptake. ↑ risk of bleeding with **aspirin, NSAIDs, clopidogrel**, or **warfarin**.
Drug-Natural Products: ↑ risk of serotonin syndrome with **St. John's wort** and **SAMe**.

Route/Dosage

PO (Adults): *Depression and GAD*—10 mg once daily, may ↑ to 20 mg once daily after 1 wk.

Hepatic Impairment

PO (Adults): 10 mg once daily.
PO (Geriatric Patients): 10 mg once daily.
PO (Children ≥12 yr): *Depression*—10 mg once daily, may ↑ to 20 mg once daily after 3 wk.

Availability (generic available)

Orally disintegrating tablets: 🍁 10 mg, 🍁 20 mg. **Oral solution (peppermint flavor):** 1 mg/mL. **Cost:** *Generic*—$190.20/240 mL. **Tablets:** 5 mg, 10 mg, 20 mg. **Cost:** *Generic*—5 mg $13.16/100, 10 mg $13.87/100, 20 mg $18.01/100.

NURSING IMPLICATIONS

Assessment

- Monitor mood changes and level of anxiety during therapy.
- Assess for suicidal tendencies, especially during early therapy. Restrict amount of drug available to patient. Risk may be increased in children, adolescents, and adults ≤24 yr. After starting therapy, children, adolescents, and young adults should be seen by health care professional at least weekly for 4 wk, every 3 wk for next 4 wk, and on advice of health care professional thereafter.
- Assess for sexual dysfunction (erectile dysfunction; decreased libido).
- Assess for serotonin syndrome (mental changes [agitation, hallucinations, coma], autonomic instability [tachycardia, labile BP, hyperthermia], neuromuscular aberrations [hyperreflexia, incoordination], and/or GI symptoms [nausea, vomiting, diarrhea]), especially in patients taking other serotonergic drugs (SSRIs, SNRIs, triptans).

Implementation

- Do not administer escitalopram and citalopram concomitantly. Taper to avoid potential withdrawal reactions. Reduce dose by 50% for 3 days, then again by 50% for 3 days, then discontinue.
- **PO:** Administer as a single dose in the morning or evening without regard to meals.

Patient/Family Teaching

- Instruct patient to take escitalopram as directed. Take missed doses on the same day as soon as remembered and consult health care professional. Resume regular dosing schedule next day. Do not double doses. Do not stop abruptly; should be discontinued gradually. Instruct patient to read *Medication Guide* before starting and with each Rx refill in case of changes.
- May cause dizziness. Caution patient to avoid driving or other activities requiring alertness until response to medication is known.
- Advise patient, family, and caregivers to look for suicidality, especially during early therapy or dose changes. Notify health care professional immediately if thoughts about suicide or dying, attempts to commit suicide, new or worse depression or anxiety, agitation or restlessness, panic attacks, insomnia, new or worse irritability, aggressiveness, acting on dangerous impulses, mania, or other changes in mood or behavior or if rash or symptoms of serotonin syndrome occur.
- Instruct patient to notify health care professional of all Rx or OTC medications, vitamins, or herbal products being taken and to consult health care professional before taking any other Rx, OTC, or herbal products, especially St. John's wort, alcohol or other CNS depressants.
- Instruct female patients to notify health care professional if pregnancy is planned or suspected or if they plan to breast feed. If used during pregnancy, should be tapered during 3rd trimester to avoid neonatal serotonin syndrome.
- Emphasize importance of follow-up exams to monitor progress.

Evaluation/Desired Outcomes

- Increased sense of well-being.
- Renewed interest in surroundings. May require 1–4 wk of therapy to obtain antidepressant effects. Full antidepressant effects occur in 4–6 wk.
- Decrease in anxiety.

REMS

esketamine (es-**ket**-a-meen)

Spravato

Classification
Therapeutic: antidepressants
Pharmacologic: N-methyl-D-aspartate antagonist

Schedule III

E

Indications

Treatment-resistant depression (in combination with an oral antidepressant).

Action

Acts as a non-competitive N-methyl-D-aspartate (NMDA) receptor antagonist; the exact mechanism by which it exerts its antidepressant effect is unknown.
Therapeutic Effects: Decreased severity of depressive symptoms and prolonged time to relapse.

Pharmacokinetics

Absorption: 48% absorbed following nasal administration.
Distribution: Extensively distributed to tissues.
Metabolism and Excretion: Primarily metabolized to noresketamine (active metabolite) in liver by CYP2B6 and CYP3A4 isoenzymes, and to lesser extent by CYP2C9 and CYP2C19 isoenzymes. Primarily excreted in urine (≥78%; <1% as unchanged drug); ≤2% excreted in feces).
Half-life: 7–12 hr.

TIME/ACTION PROFILE (plasma concentrations)

ROUTE	ONSET	PEAK	DURATION
Intranasal	unknown	20–40 min	unknown

Contraindications/Precautions

Contraindicated in: Hypersensitivity to esketamine or ketamine; Aneurysmal vascular disease (including thoracic and abdominal aorta, intracranial and peripheral arterial vessels) or arteriovenous malformation; History of intracerebral hemorrhage; Severe hepatic impairment; OB: Pregnancy (may cause fetal harm); Lactation: Lactation (↑ risk of neurotoxicity).
Use Cautiously in: History of hypertensive encephalopathy; Moderate hepatic impairment; Rep: Women of reproductive potential; Pedi: Safety and effectiveness not established; may ↑ risk of suicide attempt/ideation especially during early treatment or dose adjustment.

Adverse Reactions/Side Effects

CNS: SUICIDAL THOUGHTS/BEHAVIORS, anxiety, depersonalization, derealization, dissociative changes, dizziness, fatigue, headache, hypoesthesia, sedation, cognitive impairment, insomnia, loss of consciousness, slurred/slow speech. **CV:** ↑ BP, tachycardia. **Derm:** ↑ sweating. **EENT:** nasal irritation, throat irritation. **GI:** metallic taste, nausea, vomiting, constipation, diarrhea, dry mouth. **GU:** urinary tract infection. **Neuro:** vertigo, tremor. **Misc:** physical dependence, psychological dependence, tolerance.

Interactions

Drug-Drug: Concurrent use with **psychostimulants**, including **amphetamines**, **methylphenidate**, or **modafanil**, or **armodafanil**, as well as **monoamine oxidase inhibitors** may ↑ BP. Use with **opioids** or other **CNS depressants**, including **benzodiazepines**, **non-benzodiazepine sedative/hypnotics**, **anxiolytics**, **general anesthetics**, **muscle relaxants**, **antipsychotics**, and **alcohol** may cause profound sedation.

Route/Dosage

Intranasal (Adults): *Induction phase (Wk 1–4)*—56 mg (2 sprays in each nostril) twice weekly; may ↑ dose (after first dose) based on response and tolerability up to 84 mg (3 sprays in each nostril) twice weekly. *Maintenance phase (Wk 5–8)*—56 mg (2 sprays in each nostril) or 84 mg (3 sprays in each nostril) once weekly. *Maintenance phase (Wk 9 and beyond)*—56 mg (2 sprays in each nostril) or 84 mg (3 sprays in each nostril) once weekly or every other wk (use least frequent dosing to maintain remission/response).

Availability

Nasal spray: 28 mg/device (14 mg/spray).

NURSING IMPLICATIONS

Assessment

- Monitor patient for sedation for at least 2 hrs after each dose.
- Monitor BP before and 40 min after administration and periodically during 2 hrs after administration. If BP elevated before administration, may hold dose. If elevated following dose, continue to monitor patient.
- Monitor for worsening and emergence of suicidal thoughts and behaviors, especially during initial few mo of drug therapy and at times of dose changes.

Implementation

- Must be administered under the supervision of a health care professional.
- Due to risks of serious adverse outcomes from sedation, dissociation, and abuse and misuse, available only through a restricted program under Spravato REMS. Healthcare settings and pharmacies must be certified and patients enrolled in REMS program.
- Advise patient to avoid food for at least 2 hr and liquids for 30 min prior to administration.
- If nasal corticosteroid or nasal decongestant is administered on a dosing day, administer at least 1 hr before esketamine administration.
- Esketamine is given in conjunction with an oral antidepressant.
- **Intranasal:** Use 2 devices (for a 56 mg dose) or 3 devices (for an 84 mg dose), with a 5-min rest between use of each device. Do not prime device. Advise patient to gently blow nose before first dose. Check that indicator shows 2 or 3 green dots. Instruct patient to recline head back 45°. Have patient insert device into nostril until nose rest is between nostrils. Close opposite nostril. Sniff gently after administering dose. Take device from patient; confirm no green dots. Instruct patient to recline and rest for 5 min between doses; do not blow nose. Repeat for each dose. Discard according to institution guidelines for Schedule III drugs.

Patient/Family Teaching

- Explain purpose of esketamine, administration procedure, and Spravato REMS program to patient. Advise patient to read *Medication Guide* before starting therapy.
- May cause sedation, dissociative symptoms, perception disturbances, dizziness, vertigo, and anxiety. Caution patient to avoid driving or activities requiring alertness until next day after a restful sleep.
- Advise patient, family, and caregivers to look for changes in behavior and suicidality, especially during early therapy or dose changes. Notify health care professional immediately if thoughts about suicide or dying, attempts to commit suicide; new or worse depression or anxiety; agitation or restlessness; panic attacks; insomnia; new or worse irritability; aggressiveness; acting on dangerous impulses, mania, or other changes in mood or behavior.
- Instruct patient to notify health care professional of all Rx or OTC medications, vitamins, or herbal products being taken and to avoid concurrent use of Rx, OTC, and herbal products without consulting health care professional.
- Rep: Advise females of reproductive potential to use effective contraception during therapy and to avoid breast feeding. Notify health care professional promptly if pregnancy is planned or suspected, or if breast feeding. Encourage patients who become pregnant during therapy to enroll in pregnancy registry that monitors pregnancy outcomes in women exposed to antidepressants by contacting the National Pregnancy Registry for Antidepressants at 1-844-405-6185 or online at https://womensmentalhealth.org/clinical-and-researchprograms/pregnancyregistry/antidepressants/.

Evaluation/Desired Outcomes

- Decreased severity of depressive symptoms and prolonged time to relapse.

HIGH ALERT

esmolol (es-moe-lol)

Brevibloc

Classification

Therapeutic: antiarrhythmics (class II)
Pharmacologic: beta blockers

Indications

Management of sinus tachycardia and supraventricular arrhythmias.

Action

Blocks stimulation of $beta_1$ (myocardial)-adrenergic receptors. Does not usually affect $beta_2$ (pulmonary, vascular, or uterine)-receptor sites. **Therapeutic Effects:** Decreased heart rate. Decreased AV conduction.

Pharmacokinetics

Absorption: IV administration results in complete bioavailability.
Distribution: Rapidly and widely distributed.
Metabolism and Excretion: Metabolized by enzymes in RBCs and liver.
Half-life: 9 min.

TIME/ACTION PROFILE (antiarrhythmic effect)

ROUTE	ONSET	PEAK	DURATION
IV	within min	unknown	1–20 min

Contraindications/Precautions

Contraindicated in: Uncompensated HF; Pulmonary edema; Cardiogenic shock; Bradycardia or heart block; Known alcohol intolerance.
Use Cautiously in: Geri: ↑ sensitivity to the effects of beta blockers; Thyrotoxicosis (may mask symptoms); Diabetes mellitus (may mask symptoms of hypoglycemia); Patients with a history of severe allergic reactions (intensity of reactions may be ↑); OB, Lactation, Pedi: Safety not established; neonatal bradycardia, hypotension, hypoglycemia, and respiratory depression may occur rarely.

Adverse Reactions/Side Effects

CNS: fatigue, agitation, confusion, dizziness, drowsiness, weakness. **CV:** hypotension, peripheral ischemia. **GI:** nausea, vomiting. **Derm:** sweating. **Local:** injection site reactions.

Interactions

Drug-Drug: General anesthesia, IV **phenytoin**, and **verapamil** may cause additive myocardial depression. Additive bradycardia may occur with **digoxin**. Additive hypotension may occur with other **antihypertensives**, acute ingestion of **alcohol**, or **nitrates**. Concurrent use with **amphetamine**, **cocaine**, **ephedrine**, **epinephrine**, **norepinephrine**, **phenylephrine**, or **pseudoephedrine** may result in unopposed alpha-adrenergic stimulation (excessive hypertension, bradycardia). Concurrent **thyroid hormone** administration may ↓ effectiveness. May alter the effectiveness of **insulins** or **oral hypoglycemic agents** (dose adjustments may be necessary). May ↓ effectiveness of **theophylline**. May ↓ beneficial beta cardiovascular effects of **dopamine** or **dobutamine**. Use cautiously within 14 days of **MAO-inhibitor** therapy (may result in hypertension).

Route/Dosage

IV (Adults): *Antiarrhythmic*—500-mcg/kg loading dose over 1 min initially, followed by 50-mcg/kg/min infusion for 4 min; if no response within 5 min, give 2nd loading dose of 500 mcg/kg over 1 min, then ↑ infusion to 100 mcg/kg/min for 4 min. If no response, repeat loading dose of 500 mcg/kg over 1 min and ↑ infusion rate by 50-mcg/kg/min increments (not to exceed 200 mcg/kg/min for 48 hr). As therapeutic end point is achieved, eliminate loading doses and decrease dose increments to 25 mg/kg/min. *Intraoperative antihypertensive/antiarrhythmic*—250–500-mcg/kg loading dose over 1 min initially, followed by 50-mcg/kg/min infusion for 4 min; if no response within 5 min, give 2nd loading dose of 250–500 mcg/kg over 1 min, then ↑ infusion to 100 mcg/kg/min for 4 min. If no response, repeat loading dose of 250–500 mcg/kg over 1 min and ↑ infusion rate by 50-mcg/kg/min increments (not to exceed 200 mcg/kg/min for 48 hr).

IV (Children): *Antiarrhythmic*—50 mcg/kg/min, may be ↑ every 10 min up to 300 mcg/kg/min.

Availability (generic available)

Solution for injection (for use as loading dose): 10 mg/mL. **Premixed infusion:** 2000 mg/100 mL, 2500 mg/250 mL.

NURSING IMPLICATIONS

Assessment

- Monitor BP, ECG, and pulse frequently during dose adjustment period and periodically during therapy. The risk of hypotension is greatest within the first 30 min of initiating esmolol infusion.
- Monitor intake and output ratios and daily weights. Assess routinely for signs and symptoms of HF (dyspnea, rales/crackles, weight gain, peripheral edema, jugular venous distention).
- Assess infusion site frequently throughout therapy. Concentrations >10 mg/mL may cause redness, swelling, skin discoloration, and burning at the injection site. Do not use butterfly needles for administration. If venous irritation occurs, stop the infusion and resume at another site.
- ***Toxicity and Overdose:*** Monitor patients receiving esmolol for signs of overdose (bradycardia, severe dizziness or fainting, severe drowsiness, dyspnea, bluish fingernails or palms, seizures).
- IV glucagon and symptomatic care are used in the treatment of esmolol overdose. Because of the short action of esmolol, discontinuation of therapy may relieve acute toxicity.

Implementation

- ***High Alert:*** IV vasoactive medications are inherently dangerous. Esmolol is available in different concentrations; fatalities have occurred when loading dose vial is confused with concentrated solution for injection, which contains 2500 mg in 10 mL (250 mg/mL) and must be diluted. Before administering, have second practitioner independently check original order, dose calculations, and infusion pump settings.
- ***High Alert:*** Do not confuse Brevibloc (esmolol) with Brevital (methohexital). If both are available as floor stock, store in separate areas.
- To convert to other antiarrhythmics following esmolol administration, administer the 1st dose of the antiarrhythmic agent and decrease the esmolol dose by 50% after 30 min. If an adequate response is maintained for 1 hr following the 2nd dose of the antiarrhythmic agent, discontinue esmolol.

IV Administration

- **IV Push:** ***Diluent:*** The 10-mg/mL and 20-mg/mL vials should be used for the loading dose. These vials are already diluted. No further dilution is needed. ***Concentration:*** Avoid concentrations >10 m g/mL. ***Rate:*** Administer over 1 min.
- **Continuous Infusion:** ***Diluent:*** Premixed infusions are already diluted and ready to use. Solution is clear, colorless to light yellow. ***Concentration:*** 10 mg/mL. ***Rate:*** Based on patient's weight (see Route/Dosage section). Titration of dose is based on desired heart rate or undesired decrease in BP. Esmolol infusions should not be abruptly discontinued; the infusion rate should be tapered.
- **Y-Site Compatibility:** alfentanil, amikacin, aminophylline, amiodarone, amphotericin B liposome, anidulafungin, argatroban, ascorbic acid, atracurium, atropine, aztreonam, benztropine, bivalirudin, bleomycin, bumetanide, buprenorphine, butorphanol, calcium chloride, calcium gluconate, cangrelor, carboplatin, carmustine, caspofungin, cefazolin, cefotaxime, cefoxitin, ceftazidime, ceftriaxone, cefuroxime, chlorpromazine, cisatracurium, cisplatin, clindamycin, cyanocobalamin, cyclophosphamide, cyclosporine, cytarabine, dacarbazine, dactinomycin, daptomycin, daunorubicin, dexmedetomidine, dexrazoxane, digoxin, diltiazem, diphenhydramine, dobutamine, docetaxel, dopamine, doxorubicin, doxycycline, enalaprilat, ephedrine, epinephrine, epoetin alfa, eptifibatide, ertapenem, erythromycin, etoposide, etoposide phosphate, famotidine, fenoldopam, fentanyl, fluconazole, fludarabine, fluorouracil, folic acid, foscarnet, fosphenytoin, gemcitabine, gentamicin, glycopyrrolate, granisetron, heparin, hetastarch, hydromorphone, idarubicin, ifosfamide, imipenem/cilastatin, insulin (regular), isoproterenol, labetalol, leucovorin, levofloxacin, lidocaine, linezolid, lorazepam, magnesium sulfate, mannitol, meperidine, mesna, methotrexate, methyldopate, metoclopramide, metoprolol, metronidazole, micafungin, midazolam, mitoxantrone, morphine, moxifloxacin, multivitamins, mycophenolate, nalbuphine, naloxone, nicardipine, nitroglycerin, nitroprusside, norepinephrine, octreotide, ondansetron, oxaliplatin, oxytocin, paclitaxel, palonosetron, pancuronium, papaverine, pemetrexed, penicillin G, pentamidine, phentolamine, phenylephrine, phytonadione, piperacillin/tazobactam, potassium acetate, potassium chloride, potassium phosphates, procainamide, prochlorperazine, promethazine, propofol, propranolol, protamine, pyridoxine, quinupristin/dalfopristin, ranitidine, remifentanil, rocuronium, sodium acetate, sodium bicarbonate, streptokinase, succinylcholine, sufentanil, tacrolimus, theophylline,

thiamine, thiotepa, tigecycline, tirofiban, tobramycin, topotecan, vancomycin, vasopressin, vecuronium, verapamil, vinblastine, vincristine, voriconazole, zoledronic acid.

- **Y-Site Incompatibility:** acyclovir, amphotericin B deoxycholate, amphotericin B lipid complex, azathioprine, cefotetan, dantrolene, dexamethasone, diazepam, diazoxide, furosemide, ganciclovir, indomethacin, ketorolac, milrinone, mitomycin, oxacillin, pantoprazole, pentobarbital, phenobarbital, warfarin.

Patient/Family Teaching

- May cause drowsiness. Caution patients receiving esmolol to call for assistance during ambulation or transfer.
- Advise patients to change positions slowly to minimize orthostatic hypotension.
- Patients with diabetes should closely monitor blood glucose, especially if weakness, malaise, irritability, or fatigue occurs. Medication does not block dizziness or sweating as signs of hypoglycemia.

Evaluation/Desired Outcomes

- Control of arrhythmias without appearance of detrimental side effects.

BEERS

esomeprazole

(es-oh-**mep**-ra-zole)

NexIUM, NexIUM 24hr

Classification

Therapeutic: antiulcer agents

Pharmacologic: proton-pump inhibitors

Indications

PO, IV: GERD/erosive esophagitis (IV therapy should only be used if PO therapy is not possible/appropriate). **IV:** Reduction in risk of rebleeding following therapeutic endoscopy for acute bleeding gastric or duodenal ulcers. **PO:** Hypersecretory conditions, including Zollinger-Ellison syndrome. **PO:** With amoxicillin and clarithromycin to eradicate *Helicobacter pylori* in duodenal ulcer disease or history of duodenal ulcer disease. **PO:** Decrease risk of gastric ulcer during continuous NSAID therapy. **OTC:** Heartburn occurring ≥twice/wk.

Action

Binds to an enzyme on gastric parietal cells in the presence of acidic gastric pH, preventing the final transport of hydrogen ions into the gastric lumen. **Therapeutic Effects:** Diminished accumulation of acid in the gastric lumen with lessened gastroesophageal reflux. Healing of duodenal ulcers. Decreased incidence of gastric ulcer during continuous NSAID therapy.

Pharmacokinetics

Absorption: 90% absorbed following oral administration; food ↓ absorption.

Distribution: Unknown.

Protein Binding: 97%.

Metabolism and Excretion: Extensively metabolized by the liver (cytochrome P450 [CYP450] system, primarily CYP2C19 isoenzyme, but also the CYP3A4 isoenzyme) (the CYP2C19 enzyme system exhibits genetic polymorphism; 15–20% of Asian patients and 3–5% of Caucasian and Black patients may be poor metabolizers and may have significantly ↑ esomeprazole concentrations and an ↑ risk of adverse effects); <1% excreted unchanged in urine.

Half-life: *Children 1–11 yrs:* 0.42–0.88 hr; *Adults:* 1.0–1.5 hr.

TIME/ACTION PROFILE (blood levels*)

ROUTE	ONSET	PEAK	DURATION
PO	rapid	1.6 hr	24 hr
IV	rapid	end of infusion	24 hr

*Resolution of symptoms takes 5–8 days.

Contraindications/Precautions

Contraindicated in: Hypersensitivity to esomeprazole or related drugs (benzimidazoles); Hypersensitivity; Concurrent use of rilpivirine.

Use Cautiously in: Severe hepatic impairment; Patients using high-doses for >1 yr (↑ risk of hip, wrist, or spine fractures and fundic gland polyps); Patients using therapy for >3 yr (↑ risk of vitamin B_{12} deficiency); OB, Lactation: Use only if potential benefit outweighs potential risk.

Adverse Reactions/Side Effects

CNS: headache. **Derm:** cutaneous lupus erythematosus. **F and E:** hypomagnesemia (especially if treatment duration ≥3 mo). **GI:** CLOSTRIDIUM DIFFICILE-ASSOCIATED DIARRHEA (CDAD), abdominal pain, constipation, diarrhea, dry mouth, flatulence, fundic gland polyps, nausea. **GU:** acute interstitial nephritis. **Hemat:** vitamin B_{12} deficiency. **MS:** bone fracture. **Misc:** systemic lupus erythematosus.

Interactions

Drug-Drug: May significantly ↓ levels of **rilpivirine**; concurrent use contraindicated. May ↓ levels of **atazanavir** and **nelfinavir**; avoid concurrent use with either of these antiretrovirals. May ↑ levels and risk of toxicity of **saquinavir** (may need to ↓ dose of saquinavir). May ↓ absorption of drugs requiring acid pH, including **ketoconazole**, **itraconazole**, **ampicillin esters**, **iron salts**, **erlotinib**, and **mycophenolate mofetil**. May ↑ levels of **digoxin** and **methotrexate**. May ↑ risk of bleeding with **warfarin** (monitor INR and PT). **Vori-**

conazole may ↑ levels. May ↓ the antiplatelet effects of **clopidogrel**; avoid concurrent use. May ↑ levels of **cilostazol**; consider ↓ dose of cilostazol from 100 mg twice daily to 50 mg twice daily. **Rifampin** may ↓ levels and may ↓ response (avoid concurrent use). Hypomagnesemia ↑ risk of **digoxin** toxicity. May ↑ levels of **tacrolimus** and **methotrexate**.
Drug-Natural Products: St. John's wort may ↓ levels and may ↓ response (avoid concurrent use).

Route/Dosage

Gastroesophageal Reflux Disease

PO (Adults): *Healing of erosive esophagitis*—20 mg or 40 mg once daily for 4–8 wk; *Maintenance of healing of erosive esophagitis*—20 mg once daily; *Symptomatic GERD*—20 mg once daily for 4 wk (additional 4 wk may be considered for nonresponders); *Heartburn*—20 mg once daily for 2 wk.
PO (Children 12–17 yr): *Short-term treatment of GERD*—20–40 mg once daily for up to 8 wk.
PO (Children 1–11 yr): *Short-term treatment of GERD*—10 mg once daily for up to 8 wk; *Healing of erosive esophagitis*—<20 kg: 10 mg once daily for 8 wk; ≥20 kg: 10–20 mg once daily for 8 wk.
PO (Infants and Children 1 mo–<1 yr): *>7.5–12 kg*—10 mg once daily for up to 6 wk; *>5–7.5 kg*—5 mg once daily for up to 6 wk; *3–5 kg*—2.5 mg once daily for up to 6 wk.
IV (Adults): 20 or 40 mg once daily.
IV (Children 1–17 yr): *<55 kg*—10 mg once daily; *≥55 kg*—20 mg once daily.
IV (Children 1 mo–<1 yr): 0.5 mg/kg once daily.

Hepatic Impairment

PO, IV (Adults): *Severe hepatic impairment*—Dose should not exceed 20 mg/day.

Reduction of Risk of Rebleeding of Gastric or Duodenal Ulcers After Therapeutic Endoscopy

IV (Adults): 80 mg over 30 min, then 8 mg/hr continuous infusion for 71.5 hr.

Hepatic Impairment

IV (Adults): *Mild-to-moderate hepatic impairment*—Do not exceed continuous infusion rate of 6 mg/hr; *Severe hepatic impairment*—Do not exceed continuous infusion rate of 4 mg/hr.

H. pylori Eradication to Reduce the Risk of Duodenal Ulcer Recurrence (Triple Therapy)

PO (Adults): 40 mg once daily for 10 days with amoxicillin 1000 mg twice daily for 10 days and clarithromycin 500 mg twice daily for 10 days.

Hepatic Impairment

PO (Adults): *Severe hepatic impairment*—Dose should not exceed 20 mg/day.

Decrease Gastric Ulcer During Continuous NSAID Therapy

PO (Adults): 20 or 40 mg once daily for up to 6 mo.

Hepatic Impairment

PO (Adults): *Severe hepatic impairment*—Dose should not exceed 20 mg/day.

Pathological Hypersecretory Conditions Including Zollinger-Ellison Syndrome

PO (Adults): 40 mg twice daily.

Hepatic Impairment

PO (Adults): *Severe hepatic impairment*—Dose should not exceed 20 mg/day.

Availability (generic available)

Delayed-release capsules: 20 mg[Rx, OTC], 40 mg. **Cost:** 20 mg $713.55/90, 40 mg $731.22/90. **Delayed-release oral suspension packets:** 2.5 mg/pkt, 5 mg/pkt, 10 mg/pkt, 20 mg/pkt, 40 mg/pkt. **Cost:** All strengths $268.01/30 pkts. **Delayed-release tablets:** 20 mg[OTC]. **Powder for injection (requires reconstitution and dilution):** 40 mg/vial. ***In combination with:*** naproxen (Vimovo).

NURSING IMPLICATIONS

Assessment

- Assess routinely for epigastric or abdominal pain and frank or occult blood in the stool, emesis, or gastric aspirate.
- Monitor bowel function. Diarrhea, abdominal cramping, fever, and bloody stools should be reported to health care professional promptly as a sign of Clostridium difficile-associated diarrhea (CDAD).
- ***Lab Test Considerations:*** May cause ↑ serum creatinine, uric acid, total bilirubin, alkaline phosphatase, AST, and ALT.
- May alter hemoglobin, WBC, platelets, serum sodium, potassium, and thyroxine levels.
- May cause hypomagnesemia. Monitor serum magnesium prior to and periodically during therapy.
- May cause false positive results in diagnostic investigations for neuroendocrine tumors due to ↑ serum chromogranin A (CgA) levels secondary to drug-induced ↓ gastric acidity. Temporarily stop esomeprazole at least 14 days before assessing CgA levels and consider repeating test if initial CgA levels are high.

Implementation

- ***High Alert:*** Do not confuse Nexium (esomeprazole) with Nexavar (sorafenib).
- Antacids may be used while taking esomeprazole.
- **PO:** Administer at least 1 hr before meals. Swallow tablets and capsules whole.
- *Delayed-release capsules:* For patients with difficulty swallowing, place 1 tbsp of applesauce in an empty bowl. Open capsule and carefully empty the pellets inside onto applesauce. Mix pellets with applesauce and swallow immediately. Applesauce

should not be hot and should be soft enough to swallow without chewing. Do not store applesauce mixture for future use. Tap water, orange juice, apple juice, and yogurt have also been used. Do not crush or chew pellets.

- *For patients with an NG tube,* delayed-release capsules can be opened and intact granules emptied into a 60-mL syringe and mixed with 50 mL of water. Replace plunger and shake syringe vigorously for 15 sec. Hold syringe with tip up and check for granules in tip. Attach syringe to NG tube and administer solution. After administering, flush syringe with additional water. Do not administer if granules have dissolved or disintegrated. Administer immediately after mixing.
- For *Delayed-release oral suspension:* Mix contents of packet with 1 tbsp (15 mL) of water, leave 2–3 min to thicken, stir and drink within 30 min.
- *For Delayed-Release Oral Suspension Nasogastric or Gastric Tube:* Add 15 mL of water to a syringe and then add contents of packet. Shake the syringe, leave 2–3 min to thicken. Shake the syringe and inject through the nasogastric or gastric tube within 30 min.

IV Administration

- **IV Push:** Reconstitute each vial with 5 mL of 0.9% NaCl, LR, or D5W. Do not administer solutions that are discolored or contain a precipitate. Stable at room temperature for up to 12 hr. ***Rate:*** Administer over at least 3 min.
- **Intermittent Infusion:** ***Diluent:*** Dilute reconstituted solution to a volume of 50 mL with *D5W, 0.9% NaCl, or LR for adults* and *with 0.9% NaCl for pediatric patients.* ***Concentration:*** 0.8 mg/mL (40-mg vial) or 0.4 mg/mL (20-mg vial). Solutions diluted with 0.9% NaCl or LR are stable for 12 hr and those diluted with D5W are stable for 6 hr at room temperature. ***Rate:*** Administer over 10–30 min.
- **Continuous Infusion:** *For 80 mg Loading Dose,* reconstitute two 40 mg vials with 5 mL of 0.9% NaCl. ***Diluent:*** Further diluted in 100 mL 0.9% NaCl. ***Rate:*** Administer *loading dose* over 30 min. Follow with infusion at a rate of 8 mg/hr for 71.5 hrs.
- **Continuous Infusion:** *For 80 mg dose,* reconstitute two 40 mg vials with 5 mL of 0.9% NaCl. ***Diluent:*** Further diluted in 100 mL 0.9% NaCl. ***Rate:*** Follow loading dose with infusion at a rate of 8 mg/hr for 71.5 hrs.
- **Y-Site Compatibility:** ceftaroline, ceftolozane/tazobactam, fentanyl, furosemide, insulin,regular, meropenem/vaborbactam, metoprolol, nitroglycerin.
- **Y-Site Incompatibility:** dobutamine, dopamine, esmolol, isavuconazonium, labetalol, midazolam, morphine, tacrolimus, telavancin, tigecycline. Do not administer with other medication or solutions. Flush line with 0.9% NaCl, LR, or D5W before and after administration.

Patient/Family Teaching

- Instruct patient to take medication as directed for the full course of therapy, even if feeling better. Take missed doses as soon as remembered but not if almost time for next dose. Do not double doses. Advise patient to read the *Patient Information* sheet prior to starting therapy and with each Rx refill in case of changes.
- Advise patient to avoid alcohol, products containing aspirin or NSAIDs, and foods that may cause an increase in GI irritation.
- Advise patient to report onset of black, tarry stools; diarrhea; abdominal pain; or persistent headache to health care professional promptly.
- Instruct patient to notify health care professional of all Rx or OTC medications, vitamins, or herbal products being taken and consult health care professional before taking any new medications, especially St. John's wort.
- Advise patient to notify health care professional if signs of hypomagnesemia (seizures, dizziness, abnormal or fast heartbeat, jitteriness, jerking movements or shaking, muscle weakness, spasms of the hands and feet, cramps or muscle aches, spasm of the voice box) occur.
- Caution patient to notify health care professional if fever and diarrhea occur, especially if stool contains blood, pus, or mucus. Advise patient not to treat diarrhea without consulting health care professional.
- Advise female patient to notify health care professional if pregnancy is planned or suspected or if breast feeding.

Evaluation/Desired Outcomes

- Decrease in abdominal pain or prevention of gastric irritation and bleeding. Healing of duodenal ulcers can be seen on x-ray examination or endoscopy.
- Decrease in symptoms of GERD and erosive esophagitis. Sustained resolution of symptoms usually occurs in 5–8 days. Therapy is continued for 4–8 wk after initial episode.
- Decreased incidence of gastric ulcer during continuous NSAID therapy.
- Eradication of *H. pylori* in duodenal ulcer disease.
- Decrease in symptoms of hypersecretory conditions, including Zollinger-Ellison.

ESTRADIOL (es-tra-**dye**-ole)
Estrace

estradiol cypionate
Depo-Estradiol

estradiol valerate
Delestrogen

estradiol topical gel
Divigel, Elestrin, EstroGel

estradiol transdermal spray
EvaMist

estradiol transdermal system
Alora, Climara, ~~Estraderm~~, ✱Estradot, Menostar, Minivelle, ✱Oesclim, Vivelle-Dot

estradiol vaginal insert
Imvexxy

estradiol vaginal ring
Femring, Estring

estradiol vaginal tablet
Vagifem

Classification
Therapeutic: hormones
Pharmacologic: estrogens

Indications

PO, IM, Topical, Transdermal: Replacement of estrogen (HRT) to diminish moderate to severe vasomotor symptoms of menopause and of various estrogen deficiency states including: Female hypogonadism, Ovariectomy, Primary ovarian failure. Treatment and prevention of postmenopausal osteoporosis (not vaginal dose forms). **PO:** Inoperable metastatic postmenopausal breast or prostate carcinoma. **Vag:** Management of: Atrophic vaginitis due to menopause, Moderate to severe dyspareunia due to menopause.

Action

Estrogens promote growth and development of female sex organs and the maintenance of secondary sex characteristics in women. Metabolic effects include reduced blood cholesterol, protein synthesis, and sodium and water retention. **Therapeutic Effects:** Restoration of hormonal balance in various deficiency states, including menopause. Treatment of hormone-sensitive tumors.

Pharmacokinetics

Absorption: Well absorbed after oral administration. Readily absorbed through skin and mucous membranes.
Distribution: Widely distributed. Crosses the placenta and enters breast milk.
Metabolism and Excretion: Mostly metabolized by the liver and other tissues. Enterohepatic recirculation occurs, and more absorption may occur from the GI tract.
Half-life: Gel: 36 hr.

TIME/ACTION PROFILE (estrogenic effects)

ROUTE	ONSET	PEAK	DURATION
PO	unknown	unknown	unknown
IM	unknown	unknown	unknown
Transdermal	unknown	unknown	3–4 days (Estraderm), 7 days (Climara)
Topical	unknown	unknown	unknown
Vaginal insert	unknown	unknown	3–4 days
Vaginal ring	unknown	unknown	90 days

Contraindications/Precautions

Contraindicated in: History of anaphylaxis or angioedema to estradiol; Thromboembolic disease (e.g., DVT, PE, MI, stroke); Protein C, protein S, or antithrombin deficiency or other thrombophilic disorder; History of breast cancer; History of estrogen-dependent cancer; Hepatic impairment; Undiagnosed vaginal bleeding; OB: May cause fetal harm.
Use Cautiously in: Underlying cardiovascular disease; Severe hepatic or renal disease; History of porphyria; History of hereditary angioedema; Lactation: Usually compatible with breast feeding.

Adverse Reactions/Side Effects

CNS: headache, dizziness, lethargy. **CV:** MI, THROMBOEMBOLISM, edema, hypertension. **Derm:** oily skin, acne, pigmentation, urticaria. **EENT:** intolerance to contact lenses, worsening of myopia or astigmatism. **Endo:** gynecomastia (men), hyperglycemia. **F and E:** hypercalcemia, sodium and water retention. **GI:** nausea, weight changes, anorexia, ↑ appetite, jaundice, vomiting. **GU:** *women*—amenorrhea, dysmenorrhea, breakthrough bleeding, cervical erosions, loss of libido, vaginal candidiasis; *men*, erectile dysfunction, testicular atrophy **MS:** leg cramps. **Misc:** MALIGNANCY (BREAST, ENDOMETRIAL, OVARIAN), breast tenderness.

Interactions

Drug-Drug: May alter requirement for **warfarin**, **oral hypoglycemic agents**, or **insulins**. **Barbiturates** or **rifampin** may ↓ effectiveness. **Smoking** ↑ risk of adverse CV reactions.

Route/Dosage

Estrogens should be used in the lowest doses for the shortest period of time consistent with desired therapeutic outcome. Concurrent use of progestin is recommended during cyclical therapy to decrease the risk of endometrial carcinoma in patients with an intact uterus.

Symptoms of Menopause, Atrophic Vaginitis, Moderate-to-Severe Dyspareunia, Female Hypogonadism, Ovarian Failure/Osteoporosis

PO (Adults): 0.45–2 mg once daily or in a cycle.
IM (Adults): 1–5 mg monthly (estradiol cypionate) *or* 10–20 mg (estradiol valerate) monthly.
Topical Gel (Adults): Apply contents of one packet *(Divigel)* or one actuation from pump *(EstroGel, Elestrin)* once daily.

Topical Spray *EvaMist* (Adults): 1 spray once daily, may be ↑ to 2–3 sprays once daily.
Transdermal (Adults): *Alora*—25–50–mcg/24-hr transdermal patch applied twice weekly. *Climara*—25-mcg/24-hr transdermal patch applied weekly. *Vivelle-Dot*—25–50–mcg/24-hr transdermal patch applied twice weekly. *Menostar*—14-mcg/24-hr transdermal patch applied every 7 days. Progestin may be administered for 10–14 days of each mo. *Minivelle*—37.5–mcg/24–hr transdermal patch applied twice weekly (for treatment of vasomotor symptoms); 25–mcg/24–hr transdermal patch applied twice weekly (for prevention of postmenopausal osteoporosis).
Vag (Adults): *Cream*—2–4 g (0.2–0.4 mg estradiol) once daily for 1–2 wk, then ↓ to 1–2 g/day for 1–2 wk; then maintenance dose of 1 g 1–3 times weekly for 3 wk, then off for 1 wk; then repeat cycle once vaginal mucosa has been restored; *Vaginal ring (Estring)*—2-mg (releases 7.5 mcg estradiol/24 hr) every 3 mo; *Vaginal ring (Femring)*—12.4 mg (releases 50 mcg estradiol/24 hr) every 3 mo or 24.8 mg (releases 100 mcg estradiol/24 hr) every 3 mo (*Femring* requires concurrent progesterone); *Vaginal insert (Vagifem and Imvexxy)*—1 insert once daily for 2 wk, then 1 insert twice weekly.

Postmenopausal Breast Carcinoma
PO (Adults): 10 mg 3 times daily.

Prostate Carcinoma
PO (Adults): 1–2 mg 3 times daily.
IM (Adults): 30 mg every 1–2 wk (estradiol valerate).

Availability (generic available)

Estradiol
Tablets: 0.5 mg, 1 mg, 2 mg. **Cost:** *Generic*—0.5 mg $10.83/100, 1 mg $10.83/100, 2 mg $10.83/100.

Estradiol Cypionate
Injection (in oil): 5 mg/mL.

Estradiol Valerate
Injection (in oil): 10 mg/mL, 20 mg/mL, 40 mg/mL.

Estradiol Topical Preparations
Gel packet (Divigel): 0.25 mg/pkt, 0.5 mg/pkt, 0.75 mg/pkt, 1 mg/pkt. **Cost:** All strengths $3.45/pkt. **Gel pump (Elestrin):** 0.52 mg/actuation. **Cost:** *Elestrin (0.52 mg/actuation)*—$89.44/26 g. **Gel pump (Estrogel):** 0.75 mg/actuation. **Cost:** *EstroGel (0.75 mg/actuation)*—$103.80/50 g.

Estradiol Transdermal Preparations
Patch: 14 mcg/24-hr release rate, 25 mcg/24-hr release rate, 37.5 mcg/24-hr release rate, 50 mcg/24-hr release rate, 60 mcg/24-hr release rate, 75 mcg/24-hr release rate, 100 mcg/24-hr release rate. **Cost:** 14 mcg/24 hr $221.46/4, 25 mcg/24 hr $88.40/4, 37.5 mcg/24 hr $88.40/4, 50 mcg/24 hr $88.40/4, 60 mcg/24 hr $88.40/4, 75 mcg/24 hr $88.40/4, 100 mcg/24 hr $88.40/4. **Spray:** 1.53 mg/spray. **Cost:** $108.76/9 mL.

Estradiol Vaginal Preparations
Vaginal cream: 0.01%. **Cost:** $165.70/43 g. **Vaginal tablet (Vagifem):** 10 mcg. **Cost:** $97.05/8. **Vaginal insert (Imvexxy):** 4 mcg, 10 mcg. **Vaginal ring (Estring):** 2 mg (releases 7.5 mcg/day over 90 days). **Cost:** $252.72/1 ring. **Vaginal ring (Femring):** 12.4 mg (releases 50 mcg/day over 90 days), 24.8 mg (releases 100 mcg/day over 90 days). **Cost:** 50 mcg/day $248.98/1 ring, 100 mcg/day $259.58/1 ring. ***In combination with:*** drospirenone (Angeliq); levonorgestrel (Climara Pro); norethindrone (Activella, Combipatch); progesterone (Bijuva). See Appendix B.

E

NURSING IMPLICATIONS

Assessment
- Assess BP before and periodically during therapy.
- Monitor intake and output ratios and weekly weight. Report significant discrepancies or steady weight gain.
- **Menopause:** Assess frequency and severity of vasomotor symptoms.
- ***Lab Test Considerations:*** May cause ↑ HDL, phospholipids, and triglycerides and ↓ serum LDL and total cholesterol concentrations.
- May cause ↑ serum glucose, sodium, cortisol, prolactin, prothrombin, and factor VII, VIII, IX, and X levels. May ↓ serum folate, pyridoxine, antithrombin III, and urine pregnanediol concentrations.
- Monitor hepatic function before and periodically during therapy.
- May cause false interpretations of thyroid function tests, false ↑ in norepinephrine platelet-induced aggregability, and false ↓ in metyrapone tests.
- May cause hypercalcemia in patients with metastatic bone lesions.

Implementation
- Do not confuse Alora with Aldara.
- **PO:** Administer with or immediately after food to reduce nausea.
- **Vag:** Manufacturer provides applicator with cream. Dose is marked on the applicator. Wash applicator with mild soap and warm water after each use.
- **Transdermal:** When switching from PO form, begin transdermal therapy 1 wk after the last dose or when symptoms reappear.
- **Topical:** Apply *Divigel* individual-use once-daily packets of quick drying gel to an area measuring 5 inches by 7 inches (size of 2 palm prints) on the thigh. Do not wash area for at least 1 hr after gel has dried.
- Spray *EvaMist* on inside of forearm at the same time each day. Do not massage or rub the spray into the skin. Allow to dry for 2 min before dressing and at

least 1 hr before washing. Never spray *EvaMist* around breast or vagina. Do not use more than 56 doses, even if fluid remains in pump.

- **IM:** Injection has oil base. Roll syringe to ensure even dispersion. Administer deep IM. Avoid IV administration.

Patient/Family Teaching

- Instruct patient on correct method of administration. Instruct patient to take medication as directed. Take missed doses as soon as remembered as long as it is not just before next dose. If a dose of *EvaMist* is missed, apply if more than 12 hr before next dose; if less than 12 hr, omit dose and return to regular schedule. Do not double doses.
- Explain dose schedule and maintenance routine. Discontinuing medication suddenly may cause withdrawal bleeding.
- If nausea becomes a problem, advise patient that eating solid food often provides relief.
- Advise patient to report signs and symptoms of fluid retention (swelling of ankles and feet, weight gain), thromboembolic disorders (pain, swelling, tenderness in extremities, headache, chest pain, blurred vision), mental depression, or hepatic dysfunction (yellowed skin or eyes, pruritus, dark urine, light-colored stools) to health care professional.
- Advise patient to notify health care professional of medication regimen before treatment or surgery.
- Caution patient that cigarette smoking during estrogen therapy may cause increased risk of serious side effects, especially for women over age 35.
- Caution patient to use sunscreen and protective clothing to prevent increased pigmentation.
- Advise patient treated for osteoporosis that exercise has been found to arrest and reverse bone loss. Patient should discuss any exercise limitations with health care professional before beginning program.
- Inform patient that estrogens should not be used to decrease risk of cardiovascular disease. Estrogens may increase risk of cardiovascular disease and breast cancer.
- Instruct patient to stop taking medication and notify health care professional if pregnancy is planned or suspected, or if breast feeding.
- Emphasize the importance of routine follow-up physical exams, including BP; breast, abdomen, and pelvic examinations; Papanicolaou smears every 6–12 mo; and mammogram every 12 mo or as directed. Health care professional will evaluate possibility of discontinuing medication every 3–6 mo. If on continuous (not cyclical) therapy or without concurrent progestins, endometrial biopsy may be recommended, if uterus is intact.
- **Vag:** Instruct patient in the correct use of applicator. Patient should remain recumbent for at least 30 min after administration. May use sanitary napkin to protect clothing, but do not use tampon. If a dose is missed, do not use the missed dose, but return to regular dosing schedule.
- Instruct patient to use applicator provided with vaginal tablet. Insert as high up in the vagina as comfortable, without using force.
- **Vaginal Ring:** Instruct patient to press ring into an oval and insert into the upper third of the vaginal vault. Exact position is not critical. Once ring is inserted, patient should not feel anything. If discomfort is felt, ring is probably not in far enough; gently push farther into vagina. Leave in place continuously for 90 days. Ring does not interfere with sexual intercourse. If straining at defecation makes ring move to lower vagina, push up with finger. If expelled totally, rinse ring with lukewarm water and reinsert. To remove, hook a finger through the ring and pull it out.
- **Transdermal:** Instruct patient to wash and dry hands first. Apply disc to intact skin on hairless portion of abdomen (do not apply to breasts or waistline). Apply *Minivelle* patch to lower abdomen or buttocks. Press disc/patch for 10 sec to ensure contact with skin (especially around edges). Avoid areas where clothing may rub disc loose. Change site with each administration to prevent skin irritation. Do not reuse site for 1 wk; disc may be reapplied if it falls off.
- Advise patient referred for MRI test to discuss patch with referring health care professional and MRI facility to determine if removal of patch is necessary prior to test and for directions for replacing patch.
- *Evamist*: Caution patient to make sure children are not exposed to Evamist and do not come into contact with any skin area where the drug was applied. Women who cannot avoid contact with children should wear a garment with long sleeves to cover the application site.

Evaluation/Desired Outcomes

- Resolution of menopausal vasomotor symptoms.
- Decreased vaginal and vulvar itching, inflammation, or dryness associated with menopause.
- Normalization of estrogen levels in patients with ovariectomy or hypogonadism.
- Control of the spread of advanced metastatic breast or prostate cancer.
- Prevention of osteoporosis.

estradiol valerate/dienogest, See CONTRACEPTIVES, HORMONAL.

estrogens, conjugated

(**ess**-troe-jenz **con**-joo-gae-ted)

C.E.S, Congest, Premarin

Classification

Therapeutic: hormones

Pharmacologic: estrogens

Indications

PO: Moderate to severe vasomotor symptoms of menopause. Vulvar and vaginal atrophy associated with menopause. Estrogen deficiency states, including: Female hypogonadism, Ovariectomy, Primary ovarian failure. Prevention of postmenopausal osteoporosis. Advanced inoperable metastatic breast and prostatic carcinoma. **IM, IV:** Uterine bleeding resulting from hormonal imbalance. **Vag:** Atrophic vaginitis. Moderate to severe dyspareunia due to menopause. Concurrent use of progestin is recommended during cyclical therapy to decrease the risk of endometrial carcinoma in patients with an intact uterus.

Action

Estrogens promote the growth and development of female sex organs and the maintenance of secondary sex characteristics in women. **Therapeutic Effects:** Restoration of hormonal balance in various deficiency states and treatment of hormone-sensitive tumors.

Pharmacokinetics

Absorption: Well absorbed after oral administration. Readily absorbed through skin and mucous membranes.

Distribution: Widely distributed. Crosses placenta and enters breast milk.

Metabolism and Excretion: Mostly metabolized by liver and other tissues. Enterohepatic recirculation occurs, with more absorption from GI tract.

Half-life: Unknown.

TIME/ACTION PROFILE (estrogenic effects†)

ROUTE	ONSET	PEAK	DURATION
PO	rapid	unknown	24 hr
IM	delayed	unknown	6–12 hr
IV	rapid	unknown	6–12 hr

†Tumor response may take several wk.

Contraindications/Precautions

Contraindicated in: History of anaphylaxis or angioedema to estrogen; Thromboembolic disease (e.g., DVT, PE, MI, stroke); Undiagnosed vaginal bleeding; History of breast cancer; History of estrogen-dependent cancer; Hepatic impairment; Protein C, protein S, or antithrombin deficiency or other thrombophilic disorder; OB: May cause fetal harm; Lactation: Negatively affects quantity and quality of breast milk.

Use Cautiously in: Long-term use (more than 4–5 yr); may ↑ risk of myocardial infarction, stroke, invasive breast cancer, pulmonary emboli, deep vein thrombosis, and dementia in postmenopausal women; Underlying cardiovascular disease; Hypertriglyceridemia; History of hereditary angioedema.

Adverse Reactions/Side Effects

(Systemic use) **CNS:** headache, dizziness, insomnia, lethargy, mental depression. **CV:** MI, THROMBOEMBOLISM, edema, hypertension. **Derm:** acne, oily skin, pigmentation, urticaria. **Endo:** gynecomastia (men), hyperglycemia. **F and E:** hypercalcemia, sodium and water retention. **GI:** nausea, weight changes, anorexia, ↑ appetite, jaundice, vomiting. **GU:** *women*—amenorrhea, breakthrough bleeding, dysmenorrhea, cervical erosion, loss of libido, vaginal candidiasis; *men*, erectile dysfunction, testicular atrophy. **MS:** leg cramps. **Misc:** ANAPHYLAXIS, ANGIOEDEMA, MALIGNANCY (BREAST, ENDOMETRIAL, OVARIAN), breast tenderness.

Interactions

Drug-Drug: May alter requirement for **warfarin**, **oral hypoglycemic agents**, or **insulins**. **Barbiturates**, **carbamazepine**, or **rifampin** may ↓ effectiveness. **Smoking** ↑ risk of adverse CV reactions. **Erythromycin**, **clarithromycin**, **itraconazole**, **ketoconazole**, and **ritonavir** may ↑ risk of adverse effects.

Drug-Food: Grapefruit juice may ↑ risk of adverse effects.

Route/Dosage

Estrogens should be used in the lowest doses for the shortest period of time consistent with desired therapeutic outcome.

Ovariectomy, Primary Ovarian Failure

PO (Adults): 1.25 mg once daily administered cyclically (3 wk on, 1 wk off).

Osteoporosis/Menopausal Symptoms

PO (Adults): 0.3–1.25 mg once daily or in a cycle.

Female Hypogonadism

PO (Adults): 0.3–0.625 mg once daily administered cyclically (3 wk on, 1 wk off).

Inoperable Breast Carcinoma—Men and Postmenopausal Women

PO (Adults): 10 mg 3 times daily.

Inoperable Prostate Carcinoma

PO (Adults): 1.25–2.5 mg 3 times daily.

Uterine Bleeding

IM, IV (Adults): 25 mg, may repeat in 6–12 hr if necessary.

Atrophic Vaginitis

PO (Adults): 0.3–1.25 mg once daily.

Vag (Adults): 0.5–2 g cream (0.3125 mg–1.25 g conjugated estrogens) once daily for 3 wk, off for 1 wk, then repeat.

Moderate to Severe Dyspareunia

Vag (Adults): 0.5 g cream (0.3125 mg conjugated estrogens) twice weekly continuously or daily for 3 wk, off for 1 wk, then repeat.

Availability

Powder for injection (requires reconstitution): 25 mg/vial. **Tablets:** 0.3 mg, 0.45 mg, 0.625 mg, 0.9

mg, 1.25 mg. **Cost:** *Premarin*—0.3 mg $299.14/100, 0.45 mg $299.14/100, 0.625 mg $299.14/100, 0.9 mg $311.87/100, 1.25 mg $298.45/100. **Vaginal cream:** 0.625 mg/g. **Cost:** $208.20/30 g. ***In combination with:*** bazedoxifene (Duavee); medroxyprogesterone (Prempro and Premphase [compliance package]). See Appendix B.

NURSING IMPLICATIONS

Assessment

- Assess BP before and periodically during therapy.
- Monitor intake and output ratios and weekly weight. Report significant discrepancies or steady weight gain.
- **Menopause:** Assess frequency and severity of vasomotor symptoms.
- ***Lab Test Considerations:*** May cause ↑ HDL and triglycerides, and ↓ serum LDL and total cholesterol concentrations.
- May cause ↑ serum glucose, sodium, cortisol, prolactin, prothrombin, and factor VII, VIII, IX, and X levels. May ↓ serum folate, pyridoxine, antithrombin III, and urine pregnanediol concentrations.
- Monitor hepatic function before and periodically during therapy.
- May cause false interpretations of thyroid function tests.
- May cause hypercalcemia in patients with metastatic bone lesions.

Implementation

- Estrogens should be used in the lowest doses for the shortest period of time consistent with desired therapeutic outcome.
- **PO:** Administer with or immediately after food to reduce nausea.
- **Vag:** Manufacturer provides applicator with cream. Dose is marked on the applicator. Wash applicator with mild soap and warm water after each use.
- **IM:** To reconstitute, withdraw at least 5 mL of air from dry container and then slowly introduce the sterile diluent (bacteriostatic water for injection) against the container side. Gently agitate container to dissolve; do not shake vigorously. Solution is stable for 60 days if refrigerated. Do not use if precipitate is present or if solution is darkened.
- IV is preferred parenteral route because of rapid response.

IV Administration

- **IV Push:** ***Diluent:*** Reconstitute as for IM. Inject into distal port tubing of free-flowing IV of 0.9% NaCl, D5W, or lactated Ringer's solution. ***Concentration:*** 5 mg/mL. ***Rate:*** Administer slowly (no faster than 5 mg/min) to prevent flushing.
- **Y-Site Compatibility:** heparin, hydrocortisone sodium succinate, potassium chloride, vitamin B complex with C.
- **Y-Site Incompatibility:** pantoprazole.

Patient/Family Teaching

- Instruct patient to take oral medication as directed. Advise patient to avoid drinking grapefruit juice during therapy. Take missed doses as soon as remembered, but not just before next dose. Do not double doses.
- Explain dose schedule and maintenance routine. Discontinuing medication suddenly may cause withdrawal bleeding. Bleeding is anticipated during the wk when conjugated estrogens are withheld.
- If nausea becomes a problem, advise patient that eating solid food often provides relief. Inform patient that estrogens should not be used to decrease risk of cardiovascular disease. Estrogens may increase risk of cardiovascular disease and breast cancer.
- Advise patient to report signs and symptoms of fluid retention (swelling of ankles and feet, weight gain), thromboembolic disorders (pain, swelling, tenderness in extremities; headache; chest pain; blurred vision), depression, hepatic dysfunction (yellowed skin or eyes, pruritus, dark urine, light-colored stools), or abnormal vaginal bleeding to health care professional.
- Caution patient that cigarette smoking during estrogen therapy may increase risk of serious side effects, especially for women over age 35.
- Inform patient that *Premarin* tablet may appear in stool; this is not harmful.
- Caution patient to use sunscreen and protective clothing to prevent increased pigmentation.
- Instruct patient to notify health care professional of all Rx or OTC medications, vitamins, or herbal products being taken and to consult with health care professional before taking other medications.
- Advise patient to notify health care professional of medication regimen before treatment or surgery.
- Advise patient treated for osteoporosis that exercise has been found to arrest and reverse bone loss. The patient should discuss any exercise limitations with health care professional before beginning program.
- Contraindicated in pregnancy. Instruct patient to stop taking medication and notify health care professional if pregnancy is planned or suspected, or if breast feeding.
- Emphasize the importance of routine follow-up physical exams, including BP; breast, abdomen, and pelvic examinations; Papanicolaou (Pap) smears every 6–12 mo; and mammogram every 12 mo or as directed. Health care professional will evaluate possibility of discontinuing medication every 3–6 mo. If on continuous (not cyclical) therapy or without concurrent progestins, endometrial biopsy may be recommended if uterus is intact.
- **Vag:** Instruct patient in the correct use of applicator. Patient should remain recumbent for at least 30 min after administration. May use sanitary napkin to protect clothing, but do not use tampon. If a dose is missed, do not use the missed dose, but return to regular dosing schedule.

Evaluation/Desired Outcomes

- Resolution of menopausal vasomotor symptoms.
- Decreased vaginal and vulvar itching, inflammation, or dryness associated with menopause.
- Normalization of estrogen levels in patients with ovariectomy or hypogonadism.
- Control of the spread of advanced metastatic breast or prostate cancer.
- Prevention of osteoporosis.
- Relief of moderate to severe dyspareunia due to menopause.

BEERS

eszopiclone (es-zop-i-klone)

Lunesta

Classification

Therapeutic: sedative/hypnotics

Pharmacologic: cyclopyrrolones

Schedule IV

Indications

Insomnia.

Action

Interacts with GABA-receptor complexes; not a benzodiazepine. **Therapeutic Effects:** Improved sleep with decreased latency and increased maintenance of sleep.

Pharmacokinetics

Absorption: Rapidly absorbed after oral administration.

Distribution: Unknown.

Metabolism and Excretion: Extensively metabolized by the liver (CYP3A4 and CYP2E1 enzyme systems); metabolites are renally excreted, <10% excreted unchanged in urine.

Half-life: 6 hr.

TIME/ACTION PROFILE (blood levels)

ROUTE	ONSET	PEAK	DURATION
PO	rapid	1 hr	6 hr

Contraindications/Precautions

Contraindicated in: Hypersensitivity; History of experiencing complex sleep behaviors with zolpidem.

Use Cautiously in: Debilitated patients may have ↓ metabolism or increased sensitivity; use lower initial dose; Conditions that may alter metabolic or hemodynamic function; Severe hepatic impairment (↓ dose recommended); OB, Pedi: Safety not established; Lactation: Occasional use while breast feeding an older infant should pose little risk; Geri: ↑ risk of cognitive impairment and falls. Initial dose ↓ recommended.

Adverse Reactions/Side Effects

CNS: COMPLEX SLEEP BEHAVIORS (including sleep driving, sleep walking, or engaging in other activities while sleeping), abnormal thinking, behavior changes, depression, hallucinations, headache, next day impairment. **CV:** chest pain, peripheral edema. **Derm:** rash. **GI:** dry mouth, unpleasant taste.

Interactions

Drug-Drug: ↑ risk of CNS depression and next day impairment with other **CNS depressants** including **antihistamines, antidepressants, opioids, sedative/hypnotics,** and **antipsychotics**. ↑ levels and risk of CNS depression with **drugs that inhibit the CYP3A4 enzyme system**, including **ketoconazole, itraconazole, clarithromycin, nefazodone, ritonavir,** and **nelfinavir**. Levels and effectiveness may be ↓ by **drugs that induce the CYP3A4 enzyme system**, including **rifampin**.

Route/Dosage

PO (Adults): 1 mg immediately before bedtime; may be ↑ to 2–3 mg if needed; *Geriatric patients*—1 mg immediately before bedtime; may be ↑ to 2 mg if needed; *Concurrent use of CYP3A4 inhibitors*—1 mg immediately before bedtime; may be ↑ to 2 mg if needed.

Hepatic Impairment

PO (Adults): *Severe hepatic impairment*—1 mg immediately before bedtime; may be ↑ to 2 mg if needed.

Availability (generic available)

Tablets: 1 mg, 2 mg, 3 mg. **Cost:** 1 mg $338.76/30, 2 mg $300.85/30, 3 mg $300.85/30.

NURSING IMPLICATIONS

Assessment

- Assess sleep patterns prior to and during administration. Continued insomnia after 7–10 days of therapy may indicate primary psychiatric or mental illness.
- Assess mental status and potential for abuse prior to administration. Prolonged use of >7–10 days may lead to physical and psychological dependence. Limit amount of drug available to the patient.

Implementation

- Do not confuse Lunesta (eszopiclone) with Neulasta (pegfilgrastim).
- **PO:** Onset is rapid. Administer immediately before going to bed or after patient has gone to bed and has experienced difficulty falling asleep, only on nights when patient is able to get 8 or more hrs of sleep before being active again.
- Swallow tablet whole; do not break, crush, or chew.
- Eszopiclone is more effective if not taken with or before a high-fat, heavy meal.

Patient/Family Teaching

- Instruct patient to take eszopiclone immediately before going to bed, as directed. May result in short-term memory impairment, hallucinations, impaired coordination, and dizziness. Do not take eszopiclone if consumed alcohol that evening. Do not increase dose or discontinue without notifying health care professional. Dose may need to be decreased gradually to minimize withdrawal symptoms. Rebound insomnia and/or anxiety may occur upon discontinuation and usually resolves within 1–2 nights. Advise patient to read *Medication Guide* before starting therapy and with each Rx refill in case of changes.
- May cause daytime and next-day drowsiness. Caution patient to avoid driving or other activities requiring alertness until response to medication is known.
- Caution patient that eszopiclone may cause complex sleep behaviors (sleep walking, sleep-driving, making and eating food, talking on the phone, having sex) while unaware. Patient may not remember anything done during the night; increased risk with alcohol or other CNS depressants. Discontinue eszopiclone immediately and notify health care professional if complex sleep behaviors occur.
- Instruct patient to notify health care professional of all Rx or OTC medications, vitamins, or herbal products being taken and to consult health care professional before taking any other Rx, OTC, or herbal products.
- Caution patient to avoid concurrent use of alcohol or other CNS depressants.
- Advise patient to notify health care professional if signs and symptoms of allergic reaction (swelling of tongue or throat, trouble breathing, nausea and vomiting) occur.
- Advise patient to notify health care professional if pregnancy is planned or suspected, or if breast feeding.

Evaluation/Desired Outcomes

- Decreased sleep latency and improved sleep maintenance.

etanercept (e-tan-er-sept)

Brenzys, Enbrel, Erelzi, Eticovo

Classification
Therapeutic: antirheumatics (DMARDs)
Pharmacologic: anti-TNF agents

Indications

Enbrel, Erelzi, and Eticovo: Treatment of the following conditions: Moderately to severely active rheumatoid arthritis (may be used alone or with methotrexate), Moderate to severely active polyarticular juvenile idiopathic arthritis, Active ankylosing spondylitis. **Enbrel and Eticovo:** Treatment of the following conditions: Psoriatic arthritis (may be used alone or with methotrexate), Moderate to severe chronic plaque psoriasis in patients who are candidates for systemic therapy or phototherapy.

Action

Binds to tumor necrosis factor (TNF), making it inactive. TNF is a mediator of inflammatory response.
Therapeutic Effects: Decreased pain and swelling with decreased rate of joint destruction in patients with rheumatoid arthritis, psoriatic arthritis, juvenile idiopathic arthritis, and ankylosing spondylitis. Reduced severity of plaques.

Pharmacokinetics

Absorption: 60% absorbed after subcut administration.
Distribution: Unknown.
Metabolism and Excretion: Unknown.
Half-life: 115 hr (range 98–300 hr).

TIME/ACTION PROFILE (symptom reduction)

ROUTE	ONSET	PEAK	DURATION
Subcut	2–4 wk	unknown	unknown

Contraindications/Precautions

Contraindicated in: Hypersensitivity; Active infection (including localized); Untreated infections; Granulomatosis with polyangiitis (receiving immunosuppressive agents); Concurrent cyclophosphamide or anakinra; Lactation: Lactation.
Use Cautiously in: History of chronic or recurrent infection or underlying illness/treatment predisposing to infection (including advanced or poorly controlled diabetes); History of exposure to tuberculosis; History of opportunistic infection; History of hepatitis B; Patients residing, or who have resided, where tuberculosis, histoplasmosis, coccidioidomycoses, or blastomycosis is endemic; Pre-existing or recent demyelinating disorders (multiple sclerosis, myelitis, optic neuritis); Latex allergy (needle cover of diluent syringe contains latex); OB: Use only if needed; Pedi: Children with significant exposure to varicella virus (temporarily discontinue etanercept; consider varicella zoster immune globulin); ↑ risk of lymphoma (including hepatosplenic T-cell lymphoma [HSTCL]), leukemia, and other malignancies; Pedi: Children <2 yr (juvenile idiopathic arthritis) or <4 yr (plaque psoriasis) (safety and effectiveness not established); Geri: May have ↑ risk of infection.

Adverse Reactions/Side Effects

CNS: headache, dizziness, weakness. **Derm:** psoriasis, rash. **EENT:** rhinitis, pharyngitis. **GI:** abdominal pain, dyspepsia. **Hemat:** pancytopenia. **Local:** injection site reactions. **Resp:** upper respiratory tract infection, cough, respiratory disorder. **Misc:** INFECTION (including reactivation tuberculosis and other opportunistic infections due to bacterial, invasive fungal, viral, mycobacterial, and parasitic pathogens), MALIGNANCY (including lymphoma, HSTCL, leukemia, and skin cancer), SARCOIDOSIS.

Interactions

Drug-Drug: Concurrent use with **anakinra** ↑ risk of serious infections (not recommended). Concurrent use of **cyclophosphamide** may ↑ risk of malignancies. Concurrent use with **azathioprine** and/or **methotrexate** may ↑ risk of HSTCL. May ↓ antibody response to **live-virus vaccine** and ↑ risk of adverse reactions (do not administer concurrently).

Route/Dosage

Rheumatoid Arthritis, Psoriatic Arthritis, and Ankylosing Spondylitis

Subcut (Adults): 50 mg once weekly.

Plaque Psoriasis

Subcut (Adults): 50 mg twice weekly for 3 mo, then 50 mg once weekly, may also be given as 25–50 mg once weekly as an initial dose.
Subcut (Children ≥4 yr and ≥63 kg): 50 mg once weekly.
Subcut (Children ≥4 yr and <63 kg): 0.8 mg/kg once weekly.

Juvenile Idiopathic Arthritis

Subcut (Children ≥2 yr and ≥63 kg): 50 mg once weekly.
Subcut (Children ≥2 yr and <63 kg): 0.8 mg/kg once weekly.

Availability

Powder for injection (requires reconstitution): 25 mg/vial. **Solution for injection:** 25 mg/0.5 mL (prefilled syringe), 50 mg/mL (prefilled syringe and autoinjector).

NURSING IMPLICATIONS

Assessment

- Assess range of motion, degree of swelling, and pain in affected joints before and periodically during therapy.
- Assess patient for injection site reaction (erythema, pain, itching, swelling). Reactions are usually mild to moderate and last 3–5 days after injection.
- Monitor patients who develop a new infection while taking etanercept closely. Discontinue therapy in patients who develop a serious infection or sepsis. Do not initiate therapy in patients with active infections.
- Assess for signs and symptoms of systemic fungal infections (fever, malaise, weight loss, sweats, cough, dyspnea, pulmonary infiltrates, serious systemic illness with or without concomitant shock). Ascertain if patient lives in or has traveled to areas of endemic mycoses. Consider empiric antifungal treatment for patients at risk of histoplasmosis and other invasive fungal infections until the pathogens are identified. Consult with an infectious diseases specialist. Consider stopping etanercept until the infection has been diagnosed and adequately treated.
- ***Lab Test Considerations:*** Monitor CBC with differential periodically during therapy. May cause leukopenia, neutropenia, thrombocytopenia, and pancytopenia. Discontinue etanercept if symptoms of blood dyscrasias (persistent fever) occur.

Implementation

- Do not confuse Enbrel (etanercept) with Levbid (hyoscyamine).
- Administer a tuberculin skin test prior to administration of etanercept. Patients with active latent TB should be treated for TB prior to therapy.
- Needle cover of the prefilled syringe contains latex and should not be handled by people with latex allergies.
- **Subcut:** Prepare injection with single dose prefilled syringe or multidose vial for reconstitution.
- Solution in prefilled syringe may be allowed to reach room temperature (15–30 min); do not remove needle cap during this time.
- For multidose vial, reconstitute with 1 mL of the bacteriostatic sterile water supplied by manufacturer for a concentration of 25 mg/mL. If the vial is used for multiple doses, use a 25-gauge needle for reconstituting and withdrawing solution and apply "Mixing Date" sticker with date of reconstitution entered. Inject diluent slowly into vial to avoid foaming. Some foaming will occur. Swirl gently for dissolution; do not shake or vigorously agitate to prevent excess foaming. Solution should be clear and colorless; do not administer solution that is discolored or contains particulate matter. Dissolution usually takes <10 min. Withdraw solution into syringe. Some foam may remain in vial. Amount in syringe should approximate 1 mL. Do not filter reconstituted solution during preparation or administration. Attach a 27-gauge needle to inject. Administer as soon as possible after reconstitution; stable up to 6 hr if refrigerated. Solution and prefilled syringes are stable if refrigerated and used within 14 days.
- May be injected into abdomen, thigh, or upper arm. Rotate sites. Do not administer within 1 in. of an old site or into area that is tender, red, hard, or bruised.
- **Syringe Incompatibility:** Do not mix with other solutions or dilute with other diluents.

Patient/Family Teaching

- Instruct patient on self-administration technique, storage, and disposal of equipment. First injection should be administered under the supervision of health care professional. Provide patient with a puncture-proof container for used equipment. Advise patient to read *Medication Guide* before starting therapy and with each Rx refill in case of changes.

- Advise patient not to receive live vaccines during therapy. Parents should be advised that children should complete immunizations to date before initiation of etanercept. Patients with significant exposure to varicella virus (chickenpox) should temporarily discontinue therapy and varicella immune globulin should be considered.
- Instruct patient to notify health care professional of all Rx or OTC medications, vitamins, or herbal products being taken and to consult health care professional before taking any other Rx, OTC, or herbal products.
- Advise patient that methotrexate, analgesics, NSAIDs, corticosteroids, and salicylates may be continued during therapy.
- Instruct patient to notify health care professional if upper respiratory or other infections occur. Therapy may need to be discontinued if serious infection occurs.
- Advise patient of risk of malignancies such as hepatosplenic T-cell lymphoma. Instruct patient to report signs and symptoms (splenomegaly, hepatomegaly, abdominal pain, persistent fever, night sweats, weight loss) to health care professional promptly.
- Instruct female patients to notify health care professional if pregnancy is planned or suspected and to avoid breast feeding during therapy. Advise patients who were pregnant during therapy to notify health care professional; may limit administration of live vaccines to infant.

Evaluation/Desired Outcomes
- Reduction in symptoms of rheumatoid arthritis. Symptoms may return within 1 mo of discontinuation of therapy.
- Reduced severity of plaques in chronic plaque psoriasis.

ethambutol (e-tham-byoo-tole)
Etibi, Myambutol

Classification
Therapeutic: antituberculars

Indications
Active tuberculosis or other mycobacterial diseases (with at least one other drug).

Action
Inhibits the growth of mycobacteria. **Therapeutic Effects:** Tuberculostatic effect against susceptible organisms.

Pharmacokinetics
Absorption: Rapidly and well absorbed (80%) from the GI tract.
Distribution: Widely distributed; crosses blood-brain barrier in small amounts; crosses placenta and enters breast milk.
Protein Binding: 20–30%.
Metabolism and Excretion: 50% metabolized by the liver, 50% eliminated unchanged by the kidneys.
Half-life: 3.3 hr (increased in renal or hepatic impairment).

TIME/ACTION PROFILE (blood levels)

ROUTE	ONSET	PEAK	DURATION
PO	rapid	2–4 hr	24 hr

Contraindications/Precautions
Contraindicated in: Hypersensitivity; Optic neuritis.
Use Cautiously in: Renal and severe hepatic impairment (dosage reduction required); OB: Although safety not established, ethambutol has been used with isoniazid in pregnant women without fetal adverse effects; Lactation: Usually compatible with breast feeding (AAP).

Adverse Reactions/Side Effects
CNS: confusion, dizziness, hallucinations, headache, malaise. **EENT:** optic neuritis. **GI:** HEPATITIS, abdominal pain, anorexia, nausea, vomiting. **Metab:** hyperuricemia. **MS:** joint pain. **Neuro:** peripheral neuritis. **Resp:** pulmonary infiltrates. **Misc:** anaphylactoid reactions, fever.

Interactions
Drug-Drug: Neurotoxicity may be ↑ with other **neurotoxic agents**. **Aluminum hydroxide** may decrease absorption (space doses 4 hr apart).

Route/Dosage
PO (Adults and Children >13 yr): 15–25 mg/kg/day (maximum 2.5 g/day) *or* 50 mg/kg (up to 2.5 g) twice weekly *or* 25–30 mg/kg (up to 2.5 g) 3 times weekly.
PO (Children 1 mo—13 yr): *HIV negative*—15–20 mg/kg/day once daily (maximum: 1 g/day) or 50 mg/kg/dose twice weekly (maximum: 2.5 g/dose); *HIV-exposed/-infected*—15–25 mg/kg/day once daily (maximum: 2.5 g/day); *MAC, secondary prophylaxis, or treatment in HIV-exposed/-infected*—15–25 mg/kg/day once daily (maximum: 2.5 g/day) with clarithromycin (or azithromycin) with or without rifabutin; *Nontuberculous mycobacterial infection*—15–25 mg/kg/day once daily (maximum: 2.5 g/day).

Availability (generic available)
Tablets: 100 mg, 400 mg.

NURSING IMPLICATIONS
Assessment
- Mycobacterial studies and susceptibility tests should be performed before and periodically during therapy to detect possible resistance.
- Assess lung sounds and character and amount of sputum periodically during therapy.
- Assessments of visual function should be made frequently during therapy. Advise patient to report blur-

ring of vision, constriction of visual fields, or changes in color perception immediately. Visual impairment, if not identified early, may lead to permanent sight impairment.

- ***Lab Test Considerations:*** Monitor renal and hepatic functions, CBC, and uric acid levels routinely. Frequently causes elevated uric acid concentrations, which may precipitate an attack of gout.

Implementation

- Ethambutol is given as a single daily dose and should be taken at the same time each day. Some regimens require dosing 2–3 times/wk. Usually administered concurrently with other antitubercular medications to prevent development of bacterial resistance.
- **PO:** Administer with food or milk to minimize GI irritation.
- **PO:** Tablets may be crushed and mixed with apple juice or apple sauce.

Patient/Family Teaching

- Instruct patient to take medication as directed. Take missed doses as soon as possible unless almost time for next dose; do not double up on missed doses. A full course of therapy may take mo to yr. Do not discontinue without consulting health care professional, even though symptoms may disappear.
- Advise patient to notify health care professional if pregnancy is suspected.
- Instruct patient to notify health care professional if no improvement is seen in 2–3 wk. Health care professional should also be notified if unexpected weight gain or decreased urine output occurs.
- Emphasize the importance of routine exams to evaluate progress and ophthalmic examinations if signs of optic neuritis occur.

Evaluation/Desired Outcomes

- Resolution of clinical symptoms of tuberculosis.
- Decrease in acid-fast bacteria in sputum samples.
- Improvement seen in chest x rays. Therapy for tuberculosis is usually continued for at least 1–2 yr.

ethinyl estradiol/desogestrel, **See CONTRACEPTIVES, HORMONAL.**

ethinyl estradiol/drospirenone, **See CONTRACEPTIVES, HORMONAL.**

ethinyl estradiol/ethynodiol, **See CONTRACEPTIVES, HORMONAL.**

ethinyl estradiol/etonogestrel, **See CONTRACEPTIVES, HORMONAL.**

ethinyl estradiol/levonorgestrel, **See CONTRACEPTIVES, HORMONAL.**

ethinyl estradiol/norelgestromin, **See CONTRACEPTIVES, HORMONAL.**

ethinyl estradiol/norethindrone, **See CONTRACEPTIVES, HORMONAL.**

ethinyl estradiol/norgestimate, **See CONTRACEPTIVES, HORMONAL.**

ethinyl estradiol/norgestrel, **See CONTRACEPTIVES, HORMONAL.**

BEERS

etodolac (ee-toe-doe-lak)

~~Lodine~~, ~~Lodine XL~~

Classification

Therapeutic: antirheumatics, nonopioid analgesics

Pharmacologic: pyranocarboxylic acid

Indications

Osteoarthritis. Rheumatoid arthritis. Mild to moderate pain (not XL tablets).

Action

Inhibits prostaglandin synthesis. Also has uricosuric action. **Therapeutic Effects:** Suppression of inflammation. Decreased severity of pain.

Pharmacokinetics

Absorption: Well absorbed after oral administration.
Distribution: Widely distributed.
Protein Binding: >99%.
Metabolism and Excretion: Mostly metabolized by the liver; <1% excreted unchanged in urine.
Half-life: 6–7 hr (single dose); 7.3 hr (chronic dosing).

TIME/ACTION PROFILE (analgesic effect)

ROUTE	ONSET	PEAK	DURATION
PO (analgesic)	0.5 hr	1–2 hr	4–12 hr
PO (anti-inflammatory)	days–wk	unknown	6–12 hr†

†Up to 24 hr as XL (extended-release) tablet.

Contraindications/Precautions

Contraindicated in: Hypersensitivity; Active GI bleeding or ulcer disease; Cross-sensitivity may exist with other NSAIDs, including aspirin; Peri-operative pain from coronary artery bypass graft (CABG) surgery; OB: Use during 2nd half of pregnancy can result in premature closure of ductus arteriosis.

Use Cautiously in: Renal or hepatic disease; Cardiovascular disease or risk factors for cardiovascular disease (may ↑ risk of serious cardiovascular thrombotic events, myocardial infarction, and stroke, especially with prolonged use or use of higher doses); History of ulcer disease; Lactation: Limited information available; use other safer NSAID; Pedi: Safety not established; Geri: ↑ risk of GI bleeding.

Adverse Reactions/Side Effects

CNS: depression, dizziness, drowsiness, insomnia, malaise, nervousness, syncope, weakness. **EENT:** blurred vision, photophobia, tinnitus. **Resp:** asthma. **CV:** HF, MYOCARDIAL INFARCTION, STROKE, edema, hypertension, palpitations. **GI:** GI BLEEDING, dyspepsia, abdominal pain, constipation, diarrhea, drug-induced hepatitis, dry mouth, flatulence, gastritis, nausea, stomatitis, thirst, vomiting. **GU:** dysuria, renal failure, urinary frequency. **Derm:** EXFOLIATIVE DERMATITIS, STEVENS-JOHNSON SYNDROME, TOXIC EPIDERMAL NECROLYSIS, ecchymoses, flushing, hyperpigmentation, pruritus, rash, sweating. **Hemat:** anemia, prolonged bleeding time, thrombocytopenia. **Misc:** allergic reactions including ANAPHYLAXIS, ANGIOEDEMA, chills, fever.

Interactions

Drug-Drug: Concurrent use with **aspirin** may ↓ effectiveness. ↑ adverse GI effects with **aspirin**, other **NSAIDs**, **potassium supplements**, **corticosteroids**, **antiplatelet agents**, or **alcohol**. Chronic use with **acetaminophen** may ↑ risk of adverse renal reactions. May ↓ effectiveness of **diuretic** or **antihypertensive** therapy. May ↑ serum **lithium** levels and ↑ risk of toxicity. ↑ risk of toxicity from **methotrexate**. ↑ risk of bleeding with **cefotetan**, **valproic acid**, **thrombolytics**, **antiplatelet agents**, or **anticoagulants**. ↑ risk of adverse hematologic reactions with **antineoplastics** or **radiation therapy**. May ↑ the risk of nephrotoxicity from **cyclosporine**.

Drug-Natural Products: ↑ risk of bleeding with **arnica**, **chamomile**, **clove**, **dong quai**, **fever few**, **garlic**, **ginko**, and ***Panax ginseng***.

Route/Dosage

PO (Adults): *Analgesia*—200–400 mg every 6–8 hr (not to exceed 1200 mg/day). *Osteoarthritis/rheumatoid arthritis*—300 mg 2–3 times daily, 400 mg twice daily, or 500 mg twice daily; may also be given as 400–1200 mg once daily as XL tablets.

Availability (generic available)

Capsules: 200 mg, 300 mg. **Tablets:** 400 mg, 500 mg. **Extended-release tablets:** 400 mg, 500 mg, 600 mg.

NURSING IMPLICATIONS

Assessment

- Patients who have asthma, aspirin-induced allergy, and nasal polyps are at increased risk for developing hypersensitivity reactions. Monitor for rhinitis, asthma, and urticaria.
- Assess for rash periodically during therapy. May cause Stevens-Johnson syndrome. Discontinue therapy if severe or if accompanied with fever, general malaise, fatigue, muscle or joint aches, blisters, oral lesions, conjunctivitis, hepatitis, and/or eosinophilia.
- **Osteoarthritis/Rheumatoid Arthritis:** Assess pain and range of movement before and 1–2 hr after administration.
- **Pain:** Assess location, duration, and intensity of the pain before and 60 min after administration.
- ***Lab Test Considerations:*** May cause ↓ hemoglobin, hematocrit, leukocyte, and platelet counts.
- Monitor liver function tests within 8 wk of initiating etodolac therapy and periodically during therapy. May cause ↑ serum alkaline phosphatase, LDH, AST, and ALT concentrations.
- Monitor BUN, serum creatinine, and electrolytes periodically during therapy. May cause ↑ BUN, serum creatinine, and electrolyte concentrations and ↓ urine electrolyte concentrations.
- May cause ↓ serum and ↑ urine uric acid concentrations.

Implementation

Administration in higher-than-recommended doses does not provide increased effectiveness but may cause increased side effects.

- Use lowest effective dose for shortest period of time.
- **PO:** For rapid initial effect, administer 30 min before or 2 hr after meals. May be administered with food, milk, or antacids containing aluminum or magnesium to decrease GI irritation.
- Do not break, crush, or chew extended-release tablets.

Patient/Family Teaching

- Advise patients to take etodolac with a full glass of water and to remain in an upright position for 15–30 min after administration.
- Instruct patient to take medication as directed. Take missed doses as soon as possible within 1–2 hr if taking twice/day, or unless almost time for next dose if taking more than twice/day. Do not double doses.

- Etodolac may occasionally cause drowsiness or dizziness. Advise patient to avoid driving or other activities requiring alertness until response to the medication is known.
- Caution patient to avoid the concurrent use of alcohol, aspirin, acetaminophen, NSAIDs, or other OTC medications without consultation with health care professional.
- Advise patient to inform health care professional of medication regimen before treatment or surgery.
- Advise patient to consult health care professional if rash, itching, visual disturbances, tinnitus, weight gain, edema, black stools, persistent headache, or influenza-like syndrome (chills, fever, muscle aches, pain) occurs.
- Advise patient to notify health care professional if pregnancy is planned or suspected or if breast feeding.

Evaluation/Desired Outcomes

- Decreased severity of pain.
- Improved joint mobility. Patients who do not respond to one NSAID may respond to another. May require 2 wk or more for maximum anti-inflammatory effects.

etonogestrel, See CONTRACEPTIVES, HORMONAL.

everolimus (e-ver-**oh**-li-mus)

Afinitor, Afinitor Disperz, ~~Certican~~, Zortress

Classification

Therapeutic: antineoplastics, immunosuppressants

Pharmacologic: kinase inhibitors

Indications

Afinitor. Advanced renal cell carcinoma that has failed treatment with sunitinib or sorafenib. Subependymal giant cell astrocytoma (SEGA) associated with tuberous sclerosis complex (TSC) in patients who are not candidates for curative surgical resection. TSC-associated partial-onset seizures (adjunctive treatment). Progressive neuroendocrine tumors of pancreatic origin (PNET) in patients with unresectable, locally advanced, or metastatic disease. Progressive, well-differentiated, non-functional neuroendocrine tumors (NET) of GI or lung origin in patients with unresectable, locally advanced, or metastatic disease. Renal angiomyolipoma with TSC in patients not requiring immediate surgery. Treatment of postmenopausal women with advanced hormone receptor-positive, HER2-negative breast cancer in combination with exemestane, after failure of treatment with letrozole or anastrozole. **Zortress**. Prevention of organ rejection in patients who have received a kidney transplant and are at low-to-moderate immunologic risk. Prevention of organ rejection in patients who have received a liver transplant.

Action

Acts as a kinase inhibitor, decreasing cell proliferation. Inhibits activation and proliferation of T and B lymphocytes. **Therapeutic Effects:** Decreased spread of renal cell carcinoma and breast cancer. Improvement in progression-free survival in patients with PNET. Decreased volume of SEGA and angiomyolipoma lesions. Prevention of kidney and liver transplant rejection. Reduction in seizure frequency.

Pharmacokinetics

Absorption: Well absorbed following oral administration.

Distribution: 20% confined to plasma.

Metabolism and Excretion: Mostly metabolized by liver and other systems (CYP3A4 and P-gp; metabolites are mostly excreted in feces [80%] and urine [5%]).

Half-life: 30 hr.

TIME/ACTION PROFILE (blood levels))

ROUTE	ONSET	PEAK	DURATION
PO	unknown	1–2 hr	24 hr

Contraindications/Precautions

Contraindicated in: Hypersensitivity to everolimus or other rapamycins; Severe hepatic impairment (Child-Pugh class C); use only if benefit exceeds risk for renal cell carcinoma, PNET, breast cancer, and renal angiomyolipoma with TSC; Concurrent use with strong CYP3A4 inhibitors (i.e., ketoconazole, itraconazole, clarithromycin, atazanavir, nefazodone, saquinavir, ritonavir, indinavir, nelfinavir, voriconazole); Heart transplantation (Zortress) (↑ risk of mortality); Functional carcinoid tumors; OB: Avoid use in pregnancy (may cause fetal harm); Lactation: Avoid breast feeding.

Use Cautiously in: Mild or moderate hepatic impairment (Child-Pugh class A or B); dose ↓ required; Concurrent use of moderate CYP3A4 and/or P-gp inhibitors; dose ↓ required; Exposure to sunlight/UV light (may ↑ risk of malignant skin changes); Rep: Women of reproductive potential and men with female partners of reproductive potential; Geri: May be more sensitive to drug effects; consider age-related ↓ in hepatic function, concurrent disease states and drug therapy; Pedi: Safety not established for indications other than SEGA and TSC-associated partial-onset seizures.

Adverse Reactions/Side Effects

CNS: <u>fatigue</u>, <u>weakness</u>, headache. **CV:** <u>peripheral edema</u>. **Derm:** delayed wound healing, dry skin, pruritus, rash. **GI:** HEPATIC ARTERY THROMBOSIS, anorexia, constipation, diarrhea, mucositis, mouth ulcers, nausea, stomatitis, vomiting, dysgeusia. **GU:** acute renal failure, amenorrhea, ↓ fertility, menstrual irregularities, proteinuria. **Hemat:** HEMOLYTIC UREMIC SYNDROME, THROMBOTIC MICROANGIOPATHY, THROMBOTIC THROMBOCYTOPENIC PURPURA, anemia, leukopenia, thrombocytopenia. **Metab:** hyperglycemia, hyperlipidemia, hypertriglyceridemia. **MS:** extremity pain. **Resp:** INTERSTITIAL LUNG DISEASE, PULMONARY HYPERTENSION, cough, dyspnea, pulmonary embolism. **Misc:** HYPERSENSITIVITY REACTIONS (including anaphylaxis and angioedema), fever, infection (including activation of latent viral infections such as BK virus-associated nephropathy), kidney arterial/venous thrombosis (Zortress), ↑ risk of lymphoma/skin cancer (Zortress).

Interactions

Drug-Drug: Strong **CYP3A4 inhibitors**, including **atazanavir**, **clarithromycin**, **indinavir**, **itraconazole**, **ketoconazole**, **nefazodone**, **nelfinavir**, **ritonavir**, **saquinavir**, or **voriconazole** ↑ levels and the risk of toxicity; avoid concurrent use. Moderate inhibitors of CYP3A4, including **aprepitant**, **diltiazem**, **erythromycin**, **fluconazole**, **fosamprenavir**, and **verapamil** ↑ levels and the risk of toxicity; ↓ dose of everolimus (Afinitor). Avoid concurrent use with strong **CYP3A4 inducers** including **carbamazepine**, **dexamethasone**, **phenobarbital**, **phenytoin**, **rifabutin**, and **rifampin**; ↑ dose of everolimus may be required. **Cyclosporine**, **aprepitant**, **diltiazem**, **verapamil**, **fluconazole**, and **fosamprenavir** may ↑ levels. ↑ risk of nephrotoxicity with **aminoglycosides**, **amphotericin B**, **cisplatin**, or **cyclosporine**. **ACE inhibitors** may ↑ risk of angioedema. May ↓ antibody formation and ↑ risk of adverse reactions from **live-virus vaccines**; avoid use of live-virus vaccines during treatment.
Drug-Natural Products: **St. John's wort** may ↓ levels and efficacy; avoid concurrent use.
Drug-Food: ↑ blood levels and risk of toxicity with **grapefruit juice**; avoid concurrent use.

Route/Dosage

Advanced Renal Cell Carcinoma, Advanced PNET, Advanced NET, Advanced Hormone Receptor-Positive, HER2-Negative Breast Cancer, and Renal Angiomyolipoma with TSC (Afinitor)

PO (Adults): 10 mg once daily until disease progression or unacceptable toxicity; *Concurrent use of P-glycoprotein inhibitor and moderate CYP3A4 inhibitor*—2.5 mg once daily until disease progression or unacceptable toxicity; *Concurrent use of P-glycoprotein inducer and strong CYP3A4 inducer*—↑ dose in 5 mg increments up to 20 mg once daily; continue until disease progression or unacceptable toxicity.

Hepatic Impairment

PO (Adults): *Mild hepatic impairment (Child–Pugh Class A)*—7.5 mg once daily until disease progression or unacceptable toxicity; may ↓ to 5 mg once daily if not well tolerated; *Moderate hepatic impairment (Child–Pugh Class B)*—5 mg once daily until disease progression or unacceptable toxicity; may ↓ to 2.5 mg once daily if not well tolerated; *Severe hepatic impairment (Child–Pugh Class C)*—2.5 mg once daily until disease progression or unacceptable toxicity.

SEGA with TSC (Afinitor)

PO (Adults and Children ≥1 yr): 4.5 mg/m² once daily. Titrate, as needed, at 2-wk intervals to achieve recommended whole blood trough concentration. Continue until disease progression or unacceptable toxicity; *Concurrent use of P-glycoprotein inhibitor and moderate CYP3A4 inhibitor*—2.25 mg/m² once daily. Titrate, as needed, at 2-wk intervals to achieve recommended whole blood trough concentration. Continue until disease progression or unacceptable toxicity; *Concurrent use of P-glycoprotein inducer and strong CYP3A4 inducer*—9 mg/m² once daily. Titrate, as needed, at 2-wk intervals to achieve recommended whole blood trough concentration. Continue until disease progression or unacceptable toxicity.

Hepatic Impairment

PO (Adults and Children ≥1 yr): *Severe hepatic impairment (Child–Pugh Class C)*—2.5 mg/m² once daily. Titrate, as needed, at 2-wk intervals to achieve recommended whole blood trough concentration. Continue until disease progression or unacceptable toxicity.

TSC—Associated Partial-Onset Seizures (Afinitor)

PO (Adults and Children ≥2 yr): 5 mg/m² once daily. Titrate, as needed, at 2-wk intervals to achieve recommended whole blood trough concentration. Continue until disease progression or unacceptable toxicity; *Concurrent use of P-glycoprotein inhibitor and moderate CYP3A4 inhibitor*—2.5 mg/m² once daily. Titrate, as needed, at 2-wk intervals to achieve recommended whole blood trough concentration. Continue until disease progression or unacceptable toxicity; *Concurrent use of P-glycoprotein inducer and strong CYP3A4 inducer*—10 mg/m² once daily. Titrate, as needed, at 2-wk intervals to achieve recommended whole blood trough concentration. Continue until disease progression or unacceptable toxicity.

Hepatic Impairment

PO (Adults and Children ≥2 yr): *Severe hepatic impairment (Child–Pugh Class C)*—2.5 mg/m² once daily. Titrate, as needed, at 2-wk intervals to achieve recommended whole blood trough concentration. Continue until disease progression or unacceptable toxicity.

Kidney Transplantation (Zortress)

PO (Adults): 0.75 mg twice daily (with reduced-dose cyclosporine); titrate to achieve recommended whole blood trough concentration.

Hepatic Impairment

PO (Adults): *Mild hepatic impairment (Child–Pugh Class A)* — ↓ daily dose by 33%; *Moderate or severe hepatic impairment (Child–Pugh Class B or C)* — ↓ daily dose by 50%.

Liver Transplantation (Zortress)

PO (Adults): 1 mg twice daily (with reduced-dose tacrolimus) (start ≥30 days post-transplant); titrate to achieve recommended whole blood trough concentration.

Hepatic Impairment

PO (Adults): *Mild hepatic impairment (Child–Pugh Class A)* — ↓ daily dose by 33%; *Moderate or severe hepatic impairment (Child–Pugh Class B or C)* — ↓ daily dose by 50%.

Availability (generic available)

Tablets (Afinitor): 2.5 mg, 5 mg, 7.5 mg, 10 mg. **Tablets for oral suspension (Afinitor Disperz):** 2 mg, 3 mg, 5 mg. **Tablets (Zortress):** 0.25 mg, 0.5 mg, 0.75 mg, 1 mg.

NURSING IMPLICATIONS

Assessment

- Assess for symptoms of noninfectious pneumonitis (hypoxia, pleural effusion, cough, dyspnea) during therapy. If symptoms are mild, therapy may continue. *If Grade 2 pneumonitis occurs:* hold therapy until Grade 0–1; reinitiate everolimus at a 50% dose. Permanently discontinue if does not resolve or improve to Grade 1 within 4 wk. *If Grade 3 pneumonitis occurs:* hold therapy until Grade 0–1; resume at 50% of previous dose. Change to every other day if dose is lower than lowest available strength. Permanently discontinue if Grade 3 pneumonitis recurs. *If Grade 4 pneumonitis occurs:* permanently discontinue.
- Assess for mouth ulcers, stomatitis, or oral mucositis; usually occurs within first 8 wk of therapy. Begin dexamethasone alcohol-free oral solution as a swish and spit mouthwash when starting therapy to reduce incidence and severity of stomatitis. Topical treatments may be used; avoid peroxide-containing mouthwashes and antifungals unless fungal infection has been diagnosed. *If stomatitis Grade 2 occurs:* hold therapy until Grade 0–1; resume at previous dose. If Grade 2 recurs, withhold until Grade 0–1; resume at 50% dose. Change to every other day if dose is lower than lowest available strength. *If Grade 3 stomatitis occurs:* hold therapy until Grade 0–1; hold until Grade 0–1; resume at 50% of previous dose. Change to every other day if dose is lower than lowest available strength. *If Grade 4 stomatitis occurs:* discontinue permanently.
- Assess for signs and symptoms of systemic fungal infections (fever, malaise, weight loss, sweats, cough, dyspnea, pulmonary infiltrates, serious systemic illness with or without concomitant shock). Withold therapy until infection has been diagnosed and adequately treated.
- Monitor for signs and symptoms of hypersensitivity reactions (anaphylaxis, dyspnea, flushing, chest pain, angioedema) during therapy. Permanently discontinue therapy if severe reactions occur.
- ***Lab Test Considerations:*** Obtain a negative pregnancy test before starting therapy.
- Monitor renal function prior to and periodically during therapy. May cause ↑ BUN, serum creatinine, and proteinuria.
- Monitor fasting serum glucose and lipid profile prior to and periodically during therapy. May cause ↑ cholesterol, triglycerides, glucose. Attempt to achieve optimal glucose and lipid control prior to therapy. *If Grade 3 metabolic events (hyperglycemia, dyslipidemia) occur:* hold until improvement to Grade 0, 1, or 2. Resume at 50% of previous dose. Change to every other day if dose is lower than lowest available strength.
- Monitor CBC prior to and every 6 mo for 1st yr of therapy and annually thereafter; may cause ↓ hemoglobin, lymphocytes, neutrophils, and platelets. *If Grade 2 thrombocytopenia occurs:* hold dose until Grade 0–1; resume at same dose. *If Grade 3 or 4 thrombocytopenia occurs:* hold until improvement to Grade 0, 1, or 2. Resume at 50% of previous dose. Change to every other day if dose is lower than lowest available strength. *If Grade 3 neutropenia occurs:* hold dose until Grade 0–1; resume at same dose. *If Grade 4 neutropenia occurs:* hold until improvement to Grade 0, 1, or 2. Resume at 50% of previous dose. Change to every other day if dose is lower than lowest available strength. *If Grade 3 febrile neutropenia occurs:* hold until improvement to Grade 0, 1, or 2 and no fever. Resume at 50% of previous dose. Change to every other day if dose is lower than lowest available strength. *If Grade 4 febrile neutropenia occurs:* discontinue permanently.
- May cause ↑ AST, ALT, phosphate, and bilirubin.
- **Afinitor:** Monitor *Afinitor* trough levels 2 wk after initiation of therapy, a change in dose, a change in co-administration of CYP3A4 and/or P-gp inducers or inhibitors, change in hepatic function, or change in dose form between everolimus tablets and *Disperz.* Once at a stable dose, monitor trough concentrations every 3–6 mo in patients with changing body surface area or every 6–12 mo in patients

with stable body surface area for duration of treatment. Therapeutic blood concentrations are 5–15 ng/mL (*Afinitor*). If trough concentration is <5 ng/mL increase daily dose by 2.5 mg in patients taking tablets and 2 mg for *Disperz*. If trough concentration is >15 ng/mL decrease daily dose by 2.5 mg in patients taking tablets and 2 mg for *Disperz*. If dose reduction is required with lowest dose, administer every other day. Do not combine dose forms to achieve dose. **Zortress:** Therapeutic blood concentrations are 3–8 ng/mL via the LCMSMS assay (*Zortress*). Base dose adjustments of *Zortress* on trough concentrations obtained 4 or 5 days after a previous dosing change. Adjust dose if trough concentration is <3 ng/mL by doubling dose using available tablet strengths (0.25 mg, 0.5 mg or 0.75 mg). If trough concentration is >8 ng/mL on 2 consecutive measures; decrease dose of *Zortress* by 0.25 mg twice daily.

Implementation

- **PO:** Administer at the same time each day consistently with or without food, followed by a whole glass of water. Swallow tablets whole; do not break, crush, or chew.
- Do not combine the 2 dose forms (*Afinitor Tablets* and *Afinitor Disperz*) to achieve the desired total dose. Use one dose form or the other.
- Administer *Disperz*, dispersable tablet, as a suspension only. Wear gloves to avoid possible contact with everolimus when preparing suspensions for another person. Place dose in 10 mL syringe; do not exceed 10 mg/syringe. If higher dose required, use additional syringe. Do not break or crush tablets. Draw 5 mL water and 4 mL of air into syringe. Place filled syringe into container (tip up) for 3 min until tablets are in suspension. Invert syringe five times immediately prior to administration. Administer immediately after preparation; discard suspension if not administered within 60 min after preparation. After administration, draw 5 mL of water and 4 mL of air into same syringe, and swirl contents to suspend remaining particles. Administer entire contents of syringe. Can also be dispersed using same technique and 25 mL water in small glass.

Patient/Family Teaching

- Instruct patient to take everolimus at the same time each day as directed. Take missed doses as soon as remembered up to 6 hr after time of normal dose. If more than 6 hr after normal dose, omit dose for that day and take next dose next day; do not take two doses to make up missed dose. Do not eat grapefruit or drink grapefruit juice during therapy. Advise patient to read *Patient Information* prior to beginning therapy and with each Rx refill in case of new information.
- Advise patient to report worsening respiratory symptoms or signs of infection (new or worsening cough, shortness of breath, chest pain, difficulty breathing or wheezing, fever, chills, skin rash, joint pain and inflammation, tiredness, loss of appetite, nausea, pale stool or dark urine, yellowing of the skin, pain in upper right side) or severe allergic reaction (rash, itching, hives, flushing, trouble breathing or swallowing, chest pain, dizziness, trouble breathing, swelling of tongue, mouth, or throat) to health care professional promptly.
- Inform patient that mouth sores may occur. Consult health care professional for treatment if pain, discomfort, or open sores in mouth occur. May require special mouthwash or gel.
- Instruct patient to avoid use of live vaccines and close contact with those who have received live vaccines.
- Instruct patient to notify health care professional of all Rx or OTC medications, vitamins, or herbal products being taken and to consult with health care professional before taking other medications, especially St. John's wort.
- Rep: May have teratogenic effects and decrease male and female fertility. Advise female patients to use effective contraception during and for up to 8 wk after last dose, male patients with female partners of reproductive potential to use effective contraception during and for up to 4 wk after last dose, and to notify health care professional if pregnancy is planned or suspected. Advise female patients to avoid breast feeding for 2 wk after last dose.
- Emphasize the importance of routine blood tests to determine effectiveness and side effects.

Evaluation/Desired Outcomes

- Decreased spread of tumor. Continue treatment as long as clinical benefit is observed or until unacceptable toxicity occurs.
- Prevention of kidney or liver transplant rejection.
- Reduced seizure frequency.

evolocumab

(e-vo-**lo**-kyoo-mab)

Repatha

Classification

Therapeutic: lipid-lowering agents

Pharmacologic: proprotein convertase subtilisin kexin type 9 (PCSK9) inhibitor antibodies

Indications

Lowering of low density lipoprotein cholesterol (LDL-C) as an adjunct to diet in patients with primary hyperlipidemia (including heterozygous familial hypercholesterolemia [HeFH] as monotherapy or in combination with other lipid-lowering therapies). Additional lowering of LDL-C as an adjunct to diet and other LDL-C-lowering therapies in patients with homozygous familial hypercholesterolemia (HoFH). To reduce the risk of myocardial infarction, stroke, and coronary revascularization in patients with cardiovascular disease.

Action

A human monoclonal immunoglobulin (IgG2) produced in genetically engineered Chinese hamster ovary cells that binds to PCSK9 inhibiting its binding to the low density lipoprotein receptor (LDLR) resulting in ↑ number of LDLRs available to clear LDL from blood.

Therapeutic Effects: ↓ LDL-C. Reduction in the risk of myocardial infarction, stroke, and coronary revascularization.

Pharmacokinetics

Absorption: Well absorbed (72%) following subcut administration.

Distribution: Crosses the placenta.

Metabolism and Excretion: Eliminated by binding to PCSK9 and by proteolytic degradation.

Half-life: 11–17 days.

TIME/ACTION PROFILE (effect circulating unbound PCSK9)

ROUTE	ONSET	PEAK	DURATION
subcut	rapid	4 hr	2–4 wk

Contraindications/Precautions

Contraindicated in: History of serious hypersensitivity to evolocumab.

Use Cautiously in: Severe renal/hepatic impairment; OB: Crosses the placenta, consider fetal risks; Lactation: Consider benefits of breast feeding against possible risk to infant; Pedi: Children <13 yr (safety and effectiveness not established); Geri: Elderly patients may be more sensitive to drug effects.

Adverse Reactions/Side Effects

Local: injection site reactions. **MS:** back pain. **Misc:** HYPERSENSITIVITY REACTIONS (including angioedema, rash, urticaria).

Interactions

Drug-Drug: None noted.

Route/Dosage

Established Cardiovascular Disease or Primary Hyperlipidemia (including HeFH)

Subcut (Adults): 140 mg every 2 wk or 420 mg once monthly.

HoFH

Subcut (Adults): 420 mg once monthly.

Availability

Solution for injection (needle cover contains latex derivative): 420 mg/mL (Pushtronex system), 140 mg/mL (prefilled syringes and autoinjector).

NURSING IMPLICATIONS

Assessment

- Obtain a diet history, especially with regard to fat consumption.
- Monitor for signs and symptoms of hypersensitivity reactions (rash, urticaria) during therapy. If symptoms occur, discontinue therapy.
- Assess for latex allergy. Needle cover of the glass prefilled syringe and the autoinjector contain dry natural rubber (a derivative of latex); may cause allergic reactions.
- ***Lab Test Considerations:*** Assess LDL-C levels within 4–8 wk of initiating; response to therapy depends on degree of LDL-receptor function.

Implementation

- **Subcut:** To administer the 140 mg dose using *Single-Use Prefilled SureClick® Autoinjector*, give 3 injections, using 3 separate pens/syringes in 3 separate sites, consecutively within 30 min. When switching dose regimens, administer first dose of new regimen on next scheduled date of prior regimen. If stored in refrigerator allow solution to warm to room temperature for at least 30 min before injecting. May also be stored at room temperature, but only stable for 30 days. Solution is clear to opalescent and colorless to pale yellow; do not administer solutions that are cloudy or contain particulate matter. Do not shake. Stretch or pinch skin. Inject into thigh, abdomen, or upper arm at a 90° angle. Injection may take 15 sec. Window turns from clear to yellow when the injection is done. Rotate sites with each injection. Do not inject into areas that are tender, bruised, red, or indurated. Do not reuse prefilled pen or syringe. Do not administer other injectable drugs at same site.
- To administer the 420 mg dose using *Pushtronex on-body infusor system:* Remove on-body infusor and prefilled cartridge from refrigerator 45 min prior to use to allow to reach room temperature; do not use other sources of warming. Prepare injection site with little hair (may trim) and firm and flat skin surface by cleaning with alcohol and allowing to dry. May use thigh, abdomen (except 2 inches from umbilicus) or outer area of upper arm if not self-administered. Avoid areas that are tender, bruised, red, or hard, or areas with wrinkles, skin folds, scars, stretch marks, moles and excessive hair. Solution in cartridge should be clear and colorless to slightly yellow; do not administer solutions that are discolored or contain particular matter. Clean bottom of cartridge with alcohol and load into on-body infusor; press firmly on top of unit to secure. Administer injection within 5 min after loading the cartridge; >5 min may dry out medication. Swing door close until it snaps. Peel away both green pull tabs to show ad-

hesive. When blue light flashes, infusor is on. If using abdomen, stretch skin prior to applying; do not stretch skin for thigh placement. Apply infusor to skin making sure blue light is visible and firmly press start button. Flashing green light and click indicates infusion has begun; may beep and patient may feel a pinch. Solution is injected over 9 min. When green light changes to solid, infusion is complete. Remove from skin and check medicine window for green light to be off. Dispose of on-body infusor in a sharps container.

Patient/Family Teaching

- Instruct patient in correct technique for self-injection or on-body infusor, care and disposal of equipment. Administer missed doses within 7 days, then resume original schedule. If not administered within 7 days, wait until next dose on original schedule. Advise patient to read *Patient Information* before starting therapy and with each Rx refill in case of changes.
- Advise patient that this medication should be used in conjunction with diet restrictions (fat, cholesterol, carbohydrates, alcohol), exercise, and cessation of smoking.
- Instruct patient to notify health care professional of all Rx or OTC medications, vitamins, or herbal products being taken and to consult health care professional before taking any other Rx, OTC, or herbal products.
- Advise patient to notify health care professional of medication regimen prior to treatment or surgery.
- Advise patient to notify health care professional if pregnancy is planned or suspected or if breast feeding. Encourage pregnant patients to enroll in pregnancy exposure registry that monitors pregnancy outcomes in women exposed to evolocumab during pregnancy by contacting 1-877-311-8972 or https://mothertobaby.org/ongoing-study/repatha/.

Evaluation/Desired Outcomes

- ↓ LDL-C levels.
- Reduction in the risk of myocardial infarction, stroke, and coronary revascularization.

exemestane (ex-e-mes-tane)

Aromasin

Classification

Therapeutic: antineoplastics

Pharmacologic: aromatase inhibitors

Indications

Adjuvant treatment of breast cancer in postmenopausal women who have estrogen-receptor positive early disease and who have already received 2–3 yr of tamoxifen and are then switched to exemestane to complete a total of 5 yr of adjuvant therapy. Treatment of advanced postmenopausal breast cancer that has progressed despite tamoxifen therapy.

Action

Inhibits aromatase, an enzyme responsible for the conversion of androgen to estrogen. In postmenopausal women, the primary source of estrogen is androgen. Decreases circulating estrogen. **Therapeutic Effects:** Decreased spread of estrogen-sensitive breast cancer.

Pharmacokinetics

Absorption: 42% absorbed following oral administration.

Distribution: Extensively distributed.

Metabolism and Excretion: Mostly metabolized by the liver (CYP3A4 enzyme system); metabolites are excreted in urine (40%) and feces (40%); <1% excreted unchanged in urine.

Half-life: 24 hr.

TIME/ACTION PROFILE (suppression of circulating estrogen)

ROUTE	ONSET	PEAK	DURATION
PO	unknown	2–3 days	4–5 days

Contraindications/Precautions

Contraindicated in: Hypersensitivity; Premenopausal status; OB: Pregnancy (may cause fetal harm); Lactation: Breast feeding should be avoided.

Use Cautiously in: Rep: Women of reproductive potential; Pedi: Safety and effectiveness not established.

Adverse Reactions/Side Effects

CNS: fatigue, depression, insomnia. **CV:** THROMBOEMBOLISM, hypertension. **GI:** diarrhea, nausea. **GU:** endometrial hyperplasia, uterine polyps. **Endo:** visual disturbances. **Derm:** alopecia, hot flashes, ↑ sweating, dermatitis. **MS:** arthralgia, musculoskeletal pain, carpal tunnel syndrome, muscle cramps, osteoporosis. **Neuro:** neuropathy, paresthesia.

Interactions

Drug-Drug: Strong **CYP3A4 inducers** including **rifampin** or **phenytoin** may ↓ levels and effectiveness; ↑ daily dose to 50 mg once daily. **Estrogens** can interfere with action.

Route/Dosage

PO (Adults): 25 mg once daily; *Concurrent use with strong CYP3A4 inducers*—50 mg once daily.

Availability (generic available)

Tablets: 25 mg.

NURSING IMPLICATIONS

Assessment

- Assess patient for pain and other side effects periodically during therapy.
- ***Lab Test Considerations:*** May cause ↑ GTT, AST, ALT, alkaline phosphatase, bilirubin, and creatinine levels.
- Assess 25-hydroxy vitamin D levels prior to starting therapy. Supplement vitamin D deficiency with vita-

min D due to high prevalence of vitamin D deficiency in women with early breast cancer.

Implementation

- Take 1 tablet daily after a meal.

Patient/Family Teaching

- Instruct patient to take exemestane as directed at the same time each day. Take missed doses as soon as remembered unless it is almost time for next dose. Do not double doses. Advise patient to read the *Patient Information* leaflet before starting and with each Rx refill in case of changes.
- Advise patient not to take other estrogen-containing agents; may interfere with action of exemestane.
- Inform patient that lower level of estrogen may lead to decreased bone mineral density over time and increased risk of osteoporosis and fracture. Women with osteoporosis or at risk of osteoporosis should have their bone mineral density formally assessed by bone densitometry at end of treatment. Monitor patients for bone mineral density loss and treat as appropriate.
- Advise patient to notify health care professional immediately if chest pain or signs of heart failure or stroke occur.
- Advise patient to notify health care professional of all Rx or OTC medications, vitamins, or herbal products being taken and to consult with health care professional before taking other medications.
- Rep: Exemestane is teratogenic; advise female patients to use effective contraception during therapy and for at least 1 mo after last dose and to avoid breast feeding.
- Explain need for follow-up blood tests to check liver and kidney function.

Evaluation/Desired Outcomes

- Slowing of disease progression in women with breast cancer.

exenatide (ex-en-a-tide)

Bydureon, Bydureon BCise, Byetta

Classification

Therapeutic: antidiabetics

Pharmacologic: incretin mimetic agents

Indications

Management of type 2 diabetes as an adjunct to diet and exercise (not recommended as first-line therapy).

Action

Mimics the action of incretin which promotes endogenous insulin secretion and promotes other mechanisms of glucose-lowering. **Therapeutic Effects:** Improved control of blood glucose.

Pharmacokinetics

Absorption: Well absorbed following subcutaneous administration.

Distribution: Unknown.

Metabolism and Excretion: Excreted mostly by glomerular filtration followed by degradation.

Half-life: *Immediate-release*—2.4 hr.

TIME/ACTION PROFILE (effects on postprandial blood glucose)

ROUTE	ONSET	PEAK	DURATION
Subcut (immediate-release)	within 30 min	2.1 hr	8 hr
Subcut (extended-release)	unknown	9 wk	unknown

Contraindications/Precautions

Contraindicated in: Hypersensitivity; Type 1 diabetes or diabetic ketoacidosis; Severe renal impairment or end-stage renal disease (CCr <30 mL/min) (immediate-release); CCr <45 mL/min (extended-release); Severe gastrointestinal disease; Personal or family history of medullary thyroid carcinoma (extended-release only); Multiple Endocrine Neoplasia syndrome type 2 (extended-release only).

Use Cautiously in: History of pancreatitis; Concurrent use of prandial insulin (extended-release only); Concurrent use of ACE inhibitors, NSAIDs, or diuretics (↑ risk of renal impairment); OB: Use during pregnancy only if benefit to patient outweighs potential risk to fetus; Lactation: Use during breast feeding only if benefit to patient outweighs potential risk to infant; Pedi: Safety and effectiveness not established.

Adverse Reactions/Side Effects

CV: dizziness, headache, jitteriness, weakness. **Derm:** hyperhydrosis. **Endo:** THYROID C-CELL TUMORS (extended-release), hypoglycemia. **GI:** PANCREATITIS, diarrhea, nausea, vomiting, cholecystitis, cholelithiasis, dyspepsia, gastrointestinal reflux. **GU:** acute renal failure, renal impairment. **Metab:** ↓ appetite, weight loss. **Misc:** injection site reactions.

Interactions

Drug-Drug: Concurrent use with **sulfonylureas** or **insulin** may ↑ risk of hypoglycemia (↓ dose of **sulfonylurea** or **insulin** if hypoglycemia occurs); concomitant use of **insulin** with extended-release exenatide not recommended. Concurrent use with **nateglinide** or **repaglinide** may ↑ risk of hypoglycemia. Due to slowed gastric emptying, may ↓ absorption of **orally administered medications**, especially those requiring rapid GI absorption or require a specific level for efficacy; take oral **anti-infectives** and **oral contra-**

ceptives at least 1 hr before injecting exenatide). Concurrent use of **ACE inhibitors**, **NSAIDs**, or **diuretics** may ↑ risk of renal impairment.

Route/Dosage

Immediate Release (Byetta)

Subcut (Adults): 5 mcg within 60 min before morning and evening meal; after 1 mo, dose may be ↑ to 10 mcg depending on response.

Renal Impairment

Subcut (Adults): *CCr 30–50 mL/min*—Use caution when ↑ dose from 5 mcg to 10 mcg.

Extended Release (Bydureon and Bydureon BCise)

Subcut (Adults): 2 mg every 7 days.

Availability

Solution for injection (Byetta): 300 mcg/1.2–mL pen (delivers 5 mcg/dose), 600 mcg/2.4–mL pen (delivers 10 mcg/dose). **Suspension for injection (Bydureon):** 2 mg/vial or pen. **Suspension for injection (Bydureon BCise):** 2 mg/autoinjector pen.

NURSING IMPLICATIONS

Assessment

- Observe for signs and symptoms of hypoglycemic reactions (abdominal pain, sweating, hunger, weakness, dizziness, headache, drowsiness, tremor, tachycardia, anxiety, confusion, irritability, jitteriness), especially when combined with oral sulfonylureas.
- Assess for signs and symptoms of pancreatitis (persistent severe abdominal pain, sometimes radiating to the back, may or may not be accompanied by vomiting) at beginning of therapy and with dose increases. If suspected, promptly discontinue therapy and initiate appropriate management. If pancreatitis is confirmed, do not restart exenatide. Consider other antidiabetic therapies in patients with a history of pancreatitis.
- ***Lab Test Considerations:*** Monitor serum glucose and glycolysated hemoglobin periodically during therapy to evaluate effectiveness of therapy.
- Monitor renal function prior to and periodically during therapy. Renal dysfunction may be reversed with discontinuation of therapy.

Implementation

- Some medications may need to be taken 1 hr before exenatide.
- Patients stabilized on a diabetic regimen who are exposed to stress, fever, trauma, infection, or surgery may require administration of insulin.
- **Subcut:** *Immediate release:* Follow directions for *New Pen Setup* in *Information for Patient* prior to use of each new pen. Inject exenatide in thigh, abdomen, or upper arm at any time within the 60–min period **before** the morning and evening meals. Do not administer after a meal. Do not mix with insulin. Solution should be clear and colorless; do not administer solutions that are discolored or contain particulate matter. Refrigerate; discard pen 30 days after 1st use, even if some drug remains in pen. Do not freeze. Do not store pen with needle attached; medication may leak from pen or air bubbles may form in the cartridge.
- **Subcut:** *Extended release:* Remove from refrigerator 15 min prior to mixing. Dilute with diluent and needles included in tray. Suspension should be white or off-white and cloudy. Mix by shaking vigorously for 15 sec. Do not inject solutions that are discolored or contain particulate matter. Administer without regard to meals. Inject into upper arm, abdomen, or thigh; change site each wk. Refrigerate; each tray can be kept at room temperature if not >77°F for up to 4 wk. Store *Bydureon BCise* flat. Do not use beyond expiration date.
- Do not mix insulin in the same syringe with exenatide. Injection of *Bydureon Bcise* and insulin may be administered in the same body area, but not right next to each other.
- If switching from immediate-release to extended-release, discontinue other forms of exenatide before starting *Bydureon BCise*. When switching from another extended-release product, may change with next scheduled dose. May cause transient ↑ in blood glucose for 2–4 wk.

Patient/Family Teaching

- Instruct patient to take exenatide *immediate release* as directed within 60 min before a meal. Do not take after a meal. If a dose is missed, skip the dose and take the next dose at the prescribed time. Do not take an extra dose or increase the amount of the next dose to make up for missed dose. If a dose of exenatide *extended release* is missed, administer as soon as remembered as long as the next dose is due at least 3 days later; if 1 or 2 days later skip dose and administer next dose as scheduled. The day of weekly administration can be changed as long as the last dose was administered 3 or more days before. Advise patient to read *Medication Guide* before starting therapy and with each Rx refill.
- Instruct patient in proper technique for administration, timing of dose, and concurrent oral medications, storage of medication, and disposal of used needles. Patients should read the *Information for Patient* insert prior to initiation of therapy and with each Rx refill. Advise patient that *New Pen Setup* should be done only with each new pen, not with each dose.
- Inform patient that pen needles are not included with pen and must be purchased separately. Advise patient which needle length and gauge

should be used. Caution patient not to share pen and needles.

- Caution patient to never share pen with others, even if needle is changed. May cause transmission of bloodborne pathogens.
- Explain to patient that exenatide helps control hyperglycemia but does not cure diabetes. Therapy is usually long term.
- Encourage patient to follow prescribed diet, medication, and exercise regimen to prevent hyperglycemic or hypoglycemic episodes.
- Review signs of hypoglycemia and hyperglycemia with patient. If hypoglycemia occurs, advise patient to take a glass of orange juice or 2–3 tsp of sugar, honey, or corn syrup dissolved in water, and notify health care professional. Risk of hypoglycemia is increased if sulfonylureas are taken concurrently with exenatide.
- Advise patient to notify health care professional immediately if symptoms of pancreatitis (unexplained, persistent, severe abdominal pain which may or may not be accompanied by vomiting) occur.
- Inform patient that therapy may result in reduction of appetite, food intake, and/or body weight. Dose modification is not necessary. Nausea is more common at initiation of therapy and usually decreases over time.
- Instruct patient to notify health care professional of all Rx or OTC medications, vitamins, or herbal products being taken and to consult health care professional before taking any other Rx, OTC, or herbal products. Exenatide delays stomach emptying. Some medications (such as anti-infectives and oral contraceptives) may need to be taken 1 hr before exenatide injection.
- Instruct patient in proper testing of blood glucose and urine ketones. These tests should be monitored closely during periods of stress or illness and health care professional notified if significant changes occur.
- Advise patient to inform health care professional of medication regimen before treatment or surgery.
- Advise patient to carry a form of sugar (sugar packets, candy) and identification describing disease process and medication regimen at all times.
- Advise patient to notify health care professional if pregnancy is suspected or planned, or if breast feeding.
- Emphasize the importance of routine follow-up exams and regular testing of blood glucose and glycosylated hemoglobin.

Evaluation/Desired Outcomes

- Control of blood glucose levels without the appearance of hypoglycemic or hyperglycemic episodes.

ezetimibe (e-zet-i-mibe)

✱Ezetrol, Zetia

Classification
Therapeutic: lipid-lowering agents
Pharmacologic: cholesterol absorption inhibitors

Indications

Alone or with other agents (HMG-CoA reductase inhibitors) in the management of dyslipidemias including primary hypercholesterolemia, homozygous familial hypercholesterolemia, and homozygous sitosterolemia.

Action

Inhibits absorption of cholesterol in the small intestine. **Therapeutic Effects:** Lowering of cholesterol, a known risk factor for atherosclerosis.

Pharmacokinetics

Absorption: Following absorption, rapidly converted to ezetimibe-glucaronide, which is active. Bioavailability is variable.

Distribution: Unknown.

Metabolism and Excretion: Undergoes enterhepatic recycling, mostly eliminated in feces, minimal renal excretion.

Half-life: 22 hr.

TIME/ACTION PROFILE

ROUTE	ONSET	PEAK	DURATION
PO	unknown	unknown	unknown

Contraindications/Precautions

Contraindicated in: Hypersensitivity; Acute liver disease or unexplained laboratory evidence of liver disease (when used with HMG-CoA reductase inhibitor); Moderate or severe hepatic impairment; Concurrent use of fibrates; OB: Pregnancy (may cause fetal harm) from cholesterol; Lactation: Lactation.

Use Cautiously in: Pedi: Children <10 yr (safety and effectiveness not established).

Adverse Reactions/Side Effects

Derm: rash. **GI:** cholecystitis, cholelithiasis, ↑ liver enzymes (with HMG-CoA reductase inhibitors), nausea, pancreatitis. **Misc:** ANGIOEDEMA.

Interactions

Drug-Drug: Effects may be ↓ by **cholestyramine** or other **bile acid sequestrants**. Concurrent use of **fibrates** may ↑ levels and the risk of cholelithiasis. **Cyclosporine** may ↑ levels. May ↑ risk of rhabdomyolysis when used with **HMG CoA-reductase inhibitors**.

Route/Dosage

PO (Adults): 10 mg once daily.

Renal Impairment

PO (Adults): *CCr <60 mL/min and concurrent use with simvastatin*—Not to exceed simvastatin dose of 20 mg/day.

Availability (generic available)

Tablets: 10 mg. **Cost:** $517.89/90. ***In combination with:*** simvastatin (Vytorin); see Appendix B.

NURSING IMPLICATIONS

Assessment

- Obtain a diet history, especially with regard to fat consumption.
- ***Lab Test Considerations:*** Evaluate serum cholesterol and triglyceride levels before initiating, after 2–4 wk of therapy, and periodically thereafter.
- May cause ↑ liver transaminases when administered with HMG-CoA reductase inhibitors. Monitor liver enzymes prior to initiation and during therapy according to recommendations of HMG-CoA reductase inhibitor. Elevations are usually asymptomatic and return to baseline with continued therapy.

Implementation

- Do not confuse Zetia with Zestril (lisinopril).
- **PO:** Administer without regard to meals. May be taken at the same time as HMG-CoA reductase inhibitors.

Patient/Family Teaching

- Instruct patient to take ezetimibe as directed, at the same time each day, even if feeling well. Take missed doses as soon as remembered, but do not take more than 1 dose/day. Medication helps control but does not cure elevated serum cholesterol levels.
- Advise patient that this medication should be used in conjunction with diet restrictions (fat, cholesterol, carbohydrates, alcohol), exercise, and cessation of smoking. Ezetimibe does not assist with weight loss.
- Instruct patient to notify health care professional if unexplained muscle pain, tenderness, or weakness occur. Risk may increase when used with HMG-CoA reductase inhibitors.
- Instruct patient to notify health care professional of all Rx or OTC medications, vitamins, or herbal products being taken and to consult health care professional before taking any other Rx, OTC, or herbal products.
- Advise patient to notify health care professional of medication regimen prior to treatment or surgery.
- Instruct female patients to notify health care professional promptly if pregnancy is planned or suspected or if breast feeding. If regimen includes HMG-CoA reductase inhibitors, they are contraindicated in pregnancy.
- Emphasize the importance of follow-up exams to determine effectiveness and to monitor for side effects.

Evaluation/Desired Outcomes

- Decrease in serum LDL and total cholesterol levels.

famciclovir (fam-sye-kloe-veer)

~~Famvir~~

Classification
Therapeutic: antivirals

Indications

Acute herpes zoster infections (shingles). Treatment/suppression of recurrent herpes genitalis in immunocompetent patients. Treatment of recurrent herpes labialis (cold sores) in immunocompetent patients. Treatment of recurrent mucocutaneous herpes simplex virus (HSV) infection in HIV-infected patients.

Action

Inhibits viral DNA synthesis in herpes-infected cells only. **Therapeutic Effects:** Decreased duration of herpes zoster infection with decreased duration of viral shedding. Decreased time to healing for cold sores. Decreased lesion formation and improved healing in recurrent HSV infection.

Pharmacokinetics

Absorption: Following absorption, famciclovir is rapidly converted in the intestinal wall to penciclovir, the active compound.
Distribution: Unknown.
Metabolism and Excretion: Penciclovir is mostly excreted by the kidneys.
Half-life: *Penciclovir*—2.1–3 hr (↑ in renal impairment).

TIME/ACTION PROFILE (penciclovir blood levels)

ROUTE	ONSET	PEAK	DURATION
PO	rapid	0.9 hr	8–12 hr

Contraindications/Precautions

Contraindicated in: Hypersensitivity.
Use Cautiously in: Patients with impaired renal function (↑ dose interval/↓ dose recommended if CCr <40–60 mL/min); OB: Use during pregnancy only if benefit to patient outweighs potential risk to fetus; Lactation: Use during breast feeding only if benefit to patient outweighs potential risk to infant; Pedi: Safety and effectiveness not established; Geri: Consider age-related ↓ in renal function when prescribing.

Adverse Reactions/Side Effects

CNS: SEIZURES, headache, dizziness, fatigue. **CV:** palpitations. **Derm:** hypersensitivity vasculitis. **GI:** diarrhea, nausea, vomiting. **GU:** ↓ fertility (males). **Misc:** ANAPHYLAXIS.

Interactions

Drug-Drug: Probenecid ↑ plasma concentrations of penciclovir.

Route/Dosage

Herpes Zoster

PO (Adults): 500 mg every 8 hr for 7 days.

Renal Impairment

PO (Adults): *CCr 40–59 mL/min*—500 mg every 12 hr; *CCr 20–39 mL/min*—500 mg every 24 hr; *CCr <20 mL/min*—250 mg every 24 hr; *Hemodialysis*—250 mg after each dialysis.

Recurrent Genital Herpes Simplex Infections

PO (Adults): 1000 mg twice daily for one day.

Renal Impairment

PO (Adults): *CCr 40–59 mL/min*—500 mg twice daily for 1 day; *CCr 20–39 mL/min*—500 mg as a single dose; *CCr <20 mL/min*—250 mg as a single dose; *Hemodialysis*—250 mg as a single dose after dialysis.

Suppression of Recurrent Herpes Simplex Infections

PO (Adults): 250 mg every 12 hr for up to 1 yr.

Renal Impairment

PO (Adults): *CCr 20–39 mL/min*—125 mg every 12 hr for 5 days; *CCr <20 mL/min*—125 mg every 24 hr for 5 days; *Hemodialysis*—125 mg after each dialysis.

Recurrent Herpes Labialis Infections (cold sores)

PO (Adults): 1500 mg as a single dose.

Renal Impairment

PO (Adults): *CCr 40–59 mL/min*—750 mg as a single dose; *CCr 20–39 mL/min*—500 mg as a single dose; *CCr <20 mL/min*—250 mg as a single dose; *Hemodialysis*—250 mg as a single dose after dialysis.

Herpes Simplex in HIV-Infected Patients

PO (Adults): 500 mg every 12 hr for 7 days.

Renal Impairment

PO (Adults): *CCr 20–39 mL/min*—500 mg every 24 hr for 7 days; *CCr <20 mL/min*—250 mg every 24 hr for 7 days; *Hemodialysis*—250 mg after each dialysis.

Availability (generic available)

Tablets: 125 mg, 250 mg, 500 mg.

NURSING IMPLICATIONS

Assessment

- Assess lesions prior to and daily during therapy.
- Assess patient for postherpetic neuralgia periodically during and following therapy.

Implementation

- Famciclovir therapy should be started as soon as herpes zoster is diagnosed, at least within 72 hr, preferably within 48 hr.
- **PO:** Famciclovir may be administered without regard to meals.

Patient/Family Teaching

- Instruct patient to take famciclovir as directed for the full course of therapy. Take missed doses as soon as remembered, if not just before next dose.
- Inform patient that famciclovir does not prevent the spread of infection to others. Until all lesions have crusted, precautions should be taken around others who have not had chickenpox or varicella vaccine or people who are immunosuppressed.
- Advise patient to use condoms during sexual contact and to avoid sexual contact while lesions are present.
- May cause dizziness. Caution patient to avoid driving and other activities requiring alertness until response to medication is known.
- Advise patient to notify health care professional immediately if seizures or signs and symptoms of anaphylaxis (rash, facial swelling, difficulty breathing) occur.
- Instruct women with genital herpes to have yearly Papanicolaou (Pap) smears because of increased risk of cervical cancer.
- Rep: Advise women of childbearing potential to notify health care professional if pregnancy is planned or suspected or if breast feeding. Encourage women who become pregnant while taking famciclovir to enroll in the pregnancy reporting system to monitor maternal-fetal outcomes. Report pregnancies and pregnancy outcomes to the Novartis Adverse Event reporting line at 1-888-NOW-NOVA (669-6682). May cause decreased fertility in male patients.

Evaluation/Desired Outcomes

- Decrease in time to full crusting, loss of vesicles, loss of ulcers, and loss of crusts in patients with acute herpes zoster (shingles).
- Crusting over and healing of lesions in herpes labialis, genital herpes, and in recurrent mucocutaneous HSV infection in HIV-infected patients.
- Prevention of recurrence of herpes genitalis.
- Decreased time to healing for cold sores.

famotidine, **See HISTAMINE H_2 ANTAGONISTS.**

febuxostat (fe-bux-o-stat)

Uloric

Classification

Therapeutic: antigout agents

Pharmacologic: xanthine oxidase inhibitors

Indications

Chronic management of hyperuricemia in patients with gout who have an inadequate response to a maximally titrated dose of allopurinol, who are intolerant to allopurinol, or in whom allopurinol is not an appropriate treatment option.

Action

Decreases production of uric acid by inhibiting xanthine oxidase. **Therapeutic Effects:** Lowering of serum uric acid levels with resultant decrease in gouty attacks.

Pharmacokinetics

Absorption: Well absorbed (49%) following oral administration.

Distribution: Unknown.

Protein Binding: 99.2%.

Metabolism and Excretion: Extensively metabolized by the liver; minimal renal excretion of unchanged drug, 45% eliminated in feces as unchanged drug, remainder is eliminated in urine and feces as inactive metabolites.

Half-life: 5–8 hr.

TIME/ACTION PROFILE (blood levels)

ROUTE	ONSET	PEAK	DURATION
PO	rapid	1–1.5 hr*	24 hr

*Maximum lowering of uric acid may take 2 wk.

Contraindications/Precautions

Contraindicated in: Concurrent azathioprine or mercaptopurine.

Use Cautiously in: Cardiovascular disease (↑ risk of cardiovascular death compared to allopurinol) (consider using low-dose aspirin when using febuxostat in these patients); Severe renal impairment (CCr <30 mL/min); Severe hepatic impairment; Previous skin reaction with allopurinol; OB: Use only when potential maternal benefit outweighs potential fetal risk; Lactation: Unknown if excreted into breast milk; use caution when breast feeding; Pedi: Safety and effectiveness not established.

Adverse Reactions/Side Effects

Derm: DRUG REACTION WITH EOSINOPHILIA AND SYSTEMIC SYMPTOMS (DRESS), STEVENS-JOHNSON SYNDROME, TOXIC EPIDERMAL NECROLYSIS, rash. **GI:** ↑ liver enzymes, nausea. **MS:** gout flare, arthralgia.

Interactions

Drug-Drug: Significantly ↑ levels of and risk of serious toxicity from **azathioprine** and **mercaptopurine**; concurrent use is contraindicated. May ↑ levels of **theophylline**; use cautiously together.

Route/Dosage

PO (Adults): 40 mg once daily initially; if serum uric acid does not ↓ to <6 mg/dL, ↑ to 80 mg once daily.

Renal Impairment

PO (Adults): *CCr <30 mL/min*—Maximum dose = 40 mg/day.

Availability (generic available)

Tablets: 40 mg, 80 mg.

NURSING IMPLICATIONS

Assessment

- Assess for joint pain and swelling, especially during early therapy. Changing serum uric acid levels from mobilization of urate from tissue deposits may cause gout flares. Use prophylactic NSAID or colchicine therapy for up to 6 mo. If a gout flare occurs, continue febuxostat therapy and treat flare concurrently.
- Monitor for signs and symptoms of MI and stroke.
- Assess patient for skin reactions throughout therapy. Reactions may be severe and life threatening. Discontinue therapy if severe reactions or moderate rashes with systemic symptoms occur.
- ***Lab Test Considerations:*** Monitor serum uric acid levels prior to, 2 wk after intitiating, and periodically thereafter. *If serum uric acid levels are ≥6 mg/dL after 2 wk of daily 40 mg therapy,* increase dose to 80 mg daily.
- Monitor liver function at 2 and 4 mo of therapy and periodically thereafter. May cause ↑ AST, ALT, CPK, LDH, alkaline phosphatase, and creatine.
- May cause prolonged aPTT and PT, and ↓ hematocrit, hemoglobin, RBC, platelet count, and lymphocyte, neutrophil counts. May cause ↑ or ↓ WBC.
- May cause ↓ serum bicarbonate and ↑ serum sodium, glucose, potassium, and TSH levels.
- May cause ↑ serum cholesterol, triglycerides, amylase, and LDL levels.
- May cause ↑ BUN and serum creatinine and proteinuria.

Implementation

- **PO:** May be taken with or without food and with antacids.

Patient/Family Teaching

- Instruct patient to take febuxostat as directed. If a gout flare occurs, continue febuxostat and consult health care professional; medications to manage gout flare may be added.
- Advise patient to notify health care professional if rash, chest pain, shortness of breath, dizziness, rapid or irregular heartbeat, or stroke symptoms (weakness, blurred vision, headache, confusion, slurred speech) occur or if side effects are persistent or bothersome.
- Instruct patient to notify health care professional of all Rx or OTC medications, vitamins, or herbal products being taken and to consult health care professional before taking any other Rx, OTC, or herbal products.
- Advise female patient to notify health care professional if pregnancy is planned or suspected or if breast feeding.
- Emphasize the importance of follow-up lab tests to monitor therapy.

Evaluation/Desired Outcomes

- Reduction in serum uric acid levels and resultant gout attacks.

F

felodipine (fe-loe-di-peen)

Plendil

Classification

Therapeutic: antianginals, antihypertensives

Pharmacologic: calcium channel blockers

Indications

Management of hypertension, angina pectoris, and vasospastic (Prinzmetal's) angina.

Action

Inhibits the transport of calcium into myocardial and vascular smooth muscle cells, resulting in inhibition of excitation-contraction coupling and subsequent contraction. **Therapeutic Effects:** Systemic vasodilation resulting in decreased BP. Coronary vasodilation resulting in decreased frequency and severity of attacks of angina.

Pharmacokinetics

Absorption: Well absorbed after oral administration, but extensively metabolized, resulting in ↓ bioavailability.

Distribution: Unknown.

Protein Binding: >99%.

Metabolism and Excretion: Mostly metabolized; minimal amounts excreted unchanged by kidneys.

Half-life: 11–16 hr.

TIME/ACTION PROFILE (antihypertensive effect)

ROUTE	ONSET	PEAK	DURATION
PO	1 hr	2–4 hr	up to 24 hr

Contraindications/Precautions

Contraindicated in: Hypersensitivity (cross-sensitivity may occur); Sick sinus syndrome; 2nd- or 3rd-degree AV block (unless an artificial pacemaker is in place); Systolic BP <90 mm Hg.

Use Cautiously in: Severe hepatic impairment (dose ↓ recommended); Geri: Dose ↓ recommended; ↑ risk of hypotension; Severe renal impairment; History of serious ventricular arrhythmias or HF; OB, Lactation, Pedi: Safety not established.

Adverse Reactions/Side Effects

CNS: headache, abnormal dreams, anxiety, confusion, dizziness, drowsiness, nervousness, psychiatric disturbances, weakness. **EENT:** blurred vision, disturbed equilibrium, epistaxis, tinnitus. **Resp:** cough, dyspnea. **CV:** ARRHYTHMIAS, HF, peripheral edema, chest pain, hypotension, palpitations, syncope, tachycardia. **GI:** anorexia, constipation, diarrhea, dry mouth, dysgeusia, dyspepsia, ↑ liver enzymes, nausea, vomiting. **GU:** dysuria, nocturia, polyuria, sexual dysfunction, urinary frequency. **Derm:** dermatitis, erythema multiforme, flushing, ↑ sweating, photosensitivity, pruritus/urticaria, rash. **Endo:** gynecomastia, hyperglycemia. **Hemat:** anemia, leukopenia, thrombocytopenia. **Metab:** weight gain. **MS:** joint stiffness, muscle cramps. **Neuro:** paresthesia, tremor. **Misc:** STEVENS-JOHNSON SYNDROME, gingival hyperplasia.

Interactions

Drug-Drug: Additive hypotension may occur when used concurrently with **fentanyl**, other **antihypertensives**, **nitrates**, acute ingestion of **alcohol**, or **quinidine**. Antihypertensive effects may be ↓ by concurrent use of **NSAIDs**. **Ketoconazole**, **itraconazole**, **propranolol**, and **erythromycin** ↓ metabolism and ↑ blood levels and the risk of toxicity (dose ↓ may be necessary).

Drug-Food: **Grapefruit juice** ↑ serum levels and effect.

Route/Dosage

PO (Adults): 5 mg/day (2.5 mg/day in geriatric patients); may ↑ every 2 wk (range 5–10 mg/day; not to exceed 10 mg/day).

Availability (generic available)

Extended-release tablets: 2.5 mg, 5 mg, 10 mg.

NURSING IMPLICATIONS

Assessment

- Monitor BP and pulse before therapy, during dosage titration, and periodically during therapy. Monitor ECG periodically during prolonged therapy.
- Monitor intake and output ratios and daily weight. Assess for signs of HF (peripheral edema, rales/crackles, dyspnea, weight gain, jugular venous distention).
- Assess for rash periodically during therapy. May cause Stevens-Johnson syndrome. Discontinue therapy if severe or if accompanied with fever, general malaise, fatigue, muscle or joint aches, blisters, oral lesions, conjunctivitis, hepatitis, and/or eosinophilia.
- **Angina:** Assess location, duration, intensity, and precipitating factors of patient's anginal pain.
- **Hypertension:** Check frequency of refills to monitor adherence.
- ***Lab Test Considerations:*** Total serum calcium concentrations are not affected by calcium channel blockers.
- Monitor serum potassium periodically. Hypokalemia ↑ risk of arrhythmias and should be corrected.
- Monitor renal and hepatic functions periodically during long-term therapy. May cause ↑ in hepatic enzymes after several days of therapy, which return to normal upon discontinuation of therapy.

Implementation

- **PO:** May be administered without regard to meals. May be administered with meals if GI irritation becomes a problem.
- Swallow tablets whole; do not break, crush, or chew. Empty tablets that appear in stool are not significant.

Patient/Family Teaching

- Advise patient to take medication as directed, even if feeling well. If a dose is missed, take as soon as possible unless almost time for next dose; do not double doses. May need to be discontinued gradually.
- Instruct patient on correct technique for monitoring pulse. Instruct patient to contact health care professional if heart rate is <50 bpm.
- Advise patient to avoid grapefruit or grapefruit juice during therapy.
- Caution patient to change positions slowly to minimize orthostatic hypotension.
- May cause drowsiness or dizziness. Advise patient to avoid driving or other activities requiring alertness until response to the medication is known.
- Instruct patient on importance of maintaining good dental hygiene and seeing dentist frequently for teeth cleaning to prevent tenderness, bleeding, and gingival hyperplasia (gum enlargement).
- Instruct patient to notify health care professional of all Rx or OTC medications, vitamins, or herbal products being taken and to avoid concurrent use of alcohol or OTC medications and herbal products, especially cold preparations, without consulting health care professional.
- Advise patient to notify health care professional if rash, irregular heartbeat, dyspnea, swelling of hands and feet, pronounced dizziness, nausea, constipation, or hypotension occurs or if headache is severe or persistent.
- Caution patient to wear protective clothing and to use sunscreen to prevent photosensitivity reactions.
- Advise patient to inform health care professional of medication regimen before treatment or surgery.
- Advise patient to notify health care professional if pregnancy is planned or suspected or if breast feeding.
- **Angina:** Instruct patient on concurrent nitrate or beta-blocker therapy to continue taking both medications as directed and to use SL nitroglycerin as needed for anginal attacks.
- Advise patient to contact health care professional if chest pain does not improve or worsens after therapy; occurs with diaphoresis or shortness of breath; or if severe, persistent headache occurs.

- Caution patient to discuss exercise restrictions with health care professional before exertion.
- **Hypertension:** Encourage patient to comply with other interventions for hypertension (weight reduction, low-sodium diet, smoking cessation, moderation of alcohol consumption, regular exercise, and stress management). Medication controls but does not cure hypertension.
- Instruct patient and family in proper technique for monitoring BP. Advise patient to take BP weekly and to report significant changes.

Evaluation/Desired Outcomes

- Decrease in BP.
- Decrease in frequency and severity of anginal attacks.
- Decrease in need for nitrate therapy.
- Increase in activity tolerance and sense of well-being.

fenofibrate (fen-o-fi-brate)

Antara, Fenoglide, ✤Fenomax, ✤Lipidil EZ, ✤Lipidil Supra, Lipofen, Tricor, Triglide

Classification

Therapeutic: lipid-lowering agents

Pharmacologic: fibric acid derivatives

Indications

With dietary therapy to decrease LDL cholesterol, total cholesterol, triglycerides, and apolipoprotein B in adult patients with hypercholesterolemia or mixed dyslipidemia. With dietary management in the treatment of severe hypertriglyceridemia (types IV and V hyperlipidemia) in patients who are at risk for pancreatitis and do not respond to nondrug therapy.

Action

Fenofibric acid primarily inhibits triglyceride synthesis. **Therapeutic Effects:** Lowering of cholesterol and triglycerides with subsequent decreased risk of pancreatitis.

Pharmacokinetics

Absorption: Well absorbed (60%) after oral administration; absorption ↑ by food.

Distribution: Unknown.

Protein Binding: 99%.

Metabolism and Excretion: Rapidly converted to fenofibric acid, which is the active metabolite; fenofibric acid is metabolized by the liver. Fenofibric acid and its metabolites are primarily excreted in urine (60%).

Half-life: 20 hr.

TIME/ACTION PROFILE (lowering of triglycerides)

ROUTE	ONSET	PEAK	DURATION
PO	unknown	2 wk	unknown

Contraindications/Precautions

Contraindicated in: Hypersensitivity; Hepatic impairment (including primary biliary cirrhosis); Pre-existing gallbladder disease; Severe renal impairment; Concurrent use of HMG-CoA reductase inhibitors; Lactation: Lactation.

Use Cautiously in: Concurrent warfarin or HMG-CoA reductase inhibitor therapy; OB: Use only if potential benefits outweigh risks to the fetus; Pedi: Safety not established; Geri: Age-related ↓ in renal function may make older patients more susceptible to adverse reactions.

Adverse Reactions/Side Effects

CNS: fatigue/weakness, headache. **CV:** PULMONARY EMBOLISM, arrhythmias, deep vein thrombosis. **Derm:** DRUG REACTION WITH EOSINOPHILIA AND SYSTEMIC SYMPTOMS (DRESS), STEVENS-JOHNSON SYNDROME, TOXIC EPIDERMAL NECROLYSIS, rash, urticaria. **GI:** cholelithiasis, pancreatitis. **Metab:** ↓ HDL levels. **MS:** rhabdomyolysis. **Resp:** INTERSTITIAL LUNG DISEASE. **Misc:** HYPERSENSITIVITY REACTIONS (including anaphylaxis and angioedema).

Interactions

Drug-Drug: ↑ anticoagulant effects of **warfarin**. **HMG-CoA reductase inhibitors** ↑ risk of rhabdomyolysis (concurrent use should be avoided). Absorption is ↓ by **bile acid sequestrants** (fenofibrate should be given 1 hr before or 4–6 hr after). ↑ risk of nephrotoxicity with **cyclosporine**. Concurrent use with **colchicine** may ↑ risk of rhabdomyolysis.

Route/Dosage

Primary Hypercholesterolemia/Mixed Dyslipidemia

PO (Adults): *Antara*—90 mg once daily; *Fenoglide*—120 mg once daily; *Tricor*—145 mg once daily; *Triglide*—160 mg once daily; *Lipofen*—150 mg once daily.

Renal Impairment

PO (Adults): *CCr 30–89 mL/min—Antara*—30 mg once daily initially; may titrate, if needed, up to 90 mg once daily. *Fenoglide*—40 mg once daily initially; may titrate, if needed, up to 120 mg once daily. *Lipofen*—50 mg once daily initially; may titrate, if needed, up to 150 mg once daily. *Tricor*—48 mg once daily initially; may titrate, if needed, up to 145 mg once daily.

Hypertriglyceridemia

PO (Adults): *Antara*—30–90 mg once daily; *Fenoglide*—40–120 mg once daily; *Tricor*—48–145 mg once daily; *Triglide*—160 mg once daily; *Lipofen*—50–150 mg once daily.

Renal Impairment

PO (Adults): *CCr 30–89 mL/min—Antara*—30 mg once daily initially; may titrate, if needed, up to 90 mg once daily. *Fenoglide*—40 mg once daily initially; may titrate, if needed, up to 120 mg once daily. *Lipofen*—50 mg once daily initially; may titrate, if needed, up to 150 mg once daily. *Tricor*—48 mg once daily initially; may titrate, if needed, up to 145 mg once daily.

Availability (generic available)

Capsules (Lipofen): 50 mg, 150 mg. **Cost:** 50 mg $213.58/90, 150 mg $468.24/90. **Micronized capsules (Antara):** 30 mg, 90 mg. **Tablets (Fenoglide):** 40 mg, 120 mg. **Cost:** 40 mg $289.44/90, 120 mg $869.40/90. **Tablets (Tricor):** 48 mg, 145 mg. **Cost:** *Generic*—48 mg $171.86/90, 145 mg $515.58/90. **Tablets (Triglide):** 160 mg. **Cost:** *Generic*—160 mg $176.40/100.

NURSING IMPLICATIONS

Assessment

- Obtain a diet history, especially with regard to fat consumption. Attempt to obtain normal serum triglyceride levels with diet, exercise, and weight loss in obese patients before fenofibrate therapy is instituted.
- Assess patient for cholelithiasis. If symptoms occur, gallbladder studies are indicated. Discontinue therapy if gallstones are found.
- Assess patient for skin reactions throughout therapy. Reactions may be severe and life threatening. Discontinue therapy if severe reactions or moderate rashes with systemic symptoms occur.
- ***Lab Test Considerations:*** Monitor serum lipids before therapy to determine consistent elevations, then monitor periodically during therapy.
- Monitor serum AST and ALT periodically during therapy. May cause ↑ levels. Therapy should be discontinued if levels rise >3 times the normal limit.
- If patient develops muscle tenderness during therapy, monitor CPK levels. If CPK levels are markedly ↑ or myopathy occurs, discontinue therapy.
- May cause mild to moderate ↓ in hemoglobin, hematocrit, and WBCs. Monitor periodically during first 12 mo of therapy. Levels usually stabilize during long-term therapy.
- Monitor prothrombin levels frequently until levels stabilize in patients taking anticoagulants concurrently.

Implementation

- Do not confuse Tricor (fenofibrate) with Tracleer (bosentan).
- Place patients on a triglyceride-lowering diet before therapy and encourage them to remain on this diet throughout therapy.
- Dose may be increased after repeated serum triglyceride levels every 4–8 wk.
- Brands are not interchangeable.
- **PO:** Administer *Antara, Fenoglide, Lipofen, Lipidil Supra, Lofibra,* and *Tricor* products with meals. *Triglide* formulation may be taken without regard to meals.

Patient/Family Teaching

- Instruct patient to take medication as directed, not to skip doses or double up on missed doses. Medication helps control but does not cure elevated serum triglyceride levels.
- Advise patient that this medication should be used in conjunction with diet restrictions (fat, cholesterol, carbohydrates, alcohol), exercise, and cessation of smoking.
- Instruct patient to notify health care professional if unexplained muscle pain, tenderness, or weakness occurs, especially if accompanied by fever or malaise.
- Advise patient to notify health care professional of medication regimen before treatment or surgery.
- Instruct female patients to notify health care professional promptly if pregnancy is planned or suspected and to avoid breast feeding during and for at least 5 days after last dose of therapy.
- Emphasize the importance of follow-up exams to determine effectiveness and to monitor for side effects.

Evaluation/Desired Outcomes

- Decrease in serum triglycerides and cholesterol to normal levels. Therapy should be discontinued in patients who do not have an adequate response in 2 mo of therapy.

fenofibric acid

(feen-oh-**fye**-brik **as**-id)

Fibricor, TriLipix

Classification

Therapeutic: lipid-lowering agents

Pharmacologic: fibric acid derivatives

Indications

With a statin to reduce triglycerides (TG) and increase high density lipoprotein-C (HDL-C) in patients with mixed dyslipidemias and CHD or a CHD risk equivalent who are on statin therapy to achieve their low-density lipoprotein-C (LDL-C) goal (TriLipix only). As monotherapy to reduce TG in patients with severe hypertriglyceridemia. As monotherapy to reduce elevated LDL-C, total cholesterol (Total-C), TG, and apolipoprotein B (Apo B), and increase HDL-C in patients with primary hyperlipidemia or mixed dyslipidemia. Part of a comprehensive program to decrease cardiovascular risk factors.

Action

Activates the peroxisome proliferator activated receptor α (PPARα), resulting in increased lipolysis and elimination of triglycerides from plasma. Activation of PPARα also increases production of HDL. **Therapeutic Effects:** Improvement in lipid profile with lowered triglycerides and LDL cholesterol, and increased HDL cholesterol.

Pharmacokinetics

Absorption: Well absorbed following oral administration.

Distribution: Unknown.

Protein Binding: 99%.

Metabolism and Excretion: Fenofibric acid is the active metabolite of fenofibrate. Fenofibric acid is mostly metabolized by glucuronidation and the metabolites are mostly excreted by the kidneys.

Half-life: 20 hr.

TIME/ACTION PROFILE (effects on blood lipids)

ROUTE	ONSET	PEAK	DURATION
PO	unknown	4–5 hr†	unknown

†Blood levels.

Contraindications/Precautions

Contraindicated in: Hypersensitivity to fenofibric acid, choline fenofibrate or fenofibrate; Severe renal impairment (CCr <30 mL/min); Active liver or gallbladder disease; Lactation: Lactation.

Use Cautiously in: Mild/moderate renal impairment (dose ↓ required for CCr 30–80 mL/min); Concurrent use with statins in elderly patients, patients with diabetes, renal failure, or hypothyroidism (↑ risk of myopathy/rhabdomyolysis); OB: Use only if potential maternal benefit justifies potential fetal risk; Pedi: Safety and effectiveness not established; Geri: Consider age-related ↓ in renal function, concurrent illnesses and drug therapy.

Adverse Reactions/Side Effects

CNS: headache. **Derm:** DRUG REACTION WITH EOSINOPHILIA AND SYSTEMIC SYMPTOMS (DRESS), STEVENS-JOHNSON SYNDROME, TOXIC EPIDERMAL NECROLYSIS. **GI:** diarrhea, nausea, cholelithiasis, ↑ liver enzymes, pancreatitis. **GU:** ↑ serum creatinine. **Metab:** ↓ HDL levels. **MS:** MYOPATHY/RHABDOMYOLYSIS, myalgia, back pain. **Resp:** INTERSTITIAL LUNG DISEASE. **Misc:** HYPERSENSITIVITY REACTIONS (including anaphylaxis and angioedema).

Interactions

Drug-Drug: ↑ effects and risk of bleeding with **warfarin**; monitor prothrombin time/INR. **Bile acid sequestrants** may ↓ absorption and effectiveness; administer at least 1 hr before or 4–6 hr after a bile acid sequestrant. Concurrent use with **nephrotoxic drugs** including **cyclosporine** may impair renal function and excretion, ↑ risk of adverse reactions. Concurrent use with **colchicine** may ↑ risk of rhabdomyolysis.

Route/Dosage

Hypertriglyceridemia

PO (Adults): *Fibricor*—35–105 mg once daily; *TriLipix*—45–135 mg once daily.

Renal Impairment

PO (Adults): *CCr 30–89 mL/min—Fibricor*—35 mg once daily initially; may titrate, if needed, up to 105 mg once daily. *TriLipix*—45 mg once daily initially; may titrate, if needed, up to 135 mg once daily.

Primary Hypercholesterolemia or Mixed Dyslipidemia

PO (Adults): *Fibricor*—105 mg once daily; *TriLipix*—135 mg once daily.

Renal Impairment

PO (Adults): *CCr 30–89 mL/min—Fibricor*—35 mg once daily initially; may titrate, if needed, up to 105 mg once daily. *TriLipix*—45 mg once daily initially; may titrate, if needed, up to 135 mg once daily.

Availability (generic available)

Delayed-release capsules (Fibricor): 35 mg, 105 mg. **Delayed-release capsules (TriLipix):** 45 mg, 135 mg.

NURSING IMPLICATIONS

Assessment

- Obtain a diet history, especially with regard to fat consumption. Every attempt should be made to obtain normal serum triglyceride levels with diet, exercise, and weight loss in obese patients before fenofibric acid therapy is instituted.
- Assess patient for cholelithiasis. If symptoms occur, gallbladder studies are indicated. Discontinue therapy if gallstones are found.
- Assess patient for skin reactions throughout therapy. Reactions may be severe and life threatening. Discontinue therapy if severe reactions or moderate rashes with systemic symptoms occur.
- ***Lab Test Considerations:*** Monitor serum lipids before therapy to determine consistent elevations, then monitor periodically during therapy.
- Monitor serum AST and ALT before and periodically during therapy. May cause ↑ levels. Discontinue therapy if levels rise >3 times the normal limit.

- If patient develops muscle tenderness during therapy, CPK levels should be monitored. If CPK levels are markedly ↑ or myopathy occurs, therapy should be discontinued.
- May cause reversible ↑ in serum creatinine. Monitor renal function in patients at risk for renal insufficiency (elderly, diabetics).
- May cause mild to moderate ↓ in hemoglobin, hematocrit, and WBCs. Monitor periodically during first 12 mo of therapy. Levels usually stabilize during long-term therapy.
- Monitor prothrombin time and INR monitored frequently until levels stabilize in patients taking anticoagulants concurrently.

Implementation

- Patients should be placed on a triglyceride-lowering diet before therapy and remain on this diet throughout therapy.
- **PO:** Administer without regard to meals. Swallow capsules whole; do not open, crush, or chew. May be administered at same time as statin dose.

Patient/Family Teaching

- Instruct patient to take medication as directed. Take missed doses as soon as remembered; if time for next dose, skip dose and take next dose at regular time. Do not double doses. Medication helps control but does not cure elevated serum triglyceride levels. Advise patient to read *Medication Guide* before starting and with each Rx refill, as new information may be available.
- Advise patient that this medication should be used in conjunction with diet restrictions (fat, cholesterol, carbohydrates, alcohol), exercise, and cessation of smoking.
- Instruct patient to notify health care professional if rash or unexplained muscle pain, tenderness, weakness, tiredness, fever, nausea, vomiting, or abdominal pain occurs, especially if accompanied by fever or malaise.
- Instruct female patients to notify health care professional promptly if pregnancy is planned or suspected and to avoid breast feeding during and for at least 5 days after last dose of therapy.
- Advise patient to notify health care professional of all Rx or OTC medications, vitamins, or herbal products being taken and to consult with health care professional before taking other medications.
- Advise patient to notify health care professional of medication regimen before treatment or surgery.
- Emphasize the importance of follow-up exams to determine effectiveness and to monitor for side effects.

Evaluation/Desired Outcomes

- Decrease in serum triglycerides and LDL cholesterol to normal levels with an increase in HDL levels.

HIGH ALERT

fentaNYL (parenteral)

(fen-ta-nil)

Sublimaze

Classification

Therapeutic: opioid analgesics

Pharmacologic: opioid agonists

Schedule II

Indications

Analgesic supplement to general anesthesia; usually with other agents (ultra–short-acting barbiturates, neuromuscular blocking agents, and inhalation anesthetics) to produce balanced anesthesia. Induction/maintenance of anesthesia (with oxygen or oxygen/nitrous oxide and a neuromuscular blocking agent). Neuroleptanalgesia/neuroleptanesthesia (with or without nitrous oxide). Supplement to regional/local anesthesia. Preoperative and postoperative analgesia. **Unlabeled Use:** Continuous IV infusion as part of PCA.

Action

Binds to opiate receptors in the CNS, altering the response to and perception of pain. Produces CNS depression. **Therapeutic Effects:** Supplement in anesthesia. Decreased pain.

Pharmacokinetics

Absorption: Well absorbed after IM administration.
Distribution: Unknown.
Metabolism and Excretion: Mostly metabolized by the liver, 10–25% excreted unchanged by the kidneys.
Half-life: Children: Bolus dose—2.4 hr, long-term continuous infusion—11–36 hr; Adults: 2–4 hr (↑ after cardiopulmonary bypass and in geriatric patients).

TIME/ACTION PROFILE (analgesia*)

ROUTE	ONSET	PEAK	DURATION
IM	7–15 min	20–30 min	1–2 hr
IV	1–2 min	3–5 min	0.5–1 hr

*Respiratory depression may last longer than analgesia.

Contraindications/Precautions

Contraindicated in: Hypersensitivity; cross-sensitivity among agents may occur; Known intolerance.
Use Cautiously in: Diabetes; Severe renal, pulmonary, or hepatic disease; CNS tumors; ↑ intracranial pressure; Head trauma; Adrenal insufficiency; Undiagnosed abdominal pain; Hypothyroidism; Alcoholism; Cardiac disease (arrhythmias); OB: Use during pregnancy only if maternal benefit outweighs potential risk to fetus. Chronic maternal treatment with opioids during pregnancy may result in neonatal abstinence syndrome; Lactation: Use while breast feeding only if maternal benefit outweighs potential risk to infant (may

cause infant sedation and/or respiratory depression); Geri: Geriatric, debilitated, or critically ill patients.

Adverse Reactions/Side Effects

CNS: confusion, paradoxical excitation/delirium, postoperative depression, postoperative drowsiness. **CV:** arrhythmias, bradycardia, circulatory depression, hypotension. **Derm:** facial itching. **EENT:** blurred/double vision. **Endo:** adrenal insufficiency. **GI:** biliary spasm, nausea/vomiting. **MS:** skeletal and thoracic muscle rigidity (with rapid IV infusion). **Resp:** APNEA, LARYNGOSPASM, allergic bronchospasm, respiratory depression.

Interactions

Drug-Drug: Avoid use in patients who have received **MAO inhibitors** within the previous 14 days (may produce unpredictable, potentially fatal reactions). Concomitant use of **CYP3A4 inhibitors** including **ritonavir, ketoconazole, itraconazole, clarithromycin, nelfinavir, nefazodone, diltiazem, aprepitant, fluconazole, fosamprenavir, verapamil**, and **erythromycin** may result in ↑ levels and ↑ risk of CNS and respiratory depression. Concurrent use with **CYP3A4 inducers** including **barbiturates, carbamazepine, efavirenz, corticosteroids, modafinil, nevirapine, oxcarbazepine, phenobarbital, phenytoin, rifabutin**, or **rifampin** may ↓ levels and analgesia; if inducers are discontinued or dosage ↓, patients should be monitored for signs of opioid toxicity and necessary dose adjustments should be made. Use with **benzodiazepines** or other **CNS depressants** including other **opioids, non-benzodiazepine sedative/hypnotics, anxiolytics, general anesthetics, muscle relaxants, antipsychotics**, and **alcohol** may cause profound sedation, respiratory depression, coma, and death; reserve concurrent use for when alternative treatment options are inadequate. ↑ risk of hypotension with **benzodiazepines**. **Nalbuphine** or **buprenorphine** may ↓ analgesia. Drugs that affect serotonergic neurotransmitter systems, including **tricyclic antidepressants, SSRIs, SNRIs, MAO inhibitors, TCAs, tramadol, trazodone, mirtazapine, 5-HT_3 receptor antagonists, linezolid, methylene blue**, and **triptans** ↑ risk of serotonin syndrome.
Drug-Food: Grapefruit juice is a moderate inhibitor of the CYP3A4 enzyme system; concurrent use may ↑ blood levels and the risk of respiratory and CNS depression. Careful monitoring and dose adjustment is recommended.

Route/Dosage

Preoperative Use

IM, IV (Adults and Children >12 yr): 50–100 mcg 30–60 min before surgery.

Adjunct to General Anesthesia

IM, IV (Adults and Children >12 yr): *Low dose–minor surgery*—2 mcg/kg. *Moderate dose–major surgery*—2–20 mcg/kg. *High dose–major surgery*—20–50 mcg/kg.

Adjunct to Regional Anesthesia

IM, IV (Adults and Children >12 yr): 50–100 mcg.

Postoperative Use (Recovery Room)

IM, IV (Adults and Children >12 yr): 50–100 mcg; may repeat in 1–2 hr.

General Anesthesia

IV (Adults and Children >12 yr): 50–100 mcg/kg (up to 150 mcg/kg).
IV (Children 1–12 yr): 2–3 mcg/kg.

Sedation/Analgesia

IV (Adults and Children >12 yr): 0.5–1 mcg/kg/dose, may repeat after 30–60 min.
IV (Children 1–12 yr): *Bolus*—1–2 mcg/kg/dose, may repeat at 30–60 min intervals. *Continuous infusion*—1–5 mcg/kg/hr following bolus dose.
IV (Neonates): *Bolus*—0.5–3 mcg/kg/dose. *Continuous infusion*—0.5–2 mcg/kg/hr following bolus dose. *Continuous infusion during ECMO*—5–10 mcg/kg bolus followed by 1–5 mcg/kg/hr, may require up to 20 mcg/kg/hr after 5 days of therapy.

Availability (generic available)

Solution for injection: 50 mcg/mL.

NURSING IMPLICATIONS

Assessment

- Monitor respiratory rate and BP frequently throughout therapy. Report significant changes immediately. The respiratory depressant effects of fentanyl may last longer than the analgesic effects. Initial doses of other opioids should be reduced by 25–33% of the usually recommended dose. Monitor closely.
- Geri: Opioids have been associated with increased risk of falls in geriatric patients. Assess risk and implement fall prevention strategies.
- Assess type, location, and intensity of pain before and 30 min after IM administration or 3–5 min after IV administration when fentanyl is used to treat pain.
- ***Lab Test Considerations:*** May cause ↑ serum amylase and lipase concentrations.
- ***Toxicity and Overdose:*** Symptoms of toxicity include respiratory depression, hypotension, arrhythmias, bradycardia, and asystole. Atropine may be used to treat bradycardia. If respiratory depression persists after surgery, prolonged mechanical ventilation may be required. If an opioid antagonist is required to reverse respiratory depression or coma, naloxone (Narcan) is the antidote. Dilute the 0.4-mg

ampule of naloxone in 10 mL of 0.9% NaCl and administer 0.5 mL (0.02 mg) by IV push every 2 min. Pedi: For children and patients weighing <40 kg, dilute 0.1 mg of naloxone in 10 mL of 0.9% NaCl for a concentration of 10 mcg/mL and administer 0.5 mcg/kg every 2 min. Titrate dose to avoid withdrawal, seizures, and severe pain. Administration of naloxone in these circumstances, especially in cardiac patients, has resulted in hypertension and tachycardia, occasionally causing left ventricular failure and pulmonary edema.

Implementation

- ***High Alert:*** Accidental overdosage of opioid analgesics has resulted in fatalities. Before administering, clarify all ambiguous orders; have second practitioner independently check original order, dose calculations, route of administration, and infusion pump programming.
- Do not confuse fentanyl with sufentanil.
- Benzodiazepines may be administered before or after administration of fentanyl to reduce the induction dose requirements, decrease the time to loss of consciousness, and produce amnesia. This combination may also increase the risk of hypotension and respiratory depression.

IV Administration

- **IV Push:** ***Diluent:*** Administer undiluted. ***Concentration:*** 50 mcg/mL. ***Rate:*** Inject slowly over 1–3 min. Administer doses >5 mcg/kg over 5–10 min. Slow IV administration may reduce the incidence and severity of muscle rigidity, bradycardia, or hypotension. Neuromuscular blocking agents may be administered concurrently to decrease chest wall muscle rigidity.
- **Intermittent Infusion:** ***Diluent:*** May be diluted in D5W or 0.9% NaCl. ***Concentration:*** Up to 50 mcg/mL. ***Rate:*** see IV Push.
- **Y-Site Compatibility:** acetaminophen, acyclovir, alemtuzumab, alfentanil, alprostadil, amikacin, aminocaproic acid, aminophylline, amphotericin B deoxycholate, amphotericin B lipid complex, amphotericin B liposome, anidulafungin, argatroban, arsenic trioxide, ascorbic acid, atracurium, atropine, azathioprine, aztreonam, benztropine, bivalirudin, bleomycin, bumetanide, buprenorphine, butorphanol, calcium chloride, calcium gluconate, cangrelor, carboplatin, carmustine, caspofungin, cefazolin, cefotaxime, cefotetan, cefoxitin, ceftaroline, ceftazidime, ceftolozane/tazobactam, ceftriaxone, cefuroxime, chloramphenicol, chlorpromazine, cisatracurium, cisplatin, clindamycin, cyanocobalamin, cyclophosphamide, cyclosporine, cytarabine, dacarbazine, dactinomycin, daptomycin, daunorubicin hydrochloride, dexamethasone, dexmedetomidine, dexrazoxane, digoxin, diltiazem, diphenhydramine, dobutamine, docetaxel, dolasetron, dopamine, doxacurium, doxapram, doxorubicin, doxorubicin liposomal, doxycycline, enalaprilat, ephedrine, epinephrine, epirubicin, epoetin alfa, eptifibatide, erythromycin, esmolol, etomidate, etoposide, etoposide phosphate, famotidine, fenoldopam, fluconazole, fludarabine, fluorouracil, folic acid, foscarnet, fosphenytoin, furosemide, ganciclovir, gemcitabine, gentamicin, glycopyrrolate, granisetron, heparin, hetastarch, hydrocortisone, hydromorphone, idarubicin, ifosfamide, imipenem/cilastatin, insulin regular, irinotecan, isavuconazonium, isoproterenol, ketorolac, labetalol, leucovorin calcium, levofloxacin, lidocaine, linezolid, lorazepam, magnesium sulfate, mannitol, meperidine, meropenem/vaborbactam, mesna, metaraminol, methotrexate, methyldopate, methylpresnisolone, metoclopramide, metoprolol, midazolam, milrinone, mitomycin, mitoxantrone, morphine, multivitamins, mycophenolate, nafcillin, nalbuphine, naloxone, nicardipine, nitroglycerin, nitroprusside, norepinephrine, octreotide, ondansetron, oritavancin, oxacillin, oxaliplatin, oxytocin, paclitaxel, palonosetron, pamidronate, pancuronium, papaverine, pemetrexed, penicillin G, pentamidine, pentobarbital, phenobarbital, phentolamine, phenylephrine, phytonadione, piperacillin/tazobactam, plazomicin, potassium acetate, potassium chloride, procainamide, prochlorperazine, promethazine, propofol, propranolol, protamine, pyridoxime, quinupristin/dalfopristin, ranitidine, remifentanil, rituximab, rocuronium, sargramostim, scopolamine, sodium acetate, sodium bicarbonate, streptokinase, succinylcholine, sufentanil, tacrolimus, tedizolid, theophylline, thiamine, thiopental, thiotepa, tigecycline, tirofiban, tobramycin, tolazoline, topotecan, trastuzumab, vancomycin, vasopressin, vecuronium, verapamil, vinblastine, vincristine, vinorelbine, vitamin B complex with C, voriconazole, zoledronic acid.
- **Y-Site Incompatibility:** dantrolene, diazoxide, hydroxycobalamin, pantoprazole, phenytoin, trimethoprim/sulfamethoxazole.

Patient/Family Teaching

- Discuss the use of anesthetic agents and the sensations to expect with the patient before surgery.
- Explain pain assessment scale to patient.
- Caution patient to change positions slowly to minimize orthostatic hypotension. Geri: Geriatric patients may be at a greater risk for orthostatic hypotension and, consequently, falls. Teach patient to take precautions until drug effects have completely resolved.
- Medication causes dizziness and drowsiness. Advise patient to call for assistance during ambulation and transfer, and to avoid driving or other activities requiring alertness for 24 hr after administration during outpatient surgery.
- Instruct patient to avoid alcohol or other CNS depressants for 24 hr after administration for outpatient surgery.

Evaluation/Desired Outcomes

- General quiescence.
- Reduced motor activity.
- Pronounced analgesia.

REMS HIGH ALERT

fentaNYL (transdermal)

(fen-ta-nil)

Duragesic

Classification

Therapeutic: opioid analgesics, anesthetic adjuncts

Pharmacologic: opioid agonists

Schedule II

Indications

Moderate to severe chronic pain in opioid-tolerant patients requiring use of daily, around-the-clock long-term opioid treatment and for which alternative treatment options are inadequate (extended-release). Transdermal fentanyl is not recommended for the control of postoperative, mild, or intermittent pain, nor should it be used for short-term pain relief.

Action

Binds to opiate receptors in the CNS, altering the response to and perception of pain. **Therapeutic Effects:** Decrease in severity of chronic pain.

Pharmacokinetics

Absorption: Well absorbed (92% of dose) through skin surface under transdermal patch, creating a depot in the upper skin layers. Release from transdermal system into systemic circulation ↑ gradually to a constant rate, providing continuous delivery for 72 hr.

Distribution: Crosses the placenta; enters breast milk.

Metabolism and Excretion: Mostly metabolized by the liver (CYP3A4 enzyme system); 10–25% excreted unchanged by the kidneys.

Half-life: 17 hr after removal of a single application patch, ↑ to 21 hr after removal of multiple patches (because of continued release from deposition of drug in skin layers).

TIME/ACTION PROFILE (↓ pain)

ROUTE	ONSET	PEAK	DURATION
Transdermal	6 hr†	12–24 hr	72 hr‡

†Achievement of blood levels associated with analgesia. Maximal response and dose titration may take up to 6 days.
‡While patch is worn.

Contraindications/Precautions

Contraindicated in: Hypersensitivity to fentanyl or adhesives; Patients who are not opioid tolerant; Acute, mild, intermittent, or postoperative pain; Significant respiratory depression; Acute or severe bronchial asthma; Paralytic ileus; Severe hepatic or renal impairment; Alcohol intolerance (small amounts of alcohol released into skin); OB: Not recommended during labor and delivery; Lactation: Avoid use during breast feeding; may cause infant sedation and/or respiratory depression.

Use Cautiously in: Diabetes; Patients with severe pulmonary disease; Mild or moderate hepatic or renal impairment; CNS tumors; ↑ intracranial pressure; Head trauma; Adrenal insufficiency; Undiagnosed abdominal pain; Hypothyroidism; Alcoholism; Cardiac disease (particularly bradyarrhythmias); Fever or situations that ↑ body temperature (↑ release of fentanyl from delivery system); Titration period (additional analgesics may be required); Cachectic or debilitated patients (dose ↓ suggested because of altered drug disposition); OB: Use only if the potential benefit justifies the potential risk to the fetus. Chronic maternal treatment with opioids during pregnancy may result in neonatal abstinence syndrome; Pedi: Children <2 yr (safety not established); pediatric patients initiating therapy at 25 mcg/hr should be opioid tolerant and receiving at least 60 mg oral morphine equivalents per day; Geri: ↑ risk of respiratory depression; dose ↓ suggested.

Adverse Reactions/Side Effects

CNS: <u>confusion</u>, <u>sedation</u>, <u>weakness</u>, dizziness, restlessness. **Resp:** APNEA, bronchoconstriction, laryngospasm, RESPIRATORY DEPRESSION. **CV:** bradycardia, hypotension. **GI:** <u>anorexia</u>, <u>constipation</u>, <u>dry mouth</u>, <u>nausea</u>, <u>vomiting</u>. **Derm:** <u>sweating</u>, erythema. **Endo:** adrenal insufficiency. **Local:** application site reactions. **MS:** skeletal and thoracic muscle rigidity. **Misc:** physical dependence, psychological dependence.

Interactions

Drug-Drug: Avoid use in patients who have received **MAO inhibitors** within the previous 14 days (may produce unpredictable, potentially fatal reactions). Concomitant use of **CYP3A4 inhibitors** including **ritonavir**, **ketoconazole**, **itraconazole**, **clarithromycin**, **nelfinavir**, **nefazodone**, **amiodarone**, **diltiazem**, **aprepitant**, **fluconazole**, **fosamprenavir**, **verapamil**, and **erythromycin** may result in ↑ plasma levels and ↑ risk of CNS and respiratory depression. Levels and effectiveness may be ↓ by **CYP3A4 inducers** including **rifampin**, **carbamazepine**, and **phenytoin**. Use with **benzodiazepines** or other **CNS depressants** including other **opioids**, **non-benzodiazepine sedative/hypnotics**, **anxiolytics**, **general anesthetics**, **muscle relaxants**, **antipsychotics**, and

alcohol may cause profound sedation, respiratory depression, coma, and death; reserve concurrent use for when alternative treatment options are inadequate. Drugs that affect serotonergic neurotransmitter systems, including **tricyclic antidepressants**, **SSRIs**, **SNRIs**, **MAO inhibitors**, **TCAs**, **tramadol**, **trazodone**, **mirtazapine**, **5–HT$_3$ receptor antagonists**, **linezolid**, **methylene blue**, and **triptans** ↑ risk of serotonin syndrome.

Drug-Natural Products: Concomitant use of **kava-kava**, **valerian**, or **chamomile** can ↑ CNS depression.

Drug-Food: Grapefruit juice is a moderate inhibitor of the CYP3A4 enzyme system; concurrent use may ↑ blood levels and the risk of respiratory and CNS depression. Careful monitoring and dose adjustment is recommended.

Route/Dosage

Transdermal (Adults): 25 mcg/hr is the initial dose; patients who have not been receiving opioids should receive not more than 25 mcg/hr. To calculate the dose of transdermal fentanyl required in patients who are already receiving opioid analgesics, assess the 24-hr requirement of currently used opioid. Using the equianalgesic table in Appendix J, convert this to an equivalent amount of morphine/24 hr. Conversion to fentanyl transdermal may be accomplished by using the fentanyl conversion table (Appendix J). During dose titration, additional short-acting opioids should be available for breakthrough pain. Morphine 10 mg IM or 60 mg PO every 4 hr (60 mg/24 hr IM or 360 mg/24 hr PO) is considered to be approximately equivalent to transdermal fentanyl 100 mcg/hr. Transdermal patch lasts 72 hr in most patients. Some patients require a new patch every 48 hr.

Transdermal (Adults >60 yr, Debilitated, or Cachectic Patients): Initial dose should be 25 mcg/hr unless previous opioid use was >135 mg morphine PO/ day (or other opioid equivalent).

Hepatic Impairment

Transdermal (Adults): *Mild-to-moderate hepatic impairment*—12 mcg/hr is the initial dose.

Renal Impairment

Transdermal (Adults): *Mild-to-moderate renal impairment*—12 mcg/hr is the initial dose.

Availability (generic available)

Transdermal systems: 12.5 mcg/hr, 25 mcg/hr, 37.5 mcg/hr, 50 mcg/hr, 62.5 mcg/hr, 75 mcg/hr, 87.5 mcg/hr, 100 mcg/hr. **Cost:** *Generic*—12 mcg/hr \$101.51/5, 25 mcg/hr \$72.17/5, 50 mcg/hr \$131.92/5, 75 mcg/hr \$201.23/5, 100 mcg/hr \$267.07/5.

NURSING IMPLICATIONS

Assessment

- Assess type, location, and intensity of pain before and 24 hr after application and periodically during therapy. Monitor pain frequently during initiation of therapy and dose changes to assess need for supplementary analgesics for breakthrough pain.
- Assess BP, pulse, and respirations before and periodically during administration. If respiratory rate is <10/min, assess level of sedation. Physical stimulation may be sufficient to prevent significant hypoventilation. Dose may need to be decreased by 25–50%. Initial drowsiness will diminish with continued use.
- Prolonged use may lead to physical and psychological dependence and tolerance. This should not prevent patient from receiving adequate analgesia. Most patients who receive opioid analgesics for pain rarely develop psychological dependence.
- Progressively higher doses may be required to relieve pain with long-term therapy. It may take up to 6 days after increasing doses to reach equilibrium, so patients should wear higher dose through 2 applications before increasing dose again.
- Assess bowel function routinely. Prevent constipation with increased intake of fluids and bulk, and laxatives to minimize constipating effects. Administer stimulant laxatives routinely if opioid use exceeds 2–3 days, unless contraindicated. Consider drugs for opioid —induced constipation.
- Assess risk for opioid addiction, abuse, or misuse prior to administration. Monitor for respiratory depression, especially during initiation or following dose increase; serious, life-threatening, or fatal respiratory depression may occur. Misuse or abuse of *transdermal fentanyl* by chewing, swallowing, snorting or injecting fentanyl extracted from transdermal system will result in the uncontrolled delivery of fentanyl and risk of overdose and death.
- ***Lab Test Considerations:*** May ↑ plasma amylase and lipase levels.
- ***Toxicity and Overdose:*** If an opioid antagonist is required to reverse respiratory depression or coma, naloxone is the antidote. Dilute the 0.4-mg ampule of naloxone in 10 mL of 0.9% NaCl and administer 0.5 mL (0.02 mg) by IV push every 2 min. For patients weighing <40 kg, dilute 0.1 mg of naloxone in 10 mL of 0.9% NaCl for a concentration of 10 mcg/ mL and administer 0.5 mcg/kg every 2 min. Titrate dose to avoid withdrawal, seizures, and severe pain. Monitor patient closely; dose may need to be repeated or may need to be administered as an infusion because of long duration of action despite removal of patch.

Implementation

- Do not confuse fentanyl with sufentanil.
- ***High Alert:*** Accidental overdose of opioid analgesics has resulted in fatalities. Before administering, confirm patient is opioid tolerant and clarify ambiguous orders.
- 12-mcg patch delivers 12.5 mcg/hr of fentanyl. Use supplemental doses of short-acting opioid analgesics

to manage pain until relief is obtained with the transdermal system. Patients may continue to require supplemental opioids for breakthrough pain. If >100 mcg/hr is required, use multiple transdermal systems.

- Titrate dose based on patient's report of pain until adequate analgesia (50% reduction in patient's pain rating on numerical or visual analogue scale or patient reports satisfactory relief) is attained. Determine dose by calculating the previous 24-hr analgesic requirement and converting to the equianalgesic morphine dose using Appendix J. The conversion ratio from morphine to transdermal fentanyl is conservative; 50% of patients may require a dose increase after initial application. Increase after 3 days based on required daily doses of supplemental analgesics. Base increases on ratio of 45 mg/24 hr of oral morphine to 12.5 mcg/hr increase in transdermal fentanyl dose.
- Coadministration with nonopioid analgesics may have additive analgesic effects and permit lower opioid doses.
- To convert to another opioid analgesic, remove transdermal fentanyl system and begin treatment with half the equianalgesic dose of the new analgesic in 12–18 hr.
- Medication should be discontinued gradually after long-term use to prevent withdrawal symptoms.
- FDA strongly encourages health care professionals to complete a REMS-compliant education program that includes all the elements of the FDA Education *Blueprint for Health Care Providers Involved in the Management or Support of Patients with Pain,* available at www.fda.gov/OpioidAnalgesicREMSBlueprint. Information on programs can be found at 1-800-503-0784 or www.opioidanalgesicrems.com.
- **Transdermal:** Apply system to flat, nonirritated, and nonirradiated site such as chest, back, flank, or upper arm. If skin preparation is necessary, use clear water and clip, do not shave, hair. Allow skin to dry completely before application. Apply immediately after removing from package. Do not alter the system (i.e., cut) in any way before application. Remove liner from adhesive layer and press firmly in place with palm of hand for 30 sec, especially around the edges, to make sure contact is complete. Remove used system and fold so that adhesive edges are together. Flush system down toilet immediately on removal or follow the institutional disposal policy. Apply new system to a different site.

Patient/Family Teaching

- Instruct patient in how and when to ask for and take pain medication. Discuss safe use, risks, and proper storage and disposal of opioid analgesics with patients and caregivers with each Rx. The Patient Counseling Guide (PCG) is available at www.fda.gov/OpioidAnalgesicREMSPCG. Advise patient to read *Medication Guide* before starting therapy and with each Rx refill in case of changes.
- Instruct patient in correct method for application and disposal of transdermal system. Fatalities have occurred from children having access to improperly discarded patches. May be worn while bathing, showering, or swimming.
- Advise patient to avoid grapefruit juice during therapy.
- Advise patient that fentanyl is a drug with known abuse potential. Protect it from theft, and never give to anyone other than the individual for whom it was prescribed. Store out of sight and reach of children, and in a location not accessible by others.
- May cause drowsiness or dizziness. Caution patient to call for assistance when ambulating or smoking and to avoid driving or other activities requiring alertness until response to medication is known.
- Advise patient to change positions slowly to minimize dizziness.
- Caution patient to avoid concurrent use of alcohol or other CNS depressants with this medication.
- Caution patient that fever, electric blankets, heating pads, saunas, hot tubs, and heated water beds increase the release of fentanyl from the patch.
- Advise patient that good oral hygiene, frequent mouth rinses, and sugarless gum or candy may decrease dry mouth.
- Advise patient to notify health care professional of all Rx or OTC medications, vitamins, or herbal products being taken and to consult with health care professional before taking other medications.
- Advise patient referred for MRI test to discuss patch with referring health care professional and MRI facility to determine if removal of patch is necessary prior to test and for directions for replacing patch.
- Instruct female patient to notify health care professional if pregnancy is planned or suspected and to avoid breast feeding during therapy. Inform patient of potential for neonatal opioid withdrawal syndrome with prolonged use during pregnancy. Monitor neonate for signs and symptoms of withdrawal symptoms (irritability, hyperactivity and abnormal sleep pattern, high pitched cry, tremor, vomiting, diarrhea, and/or failure to gain weight); usually occur the first days after birth.

Evaluation/Desired Outcomes

- Decrease in severity of pain without a significant alteration in level of consciousness, respiratory status, or BP.

REMS HIGH ALERT

FENTANYL (transmucosal)
(fen-ta-nil)

fentaNYL (buccal tablet)
Fentora

fentaNYL (nasal spray)
Lazanda

fentaNYL (oral transmucosal lozenge)
Actiq

fentaNYL (sublingual spray)
Subsys

fentaNYL (sublingual tablet)
Abstral

Classification
Therapeutic: opioid analgesics
Pharmacologic: opioid agonists

Schedule II

Indications
Management of breakthrough pain in cancer patients >18 yr old already receiving opioids and tolerant to around-the-clock opioids for persistent cancer pain (60 mg/day of oral morphine or equivalent).

Action
Binds to opioid receptors in the CNS, altering the response to and perception of pain. **Therapeutic Effects:** Decrease in severity of breakthrough pain.

Pharmacokinetics
Absorption: *Buccal tablet*—65% absorbed from buccal mucosa; 50% is absorbed transmucosally, remainder is swallowed and is absorbed slowly from the GI tract. Buccal absorption is enhanced by an effervescent reaction in the dose form; *Nasal spray*—Well absorbed from nasal mucosa (bioavailability higher than that of oral transmucosal lozenge); *Oral transmucosal lozenge*—Initial rapid absorption (25%) from buccal mucosa is followed by more prolonged absorption (25%) from GI tract (combined bioavailability 50%); *Sublingual spray*—76% absorbed through sublingual mucosa; *Sublingual tablets*—54% absorbed from oral mucosa following sublingual administration.
Distribution: Readily crosses the placenta and enters breast milk.
Metabolism and Excretion: Mostly metabolized in the liver and intestinal mucosa via the CYP3A4 enzyme system; inactive metabolites are excreted in urine; <7% excreted unchanged in urine.
Half-life: *Buccal tablet*—2.6–11.7 hr (↑ with dose); *Nasal spray*—15–25 hr (↑ with dose); *Sublingual spray*—5–12 hr; *Sublingual tablet*—5–10 hr (↑ with dose); *Transmucosal lozenge*—7 hr.

TIME/ACTION PROFILE (↓ pain)

ROUTE	ONSET	PEAK	DURATION
Buccal tablet	15 min	40–60 min	60 min
Nasal spray	within 10 min	unknown	2–4 hr
Oral transmucosal lozenge	rapid	15–30 min	several hr
SL	within 30 min	30–60 min	2–4 hr

Contraindications/Precautions
Contraindicated in: Known intolerance or hypersensitivity; Acute/postoperative pain including headache/migraine, dental pain, or emergency room use; Opioid—naive (nontolerant) patients; Concurrent use of MAO inhibitors; OB: Labor and delivery; Lactation: Avoid use during breast feeding; may cause infant sedation and/or respiratory depression.
Use Cautiously in: Chronic obstructive pulmonary disease or pre-existing medical conditions predisposing to hypoventilation; Concurrent use of CNS active drugs; History of substance abuse; Severe renal/hepatic impairment (use lowest effective starting dose); Concurrent use of CYP3A4 inhibitors (use lowest effective dose); Bradyarrhythmias; OB: Use only if the potential benefit justifies the potential risk to the fetus. Chronic maternal treatment with opioids during pregnancy may result in neonatal abstinence syndrome; Geri: May be more sensitive to effects and may have an ↑ risk of adverse reactions; titrate dosage carefully; Pedi: Safety and effectiveness not established.
Exercise Extreme Caution in: Patients susceptible to intracranial effects of CO_2 retention including those with ↑ intracranial pressure, head injuries, or impaired consciousness.

Adverse Reactions/Side Effects
Opioid side effects ↑ with ↑ dosage.
CNS: dizziness, drowsiness, headache, confusion, depression, fatigue, hallucinations, headache, insomnia, weakness. **Resp:** RESPIRATORY DEPRESSION, dyspnea. **CV:** hypotension. **Endo:** adrenal insufficiency. **GI:** constipation, nausea, vomiting, abdominal pain, anorexia, dry mouth. **Misc:** allergic reaction including ANAPHYLAXIS, physical dependence, psychological dependence.

Interactions
Drug-Drug: Should not be used within 14 days of **MAO inhibitors** because of possible severe and unpredictable reactions. Concurrent use of **CYP3A4 inhibitors** including **ritonavir**, **ketoconazole**, **itraconazole**, **fluconazole**, **clarithromycin**, **erythromycin**, **nefazodone**, **diltiazem**, **verapamil**, **nelfinavir**, and **fosamprenavir** ↑ levels and risk of opioid toxicity; careful monitoring during initiation, dose changes, or discontinuation of the inhibitor is recommended. Concurrent use with **CYP3A4 inducers** including **barbiturates**, **carbamazepine**, **efavirenz**, **corticosteroids**, **modafinil**, **nevirapine**, **oxcarba-**

zepine, **phenobarbital**, **phenytoin**, **rifabutin**, or **rifampin** may ↓ fentanyl levels and analgesia; if inducers are discontinued or dosage ↓, patients should be monitored for signs of opioid toxicity and necessary dose adjustments should be made. Use with **benzodiazepines** or other **CNS depressants** including other **opioids**, **non-benzodiazepine sedative/hypnotics**, **anxiolytics**, **general anesthetics**, **muscle relaxants**, **antipsychotics**, and **alcohol** may cause profound sedation, respiratory depression, coma, and death; reserve concurrent use for when alternative treatment options are inadequate. Drugs that affect serotonergic neurotransmitter systems, including **tricyclic antidepressants**, **SSRIs**, **SNRIs**, **MAO inhibitors**, **TCAs**, **tramadol**, **trazodone**, **mirtazapine**, **5–HT_3 receptor antagonists**, **linezolid**, **methylene blue**, and **triptans** ↑ risk of serotonin syndrome.

Drug-Natural Products: St. John's wort is an inducer of CYP3A4; concurrent use may ↓ levels and analgesia; if inducers are discontinued or dosage decreased, patients should be monitored for signs of opioid toxicity and necessary dosage adjustments made.

Drug-Food: Grapefuit juice is a moderate inhibitor of CYP3A4 enzyme system; concurrent use may ↑ levels and the risk of CNS and respiratory depression. Careful monitoring and dose adjustment may be necessary.

Route/Dosage

Transmucosal Products Are Not Equivalent on a mcg-to-mcg Basis

Buccal (Adults): *Tablets*— 100 mcg, then titrate to dose that provides adequate analgesia without undue side effects.

Intranasal (Adults): One 100-mcg spray in one nostril initially, then titrate in a step-wise manner (↑ to one 100-mcg spray in each nostril [200 mcg total]), then a total of three 100–mcg sprays (one in right nostril, then one in left nostril, then last spray in right nostril), then one 400-mcg spray in one nostril (or two 100–mcg sprays in each nostril [400 mcg total]), then two 300–mcg sprays in each nostril [600 mcg total], then one 400-mcg spray in each nostril [800 mcg total] to provide adequate analgesia without undue side effects (up to a maximum of one 400-mcg spray in each nostril).

Oral transmucosal (Adults): One 200-mcg unit dissolved in mouth (see Implementation section) over 15 min; additional unit may be used 15 min after first unit is completed. If more than 1 unit is required per episode (as evaluated over several episodes), dose may be ↑ as required to control pain. Optimal usage/titration should result in using no more than 4 units/day.

SL (Adults): *Tablets*— 100 mcg initially, then titrate using 100-mcg increments to provide adequate analgesia without undue side effects (not to exceed 2 doses per episode; no more than 4 doses per day; separate by at least 2 hr); *Spray*— 100 mcg initially; if pain not relieved within 30 min, repeat 100-mcg dose (do not take more than 2 doses per breakthrough pain episode); patients must wait ≥4 hr before treating another episode of breakthrough pain. Dose may be titrated during subsequent pain episodes to 200 mcg, then 400 mcg, then 600 mcg, then 800 mcg, then 1200 mcg, and then 1600 mcg to provide adequate analgesia and undue side effects.

Availability (generic available)

Buccal tablets: 100 mcg, 200 mcg, 300 mcg, 400 mcg, 600 mcg, 800 mcg. **Cost:** 200 mcg $1,006.04/28. **Nasal spray:** 100 mcg/spray, 300 mcg/spray, 400 mcg/spray. **Oral transmucosal lozenge on a stick (berry flavor-sugar free):** 200 mcg, 400 mcg, 600 mcg, 800 mcg, 1200 mcg, 1600 mcg. **Cost:** *Generic*— 400 mcg $599.93/30, 1200 mcg $799.93/30, 1600 mcg $1,155.89/30. **Sublingual spray:** 100 mcg/spray, 200 mcg/spray, 400 mcg/spray, 600 mcg/spray, 800 mcg/spray. **Sublingual tablets:** 100 mcg, 200 mcg, 300 mcg, 400 mcg, 600 mcg, 800 mcg.

NURSING IMPLICATIONS

Assessment

- Monitor type, location, and intensity of pain before and 1 hr after administration of transmucosal fentanyl.
- Assess BP, pulse, and respirations before and periodically during administration. If respiratory rate is <10 min, assess level of sedation. Physical stimulation may be sufficient to prevent hypoventilation. Subsequent doses may need to be decreased. Patients tolerant to opioid analgesics are usually tolerant to the respiratory depressant effects also.
- Monitor for application site reactions (paresthesia, ulceration, bleeding, pain, ulcer, irritation). Reactions are usually self-limited and rarely require discontinuation.
- ***Lab Test Considerations:*** May cause anemia, neutropenia, thrombocytopenia, and leukopenia.
- May cause hypokalemia, hypoalbuminemia, hypercalcemia, hypomagnesemia, and hyponatremia.
- ***Toxicity and Overdose:*** If an opioid antagonist is required to reverse respiratory depression or coma, naloxone is the antidote. Dilute the 0.4-mg ampule of naloxone in 10 mL of 0.9% NaCl and administer 0.5 mL (0.02 mg) by IV push every 2 min. For patients weighing <40 kg, dilute 0.1 mg of naloxone in 10 mL of 0.9% NaCl for a concentration of 10 mcg/mL and administer 0.5 mcg every 2 min. Use extreme caution when titrating dose in patients physically dependent on opioid analgesics to avoid withdrawal, seizures, and severe pain. Duration of respiratory depression may be longer than duration of opioid antagonist, requiring repeated doses.

Implementation

- ***High Alert:*** Accidental overdose of opioid analgesics has resulted in fatalities. Before administering, clarify all ambiguous orders; have second practitioner independently check original order and dose calculations.
- Do not confuse fentanyl with sufentanil.
- Patients considered opioid-tolerant are those who are taking ≥60 mg of oral morphine/day, at least 25 mcg transdermal fentanyl/hr, 30 mg of oxycodone/day, 8 mg of hydromorphone/day or an equianalgesic dose of another opioid for ≥1 wk.
- ***High Alert:*** Dose may be lethal to a child; keep out of reach of children.
- Do not substitute fentanyl products; doses are not equivalent.
- **REMS:** Health care professionals who prescribe transmucosal immediate-release fentanyl (TIRF) medicines for outpatient use are required to enroll in the TIRF REMS Access program. Health care professionals already enrolled in an individual Risk Evaluation and Mitigation Strategy (REMS) program for at least one TIRF medicine, will be automatically transitioned to the shared TIRF REMS Access program, and do not need to re-enroll. Enrollment renewal in TIRF REMS program is required every 2 yr from the date of enrollment. Information can be found at www.TIRFREMSaccess.com. A TIRF REMS Access Patient-Prescriber Agreement Form must be signed with each new patient before writing the patient's first TIRF prescription and health care professionals must also provide patients with a copy of the *Medication Guide* during counseling about the proper use of their TIRF medicine. Pharmacists who dispense TIRF medicines are also required to enroll in the TIRF REMS program and re-enroll every 2 yr. Patients are enrolled in the TIRF REMS Access program by the pharmacy at the time their first prescription is filled. Patients can locate a participating pharmacy by consulting their prescriber or calling the TIRF REMS Access program at 1-866-822-1483.
- **Buccal:** *Fentora*: Do not attempt to push tablet through blister, may cause damage to tablet. Open by tearing along perforations to separate from blister card. Then bend blister unit on line where indicated. Blister backing should then be peeled to expose tablets. Use immediately; do not store, may damage integrity of tablet. Tablets are not to be sucked, chewed, or swallowed whole; this will reduce medication effectiveness. Place between cheek and gum above a molar or under tongue and allow medication to dissolve, usually 14–25 min. May cause bubbling sensation between teeth and gum while tablet dissolves. Do not attempt to split tablet. After 30 min, if remnants of tablet remain, swallow with glass of water.
- For patients not previously using transmucosal fentanyl, initial dose should be 100 mcg. Titrate to provide adequate relief while minimizing side effects. For patients switching from oral transmucosal fentanyl to fentanyl buccal, if transmucosal dose is 200–400 mcg, switch to 100 mcg buccal; if transmucosal dose is 600–800 mcg, switch to 200 mcg buccal; if transmucosal dose is 1200–1600 mcg, switch to 400 mcg buccal fentanyl.
- Dose may be repeated once during a single episode of breakthrough pain if not adequately relieved. Redose may occur 30 min after start of administration of fentanyl buccal and the same dose should be used.
- If more than 1 dose is required per breakthrough pain episode for several consecutive episodes, dose of maintenance opioid and fentanyl buccal should be adjusted. To increase dose, use multiples of 100 mcg tablet, use two 100-mcg tablets (1 on each side of mouth in buccal cavity). If unsuccessful in controlling breakthrough pain episode, two 100-mcg tablets may be placed on each side of mouth in buccal cavity (four 100-mcg tablets). Titrate above 400 mcg by 200 mcg increments. To reduce risk of overdose, patients should have only one strength available at any one time.
- Once a successful dose has been established, if more than 4 breakthrough pain episodes/day occur, reevaluate opioid dose for persistent pain.
- Inform patient if medication is no longer needed they should contact Cephalon at 1-800-896-5855 or remove from blister pack and flush any remaining product down toilet.
- **Intranasal:** *Lazanda*: Prime the device before use by spraying into the pouch (4 sprays in total). Insert nozzle of the bottle a short distance (about ½ inch or 1 cm) into nose and point toward bridge of nose, tilting the bottle slightly. Press down firmly on finger grips until a "click" is heard and the number in the counting window advances by one. Advise patients that the fine-mist spray is not always felt on the nasal mucosal membrane and to rely on the audible click and advancement of dose counter to confirm a spray has been administered.
- All patients (including those switching from another fentanyl product) must start using one 100-mcg spray of fentanyl sublingual (1 spray in 1 nostril). If adequate analgesia is obtained within 30 min of administration of the 100-mcg single spray, treat subsequent episodes of breakthrough pain with this dose. If adequate analgesia is not achieved with first 100-mcg dose, ↑ dose in a step-wise manner over consecutive episodes of breakthrough pain until adequate analgesia with tolerable side effects is achieved. Patients MUST wait at least 2 hr before treating another episode of breakthrough cancer pain with fentanyl intranasal. Confirm the dose of fentanyl intranasal that works for patient with a 2nd episode of breakthrough pain and review their experience with their health care professional to determine if that dose is appropriate, or whether a further adjustment is warranted.

- During any episode of breakthrough cancer pain, if there is inadequate pain relief after 30 min following fentanyl intranasal dosing or if a separate episode of breakthrough cancer pain occurs before the next dose of fentanyl intranasal is permitted (i.e., within 2 hr), patients may use a rescue medication as directed by their health care professional.
- For patients no longer requiring opioid therapy, consider discontinuing fentanyl sublingual along with a gradual downward titration of other opioids to minimize possible withdrawal effects. In patients who continue to take chronic opioid therapy for persistent pain but no longer require treatment for breakthrough pain, fentanyl intranasal therapy can usually be discontinued immediately.
- **Transmucosal:** *Actiq*: Open the foil package immediately before use. Instruct patient to place unit in the mouth between the cheek and lower gum, moving it from one side to the other using the handle. Patient should suck, not chew, the lozenge. If it is chewed and swallowed, lower peak concentrations and lower bioavailability may occur. Instruct patient to consume lozenge over 15-min period; longer or shorter periods may be less efficacious. If signs of excessive opioid effects occur, remove from patient's mouth immediately and decrease future doses.
- Initial dose for breakthrough pain should be 200 mcg. Six 200-mcg units should be prescribed and should be used before increasing to a higher dose. If one unit is ineffective, a 2nd unit may be started 15 min after the completion of the first unit. Do not use more than 2 units during a single episode of breakthrough pain during titration phase. With each new dose during titration, 6 units should be prescribed, allowing treatment of several episodes of breakthrough pain. Adequate dose is determined based on effective analgesia with acceptable side effects. Side effects during titration period are usually greater than after effective dose is determined.
- Once an effective dose is determined, instruct patient to limit dose to 4 units/day. If >4 units/day are required, consider increasing the dose of the long-acting opioid.
- Discontinue with a gradual decrease in dose to prevent signs and symptoms of abrupt withdrawal.
- To dispose of remaining unit, using wire-cutting pliers cut off the drug matrix end so that it falls into the toilet. Flush remaining drug matrix down toilet. Drug remaining on handle may be removed by placing under running warm water until dissolved. Dispose of drug-free handle according to institutional protocol. ***High Alert:*** Partially consumed units are no longer protected by child-resistant pouch; dose may still be fatal. A temporary child-resistant storage bottle is provided for partially consumed units that cannot be disposed of properly.
- **SL: Abstral**: Dose must start with 100 mcg initially, titrate to adequate pain relief; if initial dose is adequate, this will be the dose for subsequent breakthrough pain; if dose is inadequate within 30 min give supplemental 100-mcg dose and ↑ next breakthrough dose by 100 mcg; if inadequate continue to ↑ breakthrough dose to 300, then 400, then 600 mcg, then 800 mcg; limit treatment to 4 episodes/24 hr.
- If inadequate analgesia after first dose, a 2nd dose may be used after 30 min. No more than 2 doses may be used to treat an episode of breakthrough pain. Episodes should be separated by at least 2 hr. Other rescue medications may be used as directed.
- Once a successful dose has been established, if more than 4 breakthrough pain episodes/day occur, reevaluate opioid dose for persistent pain.
- Place tablet on the floor of the mouth directly under the tongue and allow to dissolve completely; do not chew, suck, or swallow. Do not eat or drink anything until tablet is dissolved. In patients with dry mouth, water may be used to moisten oral mucosa *before* taking sublingual fentanyl. Advise patient to dispose of unused fentanyl sublingual tablets by removing from blister pack and flushing down toilet.
- **SL: Subsys**: Dose must start with 100 mcg initially, titrate to adequate pain relief; if initial dose is adequate, this will be the dose for subsequent breakthrough pain; if dose is inadequate within 30 min give supplemental 100-mcg dose and ↑ next breakthrough dose by 100 mcg; if inadequate continue to ↑ breakthrough dose to 400, then 600 mcg, then 800 mcg, then 1600 mcg.
- If inadequate analgesia after first dose, a 2nd dose may be used after 30 min. No more than 2 doses may be used to treat an episode of breakthrough pain. Episodes should be separated by at least 4 hr. Other rescue medications may be used as directed.
- Spray contents under tongue. Follow instructions in *Medication Guide*.
- Before you throw away the *Subsys* spray units, empty all of medicine (up to 10 spray units) into charcoal-lined disposal pouch provided with each dose. Put nozzle of spray unit upside-down into opening of charcoal-lined disposal pouch. Squeeze fingers and thumb together to spray into the charcoal lined disposal pouch. Place empty spray unit into pouch. To seal used charcoal-lined disposal pouch, remove backing from adhesive strip. Fold the flap down and press to seal charcoal-lined disposal pouch. Place sealed charcoal-lined disposal pouch into a disposal bag and seal. Discard sealed disposal bag in trash

F

out of reach of children. This protects others, especially children from harm. Follow instructions for use of disposal pouch in *Medication Guide* and *Instructions for Use*.

Patient/Family Teaching

- Instruct patient to take fentanyl as directed. Do not take more often than prescribed, keep out of reach of children, protect it from being stolen, and do not share with others, even if they have the same symptoms. Open only when ready to administer. Advise patient to review *Medication Guide* before and with each Rx refill; new information may be available. Advise patient to notify health care professional if breakthrough pain is not alleviated, worsens, if >4 units/day are required to control pain, or if excessive opioid effects occur.
- Explain TIRF REMS program to patient and caregiver. Patients must sign the Patient-Prescriber Agreement Form to confirm they understand the risks, appropriate use, and storage of fentanyl transmucosal.
- Advise patient to avoid grapefruit juice during therapy.
- Caution patient to make position changes slowly to minimize orthostatic hypotension.
- Medication causes dizziness and drowsiness. Advise patient to call for assistance during ambulation and transfer, and to avoid driving or other activities requiring alertness until response to medication is known.
- Instruct patient to avoid concurrent use of alcohol or other CNS depressants, such as sleep aids.
- Advise patient to notify health care professional if sores on gums or inside cheek become a problem.
- Advise patient to notify health care professional of all Rx or OTC medications, vitamins, or herbal products being taken and to consult with health care professional before taking other medications.
- Advise patient to notify health care professional if pregnancy is planned or suspected or if breast feeding.
- *Actiq*: Inform patient that this drug may contain sugar and may cause dry mouth. Advise patient to maintain good oral hygiene regular dental exams.

Evaluation/Desired Outcomes

- Decrease in severity of pain during episodes of breakthrough pain in patients receiving and tolerant to long-acting opioids.

ferric citrate (fe-rik si-trate)

Auryxia

Classification

Therapeutic: electrolyte modifiers
Pharmacologic: phosphate binders

Indications

Treatment of hyperphosphatemia in patients with chronic kidney disease on dialysis. Treatment of iron deficiency anemia in patients with chronic kidney disease not on dialysis.

Action

Binds phosphorous and precipitates it as ferric phosphate. After being transported through enterocytes into the blood, oxidized ferric iron circulates bound to transferrin where it is incorporated into hemoglobin. **Therapeutic Effects:** Maintenance of normal phosphorous levels. Resolution of iron deficiency anemia.

Pharmacokinetics

Absorption: Some absorption follows oral administration and may lead to iron overload.
Distribution: Unknown.
Metabolism and Excretion: Following binding, precipitated ferric phosphate is excreted in stool.
Half-life: Unknown.

TIME/ACTION PROFILE (lowering of serum phosphorous)

ROUTE	ONSET	PEAK	DURATION
PO	within 1 wk	unknown	unknown

Contraindications/Precautions

Contraindicated in: Iron overload syndromes including hemochromatosis.
Use Cautiously in: GI bleeding/inflammation; OB: Use cautiously during pregnancy (consider effects on vitamins/nutrient and potential iron overload); Lactation: Consider possible iron transport into milk; Pedi: Safety and effectiveness not established.

Adverse Reactions/Side Effects

GI: diarrhea, discolored feces, nausea, constipation, vomiting. **Hemat:** iron overload.

Interactions

Drug-Drug: Binds and ↓ absorption of **doxycycline** (should be given ≥1 hr prior to ferric citrate). Binds and ↓ absorption of **ciprofloxacin** (should be given ≥2 hr prior to or after ferric citrate).

Route/Dosage

Hyperphosphatemia

PO (Adults): 2 tablets (2 g ferric citrate) 3 times daily. Adjust by 1–2 tablets/day at weekly (or longer) intervals to attain and maintain target phosphorous levels (max = 12 tablets/day).

Iron Deficiency Anemia

PO (Adults): 1 tablet (1 g ferric citrate) 3 times daily. Adjust dose as needed to attain and maintain target hemoglobin levels (max = 12 tablets/day).

Availability (generic available)

Tablets: 1 g (contains 210 mg ferric iron).

NURSING IMPLICATIONS

Assessment

- Monitor clinical responses or blood levels of concurrent medications; may decrease bioavailability of medications administered concurrently.
- ***Lab Test Considerations:*** Monitor serum phosphorous prior to starting and periodically during therapy to keep serum phosphorous at target levels.
- Assess iron parameters (serum ferritin and transferritin saturation TSAT) prior to starting and periodically during therapy. May cause ↑ serum ferritin and TSAT requiring reduced dose or discontinuation of IV iron therapy.

Implementation

- **PO:** Administer 3 times daily with meals. Swallow tablets whole; do not crush or chew; may cause discoloration of mouth and teeth. Titrate doses no less than weekly.

Patient/Family Teaching

- Instruct patient to take ferric citrate as directed and to continue with prescribed diet.
- Advise patient that ferric citrate may cause dark stools; this is normal for medications containing iron.
- Inform patient that ferric citrate may cause diarrhea, nausea, constipation, and vomiting. Notify health care professional if GI symptoms become severe or persistent.
- Advise patient to notify health care professional of all Rx or OTC medications, vitamins, or herbal products being taken and to consult with health care professional before taking other medications. Medications may need to be taken separately from ferric citrate.
- Advise patient to store ferric citrate out of the reach of children; if accidentally ingested by a child seek immediate medical attention.
- Advise female patient to notify health care professional if pregnancy is planned or suspected or if breast feeding.

Evaluation/Desired Outcomes

- Normal serum phosphorous levels.

ferrous fumarate, See IRON SUPPLEMENTS.

ferrous gluconate, See IRON SUPPLEMENTS.

ferrous sulfate, See IRON SUPPLEMENTS.

🧬 fesoterodine

(fee-soe-**ter**-o-deen)

Toviaz

Classification

Therapeutic: urinary tract antispasmodics

Pharmacologic: anticholinergics

Indications

Treatment of overactive bladder function that results in urinary frequency, urgency, or urge incontinence.

Action

Acts as a competitive muscarinic receptor antagonist resulting in inhibition of cholinergically mediated bladder contraction. **Therapeutic Effects:** Decreased urinary frequency, urgency, and urge incontinence.

Pharmacokinetics

Absorption: Rapidly absorbed following oral administration, but is rapidly converted to its active metabolite (bioavailability of metabolite 52%); further metabolism occurs in the liver via CYP2D6 and CYP3A4 enzyme systems; 🧬 the CYP2D6 enzyme system exhibits genetic polymorphism; ~7% of population may be poor metabolizers (PMs) and may have significantly ↑ fesoterodine concentrations and an ↑ risk of adverse effects. 16% of active metabolite is excreted in urine, most of the remainder of inactive metabolites are renally excreted. 7% excreted in feces.

Distribution: Unknown.

Metabolism and Excretion: Rapidly converted by esterases to active metabolite.

Half-life: 7 hr (following oral administration).

TIME/ACTION PROFILE (active metabolite)

ROUTE	ONSET	PEAK	DURATION
PO	rapid	5 hr	24 hr

Contraindications/Precautions

Contraindicated in: Hypersensitivity; Urinary retention; Gastric retention; Severe hepatic impairment; Uncontrolled narrow-angle glaucoma.

Use Cautiously in: Significant bladder outlet obstruction (↑ risk of retention); Severe renal insufficiency (dose adjustment required); ↓ GI motility including severe constipation; Treated narrow-angle glaucoma (use only if benefits outweigh risks); Myasthenia gravis; Severe renal impairment (dose should not exceed 4 mg/day); Geri: ↑ risk of anticholinergic side effects in patients >75 yr; OB, Lactation: Avoid using unless potential benefits outweighs potential risk to fetus/neonate; Pedi: Safety not established.

Adverse Reactions/Side Effects

CNS: dizziness, drowsiness, headache. **CV:** tachycardia (dose related). **GI:** <u>dry mouth</u>, constipation, nausea, upper abdominal pain. **GU:** dysuria, urinary retention. **MS:** back pain. **Misc:** ANGIOEDEMA.

Interactions

Drug-Drug: Concurrent use of **potent CYP3A4 enzyme inhibitors** including **ketoconazole**, **itraconazole**, and **clarithromycin** ↑ blood levels and risk of toxicity; daily dose should not exceed 4 mg. Use **less potent inhibitors of CYP3A4** (such as **erythromycin**) with caution; escalate dose carefully. Anticholinergic effects may alter the GI absorption of other drugs.

Route/Dosage

PO (Adults): 4 mg once daily initially may be ↑ to 8 mg/daily; *Concurrent potent CYP3A4 inhibitors or CCr <30 mL/min*—dose should not exceed 4 mg/day.

Availability (generic available)

Extended-release tablets: 4 mg, 8 mg.

NURSING IMPLICATIONS

Assessment

- Assess for urinary urgency, frequency, and urge incontinence periodically during therapy.
- Monitor for signs and symptoms of angioedema (swelling of face, lips, tongue, and/or larynx). May occur with first or subsequent doses. Discontinue therapy and prove supportive therapy. Have epinephrine, corticosteroids, and resuscitation equipment available.
- ***Lab Test Considerations:*** May cause ↑ ALT and GGT.

Implementation

- **PO:** Administer without regard to food.
- Swallow extended-release tablets whole; do not break, crush, or chew.

Patient/Family Teaching

- Instruct patient to take fesoterodine as directed. If a dose is missed, omit and begin taking again the next day; do not take 2 doses the same day. Advise patient to read the *Patient Information* sheet prior to initiation of therapy and with each Rx refill in case of changes.
- May cause drowsiness, dizziness, and blurred vision. Caution patient to avoid driving or other activities requiring alertness until response to medication is known.
- Advise patient to avoid alcohol; may increase drowsiness.
- Advise patient to use caution in hot environments; may cause decreased sweating and severe heat illness.
- Instruct patient to notify health care professional of all Rx or OTC medications, vitamins, or herbal products being taken and to consult with health care professional before taking other medications.
- Advise patient to stop medication and notify health care professional if signs and symptoms of angioedema occur.
- Advise patient to notify health care professional if pregnancy is planned or suspected or if breast feeding.

Evaluation/Desired Outcomes

- Decreased urinary frequency, urgency, and urge incontinence.

fexofenadine

(fex-oh-**fen**-a-deen)

~~Allegra~~, Allegra Allergy, Children's Allegra Allergy, ~~Children's Allegra Hives~~, ~~Mucinex Allergy~~

Classification

Therapeutic: allergy, cold, and cough remedies, antihistamines

Indications

Relief of symptoms of seasonal allergic rhinitis. Management of chronic idiopathic urticaria.

Action

Antagonizes the effects of histamine at peripheral histamine–1 (H_1) receptors, including pruritus and urticaria. Also has a drying effect on the nasal mucosa.

Therapeutic Effects: Decreased sneezing, rhinorrhea, itchy eyes, nose, and throat associated with seasonal allergies. Decreased urticaria.

Pharmacokinetics

Absorption: Rapidly absorbed after oral administration.

Distribution: Unknown.

Metabolism and Excretion: 80% excreted in urine, 11% excreted in feces.

Half-life: 14.4 hr (↑ in renal impairment).

TIME/ACTION PROFILE (antihistaminic effect)

ROUTE	ONSET	PEAK	DURATION
PO	within 1 hr	2–3 hr	12–24 hr

Contraindications/Precautions

Contraindicated in: Hypersensitivity.

Use Cautiously in: Renal impairment (↑ dosing interval recommended); OB: Use only if potential maternal benefit justifies potential fetal risk; Lactation: Safety not established.

Adverse Reactions/Side Effects

CNS: drowsiness, fatigue. **GI:** dyspepsia. **GU:** dysmenorrhea.

Interactions

Drug-Drug: Magnesium and aluminum-containing antacids ↓ absorption and may decrease effectiveness.

Drug-Food: Apple, **orange**, and **grapefruit juice** ↓ absorption and may decrease effectiveness.

Route/Dosage

PO (Adults and Children ≥12 yr): 60 mg twice daily, or 180 mg once daily.
PO (Children 2–11 yr): 30 mg twice daily.
PO (Children 6 mo–2 yr): 15 mg twice daily.

Renal Impairment

PO (Adults): 60 mg once daily as a starting dose.
PO (Children 6–11 yr): 30 mg once daily as a starting dose.

Availability (generic available)

Gelcaps: 180 mg^{OTC}. **Orally disintegrating tablets:** 30 mg^{OTC}. **Suspension (berry flavor):** 30 mg/5 mL^{OTC}. **Tablets:** 60 mg^{OTC}, ✽ 120 mg^{OTC}, 180 mg^{OTC}. ***In combination with:*** pseudoephedrine (Allegra-D). See Appendix B.

NURSING IMPLICATIONS

Assessment

- Assess allergy symptoms (rhinitis, conjunctivitis, hives) before and periodically during therapy.
- Assess lung sounds and character of bronchial secretions. Maintain fluid intake of 1500–2000 mL/day to decrease viscosity of secretions.
- ***Lab Test Considerations:*** Will cause false-negative reactions on allergy skin tests; discontinue 3 days before testing.

Implementation

- Do not confuse Allegra (fexofenadine) with Viagra (sildenafil). Do not confuse Allegra (fexofenadine) with Allegra Anti-Itch Cream (diphenhydramine/allantoin).
- **PO:** Administer with food or milk to decrease GI irritation. Administer capsules and tablets with water or milk, not juice. Shake solution bottle well before use.

Patient/Family Teaching

- Instruct patient to take medication as directed. Take missed doses as soon as remembered unless almost time for next dose. Do not take more than recommended.
- Instruct patient or parents to avoid taking fexofenadine with fruit juices (apple, orange, grapefruit) or antacids containing aluminum or magnesium; may decrease effectiveness of fexofenadine.
- Inform patient that drug may cause drowsiness, although it is less likely to occur than with other antihistamines. Avoid driving or other activities requiring alertness until response to drug is known.
- Advise females of reproductive potential to notify health care professional if pregnancy is planned or suspected or if breast feeding.
- Instruct patient to contact health care professional if symptoms persist.

Evaluation/Desired Outcomes

- Decrease in allergic symptoms.
- Decrease in urticaria.

fidaxomicin (fi-dax-oh-mye-sin)

Dificid

Classification
Therapeutic: anti-infectives
Pharmacologic: macrolides

Indications

Treatment of diarrhea associated with *Clostridium difficile*.

Action

Bactericial action mostly against clostridia; inhibits RNA synthesis. Acts locally in the GI tract to eliminate *Clostridium difficile*. **Therapeutic Effects:** Elimination of diarrhea caused by *Clostridium difficile*.

Pharmacokinetics

Absorption: Minimal systemic absorption.
Distribution: Stays primarily in the GI tract.
Metabolism and Excretion: Mostly transformed via hydrolysis in the GI tract to OP-1118, its active metabolite. Eliminated mostly (>92%) in feces: <1% excreted in urine.
Half-life: *Fidaxomicin*—11.7 hr; *OP-1118*—11.2 hr.

TIME/ACTION PROFILE

ROUTE	ONSET	PEAK	DURATION
PO	unknown	unknown	unknown

Contraindications/Precautions

Contraindicated in: Hypersensitivity to fidaxomicin or macrolides (cross-sensitivity may occur).
Use Cautiously in: OB: Use only if potential maternal benefit justifies potential fetal risk; Lactation: Use while breast feeding only if potential maternal benefit justifies potential risk to infant; Pedi: Safety and effectiveness not established.

Adverse Reactions/Side Effects

GI: GI HEMORRHAGE, <u>nausea</u>, abdominal pain. **Hemat:** anemia, neutropenia. **Misc:** HYPERSENSITIVITY REACTIONS (including angioedema).

Interactions

Drug-Drug: None reported.

Route/Dosage

PO (Adults): 200 mg twice daily for 10 days.

Availability

Tablets: 200 mg.

NURSING IMPLICATIONS

Assessment

- Monitor bowel function for diarrhea, abdominal cramping, fever, and bloody stools. May begin up to several wk following cessation of antibiotic therapy.
- Monitor for signs and symptoms of hypersensitivity reactions (dyspnea, pruritus, rash, angioedema of mouth, throat, and face) periodically during therapy. Risk increases with a macrolide allergy.
- ***Lab Test Considerations:*** May cause ↑ serum alkaline phosphatase, and hepatic enzymes.
- May cause ↓ serum bicarbonate, ↓ platelet count, anemia, and neutropenia.
- May cause hyperglycemia and metabolic acidosis.

Implementation

- **PO:** Administer twice daily, about 12 hr apart, without regard to food.

Patient/Family Teaching

- Instruct patient to take fidamoxicin twice daily, 12 hr apart, as directed for the full course of therapy, even if feeling better. Skipping doses or not completing full course of therapy may decrease effectiveness of therapy and increase risk that bacteria will develop resistance and not be treatable in the future.
- Advise patient to notify health care professional of all Rx or OTC medications, vitamins, or herbal products being taken and to consult with health care professional before taking other medications.
- Advise females of reproductive potential to notify health care professional if pregnancy is planned or suspected or if breast feeding.

Evaluation/Desired Outcomes

- Decrease in diarrhea caused by *Clostridium difficile*.

filgrastim (fil-gra-stim)

Granix, 🍁Grastofil, Neupogen, Nivestym, Zarxio

Classification
Therapeutic: colony-stimulating factors

Indications

Prevention of febrile neutropenia and associated infection in patients who have received bone marrow–depressing antineoplastics for the treatment of nonmyeloid malignancies. Reduction of time for neutrophil recovery and duration of fever in patients undergoing induction and consolidation chemotherapy for acute myelogenous leukemia. Reduction of time to neutrophil recovery and sequelae of neutropenia in patients with nonmyeloid malignancies undergoing myeloablative chemotherapy followed by bone marrow transplantation. Mobilization of hematopoietic progenitor cells into peripheral blood for collection by leukapheresis. Management of severe chronic neutropenia. Survival improvement in patients acutely exposed to myelosuppressive doses of radiation. **Unlabeled Use:** Neutropenia associated with HIV infection. Neonatal neutropenia.

Action

A glycoprotein, filgrastim binds to and stimulates immature neutrophils to divide and differentiate. Also activates mature neutrophils. **Therapeutic Effects:** Decreased incidence of infection in patients who are neutropenic from chemotherapy or other causes. Improved harvest of progenitor cells for bone marrow transplantation. Improved survival in patients exposed to myelosuppressive doses of radiation.

Pharmacokinetics

Absorption: Well absorbed after subcut administration.
Distribution: Unknown.
Metabolism and Excretion: Unknown.
Half-life: *Adults*—3.5 hr; *Neonates*—4.4 hr.

TIME/ACTION PROFILE

ROUTE	ONSET	PEAK	DURATION
IV, subcut	unknown	unknown	4 days†

†Return of neutrophil count to baseline.

Contraindications/Precautions

Contraindicated in: Hypersensitivity to filgrastim or *Escherichia coli*-derived proteins.
Use Cautiously in: Malignancy with myeloid characteristics; Pre-existing cardiac disease; OB: Use only if potential maternal benefit justifies potential fetal risk; Lactation: Use while breast feeding only if potential maternal benefit justifies potential risk to infant.

Adverse Reactions/Side Effects

CV: aortitis, vasculitis. **EENT:** hemoptysis. **GI:** SPLENIC RUPTURE, splenomegaly. **GU:** glomerulonephritis. **Hemat:** excessive leukocytosis, sickle cell crises, thrombocytopenia. **Local:** pain at injection site. **MS:** medullary bone pain. **Resp:** ACUTE RESPIRATORY DISTRESS SYNDROME, pulmonary infiltrates. **Misc:** HYPERSENSITIVITY REACTIONS (including anaphylaxis).

Interactions

Drug-Drug: Simultaneous use with **antineoplastics** may have adverse effects on rapidly proliferating neutrophils—avoid use for 24 hr before and 24 hr after chemotherapy. **Lithium** may potentiate the release of neutrophils; concurrent use should be undertaken cautiously.

Route/Dosage

After Myelosuppressive Chemotherapy

IV, Subcut (Adults and Children): 5 mcg/kg/day as a single subcut injection, by short IV infusion, or via continuous IV infusion for up to 2 wk or until ANC reaches 10,000/mm^3. Initiate at least 24 hr after chemotherapy. Dose may be ↑ by 5 mcg/kg during each cycle of chemotherapy, depending on blood counts.

After Bone Marrow Transplantation

IV (Adults): 10 mcg/kg/day as a continuous IV infusion for up to 24 hr; initiate at least 24 hr after chemotherapy and at least 24 hr after bone marrow transplantation. Subsequent dose is adjusted according to blood counts.

Peripheral Blood Progenitor Cell Collection and Therapy

Subcut (Adults): 10 mcg/kg/day for at least 4 days before first leukapheresis and continued until last leukapheresis; Discontinue if WBC >100,000 cells/mm³.

Severe Chronic Neutropenia

Subcut (Adults): *Congenital neutropenia*—6 mcg/kg twice daily. *Idiopathic/cyclical neutropenia*—5 mcg/kg daily (↓ if ANC remains >10,000/mm³).

After Myelosuppressive Radiation

Subcut (Adults): 10 mcg/kg once daily; initiate as soon as possible after exposure to radiation doses greater than 2 gray (Gy); continue until ANC remains >1000/mm³ for 3 consecutive blood counts (performed every 3 days) or is >10,000/mm³ after a radiation-induced nadir.

Neonatal Neutropenia

IV, Subcut (Neonates): 5–10 mcg/kg/day once daily for 3–5 days.

Availability

Solution for injection (prefilled syringes): 300 mcg/0.5 mL, 480 mcg/0.8 mL. **Solution for injection (vials):** 300 mcg/1 mL, 480 mcg/1.6 mL.

NURSING IMPLICATIONS

Assessment

- Monitor heart rate, BP, and respiratory status before and periodically during therapy.
- Assess bone pain throughout therapy. Pain is usually mild to moderate and controllable with nonopioid analgesics, but may require treatment with opioid analgesics, especially in patients receiving high-dose IV therapy. Loratadine 10 mg PO administered before filgrastim dose has been used to prevent bone pain.
- Monitor for signs and symptoms of allergic reactions (rash, urticaria, facial edema, wheezing, dyspnea, hypotension, tachycardia). Usually occur within 30 min of administration. Treatment includes antihistamines, steroids, bronchodilators, and/or epinephrine; may recur with rechallenge.
- Assess for signs and symptoms of acute respiratory distress syndrome (fever, lung infiltrates, or respiratory distress). If symptoms occur, withhold filgrastim until symptoms resolve or discontinue.
- Monitor for signs and symptoms of splenic enlargement or rupture (left upper abdominal or shoulder pain).
- May cause transient positive bone-imaging changes.
- ***Lab Test Considerations:*** *After chemotherapy,* obtain a CBC with differential, including examination for the presence of blast cells, and platelet count before chemotherapy and twice weekly during therapy to avoid leukocytosis. Monitor ANC. A transient rise is seen 1–2 days after initiation of therapy, but therapy should not be discontinued until ANC >10,000/mm³.
- *After bone marrow transplant,* the daily dose is titrated by the neutrophil response. When the ANC is >1000/mm³ for 3 consecutive days, reduce dose to 5 mcg/kg/day. If the ANC remains >1000/mm³ for 3 or more consecutive days, discontinue filgrastim. If the ANC decreases to <1000/mm³, resume filgrastim at 5 mcg/kg/day.
- *For chronic severe neutropenia,* monitor CBC with differential and platelet count twice weekly during initial 4 wk of therapy and during 2 wk after any dose adjustment.
- May cause ↓ platelet count and transient ↑ in uric acid, LDH, and alkaline phosphatase concentrations.

Implementation

- Administer no earlier than 24 hr after cytotoxic chemotherapy, at least 24 hr after bone marrow infusion, and not during the 24 hr before administration of chemotherapy.
- Refrigerate; do not freeze. Do not shake. May warm to room temperature for up to 6 hr before injection. Discard if left at room temperature for >6 hr. Vial is for 1-time use only.
- **Subcut:** May be administered in outer area of upper arms, abdomen, thighs, or upper outer areas of buttock. If dose requires >1 mL of solution, may be divided into 2 injection sites.
- Cap of needle contains latex; avoid administration by persons with latex allergy.
- May also be administered as a continuous subcut infusion over 24 hr after bone marrow transplantation.

IV Administration

- **Continuous Infusion:** ***Diluent:*** Dilute in D5W; do not dilute with 0.9% NaCl, will precipitate. Refrigerate; do not freeze. Do not shake. May warm to room temperature for up to 6 hr before injection. Vial is for 1-time use only. ***Concentration:*** Dilute to a final concentration of at least 15 mcg/mL. If the final concentration is <15 mcg/mL, human albumin in a concentration of 2 mg/mL must be added to D5W before filgrastim to prevent adsorption of the components of the drug delivery system. May be stored at room temperature for up to 24 hr. ***Rate:*** *After chemotherapy* dose is administered via infusion over 15–60 min.
- *After chemotherapy* dose may also be administered as a continuous infusion.
- *After bone marrow transplant,* administer dose as an infusion over 4 or 24 hr.

- **Y-Site Compatibility:** acyclovir, allopurinol, amikacin, aminophylline, ampicillin, ampicillin/sulbactam, aztreonam, bleomycin, bumetanide, buprenorphine, butorphanol, calcium gluconate, carboplatin, carmustine, cefazolin, cefotetan, ceftazidime, chlorpromazine, cisplatin, cyclophosphamide, cytarabine, dacarbazine, daunorubicin hydrochloride, dexamethasone, diphenhydramine, doxorubicin, doxycycline, droperidol, enalaprilat, famotidine, floxuridine, fluconazole, fludarabine, ganciclovir, granisetron, haloperidol, hydrocortisone, hydromorphone, idarubicin, ifosfamide, leucovorin calcium, levofloxacin, lorazepam, melphalan, meperidine, mesna, methotrexate, metoclopramide, mitoxantrone, morphine, nalbuphine, ondansetron, posaconazole, potassium chloride, promethazine, ranitidine, rituximab, sodium acetate, sodium bicarbonate, streptozocin, tobramycin, trastuzumab, trimethoprim/sulfamethoxazole, vancomycin, vinblastine, vincristine, vinorelbine, zidovudine.
- **Y-Site Incompatibility:** aminocaproic acid, cefepime, cefotaxime, cefoxitin, ceftaroline, ceftriaxone, cefuroxime, clindamycin, dactinomycin, etoposide, fluorouracil, furosemide, heparin, mannitol, methylprednisolone, metronidazole, mitomycin, prochlorperazine, thiotepa.

Patient/Family Teaching

- Explain purpose of filgrastim to patient. Instruct patient and caregiver on correct technique for injection, care and disposal of equipment. Advise patient to notify health care professional regarding when to give next dose if a dose is missed. Instruct patient and caregiver to read *Instructions for Patients and Caregivers* before starting therapy and with each Rx refill in case of changes.
- Instruct patient to notify health care professional immediately if signs and symptoms of spleen enlargement or rupture, allergic reaction, ARDS, glomerulonephritis (swelling of face or ankles, dark colored urine or blood in urine, decrease in urine production) or vasculitis (skin redness, purple spots on skin) occur. Discuss risk of sickle cell crisis with patients with sickle cell disease before administering.
- Advise patient to notify health care professional of all Rx or OTC medications, vitamins, or herbal products being taken and to consult with health care professional before taking other medications.
- Rep: Advise females of reproductive potential to notify health care professional if pregnancy is planned or suspected or if breast feeding.
- **Home Care Issues:** Instruct patient on correct technique and proper disposal for home administration. Caution patient not to reuse needle, vial, or syringe. Provide patient with a puncture-proof container for needle and syringe disposal.

Evaluation/Desired Outcomes

- Decreased incidence of infection in patients who receive bone marrow–depressing antineoplastics.
- Reduction of duration and sequelae of neutropenia after bone marrow transplantation.
- Reduction of the incidence and duration of sequelae of neutropenia in patients with severe chronic neutropenia.
- Improved harvest of progenitor cells for bone marrow transplantation.
- Improved survival in patients exposed to myelosuppressive doses of radiation.

finasteride (fi-nas-teer-ide)

Propecia, Proscar

Classification

Therapeutic: hair regrowth stimulants

Pharmacologic: androgen inhibitors

Indications

Benign prostatic hyperplasia (BPH); can be used with doxazosin. Androgenetic alopecia (male pattern baldness) in men only.

Action

Inhibits the enzyme 5-alpha-reductase, which is responsible for converting testosterone to its potent metabolite 5-alpha-dihydrotestosterone in prostate, liver, and skin; 5-alpha-dihydrotestosterone is partially responsible for prostatic hyperplasia and hair loss. **Therapeutic Effects:** Reduced prostate size with associated decrease in urinary symptoms. Decreases hair loss; promotes hair regrowth.

Pharmacokinetics

Absorption: Well absorbed after oral administration (63%).

Distribution: Enters prostatic tissue and crosses the blood-brain barrier. Remainder of distribution not known.

Protein Binding: 90%.

Metabolism and Excretion: Mostly metabolized; 39% excreted in urine as metabolites; 57% excreted in feces.

Half-life: 6 hr (range 6–15 hr; slightly ↑ in patients >70 yr).

TIME/ACTION PROFILE (↓ in dihydrotestosterone levels†)

ROUTE	ONSET	PEAK	DURATION
PO	rapid	8 hr	2 wk

†Clinical effects as noted by urinary tract symptoms and hair regrowth may not be evident for several mo and remain for 4 mo after discontinuation.

Contraindications/Precautions

Contraindicated in: Hypersensitivity; Women.

Use Cautiously in: Hepatic impairment;; Obstructive uropathy.

Adverse Reactions/Side Effects

Endo: gynecomastia. **GU:** PROSTATE CANCER (HIGH-GRADE), ↓ libido, ↓ volume of ejaculate, erectile dysfunction, infertility. **Misc:** ANGIOEDEMA, BREAST CANCER.

Interactions

Drug-Drug: None reported.

Route/Dosage

PO (Adults): *BPH*—5 mg once daily (Proscar); *Androgenetic alopecia*—1 mg once daily (Propecia).

Availability (generic available)

Tablets: 1 mg (Propecia), 5 mg (Proscar). **Cost:** *Generic*—1 mg $134.61/100, 5 mg $21.85/100.

NURSING IMPLICATIONS

Assessment

- Assess for symptoms of prostatic hyperplasia (urinary hesitancy, feeling of incomplete bladder emptying, interruption of urinary stream, impairment of size and force of urinary stream, terminal urinary dribbling, straining to start flow, dysuria, urgency) before and periodically during therapy.
- Digital rectal examinations should be performed before and periodically during therapy for BPH.
- ***Lab Test Considerations:*** Serum prostate-specific antigen (PSA) concentrations, which are used to screen for prostate cancer, may be evaluated before and periodically during therapy. Finasteride may cause a ↓ in serum PSA levels.

Implementation

- Do not confuse Proscar (finasteride) with Prograf (tacrolimus) or Provera (medroxyprogesterone).
- **PO:** Administer once daily with or without meals.

Patient/Family Teaching

- Instruct patient to take finasteride as directed, even if symptoms improve or are unchanged. At least 6–12 mo of therapy may be necessary to determine whether or not an individual will respond to finasteride. Advise patient to read the *Patient Package Insert* prior to starting therapy and with each Rx refill in case of changes.
- Inform patient that the volume of ejaculate may be decreased and erectile dysfunction and decreased libido may occur during therapy and after therapy is completed.
- Advise patient to notify health care professional promptly if changes in breasts (lumps, pain, nipple discharge) occur.
- Inform patient that there is an increased risk of high grade prostate cancer in men taking this drug.
- Rep: Caution patient that finasteride poses a potential risk to a male fetus. Women who are pregnant or may become pregnant should avoid exposure to semen of a partner taking finasteride and should not handle crushed finasteride because of the potential for absorption.
- Emphasize the importance of periodic follow-up exams to determine whether a clinical response has occurred.

Evaluation/Desired Outcomes

- Decrease in urinary symptoms of benign prostatic hyperplasia.
- Hair regrowth in androgenetic alopecia. Evidence of hair growth usually requires 3 mo or longer. Continued use is recommended to sustain benefit. Withdrawal leads to reversal of effect within 12 mo.

fingolimod (fin-go-li-mod)

Gilenya

Classification
Therapeutic: anti-multiple sclerosis agents
Pharmacologic: receptor modulators

Indications

Relapsing forms of multiple sclerosis (MS), including clinically isolated syndrome, relapsing-remitting disease, and active secondary progressive disease.

Action

Converted by sphingosine kinase to the active metabolite fingolimod-phosphate, which binds to sphingosine 1–phosphate receptors, resulting in ↓ migration of lymphocytes into peripheral blood. This may ↓ lymphocyte migration into the CNS. **Therapeutic Effects:** ↓ frequency of relapses/delayed accumulation of disability.

Pharmacokinetics

Absorption: Well absorbed (93%) following oral administration.

Distribution: Extensively distributed to body tissues; 86% of parent drug distributes into red blood cells; active metabolite uptake 17%.

Metabolism and Excretion: Converted to its active metabolite, then metabolized mostly by the CYP450 4F2 enzyme system, with further degradation by other enzyme systems. Most inactive metabolites excreted in urine (81%); <2.5% excreted as fingolimod and fingolimod-phosphate in feces.

Protein Binding: >99.7%.

Half-life: 6–9 hr.

TIME/ACTION PROFILE

ROUTE	ONSET	PEAK	DURATION
PO	unknown	1–2 mo*	2 mo†

*Time to steady state blood levels, peak blood levels after a single dose at 12–16 hr.

†Time for complete elimination.

Contraindications/Precautions

Contraindicated in: Hypersensitivity; MI, unstable angina, stroke, TIA, or class III or IV HF within previous 6 mo; 2nd- or 3rd-degree heart block or sick sinus syndrome (in the absence of a pacemaker); QT interval ≥500 msec; Cardiac arrhythmias requiring use of class Ia or III antiarrhythmics; Active acute/chronic untreated infections; Lactation: Breast feeding should be avoided.

Use Cautiously in: Concurrent use of beta blockers, diltiazem, verapamil, or digoxin (↑ risk of bradycardia/heart block); History of ischemic heart disease, MI, HF, cerebrovascular disease, uncontrolled hypertension, AV or SA heart block, symptomatic bradycardia, recurrent syncope, cardiac arrest, or severe untreated sleep apnea (↑ risk of bradycardia/heart block); QT interval prolongation before doing or during observation period (>450 msec in adult and pediatric males, >470 msec in adult females, >460 msec in pediatric females), hypokalemia, hypomagnesemia, congenital long QT syndrome, or concurrent use of QT interval prolonging medications (↑ risk of QT interval prolongation); Severe hepatic impairment (↑ blood levels and risk of adverse reactions); Diabetes mellitus/history of uveitis (↑ risk of macular edema); Negative history for chickenpox or vaccination against varicella zoster virus vaccination; Geri: Risk of adverse reactions may be ↑ consider age-related ↓ in cardiac/renal/hepatic function, chronic illnesses, and concurrent drug therapy; Pedi: Children <10 yr (safety and effectiveness not established); OB: Use only if potential benefit justifies potential risk to fetus.

Adverse Reactions/Side Effects

CNS: POSTERIOR REVERSIBLE ENCEPHALOPATHY SYNDROME (PRES), PROGRESSIVE MULTIFOCAL LEUKOENCEPHALOPATHY (PML), headache. **CV:** ASYSTOLE, BRADYCARDIA, HEART BLOCK, QT INTERVAL PROLONGATION, hypertension, syncope. **Derm:** BASAL CELL CARCINOMA, MELANOMA. **EENT:** blurred vision, eye pain, macular edema. **GI:** HEPATOTOXICITY, diarrhea, ↑ liver enzymes. **Hemat:** leukopenia, lymphopenia. **MS:** back pain. **Resp:** cough, ↓ pulmonary function. **Misc:** HYPERSENSITIVITY REACTIONS (including rash, urticaria, and angioedema), INFECTION (including bacterial, viral and fungal), LYMPHOMA.

Interactions

Drug-Drug: **Class Ia or class III antiarrhythmics** may ↑ risk of serious arrhythmias; concurrent use contraindicated. Concurrent use of **beta blockers**, **diltiazem**, **verapamil**, **ivabradine**, **clonidine**, or **digoxin** may ↑ risk of bradycardia; careful monitoring recommended. Concurrent use of **QT-interval prolonging medications** may ↑ risk of QT interval prolongation and torsade de pointes. Concurrent use of **ketoconazole** may ↑ blood levels and risk of adverse reactions. ↑ risk of immunosuppression with **antineoplastics**, **immunosuppressants**, or **immune modulating therapies**. **Live-attenuated vaccines** ↑ risk of infection.

Route/Dosage

PO (Adults and Children ≥10 yr and >40 kg): 0.5 mg once daily.
PO (Children ≥10 yr and ≤40 kg): 0.25 mg once daily.

Availability

Capsules: 0.25 mg, 0.5 mg.

NURSING IMPLICATIONS

Assessment

- Perform *first-dose monitoring* in all patients when starting therapy, when re-starting therapy after drug was discontinued for at least 14 days, when therapy is interrupted ≥1 day within first 2 wk of therapy; when therapy is interrupted for >7 days during wks 3 and 4 of therapy, and in pediatric patients when increasing dose.
- *First dose monitoring:* Monitor pulse and BP hourly for bradycardia for at least 6 hr following first dose and periodically during therapy. Obtain baseline ECG before first dose and at end of observation period. *If after 6 hrs of therapy* patient develops heart rate <45 bpm in adults, <55 bpm in pediatric patients ≥12 yrs, or <60 bpm in pediatric patients 10 or 11 yrs of age; heart rate 6 hrs postdose is at lowest value postdose, maximum pharmacodynamic effect on the heart may not have occurred; ECG 6 hrs postdose shows new onset second degree or higher AV block continue monitoring until resolves. If pharmacological treatment is required, continue monitoring overnight and repeat 6-hr monitoring after the second dose. Monitor ECG continuously overnight if pharmacologic intervention for symptomatic bradycardia required, patient has preexisting heart or cerebrovascular condition, patients has a prolonged QTc interval before dosing or during 6-hr observation, or at risk for QT prolongation, or on concurrent therapy with QT prolonging drugs.
- Monitor for signs of infection (fever, tiredness, body aches, chills, nausea, vomiting, headache, sore throat) during and for 2 mo after discontinuation of therapy. Consider suspending therapy if serious infection develops.
- Perform an ophthalmologic exam prior to starting fingolimod, at 3–4 mo after starting therapy, and if visual disturbances occur. Monitor visual acuity at baseline and during routine exams. Patients with diabetes or history of uveitis are at ↑ risk and should have regular ophthalmologic exams.
- Monitor pulmonary function tests for decline periodically during therapy. Obtain spirometry and diffusion lung capacity for carbon monoxide when indicated clinically.
- Assess for any new signs or symptoms that may be suggestive of PML, an opportunistic infection of the

brain caused by the Jakob Cruzfeldt (JC) virus, that may be fatal; hold dose and notify health care professional promptly. PML symptoms may begin gradually (hemiparesis, apathy, confusion, cognitive deficiencies, and ataxia) and may include deteriorating renal function. Monitoring MRI every 6 mo may identify PML before clinical signs and symptoms occur.

- May cause severe increase in disability upon discontinuation of therapy. Monitor patients for increase in disability 12–24 wk following discontinuation.
- ***Lab Test Considerations:*** Obtain baseline liver function tests before starting, periodically during, and for 2 mo after therapy discontinued. May cause ↑ liver transaminases and bilirubin. Monitor liver function tests if symptoms develop and discontinue therapy if liver injury is confirmed.
- Before initiating therapy, obtain a recent (within 6 mo) CBC. May cause ↓ lymphocyte counts.
- Test patients for antibodies to varicella zoster virus (VZV) before starting therapy. Administer varicella vaccine to patients who are antibody negative before starting therapy. Complete all immunizations in accordance with current immunization guidelines for pediatric patients before starting therapy.
- May cause decreased lymphocyte count for up to 2 mo following discontinuation.

Implementation

- **PO:** Administer once daily without regard to food.

Patient/Family Teaching

- Instruct patient to take fingolimod as directed. If a dose is missed, contact health care professional before taking next dose; may need to be observed by a health care professional for at least 6 hrs after taking next dose. Do not discontinue therapy without consulting health care professional, may cause severe increase in disability. Advise patient to read the *Medication Guide* prior to starting therapy and with each Rx refill in case of changes.
- Advise patient to notify health care professional if signs and symptoms of liver dysfunction (unexplained nausea, vomiting, abdominal pain, fatigue, anorexia, jaundice, dark urine), infection, PML, new onset of dyspnea, PRES (sudden headache, confusion, seizures, loss of vision, weakness), hypersensitivity reactions (rash or itchy hives, swelling of lips, tongue, or face), skin nodules (shiny pearly nodules), patches or open sores that do not heal within weeks, or changes in vision develop.
- Instruct patient not to receive live-attenuated vaccines during and for 2 mo after treatment due to risk of infection. Patients who have not had a health care professional confirmed history of chickenpox or documentation of a full course vaccination should be tested for antibodies to varicella zoster virus before starting therapy. Antibody-negative patients should receive vaccination prior to starting therapy, then postpone start of fingolimod for 1 mo to allow for full effect of vaccination.
- Advise patient to notify health care professional of all Rx or OTC medications, vitamins, or herbal products being taken and to consult with health care professional before taking other medications.
- May cause basal cell carcinoma, melanoma, and lymphoma. Caution patient to use sunscreen with a high protection factor, wear protective clothing, and limit exposure to sunlight and ultraviolet light.
- Rep: Advise female patients to use contraception during and for at least 2 mo after discontinuation of therapy and to notify health care professional immediately if pregnancy is planned or suspected or if breast feeding. Encourage pregnant patients to enroll in the pregnancy registry by calling 1-877-598-7237 or visiting www.gilenyapregnancyregistry.com.

Evaluation/Desired Outcomes

- Reduction in frequency of clinical exacerbations and delay of accumulation of physical disability in patients with relapsing forms of multiple sclerosis.

REMS

flibanserin (flib-an-ser-in)

Addyi

Classification

Therapeutic: sexual dysfunction agents

Indications

Treatment of premenopausal women with hypoactive sexual desire disorder (HSDD) unrelated to concurrent medical/psychiatric diagnoses, relationship issues, or substance abuse. Does not enhance sexual performance.

Action

May be explained by agonist activity at $5-HT_{1A}$ receptors and antagonist activity at $5-HT_{2A}$ receptors; also has moderate antagonist activity at $5-HT_{2B}$, $5-HT_{2C}$, and dopamine D_4 receptors. **Therapeutic Effects:** ↑ sexual desire with ↓ distress and interpersonal dysfunction.

Pharmacokinetics

Absorption: Moderately absorbed (33%) following oral administration.

Distribution: Unknown.

Protein Binding: 98%.

Metabolism and Excretion: Highly metabolized, mostly by the CYP3A4 enzyme system with lesser metabolized by CYP2C19; the CYP2C19 enzyme system exhibits genetic polymorphism; poor metabolizers may have significantly ↑ flibanserin concentrations and an

↑ risk of adverse effects. 44% excreted in urine, 51% in feces almost entirely as metabolites which do not appear to be pharmacologically active.
Half-life: 11 hr.

TIME/ACTION PROFILE (blood levels)

ROUTE	ONSET	PEAK	DURATION
PO	within 1 hr	1 hr	24 hr

Contraindications/Precautions

Contraindicated in: Alcohol ingestion (excess risk of hypotension/syncope); Concurrent use of strong/moderate CYP3A4 inhibitors; Concurrent use of CYP3A4 inducers; Hepatic impairment; Lactation: Breast feeding is not recommended.
Use Cautiously in: CYP2C19 poor metabolizers (↑ risk of adverse reactions including hypotension, syncope, and drowsiness); Geri: Not indicated for use in the elderly; OB: Safe use during pregnancy has not been established; Pedi: Not indicated for use in children.

Adverse Reactions/Side Effects

CNS: dizziness, drowsiness, anxiety, fatigue, insomnia, vertigo. **CV:** HYPOTENSION/SYNCOPE. **GI:** nausea, constipation, dry mouth. **Derm:** rash.

Interactions

Drug-Drug: Concurrent use of **strong or moderate CYP3A4 inhibitors** including **atazanavir**, **ciprofloxacin**, **clarithromycin**, **conivaptan**, **diltiazem**, **erythromycin**, **fluconazole**, **fosamprenavir**, **indinavir**, **itraconazole**, **ketoconazole**, **indinavir**, **nelfinavir**, **posaconazole**, **ritonavir**, **saquinavir**, and **verapamil** ↑ blood levels, effects and risk of serious adverse reactions; concurrent use is contraindicated. Wait two wk after discontinuing inhibitor before initiating fibanserin. If initiating inhibitor, wait two days after last dose of flibanserin. Concurrent use with **alcohol** ↑ risk of hypotension/syncope and excess sedation; concurrent use is contraindicated. Concurrent use of **oral hormonal contraceptives** and **weak CYP3A4 inhibitors** including **cimetidine**, **fluoxetine**, and **ranitidine** may also ↑ blood levels, effects and the risk of adverse reactions; avoid use of multiple weak CYP3A4 inhibitors. **Strong CYP2C19 inhibitors** including **proton pump inhibitors**, **SSRIs**, **benzodiazepines**, and **antifungals** ↑ blood levels, effects, and the risk of adverse reactions including hypotension, syncope, and CNS depression; concurrent use should be undertaken with caution. **CYP3A4 inducers** including **carbamazepine**, **phenobarbital**, **phenytoin**, **rifabutin**, **rifampin**, and **rifapentine** ↓ blood levels and effectiveness; concurrent use in not recommended. ↑ **digoxin** and **sirolimus** levels and risk of toxicity; careful monitoring recommended. ↑ risk of CNS depression with other **CNS depressants** including **alcohol**, **antihistamines**, **opioids**, **sedative/hypnotics**, some **antianxiety agents**, **antidepressants**, and **antipsychotics**.
Natural-Natural: Concurrent use with **ginko** may also ↑ blood levels, effects and the risk of adverse reactions; avoid use with other weak CYP3A4 inhibitors. **St. John's wort** ↓ blood levels and effectiveness; concurrent use is not recommended.
Drug-Food: Concurrent ingestion of **grapefruit juice** ↑ blood levels, effects, and risk of hypotension/syncope; concurrent ingestion is contraindicated.

Route/Dosage

PO (Adults): 100 mg once daily (at bedtime).

Availability

Tablets: 100 mg.

NURSING IMPLICATIONS

Assessment

- Assess sexual desire and related distress and interpersonal dysfunction before and periodically during therapy.
- Monitor for hypotension and syncope. Have patient lie supine if dizziness occurs.
- Assess likelihood of patient abstaining from alcohol, taking into account the patient's current and past drinking behavior, and other pertinent social and medical history. Counsel patients who are prescribed flibanserin about the importance of abstaining from alcohol use; interaction with alcohol increases risk of hypotension and syncope.

Implementation

- Administer once daily at bedtime; administration during waking hrs increases risks of hypotension, syncope, accidental injury, and central nervous system (CNS) depression.
- Only available through a restricted program, *Addyi REMS Program* due to increased risk of severe hypotension and syncope interaction with alcohol.

Patient/Family Teaching

- Instruct patient to take flibanserin as directed. If dose is missed, omit and take next dose at bedtime on next day. Advise patient to read *Patient Information* before starting therapy and with each Rx refill in case of changes.
- Advise patient to avoid grapefruit juice during therapy.
- Caution patient to avoid alcohol during therapy; increases hypotensive effects. May cause dizziness and fainting.
- Advise patient if dizziness occurs, immediately lie supine and promptly seek medical help if symptoms do not resolve.
- May cause drowsiness. Caution patient to avoid driving and other activities requiring alertness until 6 hrs after each dose or until response to medication is known.
- Instruct patient to notify health care professional of all Rx or OTC medications, vitamins, or herbal products being taken and consult health care profes-

sional before taking any new medications, especially St. John's wort.

- Advise patient to notify health care professional if pregnancy is planned or suspected and to avoid breast feeding.

Evaluation/Desired Outcomes

- Increase in sexual desire. If no improvement in 8 wk, discontinue flibanserin.

fluconazole (floo-kon-a-zole)

Canesoral, Diflucan, Diflucan One

Classification
Therapeutic: antifungals (systemic)

Indications

PO, IV: Fungal infections caused by susceptible organisms, including: Oropharyngeal or esophageal candidiasis, Serious systemic candidal infections, Urinary tract infections, Peritonitis, Cryptococcal meningitis. Prevention of candidiasis in patients who have undergone bone marrow transplantation. **PO:** Single-dose oral treatment of vaginal candidiasis. **Unlabeled Use:** Prevention of recurrent vaginal yeast infections.

Action

Inhibits synthesis of fungal sterols, a necessary component of the cell membrane. **Therapeutic Effects:** Fungistatic action against susceptible organisms. May be fungicidal in higher concentrations. **Spectrum:** *Cryptococcus neoformans*. *Candida* spp.

Pharmacokinetics

Absorption: Well absorbed after oral administration.
Distribution: Widely distributed, good penetration into CSF, saliva, sputum, vaginal fluid, skin, eye, and peritoneum. Excreted in breast milk.
Metabolism and Excretion: >80% excreted unchanged by the kidneys; <10% metabolized by the liver.
Half-life: Premature neonates: 46–74 hr; Children: 19–25 hr (PO) and 15–17 hr (IV); Adults: 30 hr (↑ in renal impairment).

TIME/ACTION PROFILE (blood levels)

ROUTE	ONSET	PEAK	DURATION
PO	unknown	2–4 hr	24 hr
IV	rapid	end of infusion	24 hr

Contraindications/Precautions

Contraindicated in: Hypersensitivity to fluconazole or other azole antifungals; Concurrent use with pimozide, erythromycin, or quinidine.
Use Cautiously in: Renal impairment (dose ↓ required if CCr <50 mL/min); Underlying liver disease; Structural heart disease, electrolyte abnormalities, or concurrent use of other QT interval-prolonging medications; OB: Safety not established; congenital defects have occurred with use of high-dose fluconazole (400–800 mg/day); Lactation: Usually compatible with breast feeding; Geri: ↑ risk of adverse reactions (rash, vomiting, diarrhea, seizures); consider age-related ↓ in renal function in determining dose.

Adverse Reactions/Side Effects

Incidence of adverse reactions is increased in HIV patients.
CNS: headache, dizziness, seizures. **CV:** TORSADE DE POINTES, QT interval prolongation. **Derm:** STEVENS-JOHNSON SYNDROME. **Endo:** adrenal insufficiency, hypokalemia, hypertriglyceridemia. **GI:** HEPATOTOXICITY, abdominal discomfort, diarrhea, nausea, vomiting.
Misc: HYPERSENSITIVITY REACTIONS (including anaphylaxis).

Interactions

Drug-Drug: May ↑ levels of **pimozide**, **erythromycin**, **amiodarone** (especially with high-dose fluconazole [800 mg]), and **quinidine** which can prolong the QT interval and ↑ the risk of torsade de pointes. May ↑ levels of and the risk of bleeding with **warfarin**. **Rifampin**, **rifabutin**, and **isoniazid** ↓ levels. Fluconazole at doses >200 mg/day may inhibit the CYP3A4 enzyme system and effect the activity of drugs metabolized by this system. ↑ hypoglycemic effects of **tolbutamide**, **glyburide**, or **glipizide**. ↑ levels and risk of toxicity from **cyclosporine**, **carbamazepine**, **celecoxib**, **rifabutin**, **tacrolimus**, **sirolimus**, **theophylline**, **zidovudine**, **alfentanil**, and **phenytoin**. ↑ levels and effects of **benzodiazepines**, **amlodipine**, **felodipine**, **isradipine**, **nifedipine**, **nisoldipine**, **verapamil**, **atorvastatin**, **fluvastatin**, **lovastatin**, **simvastatin**, **methadone**, **flurbiprofen**, **prednisone**, **saquinavir**, **tricyclic antidepressants**, and **losartan**. ↑ levels of **tofacitinib**; ↓ dose of tofacitinib to 5 mg once daily. May ↑ risk of bleeding with **warfarin**. May antagonize effects of **amphotericin B**. May ↑ **voriconazole** levels; avoid concurrent use. May ↑ **olaparib** levels; concurrent use not recommended.

Route/Dosage

Oropharyngeal Candidiasis

PO, IV (Adults): 200 mg initially, then 100 mg daily for at least 2 wk.
PO, IV (Children >14 days): 6 mg/kg initially, then 3 mg/kg/day for at least 2 wk.
PO, IV (Neonates <14 days, 30–36 wk gestation): same dose as older children except frequency is every 48 hr; Premature neonates <29 wk gestation: 5–6 mg/kg/dose every 48–72 hr.

Esophageal Candidiasis

PO, IV (Adults): 200 mg initially, then 100 mg once daily for at least 3 wk (up to 400 mg/day).

PO, IV (Children >14 days): 6 mg/kg initially, then 3–12 mg/kg/day for at least 3 wk.
PO, IV (Neonates <14 days, 30–36 wk gestation): same dose as older children except frequency is every 48 hr; Premature neonates <29 wk gestation: 5–6 mg/kg/dose every 48–72 hr.

Vaginal Candidiasis

PO (Adults): 150-mg single dose; prevention of recurrence (unlabeled)—150 mg daily for 3 days then weekly for 6 mo.

Systemic Candidiasis

PO, IV (Adults): 400 mg/day initially, then 200–800 mg/day for 28 days.
PO, IV (Children >14 days): 6–12 mg/kg/day for 28 days.
PO, IV (Neonates <14 days, 30–36 wk gestation): same dose as older children except frequency is every 48 hr; Premature neonates <29 wk gestation: 5–6 mg/kg/dose every 48–72 hr.

Cryptococcal Meningitis

PO, IV (Adults): *Treatment*—400 mg once daily until favorable clinical response, then 200–800 mg once daily for at least 10–12 wk after clearing of CSF; change to oral therapy as soon as possible. *Suppressive therapy*—200 mg once daily.
PO, IV (Children >14 days): 12 mg/kg/day initially, then 6–12 mg/kg/day for at least 10–12 wk after clearing of CSF; change to oral therapy as soon as possible. *Suppressive therapy*—6 mg/kg/day.
PO, IV (Neonates <14 days, 30–36 wk gestation): same dose as older children except frequency is every 48 hr; Premature neonates <29 wk gestation: 5–6 mg/kg/dose every 48–72 hr.

Prevention of Candidiasis after Bone Marrow Transplant

PO, IV (Adults): 400 mg once daily; begin several days before procedure if severe neutropenia is expected, and continue for 7 days after ANC >1000 /mm^3.
PO, IV (Children >14 days): 10–12 mg/kg/day, not to exceed 600 mg/day.

Renal Impairment

PO, IV (Adults): *CCr ≤50 mL/min (no hemodialysis)*—Give 50% of the usual dose (not for single-dose therapy); *Hemodialysis*—Give 100% of the usual dose after each dialysis session; give reduced dose based on CCr on non-dialysis days (not for single-dose therapy).

Availability (generic available)

Powder for oral suspension (orange flavor) (requires reconstitution): 10 mg/mL, 40 mg/mL. **Cost:** *Generic*—10 mg/mL $36.00/35 mL, 40 mg/mL $130.76/35 mL. **Premixed infusion:** 200 mg/100 mL 0.9% NaCl, 400 mg/200 mL 0.9% NaCl. **Tablets:** 50 mg, 100 mg, 150 mg, 200 mg. **Cost:** *Generic*—100 mg $88.17/30, 150 mg $6.99/1.

NURSING IMPLICATIONS

Assessment

- Assess infected area and monitor CSF cultures before and periodically during therapy.
- Specimens for culture should be taken before instituting therapy. Therapy may be started before results are obtained.
- Assess patient for rash (mild to moderate rash usually occurs in the 2nd wk of therapy and resolves within 1–2 wk of continued therapy). If rash is severe (extensive erythematous or maculopapular rash with moist desquamation or angioedema), accompanied by systemic symptoms (serum sickness-like reaction, Stevens-Johnson syndrome, toxic epidermal necrolysis), or occurs during treatment for a superficial fungal infection, therapy must be discontinued immediately.
- ***Lab Test Considerations:*** Monitor BUN and serum creatinine before and periodically during therapy; patients with renal dysfunction will require dose adjustment.
- Monitor liver function tests before and periodically during therapy. May cause ↑ AST, ALT, serum alkaline phosphate, and bilirubin concentrations.

Implementation

- Do not confuse Diflucan (fluconazole) with Diprivan (propofol).
- **PO:** Shake oral suspension well before administration.

IV Administration

- **Intermittent Infusion:** ***Diluent:*** Premixed infusions are prediluted and ready to use. Do not unwrap until ready to use. Do not administer solution that is cloudy or has a precipitate. Check for leaks by squeezing inner bag. If leaks are found, discard container as unsterile. ***Concentration:*** 2 mg/mL. ***Rate:*** Infuse over 1–2 hr. Do not exceed a rate of 200 mg/hr. Pedi: For children receiving doses >6 mg/kg/day, give over 2 hr.
- **Y-Site Compatibility:** acyclovir, aldesleukin, alemtuzumab, alfentanil, allopurinol, amifostine, amikacin, aminocaproic acid, aminophylline, amiodarone, anidulafungin, argatroban, arsenic trioxide, ascorbic acid, atracurium, atropine, azathioprine, azithromycin, aztreonam, benztropine, bivalirudin, bleomycin, bumetanide, buprenorphine, butorphanol, calcium chloride, cangrelor, carboplatin, carmustine, caspofungin, cefazolin, cefepime, cefotetan, cefoxitin, ceftaroline, chlorpromazine, cisatracurium, cisplatin, cyanocobalamin, cyclophosphamide, cyclosporine, cytarabine, dacarbazine, dactinomycin, daptomycin, daunorubicin, defibrotide, dexamethasone sodium phosphate, dexmedetomidine, dexrazoxane, diltiazem, diphenhydramine, dobutamine, docetaxel, dolasetron, dopamine, doxorubicin hydrochloride, doxorubicin liposomal, doxycycline, droperidol, enalaprilat, ephedrine, epinephrine,

epirubicin, epoetin alfa, eptifibatide, ertapenem, erythromycin, esmolol, etoposide, etoposide phosphate, famotidine, fenoldopam, fentanyl, filgrastim, fludarabine, fluorouracil, folic acid, foscarnet, fosphenytoin, ganciclovir, gemcitabine, gentamicin, glycopyrrolate, granisetron, heparin, hetastarch, hydrocortisone, hydromorphone, idarubicin, ifosfamide, immune globulin IV, indomethacin, insulin, regular, irinotecan, isoproterenol, ketorolac, labetalol, leucovorin calcium, levofloxacin, lidocaine, linezolid, lorazepam, magnesium sulfate, mannitol, melphalan, meperidine, meropenem, mesna, methotrexate, methyldopate, methylprednisolone , metoclopramide, metoprolol, midazolam, milrinone, mitomycin, mitoxantrone, morphine, multivitamins, mycophenolate, nafcillin, nalbuphine, naloxone, nicardipine, nitroglycerin, nitroprusside, norepinephrine, octreotide, ondansetron, oritavancin, oxacillin, oxaliplatin, oxytocin, paclitaxel, palonosetron, pamidronate, pancuronium, papaverine, pemetrexed, penicillin G, pentobarbital, phenobarbital, phentolamine, phenylephrine, phytonadione, piperacillin/tazobactam, plazomicin, potassium acetate, potassium chloride, procainamide, prochlorperazine, promethazine, propofol, propranolol, protamine, pyridoxine, quinupristin-dalfopristin, ranitidine, remifentanil, rituximab, rocuronium, sargramostim, sodium acetate, sodium bicarbonate, streptokinase, succinylcholine, sufentanil, tacrolimus, telavancin, theophylline, thiotepa, tigecycline, tirofiban, tobramycin, topotecan, trastuzumab, vancomycin, vasopressin, vecuronium, verapamil, vinblastine, vincristine, vinorelbine, voriconazole, zidovudine, zoledronic acid.

- **Y-Site Incompatibility:** amphotericin B deoxycholate, amphotericin B lipid complex, ampicillin, dantrolene, diazepam, pantoprazole, trimethoprim/sulfamethoxazole.

Patient/Family Teaching

- Instruct patient to take medication as directed, even if feeling better. Doses should be taken at the same time each day. Take missed doses as soon as remembered, but not if almost time for next dose. Do not double doses.
- Instruct patient to notify health care professional if skin rash, abdominal pain, fever, or diarrhea becomes pronounced, if signs and symptoms of liver dysfunction (unusual fatigue, anorexia, nausea, vomiting, jaundice, dark urine, or pale stools) occur, if unusual bruising or bleeding occur, or if no improvement is seen within a few days of therapy.
- Advise patient to notify health care professional if pregnancy is planned or suspected or if breast feeding.

Evaluation/Desired Outcomes

- Resolution of clinical and laboratory indications of fungal infections. Full course of therapy may require wk or mo of treatment after resolution of symptoms.
- Prevention of candidiasis in patients who have undergone bone marrow transplantation.
- Decrease in skin irritation and vaginal discomfort in patients with vaginal candidiasis. Diagnosis should be reconfirmed with smears or cultures before a second course of therapy to rule out other pathogens associated with vulvovaginitis. Recurrent vaginal infections may be a sign of systemic illness.

fludrocortisone

(floo-droe-**kor**-ti-sone)

🍁Florinef

Classification

Therapeutic: hormones

Pharmacologic: corticosteroids (mineralocorticoid)

Indications

Sodium loss and hypotension associated with adrenocortical insufficiency (given with hydrocortisone or cortisone). Management of sodium loss due to congenital adrenogenital syndrome (congenital adrenal hyperplasia). **Unlabeled Use:** Idiopathic orthostatic hypotension (with increased sodium intake). Type IV renal tubular acidosis.

Action

Causes sodium reabsorption, hydrogen and potassium excretion, and water retention by its effects on the distal renal tubule. **Therapeutic Effects:** Maintenance of sodium balance and BP in patients with adrenocortical insufficiency.

Pharmacokinetics

Absorption: Well absorbed following oral administration.

Distribution: Widely distributed; probably enters breast milk.

Protein Binding: High.

Metabolism and Excretion: Mostly metabolized by the liver.

Half-life: 3.5 hr.

TIME/ACTION PROFILE (mineralocorticoid activity)

ROUTE	ONSET	PEAK	DURATION
PO	unknown	unknown	1–2 days

Contraindications/Precautions

Contraindicated in: Hypersensitivity.

Use Cautiously in: HF; Addison's disease (patients may have exaggerated response); OB, Lactation, Pedi: Safety not established.

Adverse Reactions/Side Effects

CNS: dizziness, headache. **CV:** HF, arrhythmias, edema, hypertension. **Endo:** adrenal suppression, weight gain. **F and E:** hypokalemia, hypokalemic alkalosis. **GI:** anorexia, nausea. **MS:** arthralgia, muscular weakness, tendon contractures. **Neuro:** ascending paralysis. **Misc:** hypersensitivity reactions.

Interactions

Drug-Drug: Use with **thiazide or loop diuretics**, **piperacillin**, or **amphotericin B** may ↑ risk of hypokalemia. Hypokalemia may ↑ risk of **digoxin** toxicity. May produce prolonged neuromuscular blockade following the use of **nondepolarizing neuromuscular blocking agents**. **Phenobarbital** or **rifampin** may ↑ metabolism and ↓ effectiveness.

Drug-Food: Large amounts of **salt** or **sodium-containing foods** may cause excessive sodium retention and potassium loss.

Route/Dosage

PO (Adults): *Adrenocortical insufficiency*—100 mcg/day (range 100 mcg 3 times weekly—200 mcg daily). Doses as small as 50 mcg daily may be required by some patients. Use with 10–37.5 mg cortisone daily or 10–30 mg hydrocortisone daily. *Adrenogenital syndrome*—100–200 mcg/day. *Idiopathic hypotension*—50–200 mcg/day (unlabeled).

PO (Children): 50–100 mcg/day.

Availability (generic available)

Tablets: 100 mcg (0.1 mg).

NURSING IMPLICATIONS

Assessment

- Monitor BP periodically during therapy. Report significant changes. Hypotension may indicate insufficient dose.
- Monitor for fluid retention (weigh daily, assess for edema, and auscultate lungs for rales/crackles).
- Monitor patients with Addison's disease closely and stop treatment if a significant increase in weight or BP, edema, or cardiac enlargement occurs. Patients with Addison's disease are more sensitive to the action of fludrocortisone and may have an exaggerated response.
- ***Lab Test Considerations:*** Monitor serum electrolytes periodically during therapy. Fludrocortisone causes ↓ serum potassium levels.

Implementation

- ***High Alert:*** Do not confuse Florinef (fludrocortisone) with Floranex (*Lactobacillus*) or Florastor (*Saccharomyces boulardii*).
- **PO:** Tablets are scored and may be broken if dose adjustment is necessary.

Patient/Family Teaching

- Instruct patient to take medication as directed. Take missed doses as soon as remembered but not just before next dose is due. Explain that lifelong therapy may be necessary and that abrupt discontinuation may lead to Addisonian Crisis. Patient should keep an adequate supply available at all times.
- Advise patient to follow dietary modification prescribed by health care professional. Instruct patient to follow a diet high in potassium (see Appendix K). Amount of sodium allowed in diet varies with pathophysiology.
- Instruct patient to inform health care professional if weight gain or edema, muscle weakness, cramps, nausea, anorexia, or dizziness occurs.
- Advise females of reproductive potential to notify health care professional if pregnancy is planned or suspected, or if breast feeding.
- Advise patient to carry identification at all times describing disease process and medication regimen.

Evaluation/Desired Outcomes

- Normalization of fluid and electrolyte balance without the development of hypokalemia or hypertension.

flumazenil (flu-maz-e-nil)

Anexate, Romazicon

Classification

Therapeutic: antidotes

Indications

Complete/partial reversal of effects of benzodiazepines used as general anesthetics, or during diagnostic or therapeutic procedures. Management of intentional or accidental overdose of benzodiazepines.

Action

Flumazenil is a benzodiazepine derivative that antagonizes the CNS depressant effects of benzodiazepine compounds. It has no effect on CNS depression from other causes, including opioids, alcohol, barbiturates, or general anesthetics. **Therapeutic Effects:** Reversal of benzodiazepine effects.

Pharmacokinetics

Absorption: IV administration results in complete bioavailability.

Distribution: Unknown.

Protein Binding: 50% primarily to albumin.

Metabolism and Excretion: Metabolism of flumazenil occurs primarily in the liver.

Half-life: Children: 20–75 min; Adults: 41–79 min.

TIME/ACTION PROFILE (reversal of benzodiazepine effects)

ROUTE	ONSET	PEAK	DURATION
IV	1–2 min	6–10 min	1–2 hr†

†Depends on dose/concentration of benzodiazepine and dose of flumazenil.

Contraindications/Precautions

Contraindicated in: Hypersensitivity to flumazenil or benzodiazepines; Patients receiving benzodiazepines for life-threatening medical problems, including status epilepticus or ↑ intracranial pressure; Serious cyclic antidepressant overdosage.

Use Cautiously in: Mixed CNS depressant overdose (effects of other agents may emerge when benzodiazepine effect is removed); History of seizures (seizures are more likely to occur in patients who are experiencing sedative/hypnotic withdrawal, who have recently received repeated doses of benzodiazepines, or who have a previous history of seizure activity); Head injury (may ↑ intracranial pressure and risk of seizures); Severe hepatic impairment; OB, Lactation: Safety not established; Pedi: Children <1 yr (safety not established).

Adverse Reactions/Side Effects

CNS: SEIZURES, dizziness, agitation, confusion, drowsiness, emotional lability, fatigue, headache, sleep disorders. **EENT:** abnormal hearing, abnormal vision, blurred vision. **CV:** arrhythmias, chest pain, hypertension. **GI:** nausea, vomiting, hiccups. **Derm:** flushing, sweating. **Local:** pain/injection-site reactions, phlebitis. **Neuro:** paresthesia. **Misc:** rigors, shivering.

Interactions

Drug-Drug: None significant.

Route/Dosage

Reversal of Conscious Sedation or General Anesthesia

IV (Adults): 0.2 mg. Additional doses may be given at 1-min intervals until desired results are obtained, up to a total dose of 1 mg. If resedation occurs, regimen may be repeated at 20-min intervals, not to exceed 3 mg/hr.

IV (Children): 0.01 mg/kg (up to 0.2 mg); if the desired level of consciousness is not obtained after waiting an additional 45 sec, further injections of 0.01 mg/kg (up to 0.2 mg) can be administered and repeated at 60-sec intervals when necessary (up to a maximum of 4 additional times) to a maximum total dose of 0.05 mg/kg or 1 mg, whichever is lower. The dose should be individualized based on the patient's response.

Suspected Benzodiazepine Overdose

IV (Adults): 0.2 mg. Additional 0.3 mg may be given 30 sec later. Further doses of 0.5 mg may be given at 1-min intervals, if necessary, to a total dose of 3 mg. Usual dose required is 1–3 mg. If resedation occurs, additional doses of 0.5 mg/min for 2 min may be given at 20-min intervals (given no more than 1 mg at a time, not to exceed 3 mg per hr).

IV (Children): *Unlabeled*—0.01 mg/kg (maximum dose 0.2 mg) with repeat doses every min up to a cumulative dose of 1 mg. As an alternative to repeat doses, continuous infusions of 0.005–0.01 mg/kg/hr have been used.

Availability (generic available)

Injection: 0.1 mg/mL.

NURSING IMPLICATIONS

Assessment

- Assess level of consciousness and respiratory status before and during therapy. Observe patient for at least 2 hr after administration for the appearance of resedation. Hypoventilation may occur.
- **Overdose:** Attempt to determine time of ingestion and amount and type of benzodiazepine taken. Knowledge of agent ingested allows an estimate of duration of CNS depression.

Implementation

- Do not confuse flumazenil with influenza virus vaccine.
- Ensure that patient has a patent airway before administration of flumazenil.
- Observe IV site frequently for redness or irritation. Administer through a free-flowing IV infusion into a large vein to minimize pain at the injection site.
- Optimal emergence should be undertaken slowly to decrease undesirable effects including confusion, agitation, emotional lability, and perceptual distortion.
- Institute seizure precautions. Seizures are more likely to occur in patients who are experiencing sedative/hypnotic withdrawal, patients who have recently received repeated doses of benzodiazepines, or those who have a previous history of seizure activity. Seizures may be treated with benzodiazepines, barbiturates, or phenytoin. Larger than normal doses of benzodiazepines may be required.
- **Suspected Benzodiazepine Overdose:** If no effects are seen after administration of flumazenil, consider other causes of decreased level of consciousness (alcohol, barbiturates, opioid analgesics).

IV Administration

- **IV Push:** ***Diluent:*** May be administered undiluted or diluted in syringe with D5W, 0.9% NaCl, or LR. Diluted solution should be discarded after 24 hr. ***Concentration:*** Up to 0.1 mg/mL. ***Rate:*** Administer each dose over 15–30 sec into free-flowing IV in a large vein. Do not exceed 0.2 mg/min in children or 0.5 mg/min in adults.

Patient/Family Teaching

- Flumazenil does not consistently reverse the amnestic effects of benzodiazepines. Provide patient and family with written instructions for postprocedure care. Inform family that patient may appear alert at the time of discharge but the sedative effects of the benzodiazepine may recur. Instruct patient to avoid driving or other activities requiring alertness for at least 24 hr after discharge.
- Instruct patient not to take any alcohol or nonprescription drugs for at least 18–24 hr after discharge.
- Resumption of usual activities should occur only when no residual effects of the benzodiazepine remain.

Evaluation/Desired Outcomes

- Improved level of consciousness.
- Decrease in respiratory depression caused by benzodiazepines.

flunisolide, See CORTICOSTEROIDS (INHALATION) and CORTICOSTEROIDS (NASAL) .

fluocinolone, See CORTICOSTEROIDS (TOPICAL/LOCAL).

fluocinonide, See CORTICOSTEROIDS (TOPICAL/LOCAL).

FLUOROQUINOLONES
(floor-oh-**kwin**-oh-lones)

ciprofloxacin† (sip-roe-**flox**-a-sin)
Cipro, Cipro XR

delafloxacin (del-a-**floks**-a-sin)
Baxdela

gemifloxacin (gem-i-**flox**-a-sin)
Factive

levofloxacin (le-voe-**flox**-a-sin)
Levaquin

moxifloxacin† (mox-i-**flox**-a-sin)
Avelox

ofloxacin† (oh-**flox**-a-sin)
~~Floxin~~

Classification
Therapeutic: anti-infectives
Pharmacologic: fluoroquinolones

†See Appendix C for ophthalmic use

Indications

PO, IV: Treatment of the following bacterial infections: Urinary tract infections including cystitis and prostatitis (ciprofloxacin, levofloxacin, ofloxacin) (should be used for acute uncomplicated cystitis only when there are no other alternative treatment options), Gonorrhea (may not be considered first-line agents due to increasing resistance), Gynecologic infections (ciprofloxacin, ofloxacin), Respiratory tract infections including acute sinusitis, acute exacerbations of chronic bronchitis, and pneumonia (should be used for acute sinusitis or acute bacterial exacerbations of chronic bronchitis only when there are no other alternative treatment options), Skin and skin structure infections (delafloxacin, levofloxacin, moxifloxacin, ciprofloxacin, ofloxacin), Bone and joint infections (ciprofloxacin), Infectious diarrhea (ciprofloxacin), Intra-abdominal infections (ciprofloxacin, moxifloxacin). Febrile neutropenia (ciprofloxacin). Postexposure treatment of inhalational anthrax (ciprofloxacin, levofloxacin). Treatment and prophylaxis of plague (ciprofloxacin, levofloxacin, moxifloxacin).

Action

Inhibit bacterial DNA synthesis by inhibiting DNA gyrase. **Therapeutic Effects:** Death of susceptible bacteria. **Spectrum:** Broad activity includes many gram-positive pathogens: Staphylococci including methicillin-resistant *Staphylococcus aureus*, *Staphylococcus epidermidis*, *Staphylococcus saprophyticus*, *Streptococcus pneumoniae*, *Streptococcus pyogenes*, and *Bacillus anthracis*. Gram-negative spectrum notable for activity against: *Escherichia coli*, *Klebsiella*, *Enterobacter*, *Salmonella*, *Shigella*, *Proteus*, *Providencia*, *Morganella morganii*, *Pseudomonas aeruginosa*, *Serratia*, *Haemophilus*, *Acinetobacter*, *Neisseria gonorrhoeae*, *Moraxella catarrhalis*, *Campylobacter*, and *Yersinia pestis*. Additional spectrum includes: *Chlamydia pneumoniae*, *Legionella pneumoniae*, and *Mycoplasma pneumoniae*.

Pharmacokinetics

Absorption: Well absorbed after oral administration (*ciprofloxacin*—70%; *delafloxacin*—59%; *moxifloxacin*—90%; *gemifloxacin*—71%; *levofloxacin*—99%; *ofloxacin*—98%).

Distribution: Widely distributed. High tissue and urinary levels are achieved. All agents appear to cross the placenta. *Ciprofloxacin* and *ofloxacin* enter breast milk.

Metabolism and Excretion: *Ciprofloxacin*—15% metabolized by the liver, 40–50% excreted unchanged by the kidneys; *delafloxacin*—primarily undergoes glucuronidation; 50–65% excreted unchanged by the kidneys; 28–48% excreted unchanged in feces; *gemifloxacin*—minimal metabolism, 61% excreted unchanged in feces, 36% excreted unchanged in urine; *levofloxacin*—87% excreted unchanged in urine, small amounts metabolized; *moxifloxacin*—

mostly metabolized by the liver, 20% excreted unchanged in urine, 25% excreted unchanged in feces; *ofloxacin*—70–80% excreted unchanged by the kidneys.

Half-life: *Ciprofloxacin*—4 hr; *delafloxacin*—3.7 hr (IV); 4.2–8.5 hr (PO); *gemifloxacin*—7 hr; *levofloxacin*—8 hr; *moxifloxacin*—12 hr; *ofloxacin*—5–7 hr (all are ↑ in renal impairment).

TIME/ACTION PROFILE (blood levels)

ROUTE	ONSET	PEAK	DURATION
Ciprofloxacin—PO	rapid	1–2 hr	12 hr
Ciprofloxacin—PO-ER	rapid	1–4 hr	24 hr
Ciprofloxacin—IV	rapid	end of infusion	12 hr
Delafloxacin—PO	rapid	1 hr	12 hr
Delafloxacin—IV	rapid	end of infusion	12 hr
Gemifloxacin—PO	rapid	0.5–2 hr	24 hr
Levofloxacin—PO	rapid	1–2 hr	24 hr
Levofloxacin—IV	rapid	end of infusion	24 hr
Moxifloxacin—PO	within 1 hr	1–3 hr	24 hr
Moxifloxacin—IV	rapid	end of infusion	24 hr
Ofloxacin—PO	rapid	1–2 hr	12 hr
Ofloxacin—IV	rapid	end of infusion	12 hr

Contraindications/Precautions

Contraindicated in: Hypersensitivity. Cross-sensitivity among agents within class may occur; History of myasthenia gravis (may worsen symptoms including muscle weakness and breathing problems); Patients with or at ↑ risk for aortic aneurysm (use only if no alternatives); **Gemifloxacin and moxifloxacin**: Concurrent use of Class IA antiarrhythmics (disopyramide, quinidine, procainamide) or Class III antiarrhythmics (amiodarone, sotalol) (↑ risk of QTc interval prolongation and torsade de pointes); Known QT interval prolongation or concurrent use of agents causing prolongation; **Ciprofloxacin**: Concurrent use with tizanidine; **Delafloxacin**: End-stage renal disease (eGFR <15 mL/min); OB: Do not use unless potential benefit outweighs potential fetal risk; Pedi: Use only for treatment of anthrax, plague, and complicated UTIs in children 1–17 yrs due to possible arthropathy.

Use Cautiously in: Seizure disorder; Depression; Renal impairment (dose ↓ if CCr ≤50 mL/min for ciprofloxacin, levofloxacin, ofloxacin; <40 mL/min for gemifloxacin); Cirrhosis (levofloxacin, moxifloxacin); **Gemifloxacin and moxifloxacin**: Concurrent use of erythromycin, antipsychotics, and tricyclic antidepressants (↑ risk of QTc prolongation and torsades de pointes); **Gemifloxacin and moxifloxacin**: Bradycardia; **Gemifloxacin and moxifloxacin**: Acute myocardial ischemia; **Delafloxacin**: Severe renal impairment (dose ↓ if eGFR 15–29 mL/min) (IV diluent may accumulate and ↑ SCr) (↑ risk of tendon rupture in renal failure); Concurrent use of corticosteroids (↑ risk of tendinitis/tendon rupture); Kidney, heart, or lung transplant patients (↑ risk of tendinitis/tendon rupture); Rheumatoid arthritis (↑ risk of tendon rupture); Diabetes; Lactation: Safety not established except for treatment of anthrax; Geri: ↑ risk of adverse reactions.

F

Adverse Reactions/Side Effects

CNS: ELEVATED INTRACRANIAL PRESSURE (including pseudotumor cerebri), SEIZURES, SUICIDAL THOUGHTS/BEHAVIORS, dizziness, headache, insomnia, acute psychoses, agitation, confusion, depression, drowsiness, hallucinations, lightheadedness, nightmares, paranoia, toxic psychosis. **CV:** AORTIC ANURYSM/DISSECTION; *gemifloxacin, levofloxacin, moxifloxacin*, TORSADES DE POINTES, QT interval prolongation, vasodilation. **Derm:** STEVENS-JOHNSON SYNDROME, acute generalized exanthematous pustulosis, photosensitivity, rash. **Endo:** hyperglycemia, hypoglycemia. **GI:** HEPATOTOXICITY (CIPROFLOXACIN), CLOSTRIDIUM DIFFICILE-ASSOCIATED DIARRHEA (CDAD), diarrhea, nausea, abdominal pain, ↑ liver enzymes (ciprofloxacin, moxifloxacin), vomiting. **GU:** vaginitis. **Local:** phlebitis at IV site. **MS:** arthralgia, myalgia, tendinitis, tendon rupture. **Neuro:** peripheral neuropathy, tremor. **Misc:** HYPERSENSITIVITY REACTIONS (including anaphylaxis).

Interactions

Drug-Drug: Ciprofloxacin may ↑ **tizanidine** levels and risk of hypotension and sedation; concurrent use contraindicated. Concurrent use with **QT interval-prolonging medications** may ↑ risk of QT interval prolongation and torsades de pointes; avoid concurrent use. Ciprofloxacin may ↑ **theophylline** levels and risk of CNS toxicity; avoid concurrent use; if concurrent use cannot be avoided, closely monitor serum theophylline levels. Ciprofloxacin may ↑ levels and risk of toxicity of CYP1A2 substrates, including **ropinirole**, **clozapine**, **olanzapine**, and **zolpidem**; avoid concurrent use with **zolpidem**. Administration with **antacids**, **iron salts**, **bismuth subsalicylate**, **sucralfate**, **sevelemer**, **lanthanum**, **didanosine**, and **zinc salts** ↓ absorption of fluoroquinolones; separate administration of medications. May ↑ the effects of and risk of bleeding from **warfarin**. Ciprofloxacin may alter levels and the effects of **phenytoin**. Levels of fluoroquinolones may be ↓ by **antineoplastics**. **Probenecid** may ↑ levels and risk of toxicity. May ↑ risk of nephrotoxicity from

cyclosporine. Concurrent use of ciprofloxacin with **NSAIDs** may ↑ risk of seizures. Concurrent therapy with **corticosteroids** may ↑ the risk of tendon rupture. May ↑ risk of hypoglycemia when used with **antidiabetic agents**.
Drug-Natural Products: Fennel ↓ the absorption of ciprofloxacin.
Drug-Food: Absorption is impaired by **concurrent tube feeding** (because of metal cations). Absorption is ↓ if taken with **dairy products** or calcium-fortified juices.

Route/Dosage

Ciprofloxacin

PO (Adults): *Most infections*—500–750 mg every 12 hr. *Complicated urinary tract infections*—500 mg every 12 hr for 7–14 days (immediate-release); *or* 1000 mg every 24 hr for 7–14 days (extended-release). *Uncomplicated urinary tract infections*—250 mg every 12 hr for 3 days (immediate-release) *or* 500 mg every 24 hr for 3 days (extended-release). *Gonorrhea*—250-mg single dose. *Inhalational anthrax (postexposure) or cutaneous anthrax*—500 mg every 12 hr for 60 days; *Plague*—500–750 mg every 12 hr for 14 days.
PO (Children 1–17 yr): *Complicated urinary tract infections*—10–15 mg/kg every 12 hr (max = 750 mg/dose) for 10–21 days. *Inhalational anthrax (postexposure) or cutaneous anthrax*—10–15 mg/kg every 12 hr (max = 500 mg/dose) for 60 days; *Plague*—15 mg/kg every 8–12 hr (max = 500 mg/dose) for 10–21 days.
IV (Adults): *Most infections*—400 mg every 12 hr. *Complicated urinary tract infections*—400 mg every 12 hr for 7–14 days. *Uncomplicated urinary tract infections*—200 mg every 12 hr for 7–14 days. *Inhalational anthrax (post exposure)*—400 mg every 12 hr for 60 days; *Plague*—400 mg every 8–12 hr for 14 days.
IV (Children 1–17 yr): *Inhalational anthrax (post exposure)*—10 mg/kg every 12 hr (not to exceed 400 mg/dose) for 60 days; *Complicated urinary tract infections*—6–10 mg/kg every 8 hr (max = 400 mg/dose) for 10–21 days; *Plague*—10 mg/kg every 8–12 hr (max = 400 mg/dose) for 10–21 days.

Renal Impairment

PO (Adults): *CCr 30–50 mL/min*—250–500 mg every 12 hr; *CCr 5–29 mL/min*—250–500 mg every 18 hr (immediate-release) *or* 500 mg every 24 hr (extended-release).
IV (Adults): *CCr 5–29 mL/min*—200–400 mg every 18–24 hr.

Delafloxacin

IV (Adults): 300 mg every 12 hr for 5–14 days *or* 300 mg every 12 hr followed by switching to oral regimen (at dose stated below) for a total of 5–14 days.
PO (Adults): 450 mg every 12 hr for 5–14 days.

Renal Impairment

IV (Adults): *eGFR 15–29 mL/min*—200 mg every 12 hr *or* 200 mg every 12 hr followed by switching to oral regimen (450 mg every 12 hr); *eGFR <15 mL/min*—Not recommended.

Gemifloxacin

PO (Adults): *Acute bacterial exacerbation of chronic bronchitis*—320 mg once daily for 5 days; *Community-acquired pneumonia caused by* Klebsiella pneumoniae, Moraxella catarrhalis, *or multidrug-resistant strains of* Streptococcus pneumoniae—320 mg once daily for 7 days.
Community-acquired-pneumonia caused by Streptococcus pneumoniae, Haemophilus influenzae, Mycoplasma pneumoniae, *or* Chlamydia pneumoniae—320 mg once daily for 5 days.

Renal Impairment

PO (Adults): *CCr ≤40 mL/min*—160 mg once daily for 5 days.

Levofloxacin

PO, IV (Adults): *Most infections*—250–750 mg every 24 hr; *inhalational anthrax (postexposure)*—500 mg once daily for 60 days.
PO, IV (Children >50 kg): *Inhalational anthrax (postexposure)*—500 mg once daily for 60 days; *Plague*—500 mg once daily for 10–14 days.
PO, IV (Children <50 kg and ≥6 mo): *Inhalational anthrax (postexposure)*—8 mg/kg (max: 250 mg/dose) every 12 hr for 60 days. *Plague*—8 mg/kg (max: 250 mg/dose) every 12 hr for 10–14 days; *Other infections*—10 mg/kg/dose every 24 hr (max: 500 mg/dose).

Renal Impairment

PO, IV (Adults): *Normal renal function dosing of 750 mg/day: CCr 20–49 mL/min*—750 mg every 48 hr; *CCr 10–19 mL/min*—750 mg initially, then 500 mg every 48 hr; *Normal renal function dosing of 500 mg/day: CCr 20–49 mL/min*—500 mg initially then 250 mg every 24 hr; *CCr 10–19 mL/min*—500 mg initially then 250 mg every 48 hr. *Normal renal function dosing of 250 mg/day: CCr 10–19 mL/min*—250 mg every 48 hr.

Moxifloxacin

PO, IV (Adults): *Bacterial sinusitis*—400 mg once daily for 10 days; *Community-acquired pneumonia*—400 mg once daily for 7–14 days. *Acute bacterial exacerbation of chronic bronchitis*—400 mg once daily for 5 days. *Complicated intra-abdominal infection*—400 mg once daily for 5–14 days. *Skin/skin structure infections*—400 mg/day for 7–21 days. *Treatment/prevention of plague*—400 mg once daily for 10–14 days.

Ofloxacin

PO (Adults): *Most infections*—400 mg every 12 hr. *Prostatitis*—300 mg every 12 hr for 6 wk. *Uncompli-*

cated urinary tract infections—200 mg every 12 hr for 3–7 days. *Complicated urinary tract infections*—200 mg every 12 hr for 10 days. *Gonorrhea*—400-mg single dose.

Renal Impairment

PO, IV (Adults): *CCr 20–50 mL/min*—100% of the usual dose every 24 hr; *CCr <20 mL/min*—50% of the usual dose every 24 hr.

Availability

Ciprofloxacin (generic available)

Extended-release tablets: 500 mg, 1000 mg. **Cost:** *Generic*—500 mg $489.94/50, 1000 mg $557.80/50. **Oral suspension (strawberry flavor):** 250 mg/5 mL, 500 mg/5 mL. **Cost:** *Generic*—250 mg/5 mL $123.24/100 mL, 500 mg/5 mL $144.28/100 mL. **Premixed infusion:** 200 mg/100 mL D5W, 400 mg/200 mL D5W. **Solution for injection (requires dilution):** 10 mg/mL. **Tablets:** 100 mg, 250 mg, 500 mg, 750 mg. **Cost:** *Generic*—100 mg $20.22/6, 250 mg $7.51/30, 500 mg $15.38/30, 750 mg $278.41/50. ***In combination with:*** hydrocortisone (Cipro HC) (see Appendix B).

Delafloxacin

Lyophilized powder for injection (requires reconstitution and dilution): 300 mg/vial. **Tablets:** 450 mg.

Gemifloxacin (generic available)

Tablets: 320 mg. **Cost:** $239.20/5.

Levofloxacin (generic available)

Tablets: 250 mg, 500 mg, 750 mg. **Cost:** *Generic*—500 mg $13.77/50, 750 mg $24.22/20. **Oral solution:** 25 mg/mL. **Cost:** *Generic*—$579.42/480 mL. **Solution for injection (requires dilution):** 25 mg/mL. **Premixed infusion:** 250 mg/50 mL D5W, 500 mg/100 mL D5W, 750 mg/150 mL D5W.

Moxifloxacin (generic available)

Tablets: 400 mg. **Cost:** $769.58/30. **Premixed infusion:** 400 mg/250 mL 0.8% NaCl.

Ofloxacin (generic available)

Tablets: 200 mg, 300 mg, 400 mg. **Cost:** *Generic*—200 mg $239.20/50, 300 mg $284.66/50, 400 mg $600.36/100.

NURSING IMPLICATIONS

Assessment

- Assess for infection (vital signs; appearance of wound, sputum, urine, and stool; WBC; urinalysis; frequency and urgency of urination; cloudy or foul-smelling urine) prior to and during therapy.
- Obtain specimens for culture and sensitivity before initiating therapy. First dose may be given before receiving results.
- Observe for signs and symptoms of anaphylaxis (rash, pruritus, laryngeal edema, wheezing). Discontinue drug and notify health care professional immediately if these problems occur. Keep epinephrine, an antihistamine, and resuscitation equipment close by in case of an anaphylactic reaction. Patients taking gemifloxacin who are at greater risk for rash are those receiving gemifloxacin for >7 days, <40 yr of age, females, and postmenopausal females receiving hormone replacement therapy.
- Monitor bowel function. Diarrhea, abdominal cramping, fever, and bloody stools should be reported to health care professional promptly as a sign of Clostridium difficile-associated diarrhea (CDAD). May begin up to several wk following cessation of therapy.
- Assess for rash periodically during therapy. May cause Stevens-Johnson syndrome. Discontinue therapy if severe or if accompanied with fever, general malaise, fatigue, muscle or joint aches, blisters, oral lesions, conjunctivitis, hepatitis, and/or eosinophilia.
- Assess for signs and symptoms of peripheral neuropathy (pain, burning, tingling, numbness, and/or weakness or other alterations of sensation including light touch, pain, temperature, position sense, and vibratory sensation) periodically during therapy. Symptoms may be irreversible; discontinue fluoroquinolone if symptoms occur.
- Assess for suicidal tendencies, depression, or changes in behavior periodically during therapy.
- ***Lab Test Considerations:*** May cause ↑ serum AST, ALT, LDH, bilirubin, and alkaline phosphatase. May also cause ↑ or ↓ serum glucose. Monitor blood glucose in patients with diabetes taking insulin or oral hypoglycemic agents. Medication may cause hyperglycemia or hypoglycemia. Moxifloxacin may cause hyperglycemia, hyperlipidemia, and altered prothrombin time. It may also cause ↑ WBC; ↑ serum calcium, chloride, albumin, and globulin; and ↓ hemoglobin, RBCs, neutrophils, eosinophils, and basophils. Monitor prothrombin time closely in patients receiving fluoroquinolones and warfarin; may enhance the anticoagulant effects of warfarin.

Implementation

- Do not confuse levofloxacin with levetiracetam.
- **PO:** Administer *ofloxacin* on an empty stomach 1 hr before or 2 hr after meals, with a full glass of water. *Moxifloxacin, ciprofloxacin, levofloxacin,* and *gemifloxacin* may be administered without regard to meals. Should be taken at least 2 hr (3 hr for gemifloxacin, 4 hr for moxifloxacin) before or 2 hr (6 hr for *ciprofloxacin,* 8 hr for *moxifloxacin*) after antacids or other products containing calcium, iron, zinc, magnesium, or aluminum. Gemifloxacin should be taken at least 2 hr before sucralfate. *Delaf-*

loxacin may be administered without regard to food and with a full glass of water, at the same time each day. Products or foods containing calcium, magnesium, aluminum, iron, or zinc should not be ingested for 2 hr before and 6 hr after administration.
- If gastric irritation occurs, ciprofloxacin may be administered with meals.
- Ciprofloxacin 5% and 10% oral suspension should not be administered through a feeding tube (may ↓ absorption). Shake solution for 15 sec prior to administration.
- *Gemifloxacin* and *ciprofloxacin extended-release tablets;* swallow whole; do not break, crush, or chew.

Ciprofloxacin

IV Administration

- **Intermittent Infusion:** ***Diluent:*** Dilute with 0.9% NaCl or D5W. Stable for 14 days at refrigerated or room temperature. ***Concentration:*** 1–2 mg/mL. ***Rate:*** Administer over 60 min into a large vein to minimize venous irritation.
- **Y-Site Compatibility:** alemtuzumab, amifostine, amiodarone, anidulafungin, argatroban, arsenic trioxide, aztreonam, bivalirudin, bleomycin, calcium gluconate, carboplatin, carmustine, caspofungin, ceftaroline, ceftazidime, cisatracurium, cisplatin, cyclophosphamide, cytarabine, dactinomycin, daptomycin, daunorubicin, dexmedetomidine, dexrazoxane, digoxin, diltiazem, dimenhydrinate, diphenhydramine, dobutamine, docetaxel, dopamine, doxorubicin, doxorubicin liposomal, epirubicin, eptifibatide, etoposide, etoposide phosphate, fenoldopam, fludarabine, fosphenytoin, gemcitabine, gentamicin, granisetron, hetastarch, hydromorphone, idarubicin, ifosfamide, irinotecan, labetalol, leucovorin calcium, lidocaine, linezolid, lorazepam, meperidine, mesna, methotrexate, metoclopramide, midazolam, milrinone, mitomycin, mitoxantrone, mycophenolate, naloxone, nicardipine, octreotide, ondansetron, oxaliplatin, oxytocin, paclitaxel, palonosetron, pamidronate, pancuronium, posaconazole, potassium acetate, potassium chloride, promethazine, quinupristin-dalfopristin, ranitidine, remifentanil, rocuronium, tacrolimus, telavancin, thiotepa, tigecycline, tirofiban, tobramycin, topotecan, trastuzumab, vancomycin, vasopressin, vecuronium, verapamil, vinblastine, vincristine, vinorelbine, voriconazole, zoledronic acid.
- **Y-Site Incompatibility:** acyclovir, aminocaproic acid, aminophylline, amphotericin B lipid complex, amphotericin B liposome, ampicillin/sulbactam, blinatumomab, cangrelor, cefepime, dexamethasone, esmolol, fluorouracil, foscarnet, fosfomycin, furosemide, heparin, hydrocortisone, magnesium sulfate, meropenem, methylprednisolone, pantoprazole, pemetrexed, phenytoin, piperacillin/tazobactam, potassium phosphates, propofol, rituximab, sodium phosphates, warfarin.

Delafloxacin

- **Intermittent Infusion:** Reconstitute with 10.5 mL D5W or 0.9% NaCl for each 300 mg vial. Shake vigorously to completely dissolve. ***Concentration:*** 25 mg/mL. Solution is clear yellow to amber; do not administer solutions that are discolored or contain particulate matter. Reconstituted solution is stable if refrigerated or at room temperature for 24 hrs.. ***Diluent:*** Dilute to volume of 250 mL with 0.9% NaCl or D5W. ***Concentration:*** 1.2 mg/mL. Diluted solution is stable if refrigerated or at room temperature for 24 hrs. ***Rate:*** Infuse over 60 min.
- **Y-Site Incompatibility:** Do not administer with other drugs; flush line before and after each dose.

Levofloxacin

IV Administration

- **Intermittent Infusion:** ***Diluent:*** Dilute with 0.9% NaCl, D5W, or dextrose/saline combinations. Also available in premixed bottles and flexible containers with D5W, which need no further dilution. ***Concentration:*** 5 mg/mL. Discard unused solution. Diluted solution is stable for 72 hr at room temperature and 14 days if refrigerated. ***Rate:*** Administer by infusion over at least 60 min for 250 mg or 500 mg doses and over 90 min for 750 mg dose. Avoid rapid bolus injection to prevent hypotension.
- **Y-Site Compatibility:** alemtuzumab, alfentanil, amifostine, amikacin, aminocaproic acid, aminophylline, ampicillin, ampicillin/sulbactam, anidulafungin, argatroban, atracurium, aztreonam, bivalirudin, bleomycin, bumetanide, buprenorphine, busulfan, butorphanol, caffeine citrate, calcium gluconate, cangrelor, carboplatin, carmustine, caspofungin, cefepime, cefotetan, ceftaroline, ceftazidime, ceftriaxone, cefuroxime, chlorpromazine, cisatracurium, cisplatin, clindamycin, cyclophosphamide, cyclosporine, cytarabine, dacarbazine, dactomycin, daptomycin, dexamethasone, dexmedetomidine, dexrazoxane, digoxin, diltiazem, diphenhydramine, dobutamine, docetaxel, dolasetron, dopamine, doxorubicin liposome, doxycycline, droperidol, enalaprilat, ephedrine, epinephrine, epirubicin, eptifibatide, ertapenem, erythromycin, esmolol, etoposide, etoposide phosphate, famotidine, fenoldopam, fentanyl, filgrastim, fluconazole, fludarabine, foscarnet, fosphenytoin, gemcitabine, gentamicin, granisetron, haloperidol, hydrocortisone, hydromorphone, idarubicin, ifosfamide, imipenem/cilastatin, irinotecan, isoproterenol, labetalol, leucovorin, levorphanol, lidocaine, linezolid, mannitol, meperidine, mesna, methylprednisolone, metoclopramide, metronidazole, midazolam, milrinone, mitomycin, mitoxantrone, mycophenolate, nalbuphine, naloxone, nicardipine, octreotide, ondansetron, oxacillin, oxaliplatin, oxytocin, paclitaxel, palonosetron, pamidronate, pancuronium, pemetrexed, penicillin G sodium, pentamidine, phenylephrine, potassium ace-

tate, potassium chloride, promethazine, propranolol, quinupristin/dalfopristin, ranitidine, remifentanil, rocuronium, sargramostim, sodium bicarbonate, succinylcholine, sufentanil, tacrolimus, theophylline, thiotepa, tigecycline, tirofiban, tobramycin, topotecan, trimethoprim/sulfamethoxazole, vancomycin, vasopressin, vecuronium, verapamil, vinblastine, vincristine, vinorelbine, voriconazole, zidovudine, zoledronic acid.

- **Y-Site Incompatibility:** acyclovir, alprostadil, amiodarone, amphotericin B colloidal, amphotericin B lipid complex, amphotericin B liposome, cefazolin, cefoxitin, daunorubicin hydrochloride, diazepam, fluorouracil, furosemide, ganciclovir, heparin, indomethacin, ketorolac, methotrexate, micafungin, nitroglycerin, nitroprusside, pantoprazole, pentobarbital, phenytoin, piperacillin/tazobactam, prochlorperazine, propofol, rituximab, streptozocin, telavancin, thiopental, trastuzumab.

Moxifloxacin

IV Administration

- **Intermittent Infusion:** ***Diluent:*** Premixed bags are diluted in sodium chloride 0.8% and should not be further diluted. Use transfer set whose piercing pin does not require excessive force; insert with a gentle twisting motion until pin is firmly seated. ***Concentration:*** 1.6 mg/mL. ***Rate:*** Administer over 60 min. Avoid rapid or bolus infusion.
- **Y-Site Compatibility:** alemtuzumab, amifostine, aminocaproic acid, amiodarone, anidulafungin, argatroban, arsenic trioxide, atracurium, bivalirudin, bleomycin, bumetanide, busulfan, calcium acetate, calcium chloride, calcium gluconate, cangrelor, carboplatin, carmustine, caspofungin, ceftaroline, chlorpromazine, cisatracurium, cisplatin, cyclophosphamide, cyclosporine, cytarabine, dacarbazine, dactinomycin, daptomycin, daunorubicin hydrochloride, dexamethasone, dexmedetomidine, dexrazoxane, digoxin, diltiazem, diphenhydramine, dobutamine, docetaxel, dolasetron, dopamine, doxorubicin , doxorubicin liposome, droperidol, enalaprilat, epinephrine, epirubicin, ertapenem, esmolol, etoposide, etoposide phosphate, famotidine, fenoldopam, fludarabine, gemcitabine, glycopyrrolate, granisetron, haloperidol, heparin, hetastarch, hydralazine, hydrocortisone , idarubicin, ifosfamide, insulin, regular, irinotecan, isoproterenol, ketorolac, labetalol, leucovorin calcium, lidocaine, magnesium sulfate, mannitol, melphalan, mesna, methotrexate, methyldopate, methylprednisolone, metoclopramide, metoprolol, milrinone, mitomycin, mitoxantrone, mycophenolate, naloxone, nicardipine, nitroglycerin, norepinephrine, octreotide, ondansetron, oxaliplatin, oxytocin, paclitaxel, palonosetron, pamidronate, pancuronium, pemetrexed, phentolamine, phenylephrine, potassium acetate, potassium chloride, potassium phosphates, procainamide, prochlorperazine, promethazine, propranolol, ranitidine, rocuronium, sodium acetate, sodium bicarbonate, sodium phosphates, streptozocin, succinylcholine, tacrolimus, theophylline, thiotepa, tigecycline, tirofiban, topotecan, vasopressin, vecuronium, verapamil, vinblastine, vincristine, vinorelbine, zoledronic acid.
- **Y-Site Incompatibility:** allopurinol, aminophylline, amphotericin B lipid complex, dantrolene, fluorouracil, fosphenytoin, furosemide, nitroprusside, pantoprazole, phenytoin, vancomycin, voriconazole.

Patient/Family Teaching

- Instruct patient to take medication as directed at evenly spaced times and to finish drug completely, even if feeling better. Take missed doses as soon as possible, unless almost time for next dose. Do not double doses. Advise patient that sharing of this medication may be dangerous.
- Advise patients to notify health care professional immediately if they are taking theophylline.
- Encourage patient to maintain a fluid intake of at least 1500–2000 mL/day to prevent crystalluria.
- Advise patient that antacids or medications containing iron or zinc will decrease absorption. *Ciprofloxacin, levofloxacin,* and *ofloxacin* should be taken at least 2 hr before (3 hr for *gemifloxacin*, 4 hr for *moxifloxacin*) or 2 hr after (6 hrs for *ciprofloxacin,* and *delafloxacin*, 8 hr for *moxifloxacin*) these products.
- May cause dizziness and drowsiness. Caution patient to avoid driving or other activities requiring alertness until response to medication is known.
- Advise patient to notify health care professional of any personal or family history of QTc prolongation or proarrhythmic conditions such as recent hypokalemia, significant bradycardia, or recent myocardial ischemia or if fainting spells or palpitations occur. Patients with this history should not receive gemifloxacin.
- Advise patient to stop taking fluoroquinolone and notify health care professional immediately if signs and symptoms of peripheral neuropathy occur.
- Caution patient to use sunscreen and protective clothing to prevent phototoxicity reactions during and for 5 days after therapy. Notify health care professional if a sunburn-like reaction or skin eruption occurs.
- Instruct patients being treated for gonorrhea that partners also must be treated.
- Advise patient to notify health care professional of all Rx or OTC medications, vitamins, or herbal products being taken and to consult with health care professional before taking other medications.

- Advise patient to report signs of superinfection (furry overgrowth on the tongue, vaginal itching or discharge, loose or foul-smelling stools).
- Instruct patient to notify health care professional if fever and diarrhea develop, especially if stool contains blood, pus, or mucus. Advise patient not to treat diarrhea without consulting health care professional.
- Instruct patient to notify health care professional immediately if rash, jaundice, signs of hypersensitivity, or tendon (shoulder, hand, Achilles, and other) pain, swelling, or inflammation occur. If tendon symptoms occur, avoid exercise and use of the affected area. Increased risk in >65 yrs old; kidney, heart, and lung transplant recipients; and patients taking corticosteroids concurrently. Therapy should be discontinued.
- Advise patient, family, and caregivers to look for suicidality, especially during early therapy or dose changes. Notify health care professional immediately if thoughts about suicide or dying, attempts to commit suicide, new or worse depression or anxiety, agitation or restlessness, panic attacks, insomnia, new or worse irritability, aggressiveness, acting on dangerous impulses, mania, or other changes in mood or behavior.
- Advise female patient of reproductive potential to notify health care professional if pregnancy is planned or suspected or if breast feeding.

Evaluation/Desired Outcomes

- Resolution of the signs and symptoms of infection. Time for complete resolution depends on organism and site of infection.
- Post exposure treatment of inhalational anthrax or cutaneous anthrax (ciprofloxacin and levofloxacin).
- Prevention and treatment of plague (ciprofloxacin, levofloxacin, and moxifloxacin).

HIGH ALERT

fluorouracil

(flure-oh-**yoor**-a-sill)

Carac, Efudex, Fluoroplex, Tolak

Classification

Therapeutic: antineoplastics

Pharmacologic: antimetabolites

Indications

IV: Used alone and in combination with other modalities (surgery, radiation therapy, other antineoplastics) in the treatment of: Colorectal adenocarcinoma, Breast adenocarcinoma, Gastric adenocarcinoma, Pancreatic adenocarcinoma. **Topical:** Management of multiple actinic (solar) keratoses and superficial basal cell carcinomas.

Action

Inhibits DNA and RNA synthesis by preventing thymidine production (cell-cycle S-phase–specific). **Therapeutic Effects:** Death of rapidly replicating cells, particularly malignant ones.

Pharmacokinetics

Absorption: Minimal absorption (5–10%) after topical application.

Distribution: Widely distributed; concentrates and persists in tumors.

Metabolism and Excretion: Metabolized by dihydropyrimidine dehydrogenase to a less toxic compound; inactive metabolites are excreted primarily in urine.

Half-life: 20 hr.

TIME/ACTION PROFILE (IV = effects on blood counts, Top = dermatologic effects)

ROUTE	ONSET	PEAK	DURATION
IV	1–9 days	9–21 days (nadir)	30 days
Top	2–3 days	2–6 wk	1–2 mo

Contraindications/Precautions

Contraindicated in: Hypersensitivity; Dihydropyrimidine dehydrogenase deficiency (patients at ↑ risk of 5-FU toxicity); OB, Lactation: Pregnancy or lactation.

Use Cautiously in: Infections; Depressed bone marrow reserve; Other chronic debilitating illnesses; Obese patients, patients with edema or ascites (dose should be based on ideal body weight).

Adverse Reactions/Side Effects

More likely to occur with systemic use than with topical use.

CNS: acute cerebellar dysfunction. **CV:** CARDIOTOXICITY. **GI:** diarrhea, nausea, stomatitis, vomiting. **Derm:** alopecia, maculopapular rash, local inflammatory reactions (topical only), melanosis of nails, nail loss, palmar-plantar erythrodysesthesia, phototoxicity. **Endo:** sterility. **Hemat:** anemia, leukopenia, thrombocytopenia. **Local:** thrombophlebitis. **Misc:** fever.

Interactions

Drug-Drug: Combination chemotherapy with **irinotecan** may produce unacceptable toxicity (dehydration, neutropenia, sepsis). Additive bone marrow depression with other **bone marrow depressants**, including other **antineoplastics** and **radiation therapy**. May ↓ antibody response to **live-virus vaccines** and ↑ risk of adverse reactions.

Route/Dosage

Doses may vary greatly, depending on tumor, patient condition, and protocol used.

Advanced Colorectal Cancer

IV (Adults): *In combination with leucovorin alone or leucovorin + oxaliplatin or irinotecan*—400 mg/m² as IV bolus on Day 1, then 2400–3000 mg/m² continuous infusion every 2 wk; *In combination with leucovorin*—500 mg/m² as IV bolus 1 hr after leucovorin on Days 1, 8, 15, 22, 29, and 36 every 8 wk.

Breast Cancer

IV (Adults): *In combination with cyclophosphamide + epirubicin or cyclophosphamide + methotrexate*—500 mg/m² or 600 mg/m² on Days 1 and 28 every 28 days for 6 cycles .

Gastric Adenocarcinoma

IV (Adults): *As part of platinum-containing regimen*—200–1000 mg/m² as IV infusion (frequency of administration and number of cycles depends on specific regimen used).

Pancreatic Adenocarcinoma

IV (Adults): *In combination with leucovorin or as part of multidrug regimen*—400 mg/m² as IV bolus on Day 1, then 2400 mg/m² continuous infusion every 2 wk.

Actinic (Solar) Keratoses

Topical (Adults): *Carac*—Apply 0.5% cream to lesions once daily for up to 4 wk; *Efudex*—Apply 2% or 5% solution or cream to lesions twice daily for 2–4 wk; *Fluoroplex*—Apply 1% cream to lesions twice daily for 2–6 wk.

Superficial Basal Cell Carcinomas

Topical (Adults): *Efudex*—Apply 5% solution or cream to lesions twice daily for 3–6 wk (up to 12 wk).

Availability (generic available)

Solution for injection: 50 mg/mL. **Cream:** 0.5%, 1%, 4%, 5%. **Solution:** 2%, 5%.

NURSING IMPLICATIONS

Assessment

- Monitor vital signs before and frequently during therapy.
- Assess mucous membranes, number and consistency of stools, and frequency of vomiting. Assess for signs of infection (fever, chills, sore throat, cough, hoarseness, pain in lower back or side, difficult or painful urination). Assess for bleeding (bleeding gums; bruising; petechiae; and guaiac test stools, urine, and emesis). Avoid IM injections and taking rectal temperatures. Apply pressure to venipuncture sites for 10 min. Notify health care professional if symptoms of toxicity (stomatitis or esophagopharyngitis, uncontrollable vomiting, diarrhea, GI bleeding, myocardial ischemia, leukocyte count <3500/mm³, platelet count <100,000/mm³, or hemorrhage from any site) occur; drug will need to be discontinued. May be reinitiated at a lower dose when side effects have subsided.
- Assess IV site frequently for inflammation or infiltration. Patient should notify nurse if pain or irritation at injection site occurs. May cause thrombophlebitis. If extravasation occurs, infusion must be stopped and restarted in another vein to avoid damage to subcut tissue. Report immediately. Standard treatment includes application of ice compresses.
- Assess skin for palmar-plantar erythrodysesthesia (tingling of hands and feet followed by pain, erythema, swelling, desquamation) throughout therapy. Occurs more frequently with continuous infusion. Usually occurs after 8–9 wk of therapy, but may occur earlier. Withhold fluorouracil for Grades 2 or 3 and resume at lower dose when resolved or Grade 1.
- Monitor intake and output, appetite, and nutritional intake. GI effects usually occur on 4th day of therapy. Adjusting diet as tolerated may help maintain fluid and electrolyte balance and nutritional status and administering antidiarrheal agents. May cause severe diarrhea. Withhold therapy if Grade 3 or 4 diarrhea occurs and until resolved or decreased to Grade 1, then resume at reduced dose.
- Monitor patient for cerebellar dysfunction (ataxia, confusion, disorientation, visual disturbances). This may persist after discontinuation of therapy.
- Monitor for angina, myocardial infarction/ischemia, arrhythmia, and heart failure in patients with no history of coronary artery disease or myocardial dysfunction. Discontinue therapy if symptoms occur.
- Monitor for signs and symptoms of hyperammonemic encephalopathy (altered mental status, confusion, disorientation, coma, ataxia) with ↑ serum ammonia level within 72 hrs of start of infusion. Discontinue fluorouracil and initiate ammonia-lowering therapy.
- Assess for mucositis, stomatitis, and esophagopharyngitis during therapy. May lead to mucosal sloughing or ulceration. Occurs more frequently with IV bolus doses. If Grade 3 or 4 mucositis occurs, withhold dose and resume at reduced dose when resolved or reduced to Grade 1.
- **Topical:** Inspect involved skin before and throughout therapy.
- ***Lab Test Considerations:*** May cause ↓ in plasma albumin.
- Monitor hepatic (AST, ALT, LDH, and serum bilirubin), renal, and hematologic (hematocrit, hemoglobin, leukocyte, platelet count) functions before each treatment and periodically during therapy. Monitor CBC daily during IV therapy. Report WBC of <3500/mm³ or platelets <100,000/mm³ immediately; they are criteria for discontinuation. Nadir of leukopenia usually occurs in 9–14 days, with recovery by day 30. May also cause thrombocytopenia. Withhold doses if Grade 4 myelosuppression occurs. Resume at reduced dose when resolved or improved to Grade 1.
- May cause ↑ in urine excretion of 5-hydroxyindoleacetic acid (5-HIAA).

Implementation

- ***High Alert:*** Fatalities have occurred with incorrect administration of chemotherapeutic agents. Before administering, clarify all ambiguous orders; double-check single, daily, and course-of-therapy dose limits; have second practitioner independently double-check original order, calculations, and infusion pump settings. The number 5 in 5-fluorouracil is part of the drug name and does not refer to the dose.
- Prepare solution in a biologic cabinet. Wear gloves, gown, and mask while handling IV medication. Discard IV equipment in specially designated containers.

IV Administration

- **IV Push:** ***Diluent:*** May be administered undiluted. ***Concentration:*** 50 mg/mL. ***Rate:*** Rapid IV push administration (over 1–2 min) is most effective, but there is a more rapid onset of toxicity.
- **Intermittent Infusion:** ***Diluent:*** May be diluted with D5W or 0.9% NaCl.
- Use plastic IV tubing and IV bags to maintain greater stability of medication. Solution is stable for 24 hr at room temperature; do not refrigerate. Solution is colorless to faint yellow. Discard highly discolored or cloudy solution. If crystals form, dissolve by warming solution to 140°F, shaking vigorously, and cooling to body temperature. ***Concentration:*** Up to 50 mg/mL. ***Rate:*** Onset of toxicity is greatly delayed by administering an infusion over 2–8 hr.
- **Y-Site Compatibility:** acyclovir, alfentanil, allopurinol, amifostine, amikacin, aminophylline, amphotericin B lipid complex, amphotericin B liposome, ampicillin, ampicillin/sulbactam, anidulafungin, argatroban, azithromycin, aztreonam, bivalirudin, bleomycin, bumetanide, butorphanol, calcium gluconate, carboplatin, carmustine, cefazolin, cefepime, cefotaxime, cefotetan, cefoxitin, ceftazidime, ceftriaxone, cefuroxime, cisatracurium, cisplatin, clindamycin, cyclophosphamide, cyclosporine, dacarbazine, daptomycin, dexamethasone, dexmedetomidine, dexrazoxane, digoxin, docetaxel, dopamine, doxorubicin liposome, enalaprilat, ephedrine, ertapenem, erythromycin, esmolol, etoposide phosphate, famotidine, fenoldopam, fentanyl, fluconazole, fludarabine, foscarnet, fosphenytoin, furosemide, ganciclovir, gemcitabine, gentamicin, granisetron, heparin, hetastarch, hydrocortisone, hydromorphone, ifosfamide, imipenem/cilastatin, isoproterenol, ketorolac, labetalol, leucovorin, levorphanol, lidocaine, linezolid, magnesium sulfate, mannitol, melphalan, meperidine, meropenem, mesna, methohexital, methotrexate, methylprednisolone, metoprolol, metronidazole, milrinone, mitomycin, mitoxantrone, morphine, nalbuphine, naloxone, nitroglycerin, nitroprusside, octreotide, paclitaxel, palonosetron, pamidronate, pancuronium, pantoprazole, pemetrexed, pentobarbital, phenobarbital, phenylephrine, piperacillin/tazobactam, potassium acetate, potassium chloride, potassium phosphates, procainamide, propofol, propranolol, ranitidine, remifentanil, rituximab, sargramostim, sodium acetate, sodium bicarbonate, sodium phosphates, succinylcholine, sufentanil, theophylline, thiopental, thiotepa, tigecycline, tirofiban, tobramycin, trastuzumab, vasopressin, vecuronium, vinblastine, vincristine, vitamin B complex with C, voriconazole, zidovudine, zoledronic acid.
- **Y-Site Incompatibility:** aldesleukin, amiodarone, amphotericin B deoxycholate, buprenorphine, calcium chloride, caspofungin, chlorpromazine, ciprofloxacin, diazepam, diltiazem, diphenhydramine, dobutamine, doxycycline, droperidol, epinephrine, epirubicin, filgrastim, haloperidol, hydroxyzine, idarubicin, irinotecan, levofloxacin, lorazepam, midazolam, minocycline, moxifloxacin, nicardipine, pentamidine, phenytoin, prochlorperazine, promethazine, quinapristin/dalfopristin, topotecan, vancomycin, verapamil, vinorelbine.
- **Topical:** Consult health care professional before administering topical preparations to determine which skin preparation regimen should be followed. Tight occlusive dressings are not advised because of irritation to surrounding healthy tissue. A loose gauze dressing for cosmetic purposes is usually preferred. Wear gloves when applying medication. Do not use metallic applicator.

Patient/Family Teaching

- Instruct patient to notify health care professional if fever; chills; sore throat; signs of infection; yellowing of skin or eyes; abdominal pain; joint or flank pain; swelling of feet or legs; bleeding gums; bruising; petechiae; or blood in urine, stool, or emesis occurs. Caution patient to avoid crowds and persons with known infections. Instruct patient to use soft toothbrush and electric razor. Patients should be cautioned not to drink alcoholic beverages or take products containing aspirin or NSAIDs.
- Advise patient to rinse mouth with clear water after eating and drinking and to avoid flossing to minimize stomatitis. Viscous lidocaine may be used if mouth pain interferes with eating. Stomatitis pain may require treatment with opioid analgesics.
- Discuss with patient the possibility of hair loss. Explore methods of coping.
- Caution patient to use sunscreen and protective clothing to prevent phototoxicity reactions.
- Instruct patient not to receive any vaccinations without advice of health care professional.
- Rep: May be teratogenic. Advise female patients of reproductive potential and male patients with partners of reproductive potential to use effective contraception during therapy and for at least 3 mo following completion of therapy and to avoid breast feeding during therapy. Inform patients that fertility may be impaired during therapy.

- Emphasize the importance of routine follow-up lab tests to monitor progress and to check for side effects.
- **Topical:** Instruct patient in correct application of solution or cream. Emphasize importance of avoiding the eyes; caution should also be used when applying medication near mouth and nose. If patient uses clean finger to self-administer, emphasize importance of washing hands thoroughly after application. Explain that erythema, scaling, and blistering with pruritus and burning sensation are expected. Advise patient to avoid sunlight or ultraviolet light (tanning booths) as much as possible; may increase side effects. Therapy is discontinued when erosion, ulceration, and necrosis occur in 2–6 wk (10–12 wk for basal cell carcinomas). Skin heals 4–8 wk later.

Evaluation/Desired Outcomes

- Tumor regression.
- Removal of solar keratoses or superficial basal cell skin cancers.

FLUoxetine (floo-**ox**-uh-teen)

PROzac, PROzac Weekly, Sarafem, Selfemra

Classification

Therapeutic: antidepressants

Pharmacologic: selective serotonin reuptake inhibitors (SSRIs)

Indications

Major depressive disorder. Obsessive compulsive disorder (OCD). Bulimia nervosa. Panic disorder. Acute treatment of depressive episodes associated with bipolar I disorder (when used with olanzapine). Treatment-resistant depression (when used with olanzapine). **Sarafem and Selfemra:** Premenstrual dysphoric disorder (PMDD). **Unlabeled Use:** Anorexia nervosa: ADHD, Diabetic neuropathy, Fibromyalgia, Obesity, Raynaud's phenomenon, Social anxiety disorder (social phobia), Posttraumatic stress disorder (PTSD).

Action

Selectively inhibits the reuptake of serotonin in the CNS. **Therapeutic Effects:** Antidepressant action. Decreased behaviors associated with: panic disorder, bulimia. Decreased mood alterations associated with PMDD.

Pharmacokinetics

Absorption: Well absorbed after oral administration.
Distribution: Crosses the blood-brain barrier.
Protein Binding: 94.5%.
Metabolism and Excretion: Converted by the liver to norfluoxetine (primarily by CYP2D6 isoenzyme), another antidepressant compound; the CYP2D6 enzyme system exhibits genetic polymorphism (~7% of population may be poor metabolizers and may have significantly ↑ fluoxetine concentrations and an ↑ risk of adverse effects). Fluoxetine and norfluoxetine are mostly metabolized by the liver; 12% excreted by kidneys as unchanged fluoxetine, 7% as unchanged norfluoxetine.
Half-life: 1–3 days (norfluoxetine 5–7 days).

TIME/ACTION PROFILE (antidepressant effect)

ROUTE	ONSET	PEAK	DURATION
PO	1–4 wk	unknown	2 wk

Contraindications/Precautions

Contraindicated in: Hypersensitivity; Concurrent use of MAO inhibitors or MAO-like drugs (linezolid or methylene blue); Concurrent use of pimozide; Concurrent use of thioridazine (fluoxetine should be discontinued at least 5 wk before thioridazine therapy is initiated).

Use Cautiously in: History of seizures; Debilitated patients (↑ risk of seizures); Diabetes mellitus; Patients with concurrent chronic illness or multiple drug therapy (dose adjustments may be necessary); Hepatic impairment (↓ doses/↑ dosing interval may be necessary); May ↑ risk of suicide attempt/ideation especially during early treatment or dose adjustment; Congenital long QT syndrome, history of QT interval prolongation, family history of long QT syndrome or sudden cardiac death, concurrent use of QT interval prolonging drugs, hypokalemia, hypomagnesemia, recent MI, uncompensated HF, or bradycardia; Angle-closure glaucoma; OB: Use during first trimester may ↑ risk of cardiovascular malformations in infant. Use during third trimester may result in neonatal serotonin syndrome requiring prolonged hospitalization, respiratory and nutritional support. May cause sedation in infant. Use only if potential benefit justifies potential risk to fetus; Lactation: May cause sedation in infant; discontinue drug or bottle-feed; Pedi: Risk of suicide ideation or attempt may be greater in children or adolescents (safe use in children <7 yr not established); Geri: Geriatric patients are at ↑ risk for excessive CNS stimulation, sleep disturbances, and agitation.

Adverse Reactions/Side Effects

CNS: NEUROLEPTIC MALIGNANT SYNDROME, SEIZURES, SUICIDAL THOUGHTS, anxiety, drowsiness, headache, insomnia, nervousness, abnormal dreams, dizziness, fatigue, hypomania, mania, weakness. **EENT:** mydriasis, stuffy nose, visual disturbances. **Resp:** cough. **CV:** TORSADES DE POINTES, chest pain, palpitations, QT interval prolongation. **GI:** diarrhea, abdominal pain, abnormal taste, anorexia, constipation, dry mouth, dyspepsia, nausea, vomiting, weight loss. **GU:** sexual dysfunction, urinary frequency. **Derm:** ↑ sweating, pruritus, erythema nodusum, flushing, rashes. **Endo:** dysmenorrhea. **F and E:** hyponatremia. **MS:** arthralgia, back pain, myalgia. **Neuro:** tremor. **Misc:** SEROTONIN SYNDROME, allergic reactions, fever, flu-like syndrome, hot flashes, sensitivity reaction.

Interactions

Drug-Drug: Discontinue use of **MAO inhibitors** for 14 days before fluoxetine therapy; combined therapy may result in confusion, agitation, seizures, hypertension, and hyperpyrexia (serotonin syndrome). Fluoxetine should be discontinued for at least 5 wk before MAO inhibitor therapy is initiated. Concurrent use with **MAO-inhibitor-like drugs**, such as **linezolid** or **methylene blue** may ↑ risk of serotonin syndrome; concurrent use contraindicated; do not start therapy in patients receiving **linezolid** or **methylene blue**; if **linezolid** or **methylene blue** need to be started in a patient receiving fluoxetine, immediately discontinue fluoxetine and monitor for signs/symptoms of serotonin syndrome for 2 wk or until 24 hr after last dose of linezolid or methylene blue, whichever comes first (may resume fluoxetine therapy 24 hr after last dose of linezolid or methylene blue). Concurrent use with **pimozide** may ↑ risk of QT interval prolongation. ↑ levels of **thioridazine** may ↑ risk of QT interval prolongation (concurrent use contraindicated; fluoxetine should be discontinued for at least 5 wk before thioridazine is initiated). **QT interval prolonging drugs** may ↑ the risk of QT interval prolongation with arrhythmias; avoid concurrent use. Inhibits the activity of cytochrome P450 2D6 enzyme in the liver and ↑ effects of drugs metabolized by this enzyme system. **Medications that inhibit the P450 enzyme system** (including **ritonavir**, **saquinavir**, and **efavirenz**) may ↑ risk of developing the serotonin syndrome. For concurrent use with **ritonavir** ↓ fluoxetine dose by 70%; if initiating fluoxetine, start with 10 mg/day dose. ↓ metabolism and ↑ effects of **alprazolam** (decrease alprazolam dose by 50%). Drugs that affect serotonergic neurotransmitter systems, including **tricyclic antidepressants**, **SNRIs**, **fentanyl**, **buspirone**, **tramadol**, **amphetamines**, and **triptans** ↑ risk of serotonin syndrome. ↑ CNS depression with **alcohol**, **antihistamines**, other **antidepressants**, **opioid analgesics**, or **sedative/hypnotics**. ↑ risk of side effects and adverse reactions with other **antidepressants**, **risperidone**, or **phenothiazines**. May ↑ effectiveness/risk of toxicity from **carbamazepine**, **clozapine**, **digoxin**, **haloperidol**, **phenytoin**, **lithium**, or **warfarin**. May ↓ the effects of **buspirone**. **Cyproheptadine** may ↓ or reverse effects of fluoxetine. May ↑ sensitivity to **adrenergics** and increase the risk of serotonin syndrome. May alter the activity of other **drugs that are highly bound to plasma proteins**. ↑ risk of serotonin syndrome with **$5HT_1$ agonists**. ↑ risk of bleeding with **NSAIDS**, **aspirin**, **clopidogrel**, or **warfarin**.

Drug-Natural Products: ↑ risk of serotonin syndrome with **St. John's wort** and **SAMe**.

Route/Dosage

PO (Adults): *Depression, OCD*—20 mg/day in the morning. After several wk, may ↑ by 20 mg/day at weekly intervals. Doses greater than 20 mg/day should be given in 2 divided doses, in the morning and at noon (not to exceed 80 mg/day). Patients who have been stabilized on the 20 mg/day dose may be switched over to delayed-release capsules (Prozac Weekly) at dose of 90 mg weekly, initiated 7 days after the last 20-mg dose. *Panic disorder*—10 mg/day initially, may ↑ after 1 wk to 20 mg/day (usual dose is 20 mg, but may be ↑ as needed/tolerated up to 60 mg/day). *Bulimia nervosa*—60 mg/day (may need to titrate up to dosage over several days). *PMDD*—20 mg/day (not to exceed 80 mg/day) *or* 20 mg/day starting 14 days prior to expected onset on menses, continued through first full day of menstruation, repeated with each cycle. *Depressive episodes associated with bipolar I disorder*—20 mg/day with olanzapine 5 mg/day (both given in evening); may ↑ fluoxetine dose up to 50 mg/day and olanzapine dose up to 12.5 mg/day; *Treatment-resistant depression*—20 mg/day with olanzapine 5 mg/day (both given in evening); may ↑ fluoxetine dose up to 50 mg/day and olanzapine dose up to 20 mg/day.

PO (Geriatric Patients): *Depression*—10 mg/day in the morning initially, may be ↑ (not to exceed 60 mg/day).

PO (Children 7–17 yr): *Depression and OCD (adolescents and higher weight children)*—10 mg/day may be ↑ after 2 wk to 20 mg/day; additional increases may be made after several more wk (range 20–60 mg/day); *Depression and OCD (lower-weight children)*—10 mg/day initially, may be ↑ after several more wk (range 20–30 mg/day).

PO (Children 10–17 yr): *Depressive episodes associated with bipolar I disorder*—20 mg/day with olanzapine 2.5 mg/day (both given in evening); may ↑ fluoxetine dose up to 50 mg/day and olanzapine dose up to 12 mg/day.

Availability (generic available)

Tablets: 10 mg, 15 mg, 20 mg, 60 mg. **Cost:** *Generic*—20 mg $73.03/100. **Capsules:** 10 mg, 20 mg, 40 mg. **Cost:** *Generic*—10 mg $10.83/100, 20 mg $8.62/100, 40 mg $41.03/100. **Delayed-release capsules (Prozac Weekly):** 90 mg. **Cost:** *Generic*—$147.96/4. **Oral solution (mint flavor):** 20 mg/5 mL. **Cost:** *Generic*—$118.00/120 mL. ***In combination with:*** olanzapine (Symbyax; see Appendix B).

NURSING IMPLICATIONS

Assessment

- Monitor mood changes. Inform health care professional if patient demonstrates significant increase in anxiety, nervousness, or insomnia.
- Assess for suicidal tendencies, especially during early therapy. Restrict amount of drug available to

patient. Risk may be increased in children, adolescents, and adults ≤24 yr. After starting therapy, children, adolescents, and young adults should be seen by health care professional at least weekly for 4 wk, every 3 wk for next 4 wk, and on advice of health care professional thereafter.

- Monitor appetite and nutritional intake. Weigh weekly. Notify health care professional of continued weight loss. Adjust diet as tolerated to support nutritional status.
- Assess for sensitivity reaction (urticaria, fever, arthralgia, edema, carpal tunnel syndrome, rash, hives, lymphadenopathy, respiratory distress) and notify health care professional if present; symptoms usually resolve by stopping fluoxetine but may require administration of antihistamines or corticosteroids.
- Assess for sexual side effects (erectile dysfunction; decreased libido).
- Monitor for development of neuroleptic malignant syndrome (fever, respiratory distress, tachycardia, seizures, diaphoresis, arrhythmias, hypertension or hypotension, pallor, tiredness, severe muscle stiffness, loss of bladder control). Report immediately.
- Assess for serotonin syndrome (mental changes [agitation, hallucinations, coma], autonomic instability [tachycardia, labile BP, hyperthermia], neuromuscular aberrations [hyperreflexia, incoordination], and/or GI symptoms [nausea, vomiting, diarrhea]), especially in patients taking other serotonergic drugs (SSRIs, SNRIs, triptans).
- **OCD:** Assess for frequency of obsessive-compulsive behaviors. Note degree to which these thoughts and behaviors interfere with daily functioning.
- **Bulimia Nervosa:** Assess frequency of binge eating and vomiting during therapy.
- **PMDD:** Monitor mood prior to and periodically during therapy.
- ***Lab Test Considerations:*** Monitor CBC and differential periodically during therapy. Notify health care professional if leukopenia, anemia, thrombocytopenia, or increased bleeding time occurs.
- Proteinuria and mild ↑ in AST may occur during sensitivity reactions.
- May cause ↑ in serum alkaline phosphatase, ALT, BUN, creatine phosphokinase, hypouricemia, hypocalcemia, hypoglycemia or hyperglycemia, and hyponatremia.
- May cause hypoglycemia in patient with diabetes.

Implementation

- Do not confuse fluoxetine with duloxetine, paroxetine, or Loxitane (loxapine). Do not confuse Prozac with Prilosec (omeprazole), Prograf (tacrolimus), or Provera (medroxyprogesterone). Do not confuse Sarafem (fluoxetine) with Serophene (clomiphene).
- **PO:** Administer as a single dose in the morning. Some patients may require increased amounts, in divided doses, with a 2nd dose at noon.
- May be administered with food to minimize GI irritation. Do not open, dissolve, chew, or crush delayed-release capsules.
- Doses of *PROzac Weekly* may be started after last dose of *PROzac* 20 mg. Dose may be increased after several wk if improvement not clinically significant.

Patient/Family Teaching

- Instruct patient to take fluoxetine as directed. Take missed doses as soon as remembered unless almost time for next dose, then omit and return to regular schedule. Do not double doses or discontinue without consulting health care professional; discontinuation may cause anxiety, insomnia, nervousness.
- May cause drowsiness, dizziness, impaired judgment, and blurred vision. Caution patient to avoid driving and other activities requiring alertness until response to the drug is known.
- Advise patient, family, and caregivers to look for suicidality, especially during early therapy or dose changes. Notify health care professional immediately if thoughts about suicide or dying, attempts to commit suicide, new or worse depression or anxiety, agitation or restlessness, panic attacks, insomnia, new or worse irritability, aggressiveness, acting on dangerous impulses, mania, or other changes in mood or behavior, or if symptoms of serotonin syndrome occur.
- Instruct patient to notify health care professional of all Rx or OTC medications, vitamins, or herbal products being taken and consult health care professional before taking any new medications. Advise patient to avoid taking other CNS depressants or alcohol.
- Caution patient to change positions slowly to minimize dizziness.
- Inform patient that frequent mouth rinses, good oral hygiene, and sugarless gum or candy may minimize dry mouth. If dry mouth persists for more than 2 wk, consult health care professional regarding use of saliva substitute.
- Caution patient to wear protective clothing and use sunscreen to prevent photosensitivity reactions.
- Inform patient that medication may cause decreased libido.
- Advise patient to notify health care professional if symptoms of sensitivity reaction occur or if headache, nausea, anorexia, anxiety, or insomnia persists.
- Instruct female patients to inform health care professional if pregnancy is planned or suspected, or if breast feeding.
- Emphasize the importance of follow-up exams to monitor progress.

Evaluation/Desired Outcomes

- Increased sense of well-being.
- Renewed interest in surroundings. May require 1–4 wk of therapy to obtain antidepressant effects.
- Decrease in obsessive-compulsive behaviors.
- Decrease in binge eating and vomiting in patients with bulimia nervosa.
- Decreased incidence frequency of panic attacks.
- Decreased mood alterations associated with PMDD.

flurandrenolide, See CORTICOSTEROIDS (TOPICAL/LOCAL).

fluticasone, See CORTICOSTEROIDS (INHALATION), CORTICOSTEROIDS (NASAL), and CORTICOSTEROIDS (TOPICAL/LOCAL).

fluticasone/umeclidinium/vilanterol

(floo-**tik**-a-sone/ue-mek-li-**din**-ee-um/vye-**lan**-ter-ol)

Trelegy Ellipta

Classification

Therapeutic: bronchodilators

Pharmacologic: corticosteroids, anticholinergics, adrenergics

Indications

Maintenance treatment of COPD.

Action

Fluticasone—decreases airway inflammation; *umeclidinium*—acts as an anticholinergic by inhibiting M3 muscarinic receptors in bronchial smooth muscle resulting in bronchodilation; *vilanterol*—$beta_2$-adrenergic agonist that stimulates adenyl cyclase, resulting in accumulation of cyclic adenosine monophosphate and subsequent bronchodilation. **Therapeutic Effects:** Improved airflow and ↓ exacerbations in COPD.

Pharmacokinetics

Absorption: *Fluticasone*—15.2% systemically absorbed from lungs following inhalation; minimal absorption from swallowing; *umeclidinium*—mostly absorbed from lungs; minimal oral absorption; *vilanterol*—mostly absorbed from lungs; minimal oral absorption.

Distribution: Unknown.

Protein Binding: *Fluticasone*—>99%, *vilanterol*—94%.

Metabolism and Excretion: *Fluticasone*—primarily metabolized by CYP3A4 to inactive metabolites; parent drug and metabolites excreted primarily in feces, 1–2% excreted in urine; *umeclidinium*—primarily metabolized by CYP2D6 to inactive metabolites; parent drug and metabolites excreted in feces (58%) and urine (22%); *vilanterol*—primarily metabolized by CYP3A4 to inactive metabolites; parent drug and metabolites excreted in urine (70%) and feces (30%).

Half-life: *Fluticasone*—24 hr; *umeclidinium*—11 hr; *vilanterol*—11 hr.

TIME/ACTION PROFILE (bronchodilation)

ROUTE	ONSET	PEAK	DURATION
Inhalation	1 hr	2–12 hr	24 hr

Contraindications/Precautions

Contraindicated in: Hypersensitivity to any components or severe hypersensitivity to milk proteins; Asthma; Acute attack of COPD (onset of action is delayed).

Use Cautiously in: Active untreated infections; Cardiovascular disease; Prolonged immobilization, family history of osteoporosis, postmenopausal status, tobacco use, advanced age, poor nutrition, or chronic use of anticonvulsants or oral corticosteroids (↑ risk of ↓ bone mineral density); Narrow-angle glaucoma (may cause acute angle closure); Cataracts; Urinary retention, prostatic hyperplasia, bladder-neck obstruction; History of seizures, thyrotoxicosis, diabetes mellitus, or ketacidosis; Hepatic or renal impairment; OB: Safety not established; Lactation: Use while breast feeding only if maternal benefit outweighs potential risk to infant; Pedi: Safety and effectiveness not established; Geri: May be more sensitive to drug effects.

Exercise Extreme Caution in: Concurrent use of MAOIs, tricyclic antidepressants, or QTc interval prolonging drugs.

Adverse Reactions/Side Effects

CNS: headache. **CV:** ARRHYTHMIAS, hypertension, QTc interval prolongation, tachycardia. **EENT:** cataracts, dysphonia, glaucoma, oral candidiasis. **Endo:** adrenal suppression, hyperglycemia. **F and E:** hypokalemia. **GI:** constipation, diarrhea, metallic taste. **GU:** urinary retention. **MS:** arthralgia, back pain, ↓ bone mineral density. **Resp:** ↑ risk of pneumonia, paradoxical bronchospasm. **Misc:** HYPERSENSITIVITY REACTIONS (including anaphylaxis and angioedema).

Interactions

Drug-Drug: CYP3A4 inhibitors, including **clarithromycin**, **conivaptan**, **indinavir**, **itraconazole**, **ketoconazole**, **lopinavir**, **nefazodone**, **nelfinavir**, **ritonavir**, **saquinavir**, or **voriconazole** may ↑ fluticasone and vilanterol levels and the risk of corticosteroid effects or adverse cardiovascular reactions; concurrent use should be undertaken with caution. Concurrent use with **MAO inhibitors**, **tricyclic antidepressants**, or **QTc interval prolonging drugs** ↑ risk of cardiovascular reactions from vilanterol; exercise extreme caution when considering concurrent use or use within 2 wk of discontinuing above drugs. Concurrent use of **beta-blockers** may ↓ effectiveness of vilanterol and ↑ risk of severe bronchospasm; consider use of cardioselective beta-blocker. ↑ risk of hypokalemia with concurrent use of **loop diuretics** or **thiazide diuretics**. ↑ risk of anticholinergic adverse reactions when used concurrently with other **anticholinergics**; avoid concurrent use.

Route/Dosage

Inhaln (Adults): One inhalation (fluticasone 100 mcg/umeclidinium 62.5 mcg/vilanterol 25 mcg) once daily.

Availability

Powder for inhalation (contains lactose): fluticasone 100 mcg/umeclidinium 62.5 mcg/vilanterol 25 mcg in a two-strip blister per dose.

NURSING IMPLICATIONS

Assessment

- Monitor respiratory status and lung sounds. Assess pulmonary function tests periodically during and for several mo after a transfer from systemic to inhalation corticosteroids.
- Monitor for signs and symptoms of hypersensitivity reactions (rash, pruritis, swelling of face and neck, dyspnea) periodically during therapy.
- Monitor ECG BP, and pulse rate periodically during therapy. May cause ↑ pulse, ↑BP, prolonged QTc interval, ST segment depression, supraventricular tachycardia, and extra systoles.
- Observe for paradoxical bronchospasm (wheezing, dyspnea, tightness in chest) and hypersensitivity reaction (rash; urticaria; swelling of the face, lips, or eyelids). If condition occurs, withhold medication and notify health care professional immediately.
- Assess patients changing from systemic corticosteroids to inhalation corticosteroids for signs of adrenal insufficiency (anorexia, nausea, weakness, fatigue, hypotension, hypoglycemia) during initial therapy and periods of stress. If these signs appear, notify health care professional immediately; condition may be life-threatening.
- Monitor for withdrawal symptoms (joint or muscular pain, lassitude, depression) during withdrawal from oral corticosteroids.
- May cause decreased bone mineral density during prolonged therapy. Monitor patients with increased risk (prolonged immobilization, family history of osteoporosis, post-menopausal status, tobacco use, advanced age, poor nutrition, chronic use of drugs that can reduce bone mass [anticonvulsants, oral corticosteroids]) for fractures.
- ***Lab Test Considerations:*** May cause hypokalemia and hyperglycemia.

Implementation

- **Inhaln:** Administer once daily at the same time each day. Do not open cover of inhaler until you are ready to use it. If cover is closed before use, dose will be lost. Close cover after medication is inhaled. Discard dessicant; do not eat or inhale. Discard inhaler 6 wk after opening; inhaler is not reusable.
- After inhalation, rinse mouth with water without swallowing to help reduce risk of oropharyngeal candidiasis.

Patient/Family Teaching

- Advise patient to take medication as directed. If a dose is missed, take as soon as remembered unless almost time for next dose. Instruct patient to read the *Patient Information and Instructions for Use* before using and with each Rx refill, in case of new information. Advise patient not to discontinue medication without consulting health care professional; gradual decrease is required.
- Caution patient not to use medication to treat acute symptoms. A rapid-acting inhaled beta-adrenergic bronchodilator should be used for relief of acute asthma attacks. Notify health care professional immediately if symptoms get worse or more inhalations than usual are needed from rescue inhaler.
- Advise patient to stop using medication and notify health care professional immediately if signs and symptoms of hypersensitivity reactions occur.
- Instruct patient not to use additional long-acting $Beta_2$-agonists.
- Caution patient to avoid smoking, known allergens, and other respiratory irritants.
- Advise patient to notify health care professional if signs and symptoms of pneumonia (fever, chills, shortness of breath, increased cough, increased sputum production or change in mucus color), urinary retention (difficulty passing urine, painful urination), sore throat or mouth occur.
- Instruct patient to notify health care professional immediately if exposed to chickenpox or measles. Inform patients of potential worsening of existing tuberculosis; fungal, bacterial, viral, or parasitic infections; or ocular herpes simplex.
- Instruct patient to notify health care professional of all Rx or OTC medications, vitamins, or herbal products being taken and consult health care professional before taking other Rx, OTC, or herbal products.
- Advise patient to have regular eye examinations; may increase risk of cataracts and glaucoma. Instruct patient to notify health care professional immediately if signs and symptoms of glaucoma (eye pain or discomfort, blurred vision, visual halos or colored images in association with red eyes from conjunctival congestion corneal edema) occur.

- Advise female patients to notify health care professional if pregnancy is planned or suspected or if breast feeding.

Evaluation/Desired Outcomes

- Improved airflow and ↓ exacerbations in COPD.

fluvastatin, See HMG-CoA REDUCTASE INHIBITORS (statins).

fluvoxaMINE

(floo-**voks**-a-meen)

Luvox, ~~Luvox CR~~

Classification

Therapeutic: antidepressants, antiobsessive agents

Pharmacologic: selective serotonin reuptake inhibitors (SSRIs)

Indications

Obsessive-compulsive disorder (OCD). **Unlabeled Use:** Depression. Generalized anxiety disorder (GAD). Social anxiety disorder (SAD). Post-traumatic stress disorder (PTSD).

Action

Inhibits the reuptake of serotonin in the CNS. **Therapeutic Effects:** Decrease in obsessive-compulsive behaviors.

Pharmacokinetics

Absorption: 53% absorbed after oral administration.

Distribution: Excreted in breast milk; enters the CNS. Remainder of distribution not known.

Metabolism and Excretion: Mostly metabolized by the liver (CYP2D6 isoenzyme); the CYP2D6 enzyme system exhibits genetic polymorphism; ~7% of population may be poor metabolizers (PMs) and may have significantly ↑ fluvoxamine concentrations and an ↑ risk of adverse effects.

Half-life: 13.6–15.6 hr.

TIME/ACTION PROFILE (improvement on obsessive-compulsive behaviors)

ROUTE	ONSET	PEAK	DURATION
PO	within 2–3 wk	several mo	unknown

Contraindications/Precautions

Contraindicated in: Hypersensitivity to fluvoxamine or other SSRIs; Concurrent use of MAOIs (or within 14 days of discontinuing fluvoxamine), MAOI-like drugs (linezolid or methylene blue), alosetron, pimozide, thioridazine, or tizanidine.

Use Cautiously in: Impaired hepatic function; Risk of suicide (may ↑ risk of suicide attempt/ideation especially during early treatment or dose adjustment); Angle-closure glaucoma; OB: Neonates exposed to SSRI in third trimester may develop drug discontinuation syndrome including respiratory distress, feeding difficulty, and irritability; Lactation: Discontinue drug or bottle-feed; Pedi: May ↑ risk of suicide attempt/ideation especially during early treatment or dose adjustment; may be greater in children and adolescents (safety not established in children <18 yr [controlled release] and <8 yr [immediate-release]); Pedi: Safety not established in children <8 yr (for immediate-release); Geri: May have ↑ sensitivity; recommend lower initial dose and slower dosage titration.

Adverse Reactions/Side Effects

CNS: NEUROLEPTIC MALIGNANT SYNDROME, SUICIDAL THOUGHTS, sedation, dizziness, drowsiness, headache, insomnia, nervousness, weakness, agitation, anxiety, apathy, emotional lability, manic reactions, mental depression, psychotic reactions, syncope. **EENT:** sinusitis. **Resp:** cough, dyspnea. **CV:** edema, hypertension, palpitations, postural hypotension, tachycardia, vasodilation. **GI:** constipation, diarrhea, dry mouth, dyspepsia, nausea, anorexia, dysphagia, ↑ liver enzymes, flatulence, vomiting. **GU:** ↓ libido/sexual dysfunction. **Derm:** ↑ sweating. **Metab:** weight gain, weight loss. **MS:** hypertonia, myoclonus/twitching. **Neuro:** hypokinesia/hyperkinesia, tremor. **Misc:** SEROTONIN SYNDROME, allergic reactions, chills, flu-like symptoms, tooth disorder/caries, yawning.

Interactions

Drug-Drug: Concurrent use with **MAO inhibitors** may result in serious potentially fatal reactions (MAO inhibitors should be stopped at least 14 days before fluvoxamine therapy. Fluvoxamine should be stopped at least 14 days before MAO inhibitor therapy). Concurrent use with **MAO-inhibitor-like drugs**, such as **linezolid** or **methylene blue** may ↑ risk of serotonin syndrome; concurrent use contraindicated; do not start therapy in patients receiving **linezolid** or **methylene blue**; if **linezolid** or **methylene blue** need to be started in a patient receiving fluvoxamine, immediately discontinue fluvoxamine and monitor for signs/symptoms of serotonin syndrome for 2 wk or until 24 hr after last dose of linezolid or methylene blue, whichever comes first (may resume fluvoxamine therapy 24 hr after last dose of linezolid or methylene blue). **Smoking** may ↓ effectiveness of fluvoxamine. Concurrent use with **tricyclic antidepressants** may ↑ plasma levels of fluvoxamine. Drugs that affect serotonergic neurotransmitter systems, including **SSRIs**, **SNRIs**, **fentanyl**, **buspirone**, **tramadol**, **amphetamines**, and **triptans** ↑ risk of serotonin syndrome. ↓ metabolism and may ↑ effects of some **beta blockers** (**propranolol**), **alosetron** (avoid concurrent use), some **benzodiazepines** (avoid concurrent **diazepam**), **carbamazepine**, **methadone**, **lithium**, **theophylline** (↓ dose to 33% of usual dose), **ramelteon** (avoid concurrent use), **warfarin**, and **L-tryptophan**. ↑ risk of bleeding

with **NSAIDS**, **aspirin**, **clopidogrel**, or **warfarin**. ↑ blood levels and risk of toxicity from **clozapine** (dosage adjustments may be necessary).
Drug-Natural Products: Use with **St. John's wort** ↑ of serotonin syndrome.

Route/Dosage

PO (Adults): *Immediate release*— 50 mg daily at bedtime; ↑ by 50 mg every 4–7 days until desired effect is achieved. If daily dose >100 mg, give in 2 equally divided doses or give a larger dose at bedtime (not to exceed 300 mg/day); *Controlled release*— 100 mg at bedtime; ↑ by 50 mg every 7 days until desired effect is achieved, not to exceed 300 mg/day.
PO (Children 8–17 yr): *Immediate release*— 25 mg at bedtime, may ↑ by 25 mg/day every 4–7 days (not to exceed 200 mg/day; daily doses >50 mg should be given in divided doses with a larger dose at bedtime).

Hepatic Impairment

PO (Adults): *Immediate release*— 25 mg daily at bedtime initially, slower titration, and longer dosing intervals should be used.

Availability (generic available)

Tablets: 25 mg, 50 mg, 100 mg. **Controlled-release capsules:** 100 mg, 150 mg.

NURSING IMPLICATIONS

Assessment

- Monitor mood changes. Assess patient for frequency of obsessive-compulsive behaviors. Note degree to which these thoughts and behaviors interfere with daily functioning. Inform health care professional if patient demonstrates significant increase in anxiety, nervousness, or insomnia.
- Assess for suicidal tendencies, especially during early therapy. Restrict amount of drug available to patient. Risk may be increased in children, adolescents, and adults ≤24 yrs. After starting therapy, children, adolescents, and young adults should be seen by health care professional at least weekly for 4 wk, every 3 wk for next 4 wk, and on advice of health care professional thereafter.
- Monitor appetite and nutritional intake. Weigh weekly. Report significant changes in weight. Adjust diet as tolerated to support nutritional status.
- Assess for serotonin syndrome (mental changes [agitation, hallucinations, coma], autonomic instability [tachycardia, labile BP, hyperthermia], neuromuscular aberations [hyperreflexia, incoordination], and/or GI symptoms [nausea, vomiting, diarrhea]), especially in patients taking other serotonergic drugs (SSRIs, SNRIs, triptans).
- ***Toxicity and Overdose:*** Common symptoms of toxicity include drowsiness, vomiting, diarrhea, and dizziness. Coma, tachycardia, bradycardia, hypotension, ECG abnormalities, liver function abnormalities, and convulsions may also occur. Treatment is symptomatic and supportive.

Implementation

- Do not confuse fluvoxamine with fluphenazine or flavoxate. Do not confuse Luvox with Lasix (furosemide).
- Taper to avoid withdrawal effects. Reduce dose by 50% for 3 days, then reduce by 50% for 3 days, then discontinue.
- **PO:** Initial therapy is administered as a single bedtime dose. May be increased every 4–7 days as tolerated.
- Fluvoxamine may be given without regard to meals. Do not open, break, crush, or chew controlled-release capsules.

Patient/Family Teaching

- Instruct patient to take fluvoxamine as directed. Do not skip or double up on missed doses. Improvement in symptoms may be noticed in 2–3 wk, but medication should be continued as directed.
- May cause drowsiness and dizziness. Caution patient to avoid driving and other activities requiring alertness until response to medication is known.
- Advise patient, family, and caregivers to look for suicidality, especially during early therapy or dose changes. Notify health care professional immediately if thoughts about suicide or dying, attempts to commit suicide, new or worse depression or anxiety, agitation or restlessness, panic attacks, insomnia, new or worse irritability, aggressiveness, acting on dangerous impulses, mania, or other changes in mood or behavior or if symptoms of serotonin syndrome occur.
- Advise patient to notify health care professional if rash or hives occur or if headache, nausea, anorexia, anxiety, or insomnia persists.
- Instruct patient to notify health care professional of all Rx or OTC medications, vitamins, or herbal products being taken and consult health care professional before taking any new medications, especially St. John's wort. Advise patient to avoid taking other CNS depressants or alcohol.
- Advise patient to avoid use of caffeine (chocolate, tea, cola).
- Instruct female patients to notify health care professional if breast feeding or if pregnancy is planned or suspected.
- Emphasize the importance of follow-up exams to monitor progress.

Evaluation/Desired Outcomes

- Decrease in symptoms of obsessive-compulsive disorder.

HIGH ALERT

fondaparinux
(fon-da-**par**-i-nux)
Arixtra

Classification
Therapeutic: anticoagulants
Pharmacologic: active factor X inhibitors

Indications
Prevention and treatment of deep vein thrombosis and pulmonary embolism. **Unlabeled Use:** Systemic anticoagulation for other diagnoses.

Action
Binds selectively to antithrombin III (AT III). This binding potentiates the neutralization (inactivation) of active factor X (Xa). **Therapeutic Effects:** Interruption of the coagulation cascade resulting in inhibition of thrombus formation. Prevention of thrombus formation decreases the risk of pulmonary emboli.

Pharmacokinetics
Absorption: 100% absorbed following subcutaneous administration.
Distribution: Distributes mainly throughout the intravascular space.
Metabolism and Excretion: Eliminated mainly unchanged in urine.
Half-life: 17–21 hr.

TIME/ACTION PROFILE (anticoagulant effect)

ROUTE	ONSET	PEAK	DURATION
Subcut	rapid	3 hr	24 hr

Contraindications/Precautions
Contraindicated in: Hypersensitivity; Severe renal impairment (CCr <30 mL/min; ↑ risk of bleeding); Body weight <50 kg (for prophylaxis) (markedly ↑ risk of bleeding); Active major bleeding; Bacterial endocarditis; Thrombocytopenia due to fondaparinux antibodies.
Use Cautiously in: Mild-to-moderate renal impairment (CCr 30–50 mL/min); Untreated hypertension; Recent history of ulcer disease; Body weight <50 kg (for treatment of DVT or PE) (may ↑ risk of bleeding); Geri: Patients >65 yr (↑ risk of bleeding); Malignancy; History of heparin-induced thrombocytopenia; OB: Use during pregnancy only if clearly needed; Lactation, Pedi: Safety not established.
Exercise Extreme Caution in: History of congenital or acquired bleeding disorder; Severe uncontrolled hypertension; Hemorrhagic stroke; Recent CNS or ophthalmologic surgery; Active GI bleeding/ulceration; Retinopathy (hypertensive or diabetic); Neuroaxial spinal anesthesia or spinal puncture, especially if concurrent with an indwelling epidural catheter, drugs affecting hemostasis, history of traumatic/repeated spinal puncture or spinal deformity (↑ risk of spinal/epidural hematoma that may lead to long-term or permanent paralysis).

Adverse Reactions/Side Effects
CNS: confusion, dizziness, headache, insomnia. **CV:** edema, hypotension. **GI:** constipation, diarrhea, dyspepsia, ↑ liver enzymes, nausea, vomiting. **GU:** urinary retention. **Derm:** bullous eruption, hematoma, purpura, rash. **Hemat:** bleeding, thrombocytopenia. **F and E:** hypokalemia. **Misc:** hypersensitivity reactions including ANGIOEDEMA, fever, ↑ wound drainage.

Interactions
Drug-Drug: Risk of bleeding may be ↑ by concurrent use of **warfarin** or **drugs that affect platelet function**, including **aspirin**, **NSAIDs**, **dipyridamole**, some **cephalosporins**, **valproates**, **clopidogrel**, **eptifibatide**, **tirofiban**, and **dextran**.
Drug-Natural Products: ↑ risk of bleeding with **arnica**, **chamomile**, **clove**, **dong quai**, **feverfew**, **garlic**, **ginger**, **gingko**, ***Panax ginseng***, and others.

Route/Dosage

Treatment of DVT/PE
Subcut (Adults): *<50 kg*—5 mg once daily for at least 5 days until therapeutic anticoagulation with warfarin is achieved (INR >2 for 2 consecutive days); warfarin may be started within 72 hr of fondaparinux (has been used for up to 26 days); *50–100 kg*—7.5 mg once daily for at least 5 days until therapeutic anticoagulation with warfarin is achieved (INR >2 for 2 consecutive days); *>100 kg*—10 mg once daily for at least 5 days until therapeutic anticoagulation with warfarin is achieved (INR >2 for 2 consecutive days); warfarin may be started within 72 hr of fondaparinux.

Prevention of DVT/PE
Subcut (Adults): 2.5 mg once daily, starting 6–8 hr after surgery, continuing for 5–9 days (up to 11 days) following abdominal surgery or knee/hip replacement or continuing for 24 days following hip fracture surgery (up to 32 days).

Availability (generic available)
Solution for subcut injection (prefilled syringes): 2.5 mg/0.5 mL, 5 mg/0.4 mL, 7.5 mg/0.6 mL, 10 mg/0.8 mL.

NURSING IMPLICATIONS

Assessment
- Assess for signs of bleeding and hemorrhage (bleeding gums; nosebleed; unusual bruising; black, tarry stools; hematuria; fall in hematocrit; sudden drop in BP; guaiac positive stools); bleeding from surgical site. Notify health care professional if these occur.
- Assess for evidence of additional or increased thrombosis. Symptoms will depend on area of involvement. Monitor neurological status frequently for signs of impairment, especially in patients with

indwelling epidural catheters for administration of analgesia or with concomitant use of drugs affecting hemostasis (NSAIDs, platelet inhibitors, other anticoagulants). Risk is increased by traumatic or repeated epidural or spinal puncture. May require urgent treatment.

- ***Lab Test Considerations:*** Monitor platelet count closely; may cause thrombocytopenia. If platelet count is <100,000/mm^3, discontinue fondaparinux.
- Fondaparinux is not accurately measured by prothrombin time (PT), activated thromboplastin time (aPTT), or international standards of heparin or low-molecular-weight heparins. If unexpected changes in coagulation parameters or major bleeding occurs, discontinue fondaparinux.
- Monitor CBC, serum creatinine levels, and stool occult blood tests routinely during therapy.
- May cause asymptomatic ↑ in AST and ALT. Elevations are fully reversible and not associated with ↑ in bilirubin.
- May cause ↑ aPTT temporally associated with bleeding with or without concomitant administration of other anticoagulants and thrombocytopenia with thrombosis similar to heparin-induced thrombocytopenia, with or without exposure to heparin or low-molecular-weight heparins.

Implementation

- ***High Alert:*** Do not confuse Arixtra with Arista AH (absorbable hemostatic agent).
- Fondaparinux cannot be used interchangeably with heparin, low-molecular-weight heparins, or heparinoids as they differ in manufacturing process, anti-Xa and anti-IIa activity, units, and dose. Each of these medications has its own instructions for use.
- Initial dose should be administered 6–8 hr after surgery. Administration before 6 hr after surgery has been associated with risk of major bleeding.
- **Subcut:** Administer subcut only into fatty tissue, alternating sites between right and left anterolateral or posterolateral abdominal wall. Inject entire length of needle at a 45° or 90° angle into a skin fold held between thumb and forefinger; hold skin fold throughout injection. Do not aspirate or massage. Rotate sites frequently. Do not administer IM because of danger of hematoma formation. Solution should be clear; do not inject solution containing particulate matter. Do not mix with other injections.
- Fondaparinux is provided in a single-dose prefilled syringe with an automatic needle protection system. Do not expel air bubble from prefilled syringe before injection to prevent loss of drug.

Patient/Family Teaching

- Advise patient to report any symptoms of unusual bleeding or bruising, dizziness, itching, rash, fever, swelling, or difficulty breathing to health care professional immediately.
- Instruct patient not to take aspirin or NSAIDs without consulting health care professional during therapy.

Evaluation/Desired Outcomes

- Prevention and treatment of deep vein thrombosis and pulmonary embolism.

F

foscarnet (foss-**kar**-net)

Foscavir

Classification

Therapeutic: antivirals

Indications

Treatment of cytomegalovirus (CMV) retinitis in HIV-infected patients (alone or with ganciclovir). Treatment of acyclovir-resistant mucocutaneous herpes simplex virus (HSV) infections in immunocompromised patients.

Action

Prevents viral replication by inhibiting viral DNA-polymerase and reverse transcriptase. **Therapeutic Effects:** Virustatic action against susceptible viruses including CMV.

Pharmacokinetics

Absorption: IV administration results in complete bioavailability.

Distribution: Variable penetration into CSF. May concentrate in and be slowly released from bone.

Metabolism and Excretion: 80–90% excreted unchanged in urine.

Half-life: 3 hr (in patients with normal renal function); longer half-life of 90 hr may reflect release of drug from bone.

TIME/ACTION PROFILE

ROUTE	ONSET	PEAK	DURATION
IV	rapid	end of infusion	8–24 hr

Contraindications/Precautions

Contraindicated in: Hypersensitivity; HF (due to sodium content); Patients on sodium-restricted diets; Hemodialysis; Lactation: Avoid breast feeding.

Use Cautiously in: Renal impairment (dose ↓ required if CCr ≤1.4–1.6 mL/min/kg; see product information); History of seizures; History of QT interval prolongation or cardiovascular disease; Concurrent use of other QT interval prolonging medications; Hypokalemia or hypomagnesemia (must be corrected prior to therapy); OB, Pedi: Safety not established.

Adverse Reactions/Side Effects

CNS: SEIZURES, headache, anxiety, confusion, dizziness, fatigue, malaise, mental depression, weakness. **EENT:** conjunctivitis, eye pain, vision abnormalities. **Resp:** coughing, dyspnea. **CV:** TORSADE DE POINTES, chest pain, edema, palpitations, QT interval prolongation. **GI:** diarrhea, nausea, vomiting, abdominal pain, abnormal taste sensation, anorexia, constipation, dyspepsia. **GU:** renal failure, albuminuria, dysuria, nocturia, polyuria, urinary retention. **Derm:** ↑ sweating, pruritus, rash, skin ulceration. **F and E:** hypocalcemia, hypokalemia, hypomagnesemia, hyperphosphatemia, hypophosphatemia. **Hemat:** anemia, granulocytopenia, leukopenia, neutropenia. **Local:** pain/inflammation at injection site. **MS:** arthralgia, myalgia, back pain, involuntary muscle contraction. **Neuro:** ataxia, hypoesthesia, neuropathy, paresthesia, tremor. **Misc:** HYPERSENSITIVITY REACTIONS (including anaphylaxis, urticaria, and angioedema), fever, chills, flu-like syndrome, lymphoma, sarcoma.

Interactions

Drug-Drug: Avoid use of drugs known to prolong the QTc interval including **quinidine**, **procainamide**, **amiodarone**, **sotalol**, **chlorpromazine**, **thioridazine**, **moxifloxacin**, **pentamidine**, and **methadone**. Concurrent use with parenteral **pentamidine** may result in severe, life-threatening hypocalcemia. Risk of nephrotoxicity may be ↑ by concurrent use of other **nephrotoxic agents (amphotericin B, aminoglycosides, cyclosporine, acyclovir, methotrexate, tacrolimus, pentamidine (IV))**.

Route/Dosage

IV (Adults): *CMV retinitis*— 60 mg/kg every 8 hr or 90 mg/kg every 12 hr for 2–3 wk, then 90–120 mg/kg/day as a single dose. Dose ↓ required for any degree of renal impairment; *HSV*— 40 mg/kg every 8–12 hr for 2–3 wk or until healing occurs.

Availability (generic available)

Solution for injection: 24 mg/mL.

NURSING IMPLICATIONS

Assessment

- Monitor ECG periodically during therapy for QT interval prolongation.
- **CMV Retinitis:** Diagnosis of CMV retinitis should be determined by ophthalmoscopy before treatment with foscarnet. Ophthalmologic examinations should also be performed at the conclusion of induction and every 4 wk during maintenance therapy.
- Culture for CMV (urine, blood, throat) may be taken before administration. However, a negative CMV culture does not rule out CMV retinitis.
- **HSV Infections:** Assess lesions before and daily during therapy.
- ***Lab Test Considerations:*** Monitor serum creatinine before and 2–3 times weekly during induction therapy and at least once every 1–2 wk during maintenance therapy. Monitor 24-hr CCr before and periodically throughout therapy. If CCr drops below 0.4 mL/min/kg, discontinue foscarnet.
- Monitor serum calcium, magnesium, potassium, and phosphorus before and 2–3 times weekly during induction therapy and at least weekly during maintenance therapy. May cause ↓ concentrations.
- May cause anemia, granulocytopenia, leukopenia, and thrombocytopenia. May cause ↑ AST and ALT levels and abnormal A-G ratios.

Implementation

- Adequately hydrate patient with 750–1000 mL of 0.9% NaCl or D5W before first infusion to establish diuresis, then administer 750–1000 mL with 120 mg/kg of foscarnet or 500 mL with 40–60 mg/kg of foscarnet with each dose to prevent renal toxicity.

IV Administration

- **Intermittent Infusion:** ***Diluent:*** May be administered via central line undiluted. If administered via peripheral line, *must* be diluted with D5W or 0.9% NaCl to prevent vein irritation. Do not administer solution that is discolored or contains particulate matter. Do not refrigerate or freeze; stable for 24 hrs at room temperature. Use diluted solution within 24 hr. ***Concentration:*** Undiluted: 24 mg/mL; Diluted: 12 mg/mL.
- Dose is based on patient weight; excess solution may be discarded from bottle before administration to prevent overdosage.
- Patients who experience progression of CMV retinitis during maintenance therapy may be retreated with induction therapy followed by maintenance therapy. ***Rate:*** Administer at a rate not to exceed 1 mg/kg/min.
- Infuse solution via infusion pump to ensure accurate infusion rate.
- **Y-Site Compatibility:** aldesleukin, alemtuzumab, alfentanil, amifostine, amikacin, aminophylline, amphotericin B liposome, ampicillin, ampicillin/sulbactam, anidulafungin, argatroban, atracurium, azithromycin, aztreonam, bivalirudin, bleomycin, bumetanide, buprenorphine, busulfan, butorphanol, carboplatin, carmustine, cefazolin, cefotaxime, cefotetan, cefoxitin, ceftazidime, ceftriaxone, cefuroxime, chloramphenicol, cisatracurium, cisplatin, clindamycin, cyclophosphamide, cyclosporine, cytarabine, dacarbazine, dactinomycin, daptomycin, dexamethasone sodium phosphate, dexmedetomidine, dexrazoxane, diltiazem, docetaxel, dopamine, doxacurium, enalaprilat, ephedrine, epinephrine, eptifibatide, ertapenem, erythromycin lactobionate, esmolol, etoposide, etoposide phosphate, famotidine, fenoldopam, fentanyl, fluconazole, flucytosine, fludarabine, fluorouracil, fosphenytoin, furosemide, gemcitabine, gentamicin, glycopyrrolate, granisetron, heparin, hetastarch, hydrocortisone, hydromorphone, ifosfamide, imipenem-cilastatin, insulin, irinotecan, isoproterenol, ketorolac, levofloxacin,

lidocaine, linezolid, magnesium sulfate, mannitol, melphalan, meperidine, meropenem, mesna, methotrexate, metoclopramide, metoprolol, metronidazole, milrinone, mitomycin, morphine, nafcillin, nalbuphine, naloxone, nitroglycerin, nitroprusside, octreotide, oxacillin, oxaliplatin, oxytocin, paclitaxel, palonosetron, pamidronate, pancuronium, pantoprazole, pemetrexed, penicillin G potassium, pentobarbital, phenylephrine, piperacillin/tazobactam, potassium acetate, potassium chloride, potassium phosphates, procainamide, propranolol, ranitidine, remifentanil, rocuronium, sodium acetate, sodium bicarbonate, sodium phosphates, streptozocin, succinylcholine, sufentanil, tacrolimus, theophylline, thiotepa, tigecycline, tirofiban, tobramycin, vancomycin, vecuronium, vinblastine, vincristine, voriconazole, zidovudine, zoledronic acid.

- **Y-Site Incompatibility:** Manufacturer recommends that foscarnet not be administered concurrently with other drugs or solutions in the same IV catheter except D5W or 0.9% NaCl, acyclovir, allopurinol, amphotericin B deoxycholate, amphotericin B lipid complex, calcium chloride, calcium gluconate, caspofungin, chlorpromazine, ciprofloxacin, dantrolene, daunorubicin, diazepam, digoxin, diphenhydramine, dobutamine, dolasetron, doxorubicin, droperidol, epirubicin, ganciclovir, haloperidol, idarubicin, labetalol, leucovorin, methylprednisolone, midazolam, mitoxantrone, mycophenolate, nicardipine, norepinephrine, ondansetron, pentamidine, prochlorperazine, promethazine, quinupristin/dalfopristin, thiopental, topotecan, verapamil, vinorelbine.

Patient/Family Teaching

- Inform patient that foscarnet is not a cure for CMV retinitis. Progression of retinitis may continue in immunocompromised patients during and after therapy. Advise patients to have regular ophthalmologic exams.
- May cause dizziness and seizures. Caution patient to avoid driving or other activities requiring alertness until response to medication is known.
- Advise patient to notify health care professional immediately if perioral tingling or numbness in the extremities or paresthesia occurs during or after infusion. If these signs of electrolyte imbalance occur during administration, infusion should be stopped and lab samples for serum electrolyte concentrations obtained immediately.
- Emphasize the importance of frequent follow-up exams to monitor renal function and electrolytes.

Evaluation/Desired Outcomes

- Management of the symptoms of CMV retinitis in patients with AIDS.
- Crusting over and healing of skin lesions in HSV infections.

fosinopril, See ANGIOTENSIN-CONVERTING ENZYME (ACE) INHIBITORS.

fosphenytoin

(foss-**fen**-i-toyn)

Cerebyx

Classification

Therapeutic: anticonvulsants

Indications

Short-term (<5 day) parenteral management of generalized, tonic-clonic status epilepticus when use of phenytoin is not feasible. Treatment and prevention of seizures during neurosurgery when use of phenytoin is not feasible.

Action

Limits seizure propagation by altering ion transport. May also decrease synaptic transmission. Fosphenytoin is rapidly converted to phenytoin, which is responsible for its pharmacologic effects. **Therapeutic Effects:** Diminished seizure activity.

Pharmacokinetics

Absorption: Rapidly converted to phenytoin after IV administration and completely absorbed after IM administration.

Distribution: Distributes into CSF and other body tissues and fluids. Enters breast milk; crosses the placenta, achieving similar maternal/fetal levels. Preferentially distributes into fatty tissue.

Protein Binding: *Fosphenytoin*—95–99%; *phenytoin*—90–95%.

Metabolism and Excretion: Mostly metabolized by the liver; minimal amounts excreted in the urine.

Half-life: *Fosphenytoin*—15 min; *phenytoin*—22 hr (range 7–42 hr).

TIME/ACTION PROFILE (anticonvulsant effect)

ROUTE	ONSET	PEAK	DURATION
IM	unknown	30 min	up to 24 hr
IV	15–45 min	15–60 min	up to 24 hr

Contraindications/Precautions

Contraindicated in: Hypersensitivity; Sinus bradycardia, sinoatrial block, 2nd- or 3rd-degree AV heart block or Adams-Stokes syndrome; Concurrent use of delavirdine; Prior acute hepatotoxicity due to fosphenytoin or phenytoin.

Use Cautiously in: Hepatic or renal impairment (↑ risk of adverse reactions; dose ↓ recommended for hepatic impairment); OB: Pregnancy (↑ risk of congenital anomalies; ↑ risk of hemorrhage in newborn if used at term); Lactation: Present in breast milk; should weigh risk of potential adverse effects on infant versus potential benefit to mother.

Exercise Extreme Caution in: Patients positive for HLA-B*1502 allele (unless exceptional circumstances exist where benefits clearly outweigh the risks).

Adverse Reactions/Side Effects

CNS: dizziness, drowsiness, nystagmus, agitation, brain edema, headache, stupor, vertigo. **CV:** hypotension (with rapid IV administration), tachycardia. **Derm:** ACUTE GENERALIZED EXANTHEMATOUS PUSTULOSIS, DRUG REACTION WITH EOSINOPHILIA AND SYSTEMIC SYMPTOMS (DRESS), STEVENS-JOHNSON SYNDROME, TOXIC EPIDERMAL NECROLYSIS, pruritus, purple glove syndrome, rash. **EENT:** amblyopia, deafness, diplopia, tinnitus. **GI:** dry mouth, nausea, taste perversion, tongue disorder, vomiting. **MS:** back pain. **Neuro:** ataxia, dysarthria, extrapyramidal syndrome, hypesthesia, incoordination, paresthesia, tremor. **Misc:** ANGIOEDEMA, pelvic pain.

Interactions

Drug-Drug: May ↓ the effects of **delavirdine**, resulting in loss of virologic response and potential resistant (concurrent use contraindicated). **Disulfiram**, acute ingestion of **alcohol**, **amiodarone**, **capecitabine**, **chloramphenicol**, **chlordiazepoxide**, **cimetidine**, **diazepam**, **estrogens**, **ethosuximide**, **felbamate**, **fluconazole**, **fluorouracil**, **fluoxetine**, **fluvastatin**, **fluvoxamine**, **halothane**, **isoniazid**, **itraconazole**, **ketoconazole**, **methylphenidate**, **miconazole**, **omeprazole**, **oxcarbazepine**, **phenothiazines**, **salicylates**, **sertraline**, **succinamides**, **sulfonamides**, **topiramate**, **trazodone**, **voriconazole**, and **warfarin** may ↑ phenytoin blood levels. **Barbiturates**, **bleomycin**, **carbamazepine**, **carboplatin**, **cisplatin**, **diazoxide**, **doxorubicin**, **folic acid**, **fosamprenavir**, **methotrexate**, **nelfinavir**, **rifampin**, **ritonavir**, **theophylline**, **vigabatrin**, and chronic ingestion of **alcohol** may ↓ phenytoin blood levels. Phenytoin may ↓ the effects of **albendazole**, **amiodarone**, **atorvastatin**, **benzodiazepines**, **carbamazepine**, **chloramphenicol**, **clozapine**, **corticosteroids**, **cyclosporine**, **digoxin**, **disopyramide**, **doxycycline**, **efavirenz**, **estrogens**, **felbamate**, **fluconazole**, **fluvastatin**, **folic acid**, **furosemide**, **indinavir**, **irinotecan**, **itraconazole**, **ketoconazole**, **lamotrigine**, **lopinavir/ritonavir**, **methadone**, **mexiletine**, **nelfinavir**, **nifedipine**, **nimodpine**, **nisoldipine**, **oral contraceptives**, **oxcarbazepine**, **paclitaxel**, **paroxetine**, **posaconazole**, **propafenone**, **quetiapine**, **quinidine**, **rifampin**, **ritonavir**, **saquinavir**, **sertraline**, **simvastatin**, **tacrolimus**, **theophylline**, **topiramate**, **tricyclic antidepressants**, **verapamil vitamin D**, **voriconazole**, **warfarin**, and **zonisamide**.

Drug-Natural Products: **St. John's wort** may ↓ levels.

Route/Dosage

Note: Doses of fosphenytoin are expressed as phenytoin sodium equivalents [PE].

Status Epilepticus

IV (Adults and Children): 15–20 mg PE/kg.

Nonemergent and Maintenance Dosing

IV, IM (Adults and Children >16 yr): *Loading dose*—10–20 mg PE/kg. *Maintenance dose*—4–6 mg PE/kg/day.

IV (Children Birth to <17 yr): *Loading dose*—10–15 mg PE/kg. *Maintenance dose*—2–4 mg PE/kg/day.

Availability (generic available)

Solution for injection: 50 mg PE/mL, 75 mg PE/mL.

NURSING IMPLICATIONS

Assessment

- Assess location, duration, frequency, and characteristics of seizure activity. EEG may be monitored periodically during therapy.
- Monitor BP, ECG, and respiratory function continuously during administration of fosphenytoin and during period when peak serum phenytoin levels occur (15–30 min after administration).
- Observe patient for development of rash. Discontinue fosphenytoin at the first sign of skin reactions. Serious adverse reactions such as exfoliative, purpuric, or bullous rashes or the development of lupus erythematosus, Stevens-Johnson syndrome, or toxic epidermal necrolysis preclude further use of fosphenytoin. Stevens-Johnson syndrome and toxic epidermal necrolysis are significantly more common in patients with a particular human leukocyte antigen (HLA) allele, HLA-B*1502 (occurs almost exclusively in patients with Asian ancestry, including Han Chinese, Filipinos, Malaysians, South Asian Indians, and Thais). Avoid using fosphenytoin as an alternative to carbamazepine for patients who test positive. If less serious skin eruptions (measles-like or scarlatiniform) occur, fosphenytoin may be resumed after complete clearing of the rash. If rash reappears, avoid further use of fosphenytoin.
- Assess mental status (orientation, mood, behavior) before and periodically during therapy. Monitor closely for notable changes in behavior that could indicate the emergence or worsening of suicidal thoughts or behavior or depression.
- Monitor injection site for edema, discoloration, and pain distal to the site of injection (described as "purple glove syndrome") frequently during therapy. May or may not be associated with extravasation. The syndrome may not develop for several days after injection of fosphenytoin.
- ***Lab Test Considerations:*** Fosphenytoin contains 0.0037 mmol phosphate per mg PE. Monitor serum

phosphate concentrations in patients with renal insufficiency; may cause ↑ phosphate concentrations.

- May cause ↑ serum alkaline phosphatase, GTT, and glucose levels.
- Fosphenytoin therapy may be monitored using phenytoin levels. Optimal total plasma phenytoin concentrations are typically 10–20 mcg/mL (unbound plasma phenytoin concentrations of 1–2 mcg/mL).
- ***Toxicity and Overdose:*** Serum phenytoin levels should not be monitored until complete conversion from fosphenytoin to phenytoin has occurred (2 hr after IV or 4 hr after IM administration).
- Initial signs and symptoms of phenytoin toxicity include nystagmus, ataxia, confusion, nausea, slurred speech, and dizziness.

Implementation

- Do not confuse Cerebyx (fosphenytoin) with Celebrex (celecoxib) or Celexa (citalopram).
- Do not confuse concentration of fosphenytoin with total amount of drug in vial.
- Implement seizure precautions.
- When substituting *fosphenytoin* for oral *phenytoin* therapy, the same total daily dose may be given as a single dose. Unlike parenteral phenytoin, fosphenytoin may be given safely by the IM route.
- The anticonvulsant effect of fosphenytoin is not immediate. Additional measures (including parenteral benzodiazepines) are usually required in the immediate management of status epilepticus. Loading dose of *fosphenytoin* should be followed with the institution of maintenance anticonvulsant therapy.

IV Administration

- **IV Push:** ***Diluent:*** D5W or 0.9% NaCl. ***Concentration:*** 1.5–25 mg PE/mL. May be refrigerated for up to 48 hr. ***Rate:*** Administer at a rate of <150 mg PE/min in adults and <3 mg/kg/min in children to minimize risk of hypotension and arrhythmias.
- **Y-Site Compatibility:** acyclovir, alemtuzumab, alfentanil, allopurinol, amifostine, amikacin, aminocaproic acid, aminophylline, amphotericin B lipid complex, amphotericin B liposome, ampicillin, ampicillin/sulbactam, anidulafungin, argatroban, arsenic trioxide, azithromycin, aztreonam, bivalirudin, bleomycin, bumetanide, buprenorphine, busulfan, butorphanol, carboplatin, carmustine, cefazolin, cefepime, cefotaxime, cefotetan, cefoxitin, ceftazidime, ceftolozane/tazobactam, ceftriaxone, cefuroxime, chloramphenicol, ciprofloxacin, cisatracurium, cisplatin, clindamycin, cyclophosphamide, cyclosporine, cytarabine, dacarbazine, dactinomycin, daptomycin, dexamethasone, dexmedetomidine, dexrazoxane, digoxin, diltiazem, diphenhydramine, docetaxel, doxacurium, doxorubicin liposomal, doxycycline, enalaprilat, ephedrine, epinephrine, eptifibatide, ertapenem, erythromycin, esmolol, etoposide, etoposide phosphate, famotidine, fentanyl, fluconazole, fludarabine, fluorouracil, foscarnet, fosfomycin, furosemide, ganciclovir, gemcitabine, gentamicin, glycopyrrolate, granisetron, heparin, hetastarch, hydrocortisone, hydromorphone, ifosfamide, imipenem/cilastatin, insulin, regular, isoproterenol, ketotolac, labetalol, leucovorin calcium, levofloxacin, lidocaine, linezolid, lorazepam, magnesium sulfate, mannitol, mephalan, meperidine, meropenem, meropenen/vaborbactam, mesna, methotrexate, methyldopate, methylprednisolone, metoclopramide, metoprolol, milrinone, mitomycin, morphine, nalbuphine, naloxone, nitroglycerin, nitroprusside, norepinephrine, octreotide, ondansetron, oxaliplatin, oxytocin, paclitaxel, palonosetron, pamidronate, pancuronium, pantoprazole, pemetrexed, pentobarbital, phenobarbital, phentolamine, phenylephrine, piperacillin/tazobactam, plazomicin, potassium acetate, potassium chloride, potassium phosphates, procainamide, propranolol, ranitidine, remifentanil, rocuronium, sodium acetate, sodium bicarbonate, sodium phosphates, succinylcholine, sufentanil, tacrolimus, tedizolid, theophylline, thiotepa, tigecycline, tirofiban, tobramycin, trimethoprim/sulfamethoxazole, vancomycin, vasopressin, vecuronium, vinblastine, vincristine, vinorelbine, voriconazole, zidovudine, zoledronic acid.
- **Y-Site Incompatibility:** amiodarone, calcium chloride, calcium gluconate, caspofungin, chlorpromazine, dantrolene, daunorubicin hydrochloride, diazepam, dobutamine, dolasetron, doxorubicin hydrochloride, droperidol, epirubicin, fenoldopam, haloperidol, hydralazine, hydroxyzine, idarubicin, irinotecan, isavuconazonium, midazolam, mitoxantrone, moxifloxacin, mycophenolate, nicardipine, pentamidine, phenytoin, prochlorperazine, quinupristin/dalfopristin, thiopental, topotecan, verapamil.

Patient/Family Teaching

- May cause drowsiness or dizziness. Caution patient to avoid driving or other activities requiring alertness until response to medication is known. Do not resume driving until physician gives clearance based on control of seizure disorder.
- Instruct patients that behavioral changes, skin rash, fever, sore throat, mouth ulcers, easy bruising, petechiae, unusual bleeding, abdominal pain, chills, pale stools, dark urine, jaundice, severe nausea or vomiting, drowsiness, slurred speech, unsteady gait, swollen glands, or persistent headache should be reported to health care professional immediately. Advise patient and family to notify health care professional if thoughts about suicide or dying, attempts to commit suicide; new or worse depression; new or worse anxiety; feeling very agitated or restless; panic

attacks; trouble sleeping; new or worse irritability; acting aggressive; being angry or violent; acting on dangerous impulses; an extreme increase in activity and talking, other unusual changes in behavior or mood occur.
- Advise patient to notify health care professional of all Rx or OTC medications, vitamins, or herbal products being taken and to consult with health care professional before taking other medications, especially St. John's wort.
- Rep: Advise female patients to use an additional nonhormonal method of contraception during therapy and until next menstrual period. Instruct patient to notify health care professional if pregnancy is planned or suspected. Encourage patients who become pregnant to enroll in the North American Antiepileptic Drug (NAAED) Pregnancy Registry by calling 1-888-233-2334 or on the web at www.aedpregnancyregistry.org. Enrollment must be done by patients themselves.
- Advise patient to carry identification describing disease process and medication regimen at all times.
- Emphasize the importance of routine exams to monitor progress. Patient should have routine physical exams, especially monitoring skin and lymph nodes, and EEG testing.

Evaluation/Desired Outcomes
- Decrease or cessation of seizures without excessive sedation.

fremanezumab
(free-ma-**nez**-ue-mab)
Ajovy

Classification
Therapeutic: vascular headache suppressants
Pharmacologic: monoclonal antibodies, calcitonin gene-related peptide receptor antagonists

Indications
Migraine prevention.

Action
Monoclonal antibody that binds to the calcitonin gene-related peptide (CGRP) receptor, which reduces the neuroinflammatory and vasodilatory effects of CGRP. **Therapeutic Effects:** Reduction in frequency of migraines.

Pharmacokinetics
Absorption: Unknown.
Distribution: Minimal distribution to tissues.
Metabolism and Excretion: Degraded by enzymatic proteolysis into small peptides and amino acids.
Half-life: 31 days.

TIME/ACTION PROFILE (plasma concentrations)

ROUTE	ONSET	PEAK	DURATION
Subcut	unknown	5–7 days	1 mo

Contraindications/Precautions
Contraindicated in: Hypersensitivity.
Use Cautiously in: OB: Safety and effectiveness not established; Lactation: Use only if potential maternal benefit justifies potential risk to infant; Pedi: Safety and effectiveness not established.

Adverse Reactions/Side Effects
Local: injection site reactions. **Misc:** hypersensitivity reactions.

Interactions
Drug-Drug: None reported.

Route/Dosage
Subcut (Adults): 225 mg once monthly *or* 675 mg every 3 mo.

Availability
Solution for injection (prefilled syringes): 225 mg/1.5 mL.

NURSING IMPLICATIONS

Assessment
- Assess frequency and intensity of migraines.
- Monitor for signs and symptoms of hypersensitivity reactions (rash, pruritus, drug hypersensitivity, urticaria) during therapy. May occur up to 1 mo after administration. If reaction is severe, discontinue fremanezumab and treat as needed.

Implementation
- **Subcut:** Prior to use allow vial to sit at room temperature for at least 30 min, protect from direct sunlight. Do no use other methods to warm solution (hot water or microwave). Do not shake. Solution is clear to opalescent, colorless to light yellow; do not administer solutions that are discolored, cloudy, or contain particulate matter. Store in refrigerator in original carton to protect from light; do not freeze. May be stored up to 24 hr at room temperature; discard if at room temperature >24 hr.
- Inject entire contents into abdomen, thigh, or upper arm. Do not inject into areas where the skin is tender, bruised, red, or hard.

Patient/Family Teaching
- Instruct patient to take as directed. Administer missed doses as soon as possible and schedule next dose from date last dose administered. Educate patient and/or caregiver on correct technique for injection and disposal of equipment. Advise patient to read *Patient Information* before starting therapy and with each Rx refill in case of changes.
- Instruct patient to notify health care professional immediately if signs and symptoms of hypersensitivity

reaction (itching, rash, hives, swelling of face, mouth, tongue or throat, trouble breathing) occur.

- Advise patient to notify health care professional of all Rx or OTC medications, vitamins, or herbal products being taken and to consult with health care professional before taking other medications.
- Advise female patients to notify health care professional if pregnancy is planned or suspected or if breast feeding.

Evaluation/Desired Outcomes

- Decrease in frequency and intensity of migraines.

frovatriptan (froe-va-trip-tan)

Frova

Classification

Therapeutic: vascular headache suppressants

Pharmacologic: 5-HT_1 agonists

Indications

Acute treatment of migraine headache.

Action

Acts as an agonist at specific 5-HT receptor sites in intracranial blood vessels and sensory trigeminal nerves. **Therapeutic Effects:** Cranial vessel vasoconstriction with associated decrease in release of neuropeptides and resultant decrease in migraine headache.

Pharmacokinetics

Absorption: 20–30% following oral administration.

Distribution: Unknown.

Metabolism and Excretion: Mostly metabolized by the liver (P450 1A2 enzyme system); some metabolites eliminated in urine, <10% excreted unchanged.

Half-life: 26 hr.

TIME/ACTION PROFILE (blood levels)

ROUTE	ONSET	PEAK	DURATION
PO	unknown	2–4 hr	unknown

Contraindications/Precautions

Contraindicated in: Hypersensitivity; History, symptoms or findings consistent with; Cerebrovascular syndromes including; Uncontrolled hypertension; Hemiplegic or basilar migraine; Peripheral vascular disease, including ischemic bowel disease; Should not be used within 24 hr of any other 5-HT agonist or ergot-type compounds (e.g. dihydroergotamine, ergotamine); Pedi: Children <18 yr.

Use Cautiously in: Concurrent use of SSRIs or SNRIs (↑ risk of serotonin syndrome); Geri: May be more susceptible to adverse cardiovascular effects; OB, Lactation: Safety not established.

Exercise Extreme Caution in: Cardiovascular risk factors (hypertension, hypercholesterolemia, cigarette smoking, obesity, diabetes, strong family history, menopausal women or men >40 yr); use only if cardiovascular status has been evaluated and determined to be safe and first dose is administered under supervision.

Adverse Reactions/Side Effects

CNS: dizziness, drowsiness, fatigue. **CV:** CORONARY ARTERY VASOSPASM, MI, VENTRICULAR FIBRILLATION, VENTRICULAR TACHYCARDIA, chest pain, myocardial ischemia. **GI:** dry mouth, dyspepsia, nausea. **Derm:** flushing. **MS:** skeletal pain. **Neuro:** paresthesia. **Misc:** pain.

Interactions

Drug-Drug: Hormonal contraceptives or **propranolol** may ↑ levels. ↑ risk of serious vasospastic reactions with **dihydroergotamine** or **ergotamine** (concurrent use contraindicated). ↑ risk of serotonin syndrome when used with **fluoxetine**, **paroxetine**, **sertraline**, **fluvoxamine**, **citalopram**, **escitalopram**, **venlafaxine**, or **duloxetine**.

Route/Dosage

PO (Adults): 2.5 mg; if there has been initial relief, a 2nd tablet may be taken after at least 2 hr (daily dose should not exceed 3 tablets and should not be used to treat more than 4 attacks/30 day period).

Availability (generic available)

Tablets: 2.5 mg.

NURSING IMPLICATIONS

Assessment

- Assess pain location, intensity, duration, and associated symptoms (photophobia, phonophobia, nausea, vomiting) during migraine attack.

Implementation

- **PO:** Tablets may be administered at any time after the headache starts.

Patient/Family Teaching

- Inform patient that frovatriptan should be used only during a migraine attack. It is meant to be used to relieve migraine attack but not to prevent or reduce the number of attacks.
- Instruct patient to administer frovatriptan as soon as symptoms appear, but it may be administered any time during an attack. If migraine symptoms return, a 2nd dose may be used. Allow at least 2 hr between doses, and do not use more than 3 tablets in any 24-hr period.
- If dose does not relieve headache, additional frovatriptan doses are not likely to be effective; notify health care professional.
- Caution patient not to take frovatriptan within 24 hr of another vascular headache suppressant.

- Advise patient that lying down in a darkened room following frovatriptan administration may further help relieve headache.
- May cause dizziness or drowsiness. Caution patient to avoid driving or other activities requiring alertness until response to medication is known.
- Advise patient that overuse (use more than 10 days/mo) may lead to exacerbation of headache (migraine-like daily headaches, or as a marked increase in frequency of migraine attacks). May require gradual withdrawal of frovatriptan and treatment of symptoms (transient worsening of headache).
- Advise patient to notify health care professional prior to next dose of frovatriptan if pain or tightness in the chest occurs during use. If pain is severe or does not subside, notify health care professional immediately. If wheezing; heart throbbing; swelling of eyelids, face, or lips; skin rash; skin lumps; or hives occur, notify health care professional immediately and do not take more frovatriptan without approval of health care professional. If feelings of tingling, heat, flushing, heaviness, pressure, drowsiness, dizziness, tiredness, or sickness develop, discuss with health care professional at next visit.
- Advise patient to avoid alcohol, which aggravates headaches, during frovatriptan use.
- Advise patient to notify health care professional of all Rx or OTC medications, vitamins, or herbal products being taken and to consult with health care professional before taking other medications.
- Advise patient to notify health care professional immediately if signs or symptoms of serotonin syndrome occur.
- Caution patient not to use frovatriptan if pregnancy is planned or suspected, or if breast feeding. Adequate contraception should be used during therapy.

Evaluation/Desired Outcomes

- Relief of migraine attack.

furosemide (fur-**oh**-se-mide)

Lasix

Classification

Therapeutic: diuretics

Pharmacologic: loop diuretics

Indications

Edema due to heart failure, hepatic impairment, or renal disease. Hypertension.

Action

Inhibits the reabsorption of sodium and chloride from the loop of Henle and distal renal tubule. Increases renal excretion of water, sodium, chloride, magnesium, potassium, and calcium. Effectiveness persists in impaired renal function. **Therapeutic Effects:** Diuresis and subsequent mobilization of excess fluid (edema, pleural effusions). Decreased BP.

Pharmacokinetics

Absorption: 60–67% absorbed after oral administration (↓ in acute HF and in renal failure); also absorbed from IM sites.

Distribution: Crosses placenta, enters breast milk.

Protein Binding: 91–99%.

Metabolism and Excretion: Minimally metabolized by liver, some nonhepatic metabolism, some renal excretion as unchanged drug.

Half-life: 30–60 min (↑ in renal impairment).

TIME/ACTION PROFILE (diuretic effect)

ROUTE	ONSET	PEAK	DURATION
PO	30–60 min	1–2 hr	6–8 hr
IM	10–30 min	unknown	4–8 hr
IV	5 min	30 min	2 hr

Contraindications/Precautions

Contraindicated in: Hypersensitivity; Cross-sensitivity with thiazides and sulfonamides may occur; Hepatic coma or anuria; Some liquid products may contain alcohol, avoid in patients with alcohol intolerance.

Use Cautiously in: Severe liver disease (may precipitate hepatic coma; concurrent use with potassium-sparing diuretics may be necessary); Electrolyte depletion; Diabetes mellitus; Hypoproteinemia (↑ risk of ototoxicity); Severe renal impairment (↑ risk of ototoxicity); OB, Lactation: Safety not established; Pedi: ↑ risk for renal calculi and patent ductus arteriosis in premature neonates; Geri: May have ↑ risk of side effects, especially hypotension and electrolyte imbalance, at usual doses.

Adverse Reactions/Side Effects

CNS: blurred vision, dizziness, headache, vertigo. **CV:** hypotension. **Derm:** ERYTHEMA MULTIFORME, STEVENS-JOHNSON SYNDROME, TOXIC EPIDERMAL NECROLYSIS, photosensitivity, pruritis, rash, urticaria. **EENT:** hearing loss, tinnitus. **Endo:** hypercholesterolemia, hyperglycemia, hypertriglyceridemia, hyperuricemia. **F and E:** dehydration, hypocalcemia, hypochloremia, hypokalemia, hypomagnesemia, hyponatremia, hypovolemia, metabolic alkalosis. **GI:** anorexia, constipation, diarrhea, dry mouth, dyspepsia, ↑ liver enzymes, nausea, pancreatitis, vomiting. **GU:** ↑ BUN, excessive urination, nephrocalcinosis. **Hemat:** APLASTIC ANEMIA, AGRANULOCYTOSIS, hemolytic anemia, leukopenia, thrombocytopenia. **MS:** muscle cramps. **Neuro:** paresthesia. **Misc:** fever.

Interactions

Drug-Drug: ↑ risk of hypotension with **antihypertensives**, **nitrates**, or acute ingestion of **alcohol**. ↑ risk of hypokalemia with other **diuretics**, **amphotericin B**, **stimulant laxatives**, and **corticosteroids**. Hypokalemia may ↑ risk of **digoxin** toxicity and ↑ risk of arrhythmia in patients taking drugs that prolong the QT interval. ↓ **lithium** excretion, may cause **lithium** toxicity. ↑ risk of ototoxicity with **aminoglycosides** or **cisplatin**. ↑ risk of nephrotoxicity with **cisplatin**. **NSAIDS** ↓ effects of furosemide. May ↑ risk of **methotrexate** toxicity. ↓ effects when given at same time as **sucralfate**, **cholestyramine**, or **colestipol**. ↑ risk of **salicylate** toxicity (with use of high-dose **salicylate** therapy). Concurrent use with **cyclosporine** may ↑ risk of gouty arthritis.

Route/Dosage

Edema

PO (Adults): 20–80 mg/day as a single dose initially, may repeat in 6–8 hr; may ↑ dose by 20–40 mg every 6–8 hr until desired response. Maintenance doses may be given once or twice daily (doses up to 2.5 g/day have been used in patients with HF or renal disease). *Hypertension*—40 mg twice daily initially (when added to regimen, ↓ dose of other antihypertensives by 50%); adjust further dosing based on response; *Hypercalcemia*—120 mg/day in 1–3 doses.

PO (Children >1 mo): 2 mg/kg as a single dose; may be ↑ by 1–2 mg/kg every 6–8 hr (maximum dose = 6 mg/kg).

PO (Neonates): 1–4 mg/kg/dose 1–2 times/day.

IM, IV (Adults): 20–40 mg, may repeat in 1–2 hr and ↑ by 20 mg every 1–2 hr until response is obtained, maintenance dose may be given every 6–12 hr; *Continuous infusion*—Bolus 0.1 mg/kg followed by 0.1 mg/kg/hr, double every 2 hr to a maximum of 0.4 mg/kg/hr.

IM, IV (Children): 1–2 mg/kg/dose every 6–12 hr; *Continuous infusion*—0.05 mg/kg/hr, titrate to clinical effect.

IM, IV (Neonates): 1–2 mg/kg/dose every 12–24 hr.

Hypertension

PO (Adults): 40 twice daily initially (when added to regimen, ↓ dose of other antihypertensives by 50%); adjust further dosing based on response.

Availability (generic available)

Oral solution (10 mg/mL—orange flavor, 8 mg/mL—pineapple—peach flavor): 8 mg/mL, 10 mg/mL. **Cost:** *Generic*—10 mg/mL $10.40/60 mL. **Tablets:** 20 mg, 40 mg, 80 mg, 🍁 500 mg. **Cost:** *Generic*—20 mg $6.50/100, 40 mg $7.11/100, 80 mg $10.83/100. **Solution for injection:** 10 mg/mL.

NURSING IMPLICATIONS

Assessment

- Assess fluid status. Monitor daily weight, intake and output ratios, amount and location of edema, lung sounds, skin turgor, and mucous membranes. Notify health care professional if thirst, dry mouth, lethargy, weakness, hypotension, or oliguria occurs.
- Monitor BP and pulse before and during administration. Monitor frequency of prescription refills to determine compliance in patients treated for hypertension.
- Geri: Diuretic use is associated with increased risk for falls in older adults. Assess falls risk and implement fall prevention strategies.
- Assess patients receiving digoxin for anorexia, nausea, vomiting, muscle cramps, paresthesia, and confusion. Patients taking digoxin are at increased risk of digoxin toxicity because of the potassium-depleting effect of the diuretic. Potassium supplements or potassium-sparing diuretics may be used concurrently to prevent hypokalemia.
- Assess patient for tinnitus and hearing loss. Audiometry is recommended for patients receiving prolonged high-dose IV therapy. Hearing loss is most common after rapid or high-dose IV administration in patients with decreased renal function or those taking other ototoxic drugs.
- Assess for allergy to sulfonamides.
- Assess patient for skin rash frequently during therapy. Discontinue furosemide at first sign of rash; may be life-threatening. Stevens-Johnson syndrome, toxic epidermal necrolysis, or erythema multiforme may develop. Treat symptomatically; may recur once treatment is stopped.
- ***Lab Test Considerations:*** Monitor electrolytes, renal and hepatic function, serum glucose, and uric acid levels before and periodically throughout therapy. Commonly ↓ serum potassium. May cause ↓ serum sodium, calcium, and magnesium concentrations. May also cause ↑ BUN, serum glucose, creatinine, and uric acid levels.

Implementation

- Do not confuse Lasix (furosemide) with Luvox (fluvoxamine).
- If administering twice daily, give last dose no later than 5 PM to minimize disruption of sleep cycle.
- IV route is preferred over IM route for parenteral administration.
- **PO:** May be taken with food or milk to minimize gastric irritation. Tablets may be crushed if patient has difficulty swallowing.
- Do not administer discolored solution or tablets.

IV Administration

- **IV Push:** ***Diluent:*** Administer undiluted (larger doses may be diluted and administered as intermittent infusion [see below]). ***Concentration:*** 10 mg/mL. ***Rate:*** Administer at a rate of 20 mg/min. Pedi: Administer at a maximum rate of 0.5–1 mg/kg/min (for doses <120 mg) with infusion not exceeding 10 min.
- **Intermittent Infusion:** ***Diluent:*** Dilute larger doses in 50 mL of D5W, D10W, D20W, D5/0.9% NaCl, D5/LR, 0.9% NaCl, 3% NaCl, or LR. Infusion stable for 24 hr at room temperature. Do not refrig-

erate. Protect from light. ***Concentration:*** 1 mg/mL. ***Rate:*** Administer at a rate not to exceed 4 mg/min (for doses >120 mg) in adults to prevent ototoxicity. Pedi: not to exceed 1 mg/kg/min with infusion not exceeding 10 min. Use an infusion pump to ensure accurate dose.

- **Y-Site Compatibility:** acyclovir, alfentanil, allopurinol, alprostadil, amifostine, amikacin, aminocaproic acid, aminophylline, amphotericin B cholesteryl, amphotericin B lipid complex, amphotericin B liposome, anidulafungin, argatroban, ascorbic acid, atropine, azathioprine, aztreonam, bivalirudin, bleomycin, bumetanide, calcium chloride, calcium gluconate, carboplatin, carmustine, cefazolin, cefepime, cefotaxime, cefotetan, cefoxitin, ceftaroline, ceftazidime, ceftriaxone, cefuroxime, chloramphenicol, cisplatin, cladribine, clindamycin, cyanocobalamin, cyclophosphamide, cyclosporine, cytarabine, dactinomycin, daptomycin, dexamethasone, dexmedetomidine, digoxin, docetaxel, doxacurium, doxorubicin liposome, enalaprilat, ephedrine, epinephrine, epoetin alfa, ertapenem, esomeprazole, etoposide, etoposide phosphate, fentanyl, fludarabine, fluorouracil, folic acid, foscarnet, ganciclovir, granisetron, hydrocortisone sodium succinate, hydromorphone, ibuprofen, ifosfamide, imipenem/cilastatin, indomethacin, ketorolac, leucovorin calcium, lidocaine, linezolid, lorazepam, mannitol, melphalan, meropenem, methotrexate, methylprednisolone, metoprolol, metronidazole, micafungin, mitomycin, multivitamins, nafcillin, naloxone, nitroprusside, octreotide, oxacillin, oxaliplatin, oxytocin, paclitaxel, palonosetron, pamidronate, pemetrexed, penicillin G, pentobarbital, phenobarbital, phytonadione, piperacillin/tazobactam, potassium acetate, potassium chloride, procainamide, propofol, propranolol, ranitidine, remifentanil, sargramostim, sodium acetate, sodium bicarbonate, streptokinase, succinylcholine, sufentanil, theophylline, thiotepa, tigecycline, tirofiban, tobramycin, vitamin B complex with C, voriconazole, zoledronic acid.
- **Y-Site Incompatibility:** alemtuzumab, amsacrine, atracurium, benztropine, butorphanol, caspofungin, chlorpromazine, ciprofloxacin, dantrolene, dexrazoxane, diazepam, diazoxide, diltiazem, diphenhydramine, dolasetron, doxycycline, droperidol, epirubicin, eptifibitide, erythromycin, esmolol, fenoldopam, filgrastim, gemcitabine, gentamicin, glycopyrrolate, haloperidol, hydroxyzine, idarubicin, irinotecan, ketamine, levofloxacin, metaraminol, methyldopate, midazolam, milrinone, mitoxantrone, moxifloxacin, mycophenolate, nalbuphine, nicardipine, ondansetron, pancuronium, papaverine, pentamidine, phentolamine, phenylephrine, phenytoin, prochlorperazine, promethazine, protamine, pyridoxime, quinupristin/dalfopristin, rituximab, rocuronium, telavancin, thiamine, trastuzumab, trimethoprim/sulfamethoxazole, vancomycin, vecuronium, verapamil, vinblastine, vinorelbine.

Patient/Family Teaching

- Instruct patient to take furosemide as directed. Take missed doses as soon as possible; do not double doses.
- Caution patient to change positions slowly to minimize orthostatic hypotension. Caution patient that the use of alcohol, exercise during hot weather, or standing for long periods during therapy may enhance orthostatic hypotension.
- Instruct patient to consult health care professional regarding a diet high in potassium (see Appendix K).
- Advise patient to contact health care professional if weight gain more than 3 lbs in 1 day.
- Instruct patient to notify health care professional of all Rx or OTC medications, vitamins, or herbal products being taken and to consult health care professional before taking any OTC medications concurrently with this therapy.
- Instruct patient to notify health care professional of medication regimen before treatment or surgery.
- Caution patient to use sunscreen and protective clothing to prevent photosensitivity reactions.
- Advise patient to contact health care professional immediately if rash, muscle weakness, cramps, nausea, dizziness, numbness, or tingling of extremities occurs.
- Advise diabetic patients to monitor blood glucose closely; may cause increased blood glucose levels.
- Advise females of reproductive potential to notify health care professional if pregnancy is planned or suspected, or if breast feeding. Monitor fetal growth during pregnancy; increased risk for higher birth weights.
- Emphasize the importance of routine follow-up examinations.
- Geri: Caution older patients or their caregivers about increased risk for falls. Suggest strategies for fall prevention.
- **Hypertension:** Advise patients on antihypertensive regimen to continue taking medication even if feeling better. Furosemide controls but does not cure hypertension.
- Reinforce the need to continue additional therapies for hypertension (weight loss, exercise, restricted sodium intake, stress reduction, regular exercise, moderation of alcohol consumption, cessation of smoking).

Evaluation/Desired Outcomes

- Decrease in edema.
- Decrease in abdominal girth and weight.
- Increase in urinary output.
- Decrease in BP.

gabapentin (ga-ba-pen-tin)

Gralise, Horizant, Neurontin

Classification

Therapeutic: analgesic adjuncts, therapeutic, anticonvulsants, mood stabilizers

Schedule V (only schedule V in some states)

Indications

Partial seizures (adjunct treatment) (immediate-release only). Postherpetic neuralgia. Restless legs syndrome (Horizant only). **Unlabeled Use:** Neuropathic pain. Prevention of migraine headache. Bipolar disorder. Anxiety. Diabetic peripheral neuropathy.

Action

Mechanism of action is not known. May affect transport of amino acids across and stabilize neuronal membranes. **Therapeutic Effects:** Decreased incidence of seizures. Decreased postherpetic pain. Decreased leg restlessness.

Pharmacokinetics

Absorption: Well absorbed after oral administration by active transport. At larger doses, transport becomes saturated and absorption ↓ (bioavailability ranges from 60% for a 300-mg dose to 35% for a 1600-mg dose).

Distribution: Crosses blood-brain barrier; enters breast milk.

Metabolism and Excretion: Eliminated mostly by renal excretion of unchanged drug.

Half-life: *Adults*—5–7 hr (normal renal function); up to 132 hr in anuria; *Children*—4.7 hr.

TIME/ACTION PROFILE (blood levels)

ROUTE	ONSET	PEAK	DURATION
PO-IR	rapid	2–4 hr	8 hr
PO-SR	unknown	5–8 hr	24 hr

Contraindications/Precautions

Contraindicated in: Hypersensitivity.

Use Cautiously in: All patients (may ↑ risk of suicidal thoughts/behaviors); Renal impairment (↓ dose and/or ↑ dosing interval if CCr ≤60 mL/min); OB, Lactation: Safety not established; Pedi: Children <18 yr (sustained-/extended-release) or <3 yr (immediate-release) (safety and effectiveness not established); Geri: May be more susceptible to toxicity due to age-related ↓ in renal function.

Adverse Reactions/Side Effects

CNS: SUICIDAL THOUGHTS, confusion, depression, dizziness, drowsiness, sedation, anxiety, concentration difficulties (children), emotional lability (children), hostility, hyperkinesia (children), malaise, vertigo, weakness. **CV:** hypertension. **EENT:** abnormal vision, nystagmus. **GI:** weight gain, anorexia, flatulence, gingivitis. **MS:** RHABDOMYOLYSIS, arthralgia, ↑ creatine kinase. **Neuro:** ataxia, altered reflexes, hyperkinesia, paresthesia. **Misc:** HYPERSENSITIVITY REACTIONS (including anaphylaxis or angioedema).

Interactions

Drug-Drug: Antacids may ↓ absorption of gabapentin. ↑ risk of CNS depression with other **CNS depressants**, including **alcohol**, **antihistamines**, **opioids**, and **sedative/hypnotics**. May ↓ **hydrocodone** levels.

Drug-Natural Products: Kava-kava, **valerian**, or **chamomile** can ↑ CNS depression.

G

Route/Dosage

The sustained-/extended-release formulations should not be interchanged with the immediate-release products.

Epilepsy

PO (Adults and Children >12 yr): 300 mg 3 times daily initially. Titration may be continued until desired (range is 900–1800 mg/day in 3 divided doses; doses should not be more than 12 hr apart). Doses up to 2400–3600 mg/day have been well tolerated.

PO (Children ≥5–12 yr): 10–15 mg/kg/day in 3 divided doses initially titrated upward over 3 days to 25–35 mg/kg/day in 3 divided doses; dosage interval should not exceed 12 hr (doses up to 50 mg/kg/day have been used).

PO (Children 3–4 yrs): 10–15 mg/kg/day in 3 divided doses initially titrated upward over 3 days to 40 mg/kg/day in 3 divided doses; dosage interval should not exceed 12 hr (doses up to 50 mg/kg/day have been used).

Renal Impairment

PO (Adults and Children >12 yr): *CCr 30–59 mL/min*—200–700 mg twice daily; *CCr 15–29 mL/min*—200–700 mg once daily; *CCr 15 mL/min*—100–300 mg once daily; *CCr <15 mL/min*—Reduce daily dose in proportion to CCr.

Postherpetic Neuralgia

PO (Adults): *Immediate-release*—300 mg once daily on first day, then 300 mg 2 times daily on 2nd day, then 300 mg 3 times/day on day 3, may then be titrated upward as needed up to 600 mg 3 times/day; *Sustained-release (Gralise)*—300 mg once daily on first day, then 600 mg once daily on 2nd day, then 900 mg once daily on days 3–6, then 1200 mg once daily on days 7–10, then 1500 mg once daily on days 11–14, then 1800 mg once daily thereafter; *Extended-release (Horizant)*—600 mg once daily in the morning on days 1–3, then 600 mg twice daily thereafter.

Renal Impairment

PO (Adults): *CCr 30–59 mL/min*—200–700 mg twice daily (immediate-release); 600–1800 mg once daily (sustained-release [Gralise]); 300 mg once daily in the morning on days 1–3, then 300 mg twice daily thereafter (may ↑ to 600 mg twice daily, as needed) (extended-release [Horizant]); *CCr 15–29 mL/min*—200–700 mg once daily (immediate-release); sustained release (Gralise) not recommended; 300 mg in the morning on days 1 and 3, then 300 mg once daily in the morning thereafter (may ↑ to 300 mg twice daily, as needed) (extended-release [Horizant]); *CCr 15 mL/min*—100–300 mg once daily (immediate-release); sustained release (Gralise) not recommended; *CCr <15 mL/min*—↓ daily dose in proportion to CCr (immediate release); sustained release (Gralise) not recommended; 300 mg every other day in the morning (may ↑ to 300 mg once daily in the morning, as needed) (extended-release [Horizant]); *CCr <15 mL/min (on hemodialysis)*—300 mg after each dialysis session (may ↑ to 600 mg after each dialysis session, as needed) (extended-release [Horizant]).

Restless Legs Syndrome

PO (Adults): *Extended-release (Horizant)*—600 mg once daily at 5 PM.

Renal Impairment

(Adults): *CCr 30–59 mL/min*—300 mg once daily at 5 PM; may ↑ to 600 mg once daily at 5 PM as needed; *CCr 15–29 mL/min*—300 mg once daily at 5 PM; *CCr <15 mL/min*—300 mg every other day; *CCr <15 mL/min (on hemodialysis)*—Not recommended.

Neuropathic Pain (unlabeled use)

PO (Adults): 100 mg 3 times daily initially. Titrate weekly by 300 mg/day up to 900–2400 mg/day (maximum: 3600 mg/day).

PO (Children): 5 mg/kg/dose at bedtime initially then ↑ to 5 mg/kg twice daily on day 2 and 5 mg/kg 3 times daily on day 3. Titrate to effect up to 8–35 mg/kg/day in 3 divided doses.

Availability (generic available)

Capsules: 100 mg, 300 mg, 400 mg. **Cost:** *Generic*—100 mg $11.45/100, 300 mg $15.18/100, 400 mg $12.36/100. **Tablets:** 600 mg, 800 mg. **Cost:** *Generic*—600 mg $33.96/100, 800 mg $49.20/100. **Extended-release tablets (Horizant):** 300 mg, 600 mg. **Sustained-release tablets (Gralise):** 300 mg, 600 mg. **Cost:** 300 mg $99.00/30, 600 mg $329.40/90. **Oral solution (cool strawberry anise flavor):** 250 mg/5 mL, 300 mg/6 mL. **Cost:** *Generic*—$148.91/470 mL.

NURSING IMPLICATIONS

Assessment

- Monitor closely for notable changes in behavior that could indicate the emergence or worsening of suicidal thoughts or behavior or depression.
- **Seizures:** Assess location, duration, and characteristics of seizure activity.
- **Postherpetic Neuralgia & Neuropathic Pain:** Assess location, characteristics, and intensity of pain periodically during therapy.
- **Migraine Prophylaxis:** Monitor frequency and intensity of pain on pain scale.
- **Restless Leg Syndrome**: Assess frequency and intensity of restless leg syndrome prior to and periodically during therapy.
- ***Lab Test Considerations:*** May cause false-positive readings when testing for urinary protein with *Ames N-Multistix SG* dipstick test; use sulfosalicylic acid precipitation procedure.
- May cause leukopenia.

Implementation

- Do not confuse gabapentin with gemfibrozil. Do not confuse Neurontin (gabapentin) with Motrin (ibuprofen).
- Doses of *Gralise* and *Horizant* are not interchangeable with other dose forms of gabapentin.
- **PO:** May be administered without regard to meals.
- 600-mg and 800-mg tablets are scored and can be broken to administer a half-tablet. If half-tablet is used, administer other half at the next dose. Discard half-tablets not used within several days.
- Administer *Gralise* with evening meal. Swallow tablet whole; do not crush, break, or chew.
- Administer *Horizant for Restless Leg Syndrome* with evening meal at 5 PM. *Horizant for Postherpetic Neuralgia* is administered twice daily. Swallow tablet whole; do not crush, break, or chew.
- Gabapentin should be discontinued gradually over at least 1 wk. If dose is 600 mg/day, may discontinue without tapering. If >600 mg/day, titrate daily to 600 mg for 1 wk, then discontinue. If patient is taking 600 mg twice daily, taper to once daily before discontinuing. Abrupt discontinuation may cause increase in seizure frequency.

Patient/Family Teaching

- Instruct patient to take medication exactly as directed. Patients on 3 times daily dosing should not exceed 12 hr between doses. Take missed doses as soon as possible; if less than 2 hr until next dose, take dose immediately and take next dose 1–2 hr later, then resume regular dosing schedule. Do not double dose. Do not discontinue abruptly; may cause increase in frequency of seizures. Instruct patient to read the *Medication Guide* before starting and with each Rx refill, as changes may occur.
- Advise patient not to take gabapentin within 2 hr of an antacid.
- Gabapentin may cause dizziness and drowsiness. Caution patient to avoid driving or activities requiring alertness until response to medication is known. Seizure patients should not resume driving until physician gives clearance based on control of seizure disorder.

- Advise patient and family to notify health care professional if thoughts about suicide or dying, attempts to commit suicide; new or worse depression; new or worse anxiety; feeling very agitated or restless; panic attacks; trouble sleeping; new or worse irritability; acting aggressive; being angry or violent; acting on dangerous impulses; an extreme increase in activity and talking; or other unusual changes in behavior or mood occur.
- Instruct patient to notify health care professional of medication regimen before treatment or surgery.
- Rep: Advise female patient to notify health care professional if pregnancy is planned or suspected or if breast feeding. Encourage patients who become pregnant to enroll in the North American Antiepileptic Drug (NAAED) Pregnancy Registry by calling 1-888-233-2334 or on the web at www.aedpregnancyregistry.org.
- Advise patient to carry identification describing disease process and medication regimen at all times.

Evaluation/Desired Outcomes

- Decreased frequency of or cessation of seizures.
- Decreased postherpetic neuralgia pain.
- Decreased intensity of neuropathic pain.
- Decreased frequency of migraine headaches.
- Increased mood stability.
- Decreased effects of restless leg syndrome.

galantamine

(ga-**lant**-a-meen)

Razadyne, Razadyne ER

Classification

Therapeutic: anti-Alzheimer's agents

Pharmacologic: cholinergics (cholinesterase inhibitors)

Indications

Mild to moderate dementia/neurocognitive disorder of the Alzheimer's type.

Action

Enhances cholinergic function by reversible inhibition of cholinesterase. **Therapeutic Effects:** Decreased dementia/cognitive decline (temporary) associated with Alzheimer's disease. Cognitive enhancer.

Pharmacokinetics

Absorption: Well absorbed (90%) following oral administration.

Distribution: Unknown.

Metabolism and Excretion: Mostly metabolized by the liver (primarily by CYP2D6 and CYP3A4 isoenzymes); the CYP2D6 enzyme system exhibits genetic polymorphism; ~7% of population may be poor metabolizers (PMs) and may have significantly ↑ galantamine concentrations and an ↑ risk of adverse effects. 20% excreted unchanged in urine.

Half-life: 7 hr.

TIME/ACTION PROFILE (anticholinesterase activity)

ROUTE	ONSET	PEAK	DURATION
PO	unknown	1 hr	12 hr
PO-ER	unknown	1 hr	24 hr

Contraindications/Precautions

Contraindicated in: Hypersensitivity; Severe hepatic or renal impairment; Pedi, Lactation: Children or lactation.

Use Cautiously in: Patients with supraventricular cardiac conduction defects or concurrent use of drugs that may slow heart rate (↑ risk of bradycardia); History of ulcer disease/GI bleeding/concurrent NSAID use; Severe asthma or obstructive pulmonary disease; Mild to moderate renal impairment (avoid use if CCr <9 mL/min); Mild to moderate hepatic impairment (cautious dose titration recommended); May ↑ risk of cardiovascular mortality; OB: Use only if potential benefit outweighs potential risk to fetus.

Adverse Reactions/Side Effects

CNS: dizziness, fatigue, headache, syncope. **CV:** bradycardia, chest pain. **GI:** nausea, vomiting, anorexia, ↓ weight, diarrhea, dyspepsia, flatulence. **GU:** bladder outflow obstruction, incontinence. **Neuro:** tremor. **Derm:** ACUTE GENERALIZED EXANTHEMATOUS PUSTULOSIS, STEVENS-JOHNSON SYNDROME.

Interactions

Drug-Drug: Will ↑ neuromuscular blockade from **succinylcholine-type neuromuscular blocking agents**. May ↑ effects of other **cholinesterase inhibitors** or other **cholinergic agonists**, including **bethanechol**. May ↓ effectiveness of **anticholinergic medications**. Blood levels and effects may be ↑ by **ketoconazole**, **paroxetine**, **amitriptyline**, **fluvoxamine**, or **quinidine**.

Route/Dosage

PO (Adults): *Immediate-release tablets*—4 mg twice daily initially, dose increments of 4 mg should be made at 4 wk intervals, up to 12 mg twice daily. Doses up to 16 mg twice daily have been used (range 16–32 mg/day; *Extended-release capsules*—8 mg/day as a single dose in the morning, may be ↑ to 16 mg/day after 4 wk, then up to 24 mg/day after 4 wk; increments based on benefit/tolerability.

Renal Impairment

PO (Adults): *Moderate renal impairment*—Daily dose should not exceed 16 mg.

Hepatic Impairment

PO (Adults): *Moderate hepatic impairment*—Daily dose should not exceed 16 mg.

Availability (generic available)

Immediate-release tablets: 4 mg, 8 mg, 12 mg. **Extended-release capsules:** 8 mg, 16 mg, 24 mg. **Oral solution:** 4 mg/mL.

NURSING IMPLICATIONS

Assessment

- Assess cognitive function (memory, attention, reasoning, language, ability to perform simple tasks) periodically during therapy.
- Monitor heart rate periodically during therapy. May cause bradycardia.

Implementation

- Do not confuse Razadyne with Rozerem (ramelteon).
- Patient should be maintained on a stable dose for a minimum of 4 wk prior to increasing dose.
- If dose has been interrupted for several days or longer, restart at the lowest dose and escalate to the current dose.
- **PO:** Administer twice daily, preferably with morning and evening meal. Administration with food, the use of antiemetic medications, and ensuring adequate fluid intake may decrease nausea and vomiting.
- Administer extended-release capsules in the morning, preferably with food. Swallow whole; do not open, crush, or chew.
- Use pipette provided with oral solution to administer accurate amount.

Patient/Family Teaching

- Emphasize the importance of taking galantamine daily, as directed. Instruct patient and/or caregiver in correct use of pipette if using oral solution; review *Oral Solution Instruction Sheet* included with product prior to use. Skip missed doses and return to regular schedule the following day; do not double doses. If >3 days doses are missed, restart at lowest dose. Do not discontinue abruptly; although no increase in frequency of adverse events may occur, beneficial affects of galantamine are lost when the drug is discontinued.
- Caution patient and caregiver that galantamine may cause dizziness. Monitor and assist with ambulation and caution patient to avoid driving and other activities requiring alertness until response to medication is known.
- Instruct patient to maintain adequate fluid intake during therapy.
- Advise patient and caregiver to stop taking galantamine and notify health care professional immediately if rash occurs.
- Advise patient and caregiver to notify health care professional if nausea or vomiting persists beyond 7 days or if new symptoms occur or previously noted symptoms increase in severity.
- Advise patient and caregiver to notify health care professional of medication regimen prior to treatment or surgery.
- Teach patient and caregivers that improvements in cognitive functioning may take wk to mo to stabilize.
- Caution that disease is not cured and degenerative process is not reversed.
- Emphasize the importance of follow-up exams to monitor progress.

Evaluation/Desired Outcomes

- Improvement in cognitive function (memory, attention, reasoning, language, ability to perform simple tasks) in patients with Alzheimer's disease.

galcanezumab

(gal-ka-nez-ue-mab)

Emgality

Classification

Therapeutic: vascular headache suppressants

Pharmacologic: monoclonal antibodies, calcitonin gene-related peptide receptor antagonists

Indications

Migraine prevention. Treatment of episodic cluster headaches.

Action

Monoclonal antibody that binds to the calcitonin gene-related peptide (CGRP) receptor, which reduces the neuroinflammatory and vasodilatory effects of CGRP. **Therapeutic Effects:** Reduction in frequency of migraines and cluster headaches.

Pharmacokinetics

Absorption: Unknown.

Distribution: Some tissue distribution.

Metabolism and Excretion: Degraded into small peptides and amino acids via catabolic pathways.

Half-life: 27 days.

TIME/ACTION PROFILE (plasma concentrations)

ROUTE	ONSET	PEAK	DURATION
Subcut	unknown	5 days	1 mo

Contraindications/Precautions

Contraindicated in: Hypersensitivity.

Use Cautiously in: OB: Safety and effectiveness not established; Lactation: Use only if potential maternal benefit justifies potential risk to infant; Pedi: Safety and effectiveness not established.

Adverse Reactions/Side Effects

Local: injection site reactions. **Misc:** hypersensitivity reactions.

Interactions

Drug-Drug: None reported.

Route/Dosage

Migraine Prevention

Subcut (Adults): 240 mg once initially as loading dose, then 120 mg once monthly.

Episodic Cluster Headache

Subcut (Adults): 300 mg once at the onset of the cluster period, then 300 mg once monthly until the end of the cluster period.

Availability

Solution for injection (prefilled pens and prefilled syringes): 100 mg/mL, 120 mg/mL.

NURSING IMPLICATIONS

Assessment

- Assess frequency and intensity of migraines and cluster headaches.
- Monitor for signs and symptoms of hypersensitivity reactions (rash, urticaria, dyspnea) during therapy. If reaction is severe, discontinue galcanezumab and treat as needed.

Implementation

- **Subcut:** Prior to use allow vial to sit at room temperature for at least 30 min, protect from direct sunlight. Do no use other methods to warm solution (hot water or microwave). Do not shake. Solution is clear to opalescent, colorless to light yellow; do not administer solutions that are discolored, cloudy, or contain particulate matter. Store in refrigerator in original carton to protect from light; do not freeze. May be stored in original carton to protect from light up to 7 days at room temperature; discard if at room temperature >7 days. Do not put back in refrigerator.
- Inject entire contents into abdomen, thigh, or upper arm. Do not inject into areas where the skin is tender, bruised, red, or hard.

Migraines

- *Loading dose:* 240 mg (2 consecutive subcut injections of 120 mg each) once. *Monthly:* follow loading dose with monthly doses of 120 mg.

Cluster Headaches

- **Subcut:** 300 mg (3 consecutive subcut injections of 100 mg each) at onset of cluster period; then monthly until end of cluster period.

Patient/Family Teaching

- Instruct patient to take as directed. Administer missed doses as soon as possible and schedule next dose from date last dose administered. Educate patient and/or caregiver on correct technique for injection and disposal of equipment. Advise patient to read *Patient Information* before starting therapy and with each Rx refill in case of changes.
- Instruct patient to notify health care professional immediately if signs and symptoms of hypersensitivity reaction (itching, rash, hives, swelling of face, mouth, tongue or throat, trouble breathing) occur.
- Advise patient to notify health care professional of all Rx or OTC medications, vitamins, or herbal products being taken and to consult with health care professional before taking other medications.
- Advise female patients to notify health care professional if pregnancy is planned or suspected or if breast feeding.

Evaluation/Desired Outcomes

- Reduction in frequency of migraines and cluster headaches.

ganciclovir (gan-sye-kloe-vir)

Cytovene

Classification
Therapeutic: antivirals

Indications

Treatment of cytomegalovirus (CMV) retinitis in immunocompromised patients, including HIV-infected patients (may be used with foscarnet). Prevention of CMV infection in transplant patients at risk. Congenital CMV infection in neonates.

Action

CMV converts ganciclovir to its active form (ganciclovir phosphate) inside the host cell, where it inhibits viral DNA polymerase. **Therapeutic Effects:** Antiviral effect directed preferentially against CMV-infected cells.

Pharmacokinetics

Absorption: IV administration results in complete bioavailability.
Distribution: Widely distributed; enters CSF.
Protein Binding: 1–2%.
Metabolism and Excretion: 90% excreted unchanged by the kidneys.
Half-life: *Adults:* 2.9 hr; *Children 9 mo–12 yr:* 2.4 ±0.7 hr; *Neonates:* 2.4 hr (↑ in renal impairment).

TIME/ACTION PROFILE (antiviral levels)

ROUTE	ONSET	PEAK	DURATION
IV	rapid	end of infusion	12–24 hr

Contraindications/Precautions

Contraindicated in: Hypersensitivity to ganciclovir or acyclovir; Bone marrow depression or immunosuppression or thrombocytopenia (do not administer if ANC <500/mm³ or platelet count <25,000/mm³); Lactation: Avoid breast feeding.

Use Cautiously in: Renal impairment (dose ↓ required if CCr <80 mL/min); OB: Use only if potential maternal benefit justifies potential fetal risk; Rep: Women of reproductive potential and men with female partners of reproductive potential; Geri: Dose ↓ recommended.

Adverse Reactions/Side Effects

CNS: SEIZURES, abnormal dreams, coma, confusion, dizziness, drowsiness, headache, malaise, nervousness. **CV:** arrhythmias, edema, hypertension, hypotension. **Derm:** alopecia, photosensitivity, pruritus, rash, urticaria. **Endo:** hypoglycemia. **GI:** GI BLEEDING, abdominal pain, ↑ liver enzymes, nausea, vomiting. **GU:** ↓ fertility, gonadal suppression, hematuria, renal toxicity. **Hemat:** neutropenia, thrombocytopenia, anemia, eosinophilia. **Local:** pain/phlebitis at IV site. **Neuro:** ataxia, tremor. **Resp:** dyspnea. **Misc:** fever.

Interactions

Drug-Drug: Toxicity may be ↑ by **probenecid**. ↑ risk of seizures with **imipenem/cilastatin**; concurrent use not recommended. Concurrent use of other **cyclosporine** or **amphotericin B** ↑ risk of nephrotoxicity. ↑ risk of nephrotoxicity and hematological toxicity with **mycophenolate mofetil**. Concurrent use with **dapsone**, **doxorubicin**, **flucytosine**, **hydroxyurea**, **pentamidine**, **tacrolimus**, **trimethoprim/sulfamethoxazole**, **vinblastine**, **vincristine**, or **zidovudine** ↑ risk of nephrotoxicity and myelosuppression. May ↑ **didanosine** levels.

Route/Dosage

IV (Adults and Children >3 mo): *Induction*—5 mg/kg every 12 hr for 14–21 days. *Maintenance regimen*—5 mg/kg/day or 6 mg/kg for 5 days of each wk. If progression occurs, ↑ to every 12 hr regimen. *Prevention*—5 mg/kg every 12 hr for 7–14 days, then 5 mg/kg/day or 6 mg/kg for 5 days of each wk.

IV (Neonates): *Congenital CMV infection*—12 mg/kg/day divided every 12 hr x 6 wk.

Renal Impairment

IV (Adults and Children): *Induction*—CCr 50–69 mL/min: 2.5 mg/kg/dose every 12 hr; CCr 25–49 mL/min: 2.5 mg/kg/dose every 24 hr; CCr 10–24 mL/min: 1.25 mg/kg/dose every 24 hr; CCr <10 mL/min: 1.25 mg/kg 3 times/wk after hemodialysis; *Maintenance*—CCr 50–69 mL/min: 2.5 mg/kg/dose every 24 hr; CCr 25–49 mL/min: 1.25 mg/kg/dose every 24 hr; CCr 10–24 mL/min: 0.625 mg/kg/dose every 24 hr; CCr <10 mL/min: 0.625 mg/kg 3 times/wk after hemodialysis.

Availability (generic available)

Lyophilized powder for injection (requires reconstitution and dilution): 500 mg/vial. **Premixed infusion:** 500 mg/250 mL.

NURSING IMPLICATIONS

Assessment

- Diagnosis of CMV retinitis should be determined by ophthalmoscopy before treatment with ganciclovir.
- Culture for CMV (urine, blood, throat) may be taken before administration. However, a negative CMV culture does not rule out CMV retinitis. If symptoms do not respond after several wk, resistance to ganciclovir may have occurred. Ophthalmologic exams should be performed weekly during induction and every 2 wk during maintenance or more frequently if the macula or optic nerve is threatened. Progression of CMV retinitis may occur during or after ganciclovir treatment.
- Assess for signs of infection (fever, chills, cough, hoarseness, lower back or side pain, sore throat, difficult or painful urination). Notify health care professional if these symptoms occur.
- Assess for bleeding (bleeding gums, bruising, petechiae; guaiac stools, urine, and emesis). Avoid IM injections and taking rectal temperatures. Apply pressure to venipuncture sites for 10 min.
- ***Lab Test Considerations:*** Obtain a negative pregnancy test prior to starting therapy.
- Monitor neutrophil and platelet count at least every 2 days during twice daily therapy and weekly thereafter. Granulocytopenia usually occurs during the first 2 wk of treatment but may occur anytime during therapy. Do not administer if neutrophil count <500/mm³ or platelet count <25,000/mm³. Recovery begins within 3–7 days of discontinuation of therapy.
- Monitor BUN and serum creatinine at least once every 2 wk throughout therapy.
- Monitor liver function tests (AST, ALT, serum bilirubin, alkaline phosphatase) periodically during therapy. May cause ↑ levels.
- May cause ↓ blood glucose.

Implementation

- Do not confuse Cytovene (ganciclovir) with Cytosar (cytarabine).
- Do not administer subcut or IM; severe tissue irritation may result.
- **IV:** Observe infusion site for phlebitis. Rotate infusion site to prevent phlebitis.
- Maintain adequate hydration throughout therapy.

IV Administration

- Prepare solution in a biologic cabinet. Wear gloves, gown, and mask while handling medication. Discard IV equipment in specially designated containers.
- **Intermittent Infusion:** Reconstitute 500 mg with 10 mL of sterile water for injection for a concentra-

tion of 50 mg/mL. Do not reconstitute with bacteriostatic water with parabens; precipitation will occur. Shake well to dissolve completely. Discard vial if particulate matter or discoloration occurs. Reconstituted solution is stable for 12 hr at room temperature; do not refrigerate.

- ***Diluent:*** Dilute in 100 mL of D5W, 0.9% NaCl, Ringer's or LR. Once diluted for infusion, solution should be used within 24 hr. Refrigerate but do not freeze. ***Concentration:*** 10 mg/mL. ***Rate:*** Administer slowly, via infusion pump, over 1 hr using an in-line filter. Rapid administration may increase toxicity.
- **Y-Site Compatibility:** alemtuzumab, alfentanyl, allopurinol, amphotericin B deoxycholate, amphotericin B lipid complex, anidulafungin, argatroban, arsenic trioxide, atropine, azithromycin, bivalirudin, bleomycin, calcium chloride, calcium gluconate, carboplatin, carmustine, caspofungin, cisplatin, cyanocobalamin, cyclophosphamide, cyclosporine, dactinomycin, daptomycin, defibrotide, dexamethasone, dexmedetomidine, digoxin, docetaxel, doxacurium, doxorubicin liposome, enalaprilat, epoetin alfa, eptifibatide, ertapenem, etoposide, etoposide phosphate, fentanyl, filgrastim, fluconazole, fluorouracil, folic acid, fosphenytoin, furosemide, glycopyrrolate, granisetron, heparin, hetastarch, hydromorphone, ifosfamide, indomethacin, insulin, regular, labetalol, leucovorin calcium, linezolid, lorazepam, mannitol, melphalan, methotrexate, metoprolol, milrinone, mitoxantrone, nafcillin, naloxone, nitroglycerin, nitroprusside, octreotide, oxytocin, paclitaxel, pamidronate, pancuronium, pantoprazole, pemetrexed, pentobarbital, phenobarbital, phytonadione, potassium chloride, propranolol, protamine, ranitidine, remifentanil, rituximab, rocuronium, sodium acetate, sufentanil, thiotepa, tigecycline, tirofiban, trastuzumab, vasopressin, vinblastine, vincristine, voriconazole, zoledronic acid.
- **Y-Site Incompatibility:** aldesleukin, amifostine, amikacin, aminophylline, amiodarone, ampicillin, ampicillin/sulbactam, amsacrine, ascorbic acid, atracurium, azathioprine, aztreonam, benztropine, bumetanide, butorphanol, cefazolin, cefepime, cefotaxime, cefotetan, cefoxitin, ceftazidime, ceftriaxone, cefuroxime, chloramphenicol, chlorpromazine, clindamycin, cytarabine, dacarbazine, dantrolene, daunorubicin, dexrazoxane, diazepam, diazoxide, diltiazem, diphenhydramine, dobutamine, dolasetron, dopamine, doxorubicin, doxycycline, ephedrine, epinephrine, epirubicin, erythromycin, esmolol, famotidine, fenoldopam, fludarabine, foscarnet, gemcitabine, gentamicin, haloperidol, hydralazine, hydrocortisone, hydroxyzine, idarubicin, imipenem/cilastatin, irinotecan, isoproterenol, ketorolac, levofloxacin, lidocaine, magnesium sulfate, meperidine, mesna, metaraminol, methyldopate, methylprednisolone, metoclopramide, metronidazole, midazolam, minocycline, mitomycin, morphine, multivitamins, mycophenolate, nalbuphine, nicardipine, norepinephrine, ondansetron, oxacillin, palonosetron, papaverine, penicillin G, pentamidine, phentolamine, phenylephrine, phenytoin, piperacillin/tazobactam, potassium acetate, procainamide, prochlorperazine, promethazine, pyridoxime, quinupristin/dalfopristin, sargramostim, sodium bicarbonate, streptokinase, succinylcholine, tacrolimus, theophylline, thiamine, tobramycin, tolazoline, topotecan, trimethoprim/sulfamethoxazole, vancomycin, vecuronium, verapamil, vinorelbine.

Patient/Family Teaching

- Inform patient that ganciclovir is not a cure for CMV retinitis. Progression of retinitis may continue in immunocompromised patients during and after therapy. Advise patients to have regular ophthalmic exams at least every 6 wk. Duration of therapy for CMV prevention is based on the duration and degree of immunosuppression.
- Advise patient to notify health care professional if fever; chills; sore throat; other signs of infection; bleeding gums; bruising; petechiae; or blood in urine, stool, or emesis occurs. Caution patient to avoid crowds and persons with known infections. Instruct patient to use soft toothbrush and electric razor. Patient should be cautioned not to drink alcoholic beverages or take products containing aspirin or NSAIDs.
- Caution patient to use sunscreen and protective clothing to prevent photosensitivity reactions.
- Rep: May have teratogenic effects. Advise female patients of reproductive potential to use a nonhormonal method of contraception during and for at least 30 days after last dose and to avoid breast feeding during therapy. Advise male patients to use condoms during and for at least 90 days after therapy. Inform patients that ganciclovir may cause temporary or permanent female and male infertility.
- Emphasize the importance of frequent follow-up exams to monitor blood counts.

Evaluation/Desired Outcomes

- Treatment of the symptoms of CMV retinitis in immunocompromised patients.
- Prevention of CMV retinitis in transplant patients at risk.

G

gefitinib (je-fit-in-ib)

Iressa

Classification

Therapeutic: antineoplastics

Pharmacologic: enzyme inhibitors

Indications

First-line treatment of patients with metastatic non–small-cell lung cancer (NSCLC) whose tumors have epidermal growth factor receptor (EGFR) exon 19 deletions or exon 21 (L858R) substitution mutations.

Action

Inhibits activation of kinases found in transmembrane cell surface receptors, including EGFR. **Therapeutic Effects:** Prolonged progression-free survival.

Pharmacokinetics

Absorption: 60% absorbed following oral administration.
Distribution: Extensively distributed.
Metabolism and Excretion: Mostly metabolized by the liver (CYP3A4 enzyme system); excreted in feces, <4% excreted in urine.
Half-life: 48 hr.

TIME/ACTION PROFILE (plasma levels)

ROUTE	ONSET	PEAK	DURATION
PO	unknown	3–7 hr	unknown

Contraindications/Precautions

Contraindicated in: Hypersensitivity; OB: May cause fetal harm; Lactation: Safety not established; Pedi: Safety and effectiveness not established.
Use Cautiously in: Idiopathic pulmonary fibrosis (↑ risk of pulmonary toxicity); Concurrent use of strong inhibitors of the CYP3A4 enzyme system (may ↑ risk of toxicity); OB: Women with childbearing potential.

Adverse Reactions/Side Effects

EENT: aberrant eyelash growth, blepharitis, conjunctivitis, corneal erosion/ulcer, dry eye, nose bleeding. **Resp:** INTERSTITIAL LUNG DISEASE, dyspnea. **GI:** GI PERFORATION, HEPATOTOXICITY, anorexia, diarrhea, nausea, vomiting, dry mouth, mouth ulceration. **GU:** ↓ fertility (females), hematuria, ↑ serum creatinine. **Derm:** ERYTHEMA MULTIFORME, STEVENS-JOHNSON SYNDROME, TOXIC EPIDERMAL NECROLYSIS, rash, alopecia, pruritus. **F and E:** dehydration. **Metab:** weight loss. **Misc:** allergic reactions including ANGIOEDEMA, fever.

Interactions

Drug-Drug: Strong inducers of the CYP3A4 enzyme system, including **rifampin** and **phenytoin**, ↓ blood levels and effects (↑ dose of gefitinib to 500 mg/day). Strong inhibitors of the CYP3A4 enzyme system, including **ketoconazole** and **itraconazole**, ↑ blood levels and effects. Absorption and efficacy may be ↓ by **drugs that ↑ gastric pH** including **H_2 receptor antagonist**, **proton pump inhibitors**, and **antacids**; take geftinib 12 hr after last dose or 12 hr before the next dose of proton pump inhibitor; take geftinib 6 hr after last dose or 6 hr before next dose H_2 receptor antagonist or antacid. May ↑ the risk of bleeding with **warfarin**.

Route/Dosage

PO (Adults): 250 mg once daily; *Concurrent use of rifampin or phenytoin*—500 mg once daily (resume 250 mg once daily dose 7 days after discontinuing strong CYP3A4 inducer).

Availability

Tablets: 250 mg.

NURSING IMPLICATIONS

Assessment

- Assess for signs of pulmonary toxicity (dyspnea, cough, fever). Withhold gefitinib during diagnosis. If interstitial lung disease is confirmed, discontinue gefitinib and treat appropriately.
- Assess patient for eye symptoms such as pain during therapy. May require interruption of therapy and removal of aberrant eyelash. After symptoms and eye changes have resolved, may reinstate therapy.
- Monitor for rash. Interrupt or discontinue therapy if severe bullous, blistering or exfoliating conditions develop.
- ***Lab Test Considerations:*** Monitor liver function tests periodically. May cause ↑ transaminases, bilirubin, and alkaline phosphatase. Withhold gefitinib in patients with worsening liver function tests; discontinue gefitinib if elevations are severe.
- Monitor for changes in prothrombin time and INR in patients taking warfarin. May cause ↑ levels.

Implementation

- Available only through the *Iressa Access Program*. Patients must be currently on the medication or in an approved study and must sign the Patient Consent Form. Physicians and prescribers must enroll in program.
- FDA-approved test must be used to detect EGFR mutations in NSCLC. Patients must have EGFR exon 19 deletions or exon 21 substitutions to use gefitinib.
- **PO:** Administer one tablet daily without regard to food. Tablets can also be dispersed in half a glass of drinking water (noncarbonated). No other liquids should be used. Drop the tablet in the water, without crushing it, stir until the tablet is dispersed (approximately 10 min), and drink the liquid immediately. Rinse the glass with half a glass of water and drink. The liquid can also be administered through a nasogastric tube.
- May interrupt therapy briefly (14 days) for patients with poorly tolerated diarrhea with dehydration or skin adverse reactions. Follow by restarting 250 mg dose.

Patient/Family Teaching

- Instruct patient to take gefitinib as directed. Take missed doses up to 12 hrs of next dose. Advise patient to read the *Instruction Sheet* with each Rx refill; new information may be available.

- Advise patient to notify health care professional promptly if severe persistent diarrhea, nausea, vomiting, or anorexia occur; if shortness of breath or cough occur or worsen; or if eye irritation or other new symptoms develop.
- Rep: Instruct female patient to use effective contraception during and for 2 wk after last dose and notify health care professional if pregnancy is suspected or if breast feeding.

Evaluation/Desired Outcomes

- Decrease in size and spread of tumors in non–small-cell lung cancer.

HIGH ALERT

gemcitabine (jem-site-a-been)

~~Gemzar~~, Infugem

Classification

Therapeutic: antineoplastics

Pharmacologic: antimetabolites, nucleoside analogues

Indications

Pancreatic cancer (locally advanced or metastatic). Inoperable locally advanced/metastatic non–small-cell lung cancer (with cisplatin). Metastatic breast cancer after failure of prior anthracycline-containing adjuvant chemotherapy (unless anthracycline therapy contraindicated) (with paclitaxel). Advanced ovarian cancer that has relapsed 6 mo after completion of platinum-based therapy (with carboplatin).

Action

Interferes with DNA synthesis (cell-cycle phase–specific). **Therapeutic Effects:** Death of rapidly replicating cells, particularly malignant ones.

Pharmacokinetics

Absorption: IV administration results in complete bioavailability.

Distribution: Unknown.

Metabolism and Excretion: Converted in cells to active diphosphate and triphosphate metabolites; these are excreted primarily by the kidneys.

Half-life: 32–94 min.

TIME/ACTION PROFILE (effect on blood counts)

ROUTE	ONSET	PEAK	DURATION
IV	unknown	unknown	unknown

Contraindications/Precautions

Contraindicated in: Hypersensitivity; OB: Pregnancy (may cause fetal harm); Lactation: Lactation (can expose infant to serious adverse effects).

Use Cautiously in: History of cardiovascular disease; Hepatic or renal impairment (↑ risk of toxicity); Rep: Women of reproductive potential and men with female partners of reproductive potential; Pedi: Safety and effectiveness not established.

Adverse Reactions/Side Effects

CNS: POSTERIOR REVERSIBLE ENCEPHALOPATHY SYNDROME (PRES). **CV:** ARRHYTHMIAS, CAPILLARY LEAK SYNDROME, CEREBROVASCULAR ACCIDENT, MI, edema, hypertension. **Derm:** alopecia, rash. **GI:** HEPATOTOXICITY, diarrhea, ↑ liver enzymes, nausea, stomatitis, vomiting. **GU:** HEMOLYTIC UREMIC SYNDROME, hematuria, proteinuria, ↓ fertility (males), renal failure. **Hemat:** anemia, leukopenia, thrombocytopenia, thrombotic microangiopathy. **Local:** injection site reactions. **Neuro:** paresthesias. **Resp:** ADULT RESPIRATORY DISTRESS SYNDROME (ARDS), PULMONARY FIBROSIS, dyspnea, bronchospasm, pulmonary edema. **Misc:** flu-like symptoms, fever, anaphylactoid reactions.

Interactions

Drug-Drug: ↑ bone marrow depression with other **antineoplastics** or **radiation therapy**. May ↓ antibody response to **live virus vaccines** and ↑ risk of adverse reactions.

Route/Dosage

Pancreatic Cancer

IV (Adults): 1000 mg/m² once weekly for 7 wk, followed by a wk of rest, then on Days 1, 8, and 15 of each 28–day cycle.

Non–Small-Cell Lung Cancer

IV (Adults): 1000 mg/m² on Days 1, 8, and 15 of each 28-day cycle (cisplatin is also given on day 1) *or* 1250 mg/m² on Days 1 and 8 of each 21-day cycle (cisplatin is also given on Day 1).

Breast Cancer

IV (Adults): 1250 mg/m² on Days 1 and 8 of each 21-day cycle (paclitaxel is also given on Day 1).

Ovarian Cancer

IV (Adults): 1000 mg/m² on Days 1 and 8 of each 21-day cycle (carboplatin is also given on Day 1).

Availability (generic available)

Powder for injection (requires reconstitution): 200 mg/vial, 1 g/vial, 2 g/vial. **Premixed infusion:** 1200 mg/120 mL 0.9% NaCl, 1300 mg/130 mL 0.9% NaCl, 1400 mg/140 mL 0.9% NaCl, 1500 mg/150 mL 0.9% NaCl, 1600 mg/160 mL 0.9% NaCl, 1700 mg/170 mL 0.9% NaCl, 1800 mg/180 mL 0.9% NaCl, 1900 mg/190 mL 0.9% NaCl, 2000 mg/200 mL 0.9% NaCl, 2200 mg/220 mL 0.9% NaCl.

NURSING IMPLICATIONS

Assessment

- Monitor vital signs before and frequently during therapy.
- Assess injection site during administration. Although gemcitabine is not a vesicant, local reactions may occur.
- Monitor for bone marrow depression. Assess for bleeding (bleeding gums, bruising, petechiae; guaiac stools, urine, and emesis) and avoid IM injections and taking rectal temperatures if platelet count is low. Apply pressure to venipuncture sites for 10 min. Assess for signs of infection during neutropenia. Anemia may occur. Monitor for increased fatigue, dyspnea, and orthostatic hypotension.
- Monitor intake and output, appetite, and nutritional intake. Mild to moderate nausea and vomiting occur frequently. Antiemetics may be used prophylactically.
- Assess for signs and symptoms of capillary leak syndrome (severe hypotension, hypoalbuminemia, hemoconcentration). Discontinue therapy if symptoms occur.
- Monitor respiratory status during therapy. Discontinue gemcitabine if unexplained dyspnea or other evidence of severe pulmonary toxicity occurs. May occur up to 2 wk after last dose.
- Monitor for signs and symptoms of posterior reversible encephalopathy syndrome (PRES) (headache, seizure, lethargy, hypertension, confusion, blindness, and other visual and neurologic disturbances) during therapy. Confirm diagnosis of PRES with magnetic resonance imaging (MRI). Discontinue gemcitabine if PRES develops during therapy.
- ***Lab Test Considerations:*** Monitor CBC, including differential and platelet count, before each dose. Dose guidelines are based on CBC. **For single-agent use:** *If absolute granulocyte count is >1000 and platelet count is >100,000,* full dose may be administered. *If absolute granulocyte count is 500–999 or platelet count is 50,000–99,000,* 75% of dose may be given. *If absolute granulocyte count is <500 or platelet count is <50,000,* withhold further doses. **For gemcitabine with paclitaxel (breast cancer):** *If absolute granulocyte count is >1200 and platelet count is >75,000,* full dose may be administered. *If absolute granulocyte count is 1000–1199 or platelet count is 50,000–75,000,* 75% of dose may be given. *If absolute granulocyte count is 700–999 or platelet count is ≥50,000,* 50% of dose may be given. *If absolute granulocyte count is <700 or platelet count is <50,000,* withhold further doses. **For gemcitabine with carboplatin (ovarian cancer):** *If absolute granulocyte count is >1500 and platelet count is >100,000,* full dose may be administered. *If the absolute granulocyte count is 1000–1499 or platelet count is 75,000–99,000,* 75% of dose may be given. *If the absolute granulocyte count is <1000 or the platelet count is <75,000,* withhold further doses.
- Monitor serum creatinine, potassium, calcium, and magnesium in patients taking cisplatin with gemcitabine.
- Monitor hepatic and renal function before and periodically during therapy. May cause transient ↑ in serum AST, ALT, alkaline phosphatase, and bilirubin concentrations. Discontinue gemcitabine for severe hepatic toxicity or hemolytic-uremic syndrome.
- May also cause ↑ BUN and serum creatinine concentrations, proteinuria, and hematuria.

Implementation

- ***High Alert:*** Fatalities have occurred with incorrect administration of chemotherapeutic agents. Before administering, clarify all ambiguous orders; double-check single, daily, and course-of-therapy dose limits; have second practitioner independently double-check original order, calculations, and infusion pump settings.

IV Administration

- Solution should be prepared in a biologic cabinet. Wear gloves, gown, and mask while handling IV medication. Discard IV equipment in specially designated containers.
- **Intermittent Infusion:** To reconstitute, add 5 mL of 0.9% NaCl without preservatives to 200-mg vial or 25 mL of 0.9% NaCl to the 1-g vial of gemcitabine for a concentration of 40 mg/mL. Incomplete dissolution may result in concentrations greater than 40 mg/mL. ***Diluent:*** May be further diluted with 0.9% NaCl. Solution is colorless to light straw color. Do not administer solutions that are discolored or contain particulate matter. Solution is stable for 24 hr at room temperature. Discard unused portions. Do not refrigerate; crystallization may occur. ***Concentration:*** 0.1–38 mg/mL. ***Rate:*** Administer dose over 30 min. If 2 bags required, infuse total of both bags over 30 min. Infusions longer than 60 min have a greater incidence of toxicity.
- **Y-Site Compatibility:** alemtuzumab, alfentanil, allopurinol, amifostine, amikacin, aminocaproic acid, aminophylline, amiodarone, ampicillin, ampicillin/sulbactam, anidulafungin, argatroban, atracurium, azithromycin, aztreonam, bivalirudin, bleomycin, bumetanide, buprenorphine, butorphanol, calcium acetate, calcium chloride, calcium gluconate, carboplatin, carmustine, caspofungin, cefazolin, cefotetan, cefoxitin, ceftazidime, ceftriaxone, cefuroxime, chlorpromazine, ciprofloxacin, cisatracurium, cisplatin, clindamycin, cyclophosphamide, cyclosporine, cytarabine, dacarbazine, dactinomycin, daunorubicin, dexamethasone, dexmedetomidine, dexrazoxane, digoxin, diltiazem, diphenhydramine, dobutamine, docetaxel, dolasetron, dopamine, doxacurium, doxorubicin, doxycycline, droperidol, enalaprilat, ephedrine, epinephrine, epirubicin, ertape-

nem, erythromycin, esmolol, etoposide, etoposide phosphate, famotidine, fenoldopam, fentanyl, floxuridine, fluconazole, fludarabine, fluorouracil, foscarnet, fosphenytoin, gentamicin, glycopyrrolate, granisetron, haloperidol, heparin, hetastarch, hydralazine, hydrocortisone, hydromorphone, idarubicin, ifosfamide, insulin, regular, isoproterenol, labetalol, leucovorin calcium, levofloxacin, lidocaine, linezolid, lorazepam, magnesium sulfate, mannitol, meperidine, meropenem, mesna, metaraminol, methyldopate, metoclopramide, metoprolol, midazolam, milrinone, mitoxantrone, morphine, moxifloxacin, nalbuphine, naloxone, nicardipine, nitroglycerin, nitroprusside, norepinephrine, octreotide, ondansetron, oxaliplatin, paclitaxel, palonosetron, pamidronate, pancuronium, pentamidine, pentobarbital, phenobarbital, phentolamine, potassium acetate, potassium chloride, potassium phosphates, procainamide, promethazine, propranolol, quinupristin/dalfopristin, ranitidine, remifentanil, rituximab, rocuronium, sodium acetate, sodium bicarbonate, sodium phosphates, streptozocin, succinylcholine, sufentanil, tacrolimus, theophylline, thiotepa, tigecycline, tirofiban, tobramycin, tolazoline, topotecan, trastuzumab, trimethoprim/sulfamethoxazole, vancomycin, vasopressin, vecuronium, verapamil, vinblastine, vincristine, vinorelbine, voriconazole, zidovudine, zoledronic acid.

- **Y-Site Incompatibility:** acyclovir, amphotericin B lipid complex, amphotericin B liposome, cefepime, cefotaxime, chloramphenicol, dantrolene, daptomycin, diazepam, doxorubicin liposomal, furosemide, ganciclovir, imipenem-cilastatin, irinotecan, ketorolac, methotrexate, methoprednisolone, mitomycin, nafcillin, pantoprazole, pemetrexed, phenytoin, piperacillin/tazobactam, prochlorperazine, thiopental.

Patient/Family Teaching

- Instruct patient to notify health care professional if fever; chills; sore throat; signs of infection; bleeding gums; bruising; petechiae; or blood in urine, stool, or emesis occurs. Caution patient to avoid crowds and persons with known infections. Instruct patient to use soft toothbrush and electric razor. Patient should be cautioned not to drink alcoholic beverages or take products containing aspirin or NSAIDs.
- Instruct patient to inspect oral mucosa for erythema and ulceration. If ulceration occurs, advise patient to use sponge brush and rinse mouth with water after eating and drinking. Stomatitis pain may require management with opioid analgesics.
- Instruct patient to notify health care professional if flu-like symptoms (fever, anorexia, headache, cough, chills, myalgia), swelling of feet or legs, signs and symptoms of pulmonary toxicity (shortness of breath, wheezing, cough), hemolytic-uremic syndrome (changes in color or volume of urine output, increased bruising or bleeding), or hepatic toxicity (jaundice, pain/tenderness in right upper abdominal quadrant) occur.
- Discuss with patient the possibility of hair loss. Explore methods of coping.
- Instruct patient not to receive any vaccinations without advice of health care professional.
- Rep: Advise patient that medication may have teratogenic effects. Advise females of reproductive potential to use effective contraception during and for 6 mo after final dose and to avoid breast feeding during and for at least 1 wk after last dose. Advise males with female partners of reproductive potential to use effective contraception during and for 3 mo after last dose. May cause male infertility.
- Emphasize the need for periodic lab tests to monitor for side effects.

Evaluation/Desired Outcomes

- Palliative, symptomatic improvement in patients with pancreatic cancer.
- Decrease in size and spread of malignancy in lung, ovarian, and breast cancer.

gemfibrozil (gem-fye-broe-zil)

Lopid

Classification

Therapeutic: lipid-lowering agents

Pharmacologic: fibric acid derivatives

Indications

Management of type II-b hyperlipidemia (decreased HDL, increased LDL, increased triglycerides) in patients who do not yet have clinical coronary artery disease and have failed therapy with diet, exercise, weight loss, or other agents (niacin, bile acid sequestrants).

Action

Inhibits peripheral lipolysis. Decreases triglyceride production by the liver. Decreases production of the triglyceride carrier protein. Increases HDL. **Therapeutic Effects:** Decreased plasma triglycerides and increased HDL.

Pharmacokinetics

Absorption: Well absorbed after oral administration.

Distribution: Unknown.

Metabolism and Excretion: Some metabolism by the liver, 70% excreted by the kidneys (mostly unchanged), 6% excreted in feces.

Half-life: 1.3–1.5 hr.

TIME/ACTION PROFILE (triglyceride-VLDL–lowering effect)

ROUTE	ONSET	PEAK	DURATION
PO	2–5 days	4 wk	several mo

Contraindications/Precautions

Contraindicated in: Hypersensitivity; Hepatic impairment; Severe renal impairment; Primary biliary cirrhosis; Gallbladder disease; Concurrent use of simvastatin, repaglinide, dasabuvir, or selexipag.

Use Cautiously in: OB, Lactation, Pedi: Safety not established.

Adverse Reactions/Side Effects

CNS: dizziness, headache. **Derm:** alopecia, rash, urticaria. **EENT:** blurred vision. **GI:** abdominal pain, diarrhea, epigastric pain, flatulence, gallstones, heartburn, nausea, vomiting. **Hemat:** anemia, leukopenia. **MS:** myositis.

Interactions

Drug-Drug: May ↑ levels of **CYP2C8 substrates**, including **dabrafenib**, **dasabuvir**, **enzalutamide**, **loperamide**, **montelukast**, **paclitaxel**, **pioglitazone**, **rosiglitazone**, or **selexipag**; concurrent use with **dasabuvir** or **selexipag** contraindicated. May ↑ levels of **OATP1B1 substrates**, including **atorvastatin**, **bosentan**, **ezetimibe**, **fluvastatin**, **glyburide**, **olmesartan**, **pitavastatin**, **pravastatin**, **repaglinide**, **rifampin**, **rosuvastatin**, **simvastatin**, and **valsartan**; concurrent use with **simvastatin** or **repaglinide** is contraindicated; avoid concurrent use with other **HMG-CoA reductase inhibitors**. May ↑ levels and the risk of bleeding with **warfarin**. Concurrent use with **colchicine** may ↑ risk of rhabdomyolysis, especially in patients with renal dysfunction or elderly. May ↓ the effect of **cyclosporine**. **Cholestyramine** and **colestipol** may ↓ absorption; separate administration by ≥2 hr.

Route/Dosage

PO (Adults): 600 mg twice daily 30 min before breakfast and dinner.

Availability (generic available)

Capsules: 🍁 300 mg. **Tablets:** 600 mg. **Cost:** *Generic*—$24.07/100.

NURSING IMPLICATIONS

Assessment

- Obtain patient's diet history, especially regarding fat and alcohol consumption.
- ***Lab Test Considerations:*** Monitor serum triglyceride and cholesterol levels before and periodically during therapy. Assess LDL and VLDL levels before and periodically during therapy. Discontinue gemfibrozil if paradoxical ↑ in lipid levels occurs.
- Assess liver function tests before and periodically during therapy. May cause ↑ serum bilirubin, alkaline phosphatase, CK, LDH, AST, and ALT. If hepatic function tests rise significantly, discontinue therapy and do not resume.
- Evaluate CBC and electrolytes every 3–6 mo and then yearly during therapy. May cause mild ↓ in hemoglobin, hematocrit, and leukocyte counts. May cause ↓ serum potassium concentrations.
- May cause slight ↑ in serum glucose.

Implementation

- Do not confuse gemfibrozil with gabapentin.
- **PO:** Administer 30 min before breakfast or dinner.

Patient/Family Teaching

- Instruct patient to take medication as directed, not to skip doses or double up on missed doses. Take missed doses as soon as remembered unless almost time for next dose.
- Advise patient that gemfibrozil should be used in conjunction with dietary restrictions (fat, cholesterol, carbohydrates, alcohol), exercise, and cessation of smoking.
- Instruct patient to notify health care professional promptly if severe stomach pains with nausea and vomiting, fever, chills, sore throat, rash, diarrhea, muscle cramping, general abdominal discomfort, or persistent flatulence occur.
- Advise female patient to notify health care professional if pregnancy is planned or suspected or if breast feeding.

Evaluation/Desired Outcomes

- Decrease in serum triglyceride and cholesterol levels and improved HDL to total cholesterol ratios. If response is not seen within 3 mo, medication is usually discontinued.

gentamicin, See AMINOGLYCOSIDES.

glecaprevir/pibrentasvir

(glek-**a**-pre-vir/pi-**brent**-as-vir)

🍁 Maviret, Mavyret

Classification

Therapeutic: antivirals

Pharmacologic: NS5A inhibitors, protease inhibitors

Indications

Chronic hepatitis C virus (HCV) genotypes 1, 2, 3, 4, 5, or 6 infection without cirrhosis or with compensated cirrhosis (Child-Pugh A). Chronic HCV genotype 1 infection in patients who have previously received treatment with a regimen containing an HCV NS5A inhibitor or an NS3/4A protease inhibitor, but not both.

Action

Glecaprevir—inhibits the HCV NS3/4A protease, resulting in inhibition of viral replication; *Pibrentasvir*—inhibits the HCV NS5A protein, resulting in inhibition of viral replication. **Therapeutic Effects:** Decreased levels of HCV with sustained virologic response and lessened sequelae of chronic HCV infection.

Pharmacokinetics

Glevaprevir

Absorption: Well absorbed following oral administration; absorption ↑ by high-fat meal.
Distribution: Unknown.
Protein Binding: 97.5%.
Metabolism and Excretion: Partially metabolized by CYP3A4; 92% excreted in feces and <1% eliminated in urine.
Half-life: 6 hr.

Pibrentasvir

Absorption: Well absorbed following oral administration.
Distribution: Unknown.
Protein Binding: >99.9%.
Metabolism and Excretion: Not metabolized; 97% excreted in feces.
Half-life: 13 hr.

TIME/ACTION PROFILE (blood levels)

ROUTE	ONSET	PEAK	DURATION
glecaprevir (PO)	unknown	5 hr	24 hr
pibrentasvir (PO)	unknown	5 hr	24 hr

Contraindications/Precautions

Contraindicated in: Moderate or severe hepatic impairment (Child-Pugh B or C) or any prior history of hepatic decompensation (↑ risk of hepatic decompensation/failure); Concurrent use of atazanavir, carbamazepine, dabigatran, darunavir, efavirenz, lopinavir, oral contraceptives containing ethinyl estradiol, rifampin, ritonavir, or St. John's wort.

Use Cautiously in: Receiving immunosuppressant or chemotherapy medications (↑ risk of hepatitis B virus reactivation); OB: Safety not established; Lactation: Weigh benefits of breast feeding against possible adverse effects; Pedi: Children <12 yr (safety and effectiveness not established).

Adverse Reactions/Side Effects

CNS: fatigue, headache. **Derm:** pruritus. **GI:** diarrhea, hyperbilirubinemia, nausea. **Misc:** hepatitis B virus reactivation.

Interactions

Drug-Drug: **Atazanavir** may ↑ levels of glecaprevir/pibrentasvir and ↑ risk of liver enzyme elevation; concurrent use contraindicated. **Rifampin** may ↓ levels/effectiveness of glecaprevir/pibrentasvir; concurrent use contraindicated. **Strong CYP3A inducers**, including **carbamazepine** or **efavirenz** may ↓ levels/effectiveness of glecaprevir/pibrentasvir; concurrent use not recommended. **Darunavir**, **lopinavir**, or **ritonavir** may ↑ levels of glecaprevir/pibrentasvir; concurrent use not recommended. May ↑ levels of **atorvastatin, fluvastatin, lovastatin, pitavastatin, pravastatin, rosuvastatin**, and **simvastatin** and ↑ risk of myopathy; concurrent use with atorvastatin, lovastatin, and simvastatin not recommended; ↓ dose of pravastatin by 50%; do not exceed rosuvastatin dose of 10 mg/day; use lowest possible dose of fluvastatin or pitavastatin. May ↑ **dabigatran** levels; avoid concurrent use. May ↑ **digoxin** levels; ↓ digoxin dose by 50% when initiating glecaprevir/pibrentasvir therapy. Concurrent use with **ethinyl estradiol-containing oral contraceptives** may ↑ risk of liver enzyme elevation; concurrent use not recommended. **Cyclosporine** may ↑ levels/toxicity of glecaprevir/pibrentasvir; concurrent use not recommended if patients require cyclosporine dose >100 mg/day. May cause fluctuations in INR when used with **warfarin**; closely monitor INR. ↑ risk of hypoglycemia with use of certain **antidiabetic agents**.

Drug-Natural Products: **St. John's wort** may ↓ levels/effectiveness of glecaprevir/pibrentasvir; concurrent use not recommended.

Route/Dosage

PO (Adults and Children ≥12 yr or ≥45 kg): *Genotype 1, 2, 3, 4, 5, or 6: Treatment-naïve with no cirrhosis or with compensated cirrhosis (Child–Pugh A)*—3 tablets (glecaprevir 300 mg/pibrentasvir 120 mg) once daily for 8 wk; *Genotype 1: Treatment-experienced with NS5A inhibitor (with no cirrhosis or with compensated cirrhosis [Child–Pugh A])*—3 tablets (glecaprevir 300 mg/pibrentasvir 120 mg) once daily for 16 wk; *Genotype 1: Treatment-experienced with NS3/4A protease inhibitor (with no cirrhosis or with compensated cirrhosis [Child–Pugh A])*—3 tablets (glecaprevir 300 mg/pibrentasvir 120 mg) once daily for 12 wk; *Genotype 1, 2, 4, 5, or 6: Treatment-experienced with regimens containing interferon, pegylated interferon, ribavirin, and/or sofosbuvir (no cirrhosis)*—3 tablets (glecaprevir 300 mg/pibrentasvir 120 mg) once daily for 8 wk; *Genotype 1, 2, 4, 5, or 6: Treatment-experienced with regimens containing interferon, pegylated interferon, ribavirin, and/or sofosbuvir (with compensated cirrhosis [Child–Pugh A])*—3 tablets (glecaprevir 300 mg/pibrentasvir 120 mg) once daily for 12 wk; *Genotype 3: Treatment-experienced with regimens containing interferon, pegylated interferon, ribavirin, and/or sofosbuvir (with no cirrhosis or with compensated cirrhosis [Child–Pugh A])*—3 tablets (glecaprevir 300 mg/pibrentasvir 120 mg) once daily for 16 wk; *Liver or kidney transplant recipients*—3 tablets (glecaprevir 300 mg/pibrentasvir 120 mg) once daily for 12 wk (16 wk for those with Genotype 1 who are treatment experienced with NS5A inhibitor without prior treatment with an NS3/4A protease inhibitor; 16 wk for those with Genotype 3 who are treatment experienced with regimens containing interferon, pegylated interferon, ribavirin, and/or sofosbuvir).

Availability

Tablets: glecaprevir 100 mg/pibrentasvir 40 mg.

NURSING IMPLICATIONS

Assessment

- Monitor for signs and symptoms of hepatitis B reactivation or hepatitis (jaundice, dark urine, light colored stools, fatigue, weakness, loss of appetite, nausea, vomiting, stomach pain) during therapy.
- ***Lab Test Considerations:*** Test all patients for current or prior hepatitis B virus (HBV) infection before starting hepatitis C virus therapy; may cause hepatitis B virus reactivation. Measure hepatitis B surface antigen (HBsAg) and hepatitis core antibody (anti-HBc). Monitor for clinical and laboratory signs of hepatitis flare (↑ AST, ALT, bilirubin, liver failure, death) or HBV reactivation (rapid ↑ in serum HBV DNA level) during HCV treatment and post-treatment follow-up.
- Test patient with HCV genotype 1a infection for presence of virus with NS5A resistance-associated polymorphisms prior to starting therapy with Mavyret™ to determine dose regimen and duration.

Implementation

- **PO:** Administer once daily with food.

Patient/Family Teaching

- Instruct patient to take medication as directed. Do not skip or miss dose. If dose is missed, take if <18 hrs from usual time taken, then take next dose at usual time. If >18 hrs from usual time of dose, omit dose and take next dose at usual time. Do not stop medication without consulting health care professional. Advise patient to read *Patient Information* before starting therapy and with each Rx refill in case of changes.
- Advise patient to notify health care professional if they have a history of HBV. May cause reactivation.
- Instruct patient to notify health care professional of all Rx or OTC medications, vitamins, or herbal products being taken and consult health care professional before taking any new medications, especially St. John's wort.
- Rep: Advise all patients to notify health care professional if pregnancy is planned or suspected or if breast feeding.

Evaluation/Desired Outcomes

- Decreased levels of HCV with sustained virologic response and lessened sequelae of chronic HCV infection.

glimepiride, See SULFONYLUREAS.

glipiZIDE, See SULFONYLUREAS.

glucagon (gloo-ka-gon)

Baqsimi, GlucaGen, Gvoke

Classification
Therapeutic: hormones
Pharmacologic: pancreatics

Indications

Acute management of severe hypoglycemia. Facilitation of radiographic examination of the GI tract. **Unlabeled Use:** Beta-blocker overdose. Calcium channel blocker overdose.

Action

Stimulates hepatic production of glucose from glycogen stores (glycogenolysis). Relaxes the musculature of the GI tract (stomach, duodenum, small bowel, and colon), temporarily inhibiting movement. Has positive inotropic and chronotropic effects. **Therapeutic Effects:** Increase in blood glucose. Relaxation of GI musculature, facilitating radiographic examination.

Pharmacokinetics

Absorption: Well absorbed following IM, intranasal, and subcut administration; IV administration results in complete bioavailability.
Distribution: Unknown.
Metabolism and Excretion: Extensively metabolized by the liver, plasma, and kidneys.
Half-life: 8–18 min.

TIME/ACTION PROFILE

ROUTE	ONSET	PEAK	DURATION
IM (hyperglycemic action)	within 10 min	30 min	12–27 min
IV (hyperglycemic action)	1 min	5 min	9–17 min
Subcut (hyperglycemic action)	within 10 min	30–45 min	60–90 min
Intranasal (hyperglycemic action)	within 15 min	unknown	unknown
IV (effect on GI musculature)	45 sec (for 0.25–2-mg dose)	unknown	9–17 min (0.25–0.5-mg dose); 22–25 min (2-mg dose)
IM (effect on GI musculature)	8–10 min (1-mg dose); 4–7 min (2-mg dose)	unknown	9–27 min (1-mg dose); 21–32 min (2-mg dose)

Contraindications/Precautions

Contraindicated in: Hypersensitivity; Pheochromocytoma; Insulinoma.

Use Cautiously in: Prolonged fasting, starvation, adrenal insufficiency, or chronic hypoglycemia (low levels of releasable glucose); When used to inhibit GI motility, use cautiously in geriatric patient with cardiac disease or diabetics; OB: Use only if potential maternal benefit justifies potential fetal risk; Lactation: Safety not established; Pedi: Children <4 yr (safety and effectiveness of nasal powder not established).

Adverse Reactions/Side Effects

CNS: headache. **CV:** hypotension. **Derm:** necrolytic migratory erythema. **EENT:** epistaxis, eye redness, itchy eyes, itchy throat, nasal congestion, nasal discomfort, nasal itching, rhinorrhea, sneezing, watery eyes. **GI:** nausea, vomiting. **Resp:** cough. **Misc:** HYPERSENSITIVITY REACTIONS (including anaphylaxis).

Interactions

Drug-Drug: Large doses may ↑ the effect of **warfarin**. Negates the response to **insulin** or **oral hypoglycemic agents**. **Phenytoin** inhibits the stimulant effect of glucagon on insulin release. Hyperglycemic effect is intensified and prolonged by **epinephrine**. Patients on concurrent **beta blocker** therapy may have a greater ↑ in heart rate and BP.

Route/Dosage

Hypoglycemia

IV, IM, Subcut (Adults and Children >25 kg): 1 mg; may be repeated in 15 min if necessary.
Subcut (Adults and Children ≥12 yr): *Gvoke*—1 mg; may be repeated in 15 min if necessary.
IV, IM, Subcut (Children <25 kg): 0.5 mg or 0.02–0.03 mg/kg; may be repeated in 15 min if necessary.
IV, IM, Subcut (Children >6 yr and unknown weight): 1 mg; may be repeated in 15 min if necessary.
IV, IM, Subcut (Children <6 yr and unknown weight): 0.5 mg or 0.02–0.03 mg/kg; may be repeated in 15 min if necessary.
Subcut (Children 2–12 yr and ≥45 kg): *Gvoke*—1 mg; may be repeated in 15 min if necessary.
Subcut (Children 2–12 yr and <45 kg): *Gvoke*—0.5 mg; may be repeated in 15 min if necessary.
Intranasal (Adults and Children ≥4 yr): 3 mg (one actuation) in one nostril; may be repeated in 15 min if necessary.

Radiographic Examination of the GI Tract

IM, IV (Adults): 0.25–2 mg; depending on location and duration of examination (0.5 mg IV or 2 mg IM for relaxation of stomach; for examination of the colon 2 mg IM 10 min before procedure).

Antidote (unlabeled)

IV (Adults): *Beta blocker overdose*—50–150 mcg (0.05–0.15 mg)/kg, followed by 1–5 mg/hr infusion. *Calcium channel blocker overdose*—2 mg; additional doses determined by response.

Availability

Nasal powder: 3 mg/device. **Powder for injection (requires reconstitution):** 1-mg (equivalent to 1 unit) vials as an emergency kit for low blood glucose and as a diagnostic kit. **Solution for subcutaneous injection (Gvoke) (prefilled syringes and prefilled autoinjectors):** 0.5 mg/0.1 mL, 1 mg/0.2 mL.

NURSING IMPLICATIONS

Assessment

- Assess for signs of hypoglycemia (sweating, hunger, weakness, headache, dizziness, tremor, irritability, tachycardia, anxiety) prior to and periodically during therapy.
- Assess neurologic status throughout therapy. Institute safety precautions to protect patient from injury caused by seizures, falling, or aspiration. For insulin shock therapy, 0.5–1 mg is administered after 1 hr of coma; patient usually awakens in 10–25 min. If no response occurs, repeat the dose. Feed patient supplemental carbohydrates orally to replenish liver glycogen and prevent secondary hypoglycemia as soon as possible after awakening, especially pediatric patients.
- Assess nutritional status. Patients who lack liver glycogen stores (starvation, chronic hypoglycemia, adrenal insufficiency) will require glucose instead of glucagon.
- Assess for nausea and vomiting after administration of dose. Protect patients with depressed level of consciousness from aspiration by positioning on side; ensure that a suction unit is available. Notify health care professional if vomiting occurs; patient will require parenteral glucose to prevent recurrent hypoglycemia.
- ***Lab Test Considerations:*** Monitor serum glucose levels throughout episode, during treatment, and for 3–4 hr after patient regains consciousness. Use of bedside fingerstick blood glucose determination methods is recommended for rapid results. Follow-up lab results may be ordered to validate fingerstick values, but do not delay treatment while awaiting lab results, as this could result in neurologic injury or death.
- Large doses of glucagon may cause a ↓ in serum potassium concentrations.

Implementation

- May be given subcut, IM, or IV. Reconstitute with diluent supplied in kit by manufacturer. Inspect solution prior to use; use only clear, water-like solution. Solution is stable for 48 hr if refrigerated, 24 hr at room temperature. Unmixed medication should be stored at room temperature.

- Administer supplemental carbohydrates IV or orally to facilitate increase of serum glucose levels.
- **Subcut:** *Gvoke* solution is clear and colorless to pale yellow; do not administer if solution is discolored or contains particulate matter. Inject in lower abdomen, outer thigh, or outer upper arm.
- **Intranasal:** Administer by inserting tip into one nostril and pressing device plunger all the way in until green line is no longer showing. Dose does not need to be inhaled. Call for emergency assistance immediately after administering dose. When patient responds to treatment, give oral carbohydrates.

IV Administration

- **IV Push:** ***Diluent:*** Reconstitute each vial with 1 mL of an appropriate diluent. For doses ≤2 mg, use diluent provided by manufacturer. For doses >2 mg, use sterile water for injection instead of diluent supplied by manufacturer to minimize risk of thrombophlebitis, CNS toxicity, and myocardial depression from phenol preservative in diluent supplied by manufacturer. Reconstituted vials should be used immediately. ***Concentration:*** Not exceed 1 mg/mL. ***Rate:*** Administer at a rate not exceeding 1 mg/min. May be administered through IV line containing D5W.
- **Continuous Infusion:** ***Diluent:*** Reconstitute vials as per directions above (use sterile water for injection). Further dilute 10 mg of glucagon in 100 mL of D5W. ***Concentration:*** 0.1 mg/mL. ***Rate:*** See Route/Dosage section.
- **Y-Site Compatibility:** naloxone.

Patient/Family Teaching

- Teach patient and family signs and symptoms of hypoglycemia. Instruct patient to take oral glucose as soon as symptoms of hypoglycemia occur; glucagon is reserved for episodes when patient is unable to swallow because of decreased level of consciousness.
- **Home Care Issues** Instruct family on correct technique to prepare, draw up, and administer injection. Health care professional must be contacted immediately after each dose for orders regarding further therapy or adjustment of insulin dose or diet.
- Advise family that patient should receive oral glucose when alertness returns.
- Instruct family to position patient on side until fully alert. Explain that glucagon may cause nausea and vomiting. Aspiration may occur if patient vomits while lying on back.
- Instruct patient to check expiration date monthly and to replace outdated medication immediately.
- Review hypoglycemic medication regimen, diet, and exercise programs.
- Patients with diabetes mellitus should carry a source of sugar (such as a packet of sugar or candy) and identification describing disease process and treatment regimen at all times.
- Advise patient to notify health care professional if pregnancy is suspected or if breast feeding.

Evaluation/Desired Outcomes

- Increase of serum glucose to normal levels with improved level of consciousness.
- Smooth muscle relaxation of the stomach, duodenum, and small and large intestine in patients undergoing radiologic examination of the GI tract.

glyBURIDE, See SULFONYLUREAS.

glycopyrrolate

(glye-koe-**pye**-roe-late)

Cuvposa, Glyrx-PF, ~~Robinul~~

Classification

Therapeutic: antispasmodics

Pharmacologic: anticholinergics

Indications

Inhibits salivation and excessive respiratory secretions when given preoperatively. Reverses some of the secretory and vagal actions of cholinesterase inhibitors used to treat nondepolarizing neuromuscular blockade (cholinergic adjunct). Adjunctive management of peptic ulcer disease. **Oral solution:** Reduce chronic severe drooling in children with neurologic conditions associated with drooling.

Action

Inhibits the action of acetylcholine at postganglionic sites located in smooth muscle, secretory glands, and the CNS (antimuscarinic activity). Low doses decrease sweating, salivation, and respiratory secretions. Intermediate doses result in increased heart rate. Larger doses decrease GI and GU tract motility. **Therapeutic Effects:** Decreased GI and respiratory secretions.

Pharmacokinetics

Absorption: Incompletely absorbed (<10%) after oral administration. Well absorbed after IM administration.

Distribution: Distribution not fully known. Does not significantly cross the blood-brain barrier or eye. Crosses the placenta.

Metabolism and Excretion: Eliminated primarily unchanged in the urine and bile.

Half-life: 1.7 hr (0.6–4.6 hr).

TIME/ACTION PROFILE (anticholinergic effects)

ROUTE	ONSET	PEAK	DURATION
PO	1 hr	unknown	8–12 hr
IM	15–30 min	30–45 min	2–7 hr*
IV	1–10 min	unknown	2–7 hr*

*Antisecretory effect lasts up to 7 hr; vagal blockade lasts 2–3 hr.

Contraindications/Precautions

Contraindicated in: Hypersensitivity; Angle-closure glaucoma; Acute hemorrhage; Tachycardia secondary to cardiac insufficiency or thyrotoxicosis; Severe ulcerative colitis; Toxic megacolon; Myasthenia gravis; Obstructive uropathy; Paralytic ileus; Concurrent use of oral potassium chloride dosage forms (oral solution only).

Use Cautiously in: Patients who may have intra-abdominal infections; Prostatic hyperplasia; Chronic renal, hepatic, pulmonary, or cardiac disease; Hyperthyroidism; Down syndrome and children with spastic paralysis or brain damage (may be hypersensitive to antimuscarinic effects); OB, Lactation: Safety not established; Pedi: ↑ sensitivity to anticholinergic effects and adverse reactions; Geri: ↑ sensitivity to anticholinergic effects and adverse reactions.

Adverse Reactions/Side Effects

CNS: headache, confusion, drowsiness. **CV:** tachycardia, orthostatic hypotension, palpitations. **Derm:** flushing. **EENT:** nasal congestion, blurred vision, cycloplegia, dry eyes, mydriasis. **GI:** dry mouth, vomiting, constipation. **GU:** urinary hesitancy, urinary retention.

Interactions

Drug-Drug: May ↑ GI mucosal lesions in patients taking oral **potassium chloride** tablets; concurrent use with oral glycopyrrolate solution contraindicated. Additive anticholinergic effects with other **anticholinergics**, including **antihistamines**, **phenothiazines**, **meperidine**, **amantadine**, **tricyclic antidepressants**, **quinidine**, and **disopyramide**. May alter the absorption of other **orally administered drugs** by slowing motility of the GI tract. May ↑ GI transit time of oral **digoxin** and ↑ digoxin levels. **Antacids** or **adsorbent antidiarrheal agents** ↓ absorption of anticholinergics. May ↑ GI mucosal lesions in patients taking oral **potassium chloride** tablets. May ↑ **atenolol** and **metformin** levels. May ↓ levels of **haloperidol** and **levodopa**. Concurrent use may ↓ absorption of **ketoconazole** (administer 2 hr after ketoconazole).

Route/Dosage

Control of Secretions during Surgery

IM (Adults): 4.4 mcg/kg 30–60 min preop (not to exceed 0.1 mg).
IM (Children >2 yr): 4.4 mcg/kg 30–60 min preop.
IM (Children <2 yr): 4.4–8.8 mcg/kg 30–60 min preop.

Control of Secretions (chronic)

IM, IV (Children): 4–10 mcg/kg/dose every 3–4 hr.
PO (Children): 40–100 mcg/kg/dose 3–4 times/day.

Cholinergic Adjunct

IV (Adults and Children): 200 mcg for each 1 mg of neostigmine or 5 mg of pyridostigmine given at the same time.

Antiarrhythmic

IV (Adults): 100 mcg, may be repeated every 2–3 min.
IV (Children): 4.4 mcg/kg (up to 100 mcg); may be repeated every 2–3 min.

Peptic Ulcer

PO (Adults): 1–2 mg 2–3 times daily. An additional 2 mg may be given at bedtime; may be ↓ to 1 mg twice daily (not to exceed 8 mg/day).
IM, IV (Adults): 100–200 mcg every 4 hr up to 4 times daily.

Chronic Severe Drooling

PO (Children 3–16 yr): *Oral solution*—0.02 mg/kg 3 times daily; may ↑ by 0.02 mg/kg 3 times daily every 5–7 days (not to exceed 0.1 mg/kg 3 times daily or 1.5–3 mg/dose).

Availability (generic available)

Oral solution (cherry-flavor): 1 mg/5 mL. **Solution for injection:** 200 mcg (0.2 mg)/mL. **Tablets:** 1 mg, 1.5 mg, 2 mg.

NURSING IMPLICATIONS

Assessment

- Assess heart rate, BP, and respiratory rate before and periodically during parenteral therapy.
- Monitor intake and output ratios in geriatric or surgical patients; glycopyrrolate may cause urinary retention. Instruct patient to void before parenteral administration.
- Assess patient routinely for abdominal distention and auscultate for bowel sounds. If constipation becomes a problem, increasing fluids and adding bulk to the diet may help alleviate the constipating effects of the drug.
- Periodic intraocular pressure determinations should be made for patients receiving long-term therapy.
- Pedi: Monitor amount and frequency of drooling periodically during therapy.
- Assess for hyperexcitability, a paradoxical response that may occur in children.
- ***Lab Test Considerations:*** Antagonizes effects of pentagastrin and histamine during the gastric acid secretion test. Avoid administration for 24 hr preceding the test.
- May cause ↓ uric acid levels in patients with gout or hyperuricemia.
- ***Toxicity and Overdose:*** If overdose occurs, neostigmine is the antidote.

Implementation

- Do not administer cloudy or discolored solution.
- **PO:** Administer 30–60 min before meals to maximize absorption.
- For drooling: Administer at least 1 hr before or 2 hr after meals.
- Do not administer within 1 hr of antacids or antidiarrheal medications.
- Oral dose is 10 times the parenteral dose.
- **IM:** May be administered undiluted (200 mcg/mL).

IV Administration

- **IV Push:** ***Diluent:*** May be given undiluted through Y-site. ***Concentration:*** 200 mcg/mL. ***Rate:*** Administer at a maximum rate of 20 mcg over 1 min.
- **Y-Site Compatibility:** acyclovir, alemtuzumab, alfentanil, amikacin, aminophylline, amiodarone, anidulafungin, argatroban, arsenic trioxide, ascorbic acid, atracurium, atropine, azathioprine, aztreonam, benztropine, bivalirudin, bleomycin, bumetanide, buprenorphine, butorphanol, calcium chloride, calcium gluconate, carmustine, caspofungin, cefazolin, cefotaxime, cefotetan, cefoxitin, ceftazidime, ceftriaxone, cefuroxime, chloramphenicol, chlorpromazine, cisplatin, clindamycin, cyanocobalamin, cyclosporine, dacarbazine, dactinomycin, daptomycin, daunorubicin, dexamethasone, dexmedetomidine, dexrazoxane, digoxin, diltiazem, diphenhydramine, dobutamine, docetaxel, dopamine, doxorubicin liposomal, doxycycline, enalaprilat, ephedrine, epinephrine, epoetin alfa, ertapenem, erythromycin, esmolol, etoposide, etoposide phosphate, famotidine, fenoldopam, fentanyl, fluconazole, fludarabine, folic acid, foscarnet, fosphenytoin, ganciclovir, gemcitabine, gentamicin, granisetron, heparin, hetastarch, hydrocortisone, hydromorphone, idarubicin, imipenem/cilastatin, isoproterenol, ketorolac, labetalol, leucovorin calcium, lidocaine, linezolid, lorazepam, magnesium sulfate, mannitol, meperidine, mesna, metaraminol, methyldopate, methylprednisolone, metoclopramide, metoprolol, midazolam, milrinone, mitoxantrone, morphine, moxifloxcin, multivitamins, mycophenolate, nafcillin, nalbuphine, naloxone, nitroglycerin, nitroprusside, norepinephrine, octreotide, ondansetron, oxacillin, oxaliplatin, oxytocin, paclitaxel, palonosetron, pamidronate, pancuronium, papaverine, pemetrexed, penicillin G, pentamidine, pentobarbital, phenobarbital, phentolamine, phenylephrine, phytonadione, potassium acetate, potassium chloride, procainamide, promethazine, propofol, propranolol, protamine, pyridoxime, ranitidine, sodium bicarbonate, streptokinase, succinylcholine, sufentanil, tacrolimus, theophylline, thiamine, thiotepa, tigecycline, tirofiban, tobramycin, tolazoline, topotecan, vancomycin, vasopressin, vecuronium, verapamil, vinorelbine, voriconazole, zoledronic acid.
- **Y-Site Incompatibility:** amphotericin B lipid complex, dantrolene, diazepam, diazoxide, furosemide, indomethacin, insulin, regular, irinotecan, mitomycin, pantoprazole, phenytoin, piperacillin/tazobactam, trimethoprim/sulfamethoxazole.

Patient/Family Teaching

- Instruct patient to take glycopyrrolate as directed and not to take more than the prescribed amount. Take missed doses as soon as remembered if not just before next dose.
- Medication may cause drowsiness and blurred vision. Caution patient to avoid driving or other activities requiring alertness until response to the medication is known.
- Inform patient that frequent oral rinses, sugarless gum or candy, and good oral hygiene may help relieve dry mouth. Consult health care professional regarding use of saliva substitute if dry mouth persists for more than 2 wk.
- Advise patient to change positions slowly to minimize the effects of drug-induced orthostatic hypotension.
- Caution patient to avoid extremes of temperature. This medication decreases the ability to sweat and may increase the risk of heat stroke.
- Advise patient to notify health care professional immediately if eye pain or increased sensitivity to light occurs. Emphasize the importance of routine eye exams throughout therapy.
- Advise patient to consult health care professional before taking any OTC medications concurrently with this therapy.
- Advise females of reproductive potential to notify health care professional if pregnancy is planned or suspected, or if breast feeding.
- Geri: Advise geriatric patients about increased susceptibility to side effects and to call health care professional immediately if they occur.
- Pedi: Instruct parents to use a calibrated measuring device with solution for accurate dosing.
- Advise parents to stop glycopyrrolate and notify health care professional if constipation; signs of urinary retention (inability to urinate, dry diapers or undergarments, irritability, or crying); or rash, hives, or an allergic reaction occurs.
- Glycopyrrolate reduces sweating. Advise parents to avoid exposure of the patient to hot or very warm environmental temperatures to avoid overheating and heat exhaustion or heat stroke.

Evaluation/Desired Outcomes

- Mouth dryness preoperatively.
- Reversal of cholinergic medications.
- Decrease in GI motility and pain in patients with peptic ulcer disease.
- Reduce chronic severe drooling in children with neurologic conditions associated with drooling.

glycopyrrolate/formoterol

(glye-koe-**pye**-roe-late/for-**moe**-te-rol)

Bevespi Aerosphere

Classification

Therapeutic: bronchodilators

Pharmacologic: anticholinergics, long-acting beta2-adrenergic agonists (LABAs)

Indications

Maintenance treatment of COPD.

Action

Glycopyrrolate—acts as an anticholinergic by inhibiting M3 muscarinic receptors in bronchial smooth muscle resulting in bronchodilation; *Formoterol*—a $beta_2$-adrenergic agonist that stimulates adenyl cyclase, resulting in accumulation of cyclic adenosine monophosphate at $beta_2$—adrenergic receptors resulting in bronchodilation. **Therapeutic Effects:** Bronchodilation with decreased airflow obstruction.

Pharmacokinetics

Absorption: *Glycopyrrolate*—some systemic absorption from lungs and GI tract (40%). *formoterol*—majority of inhaled drug is swallowed and absorbed.

Distribution: *Glycopyrrolate*—unknown. *formoterol*—unknown.

Metabolism and Excretion: *Glycopyrrolate*—undergoes hydroxylation to inactive metabolite; eliminated primarily unchanged in the urine and bile. *formoterol*—mostly metabolized by the liver; 10–18% excreted unchanged in urine.

Half-life: *Glycopyrrolate*—33–53 hr. *formoterol*—10 hr.

TIME/ACTION PROFILE (bronchodilation)

ROUTE	ONSET	PEAK	DURATION
formoterol—Inhaln	within 3 min	15 min	unknown
glycopyrrolate—Inhaln	unknown	unknown	unknown

Contraindications/Precautions

Contraindicated in: Hypersensitivity; Asthma; Acutely deteriorating COPD or acute respiratory symptoms; Lactation: Discontinue drug or discontinue breast feeding.

Use Cautiously in: History of cardiovascular disorders (coronary insufficiency, arrhythmias, hypertension); History of seizures; Thyrotoxicosis; Narrow-angle glaucoma; Urinary retention, prostatic hyperplasia, bladder-neck obstruction; Hepatic impairment; OB: Use only if potential maternal benefit justifies potential fetal risk; formoterol may interfere with uterine contractility during labor; Pedi: Safety and effectiveness not established.

Exercise Extreme Caution in: Concurrent use of MAO inhibitors, tricyclic antidepressants or drugs that prolong the QTc interval.

Adverse Reactions/Side Effects

Combination.

CNS: anxiety, dizziness, headache. **CV:** chest pain, hypertension, tachycardia. **F and E:** hypokalemia. **GI:** dry mouth, vomiting. **GU:** urinary tract infection. **MS:** arthralgia, muscle spasms. **Resp:** cough, paradoxical bronchospasm. **Misc:** HYPERSENSITIVITY REACTIONS (including angioedema, urticaria, or rash).

Interactions

Drug-Drug: Concurrent use with other **adrenergics** may ↑ adrenergic adverse reactions (↑ heart rate, BP, jitteriness). ↑ risk of hypokalemia or ECG changes with **xanthine derivatives**, **corticosteroids**, **loop diuretics** or **thiazide diuretics**. ↑ risk of serious adverse cardiovascular effects with **MAO inhibitors**, **tricyclic antidepressants**, **QT-interval prolonging drugs**; use with extreme caution. Effectiveness may be ↓ by **beta-blockers**; use cautiously and only when necessary. ↑ risk of anticholinergic adverse reactions when used concurrently with other **anticholinergics**; avoid concurrent use.

Route/Dosage

Inhaln (Adults): 2 inhalations twice daily.

Availability

Inhalation aerosol: glycopyrrolate 9 mcg/formoterol 4.8 mcg per inhalation in 10.7-g canister (120 inhalations).

NURSING IMPLICATIONS

Assessment

- Assess lung sounds, pulse, and BP before administration and during peak of medication. Note amount, color, and character of sputum produced.
- Monitor pulmonary function tests before initiating and periodically during therapy to determine effectiveness.
- Observe for paradoxical bronchospasm (wheezing, dyspnea, tightness in chest) and hypersensitivity reaction (rash; urticaria; swelling of the face, lips, or eyelids). If condition occurs, withhold medication and notify health care professional immediately.
- Monitor ECG periodically during therapy. May cause prolonged QTc interval.
- Monitor patient for signs of hypersensitivity reactions (difficulties in breathing or swallowing, swelling of tongue, lips and face, urticaria, or skin rash)

throughout therapy. Discontinue therapy and consider alternative if reaction occurs.

- ***Lab Test Considerations:*** May cause ↑ serum glucose and decreased serum potassium.

Implementation

- **Inhaln:** Administer as 2 inhalations twice daily, morning and evening. Shake well prior to use. Prime by releasing 4 sprays into air away from face before 1st use and by releasing 2 sprays if unused for more than 7 days. See Appendix for use of metered-dose inhalers.

Patient/Family Teaching

- Instruct patient to use medication as directed. Do not discontinue therapy without discussing with health care professional, even if feeling better. If a dose is missed skip dose and take next dose at regularly scheduled time. Do not double doses. Use a rapid-acting bronchodilator if symptoms occur before next dose is due. Caution patient not to use more than 2 times a day; may cause adverse effects, paradoxical bronchospasm, or loss of effectiveness of medication. Instruct patient to review *Medication Guide* before starting therapy and with each Rx refill in case of changes.
- Caution patient not to use medication to treat acute symptoms. A rapid-acting inhaled beta-adrenergic bronchodilator should be used for relief of acute asthma attacks. Notify health care professional immediately if symptoms get worse or more inhalations than usual are needed from rescue inhaler.
- Advise patient to clean inhaler each wk so medicine will not build up and block spray through mouthpiece. Take canister out of the actuator, run warm water through actuator, and allowing actuator to air-dry overnight. Shake and re-prime with 2 sprays before use.
- Instruct patient to contact health care professional immediately if shortness of breath is not relieved by medication or nausea, vomiting, shakiness, headache, fast or irregular heartbeat, sleeplessness, or signs and symptoms of narrow angle glaucoma (eye pain or discomfort, blurred vision, visual halos or colored images, red eyes) or urinary retention (difficulty passing urine, painful urination) occur.
- Advise patient to consult health care professional before taking any Rx, OTC, or herbal products or alcohol concurrently with this therapy. Caution patient also to avoid smoking and other respiratory irritants.
- Advise patient to notify health care professional if pregnancy is planned or suspected, or if breast feeding.

Evaluation/Desired Outcomes

- Bronchodilation with decreased airflow obstruction.

golimumab (go-li-mu-mab)

Simponi, Simponi Aria, ✱Simponi IV

Classification

Therapeutic: antirheumatics

Pharmacologic: DMARDs, monoclonal antibodies, anti-TNF agents

Indications

Simponi and Simponi Aria: Treatment of the following conditions: Moderately to severely active rheumatoid arthritis (with methotrexate), Active psoriatic arthritis (alone or with methotrexate or other nonbiologic DMARD), Active ankylosing spondylitis. **Simponi:** Moderately to severely active ulcerative colitis in patients who have demonstrated corticosteroid dependence or have responded inadequately to immunosuppressants such as aminosalicylates, corticosteroids, azathioprine, or 6–mercaptopurine.

Action

Inhibits binding of TNFα to receptors inhibiting activity and resulting in anti-inflammatory and antiproliferative activity. **Therapeutic Effects:** Decreased pain and swelling with decreased joint destruction in patients with rheumatoid arthritis, psoriatic arthritis, and ankylosing spondylitis. Induction and maintenance of clinical remission of ulcerative colitis.

Pharmacokinetics

Absorption: Well absorbed following subcutaneous administration. IV administration results in complete bioavailability.

Distribution: Distributed primarily in the circulatory system with limited extravascular distribution.

Metabolism and Excretion: Unknown.

Half-life: 2 wk.

TIME/ACTION PROFILE (improvement)

ROUTE	ONSET	PEAK	DURATION
Subcut	within 3 mo	2–7 days†	unknown
IV	within 3 mo	unknown	unknown

† Blood levels.

Contraindications/Precautions

Contraindicated in: Active infection (including localized); Concurrent use of abatacept or anakinra (↑ risk of infections); Lactation: Avoid during breast feeding.

Use Cautiously in: History of chronic or recurrent infection or underlying illness/treatment predisposing to infection; History of exposure to tuberculosis; History of opportunistic infection; Patients residing, or who have resided, where tuberculosis, histoplasmosis, coccidioidomycoses, or blastomycosis is endemic; History of HF (may worsen); Pre-existing CNS demyelinating disorders (including multiple sclerosis or Guillain-Barré syndrome); History of cytopenias (may worsen);

History of psoriasis (may exacerbate); Hepatitis B virus carriers (risk of reactivation); Geri: Use cautiously in elderly patients due to ↑ risk of infection; OB: Use during pregnancy only if clearly needed; Pedi: Safety not established; ↑ risk of lymphoma (including HSTCL), leukemia, and other malignancies.

Adverse Reactions/Side Effects

CNS: CENTRAL NERVOUS SYSTEM DEMYELINATING DISORDERS, Guillain-Barre syndrome, multiple sclerosis. **EENT:** nasopharyngitis, optic neuritis. **Resp:** upper respiratory tract infection. **CV:** HF, hypertension. **GI:** ↑ liver enzymes. **Derm:** psoriasis. **Hemat:** agranulocytosis, aplastic anemia, leukopenia, neutropenia, pancytopenia, thrombocytopenia. **Local:** injection site reactions. **Neuro:** paresthesia. **Misc:** ANAPHYLAXIS, HYPERSENSITIVITY REACTIONS, INFECTIONS (including reactivation tuberculosis and other opportunistic infections due to bacterial, invasive fungal, viral, mycobacterial, and parasitic pathogens), MALIGNANCY (including lymphoma, HSTCL, leukemia, and skin cancer), fever, lupus-like syndrome.

Interactions

Drug-Drug: Abatacept, **anakinra**, **corticosteroids**, or **methotrexate** ↑ risk of serious infections; concurrent use with anakinra or abatacept is not recommended. Use of **live virus vaccines** or therapeutic infectious agents may ↑ risk of infection; avoid concurrent use. Concurrent use with **azathioprine** and/or **6–mercaptopurine** may ↑ risk of HSTCL. May normalize previously suppressed levels of CYP450 enzymes, following initiation or discontinuation of golimumab, effects of substrates of this system may be altered and should be monitored, including **warfarin**, **theophylline**, and **cyclosporine**.

Route/Dosage

Rheumatoid Arthritis

Subcut (Adults): 50 mg once monthly.
IV (Adults): 2 mg/kg initially and 4 wk later, then 2 mg/kg every 8 wk.

Psoriatic Arthritis and Ankylosing Spondylitis

Subcut (Adults): 50 mg once monthly.
IV (Adults): 2 mg/kg initially and 4 wk later, then 2 mg/kg every 8 wk.

Ulcerative Colitis

Subcut (Adults): 200 mg initially, then 100 mg 2 wk later, then 100 mg every 4 wk.

Availability

Solution for subcutaneous injection: 50 mg/0.5 mL in single-dose prefilled syringes and Smartject autoinjectors, 100 mg/mL in single-dose prefilled syringes and Smartject autoinjectors. **Solution for intravenous injection (Simponi Aria):** 12.5 mg/mL.

NURSING IMPLICATIONS

Assessment

- Assess for signs and symptoms of infection (fever, dyspnea, flu-like symptoms, frequent or painful urination, redness or swelling at the site of a wound) prior to, during, and after therapy. Discontinue therapy if serious or opportunistic infection or sepsis occurs. If new infection develops during therapy, assess patient and institute antimicrobial therapy. Patients who tested negative for latent tuberculosis (TB) prior to therapy may develop TB during therapy. Initiate treatment for latent TB prior to initiating therapy.
- Test for HBV prior to therapy and monitor carriers of HBV for signs of reactivation during and for several mo after therapy. If reactivation occurs, discontinue golimumab and institute antiviral therapy.
- Monitor patients with HF for new or worsening symptoms. Discontinue therapy if symptoms occur.
- Assess for exacerbations and new onset psoriasis. Discontinue therapy if these occur.
- Assess patient for latex allergy. Needle cover of syringe contains latex and should not be handled by persons sensitive to latex.
- Assess for signs and symptoms of systemic fungal infections (fever, malaise, weight loss, sweats, cough, dyspnea, pulmonary infiltrates, serious systemic illness with or without concomitant shock). Ascertain if patient lives in or has traveled to areas of endemic mycoses. Consider empiric antifungal treatment for patients at risk of histoplasmosis and other invasive fungal infections until the pathogens are identified. Consult with an infectious diseases specialist. Consider stopping golimumab until the infection has been diagnosed and adequately treated.
- Observe for signs and symptoms of anaphylaxis (rash, pruritus, laryngeal edema, wheezing). Discontinue drug and notify health care professional immediately if these problems occur. Keep epinephrine, an antihistamine, and resuscitation equipment close by in case of an anaphylactic reaction.
- **Rheumatoid Arthritis:** Assess pain and range of motion prior to and periodically during therapy.
- **Ulcerative Colitis:** Assess for signs and symptoms before, during, and after therapy.
- ***Lab Test Considerations:*** Monitor liver function tests periodically during therapy. May cause ↑ serum AST and ALT.
- Monitor CBC with differential periodically during therapy. May cause leukopenia, neutropenia, thrombocytopenia, and pancytopenia. Discontinue golimumab if symptoms of blood dyscrasias (persistent fever) occur.

- Monitor for HBV blood tests before starting, during, and for several mo after therapy is completed.

Implementation

- Administer a tuberculin skin test prior to administration of golimumab. Assess if treatment for latent tuberculosis is needed; an induration of 5 mm or greater is a positive tuberculin skin test, even for patients previously vaccinated with Bacille Calmette-Guerin (BCG). Consider antituberculosis therapy prior to therapy in patients with a history of latent or active tuberculosis if an adequate course of treatment cannot be confirmed, and for patients with risk factors for tuberculosis infection.
- Initial injection should be supervised by health care professional.
- Refrigerate solution; do not freeze. Allow prefilled syringe or autoinjector to sit at room temperature for 30 min prior to injection; do not warm in any other way. Do not shake. Solution is clear to slightly opalescent and colorless to light yellow. Do not administer solutions that are discolored, cloudy, or contain particulate matter. Discard unused solution.
- **Subcut:** Remove the needle cover or autoinjector cap just prior to injection. Inject into front of middle thigh, lower part of abdomen 2 inches from navel, or caregiver may administer into outer area of upper arm. Do not inject in areas where skin is tender, bruised, red, scaly, or hard; avoid scars or stretch marks. Press a cotton ball or gauze over injection site for 10 sec; do not rub.
- *Autoinjector:* Press open end of autoinjector against skin at 90° angle. Use free hand to pinch and hold skin at injection site. Press button with fingers or thumb; button will stay pressed and does not need to be held. Injection will begin following a loud click. Keep holding the autoinjector against skin until a 2nd loud click is heard (usually 3–6 sec, but may take up to 15 sec). Lift autoinjector from skin following 2nd click. Yellow indicator in viewing window indicates autoinjector worked correctly. If yellow does not appear in viewing window call 1-800-457-6399 for help.
- *Prefilled syringe:* Hold body of syringe between thumb and index finger. Do not pull back on plunger at any time. Pinch skin. Using a dart-like motion, insert needle into pinched skin at 45° angle. Inject all medication by pushing plunger until plunger head is between needle guard wings. Take needle out of skin and let go of skin. Slowly take thumb off plunger to allow empty syringe to move up until entire needle is covered by needle guard.

IV Administration

- **Intermittent Infusion:** Solution in vial is colorless to light yellow; may contain a few fine translucent particles of protein. Do not use if opaque particles, discoloration, or other particles present. ***Diluent:*** Withdraw volume of dose from 100 mL bag of 0.9% NaCl or 0.45% NaCl and discard. Add golimumab dose to infusion bag; mix gently. Solution is stable for 4 hrs at room temperature. ***Rate:*** Infuse through an in-line, sterile, non-pyrogenic, low protein-binding filter with ≤ 0.22 micrometer pore size over 30 min.

Patient/Family Teaching

- Instruct patient on correct technique for administration. Review patient information sheet, preparation of dose, administration sites and technique, and disposal of equipment into a puncture-resistant container. Advise patient of risks and benefits of golimumab therapy. Inject missed doses as soon as remembered, then return to regular schedule. Instruct patient to read *Medication Guide* before starting therapy and with each Rx refill; new information may be available.
- Caution patient not to share this medication with others, even with the same symptoms; may be harmful.
- Inform patient of increased risk of infections, malignancies, cardiac and nervous system disorders during therapy.
- Caution patient to notify health care professional promptly if any signs of infection, including TB, invasive fungal infections (fever, malaise, weight loss, sweats, cough, dyspnea, pulmonary infiltrates, serious systemic illness with or without concomitant shock), reactivation of HBV (muscle aches, clay-colored bowel movements, feeling very tired, fever, dark urine, chills, skin or eyes look yellow, stomach discomfort, little or no appetite, skin rash, vomiting), hypersensitivity reactions, or nervous system problems (vision changes, weakness in arms or legs, numbness or tingling in any part of the body) develop.
- Advise patient to examine skin periodically during therapy and notify health care professional of any changes in appearance of skin or growths on skin.
- Advise patient to notify health care professional of all Rx or OTC medications, vitamins, or herbal products being taken and to consult with health care professional before taking other medications.
- Inform patient to avoid receiving live vaccinations; other vaccinations may be given.
- Inform patient of increased risk of cancer. Advise patient of need for screening for dysplasia (colonoscopy, skin cancer examinations, biopsy) periodically during therapy.
- Advise patient to notify health care professional if pregnancy is planned or suspected or if breast feeding. Notify health care professional if you have recently had a baby while taking golimumab. Infants may have an increased chance of getting an infection for up to 6 mo after birth; vaccinations may be delayed.

Evaluation/Desired Outcomes

- Decreased pain and swelling with decreased rate of joint destruction in patients with rheumatoid arthritis.

- Decreased signs and symptoms, slowed progression of joint destruction, and improved physical function in patients with psoriatic arthritis.
- Reduced signs and symptoms of ankylosing spondylitis.
- Decreased symptoms, maintaining remission, and mucosal healing with decreased corticosteroid use in ulcerative colitis.

goserelin (goe-se-rel-lin)
Zoladex

Classification
Therapeutic: antineoplastics, hormones
Pharmacologic: gonadotropin-releasing hormones

Indications
Prostate cancer in patients who cannot tolerate orchiectomy or estrogen therapy (palliative). With flutamide and radiation therapy in the treatment of locally confined stage T2b–T4 (stage B2–C) prostate cancer. Advanced breast cancer in peri- and postmenopausal women (palliative). Endometriosis. Produces thinning of the endometrium before endometrial ablation for dysfunctional uterine bleeding.

Action
Acts as a synthetic form of luteinizing hormone–releasing hormone (LHRH, GnRH). Inhibits the production of gonadotropins by the pituitary gland. Initially, levels of luteinizing hormone (LH), follicle-stimulating hormone (FSH), and testosterone increase. Continued administration leads to decreased production of testosterone and estradiol. **Therapeutic Effects:** Decreased spread of cancer of the prostate or breast. Regression of endometriosis with decreased pain. Thinning of the endometrium.

Pharmacokinetics
Absorption: Well absorbed from subcut implant. Absorption is slower in first 8 days, then is faster and continuous for remainder of 28-day dosing cycle.
Distribution: Unknown.
Metabolism and Excretion: Some metabolism by the liver (<10%), some excretion by kidneys (>90%, only 20% as unchanged drug).
Half-life: 4.2 hr.

TIME/ACTION PROFILE (↓ in serum testosterone levels)

ROUTE	ONSET	PEAK	DURATION
Subcut	unknown	2–4 wk	length of therapy

Contraindications/Precautions
Contraindicated in: Hypersensitivity; Undiagnosed vaginal bleeding; OB, Lactation: Pregnancy or lactation.
Use Cautiously in: Congenital long QT syndrome, HF, hypokalemia, or hypomagnesemia; Concurrent use of other drugs known to prolong the QTc interval; Low BMI (↑ risk of bleeding complications); Concurrent use of anticoagulant therapy (↑ risk of bleeding complications); Pedi: Safety not established.

Adverse Reactions/Side Effects
CNS: STROKE, headache, anxiety, depression, dizziness, fatigue, insomnia, mood swings, seizures, weakness. **Resp:** dyspnea. **CV:** MYOCARDIAL INFARCTION, QT INTERVAL PROLONGATION, vasodilation, chest pain, hypertension, palpitations. **GI:** anorexia, constipation, diarrhea, nausea, ulcer, vomiting. **GU:** renal insufficiency, urinary obstruction. **Derm:** sweating, acne, rash. **Endo:** ↓ libido, erectile dysfunction, breast swelling, breast tenderness, infertility, ovarian cysts, ovarian hyperstimulation syndrome (with gonadotropins). **F and E:** peripheral edema. **Hemat:** anemia. **Metab:** gout, hyperglycemia, ↑ lipids. **MS:** ↑ bone pain, arthralgia, ↓ bone density. **Misc:** hot flashes, chills, fever, injection site/vascular injury, weight gain.

Interactions
Drug-Drug: None significant.

Route/Dosage
Subcut (Adults): 3.6 mg every 4 wk or 10.8 mg every 12 wk. *Endometrial thinning*—1 or 2 depots given 4 wk apart; if 1 depot used, surgery is performed at 4 wk; if 2 depots used, surgery is performed 2–4 wk after 2nd depot.

Availability
Implant: 3.6 mg, 10.8 mg.

NURSING IMPLICATIONS
Assessment
- Monitor for signs and symptoms of injection site injury/abdominal hemorrhage (abdominal pain, abdominal distension, dyspnea, dizziness, hypotension, and/or any altered levels of consciousness) following administration. Advise patient to report symptoms immediately to health care professional.
- **Cancer:** Monitor patients with vertebral metastases for increased back pain and decreased sensory/motor function.
- Monitor intake and output ratios and assess for bladder distention in patients with urinary tract obstruction during initiation of therapy.
- **Endometriosis:** Assess patient for signs and symptoms of endometriosis before and periodically during therapy. Amenorrhea usually occurs within 8 wk of initial administration and menses usually resume 8 wk after completion.

- ***Lab Test Considerations:*** Initially ↑, then ↓ LH and FSH. This leads to castration levels of testosterone in men 2–4 wk after initial increase in concentrations.
- Monitor serum acid phosphatase and prostate-specific antigen concentrations periodically during therapy. May cause transient ↑ in serum acid phosphatase concentrations, which usually return to baseline by the 4th wk of therapy and may ↓ to below baseline or return to baseline if elevated before therapy.
- May cause hypercalcemia in patients with breast or prostate cancer with bony metastases.
- May cause an ↑ in serum HDL, LDL, and triglycerides.
- May cause hyperglycemia. Monitor blood glucose and HbA1c periodically during therapy.

Implementation
- **Subcut:** Implant is inserted in upper subcut tissue of upper abdominal wall every 28 days. Local anesthesia may be used before injection.
- If the implant needs to be removed for any reason, it can be located by ultrasound.

Patient/Family Teaching
- Explain purpose of goserelin to patient. Emphasize importance of adhering to the schedule of monthly or every-3-mo administration.
- Advise patient that bone pain may increase at initiation of therapy. This will resolve with time. Patient should discuss use of analgesics to control pain with health care professional.
- Advise female patients to notify health care professional if regular menstruation persists.
- Inform diabetic patients of potential for hyperglycemia. Encourage close monitoring of serum glucose.
- Advise patient that medication may cause hot flashes. Notify health care professional if these become bothersome. Hormone replacement therapy may be added to decrease vasomotor symptoms and vaginal dryness without compromising beneficial effect.
- Instruct patient to notify health care professional promptly if difficulty urinating or if symptoms of myocardial infarction or stroke (chest pain, difficulty breathing, weakness, loss of consciousness) occur.
- Rep: Advise premenopausal women to notify health care professional if pregnancy is planned or suspected or if breast feeding. Effective contraception should be used during and for 12 wk after treatment ends.

Evaluation/Desired Outcomes
- Decrease in the spread of prostate cancer.
- Reduction of symptoms of advanced breast cancer in peri- and postmenopausal women.
- Decrease in the signs and symptoms of endometriosis. Symptoms are usually reduced within 4 wk of implantation.
- Thinning of the endometrium before endometrial ablation for dysfunctional uterine bleeding.

granisetron (gra-nees-e-tron)
~~Kytril~~, Sustol, ✱Kytril

granisetron (transdermal)
Sancuso

Classification
Therapeutic: antiemetics
Pharmacologic: 5-HT_3 antagonists

Indications
PO: Prevention of nausea and vomiting due to emetogenic chemotherapy or radiation therapy. Prevention and treatment of postoperative nausea and vomiting. **Subcut:** Prevention of acute and delayed nausea and vomiting due to moderately emetogenic chemotherapy or anthacycline/cyclophosphamide combination chemotherapy (with dexamethasone). **Transdermal:** Prevention of nausea and vomiting due to moderately/highly emetogenic chemotherapy.

Action
Blocks the effects of serotonin at receptor sites (selective antagonist) located in vagal nerve terminals and in the chemoreceptor trigger zone in the CNS. **Therapeutic Effects:** Decreased incidence and severity of nausea and vomiting following emetogenic chemotherapy, radiation therapy, or surgery.

Pharmacokinetics
Absorption: 50% absorbed following oral administration; transdermal enters systemic circulation via passive diffusion through intact skin.
Distribution: Distributes into erythrocytes; remainder of distribution is unknown.
Protein Binding: 65%.
Metabolism and Excretion: Mostly metabolized by the liver; 12% excreted unchanged in urine.
Half-life: *Patients with cancer*—10–12 hr (range 0.9–31.1 hr); *healthy volunteers* —3–4 hr (range 0.9–15.2 hr); *geriatric patients*—7.7 hr (range 2.6–17.7 hr); *subcutaneous*—24 hr.

TIME/ACTION PROFILE

ROUTE	ONSET	PEAK	DURATION
PO	rapid	60 min	24 hr
IV	1–3 min	30 min	up to 24 hr
TD*	unknown	48 hr	unknown
Subcut*	unknown	12 hr	7 days

*Blood levels.

Contraindications/Precautions
Contraindicated in: Hypersensitivity; Some products contain benzyl alcohol; avoid use in neonates; Severe renal impairment (subcut).
Use Cautiously in: History of arrhythmias or conduction disorders; Recent abdominal surgery (subcutaneous); Moderate renal impairment (↓ frequency of administration); OB, Lactation: Safety not established;

Pedi: Safety and effectiveness not established in children <18 yr (oral, subcut, or transdermal) or <2 yr (IV).

Adverse Reactions/Side Effects

CNS: headache, agitation, anxiety, CNS stimulation, dizziness, drowsiness, headache, insomnia, weakness. **CV:** hypertension, QT interval prolongation. **GI:** constipation, abdominal pain, diarrhea, dyspepsia, ↑ liver enzymes, taste disorder. **Derm:** *Topical*—application site reactions, photosensitivity. **Misc:** HYPERSENSITIVITY REACTIONS (including anaphylaxis), SEROTONIN SYNDROME, injection site reactions (subcutaneous) (including infection, bruising, hematoma, bleeding, pain, or nodules), fever.

Interactions

Drug-Drug: ↑ risk of extrapyramidal reactions with other **agents causing extrapyramidal reactions**. ↑ risk of QT interval prolongation with other **agents causing QT interval prolongation**. Drugs that affect serotonergic neurotransmitter systems, including **SSRIs**, **SNRIs**, **tricyclic antidepressants**, **MAOIs**, **fentanyl**, **lithium**, **buspirone**, **tramadol**, **methylene blue**, and **triptans** ↑ risk of serotonin syndrome.

Route/Dosage

Prevention of Nausea and Vomiting Due to Emetogenic Chemotherapy

PO (Adults): 1 mg twice daily; 1st dose given at least 60 min prior to chemotherapy and 2nd dose 12 hr later only on days when chemotherapy is administered; may also be given as 2 mg once daily at least 60 min prior to chemotherapy.
IV (Adults and Children 2–16 yr): 10 mcg/kg given within 30 min prior to chemotherapy or 20–40 mcg/kg/day divided once or twice daily (maximum: 3 mg/dose or 9 mg/day).
Transdermal (Adults): One 34.3-mg patch (delivers 3.1 mg/24 hr) applied up to 48 hr prior to chemotherapy, leave in place for at least 24 hr following chemotherapy, may be left in place for a total of 7 days.

Prevention of Nausea and Vomiting Associated with Radiation Therapy

PO (Adults): 2 mg taken once daily within 1 hr of radiation therapy.

Prevention and Treatment of Postoperative Nausea and Vomiting

IV (Adults): *Prevention*—1 mg prior to induction of anesthesia or just prior to reversal of anesthesia; *Treatment*—1 mg.
IV (Children ≥4 yr): 20–40 mcg/kg as a single dose (maximum: 1 mg).

Prevention of Acute and Delayed Nausea and Vomiting Due to Emetogenic Chemotherapy

Subcut (Adults): 10 mg given at least 30 min prior to chemotherapy (with dexamethasone) on Day 1 of chemotherapy; do not administer more frequently than every 7 days.

Renal Impairment

Subcut (Adults): *CCr 30–59 mL/min*—Do not administer more frequently than every 14 days.

Availability (generic available)

Tablets: 1 mg. **Solution for intravenous injection:** 0.1 mg/mL, 1 mg/mL. **Solution for subcutaneous injection (in prefilled syringes):** 10 mg/0.4 mL. **Transdermal patch:** 3.1 mg/24 hr.

NURSING IMPLICATIONS

Assessment

- Assess patient for nausea, vomiting, abdominal distention, and bowel sounds prior to and following administration.
- Assess for extrapyramidal symptoms (involuntary movements, facial grimacing, rigidity, shuffling walk, trembling of hands) during therapy. This occurs rarely and is usually associated with concurrent use of other drugs known to cause this effect.
- Monitor ECG in patients with HF, bradycardia, underlying heart disease, renal impairment, and elderly patients.
- Monitor for signs and symptoms of serotonin syndrome (mental status changes [agitation, hallucinations, delirium, and coma], autonomic instability [tachycardia, labile BP, dizziness, diaphoresis, flushing, hyperthermia], neuromuscular symptoms [tremor, rigidity, myoclonus, hyperreflexia, incoordination], seizures, with or without gastrointestinal symptoms [nausea, vomiting, diarrhea]). If symptoms occur discontinue granisetron and treat symptomatically.
- **Transdermal:** Monitor application site. If allergic, erythematous, macular, or papular rash or pruritus occurs, remove patch.
- ***Lab Test Considerations:*** May cause ↑ AST and ALT levels.

Implementation

- Correct hypokalemia and hypomagnesemia before administering.
- For chemotherapy or radiation, granisetron is administered only on the day(s) chemotherapy or radiation is given. Continued treatment when not on chemotherapy or radiation therapy has not been found to be useful.

G

- **PO:** Administer 1st dose up to 1 hr before chemotherapy or radiation therapy and 2nd dose 12 hr after the first.
- **Subcut:** Use kit and components provided by manufacturer. Injection should be administered by health care professional. Remove kit from refrigerator and allow to warm to room temperature for 60 min. Activate one syringe warming pouch, and wrap syringe in warming pouch for 5 to 6 min to warm to body temperature. Do not inject solutions that contain particulate matter. Inject in back of upper arm or in skin of abdomen at least 1 inch away from umbilicus. Avoid injecting in areas where skin is burned, hardened, inflamed, or swollen. Topical anesthesia may be used at injection site prior to injection. Solution is viscous and requires a slow, sustained injection over 20 to 30 sec. Pressing the plunger harder will NOT expel medication faster.

IV Administration

- **IV Push:** ***Diluent:*** May be administered undiluted or diluted in 20–50 mL of 0.9% NaCl or D5W. Solution should be prepared at time of administration but is stable for 24 hr at room temperature. ***Concentration:*** Up to 1 mg/mL. ***Rate:*** Administer undiluted granisetron over 30 sec or as a diluted solution over 5 min.
- **Y-Site Compatibility:** acetaminophen, alemtuzumab, alfentanil, allopurinol, amifostine, amikacin, aminocaproic acid, aminophylline, amiodarone, amphotericin B lipid complex, amphotericin B liposome, ampicillin, ampicillin/sulbactam, anidulafungin, argatroban, atracurium, azithromycin, aztreonam, bivalirudin, bleomycin, bumetanide, buprenorphine, busulfan, butorphanol, calcium acetate, calcium chloride, calcium gluconate, carboplatin, carmustine, caspofungin, cefazolin, cefepime, cefotaxime, cefotetan, cefoxitin, ceftaroline, ceftazidime, ceftriaxone, cefuroxime, chloramphenicol, chlorpromazine, ciprofloxacin, cisatracurium, cisplatin, cladribine, clindamycin, cyclophosphamide, cyclosporine, cytarabine, dacarbazine, dactinomycin, daptomycin, daunorubicin hydrochloride, dexamethasone, dexmedetomidine, dexrazoxane, digoxin, diltiazem, diphenhydramine, dobutamine, docetaxel, dopamine, doxorubicin hydrochloride, doxorubicin liposome, doxycycline, droperidol, enalaprilat, ephedrine, epinephrine, epirubicin, eptifibatide, ertapenem, erythromycin, esmolol, etoposide, etoposide phosphate, famotidine, fenoldopam, fentanyl, filgrastim, floxuridine, fluconazole, fludarabine, fluorouracil, fosaprepitant, foscarnet, fosphenytoin, furosemide, ganciclovir, gemcitabine, gentamicin, glycopyrrolate, haloperidol, heparin, hetastarch, hydralazine, hydrocortisone, hydromorphone, idarubicin, ifosfamide, imipenem/cilastatin, insulin, irinotecan, isoproterenol, ketorolac, labetalol, leucovorin, levofloxacin, lidocaine, linezolid, lorazepam, magnesium sulfate, mannitol, melphalan, meperidine, meropenem, mesna, methotrexate, methyldopate, methylprednisolone, metoclopramide, metoprolol, metronidazole, midazolam, milrinone, mitomycin, mitoxantrone, morphine, moxifloxacin, mycophenolate, nafcillin, nalbuphine, naloxone, nicardipine, nitroglycerin, nitroprusside, norepinephrine, octreotide, oxaliplatin, oxytocin, paclitaxel, pamidronate, pancuronium, pantoprazole, pemetrexed, pentamidine, pentobarbital, phenobarbital, phentolamine, phenylephrine, piperacillin/tazobactam, potassium acetate, potassium chloride, potassium phosphates, procainamide, prochlorperazine, promethazine, propofol, propranolol, quinupristin/dalfopristin, ranitidine, remifentanil, rituximab, rocuronium, sargramostim, sodium acetate, sodium bicarbonate, sodium phosphates, streptozocin, succinylcholine, sufentanil, tacrolimus, theophylline, thiopental, thiotepa, tigecycline, tirofiban, tobramycin, topotecan, trastuzumab, trimethoprim/sulfamethoxazole, vancomycin, vasopressin, vecuronium, verapamil, vinblastine, vincristine, vinorelbine, voriconazole, zidovudine, zoledronic acid.
- **Y-Site Incompatibility:** amphotericin B deoxycholate, dantrolene, diazepam, phenytoin.
- **Additive Incompatibility:** Granisetron should not be admixed with other medications.
- **Transdermal:** Apply system to clear, dry, intact healthy skin on upper outer arm 24–48 hr before chemotherapy. Do not use creams, lotions, or oils that may keep patch from sticking. Do not apply to skin that is red, irritated, or damaged. Apply immediately after removing from package. Do not cut patch into pieces. Remove liner from adhesive layer and press firmly in place with palm of hand for 30 sec, especially around the edges, to make sure contact is complete. Patch should be worn throughout chemotherapy. If patch does not stick, bandages or medical adhesive tape may be applied on edges of patch; do not cover patch with tape or bandages or wrap completely around arm. Patient may shower and wash normally while wearing patch; avoid swimming, strenuous exercise, sauna, or whirlpool during patch use. Remove patch gently at least 24 hr after completion of chemotherapy; may be worn for up to 7 days. Fold so that adhesive edges are together. Throw away in garbage out of reach of children and pets. Do not reuse patch. Use soap and water to remove remaining adhesive; do not use alcohol or acetone.

Patient/Family Teaching

- Instruct patient to take granisetron as directed.
- Advise patient to notify health care professional immediately if involuntary movement of eyes, face, or limbs occurs.
- May cause dizziness and drowsiness. Caution patient to avoid driving and other activities requiring alertness until response to medication is known.

- Advise patient to notify health care professional if symptoms of abnormal heart rate or rhythm (racing heartbeat, shortness of breath, dizziness, fainting) or serotonin syndrome occur.
- Advise patient to notify health care professional of all Rx or OTC medications, vitamins, or herbal products being taken and to consult with health care professional before taking other medications.
- Advise female patient to notify health care professional if pregnancy is planned or suspected or if breast feeding.
- **Transdermal:** Instruct patient on correct application, removal, and disposal of patch. Advise patient to read *Patient Information* sheet prior to using and with each Rx refill in case of new information. Inform patient that additional granisetron should not be taken during patch application unless directed by health care professional.
- Advise patient referred for MRI test to discuss patch with referring health care professional and MRI facility to determine if removal of patch is necessary prior to test and for directions for replacing patch.
- Advise patient to avoid using a heating pad near or over patch and to cover patch application site with clothing to avoid exposure to sunlight, sunlamp, or tanning beds during and for 10 days following removal of patch.
- Instruct patient to notify health care professional if pain or swelling in the abdomen occurs or if redness at patch removal site remains for more than 3 days.

Evaluation/Desired Outcomes

- Prevention of nausea and vomiting associated with emetogenic cancer chemotherapy or radiation therapy.
- Prevention and treatment of postoperative nausea and vomiting.

BEERS

guanFACINE (gwahn-fa-seen)

Intuniv, Intuniv XR, ~~Tenex~~

Classification

Therapeutic: antihypertensives

Pharmacologic: centrally acting antiadrenergics

Indications

Hypertension (with thiazide-type diuretics) (immediate-release). Treatment of attention-deficit hyperactivity disorder (ADHD) as monotherapy or as adjunctive therapy to stimulants (extended-release).

Action

Stimulates CNS alpha$_2$-adrenergic receptors, producing a decrease in sympathetic outflow to heart, kidneys, and blood vessels. Result is decreased BP and peripheral resistance, a slight decrease in heart rate, and no change in cardiac output. Mechanism of action in ADHD is unknown. **Therapeutic Effects:** Lowering of BP in hypertension. Increased attention span in ADHD.

Pharmacokinetics

Absorption: Immediate-release is well absorbed (80%); extended-release has lower rate and extent of absorption (↑ absorption with high-fat meals).

Distribution: Appears to be widely distributed.

Metabolism and Excretion: 50% metabolized by the liver, 50% excreted unchanged by the kidneys.

Half-life: 17 hr.

TIME/ACTION PROFILE (antihypertensive effect)

ROUTE	ONSET	PEAK	DURATION
PO (single dose)	unknown	8–12 hr	24 hr
PO (multiple doses)	within 1 wk	1–3 mo	unknown

Contraindications/Precautions

Contraindicated in: Hypersensitivity.

Use Cautiously in: Severe coronary artery disease or recent myocardial infarction; Geri: May have ↑ sensitivity, especially those with hepatic, cardiac, or renal dysfunction; Cerebrovascular disease; Severe renal or liver disease; History of hypotension, heart block, bradycardia, or cardiovascular disease; OB, Lactation, Pedi: Pregnancy, lactation, or children <6 yr (safety not established).

Adverse Reactions/Side Effects

CNS: drowsiness, headache, weakness, depression, dizziness, fatigue, insomnia, irritability. **CV:** bradycardia, chest pain, hypotension, palpitations, rebound hypertension, syncope. **EENT:** tinnitus. **GI:** constipation, dry mouth, abdominal pain, nausea. **GU:** erectile dysfunction. **Resp:** dyspnea.

Interactions

Drug-Drug: ↑ hypotension with other **antihypertensives**, **nitrates**, and acute ingestion of **alcohol**. ↑ CNS depression may occur with other **CNS depressants**, including **alcohol**, **antihistamines**, **opioid analgesics**, **tricyclic antidepressants**, and **sedative/hypnotics**. **NSAIDs** may ↓ effectiveness. **Adrenergics** may ↓ effectiveness. ↑ risk of hypotension and bradycardia with strong and moderate **CYP3A4 inhibitors**, including **ketoconazole** and **fluconazole** (a ↓ in dose of guanfacine may be needed). Strong and moderate **CYP3A4 inducers**, including **rifampin**, **efavirenz**, and **carbamazepine** may ↓ effects (an ↑ in dose of guanfacine may be needed). May ↑ levels of **valproic acid**.

Route/Dosage

Immediate-release and extended-release tablets should not be interchanged.

Hypertension

PO (Adults): 1 mg daily given at bedtime, may be ↑ if necessary at 3–4 wk intervals up to 2 mg/day; may also be given in 2 divided doses.

ADHD

PO (Adults and Children ≥6 yr): 1 mg once daily in morning or evening; may be ↑ by 1 mg/day at weekly intervals to achieve dose of 1–4 mg/day (6–12 yr) or 1–7 mg-day (13–17 yr) when used as monotherapy or 1–4 mg/day when used as adjunctive therapy. *Concurrent strong or moderate CYP3A4 inhibitor*—↓ initial and maintenance dose by 50%; *Concurrent strong or moderate CYP3A4 inducer*—Consider ↑ initial and maintenance dose up to double the recommended level (maintenance dose can be ↑ over period of 1–2 wk).

Availability (generic available)

Extended-release tablets (Intuniv): 1 mg, 2 mg, 3 mg, 4 mg. **Cost:** All strengths $884.11/100. **Tablets:** 1 mg, 2 mg. **Cost:** *Generic*—1 mg $10.34/100, 2 mg $25.67/100.

NURSING IMPLICATIONS

Assessment

- **Hypertension:** Monitor BP (lying and standing) and pulse frequently during initial dose adjustment and periodically during therapy. Report significant changes.
- Monitor frequency of prescription refills to determine adherence.
- **ADHD:** Assess attention span, impulse control, and interactions with others.
- Monitor BP and heart rate prior to starting therapy, following dose increases, and periodically during therapy. May cause hypotension, orthostatic hypotension, and bradycardia.
- ***Lab Test Considerations:*** May cause temporary, clinically insignificant ↑ in plasma growth hormone levels.
- May cause ↓ in urinary catecholamines and vanillylmandelic acid levels.

Implementation

- Do not confuse guanfacine with guaifenesin. Do not confuse Intuniv (guanfacine) with Invega (paliperidone).
- Do not substitute extended-release tablets for immediate-release tablets on a mg-mg basis. Doses are not the same.
- **PO:** *For hypertension:* Administer daily dose at bedtime to minimize daytime sedation.
- *For ADHD:* Administer once daily. Swallow extended-release tablets whole; do not crush, break, or chew. Do not administer with high fat meals, due to increased exposure.

Patient/Family Teaching

- Advise patient to notify health care professional of all Rx or OTC medications, vitamins, or herbal products being taken and to consult with health care professional before taking other medications, especially cough, cold, or allergy remedies.
- Caution patient to avoid alcohol and other CNS depressants while taking guanfacine.
- Advise patient to notify health care professional if dry mouth or constipation persists. Frequent mouth rinses, good oral hygiene, and sugarless gum or candy may minimize dry mouth. Increase in fluid and fiber intake and exercise may decrease constipation.
- Instruct patient to notify health care professional of medication regimen prior to treatment or surgery.
- Advise patient to notify health care professional if dizziness, prolonged drowsiness, fatigue, weakness, depression, headache, sexual dysfunction, mental depression, or sleep pattern disturbance occurs. Discontinuation may be required if drug-related mental depression occurs.
- Advise female patients to notify health care professional if pregnancy is planned or suspected, or if breast feeding.
- Emphasize the importance of follow-up exams to evaluate effectiveness of medication.
- **Hypertension:** Emphasize the importance of continuing to take medication as directed, even if feeling well. Medication controls but does not cure hypertension. Instruct patient to take medication at the same time each day. Take missed doses as soon as remembered; do not double doses. If 2 or more doses are missed, consult health care professional. Do not discontinue abruptly; may cause sympathetic overstimulation (nervousness, anxiety, rebound hypertension, chest pain, tachycardia, increased salivation, nausea, trembling, stomach cramps, sweating, difficulty sleeping). These effects may occur 2–7 days after discontinuation, although rebound hypertension is rare and more likely to occur with high doses.
- Advise patient to make sure enough medication is available for weekends, holidays, and vacations. A written prescription may be kept in wallet in case of emergency.
- Encourage patient to comply with additional interventions for hypertension (weight reduction, low-sodium diet, smoking cessation, moderation of alcohol consumption, regular exercise, and stress management).
- Instruct patient and family on proper technique for BP monitoring. Advise them to check BP at least weekly and to report significant changes.
- May cause drowsiness or dizziness. Advise patient to avoid driving or other activities requiring alertness until response to the medication is known.

- **ADHD:** Instruct patient to take medication as directed at the same time each day. Take missed doses as soon as possible, but should not take more than the total daily amount in any 24-hr period. Do not stop taking abruptly; discontinue gradually at no more than 1 mg every 3–7 days. Monitor heart rate and BP during discontinuation. Advise patient and parents to read the *Medication Guide* prior to starting therapy and with each Rx refill.
- Inform patient that sharing this medication may be dangerous.
- Pedi: Advise parents to notify school nurse of medication regimen.

Evaluation/Desired Outcomes

- Decrease in BP without excessive side effects.
- Improved attention span and social interactions in ADHD. Re-evaluate use if used for >9 wk.

guselkumab (gue-sel-**koo**-mab)

Tremfya

Classification

Therapeutic: antipsoriatics

Pharmacologic: interleukin antagonists, monoclonal antibodies

Indications

Moderate-to-severe plaque psoriasis in patients who are candidates for phototherapy or systemic therapy.

Action

Binds to the p19 protein subunit of the interleukin (IL)-23 cytokine to prevent its interaction with the IL-23 receptor. This cytokine is normally involved in inflammatory and immune responses. Binding to interleukins antagonizes their effects, inhibiting the release of proinflammatory cytokines and chemokines. **Therapeutic Effects:** Decrease in area and severity of psoriatic lesions.

Pharmacokinetics

Absorption: 49% absorbed following subcutaneous administration.

Distribution: Well distributed to tissues.

Metabolism and Excretion: Broken down by catabolic processes into peptides and amino acids.

Half-life: 15–18 days.

TIME/ACTION PROFILE (plasma concentrations)

ROUTE	ONSET	PEAK	DURATION
Subcut	unknown	5.5 days	8 wk

Contraindications/Precautions

Contraindicated in: Hypersensitivity; Active, untreated infection.

Use Cautiously in: History of tuberculosis (possibility of reactivation); OB: Use only if potential maternal benefit justifies potential fetal risk; Lactation: Safety not established; Pedi: Safety and effectiveness not established.

Exercise Extreme Caution in: Chronic infection or history of recurrent infection.

Adverse Reactions/Side Effects

CNS: headache. **GI:** diarrhea, ↑ liver enzymes. **Local:** injection site reactions. **MS:** arthralgia. **Misc:** HYPERSENSITIVITY REACTIONS, infection.

Interactions

Drug-Drug: May ↓ antibody response to and ↑ risk of adverse reactions from **live vaccines**; avoid use during therapy. May affect the activity of CYP450 drug-metabolizing enzymes; appropriate monitoring and dose adjustment should be carried out when treatment is started in patients receiving concurrent treatment with **CYP450 substrate**, especially those with a narrow therapeutic index, including **warfarin** and **cyclosporine**.

Route/Dosage

Subcut (Adults): 100 mg initially and 4 wk later, then 100 mg every 8 wk.

Availability

Solution for injection (prefilled syringes and patient-controlled injectors): 100 mg/mL.

NURSING IMPLICATIONS

Assessment

- Assess affected area(s) prior to and periodically during therapy.
- Assess patient for latent tuberculosis with a tuberculin skin test prior to initiation of therapy. Treatment of latent tuberculosis should be started before therapy with guselkumab.
- Assess for signs of infection (fever, dyspnea, flu-like symptoms, frequent or painful urination, redness or swelling at the site of a wound), including tuberculosis, prior to injection. Monitor new infections closely; most common are upper respiratory tract infections, bronchitis, and urinary tract infections.
- ***Lab Test Considerations:*** May cause ↑ liver enzymes.

Implementation

- Update immunizations to current prior to initiating therapy. Patients on guselkumab may receive concurrent vaccinations, except for live vaccines.
- **Subcut:** Allow syringe and solution to reach room temperature, for 30 min before injecting. Solution is clear and colorless to light yellow solution and may contain small translucent particles; do not administer solutions that are cloudy, discolored or contain

large particles. Store solution in refrigerator in original carton to protect from light; do not shake or freeze. Inject full amount (1 mL) of *One Press injector* in front of thigh, abdomen, or upper arm. Avoid areas that are tender, bruised, red, hard, thick, scaly, or affected by psoriasis.

Patient/Family Teaching

- Instruct patient on correct technique for self-injection, care and disposal of equipment. Review *Medication Guide* with patient before starting therapy and with each injection.
- Advise patient to notify health care professional if signs and symptoms of infection (fever, chills, sore throat, painful urination) occur.
- Instruct patient to avoid receiving live vaccines during therapy.
- Advise patient to notify health care professional immediately if signs and symptoms of hypersensitivity reaction (feel faint; swelling of face, eyelids, lips, mouth, tongue or throat; trouble breathing; throat tightness; chest tightness; skin rash; hives) occur.
- Instruct patient to notify health care professional of all Rx or OTC medications, vitamins, or herbal products being taken and consult health care professional before taking any new medications.
- Instruct patient to notify health care professional of medication regimen prior to treatment or surgery.
- Advise female patient to notify health care professional if pregnancy is planned or suspected, or if breast feeding.

Evaluation/Desired Outcomes

- Decrease in extent and severity of psoriatic lesions.

halcinonide, See CORTICOSTEROIDS (TOPICAL/LOCAL).

halobetasol, See CORTICOSTEROIDS (TOPICAL/LOCAL).

BEERS

haloperidol (ha-loe-**per**-i-dole)

Haldol, Haldol Decanoate

Classification

Therapeutic: antipsychotics

Pharmacologic: butyrophenones

Indications

Acute and chronic psychotic disorders including: schizophrenia, manic states, drug-induced psychoses. Patients with schizophrenia who require long-term parenteral (IM) antipsychotic therapy. Also useful in managing aggressive or agitated patients. Tourette's syndrome. Severe behavioral problems in children which may be accompanied by: unprovoked, combative, explosive hyperexcitability, hyperactivity accompanied by conduct disorders (short-term use when other modalities have failed). Considered second-line treatment after failure with atypical antipsychotic. **Unlabeled Use:** Nausea and vomiting from surgery or chemotherapy.

Action

Alters the effects of dopamine in the CNS. Also has anticholinergic and alpha-adrenergic blocking activity. **Therapeutic Effects:** Diminished signs and symptoms of psychoses. Improved behavior in children with Tourette's syndrome or other behavioral problems.

Pharmacokinetics

Absorption: Well absorbed following PO/IM administration. Decanoate salt is slowly absorbed and has a long duration of action.

Distribution: Concentrates in liver. Crosses placenta; enters breast milk.

Protein Binding: 92%.

Metabolism and Excretion: Mostly metabolized by the liver.

Half-life: 21–24 hr.

TIME/ACTION PROFILE (antipsychotic activity)

ROUTE	ONSET	PEAK	DURATION
PO	2 hr	2–6 hr	8–12 hr
IM	20–30 min	30–45 min	4–8 hr†
IM (decanoate)	3–9 days	unknown	1 mo

†Effect may persist for several days.

Contraindications/Precautions

Contraindicated in: Hypersensitivity; Angle-closure glaucoma; Bone marrow depression; CNS depression; Parkinsonism; Severe liver or cardiovascular disease (QT interval prolonging conditions); Some products contain tartrazine, sesame oil, or benzyl alcohol and should be avoided in patients with known intolerance or hypersensitivity.

Use Cautiously in: Debilitated patients (dose ↓ required); Cardiac disease (risk of QT prolongation with high doses); Diabetes; Respiratory insufficiency; Prostatic hyperplasia; CNS tumors; Intestinal obstruction; Seizures; Patients at risk for falls; OB: Neonates at ↑ risk for extrapyramidal symptoms and withdrawal after delivery when exposed during the 3rd trimester; use only if benefit outweighs risk to fetus; Lactation: Discontinue drug or bottle-feed; Geri: Dose ↓ required due to ↑ sensitivity; ↑ risk of mortality in elderly patients treated for dementia-related psychosis.

Adverse Reactions/Side Effects

CNS: SEIZURES, extrapyramidal reactions, confusion, drowsiness, restlessness, tardive dyskinesia. **EENT:** blurred vision, dry eyes. **Resp:** respiratory depression. **CV:** hypotension, tachycardia, ECG changes (QT prolongation, torsade de pointes), ventricular arrhythmias. **GI:** constipation, dry mouth, anorexia, drug-induced hepatitis, ileus, weight gain. **GU:** impotence, urinary retention. **Derm:** diaphoresis, photosensitivity, rashes. **Endo:** amenorrhea, galactorrhea, gynecomastia. **Hemat:** AGRANULOCYTOSIS, anemia, leukopenia, neutropenia. **Metab:** hyperpyrexia. **Misc:** NEUROLEPTIC MALIGNANT SYNDROME, hypersensitivity reactions.

Interactions

Drug-Drug: May enhance the QTc-prolonging effect of **QTc-prolonging agents**. ↑ hypotension with **antihypertensives**, **nitrates**, or acute ingestion of **alcohol**. ↑ anticholinergic effects with **drugs having anticholinergic properties**, including **antihistamines**, **antidepressants**, **atropine**, **phenothiazines**, **quinidine**, and **disopyramide**. ↑ CNS depression with other **CNS depressants**, including **alcohol**, **antihistamines**, **opioid analgesics**, and **sedative/hypnotics**. Concurrent use with **epinephrine** may result in severe hypotension and tachycardia. May ↓ therapeutic effects of **levodopa**. Acute encephalopathic syndrome may occur when used with **lithium**. Dementia may occur with **methyldopa**.

Drug-Natural Products: **Kava-kava**, **valerian**, or **chamomile** can ↑ CNS depression.

Route/Dosage

Haloperidol

PO (Adults): 0.5–5 mg 2–3 times daily. Patients with severe symptoms may require up to 100 mg/day.

PO (Geriatric Patients or Debilitated Patients): 0.5–2 mg twice daily initially; may be gradually ↑ as needed.
PO (Children 3–12 yr or 15–40 kg): 0.25–0.5 mg/day given in 2–3 divided doses; increase by 0.25–0.5 mg every 5–7 days; maximum dose: 0.15 mg/kg/day (up to 0.75 mg/kg/day for Tourette's syndrome or 0.15 mg/kg/day for psychoses).
IM (Adults): 2–5 mg every 1–8 hr (not to exceed 100 mg/day).
IM (Children 6–12 yr): 1–3 mg/dose every 4–8 hrs to a maximum of 0.15 mg/kg/day.
IV (Adults): 0.5–5 mg, may be repeated every 30 min (unlabeled).

Haloperidol Decanoate

IM (Adults): 10–15 times the previous daily PO dose but not to exceed 100 mg initially, given monthly (not to exceed 300 mg/mo).

Availability (generic available)

Tablets: 0.5 mg, 1 mg, 2 mg, 5 mg, 10 mg, 20 mg. **Oral concentrate:** 2 mg/mL. **Haloperidol lactate injection:** 5 mg/mL. **Haloperidol decanoate injection:** 50 mg/mL, 100 mg/mL.

NURSING IMPLICATIONS

Assessment

- Assess mental status (orientation, mood, behavior) prior to and periodically during therapy.
- Assess positive (hallucination, delusions) and negative (social isolation) symptoms of schizophrenia.
- Assess weight and BMI initially and throughout therapy. Refer as appropriate for nutritional/weight and medical management.
- Monitor BP (sitting, standing, lying) and pulse prior to and frequently during the period of dose adjustment. May cause QT interval changes on ECG.
- Observe patient carefully when administering medication, to ensure that medication is actually taken and not hoarded.
- Monitor intake and output ratios and daily weight. Assess patient for signs and symptoms of dehydration (decreased thirst, lethargy, hemoconcentration), especially in geriatric patients.
- Assess fluid intake and bowel function. Increased bulk and fluids in the diet help minimize constipating effects.
- Monitor patient for onset of akathisia (restlessness or desire to keep moving), which may appear within 6 hr of 1st dose and may be difficult to distinguish from psychotic agitation. Benztropine may be used to differentiate agitation from akathisia. Observe closely for extrapyramidal side effects (*parkinsonian*—difficulty speaking or swallowing, loss of balance control, pill rolling of hands, mask-like face, shuffling gait, rigidity, tremors; and *dystonic*—muscle spasms, twisting motions, twitching, inability to move eyes, weakness of arms or legs). Trihexyphenidyl or benzotropine may be used to control these symptoms. Benzodiazepines may alleviate akathisia.
- Monitor for tardive dyskinesia (uncontrolled rhythmic movement of mouth, face, and extremities; lip smacking or puckering; puffing of cheeks; uncontrolled chewing; rapid or worm-like movements of tongue, excessive eye blinking). Report immediately; may be irreversible.
- Monitor for symptoms related to hyperprolactinemia (menstrual abnormalities, galactorrhea, sexual dysfunction).
- Monitor for development of neuroleptic malignant syndrome (fever, respiratory distress, tachycardia, seizures, diaphoresis, hypertension or hypotension, pallor, tiredness, severe muscle stiffness, loss of bladder control). Report symptoms immediately. May also cause leukocytosis, elevated liver function tests, elevated CPK.
- Assess for falls risk. Drowsiness, orthostatic hypotension, and motor and sensory instability increase risk. Institute prevention if indicated.
- ***Lab Test Considerations:*** Monitor CBC with differential and liver function tests periodically during therapy.
- Monitor serum prolactin prior to and periodically during therapy. May cause ↑ serum prolactin levels.

Implementation

- Avoid skin contact with oral solution; may cause contact dermatitis.
- **PO:** Administer with food or full glass of water or milk to minimize GI irritation.
- Use calibrated measuring device for accurate dosage. Do not dilute concentrate with coffee or tea; may cause precipitation. May be given undiluted or mixed with water or juice.
- **IM:** Inject slowly, using 2-in., 21-gauge needle into well-developed muscle via Z-track technique. Do not exceed 3 mL per injection site. Slight yellow color does not indicate altered potency. Keep patient recumbent for at least 30 min following injection to minimize hypotensive effects.

IV Administration

- **IV:** Haloperidol decanoate should not be administered IV.
- **IV Push:** ***Diluent:*** May be administered undiluted for rapid control of acute psychosis or delirium. ***Concentration:*** 5 mg/mL. ***Rate:*** Administer at a rate of 5 mg/min.
- **Intermittent Infusion:** ***Diluent:*** May be diluted in 30–50 mL of D5W. ***Rate:*** Infuse over 30 min.
- **Y-Site Compatibility:** alemtuzumab, amifostine, aminocaproic acid, amphotericin B liposome, amsacrine, anidulafungin, argatroban, azithromycin, bleomycin, cangrelor, carboplatin, carmustine, caspofungin, ceftaroline, cisatracurium, cisplatin, cladribine, clonidine, cyclophosphamide, cytarabine, dacarbazine, dactinomycin, daptomycin, daunorubi-

cin, dexmedetomidine, dexrazoxane, diltiazem, docetaxel, doxacurium, doxorubicin hydrochloride, doxorubicin liposome, epirubicin, eptifibatide, ertapenem, etoposide, etoposide phosphate, fenoldopam, filgrastim, fludarabine, gemcitabine, granisetron, hetastarch, hydromorphone, idarubicin, ifosfamide, irinotecan, ketamine, leucovorin calcium, levofloxacin, linezolid, lorazepam, melphalan, methadone, metronidazole, milrinone, mitoxantrone, morphine, moxifloxacin, mycophenolate, nicardipine, octreotide, oxaliplatin, paclitaxel, palonosetron, pamidronate, pancuronium, pemetrexed, potassium acetate, propofol, quinupristin/dalfopristin, remifentanil, rituximab, rocuronium, sodium acetate, tacrolimus, thiotepa, tigecycline, tirofiban, trastuzumab, vecuronium, vinblastine, vincristine, vinorelbine, voriconazole, zoledronic acid.
- **Y-Site Incompatibility:** acyclovir, allopurinol, aminophylline, amphotericin B deoxycholate, amphotericin B lipid complex, ampicillin, ampicillin/sulbactam, azathioprine, bumetanide, calcium chloride, cefazolin, cefepime, cefonocid, cefotaxime, cefotetan, cefoxitin, ceftazidime, ceftriaxone, cefuroxime, chloramphenicol, clindamycin, dantrolene, dexamethasone, diazepam, diazoxide, epoetin alfa, fluorouracil, folic acid, foscarnet, fosphenytoin, furosemide, ganciclovir, heparin, hydralazine, hydrocortisone, imipenem/cilastatin, indomethacin, ketorolac, magnesium sulfate, methylprednisolone, nafcillin, oxacillin, pantoprazole, penicillin G, pentobarbital, phenobarbital, phenytoin, piperacillin/tazobactam, potassium chloride, sargramostim, sodium bicarbonate, trimethoprim/sulfamethoxazole.

Patient/Family Teaching

- Advise patient to take medication as directed. Take missed doses as soon as remembered, with remaining doses evenly spaced throughout the day. May require several wk to obtain desired effects. Do not increase dose or discontinue medication without consulting health care professional. Abrupt withdrawal may cause dizziness; nausea; vomiting; GI upset; trembling; or uncontrolled movements of mouth, tongue, or jaw.
- Inform patient of possibility of extrapyramidal symptoms, tardive dyskinesia, and neuroleptic malignant syndrome. Caution patient to report symptoms immediately.
- Advise patient to change positions slowly to minimize orthostatic hypotension. Protect from falls.
- May cause drowsiness. Caution patient to avoid driving or other activities requiring alertness until response to medication is known.
- Caution patient to avoid taking alcohol or other CNS depressants concurrently with this medication.
- Advise patient to use sunscreen and protective clothing when exposed to the sun to prevent photosensitivity reactions. Extremes of temperature should also be avoided; drug impairs body temperature regulation.
- Instruct patient to use frequent mouth rinses, good oral hygiene, and sugarless gum or candy to minimize dry mouth.
- Advise patient to notify health care professional of medication regimen prior to treatment or surgery.
- Instruct patient to notify health care professional promptly if weakness, tremors, visual disturbances, dark-colored urine or clay-colored stools, sore throat, fever, menstrual abnormalities, galactorrhea, or sexual dysfunction occur.
- Advise patient to notify health care professional if pregnancy is planned or suspected and to avoid breast feeding during therapy.
- Emphasize the importance of routine follow-up exams to monitor response to medication and detect side effects.

Evaluation/Desired Outcomes

- Decrease in hallucinations, insomnia, agitation, hostility, and delusions.
- Decreased tics and vocalization in Tourette's syndrome.
- Improved behavior in children with severe behavioral problems. If no therapeutic effects are seen in 2–4 wk, dosage may be increased.

HIGH ALERT

heparin (hep-a-rin)

Hepalean, Hep-Lock, Hep-Lock U/P

Classification
Therapeutic: anticoagulants
Pharmacologic: antithrombotics

Indications

Prophylaxis and treatment of various thromboembolic disorders including: Venous thromboembolism, Pulmonary emboli, Atrial fibrillation with embolization, Acute and chronic consumptive coagulopathies, Peripheral arterial thromboembolism. Used in very low doses (10–100 units) to maintain patency of IV catheters (heparin flush).

Action

Potentiates the inhibitory effect of antithrombin on factor Xa and thrombin. In low doses, prevents the conversion of prothrombin to thrombin by its effects on factor Xa. Higher doses neutralize thrombin, preventing the conversion of fibrinogen to fibrin. **Therapeutic Effects:** Prevention of thrombus formation. Prevention of extension of existing thrombi (full dose).

Pharmacokinetics

Absorption: Erratically absorbed following subcut or IM administration.

Distribution: Does not cross the placenta or enter breast milk.
Protein Binding: Very high (to low-density lipoproteins, globulins, and fibrinogen).
Metabolism and Excretion: Probably removed by the reticuloendothelial system (lymph nodes, spleen).
Half-life: 1–2 hr (↑ with increasing dose); affected by obesity, renal and hepatic function, malignancy, presence of pulmonary embolism, and infections.

TIME/ACTION PROFILE (anticoagulant effect)

ROUTE	ONSET	PEAK	DURATION
Heparin subcut	20–60 min	2 hr	8–12 hr
Heparin IV	immediate	5–10 min	2–6 hr

Contraindications/Precautions

Contraindicated in: Hypersensitivity; Uncontrolled bleeding; History of heparin-induced thrombocytopenia; Severe thrombocytopenia; Open wounds (full dose); Pedi: Avoid use of products containing benzyl alcohol in premature infants.
Use Cautiously in: Severe liver or kidney impairment; Retinopathy (hypertensive or diabetic); Ulcer disease; Spinal cord or brain injury; History of congenital or acquired bleeding disorder; Malignancy; OB: Use only if potential maternal benefit justifies potential fetal risk; Lactation: Use while breast feeding only if potential maternal benefit justifies potential risk to infant; Geri: Women >60 yr have ↑ risk of bleeding.
Exercise Extreme Caution in: Severe uncontrolled hypertension; Bacterial endocarditis, bleeding disorders; GI bleeding/ulceration/pathology; Hemorrhagic stroke; History of thrombocytopenia related to heparin; Recent CNS or ophthalmologic surgery; Active GI bleeding/ulceration;.

Adverse Reactions/Side Effects

Derm: alopecia (long-term use), rash, urticaria. **GI:** drug-induced hepatitis. **Hemat:** BLEEDING, HEPARIN-INDUCED THROMBOCYTOPENIA (HIT) (WITH OR WITHOUT THROMBOSIS), anemia. **Local:** pain at injection site. **MS:** osteoporosis (long-term use). **Misc:** fever, hypersensitivity reactions.

Interactions

Heparin is frequently used concurrently or sequentially with other agents affecting coagulation. The risk of potentially serious interactions is greatest with full anticoagulation.
Drug-Drug: Risk of bleeding may be ↑ by concurrent use of **drugs that affect platelet function**, including **aspirin**, **NSAIDs**, **clopidogrel**, **dipyridamole**, some **penicillins**, **eptifibitide**, **tirofiban**, and **dextran**. Risk of bleeding may be ↑ by concurrent use of **drugs that cause hypoprothrombinemia**, including **quinidine**, **cefotetan**, and **valproic acid**. Concurrent use of **thrombolytics** ↑ risk of bleeding. Heparins affect the prothrombin time used in assessing the response to **warfarin**. **Digoxin**, **tetracyclines**, **nicotine**, and **antihistamines** may ↓ anticoagulant effect of heparin. **Streptokinase** may be followed by relative resistance to heparin.
Drug-Natural Products: ↑ risk of bleeding with **arnica**, **anise**, **chamomile**, **clove**, **dong quai**, **fever few**, **garlic**, **ginger**, and **Panax ginseng**.

Route/Dosage

Therapeutic Anticoagulation

IV (Adults): *Intermittent bolus*—10,000 units, followed by 5000–10,000 units every 4–6 hr. *Continuous infusion*—5000 units (35–70 units/kg), followed by 20,000–40,000 units infused over 24 hr (approx. 1000 units/hr or 15–18 units/kg/hr).
IV (Children >1 yr): *Intermittent bolus*—50–100 units/kg, followed by 50–100 units/kg every 4 hr. *Continuous infusion*—Loading dose 75 units/kg, followed by 20 units/kg/hr, adjust to maintain aPTT of 60–85 sec.
IV (Neonates and Infants <1 yr): *Continuous infusion*—Loading dose 75 units/kg, followed by 28 units/kg/hr, adjust to maintain aPTT of 60–85 sec.
Subcut (Adults): 5000 units IV, followed by initial subcut dose of 10,000–20,000 units, then 8000–10,000 units every 8 hr or 15,000–20,000 units every 12 hr.

Prophylaxis of Thromboembolism

Subcut (Adults): 5000 units every 8–12 hr (may be started 2 hr prior to surgery).

Cardiovascular Surgery

IV (Adults): At least 150 units/kg (300 units/kg if procedure <60 min; 400 units/kg if >60 min).
Intra-arterial (Neonates , Infants, and Children): 100–150 units/kg via an artery prior to cardiac catheterization.

Line Flushing

IV (Adults and Children): 10–100 units/mL (10 units/mL for infants <10 kg, 100 units/mL for all others) solution to fill heparin lock set to needle hub; replace after each use.

Total Parenteral Nutrition

IV (Adults and Children): 0.5–1 units/mL (final solution concentration) to maintain line patency.

Arterial Line Patency

Intra-arterial (Neonates): 0.5–2 units/mL.

Availability (generic available)

Premixed infusion: 1000 units/500 mL, 2000 units/1000 mL, 12,500 units/250 mL, 25,000 units in 250 and 500 mL. **Solution for injection:** 10 units/mL, 100 units/mL, 1000 units/mL, 5000 units/mL, 7500 units/mL, 10,000 units/mL, 20,000 units/mL, 40,000 units/mL.

NURSING IMPLICATIONS

Assessment

- Assess for signs of bleeding and hemorrhage (bleeding gums; nosebleed; unusual bruising; black, tarry stools; hematuria; fall in hematocrit or BP; guaiac-positive stools). Notify health care professional if these occur.
- Assess patient for evidence of additional or increased thrombosis. Symptoms will depend on area of involvement.
- Monitor patient for hypersensitivity reactions (chills, fever, urticaria).
- **Subcut:** Observe injection sites for hematomas, ecchymosis, or inflammation.
- ***Lab Test Considerations:*** Monitor activated partial thromboplastin time (aPTT) and hematocrit prior to and periodically during therapy. When *intermittent IV* therapy is used, draw aPTT levels 30 min before each dose during initial therapy and then periodically. During *continuous* administration, monitor aPTT levels every 4 hr during early therapy. For *Subcut* therapy, draw blood 4–6 hr after injection.
- Monitor platelet count every 2–3 days during therapy. May cause mild thrombocytopenia, which appears on 4th day and resolves despite continued heparin therapy. Heparin-induced thrombocytopenia (HIT), a more severe form which necessitates discontinuing medication, may develop on 8th day of therapy; may reduce platelet count to as low as 5000/mm^3 and lead to increased resistance to heparin therapy. HIT may progress to development of venous and arterial thrombosis (HITT) and may occur up to several wk after discontinuation. Patients who have received a previous course of heparin may be at higher risk for severe thrombocytopenia for several mo after the initial course.
- May cause hyperkalemia and ↑ AST and ALT levels.
- ***Toxicity and Overdose:*** Protamine sulfate is the antidote. Due to short half-life, overdose can often be treated by withdrawing the drug.

Implementation

- ***High Alert:*** Fatal hemorrhages have occurred in pediatric patients due to errors in which heparin sodium injection vials were confused with heparin flush vials. Carefully examine all heparin sodium injection vials to confirm the correct vial choice prior to administration. Have second practitioner independently check original order, dose calculation, and infusion pump settings. Unintended concomitant use of two heparin products (unfractionated heparin and LMW heparins) has resulted in serious harm or death. Review patients' recent (emergency department, operating room) and current medication administration records before administering any heparin or LMW heparin product. Do not confuse heparin with Hespan (hetastarch in sodium chloride). Do not confuse vials of heparin with vials of insulin.
- Inform all personnel caring for patient of anticoagulant therapy. Venipunctures and injection sites require application of pressure to prevent bleeding or hematoma formation. Avoid IM injections of other medications; hematomas may develop.
- In patients requiring long-term anticoagulation, oral anticoagulant therapy should be instituted 4–5 days prior to discontinuing heparin therapy.
- Solution is colorless to slightly yellow.

IV Administration

- **Subcut:** Administer deep into subcut tissue. Alternate injection sites between arm and the left and right abdominal wall above the iliac crest. Inject entire length of needle at a 45°- or 90°-angle into a skin fold held between thumb and forefinger; hold skin fold throughout injection. Do not aspirate or massage. Rotate sites frequently. Do not administer IM because of danger of hematoma formation. Solution should be clear; do not inject solution containing particulate matter.
- **IV Push:** ***Diluent:*** Administer loading dose undiluted. ***Concentration:*** Varies depending upon vial used. ***Rate:*** Administer over at least 1 min. Loading dose given before continuous infusion.
- **Continuous Infusion:** ***Diluent:*** Dilute 25,000 units of heparin in 250–500 mL of 0.9% NaCl or D5W. Premixed infusions are already diluted and ready to use. Admixed solutions stable for 24 hr at room temperature or if refrigerated. Premixed infusion stable for 30 days once overwrap removed. ***Concentration:*** 50–100 units/mL. ***Rate:*** See Route/Dosage section. Adjust to maintain therapeutic aPTT. Use an infusion pump to ensure accuracy.
- **Flush:** To prevent clot formation in intermittent infusion (heparin lock) sets, inject dilute heparin solution of 10–100 units/0.5–1 mL after each medication injection or every 8–12 hr. To prevent incompatibility of heparin with medication, flush lock set with sterile water or 0.9% NaCl for injection before and after medication is administered.
- **Y-Site Compatibility:** acetaminophen, acetylcysteine, acyclovir, alemtuzumab, alfentanil, allopurinol, amifostine, aminocaproic acid, aminophylline, amphotericin B lipid complex, amphotericin B liposome, anidulafungin, argatroban, arsenic trioxide, ascorbic acid, atropine, azathioprine, azithromycin, aztreonam, benztropine, bivalirudin, bleomycin, bumetanide, buprenorphine, butorphanol, calcium chloride, calcium gluconate, cangrelor, carboplatin, carmustine, cefazolin, cefotaxime, cefotetan, cefoxitin, ceftaroline, ceftazidime, ceftazidime/avibactam, ceftolozane/tazobactam, ceftriaxone, cefuroxime,

H

chloramphenicol, cisplatin, cladribine, clindamycin, cyanocobalamin, cyclophosphamide, cyclosporine, cytarabine, dactinomycin, daptomycin, defibrotide, dexamethasone, dexmedetomidine, dexrazoxane, digoxin, docetaxel, dopamine, doxacurium, doxapram, doxorubicin liposome, enalaprilat, ephedrine, epinephrine, epoetin alfa, eptifibatide, ertapenem, esmolol, estrogens, conjugated, etoposide, etoposide phosphate, famotidine, fenoldopam, fentanyl, fluconazole, fludarabine, fluorouracil, folic acid, foscarnet, fosphenytoin, furosemide, ganciclovir, gemcitabine, gemtuzumab, glycopyrrolate, granisetron, hetastarch, hydrocortisone, hydromorphone, ibuprofen lysine, ifosfamide, imipenem/cilastatin, indomethacin, irinotecan, isoproterenol, ketorolac, leucovorin calcium, lidocaine, linezolid, lorazepam, magnesium sulfate, mannitol, melphalan, meropenem, meropenem/vaborbactam, mesna, metaraminol, methohexital, methotrexate, methoxamine, methyldopate, methylergonovine, metoclopramide, metoprolol, micafungin, midazolam, milrinone, mitomycin, morphine, moxifloxacin, multiple vitamins, nafcillin, nalbuphine, naloxone, neostigmine, nitroglycerin, nitroprusside, norepinephrine, octreotide, ondansetron, oxacillin, oxaliplatin, oxytocin, paclitaxel, palonosetron, pamidronate, pancuronium, pemetrexed, penicillin G, pentobarbital, phenobarbital, phentolamine, phenylephrine, phytonadione, piperacillin/tazobactam, potassium acetate, potassium chloride, procainamide, prochlorperazine, promazine, propofol, propranolol, pyridostigmine, pyridoxime, ranitidine, remifentanil, rituximab, rocuronium, sargramostim, scopolamine, sodium acetate, sodium bicarbonate, streptokinase, succinylcholine, sufentanil, tacrolimus, tedizolid, theophylline, thiamine, thiopental, thiotepa, tigecycline, tirofiban, tolazoline, tranexamic acid, trastuzumab, vasopressin, vecuronium, verapamil, vinblastine, vincristine, voriconazole, warfarin, zidovudine, zoledronic acid.

- **Y-Site Incompatibility:** alteplase, amiodarone, amphotericin B deoxycholate, amsacrine, blinatumomab, caspofungin, ciprofloxacin, dantrolene, daunorubicin hydrochloride, diazepam, diazoxide, dolasetron, doxycycline, epirubicin, filgrastim, haloperidol, hydroxyzine, idarubicin, isavuconazonium, ketamine, levofloxacin, minocycline, mitoxantrone, mycophenolate, oritavancin, palifermin, papaverine, pentamidine, phenytoin, plazomicin, protamine, quinupristin/dalfopristin, reteplase.
- **Additive Compatibility:** It is recommended that heparin not be mixed in solution with other medications when given for anticoagulation, even those that are compatible, because changes in rate of heparin infusion may be required that would also affect admixtures.

Patient/Family Teaching

- Advise patient to report any symptoms of unusual bleeding or bruising to health care professional immediately.
- Instruct patient not to take medications containing aspirin or NSAIDs while on heparin therapy.
- Caution patient to avoid IM injections and activities leading to injury and to use a soft toothbrush and electric razor during heparin therapy.
- Advise patient to inform health care professional of medication regimen prior to treatment or surgery.
- Advise females of reproductive potential to notify health care professional if pregnancy is planned or suspected, or if breast feeding.
- Patients on anticoagulant therapy should carry an identification card with this information at all times.

Evaluation/Desired Outcomes

- Prolonged partial thromboplastin time (PTT) of 1.5–2.5 times the control, without signs of hemorrhage.
- Prevention of deep vein thrombosis and pulmonary emboli.
- Patency of IV catheters.

HIGH ALERT

HEPARINS (LOW MOLECULAR WEIGHT)

dalteparin (dal-**te**-pa-rin)
Fragmin

enoxaparin (e-nox-a-**pa**-rin)
Lovenox

Classification
Therapeutic: anticoagulants
Pharmacologic: antithrombotics

Indications

Enoxaparin and dalteparin: Prevention of venous thromboembolism (VTE) (deep vein thrombosis [DVT] and/or pulmonary embolism [PE]) in surgical or medical patients. **Dalteparin only:** Extended treatment of symptomatic DVT and/or PE in patients with cancer. **Enoxaparin only:** Treatment of DVT with or without PE (with warfarin). **Enoxaparin and dalteparin:** Prevention of ischemic complications (with aspirin) from unstable angina and non-ST-segment-elevation MI. **Enoxaparin only:** Treatment of acute ST-segment-elevation MI (with thrombolytics or percutaneous coronary intervention).

Action

Potentiate the inhibitory effect of antithrombin on factor Xa and thrombin. **Therapeutic Effects:** Prevention of thrombus formation.

Pharmacokinetics

Absorption: Well absorbed after subcut administration (87% for dalteparin, 92% for enoxaparin).
Distribution: Unknown.
Metabolism and Excretion: *Dalteparin*—unknown; *enoxaparin*—primarily eliminated renally.

Half-life: *Dalteparin*—2.1–2.3 hr; *enoxaparin*—3–6 hr (all are ↑ in renal insufficiency).

TIME/ACTION PROFILE (anticoagulant effect)

ROUTE	ONSET	PEAK	DURATION
Dalteparin subcut	rapid	4 hr	up to 24 hr
Enoxaparin subcut	unknown	3–5 hr	12 hr

Contraindications/Precautions

Contraindicated in: Hypersensitivity to specific agents, unfractionated heparin, or pork products; cross-sensitivity may occur; Some products contain sulfites or benzyl alcohol and should be avoided in patients with known hypersensitivity or intolerance; Active major bleeding; *Enoxaparin*—History of immune-mediated heparin-induced thrombocytopenia (HIT) within the past 100 days or in the presence of circulating antibodies; *Dalteparin*—History of heparin-induced thrombocytopenia; *Dalteparin*—regional anesthesia during treatment for unstable angina/non–Q-wave MI.

Use Cautiously in: Severe hepatic or renal disease (adjust dose of enoxaparin if CCr <30 mL/min); Women <45 kg or men <57 kg; Retinopathy (hypertensive or diabetic); Untreated hypertension; *Enoxaparin*—History of HIT >100 days ago and no circulating antibodies present; Recent history of ulcer disease; History of congenital or acquired bleeding disorder; OB: Safety not established; should not be used in pregnant patients with prosthetic heart valves or inherited/acquired thrombophilias without careful monitoring; if enoxaparin used during pregnancy, use preservative-free formulation; Lactation: Use during breast feeding only if benefit to patient outweighs potential risk to fetus; Pedi: Safety and effectiveness not established; enoxaparin multidose vial contains benzyl alcohol which can cause potentially fatal "gasping syndrome" in neonates; Geri: May have ↑ risk of bleeding due to age-related ↓ in renal function; *Dalteparin*—Geri: ↑ mortality in patients >70 yrs with renal insufficiency.

Exercise Extreme Caution in: Spinal/epidural anesthesia (↑ risk of spinal/epidural hematomas, especially with concurrent NSAIDs, repeated or traumatic epidural puncture, or indwelling epidural catheter); Severe uncontrolled hypertension; Bacterial endocarditis; Bleeding disorders.

Adverse Reactions/Side Effects

CNS: dizziness, headache, insomnia. **CV:** edema. **Derm:** alopecia, ecchymoses, pruritus, rash, urticaria. **GI:** constipation, ↑ liver enzymes, nausea, vomiting. **GU:** urinary retention. **Hemat:** BLEEDING, anemia, eosinophilia, thrombocytopenia. **Local:** erythema at injection site, hematoma, irritation, pain. **MS:** osteoporosis. **Misc:** fever.

Interactions

Drug-Drug: Risk of bleeding may be ↑ by concurrent use of **drugs that affect platelet function and coagulation**, including **warfarin**, **aspirin**, **NSAIDs**, **dipyridamole**, **clopidogrel**, **eptifibatide**, **tirofiban**, and **thrombolytics**.

Drug-Natural Products: ↑ bleeding risk with **arnica**, **chamomile**, **clove**, **feverfew**, **garlic**, **ginger**, **ginkgo**, **Panax ginseng**, and others.

Route/Dosage

Dalteparin

Subcut (Adults): *Prophylaxis of DVT following abdominal surgery*—2500 units 1–2 hr before surgery, then once daily for 5–10 days; *Prophylaxis of VTE in high-risk patients undergoing abdominal surgery*—5000 units evening before surgery, then once daily for 5–10 days *or* in patients with malignancy, 2500 units 1–2 hr before surgery, another 2500 units 12 hr later, then 5000 units once daily for 5–10 days; *Prophylaxis of VTE in patients undergoing hip replacement surgery*—2500 units within 2 hr before surgery, then 2500 units 4–8 hr after surgery, then 5000 units once daily (start at least 6 hr after postsurgical dose) for 5–10 days *or* 5000 units evening before surgery (10–14 hr before surgery), then 5000 units 4–8 hr after surgery, then 5000 units once daily for 5–10 days *or* 2500 units 4–8 hr after surgery, then 5000 units once daily (start at least 6 hr after postsurgical dose); *Prophylaxis of VTE in medical patients with severely restricted mobility during acute illness:* 5000 units once daily for 12–14 days. *Unstable angina/non–ST-segment-elevation MI*—120 units/kg (not to exceed 10,000 units) every 12 hr for 5–8 days with concurrent aspirin; *Extended treatment of symptomatic VTE in cancer patients*—200 units/kg (not to exceed 18,000 units) once daily for first 30 days, followed by 150 units/kg (not to exceed 18,000 units) once daily for mo 2–6.

Renal Impairment

Subcut (Adults): *Cancer patients receiving extended treatment of symptomatic VTE with CCr <30 mL/min*—Monitor anti-Xa levels (target 0.5–1.5 IU/mL).

Enoxaparin

Subcut (Adults): *VTE prophylaxis in patients undergoing knee replacement surgery*—30 mg every 12 hr starting 12–24 hr postop for 7–10 days; *VTE prophylaxis in patients undergoing hip replacement surgery*—30 mg every 12 hr starting 12–24 hr postop *or* 40 mg once daily starting 12 hr before surgery (either dose may be continued for 7–14 days; continued prophylaxis with 40 mg once daily may be continued for up to 3 wk); *VTE prophylaxis following abdominal surgery*—40 mg once daily starting 2 hr before surgery and then continued for 7–12 days or until ambulatory (up to 14 days); *VTE prophylaxis in medical patients with acute illness*—40 mg once daily for 6–14 days; *Treatment of DVT/PE (outpatient)*—1 mg/kg every 12 hr. Warfarin should be started within 72 hr; enoxaparin may be continued for a minimum of 5 days and until therapeutic anticoagulation with warfarin is achieved (INR >2 for 2 consecutive days); *Treatment of DVT/PE (inpatient)*—1 mg/kg every 12 hr *or* 1.5 mg/kg once daily. Warfarin should be started within 72 hr; enoxaparin may be continued for a minimum of 5 days and until therapeutic anticoagulation with warfarin is achieved (INR >2 for two consecutive days); *Unstable angina/non–ST-segment-elevation MI*—1 mg/kg every 12 hr for 2–8 days (with aspirin).

IV, Subcut (Adults <75 yr): *Acute ST-segment-elevation MI*—Administer single IV bolus of 30 mg plus 1 mg/kg subcut dose (maximum of 100 mg for first 2 doses only), followed by 1 mg/kg subcut every12 hr. The usual duration of treatment is 2–8 days. In patients undergoing percutaneous coronary intervention, if last subcut dose was <8 hr before balloon inflation, no additional dosing needed; if last subcut dose was ≥8 hr before balloon inflation, administer single IV bolus of 0.3 mg/kg.

Subcut (Adults ≥75 yr): *Acute ST-segment-elevation MI*—0.75 mg/kg every 12 hr (no IV bolus needed) (maximum of 75 mg for first 2 doses only; no initial bolus). The usual duration of treatment is 2–8 days.

Renal Impairment

Subcut (Adults CCr <30 mL/min): *VTE prophylaxis for abdominal or knee/hip replacement surgery*—30 mg once daily. *Treatment of DVT/PE*—1 mg/kg once daily. *Unstable angina/non-ST-segment-elevation MI*—1 mg/kg once daily. *Acute ST-segment-elevation MI (patients <75 yr)*—Single IV bolus of 30 mg plus 1 mg/kg subcut dose, followed by 1 mg/kg subcut once daily. *Acute ST-segment-elevation MI (patients ≥75 yr)*—1 mg/kg once daily (no initial bolus).

Availability

Dalteparin

Solution for injection (prefilled syringes): 2500 units/0.2 mL, 5000 units/0.2 mL, 7500 units/0.3 mL, 10,000 units/1 mL, 12,500 units/0.5 mL, 15,000 units/0.6 mL, 18,000 units/0.72 mL. **Solution for injection (multidose vials):** 25,000 units/mL.

Enoxaparin (generic available)

Solution for injection (prefilled syringes): 30 mg/0.3 mL, 40 mg/0.4 mL, 60 mg/0.6 mL, 80 mg/0.8 mL, 100 mg/1 mL, 120 mg/0.8 mL, 150 mg/mL. **Solution for injection (multidose vials):** 100 mg/mL.

NURSING IMPLICATIONS

Assessment

- Assess for signs of bleeding and hemorrhage (bleeding gums; nosebleed; unusual bruising; black, tarry stools; hematuria; fall in hematocrit or BP; guaiac-positive stools); bleeding from surgical site. Notify health care professional if these occur.
- Assess patient for evidence of additional or increased thrombosis. Symptoms depend on area of involvement.
- Assess for evidence of additional or increased thrombosis. Symptoms depend on area of involvement. Monitor neurological status frequently for signs of neurological impairment. May require urgent treatment.
- Monitor for hypersensitivity reactions (chills, fever, urticaria). Report signs to health care professional.
- Monitor patients with epidural catheters frequently for signs and symptoms of neurologic impairment. Delay placement or removal of catheter for at least 12 hrs after administration of lower doses (30 mg once or twice daily or 40 mg once daily) and at least 24 hrs after administration of higher doses (0.75 mg/kg twice daily, 1 mg/kg twice daily, or 1.5 mg/kg once daily) of enoxaparin. Do not give 2nd enoxaparin dose in twice daily regimen to patients receiving 0.75 mg/kg twice daily dose or 1 mg/kg twice daily dose to allow a longer delay before catheter placement or removal, then delay next dose for at least 4 hrs. ***For patients with creatinine clearance** <30 mL/min,* double timing of removal of catheter, at least 24 hrs for lower dose (30 mg once daily) and at least 48 hrs for higher dose (1 mg/kg/day). Monitor for signs and symptoms of neurological impairment (midline back pain, sensory and motor deficits [numbness or weakness in lower limbs], bowel and/or bladder dysfunction) frequently if epidural or spinal anesthesia or lumbar puncture is done during therapy.
- **Subcut:** Observe injection sites for hematomas, ecchymosis, or inflammation.
- ***Lab Test Considerations:*** Monitor CBC, platelet count, and stools for occult blood periodically during therapy. *If thrombocytopenia occurs (platelet count <100,000/mm³)*, discontinue therapy. *If hematocrit ↓ unexpectedly,* assess patient for potential bleeding sites. For *dalteparin* use for extended treatment of symptomatic VTE in cancer patients, if platelets ↓ to 50,000–100,000/mm³, reduce dose to 2500 units once daily until recovery to ≥100,000/mm³; if platelets <50,000/mm³, discontinue until count returns to ≥50,000/mm³.
- Special monitoring of aPTT is not necessary. Monitoring of anti-Xa levels may be considered in patients who are obese or have renal dysfunction (for *enoxaparin*, obtain 4 hr after injection).
- Monitoring of antifactor Xa levels may be necessary to titrate doses in pediatric patients (therapeutic range 0.5–1 unit/mL).
- May cause ↑ in AST and ALT levels.
- ***Toxicity and Overdose:*** For *enoxaparin* overdose, protamine sulfate 1 mg for each mg of *enoxaparin* should be administered by slow IV injection. For *dalteparin* overdose, protamine sulfate 1 mg for

each 100 anti-factor Xa IU of *dalteparin* should be administered by slow IV injection. If the aPTT measured 2–4 hr after protamine administration remains prolonged, a 2nd infusion of protamine 0.5 mg/100 anti-factor Xa IU of *dalteparin* may be administered.

Implementation

- ***High Alert:*** Unintended concomitant use of two heparin products (unfractionated heparin and low molecular weight heparins) has resulted in serious harm and death. Review patients' recent and current medication administration records before administering any heparin or low-molecular-weight heparin product.
- Do not confuse Lovenox with Levemir.
- Cannot be used interchangeably (unit for unit) with unfractionated heparin or other low-molecular-weight heparins.
- **Subcut:** Administer deep into subcut tissue. Alternate injection sites daily between the left and right anterolateral and left and right posterolateral abdominal wall, the upper thigh, or buttocks. Inject entire length of needle at a 45° or 90° angle into a skin fold held between thumb and forefinger; hold skin fold throughout injection. Do not aspirate or massage. Rotate sites frequently. Do not administer IM because of danger of hematoma formation. Solution should be clear and colorless to slightly yellow; do not inject solution containing particulate matter.
- If excessive bruising occurs, ice cube massage of site before injection may lessen bruising.
- **Enoxaparin:** To avoid the loss of drug, do not expel the air bubble from the syringe before the injection.
- **Subcut:** Per manufacturer's recommendations, to enhance absorption, inject enoxaparin into left or right anterolateral or posterolateral abdominal wall only.
- To minimize risk of bleeding after vascular instrumentation for unstable angina, recommended intervals between doses should be followed closely. Leave vascular access sheath in place for 6–8 hr after enoxaparin dose. Give next enoxaparin dose ≥6–8 hr after sheath removal. Observe site for bleeding or hematoma formation.

IV Administration

- **IV Push:** (for treatment of STEMI only) Inject via IV line. Flush with 0.9% NaCl or D5W prior to and following administration to avoid mixture with other drugs and clear the port of the drug. May be administered with 0.9% NaCl or D5W. ***Rate:*** Inject as a bolus.
- **Y-Site Incompatibility:** Do not mix or co-administer with other medications.

Patient/Family Teaching

- Instruct patient in correct technique for self injection, care and disposal of equipment.
- Advise patient to report any symptoms of unusual bleeding or bruising, dizziness, itching, rash, fever, swelling, or difficulty breathing to health care professional immediately.
- Instruct patient not to take aspirin or NSAIDs without consulting health care professional while on therapy.
- Advise females of reproductive potential to notify health care professional if pregnancy is planned or suspected, or if breast feeding.

Evaluation/Desired Outcomes

- Prevention of DVT and pulmonary emboli (enoxaparin and dalteparin).
- Resolution of DVT and pulmonary embolism (enoxaparin only).
- Prevention of ischemic complications (with aspirin) in patients with unstable angina or non–ST-segment-elevation MI (enoxaparin and dalteparin).
- Treatment of acute ST-segment-elevation myocardial infarction (enoxaparin only).

HISTAMINE H_2 ANTAGONISTS

cimetidine (sye-**me**-ti-deen)
Tagamet, Tagamet HB

famotidine (fa-**moe**-ti-deen)
✱Acid Control, Pepcid, Pepcid AC, ✱Peptic Guard, ✱Ulcidine

nizatidine (ni-**za**-ti-deen)
Axid, Axid AR

raNITIdine (ra-**ni**-ti-deen)
✱Acid Reducer, Zantac, Zantac EFFERdose, Zantac 75, Zantac 150

Classification
Therapeutic: antiulcer agents
Pharmacologic: histamine H_2 antagonists

Indications

Short-term treatment of active duodenal ulcers and benign gastric ulcers. Maintenance therapy for duodenal and gastric ulcers after healing of active ulcers. Management of GERD. Treatment of heartburn, acid indigestion, and sour stomach (OTC use). **Cimetidine, famotidine, ranitidine:** Management of gastric hypersecretory states (Zollinger-Ellison syndrome). **Famotidine, ranitidine IV:** Prevention and treatment of stress-induced upper GI bleeding in critically ill patients. **Ranitidine:** Treatment of and maintenance therapy for erosive esophagitis. **Unlabeled Use:** Management of GI symptoms associated with the use of NSAIDs. Prevention of acid inactivation of supplemental pancreatic enzymes in patients with pancreatic insufficiency. Management of urticaria.

Action

Inhibits the action of histamine at the H_2-receptor site located primarily in gastric parietal cells, resulting in inhibition of gastric acid secretion. **Therapeutic Effects:** Healing and prevention of ulcers. Decreased symptoms of gastroesophageal reflux. Decreased secretion of gastric acid.

Pharmacokinetics

Absorption: *Cimetidine*—well absorbed after oral administration. *Famotidine*—40–45% absorbed after oral administration. *Nizatidine*—70–95% absorbed after oral administration. *Ranitidine*—50% absorbed after PO and IM administration.

Distribution: All agents enter breast milk and cerebrospinal fluid.

Metabolism and Excretion: *Cimetidine*—30% metabolized by the liver; remainder is eliminated unchanged by the kidneys. *Famotidine*—up to 70% excreted unchanged by the kidneys, 30–35% metabolized by the liver. *Nizatidine*—60% excreted unchanged by the kidneys; some hepatic metabolism; at least 1 metabolite has histamine-blocking activity. *Ranitidine*—metabolized by the liver, mostly on first pass; 30% excreted unchanged by the kidneys after PO administration, 70% after parenteral administration.

Half-life: *Cimetidine*—2 hr; *famotidine*—2.5–3.5 hr; *nizatidine*—1.6 hr; *ranitidine*—2–2.5 hr (all are ↑ in renal impairment).

TIME/ACTION PROFILE

ROUTE	ONSET	PEAK	DURATION
Cimetidine PO	30 min	45–90 min	4–5 hr
Famotidine PO	within 60 min	1–4 hr	6–12 hr
Famotidine IV	within 60 min	0.5–3 hr	8–15 hr
Nizatidine PO	unknown	unknown	8–12 hr
Ranitidine PO	unknown	1–3 hr	8–12 hr
Ranitidine IM	unknown	15 min	8–12 hr
Ranitidine IV	unknown	15 min	8–12 hr

Contraindications/Precautions

Contraindicated in: Hypersensitivity; Some products contain alcohol and should be avoided in patients with known intolerance; Some products contain aspartame and should be avoided in patients with phenylketonuria.

Use Cautiously in: Renal impairment (more susceptible to adverse CNS reactions; ↑ dose interval recommended for *cimetidine* and *nizatidine* if CCr ≤50 mL/min, and for *famotidine* and *ranitidine* if CCr <50 mL/min; Hepatic impairment (for *ranitidine*); Acute porphyria (for *ranitidine*); Geri: More susceptible to adverse CNS reactions; dose ↓ recommended; OB, Lactation: Pregnancy or lactation.

Adverse Reactions/Side Effects

CNS: confusion, dizziness, drowsiness, hallucinations, headache. **CV:** ARRHYTHMIAS. **GI:** constipation, diarrhea, drug-induced hepatitis (nizatidine, cimetidine), nausea. **GU:** ↓ sperm count, erectile dysfunction (cimetidine). **Endo:** gynecomastia. **Hemat:** AGRANULOCYTOSIS, APLASTIC ANEMIA, anemia, neutropenia, thrombocytopenia. **Local:** pain at IM site. **Misc:** hypersensivity reactions, vasculitis.

Interactions

Drug-Drug: Cimetidine is a moderate inhibitor of the CYP1A2, CYP2C9, CYP2D6, and CYP3A4 isoenzymes in the liver; may lead to ↑ levels and toxicity with **benzodiazepines** (especially **chlordiazepoxide**, **diazepam**, and **midazolam**), some **beta blockers (labetalol**, **metoprolol**, **propranolol)**, **caffeine**, **calcium channel blockers**, **carbamazepine**, **cyclosporine**, **dofetilide**, **lidocaine**, **metronidazole**, **mexiletine**, **nefazodone**, **pentoxifylline**, **phenytoin**, **procainamide**, **propafenone**, **quinidine**, **metformin**, **risperidone**, **ritonavir**, **ropinirole**, **selective serotonin reuptake inhibitors**, **sildenafil**, **sulfonylureas**, **tacrolimus**, **theophylline**, **tricyclic antidepressants**, **venlafaxine**, and **warfarin**. Famotidine, nizatidine, and ranitidine have a much smaller and less significant effect on the metabolism of other drugs. Cimetidine may ↑ myelosuppressive effects of **carmustine** (avoid concurrent use). All may ↓ absorption of **ketoconazole**, **itraconazole**, **atazanavir**, **delavirdine**, and **gefitinib**. Ranitidine may ↑ absorption of **triazolam**, **midazolam**, and **glipizide**. Ranitidine may ↑ **procainamide** levels. Ranitidine may ↑ the effects of **warfarin**.

Route/Dosage

Cimetidine

PO (Adults): *Short-term treatment of active ulcers*—300 mg 4 times daily *or* 800 mg at bedtime *or* 400–600 mg twice daily (not to exceed 2.4 g/day) for up to 8 wk. *Duodenal ulcer prophylaxis*—300 mg twice daily *or* 400 mg at bedtime. *GERD*—400 mg every 6 hr *or* 800 mg twice daily for 12 wk. *Gastric hypersecretory conditions*—300–600 mg every 6 hr (up to 2400 mg/day). *OTC use*—up to 200 mg may be taken twice daily (for not more than 2 wk).

PO (Children): *Short-term treatment of active ulcers*—5–10 mg/kg every 6 hr.

Renal Impairment

PO (Adults): *CCr 10–50 mL/min*—Administer 50% of normal dose; *CCr <10 mL/min*—Administer 25% of normal dose.

Renal Impairment

PO (Children): 10–15 mg/kg/day.

Famotidine

PO (Adults): *Short-term treatment of active duodenal ulcers*—40 mg/day at bedtime or 20 mg twice daily for up to 8 wk. *Treatment of benign gastric ulcers*—40 mg/day at bedtime. *Maintenance treatment of duodenal ulcers*—20 mg once daily at bedtime. *GERD*—20 mg twice daily for up to 6 wk; up to 40 mg twice daily for up to 12 wk for esophagitis with erosions, ulcerations, and continuing symptoms. *Gastric hypersecretory conditions*—20 mg every 6 hr initially, up to 160 mg every 6 hr. *OTC use*—10 mg for relief of symptoms; for prevention—10 mg 60 min before eating or take 10 mg as chewable tablet 15 min before heartburn-inducing foods or beverages (not to exceed 20 mg/24 hr for up to 2 wk).

PO, IV (Children 1–16 yr): *Peptic ulcer*—0.5 mg/kg/day as a single bedtime dose or in 2 divided doses (up to 40 mg daily); *GERD*—1 mg/kg/day in 2 divided doses (up to 80 mg twice daily).

PO (Infants >3 mo–1 yr): *GERD*—0.5 mg/kg/dose twice daily.

PO (Infants and neonates <3 mo): *GERD*—0.5 mg/kg/dose once daily.

IV (Adults): 20 mg every 12 hr.

Renal Impairment

PO (Adults): *CCr <50 mL/min*—administer normal dose every 36–48 hr *or* 50% of normal dose at normal dosing interval. *CCr <10 mL/min*—dosing interval may need to be ↑ to every 36–48 hr.

Nizatidine

PO (Adults): *Short-term treatment of active duodenal or benign gastric ulcers*—300 mg once daily at bedtime. *Maintenance treatment of duodenal ulcers*—150 mg once daily at bedtime. *GERD*—150 mg twice daily. *OTC use*—75 mg twice daily given 30–60 min before foods or beverages expected to cause symptoms.

Renal Impairment

PO (Adults): *Short-term treatment of active ulcers—CCr 20–50 mL/min*—150 mg once daily; *CCr <20 mL/min*—150 mg every other day. *Maintenance treatment of duodenal ulcers—CCr 20–50 mL/min*—150 mg every other day; *CCr <20 mL/min*—150 mg every 3 days.

Ranitidine

PO (Adults): *Short-term treatment of active duodenal or benign gastric ulcers*—150 mg twice daily *or* 300 mg once daily at bedtime. *Maintenance treatment of duodenal or gastric ulcers*—150 mg once daily at bedtime. *GERD*—150 mg twice daily. *Erosive esophagitis*—150 mg 4 times daily initially, then 150 mg twice daily as maintenance. *Gastric hypersecretory conditions*—150 mg twice daily initially; up to 6 g/day have been used. *OTC use*—75 mg 30–60 min before foods or beverages expected to cause symptoms (up to twice daily) (not to be used for more than 2 wk).

PO (Children 1 mo–16 yr): *Treatment of gastric/duodenal ulcers*—2–4 mg/kg/day in 2 divided doses (up to 300 mg/day); *Maintenance treatment of ulcers*—2–4 mg/kg once daily (up to 150 mg/day); *GERD/erosive esophagitis*—5–10 mg/kg/day in 2 divided doses (up to 300 mg/day for GERD or 600 mg/day for erosive esophagitis).

PO (Neonates): 2 mg/kg/day in 2 divided doses.

IV, IM (Adults): 50 mg every 6–8 hr. *Continuous IV infusion*—6.25 mg/hr. *Gastric hypersecretory conditions*—1 mg/kg/hr; may be ↑ by 0.5 mg/kg/hr (not to exceed 2.5 mg/kg/hr).

IV, IM (Children 1 mo–16 yr): *Treatment of gastric/duodenal ulcers*—2–4 mg/kg/day divided every 6–8 hr (up to 200 mg/day). *Continuous infusion*—1 mg/kg/dose followed by 0.08–0.17 mg/kg/hr.

IV (Neonates): 1.5 mg/kg/dose load, then in 12 hr start maintenance of 1.5–2 mg/kg/day divided every 12 hr. *Continuous IV infusion*—1.5 mg/kg/dose load followed by 0.04–0.08 mg/kg/hr infusion.

Renal Impairment

PO (Adults): *CCr <50 mL/min*—150 mg every 24 hr.

Renal Impairment

IV (Adults): *CCr <50 mL/min*—50 mg every 24 hr.

Availability

Cimetidine (generic available)

Tablets: 200 mg[Rx, OTC], 300 mg, 400 mg, 🍁 600 mg, 800 mg. **Cost:** *Generic*—200 mg $82.15/100, 300 mg $90.45/100, 400 mg $146.85/100, 800 mg $220.00/100. **Oral liquid (mint-peach flavor):** 200 mg/5 mL[OTC], 300 mg/5 mL. **Cost:** *Generic*—300 mg/5 mL $89.00/237 mL.

Famotidine (generic available)

Tablets: 10 mg[OTC], 20 mg[Rx, OTC], 40 mg. **Cost:** *Generic*—20 mg $173.50/100, 40 mg $335.00/100. **Gelcaps:** 10 mg[OTC]. **Oral suspension (cherry-banana-mint flavor):** 40 mg/5 mL. **Cost:** *Generic*—$176.95/50 mL. **Premixed infusion:** 20 mg/50 mL 0.9% NaCl. **Solution for injection:** 10 mg/mL. ***In combination with:*** ibuprofen (Duexis), calcium carbonate and magnesium hydroxide[OTC] (Pepcid Complete, see Appendix B).

Nizatidine (generic available)

Tablets: 75 mg[OTC]. **Capsules:** 150 mg, 300 mg. **Cost:** *Generic*—150 mg $143.28/60, 300 mg $142.98/30. **Oral solution (bubble gum flavor):** 15 mg/mL. **Cost:** *Generic*—$347.65/473 mL.

Ranitidine (generic available)

Tablets: 75 mg[OTC], 150 mg, 300 mg. **Cost:** *Generic*—150 mg $156.20/100, 300 mg $87.85/30. **Capsules:** 150 mg, 300 mg. **Cost:** *Generic*—150 mg $91.27/60, 300 mg $82.30/30. **Effervescent tablets (EFFERdose):** 25 mg. **Syrup (peppermint flavor):** 15 mg/mL. **Cost:** *Generic*—$350.49/473 mL. **Premixed infusion:** 50 mg/50 mL 0.45% NaCl. **Solution for injection:** 25 mg/mL.

NURSING IMPLICATIONS

Assessment

- Assess for epigastric or abdominal pain and frank or occult blood in the stool, emesis, or gastric aspirate.
- Geri: Assess geriatric and debilitated patients routinely for confusion. Report promptly.
- ***Lab Test Considerations:*** Monitor CBC with differential periodically during therapy.
- Antagonize effects of pentagastrin and histamine during gastric acid secretion testing. Avoid administration for 24 hr before the test.
- May cause false-negative results in skin tests using allergenic extracts. Histamine H_2 antagonists should be discontinued 24 hr before the test.
- May cause ↑ in serum transaminases and serum creatinine.
- Serum prolactin concentration may be ↑ after IV bolus of *cimetidine*. May also cause ↓ parathyroid concentrations.
- *Nizatidine* may cause ↑ alkaline phosphatase concentrations.
- *Ranitidine* and *famotidine* may cause false-positive results for urine protein; test with sulfosalicylic acid.

Implementation

- Do not confuse ranitidine with rimantidine. Do not confuse Zantac (ranitidine) with Xanax (alprazolam) or Zyrtec (cetirizine).
- **PO:** Administer with meals or immediately afterward and at bedtime to prolong effect.
- If antacids or sucralfate are used concurrently for relief of pain, avoid administration of antacids within 30 min–1 hr of the H_2 antagonist and take sucralfate 2 hr after H_2 antagonist; may ↓ absorption of H_2 antagonist.
- Doses administered once daily should be administered at bedtime to prolong effect.
- Shake oral suspension before administration. Discard unused suspension after 30 days.
- Remove foil from *ranitidine effervescent tablets* and dissolve in 6–8 oz water before drinking.

Famotidine

IV Administration

- **IV Push:** ***Diluent:*** 0.9% NaCl, D5W, D10W, or LR. ***Concentration:*** 4 mg/mL. ***Rate:*** Administer at a rate of 10 mg/min. Rapid administration may cause hypotension.
- **Intermittent Infusion:** ***Diluent:*** Dilute each 20 mg in 100 mL of 0.9% NaCl, D5W, D10W, or LR. Diluted solution is stable for 48 hr at room temperature. Do not use solution that is discolored or contains a precipitate. ***Concentration:*** 0.2 mg/mL. ***Rate:*** Administer over 15–30 min.
- **Y-Site Compatibility:** acyclovir, alemtuzumab, alfentanil, allopurinol, amifostine, amikacin, aminocaproic acid, aminophylline, amiodarone, amphotericin B lipid complex, amphotericin B liposome, amsacrine, anakinra, anidulafungin, argatroban, ascorbic acid, atracurium, atropine, aztreonam, benztropine, bleomycin, bumetanide, buprenorphine, butorphanol, calcium chloride, calcium gluconate, carboplatin, carmustine, caspofungin, cefotaxime, ceftaroline, ceftazidime, cefuroxime, chlorpromazine, cisatracurium, cisplatin, cladribine, clindamycin, cyanocobalamin, cyclophosphamide, cyclosporine, cytarabine, dacarbazine, dactinomycin, daptomycin, daunorubicin hydrochloride, dexamethasone, dexmedetomidine, dexrazoxane, digoxin, diltiazem, diphenhydramine, dobutamine, docetaxel, dopamine, doxacurium, doxorubicin, doxorubicin liposome, doxycycline, droperidol, enalaprilat, ephedrine, epinephrine, epirubicin, epoetin alfa, eptifibitide, ertapenem, erythromycin lactobionate, esmolol, etoposide, etoposide phosphate, fenoldopam, fentanyl, filgrastim, fluconazole, fludarabine, fluorouracil, folic acid, foscarnet, fosphenytoin, gemcitabine, gentamicin, glycopyrrolate, granisetron, heparin, hetastarch, hydrocortisone, hydromorphone, idarubicin, ifosfamide, imipenem/cilastatin, irinotecan, isoproterenol, ketorolac, labetalol, leucovorin calcium, levofloxacin, lidocaine, linezolid, lorazepam, magnesium sulfate, mannitol, melphalan, meperidine, mesna, metaraminol, methotrexate, methyldopate, methylprednisolone, metoclopramide, metoprolol, metronidazole, midazolam, milrinone, mitoxantrone, morphine, moxifloxacin, multivitamins, mycophenolate, nafcillin, nalbuphine, naloxone, nicardipine, nitroglycerin, nitroprusside, norepinephrine, octreotide, ondansetron, oxacillin, oxaliplatin, oxytocin, paclitaxel, palonosetron, pamidronate, pancuronium, papaverine, pemetrexed, penicillin G, pentamidine, pentobarbital, perphenazine, phenobarbital, phentolamine, phenylephrine, phytonadione, potassium acetate, potassium chloride, potassium phosphates, procainamide, prochlorperazine, promethazine, propofol, propranolol, protamine, pyridoxime, ranitidine, remifentanil, rituximab, sargramostim, sodium acetate, sodium bicarbonate, streptokinase, succinylcholine, sufentanil, tacrolimus, telavancin, theophylline, thiamine, thiotepa, tigecycline, tirofiban, tobramycin, tolazoline, trastuzumab, vancomycin, vasopressin, vecuronium, verapamil, vinblastine, vincristine, vinorelbine, voriconazole, zoledronic acid.
- **Y-Site Incompatibility:** amphotericin B deoxycholate, azathioprine, cefepime, chloramphenicol, dantrolene, diazepam, diazoxide, ganciclovir, indomethacin, mitomycin, pantoprazole, piperacillin/tazobactam, trimethoprim/sulfamethoxazole.

Ranitidine

IV Administration

- **IV Push:** ***Diluent:*** 0.9% NaCl or D5W for injection. ***Concentration:*** 2.5 mg/mL. ***Rate:*** Administer over at least 5 min not to exceed 10 mg/min. Rapid administration may cause hypotension and arrhythmias.

- **Intermittent Infusion:** ***Diluent:*** Dilute each 50 mg in 100 mL of 0.9% NaCl or D5W. Diluted solution is stable for 48 hr at room temperature. Do not use solution that is discolored or that contains precipitate. ***Concentration:*** 0.5 mg/mL. ***Rate:*** Administer over 15–30 min.
- **Continuous Infusion:** ***Diluent:*** D5W. ***Concentration:*** 150 mg/250 mL (no greater than 2.5 mg/mL for Zollinger-Ellison patients). ***Rate:*** Administer at a rate of 6.25 mg/hr. In patients with Zollinger-Ellison syndrome, start infusion at 1 mg/kg/hr. If gastric acid output is >10 mEq/hr or patient becomes symptomatic after 4 hr, adjust dose by 0.5 mg/kg/hr increments and remeasure gastric output.
- **Y-Site Compatibility:** acetaminophen, acyclovir, aldesleukin, alemtuzumab, alfentanil, allopurinol, amifostine, amikacin, aminocaproic acid, aminophylline, amphotericin B lipid complex, amphotericin B liposome, amsacrine, anakinra, anidulafungin, argatroban, ascorbic acid, atracurium, atropine, azithromycin, aztreonam, benztropine, bivalirudin, bleomycin, bumetanide, buprenorphine, butorphanol, calcium chloride, calcium gluconate, carboplatin, carmustine, cefazolin, cefepime, cefotaxime, cefotetan, cefoxitin, ceftaroline, ceftazidime, ceftriaxone, cefuroxime, chloramphenicol, chlorpromazine, ciprofloxacin, cisatracurium, cisplatin, cladribine, clindamycin, cyanocobalamin, cyclophosphamide, cyclosporine, cytarabine, dacarbazine, dactinomycin, daptomycin, daunorubicin, dexamethasone, dexmedetomidine, dexrazoxane, digoxin, diltiazem, diphenhydramine, dobutamine, docetaxel, dopamine, doxacurium, doxapram, doxorubicin hydrochloride, doxorubicin liposome, doxycycline, enalaprilat, ephedrine, epinephrine, epirubicin, epoetin alfa, eptifibatide, ertapenem, erythromycin, esmolol, etoposide, etoposide phosphate, famotidine, fenoldopam, fentanyl, filgrastim, fluconazole, fludarabine, fluorouacil, folic acid, foscarnet, fosphenytoin, furosemide, ganciclovir, gemcitabine, gentamicin, glycopyrrolate, granisetron, haloperidol, heparin, hydrocortisone, hydromorphone, idarubicin, ifosfamide, imipenem/cilastatin, indomethacin, irinotecan, isoproterenol, ketamine, ketorolac, labetalol, leucovorin calcium, levofloxacin, lidocaine, linezolid, lorazepam, magnesium sulfate, mannitol, melphalan, meperidine, mesna, metaraminol, methotrexate, methyldopate, methylprednisolone, metoclopramide, metoprolol, metronidazole, midazolam, milrinone, mitoxantrone, morphine, moxifloxacin, multivitamins, mycophenolate, nafcillin, nalbuphine, naloxone, nitroglycerin, nitroprusside, norepinephrine, octreotide, ondansetron, oxacillin, oxaliplatin, oxytocin, paclitaxel, palonosetron, pamidronate, pancuronium, papaverine, pemetrexed, penicillin G, pentamidine, pentobarbital, phenobarbital, phentolamine, phenylephrine, phytonadione, piperacillin/tazobactam, potassium acetate, potassium chloride, procainamide, prochlorperazine, promethazine, propofol, propranolol, protamine, pyridoxime, remifentanil, rituximab, rocuronium, sargramostim, sodium acetate, sodium bicarbonate, strepotkinase, succinylcholine, sufentanil, tacrolimus, telavancin, theophylline, thiamine, thiopental, thiotepa, tigecycline, tirofiban, tobramycin, tolazoline, trastuzumab, vancomycin, vasopressin, vecuronium, verapamil, vinblastine, vincristine, vinorelbine, warfarin, zidovudine, zoledronic acid.
- **Y-Site Incompatibility:** amiodarone, caspofungin, dacarbazine, dantrolene, diazepam, diazoxide, pantoprazole, phenytoin, quinupristin/dalfopristin, trimethoprim/sulfamethoxazole.

H

Patient/Family Teaching

- Instruct patient to take medication as directed for the full course of therapy, even if feeling better. Take missed doses as soon as remembered but not if almost time for next dose. Do not double doses.
- Advise patients taking OTC preparations not to take the maximum dose continuously for more than 2 wk without consulting health care professional. Notify health care professional if difficulty swallowing occurs or abdominal pain persists.
- Inform patient that smoking interferes with the action of histamine antagonists. Encourage patient to quit smoking or at least not to smoke after last dose of the day.
- May cause drowsiness or dizziness. Caution patient to avoid driving or other activities requiring alertness until response to the drug is known.
- Advise patient to avoid alcohol, products containing aspirin or NSAIDs, and foods that may cause an increase in GI irritation.
- Inform patient that increased fluid and fiber intake and exercise may minimize constipation.
- Advise patient to report onset of black, tarry stools; fever; sore throat; diarrhea; dizziness; rash; confusion; or hallucinations to health care professional promptly.
- Advise patient to notify health care professional if pregnancy is planned or suspected or if breast feeding.

Evaluation/Desired Outcomes

- Decrease in abdominal pain.
- Treatment and prevention of gastric or duodenal irritation and bleeding. Healing of duodenal ulcers can be seen by x-rays or endoscopy. Therapy is continued for at least 6 wk in treatment of ulcers but not usually longer than 8 wk.
- Decreased symptoms of esophageal reflux.
- Treatment of heartburn, acid indigestion, and sour stomach (OTC use).

HMG-CoA REDUCTASE INHIBITORS (statins)

atorvastatin (a-**tore**-va-stat-in)
Lipitor

fluvastatin (**floo**-va-sta-tin)
~~Lescol~~, Lescol XL

lovastatin (**loe**-va-sta-tin)
Altoprev, ~~Mevacor~~

pitavastatin (pi-**tava**-sta-tin)
Livalo, Zypitamag

pravastatin (**pra**-va-sta-tin)
Pravachol

rosuvastatin (roe-**soo**-va-sta-tin)
Crestor, Ezallor Sprinkle

simvastatin (**sim**-va-sta-tin)
FloLipid, Zocor

Classification
Therapeutic: lipid-lowering agents
Pharmacologic: HMG-CoA reductase inhibitors

Indications

Adjunctive management of primary hypercholesterolemia and mixed dyslipidemias. **Atorvastatin:** Primary prevention of cardiovascular disease (↓ risk of MI or stroke) in patients with multiple risk factors for coronary heart disease CHD or type 2 diabetes mellitus (also ↓ risk of angina or revascularization procedures in patients with multiple risk factors for CHD). **Atorvastatin and pravastatin:** Secondary prevention of cardiovascular disease (↓ risk of MI, stroke, revascularization procedures, angina, and hospitalizations for HF) in patients with clinically evident CHD. **Fluvastatin:** Secondary prevention of coronary revascularization procedures in patients with clinically evident CHD. **Fluvastatin and lovastatin:** Slow progression of coronary atherosclerosis in patients with CHD. **Lovastatin:** Primary prevention of CHD (↓ risk of MI, unstable angina, and coronary revascularization) in patients without symptomatic cardiovascular disease with ↑ total and low-density lipoprotein (LDL) cholesterol and ↓ high-density lipoprotein (HDL) cholesterol. **Pravastatin:** Primary prevention of CHD (↓ risk of MI, coronary revascularization, and cardiovascular mortality) in patients without clinically evident CHD. **Simvastatin:** Secondary prevention of cardiovascular events (↓ risk of MI, coronary revascularization, stroke, and cardiovascular mortality) in patients with clinically evident CHD or those at high-risk for CHD (history of diabetes, peripheral arterial disease, or stroke). **Rosuvastatin:** Slow progression of coronary atherosclerosis. **Rosuvastatin:** Primary prevention of cardiovascular disease (reduces risk of stroke, myocardial infarction, and revascularization) in patients without clinically evident coronary heart disease but with an increased risk of cardiovascular disease because of age (≥50 yr for men; ≥60 yr for women), hsCRP ≥2 mg/L, and the presence of ≥1 risk factor for cardiovascular disease (hypertension, low HDL-C, smoking, or premature family history of coronary heart disease). **Rosuvastatin:** Adjunctive therapy to diet and exercise for the reduction of LDL cholesterol in children 8–17 yrs with heterozygous familial hypercholesterolemia if after diet therapy fails the following still exist: LDL cholesterol remains >190 mg/dL or remains >160 mg/dL (with family history of premature cardiovascular disease or ≥2 risk factors for cardiovascular disease).

Action

Inhibit an enzyme, 3-hydroxy-3-methylglutaryl-coenzyme A (HMG-CoA) reductase, which is responsible for catalyzing an early step in the synthesis of cholesterol.
Therapeutic Effects: Lowers total and LDL cholesterol and triglycerides. Slightly increase HDL. Slows the progression of coronary atherosclerosis with resultant decrease in CHD-related events (all agents except rosuvastatin have indication for ↓ events).

Pharmacokinetics

Absorption: *Atorvastatin*—rapidly absorbed but undergoes extensive GI and hepatic metabolism, resulting in 14% bioavailability; *fluvastatin*—98% absorbed after oral administration, but undergoes extensive first-pass metabolism resulting in 24% bioavailability; *lovastatin, pravastatin*—poorly and variably absorbed after oral administration; *pitavastatin*—well absorbed (51%) after oral administration; *rosuvastatin*—20% absorbed following oral administration; *simvastatin*—85% absorbed but rapidly metabolized.
Distribution: *Atorvastatin*—probably enters breast milk. *Fluvastatin*—enters breast milk. *Lovastatin*—crosses the blood-brain barrier and placenta. *Pravastatin*—small amounts enter breast milk. *Pitavastatin, rosuvastatin, and simvastatin*—unknown.
Protein Binding: *Atorvastatin, fluvastatin, pitavastatin, and simvastatin*—>98%.
Metabolism and Excretion: All agents are extensively metabolized by the liver; amount excreted unchanged in urine: *atorvastatin*—<2%, *lovastatin*—10%, *fluvastatin*—5%, *pitavastatin*—15%, *pravastatin*—20%, and *simvastatin*—13%.
Half-life: *Atorvastatin*—14 hr; *fluvastatin*—1.2 hr; *lovastatin*—3 hr; *pitavastatin*—12 hr; *pravastatin*—1.3–2.7 hr; *rosuvastatin*—19 hr; *simvastatin*—unknown.

TIME/ACTION PROFILE (cholesterol-lowering effect)

ROUTE	ONSET	PEAK	DURATION*
Atorvastatin	unknown	unknown	20–30 hr
Fluvastatin	1–2 wk	4–6 wk	unknown
Lovastatin	2 wk	4–6 wk	6 wk
Pitavastatin	within 4 wk	4 wk	unknown
Pravastatin	several days	2–4 wk	unknown
Rosuvastatin	unknown	2–4 wk	unknown
Simvastatin	several days	2–4 wk	unknown

*After discontinuation.

Contraindications/Precautions

Contraindicated in: Hypersensitivity; Active liver disease or unexplained persistent ↑ in AST or ALT; *Simvastatin and lovastatin*—Concurrent use of strong CYP3A4 inhibitors (↑ risk of myopathy/rhabdomyolysis); *Pitavastatin*—Concurrent use of cyclosporine; *Pitavastatin*—severe renal impairment (CCr <30 mL/min); *Simvastatin*—Concurrent use of cyclosporine, gemfibrozil, or danazol (↑ risk of myopathy/rhabdomyolysis); OB: Avoid use during pregnancy (may cause fetal harm); Lactation: Avoid breast feeding if treatment is necessary.

Use Cautiously in: History of liver disease; Alcoholism; *Rosuvastatin*—patients with Asian ancestry (may have ↑ blood levels and ↑ risk of rhabdomyolysis); *Atorvastatin*—Concurrent use of gemfibrozil, azole antifungals, erythromycin, clarithromycin, protease inhibitors, niacin, or cyclosporine (higher risk of myopathy/rhabdomyolysis); *Lovastatin*—Concurrent use of gemfibrozil, niacin, cyclosporine, amiodarone, danazol, diltiazem, verapamil, colchicine, or ranolazine (higher risk of myopathy/rhabdomyolysis); *Pitavastatin*—Hypothyroidism, concurrent use of fibrates or lipid-lowering doses of niacin (higher risk of myopathy/rhabdomyolysis); *Rosuvastatin*—Concurrent use of gemfibrozil, azole antifungals, protease inhibitors, niacin, cyclosporine, amiodarone, or verapamil (higher risk of myopathy/rhabdomyolysis); *Simvastatin*—Concurrent use of amiodarone, amlodipine, diltiazem, dronedarone, verapamil, lomitapide, or ranolazine (↑ risk of myopathy/rhabdomyolysis); *Simvastatin*—Chinese patients receiving ≥1 g/day of niacin (↑ risk of myopathy; do not use simvastatin 80 mg/day in these patients); Renal impairment; Geri: *Pitavastatin*—↑ risk of myopathy (age >65 yr); Rep: Women of reproductive potential (use effective contraception); Pedi: Children <8 yr (safety and effectiveness not established); some products approved for use in older children only.

Adverse Reactions/Side Effects

CNS: amnesia, confusion, dizziness, headache, insomnia, memory loss, weakness. **CV:** chest pain, peripheral edema. **Derm:** rash, pruritus. **EENT:** rhinitis; *lovastatin*, blurred vision. **Endo:** hyperglycemia. **GI:** abdominal cramps, constipation, diarrhea, flatus, heartburn, altered taste, drug-induced hepatitis, dyspepsia, ↑ liver enzymes, nausea, pancreatitis. **GU:** erectile dysfunction. **MS:** RHABDOMYOLYSIS, arthralgia, arthritis, immune-mediated necrotizing myopathy, myalgia, myopathy (↑ with simvastatin 80 mg/day dose). **Resp:** bronchitis. **Misc:** HYPERSENSITIVITY REACTIONS (including angioedema and urticaria).

Interactions

Atorvastatin, lovastatin, simvastatin, and rosuvastatin are metabolized by the CYP3A4 metabolic pathway. Fluvastatin is metabolized by CYP 2C9. Pravastatin is not metabolized by the CYP P450 system.

Drug-Drug: Atorvastatin, lovastatin, and simvastatin may interact with **CYP3A4 inhibitors**. Risk of myopathy with lovastatin is ↑ by concurrent use of **strong CYP3A4 inhibitors**, including **ketoconazole**, **itraconazole**, **posaconazole**, **voriconazole protease inhibitors**, **clarithromycin**, **erythromycin**, **nefazodone**, and **cobicistat-containing products**; concurrent use contraindicated. Risk of myopathy with simvastatin is ↑ by concurrent use of **cyclosporine**, **gemfibrozil**, **danazol**, **erythromycin**, **clarithromycin**, **protease inhibitors**, **nefazodone**, **ketoconazole**, **itraconazole**, **voriconazole**, **posaconazole**, and **cobicistat-containing products**; concurrent use contraindicated. Risk of myopathy with pitavastatin is ↑ by concurrent use of **cyclosporine**; concurrent use contraindicated. Bioavailability and effectiveness may be ↓ by **cholestyramine** and **colestipol**. Risk of myopathy with atorvastatin is ↑ by concurrent use of **cyclosporine**, **gemfibrozil**, **itraconazole**, **colchicine**, **erythromycin**, **clarithromycin**, **nelfinavir**, **ritonavir/saquinavir**, **lopinavir/ritonavir**, **tipranavir/ritonavir**, **saquinavir/ritonavir**, **darunavir/ritonavir**, **fosamprenavir**, **fosamprenavir/ritonavir**, and large doses of **niacin**; concurrent use with gemfibrozil, cyclosporine, or tipranavir/ritonavir should be avoided; use lowest dose with lopinavir/ritonavir; use ↓ doses with nelfinavir, clarithromycin, itraconazole, saquinavir/ritonavir, darunavir/ritonavir, fosamprenavir, or fosamprenavir/ritonavir. Risk of myopathy with fluvastatin is ↑ by concurrent use of **gemfibrozil**, **erythromycin**, **colchicine**, **cyclosporine**, **azole antifungal agents**, or large doses of **niacin** may ↑ risk of myopathy; concurrent use with gemfibrozil should be avoided; use ↓ doses with cyclosporine and fluconazole. Risk of myopathy with lovastatin is ↑ by concurrent use of **amiodarone cyclosporine**, **gemfibrozil**, **diltiazem**, **verapamil**, **danazol**, and large doses of **niacin**; concurrent use with gemfibrozil or cyclosporine should be avoided; use ↓ doses with danazol, amiodarone, diltiazem, or verapamil. Risk of myopathy with pitavastatin is ↑ by concurrent use of **erythromycin**, **rifampin**,

colchicine, **fibrates**, or large doses of **niacin**; use ↓ doses with erythromycin, rifampin, and niacin; concurrent use with gemfibrozil should be avoided. Risk of myopathy with pravastatin is ↑ by concurrent use of **cyclosporine**, **fibrates**, **colchicine**, **erythromycin**, **clarithromycin**, **azithromycin**, or large doses of **niacin**; concurrent use with gemfibrozil should be avoided; consider lower dose with niacin. Risk of myopathy with rosuvastatin is ↑ by concurrent use of **cyclosporine**, **lopinavir/ritonavir**, **atazanavir/ritonavir**, **colchicine**, **fibrates**, or large doses of **niacin**; concurrent use of gemfibrozil should be avoided, if possible; use ↓ doses with cyclosporine, lopinavir/ritonavir, and atazanavir/ritonavir. Risk of myopathy with simvastatin is ↑ by concurrent use of **amiodarone**, **amlodipine**, **diltiazem**, **dronedarone**, **verapamil**, **lomitapide**, **ranolazine**, or **niacin**. Atorvastatin, fluvastatin, and simvastatin may slightly ↑ serum **digoxin** levels. Atorvastatin and rosuvastatin may ↑ levels of **hormonal contraceptives**. Atorvastatin, fluvastatin, lovastatin, rosuvastatin, and simvastatin may ↑ risk of bleeding with **warfarin**. **Alcohol**, **cimetidine**, **ranitidine**, and **omeprazole** may ↑ fluvastatin levels. **Rifampin** may ↓ fluvastatin levels. **Antacids** ↓ absorption of rosuvastatin (administer 2 hr after rosuvastatin. **Lopinavir/ritonavir** may ↑ rosuvastatin levels. Fluvastatin ↑ levels of **glyburide**.

Drug-Natural Products: St. John's wort may ↓ levels and effectiveness (lovastatin and simvastatin).

Drug-Food: Large quantities of **grapefruit juice** may ↑ blood levels and ↑ risk of rhabdomyolysis (atorvastatin, lovastatin, and simvastatin); concurrent use contraindicated. **Food** ↑ blood levels of lovastatin.

Route/Dosage

Atorvastatin

PO (Adults): 10–20 mg once daily initially; (may start with 40 mg/day if LDL-C needs to be ↓ by >45%); may ↑ every 2–4 wk up to 80 mg/day; *Concurrent nelfinavir therapy*—Dose should not exceed 40 mg/day; *Concurrent clarithromycin, itraconazole, saquinavir/ritonavir, darunavir/ritonavir, fosamprenavir, or fosamprenavir/ritonavir therapy*—Dose should not exceed 20 mg/day.

PO (Children 10–17 yr): 10 mg/day initially, may ↑ every 4 wk up to 20 mg/day; *Concurrent nelfinavir therapy*—Dose should not exceed 40 mg/day; *Concurrent clarithromycin, itraconazole, saquinavir/ritonavir, darunavir/ritonavir, fosamprenavir, or fosamprenavir/ritonavir therapy*—Dose should not exceed 20 mg/day.

Fluvastatin

PO (Adults): 20–40 mg (immediate-release) once daily at bedtime. May ↑ to 40 mg twice daily (immediate-release) or 80 mg once daily (extended-release); *Concurrent fluconazole or cyclosporine therapy*—Dose should not exceed 20 mg twice daily.

Lovastatin

PO (Adults): 20 mg once daily with evening meal. May ↑ at 4-wk intervals to a maximum of 80 mg/day (immediate-release) or 60 mg/day (extended-release); *Concurrent danazol, verapamil, or diltiazem therapy*—Initiate at 10 mg once daily; do not exceed 20 mg/day; *Concurrent amiodarone therapy*—Dose should not exceed 40 mg/day.

Renal Impairment

PO (Adults): *CCr <30 mL/min*—Dose should not exceed 20 mg/day unless carefully titrated.

PO (Children /Adolescents 10–17 yr): *Familial heterozygous hypercholesterolemia*—10–40 mg/day adjusted at 4-wk intervals.

Pitavastatin

PO (Adults): 2 mg once daily initially, may ↑ up to 4 mg once daily depending on response. *Concurrent erythromycin therapy*—Dose should not exceed 1 mg/day; *Concurrent rifampin therapy*—Dose should not exceed 2 mg/day.

Renal Impairment

PO (Adults): *CCr 30–<60 mL/min*—1 mg once daily initially, may ↑ up to 2 mg daily.

Pravastatin

PO (Adults): 40 mg once daily at bedtime, may be ↑ after 4 wk, if needed to 80 mg once daily at bedtime); *Concurrent cyclosporine therapy*—Initiate therapy with 10 mg once daily at bedtime; may be ↑ after 4 wk, if needed, to 20 mg once daily at bedtime (max dose = 20 mg/day); *Concurrent clarithromycin therapy*—Dose should not exceed 40 mg/day.

PO (Children 14–18 yrs): 40 mg once daily (max dose = 40 mg/day).

PO (Children 8–13 yrs): 20 mg once daily (max dose = 20 mg/day).

Renal Impairment

PO (Adults): *CCr<30 mL/min*—Initiate therapy with 10 mg once daily at bedtime; may titrate at 4–wk intervals as needed (max dose = 80 mg/day).

Rosuvastatin

PO (Adults): 10 mg once daily initially (range 5–20 mg initially) (20 mg initial dose may be considered for patients with LDL-C >190 mg/dL or homozygous familial hypercholesterolemia); dose may be adjusted at 2–4 wk intervals, some patients may require up to 40 mg/day, however this dose is associated with ↑ risk of rhabdomyolysis; *Patients with Asian ancestry*—initial dose should be 5 mg; *Concurrent cyclosporine therapy*—Dose should not exceed 5 mg/day; *Concurrent lopinavir/ritonavir or atazanavir/ritonavir therapy*—Dose should not exceed 10 mg/day; *Concurrent gemfibrozil therapy*—Dose should not exceed 10 mg/day (avoid if possible).

PO (Children 10–17 yr): 5–20 mg once daily.
PO (Children 8–<10 yr): 5–10 mg once daily.

Renal Impairment

PO (Adults): *CCr <30 mL/min*—5 mg once daily initially; dose may be ↑ but should not exceed 10 mg/day.

Simvastatin

The 80 mg dose should be restricted to patients who have been taking this dose for ≥12 mo without evidence of muscle toxicity.

PO (Adults): 5–40 mg once daily in the evening; if LDL goal cannot be achieved with 40 mg/day dose, add another lipid-lowering therapy (do not ↑ simvastatin dose to 80 mg/day). *Concurrent verapamil, diltiazem, or dronedarone therapy*—Dose should not exceed 10 mg/day. *Concurrent amiodarone, amlodipine, or ranolazine therapy*—Dose should not exceed 20 mg/day; *Concurrent lomitapide therapy*—↓ dose by 50% (dose should not exceed 20 mg/day or 40 mg/day for patients who previously received 80 mg/day chronically [for ≥12 mo] without evidence of myopathy).
PO (Children 10–17 yr): 10 mg once daily initially, may ↑ at 4–wk intervals up to 40 mg/day. *Concurrent verapamil or diltiazem therapy*—Dose should not exceed 10 mg/day. *Concurrent amiodarone, amlodipine, or ranolazine therapy*—Dose should not exceed 20 mg/day.

Renal Impairment

PO (Adults): *CCr <10 mL/min*—5 mg once daily initially, titrate carefully.

Availability

Atorvastatin (generic available)

Tablets: 10 mg, 20 mg, 40 mg, 80 mg. **Cost:** *Generic*—10 mg $33.25/100, 20 mg $48.75/100, 40 mg $40.42/100, 80 mg $49.20/100. ***In combination with:*** amlodipine (Caduet); see Appendix B.

Fluvastatin (generic available)

Capsules: 20 mg, 40 mg. **Cost:** *Generic*—All strengths $113.40/30. **Extended-release tablets:** 80 mg. **Cost:** $194.69/30.

Lovastatin (generic available)

Extended-release tablets (Altoprev): 20 mg, 40 mg, 60 mg. **Cost:** All strengths $555.98/30. **Tablets :** 10 mg, 20 mg, 40 mg. **Cost:** *Generic*—10 mg $10.83/100, 20 mg $10.83/100, 40 mg $16.50/100.

Pitavastatin (generic available)

Tablets: 1 mg, 2 mg, 4 mg. **Cost:** All strengths $492.48/90.

Pravastatin (generic available)

Tablets: 10 mg, 20 mg, 40 mg, 80 mg. **Cost:** *Generic*—20 mg $10.83/100, 40 mg $29.82/100, 80 mg $142.06/100.

Rosuvastatin

Sprinkle capsules (Ezallor): 5 mg, 10 mg, 20 mg, 40 mg. **Tablets (Crestor):** 5 mg, 10 mg, 20 mg, 40 mg. **Cost:** 5 mg $609.27/100, 10 mg $600.47/100, 20 mg $609.27/100, 40 mg $541.62/100.

Simvastatin (generic available)

Oral suspension (FloLipid): 20 mg/5 mL, 40 mg/5 mL. **Tablets (Zocor):** 5 mg, 10 mg, 20 mg, 40 mg, 80 mg. **Cost:** *Generic*—5 mg $7.11/100, 10 mg $10.83/100, 20 mg $10.83/100, 40 mg $10.83/100, 80 mg $9.83/100. ***In combination with:*** ezetimibe (Vytorin). See Appendix B.

NURSING IMPLICATIONS

Assessment

- Obtain a dietary history, especially with regard to fat consumption.
- ***Lab Test Considerations:*** Evaluate serum cholesterol and triglyceride levels before initiating, after 4–6 wk of therapy, and periodically thereafter.
- Monitor liver function tests, including AST and ALT, before initiating therapy and if signs of liver injury (fatigue, anorexia, right upper abdominal discomfort, dark urine, or jaundice) occur. May also cause ↑ alkaline phosphatase and bilirubin levels.
- If patient develops muscle tenderness during therapy, monitor CK levels. If CK levels are >10 times the upper limit of normal or myopathy occurs, therapy should be discontinued. Monitor for signs and symptoms of immune-mediated necrotizing myopathy (IMNM) (proximal muscle weakness and ↑ serum creatine kinase), persisting despite discontinuation of statin therapy. Perform muscle biopsy to diagnose; shows necrotizing myopathy without significant inflammation. Treat with immunosuppressive agents.

Implementation

- Do not confuse Lipitor with Zyrtec. Do not confuse Mevacor with Benicar. Do not confuse atorvastatin with atomoxetine.
- **PO:** Administer *lovastatin* with food. Administration on an empty stomach decreases absorption by approximately 30%. Initial once-daily dose is administered with the evening meal.
- Administer extended-release tablets at bedtime. Extended-release tablets should be swallowed whole, do not break, crush, chew or open capsules.
- Administer *fluvastatin, pravastatin,* and *simvastatin* once daily in the evening. Do not take two 40 mg fluvastatin tablets at one time. *Atorvastatin, pitavas-*

tatin, and *rosuvastatin* can be taken any time of day. May be administered without regard to food.

- Administer *Ezallor Sprinkle* (rosuvastatin) as a single dose at any time of day, with or without food. Swallow capsules whole; do not crush or chew. For patients who cannot swallow capsules, open capsule for administration. When initiating *Ezallor Sprinkle* therapy or switching from another HMG-CoA reductase inhibitor therapy, begin with *Ezallor Sprinkle* starting dose, and then only titrate according to patient's response. Monitor lipid levels within 2–4 wk of starting *Ezallor Sprinkle* and adjust dose as needed. Consider starting *Ezallor Sprinkle* with 5 mg once daily in Asian patients; may cause increased rosuvastatin plasma concentrations.
- Avoid large amounts of grapefruit juice during therapy; may ↑ risk of toxicity.
- If *fluvastatin* or *pravastatin* is administered in conjunction with bile acid sequestrants (cholestyramine, colestipol), administer at least 4 hr after bile acid sequestrant.
- If *rosuvastatin* is administered in conjunction with magnesium or aluminum-containing antacids, administer antacid at least 2 hr after *rosuvastatin*.

Patient/Family Teaching

- Instruct patient to take medication as directed and not to skip doses or double up on missed doses. Advise patient to avoid drinking more than 200 mL/day of grapefruit juice during therapy. Medication helps control but does not cure elevated serum cholesterol levels.
- Advise patient that this medication should be used in conjunction with diet restrictions (fat, cholesterol, carbohydrates, alcohol), exercise, and cessation of smoking.
- Instruct patient to notify health care professional if signs of liver injury or if unexplained muscle pain, tenderness, or weakness occurs, especially if accompanied by fever or malaise.
- Advise patient to notify health care professional of all Rx or OTC medications, vitamins, or herbal products being taken and to consult with health care professional before taking other medications, especially St. John's wort.
- Advise patient to notify health care professional of medication regimen before treatment or surgery.
- Rep: Instruct female patients to notify health care professional promptly if pregnancy is planned or suspected. Advise women with reproductive potential to use effective contraception during therapy and discuss plans to discontinue statins if trying to conceive. Advise patients to avoid breast feeding during therapy.
- Emphasize the importance of follow-up exams to determine effectiveness and to monitor for side effects.

Evaluation/Desired Outcomes

- Decrease in LDL and total cholesterol levels.
- Increase in HDL cholesterol levels.
- Decrease in triglyceride levels.
- Slowing of the progression of coronary artery disease.
- Prevention of cardiovascular disease.

HUMAN PAPILLOMAVIRUS VACCINE

(**hyoo**-man pa-pil-**lo**-ma)

human papillomavirus quadrivalent (types 6, 11, 16, and 18) vaccine, recombinant
Gardasil

human papillomavirus bivalent (types 16 and 18) vaccine, recombinant
Cervarix

human papillomavirus 9-valent (types 6, 11, 16, 18, 31, 33, 45, 52, and 58) vaccine, recombinant
Gardasil 9

Classification
Therapeutic: vaccines/immunizing agents

Indications

Gardasil and Gardasil 9: Prevention of cervical, vulvar, vaginal, and anal cancers and genital warts (in females) and anal cancer and genital warts (in males). **Cervarix:** Prevention of cervical cancer.

Action

Vaccination results in antibodies to HPV viruses that are causative agents for cervical, vulvar, vaginal, and anal cancers and genital warts. **Therapeutic Effects:** Prevention of cervical, vulvar, vaginal, and anal cancers and genital warts.

Pharmacokinetics

Absorption: Well absorbed following IM administration.
Distribution: Unknown.
Metabolism and Excretion: Unknown.
Half-life: Unknown.

TIME/ACTION PROFILE (antibody response)

ROUTE	ONSET	PEAK	DURATION
IM	unknown	6 mo*	unknown

*After third vaccination.

Contraindications/Precautions

Contraindicated in: Hypersensitivity; Thrombocytopenia/bleeding disorder; OB: Limited data available; use only if potential benefit justifies potential risk to fetus.

Use Cautiously in: Current/recent febrile illness; Immunosuppression may ↓ antibody response; Lactation: Excretion into breast milk unknown; Pedi: Children <9 yr (safety not established).

Adverse Reactions/Side Effects

Neuro: fainting. **Local:** injection site reactions.
Misc: ANAPHYLAXIS (RARE).

Interactions

Drug-Drug: Immunosuppressants or **antineoplastics** may ↓ antibody response.

Route/Dosage

IM (Adults and Children —males and females 9–26 yr): *Gardasil and Gardasil 9*—Three 0.5 mL doses at 0, 2, and 6 mo.
IM (Adults and Children —females 9–25 yr): *Cervarix*—Three 0.5 mL doses at 0, 2, and 6 mo.

Availability

Sterile preparation for intramuscular administration (Gardasil): 20 mcg of HPV 6 L1 protein, 40 mcg of HPV 11 L1 protein, 40 mcg of HPV 16 L1 protein, and 20 mcg of HPV 18 L1 protein/0.5-mL dose. **Sterile preparation for intramuscular administration (Gardasil 9):** 30 mcg of HPV 6 L1 protein, 40 mcg of HPV 11 L1 protein, 60 mcg of HPV 16 L1 protein, 40 mcg of HPV 18 L1 protein, 20 mcg of HPV 31 L1 protein, 20 mcg of HPV 33 L1 protein, 20 mcg of HPV 45 L1 protein, 20 mcg of HPV 52 L1 protein, and 20 mcg of HPV 58 L1 protein/0.5-mL dose. **Sterile preparation for intramuscular administration (Cervarix):** 20 mcg of HPV type 16 L1 protein and 20 mcg of HPV type 18 L1 protein.

NURSING IMPLICATIONS

Assessment

- Assess vital signs prior to administration. Do not administer to patient with a current or recent febrile illness; low grade fever (<100°F) and mild upper respiratory infection are usually not contraindicated.
- Monitor patient for 15 min following injection for fainting. Patient should remain lying down or seated to prevent falls or injury.

Implementation

- Vaccine is not intended for treatment of active genital warts or cervical cancer and will not protect from diseases not caused by HPV.
- **IM:** *Gardasil and Gardisil 9:* Prefilled syringe is for single use; do not use for more than one person. Administer as supplied; do not dilute; administer full dose. Shake well prior to administration to maintain suspension of vaccine. Solution is cloudy and white; do not administer solution that is discolored or contains particulate matter. If using single-dose vial, withdraw 0.5 mL dose and administer entire contents of syringe. Administer intramuscularly in the deltoid or in the high anterolateral area of the thigh.
- **IM:** *Cervarix:* Prefilled syringe is for single use; do not use for more than one person. Administer as supplied; do not dilute; administer full dose. Shake vial or syringe well before use. Solution is a turbid, white suspension; do not administer if it is discolored or contains particulate matter. The tip cap and rubber plunger of needleless prefilled syringes contain dry natural latex rubber; may cause allergic reactions in latex sensitive individuals. Vial stopper does not contain latex.

H

Patient/Family Teaching

- Provide information about vaccine and the importance of completing immunization series, unless contraindicated, to patient and guardian.
- Inform patient that vaccine does not replace routine cervical cancer screening or prevent other sexually transmitted diseases; such screening should be continued as usual.
- Advise patient to notify health care professional of all Rx or OTC medications, vitamins, or herbal products being taken and to consult with health care professional before taking other medications.
- Rep: Advise patient to notify health care professional if pregnancy is planned or suspected. Women exposed to *Gardasil or Gardisil 9* vaccine during pregnancy are encouraged to call manufacturer pregnancy registry at 800-986-8999. Women exposed to *Cervarix* vaccine during pregnancy are encouraged to call manufacturer pregnancy registry at 800-452-9622.
- Instruct patient to report any adverse reactions to health care professional.

Evaluation/Desired Outcomes

- Prevention of cervical cancer, genital warts, cervical adenocarcinoma in situ, cervical, vulvar, anal, and vaginal intraepithelial neoplasia caused by HPV.

hydrALAZINE

(hye-**dral**-a-zeen)
Apresoline

Classification
Therapeutic: antihypertensives
Pharmacologic: vasodilators

Indications

Moderate to severe hypertension (with a diuretic). **Unlabeled Use:** HF unresponsive to conventional therapy with digoxin and diuretics.

Action

Direct-acting peripheral arteriolar vasodilator. **Therapeutic Effects:** Lowering of BP in hypertensive patients and decreased afterload in patients with HF.

Pharmacokinetics

Absorption: Rapidly absorbed following oral administration; well absorbed from IM sites.
Distribution: Widely distributed. Crosses the placenta; enters breast milk in minimal concentrations.
Metabolism and Excretion: Mostly metabolized by the GI mucosa and liver by N-acetyltransferase (rate of acetylation is genetically determined [slow acetylators have ↑ hydralazine levels and ↑ risk of toxicity; fast acetylators have ↓ hydralazine levels and ↓ response]).
Half-life: 2–8 hr.

TIME/ACTION PROFILE (antihypertensive effect)

ROUTE	ONSET	PEAK	DURATION
PO	45 min	2 hr	2–4 hr
IM	10–30 min	1 hr	3–8 hr
IV	5–20 min	15–30 min	2–6 hr

Contraindications/Precautions

Contraindicated in: Hypersensitivity; Some products contain tartrazine and should be avoided in patients with known intolerance.
Use Cautiously in: Cardiovascular or cerebrovascular disease; Severe renal and hepatic impairment (dose modification may be necessary); OB, Lactation: Has been used safely during pregnancy.

Adverse Reactions/Side Effects

CNS: dizziness, drowsiness, headache. **CV:** tachycardia, angina, arrhythmias, edema, orthostatic hypotension. **GI:** diarrhea, nausea, vomiting. **Derm:** rash. **MS:** arthralgias, arthritis. **Neuro:** peripheral neuropathy. **Misc:** drug-induced lupus syndrome.

Interactions

Drug-Drug: ↑ hypotension with acute ingestion of **alcohol**, other **antihypertensives**, or **nitrates**. **MAO inhibitors** may exaggerate hypotension. May ↓ pressor response to **epinephrine**. **NSAIDs** may ↓ antihypertensive response. **Beta blockers** ↓ tachycardia from hydralazine (therapy may be combined for this reason). **Metoprolol** and **propranolol** ↑ levels. ↑ levels of **metoprolol** and **propranolol**.

Route/Dosage

PO (Adults): *Hypertension*—10 mg 4 times daily initially. After 2–4 days may ↑ to 25 mg 4 times daily for the rest of the 1st wk; may then ↑ to 50 mg 4 times daily (up to 300 mg/day). Once maintenance dose is established, twice-daily dosing may be used. *HF*—25–37.5 mg 4 times daily; may be ↑ up to 300 mg/day in 3–4 divided doses.
PO (Children >1 mo): Initial—0.75–1 mg/kg/day in 2–4 divided doses, not to exceed 25 mg/dose; may ↑ gradually to 5 mg/kg/day in infants and 7.5 mg/kg/day in children (not to exceed 200 mg/day) in 2–4 divided doses.
IM, IV (Adults): *Hypertension*—5–40 mg repeated as needed. *Eclampsia*—5 mg every 15–20 min; if no response after a total of 20 mg, consider an alternative agent.
IM, IV (Children >1 mo): Initial—0.1–0.2 mg/kg/dose (not to exceed 20 mg) every 4–6 hr as needed, up to 1.7–3.5 mg/kg/day in 4–6 divided doses.

Availability (generic available)

Tablets: 10 mg, 25 mg, 50 mg, 100 mg. **Injection:** 20 mg/mL. ***In combination with:*** isosorbide dinitrate (BiDil). See Appendix B.

NURSING IMPLICATIONS

Assessment

- Monitor BP and pulse frequently during initial dose adjustment and periodically during therapy. About 50–65% of Caucasians, Black, South Indians, and Mexicans are slow acetylators at risk for toxicity, while 80–90% of Eskimos, Japanese, and Chinese are rapid acetylators at risk for decreased levels and treatment failure.
- Monitor frequency of prescription refills to determine adherence.
- ***Lab Test Considerations:*** Monitor CBC, electrolytes, LE cell prep, and ANA titer prior to and periodically during prolonged therapy.
- May cause a positive direct Coombs' test result.

Implementation

- Do not confuse hydralazine with hydroxyzine or hydrochlorothiazide.
- IM or IV route should be used only when drug cannot be given orally.
- May be administered concurrently with diuretics or beta blockers to permit lower doses and minimize side effects.
- **PO:** Administer with meals consistently to enhance absorption.
- Pharmacist may prepare oral solution from hydralazine injection for patients with difficulty swallowing.

IV Administration

- **IV Push:** ***Diluent:*** Administer undiluted. Use solution as quickly as possible after drawing through needle into syringe. ***Concentration:*** 20 mg/mL. ***Rate:*** Administer over at least 1 min. Pedi: Administer at a rate of 0.2 mg/kg/min in children. Monitor BP and pulse in all patients frequently after injection.
- **Y-Site Compatibility:** alemtuzumab, amiodarone, anidulafungin, argatroban, bivalirudin, bleomycin, carmustine, cyclophosphamide, dacarbazine, dactinomycin, daptomycin, daunorubicin hydrochloride, dexrazoxane, diltiazem, docetaxel, etoposide, etoposide phosphate, fenoldopam, fludarabine, gemcitabine, granisetron, hetastarch, hydromorphone, idarubicin, irinotecan, leucovorin, linezolid, mesna,

metronidazole, milrinone, mitomycin, mitoxantrone, moxifloxacin, mycophenolate, octreotide, oxaliplatin, paclitaxel, palonosetron, pamidronate, pancuronium, prochlorperazine, tacrolimus, thiotepa, tirofiban, topotecan, vecuronium, vinblastine, vincristine, vinorelbine, vitamin B complex with C, voriconazole, zoledronic acid.

- **Y-Site Incompatibility:** acyclovir, amphotericin B deoxycholate, amphotericin B lipid complex, ampicillin/sulbactam, ascorbic acid, azathioprine, cefazolin, cefotaxime, cefotetan, cefoxitin, ceftazidime, ceftriaxone, cefuroxime, dantrolene, diazepam, doxorubicin liposomal, ertapenem, folic acid, foscarnet, fosphenytoin, ganciclovir, haloperidol, indomethacin, lorazepam, methylprednisolone, multivitamins, nafcillin, nitroprusside, oxacillin, pantoprazole, pemetrexed, pentobarbital, phenytoin, piperacillin/tazobactam, potassium acetate, sodium acetate, tigecycline, trimethoprim/sulfamethoxazole.

Patient/Family Teaching

- Emphasize the importance of continuing to take this medication, even if feeling well. Instruct patient to take medication at the same time each day; last dose of the day should be taken at bedtime. Take missed doses as soon as remembered; do not double doses. If more than 2 doses in a row are missed, consult health care professional. Must be discontinued gradually to avoid sudden increase in BP. Hydralazine controls but does not cure hypertension.
- Encourage patient to comply with additional interventions for hypertension (weight reduction, low-sodium diet, smoking cessation, moderation of alcohol intake, regular exercise, and stress management). Instruct patient and family on proper technique for BP monitoring. Advise them to check BP at least weekly and report significant changes.
- Patients should weigh themselves twice weekly and assess feet and ankles for fluid retention.
- May occasionally cause drowsiness. Advise patient to avoid driving or other activities requiring alertness until response to medication is known.
- Caution patient to avoid sudden changes in position to minimize orthostatic hypotension.
- Advise patient to notify health care professional of all Rx or OTC medications, vitamins, or herbal products being taken and to consult with health care professional before taking other medications, especially cough, cold, or allergy remedies.
- Instruct patient to notify health care professional of medication prior to treatment or surgery.
- Advise patient to notify health care professional immediately if general tiredness; fever; muscle or joint aching; chest pain; skin rash; sore throat; or numbness, tingling, pain, or weakness of hands and feet occurs. Vitamin B_6 (pyridoxine) may be used to treat peripheral neuritis.
- Advise patient to notify health care professional if pregnancy is planned or suspected or if breast feeding.
- Emphasize the importance of follow-up exams to evaluate effectiveness of medication.

Evaluation/Desired Outcomes

- Decrease in BP without appearance of side effects.
- Decreased afterload in patients with HF.

hydralazine/isosorbide dinitrate

(hye-**dral**-a-zeen eye-so-**sor**-bide di-**ni**-trate)

BiDil

Classification

Therapeutic: vasodilators

Pharmacologic: vasodilators, nitrates

Indications

Management of heart failure in black patients.

Action

BiDil is a fixed-dose combination of **isosorbide dinitrate**, a vasodilator with effects on both arteries and veins, and **hydralazine**, a predominantly arterial vasodilator. **Therapeutic Effects:** Improved survival, increased time to hospitalization and decreased symptoms of heart failure in black patients.

Pharmacokinetics

See pharmacokinetic sections in hydralazine and isosorbide dinitrate monographs of Davis's Drug Guide for Nurses for more information.

Absorption: *Hydralazine*— 10–26% absorbed in HF patients, absorption can be saturated leading to large ↑ in absorption with higher doses; *isosorbide dinitrate*—variable absorbed (10–90%) reflecting first-pass hepatic metabolism.

Distribution: *Hydralazine*—widely distributed, crosses the placenta, minimal amounts in breast milk; *isosorbide dinitrate*—accumulates in muscle and venous wall.

Metabolism and Excretion: *Hydralazine*—mostly metabolized by GI mucosa and liver; *isosorbide dinitrate*—undergoes extensive first-pass metabolism in the liver, mostly metabolized by the liver, some metabolites are vasodilators.

Half-life: *Hydralazine*—4 hr; *isosorbide dinitrate*—2 hr.

TIME/ACTION PROFILE (effect on BP)

ROUTE	ONSET	PEAK	DURATION
hydralazine	45 min	2 hr	2–4 hr
isosorbide	15–40 min	unknown	4 hr

Contraindications/Precautions

Contraindicated in: Hypersensitivity to either component; Concurrent use of PDE-5 inhibitor (avanafil, sildenafil, tadalafil, vardenafil) or riociguat.

Use Cautiously in: Severe renal/hepatic impairment (dose modification may be necessary); Head trauma or cerebral hemorrhage; OB: Safety not established; Lactation: Use while breast feeding only if potential maternal benefit justifies potential risk to infant; Pedi: Safety and effectiveness not established; Geri: Start with lower doses.

Adverse Reactions/Side Effects

Hydralazine **CNS:** dizziness, drowsiness, headache. **CV:** tachycardia, angina, arrhythmias, edema, orthostatic hypotension. **Derm:** rash. **F and E:** sodium retention. **GI:** diarrhea, nausea, vomiting. **MS:** arthralgias, arthritis. **Neuro:** peripheral neuritis. **Misc:** drug-induced lupus syndrome.

Isosorbide Dinitrate

CNS: dizziness, headache, apprehension, weakness. **CV:** hypotension, tachycardia, paradoxic bradycardia, syncope. **GI:** abdominal pain, nausea, vomiting. **Misc:** flushing, tolerance.

Interactions

Drug-Drug: Concurrent use of **avanafil**, **sildenafil**, **tadalafil**, or **vardenafil** may result in severe hypotension; concurrent use contraindicated. Concurrent use of **riociguat** may result in severe hypotension; concurrent use contraindicated. ↑ risk of hypotension with other **antihypertensives**, acute ingestion of **alcohol**, and **phenothiazines**. **MAO inhibitors** may exaggerate hypotension. May ↓ the pressor response to **epinephrine**. **Beta blockers** ↓ tachycardia from hydralazine (therapy may be combined for this reason). **Metoprolol** and **propranolol** may ↑ hydralazine levels. Hydralazine ↑ levels of **metoprolol** and **propranolol**.

Route/Dosage

PO (Adults): 1 tablet 3 times daily, may be ↑ to 2 tablets 3 times daily.

Availability

Tablets: hydralazine 37.5 mg/isosorbide dinitrate 20 mg.

NURSING IMPLICATIONS

Assessment

- Monitor BP and pulse routinely during period of dose adjustment. Symptomatic hypotension may occur even with small doses. Use caution with patients who are volume depleted or hypotensive.
- Assess for signs and symptoms of peripheral neuritis (paresthesia, numbness, tingling) periodically during therapy. Adding pyridoxine may cause symptoms to decrease.
- ***Lab Test Considerations:*** If symptoms of systemic lupus erythematosus (SLE) occur obtain a CBC and ANA titer. If positive for SLE, carefully weigh risks/benefits of continued therapy.

Implementation

- Dose may be titrated rapidly over 3–5 days, but may need to decrease if side effects occur. May decrease to one-half tablet 3 times daily if intolerable side effects occur. Titrate up as soon as side effects subside.

Patient/Family Teaching

- Instruct patient to take medication as directed on a regular schedule.
- Caution patient to make position changes slowly to minimize orthostatic hypotension.
- May cause dizziness. Caution patient to avoid driving or other activities requiring alertness until response to medication is known.
- Advise patient to avoid concurrent use of alcohol or medications for erectile dysfunction with this medication. Patient should also consult health care professional before taking Rx, OTC, or herbal products while taking this medication.
- Caution patient that inadequate fluid intake or excessive fluid loss from perspiration, diarrhea, or vomiting may lead to a fall in BP, dizziness, or syncope. If syncope occurs, discontinue medication and notify health care professional promptly.
- Inform patient that headache is a common side effect that should decrease with continuing therapy. Aspirin or acetaminophen may be ordered to treat headache. Notify health care professional if headache is persistent or severe. Do not alter dose to avoid headache.
- Advise patient to notify health care professional if symptoms of systemic lupus erythematosus occur (arthralgia, fever, chest pain, prolonged malaise, or other unexplained symptoms).
- Advise female patient to notify health care professional if pregnancy is planned or suspected or if breast feeding.

Evaluation/Desired Outcomes

- Improved survival, increased time to hospitalization, and decreased symptoms of heart failure in black patients.

hydroCHLOROthiazide, See DIURETICS (THIAZIDE).

REMS HIGH ALERT

HYDROcodone

(hye-droe-**koe**-done)

Hysingla ER, Zohydro ER

HYDROcodone/Acetaminophen

Anexsia, Norco

HYDROcodone/Ibuprofen

Reprexain

Classification

Therapeutic: allergy, cold, and cough remedies (antitussive), opioid analgesics
Pharmacologic: opioid agonists/nonopioid analgesic combinations

Schedule II

For information on the acetaminophen and ibuprofen components of these formulations, see the acetaminophen and ibuprofen monographs

Indications

Extended-release product: Management of pain that is severe enough to warrant daily, around-the-clock, long-term opioid treatment where alternative treatment options are inadequate. **Combination products**: Management of moderate to severe pain. Antitussive (usually in combination products with decongestants).

Action

Bind to opiate receptors in the CNS. Alter the perception of and response to painful stimuli while producing generalized CNS depression. Suppress the cough reflex via a direct central action. **Therapeutic Effects:** Decrease in severity of moderate pain. Suppression of the cough reflex.

Pharmacokinetics

Absorption: Well absorbed following oral administration.
Distribution: Unknown.
Metabolism and Excretion: Mostly metabolized by the liver; eliminated in the urine (50–60% as metabolites, 10% as unchanged drug).
Half-life: 2.2 hr; *Extended-release*—8 hr.

TIME/ACTION PROFILE (analgesic effect)

ROUTE	ONSET	PEAK	DURATION
PO	10–30 min	30–60 min	4–6 hr
PO-ER	unknown	unknown	unknown

Contraindications/Precautions

Contraindicated in: Hypersensitivity to hydrocodone (cross-sensitivity may exist to other opioids); Significant respiratory depression; Paralytic ileus; Acute or severe bronchial asthma or hypercarbia; Congenital long QT syndrome (Hysingla only); Hypersensitivity to acetaminophen/ibuprofen (for combination products); Ibuprofen-containing products should be avoided in patients with bleeding disorders or thrombocytopenia; Acetaminophen-containing products should be avoided in patients with severe hepatic or renal disease; Ibuprofen-containing products should be avoided in patients undergoing coronary artery bypass graft surgery; OB, Lactation: Avoid chronic use; Products containing alcohol, aspartame, saccharin, sugar, or tartrazine (FDC yellow dye #5) should be avoided in patients who have hypersensitivity or intolerance to these compounds.
Use Cautiously in: Head trauma; ↑ intracranial pressure; Severe renal, hepatic, or pulmonary disease; Cardiovascular disease (ibuprofen-containing products only); History of peptic ulcer disease (ibuprofen-containing products only); Alcoholism; Difficulty swallowing; Patients with undiagnosed abdominal pain; Prostatic hyperplasia; OB: Labor and delivery; OB, Lactation: Avoid chronic use; prolonged use of opioids during pregnancy can result in neonatal opioid withdrawal syndrome; Geri: Geriatric or debilitated patients (initial dose ↓ required; more prone to CNS depression, constipation).

H

Adverse Reactions/Side Effects

Noted for hydrocodone only; see acetaminophen/ibuprofen monographs for specific information on individual components.
CNS: confusion, dizziness, sedation, euphoria, hallucinations, headache, unusual dreams. **EENT:** blurred vision, diplopia, miosis. **CV:** hypotension, bradycardia, QT interval prolongation (Hysingla only). **GI:** constipation, dyspepsia, nausea, choking, dysphagia, esophageal obstruction, vomiting. **GU:** urinary retention. **Endo:** adrenal insufficiency. **Derm:** sweating. **Resp:** RESPIRATORY DEPRESSION. **Misc:** physical dependence, psychological dependence, tolerance.

Interactions

Drug-Drug: Use with extreme caution in patients receiving **MAO inhibitors**; may produce severe, unpredictable reactions—do not use within 14 days of each other. Concurrent use of **CYP3A4 inhibitors** including **ritonavir**, **ketoconazole**, **itraconazole**, **fluconazole**, **clarithromycin**, **erythromycin**, **nefazodone**, **diltiazem**, **verapamil**, **nelfinavir**, and **fosamprenavir** ↑ levels and risk of opioid toxicity; careful monitoring during initiation, dose changes, or discontinuation of the inhibitor is recommended. Concurrent use with **CYP3A4 inducers** including **barbiturates**, **carbamazepine**, **efavirenz**, **corticosteroids**, **modafinil**, **nevirapine**, **oxcarbazepine**, **phenobarbital**, **phenytoin**, **rifabutin**, or **rifampin** may ↓ fentanyl levels and analgesia; if inducers are discontinued or dosage ↓, patients should be monitored for signs of opioid toxicity and necessary dose adjustments should be made. Use with **benzodiazepines** or other **CNS depressants** including other**opioids**, **non-benzodiazepine sedative/hypnotics**, **anxiolytics**, **general anesthetics**, **muscle relaxants**, **antipsychotics**, and **alcohol** may cause profound sedation, respiratory depression, coma, and death; reserve concurrent use for when alternative treatment options are inadequate. Administration of partial antagonist opioids (**buprenorphine**, **butorphanol**, or **nalbuphine**) may ↓ analgesia or precipitate opioid withdrawal in physically dependent patients. **Anticholinergic drugs** may ↑ risk of urinary retention and constipation. Drugs that affect serotonergic neurotransmitter systems, including **tricyclic antidepressants**, **SSRIs**, **SNRIs**, **MAO inhibitors**, **TCAs**, **tramadol**, **trazodone**, **mirtazapine**, **5–HT_3 receptor antagonists**, **linezolid**, **methylene blue**, and **triptans** ↑ risk of serotonin syndrome.

Drug-Natural Products: Concomitant use of **kava-kava**, **valerian**, **skullcap**, **chamomile**, or **hops** can ↑ CNS depression.

Route/Dosage

PO (Adults): *Analgesic (in combo products)*—2.5–10 mg every 3–6 hr as needed; if using combination products, acetaminophen dosage should not exceed 4 g/day and should not exceed 5 tablets/day of ibuprofen-containing products; *Antitussive*—5 mg every 4–6 hr as needed; *Extended-release (Zohydro ER)*—10 mg every 12 hr; may ↑ as needed in increments of 10 mg every 12 hr every 3–7 days; *Extended-release (Hysingla)*—20 mg once daily; may ↑ as needed in increments of 10–20 mg/day every 3–5 days.

Renal Impairment

PO (Adults): *CCr <45 mL/min*—Extended-release (Hysingla): ↓ initial dose by 50%.

Hepatic Impairment

PO (Adults): *Extended-release (Hysingla)*—↓ initial dose by 50%.

Availability

Hydrocodone (generic available)

Extended-release capsules (Zohydro ER) (abuse deterrent): 10 mg, 15 mg, 20 mg, 30 mg, 40 mg, 50 mg. **Extended-release tablets (Hysingla ER) (abuse deterrent):** 20 mg, 30 mg, 40 mg, 60 mg, 80 mg, 100 mg, 120 mg. **Syrup:** 🍁 1 mg/mL. ***In combination with:*** chlorpheniramine (Tussicaps, Tussionex, Vituz); chlorpheniramine and pseudoephedrine (Zutripro); guaifenesin (Obredon, Xtrelus); guaifenesin and pseudoephedrine (Hycofenix); pseudoephedrine (Rezira). See Appendix B.

Hydrocodone/Acetaminophen (generic available)

Tablets: 2.5 mg hydrocodone/325 mg acetaminophen, 5 mg hydrocodone/325 mg acetaminophen (Anexsia 5/325, Norco), 7.5 mg hydrocodone/325 mg acetaminophen (Anexsia 7.5/325, Norco), 10 mg hydrocodone/325 mg acetaminophen (Norco). **Cost:** *Generic*—5 mg/325 mg $15.08/100, 7.5 mg/325 mg $30.93/100, 10 mg/325 mg $41.59/100. **Elixir/oral solution:** 7.5 mg hydrocodone plus 325 mg acetaminophen/15 mL, 10 mg hydrocodone plus 325 mg acetaminophen/15 mL. **Cost:** *Generic*—$58.12/473 mL.

Hydrocodone/Ibuprofen (generic available)

Tablets: 2.5 mg hydrocodone/200 mg ibuprofen (Reprexain), 5 mg hydrocodone/200 mg ibuprofen, 7.5 mg hydrocodone/200 mg ibuprofen, 10 mg hydrocodone/200 mg ibuprofen (Reprexain). **Cost:** *Generic*—7.5 mg/200 mg $48.40/100.

NURSING IMPLICATIONS

Assessment

- Assess BP, pulse, and respirations before and periodically during administration. If respiratory rate is <10/min, assess level of sedation. Physical stimulation may be sufficient to prevent significant hypoventilation. Dose may need to be decreased by 25–50%. Initial drowsiness will diminish with continued use.
- Assess bowel function routinely. Prevention of constipation should be instituted with increased intake of fluids and bulk, and laxatives to minimize constipating effects. Stimulant laxatives should be administered routinely if opioid use exceeds 2–3 days, unless contraindicated. Consider drugs for opioid-induced constipation.
- **Pain:** Assess type, location, and intensity of pain prior to and 1 hr (peak) following administration. When titrating opioid doses, increases of 25–50% should be administered until there is either a 50% reduction in the patient's pain rating on a numerical or visual analogue scale or the patient reports satisfactory pain relief. A repeat dose can be safely administered at the time of the peak if previous dose is ineffective and side effects are minimal.
- Patients taking extended-release hydrocodone may require additional short-acting or rapid-onset opioid doses for breakthrough pain. Doses of short-acting opioids should be equivalent to 10–20% of 24 hr total and given every 2 hr as needed.
- An equianalgesic chart (see Appendix J) should be used when changing routes or when changing from one opioid to another.
- Prolonged use may lead to physical and psychological dependence and tolerance. This should not prevent patient from receiving adequate analgesia. Patients who receive opioids for pain rarely develop psychological dependence. If progressively higher doses are required, consider conversion to a stronger opioid.
- Assess risk for opioid addiction, abuse, or misuse prior to administration. Abuse or misuse of extended-release preparations by crushing, chewing, snorting, or injecting dissolved product will result in uncontrolled delivery of hydrocodone and can result in overdose and death. Hysingla ER and Zohydro ER are abuse deterrent formulations that are difficult to crush and, if crushed, result in a gel.
- **Cough:** Assess cough and lung sounds during antitussive use.

- ***Lab Test Considerations:*** May cause ↑ plasma amylase and lipase concentrations.
- ***Toxicity and Overdose:*** If an opioid antagonist is required to reverse respiratory depression or coma, naloxone is the antidote. Dilute the 0.4-mg ampule of naloxone in 10 mL of 0.9% NaCl and administer 0.5 mL (0.02 mg) by IV push every 2 min. For children and patients weighing <40 kg, dilute 0.1 mg of naloxone in 10 mL of 0.9% NaCl for a concentration of 10 mcg/mL and administer 0.5 mcg/kg every 2 min. Titrate dose to avoid withdrawal, seizures, and severe pain.

Implementation

- ***High Alert:*** Do not confuse hydrocodone with oxycodone. Do not confuse Reprexain (hydrocodone/ibuprofen) with Zyprexa (olanzapine).
- Explain therapeutic value of medication prior to administration to enhance the analgesic effect.
- Regularly administered doses may be more effective than prn administration. Analgesic is more effective if given before pain becomes severe.
- Combination with nonopioid analgesics may have additive analgesic effects and permit lower doses. Maximum doses of nonopioid agents limit the titration of hydrocodone doses.
- Medication should be discontinued gradually after long-term use to prevent withdrawal symptoms. For patients on long-acting agents who are physically opioid-dependent, initiate the taper by a small enough increment (e.g., no greater than 10% to 25% of total daily dose) to avoid withdrawal symptoms, and proceed with dose-lowering at an interval of every 2–4 wk. Patients who have been taking opioids for briefer periods of time may tolerate a more rapid taper.
- FDA strongly encourages health care professionals to complete a REMS-compliant education program that includes all the elements of the FDA Education *Blueprint for Health Care Providers Involved in the Management or Support of Patients with Pain,* available at www.fda.gov/OpioidAnalgesicREMSBlueprint. Information on programs can be found at 1-800-503-0784 or www.opioidanalgesicrems.com.
- **PO:** May be administered with food or milk to minimize GI irritation.
- Swallow extended-release capsules whole; do not open, crush, dissolve, or chew.

Patient/Family Teaching

- Advise patient to take medication as directed and not to take more than the recommended amount. Severe and permanent liver damage may result from prolonged use or high doses of acetaminophen. Renal damage may occur with prolonged use of acetaminophen or ibuprofen. Doses of nonopioid agents should not exceed the maximum recommended daily dose. Do not stop taking without discussing with health care professional; may cause withdrawal symptoms if discontinued abruptly after prolonged use. Discuss safe use, risks, and proper storage and disposal of opioid analgesics with patients and caregivers with each Rx. The Patient Counseling Guide (PCG) is available at www.fda.gov/OpioidAnalgesicREMSPCG.
- Instruct patient on how and when to ask for and take pain medication.
- Advise patient that hydrocodone is a drug with known abuse potential. Protect it from theft, and never give to anyone other than the individual for whom it was prescribed. Store out of sight and reach of children, and in a location not accessible by others.
- May cause drowsiness or dizziness. Advise patient to call for assistance when ambulating or smoking. Caution patient to avoid driving or other activities requiring alertness until response to the medication is known.
- Advise patient to notify health care professional if pain control is not adequate or if severe or persistent side effects occur.
- Advise patient to change positions slowly to minimize orthostatic hypotension.
- Caution patient to avoid concurrent use of alcohol or other CNS depressants with this medication.
- Instruct patient to notify health care professional of all Rx or OTC medications, vitamins, or herbal products being taken and consult health care professional before taking any new medications.
- Emphasize the importance of aggressive prevention of constipation with the use of hydrocodone.
- Encourage patient to turn, cough, and breathe deeply every 2 hr to prevent atelectasis.
- Advise patient that good oral hygiene, frequent mouth rinses, and sugarless gum or candy may decrease dry mouth.
- Rep: Advise patient to notify health care professional if pregnancy is planned or suspected, or if breast feeding. Inform patient of potential for neonatal opioid withdrawal syndrome with prolonged use during pregnancy. Monitor neonate for signs and symptoms of withdrawal symptoms (irritability, hyperactivity and abnormal sleep pattern, high pitched cry, tremor, vomiting, diarrhea, and/or failure to gain weight); usually occur the first days after birth.

Evaluation/Desired Outcomes

- Decrease in severity of pain without a significant alteration in level of consciousness or respiratory status.
- Suppression of nonproductive cough.

hydrocortisone, See CORTICOSTEROIDS (SYSTEMIC).

hydrocortisone, See CORTICOSTEROIDS (TOPICAL/LOCAL).

REMS HIGH ALERT

HYDROmorphone

(hye-droe-**mor**-fone)

Dilaudid, ~~Dilaudid-HP~~, ~~Exalgo~~,

🍁Hydromorph Contin

Classification

Therapeutic: allergy, cold, and cough remedies (antitussives), opioid analgesics

Pharmacologic: opioid agonists

Schedule II

Indications

Moderate to severe pain (alone and in combination with nonopioid analgesics). Moderate to severe chronic pain in opioid-tolerant patients requiring use of daily, around-the-clock long-term opioid treatment and for which alternative treatment options are inadequate (extended-release). Antitussive (lower doses).

Action

Binds to opiate receptors in the CNS. Alters the perception of and response to painful stimuli while producing generalized CNS depression. Suppresses the cough reflex via a direct central action. **Therapeutic Effects:** Decrease in moderate to severe pain. Suppression of cough.

Pharmacokinetics

Absorption: Well absorbed following oral, rectal, subcut, and IM administration. Extended-release product results in an initial release of drug, followed by a 2nd sustained phase of absorption.

Distribution: Widely distributed. Crosses the placenta; enters breast milk.

Metabolism and Excretion: Mostly metabolized by the liver.

Half-life: *Oral (immediate-release), or injection*—2–4 hr; *Oral (extended-release)*—8–15 hr.

TIME/ACTION PROFILE (analgesic effect)

ROUTE	ONSET	PEAK	DURATION
PO-IR	30 min	30–90 min	4–5 hr
PO-ER	unknown	unknown	unknown
Subcut	15 min	30–90 min	4–5 hr
IM	15 min	30–60 min	4–5 hr
IV	10–15 min	15–30 min	2–3 hr
Rect	15–30 min	30–90 min	4–5 hr

Contraindications/Precautions

Contraindicated in: Hypersensitivity; Some products contain bisulfites and should be avoided in patients with known hypersensitivity; Severe respiratory depression (in absence of resuscitative equipment) (extended-release only); Acute or severe bronchial asthma (extended-release only); Paralytic ileus (extended-release only); Acute, mild, intermittent, or postoperative pain (extended-release only); Prior GI surgery or narrowing of GI tract (extended-release only); Opioid non-tolerant patients (extended-release only); Severe hepatic impairment (extended-release only).

Use Cautiously in: Head trauma; ↑ intracranial pressure; Severe pulmonary disease; Moderate or severe renal disease (extended-release only) (dose ↓ recommended); Moderate hepatic impairment (extended-release only) (dose ↓ recommended); Hypothyroidism; Seizure disorder; Adrenal insufficiency; Alcoholism; Undiagnosed abdominal pain; Prostatic hypertrophy; Biliary tract disease (including pancreatitis); OB: Labor and delivery; OB, Lactation: Avoid chronic use; prolonged use of opioids during pregnancy can result in neonatal opioid withdrawal syndrome; Geri: Geriatric or debilitated patients (↑ risk of respiratory depression; dose ↓ suggested).

Adverse Reactions/Side Effects

CNS: confusion, sedation, dizziness, dysphoria, euphoria, floating feeling, hallucinations, headache, unusual dreams. **CV:** hypotension, bradycardia. **Derm:** flushing, sweating. **EENT:** blurred vision, diplopia, miosis. **Endo:** adrenal insufficiency. **GI:** constipation, dry mouth, nausea, vomiting. **GU:** urinary retention. **Resp:** RESPIRATORY DEPRESSION. **Misc:** physical dependence, psychological dependence, tolerance.

Interactions

Drug-Drug: Exercise extreme caution with **MAO inhibitors** (may produce severe, unpredictable reactions—reduce initial dose of hydromorphone to 25% of usual dose, discontinue MAO inhibitors 2 wk prior to hydromorphone). Use with **benzodiazepines** or other **CNS depressants** including other **opioids**, **non-benzodiazepine sedative/hypnotics**, **anxiolytics**, **general anesthetics**, **muscle relaxants**, **antipsychotics**, and **alcohol** may cause profound sedation, respiratory depression, coma, and death; reserve concurrent use for when alternative treatment options are inadequate. Administration of partial antagonists (**buprenorphine**, **butorphanol**, or **nalbuphine**) may precipitate opioid withdrawal in physically dependent patients. **Nalbuphine** may ↓ analgesia. Drugs that affect serotonergic neurotransmitter systems, including **tricyclic antidepressants**, **SSRIs**, **SNRIs**, **MAO inhibitors**, **TCAs**, **tramadol**, **trazodone**, **mirtazapine**, **5-HT$_3$ receptor antagonists**, **linezolid**, **methylene blue**, and **triptans** ↑ risk of serotonin syndrome.

Drug-Natural Products: Concomitant use of **kava-kava**, **valerian**, **chamomile**, or **hops** can ↑ CNS depression.

Route/Dosage

Doses depend on level of pain and tolerance. Larger doses may be required during chronic therapy.

Analgesic

PO (Adults ≥50 kg): *Immediate-release*—4–8 mg every 3–4 hr initially (some patients may respond to doses as small as 2 mg initially); *or* once 24-hr opioid requirement is determined, convert to *extended-release* by administering total daily oral dose once daily.
PO (Adults and Children <50 kg): 0.06 mg/kg every 3–4 hr initially, younger children may require smaller initial doses of 0.03 mg/kg. Maximum dose 5 mg.
IV, IM, Subcut (Adults ≥50 kg): 1.5 mg every 3–4 hr as needed initially; may be ↑.
IV, IM, Subcut (Adults and Children <50 kg): 0.015 mg/kg mg every 3–4 hr as needed initially; may be ↑.
IV (Adults): *Continuous infusion (unlabeled)*—0.2–3 mg/hr depending on previous opioid use. An initial bolus of twice the hourly rate in mg may be given with subsequent breakthrough boluses of 50–100% of the hourly rate in mg.
Rect (Adults): 3 mg every 6–8 hr initially as needed.

Hepatic Impairment

PO (Adults): *Moderate hepatic impairment (extended–release)*—↓ initial dose by 75%.

Renal Impairment

PO (Adults): *Moderate renal impairment (extended–release)*—↓ initial dose by 50%; *Severe renal impairment (extended–release)*—↓ initial dose by 75%.

Antitussive

PO (Adults and Children >12 yr): 1 mg every 3–4 hr.
PO (Children 6–12 yr): 0.5 mg every 3–4 hr.

Availability (generic available)

Controlled-release capsules: 🍁3 mg, 🍁4.5 mg, 🍁6 mg, 🍁9 mg, 🍁12 mg, 🍁18 mg, 🍁24 mg, 🍁30 mg. **Extended-release tablets (abuse-deterrent):** 8 mg, 12 mg, 16 mg, 32 mg. **Oral solution:** 1 mg/mL. **Rectal suppositories:** 3 mg. **Solution for injection (requires dilution):** 1 mg/mL, 2 mg/mL, 4 mg/mL, 10 mg/mL. **Tablets:** 2 mg, 4 mg, 8 mg.

NURSING IMPLICATIONS

Assessment

- Assess BP, pulse, and respirations before and periodically during administration. If respiratory rate is <10/min, assess level of sedation. Dose may need to be decreased by 25–50%. Initial drowsiness will diminish with continued use. Geri, Pedi: Assess geriatric and pediatric patients frequently; more sensitive to the effects of opioid analgesics and may experience side effects and respiratory complications more frequently.
- Assess bowel function routinely. Institute prevention of constipation with increased intake of fluids and bulk, and laxatives to minimize constipating effects. Administer stimulant laxatives routinely if opioid use exceeds 2–3 days, unless contraindicated. Consider drugs for opioid induced constipation.
- **Pain:** Assess type, location, and intensity of pain prior to and 1 hr following IM or PO and 5 min (peak) following IV administration. When titrating opioid doses, increases of 25–50% should be administered until there is either a 50% reduction in the patient's pain rating on a numerical or visual analogue scale or the patient reports satisfactory pain relief. When titrating doses of short-acting hydromorphone, a repeat dose can be safely administered at the time of the peak if previous dose is ineffective and side effects are minimal.
- Patients on a continuous infusion should have additional bolus doses provided every 15–30 min, as needed, for breakthrough pain. The bolus dose is usually set to the amount of drug infused each hr by continuous infusion.
- Patients taking extended-release hydromorphone may require additional short-acting or rapid-onset opioid doses for breakthrough pain. Doses of short-acting opioids should be equivalent to 10–20% of 24 hr total and given every 2 hr as needed.
- An equianalgesic chart (see Appendix J) should be used when changing routes or when changing from one opioid to another.
- Prolonged use may lead to physical and psychological dependence and tolerance. This should not prevent patient from receiving adequate analgesia. Patients who receive hydromorphone for pain rarely develop psychological dependence. Progressively higher doses may be required to relieve pain with long-term therapy.
- Assess risk for opioid addiction, abuse, or misuse prior to administration. Abuse or misuse of extended-release preparations by crushing, chewing, snorting, or injecting dissolved product will result in uncontrolled delivery of hydromorphone and can result in overdose and death.
- **Cough:** Assess cough and lung sounds during antitussive use.
- ***Lab Test Considerations:*** May ↑ plasma amylase and lipase concentrations.
- ***Toxicity and Overdose:*** If an opioid antagonist is required to reverse respiratory depression or coma,

naloxone (Narcan) is the antidote. Dilute the 0.4-mg ampule of naloxone in 10 mL of 0.9% NaCl and administer 0.5 mL (0.02 mg) by IV push every 2 min. For children and patients weighing <40 kg, dilute 0.1 mg of naloxone in 10 mL of 0.9% NaCl for a concentration of 10 mcg/mL and administer 0.5 mcg every 2 min. Titrate dose to avoid withdrawal, seizures, and severe pain.

Implementation

- ***High Alert:*** Accidental overdose of opioid analgesics has resulted in fatalities. Before administering, check infusion pump settings. Pedi: Medication errors with opioid analgesics are common in pediatric patients; calculate doses carefully. Use appropriate measuring devices.
- ***High Alert:*** Do not confuse hydromorphone with buprenorphine, morphine, or oxymorphone; fatalities have occurred. Do not confuse high-potency (HP) dose forms with regular dose forms.
- Explain therapeutic value of medication prior to administration to enhance the analgesic effect.
- Regularly administered doses may be more effective than prn administration. Analgesic is more effective if given before pain becomes severe.
- Coadministration with nonopioid analgesics may have additive analgesic effects and permit lower opioid doses.
- Medication should be discontinued gradually after long-term use to prevent withdrawal symptoms. For patients on long-acting agents who are physically opioid-dependent, initiate the taper by a small enough increment (e.g., no greater than 10% to 25% of total daily dose) to avoid withdrawal symptoms, and proceed with dose-lowering at an interval of every 2–4 wks. Patients who have been taking opioids for briefer periods of time may tolerate a more rapid taper.
- When converting from immediate-release to extended-release hydromorphone administer total daily oral hydromorphone dose once daily; dose of extended-release product can be titrated every 3–4 days. To convert from another opioid to extended-release hydromorphone, convert to total daily dose of hydromorphone and then administer 50% of this dose as extended-release hydromorphone once daily; can then titrate dose every 3–4 days. When converting from transdermal fentanyl, initiate extended-release hydromorphone 18 hr after removing transdermal fentanyl patch; for each 25 mcg/hr fentanyl transdermal dose, the equianalgesic dose of extended-release hydromorphone is 12 mg once daily (should initiate at 50% of this calculated total daily dose given once daily).
- **PO:** May be administered with food or milk to minimize GI irritation.
- Swallow extended-release tablets whole; do not break, crush, dissolve, or chew.
- FDA strongly encourages health care professionals to complete a REMS-compliant education program that includes all the elements of the FDA Education *Blueprint for Health Care Providers Involved in the Management or Support of Patients with Pain,* available at www.fda.gov/OpioidAnalgesicREMSBlueprint. Information on programs can be found at 1-800-503-0784 or www.opioidanalgesicrems.com.

IV Administration

- **IV Push:** ***Diluent:*** Dilute with at least 5 mL of sterile water or 0.9% NaCl for injection. Inspect solution for particulate matter. Slight yellow color does not alter potency. Store at room temperature. ***Rate:*** Administer slowly, at a rate not to exceed 2 mg over 3–5 min. ***High Alert:*** Rapid administration may lead to increased respiratory depression, hypotension, and circulatory collapse.
- **Y-Site Compatibility:** acetaminophen, acyclovir, alemtuzumab, allopurinol, amifostine, amikacin, aminocaproic acid, aminophylline, amiodarone, amphotericin B lipid complex, amphotericin B liposome, ampicillin/sulbactam, amsacrine, anidulafungin, argatroban, arsenic trioxide, atracurium, atropine, azithromycin, aztreonam, bivalirudin, bleomycin, bumetanide, busulfan, calcium chloride, calcium gluconate, cangrelor, carboplatin, carmustine, caspofungin, cefepime, cefotaxime, cefotetan, cefoxitin, ceftaroline, ceftazidime, ceftolozane/tazobactam, ceftriaxone, cefuroxime, chloramphenicol, chlorpromazine, ciprofloxacin, cisatracurium, cisplatin, cladribine, clindamycin, cyclophosphamide, cyclosporine, cytarabine, dacarbazine, dactinomycin, daptomycin, daunorubicin hydrochloride, dexamethasone, dexmedetomidine, dexrazoxane, digoxin, diltiazem, diphenhydramine, dobutamine, docetaxel, dolasetron, dopamine, doxorubicin, doxorubicin liposome, doxycycline, droperidol, enalaprilat, ephedrine, epinephrine, epirubicin, eptifibatide, ertapenem, erythromycin, esmolol, etoposide, etoposide phosphate, famotidine, fenoldopam, fentanyl, filgrastim, fluconazole, fludarabine, fluorouracil, foscarnet, fosphenytoin, furosemide, ganciclovir, gemcitabine, gemtuzumab, gentamicin, glycopyrrolate, granisetron, haloperidol, heparin, hetastarch, hydralazine, hydrocortisone, idarubicin, ifosfamide, imipenem/cilastatin, insulin, regular, irinotecan, isavuconazonium, isoproterenol, ketorolac, labetalol, leucovorin calcium, levofloxacin, lidocaine, linezolid, lorazepam, magnesium sulfate, mannitol, melphalan, meropenem, meropenem/vaborbactam, mesna, methohexital, methotrexate, methyldopate, methylprednisolone, metoclopramide, metoprolol, micafungin, midazolam, milrinone, mitomycin, mitoxantrone, morphine, mycophenolate, nafcillin, naloxone, nicardipine, nitroglycerin, nitroprusside, norepinephrine, octreotide, ondansetron, oxacillin, oxaliplatin, oxytocin, paclitaxel, palonosetron, pamidronate, pancuronium, pemetrexed, penicillin G potassium, pentamidine, pentobarbital, phenylephrine,

piperacillin/tazobactam, plazomicin, posaconazole, potassium acetate, potassium chloride, potassium phosphates, procainamide, prochlorperazine, promethazine, propofol, propranolol, quinupristin/dalfopristin, ranitidine, remifentanil, rituximab, rocuronium, scopolamine, sodium acetate, sodium phosphates, streptozocin, succinylcholine, tacrolimus, tedizolid, theophylline, thiotepa, tigecycline, tirofiban, tobramycin, topotecan, trastuzumab, trimethoprim/sulfamethoxazole, vancomycin, vasopressin, vecuronium, verapamil, vinblastine, vincristine, vinorelbine, zidovudine, zoledronic acid.

- **Y-Site Incompatibility:** amphotericin B deoxycholate, dantrolene, dimenhydrinate, minocycline, phenytoin, sargramostim, thiopental.

Patient/Family Teaching

- Instruct patient on how and when to ask for pain medication. Do not stop taking without discussing with health care professional; may cause withdrawal symptoms if discontinued abruptly after prolonged use. Discuss safe use, risks, and proper storage and disposal of opioid analgesics with patients and caregivers with each Rx. The Patient Counseling Guide (PCG) is available at www.fda.gov/OpioidAnalgesicREMSPCG.
- Advise patient that hydromorphone is a drug with known abuse potential. Protect it from theft, and never give to anyone other than the individual for whom it was prescribed. Store out of sight and reach of children, and in a location not accessible by others.
- May cause drowsiness or dizziness. Advise patient to call for assistance when ambulating or smoking. Caution patient to avoid driving or other activities requiring alertness until response to medication is known.
- Advise patient to notify health care professional if pain control is not adequate or if side effects occur.
- Advise patient to change positions slowly to minimize orthostatic hypotension.
- Instruct patient to avoid concurrent use of alcohol or other CNS depressants.
- Instruct patient to notify health care professional of all Rx or OTC medications, vitamins, or herbal products being taken and consult health care professional before taking any new medications.
- Encourage patient to turn, cough, and breathe deeply every 2 hr to prevent atelectasis.
- Rep: Advise patient to notify health care professional if pregnancy is planned or suspected, or if breast feeding. Inform patient of potential for neonatal opioid withdrawal syndrome with prolonged use during pregnancy. Monitor neonate for signs and symptoms of withdrawal symptoms (irritability, hyperactivity and abnormal sleep pattern, high pitched cry, tremor, vomiting, diarrhea, and/or failure to gain weight); usually occur the first days after birth.
- **Home Care Issues:** Explain to patient and family how and when to administer hydromorphone, discuss safe storage of medication, and how to care for infusion equipment properly. Pedi: Teach parents or caregivers how to accurately measure liquid medication and to use only measuring device dispensed with medication.
- Emphasize the importance of aggressive prevention of constipation with the use of hydromorphone.

Evaluation/Desired Outcomes

- Decrease in severity of pain without a significant alteration in level of consciousness or respiratory status.
- Suppression of cough.

hydroxocobalamin, See VITAMIN B_{12} PREPARATIONS.

hydroxychloroquine

(hye-drox-ee-**klor**-oh-kwin)

Plaquenil

Classification

Therapeutic: antimalarials, antirheumatics (DMARDs)

Indications

Treatment of uncomplicated malaria in geographic areas where chloroquine-resistance is not reported. Prophylaxis of malaria in geographic areas where chloroquine-resistance is not reported. Treatment of acute and chronic rheumatoid arthritis. Treatment of chronic discoid lupus erythematosus and systemic lupus erythematosus.

Action

Inhibits protein synthesis in susceptible organisms by inhibiting DNA and RNA polymerase. **Therapeutic Effects:** Death of plasmodia responsible for causing malaria. Also has anti-inflammatory properties. **Spectrum:** Active against chloroquine-sensitive strains of: *Plasmodium falciparum*, *Plasmodium malariae*, a-*Plasmodium ovale*, and *Plasmodium vivax*.

Pharmacokinetics

Absorption: Highly variable (31–100%) following oral administation.

Distribution: Widely distributed; high concentrations in RBCs; crosses the placenta; excreted into breast milk.

Metabolism and Excretion: Partially metabolized by the liver to active metabolites; partially excreted unchanged by the kidneys.

Half-life: 40 days.

TIME/ACTION PROFILE (blood levels)

ROUTE	ONSET	PEAK	DURATION
PO	rapid†	1–2 hr	days–wk

†Onset of antirheumatic action may take 6 wk.

Contraindications/Precautions

Contraindicated in: Hypersensitivity to hydroxychloroquine or chloroquine; Previous visual damage from hydroxychloroquine or chloroquine.

Use Cautiously in: Concurrent use of hepatotoxic drugs; Hepatic impairment or alcoholism; Use of high doses (>5 mg/kg base), duration of use >5 yr, renal impairment, concurrent use of tamoxifen or macular disease (↑ risk of retinopathy); G6PD deficiency; Psoriasis; Porphyria; Bone marrow depression; Obesity (determine dose by ideal body weight); OB, Lactation: Avoid use unless treating/preventing malaria or treating amebic abscess; Pedi: Safety and effectiveness for chronic use not established; Geri: ↓ renal function may ↑ risk of adverse reactions.

Adverse Reactions/Side Effects

CNS: SEIZURES, SUICIDAL THOUGHTS/BEHAVIORS, aggressiveness, anxiety, dizziness, fatigue, headache, irritability, nightmares, personality changes, psychoses. **CV:** HF, TORSADE DE POINTES, heart block, QT interval prolongation. **Derm:** DRUG REACTION WITH EOSINOPHILIA AND SYSTEMIC SYMPTOMS (DRESS), ERYTHEMA MULTIFORME, STEVENS-JOHNSON SYNDROME, TOXIC EPIDERMAL NECROLYSIS, acute generalized exanthematous pustulosis, alopecia, hair color changes, hyperpigmentation, photosensitivity, pruritus, rash, urticaria. **EENT:** corneal deposits, nystagmus, retinopathy, tinnitus, vertigo, visual disturbances. **Endo:** hypoglycemia. **GI:** HEPATOTOXICITY, abdominal pain, anorexia, diarrhea, ↑ liver enzymes, nausea, vomiting. **Hemat:** AGRANULOCYTOSIS, APLASTIC ANEMIA, leukopenia, thrombocytopenia. **Metab:** ↓ weight. **Neuro:** ataxia, dyskinesia, dystonia, neuromyopathy, peripheral neuritis, tremor. **Resp:** PULMONARY HYPERTENSION, bronchospasm. **Misc:** ANGIOEDEMA.

Interactions

Drug-Drug: Concurrent use of other **QT interval-prolonging drugs** may ↑ risk of torsade de pointes. May ↑ the risk of hepatotoxicity when administered with **hepatotoxic drugs**. May ↑ risk of hypoglycemia when used with **antidiabetic agents**. Use with **mefloquine** may ↑ risk of seizures. **Antacids** may bind to and ↓ the absorption of hydroxychloroquine; separate administration by ≥4 hr. **Cimetidine** may ↑ levels; avoid concurrent use. **Urinary acidifiers** may ↑ renal excretion. May ↑ levels of **digoxin** or **cyclosporine**.

Route/Dosage

200 mg hydroxychloroquine sulfate = 155 mg of hydroxychloroquine base.

Malaria

PO (Adults): *Prophylaxis*—400 mg sulfate (310 mg base) once weekly; start 2 wk prior to entering malarious area; continue for 4 wk after leaving area. *Treatment*—800 mg sulfate (620 mg base), then 400 mg sulfate (310 mg base) at 6 hr, 24 hr, and 48 hr after initial dose.

PO (Children ≥31 kg): *Prophylaxis*—6.5 mg/kg sulfate (5 mg/kg base) (not to exceed 400 mg sulfate [310 mg base]) once weekly; start 2 wk prior to entering malarious area; continue for 4 wk after leaving area. *Treatment*—13 mg/kg sulfate (10 mg/kg base) (not to exceed 800 mg sulfate [620 mg base]) initially, then 6.5 mg/kg sulfate (5 mg/kg base) (not to exceed 400 mg sulfate [310 mg base]) at 6 hr, 24 hr, and 48 hr after initial dose.

Rheumatoid Arthritis

PO (Adults): 400–600 mg sulfate (310–465 mg base) per day in 1–2 divided doses; once adequate response obtained, may ↓ dose to maintenance dose of 200–400 mg sulfate (155–310 mg base) per day in 1–2 divided doses.

Lupus Erythematosus

PO (Adults): 200–400 mg sulfate (155–310 mg base) per day in 1–2 divided doses.

Availability (generic available)

Tablets: 200 mg sulfate (155 mg base). **Cost:** *Generic*—$14.88/100.

NURSING IMPLICATIONS

Assessment

- Assess deep tendon reflexes periodically to determine muscle weakness. Therapy may be discontinued should this occur.
- Obtain baseline occular exam within first yr of therapy. Patients on prolonged high-dose therapy should have eye exams prior to and every 3–6 mo during therapy to detect retinal damage. Monitor patients without risk factors every 5 yrs. Retinal changes may progress even after therapy is completed.
- Monitor ECG for cardiomyopathy and QT prolongation periodically during therapy.
- Monitor for signs and symptoms of DRESS (fever, rash, lymphadenopathy, and/or facial swelling, associated with involvement of other organ systems (hepatitis, nephritis, hematologic abnormalities, myocarditis, myositis) during therapy. May resemble an acute viral infection. Eosinophilia is often present. Discontinue therapy if signs occur.
- Assess for rash periodically during therapy. May cause Stevens-Johnson syndrome. Discontinue therapy if severe or if accompanied with fever, general malaise, fatigue, muscle or joint aches, blisters, oral lesions, conjunctivitis, hepatitis and/or eosinophilia.
- Assess for suicidal tendencies, depression, or changes in behavior periodically during therapy.

- **Malaria or Lupus Erythematosus:** Assess patient for improvement in signs and symptoms of condition daily throughout course of therapy.
- **Rheumatoid Arthritis:** Assess patient monthly for pain, swelling, and range of motion.
- ***Lab Test Considerations:*** Monitor CBC and platelet count periodically throughout therapy. May cause decreased RBC, WBC, and platelet counts. If severe decreases occur that are not related to the disease process, hydroxychloroquine should be discontinued.
- Monitor liver function tests periodically during therapy.
- May cause hypoglycemia.

Implementation

- Do not confuse hydroxychloroquine with hydroxyurea.
- **PO:** Administer with milk or meals to minimize GI distress.
- Tablets may be crushed and placed inside empty capsules for patients with difficulty swallowing. Contents of capsules may also be mixed with a teaspoonful of jam, jelly, or Jell-O prior to administration.
- **Malaria Prophylaxis:** Hydroxychloroquine therapy should be started 2 wk prior to potential exposure and continued for 4–6 wk after leaving the malarious area.

Patient/Family Teaching

- Instruct patient to take medication exactly as directed and continue full course of therapy even if feeling better. Missed doses should be taken as soon as remembered unless it is almost time for next dose. Do not double doses.
- Advise patients to avoid use of alcohol while taking hydroxychloroquine.
- Caution patient to keep hydroxychloroquine out of reach of children; fatalities have occurred with ingestion of 3 or 4 tablets.
- Explain need for periodic ophthalmic exams for patients on prolonged high-dose therapy. Advise patient that the risk of ocular damage may be decreased by the use of dark glasses in bright light. Protective clothing and sunscreen should also be used to reduce risk of dermatoses.
- Advise patient to notify health care professional promptly if sore throat, fever, unusual bleeding or bruising, blurred vision, visual changes, ringing in the ears, difficulty hearing, or muscle weakness occurs.
- Advise female patient to notify health care professional if pregnancy is planned or suspected, or if breast feeding.
- **Malaria Prophylaxis:** Review methods of minimizing exposure to mosquitoes with patients receiving hydroxychloroquine prophylactically (use repellent, wear long-sleeved shirt and long trousers, use screen or netting).
- Advise patient to notify health care professional if fever develops while traveling or within 2 mo of leaving an endemic area.
- **Rheumatoid Arthritis:** Instruct patient to contact health care professional if no improvement is noticed within a few days. Treatment for rheumatoid arthritis may require up to 6 mo for full benefit.

Evaluation/Desired Outcomes

- Prevention or resolution of malaria.
- Improvement in signs and symptoms of rheumatoid arthritis.
- Improvement in symptoms of lupus erythematosus.

HYDROXYprogesterone caproate
(hye-drox-ee-pro-**jess**-te-rone **kap**-roe-ate)
Makena

Classification
Therapeutic: hormones
Pharmacologic: progestins

Indications

To ↓ the risk of preterm birth in women with a singleton pregnancy who have a history of previous singleton preterm birth.

Action

A synthetic analog of progesterone. Produces secretory changes in the endometrium. ↑s basal temperature. Produces changes in the vaginal epithelium. Relaxes uterine smooth muscle. Stimulates mammary alveolar growth. Inhibits pituitary function. Action in reducing risk of recurrent preterm birth is unknown. **Therapeutic Effects:** ↓ risk of preterm birth in women at risk.

Pharmacokinetics

Absorption: Slowly absorbed following IM administration.
Distribution: Unknown.
Protein Binding: Extensively bound to plasma proteins.
Metabolism and Excretion: Extensively metabolized by the liver.
Half-life: 7.8 days.

TIME/ACTION PROFILE (blood levels)

ROUTE	ONSET	PEAK	DURATION
IM	unknown	4.6 days	7 days

Contraindications/Precautions

Contraindicated in: Hypersensitivity to hydroxyprogesterone or castor oil; History of or known thrombosis/thromboembolic disorder; History of or known/suspected breast cancer or other hormone-sensitive cancer; Unexplained abnormal vaginal bleeding unrelated to pregnancy; Cholestatic jaundice of pregnancy; Benign/malignant liver tumors or active liver disease; Uncontrolled hypertension.

Use Cautiously in: Risk factors for thromboembolic disorders (may ↑ risk); Diabetes mellitus or risk factors for diabetes mellitus (may impair glucose tolerance); History of preeclampsia, epilepsy, cardiac or renal impairment (may be adversely affected by fluid retention); History of depression (may worsen); Safe and effective use in children <16 yr has not been established.

Adverse Reactions/Side Effects

CNS: depression. **CV:** hypertension. **Derm:** urticaria, pruritus. **F and E:** fluid retention. **GI:** diarrhea, jaundice, nausea. **Hemat:** THROMBOEMBOLISM. **Local:** injections site reactions. **Misc:** HYPERSENSITIVITY REACTIONS (including angioedema).

Interactions

Drug-Drug: May ↑ metabolism and ↓ blood levels and effectiveness of **drugs metabolized by the CYP1A2, CYP2A6, and CYP2B6 enzyme systems**.

Route/Dosage

IM (Adults): 250 mg once weekly starting between 16 wk, 0 days and 20 wk, 6 days continuing until wk 37 of gestation or delivery, whichever occurs first.

Subcut (Adults): 275 mg once weekly starting between 16 wk, 0 days and 20 wk, 6 days continuing until wk 37 of gestation or delivery, whichever occurs first.

Availability (generic available)

Solution for IM injection (contains castor oil; multidose vial also contains benzyl alcohol): 250 mg/mL. **Solution for subcut injection (auto-injectors; contains castor oil):** 250 mg/mL.

NURSING IMPLICATIONS

Assessment

- Monitor for signs and symptoms of thromboembolic disorders during therapy.
- Monitor vital signs during therapy. If hypertension occurs, consider discontinuation of therapy.
- Assess for signs and symptoms of allergic reactions (urticaria, pruritus, angioedema) during therapy. Consider discontinuation if allergic reactions occur.
- Monitor for fluid retention during therapy, especially in patients at ↑ risk for complications (preeclampsia, epilepsy, migraine, asthma, cardiac or renal dysfunction).
- Assess mental status and mood changes, especially in women with a history of depression. Discontinue hydroxyprogesterone if depression recurs or worsens.
- ***Lab Test Considerations:*** May ↓ glucose tolerance. Monitor serum glucose in prediabetic and diabetic women during therapy.

Implementation

- Do not confuse hydroxyprogesterone with medroxyprogesterone.
- **Subcut:** Administer via auto-injector in back of upper arm. Rotate sites. Avoid areas where skin is tender, bruised, red, scaly, raised, thick, or hard. Avoid areas with scars, tattoos, or stretch marks. Solution is clear, yellow, viscous and oily. Do not administer solutions that are cloudy or contain particles. Store at room temperature in box to protect from light.
- **IM:** Draw up 1 mL of solution into a 3 mL syringe with an 18 gauge needle. Solution is clear, yellow, viscous and oily. Do not administer solutions that are cloudy or contain particles. Change needle to 21 gauge 1 1/2 inch needle. Inject into upper outer quadrant of gluteus maximus slowly, over 1 min or longer. Apply pressure to injection site to minimize bruising and swelling. Store hydroxyprogesterone in original box, at room temperature, protected from light. Discard unused product after 5 wk from first use.

Patient/Family Teaching

- Instruct patient to continue to receive injection weekly from health care professional. If a dose is missed, consult health care professional for instructions regarding returning to schedule.
- Advise patient to notify health care professional if signs and symptoms of blood clots (leg swelling, redness in leg, a spot on leg that is warm to touch, leg pain that worsens when foot is bended), allergic reactions (hives, itching, swelling of face), depression, or yellowing of skin and whites of the eyes occur.
- Inform patient that injection site reactions (pain, swelling, itching, bruising, nodule formation) may occur. If ↑ pain over time, oozing of blood or fluid, or swelling occur, notify health care professional.
- Advise patient to notify health care professional of all Rx or OTC medications, vitamins, or herbal products being taken and to consult with health care professional before taking other medications.
- Advise patient to notify health care professional if breast feeding.

Evaluation/Desired Outcomes

- ↓ risk of preterm birth in women at risk.

ibandronate (i-ban-dro-nate)
Boniva

Classification
Therapeutic: bone resorption inhibitors
Pharmacologic: biphosphonates

Indications
Treatment/prevention of postmenopausal osteoporosis.

Action
Inhibits resorption of bone by inhibiting osteoclast activity. **Therapeutic Effects:** Reversal/prevention of progression of osteoporosis with decreased fractures.

Pharmacokinetics
Absorption: 0.6% absorbed following oral administration (significantly ↓ by food).
Distribution: Rapidly binds to bone.
Protein Binding: 90.9–99.5%.
Metabolism and Excretion: 50–60% excreted in urine; unabsorbed drug is eliminated in feces.
Half-life: *PO*—10–60 hr; *IV*—4.6–25.5 hr.

TIME/ACTION PROFILE

ROUTE	ONSET	PEAK	DURATION
PO	unknown	0.5–2 hr	up to 1 mo
IV	unknown	3 hr	up to 3 mo

Contraindications/Precautions
Contraindicated in: Hypersensitivity; Abnormalities of the esophagus which delay esophageal emptying (i.e. strictures, achalasia); Uncorrected hypocalcemia; Inability to stand/sit upright for at least 60 min; CCr <30 mL/min.
Use Cautiously in: History of upper GI disorders; Concurrent use of NSAIDs or aspirin; Invasive dental procedures, cancer, receiving chemotherapy, corticosteroids, or angiogenesis inhibitors, poor oral hygiene, periodontal disease, dental disease, anemia, coagulopathy, infection, or poorly-fitting dentures (may ↑ risk of jaw osteonecrosis); OB: Use only if potential benefit outweighs risks to mother and fetus; Lactation: Lactation; Pedi: Children <18 yr (safety not established); Geri: Consider age related ↓ in body mass, renal and hepatic function, concurrent disease states, and drug therapy.

Adverse Reactions/Side Effects
GI: diarrhea, dyspepsia, dysphagia, esophageal cancer, esophagitis, esophageal/gastric ulcer. **MS:** musculoskeletal pain, pain in arms/legs, femur fractures, osteonecrosis (primarily of jaw). **Derm:** ERYTHEMA MULTIFORME, STEVENS-JOHNSON SYNDROME. **Resp:** asthma exacerbation. **Misc:** ANAPHYLAXIS, injection site reactions.

Interactions
Drug-Drug: Calcium-, aluminum-, magnesium-, and **iron**-containing products, including **antacids** ↓ absorption (ibandronate should be taken 60 min before). Concurrent use of **NSAIDs** including **aspirin**, may ↑ risk of gastric irritation.
Drug-Food: Milk and other foods ↓ absorption.

Route/Dosage
PO (Adults): 150 mg once monthly.
IV (Adults): 3 mg every 3 mo.

Availability (generic available)
Tablets: 150 mg. **Injection:** 3 mg/3 mL in prefilled single-use syringe.

NURSING IMPLICATIONS

Assessment
- **Osteoporosis:** Assess patients for low bone mass before and periodically during therapy.
- **IV:** Monitor for signs and symptoms of anaphylactic reactions (swelling of face, lips, mouth or tongue; trouble breathing; wheezing; severe itching; skin rash, redness or swelling; dizziness or fainting; fast heartbeat or pounding in chest; sweating) during therapy. Discontinue injection immediately and begin supportive treatment if symptoms occur.
- Perform a routine oral exam prior to initiation of therapy. Dental exam with appropriate preventative dentistry should be considered prior to therapy. Patients with history of tooth extraction, poor oral hygiene, gingival infections, diabetes, or use of a dental appliance or those taking immunosuppressive therapy, angiogenesis inhibitors, or systemic corticosteroids are at greater risk for osteonecrosis of the jaw.
- ***Lab Test Considerations:*** Assess serum calcium before and periodically during therapy. Hypocalcemia and vitamin D deficiency should be treated before initiating ibandronate therapy.
- May cause ↓ total alkaline phosphatase levels.
- May cause hypercholesterolemia.

Implementation
- **PO:** Administer first thing in the morning with 6–8 oz plain water 30 min before other medications, beverages, or food. Tablet should be swallowed whole; do not break, crush, or chew.
- *Once-monthly tablet* should be administered on the same date each mo.

IV Administration
- **IV:** Administer using prefilled syringe. Do not administer solution that is discolored or contains particulate matter. Administer IV only; other routes may cause tissue damage.
- ***Rate:*** Administer as a 15–30 sec bolus.
- **Y-Site Incompatibility:** Do not administer with calcium-containing solutions or other IV drugs.

Patient/Family Teaching

- Advise patient to eat a balanced diet and consult health care professional about the need for supplemental calcium and vitamin D. Wait at least 60 min after administration before taking supplemental calcium and vitamin D.
- Encourage patient to participate in regular exercise and to modify behaviors that increase the risk of osteoporosis (stop smoking, reduce alcohol consumption).
- Inform patient that severe musculoskeletal pain may occur within days, mo, or yr after starting ibandronate. Symptoms may resolve completely after discontinuation or slow or incomplete resolution may occur. Notify health care professional if severe pain occurs.
- Advise patient to notify health care professional if rash or signs and symptoms of osteonecrosis of the jaw (pain, numbness, swelling of or drainage from the jaw, mouth, or teeth) occur.
- Instruct patient to notify health care professional if swallowing difficulties, chest pain, new or worsening heartburn, or trouble or pain when swallowing occurs; may be signs of problems of the esophagus.
- Advise patient to inform health care professional of ibandronate therapy prior to dental surgery.
- Advise female patient to notify health care professional if pregnancy is planned or suspected or if breast feeding.
- **PO:** Instruct patient on the importance of taking as directed, first thing in the morning, 60 min before other medications, beverages, or food. Ibandronate should be taken with 6–8 oz plain water (mineral water, orange juice, coffee, and other beverages decrease absorption). Do not chew or suck on tablet. If a dose is missed, skip dose and resume the next morning; do not double doses or take later in the day. If a once-monthly dose is missed and the next scheduled dose is >7 days away, take in the morning following the date it is remembered. Resume original schedule the following mo. If the next dose is <7 days away, omit dose and take next scheduled dose. Do not discontinue without consulting health care professional.
- Caution patient to remain upright for 60 min following dose to facilitate passage to stomach and minimize risk of esophageal irritation. Advise patient to stop taking ibandronate and contact health care professional if symptoms of esophageal irritation (new or worsening dysphagia, pain on swallowing, retrosternal pain, or heartburn) occur.
- **IV:** Advise patient that IV doses should not be administered sooner that every 3 mo. If a dose is missed, have health care professional administer as soon as possible; next injection should be scheduled 3 mo from last injection.

Evaluation/Desired Outcomes

- Prevention of or decrease in the progression of osteoporosis in postmenopausal women. Discontinuation after 3–5 yr should be considered for women with low risk for fractures.

BEERS

ibuprofen (eye-byoo-**proe**-fen)

Advil, Advil Infants, Advil Junior Strength, Advil Migraine, Children's Advil, ✱Children's Europrofen, Children's Motrin, ✱Motrin, Motrin IB, Motrin Infants Drops, Motrin Junior Strength, PediaCare IB Ibuprofen

ibuprofen (injection)

Caldolor, NeoProfen (ibuprofen lysine)

Classification

Therapeutic: antipyretics, antirheumatics, nonopioid analgesics, nonsteroidal anti-inflammatory agents

Pharmacologic: nonopioid analgesics

Indications

PO, IV: Treatment of: Mild to moderate pain, Fever. **PO:** Treatment of: Inflammatory disorders including rheumatoid arthritis (including juvenile) and osteoarthritis, Dysmenorrhea. **IV:** Moderate to severe pain with opioid analgesics. Closure of a clinically significant PDA in neonates weighing 500–1500 g and ≤32 wk gestational age (ibuprofen lysine only)

Action

Inhibits prostaglandin synthesis. **Therapeutic Effects:** Decreased pain and inflammation. Reduction of fever.

Pharmacokinetics

Absorption: Oral formulation is well absorbed (80%) from the GI tract; IV administration results in complete bioavailability.

Distribution: Does not enter breast milk in significant amounts.

Protein Binding: 99%.

Metabolism and Excretion: Mostly metabolized by the liver; small amounts (1%) excreted unchanged by the kidneys.

Half-life: Neonates: 26–43 hr; Children: 1–2 hr; Adults: 2–4 hr.

TIME/ACTION PROFILE

ROUTE	ONSET	PEAK	DURATION
PO (antipyretic)	0.5–2.5 hr	2–4 hr	6–8 hr
PO (analgesic)	30 min	1–2 hr	4–6 hr
PO (anti-inflammatory)	≤7 days	1–2 wk	unknown
IV (analgesic)	unknown	unknown	6 hr
IV (antipyretic)	within 2 hr	10–12 hr†	4–6 hr

†With repeated dosing.

Contraindications/Precautions

Contraindicated in: Hypersensitivity (cross-sensitivity may exist with other NSAIDs, including aspirin); Active GI bleeding or ulcer disease; Chewable tablets contain aspartame and should not be used in patients with phenylketonuria; Coronary artery bypass graft (CABG) surgery; History of recent MI; Severe HF; OB: Avoid after 30 wk gestation (may cause premature closure of fetal ductus arteriosus); Pedi: Ibuprofen lysine: Preterm neonates with untreated infection, congenital heart disease where patency of PDA is necessary for pulmonary or systemic blood flow, bleeding, thrombocytopenia, coagulation defects, necrotizing enterocolitis, significant renal dysfunction.

Use Cautiously in: Cardiovascular disease or risk factors for cardiovascular disease (may ↑ risk of serious cardiovascular thrombotic events, MI, and stroke, especially with prolonged use or use of higher doses); avoid use in patients with recent MI or HF; Renal or hepatic disease, dehydration, or patients on nephrotoxic drugs (may ↑ risk of renal toxicity); Aspirin triad patients (asthma, nasal polyps, and aspirin intolerance); can cause fatal anaphylactoid reactions; Chronic alcohol use/abuse; Geri: ↑ risk of adverse reactions secondary to age-related ↓ in renal and hepatic function, concurrent illnesses, and medications; Coagulation disorders; OB: Use cautiously up to 30 wk gestation; avoid after that; Lactation: Use cautiously; Pedi: Safety not established for infants <6 mo (oral and IV Caldolor); hyperbilirubinemia in neonates (may displace bilirubin from albumin-binding sites); safety and effectiveness of ibuprofen lysine only established in premature infants.

Exercise Extreme Caution in: History of GI bleeding or GI ulcer disease.

Adverse Reactions/Side Effects

CNS: headache, dizziness, drowsiness, intraventricular hemorrhage (ibuprofen lysine), psychic disturbances. **CV:** HF, MYOCARDIAL INFARCTION, STROKE, arrhythmias, edema, hypertension. **Derm:** EXFOLIATIVE DERMATITIS, STEVENS-JOHNSON SYNDROME, TOXIC EPIDERMAL NECROLYSIS, rash, injection site reaction. **EENT:** amblyopia, blurred vision, tinnitus. **F and E:** hyperkalemia. **GI:** GI BLEEDING, HEPATITIS, constipation, dyspepsia, nausea, necrotizing enterocolitis (ibuprofen lysine), vomiting, abdominal discomfort. **GU:** cystitis, hematuria, renal failure. **Hemat:** anemia, blood dyscrasias, prolonged bleeding time. **Misc:** HYPERSENSITIVITY REACTIONS (including anaphylaxis).

Interactions

Drug-Drug: May limit the cardioprotective (antiplatelet) effects of low-dose **aspirin**. Concurrent use with **aspirin** may ↓ effectiveness of ibuprofen. Additive adverse GI side effects with **aspirin**, **oral potassium**, other **NSAIDs**, **corticosteroids**, or **alcohol**. Chronic use with **acetaminophen** may ↑ risk of adverse renal reactions. May ↓ effectiveness of **diuretics**, **ACE inhibitors**, or other **antihypertensives**. May ↑ hypoglycemic effects of **insulin** or **oral hypoglycemic agents**. May ↑ serum **lithium** levels and risk of toxicity. ↑ risk of toxicity from **methotrexate**. **Probenecid** ↑ risk of toxicity from ibuprofen. ↑ risk of bleeding with **cefotetan**, **corticosteroids**, **valproic acid**, **thrombolytics**, **warfarin**, and **drugs affecting platelet function** including **clopidogrel**, **eptifibatide**, or **tirofiban**. ↑ risk of adverse hematologic reactions with **antineoplastics** or **radiation therapy**. ↑ risk of nephrotoxicity with **cyclosporine**. May ↓ the clearance and ↑ levels of **amikacin**.

Drug-Natural Products: ↑ bleeding risk with **arnica**, **chamomile**, **feverfew**, **garlic**, **ginger**, **ginkgo**, **Panax ginseng**, and others.

Route/Dosage

Analgesia/Anti-Inflammatory/Antipyretic

PO (Adults): *Anti-inflammatory*—400–800 mg 3–4 times daily (not to exceed 3200 mg/day). *Analgesic/antidysmenorrheal/antipyretic*—200–400 mg every 4–6 hr (not to exceed 1200 mg/day).

PO (Children 6 mo–12 yr): *Anti-inflammatory*—30–50 mg/kg/day in 3–4 divided doses (maximum dose: 2.4 g/day). *Antipyretic*—5 mg/kg for temperature <102.5°F (39.17°C) or 10 mg/kg for higher temperatures (not to exceed 40 mg/kg/day); may be repeated every 4–6 hr.

PO (Infants and Children): *Analgesic*—4–10 mg/kg/dose every 6–8 hr.

IV (Adults): *Analgesic*—400–800 mg every 6 hr as needed (not to exceed 3200 mg/day); *Antipyretic*—400 mg initially, then 400 mg every 4–6 hr or 100–200 mg every 4 hr as needed (not to exceed 3200 mg/day).

IV (Children 12–17 yr): *Analgesic and antipyretic*—400 mg every 4–6 hr as needed (not to exceed 2400 mg/day).

IV (Children 6 mo–12 yr): *Analgesic and antipyretic*—10 mg/kg (not to exceed 400 mg) every 4–6 hr as needed (not to exceed 40 mg/kg/day or 2400 mg/day, whichever is less).

Pediatric OTC Dosing

PO (Children 11 yr/72–95 lb): 300 mg every 6–8 hr.

PO (Children 9–10 yr/60–71 lb): 250 mg every 6–8 hr.

PO (Children 6–8 yr/48–59 lb): 200 mg every 6–8 hr.

PO (Children 4–5 yr/36–47 lb): 150 mg every 6–8 hr.

PO (Children 2–3 yr/24–35 lb): 100 mg every 6–8 hr.
PO (Children 12–23 mo/18–23 lb): 75 mg every 6–8 hr.
PO (Infants 6–11 mo/12–17 lb): 50 mg every 6–8 hr.

PDA Closure

IV (Neonates Gestational age ≤32 wk, 500–1500 g): 10 mg/kg followed by two doses of 5 mg/kg at 24 and 48 hr after initial dose.

Availability (generic available)

Capsules (liquigels): 200 mg[OTC]. **Chewable tablets (fruit, grape, orange, and citrus flavor):** 100 mg[OTC]. **Oral solution (berry flavor):** 50 mg/1.25 mL[OTC]. **Oral suspension (fruit, berry, grape flavor):** 100 mg/5 mL[OTC]. **Solution for injection (requires dilution):** 100 mg/mL (Caldolor) 10 mg/mL (NeoProfen). **Tablets:** 200 mg[OTC], 400 mg, 600 mg, 800 mg. ***In combination with:*** decongestants[OTC], hydrocodone (Reprexain), famotidine (Duexis). See Appendix B.

NURSING IMPLICATIONS

Assessment

- Patients who have asthma, aspirin-induced allergy, and nasal polyps are at increased risk for developing hypersensitivity reactions. Assess for rhinitis, asthma, and urticaria.
- Assess for signs and symptoms of GI bleeding (tarry stools, light-headedness, hypotension), renal dysfunction (elevated BUN and serum creatinine levels, decreased urine output), and hepatic impairment (elevated liver enzymes, jaundice). Geri: Higher risk for poor outcomes or death from GI bleeding. Age-related renal impairment increases risk of hepatic and renal toxicity.
- Assess patient for skin rash frequently during therapy. Discontinue ibuprofen at first sign of rash; may be life-threatening. Stevens-Johnson syndrome or toxic epidermal necrolysis may develop. Treat symptomatically; may recur once treatment is stopped.
- **Pain:** Assess pain (note type, location, and intensity) prior to and 1–2 hr following administration.
- **Arthritis:** Assess pain and range of motion prior to and 1–2 hr following administration.
- **Fever:** Monitor temperature; note signs associated with fever (diaphoresis, tachycardia, malaise).
- **PDA Closure:** Monitor preterm neonates for signs of bleeding, infection and decreased urine output. Monitor IV site for signs of extravasation. If ductus arteriosus closes or size significantly decreases, 2nd and 3rd doses are unnecessary.
- ***Lab Test Considerations:*** BUN, serum creatinine, CBC, and liver function tests should be evaluated periodically in patients receiving prolonged therapy.
- Serum potassium, BUN, serum creatinine, alkaline phosphatase, LDH, AST, and ALT may show ↑ levels. Blood glucose, hemoglobin, and hematocrit concentrations, leukocyte and platelet counts, and CCr may be ↓.
- May cause prolonged bleeding time; may persist for <1 day following discontinuation.
- **PDA Closure:** If urinary output <0.6 mL/kg/hr at time of 2nd or 3rd dose, hold dose until renal function has returned to normal.

Implementation

- Do not confuse Motrin (ibuprofen) with Neurontin (gabapentin).
- Administration of higher than recommended doses does not provide increased pain relief but may increase incidence of side effects.
- Patient should be well hydrated before administration to prevent renal adverse reactions. Do not give to neonates with urine output <0.6 mL/kg/hr.
- Use lowest effective dose for shortest period of time, especially in the elderly, to minimize risk of cardiovascular thrombotic events.
- Coadministration with opioid analgesics may have additive analgesic effects and may permit lower opioid doses.
- **PO:** For rapid initial effect, administer 30 min before or 2 hr after meals. May be administered with food, milk, or antacids to decrease GI irritation. Tablets may be crushed and mixed with fluids or food; 800-mg tablet can be dissolved in water.
- **Dysmenorrhea:** Administer as soon as possible after the onset of menses. Prophylactic treatment has not been shown to be effective.

IV Administration

- **Intermittent Infusion:** ***Diluent:*** 0.9% NaCl, D5W, or LR. ***Concentration:*** *Ibuprofen injection:* Dilute the 800 mg dose in at least 200 mL and the 100 mg, 200 mg, and 400 mg doses in at least 100 mL for a concentration of 4 mg/mL or less. *Ibuprofen lysine:* Dilute in appropriate volume of D5W or 0.9% NaCl and infuse over 15 min. Do not administer solutions that are discolored or contain particulate matter. Stable for up to 24 hr at room temperature. Discard remaining solution; does not contain preservatives. ***Rate:*** Infuse over at least 30 min for adults and at least 10 min for children for *Caldolor* or over 15 min for *NeoProfen*.

Ibuprofen

- **Y-Site Compatibility:** metoprolol.
- **Y-Site Incompatibility:** esmolol, labetalol.

Ibuprofen Lysine

- **Y-Site Compatibility:** ceftazidime, epinephrine, furosemide, heparin, insulin, regular, phenobarbital, potassium chloride, sodium bicarbonate.
- **Y-Site Incompatibility:** amikacin, amino acids, caffeine citrate, dobutamine, dopamine, isoproterenol, midazolam, multi-electrolyte concentrate, vancomycin, vecuronium.

Patient/Family Teaching

- Advise patients to take ibuprofen with a full glass of water and to remain in an upright position for 15–30 min after administration.
- Instruct patient to take medication as directed. Take missed doses as soon as remembered but not if almost time for next dose. Do not double doses. Pedi: Teach parents and caregivers to calculate and measure doses accurately and to use measuring device supplied with product.
- May cause drowsiness or dizziness. Advise patient to avoid driving or other activities requiring alertness until response to medication is known.
- Caution patient to avoid the concurrent use of alcohol, aspirin including low dose aspirin, acetaminophen, and other OTC or herbal products without consulting health care professional.
- Advise patient to inform health care professional of medication regimen prior to treatment or surgery.
- Instruct patients not to take OTC ibuprofen preparations for more than 10 days for pain or more than 3 days for fever, and to consult health care professional if symptoms persist or worsen. Many OTC products contain ibuprofen; avoid duplication.
- Caution patient that use of ibuprofen with 3 or more glasses of alcohol per day may increase the risk of GI bleeding.
- Advise patient to consult health care professional if rash, itching, visual disturbances, tinnitus, weight gain, edema, epigastric pain, dyspepsia, black stools, hematemesis, persistent headache, or influenza-like syndrome (chills, fever, muscle aches, pain), or cardiovascular events (chest pain, shortness of breath, weakness, slurring of speech) occurs.
- Pedi: Advise parents or caregivers not to administer ibuprofen to children who may be dehydrated (can occur with vomiting, diarrhea, or poor fluid intake); dehydration increases risk of renal dysfunction.
- Rep: Advise females of reproductive potential to notify health care professional if pregnancy is planned or suspected and to avoid ibuprofen starting at 30 wk gestation because of risk of premature closing of the fetal ductus arteriosus. May cause temporary infertility in women.

Evaluation/Desired Outcomes

- Decrease in severity of pain.
- Improved joint mobility. Partial arthritic relief is usually seen within 7 days, but maximum effectiveness may require 1–2 wk of continuous therapy. Patients who do not respond to one NSAID may respond to another.
- Reduction in fever.
- Closure of PDA.

idaruCIZUmab

(eye-da-roo-**siz**-ue-mab)
Praxbind

Classification
Therapeutic: antidotes
Pharmacologic: monoclonal antibodies

Indications

To counteract the anticoagulant effect of dabigatran for emergency surgery/urgent procedures or life-threatening uncontrolled bleeding.

Action

Human monoclonal antibody fragment (Fab) that selectively binds to dabigatran and its metabolites, preventing its binding to thrombin and negating its anticoagulant effects. Does not reverse any other anticoagulants. **Therapeutic Effects:** Reversal of the anticoagulant effect of dabigatran.

Pharmacokinetics

Absorption: IV administration results in complete bioavailability.
Distribution: Unknown.
Metabolism and Excretion: Biodegraded to smaller molecules. 60% excreted in urine, remainder via protein catabolism primarily in the kidneys.
Half-life: 10.3 hr.

TIME/ACTION PROFILE

ROUTE	ONSET	PEAK	DURATION
IV	immediate	unknown	24 hr

Contraindications/Precautions

Contraindicated in: None noted.
Use Cautiously in: Geri: Elderly patients may be more sensitive to drug effects; OB: Safety not established. Consider maternal benefits and fetal risks; Lactation: Safety not established, consider beneficial effects of breast feeding and possible adverse effects in infant; Pedi: Safety and effectiveness not established.
Exercise Extreme Caution in: Hereditary fructose intolerance (risk of serious adverse reactions due to sorbitol excipient); History of serious hypersensitivity (including anaphylactoid reactions) to idarucizumab.

Adverse Reactions/Side Effects

CNS: delirium. **CV:** THROMBOEMBOLISM. **F and E:** hypokalemia. **GI:** constipation. **Misc:** fever, hypersensitivity reactions.

Interactions

Drug-Drug: None noted.

Route/Dosage

IV (Adults): 5 g as single dose.

Availability
Solution for injection (contains sorbitol): 2.5 g/50 mL.

NURSING IMPLICATIONS

Assessment
- Reversal of dabigatran exposes patient to thrombotic risk of their underlying disease; may cause thromboembolism. Resume anticoagulant therapy as soon as medically appropriate. Dabigatran therapy can be reinstituted 24 hr after idarucizumab infusion.
- Monitor for signs and symptoms of hypersensitivity reactions (rash, urticaria, fever, pruritus, dyspnea, orofacial swelling). Contains sorbitol; reactions in patients with hereditary fructose intolerance have included hypoglycemia, hypophosphatemia, metabolic acidosis, increase in uric acid, acute liver failure. If symptoms occur discontinue therapy and treat symptomatically.
- ***Lab Test Considerations:*** Monitor coagulation parameters (activated partial thromboplastin time [aPTT], ecarin clotting time [ECT]) 12–24 hrs after infusion.
- May cause hypokalemia.

Implementation
- Do not confuse idarucizumab with idarubicin.

IV Administration
- **Intermittent Infusion:** Flush IV line with 0.9% NaCl prior to and following infusion. Solution is clear to opalescent, colorless to slightly yellow; do not administer solutions that are discolored or contain precipitates. Administer as 2 consecutive infusion or inject both vials consecutively via syringe. Must be administered within 1 hr when removed from vial. Store at room temperature and use within 6 hr if exposed to light.

Patient/Family Teaching
- Explain purpose of idarucizumab to patient.
- Instruct patient to notify health care professional immediately if bleeding or signs and symptoms of hypersensitivity occur.
- Advise patient to notify health care professional if pregnancy is planned or suspected, or if breast feeding.

Evaluation/Desired Outcomes
- Reversal of the anticoagulant effect of dabigatran.

ifosfamide (eye-foss-fam-ide)
Ifex

Classification
Therapeutic: antineoplastics
Pharmacologic: alkylating agents

Indications
Germ cell testicular carcinoma (with other agents). Used with mesna, which prevents ifosfamide-induced hemorrhagic cystitis.

Action
Following conversion to active compounds, interferes with DNA replication and RNA transcription, ultimately disrupting protein synthesis (cell-cycle phase–nonspecific). **Therapeutic Effects:** Death of rapidly replicating cells, particularly malignant ones.

Pharmacokinetics
Absorption: Administered IV only; inactive prior to conversion to metabolites.
Distribution: Excreted in breast milk.
Metabolism and Excretion: Metabolized by the liver to active antineoplastic compounds.
Half-life: 15 hr.

TIME/ACTION PROFILE (effects on blood counts)

ROUTE	ONSET	PEAK	DURATION
IV	unknown	7–14 days	21 days

Contraindications/Precautions
Contraindicated in: Hypersensitivity; OB, Lactation: Pregnancy or lactation.
Use Cautiously in: Patients with childbearing potential; Active infections; ↓ bone marrow reserve; Geri: Geriatric patients; Other chronic debilitating illness; Renal impairment; Pedi: Children.

Adverse Reactions/Side Effects
CNS: CNS toxicity (somnolence, confusion, hallucinations, coma), cranial nerve dysfunction, disorientation, dizziness. **CV:** cardiotoxicity. **GI:** nausea, vomiting, anorexia, constipation, diarrhea, hepatotoxicity. **GU:** hemorrhagic cystitis, dysuria, sterility, renal toxicity. **Derm:** alopecia. **Hemat:** ANEMIA, LEUKOPENIA, THROMBOCYTOPENIA. **Local:** phlebitis. **Misc:** allergic reactions.

Interactions
Drug-Drug: CYP3A4 inhibitors, including **ketoconazole, fluconazole, itraconazole, sorafenib,** and **aprepitant** may ↓ its effectiveness. **CYP3A4 inducers**, including **carbamazepine, phenytoin, phenytoin, phenobarbital**, and **rifampin** may ↑ the formation of a toxic metabolite and may ↑ risk of toxicity. ↑ myelosuppression with other **antineoplastics** or **radiation therapy**. Toxicity may be ↑ by **allopurinol** or **phenobarbital**. May ↓ antibody response to and ↑ risk of adverse reactions from **live-virus vaccines**.
Drug-Food: Grapefruit juice may ↑ levels; avoid concurrent use.

Route/Dosage

Other Regimens are Used

IV (Adults): 1.2 g/m²/day for 5 days; coadminister with mesna. May repeat cycle every 3 wk.

Availability (generic available)

Powder for injection (requires reconstitution): 1 g/vial, 3 g/vial. **Solution for injection:** 50 mg/mL.

NURSING IMPLICATIONS

Assessment

- Monitor BP, pulse, respiratory rate, and temperature frequently during administration. Report significant changes.
- Monitor urinary output frequently during therapy. Notify health care professional if hematuria occurs. To reduce the risk of hemorrhagic cystitis, fluid intake should be at least 3000 mL/day for adults and 1000–2000 mL/day for children. Mesna is given concurrently to prevent hemorrhagic cystitis.
- Monitor neurologic status. Ifosfamide should be discontinued if severe CNS symptoms (agitation, confusion, hallucinations, unusual tiredness) occur. Symptoms usually abate within 3 days of discontinuation of ifosfamide but may persist for longer; fatalities have been reported.
- Assess nausea, vomiting, and appetite. Weigh weekly. Premedication with an antiemetic may be used to minimize GI effects. Adjust diet as tolerated.
- Monitor for bone marrow depression. Assess for bleeding (bleeding gums, bruising, petechiae, guaiac stools, urine, and emesis) and avoid IM injections and taking rectal temperatures if platelet count is low. Apply pressure to venipuncture sites for 10 min. Assess for signs of infection during neutropenia. Anemia may occur. Monitor for increased fatigue, dyspnea, and orthostatic hypotension.
- ***Lab Test Considerations:*** Monitor CBC, differential, and platelet count prior to and periodically during therapy. Withhold dose if WBC <2000/mm³ or platelet count is <50,000/mm³. Nadir of leukopenia and thrombocytopenia occurs within 7–14 days and usually recovers within 21 days of therapy.
- Urinalysis should be evaluated before each dose. Withhold dose until recovery if urinalysis shows >10 RBCs per high-power field.
- May cause ↑ in liver enzymes and serum bilirubin.
- Monitor AST, ALT, serum alkaline phosphatase, bilirubin, and LDH prior to and periodically during therapy. May cause ↑ in liver enzymes and serum bilirubin.
- Monitor BUN, serum creatinine, phosphate, and potassium periodically during therapy. May cause hypokalemia.

Implementation

- Prepare solution in a biologic cabinet. Wear gloves, gown, and mask while handling IV medication. Discard IV equipment in specially designated containers.

IV Administration

- **IV:** Prepare solution by diluting each 1-g vial with 20 mL of sterile water or bacteriostatic water for injection containing parabens. Use solution prepared without bacteriostatic water within 6 hr. Solution prepared with bacteriostatic water is stable for 1 wk at 30°C or 6 wk at 5°C.
- **Intermittent Infusion:** ***Diluent:*** May be further diluted in D5W, 0.9% NaCl, LR, or sterile water for injection. ***Concentration:*** 0.6 to 20 mg/mL (maximum 40 mg/mL). Dilute solution is stable for 7 days at room temperature or 6 wk if refrigerated. ***Rate:*** Administer over at least 30 min.
- **Continuous Infusion:** Has also been administered as a continuous infusion over 72 hr.
- **Y-Site Compatibility:** acyclovir, alemtuzumab, alfentanil, allopurinol, amifostine, amikacin, aminocaproic acid, aminophylline, amiodarone, amphotericin B cholesteryl, amphotericin B deoxycholate, amphotericin B lipid complex, amphotericin B liposome, ampicillin, ampicillin/sulbactam, anidulafungin, argatroban, azithromycin, aztreonam, bivalirudin, bleomycin, bumetanide, buprenorphine, butorphanol, calcium chloride, calcium gluconate, carboplatin, caspofungin, cefazolin, cefotaxime, cefotetan, cefoxitin, ceftazidime, ceftriaxone, cefuroxime, chlorpromazine, ciprofloxacin, cisatracurium, cisplatin, clindamycin, cyclosporine, cytarabine, dacarbazine, dactinomycin, daptomycin, dexamethasone, dexmedetomidine, dexrazoxane, digoxin, diltiazem, diphenhydramine, dobutamine, docetaxel, dolasetron, dopamine, doxorubicin hydrochloride, doxorubicin liposome, doxycycline, droperidol, enalaprilat, ephedrine, epinephrine, epirubicin, ertapenem, erythromycin, esmolol, etoposide, etoposide phosphate, famotidine, fenoldopam, fentanyl, filgrastim, fluconazole, fludarabine, fluorouracil, foscarnet, fosphenytoin, furosemide, ganciclovir, gemcitabine, gentamicin, granisetron, haloperidol, heparin, hetastarch, hydrocortisone, hydromorphone, idarubicin, imipenem/cilastatin, insulin, isoproterenol, ketorolac, labetalol, leucovorin calcium, levofloxacin, levorphanol, lidocaine, linezolid, lorazepam, magnesium sulfate, mannitol, melphalan, meperidine, meropenem, mesna, methylprednisolone, metoclopramide, metoprolol, metronidazole, midazolam, milrinone, minocycline, mitomycin, mitoxantrone, morphine, moxifloxacin, nalbuphine, naloxone, nicardipine, nitroglycerin, nitroprusside, norepinephrine, octreotide, ondansetron, oxalipla-

tin, paclitaxel, palonosetron, pamidronate, pancuronium, pemetrexed, pentamidine, pentobarbital, phenobarbital, phenylephrine, piperacillin/tazobactam, potassium acetate, potassium chloride, procainamide, prochlorperazine, promethazine, propofol, propranolol, quinupristin/dalfopristin, ranitidine, remifentanil, rituximab, rocuronium, sargramostim, sodium acetate, sodium bicarbonate, sodium phosphates, succinylcholine, sufentanil, tacrolimus, theophylline, thiopental, thiotepa, tigecycline, tirofiban, tobramycin, topotecan, trastuzumab, trimethoprim/sulfamethoxazole, vancomycin, vasopressin, vecuronium, verapamil, vinblastine, vincristine, vinorelbine, voriconazole, zidovudine, zoledronic acid.
- **Y-Site Incompatibility:** cefepime, diazepam, methotrexate, pantoprazole, phenytoin, potassium phosphates.

Patient/Family Teaching

- Emphasize need for adequate fluid intake throughout therapy. Patient should void frequently to decrease bladder irritation from metabolites excreted by the kidneys. Notify health care professional immediately if hematuria is noted.
- Instruct patient to drink at least 8 glasses of water/day during and for 3 days after completion of therapy.
- Advise patient to avoid grapefruit and grapefruit juice during therapy.
- Instruct patient to notify health care professional promptly if fever; chills; cough; hoarseness; sore throat; signs of infection; lower back or side pain; painful or difficult urination; bleeding gums; bruising; petechiae; blood in urine, stool, or emesis; or confusion occurs.
- Caution patient to avoid crowds and persons with known infections. Instruct patient to use soft toothbrush and electric razor and to avoid falls. Patients should also be cautioned not to drink alcoholic beverages or to take products containing aspirin or NSAIDs, as these may precipitate GI hemorrhage.
- Discuss with patient the possibility of hair loss. Explore methods of coping.
- Instruct patient to notify health care professional of all Rx or OTC medications, vitamins, or herbal products being taken and to consult with health care professional before taking other medications.
- Instruct patient not to receive any vaccinations without advice of health care professional; ifosfamide may decrease antibody response to and increase risk of adverse reactions from live-virus vaccines.
- Review with patient the need for contraception during therapy and for at least 6 mo after therapy. Women should avoid pregnancy and breast feeding and men should avoid fathering a child during and for at least 6 mo after end of therapy.
- Rep: Caution patient about the potential for amenorrhea, premature menopause, and sterility from this medication.

Evaluation/Desired Outcomes

- Decrease in size or spread of malignant germ cell testicular carcinoma.

BEERS

iloperidone

(eye-loe-**per**-i-done)

Fanapt

Classification

Therapeutic: antipsychotics

Pharmacologic: benzisoxazoles

Indications

Schizophrenia.

Action

May act by antagonizing dopamine and serotonin in the CNS. **Therapeutic Effects:** Decreased symptoms of schizophrenia.

Pharmacokinetics

Absorption: Well absorbed (96%) following oral administration.

Distribution: Unknown.

Metabolism and Excretion: Extensively metabolized by the liver. Metabolism is genetically determined; primarily by CYP3A4 and CYP2D6 enzyme systems, with individual variability in metabolism via CYP2D6 (extensive metabolizers [EM] and poor metabolizers [PM] and some in-between; 7–10% of Caucasians and 3–8% of Black/African Americans are considered PM). Two major metabolites (P88 and P95) may be partially responsible for pharmacologic activity. 58% excreted in urine as metabolites in EM and 45% in PM; 20% eliminated in feces in EM and 22.1% in PM.

Half-life: *EMs*—iloperidone–18 hr, P88–26 hr, P95–23 hr; *PMs*—iloperidone–33 hr, P88–37 hr, P95–31 hr.

TIME/ACTION PROFILE (antipsychotic effect)

ROUTE	ONSET	PEAK	DURATION
PO	2–4 wk	2–4 hr†	unknown

†Blood level.

Contraindications/Precautions

Contraindicated in: Hypersensitivity; Concurrent use of drugs known to prolong QTc interval; Bradycardia, recent MI or uncompensated heart failure (↑ risk of serious arrhythmias); Congenital long QT syndrome, QTc interval >500 msec or history of cardiac arrhythmias; Electrolyte abnormalities, especially hypomagnesemia or hypokalemia (correct prior to therapy); Severe hepatic impairment; Lactation: Breast feeding should be avoided.

Use Cautiously in: Known cardiovascular disease including heart failure, history of MI/ischemia, conduction abnormalities, cerebrovascular disease, or other conditions known to predispose to hypotension including dehydration, hypovolemia, concurrent antihypertensive therapy (↑ risk of orthostatic hypotension); Concurrent use of CYP3A4 or CYP2D6 inhibitors; Known ↓ WBC or history of drug-induced leukopenia/neutropenia; Circumstances that may result in ↑ body temperature, including strenuous exercise, exposure to extreme heat, concurrent anticholinergic activity, or dehydration (may impair thermoregulation); Patients at risk for aspiration or falls; Moderate hepatic impairment; OB: Neonates at ↑ risk for extrapyramidal symptoms and withdrawal after delivery when exposed during the 3rd trimester; use only if potential maternal benefit justifies potential fetal risk; Pedi: Safety and effectiveness not established; Geri: Elderly patients with dementia-related psychoses (↑ risk of death, CVA or TIA).

Adverse Reactions/Side Effects

CNS: NEUROLEPTIC MALIGNANT SYNDROME, SUICIDAL THOUGHTS, dizziness, drowsiness, fatigue, agitation, delusion, restlessness, extrapyramidal disorders. **CV:** orthostatic hypotension, tachycardia, palpitations, QTc interval prolongation. **EENT:** nasal congestion. **Endo:** dyslipidemia, hyperglycemia, hyperprolactinemia. **GI:** dry mouth, nausea, abdominal discomfort, diarrhea. **GU:** priapism, urinary incontinence. **Metab:** weight gain, weight loss. **MS:** ↓ bone density, musculoskeletal stiffness. **Neuro:** tardive dyskinesia. **Misc:** ANAPHYLAXIS, ANGIOEDEMA.

Interactions

Drug-Drug: Avoid concurrent use of drugs known to prolong the QTc interval including **quinidine**, **procainamide**, **amiodarone**, **sotalol**, **chlorpromazine**, **thioridazine**, **moxifloxacin**, **pentamidine**, and **methadone**. Concurrent use of strong **CYP2D6 inhibitors** including **fluoxetine** and **paroxetine** ↑ levels and the risk of toxicity; dose ↓ is required. Concurrent use of strong **CYP3A4 inhibitors** including **ketoconazole** and **clarithromycin** ↑ levels and the risk of toxicity; dosage ↓ is required. Concurrent use of **antihypertensives** including **diuretics** may ↑ risk of orthostatic hypotension. Concurrent use of **anticholinergics** may ↑ risk of impaired thermoregulation.

Route/Dosage

PO (Adults): Initiate treatment with 1 mg twice daily on the first day, then 2 mg twice daily the 2nd day, then ↑ by 2 mg/day every day until a target dose of 12–24 mg/day given in two divided doses is reached; *Concurrent use of strong CYP2D6 or CYP3A4 inhibitors*—↓ dose by 50%, if inhibitor is withdrawn ↑ dose to previous amount. Retitration is required if iloperidone is discontinued >300 days; *Poor metabolizers of CYP2D6*—↓ dose by 50%.

Availability (generic available)

Tablets: 1 mg, 2 mg, 4 mg, 6 mg, 8 mg, 10 mg, 12 mg.

NURSING IMPLICATIONS

Assessment

- Monitor patient's mental status (delusions, hallucinations, and behavior) before and periodically during therapy.
- Monitor mood changes. Assess for suicidal tendencies, especially during early therapy. Restrict amount of drug available to patient.
- Monitor BP (sitting, standing, lying down) and pulse before and periodically during therapy. May cause prolonged QT interval, tachycardia, and orthostatic hypotension. Protect patient from falls.
- Observe patient when administering medication to ensure that medication is actually swallowed and not hoarded.
- Monitor patient for onset of extrapyramidal side effects (*akathisia*—restlessness; *dystonia*—muscle spasms and twisting motions; or *pseudoparkinsonism*—mask-like face, rigidity, tremors, drooling, shuffling gait, dysphagia). Report these symptoms; reduction of dose or discontinuation of medication may be necessary.
- Monitor for tardive dyskinesia (involuntary rhythmic movement of mouth, face, and extremities). Report immediately and discontinue therapy; may be irreversible.
- Monitor for development of neuroleptic malignant syndrome (fever, respiratory distress, tachycardia, seizures, diaphoresis, hypertension or hypotension, pallor, tiredness). Discontinue iloperidone and notify health care professional immediately if these symptoms occur.
- Monitor for symptoms related to hyperprolactinemia (menstrual abnormalities, galactorrhea, sexual dysfunction).
- Assess weight and BMI initially and during therapy. Refer as appropriate for nutritional/weight and medical management.
- Assess for falls risk. Drowsiness, orthostatic hypotension, and motor and sensory instability increase risk. Institute prevention if indicated.
- ***Lab Test Considerations:*** Monitor fasting blood glucose before and periodically during therapy in diabetic patients.
- Monitor CBC frequently during initial mo of therapy in patients with pre-existing or history of low WBC. May cause leukopenia, neutropenia, or agranulocytosis. Discontinue therapy if this occurs.
- Monitor serum potassium and magnesium levels in patients at risk for electrolyte disturbances.
- Monitor serum prolactin prior to and periodically during therapy. May cause ↑ serum prolactin levels.

Implementation

- Do not confuse Fanapt (iloperidone) with Xanax (alprazolam).
- **PO:** Administer twice daily without regard to food.

Patient/Family Teaching

- Instruct patient to take medication exactly as directed. If doses are missed for >3 days, restart at initiation dose. Advise patient that appearance of tablets in stool is normal and not of concern.
- Inform patient of the possibility of extrapyramidal symptoms, neuroleptic malignant syndrome, and tardive dyskinesia. Instruct patient to report these symptoms immediately to health care professional.
- Advise patient to change positions slowly to minimize orthostatic hypotension. Protect from falls.
- Inform patient of potential for weight gain and hyperglycemia, and the need for monitoring weight and blood glucose periodically during therapy.
- May cause drowsiness. Caution patient to avoid driving or other activities requiring alertness until response to medication is known.
- Extremes in temperature should also be avoided; this drug impairs body temperature regulation.
- Instruct patient to notify health care professional promptly if sore throat, fever, unusual bleeding or bruising, rash, tremors, palpitations, fainting, menstrual abnormalities, galactorrhea, or sexual dysfunction occur.
- Advise patient and family to notify health care professional if thoughts about suicide or dying, attempts to commit suicide; new or worse depression; new or worse anxiety; feeling very agitated or restless; panic attacks; trouble sleeping; new or worse irritability; acting aggressive; being angry or violent; acting on dangerous impulses; an extreme increase in activity and talking; other unusual changes in behavior or mood occur.
- Caution patient to avoid concurrent use of alcohol and other CNS depressants.
- Advise patient to notify health care professional of all Rx or OTC medications, vitamins, or herbal products being taken and to consult with health care professional before taking other medications.
- Advise patient to notify health care professional of medication regimen before treatment or surgery.
- Rep: Advise female patients to notify health care professional if pregnancy is planned or suspected, and to avoid breast feeding. Encourage women who become pregnant while taking iloperidone to enroll in the National Pregnancy Registry for Atypical Antipsychotics at 1-866-961-2388 or visit http://womensmentalhealth.org/clinical-and-research-programs/pregnancyregistry/. Monitor neonates for extrapyramidal and/or withdrawal symptoms and manage symptoms appropriately.
- Emphasize the need for continued follow-up for psychotherapy and monitoring for side effects.

Evaluation/Desired Outcomes

- Decrease in excited, paranoid, or withdrawn behavior.

HIGH ALERT

imatinib (i-mat-i-nib)

Gleevec

Classification

Therapeutic: antineoplastics
Pharmacologic: enzyme inhibitors

Indications

Newly diagnosed Philadelphia positive (Ph+) chronic myeloid leukemia (CML). CML in blast crisis, accelerated phase, or in chronic phase after failure of interferon-alpha treatment. Kit (CD117) positive metastatic/unresectable malignant gastrointestinal stomal tumors (GIST). Adjuvant treatment following resection of Kit (CD117) positive GIST. Pediatric patients with Ph+ CML after failure of bone marrow transplant or resistance to interferon-alpha. Adult patients with relapsed or refractory Ph+ acute lymphoblastic leukemia (ALL). Newly diagnosed Ph+ ALL (in combination with chemotherapy). Myelodysplastic/myeloproliferative disease (MDS/MPD) associated with platelet-derived growth factor receptor (PDGFR) gene re-arrangements. Aggressive systemic mastocytosis (ASM) without the D816V c-Kit mutation or with c-Kit mutational status unknown. Hypereosinophilic syndrome and/or chronic eosinophilic leukemia (HES/CEL). Unresectable, recurrent, or metastatic dermatofibrosarcoma protuberans (DFSP).

Action

Inhibits kinases which may be produced by malignant cell lines. **Therapeutic Effects:** Inhibits production of malignant cell lines with decreased proliferation of leukemic cells in CML, HES/CEL, and ALL and malignant cells in GIST, MDS/MPD, ASM, and DFSP.

Pharmacokinetics

Absorption: Well absorbed (98%) following oral administration.

Distribution: Unknown.

Protein Binding: 95%.

Metabolism and Excretion: Mostly metabolized by the CYP3A4 enzyme system to N-demethyl imatinib, which is as active as imatinib. Excreted mostly in feces as metabolites. 5% excreted unchanged in urine.

Half-life: *Imatinib*—18 hr; *N-desmethyl imatinib*—40 hr.

TIME/ACTION PROFILE (blood levels of imatinib)

ROUTE	ONSET	PEAK	DURATION
PO	unknown	2–4 hr	24 hr

Contraindications/Precautions

Contraindicated in: Hypersensitivity; OB: Potential for fetal harm; Lactation: Potential for serious adverse reactions in nursing infants; breast feeding should be avoided.

Use Cautiously in: Hepatic impairment (dose ↓ recommended if bilirubin >3 times normal or liver transaminases >5 times normal); Cardiac disease (severe HF and left ventricular dysfunction may occur); Renal impairment, diabetes, hypertension, HF (↑ risk of nephrotoxicity); Rep: Women of reproductive potential; Pedi: Children <1 yr (safety not established); Geri: ↑ risk of edema.

Adverse Reactions/Side Effects

CNS: fatigue, headache, weakness, dizziness, somnolence. **CV:** HF. **EENT:** epistaxis, nasopharyngitis, blurred vision. **GU:** nephrotoxicity. **Resp:** cough, dyspnea, pneumonia. **GI:** HEPATOTOXICITY, abdominal pain, anorexia, constipation, diarrhea, dyspepsia, nausea, vomiting. **Derm:** DRUG RASH WITH EOSINOPHILIA AND SYSTEMIC SYMPTOMS (DRESS), petechiae, pruritus, skin rash. **F and E:** edema (including pleural effusion, pericardial infusion, pulmonary edema, and superficial edema), hypokalemia. **Endo:** ↓ growth (in children), hypothyroidism. **Hemat:** BLEEDING, NEUTROPENIA, THROMBOCYTOPENIA. **Metab:** weight gain. **MS:** arthralgia, muscle cramps, musculoskeletal pain, myalgia. **Misc:** TUMOR LYSIS SYNDROME, fever, night sweats.

Interactions

Drug-Drug: Blood levels and effects are ↑ by concurrent use of potent CYP3A4 inhibitors (e.g., **ketoconazole**, **itraconazole**, **clarithromycin**, **atazanavir**, **indinavir**, **nefazodone**, **nelfinavir**, **ritonavir**, **saquinavir**, or **voriconazole**). Blood levels and effects may be ↓ by potent CYP3A4 inducers (e.g., **dexamethasone**, **phenytoin**, **carbamazepine**, **rifampin**, **rifabutin**, and **phenobarbital**; if used concurrently, ↑ dose of imatinib by 50%. ↑ blood levels of **simvastatin**. Imatinib inhibits the following enzyme systems: CYP2C9, CYP2D6, CYP3A4/5 and may be expected to alter the effects of other drugs metabolized by these systems.

Drug-Food: Blood levels and effects are ↑ by **grapefruit juice**; concurrent use should be avoided.

Route/Dosage

Chronic Myeloid Leukemia

PO (Adults): *Chronic phase*—400 mg once daily, may be ↑ to 600 mg once daily; *accelerated phase or blast crisis*—600 mg once daily; may be ↑ to 800 mg/day given as 400 mg twice daily based on response and circumstances.

PO (Children): *Newly diagnosed Ph+ CML*—340 mg/m² once daily (not to exceed 600 mg); *CML recurrent after failure of bone marrow transplant or resistance to interferon-alpha*—260 mg/m² once daily.

Gastrointestinal Stromal Tumors

PO (Adults): *Metastatic or unresectable*—400 mg once daily; may be ↑ to 400 mg twice daily if well tolerated and response insufficient; *Adjuvant treatment after resection*—400 mg once daily.

Ph+ Acute Lymphoblastic Leukemia

PO (Adults): 600 mg once daily.

PO (Children): 340 mg/m² once daily (not to exceed 600 mg).

Myelodysplastic/Myeloproliferative Diseases

PO (Adults): 400 mg once daily.

Aggressive Systemic Mastocytosis

PO (Adults): 400 mg once daily. *For patients with eosinophilia*—100 mg once daily; ↑ to 400 mg once daily if well tolerated and response insufficient.

Hypereosinophilic Syndrome and/or Chronic Eosinophilic Leukemia

PO (Adults): 400 mg once daily. *For patients with FIP1L1–PDGFRa fusion kinase*—100 mg once daily; ↑ to 400 mg once daily if well tolerated and response insufficient.

Dermatofibrosarcoma Protuberans

PO (Adults): 400 mg twice daily.

Hepatic Impairment

PO (Adults): ↓ dose by 25% in severe hepatic impairment.

Renal Impairment

PO (Adults): *CCr 40–59 mL/min*—Do not exceed dose of 600 mg/day; *CCr 20–39 mL/min*—↓ initial dose by 50%; ↑ as tolerated.

Availability (generic available)

Tablets: 100 mg, 400 mg.

NURSING IMPLICATIONS

Assessment

- Monitor for fluid retention. Weigh regularly, and assess for signs of pleural effusion, pericardial effusion, pulmonary edema, ascites (dyspnea, periorbital edema, swelling in feet and ankles, weight gain). Evaluate unexpected weight gain. Edema is usually managed with diuretics. General fluid retention is usually dose related, more common in accelerated phase or blast crisis, and is more common in the elderly. Treatment usually involves diuretics, supportive therapy, and interruption of imatinib.
- Monitor growth rate in children and adolescents; may cause decrease in growth.

- Monitor vital signs; may cause fever.
- Monitor for tumor lysis syndrome (malignant disease progression, high WBC counts, hyperuricemia, hyperkalemia, hyperphosphatemia, hypocalcemia, and/or dehydration). Prevent by maintain adequate hydration and correcting uric acid levels prior to starting imatinib.
- Monitor for signs and symptoms of DRESS (fever, rash, lymphadenopathy, and/or facial swelling, associated with involvement of other organ systems (hepatitis, nephritis, hematologic abnormalities, myocarditis, myositis) during therapy. May resemble an acute viral infection. Eosinophilia is often present. Discontinue therapy if signs occur.
- ***Lab Test Considerations:*** Monitor liver function before and monthly during treatment or when clinically indicated. May cause ↑ transaminases and bilirubin which usually lasts 1 wk and may require dose reduction or interruption. If bilirubin is >3 times the upper limit of normal or transaminases are >5 times the upper limit of normal, withhold dose until bilirubin levels return to <1.5 times the upper limit of normal and transaminase levels to <2.5 times the upper limit of normal. Treatment may then be continued at reduced levels (patients on 400 mg/day should receive 300 mg/day and patients receiving 600 mg/day should receive 400 mg/day).
- Monitor CBC weekly for the first mo, biweekly for the 2nd mo, and periodically during therapy. May cause neutropenia and thrombocytopenia, usually lasting 2–3 wk or 3–4 wk, respectively, and anemia. Usually requires dose reduction, but may require discontinuation (see Implementation).
- Patients receiving *chronic phase, myelodysplastic/myeloproliferative disease, aggressive systemic mastocytosis, and hypereosinophilic syndrome and/or chronic eosinophilic leukemia* treatment who develop an ANC $<1.0 \times 10^9$/L and/or platelets $<50 \times 10^9$/L should stop imatinib until ANC $\geq 1.5 \times 10^9$/L and platelets are $\geq 75 \times 10^9$/L. Then resume imatinib treatment at 400 mg or 600 mg/day.
- *Patients receiving accelerated phase and blast crisis treatment or Ph+ acute lymphoblastic leukemia* who develop an ANC $<0.5 \times 10^9$/L and/or platelets $<10 \times 10^9$/L should determine if cytopenia is related to leukemia via marrow aspirate or biopsy. If cytopenia is unrelated to leukemia, reduce dose to 400 mg/day. If cytopenia persists for 2 wk, reduce dose to 300 mg/day. If cytopenia persists for 4 wk and is still unrelated to leukemia, stop imatinib until ANC $\geq 1 \times 10^9$/L and platelets are $\geq 20 \times 10^9$/L. Then resume imatinib treatment at 300 mg/day.
- *Patients receiving aggressive systemic mastocytosis with eosinophilia or hypereosinophilic syndrome and/or chronic eosinophilic leukemia with FIP1L1–PDGFRa fusion kinase* who develop ANC $<1.0 \times 10^9$/L and platelets $<50 \times 10^9$/L should stop imatinib until ANC $\geq 1.5 \times 10^9$/L and platelets $\geq 75 \times 10^9$/L. Resume treatment at previous dose.
- May cause hypokalemia.
- Verify pregnancy status in females with reproductive potential before starting therapy.

Implementation

- ***High Alert:*** Fatalities have occurred with incorrect administration of chemotherapeutic agents. Before administering, clarify all ambiguous orders; double check single, daily, and course-of-therapy dose limits; have second practitioner independently double check original order and dose calculations. Therapy should be initiated by physician experienced in the treatment of patients with chronic myeloid leukemia.
- Patients requiring anticoagulation should receive low-molecular-weight or standard heparin, not warfarin.
- Treatment should be continued as long as patient continues to benefit.
- **PO:** Administer with food and a full glass of water to minimize GI irritation.
- Tablets may be dispersed in water or apple juice (50 mL for the 100 mg and 100 mL for the 400 mg tablet) and stirred with a spoon for patients unable to swallow pills. Administer immediately after suspension.
- Doses for children may be given once daily or divided into two doses, one in morning and one in evening.
- Administer doses >800 m g/day as 400 mg twice daily to decrease exposure to iron.

Patient/Family Teaching

- Explain purpose of imatinib to patient. Instruct patient to take imatinib as directed. If a dose is missed, take next dose at regular scheduled time. Do not double doses.
- Advise patient to avoid grapefruit and grapefruit juice during therapy.
- May cause drowsiness or dizziness. Caution patient to avoid driving or other activities requiring alertness until response to medication is known.
- Inform patient of possibility of edema and fluid retention. Advise patient to notify health care professional if unexpected rapid weight gain occurs.
- Advise patient to notify health care professional if signs and symptoms of liver failure (jaundice, anorexia, bleeding or bruising) or DRESS occur.
- Rep: Advise female patient with reproductive potential to use effective contraception during and for at least 14 days after last dose of imatinib. Advise patient to notify health care professional if pregnancy is planned or suspected; avoid breast feeding for at least 1 mo after last dose of imatinib.

Evaluation/Desired Outcomes

- Decrease in production of leukemic cells in patients with CML, HES/CEL, and ALL and malignant cells in GIST, MDS/MPD, ASM, and DFSP.

imipenem/cilastatin
(i-me-**pen**-em/sye-la-**stat**-in)
Primaxin

Classification
Therapeutic: anti-infectives
Pharmacologic: carbapenems

Indications
Treatment of: Lower respiratory tract infections, Urinary tract infections, Abdominal infections, Gynecologic infections, Skin and skin structure infections, Bone and joint infections, Bacteremia, Endocarditis, Polymicrobic infections.

Action
Imipenem binds to the bacterial cell wall, resulting in cell death. Combination with cilastatin prevents renal inactivation of imipenem, resulting in high urinary concentrations. Imipenem resists the actions of many enzymes that degrade most other penicillins and penicillin-like anti-infectives. **Therapeutic Effects:** Bactericidal action against susceptible bacteria. **Spectrum:** Spectrum is broad. Active against most gram-positive aerobic cocci: *Streptococcus pneumoniae*, Group A beta-hemolytic streptococci, *Enterococcus*, *Staphylococcus aureus*. Active against many gram-negative bacillary organisms: *Escherichia coli*, *Klebsiella*, *Acinetobacter*, *Proteus*, *Serratia*, *Pseudomonas aeruginosa*. Also displays activity against: *Salmonella*, *Shigella*, *Neisseria gonorrhoeae*, Numerous anaerobes.

Pharmacokinetics
Absorption: IV administration results in complete bioavailability.
Distribution: Widely distributed. Crosses the placenta; enters breast milk.
Metabolism and Excretion: *Imipenem and cilastatin*—70% excreted unchanged by the kidneys.
Half-life: *Imipenem and cilastatin*—1 hr (↑ in renal impairment).

TIME/ACTION PROFILE (blood levels)

ROUTE	ONSET	PEAK	DURATION
IV	rapid	end of infusion	6–8 hr

Contraindications/Precautions
Contraindicated in: Hypersensitivity; Cross-sensitivity may occur with penicillins and cephalosporins.
Use Cautiously in: Previous history of multiple hypersensitivity reactions; Seizure disorders; Renal impairment (dose ↓ required if CCr ≤70 mL/min/1.73 m²); OB: Safety not established; Lactation: Use during breast feeding only if benefit to patient outweighs potential risk to infant; Pedi: Children with CNS infections (↑ risk of seizures) or children <30 kg with renal impairment (safety not established); Geri: May be at ↑ risk for toxic reactions due to age-related ↑ in renal function.

Adverse Reactions/Side Effects
CNS: SEIZURES, dizziness, somnolence. **CV:** hypotension. **Derm:** rash, pruritus, sweating, urticaria. **GI:** CLOSTRIDIUM DIFFICILE-ASSOCIATED DIARRHEA (CDAD), diarrhea, nausea, vomiting. **Hemat:** eosinophilia. **Local:** phlebitis at IV site. **Misc:** HYPERSENSITIVITY REACTIONS (including anaphylaxis), fever, superinfection.

Interactions
Drug-Drug: Do not admix with **aminoglycosides** (inactivation may occur). **Probenecid** ↓ renal excretion and ↑ blood levels. ↑ risk of seizures with **ganciclovir** or **cyclosporine** (avoid concurrent use of ganciclovir). May ↓ serum **valproate** levels (↑ risk of seizures).

Route/Dosage
IV (Adults): *Mild infections*—250–500 mg every 6 hr; *Moderate infections*—500 mg every 6–8 hr *or* 1 g every 8 hr; *Serious infections*—500 mg every 6 hr to 1 g every 6–8 hr.
IV (Children ≥3 mo): 15–25 mg/kg every 6 hr; higher doses have been used in older children with cystic fibrosis.
IV (Children 4 wk–3 mo): 25 mg/kg every 6 hr.
IV (Children 1–4 wk): 25 mg/kg every 8 hr.
IV (Children <1 wk): 25 mg/kg every 12 hr.

Renal Impairment
IV (Adults): If dose for normal renal function is 1 g/day *CCr 41–70 mL/min*—125–250 mg every 6–8 hr, *CCr 21–40 mL/min*—125–250 mg every 8–12 hr, *CCr 6–20 mL/min*—125–250 mg every 12 hr; **If dose for normal renal function is 1.5 g/day** *CCr 41–70 mL/min*—125–250 mg every 6–8 hr, *CCr 21–40 mL/min*—125–250 mg every 8–12 hr, *CCr 6–20 mL/min*—125–250 mg every 12 hr; **If dose for normal renal function is 2 g/day** *CCr 41–70 mL/min*—125–500 mg every 6–8 hr, *CCr 21–40 mL/min*—125–250 mg every 8–12 hr, *CCr 6–20 mL/min*—125–250 mg every 12 hr; **If dose for normal renal function is 3 g/day** *CCr 41–70 mL/min*—250–500 mg every 6–8 hr, *CCr 21–40 mL/min*—250–500 mg every 6–8 hr, *CCr 6–20 mL/min*—250–500 mg every 12 hr; **If dose for normal renal function is 4 g/day** *CCr 41–70 mL/min*—250–750 mg every 6–8 hr, *CCr 21–40 mL/min*—250–500 mg every 6–8 hr, *CCr 6–20 mL/min*—250–250 mg every 12 hr.

Availability (generic available)

Powder for injection (requires reconstitution and dilution): 250 mg imipenem/250 mg cilastatin, 500 mg imipenem/500 mg cilastatin.

NURSING IMPLICATIONS

Assessment

- Assess patient for infection (vital signs; appearance of wound, sputum, urine, and stool; WBC) at beginning of and throughout therapy.
- Obtain a history before initiating therapy to determine previous use of and reactions to penicillins. Persons with a negative history of penicillin sensitivity may still have an allergic response.
- Obtain specimens for culture and sensitivity before initiating therapy. First dose may be given before receiving results.
- Observe patient for signs and symptoms of anaphylaxis (rash, pruritus, laryngeal edema, wheezing). Discontinue the drug and notify the physician immediately if these occur. Have epinephrine, an antihistamine, and resuscitative equipment close by in the event of an anaphylactic reaction.
- ***Lab Test Considerations:*** BUN, AST, ALT, LDH, serum alkaline phosphatase, bilirubin, and creatinine may be transiently ↑.
- Hemoglobin and hematocrit concentrations may be ↓.
- May cause positive direct Coombs' test.

Implementation

IV Administration

- **Intermittent Infusion:** Reconstitute each 250- or 500-mg vial with 10 mL of D5W, D5/0.9% NaCl, 0.9% NaCl, or D5/0.45% NaCl and shake well. ***Diluent:*** Further dilute in 100 mL of D5W or 0.9% NaCl. Solution may range from clear to yellow in color. Infusion is stable for 4 hr at room temperature and 24 hr if refrigerated. ***Concentration:*** 2.5 mg/mL (with 250–mg vial); 5 mg/mL (with 500-mg vial). ***Rate:*** Infuse doses ≤500 mg over 20–30 min. Infuse doses ≥750 mg over 40–60 min. Pedi: Infuse doses ≤500 mg over 15–30 min. Infuse doses >500 m g over 40–60 min.
- Rapid infusion may cause nausea and vomiting. If these symptoms develop, slow infusion.
- **Y-Site Compatibility:** acyclovir, alfentanil, amifostine, amikacin, aminocaproic acid, anidulafungin, argatroban, arsenic trioxide, ascorbic acid, atracurium, atropine, benztropine, bivalirudin, bleomycin, bumetanide, buprenorphine, butorphanol, carboplatin, carmustine, caspofungin, cefazolin, cefepime, cefotaxime, cefotetan, cefoxitin, ceftazidime, ceftazidime/avibactam, cefuroxime, chloramphenicol, cisatracurium, cisplatin, clindamycin, cyanocobalamin, cyclophosphamide, cyclosporine, cytarabine, dactinomycin, daunorubicin, dexamethasone, dexmedetomidine, dexrazoxane, digoxin, diltiazem, diphenhydramine, docetaxel, dolasetron, dopamine, doxacurium, doxorubicin, doxorubicin liposomal, doxycycline, enalaprilat, ephedrine, epinephrine, epirubicin, epoetin alfa, eptifibatide, erythromycin, esmolol, etoposide, famotidine, fenoldopam, fentanyl, fludarabine, fluorouracil, folic acid, foscarnet, fosphenytoin, furosemide, gemtuzumab, gentamicin, glycopyrrolate, granisetron, heparin, hydrocortisone, hydromorphone, idarubicin, ifosfamide, indomethacin, insulin regular, irinotecan, isavuconazonium, isoproterenol, ketorolac, labetalol, leucovorin calcium, levofloxacin, lidocaine, linezolid, magnesium sulfate, melphalan, meropenem/vaborbactam, mesna, methotrexate, methylprednisolone, metoclopramide, metoprolol, mitomycin, mitoxantrone, morphine, multivitamins, nafcillin, naloxone, nitroglycerin, norepinephrine, octreotide, ondansetron, oxacillin, oxaliplatin, oxytocin, paclitaxel, pamidronate, pancuronium, pantoprazole, pemetrexed, penicillin G, pentobarbital, phentolamine, phenylephrine, phytonadione, plazomicin, potassium acetate, potassium chloride, propofol, propranolol, protamine, ranitidine, remifentanil, rituximab, rocuronium, sodium acetate, streptokinase, succinylcholine, sufentanil, tacrolimus, tedizolid, theophylline, thiotepa, tigecycline, tirofiban, tobramycin, tolazoline, trastuzumab, vasopressin, verapamil, vinblastine, vincristine, vinorelbine, voriconazole, zidovudine, zoledronic acid.
- **Y-Site Incompatibility:** alemtuzumab, allopurinol, amiodarone, amphotericin B deoxycholate, amphotericin B lipid complex, amphotericin B liposome, azathioprine, blinatumomab, ceftriaxone, chlorpromazine, dacarbazine, dantrolene, daptomycin, diazepam, diazoxide, etoposide phosphate, ganciclovir, gemcitabine, haloperidol, lorazepam, mannitol, metaraminol, methyldopate, milrinone, mycophenolate, nalbuphine, nicardipine, palonosetron, phenytoin, prochlorperazine, pyridoxime, quinupristin/dalfopristin, sargramostim, sodium bicarbonate, thiamine, topotecan, trimethoprim/sulfamethoxazole, vecuronium.
- **Additive Incompatibility:** May be inactivated if administered concurrently with aminoglycosides. If administered concurrently, administer in separate sites, if possible, at least 1 hr apart. If second site is unavailable, flush lines between medications.

Patient/Family Teaching

- Advise patient to report the signs of superinfection (black, furry overgrowth on the tongue; vaginal itching or discharge; loose or foul-smelling stools) and allergy. Consult health care professional before treating with antidiarrheals.
- Caution patient to notify health care professional if fever and diarrhea occur, especially if stool contains blood, pus, or mucus. Advise patient not to treat diarrhea without consulting health care professional. May occur up to several wk after discontinuation of medication.

Evaluation/Desired Outcomes

- Resolution of the signs and symptoms of infection. Length of time for complete resolution depends on the organism and site of infection.

BEERS

imipramine (im-ip-ra-meen)

Impril, Tofranil, Tofranil PM

Classification

Therapeutic: antidepressants

Pharmacologic: tricyclic antidepressants

Indications

Various forms of depression. Enuresis in children. **Unlabeled Use:** Adjunct in the management of chronic pain, incontinence (in adults), vascular headache prophylaxis, cluster headache, insomnia.

Action

Potentiates the effect of serotonin and norepinephrine. Has significant anticholinergic properties. **Therapeutic Effects:** Antidepressant action that develops slowly over several weeks.

Pharmacokinetics

Absorption: Well absorbed from the GI tract.

Distribution: Widely distributed. Probably crosses the placenta and enters breast milk.

Protein Binding: 89–95%.

Metabolism and Excretion: Mostly metabolized by the liver (CYP2D6 isoenzyme) to desipramine; the CYP2D6 enzyme system exhibits genetic polymorphism; ~7% of population may be poor metabolizers (PMs) and may have significantly ↑ imipramine concentrations and an ↑ risk of adverse effects.

Half-life: 8–16 hr.

TIME/ACTION PROFILE (antidepressant effect)

ROUTE	ONSET	PEAK	DURATION
PO	hrs	2–6 wk	wk

Contraindications/Precautions

Contraindicated in: Hypersensitivity; Cross-sensitivity with other antidepressants may occur; Angle-closure glaucoma; Hypersensitivity to tartrazine or sulfites (in some preparations); Recent MI, known history of QTc interval prolongation, heart failure; Concurrent use of MAO inhibitors or MAO-like drugs (linezolid or methylene blue).

Use Cautiously in: Pre-existing cardiovascular disease; Seizures or history of seizure disorder; May ↑ risk of suicide attempt/ideation especially during early treatment or dose adjustment; Lactation: Drug is present in breast milk; discontinue imipramine or bottle feed; Pedi: Suicide risk may be greater in children or adolescents. Safety not established in children <6 yr; Geri: More susceptible to adverse reactions. Geriatric males with prostatic hyperplasia are more susceptible to urinary retention.

Adverse Reactions/Side Effects

CNS: SUICIDAL THOUGHTS, drowsiness, fatigue, agitation, confusion, hallucinations, insomnia. **EENT:** blurred vision, dry eyes. **CV:** ARRHYTHMIAS, hypotension, ECG changes. **GI:** constipation, dry mouth, nausea, paralytic ileus, weight gain. **GU:** urinary retention, ↓ libido. **Derm:** photosensitivity. **Endo:** gynecomastia. **Hemat:** blood dyscrasias.

Interactions

Drug-Drug: Concurrent use with **MAO inhibitors** may result in serious potentially fatal reactions (MAO inhibitors should be stopped at least 14 days before imipramine therapy. Imipramine should be stopped at least 14 days before MAO inhibitor therapy). Concurrent use with **MAO-inhibitor like drugs**, such as **linezolid** or **methylene blue** may ↑ risk of serotonin syndrome; concurrent use contraindicated; do not start therapy in patients receiving **linezolid** or **methylene blue**; if **linezolid** or **methylene blue** need to be started in a patient receiving imipramine, immediately discontinue imipramine and monitor for signs/symptoms of serotonin syndrome for 2 wk or until 24 hr after last dose of linezolid or methylene blue, whichever comes first (may resume imipramine therapy 24 hr after last dose of linezolid or methylene blue). Concurrent use with **SSRI antidepressants** may result in ↑ toxicity and should be avoided (**fluoxetine** should be stopped 5 wk before). Hypertensive crisis may occur with **clonidine**. Imipramine is metabolized in the liver by the **cytochrome P450 2D6 enzyme** and its action may be affected by drugs that compete for metabolism by this enzyme including **other antidepressants**, **phenothiazines**, **carbamazepine**, **class 1C antiarrhythmics (propafenone, flecainide)**; when used concurrently, dose reduction of one or the other or both may be necessary. Concurrent use of other drugs that inhibit the activity of the enzyme, including **cimetidine**, **quinidine**, **amiodarone**, and **ritonavir**, may result in ↑ effects of imipramine. Concurrent use with **levodopa** may result in delayed/↓ absorption of levodopa or hypertension. Blood levels and effects may be ↓ by **rifamycins**. ↑ CNS depression with other **CNS depressants** including **alcohol**, **antihistamines**, **clonidine**, **opioids**, and **sedative/hypnotics**. **Barbiturates** may alter blood levels and effects. **Adrenergic** and **anticholinergic** side effects may be ↑ with other **agents having these properties**. **Phenothiazines** or **hormonal contraceptives** ↑ levels and may cause toxicity. **Cigarette smoking (nicotine)** may ↑ metabolism and alter effects. Drugs that affect serotonergic neurotransmitter systems, including **SSRIs**, **SNRIs**,

fentanyl, **buspirone**, **tramadol**, and **triptans** ↑ risk of serotonin syndrome.

Drug-Natural Products: Use with **St. John's wort** ↑ risk of serotonin syndrome. Concomitant use of **kava-kava**, **valerian**, or **chamomile** can ↑ CNS depression. ↑ anticholinergic effects with **jimson weed** and **scopolia**.

Route/Dosage

PO (Adults): 25–50 mg 3–4 times daily (not to exceed 300 mg/day); total daily dose may be given at bedtime.

PO (Geriatric Patients): 25 mg at bedtime initially, up to 100 mg/day in divided doses.

PO (Children >12 yr): *Antidepressant*—25–50 mg/day in divided doses (not to exceed 100 mg/day).

PO (Children 6–12 yr): *Antidepressant*—10–30 mg/day in 2 divided doses.

PO (Children ≥6 yr): *Enuresis*—25 mg once daily 1 hr before bedtime; ↑ if necessary by 25 mg at weekly intervals to 50 mg in children <12 yr, up to 75 mg in children >12 yr.

Availability (generic available)

Tablets: 10 mg, 25 mg, 50 mg, 🍁 75 mg. **Capsules:** 75 mg, 100 mg, 125 mg, 150 mg.

NURSING IMPLICATIONS

Assessment

- Monitor BP and pulse rate prior to and during initial therapy.
- Monitor plasma levels in treatment-resistant patients.
- Monitor weight and BMI initially and periodically throughout therapy.
- For overweight/obese individuals, obtain FBS and cholesterol levels. Refer as appropriate for nutrition/weight management and medical management.
- Obtain weight and BMI initially and regularly throughout therapy.
- Assess for sexual dysfunction (decreased libido; erectile dysfunction).
- Assess for suicidal tendencies, especially during early therapy. Restrict amount of drug available to patient. Risk may be increased in children, adolescents, and adults ≤24 yrs. After starting therapy, children, adolescents, and young adults should be seen by health care professional at least weekly for 4 wk, every 3 wk for next 4 wk, and on advice of health care professional thereafter.
- Pedi, Geri: Monitor baseline and periodic ECGs in elderly patients or patients with heart disease and before increasing dose with children treated for enuresis. May cause prolonged PR and QT intervals and may flatten T waves.
- **Depression:** Assess mental status (orientation, mood, behavior) frequently. Confusion, agitation, and hallucinations may occur during initiation of therapy and may require dosage reduction. Assess for suicidal tendencies, especially during early therapy. Restrict amount of drug available to patient.
- **Enuresis:** Assess frequency of bedwetting during therapy. Ask patient or caretaker to maintain diary.
- **Pain:** Assess location, duration, and severity of pain periodically during therapy. Use pain scale to monitor effectiveness of therapy.
- ***Lab Test Considerations:*** Assess leukocyte and differential blood counts and renal and hepatic functions prior to and periodically during prolonged or high-dose therapy.
- Serum levels may be monitored in patients who fail to respond to usual therapeutic dose. Therapeutic plasma concentration range for depression is 150–300 ng/mL.
- May cause alterations in blood glucose levels.
- ***Toxicity and Overdose:*** Symptoms of acute overdose include disturbed concentration, confusion, restlessness, agitation, seizures, drowsiness, mydriasis, arrhythmias, fever, hallucinations, vomiting, and dyspnea.
- Treatment of overdose includes gastric lavage, activated charcoal, and a stimulant cathartic. Maintain respiratory and cardiac function (monitor ECG for at least 5 days) and temperature. Medications may include digoxin for HF, antiarrhythmics, and anticonvulsants.

Implementation

- Dose increases should be made at bedtime because of sedation. Dose titration is a slow process; may take wk to mo. May be given as a single dose at bedtime to minimize sedation during the day.
- Taper to avoid withdrawal effects. Reduce by 50% for 3 days, then reduce by 50% for 3 days, then discontinue.
- **PO:** Administer medication with or immediately following a meal to minimize gastric irritation.
- **IM:** May be slightly yellow or red in color. Crystals may develop if solution is cool; place ampule under warm running water for 1 min to dissolve.

Patient/Family Teaching

- Instruct patient to take medication as directed. Take missed doses as soon as possible unless almost time for next dose; if regimen is a single dose at bedtime, do not take in the morning because of side effects. Advise patient that drug effects may not be noticed for at least 2 wk. Abrupt discontinuation may cause nausea, vomiting, diarrhea, headache, trouble sleeping with vivid dreams, and irritability.
- May cause drowsiness and blurred vision. Caution patient to avoid driving and other activities requiring alertness until response to drug is known.
- Instruct patient to notify health care professional if visual changes occur. Inform patient that periodic glaucoma testing may be needed during long-term therapy.
- Caution patient to change positions slowly to minimize orthostatic hypotension. Advise patient, family,

and caregivers to look for suicidality, especially during early therapy or dose changes. Notify health care professional immediately if thoughts about suicide or dying, attempts to commit suicide, new or worse depression or anxiety, agitation or restlessness, panic attacks, insomnia, new or worse irritability, aggressiveness, acting on dangerous impulses, mania, or other changes in mood or behavior or if symptoms of serotonin syndrome occur.

- Advise patient to avoid alcohol or other CNS depressant drugs during therapy and for at least 3–7 days after therapy has been discontinued.
- Instruct patient to notify health care professional if urinary retention, dry mouth, or constipation persists. Sugarless candy or gum may diminish dry mouth and an increase in fluid intake or bulk may prevent constipation. If symptoms persist, dose reduction or discontinuation may be necessary. Consult health care professional if dry mouth persists for more than 2 wk.
- Caution patient to use sunscreen and protective clothing to prevent photosensitivity reactions.
- Alert patient that urine may turn blue-green in color.
- Inform patient of need to monitor dietary intake, as possible increase in appetite may lead to undesired weight gain. Inform patient that increased amounts of riboflavin in the diet may be required; consult health care professional.
- Advise patient to notify health care professional of medication regimen prior to treatment or surgery.
- Therapy for depression is usually prolonged. Emphasize the importance of follow-up exams to evaluate progress and improve coping skills.
- Instruct female patients to notify health care professional if pregnancy is planned or suspected, or if breast feeding.
- Pedi: Inform parents that the side effects most likely to occur include nervousness, insomnia, unusual tiredness, and mild nausea and vomiting. Notify health care professional if these symptoms become pronounced.
- Advise parents to keep medication out of reach of children to prevent inadvertent overdose.

Evaluation/Desired Outcomes

- Increased sense of well-being.
- Renewed interest in surroundings.
- Increased appetite.
- Improved energy level.
- Pain relief.
- Diminished incidence of enuresis.
- Improved sleep in patients treated for depression. Patient may require 2–6 wk of therapy before full therapeutic effects of medication are noticeable.
- Control of bedwetting in children >6 yr.
- Decrease in chronic neurogenic pain.

indacaterol (in-da-kat-e-role)

Arcapta Neohaler, ✤Onbrez Breezhaler

Classification

Therapeutic: bronchodilators, COPD agents

Pharmacologic: adrenergics

Indications

Long-term maintenance treatment of airflow obstruction associated with chronic obstructive pulmonary disease (COPD), including chronic bronchitis and/or emphysema.

Action

Produces accumulation of cyclic adenosine monophosphate (cAMP) at beta$_2$-adrenergic receptors. Relatively specific for pulmonary receptors. Acts as a long-acting beta-agonist (LABA). **Therapeutic Effects:** Bronchodilation, with improvement in symptoms of COPD.

Pharmacokinetics

Absorption: Some systemic absorption from lungs and GI tract (43–45%).

Distribution: Extensively distributed.

Metabolism and Excretion: 54% excreted unchanged in feces; absorbed drug is mostly metabolized; 23% excreted in feces as metabolites.

Half-life: 45.5–126 hr.

TIME/ACTION PROFILE (blood levels)

ROUTE	ONSET	PEAK	DURATION
Inhaln	unknown	15 min	24 hr†

†Bronchodilation.

Contraindications/Precautions

Contraindicated in: Hypersensitivity; Acutely deteriorating COPD or acute respiratory symptoms; Asthma.

Use Cautiously in: OB: Use only if potential maternal benefit justifies potential fetal risk; may interfere with uterine contractility during labor; Lactation: Use while breast feeding only if potential maternal benefit justifies potential risk to infant; Pedi: Safety and effectiveness not established.

Exercise Extreme Caution in: Concurrent use of MAO inhibitors, tricyclic antidepressants or drugs that prolong the QTc interval (↑ risk of adverse cardiovascular reactions).

Adverse Reactions/Side Effects

CNS: headache. **EENT:** nasopharyngitis, oropharyngeal pain. **GI:** nausea. **Resp:** PARADOXICAL BRONCHOSPASM, cough. **Misc:** HYPERSENSITIVITY REACTIONS (including angioedema).

Interactions

Drug-Drug: ↑ risk of serious adverse cardiovascular effects with **MAO inhibitors, tricyclic antidepres-**

sants, drugs that prolong the QTc interval; use with extreme caution. Effectiveness may be ↓ by beta-blockers; use cautiously and only when necessary. Concurrent use with other **adrenergics** may ↑ adrenergic adverse reactions (↑ heart rate, BP, jitteriness). ↑ risk of hypokalemia or ECG changes with **xanthine derivatives, corticosteroids, diuretics**, or **non-potassium sparing diuretics**.

Drug-Natural Products: Use with **caffeine-containing herbs (cola nut, guarana, mate, tea, coffee)** ↑ stimulant effect.

Route/Dosage

Inhaln (Adults): 75 mcg once daily.

Availability

Capsules for inhalation: 75 mcg.

NURSING IMPLICATIONS

Assessment

- Assess respiratory status (rate, breath sounds, degree of dyspnea, pulse) before administration and at peak of medication. Consult health care professional about alternative medication if severe bronchospasm is present; onset of action is too slow for patients in acute distress. If paradoxical bronchospasm (wheezing) occurs, withhold medication and notify health care professional immediately.
- Monitor for signs and symptoms of allergic reactions (difficulties in breathing or swallowing, swelling of tongue, lips and face, urticaria, skin rash). Discontinue therapy if symptoms occur.
- ***Lab Test Considerations:*** May cause transient hypokalemia and hyperglycemia.

Implementation

- **Inhaln:** Pull cap off *Neohaler*. Open inhaler by holding the base and tilting the mouthpiece. Tear perforation to separate one blister from blister card; peal away protective back to expose foil. With dry hands, push capsule through foil to remove. Insert capsule into capsule chamber; do not swallow capsule or place directly into mouthpiece. Close inhaler until it clicks. Press both buttons fully 1 time; click is heard as capsule is pierced; do not press piercing buttons more than 1 time. Release buttons fully. Breathe out; do not blow into mouthpiece. Close lips around mouthpiece; hold inhaler with buttons left and right (not up and down). Breathe in rapidly and steadily, as deep as possible, a whirring noise is heard. Continue to hold breath as long as possible while removing inhaler from mouth. Open inhaler, if powder remains in capsule, close inhaler and inhale again. Usually requires 1–2 breaths. Remove capsule.

Patient/Family Teaching

- Instruct patient in the correct use of capsules and *Neohaler*. Advise patient not to discontinue without consulting health care professional; symptoms may recur.
- Inform patient that indacaterol is not a bronchodilator and should not be used for treating sudden breathing problems.
- Advise patient to notify health care professional if signs and symptoms of allergic reaction, worsening symptoms; decreasing effectiveness of inhaled, short-acting beta$_2$-agonists; need for more inhalations than usual of inhaled, short-acting beta$_2$-agonists; or significant decrease in lung function occur.
- Instruct patient to notify health care professional of all Rx or OTC medications, vitamins, or herbal products being taken and to avoid concurrent use of Rx, OTC, and herbal products without consulting health care professional.
- Advise female patient to notify health care professional if pregnancy is planned or suspected, or if breast feeding.

Evaluation/Desired Outcomes

- Decrease in the number of flare-ups or the worsening of COPD symptoms (exacerbations).

BEERS

indomethacin

(in-doe-**meth**-a-sin)

Indocin, Tivorbex

Classification

Therapeutic: antirheumatics, ductus arteriosus patency adjuncts (IV only), nonsteroidal anti-inflammatory agents

Indications

PO: Inflammatory disorders including: Rheumatoid arthritis, Gouty arthritis, Osteoarthritis, Ankylosing spondylitis. Mild-to-moderate acute pain. **IV:** Alternative to surgery in the management of patent ductus arteriosus (PDA) in premature neonates.

Action

Inhibits prostaglandin synthesis. In the treatment of PDA, decreased prostaglandin production allows the ductus to close. **Therapeutic Effects: PO:** Suppression of pain and inflammation. **IV:** Closure of PDA.

Pharmacokinetics

Absorption: Well absorbed after oral administration in adults, incomplete oral absorption in neonates.

Distribution: Crosses the blood-brain barrier and the placenta. Enters breast milk.

Protein Binding: 99%.

Metabolism and Excretion: Mostly metabolized by the liver.

Half-life: Neonates <2 wk: 20 hr; >2 wk: 11 hr; Adults: 2.6–11 hr.

TIME/ACTION PROFILE

ROUTE	ONSET	PEAK	DURATION
PO (analgesic)	30 min	0.5–2 hr	4–6 hr
PO-ER (analgesic)	30 min	unknown	4–6 hr
PO (anti-inflammatory)	up to 7 days	1–2 wk	4–6 hr
PO-ER (anti-inflammatory)	up to 7 days	1–2 wk	4–6 hr
IV (closure of PDA)	up to 48 hr	unknown	unknown

Contraindications/Precautions

Contraindicated in: Hypersensitivity; Known alcohol intolerance (suspension); Cross-sensitivity may exist with other NSAIDs, including aspirin; Active GI bleeding; Ulcer disease; Proctitis or recent history of rectal bleeding; Intraventricular hemorrhage; Thrombocytopenia; Coronary artery bypass graft (CABG) surgery; Pedi: ↑ risk of necrotizing enterocolitis and bowel perforation in premature infants with PDA.

Use Cautiously in: Severe renal or hepatic impairment; Cardiovascular disease or risk factors for cardiovascular disease (may ↑ risk of serious cardiovascular thrombotic events, myocardial infarction, and stroke, especially with prolonged use or use of higher doses); avoid use in patients with recent MI or HF; History of ulcer disease; Seizure disorders; Hypertension; OB: Not recommended starting at 30 wk gestation (potential for causing premature closure of ductus arteriosus); Lactation: Usually compatible with breast feeding; Geri: ↑ risk of adverse reactions.

Adverse Reactions/Side Effects

CNS: dizziness, drowsiness, headache, psychic disturbances. **CV:** HF, MYOCARDIAL INFARCTION, STROKE, edema, hypertension. **Derm:** rash. **EENT:** blurred vision, tinnitus. **F and E:** hyperkalemia; *IV*, dilutional hyponatremia; *IV*, hypoglycemia. **GI:** *PO*—GI BLEEDING, HEPATOTOXICITY, PANCREATITIS, constipation, dyspepsia, nausea, vomiting, discomfort, necrotizing enterocolitis. **GU:** cystitis, hematuria, renal failure. **Hemat:** thrombocytopenia, blood dyscrasias, prolonged bleeding time. **Local:** phlebitis at IV site. **Misc:** HYPERSENSITIVITY REACTIONS (including anaphylaxis).

Interactions

Drug-Drug: Concurrent use with **aspirin** may ↓ effectiveness. Additive adverse GI effects with **aspirin**, other **NSAIDs**, **corticosteroids**, or **alcohol**. Chronic use of **acetaminophen** ↑ risk of adverse renal reactions. May ↓ effectiveness of **diuretics** or **antihypertensives**. May ↑ hypoglycemia from **insulins** or **oral hypoglycemic agents**. May ↑ risk of toxicity from **lithium** or **zidovudine** (avoid concurrent use with zidovudine). ↑ risk of toxicity from **methotrexate**. **Probenecid** ↑ risk of toxicity from indomethacin. ↑ risk of bleeding with **anticoagulants**, **aspirin**, **clopidogrel**, **ticagrelor**, **prasugrel**, **corticosteroids**, **fibrinolytics**, **SNRIs**, or **SSRIs**. ↑ risk of adverse hematologic reactions with **antineoplastics** or **radiation therapy**. ↑ risk of nephrotoxicity with **cyclosporine**. Concurrent use with **potassium-sparing diuretics** may result in hyperkalemia. May ↑ levels of **digitalis glycosides**, **methotrexate**, **lithium**, and **aminoglycosides** when used IV in neonates.

Drug-Natural Products: ↑ bleeding risk with **anise**, **arnica**, **chamomile**, **clove**, **dong quai**, **feverfew**, **garlic**, **ginger**, **ginkgo**, **Panax ginseng**.

Route/Dosage

Anti-inflammatory

PO (Adults): *Antiarthritic*—25–50 mg 2–4 times daily *or* 75-mg extended-release capsule once or twice daily (not to exceed 200 mg or 150 mg of SR/day). A single bedtime dose of 100 mg may be used. *Antigout*—100 mg initially, followed by 50 mg 3 times daily for relief of pain, then ↓ further. *Mild-to-moderate acute pain (Tivorbex)*—20 mg 3 times daily or 40 mg 2–3 times daily.

PO (Children >2 yr): 1–2 mg/kg/day in 2–4 divided doses (not to exceed 4 mg/kg/day or 150–200 mg/day).

PDA Closure

IV (Neonates): *Treatment*—0.2 mg/kg initially, then 2 subsequent doses at 12–24 hr intervals of 0.1 mg/kg if age <48 hr at time of initial dose; 0.2 mg/kg if 2–7 days at initial dose; 0.25 mg/kg if age >7 days at initial dose. *Prophylaxis*—0.1–0.2 mg/kg initially, then 0.1 mg/kg every 12–24 hr for 2 doses.

Availability (generic available)

Capsules: 25 mg, 50 mg. **Capsules (Tivorbex):** 20 mg, 40 mg. **Oral suspension (fruit mint, pineapple coconut mint flavors):** 5 mg/mL. **Powder for injection (requires reconstitution):** 1 mg/vial. **Rectal suppository:** 50 mg, 🍁100 mg. **Sustained-release capsules:** 75 mg.

NURSING IMPLICATIONS

Assessment

- Patients who have asthma, aspirin-induced allergy, and nasal polyps are at increased risk for developing hypersensitivity reactions. Monitor for rhinitis, asthma, and urticaria.
- Assess patient for skin rash frequently during therapy. Discontinue ibuprofen at first sign of rash; may be life-threatening. Stevens-Johnson syndrome or toxic epidermal necrolysis may develop. Treat symptomatically; may recur once treatment is stopped.

- Monitor BP during initiation periodically during therapy. May cause fluid retention and edema, leading to new onset or worsening hypertension.
- **Arthritis:** Assess limitation of movement and pain—note type, location, and intensity before and 1–2 hr after administration.
- **PDA:** Monitor respiratory status, heart rate, BP, echocardiogram, and heart sounds routinely throughout therapy.
- Monitor intake and output. Fluid restriction is usually instituted throughout therapy.
- **Acute pain:** Assess type, location, and intensity of pain prior to and 2 hrs (peak) following administration.
- ***Lab Test Considerations:*** Evaluate BUN, serum creatinine, CBC, serum potassium levels, and liver function tests periodically in patients receiving prolonged therapy.
- Serum potassium, BUN, serum creatinine, AST, and ALT tests may show ↑ levels. Blood glucose concentrations may be altered. Hemoglobin and hematocrit concentrations, leukocyte and platelet counts, and CCr may be ↓.
- Urine glucose and urine protein concentrations may be ↑.
- Leukocyte and platelet count may be ↓. Bleeding time may be prolonged for several days after discontinuation.

Implementation

- If prolonged therapy is used, dose should be reduced to the lowest level that controls symptoms to minimize risk of cardiovascular thrombotic events.
- **PO:** Administer after meals, with food, or with antacids to decrease GI irritation. Do not break, crush, or chew sustained-release capsules.
- Shake suspension before administration. Do not mix with antacid or any other liquid.

IV Administration

- **IV Push:** ***Diluent:*** Preservative-free 0.9% NaCl or preservative-free sterile water. Reconstitute with 1 or 2 mL of diluent. ***Concentration:*** 0.5–1 mg/mL. Reconstitute immediately before use and discard any unused solution. Do not dilute further or admix. Do not administer via umbilical catheter into vessels near the superior mesenteric artery, as these can cause vasoconstriction and compromise blood flow to the intestines. Do not administer intra-arterially. ***Rate:*** Administer over 20–30 min. Avoid extravasation, as solution is irritating to tissues.
- **Y-Site Compatibility:** aminophylline, ascorbic acid, atropine, bumetanide, cefazolin, cefotaxime, cefoxitin, ceftazidime, ceftriaxone, cefuroxime, chloramphenicol, cisplatin, clindamycin, cyanocobalamin, cyclosporine, dexamethasone, digoxin, enalaprilat, ephedrine, epoetin alfa, fentanyl, fluconazole, folic acid, furosemide, ganciclovir, heparin, hydrocortisone, imipenem/cilastatin, insulin, regular, ketorolac, lidocaine, mannitol, metoclopramide, metoprolol, multivitamins, nafcillin, nitroglycerin, nitroprusside, penicillin G, pentobarbital, phenobarbital, phytonadione, potassium chloride, procainamide, ranitidine, sodium bicarbonate, streptokinase, theophylline.
- **Y-Site Incompatibility:** amikacin, amino acid injection, atracurium, aztreonam, benztropine, buprenorphine, butorphanol, calcium chloride, calcium gluconate, cefotetan, chlorpromazine, dactinomycin, dantrolene, daunorubicin hydrochloride, diazepam, diphenhydramine, dobutamine, dopamine, doxycycline, epinephrine, erythromycin, esmolol, etoposide, famotidine, gentamicin, glycopyrrolate, haloperidol, hydralazine, isoproterenol, labetalol, levofloxacin, magnesium sulfate, meperidine, methyldopate, midazolam, minocycline, morphine, nalbuphine, norepinephrine, ondansetron, oxytocin, paclitaxel, pantoprazole, papaverine, pentamidine, phenylephrine, phenytoin, prochlorperazine, promethazine, propranolol, protamine, pyridoxine, succinylcholine, sufentanil, thiamine, tobramycin, tolazoline, trimethoprim/sulfamethoxazole, vancomycin, vasopressin, verapamil.

Patient/Family Teaching

- Advise patient to take this medication with a full glass of water and to remain in an upright position for 15–30 min after administration.
- Instruct patient to take medication as directed. Take missed doses as soon as remembered if not almost time for next dose. Do not double doses.
- May cause drowsiness or dizziness. Advise patient to avoid driving or other activities requiring alertness until response to medication is known.
- Caution patient to avoid the concurrent use of alcohol, aspirin, other NSAIDs, acetaminophen, or other OTC medications without consulting health care professional.
- Caution patient to wear sunscreen and protective clothing to prevent photosensitivity reactions.
- Advise patient to inform health care professional of medication regimen before treatment or surgery.
- Instruct patient to notify health care professional immediately if signs and symptoms of cardiovascular thrombotic events (shortness of breath or trouble breathing, chest pain, weakness in one part or side of body, slurred speech); hepatotoxicity (nausea, fatigue, lethargy, diarrhea, pruritus, jaundice, right upper quadrant tenderness, "flu-like" symptoms) occur or if rash, itching, chills, fever, muscle aches, visual disturbances, weight gain, edema, abdominal pain, black stools, or persistent headache occurs.
- Rep: Advise females of reproductive potential to notify health care professional if pregnancy is planned or suspected and to avoid indomethacin starting at 30 wk gestation because of risk of premature closing of the fetal ductus arteriosus. May cause temporary infertility in women.
- **PDA:** Explain to parents the purpose of medication and the need for frequent monitoring.

Evaluation/Desired Outcomes

- Decrease in severity of mild to moderate pain.
- Improved joint mobility. Partial arthritic relief is usually seen within 2 wk, but maximum effectiveness may require up to 1 mo of continuous therapy. Patients who do not respond to one NSAID may respond to another.
- Successful PDA closure.

inFLIXimab (in-flix-i-mab)

Inflectra, Ixifi, Remicade, Renflexis, Remsima

Classification

Therapeutic: antirheumatics (DMARDs), gastrointestinal anti-inflammatories

Pharmacologic: monoclonal antibodies

Indications

Moderately to severely active rheumatoid arthritis (in combination with methotrexate). Moderately to severely active Crohn's disease in patients with an inadequate response to conventional therapy. Active psoriatic arthritis. Active ankylosing spondylitis. Moderately to severely active ulcerative colitis in patients with an inadequate response to conventional therapy. Chronic severe plaque psoriasis in patients who are candidates for systemic therapy and when other systemic therapies are less appropriate.

Action

Neutralizes and prevents the activity of tumor necrosis factor-alpha (TNF-alpha), resulting in anti-inflammatory and antiproliferative activity. **Therapeutic Effects:** Decreased signs and symptoms, decreased rate of joint destruction and improved physical function in rheumatoid arthritis and psoriatic arthritis. Decreased signs and symptoms and induction and maintenance of clinical remission in Crohn's disease. Reduction in number of fistulas and maintenance of closure of fistulae in Crohn's disease. Decreased signs and symptoms in ankylosing spondylitis. Decreased signs and symptoms, maintenance of clinical remission and mucosal healing, and eliminating corticosteroid use in ulcerative colitis. Decreased induration, scaling, and erythema of psoriatic lesions.

Pharmacokinetics

Absorption: IV administration results in complete bioavailability.

Distribution: Predominantly distributed within the vascular compartment.

Metabolism and Excretion: Unknown.

Half-life: 9.5 days.

TIME/ACTION PROFILE (symptoms of Crohn's disease)

ROUTE	ONSET	PEAK	DURATION
IV	1–2 wk	unknown	12–48 wk†

†After infusion.

Contraindications/Precautions

Contraindicated in: Hypersensitivity to infliximab, murine (mouse) proteins, or other components in the formulation; Moderate to severe HF (doses >5 mg/kg); Concurrent anakinra or abatacept; Lactation: Lactation.

Use Cautiously in: History of chronic or recurrent infection or underlying illness/treatment predisposing to infection; Patients being retreated after 2 yr without treatment (↑ risk of adverse reactions); History of tuberculosis or exposure (latent tuberculosis should be treated prior to infliximab therapy); History of opportunistic infection; Patients residing, or who have resided, where tuberculosis, histoplasmosis, coccidioidomycoses, or blastomycosis is endemic; Chronic obstructive pulmonary disease (↑ risk of malignancy); Geri: Geriatric patients; OB: Use only if clearly needed; infants exposed *in-utero* may be at ↑ risk for infection or agranulocytosis; Pedi: Children <6 yr (safety not established); ↑ risk of lymphoma (including hepatosplenic T-cell lymphoma [HSTCL] in patients with Crohn's disease or ulcerative colitis), leukemia, and other malignancies.

Adverse Reactions/Side Effects

CNS: STROKE, fatigue, headache, anxiety, depression, dizziness, insomnia. **EENT:** conjunctivitis, vision loss. **Resp:** upper respiratory tract infection, bronchitis, cough, dyspnea, laryngitis, pharyngitis, respiratory tract allergic reaction, rhinitis, sinusitis. **CV:** ARRHYTHMIAS, MYOCARDIAL ISCHEMIA/INFARCTION, chest pain, hypertension, hypotension, pericardial effusion, tachycardia, HF. **GI:** abdominal pain, nausea, vomiting, constipation, diarrhea, dyspepsia, flatulence, hepatotoxicity, intestinal obstruction, oral pain, tooth pain, ulcerative stomatitis. **GU:** dysuria, urinary frequency, urinary tract infection. **Derm:** acne, alopecia, dry skin, ecchymosis, eczema, erythema, flushing, hematoma, hot flashes, pruritus, psoriasis, rash, sweating, urticaria. **Hemat:** neutropenia. **MS:** arthralgia, arthritis, back pain, involuntary muscle contractions, myalgia. **Neuro:** paresthesia. **Misc:** INFECTIONS (including reactivation tuberculosis and other opportunistic infections due to bacterial, invasive fungal, viral, mycobacterial, and parasitic pathogens), MALIGNANCY (including lymphoma, HSTCL, leukemia, skin cancer, and cervical cancer), fever, SARCOIDOSIS, infusion reactions, chills, flu-like syndrome, herpes simplex, herpes zoster, hypersensitivity reactions, lupus-like syndrome, moniliasis, pain, peripheral edema, vasculitis.

Interactions

Drug-Drug: Concurrent use with **anakinra** or **abatacept** ↑ risk of serious infections (not recommended). Concurrent use with **azathioprine** and/or **methotrexate** may ↑ risk of HSTCL. Use of **live virus vaccines** or therapeutic infectious agents may ↑ risk of infection; avoid concurrent use; wait for ≥6 mo before administering any live vaccines to infants exposed *in-utero.*

Route/Dosage

Rheumatoid Arthritis

IV (Adults): 3 mg/kg initially, then repeat at 2 and 6 wk after initial infusion, then repeat every 8 wk; dose may be adjusted in partial responders up to 10 mg/kg or treatment as often as every 4 wk (to be used with methotrexate).

Crohn's Disease

IV (Adults): 5 mg/kg initially, then repeat at 2 and 6 wk after initial infusion, then maintenance dose of 5 mg/kg every 8 wk; dose may be adjusted up to 10 mg/kg in patients who initially respond and then lose their response.
IV (Children): 5 mg/kg initially, then repeat at 2 and 6 wk after initial infusion, then maintenance dose of 5 mg/kg every 8 wk.

Ankylosing Spondylitis

IV (Adults): 5 mg/kg initially, then repeat at 2 and 6 wk after initial infusion, then maintenance dose of 5 mg/kg every 6 wk.

Psoriatic Arthritis

IV (Adults): 5 mg/kg initially, then repeat at 2 and 6 wk after initial infusion, then maintenance dose of 5 mg/kg every 8 wk (to be used with or without methotrexate).

Ulcerative Colitis

IV (Adults and Children ≥6 yr): 5 mg/kg initially, then repeat at 2 and 6 wk after initial infusion, then maintenance dose of 5 mg/kg every 8 wk.

Plaque Psoriasis

IV (Adults): 5 mg/kg initially, then repeat at 2 and 6 wk after initial infusion, then maintenance dose of 5 mg/kg every 8 wk.

Availability

Powder for injection: 100 mg/vial.

NURSING IMPLICATIONS

Assessment

- Assess for infusion-related reactions (fever, chills, urticaria, pruritus) during and for 2 hr after infusion. Symptoms usually resolve when infusion is discontinued. Reactions are more common after 1st or 2nd infusion. Frequency of reactions may be reduced with immunosuppressant agents.
- Monitor patients who develop a new infection while taking infliximab closely. Discontinue therapy in patients who develop a serious infection or sepsis. Do not initiate therapy in patients with active infections.
- Assess for signs and symptoms of systemic infections (fever, malaise, weight loss, sweats, cough, dyspnea, pulmonary infiltrates, serious systemic illness with or without concomitant shock). Ascertain if patient lives in or has traveled to areas of endemic mycoses. Consider empiric antifungal treatment for patients at risk of histoplasmosis and other invasive fungal infections until the pathogens are identified. Consult with an infectious diseases specialist. Consider stopping infliximab until the infection has been diagnosed and adequately treated.
- Assess for latent tuberculosis with a tuberculin skin test prior to initiation of and during therapy. Treatment of latent tuberculosis should be initiated prior to therapy with infliximab.
- Observe patient for hypersensitivity reactions (urticaria, dyspnea, hypotension) during infusion. Discontinue infliximab if severe reaction occurs. Have medications (antihistamines, acetaminophen, corticosteroids, epinephrine) and equipment readily available in the event of a severe reaction.
- **Rheumatoid Arthritis:** Assess pain and range of motion prior to and periodically during therapy.
- **Crohn's Disease and Ulcerative Colitis:** Assess for signs and symptoms before, during, and after therapy.
- **Psoriasis:** Assess lesions periodically during therapy.
- ***Lab Test Considerations:*** May cause ↑ in positive ANA. Frequency may be decreased with baseline immunosuppressant therapy.
- Monitor liver function tests periodically during therapy. May cause mild to moderate AST and ALT ↑ without progressing to liver dysfunction. If patient develops jaundice or liver enzyme elevations ≥5 times the upper limits of normal, discontinue infliximab.
- Monitor CBC with differential periodically during therapy. May cause leukopenia, neutropenia, thrombocytopenia, and pancytopenia. Discontinue infliximab if symptoms of blood dyscrasias (persistent fever) occur.

Implementation

- Do not confuse infliximab with rituximab.

IV Administration

- **Intermittent Infusion:** Calculate the total number of vials needed. Reconstitute each vial with 10 mL of sterile water for injection using a syringe with a 21-gauge needle or smaller. Direct stream to sides of vial. Do not use if vacuum is not present in vial. Gently swirl solution by rotating vial to dilute; do not shake. May foam on reconstitution; allow to stand for 5 min. Solution is colorless to light yellow and opalescent; a few translucent particles may develop because infliximab is a protein. Do not use if opaque particles, discoloration, or other particles occur. *Diluent:* Withdraw volume of total infliximab dose from infusion container containing 250 mL with 0.9% NaCl. Slowly add total dose of infliximab. Do not dilute with other solutions. *Concentration:* 0.4 to 4 mg/mL. Mix gently. Infusion should begin within 3 hr of preparation. Solution is incompatible with polyvinyl chloride equipment. Prepare in glass infusion bottle or polypropylene or polyolefin bags. Do not reuse or store any portion of infusion solution. *Rate:* Administer over at least 2 hr through polyethylene-lined administration set with an in-line, sterile, nonpyrogenic, low protein-building filter with ≤1.2-micron pore size.

- **Y-Site Incompatibility:** Do not administer concurrently in the same line with any other agents.

Patient/Family Teaching

- Advise patient that adverse reactions (myalgia, rash, fever, polyarthralgia, pruritus) may occur 3–12 days after delayed (>2 yr) retreatment with infliximab. Symptoms usually decrease or resolve within 1–3 days. Instruct patient to notify health care professional if symptoms occur.
- May cause dizziness. Caution patient to avoid driving or other activities requiring alertness until response to medication is known.
- Advise patient to notify health care professional promptly if symptoms of fungal infection occur.
- Advise patient of risk of malignancies such as hepatosplenic T-cell lymphoma. Instruct patient to report signs and symptoms (splenomegaly, hepatomegaly, abdominal pain, persistent fever, night sweats, weight loss) to health care professional promptly.
- Advise patient to examine skin periodically during therapy and notify health care professional of any changes in appearance of skin or growths on skin.
- Instruct patient not to receive live vaccines during therapy.
- Rep: Advise female patient to notify health care professional if pregnancy is planned or suspected and to avoid breast feeding. Infants exposed to infliximab in utero should wait at least 6 mo before receiving any live vaccine; may be at increased risk of infection.

Evaluation/Desired Outcomes

- Decreased pain and swelling with decreased rate of joint destruction and improved physical function in patients with ankylosing spondylitis, psoriatic, or rheumatoid arthritis.
- Decrease in the signs and symptoms of Crohn's disease and a decrease in the number of draining enterocutaneous fistulas. Decreased symptoms, maintaining remission, and mucosal healing with decreased corticosteroid use in ulcerative colitis.
- Decrease in induration, scaling, and erythema of psoriatic lesions.

insulin degludec

(in-soo-lin **deg**-lu-dek)

Tresiba

Classification

Therapeutic: antidiabetics, hormones

Pharmacologic: pancreatics

See Appendix L for more information concerning insulins

Indications

Improvement of glycemic control in adults with diabetes mellitus.

Action

Lowers blood glucose by: stimulating glucose uptake in skeletal muscle and fat, inhibiting hepatic glucose production. Other actions: inhibition of lipolysis and proteolysis, enhanced protein synthesis. **Therapeutic Effects:** Control of hyperglycemia in diabetic patients.

Pharmacokinetics

Absorption: Absorption is slow and delayed.

Distribution: Widely distributed.

Protein Binding: >99%.

Metabolism and Excretion: Metabolized by liver, spleen, kidney, and muscle.

Half-life: 25 hr (as a result of rate of absorption).

TIME/ACTION PROFILE (effect on blood sugar)

ROUTE	ONSET	PEAK	DURATION
subcut	within 2 hr	12 hr	up to 42 hr†

†Following discontinuation after chronic use.

Contraindications/Precautions

Contraindicated in: Hypersensitivity to insulin degludec; Hypoglycemia.

Use Cautiously in: Stress and infection (may temporarily ↑ insulin requirements); Renal/hepatic impairment (may ↓ insulin requirements); Concomitant use with pioglitazone or rosiglitazone (↑ risk of fluid retention and worsening HF); Effects may be ↓ in obese patients; Patients with visual impairment who may rely on audible clicks to dial their dose; Geri: Elderly may be ↑ sensitive to drug effects; OB: Pregnancy may temporarily ↑ insulin requirements; Lactation: Consider possible effects on infant (lactating females may require adjustments in insulin dose and/or meal plan); Pedi: Children <1 yr (safety and effectiveness not established).

Adverse Reactions/Side Effects

Endo: HYPOGLYCEMIA. **F and E:** hypokalemia. **Local:** lipodystrophy, pruritus, erythema, swelling. **Misc:** HYPERSENSITIVITY REACTIONS (including anaphylaxis).

Interactions

Drug-Drug: Beta blockers and **clonidine** may mask some of the signs and symptoms of hypoglycemia. **Corticosteroids**, **thyroid supplements**, **estrogens**, **isoniazid**, **niacin**, **phenothiazines**, and **rifampin** may ↑ insulin requirements. **Alcohol**, **ACE inhibitors**, **MAO inhibitors**, **octreotide**, **oral hypoglycemic agents**, and **salicylates** may ↓ insulin requirements. Concurrent use with **pioglitazone** or **rosiglitazone** may ↑ risk of fluid retention and worsening HF.
Drug-Natural Products: Glucosamine may worsen blood glucose control. **Fenugreek**, **chromium**, and **coenzyme Q-10** may produce additive hypoglycemic effects.

Route/Dosage

Subcut (Adults): *Type 1 diabetes (insulin naïve)*—⅓–½ of the total daily insulin dose given once daily, then adjust on the basis of patient's needs (remainder of insulin dose should be given as a short-acting insulin and divided between each daily meal) (usual starting total daily insulin dose = 0.2–0.4 units/kg); *Type 2 diabetes (insulin naïve)*—10 units once daily, then adjust on the basis of patient's needs; *Type 1 or 2 diabetes (and already on insulin)*—Give the same dose as the total daily dose of the long-acting or intermediate-acting insulin once daily, then adjust on the basis of patient's needs.
Subcut (Children ≥1 yr): *Type 1 or 2 diabetes (and already on insulin)*—Give 80% of the total daily dose of the long-acting or intermediate-acting insulin once daily, then adjust on the basis of patient's needs.

Availability

Solution for injection: 100 units/mL (prefilled pens and vials), 200 units/mL (prefilled pens). ***In combination with:*** insulin aspart (Rysodeg 70/30); liraglutide (Xultophy). See Appendix B.

NURSING IMPLICATIONS

Assessment

- Assess patient for signs and symptoms of hypoglycemia (anxiety; restlessness; tingling in hands, feet, lips, or tongue; chills; cold sweats; confusion; cool, pale skin; difficulty in concentration; drowsiness; nightmares or trouble sleeping; excessive hunger; headache; irritability; nausea; nervousness; tachycardia; tremor; weakness; unsteady gait) and hyperglycemia (confusion, drowsiness; flushed, dry skin; fruit-like breath odor; rapid, deep breathing, polyuria; loss of appetite; nausea; vomiting; unusual thirst) periodically during therapy.
- Monitor body weight periodically. Changes in weight may necessitate changes in insulin dose.
- Monitor for signs and symptoms of hypersensitivity reactions (swelling of tongue and lips, diarrhea, nausea, tiredness, itching, urticaria). Discontinue insulin degludec and treat symptomatically.
- ***Lab Test Considerations:*** Monitor blood glucose during therapy, more frequently in ketoacidosis and times of stress. Hemoglobin A_{1C} may be monitored every 3–6 mo to determine effectiveness.
- Monitor serum potassium periodically during therapy, especially in patients at risk (patients using potassium-lowering medications, patients taking medications sensitive to serum potassium concentrations). May cause hypokalemia.
- ***Toxicity and Overdose:*** Overdose is manifested by symptoms of hypoglycemia. Mild hypoglycemia may be treated by ingestion of oral glucose. Severe hypoglycemia is a life-threatening emergency; treatment consists of IV glucose, glucagon, or epinephrine.

Implementation

- ***High Alert:*** Insulin-related medication errors have resulted in patient harm and death. Clarify ambiguous orders; do not accept orders using the abbreviation "u" for units (can be misread as a zero or the numeral 4; has resulted in tenfold overdoses). Insulins are available in different types, strengths. Check type, dose, and expiration date. Do not interchange insulins without consulting health care professional. Do not confuse Tresiba (insulin degludec) with Tarceva (erlotinib), Toujeo (insulin glargine), Tradjenta (linagliptin), or Trulicity (dulaglutide).
- Use U-100 vial for pediatric patients requiring <5 units of insulin degludec each day.
- **Subcut:** Inject once daily at the same time each day. Administer into thigh, upper arm, or abdomen. Press and hold down the dose button until dose counter shows 0 and then keep needle in the skin and count slowly to 6. When dose counter returns to 0, prescribed dose is not completely delivered until 6 sec later. If the needle is removed earlier, a stream of insulin may be seen coming from the needle tip. If so, full dose will not be delivered; frequently check blood glucose levels, may need additional insulin. Use a new needle for each dose; do not reuse needles. Rotate injection sites to reduce risk of lipodystrophy. Do not administer IV, IM, or in an insulin infusion pump. Solution is clear and colorless; do not administer solutions that are discolored or contain a precipitate. Store unopened prefilled pens in refrigerator; do not freeze. Do not store opened (in-use) prefilled pens in refrigerator; stable at controlled room temperature, protected from light for 56 days (8 wk).
- Do not mix with other insulins or solutions.
- Do not transfer from pen into a syringe for administration.
- Dose increases should be made every 3–4 days as needed.
- Do not perform dose conversion when using the *Tresiba* U-100 or U-200 *FlexTouch* pens. Dose window for both the *Tresiba* U-100 and U-200 *FlexTouch* pens shows number of insulin units to be delivered and no conversion is needed.
- **Starting Dose in Insulin Naïve Patients :** *Type 1 Diabetes Mellitus:* Starting dose is one-third to one-

half total daily insulin dose. Administer remainder of total daily insulin dose as short-acting insulin divided between daily meals. Generally, 0.2 to 0.4 units of insulin/kg can be used to calculate initial total daily insulin dose in insulin naïve patients with type 1 diabetes. *Type 2 Diabetes Mellitus:* 10 units once daily.

- **Starting Dose in Patients Already on Insulin Therapy :** *Type 1 and Type 2 Diabetes Mellitus:* Start insulin degludec at same unit dose as total daily long or intermediate-acting insulin unit dose.

Patient/Family Teaching

- Instruct patient on proper technique for administration. Include type of insulin, equipment (syringe, cartridge pens, alcohol swabs), storage, and place to discard syringes. If a dose is missed, inject daily dose during waking hrs upon discovering missed dose. Ensure that at least 8 hrs have elapsed between consecutive injections. Discuss importance of not changing brands of insulin or syringes, selection and rotation of injection sites, and compliance with therapeutic regimen. Advise patient to read *Patient Information* before starting therapy and with each Rx refill in case of changes.
- Caution patient not to share pen device with another person, even if needle is changed; may risk transmission of bloodborne pathogens.
- Explain to patient that this medication controls hyperglycemia but does not cure diabetes. Therapy is long term.
- Instruct patient in proper testing of serum glucose and ketones. These tests should be closely monitored during periods of stress or illness, and health care professional notified of significant changes.
- Emphasize the importance of compliance with nutritional guidelines and regular exercise as directed by health care professional.
- Instruct patient to notify health care professional of all Rx or OTC medications, vitamins, or herbal products being taken and to consult health care professional before taking other Rx, OTC, herbal products, or alcohol.
- Advise patient to notify health care professional of medication regimen prior to treatment or surgery.
- Advise patient to notify health care professional if nausea, vomiting, or fever develops, if unable to eat regular diet, or if blood glucose levels are not controlled.
- Instruct patient and caregiver on signs and symptoms of hypoglycemia and hyperglycemia and what to do if they occur.
- Patients with diabetes mellitus should carry a source of sugar (candy, glucose gel) and identification describing their disease and treatment regimen at all times.
- Advise patient to notify health care professional if pregnancy is planned or suspected or if breast feeding.
- Emphasize the importance of regular follow-up, especially during first few wk of therapy.

Evaluation/Desired Outcomes

- Control of blood glucose levels in diabetic patients without the appearance of hypoglycemic or hyperglycemic episodes.

HIGH ALERT

INSULIN (mixtures) (in-su-lin)

insulin lispro protamine suspension/insulin lispro injection mixtures, rDNA origin
HumaLOG Mix 75/25, HumaLOG Mix 50/50

insulin aspart protamine suspension/insulin aspart injection mixtures, rDNA origin
NovoLOG Mix 70/30

NPH/regular insulin mixtures
HumuLIN 70/30, NovoLIN 70/30

Classification
Therapeutic: antidiabetics, hormones
Pharmacologic: pancreatics

See Appendix L for more information concerning insulins

Indications

Control of hyperglycemia in patients with type 1 or type 2 diabetes mellitus.

Action

Lower blood glucose by: stimulating glucose uptake in skeletal muscle and fat, inhibiting hepatic glucose production. Other actions: inhibition of lipolysis and proteolysis, enhanced protein synthesis. **Therapeutic Effects:** Control of hyperglycemia in diabetic patients.

Pharmacokinetics

Absorption: Well absorbed from subcutaneous administration sites. Absorption rate is determined by type of insulin, injection site, volume of injectate, and other factors.
Distribution: Widely distributed.
Metabolism and Excretion: Metabolized by liver, spleen, kidney, and muscle.
Half-life: 5–6 min (prolonged in patients with diabetes; biologic half-life is 1–1.5 hr).

TIME/ACTION PROFILE (hypoglycemic effect)

ROUTE	ONSET	PEAK	DURATION
insulin lispro protamine suspension/ insulin lispro injection mixture subcut	15–30 min	2.8 hr	24 hr
insulin aspart protamine suspension/ insulin aspart injection mixture subcut	15 min	1–4 hr	18–24 hr
NPH/Regular Insulin mixture subcutaneous	30 min	2–12 hr	24 hr

Contraindications/Precautions

Contraindicated in: Hypoglycemia; Allergy or hypersensitivity to a particular type of insulin, preservatives, or other additives.

Use Cautiously in: Stress and infection (may temporarily ↑ insulin requirements); Renal/hepatic impairment (may ↓ insulin requirements); Concomitant use with pioglitazone or rosiglitazone (↑ risk of fluid retention and worsening HF); OB: Pregnancy may temporarily ↑ insulin requirements; Lactation: Use while breast feeding only if potential maternal benefit justifies potential risk to infant; Pedi: Safety of Humalog not established.

Adverse Reactions/Side Effects

Endo: HYPOGLYCEMIA. **F and E:** hypokalemia. **Local:** erythema, lipodystrophy, pruritis, swelling. **Misc:** HYPERSENSITIVITY REACTIONS (including anaphylaxis).

Interactions

Drug-Drug: Beta blockers and **clonidine** may mask some of the signs and symptoms of hypoglycemia. **Corticosteroids**, **thyroid supplements**, **estrogens**, **isoniazid**, **niacin**, **phenothiazines**, and **rifampin** may ↑ insulin requirements. **Alcohol**, **ACE inhibitors**, **MAO inhibitors**, **octreotide**, **oral hypoglycemic agents**, and **salicylates** may ↓ insulin requirements. Concurrent use with **pioglitazone** or **rosiglitazone** may ↑ risk of fluid retention and worsening HF.

Drug-Natural Products: Glucosamine may worsen blood glucose control. **Fenugreek**, **chromium**, and **coenzyme Q-10** may produce additive hypoglycemic effects.

Route/Dosage

Dose depends on blood glucose, response, and many other factors.

Subcut (Adults and Children): 0.5–1 unit/kg/day. *Adolescents during rapid growth*—0.8–1.2 units/kg/day.

Availability

Insulin aspart protamine suspension/insulin aspart injection mixture: 70% insulin aspart protamine suspension and 30% insulin aspart inection—NovoLog Mix 70/30 100 units/mL (vials and prefilled pens). **Insulin lispro protamine suspension/insulin lispro injection mixture:** 75% insulin lispro protamine suspension and 25% insulin lispro injection—Humalog Mix 75/25 100 units/mL (vials and prefilled pens), 50% insulin lispro protamine suspension and 50% insulin lispro injection—Humalog Mix 50/50 100 units/mL (vials and prefilled pens). **NPH insulin/regular insulin suspension mixture:** 70 units NPH/30 units regular insulin/mL—Novolin 70/30, Humulin 70/30 (100 units/mL total) (vials and prefilled pens)OTC.

NURSING IMPLICATIONS

Assessment

- Assess for symptoms of hypoglycemia (anxiety; restlessness; tingling in hands, feet, lips, or tongue; chills; cold sweats; confusion; cool, pale skin; difficulty in concentration; drowsiness; excessive hunger; headache; irritability; nightmares or trouble sleeping; nausea; nervousness; tachycardia; tremor; weakness; unsteady gait) and hyperglycemia (confusion, drowsiness; flushed, dry skin; fruit-like breath odor; rapid, deep breathing, polyuria; loss of appetite; nausea; vomiting; unusual thirst) periodically during therapy.
- Monitor body weight periodically. Changes in weight may necessitate changes in insulin dose.
- ***Lab Test Considerations:*** Monitor blood glucose every 6 hr during therapy, more frequently in ketoacidosis and times of stress. Hemoglobin A_{1C} may also be monitored every 3–6 mo to determine effectiveness.
- Monitor serum potassium in patients at risk for hypokalemia (those using potassium-lowering agents, those receiving IV insulin) periodically during therapy.
- ***Toxicity and Overdose:*** Overdose is manifested by symptoms of hypoglycemia. Mild hypoglycemia may be treated by ingestion of oral glucose. Severe hypoglycemia is a life-threatening emergency; treatment consists of IV glucose, glucagon, or epinephrine.

Implementation

- ***High Alert:*** Insulin-related medication errors have resulted in patient harm and death. Clarify ambiguous orders; do not accept orders using the abbreviation "u" for units (can be misread as a zero or the numeral 4; has resulted in tenfold overdoses).
- Insulins are available in different types and strengths. Check type, dose, and expiration date with another licensed nurse. Do not interchange insulins without consulting health care professional.
- Do not confuse Humalog with Humulin. Do not confuse Humulin 70/30 with Humalog Mix 75/25. Do not confuse Novolin with Novolog.
- Use *only* insulin syringes to draw up dose. The unit markings on the insulin syringe must match the insulin's units/mL.

- Insulin should be stored in a cool place but does not need to be refrigerated. Follow manufacturer's instructions regarding storage of insulin and insulin pens before and after use. Do not use if cloudy, discolored, or unusually viscous.
- NPH insulins should not be used in the management of ketoacidosis.
- **Subcut:** Rotate injection sites.
- Administer into abdominal wall, thigh, or upper arm subcutaneously.

Patient/Family Teaching

- Instruct patient on proper technique for administration. Include type of insulin, equipment (syringe, cartridge pens, alcohol swabs), storage, and place to discard syringes. Discuss the importance of not changing brands of insulin or syringes, selection and rotation of injection sites, and compliance with therapeutic regimen. Caution patient that insulin pens should not be shared with others, even if clean needles are used.
- Caution patient not to share pen device with another person, even if needle is changed; may risk transmission of bloodborne pathogens.
- Explain to patient that this medication controls hyperglycemia but does not cure diabetes. Therapy is long term.
- Instruct patient in proper testing of serum glucose and ketones. These tests should be closely monitored during periods of stress or illness and health care professional notified of significant changes.
- Emphasize the importance of compliance with nutritional guidelines and regular exercise as directed by health care professional.
- Instruct patient to notify health care professional of all Rx or OTC medications, vitamins, or herbal products being taken and to consult health care professional before taking other Rx, OTC, herbal products, or alcohol.
- Advise patient to notify health care professional of medication regimen prior to treatment or surgery.
- Advise patient to notify health care professional if nausea, vomiting, or fever develops, if unable to eat regular diet, or if blood glucose levels are not controlled.
- Instruct patient on signs and symptoms of hypoglycemia and hyperglycemia and what to do if they occur.
- Patients with diabetes mellitus should carry a source of sugar (candy, glucose gel) and identification describing their disease and treatment regimen at all times.
- Advise patient to notify health care professional if pregnancy is planned or suspected, or if breast feeding.
- Emphasize the importance of regular follow-up, especially during first few wk of therapy.

Evaluation/Desired Outcomes

- Control of blood glucose levels in diabetic patients without the appearance of hypoglycemic or hyperglycemic episodes.

HIGH ALERT

NPH insulin (isophane insulin suspension)

HumuLIN N, NovoLIN N

Classification

Therapeutic: antidiabetics, hormones

Pharmacologic: pancreatics

See Appendix L for more information concerning insulins

Indications

Control of hyperglycemia in patients with diabetes mellitus.

Action

Lowers blood glucose by: stimulating glucose uptake in skeletal muscle and fat, inhibiting hepatic glucose production. Other actions of insulin: inhibition of lipolysis and proteolysis, enhanced protein synthesis. **Therapeutic Effects:** Control of hyperglycemia in diabetic patients.

Pharmacokinetics

Absorption: Rapidly absorbed from subcutaneous administration sites. Presence of protamine delays peak effect and prolongs action.

Distribution: Identical to endogenous insulin.

Metabolism and Excretion: Metabolized by liver, spleen, kidney, and muscle.

Half-life: Unknown.

TIME/ACTION PROFILE (hypoglycemic effect)

ROUTE	ONSET	PEAK	DURATION
NPH subcutaneous	2–4 hr	4–10 hr	10–16 hr
70% NPH/30% Regular Insulin mixture	30 min	2–12 hr	24 hr

Contraindications/Precautions

Contraindicated in: Hypoglycemia; Allergy or hypersensitivity to a particular type of insulin, preservatives, or other additives.

Use Cautiously in: Stress or infection (may temporarily ↑ insulin requirements); Renal/hepatic impairment (may ↓ insulin requirements); Concomitant use with pioglitazone or rosiglitazone (↑ risk of fluid retention and worsening HF); OB: Pregnancy may temporarily ↑ insulin requirements; Lactation: Use while breast feeding only if potential maternal benefit justifies potential risk to infant.

Adverse Reactions/Side Effects

Endo: HYPOGLYCEMIA. **F and E:** hypokalemia. **Local:** lipodystrophy, pruritus, erythema, swelling. **Misc:** HYPERSENSITIVITY REACTIONS (including anaphylaxis).

Interactions

Drug-Drug: Beta blockers and **clonidine** may mask some of the signs and symptoms of hypoglycemia. **Corticosteroids**, **thyroid supplements**, **estrogens**, **isoniazid**, **niacin**, **phenothiazines**, and **rifampin** may ↑ insulin requirements. **Alcohol**, **ACE inhibitors**, **MAO inhibitors**, **octreotide**, **oral hypoglycemic agents**, and **salicylates** may ↓ insulin requirements. Concurrent use with **pioglitazone** or **rosiglitazone** may ↑ risk of fluid retention and worsening HF.
Drug-Natural Products: Glucosamine may worsen blood glucose control. **Fenugreek**, **chromium**, and **coenzyme Q-10** may produce additive hypoglycemic effects.

Route/Dosage

Dose depends on blood glucose, response, and many other factors.
Subcut (Adults and Children): 0.5–1 unit total insulin/kg/day. *Adolescents during rapid growth*—0.8–1.2 units total insulin/kg/day.

Availability

Solution for injection: 100 units/mL (vials and prefilled pens).

NURSING IMPLICATIONS

Assessment

- Assess patient periodically for symptoms of hypoglycemia (anxiety; restlessness; tingling in hands, feet, lips, or tongue; chills; cold sweats; confusion; cool, pale skin; difficulty in concentration; drowsiness; nightmares or trouble sleeping; excessive hunger; headache; irritability; nausea; nervousness; tachycardia; tremor; weakness; unsteady gait) and hyperglycemia (confusion, drowsiness; flushed, dry skin; fruit-like breath odor; rapid, deep breathing, polyuria; loss of appetite; unusual thirst) during therapy.
- Monitor body weight periodically. Changes in weight may necessitate changes in insulin dose.
- ***Lab Test Considerations:*** Monitor blood glucose every 6 hr during therapy, more frequently in changes to insulin regimen, ketoacidosis, and times of stress. A1C may be monitored every 3–6 mo to determine effectiveness.
- Monitor serum potassium in patients at risk for hypokalemia (those using potassium-lowering agents, those receiving IV insulin) periodically during therapy.
- ***Toxicity and Overdose:*** Overdose is manifested by symptoms of hypoglycemia. Mild hypoglycemia may be treated by ingestion of oral glucose. Severe hypoglycemia is a life-threatening emergency; treatment consists of IV glucose, glucagon, or epinephrine.

Implementation

- ***High Alert:*** Medication errors involving insulins have resulted in serious patient harm and death. Clarify all ambiguous orders and do not accept orders using the abbreviation "u" for units, which can be misread as a zero or the numeral 4 and has resulted in tenfold overdoses. Insulins are available in different types and strengths. Check type, dose, and expiration date with another licensed nurse. Do not interchange insulins without consulting physician or other health care professional.
- Do not confuse Humulin N (NPH insulin) with Humalog (insulin lispro) or Novolin N (NPH insulin). Do not confuse Novolin N (NPH insulin) with Novolog (insulin aspart).
- Use *only* insulin syringes to draw up dose. The unit markings on the insulin syringe must match the insulin's units/mL. Special syringes for doses <50 units are available. Prior to withdrawing dose, rotate vial between palms to ensure uniform solution; do not shake.
- When mixing insulins, draw regular insulin or insulin lispro into syringe first to avoid contamination of regular insulin vial.
- Insulin should be stored in a cool place but does not need to be refrigerated. Once opened, store at room temperature. Follow manufacturer's instructions regarding storage of insulin and insulin pens before and after use.
- When transferring from once-daily NPH human insulin to *insulin glargine*, the dose usually remains unchanged. When transferring from twice-daily NPH human insulin to insulin glargine, the initial dose of insulin glargine is usually reduced by 20%.
- NPH insulin should not be used in the management of ketoacidosis.
- **Subcut:** Administer NPH insulin within 30–60 min before a meal. Inject subcut in abdomen, thigh, upper arm, or buttocks. Rotate injection sites to reduce risk of lipodystrophy.

Patient/Family Teaching

- Instruct patient on proper technique for administration. Include type of insulin, equipment (syringe, cartridge pens, alcohol swabs), storage, and place to discard syringes. Discuss the importance of not changing brands of insulin or syringes, selection and rotation of injection sites, and compliance with therapeutic regimen. Caution patient that insulin pens should not be shared with others, even if clean needles are used.
- Demonstrate technique for mixing insulins by drawing up regular insulin or insulin lispro first and rolling intermediate-acting insulin vial between palms to mix, rather than shaking (may cause inaccurate dose).

- Caution patient not to share pen device with another person, even if needle is changed; may risk transmission of bloodborne pathogens.
- Explain to patient that this medication controls hyperglycemia but does not cure diabetes. Therapy is long term.
- Instruct patient in proper testing of serum glucose and ketones. These tests should be closely monitored during periods of stress or illness and health care professional notified of significant changes.
- Emphasize the importance of compliance with nutritional guidelines and regular exercise as directed by health care professional.
- Instruct patient to notify health care professional of all Rx or OTC medications, vitamins, or herbal products being taken and to consult health care professional before taking other Rx, OTC, herbal products, or alcohol.
- Advise patient to notify health care professional of medication regimen prior to treatment or surgery.
- Advise patient to notify health care professional if nausea, vomiting, or fever develops, if unable to eat regular diet, or if blood glucose levels are not controlled.
- Instruct patient on signs and symptoms of hypoglycemia and hyperglycemia and what to do if they occur.
- Patients with diabetes mellitus should carry a source of sugar (candy, glucose gel) and identification describing their disease and treatment regimen at all times.
- Advise females of reproductive potential to notify health care professional if pregnancy is planned or suspected, or if breast feeding.
- Emphasize the importance of regular follow-up, especially during first few wk of therapy.

Evaluation/Desired Outcomes

- Control of blood glucose levels in diabetic patients without the appearance of hypoglycemic or hyperglycemic episodes.

HIGH ALERT

insulin, regular (in-su-lin)

🍁Entuzity, HumuLIN R, Myxredlin, NovoLIN R, HumuLIN R U-500 (Concentrated)

Classification

Therapeutic: antidiabetics, hormones
Pharmacologic: pancreatics

See Appendix L for more information concerning insulins

Indications

Control of hyperglycemia in patients with diabetes mellitus. **Concentrated regular insulin U-500:** Only for use in patients with insulin requirements >200 units/day. **Unlabeled Use:** Treatment of hyperkalemia.

Action

Lowers blood glucose by: stimulating glucose uptake in skeletal muscle and fat, inhibiting hepatic glucose production. Other actions of insulin: inhibition of lipolysis and proteolysis, enhanced protein synthesis. **Therapeutic Effects:** Control of hyperglycemia in diabetic patients.

Pharmacokinetics

Absorption: Rapidly absorbed from subcutaneous administration sites. U-100 regular insulin is absorbed slightly more quickly than U-500.
Distribution: Identical to endogenous insulin.
Metabolism and Excretion: Metabolized by liver, spleen, kidney, and muscle.
Half-life: 30–60 min.

TIME/ACTION PROFILE (hypoglycemic effect)

ROUTE	ONSET	PEAK	DURATION
Regular insulin IV	10–30 min	15–30 min	30–60 min
Regular insulin subcutaneous	30–60 min	2–4 hr	5–7 hr

Contraindications/Precautions

Contraindicated in: Hypoglycemia; Allergy or hypersensitivity to a particular type of insulin, preservatives, or other additives.
Use Cautiously in: Stress or infection—may temporarily ↑ insulin requirements; Renal/hepatic impairment—may ↓ insulin requirements; Concomitant use with pioglitazone or rosiglitazone (↑ risk of fluid retention and worsening HF); OB: Pregnancy may temporarily ↑ insulin requirements; Lactation: Use while breast feeding only if maternal benefit justifies potential risk to infant.

Adverse Reactions/Side Effects

Endo: HYPOGLYCEMIA. **F and E:** hypokalemia. **Local:** lipodystrophy, pruritus, erythema, swelling. **Misc:** HYPERSENSITIVITY REACTIONS (including anaphylaxis).

Interactions

Drug-Drug: Beta blockers and **clonidine** may mask some of the signs and symptoms of hypoglycemia. **Corticosteroids**, **thyroid supplements**, **estrogens**, **isoniazid**, **niacin**, **phenothiazines**, and **rifampin** may ↑ insulin requirements. **Alcohol**, **ACE inhibitors**, **MAO inhibitors**, **octreotide**, **oral hypoglycemic agents**, and **salicylates** may ↓ insulin requirements.

Concurrent use with **pioglitazone** or **rosiglitazone** may ↑ risk of fluid retention and worsening HF.

Drug-Natural Products: Glucosamine may worsen blood glucose control. **Fenugreek, chromium**, and **coenzyme Q-10** may produce additive hypoglycemic effects.

Route/Dosage

Dose depends on blood glucose, response, and many other factors.

Ketoacidosis—Regular (100 units/mL) Insulin Only

IV (Adults): 0.1 unit/kg/hr as a continuous infusion.
IV (Children): Loading dose—0.1 unit/kg, then maintenance continuous infusion 0.05–0.2 unit/kg/hr, titrate to optimal rate of ↓ of serum glucose of 80–100 mg/dL/hr.

Maintenance Therapy

Subcut (Adults and Children): 0.5–1 unit/kg/day in divided doses. *Adolescents during rapid growth*—0.8–1.2 unit/kg/day in divided doses.

Treatment of Hyperkalemia

Subcut, IV (Adults and Children): Dextrose 0.5–1 g/kg combined with insulin 1 unit for every 4–5 g dextrose given.

Availability

Premixed infusion: 100 units/100 mL 0.9% NaCl. **Solution for injection:** 100 units/mL (vials and prefilled pens)[OTC]. **Solution for injection (concentrated):** 500 units/mL (vials and prefilled pens). ***In combination with:*** NPH insulins (Humulin 70/30, Novolin 70/30).

NURSING IMPLICATIONS

Assessment

- Assess patient periodically for symptoms of hypoglycemia (anxiety; restlessness; tingling in hands, feet, lips, or tongue; chills; cold sweats; confusion; cool, pale skin; difficulty in concentration; drowsiness; nightmares or trouble sleeping; excessive hunger; headache; irritability; nausea; nervousness; tachycardia; tremor; weakness; unsteady gait) and hyperglycemia (confusion, drowsiness; flushed, dry skin; fruit-like breath odor; rapid, deep breathing, polyuria; loss of appetite; unusual thirst) during therapy.
- Monitor body weight periodically. Changes in weight may necessitate changes in insulin dose.
- ***Lab Test Considerations:*** Monitor blood glucose every 6 hr during therapy, more frequently in ketoacidosis and times of stress. A1C may be monitored every 3–6 mo to determine effectiveness.
- Monitor serum potassium in patients at risk for hypokalemia (those using potassium-lowering agents, those receiving IV insulin) periodically during therapy.
- ***Toxicity and Overdose:*** Overdose is manifested by symptoms of hypoglycemia. Mild hypoglycemia may be treated by ingestion of oral glucose. Severe hypoglycemia is a life-threatening emergency; treatment consists of IV glucose, glucagon, or epinephrine.

Implementation

- ***High Alert:*** Medication errors involving insulins have resulted in serious patient harm and death. Clarify all ambiguous orders and do not accept orders using the abbreviation "u" for units, which can be misread as a zero or the numeral 4 and has resulted in tenfold overdoses. Insulins are available in different types and strengths. Check type, dose, and expiration date with another licensed nurse. Do not interchange insulins without consulting health care professional. Do not confuse regular **concentrated (U-500)** insulin with regular insulin.To prevent errors between regular U-100 insulin and concentrated U-500 insulin, concentrated U-500 insulin is marked with a band of diagonal brown strips and "U-500" is highlighted in red on the label and a conversion chart should always be available.
- Do not confuse Humulin with Humalog (insulin lispro). Do not confuse Novolin with Novolog.
- Use ***only*** insulin syringes to draw up dose. The unit markings on the insulin syringe must match the insulin's units/mL. Special syringes for doses <50 units and U-500 insulin are available. Prior to withdrawing dose, rotate vial between palms to ensure uniform solution; do not shake.
- When mixing insulins, draw regular insulin into syringe first to avoid contamination of regular insulin vial.
- Insulin should be stored in a cool place but does not need to be refrigerated. Once opened, store at room temperature. Follow manufacturer's instructions regarding storage of insulin and insulin pens before and after use.
- **Subcut:** Administer regular insulin within 15–30 min before a meal.

IV Administration

- **IV:** Do not use if cloudy, discolored, or unusually viscous. ***High Alert:*** Do not administer regular (concentrated) insulin U-500 IV.
- **IV Push:** ***Diluent:*** May be administered IV undiluted directly into vein or through Y-site. ***Rate:*** Administer up to 50 units over 1 min.
- **Continuous Infusion:** ***Diluent:*** May be diluted in 0.9% NaCl using polyvinyl chloride infusion bags. ***Concentration:*** 0.1 unit/mL to 1 unit/mL in infusion systems with the infusion fluids. ***Rate:*** Rate should be ordered by health care professional, and infusion placed on an IV pump for accurate administration.
- Rate of administration should be decreased when serum glucose level reaches 250 mg/dL.
- **Y-Site Compatibility:** acyclovir, alfentanil, aminophylline, amphotericin B lipid complex, anidulafungin, argatroban, ascorbic acid, atropine, azathio-

prine, aztreonam, benztropine, bivalirudin, bleomycin, bumetanide, buprenorphine, calcium chloride, calcium gluconate, carboplatin, carmustine, caspofungin, cefazolin, cefepime, ceftaroline, ceftazidime, ceftriaxone, cefuroxime, chloramphenicol, clindamycin, cyanocobalamin, cyclophosphamide, cytarabine, dacarbazine, dactinomycin, daptomycin, daunorubicin hydrochloride, dexamethasone, dexmedetomidine, dexrazoxane, docetaxel, doxorubicin liposomal, doxycycline, enalapril, ephedrine, epirubicin, epoetin alfa, ertapenem, erythromycin, esmolol, esomeprazole, etoposide, etoposide phosphate, fenoldopam, fentanyl, fluconazole, fludarabine, folic acid, foscarnet, fosphenytoin, ganciclovir, gemcitabine, granisetron, hetastarch, hydrocortisone, hydromorphone, ibuprofen lysine, idarubicin, ifosfamide, imipenem/cilastatin, indomethacin, irinotecan, ketorolac, leucovorin calcium, lidocaine, linezolid, lorazepam, magnesium sulfate, mannitol, meperidine, meropenem, mesna, methotrexate, methyldopate, methylprednisolone, metoclopramide, metoprolol, metronidazole, milrinone, mitoxantrone, moxifloxacin, mycophenolate, nalbuphine, naloxone, nitroglycerin, nitroprusside, octreotide, oxacillin, oxaliplatin, paclitaxel, palonosetron, pamidronate, pancuronium, papaverine, pemetrexed, penicillin G, pentobarbital, phenobarbital, phytonadione, potassium acetate, potassium chloride, procainamide, promethazine, propofol, pyridoxine, remifentanil, sodium bicarbonate, streptokinase, sufentanil, tacrolimus, terbutaline, theophylline, thiamine, thiotepa, tigecycline, tirofiban, topotecan, vancomycin, vecuronium, verapamil, vinblastine, vincristine, vinorelbine, vitamin B complex with C, voriconazole, zoledronic acid.

- **Y-Site Incompatibility:** alemtuzumab, butorphanol, cefoxitin, chlorpromazine, cisplatin, dantrolene, diazepam, diphenhydramine, glycopyrrolate, hydroxyzine, isoproterenol, ketamine, labetalol, micafungin, mitomycin, pentamidine, phentolamine, phenylephrine, phenytoin, piperacillin/tazobactam, prochlorperazine, propranolol, protamine, quinupristin/dalfopristin, rocuronium, trimethoprim/sulfamethoxazole.
- **Additive Compatibility:** May be added to total parenteral nutrition (TPN) solutions.

Patient/Family Teaching

- Instruct patient on proper technique for administration. Include type of insulin, equipment (syringe, cartridge pens, alcohol swabs), storage, and place to discard syringes. Discuss the importance of not changing brands of insulin or syringes, selection and rotation of injection sites, and compliance with therapeutic regimen. Opened, unused insulin vials should be discarded 1 mo after opening.
- Demonstrate technique for mixing insulins by drawing up regular insulin first and rolling intermediate-acting insulin vial between palms to mix, rather than shaking (may cause inaccurate dose).
- Caution patient not to share pen device with another person, even if needle is changed; may risk transmission of bloodborne pathogens.
- Explain to patient that this medication controls hyperglycemia but does not cure diabetes. Therapy is long term.
- Instruct patient in proper testing of serum glucose and ketones. These tests should be closely monitored during periods of stress or illness and health care professional notified of significant changes.
- Emphasize the importance of compliance with nutritional guidelines and regular exercise as directed by health care professional.
- Instruct patient to notify health care professional of all Rx or OTC medications, vitamins, or herbal products being taken and to consult health care professional before taking other Rx, OTC, herbal products, or alcohol.
- Advise patient to notify health care professional of medication regimen prior to treatment or surgery.
- Advise patient to notify health care professional if nausea, vomiting, or fever develops, if unable to eat regular diet, or if blood glucose levels are not controlled.
- Instruct patient on signs and symptoms of hypoglycemia and hyperglycemia and what to do if they occur.
- Advise patient to notify health care professional if pregnancy is planned or suspected or if breast feeding or planning to breast feed.
- Patients with diabetes mellitus should carry a source of sugar (candy, glucose gel) and identification describing their disease and treatment regimen at all times.
- Emphasize the importance of regular follow-up, especially during first few wk of therapy.

Evaluation/Desired Outcomes

- Control of blood glucose levels in diabetic patients without the appearance of hypoglycemic or hyperglycemic episodes.

HIGH ALERT

INSULINS (long-acting)

(in-su-lin)

insulin degludec

Tresiba

insulin detemir

Levemir

insulin glargine
Basaglar, Lantus, Toujeo

Classification
Therapeutic: antidiabetics, hormones
Pharmacologic: pancreatics

See Appendix L for more information concerning insulins

Indications
Control of hyperglycemia in patients with type 1 or type 2 diabetes mellitus.

Action
Lower blood glucose by: stimulating glucose uptake in skeletal muscle and fat, inhibiting hepatic glucose production. Other actions: inhibition of lipolysis and proteolysis, enhanced protein synthesis. **Therapeutic Effects:** Control of hyperglycemia in diabetic patients.

Pharmacokinetics
Absorption: Physiochemical characteristics of long-acting insulins result in delayed and prolonged absorption.
Distribution: Widely distributed.
Metabolism and Excretion: Metabolized by liver, spleen, kidney, and muscle.
Half-life: 5–6 min (prolonged in patients with diabetes); biologic half-life is 1–1.5 hr; *insulin degludec* 25 hr; *insulin detemir* 5–7 hr (dose-dependent).

TIME/ACTION PROFILE (hypoglycemic effect)

ROUTE	ONSET	PEAK	DURATION
Insulin degludec	within 2 hr	12 hr	up to 42 hr*
Insulin detemir	3–4 hr	3–14 hr†	6–24 hr‡
Insulin glargine	3–4 hr	none†	24 hr

*Following discontinuation after chronic use.
†Small amounts of insulin glargine and insulin detemir are slowly released resulting in a relatively constant effect over time.
‡Duration is dose dependent; duration ↑ as dose ↑.

Contraindications/Precautions
Contraindicated in: Hypoglycemia; Allergy or hypersensitivity to a particular type of insulin, preservatives, or other additives.
Use Cautiously in: Stress and infection (may temporarily ↑ insulin requirements); Renal/hepatic impairment (may ↓ insulin requirements); Concomitant use with pioglitazone or rosiglitazone (↑ risk of fluid retention and worsening HF); Patients with visual impairment who may rely on audible clicks to dial their dose (Toujeo and Tresiba); OB: Pregnancy may temporarily ↑ insulin requirements; Pedi: Children <18 yr (Toujeo), <6 yr (Basaglar or Lantus), <2 yr (detemir), or <1 yr (degludec) (safety not established).

Adverse Reactions/Side Effects
Endo: HYPOGLYCEMIA. **F and E:** hypokalemia. **Local:** lipodystrophy, pruritus, erythema, swelling. **Misc:** HYPERSENSITIVITY REACTIONS (including anaphylaxis).

Interactions
Drug-Drug: Beta blockers and **clonidine** may mask some of the signs and symptoms of hypoglycemia. **Corticosteroids, thyroid supplements, estrogens, isoniazid, niacin, phenothiazines,** and **rifampin** may ↑ insulin requirements. **Alcohol, ACE inhibitors, MAO inhibitors, octreotide, oral hypoglycemic agents,** and **salicylates** may ↓ insulin requirements. Concurrent use with **pioglitazone** or **rosiglitazone** may ↑ risk of fluid retention and worsening HF.
Drug-Natural Products: Glucosamine may worsen blood glucose control. **Fenugreek, chromium,** and **coenzyme Q-10** may produce additive hypoglycemic effects.

Route/Dosage
Toujeo has a lower glucose lowering effect than Basaglar or Lantus on a unit-to-unit basis.

Insulin Degludec
Subcut (Adults): *Type 1 diabetes (insulin naïve)*—⅓–½ of the total daily insulin dose given once daily, then adjust on the basis of patient's needs (remainder of insulin dose should be given as a short-acting insulin and divided between each daily meal) (usual starting total daily insulin dose = 0.2–0.4 units/kg); *Type 2 diabetes (insulin naïve)*—10 units once daily, then adjust on the basis of patient's needs; *Type 1 or 2 diabetes (and already on insulin)*—Give the same dose as the total daily dose of the long-acting or intermediate-acting insulin once daily, then adjust on the basis of patient's needs.
Subcut (Children ≥1 yr): *Type 1 or 2 diabetes (and already on insulin)*—Give 80% of the total daily dose of the long-acting or intermediate-acting insulin once daily, then adjust on the basis of patient's needs.

Insulin Detemir
Subcut (Adults and Children ≥6 yr): *Type 2 diabetes patients who are insulin-naive*—0.1–0.2 units/kg once daily in the evening (or divided into a twice daily regimen) *or* 10 units once daily in the evening (or divided into a twice daily regimen). *Patients with type 1 or 2 diabetes receiving basal insulin or basal bolus therapy*—May substitute on an equivalent unit-per-unit basis.

Insulin Glargine (Basaglar or Lantus)
Subcut (Adults and Children ≥6 yr): *Type 1 diabetes (insulin naïve)*—⅓ of the total daily insulin dose given once daily, then adjust on the basis of patient's needs (remainder of insulin dose should be given as a short-acting insulin) (usual starting total daily insulin dose = 0.2–0.4 units/kg); *Type 2 diabetes (insulin naïve)*—0.2 units/kg or up to 10 units once daily;

then adjust on the basis of patient's needs; *Type 1 or 2 diabetes (and converting from Toujeo)*—Give 80% of Toujeo dose as Basaglar or Lantus once daily, then adjust on the basis of patient's needs; *Type 1 or 2 diabetes (and converting from once daily NPH)*—Give the same dose once daily, then adjust on the basis of patient's needs; *Type 1 or 2 diabetes (and converting from twice daily NPH)*—Give 80% of the total daily NPH dose once daily, then adjust on the basis of patient's needs.

Insulin Glargine (Toujeo)

Subcut (Adults): *Type 1 diabetes (insulin naïve)*—⅓ to ½ of the total daily insulin dose given once daily, then adjust on the basis of patient's needs (range = 1–80 units/day), (remainder of insulin dose should be given as a short-acting insulin) (usual starting total daily insulin dose = 0.2–0.4 units/kg); *Type 2 diabetes (insulin naïve)*—0.2 units/kg once daily, then adjust on the basis of patient's needs; *Type 1 or 2 diabetes (and converting from intermediate or long-acting insulin)*—Use same total daily dose and give once daily, then adjust on the basis of patient's needs; *Type 1 or 2 diabetes (and converting from NPH insulin)*—Use 80% of the total daily NPH and give once daily, then adjust on the basis of patient's needs.

Availability

Insulin Degludec

Solution for injection: 100 units/mL (prefilled pens and vials), 200 units/mL (prefilled pens). ***In combination with:*** insulin aspart (Rysodeg 70/30); liraglutide (Xultophy). See Appendix B.

Insulin Detemir

Solution for injection: 100 units/mL (prefilled pens and vials). **Cost:** $177.61/10-mL vial; *Levemir Flexpen (3 mL)*—$290.07/5 pens.

Insulin Glargine

Solution for injection (Basaglar): 100 units/mL (prefilled pens). **Solution for injection (Lantus):** 100 units/mL (prefilled pens and vials). **Cost:** $180.34/10-mL vial; *Lantus Solostar (3 mL)*—$306.22/5 pens. **Solution for injection (Toujeo):** 300 units/mL (prefilled pens). ***In combination with:*** lixisenatide (Soliqua). See Appendix B.

NURSING IMPLICATIONS

Assessment

- Assess patient for signs and symptoms of hypoglycemia (anxiety; restlessness; mood changes; tingling in hands, feet, lips, or tongue; chills; cold sweats; confusion; cool, pale skin; difficulty in concentration; drowsiness; nightmares or trouble sleeping; excessive hunger; headache; irritability; nausea; nervousness; tachycardia; tremor; weakness; unsteady gait) and hyperglycemia (confusion, drowsiness; flushed, dry skin; fruit-like breath odor; rapid, deep breathing, polyuria; loss of appetite; nausea; vomiting; tiredness; unusual thirst) periodically during therapy.
- Monitor body weight periodically. Changes in weight may necessitate changes in insulin dose.
- ***Lab Test Considerations:*** Monitor blood glucose every 6 hr during therapy, more frequently in ketoacidosis and times of stress. Hemoglobin A_{1C} may also be monitored every 3–6 mo to determine effectiveness.
- Monitor serum potassium in patients at risk for hypokalemia (those using potassium-lowering agents, those receiving IV insulin) periodically during therapy.
- ***Toxicity and Overdose:*** Overdose is manifested by symptoms of hypoglycemia. Mild hypoglycemia may be treated by ingestion of oral glucose. Severe hypoglycemia is a life-threatening emergency; treatment consists of IV glucose, glucagon, or epinephrine. Recovery from hypoglycemia may be delayed due to the prolonged effect of long-acting insulins.

Implementation

- ***High Alert:*** Insulin-related medication errors have resulted in patient harm and death. Clarify ambiguous orders; do not accept orders using the abbreviation "u" for units (can be misread as a zero or the numeral 4; has resulted in tenfold overdoses).
- Insulins are available in different types and strengths. Check type, dose, and expiration date with another licensed nurse. Do not interchange insulins without consulting health care professional.
- Do not confuse Levemir (insulin detemir) with Lovenox (enoxaparin).
- Use *only* insulin syringes to draw up dose. The unit markings on the insulin syringe must match the insulin's units/mL. Special syringes for doses <50 units are available. Prior to withdrawing dose, rotate vial between palms to ensure uniform solution; do not shake.
- Use U-100 vial for pediatric patients requiring <5 units of insulin degludec each day.
- ***High Alert:*** Do not mix *insulin glargine or insulin detemir* with any other insulin or solution, or use syringes containing any other medicinal product or residue. If giving with a short-acting insulin, use separate syringes and different injection sites. Solution should be clear and colorless with no particulate matter.
- Do not use if cloudy, discolored, or unusually viscous. Store unopened vials and cartridges of *insulin glargine and insulin detemir* in the refrigerator; do not freeze. If unable to refrigerate, the 10-mL vial of

insulin glargine can be kept in a cool place unrefrigerated for up to 28 days. Once the cartridge is placed in a pen, do not refrigerate. After initial use, *insulin detemir* vials, cartridges, or a prefilled syringe may be stored in a cool place for 42 days. *Insulin degludec* pens may be stored in the refrigerator or kept at room temperature for up to 56 days. Do not store in-use cartridges and pre-filled syringes in refrigerator or with needle in place. Keep away from direct heat and sunlight.

- When transferring from once-daily NPH human insulin to *insulin glargine*, the dose usually remains unchanged. When transferring from twice-daily NPH human insulin to insulin glargine, the initial dose of insulin glargine is usually reduced by 20%.
- **Subcut:** Rotate injection sites.
- Administer *insulin glargine* and *insulin degludec* once daily at the same time each day.
- Administer *daily insulin detemir* with evening meal or at bedtime. With *twice daily insulin detemir*, administer evening dose with evening meal, at bedtime, or 12 hr after morning dose.
- Do not administer *insulin detemir, insulin degludec,* or *insulin glargine* IV or in insulin pumps.

Patient/Family Teaching

- Instruct patient on proper technique for administration. Include type of insulin, equipment (syringe, cartridge pens, alcohol swabs), storage, and place to discard syringes. Discuss the importance of not changing brands of insulin or syringes, selection and rotation of injection sites, and compliance with therapeutic regimen. Patients taking insulin detemir and *insulin degludec* should be given the *Patient Information* circular for this product.
- Caution patient not to share pen device with another person, even if needle is changed; may risk transmission of bloodborne pathogens.
- Explain to patient that this medication controls hyperglycemia but does not cure diabetes. Therapy is long term.
- Instruct patient in proper testing of serum glucose and ketones. These tests should be closely monitored during periods of stress or illness and health care professional notified of significant changes.
- Emphasize the importance of compliance with nutritional guidelines and regular exercise as directed by health care professional.
- Instruct patient to notify health care professional of all Rx or OTC medications, vitamins, or herbal products being taken and to consult health care professional before taking other Rx, OTC, herbal products, or alcohol.
- Advise patient to notify health care professional of medication regimen prior to treatment or surgery.
- Advise patient to notify health care professional if nausea, vomiting, or fever develops, if unable to eat regular diet, or if blood glucose levels are not controlled.
- Instruct patient on signs and symptoms of hypoglycemia and hyperglycemia and what to do if they occur.
- Patients with diabetes mellitus should carry a source of sugar (candy, glucose gel) and identification describing their disease and treatment regimen at all times.
- Advise patient to notify health care professional if pregnancy is planned or suspected or if breast feeding or planning to breast feed.
- Emphasize the importance of regular follow-up, especially during first few wk of therapy.

Evaluation/Desired Outcomes

- Control of blood glucose levels in diabetic patients without the appearance of hypoglycemic or hyperglycemic episodes.

HIGH ALERT

INSULINS (rapid acting)
(in-su-lin)

insulin aspart, rDNA origin
Fiasp, NovoLOG, NovoRapid

insulin glulisine
Apidra, Apidra Solostar

insulin lispro, rDNA origin
Admelog, HumaLOG

Classification
Therapeutic: antidiabetics, hormones
Pharmacologic: pancreatics

See Appendix L for more information concerning insulins

Indications

Control of hyperglycemia in patients with type 1 or type 2 diabetes mellitus.

Action

Lower blood glucose by: stimulating glucose uptake in skeletal muscle and fat, inhibiting hepatic glucose production. Other actions: inhibition of lypolysis and proteolysis, enhanced protein synthesis. These are rapid-acting insulins with a more rapid onset and shorter duration than regular insulin; should be used with an intermediate- or long-acting insulin. **Therapeutic Effects:** Control of hyperglycemia in diabetic patients.

Pharmacokinetics

Absorption: Very rapidly absorbed from subcut administration sites.

Distribution: Widely distributed.

Metabolism and Excretion: Metabolized by liver, spleen, kidney, and muscle.

Half-life: *Insulin aspart*—1–1.5 hr; *Insulin lispro*—1 hr; *insulin glulisine*—42 min.

TIME/ACTION PROFILE (hypoglycemic effect)

ROUTE	ONSET	PEAK	DURATION
Insulin aspart	within 15 min	1–2 hr	3–4 hr
Insulin glulisine	within 15 min	1–2 hr	3–4 hr
Insulin lispro	within 15 min	1–2 hr	3–4 hr

Contraindications/Precautions

Contraindicated in: Hypoglycemia; Allergy or hypersensitivity to a particular type of insulin, preservatives, or other additives.

Use Cautiously in: Stress and infection (may temporarily ↑ insulin requirements); Renal/hepatic dysfunction (may ↓ insulin requirements); Concomitant use with pioglitazone or rosiglitazone (↑ risk of fluid retention and worsening HF); OB: Pregnancy may temporarily ↑ insulin requirements; Pedi: Safety not established in children <3 yr (for insulin lispro), <4 yr (insulin glulisine), <6 yr (for insulin aspart).

Adverse Reactions/Side Effects

Endo: HYPOGLYCEMIA. **F and E:** hypokalemia. **Local:** erythema, lipodystrophy, pruritus, swelling. **Misc:** allergic reactions including ANAPHYLAXIS.

Interactions

Drug-Drug: Beta blockers and **clonidine** may mask some of the signs and symptoms of hypoglycemia. **Corticosteroids**, **thyroid supplements**, **estrogens**, **isoniazid**, **niacin**, **phenothiazines**, and **rifampin** may ↑ insulin requirements. **Alcohol**, **ACE inhibitors**, **MAO inhibitors**, **octreotide**, **oral hypoglycemic agents**, and **salicylates** may ↓ insulin requirements. Concurrent use with **pioglitazone** or **rosiglitazone** may ↑ risk of fluid retention and worsening HF.

Drug-Natural Products: Glucosamine may worsen blood glucose control. **Fenugreek**, **chromium**, and **coenzyme Q-10** may produce additive hypoglycemic effects.

Route/Dosage

Dose depends on blood glucose, response, and many other factors. Only insulin aspart and insulin glulisine can be administered IV.

Subcut (Adults and Children): Total insulin dose determined by needs of patient; generally 0.5–1 unit/kg/day; 50–70% of this dose may be given as meal-related boluses of rapid-acting insulin, and the remainder as an intermediate or long-acting insulin. *Subcutaneous infusion pump*—~50% of total dose can be given as meal-related boluses and ~50% of total dose can be given as basal infusion.

Availability

Insulin aspart: 100 units/mL in 10-mL vials and 3-mL prefilled cartridges or pens. **Cost:** $163.68/10-mL vial, *NovoLog Flexpen (3 mL)*—$310.56/5 pens; *NovoLog Pen Fill (3 mL)*—$298.95/5 cartridges. **Insulin aspart 70/30 mix (Novolog Mix 70/30):** 70% insulin aspart protamine suspension and 30% insulin aspart solution mix 100 units/mL in 10-mL vials and 3-mL prefilled pens. **Cost:** $169.64/10–mL vial, *NovoLog Mix 70/30 Flexpen (3 mL)*—$310.56/5 pens. **Insulin glulisine:** 100 units/mL in 10-mL vials and 3-mL prefilled pens. **Cost:** $158.53/10–mL vial, *Apidra Solostar (3 mL)*—$294.61/5 pens. **Insulin lispro:** 100 units/mL in 10-mL vials and 3-mL prefilled cartridges and pens, 200 units/mL in 3-mL prefilled cartridges and pens. **Cost:** $163.56/10-mL vial, *Humalog Kwikpen (3 mL)*—$309.53/5 pens. **Insulin lispro 75/25 mix (Humalog Mix 75/25):** 75% lispro insulin protamine suspension and 25% insulin lispro mix 100 units/mL in 10-mL vials and 3-mL prefilled pens. **Cost:** $165.07/10-mL vial. **Insulin lispro 50/50 mix (Humalog Mix 50/50):** 50% lispro insulin protamine suspension and 50% insulin lispro mix 100 units/mL in 10-mL vials and 3-mL prefilled pens. **Cost:** *Humalog Mix 50/50 Kwikpen (3 mL)*—$303.58/5 pens.

NURSING IMPLICATIONS

Assessment

- Assess for symptoms of hypoglycemia (anxiety; restlessness; tingling in hands, feet, lips, or tongue; chills; cold sweats; confusion; cool, pale skin; difficulty in concentration; drowsiness; nightmares or trouble sleeping; excessive hunger; headache; irritability; nausea; nervousness; tachycardia; tremor; weakness; unsteady gait) and hyperglycemia (confusion, drowsiness; flushed, dry skin; fruit-like breath odor; rapid, deep breathing, polyuria; loss of appetite; nausea; vomiting; unusual thirst) periodically during therapy.
- Monitor body weight periodically. Changes in weight may necessitate changes in insulin dose.
- Assess patient for signs of allergic reactions (rash, shortness of breath, wheezing, rapid pulse, sweating, low BP) during therapy.
- ***Lab Test Considerations:*** Monitor blood glucose every 6 hr during therapy, more frequently in ketoacidosis and times of stress. HbA_{1C} may also be monitored every 3–6 mo to determine effectiveness.
- Monitor serum potassium in patients at risk for hypokalemia (those using potassium-lowering agents, those receiving IV insulin) periodically during therapy.
- ***Toxicity and Overdose:*** Overdose is manifested by symptoms of hypoglycemia. Mild hypoglycemia may be treated by ingestion of oral glucose. Severe hypoglycemia is a life-threatening emergency; treatment consists of IV glucose, glucagon, or epinephrine. Early signs of hypoglycemia may be less pronounced by long duration of diabetes, diabetic nerve disease, and use of beta blockers; may result in loss

of consciousness prior to patient's awareness of hypoglycemia.

Implementation

- ***High Alert:*** Insulin-related medication errors have resulted in patient harm and death. Clarify ambiguous orders; do not accept orders using the abbreviation "u" for units (can be misread as a zero or the numeral 4; has resulted in tenfold overdoses).
- Insulins are available in different types and strengths. Check type, dose, and expiration date with another licensed nurse. Do not interchange insulins without consulting health care professional.
- Do not confuse Humalog with Humulin. Do not confuse Novolog with Novolin. Do not confuse Apidra with Spiriva (tiotropium).
- Use *only* insulin syringes to draw up dose. The unit markings on the insulin syringe must match the insulin's units/mL. Special syringes for doses <50 units are available. Do not draw up dose into a syringe from the Kwik Pens; syringe markings do not match-up and could lead to a medication error. Use *only* U-100 insulin syringes to draw up *insulin lispro* dose. Prior to withdrawing dose, rotate vial between palms to ensure uniform solution; do not shake.
- *Insulin aspart, insulin glulisine,* and *insulin lispro* may be mixed with NPH insulin. When mixing insulins, draw insulin aspart, insulin glulisine, or insulin lispro into syringe first to avoid contamination of rapid-acting insulin vial. Mixed insulins should never be used in a pump or for IV infusion.
- Store vials in refrigerator. Vials may also be kept at room temperature for up to 28 days. Do not use if cloudy, discolored, or unusually viscous. Store cartridges and pens at room temperature and use within 28 days. Never use the *PenFill* cartridge after the expiration date on the *PenFill* cartridge or on the box.
- Because of their short duration, *insulin lispro, insulin glulisine,* and *insulin aspart* must be used with a longer-acting insulin or insulin infusion pump. In patients with type 2 diabetes, *insulin lispro* may be used without a longer-acting insulin when used in combination with an oral sulfonylurea agent.
- Humalog U-200 should not be mixed with other insulins, administered IV, or used in insulin pumps.
- **Subcut:** Administer into abdominal wall, thigh, or upper arm subcut. Rotate injection sites.
- Administer *insulin aspart* within 5–10 min before a meal.
- When used as meal time insulin, administer *insulin glulisine* 15 min before or within 20 min after starting a meal.
- Administer *insulin lispro* within 15 min before or immediately after a meal.
- May also be administered subcut via external insulin pump. Do not mix with other insulins or solution when used with a pump. Change the solution in the reservoir at least every 6 days, change the infusion set, and the infusion set insertion site at least every 3 days. Do not mix with other insulins or with a diluent when used in the pump.
- **IV:** *Insulin aspart* and *insulin glulisine* may be administered IV in selected situations under appropriate medical supervision. ***Diluent:*** Dilute *insulin aspart* with 0.9% NaCl or D5W in infusion systems using polypropylene infusion bags. Dilute *insulin glulisine* with 0.9% NaCl, using polyvinyl chloride (PVC) Viaflex infusion bags and Polyvinyl chloride (PVC) tubing (Clearlink System Continu-Flo solution set) with a dedicated infusion line. ***Concentration:*** 0.05–1 unit/mL. *Insulin lispro Humalog U-100* can be administered IV under medical supervision ONLY with close monitoring of blood glucose and potassium levels to avoid hypoglycemia and hypokalemia. ***Concentration:*** 0.1 unit/mL to 1 unit/mL. ***Diluent:*** 0.9% NaCl. Solutions of insulin lispro and 0.9% NaCl can be stored for 48 hrs in refrigerator, then used at room temperature for another 48 hr.

Patient/Family Teaching

- Instruct patient on proper technique for administration. Include type of insulin, equipment (syringe, cartridge pens, external pump, alcohol swabs), storage, and place to discard syringes. Discuss the importance of not changing brands of insulin or syringes, selection and rotation of injection sites, and compliance with therapeutic regimen. Caution patient that insulin pens should not be shared with others, even if clean needles are used.
- Demonstrate technique for mixing insulins by drawing up insulin aspart, insulin glulisine, or insulin lispro first. Roll intermediate-acting insulin vial between palms to mix, rather than shaking (may cause inaccurate dose).
- Caution patient not to share pen device with another person, even if needle is changed; may risk transmission of bloodborne pathogens.
- Explain to patient that this medication controls hyperglycemia but does not cure diabetes. Therapy is long term.
- Instruct patient in proper testing of serum glucose and ketones. These tests should be closely monitored during periods of stress or illness and health care professional notified of significant changes.
- Emphasize the importance of compliance with nutritional guidelines and regular exercise as directed by health care professional.
- Advise patient to notify health care professional of all Rx or OTC medications, vitamins, or herbal products being taken and to consult with health care professional before taking other medications or alcohol.
- Advise patient to notify health care professional of medication regimen prior to treatment or surgery.
- Advise patient to notify health care professional if nausea, vomiting, or fever develops, if unable to eat

regular diet, or if blood glucose levels are not controlled.

- Instruct patient on signs and symptoms of hypoglycemia and hyperglycemia and what to do if they occur.
- Advise patient to notify health care professional if pregnancy is planned or suspected or if breast feeding or planning to breast feed.
- Patients with diabetes mellitus should carry a source of sugar (candy, glucose gel) and identification describing their disease and treatment regimen at all times.
- Emphasize the importance of regular follow-up, especially during first few wk of therapy.

Evaluation/Desired Outcomes

- Control of blood glucose levels without the appearance of hypoglycemic or hyperglycemic episodes.

INTERFERONS, BETA
(in-ter-**feer**-on)

interferon beta-1a
Avonex, Rebif

interferon beta-1b
Betaseron, Extavia

Classification
Therapeutic: anti-multiple sclerosis agents, immune modifiers
Pharmacologic: interferons

Indications
Relapsing forms of multiple sclerosis, including clinically isolated syndrome, relapsing-remitting disease, and active secondary progressive disease.

Action
Antiviral and immunoregulatory properties produced by interacting with specific receptor sites on cell surfaces may explain beneficial effects. Produced by recombinant DNA technology. **Therapeutic Effects:** Reduce incidence of relapse (neurologic dysfunction) and slow physical disability.

Pharmacokinetics
Absorption: *Interferon beta-1b*—50% absorbed following subcut administration.
Distribution: Unknown.
Metabolism and Excretion: Unknown.
Half-life: *Interferon beta-1a*—69 hr (subcut), 10 hr (IM); *interferon beta-1b*—8 min–4.3 hr.

TIME/ACTION PROFILE (serum concentrations)

ROUTE	ONSET	PEAK	DURATION
Interferon beta-1a IM, subcut	unknown	3–15 h	unknown
Interferon beta-1b subcut	rapid	16 h	unknown

Contraindications/Precautions
Contraindicated in: Hypersensitivity to natural or recombinant interferon beta or human albumin.
Use Cautiously in: History of suicide attempt or depression; History of seizures (interferon beta-1a); Cardiovascular disease; Congestive HF (may worsen HF); Liver disease (interferon beta-1a); History of alcohol abuse (interferon beta-1a); Latex sensitivity (Extavia only); OB: May ↑ risk of spontaneous abortion; use only if potential maternal benefit outweighs potential fetal risk; Lactation: Safety not established; Rep: Women of reproductive potential; Pedi: Safety and effectiveness not established.

Adverse Reactions/Side Effects
CNS: SEIZURES (↑ WITH INTERFERON BETA-1A), depression, dizziness, fatigue, headache, insomnia, drowsiness, incoordination, rigors, suicidal ideation. **CV:** chest pain, edema, hypertension. **Derm:** ERYTHEMA MULTIFORME, STEVENS-JOHNSON SYNDROME, rash, alopecia, ↑ sweating. **EENT:** sinusitis, vision abnormalities. **GI:** constipation, nausea, vomiting, abdominal pain, autoimmune hepatitis, dry mouth, ↑ liver enzymes. **GU:** cystitis, erectile dysfunction, polyuria, urinary incontinence. **Hemat:** THROMBOTIC THROMBOCYTOPENIC PURPURA, HEMOLYTIC UREMIC SYNDROME, neutropenia, anemia, eosinophilia, thrombocytopenia. **Local:** injection-site reactions, injection site necrosis. **MS:** myalgia, arthralgia, drug-induced lupus erythematosis, muscle spasm. **Resp:** dyspnea, upper respiratory tract infection. **Misc:** HYPERSENSITIVITY REACTIONS (including anaphylaxis and angioedema), chills, fever, flu-like symptoms, pain.

Interactions
(All interactions below are for Interferon beta-1b).
Drug-Drug: ↑ myelosuppression may occur with other myelosuppressives including **antineoplastics**. Concurrent use of **hepatotoxic agents** may ↑ the risk of hepatotoxicity (↑ liver enzymes).
Drug-Natural Products: Avoid concomitant use with immmunomodulating natural products such as **astragalus**, **echinacea**, and **melatonin**.

Route/Dosage

Interferon Beta-1a

IM (Adults): *Avonex*—30 mcg once weekly.
Subcut (Adults): *Rebif (target dose of 22 mcg 3 times/wk)*—Start with 4.4 mcg 3 times/wk for 2 wk, then ↑ to 11 mcg 3 times/wk for 2 wk, then ↑ to maintenance dose of 22 mcg 3 times/wk. *Rebif (target dose of 44 mcg 3 times/wk)*—Start with 8.8 mcg 3 times/wk for 2 wk, then ↑ to 22 mcg 3 times/wk for 2 wk, then ↑ to maintenance dose of 44 mcg 3 times/wk.

Interferon Beta-1b

Subcut (Adults): Initiate with 0.0625 mg (2 million units) every other day and then ↑ dose by 0.0625 mg every 2 wk over a 6-wk period up to target dose of 0.25 mg (8 million units) every other day.

Availability

Interferon Beta-1a

Lyophilized powder for injection (Avonex): 30 mcg/vial. **Solution for injection (prefilled syringes and prefilled pens) (Avonex):** 30 mcg/0.5 mL. **Solution for injection (prefilled syringes) (Rebif):** 22 mcg/0.5 mL, 44 mcg/0.5 mL, titration pack of 6 syringes prefilled with 8.8 mcg/0.2 mL and 6 syringes prefilled with 22 mcg/0.5 mL.

Interferon Beta-1b

Lyophilized powder for injection: 0.3 mg/vial.

NURSING IMPLICATIONS

Assessment

- Assess frequency of exacerbations of symptoms of multiple sclerosis periodically during therapy.
- Monitor patient for signs of depression during therapy. If depression occurs, notify health care professional immediately; discontinuation of therapy should be considered.
- ***Lab Test Considerations:*** Monitor hemoglobin, WBC, platelets, and blood chemistries including liver function tests prior to and 1, 3, and 6 mo after initiation of therapy and periodically thereafter. Therapy may be temporarily discontinued if the absolute neutrophil count is $<750/mm^3$, if AST or ALT exceeds 10 times the upper limit of normal, or if serum bilirubin exceeds 5 times the upper limit of normal. Once the absolute neutrophil count is $>750/mm^3$ or the hepatic enzymes have returned to normal, therapy can be restarted at 50% of the original dose.
- Thyroid function tests should be monitored every 6 mo, especially in patients with a history of thyroid abnormalities.

Implementation

- Do not confuse products. Interferon beta-1a and interferon beta-1b are not interchangeable.
- **Interferon Beta-1a:** *Avonex:* Reconstitute with 1.1 mL of diluent and swirl gently to dissolve. Do not shake the vial. Inject into the thigh or upper arm. Keep reconstituted solution in refrigerator; inject within 6 hr of reconstitution.
- *Rebif:* Administer subcut via prefilled, single-use syringe at the same time (afternoon or evening) on the same days (Monday, Wednesday, Friday) at least 48 hr apart each wk. Rotate sites with each injection to minimize risk of injection site reactions (pain, erythema, edema, cellulitis, abscess, necrosis). Avoid areas that are inflamed, edematous, erythematous, ecchymotic, or have signs of infection. Discard unused portions. Store in refrigerator.
- **Interferon Beta-1b:** To reconstitute, inject 1.2 mL of diluent supplied into interferon beta-1b vial for a concentration of 0.25 mg/mL. Swirl gently to dissolve completely; do not shake. Do not use solutions that are discolored or contain particulate matter. Keep reconstituted solution refrigerated; inject within 3 hr of reconstitution. Rubber cap of diluent prefilled syringe of Extavia contains latex and should not be handled by individuals allergic to latex.
- Following reconstitution, withdraw 1 mL into a syringe with a 27-gauge needle and inject subcut into arm, abdomen, hip, or thigh. Pinch skin during injection and inject at a 90° angle. Gently massage injection site. Rotate sites with each injection to minimize risk of injection site reactions. Discard unused portion; vials are for single dose only.

Patient/Family Teaching

- **Home Care Issues:** Instruct patient in correct technique for injection and care and disposal of equipment. Caution patient not to reuse needles or syringes and provide patient with a puncture-resistant container for disposal.
- Instruct patient to take medication as directed; do not change dose or schedule without consulting health care professional. Patients should receive a medication guide with each product.
- Advise patient and family to notify health care professional if thoughts about suicide or dying, attempts to commit suicide; new or worse depression; new or worse anxiety; feeling very agitated or restless; panic attacks; trouble sleeping; new or worse irritability; acting aggressive; being angry or violent; acting on dangerous impulses; an extreme increase in activity and talking, other unusual changes in behavior or mood occur.
- Inform patient that flu-like symptoms (fever, chills, myalgia, sweating, malaise) may occur during therapy. Acetaminophen may be used for relief of fever and myalgias.
- Advise patient to notify health care professional if pregnancy is planned or suspected or if breast feeding. May cause spontaneous abortion.

Evaluation/Desired Outcomes

- Decrease in the frequency of relapse (neurologic dysfunction) in patients with relapsing-remitting multiple sclerosis.

ipilimumab (i-pil-li-moo-mab)

Yervoy

Classification

Therapeutic: antineoplastics

Pharmacologic: monoclonal antibodies

Indications

Treatment of unresectable/metastatic melanoma. Adjuvant treatment of cutaneous melanoma with pathologic involvement of regional lymph nodes >1 mm in patients who have undergone complete resection, including total lymphadenectomy. Treatment of previously untreated, advanced renal cell carcinoma in patients who are at intermediate or poor risk (with nivolumab). Microsatellite instability-high (MSI-H) or mismatch repair deficient (dMMR) metastatic colorectal cancer that has progressed following treatment with a fluoropyrimidine, oxaliplatin, and irinotecan.

Action

Binds to cytotoxic T-lymphocyte-associated antigen 4 (CTLA-4) and prevents it from binding to CD80/CD86 ligands. CTLA-4 is a negative regulator of T-cell activation; binding results in augmented T-cell activation and proliferation as well as enhanced T-cell responsiveness. **Therapeutic Effects:** ↓ spread or recurrence of melanoma and improved survival. Improved survival with renal cell carcinoma. ↓ progression of MSI-H or dMMR metastatic colorectal cancer.

Pharmacokinetics

Absorption: IV administration results in complete bioavailability.

Distribution: Crosses the placenta.

Metabolism and Excretion: Unknown.

Half-life: 14.7 days.

TIME/ACTION PROFILE

ROUTE	ONSET	PEAK	DURATION
IV	unknown	unknown	unknown

Contraindications/Precautions

Contraindicated in: Lactation: Avoid breast feeding.

Use Cautiously in: Patients undergoing allogeneic hematopoietic stem cell transplantation (↑ risk of graft-versus-host disease; OB: Use only if potential maternal benefit justifies potential risk to the fetus; may cause fetal harm; Rep: Women of reproductive potential; Pedi: Children <12 yr (safety and effectiveness not established).

Adverse Reactions/Side Effects

CNS: IMMUNE-MEDIATED ENCEPHALITIS, fatigue. **Derm:** IMMUNE-MEDIATED DERMATITIS (INCLUDING STEPHENS-JOHNSON SYNDROME AND TOXIC EPIDERMAL NECROLYSIS, pruritus, rash. **EENT:** IMMUNE-MEDIATED OCULAR DISEASE, hearing loss. **Endo:** IMMUNE-MEDIATED ENDROCRINOPATHIES (INCLUDING HYPOPITUITARISM, HYPOTHYROIDISM, HYPERTHYROIDISM, ADRENAL INSUFFICIENCY, CUSHING'S SYNDROME, AND HYPOGONADISM). **GI:** IMMUNE-MEDIATED COLITIS, IMMUNE-MEDIATED HEPATITIS, colitis, diarrhea. **GU:** IMMUNE-MEDIATED NEPHRITIS, renal impairment. **MS:** myositis. **Neuro:** IMMUNE-MEDIATED NEUROPATHY. **Resp:** IMMUNE-MEDIATED PNEUMONITIS. **Misc:** INFUSION REACTIONS, SARCOIDOSIS.

Interactions

Drug-Drug: Concurrent use with **vemurafenib** may ↑ risk of hepatic dysfunction.

Route/Dosage

Unresectable/Metastatic Melanoma

IV (Adults and Children ≥12 yr): 3 mg/kg every 3 wk for a total of 4 doses.

Adjuvant Treatment of Melanoma

IV (Adults and Children ≥12 yr): 10 mg/kg every 3 wk for 4 doses, then 10 mg/kg every 12 wk for up to 3 yr.

Renal Cell Carcinoma

IV (Adults): 1 mg/kg every 3 wk for 4 doses (administer after nivolumab on same day), then give nivolumab alone.

Colorectal Cancer

IV (Adults): 1 mg/kg every 3 wk for up to 4 doses (administer after nivolumab on same day) or until disease progression or unacceptable toxicity.

Availability

Solution for injection (requires dilution): 5 mg/mL.

NURSING IMPLICATIONS

Assessment

- Monitor for signs and symptoms of enterocolitis (diarrhea, abdominal pain, mucus or blood in stool, with or without fever) and bowel perforation (peritoneal signs, ileus). Rule out infection and consider endoscopic evaluation. If severe enterocolitis occurs, discontinue ilipimumab and start systemic corticosteroids at doses of 1–2 mg/kg/day of prednisone or equivalents. At improvement to Grade 1 or less, taper corticosteroid over at least 1 mo. Consider adding anti-TNF therapy or other immunosuppressive therapy if signs and symptoms of enterocolitis persist despite systemic corticosteroid therapy within 3–5 days or if they recur after symptomatic improvement. Hold dose for moderate enterocolitis; administer anti-diarrheal treatment and if persists for >1 wk, start corticosteroids at a dose of 0.5 mg/kg/day of prednisone or equivalent.

- Assess for signs and symptoms of hepatotoxicity (yellowing of skin or whites of eyes, unusual darkening of urine, unusual tiredness, pain in right upper stomach) before each dose. If hepatotoxicity occurs, rule out infectious or malignant causes. Permanently discontinue ipilimumab if Grade 3–5 hepatotoxicity occurs and start systemic corticosteroids at a dose of 1–2 mg/kg/day of prednisone or equivalent. When liver function tests show sustained improvement or return to baseline, start corticosteroid taper over 1 mo. May administer mycophenolate in patients with persistent severe hepatitis despite high-dose corticosteroids. Hold ipilimumab in patients with Grade 2 hepatotoxicity.
- Monitor for signs and symptoms of dermatitis (rash, pruritus). Unless other causes are identified, assume immune-mediated dermatitis. Permanently discontinue ipilimumab in patients with Stevens-Johnson syndrome, toxic epidermal necrolysis, or rash complicated by full thickness dermal ulceration, or necrotic, bullous, or hemorrhagic manifestations. Administer corticosteroids at a dose of 1–2 mg/kg/day of prednisone or equivalent. When dermatitis is controlled, taper corticosteroids over at least 1 mo. Hold ipilimumab in patients with moderate to severe signs and symptoms. Treat mild to moderate dermatitis symptomatically. Administer topical or systemic corticosteroids if there is no improvement of symptoms within 1 wk.
- Monitor for symptoms of motor or sensory neuropathy (unilateral or bilateral weakness, sensory alterations, paresthesia). Permanently discontinue ipilimumab in patients with severe neuropathy (interfering with daily activities). Institute treatment as needed. Consider systemic corticosteroids of 1–2 mg/kg/day of prednisone or equivalent for severe neuropathy. Hold dose of ipilimumab in patients with moderate neuropathy (not interfering with daily activities).
- Monitor for clinical signs and symptoms of hypophysitis, adrenal insufficiency (including adrenal crisis), and hyper- or hypothyroidism (fatigue, headache, mental status changes, abdominal pain, unusual bowel habits, hypotension). Unless other causes are determined, consider signs and symptoms as immune-mediated endocrinopathies. Hold ipilimumab in symptomatic patients and initiate corticosteroids at 1–2 mg/kg/day of prednisone or equivalents. Initiate hormone replacement therapy as needed.
- Monitor for signs and symptoms of immune-mediated encephalitis (new-onset moderate to severe neurologic signs or symptoms). Hold ipilimumab and rule out infections and other potential causes. If other causes are ruled out, administer corticosteroids at a dose of 1–2 mg/kg/day prednisone equivalents, followed by corticosteroid taper. Permanently discontinue ipilimumab for immune-mediated encephalitis.
- Assess eyes for signs and symptoms of uveitis, iritis, or episcleritis. Administer corticosteroid eyedrops if these occur. Permanently discontinue ipilimumab for immune-mediated ocular disease unresponsive to local immunosuppressive therapy. Consider Vogt Koyanagi-Harada-like syndrome if uveitis occurs with other immune-mediated adverse reactions. May require treatment with systemic steroids to reduce the risk of permanent vision loss.
- ***Lab Test Considerations:*** Monitor liver function tests (AST, ALT, bilirubin) prior to each dose of ipilimumab; ↑ frequency of monitoring if levels ↑. Hold ipilimumab in patients with Grade 2 hepatotoxicity. With complete or partial resolution (Grade 0–1), and patient receiving <7.5 mg prednisone, resume at a dose of 3 mg/kg every 3 wk until administration of all 4 planned doses or 16 wk from first dose, whichever occurs earlier. Discontinue ipilimumab permanently with Grade 3–5 hepatotoxicity and administer systemic corticosteroids at a dose of 1–2 mg/kg/day of prednisone or equivalent. Initiate corticosteroid taper when liver function tests show sustained improvement or return to baseline; continue to taper over 1 mo.
- Monitor thyroid function tests and serum chemistries at start of therapy, before each dose, and as clinically indicated.

Implementation

- For unresectable/metastatic melanoma, doses may be delayed in the event of toxicity, but must be administered within 16 wk from 1st dose. For adjuvant treatment of melanoma, doses can be omitted, but not delayed in the event of toxicity.
- Hold dose for any moderate immune-mediated adverse reactions or for symptomatic endocrinopathy. For patients with complete or partial resolution of adverse reactions (Grade 0–1), who are receiving equivalents of <7.5 mg prednisone/day, resume ipilimumab therapy.
- Permanently discontinue if persistent moderate adverse reactions or inability to reduce corticosteroid dose to equivalent of prednisone 7.5 mg/day, failure to complete full treatment course within 16 wk from infusion of 1st dose, or severe or life threatening adverse reactions occur including: Colitis with abdominal pain, fever, or peritoneal signs; ↑ in stool frequency of 7 or more over baseline, stool incontinence. Need for IV hydration for >24 hrs, GI hemorrhage and GI perforation; AST or ALT >5 times the upper limits of normal or total bilirubin >3 times the upper limit of normal; Stevens-Johnson syndome, toxic epidermal necrolysis, or rash complicated by full-thickness dermal ulceration, or necrotic, bullous, or hemorrhagic manifestations; Severe motor or sensory neuropathy, Guillian-Barre syndrome, or myasthenia gravis; Severe immune-

mediated reactions involving any organ system (nephritis, pneumonitis, pancreatitis, non-infectious myocarditis); and Immune-mediated ocular disease that is unresponsive to topical immunosuppressive therapy.

- Allow vial to stand at room temperature for 5 min prior to preparation of infusion. Withdraw amount of ipilimumab required and transfer to IV bag. ***Diluent:*** Dilute with 0.9% NaCL or D5W. ***Concentration:*** 1 mg/mL to 2 mg/mL. Mix slowly by gentle inversion; do not shake. Solution is clear, pale yellow, and may contain translucent-to-white amorphous particles; do not administer if cloudy, discolored, or contains particulate matter. Store for up to 24 hr at room temperature or refrigerated; do not freeze, protect from light. Discard partially used vials. ***Rate:*** **Melanoma**: Infuse over 90 min through a sterile, non-pyrogenic, low-protein-binding in-line filter. Flush the IV line with 0.9% NaCl or D5W after each dose. **Renal cell carcinoma or colorectal cancer**: Infuse over 30 min immediately following niovolumab infusion through a sterile, non-pyrogenic, low-protein-binding in-line filter. Flush the IV line with 0.9% NaCl or D5W after each dose.
- **Y-Site Incompatibility:** Do not mix with or infuse with other solutions or products.

Patient/Family Teaching

- Inform patient of the risk of immune-mediated reactions due to T-cell activation and proliferation. Advise patients these may be severe and fatal. Instruct patient to notify health care professional immediately if signs and symptoms occur.
- Instruct patient to read the *Medication Guide* before starting therapy and with each Rx refill in case of changes.
- Advise patient to notify health care professional if signs and symptoms of enterocolitis, hepatitis, skin reactions, neuropathies, endocrinopathies, pneumonitis, nephritis, or encephalitis occur.
- Rep: Inform female patient to use effective contraception and avoid breast feeding during and for at least 3 mo following therapy. Women must choose to discontinue breast feeding or ipilimumab. Advise female patients to notify health care professional if pregnancy is planned or suspected. Encourage women who become pregnant during therapy to enroll in a Pregnancy Safety Surveillance Study by calling 1-844-593-7869.

Evaluation/Desired Outcomes

- ↓ spread or recurrence of melanoma.
- Improved survival with renal cell carcinoma.
- ↓ progression of MSI-H or dMMR metastatic colorectal cancer.

ipratropium (i-pra-**troe**-pee-um)

Atrovent, Atrovent HFA

Classification
Therapeutic: allergy, cold, and cough remedies, bronchodilators
Pharmacologic: anticholinergics

Indications

Inhaln: Maintenance therapy of reversible airway obstruction due to COPD, including chronic bronchitis and emphysema. **Intranasal:** Rhinorrhea associated with allergic and nonallergic perennial rhinitis (0.03% solution) or the common cold (0.06% solution). **Unlabeled Use: Inhaln:** Adjunctive management of bronchospasm caused by asthma.

Action

Inhaln: Inhibits cholinergic receptors in bronchial smooth muscle, resulting in decreased concentrations of cyclic guanosine monophosphate (cGMP). Decreased levels of cGMP produce local bronchodilation. **Intranasal:** Local application inhibits secretions from glands lining the nasal mucosa. **Therapeutic Effects: Inhaln:** Bronchodilation without systemic anticholinergic effects. **Intranasal:** Decreased rhinorrhea.

Pharmacokinetics

Absorption: Minimal systemic absorption (2% for inhalation solution; 20% for inhalation aerosol; <20% following nasal use).
Distribution: 15% of dose reaches lower airways after inhalation.
Metabolism and Excretion: Small amounts absorbed are metabolized by the liver.
Half-life: 2 hr.

TIME/ACTION PROFILE (bronchodilation)

ROUTE	ONSET	PEAK	DURATION
Inhalation	1–3 min	1–2 hr	4–6 hr
Intranasal	15 min	unknown	6–12 hr

Contraindications/Precautions

Contraindicated in: Hypersensitivity to ipratropium, atropine, belladonna alkaloids, or bromide; Avoid use during acute bronchospasm; **Note: Atrovent HFA has replaced the discontinued Atrovent CFC (chlorofluorocarbon). Soy and CFC-allergic patients can now safely use the Atrovent HFA formulation. However, Combivent (ipratropium/albuterol combination) MDI does contain soya lecithin and is contraindicated in patients with a history of hypersensitivity to soy and peanuts.**
Use Cautiously in: Patients with bladder neck obstruction, prostatic hyperplasia, glaucoma, or urinary retention; Geri: May be more sensitive to effects.

Adverse Reactions/Side Effects

CNS: dizziness, headache, nervousness. **EENT:** blurred vision, sore throat; *nasal only*, epistaxis, nasal dryness/irritation. **Resp:** bronchospasm, cough. **CV:** hypotension, palpitations. **GI:** GI irritation, nausea. **Derm:** rash. **Misc:** allergic reactions.

Interactions

Drug-Drug: ↑ anticholinergic effects with other **drugs having anticholinergic properties (antihistamines, phenothiazines, disopyramide)**.

Route/Dosage

Inhaln (Adults and Children >12 yr): *Metered-dose inhaler (nonacute)*—2 inhalations 4 times daily (not to exceed 12 inhalations/24 hr or more frequently than every 4 hr). *Acute exacerbations*—4–8 puffs using a spacer device as needed. *Via nebulization (nonacute)*—500 mcg 3–4 times daily. *Via nebulization (acute exacerbations)*—500 mcg every 30 min for 3 doses then every 2–4 hr as needed.
Inhaln (Children 5–12 yr): *Metered-dose inhaler (nonacute)*—1–2 inhalations every 6 hr as needed (not to exceed 12 inhalations/24 hr). *Acute exacerbations*—4–8 puffs as needed. *Via nebulization (nonacute)*—250–500 mcg 4 times daily given every 6 hr. *Acute exacerbations*—250 mcg every 20 min for 3 doses then every 2–4 hr as needed.
Inhaln (Infants): *Nebulization*—125–250 mcg 3 times a day.
Inhaln (Neonates): *Nebulization*—25 mcg/kg/dose 3 times a day.
Intranasal (Adults and Children >6 yr): *0.03% solution*—2 sprays in each nostril 2–3 times daily (21 mcg/spray).
Inhaln (Adults and Children >5 yr): *0.06% solution*—2 sprays in each nostril 3–4 times daily (42 mcg/spray).

Availability (generic available)

Aerosol inhaler (HFA) (chlorofluorocarbon-free): 17 mcg/spray in 12.9-g canister (200 inhalations). **Inhalation solution:** 🍁 0.0125%, 0.02% in single-dose vials containing 500 mcg, 🍁 0.025%. **Nasal spray:** 0.03% solution—21 mcg/spray in 30-mL bottle (345 sprays/bottle), 0.06% solution—42 mcg/spray in 15-mL bottle (165 sprays). ***In combination with:*** albuterol (Combivent). See Appendix B.

NURSING IMPLICATIONS

Assessment

- Assess for allergy to atropine and belladonna alkaloids; patients with these allergies may also be sensitive to ipratropium. Atrovent HFA MDI does not contain CFC or soy and may be used safely in soy or CFC-allergic patients. However, Combivent MDI should be avoided in soy or peanut-allergic patients.
- **Inhaln:** Assess respiratory status (rate, breath sounds, degree of dyspnea, pulse) before administration and at peak of medication. Consult health care professional about alternative medication if severe bronchospasm is present; onset of action is too slow for patients in acute distress. If paradoxical bronchospasm (wheezing) occurs, withhold medication and notify health care professional immediately.
- **Nasal Spray:** Assess patient for rhinorrhea.

Implementation

- **Inhaln:** See Appendix D for administration of inhalation medications.
- When ipratropium is administered concurrently with other inhalation medications, administer adrenergic bronchodilators first, followed by ipratropium, then corticosteroids. Wait 5 min between medications.
- Solution for *nebulization* can be diluted with preservative-free 0.9% NaCl. Diluted solution should be used within 24 hr at room temperature or 48 hr if refrigerated. Solution can be mixed with preservative-free albuterol, cromolyn, or metaproterenol if used within 1 hr of mixing.

Patient/Family Teaching

- Instruct patient in proper use of inhaler, nebulizer, or nasal spray and to take medication as directed. Take missed doses as soon as remembered unless almost time for the next dose; space remaining doses evenly during day. Do not double doses.
- Advise patient that rinsing mouth after using inhaler, good oral hygiene, and sugarless gum or candy may minimize dry mouth. Health care professional should be notified if stomatitis occurs or if dry mouth persists for more than 2 wk.
- **Inhalation:** Caution patient not to exceed 12 doses within 24 hr. Patient should notify health care professional if symptoms do not improve within 30 min after administration of medication or if condition worsens.
- Explain need for pulmonary function tests prior to and periodically during therapy to determine effectiveness of medication.
- Caution patient to avoid spraying medication in eyes; may cause blurring of vision or irritation.
- Advise patient to inform health care professional if cough, nervousness, headache, dizziness, nausea, or GI distress occurs.
- **Nasal Spray:** Instruct patient in proper use of nasal spray. Clear nasal passages gently before administration. Do not inhale during administration, so medication remains in nasal passages. Prime pump initially with 7 actuations. If used regularly, no further priming is needed. If not used in 24 hr, prime with 2 actuations. If not used for >7 days, prime with 7 actuations.
- Advise patient to contact health care professional if symptoms do not improve within 1–2 wk or if condition worsens.

Evaluation/Desired Outcomes

- Decreased dyspnea.
- Improved breath sounds.
- Decrease in rhinorrhea from perennial rhinitis or the common cold.

irbesartan, See ANGIOTENSIN II RECEPTOR ANTAGONISTS.

irinotecan

(eye-ri-noe-**tee**-kan)

Camptosar

Classification

Therapeutic: antineoplastics

Pharmacologic: enzyme inhibitors

Indications

Metastatic colorectal cancer (with 5-fluorouracil and leucovorin).

Action

Interferes with DNA synthesis by inhibiting the enzyme topoisomerase. **Therapeutic Effects:** Death of rapidly replicating cells, particularly malignant ones.

Pharmacokinetics

Absorption: IV administration results in complete bioavailability.

Distribution: Unknown.

Protein Binding: *Irinotecan*—30–68%; *SN-38 (active metabolite)*—95%.

Metabolism and Excretion: Converted by the liver to SN-38, its active metabolite, which is metabolized by the liver by UDP-glucuronosyl 111 transferase 1A1 (UGT1A1) and CYP3A4. Small amounts excreted by kidneys.

Half-life: 6 hr.

TIME/ACTION PROFILE (hematologic effects)

ROUTE	ONSET	PEAK	DURATION
IV	unknown	21–29 days	27–34 days

Contraindications/Precautions

Contraindicated in: Hypersensitivity; Hereditary fructose intolerance (contains sorbitol); Concurrent use of ketoconazole and St. John's wort; OB, Lactation: Pregnancy or lactation.

Use Cautiously in: Previous pelvic or abdominal irradiation or age ≥65 yr (↑ risk of myelosuppression); Presence of infection, underlying bone marrow depression, or concurrent chronic illness; History of prior pelvic/abdominal irradiation and serum bilirubin >1–2 mg/dL (initial dose reduction recommended); Hepatic impairment; Previous severe myelosuppression or diarrhea (reinstitute at lower dose following resolution); Patients with genetically reduced UGT1A1 activity (↑ risk of neutropenia); Rep: Women of reproductive potential; Pedi: Safety not established; Geri: ↑ sensitivity to adverse effects (myelosuppression); initiate at lower dose.

Adverse Reactions/Side Effects

CNS: dizziness, headache, insomnia, weakness. **CV:** edema, vasodilation. **Derm:** alopecia, rash, sweating. **EENT:** rhinitis. **F and E:** dehydration. **GI:** DIARRHEA, ↑ LIVER ENZYMES, abdominal pain/cramping, anorexia, constipation, dyspepsia, flatulence, nausea, stomatitis, vomiting, abdominal enlargement, colonic ulceration. **Hemat:** NEUTROPENIA, anemia, leukopenia, thrombocytopenia. **Local:** injection site reactions. **Metab:** weight loss. **MS:** INFECTION, back pain. **Resp:** INTERSTITIAL LUNG DISEASE, coughing, dyspnea. **Misc:** chills, fever.

Interactions

Drug-Drug: Combination with **fluorouracil** may result in serious toxicity (dehydration, neutropenia, sepsis). ↑ bone marrow depression may occur with other **antineoplastics** or **radiation therapy**. Strong **CYP3A4 inhibitors (ketoconazole, clarithromycin, indinavir, itraconazole, lopinavir, nefazodone, nelfinavir, ritonavir, saquinavir,** and **voriconazole**) and strong **UGT1A1 inhibitors (atazanavir, gemfibrozil,** and **indinavir**) may ↑ levels of irinotecan and its active metabolite; should be discontinued ≥1 wk before initiating irinotecan. **Phenobarbital, phenytoin, carbamazepine, rifampin,** or **rifabutin** may ↓ levels of irinotecan and its active metabolite; consider using an alternative anticonvulsant at least 2 wk before initiating irinotecan. **Laxatives** should be avoided (diarrhea may be ↑). **Diuretics** ↑ risk of dehydration (may discontinue during therapy). **Dexamethasone** may ↑ risk of hyperglycemia and lymphocytopenia. **Prochlorperazine** given on the same day as irinotecan ↑ risk of akathisia. May ↓ antibody response to and ↑ risk of adverse reactions from **live virus vaccines**.

Drug-Natural Products: St. John's wort ↓ levels of the active metabolite; concurrent use is contraindicated; should be discontinued at least 2 wk before initiating irinotecan.

Route/Dosage

Other regimens are used; careful modification required for all levels of toxicity/tolerance.

Single Agent

IV (Adults): *Weekly dosage schedule*—125 mg/m² once weekly for 4 wk, followed by a 2-wk rest period. Cycle may be repeated using doses which depend on patient tolerance and degree of toxicity encountered. *Once-every-3-wk schedule*—350 mg/m² once every 3 wk. Cycle may be repeated using doses which depend on patient tolerance and degree of toxicity encountered.

IV (Geriatric Patients >70 yr): *Weekly dosage schedule*—125 mg/m² once weekly for 4 wk, followed by a 2-wk rest period. Cycle may be repeated using doses which depend on patient tolerance and degree of toxicity encountered. *Once-every-3-wk schedule*—300 mg/m² once every 3 wk. Cycle may be repeated using doses which depend on patient tolerance and degree of toxicity encountered.

IV (Adult Patients with Reduced UGT1A1 Activity): *Weekly dosage schedule*—100 mg/m² once weekly for 4 wk, followed by a 2-wk rest period. Cycle may be repeated using doses which depend on patient tolerance and degree of toxicity encountered. *Once-every-3-wk schedule*—300 mg/m² once every 3 wk. Cycle may be repeated using doses which depend on patient tolerance and degree of toxicity encountered.

Hepatic Impairment

IV (Adults): *Bilirubin 1–2 mg/dL and history of prior pelvic/abdominal irradiation— Weekly dosage schedule*—Initiate therapy at lower dose (100 mg/m²); once weekly for 4 wk, followed by a 2-wk rest period. Cycle may be repeated with dose adjusted as tolerated. *Once-every-3-wk schedule*—300 mg/m² once every 3 wk. Cycle may be repeated with dose adjusted as tolerated.

As Part of Combination Therapy with Leucovorin and 5-Fluorouracil

IV (Adults): *Regimen 1 (Bolus regimen)*—125 mg/m² once weekly for 4 wk, followed by a 2-wk rest period. Cycle may be repeated using doses that depend on patient tolerance and degree of toxicity encountered; *Regimen 2 (Infusional regimen)*—180 mg/m² every 2 wk for 3 doses, followed by a 3-wk rest period. Cycle may be repeated using doses that depend on patient tolerance and degree of toxicity encountered.

IV (Adult Patients with Reduced UGT1A1 Activity): *Regimen 1 (Bolus regimen)*—100 mg/m² once weekly for 4 wk, followed by a 2-wk rest period. Cycle may be repeated using doses that depend on patient tolerance and degree of toxicity encountered; *Regimen 2 (Infusional regimen)*—150 mg/m² every 2 wk for 3 doses, followed by a 3-wk rest period. Cycle may be repeated using doses that depend on patient tolerance and degree of toxicity encountered.

Availability (generic available)

Solution for injection: 20 mg/mL.

NURSING IMPLICATIONS

Assessment

- Monitor vital signs frequently during administration.
- Monitor for bone marrow depression. Assess for bleeding (bleeding gums, bruising, petechiae, guaiac stools, urine, and emesis) and avoid IM injections and taking rectal temperatures if platelet count is low. Apply pressure to venipuncture sites for 10 min. Assess for signs of infection during neutropenia. Anemia may occur. Monitor for increased fatigue, dyspnea, and orthostatic hypotension.
- Monitor closely for the development of diarrhea. Two types may occur. The early type occurs within 24 hr of administration and may be preceded by cramps and sweating. Atropine 0.25–1 mg IV may be given to decrease symptoms. Potentially life-threatening diarrhea may occur more than 24 hr after a dose and may be accompanied by severe dehydration and electrolyte imbalance. Loperamide 4 mg initially, followed by 2 mg every 2 hr until diarrhea ceases for at least 12 hr (or 4 mg every 4 hr if given during sleeping hours) should be administered promptly to treat late-occurring diarrhea. Do not administer loperamide at these doses for >48 hr. Careful fluid and electrolyte replacement should be instituted to prevent complications. *If diarrhea of 2–3 stools/day pretreatment occurs,* maintain dose. *If diarrhea of 4–6 stools/day pretreatment occurs during a cycle,* ↓ by 25 mg/m². *If diarrhea of 4–6 stools/day pretreatment occurs at the beginning of a weekly cycle or at the beginning of a once every 3 wk cycle,* maintain dose. *If diarrhea of 7–9 stools/day pretreatment occurs during a cycle,* hold dose until resolved to ≤grade 2, then ↓ by 25 mg/m². *If diarrhea of 7–9 stools/day pretreatment occurs at the beginning of a weekly cycle,* ↓ by 25 mg/m². *If diarrhea of 7–9 stools/day pretreatment occurs at the beginning of a once every 3 wk cycle,* ↓ by 50 mg/m². *If diarrhea ≥10 stools/day pretreatment occurs during a cycle,* hold dose until resolved to ≤grade 2, then ↓ by 50 mg/m². *If diarrhea ≥10 stools/day pretreatment occurs at the beginning of a weekly cycle or at the beginning of a once every 3 wk cycle,* ↓ by 50 mg/m².
- Nausea and vomiting are common. Pretreatment with dexamethasone 10 mg along with agents such as ondansetron or granisetron should be started on the same day as irinotecan at least 30 min before administration. Prochlorperazine may be used on subsequent days but may increase risk of akathisia if given on the same day as irinotecan.
- Assess IV site frequently for inflammation. Avoid extravasation. If extravasation occurs, infusion must be stopped and restarted in another vein to avoid damage to subcut tissue. Flushing site with sterile water and application of ice over the extravasated site are recommended.
- If signs of pulmonary toxicity (dyspnea, cough, fever) occur, interrupt therapy. If interstitial pulmonary disease is determined, discontinue irinotecan.
- Assess for cholinergic symptoms (rhinitis, increased salivation, miosis, lacrimation, diaphoresis, flushing, abdominal cramping, diarrhea) during therapy. Atropine 0.25–1 mg subcut or IV may be used to prevent or treat symptoms.
- ***Lab Test Considerations:*** Consider laboratory test to determine the UGT1A1 status. Testing can detect the UGT1A1 6/6, 6/7 and 7/7 genotypes.
- Monitor CBC with differential and platelet count prior to each dose. *If neutropenia, ANC 1500–1999/mm³ occurs,* maintain dose. *If ANC 1000–*

1499/mm³ occurs during a cycle, ↓ dose by 25 mg/m². *If ANC 1000–1499/mm³ occurs at beginning of cycle,* maintain dose. *If ANC 500–999/mm³ occurs during a cycle,* hold dose until resolved to ≤grade 2, then ↓ by 25 mg/m². *If ANC 500–999/mm³ occurs at the beginning of a weekly cycle,* ↓ dose by 25 mg/m². *If ANC 500–999/mm³ occurs at the beginning of a once every 3 wk cycle,* ↓ dose by 50 mg/m². *If ANC <500/mm³ occurs during a cycle,* hold dose until resolved to ≤grade 2, then ↓ by 50 mg/m². *If ANC 500–999/mm³ occurs at the beginning of a weekly cycle or at the beginning of a once every 3 wk cycle,* ↓ dose by 50 mg/m². *If neutropenic fever occurs during a cycle,* hold dose until resolved, then ↓ by 50 mg/m² when resolved. *If neutropenic fever occurs at the beginning of a weekly cycle or at the beginning of a once every 3 wk cycle,* ↓ by 50 mg/m². Administration of a colony-stimulating factor may be considered if clinically significant decreases in WBC (<2000/mm³), neutrophil count (<1000/mm³), hemoglobin (<9 g/dL), or platelet count (<100,000 cells/mm³) occur.

- May cause ↑ serum alkaline phosphatase and AST concentrations.

Implementation

IV Administration

- Prepare solution in a biologic cabinet. Wear gloves, gown, and mask while handling IV medication. Discard IV equipment in specially designated containers.
- **Intermittent Infusion:** ***Diluent:*** Dilute before infusion with D5W or 0.9% NaCl. Usual diluent is 500 mL of D5W. ***Concentration:*** 0.12–2.8 mg/mL. Solution is pale yellow. Do not administer solutions that are cloudy or contain particulate matter. Solution is stable for 24 hr at room temperature or 48 hr if refrigerated. To prevent microbial contamination, solutions should be used within 24 hr of dilution if refrigerated or 6 hr at room temperature. Do not refrigerate solutions diluted with 0.9% NaCl. ***Rate:*** Administer dose over 90 min.
- **Y-Site Compatibility:** alemtuzumab, alfentanil, amifostine, amikacin, aminocaproic acid, aminophylline, amiodarone, ampicillin, ampicillin/sulbactam, anidulafungin, argatroban, atracurium, azithromycin, aztreonam, bivalirudin, bleomycin, bumetanide, buprenorphine, butorphanol, calcium chloride, calcium gluconate, carboplatin, caspofungin, cefazolin, cefotetan, cefoxitin, ceftazidime, cefuroxime, ciprofloxacin, cisatracurium, cisplatin, clindamycin, cyclophosphamide, cyclosporine, cytarabine, dacarbazine, daptomycin, daunorubicin, dexamethasone, dexrazoxane, digoxin, diltiazem, diphenhydramine, dobutamine, docetaxel, dolasetron, dopamine, doxacurium, doxorubicin, doxorubicin liposomal, doxycycline, enalaprilat, ephedrine, epinephrine, ertapenem, erythromycin, esmolol, etoposide, etoposide phosphate, famotidine, fenoldopam, fentanyl, fluconazole, foscarnet, gentamicin, granisetron, haloperidol, heparin, hetastarch, hydralazine, hydrocortisone, hydromorphone, idarubicin, imipenem/cilastatin, insulin, regular, isoproterenol, ketorolac, labetalol, leucovorin calcium, levofloxacin, levoleucovorin, levorphanol, lidocaine, linezolid, lorazepam, magnesium sulfate, mannitol, meperidine, meropenem, mesna, metaraminol, methyldopate, metoclopramide, metoprolol, metronidazole, midazolam, milrinone, mitoxantrone, morphine, moxifloxacin, nalbuphine, naloxone, nicardipine, nitroglycerin, norepinephrine, octreotide, ondansetron, oxaliplatin, paclitaxel, palonosetron, pancuronium, pantoprazole, pentamidine, pentobarbital, phenobarbital, phentolamine, phenylephrine, potassium acetate, potassium chloride, potassium phosphates, procainamide, prochlorperazine, promethazine, propranolol, quinupristin/dalfopristin, ranitidine, remifentanyl, rituximab, rocuronium, sodium acetate, sodium bicarbonate, sodium phosphates, succinylcholine, sufentanil, tacrolimus, theophylline, thiotepa, tigecycline, tirofiban, tobramycin, tolazoline, trimethoprim/sulfamethoxazole, vancomycin, vasopressin, vecuronium, verapamil, vinblastine, vinorelbine, voriconazole, zidovudine, zoledronic acid.
- **Y-Site Incompatibility:** acyclovir, allopurinol, amphotericin B lipid complex, amphotericin B liposome, cefepime, cefotaxime, ceftriaxone, chloramphenicol, chlorpromazine, dantrolene, dexmedetomidine, diazepam, droperidol, fluorouracil, fosphenytoin, furosemide, ganciclovir, gemcitabine, glycopyrrolate, methohexital, methylprednisolone, mitomycin, nafcillin, nitroprusside, pemetrexed, phenytoin, piperacillin/tazobactam, thiopental, trastuzumab.

Patient/Family Teaching

- Instruct patient to report occurrence of diarrhea to health care professional immediately if diarrhea occurs for first time during treatment; black or bloody stools; symptoms of dehydration such as lightheadedness, dizziness, or faintness; inability to take fluids by mouth due to nausea or vomiting; or inability to get diarrhea under control within 24 hrs. Diarrhea may be accompanied by severe dehydration and electrolyte imbalance. It may be life-threatening; treat promptly. Loperamide may be used for treatment up to 48 hrs.
- Instruct patient to notify health care professional promptly if fever; chills; sore throat; signs of infection; bleeding gums; bruising; petechiae; blood in

I

urine, stool, or emesis occurs. Caution patient to avoid crowds and persons with known infections. Instruct patient to monitor temperature frequently, use soft toothbrush and electric razor. Caution patient not to drink alcoholic beverages or take products containing aspirin or other NSAIDs.

- Instruct patient to notify nurse of pain at injection site immediately.
- Instruct patient to notify health care professional if vomiting, fainting, or dizziness occurs.
- Discuss with patient possibility of hair loss. Explore methods of coping.
- Instruct patient not to receive any vaccinations without consulting health care professional.
- Rep: Advise patient that this medication may have teratogenic effects. Advise patient to use effective contraception during therapy.
- Emphasize the need for periodic lab tests to monitor for side effects.

Evaluation/Desired Outcomes

- Decrease in size and spread of malignancy.

IRON SUPPLEMENTS

carbonyl iron (100%)
(kar-bo-nil **eye**-ern)
Feosol, Icar

ferrous fumarate (33% elemental iron) (**fer**-us **fyoo**-ma-rate)
Ferretts, Ferrimin 150, Hemocyte

ferrous gluconate (12% elemental iron) (**fer**-us **gloo**-koe-nate)
Ferate

ferrous sulfate (30% elemental iron) (**fer**-us **sul**-fate)
Fer-In-Sol, FeroSul, Slow Fe, Slow Iron

iron dextran (**eye**-ern **dex**-tran)
DexFerrum, ✦Dexiron, InFeD, ✦Infufer

iron polysaccharide
(**eye**-ern poll-ee-**sak**-a-ride)
Ferrex 150, IFerex 150, Myferon 150, NovaFerrum, Nu-Iron, Poly-Iron 150

iron sucrose (**eye**-ern **su**-krose)
Venofer

sodium ferric gluconate complex
(**so**-dee-yum **ferr**-ic **gloo**-ko-nate)
Ferrlecit

Classification
Therapeutic: antianemics
Pharmacologic: iron supplements

Indications

PO: Prevention/treatment of iron-deficiency anemia. **IM, IV:** *Iron dextran*—Treatment of iron-deficiency anemia in patients who cannot tolerate or receive oral iron. *Sodium ferric gluconate complex*—Treatment of iron deficiency in patients undergoing chronic hemodialysis or peritoneal dialysis who are concurrently receiving erythropoietin. Treatment of iron-deficiency anemia in patients with chronic kidney disease including patients who are not on dialysis (with or without erythropoietin) and patients dependent on dialysis (with erythropoietin).

Action

An essential mineral found in hemoglobin, myoglobin, and many enzymes. Enters the bloodstream and is transported to the organs of the reticuloendothelial system (liver, spleen, bone marrow), where it is separated out and becomes part of iron stores. **Therapeutic Effects:** Prevention/treatment of iron deficiency.

Pharmacokinetics

Absorption: 5–10% of dietary iron is absorbed (up to 30% in deficiency states). Therapeutically administered PO iron may be 60% absorbed via an active and passive transport process. Well absorbed following IM administration.
Distribution: Remains in the body for many mo. Crosses the placenta; enters breast milk.
Protein Binding: ≥90%.
Metabolism and Excretion: Mostly recycled; small daily losses occurring via desquamation, sweat, urine, and bile.
Half-life: *Iron dextran, iron sucrose*—6 hr.

TIME/ACTION PROFILE (effects on erythropoiesis)

ROUTE	ONSET	PEAK	DURATION
PO	4 days	7–10 days	2–4 mo
IM, IV	4 days	1–2 wk	wk–mos

Contraindications/Precautions

Contraindicated in: Hemochromatosis, hemosiderosis, or other evidence of iron overload; Anemias not due to iron deficiency; Some products contain alcohol, tartrazine, or sulfites and should be avoided in patients with known intolerance or hypersensitivity.
Use Cautiously in: Peptic ulcer; Ulcerative colitis or regional enteritis (condition may be aggravated); Alcoholism; Severe hepatic impairment; Severe renal impairment (oral products); Pre-existing cardiovascular disease (iron dextran) (may be exacerbated by adverse reactions to this drug); Significant allergies or asthma (iron dextran); History of drug allergy or multiple drug allergies (iron dextran) (may be at ↑ risk for anaphylactic reaction); Rheumatoid arthritis (iron dextran) (may have exacerbation of joint swelling); OB, Lactation: Pregnancy or lactation (safety of some parenteral products not established); Pedi: Safety not established

for infants <4 mo (iron dextran), children <2 yr (iron sucrose), or children <6 yr (sodium ferric gluconate complex); safety may not be established for other products in the pediatric population.

Adverse Reactions/Side Effects

CNS: *IM, IV*— SEIZURES, dizziness, headache, syncope. **CV:** *IM, IV*—hypotension, hypertension, tachycardia. **Derm:** *IM, IV*—flushing, urticaria. **GI:** nausea; *PO*, constipation, dark stools, diarrhea, epigastric pain, GI bleeding; *IM, IV*, taste disorder, vomiting. **Local:** pain at IM site (iron dextran), phlebitis at IV site, skin staining at IM site (iron dextran). **MS:** *IM, IV*—arthralgia, myalgia. **Resp:** *IV*—cough, dyspnea. **Misc:** *PO*—staining of teeth (liquid preparations); *IM, IV*, HYPERSENSITIVITY REACTIONS (including anaphylaxis), fever, lymphadenopathy, sweating.

Interactions

Drug-Drug: Oral iron supplements ↓ absorption of **tetracyclines**, **bisphosphonates**, **fluoroquinolones**, **levothyroxine**, **mycophenolate mofetil**, and **penicillamine** (simultaneous administration should be avoided). ↓ absorption of and may ↓ effects of **levodopa** and **methyldopa**. Concurrent administration of **H_2 antagonists**, **proton pump inhibitors**, and **cholestyramine** may ↓ absorption of iron. Doses of **ascorbic acid** ≥200 mg may ↑ absorption of iron up to ≥30%. **Chloramphenicol** and **vitamin E** may ↓ hematologic response to iron therapy. **ACE inhibitors** may ↑ risk of anaphylactic reaction with iron dextran.
Drug-Food: Iron absorption is ↓ 33–50% by concurrent administration of food.

Route/Dosage

Oral Iron Dosage for Iron Deficiency (expressed as mg elemental iron, note individual salt forms, multiple ones exist—see approximate equivalent doses below for dose conversions).

Approximate Equivalent Doses (mg of iron salt): *Ferrous fumarate*—197; *Ferrous gluconate*—560; *Ferrous sulfate*—324; *Ferrous sulfate, exsiccated*—217.

PO (Adults): *Deficiency*—120–240 mg/day (2–3 mg/kg/day) in 2–4 divided doses. *Prophylaxis*—60–100 mg/day.
PO (Infants and Children): *Severe deficiency*—4–6 mg/kg/day in 3 divided doses. *Mild to moderate deficiency*—3 mg/kg/day in 1–2 divided doses. *Prophylaxis*—1–2 mg/kg/day in 1–2 divided dose (maximum: 15 mg/day).
PO (Neonates, premature): 2–4 mg/kg/day in 1–2 divided doses, maximum: 15 mg/day.

Iron Dextran

IM, IV (Adults and Children): Test dose of 0.5 mL (25 mg) is given 1 hr prior to therapy.
IM, IV (Infants): Test dose of 0.25 mL (12.5 mg) is given 1 hr prior to therapy.
IM, IV (Adults and Children >15 kg): *Iron deficiency*—Total dose (mL) = 0.0442 × (desired Hgb − actual Hgb) × lean body weight (kg) + [0.26 × lean body weight (kg)]. Divided up and given in small daily doses until total is reached; not to exceed 100 mg/day. *Total dose IV infusion*—Total dose may be diluted and infused over 4–5 hr following a test dose of 10 drops (unlabeled).
IM, IV (Adults): *Blood loss*—Dose (mL) = (Blood loss [mL] × hematocrit) × 0.02.
IM, IV (Children 5–15 kg): *Iron deficiency*—Total dose (mL) = 0.042 (desired Hgb − actual Hgb) × weight (kg) + [0.26 × weight (kg)]. Divided up and given in small daily doses until total is reached; not to exceed 25 mg/day in children <5 kg; 50 mg/day in children 5–10 kg; or 100 mg/day in children >10 kg.

Iron Polysaccharide Complex

PO (Adults): 50–100 mg twice daily of tablets/elixir or 150–300 mg/day of the capsules.
PO (Children >6 yr): 50–100 mg/day (may be given in divided doses).
PO (Infants): 1–2 mg/kg/day.
PO (Adults—Pregnant Women): 30–60 mg/day.

Iron Sucrose

IV (Adults): *Hemodialysis dependent patients*—100 mg during each dialysis session for 10 doses (total of 1000 mg); may repeat if iron deficiency recurs; *Non-dialysis dependent patients*—200 mg on 5 different days within a 14 day period to a total of 1000 mg; may also be given as infusion of 500 mg on day 1 and day 14; may repeat if iron deficiency recurs; *Peritoneal dialysis patients*—administered in a total cumulative dose of 1000 mg in 3 divided doses, 14 days apart within a 28 day period with first 2 doses of 300 mg and third dose of 400 mg; may repeat if iron deficiency recurs.
IV (Children ≥2 yr): *Hemodialysis dependent patients (for iron maintenance therapy)*—0.5 mg/kg (max = 100 mg/dose) every 2 wk for 12 wk; may repeat if necessary; *Non-dialysis dependent patients or peritoneal dialysis patients who are receiving erythropoietin for iron maintenance therapy*—0.5 mg/kg (max = 100 mg/dose) every 4 wk for 12 wk; may repeat if necessary.

Sodium Ferric Gluconate Complex

IV (Adults): 10 mL (125 mg elemental iron) repeated during 8 sequential dialysis treatments to a total cumulative dose of 1 g.
IV (Children >6 yr): 0.12 mL/kg (not to exceed 125 mg/dose) repeated during 8 sequential dialysis treatments.

Availability

Carbonyl Iron (100% Iron)

Oral suspension: 15 mg/1.25 mL^{OTC}. **Tablets:** 50 mg^{OTC}.

Ferrous Fumarate (33% Elemental Iron) (generic available)

Tablets: 324 mg^{OTC}, 325 mg^{OTC}.

Ferrous Gluconate (11.6% Elemental Iron) (generic available)

Tablets: 240 mg^{OTC}, 324 mg^{OTC}.

Ferrous Sulfate (20–30% Elemental Iron)

Delayed-release tablets: 324 mg^{OTC}, 325 mg^{OTC}. **Extended-release tablets:** 140 mg^{OTC}, 142 mg^{OTC}, 160 mg^{OTC}. **Oral solution:** 75 mg/mL^{OTC}. **Syrup:** 300 mg/5 mL^{OTC}. **Tablets:** 325 mg^{OTC}.

Iron Dextran

Solution for injection: 50 mg/mL.

Iron Polysaccharide (mg Iron)

Capsules: 50 mg ^{OTC}, 150 mg ^{OTC}, 200 mg^{OTC}. **Oral solution:** 15 mg/mL ^{OTC}, 125 mg/5 mL ^{OTC}.

Iron Sucrose

Aqueous complex for injection: 20 mg/mL.

Sodium Ferric Gluconate Complex (generic available)

Solution for injection (requires dilution): 12.5 mg/mL.

NURSING IMPLICATIONS

Assessment

- Assess nutritional status and dietary history to determine possible cause of anemia and need for patient teaching.
- Assess bowel function for constipation or diarrhea. Notify health care professional and use appropriate nursing measures should these occur.
- **Iron Dextran, Iron Sucrose, and Sodium Ferric Gluconate Complex:** Monitor BP and heart rate frequently following IV administration until stable. Rapid infusion rate may cause hypotension and flushing.
- Assess patient for signs and symptoms of anaphylaxis (rash, pruritus, laryngeal edema, wheezing) for at least 30 min following injection. Notify health care professional immediately if these occur. Keep epinephrine and resuscitation equipment close by in the event of an anaphylactic reaction.
- ***Lab Test Considerations:*** Monitor hemoglobin, hematocrit, and reticulocyte values prior to and every 3 wk during the first 2 mo of therapy and periodically thereafter. Serum ferritin and iron levels may also be monitored to assess effectiveness of therapy.
- Occult blood in stools may be obscured by black coloration of iron in stool. Guaiac test results may occasionally be false-positive.
- **Iron Dextran:** Monitor hemoglobin, hematocrit, reticulocyte values, transferrin, ferritin, total iron-binding capacity, and plasma iron concentrations periodically during therapy. Serum ferritin levels peak in 7–9 days and return to normal in 3 wk. Serum iron determinations may be inaccurate for 1–2 wk after therapy with large doses; therefore, hemoglobin and hematocrit are used to gauge initial response.
- May impart a brownish hue to blood drawn within 4 hr of administration. May cause false ↑ in serum bilirubin and false decrease in serum calcium values.
- Prolonged PTT may be calculated when blood sample is anticoagulated with citrate dextrose solution; use sodium citrate instead.
- **Iron Sucrose:** Monitor hemoglobin, hematocrit, serum ferritin, and transferritin saturation prior to and periodically during therapy. Transferrin saturation values increase rapidly after IV administration; therefore, serum iron values may be reliably obtained 48 hr after IV administration. Withhold iron therapy if evidence of iron overload occurs.
- May cause ↑ liver enzymes.
- ***Toxicity and Overdose:*** Early symptoms of overdose include stomach pain, fever, nausea, vomiting (may contain blood), and diarrhea. Late symptoms include bluish lips, fingernails, and palms; drowsiness; weakness; tachycardia; seizures; metabolic acidosis; hepatic injury; and cardiovascular collapse. Patient may appear to recover prior to the onset of late symptoms. Hospitalization continues for 24 hr after patient becomes asymptomatic to monitor for delayed onset of shock or GI bleeding. Late complications of overdose include intestinal obstruction, pyloric stenosis, and gastric scarring.
- If patient is comatose or seizing, gastric lavage with sodium bicarbonate is performed. Deferoxamine is the antidote. Additional supportive treatments to maintain fluid and electrolyte balance and correction of metabolic acidosis are also indicated.
- If signs of overdose occur during IV administration of iron sucrose, treatment includes IV fluids, corticosteroids, and/or antihistamines. Administering at a slower rate usually relieves symptoms.

Implementation

- Discontinue oral iron preparations prior to parenteral administration.
- Sodium ferric gluconate and iron sucrose are for IV use only.
- **PO:** Oral preparations are most effectively absorbed if administered 1 hr before or 2 hr after meals. If gastric irritation occurs, administer with meals. Take tablets and capsules with a full glass of water or juice. Do not crush or chew enteric-coated tablets and do not open capsules.
- Liquid preparations may stain teeth. Dilute in water or fruit juice, full glass (240 mL) for adults and ½ glass (120 mL) for children, and administer with a straw or place drops at back of throat.

- Avoid using antacids, coffee, tea, dairy products, eggs, or whole-grain breads with or within 1 hr after administration of ferrous salts. Iron absorption is decreased by 33% if iron and calcium are given with meals. If calcium supplementation is needed, calcium carbonate does not decrease absorption of iron salts if supplements are administered between meals.
- **Iron Dextran:** The 2-mL ampule may be used for IM or IV administration.
- Prior to initial IM or IV dose, a test dose of 25 mg should be given by the same route as the dose will be given, to determine reaction. The IV test dose should be administered over at least 30 sec. The IM dose should be administered in the same injection site and by same technique as the therapeutic dose. The remaining portion may be administered after 1 hr, if no adverse symptoms have occurred.
- **IM:** Inject deeply via Z-track technique into upper outer quadrant of buttock, never into arm or other exposed areas. Use a 2–3 in., 19- or 20-gauge needle. Change needles between withdrawal from container and injection to minimize staining of subcut tissues. Stains are usually permanent.

IV Administration

- **IV: Iron Dextran**: Following IV administration, patient should remain recumbent for at least 30 min to prevent orthostatic hypotension.
- **IV Push:** ***Diluent:*** May administer undiluted or dilute in 0.9% NaCl or D5W. ***Concentration:*** 50 mg/mL. ***Rate:*** Administer slowly at a rate of 50 mg (1 mL) over at least 1 min.
- **Intermittent Infusion:** May be diluted in 200–1000 mL of 0.9% NaCl or D5W; 0.9% NaCl is the preferred diluent; dilution in D5W increases incidence of pain and phlebitis. ***Rate:*** Administer over 1–6 hr following a test dose of 10 drops/min for 10 min. Flush line with 10 mL of 0.9% NaCl at completion of infusion.
- **Y-Site Incompatibility:** Discontinue other IV solutions during infusion.
- **Additive Incompatibility:** Manufacturers recommend that iron dextran not be mixed with other solutions; however, iron dextran has been added to total parenteral nutrition solutions.
- **Sodium Ferric Gluconate Complex:** ***Diluent:*** To administer therapeutic dose of 10 mL (125 mg of elemental iron) dilute in 100 mL of 0.9% NaCl. ***Rate:*** Administer at a maximum rate of 12.5 mg/min.
- **Iron Sucrose:** Each 5-mL vial contains 100 mg of elemental iron.
- Solution is brown. Inspect for particulate matter or discoloration. Do not administer solutions that contain particulate matter or are discolored. Solution is stable for 7 days at room temperature or if refrigerated in syringe, or 7 days at room temperature diluted in IV bag.

Hemodialysis Dependent Patients:

- Most patients require a minimum cumulative dose of 1000 mg of elemental iron, administered over 10 sequential dialysis sessions, to achieve a favorable hemoglobin or hematocrit response.
- **IV Push:** May be administered undiluted by slow injection. ***Rate:*** Inject at a rate of 100 mg over 2–5 min into dialysis line early during the dialysis session (generally within the first hr), not to exceed one vial per injection. Discard any unused portion.
- **Intermittent Infusion:** May be administered as an infusion of 100 mg diluted in a maximum of 100 mL of 0.9% NaCl. ***Rate:*** Infuse over at least 15 min, per consecutive hemodialysis session.

Non-dialysis Dependent Patients:

- **IV Push:** May be administered as a slow injection of 200 mg undiluted. ***Rate:*** Administer over 2–5 min.
- **Intermittent Infusion:** Dilute 200 mg in 100 mL 0.9% NaCl. Has also been given as 500 mg diluted in 250 mL 0.9% NaCl. ***Rate:*** Infuse 15 min. Infuse 500 mg dose over 3.5–4 hr on days 1 and 14. May cause hypotension; monitor closely.
- **Additive Incompatibility:** Iron sucrose should not be admixed with any other medications or parenteral nutrition solutions.

Peritoneal Dialysis Patients

- **Intermittent Infusion:** ***Diluent:*** Dilute each dose in a maximum of 250 mL of 0.9% NaCl. ***Rate:*** Administer doses of 300 mg over 1.5 hrs and doses of 400 mg over 2.5 hrs.

Pediatric Patients

- **IV Push:** May be administered undiluted as 0.5 mg/kg, not to exceed 100 mg per dose. ***Rate:*** Inject over 5 min.
- **Intermittent Infusion:** Dilute in 0.9% NaCl at a concentration of 1–2 mg/mL. Do not dilute to concentrations below 1 mg/mL. ***Rate:*** Infuse over 5–60 min.
- **Additive Incompatibility:** Do not mix iron sucrose with other medications or add to parenteral nutrition solutions for IV infusion.

Patient/Family Teaching

- Explain purpose of iron therapy to patient.
- Encourage patient to comply with medication regimen. Take missed doses as soon as remembered within 12 hr; otherwise, return to regular dosing schedule. Do not double doses.
- Advise patient that stools may become dark green or black and that this change is harmless.
- Instruct patient to follow a diet high in iron (see Appendix K).

- Discuss with parents the risk of children's overdosing on iron. Medication should be stored in the original childproof container and kept out of reach of children. Do not refer to vitamins as candy. In the event of a suspected overdose, parents or guardians should contact the poison control center (1-800-222-1222) or emergency medical services (911) immediately.
- Advise females of reproductive potential to notify health care professional if pregnancy is planned or suspected or if breast feeding.
- **Iron Dextran:** Delayed reaction may occur 1–2 days after administration and last 3–4 days if IV route used, 3–7 days with IM route. Instruct patient to contact physician if fever, chills, malaise, muscle and joint aches, nausea, vomiting, dizziness, and backache occur.
- **Iron sucrose and sodium ferric gluconate complex:** Instruct patient to immediately report symptoms of hypersensitivity reaction to health care professional.

Evaluation/Desired Outcomes

- Increase in hemoglobin, which may reach normal parameters after 1–2 mo of therapy. May require 3–6 mo for normalization of body iron stores.
- Improvement in iron deficiency anemia or anemia of chronic renal failure.

isavuconazonium

(eye-sa-vue-kon-a-**zoe**-nee-um)

Cresemba

Classification

Therapeutic: antifungals

Pharmacologic: azoles

Indications

Treatment of invasive aspergillosis and mucormycosis.

Action

A prodrug that is converted (rapidly hydrolyzed) to isavuconazole. Inhibits the synthesis of ergosterol, a key component of fungal cell walls. **Therapeutic Effects:** Resolution of invasive fungal infections. **Spectrum:** Active against *Aspergillus flavus*, *Aspergillus fumigatus*, *Aspergillus niger*, and Mucormycetes species including *Rhizopus oryzae*.

Pharmacokinetics

Absorption: Prodrug is rapidly converted to isavuconazole, the active component. 98% absorbed following oral administration. Similar conversion follows intravenous administration, resulting in complete bioavailability.

Distribution: Extensively distributed.

Protein Binding: >99%.

Metabolism and Excretion: Extensively metabolized (mostly by CYP3A4 and CYPA5); inactive metabolites are mostly renally eliminated, <1% excreted unchanged in urine.

Half-life: 130 hr.

TIME/ACTION PROFILE (blood levels)

ROUTE	ONSET	PEAK	DURATION
PO	unknown	2 hr	unknown
IV	unknown	end of infusion	unknown

Contraindications/Precautions

Contraindicated in: Known hypersensitivity; Strong CYP3A4 inhibitors; Familial short QT syndrome; Strong CYP3A4 inducers; Lactation: Discontinue breast feeding.

Use Cautiously in: Severe hepatic impairment (use only if benefits outweigh risks, monitor carefully for adverse reactions); OB: Use during pregnancy only if maternal benefits outweigh risks to the fetus; Pedi: Safe and effective use in children <18 yr has not been established.

Adverse Reactions/Side Effects

CNS: fatigue, insomnia, headache, anxiety, delerium. **Resp:** cough, dyspnea, respiratory failure. **CV:** peripheral edema, chest pain, hypotension. **GI:** constipation, diarrhea, ↑ liver enzymes, nausea, vomiting, ↓ appetite, dyspepsia. **GU:** renal failure. **Derm:** pruritus, rash. **F and E:** hypokalemia, hypomagnesemia. **Local:** injection site reactions. **MS:** back pain. **Misc:** infusion-related reactions.

Interactions

Drug-Drug: ↑ levels and risk of toxicity with **strong inhibitors of CYP3A4**, including **ketoconazole** or high-dose **ritonavir**; concurrent use is contraindicated. **Lopinavir/ritonavir** significantly ↑ levels and risk of toxicity; concurrent use should be undertaken with caution. Isavuconazonium ↓ levels and effectiveness of **lopinavir/ritonavir**. Isavuconazonium ↑ levels and risk of toxicity with **atorvastatin**, **cyclosporine**, **digoxin**, **midazolam**, **mycophenolate**, **sirolimus**, **tacrolimus**; undertake concurrent use with caution, monitoring drug effects and making adjustments if necessary. **Strong inducers of CYP3A4** including long-acting **barbiturates**, **carbamazepine**, or **rifampin** ↓ levels and effectiveness; concurrent use is contraindicated. ↓ levels and effectiveness of **bupropion**; bupropion dose may need to be ↑ but should not exceed maximum recommended dose.

Drug-Natural Products: St. John's wort ↓ blood levels and effectiveness; concurrent use is contraindicated.

Route/Dosage

186 mg isavuconazonium = 100 mg isavuconazole; doses expressed as isavuconazole.

PO, IV (Adults ≥18 yr): *Loading dose*—200 mg every 8 hr for six doses; *maintenance dose*—200 mg once daily starting 12–24 hr after last loading dose.

Availability

186 mg isavuconazonium = 100 mg isavuconazole; strength expressed as isavuconazole

Capsules: 100 mg. **Lyophilized powder for intravenous injection (requires reconstitution):** 200 mg.

NURSING IMPLICATIONS

Assessment

- Obtain specimens for culture and sensitivity prior to therapy. First dose may be given before receiving results.
- Monitor for signs and symptoms of infusion-related reactions (hypotension, dyspnea, chills, dizziness, paresthesia, hypoesthesia) periodically during therapy. Discontinue infusion if symptoms occur.
- Monitor skin for hypersensitivity reactions during therapy.
- ***Lab Test Considerations:*** Monitor liver function tests prior to and periodically during therapy. Discontinue therapy if clinical signs of liver disease occur.
- May cause hypokalemia and hypomagnesemia.

Implementation

- Oral and IV formulations are bioequivalent; may be used interchangeably. Loading dose is not needed when switching.
- **PO:** Administer without regard to food. Swallow capsule whole; do not open, dissolve, crush or chew.

IV Administration

- Reconstitute by adding 5 mL sterile water to vial. Shake gently to dissolve powder completely. Solution should be clear and colorless; do not administer solutions that are discolored or contain particulate matter. Solution is stable for 1 hr at room temperature.
- **Intermittent Infusion:** ***Diluent:*** Remove 5 mL of reconstituted solution from vial and add to 250 mL 0.9% NaCl or D5W. ***Concentration:*** 1.5 mg isavuconazonium/mL. Diluted solution may show visible translucent to white particulates; removed with in-line filter. Roll bag to mix gently; avoid shaking. Solution is stable if infused at room temperature within 6 hrs; may refrigerate for up to 24 hrs; do not freeze. Flush line with 0.9% NaCl or D5W prior to and following infusion. ***Rate:*** Infuse over at least 1 hr to minimize infusion-related reactions. Infuse through a 0.2–1.2 micron in-line filter. Do not administer as a bolus injection.
- **Y-Site Incompatibility:** Do not infuse with other medication.

Patient/Family Teaching

- Instruct patient to take isavuconazonium as directed. Do not stop taking isavuconazonium without consulting heath care professional. Advise patient to read *Patient Information* before starting and with each Rx refill in case of changes.
- Advise patient to notify health care professional promptly of signs and symptoms of liver disease (itchy skin, nausea, vomiting, yellowing of eyes, feeling very tired, flu-like symptoms), infusion-related reactions, or rash occur.
- Instruct patient to notify health care professional of all Rx or OTC medications, vitamins, or herbal products being taken and consult health care professional before taking any new medications.
- Advise female patient to notify health care professional if pregnancy is planned or suspected or if breast feeding.
- Emphasize the importance of lab tests to monitor for side effects during therapy.

Evaluation/Desired Outcomes

- Resolution of signs and symptoms of invasive fungal infection.

isoniazid (eye-soe-**nye**-a-zid)

INH, Isotamine

Classification
Therapeutic: antituberculars

Indications

First-line therapy of active tuberculosis, in combination with other agents. Prevention of tuberculosis in patients exposed to active disease (alone).

Action

Inhibits mycobacterial cell wall synthesis and interferes with metabolism. **Therapeutic Effects:** Bacteriostatic or bactericidal action against susceptible mycobacteria.

Pharmacokinetics

Absorption: Well absorbed following PO/IM administration.

Distribution: Widely distributed; readily crosses the blood-brain barrier. Crosses the placenta; enters breast milk in concentrations equal to plasma.

Protein Binding: 10–15%.

Metabolism and Excretion: 50% metabolized by the liver by N-acetyltransferase (rate of acetylation is genetically determined [slow acetylators have ↑ isoniazid levels and ↑ risk of toxicity; fast acetylators have ↓ isoniazid levels and ↑ risk for treatment failure]); 50% excreted unchanged by the kidneys.

Half-life: 1–4 hr in patients with normal renal and hepatic function; 0.5–1.6 hr in fast acetylators; 2–5 hr in slow acetylators.

TIME/ACTION PROFILE (blood levels)

ROUTE	ONSET	PEAK	DURATION
PO	rapid	1–2 hr	up to 24 hr
IM	rapid	1–2 hr	up to 24 hr

Contraindications/Precautions

Contraindicated in: Hypersensitivity; Acute liver disease; History of hepatitis from previous use.

Use Cautiously in: History of liver damage or chronic alcohol ingestion; Black and Hispanic women, women in the postpartum period, or patients >50 yr (↑ risk of drug-induced hepatitis); Severe renal impairment (dose ↓ may be necessary); Malnourished patients, patients with diabetes, or chronic alcoholics (↑ risk of neuropathy); OB, Lactation: Although safety is not established, isoniazid has been used with ethambutol to treat tuberculosis in pregnant women without harm to the fetus.

Adverse Reactions/Side Effects

CNS: psychosis, seizures. **EENT:** visual disturbances. **GI:** DRUG-INDUCED HEPATITIS, nausea, vomiting. **Derm:** DRUG REACTION WITH EOSINOPHILIA AND SYSTEMIC SYMPTOMS (DRESS), TOXIC EPIDERMAL NECROLYSIS, rash. **Endo:** gynecomastia. **GI:** PANCREATITIS. **Hemat:** blood dyscrasias. **Neuro:** peripheral neuropathy. **Misc:** fever.

Interactions

Drug-Drug: Additive CNS toxicity with other **antituberculars**. **BCG vaccine** may not be effective during isoniazid therapy. Isoniazid ↓ metabolism of and may ↑ levels of **phenytoin**. **Aluminum-containing antacids** may ↓ absorption. Psychotic reactions and coordination difficulties may result with **disulfiram**. Concurrent administration of **pyridoxine** may prevent neuropathy. ↑ risk of hepatotoxicity with other **hepatotoxic agents** including **alcohol**, **acetaminophen**, and **rifampin**. Isoniazid may ↓ blood levels and effectiveness of **ketoconazole**. May ↑ **carbamazepine** levels and risk of hepatotoxicity. May ↓ effectiveness of **clopidogrel** (avoid concurrent use).

Drug-Food: Severe reactions may occur with ingestion of foods containing high concentrations of **tyramine** (see Appendix K).

Route/Dosage

PO, IM (Adults): 300 mg/day (5 mg/kg) *or* 15 mg/kg (up to 900 mg) 2–3 times weekly.

PO, IM (Children <40 kg): *Latent TB infection*—10–20 mg/kg/day (up to 300 mg/day) *or* 20–40 mg/kg (up to 900 mg) 2 times weekly; *Active TB infection*—10–15 mg/kg/day (up to 300 mg/day) *or* 20–40 mg/kg (up to 900 mg) 2 times weekly.

Availability (generic available)

Tablets: 100 mg, 300 mg. **Oral solution (orange, raspberry flavor):** 50 mg/5 mL. **Solution for injection:** 100 mg/mL. ***In combination with:*** rifampin (Rifamate); rifampin and pyrazinamide (Rifater). See Appendix B.

NURSING IMPLICATIONS

Assessment

- Mycobacterial studies and susceptibility tests should be performed prior to and periodically throughout therapy to detect possible resistance. About 50 to 65% of Caucasians, Black, South Indians, and Mexicans are slow acetylators at risk for toxicity, while 80 to 90% of Eskimos, Japanese, and Chinese are rapid acetylators at risk for decreased levels and treatment failure.
- Monitor for signs and symptoms of DRESS (fever, rash, lymphadenopathy, and/or facial swelling, associated with involvement of other organ systems (hepatitis, nephritis, hematologic abnormalities, myocarditis, myositis) during therapy. May resemble an acute viral infection. Eosinophilia is often present. Discontinue therapy if signs occur.
- Assess for rash periodically during therapy. May cause Stevens-Johnson syndrome. Discontinue therapy if severe or if accompanied with fever, general malaise, fatigue, muscle or joint aches, blisters, oral lesions, conjunctivitis, hepatitis, and/or eosinophilia.
- ***Lab Test Considerations:*** Hepatic function should be evaluated prior to and monthly throughout therapy. Increased AST, ALT, and serum bilirubin may indicate drug-induced hepatitis. Black and Hispanic women, postpartal women, and patients >50 yr are at highest risk. Risk is lower in children; therefore, liver function tests are usually ordered less frequently for children.
- ***Toxicity and Overdose:*** If isoniazid overdosage occurs, treatment with pyridoxine (vitamin B) is instituted.

Implementation

- **PO:** May be administered with food or antacids if GI irritation occurs, although antacids containing aluminum should not be taken within 1 hr of administration.
- **IM:** Medication may cause discomfort at injection site. Massage site after administration and rotate injection sites.
- Solution may form crystals at low temperatures; crystals will redissolve upon warming to room temperature.

Patient/Family Teaching

- Advise patient to take medication as directed. Take missed doses as soon as possible unless almost time for next dose; do not double up on missed doses. Emphasize the importance of continuing therapy even after symptoms have subsided. Therapy may be continued for 6 mo–2 yr.

- Advise patient to notify health care professional promptly if signs and symptoms of hepatitis (yellow eyes and skin, nausea, vomiting, anorexia, dark urine, unusual tiredness, or weakness) or peripheral neuritis (numbness, tingling, paresthesia) occur. Pyridoxine may be used concurrently to prevent neuropathy. Any changes in visual acuity, eye pain, or blurred vision should also be reported immediately.
- Caution patient to avoid the use of alcohol during this therapy, as this may increase the risk of hepatotoxicity. Ingestion of Swiss or Cheshire cheeses, fish (tuna, skipjack, and sardinella), and possibly tyramine-containing foods (see Appendix K) should also be avoided, as they may result in redness or itching of the skin; hot feeling; rapid or pounding heartbeat; sweating; chills; cold, clammy feeling; headache; or light-headedness.
- Emphasize the importance of regular follow-up physical and ophthalmologic exams to monitor progress and to check for side effects.

Evaluation/Desired Outcomes

- Resolution of signs and symptoms of tuberculosis.
- Negative sputum cultures.
- Prevention of activation of tuberculosis in persons known to have been exposed.

ISOSORBIDE

isosorbide dinitrate

(eye-soe-**sor**-bide dye-**nye**-trate)
Dilatrate-SR, Isordil

isosorbide mononitrate

(eye-soe-**sor**-bide mo-noe-**nye**-trate)
~~Imdur~~, ✦Imdur, ~~Ismo~~, Monoket

Classification
Therapeutic: antianginals
Pharmacologic: nitrates

Indications

Prophylactic management of angina pectoris. **Unlabeled Use:** Treatment of chronic heart failure (unlabeled).

Action

Produce vasodilation (venous greater than arterial). Decrease left ventricular end-diastolic pressure and left ventricular end-diastolic volume (preload). Net effect is reduced myocardial oxygen consumption. Increase coronary blood flow by dilating coronary arteries and improving collateral flow to ischemic regions. **Therapeutic Effects:** Prevention of anginal attacks.

Pharmacokinetics

Absorption: Isosorbide dinitrate undergoes extensive first-pass metabolism by the liver, resulting in 25% bioavailability; isosorbide mononitrate has 100% bioavailability (does not undergo first-pass metabolism).
Distribution: Unknown.
Metabolism and Excretion: Isosorbide dinitrate is metabolized by the liver to 2 active metabolites (5–mononitrate and 2–mononitrate). Isosorbide mononitrate is primarily metabolized by the liver to inactive metabolites; primarily excreted in urine as metabolites.
Half-life: *Isosorbide dinitrate*—1 hr; *isosorbide mononitrate*—5 hr.

TIME/ACTION PROFILE (cardiovascular effects)

ROUTE	ONSET	PEAK	DURATION
ISDN-PO	45–60 min	unknown	4 hr
ISDN-PO-ER	30 min	unknown	up to 12 hr
ISMN-PO	30–60 min	unknown	7 hr
ISMN-ER	unknown	unknown	12 hr

Contraindications/Precautions

Contraindicated in: Hypersensitivity; Concurrent use of PDE-5 inhibitor or riociguat.
Use Cautiously in: Volume depleted patients; Right ventricular infarction; Hypertrophic cardiomyopathy; OB: May compromise maternal/fetal circulation; Lactation: No data available; Pedi: Safety not established; Geri: Initial dose ↓ required due to ↑ potential for hypotension.

Adverse Reactions/Side Effects

CNS: dizziness, headache. **CV:** hypotension, tachycardia, paradoxic bradycardia, syncope. **Derm:** flushing. **GI:** nausea, vomiting. **Misc:** tolerance.

Interactions

Drug-Drug: Concurrent use of **avanafil**, **sildenafil**, **tadalafil**, or **vardenafil** may result in severe hypotension (do not use within 24 hr of isosorbide dinitrate or mononitrate); concurrent use contraindicated. Concurrent use of **riociguat** may result in severe hypotension; concurrent use contraindicated. Additive hypotension with **antihypertensives**, acute ingestion of **alcohol**, **beta blockers**, **calcium channel blockers**, and **phenothiazines**.

Route/Dosage

Isosorbide Dinitrate

PO (Adults): *Prophylaxis of angina pectoris*—5–20 mg 2–3 times daily; usual maintenance dose is 10–40 mg every 6 hr (immediate-release) or 40–80 mg every 8–12 hr (sustained-release).

Isosorbide Mononitrate

PO (Adults): *ISMO, Monoket*—5–20 mg twice daily with the 2 doses given 7 hr apart. *Imdur*—30–60 mg once daily; may ↑ to 120 mg once daily (maximum dose = 240 mg/day).

Availability

Isosorbide Dinitrate (generic available)

Tablets: 5 mg, 10 mg, 20 mg, 30 mg, 40 mg. **Cost:** *Isordil*—40 mg $191.65/100; *Generic*—5 mg $15.54/100, 10 mg $32.96/100, 20 mg $18.85/100, 30 mg $23.32/100. **Extended-release tablets:** 40 mg. **Sustained-release capsules:** 40 mg. ***In combination with:*** hydralazine (BiDil). See Appendix B.

Isosorbide Mononitrate (generic available)

Tablets (Monoket): 10 mg, 20 mg. **Cost:** *Generic*—10 mg $55.97/180, 20 mg $48.99/180. **Extended-release tablets:** 30 mg, 60 mg, 120 mg. **Cost:** *Generic*—30 mg $10.00/90, 60 mg $10.00/90, 120 mg $61.18/90.

NURSING IMPLICATIONS

Assessment

- Assess location, duration, intensity, and precipitating factors of anginal pain.
- Monitor BP and pulse routinely during period of dose adjustment.
- ***Lab Test Considerations:*** Excessive doses may ↑ methemoglobin concentrations.

Implementation

Isosorbide Dinitrate

- **PO:** Swallow extended-release capsules whole; do not break, crush, or chew.

Isosorbide Mononitrate

- **PO:** Swallow extended-release tablets whole; do not break, crush, or chew.

Patient/Family Teaching

- Instruct patient to take medication as directed, even if feeling better. Take missed doses as soon as remembered; doses of isosorbide dinitrate should be taken at least 2 hr apart (6 hr with extended-release preparations); daily doses of isosorbide mononitrate should be taken 7 hr apart. Do not double doses. Do not discontinue abruptly.
- Caution patient to make position changes slowly to minimize orthostatic hypotension.
- May cause dizziness. Caution patient to avoid driving or other activities requiring alertness until response to medication is known.
- Instruct patient to take last dose of day (when taking 2–4 doses/day) no later than 7 pm to prevent the development of tolerance.
- Advise patient to avoid concurrent use of alcohol with this medication. Instruct patient to notify health care professional of all Rx or OTC medications, vitamins, or herbal products being taken and to consult health care professional before taking other Rx, OTC, or herbal products.
- Inform patient that headache is a common side effect that should decrease with continuing therapy. Aspirin or acetaminophen may be ordered to treat headache. Notify health care professional if headache is persistent or severe. Do not alter dose to avoid headache.
- Advise patient to notify health care professional if dry mouth or blurred vision occurs.
- Advise females of reproductive potential to notify health care professional if pregnancy is planned or suspected, or if breast feeding.

Evaluation/Desired Outcomes

- Decrease in frequency and severity of anginal attacks.
- Increase in activity tolerance.

REMS

ISOtretinoin

(eye-soe-**tret**-i-noyn)

Absorica, ~~Accutane~~, ✦Accutane, Amnesteem, Claravis, ✦Clarus, ✦Epuris, Myorisan, Zenatane

Classification

Therapeutic: antiacne agents

Pharmacologic: retinoids

Indications

Management of severe nodular acne resistant to more conventional therapy, including topical therapy and systemic antibiotics. Not to be used under any circumstances in pregnant patients.

Action

A metabolite of vitamin A (retinol); reduces sebaceous gland size and differentiation. **Therapeutic Effects:** Diminution and resolution of severe acne. May also prevent abnormal keratinization.

Pharmacokinetics

Absorption: Rapidly absorbed following (23–25%) oral administration; absorption ↑ when taken with a high-fat meal.

Distribution: Appears to be widely distributed; crosses the placenta.

Protein Binding: 99.9%.

Metabolism and Excretion: Metabolized by the liver and excreted in the urine and feces.

Half-life: 10–20 hr.

TIME/ACTION PROFILE (diminution of acne)

ROUTE	ONSET	PEAK	DURATION
PO	unknown	up to 8 wk	unknown

Contraindications/Precautions

Contraindicated in: Hypersensitivity to retinoids, glycerin, soybean oil, or parabens; OB, Lactation: Pregnancy and lactation; Rep: Women of childbearing age who may become or who intend to become pregnant; Patients planning to donate blood.

Use Cautiously in: Pre-existing hypertriglyceridemia; Diabetes mellitus; History of alcohol abuse, psychosis, depression, or suicide attempt; Obese patients; Inflammatory bowel disease; Pedi: Children <12 yr (safety not established).

Adverse Reactions/Side Effects

CNS: SUICIDE ATTEMPT, behavior changes, depression, PSEUDOTUMOR CEREBRI, psychosis, suicidal ideation. **CV:** edema. **Derm:** STEVENS-JOHNSON SYNDROME, TOXIC EPIDERMAL NECROLYSIS, pruritus, palmar desquamation, photosensitivity, skin infections, thinning of hair. **EENT:** conjunctivitis, epistaxis, blurred vision, contact lens intolerance, corneal opacities, ↓ night vision, dry eyes. **GI:** cheilitis, dry mouth, nausea, vomiting, abdominal pain, anorexia, hepatitis, pancreatitis, ↑ appetite. **Hemat:** anemia. **Metab:** ↓ high-density lipoprotein cholesterol, hypercholesterolemia, hypertriglyceridemia, hyperglycemia, hyperuricemia. **MS:** arthralgia, back pain, muscle/bone pain (↑ in adolescents), hyperostosis. **Misc:** SEVERE BIRTH DEFECTS, ↑ thirst.

Interactions

Drug-Drug: Additive toxicity with **vitamin A** and **drugs having anticholinergic properties**. ↑ risk of pseudotumor cerebri with **tetracycline** or **minocycline**. Concurrent use with **alcohol** ↑ risk of hypertriglyceridemia. Drying effects ↑ by concurrent use of **benzoyl peroxide**, **sulfur**, **tretinoin**, and **other topical agents**.

Drug-Food: Excessive ingestion of **foods high in vitamin A** may result in additive toxicity.

Route/Dosage

PO (Adults and Children ≥12 yr): 0.5–1 mg/kg/day (up to 2 mg/kg/day) in 2 divided doses for 15–20 wk. Once discontinued, if relapse occurs, therapy may be reinstituted after an 8-wk rest period.

Availability (generic available)

Capsules: 10 mg, 20 mg, 25 mg, 30 mg, 35 mg, 40 mg.

NURSING IMPLICATIONS

Assessment

- Verify that patient receiving isotretinoin is registered with the *iPLEDGE program* and is completing all required interactions with their health care provider.
- Assess skin prior to and periodically during therapy. Transient worsening of acne may occur at initiation of therapy. Note number and severity of cysts, degree of skin dryness, erythema, and itching.
- Assess for allergy to parabens; capsules contain parabens as a preservative.
- Monitor patient for behavioral changes throughout therapy. May cause depression, psychosis, and suicide ideation. If behavioral changes occur, they usually resolve with discontinuation of therapy.
- Assess for rash periodically during therapy. May cause Stevens-Johnson syndrome or toxic epidermal necrolysis. Discontinue therapy if severe or if accompanied with fever, general malaise, fatigue, muscle or joint aches, blisters, oral lesions, conjunctivitis, hepatitis, and/or eosinophilia.
- ***Lab Test Considerations:*** Obtain 2 negative sequential serum or urine pregnancy tests with a sensitivity ≥25 mIU/mL before receiving initial prescription and monthly before each new Rx.
- Monitor liver function (AST, ALT, and LDH) prior to therapy, after 1 mo of therapy, and periodically thereafter. Inform health care professional if these values become ↑ therapy may need to be discontinued.
- Monitor blood lipids (cholesterol, HDL, triglycerides) under fasting conditions prior to beginning therapy, at 1–2 wk intervals until lipid response to isotretinoin is established (usually within 1 mo), and periodically thereafter. Report ↑ cholesterol and triglyceride levels or ↓ HDL.
- Obtain baseline and periodic CBC, urinalysis, and SMA-12. May cause ↑ blood glucose, CPK, platelet counts, and sedimentation rate. May ↓ RBC and WBC parameters. May cause proteinuria, red and white blood cells in urine, and ↑ uric acid.

Implementation

- Do not confuse isotretinoin with tretinoin.
- Isotretinoin is approved for marketing only under the *iPLEDGE program*, a special restricted distribution program approved by the FDA.
- Only patients who meet all requirements of the *iPLEDGE program* may receive isotretinoin.
- Isotretinoin may only be prescribed by health care providers registered and activated with the *iPLEDGE program*.
- Isotretinoin may only be dispensed by pharmacies registered with the *iPLEDGE program*.
- **PO:** Administer with meals. Do not crush or open capsules.

Patient/Family Teaching

- Explain the *iPLEDGE program* and its requirements to patient and parent.
- Instruct patient to take isotretinoin as directed. Do not take more than the amount prescribed. Take missed doses as soon as remembered if not almost time for next dose. Do not double doses. Patients must read *Medication Guide* and sign consent form prior to initiation of therapy.

- Explain to patient that a temporary worsening of acne may occur at beginning of therapy.
- Rep: Instruct female patients of reproductive potential to use 2 forms of contraception 1 mo before therapy, throughout therapy, and for at least 1 mo after discontinuation of drug. This drug is contraindicated during pregnancy and may cause birth defects. Patient who can become pregnant must have 2 negative serum or urine pregnancy tests with a sensitivity ≥25 mIU/mL before receiving initial prescription. First test is obtained by prescriber when decision is made to prescribe isotretinoin. Second pregnancy test should be done after patient has used 2 forms of contraception for 1 mo and during first 5 days of menstrual period immediately preceding beginning of therapy. For patients with amenorrhea, second test should be done 11 days after last act of unprotected sexual intercourse. Each mo of therapy patient must have a negative result from a urine or serum pregnancy test. Pregnancy test must be repeated every mo prior to receiving prescription in patients who can become pregnant. Patient should discontinue medication and inform health care professional immediately if pregnancy is suspected. Recommended consent form prepared by manufacturer stresses fetal risk. Parents of minors should also read and sign form. Yellow self-adhesive qualification stickers completed by prescriber must accompany prescription. Advise patient to avoid breast feeding during and for at least 8 days after last dose.
- Advise patient and family to notify health care professional if rash or thoughts about suicide or dying, attempts to commit suicide; new or worse depression; new or worse anxiety; feeling very agitated or restless; panic attacks; trouble sleeping; new or worse irritability; acting aggressive; being angry or violent; acting on dangerous impulses; an extreme increase in activity and talking; other unusual changes in behavior or mood occur.
- May cause sudden decrease in night vision. Caution patient to avoid driving at night until response to the medication is known.
- Advise patient to consult with health care professional before using other acne preparations while taking isotretinoin. Soaps, cosmetics, and shaving lotion may also worsen dry skin.
- Advise patient to notify health care professional of all Rx or OTC medications, vitamins, or herbal products being taken and to consult with health care professional before taking other medications, especially St. John's wort.
- Inform patient that dry skin and chapped lips will occur. Lubricant to lips may help cheilitis.
- Instruct patient that oral rinses, good oral hygiene, and sugarless gum or candy may help minimize dry mouth. Notify health care professional if dry mouth persists for more than 2 wk.
- Discuss possibility of excessively dry eyes with patients who wear contact lenses. Patient should contact health care professional about eye lubricant. Patient may need to switch to glasses during course of therapy and for up to 2 wk following discontinuation.
- Advise patient to avoid alcoholic beverages while taking isotretinoin, as this may further increase triglyceride levels.
- Caution patient to use sunscreen and protective clothing to prevent photosensitivity reactions. Health care professional should be consulted about sunscreen, as some sunscreens may worsen acne.
- Instruct patient not to take vitamin A supplements and to avoid excessive ingestion of foods high in vitamin A (liver; fish liver oils; egg yolks; yellow-orange fruits and vegetables; dark green, leafy vegetables; whole milk; vitamin A–fortified skim milk; butter; margarine) while taking isotretinoin; this may result in hypervitaminosis.
- Advise patient not to donate blood while receiving this medication. After discontinuing isotretinoin, wait at least 1 mo before donating blood to prevent the possibility of a pregnant patient receiving the blood.
- Inform diabetic patients that difficulty controlling blood glucose may occur.
- Instruct patient to report burning of eyes, visual changes, rash, abdominal pain, diarrhea, headache, nausea, and vomiting to health care professional.
- Inform patient of need for medical follow-up. Periodic lab tests may be required.

Evaluation/Desired Outcomes

- Decrease in the number and severity of cysts in severe acne. Therapy may take 4–5 mo before full effects are seen. Therapy is discontinued when the number of cysts is reduced by 70% or after 5 mo. Improvement may occur after discontinuation of therapy; therefore, a delay of at least 8 wk is recommended before a second course of therapy is considered.

istradefylline (is-tra-**def**-i-lin)

Nourianz

Classification

Therapeutic: antiparkinson agents

Pharmacologic: adenosine receptor antagonist

Indications

Adjunctive treatment to levodopa/carbidopa in patients with Parkinson's disease experiencing "off" episodes.

Action

Acts as an adenosine receptor antagonist; the mechanism by which these effects exert beneficial effects in patients with Parkinson's disease is unknown. **Therapeutic Effects:** Reduction in "off" time.

Pharmacokinetics

Absorption: Unknown.

Distribution: Extensively distributed to tissues.

Protein Binding: 98%.

Metabolism and Excretion: Primarily metabolized in liver via CYP1A1 and CYP3A4 isoenzymes. 48% excreted in feces, 39% in urine.
Half-life: 83 hr.

TIME/ACTION PROFILE (plasma concentrations)

ROUTE	ONSET	PEAK	DURATION
PO	unknown	4 hr	24 hr

Contraindications/Precautions

Contraindicated in: Severe psychotic disorders (may worsen psychosis); Severe hepatic impairment; OB: Pregnancy (may cause fetal harm).
Use Cautiously in: End-stage renal disease; Moderate hepatic impairment; Lactation: Use while breast feeding only if potential maternal benefit justifies potential risk to infant; Rep: Women of reproductive potential; Pedi: Safety and effectiveness not established.

Adverse Reactions/Side Effects

CNS: dyskinesia, aggression, agitation, confusion, delusions, delirium, disorientation, dizziness, hallucinations, impulse control disorders (gambling, sexual), insomnia, mania, paranoid ideation. **Derm:** rash. **Endo:** hyperglycemia, hyperuricemia. **GI:** constipation, diarrhea, nausea. **Metab:** ↓ appetite.

Interactions

Drug-Drug: Concurrent use with **levodopa** may cause or exacerbate dyskinesia. **Cigarette smoking** may ↓ levels; if patient smokes ≥20 cigarettes/day, ↑ dose to 40 mg once daily. **Strong CYP3A4 inhibitors**, including **clarithromycin**, **itraconazole**, **ketoconazole**, may significantly ↑ levels. **Strong CYP3A4 inducers**, including **carbamazepine**, **phenytoin**, **rifampin**, may significantly ↓ levels; avoid concurrent use. Higher doses (40 mg/day) may ↑ levels of **CYP3A4 substrates**, including **atorvastatin**. May ↑ levels of **P-glycoprotein substrates**, including **digoxin**.
Drug-Natural Products: St. John's wort may significantly ↓ levels; avoid concurrent use.

Route/Dosage

PO (Adults): 20 mg once daily; may ↑ to 40 mg once daily, if needed, based on clinical response. *Concurrent use of strong CYP3A4 inhibitors*—Do not exceed 20 mg/day.

Hepatic Impairment

PO (Adults): *Moderate hepatic impairment (Child-Pugh B)*—Do not exceed 20 mg/day.

Availability

Tablets: 20 mg, 40 mg.

NURSING IMPLICATIONS

Assessment

- Assess parkinsonian symptoms (akinesia, rigidity, tremors, pill rolling, shuffling gait, mask-like face, twisting motions, and drooling) during therapy. "On-off phenomenon" may cause symptoms to appear or improve suddenly.
- Assess for signs and symptoms of dyskinesia (abnormal movements, uncontrolled sudden movements) before and during therapy.
- Monitor for signs and symptoms of behavior changes (hallucinations, psychotic behavior, paranoid ideation, delusions, confusion, mania, disorientation, aggressive behavior, agitation, delirium) during therapy. Consider reducing dose or discontinuing therapy.

Implementation

- **PO:** Administer once daily without regard for food.

Patient/Family Teaching

- Instruct patient to take medication at regular intervals as directed. Advise patient to read *Patient Information* before starting therapy and with each Rx refill in case of changes.
- Advise patient to notify health care professional of all Rx or OTC medications, vitamins, or herbal products being taken and to consult with health care professional before taking other medications.
- Advise patient and family to notify health care professional if signs and symptoms of hallucinations or psychosis (being overly suspicious or feeling people want to harm you, disorientation, believing things that are not real, aggressive behavior, seeing or hearing things that are not real, agitation, confusion, delirium, increase activity or talking, or if new or increased gambling, sexual, or other intense urges occur). Dose reduction may be required.
- Advise females of reproductive potential to use effective contraception and avoid breast feeding during therapy. Advise patient to notify health care professional if pregnancy is planned or suspected, or if breast feeding.

Evaluation/Desired Outcomes

- Decreased "off" time in patients with Parkinson's disease.

ivabradine (eye-vab-ra-deen)

Corlanor, ✱Lancora

Classification
Therapeutic: heart failure agents
Pharmacologic: hyperpolarization-activated cyclic nucleotide-gated channel blockers

Indications

To decrease the need for hospitalization due to worsening HF in patients with stable, but symptomatic chronic HF (ejection fraction <35%, sinus rhythm ≥70 bpm, receiving highest tolerated doses of beta-blockers or are unable to tolerate beta-blockers). Treatment of stable, symptomatic HF due to dilated cardiomyopathy in pediatric patients ≥6 mo old who are in sinus rhythm with an elevated heart rate.

Action

Inhibits the cardiac pacemaker I_f-current by acting as a hyperpolarization-activated cyclic nucleoside-gated channel blocker, resulting in ↓ spontaneous pacemaker activity of sinus node. Decreases heart rate without affecting contractility or ventricular repolarization.
Therapeutic Effects: Lowering of heart rate with reduced need for hospitalization in HF patients.

Pharmacokinetics

Absorption: 40% absorbed following oral administration (undergoes first pass metabolism); food delays absorption and ↑ blood levels.
Distribution: Unknown.
Metabolism and Excretion: Extensively metabolized, primarily by the CYP3A4 enzyme system. The major metabolite is pharmacologically active and has the same potency as ivabradine. Metabolites excreted equally in urine and feces; 4% excreted unchanged in urine.
Half-life: 6 hr.

TIME/ACTION PROFILE (blood levels)

ROUTE	ONSET	PEAK	DURATION
PO	unknown	1 hr	12 hr

Contraindications/Precautions

Contraindicated in: Acute decompensated heart failure; Clinically significant hypotension; Sick sinus syndrome, sinoatrial block, or 2nd or 3rd degree heart block (unless a functioning demand pacemaker is in place, ↑ risk of bradycardia); Clinically significant bradycardia; Severe hepatic impairment; Pacemaker dependence; Concurrent use of strong CYP3A4 inhibitors; OB: Pregnancy (may cause fetal harm); Lactation: Discontinue ivabradine or discontinue breast feeding.
Use Cautiously in: Rep: Women of reproductive potential; Pedi: Children <6 mo (safety and effectiveness not established).

Adverse Reactions/Side Effects

CV: TORSADE DE POINTES, atrial fibrillation, bradycardia, heart block, hypertension, QT interval prolongation, sinus arrest. **EENT:** phosphenes (luminous phenomena).

Interactions

Drug-Drug: Strong CYP3A4 inhibitors, including **azole antifungals**, **macolide anti-infectives**, **HIV protease inhibitors**, and **nefazodone** may ↑ levels; concurrent use contraindicated. **Moderate CYP3A4 inhibitors**, including **diltiazem** and **verapamil**, may ↑ levels and ↑ risk of bradycardia; avoid concurrent use. **CYP3A4 inducers**, including **barbiturates**, **phenytoin**, and **rifampicin** may ↓ levels; avoid concurrent use. ↑ risk of bradycardia with concurrent use of **negative chronotropes** including **amiodarone**, **beta-blockers**, and **digoxin**; monitor heart rate. Concurrent use of **QT-interval prolonging drugs** may ↑ risk of QT interval prolongation and torsade de pointes.
Drug-Natural Products: Concurrent use of **St. John's wort** may ↓ blood levels and effectiveness and should be avoided.
Drug-Food: Concurrent ingestion of **grapefruit juice** may ↑ blood levels and the risk of adverse effects and should be avoided.

Route/Dosage

PO (Adults): 5 mg twice daily for 2 wk; dose may then be adjusted based on heart rate, not to exceed 7.5 mg twice daily; *Patients with conduction defects or bradycardia*—2.5 mg twice daily initially.
PO (Children ≥6 mo and ≥40 kg): *Tablets*—2.5 mg twice daily; adjust dose at 2–wk intervals by 2.5 mg twice daily to achieve a heart rate reduction of ≥20%; not to exceed 7.5 mg twice daily.
PO (Children ≥6 mo and <40 kg): *Oral solution*—0.05 mg/kg twice daily; adjust dose at 2–wk intervals by 0.05 mg/kg twice daily to achieve a heart rate reduction of ≥20%; not to exceed 0.2 mg/kg twice daily (6 mo–<1 yr) or 0.3 mg/kg twice daily (≥1 yr) up to max of 7.5 mg twice daily.

Availability

Oral solution: 1 mg/mL. **Tablets:** 5 mg, 7.5 mg.

NURSING IMPLICATIONS

Assessment

- Assess heart rate prior to, after 2 wk, and periodically during therapy. Adjust dose for a resting heart rate 50–60 bpm. *If heart rate >60 bpm,* increase dose by 2.5 mg given twice daily up to 7.5 mg twice daily. *If heart rate 50–60 bpm,* maintain dose. *If heart rate <50 bpm or signs and symptoms of bradycardia (dizziness, fatigue, hypotension) occur,* decrease dose by 2.5 mg given twice daily; if current dose is 2.5 mg given twice daily, discontinue ivabradine.
- Monitor ECG periodically during therapy. May cause atrial fibrillation and torsade de pointes. Discontinue ivabradine if atrial fibrillation occurs.

Implementation

- **PO:** Administer twice daily with meals.
- For oral solution, empty entire contents of ampule(s) into a medication cup. With a calibrated oral syringe, measure prescribed dose and administer orally. Discard unused oral solution; do not store or reuse. Solution is colorless.

Patient/Family Teaching

- Instruct patient to take ivabradine as directed. If dose is missed or patient spits out drug omit dose; do not double doses.
- Advise patient to avoid taking grapefruit juice during therapy; may increase risk of side effects.
- Advise patient to notify health care professional if signs and symptoms of irregular or rapid heartbeat (heart pounding or racing, chest pressure, worsened shortness of breath, near fainting or fainting) or slower than normal heart rate (dizziness, fatigue, lack of energy) occur. In young children signs and symptoms of slow heart rate (poor feeding, difficulty breathing, turning blue).
- Inform patient that ivabradine may cause phosphenes or luminous phenomena, a transiently enhanced brightness in a limited area of the visual field, halos, image decomposition, colored bright lights, or multiple images. Phosphenes are usually triggered by sudden variations in light intensity. Usually begin within first 2 mo of therapy, may occur repeatedly of mild to moderate intensity, and resolve after therapy is discontinued.
- Instruct patient to notify health care professional of all Rx or OTC medications, vitamins, or herbal products being taken and to consult health care professional before taking any other Rx, OTC, or herbal products, especially St. John's wort.
- May be teratogenic. Advise female patient of reproductive potential to use effective contraception during therapy and to avoid breast feeding during therapy. Advise patient to notify health care professional immediately if pregnancy is suspected.

Evaluation/Desired Outcomes

- Lowering of heart rate to prevent hospitalization in patients with HF.

ixabepilone (icks-a-**bep**-i-lone)
Ixempra

Classification
Therapeutic: antineoplastics
Pharmacologic: epothilone B analogues

Indications

Combination use with capecitabine for the treatment of metastatic or locally advanced breast cancer currently resistant to a taxane and anthracycline or resistant to a taxane and cannot tolerate further anthracycline. May also be used as monotherapy for breast cancers that are not responding to anthracyclines, taxane, or capecitabine.

Action

Binds to β-tubulin subunits on microtubules; this action blocks cells in mitosis, leading to cell death. Also has antiangiogenic activity. **Therapeutic Effects:** Decreased spread of breast cancer.

Pharmacokinetics

Absorption: IV administration results in complete bioavailablity.
Distribution: Unknown.
Metabolism and Excretion: Extensively metabolized by the liver, primarily by the CYP3A4 enzyme system. Metabolites are not active and are excreted mainly by the kidneys.
Half-life: 52 hr.

TIME/ACTION PROFILE (blood levels)

ROUTE	ONSET	PEAK	DURATION
IV	unknown	end of infusion	unknown

Contraindications/Precautions

Contraindicated in: Previous hypersensitivity to any medications containing Cremophor EL or similar derivatives (polyoxyethylated castor oil); Neutrophils <1500 cells/m^3 or platelets <100,000 cells/m^3; Severe hepatic impairment; Use with capecitabine is contraindicated for hepatic impairment (AST or ALT >2.5 × upper limits of normal or bilirubin >1 × upper limit of normal) due to ↑ risk of toxicity and death associated with neutropenia; OB, Lactation: Pregnancy or lactation.

Use Cautiously in: Toxicity; dose adjustments may be required for neuropathy/arthralgia/myalgia/fatigue, neutropenia, thrombocytopenia, moderate hepatic impairment or palmar-plantar erythrodysesthesia; Diluent contains dehydrated alcohol; consider possible CNS effects; Diabetes or history of neuropathy (↑ risk of severe neuropathy); History of cardiac disease (may ↑ risk of myocardial ischemia or ventricular dysfunction; OB: Patients with childbearing potential; Pedi: Effectiveness not established.

Adverse Reactions/Side Effects

CNS: fatigue, weakness, dizziness, headache, insomnia. **EENT:** ↑ lacrimation. **CV:** chest pain, edema, left ventricular dysfunction, myocardial ischemia. **Resp:** dyspnea. **GI:** abdominal pain, anorexia, constipation, diarrhea, mucositis, nausea, stomatitis, vomiting, altered taste. **Derm:** alopecia, hyperpigmentation, nail disorder, palmar-plantar erythrodysesthesia (combination therapy with capecitabine), exfoliation, pruritus, rash, hot flushes. **Hemat:** MYELOSUPPRESSION. **MS:** arthralgia, musculoskeletal pain, myalgia. **Neuro:** peripheral neuropathy. **Misc:** hypersensitivity reactions.

Interactions

Drug-Drug: Strong CYP3A4 inhibitors including **ketoconazole, itraconazole, voriconazole, clarithromycin, atazanavir, delavirdine, ritonavir,**

saquinavir, **nefazodone** ↑ blood levels and the risk of serious toxicities; concurrent use should be avoided if possible. If concurrent use is required, dose reduction of ixabepilone is recommended. Inducers of the **CYP3A4 enzyme system** including **dexamathasone**, **phenytoin**, **carbamazepine**, **phenobarbital**, **rifampin**, **rifampicin**, or **rifabutin** may ↓ levels and effectiveness, avoid if possible.

Drug-Natural Products: St. John's wort may ↓ blood levels and should be avoided.

Drug-Food: Grapefruit juice may ↑ blood levels and toxicity; avoid concurrent use.

Route/Dosage

IV (Adults): 40 mg/m² every 3 wk; not to exceed dose greater than that calculated for 2.2 m² (88 mg/dose).

Hepatic Impairment

IV (Adults): *Moderate Impairment*—20 mg/m² every 3 wk; not to exceed 30 mg/m².

Availability

Powder for injection (requires specific diluent for initial reconstitution): 15-mg vial (contains 16 mg ixabepilone to allow for withdrawal losses) with 8 mL of diluent in a separate vial as a kit, 45-mg vial (contains 47 mg ixabepilone to allow for withdrawal losses) with 23.5 mL of diluent in a separate vial.

NURSING IMPLICATIONS

Assessment

- Monitor for hypersensitivity reaction (flushing, rash, dyspnea, bronchospasm). If severe reactions occur stop infusion and provide aggressive supportive treatment with epinephrine and corticosteroids. In subsequent cycles, add corticosteroids to the premedication regimen.
- Monitor for myelosuppression frequently during therapy. Assess for signs of infection during neutropenia. Assess for bleeding (bleeding gums, bruising, petechiae, blood in stools, urine, and emesis) and avoid IM injections and taking rectal temperatures if platelet count is low. Apply pressure to venipuncture sites for 10 min.
- Assess patient for signs of peripheral neuropathy (burning sensation, hyperesthesia, hypoesthesia, paresthesia, discomfort, neuropathic pain); may occur early during treatment within the first 3 cycles. Patients experiencing new or worsening symptoms may require a reduction or delay in dose of ixabepilone. If neuropathy is Grade 2 (moderate) lasting for ≥7 days or Grade 3 (severe) lasting for <7 days decrease dose by 20%. If neuropathy is Grade 3 lasting ≥7 days or is disabling discontinue treatment.
- ***Lab Test Considerations:*** Monitor CBC and platelets frequently during therapy. If neutrophil count is <500 cells/mm³ for ≥7 days or patient has febrile neutropenia or if platelet count is <25,000/mm³ or platelets are <50,000/mm³ with bleeding, decrease the dose by 20%. Begin new treatment cycle only if neutrophil count is at least 1500 cells/mm³ and nonhematologic toxicities have improved to Grade 1 (mild) or resolved. May also cause leukopenia and anemia.
- Monitor hepatic function prior to therapy. Patients with decreased hepatic function require a decreased dose. If AST and ALT ≤2.5 × the upper limits of normal (ULN) and bilirubin ≤1 × ULN, administer ixabepilone at 40 mg/m². If AST and ALT ≤10 × ULN and bilirubin ≤1 × ULN, administer ixabepilone at 32 mg/m². If AST and ALT ≤10 × ULN and bilirubin >1.5–≤3 × ULN, administer ixabepilone at 20–30 mg/m².

Implementation

- Premedicate patient with an H_1 and an H_2 antagonist approximately 1 hr before ixabepilone infusion. Patients who experienced a hypersensitivity reaction in a previous ixabepilone cycle should also be premedicated with corticosteroids and extension of the infusion time should be considered.
- To minimize risk of dermal exposure, wear impervious gloves when handling ixabepilone vials regardless of setting (unpacking and inspection, transport within a facility, dose preparation and administration).

IV Administration

- **Intermittent Infusion:** Remove *Ixempra kit* (containing ixabepilone vial and diluent vial) from refrigerator and allow to stand at room temperature for 30 min prior to diluting. *Ixempra kit* must be stored in refrigerator. When vials are first removed from refrigerator, a white precipitate may be observed in the diluent vial; precipitate will dissolve to form a clear solution once diluent warms to room temperature. Use only diluent supplied in kit for reconstitution. Reconstitute 15-mg vial with 8 mL and 45-mg vial with 23.5 mL of diluent. Gently swirl and invert vial until powder is completely dissolved. ***Diluent:*** Prior to administration, dilute constituted solution further with only LR supplied in DEHP-free bags. Dilute as soon as possible after constitution, but may be stored at room temperature and room light for up to 1 hr. For most doses use 250 mL bag of LR, 0.9% NaCl (pH adjusted 6.0–9.0 with sodium bicarbonate), or Plasma-lyte A injection (pH 7.4). ***Concentration:*** If final concentration is not between 0.2 mg/mL and 0.6 mg/mL, add to appropriate size bag of LR. Thoroughly mix infusion bag by manual rotation. Diluted solution is stable for up to 6 hr at room temperature and room light; must complete infusion during 6-hr period. Administer through an in-line filter with a microporous membrane of 0.2–1.2 microns. DEHP-free infusion containers and administration sets must be used. Discard remaining solution. ***Rate:*** Infuse over 3 hr.

Patient/Family Teaching

- Advise patient to avoid grapefruit juice during therapy; may lead to increased levels and side effects.
- Solution contains alcohol and may cause drowsiness or dizziness. Caution patient to avoid driving and other activities requiring alertness until response to medication is known.
- Instruct patient to notify health care professional promptly if fever >100.5°F; chills; cough; hoarseness; sore throat; signs of infection; lower back or side pain; burning, painful or difficulty urination; bleeding gums; bruising; petechiae; blood in stools, urine, or emesis; increased fatigue; dyspnea; or orthostatic hypotension occurs. Caution patient to avoid crowds and persons with known infections. Instruct patients to use a soft toothbrush and electric razor and to avoid falls. Caution patient not to drink alcoholic beverages or take medication containing aspirin or NSAIDs; may precipitate bleeding.
- Instruct patient to notify health care professional promptly if signs and symptoms of hypersensitivity (hives, urticaria, pruritus, rash, flushing, swelling, dyspnea, chest tightness), peripheral neuropathy (numbness and tingling in hands and feet), or cardiac adverse reactions (chest pain, difficulty breathing, palpitations, unusual weight gain) occur.
- Advise patient to notify health care professional of all Rx or OTC medications, vitamins, or herbal products being taken and to consult health care professional before taking other Rx, OTC, or herbal products, especially St. John's wort.
- Instruct patient not to receive any vaccinations without advice of health care professional.
- Discuss the possibility of hair loss with patient. Explore methods of coping. Regrowth usually occurs 2–3 mo after discontinuation of therapy.
- Advise women of childbearing potential to use effective contraception during therapy and to avoid breast feeding during therapy.

Evaluation/Desired Outcomes

- Decreased progression of breast cancer.

ixazomib (ix-az-oh-mib)

Ninlaro

Classification

Therapeutic: antineoplastics

Pharmacologic: proteasome inhibitors

Indications

Treatment of multiple myeloma in patients whose disease has relapsed despite receiving ≥1 previous drug therapy (in combination with lenalidomide and dexamethasone).

Action

Acts as a proteasome inhibitor by binding to sites on the 20s proteasome. Has antiproliferative and proapoptotic activity. **Therapeutic Effects:** Delayed progression of multiple myeloma.

Pharmacokinetics

Absorption: 58% absorbed following oral administration; bioavailability ↓ by high-fat foods.

Distribution: Extensively distributed to tissues.

Protein Binding: 99%.

Metabolism and Excretion: Metabolized by multiple CYP450 enzymes (including CYP1A2, CYP2B6, CYP2C8, CYP2C9, CYP2C19, CYP2D6, and CYP3A4). 62% excreted in urine (<3.5% as unchanged drug), 22% excreted in feces.

Half-life: 9.5 days.

TIME/ACTION PROFILE (blood levels)

ROUTE	ONSET	PEAK	DURATION
PO	unknown	1 hr	unknown

Contraindications/Precautions

Contraindicated in: Concurrent use of strong CYP3A inducers; OB: May cause fetal harm; Lactation: Avoid breast feeding.

Use Cautiously in: Moderate or severe hepatic impairment (↓ dose recommended); Severe renal impairment or end stage renal disease (↓ dose recommended); Rep: Women and men of reproductive potential; Pedi: Safety and effectiveness not established.

Adverse Reactions/Side Effects

CV: edema. **Derm:** rash. **EENT:** blurred vision, conjunctivitis, dry eye. **GI:** HEPATOTOXICITY, constipation, diarrhea, nausea, vomiting. **Hemat:** NEUTROPENIA, THROMBOCYTOPENIA. **MS:** back pain. **Neuro:** peripheral neuropathy. **Misc:** herpes zoster infection.

Interactions

Drug-Drug: Strong CYP3A4 inducers, including **carbamazepine**, **phenytoin**, and **rifampin**, may ↓ levels and effectiveness; avoid concurrent use.

Drug-Natural Products: St. John's wort may ↓ levels and effectiveness; avoid concurrent use.

Route/Dosage

PO (Adults): 4 mg once a wk on Days 1, 8, and 15 of a 28–day treatment cycle.

Renal Impairment

(Adults): *CCr <30 mL/min or requiring dialysis*—3 mg once a wk on Days 1, 8, and 15 of a 28-day treatment cycle.

Hepatic Impairment

(Adults): *Moderate or severe hepatic impairment (total bilirubin >1.5 × ULN)*—3 mg once a wk on Days 1, 8, and 15 of a 28–day treatment cycle.

Availability

Capsules: 2.3 mg, 3 mg, 4 mg.

NURSING IMPLICATIONS

Assessment

- Assess for rash (usually maculopapular or macular) periodically during therapy. *If Grade 2 or 3 rash occurs,* withhold lenalidomide until rash recovers to ≤Grade 1, then resume lenalidomide at next lower dose. *If Grade 2 or 3 rash occurs again,* withhold ixazomib and lenalidomide until rash ≤Grade 1, then resume ixazomib at next lower dose and resume lenalidomide at most recent dose. *If Grade 4 rash occurs,* discontinue therapy.
- Assess for signs and symptoms of peripheral neuropathy (numbness, tingling, burning, pain in feet or hands, or weakness in arms or legs) periodically during therapy. *If Grade 1 peripheral neuropathy with pain or Grade 2 peripheral neuropathy occurs,* withhold ixazomib until peripheral neuropathy recovers to ≤Grade 1 without pain or patient's baseline, then resume ixazomib at most recent dose. *If Grade 2 peripheral neuropathy with pain or Grade 3 peripheral neuropathy occurs,* withhold ixazomib until return to patient's baseline condition or ≤Grade 1 peripheral neuropathy, then resume ixazomib at next lower dose. *If Grade 4 peripheral neuropathy occurs,* discontinue therapy.
- ***Lab Test Considerations:*** Prior to each 28–day cycle, absolute neutrophil count (ANC) should be ≥1,000/mm³, platelet count should be ≥75,000/mm³, and non-hematologic toxicities should be recovered to patient's baseline condition or ≤Grade 1. For patients taking ixazomib, lenalidomide, and dexamethasone, *if ANC <500/mm³,* withhold ixazomib and lenalidomide until ANC ≥500/mm³, then resume lenalidomide at next lower dose and resume ixazomib at most recent dose. Consider adding granulocyte stimulating factor (G-CSF) as per clinical guidelines. *If ANC <500/mm³ again,* withhold ixazomib and lenalidomide until ANC ≥500/mm³, then resume ixazomib at next lower dose and resume lenalidomide at most recent dose.
- Monitor platelet counts at least monthly during therapy and more frequently during 1st three cycles. Nadir of thrombocytopenia usually occurs Days 14-21 of each 28-day cycle and recovery to baseline by start of next cycle. *If platelet count ≤30,000/mm³,* withhold ixazomib and lenalidomide until platelet count is ≥30,000/mm³, then resume lenalidomide at next lower dose and resume ixazomib at most recent dose. *If platelet count <30,000/mm³ again,* withhold ixazomib and lenalidomide until platelet count is ≥30,000/mm³, then resume ixazomib at next lower dose and resume lenalidomide at most recent dose.
- Monitor hepatic enzymes periodically during therapy and adjust dosing for Grade 3 or 4 symptoms.

Implementation

- Consider starting antiviral prophylaxis prior therapy to decrease risk of herpes zoster infection.
- **PO:** Administer once weekly on same day and at same time for first 3 wk of four wk cycle. Take capsules at least 1 hr before or at least 2 hrs after food. Swallow capsule whole with water; do not open, crush, or chew.
- Dexamethasone should be taken with food and not with ixazomib.

Patient/Family Teaching

- Instruct patient to take ixazomib as directed. Take delayed or missed doses only if next scheduled dose is ≥72 hrs away. Do not take within 72 hrs of next scheduled dose and do not double doses. If vomiting occurs after taking dose, omit dose and resume dosing at time of next scheduled dose. Advise patient to read *Patient Information* sheet prior to starting therapy and with each Rx refill in case of changes.
- Caution patient to avoid direct contact with capsule contents. If powder accidentally gets on skin, wash area well with soap and water. If in eyes, flush eyes well with water.
- Advise patient to notify health care professional if signs and symptoms of thrombocytopenia (bleeding, easy bruising), GI problems (diarrhea, constipation, nausea, vomiting), peripheral neuropathy (tingling, numbness, pain, burning in feet or hands, weakness in arms or legs), liver problems (yellowing of skin or whites of eyes, pain in right upper abdomen), swelling in arms, hands, legs, ankles, or feet, or weight gain from swelling, new or worsening rash, or back pain occurs.
- Advise patient to notify health care professional of all Rx or OTC medications, vitamins, or herbal products being taken and to consult with health care professional before taking other medications, especially St. John's wort.
- Rep: May be teratogenic. Advise male and female patients to avoid pregnancy and breast feeding and use effective nonhormonal contraception during and for at least 90 days following therapy.

Evaluation/Desired Outcomes

- Delayed progression of multiple myeloma signs and symptoms.

ixekizumab (ix-ee-kiz-ue-mab)

Taltz

Classification
Therapeutic: antipsoriatics
Pharmacologic: interleukin antagonists

Indications

Moderate-to-severe plaque psoriasis in patients who are candidates for systemic therapy or phototherapy. Active psoriatic arthritis (alone or with a nonbiologic DMARD). Active ankylosing spondylitis.

Action

A monoclonal antibody that acts as an antagonist of interleukin (IL)–17A by selectively binding to it and preventing its interaction with the IL–17 receptor. Antagonism prevents the production of inflammatory cytokines and chemokines. **Therapeutic Effects:** Decreased plaque formation and spread in plaque psoriasis. Decreased pain and swelling with decreased joint destruction in psoriatic arthritis. Decreased disease activity in ankylosing spondylitis.

Pharmacokinetics

Absorption: Well absorbed (60–81%) following subcut administration.
Distribution: Minimally distributed to tissues.
Metabolism and Excretion: Catabolized into small peptides and amino acids.
Half-life: 13 days.

TIME/ACTION PROFILE (blood levels)

ROUTE	ONSET	PEAK	DURATION
Subcut	unknown	4 days	unknown

Contraindications/Precautions

Contraindicated in: Hypersensitivity; Active tuberculosis.
Use Cautiously in: Inflammatory bowel disease (may lead to exacerbations); OB: Safety not established; Lactation: Use while breast feeding only if potential maternal risk justifies potential risk to infant; Pedi: Safety and effectiveness not established.

Adverse Reactions/Side Effects

GI: inflammatory bowel disease, nausea. **Hemat:** neutropenia, thrombocytopenia. **Local:** injection site reactions. **Misc:** HYPERSENSITIVITY REACTIONS (including anaphylaxis, angioedema, and urticaria), INFECTION (including reactivation tuberculosis).

Interactions

Drug-Drug: May ↓ antibody response to **live-virus vaccine** and ↑ risk of adverse reactions (do not administer concurrently). May affect activity of CYP450 enzymes and may alter the effectiveness/toxicity of drugs that are substrates of CYP450 (including **warfarin** and **cyclosporine**; close monitoring is recommended to make any necessary dose modifications.

Route/Dosage

Plaque Psoriasis

Subcut (Adults): 160 mg (as two 80–mg injections) at Wk 0, then 80 mg at Wks 2, 4, 6, 8, 10, and 12, then 80 mg every 4 wk.

Psoriatic Arthritis and Ankylosing Spondylitis

Subcut (Adults): 160 mg (as two 80–mg injections) initially, then 80 mg every 4 wk.

Availability

Solution for injection (prefilled autoinjectors and syringes): 80 mg/mL.

NURSING IMPLICATIONS

Assessment

- Assess for tuberculosis infection before starting therapy; do not administer to patient with active TB infection. Initiate treatment of latent TB before administering ixekizumab. In patient with previous history of TB in whom adequate course cannot be confirmed, consider anti-TB therapy before starting ixekizumab.
- Monitor for signs and symptoms of infection (fever, sweats, chills, muscle aches, cough, dyspnea, blood in mucus, weight loss, warm, red, or painful skin or sores, diarrhea or stomach pain, burning or frequency of urination) before and periodically during therapy.
- Monitor for signs and symptoms of hypersensitivity (urticaria, feeling faint, swelling of face, eyelids, lips, mouth, tongue, or throat, dyspnea, throat tightness, chest tightness, rash) during therapy. If hypersensitivity reaction occurs, discontinue ixekizumab immediately and begin supportive therapy.
- Monitor for onset or exacerbation of inflammatory bowel disease (abdominal pain, diarrhea with or without blood, weight loss) during therapy.
- ***Lab Test Considerations:*** May cause neutropenia and thrombocytopenia.

Implementation

- Consider completing all age appropriate immunizations prior to starting therapy.
- **Subcut:** Allow to reach room temperature (30 min) before injection; do not microwave, run under hot water, or leave in sunlight to warm. Solution is clear and colorless to slightly yellow; do not administer solutions that are discolored or contain a precipitate. For *prefilled syringe,* pinch skin and inject into upper arm, thigh, or abdomen at a 45° angle, let go of skin pinch before injecting. Place *autoinjector*

flat against skin at injection site before injecting. Avoid areas where skin is bruised, tender, erythematous, indurated, or affected by psoriasis. Rotate injection sites. Store in refrigerator in original box to protect from light; may be stored at room temperature for up to 5 days. Do not return to refrigerator once stored at room temperature.

Patient/Family Teaching

- Instruct patient and caregiver in proper technique for self-injection and care and disposal of equipment. Administer missed doses as soon as possible and resume regular dosing schedule. Advise patient to read *Medication Guide and Instructions for Use* prior to starting therapy and with each Rx refill in case of changes.
- Advise patient to notify health care professional if signs and symptoms of allergic reaction, infection, or inflammatory bowel disease occur.
- Advise patient to avoid use of live vaccines during therapy.
- Instruct patient to notify health care professional of all Rx or OTC medications, vitamins, or herbal products being taken and consult health care professional before taking any new medications.
- Rep: Advise female patients of reproductive potential to notify health care professional if pregnancy is planned or suspected, or if breast feeding.

Evaluation/Desired Outcomes

- Decreased plaque formation and spread in patients with plaque psoriasis.
- Decreased pain and swelling with decreased joint destruction in psoriatic arthritis.
- Decreased disease activity in ankylosing spondylitis.

ketoconazole, See ANTIFUNGALS (TOPICAL).

BEERS

ketorolac† (kee-toe-role-ak)

Sprix, ~~Toradol~~, ✱Toradol

Classification

Therapeutic: nonsteroidal anti-inflammatory agents, nonopioid analgesics

Pharmacologic: pyrroziline carboxylic acid

†See Appendix C for ophthalmic use

Indications

Short-term management of pain (not to exceed 5 days total for all routes combined).

Action

Inhibits prostaglandin synthesis, producing peripherally mediated analgesia. Also has antipyretic and anti-inflammatory properties. **Therapeutic Effects:** Decreased pain.

Pharmacokinetics

Absorption: Rapidly and completely absorbed following all routes of administration.

Distribution: Enters breast milk in low concentrations.

Protein Binding: 99%.

Metabolism and Excretion: Primarily metabolized by the liver. Ketorolac and its metabolites are excreted primarily by the kidneys (92%); 6% excreted in feces.

Half-life: 4.5 hr (range 3.8–6.3 hr; ↑ in geriatric patients and patients with impaired renal function).

TIME/ACTION PROFILE (analgesic effects)

ROUTE	ONSET	PEAK	DURATION
PO	unknown	2–3 hr	4–6 hr or longer
IM, IV	10 min	1–2 hr	6 hr or longer
IN	unknown	unknown	6–8 hr or longer

Contraindications/Precautions

Contraindicated in: Hypersensitivity; Cross-sensitivity with other NSAIDs may exist; Preoperative use; Active or history of peptic ulcer disease or GI bleeding; Known alcohol intolerance (injection only); Coronary artery bypass graft (CABG) surgery; Cerebrovascular bleeding; Advanced renal impairment or at risk for renal failure due to volume depletion; Concurrent use of pentoxifylline or probenecid; OB: Chronic use in 3rd trimester may cause constriction of ductus arteriosus. May inhibit labor and ↑ maternal bleeding at delivery.

Use Cautiously in: Cardiovascular disease or risk factors for cardiovascular disease (may ↑ risk of serious cardiovascular thrombotic events, myocardial infarction, and stroke, especially with prolonged use or use of higher doses); avoid use in patients with recent MI or HF; Heart failure; Coagulation disorders; Mild-to-moderate renal impairment (↓ dose may be required); Hepatic impairment; Pedi: Safety not established in neonates; Geri: Appears on Beers list; ↑ risk of GI bleeding; Lactation: Lactation.

Adverse Reactions/Side Effects

CNS: <u>drowsiness</u>, abnormal thinking, dizziness, euphoria, headache. **CV:** HF, MYOCARDIAL INFARCTION, STROKE, edema, pallor, vasodilation. **Derm:** EXFOLIATIVE DERMATITIS, STEVENS-JOHNSON SYNDROME, TOXIC EPIDERMAL NECROLYSIS, pruritus, purpura, sweating, urticaria. **EENT:** ↑ lacrimation (spray), nasal discomfort (spray), throat irritation (spray). **F and E:** hyperkalemia. **GI:** GI BLEEDING, abnormal taste, diarrhea, dry mouth, dyspepsia, GI pain, ↑ liver enzymes, nausea. **GU:** oliguria, renal toxicity, urinary frequency. **Hemat:** prolonged bleeding time. **Local:** injection site pain. **Neuro:** paresthesia. **Resp:** asthma, dyspnea. **Misc:** HYPERSENSITIVITY REACTIONS (including anaphylaxis).

Interactions

Drug-Drug: **Probenecid** ↑ levels and the risk of adverse reactions; concurrent use is contraindicated. ↑ risk of bleeding when used with **pentoxifylline**; concurrent use is contraindicated. Concurrent use with **aspirin** may ↓ effectiveness. ↑ adverse GI effects with **aspirin**, other **NSAIDs**, **potassium supplements**, **corticosteroids**, or **alcohol**. May ↓ effectiveness of **diuretics** or **antihypertensives**. May ↑ serum **lithium** levels and ↑ risk of toxicity. ↑ risk of toxicity from **methotrexate**. ↑ risk of bleeding with **anticoagulants**, **aspirin**, **clopidogrel**, **ticagrelor**, **prasugrel**, **corticosteroids**, **fibrinolytics**, **SNRIs**, or **SSRIs**. ↑ risk of adverse hematologic reactions with **antineoplastics** or **radiation therapy**. May ↑ risk of nephrotoxicity from **cyclosporine**.

Drug-Natural Products: ↑ bleeding risk with **arnica**, **chamomile**, **clove**, **dong quai**, **feverfew**, **garlic**, **ginger**, **ginkgo**, **Panax ginseng**.

Route/Dosage

Oral therapy is indicated only as a continuation of parenteral therapy. Total duration of therapy by all routes should not exceed 5 days.

PO (Adults <65 yr): 20 mg initially, followed by 10 mg every 4–6 hr (not to exceed 40 mg/day).

PO (Adults ≥65 yr, <50 kg, or with renal impairment): 10 mg every 4–6 hr (not to exceed 40 mg/day).

K

PO (Children 2–16 yr, <50 kg): 1 mg/kg as a single dose. No data available for multiple doses.
IM (Adults <65 yr): *Single dose*—60 mg. *Multiple dosing*—30 mg every 6 hr (not to exceed 120 mg/day).
IM (Adults ≥65 yr, <50 kg, or with renal impairment): *Single dose*—30 mg. *Multiple dosing*—15 mg every 6 hr (not to exceed 60 mg/day).
IM (Children 2–16 yr, <50 kg): *Single dose*—0.4–1 mg/kg (maximum: 30 mg/dose). *Multiple dosing*—0.5 mg/kg every 6 hr.
IV (Adults <65 yr): *Single dose*—30 mg. *Multiple dosing*—30 mg every 6 hr (not to exceed 120 mg/day).
IV (Adults ≥65 yr, <50 kg, or with renal impairment): *Single dose*—15 mg. *Multiple dosing*—15 mg every 6 hr (not to exceed 60 mg/day).
IV (Children 2–16 yr, <50 kg): *Single dose*—0.4–1 mg/kg (maximum: 15 mg/dose). *Multiple dosing*—0.5 mg/kg every 6 hr.
Intranasal (Adults <65 yr): 1 spray in each nostril every 6–8 hr (not to exceed 4 sprays in each nostril/day).
Intranasal (Adults ≥65 yr, <50 kg, or with renal impairment): 1 spray in only one nostril every 6–8 hr (not to exceed 4 sprays in one nostril/day).

Availability (generic available)

Nasal spray (Sprix): 15.75 mg/spray in 1.7–g bottle (delivers 8 sprays). **Solution for injection:** 15 mg/mL, 30 mg/mL. **Tablets:** 10 mg.

NURSING IMPLICATIONS

Assessment

- Patients who have asthma, aspirin-induced allergy, and nasal polyps are at increased risk for developing hypersensitivity reactions. Assess for rhinitis, asthma, and urticaria.
- Assess for rash periodically during therapy. May cause Stevens-Johnson syndrome or toxic epidermal necrolysis. Discontinue therapy if severe or if accompanied with fever, general malaise, fatigue, muscle or joint aches, blisters, oral lesions, conjunctivitis, hepatitis, and/or eosinophilia.
- Monitor BP during initiation and periodically during therapy. May cause fluid retention and edema leading to new onset or worsening hypertension.
- **Pain:** Assess pain (note type, location, and intensity) prior to and 1–2 hr following administration.
- ***Lab Test Considerations:*** Evaluate liver function tests, especially AST and ALT, periodically in patients receiving prolonged therapy. May cause ↑ levels.
- May cause prolonged bleeding time that may persist for 24–48 hr following discontinuation of therapy.
- May cause ↑ BUN, serum creatinine, or potassium concentrations.

Implementation

- Do not confuse ketorolac with Ketalar (ketamine) or methadone.
- Administration in higher-than-recommended doses does not provide increased effectiveness but may cause increased side effects. Duration of ketorolac therapy, by all routes combined, should not exceed 5 days. Use lowest effective dose for shortest period of time to minimize risk of cardiovascular thrombotic events.
- Coadministration with opioid analgesics may have additive analgesic effects and may permit lower opioid doses.
- **PO:** Ketorolac therapy should always be given initially by the IM or IV route. Use oral therapy *only* as a continuation of parenteral therapy.

IV Administration

- **IV Push:** Administer undiluted. ***Concentration:*** 15–30 mg/mL. ***Rate:*** Administer over at least 15 sec.
- **Y-Site Compatibility:** acetaminophen, alfentanil, amikacin, aminocaproic acid, aminophylline, amphotericin B lipid complex, amphotericin B liposome, anidulafungin, argatroban, ascorbic acid, atracurium, atropine, aztreonam, benztropine, bivalirudin, bleomycin, bumetanide, buprenorphine, butorphanol, carboplatin, carmustine, cefazolin, cefotaxime, cefotetan, cefoxitin, ceftazidime, ceftriaxone, cefuroxime, chloramphenicol, cisatracurium, cisplatin, clindamycin, cyanocobalamin, cyclophosphamide, cyclosporine, cytarabine, dactinomycin, daptomycin, dexamethasone, dexmedetomidine, dexrazoxane, digoxin, docetaxel, dopamine, doxorubicin hydrochloride, doxorubicin liposomal, enalaprilat, ephedrine, epinephrine, epoetin alfa, eptifibatide, ertapenem, etoposide, etoposide phosphate, famotidine, fentanyl, fluconazole, fludarabine, fluorouracil, folic acid, foscarnet, fosphenytoin, furosemide, gentamicin, glycopyrrolate, granisetron, heparin, hetastarch, hydrocortisone, hydromorphone, ifosfamide, imipenem/cilastatin, indomethacin, insulin, regular, irinotecan, isoproterenol, leucovorin calcium, lidocaine, linezolid, lorazepam, magnesium sulfate, mannitol, meperidine, mesna, methotrexate, methylprednisolone, metoclopramide, metoprolol, milrinone, mitoxantrone, mivacurium, morphine, moxifloxacin, multivitamins, nafcillin, naloxone, nitroglycerin, nitroprusside, norepinephrine, octreotide, ondansetron, oxacillin, oxaliplatin, oxytocin, paclitaxel, palonosetron, pamidronate, pancuronium, pemetrexed, penicillin G, phenobarbital, phenylephrine, phytonadione, piperacillin/tazobactam, potassium acetate, potassium chloride, procainamide, propranolol, ranitidine, remifentanil, sodium acetate, sodium bicarbonate, streptokinase, succinylcholine, sufentanil, tacrolimus, theophylline, thiotepa, tigecycline, tirofiban, tobramycin, vasopressin, verapamil, vinblastine, vincristine, voriconazole, zoledronic acid.
- **Y-Site Incompatibility:** acyclovir, alemtuzumab, amiodarone, azithromycin, calcium chloride, caspo-

fungin, chlorpromazine, dacarbazine, dantrolene, daunorubicin hydrochloride, diazepam, diltiazem, diphenhydramine, dobutamine, dolasetron, doxycycline, epirubicin, erythromycin, esmolol, fenoldopam, ganciclovir, gemcitabine, gemtuzumab, haloperidol, hydroxyzine, idarubicin, labetalol, levofloxacin, metaraminol, midazolam, minocycline, mycophenolate, nalbuphine, nicardipine, pantoprazole, papaverine, pentamidine, phentolamine, phenytoin, prochlorperazine, promethazine, protamine, pyridoxine, quinupristin/dalfopristin, rocuronium, topotecan, trimethoprim/sulfamethoxazole, vancomycin, vecuronium, vinorelbine.

- **Intranasal:** Activate pump before first use by holding bottle arm's length away with index finger and middle finger resting on top of finger flange and thumb supporting base. Press down evenly and release pump 5 times to activate. Prior to each use, blow nose gently to clear nostrils. Sit up straight or stand. Tilt head slightly forward. Insert tip of container into nostril. Point container away from center of nose. Push down to spray. Bottles are for 24 hr use; discard bottle no more than 24 hrs after taking first dose, even if the bottle still contains some liquid.

Patient/Family Teaching

- Instruct patient on how and when to ask for and take pain medication. Advise patient to read *Medication Guide* and *Instructions for Use* before starting and with each Rx refill in case of changes.
- Instruct patient to take medication exactly as directed. Take missed doses as soon as remembered if not almost time for next dose. Do not double doses. Do not take more than prescribed or for longer than 5 days.
- May cause drowsiness or dizziness. Advise patient to avoid driving or other activities requiring alertness until response to the medication is known.
- Instruct patient to notify health care professional of all Rx or OTC medications, vitamins, or herbal products being taken and consult health care professional before taking any new medications.
- Caution patient to avoid the concurrent use of alcohol, aspirin, NSAIDs, acetaminophen, or other OTC medications without consulting health care professional.
- Advise patient to inform health care professional of medication regimen prior to treatment or surgery.
- Advise patient to consult health care professional if rash, itching, visual disturbances, tinnitus, weight gain, edema, black stools, persistent headache, or influenza-like syndrome (chills, fever, muscle aches, pain) occurs.
- Rep: Advise female patient to notify health care professional if pregnancy is planned or suspected, or if breast feeding. Advise patient to avoid use during pregnancy starting at 30 wk; increases risk of premature closure of ductus arteriosus. May cause temporary infertility in women.
- **Intranasal:** Instruct patient on correct technique for administration, need to open a new bottle every 24 hr, and the 5 day limit for use.

Evaluation/Desired Outcomes

- Decrease in severity of pain. Patients who do not respond to one NSAID may respond to another.

K

HIGH ALERT

labetalol (la-bet-a-lole)

Trandate

Classification

Therapeutic: antianginals, antihypertensives

Pharmacologic: beta blockers

Indications

Hypertension.

Action

Blocks stimulation of $beta_1$ (myocardial)- and $beta_2$ (pulmonary, vascular, and uterine)-adrenergic receptor sites. Also has $alpha_1$-adrenergic blocking activity, which may result in more orthostatic hypotension. **Therapeutic Effects:** Decreased BP.

Pharmacokinetics

Absorption: Well absorbed but rapidly undergoes extensive first-pass hepatic metabolism, resulting in 25% bioavailability.

Distribution: Some CNS penetration; crosses the placenta.

Protein Binding: 50%.

Metabolism and Excretion: Undergoes extensive hepatic metabolism.

Half-life: 3–8 hr.

TIME/ACTION PROFILE (cardiovascular effects)

ROUTE	ONSET	PEAK	DURATION
PO	20 min–2 hr	1–4 hr	8–12 hr
IV	2–5 min	5 min	16–18 hr

Contraindications/Precautions

Contraindicated in: Decompensated HF; Pulmonary edema; Cardiogenic shock; Bradycardia or heart block.

Use Cautiously in: Renal or hepatic impairment; Pulmonary disease (including asthma); Diabetes mellitus (may mask signs of hypoglycemia); Thyrotoxicosis (may mask symptoms); Patients with a history of severe allergic reactions (intensity of reactions may be ↑); OB: May cause fetal/neonatal bradycardia, hypotension, hypoglycemia, or respiratory depression; Lactation: Use while breast feeding only if potential maternal benefit justifies potential risk to infant; Pedi: Safety and effectiveness not established; Geri: ↑ sensitivity to beta blockers (↑ risk of orthostatic hypotension); initial dosage ↓ recommended.

Adverse Reactions/Side Effects

CNS: fatigue, weakness, anxiety, depression, dizziness, drowsiness, insomnia, memory loss, mental status changes, nightmares. **CV:** ARRHYTHMIAS, BRADYCARDIA, CHF, orthostatic hypotension. **Derm:** itching, rash. **EENT:** blurred vision, dry eyes, intraoperative floppy iris syndrome, nasal stuffiness. **Endo:** hyperglycemia, hypoglycemia. **GI:** constipation, diarrhea, nausea. **GU:** erectile dysfunction, ↓ libido. **MS:** arthralgia, back pain, muscle cramps. **Neuro:** paresthesia. **Resp:** PULMONARY EDEMA, bronchospasm, wheezing.

Interactions

Drug-Drug: General anesthesia and **verapamil** may cause additive myocardial depression. Additive bradycardia may occur with **digoxin**, **verapamil**, or **diltiazem**. Additive hypotension may occur with other **antihypertensives**, acute ingestion of **alcohol**, or **nitrates**. Concurrent **thyroid** administration may ↓ effectiveness. May alter the effectiveness of **insulin** or **oral hypoglycemic agents** (dose adjustments may be necessary). May ↓ the effectiveness of **adrenergic bronchodilators** and **theophylline**. May ↓ beneficial beta cardiovascular effects of **dopamine** or **dobutamine**. Use cautiously within 14 days of **MAO inhibitor** therapy (may result in hypertension). Effects may be ↑ by **propranolol** or **cimetidine**. Concurrent **NSAIDs** may ↓ antihypertensive action.

Route/Dosage

PO (Adults): 100 mg twice daily initially, may ↑ by 100 mg twice daily every 2–3 days as needed (usual range 400–800 mg/day in 2–3 divided doses; doses up to 1.2–2.4 g/day have been used).

IV (Adults): 20 mg (0.25 mg/kg) initially, additional doses of 40–80 mg may be given every 10 min as needed (not to exceed 300 mg total dose) *or* 2 mg/min infusion (range 50–300 mg total dose required).

Availability (generic available)

Solution for injection: 5 mg/mL. **Tablets:** 100 mg, 200 mg, 300 mg.

NURSING IMPLICATIONS

Assessment

- Monitor BP and pulse frequently during dose adjustment and periodically during therapy. Assess for orthostatic hypotension when assisting patient up from supine position.
- Check frequency of refills to determine compliance.
- Patients receiving *labetalol IV* must be supine during and for 3 hr after administration. Vital signs should be monitored every 5–15 min during and for several hrs after administration.
- Monitor intake and output ratios and daily weight. Assess patient routinely for evidence of fluid overload (peripheral edema, dyspnea, rales/crackles, fatigue, weight gain, jugular venous distention).
- ***Lab Test Considerations:*** May cause ↑ BUN, serum lipoprotein, potassium, triglyceride, and uric acid levels.

L

- May cause ↑ ANA titers.
- May cause ↑ in blood glucose levels.
- May cause ↑ serum alkaline phosphatase, LDH, AST, and ALT levels. Discontinue if jaundice or laboratory signs of hepatic function impairment occur.
- ***Toxicity and Overdose:*** Monitor patients receiving beta blockers for signs of overdose (bradycardia, severe dizziness or fainting, severe drowsiness, dyspnea, bluish fingernails or palms, seizures). Notify health care professional immediately if these signs occur.
- Glucagon has been used to treat bradycardia and hypotension.

Implementation

- ***High Alert:*** IV vasoactive medications are inherently dangerous. Before administering intravenously, have second practitioner independently check original order, dosage calculations, and infusion pump settings.
- Do not confuse labetalol with Lamictal or lamotrigine.
- Discontinuation of concurrent clonidine should take place gradually, with beta blocker discontinued first. Then, after several days, discontinue clonidine.
- **PO:** Take apical pulse prior to administering. If <50 bpm or if arrhythmia occurs, withhold medication and notify health care professional.
- Administer with meals or directly after eating to enhance absorption.

IV Administration

- **IV Push:** ***Diluent:*** Administer undiluted. ***Concentration:*** 5 mg/mL. ***Rate:*** Administer slowly over 2 min.
- **Continuous Infusion:** ***Diluent:*** Add 200 mg of labetalol to 160 mL of diluent. May also be administered as undiluted drug. Compatible diluents include D5W, 0.9% NaCl, D5/0.9% NaCl, and LR. ***Concentration:*** Diluted: 1 mg/mL; Undiluted: 5 mg/mL. ***Rate:*** Administer at a rate of 2 mg/min. Titrate for desired response. Infuse via infusion pump to ensure accurate dose.
- **Y-Site Compatibility:** alemtuzumab, alfentanil, amikacin, aminocaproic acid, aminophylline, amiodarone, anidulafungin, argatroban, ascorbic acid, atracurium, atropine, aztreonam, bivalirudin, bleomycin, bumetanide, buprenorphine, butorphanol, calcium chloride, calcium gluconate, carboplatin, carmustine, caspofungin, cefazolin, ceftazidime, chlorpromazine, cisplatin, clonidine, cyanocobalamin, cyclophosphamide, cyclosporine, dactinomycin, daptomycin, dexmedetomidine, digoxin, diltiazem, diphenhydramine, dobutamine, docetaxel, dopamine, doxorubicin hydrochloride, doxycycline, enalaprilat, ephedrine, epinephrine, epirubicin, epoetin alfa, eptifibatide, ertapenem, erythromycin lactobionate, esmolol, etoposide, etoposide phosphate, famotidine, fenoldopam, fentanyl, fluconazole, fludarabine, fluorouracil, folic acid, ganciclovir, gemcitabine, gentamicin, glycopyrrolate, granisetron, hydromorphone, idarubicin, ifosfamide, imipenem/cilastatin, irinotecan, isoproterenol, levofloxacin, lidocaine, linezolid, lorazepam, magnesium sulfate, mannitol, meperidine, methoxamine, methyldopate, methylprednisolone sodium succinate, metoclopramide, metoprolol, metronidazole, midazolam, milrinone, mitoxantrone, morphine, multivitamins, mycophenolate, nalbuphine, naloxone, nicardipine, nitroglycerin, nitroprusside, norepinephrine, octreotide, ondansetron, oxacillin, oxaliplatin, oxytocin, palonosetron, pamidronate, pancuronium, papaverine, pemetrexed, pentamidine, pentobarbital, phenobarbital, phentolamine, phenylephrine, phytonadione, potassium acetate, potassium chloride, potassium phosphates, procainamide, prochlorperazine, promethazine, propofol, propranolol, protamine, pyridoxime, quinupristin/dalfopristin, ranitidine, rocuronium, sodium acetate, sodium bicarbonate, streptokinase, succinylcholine, sufentanil, tacrolimus, telavancin, theophylline, thiamine, thiotepa, tigecycline, tirofiban, tobramycin, tolazoline, trimetaphan, vancomycin, vasopressin, vecuronium, verapamil, vincristine, vinorelbine, voriconazole, zoledronic acid.
- **Y-Site Incompatibility:** acyclovir, amphotericin B deoxycholate, amphotericin B lipid complex, amphotericin B liposome, azathioprine, cefotaxime, cefotetan, cefoxitin, ceftaroline, ceftriaxone, cefuroxime, dantrolene, dexamethasone sodium phosphate, diazepam, diazoxide, hydrocortisone sodium succinate, indomethacin, insulin, ketorolac, micafungin, paclitaxel, pantoprazole, penicillin G, phenytoin, piperacillin/tazobactam, thiopental, warfarin.

Patient/Family Teaching

- Instruct patient to take medication as directed, at the same time each day, even if feeling well; do not skip or double up on missed doses. Take missed doses as soon as possible up to 8 hr before next dose. Abrupt withdrawal may precipitate life-threatening arrhythmias, hypertension, or myocardial ischemia.
- Advise patient to make sure enough medication is available for weekends, holidays, and vacations. A written prescription may be kept in wallet in case of emergency.
- Teach patient and family how to check pulse and BP. Instruct them to check pulse daily and BP biweekly. Advise patient to hold dose and contact health care professional if pulse is <50 bpm or BP changes significantly.
- May cause drowsiness or dizziness. Caution patients to avoid driving or other activities that require alertness until response to the drug is known. Caution patients receiving labetalol IV to call for assistance during ambulation or transfer.
- Advise patients to make position changes slowly to minimize orthostatic hypotension, especially during initiation of therapy or when dose is increased. Pa-

tients taking oral labetalol should be especially cautious when drinking alcohol, standing for long periods, or exercising, and during hot weather, because orthostatic hypotension is enhanced.

- Caution patient that this medication may increase sensitivity to cold.
- Instruct patient to notify health care professional of all Rx or OTC medications, vitamins, or herbal products being taken and to consult health care professional before taking any Rx, OTC, or herbal products, especially cold preparations, concurrently with this medication. Patients on antihypertensive therapy should also avoid excessive amounts of coffee, tea, and cola.
- Patients with diabetes should closely monitor blood glucose, especially if weakness, malaise, irritability, or fatigue occurs. Medication may mask tachycardia and increased BP as signs of hypoglycemia, but dizziness and sweating may still occur.
- Advise patient to notify health care professional if slow pulse, difficulty breathing, wheezing, cold hands and feet, dizziness, light-headedness, confusion, depression, rash, fever, sore throat, unusual bleeding, or bruising occurs.
- Instruct patient to inform health care professional of medication regimen prior to treatment or surgery.
- Advise females of reproductive potential to notify health care professional if pregnancy is planned or suspected, or if breast feeding.
- Advise patient to carry identification describing disease process and medication regimen at all times.
- **Hypertension:** Reinforce the need to continue additional therapies for hypertension (weight loss, sodium restriction, stress reduction, regular exercise, moderation of alcohol consumption, and smoking cessation). Medication controls but does not cure hypertension.

Evaluation/Desired Outcomes

- Decrease in BP.

lacosamide (la-kose-a-mide)

Vimpat

Classification

Therapeutic: anticonvulsants

Schedule V

Indications

Treatment of partial-onset seizures as either monotherapy or adjunctive therapy.

Action

Mechanism is not known, but may involve enhancement of slow inactivation of sodium channels with resultant membrane stabilization. **Therapeutic Effects:** Decreased incidence and severity of partial-onset seizures.

Pharmacokinetics

Absorption: 100% absorbed following oral administration; IV administration results in complete bioavailability.

Distribution: Unknown.

Protein Binding: <15%.

Metabolism and Excretion: Partially metabolized by the liver; 40% excreted in urine as unchanged drug, 30% as a metabolite.

Half-life: 13 hr.

TIME/ACTION PROFILE (blood levels)

ROUTE	ONSET	PEAK	DURATION
PO	unknown	1–4 hr	12 hr
IV	unknown	end of infusion	12 hr

Contraindications/Precautions

Contraindicated in: Hypersensitivity; Severe hepatic impairment; Lactation: Lactation.

Use Cautiously in: CCr <30 mL/min (use lower daily dose); All patients (may ↑ risk of suicidal thoughts/behaviors); Hepatic or renal impairment and taking strong inhibitor of CYP3A4 or CYP2C9 (dose ↓ may be needed); Mild to moderate hepatic impairment; titrate dose carefully, use lower daily dose; Known cardiac conduction problems (heart block or sick sinus syndrome without a pacemaker), severe cardiac disease (MI or HF), Brugada syndrome, or taking medications that affect cardiac conduction; Diabetic neuropathy or cardiac disease (↑ risk for atrial fibrillation/flutter); OB: Use only if potential benefit justifies risk to the fetus; Pedi: Children <4 yr (safety and effectiveness not established); Geri: Titrate dose carefully.

Adverse Reactions/Side Effects

CNS: SUICIDAL THOUGHTS, dizziness, headache, hallucinations, syncope, vertigo. **CV:** VENTRICULAR ARRHYTHMIAS, atrial fibrillation/flutter, bradycardia, heart block, syncope. **Derm:** DRUG REACTION WITH EOSINOPHILIA AND SYSTEMIC SYMPTOMS (DRESS), STEVENS-JOHNSON SYNDROME, TOXIC EPIDERMAL NECROLYSIS, rash. **EENT:** diplopia. **GI:** nausea, vomiting. **Hemat:** AGRANULOCYTOSIS. **Neuro:** ataxia. **Misc:** physical dependence, psychological dependence.

Interactions

Drug-Drug: Use cautiously with other drugs that affect cardiac conduction, including **sodium channel blockers**, **beta blockers**, **diltiazem**, **verapamil**, **potassium channel blockers**, and **PR-interval prolonging medications**.

Route/Dosage

PO, IV (Adults): *Monotherapy*— 100 mg twice daily; may ↑ weekly by 100 mg/day in 2 divided doses up to a maintenance dose of 150–200 mg twice daily; may also initiate therapy with 200-mg single loading dose followed 12 hr later by 100 mg twice daily; may ↑ weekly by 100 mg/day in 2 divided doses up to a maintenance dose of 150–200 mg twice daily; *Adjunctive therapy*— 50 mg twice daily; may ↑ weekly by 100 mg/day in 2 divided doses up to a maintenance dose of 100–200 mg twice daily; may also initiate therapy with 200-mg single loading dose followed 12 hr later by 100 mg twice daily for 1 wk; may ↑ weekly by 100 mg/day in 2 divided doses up to a maintenance dose of 4200 mg twice daily.

PO (Children 4–<17 yr and >50 kg): *Monotherapy*— 50 mg twice daily; may ↑ weekly by 100 mg/day in 2 divided doses up to a maintenance dose of 150–200 mg twice daily; *Adjunctive therapy*— 50 mg twice daily; may ↑ weekly by 100 mg/day in 2 divided doses up to a maintenance dose of 100–200 mg twice daily.

PO (Children 4–<17 yr and 30–<50 kg): *Monotherapy or adjunctive therapy*— 1 mg/kg twice daily; may ↑ weekly by 2 mg/kg/day in 2 divided doses up to a maintenance dose of 2–4 mg/kg twice daily.

PO (Children 4–<17 yr and 11–<30 kg): *Monotherapy or adjunctive therapy*— 1 mg/kg twice daily; may ↑ weekly by 2 mg/kg/day in 2 divided doses up to a maintenance dose of 3–6 mg/kg twice daily.

Hepatic/Renal Impairment

PO, IV (Adults): *CCr ≤30 mL/min or mild to moderate hepatic impairment*—Do not exceed 300 mg/day.

Availability

Oral solution: 10 mg/mL. **Solution for injection:** 10 mg/mL. **Tablets:** 50 mg, 100 mg, 150 mg, 200 mg.

NURSING IMPLICATIONS

Assessment

- Assess location, duration, and characteristics of seizure activity. Institute seizure precautions.
- Monitor closely for notable changes in behavior that could indicate the emergence or worsening of suicidal thoughts or behavior or depression.
- Assess patient for skin rash frequently during therapy. Discontinue at first sign of rash; may be life-threatening. Stevens-Johnson syndrome may develop. Treat symptomatically; may recur once treatment is stopped.
- Monitor for signs and symptoms of DRESS (fever, rash, lymphadenopathy, and/or facial swelling, associated with involvement of other organ systems (hepatitis, nephritis, hematologic abnormalities, myocarditis, myositis) during therapy. May resemble an acute viral infection. Eosinophilia is often present. Discontinue therapy if signs occur.
- **IV:** Assess ECG prior to therapy in patients with pre-existing cardiac disease before starting after titration to steady-state maintence. Monitor patients with cardiac conduction problems, on medications that prolong PR interval, or with severe cardiac disease (myocardial ischemia, heart failure) closely, as IV lacosamide may cause bradycardia or AV block.
- ***Lab Test Considerations:*** May cause ↑ ALT, which may return to normal without treatment.
- Monitor CBC and platelets periodically during therapy.

Implementation

- Do not confuse Vimpat (lacosamide) with Venofer (iron sucrose) or Vfend (voriconazole).
- IV administration is indicated for short term replacement (up to 5 days) when PO administration is not feasible. When switching from PO to IV, initial total daily dose should be equivalent to total daily dose and frequency of PO therapy. At end of IV period, may switch to PO at equivalent daily dose and frequency of IV therapy.
- When switching from another antiepileptic drug to lacosamide, administer 150 mg–200 mg twice daily for at least 3 days before beginning withdrawal of other antiepileptic drug. Gradually decrease other antiepileptic drug over 6 wk.
- When administering loading dose, monitor for CNS adverse reactions (dizziness, headache, nausea, somnolence, fatigue). May occur more frequently.
- When discontinuing lacosamide, gradually decrease dose over 1 wk.
- **PO:** May be administered with or without food. Swallow tablets whole with liquid; do not crush, break, or chew.
- Use a calibrated measuring device for accurate dosing of oral solution; household measures are not accurate. Discard any unused solution 7 wk after opening bottle.
- Oral solution may also be given via nasogastric tube or gastrostomy tube.

IV Administration

- **Intermittent Infusion:** ***Diluent:*** May be administered undiluted or diluted with 0.9% NaCl, D5W, or LR. ***Concentration:*** 10 mg/mL. Solution is clear and colorless; do not administer solutions that are discolored or contain a precipitate. Solution is stable for 4 hr at room temperature. Discard unused portion. ***Rate:*** Infuse over 15–60 min, preferably 30–60 min.

Patient/Family Teaching

- Instruct patient to take lacosamide around the clock, as directed. Medication should be gradually discontinued over at least 1 wk to prevent seizures. Advise patient to read the *Medication Guide* before starting therapy and with each Rx refill.
- May cause dizziness, ataxia, and syncope. Caution patient to avoid driving or other activities requiring alertness until response to medication is known. Tell patient not to resume driving until physician gives

clearance based on control of seizure disorder. If syncope occurs, advise patient to lay down with legs raised until recovered and notify health care professional.

- Inform patients and families of risk of suicidal thoughts and behavior and advise that behavioral changes, emergency or worsening signs and symptoms of depression, unusual changes in mood, or emergence of suicidal thoughts, behavior, or thoughts of self-harm, rash, or signs and symptoms of DRESS should be reported to health care professional immediately.
- Instruct patient to notify health care professional if signs of multiorgan hypersensitivity reactions (fever, rash, fatigue, jaundice, dark urine) occur.
- Advise patient to consult health care professional before taking other Rx, OTC, or herbal preparation and to avoid taking alcohol or other CNS depressants concurrently with lacosamide.
- Rep: Advise female patients to notify health care professional if pregnancy is planned or suspected or if breast feeding. Encourage pregnant patients to enroll in the North American Anticpileptic Drug (NAAED) pregnancy registry by calling 1-888-233–2334, call must be made by patient. Information on registry can be found at the website http://www.aedpregnancyregistry.org/.

Evaluation/Desired Outcomes

- Decreased seizure activity.

lactulose (lak-tyoo-lose)

Cholac, Constilac, Constulose, Enulose, Generlac, Kristalose

Classification
Therapeutic: laxatives
Pharmacologic: osmotics

Indications

Treatment of chronic constipation. Adjunct in the management of portal-systemic (hepatic) encephalopathy (PSE).

Action

Increases water content and softens the stool. Lowers the pH of the colon, which inhibits the diffusion of ammonia from the colon into the blood, thereby reducing blood ammonia levels. **Therapeutic Effects:** Relief of constipation. Decreased blood ammonia levels with improved mental status in PSE.

Pharmacokinetics

Absorption: Less than 3% absorbed after oral administration.
Distribution: Unknown.
Metabolism and Excretion: Absorbed lactulose is excreted unchanged in the urine. Unabsorbed lactulose is metabolized by colonic bacteria to lactic, acetic, and formic acids.
Half-life: Unknown.

TIME/ACTION PROFILE (relief of constipation)

ROUTE	ONSET	PEAK	DURATION
PO	24–48 hr	unknown	unknown

Contraindications/Precautions

Contraindicated in: Patients on low-galactose diets.
Use Cautiously in: Diabetes mellitus; Excessive or prolonged use (may lead to dependence); OB, Lactation: Safety not established.

Adverse Reactions/Side Effects

GI: belching, cramps, distention, flatulence, diarrhea.
Endo: hyperglycemia (diabetic patients).

Interactions

Drug-Drug: Should not be used with other **laxatives** in the treatment of hepatic encephalopathy (leads to inability to determine optimal dose of lactulose). **Anti-infectives** may ↓ effectiveness in treatment of hepatic encephalopathy.

Route/Dosage

Constipation

PO (Adults): 15–30 mL/day up to 60 mL/day as liquid or 10–20 g as powder for oral solution (up to 40 g/day has been used).
PO (Children): 7.5 mL daily after breakfast (unlabeled).

PSE

PO (Adults): 30–45 mL 3–4 times/day; may be given every 1–2 hr initially to induce laxation.
PO (Infants): 2.5–10 mL daily in 3–4 divided doses (unlabeled).
PO (Children and Adolescents): 40–90 mL daily in 3–4 divided doses (unlabeled).
Rect (Adults): 300 mL diluted and administered as a retention enema every 4–6 hr.

Availability (generic available)

Oral solution: 10 g lactulose/15 mL. **Rectal solution:** 10 g lactulose/15 mL. **Single-use packets (Kristalose):** 10 g (equal to 15 mL liquid lactulose), 20 g (equal to 30 mL liquid lactulose).

NURSING IMPLICATIONS

Assessment

- Assess patient for abdominal distention, presence of bowel sounds, and normal pattern of bowel function.

- Assess color, consistency, and amount of stool produced.
- **PSE:** Assess mental status (orientation, level of consciousness) before and periodically throughout course of therapy.
- ***Lab Test Considerations:*** ↓ blood ammonia concentrations by 25–50%.
- May cause ↑ blood glucose levels in diabetic patients.
- Monitor serum electrolytes periodically when used chronically. May cause diarrhea with resulting hypokalemia and hypernatremia.

Implementation

- When used in hepatic encephalopathy, adjust dose until patient averages 2–3 soft bowel movements per day. During initial therapy, 30–45 mL may be given hourly to induce rapid laxation.
- Darkening of solution does not alter potency.
- **PO:** Mix with fruit juice, water, milk, or carbonated citrus beverage to improve flavor. Administer with a full glass (240 mL) of water or juice. May be administered on an empty stomach for more rapid results.
- Dissolve single dose packets (Kristalose) in 4 oz of water. Solution should be colorless to slightly pale yellow.
- **Rect:** To administer enema, use rectal balloon catheter. Mix 300 mL of lactulose with 700 mL of water or 0.9% NaCl. Enema should be retained for 30–60 min. If inadvertently evacuated, may repeat administration.

Patient/Family Teaching

- Encourage patients to use other forms of bowel regulation, such as increasing bulk in the diet, increasing fluid intake, and increasing mobility. Normal bowel habits are individualized and may vary from 3 times/day to 3 times/wk.
- Caution patients that this medication may cause belching, flatulence, or abdominal cramping. Health care professional should be notified if this becomes bothersome or if diarrhea occurs.

Evaluation/Desired Outcomes

- Passage of a soft, formed bowel movement, usually within 24–48 hr.
- Clearing of confusion, apathy, and irritation, and improved mental status in PSE. Improvement may occur within 2 hr after enema and 24–48 hr after oral administration.

lamiVUDine (la-mi-vyoo-deen)

3TC, Epivir, Epivir-HBV, Heptovir

Classification

Therapeutic: antiretrovirals, antivirals

Pharmacologic: nucleoside reverse transcriptase inhibitors

Indications

HIV infection (with other antiretrovirals). Chronic hepatitis B infection. **Unlabeled Use:** Part of HIV-post-exposure prophylaxis with zidovudine and indinavir.

Action

After intracellular conversion to its active form (lamivudine-5-triphosphate), inhibits viral DNA synthesis by inhibiting the enzyme reverse transcriptase. **Therapeutic Effects:** Slows the progression of HIV infection and decreases the occurrence of its sequelae. Increases CD4 cell counts and decreases viral load. Protection from liver damage caused by chronic hepatitis B infection; decreases viral load.

Pharmacokinetics

Absorption: Well absorbed after oral administration (86% in adults, 66% in infants and children).

Distribution: Distributes into the extravascular space. Some penetration into CSF; remainder of distribution unknown.

Metabolism and Excretion: Mostly excreted unchanged in urine; <5% metabolized by the liver.

Half-life: *Adults*—3.7 hr; *children*—2 hr.

TIME/ACTION PROFILE (blood levels)

ROUTE	ONSET	PEAK	DURATION
PO	unknown	0.9 hr†	12 hr

†On an empty stomach; peak levels occur at 3.2 hr if lamivudine is taken with food. Food does not affect total amount of drug absorbed.

Contraindications/Precautions

Contraindicated in: Hypersensitivity; Concurrent use of antiretroviral combination products containing lamivudine or emtricitabine; Lactation: Breast feeding not recommended for HIV positive mothers.

Use Cautiously in: Impaired renal function (↑ dosing interval/↓ dose if CCr <50 mL/min); Women and obesity (↑ risk of lactic acidosis and severe hepatomegaly with steatosis); Coinfection with hepatitis B (hepatitis may recur after discontinuation of lamivudine; Epivir HBV is not indicated for treatment of HIV because lamivudine dosage is subtherapeutic); OB, Pedi: Pregnancy or children <3 mo (safety not established); Geri: ↓ dose may be necessary due to age-related ↓ in renal function.

Exercise Extreme Caution in: Pedi: Pediatric patients with a history of or significant risk factors for pancreatitis (use only if no alternative).

Adverse Reactions/Side Effects

Noted for combination of lamivudine plus zidovudine.

CNS: SEIZURES, fatigue, headache, insomnia, malaise, depression, dizziness. **Derm:** alopecia, erythema multiforme, rash, urticaria. **Endo:** hyperglycemia. **F and E:** lactic acidosis. **GI:** HEPATOMEGALY WITH STEATOSIS, PANCREATITIS (↑ in pediatric patients), anorexia, diarrhea, nausea, vomiting, abdominal discomfort, ↑ liver enzymes, dyspepsia. **Hemat:** anemia, neutropenia, pure red cell aplasia. **MS:** musculoskeletal pain, arthralgia, muscle weakness, myalgia, rhabdomyolysis. **Neuro:** neuropathy. **Resp:** cough. **Misc:** HYPERSENSITIVITY REACTIONS (including anaphylaxis), immune reconstitution syndrome.

Interactions

Drug-Drug: Trimethoprim/sulfamethoxazole may ↑ levels (dose alteration may be necessary in renal impairment). ↑ risk of pancreatitis with concurrent use of other **drugs causing pancreatitis.** ↑ risk of neuropathy with concurrent use of other **drugs causing neuropathy.** Combination therapy with **tenofovir** and **abacavir** may lead to virologic nonresponse and should not be used. **Sorbitol** may ↓ levels; avoid concurrent use.

Route/Dosage

HIV infection

PO (Adults): 150 mg twice daily or 300 mg once daily.
PO (Children ≥3 mo): *Oral solution*—5 mg/kg twice daily or 10 mg/kg once daily (max dose = 300 mg/day); *Tablets*—14–19 kg: 75 mg twice daily or 150 mg once daily; 20–24 kg: 75 mg in AM, 150 mg in PM or 225 mg once daily; ≥25 kg: 150 mg twice daily or 300 mg once daily.

Renal Impairment

(Adults and Children ≥25 kg): *CCr 30–49 mL/min*—150 mg once daily; *CCr 15–29 mL/min*—150 mg initially, then 100 mg once daily; *CCr 5–14 mL/min*—150 mg initially, then 50 mg once daily; *CCr <5 mL/min*—50 mg initially, then 25 mg once daily.

Chronic Hepatitis B

PO (Adults): 100 mg once daily.

Renal Impairment

PO (Adults): *CCr 30–49 mL/min*—100 mg first dose, then 50 mg once daily; *CCr 15–29 mL/min*—100 mg first dose, then 25 mg once daily; *CCr 5–14 mL/min*—35 mg first dose, then 15 mg once daily; *CCr <5 mL/min*—35 mg first dose, then 10 mg once daily.
PO (Children 2–17 yr): 3 mg/kg once daily (up to 100 mg/day).

Availability (generic available)

Epivir

Oral solution (strawberry-banana flavor): 10 mg/mL. **Tablets:** 150 mg, 300 mg. ***In combination with:*** abacavir (Epzicom); abacavir and dolutegravir (Triumeq); efavirenz and tenofovir disoproxil fumarate (Symfi); lamivudine (Dovato); tenofovir disoproxil fumarate (Cimduo, Temixys); zidovudine (Combivir); zidovudine and abacavir (Trizivir). See Appendix B.

Epivir-HBV

Oral solution (strawberry-banana flavor): 5 mg/mL. **Tablets:** 100 mg.

NURSING IMPLICATIONS

Assessment

- Assess patient, especially pediatric patients, for signs of pancreatitis (nausea, vomiting, abdominal pain) periodically during therapy. May require discontinuation of therapy.
- **HIV:** Assess patient for change in severity of symptoms of HIV infection and for symptoms of opportunistic infection during therapy.
- Monitor patient for signs and symptoms of peripheral neuropathy (tingling, burning, numbness, or pain in hands or feet); may be difficult to differentiate from peripheral neuropathy of severe HIV disease. May require discontinuation of therapy.
- **Chronic Hepatitis B Infection:** Monitor signs of hepatitis (jaundice, fatigue, anorexia, pruritus) during therapy.
- ***Lab Test Considerations:*** Monitor viral load and CD4 levels before and periodically during therapy.
- Monitor serum amylase, lipase, and triglycerides periodically during therapy. Elevated serum levels may indicate pancreatitis and require discontinuation.
- Monitor liver function. May cause ↑ levels of AST, ALT, CPK, bilirubin, and alkaline phosphatase, which usually resolve after interruption of therapy. Lactic acidosis may occur with hepatic toxicity causing hepatic steatosis; may be fatal, especially in women.
- May rarely cause neutropenia and anemia.

Implementation

- Do not confuse lamivudine with lamotrigine. Do not confuse Epivir tablets and oral solution with Epivir-HBV tablets and oral solutions. Epivir Tablets and Oral Solution contain a higher dose of the same active ingredient (lamivudine) as Epivir-HBV Tablets and Oral Solution. Epivir-HBV was developed for patients with hepatitis B; do not use for patients dually infected with HIV and hepatitis B; use may lead to lamivudine-resistant HIV due to subtherapeutic dose.
- **PO:** May be administered without regard to food.
- Epivir scored tablet is preferred for HIV-1-infected pediatric patients weighing at least 14 kg and able to swallow pill; solution is associated with higher resistance rates. Before prescribing, assess for ability to swallow tablets. For patients unable to safely and reliably swallow tablets, oral solution may be used.

Patient/Family Teaching

- Instruct patient to take lamivudine as directed, every 12 hr. Explain the difference between Epivir and Epivir-HBV to patients. Emphasize the importance of compliance with full course of therapy, not taking more than the prescribed amount, and not discon-

L

tinuing without consulting health care professional; discontinuation may lead to deterioration of liver disease. Take missed doses as soon as possible unless almost time for next dose. Do not double doses. Caution patient not to share medication with others. Advise patient to read *Patient Information* before starting and with each Rx refill in case of changes.

- Inform patient that lamivudine does not cure HIV disease or prevent associated or opportunistic infections. Lamivudine does not reduce the risk of transmission of HIV to others through sexual contact or blood contamination. Caution patient to use a condom during sexual contact and avoid sharing needles or donating blood to prevent spreading HIV to others. Advise patient that the long-term effects of lamivudine are unknown at this time.
- Instruct patient to notify health care professional promptly if signs of peripheral neuropathy, pancreatitis, lactic acidosis (feel very weak or tired; feel cold, especially in arms and legs; unusual muscle pain; feel dizzy or light-headed; trouble breathing; fast or irregular heartbeat; stomach pain with nausea and vomiting), liver problems (yellowing of skin or white part of eyes; loss of appetite; nausea; dark or "tea-colored" urine; pain, aching, or tenderness on right side of abdomen; light-colored stools) or Immune Reconstitution Syndrome (signs and symptoms of an infection, Mycobacterium avium infection, cytomegalovirus, Pneumocystis jirovecii pneumonia, tuberculosis) occur.
- Inform patient that redistribution and accumulation of body fat may occur, causing central obesity, dorsocervical fat enlargement (buffalo hump), peripheral wasting, breast enlargement, and cushingoid appearance. The cause and long-term effects are not known.
- Instruct patient to notify health care professional of all Rx or OTC medications, vitamins, or herbal products being taken and to consult health care professional before taking other Rx, OTC, or herbal products.
- Rep: Instruct females using hormonal contraceptives to use an alternative nonhormonal method of contraception. Advise patient to notify health care professional if pregnancy is planned or suspected and to avoid breast feeding. If pregnant patient is exposed to lamivudine, register patient in *Antiretroviral Pregnancy Registry* by calling 1-800-258-4263.
- Emphasize the importance of regular follow-up exams and blood tests to determine progress and monitor for side effects.

Evaluation/Desired Outcomes

- Slowing of the progression of HIV infection and its sequelae.
- Decrease in viral load and improvement in CD4 levels in patients with advanced HIV infection.
- Protection from liver damage caused by chronic hepatitis B infection; decreases viral load.

lamoTRIgine (la-moe-tri-jeen)

LaMICtal, LaMICtal ODT, LaMICtal XR

Classification
Therapeutic: anticonvulsants

Indications

Adjunct treatment of partial seizures in adults and children with epilepsy (immediate-release, extended-release, chewable, and orally disintegrating tablets). Lennox-Gastaut syndrome (immediate-release, chewable, and orally disintegrating tablets only). Adjunct treatment of primary generalized tonic-clonic seizures in adults and children (immediate-release, extended-release, chewable, and orally disintegrating tablets). Conversion to monotherapy in adults with partial seizures receiving carbamazepine, phenytoin, phenobarbital, primidone, or valproate as the single antiepileptic drug (immediate-release, extended-release, chewable, and orally disintegrating tablets only). Maintenance treatment of bipolar disorder (immediate-release, chewable, and orally disintegrating tablets only).

Action

Stabilizes neuronal membranes by inhibiting sodium transport. **Therapeutic Effects:** Decreased incidence of seizures. Delayed time to recurrence of mood episodes in bipolar disorder.

Pharmacokinetics

Absorption: 98% absorbed following oral administration.
Distribution: Enters breast milk. Highly bound to melanin-containing tissues (eyes, pigmented skin).
Metabolism and Excretion: Mostly metabolized by the liver via glucuronidation to inactive metabolites; 10% excreted unchanged by the kidneys.
Half-life: Children taking enzyme–inducing antiepileptic drugs (AEDs): 7–10 hr; Children taking enzyme inducers and valproic acid: 15–27 hr; Children taking valproic acid: 44–94 hr; Adults: 25.4 hr (during chronic therapy of lamotrigine alone).

TIME/ACTION PROFILE (blood levels)

ROUTE	ONSET	PEAK	DURATION
PO	unknown	1.4–4.8 hr; 4–10 hr (XR)	unknown

Contraindications/Precautions

Contraindicated in: Hypersensitivity; Acute manic or mixed episodes.
Use Cautiously in: All patients (may ↑ risk of suicidal thoughts/behaviors); Patients with renal impairment, impaired cardiac function, and hepatic impairment (lower maintenance doses may be required); Prior history of rash to lamotrigine; OB: Exposure during first trimester may ↑ risk of cleft lip/palate; Lactation: Enters breast milk; use while breast feeding only if

potential maternal benefit justifies potential risk to infant; Pedi: Immediate-release, chewable, and orally disintegrating tablets not safe for children <2 yr; extended-release tablets not approved for use in children <13 yr.

Adverse Reactions/Side Effects

CNS: ASEPTIC MENINGITIS, SUICIDAL THOUGHTS, ataxia, dizziness, headache, behavior changes, depression, drowsiness, insomnia, tremor. **Derm:** DRUG REACTION WITH EOSINOPHILIA AND SYSTEMIC SYMPTOMS (DRESS), STEVENS-JOHNSON SYNDROME, photosensitivity, rash (higher incidence in children, patients taking valproic acid, high initial doses, or rapid dose increases). **EENT:** blurred vision, double vision, rhinitis. **GI:** HEPATIC FAILURE, nausea, vomiting. **GU:** vaginitis. **Hemat:** HEMOPHAGOCYTIC LYMPHOHISTIOCYTOSIS. **MS:** arthralgia.

Interactions

Drug-Drug: Concurrent use with **carbamazepine** may ↑ levels of an active metabolite of carbamazepine. Concurrent use with drugs that induce glucuronidation, including **phenobarbital**, **phenytoin**, **primidone**, **carbamazepine**, **estrogen-containing oral contraceptives**, **rifampin**, **lopinavir/ritonavir**, or **atazanavir/ritonavir** may ↓ levels; lamotrigine dose adjustments may be necessary when starting and stopping oral contraceptive or atazanavir/ritonavir therapy. Concurrent use with drugs that inhibit glucuronidation, including **valproic acid**, may ↑ levels and ↑ incidence of rash; may also ↓ valproic acid levels (↓ lamotrigine dose by at least 50%).

Route/Dosage

Epilepsy

In Combination with Other Antiepileptic Agents

PO (Adults and Children >12 yr; Immediate-release, chewable, or orally disintegrating tablets): *Patients taking anti-epileptic drugs other than carbamazepine, phenobarbital, phenytoin, primidone, or valproate*— 25 mg once daily for first 2 wk, then 50 mg once daily for next 2 wk; then ↑ by 50 mg/day every 1–2 wk to maintenance dose of 225–375 mg/day (in 2 divided doses); *Patients taking carbamazepine, phenobarbital, phenytoin, or primidone (and not valproate)* — 50 mg once daily for first 2 wk, then 50 mg twice daily for next 2 wk; then ↑ by 100 mg/day every 1–2 wk to maintenance dose of 300–500 mg/day (in 2 divided doses); *Patients taking regimen containing valproate*— 25 mg every other day for first 2 wk, then 25 mg once daily for next 2 wk; then ↑ by 25–50 mg/day every 1–2 wk to maintenance dose of 100–400 mg/day (in 1–2 divided doses) (maintenance dose of 100–200 mg/day if receiving valproate alone).

PO (Adults and Children ≥13 yr; Extended-release tablets): *Patients taking anti-epileptic drugs other than carbamazepine, phenobarbital, phenytoin, primidone, or valproate*— 25 mg once daily for first 2 wk, then 50 mg once daily for next 2 wk; then 100 mg once daily for 1 wk, then 150 mg once daily for 1 wk, then 200 mg once daily for 1 wk, then ↑ by 100 mg/day every wk to maintenance dose of 300–400 mg once daily; *Patients taking carbamazepine, phenobarbital, phenytoin, or primidone (and not valproate)* — 50 mg once daily for first 2 wk, then 100 mg once daily for next 2 wk, then 200 mg once daily for 1 wk, then 300 mg once daily for 1 wk, then 400 mg once daily for 1 wk, then ↑ by 100 mg/day every wk to maintenance dose of 400–600 mg once daily; *Patients taking regimen containing valproate*— 25 mg every other day for first 2 wk, then 25 mg once daily for next 2 wk, then 50 mg once daily for 1 wk, then 100 mg once daily for 1 wk, then 150 mg once daily for 1 wk, then maintenance dose of 200–250 mg once daily.

PO (Children 2–12 yr; Immediate-release, chewable, or orally disintegrating tablets): *Patients taking anti-epileptic drugs other than carbamazepine, phenobarbital, phenytoin, primidone, or valproate* — 0.3 mg/kg/day in 1–2 divided doses (rounded down to nearest whole tablet) for first 2 wk, then 0.6 mg/kg/day in 2 divided doses (rounded down to nearest whole tablet) for next 2 wk; then ↑ by 0.6 mg/kg/day (rounded down to nearest whole tablet) every 1–2 wk to maintenance dose of 4.5–7.5 mg/kg/day (not to exceed 300 mg/day in 2 divided doses); *Patients taking carbamazepine, phenobarbital, phenytoin, or primidone (and not valproate)*— 0.6 mg/kg/day in 2 divided doses (rounded down to nearest whole tablet) for first 2 wk, then 1.2 mg/kg/day in 2 divided doses (rounded down to nearest whole tablet) for next 2 wk; then ↑ by 1.2 mg/kg/day (rounded down to nearest whole tablet) every 1–2 wk to maintenance dose of 5–15 mg/kg/day (not to exceed 400 mg/day in 2 divided doses). *Patients taking regimen containing valproate*— 0.15 mg/kg/day in 1–2 divided doses (rounded down to nearest whole tablet) for first 2 wk, then 0.3 mg/kg in 1–2 divided doses (rounded down to nearest whole tablet) for next 2 wk; then ↑ by 0.3 mg/kg/day (rounded down to nearest whole tablet) every 1–2 wk to maintenance dose of 1–5 mg/kg/day (not to exceed 200 mg/day in 1–2 divided doses) (maintenance dose of 1–3 mg/kg/day if receiving valproate alone).

Conversion to Monotherapy

PO (Adults and Children ≥16 yr; Immediate-release, chewable, or orally disintegrating tablets): *Patients taking carbamazepine, phenobarbital, phenytoin, or primidone (and not valproate)*—After achieving a dose of 500 mg/day (as per dosing guide-

L

lines above), ↓ dose of other antiepileptic by 20% weekly over 4 wk; *Patients taking regimen containing valproate*—After achieving a dose of 200 mg/day (as per dosing guidelines above), ↓ valproate dose by 500 mg/day on a weekly basis until a dose of 500 mg/day is achieved. Maintain the valproate dose of 500 mg/day and the lamotrigine dose of 500 mg/day for 1 wk. Then ↑ lamotrigine dose to 300 mg/day and ↓ valproate dose to 250 mg/day, and maintain these doses for 1 wk. Then discontinue valproate and ↑ lamotrigine dose by 100 mg/day every wk until maintenance dose of 500 mg/day is achieved.

PO (Adults and Children ≥13 yr; Extended-release tablets): *Patients taking carbamazepine, phenobarbital, phenytoin, or primidone (and not valproate)*—After achieving a dose of 500 mg/day (as per dosing guidelines above), ↓ dose of other antiepileptic by 20% weekly over 4 wk. Two wk later, ↓ dose of lamotrigine by 100 mg/day every wk to achieve maintenance dose of 250–300 mg/day; *Patients taking regimen containing valproate*—After achieving a dose of 150 mg/day (as per dosing guidelines above), ↓ valproate dose by 500 mg/day on a weekly basis until a dose of 500 mg/day is achieved. Maintain the valproate dose of 500 mg/day and the lamotrigine dose of 150 mg/day for 1 wk. Then ↑ lamotrigine dose to 200 mg/day and ↓ valproate dose to 250 mg/day, and maintain these doses for 1 wk. Then discontinue valproate and ↑ lamotrigine dose to 250–300 mg/day; *Patients taking anti-epileptic drugs other than carbamazepine, phenobarbital, phenytoin, primidone, or valproate* —After achieving a dose of 250–300 mg/day (as per dosing guidelines above), ↓ dose of other antiepileptic by 20% weekly over 4 wk.

Bipolar Disorder

Escalation Regimen

PO (Adults): *Patients not taking cabamazepine, phenobarbital, phenytoin, primidone, rifampin, or valproate*—25 mg once daily for first 2 wk, then 50 mg once daily for next 2 wk, then 100 mg once daily for 1 wk, then 200 mg once daily; *Patients taking valproate*—25 mg every other day for first 2 wk, then 25 mg once daily for next 2 wk, then 50 mg once daily for 1 wk, then 100 mg once daily; *Patients taking carbamazepine, phenobarbital, phenytoin, primidone, or rifampin (and not valproate)* 50 mg once daily for first 2 wk, then 100 mg/day (in divided doses) for next 2 wk, then 200 mg/day (in divided doses) for one wk, then 300 mg/day (in divided doses) for 1 wk, then up to 400 mg/day (in divided doses).

Dosage Adjustment Following Discontinuation of Other Psychotropics

PO (Adults): *Following discontinuation of valproate (if current dose 100 mg/day)*—↑ to 150 mg/day for 1 wk, then 200 mg/day; *Following discontinuation of carbamazepine, phenobarbital, phenytoin, primidone, or rifampin (if current dose 400 mg/day)*—400 mg/day for 1 wk, then 300 mg/day for 1 wk, then 200 mg/day; *Following discontinuation of other psychotropics*—maintain previous dose.

Availability (generic available)

Chewable dispersible tablets: 2 mg, 5 mg, 25 mg. **Cost:** *Generic*—5 mg $305.33/100, 25 mg $319.80/100. **Extended-release tablets:** 25 mg, 50 mg, 100 mg, 200 mg, 250 mg, 300 mg. **Cost:** *Generic*—25 mg $196.43/30, 50 mg $392.81/30, 100 mg $420.77/30, 200 mg $448.70/30, 250 mg $611.88/30, 300 mg $673.07/30. **Immediate-release tablets:** 25 mg, 100 mg, 150 mg, 200 mg. **Cost:** *Generic*—25 mg $415.96/100, 100 mg $475.12/100, 150 mg $312.44/100, 200 mg $340.15/100. **Orally disintegrating tablets:** 25 mg, 50 mg, 100 mg, 200 mg. **Cost:** 25 mg $218.27/30, 50 mg $233.78/30, 100 mg $249.29/30, 200 mg $297.47/30.

NURSING IMPLICATIONS

Assessment

- Monitor closely for notable changes in behavior that could indicate the emergence or worsening of suicidal thoughts or behavior or depression.
- Assess patient for skin rash frequently during therapy. Discontinue lamotrigine at first sign of rash; may be life-threatening. Stevens-Johnson syndrome or toxic epidermal necrolysis may develop. Rash usually occurs during the initial 2–8 wk of therapy and is more frequent in patients taking multiple antiepileptic agents, especially valproic acid, and much more frequent in patients <16 yr.
- Monitor for signs and symptoms of multiorgan hypersensitivity reactions—DRESS (rash, fever, lymphadenopathy). May be associated with other organ involvement (hepatitis, hepatic failure, blood dyscrasias, acute multiorgan failure). If cause cannot be determined, discontinue lamotrigine immediately.
- **Seizures:** Assess location, duration, and characteristics of seizure activity.
- **Bipolar disorders:** Assess mood, ideation, and behaviors frequently. Initiate suicide precautions if indicated.
- ***Lab Test Considerations:*** Lamotrigine plasma concentrations may be monitored periodically during therapy, especially in patients concurrently taking other anticonvulsants. Therapeutic plasma concentration range has not been established, proposed therapeutic range: 1–5 mcg/mL.
- May cause false-positive results for phencyclidine (PCP) in some rapid urine drug screens. Use a more specific analytical method to confirm results.

Implementation

- Do not confuse lamotrigine with labetalol, lamivudine, levetiracetam, or levothyroxine. Do not confuse Lamical with labetalol or Lamisil (terbinafine).
- When converting from immediate-release to XR form, initial dose of XR should match the total daily

dose of immediate-release lamotrigine; monitor closely and adjust as needed.

- **PO:** May be administered without regard to meals. Swallow XR tablets whole; do not break, crush, or chew.
- Lamotrigine should be discontinued gradually over at least 2 wk, unless safety concerns require a more rapid withdrawal. Abrupt discontinuation may cause increase in seizure frequency.
- **Orally Disintegrating Tablets:** Place on the tongue and move around the mouth. Tablet will rapidly disintegrate, can be swallowed with or without water, and can be taken with or without food.
- **Chewable/Dispersible Tablets:** May be swallowed whole, chewed, or dispersed in water or dispersed in fruit juice. If chewed, follow with water or fruit juice to aid in swallowing. Only use whole tablets, do not attempt to administer partial quantities of dispersible tablets.

Patient/Family Teaching

- Instruct patient to take medication exactly as directed. Take missed doses as soon as possible unless almost time for next dose. Do not double doses. Do not discontinue abruptly; may cause increase in frequency of seizures. Instruct patient to read the *Medication Guide* before starting and with each Rx refill, changes may occur.
- Advise patient to notify health care professional immediately if skin rash, fever, or swollen lymph glands occur or if frequency of seizures increases.
- May cause dizziness, drowsiness, and blurred vision. Caution patient to avoid driving or activities requiring alertness until response to medication is known. Do not resume driving until physician gives clearance based on control of seizure disorder.
- Caution patient to wear sunscreen and protective clothing to prevent photosensitivity reactions.
- Advise patient and family to notify health care professional if thoughts about suicide or dying, attempts to commit suicide; new or worse depression; new or worse anxiety; feeling very agitated or restless; panic attacks; trouble sleeping; new or worse irritability; acting aggressive; being angry or violent; acting on dangerous impulses; an extreme increase in activity and talking; other unusual changes in behavior or mood or if symptoms of aseptic meningitis (headache, fever, nausea, vomiting, and nuchal rigidity, rash, photophobia, myalgia, chills, altered consciousness, somnolence) occur.
- Instruct patient to notify health care professional of medication regimen prior to treatment or surgery.
- Advise patient to notify health care professional immediately if signs and symptoms of hemophagocytic lymphohistiocytosis (fever, hepatosplenomegaly, rash, lymphadenopathy, neurologic symptoms, cytopenias, high serum ferritin, hypertriglyceridemia, liver function, coagulation abnormalities) occur. Symptoms usually occur between 8 and 24 days. May be fatal.
- Rep: Advise female patients to use a nonhormonal form of contraception while taking lamotrigine, to avoid breast feeding, and to notify health care professional if pregnancy is planned or suspected. Encourage patients who become pregnant to enroll in the North American Antiepileptic Drug Pregnancy Registry. Must be done by patients themselves by calling 1-888-233-2334 or on the website http://www.aedpregnancyregistry.org.
- Advise patient to carry identification at all times describing disease process and medication regimen.

Evaluation/Desired Outcomes

- Decrease in the frequency of or cessation of seizures.
- Delay in time to occurrence of mood episodes (depression, mania, hypomania, mixed episodes) in patients with Bipolar I disorder.

BEERS

lansoprazole (lan-soe-pra-zole)

Prevacid, Prevacid 24 Hr, Prevacid SoluTab

Classification

Therapeutic: antiulcer agents

Pharmacologic: proton-pump inhibitors

Indications

Erosive esophagitis. Duodenal ulcers (with or without anti-infectives for *Helicobacter pylori*). Active benign gastric ulcer. Short-term treatment of symptomatic GERD. Healing and risk reduction of NSAID-associated gastric ulcer. Pathologic hypersecretory conditions, including Zollinger-Ellison syndrome. **OTC:** Heartburn occurring ≥twice/wk.

Action

Binds to an enzyme in the presence of acidic gastric pH, preventing the final transport of hydrogen ions into the gastric lumen. **Therapeutic Effects:** Diminished accumulation of acid in the gastric lumen, with lessened acid reflux. Healing of duodenal ulcers and esophagitis.

Pharmacokinetics

Absorption: 80% absorbed after oral administration.

Distribution: Unknown.

Protein Binding: 97%.

Metabolism and Excretion: Extensively metabolized by the liver to inactive compounds. Converted in-

tracellularly to at least two other antisecretory compounds.
Half-life: Children: 1.2–1.5 hr; Adults: 1.3–1.7 hr (↑ in geriatric patients and patients with impaired hepatic function).

TIME/ACTION PROFILE (acid suppression)

ROUTE	ONSET	PEAK	DURATION
PO	rapid	1.7 hr	more than 24 hr

Contraindications/Precautions

Contraindicated in: Hypersensitivity; Concurrent use of rilpivirine-containing products.
Use Cautiously in: Solutabs contain aspartame; use caution in patients with phenylketonuria; Severe hepatic impairment (not to exceed 30 mg/day in these patients); Patients using high-doses for >1 yr (↑ risk of hip, wrist, or spine fractures and fundic gland polyps); Patients using therapy for >3 yr (↑ risk of vitamin B_{12} deficiency); OB, Lactation: Safety not established; Geri: Maintenance dose not to exceed 30 mg/day unless additional acid suppression is required; Pedi: Children <1 yr (safety not established).

Adverse Reactions/Side Effects

CNS: dizziness, headache. **Derm:** cutaneous lupus erythematosus, rash. **F and E:** hypomagnesemia (especially if treatment duration ≥3 mo). **GI:** CLOSTRIDIUM DIFFICILE-ASSOCIATED DIARRHEA (CDAD), diarrhea, abdominal pain, fundic gland polyps, nausea. **GU:** acute interstitial nephritis. **Hemat:** vitamin B_{12} deficiency. **MS:** bone fracture. **Misc:** systemic lupus erythematosus.

Interactions

Drug-Drug: May ↓ **rilpivirine** levels and ↑ risk of resistance; concurrent use contraindicated. **Sucralfate** ↓ absorption of lansoprazole (take 30 min before sucralfate). May ↓ absorption of drugs requiring acid pH, including **ketoconazole**, **itraconazole**, **atazanavir**, **nelfinavir**, **ampicillin esters**, **iron salts**, **erlotinib**, and **mycophenolate mofetil**; avoid concurrent use with **atazanavir** and **nelfinavir**. May ↑ levels of **digoxin tacrolimus**, and **methotrexate**. May ↑ risk of bleeding with **warfarin** (monitor INR/PT). Hypomagnesemia ↑ risk of **digoxin** toxicity.

Route/Dosage

PO (Adults): *Short-term treatment of duodenal ulcer*—15 mg once daily for 4 wk; *H. pylori eradication to reduce the risk of duodenal ulcer recurrence*—30 mg twice daily with clarithromycin 500 mg twice daily and amoxicillin 1000 mg twice daily for 10–14 days (triple therapy) or 30 mg 3 times daily with 1000 mg amoxicillin 3 times daily for 14 days (dual therapy); *Maintenance of healed duodenal ulcers*—15 mg once daily; *Short-term treatment of gastric ulcers/healing of NSAID-associated gastric ulcer*—30 mg once daily for up to 8 wk; *Risk reduction of NSAID-associated gastric ulcer*—15 mg once daily for up to 12 wk; *Short-term treatment of symptomatic GERD*—15 mg once daily for up to 8 wk; *Short-term treatment of erosive esophagitis*—30 mg once daily for up to 8 wk (8 additional wk may be necessary); *Maintenance of healing of erosive esophagitis*—15 mg once daily; *Pathologic hypersecretory conditions*—60 mg once daily intially, up to 90 mg twice daily (daily dose >120 mg should be given in divided doses).
PO (Adults): *OTC*—15 mg once daily for up to 14 days (14 day course may be repeated every 4 mo).
PO (Children 12–17 yr): *Non-erosive GERD*—15 mg once daily for up to 8 wk; *Erosive esophagitis*—30 mg once daily for up to 8 wk.
PO (Children 1–11 yr and >30 kg): *GERD and Erosive Esophagitis*—30 mg once daily for up to 12 wk.
PO (Children 1–11 yr and ≤30 kg): *GERD and Erosive Esophagitis*—15 mg once daily for up to 12 wk.

Availability (generic available)

Delayed-release capsules: 15 mg[Rx, OTC], 30 mg. **Delayed-release orally disintegrated tablets (SoluTabs):** 15 mg[Rx, OTC], 30 mg. ***In combination with:*** amoxicillin and clarithromycin as part of a compliance package (Prevpac). See Appendix B.

NURSING IMPLICATIONS

Assessment

- Assess patient routinely for epigastric or abdominal pain and for frank or occult blood in stool, emesis, or gastric aspirate.
- Monitor bowel function. Diarrhea, abdominal cramping, fever, and bloody stools should be reported to health care professional promptly as a sign of Clostridium difficile-associated diarrhea (CDAD). May begin up to several wk following cessation of therapy.
- ***Lab Test Considerations:*** May cause abnormal liver function tests, including ↑ AST, ALT, alkaline phosphatase, LDH, and bilirubin.
- May cause ↑ serum creatinine and ↑ or ↓ electrolyte levels.
- May alter RBC, WBC, and platelet levels.
- May also cause ↑ gastrin levels, abnormal A/G ratio, hyperlipidemia, and ↑ or ↓ cholesterol.
- Monitor INR and prothrombin time in patients taking warfarin.
- May cause hypomagnesemia. Monitor serum magnesium prior to and periodically during therapy.
- May cause vitamin B_{12} deficiency with long term use (>3 yrs).
- May ↑ serum chromogranin levels which may interfere with diagnosis of neuroendocrine tumors.

Implementation

- **PO:** *Delayed-release capsules:* Administer before meals. Swallow whole; do not crush or chew capsule contents. Capsules may be opened and sprinkled on 1 tbsp of applesauce, *Ensure,* pudding, cottage cheese, yogurt, or strained pears and swallowed immediately for patients with difficulty swallowing.

- For patients with an NG tube, capsules may be opened and intact granules may be mixed in 40 mL of apple juice and injected through the NG tube into stomach. Flush NG tube with additional apple juice to clear tube.
- *Orally disintegrating tablets* may be placed on tongue, allowed to disintegrate and swallowed with or without water. Do not cut or break tablet. For administration via oral syringe or nasogastric tube, *Prevacid SoluTab* can be administered by placing a 15-mg tablet in oral syringe and drawing up 4 mL of water, or a 30-mg tablet in oral syringe and drawing up 10 mL of water. Shake gently to allow for a quick dispersal. After tablet has dispersed, administer the contents within 15 min. Refill syringe with 2 mL (5 mL for the 30-mg tablet) of water, shake gently, and administer any remaining contents and flush nasogastric tube.
- Antacids may be used concurrently.

Patient/Family Teaching

- Instruct patient to take medication as directed for the full course of therapy, even if feeling better. Take missed doses as soon as remembered unless almost time for next dose; do not double doses. Advise patient to read *Medication Guide* before starting and with each Rx refill in case of changes.
- May occasionally cause dizziness. Caution patient to avoid driving and other activities that require alertness until response to medication is known.
- Advise patient to avoid alcohol, products containing aspirin or NSAIDs, and foods that may cause an increase in GI irritation.
- Advise patient to report onset of black, tarry stools; diarrhea; or abdominal pain to health care professional promptly. Instruct patient to notify health care professional immediately if rash, diarrhea, abdominal cramping, fever, or bloody stools occur and not to treat with antidiarrheals without consulting health care professional.
- Instruct patient to notify health care professional of all Rx or OTC medications, vitamins, or herbal products being taken and consult health care professional before taking any new medications.
- Advise female patient to notify health care professional if pregnancy is planned or suspected or if breast feeding.

Evaluation/Desired Outcomes

- Decrease in abdominal pain or prevention of gastric irritation and bleeding. Healing of duodenal ulcers can be seen on x-ray examination or endoscopy. Therapy is continued for at least 2–4 wk. Therapy for pathologic hypersecretory conditions may be long term.
- Healing in patients with erosive esophagitis. Therapy is continued for up to 8 wk, and an additional 8-wk course may be used for patients who do not heal in 8 wk or whose ulcer recurs.

lanthanum carbonate
(lan-than-um)
Fosrenol

Classification
Therapeutic: hypophosphatemics
Pharmacologic: phosphate binders

Indications

Reduction of serum phosphate levels associated with end-stage renal disease.

Action

Dissociates in the upper GI tract forming lanthanate ions, which form an insoluble complex with phosphate. **Therapeutic Effects:** Decreased serum phosphate levels.

Pharmacokinetics

Absorption: Negligible absorption.
Distribution: Stays within the GI tract.
Metabolism and Excretion: Eliminated almost entirely in feces.
Half-life: 53 hr (in plasma).

TIME/ACTION PROFILE (effect on phosphate levels)

ROUTE	ONSET	PEAK	DURATION
PO	unknown	2–3 wk	unknown

Contraindications/Precautions

Contraindicated in: Bowel obstruction; Ileus; Fecal impaction; OB: Congenital abnormalities noted in animal studies; Pedi: Potential negative effect on developing bone.
Use Cautiously in: Patients with risk factors for GI obstruction or perforation, including history of GI surgery, colon cancer, or GI ulceration, diverticular disease, peritonitis, constipation, ileus, diabetic gastroparesis, or taking medications that cause constipation; Lactation: Safety not established.

Adverse Reactions/Side Effects

GI: nausea, vomiting, diarrhea, fecal impaction, GI obstruction, GI perforation, ileus. **F and E:** hypocalcemia.

Interactions

Drug-Drug: May ↓ absorption of **fluoroquinolones**, **tetracyclines**, and **levothyroxine**; administer at least 1 hr before or 3 hr after lanthanum carbonate.

Route/Dosage

PO (Adults): 1500 mg/day in divided doses; may be titrated upward every 2–3 wk in increments of 750 mg/day up to 4500 mg/day (usual range 1500–3000 mg/day).

Availability (generic available)

Chewable tablets: 250 mg, 500 mg, 750 mg, 1000 mg. **Oral powder:** 750 mg/pkt, 1000 mg/pkt.

NURSING IMPLICATIONS

Assessment

- Assess patient for nausea and vomiting during therapy.
- ***Lab Test Considerations:*** Monitor serum phosphate levels prior to and periodically during therapy.

Implementation

- Do not confuse lanthanum carbonate with lithium carbonate.
- Divide total daily dose and administer with meals.
- **PO:** Administer with or immediately after meals. Tablets should be crushed or chewed completely before swallowing; intact tablets should not be swallowed.
- Sprinkle powder on small quantity of applesauce or other similar food; consume immediately. Consider powder formulation for patients with poor dentition or who have difficulty chewing tablets.

Patient/Family Teaching

- Instruct patient to take lanthanum as directed.

Evaluation/Desired Outcomes

- Decrease in serum phosphate to below than 6.0 mg/dL in patients with end stage renal disease.

lapatinib (la-pat-i-nib)

Tykerb

Classification

Therapeutic: antineoplastics

Pharmacologic: enzyme inhibitors, kinase inhibitors

Indications

Advanced or metastatic breast cancer with tumor overexpression of the Human Epidermal Receptor Type 2 (HER2) and past therapy with an anthracycline, a taxane and trastuzumab (used in combination with capecitabine). Postmenopausal women with hormone-receptor positive metastatic breast cancer that overexpresses HER2 for whom hormonal therapy is indicated (used in combination with letrozole).

Action

Acts as an inhibitor of intracellular tyrosine kinase affecting Epidermal Growth Factor (EGFR, ErbB1) and HER2 (ErbB2). Inhibits the growth of ErbB-driven tumors. Effect is additive with capecitabine. **Therapeutic Effects:** Decreased/slowed spread of metastatic breast cancer.

Pharmacokinetics

Absorption: Incompletely and variably absorbed following oral administration; blood levels ↑ by food.

Distribution: Unknown.

Protein Binding: >99%.

Metabolism and Excretion: Extensively metabolized by, mostly by CYP3A4 and CYP3A5 enzyme systems; <2% excreted by kidneys.

Half-life: 24 hr.

TIME/ACTION PROFILE (blood levels)

ROUTE	ONSET	PEAK	DURATION
PO	unknown	4 hr	24 hr

Contraindications/Precautions

Contraindicated in: Hypersensitivity; ↓ left ventricular ejection fraction (Grade 2 or greater); OB, Lactation: Pregnancy or lactation.

Use Cautiously in: Concurrent use of CYP3A4 inhibitors including ketoconazole, itraconazole, clarithromycin, atazanavir, indinavir, nefazodone, nelfinavir, ritoanvir, saquinavir, and voriconazole should be avoided (if necessary, ↓ lapatinib dose); Concurrent use of CYP3A4 inducers including dexamathasone, phenytoin, carbamazepine, rifampin, rifabutin, rifapentin, phenobarbital, and St. John's wort should be avoided (if necessary, ↑ lapatinib dose; Severe hepatic impairment (dose ↓ recommended for Child-Pugh Class C); Known QTc interval prolongation or co-existing risk factors for QTc interval prolongation including hypokalemia, hypomagnesemia, concurrent antiarrhythmics or medications that are known to prolong the QTc interval; Geri: May be more sensitive to effects; Pedi: Safety not established.

Adverse Reactions/Side Effects

CNS: fatigue, insomnia. **Resp:** dyspnea, interstitial lung disease, pneumonitis. **CV:** ↓ left ventricular ejection fraction, QT interval prolongation. **GI:** DIARRHEA, HEPATOTOXICITY, nausea, vomiting, dyspepsia, ↑ liver enzymes, stomatitis. **Derm:** ERYTHEMA MULTIFORM, STEVENS-JOHNSON SYNDROME, TOXIC EPIDERMAL NECROLYSIS, palmar-plantar erythrodysesthesia, rash, dry skin, nail disorders. **Hemat:** neutropenia. **MS:** back pain, extremity pain.

Interactions

Drug-Drug: Lapatinib inhibits CYP3A4, CYP28, and P-glycoprotein; concurrent use of drugs which are substrates for these enzymes should be undertaken with caution. May ↑ effects of **midazolam**, **paclitaxel**, and

digoxin. Concurrent use of **strong CYP3A4 inhibitors** including **ketoconazole**, **itraconazole**, **clarithromycin**, **atazanavir**, **indinavir**, **nefazodone**, **nelfinavir**, **ritonavir**, **saquinavir**, and **voriconazole** may ↑ blood levels and the risk of toxicity. Concurrent use should be avoided, but if necessary, dose of lapatinib should be ↓. Concurrent use of **strong CYP3A4 inducers** including **dexamethasone**, **phenytoin**, **carbamazepine**, **rifampin**, **rifabutin**, **rifapentin**, and **phenobarbital** may ↓ blood levels and effectiveness. Concurrent use should be avoided, but if necessary, dose of lapatinib should be ↑.

Drug-Natural Products: Concurrent use of **St. John's wort** may ↓ blood levels and effectiveness. Concurrent use should be avoided, but if necessary dose of lapatinib should be ↑.

Drug-Food: Concurrent **grapefruit juice** may ↑ blood levels and the risk of toxicity and should be avoided.

Route/Dosage

PO (Adults): *HER2 positive metastatic breast cancer*—1250 mg once daily for 21 days; *Hormone receptor positive, HER2 positive metastatic breast cancer*—1500 mg once daily; *Concurrent use of strong CYP3A4 inhibitor*—↓ dose to 500 mg once daily; *Concurrent use of strong CYP3A4 inducer*—HER2 positive metastatic breast cancer: Gradually titrate dose from 1250 mg once daily up to 4500 mg once daily as tolerated; Hormone receptor positive, HER2 positive metastatic breast cancer: Gradually titrate dose from 1500 mg once daily up to 5500 mg once daily as tolerated.

Hepatic Impairment

PO (Adults): *Severe hepatic impairment*—HER2 positive metastatic breast cancer: 750 mg/day; Hormone receptor positive, HER2 positive metastatic breast cancer: 1000 mg/day.

Availability

Tablets: 250 mg.

NURSING IMPLICATIONS

Assessment

- Evaluate left ventricular ejection fraction (LVEF) prior to therapy to determine if within institution's normal limits. Continue to monitor periodically during therapy to ensure it does not fall below limits. If LVEF decreases to Grade 2 or greater discontinue therapy. If returns to normal and patient is asymptomatic after 2 wk, may restart therapy at a reduced dose of 1000 mg/day (with cabcitabine) or 1250 mg/day (with letrazole).
- Monitor for diarrhea; usually occurs within first 6 days of therapy and lasts 4–5 days. Treat with antidiarrheals (loperamide) after first loose stool. If diarrhea is severe, treat with oral or intravenous fluids, antibiotics (fluoroquinolones) especially if diarrhea persists >24 hrs or accompanied by fever; may require interruption or discontinuation of therapy. If accompanied by moderate to severe abdominal cramping, nausea or vomiting, decreased performance status, fever, sepsis, neutropenia, frank bleeding, or dehydration, interrupt therapy and reintroduce at lower dose (from 1,250 mg/day to 1,000 mg/day or from 1,500 mg/day to 1,250 mg/day) when diarrhea <Grade 1. If Grade 4 diarrhea occurs, discontinue therapy.
- Monitor ECG prior to and periodically during therapy to monitor QT.
- Monitor for respiratory status for symptoms of interstitial lung disease and pneumonitis (dyspnea, cough); may require discontinuation of therapy.
- Monitor for signs and symptoms of skin reactions (progressive skin rash often with blisters or mucosal lesions). Discontinue lapatinib if erythema multiforme, Stevens-Johnson syndrome, or toxic epidermal necrolysis are suspected.
- ***Lab Test Considerations:*** Monitor liver function tests prior to initiation and every 4–6 wk during therapy and as clinically indicated. Discontinue and do not restart lapatinib if patients experience severe changes in liver function tests.
- Monitor serum potassium and magnesium prior to and periodically during therapy.

Implementation

- Correct hypokalemia and hypomagnesemia prior to therapy.
- **PO:** Administer tablets once daily at least 1 hr before or 1 hr after a meal for 21 days. Do not divide daily dose.

Patient/Family Teaching

- Instruct patient to take lapatinib as directed and to review the *Patient Information Sheet* prior to therapy and with each refill for new information. If a dose is missed take as soon remembered that day. If a day is missed, skip the dose; do not double doses. Caution patient not to share this medication with others, even with same condition; may be harmful.
- Advise patient to avoid drinking grapefruit juice or eating grapefruit during therapy.
- Advise patient to report signs or decreased LVEF (shortness of breath, palpitations, fatigue) and skin rash to health care professional promptly.
- Instruct patient to notify health care professional of all Rx or OTC medications, vitamins, or herbal products being taken and consult health care professional before taking any new medications, especially St. John's wort.
- Advise patient that lapatinib may cause diarrhea, which may become severe. Instruct patient in how to

L

prevent and manage diarrhea and to notify health care professional if severe.

- Advise female patients to notify health care professional if pregnancy is planned or suspected; therapy may be teratogenic.

Evaluation/Desired Outcomes

- Decreased/slowed spread of metastatic breast cancer.

ledipasvir/sofosbuvir

(led-i-**pas**-vir/soe-**fos**-bue-vir)

Harvoni

Classification

Therapeutic: antivirals

Pharmacologic: NS5A inhibitors, polymerase inhibitors

Indications

Chronic hepatitis C virus (HCV) infection (genotypes 1, 4, 5, or 6) in patients without cirrhosis or with compensated cirrhosis. Chronic HCV infection (genotype 1) in patients with decompensated cirrhosis (in combination with ribavirin). Chronic HCV infection (genotypes 1 or 4) in patients who are liver transplant recipients without cirrhosis or with compensated cirrhosis (in combination with ribavirin).

Action

Ledipasvir—inhibits NS5A, a protein required for viral replication. *Sofosbuvir*—inhibits RNA-dependent RNA polymerase, resulting in inhibition of viral replication.
Therapeutic Effects: Decreased HCV RNA levels with decreased severity and sequelae of CHC.

Pharmacokinetics

Ledipasvir
Absorption: Well absorbed following oral administration.
Distribution: Unknown.
Protein Binding: >99.8%.
Metabolism and Excretion: Minimal metabolism, undergoes biliary excretion. Mostly excreted unchanged in feces (86%), 1% eliminated in urine.
Half-life: 47 hr.
Sofosbuvir
Absorption: Rapidly metabolized following absorption (extensive first-pass effect).
Distribution: Unknown.
Protein Binding: 61–65%.
Metabolism and Excretion: Extensively metabolized with much conversion to GS-461203, an active antiviral moiety, then converted GS-331007, which does not have antiviral activity. 80% excreted in urine mostly as GS-331007 (3.5% as unchanged drug), 14% excreted in feces, 2.5% excreted in expired air.
Half-life: *Sofosbuvir*—0.4 hr; *GS-331007*—27 hr.

TIME/ACTION PROFILE (blood levels)

ROUTE	ONSET	PEAK	DURATION
ledipasvir	unknown	4–5 hr	24 hr
sofosbuvir	unknown	0.8–1 hr†	24 hr

†Sofosbuvir (2–4 hr for GS-331007).

Contraindications/Precautions

Contraindicated in: Should not be used with other drugs/regimens that already containing sofosbuvir; Concurrent use of P-gp inducers, some anticonvulsants, some antivirals and rosuvastatin; Severe renal impairment (eGFR <30 mL/min/1.73 m^2) or end stage renal disease (no dose recommendation); Any condition in which ribavirin is contraindicated.
Use Cautiously in: Receiving immunosuppressant or chemotherapy medications (↑ risk of hepatitis B virus reactivation); Geri: May be more sensitive to drug effects; Lactation: Weigh benefits of breast feeding against possible adverse effects; OB: Use only if potential benefit justifies fetal risk; Pedi: Children <3 yr (safety and effectiveness not established).

Adverse Reactions/Side Effects

CNS: fatigue, headache, insomnia. **GI:** diarrhea, hepatitis B virus reactivation, nausea.

Interactions

Drug-Drug: Concurrent use of **P-gp inducers** including **rifampin** ↓ levels and effectiveness of both ledipasvir and sofosbuvir; concurrent use contraindicated. Ledipasvir inhibits P-gp and may ↑ levels of **substrates of P-gp**. **Amiodarone** may ↑ risk of symptomatic bradycardia; concurrent use not recommended; if amiodarone necessary, monitor patients in inpatient setting for first 48 hr of concomitant use and then monitor heart rate on outpatient basis for at least the first 2 wk of treatment (follow same monitoring procedure if discontinuing amiodarone immediately before initiation of ledipasvir/sofosbuvir therapy). **Acid-reducing agents** may ↓ levels of ledipasvir; separate **antacids** including **magnesium and aluminum hydroxide** by 4 hr, administer **H_2-receptor antagonists** including **famotidine** simultaneously or 12 hr apart (dose of antagonist should not exceed famotidine 40 mg twice daily or equivalent), **proton-pump inhibitors** including **omeprazole** 20 mg daily or equivalent may be given simultaneously. May ↑ levels/effects/risk of toxicity with **digoxin** (therapeutic monitoring recommended). Level and effectiveness ↓ by **carbamazepine**, **phenytoin**, **phenobarbital**, and **oxcarbazepine** concurrent use is not recommended. Levels and effectiveness may be ↓ by concurrent use of **rifabutin** and **rifapentine**; concurrent use not recommended. ↑ levels and risk of adverse reactions from **tenofovir** and **tenofovir-containing combinations** (dosage adjustments may be necessary, consider alternative regimens). Levels and effectiveness are ↓ by **tipranavir/ritonavir**; concurrent use not recommended. May ↑ levels/toxicity of **rosuvastatin** and **atorvastatin**; concurrent use with rosuvastatin not recommended; monitor closely for atorvastatin-induced myopathy or rhabdomyolysis. May cause fluctuations in INR when used with **warfarin**; closely monitor INR. May ↑ risk of hypoglycemia when used with certain **antidiabetic agents**.

Drug-Natural Products: Concurrent use with **St. John's wort** ↓ blood levels and effectiveness; concurrent use contraindicated.

Route/Dosage

PO (Adults): *Genotype 1 (treatment-naïve without cirrhosis or with compensated cirrhosis [Child-Pugh A])*—Ledipasvir 90 mg/sofosbuvir 400 mg (one tablet) once daily for 12 wk; *Genotype 1 (treatment-experienced without cirrhosis)*—Ledipasvir 90 mg/sofosbuvir 400 mg (one tablet) once daily for 12 wk; *Genotype 1 (treatment-experienced with compensated cirrhosis [Child-Pugh A])*—Ledipasvir 90 mg/sofosbuvir 400 mg (one tablet) once daily for 24 wk; *Genotype 1 (treatment-naïve or treatment-experienced with decompensated cirrhosis [Child-Pugh B or C])*—Ledipasvir 90 mg/sofosbuvir 400 mg (one tablet) once daily with ribavirin for 12 wk; *Genotype 1 or 4 (treatment-naïve or treatment-experienced liver transplant recipients without cirrhosis or with compensated cirrhosis [Child-Pugh A])*—Ledipasvir 90 mg/sofosbuvir 400 mg (one tablet) once daily with ribavirin for 12 wk; *Genotype 4, 5, or 6 (treatment-naïve or treatment-experienced without cirrhosis or with compensated cirrhosis [Child-Pugh A])*—Ledipasvir 90 mg/sofosbuvir 400 mg (one tablet) once daily for 12 wk.

PO (Children ≥3 yr and ≥35 kg): *Genotype 1 (treatment-naïve without cirrhosis or with compensated cirrhosis [Child-Pugh A])*—Ledipasvir 90 mg/sofosbuvir 400 mg (as one 90 mg/400 mg tablet, two 45 mg/200 mg tablets, or two 45 mg/200 mg packets of oral pellets) once daily for 12 wk; *Genotype 1 (treatment-experienced without cirrhosis)*—Ledipasvir 90 mg/sofosbuvir 400 mg (as one 90 mg/400 mg tablet, two 45 mg/200 mg tablets, or two 45 mg/200 mg packets of oral pellets) once daily for 12 wk; *Genotype 1 (treatment-experienced with compensated cirrhosis [Child-Pugh A])*—Ledipasvir 90 mg/sofosbuvir 400 mg (as one 90 mg/400 mg tablet, two 45 mg/200 mg tablets, or two 45 mg/200 mg packets of oral pellets) once daily for 24 wk; *Genotype 1 (treatment-naïve or treatment-experienced with decompensated cirrhosis [Child-Pugh B or C])*—Ledipasvir 90 mg/sofosbuvir 400 mg (as one 90 mg/400 mg tablet, two 45 mg/200 mg tablets, or two 45 mg/200 mg packets of oral pellets) once daily with ribavirin for 12 wk; *Genotype 1 or 4 (treatment-naïve or treatment-experienced liver transplant recipients without cirrhosis or with compensated cirrhosis [Child-Pugh A])*—Ledipasvir 90 mg/sofosbuvir 400 mg (as one 90 mg/400 mg tablet, two 45 mg/200 mg tablets, or two 45 mg/200 mg packets of oral pellets) once daily with ribavirin for 12 wk; *Genotype 4, 5, or 6 (treatment-naïve or treatment-experienced without cirrhosis or with compensated cirrhosis [Child-Pugh A])*—Ledipasvir 90 mg/sofosbuvir 400 mg (as one 90 mg/400 mg tablet, two 45 mg/200 mg tablets, or two 45 mg/200 mg packets of oral pellets) once daily for 12 wk.

PO (Children ≥3 yr and 17–<35 kg): *Genotype 1 (treatment-naïve without cirrhosis or with compensated cirrhosis [Child-Pugh A])*—Ledipasvir 45 mg/sofosbuvir 200 mg (as one 45 mg/200 mg tablet or one 45 mg/200 mg packet of oral pellets) once daily for 12 wk; *Genotype 1 (treatment-experienced without cirrhosis)*—Ledipasvir 45 mg/sofosbuvir 200 mg (as one 45 mg/200 mg tablet or one 45 mg/200 mg packet of oral pellets) once daily for 12 wk; *Genotype 1 (treatment-experienced with compensated cirrhosis [Child-Pugh A])*—Ledipasvir 45 mg/sofosbuvir 200 mg (as one 45 mg/200 mg tablet or one 45 mg/200 mg packet of oral pellets) once daily for 24 wk; *Genotype 1 (treatment-naïve or treatment-experienced with decompensated cirrhosis [Child-Pugh B or C])*—Ledipasvir 45 mg/sofosbuvir 200 mg (as one 45 mg/200 mg tablet or one 45 mg/200 mg packet of oral pellets) once daily with ribavirin for 12 wk; *Genotype 1 or 4 (treatment-naïve or treatment-experienced liver transplant recipients without cirrhosis or with compensated cirrhosis [Child-Pugh A])*—Ledipasvir 45 mg/sofosbuvir 200 mg (as one 45 mg/200 mg tablet or one 45 mg/200 mg packet of oral pellets) once daily with ribavirin for 12 wk; *Genotype 4, 5, or 6 (treatment-naïve or treatment-experienced without cirrhosis or with compensated cirrhosis [Child-Pugh A])*—Ledipasvir 45 mg/sofosbuvir 200 mg (as one 45 mg/200 mg tablet or one 45 mg/200 mg packet of oral pellets) once daily for 12 wk.

PO (Children ≥3 yr and <17 kg): *Genotype 1 (treatment-naïve without cirrhosis or with compensated cirrhosis [Child-Pugh A])*—Ledipasvir 33.75 mg/sofosbuvir 150 mg (as one 33.75 mg/150 mg packet of oral pellets) once daily for 12 wk; *Genotype 1 (treatment-experienced without cirrhosis)*—Ledipasvir 45 mg/sofosbuvir 200 mg (as one 33.75 mg/150 mg packet of oral pellets) once daily for 12 wk; *Genotype 1 (treatment-experienced with compensated cirrhosis [Child-Pugh A])*—Ledipasvir 45 mg/sofosbuvir 200 mg (as one 33.75 mg/150 mg packet of oral pellets) once daily for 24 wk; *Genotype 1 (treatment-naïve or treatment-experienced with decompensated cirrhosis [Child-Pugh B or C])*—Ledipasvir 45 mg/sofosbuvir 200 mg (as one 33.75 mg/150 mg packet of oral pellets) once daily with ribavirin for 12

L

wk; *Genotype 1 or 4 (treatment-naïve or treatment-experienced liver transplant recipients without cirrhosis or with compensated cirrhosis [Child-Pugh A])*—Ledipasvir 45 mg/sofosbuvir 200 mg (as one 33.75 mg/150 mg packet of oral pellets) once daily with ribavirin for 12 wk; *Genotype 4, 5, or 6 (treatment-naïve or treatment-experienced without cirrhosis or with compensated cirrhosis [Child-Pugh A])*—Ledipasvir 45 mg/sofosbuvir 200 mg (as one 33.75 mg/150 mg packet of oral pellets) once daily for 12 wk.

Availability

Oral pellets: ledipasvir 33.75 mg/sofosbuvir 150 mg/pkt, ledipasvir 45 mg/sofosbuvir 200 mg/pkt. **Tablets:** ledipasvir 45 mg/sofosbuvir 200 mg, ledipasvir 90 mg/sofosbuvir 400 mg.

NURSING IMPLICATIONS

Assessment

- Monitor symptoms of hepatitis during therapy.
- ***Lab Test Considerations:*** Determine current or prior HBV infection by measuring hepatitis B surface antigen (HBsAg) and hepatitis B core antibody (anti-HBc) before initiating HCV therapy.
- May cause ↑ serum bilirubin and lipase levels.

Implementation

- **PO:** Administer once daily with or without food.
- Administer pellets within 30 min of gently mixing with food and swallow entire contents without chewing to avoid a bitter aftertaste. If pellets are administered with food, sprinkle the pellets on one or more spoonfuls of non-acidic soft food (pudding, chocolate syrup, mashed potato, ice cream) at or below room temperature.

Patient/Family Teaching

- Instruct patient to take ledipasvir/sofosbuvir at the same time each day for the full course of therapy. Take missed doses as soon as remembered on same day; do not take more than 1 tablet in a day. Do not stop taking ledipasvir/sofosbuvir without consulting health care professional. Advise patient to read *Patient Information* prior to starting therapy and with each Rx refill in case of changes.
- Inform patient that ledipasvir/sofosbuvir may not reduce the risk of transmission of CHC to others; use appropriate precautions to prevent transmission.
- Instruct patient that ledipasvir/sofosbuvir should not be shared with others; may be harmful.
- Advise patient to notify health care professional of all Rx or OTC medications, vitamins, or herbal products being taken and consult health care professional before taking any new medications, especially St. John's wort.
- Instruct patient to take antacids containing aluminum or magnesium 4 hrs before or 4 hrs after ledipasvir/sofosbuvir.
- Advise female patient to notify health care professional if pregnancy is planned or suspected and to avoid breast feeding.

Evaluation/Desired Outcomes

- Decreased HCV RNA levels with decreased severity and sequelae of CHC.

lefamulin (le-fam-ue-lin)

Xenleta

Classification

Therapeutic: anti-infectives

Pharmacologic: pleuromutilins

Indications

Community-acquired bacterial pneumonia.

Action

Acts as a pleuromutilin that ultimately interferes with bacterial protein synthesis at the level of the 50S ribosome. **Therapeutic Effects:** Resolution of pneumonia. **Spectrum:** Active against gram-positive pathogens, including: *Staphylococcus aureus* (methicillin-sensitive strains only), *Streptococcus pneumoniae*. Also active against the following gram-negative pathogen: *Haemophilus influenzae*. Also active against several other pathogens, including: *Legionella pneumophilia*, *Chlamydia pneumoniae*, *Mycoplasma pneumoniae*.

Pharmacokinetics

Absorption: 25% absorbed following oral administration; IV administration results in complete bioavailability.

Distribution: Extensively distributed to tissues.

Protein Binding: 94–97%.

Metabolism and Excretion: Primarily metabolized in the liver via the CYP3A4 isoenzyme. Primarily excreted in feces (77%; 4–9% as unchanged drug), with 15% excreted in urine (9–14% as unchanged drug).

Half-life: 8 hr.

TIME/ACTION PROFILE (plasma concentrations)

ROUTE	ONSET	PEAK	DURATION
IV	unknown	at end of infusion	12 hr
PO	unknown	0.88–2 hr	12 hr

Contraindications/Precautions

Contraindicated in: Hypersensitivity to lefamulin or retapamulin; Concurrent use of CYP3A4 substrates that prolong the QT interval; QT interval prolongation or a history of ventricular arrhythmias (including torsades de pointes); Concurrent use of QT interval prolonging medications; Moderate or severe hepatic impairment (oral tablets only); OB: Pregnancy (may cause fetal harm); Lactation: Lactation (may cause fetal harm).

Use Cautiously in: Severe hepatic impairment (↑ dosing interval for IV injection); Rep: Women of reproductive potential; Pedi: Safety and effectiveness not established.

Adverse Reactions/Side Effects

CNS: headache, insomnia. **CV:** QT INTERVAL PROLONGATION. **F and E:** hypokalemia. **GI:** CLOSTRIDIUM DIFFICILE ASSOCIATED DIARRHEA (CDAD), diarrhea, ↑ liver enzymes, nausea, vomiting. **Local:** injection site reactions.

Interactions

Drug-Drug: **CYP3A4 substrates** that prolong the QT interval, including **pimozide**, may ↑ the risk of QT interval prolongation and torsades de pointes; concurrent use contraindicated. **Class Ia antiarrhythmics** or **Class III antiarrhythmics** may ↑ the risk of QT interval prolongation and torsades de pointes; avoid concurrent use. **QT interval prolonging medications**, including **antipsychotics**, **erythromycin**, **moxifloxacin**, or **tricyclic antidepressants** may ↑ the risk of QT interval prolongation and torsades de pointes; avoid concurrent use. **Strong CYP3A4 inhibitors** or **P-gp inhibitors** may ↑ levels of oral lefamulin; avoid concurrent use. **Moderate or strong CYP3A4 inducers** or **P-gp inducers** may ↓ levels of either oral or IV lefamulin; avoid concurrent use. Lefamulin tablets may ↑ levels of **CYP3A4 substrates**, including **benzodiazepines**, **diltiazem**, **lovastatin**, **PDE5 inhibitors**, **simvastatin**, and **verapamil**; monitor closely for adverse reactions.

Route/Dosage

IV (Adults): 150 mg every 12 hr for 5–7 days; may switch at any time to oral regimen to complete the treatment course.

PO (Adults): 600 mg every 12 hr for 5 days.

Hepatic Impairment

IV (Adults): *Severe hepatic impairment (Child-Pugh C)*—150 mg every 24 hr for 5–7 days.

Availability

Film-coated tablets: 600 mg. **Solution for injection (requires dilution):** 10 mg/mL.

NURSING IMPLICATIONS

Assessment

- Assess for infection (vital signs; appearance of wound, sputum, urine, and stool; WBC) at beginning of and during therapy, especially in geriatric patients.
- Obtain specimens for culture and sensitivity before initiating therapy. First dose may be given before receiving results.
- Monitor bowel function. Diarrhea, abdominal cramping, fever, and bloody stools should be reported to health care professional promptly as a sign of Clostridium difficile-associated diarrhea (CDAD). May begin up to several wk following cessation of therapy.
- Monitor ECG for QT prolongation in patients with ventricular arrhythmias or those on other drugs that prolong QT interval.
- Monitor for signs and symptoms of hypersensitivity reactions (rash, hives, swelling of face or throat) during therapy.
- ***Lab Test Considerations:*** Obtain a negative pregnancy test before starting therapy.

Implementation

- **PO:** Administer at least 1 hr before or 2 hr after a meal. Swallow tablets whole with 6–8 oz of water; do not crush, break, or chew.
- **Intermittent Infusion:** Dilute entire 15 mL vial into diluent bag supplied containing 250 mL of 10 mM citrate buffered 0.9% NaCl. Mix thoroughly. Solution is clear and colorless; do not administer solutions that are discolored or contain particulate matter. Solution is stable for 24 hr at room temperature or 48 hr if refrigerated. ***Rate:*** Infuse over 60 min.

Patient/Family Teaching

- Instruct patient to take lefamulin as directed. Take missed doses as soon as remembered up to 8 hr before next dose. If less than 8 hr before next dose, omit dose, and resume dosing at next scheduled dose.
- Instruct patient to notify health care professional immediately if rash, diarrhea, abdominal cramping, fever, or bloody stools occur and not to treat with antidiarrheals without consulting health care professionals.
- Advise patient to report the signs of superinfection (black, furry overgrowth on the tongue, vaginal itching or discharge, loose or foul-smelling stools) to health care professional.
- Advise patient to notify health care professional of all Rx or OTC medications, vitamins, or herbal products being taken and to consult with health care professional before taking other medications.
- Advise females of reproductive potential to use effective contraception and avoid breast feeding during and for 2 days after final dose. If patient becomes pregnant while taking lefamulin, encourage patient to enrol in registry to monitor pregnancy outcomes by calling 1-855-5NABRIVA to enroll.

Evaluation/Desired Outcomes

- Resolution of the signs and symptoms of infection. Length of time for complete resolution depends on the organism and site of infection.

leflunomide (le-flu-noe-mide)

Arava

Classification

Therapeutic: antirheumatics (DMARDs)

Pharmacologic: immune response modifiers, pyrimidine synthesis inhibitors

Indications

Rheumatoid arthritis (disease-modifying agent).

Action

Inhibits an enzyme required for pyrimidine synthesis; has antiproliferative and anti-inflammatory effects. **Therapeutic Effects:** Decreased pain and inflammation, slowed structural progression and improved physical function.

Pharmacokinetics

Absorption: Tablets are 80% absorbed following oral administration; rapidly converted to the M1 metabolite, which is responsible for pharmacologic activity.

Distribution: Crosses the placenta.

Protein Binding: 99%.

Metabolism and Excretion: Extensively metabolized with metabolites excreted in urine (43%) and feces (48%). Also undergoes biliary recycling.

Half-life: 14–18 days.

TIME/ACTION PROFILE (antirheumatic effect)

ROUTE	ONSET	PEAK	DURATION
PO	1 mo	3–6 mo	wk–mos†

†Due to persistence of active metabolite.

Contraindications/Precautions

Contraindicated in: Hypersensitivity to leflunomide or teriflunomide; Compromised immune function, including bone marrow dysplasia or severe uncontrolled infection; Concurrent vaccination with live vaccines; Hepatic impairment; OB: May cause fetal abnormalities or death. Contact Pregnancy Registry if accidental exposure occurs; Lactation: Lactation.

Use Cautiously in: Renal insufficiency; History of interstitial lung disease; Patients >60 yr, with diabetes, or taking neurotoxic medications (↑ risk of peripheral neuropathy); Pedi: Safety and effectiveness not established; OB: Women with childbearing potential must use two forms of birth control. Should not be used in men attempting to father a child.

Exercise Extreme Caution in: Concurrent use of other hepatotoxic agents (↑ risk of hepatotoxicity).

Adverse Reactions/Side Effects

CNS: headache, dizziness, weakness. **Resp:** INTERSTITIAL LUNG DISEASE, bronchitis, cough, pharyngitis, pneumonia, respiratory infection, rhinitis, sinusitis. **CV:** chest pain, hypertension. **GI:** HEPATOTOXICITY, diarrhea, nausea, abdominal pain, anorexia, dyspepsia, gastroenteritis, ↑ liver enzymes, mouth ulcers, vomiting. **GU:** urinary tract infection. **Derm:** STEVENS-JOHNSON SYNDROME, TOXIC EPIDERMAL NECROLYSIS, alopecia, rash, dry skin, eczema, pruritus. **F and E:** hypokalemia. **Metab:** weight loss. **MS:** arthralgia, back pain, joint disorder, leg cramps, synovitis, tenosynovitis. **Neuro:** paresthesia, peripheral neuropathy. **Misc:** DRUG REACTION WITH EOSINOPHILIA AND SYSTEMIC SYMPTOMS (DRESS), allergic reactions, flu syndrome, infections including sepsis and tuberculosis reactivation, pain.

Interactions

Drug-Drug: Cholestyramine and **activated charcoal** cause a rapid and significant ↓ in blood levels of active metabolite. Concurrent use of **methotrexate** and other **hepatotoxic drugs** ↑ risk of hepatotoxicity. Concurrent administration of **rifampin** ↑ blood levels of the active metabolite. May ↑ risk of bleeding with **warfarin**.

Route/Dosage

PO (Adults): *Loading dose*—100 mg daily for 3 days; *maintenance dosing*—20 mg/day (if intolerance occurs, dose may be ↓ to 10 mg/day).

Availability (generic available)

Tablets: 10 mg, 20 mg, 100 mg.

NURSING IMPLICATIONS

Assessment

- Assess range of motion and degree of swelling and pain in affected joints before and periodically during therapy.
- Monitor for signs and symptoms of interstitial lung disease (new onset or worsening cough or dyspnea, associated with fever). May require discontinuation of therapy; consider drug elimination procedure if needed.
- Assess for rash periodically during therapy. May cause Stevens-Johnson syndrome or toxic epidermal necrolysis. Discontinue therapy if severe or if accompanied with fever, general malaise, fatigue, muscle or joint aches, blisters, oral lesions, conjunctivitis, hepatitis, and/or eosinophilia.
- ***Lab Test Considerations:*** Monitor liver function throughout therapy. Assess ALT at baseline, then monthly during initial 6 mo of therapy, then every 6–8 wk. If given concurrently with methotrexate, monitor ALT, AST, and serum albumin monthly. May cause ↑ ALT and AST, which are usually reversible with reduction in dose or discontinuation, but may be fatal. If ALT is 2–3 times the upper limit of normal, reduce dose to 10 mg/day and continue therapy. Monitor closely after dose reduction; plasma levels may not ↓ for several wk due to long half-life. If ALT ↑ of 2–3 times the upper limit of normal persists despite dose reduction or if ALT >3 times the upper limit of normal occurs, discontinue leflunomide and administer cholestyramine (see Toxicity and

Overdose). Monitor closely and readminister cholestyramine as indicated.

- Monitor CBC with platelets monthly for 6 mo following initiation of therapy and every 6–8 wk thereafter. If used with methotrexate or other immunosuppressive therapy continue monitoring monthly. If bone marrow depression occurs, discontinue leflunomide and begin decreasing levels with cholestyramine (see Implementation).
- May rarely cause ↑ of alkaline phosphatase and bilirubin.
- ***Toxicity and Overdose:*** If overdose or significant toxicity occurs, cholestyramine 8 g 3 times a day for 24 hr, or activated charcoal orally or via nasogastric tube, 50 g every 6 hr for 24 hr, is recommended to accelerate elimination.

Implementation

- Administer a tuberculin skin test prior to administration of leflunomide. Patients with active latent TB should be treated for TB prior to therapy.
- **PO:** Initiate therapy with loading dose of 100 mg/day for 3 days, followed by 20 mg/day dose. May decrease to 10 mg/day if not well tolerated.
- **Drug Elimination Procedure:** Recommended to achieve nondetectable plasma levels <0.02 mg/L after stopping treatment with leflunomide. Administer cholestyramine 8 g 3 times daily for 11 days. (Days do not need to be consecutive unless rapid lowering of levels is desired.) Verify plasma levels <0.02 mg/L by 2 separate tests at least 14 days apart. If plasma levels >00.02 mg/L, consider additional cholestyramine treatment. Plasma levels may take up to 2 yr to reach nondetectable levels without drug elimination procedure.

Patient/Family Teaching

- Instruct patient to take leflunomide as directed.
- May cause dizziness. Caution patient to avoid driving or other activities requiring alertness until response to medication is known.
- Advise patient to consult health care professional prior to taking other Rx, OTC, or herbal products concurrently with leflunomide. Aspirin, NSAIDs, or low-dose corticosteroids may be continued during therapy, but other agents for treatment of rheumatoid arthritis may require discontinuation.
- Discuss the possibility of hair loss with patient. Explore methods of coping.
- Advise patient to notify health care professional if rash, mucous membrane lesions, unusual tiredness, abdominal pain, jaundice, or symptoms of interstitial lung disease occur.
- Instruct patient to avoid vaccinations with live vaccines during and following therapy without consulting health care professional.
- Rep: Caution patients of childbearing age that leflunomide has teratogenic effects. Women wishing to become pregnant must undergo the drug elimination procedure (see Implementation) and verify that the M1 metabolite plasma levels are <0.02 mg/L. Men wishing to father a child should also take cholestyramine 8 g 3 times daily for 11 days to minimize any possible risk.
- Emphasize the importance of routine lab tests to monitor for side effects.

Evaluation/Desired Outcomes

- Decrease in signs and symptoms of rheumatoid arthritis and slowing of structural damage as evidenced by x-ray erosions and joint narrowings.
- Improved physical function.

REMS

lenalidomide
(le-na-**lid**-o-mide)
Revlimid

Classification
Therapeutic: antineoplastics
Pharmacologic: immunomodulatory agents

Indications

Transfusion-dependent anemia due to specific myelodysplastic syndromes (MDS) associated with deletion 5q cytogenetic abnormality. Multiple myeloma (MM) (in combination with dexamethasone). Maintenance therapy in patients with MM after autologous hematopoietic stem cell transplantation (auto-HSCT). Mantle cell lymphoma (MCL) patients whose disease has relapsed or progressed after 2 prior therapies including bortezomib. Previously treated follicular lymphoma (FL) (in combination with rituximab). Previously treated marginal zone lymphoma (MZL) (in combination with rituximab).

Action

Lenalidomide is a structural analog of thalidomide. Inhibits secretion of pro-inflammatory cytokines and increases secretion of anti-inflammatory cytokines.
Therapeutic Effects: Decreased anemia in certain MDS with a decreased requirement for transfusions. Slowed progression of MM and MCL. Improved progression-free survival in FL and MZL.

Pharmacokinetics

Absorption: Well absorbed following oral administration. Levels are higher in patients with MM.
Distribution: Crosses the placenta.
Metabolism and Excretion: 66% excreted unchanged in urine, some renal excretion involves active secretion.
Half-life: 3 hr.

TIME/ACTION PROFILE (↓ need for transfusions)

ROUTE	ONSET	PEAK	DURATION
PO	within 3 mo	unknown	unknown

Contraindications/Precautions

Contraindicated in: Hypersensitivity; Chronic lymphocytic leukemia (↑ risk of mortality); Concurrent use of pembrolizumab in patients with MM (↑ risk of mortality); OB: Pregnancy (contraception must be used in males and females); Lactation: Lactation.
Use Cautiously in: Renal impairment (may ↑ risk of adverse reactions; dose ↓ recommended if CCr <60 mL/min); Patients with MCL with high tumor burden, high MCL International Prognostic Index at diagnosis, and high white blood cell count at baseline (↑ risk of early mortality); Rep: Women of reproductive potential and men with female partners of reproductive potential; Geri: Consider age-related ↓ in renal function; Pedi: Safety not established.

Adverse Reactions/Side Effects

CNS: dizziness, fatigue, headache, insomnia, depression. **CV:** DVT, MI, PULMONARY EMBOLISM, STROKE, edema, chest pain, deep vein thrombosis, palpitations. **Derm:** DRUG REACTION WITH EOSINOPHILIA AND SYSTEMIC SYMPTOMS (DRESS), STEVENS-JOHNSON SYNDROME, TOXIC EPIDERMAL NECROLYSIS, pruritus, rash, dry skin, sweating. **Endo:** hyperthyroidism, hypothyroidism. **F and E:** hypokalemia, hypomagnesemia. **GI:** HEPATOTOXICITY, abdominal pain, constipation, diarrhea, nausea, vomiting, abnormal taste, anorexia, dry mouth. **Hemat:** NEUTROPENIA, THROMBOCYTOPENIA. **MS:** arthralgia, myalgia. **Resp:** cough, pharyngitis. **Misc:** ANGIOEDEMA, MALIGNANCY, fever, chills, tumor flare reaction, tumor lysis syndrome.

Interactions

Drug-Drug: Risk of neutropenia and thrombocytopenia may ↑ with **antineoplastics**, **immunosuppressants**, and **radiation therapy**. May ↑ **digoxin** levels. **Erythropoeitin**, **darbepoeitin**, and **estrogens** may ↑ risk of thromboembolic events.

Route/Dosage

MDS

PO (Adults): 10 mg once daily.

Renal Impairment

PO (Adults): *CCr 30–60 mL/min*—5 mg once daily; *CCr <30 mL/min (not on dialysis)*—2.5 mg once daily; *CCr <30 mL/min (requiring dialysis)*—2.5 mg once daily (give after dialysis on dialysis days).

MM

PO (Adults): 25 mg once daily on days 1–21 of repeated 28-day cycles (with dexamethasone); if patients not eligible for auto-HSCT, continue treatment until disease progression or unacceptable toxicity; for patients eligible for auto-HSCT, hematopoietic stem cell mobilization should take place within 4 cycles.

Renal Impairment

PO (Adults): *CCr 30–50 mL/min*—10 mg once daily; if patient tolerates initial dose, may ↑ to 15 mg once daily after 2 cycles; *CCr <30 mL/min (not on dialysis)*—15 mg every 48 hr; *CCr <30 mL/min (requiring dialysis)*—5 mg once daily (give after dialysis on dialysis days).

Maintenance Therapy for MM Following Auto-HSCT

PO (Adults): After adequate hematologic recovery (ANC ≥ 1000/mcL and/or platelet counts ≥75,000/mcL), initiate therapy with 10 mg once daily continuously on Days 1–28 of repeated 28–day cycles); after 3 cycles, dose may be ↑ to 15 mg once daily, if tolerated; continue treatment until disease progression or unacceptable toxicity.

Renal Impairment

PO (Adults): *CCr 30–60 mL/min*—5 mg once daily; *CCr <30 mL/min (not on dialysis)*—2.5 mg once daily; *CCr <30 mL/min (requiring dialysis)*—2.5 mg once daily (give after dialysis on dialysis days).

MCL

PO (Adults): 25 mg once daily on days 1–21 of repeated 28–day cycles; continue treatment until disease relapse or unacceptable toxicity develops.

Renal Impairment

PO (Adults): *CCr 30–60 mL/min*—10 mg once daily; *CCr <30 mL/min (not on dialysis)*—15 mg every 48 hr; *CCr <30 mL/min (requiring dialysis)*—5 mg once daily (give after dialysis on dialysis days).

FL or MZL

PO (Adults): 20 mg once daily on days 1–21 of repeated 28–day cycles for up to 12 cycles (with rituximab).

Renal Impairment

PO (Adults): *CCr 30–60 mL/min*—10 mg once daily; if patient tolerates initial dose, may ↑ to 15 mg once daily after 2 cycles; *CCr <30 mL/min (not on dialysis)*—5 mg once daily; *CCr <30 mL/min (requiring dialysis)*—5 mg once daily (give after dialysis on dialysis days).

Availability

Capsules: 2.5 mg, 5 mg, 10 mg, 15 mg, 20 mg, 25 mg.

NURSING IMPLICATIONS

Assessment

- Assess for signs of deep venous thrombosis and pulmonary edema (dyspnea, chest pain, arm or leg swelling) periodically during therapy; risk is greater when lenalidomide is administered with dexamethasone.

- Assess for skin rash. Discontinue lenalidomide if rash occurs; may cause Stevens-Johnson syndrome or toxic epidermal necrolysis.
- Monitor for signs and symptoms of tumor flare reaction (tender lymph node swelling, low-grade fever, pain rash) in patients with MCL; may mimic disease progression. *Grade 1 and 2 tumor flare reaction (TFR):* Lenalidomide may be continued in patients without interruption or modification, at health care professional's discretion. May also be treated with corticosteroids, nonsteroidal anti-inflammatory drugs (NSAIDs) and/or opioid analgesics. *Grade 3 or 4 TFR:* withhold treatment with lenalidomide until TFR resolves to ≤ Grade 1. May be treated for management of symptoms per the guidance for treatment of Grade 1 and 2 TFR.
- ***Lab Test Considerations:*** Assess pregnancy status prior to starting therapy. Pregnancy tests with a sensitivity of at least 50 mIU/mL must be done within 10–14 days and within 24 hrs of starting therapy. Once treatment has started pregnancy tests should occur weekly during first 4 wk of use, then every 4 wk in females with a regular menstrual cycle and every 2 wk in females with an irregular cycle.
- *Patients taking lenalidomide for MM with dexamethasone or as maintenance therapy:* Monitor CBC every 7 days for first 2 cycles, on days 1 and 15 of Cycle 3, and every 28 days thereafter. *Patients taking lenalidomide for MDS:* Monitor CBC with differential, platelet count, hemoglobin, and hematocrit weekly for first 8 wk of therapy and at least monthly thereafter. *Patients taking lenalidomide for MCL:* Monitor CBC weekly for first 28 days, every 2 wk during Cycles 2–4, and monthly thereafter. May require dose interruption and/or reduction and use of blood support and/or growth factors.
- May cause neutropenia with an onset of 42 days (range 4–411 days) and recovery time of 17 days (range 2–170 days). *For MM:* starting dose is 25 mg/day—If neutropenia develops and neutrophils fall to <1000/mcl interrupt therapy, follow CBC weekly. When neutrophils return to ≥1000/mcl and neutropenia is the only toxicity, resume lenalidomide at 25 mg daily. If neutrophils return to ≥1000/mcl and if other toxicity, resume lenalidomide at next lower dose. For each subsequent drop <1000/mcl interrupt therapy. If neutrophils return to ≥1000/mcl, resume at next lower dose. Do not administer doses below 2.5 mg. *For MDS, MZL, or FL:* starting dose is 10 mg/day—if neutropenia develops within 4 wk of starting at a 10 mg/day dose in a patient with a baseline neutrophil count (ANC) ≥1000/mcL and ANC falls to <750/mcL interrupt lenalidomide therapy and resume at 5 mg/day dose when ANC returns to ≥1000/mcL. If baseline ANC is <1000/mcL and ANC falls to <500/mcL, interrupt therapy and resume at 5 mg/day dose when ANC returns to ≥500/mcL. If neutropenia develops after 4 wk of therapy at 10 mg/day dose, and ANC <500/mcL for ≥7 days or <500/mcL associated with fever ≥38.5°C, interrupt therapy and resume at 5 mg/day when ANC returns to ≥500/mcL. If neutropenia develops at 5 mg/day dose and ANC <500/mcL for ≥7 days or <500/mcL associated with fever ≥38.5°C, interrupt therapy and resume at 2.5 mg daily when ANC returns to ≥500/mcL. *For MCL:* starting dose is 25 mg/day on days 1–21 of repeated 28-day cycles—If neutrophils fall to <1000/mcl for at least 7 days or fall to <1000/mcl with fever ≥38.5°C or fall to <500/mcl, interrupt therapy and follow CBC weekly. If neutrophils return to ≥1000/mcl resume at 5 mg less than previous dose. Do not administer doses below 5 mg. *For MZL or FL:* If neutrophils return to ≥1000/mcl and patient starting dose was 20 mg daily, resume at 5 mg less than previous dose. Do not administer doses below 5 mg. If neutrophils return to ≥1000/mcl patient starting dose was 10 mg daily, resume at 5 mg less than previous dose. Do not administer doses below 2.5 mg.
- May cause thrombocytopenia with an onset of 28 days (range 8–290 days) and a recovery in 22 days (range 5–224 days). *For MM:* starting dose is 25 mg/day—If platelets fall to <30,000/mcl interrupt therapy and follow CBC weekly. When platelets return to ≥30,000/mcl restart lenalidomide at next lower dose. For each subsequent drop <30,000/mcl interrupt therapy. When platelets return to ≥30,000/mcl resume at next lower dose. Do not administer doses below 2.5 mg. *For MDS, MZL, or FL:* starting dose is 10 mg/day—If thrombocytopenia develops within 4 wk of starting a 10 mg dose in a patient with a baseline of ≥100,000/mcL, and platelets fall to <50,000/mcL interrupt lenalidomide therapy and resume at 5 mg/day dose when platelets return to >50,000/mcL. If baseline was <100,000/mcL and platelets fall to 50% of baseline value interrupt therapy. If baseline ≥60,000/mcL and returns to ≥50,000/mcL or if baseline is <60,000/mcL and returns to ≥30,000/mcL resume therapy at 5 mg/day. If thrombocytopenia develops after 4 wk of treatment at 10 mg/day and platelets are <30,000/mcL or <50,000/mcL with platelet transfusions, interrupt therapy. When platelets return to ≥30,000/mcL without hemostatic failure resume therapy at 2.5 mg/day. *For MCL:* starting dose is 25 mg/day on days 1–21 of repeated 28–day cycles—If platelets fall to <50,000/mcl interrupt therapy and follow CBC weekly. If platelets return to ≥50,000/mcl resume at 5 mg less than previous dose. Do not administer doses below 5 mg.

- Monitor liver enzymes periodically during therapy. Stop therapy if enzymes are elevated; may resume when return to normal or decrease dose.
- May cause anemia and leukopenia.
- May cause hypokalemia, hypomagnesemia, and ↑ ALT levels.
- Monitor thyroid function before starting and periodically during therapy.

Implementation

- Patients must meet the following conditions before receiving therapy: they must understand the risks and be able to carry out instructions, must be capable of complying with patient registration and patient survey in the *Revlimid REMS program*, must comply with contraceptive measures, have received both oral and written warnings of the risks of contraception failure and the need for two reliable forms of contraception (females) or the risks of exposing a fetus to the drug and the need to use a latex condom during sexual conduct with a female with childbearing potential (male), acknowledge understanding of these warnings in writing, and if the patient is between 12 and 18 yr of age, their parent or legal guardian is to read the educational materials and agree to try to ensure compliance with conditions.
- Lenalidomide can only be prescribed by health care providers registered in the *Revlimide REMS program* and only be dispensed by a pharmacy that is registered in the *Revlimid REMS program*.
- Patients with multiple myeloma who are eligible for autologous stem cell transplantation should have stem cell mobilization performed within 4 cycles of therapy.
- **PO:** Administer once daily without regard to food, at the same time each day, with water. Capsules should be swallowed whole; do not open, break, or chew.

Patient/Family Teaching

- Instruct patient to take lenalidomide as directed and to comply with all aspects of the *Revlimid REMS program*. Take missed doses as soon as remembered within 12 hr of dose missed. If more than 12 hrs, skip dose and return to next scheduled dose; do not administer 2 doses within 12 hrs. Inform patient that they are required to participate in a telephone survey and patient registry while taking lenalidomide. Details are available at www.REVLIMID.com. Advise patient to read *Medication Guide* before starting and with each Rx refill in case of changes.
- Caution patient not to share lenalidomide with anyone, even someone who has similar symptoms.
- Advise patient to notify health care professional if rash, shortness of breath, chest pain, or arm or leg swelling, signs of infection (fever, dyspnea), rash, signs and symptoms of liver failure (yellowing of skin or white part of eyes; dark or brown (tea-colored) urine; pain on upper right side of your abdomen; feeling tired; unusual bleeding or bruising), hypersensitivity (swelling of lips, mouth, tongue, or throat; trouble breathing or swallowing; hives; very fast heartbeat; feeling dizzy or faint) occur.
- May cause dizziness. Caution patient to avoid driving and other activities requiring alertness until response to medication is known.
- Inform patient that lenalinomide may cause an increased risk of death in patients with MCL and may increase risk of new cancers.
- Instruct patient to notify health care professional of all Rx or OTC medications, vitamins, or herbal products being taken and consult health care professional before taking any new medications.
- Advise patient that they cannot donate blood during and for 1 mo following therapy and male patients cannot donate sperm while taking lenalidomide.
- Inform patient of risk of new cancers during therapy.
- Rep: Inform female patients of reproductive potential that they must use one highly effective method (IUD, hormonal contraceptive, tubal ligation, partner's vasectomy) and one additional method (latex condom, diaphragm, cervical cap) AT THE SAME TIME for at least 4 wk before, during therapy and interruptions of therapy, and for 4 wk following discontinuation of therapy, even with a history of infertility unless due to a hysterectomy or patient has been postmenopausal naturally for 24 consecutive mo. Advise female patients to avoid breast feeding during therapy. Males with female partners of reproductive potential receiving lenalidomide must always use a latex condom during and for up to 4 wk following discontinuation, even if they have undergone a successful vasectomy. Lenalidomide must be discontinued if pregnancy is suspected or confirmed. Suspected fetal exposure must be reported to FDA via MedWatch at 1-800-FDA-1088 and to manufacturer at 1-888-668-2528. Inform females there is a Pregnancy Exposure Registry that monitors pregnancy outcomes in females exposed to REVLIMID during pregnancy and that they can contact the Pregnancy Exposure Registry by calling 1-888-423-5436 [see Use in Specific Populations (8.1)].

Evaluation/Desired Outcomes

- Decreased anemia in MDS with a decreased requirement for transfusions.
- Slowing of MM progression.
- Slowing progression of MCL.
- Improved progression-free survival in FL and MZL.

lenvatinib (len-va-ti-nib)

Lenvima

Classification

Therapeutic: antineoplastics
Pharmacologic: kinase inhibitors

Indications

Locally recurrent or metastatic/progressive, radioactive-iodine-refractory differentiated thyroid cancer. Advanced renal cell carcinoma following one previous anti-angiogenic therapy (in combination with everolimus). Unresectable hepatocellular carcinoma. Advanced endometrial carcinoma that is not microsatellite instability-high or mismatch repair deficient, in patients who have disease progression following prior systemic therapy and are not candidates for curative surgery or radiation (in combination with pembrolizumab).

Action

Acts as a receptor tyrosine kinase inhibitor; inhibits kinase activities of various vascular endoethelial growth factor receptors, resulting in decreased pathogenic angiogenesis, tumor growth and spread. **Therapeutic Effects:** Decreased progression and improved survival of differentiated thyroid cancer, endometrial cancer, renal cell carcinoma, and hepatocellular carcinoma.

Pharmacokinetics

Absorption: Well absorbed following oral administration.

Distribution: Unknown.

Protein Binding: 98–99%.

Metabolism and Excretion: Metabolized by CYP3A and aldehyde oxidase; 64% eliminated in feces, 25% in urine.

Half-life: 28 hr.

TIME/ACTION PROFILE (improvement in progression-free survival)

ROUTE	ONSET	PEAK	DURATION
PO	within 2 mo	8 mo	throughout treatment

Contraindications/Precautions

Contraindicated in: Lactation: Discontinue lenvatinib or discontinue breast feeding; OB: Pregnancy (may cause fetal harm).

Use Cautiously in: Hypertension (control BP before initiating treatment, may need to withhold/discontinue for life-threatening elevation); History of heart failure (may need to withhold/discontinue for worsening HF); History of congenital long QTc syndrome, HF, bradyarrhythmias, concurrent use of drugs that prolong QTc, including Class Ia and III antiarrhythmics (↑ risk of further QTc prolongation and serious arrthythmias, may require interruption/discontinuation of lenvatinib); Severe hepatic or renal impairment (lower dose required); Dehydration/volume depletion (↑ risk of renal impairment, may need to withhold/discontinue for worsening renal function); Hypocalcemia (replace calcium, if persistent may require dose adjustment/interruption); History of reversible posterior leukencephalopathy syndrome (may require dose adjustment/interruption); May damage male reproductive tissue resulting in decreased fertility; Rep: Women of reproductive potential; Pedi: Safe and effective use in children has not been established.

Adverse Reactions/Side Effects

CNS: CAROTID ARTERY HEMORRHAGE, REVERSIBLE POSTERIOR LEUKOENCEPHALOPATHY SYNDROME (RPLS), fatigue, insomnia, headache. **CV:** ARTERIAL THROMBOEMBOLIC EVENTS, HF, QTC PROLONGATION, hypertension, hypotension. **Derm:** alopecia, palmar-plantar erythrodysesthesia syndrome, rash, hyperkeratosis, impaired wound healing. **EENT:** dysphonia, epistaxis. **Endo:** hypothyroidism. **F and E:** dehydration, hypocalcemia, hypokalemia. **GI:** GASTROINTESTINAL PERFORATION/FISTULA FORMATION, HEPATOTOXICITY, abdominal pain, ↓ appetite, diarrhea, dry mouth, dysgeusia, nausea, stomatitis, vomiting, ↑ liver enzymes. **GU:** NEPHROTIC SYNDROME, proteinuria, renal impairment, ↓ fertility. **Hemat:** hemorrhagic events, thrombocytopenia. **Metab:** ↓ weight. **MS:** arthralgia/myalgia. **Resp:** cough.

Interactions

Drug-Drug: Concurrent use of drugs that prolong QTc, including Class Ia and III antiarrhythmics may ↑ risk of further QTc prolongation and serious arrhythmias (may require interruption/discontinuation of lenvatinib).

Route/Dosage

Differentiated Thyroid Cancer

PO (Adults): 24 mg once daily until disease progression or unacceptable toxicity.

Renal Impairment

PO (Adults): *CCr <30 mL/min*— 14 mg once daily until disease progression or unacceptable toxicity.

Hepatic Impairment

PO (Adults): *Child–Pugh C*— 14 mg once daily until disease progression or unacceptable toxicity.

Renal Cell Carcinoma

PO (Adults): 18 mg once daily until disease progression or unacceptable toxicity.

Renal Impairment

PO (Adults): *CCr <30 mL/min*— 10 mg once daily until disease progression or unacceptable toxicity.

Hepatic Impairment

PO (Adults): *Child–Pugh C*— 10 mg once daily until disease progression or unacceptable toxicity.

Hepatocellular Carcinoma

PO (Adults ≥60 kg): 12 mg once daily until disease progression or unacceptable toxicity.

PO (Adults <60 kg): 8 mg once daily until disease progression or unacceptable toxicity.

Endometrial Carcinoma

PO (Adults): 20 mg once daily until disease progression or unacceptable toxicity.

Renal Impairment

PO (Adults): *CCr <30 mL/min*—10 mg once daily until disease progression or unacceptable toxicity.

Hepatic Impairment

PO (Adults): *Child–Pugh C*—10 mg once daily until disease progression or unacceptable toxicity.

Availability

Capsules: 4 mg, 10 mg.

NURSING IMPLICATIONS

Assessment

- Assess BP prior to and after 1 wk, then every 2 wk for first 2 mo, and then at least monthly thereafter during therapy. Initiate or adjust medication management to control BP. Hold lenvatinib for Grade 3 hypertension that persists despite antihypertensive therapy. Resume at a reduced dose (*1st occurrence*—20 mg/day; *2nd occurrence*—14 mg/day; *3rd occurrence*—10 mg/day) when hypertension is controlled or ≤Grade 2. Discontinue lenvatinib for life-threatening hypertension.
- Monitor for clinical signs and symptoms of cardiac dysfunction (shortness of breath, swollen ankles) during therapy. Hold lenvatinib for Grade 3 cardiac dysfunction until improved to Grade 0 or 1 or baseline. Resume at reduced dose (*1st occurrence*—20 mg/day; *2nd occurrence*—14 mg/day; *3rd occurrence*—10 mg/day) or discontinue depending on severity and persistence of cardiac dysfunction.
- Monitor for signs and symptoms of arterial thromboembolic events (chest pain, acute neurologic symptoms of MI or stroke) during therapy. Discontinue lenvatinib if event occurs.
- Assess for signs and symptoms of gastrointestinal perforation or fistula formation (severe abdominal pain) during therapy. Discontine lenvatinib if gastrointestinal perforation or fistula occurs.
- Monitor ECG for patients with congential long QT syndrome, congestive heart failure, bradyarrhythmias, or those taking drugs known to prolong QT interval. Hold lenvatinib for development of QT interval prolongation >500 ms or >60 ms increase from baseline. Hold until improves to ≤480 ms or baseline. Resume at reduced dose (*1st occurrence*—20 mg/day; *2nd occurrence*—14 mg/day; *3rd occurrence*—10 mg/day) when QT prolongation resolves to Grade 0 or 1.
- Monitor for signs and symptoms of reversible posterior leukoencephalopathy syndrome (RPLS) (severe headache, seizures, weakness, confusion, blindness or change in vision) during therapy. If symptoms occur, confirm diagnosis with MRI. Hold lenvatinib for RPLS until fully resolved. Resume at reduced dose (*1st occurrence*—20 mg/day; *2nd occurrence*—14 mg/day; *3rd occurrence*—10 mg/day) or discontinue depending on severity and persistence of neurologic symptoms.
- Monitor for bleeding (severe and persistent nose bleeds, vomiting blood, red or black stools, coughing up blood or blood clots, heavy or new onset vaginal bleeding) during therapy. Hold lenvatinib for Grade 3 hemorrhage until resolved to Grade 0 or 1. Resume at reduced dose (*1st occurrence*—20 mg/day; *2nd occurrence*—14 mg/day; *3rd occurrence*—10 mg/day) or discontinue depending on severity and persistence of hemorrhage. Discontinue lenvatinib if Grade 4 hemorrhage occurs.
- ***Lab Test Considerations:*** Obtain a negative pregnancy test before starting therapy.
- Monitor serum ALT and AST levels for hepatotoxicity prior to and every 2 wk for first 2 mo, and at least monthly thereafter during therapy. Hold lenvatinib for Grade 3 cardiac dysfunction until improved to Grade 0 or 1 or baseline. Resume at reduced dose (*1st occurrence*—20 mg/day; *2nd occurrence*—14 mg/day; *3rd occurrence*—10 mg/day) or discontinue depending on severity and persistence of hepatotoxicity. May cause hypoalbuminemia, ↑ alkaline phosphatase, and hyperbilirubinemia.
- Monitor for proteinuria prior to and periodically during therapy. If urine dipstick proteinuria ≥2+ is detected, obtain 24 hr urine protein. Hold lenvatinib for ≥2 g proteinuria/24 hrs and resume at reduced dose (*1st occurrence*—20 mg/day; *2nd occurrence*—14 mg/day; *3rd occurrence*—10 mg/day) when proteinuria <2 g/24 hrs. Discontinue lenvatinib for nephrotic syndrome.
- Monitor BUN and creatinine prior to and periodically during therapy. Hold lenvatinib for Grade 3 or 4 renal failure/impairment until resolved to Grade 0 or 1 or baseline. Resume at reduced dose (*1st occurrence*—20 mg/day; *2nd occurrence*—14 mg/day; *3rd occurrence*—10 mg/day) or discontinue depending on severity and persistence of renal impairment.
- Monitor and correct electrolyte abnormalities. Monitor serum calcium levels at least monthly and replace calcium as needed during therapy. Interrupt and adjust lenvatinib dose based on severity, presence of ECG changes, and persistence of hypocalcemia. May cause hypokalemia, hypomagnesemia, hypoglycemia, hypercalcemia, and hyperkalemia.
- Monitor TSH levels monthly and adjust thyroid replacement medication as needed in patients with ↓ thyroid levels.
- May cause ↑ serum lipase and amylase, hypercholesterolemia, and ↓ platelet count.

Implementation

- **PO:** Administer two 10-mg capsules and one 4-mg capsule to make 24 mg at the same time each day without regard to food. Swallow capsules whole; do not open, crush, or chew. For patients with difficulty swallowing, open capsule and dissolve capsule in small glass of liquid. Measure 1 tablespoon of water or apple juice and put capsule in liquid without breaking or crushing. Leave capsule in liquid for at least 10 min. Stir for at least 3 min, then drink mixture. After drinking, add same amount (1 tablespoon) of water or apple juice to glass. Swirl contents and swallow additional liquid.

Patient/Family Teaching

- Instruct patient to take lenvatinib as directed at the same time each day. Take missed dose within 12 hrs or omit and take next dose at usual time; do not double doses. Advise patient to read *Patient Information* before starting therapy and with each Rx refill in case of changes.
- Advise patient to notify health care professional promptly if signs and symptoms of high BP, heart problems, blood clots (severe chest pain or pressure; pain in arms, back, or jaw; shortness of breath; numbness or weakness on 1 side of body; trouble talking; sudden severe headache; sudden vision changes), liver problems (yellow skin or whites of eyes, dark tea colored urine, light-colored bowel movements), severe stomach pain, RPLS, or bleeding occur.
- Advise patient to notify health care professional of all Rx or OTC medications, vitamins, or herbal products being taken and to consult with health care professional before taking other medications.
- Rep: May be teratogenic. Advise females of reproductive potential to use effective contraception during and for at least 30 days following last dose of therapy and to notify health care professional if pregnancy is suspected. Advise patient to avoid breast feeding during and for at least 1 wk after last dose. May cause infertility in males and females.
- Emphasize importance of lab tests to monitor for adverse reactions.

Evaluation/Desired Outcomes

- Decreased progression and improved survival of differentiated thyroid cancer, endometrial cancer, renal cell carcinoma, and hepatocellular carcinoma.

letrozole (let-roe-zole)

Femara

Classification

Therapeutic: antineoplastics

Pharmacologic: aromatase inhibitors

Indications

First-line or second-line treatment of postmenopausal women with hormone receptor positive or hormone receptor unknown advanced breast cancer. Adjuvant treatment of postmenopausal women with hormone receptor positive early breast cancer. Extended adjuvant treatment of postmenopausal early breast cancer already treated with 5 yr of tamoxifen.

Action

Inhibits the enzyme aromatase, which is partially responsible for conversion of precursors to estrogen. **Therapeutic Effects:** Lowers levels of circulating estrogen, which may halt progression of estrogen-sensitive breast cancer. Decreased risk of recurrence/metastatic disease.

Pharmacokinetics

Absorption: Rapidly and completely absorbed.

Distribution: Unknown.

Metabolism and Excretion: Mostly metabolized by the liver.

Half-life: 2 days.

TIME/ACTION PROFILE (effect on lowering of serum estradiol levels)

ROUTE	ONSET	PEAK	DURATION
PO	unknown	2–3 days	unknown

Contraindications/Precautions

Contraindicated in: Hypersensitivity; Premenopausal women; OB: Potential for fetal harm.

Use Cautiously in: Severe hepatic impairment; Rep: Women of reproductive potential; Lactation, Pedi: Safety not established.

Adverse Reactions/Side Effects

CNS: anxiety, depression, dizziness, drowsiness, fatigue, headache, vertigo, weakness. **CV:** cerebrovascular events, chest pain, edema, hypertension, thromboembolic events. **Derm:** alopecia, hot flashes, ↑ sweating, pruritus, rash. **F and E:** hypercalcemia. **GI:** nausea, abdominal pain, anorexia, constipation, diarrhea, dyspepsia, vomiting. **GU:** ↓ fertility. **Metab:** hypercholesterolemia, weight gain. **MS:** musculoskeletal pain, arthralgia, ↓ bone density, fracture. **Resp:** cough, dyspnea, pleural effusion.

Interactions

Drug-Drug: None reported.

Route/Dosage

PO (Adults): 2.5 mg once daily.

Hepatic Impairment

PO (Adults): *Severe hepatic impairment*—2.5 mg every other day.

Availability (generic available)

Tablets: 2.5 mg.

NURSING IMPLICATIONS

Assessment
- Assess patient for pain and other side effects periodically throughout therapy.
- Monitor bone mineral density periodically during therapy.
- ***Lab Test Considerations:*** Obtain a negative pregnancy test before starting therapy.
- May cause elevated AST, ALT, alkaline phosphatase, bilirubin, GGT and cholesterol levels.

Implementation
- Do not confuse Femara (letrozole) with Femhrt (ethinyl estradiol/norethindrone).
- **PO:** May be taken without regard to food.

Patient/Family Teaching
- Instruct patient to take medication as directed.
- May cause dizziness and fatigue. Caution patient to avoid driving and other activities requiring awareness until response to medication is known.
- Inform patient of potential for adverse reactions and advise her to notify health care professional if side effects are problematic.
- Advise females of reporductive potential to use effective contraception and to avoid breast feeding during and for 3 wk after last dose of letrozole. May impair fertility in males and females. Caution women who are perimenopausal or who recently became menopausal to use adequate contraception during therapy; letrozole may cause fetal harm.

Evaluation/Desired Outcomes
- Slowing of disease progression in women with advanced breast cancer.
- Decreased risk of recurrence/metastatic disease.

leucovorin calcium
(loo-koe-**vor**-in)

Classification
Therapeutic: antidotes (for methotrexate), vitamins
Pharmacologic: folic acid analogues

Indications
Minimizes hematologic effects of high-dose methotrexate therapy (leucovorin rescue). Advanced colorectal carcinoma (with 5-fluorouracil). Management of overdoses/prevention of toxicity from folic acid antagonists (pyrimethamine, trimethoprim). Folic acid deficiency (megaloblastic anemia) unresponsive to oral replacement.

Action
The reduced form of folic acid that serves as a cofactor in the synthesis of DNA and RNA. **Therapeutic Effects:** Reversal of toxic effects of folic acid antagonists. Reversal of folic acid deficiency.

Pharmacokinetics
Absorption: Well absorbed (38%) following PO administration. ↓ bioavailability with larger doses. Oral absorption is saturated at doses >25 mg.
Distribution: Widely distributed. Concentrates in the CNS and liver.
Metabolism and Excretion: Extensively converted to tetrahydrofolic derivatives, including 5-methyltetrahydrofolate, a major storage form.
Half-life: 3.5 hr.

TIME/ACTION PROFILE (serum folate levels)

ROUTE	ONSET	PEAK	DURATION
PO	20–30 min	unknown	3–6 hr
IM	10–20 min	unknown	3–6 hr
IV	<5 min	unknown	3–6 hr

Contraindications/Precautions
Contraindicated in: Hypersensitivity; Pedi: Preparations containing benzyl alcohol should not be used in neonates.
Use Cautiously in: Undiagnosed anemia (may mask the progression of pernicious anemia); Ascites; Renal failure; Dehydration; Pleural effusions; Urine pH <7; OB, Lactation: Safety not established but has been used safely to treat megaloblastic anemia in pregnancy.

Adverse Reactions/Side Effects
Hemat: thrombocytosis. **Misc:** allergic reactions (rash, urticaria, wheezing).

Interactions
Drug-Drug: May ↓ anticonvulsant effect of **barbiturates, phenytoin,** or **primidone**. High doses of the liquid contain significant **alcohol** and may cause ↑ CNS depression when used with **CNS depressants**. Concurrent use with **trimethoprim/sulfamethoxazole** may result in ↓ anti-infective efficacy and poor therapeutic outcome when used to treat *Pneumocystis jirovecii* pneumonia in HIV patients. May ↑ therapeutic effects and toxicity of **fluorouracil**; therapy may be combined for this purpose.

Route/Dosage

High-Dose Methotrexate—Leucovorin Rescue. Must start within 24 hr of methotrexate.

PO, IM, IV (Adults and Children): *Normal methotrexate elimination*— 10 mg/m² every 6 hr (1st dose IV/IM, then change to PO) until methotrexate level is $<5 \times 10^{-8}$ M (0.05 micromolar). Larger doses/longer duration may be required in patients with aciduria, ascites, dehydration, renal impairment, GI obstruction, pleural/peritoneal effusions. Dose of leucovorin should be determined on the basis of plasma methotrexate levels.

Advanced Colorectal Cancer

IV (Adults): 200 mg/m² followed by 5-fluorouracil 370 mg/m² or leucovorin 20 mg/m² is followed by 5-

fluorouracil 425 mg/m². Regimen is given daily for 5 days every 4–5 wk.

Prevention of Hematologic Toxicity from Pyrimethamine

PO, IV (Adults and Children): 5–15 mg/day.

Inadvertent Overdose of Folic Acid Antagonists

IM, IV (Adults and Children): *Methotrexate–large doses*—75 mg IV followed by 12 mg IM every 6 hr for 4 doses; *methotrexate–average doses*—6–12 mg IM every 6 hr for 4 doses; *other folic acid antagonists*—amount equal in mg to folic acid antagonist.

Megaloblastic Anemia

PO, IM, IV (Adults and Children): Up to 1 mg/day (up to 6 mg/day for dihydrofolate reductase deficiency).

Availability (generic available)

Powder for injection: 50 mg/vial, 100 mg/vial, 200 mg/vial, 350 mg/vial, 500 mg/vial. **Solution for injection (preservative-free):** 10 mg/mL. **Tablets:** 5 mg, 10 mg, 15 mg, 25 mg.

NURSING IMPLICATIONS

Assessment

- Assess patient for nausea and vomiting secondary to methotrexate therapy or folic acid antagonists (pyrimethamine and trimethoprim) overdose. Parenteral route may be necessary to ensure that patient receives dose.
- Monitor for development of allergic reactions (rash, urticaria, wheezing). Notify health care professional if these occur.
- **Megaloblastic Anemia:** Assess degree of weakness and fatigue.
- ***Lab Test Considerations:* Leucovorin rescue:** Monitor serum methotrexate levels to determine dose and effectiveness of therapy. Leucovorin calcium levels should be equal to or greater than methotrexate level. Rescue continues until serum methotrexate level is $<5 \times 10$ M.
- Monitor CCr and serum creatinine prior to and every 24 hr during therapy to detect methotrexate toxicity. An increase >50% over the pretreatment concentration at 24 hr is associated with severe renal toxicity.
- Monitor urine pH every 6 hr during therapy; pH should be maintained >7 to decrease nephrotoxic effects of high-dose methotrexate. Sodium bicarbonate or acetazolamide may be ordered to alkalinize urine.
- *Megaloblastic anemia*—Monitor plasma folic acid levels, hemoglobin, hematocrit, and reticulocyte count prior to and periodically during therapy.

Implementation

- Do not confuse leucovorin calcium with levoleucovorin. Do not confuse leucovorin calcium with Leukeran (chlorambucil).
- Make sure leucovorin calcium is available before administering high-dose methotrexate. Administration must be initiated within 24 hr of methotrexate therapy.
- Administer as soon as possible after toxic dose of folic acid antagonists (pyrimethamine and trimethoprim). Effectiveness of therapy begins to decrease 1 hr after overdose.
- **PO:** Parenteral therapy should be used in patients with GI toxicity, with nausea and vomiting, or with doses >25 mg.
- **IM:** IM route is preferred for treatment of megaloblastic anemia. Ampules of leucovorin calcium injection for IM use do not require reconstitution.

IV Administration

- **IV Push:** Bacteriostatic water or sterile water. Do not use product containing benzyl alcohol. Use immediately if reconstituted with sterile water for injection. Stable for 7 days when reconstituted with bacteriostatic water. ***Concentration:*** reconstitute 50-mg, 100-mg, and 200-mg vials to a concentration of 10 mg/mL; reconstitute 350-mg vial to a concentration of 20 mg/mL. ***Rate:*** Administer by slow injection over a minimum of 3 min; not to exceed 160 mg/min.
- **Intermittent Infusion:** ***Diluent:*** May be diluted in 100–500 mL of D5W, D10W, 0.9% NaCl, Ringer's, or LR. Stable for 24 hr.
- **Y-Site Compatibility:** acyclovir, alemtuzumab, alfentanil, allopurinol, amifostine, amikacin, aminocaproic acid, aminophylline, ampicillin, ampicillin/sulbactam, anidulafungin, argatroban, azithromycin, aztreonam, bivalirudin, bleomycin, bumetamide, buprenorphine, busulfan, butorphanol, calcium acetate, calcium chloride, calcium gluconate, carmustine, caspofungin, cefepime, cefotaxime, cefotetan, cefoxitin, ceftazidime, cefuroxime, chloramphenicol, ciprofloxacin, cisatracurium, cisplatin, cladribine, clindamycin, cyclophosphamide, cyclosporine, cytarabine, dacarbazine, dactinomycin, daptomycin, daunorubicin hydrochloride, dexamethasone, dexamedetomidine, dexrazoxane, digoxin, diltiazem, diphenhydramine, dobutamine, docetaxel, dolasetron, dopamine, doxorubicin hydrochloride, doxorubicin liposomal, doxycycline, enalaprilat, ephedrine, epinephrine, eptifibatide, ertapenem, erythromycin, esmolol, etoposide, etoposide phosphate, famotidine, fenoldopam, fentanyl, filgrastim, fluconazole, fludarabine, fluorouracil, fospheny-

L

toin, furosemide, ganciclovir, gemcitabine, gentamicin, glycopyrrolate, granisetron, haloperidol, heparin, hetastarch, hydralazine, hydrocortisone, hydromorphone, idarubicin, ifosfamide, imipenem/cilastatin, insulin, irinotecan, isoproterenol, ketorolac, labetalol, levofloxacin, lidocaine, linezolid, lorazepam, magnesium sulfate, mannitol, melphalan, meperidine, meropenem, mesna, methotrexate, methyldopate, metoclopramide, metoprolol, metronidazole, midazolam, milrinone, mitomycin, mitoxantrone, morphine, moxifloxacin, mycophenolate, nafcillin, nalbuphine, nicardipine, nitroglycerin, nitroprusside, norepinephrine, octreotide, ondansetron, oxaliplatin, oxytocin, paclitaxel, palonosetron, pancuronium, pemetrexed, pentobarbital, phenobarbital, phenylephrine, piperacillin/tazobactam, potassium acetate, potassium chloride, procainamide, prochlorperazine, promethazine, propranolol, ranitidine, remifentanil, rituximab, rocuronium, sodium acetate, sodium phosphates, streptozocin, succinylcholine, sufentanil, tacrolimus, theophylline, thiotepa, tigecycline, tirofiban, tobramycin, topotecan, trastuzumab, trimethoprim/sulfamethoxazole, vasopressin, vecuronium, verapamil, vinblastine, vincristine, vinorelbine, voriconazole, zidovudine.

- **Y-Site Incompatibility:** amiodarone, amphotericin B deoxycholate, amphotericin B lipid complex, amphotericin B liposome, carboplatin, ceftriaxone, chlorpromazine, dantrolene, diazepam, droperidol, epirubicin, foscarnet, methylprednisolone, naloxone, pamidronate, pantoprazole, pentamidine, phenytoin, potassium phosphates, quinupristin/dalfopristin, sodium bicarbonate, thiopental, vancomycin.

Patient/Family Teaching

- Explain purpose of medication to patient. Emphasize need to take exactly as ordered. Advise patient to contact health care professional if a dose is missed.
- Advise females of reproductive potential to notify health care professional if pregnancy is planned or suspected, or if breast feeding.
- **Leucovorin Rescue:** Instruct patient to drink at least 3 liters of fluid each day during leucovorin rescue.
- **Folic Acid Deficiency:** Encourage patient to eat a diet high in folic acid (meat proteins; bran; dried beans; and green, leafy vegetables).

Evaluation/Desired Outcomes

- Reversal of bone marrow and GI toxicity in patients receiving methotrexate or in overdose of folic acid antagonists.
- Increased sense of well-being and increased production of normoblasts in patients with megaloblastic anemia.

leuprolide (loo-**proe**-lide)

Eligard, ~~Lupron~~, 🍁 Lupron, Lupron Depot, Lupron Depot-Ped

Classification

Therapeutic: antineoplastics

Pharmacologic: hormones, gonadotropin-releasing hormones

Indications

Advanced prostate cancer in patients who are unable to tolerate orchiectomy or estrogen therapy (may be used in combination with flutamide or bicalutamide). Central precocious puberty (CPP). Endometriosis. Uterine fibroids (with iron therapy).

Action

A synthetic analogue of luteinizing hormone–releasing hormone (LHRH). Initially causes a transient increase in testosterone; however, with continuous administration, testosterone levels are decreased. Reduces gonadotropins, testosterone, and estradiol. **Therapeutic Effects:** Decreased testosterone levels and resultant decrease in spread of prostate cancer. Reduction of pain/lesions in endometriosis. Decreased growth of fibroids. Delayed puberty.

Pharmacokinetics

Absorption: Rapidly and almost completely absorbed following subcut administration. More slowly absorbed following IM administration of depot form.

Distribution: Unknown.

Metabolism and Excretion: Unknown.

Half-life: 3 hr.

TIME/ACTION PROFILE (effect on hormone levels)

ROUTE	ONSET†	PEAK‡	DURATION§
Subcut	within 1st wk	2–4 wk	4–12 wk
IM	within 1st wk	2–4 wk	4–12 wk
IM-depot	within 1st wk	2–4 wk	4–12 wk

†Initial transient ↑ in testosterone and estradiol levels.

‡Maximum decline in testosterone and estradiol levels.

§Restoration of normal pituitary–gonadal function; in amenorrheic patients, normal menses usually returns 60–90 days after treatment is discontinued.

Contraindications/Precautions

Contraindicated in: Hypersensitivity to synthetic analogues of LHRH (GnRH); OB: Pregnancy (may cause fetal harm); Lactation: Lactation.

Use Cautiously in: Hypersensitivity to benzyl alcohol (results in induration and erythema at subcut site); Congenital long QT syndrome, HF, electrolyte abnormalities, or concurrent use of other drugs known to prolong the QT interval; Seizures, cerebrovascular disorders, CNS tumor, or concurrent use of bupropion or selective serotonin reuptake inhibitors.

Adverse Reactions/Side Effects

CNS: SEIZURES, STROKE, aggression, anger, dizziness, headache, impatience, irritability, syncope; *Depot*, depression, drowsiness, personality disorder; *Subcut*, anxiety, blurred vision, lethargy, memory disorder, mood swings. **EENT:** blurred vision; *Subcut*, hearing disorder. **CV:** MYOCARDIAL INFARCTION, PULMONARY EMBOLI, angina, arrhythmias; *Depot*, QT INTERVAL PROLONGATION, vasodilation. **Derm:** *Depot*—hair growth, rash; *Subcut*, dry skin, hair loss, pigmentation, skin cancer, skin lesions. **Endo:** breast swelling, breast tenderness, hyperglycemia. **F and E:** hypercalcemia, lower extremity edema. **GI:** anorexia, diarrhea, dysphagia, nausea, vomiting; *Depot*, HEPATOTOXICITY, gingivitis; *Subcut*, GI BLEEDING, hepatic dysfunction, peptic ulcer, rectal polyps, taste disorders. **GU:** ↓ fertility (males), ↓ testicular size, dysuria, incontinence, testicular pain; *Depot*, cervix disorder; *Subcut*, bladder spasm, penile swelling, prostate pain, urinary obstruction. **Local:** burning, itching, swelling at injection site. **Metab:** *Depot*—hyperuricemia, ↓ bone density. **MS:** fibromyalgia, transient ↑ in bone pain (prostate cancer only); *Subcut*, ankylosing spondylitis, joint pain, pelvic fibrosis, temporal bone pain. **Neuro:** *Subcut*—peripheral neuropathy. **Resp:** hemoptysis; *Depot*, epistaxis, throat nodules; *Subcut*, cough, pleural rub, pulmonary fibrosis, pulmonary infiltrate. **Misc:** hot flashes, chills, ↓ libido, fever; *Depot*, body odor, epistaxis.

Interactions

Drug-Drug: ↑ antineoplastic effects with **antiandrogens (megestrol, flutamide)**. Concurrent use with **bupropion** or **SSRIs** may ↑ risk of seizures.

Route/Dosage

Advanced Prostate Cancer

Subcut (Adults): *Leuprolide acetate*—1 mg/day; *Eligard*—7.5 mg once monthly, 22.5 mg every 3 mo, 30 mg every 4 mo, or 45 mg every 6 mo.

IM (Adults): *Lupron Depot*—7.5 mg once monthly *or* 22.5 mg every 3 mo *or* 30 mg every 4 mo *or* 45 mg every 6 mo.

Endometriosis

IM (Adults): *Lupron Depot*—3.75 mg once monthly for up to 6 mo *or* 11.25 mg every 3 mo for up to 2 doses.

Uterine Fibroids (with iron therapy)

IM (Adults): *Lupron Depot*—3.75 mg once monthly for up to 3 mo *or* 11.25 mg single injection.

Central Precocious Puberty (CPP)

Subcut (Children): *Leuprolide acetate*—50 mcg/kg/day, may ↑ by 10 mcg/kg/day as required.

IM (Children >37.5 kg): *Lupron Depot-Ped*—15 mg every 4 wk; may ↑ by 3.75 mg every 4 wk as required.

IM (Children 26–37.5 kg): *Lupron Depot-Ped*—11.25 mg every 4 wk; may ↑ by 3.75 mg every 4 wk as required.

IM (Children ≤25 kg): *Lupron Depot-Ped*—7.5 mg every 4 wk; may ↑ by 3.75 mg every 4 wk as required.

IM (Children): *Lupron Depot-Ped*—11.25 or 30 mg every 3 mo.

Availability (generic available)

Lyophilized microspheres for depot injection (Lupron Depot): 3.75 mg, 7.5 mg, 11.25 mg, 22.5 mg, 30 mg, 45 mg. **Lyophilized microspheres for depot injection (Lupron Depot-Ped):** 7.5 mg, 11.25 mg, 15 mg, 30 mg. **Polymeric matrix injectable formulation for injection (Eligard):** 7.5 mg, 22.5 mg, 30 mg, 45 mg. **Solution for injection (leuprolide acetate):** 1 mg/0.2 mL.

L

NURSING IMPLICATIONS

Assessment

- Monitor ECG periodically in patients at risk for QT interval prolongation.
- **Prostate Cancer:** Assess for an increase in bone pain, especially during the first few wk of therapy. Monitor patients with vertebral metastases for increased back pain and decreased sensory/motor function.
- Monitor intake and output ratios; assess for bladder distention in patients with urinary tract obstruction during initiation of therapy.
- **Fibroids:** Assess for severity of symptoms (bloating, pelvic pain, pressure, excessive vaginal bleeding) periodically during therapy.
- **Endometriosis:** Assess for endometrial pain prior to and periodically during therapy.
- **CPP:** Prior to therapy, diagnosis of CPP should be confirmed by onset of secondary sex characteristics in girls <8 yr or boys <9 yr; a complete physical and endocrinologic examination, including height, weight, hand and wrist x-ray; total sex steroid level (estradiol or testosterone); adrenal steroid level; beta human chorionic gonadotropin level; GnRH stimulation test; and computerized tomography of the head must be performed. These parameters are monitored after 1–2 mo and every 6–12 mo during therapy.
- Assess for signs of precocious puberty (menses, breast development, testicular growth) periodically during therapy. Dose is increased until no progression of the disease is noted either clinically or by lab test parameters, then usually maintained throughout therapy. Discontinuation of therapy

should be considered before age 11 in girls and age 12 in boys.

- ***Lab Test Considerations:*** Initially ↑, then ↓ luteinizing hormone (LH) and follicle-stimulating hormone (FSH). This leads to castration levels of testosterone in boys 2–4 wk after initial increase in concentrations.
- Monitor testosterone, prostatic acid phosphate, and prostate-specific antigen (PSA) levels to evaluate response to therapy. Transient ↑ in levels may occur during the 1st mo of therapy for prostate cancer.
- Monitor electrolytes before starting and periodically during therapy. May cause ↑ BUN, serum calcium, uric acid, hypoproteinemia, LDH, alkaline phosphatase, AST, hyperglycemia, hyperlipidemia, hyperphosphatemia, WBC, PT, or PTT. May also cause ↓ platelets and serum potassium.
- Monitor blood sugar and glycosylated hemoglobin periodically during therapy.

Implementation

- Do not confuse Lupron Depot with Lupron Depot-Ped.
- Norethindrone acetate 5 mg daily may be used to prevent bone density loss from leuprolide.
- Correct electrolyte abnormalities before starting therapy.
- **Subcut:** ***Eligard subcut formulation:*** **Bring to room temperature before mixing. Assemble the Eligard kit and reconstitute solution using syringes provided, as directed by manufacturer. Wearing gloves, mix in syringes as directed by manufacturer, do not shake. Solution must reach room temperature before administration and must be administered within 30 min of mixing, or be discarded. Solution is light tan to tan in color. Inject into abdomen, upper buttocks, or anywhere that has adequate amounts of subcut tissue without excessive pigment, nodules, lesions, or hair. Vary site with each injection. Store in refrigerator; may also be stored at room temperature in original packing for up to 8 wk before mixing.**
- **IM:** Use syringe supplied by manufacturer. Rotate sites.
- Leuprolide depot is *only* for IM injection.
- *Lupron Depot formulation:* To prepare for injection screw white plunger into end stopper until stopper begins to turn. Hold syringe upright; release diluent by slowly pushing, over 6–8 sec, until the first stopper is at the blue line in the middle of the barrel. Keep syringe upright. Mix microspheres by shaking syringe until power forms a unified suspension. Tap syringe if caking or clumping occurs. Suspension will appear milky. Do not use if powder does not go into suspension. Keep syringe upright, remove cap and expel air. Inject at 90° angle in gluteal area, anterior thigh, or deltoid; rotate injection sites. Suspension settles very quickly; mix and administer immediately.
- Store at room temperature; stable for 24 hr following reconstitution.

Patient/Family Teaching

- Advise patient that medication may cause hot flashes. Notify health care professional if these become bothersome.
- Leuprolide depot usually causes a temporary discontinuation of menstruation. Advise patient to notify health care professional if menstruation persists or if intermittent bleeding occurs.
- Inform patient of the possibility of the development or worsening of depression and occurrence of memory disorders.
- **Prostate Cancer:** Instruct patient and family on subcut injection technique. Review patient insert provided with leuprolide patient-administration kit.
- Instruct patient to take medication exactly as directed. Take missed doses as soon as remembered unless not remembered until next day.
- Advise patient that bone pain may increase at initiation of therapy, but will resolve with time. Patient should discuss with health care professional use of analgesics to control pain.
- Instruct patient to notify health care professional promptly if difficulty urinating, weakness, or numbness occurs.
- **Endometriosis:** Advise patient to use a form of contraception other than oral contraceptives during therapy. Inform patient that amenorrhea is expected but does not guarantee contraception. Advise patient that breast feeding should be avoided during therapy.
- **Central Precocious Puberty:** Instruct patient and family on the proper technique for subcut injection. Emphasize the importance of administering the medication at the same time each day. Rotate injection sites periodically.
- Inform patient and parents that if injections are not given daily, pubertal process may be reactivated.
- Advise patient and parents that during the first 2 mo of therapy patient may experience a light menstrual flow or spotting. Health care professional should be notified if this continues beyond 2nd mo.
- Instruct patient and parents to notify health care professional immediately if irritation at the injection site or unusual signs or symptoms occur.

Evaluation/Desired Outcomes

- Decrease in the spread of prostate cancer.
- Decrease in lesions and pain in endometriosis.
- Resolution of the signs of CPP.
- Improvement in preoperative hematologic parameters in patients with anemia from uterine fibroids.

levalbuterol

(leev-al-**byoo**-ter-ole)

Xopenex, Xopenex HFA

Classification

Therapeutic: bronchodilators

Pharmacologic: adrenergics

Indications

Bronchospasm due to reversible airway disease (short-term control agent).

Action

R-enantiomer of racemic albuterol. Binds to beta-2 adrenergic receptors in airway smooth muscle leading to activation of adenylcyclase and increased levels of cyclic-3′, 5′-adenosine monophosphate (cAMP). Increases in cAMP activate kinases, which inhibit the phosphorylation of myosin and decrease intracellular calcium. Decreased intracellular calcium relaxes bronchial smooth muscle. **Therapeutic Effects:** Relaxation of airway smooth muscle with subsequent bronchodilation. Relatively selective for beta-2 (pulmonary) receptors.

Pharmacokinetics

Absorption: Some absorption occurs following inhalation.

Distribution: Unknown.

Metabolism and Excretion: Metabolized in the liver to an inactive sulfate and 3–6% excreted unchanged in the urine.

Half-life: 3.3–4 hr.

TIME/ACTION PROFILE (bronchodilation)

ROUTE	ONSET	PEAK	DURATION
Inhaln	10–17 min	90 min	5–6 hr

Contraindications/Precautions

Contraindicated in: Hypersensitivity to levalbuterol or albuterol.

Use Cautiously in: Cardiovascular disorders (including coronary insufficiency, hypertension, and arrhythmias); History of seizures; Hypokalemia; Hyperthyroidism; Diabetes mellitus; Unusual sensitivity to adrenergic amines; OB: Safety not established; Lactation: Use while breast feeding only if maternal benefit outweighs potential risk to infant; Pedi: Children <6 yr (nebulized solution) or <4 yr (metered-dose inhaler) (safety not established).

Exercise Extreme Caution in: Concurrent use or use within 2 wk of **tricyclic antidepressants** or **MAO inhibitors** (may ↑ risk of adverse cardiovascular reactions).

Adverse Reactions/Side Effects

CNS: anxiety, dizziness, headache, nervousness. **CV:** tachycardia. **Endo:** hyperglycemia. **F and E:** hypokalemia. **GI:** dyspepsia, vomiting. **Neuro:** tremor. **Resp:** PARADOXICAL BRONCHOSPASM (excessive use of inhalers), cough, turbinate edema.

Interactions

Drug-Drug: Concurrent use or use within 2 wk of **tricyclic antidepressants** or **MAO inhibitors** may ↑ risk of adverse cardiovascular reactions (use with extreme caution). **Beta blockers** block the beneficial pulmonary effects of adrenergic bronchodilators (choose cardioselective beta blockers if necessary and with caution). May ↑ risk of hypokalemia from **potassium-losing diuretics**. May ↓ serum **digoxin** levels. May ↑ risk of arrhythmias with **hydrocarbon inhalation anesthetics** or **cocaine**.

Drug-Natural Products: Use with caffeine-containing herbs **(guarana, tea, coffee)** ↑ stimulant effect.

Route/Dosage

Inhaln (Adults and Children ≥4 yr): 2 inhalations every 4–6 hr; some patients may respond to 1 inhalation every 4 hr.

Inhaln (Adults and Children >12 yr): 0.63 mg via nebulization 3 times daily (every 6–8 hr); may be ↑ to 1.25 mg 3 times daily (every 6–8 hr).

Inhaln (Children 6–11 yr): 0.31 mg via nebulization 3 times daily (not to exceed 0.63 mg 3 times daily).

Availability (generic available)

Inhalation aerosol: 45 mcg/actuation in 15-g canisters (200 metered actuations). **Cost:** $54.23/15 g. **Inhalation solution:** 0.31 mg/3 mL, 0.63 mg/3 mL, 1.25 mg/3 mL, 1.25 mg/0.5 mL. **Cost:** *Generic*—All strengths $6.71/3 mL.

NURSING IMPLICATIONS

Assessment

- Assess lung sounds, pulse, and BP before administration and during peak of medication. Note amount, color, and character of sputum produced. Closely monitor patients on higher dose for adverse effects.
- Monitor pulmonary function tests before initiating therapy and periodically during course to determine effectiveness of medication.
- Observe for paradoxical bronchospasm (wheezing, dyspnea, tightness in chest). If condition occurs, withhold medication and notify health care provider immediately.
- ***Lab Test Considerations:*** May cause ↑ serum glucose and ↓ serum potassium.

Implementation

- **Inhaln:** Allow at least 1 min between inhalations of aerosol medication.
- For nebulization, levalbuterol solution does not require dilution prior to administration. Once the foil

pouch is opened, vials must be used within 2 wk; open vials may be stored for 1 wk. Discard vial if solution is not clear or colorless.

Patient/Family Teaching

- Instruct patient in the proper use of inhalation aerosol nebulizer (see Appendix D) and to take levalbuterol as directed. Caution patient not to exceed recommended dose; may cause adverse effects, paradoxical bronchospasm, or loss of effectiveness of medication.
- Instruct patient to notify health care professional of all Rx or OTC medications, vitamins, or herbal products being taken and to consult health care professional before taking any OTC medications or alcoholic beverages concurrently with this therapy. Caution patient also to avoid smoking and other respiratory irritants.
- Instruct patient to contact health care professional immediately if shortness of breath is not relieved by medication or is accompanied by diaphoresis, dizziness, palpitations, or chest pain.
- Advise patients to use levalbuterol first if using other inhalation medications, and allow 5 min to elapse before administering other inhalant medications unless otherwise directed.
- Advise patient to rinse mouth with water after each inhalation dose to minimize dry mouth.
- Advise females of reproductive potential to notify health care professional if pregnancy is planned or suspected, or if breast feeding. Encourage women who become pregnant while taking levalbuterol to enroll in the Asthma & Pregnancy Study to monitor pregnancy outcomes in women exposed to asthma medications by calling 1-877-311-8972 or visiting www.mothertobaby.org/ongoing-study/asthma.
- Instruct patient to notify health care professional if no response to the usual dose of levalbuterol.

Evaluation/Desired Outcomes

- Prevention or relief of bronchospasm.

levETIRAcetam

(le-ve-teer-**a**-se-tam)

Elepsia XR, Keppra, Keppra XR, ~~Roweepra~~, Spritam

Classification

Therapeutic: anticonvulsants

Pharmacologic: pyrrolidines

Indications

Partial onset seizures (adjunct). Primary generalized tonic-clonic seizures (adjunct) (immediate-release and injection only). Myoclonic seizures in patients with juvenile myoclonic epilepsy (adjunct) (immediate-release and injection only). **Unlabeled Use:** Status epilepticus.

Action

Appears to inhibit burst firing without affecting normal neuronal excitability and may selectively prevent hypersynchronization of epileptiform burst firing and propagation of seizure activity. **Therapeutic Effects:** Decreased incidence and severity of seizures.

Pharmacokinetics

Absorption: Rapidly and completely absorbed following oral administration.

Distribution: Unknown.

Protein Binding: <10%.

Metabolism and Excretion: 66% excreted unchanged by the kidneys; some metabolism by the liver (metabolites inactive).

Half-life: 7.1 hr (↑ in renal impairment).

TIME/ACTION PROFILE (blood levels)

ROUTE	ONSET	PEAK	DURATION
PO	rapid	1–1.5 hr†‡	12 hr

†1 hr in the fasting state, 1.5 hr when taken with food.
‡4 hr with extended-release.

Contraindications/Precautions

Contraindicated in: Hypersensitivity; Lactation: Lactation.

Use Cautiously in: All patients (may ↑ risk of suicidal thoughts/behaviors); Renal impairment (dose ↓ recommended if CCr ≤80 mL/min); Pedi: Safety and effectiveness not established in children <16 yr (injection), <12 yr (extended-release); OB: Use only if potential benefit justifies potential risk to fetus; blood levels may be ↓ during pregnancy (especially during 3rd trimester); Geri: ↓ renal elimination (dose ↓ may be necessary).

Adverse Reactions/Side Effects

CNS: SUICIDAL THOUGHTS, aggression, agitation, anger, anxiety, apathy, depersonalization, depression, dizziness, drowsiness, fatigue, hostility, irritability, personality disorder, psychosis, weakness, hyperkinesia. **CV:** hypertension. **Derm:** DRUG REACTION WITH EOSINOPHILIA AND SYSTEMIC SYMPTOMS (DRESS), STEVENS-JOHNSON SYNDROME, TOXIC EPIDERMAL NECROLYSIS. **Hemat:** AGRANULOCYTOSIS, anemia, eosinophilia, neutropenia, thrombocytopenia. **Neuro:** coordination difficulties (adults only). **Misc:** HYPERSENSITIVITY REACTIONS (including anaphylaxis and angioedema).

Interactions

Drug-Drug: None noted.

Route/Dosage

Only the oral solution should be used in patients ≤20 kg.

Partial Onset Seizures

PO, IV (Adults and Children ≥16 yr): 500 mg twice daily initially; may ↑ by 1000 mg/day at 2-wk intervals up to 3000 mg/day (in 2 divided doses).

PO (Adults and Children ≥12 yr): *Extended-release*—1000 mg once daily; may ↑ by 1000 mg/day at 2-wk intervals up to 3000 mg/day.
PO (Adults and Children ≥4 yr and >40 kg): *Tablets for oral suspension*—500 mg twice daily; may ↑ by 1000 mg/day at 2-wk intervals up to 3000 mg/day in 2 divided doses.
PO, IV (Children 4–15 yr): 10 mg/kg twice daily; ↑ by 20 mg/kg/day at 2-wk intervals to recommended dose of 30 mg/kg twice daily (maximum dose: 3000 mg/day in 2 divided doses).
PO (Children ≥4 yr and 20–40 kg): *Tablets for oral suspension*—250 mg twice daily; may ↑ by 500 mg/day at 2-wk intervals up to 1500 mg/day in 2 divided doses.
PO, IV (Children 6 mo–3 yr): 10 mg/kg twice daily; ↑ by 20 mg/kg/day at 2-wk intervals to recommended dose of 25 mg/kg twice daily.
PO, IV (Children 1–5 mo): 7 mg/kg twice daily; ↑ by 14 mg/kg/day at 2-wk intervals to recommended dose of 21 mg/kg twice daily.

Primary Generalized Tonic-Clonic Seizures

PO, IV (Adults and Children ≥16 yr): 500 mg twice daily initially; ↑ by 1000 mg/day at 2-wk intervals to recommended dose of 3000 mg/day.
PO (Adults and Children ≥6 yr and >40 kg): *Tablets for oral suspension*—500 mg twice daily; may ↑ by 1000 mg/day at 2-wk intervals up to 3000 mg/day in 2 divided doses.
PO, IV (Children 6–15 yr): 10 mg/kg twice daily; ↑ by 20 mg/kg/day at 2-wk intervals to recommended dose of 30 mg/kg twice daily.
PO (Children ≥6 yr and 20–40 kg): *Tablets for oral suspension*—250 mg twice daily; may ↑ by 500 mg/day at 2-wk intervals up to 1500 mg/day in 2 divided doses.

Myoclonic Seizures

PO, IV (Adults and Children ≥12 yr): 500 mg twice daily initially; ↑ by 1000 mg/day at 2-wk intervals to recommended dose of 3000 mg/day (in 2 divided doses).

Status Epilepticus

IV (Infants and Children <16 yr): 50 mg/kg as a loading dose followed by maintenance dose of 30–55 mg/kg/day IV/PO in 2 divided doses.
IV (Neonates): 20–30 mg/kg as a loading dose followed by neonatal seizure dosing.

Renal Impairment

PO, IV (Adults): *CCr 50–80 mL/min*—500–1000 mg twice daily (1000–2000 mg once daily for extended-release); *CCr 30–50 mL/min*—250–750 mg twice daily (500–1500 mg once daily for extended-release); *CCr <30 mL/min*—250–500 mg twice daily (500–1000 mg once daily for extended-release); *Dialysis (immediate-release and injection)*—500–1000 mg once daily with a 250–500-mg supplemental dose after dialysis.

Availability (generic available)

Extended-release tablets: 500 mg, 750 mg, 1000 mg, 1500 mg. **Cost:** *Generic*—500 mg $266.82/60, 750 mg $400.64/60. **Oral solution (grape-flavored):** 100 mg/mL. **Cost:** *Generic*—$307.74/473 mL. **Premixed infusion:** 500 mg/100 mL 0.82% NaCl, 1000 mg/100 mL 0.75% NaCl, 1500 mg/100 mL 0.54% NaCl. **Solution for injection (requires dilution):** 100 mg/mL. **Tablets:** 250 mg, 500 mg, 750 mg, 1000 mg. **Cost:** *Generic*—250 mg $29.94/100, 500 mg $43.36/100, 750 mg $55.11/100, 1000 mg $148.42/180. **Tablets for oral suspension (Spritam) (spearmint-flavored):** 250 mg, 500 mg, 750 mg, 1000 mg.

L

NURSING IMPLICATIONS

Assessment

- Assess location, duration, and characteristics of seizure activity.
- Assess patient for CNS adverse effects throughout therapy. These adverse effects are categorized as somnolence and fatigue (asthenia), coordination difficulties (ataxia, abnormal gait, or incoordination), and behavioral abnormalities (agitation, hostility, anxiety, apathy, emotional lability, depersonalization, depression) and usually occur during the first 4 wk of therapy.
- Monitor mood changes. Assess for suicidal tendencies, especially during early therapy. Restrict amount of drug available to patient.
- Assess for rash periodically during therapy. May cause Stevens-Johnson syndrome. Discontinue therapy if severe or if accompanied with fever, general malaise, fatigue, muscle or joint aches, blisters, oral lesions, conjunctivitis, hepatitis, and/or eosinophilia.
- Monitor for signs and symptoms of DRESS (fever, rash, lymphadenopathy, and/or facial swelling, associated with involvement of other organ systems (hepatitis, nephritis, hematologic abnormalities, myocarditis, myositis) during therapy. May resemble an acute viral infection. Eosinophilia is often present. Discontinue therapy if signs occur.
- Monitor for signs and symptoms of anaphylaxis (dyspnea, wheezing, facial swelling). Discontinue levetiracetam if symptoms occur.
- Pedi: Monitor patients 1 mo to <4 yr of age for increases in diastolic BP.
- ***Lab Test Considerations:*** May cause ↓ RBC and WBC and abnormal liver function tests.

Implementation

- Do not confuse Keppra (levetiracetam) with Kaletra (lopinavir/ritonavir) or Keflex (cephalexin). Do not confuse levetiracetam with lamotrigine, levocarnitine, or levofloxacin.
- IV doses should be used temporarily when oral route is not feasible. To convert IV to PO, equivalent dose and frequency may be used.
- **PO:** May be administered without regard to meals.
- Administer tablets whole; do not administer partial tablets. Do not break, crush, or chew XR tablets.
- Pedi: Patients <20 kg should receive oral solution. Administer with calibrated measuring device for accurate dose.
- Discontinue gradually to minimize the risk of increase in seizure frequency.

IV Administration

- **Intermittent Infusion:** ***Diluent:*** Dilute dose in 100 mL of 0.9% NaCl, D5W, or LR. If a smaller volume is required (e.g. pediatric patients), concentration should not exceed 15 mg/mL. Do not administer solutions that are cloudy or contain particulate matter. ***Rate:*** Infuse over 15 min.
- **Y-Site Compatibility:** diazepam, lorazepam, valproate.

Patient/Family Teaching

- Instruct patient to take medication as directed. Pedi: Explain to parents the importance of using calibrated measuring device for accurate dosing. Take missed doses as soon as possible unless almost time for next dose. Do not double doses. Do not discontinue abruptly; may cause increase in frequency of seizures. Advise patient to read the *Medication Guide* prior to starting therapy and with each Rx refill in case of changes.
- May cause dizziness and somnolence. Caution patient to avoid driving or activities requiring alertness until response to medication is known. Do not resume driving until physician gives clearance based on control of seizure disorder.
- Advise patient and family to notify health care professional if thoughts about suicide or dying, attempts to commit suicide; new or worse depression; new or worse anxiety; feeling very agitated or restless; panic attacks; trouble sleeping; new or worse irritability; acting aggressive; being angry or violent; acting on dangerous impulses; an extreme increase in activity and talking; other unusual changes in behavior or mood, or if skin rash occur.
- Advise patient to notify health care professional of all Rx or OTC medications, vitamins, or herbal products being taken and to consult with health care professional before taking other medications.
- Instruct patient to notify health care professional of medication regimen prior to treatment or surgery.
- Rep: Advise female patients to notify health care professional if pregnancy is planned or suspected or if breast feeding. Encourage pregnant patients to enroll in the North American Antiepileptic Drug (NAAED) Pregnancy Registry by calling 1-888-233-2334; information is available at www.aedpregnancyregistry.org.
- Advise patient to carry identification describing disease process and medication regimen at all times.

Evaluation/Desired Outcomes

- Decrease in the frequency of or cessation of seizures.

levodopa (lee-voe-**doe**-pa)

Inbrija

Classification

Therapeutic: antiparkinson agents

Pharmacologic: dopamine agonists

Indications

Intermittent treatment of "off" episodes in patients with Parkinson's disease treated with carbidopa/levodopa.

Action

Converted to dopamine in the CNS, where it serves as a neurotransmitter. **Therapeutic Effects:** Reduction in "off" episodes.

Pharmacokinetics

Absorption: 70% absorbed following oral inhalation.

Distribution: Extensively distributed to tissues.

Metabolism and Excretion: Primarily metabolized in liver by decarboxylation (via dopa decarboxylase) and O-methylation (by catechol-O-methyltransferase [COMT]).

Half-life: 2.3 hr.

TIME/ACTION PROFILE (plasma concentrations)

ROUTE	ONSET	PEAK	DURATION
Inhaln	unknown	30 min	unknown

Contraindications/Precautions

Contraindicated in: Concurrent or recent (within past 2 wk) use of nonselective MAO inhibitor therapy; Major psychotic disorders; Asthma, COPD, or underlying lung disease (may ↑ risk of bronchospasm).

Use Cautiously in: Glaucoma (may ↑ intraocular pressure); OB: Safety not established; Lactation: Use while breast feeding only if potential maternal benefit justifies potential risk to infant; Pedi: Safety and effectiveness not established; Geri: ↑ risk of adverse reactions.

Adverse Reactions/Side Effects

CNS: aggression, agitation, confusion, delirium, delusions, disorientation, hallucinations, headache, insomnia, paranoid ideation, psychosis, sedation, urges (gambling, sexual), vivid dreams. **CV:** orthostatic hypotension. **EENT:** ↑ intraocular pressure, nasal discharge discoloration, nasopharyngitis. **GI:** hyperbilirubinemia, ↑ liver enzymes, nausea, vomiting. **MS:** dyskinesias. **Resp:** cough, upper respiratory tract infection, sputum discoloration. **Misc:** falls.

Interactions

Drug-Drug: **Nonselective MAO inhibitors**, including **phenelzine** or **tranylcypromine**, can ↑ risk of severe hypertension; concurrent use contraindicated (MAO inhibitor must be discontinued ≥2 wk before initiating levodopa). **Selective MAO inhibitors**, including **rasagiline** or **selegiline** may ↑ risk of orthostatic hypotension. **Haloperidol**, **isoniazid metoclopramide**, **phenothiazines**, or **risperidone** may ↓ effectiveness. **Iron** or **multivitamins** containing iron may ↓ absorption of levodopa.

Route/Dosage

Should be used in patients already taking carbidopa/levodopa.
Inhaln (Adults): 84 mg as needed for "off" episodes up to 5 times per day (max = 420 mg/day).

Availability

Capsules for oral inhalation: 42 mg.

NURSING IMPLICATIONS

Assessment

- Assess parkinsonian symptoms (akinesia, rigidity, tremors, pill rolling, shuffling gait, mask-like face, twisting motions, and drooling) during therapy. "On-off phenomenon" may cause symptoms to appear or improve suddenly.
- Assess for signs and symptoms of dyskinesia (abnormal movements, uncontrolled sudden movements of face, tongue, or other body parts) before and during therapy. May increase during therapy requiring dose adjustment or discontinuation.
- Monitor for signs and symptoms of behavior changes (hallucinations, psychotic behavior, paranoid ideation, delusions, confusion, mania, disorientation, aggressive behavior, agitation, delirium) during therapy. Consider reducing dose or discontinuing therapy.
- ***Lab Test Considerations:*** May cause ↑ alkaline phosphatase, AST, ALT, lactic dehydrogenase (LDH), and bilirubin.
- May cause ↑ blood urea nitrogen (BUN), hemolytic anemia and positive direct antibody test.

Implementation

- **Inhaln:** Administer up to 5 times daily when symptoms of an OFF period start to return. Capsules are for oral inhalation only; use only with the Inbrija inhaler.

Patient/Family Teaching

- Instruct patient to take medication when their Parkinson's symptoms (OFF periods) first occurs as directed. Instruct patient in correct use of Imbrija inhaler and that each dose is 2 capsules. Capsules are for use in inhaler; do not take orally. Discontinue slowly; abrupt discontinuation may cause fever, confusion, stiff muscles, changes in breathing and heartbeat. Advise patient to read *Patient Information* before starting therapy and with each Rx refill in case of changes.
- May cause sudden onset of sleep, drowsiness, or dizziness. Advise patient to avoid driving and other activities that require alertness until response to drug is known.
- Inform patient that medication may cause dark color bodily fluids (saliva, sputum, urine, sweat).
- Advise patient to notify health care professional if abnormal involuntary movements appear or get worse during therapy.
- Caution patient to change positions slowly to minimize orthostatic hypotension. Health care professional should be notified if orthostatic hypotension occurs.
- Advise patient to notify health care professional of all Rx or OTC medications, vitamins, or herbal products being taken and to consult with health care professional before taking other medications.
- Advise patient and family to notify health care professional if signs and symptoms of hallucinations or psychosis (being overly suspicious or feeling people want to harm you, disorientation, believing things that are not real, aggressive behavior, seeing or hearing things that are not real, agitation, confusion, delirium, increase activity or talking), or if new or increased gambling, sexual, or other intense urges occur. Dose reduction may be required.
- Advise females of reproductive potential to use effective contraception and avoid breast feeding during therapy. Advise patient to notify health care professional if pregnancy is planned or suspected, or if breast feeding.

Evaluation/Desired Outcomes

- Decreased "off" time in patients with Parkinson's disease.

levomilnacipran

(lee-voe-mil-**na**-si-pran)
Fetzima

Classification
Therapeutic: antidepressants
Pharmacologic: selective serotonin/norepinephrine reuptake inhibitors

Indications

Treatment of major depressive disorder.

Action

Inhibits neuronal reuptake of norepinephrine and serotonin in the CNS (SNRI). **Therapeutic Effects:** Decrease in depressive symptomatology, with fewer relapses/recurrences.

Pharmacokinetics

Absorption: Well absorbed (92%) following oral administration.

Distribution: Widely distributed.

Metabolism and Excretion: 58% eliminated unchanged in urine; 42% metabolized, primarily by the CYP3A4 enzyme system; metabolites are renally eliminated.

Half-life: 12 hr.

TIME/ACTION PROFILE

ROUTE	ONSET	PEAK	DURATION
PO	Unknown	6–8 hr (blood level)	Unknown

Contraindications/Precautions

Contraindicated in: Hypersensitivity to levomilnacipran or milnacipran; Uncontrolled narrow-angle glaucoma; Concurrent use of or in close temporal proximity to MAO inhibitors, linezolid or methylene blue (risk of serotonin syndrome); Concurrent use of alcohol; Lactation: Lactation.

Use Cautiously in: History of hypertension, cardiovascular or cerebrovascular disease (BP should be controlled prior to treatment); History of bipolar disorder (may activate mania/hypomania); Renal impairment (dose ↓ required for CCr <60 mL/min); OB: Use only if potential maternal benefit justifies potential fetal risk; Pedi: ↑ risk of suicidal thinking and behavior (suicidality) in adolescents and young adults up to 24 yrs with major depressive disorder; Geri: Consider age-related ↓ in renal function, chronic disease state and concurrent drug therapy; may have ↑ risk of hyponatremia.

Exercise Extreme Caution in: Concurrent use with other serotonergic drugs (↑ risk of serotonin syndrome especially during initiation and dose adjustment).

Adverse Reactions/Side Effects

CNS: activation of mania/hypomania. **CV:** hypertension, hypotension, palpitations, tachycardia. **Derm:** hot flush, hyperhydrosis, rash. **EENT:** mydrasis. **F and E:** hyponatremia (in association with syndrome of inappropriate antidiuretic hormone [SIADH]). **GI:** nausea, ↓ appetite, constipation, vomiting. **GU:** ejaculation disorder, erectile dysfunction, testicular pain, urinary hesitation/retention. **Hemat:** bleeding. **Misc:** SEROTONIN SYNDROME.

Interactions

Drug-Drug: Concurrent use with **MAO inhibitors used for psychiatric disorders** may result in serious, potentially fatal reactions; wait at least 14 days following discontinuation of MAO inhibitor before initiation of levomilnacipran. Wait at least 7 days after discontinuing levomilnacipran before initiation of MAO inhibitor. Concurrent use with **MAO-inhibitor like drugs**, such as **linezolid** or **methylene blue**, may ↑ risk of serotonin syndrome; concurrent use contraindicated; do not start therapy in patients receiving **linezolid** or **methylene blue**; if **linezolid** or **methylene blue** need to be started in a patient receiving levomilnacipran, immediately discontinue levomilnacipran and monitor for signs/symptoms of serotonin syndrome for 2 wk or until 24 hr after last dose of linezolid or methylene blue, whichever comes first (may resume levomilnacipran therapy 24 hr after last dose of linezolid or methylene blue). Drugs that affect serotonergic neurotransmitter systems, including **tricyclic antidepressants, SNRIs, fentanyl, buspirone, tramadol, amphetamines,** and **triptans**, ↑ risk of serotonin syndrome. Concurrent use of **NSAIDs, aspirin, warfarin** or other **drugs that affect coagulation** may ↑ the risk of bleeding. Blood levels and risk of toxicity ↑ by concurrent use of **CYP3A4 inhitors** including **ketoconazole, clarithromycin, ritonavir**; daily dose should not exceed 80 mg. Concurrent use of other **medications that may ↑ BP** may ↑ risk of hypertension. Concurrent use with **alcohol** may cause a rapid release of drug and should be avoided. Concurrent use with other **CNS-active medications**, especially other **NSRIs**.

Drug-Natural Products: Concurrent use with **St. John's wort** or **tryptophan** may ↑ the risk of serotinin syndrome; also ↑ risk of coronary vasoconstriction and hypertension.

Route/Dosage

PO (Adults): 20 mg once daily for 2 days, then ↑ to 40 mg once daily, may then ↑ by 40 mg every two or more days; may ↑ up to 120 mg/day; *Concurrent use of CYP3A4 inhibitors (including ketoconazole, clarithromycin, ritonavir)*—not to exceed 80 mg/day.

Renal Impairment

PO (Adults): *CCr 30–59 mL/min*—not to exceed 80 mg/day; *CCr 15–29 mL/min*—not to exceed 40 mg/day.

Availability

Extended-release capsules: 20 mg, 40 mg, 80 mg, 120 mg.

NURSING IMPLICATIONS

Assessment

- Monitor BP and heart rate before and periodically during therapy. Treat pre-existing hypertension and cardiac disease prior to therapy. Sustained hypertension may require discontinuation of therapy.

- Monitor closely for notable changes in behavior that could indicate the emergence or worsening of suicidal thoughts or behavior or depression.
- Assess for serotonin syndrome (mental changes [agitation, hallucinations, coma], autonomic instability [tachycardia, labile BP, hyperthermia], neuromuscular aberrations [hyperreflexia, incoordination], and/or GI symptoms [nausea, vomiting, diarrhea]), especially in patients taking other serotonergic drugs (SSRIs, SNRIs, triptans).
- ***Lab Test Considerations:*** May cause hyponatremia.

Implementation

- ***High Alert:*** Do not confuse Fetzima (levomilnacipran) with Farxiga (dapagliflozin).
- **PO:** Administer daily without regard to food. Swallow capsule whole; do not open, crush, or chew.

Patient/Family Teaching

- Instruct patient to take levomilnacipran as directed at the same time each day. Take missed doses as soon as possible unless time for next dose; do not double dose. Do not stop abruptly; must be decreased gradually. Abrupt discontinuation may cause dysphoric mood, irritability, agitation, dizziness, paresthesia, electric shock sensation, anxiety, confusion, headache, lethargy, emotional lability, insomnia, hypomania, tinnitus, and seizures. Advise patient to read *Medication Guide* prior to therapy and with each Rx refill in case of changes.
- May cause drowsiness and may affect ability to make decisions or react quickly. Caution patient to avoid driving or other activities requiring alertness until response to medication is known.
- Advise patient, family, and caregivers to look for activation of mania/hypomania and suicidality, especially during early therapy or dose changes. Notify health care professional immediately if thoughts about suicide or dying, attempts to commit suicide; new or worse depression or anxiety; agitation or restlessness; panic attacks; insomnia; new or worse irritability; aggressiveness; acting on dangerous impulses, mania, or other changes in mood or behavior or if symptoms of serotonin syndrome occur.
- Caution patient of the risk or serotonin syndrome (agitation, hallucinations, changes in mental status, muscle twitching, fast heartbeat, high or low BP, sweating or fever, nausea or vomiting, diarrhea, muscle stiffness or tightness), especially when taking triptans, tramadol, tryptophan supplements and other serotonergic or antipsychotic agents.
- Instruct patient to notify health care professional of all Rx or OTC medications, vitamins, or herbal products being taken and to avoid concurrent use of Rx, OTC, and herbal products, especially NSAIDs, aspirin, and warfarin, without consulting health care professional; may increase bleeding.
- Instruct patient to notify health care professional if signs of hyponatremia (headache, difficulty concentrating, memory impairment, confusion, weakness, unsteadiness) occur.
- Advise patient to avoid taking alcohol during levomilnacipran therapy.
- Instruct patient to notify health care professional if pregnancy is planned or suspected, and to avoid breast feeding during therapy.
- Encourage patient to maintain routine follow-up visits with health care provider to determine effectiveness.

Evaluation/Desired Outcomes

- Increased sense of well-being.
- Renewed interest in surroundings. Need for therapy should be periodically reassessed.

L

levonorgestrel, **See CONTRACEPTIVES, HORMONAL.**

levothyroxine

(lee-voe-thye-**rox**-een)

Eltroxin, Euthyrox, Levo-T, Levoxyl, Synthroid, Thyro-Tabs, Tirosint, Tirosint-SOL, Unithroid

Classification

Therapeutic: hormones

Pharmacologic: thyroid preparations

Indications

Thyroid supplementation in hypothyroidism. Treatment or suppression of euthyroid goiters. Adjunctive treatment for thyrotropin-dependent thyroid cancer.

Action

Synthetic form of thyroxine (T_4). Replacement of or supplementation to endogenous thyroid hormones. Principal effect is increasing metabolic rate of body tissues: Promote gluconeogenesis, Increase utilization and mobilization of glycogen stores, Stimulate protein synthesis, Promote cell growth and differentiation, Aid in the development of the brain and CNS. **Therapeutic Effects:** Replacement in hypothyroidism to restore normal hormonal balance. Suppression of thyroid cancer.

Pharmacokinetics

Absorption: Levothyroxine is variably (40–80%) absorbed from the GI tract.

Distribution: Distributed into most body tissues. Thyroid hormones do not readily cross the placenta; minimal amounts enter breast milk.
Protein Binding: >99%.
Metabolism and Excretion: Metabolized by the liver and other tissues to active T3. Thyroid hormone undergoes enterohepatic recirculation and is excreted in the feces via the bile.
Half-life: 6–7 days.

TIME/ACTION PROFILE

ROUTE	ONSET	PEAK	DURATION
Levothyroxine PO	unknown	1–3 wk	1–3 wk
Levothyroxine IV	6–8 hr	24 hr	unknown

Contraindications/Precautions

Contraindicated in: Hypersensitivity; Recent MI; Hyperthyroidism.
Use Cautiously in: Cardiovascular disease (initiate therapy with lower doses); Severe renal insufficiency; Uncorrected adrenocortical disorders; Pedi: Monitor neonates and infants for cardiac overload, arrhythmias, and aspiration during first 2 wk of therapy; Geri: Extremely sensitive to thyroid hormones; initial dose should be ↓.

Adverse Reactions/Side Effects

Usually only seen when excessive doses cause iatrogenic hyperthyroidism.
CNS: headache, insomnia, irritability. **CV:** angina pectoris, arrhythmias, tachycardia. **Derm:** sweating. **Endo:** hyperthyroidism, menstrual irregularities. **GI:** abdominal cramps, diarrhea, vomiting. **Metab:** heat intolerance, weight loss. **MS:** accelerated bone maturation in children.

Interactions

Drug-Drug: Cholestyramine, **colesevelam**, **colestipol**, **sodium polystyrene sulfonate**, and **sevelemer** may bind to and ↓ absorption of orally administered levothyroxine; administer levothyroxine ≥4 hr prior to these medications. Absorption may be ↓ by **orlistat**, **proton pump inhibitors**, **sucralfate**, **antacids**, and **simethicone**. May ↑ the effects of **warfarin**. May ↑ requirement for **insulin** or **oral hypoglycemic agents** in diabetics. Concurrent **estrogen** therapy may ↑ thyroid replacement requirements. ↑ cardiovascular effects with **adrenergics** (sympathomimetics).
Drug-Food: Foods or supplements containing calcium, iron, magnesium, or zinc may bind levothyroxine and prevent complete absorption.

Route/Dosage

PO (Adults): *Hypothyroidism*—50 mcg as a single dose initially; may be ↑ every 2–3 wk by 25 mcg/day; usual maintenance dose is 75–125 mcg/day (1.5 mcg/kg/day).
PO (Geriatric Patients and Patients with Increased Sensitivity to Thyroid Hormones): 12.5–25 mcg as a single dose initially; may be ↑ every 6–8 wk; usual maintenance dose is 75 mcg/day.
PO (Children >12 yr): 2–3 mcg/kg/day (≥150 mcg/day).
PO (Children 6–12 yr): 4–5 mcg/kg/day (100–125 mcg/day).
PO (Children 1–5 yr): 5–6 mcg/kg/day (75–100 mcg/day).
PO (Children 6–12 mo): 6–8 mcg/kg/day (50–75 mcg/day).
PO (Infants 3–6 mo): 8–10 mcg/kg/day (25–50 mcg/day).
PO (Infants 0–3 mo or Infants at Risk for Cardiac Failure): 10–15 mcg/kg/day or 25 mcg/day; may be ↑ after 4–6 wk to 50 mcg.
IM, IV (Adults): *Hypothyroidism*—50–100 mcg/day as a single dose. *Myxedema coma/stupor*—300–500 mcg IV; additional 100–300 mcg may be given on 2nd day, followed by daily administration of smaller doses.
IM, IV (Children): *Hypothyroidism*—50–80% of the oral dose.

Availability (generic available)

Capsules (Tirosint): 13 mcg, 25 mcg, 50 mcg, 75 mcg, 88 mcg, 100 mcg, 112 mcg, 125 mcg, 137 mcg, 150 mcg, 175 mcg, 200 mcg. **Oral solution :** 13 mcg/mL, 25 mcg/mL, 50 mcg/mL, 75 mcg/mL, 88 mcg/mL, 100 mcg/mL, 112 mcg/mL, 125 mcg/mL, 137 mcg/mL, 150 mcg/mL, 175 mcg/mL, 200 mcg/mL. **Powder for injection (requires reconstitution):** 100 mcg/vial, 200 mcg/vial, 500 mcg/vial. **Solution for injection:** 20 mcg/mL, 40 mcg/mL, 100 mcg/mL. **Tablets:** 25 mcg, 50 mcg, 75 mcg, 88 mcg, 100 mcg, 112 mcg, 125 mcg, 137 mcg, 150 mcg, 175 mcg, 200 mcg, 300 mcg.

NURSING IMPLICATIONS

Assessment

- Assess apical pulse and BP prior to and periodically during therapy. Assess for tachyarrhythmias and chest pain.
- **Children:** Monitor height, weight, and psychomotor development.
- ***Lab Test Considerations:*** Monitor thyroid function studies prior to and during therapy. Monitor thyroid-stimulating hormone serum levels in adults 8–12 wk after changing from one brand to another.
- Monitor blood and urine glucose in diabetic patients. Insulin or oral hypoglycemic dose may need to be increased.
- ***Toxicity and Overdose:*** Overdose is manifested as hyperthyroidism (tachycardia, chest pain, nervousness, insomnia, diaphoresis, tremors, weight loss). Usual treatment is to withhold dose for 2–6 days then resume at a lower dose. Acute overdose is treated by induction of emesis or gastric lavage, followed by activated charcoal. Sympathetic overstimu-

lation may be controlled by antiadrenergic drugs (beta blockers), such as propranolol. Oxygen and supportive measures to control symptoms are also used.

Implementation

- ***High Alert:*** Do not confuse levothyroxine with lamotrigine, Lanoxin (digoxin), or liothyronine.
- **PO:** Administer with a full glass of water, on an empty stomach, 30–60 min before breakfast, to prevent insomnia.
- Initial dose is low, especially in geriatric and cardiac patients. Dose is increased gradually, based on thyroid function tests.
- For patients with difficulty swallowing, tablets can be crushed and placed in 5–10 mL of water and administered immediately via dropper or spoon; do not store suspension.

IV Administration

- **IV Push:** Reconstitute the 200-mcg and 500-mcg vials with 2 or 5 mL, respectively, of 0.9% NaCl without preservatives (diluent usually provided). ***Concentration:*** 100 mcg/mL. Shake well to dissolve completely. Administer solution immediately after preparation; discard unused portion. ***Rate:*** Administer at a rate of 100 mcg over 1 min. Do not add to IV infusions; may be administered through Y-tubing.
- **Y-Site Incompatibility:** Do not admix with other IV solutions.

Patient/Family Teaching

- Instruct patient to take medication as directed at the same time each day. Take missed doses as soon as remembered unless almost time for next dose. If more than 2–3 doses are missed, notify health care professional. Do not discontinue without consulting health care professional.
- Explain to patient that medication does not cure hypothyroidism; it provides a thyroid hormone supplement. Therapy is lifelong.
- Advise patient to notify health care professional if headache, nervousness, diarrhea, excessive sweating, heat intolerance, chest pain, increased pulse rate, palpitations, weight loss >2 lb/wk, or any unusual symptoms occur.
- Caution patient to avoid taking other medications concurrently with thyroid preparations unless instructed by health care professional. Advise patient to take 4 hrs apart from antacids, iron, and calcium supplements.
- Instruct patient to inform health care professionals of thyroid therapy.
- Advise females of reproductive potential to notify health care professional if pregnancy is planned or suspected, or if breast feeding. Pregnancy may increase thyroid requirements.
- Emphasize importance of follow-up exams to monitor effectiveness of therapy. Thyroid function tests are performed at least yearly.
- Pedi: Discuss with parents the need for routine follow-up studies to ensure correct development. Inform patient that partial hair loss may be experienced by children on thyroid therapy. This is usually temporary.

Evaluation/Desired Outcomes

- Resolution of symptoms of hypothyroidism and normalization of hormone levels.

HIGH ALERT

LIDOCAINE

lidocaine (parenteral)
(**lye**-doe-kane)
Xylocaine, ✱Xylocard

lidocaine (local anesthetic)
Xylocaine

lidocaine (mucosal)
✱Jampocaine Viscous, Xylocaine Viscous

lidocaine (transdermal)
Lidoderm, ZTLido

lidocaine (topical)
✱Betacaine, ✱Cathejell, Glydo, ✱Lidodan, L-M-X 4, L-M-X 5, ✱Lyracaine, ✱Maxilene, ✱Stallion, ✱Topicaine, Xylocaine

Classification
Therapeutic: anesthetics (topical/local), antiarrhythmics (class IB)

Indications

IV: Ventricular arrhythmias. **IM:** Self-injected or when IV unavailable (during transport to hospital facilities). **Local:** Infiltration/mucosal/topical anesthetic. **Transdermal:** Pain due to post-herpetic neuralgia.

Action

IV, IM: Suppresses automaticity and spontaneous depolarization of the ventricles during diastole by altering the flux of sodium ions across cell membranes with little or no effect on heart rate. **Local:** Produces local anesthesia by inhibiting transport of ions across neuronal membranes, thereby preventing initiation and conduction of normal nerve impulses. **Therapeutic Effects:** Control of ventricular arrhythmias. Local anesthesia.

Pharmacokinetics

Absorption: Well absorbed after administration into the deltoid muscle; some absorption follows local use.
Distribution: Widely distributed. Concentrates in adipose tissue. Crosses the blood-brain barrier and placenta; enters breast milk.
Metabolism and Excretion: Mostly metabolized by the liver; <10% excreted in urine as unchanged drug.
Half-life: Biphasic—initial phase, 7–30 min; terminal phase, 90–120 min; ↑ in HF and liver impairment.

TIME/ACTION PROFILE (IV, IM = antiarrhythmic effects; local = anesthetic effects)

ROUTE	ONSET	PEAK	DURATION
IV	immediate	immediate	10–20 min (up to several hrs after continuous infusion)
IM	5–15 min	20–30 min	60–90 min
Local	rapid	unknown	1–3 hr

Contraindications/Precautions

Contraindicated in: Hypersensitivity; cross-sensitivity may occur; Third-degree heart block; Wolff-Parkinson-White syndrome; Pedi: Children <3 yr (↑ risk of seizures, cardiac arrest and death with viscous lidocaine); viscous lidocaine should not be used for teething pain; should only be used for other indications when safer alternatives are not available or have failed.
Use Cautiously in: Glucose–6–phosphate dehydrogenase deficiency, history of methemoglobinemia, cardiac or pulmonary disease, or concurrent exposure to oxidizing agents (or metabolites of these agents) (↑ risk of methemoglobinemia); Liver disease, HF, patients weighing <50 kg, and geriatric patients (↓ bolus and/or maintenance dose); Respiratory depression; Shock; Heart block; OB, Lactation: Use only if the potential benefit justifies the potential risk to the fetus; Pedi: Infants <6 mo (↑ risk of methemoglobinemia); safety of transdermal patch not established in children.

Adverse Reactions/Side Effects

CNS: SEIZURES, confusion, drowsiness, agitation, blurred vision, dizziness, slurred speech. **CV:** CARDIAC ARREST, arrhythmias, bradycardia, heart block, hypotension. **EENT:** *mucosal use*—↓ or absent gag reflex. **GI:** nausea, vomiting. **Hemat:** methemoglobinemia. **Local:** stinging, burning, contact dermatitis, erythema. **MS:** chondrolysis. **Neuro:** paresthesia, tremor. **Resp:** bronchospasm. **Misc:** allergic reactions, including ANAPHYLAXIS.

Interactions

Drug-Drug: Concurrent use of **acetaminophen**, **benzocaine**, **bupivacaine**, **chloroquine**, **cyclophosphamide**, **dapsone**, **flutamide**, **hydroxyurea**, **ifosfamide**, **metoclopramide**, **nitrofurantoin**, **nitroglycerin**, **nitroprusside**, **nitrous oxide**, **phenobarbital**, **phenytoin**, **prilocaine**, **primaquine**, **procaine**, **quinine**, **rasburicase**, **ropivacaine**, **sulfonamides**, **tetracaine**, and **valproate** may ↑ risk of methemoglobinemia; monitor closely. ↑ cardiac depression and toxicity with **phenytoin**, **amiodarone**, **quinidine**, **procainamide**, or **propranolol**. **Cimetidine**, **azole antifungals**, **clarithromycin**, **erythromycin**, **fluoxetine**, **fluvoxamine**, **nefazodone**, **paroxetine**, **protease inhibitors**, **propofol**, **ritonavir**, **verapamil**, and **propranolol** may ↓ metabolism and ↑ risk of toxicity. Lidocaine may ↑ levels of **calcium channel blockers**, certain **benzodiazepines**, **cyclosporine**, **fluoxetine**, **lovastatin**, **simvastatin**, **mirtazapine**, **paroxetine**, **ritonavir**, **tacrolimus**, **theophylline**, **tricyclic antidepressants**, and **venlafaxine**. Effects of lidocaine may be ↓ by **carbamazepine**, **phenobarbital**, **phenytoin**, and **rifampin**.

Route/Dosage

Ventricular Tachycardia (with a Pulse) or Pulseless Ventricular Tachycardia/Ventricular Fibrillation

IV (Adults): 1–1.5 mg/kg bolus; may repeat doses of 0.5–0.75 mg/kg every 5–10 min up to a total dose of 3 mg/kg; may then start continuous infusion of 1–4 mg/min.
Endotracheal (Adults): Give 2–2.5 times the IV loading dose down the endotracheal tube, followed by a 10 mL saline flush.
IV (Children): 1 mg/kg bolus (not to exceed 100 mg), followed by 20–50 mcg/kg/min continuous infusion (range 20–50 mcg/kg/min); may administer 2nd bolus of 0.5–1 mg/kg if delay between bolus and continuous infusion.
Endotracheal (Children): Give 2–3 mg/kg down the endotracheal tube followed by a 5 mL saline flush.
IM (Adults and Children ≥50 kg): 300 mg (4.5 mg/kg); may be repeated in 60–90 min.

Local

Infiltration (Adults and Children): Infiltrate affected area as needed (increased amount and frequency of use increases likelihood of systemic absorption and adverse reactions).
Topical (Adults): Apply to affected area 2–3 times daily.
Mucosal (Adults): *For anesthetizing oral surfaces*—20 mg as 2 sprays/quadrant (not to exceed 30 mg/quadrant) may be used. 15 mL of the viscous solution may be used every 3 hr for oral or pharyngeal pain. *For anesthetizing the female urethra*—3–5 mL of the jelly or 20 mg as 2% solution may be used. *For anesthetizing the male urethra*—5–10 mL of the jelly or 5–15 mL of 2% solution may be used before cathe-

terization or 30 mL of jelly before cystoscopy or similar procedures. Topical solutions may be used to anesthetize mucous membranes of the larynx, trachea, or esophagus.

Mucosal (Children ≥3 yr): Do not exceed 4.5 mg/kg/dose (or 300 mg/dose) of viscous solution; swish in the mouth and spit out no more frequently than every 3 hr (maximum: 4 doses per 12-hr period).

Mucosal (Children <3 yr): ≤1.2 mL applied to area with a cotton-tipped applicator no more frequently than every 3 hr (maximum: 4 doses per 12-hr period); use only if the underlying condition requires treatment with product volume of ≤1.2 mL.

Transdermal (Adults): Up to 3 patches may be applied once for up to 12 hr in any 24-hr period; consider smaller areas of application in geriatric or debilitated patients.

Availability (generic available)

Autoinjector for IM injection: 300 mg/3 mL. **IV push injection:** 5 mg/mL (0.5%), 10 mg/mL (1%), 15 mg/mL (1.5%), 20 mg/mL (2%). **For IV admixture:** 100 mg/mL (10%). **Premixed solution for IV infusion:** 200 mg/100 mL D5W (0.2%), 400 mg/100 mL D5W (0.4%), 1000 mg/250 mL D5W (0.4%), 2000 mg/500 mL D5W (0.4%), 800 mg/100 mL D5W (0.8%), 2000 mg/250 mL D5W (0.8%). **Injection for local infiltration/nerve block:** 0.5%, 1%, 2%, 4%. ***In combination with:*** epinephrine for local infiltration. **Cream:** 4%^OTC. **Gel:** 0.5%^OTC, 2.5%^OTC, 🍁5%^OTC. **Jelly:** 2%. **Liquid:** 5%. **Ointment:** 5%. **Transdermal system:** 1.8%, 5%. **Cost:** $309.45/30. **Solution:** 4%. **Spray:** 10%. **Viscous solution:** 2%. ***In combination with:*** prilocaine (as EMLA cream, Oraquix); with tetracaine (Synera); with bupivacaine (Duocaine); with epinephrine (LidoSite).

NURSING IMPLICATIONS

Assessment

- **Antiarrhythmic:** Monitor ECG continuously and BP and respiratory status frequently during administration.
- **Anesthetic:** Assess degree of numbness of affected part.
- **Transdermal:** Monitor for pain intensity in affected area periodically during therapy.
- ***Lab Test Considerations:*** Serum electrolyte levels should be monitored periodically during prolonged therapy.
- IM administration may cause ↑ CPK levels.
- ***Toxicity and Overdose:*** Monitor serum lidocaine levels periodically during prolonged or high-dose IV therapy. Therapeutic serum lidocaine levels range from 1.5–5 mcg/mL.
- Signs and symptoms of toxicity include confusion, excitation, blurred or double vision, nausea, vomiting, ringing in ears, tremors, twitching, seizures, difficulty breathing, severe dizziness or fainting, and unusually slow heart rate.
- If symptoms of overdose occur, stop infusion and monitor patient closely.

Implementation

- ***High Alert:*** Lidocaine is readily absorbed through mucous membranes. Inadvertent overdose of lidocaine jelly and spray has resulted in patient harm or death from neurologic and/or cardiac toxicity. Do not exceed recommended doses.
- **Throat Spray:** Ensure that gag reflex is intact before allowing patient to drink or eat.
- **IM:** IM injections are recommended only when ECG monitoring is not available and benefits outweigh risks. Administer IM injections only into deltoid muscle while frequently aspirating to prevent IV injection.

IV Administration

- **IV Push:** Only 1% and 2% solutions are used for IV push injection. ***Diluent:*** Administer undiluted. ***Rate:*** Administer loading dose over 2–3 min. Follow by IV continuous infusion.
- **Continuous Infusion:** ***Diluent:*** Lidocaine vials need to be further diluted. Dilute 2 g of lidocaine in 250 mL or 500 mL of D5W or 0.9% NaCl. Admixed infusion stable for 24 hr at room temperature. Premixed infusions are already diluted and ready to use. ***Concentration:*** 4–8 mg/mL. ***Rate:*** See Route/Dosage section. Administer via infusion pump for accurate dose.
- **Y-Site Compatibility:** acetaminophen, acyclovir, alemtuzumab, alfentanil, alteplase, amikacin, aminocaproic acid, aminophylline, amiodarone, amphotericin B lipid complex, amphotericin B liposome, anidulafungin, argatroban, ascorbic acid, atropine, azithromycin, aztreonam, benztropine, bivalirudin, bleomycin, bumetanide, buprenorphine, butorphanol, calcium chloride, calcium gluconate, cangrelor, carboplatin, carmustine, caspofungin, cefazolin, cefotaxime, cefoxitin, ceftaroline, ceftazidime, ceftriaxone, cefuroxime, chloramphenicol, chlorpromazine, ciprofloxacin, cisatracurium, cisplatin, clindamycin, cyanocobalamin, cyclophosphamide, cyclosporine, cytarabine, dacarbazine, dactinomycin, daptomycin, daunorubicin hydrochloride, dexamethasone, dexmedetomidine, dexrazoxane, digoxin, diltiazem, diphenhydramine, dobutamine, docetaxel, dopamine, doxorubicin hydrochloride, doxorubicin liposomal, doxycycline, enalaprilat, ephedrine, epinephrine, epirubicin, epoetin alfa, eptifibatide, ertapenem, erythromycin, esmolol, etomidate, etoposide, etoposide phosphate, famotidine, fenoldopam, fentanyl, fluconazole, fludarabine, fluorouracil, folic acid, foscarnet, fosphenytoin, furo-

semide, gemcitabine, gentamicin, glycopyrrolate, granisetron, heparin, hetastarch, hydrocortisone, hydromorphone, idarubicin, ifosfamide, imipenem/cilastatin, indomethacin, insulin, irinotecan, isoproterenol, ketorolac, labetalol, levofloxacin, linezolid, lorazepam, magnesium sulfate, mannitol, meperidine, mesna, methotrexate, methyldopate, methylprednisolone, metoclopramide, metronidazole, micafungin, midazolam, mitoxantrone, morphine, moxifloxacin, multivitamins, mycophenolate, nafcillin, nalbuphine, naloxone, nicardipine, nitroglycerin, nitroprusside, norepinephrine, octreotide, ondansetron, oxacillin, oxaliplatin, oxytocin, paclitaxel, palonosetron, pamidronate, pancuronium, papaverine, pemetrexed, penicillin G, pentamidine, phentolamine, phenylephrine, phytonadione, piperacillin/tazobactam, potassium acetate, potassium chloride, procainamide, prochlorperazine, promethazine, propofol, propranolol, protamine, pyridoxine, quinupristin/dalfopristin, ranitidine, remifentanil, rocuronium, sodium acetate, sodium bicarbonate, streptokinase, succinylcholine, sufentanil, tacrolimus, theophylline, thiamine, thiotepa, tigecycline, tirofiban, tobramycin, trimetaphan, vancomycin, vasopressin, vecuronium, verapamil, vinblastine, vincristine, vinorelbine, vitamin B complex with C, voriconazole, warfarin, zoledronic acid.

- **Y-Site Incompatibility:** acyclovir, amphotericin B colloidal, azathioprine, caspofungin, dantrolene, diazepam, ganciclovir, milrinone, pantoprazole, pentobarbital, phenobarbital, phenytoin, thiopental, trimethoprim/sulfamethoxazole.
- **Infiltration:** Lidocaine with epinephrine may be used to minimize systemic absorption and prolong local anesthesia.
- **Transdermal:** When used concomitantly with other products containing local anesthetic agents, consider amount absorbed from all formulations.

Patient/Family Teaching

- Explain purpose of lidocaine to patient.
- May cause drowsiness and dizziness. Advise patient to call for assistance during ambulation and transfer.
- Advise females of reproductive potential to notify health care professional if pregnancy is planned or suspected, or if breast feeding.
- **IM:** Available in LidoPen Auto-Injector for use outside the hospital setting. Advise patient to telephone health care professional immediately if symptoms of a heart attack occur. Do not administer unless instructed by health care professional. To administer, remove safety cap and place back end on thickest part of thigh or deltoid muscle. Press hard until needle prick is felt. Hold in place for 10 sec, then massage area for 10 sec. Do not drive after administration unless absolutely necessary.
- **Topical:** Apply *Lidoderm Patch* to intact skin to cover the most painful area. Patch may be cut to smaller sizes with scissors before removing release liner. Clothing may be worn over patch. Avoid contact with water (bathing, swimming, showering), may not stick if it gets wet. If irritation or burning sensation occurs during application, remove patch until irritation subsides. Wash hands after application; avoid contact with eyes. Dispose of used patch to avoid access by children or pets.
- Caution women to consult health care professional before using a topical anesthetic for a mammogram or other procedures. If recommended, use lowest drug concentration, and apply sparingly. Do not apply to broken or irritated skin, do not wrap skin, and do not apply heat to area (heating pad/electric blanket), to decrease chance that drug may be absorbed into the body. May result in seizures, cardiac arrhythmias, respiratory failure, coma, and death.
- Advise patient referred for MRI test to discuss patch with referring health care professional and MRI facility to determine if removal of patch is necessary prior to test and for directions for replacing patch.
- **Mucosal:** Caution parent to administer as directed, not to use more or more often than directed, and to use measuring device for accurate dose in children younger than 3 yrs. Advise parent that if signs and symptoms of toxicity (lethargy, shallow breathing, seizure activity) occur to seek emergency attention and not to administer more lidocaine.
- Caution parents that oral lidocaine causes numbness and may impair swallowing; do not administer food and/or chewing gum for at least 60 min after administration.

Evaluation/Desired Outcomes

- Decrease in ventricular arrhythmias.
- Local anesthesia.

linaGLIPtin (lin-a-**glip**-tin)

Tradjenta, Trajenta

Classification

Therapeutic: antidiabetics

Pharmacologic: dipeptidyl peptidase-4 (DDP-4) inhibitors, enzyme inhibitors

Indications

Adjunct to diet and exercise in the management of type 2 diabetes mellitus.

Action

Inhibits the enzyme dipeptidyl peptidase-4 (DPP-4), which slows the inactivation of incretin hormones, resulting in increased levels of active incretin hormones. These hormones are released by the intestine throughout the day, and are involved in regulation of glucose. Increased/prolonged incretin levels increase insulin release and decrease glucagon levels. **Therapeutic Effects:** Improved control of blood glucose.

Pharmacokinetics

Absorption: 30% absorbed following oral administration.

Distribution: Extensively distributed to tissues.

Metabolism and Excretion: Approximately 90% excreted unchanged in urine; minimally metabolized.

Half-life: >100 hr (due to saturable binding to DPP-4).

TIME/ACTION PROFILE

ROUTE	ONSET	PEAK	DURATION
PO	unknown	1.5 hr†	24 hr

†Blood level.

Contraindications/Precautions

Contraindicated in: Hypersensitivity. Cross-sensitivity may exist with sitagliptin, alogliptin, or saxagliptin; Type 1 diabetes mellitus; Diabetic ketoacidosis.

Use Cautiously in: History of pancreatitis; History of HF or renal impairment (↑ risk of HF); OB: Use only if potential maternal benefit justifies potential fetal risk; Lactation: Use while breast feeding only if potential maternal benefit justifies potential risk to infant; Pedi: Safety and effectiveness not established; Geri: Elderly may have greater sensitivity to drug effects.

Adverse Reactions/Side Effects

CV: HF. **Derm:** bullous pemphigoid, localized exfoliation, urticaria. **GI:** PANCREATITIS, ↑ lipase. **Metab:** hypoglycemia, hypertriglyceridemia. **MS:** RHABDOMYOLYSIS, arthralgia. **Resp:** bronchial hyperreactivity. **Misc:** HYPERSENSITIVITY REACTIONS (including anaphylaxis, angioedema, and exfoliative skin conditions).

Interactions

Drug-Drug: ↑ risk of hypoglycemia with **sulfonylureas** or **insulin**; dose ↓ of sulfonylurea or insulin may be necessary. Concurrent use of P-glycoprotein or CYP3A4 inducers, including **rifampin**, may ↓ blood levels and effectiveness and should be avoided.

Route/Dosage

PO (Adults): 5 mg once daily.

Availability

Tablets: 5 mg. ***In combination with:*** empagliflozin (Glyxambi); metformin (Jentadueto); metformin XR (Jentadueto XR). See Appendix B.

NURSING IMPLICATIONS

Assessment

- Observe patient for signs and symptoms of hypoglycemic reactions (abdominal pain, sweating, hunger, weakness, dizziness, headache, tremor, tachycardia, anxiety).
- Monitor for signs of pancreatitis (nausea, vomiting, anorexia, persistent severe abdominal pain, sometimes radiating to the back) during therapy. If pancreatitis occurs, discontinue linagliptin and monitor serum and urine amylase, amylase/creatinine clearance ratio, electrolytes, serum calcium, glucose, and lipase.
- Monitor for arthralgia. Severe joint pain usually disappears with discontinuation of linagliptin.
- ***Lab Test Considerations:*** Monitor hemoglobin A1C prior to and periodically during therapy.
- May cause ↑ uric acid levels.

Implementation

- Do not confuse linagliptin with linaclotide. Do not confuse Tradjenta (linagliptin) with Toujeo (insulin glargine), Tresiba (insulin degludec), or Trulicity (dulaglutide).
- Patients stabilized on a diabetic regimen who are exposed to stress, fever, trauma, infection, or surgery may require administration of insulin.
- **PO:** May be administered without regard to food.

Patient/Family Teaching

- Instruct patient to take linagliptin as directed. Take missed doses as soon as remembered, unless it is almost time for next dose; do not double doses. Advise patient to read the *Medication Guide* before starting and with each Rx refill in case of changes.
- Explain to patient that linagliptin helps control hyperglycemia but does not cure diabetes. Therapy is usually long term.
- Instruct patient not to share this medication with others, even if they have the same symptoms; it may harm them.
- Encourage patient to follow prescribed diet, medication, and exercise regimen to prevent hyperglycemic or hypoglycemic episodes.
- Review signs of hypoglycemia and hyperglycemia with patient. If hypoglycemia occurs, advise patient to take a glass of orange juice or 2–3 tsp of sugar, honey, or corn syrup dissolved in water, and notify health care professional.
- Instruct patient in proper testing of blood glucose and urine ketones. These tests should be monitored closely during periods of stress or illness and health care professional notified if significant changes occur.
- Advise patient to notify health care professional promptly if signs and symptoms of pancreatitis or if rash; hives; blisters; or swelling of face, lips, or throat occur.
- Advise patient to notify health care professional of all Rx or OTC medications, vitamins, or herbal products being taken and to consult with health care professional before taking other medications, especially other oral hypoglycemic medications.

- Advise females of reproductive potential to notify health care professional if pregnancy is planned or suspected, or if breast feeding.

Evaluation/Desired Outcomes

- Improved hemoglobin A1C, fasting plasma glucose and 2-hr post-prandial glucose levels.

linezolid (li-nez-o-lid)

Zyvox, Zyvoxam

Classification
Therapeutic: anti-infectives
Pharmacologic: oxazolidinones

Indications

Treatment of: Infections caused by vancomycin-resistant *Enterococcus faecium*, Nosocomial pneumonia caused by *Staphylococcus aureus* (methicillin-susceptible and -resistant strains), Complicated skin/skin structure infections caused by *Staphylococcus aureus* (methicillin-susceptible and -resistant strains), *Streptococcus pyogenes* or *Streptococcus agalactiae* (including diabetic foot infections), Uncomplicated skin/skin structure infections caused by *Staphylococcus aureus* (methicillin-susceptible and -resistant strains), *Streptococcus pyogenes*, Community-acquired pneumonia caused by *Streptococcus pneumoniae* (including multi-drug resistant strains) or *Staphylococcus aureus* (methicillin-susceptible strains only).

Action

Inhibits bacterial protein synthesis at the level of the 23S ribosome of the 50S subunit. **Therapeutic Effects:** Bactericidal action against streptococci; bacteriostatic action against enterococci and staphylococci.

Pharmacokinetics

Absorption: Rapidly and extensively (100%) absorbed following oral administration.
Distribution: Readily distributes to well-perfused tissues.
Metabolism and Excretion: 65% metabolized, mostly by the liver; 30% excreted unchanged by the kidneys.
Half-life: 6.4 hr.

TIME/ACTION PROFILE

ROUTE	ONSET	PEAK	DURATION
PO	rapid	1–2 hr	12 hr
IV	rapid	end of infusion	12 hr

Contraindications/Precautions

Contraindicated in: Hypersensitivity; Phenylketonuria (suspension contains aspartame); Uncontrolled HTN, pheochromocytoma, thyrotoxicosis, or concurrent use of sympathomimetic agents, vasopressors, or dopaminergic agents (↑ risk of hypertensive response); Concurrent or recent (<2 wk) use of monoamine oxidase (MAO) inhibitors (↑ risk of hypertensive response); Carcinoid syndrome or concurrent use of SSRIs, TCAs, triptans, meperidine, or buspirone (↑ risk of serotonin syndrome).
Use Cautiously in: Thrombocytopenia, concurrent use of antiplatelet agents or bleeding diathesis (platelet counts should be monitored more frequently); Diabetes (↑ risk of hypoglycemia); OB: Safety not established; use only if maternal benefit outweighs potential risk to fetus; Lactation: Lactation.

Adverse Reactions/Side Effects

CV: headache, insomnia. **Derm:** TOXIC EPIDERMAL NECROLYSIS. **EENT:** teeth discoloration, tongue discoloration. **GI:** CLOSTRIDIUM DIFFICILE-ASSOCIATED DIARRHEA (CDAD), diarrhea, ↑ liver enzymes, nausea, taste alteration, vomiting. **Endo:** hypoglycemia. **F and E:** lactic acidosis. **Hemat:** thrombocytopenia. **Neuro:** optic neuropathy, peripheral neuropathy. **Misc:** SEROTONIN SYNDROME.

Interactions

Drug-Drug: ↑ risk of hypertensive response with **MAO inhibitors**, **sympathomimetics** (e.g., **pseudoephedrine**), **vasopressors** (e.g., **epinephrine**, **norepinephrine**), and **dopaminergic agents** (e.g., **dopamine**, **dobutamine**); concurrent or recent use should be avoided. ↑ risk of serotonin syndrome with **SSRIs**, **SNRIs**, **TCAs**, **triptans**, **meperidine**, **bupropion**, or **buspirone**; avoid concurrent use. **Rifampin**, **carbamazepine**, **phenytoin**, and **phenobarbital** may ↓ levels. Concurrent use with **oral hypoglycemics** or **insulin** may ↑ risk of hypoglycemia.
Drug-Food: Because of monoamine oxidase inhibitory properties, consumption of large amounts of foods or beverages containing tyramine should be avoided (↑ risk of pressor response. See Appendix K).

Route/Dosage

Vancomycin-Resistant *Enterococcus faecium* Infections

PO, IV (Adults): 600 mg every 12 hr for 14–28 days.
PO, IV (Children birth–11 yr): Iin the first wk of life, pre-term neonates may initially receive 10 mg/kg every 12 hr.

Pneumonia, Complicated Skin/Skin Structure Infections

PO, IV (Adults): 600 mg every 12 hr for 10–14 days.
PO, IV (Children birth–11 yr): 10 mg/kg every 8 hr for 10–14 days (in the first wk of life, pre-term neonates may initially receive 10 mg/kg every 12 hr).

Uncomplicated Skin/Skin Structure Infections

PO (Adults): 400 mg every 12 hr for 10–14 days.
PO, IV (Children 5–11 yr): 10 mg/kg every 12 hr for 10–14 days.

PO, IV (Children <5 yr): 10 mg/kg every 8 hr for 10–14 days (in the first wk of life, pre-term neonates may initially receive 10 mg/kg every 12 hr).

Availability (generic available)

Oral suspension: (orange-flavored): 100 mg/5 mL. **Premixed infusion:** 200 mg/100 mL, 600 mg/300 mL. **Tablets:** 600 mg.

NURSING IMPLICATIONS

Assessment

- Assess for infection (vital signs; appearance of wound, sputum, urine, and stool; WBC) at beginning of and during therapy.
- Obtain specimens for culture and sensitivity prior to initiating therapy. First dose may be given before receiving.
- May cause lactic acidosis. Notify health care professional if recurrent nausea and vomiting, unexplained acidosis, or low bicarbonate levels occur.
- Monitor visual function in patients receiving linezolid for ≥3 mo or who report visual symptoms (changes in acuity or color vision, blurred vision, visual field defect) regardless of length of therapy. If optic neuropathy occurs, therapy should be reconsidered.
- Monitor bowel function. Diarrhea, abdominal cramping, fever, and bloody stools should be reported to health care professional promptly as a sign of Clostridium difficile-associated diarrhea (CDAD). May begin up to several wk following cessation of therapy.
- Monitor patient taking serotonergic drugs for signs of serotonin syndrome (hyperthermia, rigidity, myoclonus, autonomic instability, mental status changes (extreme agitation progressing to delirium and coma) for 2 wk (5 wk if fluoxetine was taken) or until 24 hrs after the last dose of linezolid, whichever comes first.
- ***Lab Test Considerations:*** May cause bone marrow suppression, anemia, leukopenia, pancytopenia. Monitor CBC and platelet count weekly, especially in patients at risk for increased bleeding, having pre-existing bone marrow suppression, receiving concurrent medications that may cause myelosuppression, or requiring >2 wk of therapy. Discontinue therapy if bone marrow suppression occurs or worsens.
- May cause ↑ AST, ALT, LDH, alkaline phosphatase, and BUN.
- May cause hypoglycemia requiring decrease in dose of antidiabetic agent or discontinuation of linezolid.

Implementation

- ***High Alert:*** Do not confuse Zyvox with Zovirax (acyclovir).
- Dose adjustment is not necessary when switching from IV to oral dose.
- **PO:** May be administered with or without food.
- Before using oral solution gently invert 3–5 times to mix; do not shake. Store at room temperature.

IV Administration

- **Intermittent Infusion:** ***Diluent:*** Premixed infusions are already diluted and ready to use. Solution is yellowish in color which may intensify over time without affecting its potency. ***Concentration:*** 2 mg/mL. ***Rate:*** Infuse over 30–120 min. Flush line before and after infusion.
- **Y-Site Compatibility:** acyclovir, alemtuzumab, alfentanil, allopurinol, amifostine, amikacin, aminocaproic acid, aminophylline, amiodarone, amphotericin B lipid complex, amphotericin B liposome, ampicillin, ampicillin/sulbactam, anidulafungin, argatroban, azithromycin, aztreonam, bivalirudin, bleomycin, bumetanide, buprenorphine, busulfan, butorphanol, calcium acetate, calcium chloride, calcium gluconate, cangrelor, carboplatin, carmustine, caspofungin, cefazolin, cefepime, cefotaxime, cefotetan, cefoxitin, ceftazidime, ceftriaxone, cefuroxime, chloramphenicol, ciprofloxacin, cisatracurium, cisplatin, clindamycin, cyclophosphamide, cyclosporine, cytarabine, dacarbazine, dactinomycin, daptomycin, daunorubicin hydrochloride, dexamethasone, dexmedetomidine, dexrazoxane, digoxin, diltiazem, diphenhydramine, dobutamine, docetaxel, dolasetron, dopamine, doxorubicin hydrochloride, doxorubicin liposomal, doxycycline, droperidol, enalaprilat, ephedrine, epinephrine, epirubicin, eptifibatide, ertapenem, esmolol, etoposide, etoposide phosphate, famotidine, fenoldopam, fentanyl, fluconazole, fludarabine, fluorouracil, foscarnet, fosphenytoin, furosemide, ganciclovir, gemcitabine, gentamicin, glycopyrrolate, granisetron, haloperidol, heparin, hydralazine, hydrocortisone, hydromorphone, idarubicin, ifosfamide, imipenem/cilastatin, insulin, irinotecan, isoproterenol, ketorolac, labetalol, leucovorin, levofloxacin, lidocaine, lorazepam, magnesium sulfate, mannitol, melphalan, meperidine, meropenem, mesna, methotrexate, methyldopate, methylprednisolone, metoclopramide, metoprolol, metronidazole, midazolam, milrinone, mitomycin, mitoxantrone, morphine, mycophenolate, nafcillin, nalbuphine, naloxone, nicardipine, nitroglycerin, nitroprusside, norepinephrine, octreotide, ondansetron, oxaliplatin, oxytocin, paclitaxel, palonosetron, pamidronate, pancuronium, pemetrexed, pentobarbital, phenobarbital, phenylephrine, piperacillin/tazobactam, potassium acetate, potassium chloride, potassium phosphates, procainamide, prochlorperazine, promethazine, propranolol, quinupristin/dalfopristin, ranitidine, remifentanil, rocuronium, sodium acetate, sodium

L

bicarbonate, sodium phosphates, streptozocin, succinylcholine, sufentanil, tacrolimus, theophylline, thiotepa, tigecycline, tirofiban, tobramycin, topotecan, trimethoprim/sulfamethoxazole, vancomycin, vasopressin, vecuronium, verapamil, vinblastine, vincristine, vinorelbine, voriconazole, zidovudine, zoledronic acid.

- **Y-Site Incompatibility:** chlorpromazine, dantrolene, diazepam, pantoprazole, pentamidine, phenytoin, thiopental.

Patient/Family Teaching

- Advise patients taking oral linezolid to take as directed, for full course of therapy, even if feeling better. Take missed doses as soon as remembered unless almost time for next dose; do not double dose.
- Instruct patient to avoid large quantities of foods or beverages containing tyramine (See Appendix K). May cause hypertensive response.
- Instruct patient to notify health care professional if patient has a history of hypertension or seizures.
- Advise patient to notify health care professional of all Rx or OTC medications, vitamins, or herbal products being taken and to consult with health care professional before taking other medications, especially cold remedies, decongestants, or antidepressants.
- Instruct patient to notify health care professional if changes in vision occur or immediately if diarrhea, abdominal cramping, fever, or bloody stools occur and not to treat with antidiarrheals without consulting health care professionals.
- Advise female patient to notify health care professional if pregnancy is planned or suspected or if breast feeding.
- Advise patient to notify health care professional if no improvement is seen in a few days.

Evaluation/Desired Outcomes

- Resolution of signs and symptoms of infection. Length of time for complete resolution depends on organism and site of infection.

liraglutide (lir-a-gloo-tide)

Saxenda, Victoza

Classification

Therapeutic: antidiabetics

Pharmacologic: glucagon-like peptide-1 (GLP-1) receptor agonists

Indications

Victoza: Type 2 diabetes mellitus (as adjunct to diet and exercise). To reduce the risk of major adverse cardiovascular events (cardiovascular death, non-fatal myocardial infarction, or non-fatal stroke) in patients with type 2 diabetes mellitus and established cardiovascular disease. **Saxenda**: Chronic weight management in patients who are obese (body mass index [BMI] ≥30 kg/m²) or are overweight (BMI ≥27 kg/m²) with ≥1 weight-related comorbid condition (e.g. hypertension, dyslipidemia, type 2 diabetes).

Action

Acts as an acylated human glucagon-like peptide-1 (GLP-1, an incretin) receptor agonist; increases intracellular cyclic AMP (cAMP) leading to insulin release when glucose is elevated, which then subsides as blood glucose decreases toward euglycemia. Also decreases glucagon secretion and delays gastric emptying. Also helps to suppress appetite, leading to decreased caloric intake. **Therapeutic Effects:** Improved glycemic control. Reduction in body weight. Reduction in cardiovascular death, non-fatal myocardial infarction, or non-fatal stroke.

Pharmacokinetics

Absorption: 55% absorbed following subcutaneous injection.
Distribution: Unknown.
Protein Binding: >98%.
Metabolism and Excretion: Endogenously metabolized.
Half-life: 13 hr.

TIME/ACTION PROFILE

ROUTE	ONSET	PEAK	DURATION
Subcut	within 4 wk† within 2 wk‡	8 wk† 40 wk‡	unk†‡

†↓ in HbA1c.
‡↓ in body weight.

Contraindications/Precautions

Contraindicated in: Hypersensitivity; Personal or family history of medullary thyroid carcinoma; Multiple Endocrine Neoplasia syndrome type 2; Type 1 diabetes (Victoza only); Diabetic ketoacidosis (Victoza only); Concurrent use with insulin or other weight-loss products (Saxenda only); History of suicidal attempts or suicidal thoughts (Saxenda only); OB: Weight loss not recommended during pregnancy (Saxenda only); Lactation: Avoid use.
Use Cautiously in: History of pancreatitis; History of angioedema or anaphylaxis to another GLP-1 receptor agonist; Hepatic/renal impairment; OB: Use only if potential benefit justifies potential risk to fetus (Victoza only); Pedi: Children <10 yr (safety and effectiveness not established).

Adverse Reactions/Side Effects

CNS: SUICIDAL BEHAVIOR/IDEATION (Saxenda only), headache. **CV:** tachycardia. **Derm:** pruritis, rash. **Endo:** THYROID C-CELL TUMORS. **GI:** PANCREATITIS, diarrhea, nausea, vomiting, cholecystitis, cholelithiasis (Saxenda only), constipation. **GU:** acute renal failure. **Local:** injection site reactions. **Misc:** HYPERSENSITIVITY REACTIONS (including anaphylaxis and angioedema).

Interactions

Drug-Drug: Concurrent use with **agents that increase insulin secretion**, including **sulfonylureas**, may ↑ the risk of serious hypoglycemia, use cautiously and consider dose ↓ of agent increasing insulin secretion. May alter absorption of concomitantly administered **oral medications** due to delayed gastric emptying.

Route/Dosage

Victoza

Type 2 DM

Subcut (Adults): 0.6 mg once daily for 1 wk, then 1.2 mg once daily for 1 wk; may then ↑ dose, if needed, up to 1.8 mg once daily.

Subcut (Children ≥10 yr): 0.6 mg once daily for 1 wk; may then ↑ dose, if needed, to 1.2 mg once daily; after 1 wk, if additional glycemic control needed, may then ↑ dose to 1.8 mg once daily.

Reduction in Risk of Major Adverse Cardiovascular Events

Subcut (Adults): 0.6 mg once daily for 1 wk, then 1.2 mg once daily for 1 wk; may then ↑ dose, if needed, up to 1.8 mg once daily.

Saxenda

Subcut (Adults): 0.6 mg once daily for 1 wk (Wk 1), then 1.2 mg once daily for 1 wk (Wk 2), then 1.8 mg once daily for 1 wk (Wk 3), then 2.4 mg once daily for 1 wk (Wk 4), then 3 mg once daily.

Availability

Solution for injection (Saxenda) (prefilled pens): 18 mg/3 mL (delivers doses of 0.6 mg, 1.2 mg, 1.8 mg, 2.4 mg, or 3 mg). **Solution for injection (Victoza) (prefilled pens):** 18 mg/3 mL (delivers doses of 0.6 mg, 1.2 mg, or 1.8 mg). ***In combination with:*** insulin degludec (Xultophy). See Appendix B.

NURSING IMPLICATIONS

Assessment

- If thyroid nodules or elevated serum calcitonin are noted, patient should be referred to an endocrinologist.
- Monitor for pancreatitis (persistent severe abdominal pain, sometimes radiating to the back, with or without vomiting). If pancreatitis is suspected, discontinue liraglutide; if confirmed, do not restart liraglutide.
- **Victoza:** Observe patient taking concurrent insulin for signs and symptoms of hypoglycemic reactions (sweating, hunger, weakness, dizziness, tremor, tachycardia, anxiety).
- **Saxenda:** Monitor patients for weight loss and adjust concurrent medications (antihypertensives, antidiabetics, lipid-lowering agents) as needed.
- ***Lab Test Considerations:*** Monitor serum HbA1c periodically during therapy to evaluate effectiveness.

Implementation

- Patients stabilized on a diabetic regimen who are exposed to stress, fever, trauma, infection, or surgery may require administration of insulin.
- **Subcut:** Administer once daily at any time of the day, without regard to food. Inject into abdomen, thigh, or upper arm. Solution should be clear and colorless; do not administer solutions that are discolored or contain particulate matter.
- Initial dose of 0.6 mg/day is increased after 1 wk to 1.2 mg/day. If glycemic control is not acceptable, increase to 1.8 mg/day. Available in a prefilled pen without needle; patient may require Rx for needles.
- *First Time Use for Each New Pen*—Follow manufacturer's instructions only once with each new pen or if pen is dropped.

Patient/Family Teaching

- Instruct patient on use of pen injector and to take liraglutide as directed. If a dose is missed, omit and take next dose as scheduled; do not double doses. If >3 days dosing missed, reinitiate with 0.6 mg dose; titrate at direction of health care professional. Pen should never be shared between patients, even if needle is changed. Store pen in refrigerator; do not freeze. After initial use, pen may be stored at room temperature or refrigerated up to 30 days. Keep pen cap on when not in use. Protect from excessive heat and sunlight. Remove and safely discard needle after each injection and store pen without needle attached. Advise patient to read the *Patient Medication Guide* before starting liraglutide and with each Rx refill.
- If a dose is missed do not make up, skip and take next scheduled dose the next day. If more than 3 days are missed, reinitiate at 0.6 mg to minimize GI effects. Notify health care professional and increase dose as directed.
- Inform patient that nausea is the most common side effect, but usually decreases over time.
- Advise patient taking insulin and liraglutide to never mix insulin and liraglutide together. Give as 2 separate injections. Both injections may be given in the same body area, but should not be given right next to each other.
- Explain to patient that this medication controls hyperglycemia but does not cure diabetes. Therapy is long-term.
- Review signs of hypoglycemia and hyperglycemia with patient. If hypoglycemia occurs, advise patient to take a glass of orange juice or 2–3 tsp of sugar,

honey, or corn syrup dissolved in water and notify health care professional.

- Encourage patient to follow prescribed diet, medication, and exercise regimen to prevent hypoglycemic or hyperglycemic episodes.
- Instruct patient in proper testing of serum glucose and ketones. These tests should be closely monitored during periods of stress or illness, and health care professional should be notified if significant changes occur.
- Advise patient to tell health care professional what medications they are taking and to avoid taking new Rx, OTC, vitamins, or herbal products without consulting health care professional.
- Advise patient to discontinue liraglutide and notify health care professional immediately if signs of pancreatitis (nausea, vomiting, abdominal pain) occur.
- Advise patient to inform health care professional of medication regimen before treatment or surgery.
- Inform patient of risk of benign and malignant thyroid C-cell tumors. Advise patient to notify health care professional if symptoms of thyroid tumors (lump in neck, hoarseness, trouble swallowing, shortness of breath) or if signs of allergic reaction (swelling of face, lips, tongue, or throat; fainting or feeling dizzy; very rapid heartbeat; problems breathing or swallowing; severe rash or itching) occur.
- Insulin is the preferred method of controlling blood glucose during pregnancy. Counsel female patients to notify health care professional if pregnancy is planned or suspected, or if breast feeding.
- Advise patient to carry a form of sugar (sugar packets, candy) and identification describing disease process and medication regimen at all times.
- Emphasize the importance of routine follow-up exams.

Evaluation/Desired Outcomes

- Improved glycemic control.
- Reduction in body weight. If patient has not lost at least 4% of body weight after 16 wk of therapy, it is unlikely that patient will achieve and sustain clinically meaningful weight loss with continued treatment.
- Reduction in cardiovascular death, non-fatal myocardial infarction, or non-fatal stroke.

lisdexamfetamine

(lis-dex-am-**fet**-a-meen)

Vyvanse

Classification

Therapeutic: central nervous system stimulants

Pharmacologic: sympathomimetics

Schedule II

Indications

Attention deficit hyperactivity disorder (ADHD). Moderate to severe binge eating disorder.

Action

Blocks reuptake and increases release of norepinephrine and dopamine resulting in increased levels in extraneuronal space. **Therapeutic Effects:** Improved attention span in ADHD. Reduction in number of binge eating days per wk.

Pharmacokinetics

Absorption: Rapidly absorbed and converted to dextroamphetamine, the active drug.

Distribution: Unknown.

Metabolism and Excretion: 42% excreted in urine as amphetamine.

Half-life: less than 1 hr for lisdexamfetamine.

TIME/ACTION PROFILE

ROUTE	ONSET	PEAK	DURATION
PO	rapid	1 hr	24 hr

Contraindications/Precautions

Contraindicated in: Hypersensitivity to lisdexamfetamine or other sympathomimetic amines; Advanced arteriosclerosis; Symptomatic cardiovascular disease including known structural cardiac abnormalities (may ↑ the risk of sudden death); Moderate to severe hypertension; Glaucoma; Agitation; History of substance abuse; Concurrent use or use within 14 days of MAO inhibitors or MAO-like drugs (linezolid or methylene blue); Lactation: Lactation.

Use Cautiously in: History of pre-existing psychosis, bipolar disorder, aggression, tics, Tourette's syndrome or seizures (may exacerbate condition); Severe renal impairment (↓ maximum daily dose); OB: Use only if maternal benefit outweighs fetal risk; Pedi: Children <6 yr (safety and effectiveness not established).

Adverse Reactions/Side Effects

CNS: behavioral disturbances, dizziness, hallucinations, insomnia, irritability, mania, psychomotor hyperactivity, thought disorder, tics. **CV:** SUDDEN DEATH, Raynaud's phenomenon. **EENT:** blurred vision, poor accommodation. **GI:** abdominal pain, ↓ appetite, dry mouth, nausea, vomiting. **Derm:** alopecia, rash. **GU:** ↓ libido, priapism. **Metab:** ↓ weight. **MS:** RHABDOMYOLYSIS. **Neuro:** paresthesia. **Misc:** SEROTONIN SYNDROME, long-term growth suppression.

Interactions

Drug-Drug: Concurrent use with **MAO inhibitors** or **MAO-inhibitor-like drugs**, such as **linezolid** or **methylene blue** may result in serious, potentially fatal reactions; wait at least 14 days following discontinuation of MAO inhibitor before initiation of amphetamine mixtures. Drugs that affect serotonergic neurotransmitter systems, including **MAO inhibitors**, **tricyclic antidepressants**, **SSRIs**, **SNRIs**, **fentanyl**, **buspirone**,

tramadol, **lithium**, and **triptans** ↑ risk of serotonin syndrome. Concurrent use of other **sympathomimetic amines** may result in additive effects and ↑ risk of adverse reactions. **Urinary acidifying agents** including **sodium acid phosphate** ↑ excretion and ↓ blood levels and may result in ↓ effectiveness. May ↓ effectiveness of **adrenergic blockers**. ↑ risk of adverse cardiovascular reactions with **tricyclic antidepressants**. May ↓ sedating effects of **antihistamines**. May ↓ effectiveness of **antihypertensives**. Effects may be ↓ by **haloperidol**, **lithium**, or **chlorpromazine**. May ↓ absorption of **phenobarbital** or **phenytoin**.

Route/Dosage

ADHD

PO (Adults and Children 6–17 yr): 30 mg once daily; may ↑ by 10–20 mg/day at weekly intervals, up to 70 mg/day.

Binge Eating Disorder

PO (Adults): 30 mg once daily; may ↑ by 20 mg/day at weekly intervals, up to target dose of 50–70 mg/day.

Renal Impairment

PO (Adults and Children 6–17 yr): *CCr 15–29 mL/min*—Do not exceed 50 mg/day; *CCr <15 mL/min*—Do not exceed 30 mg/day.

Availability

Capsules: 10 mg, 20 mg, 30 mg, 40 mg, 50 mg, 60 mg, 70 mg. **Cost:** 20 mg $531.93/90, 30 mg $566.90/90, 40 mg $509.91/90, 50 mg $514.34/90, 60 mg $529.67/90, 70 mg $500.01/90. **Chewable tablets:** 10 mg, 20 mg, 30 mg, 40 mg, 50 mg, 60 mg.

NURSING IMPLICATIONS

Assessment

- Monitor BP, pulse, and respiration before administering and periodically during therapy. Obtain a history (including assessment of family history of sudden death or ventricular arrhythmia), physical exam to assess for cardiac disease, and further evaluation (ECG and echocardiogram), if indicated. If exertional chest pain, unexplained syncope, or other cardiac symptoms occur, evaluate promptly.
- Assess risk of abuse prior to prescribing. After prescribing, keep accurate prescription records, educate patient and family about risk of abuse, monitor for signs of abuse and overdose, and evaluate need for use periodically during therapy.
- Screen patients with bipolar disorder for risk of manic episode (comorbid or history of depressive symptoms or a family history of suicide, bipolar disorder, depression) prior to starting therapy.
- Monitor growth, both height and weight, in children on long-term therapy.
- Monitor closely for behavior change.
- Assess for serotonin syndrome (mental changes [agitation, hallucinations, coma], autonomic instability [tachycardia, labile BP, hyperthermia], neuromuscular aberrations [hyperreflexia, incoordination], and/or GI symptoms [nausea, vomiting, diarrhea]), especially in patients taking other serotonergic drugs (SSRIs, SNRIs, triptans).
- **ADHD:** Assess child's attention span, impulse control, and interactions with others. Therapy may be interrupted at intervals to determine whether symptoms are sufficient to continue therapy.
- **Binge Eating Disorder:** Monitor frequency and amount of binge eating.
- ***Lab Test Considerations:*** May cause ↑ plasma corticosteroid levels interfering with urinary steroid determinations.

Implementation

- **PO:** Administer in the morning without regard to meals. Afternoon doses should be avoided due to potential for insomnia. Capsules may be swallowed whole or opened and the entire contents dissolved in yogurt, water, or orange juice. If solution method is used, consume immediately; do not store for future use. Do not divide capsules or take less than one capsule per day. Chewable tablets must be chewed thoroughly. Tablets and chewable tablets can be substituted on a unit per unit/mg per mg basis.

Patient/Family Teaching

- Instruct patient to take medication as directed. Advise patient and parents to read *Medication Guide* prior to initiation of therapy and with each renewal of Rx refill. If more than prescribed amount is taken notify health care professional immediately. Instruct patient not to alter dose without consulting health care professional.
- Inform patient that sharing this medication may be dangerous.
- Advise patient to check weight 2–3 times weekly and report weight loss to health care professional. Pedi: If reduced appetite and weight loss are a problem, advise parents to provide high calorie meals when drug levels are low (at breakfast and or bedtime).
- Inform patients starting therapy of risk of peripheral vasculopathy. Instruct patients to notify health care professional of any new numbness; pain; skin color change from pale, to blue, to red; or coolness or sensitivity to temperature in fingers or toes, and call if unexplained wounds appear on fingers or toes. May require rheumatology consultation.
- Advise parents to notify health care professional immediately if child has signs of heart problems (chest pain, shortness of breath, fainting) or if new or worsening mental symptoms or problems, especially seeing or hearing things that are not real, believing things that are not real, or are suspicious occur.

L

- May cause dizziness or blurred vision. Caution patient to avoid driving or activities requiring alertness until response to medication is known.
- Advise patient to notify health care professional if nervousness, restlessness, insomnia, dizziness, anorexia, or dry mouth becomes severe.
- Advise patient to notify health care professional of all Rx or OTC medications, vitamins, or herbal products being taken and to consult with health care professional before taking other medications.
- Inform patient that health care professional may order periodic holidays from the drug to assess progress and to decrease dependence.
- Advise patient to notify health care professional if pregnancy is planned or suspected, and to avoid breast feeding.
- Emphasize the importance of routine follow-up exams to monitor progress.
- **Home Care Issues:** Advise parents to notify school nurse of medication regimen.

Evaluation/Desired Outcomes

- Improved attention span, decreased impulsiveness and hyperactivity in ADHD.
- Reduction in number of binge eating days per wk.

lisinopril, See ANGIOTENSIN-CONVERTING ENZYME (ACE) INHIBITORS.

lithium (lith-ee-um)

Carbolith, Lithane, Lithmax, Lithobid

Classification
Therapeutic: mood stabilizers

Indications

Treatment of acute manic and mixed episodes associated with bipolar I disorder. Maintenance treatment of bipolar I disorder.

Action

Alters cation transport in nerve and muscle. May also influence reuptake of neurotransmitters. **Therapeutic Effects:** Prevents/decreases incidence of acute manic episodes.

Pharmacokinetics

Absorption: Completely absorbed after oral administration.
Distribution: Widely distributed into many tissues and fluids; CSF levels are 50% of plasma levels. Crosses the placenta; enters breast milk.
Metabolism and Excretion: Excreted almost entirely unchanged by the kidneys.
Half-life: 20–27 hr.

TIME/ACTION PROFILE (antimanic effects)

ROUTE	ONSET	PEAK	DURATION
PO, PO–ER	5–7 days	10–21 days	days

Contraindications/Precautions

Contraindicated in: Hypersensitivity; Brugada syndrome; Some products contain alcohol or tartrazine and should be avoided in patients with known hypersensitivity or intolerance; OB: Pregnancy (may cause fetal harm); Lactation: Lactation.
Use Cautiously in: Significant cardiovascular disease, renal impairment, dehydration, fever, or hyponatremia (↑ risk of lithium toxicity); Diabetes mellitus; Pedi: Children <7 yr (safety and effectiveness not established); Geri: Initial dosage ↓ recommended.

Adverse Reactions/Side Effects

CNS: PSEUDOTUMOR CEREBRI, SEIZURES, fatigue, headache, impaired memory, ataxia, sedation, confusion, dizziness, drowsiness, psychomotor retardation, restlessness, stupor. **CV:** ECG changes, arrhythmias, edema, hypotension, unmasking of Brugada syndrome. **Derm:** acneiform eruption, folliculitis, alopecia, diminished sensation, pruritus. **EENT:** aphasia, blurred vision, dysarthria, tinnitus. **Endo:** hypothyroidism, goiter, hyperglycemia, hyperparathyroidism, hyperthyroidism. **F and E:** hypercalcemia, hyponatremia. **GI:** abdominal pain, anorexia, bloating, diarrhea, nausea, dry mouth, metallic taste. **GU:** polyuria, glycosuria, nephrogenic diabetes insipidus, renal impairment. **Hemat:** leukocytosis. **Metab:** weight gain. **MS:** muscle weakness, hyperirritability, rigidity. **Neuro:** tremors. **Misc:** SEROTONIN SYNDROME.

Interactions

Drug-Drug: May prolong the action of **neuromuscular blocking agents**. ↑ risk of neurologic toxicity with **calcium channel blockers**, **methyldopa**, **phenytoin**, or **carbamazepine**. **Diuretics**, **NSAIDs**, **ACE inhibitors**, **angiotensin II receptor blockers**, and **metronidazole** may ↑ levels and risk of toxicity. Hypothyroid effects may be additive with **potassium iodide** or **antithyroid agents**. **Aminophylline**, **acetazolamide**, **theophylline**, and **sodium bicarbonate** ↑ renal elimination and ↓ effectiveness. **Psyllium** can ↓ **lithium** levels. Drugs that affect serotonergic neurotransmitter systems, including **tricyclic antidepressants**, **SSRIs**, **SNRIs**, **fentanyl**, **buspirone**, **tramadol**, **amphetamines**, and **triptans** ↑ risk of serotonin syndrome. Concurrent use with **antipsychotics** may ↑ risk of developing an encephalopathic syndrome (i.e., weakness, lethargy, fever, tremulousness and confusion, extrapyramidal symptoms, leukocytosis, ↑ BUN, and ↑ fasting blood glucose); monitor closely.

Drug-Natural Products: Caffeine-containing herbs (**cola nut**, **guarana**, **mate**, **tea**, **coffee**) may ↓ **lithium** serum levels and efficacy. ↑ risk of serotonergic side effects including serotonin syndrome with **St. John's wort**.
Drug-Food: Large changes in **sodium** intake may alter the renal elimination of lithium. ↑ sodium intake will ↑ renal excretion.

Route/Dosage

Precise dosing is based on serum lithium levels. 300 mg lithium carbonate contains 8–12 mEq lithium.
PO (Adults and Children ≥7 yr and >30 kg): *Tablets/capsules/liquid*—300 mg 3 times daily initially; ↑ by 300 mg/day every 3 days; usual dose for treatment of acute manic and mixed episodes = 600 mg 2–3 times daily; usual maintenance dose = 300–600 mg 2–3 times daily.
PO (Adults and Children >12 yr): *Extended-release tablets*—450–900 mg twice daily *or* 300–600 mg 3 times daily initially; usual maintenance dose is 450 mg twice daily *or* 300 mg 3 times daily.
PO (Children ≥7 yr and 20–30 kg): *Tablets/capsules/liquid*—300 mg twice daily initially; ↑ by 300 mg/wk; usual dose for treatment of acute manic and mixed episodes = 600–1500 mg/day in divided doses; usual maintenance dose = 600–1200 mg/day in divided doses.

Availability (generic available)

Capsules: 150 mg, 300 mg, 600 mg. **Cost:** *Generic*—150 mg $13.97/100, 300 mg $17.91/100, 600 mg $39.11/100. **Extended-release tablets:** 300 mg, 450 mg. **Cost:** *Generic*—300 mg $46.52/100, 450 mg $50.05/100. **Oral solution:** 300 mg (8 mEq lithium)/5 mL. **Tablets:** 300 mg. **Cost:** *Generic*—$21.52/100.

NURSING IMPLICATIONS

Assessment

- Assess mental status (orientation, mood, behavior) initially and periodically. Initiate suicide precautions if indicated.
- Monitor intake and output ratios. Report significant changes in totals. Unless contraindicated, fluid intake of at least 2000–3000 mL/day should be maintained. Weight should also be monitored at least every 3 mo.
- ***Lab Test Considerations:*** Evaluate renal and thyroid function, WBC with differential, serum electrolytes, and glucose periodically during therapy.
- ***Toxicity and Overdose:*** Monitor serum lithium levels twice weekly during initiation of therapy and every 2 mo during chronic therapy. Draw blood samples in the morning immediately before next dose. Therapeutic levels range from 0.5–1.5 mEq/L for acute mania and 0.6–1.2 mEq/L for long term control. Serum concentrations should not exceed 2.0 mEq/L.
- Assess patient for signs and symptoms of lithium toxicity (vomiting, diarrhea, slurred speech, lightheadedness, decreased coordination, drowsiness, muscle weakness, tremor, or twitching). If these occur, report before administering next dose.

Implementation

- Do not confuse lithium carbonate with lanthanum carbonate. Do not confuse lithium with Ultram (tramadol).
- **PO:** Administer with food or milk to minimize GI irritation. Extended-release preparations should be swallowed whole; do not break, crush, or chew.

Patient/Family Teaching

- Instruct patient to take medication as directed, even if feeling well. Take missed doses as soon as remembered unless within 2 hr of next dose (6 hr if extended release).
- Lithium may cause dizziness or drowsiness. Caution patient to avoid driving or other activities requiring alertness until response to medication is known.
- Low sodium levels may predispose patient to toxicity. Advise patient to drink 2000–3000 mL fluid each day and eat a diet with consistent and moderate sodium intake. Excessive amounts of coffee, tea, and cola should be avoided because of diuretic effect. Avoid activities that cause excess sodium loss (heavy exertion, exercise in hot weather, saunas). Notify health care professional of fever, vomiting, and diarrhea, which also cause sodium loss.
- Advise patient that weight gain may occur. Review principles of a low-calorie diet.
- Advise patient to notify health care professional of all Rx or OTC medications, vitamins, or herbal products being taken and to consult with health care professional before taking other medications, especially NSAIDs.
- Review side effects and symptoms of toxicity with patient. Instruct patient to stop medication and report signs of toxicity to health care professional promptly.
- Advise patient to notify health care professional if fainting, irregular pulse, or difficulty breathing occurs.
- Lithium may be teratogenic. Advise female patients of reproductive potential to use contraception during therapy and to consult health care professional if

pregnancy is planned or suspected, and to avoid breast feeding. Monitor breast-fed infants for signs and symptoms of lithium toxicity (hypertonia, hypothermia, cyanosis, ECG changes).
- Emphasize the importance of periodic lab tests to monitor for lithium toxicity.

Evaluation/Desired Outcomes
- Resolution of the symptoms of mania (hyperactivity, pressured speech, poor judgment, need for little sleep).
- Decreased incidence of mood swings in bipolar disorders.
- Improved affect in unipolar disorders. Improvement in condition may require 1–3 wk.
- Decreased incidence of acute manic episodes.

lixisenatide (lix-i-**sen**-a-tide)
Adlyxin

Classification
Therapeutic: antidiabetics
Pharmacologic: glucagon-like peptide-1 (GLP-1) receptor agonists

Indications
Adjunct to diet and exercise in the treatment of type 2 diabetes mellitus.

Action
Acts as an agonist at the glucagon-like peptide-1 (GLP-1) receptor resulting in augmented glucose-dependent insulin secretion and slowing of gastric emptying. **Therapeutic Effects:** Improved glycemic control.

Pharmacokinetics
Absorption: Bioavailability following subcut injection unknown.
Distribution: Extensively distributed to tissues.
Metabolism and Excretion: Degraded by proteolytic enzymes and excreted primarily through urine.
Half-life: 3 hr.

TIME/ACTION PROFILE (effect on postprandial blood glucose)

ROUTE	ONSET	PEAK	DURATION
Subcut	unknown	1–3 hr	unknown

Contraindications/Precautions
Contraindicated in: Hypersensitivity; End-stage renal disease.
Use Cautiously in: Renal impairment (monitor renal function during initiation and dose escalation); History of cholelithiasis or alcohol abuse (↑ risk of pancreatitis); Geri: May be more sensitive to drug effects; OB: Use only if potential benefit to mother exceeds risk to fetus; Lactation: Consider breast feeding only if potential benefit outweighs risks to infant; Pedi: Safety and effectiveness not established.

Adverse Reactions/Side Effects
CNS: dizziness, headache. **Endo:** hypoglycemia. **GI:** PANCREATITIS, nausea, vomiting, abdominal distention, abdominal pain, constipation, diarrhea, dyspepsia. **GU:** renal impairment (in association with nausea, vomiting, diarrhea, or dehydration). **Local:** injection site reactions. **Misc:** HYPERSENSITIVITY REACTIONS.

Interactions
Drug-Drug: ↑ risk of hypoglycemia with other **antidiabetic agents**, especially **insulin** and **sulfonylureas** (dose ↓ of insulin or sulfonylureas may be warranted). May alter the absorption of concurrently administered **oral medications** (take **oral contraceptives** ≥1 hr before or ≥11 hr after lixisenatide).

Route/Dosage
Subcut (Adults): 10 mcg once daily for 14 days, then ↑ to 20 mcg once daily starting on Day 15.

Availability
Solution for subcut injection (in prefilled pens): 50 mcg/mL (10 mcg/dose), 100 mcg/mL (20 mcg/dose). ***In combination with:*** insulin glargine (Soliqua). See Appendix B.

NURSING IMPLICATIONS

Assessment
- Observe for signs and symptoms of hypoglycemic reactions (abdominal pain, sweating, hunger, weakness, dizziness, headache, drowsiness, tremor, tachycardia, anxiety, confusion, irritability, jitteriness), especially when combined with oral sulfonylureas or basal infusion. May require dose ↓ of sulfonylurea or basal infusion.
- Monitor for signs and symptoms of hypersensitivity reactions (rash, swelling of face, lips, tongue or throat, difficulty breathing or swallowing, feeling faint or dizzy, tachycardia, hypotension, laryngeal edema, bronchospasm), especially in patient with history of anaphylaxis or angioedema with another GLP-1 receptor agonist.
- Monitor for signs and symptoms of pancreatitis (persistent severe abdominal pain, sometimes radiating to back and may or may not be accompanied by vomiting). Promptly discontinue lixisenatide and initiate treatment if pancreatitis is suspected. Do not restart lixisenatide if pancreatitis is confirmed. Consider other antidiabetic therapies in patients with a history of pancreatitis.
- ***Lab Test Considerations:*** Monitor serum glucose and glycolysated hemoglobin periodically during therapy to evaluate effectiveness of therapy.

- Monitor renal function when starting or ↑ lixisenatide dose in patients with renal impairment and in patients with severe GI reactions.

Implementation

- Patients stabilized on a diabetic regimen who are exposed to stress, fever, trauma, infection, or surgery may require administration of insulin.
- **Subcut:** Activate pen before first use. Administer within 1 hr before first meal of day, preferably the same meal each day. Pinch skin and inject in abdomen, thigh, or upper arm; slowly count to 2 before removing needle from skin. Rotate injection sites with each dose. Solution is clear and colorless; do not administer solutions that are discolored or contain particulate matter. Keep pen in original packaging; discard 14 days after 1st use.

Patient/Family Teaching

- Instruct patient in proper technique for administration, timing of dose and concurrent oral medications, storage of medication, and disposal of used needles. Training should include a practice injection. Administer missed doses within 1 hr of next meal. Advise patient to read *Medication Guide and Instructions for Use* before starting therapy and with each Rx refill in case of changes.
- Inform patient that pen needles are not included with pen and must be purchased separately. Advise patient which needle length and gauge should be used. Caution patient not to share pen and needles, even if needle is changed. May cause transmission of bloodborne pathogens.
- Advise patient to stop taking lixisenatide and notify health care professional immediately if signs and symptoms of hypersensitivity or pancreatitis occur.
- Explain to patient that lixisenatide helps control hyperglycemia but does not cure diabetes. Therapy is usually long term.
- Encourage patient to follow prescribed diet, medication, and exercise regimen to prevent hyperglycemic or hypoglycemic episodes.
- Review signs of hypoglycemia and hyperglycemia with patient. If hypoglycemia occurs, advise patient to take a glass of orange juice or 2–3 tsp of sugar, honey, or corn syrup dissolved in water, and notify health care professional. Risk of hypoglycemia is ↑ if sulfonylureas or basal infusion are taken concurrently with lixisenatide.
- Caution patient to maintain adequate hydration (2 L liquid/day) to minimize risk of renal failure.
- Instruct patient to notify health care professional of all Rx or OTC medications, vitamins, or herbal products being taken and consult health care professional before taking any new medications.
- Rep: Advise female patient taking oral contraceptives to take them at ≥1 hr before or 11 hr after lixisenatide dose. Advise patient to notify health care professional if pregnancy is planned or suspected or if breast feeding.

Evaluation/Desired Outcomes

- Improved glycemic control in patients with type 2 diabetes.

⧖ lofexidine (loe-fex-i-deen)

Lucemyra

Classification

Therapeutic: none assigned

Pharmacologic: adrenergics (centrally acting)

Indications

Mitigation of opioid withdrawal symptoms to facilitate abrupt opioid discontinuation in adults.

Action

Stimulates alpha$_2$-adrenergic receptors in the CNS, which results in decreased sympathetic outflow. **Therapeutic Effects:** Reduction in severity of opioid withdrawal symptoms.

Pharmacokinetics

Absorption: Well absorbed (72%) following oral administration.

Distribution: Extensively distributed to tissues, including CNS.

Metabolism and Excretion: Metabolized by the liver (primarily by CYP2D6, but also CYP1A2 and CYP2C19 to some extent) to inactive metabolites; primarily excreted in urine (15–20% as unchanged drug); ⧖ ~7% of population may be poor metabolizers and may have significantly ↑ lofexidine concentrations and an ↑ risk of adverse effects.

Half-life: 17–22 hr.

TIME/ACTION PROFILE (plasma concentrations)

ROUTE	ONSET	PEAK	DURATION
PO	unknown	3–5 hr	unknown

Contraindications/Precautions

Contraindicated in: Concurrent use with medications that lower blood pressure or heart rate; Congenital long QT syndrome.

Use Cautiously in: Severe cardiac or cerebrovascular disease, recent MI, chronic renal failure, severe bradycardia; HF, bradyarrhythmias, hepatic impairment, renal impairment, hypokalemia, or hypomagnesemia; Concurrent use of QT-interval prolonging medications; CYP2D6 poor metabolizers; Geri: ↑ risk of orthostatic hypotension and adverse CNS effects in older adults (↓ dose recommended); OB: Safety not established; Lactation: Use only if potential maternal benefit justifies potential risk to infant; Pedi: Safety and effectiveness not established.

Adverse Reactions/Side Effects

CNS: drowsiness, dizziness, insomnia. **CV:** TORSADES DE POINTES, bradycardia, hypotension, palpitations, QT interval prolongation, syncope. **EENT:** tinnitus. **GI:** dry mouth.

Interactions

Drug-Drug: Additive hypotension with other **antihypertensives** and **nitrates**; avoid concurrent use. Additive bradycardia with **beta blockers**, **diltiazem**, **verapamil**, **digoxin**, or **ivabradine**; avoid concurrent use. Additive sedation with **CNS depressants**, including **alcohol**, **antihistamines**, **opioid analgesics**, and **sedative/hypnotics**. Concurrent use with **QT interval-prolonging medications**, including **methadone**, may ↑ risk of QT interval prolongation and torsades de pointes. May ↓ **naltrexone (PO)** levels; separate administration by >2 hr. **CYP2D6 inhibitors**, including **paroxetine** may ↑ levels.

Route/Dosage

PO (Adults): 0.54 mg 4 times daily (with 5–6 hr between each dose) during the period of peak withdrawal symptoms (usually the first 5–7 days after the last opioid dose); may adjust dose based on symptoms (max dose = 2.88 mg/day or 0.72 mg/dose); may be continued for up to 14 days. Must taper therapy upon discontinuation (gradually ↓ dose over 2–4-day period).

Hepatic Impairment

PO (Adults): *Moderate hepatic impairment (Child-Pugh B)*—0.36 mg 4 times daily (with 5–6 hr between each dose) during the period of peak withdrawal symptoms (usually the first 5–7 days after the last opioid dose); *Severe hepatic impairment (Child-Pugh C)*—0.18 mg 4 times daily (with 5–6 hr between each dose) during the period of peak withdrawal symptoms (usually the first 5–7 days after the last opioid dose).

Renal Impairment

PO (Adults): *CCr 30–<90 mL/min*—0.36 mg 4 times daily (with 5–6 hr between each dose) during the period of peak withdrawal symptoms (usually the first 5–7 days after the last opioid dose); *CCr <30 mL/min*—0.18 mg 4 times daily (with 5–6 hr between each dose) during the period of peak withdrawal symptoms (usually the first 5–7 days after the last opioid dose).

Availability

Tablets: 0.18 mg.

NURSING IMPLICATIONS

Assessment

- Assess vital signs and symptoms of bradycardia and orthostatic hypotension (low blood pressure, slow heartbeat, dizziness, lightheadedness, feeling faint at rest or when standing up) before dose and as needed during therapy.
- Monitor ECG when starting therapy and in patients with HF, bradyarrhythmias, hepatic impairment, renal impairment, or those taking medications (methadone) that lead to QT prolongation.
- ***Lab Test Considerations:*** Monitor electrolytes before starting and during therapy. Correct electrolyte abnormalities (hypokalemia, hypomagnesemia) before starting therapy.

Implementation

- **PO:** Administer 3 tablets four times daily without regard to food, with 5–6 hrs between doses.

Patient/Family Teaching

- Instruct patient to take lofexidine as directed and not to stop without consulting health care professional. Abrupt discontinuation can cause diarrhea, insomnia, anxiety, chills, hyperhidrosis, and extremity pain. Reduce dose gradually.
- Caution patients that after a period of not using opioids, they may be more sensitive to the effects of opioids and at greater risk of overdosing.
- May cause dizziness and sedation. Caution patient to avoid driving and activities requiring alertness until response to medication is known.
- Caution patient to avoid sudden changes in position to decrease orthostatic hypotension. Use of alcohol, standing for long periods, exercising, dehydration, and hot weather may increase orthostatic hypotension.
- Instruct patient to notify health care professional of all Rx or OTC medications, vitamins, or herbal products being taken and to consult health care professional before taking any other Rx, OTC, or herbal products, especially benzodiazepines, barbiturates, tranquilizers, or sleeping pills.
- Caution patient to avoid concurrent use of alcohol or other CNS depressants with lofexidine.
- Advise female patients to notify health care professional if pregnancy is planned or suspected or if breast feeding.

Evaluation/Desired Outcomes

- Reduction in severity of opioid withdrawal symptoms.

loperamide (loe-per-a-mide)

✱Imodium, Imodium A-D

Classification

Therapeutic: antidiarrheals

Indications

Adjunctive therapy of acute diarrhea. Chronic diarrhea associated with inflammatory bowel disease. Decreases the volume of ileostomy drainage.

Action

Inhibits peristalsis and prolongs transit time by a direct effect on nerves in the intestinal muscle wall. Reduces fecal volume, increases fecal viscosity and bulk while diminishing loss of fluid and electrolytes. **Therapeutic Effects:** Relief of diarrhea.

Pharmacokinetics

Absorption: Not well absorbed following oral administration.

Distribution: Unknown. Does not cross the blood-brain barrier.

Protein Binding: 97%.

Metabolism and Excretion: Metabolized partially by the liver, undergoes enterohepatic recirculation; 30% eliminated in the feces. Minimal excretion in the urine.

Half-life: 10.8 hr.

TIME/ACTION PROFILE (relief of diarrhea)

ROUTE	ONSET	PEAK	DURATION
PO	1 hr	2.5–5 hr	10 hr

Contraindications/Precautions

Contraindicated in: Hypersensitivity; Patients in whom constipation must be avoided; Abdominal pain of unknown cause, especially if associated with fever; Alcohol intolerance (liquid only).

Use Cautiously in: Hepatic dysfunction; Lactation: Usually compatible with breast feeding; OB: Safety not established; Pedi: Children <2 yr (safety not established); Geri: ↑ sensitivity to effects.

Adverse Reactions/Side Effects

CNS: drowsiness, dizziness. **CV:** CARDIAC ARREST, QT INTERVAL PROLONGATION, TORSADES DE POINTES, VENTRICULAR ARRHYTHMIAS, syncope. **GI:** constipation, abdominal pain/distention/discomfort, dry mouth, nausea, vomiting. **Misc:** allergic reactions.

Interactions

Drug-Drug: ↑ CNS depression with other **CNS depressants**, including **alcohol**, **antihistamines**, **opioid analgesics**, and **sedative/hypnotics**. ↑ anticholinergic properties with other **drugs having anticholinergic properties**, including **antidepressants** and **antihistamines**. Concurrent use of **cimetidine**, **clarithromycin**, **erythromycin**, **gemfibrozil**, **itraconazole**, **ketoconazole**, **quinidine**, **quinine**, **ranitidine**, or **ritonavir** may ↑ levels and risk of cardiac arrhythmias.

Drug-Natural Products: Kava-kava, **valerian**, **skullcap**, **chamomile**, or **hops** can ↑ CNS depression.

Route/Dosage

Acute and Chronic Diarrhea

PO (Adults and Children >12 yr): 4 mg initially, then 2 mg after each loose stool. Maintenance dose usually 4–8 mg/day in divided doses (not to exceed 8 mg/day for OTC use or 16 mg/day for Rx use).

Acute Diarrhea

PO (Children 9–11 yr or 30–47 kg): 2 mg initially; then 1 mg after each loose stool (not to exceed 6 mg/24 hr; OTC use should not exceed 2 days).

PO (Children 6–8 yr or 24–30 kg): 1 mg initially, then 1 mg after each loose stool (not to exceed 4 mg/24 hr; OTC use should not exceed 2 days).

PO (Children 2–5 yr or 13–20 kg): 1 mg initially, then 0.1 mg/kg after each loose stool (not to exceed 3 mg/24 hr; OTC use should not exceed 2 days).

Chronic Diarrhea

PO (Children): 0.08–0.24 mg/kg/day divided 2–3 times/day (not to exceed 2 mg/dose).

Availability (generic available)

Tablets: 2 mg^{OTC}. **Capsules:** 2 mg. **Oral liquid (mint):** 1 mg/5 mL^{OTC}, 1 mg/7.5 mL^{OTC}. ***In combination with:*** simethicone (Imodium Multi-Symptom Relief^{OTC}, see Appendix B).

NURSING IMPLICATIONS

Assessment

- Assess frequency and consistency of stools and bowel sounds prior to and during therapy.
- Assess fluid and electrolyte balance and skin turgor for dehydration.

Implementation

- **PO:** Administer with clear fluids to help prevent dehydration, which may accompany diarrhea.

Patient/Family Teaching

- Instruct patient to take medication as directed. Do not take missed doses, and do not double doses. In acute diarrhea, medication may be ordered after each unformed stool. Advise patient not to exceed the maximum number of doses.

L

- May cause drowsiness. Advise patient to avoid driving or other activities requiring alertness until response to drug is known.
- Advise patient that frequent mouth rinses, good oral hygiene, and sugarless gum or candy may relieve dry mouth.
- Caution patient to avoid using alcohol and other CNS depressants concurrently with this medication.
- Instruct patient to notify health care professional if diarrhea persists or if fever, abdominal pain, or distention occurs.

Evaluation/Desired Outcomes

- Decrease in diarrhea.
- In acute diarrhea, treatment should be discontinued if no improvement is seen in 48 hr.
- In chronic diarrhea, if no improvement has occurred after at least 10 days of treatment with maximum dose, loperamide is unlikely to be effective.

lopinavir/ritonavir

(loe-**pin**-a-veer/ri-**toe**-na-veer)
Kaletra

Classification
Therapeutic: antiretrovirals
Pharmacologic: protease inhibitors, metabolic inhibitors

Indications

HIV infection (with other antiretrovirals).

Action

Lopinavir: Inhibits HIV viral protease. **Ritonavir:** Although ritonavir has antiretroviral activity of its own (inhibits the action of HIV protease and prevents the cleavage of viral polyproteins), it is combined with lopinavir to inhibit the metabolism of lopinavir thus increasing its plasma levels. **Therapeutic Effects:** Increased CD4 cell counts and decreased viral load with subsequent slowed progression of HIV infection and its sequelae.

Pharmacokinetics

Absorption: Well absorbed following oral administration; food enhances absorption.
Distribution: *Ritonavir*—poor CNS penetration.
Protein Binding: *Lopinavir*—98–99% bound to plasma proteins.
Metabolism and Excretion: *Lopinavir*—completely metabolized in the liver by cytochrome P450 3A (CYP450 3A); ritonavir is a potent inhibitor of this enzyme. *Ritonavir*—highly metabolized by the liver (by CYP450 3A and CYP2D6 enzymes); one metabolite has antiretroviral activity; 3.5% excreted unchanged in urine.
Half-life: *Lopinavir*—5–6 hr *Ritonavir*—3–5 hr.

TIME/ACTION PROFILE (blood levels)

ROUTE	ONSET	PEAK	DURATION
Lopinavir PO	rapid	4 hr	12 hr
Ritonavir PO	rapid	4 hr*	12 hr

*Non-fasting.

Contraindications/Precautions

Contraindicated in: Hypersensitivity (including toxic epidermal necrolysis, Stevens-Johnson syndrome, or erythema multiforme); Concurrent use of alfuzosin, colchicine, dihydroergotamine, dronedarone, elbasvir/grazoprevir, ergotamine, lomitapide, lovastatin, lurasidone, methylergonovine, midazolam (PO), pimozide, ranolazone, sildenafil (Revatio), simvastatin, and triazolam (may result in serious and/or life-threatening events); Concurrent use with St. John's wort or rifampin (may lead to ↓ virologic response and possible resistance); Hypersensitivity or intolerance to alcohol or castor oil (present in liquid); Congenital long QT syndrome, concurrent use of QT-interval prolonging drugs, or hypokalemia (↑ risk of QT interval prolongation); OB: Not recommended in pregnancy if ≥1 lopinavir resistance-associated substitution present; Lactation: Breast feeding not recommended in HIV-infected patients; Pedi: Preterm infants (should be avoided until 14 days after their due date) or full-term infants <14 days old (↑ risk of toxicity from alcohol and propylene glycol in oral solution).
Use Cautiously in: Known alcohol intolerance (oral solution contains alcohol); Impaired hepatic function, history of hepatitis (for ritonavir content); Pre-existing conduction system disease (marked first-degree AV block or second- or third-degree AV block), ischemic heart disease, or concurrent use of other drugs that increase the PR interval (especially those metabolized by CYP3A4 including verapamil or diltiazem); OB: Once daily regimen should not be used in pregnancy; Pedi: Children ≤6 mo (↑ risk of toxicity from alcohol and propylene glycol in oral solution); should not be used once daily in children.

Adverse Reactions/Side Effects

CNS: headache, insomnia, weakness. **CV:** TORSADES DE POINTES, ↑ PR interval, heart block, QT interval prolongation. **Derm:** ERYTHEMA MULTIFORME, STEVENS JOHNSON SYNDROME, TOXIC EPIDERMAL NECROLYSIS, rash. **Endo:** hyperglycemia. **GI:** HEPATOTOXICITY, PANCREATITIS, diarrhea (↑ in children), abdominal pain, nausea, taste aversion (in children), vomiting (↑ in children). **Misc:** immune reconstitution syndrome.

Interactions

Drug-Drug: May ↑ levels and risk of toxicity of **alfuzosin, dronedarone, ergot derivatives (dihy-**

droergotamine, **ergotamine**, **methylergonovine**), **elbasvir/grazoprevir**, **lomitapide**, **lovastatin**, **lurasidone**, **midazolam (oral)**, **pimozide**, **sildenafil (Revatio)**, **simvastatin**, and **triazolam**; concurrent use contraindicated. May ↑ **colchicine** levels; concurrent use in patients with renal or hepatic impairment contraindicated; ↓ dose of colchicine in patients without renal or hepatic impairment. Concurrent use of **Rifampin** ↓ levels and effectiveness; concurrent use contraindicated. ↑ risk of myopathy with **atorvastatin** or **rosuvastatin**; use lowest possible dose of statin; do not exceed rosuvastatin dose of 10 mg/day. Concurrent use with **efavirenz** or **nevirapine** ↓ lopinavir/ritonavir levels and effectiveness; dose ↑ recommended; once daily lopinavir/ritonavir regimen not recommended when these drugs are used. **Delavirdine** ↑ lopinavir levels. May ↑ **tenofovir** and **rilpivirine** levels. May ↓ **abacavir**, **etravirine**, and **zidovudine** levels. Concurrent use with **fosamprenavir** ↓ lopinavir and **fosamprenavir** levels. Concurrent use with **nelfinavir** ↓ lopinavir levels and ↑ **nelfinavir** levels; ↑ dose of lopinavir/ritonavir; once daily lopinavir/ritonavir regimen not recommended when these drugs are used. ↑ **indinavir** levels; indinavir dose should be ↓. ↑ **saquinavir** levels. **Tipranavir** ↓ lopinavir levels. ↑ **maraviroc** levels; maraviroc dose should be ↓ to 150 mg twice daily. ↑ levels of **amiodarone**, **lidocaine**, and **quinidine** (blood level monitoring recommended, if possible). Concurrent use of **carbamazepine**, **phenobarbital**, or **phenytoin** may ↓ effectiveness of lopinavir (blood level monitoring recommended; once daily lopinavir/ritonavir regimen not recommended when these drugs are used); lopinavir may also ↓ **phenytoin** levels. May ↓ **bupropion** levels/effects. ↑ levels/effects of **trazodone**. ↑ levels of dihydropyridine calcium channel blockers including **felodipine**, **nifedipine**, **amlodipine**, and **nicardipine**. May alter levels and effectiveness of **warfarin**. ↑ levels of **clarithromycin** (dose ↓ recommended for patients with CCr ≤60 mL/min. ↑ levels of **itraconazole**, **ketoconazole**, and **isavuconazonium**; high doses of itraconazole or ketoconazole not recommended. ↓ levels of **voriconazole**; concurrent use not recommended. ↑ levels of **rifabutin** (dose ↓ recommended). ↓ levels of **atovaquone** (may require dose ↑). May ↑ levels of **bedaquiline**. **Dexamethasone** may ↓ levels/effectiveness of lopinavir; consider use of alternative corticosteroid, such as beclomethasone or prednisolone. Oral solution contains alcohol, may produce intolerance when administered with **disulfiram** or **metronidazole**. May ↑ levels and risk of toxicity with immunosuppressants including **cyclosporine**, **tacrolimus**, or **sirolimus** (blood level monitoring recommended). May ↓ levels and effects of **methadone** (dose of **methadone** may need to be ↑). May ↑ levels and effects of **fentanyl**; monitor for respiratory depression. May ↓ levels and contraceptive efficacy of some estrogen-based **hormonal contraceptives** including **ethinyl estradiol** (alternative or additional methods of contraception recommended). May ↑ levels of systemic, inhaled, nasal, or ophthalmic **corticosteroids** (**betamethasone**, **budesonide**, **ciclesonide**, **dexamethasone**, **fluticasone**, **methylprednisolone**, **mometasone**, **prednisone**, or **triamcinolone**; consider alternative corticosteroid such as beclomethasone or prednisolone. May ↑ **vincristine** and **vinblastine** levels; consider holding or switching to another antiretroviral regimen that does not contain a CYP3A or P-glycoprotein inhibitor. May ↑ **dasatinib** and **nilotinib** levels; may need to ↓ doses of dasatinib and nilotinib. May ↑ **venetoclax** and **ibrutinib** levels and ↑ risk of tumor lysis syndrome; avoid concurrent use. May ↑ **abemaciclib** and **neratinib** levels and risk of toxicity; avoid concurrent use. Concurrent use of other **drugs known to ↑ PR interval** may ↑ risk of heart block. Concurrent use of other **drugs known to ↑ QT interval** should be avoided. May ↑ risk of adverse effects with **salmeterol**; concurrent use not recommended. May ↑ **bosentan** levels; initiate bosentan at 62.5 mg once daily or every other day; if patient already receiving bosentan, discontinue bosentan at least 36 hr before initiation of tipranavir and then restart bosentan at least 10 days later at 62.5 mg once daily or every other day. May ↑ levels of **sildenafil** (Viagra), **vardenafil**, **tadalafil** (Cialis) or **avanafil**; may result in hypotension, syncope, visual changes, and prolonged erection (↓ dose of sildenafil to 25 mg every 48 hr, vardenafil to 2.5 mg every 72 hr, and tadalafil to 10 mg every 72 hr recommended; do not use with avanafil). May ↑ **tadalafil (Adcirca)** levels; initiate tadalafil (Adcirca) at 20 mg once daily; if patient already receiving tadalfil (Adcirca), discontinue tadalafil (Adcirca) at least 24 hr before initiation of tipranavir and then restart tadalafil (Adcirca) at least 7 days later at 20 mg once daily. May ↑ levels of, **glecaprevir/pibrentasvir**, and **sofosbuvir/velpatasvir/voxilaprevir**, **ombitasvir**, and **paritaprevir**; avoid concurrent use. May ↓ levels of **valproate** and **lamotrigine**; may need to ↑ dose of valproate or lamotrigine. May ↑ levels of **rivaroxaban**; avoid concurrent use. May ↑ **quetiapine** levels; ↓ quetiapine dose to ⅙ of current dose.

Drug-Natural Products: Concurrent use with **St. John's wort** may ↓ levels and beneficial effect of lopinavir/ritonavir (contraindicated).

Route/Dosage

Without Concurrent Efavirenz, Nevirapine, or Nelfinavir

PO (Adults): *Patients with <3 lopinavir resistance-associated substitutions*—400/100 mg (two 200/50-mg tablets or 5 mL oral solution) twice daily *or* 800/

200 mg (four 200/50-mg tablets or 10 mL oral solution) once daily; *Patients with ≥3 lopinavir resistance-associated substitutions*—400/100 mg (two 200/50-mg tablets or 5 mL oral solution) twice daily; *Pregnant women with no lopinavir resistance-associated substitutions*—400/100 mg (two 200/50-mg tablets) twice daily; *Pregnant women with ≥1 lopinavir resistance-associated substitution*—Not recommended.

PO (Children 14 days–6 mo): *Oral solution*—16/4 mg/kg lopinavir/ritonavir content twice daily.

PO (Children ≥6 mo and <15 kg): *Oral solution*—12/3 mg/kg lopinavir/ritonavir twice daily.

PO (Children ≥6 mo and 15–40 kg): *Oral solution*—10/2.5 mg/kg lopinavir/ritonavir twice daily.

PO (Children ≥6 mo): *Tablets*—15–25 kg: 200/50 mg (two 100/25-mg tablets) twice daily; 26–35 kg: 300/75 mg (three 100/25-mg tablets) twice daily; >35 kg: 400/100 mg (four 100/25-mg tablets or two 200/50-mg tablets) twice daily.

With Concurrent Efavirenz, Nevirapine, or Nelfinavir

PO (Adults): *Therapy-naive or therapy-experienced*—500/125 mg (two 200/50-mg tablets and one 100/25-mg tablet or 6.5 mL oral solution) twice daily.

PO (Children 14 days–6 mo): Not recommended for concomitant administration with these drugs.

PO (Children ≥6 mo and <15 kg): *Oral solution*—13/3.25 mg/kg lopinavir/ritonavir twice daily.

PO (Children ≥6 mo and 15–45 kg): *Oral solution*—11/2.75 mg/kg lopinavir/ritonavir twice daily.

PO (Children ≥6 mo): *Tablets*—15–20 kg: 200/50 mg (two 100/25-mg tablets) twice daily; 21–30 kg: 300/75 mg (three 100/25-mg tablets) twice daily; 31–45 kg: 400/100 mg (four 100/25-mg tablets or two 200/50-mg tablets) twice daily.

Availability (generic available)

Oral solution: 80 mg lopinavir/20 mg ritonavir per mL (contains 42.4% alcohol). **Tablets:** 100 mg lopinavir/25 mg ritonavir, 200 mg lopinavir/50 mg ritonavir.

NURSING IMPLICATIONS

Assessment

- Assess for change in severity of HIV symptoms and for symptoms of opportunistic infections during therapy.
- Assess patient for signs of pancreatitis (nausea, vomiting, abdominal pain, increased serum lipase or amylase) periodically during therapy. May require discontinuation of therapy.
- Assess patient for rash (mild to moderate rash usually occurs in the 2nd wk of therapy and resolves within 1–2 wk of continued therapy). If rash is severe (extensive erythematous or maculopapular rash with moist desquamation or angioedema) or accompanied by systemic symptoms (serum sickness-like reaction, Stevens-Johnson syndrome, toxic epidermal necrolysis), therapy must be discontinued immediately.
- ***Lab Test Considerations:*** Monitor viral load and CD4 counts regularly during therapy.
- Monitor triglyceride and cholesterol levels prior to initiating therapy and periodically during therapy.
- May cause hyperglycemia.
- Monitor liver function before and during therapy, especially in patients with underlying hepatic disease, including hepatitis B and hepatitis C, or marked transaminase elevations. May cause ↑ serum AST, ALT, GGT, and total bilirubin concentrations.
- Monitor serum lipase and amylase levels during therapy.
- Monitor blood glucose during therapy. May cause hyperglycemia.

Implementation

- Do not confuse Kaletra (lopinavir/ritonavir) with Keppra (levetiracetam).
- Patients taking didanosine with *Kaletra* solution should take didanosine 1 hr before or 2 hr after taking lopinavir/ritonavir.
- **PO:** Tablets may be administered with or without food. Swallow whole, do not break, crush, or chew.
- Oral solution must be taken with food. Oral solution is light yellow to orange. Solution is stable if refrigerated until expiration date on label or 2 mo at room temperature. Oral solution should be avoided in premature babies until 14 days after their due date, or in full-term babies younger than 14 days of age unless a health care professional believes that the benefit of using *Kaletra* oral solution to treat HIV infection immediately after birth outweighs the potential risks. If oral solution is used in babies younger than 14 days, monitor for increases in serum osmolality, serum creatinine, and other signs of toxicity.
- *Feeding Tube:* Oral solution contains ethanol and propylene glycol. Use only compatible feeding tubes (silicone and polyvinyl chloride [PVC]); avoid use with polyurethane feeding tubes due to potential incompatibility. Follow instructions for use of the feeding tube to administer the medicine.

Patient/Family Teaching

- Emphasize the importance of taking lopinavir/ritonavir as directed, at evenly spaced times throughout day. Do not take more than prescribed amount, and do not stop taking this or other antiretrovirals without consulting health care professional. Take missed doses as soon as remembered; do not double doses. Advise patient to read the *Patient Information* prior to taking this medication and with each Rx refill in case of changes.
- Instruct parent/patient to measure oral solution carefully.
- Instruct patient that lopinavir/ritonavir should not be shared with others.

- Advise patient to notify health care professional of all Rx or OTC medications, vitamins, or herbal products being taken and to consult with health care professional before taking other medications, especially St. John's wort.
- Inform patient that lopinavir/ritonavir does not cure AIDS or prevent associated or opportunistic infections. Lopinavir/ritonavir does not reduce the risk of transmission of HIV to others through sexual contact or blood contamination. Caution patient to use a condom during sexual contact and to avoid sharing needles or donating blood to prevent spreading the AIDS virus to others. Advise patient that the long-term effects of lopinavir/ritonavir are unknown at this time.
- Instruct patient to notify health care professional immediately if rash, symptoms of lactic acidosis (tiredness or weakness, unusual muscle pain, trouble breathing, stomach pain with nausea and vomiting, cold especially in arms or legs, dizziness, fast or irregular heartbeat) or if signs of hepatotoxicity (yellow skin or whites of eyes, dark urine, light-colored stools, lack of appetite for several days or longer, nausea, abdominal pain) occur.
- Inform patient that lopinavir/ritonavir may cause hyperglycemia. Advise patient to notify health care professional if increased thirst or hunger; unexplained weight loss; or increased urination occurs.
- Caution patients taking sildenafil, vardenafil, or tadalafil of increased risk of associated side effects (hypotension, visual changes, sustained erection). Notify health care professional promptly if these occur.
- Inform patient that redistribution and accumulation of body fat may occur causing central obesity, dorsocervical fat enlargement (buffalo hump), peripheral wasting, breast enlargement, and cushingoid appearance. The cause and long-term effects are not known.
- Rep: Advise patients taking oral contraceptives to use a nonhormonal method of birth control during lopinavir/ritonavir therapy. Instruct patient to notify health care professional if pregnancy is planned or suspected and to avoid breast feeding. Encourage pregnant women exposed to lopinavir/ritonavir to enroll in the Antiviral Pregnancy Registry by calling 1-800-258-4263 to monitor maternal/fetal outcomes.
- Emphasize the importance of regular follow-up exams and blood counts to determine progress and monitor for side effects.

Evaluation/Desired Outcomes

- Delayed progression of AIDS and decreased opportunistic infections in patients with HIV.
- Decrease in viral load and improvement in CD4 cell counts.

loratadine (lor-**a**-ta-deen)

Alavert, Claritin, Claritin Allergy Childrens, Claritin Childrens, Claritin Reditabs, Loradamed

Classification
Therapeutic: antihistamines

Indications

Relief of symptoms of seasonal allergies. Management of chronic idiopathic urticaria. Management of hives.

Action

Blocks peripheral effects of histamine released during allergic reactions. **Therapeutic Effects:** Decreased symptoms of allergic reactions (nasal stuffiness; red, swollen eyes, itching).

Pharmacokinetics

Absorption: Rapidly absorbed after oral administration (80%).
Distribution: Unknown.
Protein Binding: *Loratadine*—97%; *descarboethoxyloratadine*—73–77%.
Metabolism and Excretion: Rapidly and extensively metabolized during first pass through the liver. Much is converted to descarboethoxyloratadine, an active metabolite.
Half-life: *Loratadine*—8.4 hr; *descarboethoxyloratadine*—28 hr.

TIME/ACTION PROFILE (antihistaminic effects)

ROUTE	ONSET	PEAK	DURATION
PO	1–3 hr	8–12 hr	>24 hr

Contraindications/Precautions

Contraindicated in: Hypersensitivity.
Use Cautiously in: Hepatic impairment or CCr <30 mL/min (↓ dose to 10 mg every other day); Lactation: Usually compatible with breast feeding (AAP); OB, Pedi: Pregnancy or children <2 yr (safety not established). Syrup contains sodium benzoate, avoid use in neonates; Geri: ↑ risk of adverse reactions.

Adverse Reactions/Side Effects

CNS: confusion, drowsiness (rare), paradoxical excitation. **Derm:** photosensitivity, rash. **EENT:** blurred vision. **GI:** dry mouth, GI upset. **Metab:** weight gain.

Interactions

Drug-Drug: The following interactions may occur, but are less likely to occur with loratidine than with more sedating antihistamines. **MAO inhibitors** may intensify and prolong effects of antihistamines. ↑ CNS depression may occur with other **CNS depressants**, including **alcohol**, **antidepressants**, **opioid analgesics**, and **sedative/hypnotics**. **Amiodarone** may ↑ loratadine levels and ↑ risk of QTc interval prolongation.

Drug-Natural Products: Kava-kava, **valerian**, or **chamomile** can ↑ CNS depression.

Route/Dosage

PO (Adults and Children ≥6 yr): 10 mg once daily.
PO (Children ≥2–5 yr): 5 mg once daily.

Renal Impairment

PO (Adults): *CCr <30 mL/min*—10 mg every other day.

Hepatic Impairment

PO (Adults): 10 mg every other day.

Availability (generic available)

Capsules: 10 mg[OTC]. **Chewable tablets (grape-flavor, bubblegum-flavor):** 5 mg[OTC], 10 mg[OTC]. **Oral solution (grape-flavor, fruit-flavor):** 5 mg/5 mL[OTC]. **Orally disintegrating tablets (mint):** 5 mg[OTC], 10 mg[OTC]. **Tablets:** 10 mg[OTC]. ***In combination with:*** pseudoephedrine (Claritin-D)[OTC]. See Appendix B.

NURSING IMPLICATIONS

Assessment

- Assess allergy symptoms (rhinitis, conjunctivitis, hives) before and periodically during therapy.
- Assess lung sounds and character of bronchial secretions. Maintain fluid intake of 1500–2000 mL/day to decrease viscosity of secretions.
- ***Lab Test Considerations:*** May cause false-negative result on allergy skin testing.

Implementation

- Do not confuse Claritin (loratadine) with Claritin Eye (ketotifen fumarate).
- **PO:** Administer once daily.
- *For rapidly disintegrating tablets (Alavert, Claritin Reditabs)*—place on tongue. Tablet disintegrates rapidly. May be taken with or without water.

Patient/Family Teaching

- Instruct patient to take medication as directed.
- May cause dizziness or drowsiness. Caution patient to avoid driving or other activities requiring alertness until response to medication is known.
- Caution patient to use sunscreen and protective clothing to prevent photosensitivity reactions.
- Advise patient to avoid taking alcohol or other CNS depressants concurrently with this drug.
- Advise patient that good oral hygiene, frequent rinsing of mouth with water, and sugarless gum or candy may minimize dry mouth. Patient should notify dentist if dry mouth persists >2 wk.
- Instruct patient to contact health care professional immediately if dizziness, fainting, or fast or irregular heartbeat occurs or if symptoms persist.
- Advise females of reproductive potential to notify health care professional if pregnancy is planned or suspected, or if breast feeding.

Evaluation/Desired Outcomes

- Decrease in allergic symptoms.
- Management of chronic idiopathic urticaria.
- Management of hives.

BEERS

LORazepam (lor-az-e-pam)
Ativan

Classification
Therapeutic: anesthetic adjuncts, antianxiety agents, sedative/hypnotics
Pharmacologic: benzodiazepines

Schedule IV

Indications

PO: Anxiety disorder. **IM, IV: Status epilepticus, Preanesthetic to produce sedation, decrease preoperative anxiety and induce amnesia.**

Action

Depresses the CNS, probably by potentiating GABA, an inhibitory neurotransmitter. **Therapeutic Effects:** Sedation. Decreased anxiety. Decreased seizures.

Pharmacokinetics

Absorption: Well absorbed following oral administration. Rapidly and completely absorbed following IM administration. Sublingual absorption is more rapid than oral and is similar to IM.

Distribution: Widely distributed. Crosses the blood-brain barrier. Crosses the placenta; enters breast milk.

Metabolism and Excretion: Highly metabolized by the liver.

Half-life: Full-term neonates: 18–73 hr; Older children: 6–17 hr; Adults: 10–16 hr.

TIME/ACTION PROFILE (sedation)

ROUTE	ONSET	PEAK	DURATION
PO	15–60 min	1–6 hr	8–12 hr
IM	30–60 min	1–2 hr†	8–12 hr
IV	15–30 min	15–20 min	8–12 hr

†Amnestic response.

Contraindications/Precautions

Contraindicated in: Hypersensitivity; Cross-sensitivity with other benzodiazepines may exist; Comatose patients or those with pre-existing CNS depression; Uncontrolled severe pain; Angle-closure glaucoma; Severe hypotension; Sleep apnea; OB: Use in pregnancy may

cause CNS depression, flaccidity, feeding difficulties, hypothermia, seizures, and respiratory problems in the neonate; IV use may affect child's brain development when used during 3rd trimester; Lactation: Lactation.
Use Cautiously in: Severe hepatic/renal/pulmonary impairment; Myasthenia gravis; Depression; Psychosis; History of suicide attempt or drug abuse/substance use disorder; COPD; Sleep apnea; Pedi: Safety and effectiveness not established in children <18 yr (IV) or <12 yr (PO); in ↑ doses, benzyl alcohol in injection may cause potentially fatal "gasping syndrome" in neonates; IV use may affect brain development in children <3 yr; Geri: Lower doses recommended for geriatric or debilitated patients.

Adverse Reactions/Side Effects

CNS: dizziness, drowsiness, lethargy, hangover, headache, ataxia, slurred speech, forgetfulness, confusion, mental depression, rhythmic myoclonic jerking in preterm infants, paradoxical excitation. **CV:** *rapid IV use only*—APNEA, CARDIAC ARREST, bradycardia, hypotension. **Derm:** rash. **EENT:** blurred vision. **GI:** constipation, diarrhea, nausea, vomiting, weight gain (unusual). **Resp:** respiratory depression. **Misc:** physical dependence, psychological dependence, tolerance.

Interactions

Drug-Drug: Use with **opioids** or other **CNS depressants**, including other **benzodiazepines**, **nonbenzodiazepine sedative/hypnotics**, **anxiolytics**, **general anesthetics**, **muscle relaxants**, **antipsychotics**, and **alcohol** may cause profound sedation, respiratory depression, coma, and death; reserve concurrent use for when alternative treatment options are inadequate. May ↓ the efficacy of **levodopa**. **Smoking** may ↑ metabolism and ↓ effectiveness. **Valproate** and **probenecid** can ↑ levels; ↓ dose by 50%. **Oral contraceptives** may ↓ levels.
Drug-Natural Products: Concomitant use of **kava-kava**, **valerian**, or **chamomile** can ↑ CNS depression.

Route/Dosage

Status Epilepticus

IV, IM (Adults): 4 mg; may be repeated after 10–15 min.

Preanesthetic

IM (Adults): 0.05 mg/kg (not to exceed 4 mg) ≥2 hr before surgery.
IV (Adults): 0.044 mg/kg (not to exceed 2 mg) 15–20 min before surgery.

Anxiety

PO (Adults): *Anxiety*—1–3 mg 2–3 times daily (up to 10 mg/day). *Insomnia*—2–4 mg at bedtime.
PO (Geriatric Patients or Debilitated Patients): *Anxiety*—0.5–2 mg/day in divided doses initially. *Insomnia*—0.25–1 mg initially, ↑ as needed.

Availability (generic available)

Concentrated oral solution: 2 mg/mL. **Cost:** *Generic*—$39.80/30 mL. **Solution for injection:** 2 mg/mL, 4 mg/mL. **Sublingual tablets:** ✱0.5 mg, ✱1 mg, ✱2 mg. **Tablets:** 0.5 mg, 1 mg, 2 mg. **Cost:** *Generic*—0.5 mg $6.99/100, 1 mg $9.73/100, 2 mg $10.34/100.

NURSING IMPLICATIONS

Assessment

- Conduct regular assessment of continued need for treatment.
- Pedi: Assess neonates for prolonged CNS depression related to inability to metabolize lorazepam.
- Geri: Assess geriatric patients carefully for CNS reactions as they are more sensitive to these effects. Assess falls risk.
- **Anxiety:** Assess degree and manifestations of anxiety and mental status (orientation, mood, behavior) prior to and periodically throughout therapy.
- Prolonged high-dose therapy may lead to psychological or physical dependence. Restrict amount of drug available to patient.
- **Status Epilepticus:** Assess location, duration, characteristics, and frequency of seizures. Institute seizure precautions.
- ***Lab Test Considerations:*** Patients on high-dose therapy should receive routine evaluation of renal, hepatic, and hematologic function.
- ***Toxicity and Overdose:*** If overdose occurs, flumazenil (Romazicon) is the antidote. Do not use with patients with seizure disorder. May induce seizures.

Implementation

- Do not confuse lorazepam with alprazolam, clonazepam, or Lovaza (omega-3–acid ethyl esters).
- Following parenteral administration, keep patient supine for at least 8 hr and observe closely.
- **PO:** Tablet may also be given sublingually (unlabeled) for more rapid onset.
- Take concentrated liquid solution with water, soda, pudding, or applesauce.
- **IM:** Administer IM doses deep into muscle mass at least 2 hr before surgery for optimum effect.

IV Administration

- **IV Push:** ***Diluent:*** Dilute immediately before use with an equal amount of sterile water for injection, D5W, or 0.9% NaCl for injection. Pedi: To decrease the amount of benzyl alcohol delivered to neonates, dilute the 4 mg/mL injection with preservative-free sterile water for injection to make a 0.4 mg/mL dilution for IV use. Do not use if solution is colored or contains a precipitate. ***Rate:*** Administer at a rate not to exceed 2 mg/min or 0.05 mg/kg over 2–5 min. Rapid IV administration may result in apnea, hypotension, bradycardia, or cardiac arrest.

- **Y-Site Compatibility:** acetaminophen, acyclovir, albumin, alemtuzumab, alfentanil, allopurinol, amifostine, amikacin, aminocaproic acid, aminophylline, amiodarone, amphotericin B cholesteryl, amphotericin B deoxycholate, amphotericin B lipid complex, amsacrine, anakinra, anidulafungin, argatroban, atracurium, azithromycin, bleomycin, bumetanide, buprenorphine, bulsulfan, butorphanol, calcium chloride, calcium gluconate, cangrelor, carboplatin, carmustine, cefazolin, cefepime, cefotaxime, cefotetan, cefoxitin, ceftaroline, ceftazidime, ceftriaxone, cefuroxime, chloramphenicol, ciprofloxacin, cisatracurium, cisplatin, cladribine, clindamycin, cyclophosphamide, cyclosporine, cytarabine, dactinomycin, daptomycin, dexamethasone, dexmedetomidine, dexrazoxane, digoxin, diltiazem, diphenhydramine, dobutamine, docetaxel, dopamine, doxorubicin, doxorubicin liposome, doxycycline, droperidol, enalaprilat, ephedrine, epinephrine, epirubicin, eptifibatide, ertapenem, erythromycin lactobionate, esmolol, etomidate, etoposide phosphate, famotidine, fenoldopam, fentanyl, filgrastim, fluconazole, fludarabine, fosphenytoin, furosemide, gemcitabine, gentamicin, glycopyrrolate, granisetron, haloperidol, heparin, hydrocortisone sodium succinate, hydromorphone, ifosfamide, insulin, irinotecan, isoproterenol, ketorolac, labetalol, lidocaine, linezolid, magnesium sulfate, mannitol, melphalan, meropenem, metaraminol, methadone, methotrexate, methyldopate, methylprednisolone, metoclopramide, metoprolol, metronidazole, micafungin, midazolam, milrinone, mitoxantrone, morphine, mycophenolate, nafcillin, nalbuphine, naloxone, nicardipine, nitroglycerin, nitroprusside, norepinephrine, octreotide, oxaliplatin, oxytocin, paclitaxel, palonosetron, pamidronate, pancuronium, pemetrexed, pentamidine, pentobarbital, phentolamine, phenobarbital, phenylephrine, piperacillin/tazobactam, potassium acetate, potassium chloride, procainamide, prochlorperazine, promethazine, propofol, propranolol, quinupristin/dalfopristin, ranitidine, remifentanil, rituximab, sodium acetate, sodium bicarbonate, sodium phosphates, streptozocin, succinylcholine, tacrolimus, theophylline, thiotepa, tigecycline, tirofiban, tobramycin, trastuzumab, trimethoprim/sulfamethoxazole, vancomycin, vasopressin, vecuronium, verapamil, vinblastine, vincristine, vinorelbine, voriconazole, zidovudine, zoledronic acid.
- **Y-Site Incompatibility:** aldesleukin, amphotericin B liposome, ampicillin, ampicillin/sulbactam, aztreonam, dantrolene, doxacurium, fluorouracil, hydralazine, idarubicin, imipenem/cilastatin, meperidine, mitomycin, omeprazole, ondansetron, pantoprazole, phenytoin, potassium phosphates, rocuronium, sargramostim, sufentanil.

Patient/Family Teaching

- Instruct patient to take medication exactly as directed and not to skip or double up on missed doses. If medication is less effective after a few wk, check with health care professional; do not increase dose.
- Advise patient that lorazepam is usually prescribed for short-term use and does not cure underlying problem.
- Advise patient to decrease lorazepam dose gradually to minimize withdrawal symptoms; abrupt withdrawal may cause tremors, nausea, vomiting, and abdominal and muscle cramps.
- Teach other methods to decrease anxiety, such as increased exercise, support groups, relaxation techniques. Emphasize that psychotherapy is beneficial in addressing source of anxiety and improving coping skills.
- May cause drowsiness or dizziness. Advise patient to avoid driving or other activities requiring alertness until response to medication is known.
- Caution patient to avoid taking alcohol or other CNS depressants concurrently with this medication.
- Advise patient that ativan is a drug with known abuse potential. Protect it from theft, and never give to anyone other than the individual for whom it was prescribed. Store out of sight and reach of children, and in a location not accessible by others.
- Instruct patient to contact health care professional immediately if pregnancy is planned or suspected. Monitor infants of women who have taken lorazepam for several wks or more prior to delivery for signs and symptoms of withdrawal (hypoactivity, hypotonia, hypothermia, respiratory depression, apnea, feeding problems, impaired metabolic response to cold stress). Avoid breast feeding during therapy; may cause infant sedation and inability to suckle.
- Emphasize the importance of follow-up exams to determine effectiveness of the medication.

Evaluation/Desired Outcomes

- Increase in sense of well-being.
- Decrease in subjective feelings of anxiety without excessive sedation.
- Reduction of preoperative anxiety.
- Postoperative amnesia.
- Improvement in sleep patterns.

losartan, See ANGIOTENSIN II RECEPTOR ANTAGONISTS.

lovastatin, See HMG-CoA REDUCTASE INHIBITORS (statins).

luliconazole, See ANTIFUNGALS (TOPICAL).

lumacaftor/ivacaftor

(loo-ma-**kaf**-tor/**eye**-va-**kaf**-tor)

Orkambi

Classification

Therapeutic: cystic fibrosis therapy adjuncts

Pharmacologic: transmembrane conductance regulator potentiators

Indications

Treatment of cystic fibrosis (CF) in patients who are homozygous for the *F508del* mutation in the *CFTR* gene.

Action

Ivacaftor—acts as a potentiator of the CFTR protein (a chloride channel on the surface of endothelial cells) facilitating chloride transport by increasing the channel-open probability (gating). *Lumacaftor*—improves the conformational stability of *F508del-CFTR* which results in increased processing and trafficking of mature protein to the cell surface. **Therapeutic Effects:** Improved lung function with increased weight, decreased exacerbations and CF symptoms.

Pharmacokinetics

Lumacaftor

Absorption: Some absorption follows oral administration; absorption is enhanced 2-fold by fat-containing foods.

Distribution: Widely distributed.

Protein Binding: >99%.

Metabolism and Excretion: Minimally metabolized via oxidation and glucuronidation; 51% excreted unchanged in feces; <1% excreted unchanged in urine.

Half-life: 26 hr.

Ivacaftor

Absorption: Some absorption follows oral administration; absorption is enhanced 3-fold by fat-containing foods.

Distribution: Unknown.

Protein Binding: >99%.

Metabolism and Excretion: Extensively metabolized, mostly by the CYP3A enzyme system; one metabolite (M1) is pharmacologically active; 87.8% eliminated in feces; negligible urinary elimination.

Half-life: 9 hr.

TIME/ACTION PROFILE (blood levels)

ROUTE	ONSET	PEAK	DURATION
Lumacaftor (PO)	within 1 wk	4 hr	12 hr
Ivacaftor (PO)	within 1 wk	4 hr	12 hr

Contraindications/Precautions

Contraindicated in: Concurrent use of strong CYP3A inducers; Concurrent use of sensitive CYP3A substrates or those with a narrow therapeutic index.

Use Cautiously in: Concurrent use of CYP3A inhibitors; Moderate or severe hepatic impairment (dose ↓ recommended); Severe renal impairment (CCr <30 mL/min) or end stage renal disease; Advanced lung disease (↑ risk of respiratory events); OB: Use in pregnancy only if clearly needed; Lactation: Use cautiously during breast feeding; Pedi: Children <2 yr (safety and effectiveness not established).

Adverse Reactions/Side Effects

CNS: fatigue. **CV:** ↑ blood pressure. **Derm:** rash. **EENT:** cataracts, rhinorrhea. **GI:** diarrhea, nausea, flatulence, ↑ bilirubin, ↑ liver enzymes. **GU:** amenorrhea, dysmenorrhea, menorrhagia. **MS:** ↑ creatine kinase. **Resp:** dyspnea, chest discomfort.

Interactions

Drug-Drug: Lumacaftor is a strong inducer of CYP3A4. Ivacaftor is a CYP3A substrate. **Strong CYP3A inducers** including **rifampin**, **rifabutin**, **phenobarbital**, **carbamazepine** and **phenytoin** may ↓ ivacaftor levels and effectiveness; avoid concurrent use. Lumacaftor may ↓ levels of **CYP3A substrates**, including **hormonal contraceptive agents**; avoid concurrent use with sensitive CYP3A substrates or those with a narrow therapeutic index, including **cyclosporine**, **everolimus**, **midazolam**, **sirolimus**, **tacrolimus**, or **triazolam**. **Strong CYP3A inhibitors** including **ketoconazole**, **itraconazole**, **posaconazole**, **voriconazole**, and **clarithromycin** may ↑ ivacaftor levels; no dose adjustment required when initiating CYP3A inhibitor in patients currently receiving ivacaftor/lumacaftor; ↓ initial ivacaftor/lumacaftor dose for 1 wk when starting therapy in patient currently receiving strong CYP3A4 inhibitor and then proceed with recommended dose. Lumacaftor may ↓ levels of **CYP2B6 substrates**, **CYP2C8 substrates**, **CYP2C9 substrates**, and **CYP2C19 substrates**. Ivacaftor may ↑ levels of **CYP2C9 substrates**. May ↑ or ↓ **digoxin** or **warfarin** levels. May ↓ levels of **citalopram**, **clarithromycin**, **corticosteroids**, **erythromycin**, **escitalopram**, **ibuprofen**, **itraconazole**, **ketoconazole**, **montelukast**, **posaconazole**, **proton pump inhibitors**, **raniti-**

dine, repaglinide, sertraline, sulfonylureas, voriconazole.
Drug-Natural Products: St. John's wort may ↓ ivacaftor levels and effectiveness; avoid concurrent use.

Route/Dosage

PO (Adults and Children ≥12 yr): Two lumacaftor 200 mg/ivacaftor 125 mg tablets every 12 hr with fat-containing food; *Initiation of therapy in patients receiving strong CYP3A inhibitor*—One lumacaftor 200 mg/ivacaftor 125 mg tablet once daily for 1 wk, then ↑ to two lumacaftor 200 mg/ivacaftor 125 mg tablets every 12 hr.
PO (Children 6–11 yr): Two lumacaftor 100 mg/ivacaftor 125 mg tablets every 12 hr with fat-containing food; *Initiation of therapy in patients receiving strong CYP3A inhibitor*—One lumacaftor 100 mg/ivacaftor 125 mg tablet once daily for 1 wk, then ↑ to two lumacaftor 200 mg/ivacaftor 125 mg tablets every 12 hr.
PO (Children 2–5 yr and ≥14 kg): One lumacaftor 150 mg/ivacaftor 188 mg granule packet every 12 hr with fat-containing food; *Initiation of therapy in patients receiving strong CYP3A inhibitor*—One lumacaftor 150 mg/ivacaftor 188 mg granule packet every other day for 1 wk, then ↑ to one lumacaftor 150 mg/ivacaftor 188 mg granule packet every 12 hr.
PO (Children 2–5 yr and <14 kg): One lumacaftor 100 mg/ivacaftor 125 mg granule packet every 12 hr with fat-containing food; *Initiation of therapy in patients receiving strong CYP3A inhibitor*—One lumacaftor 100 mg/ivacaftor 125 mg granule packet every other day for 1 wk, then ↑ to one lumacaftor 100 mg/ivacaftor 125 mg granule packet every 12 hr.

Hepatic Impairment

(Adults and Children ≥12 yr): *Moderate hepatic impairment (Child-Pugh Class B)*—Two lumacaftor 200 mg/ivacaftor 125 mg tablets in AM and one lumacaftor 200 mg/ivacaftor 125 mg tablet in PM; *Severe hepatic impairment (Child-Pugh Class C)*—One lumacaftor 200 mg/ivacaftor 125 mg tablet in AM and one lumacaftor 200 mg/ivacaftor 125 mg tablet in PM.

Hepatic Impairment

(Children 6–11 yr): *Moderate hepatic impairment (Child-Pugh Class B)*—Two lumacaftor 100 mg/ivacaftor 125 mg tablets in AM and one lumacaftor 100 mg/ivacaftor 125 mg tablet in PM; *Severe hepatic impairment (Child-Pugh Class C)*—One lumacaftor 100 mg/ivacaftor 125 mg tablet in AM and one lumacaftor 100 mg/ivacaftor 125 mg tablet in PM.

Hepatic Impairment

(Children 2–5 yr and ≥14 kg): *Moderate hepatic impairment (Child-Pugh Class B)*—One lumacaftor 150 mg/ivacaftor 188 mg granule packet in AM and one lumacaftor 150 mg/ivacaftor 188 mg granule packet every other PM; *Severe hepatic impairment (Child-Pugh Class C)*—One lumacaftor 150 mg/ivacaftor 188 mg granule packet in AM.

Hepatic Impairment

(Children 2–5 yr and <14 kg): *Moderate hepatic impairment (Child-Pugh Class B)*—One lumacaftor 100 mg/ivacaftor 125 mg granule packet in AM and one lumacaftor 100 mg/ivacaftor 125 mg granule packet every other PM; *Severe hepatic impairment (Child-Pugh Class C)*—One lumacaftor 100 mg/ivacaftor 125 mg granule packet in AM.

Availability

Oral granules: lumacaftor 100 mg/ivacaftor 125 mg/pkt, lumacaftor 150 mg/ivacaftor 188 mg/pkt. **Tablets:** lumacaftor 100 mg/ivacaftor 125 mg, lumacaftor 200 mg/ivacaftor 125 mg.

NURSING IMPLICATIONS

Assessment

- Assess respiratory status (chest discomfort, dyspnea, respiration abnormal) prior to and periodically during therapy.
- Monitor BP periodically during therapy; may cause hypertension.
- Obtain baseline and periodic ophthalmological exams on pediatric patients starting therapy; may cause cataracts.
- ***Lab Test Considerations:*** Determine patient's genotype prior to starting therapy. If genotype is unknown, use an FDA-cleared CF mutation test to detect presence of the F508del mutation on both alleles of the CFTR gene.
- Monitor ALT, AST, and bilirubin prior to starting therapy, every 3 mo during 1st yr of therapy, and annually thereafter. Monitor patients with a history of ALT, AST, or bilirubin ↑ more frequently. If ↑ ALT, AST, or bilirubin occur, monitored closely until resolved. *If ALT or AST >5 × upper limit of normal (ULN) when not associated ↑ bilirubin,* withhold therapy. *If ALT or AST >3 × ULN when associated with bilirubin >2 × ULN,* withhold therapy. Consider benefits and risks of resuming dosing, once ↑ levels resolve.

Implementation

- **PO:** Administer 2 tablets every 12 hrs with fat-containing food (eggs, avocados, nuts, butter, peanut butter, cheese pizza, whole-milk dairy products [whole milk, cheese, yogurt], etc).
- To administer granules, mix entire content of single-use packet with 1 tsp (5 mL) of age-appropriate soft food or liquid (puréed fruits, flavored yogurt or pudding, milk or juice). Food should be at room temperature or below. Mixture is stable for 1 hr.

Patient/Family Teaching

- Instruct patient to take medication as directed. Take missed doses within 6 hrs with fat-containing food. If >6 hrs after usual dosing time, omit dose and resume normal schedule for following dose; do not double doses. Advise patient to read *Patient Information* prior to starting and with each Rx refill in case of changes.

- May cause dizziness. Avoid driving and other activities requiring alertness until response to medication is known.
- Advise patient to notify health care professional if signs and symptoms of liver problems (pain or discomfort in upper right abdomen, yellowing of skin or white of eyes, loss of appetite, nausea or vomiting, dark, amber-colored urine, confusion) or respiratory problems (shortness of breath, chest tightness) occur.
- Advise patient to notify health care professional of all Rx or OTC medications, vitamins, or herbal products being taken and to consult with health care professional before taking other medications, especially St. John's wort.
- Advise female patients of reproductive potential to notify health care professional if pregnancy is planned or suspected, or if breast feeding. Use a nonhormonal contraceptive during therapy.
- Pedi: Advise patient of childbearing age to use nonhormonal contraception. Ivacaftor/lumacaftor may ↓ hormonal contraceptive exposure (oral, injectable, transdermal, implantable) ↓ effectiveness; do not rely upon as effective method of contraception.

Evaluation/Desired Outcomes

- Improved lung function with ↑ weight, decreased exacerbations and fewer CF symptoms.

BEERS

lurasidone (loo-**ras**-i-done)

Latuda

Classification

Therapeutic: antipsychotics

Pharmacologic: benzoisothiazole

Indications

Treatment of schizophrenia. Depressive episodes associated with bipolar I disorder (as monotherapy or with lithium or valproate).

Action

Effect may be mediated via effects on central dopamine Type 2 (D_2) and serotonin Type 2 ($5HT_{2A}$) receptor antagonism. **Therapeutic Effects:** ↓ schizophrenic behavior. ↓ depressive episodes in bipolar I disorder.

Pharmacokinetics

Absorption: 9–19% absorbed following oral administration.

Distribution: Unknown.

Protein Binding: >99%.

Metabolism and Excretion: Mostly metabolized by the CYP3A4 enzyme system. Two metabolites are pharmacologically active; 80% eliminated in feces, 8% in urine primarily as metabolites.

Half-life: 18 hr.

TIME/ACTION PROFILE

ROUTE	ONSET	PEAK	DURATION
PO	unknown	1–3 hr*	24 hr

*Blood level.

Contraindications/Precautions

Contraindicated in: Hypersensitivity; Concurrent use of strong CYP3A4 inhibitors or inducers.

Use Cautiously in: Moderate or severe renal impairment (dose adjustment recommended); Moderate or severe hepatic impairment (dose adjustment recommended); History of suicide attempt; Diabetes mellitus; Overheating/dehydration (may ↑ risk of serious adverse reactions); Patients at risk for falls; History of leukopenia or previous drug-induced leukopenia/neutropenia; Geri: ↑ risk of seizures; ↑ risk of mortality and stroke in elderly patients treated for dementia-related psychosis; use cautiously in elderly females (↑ risk of tardive dyskinesia); OB: Use in pregnancy only if potential benefit justifies potential risk to fetus; Lactation: Breast feeding should only be considered if potential benefit justifies risk to child; Pedi: May ↑ risk of suicide attempt/ideation especially during dose early treatment or dose adjustment; risk may be greater in children, adolescents, and young adults taking antidepressants; safety and effectiveness not established in children <10 yr.

Adverse Reactions/Side Effects

CNS: NEUROLEPTIC MALIGNANT SYNDROME, SEIZURES, SUICIDAL THOUGHTS, akathisia, drowsiness, parkinsonism, agitation, anxiety, cognitive/motor impairment, dizziness, dystonia, tardive dyskinesia. **CV:** bradycardia, orthostatic hypotension, syncope, tachycardia. **Derm:** pruritus, rash. **EENT:** blurred vision. **Endo:** hyperglycemia, hyperprolactinemia. **GI:** nausea, esophageal dysmotility. **Hemat:** AGRANULOCYTOSIS, anemia, leukopenia. **Metab:** dyslipidemia, weight gain.

Interactions

Drug-Drug: Strong CYP3A4 inhibitors, including **ketoconazole**, **clarithromycin**, **ritonavir**, and **voriconazole** ↑ blood levels and risk of adverse reactions; concurrent use contraindicated. **Strong CYP3A4 inducers**, including **rifampin**, **phenytoin**, and **carbamazepine** ↓ blood levels and effectiveness; concurrent use contraindicated. **Moderate inhibitors of the CYP3A4 enzyme system**, including **diltiazem**, **atazanavir**, **erythromycin**, **fluconazole**, and **verapamil** ↑ blood levels; if used concurrently, dose of lurasi-

done should not exceed 40 mg/day. ↑ sedation may occur with other **CNS depressants**, including **alcohol**, **sedative/hypnotics**, **opioids**, some **antidepressants** and **antihistamines**.
Drug-Natural Products: **St. John's wort** ↓ blood levels and effectiveness; concurrent use contraindicated.
Drug-Food: **Grapefruit juice** ↑ blood levels and risk of adverse reactions; concurrent use contraindicated.

Route/Dosage

Schizophrenia

PO (Adults): 40 mg once daily (not to exceed 160 mg once daily); *Addition of moderate CYP3A4 inhibitor to existing lurasidone therapy*— ↓ lurasidone dose by 50%; *Addition of lurasidone to existing moderate CYP3A4 inhibitor therapy*— 20 mg once daily (not to exceed 80 mg once daily).
PO (Children 13–17 yr): 40 mg once daily (not to exceed 80 mg once daily); *Addition of moderate CYP3A4 inhibitor to existing lurasidone therapy*— ↓ lurasidone dose by 50%; *Addition of lurasidone to existing moderate CYP3A4 inhibitor therapy*— 20 mg once daily (not to exceed 80 mg once daily).

Renal Impairment

PO (Adults and Children 13–17 yr): *CCr <50 mL/min*— 20 mg once daily (not to exceed 80 mg once daily).

Hepatic Impairment

(Adults and Children 13–17 yr): *Child-Pugh Class B*— 20 mg once daily (not to exceed 80 mg once daily); *Child-Pugh Class C*— 20 mg once daily (not to exceed 40 mg once daily).

Depressive Episodes Associated with Bipolar I Disorder

PO (Adults): 20 mg once daily (not to exceed 120 mg once daily); *Addition of moderate CYP3A4 inhibitor to existing lurasidone therapy*— ↓ lurasidone dose by 50%; *Addition of lurasidone to existing moderate CYP3A4 inhibitor therapy*— 20 mg once daily (not to exceed 80 mg once daily).
PO (Children 10–17 yr): 20 mg once daily (not to exceed 80 mg once daily); *Addition of moderate CYP3A4 inhibitor to existing lurasidone therapy*— ↓ lurasidone dose by 50%; *Addition of lurasidone to existing moderate CYP3A4 inhibitor therapy*— 20 mg once daily (not to exceed 80 mg once daily).

Renal Impairment

PO (Adults and Children 10–17 yr): *CCr <50 mL/min*— 20 mg once daily (not to exceed 80 mg once daily).

Hepatic Impairment

PO (Adults and Children 10–17 yr): *Child-Pugh Class B*— 20 mg once daily (not to exceed 80 mg once daily); *Child-Pugh Class C*— 20 mg once daily (not to exceed 40 mg once daily).

Availability (generic available)

Tablets: 20 mg, 40 mg, 60 mg, 80 mg, 120 mg.

NURSING IMPLICATIONS

Assessment

- Monitor patient's mental status (orientation, mood, behavior) before and periodically during therapy.
- Assess weight and BMI initially and during therapy. Refer as appropriate for nutritional/weight and medical management.
- Monitor mood changes. Assess for suicidal tendencies, especially during early therapy. Restrict amount of drug available to patient.
- Monitor BP (sitting, standing, lying down) and pulse before and frequently during initial dose titration. May cause tachycardia and orthostatic hypotension. If hypotension occurs, dose may need to be ↓.
- Observe patient when administering medication to ensure medication is swallowed and not hoarded or cheeked.
- Monitor patient for onset of extrapyramidal side effects (*akathisia*— restlessness; *dystonia*— muscle spasms and twisting motions; or *pseudoparkinsonism*— mask-like face, rigidity, tremors, drooling, shuffling gait, dysphagia). Report these symptoms; reduction of dose or discontinuation may be necessary. Trihexyphenidyl or benztropine may be used to control symptoms.
- Monitor for tardive dyskinesia (involuntary rhythmic movement of mouth, face, and extremities). Report immediately; may be irreversible.
- Monitor for symptoms related to hyperprolactinemia (menstrual abnormalities, galactorrhea, sexual dysfunction).
- Monitor for development of neuroleptic malignant syndrome (fever, respiratory distress, tachycardia, seizures, diaphoresis, hypertension or hypotension, pallor, tiredness). Notify health care professional immediately if these symptoms occur.
- Monitor for symptoms of hyperglycemia (polydipsia, polyuria, polyphagia, weakness) periodically during therapy.
- Assess for falls risk. Drowsiness, orthostatic hypotension, and motor and sensory instability increase risk. Institute prevention if indicated.
- ***Lab Test Considerations:*** May cause ↑ serum prolactin levels.
- May cause ↑ CPK.
- Obtain fasting blood glucose and cholesterol levels initially and periodically during therapy.
- Monitor CBC frequently during initial mo of therapy in patients with pre-existing or history of low WBC. May cause leukopenia, neutropenia, or agranulocytosis. Discontinue therapy if this occurs.

Implementation

- ***High Alert:*** Do not confuse Latuda (lurasidone) with Lantus (insulin glargine).
- **PO:** Administer once daily with food of at least 350 calories. Use beyond 6 wk has not been studied.

Patient/Family Teaching

- Instruct patient to take medication as directed. Emphasize the caloric food needs for taking medication.
- Inform patient of the possibility of extrapyramidal symptoms. Instruct patient to report these symptoms immediately to health care professional.
- Advise patient to change positions slowly to minimize orthostatic hypotension. Protect from falls.
- May cause drowsiness and cognitive and motor impairment. Caution patient to avoid driving or other activities requiring alertness until response to medication is known.
- Advise patient and family to notify health care professional if thoughts about suicide or dying, attempts to commit suicide; new or worse depression; new or worse anxiety; feeling very agitated or restless; panic attacks; trouble sleeping; new or worse irritability; acting aggressive; being angry or violent; acting on dangerous impulses; an extreme ↑ in activity and talking, other unusual changes in behavior or mood occur.
- Advise patient to avoid extremes in temperature; this drug impairs body temperature regulation.
- Advise patient to tell health care professional what medications they are taking and to avoid taking new Rx, OTC, vitamins, or herbal products without consulting health care professional, especially alcohol and other CNS depressants.
- Advise patient to notify health care professional of medication regimen before treatment or surgery.
- Instruct patient to notify health care professional promptly if sore throat, fever, unusual bleeding or bruising, rash, or tremors occur.
- Rep: Advise female patients to notify health care professional if pregnancy is planned or suspected, and to avoid breast feeding. Encourage women who become pregnant while taking lurasidone to enroll in the National Pregnancy Registry for Atypical Antipsychotics at 1-866-961-2388 or visit http://womensmentalhealth.org/clinical-and-research-programs/pregnancyregistry/. Monitor neonates for extrapyramidal and/or withdrawal symptoms and manage symptoms appropriately.
- Emphasize the importance of routine follow up exams to monitor side effects.

Evaluation/Desired Outcomes

- ↓ in symptoms of schizophrenia (delusions, hallucinations, social withdrawal, flat, blunted affects).
- ↓ depressive episodes in bipolar I disorder.

L

magaldrate, See MAGNESIUM AND ALUMINUM SALTS.

MAGNESIUM AND ALUMINUM SALTS

magaldrate (with simethicone)
(**mag**-al-drate)
Riopan Plus

magnesium hydroxide/aluminum hydroxide
(mag-**nee**-zhum hye-**drox**-ide/ a-**loo**-mi-num hye-**drox**-ide)
Alamag, ✱Diovol Plus, Maalox, Rulox

Classification
Therapeutic: antiulcer agents
Pharmacologic: antacids

Indications
Useful in a variety of GI complaints, including: Hyperacidity, Indigestion, GERD, Heartburn.

Action
Neutralize gastric acid following dissolution in gastric contents. Inactivate pepsin if pH is raised to ≥4. **Therapeutic Effects:** Neutralization of gastric acid with healing of ulcers and decrease in associated pain.

Pharmacokinetics
Absorption: During routine use, antacids are nonabsorbable. With chronic use, 15–30% of magnesium and smaller amounts of aluminum may be absorbed.
Distribution: Small amounts absorbed are widely distributed, cross the placenta, and appear in breast milk. Aluminum concentrates in the CNS.
Metabolism and Excretion: Excreted by the kidneys.
Half-life: Unknown.

TIME/ACTION PROFILE (effect on gastric pH)

ROUTE	ONSET	PEAK	DURATION
Aluminum PO	slightly delayed	30 min	30 min–1 hr (empty stomach); 3 hr (after meals)
Magnesium PO	slightly delayed	30 min	30 min–1 hr (empty stomach); 3 hr (after meals)

Contraindications/Precautions
Contraindicated in: Severe abdominal pain of unknown cause, especially if accompanied by fever; Renal failure (CrCl <30 mL/min); Products containing tartrazine or sugar in patients with known intolerance.
Use Cautiously in: Antacids containing magnesium in patients with any degree of renal insufficiency; ↓ bowel motility; Dehydration; Upper GI hemorrhage; Pedi: Children <12 yr (safety not established).

Adverse Reactions/Side Effects
GI: *aluminum salts*—constipation; *magnesium salts*, diarrhea. **F and E:** *magnesium salts*—hypermagnesemia; *aluminum salts*, hypophosphatemia.

Interactions
Drug-Drug: Absorption of **tetracyclines**, **phenothiazines**, **ketoconazole**, **itraconazole**, **iron salts**, **fluoroquinolones**, and **isoniazid** may be ↓ (separate by at least 2 hr).

Route/Dosage
Magaldrate/Simethicone
PO (Adults): 5–10 mL (540–1080 mg) between meals and at bedtime.

Magnesium Hydroxide/Aluminum Hydroxide
PO (Adults and Children ≥12 yr): 5–30 mL or 1–2 tablets 1–3 hr after meals and at bedtime.

Availability
Magaldrate/Simethicone (generic available)
Suspension: 540 mg magaldrate/20 mg simethicone/5 mL^OTC^, 1080 mg magaldrate/40 mg simethicone/5 mL^OTC^.

Magnesium Hydroxide/Aluminum Hydroxide (generic available)
Chewable Tablets: 300 mg aluminum hydroxide/150 mg magnesium hydroxide^OTC^. **Suspension:** 225 mg aluminum hydroxide/200 mg magnesium hydroxide/5 mL^OTC^, 500 mg aluminum hydroxide/500 mg magnesium hydroxide/5 mL^OTC^. ***In combination with:*** simethicone^OTC^. See Appendix B.

NURSING IMPLICATIONS
Assessment
- **Antacid:** Assess for heartburn and indigestion as well as location, duration, character, and precipitating factors of gastric pain.
- ***Lab Test Considerations:*** Monitor serum phosphate, potassium, and calcium levels periodically during chronic use. May cause ↑ serum calcium and ↓ serum phosphate concentrations.

M

Implementation

- Magnesium and aluminum are combined as antacids to balance the constipating effects of aluminum with the laxative effects of magnesium.
- **PO:** To prevent tablets from entering small intestine in undissolved form, they must be chewed thoroughly before swallowing. Follow with at least ½ glass of water.
- Shake suspensions well before administration.
- For an antacid effect, administer 1–3 hr after meals and at bedtime.

Patient/Family Teaching

- Caution patient to consult health care professional before taking antacids for more than 2 wk if problem is recurring, if relief is not obtained, or if symptoms of gastric bleeding (black, tarry stools; coffee-ground emesis) occur.
- Advise patient not to take this medication within 2 hr of taking other medications.
- Pedi: Aluminum- or magnesium-containing medicines can cause serious side effects in children, especially when given to children with renal disease or dehydration. Advise parents or caregivers not to administer OTC antacids to children without consulting health care professional.

Evaluation/Desired Outcomes

- Relief of gastric pain and irritation.

magnesium salicylate, See SALICYLATES.

MAGNESIUM SALTS (ORAL)

magnesium chloride (12% Mg; 9.8 mEq Mg/g)
(mag-**nee**-zhum **klor**-ide)
Chloromag, Slo-Mag

magnesium citrate (16.2% Mg; 4.4 mEq Mg/g)
(mag-**nee**-zhum **si**-trate)
Citrate of Magnesia, Citroma, ✱Citromag

magnesium gluconate (5.4% Mg; 4.4 mEq/g)
(mag-**nee**-zhum **gloo**-con-ate)
Magtrate, Magonate

magnesium hydroxide (41.7% Mg; 34.3 mEq Mg/g)
(mag-**nee**-zhum hye-**drox**-ide)
Dulcolax Magnesia Tablets, Phillips Magnesia Tablets, Phillips Milk of Magnesia, MOM

magnesium oxide (60.3% Mg; 49.6 mEq Mg/g)
(mag-**nee**-zhum **ox**-ide)
Mag-Ox 400, Uro-Mag

Classification
Therapeutic: mineral and electrolyte replacements/supplements, laxatives
Pharmacologic: salines

Indications

Treatment/prevention of hypomagnesemia. As a: Laxative, Bowel evacuant in preparation for surgical/radiographic procedures. Milk of Magnesia has also been used as an antacid.

Action

Essential for the activity of many enzymes. Play an important role in neurotransmission and muscular excitability. Are osmotically active in GI tract, drawing water into the lumen and causing peristalsis. **Therapeutic Effects:** Replacement in deficiency states. Evacuation of the colon.

Pharmacokinetics

Absorption: Up to 30% may be absorbed orally.
Distribution: Widely distributed. Cross the placenta and are present in breast milk.
Metabolism and Excretion: Excreted primarily by the kidneys.
Half-life: Unknown.

TIME/ACTION PROFILE (laxative effect)

ROUTE	ONSET	PEAK	DURATION
PO	3–6 hr	unknown	unknown

Contraindications/Precautions

Contraindicated in: Hypermagnesemia; Hypocalcemia; Anuria; Heart block; OB: Unless used for preterm labor, use during active labor or within 2 hr of delivery may ↑ potential for magnesium toxicity in newborn.
Use Cautiously in: Any degree of renal insufficiency.

Adverse Reactions/Side Effects

GI: diarrhea. **Derm:** flushing, sweating.

Interactions

Drug-Drug: Potentiates **neuromuscular blocking agents**. May ↓ absorption of **fluoroquinolones**, **nitrofurantoin**, and **tetracyclines** and **penicillamine**.

Route/Dosage

Prevention of Deficiency (in mg of Magnesium)

PO (Adults and Children >10 yr): *Adolescent and adult men*—270–400 mg/day; *adolescent and adult women*—280–300 mg/day; *pregnant women*—320 mg/day; *breast-feeding women*—340–355 mg/day.

PO (Children 7–10 yr): 170 mg/day.
PO (Children 4–6 yr): 120 mg/day.
PO (Children birth–3 yr): 40–80 mg/day.

Treatment of Deficiency (Expressed as mg of Magnesium)

PO (Adults): 200–400 mg/day in 3–4 divided doses.
PO (Children 6–11 yr): 3–6 mg/kg/day in 3–4 divided doses.

Laxative

PO (Adults): *Magnesium citrate*—240 mL; *magnesium hydroxide (Milk of Magnesia)*—30–60 mL single or divided dose or 10–20 mL as concentrate.
PO (Children 6–12 yr): *Magnesium citrate*—100 mL; *magnesium hydroxide (Milk of Magnesia)*—15–30 mL single or divided dose.
PO (Children 2–5 yr): *magnesium hydroxide (Milk of Magnesia)*—5–15 mL single or divided dose.

Availability

Magnesium Chloride (generic available)

Sustained-release tablets: 535 mg (64 mg magnesium)OTC. **Enteric-coated tablets:** 833 mg (100 mg magnesium)OTC.

Magnesium Citrate (generic available)

Oral solution: 240-, 296-, and 300-mL bottles (77 mEq magnesium/100 mL)OTC.

Magnesium Gluconate (generic available)

Tablets: 500 mgOTC. **Liquid:** 54 mg/5 mLOTC.

Magnesium Hydroxide (generic available)

Liquid: 400 mg/5 mL (164 mg magnesium/5 mL)OTC. **Concentrated liquid:** 800 mg/5 mL (328 mg magnesium/5 mL)OTC. **Chewable tablets:** 300 mg (130 mg magnesium)OTC, 600 mg (260 mg magnesium)OTC.

Magnesium Oxide (generic available)

Tablets: 400 mg (241.3 mg magnesium)OTC. **Capsules:** 140 mg (84.5 mg magnesium)OTC.

NURSING IMPLICATIONS

Assessment

- **Laxative:** Assess patient for abdominal distention, presence of bowel sounds, and usual pattern of bowel function.
- Assess color, consistency, and amount of stool produced.
- **Antacid:** Assess for heartburn and indigestion as well as location, duration, character, and precipitating factors of gastric pain.

Implementation

- **PO:** To prevent tablets entering small intestine in undissolved form, they must be chewed thoroughly before swallowing. Follow with ½ glass of water.
- *Magnesium citrate:* Refrigerate solutions to ensure they retain potency and palatability. May be served over ice. Magnesium citrate in an open container will lose carbonation upon standing; this will not affect potency but may reduce palatability.
- *Magnesium hydroxide:* Shake solution well before administration.
- **Antacid:** Administer 1–3 hr after meals and at bedtime.
- Powder and liquid forms are considered more effective than tablets.
- **Laxative:** Administer on empty stomach for more rapid results. Follow all oral laxative doses with a full glass of liquid to prevent dehydration and for faster effect. Do not administer at bedtime or late in the day.

Patient/Family Teaching

- Advise patient not to take this medication within 2 hr of taking other medications, especially fluoroquinolones, nitrofurantoin, and tetracyclines.
- **Antacids:** Caution patient to consult health care professional before taking antacids for more than 2 wk if problem is recurring, if relief is not obtained, or if symptoms of gastric bleeding (black, tarry stools; coffee-ground emesis) occur.
- **Laxatives:** Advise patient that laxatives should be used only for short-term therapy. Long-term therapy may cause electrolyte imbalance and dependence.
- Encourage patient to use other forms of bowel regulation, such as increasing bulk in the diet, fluid intake, and mobility. Normal bowel habits are individualized; frequency of bowel movement may vary from 3 times/day to 3 times/wk.
- Advise patient to notify health care professional if unrelieved constipation, rectal bleeding, or symptoms of electrolyte imbalance (muscle cramps or pain, weakness, dizziness) occur.

Evaluation/Desired Outcomes

- Relief of gastric pain and irritation.
- Passage of a soft, formed bowel movement, usually within 3–6 hr.
- Prevention and treatment of magnesium deficiency.

HIGH ALERT

magnesium sulfate (IV, parenteral) (9.9% Mg; 8.1 mEq Mg/g)

(mag-**nee**-zhum **sul**-fate)

Classification
Therapeutic: mineral and electrolyte replacements/supplements
Pharmacologic: minerals/electrolytes

Indications

Treatment/prevention of hypomagnesemia. Treatment of hypertension. Prevention of seizures associated with severe eclampsia, pre-eclampsia, or acute nephritis. **Unlabeled Use:** Preterm labor. Treatment of torsade de pointes. Adjunctive treatment for bronchodilation in moderate to severe acute asthma.

Action

Essential for the activity of many enzymes. Plays an important role in neurotransmission and muscular excitability. **Therapeutic Effects:** Replacement in deficiency states. Resolution of eclampsia.

Pharmacokinetics

Absorption: IV administration results in complete bioavailability; well absorbed from IM sites.
Distribution: Widely distributed. Crosses the placenta and is present in breast milk.
Metabolism and Excretion: Excreted primarily by the kidneys.
Half-life: Unknown.

TIME/ACTION PROFILE (anticonvulsant effect)

ROUTE	ONSET	PEAK	DURATION
IM	60 min	unknown	3–4 hr
IV	immediate	unknown	30 min

Contraindications/Precautions

Contraindicated in: Hypermagnesemia; Hypocalcemia; Anuria; Heart block; OB: Avoid using for more than 5–7 days for preterm labor (may ↑ risk of hypocalcemia and bone changes in newborn); avoid continuous use during active labor or within 2 hr of delivery due to potential for magnesium toxicity in newborn.
Use Cautiously in: Any degree of renal insufficiency; Geri: May require ↓ dosage due to age-related ↓ in renal function.

Adverse Reactions/Side Effects

CNS: drowsiness. **Resp:** ↓ respiratory rate. **CV:** arrhythmias, bradycardia, hypotension. **GI:** diarrhea. **MS:** muscle weakness. **Derm:** flushing, sweating. **Metab:** hypothermia.

Interactions

Drug-Drug: May potentiate **calcium channel blockers** and **neuromuscular blocking agents**.

Route/Dosage

Treatment of Deficiency (Expressed as mg of Magnesium)

IM, IV (Adults): *Severe deficiency*—8–12 g/day in divided doses; *mild deficiency*—1 g every 6 hr for 4 doses or 250 mg/kg over 4 hr.
IM, IV (Children >1 mo): 25–50 mg/kg/dose every 4–6 hr for 3–4 doses, maximum single dose: 2 g.
IV (Neonates): 25–50 mg/kg/dose every 8–12 hr for 2–3 doses.

Seizures/Hypertension

IM, IV (Adults): 1 g every 6 hr for 4 doses as needed.
IM, IV (Children): 20–100 mg/kg/dose every 4–6 hr as needed, may use up to 200 mg/kg/dose in severe cases.

Torsade de Pointes

IV (Infants and Children): 25–50 mg/kg/dose, maximum dose: 2 g.

Bronchodilation

IV (Adults): 2 g single dose.
IV (Children): 25 mg/kg/dose, maximum dose: 2 g.

Eclampsia/Pre-Eclampsia

IV, IM (Adults): 4–5 g by IV infusion, concurrently with up to 5 g IM in each buttock; then 4–5 g IM every 4 hr *or* 4 g by IV infusion followed by 1–2 g/hr continuous infusion (not to exceed 40 g/day or 20 g/48 hr in the presence of severe renal insufficiency).

Part of Parenteral Nutrition

IV (Adults): 4–24 mEq/day.
IV (Children): 0.25–0.5 mEq/kg/day.

Availability (generic available)

Injection: 500 mg/mL (50%). **Premixed infusion:** 1 g/100 mL, 2 g/100 mL, 4 g/50 mL, 4 g/100 mL, 20 g/500 mL, 40 g/1000 mL.

NURSING IMPLICATIONS

Assessment

- **Hypomagnesemia/Anticonvulsant:** Monitor pulse, BP, respirations, and ECG frequently throughout administration of parenteral magnesium sulfate. Respirations should be at least 16/min before each dose.
- Monitor neurologic status before and throughout therapy. Institute seizure precautions. Patellar reflex (knee jerk) should be tested before each parenteral dose of magnesium sulfate. If response is absent, no additional doses should be administered until positive response is obtained.
- Monitor newborn for hypotension, hyporeflexia, and respiratory depression if mother has received magnesium sulfate.
- Monitor intake and output ratios. Urine output should be maintained at a level of at least 100 mL/4 hr.
- ***Lab Test Considerations:*** Monitor serum magnesium levels and renal function periodically throughout administration of parenteral magnesium sulfate.

Implementation

- ***High Alert:*** Accidental overdosage of IV magnesium has resulted in serious patient harm and death. Have second practitioner independently double-check original order, dose calculations, and infusion pump settings. Do not confuse milligram (mg), gram (g), or millequivalent (mEq) dosages.

- **IM:** Administer deep IM into gluteal sites. Administer subsequent injections in alternate sides. Dilute to a concentration of 200 mg/mL prior to injection.

IV Administration

- **IV Push:** ***Diluent:*** 50% solution must be diluted in 0.9% NaCl or D5W to a concentration of ≤20% prior to administration. ***Concentration:*** ≤20%. ***Rate:*** Administer at a rate not to exceed 150 mg/min.
- **Continuous Infusion:** ***Diluent:*** Dilute in D5W, 0.9% NaCl, or LR. ***Concentration:*** 0.5 mEq/mL (60 mg/mL) (may use maximum concentration of 1.6 mEq/mL) (200 mg/mL) in fluid-restricted patients. ***Rate:*** Infuse over 2–4 hr. Do not exceed a rate of 1 mEq/kg/hr (125 mg/kg/hr). When rapid infusions are needed (severe asthma or torsade de pointes) may infuse over 10–20 min.
- **Y-Site Compatibility:** acyclovir, aldesleukin, alemtuzumab, alfentanil, amifostine, amikacin, argatroban, ascorbic acid, atropine, azithromycin, aztreonam, benztropine, bivalirudin, bleomycin, bumetanide, buprenorphine, butorphanol, calcium gluconate, carboplatin, carmustine, caspofungin, cefotaxime, cefoxitin, ceftazidime, chloramphenicol, chlorpromazine, cisatracurium, cisplatin, clindamycin, clonidine, cyanocobalamin, cyclophosphamide, cytarabine, dactinomycin, daptomycin, dexmedetomidine, dexrazoxane, digoxin, diltiazem, diphenhydramine, dobutamine, docetaxel, dolasetron, dopamine, doxacurium, doxorubicin liposome, doxycycline, enalaprilat, ephedrine, epinephrine, epoetin alfa, eptifibatide, ertapenem, esmolol, etoposide, etoposide phosphate, famotidine, fenoldopam, fentanyl, fluconazole, fludarabine, fluorouracil, folic acid, foscarnet, gemcitabine, gentamicin, glycopyrrolate, granisetron, heparin, hetastarch, hydromorphone, idarubicin, ifosfamide, imipenem/cilastatin, insulin, irinotecan, isoproterenol, ketamine, ketorolac, labetalol, calcium, lidocaine, linezolid, lorazepam, mannitol, methotrexate, methyldopate, metoclopramide, metoprolol, metronidazole, micafungin, midazolam, milrinone, mitoxantrone, morphine, moxifloxacin, multivitamins, mycophenolate, nafcillin, nalbuphine, nicardipine, nitroglycerin, nitroprusside, norepinephrine, octreotide, ondansetron, oxaliplatin, oxytocin, paclitaxel, palonosetron, pamidronate, pancuronium, pantoprazole, papaverine, pemetrexed, penicillin G, pentobarbital, phenobarbital, phentolamine, phenylephrine, piperacillin/tazobactam, potassium acetate, potassium chloride, procainamide, prochlorperazine, promethazine, propranolol, propofol, propranolol, pyridoxime, quinupristin/dalfopristin, ranitidine, remifentanil, rituximab, rocuronium, sargramostim, sodium acetate, sodium bicarbonate, streptokinase, succinylcholine, sufentanil, tacrolimus, telavancin, theophylline, thiamine, thiotepa, tigecycline, tirofiban, tobramycin, tolazoline, trastuzumab, trimetaphan, vancomycin, vasopressin, vecuronium, verapamil, vinblastine, vincristine, vinorelbine, vitamin B complex with C, voriconazole, zoledronic acid.
- **Y-Site Incompatibility:** aminophylline, amphotericin B cholesteryl sulfate, amphotericin B lipid complex, amphotericin B liposome, anidulafungin, azathioprine, calcium chloride, cefepime, ceftriaxone, cefuroxime, ciprofloxacin, dantrolene, dexamethasone sodium phosphate, diazepam, diazoxide, doxorubicin hydrochloride, epirubicin, ganciclovir, haloperidol, indomethacin, methylprednisolone sodium succinate, pentamidine, phenytoin, phytonadione.

Patient/Family Teaching

- Explain purpose of medication to patient and family.

Evaluation/Desired Outcomes

- Normal serum magnesium concentrations.
- Control of seizures associated with toxemias of pregnancy.

BEERS

meclizine (mek-li-zeen)

Antivert, Bonine, Dramamine Less Drowsy

Classification

Therapeutic: antiemetics, antihistamines

Indications

Management/prevention of: Motion sickness, Vertigo associated with diseases of vestibular system.

Action

Has central anticholinergic, CNS depressant, and antihistaminic properties. Decreases excitability of the middle ear labyrinth and depresses conduction in middle ear vestibular-cerebellar pathways. **Therapeutic Effects:** Decreased motion sickness. Decreased vertigo from vestibular pathology.

Pharmacokinetics

Absorption: Absorbed after oral administration.
Distribution: Unknown.
Metabolism and Excretion: Unknown.
Half-life: 6 hr.

TIME/ACTION PROFILE (antihistaminic effects)

ROUTE	ONSET	PEAK	DURATION
PO	1 hr	unknown	8–24 hr

Contraindications/Precautions

Contraindicated in: Hypersensitivity; OB: Has caused congenital malformations (cleft palate) in animal studies.

Use Cautiously in: Prostatic hyperplasia; Angle-closure glaucoma; Lactation: Occasional use may be acceptable; prolonged use may expose infant to drug effects or may interfere with milk supply; Pedi: Children <12 yr (safety not established); Geri: ↑ sensitivity and risk of adverse reactions.

Adverse Reactions/Side Effects

CNS: drowsiness, fatigue. **EENT:** blurred vision. **GI:** dry mouth.

Interactions

Drug-Drug: Additive CNS depression with other **CNS depressants**, including **alcohol**, other **antihistamines**, **opioid analgesics**, and **sedative/hypnotics**. Additive anticholinergic effects with other **drugs possessing anticholinergic properties**, including some **antihistamines**, **antidepressants**, **atropine**, **haloperidol**, **phenothiazines**, **quinidine**, and **disopyramide**. **CYP2D6 inhibitors** may ↑ levels.

Route/Dosage

PO (Adults and Children ≥12 yr): *Motion sickness*—25–50 mg 1 hr before exposure; may repeat in 24 hr; *vertigo*—25–100 mg/day in divided doses.

Availability (generic available)

Chewable tablets (raspberry flavor): 25 mg^{OTC}. **Tablets:** 12.5 mg, 25 mg$^{Rx,\ OTC}$, 50 mg.

NURSING IMPLICATIONS

Assessment

- Assess patient for level of sedation after administration.
- **Motion Sickness:** Assess patient for nausea and vomiting before and 60 min after administration.
- **Vertigo:** Assess degree of vertigo periodically in patients receiving meclizine for labyrinthitis.
- ***Lab Test Considerations:*** May cause false-negative results in skin tests using allergen extracts. Discontinue meclizine 72 hr before testing.

Implementation

- Do not confuse Dramamine (meclizine) with Dramamine (dimenhydrinate).
- **PO:** Administer oral doses with food, water, or milk to minimize GI irritation.

Patient/Family Teaching

- Instruct patient to take meclizine exactly as directed. If a dose is missed, take as soon as possible unless almost time for next dose. Do not double doses.
- May cause drowsiness. Caution patient to avoid driving or other activities requiring alertness until response to the medication is known.
- Advise patient that frequent mouth rinses, good oral hygiene, and sugarless gum or candy may decrease dryness of mouth.
- Caution patient to avoid concurrent use of alcohol and other CNS depressants with this medication.
- Advise females of reproductive potential to notify health care professional if pregnancy is planned or suspected, or if breast feeding.
- **Motion Sickness:** When used as prophylaxis for motion sickness, advise patient to take medication at least 1 hr before exposure to conditions that may cause motion sickness.

Evaluation/Desired Outcomes

- Prevention and relief of symptoms in motion sickness.
- Prevention and treatment of vertigo due to vestibular pathology.

medroxyPROGESTERone†

(me-**drox**-ee-proe-**jess**-te-rone)

Depo-Provera, Depo-Sub Q Provera 104, Medroxy, Provera

Classification

Therapeutic: antineoplastics, contraceptive hormones

Pharmacologic: hormones, progestins

†For contraceptive use see Contraceptives, Hormonal monograph.

Indications

To decrease endometrial hyperplasia in postmenopausal women receiving concurrent estrogen (0.625 mg/day conjugated estrogens). Treatment of secondary amenorrhea and abnormal uterine bleeding caused by hormonal imbalance. **IM:** Treatment of advanced unresponsive endometrial or renal carcinoma. †Prevention of pregnancy. Management of endometriosis-associated pain (Depo-Sub Q Provera 104 only). **Unlabeled Use:** Obesity-hypoventilation (pickwickian) syndrome. Sleep apnea. Hypersomnolence.

Action

A synthetic form of progesterone—actions include secretory changes in the endometrium, increases in basal body temperature, histologic changes in vaginal epithelium, relaxation of uterine smooth muscle, mammary alveolar tissue growth, pituitary inhibition, and withdrawal bleeding in the presence of estrogen. **Therapeutic Effects:** Decreased endometrial hyperplasia in postmenopausal women receiving concurrent estrogen (combination with estrogen decreases vasomotor symptoms and prevents osteoporosis). Restoration of hormonal balance with control of uterine bleeding. Management of endometrial or renal cancer. Prevention of pregnancy.

Pharmacokinetics

Absorption: 0.6–10% absorbed after oral administration.

Distribution: Enters breast milk.

Metabolism and Excretion: Metabolized by the liver.

Half-life: *1st phase*—52 min; *2nd phase*—230 min; *biological*—14.5 hr.

TIME/ACTION PROFILE (IM = antineoplastic effects)

ROUTE	ONSET	PEAK	DURATION
PO	unknown	unknown	unknown
IM	wk–mos	mo	unknown†
SC	unknown	1 wk	3 mo

†Contraceptive effect lasts 3 mo.

Contraindications/Precautions

Contraindicated in: Hypersensitivity; Hypersensitivity to parabens (IM suspension only); Missed abortion; Thromboembolic disease; Cerebrovascular disease; Severe liver disease; Breast or genital cancer; Porphyria; OB: May ↑ risk of fetal genitourinary malformation.

Use Cautiously in: History of liver disease; Renal disease; Cardiovascular disease; Seizure disorders; Mental depression; Lactation: If used as a contraceptive, wait 6 wk after delivery if breast feeding.

Adverse Reactions/Side Effects

CNS: depression. **CV:** DEEP VEIN THROMBOSIS, thrombophlebitis. **Derm:** chloasma, melasma, rash. **EENT:** retinal thrombosis. **Endo:** amenorrhea, breakthrough bleeding, breast tenderness, changes in menstrual flow, galactorrhea, hyperglycemia, spotting. **F and E:** edema. **GI:** drug-induced hepatitis, gingival bleeding. **GU:** cervical erosions, dysmenorrhea. **Local:** injection site reactions. **Metab:** bone loss, ↓ weight, ↑ weight. **Resp:** PULMONARY EMBOLISM. **Misc:** BREAST CANCER, HYPERSENSITIVITY REACTIONS (including anaphylaxis or angioedema).

Interactions

Drug-Drug: Strong **CYP3A4 inhibitors**, including **ketoconazole**, **itraconazole**, **clarithromycin**, **atazanavir**, **indinavir**, **nefazodone**, **nelfinavir**, **ritonavir**, **saquinavir**, and **voriconazole** may ↑ levels; avoid concurrent use. Strong **CYP3A4 inducers**, including **phenytoin**, **carbamazepine**, **rifampin**, **rifabutin**, **rifapentin**, and **phenobarbital** may ↓ levels; avoid concurrent use. May ↓ effectiveness of **bromocriptine** when used concurrently for galactorrhea/amenorrhea. Contraceptive effectiveness may be ↓ by **carbamazepine**, **phenobarbital**, **phenytoin**, **rifampin**, or **rifabutin**.

Drug-Natural Products: St. John's wort may ↓ levels; avoid concurrent use.

Route/Dosage

Postmenopausal Women Receiving Concurrent Estrogen

PO (Adults): 2.5–5 mg daily concurrently with 0.625 mg conjugated estrogens (monophasic regimen) *or* 5 mg daily on days 15–28 of the cycle with 0.625 mg conjugated estrogens taken daily throughout cycle (biphasic regimen).

Secondary Amenorrhea

PO (Adults): 5–10 mg/day for 5–10 days; start at any time in cycle.

Dysfunctional Uterine Bleeding/Induction of Menses

PO (Adults): 5–10 mg/day for 5–10 days, starting on day 16 or day 21 of menstrual cycle.

Renal or Endometrial Carcinoma

IM (Adults): 400–1000 mg, may be repeated weekly; if improvement occurs, attempt to decrease dose to 400 mg monthly.

Endometriosis-Associated Pain

Subcut (Adults): 104 mg every 12–14 wk (3 mo), beginning on day 5 of normal menses (not recommended for more than 2 yr).

Availability (generic available)

Suspension for depot injection: 🍁50 mg/mL, 150 mg/mL, 400 mg/mL. **Suspension for subcutaneous injection (Depo-Sub Q Provera 104):** 104 mg/0.65 mL. **Tablets:** 2.5 mg, 5 mg, 10 mg, 🍁100 mg. ***In combination with:*** conjugated estrogens as Prempro (single combination tablet of 0.626 mg conjugated estrogens plus 2.5 or 5 mg medroxyprogesterone) or Premphase (0.625 mg conjugated estrogens tablet for 14 days followed by combination tablet of 0.625 mg conjugated estrogens plus 5 mg medroxyprogesterone for days 15–28) in convenience packages. See Appendix B.

NURSING IMPLICATIONS

Assessment

- Monitor BP periodically during therapy.
- Assess patient's usual menstrual history. Administration of drug may begin on any day of cycle in patients with amenorrhea and on day 16 or 21 of cycle in patients with dysfunctional bleeding.
- Monitor intake and output ratios and weekly weight. Report significant discrepancies or steady weight gain.
- ***Lab Test Considerations:*** Monitor hepatic function before and periodically during therapy.
- May cause ↑ alkaline phosphatase levels. May ↓ pregnanediol excretion concentrations.
- May cause ↑ serum LDL concentrations or ↓ HDL concentrations.
- May alter thyroid hormone assays.

Implementation

- Do not confuse Depo-Provera with Depo-subQ Provera 104. Do not confuse Provera (medroxyprogesterone) with Proscar (finasteride) or Prozac (fluoxetine). Do not confuse medroxyprogesterone with methylprednisolone, or methyltestosterone.

- Only the 150 mg/mL vial or prefilled syringe should be used for contraception.
- Injectable medroxyprogesterone may lead to bone loss, especially in women younger than 21 yr. Injectable medroxyprogesterone should be used for >2 yr only if other methods of contraception are inadequate. If used long term, women should use supplemental calcium and vitamin D, and monitor bone mineral density.
- **Subcut:** Shake vigorously before use to form a uniform suspension. Inject slowly (over 5–7 sec) at a 45° angle into fatty area of anterior thigh or abdomen every 12 to 14 wk. If more than 14 wk elapse between injections, rule out pregnancy prior to administration. **Do not rub area after injection**.
- When switching from other hormonal contraceptives, administer within dosing period (7 days after taking last active pill, removing patch or ring, or within the dosing period for IM injection).
- **IM:** Shake vial or prefilled syringe vigorously before preparing IM dose. Administer deep IM into gluteal or deltoid muscle. Rotate sites with each injection. If period between injections is >14 wk, determine that patient is not pregnant before administering the drug.
- In patients with cancer, IM dose may initially be required weekly. Once stabilized, IM dose may be required only monthly.

Patient/Family Teaching

- Explain the dose schedule. Instruct patient to take medication at the same time each day. Take missed doses as soon as remembered, but do not double doses.
- Advise patients receiving medroxyprogesterone for menstrual dysfunction to anticipate withdrawal bleeding 3–7 days after discontinuing medication.
- Review patient package insert (PPI) with patient. Emphasize the importance of notifying health care professional if the following side effects occur: visual changes, sudden weakness, incoordination, difficulty with speech, headache, leg or calf pain, shortness of breath, chest pain, changes in vaginal bleeding pattern, yellow skin, swelling of extremities, depression, or rash. Patients receiving medroxyprogesterone for cancer may not receive PPI.
- Advise patient to keep a 1-mo supply of medroxyprogesterone available at all times.
- Instruct patient in correct method of monthly breast self-examination. Increased breast tenderness may occur.
- Advise patient that gingival bleeding may occur. Instruct patient to use good oral hygiene and to receive regular dental care and examinations.
- Medroxyprogesterone may cause melasma (brown patches of discoloration) on face when patient is exposed to sunlight. Advise patient to avoid sun exposure and to wear sunscreen or protective clothing when outdoors.
- Rep: Instruct patient to notify health care professional if menstrual period is missed or if pregnancy is suspected. Patient should not attempt conception for 3 mo after discontinuing medication in order to decrease risk to fetus.
- Emphasize the importance of routine follow-up physical exams, including BP; breast, abdomen, and pelvic exams; and Papanicolaou smears every 6–12 mo.
- **IM Subcut:** Advise patient to maintain adequate amounts of dietary calcium and vitamin D to help prevent bone loss.

Evaluation/Desired Outcomes

- Regular menstrual periods.
- Decrease in endometrial hyperplasia in postmenopausal women receiving concurrent estrogen.
- Control of the spread of endometrial or renal cancer.
- Prevention of pregnancy.

medroxyprogesterone, See CONTRACEPTIVES, HORMONAL.

BEERS

megestrol (me-jess-trole)

~~Megace~~, Megace ES

Classification

Therapeutic: antineoplastics, hormones

Pharmacologic: progestins

Indications

Palliative treatment of endometrial and breast carcinoma, either alone or with surgery or radiation (tablets only). Treatment of anorexia, weight loss, and cachexia associated with AIDS (oral suspension only).

Action

Antineoplastic effect may result from inhibition of pituitary function. **Therapeutic Effects:** Regression of tumor. Increased appetite and weight gain in patients with AIDS.

Pharmacokinetics

Absorption: Well absorbed from the GI tract.

Distribution: Unknown.

Protein Binding: ≥90%.

Metabolism and Excretion: Completely metabolized by the liver.

Half-life: 38 hr (range 13–104 hr).

TIME/ACTION PROFILE (antineoplastic activity)

ROUTE	ONSET	PEAK	DURATION
PO	wk–mos	2 mo	unknown

Contraindications/Precautions

Contraindicated in: Hypersensitivity; Undiagnosed vaginal bleeding; Severe liver disease; Suspension contains alcohol and should be avoided in patients with known intolerance; OB: Pregnancy (may cause fetal harm); Lactation: Lacation (may cause harm to infant).
Use Cautiously in: Diabetes; Mental depression; Renal disease; History of thrombophlebitis; Cardiovascular disease; Seizures; Rep: Women of reproductive potential; Pedi: Safety and effectiveness not established.

Adverse Reactions/Side Effects

CV: THROMBOEMBOLISM, edema. **Derm:** alopecia. **Endo:** asymptomatic adrenal suppression (chronic therapy). **GI:** GI irritation. **GU:** vaginal bleeding. **Hemat:** thrombophlebitis. **MS:** carpal tunnel syndrome.

Interactions

Drug-Drug: May ↑ INR and risk of bleeding when used with **warfarin**.

Route/Dosage

PO (Adults): *Breast carcinoma*—160 mg/day as a single dose or divided doses; *Endometrial/ovarian carcinoma*—40–320 mg/day in divided doses; *Anorexia associated with AIDS*—Megace: 800 mg once daily; may ↓ to 400 mg/day after 1 mo (range 400–800 mg/day); Megace ES: 625 mg once daily.

Availability (generic available)

Oral suspension (lemon-lime flavor): 40 mg/mL, 125 mg/mL (Megace ES). **Tablets:** 20 mg, 40 mg, ✱ 160 mg.

NURSING IMPLICATIONS

Assessment

- Assess for swelling, pain, or tenderness in legs. Report these signs of deep vein thrombophlebitis.
- **Anorexia:** Monitor weight, appetite, and nutritional intake in patients with AIDS.
- ***Lab Test Considerations:*** Obtain a negative pregnancy test prior to starting therapy.

Implementation

- Because of high dose, suspension is most convenient form for patients with AIDS.
- Do not confuse *Megace* 40 mg/mL with *Megace ES* 125 mg/mL.
- **PO:** May be administered with meals if GI irritation becomes a problem.
- Shake suspension well before administering.

Patient/Family Teaching

- Instruct patient to take megestrol as directed; do not skip or double up on missed doses. Missed doses may be taken as long as not right before next dose. Gradually decrease dose prior to discontinuation.
- Advise patient to report to health care professional any unusual vaginal bleeding or signs of deep vein thrombophlebitis.
- Discuss with patient the possibility of hair loss. Explore methods of coping.
- Rep: Advise patient that this medication may have teratogenic effects. Advise females of reproductive potential to use effective contraception during and for at least 4 mo after therapy is completed. Advise patient to notify health care professional immediately if pregnancy is planned or suspected, and to avoid breast feeding.

Evaluation/Desired Outcomes

- Slowing or arresting the spread of endometrial or breast malignancy. Therapeutic effects usually occur within 2 mo of initiating therapy.
- Increased appetite and weight gain in patients with AIDS.

M

BEERS

meloxicam (me-lox-i-kam)

Mobic, Qmiiz ODT, Vivlodex

Classification
Therapeutic: nonsteroidal anti-inflammatory agents
Pharmacologic: nonopioid analgesics

Indications

Relief of signs and symptoms of osteoarthritis and rheumatoid arthritis (including juvenile rheumatoid arthritis).

Action

Inhibits prostaglandin synthesis, probably by inhibiting the enzyme cyclooxygenase. **Therapeutic Effects:** Decreased pain and inflammation associated with osteoarthritis. Also decreases fever.

Pharmacokinetics

Absorption: Well absorbed following oral administration.
Distribution: Unknown.
Protein Binding: 99.4%.
Metabolism and Excretion: Mostly metabolized to inactive metabolites by the liver via the P450 enzyme system; metabolites are excreted in urine and feces.
Half-life: 20.1 hr.

TIME/ACTION PROFILE

ROUTE	ONSET	PEAK†	DURATION
PO	unknown	5–6 hr	24 hr

†Blood levels.

Contraindications/Precautions

Contraindicated in: Hypersensitivity; Cross-sensitivity may occur with other NSAIDs, including aspirin; Severe renal impairment (CCr ≤15 mL/min); Concurrent use of aspirin (↑ risk of adverse reactions); Coronary artery bypass graft (CABG) surgery; OB: Can cause premature closure of ductus arteriosus if used during third trimester; Phenylketonuria (orally disintegrating tablets [ODTs] only).

Use Cautiously in: Cardiovascular disease or risk factors for cardiovascular disease (may ↑ risk of serious cardiovascular thrombotic events, myocardial infarction, and stroke, especially with prolonged use or use of higher doses); avoid use in patients with recent MI or HF; Dehydration (correct deficits before initiating therapy); Impaired renal function, heart failure, liver dysfunction, concurrent ACE inhibitor or diuretic therapy (↑ risk of renal dysfunction); Coagulation disorders or concurrent anticoagulant therapy (may ↑ risk of bleeding); Lactation: Safety not established; Pedi: Children <2 yr or <60 kg (safety and effectiveness of tablets and ODTs not established); safety and effectiveness of capsules not established in children; Geri: ↑ risk of GI bleeding and renal dysfuntion.

Adverse Reactions/Side Effects

CV: HF, MYOCARDIAL INFARCTION, STROKE, edema, hypertension. **Derm:** EXFOLIATIVE DERMATITIS, STEVENS-JOHNSON SYNDROME, TOXIC EPIDERMAL NECROLYSIS, pruritus. **F and E:** hyperkalemia. **GI:** GI BLEEDING, ↑ liver enzymes, diarrhea, dyspepsia, nausea. **GU:** delayed ovulation. **Hemat:** anemia, leukopenia, thrombocytopenia.

Interactions

Drug-Drug: May ↓ antihypertensive effects of **ACE inhibitors**. May ↓ diuretic effects of **furosemide** or **thiazide diuretics**. Concurrent use with **aspirin** ↑ meloxicam blood levels and may ↑ risk of adverse reactions. Concurrent use with **cholestyramine** ↓ blood levels. ↑ plasma **lithium** levels (close monitoring recommended when meloxicam is introduced or withdrawn). ↑ risk of bleeding with **anticoagulants**, **aspirin**, **clopidogrel**, **ticagrelor**, **prasugrel**, **corticosteroids**, **fibrinolytics**, **SNRIs**, or **SSRIs**. Concurrent use with **sodium polystyrene sulfonate** may ↑ risk of colonic necrosis; concurrent use should be avoided.

Route/Dosage

ODTs are NOT interchangeable with the tablets or capsules.

PO (Adults): *Capsules*—5 mg once daily; may ↑ to 10 mg once daily, if needed; *Tablets and ODTs*—7.5 mg once daily; may ↑ to 15 mg once daily, if needed.

PO (Children 2–17 yr and ≥60 kg): *Tablets and orally disintegrating tablets (ODTs)*—7.5 mg once daily.

Availability (generic available)

Capsules: 5 mg, 10 mg. **Orally disintegrating tablets (contain phenylalanine):** 7.5 mg, 15 mg. **Tablets:** 7.5 mg, 15 mg. **Cost:** *Generic*—7.5 mg $9.02/100, 15 mg $7.41/100.

NURSING IMPLICATIONS

Assessment

- Patients who have asthma, aspirin-induced allergy, and nasal polyps are at increased risk for developing hypersensitivity reactions. Assess for rhinitis, asthma, and urticaria.
- Assess pain and range of motion prior to and 1–2 hr following administration.
- Assess for rash periodically during therapy. May cause Stevens-Johnson syndrome or toxic epidermal necrolysis. Discontinue therapy if severe or if accompanied with fever, general malaise, fatigue, muscle or joint aches, blisters, oral lesions, conjunctivitis, hepatitis, and/or eosinophilia.
- Monitor BP during initiation and periodically during therapy. May cause fluid retention and edema leading to new onset or worsening hypertension.
- ***Lab Test Considerations:*** Evaluate BUN, serum creatinine, CBC, and liver function periodically in patients receiving prolonged therapy. May cause anemia, thrombocytopenia, leukopenia, and abnormal liver or renal function tests.
- Bleeding time may be prolonged.

Implementation

- Administration in higher than recommended doses does not provide increased effectiveness but may cause increased side effects. Use lowest effective dose for shortest period of time to minimize risk of cardiovascular thrombotic events.
- **PO:** May be administered without regard to food.
- Orally disintegrating tablets can be taken without regard to food or water. With dry hands, open carton and peel back foil on the blister. Do not push tablet through foil as this could damage the tablet. Gently remove tablet from blister and place it in mouth, or onto the tongue, immediately after removing from blister. Tablet disintegrates quickly in saliva and can be swallowed with or without drinking liquid.

Patient/Family Teaching

- Advise patient to take this medication with a full glass of water and to remain in an upright position for 15–30 min after administration.
- Instruct patient to take medication as directed. Take missed doses as soon as remembered but not if almost time for the next dose. Do not double doses. Instruct parent/caregiver to read the *Medication Guide* prior to use and with each Rx refill in case of changes.
- Caution patient to avoid the concurrent use of alcohol, aspirin, acetaminophen, or other OTC medications without consulting health care professional.

- Inform patient that meloxicam may increase the risk for heart attack and stroke; risk increases with longer use or in patients with heart disease.
- Advise patient to inform health care professional of medication regimen prior to treatment or surgery, especially right before or after coronary artery bypass graft (CABG).
- Advise patient to consult health care professional if rash, itching, visual disturbances, weight gain, edema, black stools, or signs of hepatotoxicity (nausea, fatigue, lethargy, jaundice, upper right quadrant tenderness, flu-like symptoms) occur.
- Rep: Advise females of reproductive potential to notify health care professional if pregnancy is planned or suspected and to avoid meloxicam starting at 30 wk gestation because of risk of premature closing of the fetal ductus arteriosus. May cause infertility in men and temporary infertility in women.

Evaluation/Desired Outcomes

- Relief of pain.
- Improved joint mobility. Patients who do not respond to one NSAID may respond to another.

melphalan (mel-fa-lan)

Alkeran, Evomela

Classification
Therapeutic: antineoplastics
Pharmacologic: alkylating agents

Indications

IV: High-dose conditioning treatment prior to hematopoietic stem cell transplantation (Evomela only). **IV and PO:** Palliative treatment of multiple myeloma when oral therapy is not appropriate (Alkeran and Evomela). **PO:** Palliative treatment of nonresectable epithelial ovarian carcinoma (Alkeran).

Action

Inhibits DNA and RNA synthesis by alkylation (cell-cycle phase–nonspecific). **Therapeutic Effects:** Death of rapidly replicating cells, particularly malignant ones. Also has immunosuppressive properties.

Pharmacokinetics

Absorption: Incompletely and variably absorbed following oral administration. IV administration results in complete bioavailability.
Distribution: Rapidly distributed throughout total body water.
Protein Binding: ≤30%.
Metabolism and Excretion: Rapidly metabolized in the bloodstream. Small amounts (10%) excreted unchanged by the kidneys.
Half-life: 1.5 hr.

TIME/ACTION PROFILE (effects on blood counts)

ROUTE	ONSET	PEAK	DURATION
IV	unknown	2–3 wk	4–5 wk
PO	5 days	2–3 wk	5–6 wk

Contraindications/Precautions

Contraindicated in: Hypersensitivity to melphalan; OB, Lactation: Pregnancy or lactation.
Use Cautiously in: Active infections; ↓ bone marrow reserve; Renal impairment (dose ↓ recommended for IV for palliative treatment only if BUN ≥30 mg/dL; dose ↓ may be needed when using PO therapy); Rep: Women of reproductive potential and men with female sexual partners of reproductive potential; Pedi: Safety and effectiveness not established; Geri: Begin at lower end of dosing range due to potential for age-related ↓ in renal, hepatic, or cardiac function.

Adverse Reactions/Side Effects

CNS: dizziness. **CV:** peripheral edema. **Derm:** alopecia, pruritus, rash. **Endo:** menstrual irregularities. **F and E:** hypokalemia, hypophosphatemia. **GI:** constipation, diarrhea, mucositis, nausea, vomiting, hepatotoxicity. **GU:** infertility. **Hemat:** leukopenia, thrombocytopenia, anemia. **Metab:** hyperuricemia. **Misc:** HYPERSENSITIVITY REACTIONS (including anaphylaxis) (more common with IV), MALIGNANCY, fever.

Interactions

Drug-Drug: ↑ bone marrow depression with other **antineoplastics** or **radiation therapy**. May ↓ antibody response to **live-virus vaccines** and ↑ risk of adverse reactions. Concurrent IV use with **cyclosporine** may ↑ risk of renal failure.

Route/Dosage

Multiple Myeloma (Palliative Treatment)

PO (Adults): 6 mg once daily for 2–3 wk followed by up to 4 wk rest, then 2 mg once daily *or* 10 mg once daily for 7–10 days, then 2 mg once daily once WBC >4000/mm³ and platelets >100,000/mm³ *or* 0.15 mg/kg/day for 7 days, followed by 2–6 wk rest, then 0.05 mg/kg/day maintenance dose *or* 0.25 mg/kg/day for 4 days every 4–6 wk *or* 0.2 mg/kg/day for 5 days every 4–6 wk.
IV (Adults): 16 mg/m² every 2 wk for 4 doses, then every 4 wk.

Renal Impairment

IV (Adults): *BUN ≥30 mg/dL*—↓ dose by up to 50%.

Multiple Myeloma (Conditioning Treatment)

IV (Adults): 100 mg/m²/day on Day 3 and Day 2 prior to autologous stem cell transplantation on Day 0.

Ovarian Carcinoma

PO (Adults): 0.2 mg/kg/day for 5 days every 4–5 wk.

Availability (generic available)

Tablets: 2 mg. **Powder for injection (requires reconstitution and dilution):** 50 mg/vial.

NURSING IMPLICATIONS

Assessment

- Assess for signs of infection (fever, chills, sore throat, cough, hoarseness, lower back or side pain, difficult or painful urination). Notify health care professional if these symptoms occur.
- Assess for bleeding (bleeding gums, bruising, petechiae, guaiac stools, urine, and emesis). Avoid IM injections and taking rectal temperatures. Apply pressure to venipuncture sites for 10 min.
- May cause nausea and vomiting. Monitor intake and output, appetite, and nutritional intake. Prophylactic antiemetics may be used. Adjust diet as tolerated.
- Monitor for symptoms of gout (increased uric acid, joint pain, edema). Encourage patient to drink at least 2 L of fluid per day. Allopurinol may be given to decrease uric acid levels.
- Anemia may occur. Monitor for increased fatigue and dyspnea.
- Assess patient for allergy to chlorambucil. Patients may have cross-sensitivity.
- ***Lab Test Considerations:*** Monitor CBC and differential weekly during therapy. The nadir of leukopenia occurs in 2–3 wk. Notify physician if leukocyte count is <3000/mm³. The nadir of thrombocytopenia occurs in 2–3 wk. Notify physician if platelet count is <100,000/mm³. Recovery of leukopenia and thrombocytopenia occurs in 5–6 wk.
- Monitor liver function studies (AST, ALT, LDH, bilirubin) and renal function studies (BUN, creatinine) prior to and periodically during therapy to detect hepatotoxicity and nephrotoxicity.
- May cause ↑ uric acid. Monitor periodically during therapy.
- May cause ↑ 5-hydroxyindoleacetic acid (5-HIAA) concentrations as a result of tumor breakdown.

Implementation

- Do not confuse Alkeran (melphalan) with Leukeran (chlorambucil) or Myleran (busulfan).
- **PO:** May be ordered in divided doses or as a single daily dose.

IV Administration

- Solution should be prepared in a biologic cabinet. Wear gloves, gown, and mask while handling medication. Discard IV equipment in specially designated container.
- If solution contacts skin or mucosa, immediately wash skin or mucosa with soap and water.
- **Alkeran Intermittent Infusion:** Reconstitute with 10 mL of diluent supplied for a concentration of 5 mg/mL and shake vigorously until solution is clear. ***Diluent:*** Dilute dose immediately with 0.9% NaCl. ***Concentration:*** Not to exceed 0.45 mg/mL. Administer within 60 min of reconstitution. Store at room temperature and protect from light; do not refrigerate reconstituted solution. ***Rate:*** Administer over 15–30 min. Keep time between reconstitution/dilution and administration of *Alkeran* to a minimum; reconstituted and diluted solutions are unstable.
- **Evomela Intermittent Infusion:** Reconstitute with 8.6 mL 0.9% NaCl for 5 mg/mL solution. Reconstituted solution is stable for 1 hr at room temperature and 24 hr if refrigerated. Solution is clear and colorless to light yellow; do not administer solutions that are discolored or contain particulate matter. ***Diluent:*** Dilute further in 0.9% NaCl. ***Concentration:*** 0.45 mg/mL. Diluted solution is stable for an additional 4 hrs at room temperature. ***Rate:*** Infuse over 30 min via injection port or central venous catheter; may cause local tissue damage if extravasation occurs. Do not administer IV push into a peripheral vein. Administer *Evomela* by injecting slowly into a fast-running IV infusion via a central venous access line.
- **Y-Site Compatibility:** acyclovir, alemtuzumab, amikacin, aminophylline, amphotericin B lipid complex, ampicillin, anidulafungin, argatroban, aztreonam, bivalirudin, bleomycin, bumetanide, buprenorphine, butorphanol, calcium gluconate, carboplatin, carmustine, caspofungin, cefazolin, cefepime, cefotaxime, ceftazidime, ceftriaxone, cefuroxime, cisplatin, clindamycin, cyclophosphamide, cytarabine, dacarbazine, dactinomycin, daunorubicin, dexamethasone, dexrazoxane, diltiazem, diphenhydramine, doxorubicin, doxycycline, droperidol, enalaprilat, ertapenem, etoposide, famotidine, filgrastim, floxuridine, fluconazole, fludarabine, fluorouracil, furosemide, ganciclovir, gentamicin, granisetron, haloperidol, heparin, hetastarch, hydrocortisone, hydromorphone, idarubicin, ifosfamide, imipenem/cilastatin, linezolid, lorazepam, mannitol, meperidine, mesna, methotrexate, methylprednisolone, metoclopramide, metronidazole, milrinone, mitomycin, mitoxantrone, morphine, moxifloxacin, nalbuphine, octreotide, ondansetron, palonosetron, pamidronate, pancuronium, pentostatin, piperacillin/tazobactam, potassium acetate, potassium chloride, prochlorperazine, promethazine, ranitidine, sodium bicarbonate, streptozocin, thiotepa, tigecycline, tirofiban, tobramycin, trimethoprim/sulfamethoxazole, vancomycin, vasopressin, vecuronium, vinblastine, vincristine, vinorelbine, voriconazole, zidovudine, zoledronic acid.
- **Y-Site Incompatibility:** amiodarone, chlorpromazine, pantoprazole.

Patient/Family Teaching

- Instruct patient to take melphalan as directed, even if nausea and vomiting occur. If vomiting occurs shortly after dose is taken, consult health care professional. If a dose is missed, do not take at all. Advise patient to read *Patient Information* before starting therapy and with each Rx refill in case of changes.

- Advise patient to notify health care professional if fever; chills; dyspnea; persistent cough; sore throat; signs of infection; bleeding gums; bruising; petechiae; or blood in urine, stool, or emesis occurs. Caution patient to avoid crowds and persons with known infections. Instruct patient to use soft toothbrush and electric razor. Caution patient not to drink alcoholic beverages or take products containing aspirin or other NSAIDs.
- Instruct patient to notify health care professional if skin rash, vasculitis, bleeding, fever, persistent cough, nausea, vomiting, amenorrhea, weight loss, or unusual lumps/masses occur.
- Instruct patient to inspect oral mucosa for redness and ulceration. If ulceration occurs, advise patient to use sponge brush and to rinse mouth with water after eating and drinking. Consult health care professional if pain interferes with eating. Stomatitis pain may require treatment with opioid analgesics.
- Advise patient to notify health care professional immediately if signs and symptoms of allergic reactions (skin reactions, including welts, rash, itching, and redness; fast heartbeat; shortness of breath or trouble breathing; feel lightheaded or dizzy; blurry vision; swelling of face, tongue, or throat) occurs.
- Instruct patient not to receive any vaccinations without advice of health care professional.
- Inform patient that melphalan may cause new cancers.
- Rep: May be teratogenic. Advise females of reproductive potential to use effective contraception and avoid breast feeding during and after therapy. Advise males with a female partner of reproductive potential to use effective contraception during and after therapy. May cause female and male infertility.
- Emphasize need for periodic lab tests to monitor for side effects.

Evaluation/Desired Outcomes

- Decrease in size and spread of malignant tissue.

memantine (me-man-teen)

Ebixa, Namenda, Namenda XR

Classification

Therapeutic: anti-Alzheimer's agents

Pharmacologic: N-methyl-D-aspartate antagonist

Indications

Moderate to severe dementia/neurocognitive disorder associated with Alzheimer's disease.

Action

Binds to CNS N-methyl-D-aspartate (NMDA) receptor sites, preventing binding of glutamate, an excitatory neurotransmitter. **Therapeutic Effects:** Decreased symptoms of dementia/cognitive decline. Does not slow progression. Cognitive enhancement. Does not cure disease.

Pharmacokinetics

Absorption: Well absorbed after oral administration.

Distribution: Unknown.

Metabolism and Excretion: 57–82% excreted unchanged in urine by active tubular secretion moderated by pH dependent tubular reabsorption. Remainder metabolized; metabolites are not pharmacologically active.

Half-life: 60–80 hr.

TIME/ACTION PROFILE (blood levels)

ROUTE	ONSET	PEAK	DURATION
PO	unknown	3–7 hr	12 hr
PO-ER	unknown	9–12 hr	24 hr

Contraindications/Precautions

Contraindicated in: Hypersensitivity.

Use Cautiously in: Severe renal impairment (↓ dose); Severe hepatic impairment; Concurrent use of other NMDA antagonists (amantadine, rimantadine, ketamine, dextromethorphan); Concurrent use of drugs or diets that cause alkaline urine; Conditions that ↑ urine pH including severe urinary tract infections or renal tubular acidosis (lead to ↓ excretion and ↑ levels); OB, Lactation: Safety not established; Pedi: Safety and effectiveness not established.

Adverse Reactions/Side Effects

CNS: dizziness, fatigue, headache, sedation. **CV:** hypertension. **Derm:** rash. **GI:** diarrhea, weight gain. **GU:** urinary frequency. **Hemat:** anemia.

Interactions

Drug-Drug: Medications that ↑ urine pH (e.g. **carbonic anhydrase inhibitors, sodium bicarbonate**) may ↓ excretion and ↑ blood levels.

Route/Dosage

PO (Adults): *Immediate-release*—5 mg once daily initially, ↑ at weekly intervals to 10 mg/day (5 mg twice daily), then 15 mg/day (5 mg once daily, 10 mg once daily as separate doses), then to target dose of 20 mg/day (10 mg twice daily); *Extended-release*—7 mg once daily, ↑ at weekly intervals by 7 mg/day to target dose of 28 mg once daily.

Renal Impairment
(Adults): *CCr 5–29 mL/min*—Immediate-release (solution): Target dose is 10 mg/day (5 mg twice daily); Extended-release: Target dose is 14 mg once daily.

Availability (generic available)
Extended-release capsules: 7 mg, 14 mg, 21 mg, 28 mg. **Cost:** 7 mg $302.62/30, 14 mg $907.85/90, 21 mg $302.62/30, 28 mg $907.85/90. **Immediate-release tablets:** 5 mg, 10 mg. **Cost:** 5 mg $887.69/180. **Oral solution, sugar-free, alcohol-free (peppermint):** 2 mg/mL. **Cost:** $668.50/360 mL. ***In combination with:*** donepezil (Namzaric). See Appendix B.

NURSING IMPLICATIONS

Assessment
- Assess cognitive function (memory, attention, reasoning, language, ability to perform simple tasks) periodically during therapy.
- ***Lab Test Considerations:*** May cause anemia.

Implementation
- Do not confuse memantine with methadone.
- Dose increases should occur no more frequently than weekly.
- To switch from *Namenda* to *Namenda XR*, patients taking 10 mg twice daily of *Namenda* tablets may be switched to *Namenda XR* 28 mg once daily capsules the day following the last dose of a 10 mg *Namenda* tablet. Patients with renal impairment may use the same procedure to switch from *Namenda* 5 mg twice daily to *Namenda XR* 14 mg once daily.
- **PO:** May be administered without regard to food.
- Administer oral solution using syringe provided. Do not dilute or mix with other fluids.
- Swallow extended release capsules whole; do not crush, chew, or divide. Capsules may be opened, sprinkled on applesauce, and swallowed. Entire contents of each capsule should be consumed; do not divide dose.

Patient/Family Teaching
- Instruct patient and caregiver on how and when to administer memantine and how to titrate dose. Take missed doses as soon as remembered but not just before next dose; do not double doses. If several days doses are missed, may need to resume at a lower dose and re-titrate up to previous dose; consult health care professional. Advise patient and caregiver to read *Patient Instructions* before starting and with each Rx refill in case of changes.
- Caution patient and caregiver that memantine may cause dizziness. Monitor and assist with ambulation and caution patient to avoid driving and other activities requiring alertness until response to medication is known.
- Advise patient and caregiver to notify health care professional of all Rx or OTC medications, vitamins, or herbal products being taken and to consult with health care professional before taking other medications.
- Teach patient and caregivers that improvement in cognitive functioning may take months; degenerative process is not reversed.
- Advise females of reproductive potential to notify health care professional if pregnancy is planned or suspected, or if breast feeding.

Evaluation/Desired Outcomes
- Improvement in neurocognitive decline (memory, attention, reasoning, language, ability to perform simple tasks) in patients with Alzheimer's disease.

BEERS REMS HIGH ALERT

meperidine (me-**per**-i-deen)
Demerol

Classification
Therapeutic: opioid analgesics
Pharmacologic: opioid agonists

Schedule II

Indications
Moderate or severe pain (alone or with nonopioid agents). Anesthesia adjunct. Analgesic during labor. Preoperative sedation. **Unlabeled Use:** Rigors.

Action
Binds to opiate receptors in the CNS. Alters the perception of and response to painful stimuli, while producing generalized CNS depression. **Therapeutic Effects:** Decrease in severity of pain.

Pharmacokinetics
Absorption: 50% from the GI tract; well absorbed from IM sites. Oral doses are about half as effective as parenteral doses.
Distribution: Widely distributed. Crosses the placenta; enters breast milk.
Protein Binding: Neonates: 52%; Infants 3–18 mo: 85%; Adults: 60–80%.
Metabolism and Excretion: Mostly metabolized by the liver; some converted to normeperidine, which may accumulate and cause seizures. 5% excreted unchanged by the kidneys.
Half-life: Neonates: 12–39 hr; Infants 3–18 mo: 2.3 hr; Children 5–8 yr: 3 hr; Adults: 2.5–4 hr (↑ in impaired renal or hepatic function [7–11 hr]).

TIME/ACTION PROFILE (analgesia)

ROUTE	ONSET	PEAK	DURATION
PO	15 min	60 min	2–4 hr
IM	10–15 min	30–50 min	2–4 hr
Subcut	10–15 min	40–60 min	2–4 hr
IV	immediate	5–7 min	2–3 hr

Contraindications/Precautions
Contraindicated in: Hypersensitivity; Hypersensitivity to bisulfites (some injectable products); Recent

(within 14 days) MAO inhibitor therapy; Severe respiratory insufficiency; OB: Labor and delivery; Lactation: Excreted in breast milk and can cause respiratory depression in the infant.

Use Cautiously in: Head trauma; ↑ intracranial pressure; Severe renal or hepatic impairment; Acute asthma attack, COPD, hypoxia, or hypercapnea; Hypothyroidism; Adrenal insufficiency; Alcoholism; Debilitated patients (dose ↓ suggested); Undiagnosed abdominal pain or prostatic hyperplasia; Patients with renal impairment, or extensive burns; High-dose or prolonged therapy (>600 mg/day or >2 days; ↑ risk of CNS stimulation and seizures due to accumulation of normeperidine); Sickle cell anemia (may require ↓ initial doses); OB: Avoid chronic use during pregnancy as can result in neonatal opioid withdrawal syndrome; Pedi: Syrup contains benzyl alcohol, which can cause "gasping syndrome" in neonates. Children have ↑ risk of seizures due to accumulation of normeperidine; Geri: Appears on Beers list; morphine recommended.

Adverse Reactions/Side Effects

CNS: SEIZURES, confusion, sedation, dysphoria, euphoria, floating feeling, hallucinations, headache, unusual dreams. **CV:** hypotension, bradycardia. **Derm:** flushing, sweating. **EENT:** blurred vision, diplopia, miosis. **Endo:** adrenal insufficiency. **GI:** constipation, nausea, vomiting. **GU:** urinary retention. **Resp:** respiratory depression. **Misc:** HYPERSENSITIVITY REACTIONS (including anaphylaxis), physical dependence, psychological dependence, tolerance.

Interactions

Drug-Drug: Do not use in patients receiving **MAO inhibitors** or **procarbazine** (may cause fatal reaction—contraindicated within 14 days of MAO inhibitor therapy). Use with **benzodiazepines** or other **CNS depressants** including other **opioids**, **non-benzodiazepine sedative/hypnotics**, **anxiolytics**, **general anesthetics**, **muscle relaxants**, **antipsychotics**, and **alcohol** may cause profound sedation, respiratory depression, coma, and death; reserve concurrent use for when alternative treatment options are inadequate. Administration of **agonist/antagonist opioid analgesics** may precipitate opioid withdrawal in physically dependent patients. Concurrent use of **CYP3A4 inhibitors** including **ritonavir**, **ketoconazole**, **itraconazole**, **fluconazole**, **clarithromycin**, **erythromycin**, **nefazodone**, **diltiazem**, **verapamil**, **nelfinavir**, and **fosamprenavir** ↑ levels and risk of opioid toxicity; careful monitoring during initiation, dose changes, or discontinuation of the inhibitor is recommended. Concurrent use with **CYP3A4 inducers** including **barbiturates**, **carbamazepine**, **efavirenz**, **corticosteroids**, **modafinil**, **nevirapine**, **oxcarbazepine**, **phenobarbital**, **phenytoin**, **rifabutin**, or **rifampin** may ↓ levels and analgesia; if inducers are discontinued or dosage ↓, patients should be monitored for signs of opioid toxicity and necessary dose adjustments should be made. **Nalbuphine** may ↓ analgesia. **Protease inhibitors** may ↑ effects and adverse reactions (concurrent use should be avoided). **Phenytoin** ↑ metabolism and may ↓ effects. **Chlorpromazine** and **thioridazine** may ↑ the risk of adverse reactions (concurrent use should be avoided). May aggravate side effects of **isoniazid**. **Acyclovir** may ↑ plasma concentrations of meperidine and normeperidine. Drugs that affect serotonergic neurotransmitter systems, including **tricyclic antidepressants**, **SSRIs**, **SNRIs**, **MAO inhibitors**, **TCAs**, **tramadol**, **trazodone**, **mirtazapine**, **5-HT$_3$ receptor antagonists**, **linezolid**, **methylene blue**, and **triptans** ↑ risk of serotonin syndrome.

Drug-Natural Products: Concomitant use of **kava-kava**, **valerian**, or **chamomile** can ↓ CNS depression. **St. John's wort** may ↑ serious side effects, concurrent use is not recommended.

Route/Dosage

PO, IM, Subcut (Adults): *Analgesia*—50 mg every 3–4 hr; may be ↑ as needed (not to exceed 600 mg/24 hr). *Analgesia during labor*—50–100 mg IM or subcut when contractions become regular; may repeat every 1–3 hr. *Preoperative sedation*—50–100 mg IM or subcut 30–90 min before anesthesia.

PO, IM, Subcut (Children): *Analgesia*—1–1.5 mg/kg every 3–4 hr (should not exceed 100 mg/dose). *Preoperative sedation*—1–2 mg/kg 30–90 min before anesthesia (not to exceed adult dose).

IV (Adults): 15–35 mg/hr as a continuous infusion; *PCA*—10 mg initially; with a range of 1–5 mg/incremental dose, recommended lockout interval is 6–10 min (minimum 5 min).

IV (Children): *Continuous infusion*—0.5–1 mg/kg loading dose followed by 0.3 mg/kg/hr, titrate to effect up to 0.5–0.7 mg/kg/hr.

Availability (generic available)

Oral solution (banana flavor): 50 mg/5 mL. **Solution for injection (requires dilution):** 10 mg/mL, 25 mg/mL, 50 mg/mL, 75 mg/mL, 100 mg/mL. **Tablets:** 50 mg, 100 mg.

NURSING IMPLICATIONS

Assessment

- Assess type, location, and intensity of pain prior to and 1 hr following PO, subcut, and IM doses and 5 min (peak) following IV administration. When titrating opioid doses, increases of 25–50% should be administered until there is either a 50% reduction in the patient's pain rating on a numerical or visual analogue scale or the patient reports satisfactory pain relief. A repeat dose can be safely administered at the time of the peak if previous dose is ineffective and side effects are minimal.

M

- An equianalgesic chart (see Appendix J) should be used when changing routes or when changing from one opioid to another.
- Assess BP, pulse, and respirations before and periodically during administration. If respiratory rate is <10/min, assess level of sedation. Dose may need to be decreased by 25–50%. Initial drowsiness will diminish with continued use.
- Assess bowel function routinely. Prevention of constipation should be instituted with increased intake of fluids and bulk and with laxatives to minimize constipating effects. Stimulant laxatives should be administered routinely if opioid use exceeds 2–3 days, unless contraindicated. Consider drugs for opioid induced constipation.
- Prolonged use may lead to physical and psychological dependence and tolerance. This should not prevent patient from receiving adequate analgesia. Patients who receive meperidine for pain rarely develop psychological dependence. Progressively higher doses may be required to relieve pain with long-term therapy.
- Monitor patients on chronic or high-dose therapy for CNS stimulation (restlessness, irritability, seizures) due to accumulation of normeperidine metabolite. Risk of toxicity increases with doses >600 mg/24 hr, chronic administration (>2 days), and renal impairment.
- Assess risk for opioid addiction, abuse, or misuse prior to administration.
- Geri: Meperidine has been reported to cause delirium in the elderly; older adults are at increased risk for normeperidine toxicity. Monitor frequently.
- Pedi: Assess pediatric patient frequently; neonates, infants, and children are more sensitive to the effects of opioid analgesics and may experience respiratory complications, excitability, and restlessness more frequently.
- ***Lab Test Considerations:*** May ↑ plasma amylase and lipase concentrations.
- ***Toxicity and Overdose:*** If an opioid antagonist is required to reverse respiratory depression or coma, naloxone (Narcan) is the antidote. Dilute the 0.4-mg ampule of naloxone in 10 mL of 0.9% NaCl and administer 0.5 mL (0.02 mg) by IV push every 2 min. For children and patients weighing <40 kg, dilute 0.1 mg of naloxone in 10 mL of 0.9% NaCl for a concentration of 10 mcg/mL and administer 0.5 mcg/kg every 2 min. Titrate dose to avoid withdrawal, seizures, and severe pain. In patients receiving meperidine chronically, naloxone may precipitate seizures by eliminating the CNS depressant effects of meperidine, allowing the convulsant activity of normeperidine to predominate. Monitor patient closely.

Implementation

- ***High Alert:*** Accidental overdose of opioid analgesics has resulted in fatalities. Before administering, clarify all ambiguous orders; have second practitioner independently check original order, dose calculations, and infusion pump settings. Pedi: Medication errors with opioid analgesics are common in the pediatric population and include misinterpretation or miscalculation of doses and use of inappropriate measuring devices.
- Explain therapeutic value of medication prior to administration to enhance the analgesic effect.
- Regularly administered doses may be more effective than prn administration. Analgesic is more effective if given before pain becomes severe.
- Coadministration with nonopioid analgesics may have additive analgesic effects and permit lower doses.
- Oral dose is <50% as effective as parenteral. When changing to oral administration, dose may need to be increased (see Appendix J).
- Medication should be discontinued gradually after long-term use to prevent withdrawal symptoms.
- May be administered via PCA pump.
- **PO:** Doses may be administered with food or milk to minimize GI irritation. Syrup should be diluted in half-full glass of water.
- **IM:** Administration of repeated subcut doses may cause local irritation.
- FDA strongly encourages health care professionals to complete a REMS-compliant education program that includes all the elements of the FDA Education *Blueprint for Health Care Providers Involved in the Management or Support of Patients with Pain,* available at www.fda.gov/OpioidAnalgesicREMSBlueprint. Information on programs can be found at 1-800-503-0784 or www.opioidanalgesicrems.com.

IV Administration

- **IV Push:** ***Diluent:*** Dilute with sterile water or 0.9% NaCl for injection. ***Concentration:*** ≤10 mg/mL. ***Rate: High Alert:*** Administer slowly over at least 5 min. Rapid administration may lead to increased respiratory depression, hypotension, and circulatory collapse.
- **Intermittent Infusion:** ***Diluent:*** Dilute with D5W, D10W, dextrose/saline combinations, dextrose/Ringer's or lactated Ringer's injection combinations, 0.45% NaCl, 0.9% NaCl, or Ringer's or LR. Administer via infusion pump. ***Concentration:*** 1 mg/mL. ***Rate:*** Administer over 15–30 min.
- **Y-Site Compatibility:** acetaminophen, alemtuzumab, alfentanil, amifostine, amikacin, aminocaproic acid, aminophylline, amiodarone, amphotericin B lipid complex, anidulafungin, argatroban, ascorbic acid, atracurium, atropine, azithromycin, aztreonam, benztropine, bivalirudin, bleomycin, bumetanide, busulfan, calcium chloride, calcium gluconate, carboplatin, cangrelor, carmustine, caspofungin, cefazolin, cefotaxime, cefoxitin, ceftaroline, ceftazidime, ceftriaxone, cefuroxime, chlorpromazine, ciprofloxacin, cisatracurium, cisplatin,

cladribine, clindamycin, cyanocobalamin, cyclophosphamide, cyclosporine, cytarabine, dactinomycin, daptomycin, daunorubicin, daunorubicin liposome, dexmedetomidine, dexrazoxane, digoxin, diltiazem, diphenhydramine, dobutamine, docetaxel, dopamine, doxacurium, doxorubicin hydrochloride, doxycycline, droperidol, enalaprilat, ephedrine, epinephrine, epirubicin, epoetin alfa, eptifibatide, ertapenem, erythromycin, esmolol, etoposide, etoposide phosphate, famotidine, fenoldopam, fentanyl, filgrastim, floxuridine, fluconazole, fludarabine, fluorouracil, folic acid, fosphenytoin, gemcitabine, gentamicin, glycopyrrolate, granisetron, hetastarch, hydrocortisone, ifosfamide, insulin, regular, irinotecan, isoproterenol, ketamine, ketorolac, labetalol, leucovorin calcium, levofloxacin, lidocaine, linezolid, mannitol, melphalan, mesna, metaraminol, methotrexate, methyldopate, metoclopramide, metoprolol, metronidazole, midazolam, milrinone, mitomycin, mitoxantrone, morphine, multivitamins, mycophenolate, naloxone, nitroglycerin, nitroprusside, norepinephrine, octreotide, ondansetron, oxacillin, oxaliplatin, oxytocin, paclitaxel, palonosetron, pamidronate, pancuronium, papaverine, pemetrexed, penicillin G, pentamidine, phentolamine, phenylephrine, phytonadione, piperacillin/tazobactam, potassium acetate, potassium chloride, procainamide, prochlorperazine, promethazine, propofol, propranolol, protamine, pyridoxime, quinupristin/dalfopristin, ranitidine, remifentanil, rituximab, rocuronium, sargramostim, sodium acetate, streptokinase, streptozocin, succinylcholine, sufentanil, tacrolimus, theophylline, thiamine, thiotepa, tigecycline, tirofiban, tobramycin, tolazoline, topotecan, trastuzumab, trimetaphan, vancomycin, vasopressin, vecuronium, verapamil, vinblastine, vincristine, vinorelbine, voriconazole, zidovudine, zoledronic acid.

- **Y-Site Incompatibility:** allopurinol, amphotericin B liposome, azathioprine, cefepime, dantrolene, diazepam, diazoxide, ganciclovir, idarubicin, indomethacin, lorazepam, micafungin, nafcillin, pantoprazole, pentobarbital, phenobarbital, phenytoin, sodium bicarbonate, thiopental.

Patient/Family Teaching

- Instruct patient on how and when to ask for and take pain medication.
- Instruct patient to take meperidine as directed. If dose is less effective after a few wk, do not increase dose without consulting health care professional. Discuss safe use, risks, and proper storage and disposal of opioid analgesics with patients and caregivers with each Rx. The Patient Counseling Guide (PCG) is available at www.fda.gov/OpioidAnalgesicREMSPCG. Pedi: Teach parents or caregivers how to accurately measure liquid medication and to use only the measuring device dispensed with the medication.
- May cause drowsiness or dizziness. Advise patient to call for assistance when ambulating or smoking. Caution patient to avoid driving or other activities requiring alertness until response to medication is known.
- Advise patient that meperidine is a drug with known abuse potential. Protect it from theft, and never give to anyone other than the individual for whom it was prescribed. Store out of sight and reach of children, and in a location not accessible by others.
- Advise patient to change positions slowly to minimize orthostatic hypotension.
- Instruct patient to avoid concurrent use of alcohol or other CNS depressants.
- Advise ambulatory patients that nausea and vomiting may be decreased by lying down.
- Encourage patient to turn, cough, and breathe deeply every 2 hr to prevent atelectasis.
- Rep: Advise patient to notify health care professional if pregnancy is planned or suspected, or if breast feeding. Inform patient of potential for neonatal opioid withdrawal syndrome with prolonged use during pregnancy. Monitor neonate for signs and symptoms of withdrawal symptoms (irritability, hyperactivity and abnormal sleep pattern, high pitched cry, tremor, vomiting, diarrhea, and/or failure to gain weight); usually occur the first days after birth.

Evaluation/Desired Outcomes

- Decrease in severity of pain without a significant alteration in level of consciousness or respiratory status.
- Resolution of rigors.

mepolizumab
(me-poe-liz-ue-mab)
Nucala

Classification
Therapeutic: antiasthmatics
Pharmacologic: monoclonal antibodies, interleukin antagonists

Indications

Add-on maintenance treatment of severe asthma that is of an eosinophilic phenotype. Treatment of eosinophilic granulomatosis with polyangiitis.

Action

Interleukin-5 (IL-5) antagonist that inhibits binding of IL-5 to the surface of the eosinophil, which reduces the production and survival of eosinophils. **Therapeutic Effects:** Decreased incidence of asthma exacerba-

M

tions. Reduction in use of maintenance oral corticosteroid therapy. Prolonged duration of remission and reduction in use of maintenance oral corticosteroid therapy.

Pharmacokinetics

Absorption: 80% absorbed following subcut administration.
Distribution: Minimally distributed to tissues.
Metabolism and Excretion: Degraded by proteolytic enzymes located throughout the body.
Half-life: 16–22 days.

TIME/ACTION PROFILE (blood levels)

ROUTE	ONSET	PEAK	DURATION
Subcut	unknown	unknown	unknown

Contraindications/Precautions

Contraindicated in: Hypersensitivity; Acute bronchospasm or status asthmaticus.
Use Cautiously in: OB: Pregnancy; expected to cross the placenta (potential effects likely to be greater during 2nd and 3rd trimesters); Lactation: No information regarding presence of drug in human breast milk; benefits of breast feeding need to be evaluated against any potential risks to infant; Pedi: Safety and effectiveness not established in children <18 yr (eosinophilic granulomatosis with polyangiitis) or <6 yr (severe asthma of an eosinophilic phenotype).

Adverse Reactions/Side Effects

CNS: headache. **Derm:** flushing, rash. **MS:** back pain, myalgia. **Misc:** HYPERSENSITIVITY REACTIONS (including anaphylaxis and angioedema), fatigue, herpes zoster infection, injection site reactions.

Interactions

Drug-Drug: None known.

Route/Dosage

Severe Asthma

Subcut (Adults and Children ≥12 yr): 100 mg every 4 wk.
Subcut (Children 6–11 yr): 40 mg every 4 wk.

Eosinophilic Granulomatosis with Polyangiitis

Subcut (Adults): 300 mg every 4 wk.

Availability

Lyophilized powder for injection (requires reconstitution): 100 mg/vial. **Solution for injection (prefilled autoinjectors and prefilled syringes):** 100 mg/mL.

NURSING IMPLICATIONS

Assessment

- Assess respiratory status (rate, breath sounds, degree of dyspnea, pulse) periodically during therapy.
- Monitor for signs and symptoms of hypersensitivity reactions (anaphylaxis, angioedema, bronchospasm, urticaria, rash) following injection. Reactions usually occur within hrs, but may have a delayed onset (days). Discontinue mepolizumab if hypersensitivity reaction occurs.
- Assess for and treat parasitic infections prior to therapy. If infected during therapy and unresponsive to anti-helminth treatment, discontinue mepolizumab until infection resolves.

Implementation

- Only administer in a health care setting by a health care professional able to manage anaphylaxis. Mepolizumab is for prevention; do not use to treat acute bronchospasm or status asthmaticus.
- Consider administration of varicella vaccination prior to starting therapy.
- Do not abruptly stop systemic or inhaled corticosteroids when starting therapy. May ↓ corticosteroid doses gradually under direct supervision of health care professional. Corticosteroid ↓ may lead to systemic withdrawal symptoms and/or unmask conditions previously suppressed.
- Reconstitute in vial with 1.2 mL of sterile water for injection using a 2- or 3-mL syringe and a 21-gauge needle for a concentration of 100 mg/mL. Direct stream into center of cake. Swirl gently for 10 sec until powder is dissolved; do not shake. Reconstitution takes 5 min or more. Solution is clear to opalescent and colorless to pale yellow or pale brown; do not administer if solution is discolored, cloudy, or contains particles. Stable for 8 hr if refrigerated.
- **Subcut:** Administer 1 mL for the 100 mg dose or 0.4 mg for the 40 mg dose once every 4 wk into upper arm, thigh, or abdomen.

Patient/Family Teaching

- Explain purpose of mepolizumab to patient. Administer missed doses as soon as possible, if next dose is already due administer as planned. Instruct patient to read *Patient Information* before starting therapy.
- May be self-administered by adults and adolescents 12 yrs or older using the prefilled auto-injector and prefilled syringe. Remove autoinjector from refrigerator 30 min before injection; do not warm in any other way. Inspect window of autoinjector; solution is clear to opalescent, colorless to pale yellow to pale brown in color. Do not administer solutions that are discolored or contain particulate matter. Inject into thigh or abdomen, 2 inches from navel, or upper arm if administered by caregiver. If multiple injections are needed, separate each injection by at least 2 inches. Avoid areas that are tender, bruised, red, or hard.
- Inform patient of risk and signs and symptoms of anaphylaxis. Instruct patient to notify health care professional immediately if signs and symptoms of hy-

persensitivity reactions (swelling of face, mouth, tongue, fainting, dizziness, feeling lightheaded, hives, breathing problems, rash) occur.
- Advise patient to notify health care professional if asthma remains uncontrolled or worsens after starting therapy.
- Caution patient not to reduce corticosteroid dose unless instructed by health care professional.
- Instruct patient to notify health care professional of all Rx or OTC medications, vitamins, or herbal products being taken and consult health care professional before taking any new medications.
- Rep: Advise females of reproductive potential to notify health care professional if pregnancy is planned or suspected or if breast feeding. Encourage women who become pregnant while taking mepolizumab to enroll in the Pregnancy Exposure Registry by calling 1-877-311-8972 or visiting www.mothertobaby.org/asthma.

Evaluation/Desired Outcomes
- Decreased incidence of asthma exacerbations and reduction in use of maintenance oral corticosteroid therapy.

meropenem (mer-oh-pen-nem)
Merrem

Classification
Therapeutic: anti-infectives
Pharmacologic: carbapenems

Indications
Complicated skin and skin structure infections. Complicated intra-abdominal infections. Bacterial meningitis. **Unlabeled Use:** Febrile neutropenia. Hospital-acquired pneumonia and sepsis.

Action
Binds to bacterial cell wall, resulting in cell death. Meropenem resists the actions of many enzymes that degrade most other penicillins and penicillin-like anti-infectives. **Therapeutic Effects:** Bactericidal action against susceptible bacteria. **Spectrum:** Active against the following gram-positive organisms: *Staphylococcus aureus*, *Streptococcus agalactiae*, *Streptococcus pneumoniae*, *Streptococcus pyogenes*, viridans group streptococci, *Enterococcus faecalis*. Also active against the following gram-negative pathogens: *Escherichia coli*, *Haemophilus influenzae*, *Klebsiella pneumoniae*, *Neisseria meningitidis*, *Proteus mirabilis*, *Pseudomonas aeruginosa*. Active against the following anaerobes: *Bacteroides fragilis*, *Bacteroides thetaiotaomicron*, *Peptostreptococcus spp.*

Pharmacokinetics
Absorption: IV administration results in complete bioavailability.
Distribution: Widely distributed into body tissues and fluids; enters CSF when meninges are inflamed.
Metabolism and Excretion: 50–75% excreted unchanged by the kidneys.
Half-life: Premature neonates: 3 hr; Term neonates: 2 hr; Infants 3 mo–2 yr: 1.4 hr; Children >2 yr and Adults: 1 hr (↑ in renal impairment).

TIME/ACTION PROFILE (blood levels)

ROUTE	ONSET	PEAK	DURATION
IV	rapid	end of infusion	8 hr

Contraindications/Precautions
Contraindicated in: Hypersensitivity to meropenem or imipenem; Serious hypersensitivity to other beta-lactams (penicillins or cephalosporins; cross-sensitivity may occur).
Use Cautiously in: Renal impairment (↑ risk of thrombocytopenia and seizures; dose ↓ recommended if CCr <50 mL/min); History of seizures, brain lesions, or meningitis; OB: Safety not established in pregnancy; Lactation: Use during breast feeding only if potential maternal benefit outweighs risk to infant; Pedi: Children <3 mo (safety and effectiveness not established for complicated skin/skin structure infections and meningitis).

Adverse Reactions/Side Effects
CNS: SEIZURES, dizziness, headache. **Derm:** acute generalized exanthematous pustulosis, DRUG REACTION WITH EOSINOPHILIA AND SYSTEMIC SYMPTOMS (DRESS), ERYTHEMA MULTIFORME, STEVENS-JOHNSON SYNDROME, TOXIC EPIDERMAL NECROLYSIS, moniliasis (children only), pruritus, rash. **GI:** CLOSTRIDIUM DIFFICILE-ASSOCIATED DIARRHEA (CDAD), constipation, diarrhea, glossitis (↑ in children), nausea, thrush (↑ in children), vomiting. **Hemat:** thrombocytopenia (↑ in renal impairment). **Local:** inflammation at injection site, phlebitis. **Neuro:** paresthesias. **Resp:** APNEA. **Misc:** HYPERSENSITIVITY REACTIONS (including anaphylaxis).

Interactions
Drug-Drug: Probenecid ↓ renal excretion and ↑ levels; concurrent use not recommended. May ↓ serum **valproate** levels and ↑ the risk of seizures.

Route/Dosage
Complicated Skin/Skin Structure Infections
IV (Adults): 500 mg every 8 hr or 1 g every 8 hr (if caused by *Pseudomonas aeruginosa*).
IV (Children ≥3 mo–12 yr): 10 mg/kg (max dose = 500 mg) every 8 hr or 20 mg/kg (max dose = 1 g) every 8 hr (if caused by *Pseudomonas aeruginosa*).

Renal Impairment

IV (Adults): *CCr 26–50 mL/min*—500 mg every 12 hr; *CCr 10–25 mL/min*—250 mg every 12 hr; *CCr <10 mL/min*—250 mg every 24 hr.

Intra-abdominal Infections

IV (Adults): 1 g every 8 hr.
IV (Children ≥3 mo–12 yr): 20 mg/kg (max dose = 1 g) every 8 hr.
IV (Children <3 mo): *<32 wk gestational age (GA) and postnatal age (PNA) <2 wk*—20 mg/kg every 12 hr; *<32 wk GA and PNA ≥2 wk*—20 mg/kg every 8 hr; *≥32 wk GA and PNA <2 wk*—20 mg/kg every 8 hr; *≥32 wk GA and PNA ≥2 wk*—30 mg/kg every 8 hr.

Renal Impairment

IV (Adults): *CCr 26–50 mL/min*—1 g every 12 hr; *CCr 10–25 mL/min*—500 mg every 12 hr; *CCr <10 mL/min*—500 mg every 24 hr.

Bacterial Meningitis

IV (Children ≥3 mo): 40 mg/kg (max dose = 2 g) every 8 hr.

Availability (generic available)

Powder for injection (requires reconstitution): 500 mg, 1 g. **Premixed infusion:** 500 mg/50 mL 0.9% NaCl, 1 g/50 mL 0.9% NaCl.

NURSING IMPLICATIONS

Assessment

- Assess for infection (vital signs; appearance of wound, sputum, urine, and stool; WBC) at beginning of and throughout therapy.
- Obtain a history before initiating therapy to determine previous use of and reactions to penicillins. Persons with a negative history of penicillin sensitivity may still have an allergic response.
- Obtain specimens for culture and sensitivity prior to initiating therapy. First dose may be given before receiving results.
- Monitor bowel function. Diarrhea, abdominal cramping, fever, and bloody stools should be reported to health care professional promptly as a sign of Clostridium difficile-associated diarrhea (CDAD). May begin up to several wk following cessation of therapy.
- Observe for signs and symptoms of anaphylaxis (rash, pruritus, laryngeal edema, wheezing). Discontinue the drug and notify physician immediately if these symptoms occur. Have epinephrine, an antihistamine, and resuscitative equipment close by in the event of an anaphylactic reaction.
- Assess injection site for phlebitis, pain, and swelling periodically during administration.
- Monitor for signs and symptoms of DRESS (fever, rash, lymphadenopathy, and/or facial swelling, associated with involvement of other organ systems (hepatitis, nephritis, hematologic abnormalities, myocarditis, myositis) during therapy. May resemble an acute viral infection. Eosinophilia is often present. Discontinue therapy if signs occur.
- Assess patient for skin rash frequently during therapy. Discontinue meropenem at first sign of rash; may be life-threatening. Stevens-Johnson syndrome or toxic epidermal necrolysis may develop. Treat symptomatically; may recur once treatment is stopped.
- ***Lab Test Considerations:*** Monitor hematologic, hepatic, and renal functions periodically during therapy.
- BUN, AST, ALT, LDH, serum alkaline phosphatase, bilirubin, and creatinine may be transiently ↑.
- Hemoglobin and hematocrit concentrations may be ↓.
- May cause positive direct or indirect Coombs' test.

Implementation

IV Administration

- **IV Push:** Reconstitute 500-mg and 1-g vials with 10 mL and 20 mL, respectively, of sterile water for injection. ***Concentration:*** 50 mg/mL. ***Rate:*** Administer over 3–5 min.
- **Intermittent Infusion:** Reconstitute 500-mg and 1-g vials with 10 mL and 20 mL, respectively, of sterile water for injection, 0.9% NaCl, or D5W. Vials reconstituted with sterile water for injection are stable for 3 hr at room temperature and 13 hr if refrigerated; if reconstituted with 0.9% NaCl, stable for 1 hr at room temperature and 15 hr if refrigerated; if reconstituted with D5W, should be used immediately. ***Diluent:*** Further dilute in 0.9% NaCl or D5W to achieve concentration below. Infusions further diluted in 0.9% NaCl are stable for 4 hr at room temperature and 24 hr if refrigerated. Infusions further diluted in D5W are stable for 1 hr at room temperature and 4 hr if refrigerated. ***Concentration:*** 1–20 mg/mL. ***Rate:*** Infuse over 15–30 min.
- **Y-Site Compatibility:** acyclovir, alemtuzumab, aminocaproic acid, aminophylline, anidulafungin, argatroban, atropine, azithromycin, bivalirudin, bleomycin, calcium gluconate, cangrelor, carboplatin, carmustine, caspofungin, cisplatin, cyclophosphamide, cyclosporine, cytarabine, dactinomycin, daptomycin, daunorubicin hydrochloride, dexamethasone, dexmedetomidine, dexrazoxane, digoxin, diltiazem, diphenhydramine, docetaxel, doxorubicin liposomal, enalaprilat, eptifibatide, etoposide, etoposide phosphate, fluconazole, fludarabine, fluorouracil, foscarnet, fosphenytoin, furosemide, gemcitabine, gentamicin, granisetron, heparin, hetastarch, hydromorphone, ifosfamide, insulin, regular, irinotecan, labetalol, leucovorin calcium, linezolid, lorazepam, mesna, methotrexate, metoclopramide, metronidazole, milrinone, mitomycin, mitoxantrone, morphine, naloxone, norepinephrine, octreotide, ondansetron, oxaliplatin, oxytocin, paclitaxel, palonosetron, pamidronate, pancuronium, pemetrexed,

phenobarbital, potassium acetate, potassium chloride, rocuronium, tacrolimus, telavancin, thiotepa, tigecycline, tirofiban, vancomycin, vasopressin, vecuronium, vinblastine, vincristine, vinorelbine, voriconazole, zoledronic acid.

- **Y-Site Incompatibility:** amiodarone, amphotericin B lipid complex, amphotericin B liposome, ciprofloxacin, dacarbazine, diazepam, doxorubicin hydrochloride, epirubicin, fenoldopam, idarubicin, ketamine, mycophenolate, nicardipine, pantoprazole, quinupristin/dalfopristin, topotecan.

Patient/Family Teaching

- Advise patient to report the signs of superinfection (black, furry overgrowth on the tongue; vaginal itching or discharge; loose or foul-smelling stools) and allergy.
- May cause dizziness. Caution patient to avoid driving or other activities requiring alertness until response to drug is known.
- Caution patient to notify health care professional if rash or fever and diarrhea occur, especially if stool contains blood, pus, or mucus. Advise patient not to treat diarrhea without consulting health care professional. May occur up to several wk after discontinuation of medication.
- Advise patient to notify health care professional of all Rx or OTC medications, vitamins, or herbal products being taken and to consult with health care professional before taking other medications.
- Advise female patient to notify health care professional if pregnancy is planned or suspected, or if breast feeding.

Evaluation/Desired Outcomes

- Resolution of the signs and symptoms of infection. Length of time for complete resolution depends on the organism and site of infection.

meropenem/vaborbactam

(mer-oh-**pen**-nem/va-bor-**bak**-tam)

Vabomere

Classification

Therapeutic: anti-infectives

Pharmacologic: carbapenems beta-lactamase inhibitors

Indications

Treatment of complicated urinary tract infections, including pyelonephritis.

Action

Binds to bacterial cell wall, resulting in cell death. Addition of vaborbactam protects meropenem from being degraded by certain serine beta-lactamases such as *Klebsiella pneumoniae* carbapenemase (KPC). **Therapeutic Effects:** Bactericidal action against susceptible bacteria. **Spectrum:** Active against the following gram-negative pathogens: *Escherichia coli*, *Enterobacter cloacae*, *Klebsiella pneumoniae*.

Pharmacokinetics

Absorption: IV administration results in complete bioavailability.

Distribution: Well distributed into body tissues and fluids.

Metabolism and Excretion: Meropenem undergoes hydrolysis; vaborbactam is not metabolized. Both meropenem and vaborbactam are primarily excreted by the kidneys (40–60% of meropenem and 75–95% of vaborbactam excreted unchanged in the urine).

Half-life: Meropenem: 1.22 hr; vaborbactam: 1.68 hr.

TIME/ACTION PROFILE (blood levels)

ROUTE	ONSET	PEAK	DURATION
IV	rapid	end of infusion	8 hr

Contraindications/Precautions

Contraindicated in: Hypersensitivity to any of the carbapenems (ertapenem, imipenem, meropenem); Anaphylactic reactions to other beta-lactams (cross-sensitivity may occur); OB: May cause fetal harm.

Use Cautiously in: Renal impairment (↑ risk of thrombocytopenia and seizures; ↓ dose if eGFR <50 mL/min); History of seizures, brain lesions, or meningitis; Lactation: Consider benefits of breast feeding against possible risk to infant; Pedi: Safety and effectiveness not established.

Adverse Reactions/Side Effects

CNS: SEIZURES, delirium, headache. **GI:** CLOSTRIDIUM DIFFICILE-ASSOCIATED DIARRHEA (CDAD), diarrhea. **Neuro:** paresthesias. **Misc:** HYPERSENSITIVITY REACTIONS (including anaphylaxis), infusion site reactions, phlebitis.

Interactions

Drug-Drug: Probenecid ↓ renal excretion of meropenem and ↑ its blood levels; concurrent use not recommended. May ↓ **valproate** levels and ↑ risk of seizures; concurrent use not recommended.

Route/Dosage

IV (Adults): 4 g (meropenem 2 g/vaborbactam 2 g) every 8 hr for up to 14 days.

Renal Impairment

IV (Adults): *eGFR 30–49 mL/min*—2 g (meropenem 1 g/vaborbactam 1 g) every 8 hr for up to 14 days; *eGFR 15–29 mL/min*—2 g (meropenem 1 g/vaborbactam 1 g) every 12 hr for up to 14 days; *eGFR <15 mL/min*—1 g (meropenem 0.5 g/vaborbactam 0.5 g) every 12 hr for up to 14 days.

Availability

Powder for injection (requires reconstitution and dilution): 2 g/vial (1 g meropenem/1 g vaborbactam).

NURSING IMPLICATIONS

Assessment

- Assess for infection (vital signs; appearance of wound, sputum, urine, and stool; WBC) at beginning of and throughout therapy.
- Obtain a history before initiating therapy to determine previous use of and reactions to penicillins. Persons with a negative history of penicillin sensitivity may still have an allergic response.
- Obtain specimens for culture and sensitivity prior to initiating therapy. First dose may be given before receiving results.
- Monitor bowel function. Diarrhea, abdominal cramping, fever, and bloody stools should be reported to health care professional promptly as a sign of Clostridium difficile-associated diarrhea (CDAD). May begin up to several wk following cessation of therapy.
- Observe for signs and symptoms of anaphylaxis (rash, pruritus, laryngeal edema, wheezing). Discontinue the drug and notify health care professional immediately if these symptoms occur. Have epinephrine, an antihistamine, and resuscitative equipment close by in the event of an anaphylactic reaction.
- ***Lab Test Considerations:*** May cause hyperkalemia, hyperglycemia, and hypoglycemia.

Implementation

- **Intermittent Infusion:** Reconstitute each vial with 20 mL 0.9% NaCl withdrawn from infusion bag. Mix gently to dissolve. ***Diluent:*** Dilute further in 250 mL to 1000 mL infusion bag of 0.9% NaCl. ***Concentration:*** 2 mg/mL to 16 mg/mL. Solution is clear to light yellow; do not infuse solutions that are discolored or contain particulate matter. Infusion must be completed within 4 hrs if stored at room temperature or 22 hrs if refrigerated. ***Rate:*** Infuse over 3 hrs.

Patient/Family Teaching

- Advise patient to report the signs of superinfection (black, furry overgrowth on the tongue; vaginal itching or discharge; loose or foul-smelling stools) and allergy.
- May cause seizures, delirium, headaches, and/or paresthesias. Caution patient to avoid driving or other activities requiring alertness until response to medication is known.
- Caution patient to notify health care professional if fever and diarrhea occur, especially if stool contains blood, pus, or mucus. Advise patient not to treat diarrhea without consulting health care professional. May occur up to several wk after discontinuation of medication.
- Advise patient to notify health care professional of all Rx or OTC medications, vitamins, or herbal products being taken and to consult with health care professional before taking other medications.
- Advise female patient to notify health care professional if pregnancy is planned or suspected, or if breast feeding.

Evaluation/Desired Outcomes

- Resolution of the signs and symptoms of infection. Length of time for complete resolution depends on the organism and site of infection.

mesalamine (me-sal-a-meen)

Apriso, ~~Asacol~~, ✱Asacol, ✱Asacol 800, Asacol HD, Canasa, Delzicol, Lialda, ✱Mezavant, ✱Mezera, Pentasa, Rowasa, ✱Salofalk, ✱Teva 5-ASA

Classification

Therapeutic: gastrointestinal anti-inflammatories

Indications

Delzicol, Lialda, and Pentasa: Treatment and maintenance of remission of mildly-to-moderately-active ulcerative colitis. **Apriso:** Maintenance of remission of ulcerative colitis. **Asacol HD:** Treatment of moderately-active ulcerative colitis. **Canasa**: Treatment of active ulcerative proctitis. **Rowasa**: Treatment of active mild-to-moderate distal ulcerative colitis, proctosigmoiditis, or proctitis.

Action

Locally acting anti-inflammatory action in the colon, where activity is probably due to inhibition of prostaglandin synthesis. **Therapeutic Effects:** Reduction in the symptoms of ulcerative colitis, proctosigmoiditis, and proctitis.

Pharmacokinetics

Absorption: 28% absorbed following oral administration; 10–30% absorbed from the colon, depending on retention time, following rectal administration.

Distribution: Unknown.

Metabolism and Excretion: Some metabolism occurs, site unknown; mostly eliminated unchanged in the feces.

Half-life: *Oral*—12 hr (range 2–15 hr); *Rectal*—0.5–1.5 hr.

TIME/ACTION PROFILE (clinical improvement)

ROUTE	ONSET	PEAK	DURATION
PO	unknown	unknown	6–8 hr
ER	2 hr	9–12 hr	24 hr
Rectal	3–21 days	unknown	24 hr

Contraindications/Precautions

Contraindicated in: Hypersensitivity reactions to sulfonamides, salicylates, mesalamine, or sulfasalazine; Cross-sensitivity with furosemide, sulfonylurea hypoglycemic agents, or carbonic anhydrase inhibitors may exist; G6PD deficiency; Hypersensitivity to bisulfites (mesalamine enema only); Urinary tract or intestinal obstruction; Porphyria.

Use Cautiously in: Severe hepatic or renal impairment; Atopic dermatitis or atopic eczema (↑ risk of photosensitivity); Phenylketonuria (Apriso contains phenylalanine); OB: Use only if potential maternal benefit justifies potential fetal risk; use tablets only if potential benefits outweigh risk to fetus (enteric coating contains dibutyl phthalate, which has been shown to cause congenital malformations in animals); Lactation: Has caused diarrhea in some infants; careful observation required.

Adverse Reactions/Side Effects

CNS: headache, dizziness, malaise, weakness. **CV:** pericarditis. **Derm:** DRUG REACTION WITH EOSINOPHILIA AND SYSTEMATIC SYMPTOMS (DRESS), STEVENS-JOHNSON SYNDROME, hair loss, photosensitivity, rash. **EENT:** pharyngitis, rhinitis. **GI:** diarrhea, eructation (PO), flatulence, nausea, vomiting. **GU:** interstitial nephritis, pancreatitis, renal failure. **Local:** anal irritation (enema, suppository). **MS:** back pain, myalgia. **Misc:** HYPERSENSITIVITY REACTIONS (including anaphylaxis and angioedema), acute intolerance syndrome, fever.

Interactions

Drug-Drug: May ↓ metabolism and ↑ effects/toxicity of **mercaptopurine** or **thioguanine**.

Route/Dosage

One Asacol HD 800-mg tablet is NOT bioequivalent to two Delzicol 400-mg capsules.

Treatment of Ulcerative Colitis

PO (Adults): *Delzicol*—800 mg (two 400-mg capsules) 3 times daily for 6 wk; *Asacol HD*—1.6 g (two 800-mg tablets) 3 times daily for 6 wk; *Lialda*—2.4–4.8 g (two to four 1.2-g tablets) once daily for up to 8 wk; *Pentasa*—1 g (four 250-mg capsules or two 500-mg capsules) 4 times daily for up to 8 wk.

Rect (Adults): *Rowasa*—4-g enema (60 mL) at bedtime, retained for 8 hr for 3–6 wk.

PO (Children ≥12 yr and 54–90 kg): *Delzicol*—27–44 mg/kg/day in 2 divided doses (max dose = 2.4 g/day) for 6 wk.

PO (Children ≥12 yr and 33–53 kg): *Delzicol*—37–61 mg/kg/day in 2 divided doses (max dose = 2 g/day) for 6 wk.

PO (Children ≥12 yr and 17–32 kg): *Delzicol*—36–71 mg/kg/day in 2 divided doses (max dose = 1.2 g/day) for 6 wk.

Maintenance of Remission of Ulcerative Colitis

PO (Adults): *Apriso*—1.5 g (four 375-mg capsules) once daily in the morning; *Delzicol*—800 mg (two 400-mg capsules) 2 times daily; *Lialda*—2.4 g (two 1.2-g tablets) once daily; *Pentasa*—1 g (four 250-mg capsules or two 500-mg capsules) 4 times daily.

Treatment of Ulcerative Proctosigmoiditis

Rect (Adults): *Rowasa*—4-g enema (60 mL) at bedtime, retained for 8 hr (treatment duration = 3–6 wk).

Treatment of Ulcerative Proctitis

Rect (Adults): *Rowasa*—4-g enema (60 mL) at bedtime, retained for 8 hr (treatment duration = 3–6 wk); *Canasa*—Insert a 1-g suppository at bedtime, retain for at least 1–3 hr (treatment duration = 3–6 wk).

Availability (generic available)

Controlled-release capsules (Pentasa): 250 mg, 500 mg. **Delayed-release capsules (Delzicol):** 400 mg. **Delayed-release tablets:** 🍁 400 mg, 🍁 500 mg, 800 mg (Asacol HD), 🍁 1 g, 1.2 g (Lialda). **Extended-release capsules (Apriso) (contain phenylalanine):** 375 mg. **Rectal enema (Rowasa):** 🍁 1 g/100 mL, 🍁 2 g/60 mL, 4 g/60 mL, 🍁 4 g/100 mL. **Rectal foam:** 🍁 1 g/actuation. **Rectal suppository (Canasa):** 🍁 500 mg, 1 g.

M

NURSING IMPLICATIONS

Assessment

- Assess abdominal pain and frequency, quantity, and consistency of stools at the beginning of and during therapy.
- Assess for allergy to sulfonamides and salicylates. Patients allergic to sulfasalazine may take mesalamine or olsalazine without difficulty, but therapy should be discontinued if rash or fever occurs.
- Monitor intake and output ratios. Fluid intake should be sufficient to maintain a urine output of at least 1200–1500 mL daily to prevent crystalluria and stone formation.
- ***Lab Test Considerations:*** Monitor urinalysis, BUN, and serum creatinine prior to and periodically during therapy. Mesalamine may cause renal toxicity.
- Mesalamine may cause ↑ AST and ALT levels, serum alkaline phosphatase, GGTP, LDH, amylase, and lipase.

Implementation

- Do not confuse Asacol (mesalamine) with Os-Cal (calcium carbonate).
- **PO:** Administer with a full glass of water. Tablets should be swallowed whole; do not break the outer coating, which is designed to remain intact. Take *Lialda* tablets with a meal. Take *Apriso* capsules in the

morning without regard to meals. Do not co-administer with antacids; may affect dissolution of the coating of the granules in *Apriso* capsules. Intact or partially intact tablets may occasionally be found in the stool. If this occurs repeatedly, advise patient to notify health care professional. Swallow *Delzicol* capsules whole; do not break, crush, or chew. Administer without regard to meals. If unable to swallow capsules, may open capsule and swallow inner tablets. Intact or partially intact tablets may occasionally be found in the stool. If this occurs repeatedly, advise patient to notify health care professional. Two *Delzicol* 400-mg capsules are not equal to one *Asacol HD* (mesalamine) delayed-release 800-mg tablet. *Pentasa* capsules may be swallowed whole or opened and sprinkled onto applesauce or yogurt. Consume entire contents immediately. Avoid crushing or chewing capsules and capsule contents.

- **Rect:** Patient should empty bowel prior to administration of rectal dose forms.
- Avoid excessive handling of *suppository*. Remove foil wrapper and insert pointed end first into rectum with gentle pressure. Do not cut or break suppository. Retain suppository for 1–3 hr or more for maximum benefit.
- Administer 60-mL retention enema once daily at bedtime. Solution should be retained for approximately 8 hr. Prior to administration of *rectal suspension*, shake bottle well and remove the protective cap. Have patient lie on left side with the lower leg extended and the upper leg flexed for support or place the patient in knee-chest position. Gently insert the applicator tip into the rectum, pointing toward the umbilicus. Squeeze the bottle steadily to discharge most of the preparation.

Patient/Family Teaching

- Instruct patient on the correct method of administration. Advise patient to take medication as directed, even if feeling better. Take missed doses as soon as remembered unless almost time for next dose. Advise patient to read *Patient Information* before starting therapy and with each Rx refill in case of changes.
- Advise patient not to change brands of mesalamine without consulting health care professional.
- May cause dizziness. Caution patient to avoid driving or other activities that require alertness until response to medication is known.
- Advise patient to notify health care professional if skin rash, sore throat, fever, mouth sores, unusual bleeding or bruising, wheezing, fever, or hives occur.
- Instruct patient to notify health care professional if symptoms do not improve after 1–2 mo of therapy.
- Instruct patient to notify health care professional if symptoms worsen or do not improve. If symptoms of acute intolerance (cramping, acute abdominal pain, bloody diarrhea, fever, headache, rash) occur, discontinue therapy and notify health care professional immediately.
- Inform patient that proctoscopy and sigmoidoscopy may be required periodically during treatment to determine response.
- Advise female patient of reproductive potential to notify health care professional if pregnancy is planned or suspected, or if breast feeding. Monitor breast-fed infants for diarrhea.
- **Rect:** Instruct patient to use *rectal suspension* at bedtime and retain suspension all night for best results.

Evaluation/Desired Outcomes

- Decrease in diarrhea and abdominal pain.
- Return to normal bowel pattern in patients with inflammatory bowel disease. Effects may be seen within 3–21 days. The usual course of therapy is 3–6 wk.
- Maintenance of remission in patients with inflammatory bowel disease.

mesna (mes-na)

Mesnex, ✱Uromitexan

Classification

Therapeutic: antidotes

Pharmacologic: ifosfamide detoxifying agents

Indications

Prevention of ifosfamide-induced hemorrhagic cystitis (see Ifosfamide monograph). **Unlabeled Use:** May also prevent hemorrhagic cystitis from cyclophosphamide.

Action

Binds to the toxic metabolites of ifosfamide in the kidneys. **Therapeutic Effects:** Prevents hemorrhagic cystitis from ifosfamide.

Pharmacokinetics

Absorption: IV administration results in complete bioavailability; 45–79% absorbed after oral administration. Following IV with PO dosing ↑ systemic exposure.

Distribution: Unknown.

Metabolism and Excretion: Rapidly converted to mesna disulfide, then back to mesna in the kidneys, where it binds to toxic metabolites of ifosfamide (18–26% excreted as free mesna in urine after IV and PO dosing).

Half-life: *Mesna*—0.36 hr (IV); 1.2—8.3 hr (IV followed by PO); *mesna disulfide*—1.17 hr.

TIME/ACTION PROFILE (detoxifying action)

ROUTE	ONSET	PEAK	DURATION
PO, IV	rapid	unknown	4 hr

Contraindications/Precautions

Contraindicated in: Hypersensitivity to mesna or other thiol (rubber) compounds; Lactation: Lactation (may cause harm to infant).

Use Cautiously in: OB: Safety not established; Pedi: Injection contains benzyl alcohol which can cause potentially fatal "gasping syndrome" in neonates.

Adverse Reactions/Side Effects

CNS: dizziness, drowsiness, headache. **Derm:** flushing. **GI:** anorexia, diarrhea, nausea, unpleasant taste, vomiting. **Local:** injection site reactions. **Misc:** flu-like symptoms.

Interactions

Drug-Drug: None significant.

Route/Dosage

IV (Adults): Give a dose of mesna equal to 20% of the ifosfamide dose at the same time as ifosfamide and 4 and 8 hr after.

PO, IV (Adults): Give a dose of IV mesna equal to 20% of the ifosfamide dose at the same time as ifosfamide; then give PO mesna equal to 40% of the ifosfamide dose 2 and 6 hr after ifosfamide (total mesna dose is 100% of ifosfamide dose).

Availability (generic available)

Solution for injection (requires dilution): 100 mg/mL. **Tablets:** 400 mg.

NURSING IMPLICATIONS

Assessment

- Monitor for development of hemorrhagic cystitis in patients receiving ifosfamide.
- ***Lab Test Considerations:*** Obtain a negative pregnancy test before starting when mesna is given with ifosfamide.
- Causes a false-positive result when testing urinary ketones.

Implementation

- Initial IV bolus is to be given at time of ifosfamide administration.
- **PO:** If second and third doses are given orally, administer 2 and 6 hr after IV dose.
- If PO mesna is vomited within 2 hr of administration, repeat dose or use IV mesna.

IV Administration

- **Intermittent Infusion:** 2nd IV dose is given 4 hr later, 3rd dose is given 8 hr after initial dose. This schedule must be repeated with each subsequent dose of ifosfamide. ***Diluent:*** Dilute 2-, 4-, and 10-mL ampules, containing a concentration of 100 mg/mL in 8 mL, 16 mL, or 50 mL, respectively, of D5W, 0.9% NaCl, D5/0.9% NaCl, D5/0.2% NaCl, D5/0.33% NaCl, or LR. ***Concentration:*** 20 mg/mL. Refrigerate to store. Use within 6 hr. Discard unused solution. ***Rate:*** Administer over 15–30 min or as a continuous infusion.
- **Syringe Compatibility:** ifosfamide.
- **Y-Site Compatibility:** alemtuzumab, alfentanil, allopurinol, amifostine, amikacin, aminocaproic acid, aminophylline, amiodarone, amphotericin B liposome, ampicillin, ampicillin/sulbactam, anidulafungin, argatroban, azithromycin, aztreonam, bivalirudin, bleomycin, bumetanide, buprenorphine, butorphanol, calcium acetate, calcium chloride, calcium gluconate, carmustine, caspofungin, cefazolin, cefepime, cefotaxime, cefotetan, cefoxitin, ceftriaxone, cefuroxime, chloramphenicol, chlorpromazine, ciprofloxacin, cisatracurium, cladribine, clindamycin, cyclophosphamide, cytarabine, dactinomycin, dexamethasone, dexmedetomidine, dexrazoxane, digoxin, diltiazem, diphenhydramine, dobutamine, docetaxel, dolasetron, dopamine, doxorubicin hydrochloride, doxorubicin liposomal, doxycycline, droperidol, enalaprilat, ephedrine, epinephrine, epirubicin, ertapenem, erythromycin, esmolol, etoposide, etoposide phosphate, famotidine, fentanyl, filgrastim, fluconazole, fludarabine, fluorouracil, foscarnet, fosphenytoin, furosemide, gemcitabine, gentamicin, glycopyrrolate, granisetron, haloperidol, heparin, hetastarch, hydralazine, hydrocortisone, hydromorphone, idarubicin, ifosfamide, imipenem/cilastatin, insulin, regular, irinotecan, isoproterenol, ketorolac, labetalol, leucovorin, levofloxacin, lidocaine, linezolid, lorazepam, magnesium sulfate, mannitol, melphalan, meperidine, meropenem, methotrexate, methyldopate, methylprednisolone, metoclopramide, metoprolol, metronidazole, micafungin, midazolam, milrinone, mitomycin, mitoxantrone, morphine, moxifloxacin, mycophenolate, nafcillin, nalbuphine, naloxone, nitroglycerin, norepinephrine, octreotide, ondansetron, oxaliplatin, paclitaxel, palonosetron, pamidronate, pancuronium, pantoprazole, pemetrexed, pentamidine, pentobarbital, phenobarbital, phenylephrine, piperacillin/tazobactam, potassium acetate, potassium chloride, potassium phosphates, procainamide, prochlorperazine, promethazine, propranolol, ranitidine, remifentanil, rituximab, rocuronium, sargramostim, sodium acetate, sodium bicarbonate, sodium phosphates, streptozocin, succinylcholine, sufentanil, tacrolimus, theophylline, thiotepa, tigecycline, tirofiban, tobramycin, topotecan, trastuzumab, vancomycin, vasopressin, vecuronium, verapamil, vinblastine, vincristine, vinorelbine, voriconazole, zidovudine, zoledronic acid.
- **Y-Site Incompatibility:** acyclovir, amphotericin B deoxycholate, amphotericin B lipid complex, dacarbazine, dantrolene, diazepam, fenoldopam, ganciclovir, nicardipine, nitroprusside, phenytoin, quinupristin/dalfopristin, thiopental.

Patient/Family Teaching

- Inform patient that unpleasant taste may occur during administration.
- Advise patient to notify health care professional if nausea, vomiting, or diarrhea persists or is severe.
- Rep: Advise female patients of reproductive potential to use effective contraception during and for 6 mo after last dose and to avoid breast feeding during and for 1 wk after last dose of mesna. Advise males with female partners of reproductive potential to use effective contraception during and for 3 mo after last dose. Advise patient to notify health care professional immediately if pregnancy is suspected.

Evaluation/Desired Outcomes

- Prevention of hemorrhagic cystitis associated with ifosfamide therapy.

mestranol/norethindrone, **See CONTRACEPTIVES, HORMONAL.**

BEERS

metaxalone (me-**tax**-a-lone)

Skelaxin

Classification

Therapeutic: skeletal muscle relaxants (centrally acting)

Indications

Muscle spasm associated with acute painful musculoskeletal conditions (with rest and physical therapy).

Action

Skeletal muscle relaxation, probably as a result of CNS depression. **Therapeutic Effects:** Skeletal muscle relaxation.

Pharmacokinetics

Absorption: Well absorbed following oral administration.

Distribution: Unknown.

Metabolism and Excretion: Mostly metabolized by the liver; metabolites excreted in urine.

Half-life: 2–3 hr.

TIME/ACTION PROFILE

ROUTE	ONSET	PEAK	DURATION
PO	1 hr	2 hr	4–6 hr

Contraindications/Precautions

Contraindicated in: Hypersensitivity; Significant hepatic/renal impairment; History of drug-induced hemolytic anemia or other anemia.

Use Cautiously in: Hepatic impairment; History of seizures; OB, Lactation, Pedi: Pregnancy, lactation or children ≤12 yr (safety not established); Geri: Appears on Beers list. Poorly tolerated due to anticholinergic effects.

Adverse Reactions/Side Effects

CNS: drowsiness, dizziness, confusion, headache, irritability, nervousness. **GI:** nausea, anorexia, dry mouth, GI upset, vomiting. **GU:** urinary retention. **Misc:** SEROTONIN SYNDROME.

Interactions

Drug-Drug: ↑ CNS depression with other **CNS depressants** including **alcohol**, **antihistamines**, **opioid analgesics**, and **sedative/hypnotics**. Drugs that affect serotonergic neurotransmitter systems, including **SSRIs**, **tricyclic antidepressants**, **SNRIs**, **MAOIs**, **fentanyl**, **buspirone**, **tramadol**, **amphetamines**, **linezolid**, **methylene blue**, and **triptans**, ↑ risk of serotonin syndrome.

Drug-Natural Products: Concomitant use of **kava-kava**, **valerian**, or **chamomile** can ↑ CNS depression.

Route/Dosage

PO (Adults): 800 mg 3–4 times daily.

Availability (generic available)

Tablets: 400 mg, 800 mg. **Cost:** *Generic*—$409.39/100.

NURSING IMPLICATIONS

Assessment

- Assess for pain, muscle stiffness, and range of motion before and periodically during therapy.
- Geri: Assess geriatric patients for anticholinergic effects (sedation and weakness).
- ***Lab Test Considerations:*** Monitor hepatic function tests closely in patients with pre-existing liver damage.
- May cause false-positive Benedict's tests.

Implementation

- Provide safety measures as indicated. Supervise ambulation and transfer.
- **PO:** Administer 3–4 times daily.

Patient/Family Teaching

- Instruct patient to take medication as directed. Take missed doses within 1 hr; if not, return to regular dosing schedule. Do not double doses.
- Encourage patient to comply with additional therapies prescribed for muscle spasm (rest, physical therapy, heat).
- Medication may cause dizziness, drowsiness, and blurred vision. Advise patient to avoid driving and other activities requiring alertness until response to drug is known.
- Instruct patient to make position changes slowly to minimize orthostatic hypotension.
- Advise patient to avoid concurrent use of alcohol and other CNS depressants while taking this medication.

- Instruct patient to notify health care professional if skin rash or yellowish discoloration of the skin or eyes occurs.
- Advise females of reproductive potential to notify health care professional if pregnancy is planned or suspected, or if breast feeding.
- Emphasize the importance of routine follow-up exams to monitor progress.

Evaluation/Desired Outcomes

- Decreased musculoskeletal pain and muscle spasticity.
- Increased range of motion.

metFORMIN (met-for-min)

Glucophage, Glucophage XR, Glumetza, ✽Glycon, Riomet, Riomet ER

Classification

Therapeutic: antidiabetics

Pharmacologic: biguanides

Indications

Management of type 2 diabetes mellitus; may be used with diet, insulin, or sulfonylurea oral hypoglycemics.

Action

Decreases hepatic glucose production. Decreases intestinal glucose absorption. Increases sensitivity to insulin. **Therapeutic Effects:** Maintenance of blood glucose.

Pharmacokinetics

Absorption: 50–60% absorbed after oral administration.

Distribution: Enters breast milk in concentrations similar to plasma.

Metabolism and Excretion: Eliminated almost entirely unchanged by the kidneys.

Half-life: 17.6 hr.

TIME/ACTION PROFILE (blood levels)

ROUTE	ONSET	PEAK	DURATION
PO	unknown	unknown	12 hr
XR	unknown	4–8 hr	24 hr

Contraindications/Precautions

Contraindicated in: Hypersensitivity; Metabolic acidosis (including diabetic ketoacidosis); Severe renal impairment (CCr <30 mL/min); Iodinated contrast imaging procedure in patients with CCr 30–60 mL/min, a history of liver disease, alcoholism or heart failure, or in those who will be administered intra-arterial iodinated contrast (discontinue metformin and reevaluate renal function 48 hr after imaging procedure; may restart therapy if renal function stable); Hepatic impairment.

Use Cautiously in: Mild to moderate renal impairment (initiation of therapy not recommended if CCr 30–45 mL/min; if CCr becomes <45 mL/min during therapy, assess risk-to-benefit of continuing therapy); Chronic alcohol use/abuse; Hypoxic states (acute HF, shock, MI, sepsis; discontinue metformin); Surgery (temporarily discontinue metformin when food and/or fluid intake is restricted); Pituitary deficiency or hyperthyroidism; OB, Lactation, Pedi: Pregnancy, lactation, or children <10 yr (safety not established; extended release for use in patients >17 yr only); Geri: May be at ↑ risk of lactic acidosis .

Adverse Reactions/Side Effects

F and E: LACTIC ACIDOSIS. **GI:** abdominal bloating, diarrhea, nausea, vomiting, unpleasant metallic taste. **Hemat:** ↓ vitamin B_{12} levels.

Interactions

Drug-Drug: Acute or chronic **alcohol** ingestion or **iodinated contrast media** ↑ risk of lactic acidosis. **Amiloride**, **digoxin**, **morphine**, **procainamide**, **quinidine**, **ranitidine**, **triamterene**, **trimethoprim**, **calcium channel blockers**, and **vancomycin** may compete for elimination pathways with metformin. Altered responses may occur. **Cimetidine** and **furosemide** may ↑ effects of metformin. **Nifedipine** ↑ absorption and effects.

Drug-Natural Products: Glucosamine may worsen blood glucose control. **Chromium** and **coenzyme Q-10** may produce ↑ hypoglycemic effects.

Route/Dosage

PO (Adults): 500 mg twice daily; may ↑ by 500 mg at weekly intervals up to 2000 mg/day. If doses >2000 mg/day are required, give in 3 divided doses (not to exceed 2500 mg/day) or 850 mg once daily; may ↑ by 850 mg at 2-wk intervals (in divided doses) up to 2550 mg/day in divided doses (up to 850 mg 3 times daily); *Extended-release tablets or suspension*—500 mg once daily with evening meal, may ↑ by 500 mg at weekly intervals up to 2000 mg once daily.

PO (Children 10–17 yr): 500 mg twice daily, may be ↑ by 500 mg/day at 1-wk intervals, up to 2000 mg/day in 2 divided doses. *Extended-release suspension*—500 mg once daily with evening meal, may ↑ by 500 mg at weekly intervals up to 2000 mg once daily.

Availability (generic available)

Extended-release oral suspension (Riomet ER) (strawberry flavor): 500 mg/5 mL. **Extended-release tablets (Glucophage XR, Glumetza):** 500 mg, 750 mg, 1000 mg. **Cost:** *Generic*—500 mg $74.50/100, 750 mg $119.70/100. **Oral solution (Riomet) (cherry flavor):** 500 mg/5 mL. **Cost:** $59.30/118 mL. **Tablets:** 500 mg, 850 mg, 1000 mg. **Cost:** *Generic*—500 mg $6.99/100, 850 mg $7.18/100, 1000 mg $7.01/100. ***In combination with:*** alogliptin (Kazano); canagliflozin (Invokamet, Invokamet XR); dapagliflozin (Xigduo XR); dapagliflozin and saxagliptin (Qternmet XR); empagliflozin (Synjardy); glipizide (Metaglip); glyburide (Glucovance); linagliptin (Jentadueto, Jentadueto XR); pioglitazone (Actoplus Met, Actoplus Met XR); repaglinide (PrandiMet); rosiglitazone (generic only); saxagliptin (Kombiglyze XR); and sitagliptin (Janumet, Janumet XR). See Appendix B.

NURSING IMPLICATIONS

Assessment

- When combined with oral sulfonylureas, observe for signs and symptoms of hypoglycemic reactions (abdominal pain, sweating, hunger, weakness, dizziness, headache, tremor, tachycardia, anxiety).
- Patients who have been well controlled on metformin who develop illness or laboratory abnormalities should be assessed for ketoacidosis or lactic acidosis. Assess serum electrolytes, ketones, glucose, and, if indicated, blood pH, lactate, pyruvate, and metformin levels. If either form of acidosis is present, discontinue metformin immediately and treat acidosis. Patients with severe renal impairment are at greatest risk for lactic acidosis.
- ***Lab Test Considerations:*** Monitor serum glucose and glycosylated hemoglobin periodically during therapy to evaluate effectiveness of therapy. May cause false-positive results for urine ketones.
- Assess renal function before initiating and at least annually during therapy. Monitor patients at risk for renal impairment (e.g., elderly) more frequently. Discontinue metformin if renal impairment occurs.
- Monitor serum folic acid and vitamin B_{12} every 1–2 yr in long-term therapy. Metformin may interfere with absorption.

Implementation

- Do not confuse metformin with metronidazole.
- Patients stabilized on a diabetic regimen who are exposed to stress, fever, trauma, infection, or surgery may require administration of insulin. Withhold metformin and reinstitute after resolution of acute episode.
- Temporarily discontinue metformin in patients requiring surgery involving restricted intake of food and fluids. Resume metformin when oral intake has resumed and renal function is normal.
- Withhold metformin before or at the time of studies requiring IV administration of iodinated contrast media and for 48 hr after study.
- **PO:** Administer metformin with meals to minimize GI effects.
- XR tablets must be swallowed whole; do not crush, dissolve, or chew. Administer *Glumetza* with the evening meal.

Patient/Family Teaching

- Instruct patient to take metformin at the same time each day, as directed. Take missed doses as soon as possible unless almost time for next dose. Do not double doses. Instruct parent/caregiver to read the *Medication Guide* prior to use and with each Rx refill; new information may be available.
- Explain to patient that metformin helps control hyperglycemia but does not cure diabetes. Therapy is usually long term.
- Encourage patient to follow prescribed diet, medication, and exercise regimen to prevent hyperglycemic or hypoglycemic episodes.
- Review signs of hypoglycemia and hyperglycemia with patient. If hypoglycemia occurs, advise patient to take a glass of orange juice or 2–3 tsp of sugar, honey, or corn syrup dissolved in water, and notify health care professional.
- Instruct patient in proper testing of blood glucose and urine ketones. These tests should be monitored closely during periods of stress or illness and health care professional notified if significant changes occur.
- Explain to patient the risk of lactic acidosis and the potential need for discontinuation of metformin therapy if a severe infection, dehydration, or severe or continuing diarrhea occurs or if medical tests or surgery is required. Symptoms of lactic acidosis (chills, diarrhea, dizziness, low BP, muscle pain, abdominal pain, sleepiness, slow heartbeat or pulse, dyspnea, or weakness) should be reported to health care professional immediately.
- Advise patient to notify health care professional of all Rx or OTC medications, vitamins, or herbal products being taken and to consult with health care professional before taking other medications or alcohol.
- Inform patient that metformin may cause an unpleasant or metallic taste that usually resolves spontaneously.
- Inform patients taking XR tablets that inactive ingredients resembling XR tablet may appear in stools.
- Advise patient to inform health care professional of medication regimen before treatment or surgery.
- Advise patient to report the occurrence of diarrhea, nausea, vomiting, and stomach pain or fullness to health care professional.
- Rep: Insulin is the recommended method of controlling blood glucose during pregnancy. Counsel female patients to use a form of contraception other than oral contraceptives and to notify health care professional promptly if pregnancy is planned or suspected, or if breast feeding.
- Advise patient to carry a form of sugar (sugar packets, candy) and identification describing disease process and medication regimen at all times.
- Emphasize the importance of routine follow-up exams and regular testing of blood glucose, glycosylated hemoglobin, renal function, and hematologic parameters.

Evaluation/Desired Outcomes

- Control of blood glucose levels without the appearance of hypoglycemic or hyperglycemic episodes.

Control may be achieved within a few days, but full effect of therapy may be delayed for up to 2 wk. If patient has not responded to metformin after 4 wk of maximum dose therapy, an oral sulfonylurea may be added. If satisfactory results are not obtained with 1–3 mo of concurrent therapy, oral agents may be discontinued and insulin therapy instituted.

REMS HIGH ALERT

methadone (meth-a-done)

Dolophine, ✱Metadol, ✱Metadol-D, Methadose

Classification

Therapeutic: opioid analgesics

Pharmacologic: opioid agonists

Schedule II

Indications

Moderate to severe chronic pain in opioid-tolerant patients requiring use of daily, around-the-clock long-term opioid treatment and for which alternative treatment options are inadequate (extended-release). Detoxification and maintenance therapy for opioid use disorder. **Unlabeled Use:** Neonatal abstinence syndrome.

Action

Binds to opiate receptors in the CNS. Alters the perception of and response to painful stimuli, while producing generalized CNS depression. **Therapeutic Effects:** Decrease in severity of pain. Suppression of withdrawal symptoms during detoxification and maintenance from heroin and other opioids.

Pharmacokinetics

Absorption: Well absorbed from all sites (50% absorbed following oral administration).

Distribution: Widely distributed. Crosses the placenta; enters breast milk.

Protein Binding: High.

Metabolism and Excretion: Mostly metabolized by the liver; some metabolites are active and may accumulate with chronic administration.

Half-life: 15–25 hr; ↑ with chronic use.

TIME/ACTION PROFILE (analgesic effect)

ROUTE	ONSET	PEAK	DURATION
PO	30–60 min	90–120 min	4–12 hr
IM, subcut	10–20 min	60–120 min	4–6 hr

Contraindications/Precautions

Contraindicated in: Hypersensitivity; Significant respiratory depression; Acute or severe bronchial asthma; Paralytic ileus; Known alcohol intolerance (some oral solutions); Concurrent MAO inhibitor therapy.

Use Cautiously in: Structural heart disease, concomitant diuretic use, hypokalemia, hypomagnesemia, history of arrhythmia/syncope, or other risk factors for arrhythmias; Concurrent use of drugs that prolong the QTc interval or are CYP3A4 inhibitors; Head trauma; Seizure disorders; ↑ intracranial pressure; Severe renal, hepatic, or pulmonary disease; Hypothyroidism; Adrenal insufficiency; Alcoholism; Undiagnosed abdominal pain; Prostatic hyperplasia or ureteral stricture; OB: Use with addiction control: weigh risk against potential for illicit drug use. Counsel mother about potential harm to fetus. Prolonged use of methadone during pregnancy can result in neonatal opioid withdrawal syndrome; Lactation: Appears in breast milk. Weigh risks against potential for illicit drug use. Counsel mother about potential harm to infant and to wean breast feeding slowly to prevent abstinence syndrome; Geri: ↑ risk of respiratory depression (dose ↓ suggested).

M

Adverse Reactions/Side Effects

CNS: confusion, sedation, dizziness, dysphoria, euphoria, floating feeling, hallucinations, headache, unusual dreams. **CV:** TORSADES DE POINTES, hypotension, bradycardia, QT interval prolongation. **Derm:** flushing, sweating. **EENT:** blurred vision, diplopia, miosis. **Endo:** adrenal insufficiency. **GI:** constipation, nausea, vomiting. **GU:** urinary retention. **Resp:** RESPIRATORY DEPRESSION. **Misc:** physical dependence, psychological dependence, tolerance.

Interactions

Drug-Drug: Use with extreme caution in patients receiving **MAO inhibitors** (may result in severe, unpredictable reactions—↓ initial dose of methadone to 25% of usual dose). Use with extreme caution with any drug known to potentially prolong QT interval, including **class I and III antiarrhythmics**, some **neuroleptics** and **tricyclic antidepressants**, and **calcium channel blockers**. Use with extreme caution with CYP3A4 inhibitors, including **ketoconazole**, **itraconazole**, **erythromycin**, **clarithromycin**, **calcium channel blockers**, or **voriconazole**. Concurrent use with **laxatives**, **diuretics**, or **mineralocorticoids** may ↑ risk of hypomagnesemia or hypokalemia and ↑ risk of arrhythmias. Drugs that affect serotonergic neurotransmitter systems, including **tricyclic antidepressants**, **SSRIs**, **SNRIs**, **MAO inhibitors**, **TCAs**, **tramadol**, **trazodone**, **mirtazapine**, **5–HT$_3$ receptor antagonists**, **linezolid**, **methylene blue**, and **triptans** ↑ risk of serotonin syndrome. Concurrent use of **CYP3A4 inhibitors**, **CYP2C9 inhibitors**, **CYP2C19 inhibitors**, or **CYP2D6 inhibitors** including **ritonavir**, **ketoconazole**, **itraconazole**, **fluconazole**, **clarithromycin**, **erythromycin**, **nefazodone**, **dilti-**

azem, **verapamil**, **nelfinavir**, **fosamprenavir**, and **fluvoxamine** ↑ levels and risk of opioid toxicity; careful monitoring during initiation, dose changes, or discontinuation of the inhibitor is recommended. Concurrent use with **CYP3A4 inducers**, **CYP2C9 inducers**, or **CYP2C19 inducers** including **barbiturates**, **carbamazepine**, **efavirenz**, **corticosteroids**, **modafinil**, **nevirapine**, **oxcarbazepine**, **phenobarbital**, **phenytoin**, **rifabutin**, or **rifampin** may ↓ levels and analgesia; if inducers are discontinued or dosage ↓, patients should be monitored for signs of opioid toxicity and necessary dose adjustments should be made. Use with **benzodiazepines** or other **CNS depressants** including other **opioids**, **non-benzodiazepine sedative/hypnotics**, **anxiolytics**, **general anesthetics**, **muscle relaxants**, **antipsychotics**, and **alcohol** may cause profound sedation, respiratory depression, coma, and death; reserve concurrent use for when alternative treatment options are inadequate. Administration of **agonist/antagonist opioids** may precipitate opioid withdrawal in physically dependent patients. **Nalbuphine** may ↓ analgesia. **Interferons (alpha)** may ↓ metabolism and ↑ effects. May ↑ blood levels and effects of **zidovudine** and **desipramine**. May ↓ level and effects of **didanosine** and **stavudine**. Concurrent abuse of methadone with **benzodiazepines** has resulted in death.

Drug-Natural Products: St. John's wort ↑ metabolism and ↓ blood levels, concurrent use may result in withdrawal. **Kava-kava**, **valerian**, or **chamomile** can ↑ CNS depression.

Route/Dosage

Larger doses may be required for analgesia during chronic therapy; interval may be ↓/dose ↑ if pain recurs.

PO (Adults and Children ≥50 kg): *Usual starting dose for moderate to severe pain in opioid-naive patients*—2.5 mg every 8–12 hr; *Opioid detoxification*—15–40 mg once daily or amount needed to prevent withdrawal. Dose may be ↓ every 1–2 days; maintenance dose is determined on an individual basis.

PO (Adults and Children <50 kg): *Analgesic*—0.1 mg/kg/dose every 4 hr for 2–3 doses then every 6–8 hr prn; maximum: 10 mg/dose. *Iatrogenic narcotic dependency*—0.05–0.1 mg/kg/dose every 6 hr; ↑ by 0.05 mg/kg/dose until withdrawal symptoms controlled; after 1–2 days lengthen dosing interval to every 12–24 hr; taper by ↓ dose by 0.05 mg/kg/day.

PO, IV (Neonates): Initial 0.05–0.2 mg/kg/dose every 12–24 hr or 0.5 mg/kg/day divided every 8 hr; taper dose by 10–20% per wk over 1–1.5 mo.

IV, IM, Subcut (Adults and Children ≥50 kg): *Analgesic*—10 mg every 6–8 hr. *Opioid detoxification*—15–40 mg once daily or amount needed to prevent withdrawal. Dose may be ↓ every 1–2 days; maintenance dose is determined on an individual basis.

IV, IM, Subcut (Adults and Children <50 kg): *Analgesic*—0.1 mg/kg every 6–8 hr; maximum: 10 mg/dose.

Availability (generic available)

Oral concentrate (cherry and unflavored): 10 mg/mL. **Oral solution (contains alcohol) (citrus):** 5 mg/5 mL, 10 mg/5 mL. **Solution for injection:** 10 mg/mL. **Tablets:** 🍁 1 mg, 5 mg, 10 mg, 🍁 25 mg. **Tablets for oral suspension:** 40 mg (available only to licensed detoxification/maintenance programs).

NURSING IMPLICATIONS

Assessment

- **Pain:** Assess type, location, and intensity of pain prior to and 1–2 hr (peak) following administration. When titrating opioid doses, increases of 25–50% should be administered until there is either a 50% reduction in the patient's pain rating on a numeric or visual analogue scale or the patient reports satisfactory pain relief. Dose increases should be made no more frequently than every 3–5 days because of variability in half-life between patients. Cumulative effects of this medication may require periodic dose adjustments.
- Doses of methadone for patients on methadone maintenance only prevent withdrawal symptoms; *no analgesia is provided*. Additional opioid doses are required for treatment of pain.
- An equianalgesic chart (see Appendix J) should be used when changing routes or when changing from one opioid to another.
- Assess BP, pulse, and respirations before and periodically during administration. If respiratory rate is <10/min, assess level of sedation. Dose may need to be decreased by 25–50%. Initial drowsiness will diminish with continued use.
- Assess bowel function routinely. Prevention of constipation should be instituted with increased intake of fluids and bulk and with laxatives to minimize constipating effects. Stimulant laxatives should be administered routinely if opioid use exceeds 2–3 days, unless contraindicated. Consider drugs for opioid induced constipation.
- Prolonged use may lead to physical and psychological dependence and tolerance. This should not prevent patient from receiving adequate analgesia. Patients who receive methadone for pain rarely develop psychological dependence. Progressively higher doses may be required to relieve pain with long-term therapy.
- Assess for history of structural heart disease, arrhythmia, and syncope. Obtain a pretreatment ECG to measure QTc interval and follow-up ECG within 30 days and annually. Additional ECGs recommended if dose >100 m g/day or if patients have unexplained syncope or seizures. If QTc interval is >450 ms but <500 ms, discuss potential risks and benefits with patients and monitor more frequently. If the QTc interval >500 ms, consider discontinuing or reducing dose; eliminating contributing factors (drugs that promote hypokalemia) or using an alternative therapy.

- Assess risk for opioid addiction, abuse, or misuse prior to administration. Abuse or misuse by crushing, chewing, snorting, or injecting dissolved product will result in uncontrolled delivery of methadone and can result in overdose and death.
- **Opioid Detoxification:** Assess patient for signs of opioid withdrawal (irritability, runny nose and eyes, abdominal cramps, body aches, sweating, loss of appetite, shivering, unusually large pupils, trouble sleeping, weakness, yawning). Methadone maintenance is undertaken only by federally approved treatment centers. This does not preclude maintenance for addicts hospitalized for other conditions and who require temporary maintenance during their care.
- ***Lab Test Considerations:*** May ↑ plasma amylase and lipase levels.
- ***Toxicity and Overdose:*** If an opioid antagonist is required to reverse respiratory depression or coma, naloxone is the antidote. Dilute the 0.4-mg ampule of naloxone in 10 mL of 0.9% NaCl and administer 0.5 mL (0.02 mg) by IV push every 2 min. For children and patients weighing <40 kg, dilute 0.1 mg of naloxone in 10 mL of 0.9% NaCl for a concentration of 10 mcg/mL and administer 0.5 mcg/kg every 2 min. Titrate dose to avoid withdrawal, seizures, and severe pain.

Implementation

- ***High Alert:*** Do not confuse methadone with dexmethylphenidate, ketorolac, memantine, Mephyton (phytonadione), methylphenidate, or metolazone.
- Explain therapeutic value of medication prior to administration to enhance the analgesic effect.
- Regularly administered doses may be more effective than prn administration. Analgesic is more effective if administered before pain becomes severe. For patients in chronic severe pain, the oral solution containing 5 or 10 mg/5 mL is recommended on a fixed dose schedule.
- Coadministration with nonopioid analgesics may have additive analgesic effects and may permit lower doses.
- Medication should be discontinued gradually after long-term use to prevent withdrawal symptoms. For patients on long-acting agents who are physically opioid-dependent, initiate the taper by a small enough increment (e.g., no greater than 10% to 25% of total daily dose) to avoid withdrawal symptoms, and proceed with dose-lowering at an interval of every 2 to 4 wk. Patients who have been taking opioids for briefer periods of time may tolerate a more rapid taper.
- FDA strongly encourages health care professionals to complete a REMS-compliant education program that includes all the elements of the FDA Education *Blueprint for Health Care Providers Involved in the Management or Support of Patients with Pain,* available at www.fda.gov/OpioidAnalgesicREMSBlueprint. Information on programs can be found at 1-800-503-0784 or www.opioidanalgesicrems.com.
- **PO:** Doses may be administered with food or milk to minimize GI irritation.
- Dilute each dose of 10 mg/mL oral concentrate with at least 30 mL of water or other liquid prior to administration.
- Diskettes (dispersible tablets) are to be dissolved and used for detoxification and maintenance treatment only. Available only to licensed detoxification/maintenance programs.
- **Subcut, IM:** IM is the preferred parenteral route for repeated doses. Subcut administration may cause tissue irritation.

Patient/Family Teaching

- Instruct patient on how and when to ask for and take pain medication.
- Instruct patient to take methadone exactly as directed. If dose is less effective after a few wk, do not increase dose without consulting health care professional. Discuss safe use, risks, and proper storage and disposal of opioid analgesics with patients and caregivers with each Rx. The Patient Counseling Guide (PCG) is available at www.fda.gov/OpioidAnalgesicREMSPCG.
- Advise patient that methadone is a drug with known abuse potential. Protect it from theft, and never give to anyone other than the individual for whom it was prescribed. Store out of sight and reach of children, and in a location not accessible by others.
- May cause drowsiness or dizziness. Advise patient to call for assistance when ambulating or smoking and to avoid driving or other activities requiring alertness until response to medication is known.
- Inform patient of the potential for arrhythmias and emphasize the importance of regular ECGs.
- Caution patient to notify health care professional if signs of overdose (difficult or shallow breathing, extreme tiredness or sleepiness, blurred vision, inability to think, talk, or walk normally, and feelings of faintness, dizziness, or confusion) occur. Methadone has a prolonged action causing increased risk of overdose.
- Advise patient to change positions slowly to minimize orthostatic hypotension.
- Advise patient to tell health care professional what medications they are taking and to avoid taking new Rx, OTC, vitamins, or herbal products without consulting health care professional. Caution patient to avoid concurrent use of alcohol or other CNS depressants with this medication.

- Encourage patient to turn, cough, and breathe deeply every 2 hr to prevent atelectasis.
- Rep: Advise patient to notify health care professional if pregnancy is planned or suspected, or if breast feeding. Inform patient of potential for neonatal opioid withdrawal syndrome with prolonged use during pregnancy. Monitor neonate for signs and symptoms of withdrawal symptoms (irritability, hyperactivity and abnormal sleep pattern, high pitched cry, tremor, vomiting, diarrhea, and/or failure to gain weight); usually occur the first days after birth.

Evaluation/Desired Outcomes

- Decrease in severity of pain without a significant alteration in level of consciousness or respiratory status.
- Prevention of withdrawal symptoms in detoxification from heroin and other opioid analgesics.

methIMAzole (meth-**im**-a-zole)

Tapazole

Classification

Therapeutic: antithyroid agents

Indications

Palliative treatment of hyperthyroidism. Used as an adjunct to control hyperthyroidism in preparation for thyroidectomy or radioactive iodine therapy.

Action

Inhibits the synthesis of thyroid hormones. **Therapeutic Effects:** Decreased signs and symptoms of hyperthyroidism.

Pharmacokinetics

Absorption: Rapidly absorbed following oral administration.

Distribution: Crosses the placenta and enters breast milk in high concentrations.

Metabolism and Excretion: Mostly metabolized by the liver; <10% eliminated unchanged by the kidneys.

Half-life: 3–5 hr.

TIME/ACTION PROFILE (effect on thyroid function)

ROUTE	ONSET	PEAK	DURATION
PO	1 wk	4–10 wk	wk

Contraindications/Precautions

Contraindicated in: Hypersensitivity.

Use Cautiously in: Patients with ↓ bone marrow reserve; Patients >40 yr (↑ risk of agranulocytosis); OB: May cause congenital malformations (especially if used during 1st trimester; use during pregnancy only if maternal benefit outweighs potential risk to fetus; Lactation: May be used while breast feeding.

Adverse Reactions/Side Effects

CNS: drowsiness, headache, vertigo. **Derm:** rash, skin discoloration, urticaria. **GI:** HEPATOTOXICITY, diarrhea, loss of taste, nausea, parotitis, vomiting. **Hemat:** AGRANULOCYTOSIS, anemia, leukopenia, thrombocytopenia. **MS:** arthralgia. **Misc:** fever, lymphadenopathy.

Interactions

Drug-Drug: Additive bone marrow depression with **antineoplastics** or **radiation therapy**. Antithyroid effect may be ↓ by **potassium iodide** or **amiodarone**. ↑ risk of agranulocytosis with **phenothiazines**. May alter response to **warfarin** and **digoxin**.

Route/Dosage

PO (Adults): *Initial*—15–60 mg/day in 3 divided doses. *Maintenance*—5–15 mg once daily.

PO (Children): *Initial*—0.4 mg/kg/day in 3 divided doses. *Maintenance*—0.2 mg/kg/day in single dose or 2 divided doses.

Availability (generic available)

Tablets: 5 mg, 10 mg.

NURSING IMPLICATIONS

Assessment

- Monitor response for symptoms of hyperthyroidism or thyrotoxicosis (tachycardia, palpitations, nervousness, insomnia, fever, diaphoresis, heat intolerance, tremors, weight loss, diarrhea).
- Assess for development of hypothyroidism (intolerance to cold, constipation, dry skin, headache, listlessness, tiredness, or weakness). Dose adjustment may be required.
- Assess for skin rash or swelling of cervical lymph nodes. Treatment may be discontinued if this occurs.
- ***Lab Test Considerations:*** Monitor thyroid function studies prior to therapy, monthly during initial therapy, and every 2–3 mo during therapy.
- Monitor WBC and differential counts periodically during therapy. Agranulocytosis may develop rapidly; usually occurs during the first 2 mo and is more common in patients over 40 yr and those receiving >40 mg/day. This necessitates discontinuation of therapy.
- May cause ↑ AST, ALT, LDH, alkaline phosphatase, serum bilirubin, and prothrombin time.

Implementation

- Do not confuse methimazole with metolazone or methazolamide.
- **PO:** Administer at same time in relation to meals every day. Food may either increase or decrease absorption.

Patient/Family Teaching

- Instruct patient to take medication as directed, around the clock. Take missed doses as soon as remembered; take both doses together if almost time for next dose; check with health care professional if more than 1 dose is missed. Consult health care professional prior to discontinuing medication.

- Instruct patient to monitor weight 2–3 times weekly. Notify health care professional of significant changes.
- May cause drowsiness. Caution patient to avoid driving or other activities requiring alertness until response to medication is known.
- Advise patient to consult health care professional regarding dietary sources of iodine (iodized salt, shellfish).
- Advise patient to report sore throat, fever, chills, headache, malaise, weakness, yellowing of eyes or skin, unusual bleeding or bruising, rash, or symptoms of hyperthyroidism or hypothyroidism promptly.
- Instruct patient to notify health care professional of all Rx or OTC medications, vitamins, or herbal products being taken and to consult with health care professional before taking other medications.
- Advise patient to carry identification describing medication regimen at all times.
- Advise patient to notify health care professional of medication regimen prior to treatment or surgery.
- Rep: Advise female patients of reproductive potential to notify health care professional if pregnancy is planned or suspected or if breast feeding. May cause fetal harm, especially during 1st trimester. If breast feeding, monitor infant thyroid levels weekly or biweekly.
- Emphasize the importance of routine exams to monitor progress and to check for side effects.

Evaluation/Desired Outcomes

- Decrease in severity of symptoms of hyperthyroidism (lowered pulse rate and weight gain).
- Return of thyroid function studies to normal.
- May be used as short-term adjunctive therapy to prepare patient for thyroidectomy or radiation therapy or may be used in treatment of hyperthyroidism. Treatment from 6 mo to several yr may be necessary, usually averaging 1 yr.

HIGH ALERT

methotrexate (meth-o-**trex**-ate)

Metoject, Otrexup, Rasuvo, ~~Rheumatrex~~, Trexall, Xatmep

Classification

Therapeutic: antineoplastics, antirheumatics (DMARDs), immunosuppressants

Pharmacologic: antimetabolites

Indications

Alone or with other treatment modalities in the treatment of: Trophoblastic neoplasms (choriocarcinoma, chorioadenoma destruens, hydatidiform mole), Leukemias, Breast carcinoma, Head carcinoma, Neck carcinoma, Lung carcinoma. Severe psoriasis, rheumatoid arthritis, and polyarticular juvenile idiopathic arthritis unresponsive to conventional therapy. Treatment of mycosis fungoides (cutaneous T-cell lymphoma).

Action

Interferes with folic acid metabolism. Result is inhibition of DNA synthesis and cell reproduction (cell-cycle S-phase–specific). Also has immunosuppressive activity. **Therapeutic Effects:** Death of rapidly replicating cells, particularly malignant ones, and immunosuppression.

Pharmacokinetics

Absorption: Small doses are well absorbed from the GI tract. Larger doses incompletely absorbed.

Distribution: Actively transported across cell membranes, widely distributed. Does not reach therapeutic concentrations in the CSF. Crosses placenta; enters breast milk in low concentrations. Absorption in children is variable (23–95%) and dose-dependent.

Metabolism and Excretion: Excreted mostly unchanged by the kidneys.

Half-life: *Low dose*—3–10 hr; *high dose*—8–15 hr (↑ in renal impairment).

TIME/ACTION PROFILE (effects on blood counts)

ROUTE	ONSET	PEAK	DURATION
PO, IM, IV	4–7 days	7–14 days	21 days
Subcut	unknown	unknown	unknown

Contraindications/Precautions

Contraindicated in: Hypersensitivity; Alcoholism or hepatic impairment; Immunosuppression; ↓ bone marrow reserve; OB, Lactation: Pregnancy or lactation; Pedi: Products containing benzyl alcohol should not be used in neonates.

Use Cautiously in: Renal impairment (CCr must be ≥60 mL/min prior to therapy); Patients with childbearing potential; Active infections; Geri: May be more sensitive to toxicity and adverse events.

Adverse Reactions/Side Effects

CNS: arachnoiditis (IT use only), dizziness, drowsiness, headache, malaise, seizures. **Derm:** ERYTHEMA MULTIFORME, STEVENS-JOHNSON SYNDROME, TOXIC EPIDERMAL NECROLYSIS, alopecia, painful plaque erosions (during psoriasis treatment), photosensitivity, pruritus, rash, skin ulceration, soft tissue necrosis, urticaria. **EENT:** blurred vision, dysarthria, transient blindness. **GI:** HEPATOTOXICITY, anorexia, diarrhea, nausea, stomatitis, vomiting. **GU:** nephropathy, acute renal failure, infertility. **Hemat:** APLASTIC ANEMIA, anemia, leukopenia, thrombocytopenia. **Metab:** hy-

peruricemia. **MS:** osteonecrosis, stress fracture.
Resp: PULMONARY FIBROSIS, interstitial pneumonitis.
Misc: chills, fever.

Interactions

Drug-Drug: The following drugs may ↑ hematologic toxicity of methotrexate: high-dose **salicylates**, **NSAIDs**, **oral hypoglycemic agents (sulfonylureas)**, **phenytoin**, **tetracyclines**, **probenecid**, **trimethoprim/sulfamethoxazole**, **pyrimethamine**, **proton pump inhibitors** and **chloramphenicol**. ↑ hepatotoxicity with other **hepatotoxic drugs** including **azathioprine**, **sulfasalazine**, and **retinoids**. ↑ nephrotoxicity with other **nephrotoxic drugs**. ↑ bone marrow depression with other **antineoplastics** or **radiation therapy**. **Radiation therapy** ↑ risk of soft tissue necrosis and osteonecrosis. May ↓ antibody response to **live-virus vaccines** and ↑ risk of adverse reactions. ↑ risk of neurologic reactions with **acyclovir** (IT methotrexate only). **Asparaginase** may ↓ effects of methotrexate. **Nitrous oxide** may ↑ risk of toxicity; avoid concurrent use.

Drug-Natural Products: Concomitant use with **echinacea** and **melatonin** may interfere with immunosuppression. **Caffeine** may ↓ efficacy of methotrexate, similar effect may occur with **guarana**.

Route/Dosage

Trophoblastic Neoplasms

PO, IM (Adults): 15–30 mg/day for 5 days; repeat after 1 or more wk for 3–5 courses.

Breast Cancer

IV (Adults): 40 mg/m² on days 1 and 8 (with other agents; many regimens are used).

Leukemia

PO (Adults): *Induction*—3.3 mg/m²/day, usually with prednisone.
PO, IM (Adults): *Maintenance*—20–30 mg/m² twice weekly.
PO (Children): *Oral solution*—20 mg/m² once weekly.
IV (Adults): 2.5 mg/kg every 2 wk.
IT (Adults): 12 mg/m² or 15 mg.
IT (Children ≥3 yr): 12 mg.
IT (Children 2 yr): 10 mg.
IT (Children 1 yr): 8 mg.
IT (Children <1 yr): 6 mg.

Osteosarcoma

IV (Adults): 12 g/m² as a 4-hr infusion followed by leucovorin rescue, usually as part of a combination chemotherapeutic regimen (or ↑ dose until peak serum methotrexate level is 1×10^{-3} M/L but not to exceed 15 g/m²; 12 courses are given starting 4 wk after surgery and repeated at scheduled intervals.

Psoriasis

Therapy may be preceded by a 5–10-mg test dose.
PO, IM, Subcut, IV (Adults): 10–25 mg/weekly (not to exceed 30 mg/wk); Otrexup may be used when dose is 10–25 mg/wk.

Rheumatoid Arthritis

PO, Subcut (Adults): 7.5 mg weekly (not to exceed 20 mg/wk); when response is obtained, dose should be ↓. Otrexup may be used when dose is 10–20 mg/wk.

Polyarticular Juvenile Idiopathic Arthritis

PO (Children): 10 mg/m² once weekly initially, may be ↑ up to 20–30 mg/m², however response may be better if doses >20 mg/m² are given IM or subcut; Otrexup may be used when dose is 10–25 mg/wk.

Mycosis Fungoides

PO, IM, Subcut (Adults): 5–50 mg once weekly, if response is poor, dose may be changed to 15–37.5 mg twice weekly.
IM (Adults): 50 mg once weekly or 25 mg twice weekly.

Availability (generic available)

Oral solution: 2.5 mg/mL. **Powder for injection (requires reconstitution):** 1 g/vial. **Solution for injection:** 25 mg/mL. **Cost:** *Generic*—$115.02/30 mL. **Solution for injection (preservative free):** 25 mg/mL. **Solution for subcutaneous injection (Otrexup):** 10 mg/0.4 mL, 12.5 mg/0.4 mL, 15 mg/0.4 mL, 17.5 mg/0.4 mL, 20 mg/0.4 mL, 22.5 mg/0.4 mL, 25 mg/0.4 mL. **Solution for subcutaneous injection (Rasuvo):** 7.5 mg/0.15 mL, 10 mg/0.2 mL, 12.5 mg/0.25 mL, 15 mg/0.3 mL, 17.5 mg/0.35 mL, 20 mg/0.4 mL, 22.5 mg/0.45 mL, 25 mg/0.5 mL, 30 mg/0.6 mL. **Tablets:** 2.5 mg, 5 mg, 7.5 mg, 10 mg, 15 mg. **Cost:** 2.5 mg $96.36/30, 5 mg $352.75/30, 7.5 mg $529.13/30, 10 mg $705.50/30, 15 mg $1,058.27/30.

NURSING IMPLICATIONS

Assessment

- Monitor vital signs periodically during administration. Report significant changes.
- Monitor for abdominal pain, diarrhea, or stomatitis; therapy may need to be discontinued.
- Monitor for bone marrow depression. Assess for bleeding (bleeding gums, bruising, petechiae, guaiac stools, urine, and emesis) and avoid IM injections and taking rectal temperatures if platelet count is low. Apply pressure to venipuncture sites for 10 min. Assess for signs of infection during neutropenia. Anemia may occur. Monitor for increased fatigue, dyspnea, and orthostatic hypotension.
- Monitor intake and output ratios and daily weights. Report significant changes in totals.
- Monitor for symptoms of pulmonary toxicity, which may manifest early as a dry, nonproductive cough.
- Monitor for symptoms of gout (increased uric acid, joint pain, edema). Encourage patient to drink at

least 2 L of fluid each day. Allopurinol and alkalinization of urine may be used to decrease uric acid levels.

- Assess nutritional status. Administering an antiemetic prior to and periodically during therapy and adjusting diet as tolerated may help maintain fluid and electrolyte balance and nutritional status.
- Assess for rash periodically during therapy. May cause Stevens-Johnson syndrome. Discontinue therapy if severe or if accompanied with fever, general malaise, fatigue, muscle or joint aches, blisters, oral lesions, conjunctivitis, hepatitis, and/or eosinophilia.
- **IT:** Assess for development of nuchal rigidity, headache, fever, confusion, drowsiness, dizziness, weakness, or seizures.
- **Rheumatoid Arthritis:** Assess patient for pain and range of motion prior to and periodically during therapy.
- **Psoriasis:** Assess skin lesions prior to and periodically during therapy.
- ***Lab Test Considerations:*** Obtain a negative pregnancy test prior to starting therapy.
- Monitor CBC and differential prior to and frequently during therapy. The nadir of leukopenia and thrombocytopenia occurs in 7–14 days. Leukocyte and thrombocyte counts usually recover 7 days after the nadirs. Notify health care professional of any sudden drop in values.
- Monitor renal (BUN and creatinine) and hepatic function (AST, ALT, bilirubin, and LDH) prior to and every 1–2 mo during therapy. Urine pH should be monitored prior to high-dose methotrexate therapy and every 6 hr during leucovorin rescue. Urine pH should be kept above 7.0 to prevent renal damage.
- May cause ↑ serum uric acid concentrations, especially during initial treatment of leukemia and lymphoma.
- ***Toxicity and Overdose:*** Monitor serum methotrexate levels every 12–24 hr during high-dose therapy until levels are $<5 \times 10$ M. This monitoring is essential to plan correct leucovorin dose and determine duration of rescue therapy.
- With high-dose therapy, patient must receive leucovorin rescue within 24–48 hr to prevent fatal toxicity. Glucarpidase may be used for patients with impaired renal function. In cases of massive overdose, hydration and urinary alkalization with sodium bicarbonate are required to prevent renal tubule damage. Monitor fluid and electrolyte status; patients must be well hydrated. Intermittent hemodialysis using a high-flux dialyzer may be used for clearance until levels are <0.05 micromolar. Methotrexate should be delayed until recovery if WBC <1500/microliter, neutrophil count <200/microliter, platelet count <75,000/microliter, serum bilirubin level >1.2m g/dL, AST level >450 U, mucositis is present, until evidence of healing, persistent pleural effusion is present, should be drained dry prior to infusion. Adequate renal function is required. Serum creatinine must be normal, creatinine clearance must be >60 mL/min, before initiation of therapy. Serum creatinine must be measured before each course of therapy. If ↑ by ≥50% of a prior value, creatinine clearance must be >60 mL/min, even if serum creatinine is within normal range.

Implementation

- ***High Alert:*** Fatalities have occurred with chemotherapeutic agents. Before administering, clarify all ambiguous orders; double-check single, daily, and course-of-therapy dose limits; have second practitioner independently double-check original order, calculations and infusion pump settings. Methotrexate for non-oncologic use is given at a much lower dose and frequency—often just once a wk. Do not confuse non-oncologic dosing regimens with dosing regimens for cancer patients. Do not confuse methotrexate with metolazone.
- Solutions for injection should be prepared in a biologic cabinet. Wear gloves, gown, and mask while handling medication. Discard equipment in specially designated containers.
- *Otrexup* and *Rasuvo* are not indicated for treatment of neoplastic diseases. Not for patients requiring oral, IM, IV, intra-arterial, or IT dosing, doses <10 mg/wk, doses >25 mg/wk, high-dose regimens, or dose adjustments of less than 5 mg increments.
- **Subcut:** *Otrexup* and *Rasuvo* are single-dose autoinjectors. Inject once weekly in abdomen or upper thigh. Avoid areas where skin is tender, bruised, red, scaly, hard, or has scars or stretch marks. Solution is clear and yellow; do not inject solutions that are discolored or contain particulate matter.

IV Administration

- **IV Push:** ***Diluent:*** Reconstitute each vial with 25 mL of 0.9% NaCl. Use sterile preservative-free diluents for high-dose regimens to prevent complications from large amounts of benzyl alcohol. Do not use preparations that are discolored or that contain a precipitate. Reconstitute immediately before use. Discard unused portion. ***Concentration:*** <25 mg/mL for IV push and intermittent/continuous infusions. ***Rate:*** Administer at a rate of 10 mg/min into Y-site of a free-flowing IV.
- **Intermittent/Continuous Infusion:** ***Diluent:*** Doses >100–300 mg/m² may also be diluted in D5W, D5/0.9% NaCl, or 0.9% NaCl and infused as intermittent or continuous infusion. ***Rate:*** Administration rates of 4–20 mg/hr have been used.

- **Y-Site Compatibility:** acyclovir, alemtuzumab, alfentanil, allopurinol, amifostine, amikacin, aminophylline, amiodarone, amphotericin B lipid complex, amphotericin B liposome, ampicillin, ampicillin/sulbactam, anidulafungin, argatroban, azithromycin, aztreonam, bivalirudin, bleomycin, bumetanide, buprenorphine, butorphanol, calcium chloride, calcium gluconate, carboplatin, carmustine, cefazolin, cefepime, cefotaxime, cefotetan, cefoxitin, ceftazidime, ceftriaxone, cefuroxime, ciprofloxacin, cisatracurium, cisplatin, clindamycin, cyclophosphamide, cyclosporine, cytarabine, dactinomycin, daunorubicin hydrochloride, dexmedetomidine, digoxin, diphenhydramine, docetaxel, doxorubicin hydrochloride, doxorubicin liposomal, enalaprilat, ephedrine, epinephrine, epirubicin, ertapenem, erythromycin, esmolol, etoposide, etoposide phosphate, famotidine, fenoldopam, fentanyl, filgrastim, fluconazole, fludarabine, fluorouracil, foscarnet, fosphenytoin, furosemide, ganciclovir, granisetron, heparin, hydrocortisone, hydromorphone, imipenem/cilastatin, insulin, regular, isoproterenol, ketorolac, leucovorin, levorphanol, lidocaine, linezolid, lorazepam, magnesium sulfate, mannitol, melphalan, meperidine, meropenem, mesna, methohexital, methylprednisolone, metoclopramide, metoprolol, metronidazole, milrinone, mitomycin, mitoxantrone, morphine, moxifloxacin, naloxone, nitroglycerin, norepinephrine, octreotide, ondansetron, oxacillin, paclitaxel, palonosetron, pamidronate, pancuronium, pentobarbital, phenobarbital, phenylephrine, piperacillin/tazobactam, potassium acetate, potassium chloride, potassium phosphate, procainamide, prochlorperazine, propranolol, ranitidine, remifentanil, rituximab, rocuronium, sargramostim, sodium acetate, sodium bicarbonate, sodium phosphate, succinylchloride, sufentanil, tacrolimus, theophylline, thiopental, thiotepa, tigecycline, tirofiban, tobramycin, trastuzumab, trimethoprim/sulfamethoxazole, vasopressin, vecuronium, verapamil, vinblastine, vincristine, vinorelbine, voriconazole, zidovudine, zoledronic acid.
- **Y-Site Incompatibility:** amiodarone, caspofungin, chlorpromazine, dacarbazine, daptomycin, dexrazoxane, diazepam, diltiazem, dobutamine, dopamine, doxycycline, gemcitabine, gentamicin, idarubicin, ifosfamide, levofloxacin, midazolam, mycophenolate, nalbuphine, nicardipine, pantoprazole, pentamidine, phenytoin, propofol, quinupristin/dalfopristin.
- **IT:** Reconstitute preservative-free methotrexate with preservative-free 0.9% NaCl, Elliot's B solution, or patient's CSF to a concentration not greater than 2 mg/mL. May be administered via lumbar puncture or Ommaya reservoir. To prevent bacterial contamination, use immediately.

Patient/Family Teaching

- Instruct patient to take medication as directed. If a dose is missed, it should be omitted. Consult health care professional if vomiting occurs shortly after a dose is taken.
- Instruct patient to notify health care professional promptly if rash, fever; chills; cough; hoarseness; sore throat; signs of infection; lower back or side pain; painful or difficult urination; bleeding gums; bruising; petechiae; blood in stools, urine, or emesis; increased fatigue; dyspnea; or orthostatic hypotension occurs. Caution patient to avoid crowds and persons with known infections. Instruct patient to use soft toothbrush and electric razor and to avoid falls. Caution patient not to drink alcoholic beverages or take medication containing aspirin or other NSAIDs; may precipitate gastric bleeding.
- Instruct patient to inspect oral mucosa for erythema and ulceration. If ulceration occurs, advise patient to use sponge brush and to rinse mouth with water after eating and drinking. Topical therapy may be used if mouth pain interferes with eating. Stomatitis pain may require treatment with opioid analgesics.
- Advise patient to tell health care professional what medications they are taking and to avoid taking new Rx, OTC, vitamins, or herbal products without consulting health care professional.
- Discuss the possibility of hair loss with patient. Explore methods of coping.
- Instruct patient not to receive any vaccinations without advice of health care professional.
- Caution patient to use sunscreen and protective clothing to prevent photosensitivity reactions.
- Rep: May be teratogenic. Advise Female patients of reproductive potential to use effective contraception during and for at least 1 menstrual cycle after last dose and avoid breast feeding during therapy. Advise males with female partners of reproductive potential to use effective contraception during and for at least 3 mo after therapy. May impair fertility in both men and women.
- Emphasize the need for periodic lab tests to monitor for side effects.
- **Subcut:** Instruct patient on correct technique for injection and care and disposal of equipment.

Evaluation/Desired Outcomes

- Improvement of hematopoietic values in leukemia.
- Decrease in symptoms of meningeal involvement in leukemia.
- Decrease in size and spread of non-Hodgkin's lymphomas and other solid cancers.
- Resolution of skin lesions in severe psoriasis.
- Decreased joint pain and swelling.
- Improved mobility in patients with rheumatoid arthritis.
- Regression of lesions in mycosis fungoides.

BEERS

methyldopa (meth-ill-doe-pa)

~~Aldomet~~

Classification
Therapeutic: antihypertensives
Pharmacologic: centrally acting antiadrenergics

Indications

Management of moderate to severe hypertension (with other agents).

Action

Stimulates CNS alpha-adrenergic receptors, producing a decrease in sympathetic outflow to heart, kidneys, and blood vessels. Result is decreased BP and peripheral resistance, a slight decrease in heart rate, and no change in cardiac output. **Therapeutic Effects:** Lowering of BP.

Pharmacokinetics

Absorption: 50% absorbed from the GI tract.
Distribution: Crosses the blood-brain barrier. Crosses the placenta; small amounts enter breast milk.
Metabolism and Excretion: Partially metabolized by the liver, partially excreted unchanged by the kidneys.
Half-life: 1.7 hr.

TIME/ACTION PROFILE (antihypertensive effect)

ROUTE	ONSET	PEAK	DURATION
PO	4–6 hr	12–24 hr	24–48 hr

Contraindications/Precautions

Contraindicated in: Hypersensitivity; Active liver disease.
Use Cautiously in: Previous history of liver disease; OB: Has been used safely (may be used for treatment of hypertension in pregnancy); Lactation: Usually compatible with breast feeding; Geri: ↑ risk of adverse reactions; consider age-related impairment of hepatic, renal and cardiovascular function as well as other chronic illnesses. Appears on Beers list. May cause bradycardia and exacerbate depression.

Adverse Reactions/Side Effects

CNS: sedation, ↓ mental acuity, depression. **CV:** MYOCARDITIS, bradycardia, edema, orthostatic hypotension. **EENT:** nasal stuffiness. **GI:** HEPATITIS, diarrhea, dry mouth. **GU:** erectile dysfunction. **Hemat:** eosinophilia, hemolytic anemia. **Misc:** fever.

Interactions

Drug-Drug: Additive hypotension with other **antihypertensives**, acute ingestion of **alcohol**, **anesthesia**, and **nitrates**. **Amphetamines**, **barbiturates**, **tricyclic antidepressants**, **NSAIDs**, and **phenothiazines** may ↓ antihypertensive effect of methyldopa. ↑ effects and risk of psychoses with **haloperidol**. Excess sympathetic stimulation may occur with concurrent use of **MAO inhibitors** or other **adrenergics**. May ↑ **lithium** toxicity. Additive hypotension and CNS toxicity with **levodopa**. Additive CNS depression may occur with **alcohol**, **antihistamines**, **sedative/hypnotics**, some **antidepressants**, and **opioid analgesics**. Concurrent use with **nonselective beta blockers** may rarely cause paradoxical hypertension.

Route/Dosage

PO (Adults): 250–500 mg 2–3 times daily (not to exceed 500 mg/day if used with other agents); may be ↑ every 2 days as needed; usual maintenance dose is 500 mg–2 g/day (not to exceed 3 g/day).
PO (Children): 10 mg/kg/day (300 $mg/m^2/day$); may be ↑ every 2 days up to 65 mg/kg/day in divided doses (not to exceed 3 g/day).

Availability (generic available)

Tablets: 250 mg, 500 mg. ***In combination with:*** hydrochlorothiazide. See Appendix B.

NURSING IMPLICATIONS

Assessment

- Monitor BP and pulse frequently during initial dose adjustment and periodically during therapy. Report significant changes.
- Monitor frequency of prescription refills to determine compliance.
- Monitor intake and output ratios and weight and assess for edema daily, especially at beginning of therapy. Report weight gain or edema; sodium and water retention may be treated with diuretics.
- Assess patient for depression or other alterations in mental status. Notify health care professional promptly if these symptoms develop.
- Monitor temperature during therapy. Drug fever may occur shortly after initiation of therapy and may be accompanied by eosinophilia and hepatic function changes. Monitor hepatic function test if unexplained fever occurs.
- ***Lab Test Considerations:*** Monitor renal and hepatic function and CBC before and periodically during therapy.
- Monitor direct Coombs' test before and after 6 and 12 mo of therapy. May cause a positive direct Coombs' test, rarely associated with hemolytic anemia.

- May cause ↑ BUN, serum creatinine, potassium, sodium, prolactin, uric acid, AST, ALT, alkaline phosphatase, and bilirubin concentrations.
- May cause prolonged prothrombin times.
- May interfere with serum creatinine and AST measurements.

Implementation

- **PO:** Fluid retention and expanded volume may cause tolerance to develop within 2–3 mo after initiation of therapy. Diuretics may be added to regimen at this time to maintain control.
- Dose increases should be made with the evening dose to minimize drowsiness.

Patient/Family Teaching

- Emphasize the importance of continuing to take this medication, even if feeling well. Instruct patient to take medication at the same time each day; last dose of the day should be taken at bedtime. Take missed doses as soon as remembered but not if almost time for next dose. Do not double doses.
- Encourage patient to comply with additional interventions for hypertension (weight reduction, low-sodium diet, smoking cessation, moderation of alcohol consumption, regular exercise, and stress management). Methyldopa controls but does not cure hypertension.
- Instruct patient and family on proper technique for monitoring BP. Advise them to check BP at least weekly and to report significant changes.
- Instruct patient to notify health care professional if fever, muscle aches, or flu-like syndrome occurs.
- Inform patient that urine may darken or turn red-black when left standing.
- May cause drowsiness. Advise patient to avoid driving or other activities requiring alertness until response to medication is known. Drowsiness usually subsides after 7–10 days of continuous use.
- Caution patient to avoid sudden changes in position to decrease orthostatic hypotension.
- Advise patient that frequent mouth rinses, good oral hygiene, and sugarless gum or candy may minimize dry mouth. Notify health care professional if dry mouth continues for >2 wk.
- Caution patient to avoid concurrent use of alcohol or other CNS depressants.
- Advise patient to notify health care professional of all Rx or OTC medications, vitamins, or herbal products being taken and to consult with health care professional before taking other medications, especially cough, cold, or allergy remedies.
- Advise patient to notify health care professional of medication regimen before treatment or surgery.
- Advise patient to notify health care professional if pregnancy is planned or suspected, or if breast feeding.

Evaluation/Desired Outcomes

- Decrease in BP without appearance of side effects.

methylergonovine

(meth-ill-er-goe-**noe**-veen)

Methergine

Classification

Therapeutic: oxytocic

Pharmacologic: ergot alkaloids

Indications

Prevention and treatment of postpartum or postabortion hemorrhage caused by uterine atony or subinvolution.

Action

Directly stimulates uterine and vascular smooth muscle. **Therapeutic Effects:** Uterine contraction.

Pharmacokinetics

Absorption: Well absorbed following oral or IM administration.

Distribution: Unknown. Enters breast milk in small quantities.

Metabolism and Excretion: Probably metabolized by the liver.

Half-life: 30–120 min.

TIME/ACTION PROFILE (effects on uterine contractions)

ROUTE	ONSET	PEAK	DURATION
PO	5–15 min	unknown	3 hr
IM	2–5 min	unknown	3 hr
IV	immediate	unknown	45 min–3 hr

Contraindications/Precautions

Contraindicated in: Hypersensitivity; OB: Should not be used to induce labor; Lactation: Do not breast feed during treatment and for 12 hrs after the last dose; Concurrent use of potent CYP3A4 inhibitors.

Use Cautiously in: Hypertensive or eclamptic patients (more susceptible to hypertensive and arrhythmogenic side effects); History of or risk factors for coronary artery disease; Severe hepatic or renal disease; Sepsis; Concurrent use of moderat CYP3A4 inhibitors.

Exercise Extreme Caution in: OB: Third stage of labor.

Adverse Reactions/Side Effects

CNS: STROKE, dizziness, headache. **EENT:** tinnitus. **Resp:** dyspnea. **CV:** HYPERTENSION, arrhythmias, AV block, chest pain, palpitations. **GI:** nausea, vomiting. **GU:** cramps. **Derm:** diaphoresis. **Neuro:** paresthesia. **Misc:** allergic reactions.

Interactions

Drug-Drug: Excessive vasoconstriction may result when used with heavy cigarette smoking (**nicotine**), other **vasopressors**, such as **dopamine**, or **beta-blockers**. Potent **CYP3A4 inhibitors**, including **erythromycin**, **clarithromycin**, **troleandomycin**, **ritonavir**, **indinavir**, **nelfinavir**, **delavirdine**, **ketoconazole**, **itracona-**

zole, or **voriconazole** may ↑ levels and ↑ risk of ischemia; concurrent use contraindicated. Moderate **CYP3A4 inhibitors** including **saquinavir**, **nefazodone**, **fluconazole**, **fluoxetine**, **fluvoxamine**, **zileuton**, or **clotrimazole** may ↑ levels; use with caution. **CYP3A4 inducers** including **nevirapine** and **rifampin** may ↓ levels. **Anesthetics** may ↓ its oxytocic properties. May ↓ the antianginal effects of **nitrates**.

Drug-Food: Grapefruit juice may ↑ levels; use with caution.

Route/Dosage

PO (Adults): 200–400 mcg (0.2–0.4 mg) every 6–12 hr for 2–7 days.

IM, IV (Adults): 200 mcg (0.2 mg) every 2–4 hr for up to 5 doses.

Availability (generic available)

Tablets: 200 mcg (0.2 mg). **Injection:** 200 mcg (0.2 mg)/mL.

NURSING IMPLICATIONS

Assessment

- Monitor BP, heart rate, and uterine response frequently during medication administration. Notify health care professional promptly if uterine relaxation becomes prolonged or if character of vaginal bleeding changes.
- Assess for signs of ergotism (cold, numb fingers and toes, chest pain, nausea, vomiting, headache, muscle pain, weakness).
- ***Lab Test Considerations:*** If no response to methylergonovine, calcium levels may need to be assessed. Effectiveness of medication is ↓ with hypocalcemia.
- May cause ↓ serum prolactin levels.

Implementation

IV Administration

- **IV:** IV administration is used for emergencies only. Oral and IM routes are preferred.
- **IV Push:** ***Diluent:*** May be given undiluted or diluted in 5 mL of 0.9% NaCl and administered through Y site. Do not add to IV solutions. Do not mix in syringe with any other drug. Refrigerate; stable for storage at room temperature for 60 days; deteriorates with age. Use only solution that is clear and colorless and that contains no precipitate. ***Concentration:*** 0.2 mg/mL. ***Rate:*** Administer at a rate of 0.2 mg over at least 1 min.
- **Y-Site Compatibility:** heparin, hydrocortisone sodium succinate, potassium chloride, vitamin B complex with C.

Patient/Family Teaching

- Instruct patient to take medication as directed; do not skip or double up on missed doses. If a dose is missed, omit it and return to regular dose schedule.
- Advise patient that medication may cause menstrual-like cramps.
- Caution patient to avoid smoking, because nicotine constricts blood vessels.
- Instruct patient to notify health care professional if infection develops, as this may cause increased sensitivity to the medication.
- Advise patient to notify health care professional of all Rx or OTC medications, vitamins, or herbal products being taken and to consult with health care professional before taking other medications.

Evaluation/Desired Outcomes

- Contractions that maintain uterine tone and prevent postpartum hemorrhage.

methylnaltrexone

(me-thil-nal-**trex**-one)

Relistor

Classification

Therapeutic: laxatives

Pharmacologic: opioid antagonists

M

Indications

Subcut: Treatment of opioid-induced constipation (OIC) in patients with advanced illness or pain caused by active cancer who require opioid dose escalation for palliative care. **Subcut, PO:** Treatment of OIC in patients with chronic, non-cancer pain, including those with chronic pain related to prior cancer or its treatment who do not require frequent (e.g. weekly) opioid dose escalation.

Action

Acts peripherally as mu-opioid receptor antagonist, blocking opioid effects on the GI tract. **Therapeutic Effects:** Blocks constipating effects of opioids on the GI tract without loss of analgesia.

Pharmacokinetics

Absorption: Rapidly absorbed after subcutaneous and oral administration; oral absorption delayed by high-fat meal by 2 hr.

Distribution: Moderate tissue distribution, does not cross the blood-brain barrier.

Metabolism and Excretion: Some metabolism; 85% excreted unchanged in urine.

Half-life: 15 hr (oral).

TIME/ACTION PROFILE (plasma concentrations)

ROUTE	ONSET	PEAK	DURATION
Subcut	rapid	0.5 hr	24–48 hr
PO	rapid	1.5 hr	unknown

Contraindications/Precautions

Contraindicated in: Known/suspected mechanical GI obstruction.

Use Cautiously in: Known/suspected lesions of GI tract (↑ risk for GI perforation); Moderate-severe renal impairment (dose ↓ required); Moderate-severe hepatic impairment (dose ↓ may be required); OB, Lactation: Use in pregnancy only if clearly needed; use cautiously during lactation; Pedi: Safety and effectiveness not established.

Adverse Reactions/Side Effects

CNS: dizziness. **Derm:** hyperhidrosis. **GI:** GI PERFORATION, abdominal pain, flatulence, nausea, diarrhea. **Misc:** opioid withdrawal.

Interactions

Drug-Drug: None noted.

Route/Dosage

OIC in Patients with Advanced Illness

Subcut (Adults): *38–<62 kg*—8 mg every other day, not to exceed every 24 hr; *62–114 kg*—12 mg every other day, not to exceed every 24 hr; *>114 kg*—0.15 mg/kg every other day, not to exceed every 24 hr.

Renal Impairment

(Adults): *CCr <60 mL/min*—use 50% of recommended dose based on weight.

OIC in Patients with Non-Cancer Pain

Subcut (Adults): 12 mg once daily.

Renal Impairment

Subcut (Adults): *CCr <60 mL/min*—6 mg once daily.

Hepatic Impairment

Subcut (Adults): *Severe hepatic impairment (Child–Pugh Class C)*—<38 kg: 0.075 mg/kg once daily; 38–<62 kg: 4 mg once daily; 62–114 kg: 6 mg once daily: >114 kg: 0.075 mg/kg once daily.

PO (Adults): 450 mg once daily.

Renal Impairment

PO (Adults): *CCr <60 mL/min*—150 mg once daily.

Hepatic Impairment

PO (Adults): *Moderate or severe hepatic impairment (Child–Pugh Class B or C)*—150 mg once daily.

Availability

Solution for injection (prefilled syringes): 8 mg/0.4 mL, 12 mg/0.6 mL. **Cost:** All strengths $71.46/syringe. **Tablets:** 150 mg.

NURSING IMPLICATIONS

Assessment

- Assess bowel sounds and frequency, quantity, and consistency of stools periodically during therapy.
- Monitor pain intensity during therapy. Methylnaltrexone does not affect pain or effects of opioid analgesics on pain control.

Implementation

- Maintenance laxative must be stopped prior to administration of methylnaltrexone. If response is not sufficient after 3 days, laxatives may be restarted.
- **PO:** Administer with water on an empty stomach at least 30 min before first meal of the day.
- **Subcut:** Pinch skin and administer in upper arm, abdomen, or thigh at a 45° angle using a 1-mL syringe with a 27-gauge needle inserted the full length of the needle. Do not rub the injection site. Solution is clear and colorless to pale yellow. Do not administer solutions that are discolored or contain a precipitate. Solution is stable for 24 hr at room temperature. Protect vials from light. Do not freeze. Do not use single-use vials for more than 1 dose.

Patient/Family Teaching

- Instruct patient to take methylnaltrexone as directed and on correct technique for administration of methylnaltrexone and disposal of supplies. Usual schedule is one dose every other day, as needed, but no more than one dose in a 24-hr period. Advise patient to read the *Patient Information* prior to starting therapy and with each Rx refill in case of changes.
- Advise patient that laxation may occur within 30 min of subcut injection, so toilet facilities should be available following administration.
- Advise patient to discontinue all maintenance laxatives; can be added if inadequate response to methylnaltrexone.
- May cause dizziness. Caution patient to avoid driving and other activities requiring alertness until response to medication is known.
- Advise patient to notify health care professional and discontinue therapy if severe or persistent diarrhea occurs or if abdominal pain, nausea, or vomiting persists or worsens.
- Instruct patient to stop taking methylnaltrexone if they stop taking opioid medications.
- Advise patient to consult health care professional prior to taking other Rx, OTC, or herbal products.
- Advise female patients to notify health care professional if pregnancy is planned or suspected, and to avoid breast feeding; may cause opioid withdrawal in infant.

Evaluation/Desired Outcomes

- Laxation and relief of OIC.

methylphenidate (oral)

(meth-ill-**fen**-i-date)

Adhansia XR, Aptensio XR, ✱Biphentin, Concerta, Cotempla XR-ODT, ✱Foquest, Jornay PM, Metadate

CD, Methylin, Methylin ER, Quillichew ER, Quillivant XR, Ritalin, Ritalin LA, ✱Ritalin SR

methylphenidate (transdermal)

Daytrana

Classification
Therapeutic: central nervous system stimulants

Schedule II

Indications

Oral, orally distintegrating tablets, and transdermal: Treatment of ADHD (adjunct). **Oral only**: Symptomatic treatment of narcolepsy.

Action

Produces CNS and respiratory stimulation with weak sympathomimetic activity. **Therapeutic Effects:** Increased attention span in ADHD. Increased motor activity, mental alertness, and diminished fatigue in narcolepsy.

Pharmacokinetics

Absorption: Slow and incomplete after oral administration; absorption of sustained or extended-release tablet (SR) is delayed and provides continuous release; well absorbed from skin. *Aptensio XR, Metadate CD, Concerta, Ritalin LA*—provides initial rapid release followed by a second continuous release (biphasic release).

Distribution: Unknown.

Metabolism and Excretion: Mostly metabolized (80%) by the liver.

Half-life: 2–4 hr.

TIME/ACTION PROFILE (CNS stimulation)

ROUTE	ONSET	PEAK	DURATION
PO	unknown	1–3 hr	4–6 hr
PO-ER	unknown	4–7 hr	3–12 hr†
Transdermal	unknown	unknown	12 hr

†Depends on formulation.

Contraindications/Precautions

Contraindicated in: Hypersensitivity; Hyperexcitable states; Hyperthyroidism; Patients with psychotic personalities or suicidal or homicidal tendencies; Personal or family history of Tourette's syndrome; Glaucoma; Motor tics; Concurrent use or use within 14 days of MAO inhibitors or MAO-like drugs (linezolid or methylene blue); Fructose intolerance, glucose-galactose malabsorption, or sucrose-isomaltase insufficiency; Surgery.

Use Cautiously in: History of cardiovascular disease (sudden death has occurred in children with structural cardiac abnormalities or other serious heart problems); Hypertension; Diabetes mellitus; History of contact sensitization with transdermal product (may be at ↑ risk for systemic sensitization reactions with oral products); History or family history of vitiligo (may be at ↑ risk for loss of skin pigmentation with transdermal product); Continual use (may result in psychological or physical dependence); Seizure disorders (may lower seizure threshold); Concerta product should be used cautiously in patients with esophageal motility disorders or severe GI narrowing (may ↑ the risk of obstruction); OB: Use during pregnancy only if maternal benefit outweighs potential risk to fetus; Lactation: Use while breast feeding only if maternal benefit outweighs potential risk to infant; Pedi: Growth suppression may occur in children with long-term use; children <6 yr (↑ risk of adverse reactions, particularly weight loss in children 4–<6 yr); Geri: Safety and effectiveness of many of the products have not been evaluated in patients >65 yrs.

M

Adverse Reactions/Side Effects

CNS: hyperactivity, insomnia, restlessness, tremor, behavioral disturbances, dizziness, hallucinations, headache, irritability, mania, thought disorder. **CV:** SUDDEN DEATH, hypertension, palpitations, tachycardia, hypotension, peripheral vasculopathy. **Derm:** contact sensitization (erythema, edema, papules, vesicles) (transdermal), erythema, loss of skin pigmentation (transdermal), rash. **EENT:** blurred vision, teeth grinding. **GI:** anorexia, constipation, cramps, diarrhea, dry mouth, metallic taste, nausea, vomiting. **GU:** priapism. **Metab:** growth suppression (especially with prolonged use), weight loss (especially with prolonged use). **MS:** RHABDOMYOLYSIS. **Neuro:** akathisia, dyskinesia, tics. **Misc:** HYPERSENSITIVITY REACTIONS (including anaphylaxis and angioedema), fever, physical dependence, psychological dependence, tolerance.

Interactions

Drug-Drug: Concurrent use with **MAO inhibitors** or **MAO-inhibitor-like drugs**, such as **linezolid** or **methylene blue** may result in serious, potentially fatal reactions; wait at least 14 days following discontinuation of MAO inhibitor before initiation of amphetamine mixtures. Drugs that affect serotonergic neurotransmitter systems, including **MAO inhibitors**, **tricyclic antidepressants**, **SSRIs**, **SNRIs**, **fentanyl**, **buspirone**, **tramadol**, **lithium**, and **triptans** ↑ risk of serotonin syndrome. ↑ sympathomimetic effects with other **adrenergics**, including **vasoconstrictors**, **decongestants**, and **halogenated anesthetics**. Metabolism of **warfarin**, **phenytoin**, **phenobarbital**, **primidone**, **phenylbutazone**, **selective serotonin reuptake inhibitors**, and **tricyclic antidepressants** may be ↓ and effects ↑. Avoid concurrent use with **pimozide** (may mask cause of tics). May ↓ the effectiveness of

antihypertensives. **Alcohol** may ↑ rate of release of drug from some methylphenidate formulations (Metadate CD, Ritalin LA).

Drug-Natural Products: Use with caffeine-containing herbs (**guarana**, **tea**, **coffee**) ↑ stimulant effect. **St. John's wort** may ↑ risk of serotonin syndrome.

Drug-Food: Excessive use of **caffeine**-containing foods or beverages (**coffee**, **cola**, **tea**) may cause ↑ CNS stimulation.

Route/Dosage

ADHD

PO (Adults <65 yr): *Immediate-release tablets*—5–20 mg 2–3 times daily. When maintenance dose is determined, may change to extended-release formulation. *Methylphenidate SR*—may be used in place of the immediate-release tablets when the 8-hr dose corresponds to the titrated 8-hr dosage of the immediate-release tablets; *Concerta (patients who have not taken methylphenidate previously)*—18–36 mg once daily in the morning initially, may be titrated as needed up to 72 mg/day. *Concerta (patients are currently taking other forms of methylphenidate)*—18 mg once daily in the morning if previous dose was 5 mg 2–3 times daily; 36 mg once daily in the morning if previous dose was 10 mg 2–3 times daily; 54 mg once daily in the morning if previous dose was 15 mg 2–3 times daily; 72 mg once daily in the morning if previous dose was 20 mg 2–3 times daily. *Aptensio XR*—10 mg once daily; may ↑ dose in 10-mg increments at weekly intervals (maximum dose = 60 mg/day). *Quillivant XR and Quillichew ER*—20 mg once daily; may ↑ dose in 10–20-mg increments at weekly intervals (maximum dose = 60 mg/day). *Adhansia XR*—25 mg once daily; may ↑ dose in 10–15-mg increments at weekly intervals (maximum dose = 100 mg/day). *Jornay PM*—20 mg once daily in the evening; may ↑ dose in 20-mg increments at weekly intervals (maximum dose = 100 mg/day).

PO (Children ≥6 yr [Ritalin LA for children 6–12 yr]): *Immediate-release tablets*—0.3 mg/kg/dose or 2.5–5 mg before breakfast and lunch; may ↑ dose by 0.1 mg/kg/dose or by 5–10 mg/day at weekly intervals (not to exceed 60 mg/day or 2 mg/kg/day). When maintenance dose is determined, may change to extended-release formulation. *Methylphenidate SR*—may be used in place of the immediate-release tablets when the 8-hr dose corresponds to the titrated 8-hr dosage of the immediate-release tablets; *Ritalin LA (patients who have not taken methylphenidate previously)*—20 mg once daily; may ↑ by 10 mg/day at weekly intervals (max = 60 mg/day); *Ritalin LA (patients currently taking other forms of methylphenidate)*—can be used in place of immediate-release twice daily regimen given once daily at same total dose, or in place of SR product at same dose; *Concerta (patients who have not taken methylphenidate previously)*—18 mg once daily in the morning initially, may be titrated as needed up to 54 mg/day (children 6–12 yrs old) or up to 72 mg/day (children 13–17 yrs old). *Concerta (patients are currently taking other forms of methylphenidate)*—18 mg once daily in the morning if previous dose was 5 mg 2–3 times daily; 36 mg once daily in the morning if previous dose was 10 mg 2–3 times daily; 54 mg once daily in the morning if previous dose was 15 mg 2–3 times daily; 72 mg once daily in the morning if previous dose was 20 mg 2–3 times daily. *Aptensio XR*—10 mg once daily; may ↑ dose in 10-mg increments at weekly intervals (maximum dose = 60 mg/day). *Metadate CD*—20 mg once daily; may ↑ dose in 20-mg increments at weekly intervals (maximum dose = 60 mg/day). *Quillivant XR and Quillichew ER*—20 mg once daily; may ↑ dose in 10–20-mg increments at weekly intervals (maximum dose = 60 mg/day). *Adhansia XR*—25 mg once daily; may ↑ dose in 10–15-mg increments at weekly intervals (maximum dose = 85 mg/day). *Jornay PM*—20 mg once daily in the evening; may ↑ dose in 20-mg increments at weekly intervals (maximum dose = 100 mg/day). *Cotempla XR-ODT*—17.3 mg once daily in the morning; may ↑ dose in 8.6–17.3-mg increments at weekly intervals (maximum dose = 51.8 mg/day).

Transdermal (Children ≥6 yr): Apply one 10-mg patch initially (should be applied 2 hr before desired effect and removed 9 hr after application); may be titrated based on response and tolerability; may ↑ to 15-mg patch after 1 wk, and then to 20-mg patch after another wk, and then to 30-mg patch after another wk.

Narcolepsy

PO (Adults): *Immediate-release tablets*—10 mg 2–3 times/day; maximum dose 60 mg/day.

Availability (generic available)

Chewable tablets (Methylin) (grape flavor): 2.5 mg, 5 mg, 10 mg. **Cost:** 2.5 mg $351.16/100, 5 mg $501.16/100, 10 mg $715.09/100. **Extended-release capsules (Adhansia XR):** 25 mg, 35 mg, 45 mg, 55 mg, 70 mg, 85 mg, 100 mg. **Extended-release capsules (Aptensio XR):** 10 mg, 15 mg, 20 mg, 30 mg, 40 mg, 50 mg, 60 mg. **Extended-release capsules (Jornay PM):** 20 mg, 40 mg, 60 mg, 80 mg, 100 mg. **Extended-release capsules (Metadate CD):** 10 mg, 20 mg, 30 mg, 40 mg, 50 mg, 60 mg. **Cost:** *Generic*—10 mg $560.21/100, 20 mg $560.21/100, 30 mg $560.21/100, 40 mg $711.52/100, 50 mg $944.19/100, 60 mg $944.19/100. **Extended-release capsules (Ritalin LA):** 10 mg, 20 mg, 30 mg, 40 mg, 60 mg. **Cost:** *Generic*—10 mg $630.47/100, 20 mg $630.47/100, 30 mg $644.82/100, 40 mg $66.274/100. **Extended-release chewable tablets (Quillichew ER):** 20 mg, 30 mg, 40 mg. **Extended-release oral suspension (Quillivant XR) (banana flavor):** 25 mg/5 mL. **Extended-release orally-disintegrating tablets (Cotempla XR-ODT):** 8.6 mg, 17.3 mg, 25.9 mg. **Extended-release tablets (Concerta):** 18

mg, 27 mg, 36 mg, 54 mg. **Cost:** *Generic*—18 mg $622.18/100, 27 mg $637.78/100, 36 mg $657.86/100, 54 mg $715.83/100. **Extended-release tablets (Metadate ER):** 20 mg. **Extended-release tablets (Methylin ER):** 10 mg, 20 mg. **Cost:** *Generic*—10 mg $171.91/100, 20 mg $247.21/100. **Oral solution (Methylin) (grape flavor):** 5 mg/5 mL, 10 mg/5 mL. **Cost:** *Generic*—5 mg/5 mL $451.61/500 mL, 10 mg/5 mL $643.82/500 mL. **Sustained-release tablets (Ritalin SR):** ✱20 mg. **Cost:** $266.65/100. **Tablets (Ritalin):** 5 mg, 10 mg, 20 mg. **Cost:** *Generic*—5 mg $73.08/100, 10 mg $104.19/100, 20 mg $149.81/100. **Transdermal patch:** 10 mg/9 hr, 15 mg/9 hr, 20 mg/9 hr, 30 mg/9 hr. **Cost:** All strengths $249.35/30.

NURSING IMPLICATIONS

Assessment

- Monitor BP, pulse, and respiration before administering and periodically during therapy. Obtain a history (including assessment of family history of sudden death or ventricular arrhythmia), physical exam to assess for cardiac disease, and further evaluation (ECG and echocardiogram), if indicated. If exertional chest pain, unexplained syncope, or other cardiac symptoms occur, evaluate promptly.
- Monitor closely for behavior change.
- Assess risk of abuse prior to prescribing. After prescribing, keep accurate prescription records, educate patient and family about risk of abuse, monitor for signs of abuse and overdose, and evaluate need for use periodically during therapy.
- Screen patients with bipolar disorder for risk of manic episode (comorbid or history of depressive symptoms or a family history of suicide, bipolar disorder, depression) prior to starting therapy.
- Monitor for signs and symptoms of peripheral vasculopathy (numbness and burning in fingers, digital changes). May require reduction in dose or discontinuation.
- Pedi: Monitor growth, both height and weight, in children on long-term therapy.
- May produce a false sense of euphoria and well-being. Provide frequent rest periods and observe patient for rebound depression after the effects of the medication have worn off.
- **ADHD:** Assess children for attention span, impulse control, and interactions with others. Therapy may be interrupted at intervals to determine whether symptoms are sufficient to continue therapy.
- **Narcolepsy:** Observe and document frequency of episodes.
- **Transdermal:** Assess skin for signs of contact sensitization (erythema with edema, papules, or vesicles that does not improve within 48 hr or spreads beyond patch site) during therapy. May lead to systemic sensitization to other forms of methylphenidate (flare-up of previous dermatitis or prior positive patch-test sites, generalized skin eruptions, headache, fever, malaise, arthralgia, diarrhea, vomiting). If contact sensitization develops and oral methylphenidate is instituted, monitor closely.
- Monitor for signs of skin depigmentation. May cause persistent loss of skin pigmentation at and around the application site and at other sites distant from application site. Discontinue transdermal if depigmentation occurs.
- ***Lab Test Considerations:*** Monitor CBC, differential, and platelet count periodically in patients receiving prolonged therapy.

Implementation

- Do not confuse Metadate ER/CD (methylphenidate), or methylphenidate with methadone. Do not confuse Metadate CD with Metadate ER.
- **PO:** Administer immediate and sustained-release tablets on an empty stomach (30–45 min before a meal). Sustained-release tablets should be swallowed whole; do not break, crush, or chew. *Quillichew ER* chewable tablets may be broken in half. *Aptensio XL, Metadate CD* and *Ritalin LA* capsules may be opened and sprinkled on cool applesauce; entire mixture should be ingested immediately and followed by a drink of water. Do not store for future use. *Concerta* may be administered without regard to food, but must be taken with water, milk, or juice.
- Shake extended-release oral suspension for 10 sec before administering. May be given with or without food.
- **Transdermal:** Apply patch to a clean, dry site on the hip which is not oily, damaged, or irritated; do not apply to waistline where tight clothing may rub it. Press firmly in place with palm of hand for 30 sec to make sure of good contact with skin, especially around edges. Alternate site daily. Apply patch 2 hr before desired effect and remove 9 hr after applied; effects last several more hrs. Do not apply or reapply with dressings, tape, or other adhesives. Do not cut patches.
- If difficulty in separating patch from release liner, tearing, or other damage occurs during removal from liner, discard patch and apply a new patch. Inspect release liner to ensure no adhesive containing medication has transferred to liner; if transfer has occurred, discard patch. Avoid touching adhesive during application; wash hands immediately after application.
- If patch does not fully adhere or partially detaches, remove and replace with another patch. Wear patch for a total of 9 hr, regardless of number used. Exposure to water during bathing, swimming, or showering may affect patch adherence.

- Patches may be removed earlier before decreasing dose if an unacceptable loss of appetite or insomnia occurs.
- Store patches at room temperature in a safe place to prevent abuse and misuse; do not refrigerate or freeze.
- To remove patch, peel off slowly. An oil-based product (petroleum jelly, olive oil, mineral oil) may be applied gently to facilitate removal. Upon removal, fold so that adhesive side of patch adheres to itself and flush down toilet or dispose of in an appropriate lidded container.

Patient/Family Teaching

- Instruct patient to take medication as directed. If an oral dose is missed, take the remaining doses for that day at regularly spaced intervals; do not double doses. Take the last dose before 6 PM to minimize the risk of insomnia. Instruct patient not to alter dose without consulting health care professional. Abrupt cessation of high doses may cause extreme fatigue and mental depression. Instruct parent/caregiver to read the *Medication Guide* prior to use and with each Rx refill; new information may be available.
- Advise patient to check weight 2–3 times weekly and report weight loss to health care professional.
- Advise patient that methylphenidate is a drug with known abuse potential. Protect it from theft, and never give to anyone other than the individual for whom it was prescribed. Store out of sight and reach of children, and in a location not accessible by others.
- May cause dizziness or blurred vision. Caution patient to avoid driving or activities requiring alertness until response to medication is known.
- Inform patient and/or parents that shell of *Concerta* tablet may appear in the stool. This is no cause for concern.
- Advise patient to avoid using caffeine-containing beverages concurrently with this therapy.
- Advise patient to notify health care professional if nervousness, insomnia, palpitations, vomiting, skin rash, fever, painful and prolonged erections, or circulation problems (fingers or toes feel numb, cool, painful; fingers or toes change color from pale, to blue, to red) occur.
- Advise patient and/or parents to notify health care professional of behavioral changes.
- Advise patient to notify health care professional of all Rx or OTC medications, vitamins, or herbal products being taken and to consult with health care professional before taking other medications.
- Inform patient that health care professional may order periodic holidays from the drug to assess progress and to decrease dependence.
- Rep: Advise females of reproductive potential to notify health care professional if pregnancy is planned or suspected or if breast feeding. Encourage patients who become pregnant while taking methylphenidate to enroll in registry with the National Pregnancy Registry of ADHD Medications at 1-866-961-2388 or visit online at https://womensmentalhealth.org/adhd-medications/. Registry collects information about the health of females exposed to methylphenidate and their baby.
- Emphasize the importance of routine follow-up exams to monitor progress.
- **Transdermal:** Encourage parent or caregiver to use the administration chart included in package to monitor application and removal time and disposal method.
- Caution patient to avoid exposing patch to direct external heat sources (hair dryers, heating pads, electric blankets, heated water beds, etc.). May increase rate and extent of absorption.
- Inform parent/caregiver that skin redness, itching and small bumps on the skin are common. If swelling or blistering occurs, the patch should not be worn and health care professional notified. Caution parent/caregiver not to apply hydrocortisone or other solutions, creams, ointments, or emollients prior to application.
- Advise patient referred for MRI test to discuss patch with referring health care professional and MRI facility to determine if removal of patch is necessary prior to test and for directions for replacing patch.
- **Home Care Issues:** Pedi: Advise parents to notify school nurse of medication regimen.

Evaluation/Desired Outcomes

- Improved attention span and social interactions in ADHD.
- Decreased frequency of narcoleptic symptoms.

methylPREDNISolone, See CORTICOSTEROIDS (SYSTEMIC).

BEERS

metoclopramide

(met-oh-**kloe**-pra-mide)

Metonia, Reglan

Classification

Therapeutic: antiemetics

Indications

Prevention of chemotherapy-induced emesis. Treatment of acute and recurrent diabetic gastroparesis. Facilitation of small bowel intubation in radiographic procedures. Management of gastroesophageal reflux. Treatment and prevention of postoperative nausea and vomiting when nasogastric suctioning is undesirable. **Unlabeled Use:** Treatment of hiccups. Adjunct management of migraine headaches.

Action

Blocks dopamine receptors in chemoreceptor trigger zone of the CNS. Stimulates motility of the upper GI tract and accelerates gastric emptying. **Therapeutic Effects:** Decreased nausea and vomiting. Decreased symptoms of gastric stasis. Easier passage of nasogastric tube into small bowel.

Pharmacokinetics

Absorption: Well absorbed from the GI tract, from rectal mucosa, and from IM sites.

Distribution: Widely distributed into body tissues and fluids. Crosses blood-brain barrier and placenta. Enters breast milk in concentrations greater than plasma.

Metabolism and Excretion: Partially metabolized by the liver (primarily by CYP2D6; the CYP2D6 enzyme system exhibits genetic polymorphism); ~7% of population may be poor metabolizers and may have significantly ↑ metoprolol concentrations and an ↑ risk of adverse effects. 25% eliminated unchanged in the urine.

Half-life: 2.5–6 hr.

TIME/ACTION PROFILE (effects on peristalsis)

ROUTE	ONSET	PEAK	DURATION
PO	30–60 min	unknown	1–2 hr
IM	10–15 min	unknown	1–2 hr
IV	1–3 min	immediate	1–2 hr

Contraindications/Precautions

Contraindicated in: Hypersensitivity; Possible GI obstruction, perforation, or hemorrhage; Seizure disorders; Pheochromocytoma; History of tardive dyskinesia; Parkinson's disease.

Use Cautiously in: History of depression; Diabetes (may alter response to insulin); Renal impairment (↓ dose in CCr <50 mL/min); Chronic use >12 wk (↑ risk for tardive dyskinesia); CYP2D6 poor metabolizers (↑ risk for tardive dyskinesia); OB, Lactation: Safety not established; Pedi: Prolonged clearance in neonates can result in high serum concentrations and ↑ the risk for methemoglobinemia. Side effects are more common in children, especially extrapyramidal reactions. Avoid use of tablets because of ↑ risk of tardive dyskinesia and methemoglobinemia (in neonates); Geri: More susceptible to oversedation, extrapyramidal reactions, and tardive dyskinesia (↓ dose).

Adverse Reactions/Side Effects

CNS: drowsiness, extrapyramidal reactions, restlessness, NEUROLEPTIC MALIGNANT SYNDROME, anxiety, bradykinesia, cog-wheel rigidity, depression, irritability, tardive dyskinesia, tremor. **CV:** arrhythmias (supraventricular tachycardia, bradycardia), hypertension, hypotension. **Endo:** gynecomastia, hyperprolactinemia. **GI:** constipation, diarrhea, dry mouth, nausea. **Hemat:** methemoglobinemia, neutropenia, leukopenia, agranulocytosis.

Interactions

Drug-Drug: Additive CNS depression with other **CNS depressants**, including **alcohol**, **antidepressants**, **antihistamines**, **opioid analgesics**, and **sedative/hypnotics**. May ↑ absorption and risk of toxicity from **cyclosporine**. May affect the GI absorption of other **orally administered drugs** as a result of effect on GI motility. May exaggerate hypotension during **general anesthesia**. ↑ risk of tardive dyskinesia, extrapyramidal reactions, or neuromalignant syndrome with **antipsychotic agents**; avoid concurrent use. **Strong CYP2D6 inhibitors**, including **bupropion**, **fluoxetine**, **paroxetine**, or **quinidine** may ↑ levels and risk of extrapyramidal reactions; ↓ metoclopramide dose. **Opioids** and **anticholinergics** may antagonize the GI effects of metoclopramide. Use cautiously with **MAO inhibitors** (causes release of catecholamines). May ↑ neuromuscular blockade from **succinylcholine**. May ↓ effectiveness of **levodopa**. May ↑ **tacrolimus** serum levels.

Route/Dosage

Prevention of Chemotherapy-Induced Vomiting

IV (Adults and Children): 1–2 mg/kg 30 min before chemotherapy. Additional doses of 1–2 mg/kg may be given every 2–4 hr, pretreatment with diphenhydramine will ↓ the risk of extrapyramidal reactions to this dose.

Facilitation of Small Bowel Intubation

IV (Adults and Children >14 yr): 10 mg over 1–2 min.

IV (Children 6–14 yr): 2.5–5 mg (dose should not exceed 0.5 mg/kg) over 1–2 min.

IV (Children <6 yr): 0.1 mg/kg over 1–2 min.

Diabetic Gastroparesis

PO, IV, IM (Adults): 10 mg 30 min before meals and at bedtime for 2–8 wk (not to exceed 40 mg/day). *CYP2D6 poor metabolizers*—5 mg 30 min before meals and at bedtime for 2–8 wk (not to exceed 20 mg/day). *Concurrent use of strong CYP2D6 inhibitor*—5 mg 30 min before meals and at bedtime for 2–8 wk (not to exceed 20 mg/day).

PO, IV, IM (Geriatric Patients): 5 mg 30 min before meals and at bedtime for 2–8 wk; may titrate up to 10 mg 30 min before each meal and at bedtime based on response and tolerability (not to exceed 40 mg/day).

Renal Impairment

PO (Adults): *CCr ≤60 mL/min*—5 mg 30 min before meals and at bedtime for 2–8 wk (not to exceed 20 mg/day). *ESRD (including hemodialysis and peritoneal dialysis)*—5 mg twice daily for 2–8 wk (not to exceed 10 mg/day).

Hepatic Impairment

PO, IV, IM (Adults): *Mild hepatic impairment (Child-Pugh A)*—10 mg 30 min before meals and at bedtime for 2–8 wk (not to exceed 40 mg/day). *Moderate or severe hepatic impairment (Child-Pugh B or C)*—5 mg 30 min before meals and at bedtime for 2–8 wk (not to exceed 20 mg/day).

Gastroesophageal Reflux

PO (Adults): 10–15 mg 30 min before each meal and at bedtime (not to exceed 60 mg/day). *CYP2D6 poor metabolizers*—5 mg 30 min before each meal and at bedtime or 10 mg 3 times daily (not to exceed 30 mg/day). *Concurrent use of strong CYP2D6 inhibitor*—5 mg 30 min before each meal and at bedtime or 10 mg 3 times daily (not to exceed 30 mg/day).

PO (Geriatric Patients): 5 mg 30 min before each meal and at bedtime; may titrate up to 10–15 mg 30 min before each meal and at bedtime based on response and tolerability (not to exceed 60 mg/day).

Renal Impairment

PO (Adults): *CCr ≤60 mL/min*—5 mg 30 min before each meal and at bedtime or 10 mg 3 times daily (not to exceed 30 mg/day). *ESRD (including hemodialysis and peritoneal dialysis)*—5 mg 30 min before each meal and at bedtime or 10 mg twice daily (not to exceed 20 mg/day).

Hepatic Impairment

PO (Adults): *Mild hepatic impairment (Child-Pugh A)*—10–15 mg 30 min before each meal and at bedtime (not to exceed 60 mg/day). *Moderate or severe hepatic impairment (Child-Pugh B or C)*—5 mg 30 min before each meal and at bedtime or 10 mg 3 times daily (not to exceed 30 mg/day).

Postoperative Nausea/Vomiting

IM, IV (Adults): 10 mg at the end of surgical procedure, repeat in 6–8 hr if needed.

Treatment of Hiccups

PO, IM (Adults): 10–20 mg 4 times daily PO; may be preceded by a single 10-mg dose IM (unlabeled).

Availability (generic available)

Oral solution (apricot-peach flavor): 5 mg/5 mL. **Orally disintegrating tablets:** 5 mg, 10 mg. **Cost:** $26.40/10. **Solution for injection:** 5 mg/mL. **Tablets:** 5 mg, 10 mg. **Cost:** *Generic*—5 mg $11.04/100, 10 mg $7.18/100.

NURSING IMPLICATIONS

Assessment

- Assess for nausea, vomiting, abdominal distention, and bowel sounds before and after administration.
- Assess for extrapyramidal side effects (*parkinsonian*—difficulty speaking or swallowing, loss of balance control, pill rolling, mask-like face, shuffling gait, rigidity, tremors; and *dystonic*—muscle spasms, twisting motions, twitching, inability to move eyes, weakness of arms or legs) periodically throughout course of therapy. May occur wk to mo after initiation of therapy and are reversible on discontinuation. Dystonic reactions may occur within min of IV infusion and stop within 24 hr of discontinuation of metoclopramide. May be treated with 50 mg of IM diphenhydramine or diphenhydramine 1 mg/kg IV may be administered prophylactically 15 min before metoclopramide IV infusion.
- Monitor for tardive dyskinesia (uncontrolled rhythmic movement of mouth, face, and extremities; lip smacking or puckering; puffing of cheeks; uncontrolled chewing; rapid or worm-like movements of tongue). Usually occurs after a yr or more of continued therapy; risk of tardive dyskinesia increases with total cumulative dose. Report immediately and discontinue metoclopramide; may be irreversible.
- Monitor for neuroleptic malignant syndrome (hyperthermia, muscle rigidity, altered consciousness, irregular pulse or BP, tachycardia, and diaphoresis).
- Assess for signs of depression periodically throughout therapy.
- Monitor for symptoms related to hyperprolactinemia (menstrual abnormalities, galactorrhea, sexual dysfunction).
- ***Lab Test Considerations:*** May alter hepatic function test results.
- May cause ↑ serum prolactin and aldosterone concentrations.

Implementation

- **PO:** Administer doses 30 min before meals and at bedtime.
- Do not remove *orally disintegrating tablets* from the bottle until just prior to dosing. Remove tablet from bottle with dry hands and immediately place on tongue to disintegrate and swallow with saliva. Tablet typically disintegrates in 1–1.5 min. Administration with liquid is not necessary.
- **IM:** For prevention of postoperative nausea and vomiting, inject IM near the end of surgery.

IV Administration

- **IV Push:** Administer IV dose 30 min before administration of chemotherapeutic agent. ***Rate:*** Doses may be given slowly over 1–2 min. Rapid administration causes a transient but intense feeling of anxiety and restlessness followed by drowsiness.
- **Intermittent Infusion:** ***Diluent:*** May be diluted for IV infusion in 50 mL of D5W, 0.9% NaCl, D5/0.45% NaCl, Ringer's solution, or LR. Diluted solution is stable for 48 hr if protected from light or 24 hr under normal light. ***Concentration:*** May dilute to 0.2 mg/mL or give undiluted at 5 mg/mL. ***Rate:*** Infuse slowly (maximum rate 5 mg/min) over at least 15–30 min.

- **Y-Site Compatibility:** aldesleukin, alemtuzumab, alfentanil, amifostine, amikacin, aminophylline, amphotericin B lipid complex, anidulafungin, argatroban, ascorbic acid, atropine, aztreonam, benztropine, bivalirudin, bleomycin, bumetanide, buprenorphine, butorphanol, calcium chloride, calcium gluconate, carboplatin, caspofungin, cefazolin, cefotaxime, cefotetan, cefoxitin, ceftaroline, ceftazidime, ceftriaxone, cefuroxime, chloramphenicol, chlorpromazine, ciprofloxacin, cisatracurium, cisplatin, cladribine, clindamycin, cyanocobalamin, cyclophosphamide, cyclosporine, cytarabine, dactinomycin, daptomycin, dexamethasone, dexmedetomidine, digoxin, diltiazem, diphenhydramine, dobutamine, docetaxel, dopamine, doxorubicin hydrochloride, doxycycline, droperidol, enalaprilat, ephedrine, epinephrine, epirubicin, epoetin alfa, eptifibatide, ertapenem, erythromycin, esmolol, etoposide, etoposide phosphate, famotidine, fenoldopam, fentanyl, filgrastim, fluconazole, fludarabine, folic acid, foscarnet, gemcitabine, gentamicin, glycopyrrolate, granisetron, heparin, hetastarch, hydrocortisone, hydromorphone, idarubicin, ifosfamide, imipenem/cilastatin, indomethacin, insulin, regular, irinotecan, isoproterenol, ketamine, ketorolac, labetalol, leucovorin, levofloxacin, lidocaine, linezolid, lorazepam, magnesium sulfate, mannitol, melphalan, meperidine, meropenem, methadone, methotrexate, methyldopate, methylprednisolone, metoprolol, metronidazole, midazolam, milrinone, mitomycin, mitoxantrone, morphine, multiple vitamins, mycophenolate, nafcillin, nalbuphine, naloxone, nitroglycerin, nitroprusside, norepinephrine, octreotide, ondansetron, oxacillin, oxaliplatin, oxytocin, paclitaxel, palonosetron, pamidronate, pancuronium, pantoprazole, papaverine, pemetrexed, penicillin G, pentamidine, pentobarbital, phenobarbital, phenylephrine, phytonadione, piperacillin/tazobactam, potassium acetate, potassium chloride, procainamide, prochlorperazine, promethazine, propranolol, protamine, pyridoxine, quinupristin/dalfopristin, ranitidine, remifentanil, rituximab, rocuronium, sargramostim, sodium acetate, sodium bicarbonate, streptokinase, succinylcholine, sufentanil, tacrolimus, telavancin, theophylline, thiamine, thiotepa, tigecycline, tirofiban, tobramycin, topotecan, trastuzumab, vancomycin, vasopressin, vecuronium, verapamil, vinblastine, vincristine, vinorelbine, voriconazole, zidovudine, zoledronic acid.
- **Y-Site Incompatibility:** amphotericin B deoxycholate, amphotericin B liposome, carmustine, cefepime, dantrolene, diazepam, doxorubicin liposome, ganciclovir, phenytoin, propofol, trimethoprim/sulfamethoxazole.

Patient/Family Teaching

- Instruct patient to take metoclopramide as directed. Take missed doses as soon as remembered if not almost time for next dose. Advise patient to read the *Medication Guide* before starting therapy and with each Rx refill in case of changes.
- Pedi: Unintentional overdose has been reported in infants and children with the use of metoclopramide oral solution. Teach parents how to accurately read labels and administer medication.
- May cause drowsiness. Caution patient to avoid driving or other activities requiring alertness until response to medication is known.
- Advise patient to avoid concurrent use of alcohol and other CNS depressants while taking this medication.
- Inform patient of risk of extrapyramidal symptoms, tardive dyskinesia, and neuroleptic malignant syndrome. Advise patient to notify health care professional immediately if involuntary or repetitive movements of eyes, face, or limbs occur.
- Advise females of reproductive potential to notify health care professional if pregnancy is planned or suspected, or if breast feeding. Monitor neonates for extrapyramidal signs and methemoglobinemia.

Evaluation/Desired Outcomes

- Prevention or relief of nausea and vomiting.
- Decreased symptoms of gastric stasis.
- Facilitation of small bowel intubation.
- Decreased symptoms of esophageal reflux.
- Metoclopramide should not be used for more than 12 wk due to risk of tardive dyskinesia.

metOLazone (me-**tole**-a-zone)

Zaroxolyn

Classification

Therapeutic: antihypertensives, diuretics
Pharmacologic: thiazide-like diuretics

Indications

Mild to moderate hypertension. Edema associated with HF or the nephrotic syndrome.

Action

Increases excretion of sodium and water by inhibiting sodium reabsorption in the distal tubule. Promotes excretion of chloride, potassium, magnesium, and bicarbonate. May produce arteriolar dilation. **Therapeutic Effects:** Lowering of BP in hypertensive patients. Diuresis with subsequent mobilization of edema. Effect may continue in renal impairment.

Pharmacokinetics

Absorption: Absorption is variable.
Distribution: Unknown.

M

Protein Binding: 95%.
Metabolism and Excretion: Excreted mainly unchanged by the kidneys.
Half-life: 6–20 hr.

TIME/ACTION PROFILE (diuretic effect†)

ROUTE	ONSET	PEAK	DURATION
PO	1 hr	2 hr	12–24 hr

†Full antihypertensive effect may take days–wk.

Contraindications/Precautions

Contraindicated in: Hypersensitivity; Cross-sensitivity with other sulfonamides may exist; Anuria; Lactation: Lactation.
Use Cautiously in: Severe hepatic impairment; OB: Safety not established; Geri: ↑ sensitivity to drug effects.

Adverse Reactions/Side Effects

CNS: drowsiness, lethargy. **CV:** chest pain, hypotension, palpitations. **Derm:** photosensitivity, rash. **Endo:** hyperglycemia. **F and E:** hypokalemia, dehydration, hypercalcemia, hypochloremic alkalosis, hypomagnesemia, hyponatremia, hypophosphatemia, hypovolemia. **GI:** anorexia, bloating, cramping, drug-induced hepatitis, nausea, pancreatitis, vomiting. **Hemat:** blood dyscrasias. **Metab:** hyperuricemia. **MS:** muscle cramps.

Interactions

Drug-Drug: ↑ risk of hypotension with **nitrates**, acute ingestion of **alcohol**, or other **antihypertensives**. ↑ risk of hypokalemia with **corticosteroids**, **amphotericin B**, or **piperacillin/tazobactam**. May ↑ the risk of **digoxin** toxicity. ↓ the excretion of **lithium**; may cause toxicity. May ↓ the effectiveness of **methenamine**. **Stimulant laxatives** (including **aloe**, **senna**) may ↑ risk of potassium depletion.
Drug-Food: **Food** may ↑ extent of absorption.

Route/Dosage

PO (Adults): *Hypertension*—2.5–5 mg/day; *edema*—5–20 mg/day.
PO (Children): 0.2–0.4 mg/kg/day divided every 12–24 hr.

Availability (generic available)

Tablets: 2.5 mg, 5 mg, 10 mg.

NURSING IMPLICATIONS

Assessment

- Monitor BP, intake and output, and daily weight, and assess feet, legs, and sacral area for edema daily.
- Assess patient, especially if taking digoxin, for anorexia, nausea, vomiting, muscle cramps, paresthesia, and confusion. Notify health care professional if these signs of electrolyte imbalance occur. Patients taking digoxin are at risk of digoxin toxicity because of the potassium-depleting effect of the diuretic.
- Assess patient for allergy to sulfonamides.
- **Hypertension:** Monitor BP before and periodically during therapy.
- Monitor frequency of prescription refills to determine compliance.
- ***Lab Test Considerations:*** Monitor electrolytes (especially potassium), blood glucose, BUN, and serum creatinine and uric acid levels before and periodically during therapy.
- May cause ↑ in serum and urine glucose in diabetic patients.
- May cause an ↑ in serum bilirubin, calcium, creatinine, and uric acid, and a ↓ in serum magnesium, potassium, and sodium and urinary calcium concentrations.
- May cause ↓ serum protein-bound iodine (PBI) concentrations.
- May cause ↑ serum cholesterol, low-density lipoprotein, and triglyceride concentrations.

Implementation

- Do not confuse metolazone with methimazole, methazolamide, methadone, or methotrexate.
- Administer in the morning to prevent disruption of sleep cycle.
- Intermittent dose schedule may be used for continued control of edema.
- **PO:** May give with food or milk to minimize GI irritation.

Patient/Family Teaching

- Instruct patient to take metolazone at the same time each day. Take missed doses as soon as remembered but not just before next dose is due. Do not double doses.
- Instruct patient to monitor weight biweekly and notify health care professional of significant changes.
- Caution patient to change positions slowly to minimize orthostatic hypotension; may be potentiated by alcohol.
- Advise patient to use sunscreen and protective clothing in the sun to prevent photosensitivity reactions.
- Instruct patient to discuss dietary potassium requirements with health care professional (see Appendix K).
- Instruct patient to notify health care professional of medication regimen before treatment or surgery.
- Advise patient to report muscle weakness, cramps, nausea, vomiting, diarrhea, or dizziness to health care professional.
- Emphasize the importance of routine follow-up exams.
- **Hypertension:** Advise patient to continue taking the medication even if feeling better. Medication controls but does not cure hypertension.
- Encourage patient to comply with additional interventions for hypertension (weight reduction, low-sodium diet, regular exercise, smoking cessation, moderation of alcohol consumption, and stress management).

- Instruct patient and family in correct technique for monitoring weekly BP.
- Advise patient to notify health care professional of all Rx or OTC medications, vitamins, or herbal products being taken and to consult with health care professional before taking other medications, especially cough or cold preparations, concurrently with this therapy.
- Advise females of reproductive potential to notify health care professional if pregnancy is planned or suspected, or if breast feeding.

Evaluation/Desired Outcomes

- Decrease in BP.
- Increase in urine output.
- Decrease in edema.

HIGH ALERT

metoprolol (me-**toe**-proe-lole)

Kapspargo Sprinkle, Lopresor, Lopresor SR, Lopressor, Toprol-XL

Classification

Therapeutic: antianginals, antihypertensives

Pharmacologic: beta blockers

Indications

Hypertension. Angina pectoris. Prevention of MI and decreased mortality in patients with recent MI. Management of stable, symptomatic (class II or III) heart failure due to ischemic, hypertensive or cardiomyopathic origin (may be used with ACE inhibitors, diuretics and/or digoxin; Toprol XL only). **Unlabeled Use:** Ventricular arrhythmias/tachycardia. Migraine prophylaxis. Tremors. Aggressive behavior. Drug-induced akathisia. Anxiety.

Action

Blocks stimulation of $beta_1$ (myocardial)-adrenergic receptors. Does not usually affect $beta_2$ (pulmonary, vascular, uterine)-adrenergic receptor sites. **Therapeutic Effects:** Decreased BP and heart rate. Decreased frequency of attacks of angina pectoris. Decreased rate of cardiovascular mortality and hospitalization in patients with heart failure.

Pharmacokinetics

Absorption: Well absorbed after oral administration.
Distribution: Crosses the blood-brain barrier, crosses the placenta; small amounts enter breast milk.
Metabolism and Excretion: Mostly metabolized by the liver (primarily by CYP2D6; the CYP2D6 enzyme system exhibits genetic polymorphism); ~7% of population may be poor metabolizers and may have significantly ↑ metoprolol concentrations and an ↑ risk of adverse effects.
Half-life: 3–7 hr.

TIME/ACTION PROFILE (cardiovascular effects)

ROUTE	ONSET	PEAK	DURATION
PO†	15 min	unknown	6–12 hr
PO–ER	unknown	6–12 hr	24 hr
IV	immediate	20 min	5–8 hr

†Maximal effects on BP (chronic therapy) may not occur for 1 wk. Hypotensive effects may persist for up to 4 wk after discontinuation.

Contraindications/Precautions

Contraindicated in: Uncompensated HF; Pulmonary edema; Cardiogenic shock; Bradycardia, heart block, or sick sinus syndrome (in absence of a pacemaker).
Use Cautiously in: Renal impairment; Hepatic impairment; Geri: ↑ sensitivity to beta blockers; initial dose reduction recommended; Pulmonary disease (including asthma; $beta_1$ selectivity may be lost at higher doses); Diabetes mellitus (may mask signs of hypoglycemia); Thyrotoxicosis (may mask symptoms); Patients with a history of severe allergic reactions (intensity of reactions may be increased); Untreated pheochromocytoma (initiate only after alpha blocker therapy started); OB: Safety not established; crosses the placenta and may cause fetal/neonatal bradycardia, hypotension, hypoglycemia, or respiratory depression; Lactation: Safety not established; Pedi: Safety and effectiveness not established in children <18 yr (tablets, extended-release tablets, and injection) or children <6 yr (extended-release capsules).

Adverse Reactions/Side Effects

CNS: fatigue, weakness, anxiety, depression, dizziness, drowsiness, insomnia, memory loss, mental status changes, nervousness, nightmares. **CV:** BRADYCARDIA, HF, PULMONARY EDEMA, hypotension, peripheral vasoconstriction. **Derm:** rash. **EENT:** blurred vision, stuffy nose. **Endo:** hyperglycemia, hypoglycemia. **GI:** constipation, diarrhea, drug-induced hepatitis, dry mouth, flatulence, gastric pain, heartburn, ↑ liver enzymes, nausea, vomiting. **GU:** erectile dysfunction, ↓ libido, urinary frequency. **MS:** arthralgia, back pain, joint pain. **Resp:** bronchospasm, wheezing. **Misc:** drug-induced lupus syndrome.

Interactions

Drug-Drug: General anesthesia, **IV phenytoin**, and **verapamil** may cause ↑ myocardial depression. ↑ risk of bradycardia when used with **digoxin**, **verapamil**, **diltiazem**, or **clonidine**. ↑ hypotension may occur with other **antihypertensives**, acute ingestion of **alcohol**, or **nitrates**. Concurrent use with **amphetamines**, **cocaine**, **ephedrine**, **epinephrine**, **norepinephrine**, **phenylephrine**, or **pseudoephedrine** may result in unopposed alpha-adrenergic stimulation (excessive hypertension, bradycardia). Concurrent administration of **thyroid** administration may ↓ effectiveness. May alter the effectiveness of **insulins** or **oral hypoglycemic agents** (dose adjustments may be necessary). May ↓ the effectiveness of **theophylline**. May ↓ the beneficial $beta_1$-cardiovascular effects of **dopamine** or **dobutamine**. Use cautiously within 14 days of **MAO inhibitor** therapy (may result in hypertension).

Route/Dosage

When switching from immediate-release to extended-release product, the same total daily dose can be used

PO (Adults): *Hypertension/angina*—25–100 mg/day as a single dose initially or 2 divided doses; may be ↑ every 7 days as needed up to 450 mg/day (immediate-release) or 400 mg/day (extended-release) (for angina, give in divided doses). Extended-release products are given once daily. *MI*—25–50 mg (starting 15 min after last IV dose) every 6 hr for 48 hr, then 100 mg twice daily. *Heart failure*—12.5–25 mg once daily (of extended-release), can be doubled every 2 wk up to 200 mg/day. *Migraine prevention*—50–100 mg 2–4 times daily (unlabeled).
IV (Adults): *MI*—5 mg every 2 min for 3 doses, followed by oral dosing.
PO (Children ≥6 yr): *Hypertension*—1 mg/kg once daily (extended-release capsules); may be titrated, as needed (not to exceed 50 mg/day).

Availability (generic available)

Extended-release capsules (succinate; Kapspargo Sprinkle): 25 mg, 50 mg, 100 mg, 200 mg. **Extended-release tablets (succinate; Toprol XL):** 25 mg, 50 mg, 100 mg, 200 mg. **Cost:** *Generic*—25 mg $35.68/100, 50 mg $41.93/100, 100 mg $53.95/100, 200 mg $84.54/100. **Solution for injection:** 1 mg/mL. **Tablets (tartrate):** 25 mg, 37.5 mg, 50 mg, 75 mg, 100 mg. **Cost:** *Generic*—All strengths $7.18/100. ***In combination with:*** hydrochlorothiazide (Dutoprol, Lopressor HCT). See Appendix B.

NURSING IMPLICATIONS

Assessment

- Monitor BP, ECG, and pulse frequently during dose adjustment and periodically during therapy.
- Monitor frequency of prescription refills to determine compliance.
- Monitor vital signs and ECG every 5–15 min during and for several hrs after parenteral administration. If heart rate <40 bpm, especially if cardiac output is also decreased, administer atropine 0.25–0.5 mg IV.
- Monitor intake and output ratios and daily weights. Assess routinely for signs and symptoms of HF (dyspnea, rales/crackles, weight gain, peripheral edema, jugular venous distention).
- **Angina:** Assess frequency and characteristics of anginal attacks periodically during therapy.
- ***Lab Test Considerations:*** May cause ↑ BUN, serum lipoprotein, potassium, triglyceride, and uric acid levels.
- May cause ↑ ANA titers.
- May cause ↑ in blood glucose levels.
- May cause ↑ serum alkaline phosphatase, LDH, AST, and ALT levels.

Implementation

- ***High Alert:*** IV vasoactive medications are inherently dangerous. Before administering intravenously, have second practitioner independently check original order and dose calculations.
- ***High Alert:*** Do not confuse Toprol-XL (metoprolol succinate) with Topamax (topiramate). Do not confuse Lopressor (metoprolol tartrate) with Lyrica (pregabalin). Do not confuse metoprolol tartrate with metoprolol succinate.
- **PO:** Take apical pulse before administering. If <50 bpm or if arrhythmia occurs, withhold medication and notify health care professional.
- Administer metoprolol with meals or directly after eating.
- Extended-release tablets should be swallowed whole; do not break, crush, or chew.
- Swallow *Kapspargo Sprinkle* whole. If unable to swallow a capsule, may be opened and contents sprinkled over soft food (applesauce, pudding, yogurt). Swallow contents of capsule along with a small amount (tsp) of soft food. Swallow drug/food mixture within 60 min; do not store for future use. May also be administered via NG tube by opening and adding capsule contents to an all plastic oral tip syringe and adding 15 mL of water. Gently shake syringe for about 10 sec. Promptly administer through a 12 French or larger NG tube. Rinse with additional water to ensure no granules are left in syringe.

IV Administration

- **IV Push:** ***Diluent:*** Administer undiluted. ***Concentration:*** 1 mg/mL. ***Rate:*** Administer over 1 min.
- **Y-Site Compatibility:** acyclovir, alemtuzumab, alfentanil, alteplase, amikacin, aminocaproic acid, aminophylline, amiodarone, amphotericin B liposome, anidulafungin, argatroban, ascorbic acid, atropine, aztreonam, benztropine, bivalirudin, bleomycin, bumetanide, buprenorphine, butorphanol, calcium chloride, calcium gluconate, cangrelor, carboplatin, carmustine, caspofungin, cefazolin, cefonocid, cefotaxime, cefotetan, cefoxitin, ceftaroline, ceftazidime, ceftriaxone, cefuroxime, chloramphenicol, chlorpromazine, cisplatin, clindamycin, cyanocobalamin, cyclophosphamide, cyclosporine, cytarabine, dactinomycin, daptomycin, dexamethasone, dexmedetomidine, digoxin, diltiazem, diphenhydramine, dobutamine, docetaxel, dopamine, doxorubicin hydrochloride, doxycycline, enalaprilat, ephedrine, epinephrine, epirubicin, epoetin alfa, eptifibatide, esmolol, etoposide, etoposide phos-

phate, famotidine, fenoldopam, fentanyl, fluconazole, fludarabine, fluorouracil, folic acid, foscarnet, fosphenytoin, furosemide, ganciclovir, gemcitabine, gentamicin, glycopyrrolate, granisetron, heparin, hetastarch, hydrocortisone, hydromorphone, idarubicin, ifosfamide, imipenem/cilastatin, indomethacin, insulin, regular, irinotecan, isoproterenol, ketorolac, labetalol, leucovorin, linezolid, lorazepam, magnesium sulfate, mannitol, meperidine, methotrexate, methyldopate, methylprednisolone, metoclopramide, metronidazole, midazolam, milrinone, mitoxantrone, morphine, multivitamins, mycophenolate, nafcillin, nalbuphine, naloxone, nitroprusside, norepinephrine, octreotide, ondansetron, oxacillin, oxaliplatin, oxytocin, paclitaxel, palonosetron, pamidronate, pancuronium, papaverine, pemetrexed, penicillin G, pentamidine, pentobarbital, phenobarbital, phenylephrine, phytonadione, piperacillin/tazobactam, potassium acetate, potassium chloride, procainamide, prochlorperazine, promethazine, propranolol, protamine, pyridoxine, quinupristin/dalfopristin, ranitidine, rocuronium, sodium bicarbonate, streptokinase, succinylcholine, sufentanil, tacrolimus, theophylline, thiamine, thiotepa, tigecycline, tirofiban, tobramycin, vancomycin, vasopressin, vecuronium, verapamil, vincristine, vinorelbine, voriconazole, zoledronic acid.

- **Y-Site Incompatibility:** allopurinol, amphotericin B lipid complex, dantrolene, diazepam, pantoprazole, phenytoin, trimethoprim/sulfamethoxazole.

Patient/Family Teaching

- Instruct patient to take medication as directed, at the same time each day, even if feeling well; do not skip or double up on missed doses. Take missed doses as soon as possible up to 8 hr before next dose. Abrupt withdrawal may precipitate life-threatening arrhythmias, hypertension, or myocardial ischemia.
- Teach patient and family how to check pulse daily and BP biweekly and to report significant changes to health care professional.
- May cause drowsiness. Caution patient to avoid driving or other activities that require alertness until response to the drug is known.
- Advise patient to change positions slowly to minimize orthostatic hypotension.
- Caution patient that this medication may increase sensitivity to cold.
- Instruct patient to notify health care professional of all Rx or OTC medications, vitamins, or herbal products being taken and to consult health care professional before taking any Rx, OTC, or herbal products, especially cold preparations, concurrently with this medication. Patients on antihypertensive therapy should also avoid excessive amounts of coffee, tea, and cola.
- Diabetics should closely monitor blood glucose, especially if weakness, malaise, irritability, or fatigue occurs. Medication does not block sweating as a sign of hypoglycemia.
- Advise patient to notify health care professional if slow pulse, difficulty breathing, wheezing, cold hands and feet, dizziness, light-headedness, confusion, depression, rash, fever, sore throat, unusual bleeding, or bruising occurs.
- Instruct patient to inform health care professional of medication regimen before treatment or surgery.
- Advise females of reproductive potential to notify health care professional if pregnancy is planned or suspected, or if breast feeding. Monitor neonates of women taking metoprolol for symptoms of hypotension, bradycardia, hypoglycemia, and respiratory depression and manage accordingly. Monitor breast-fed infants for bradycardia, dry mouth, skin or eyes, and diarrhea or constipation.
- Advise patient to carry identification describing disease process and medication regimen at all times.
- **Hypertension:** Reinforce the need to continue additional therapies for hypertension (weight loss, sodium restriction, stress reduction, regular exercise, moderation of alcohol consumption, and smoking cessation). Medication controls but does not cure hypertension.

Evaluation/Desired Outcomes

- Decrease in BP.
- Reduction in frequency of anginal attacks.
- Increase in activity tolerance.
- Prevention of MI.

metroNIDAZOLE

(me-troe-**ni**-da-zole)

Flagyl, MetroCream, MetroGel, MetroGel-Vaginal, MetroLotion, Metro IV, ✱Nidagel, Noritate, Nuvessa, Vandazole

Classification

Therapeutic: anti-infectives, antiprotozoals, antiulcer agents

Indications

PO, IV: Treatment of the following anaerobic infections: Intra-abdominal infections (may be used with a cephalosporin), Gynecologic infections, Skin and skin structure infections, Lower respiratory tract infections, Bone and joint infections, CNS infections, Septicemia, Endocarditis. **IV:** Perioperative prophylactic agent in colorectal surgery. **PO:** Amebicide in the management of amebic dysentery, amebic liver abscess, and trichomoniasis: Treatment of peptic ulcer disease caused by

M

Helicobacter pylori. **Topical:** Treatment of acne rosacea. **Vag:** Management of bacterial vaginosis. **Unlabeled Use:** Treatment of giardiasis. Treatment of anti-infective associated Clostridium difficile-associated diarrhea (CDAD).

Action

Disrupts DNA and protein synthesis in susceptible organisms. **Therapeutic Effects:** Bactericidal, trichomonacidal, or amebicidal action. **Spectrum:** Most notable for activity against anaerobic bacteria, including: *Bacteroides*, *Clostridium*. In addition, is active against: *Trichomonas vaginalis*, *Entamoeba histolytica*, *Giardia lamblia*, *H. pylori*, *Clostridium difficile*.

Pharmacokinetics

Absorption: 80% absorbed after oral administration. Minimal absorption after topical or vaginal application.

Distribution: Widely distributed into most tissues and fluids, including CSF. Crosses the placenta and enters fetal circulation rapidly; enters breast milk in concentrations equal to plasma levels.

Metabolism and Excretion: Partially metabolized by the liver (30–60%), partially excreted unchanged in the urine, 6–15% eliminated in the feces.

Half-life: Neonates: 25–75 hr; Children and adults: 6–12 hr.

TIME/ACTION PROFILE (PO, IV = blood levels; topical = improvement in rosacea)

ROUTE	ONSET	PEAK	DURATION
PO	rapid	1–3 hr	8 hr
PO-ER	rapid	unknown	up to 24 hr
IV	rapid	end of infusion	6–8 hr
Topical	3 wk	9 wk	12 hr
Vaginal	unknown	6–12 hr	12 hr

Contraindications/Precautions

Contraindicated in: Hypersensitivity; Hypersensitivity to parabens (topical only); OB: First trimester of pregnancy.

Use Cautiously in: History of blood dyscrasias; History of seizures or neurologic problems; Severe hepatic impairment (dose ↓ suggested); Cockayne syndrome (↑ risk of hepatotoxicity and death); OB: Although safety not established, has been used to treat trichomoniasis in 2nd- and 3rd-trimester pregnancy—but not as single-dose regimen; Lactation: If needed, use single dose and interrupt nursing for 24 hr thereafter; Patients receiving corticosteroids or predisposed to edema (injection contains 28 mEq sodium/g metronidazole).

Adverse Reactions/Side Effects

CNS: SEIZURES, dizziness, headache, aseptic meningitis (IV), encephalopathy (IV), psychosis. **Derm:** STEVENS-JOHNSON SYNDROME, rash, urticaria; *topical only*, burning, mild dryness, skin irritation, transient redness. **EENT:** optic neuropathy, tearing (topical only). **GI:** abdominal pain, anorexia, nausea, diarrhea, dry mouth, furry tongue, glossitis, unpleasant taste, vomiting. **Hemat:** leukopenia. **Local:** phlebitis at IV site. **Neuro:** peripheral neuropathy. **Misc:** superinfection.

Interactions

Drug-Drug: Cimetidine may ↓ metabolism. **Phenobarbital** and **rifampin** ↑ metabolism and may ↓ effectiveness. Metronidazole ↑ the effects of **phenytoin**, **lithium**, and **warfarin**. Disulfiram-like reaction may occur with **alcohol** ingestion. May cause acute psychosis and confusion with **disulfiram**. ↑ risk of leukopenia with **fluorouracil** or **azathioprine**.

Route/Dosage

PO (Adults): *Anaerobic infections*—7.5 mg/kg every 6 hr (not to exceed 4 g/day). *Trichomoniasis*—250 mg every 8 hr for 7 days *or* single 2-g dose *or* 1 g twice daily for 1 day. *Amebiasis*—500–750 mg every 8 hr for 5–10 days. *H. pylori*—250 mg 4 times daily *or* 500 mg twice daily for 1–2 wk (with other agents). *Antibiotic associated Clostridium difficile-associated diarrhea (CDAD)*—250–500 mg 3–4 times/day for 10–14 days.

PO (Infants and Children): *Anaerobic infections*—30 mg/kg/day divided every 6 hr, maximum dose: 4 g/day *Trichomoniasis*—15–30 mg/kg/day divided every 8 hr for 7–10 days. *Amebiasis*—35–50 mg/kg/day divided every 8 hr for 5–10 days (not to exceed 750 mg/dose). *Clostridium difficile-associated diarrhea (CDAD)*—30 mg/kg/day divided every 6 hr for 7–10 days. *H. pylori*—15–20 mg/kg/day divided twice daily for 4 wk.

IV, PO (Neonates 0–4 wk, <1200 g): 7.5 mg/kg every 48 hr. *Postnatal age <7 days, 1200–2000 g*—7.5 mg/kg/day every 24 hr. *Postnatal age <7 days, >2000 g*—15 mg/kg/day divided every 12 hr. *Postnatal age >7 days, 1200–2000 g*—15 mg/kg/day divided every 12 hr. *Postnatal age >7 days, >2000 g*—30 mg/kg/day divided every 12 hr.

IV (Adults): *Anaerobic infections*—Initial dose 15 mg/kg, then 7.5 mg/kg every 6–8 hr *or* 500 mg every 6–8 hr (not to exceed 4 g/day). *Perioperative prophylaxis*—Initial dose 15 mg/kg 1 hr before surgery, then 7.5 mg/kg 6 and 12 hr later. *Amebiasis*—500–750 mg every 8 hr for 5–10 days.

IV (Children): *Anaerobic infections*—30 mg/kg/day divided every 6 hr, maximum dose: 4 g/day.

Topical (Adults): *Acne rosacea*—Apply thin film to affected area bid.

Vag (Adults): *Bacterial vaginosis*—*MetroGel Vaginal*—One applicatorful (37.5 mg) of 0.75% gel 1–2 times daily for 5 days; *Nuvessa*—One applicatorful (65 mg) of 1.3% gel as a single dose at bedtime; *Vandazole*—One applicatorful (37.5 mg) of 0.75% gel once daily for 5 days.

Vag (Children ≥12 yr): *Nuvessa*—One applicatorful (65 mg) of 1.3% gel as a single dose at bedtime.

Availability (generic available)

Capsules: 375 mg, 🍁500 mg. **Premixed infusion:** 500 mg/100 mL. **Tablets:** 250 mg, 500 mg. **Topical cream:** 0.75%, 1%. **Topical gel:** 0.75%, 1%. **Topical lotion:** 0.75%. **Vaginal cream:** 🍁10% (500 mg/applicatorful). **Vaginal gel:** 0.75% (37.5 mg/5 g applicatorful), 1.3% (65 mg/5 g applicatorful). ***In combination with:*** bismuth subcitrate potassium and tetracycline (Pylera). See Appendix B.

NURSING IMPLICATIONS

Assessment

- Assess for infection (vital signs; appearance of wound, sputum, urine, and stool; WBC) at beginning of and throughout therapy.
- Obtain specimens for culture and sensitivity before initiating therapy. First dose may be given before receiving results.
- Monitor neurologic status during and after IV infusions. Inform health care professional if numbness, paresthesia, weakness, ataxia, or seizures occur.
- Monitor intake, output, and daily weight, especially for patients on sodium restriction. Each 500 mg of premixed injection for dilution contains 14 mEq of sodium.
- Assess for rash periodically during therapy. May cause Stevens-Johnson syndrome. Discontinue therapy if severe or if accompanied with fever, general malaise, fatigue, muscle or joint aches, blisters, oral lesions, conjunctivitis, hepatitis, and/or eosinophilia.
- **Giardiasis:** Monitor three stool samples taken several days apart, beginning 3–4 wk after treatment.
- ***Lab Test Considerations:*** May alter results of serum AST, ALT, and LDH tests.

Implementation

- Do not confuse metronidzole with metformin.
- **PO:** Administer on an empty stomach, or may administer with food or milk to minimize GI irritation. Tablets may be crushed for patients with difficulty swallowing. Swallow extended-release tablets whole; do not break, crush, or chew.

IV Administration

- **Intermittent Infusion:** ***Diluent:*** Administer premixed injection (500 mg/100 mL) undiluted. Do not refrigerate. Once taken out of overwrap, premixed infusion stable for 30 days at room temperature. ***Concentration:*** 5 mg/mL. ***Rate:*** Infuse over 30–60 min.
- **Y-Site Compatibility:** acyclovir, alemtuzumab, alfentanil, allopurinol, amifostine, amikacin, aminocaproic acid, aminophylline, amiodarone, ampicillin, ampicillin/sulbactam, anidulafungin, argatroban, azithromycin, bivalirudin, bleomycin, bumetanide, buprenorphine, busulfan, butorphanol, calcium acetate, calcium chloride, calcium gluconate, cangrelor, carboplatin, carmustine, cefazolin, cefepime, cefotaxime, cefotetan, cefoxitin, ceftaroline, ceftazidime, ceftriaxone, cefuroxime, chloramphenicol, chlorpromazine, ciprofloxacin, cisatracurium, cisplatin, clindamycin, cyclophosphamide, cyclosporine, cytarabine, dacarbazine, dactinomycin, dexamethasone, dexmedetomidine, dexrazoxane, digoxin, diltiazem, dimenhydrinate, diphenhydramine, dobutamine, docetaxel, dopamine, doxorubicin hydrochloride, doxorubicin liposomal, doxycycline, droperidol, enalaprilat, ephedrine, epinephrine, epirubicin, eptifibatide, ertapenem, erythromycin, esmolol, etoposide, etoposide phosphate, famotidine, fenoldopam, fentanyl, fluconazole, fludarabine, fluorouracil, foscarnet, fosphenytoin, furosemide, gemcitabine, gentamicin, glycopyrrolate, granisetron, haloperidol, heparin, hetastarch, hydralazine, hydrocortisone, hydromorphone, idarubicin, ifosfamide, imipenem/cilastatin, insulin, regular, irinotecan, isoproterenol, ketamine, ketorolac, labetalol, leucovorin, levofloxacin, lidocaine, linezolid, lorazepam, magnesium sulfate, mannitol, melphalan, meperidine, meropenem, mesna, methotrexate, methyldopate, methylprednisolone, metoclopramide, metoprolol, midazolam, milrinone, mitoxantrone, morphine, mycophenolate, nafcillin, nalbuphine, naloxone, nicardipine, nitroglycerin, nitroprusside, norepinephrine, octreotide, ondansetron, oxaliplatin, oxytocin, paclitaxel, palonosetron, pamidronate, pancuronium, pentamidine, pentobarbital, phenylephrine, piperacillin/tazobactam, potassium acetate, potassium chloride, potassium phosphates, prochlorperazine, promethazine, propranolol, ranitidine, remifentanil, rituximab, rocuronium, sargramostim, sodium acetate, sodium bicarbonate, sodium phosphates, streptozocin, succinylcholine, sufentanil, tacrolimus, theophylline, thiopental, thiotepa, tigecycline, tirofiban, tobramycin, topotecan, trastuzumab, trimethoprim/sulfamethoxazole, vancomycin, vasopressin, vecuronium, verapamil, vincristine, vinorelbine, voriconazole, zidovudine, zoledronic acid.
- **Y-Site Incompatibility:** acetaminophen, amphotericin B lipid complex, amphotericin B liposome, aztreonam, dantrolene, daptomycin, diazepam, filgrastim, ganciclovir, pantoprazole, pemetrexed, phenytoin, procainamide, quinupristin/dalfopristin.
- **Topical:** Cleanse affected area before application. Apply and rub in a thin film twice daily, morning and evening. Avoid contact with eyes.
- **Vag:** Administer once daily dosing at bedtime.

Patient/Family Teaching

- Instruct patient to take medication as directed with evenly spaced times between doses, even if feeling better. Do not skip doses or double up on missed

M

doses. Take missed doses as soon as remembered if not almost time for next dose.

- Advise patients treated for trichomoniasis that sexual partners may be asymptomatic sources of reinfection and should be treated concurrently. Patient should also refrain from intercourse or use a condom to prevent reinfection.
- Caution patient to avoid intake of alcoholic beverages or preparations containing alcohol during and for at least 3 days after treatment with metronidazole, including vaginal gel. May cause a disulfiram-like reaction (flushing, nausea, vomiting, headache, abdominal cramps).
- May cause dizziness or light-headedness. Caution patient to avoid driving or other activities requiring alertness until response to medication is known.
- Instruct patient to notify health care professional promptly if rash occurs.
- Inform patient that medication may cause an unpleasant metallic taste.
- Advise patient to notify health care professional of all Rx or OTC medications, vitamins, or herbal products being taken and to consult with health care professional before taking other medications.
- Advise patient that frequent mouth rinses, good oral hygiene, and sugarless gum or candy may minimize dry mouth. Notify health care professional if dry mouth persists for more than 2 wk.
- Inform patient that medication may cause urine to turn dark.
- Advise patient to consult health care professional if no improvement in a few days or if signs and symptoms of superinfection (black, furry overgrowth on tongue; vaginal itching or discharge; loose or foul-smelling stools) develop.
- Advise patient to inform health care professional if pregnancy is planned or suspected or if breast feeding.
- **Vag:** Instruct patient in correct technique for intravaginal instillation. Advise patient to avoid intercourse during treatment with vaginal gel.
- **Topical:** Instruct patient on correct technique for application of topical gel. Cosmetics may be used after application of gel.

Evaluation/Desired Outcomes

- Resolution of the signs and symptoms of infection. Length of time for complete resolution depends on organism and site of infection.
- Significant results should be seen within 3 wk of application of topical gel. Application may be continued for 9 wk.

micafungin (my-ka-**fun**-gin)

Mycamine

Classification

Therapeutic: antifungals
Pharmacologic: echinocandins

Indications

Esophageal candidiasis. Candidemia/acute disseminated candidiasis/Candidal peritonitis and abscesses. Prophylaxis of *Candida* infections during hematopoetic stem cell transplantation.

Action

Inhibits synthesis of glucan required for the formation of fungal cell wall. **Therapeutic Effects:** Death of susceptible fungi. **Spectrum:** Active against the following *Candida* spp.: *C. albicans*, *C. glabrata*, *C. krusei*, *C. parapsilosis*, *C. tropicalis*.

Pharmacokinetics

Absorption: IV administration results in complete bioavailability.
Distribution: Unknown.
Protein Binding: >99 %.
Metabolism and Excretion: Mostly metabolized; 71% fecal elimination.
Half-life: 15 hr.

TIME/ACTION PROFILE

ROUTE	ONSET	PEAK	DURATION
IV	rapid	end of infusion	24 hr

Contraindications/Precautions

Contraindicated in: Hypersensitivity.
Use Cautiously in: Severe hepatic impairment; OB: Use only if potential maternal benefit justifies potential fetal risk; Lactation: Use while breast feeding only if potential maternal benefit justifies potential risk to infant; Pedi: Children <4 mo (safety and effectiveness not established).

Adverse Reactions/Side Effects

GI: worsening hepatic function/hepatitis. **GU:** renal impairment. **Hemat:** hemolysis/hemolytic anemia. **Local:** injection site reactions. **Misc:** HYPERSENSITIVITY REACTIONS (including anaphylaxis).

Interactions

Drug-Drug: ↑ blood levels and risk of toxicity with **sirolimus** and **nifedipine** (dose adjustments may be necessary).

Route/Dosage

IV (Adults): *Esophageal candidiasis*— 150 mg once daily for 15 days (range 10–30 days); *Candidemia/acute disseminated candidiasis/Candida peritonitis and abscesses*— 100 mg once daily for 15 days (range 10–47 days); *Prevention of Candida infections in stem cell transplantation*— 50 mg once daily (duration range 6–51 days).
IV (Children ≥4 mo and >30 kg): *Esophageal candidiasis*— 2.5 mg/kg once daily (max daily dose = 150 mg); *Candidemia/acute disseminated candidiasis/Candida peritonitis and abscesses*— 2 mg/kg once daily (max daily dose = 100 mg); *Prevention of*

Candida infections in stem cell transplantation—1 mg/kg once daily (max daily dose = 50 mg).
IV (Children ≥4 mo and ≤30 kg): *Esophageal candidiasis*—3 mg/kg once daily; *Candidemia/acute disseminated candidiasis/Candida peritonitis and abscesses*—2 mg/kg once daily; *Prevention of Candida infections in stem cell transplantation*—1 mg/kg once daily.
IV (Neonates): 7–10 mg/kg once daily. Higher dose should be used in neonates <27 wk gestation and those with meningitis.

Availability (generic available)

Lyophilized powder for injection (requires reconstitution and dilution): 50 mg/vial, 100 mg/vial.

NURSING IMPLICATIONS

Assessment

- Assess symptoms of esophageal candidiasis (dysphagia, odynophagia, retrosternal pain) prior to and during therapy.
- Monitor for signs of anaphylaxis (rash, pruritus, wheezing, laryngeal edema, abdominal pain). Discontinue micafungin and notify health care professional immediately if these occur.
- Assess for injection site reactions (phlebitis, thrombophlebitis) during therapy. These occur more frequently in patients receiving micafungin via peripheral IV infusion.
- ***Lab Test Considerations:*** May cause ↑ serum alkaline phosphatase, bilirubin, ALT, AST, and LDH levels. If elevations occur, monitor for worsening liver function; may require discontinuation of therapy.
- May cause ↑ BUN and serum creatinine.
- May cause leukopenia, neutropenia, thrombocytopenia, and anemia. Monitor for worsening levels; may require discontinuation of therapy.
- May cause hypokalemia, hypocalcemia, and hypomagnesemia.

Implementation

IV Administration

- **Intermittent Infusion:** ***Diluent:*** *For Adults:* Reconstitute each 50-mg vial with 5 mL of 0.9% NaCl or D5W to achieve concentration of 10 mg/mL. Reconstitute each 100-mg vial with 5 mL of 0.9% NaCl or D5W to achieve concentration of 20 mg/mL. Dissolve by gently swirling vial; do not shake vigorously. Directions for further dilution based on indication for use. For prophylaxis of *Candida* infections, add 50 mg of micafungin to 100 mL of 0.9% NaCl or D5W. For treatment of esophageal candidiasis, add 150 mg of micafungin to 100 mL of 0.9% NaCl or D5W. Reconstituted vials and infusion are stable for 24 hr at room temperature. Protect diluted solution from light. ***Concentration:*** 0.5–1.5 mg/mL.
- *For Children:* Determine dose and divide by final concentration (10 or 20 mg/mL). Add withdrawn volume to 0.9% NaCl or D5W in IV bag or syringe. ***Concentration:*** 0.5–4 mg/mL. Concentrations >1.5 mg/mL should be administered via central venous catheter to minimize infusion reactions. Discard unused vials. ***Rate:*** Flush line with 0.9% NaCl prior to administration. Infuse over 1 hr. More rapid infusions may result in more frequent histamine mediated reactions.
- **Y-Site Compatibility:** aminophylline, bumetanide, calcium chloride, calcium gluconate, carboplatin, cyclosporine, dopamine, eptifibatide, esmolol, etoposide, fenoldopam, furosemide, heparin, hydromorphone, lidocaine, lorazepam, magnesium sulfate, mesna, milrinone, nitroglycerin, nitroprusside, norepinephrine, phenylephrine, potassium chloride, potassium phosphates, sodium phosphates, tacrolimus, theophylline, vasopressin.
- **Y-Site Incompatibility:** amiodarone, cisatracurium, diltiazem, dobutamine, epinephrine, insulin, labetalol, levofloxacin, meperidine, midazolam, morphine, mycophenolate mofetil, nicardipine, octreotide, ondansetron, phenytoin, rocuronium, telavancin, vecuronium.

Patient/Family Teaching

- Inform patient of the purpose of micafungin.
- Advise patient to notify health care professional immediately if signs of anaphylaxis occur.

Evaluation/Desired Outcomes

- Resolution of signs and symptoms of esophageal candidiasis, candidemia, acute disseminated candidiasis, candidal peritonitis, and abscesses.
- Prevention of *Candida* infections during hematopoetic stem cell transplantation.

---

miconazole, **See ANTIFUNGALS (TOPICAL) and ANTIFUNGALS (VAGINAL).**

HIGH ALERT

midazolam (mid-ay-zoe-lam)

Nayzilam, Seizalam, ~~Versed~~

Classification
Therapeutic: antianxiety agents, anticonvulsants, sedative/hypnotics
Pharmacologic: benzodiazepines

Schedule IV

Indications

PO: Preprocedural sedation and anxiolysis in pediatric patients. **IM, IV:** Preoperative sedation/anxiolysis/amnesia. Status epilepticus. **IV:** Provides sedation/anxiolysis/amnesia during therapeutic, diagnostic, or radiographic procedures (conscious sedation). Aids in the induction of anesthesia and as part of balanced anesthesia. As a continuous infusion, provides sedation of mechanically ventilated patients during anesthesia or in a critical care setting. **Intranasal:** Acute treatment of intermittent, stereotypic episodes of frequent seizure activity (i.e., seizure clusters, acute repetitive seizures) that are distinct from a patient's usual seizure pattern in patients with epilepsy.

Action

Acts at many levels of the CNS to produce generalized CNS depression. Effects may be mediated by GABA, an inhibitory neurotransmitter. **Therapeutic Effects:** Short-term sedation. Postoperative amnesia. Termination of seizure activity.

Pharmacokinetics

Absorption: Rapidly absorbed following oral and nasal administration; undergoes substantial intestinal and first-pass hepatic metabolism. Well absorbed following IM administration; IV administration results in complete bioavailability.

Distribution: Crosses the blood-brain barrier and placenta; excreted in breast milk.

Protein Binding: 97%.

Metabolism and Excretion: Almost exclusively metabolized by the liver, resulting in conversion to hydroxymidazolam, an active metabolite, and 2 other inactive metabolites (metabolized by cytochrome P450 3A4 enzyme system); metabolites are excreted in urine.

Half-life: Preterm neonates: 2.6–17.7 hr; Neonates: 4–12 hr; Children: 3–7 hr; Adults: 2–6 hr (increased in renal impairment, HF, or cirrhosis).

TIME/ACTION PROFILE (sedation)

ROUTE	ONSET	PEAK	DURATION
IN	5 min	10 min	30–60 min
IM	15 min	30–60 min	2–6 hr
IV	1.5–5 min	rapid	2–6 hr

Contraindications/Precautions

Contraindicated in: Hypersensitivity; Cross-sensitivity with other benzodiazepines may occur; Shock; Comatose patients or those with pre-existing CNS depression; Uncontrolled severe pain; Acute angle-closure glaucoma; OB: Benzodiazepine drugs may ↑ risk of congenital malformations; use in the last wk of pregnancy has caused CNS depression in the neonate; may affect child's brain development when used during 3rd trimester; Lactation: Lactation; Pedi: Products containing benzyl alcohol should not be used in neonates.

Use Cautiously in: All patients (may ↑ risk of suicidal thoughts/behaviors); Pulmonary disease; HF; Renal impairment; Severe hepatic impairment; Obese pediatric patients (calculate dose on the basis of ideal body weight); Open-angle glaucoma; Pedi: Rapid injection in neonates has caused severe hypotension and seizures, especially when used with fentanyl; may affect brain development in children <3 yr; safety and effectiveness of nasal spray has not been established in children <12 yr; Geri: Older patients (especially >70 yr) are more susceptible to cardiorespiratory depressant effects; dosage ↓ required.

Adverse Reactions/Side Effects

CNS: SUICIDAL THOUGHTS, agitation, drowsiness, excess sedation, headache. **CV:** CARDIAC ARREST, arrhythmias. **Derm:** rashes. **EENT:** blurred vision. **GI:** hiccups, nausea, vomiting. **Local:** phlebitis at IV site, pain at IM site. **Resp:** APNEA, LARYNGOSPASM, RESPIRATORY DEPRESSION, bronchospasm, cough.

Interactions

Drug-Drug: ↑ CNS depression with **alcohol**, **antihistamines**, **opioid analgesics**, and other **sedative/hypnotics** (↓ midazolam dose by 30–50% if used concurrently). ↑ risk of hypotension with **antihypertensives**, **opioid analgesics**, acute ingestion of **alcohol**, or **nitrates**. **Moderate CYP3A4 inhibitors** and **strong CYP3A4 inhibitors**, including **clarithromycin**, **diltiazem**, **erythromycin**, **itraconazole**, **ketoconazole**, and **verapamil** may ↑ levels and the risk of toxicity; avoid concurrent use. **Strong CYP3A4 inducers**, including **carbamazepine**, **phenobarbital**, **phenytoin**, **rifampin**, and **rifabutin** may ↓ levels.

Drug-Natural Products: Concomitant use of **kava-kava**, **valerian**, or **chamomile** can ↑ CNS depression. Long-term use of **St. John's wort** may significantly ↓ levels.

Drug-Food: **Grapefruit juice** ↓ metabolism and may ↑ risk of toxicity.

Route/Dosage

Dose must be individualized, taking caution to reduce dose in geriatric patients and in those who are already sedated.

Preoperative Sedation/Anxiolysis/Amnesia

PO (Children 6 mo–16 yr): 0.25–0.5 mg/kg, may require up to 1 mg/kg (dose should not exceed 20 mg); *patients with cardiac/respiratory compromise or concurrent CNS depressants*—0.25 mg/kg.

IM (Adults Otherwise Healthy and <60 yr): 0.07–0.08 mg/kg 1 hr before surgery (usual dose 5 mg).

IM (Adults ≥60 yr, Debilitated or Chronically Ill): 0.02–0.03 mg/kg 1 hr before surgery (usual dose 1–3 mg).

IM (Children): 0.1–0.15 mg/kg up to 0.5 mg/kg 30–60 min prior to procedure; not to exceed 10 mg/dose.

Conscious Sedation for Short Procedures

IV (Adults and Children Otherwise Healthy >12 yr and <60 yr): 1–2.5 mg initially; dosage may be ↑ further as needed. Total doses >5 mg are rarely needed (↓ dose by 50% if other CNS depressants are used).

Maintenance doses of 25% of the dose required for initial sedation may be given as necessary.
IV (Children 6–12 yr): 0.025–0.05 mg/kg initially, then titrate dose carefully, may need up to 0.4 mg/kg total, maximum dose 10 mg.
IV (Children 6 mo–5 yr): 0.05 mg/kg initially, then titrate dose carefully, may need up to 0.6 mg/kg total, maximum dose 6 mg.
IV (Geriatric Patients ≥60 yr, Debilitated or Chronically Ill): 1–1.5 mg initially; dose may be ↑ further as needed. Total doses >3.5 mg are rarely needed (↓ dose by 30% if other CNS depressants are used). Maintenance doses of 25% of the dose required for initial sedation may be given as necessary.
Intranasal (Children): 0.2–0.3 mg/kg, may repeat in 5–15 min.

Status Epilepticus

IM (Adults): 10 mg single dose.
IV (Children >2 mo): 0.15 mg/kg load followed by a continuous infusion of 1 mcg/kg/min. Titrate dose upward every 5 min until seizure controlled, range: 1–18 mcg/kg/min.

Seizure Clusters

Intranasal (Adults and Children ≥12 yr): One spray (5 mg) into one nostril initially; if inadequate response after 10 min, administer one spray (5 mg) into other nostril. Not to exceed 2 doses for a single seizure episode. Should not be used to treat more than one episode every 3 days and no more than 5 episodes per mo.

Induction of Anesthesia (Adjunct)

IV (Adults Otherwise Healthy and <55 yr): 300–350 mcg/kg initially (up to 600 mcg/kg total). May give additional dose of 25% of initial dose if needed. If patient is premedicated, initial dose should be further ↓.
IV (Geriatric Patients >55 yr): 150–300 mcg/kg as initial dose. May give additional dose of 25% of initial dose if needed. If patient is premedicated, initial dose should be further ↓.
IV (Adults —Debilitated): 150–250 mcg/kg initial dose. May give additional dose of 25% of initial dose if needed. If patient is premedicated, initial dose should be further ↓.

Sedation in Critical Care Settings

IV (Adults): 0.01–0.05 mg/kg (0.5–4 mg in most adults) initially if a loading dose is required; may repeat every 10–15 min until desired effect is obtained; may be followed by infusion at 0.02–0.1 mg/kg/hr (1–7 mg/hr in most adults).
IV (Children): *Intubated patients only*—0.05–0.2 mg/kg initially as a loading dose; follow with infusion at 0.06–0.12 mg/kg/hr (1–2 mcg/kg/min), titrate to effect, range: 0.4–6 mcg/kg/min.
IV (Neonates >32 wk): *Intubated patients only*—0.06 mg/kg/hr (1 mcg/kg/min).
IV (Neonates <32 wk): *Intubated patients only*—0.03 mg/kg/hr (0.5 mcg/kg/min).

Availability (generic available)

Nasal spray (Nayzilam): 5 mg/0.01 mL single-dose unit. **Oral syrup (cherry flavor):** 2 mg/mL. **Solution for injection:** 1 mg/mL, 5 mg/mL.

NURSING IMPLICATIONS

Assessment

- Assess level of sedation and level of consciousness throughout and for 2–6 hr following administration.
- Monitor BP, pulse, and respiration continuously during administration, especially if co-administering opioid analgesics. Oxygen and resuscitative equipment should be immediately available during IV administration.
- ***Toxicity and Overdose:*** If overdose occurs, monitor pulse, respiration, and BP continuously. Maintain patent airway and assist ventilation as needed. If hypotension occurs, treatment includes IV fluids, repositioning, and vasopressors.
- The effects of midazolam can be reversed with flumazenil (Romazicon).

Implementation

- ***High Alert:*** Accidental overdose of oral midazolam syrup in children has resulted in serious harm or death. Do not accept orders prescribed by volume (5 mL or 1 tsp); instead, request dose be expressed in milligrams. Have second practitioner independently check original order and dose calculations. Midazolam syrup should only be administered by health care professionals authorized to administer conscious sedation.
- **PO:** To use the *Press-in Bottle Adaptor (PIBA)*, remove the cap and push bottle adaptor into neck of bottle. Close bottle tightly with cap. Solution is a clear red to purplish-red, cherry-flavored syrup. Then remove cap and insert tip of oral dispenser in bottle adaptor. Push the plunger completely down toward tip of oral dispenser and insert firmly into bottle adaptor. Turn entire unit (bottle and oral dispenser) upside down. Pull plunger out slowly until desired amount of medication is withdrawn into oral dispenser. Turn entire unit right side up and slowly remove oral dispenser from the bottle. Tip of dispenser may be covered with tip of cap until time of use. Close bottle with cap after each use.
- Dispense directly into mouth. Do not mix with any liquid prior to dispensing.
- **Intranasal:** Administer 1 spray into one nostril. If no response to initial dose after 10 min, may administer 1 spray into other nostril.
- **IM:** Administer IM doses deep into mid-outer thigh (vastus lateralis muscle), maximum concentration 1 mg/mL. Solution is clear, colorless to light yellow.

Do not administer solutions that are discolored or contain particulate matter.

IV Administration

- **IV Push:** ***Diluent:*** Administer undiluted or diluted with D5W or 0.9% NaCl. ***Concentration:*** Undiluted: 1 mg/mL or 5 mg/mL. Diluted: 0.03–3 mg/mL. ***Rate:*** Administer slowly over at least 2–5 min. Titrate dose to patient response. Rapid injection, especially in neonates, has caused severe hypotension.
- **Continuous Infusion:** ***Diluent:*** Dilute with 0.9% NaCl or D5W. ***Concentration:*** 0.5–1 mg/mL. ***Rate:*** Based on patient's weight (see Route/Dosage section). Titrate to desired level of sedation. Assess sedation at regular intervals and adjust rate up or down by 25–50% as needed. Dose should also be decreased by 10–25% every few hrs to find minimum effective infusion rate, which prevents accumulation of midazolam and provides more rapid recovery upon termination.
- **Y-Site Compatibility:** acetaminophen, alemtuzumab, alfentanil, amikacin, amiodarone, anidulafungin, argatroban, atracurium, atropine, aztreonam, benztropine, bivalirudin, bleomycin, buprenorphine, calcium chloride, calcium gluconate, carboplatin, carmustine, caspofungin, cefazolin, cefotaxime, cefoxitin, ceftaroline, ceftriaxone, ciprofloxacin, cisatracurium, cisplatin, cyanocobalamin, cyclophosphamide, cyclosporine, cytarabine, dacarbazine, dactinomycin, daptomycin, daunorubicin hydrochloride, dexmedetomidine, dezrazoxane, digoxin, diltiazem, diphenhydramine, docetaxel, dopamine, doxacurium, doxarubicin hydrochloride, doxycycline, enalaprilat, epinephrine, epirubicin, eptifibatide, erythromycin lactobionate, esmolol, etomidate, etoposide, etoposide phosphate, famotidine, fenoldopam, fentanyl, fluconazole, fludarabine, folic acid, gemcitabine, gentamicin, glycopyrrolate, granisetron, heparin, hydromorphone, idarubicin, ifosfamide, irinotecan, isoproterenol, labetalol, levofloxacin, lidocaine, linezolid, lorazepam, magnesium sulfate, mannitol, meperidine, mesna, metaraminol, methadone, methoxamine, methyldopate, metoclopramide, metoprolol, metronidazole, milrinone, mitoxantrone, morphine, mycophenolate, multivitamins, mycophenolate, nalbuphine, naloxone, nicardipine, nitroglycerin, nitroprusside, norepinephrine, octreotide, ondansetron, oxacillin, oxaliplatin, oxytocin, paclitaxel, palonosetron, pamidronate, pancuronium, papaverine, pemetrexed, penicillin G potassium, pentamidine, phentolamine, phenylephrine, phytonadione, potassium chloride, procainamide, promethazine, propranolol, protamine, pyridoxime, quinupristin/dalfopristin, ranitidine, remifentanil, rifampin, rocuronium, streptokinase, succinylcholine, sufentanil, tacrolimus, theophylline, thiotepa, tigecycline, tirofiban, tobramycin, tolazoline, trimetaphan, vancomycin, vasopressin, vecuronium, verapamil, vinblastine, vincristine, vinorelbine, voriconazole, zoledronic acid.
- **Y-Site Incompatibility:** acyclovir, aminocaproic acid, aminophylline, amphotericin B deoxycholate, amphotericin B lipid complex, amphotericin B liposome, ampicillin, ampicillin/sulbactam, ascorbic acid, azathioprine, cefepime, ceftazidime, cefuroxime, chloramphenicol, dantrolene, dexamethasone, diazepam, diazoxide, epoetin alfa, ertapenem, fluorouracil, foscarnet, fosphenytoin, furosemide, ganciclovir, hydrocortisone, ibuprofen, indomethacin, ketorolac, methotrexate, micafungin, omeprazole, pantoprazole, pentobarbital, phenobarbital, phenytoin, piperacillin/tazobactam, potassium acetate, prochlorperazine, sodium bicarbonate, thiopental, trimethoprim/sulfamethoxazole.

Patient/Family Teaching

- Inform patient that this medication will decrease mental recall of the procedure.
- Advise patient to avoid grapefruit juice during therapy.
- May cause drowsiness or dizziness. Advise patient to request assistance prior to ambulation and transfer and to avoid driving or other activities requiring alertness for 24 hr following administration.
- Instruct patient to notify health care professional of all Rx or OTC medications, vitamins, or herbal products being taken and to consult health care professional before taking any Rx, OTC, or herbal products, especially blood pressure medicine, antibiotics, and St. John's wort.
- Advise patient to avoid alcohol or other CNS depressants for 24 hr following administration of midazolam.
- Advise patient and family to notify health care professional if thoughts about suicide or dying, attempts to commit suicide; new or worse depression; new or worse anxiety; feeling very agitated or restless; panic attacks; trouble sleeping; new or worse irritability; acting aggressive; being angry or violent; acting on dangerous impulses; an extreme increase in activity and talking; other unusual changes in behavior or mood, or skin rash occur.
- Advise patient that midazolam is a drug with known abuse potential. Protect it from theft, and never give to anyone other than the individual for whom it was prescribed. Store out of sight and reach of children, and in a location not accessible by others.
- Rep: Advise female patients to notify health care professional if pregnancy is planned or suspected or if breast feeding. Encourage pregnant patients to enroll in the North American Antiepileptic Drug (NAAED) Pregnancy Registry by calling 1-888-233-2334; information is available at www.aedpregnancyregistry.org.
- **Nayzilam:** Instruct individual administering *Nayzilam* on how to identify seizure clusters and use product appropriately. Advise patients and caregivers to read *Medication Guide* before starting and with each Rx refill in case of changes. Discuss safe

use, risks, and proper storage and disposal of midazolam with patients and caregivers with each Rx refill.

Evaluation/Desired Outcomes

- Sedation during and amnesia following surgical, diagnostic, and radiologic procedures.
- Sedation and amnesia for mechanically ventilated patients in a critical care setting.
- Termination of seizure activity.

REMS

miFEPRIStone
(mi-fe-**priss**-tone)
Korlym, Mifeprex

Classification
Therapeutic: abortifacients, antidiabetics
Pharmacologic: antiprogestational agents

Indications

Mifeprex: Medical termination of intrauterine pregnancy up to day 70 of pregnancy (in combination with misoprostol). **Korlym**: Hyperglycemia secondary to hypercortisolism in patients with endogenous Cushing's syndrome who have type 2 diabetes or glucose intolerance and have failed or are not candidates for surgery.

Action

Antagonizes endometrial and myometrial effects of progesterone. Sensitizes the myometrium to contraction-inducing activity of prostaglandins. Antagonizes the glucocorticoid receptor. **Therapeutic Effects:** Termination of pregnancy. Improved control of blood glucose.

Pharmacokinetics

Absorption: Rapidly absorbed following oral administration (69% bioavailability); absorption enhanced with food.
Distribution: Unknown.
Protein Binding: 98%.
Metabolism and Excretion: Mostly metabolized by the liver (CYP3A4 enzyme system); primarily excreted in the feces.
Half-life: 18 hr.

TIME/ACTION PROFILE (termination of pregnancy)

ROUTE	ONSET	PEAK	DURATION
PO	unknown	within 2 days	unknown

Contraindications/Precautions

Contraindicated in: Hypersensitivity; Presence of an intrauterine device (IUD) (Mifeprex); OB: Confirmed or suspected ectopic pregnancy (Mifeprex); Undiagnosed adnexal mass (Mifeprex); Chronic adrenal failure (Mifeprex); Concurrent long-term corticosteroid therapy; Bleeding disorders or concurrent anticoagulant therapy (Mifeprex); Inherited porphyrias (Mifeprex); Severe hepatic impairment (Korlym); OB: Pregnancy (Korlym); Concurrent use with simvastatin, lovastatin, cyclosporine, dihydroergotamine, ergotamine, fentanyl, pimozide, quinidine, sirolimus, or tacrolimus (Korlym); Vaginal bleeding; Endometrial hyperplasia with atypia or endometrial carcinoma (Korlym).
Use Cautiously in: Chronic medical conditions such as cardiovascular, hypertensive, hepatic, renal, or respiratory disease (safety and efficacy not established) (Mifeprex); Women >35 yrs old or who smoke ≥10 cigarettes/day (Mifeprex); Concurrent use with moderate CYP3A4 inhibitors; Bleeding disorders or concurrent anticoagulant therapy (Korlym).
Exercise Extreme Caution in: Concurrent use with strong CYP3A4 inhibitors (Korlym).

M

Adverse Reactions/Side Effects

CNS: anxiety (Korlym), headache, dizziness, fainting (Mifeprex), fatigue (Korlym), weakness (Mifeprex). **CV:** peripheral edema (Korlym), hypertension (Korlym), QT interval prolongation (Korlym). **Derm:** rash (Korlym). **Endo:** hypothyroidism (Korlym), adrenal insufficiency (Korlym), ↓ HDL cholesterol (Korlym). **F and E:** hypokalemia (Korlym). **GI:** abdominal pain (Mifeprex), anorexia (Korlym), constipation (Korlym), diarrhea, dry mouth (Korlym), nausea, vomiting. **GU:** uterine bleeding, uterine cramping (Mifeprex), ruptured ectopic pregnancy (Mifeprex), pelvic pain (Mifeprex). **MS:** arthralgia (Korlym), myalgia (Korlym). **Resp:** dyspnea (Korlym), *Pneumocystis jiroveci* pneumonia. **Misc:** ANGIOEDEMA.

Interactions

Drug-Drug: Mifeprisone is a substrate and inhibitor of the **CYP3A4** enzyme system. ↑ blood levels and risk of toxicity from **dihydroergotamine**, **ergotamine**, **lovastatin**, **simvastatin**, **cyclosporine**, **fentanyl**, **pimozide**, **quinidine**, **sirolimus**, or **tacrolimus**; concurrent use with Korlym is contraindicated. **Strong CYP3A4 inhibitors**, including **ketoconazole**, **itraconazole**, **nefazodone**, **ritonavir**, **nelfinavir**, **indinavir**, **atazanavir**, **fosamprenavir**, **clarithromycin**, **conivaptan**, **lopinavir/ritonavir**, **posaconazole**, **saquinavir**, or **voriconazole** may ↑ levels; adjust dose of Korlym. **Moderate CYP3A4 inhibitors**, including **aprepitant**, **diltiazem**, **fluconazole**, **imatinib**, or **verapamil** may ↑ levels; caution with concurrent use of Korlym. Blood levels and effects may be ↓ by **rifampin**, **rifabutin dexamethasone**, **phenytoin**, **phenobarbital**, and **carbamazepine**; avoid concurrent use with Korlym.

Drug-Natural Products: Blood levels and effects may be ↓ by **St. John's wort**; avoid concurrent use with Korlym.

Drug-Food: Blood levels and effects may be ↑ by **grapefruit juice**; caution with concurrent use of Korlym.

Route/Dosage

Mifeprex

PO (Adults): *Day 1*—200 mg as a single dose, followed on *Day 2 or Day 3 (within 24–48 hr of taking Mifeprex)* by misoprostol 800 mcg (given as four 200-mcg tablets) given buccally.

Korlym

PO (Adults): 300 mg once daily; may ↑ by 300 mg/day every 2–4 wk (maximum dose = 1200 mg/day or 20 mg/kg/day); *Initiation of Korlym in patients already being treated with strong CYP3A4 inhibitor*—300 mg once daily; may titrate up to 600 mg once daily, if needed; *Initiation of strong CYP3A4 inhibitor in patients already being treated with Korlym*—Current dose of Korlym = 300 mg once daily: No change; Current dose of Korlym = 600 mg once daily: ↓ dose to 300 mg once daily (may titrate up to 600 mg once daily, if needed); Current dose of Korlym = 900 mg or 1200 mg once daily: ↓ dose to 600 mg once daily.

Renal Impairment

PO (Adults): 300 mg once daily; may ↑ by 300 mg/day every 2–4 wk (maximum dose = 600 mg/day).

Hepatic Impairment

PO (Adults): 300 mg once daily; may ↑ by 300 mg/day every 2–4 wk (maximum dose = 600 mg/day).

Availability (generic available)

Tablets (Korlym): 300 mg. **Tablets (Mifeprex):** 200 mg.

NURSING IMPLICATIONS

Assessment

- **Mifeprex**: Determine duration of pregnancy. Pregnancy is dated from the first day of the last menstrual period in a presumed 28-day cycle with ovulation occurring at mid-cycle and can be determined by menstrual history and clinical examination; use ultrasound if duration is uncertain or if ectopic pregnancy is suspected. Assess women who became pregnant with an IUD in place for ectopic pregnancy.
- Assess amount of bleeding and cramping during treatment. Determine if termination is complete on day 14.
- **Korlym:** Monitor for changes in cushingoid appearance (acne, hirsutism, striae, body weight) during therapy.
- Monitor for signs and symptoms of adrenal insufficiency (weakness, nausea, increased fatigue, hypotension, hypoglycemia) during therapy. If adrenal insufficiency is suspected, discontinue Korlym and administer glucortocoids immediately.
- ***Lab Test Considerations:*** **Mifeprex:** ↓ hemoglobin, hematocrit, and RBCs may occur in women who bleed heavily.
- Changes in quantitative human chorionic gonadotropin (hCG) levels are not accurate until at least 10 days after mifepristone administration; complete termination of pregnancy must be confirmed by clinical examination.
- **Korlym:** Obtain a negative pregnancy test in women prior to starting therapy or before restarting therapy if stopped for more than 14 days. Correct hypokalemia prior to initiating therapy. Assess serum potassium 1–2 wk after starting or increasing dose of Korlym and periodically thereafter.
- Monitor Hemoglobin A_{1c} periodically during therapy.

Implementation

- Do not confuse mifepristone with misoprostol.
- Mifepristone is only available through a restricted program, mifepristone REMS program. Prescribers must be certified by the program, patients must sign an agreement form, and mifepristone is dispensed to patients only in certain healthcare settings.
- **Mifeprex:** Mifepristone should be administered only by health care professionals who have read and understood the prescribing information, are able to assess gestational age of an embryo and diagnose ectopic pregnancies, and who are able to provide surgical intervention in cases of incomplete abortion or severe bleeding.
- Any IUD should be removed prior to mifepristone administration.
- Measures to prevent rhesus immunization, similar to those of surgical abortion, should be taken.
- **PO:** On *day 1*, after the patient has read the *Medication Guide* and signed the Patient Agreement, administer one 200 mg tablets of mifepristone as a single dose. On *day 2 or 3*, unless abortion has occurred and been confirmed by clinical examination or ultrasound, administer four 200-mcg tablets of misoprostol buccally between 24 and 48 hrs after taking mifepristone. Expulsion of pregnancy usually happens within 2–24 hrs of taking misoprostil. On *day 7–14*, confirm that termination of pregnancy has occurred by clinical examination or ultrasound. If complete expulsion has not occurred, administer another dose of misoprostil 800 mcg buccally.
- **Korlym:** Administer with a meal. Swallow tablet whole; do not crush, break, or chew.
- If Korlym therapy is interrupted, reinitiate at lowest dose (300 mg).

Patient/Family Teaching

- **Mifeprex:** Advise patient of the treatment and its effects. Patients must be given a copy of the *Medication Guide and Patient Agreement.* Patient must understand the necessity of completing the treatment schedule of three office visits (day 1, day 2–3, and day 7–14).

- Inform patient that vaginal bleeding and uterine cramping will probably occur and that prolonged or heavy vaginal bleeding is not proof of complete expulsion. Bleeding or spotting occurs for an average of 9–16 days; but may continue for more than 30 days. Advise patient that if the treatment fails, there is a risk of fetal malformation; medical abortion failures are managed by surgical termination.
- Caution patient to notify health care professional immediately if heavy bleeding (soak through 2 thick full-size sanitary pads per hr for 2 consecutive hrs or are concerned about heavy bleeding); abdominal pain or feeling sick (weakness, nausea, vomiting, diarrhea, with or without abdominal pain or fever more than 24 hr after taking mifepristone); or fever (≥100.4°F that lasts >4 hrs, may indicate life-threatening sepsis) occurs.
- Instruct patient in the steps to take in an emergency situation, including precise instructions and a telephone number to call if she has problems or concerns.
- May cause dizziness or fainting. Caution patient to avoid driving or other activities requiring alertness until response to medication is known.
- Caution patient that pregnancy can occur following termination of pregnancy and before resumption of normal menses. Contraception can be initiated as soon as pregnancy termination is confirmed, or before sexual intercourse is resumed.
- Advise patient to notify health care professional if she smokes at least 10 cigarettes a day.
- **Korlym:** Instruct patient to take Korlym as directed. Advise patient to read *Medication Guide* prior to starting therapy and with each refill in case of changes.
- Caution patient to avoid drinking grapefruit juice during therapy; may increase risk of side effects.
- Instruct patient to notify health care professional if signs and symptoms of adrenal insufficiency, abnormal vaginal bleeding, or low potassium (muscle weakness, aches, cramps, palpitations) occur.
- Advise patient to notify health care professional of all Rx or OTC medications, vitamins, or herbal products being taken and to consult with health care professional before taking other medications.
- Rep: Advise female patient to use a nonhormonal form of contraception during and for at least 1 mo after therapy. Notify health care professional immediately if pregnancy is suspected; Korlym is teratogenic. Advise female patient to avoid breast feeding during therapy.

Evaluation/Desired Outcomes

- **Mifeprex:** Termination of an intrauterine pregnancy of less than 70 days duration.
- **Korlym:** Improved control of blood glucose.

milnacipran (mil-na-**sip**-ran)

Savella

Classification

Therapeutic: antifibromyalgia agents

Pharmacologic: selective norepinephrine reuptake inhibitors

Indications

Management of fibromyalgia.

Action

Inhibits neuronal reuptake of norepinephrine and serotonin. **Therapeutic Effects:** Decreased pain associated with fibromyalgia.

Pharmacokinetics

Absorption: 85–90% absorbed following oral administration.

Distribution: Unknown.

Metabolism and Excretion: Mostly excreted urine as unchanged drug (55%) and inactive metabolites.

Half-life: *D*—isomer 8–10 hr; *L*—isomer 4–6 hr.

TIME/ACTION PROFILE (↓ in pain)

ROUTE	ONSET	PEAK	DURATION
PO	1 wk	unknown	unknown

Contraindications/Precautions

Contraindicated in: Concurrent use of MAO inhibitors or MAO-like drugs (linezolid or methylene blue); End-stage renal disease; Significant history of alcohol use/abuse; Chronic liver disease.

Use Cautiously in: History of suicide risk or attempt; History of seizures; Moderate-to-severe renal impairment (↓ dose if CCr <30 mL/min); Hypertension; Severe hepatic impairment; Obstructive uropathy (↑ risk of adverse genitourinary effects); Angle-closure glaucoma; Geri: Consider age-related ↓ in renal function, chronic disease state and concurrent drug therapy; OB: Use only if clearly required during pregnancy weighing benefit to mother versus potential harm to fetus; Lactation: Potential for serious adverse reactions in infant; discontinue drug or discontinue breast feeding; Pedi: ↑ risk of suicidal thinking and behavior (suicidality) in adolescents and young adults up to 24 yr with Major Depressive Disorder (MDD) and other psychiatric disorders.

Adverse Reactions/Side Effects

CNS: NEUROLEPTIC MALIGNANT SYNDROME, SUICIDAL THOUGHTS, dizziness, headache, insomnia. **CV:** hypertension, tachycardia. **F and E:** hyponatremia. **GI:** PANCREATITIS, constipation, dry mouth, ↑ liver enzymes, nausea, vomiting. **Derm:** hot flushes, hyperhidrosis. **Misc:** SEROTONIN SYNDROME.

M

Interactions

Drug-Drug: Concurrent use with **MAO inhibitors** may result in serious, potentially fatal reactions; wait at least 14 days following discontinuation of MAO inhibitor before initiation of milnacipran. Wait at least 5 days after discontinuing milnacipran before initiation of MAO inhibitor. Concurrent use with **MAO-inhibitor-like drugs**, such as **linezolid** or **methylene blue** may ↑ risk of serotonin syndrome; concurrent use contraindicated; do not start therapy in patients receiving **linezolid** or **methylene blue**; if **linezolid** or **methylene blue** need to be started in a patient receiving milnacipran, immediately discontinue milnacipran and monitor for signs/symptoms of serotonin syndrome for 5 days or until 24 hr after last dose of linezolid or methylene blue, whichever comes first (may resume milnacipran therapy 24 hr after last dose of linezolid or methylene blue). Drugs that affect serotonergic neurotransmitter systems, including **tricyclic antidepressants**, **SSRIs**, **fentanyl**, **buspirone**, **tramadol**, **amphetamines**, and **triptans** ↑ risk of serotonin syndrome. Concurrent use of **NSAIDs**, **aspirin**, or other **drugs that affect coagulation** may ↑ the risk of bleeding. May ↓ antihypertensive effectiveness of **clonidine**. ↑ risk of hypertension and arrhythmias with **epinephrine** or **norepinephrine**. ↑ risk of euphoria and hypotension when switching from **clomipramine**. Concurrent use with **digoxin** may result in adverse hemodynamics, including hypotension and tachycardia; avoid concurrent use with IV digoxin.

Drug-Natural Products: Use with **St. John's wort** ↑ serotonin syndrome.

Route/Dosage

PO (Adults): *Day 1*—12.5 mg; *Day 2–3*—12.5 mg twice daily; *Day 4–7*—25 mg twice daily; *After Day 7*—50 mg twice daily. Some patients may require up to 100 mg twice daily depending on response.

Renal Impairment

PO (Adults): *CCr 5–29 mL/min*—maintenance dose is 25 mg twice daily; some patients may require up to 50 mg twice daily depending on response.

Availability (generic available)

Tablets (contain tartrazine): 12.5 mg, 25 mg, 50 mg, 100 mg.

NURSING IMPLICATIONS

Assessment

- Assess intensity, quality, and location of pain periodically during therapy. May require several wk for effects to be seen.
- Monitor BP and heart rate before and periodically during therapy. Treat pre-existing hypertension and cardiac disease prior to therapy. Sustained hypertension may be dose related; decrease dose or discontinue therapy if this occurs.
- Monitor closely for changes in behavior that could indicate the emergence or worsening of suicidal thoughts or behavior or depression.
- Monitor for development of neuroleptic malignant syndrome (fever, respiratory distress, tachycardia, convulsions, diaphoresis, hypertension or hypotension, pallor, tiredness, severe muscle stiffness, loss of bladder control). Report symptoms immediately.
- ***Lab Test Considerations:*** May cause ↑ ALT, AST, and bilirubin.
- May cause hyponatremia.

Implementation

- **PO:** May be administered without regard to meals; may be more tolerable if taken with food.

Patient/Family Teaching

- Instruct patient to take milnacipran as directed at the same time each day. Take missed doses as soon as possible unless time for next dose. Do not stop abruptly; must be decreased gradually. Advise patient to read the *Medication Guide* prior to therapy and with each Rx refill.
- Encourage patient and family to be alert for emergence of anxiety, agitation, panic attacks, insomnia, irritability, hostility, impulsivity, akathisia, hypomania, mania, worsening of depression and suicidal ideation, especially during early antidepressant therapy. Assess symptoms on a day-to-day basis as changes may be abrupt. If these symptoms occur, notify health care professional.
- May cause dizziness. Caution patient to avoid driving or other activities requiring alertness until response to medication is known.
- Advise patient to notify health care professional of all Rx or OTC medications, vitamins, or herbal products being taken and to consult with health care professional before taking other medications, especially St. John's wort. Avoid use of aspirin, NSAIDs, and warfarin due to increased risk for bleeding.
- Instruct patient to notify health care professional if signs of liver damage (pruritus, dark urine, jaundice, right upper quadrant tenderness, unexplained "flu-like" symptoms) or hyponatremia (headache, difficulty concentrating, memory impairment, confusion, weakness, unsteadiness, falls), rash, or serotonin syndrome (mental status changes: agitation, hallucinations, coma; autonomic instability: tachycardia, labile BP, hyperthermia; neuromuscular aberrations: hyperreflexia, incoordination; and/or gastrointestinal symptoms: nausea, vomiting, diarrhea) occur.
- Advise patient to avoid taking alcohol during milnacipran therapy.
- Rep: Instruct patient to notify health care professional if pregnancy is planned or suspected or if breast feeding. Encourage patients who become pregnant while taking milnacipran to enroll in the

pregnancy registry by calling 1-800-643-3010 or at www.savellapregnancyregistry.com.

- Encourage patient to maintain routine follow-up visits with health care provider to determine effectiveness.

Evaluation/Desired Outcomes

- Reduction in pain and soreness associated with fibromyalgia.

HIGH ALERT

milrinone (mill-ri-none)

~~Primacor~~

Classification

Therapeutic: inotropics

Indications

Short-term treatment of HF unresponsive to conventional therapy with digoxin, diuretics, and vasodilators.

Action

Increases myocardial contractility. Decreases preload and afterload by a direct dilating effect on vascular smooth muscle. **Therapeutic Effects:** Increased cardiac output (inotropic effect).

Pharmacokinetics

Absorption: IV administration results in complete bioavailability.

Distribution: Unknown.

Metabolism and Excretion: 80–90% excreted unchanged by the kidneys.

Half-life: 2.3 hr (↑ in renal impairment).

TIME/ACTION PROFILE (hemodynamic effects)

ROUTE	ONSET	PEAK	DURATION
IV	5–15 min	unknown	3–6 hr

Contraindications/Precautions

Contraindicated in: Hypersensitivity; Severe aortic or pulmonic valvular heart disease; Hypertrophic subaortic stenosis (may ↑ outflow tract obstruction).

Use Cautiously in: History of arrhythmias, electrolyte abnormalities, abnormal digoxin levels, or insertion of vascular catheters (↑ risk of ventricular arrhythmias); Renal impairment (↓ infusion rate if CCr is <50 mL/min); OB, Lactation: Pregnancy or lactation.

Adverse Reactions/Side Effects

CNS: headache, tremor. **CV:** VENTRICULAR ARRHYTHMIAS, angina pectoris, chest pain, hypotension, supraventricular arrhythmias. **CV:** skin rash. **GI:** ↑ liver enzymes. **F and E:** hypokalemia. **Hemat:** thrombocytopenia.

Interactions

Drug-Drug: None significant.

Route/Dosage

IV (Adults): *Loading dose*—50 mcg/kg followed by *continuous infusion* at 0.5 mcg/kg/min (range 0.375–0.75 mcg/kg/min).

IV (Infants and Children): *Loading dose*—50 mcg/kg over 10 min followed by *continuous infusion* at 0.5 mcg/kg/min (range 0.25–0.75 mcg/kg/min).

Availability (generic available)

Injection: 1 mg/mL. **Premixed infusion:** 20 mg/100 mL, 40 mg/200 mL.

NURSING IMPLICATIONS

Assessment

- Monitor heart rate and BP continuously during administration. Slow or discontinue if BP drops excessively.
- Monitor intake and output and daily weight. Assess patient for resolution of signs and symptoms of HF (peripheral edema, dyspnea, rales/crackles, weight gain) and improvement in hemodynamic parameters (increase in cardiac output and cardiac index, decrease in pulmonary capillary wedge pressure). Correct effects of previous aggressive diuretic therapy to allow for optimal filling pressure.
- Monitor ECG continuously during infusion. Arrhythmias are common and may be life threatening. The risk of ventricular arrhythmias is increased in patients with a history of arrhythmias, electrolyte abnormalities, abnormal digoxin levels, or insertion of vascular catheters.
- ***Lab Test Considerations:*** Monitor electrolytes and renal function frequently during administration. Correct hypokalemia prior to administration to decrease the risk of arrhythmias.
- Monitor platelet count during therapy.
- ***Toxicity and Overdose: High Alert:*** Overdose manifests as hypotension. Dose should be decreased or discontinued. Supportive measures may be necessary.

Implementation

- ***High Alert:*** Accidental overdose of milrinone can cause patient harm or death. Have second practitioner independently check original order, dose calculations, and infusion pump settings.

IV Administration

- **IV Push:** ***Diluent:*** Loading dose may be administered undiluted. May also be diluted in 0.9% NaCl, 0.45% NaCl, or D5W for ease of administration. ***Concentration:*** 1 mg/mL. ***Rate:*** Administer the loading dose over 10 min.
- **Continuous Infusion:** ***Diluent:*** Milrinone drawn from vials must be diluted. Dilute 10 mg (10 mL) of

M

milrinone in 40 mL of diluent or 20 mg (20 mL) of milrinone in 80 mL of diluent. Compatible diluents include 0.45% NaCl, 0.9% NaCl, and D5W. Premixed infusions are already diluted and ready to use. Admixed solutions are stable for 72 hr at room temperature. Stability of premixed infusions based on manufacturer's expiration date. Do not use solutions that are discolored or contain particulate matter. ***Concentration:*** 200 mcg/mL. ***Rate:*** Based on patient's weight (see Route/Dosage section). Titrate according to hemodynamic and clinical response.

- **Y-Site Compatibility:** acyclovir, alfentanil, allopurinol, amifostine, amikacin, aminophylline, amiodarone, amphotericin B liposome, ampicillin, anidulafungin, argatroban, atracurium, aztreonam, bivalirudin, bleomycin, bumetanide, buprenorphine, busulfan, butorphanol, calcium chloride, calcium gluconate, carboplatin, carmustine, caspofungin, cefazolin, cefepime, cefotaxime, cefotetan, cefoxitin, ceftaroline, ceftazidime, ceftriaxone, cefuroxime, chloramphenicol, chlorpromazine, ciprofloxacin, cisatracurium, cisplatin, clindamycin, cyclophosphamide, cyclosporine, cytarabine, dactinomycin, daptomycin, dexamethasone sodium phosphate, dexmedetomidine, digoxin, diltiazem, dobutamine, docetaxel, dopamine, doxacurium, doxorubicin, doxycycline, droperidol, enalaprilat, ephedrine, epinephrine, epirubicin, eptifibatide, ertapenem, erythromycin, etoposide, etoposide phosphate, fenoldopam, fentanyl, fluconazole, fludarabine, fluorouracil, ganciclovir, gemcitabine, gentamicin, glycopyrrolate, granisetron, haloperidol, heparin, hetastarch, hydralazine, hydrocortisone, hydromorphone, idarubicin, ifosfamide, insulin, irinotecan, isoproterenol, ketamine, ketorolac, labetalol, levofloxacin, linezolid, lorazepam, magnesium sulfate, mannitol, melphalan, meperidine, meropenem, methohexital, methotrexate, methyldopate, methylprednisolone sodium succinate, metoclopramide, metoprolol, metronidazole, micafungin, midazolam, mitoxantrone, morphine, mycophenolate, nafcillin, nalbuphine, naloxone, nicardipine, nitroglycerin, nitroprusside, norepinephrine, octreotide, oxacillin, oxaliplatin, oxytocin, paclitaxel, palonosetron, pamidronate, pancuronium, pemetrexed, pentobarbital, phenobarbital, phenylephrine, piperacillin/tazobactam, potassium acetate, potassium chloride, potassium phosphates, prochlorperazine, promethazine, propofol, propranolol, quinupristin/dalfopristin, ranitidine, remifentanil, rocuronium, sodium acetate, sodium bicarbonate, sodium phosphates, streptozocin, succinylcholine, sufentanil, tacrolimus, telavancin, theophylline, thiopental, thiotepa, tigecycline, tirofiban, tobramycin, torsemide, vancomycin, vasopressin, vecuronium, verapamil, vincristine, vinorelbine, voriconazole, zidovudine, zoledronic acid.
- **Y-Site Incompatibility:** amphotericin B deoxycholate, amphotericin B lipid complex, dantrolene, diazepam, diphenhydramine, esmolol, furosemide, hydroxyzine, imipenem/cilastatin, lidocaine, ondansetron, pantoprazole, phenytoin, procainamide.

Patient/Family Teaching

- Inform patient and family of reasons for administration. Milrinone is not a cure but is a temporary measure to control the symptoms of HF.

Evaluation/Desired Outcomes

- Decrease in the signs and symptoms of HF.
- Improvement in hemodynamic parameters.

minocycline, See TETRACYCLINES.

mirabegron (mye-ra-**beg**-ron)

Myrbetriq

Classification

Therapeutic: urinary tract antispasmodics
Pharmacologic: beta-adrenergic agonists

Indications

Treatment of symptoms of overactive bladder (OAB) including urge urinary incontinence, urgency, and frequency (either alone or with solifenacin).

Action

Acts as a selective beta-3 adrenergic agonist. Increases bladder capacity by relaxing detusor smooth muscle during storage phase of bladder fill-void cycle. **Therapeutic Effects:** Decreased symptoms of OAB.

Pharmacokinetics

Absorption: 29–35% absorbed following oral administration.

Distribution: Widely distributed.

Metabolism and Excretion: Extensively metabolized, 6% excreted unchanged in urine (25 mg dose), remainder excreted in urine and feces as metabolites.

Half-life: 50 hr.

TIME/ACTION PROFILE (effects on bladder)

ROUTE	ONSET	PEAK	DURATION
PO	unknown	3.5 hr†	24 hr

†Blood level.

Contraindications/Precautions

Contraindicated in: Hypersensitivity; Severe uncontrolled hypertension; End-stage renal disease or severe hepatic impairment (Child-Pugh Class C); Lactation: Probably enters breast milk and may cause adverse reactions in infant.

Use Cautiously in: Hypertension; Bladder outlet obstruction/concurrent antimuscarics (↑ risk of urinary retention); Concurrent use of antimuscarinics used to treat OAB; OB: Use only if potential maternal benefit outweighs risk to fetus; Pedi: Safety and effectiveness not established.

Adverse Reactions/Side Effects

CNS: dizziness, headache. **CV:** ↑ BP, tachycardia. **EENT:** nasopharyngitis. **GI:** constipation, diarrhea, nausea. **GU:** urinary tract infection. **Misc:** ANGIOEDEMA.

Interactions

Drug-Drug: Acts as a moderate inhibitor of the CYP2D6 enzyme system. May ↑ levels and risk of adverse reactions of **drugs metabolized by the CYP2D6 enzyme system** including **desipramine**, **flecainide**, **metoprolol**, **propafenone**, and **thioridazine**. May ↑ levels and risk of toxicity with **digoxin**; use lowest effective level of digoxin/monitor serum levels).

Route/Dosage

PO (Adults): 25 mg once daily; may be ↑ to 50 mg once daily based on need/tolerance after 8 wk.

Renal Impairment

PO (Adults): *CCr 15–20 mL/min*—Should not exceed 25 mg/day.

Hepatic Impairment

PO (Adults): *Moderate hepatic impairment (Child-Pugh Class B)*—Should not exceed 25 mg/day.

Availability

Extended-release tablets: 25 mg, 50 mg.

NURSING IMPLICATIONS

Assessment

- Assess patient for urinary urgency, frequency, and urge incontinence periodically during therapy.
- Monitor BP prior to starting and periodically during therapy; may cause ↑ BP.
- Monitor for signs and symptoms of angioedema (swelling of face, lips, tongue and/or larynx). Discontinue mirabegron and treat symptomatically.

Implementation

- **PO:** Administer without regard to food.
- Swallow tablets whole with water; do not break, crush, or chew.

Patient/Family Teaching

- Instruct patient to take mirabegron as directed. If a dose is missed, omit dose and begin taking next day; do not take 2 doses on the same day. Advise patient to read *Patient Information* sheet prior to starting and with each Rx refill in case of changes.
- Inform patient that mirabegron may cause an increase in BP. Advise patient to have BP checked periodically during therapy.
- May cause dizziness. Caution patient to avoid driving or other activities requiring alertness until response to medication is known.
- Advise patient to notify health care professional if difficulty emptying bladder occurs.
- Advise patient to notify health care professional of all Rx or OTC medications, vitamins, or herbal products being taken and to consult with health care professional before taking other medications.
- Advise female patients to notify health care professional if pregnancy is planned or suspected or if breast feeding.

Evaluation/Desired Outcomes

- Decreased urinary frequency, urgency, and urge incontinence.

mirtazapine (meer-**taz**-a-peen)

Remeron, ✱Remeron RD, Remeron SolTab

Classification

Therapeutic: antidepressants

Pharmacologic: tetracyclic antidepressants

Indications

Major depressive disorder. **Unlabeled Use:** Panic disorder. Generalized anxiety disorder (GAD). Post-traumatic stress disorder (PTSD).

Action

Potentiates the effects of norepinephrine and serotonin. **Therapeutic Effects:** Antidepressant action, which may develop only after several wk.

Pharmacokinetics

Absorption: Well absorbed but rapidly metabolized, resulting in 50% bioavailability.

Distribution: Unknown.

Protein Binding: 85%.

Metabolism and Excretion: Extensively metabolized by the liver (P450 2D6, 1A2, and 3A enzymes involved); metabolites excreted in urine (75%) and feces (15%).

Half-life: 20–40 hr.

TIME/ACTION PROFILE (antidepressant effect)

ROUTE	ONSET	PEAK	DURATION
PO	1–2 wk	6 wk or more	unknown

Contraindications/Precautions

Contraindicated in: Hypersensitivity; Concurrent use of MAO inhibitors or MAO-like drugs (linezolid or methylene blue).

Use Cautiously in: History of seizures; History of suicide attempt; May ↑ risk of suicide attempt/ideation

M

especially during early treatment or dose adjustment; History of mania/hypomania; Patients with hepatic or renal impairment; Angle-closure glaucoma; OB: Safety not established; Lactation: Discontinue drug or bottle-feed; Pedi: Safety not established. Suicide risk may be greater in children or adolescents; Geri: ↑ sensitivity to CNS effects and oversedation. Begin at lower doses and titrate carefully.

Adverse Reactions/Side Effects

CNS: NEUROLEPTIC MALIGNANT SYNDROME, SUICIDAL THOUGHTS, drowsiness, abnormal dreams, abnormal thinking, agitation, akathisia, anxiety, apathy, confusion, dizziness, malaise, weakness. **EENT:** sinusitis. **Resp:** dyspnea, cough. **CV:** edema, hypotension, vasodilation. **GI:** constipation, dry mouth, ↑ appetite, abdominal pain, anorexia, ↑ liver enzymes, nausea, vomiting. **GU:** urinary frequency. **Derm:** pruritus, rash. **F and E:** ↑ thirst. **Hemat:** AGRANULOCYTOSIS. **Metab:** weight gain, hypercholesterolemia, hyponatremia, ↑ triglycerides. **MS:** arthralgia, back pain, myalgia. **Neuro:** hyperkinesia, hypesthesia, twitching. **Misc:** SEROTONIN SYNDROME, flu-like syndrome.

Interactions

Drug-Drug: May cause hypertension, seizures, and death when used with **MAO inhibitors**; do not use within 14 days of MAO inhibitor therapy. Concurrent use with **MAO-inhibitor like drugs**, such as **linezolid** or **methylene blue** may ↑ risk of serotonin syndrome; concurrent use contraindicated; do not start therapy in patients receiving **linezolid** or **methylene blue**; if **linezolid** or **methylene blue** need to be started in a patient receiving mirtazapine, immediately discontinue mirtazapine and monitor for signs/symptoms of serotonin syndrome for 2 wk or until 24 hr after last dose of linezolid or methylene blue, whichever comes first (may resume mirtazapine therapy 24 hr after last dose of linezolid or methylene blue). Drugs that affect serotonergic neurotransmitter systems, including **tricyclic antidepressants**, **SNRIs**, **fentanyl**, **buspirone**, **tramadol**, and **triptans** ↑ risk of serotonin syndrome. ↑ CNS depression with other **CNS depressants**, including **alcohol** and **benzodiazepines**. **Ketoconazole**, **cimetidine**, **clarithromycin**, **erythromycin**, **indinavir**, **itraconazole**, **ketoconazole**, **nefazodone**, **nelfinavir**, **ritonavir**, or **saquinavir** may ↑ levels. **Phenobarbital**, **phenytoin**, **carbamazepine**, **rifampin**, or **rifabutin** may ↓ levels; may need to ↑ mirtazapine dose. May ↑ the effects and risk of bleeding from **warfarin**.

Drug-Natural Products: Concomitant use of **kava-kava**, **valerian**, **skullcap**, **chamomile**, or **hops** can ↑ CNS depression. ↑ risk of serotonin syndrome with **St. John's wort** and **SAMe**.

Route/Dosage

PO (Adults): 15 mg/day as a single bedtime dose initially; may be ↑ every 1–2 wk up to 45 mg/day.

Availability (generic available)

Tablets: 7.5 mg, 15 mg, 30 mg, 45 mg. **Cost:** *Generic*—7.5 mg $158.00/60, 15 mg $81.40/30, 30 mg $83.00/30, 45 mg $85.50/30. **Orally disintegrating tablets (orange flavor):** 15 mg, 30 mg, 45 mg. **Cost:** *Generic*—15 mg $77.90/30, 30 mg $80.27/30, 45 mg $85.53/30.

NURSING IMPLICATIONS

Assessment

- Assess mental status (orientation, mood, behavior) frequently. Assess for suicidal tendencies, especially during early therapy. Restrict amount of drug available to patient.
- Monitor closely for changes in behavior that could indicate the emergence or worsening of suicidal thoughts or behavior or depression.
- Assess weight and BMI initially and throughout therapy. For overweight/obese individuals, obtain fasting blood glucose and cholesterol levels. Refer as appropriate for nutritional/weight management and medical management.
- Monitor BP and pulse rate periodically during initial therapy. Report significant changes.
- Monitor for seizure activity in patients with a history of seizures or alcohol abuse. Institute seizure precautions.
- Assess for serotonin syndrome (mental changes [agitation, hallucinations, coma], autonomic instability [tachycardia, labile BP, hyperthermia], neuromuscular aberations [hyper reflexia, incoordination], and/or GI symptoms [nausea, vomiting, diarrhea]), especially in patients taking other serotonergic drugs (SSRIs, SNRIs, triptans).
- Monitor for development of neuroleptic malignant syndrome (fever, respiratory distress, tachycardia, seizures, diaphoresis, hypertension or hypotension, pallor, tiredness). Discontinue mirtazapine and notify health care professional immediately if these symptoms occur.
- ***Lab Test Considerations:*** Assess CBC and hepatic function before and periodically during therapy.

Implementation

- May be given as a single dose at bedtime to minimize excessive drowsiness or dizziness.
- May be taken without regard to food.
- For *orally disintegrating tablets*, do not attempt to push through foil backing; with dry hands, peal back backing and remove tablet. Immediately place tablet on tongue; tablet will dissolve in sec, then swallow with saliva. Administration with liquid is not necessary.

Patient/Family Teaching

- Instruct patient to take mirtazapine as directed. Take missed doses as soon as remembered; if almost time for next dose, skip missed dose and return to regu-

lar schedule. If single bedtime dose regimen is used, do not take missed dose in morning, but consult health care professional. Do not discontinue abruptly; gradual dose reduction may be required.
- May cause drowsiness and dizziness. Caution patient to avoid driving and other activities requiring alertness until response to drug is known.
- Encourage patient and family to be alert for emergence of anxiety, agitation, panic attacks, insomnia, irritability, hostility, impulsivity, akathisia, hypomania, mania, worsening of depression and suicidal ideation, especially during early antidepressant therapy. Assess symptoms on a day-to-day basis as changes may be abrupt. If these symptoms occur, notify health care professional.
- Caution patient to change positions slowly to minimize orthostatic hypotension.
- Advise patient to avoid alcohol or other CNS depressant drugs during and for at least 3–7 days after therapy has been discontinued.
- Instruct patient to notify health care professional of signs and symptoms of serotonin syndrome (mental status changes: agitation, hallucinations, coma; autonomic instability: tachycardia, labile BP, hyperthermia; neuromuscular aberrations: hyperreflexia, incoordination; and/or gastrointestinal symptoms: nausea, vomiting, diarrhea) occur.
- Advise patient to notify health care professional if dry mouth, urinary retention, or constipation occurs. Frequent rinses, good oral hygiene, and sugarless candy or gum may diminish dry mouth. An increase in fluid intake, fiber, and exercise may prevent constipation.
- Inform patient of need to monitor dietary intake. Increase in appetite may lead to undesired weight gain.
- Advise patient to notify health care professional of all Rx or OTC medications, vitamins, or herbal products being taken and to consult with health care professional before taking other medications, especially St. John's wort.
- Advise patient to notify health care professional of medication regimen before treatment or surgery.
- Advise female patient to notify health care professional if pregnancy is planned or suspected or if breast feeding.
- Therapy for depression may be prolonged. Emphasize the importance of follow-up exam to monitor effectiveness and side effects.

Evaluation/Desired Outcomes
- Resolution of the symptoms of depression.
- Increased sense of well-being.
- Renewed interest in surroundings.
- Increased appetite.
- Improved energy level.
- Improved sleep.
- Therapeutic effects may be seen within 1 wk, although several wk are usually necessary before improvement is observed.

miSOPROStol
(mye-soe-**prost**-ole)
Cytotec

Classification
Therapeutic: antiulcer agents, cytoprotective agents
Pharmacologic: prostaglandins

Indications
Prevention of gastric mucosal injury from NSAIDs, including aspirin, in high-risk patients (geriatric patients, debilitated patients, or those with a history of ulcers). With mifepristone for termination of pregnancy. **Unlabeled Use:** Treatment of duodenal ulcers. Cervical ripening and labor induction.

Action
Acts as a prostaglandin analogue, decreasing gastric acid secretion (antisecretory effect) and increasing the production of protective mucus (cytoprotective effect). Causes uterine contractions. **Therapeutic Effects:** Prevention of gastric ulceration from NSAIDs. With mifepristone terminates pregnancy of less than 49 days.

Pharmacokinetics
Absorption: Well absorbed following oral administration and rapidly converted to its active form (misoprostol acid).
Distribution: Unknown.
Protein Binding: 85%.
Metabolism and Excretion: Undergoes some metabolism and is then excreted by the kidneys.
Half-life: 20–40 min.

TIME/ACTION PROFILE (effect on gastric acid secretion)

ROUTE	ONSET	PEAK	DURATION
PO	30 min	unknown	3–6 hr

Contraindications/Precautions
Contraindicated in: Hypersensitivity to prostaglandins; OB: Should not be used to prevent NSAID-induced gastric injury due to potential for fetal harm or death; Lactation: May cause severe diarrhea in the nursing infant.
Use Cautiously in: OB: Patients with childbearing potential should be counseled to avoid pregnancy during misoprostol therapy for prevention of NSAID-induced gastric injury. Pregnancy status should be determined before initiating therapy; Pedi: Safety not established.

Exercise Extreme Caution in: When used for cervical ripening (unlabeled use) or to induce abortion, may cause uterine rupture (risk factors are late trimester pregnancy, previous Cesarian section or uterine surgery, advanced gestational age, or ≥5 previous pregnancies).

Adverse Reactions/Side Effects

CNS: headache. **GI:** abdominal pain, diarrhea, constipation, dyspepsia, flatulence, nausea, vomiting. **GU:** miscarriage, menstrual disorders.

Interactions

Drug-Drug: ↑ risk of diarrhea with **magnesium-containing antacids**.

Route/Dosage

PO (Adults): *Antiulcer*—200 mcg 4 times daily with or after meals and at bedtime, *or* 400 mcg twice daily, with the last dose at bedtime. If intolerance occurs, dose may be ↓ to 100 mcg 4 times daily. *Termination of pregnancy*—400 mcg single dose 2 days after mifepristone if abortion has not occurred.

Intravaginally (Adults): 25 mcg (¼ of 100–mcg tablet); may repeat every 3–6 hr, if needed.

Availability (generic available)

Tablets: 100 mcg, 200 mcg. ***In combination with:*** diclofenac (Arthrotec). See Appendix B.

NURSING IMPLICATIONS

Assessment

- Assess patient routinely for epigastric or abdominal pain and for frank or occult blood in the stool, emesis, or gastric aspirate.
- Assess women of childbearing age for pregnancy. Misoprostol is usually begun on 2nd or 3rd day of menstrual period following a negative pregnancy test result.
- **Termination of pregnancy:** Monitor uterine cramping and bleeding during therapy.
- **Cervical Ripening:** Assess dilation of cervix periodically during therapy.

Implementation

- Do not confuse misoprostol with mifepristone.
- Misoprostol therapy should be started at the onset of treatment with NSAIDs.
- **PO:** Administer medication with meals and at bedtime to reduce severity of diarrhea.
- Antacids may be administered before or after misoprostol for relief of pain. Avoid those containing magnesium, because of increased diarrhea with misoprostol.

Patient/Family Teaching

- Instruct patient to take medication as directed for the full course of therapy, even if feeling better. Take missed doses as soon as possible unless next dose is due within 2 hr; do not double doses. Emphasize that sharing of this medication may be dangerous.
- Advise patient not to share misoprostol with others, even if they have similar symptoms; may be dangerous.
- Inform patient that misoprostol will cause spontaneous abortion. Women of childbearing age must be informed of this effect through verbal and written information and must use contraception throughout therapy. If pregnancy is suspected, the woman should stop taking misoprostol and immediately notify her health care professional.
- Inform patient that diarrhea may occur. Health care professional should be notified if diarrhea persists for more than 1 wk. Also advise patient to report onset of black, tarry stools or severe abdominal pain.
- Advise patient to avoid alcohol and foods that may cause an increase in GI irritation.

Evaluation/Desired Outcomes

- The prevention of gastric ulcers in patients receiving chronic NSAID therapy.
- Termination of pregnancy.
- Cervical ripening and induction of labor.

mitoMYcin (mye-toe-**mye**-sin)

~~Mutamycin~~

Classification
Therapeutic: antineoplastics
Pharmacologic: antitumor antibiotics

Indications

Used with other agents in the management of disseminated adenocarcinoma of the stomach or pancreas. **Unlabeled Use:** Palliative treatment of: Carcinoma of the colon or breast, Head and neck tumors, Advanced biliary, lung, and cervical squamous cell carcinomas.

Action

Primarily inhibits DNA synthesis by causing cross-linking; also inhibits RNA and protein synthesis (cell-cycle phase–nonspecific but is most active in S and G phases). **Therapeutic Effects:** Death of rapidly replicating cells, particularly malignant ones.

Pharmacokinetics

Absorption: IV administration results in complete bioavailability.

Distribution: Widely distributed, concentrates in tumor tissue. Does not enter CSF.

Metabolism and Excretion: Mostly metabolized by the liver. Small amounts (<10%) excreted unchanged by the kidneys and in bile.

Half-life: 50 min.

TIME/ACTION PROFILE (effects on blood counts)

ROUTE	ONSET	PEAK	DURATION
IV	3–8 wk	4–8 wk	up to 3 mo

Contraindications/Precautions

Contraindicated in: Hypersensitivity; Pregnancy or lactation.

Use Cautiously in: Active infections; ↓ bone marrow reserve; Hepatic dysfunction; History of pulmonary problems; OB: Patients with childbearing potential should be counseled to avoid pregnancy during treatment; Geri: May have ↑ sensitivity to drug effects.

Adverse Reactions/Side Effects

Resp: PULMONARY TOXICITY. **CV:** edema. **GI:** nausea, vomiting, anorexia, stomatitis. **GU:** infertility, renal failure. **Derm:** alopecia, desquamation. **Hemat:** leukopenia, thrombocytopenia, anemia. **Local:** phlebitis at IV site. **Misc:** HEMOLYTIC UREMIC SYNDROME, fever, prolonged malaise.

Interactions

Drug-Drug: Additive bone marrow depression with other **antineoplastics** or **radiation therapy**. May ↓ antibody response to **live-virus vaccines** and ↑ risk of adverse reactions. Concurrent or sequential use with **vinca alkaloids** may result in respiratory toxicity.

Route/Dosage

IV (Adults): 20 mg/m² every 6–8 wk.

Availability (generic available)

Powder for injection (requires reconstitution): 5 mg/vial, 20 mg/vial, 40 mg/vial.

NURSING IMPLICATIONS

Assessment

- Monitor vital signs periodically during administration.
- Monitor for bone marrow depression. Assess for bleeding (bleeding gums, bruising, petechiae, guaiac stools, urine, and emesis) and avoid IM injections and taking rectal temperatures if platelet count is low. Apply pressure to venipuncture sites for 10 min. Assess for signs of infection during neutropenia. Anemia may occur. Monitor for increased fatigue, dyspnea, and orthostatic hypotension.
- Monitor intake and output, appetite, and nutritional intake. Nausea and vomiting usually occur within 1–2 hr. Vomiting may stop within 3–4 hr; nausea may persist for 2–3 days. Antiemetics may be administered prophylactically. Adjust diet as tolerated to help maintain fluid and electrolyte balance and nutritional status.
- Assess respiratory status and chest x-ray examination prior to and periodically throughout course of therapy. Cough, bronchospasm, hemoptysis, or dyspnea usually occurs after several doses and may be indicative of pulmonary toxicity, which may be life threatening.
- Monitor for potentially fatal hemolytic uremic syndrome in patients receiving long-term therapy. Symptoms include microangiopathic hemolytic anemia, thrombocytopenia, renal failure, and hypertension.
- ***Lab Test Considerations:*** Monitor CBC with differential, platelet count, and observation for fragmented RBCs on peripheral blood smears prior to and periodically throughout therapy and for several mo following therapy.
- The nadirs of leukopenia and thrombocytopenia occur in 4–8 wk. Notify health care professional if leukocyte count is <4000/mm³ or if platelet count is <150,000/mm³ or is progressively declining. Recovery from leukopenia and thrombocytopenia occurs within 10 wk after cessation of therapy. Myelosuppression is cumulative and may be irreversible. Repeat courses of therapy are held until leukocyte count is >4000/mm³ and platelet count is >100,000/mm³.
- Monitor liver function studies (AST, ALT, LDH, bilirubin) and renal function studies (BUN, creatinine) prior to and periodically throughout therapy to detect hepatotoxicity and nephrotoxicity. Notify health care professional if creatinine is >1.7 m g/dL.

Implementation

- Do not confuse mitomycin with mitoxantrone.
- Solution should be prepared in a biologic cabinet. Wear gloves, gown, and mask while handling medication. Discard equipment in designated containers.
- Ensure patency of IV. Extravasation may cause severe tissue necrosis. If patient complains of discomfort at IV site, discontinue immediately and restart infusion at another site. Promptly notify physician of extravasation.

IV Administration

- **IV Push:** Reconstitute 5-mg vial with 10 mL and 10-mg vial with 40 mL of sterile water for injection. Shake the vial; may need to stand at room temperature for additional time to dissolve. Final solution is blue-gray. Reconstituted solution is stable for 7 days at room temperature, 14 days if refrigerated. ***Diluent:*** 0.9% NaCl. ***Concentration:*** 20–40 mcg/mL for administration. ***Rate:*** May be administered IV push over 5–10 min through free-flowing IV of 0.9% NaCl or D5W.
- **Y-Site Compatibility:** alfentanil, amifostine, amphotericin B lipid complex, amphotericin B liposome, ampicillin, ampicillin/sulbactam, anidulafungin, argatroban, bivalirudin, bleomycin, bumetamide, buprenorphine, butorphanol, calcium chloride, calicum gluconate, carboplatin, caspofungin, cefoxitin, ceftazidime, ceftriaxone, chloramphenicol, chlorpromazine, ciprofloxacin, cisplatin, cyclophosphamide, cyclosporine, dactinomycin, dexamethasone, dexmedetomidine, doxorubicin hydrochloride, droperidol, epirubicin, ertapenem,

fentanyl, fluconazole, fludarabine, fluorouracil, foscarnet, fosphenytoin, furosemide, granisetron, heparin, hydrocortisone, hydromorphone, ifosfamide, imipenem/cilastatin, ketorolac, leucovorin calcium, levofloxacin, linezolid, magnesium sulfate, mannitol, melphalan, meperidine, methotrexate, methylprednisolone, metoclopramide, metronidazole, moxifloxacin, nitroglycerin, octreotide, ondansetron, oxaliplatin, paclitaxel, palonosetron, pemetrexed, potassium chloride, procainamide, quinupristin/dalfopristin, ranitidine, rituximab, sodium bicarbonate, tacrolimus, thiotepa, tigecycline, tirofiban, tobramycin, trastuzumab, vasopressin, verapamil, vinblastine, vincristine, voriconazole, zidovudine, zoledronic acid.

- **Y-Site Incompatibility:** acyclovir, allopurinol, amikacin, aminophylline, amiodarone, amphotericin B deoxycholate, aztreonam, cefepime, cefotaxime, cefotetan, cefuroxime, clindamycin, dacarbazine, daptomycin, dexrazoxane, diazepam, dobutamine, docetaxel, dopamine, doxycycline, esmolol, etoposide, etoposide phosphate, famotidine, fenoldopam, filgrastim, gemcitabine, gentamicin, glycopyrrolate, haloperidol, idarubicin, insulin, irinotecan, isoproterenol, labetalol, lorazepam, midazolam, milrinone, morphine, naloxone, pantoprazole, phenytoin, piperacillin/tazobactam, promethazine, propranolol, sargramostim, succinylcholine, topotecan, vancomycin, vecuronium, vinorelbine.

Patient/Family Teaching

- Instruct patient to notify health care professional promptly if fever; chills; cough; hoarseness; sore throat; signs of infection; lower back or side pain; painful or difficult urination; bleeding gums; bruising; petechiae; blood in stools, urine, or emesis; increased fatigue; dyspnea; or orthostatic hypotension occurs. Caution patient to avoid crowds and persons with known infections. Instruct patient to use soft toothbrush and electric razor and to avoid falls. Caution patient not to drink alcoholic beverages or take medication containing aspirin or NSAIDs; may precipitate gastric bleeding.
- Instruct patient to notify health care professional if decreased urine output, edema in lower extremities, shortness of breath, skin ulceration, or persistent nausea occurs.
- Instruct patient to inspect oral mucosa for redness and ulceration. If ulceration occurs, advise patient to use sponge brush and rinse mouth with water after eating and drinking. Topical agents may be used if pain interferes with eating. Stomatitis pain may require treatment with opioid analgesics.
- Discuss with patient the possibility of hair loss. Explore coping strategies.
- Instruct patient not to receive any vaccinations without advice of health care professional.
- Rep: Advise patient that, although mitomycin may cause infertility, contraception during therapy is necessary because of teratogenic effects.
- Emphasize need for periodic lab tests to monitor for side effects.

Evaluation/Desired Outcomes

- Decrease in size and spread of malignant tissue.

mitoXANTRONE
(mye-toe-**zan**-trone)
~~Novantrone~~

Classification
Therapeutic: antineoplastics, immune modifiers
Pharmacologic: antitumor antibiotics

Indications

Acute nonlymphocytic leukemia (ANLL) in adults (with other antineoplastics). Initial chemotherapy for patients with pain associated with advanced hormone-refractory prostate cancer. Secondary (chronic) progressive, progressive relapsing, or worsening relapsing-remitting multiple sclerosis (MS). **Unlabeled Use:** Breast cancer, liver cancer, and non-Hodgkin's lymphoma.

Action

Inhibits DNA synthesis (cell-cycle phase–nonspecific). **Therapeutic Effects:** Death of rapidly replicating cells, particularly malignant ones. Decreased pain in patients with advanced prostate cancer. Decreased disability and slowed progression of MS.

Pharmacokinetics

Absorption: IV administration results in complete bioavailability.
Distribution: Widely distributed; limited penetration of CSF.
Metabolism and Excretion: Mostly eliminated by hepatobiliary clearance; <10% excreted unchanged by the kidneys.
Half-life: 5.8 days.

TIME/ACTION PROFILE (effects on blood counts)

ROUTE	ONSET	PEAK	DURATION
IV	unknown	10 days	21 days

Contraindications/Precautions

Contraindicated in: Hypersensitivity; OB, Lactation: Pregnancy or lactation.
Use Cautiously in: Presence or history of cardiovascular disease (↑ risk of heart failure); Active infection; ↓ bone marrow reserve; Previous mediastinal radiation or use of anthracyclines (↑ risk of heart failure); Impaired hepatobiliary function; Rep: Women of reproductive potential; Geri: May have ↑ sensitivity to drug effects; Pedi: Safety not established.

Adverse Reactions/Side Effects

CNS: SEIZURES, headache. **EENT:** blue-green sclera, conjunctivitis. **Resp:** cough, dyspnea. **CV:** CARDIOTOXICITY, arrhythmias, ECG changes. **GI:** HEPATOTOXICITY, abdominal pain, diarrhea, nausea, stomatitis, vomiting. **GU:** blue-green urine, gonadal suppression, renal failure. **Derm:** alopecia, rash. **Hemat:** anemia, leukopenia, secondary leukemia, thrombocytopenia. **Metab:** hyperuricemia. **Misc:** HYPERSENSITIVITY REACTIONS, fever.

Interactions

Drug-Drug: ↑ bone marrow depression with other **antineoplastics** or **radiation therapy**. Risk of cardiomyopathy ↑ by previous **anthracycline antineoplastics (daunorubicin, doxorubicin, idarubicin)** or **mediastinal radiation**. May ↓ antibody response to **live-virus vaccines** and ↑ risk of adverse reactions.

Route/Dosage

Acute Nonlymphatic Leukemia

IV (Adults): *Induction*—12 mg/m²/day for 3 days (usually given with cytosine arabinoside 100 mg/m²/day for 7 days); if incomplete remission occurs, a 2nd induction may be given. *Consolidation*—12 mg/m²/day for 2 days (usually given with cytosine arabinoside 100 mg/m²/day for 5 days), given 6 wk after induction with another course 4 wk later.

Advanced Prostate Cancer

IV (Adults): 12–14 mg/m² single dose as a short infusion (with corticosteroids).

Multiple Sclerosis

IV (Adults): 12 mg/m² every 3 mo.

Availability (generic available)

Solution for injection: 2 mg/mL.

NURSING IMPLICATIONS

Assessment

- Monitor for hypersensitivity reaction (rash, urticaria, bronchospasm, tachycardia, hypotension). If these occur, stop infusion and notify physician. Keep epinephrine, an antihistamine, and resuscitation equipment close by in the event of an anaphylactic reaction.
- Monitor for bone marrow depression. Assess for bleeding (bleeding gums, bruising, petechiae, guaiac stools, urine, and emesis) and avoid IM injections and taking rectal temperatures if platelet count is low. Apply pressure to venipuncture sites for 10 min. Assess for signs of infection during neutropenia. Anemia may occur. Monitor for increased fatigue, dyspnea, and orthostatic hypotension.
- Monitor intake and output, appetite, and nutritional intake. Assess patient for nausea and vomiting. Antiemetics may be administered prophylactically. Adjust diet as tolerated to help maintain fluid and electrolyte balance and nutritional status.
- Monitor chest x-ray, ECG, echocardiography or MUGA, and radionuclide angiography to determine ejection fraction prior to and periodically during therapy. Multiple sclerosis patients with baseline left ventricular ejection fraction (LVEF)<50% should not receive mitoxantrone. May cause cardiotoxicity, especially in patients who have received daunorubicin or doxorubicin. Assess for rales/crackles, dyspnea, edema, jugular vein distention, ECG changes, arrhythmias, and chest pain. Monitor LVEF with echocardiogram or MUGA if signs of HF occur, prior to each dose, and yearly after stopping therapy in patients with multiple sclerosis. Potentially fatal HF may occur during or for mo or years after therapy. Risk is greater in patients receiving a cumulative dose >140 mg/m².
- Monitor for symptoms of gout (↑ uric acid levels and joint pain and swelling). Encourage patient to drink at least 2 L of fluid per day. Allopurinol may be given to decrease serum uric acid levels.
- **Multiple sclerosis:** Asses frequency of exacerbations of symptoms of multiple sclerosis periodically during therapy.
- ***Lab Test Considerations:*** Monitor CBC with differential and platelet count prior to and periodically during therapy. The nadir of leukopenia usually occurs within 10 days, and recovery usually occurs within 21 days.
- Monitor liver function studies (AST, ALT, LDH, bilirubin) and renal function studies (BUN, creatinine) prior to and periodically during therapy to detect hepatotoxicity and nephrotoxicity.
- May cause ↑ uric acid concentrations. Monitor periodically during therapy.

Implementation

- Do not confuse mitoxantrone with mitomycin.
- Solution should be prepared in a biologic cabinet. Wear gloves, gown, and mask while handling medication. Discard equipment in designated containers.
- Avoid contact with skin. Use Luer-Lok tubing to prevent accidental leakage. If contact with skin occurs, immediately wash skin with soap and water.
- Clean all spills with an aqueous solution of calcium hypochlorite. Mix solution by adding 5.5 parts (per weight) of calcium hypochlorite to 13 parts water.

IV Administration

- **IV:** Monitor IV site. If extravasation occurs, discontinue IV and restart at another site. Elevate extremity with extravasation and place ice packs over area. Monitor closely and obtain surgical consultation if local reaction occurs. Mitoxantrone is not a vesicant.

- **IV Push:** ***Diluent:*** Dilute dark blue mitoxantrone solution in at least 50 mL of 0.9% NaCl or D5W. Discard unused solution appropriately. ***Rate:*** Administer slowly over at least 3 min into the tubing of a free-flowing IV of 0.9% NaCl or D5W.
- **Intermittent Infusion:** May be further diluted in D5W, 0.9% NaCl, or D5/0.9% NaCl and used immediately. ***Concentration:*** 0.02–0.5 mg/mL. ***Rate:*** Administer over 15–30 min.
- **Continuous Infusion:** May also be administered over 24 hr.
- **Y-Site Compatibility:** acyclovir, alemtuzumab, alfentanil, allopurinol, amikacin, aminophylline, amindarone, anidulafungin, argatroban, atracurium, bivalirudin, bleomycin, bumetanide, buprenorphine, butorphanol, calcium chloride, calcium gluconate, carboplatin, carmustine, caspofungin, chloramphenicol, chrlopromazine, ciprofloxacin, cisatracurium, cisplatin, cladribine, cyclophosphamide, cyclosporine, cytarabine, dacarbazine, dactinomycin, daptomycin, daunorubicin hydrochloride, dexmedetomidine, dexrazoxane, diltiazem, diphenhydramine, dobutamine, docetaxel, dopamine, doxacurium, doxycycline, droperidol, enalaprilat, ephedrine, epinephrine, erythromycin, esmolol, etoposide, etoposide phosphate, famotidine, fenoldopam, fentanyl, filgrastim, fluconazole, fludarabine, fluorouracil, ganciclovir, gemcitabine, gentamicin, glycopyrrolate, granisetron, haloperidol, hydralazine, hydrocortisone, hydromorphone, ifosfamide, imipenem/cilastatin, insulin, irinotecan, isoproterenol, ketorolac, labetalol, leucovorin, levofloxacin, levorphanol, lidocaine, linezolid, lorazepam, magnesium sulfate, mannitol, melphalan, meperidine, meropenem, mesna, metaraminol, methohexital, methotrexate, methyldopate, metoclopramide, metoprolol, metronidazole, midazolam, milrinone, morphine, moxifloxacin, nalbuphine, naloxone, nicardipine, nitroglycerin, norepinephrine, octreotide, ondansetron, oxaliplatin, palonosetron, pamidronate, pancuronium, pantamidine, pentobarbital, phenobarbital, phentolamine, phenylephrine, potassium acetate, potassium chloride, procainamide, prochlorperazine, promethazine, propranolol, quinupristin/dalfopristin, ranitidine, remifentanil, rituximab, rocuronium, sargramostim, sodium acetate, sodium bicarbonate, succinylcholine, sufentanil, tacrolimus, theophylline, thiopental, thiotepa, tigecycline, tirofiban, tobramycin, tolazoline, topotecan, trastuzumab, trimethiprom/sulfamethoxazole, vancomycin, vasopressin, vecuronium, verapamil, vinblastine, vincristine, vinorelbine, zidovudine, zoledronic acid.
- **Y-Site Incompatibility:** amphotericin B deoxycholate, amphotericin B lipid complex, amphotericin B liposome, ampicillin, ampicillin/sulbactam, azithromycin, aztreonam, cefazolin, cefepime, cefotaxime, cefoxitin, ceftazidime, ceftriaxone, cefuroxime, clindamycin, dantrolene, dexamethasone, diazepam, digoxin, doxorubicin liposome, ertapenem, foscarnet, fosphenytoin, furosemide, heparin, idarubicin, methylprednisolone, nafcillin, nitroprusside, paclitaxel, pantoprazole, pemetrexed, phenytoin, piperacillin/tazobactam, potassium phosphates, propofol, sodium phosphates, voriconazole.

Patient/Family Teaching

- Advise patient to read the *Patient Package Insert* before starting therapy and before each dose in case of changes.
- Instruct patient to notify health care professional promptly if fever; chills; cough; hoarseness; sore throat; signs of infection; lower back or side pain; painful or difficult urination; bleeding gums; bruising; petechiae; blood in stools, urine, or emesis; increased fatigue; dyspnea; or orthostatic hypotension occurs. Caution patient to avoid crowds and persons with known infections. Instruct patient to use soft toothbrush and electric razor and to avoid falls. Caution patient not to drink alcoholic beverages or take medication containing aspirin or NSAIDS; may precipitate gastric bleeding.
- Instruct patient to notify health care professional if abdominal pain, yellow skin, cough, diarrhea, or decreased urine output occurs.
- Inform patient that medication may cause the urine and sclera to turn blue-green.
- Instruct patient to inspect oral mucosa for redness and ulceration. If mouth sores occur, advise patient to use sponge brush and rinse mouth with water after eating and drinking. Topical agents may be used if pain interferes with eating. Stomatitis pain may require treatment with opioid analgesics.
- Discuss with patient the possibility of hair loss. Explore coping strategies.
- Instruct patient not to receive any vaccinations without advice of health care professional.
- Advise patient that, although mitoxantrone may cause infertility, contraception during therapy is necessary because of possible teratogenic effects.
- Emphasize need for periodic lab tests to monitor for side effects.

Evaluation/Desired Outcomes

- Decrease in the production and spread of leukemic cells.
- Decreased pain in patients with prostate cancer.
- Decrease in the frequency of relapse (neurologic dysfunction) in patients with relapsing-remitting multiple sclerosis.

modafinil (mo-daf-i-nil)

Alertec, Provigil

Classification

Therapeutic: central nervous system stimulants

Schedule IV

Indications

To improve wakefulness in patients with excessive daytime drowsiness due to narcolepsy, obstructive sleep apnea, or shift work sleep disorder.

Action

Produces CNS stimulation. **Therapeutic Effects:** Decreased daytime drowsiness in patients with narcolepsy and obstructive sleep apnea. Decreased drowsiness during work in patients with shift work sleep disorder.

Pharmacokinetics

Absorption: Rapidly absorbed; bioavailability unknown.
Distribution: Well distributed; moderately (60%) bound to plasma proteins.
Metabolism and Excretion: Highly (90%) metabolized by the liver; <10% eliminated unchanged.
Half-life: 15 hr.

TIME/ACTION PROFILE (blood levels)

ROUTE	ONSET	PEAK	DURATION
PO	rapid	2–4 hr	24 hr

Contraindications/Precautions

Contraindicated in: Hypersensitivity; History of left ventricular hypertrophy or ischemic ECG changes, chest pain, arrhythmia, or other significant manifestations of mitral valve prolapse in association with CNS stimulant use.
Use Cautiously in: History of MI or unstable angina; Severe hepatic impairment with or without cirrhosis (dosage ↓ recommended); Concurrent use of MAO inhibitors; OB, Lactation, Pedi: Safety not established; Geri: Lower doses may be necessary due to ↑ sensitivity to drug effects.

Adverse Reactions/Side Effects

CNS: SUICIDAL IDEATION, headache, aggression, amnesia, anxiety, cataplexy, confusion, delusions, depression, dizziness, hallucinations, insomnia, mania, nervousness, seizures. **CV:** arrhythmias, chest pain, hypertension, hypotension, syncope, vasodilation. **Derm:** STEVENS-JOHNSON SYNDROME, dry skin, herpes simplex, rash. **EENT:** rhinitis, abnormal vision, amblyopia, epistaxis, pharyngitis. **Endo:** hyperglycemia. **GI:** ↑ liver enzymes, nausea, anorexia, diarrhea, gingivitis, mouth ulcers, thirst, vomiting. **GU:** abnormal ejaculation, albuminuria, urinary retention. **Hemat:** eosinophilia. **MS:** joint disorder, neck pain. **Neuro:** ataxia, dyskinesia, hypertonia, paresthesia, tremor. **Resp:** dyspnea, lung disorder. **Misc:** infection.

Interactions

Drug-Drug: May ↓ the metabolism and ↑ the effects of **diazepam**, **phenytoin**, **propranolol**, or **tricyclic antidepressants** (dosage adjustments may be necessary). May ↑ the metabolism and ↓ the effects of **hormonal contraceptives**, **cyclosporine**, and **theophylline** (dosage adjustments or additional methods of contraception may be necessary).
Drug-Natural Products: Use with caffeine-containing herbs (**cola nut**, **guarana**, **mate**, **tea**, **coffee**) may ↑ stimulant effect.

Route/Dosage

PO (Adults): 200 mg once daily.

Hepatic Impairment

PO (Adults): *Severe hepatic impairment*— 100 mg once daily.

Availability (generic available)

Tablets: 100 mg, 200 mg.

NURSING IMPLICATIONS

Assessment

- Observe and document frequency of narcoleptic episodes.
- Monitor closely for changes in behavior that could indicate the emergence or worsening of suicidal thoughts or behavior or depression.
- Assess for rash periodically during therapy. May cause Stevens-Johnson syndrome. Discontinue therapy if severe or if accompanied with fever, general malaise, fatigue, muscle or joint aches, blisters, oral lesions, conjunctivitis, hepatitis and/or eosinophilia.
- Monitor for signs and symptoms of angioedema or anaphylaxis (rash, swelling of face, eyes, lips, tongue or larynx; difficulty in swallowing or breathing; hoarseness).
- ***Lab Test Considerations:*** May cause elevated liver enzymes.

Implementation

- **PO:** Administer as a single dose in the morning for patients with narcolepsy or obstructive sleep apnea. Administer 1 hr before the start of work shift for patients with shift work sleep disorder.

Patient/Family Teaching

- Instruct patient to take medication as directed. Advise patient to read the *Medication Guide* prior to starting therapy and with each Rx refill, in case of changes.
- Medication may impair judgment. Advise patient to use caution when driving or during other activities requiring alertness.
- Advise patient that modafinil is a drug with known abuse potential. Advise patient that sharing this medication with others, even those with the same symptoms, is dangerous and illegal. Protect it from theft; store out of sight and reach of children, and in a location not accessible by others.

- Encourage patient and family to be alert for emergence of anxiety, agitation, panic attacks, insomnia, irritability, hostility, impulsivity, akathisia, hypomania, mania, worsening of depression and suicidal ideation, especially during early antidepressant therapy. Assess symptoms on a day-to-day basis as changes may be abrupt. If these symptoms occur, notify health care professional.
- Advise patient to notify health care professional immediately if rash or symptoms of anaphylaxis occur.
- Advise patient to notify health care professional of all Rx or OTC medications, vitamins, or herbal products being taken and to consult with health care professional before taking other medications. If alcohol is used during therapy, intake should be limited to moderate amounts.
- Rep: Advise females of reproductive potential to use effective nonhormonal methods of contraception during and for 1 mo following discontinuation of therapy. Instruct patient to notify health care professional promptly if pregnancy is planned or suspected, or if breast feeding. Encourage women who become pregnant to enroll in the registry by calling 1-866-404-4106. Registry collects information about the safety of modafinil during pregnancy.

Evaluation/Desired Outcomes

- Decrease in narcoleptic symptoms and an enhanced ability to stay awake.

moexipril, See ANGIOTENSIN-CONVERTING ENZYME (ACE) INHIBITORS.

mometasone, See CORTICOSTEROIDS (INHALATION), CORTICOSTEROIDS (NASAL), and CORTICOSTEROIDS (TOPICAL/LOCAL).

montelukast (mon-te-loo-kast)

Singulair

Classification

Therapeutic: allergy, cold, and cough remedies, bronchodilators

Pharmacologic: leukotriene antagonists

Indications

Prevention and chronic treatment of asthma. Management of seasonal allergic rhinitis. Prevention of exercise-induced bronchoconstriction (EIB).

Action

Antagonizes the effects of leukotrienes, which mediate the following: Airway edema, Smooth muscle constriction, Altered cellular activity. Result is decreased inflammatory process, which is part of asthma and allergic rhinitis. **Therapeutic Effects:** Decreased frequency and severity of acute asthma attacks. Decreased severity of allergic rhinitis. Decreased attacks of EIB.

Pharmacokinetics

Absorption: Rapidly absorbed (63–73%) following oral administration.

Distribution: Unknown.

Protein Binding: 99%.

Metabolism and Excretion: Mostly metabolized by the liver (by P450 3A4 and 2C9 enzyme systems); metabolites eliminated in feces via bile; negligible renal excretion.

Half-life: 2.7–5.5 hr.

TIME/ACTION PROFILE (improved symptoms of asthma)

ROUTE	ONSET	PEAK†	DURATION
PO (swallow)	within 24 hr	3–4 hr	24 hr
PO (chew)	within 24 hr	2–2.5 hr	24 hr

†Blood levels.

Contraindications/Precautions

Contraindicated in: Hypersensitivity.

Use Cautiously in: Acute attacks of asthma; Phenylketonuria (chewable tablets contain aspartame); Hepatic impairment (may need ↓ doses); Reduction of corticosteroid therapy (may ↑ the risk of eosinophilic conditions); OB: Use during pregnancy only if benefit to patient outweighs potential risk to fetus; Lactation: Use while breast feeding only if benefit to patient outweighs potential risk to infant; Pedi: Children <6 yr (EIB), <2 yr (seasonal allergic rhinitis), <12 mo (asthma), <6 mo (perennial allergic rhinitis) (safety and effectiveness not established).

Adverse Reactions/Side Effects

CNS: SUICIDAL BEHAVIORS/THOUGHTS, agitation, aggression, anxiety, attention disturbance, depression, disorientation, dream abnormalities, fatigue, hallucinations, headache, insomnia, irritability, memory impairment, obsessive-compulsive symptoms, restlessness, sleep walking, stuttering, weakness . **Derm:** STEVENS-JOHNSON SYNDROME, TOXIC EPIDERMAL NECROLYSIS, rash. **EENT:** nosebleed, otitis (children), sinusitis (children). **GI:** abdominal pain, diarrhea (children), dyspepsia, nausea (children), ↑ liver enzymes. **Neuro:** tics, tremor. **Resp:** cough, rhinorrhea. **Misc:** EOSINOPHILIC CONDITIONS (including Churg-Strauss syndrome), fever.

Interactions

Drug-Drug: Drugs which induce the CYP450 enzyme system (**phenobarbital** and **rifampin**) may ↓ the effects of montelukast.

Route/Dosage

Asthma

PO (Adults and Children ≥15 yr): 10 mg once daily.
PO (Children 6–14 yr): 5 mg once daily (as chewable tablet).
PO (Children 2–5 yr): 4 mg once daily (as chewable tablet or granules).
PO (Children 12–23 mo): 4 mg once daily (as oral granules).

Exercise-Induced Bronchoconstriction

PO (Adults and Children ≥15 yrs): 10 mg ≥2 hr before exercise. Do not take within 24 hr of another dose; if taking daily doses, do not take dose for EIB.
PO (Children 6–14 yr): 5 mg (as chewable tablet) ≥2 hr before exercise. Do not take within 24 hr of another dose; if taking daily doses, do not take dose for EIB.

Allergic Rhinitis

PO (Adults and Children ≥15 yr): *Seasonal or perennial*—10 mg once daily.
PO (Children 6–14 yr): *Seasonal or perennial*—5 mg once daily (as chewable tablet).
PO (Children 2–5 yr): *Seasonal or perennial*—4 mg once daily (as chewable tablet or granules).
PO (Children 6–23 mo): *Perennial only*—4 mg once daily (as oral granules).

Availability (generic available)

Chewable tablets (cherry flavor): 4 mg, 5 mg. **Cost:** *Generic*—All strengths $169.72/30. **Oral granules:** 4 mg/pkt. **Cost:** *Generic*—$169.72/30 pkts. **Tablets:** 10 mg. **Cost:** *Generic*—$169.72/30.

NURSING IMPLICATIONS

Assessment

- Assess lung sounds and respiratory function prior to and periodically during therapy.
- Assess allergy symptoms (rhinitis, conjunctivitis, hives) before and periodically during therapy.
- Monitor closely for changes in behavior that could indicate the emergence or worsening of depression or suicidal thoughts.
- Assess for rash periodically during therapy. May cause Stevens-Johnson syndrome. Discontinue therapy if severe or if accompanied with fever, general malaise, fatigue, muscle or joint aches, blisters, oral lesions, conjunctivitis, hepatitis, and/or eosinophilia.
- ***Lab Test Considerations:*** May cause ↑ AST and ALT concentrations.

Implementation

- Doses of inhaled corticosteroids may be gradually decreased with supervision of health care professional; do not discontinue abruptly.
- **PO:** For asthma, administer once daily in the evening. For allergic rhinitis, may be administered at any time of day.
- Administer granules directly into mouth or mixed in a spoonful of cold or room temperature foods (use only applesauce, mashed carrots, rice, or ice cream). Do not open packet until ready to use. After opening packet, administer full dose within 15 min. Do not store mixture. Discard unused portion. Do not dissolve granules in fluid, but fluid may be taken following administration. Granules may be administered without regard to meals.
- *For Exercise Induced Bronchoconstriction:* Administer one tablet at least 2 hrs before exercise; do not take within 24 hr of another dose.

Patient/Family Teaching

- Instruct patient to take medication daily in the evening or at least 2 hr before exercise, even if not experiencing symptoms of asthma. Do not double doses. Do not discontinue therapy without consulting health care professional. Advise patient to read *Patient Information* before starting therapy and with each Rx refill in case of changes.
- Instruct patient not to discontinue or reduce other asthma medications without consulting health care professional.
- Advise patient that montelukast is not used to treat acute asthma attacks, but may be continued during an acute exacerbation. Patient should carry rapid-acting therapy for bronchospasm at all times. Advise patient to notify health care professional if more than the maximum number of short-acting bronchodilator treatments prescribed for a 24-hr period are needed.
- Advise patient to notify health care professional of all Rx or OTC medications, vitamins, or herbal products being taken and to consult health care professional before taking any new medications.
- Encourage patient and family to be alert for emergence of anxiety, agitation, panic attacks, insomnia, irritability, hostility, impulsivity, akathisia, hypomania, mania, worsening of depression and suicidal ideation, especially during early antidepressant therapy. Assess symptoms on a day-to-day basis as changes may be abrupt. If these symptoms or rash occurs, notify health care professional.
- Advise patient to notify health care professional if pregnancy is planned or suspected, or if breast feeding.

Evaluation/Desired Outcomes

- Prevention of and reduction in symptoms of asthma.
- Decrease in severity of allergic rhinitis.
- Prevention of exercise-induced bronchoconstriction.

REMS HIGH ALERT

morphine (mor-feen)

~~AVINza~~, Doloral, Duramorph, Embeda, Infumorph, Kadian, M-Ediat, M-Eslon, Mitigo, Morphabond ER, Morphine EPD, Morphine Extra Forte, Morphine HP, Morphine LP Epidural, MS Contin, MS Contin SRT, ~~Roxanol~~, Statex

Classification
Therapeutic: opioid analgesics
Pharmacologic: opioid agonists

Schedule II

Indications

Severe pain (the 20 mg/mL oral solution concentration should only be used in opioid-tolerant patients). Pain severe enough to require daily, around-the-clock long-term opioid treatment and for which alternative treatment options are inadequate (extended-release). Pulmonary edema. Pain associated with MI.

Action

Binds to opiate receptors in the CNS. Alters the perception of and response to painful stimuli while producing generalized CNS depression. **Therapeutic Effects:** Decrease in severity of pain. Addition of naltrexone in *Embeda* product is designed to prevent abuse or misuse by altering the formulation. Naltrexone has no effect unless the capsule is crushed or chewed.

Pharmacokinetics

Absorption: Variably absorbed (about 30%) following oral administration. More reliably absorbed from rectal, subcut, and IM sites. Following epidural administration, systemic absorption and absorption into the intrathecal space via the meninges occurs.
Distribution: Widely distributed. Crosses the placenta; enters breast milk in small amounts.
Protein Binding: Premature infants: <20%; Adults: 35%.
Metabolism and Excretion: Mostly metabolized by the liver. Active metabolites excreted renally.
Half-life: Premature neonates: 10–20 hr; Neonates: 7.6 hr; Infants 1–3 mo: 6.2 hr; Children 6 mo–2.5 yr: 2.9 hr; Children 3–6 yr: 1–2 hr; Children 6–19 yr with sickle cell disease: 1.3 hr; Adults: 2–4 hr.

TIME/ACTION PROFILE (analgesia)

ROUTE	ONSET	PEAK	DURATION
PO	unknown	60 min	4–5 hr
PO-ER	unknown	3–4 hr	8–24 hr
IM	10–30 min	30–60 min	4–5 hr
Subcut	20 min	50–90 min	4–5 hr
Rect	unknown	20–60 min	3–7 hr
IV	rapid	20 min	4–5 hr
Epidural	6–30 min	1 hr	up to 24 hr
IT	rapid (min)	unknown	up to 24 hr

Contraindications/Precautions

Contraindicated in: Hypersensitivity; Some products contain tartrazine, bisulfites, or alcohol and should be avoided in patients with known hypersensitivity; Acute, mild, intermittent, or postoperative pain (extended/sustained-release); Significant respiratory depression (extended-release); Acute or severe bronchial asthma (extended-release); Paralytic ileus (extended-release).
Use Cautiously in: Head trauma; ↑ intracranial pressure; Severe renal, hepatic, or pulmonary disease; Hypothyroidism; Seizure disorder; Adrenal insufficiency; History of substance abuse; Undiagnosed abdominal pain; Prostatic hyperplasia; Patients undergoing procedures that rapidly ↓ pain (cordotomy, radiation); long-acting agents should be discontinued 24 hr before and replaced with short-acting agents; Geri: Geriatric or debilitated patients (↑ risk of respiratory depression; dose ↓ suggested); OB, Lactation: Avoid chronic use; has been used during labor but may cause respiratory depression in the newborn; prolonged use of extended-release morphine during pregnancy can result in neonatal opioid withdrawal syndrome; Pedi: Neonates and infants <3 mo (more susceptible to respiratory depression); Pedi: Neonates (oral solution contains sodium benzoate which can cause potentially fatal gasping syndrome).

Adverse Reactions/Side Effects

CNS: confusion, sedation, dizziness, dysphoria, euphoria, floating feeling, hallucinations, headache, unusual dreams. **CV:** hypotension, bradycardia. **Derm:** flushing, itching, sweating. **EENT:** blurred vision, diplopia, miosis. **Endo:** adrenal insufficiency. **GI:** constipation, nausea, vomiting. **GU:** urinary retention. **Resp:** RESPIRATORY DEPRESSION. **Misc:** physical dependence, psychological dependence, tolerance.

Interactions

Drug-Drug: Use with **extreme caution** in patients receiving **MAO inhibitors** within 14 days prior (may result in unpredictable, severe reactions—↓ initial dose of morphine to 25% of usual dose). Use with **benzodiazepines** or other **CNS depressants** including other **opioids**, **nonbenzodiazepine sedative/hypnotics**, **anxiolytics**, **general anesthetics**, **muscle relaxants**, **antipsychotics**, and **alcohol** may cause profound sedation, respiratory depression, coma, and death; reserve concurrent use for when alternative treatment options are inadequate. Drugs that affect serotonergic neurotransmitter systems, including **tricyclic antidepressants**, **SSRIs**, **SNRIs**, **MAO inhibitors**, **TCAs**, **tramadol**, **trazodone**, **mirtazapine**, **5–HT_3 receptor antagonists**, **linezolid**, **methylene blue**, and **triptans** ↑ risk of serotonin syndrome. Administration of **partial-antagonist opioid analgesics** may precipitate opioid withdrawal in physically dependent patients. **Buprenorphine**, **nalbuphine**, or **butorphanol** may ↓ analgesia. May ↑ the anticoagulant effect of **warfarin**. **Cimetidine** ↓ metabolism and may ↑ effects.

Drug-Natural Products: Concomitant use of **kava-kava**, **valerian**, or **chamomile** can ↑ CNS depression.

Route/Dosage

Larger doses may be required during chronic therapy.

PO, Rect (Adults ≥50 kg): *Usual starting dose for moderate to severe pain in opioid-naive patients*—30 mg every 3–4 hr initially *or* once 24-hr opioid requirement is determined, convert to extended-release morphine by administering total daily oral morphine dose every 24 hr (as *Kadian* or other ER capsules), 50% of the total daily oral morphine dose every 12 hr (as *Kadian, Morphabond, MS Contin*), or 33% of the total daily oral morphine dose every 8 hr (as *Morphabond, MS Contin*). See equianalgesic chart, Appendix J. Dose of ER capsules (not *Kadian*) should not exceed 1600 mg/day because of fumaric acid in formulation.

PO, Rect (Adults and Children <50 kg): *Usual starting dose for moderate to severe pain in opioid-naive patients*—0.3 mg/kg every 3–4 hr initially.

PO (Children >1 mo): *Prompt-release tablets and solution*—0.2–0.5 mg/kg every 4–6 hr as needed. *Controlled-release tablet*—0.3–0.6 mg/kg every 12 hr.

IM, IV, Subcut (Adults ≥50 kg): *Usual starting dose for moderate to severe pain in opioid-naive patients*—4–10 mg every 3–4 hr. *MI*—8–15 mg, for very severe pain additional smaller doses may be given every 3–4 hr.

IM, IV, Subcut (Adults and Children <50 kg): *Usual starting dose for moderate to severe pain in opioid-naive patients*—0.05–0.2 mg/kg every 3–4 hr, maximum: 15 mg/dose.

IM, IV, Subcut (Neonates): 0.05 mg/kg every 4–8 hr, maximum dose: 0.1 mg/kg. Use preservative-free formulation.

IV, Subcut (Adults): *Continuous infusion*—0.8–10 mg/hr; may be preceded by a bolus of 15 mg (infusion rates vary greatly; up to 80 mg/hr have been used).

IV, Subcut (Children >1 mo): *Continuous infusion, postoperative pain*—0.01–0.04 mg/kg/hr. *Continuous infusion, sickle cell or cancer pain*—0.02–2.6 mg/kg/hr.

IV (Neonates): *Continuous infusion*—0.01–0.03 mg/kg/hr.

Epidural (Adults): *Intermittent injection*—5 mg/day (initially); if relief is not obtained at 60 min, 1–2 mg increments may be made (total dose not to exceed 10 mg/day). *Continuous infusion*—2–4 mg/24 hr; may ↑ by 1–2 mg/day (up to 30 mg/day).

Epidural (Children >1 mo): 0.03–0.05 mg/kg, maximum dose: 0.1 mg/kg or 5 mg/24 hr. Use preservative-free formulation.

IT (Adults): 0.2–1 mg. Use preservative-free formulation.

Availability (generic available)

Extended-release capsules: 30 mg, 45 mg, 60 mg, 75 mg, 90 mg, 120 mg. **Cost:** 30 mg $606.31/100, 45 mg $898.99/100, 60 mg $1,177.88/100, 75 mg $1,498.31/100, 90 mg $1,770.29/100, 120 mg $2,088.66/100. **Extended-release capsules (Kadian):** 10 mg, 20 mg, 30 mg, 40 mg, 50 mg, 60 mg, 70 mg, 80 mg, 100 mg, 130 mg, 150 mg, 200 mg. **Cost:** 10 mg $609.60/100, 20 mg $673.20/100, 30 mg $732.00/100, 40 mg $976.80/100, 50 mg $1,224.00/100, 60 mg $1,465.20/100, 70 mg $1,708.80/100, 80 mg $1,951.20/100, 100 mg $2,407.20/100, 130 mg $3,182.40/100, 150 mg $3,672.00/100, 200 mg $4,946.40/100. **Extended-release tablets (Morphabond ER, abuse deterrent):** 15 mg, 30 mg, 60 mg, 100 mg. **Extended-release tablets (MS Contin):** 15 mg, 30 mg, 60 mg, 100 mg, 200 mg. **Cost:** *Generic*—15 mg $167.57/100, 30 mg $317.19/100, 60 mg $532.39/100, 100 mg $763.63/100, 200 mg $1,838.19/100. **Oral solution:** 🍁1 mg/mL, 10 mg/5 mL, 20 mg/5 mL, 🍁5 mg/mL, 100 mg/5 mL. **Cost:** *Generic*—4 mg/mL $17.51/100 mL, 20 mg/mL $25.20/30 mL. **Rectal suppositories:** 5 mg, 10 mg, 20 mg, 30 mg. **Cost:** *Generic*—5 mg $60.00/12, 10 mg $75.00/12, 20 mg $90.00/12, 30 mg $112.50/12. **Solution for epidural, IV injection (preservative-free):** 0.5 mg/mL, 1 mg/mL. **Solution for epidural or IT use (continuous microinfusion device; preservative-free):** 10 mg/mL, 25 mg/mL. **Solution for IM, subcut, IV injection:** 1 mg/mL, 2 mg/mL, 4 mg/mL, 5 mg/mL, 8 mg/mL, 10 mg/mL, 25 mg/mL, 50 mg/mL. **Solution for IV injection (PCA device):** 1 mg/mL, 2 mg/mL, 3 mg/mL, 5 mg/mL. **Tablets:** 15 mg, 30 mg. **Cost:** *Generic*—15 mg $22.17/100, 30 mg $37.77/100.

NURSING IMPLICATIONS

Assessment

- Assess type, location, and intensity of pain prior to and 1 hr following PO, subcut, IM, and 20 min (peak) following IV administration. When titrating opioid doses, increases of 25–50% should be administered until there is either a 50% reduction in the patient's pain rating on a numerical or visual analogue scale or the patient reports satisfactory pain relief. When titrating doses of short-acting morphine, a repeat dose can be safely administered at the time of the peak if previous dose is ineffective and side effects are minimal.
- Patients on a continuous infusion should have additional bolus doses provided every 15–30 min, as needed, for breakthrough pain. The bolus dose is usually set to the amount of drug infused each hr by continuous infusion.

M

- Patients taking extended-release morphine may require additional short-acting opioid doses for breakthrough pain. Doses of short-acting opioids should be equivalent to 10–20% of 24 hr total and given every 2 hr as needed.
- An equianalgesic chart (see Appendix J) should be used when changing routes or when changing from one opioid to another.
- ***High Alert:*** Assess level of consciousness, BP, pulse, and respirations before and periodically during administration. If respiratory rate is <10/min, assess level of sedation. Physical stimulation may be sufficient to prevent significant hypoventilation. Subsequent doses may need to be decreased by 25–50%. Initial drowsiness will diminish with continued use. Geri: Assess geriatric patients frequently; older adults are more sensitive to the effects of opioid analgesics and may experience side effects and respiratory complications more frequently. Pedi: Assess pediatric patient frequently; children are more sensitive to the effects of opioid analgesics and may experience respiratory complications, excitability, and restlessness more frequently.
- Prolonged use may lead to physical and psychological dependence and tolerance. This should not prevent patient from receiving adequate analgesia. Patients who receive morphine for pain rarely develop psychological dependence. Progressively higher doses may be required to relieve pain with long-term therapy.
- Assess bowel function routinely. Institute prevention of constipation with increased intake of fluids and bulk and with laxatives to minimize constipating effects. Administer stimulant laxatives routinely if opioid use exceeds 2–3 days, unless contraindicated. Consider drugs for opioid-induced constipation.
- Assess risk for opioid addiction, abuse, or misuse prior to administration. Abuse or misuse of extended-release preparations by crushing, chewing, snorting, or injecting dissolved product will result in uncontrolled delivery of morphine and can result in overdose and death.
- ***Lab Test Considerations:*** May ↑ plasma amylase and lipase levels.
- ***Toxicity and Overdose:*** If an opioid antagonist is required to reverse respiratory depression or coma, naloxone is the antidote. Dilute the 0.4-mg ampule of naloxone in 10 mL of 0.9% NaCl and administer 0.5 mL (0.02 mg) by IV push every 2 min. For children and adults weighing <40 kg, dilute 0.1 mg of naloxone in 10 mL of 0.9% NaCl for a concentration of 10 mcg/mL and administer 0.5 mcg/kg every 2 min. Titrate dose to avoid withdrawal, seizures, and severe pain.

Implementation

- ***High Alert:*** Do not confuse MS Contin (morphine sulfate) with Oxycontin (oxycodone). Do not confuse morphine (nonconcentrated oral liquid) with morphine (concentrated oral liquid).
- ***High Alert:*** Do not confuse morphine with hydromorphone—errors have resulted in death. Use only preservative-free formulations for neonates, and for epidural and intrathecal routes in all patients.
- Abuse deterrent: *Embeda* is an abuse deterrent formulation that contains naltrexone which remains inactive unless the product is crushed or diluted. *Morphabond ER* is an abuse deterrent formulation that is difficult to crush and, if crushed results in a gel.
- Explain therapeutic value of medication prior to administration to enhance the analgesic effect.
- Regularly administered doses may be more effective than prn administration. Analgesic is more effective if given before pain becomes severe.
- Coadministration with nonopioid analgesics may have additive analgesic effects and may permit lower doses.
- When transferring from other opioids or other forms of morphine to extended-release tablets, administer a total daily dose of oral morphine equivalent to previous daily dose (see Appendix J) and divided every 8 hr (MS Contin), every 12 hr (Embeda, Kadian, MS Contin), every 24 hr (Kadian).
- Morphine should be discontinued gradually to prevent withdrawal symptoms after long-term use. For patients on long-acting agents who are physically opioid-dependent, initiate the taper by a small enough increment (no greater than 10% to 25% of total daily dose) to avoid withdrawal symptoms, and proceed with dose-lowering at an interval of every 2 to 4 wk. Patients who have been taking opioids for briefer periods of time may tolerate a more rapid taper.
- **PO:** Doses may be administered with food or milk to minimize GI irritation.
- Administer oral solution with properly calibrated measuring device; may be diluted in a glass of fruit juice just prior to administration to improve taste. Verify correct dose (mg) and correct volume (mL) prior to administration. Use an oral syringe when using 20 mg/mL concentration of oral solution.
- Swallow extended-release tablets whole; do not break, crush, dissolve, or chew (could result in rapid release and absorption of a potentially toxic dose).
- *Embeda and Kadian* capsules may be opened and the pellets sprinkled onto applesauce immediately prior to administration. Patients should rinse mouth and swallow to assure ingestion of entire dose. Pellets should not be chewed, crushed, or dissolved. *Kadian* capsules may also be opened and sprinkled on approximately 10 mL of water and flushed while swirling through a pre-wetted 16 French gastrostomy tube fitted with a funnel at the port end. Additional water should be used to transfer and flush any remaining pellets. *Kadian* should not be administered via a nasogastric tube.

- **Rect:** *MS Contin* has been administered rectally.
- **IM, Subcut:** Use IM route for repeated doses, because morphine is irritating to subcut tissues.
- FDA strongly encourages health care professionals to complete a REMS-compliant education program that includes all the elements of the FDA Education *Blueprint for Health Care Providers Involved in the Management or Support of Patients with Pain,* available at www.fda.gov/OpioidAnalgesicREMSBlueprint. Information on programs can be found at 1-800-503-0784 or www.opioidanalgesicrems.com.

IV Administration

- **IV:** Solution is colorless; do not administer discolored solution.
- **IV Push:** ***Diluent:*** Dilute with at least 5 mL of sterile water or 0.9% NaCl for injection. ***Concentration:*** 0.5–5 mg/mL. ***Rate: High Alert:*** Administer 2.5–15 mg over 5 min. Rapid administration may lead to increased respiratory depression, hypotension, and circulatory collapse.
- **Continuous Infusion:** ***Diluent:*** May be added to D5W, D10W, 0.9% NaCl, 0.45% NaCl, Ringer's or LR, dextrose/saline solution, or dextrose/Ringer's or LR. ***Concentration:*** 0.1–1 mg/mL or greater for continuous infusion. ***Rate:*** Administer via infusion pump to control the rate. Dose should be titrated to ensure adequate pain relief without excessive sedation, respiratory depression, or hypotension. May be administered via patient-controlled analgesia (PCA) pump.
- **Y-Site Compatibility:** acetaminophen, aldesleukin, alfentanil, allopurinol, amifostine, amikacin, aminocaproic acid, aminophylline, amiodarone, amsacrine, anakinra, anidulafungin, argatroban, ascorbic acid, atropine, aztreonam, benztropine, bivalirudin, bleomycin, bumetanide, buprenorphine, butorphanol, calcium chloride, calcium gluconate, cangrelor, carboplatin, carmustine, caspofungin, cefazolin, cefotaxime, cefotetan, cefoxitin, ceftaroline, ceftazidime, ceftriaxone, cefuroxime, chloramphenicol, chlorpromazine, cisatracurium, cladribine, clindamycin, cyanocobalamin, cyclophosphamide, cyclosporine, cytarabine, dacarbazine, dactinomycin, daptomycin, dexamethasone, dexmedetomidine, dexrazoxane, digoxin, diltiazem, diphenhydramine, dobutamine, docetaxel, dopamine, doxorubicin hydrochloride, doxycycline, droperidol, enalaprilat, ephedrine, epinephrine, epirubicin, epoetin alfa, eptifibatide, ertapenem, erythromycin, esmolol, etomidate, etoposide, etoposide phosphate, famotidine, fenoldopam, fentanyl, filgrastim, fluconazole, fludarabine, fluorouracil, foscarnet, fosphenytoin, gemcitabine, gentamicin, glycopyrrolate, granisetron, heparin, hydrocortisone, hydromorphone, idarubicin, ifosfamide, imipenem/cilastatin, irinotecan, isoproterenol, ketorolac, labetalol, leucovorin calcium, lidocaine, linezolid, lorazepam, magnesium sulfate, mannitol, melphalan, meperidine, meropenem, mesna, methotrexate, methyldopate, methylprednisolone, metoclopramide, metoprolol, metronidazole, midazolam, milrinone, mitoxantrone, multivitamins, mycophenolate, nafcillin, nalbuphine, naloxone, nicardipine, nitroglycerin, nitroprusside, norepinephrine, octreotide, ondansetron, oxacillin, oxaliplatin, oxytocin, paclitaxel, palonosetron, pamidronate, pancuronium, papaverine, pemetrexed, penicillin G, phenobarbital, phentolamine, phenylephrine, phytonadione, piperacillin/tazobactam, potassium acetate, potassium chloride, procainamide, prochlorperazine, promethazine, propranolol, protamine, pyridoxine, quinupristin/dalfopristin, ranitidine, remifentanil, rituximab, rocuronium, sodium acetate, sodium bicarbonate, streptokinase, succinylcholine, sufentanil, tacrolimus, theophylline, thiamine, thiotepa, tigecycline, tirofiban, tobramycin, topotecan, vancomycin, vasopressin, vecuronium, verapamil, vinblastine, vincristine, vinorelbine, vitamin B complex with C, voriconazole, warfarin, zidovudine, zoledronic acid.
- **Y-Site Incompatibility:** alemtuzumab, amphotericin B lipid complex, amphotericin B liposome, azathioprine, dantrolene, doxorubicin liposomal, folic acid, ganciclovir, indomethacin, micafungin, mitomycin, pentamidine, pentobarbital, phenytoin, sargramostim, trastuzumab.
- **Epidural:** Administer undiluted. Do not use an in-line filter. Do not admix or administer other medications in epidural space for 48 hr after administration. Administer within 4 hr after removing from vial. Store in refrigerator; do not freeze.

Patient/Family Teaching

- Instruct patient how and when to ask for pain medication. Do not stop taking without discussing with health care professional; may cause withdrawal symptoms if discontinued abruptly after prolonged use.Discuss safe use, risks, and proper storage and disposal of opioid analgesics with patients and caregivers with each Rx. The Patient Counseling Guide (PCG) is available at www.fda.gov/OpioidAnalgesicREMSPCG.
- May cause drowsiness or dizziness. Caution patient to call for assistance when ambulating or smoking and to avoid driving or other activities requiring alertness until response to medication is known.
- Advise patient that morphine is a drug with known abuse potential. Protect it from theft, and never give to anyone other than the individual for whom it was prescribed. Store out of sight and reach of children, and in a location not accessible by others.

M

- Advise patient to change positions slowly to minimize orthostatic hypotension.
- Caution patient to avoid concurrent use of alcohol or other CNS depressants with this medication.
- Encourage patients who are immobilized or on prolonged bedrest to turn, cough, and breathe deeply every 2 hr to prevent atelectasis.
- Rep: Advise patient to notify health care professional if pregnancy is planned or suspected, or if breast feeding. Inform patient of potential for neonatal opioid withdrawal syndrome with prolonged use during pregnancy. Monitor neonate for signs and symptoms of withdrawal (irritability, hyperactivity and abnormal sleep pattern, high pitched cry, tremor, vomiting, diarrhea, and/or failure to gain weight); usually occur the first days after birth.
- **Home Care Issues:** ***High Alert:*** Explain to patient and family how and when to administer morphine and how to care for infusion equipment properly. Pedi: Teach parents or caregivers how to accurately measure liquid medication and to use only the measuring device dispensed with the medication.
- Emphasize the importance of aggressive prevention of constipation with the use of morphine.

Evaluation/Desired Outcomes

- Decrease in severity of pain without a significant alteration in level of consciousness or respiratory status.
- Decrease in symptoms of pulmonary edema.

mupirocin (myoo-peer-oh-sin)

~~Bactroban~~, Centany

Classification

Therapeutic: anti-infectives

Indications

Topical: Treatment of: Impetigo, Secondarily infected traumatic skin lesions (up to 10 cm in length or 100 cm^2 area) caused by *Staphylococcus aureus* and *Streptococcus pyogenes*.

Action

Inhibits bacterial protein synthesis. **Therapeutic Effects:** Inhibition of bacterial growth and reproduction. **Spectrum:** Greatest activity against gram-positive organisms, including: *S. aureus*, Beta-hemolytic streptococci. Resolution of impetigo. Eradication of *S. aureus* carrier state.

Pharmacokinetics

Absorption: Minimal systemic absorption.
Distribution: Remains in the stratum corneum after topical use for prolonged periods of time (72 hr).
Metabolism and Excretion: Metabolized in the skin, removed by desquamation.
Half-life: 17–36 min.

TIME/ACTION PROFILE (anti-infective effect)

ROUTE	ONSET	PEAK	DURATION
Topical†	unknown	3–5 days	72 hr

†Resolution of lesions.

Contraindications/Precautions

Contraindicated in: Hypersensitivity to mupirocin or polyethylene glycol.
Use Cautiously in: Renal impairment; Burn patients; OB, Lactation: Safety not established.

Adverse Reactions/Side Effects

Derm: burning, itching, pain, stinging.

Interactions

Drug-Drug: None reported.

Route/Dosage

Topical (Adults and Children ≥2 mo): Ointment: Apply 3–5 times daily for 5–14 days.
Topical (Adults and Children ≥3 mo): Cream: Apply small amount 3 times/day for 10 days.

Availability (generic available)

Cream: 2%. **Cost:** *Generic*—$69.25/15 g. **Ointment:** 2%. **Cost:** *Generic*—$17.20/22 g.

NURSING IMPLICATIONS

Assessment

- Assess lesions before and daily during therapy.

Implementation

- **Topical:** Wash affected area with soap and water and dry thoroughly. Apply a small amount of mupirocin to the affected area 3 times daily and rub in gently. Treated area may be covered with gauze if desired.

Patient/Family Teaching

- Instruct patient on the correct application of mupirocin. Advise patient to apply medication exactly as directed for the full course of therapy. If a dose is missed, apply as soon as possible unless almost time for next dose. Avoid contact with eyes.
- **Topical:** Teach patient and family appropriate hygienic measures to prevent spread of impetigo.
- Instruct parents to notify school nurse for screening and prevention of transmission.
- Advise females of reproductive potential to notify health care professional if pregnancy is planned or suspected or if breast feeding.
- Patient should consult health care professional if symptoms have not improved in 3–5 days.

Evaluation/Desired Outcomes

- Healing of skin lesions. If no clinical response is seen in 3–5 days, condition should be re-evaluated.

REMS

mycophenolate mofetil
(mye-koe-**fee**-noe-late **moe**-fe-til)
CellCept

mycophenolic acid
(mye-koe-**fee**-noe-lik)
Myfortic

Classification
Therapeutic: immunosuppressants

Indications

Mycophenolate mofetil: Prevention of rejection in allogenic renal, hepatic, and cardiac transplantation (used concurrently with cyclosporine and corticosteroids). **Mycophenolic acid**: Prevention of rejection in allogenic renal transplantation (used concurrently with cyclosporine and corticosteroids). **Unlabeled Use:** Nephrotic syndrome.

Action

Inhibits the enzyme inosine monophosphate dehydrogenase, which is involved in purine synthesis. This inhibition results in suppression of T- and B-lymphocyte proliferation. **Therapeutic Effects:** Prevention of heart, kidney, or liver transplant rejection.

Pharmacokinetics

Absorption: Following oral and IV administration, mycophenolate mofetil is rapidly hydrolyzed to mycophenolic acid (MPA), the active metabolite. Absorption of enteric-coated mycophenolic acid (Myfortic) is delayed compared with mycophenolate mofetil (CellCept).

Distribution: Cross the placenta and enter breast milk.

Protein Binding: *MPA*—97%.

Metabolism and Excretion: MPA is extensively metabolized; <1% excreted unchanged in urine. Some enterohepatic recirculation of MPA occurs.

Half-life: *MPA*—8–18 hr.

TIME/ACTION PROFILE (blood levels of MPA)

ROUTE	ONSET	PEAK	DURATION
mycophenolate mofetil-PO	rapid	0.25–1.25 hr	N/A
mycophenolic acid	rapid	1.5–2.75 hr	N/A

Contraindications/Precautions

Contraindicated in: Hypersensitivity; Hypersensitivity to polysorbate 80 (for IV mycophenolate mofetil); OB: Avoid use during pregnancy (↑ risk of congenital anomalies or spontaneous abortion).

Use Cautiously in: Active serious pathology of the GI tract (including history of ulcer disease or GI bleeding); Phenylketonuria (oral suspension contains aspartame); Severe chronic renal impairment (dose not to exceed 1 g twice daily (CellCept) if CCr <25 mL/min/1.73 m^2); careful monitoring recommended; Delayed graft function following transplantation (observe for ↑ toxicity); Lactation: Safety not established (consider beneficial effects of breast feeding and possible adverse effects in infant); Rep: Women of reproductive potential; Geri: ↑ risk of adverse reactions related to immunosuppression; Pedi: Mycophenolate mofetil approved in children ≥3 mo for renal transplant; mycophenolic acid approved in children ≥5 yr for renal transplant; safety not established for other age groups.

Adverse Reactions/Side Effects

CNS: PROGRESSIVE MULTIFOCAL LEUKOENCEPHALOPATHY (PML), anxiety, confusion, dizziness, headache, insomnia, paresthesia, sedation, tremor. **CV:** edema, hypertension, hypotension, tachycardia. **Derm:** rash. **Endo:** hypercholesterolemia, hyperglycemia, hyperkalemia, hypocalcemia, hypokalemia, hypomagnesemia. **GI:** GI BLEEDING, anorexia, constipation, diarrhea, nausea, vomiting, abdominal pain. **GU:** renal dysfunction. **Hemat:** leukocytosis, leukopenia, thrombocytopenia, anemia, pure red cell aplasia. **Neuro:** tremor. **Resp:** cough, dyspnea. **Misc:** fever, infection (including activation of latent viral infections such as Polyomavirus-associated nephropathy or Hepatitis B/C), ↑ risk of malignancy.

Interactions

Drug-Drug: Combined use with **azathioprine** is not recommended (effects unknown). **Acyclovir** and **ganciclovir** compete with MPA for renal excretion and, in patients with renal dysfunction, may ↑ each other's toxicity. **Magnesium and aluminum hydroxide** antacids ↓ the absorption of MPA (avoid simultaneous administration). **Proton pump inhibitors**, including **dexlansoprazole**, **esomeprazole**, **lansoprazole**, **omeprazole**, **pantoprazole**, and **rabeprazole** may ↓ levels. **Cholestyramine** and **colestipol** ↓ the absorption of MPA (avoid concurrent use). May ↓ the effectiveness of **oral contraceptives** (additional contraceptive method should be used). May ↓ the antibody response to and ↑ risk of adverse reactions from **live-virus vaccines**, although influenza vaccine may be useful. **Amoxicillin/clavulanic acid** or **ciprofloxacin** may ↓ MPA trough levels. **Cyclosporine** may ↓ levels; use caution when discontinuing cyclosporine (may ↑ mycophenolate levels) or when switching from cyclosporine to another immunosupressant, such as tacrolimus or belatacept. **Telmisartan** may ↓ levels.

Drug-Food: When administered with food, peak blood levels of MPA are significantly ↓ (should be administered on an empty stomach).

M

Route/Dosage

Mycophenolate Mofetil

Renal Transplantation

PO, IV (Adults): 1 g twice daily; IV should be started ≤24 hr after transplantation and switched to PO as soon as possible (IV not recommended for ≥14 days).
PO (Children 3 mo–18 yr): 600 mg/m² twice daily (not to exceed 2 g/day).

Hepatic Transplantation

PO, IV (Adults): 1 g twice daily IV, or 1.5 g twice daily PO. IV should be started ≤24 hr after transplantation and switched to PO as soon as possible (IV not recommended for ≥14 days).

Cardiac Transplantation

PO, IV (Adults): 1.5 g twice daily; IV should be started ≤24 hr after transplantation and switched to PO as soon as possible (IV not recommended for ≥14 days).

Nephrotic Syndrome

PO (Children): *Frequent relapses*—12.5–18 mg/kg/dose twice daily; maximum: 2 g/day. *Steroid-dependent*—12–18 mg/kg/dose or 600 mg/m² twice daily; maximum: 2 g/day.

Renal Impairment

PO, IV (Adults): *CCr <25 mL/min*—daily dose should not exceed 2 g.

Mycophenolic Acid

Mycophenolate mofetil and mycophenolic acid should not be used interchangeably without the advice of a health care professional.

Renal Transplantation

PO (Adults): 720 mg twice daily.
PO (Children 5–16 yr and ≥1.19 m²): 400–450 mg/m² twice daily (not to exceed 720 mg twice daily).

Availability (generic available)

Mycophenolate Mofetil

Capsules: 250 mg. **Oral suspension (fruit flavor):** 200 mg/mL. **Powder for injection (requires reconstitution and dilution):** 500 mg/vial. **Tablets:** 500 mg.

Mycophenolic Acid

Delayed-release tablets: 180 mg, 360 mg.

NURSING IMPLICATIONS

Assessment

- Assess for symptoms of organ rejection throughout therapy.
- Assess for signs of PML (hemiparesis, apathy, confusion, cognitive deficiencies, and ataxia) periodically during therapy.
- ***Lab Test Considerations:*** Obtain a urine pregnancy test with a specificity of 25 mIU/mL immediately prior to beginning therapy and again 8–10 days later. Repeat pregnancy tests should be preformed during routine follow-up visits.
- Monitor CBC with differential weekly during the 1st mo, twice monthly for the 2nd and 3rd mo of therapy, and then monthly during the 1st yr. Neutropenia occurs most frequently from 31–180 days post-transplant. If ANC is <1000/mm³, dose should be reduced or discontinued.
- Monitor hepatic and renal status and electrolytes periodically during therapy. May cause ↑ serum alkaline phosphatase, AST, ALT, LDH, BUN, and creatinine. May also cause hyperkalemia, hypokalemia, hypocalcemia, hypomagnesemia, hyperglycemia, and hyperlipidemia.

Implementation

- The initial dose of mycophenolate should be given within 24 hr of transplant.
- Mycophenolate mofetil (Cellcept) and mycophenolic acid (Myfortic) are not interchangeable; rate of absorption is different.
- **PO:** Administer on an empty stomach, 1 hr before or 2 hr after meals. Swallow capsules and delayed-release tablets whole; do not open, crush, or chew. Mycophenolate may be teratogenic; wear gloves and avoid contact with skin or mucous membranes or inhalation of contents of capsules or oral suspension powder. Oral solution can be administered by nasogastric tube (minimum size of 8 French). Oral solution is stable for 60 days if refrigerated.
- Do not administer mycophenolate concurrently with antacids containing magnesium or aluminum.

IV Administration

- **IV:** IV route should only be used for patients unable to take oral medication and should be switched to oral dose form as soon as patient can tolerate capsules or tablets.
- **Intermittent Infusion:** ***Diluent:*** Reconstitute each vial with 14 mL of D5W. Shake gently to dissolve. Solution is slightly yellow; discard if solution is discolored or contains particulate matter. Dilute contents of 2 vials (1-g dose) further with 140 mL of D5W or 3 vials (1.5-g dose) with 210 mL of D5W. ***Concentration:*** 6 mg/mL. Solution is stable for 4 hr. ***Rate:*** Administer via slow IV infusion over at least 2 hr. Do not administer as a bolus or via rapid infusion; increases risk of phlebitis and thrombosis.
- **Y-Site Compatibility:** alemtuzumab, alfentanil, amakacin, amiodarone, anidulafungin, argatroban, atracurium, bivalirudin, bumetanide, buprenorphine, butorphanil, calcium chloride, caspofungin, ceftolozane/tazobactam, chlorpromazine, ciprofloxacin, cisatracurium, daptomycin, dexmedetomidine, dexrazoxane , digoxin, diltiazem, diphenhydramine, dobutamine, dolasetron, dopamine, doxorubicin liposomal, doxyxycline, droperidol, enalaprilat, ephedrine, epinephrine, erythromycin, esmolol, famotidine, fenoldopam, fentanyl, fluconazole, gentamicin, glycopyrrolate, granesetron, haloperidol,

hydralazine, hydromorphone, insulin, regular, isavuconazonium, isoproterenol, labetalol, leucovorin calcium, levofloxacin, linezolid, lorazepam, magnesium sulfate, mannitol, meperidine, mesna, methyldopate, metoclopramide, metoprolol, metronidazole, midazolam, milrinone, minocycline, morphine, moxifloxacin, nalbuphine, naloxone, nicardipine, nitroglycerin, norepinephrine, octreotide, ondansetron, oxytocin, pamidronate, pancuronium, pentamidine, phenylephrine, phentolamine, potassium chloride, procainamide, prochlorperazine, promazine, propranolol, quinupristin/dalfopristin, ranitidine, remifentanil, rocuronium, succinylcholine, sufentanil, tacrolimus, theophylline, tigecycline, tirofiban, tobramycin, vancomycin, vasopressin, vecuronium, verapamil, voriconazole, zidovudine, zoledronic acid.

- **Y-Site Incompatibility:** acyclovir, allopurinol, amifostine, aminocaproic acid, aminophylline, amphotericin B deoxycholate, amphotericin B lipid complex, amphotericin B liposome, ampicillin, ampicillin/sulbactam, azithromycin, aztreonam, calcium gluconate, cangrelor, cefazolin, cefotaxime, cefotetan, cefoxotin, ceftazidime, ceftriaoxone, cefuroxime, chloramphenicol, clindamycin, dantrolene, defibrotide, dexamethasone, diazepam, eftifibatide, foscarnet, fosphenytoin, furosemide, ganciclovir, gemtuzumab, heparin, hydrocortisone, imipenem/cilastatin, ketorolac, letermovir, meropenem, methotrexate, methylprednisolone, micafungin, nafcillin, nitroprusside, pantoprazole, pentobarbital, phenobarbital, phenytoin, piperacillin/tazobacatam, potassium acetate, potassium phosphates, sodium acetate, sodium phosphates, trimethoprin/sulfamethoxazole.

Patient/Family Teaching

- Instruct patient to take medication as directed, at the same time each day. Take missed dose as soon as remembered, but not if within 2 hrs before next dose. Do not skip or double up on missed doses. Do not discontinue without consulting health care professional. Advise patient to read *Medication Guide* before starting therapy and with each Rx refill in case of changes.
- Reinforce the need for lifelong therapy to prevent transplant rejection. Review symptoms of rejection for the transplanted organ, and stress need to notify health care professional immediately if signs of rejection or infection occur.
- May cause somnolence, confusion, dizziness, tremor, or hypotension. Caution patient to avoid driving and other activities requiring alertness until response from medication is known.
- Instruct patient to notify health care professional immediately if signs and symptoms of infection (temperature ≥100.5°F, cold symptoms [runny nose, sore throat], flu symptoms [upset stomach, stomach pain, vomiting, diarrhea], earache or headache, pain during urination, frequent urination, white patches in mouth or throat, unexpected bruising or bleeding, cuts, scrapes, or incisions that are red, warm, and oozing pus) or PML.
- Advise patient to avoid contact with persons with contagious diseases.
- Advise patient to avoid vaccinations with live attenuated virus during therapy.
- Inform patient of the increased risk of lymphoma and other malignancies. Advise patient to use sunscreen and wear protective clothing to decrease risk of skin cancer.
- Advise patient to notify health care professional of all Rx or OTC medications, vitamins, or herbal products being taken and to consult with health care professional before taking other medications.
- Instruct patient to avoid donating blood during and for at least 6 wk after discontinuation of therapy.
- Rep: Inform females of reproductive potential of the potential for pregnancy loss and teratogenic effects. Discuss importance of simultaneously using two reliable nonhormonal forms of contraception, unless abstinence is the chosen method, prior to beginning, during, and for 6 wk following discontinuation of therapy and to avoid breast feeding. Discuss acceptable forms of contraception with health care professional. Mycophenolate may decrease effectiveness of hormonal contraceptives. Encourage patients who become pregnant during or within 6 wk after therapy to enroll in the Pregnancy Registry by calling 1–800–617–8191 or www.mycophenolateREMS.com to monitor pregnancy outcomes in women exposed to mycophenolate during pregnancy. Instruct male patients with female partners of reproductive potential to use effective contraception during and for at least 90 days after discontinuing therapy. Advise male patients to avoid semen donation during and for at least 90 days after discontinuing therapy.
- Emphasize the importance of routine follow-up laboratory tests.

Evaluation/Desired Outcomes

- Prevention of rejection of transplanted organs.

M

nafarelin (na-fare-e-lin)
Synarel

Classification
Therapeutic: hormones
Pharmacologic: gonadotropin-releasing hormones

Indications
Endometriosis. Central precocious puberty (gonadotropin-dependent) in children.

Action
Acts as a synthetic analogue of gonadotropin-releasing hormone (GnRH). Initially increases pituitary production of luteinizing hormone (LH) and follicle-stimulating hormone (FSH), which cause ovarian steroid production. Chronic administration leads to decreased production of gonadotropins. Endometriotic lesions are sensitive to ovarian hormones. **Therapeutic Effects:** Reduction in lesions and associated pain in endometriosis. Arrest and regression of puberty in children with central precocious puberty.

Pharmacokinetics
Absorption: Well absorbed following intranasal administration.
Distribution: Unknown.
Metabolism and Excretion: 20–40% excreted in feces; 3% excreted unchanged by the kidneys.
Half-life: 3 hr.

TIME/ACTION PROFILE (↓ ovarian steroid production)

ROUTE	ONSET	PEAK	DURATION
Intranasal	within 4 wk	3–4 wk	3–6 mo†

†Relief of symptoms of endometriosis following discontinuation.

Contraindications/Precautions
Contraindicated in: Hypersensitivity to GnRH, its analogues, or sorbitol; OB, Lactation: Pregnancy or lactation.
Use Cautiously in: Rhinitis; Seizures, cerebrovascular disorders, CNS tumor, or concurrent use of bupropion or selective serotonin reuptake inhibitors.

Adverse Reactions/Side Effects
CNS: SEIZURES, STROKE, headaches, aggression, anger, depression, impatience, irritability, insomnia. **EENT:** nasal irritation. **CV:** MYOCARDIAL INFARCTION, edema. **GU:** vaginal dryness. **Derm:** acne, hirsutism, seborrhea. **Endo:** cessation of menses, impaired fertility, ↓ breast size. **Metab:** hyperglycemia. **MS:** ↓ bone density, myalgia. **Misc:** ↓ libido, hot flashes, hypersensitivity reactions, weight gain.

Interactions
Drug-Drug: Concurrent **topical nasal decongestants** may ↓ absorption of nafarelin (administer decongestant at least 2 hr after nafarelin). Concurrent use with **bupropion** or **SSRIs** may ↑ risk of seizures.

Route/Dosage
Intranasal (Adults): *Endometriosis*—1 spray (200 mcg) in 1 nostril in the morning and 1 spray in the other nostril in the evening (400 mcg/day). May ↑ to 1 spray in each nostril in the morning and evening (800 mcg/day).
Intranasal (Children): *Central precocious puberty*—2 sprays in each nostril in the morning and in the evening (1600 mcg/day); may ↑ up to 1800 mcg/day (3 sprays in alternating nostrils 3 times daily).

Availability
Nasal spray: 2 mg/mL (200 mcg/spray).

NURSING IMPLICATIONS

Assessment
- **Endometriosis:** Assess patient for endometriotic pain periodically during therapy.
- **Central Precocious Puberty:** Prior to therapy, a complete physical and endocrinologic examination including height, weight, hand and wrist x-ray, total sex steroid level (estradiol or testosterone), adrenal steroid level, beta human chorionic gonadotropin level, GnRH stimulation test, pelvic/adrenal/testicular ultrasound, and CT of the head must be performed. These parameters are monitored after 6–8 wk and every 3–6 mo during therapy.
- Assess patient for signs of precocious puberty (menses, breast development, testicular growth) periodically during therapy.
- Nafarelin is discontinued when the onset of normal puberty is desired. Monitor the onset of normal puberty and assess menstrual cycle, reproductive function, and final adult height.

Implementation
- **Endometriosis:** Treatment should be started between days 2 and 4 of the menstrual cycle and continued for up to 6 mo.

Patient/Family Teaching
- Instruct patient on the correct technique for nasal spray: The head should be tilted back slightly; wait 30 sec between sprays.
- Advise patient to consult health care professional if rhinitis occurs during therapy. If a topical decongestant is needed, do not use decongestant until 2 hr after nafarelin dosing. If possible, avoid sneezing during and immediately after nafarelin dose.
- **Endometriosis:** Inform patient that 1 spray should be administered into 1 nostril in the morning and 1 spray into the other nostril in the evening for the 400

mcg/day dose. If dose is increased to 800 mcg/day, administer 1 spray to each nostril (2 sprays) morning and evening; 1 bottle should provide a 30-day supply at the 400 mcg/day dose.

- Advise patient to use a form of contraception other than oral contraceptives during therapy. Inform patient that amenorrhea is expected. Instruct patient to notify health care professional if regular menstruation persists or if successive doses are missed.
- Advise patient that medication may cause hot flashes. Notify health care professional if these become bothersome.
- **Central Precocious Puberty:** Instruct patient on correct timing and number of sprays. The 1600 mcg/day dose is achieved by 2 sprays to each nostril in the morning (4 sprays) and 2 sprays to each nostril in the evening (4 sprays), for a total of 8 sprays. The 1800 mcg/day dose is achieved by 3 sprays into alternating nostrils 3 times per day, for a total of 9 sprays. Inform patient and parents that if doses are not taken as directed pubertal process may be reactivated. One bottle should provide a 7-day supply at the 1600 mcg/day dose.
- Advise patient and parents that during 1st mo of therapy some signs of puberty (vaginal bleeding, breast enlargement) may occur. These should resolve after the 1st mo of therapy. If these signs persist after the 2nd mo of therapy, notify health care professional.

Evaluation/Desired Outcomes

- Reduction in lesions and associated pain in endometriosis.
- Resolution of the signs of precocious puberty.

nafcillin, See PENICILLINS, PENICILLINASE RESISTANT.

naftifine, See ANTIFUNGALS (TOPICAL).

HIGH ALERT

nalbuphine (nal-byoo-feen)

Nubain

Classification
Therapeutic: opioid analgesics
Pharmacologic: opioid agonists/analgesics

Indications

Moderate to severe pain. Also provides: Analgesia during labor, Sedation before surgery, Supplement to balanced anesthesia.

Action

Binds to opiate receptors in the CNS. Alters the perception of and response to painful stimuli while producing generalized CNS depression. In addition, has partial antagonist properties, which may result in opioid withdrawal in physically dependent patients. **Therapeutic Effects:** Decreased pain.

Pharmacokinetics

Absorption: Well absorbed after IM and subcut administration.
Distribution: Probably crosses the placenta and enters breast milk.
Protein Binding: 50%.
Metabolism and Excretion: Mostly metabolized by the liver and eliminated in the feces via biliary excretion. Minimal amounts excreted unchanged by the kidneys.
Half-life: Children 1–8 yrs: 0.9 hr; Adults: 3.5–5 hr.

TIME/ACTION PROFILE (analgesia)

ROUTE	ONSET	PEAK	DURATION
IM	<15 min	60 min	3–6 hr
Subcut	<15 min	unknown	3–6 hr
IV	2–3 min	30 min	3–6 hr

Contraindications/Precautions

Contraindicated in: Hypersensitivity to nalbuphine or bisulfites; Patients physically dependent on opioids and who have not been detoxified (may precipitate withdrawal).
Use Cautiously in: Head trauma; ↑ intracranial pressure; Severe renal, hepatic, or pulmonary disease; Hypothyroidism; Adrenal insufficiency; Alcoholism; Undiagnosed abdominal pain; Prostatic hyperplasia; Patients who have recently received opioid agonists; OB: Has been used during labor but may cause respiratory depression in the newborn; prolonged use of opioids during pregnancy can result in neonatal opioid withdrawal syndrome; Lactation: May cause respiratory depression and excessive sedation in infant; Geri: Dose ↓ suggested; Pedi: Safety and effectiveness not established.

Adverse Reactions/Side Effects

CNS: dizziness, headache, sedation, confusion, dysphoria, euphoria, floating feeling, hallucinations, unusual dreams. **Endo:** adrenal insufficiency. **EENT:** blurred vision, diplopia, miosis (high doses). **Resp:** respiratory depression. **CV:** hypertension, orthostatic hypotension, palpitations. **GI:** dry mouth, nausea, vomiting, constipation, ileus. **GU:** urinary urgency. **Derm:** clammy feeling, sweating. **Misc:** physical dependence, psychological dependence, tolerance.

Interactions

Drug-Drug: Use with extreme caution in patients receiving **MAO inhibitors** (may result in unpredictable, severe reactions—↓ initial dose of nalbuphine to 25% of usual dose). Use with **benzodiazepines** or other **CNS depressants** including other**opioids**, **non-benzodiazepine sedative/hypnotics**, **anxiolytics**, **general anesthetics**, **muscle relaxants**, **antipsychotics**, and **alcohol** may cause profound sedation, respiratory depression, coma, and death; reserve concurrent use for when alternative treatment options are inadequate. May precipitate withdrawal in patients who are physically dependent on **opioid agonists**. Avoid concurrent use with other **opioid analgesic agonists** (may diminish analgesic effect). Drugs that affect serotonergic neurotransmitter systems, including **tricyclic antidepressants, SSRIs, SNRIs, MAO inhibitors, TCAs, tramadol, trazodone, mirtazapine, 5-HT$_3$ receptor antagonists, linezolid, methylene blue,** and **triptans** ↑ risk of serotonin syndrome.

Drug-Natural Products: Concomitant use of **kava-kava, valerian, skullcap, chamomile,** or **hops** can ↑ CNS depression.

Route/Dosage

Analgesia

IM, Subcut, IV (Adults): Usual dose is 10 mg every 3–6 hr (maximum: 20 mg/dose or 160 mg/day).

IM, Subcut, IV (Children): 0.1–0.15 mg/kg every 3–6 hr (maximum: 20 mg/dose or 160 mg/day).

Supplement to Balanced Anesthesia

IV (Adults): *Initial*—0.3–3 mg/kg over 10–15 min. *Maintenance*—0.25–0.5 mg/kg as needed.

Availability (generic available)

Solution for injection: 10 mg/mL, 20 mg/mL.

NURSING IMPLICATIONS

Assessment

- Assess type, location, and intensity of pain before and 1 hr after IM or 30 min (peak) after IV administration. When titrating opioid doses, increases of 25–50% should be administered until there is either a 50% reduction in the patient's pain rating on a numeric or visual analogue scale or the patient reports satisfactory pain relief. A repeat dose can be safely administered at the time of the peak if previous dose is ineffective and side effects are minimal. Patients requiring doses higher than 20 mg should be converted to an opioid agonist. Nalbuphine is not recommended for prolonged use or as first-line therapy for acute or cancer pain.
- An equianalgesic chart (see Appendix J) should be used when changing routes or when changing from one opioid to another.
- Assess BP, pulse, and respirations before and periodically during administration. If respiratory rate is <10/min, assess level of sedation. Physical stimulation may be sufficient to prevent significant hypoventilation. Dose may need to be decreased by 25–50%. Nalbuphine produces respiratory depression, but this does not markedly increase with increased doses.
- Assess previous analgesic history. Antagonistic properties may induce withdrawal symptoms (vomiting, restlessness, abdominal cramps, and increased BP and temperature) in patients physically dependent on opioids.
- Although this drug has a low potential for dependence, prolonged use may lead to physical and psychological dependence and tolerance. This should not prevent patient from receiving adequate analgesia. Most patients who receive nalbuphine for pain do not develop psychological dependence. If tolerance develops, changing to an opioid agonist may be required to relieve pain.
- Assess risk for opioid addiction, abuse, or misuse prior to administration.
- ***Lab Test Considerations:*** May cause ↑ serum amylase and lipase concentrations.
- ***Toxicity and Overdose:*** If an opioid antagonist is required to reverse respiratory depression or coma, naloxone (Narcan) is the antidote. Dilute the 0.4-mg ampule of naloxone in 10 mL of 0.9% NaCl and administer 0.5 mL (0.02 mg) by IV push every 2 min. For children and patients weighing <40 kg, dilute 0.1 mg of naloxone in 10 mL of 0.9% NaCl for a concentration of 10 mcg/mL and administer 0.5 mcg/kg every 2 min. Titrate dose to avoid withdrawal, seizures, and severe pain.

Implementation

- ***High Alert:*** Do not confuse nalbuphine with naloxone.
- Explain therapeutic value of medication before administration to enhance the analgesic effect.
- Regularly administered doses may be more effective than prn administration. Analgesic is more effective if administered before pain becomes severe.
- Coadministration with nonopioid analgesics may have additive effects and permit lower opioid doses.
- **IM:** Administer deep into well-developed muscle. Rotate sites of injections.

IV Administration

- **IV Push:** May give IV undiluted.
- ***Concentration:*** 10–20 mg/mL. ***Rate:*** Administer slowly, each 10 mg over 3–5 min.
- **Y-Site Compatibility:** acetaminophen, alfentanil, amifostine, amikacin, aminocaproic acid, aminophylline, amiodarone, argatroban, atropine, azithromycin, aztreonam, benztropine, bivalirudin, bleomycin, bumetanide, buprenorphine, butorphanol, calcium chloride, calcium gluconate, cangrelor, carboplatin, carmustine, cefazolin, cefotaxime, cefoxitin, ceftazidime, ceftriaxone, cefuroxime, chlorpromazine, cisatracurium, cladribine, clindamycin, cyanocobalamin, cyclophosphamide, cytarabine, dacarbazine, dactinomycin, daptomycin, daunorubicin hydrochloride, dexamethasone, dexmedetomidine, dexrazoxane, digoxin, diltiazem, diphenhydramine, dobutamine, dolasetron, dopamine, doxorubicin hy-

N

drochloride, doxorubicin liposomal, enalaprilat, ephedrine, epinephrine, epirubicin, epoetin alfa, eptifibatide, ertapenem, erythromycin, esmolol, etoposide, etoposide phosphate, famotidine, fenoldopam, fentanyl, filgrastim, fluconazole, fludarabine, fluorouracil, foscarnet, fosphenytoin, gemcitabine, gentamicin, glycopyrrolate, granisetron, heparin, hetastarch, idarubicin, ifosfamide, insulin, irinotecan, isoproterenol, labetalol, leucovorin, levofloxacin, lidocaine, linezolid, lorazepam, magnesium sulfate, mannitol, melphalan, meperidine, mesna, methyldopate, metoclopramide, metoprolol, midazolam, milrinone, mitoxantrone, morphine, multivitamins, mycophenolate, naloxone, nicardipine, nitroglycerin, nitroprusside, norepinephrine, octreotide, ondansetron, oxaliplatin, oxytocin, paclitaxel, palosetron, pamidronate, pancuronium, papaverine, penicillin G, phentolamine, phenylephrine, phytonadione, potassium acetate, potassium chloride, procainamide, prochlorperazine, promethazine, propofol, propranolol, protamine, pyridoxine, ranitidine, remifentanil, rituximab, rocuronium, sodium acetate, succinylcholine, sufentanil, tacrolimus, theophylline, thiamine, thiotepa, tigecycline, tirofiban, tobramycin, topotecan, vancomycin, vasopressin, vecuronium, verapamil, vinblastine, vincristine, vinorelbine, voriconazole, zoledronic acid.

- **Y-Site Incompatibility:** alemtuzumab, allopurinol, amphotericin B deoxycholate, amphotericin B lipid complex, amphotericin B liposome, anidulafungin, cefepime, chloramphenicol, cyclosporine, dantrolene, diazepam, docetaxel, folic acid, furosemide, ganciclovir, hydrocortisone, imipenem/cilastatin, indomethacin, ketorolac, methotrexate, methylprednisolone, mitomycin, pantoprazole, pemetrexed, pentamidine, pentobarbital, phenobarbital, phenytoin, piperacillin/tazobactam, sargramostim, sodium bicarbonate, streptokinase, trastuzumab, trimethoprim/sulfamethoxazole.

Patient/Family Teaching

- Instruct patient on how and when to ask for pain medication.
- May cause drowsiness or dizziness. Advise patient to call for assistance when ambulating and to avoid driving or other activities requiring alertness until response to the medication is known.
- Caution patient to change positions slowly to minimize orthostatic hypotension.
- Advise patient that frequent mouth rinses, good oral hygiene, and sugarless gum or candy may decrease dry mouth.
- Encourage patient to turn, cough, and breathe deeply every 2 hr to prevent atelectasis.
- Advise patient to avoid concurrent use of alcohol or other CNS depressants with this medication.
- Advise patient to notify health care professional if pregnancy is planned or suspected, or if breast feeding.

Evaluation/Desired Outcomes

- Decrease in severity of pain without significant alteration in level of consciousness or respiratory status.

naldemedine (nal-**dem**-e-deen)

Symproic

Classification

Therapeutic: laxatives

Pharmacologic: opioid antagonists

Indications

Treatment of opioid-induced constipation (OIC) in patients with chronic non-cancer pain, including those with chronic pain related to prior cancer or its treatment who do not require frequent (e.g., weekly) opioid dosage escalation.

Action

Acts peripherally as a mu-opioid receptor antagonist, blocking opioid effects on the GI tract. **Therapeutic Effects:** Blocks constipating effects of opioids on the GI tract without loss of analgesia.

Pharmacokinetics

Absorption: Rapidly absorbed; absorption delayed by high-fat meal by 2 hr.

Distribution: Moderate tissue distribution, does not cross the blood-brain barrier.

Protein Binding: 93–94%.

Metabolism and Excretion: Primarily metabolized by CYP3A to an active metabolite (nor-naldemedine); 57% excreted in urine (16–18% as unchanged drug), 35% excreted in feces.

Half-life: 11 hr.

TIME/ACTION PROFILE (blood levels)

ROUTE	ONSET	PEAK	DURATION
PO	unknown	0.75 hr	unknown

Contraindications/Precautions

Contraindicated in: Hypersensitivity; Known/suspected mechanical GI obstruction; ↑ risk of recurrent GI obstruction; Severe hepatic impairment; Lactation: Discontinue breast feeding or the naldemedine.

Use Cautiously in: Known/suspected lesions of GI tract (↑ risk for GI perforation); Receiving opioids for <4 wk (may be less responsive to naldemedine); OB: Use only if potential benefit outweighs potential risk to fetus; may cause opioid withdrawal in fetus; Pedi: Safety and effectiveness not established.

Adverse Reactions/Side Effects

GI: GI PERFORATION, abdominal pain, diarrhea, gastroenteritis, nausea, vomiting. **Misc:** opioid withdrawal.

Interactions

Drug-Drug: Strong CYP3A inducers, including **carbamazepine**, **phenytoin**, or **rifampin**, may ↓

naldemedine levels and its effectiveness; avoid concurrent use. Other **opioid antagonists** may cause additive effects and ↑ risk of opioid withdrawal. **Moderate CYP3A inhibitors** and **strong CYP3A inhibitors**, including **aprepitant**, **atazanavir**, **clarithromycin**, **diltiazem**, **erythromycin**, **fluconazole**, **itraconazole**, **ketoconazole**, **ritonavir**, or **saquinavir** may ↑ naldemedine levels and risk of toxicity; monitor for potential adverse effects. **P-glycoprotein inhibitors**, including **amiodarone**, **captopril**, **cyclosporine**, **quinidine**, or **verapamil** may ↑ naldemedine levels and risk of toxicity; monitor for potential adverse effects.
Drug-Natural Products: St. John's wort may ↓ naldemedine levels and its effectiveness; avoid concurrent use.

Route/Dosage

PO (Adults): 0.2 mg once daily.

Availability

Tablets: 0.2 mg.

NURSING IMPLICATIONS

Assessment

- Assess bowel sounds and frequency, quantity, and consistency of stools periodically during therapy.
- Monitor pain intensity during therapy. Naldemedine does not affect pain or effects of opioid analgesics on pain control. Discontinue naldemedine if opioid analgesic is discontinued. Patients receiving opioids for <4 wk may be less responsive to naldemedine.
- Monitor for signs and symptoms of gastrointestinal perforation (severe, persistent or worsening abdominal pain) periodically during therapy. Discontinue naldemedine if symptoms occur.

Implementation

- **PO:** Administer once daily without regard to food.

Patient/Family Teaching

- Instruct patient to take naldemedine as directed. Advise patient to read *Medication Guide* prior to starting therapy and with each refill in case of changes.
- Advise patient to notify health care professional immediately if stomach pain that does not go away occurs.
- Advise patient to notify health care professional if signs and symptoms of opioid withdrawal (sweating, chills, diarrhea, stomach pain, anxiety, irritability, yawning) occur. Patients taking methadone for pain are at increased risk for stomach pain and diarrhea.
- Instruct patient to stop taking naldemedine if they stop taking opioid medications.
- Instruct patient to notify health care professional of all Rx or OTC medications, vitamins, or herbal products being taken and consult health care professional before taking any new medications.
- Advise female patients to notify health care professional if pregnancy is planned or suspected and avoid breast feeding during and for 3 days after last dose of therapy.

Evaluation/Desired Outcomes

- Relief of opioid induced constipation, especially if opioid therapy has been for 4 wk or more.

naloxegol (nal-ox-ee-gol)

Movantik

Classification
Therapeutic: laxatives
Pharmacologic: opioid antagonists

Indications

Treatment of opioid-induced constipation (OIC) in patients with chronic non-cancer pain, including those with chronic pain related to prior cancer or its treatment who do not require frequent (e.g., weekly) opioid dose escalation.

Action

Acts peripherally as a mu receptor antagonist, blocking opioid receptors in the GI tract. **Therapeutic Effects:** Blocks constipating effects of opioids on the GI tract without loss of analgesia.

Pharmacokinetics

Absorption: Systemic absorption follows oral administration. A high-fat meal ↑ absorption.
Distribution: Does not cross the blood-brain barrier.
Metabolism and Excretion: Metabolized primarily by the CYP3A4 enzyme system; 68% excreted in feces, 16% in urine mostly as metabolites.
Half-life: 6–11 hr.

TIME/ACTION PROFILE (spontaneous bowel movement)

ROUTE	ONSET	PEAK	DURATION
PO	within 24 hr	unknown	unknown

Contraindications/Precautions

Contraindicated in: Hypersensitivity; Known/suspected/history of GI obstruction; Severe hepatic impairment; Concurrent use of strong CYP3A4 inhibitors, strong CYP3A4 inducers, or other opioid antagonists; Severe hepatic impairment; Lactation: May precipitate opioid withdrawal in infant.
Use Cautiously in: Patients with disruption of the blood-brain barrier (may precipitate opioid withdrawal); OB: Use only if potential maternal benefit justifies potential fetal risk (may precipitate fetal opioid withdrawal); Pedi: Safety and effectiveness not established; Geri: Blood levels are ↑ in elderly Japanese patients.

N

Adverse Reactions/Side Effects

CNS: headache. **Derm:** sweating. **GI:** GASTROINTESTINAL PERFORATION, abdominal pain, diarrhea, flatulence, nausea, vomiting. **Misc:** HYPERSENSITIVITY REACTIONS (including angioedema), opioid withdrawal.

Interactions

Drug-Drug: **Strong CYP3A4 inhibitors**, including **clarithromycin** and **ketoconazole** may ↑ risk of toxicity/adverse reactions; concurrent use contraindicated. **Strong CYP3A4 inducers**, including **rifampin**, may ↓ blood levels/effectiveness; concurrent use contraindicated. Other **opioid antagonists** may precipitate opioid withdrawal; concurrent use contraindicated. **Moderate CYP3A4 inhibitors**, including **diltiazem**, **erythromycin**, and **verapamil**, may ↑ risk of toxicity/adverse reactions; ↓ dose of methylnaltrexone. Concurrent use of **methadone** for pain ↑ risk of stomach pain and diarrhea.

Drug-Food: **Grapefruit/grapefruit juice** may ↑ blood levels and the risk of toxicity/adverse reactions; avoid concurrent use.

Route/Dosage

PO (Adults): 25 mg once daily; if poorly tolerated ↓ dose to 12.5 mg once daily; *Concurrent use of moderate CYP3A4 inhibitors*— 12.5 mg once daily (careful monitoring recommended).

Renal Impairment

PO (Adults): *CCr <60 mL/min*— 12.5 mg once daily initially; may cautiously ↑ to 25 mg once daily, if necessary, with careful monitoring.

Availability

Tablets: 12.5 mg, 25 mg.

NURSING IMPLICATIONS

Assessment

- Assess bowel sounds and frequency, quantity, and consistency of stools periodically during therapy.
- Monitor pain intensity during therapy. Naloxegol does not affect pain or effects of opioid analgesics on pain control. Discontinue naloxegol if opioid analgesic is discontinued.
- Monitor for signs and symptoms of gastrointestinal perforation (severe, persistent or worsening abdominal pain) periodically during therapy. Discontinue naloxegol if symptoms occur.

Implementation

- Discontinue all maintenance laxative therapy before starting naloxegol. If a suboptimal response occurs with naloxegol, laxatives may be used after 3 days.
- **PO:** Administer on an empty stomach at least 1 hr before first meal in morning or 2 hrs after meal. Tablet may be crushed to a powder, mixed with 4 oz of water (120 mL) for patients with difficulty swallowing. Drink mixture immediately; refill glass with 120 mL water, stir and drink contents.
- May be administered by NG tube. Flush the NG tube with 1 oz (30 mL) of water using a 60 mL syringe. Crush tablet to a powder and mix with 2 oz (60 mL) of water. Draw up mixture using the 60 mL syringe and administer through the NG tube. Add 2 oz (60 mL) of water to rinse container and administer to flush NG tube and any remaining medicine from NG tube into stomach.
- Avoid grapefruit and grapefruit juice during therapy.

Patient/Family Teaching

- Instruct patient to take naloxegol on an empty stomach as directed. Laxatives should be stopped before starting naloxegol, but may be restarted after 3 days if needed. Advise patient to read the *Medication Guide* prior to starting therapy and with each Rx refill in case of changes.
- Caution patient to avoid grapefruit and grapefruit juice during therapy.
- Advise patient to notify health care professional immediately if stomach pain that does not go away occurs.
- Advise patient to notify health care professional if signs and symptoms of opioid withdrawal (sweating, chills, diarrhea, stomach pain, anxiety, irritability, yawning) occur. Patients taking methadone for pain are at increased risk for stomach pain and diarrhea.
- Instruct patient to stop taking naloxegol if they stop taking opioid medications.
- Instruct patient to notify health care professional of all Rx or OTC medications, vitamins, or herbal products being taken and consult health care professional before taking any new medications.
- Advise female patients to notify health care professional if pregnancy is planned or suspected and avoid breast feeding during therapy; may cause opioid withdrawal in infant.

Evaluation/Desired Outcomes

- Relief of OIC, especially if opioid therapy has been for 4 wk or more.

naloxone (nal-ox-one)

Evzio, Narcan

Classification

Therapeutic: antidotes (for opioids)
Pharmacologic: opioid antagonists

Indications

Reversal of CNS depression and respiratory depression because of suspected opioid overdose. **Unlabeled Use:** Opioid-induced pruritus (low-dose IV infusion). Management of refractory circulatory shock.

Action

Competitively blocks the effects of opioids, including CNS and respiratory depression, without producing any agonist (opioid-like) effects. **Therapeutic Effects:** Reversal of signs of opioid excess.

Pharmacokinetics

Absorption: Well absorbed after IM or subcut administration. Rapidly absorbed from nasal mucosa.
Distribution: Rapidly distributed to tissues. Crosses the placenta.
Metabolism and Excretion: Metabolized by the liver.
Half-life: 30–90 min (IM, IV, subcut) (up to 3 hr in neonates); 2 hr (intranasal).

TIME/ACTION PROFILE (reversal of opioid effects)

ROUTE	ONSET	PEAK	DURATION
IV	1–2 min	unknown	45 min
IM, Subcut	2–5 min	unknown	>45 min
Intranasal	8–13 min	unknown	unknown

Contraindications/Precautions

Contraindicated in: Hypersensitivity.
Use Cautiously in: Cardiovascular disease; Patients physically dependent on opioids (may precipitate severe withdrawal); OB: May cause acute withdrawal syndrome in mother and fetus if mother is opioid dependent; Lactation: Safety not established; Pedi: May cause acute withdrawal syndrome in neonates of opioid-dependent mothers.

Adverse Reactions/Side Effects

CV: VENTRICULAR ARRHYTHMIAS, hypertension, hypotension. **GI:** nausea, vomiting.

Interactions

Drug-Drug: Can precipitate withdrawal in patients physically dependent on **opioid analgesics**. Larger doses may be required to reverse the effects of **buprenorphine**, **butorphanol**, or **nalbuphine**. Antagonizes postoperative **opioid analgesics**.

Route/Dosage

Postoperative Opioid-Induced Respiratory Depression

IV (Adults): 0.02–0.2 mg every 2–3 min until response obtained; repeat every 1–2 hr if needed.
IV (Children): 0.01 mg/kg; may repeat every 2–3 min until response obtained. Additional doses may be given every 1–2 hr if needed.
IM, IV, Subcut (Neonates): 0.01 mg/kg; may repeat every 2–3 min until response obtained. Additional doses may be given every 1–2 hr if needed.

Opioid-Induced Respiratory Depression During Chronic (>1 wk) Opioid Use

IV, IM, Subcut (Adults >40 kg): 20–40 mcg (0.02–0.04 mg) given as small, frequent (every min) boluses or as an infusion titrated to improve respiratory function without reversing analgesia.
IV, IM, Subcut (Adults and Children <40 kg): 0.005–0.02 mg/dose given as small, frequent (every min) boluses or as an infusion titrated to improve respiratory function without reversing analgesia.

Overdose of Opioids

IV, IM, Subcut (Adults): *Patients not suspected of being opioid dependent*—0.4 mg (10 mcg/kg); may repeat every 2–3 min (IV route is preferred). Some patients may require up to 2 mg. *Patients suspected to be opioid dependent*—Initial dose should be ↓ to 0.1–0.2 mg every 2–3 min. May also be given by IV infusion at rate adjusted to patient's response.
IM, Subcut (Adults and Children): *Evzio*—0.4 mg; may repeat every 2–3 min until emergency medical assistance arrives.
IV, IM, Subcut (Children >5 yr or >20 kg): 2 mg/dose, may repeat every 2–3 min.
IV, IM, Subcut (Infants up to 5 yr or 20 kg): 0.1 mg/kg, may repeat every 2–3 min.
Intranasal (Adults and Children): 1 spray (2 mg or 4 mg) in one nostril; may repeat dose every 2–3 min (with each subsequent dose being administered in alternate nostril).

Opioid-Induced Pruritus

IV (Children): 2 mcg/kg/hr continuous infusion, may ↑ by 0.5 mcg/kg/hr every few hrs if pruritus continues.

Availability (generic available)

Nasal spray: 4 mg/0.1 mL. **Solution for injection:** 0.4 mg/mL, 2 mg/0.4 mL (auto-injector), 2 mg/2 mL (prefilled syringe), 4 mg/10 mL. ***In combination with:*** buprenorphine (Suboxone, Zubsolv). See Appendix B.

NURSING IMPLICATIONS

Assessment

- Monitor respiratory rate, rhythm, and depth; pulse, ECG, BP; and level of consciousness frequently for 3–4 hr after the expected peak of blood concentrations. After a moderate overdose of a short half-life opioid, physical stimulation may be enough to prevent significant hypoventilation. The effects of some opioids may last longer than the effects of naloxone, and repeat doses may be necessary.
- Patients who have been receiving opioids for >1 wk are extremely sensitive to the effects of naloxone. Dilute and administer in slow increments.
- Assess patient for level of pain after administration when used to treat postoperative respiratory depression. Naloxone decreases respiratory depression but also reverses analgesia.
- Assess patient for signs and symptoms of opioid withdrawal (vomiting, restlessness, abdominal cramps, increased BP, and temperature). Symptoms

N

may occur within a few min to 2 hr. Severity depends on dose of naloxone, the opioid involved, and degree of physical dependence.

- Lack of significant improvement indicates that symptoms are caused by a disease process or other non-opioid CNS depressants not affected by naloxone.
- ***Toxicity and Overdose:*** Naloxone is a pure antagonist with no agonist properties and minimal toxicity.

Implementation

- Do not confuse naloxone with Lanoxin (digoxin) or nalbuphine. Do not confuse Narcan (naloxone) with Norcuron (vecuronium).
- Larger doses of naloxone may be necessary when used to antagonize the effects of buprenorphine, butorphanol, and nalbuphine.
- Resuscitation equipment, oxygen, vasopressors, and mechanical ventilation should be available to supplement naloxone therapy as needed.
- Doses should be titrated carefully in postoperative patients to avoid interference with control of postoperative pain.
- **Evzio:** A take-home naloxone auto-injector that patients, family members, and other caregivers can have close by in case an opioid overdose occurs. Has visual and voice instructions.
- Inject into upper outer thigh.
- **Intranasal:** Administer a single spray into 1 nostril. If patient does not respond or responds and relapses into respiratory depression, additional doses may be given every 2–3 min in alternating nostrils until emergency medical assistance arrives. Naloxone is not a substitute for emergency medical care.

IV Administration

- **IV Push:** ***Diluent:*** Administer undiluted for *suspected opioid overdose*. For *opioid-induced respiratory depression*, dilute with sterile water for injection. For children or adults weighing <40 kg, dilute 0.1 mg of naloxone in 10 mL of sterile water or 0.9% NaCl for injection. ***Concentration:*** 0.4 mg/mL, 1 mg/mL, or 10 mcg/mL (depending on preparation used). ***Rate:*** Administer over 30 sec for patients with a *suspected opioid overdose*. For patients who develop *opioid-induced respiratory depression*, administer dilute solution of 0.4 mg/10 mL at a rate of 0.5 mL (0.02 mg) IV push every 2 min. Titrate to avoid withdrawal and severe pain. Excessive dose in postoperative patients may cause excitement, pain, hypotension, hypertention, pulmonary edema, ventricular tachycardia and fibrillation, and seizures. For children and adults weighing <40 kg, administer 10 mcg/mL solution at a rate of 0.5 mcg/kg every 1–2 min.
- **Continuous Infusion:** ***Diluent:*** Dilute 2 mg of naloxone in 500 mL of 0.9% NaCl or D5W. Infusion is stable for 24 hr. ***Concentration:*** 4 mcg/mL. ***Rate:*** Titrate dose according to patient response.
- **Y-Site Compatibility:** alfentanil, amikacin, aminocaproic acid, amiodarone, anidulafungin, argatroban, ascorbic acid, atropine, azithromycin, aztreonam, benztropine, bivalirudin, bleomycin, bumetanide, buprenorphine, butorphanol, calcium chloride, calcium gluconate, carboplatin, carmustine, caspofungin, cefazolin, cefotaxime, cefotetan, cefoxitin, ceftazidime, ceftriaxone, cefuroxime, chloramphenicol, chlorpromazine, cisplatin, clindamycin, cyanocobalamin, cyclophosphamide, cyclosporine, cytarabine, dactinomycin, daptomycin, daunorubicin hydrochloride, desmopressin, dexamethasone, dexmedetomidine, dexrazoxane, digoxin, diltiazem, dimenhydrinate, diphenhydramine, dobutamine, docetaxel, dopamine, doxorubicin hydrochloride, doxorubicin liposomal, doxycycline, enalaprilat, ephedrine, epinephrine, epirubicin, epoetin alfa, eptifibatide, ertapenem, erythromycin, esmolol, etoposide, etoposide phosphate, famotidine, fenoldopam, fentanyl, fluconazole, fludarabine, fluorouracil, folic acid, foscarnet, fosphenytoin, furosemide, ganciclovir, gemcitabine, gentamicin, glycopyrrolate, granisetron, heparin, hetastarch, hydrocortisone, hydromorphone, idarubicin, ifosfamide, imipenem/cilastatin, indomethacin, insulin, irinotecan, isoproterenol, ketamine, ketorolac, labetalol, levofloxacin, lidocaine, linezolid, lorazepam, mannitol, meperidine, meropenem, mesna, methotrexate, methyldopate, methylprednisolone, metoclopramide, metoprolol, metronidazole, midazolam, milrinone, mitoxantrone, morphine, moxifloxacin, multivitamins, mycophenolate, nafcillin, nalbuphine, nitroglycerin, nitroprusside, norepinephrine, octreotide, ondansetron, oxacillin, oxaliplatin, oxytocin, paclitaxel, palonosetron, pamidronate, pancuronium, papaverine, pemetrexed, penicillin G, pentamidine, pentobarbital, phenobarbital, phentolamine, phenylephrine, phytonadione, piperacillin/tazobactam, potassium acetate, potassium chloride, procainamide, prochlorperazine, promethazine, propofol, propranolol, protamine, pyridoxine, quinupristin/dalfopristin, ranitidine, rocuronium, sodium acetate, sodium bicarbonate, streptokinase, succinylcholine, sufentanil, tacrolimus, theophylline, thiamine, tigecycline, tirofiban, tobramycin, topotecan, vancomycin, vasopressin, vecuronium, verapamil, vinblastine, vincristine, vinorelbine, voriconazole, zoledronic acid.
- **Y-Site Incompatibility:** alemtuzumab, amphotericin B lipid complex, amphotericin B liposome, dantrolene, diazepam, leucovorin, mitomycin, pantoprazole, phenytoin, thiotepa.
- **Additive Incompatibility:** Incompatible with preparations containing bisulfite, sulfite, and solutions with an alkaline pH.

Patient/Family Teaching

- As medication becomes effective, explain purpose and effects of naloxone to patient.

- **Intranasal:** Instruct parents and caregivers in the correct technique for use.
- **Evzio:** Explain purpose and instructions for use to caregiver. Advise to continue monitoring patient after injection and notify emergency medical assistance. Repeated doses may be required due to duration of naloxone.

Evaluation/Desired Outcomes

- Adequate ventilation following opioid excess.
- Alertness without significant pain or withdrawal symptoms.

BEERS

naproxen (na-prox-en)

Aleve, Anaprox, Anaprox DS, ✱Maxidol, EC-Naprosyn, Naprelan, Naprosyn

Classification

Therapeutic: nonopioid analgesics, nonsteroidal anti-inflammatory agents, antipyretics

Indications

Mild to moderate pain. Dysmenorrhea. Fever. Inflammatory disorders, including: Rheumatoid arthritis (adults and children), Osteoarthritis.

Action

Inhibits prostaglandin synthesis. **Therapeutic Effects:** Decreased pain. Reduction of fever. Suppression of inflammation.

Pharmacokinetics

Absorption: Completely absorbed from the GI tract. Sodium salt is more rapidly absorbed.
Distribution: Crosses the placenta; enters breast milk in low concentrations.
Protein Binding: >99%.
Metabolism and Excretion: Mostly metabolized by the liver.
Half-life: Children <8 yr: 8–17 hr; Children 8–14 yr: 8–10 hr; Adults: 10–20 hr.

TIME/ACTION PROFILE

ROUTE	ONSET	PEAK	DURATION
PO (analgesic)	1 hr	unknown	8–12 hr
PO (anti-inflammatory)	14 days	2–4 wk	unknown

Contraindications/Precautions

Contraindicated in: Hypersensitivity; Cross-sensitivity may occur with other NSAIDs, including aspirin; Active GI bleeding; Ulcer disease; Coronary artery bypass graft (CABG) surgery; Lactation: Passes into breast milk and should not be used by nursing mothers.
Use Cautiously in: Severe renal or hepatic impairment; Cardiovascular disease or risk factors for cardiovascular disease (may ↑ risk of serious cardiovascular thrombotic events, myocardial infarction, and stroke, especially with prolonged use or use of higher doses); avoid use in patients with recent MI or HF; History of ulcer disease or any other history of gastrointestinal bleeding (may ↑ risk of GI bleeding); Chronic alcohol use/abuse; OB: Avoid using during third trimester; may cause premature closure of the ductus arteriosus; Pedi: Children <2 yr (safety not established); Geri: ↑ risk of adverse reactions.

Adverse Reactions/Side Effects

CNS: dizziness, drowsiness, headache. **CV:** HF, MYOCARDIAL INFARCTION, STROKE, edema, hypertension, palpitations, tachycardia. **Derm:** STEVENS-JOHNSON SYNDROME, TOXIC EPIDERMAL NECROLYSIS, photosensitivity, rash, sweating, pseudoporphyria (12% incidence in children with juvenile rheumatoid arthritis—discontinue therapy if this occurs). **EENT:** tinnitus, visual disturbances. **F and E:** hyperkalemia. **GI:** DRUG-INDUCED HEPATITIS, GI BLEEDING, constipation, dyspepsia, nausea, anorexia, diarrhea, discomfort, flatulence, vomiting. **GU:** cystitis, hematuria, renal failure. **Hemat:** blood dyscrasias, prolonged bleeding time. **Resp:** dyspnea. **Misc:** HYPERSENSITIVITY REACTIONS (including anaphylaxis).

Interactions

Drug-Drug: May limit the cardioprotective (antiplatelet) effects of **aspirin**. ↑ risk of bleeding with **anticoagulants, aspirin, clopidogrel, ticagrelor, prasugrel, corticosteroids, fibrinolytics, SNRIs**, or **SSRIs**. Additive adverse GI side effects with **aspirin, corticosteroids, alcohol**, and other **NSAIDs**. **Probenecid** ↑ blood levels and may ↑ toxicity. May ↑ risk of toxicity from **methotrexate, antineoplastics**, or **radiation therapy**. May ↑ serum levels and risk of toxicity from **lithium**. ↑ risk of adverse renal effects with **cyclosporine, ACE inhibitors, angiotensin II antagonists**, or chronic use of **acetaminophen**. May ↓ response to **antihypertensives** or **diuretics**. May ↑ risk of hypoglycemia with **insulin** or **oral hypoglycemic agents**. **Oral potassium supplements** may ↑ GI adverse effects.
Drug-Natural Products: ↑ anticoagulant effect and bleeding risk with **anise, arnica, chamomile, clove, dong quai, feverfew, garlic, ginger, ginkgo, Panax ginseng, licorice**, and others.

Route/Dosage

275 mg naproxen sodium is equivalent to 250 mg naproxen.

N

Anti-Inflammatory/Analgesic/Antidysmenorrheal

PO (Adults): *Naproxen*—250–500 mg twice daily (up to 1.5 g/day). *Delayed-release naproxen*—375–500 mg twice daily. *Naproxen sodium*—275–550 mg twice daily (up to 1.65 g/day).

PO (Children >2 yr): *Analgesia:* 5–7 mg/kg/dose every 8–12 hr. *Inflammatory disease:* 10–15 mg/kg/day divided every 12 hr, maximum: 1000 mg/day.

Antigout

PO (Adults): *Naproxen*—750 mg naproxen initially, then 250 mg every 8 hr. *Naproxen sodium*—825 mg initially, then 275 mg every 8 hr.

OTC Use (naproxen sodium)

PO (Adults): 200 mg every 8–12 hr or 400 mg followed by 200 mg every 12 hr (not to exceed 600 mg/24 hr).

PO (Geriatric Patients >65 yr): Not to exceed 200 mg every 12 hr.

Availability

Naproxen (generic available)

Delayed-release tablets (EC-Naprosyn): 375 mg, 500 mg. **Extended-release tablets:** 🍁 750 mg. **Oral suspension (Naprosyn):** 125 mg/5 mL. **Rectal suppositories:** 🍁 500 mg. **Tablets (Naprosyn):** 🍁 125 mg, 250 mg, 375 mg, 500 mg. ***In combination with:*** esomeprazole (Vimovo).

Naproxen Sodium (generic available)

Capsules (Maxidol): 🍁 220 mg^{OTC}. **Extended-release tablets (Naprelan):** 375 mg, 500 mg, 750 mg. **Tablets (Aleve, Anaprox, Anaprox DS):** 220 mg^{OTC}, 275 mg, 550 mg. ***In combination with:*** pseudoephedrine (Aleve-D Sinus and Cold), sumatriptan (Treximet). See Appendix B.

NURSING IMPLICATIONS

Assessment

- Patients who have asthma, aspirin-induced allergy, and nasal polyps are at increased risk for developing hypersensitivity reactions. Assess for rhinitis, asthma, and urticaria.
- Monitor BP during initiation and periodically during therapy. May cause fluid retention and edema leading to new onset or worsening hypertension.
- Assess for rash periodically during therapy. May cause Stevens-Johnson syndrome. Discontinue therapy if severe or if accompanied with fever, general malaise, fatigue, muscle or joint aches, blisters, oral lesions, conjunctivitis, hepatitis and/or eosinophilia.
- **Pain:** Assess pain (note type, location, and intensity) prior to and 1–2 hr following administration.
- **Arthritis:** Assess pain and range of motion prior to and 1–2 hr following administration.
- **Fever:** Monitor temperature; note signs associated with fever (diaphoresis, tachycardia, malaise).
- ***Lab Test Considerations:*** Evaluate BUN, serum creatinine, CBC, and liver function tests periodically in patients receiving prolonged therapy.
- May ↑ serum potassium, BUN, serum creatinine, alkaline phosphatase, LDH, AST, and ALT tests levels. May ↓ blood glucose, hemoglobin, and hematocrit concentrations, leukocyte and platelet counts, and CCr.
- Bleeding time may be prolonged up to 4 days following discontinuation of therapy.
- May alter test results for urine 5-HIAA and urine steroid determinations.

Implementation

- Administration in higher than recommended doses does not provide increased effectiveness but may cause increased side effects. Use lowest effective dose for the shortest duration possible to minimize risk of cardiovascular thrombotic events.
- Coadministration with opioid analgesics may have additive analgesic effects and may permit lower opioid doses.
- Analgesic is more effective if given before pain becomes severe.
- **PO:** For rapid initial effect, administer 30 min before or 2 hr after meals. May be administered with food, milk, or antacids to decrease GI irritation. Food slows but does not reduce the extent of absorption. Do not mix suspension with antacid or other liquid prior to administration. Swallow extended-release, delayed-release, and controlled-release tablets whole; do not break, crush, or chew.
- **Dysmenorrhea:** Administer as soon as possible after the onset of menses. Prophylactic treatment has not been shown to be effective.

Patient/Family Teaching

- Instruct patient to take medication as directed. Take missed doses as soon as remembered but not if almost time for the next dose. Do not double doses.
- Advise patient to take this medication with a full glass of water and to remain in an upright position for 15–30 min after administration.
- May cause drowsiness or dizziness. Advise patient to avoid driving or other activities requiring alertness until response to the medication is known.
- Caution patient to avoid the concurrent use of alcohol, aspirin, acetaminophen, or other OTC medications without consulting health care professional. Use of naproxen with 3 or more glasses of alcohol per day may increase risk of GI bleeding.
- Advise patient to inform health care professional of medication regimen prior to treatment or surgery.
- Caution patient to wear sunscreen and protective clothing to prevent photosensitivity reactions (especially in children with JRA).
- Instruct patients not to take OTC naproxen preparations for more than 3 days for fever and to consult health care professional if symptoms persist or worsen.

- Advise patient to consult health care professional if rash, itching, visual disturbances, tinnitus, weight gain, edema, black stools, persistent headache, or influenza-like syndrome (chills, fever, muscle aches, pain) occurs.
- Rep: Advise females of reproductive potential to notify health care professional if pregnancy is planned or suspected and to avoid naproxen starting at 30 wk gestation because of risk of premature closing of the fetal ductus arteriosus. May cause infertility in men and temporary infertility in women.

Evaluation/Desired Outcomes

- Relief of pain.
- Improved joint mobility. Partial arthritic relief is usually seen within 2 wk, but maximum effectiveness may require 2–4 wk of continuous therapy. Patients who do not respond to one NSAID may respond to another.
- Reduction of fever.

naratriptan (nar-a-trip-tan)

Amerge

Classification

Therapeutic: vascular headache suppressants

Pharmacologic: 5-HT_1 agonists

Indications

Acute treatment of migraine headache.

Action

Acts as an agonist at specific 5-HT_1 receptor sites in intracranial blood vessels and sensory trigeminal nerves. **Therapeutic Effects:** Cranial vessel vasoconstriction with resultant decrease in migraine headache.

Pharmacokinetics

Absorption: Well absorbed (70%) following oral administration.

Distribution: Unknown.

Metabolism and Excretion: 60% excreted unchanged in urine; 30% metabolized by the liver.

Half-life: 6 hr (↑ in renal impairment).

TIME/ACTION PROFILE (↓ migraine pain)

ROUTE	ONSET	PEAK	DURATION
PO	30–60 min	2–3 hr†	up to 24 hr

†3–4 hr during migraine attack.

Contraindications/Precautions

Contraindicated in: Hypersensitivity; Ischemic heart disease or Prinzmetal's angina; Uncontrolled hypertension; Wolff-Parkinson-White syndrome, or other arrhythmias involving conduction pathways; Hemiplegic or basilar migraine; Stroke or transient ischemic attack; Peripheral vascular disease; Ischemic bowel disease; Severe renal impairment (CCr <15 mL/min); Severe hepatic impairment; Should not be used within 24 hr of other 5-HT_1 agonists or ergot-type compounds (dihydroergotamine); Geri: Age-related ↓ in renal function and ↑ likelihood of CAD greatly ↑ risk of fatal adverse events.

Use Cautiously in: Mild to moderate renal or hepatic impairment (dose should not exceed 2.5 mg/24 hr; initial dose should be ↓); OB, Lactation, Pedi: Safety not established.

Exercise Extreme Caution in: Cardiovascular risk factors (hypertension, hypercholesterolemia, cigarette smoking, obesity, diabetes, strong family history, menopausal women or men >40 yr); use only if cardiovascular status has been evaluated and determined to be safe and 1st dose is administered under supervision.

Adverse Reactions/Side Effects

CNS: dizziness, drowsiness, malaise/fatigue. **CV:** CORONARY ARTERY VASOSPASM, MI, VENTRICULAR FIBRILLATION, VENTRICULAR TACHYCARDIA, myocardial ischemia. **GI:** nausea. **Neuro:** paresthesia. **Misc:** pain/pressure sensation in throat/neck.

N

Interactions

Drug-Drug: ↑ risk of serotonin syndrome when used with **SSRI or SNRI antidepressants**. **Cigarette smoking** ↑ the metabolism of naratriptan. Blood levels and effects are ↑ by **hormonal contraceptives**. Avoid concurrent use (within 24 hr of each other) with **ergot-containing drugs (dihydroergotamine)** may result in prolonged vasospastic reactions. Avoid concurrent (within 2 wk) use with **MAO inhibitors**; produces ↑ systemic exposure and risk of adverse reactions to naratriptan.

Drug-Natural Products: ↑ risk of serotinergic side effects including serotonin syndrome with **St. John's wort** and **SAMe**.

Route/Dosage

PO (Adults): 1 or 2.5 mg; dose may be repeated in 4 hr if response is inadequate (not to exceed 5 mg/24 hr or treatment of more than 4 headaches/mo).

Availability (generic available)

Tablets: 1 mg, 2.5 mg.

NURSING IMPLICATIONS

Assessment

- Assess pain location, character, intensity, and duration and associated symptoms (photophobia, phonophobia, nausea, vomiting) during migraine attack.
- Monitor for serotonin syndrome in patients taking SSRIs or SNRIs concurrently with naratriptan.

Implementation

- **PO:** Tablets may be administered at any time after the headache starts.

Patient/Family Teaching

- Inform patient that naratriptan should be used only during a migraine attack. It is meant to be used for relief of migraine attacks but not to prevent or reduce the number of attacks.
- Instruct patient to administer naratriptan as soon as symptoms of a migraine attack appear, but it may be administered any time during an attack. If migraine symptoms return, a 2nd dose may be used. Allow at least 4 hr between doses, and do not use more than 2 tablets in any 24-hr period. Do not use to treat more than 4 headaches per mo.
- Advise patient that lying down in a darkened room following naratriptan administration may further help relieve headache.
- Advise patient that overuse (use more than 10 days/mo) may lead to exacerbation of headache (migraine-like daily headaches, or as a marked increase in frequency of migraine attacks). May require gradual withdrawal of naratriptan and treatment of symptoms (transient worsening of headache).
- Advise patient to notify health care professional prior to next dose of naratriptan if pain or tightness in the chest occurs during use. If pain is severe or does not subside, notify health care professional immediately. If wheezing; heart throbbing; swelling of eyelids, face, or lips; skin rash; skin lumps; or hives occur, notify health care professional immediately and do not take more naratriptan without approval of health care professional. If feelings of tingling, heat, flushing, heaviness, pressure, drowsiness, dizziness, tiredness, or sickness develop, discuss with health care professional at next visit.
- Instruct patient not to take additional naratriptan if no response is seen with initial dose without consulting health care professional. There is no evidence that 5 mg provides greater relief than 2.5-mg dose. Additional naratriptan doses are not likely to be effective, and alternative medications, as previously discussed with health care professional, may be used.
- Naratriptan may cause dizziness or drowsiness. Caution patient to avoid driving or other activities requiring alertness until response to medication is known.
- Advise patient to avoid alcohol, which aggravates headaches, during naratriptan use.
- Advise patient to notify health care professional of all Rx or OTC medications, vitamins, or herbal products being taken and to consult with health care professional before taking other medications. Patients concurrently taking SSRI or SNRI antidepressants should notify health care professional promptly if signs of serotonin syndrome (mental status changes: agitation, hallucinations, coma; autonomic instability: tachycardia, labile BP, hyperthermia; neuromuscular aberrations: hyperreflexia, incoordination; and/or gastrointestinal symptoms: nausea, vomiting, diarrhea) occur.
- Caution patient not to use naratriptan if pregnancy is planned or suspected or if breast feeding. Adequate contraception should be used during therapy.

Evaluation/Desired Outcomes

- Relief of migraine attack.

nebivolol (ne-**bi**-vi-lole)

Bystolic

Classification

Therapeutic: antihypertensives

Pharmacologic: beta blockers (selective)

Indications

Hypertension (alone and with other antihypertensives).

Action

Blocks stimulation of beta adrenergic receptor sites; selective for $beta_1$ (myocardial) receptors in most patients. In some patients (poor metabolizers, higher blood levels may result in some $beta_2$ [pulmonary, vascular, uterine] adrenergic) blockade. **Therapeutic Effects:** Lowering of BP.

Pharmacokinetics

Absorption: Well absorbed following oral administration.

Distribution: Unknown.

Protein Binding: 98%.

Metabolism and Excretion: Mostly metabolized by the liver, including the CYP2D6 enzyme system; some have antihypertensive action; minimal excretion of unchanged drug.

Half-life: *Extensive metabolizers*— 12 hr; *poor metabolizers*— 19 hr.

TIME/ACTION PROFILE (blood levels)

ROUTE	ONSET	PEAK	DURATION
PO	unknown	1.5–4 hr	24 hr

Contraindications/Precautions

Contraindicated in: Hypersensitivity; Severe bradycardia, heart block greater than first degree cardiogenic shock, decompensated heart failure, or sick sinus syndrome (without pacemaker); Severe hepatic impairment (Child-Pugh >B); Bronchospastic disease; OB: Lactation.

Use Cautiously in: Coronary artery disease (rapid cessation should be avoided); Compensated HF; Major surgery (anesthesia may augment myocardial depression); Diabetes mellitus (may mask signs of hypoglycemia); Thyrotoxicosis (may mask symptoms); Moderate hepatic impairment (↓ metabolism); Severe renal impairment (↓ initial dose if CCr <30 mL/min); History of severe allergic reactions (↑ intensity of reactions); Pheochromocytoma (alpha blockers required prior to beta blockers); Geri: Consider increased sensitivity, concurrent chronic diseases, medications and presence of age-related decrease in clearance; OB: Use in pregnancy only if maternal benefit outweighs fetal risk; Pedi: Safe use in children <18 yr not established.

Adverse Reactions/Side Effects

CNS: dizziness, fatigue, headache.

Interactions

Drug-Drug: Drugs that affect the CYP2D6 enzyme system are expected to alter levels and possibly effects of nebivolol; dose alterations may be required. **Fluoxetine**, a known inhibitor of CYP2D6, ↑ levels and effects; similar effects may be expected from **quinidine**, **propafenone**, and **paroxetine**. Blood levels are also ↑ by **cimetine**. **Anesthetic agents** including **ether**, **trichloroethylene**, and **cyclopropane** as well as **other myocardial depressants** or **inhibitors of AV conduction**, such as **diltiazem** and **verapamil**, may ↑ risk of myocardial depression and bradycardia. Avoid concurrent use with **beta blockers**. If used concurrently with **clonidine**, nebivolol should be tapered and discontinued several days prior to gradual withdrawal of clonidine.

Route/Dosage

PO (Adults): 5 mg once daily initially, may increase at 2 wk intervals up to 40 mg/day.

Hepatic/Renal Impairment

PO (Adults): 2.5 mg once daily initially; titrate upward cautiously.

Availability

Tablets: 2.5, 5 mg, 10 mg.

NURSING IMPLICATIONS

Assessment

- Monitor BP, ECG, and pulse prior to and periodically during therapy.
- Monitor intake and output ratios and daily weights. Assess routinely for signs and symptoms of HF (dyspnea, rales/crackles, weight gain, peripheral edema, jugular venous distention).
- ***Lab Test Considerations:*** May cause ↑ BUN, uric acid, triglycerides and ↓ HDL cholesterol and platelet count.

Implementation

- **PO:** May be administered without regard to food.
- When discontinuation is planned, observe patient carefully and advise to minimize physical activity. Taper over 1–2 wk when possible. If angina worsens or acute coronary insufficiency develops, reinstitute nebivolol promptly, at least temporarily.

Patient/Family Teaching

- Instruct patient to take nebivolol as directed, at the same time each day, even if feeling well. If a dose is missed, skip missed dose and take next scheduled dose; do not double doses. Do not discontinue without consulting health care professional. Abrupt withdrawal may precipitate life-threatening arrhythmias, hypertension, or myocardial ischemia.
- Advise patient to ensure that enough medication is available for weekends, holidays, and vacations. A written prescription may be kept in the wallet for emergencies.
- Reinforce the need to continue additional therapies for hypertension (weight loss, sodium restriction, stress reduction, regular exercise, moderation of alcohol consumption, and smoking cessation). Medication controls but does not cure hypertension.
- Teach patient and family how to check pulse and BP. Instruct them to check pulse daily and BP biweekly and to report significant changes to health care professional.
- Instruct patient to consult health care professional before taking any Rx, OTC, or herbal products, especially cold preparations, concurrently with this medication. Patients on antihypertensive therapy should also avoid excessive amounts of coffee, tea, and cola.
- May mask some signs of hypoglycemia, especially tachycardia. Diabetics should closely monitor blood sugar, especially if weakness, malaise, irritability, or fatigue occurs. Medication does not block dizziness or sweating as signs of hypoglycemia.
- May cause dizziness. Caution patients to avoid driving or other activities requiring alertness until response to medication is known.
- Advise patient to notify health care professional if difficulty breathing or signs and symptoms of worsening HF (weight gain, increasing shortness of breath, excessive bradycardia) occur.
- Instruct patient to inform health care professional of medication regimen before treatment or surgery.
- Advise patient to carry identification describing disease process and medication regimen at all times.
- Advise female patients that breast feeding should be avoided during nebivolol therapy.

Evaluation/Desired Outcomes

- Decrease in BP.

neomycin, See AMINOGLYCOSIDES.

🧬 neratinib (ne-ra-ti-nib)

Nerlynx

Classification

Therapeutic: antineoplastics

Pharmacologic: enzyme inhibitors, kinase inhibitors

Indications

Extended adjuvant treatment of early stage Human Epidermal Receptor Type 2 (HER2)-overexpressed/amplified breast cancer following adjuvant trastuzumab-based therapy.

Action

Irreversibly binds to Epidermal Growth Factor Receptor (EGFR), HER2, and HER4 to inhibit growth of tumors that express HER2 and EGFR. **Therapeutic Effects:** Decreased progression of breast cancer and improved survival.

Pharmacokinetics

Absorption: Blood levels ↑ by high-fat foods.
Distribution: Extensively distributed to tissues.
Protein Binding: >99%.
Metabolism and Excretion: Primarily metabolized in liver via CYP3A4 into active metabolites (M3, M6, M7, and M11); 97% excreted in feces, <2% excreted by kidneys.
Half-life: 7–17 hr.

TIME/ACTION PROFILE (blood levels)

ROUTE	ONSET	PEAK	DURATION
PO	unknown	2–8 hr	24 hr

Contraindications/Precautions

Contraindicated in: OB: May cause fetal harm; Lactation: Avoid breast feeding.
Use Cautiously in: Severe hepatic impairment (Child-Pugh C) (↓ dose); Rep: Women of reproductive potential and men with female partners of reproductive potential; Geri: ↑ risk of adverse reactions/side effects; Pedi: Safety and effectiveness not established.

Adverse Reactions/Side Effects

CNS: fatigue. **CV:** hypotension. **Derm:** rash, dry skin, nail disorder. **EENT:** epistaxis. **GI:** DIARRHEA, HEPATOTOXICITY, abdominal pain, ↓ appetite, dyspepsia, nausea, stomatitis, vomiting, abdominal distention, dry mouth. **GU:** renal failure, urinary tract infection. **Metab:** ↓ weight. **MS:** muscle spasms.

Interactions

Drug-Drug: ↓ levels with **proton pump inhibitors**, **H_2 blockers**, and **antacids**; avoid concurrent use with **proton pump inhibitors**; take ≥2 hr before next dose of **H_2 antagonist** or 10 hr after the **H_2 antagonist**; take 3 hr after **antacids**. **Strong or moderate CYP3A4 inhibitors**, including **aprepitant**, **cimetidine**, **ciprofloxacin**, **clarithromycin**, **clotrimazole**, **cobicistat**, **conivaptan**, **crizotinib**, **cyclosporine**, **diltiazem**, **dronedarone**, **erythromycin**, **fluconazole**, **fluvoxamine**, **idelalisib**, **imatinib**, **indinavir**, **itraconazole**, **ketoconazole**, **lopinavir**, **nefazodone**, **nelfinavir**, **posaconazole**, **ritonavir**, **saquinavir**, **tipranavir**, **verapamil**, and **voriconazole** may ↑ levels/toxicity of neratinib; avoid concurrent use. **Strong or moderate CYP3A4 inducers**, including **bosentan**, **carbamazepine**, **efavirenz**, **enzalutamide**, **mitotane**, **modafanil**, **phenytoin**, and **rifampin** may ↓ levels of neratinib and its effectiveness; avoid concurrent use. May ↑ **digoxin** levels.
Drug-Natural Products: St. John's wort may ↓ levels of neratinib and its effectiveness; avoid concurrent use.

Route/Dosage

PO (Adults): 240 mg once daily for 1 yr.

Hepatic Impairment

PO (Adults): *Severe hepatic impairment (Child-Pugh C)*—80 mg once daily for 1 yr.

Availability

Tablets: 40 mg.

NURSING IMPLICATIONS

Assessment

- Monitor for diarrhea. Use antidiarrheal prophylaxis with first dose and for first 2 cycles (56 days). *If Grade 1 diarrhea (increase of < 4 stools per day over baseline), Grade 2 diarrhea (increase of 4-6 stools per day over baseline) lasting < 5 days, Grade 3 diarrhea (increase of ≥ 7 stools per day over baseline; incontinence; hospitalization indicated; limiting self-care activities of daily living) lasting < 2 days occurs,* modify antidiarrheal therapy, modify diet, and maintain fluid intake of 2L to avoid dehydration. Once event resolves to ≤ Grade 1 or baseline, start loperamide 4 mg with each subsequent neratinib administration. *If any grade diarrhea with dehydration, fever, hypotension, renal failure, neutropenia, Grade 2 diarrhea lasting ≥ 5 days, Grade 3 diarrhea lasting >2 days despite medical therapy occurs,* hold therapy, modify diet, and maintain fluid intake of 2L to avoid dehydration. If diarrhea resolves to Grade 0-1 in ≤1 wk, resume therapy at same dose. If diarrhea resolves to Grade 0-1 in >1 wk, resume therapy at reduced dose. Once diarrhea resolves to ≤Grade 1 or baseline, start loperamide 4 mg with each subsequent neratinib administration. *If Grade 4 diarrhea (Life-threatening consequences; urgent intervention indicated) occurs,* permanently discontinue neratinib. *If diarrhea recurs to ≥Grade 2 at 120 mg neratinib per day,* permanently discontine neratinib. Obtain stool cultures to determine infectious causes of Grade 3 or 4 or with dehydration, fever, or neutropenia.
- Monitor or signs and symptoms of hepatotoxicity (worsening of fatigue, nausea, vomiting, right upper quadrant tenderness, fever, rash, eosinophilia, Grade 3 diarrhea) periodically during therapy. If symptoms occur, obtain liver function test levels to measure changes.
- ***Lab Test Considerations:*** Verify negative pregnancy test in women of reproductive potential before starting therapy.

- Monitor total bilirubin, AST, ALT, and alkaline phosphatase before starting therapy, monthly for first 3 mo, and every 3 mo during therapy. If evaluating hepatotoxicity, also obtain fractionated bilirubin and prothrombin time. *If Grade 3 ALT (>5–20 × upper limit of normal (ULN)) or Grade 3 bilirubin (>3–10 × ULN),* withhold dose until recovery to ≤ Grade 1, evaluate alternative causes, resume neratinib at next lower dose if recovery to ≤Grade 1 occurs within 3 wk. If Grade 3 ALT or bilirubin occurs again despite one dose reduction, permanently discontinue neratinib. If Grade 4 ALT (>20 × ULN) or Grade 4 bilirubin (>10 × ULN), discontinue neratinib permanently and evaluate alternative causes.

Implementation

- Do not confuse neratinib with nilotinib or niraparib.
- **PO:** Administer once daily, at same time each day, with food, continuously for 1 yr. Swallow tablets whole; do not crush, break, or chew.

Patient/Family Teaching

- Instruct patient to take neratinib as directed. If dose is missed, omit and take next scheduled dose next day. Advise patient to read *Patient Information* before starting therapy and with each Rx refill in case of changes.
- Advise patient to avoid taking grapefruit or grapefruit juice during therapy.
- Instruct patient to take loperamide according to schedule and titrate to 1–2 bowel movements/day: *For days 1–14 (wk 1–2),* take 4 mg three times daily. *Days 15–56 (wk 3–8),* take 4 mg twice daily. *Days 57–365 (wk 9–52),* take 4 mg as needed up to 16 mg/day. May require additional antidiarrheal agents and dose reduction.
- Caution patient to avoid proton pump inhibitors and H_2 antagonists during therapy and to avoid taking antacids within 3 hrs of neratinib.
- Instruct patient to notify health care professional of all Rx or OTC medications, vitamins, or herbal products being taken and consult health care professional before taking any new medications, especially St. John's wort.
- Advise patient to notify health care professional immediately if severe (≥ Grade 3) diarrhea or diarrhea associated with weakness, dizziness, or fever or if signs and symptoms of liver dysfunction occur.
- Rep: May be teratogenic. Advise female patients of reproductive potential to use effective contraception and avoid breast feeding during and for at least 1 mo after last dose. Advise male patients with partners of reproductive potential to use effective contraception during and for 3 mo after last dose.

Evaluation/Desired Outcomes

- Decreased progression of breast cancer.

netupitant/palonosetron (oral)

(ne-**too**-pi-tant/pa-lone-**o**-se-tron)
Akynzeo

fosnetupitant/palonosetron (injection)

(fos-ne-**too**-pi-tant/pa-lone-**o**-se-tron)
Akynzeo

Classification
Therapeutic: antiemetics
Pharmacologic: neurokinin antagonists, 5-HT_3 antagonists

Indications

PO: Prevention of acute and delayed nausea and vomiting associated with initial and repeat courses of cancer chemotherapy, including, but not limited to highly emetogenic chemotherapy (in combination with dexamethasone). **IV:** Prevention of acute and delayed nausea and vomiting associated with initial and repeat courses of highly emetogenic chemotherapy (in combination with dexamethasone).

Action

Netupitant—Acts as a selective antagonist at substance P/neurokinin 1 (NK1) receptors in the CNS; prevents nausea and vomiting in the acute and delayed phases after chemotherapy. *Palonosetron*—Blocks the effects of serotonin at receptor sites (selective antagonist) located in vagal nerve terminals and in the chemoreceptor trigger zones in the CNS; prevents nausea and vomiting in the acute phase. **Therapeutic Effects:** Decreased incidence and severity of nausea and vomiting following emetogenic chemotherapy.

Pharmacokinetics

Absorption: *Netupitant*—Extent of absorption following oral administration unknown; *Fosnetupitant*—Following IV administration, fosnetupitant is rapidly converted to netupitant, the active component. IV administration results in complete bioavailability; *Palonosetron*—97% absorbed following oral administration.
Distribution: *Netupitant, fosnetupitant, and palonosetron*—Extensively distributed to tissues.
Protein Binding: *Netupitant*—>99.5%; *Fosnetupitant*—92–95%.
Metabolism and Excretion: *Netupitant*—Primarily metabolized in the liver (mostly by CYP3A4, and to a lesser extent by CYP2C9 and CYP2D6) to three metabolites that have anti-emetic activity; <1% excreted unchanged in urine; *Palonosetron*—50% metabolized (mostly by CYP2D6, and to a lesser extent by CYP3A4 and CYP1A2); 40% excreted unchanged in urine.

N

Half-life: *Netupitant*—80 hr; *Palonosetron*—40 hr.

TIME/ACTION PROFILE (plasma concentrations)

ROUTE	ONSET	PEAK	DURATION
PO	within 1 hr	5 hr	unknown
IV	rapid	30 min	unknown

Contraindications/Precautions

Contraindicated in: Cross-sensitivity may occur with other 5–HT_3 antagonists; Severe hepatic or renal impairment.

Use Cautiously in: Geri: Consider age-related ↓ in renal, hepatic and cardiac function, concurrent disease states and drug therapies; OB: Use only if potential benefit justifies potential risk to fetus; Lactation: Use only if potential benefit justifies potential risk to infant; Pedi: Safety and effectiveness not established.

Adverse Reactions/Side Effects

CNS: fatigue, headache, weakness. **Derm:** erythema. **GI:** constipation, dyspepsia. **Misc:** HYPERSENSITIVITY REACTIONS (including anaphylaxis), SEROTONIN SYNDROME.

Interactions

Drug-Drug: Netupitant is a moderate inhibitor of CYP3A4 and can ↑ levels of drugs that are **CYP3A4 substrates**, including **alprazolam**, **cyclophosphamide**, **dexamethasone**, **docetaxel**, **etoposide**, **ifosfamide**, **imatinib**, **irinotecan**, **midazolam**, **erythromycin**, **paclitaxel**, **triazolam**, **vinorelbine**, **vinblastine**, and **vincristine**; avoid concomitant use for one wk; if avoiding use not feasible, ↓ dose of CYP3A4 substrate. **CYP3A4 inducers** including **rifampin** may ↓ netupitant levels and effectiveness; avoid concurrent use. Drugs that affect serotonergic neurotransmitter systems, including **tricyclic antidepressants**, **SNRIs**, **fentanyl**, **buspirone**, **tramadol**, **amphetamines**, and **triptans** ↑ risk of serotonin syndrome.

Route/Dosage

Netupitant/Palonosetron

PO (Adults): *Highly emetogenic chemotherapy (included cisplatin-based)*—One capsule (netupitant 300 mg/palonosetron 0.5 mg) 1 hr before chemotherapy on Day 1. *Anthracycline and cyclophosphamide–based chemotherapy and other chemotherapy not considered highly emetogenic*—One capsule (netupitant 300 mg/palonosetron 0.5 mg) 1 hr before chemotherapy on Day 1.

Fosnetupitant/Palonosetron

IV (Adults): *Highly emetogenic chemotherapy (included cisplatin-based)*—One vial (fosnetupitant 235 mg/palonosetron 0.25 mg) administered 30 min before chemotherapy on Day 1.

Availability

Capsules: netupitant 300 mg/palonosetron 0.5 mg. **Lyophilized powder for injection (requires reconstitution and dilution):** netupitant 235 mg/palonosetron 0.25 mg/vial.

NURSING IMPLICATIONS

Assessment

- Assess patient for nausea, vomiting, abdominal distention, and bowel sounds prior to and following administration.
- Assess for serotonin syndrome (mental changes [agitation, hallucinations, delirium, coma], autonomic instability [tachycardia, labile BP, dizziness, diaphoresis, flushing, hyperthermia], neuromuscular aberrations [tremor, rigidity, myoclonus, hyperreflexia, incoordination], seizure, and/or GI symptoms [nausea, vomiting, diarrhea]), especially in patients taking other serotonergic drugs (SSRIs, SNRIs, triptans).
- ***Lab Test Considerations:*** May cause transient ↑ in serum bilirubin, AST, and ALT levels.

Implementation

- *For highly emetogenic chemotherapy,* administer with dexamethasone PO 12 mg 30 min prior to chemotherapy on day 1 and 8 mg PO on days 2 and 4. *For chemotherapy not considered highly emetogenic,* administer dexamethasone 30 min prior to chemotherapy on Day 1 (day 2 and 4 not needed).
- **PO:** Administer netupitant/palonosetron 1 hr prior to start of chemotherapy without regard to food.

IV Administration

- **Intermittent Infusion:** Reconstitute with 20 mL D5W or 0.9% NaCl into vial along vial wall to prevent foaming; swirl gently to mix. Prepare an infusion vial or bag filled with 30 mL D5W or NaCl. Withdraw entire volume of reconstituted solution and transfer it into infusion vial or bag containing 30 mL of D5W or 0.9% NaCl for a total volume of 50 mL. Gently invert bag until complete dissolution. Do not administer solutions that are discolored or contain particulate matter. Total time from reconstitution to the start of infusion should not exceed 3 hrs. Store reconstituted solution and final diluted solution at room temperature. ***Rate:*** Infuse over 30 min starting 30 min before chemotherapy. Flush line with D5W or 0.9% NaCl at end of infusion.

Patient/Family Teaching

- Instruct patient to take netupitant/palonosetron as directed. Advise patient to read *Patient Information* prior to starting therapy and with each Rx refill in case of changes.
- Advise patient to notify health care professional promptly if signs and symptoms of anaphylaxis (shortness of breath, rash, hives, swelling of mouth, throat, and lips) or serotonin syndrome occur.
- Instruct patient to notify health care professional of all Rx or OTC medications, vitamins, or herbal products being taken and consult health care professional before taking any new medications.

- Advise female patient to notify health care professional if pregnancy is planned or suspected, or if breast feeding.

Evaluation/Desired Outcomes

- Decrease in frequency and severity of nausea and vomiting.

niCARdipine (nye-kar-di-peen)

~~Cardene~~, Cardene IV

Classification

Therapeutic: antianginals, antihypertensives
Pharmacologic: calcium channel blockers

Indications

Management of: Hypertension, Angina pectoris, Vasospastic (Prinzmetal's) angina.

Action

Inhibits the transport of calcium into myocardial and vascular smooth muscle cells, resulting in inhibition of excitation-contraction coupling and subsequent contraction. **Therapeutic Effects:** Systemic vasodilation resulting in decreased BP. Coronary vasodilation resulting in decreased frequency and severity of attacks of angina.

Pharmacokinetics

Absorption: Well absorbed following oral administration but extensively metabolized, resulting in ↓ bioavailability.
Distribution: Unknown.
Metabolism and Excretion: Mostly metabolized by the liver; ≤10% excreted unchanged by kidneys.
Half-life: 2–4 hr.

TIME/ACTION PROFILE (cardiovascular effects)

ROUTE	ONSET	PEAK	DURATION
PO	20 min	0.5–2 hr	8 hr
IV	within min	45 min	50 hr†

†Following discontinuation.

Contraindications/Precautions

Contraindicated in: Hypersensitivity; Sick sinus syndrome; 2nd- or 3rd-degree AV block (unless an artificial pacemaker is in place); SBP <90 mm Hg; Advanced aortic stenosis.
Use Cautiously in: Severe hepatic impairment (dose ↓ recommended); Severe renal impairment (dose ↓ may be necessary); History of serious ventricular arrhythmias or HF; OB, Lactation, Pedi: Safety not established; Geri: Dose ↓/slower IV infusion rates recommended due to↑ risk of hypotension.

Adverse Reactions/Side Effects

CNS: abnormal dreams, anxiety, confusion, dizziness, drowsiness, headache, jitteriness, nervousness, psychiatric disturbances, weakness. **EENT:** blurred vision, disturbed equilibrium, epistaxis, tinnitus. **Resp:** cough, dyspnea, shortness of breath. **CV:** ARRHYTHMIAS, HF, <u>peripheral edema</u>, bradycardia, chest pain, hypotension, palpitations, syncope, tachycardia. **GI:** ↑ liver function tests, anorexia, constipation, diarrhea, dry mouth, dysgeusia, dyspepsia, nausea, vomiting. **GU:** dysuria, nocturia, polyuria, sexual dysfunction, urinary frequency. **Derm:** dermatitis, erythema multiforme, flushing, ↑ sweating, photosensitivity, pruritus/urticaria, rash. **Endo:** gynecomastia, hyperglycemia. **Hemat:** anemia, leukopenia, thrombocytopenia. **Metab:** weight gain. **MS:** joint stiffness, muscle cramps. **Neuro:** paresthesia, tremor. **Misc:** STEVENS-JOHNSON SYNDROME, gingival hyperplasia.

Interactions

Drug-Drug: Additive hypotension may occur when used concurrently with **fentanyl**, other **antihypertensives**, **nitrates**, acute ingestion of **alcohol**, or **quinidine**. Antihypertensive effects may be ↓ by concurrent use of **NSAIDs**. **Cimetidine** and **propranolol** may ↓ metabolism and ↑ risk of toxicity. May ↓ the metabolism of and ↑ risk of toxicity from **cyclosporine**, **prazosin**, **quinidine**, **tacrolimus**, or **carbamazepine**.
Drug-Food: Grapefruit and grapefruit juice ↑ serum levels and effect.

Route/Dosage

PO (Adults): 20 mg 3 times daily, may ↑ every 3 days (range 20–40 mg 3 times daily).
IV (Adults): *Substitute for PO nicardipine*—if PO dose is 20 mg every 8 hr, then infusion rate is 0.5 mg/hr; if PO dose is 30 mg every 8 hr, then infusion rate is 1.2 mg/hr; if PO dose is 40 mg every 8 hr, then infusion rate is 2.2 mg/hr. *Patients not receiving PO nicardipine*—initiate therapy at 5 mg/hr, may be increased by 2.5 mg every 5–15 min as needed (up to 15 mg/hr).

Availability (generic available)

Capsules: 20 mg, 30 mg. **Injection:** 2.5 mg/mL. **Premixed infusion:** 20 mg/200 mL D5W or 0.9% NaCl, 40 mg/200 mL 0.9% NaCl.

NURSING IMPLICATIONS

Assessment

- Monitor BP and pulse prior to therapy, during dose titration, and periodically throughout therapy. Monitor ECG periodically during prolonged therapy.
- Monitor intake and output ratios and daily weight. Assess for signs of HF (peripheral edema, rales/crackles, dyspnea, weight gain, jugular venous distention).
- Assess for rash periodically during therapy. May cause Stevens-Johnson syndrome. Discontinue therapy if severe or if accompanied with fever, general

N

malaise, fatigue, muscle or joint aches, blisters, oral lesions, conjunctivitis, hepatitis, and/or eosinophilia.

- **Angina:** Assess location, duration, intensity, and precipitating factors of patient's anginal pain.
- ***Lab Test Considerations:*** Total serum calcium concentrations are not affected by calcium channel blockers.
- Monitor serum potassium periodically. Hypokalemia ↑ risk of arrhythmias; should be corrected.
- Monitor renal and hepatic functions periodically during long-term therapy. Several days of therapy may cause ↑ hepatic enzymes, which return to normal upon discontinuation of therapy.

Implementation

- Do not confuse Cardene with Cardizem. Do not confuse nicardipine with nifedipine or nimodipine.
- To transfer from IV nicardipine infusion to oral therapy with other antihypertensive, start oral therapy simultaneously with discontinuation of nicardipine infusion. If transferring to oral nicardipine therapy, administer first dose of a 3-times-a-day regimen 1 hr prior to discontinuation of infusion.
- Dose adjustments of nicardipine should be made no more frequently than every 3 days.
- **PO:** May be administered without regard to meals. May be administered with meals if GI irritation becomes a problem.

IV Administration

- **Continuous Infusion:** ***Diluent:*** Dilute each 25-mg ampule with 240 mL of D5W, D5/0.45% NaCl, D5/0.9% NaCl, 0.45% NaCl, or 0.9% NaCl. Infusion is stable for 24 hr at room temperature. ***Concentration:*** 0.1 mg/mL. ***Rate:*** Titrate rate according to BP response. Administer through large peripheral veins or central veins to reduce risk of venous thrombosis, phlebitis, local irritation, swelling, extravasation, and vascular impairment. Change infusion site every 12 hrs to minimize risk of peripheral venous irritation.
- **Y-Site Compatibility:** alemtuzumab, alfentanil, amikacin, amiodarone, anidulafungin, argatroban, atracurium, aztreonam, bivalirudin, bleomycin, bumetanide, buprenorphine, butorphanol, calcium chloride, calcium gluconate, carboplatin, carmustine, caspofungin, cefazolin, cefotaxime, cefotetan, cefoxitin, ceftriaxone, chloramphenicol, chlorpromazine, ciprofloxacin, cisatracurium, cisplatin, cyclophosphamide, cyclosporine, cytarabine, dacarbazine, daptomycin, dexmedetomidine, dexrazoxane, digoxin, diltiazem, diphenhydramine, dobutamine, docetaxel, dolasetron, dopamine, doxorubicin, doxorubicin liposomal, doxycycline, droperidol, enalaprilat, ephedrine, epinephrine, epirubicin, eptifibatide, erythromycin, esmolol, etoposide, etoposide phosphate, famotidine, fenoldopam, fentanyl, fluconazole, gemcitabine, gentamicin, granisetron, haloperidol, hetastarch, hydromorphone, idarubicin, ifosfamide, irinotecan, isoproterenol, labetalol, leucovorin, levofloxacin, levorphanol, lidocaine, linezolid, magnesium sulfate, mannitol, meperidine, metoclopramide, metoprolol, metronidazole, midazolam, milrinone, mitoxantrone, morphine, moxifloxacin, mycophenolate, nafcillin, nalbuphine, naloxone, nitroglycerin, nitroprusside, norepinephrine, octreotide, ondansetron, oxaliplatin, oxytocin, paclitaxel, palonosetron, pamidronate, pancuronium, penicillin G potassium, pentamidine, phenylephrine, potassium chloride, procainamide, prochlorperazine, promethazine, propranolol, quinupristin/dalfopristin, remifentanil, rocuronium, sodium phosphates, succinylcholine, sufentanil, tacrolimus, theophylline, tirofiban, tobramycin, vancomycin, vasopressin, vecuronium, vincristine, voriconazole, zidovudine, zoledronic acid.
- **Y-Site Incompatibility:** acyclovir, aminocaproic acid, amphotericin B deoxycholate, amphotericin B lipid complex, amphotericin B liposome, ampicillin, ampicillin/sulbactam, azithromycin, ceftazidime, cefuroxime, dexamethasone, diazepam, ertapenem, fludarabine, fluorouracil, foscarnet, fosphenytoin, furosemide, ganciclovir, hydrocortisone sodium phosphate, imipenem/cilastatin, ketorolac, meropenem, mesna, methotrexate, micafungin, pantoprazole, pemetrexed, pentobarbital, phenobarbital, phenytoin, piperacillin/tazobactam, potassium acetate, sodium bicarbonate, thiopental, thiotepa, tigecycline.

Patient/Family Teaching

- Advise patient to take medication exactly as directed, even if feeling well. Take missed doses as soon as possible unless almost time for next dose; do not double doses. May need to be discontinued gradually.
- Instruct patient on technique for monitoring pulse. Instruct patient to contact health care professional if heart rate is <50 bpm.
- Advise patient to avoid grapefruit or grapefruit juice during therapy.
- Caution patient to change positions slowly to minimize orthostatic hypotension.
- May cause drowsiness or dizziness. Advise patient to avoid driving or other activities requiring alertness until response to the medication is known.
- Instruct patient to notify health care professional of all Rx or OTC medications, vitamins, or herbal products being taken and to avoid concurrent use of alcohol or OTC medications and herbal products, especially NSAIDs and cold preparations, without consulting health care professional.
- Advise patient to notify health care professional if rash, irregular heartbeat, dyspnea, swelling of hands and feet, pronounced dizziness, nausea, constipation, or hypotension occurs or if headache is severe or persistent.
- Caution patient to wear protective clothing and to use sunscreen to prevent photosensitivity reactions.
- Advise female patient to notify health care professional if pregnancy is planned or suspected or if breast feeding.

- **Angina:** Instruct patient on concurrent nitrate or beta-blocker therapy to continue taking both medications as directed and to use SL nitroglycerin as needed for anginal attacks.
- Advise patient to contact health care professional if chest pain does not improve, worsens after therapy, or occurs with diaphoresis; if shortness of breath; or if persistent headache occurs.
- Caution patient to discuss exercise restrictions with health care professional prior to exertion.
- **Hypertension:** Encourage patient to comply with other interventions for hypertension (weight reduction, low-sodium diet, smoking cessation, moderation of alcohol consumption, regular exercise, and stress management). Medication controls but does not cure hypertension.
- Instruct patient and family in proper technique for monitoring BP. Advise patient to take BP weekly and to report significant changes to health care professional.

Evaluation/Desired Outcomes

- Decrease in BP.
- Decrease in frequency and severity of anginal attacks.
- Decrease in need for nitrate therapy.
- Increase in activity tolerance and sense of well-being.

NICOTINE (nik-o-teen)

nicotine chewing gum
Nicorette, Thrive

nicotine inhaler
Nicotrol

nicotine lozenge
Nicorette

nicotine nasal spray
Nicotrol NS

nicotine transdermal patch
Nicoderm CQ

Classification
Therapeutic: smoking deterrents

Indications

Adjunct therapy (with behavior modification) in the management of nicotine withdrawal in patients desiring to give up cigarette smoking.

Action

Provides a source of nicotine during controlled withdrawal from cigarette smoking. **Therapeutic Effects:** Lessened sequelae of nicotine withdrawal (irritability, insomnia, somnolence, headache, and increased appetite).

Pharmacokinetics

Absorption: *Gum, lozenge*—Slowly absorbed from buccal mucosa during chewing/sucking. *Inhaler*—50% of dose is systemically absorbed; most of nicotine released from inhaler is deposited in the mouth; absorption from buccal mucosa is slow. *Nasal spray*—53% absorbed from nasal mucosa. *Transdermal*—70% of nicotine released from the system is absorbed through the skin.

Distribution: Enter breast milk.

Metabolism and Excretion: Mostly metabolized by the liver. Small amounts are metabolized by kidneys and lungs; 10–20% excreted unchanged by kidneys.

Half-life: 1–2 hr.

TIME/ACTION PROFILE (nicotine blood levels)

ROUTE	ONSET	PEAK	DURATION
gum	rapid	15–30 min	unknown
inhaler	slow	within 15 min	unknown
lozenge	unknown	unknown	unknown
nasal spray	rapid	4–15 min	unknown
transdermal	rapid	2–4 hr	unknown

Contraindications/Precautions

Contraindicated in: Hypersensitivity; Recent history of MI (inhaler or nasal spray); Arrhythmias (inhaler or nasal spray); Severe or worsening angina (inhaler or nasal spray); Severe cardiovascular disease; OB: Effects on fetus unknown; spontaneous abortion has been reported. Encourage behavioral approaches to smoking cessation. Lactation: Excreted in breast milk; weigh risks of nicotine product use against risk of continued smoking. Pedi: Safety not established.

Use Cautiously in: Cardiovascular disease (including hypertension); Recent history of MI (gum, lozenge, patch); Arrhythmias (gum, lozenge, patch); Severe or worsening angina (gum, lozenge, patch); Diabetes mellitus; Pheochromocytoma; Peripheral vascular diseases; Hyperthyroidism; Continued smoking; Peptic ulcer disease; Seizures; Hepatic disease; Bronchospastic lung disease (inhaler or nasal spray); Allergic reaction to adhesive tape (patch); Geri: Begin at lower dosages.

Adverse Reactions/Side Effects

CNS: headache, insomnia, abnormal dreams, dizziness, drowsiness, impaired concentration, nervousness, seizures, weakness. **CV:** tachycardia, chest pain, hypertension. **Derm:** *transdermal*—burning at patch site, erythema, pruritus, cutaneous hypersensitivity, rash, sweating. **EENT:** sinusitis; *gum*, pharyngitis; *nasal spray*, nasopharyngeal irritation, sneezing, watering eyes, change in smell, earache, epistaxis, eye irritation, hoarseness; *inhaler*, local mouth/throat irritation. **Endo:** dysmenorrhea. **GI:** abdominal pain, abnormal taste, constipation, diarrhea, dry mouth, dyspepsia, hiccups, nausea, vomiting; *gum*, belching, ↑ appetite, ↑ salivation, oral injury, sore mouth. **MS:** arthralgia, back pain, myalgia; *gum*, jaw muscle ache. **Neuro:** paresthesia. **Resp:** *Nasal spray, inhaler*—cough, dyspnea.

Interactions

Drug-Drug: Effects of **acetaminophen**, **caffeine**, **imipramine**, **insulin**, **oxazepam**, **propranolol**, or other **beta blockers**, **adrenergic antagonists** (**prazosin**, **labetalol**), and **theophylline** may be ↑ upon smoking cessation; dose ↓ at cessation may be necessary. Effects of adrenergic agonists (e.g., **isoproterenol**, **phenylephrine**) may be ↓ upon smoking cessation; dose ↑ at cessation may be necessary. Concurrent treatment with **bupropion** may cause treatment-emergent hypertension.

Route/Dosage

Gum (Adults): If first cigarette is desired >30 min after awakening, start with 2 mg gum, if first cigarette is desired <30 min after awakening, start with 4 mg gum. Patients should chew one piece of gum every 1–2 hr for 6 wk, then one piece of gum every 2–4 hr for 3 wk, then one piece of gum every 4–8 hr for 3 wk, then discontinue. Should not exceed 24 pieces of gum/day.

Lozenge (Adults): If first cigarette is desired >30 min after awakening, start with 2 mg lozenge, if first cigarette is desired <30 min after awakening, start with 4 mg lozenge. Patients should use one lozenge every 1–2 hr for 6 wk, then one lozenge every 2–4 hr for 3 wk, then one lozenge every 4–8 hr for 3 wk, then discontinue. Should not exceed 20 lozenges/day or more than 5 lozenges in 6 hr.

Intranasal (Adults): One spray in each nostril 1–2 times/hr (up to 5 times/hr); may be ↑ up to maximum of 40 times/day (should not exceed 3 mo of therapy).

Inhaln (Adults): Patients are encouraged to use at least 6 cartridges/day for first 3–6 wk, with additional cartridges as necessary (up to 16/day) for 12 wk. Patients are self-titrated to level of nicotine they require (usual usage 6–16 cartridges/day) followed by gradual withdrawal over 6–12 wk (maximum duration of use = 6 mo).

Transdermal (Adults): *Patients smoking >10 cigarettes/day*—Begin with Step 1 (21 mg/day) for 6 wk, followed by Step 2 (14 mg/day) for 2 wk, and then Step 3 (7 mg/day) for 2 wk, then stop (total of 10 wk) (new patch should be applied every 24 hr); *Patients smoking ≤10 cigarettes/day*—Begin with Step 2 (14 mg/day) for 6 wk, followed by Step 3 (7 mg/day) for 2 wk, then stop (total of 8 wk) (new patch should be applied every 24 hr).

Availability (generic available)

Chewing gum (cinnamon, mint, spearmint, white ice, and fruit chill flavors): 2 mg^{OTC}, 4 mg^{OTC}. **Oral inhalation:** 10 mg/cartridge (delivers 4 mg). **Lozenges (original, mint, cherry, and cappuccino flavors):** 2 mg^{OTC}, 4 mg^{OTC}. **Nasal spray:** 0.5 mg/spray in 10-mL bottles (200 sprays). **Transdermal patch:** 7 mg/day^{OTC}, 14 mg/day^{OTC}, 21 mg/day^{OTC}.

NURSING IMPLICATIONS

Assessment

- Prior to therapy, assess smoking history (number of cigarettes smoked daily, smoking patterns, nicotine content of preferred brand, degree to which patient inhales smoke).
- Assess patient for symptoms of smoking withdrawal (irritability, drowsiness, fatigue, headache, nicotine craving) periodically during nicotine replacement therapy (NRT).
- Evaluate progress in smoking cessation periodically during therapy.
- ***Toxicity and Overdose:*** Monitor for nausea, vomiting, diarrhea, increased salivation, abdominal pain, headache, dizziness, auditory and visual disturbances, weakness, dyspnea, hypotension, and irregular pulse.

Implementation

- **Gum:** Protect gum from light; exposure to light causes gum to turn brown.
- **Lozenge:** Lozenge should be allowed to dissolve slowly in the mouth; it should not be chewed or swallowed.
- **Transdermal:** Patch can be worn for 16 or 24 hr; the patch can be removed before the patient goes to bed (especially if patient has vivid dreams or sleep disturbances) or can remain on while the patient sleeps (especially if patient craves cigarettes upon awakening).
- **Nasal Spray and Inhaler:** Regular use of the spray or inhaler during the first wk of therapy may help patient adjust to irritant effects of the spray.

Patient/Family Teaching

- Encourage patient to participate in a smoking cessation program while using this product.
- Review the patient instruction sheet enclosed in the package.
- Instruct patient in proper method of disposal of unit. Emphasize need to keep out of the reach of children or pets.
- Nicotine in any form can be harmful to a pregnant woman and/or the fetus. Assist patient in determining risk/benefit of nicotine replacement therapy (NRT) and harm to the fetus versus the likelihood of stopping smoking without NRT.
- Emphasize the importance of regular visits to health care professional to monitor progress of smoking cessation.
- **Gum:** Explain purpose of nicotine gum to patient. Patient should chew 1 piece of gum whenever a craving for nicotine occurs or according to a fixed schedule (every 1–2 hr while awake) as directed. Chew gum slowly until a tingling sensation is felt (about 15 chews). Then, patient should stop chew-

ing and store the gum between the cheek and gums until the tingling sensation disappears (about 1 min). Process of stopping, then resuming chewing should be repeated for approximately 30 min until most of the tingle has disappeared. Rapid, vigorous chewing may result in side effects similar to those of smoking too many cigarettes (headache, dizziness, nausea, increased salivation, heartburn, and hiccups). For best chances of quitting, chew at least 9 piece of gum/day during 1st 6 wk.

- Inform patient that the gum has a slight tobacco/pepper-like taste. Many patients initially find it unpleasant and slightly irritating to the mouth. This usually resolves after several days of therapy.
- Advise patient to carry gum at all times during therapy.
- Advise patient to avoid eating or drinking for 15 min before and during chewing of nicotine gum; these interfere with buccal absorption of nicotine.
- The gum usually can be chewed by denture wearers. Contact dentist if the gum adheres to bridgework.
- Inform patient that if they still feel need to use gum after completion of treatment period, advise them to contact a health care professional.
- Instruct patient not to swallow gum.
- Dispose of the gum by wrapping in wrapper to prevent ingestion by children and animals. Call the poison control center, emergency department, or health care professional immediately if a child ingests the gum.
- Emphasize the need to discontinue the gum and to inform health care professional if pregnancy occurs.
- **Transdermal:** Instruct patient in application and use of patch. Apply patch at the same time each day. Keep patch in sealed pouch until ready to apply. Apply to clean, dry skin of upper arm or torso free of oil, hair, scars, cuts, burns, or irritation. Press patch firmly in place with palm for 10 sec, making sure there is good contact, especially around the edges. Keep patch in place during showering, bathing, or swimming; replace patches that have fallen off. Wash hands with soap and water after handling patches. Do not trim or cut patch. No more than 1 patch should be worn at a time. Alternate application sites. Dispose of used patches by folding adhesive sides together and replacing in protective pouch or aluminum foil; keep out of reach of children.
- Advise patient that redness, itching, and burning at application site usually subside within 1 hr. Instruct patient to notify health care professional and not apply new patch if signs of allergic reaction (urticaria, generalized rash, hives) or persistent local skin reactions (severe erythema, pruritus, edema) occur.
- May cause drowsiness or dizziness. Caution patient to avoid driving or other activities requiring alertness until response to medication is known.
- Advise patient referred for MRI test to discuss patch with referring health care professional and MRI facility to determine if removal of patch is necessary prior to test and for directions for replacing patch.
- **Nasal Spray:** Instruct patient in proper use of spray. Tilt head back slightly. Do not sniff, swallow, or inhale through nose as spray is being administered. Patients who have successfully stopped smoking should continue to use the same dose for up to 8 wk, after which the spray should be discontinued over the next 4–6 wk.
- Discontinue nasal spray by using ½ dose (1 spray at a time), using the spray less frequently, skipping a dose by not using every hr, or setting a planned stop date for use of the spray.
- Treatment should be discontinued in patients who are unable to stop smoking by the 4th wk of therapy (patient is unlikely to quit on that attempt).
- Patients who fail to stop smoking should be given a therapy holiday before another attempt.
- Instruct patient to replace childproof cap after using and before disposal.
- **Inhalation:** Inhalation regimens should consist of frequent, continuous puffing for 20 min.
- Treatment should be discontinued in patients who are unable to stop smoking by the 4th wk of therapy (patient is unlikely to quit on that attempt).
- Patients who fail to stop smoking should be given a therapy holiday before another attempt.
- **Lozenge:** Instruct patient to place lozenge in mouth and allow it to slowly dissolve (20–30 min). Minimize swallowing; advise patient not to chew or swallow lozenge. May cause a warm tingling sensation in mouth. Advise patient to occasionally move lozenge from side to side of mouth until completely dissolved. Instruct patient not to eat or drink 15 min before or while lozenge is in mouth. For best chances of quitting, use at least 9 lozenges/day during 1st 6 wk. Do not use more than 1 lozenge at a time or use continuously one after the another. Lozenge should not be used after 12 wk without consulting health care professional.

Evaluation/Desired Outcomes

- Lessened sequelae of nicotine withdrawal (irritability, insomnia, somnolence, headache, and increased appetite) during smoking cessation.

BEERS

NIFEdipine (nye-**fed**-i-peen)

Adalat CC, ♣Adalat XL, Afeditab CR, Procardia, Procardia XL

Classification

Therapeutic: antianginals, antihypertensives
Pharmacologic: calcium channel blockers

N

Indications

Management of: Hypertension (extended-release only), Angina pectoris, Vasospastic (Prinzmetal's) angina. **Unlabeled Use:** Prevention of migraine headache. Management of HF or cardiomyopathy.

Action

Inhibits calcium transport into myocardial and vascular smooth muscle cells, resulting in inhibition of excitation-contraction coupling and subsequent contraction. **Therapeutic Effects:** Systemic vasodilation, resulting in decreased BP. Coronary vasodilation, resulting in decreased frequency and severity of attacks of angina.

Pharmacokinetics

Absorption: Well absorbed after oral administration, but large amounts are rapidly metabolized (primarily by CYP3A4 enzyme system), resulting in ↓ bioavailability (45–70%); bioavailability is ↑ (80%) with long-acting (CC, PA, XL) forms.
Distribution: Unknown.
Protein Binding: 92–98%.
Metabolism and Excretion: Mostly metabolized by the liver.
Half-life: 2–5 hr.

TIME/ACTION PROFILE

ROUTE	ONSET	PEAK	DURATION
PO	20 min	unknown	6–8 hr
PO–PA	unknown	4 hr	12 hr
PO–CC, PA, XL	unknown	6 hr	24 hr

Contraindications/Precautions

Contraindicated in: Hypersensitivity; Sick sinus syndrome; 2nd- or 3rd-degree AV block (unless an artificial pacemaker is in place); Systolic BP <90 mm Hg; Coadministration with grapefruit juice, rifampin, rifabutin, phenobarbital, phenytoin, carbamazepine, or St. John's wort.
Use Cautiously in: Severe hepatic impairment (↓ dose recommended); History of porphyria; Severe renal impairment (↓ dose may be necessary); History of serious ventricular arrhythmias or HF; OB, Lactation: Use only if potential benefit justifies potential risks; Pedi: Safety not established; Geri: Short-acting forms appear on Beers list due to ↑ risk of hypotension and constipation (↓ dose recommended); also associated with ↑ incidence of falls.

Adverse Reactions/Side Effects

CNS: headache, abnormal dreams, anxiety, confusion, dizziness, drowsiness, jitteriness, nervousness, psychiatric disturbances, weakness. **EENT:** blurred vision, disturbed equilibrium, epistaxis, tinnitus. **Resp:** cough, dyspnea, shortness of breath. **CV:** ARRHYTHMIAS, HF, peripheral edema, bradycardia, chest pain, hypotension, palpitations, syncope, tachycardia. **GI:** ↑ liver enzymes, anorexia, constipation, diarrhea, dry mouth, dysgeusia, dyspepsia, GI obstruction, nausea, ulcer, vomiting. **GU:** dysuria, nocturia, polyuria, sexual dysfunction, urinary frequency. **Derm:** flushing, dermatitis, erythema multiforme, ↑ sweating, photosensitivity, pruritus/urticaria, rash. **Endo:** gynecomastia, hyperglycemia. **Hemat:** anemia, leukopenia, thrombocytopenia. **Metab:** weight gain. **MS:** joint stiffness, muscle cramps. **Neuro:** paresthesia, tremor. **Misc:** STEVENS-JOHNSON SYNDROME, gingival hyperplasia.

Interactions

Drug-Drug: **Rifampin**, **rifabutin**, **phenobarbital**, **phenytoin**, or **carbamazepine** may significantly ↓ levels and effects; concurrent use is contraindicated. **Ketoconazole**, **fluconazole**, **itraconazole**, **clarithromycin**, **erythromycin**, **nefazodone**, **saquinavir**, **indinavir**, **nelfinavir**, or **ritonavir** may ↑ levels and effects; consider initiating nifedipine at lowest dose. Additive hypotension may occur when used concurrently with **fentanyl**, other **antihypertensives**, **nitrates**, acute ingestion of **alcohol**, or **quinidine**. Antihypertensive effects may be ↓ by concurrent use of **NSAIDs**. May ↑ serum levels and risk of toxicity from **digoxin**. Concurrent use with **beta blockers**, **digoxin**, or **disopyramide** may result in bradycardia, conduction defects, or HF. **Cimetidine** and **propranolol** may ↓ metabolism and ↑ risk of toxicity. May ↓ metabolism of and ↑ risk of toxicity from **cyclosporine**, **tacrolimus**, **prazosin**, **quinidine**, or **carbamazepine**. ↑ risk of GI obstruction when used concurrently with **H_2 blockers**, **opioids**, **NSAIDs**, **laxatives**, **anticholinergic drugs**, **levothyroxine**, or **neuromuscular blockers**. **Strong CYP3A4 inducers**, including **carbamazepine**, **phenobarbital**, **phenytoin**, and **rifampin** may ↓ levels and effects; avoid concurrent use.
Drug-Natural Products: **St. John's wort** may significantly ↓ levels and effects; concurrent use is contraindicated.
Drug-Food: **Grapefruit** and **grapefruit juice** ↑ serum levels and effect; avoid concurrent use.

Route/Dosage

PO (Adults): 10–30 mg 3 times daily (not to exceed 180 mg/day), *or* 10–20 mg twice daily as immediate-release form, *or* 30–90 mg once daily as sustained-release (CC, XL) form (not to exceed 90–120 mg/day).

Availability (generic available)

Capsules: 🍁5 mg, 10 mg, 20 mg. **Tablets:** 🍁10 mg. **Extended-release tablets (Adalat CC, Afeditab CR, Nifedical XL, Procardia XL):** 🍁10 mg, 🍁20 mg, 30 mg, 60 mg, 90 mg.

NURSING IMPLICATIONS

Assessment

- Monitor BP and pulse before therapy, during dose titration, and periodically during therapy. Monitor ECG periodically during prolonged therapy.
- Monitor intake and output ratios and daily weight. Assess for signs of HF (peripheral edema, rales/crackles, dyspnea, weight gain, jugular venous distention).

- Patients receiving digoxin concurrently with nifedipine should have routine tests of serum digoxin levels and be monitored for signs and symptoms of digoxin toxicity.
- Assess for rash periodically during therapy. May cause Stevens-Johnson syndrome. Discontinue therapy if severe or if accompanied with fever, general malaise, fatigue, muscle or joint aches, blisters, oral lesions, conjunctivitis, hepatitis, and/or eosinophilia.
- **Angina:** Assess location, duration, intensity, and precipitating factors of patient's anginal pain.
- ***Lab Test Considerations:*** Total serum calcium concentrations are not affected by calcium channel blockers.
- Monitor serum potassium periodically. Hypokalemia increases risk of arrhythmias; should be corrected.
- Monitor renal and hepatic functions periodically during long-term therapy. Several days of therapy may cause ↑ hepatic enzymes, which return to normal upon discontinuation of therapy.
- Nifedipine may cause positive ANA and direct Coombs' test results.

Implementation

- Do not confuse with nicardipine or nimodipine.
- **PO:** May be administered without regard to meals. May be administered with meals if GI irritation becomes a problem.
- Do not open, break, crush, or chew extended-release tablets. Empty tablets that appear in stool are not significant.
- Avoid administration with grapefruit juice.
- Sublingual use is not recommended due to serious adverse drug reactions.

Patient/Family Teaching

- Advise patient to take medication as directed, even if feeling well. Take missed doses as soon as possible unless almost time for next dose; do not double doses. May need to be discontinued gradually.
- Instruct patient on technique for monitoring pulse. Instruct patient to contact health care professional if heart rate is <50 bpm.
- Advise patient to avoid grapefruit or grapefruit juice during therapy.
- Caution patient to change positions slowly to minimize orthostatic hypotension.
- May cause drowsiness or dizziness. Advise patient to avoid driving or other activities requiring alertness until response to the medication is known.
- Geri: Teach patients and family about risk for falls and how to reduce risk in the home.
- Instruct patient on importance of maintaining good dental hygiene and seeing dentist frequently for teeth cleaning to prevent tenderness, bleeding, and gingival hyperplasia (gum enlargement).
- Instruct patient to notify health care professional of all Rx or OTC medications, vitamins, or herbal products being taken and to avoid concurrent use of alcohol or OTC medications and herbal products, especially cold preparations, without consulting health care professional.
- Advise patient to notify health care professional if rash, irregular heartbeat, dyspnea, swelling of hands and feet, pronounced dizziness, nausea, constipation, or hypotension occurs or if headache is severe or persistent.
- Caution patient to wear protective clothing and use sunscreen to prevent photosensitivity reactions.
- **Angina:** Instruct patient on concurrent nitrate or beta-blocker therapy to continue taking both medications as directed and use SL nitroglycerin as needed for anginal attacks.
- Inform patient that anginal attacks may occur 30 min after administration because of reflex tachycardia. This is usually temporary and is not an indication for discontinuation.
- Advise patient to contact health care professional if chest pain does not improve, worsens after therapy, or occurs with diaphoresis; if shortness of breath occurs; or if persistent headache occurs.
- Caution patient to discuss exercise restrictions with health care professional before exertion.
- **Hypertension:** Encourage patient to comply with other interventions for hypertension (weight reduction, low-sodium diet, smoking cessation, moderation of alcohol consumption, regular exercise, and stress management). Medication controls but does not cure hypertension.
- Instruct patient and family in proper technique for monitoring BP. Advise patient to take BP weekly and to report significant changes to health care professional.

Evaluation/Desired Outcomes

- Decrease in BP.
- Decrease in frequency and severity of anginal attacks.
- Decrease in need for nitrate therapy.
- Increase in activity tolerance and sense of well-being.

nilotinib (ni-lo-ti-nib)

Tasigna

Classification

Therapeutic: antineoplastics

Pharmacologic: enzyme inhibitors, kinase inhibitors

Indications

Newly diagnosed Philadelphia chromosome positive (Ph+) chronic myelogenous leukemia (CML) in chronic phase. Chronic or accelerated phase Ph+

N

CML in patients who are resistant or intolerant to prior treatment, including imatinib. Chronic phase Ph+ CML in patients who are resistant or intolerant to prior tyrosine-kinase inhibitor treatment.

Action

Inhibits kinases which may be produced by malignant cell lines. **Therapeutic Effects:** Inhibits production of malignant cells lines with decreased proliferation of leukemic cells.

Pharmacokinetics

Absorption: Well absorbed following oral administration. Blood levels are significantly ↑ by food.
Distribution: Unknown.
Metabolism and Excretion: Mostly metabolized by the liver; metabolites are not active.
Half-life: 17 hr.

TIME/ACTION PROFILE (blood levels)

ROUTE	ONSET	PEAK	DURATION
PO	unknown	3 hr	12 hr

Contraindications/Precautions

Contraindicated in: Hypokalemia or hypomagnesemia; Long QT syndrome; Concurrent use of QT interval prolonging medications; Concurrent use of strong CYP3A4 inhibitors (e.g. ketoconazole, itraconazole, clarithromycin, atazanavir, indinavir, nefazodone, nelfinavir, ritonavir, saquinavir, voriconazole, grapefruit juice); Concurrent use of strong CYP3A4 inducers (e.g. dexamethasone, phenytoin, carbamazepine, rifampin, rifabutin, rifapentine, phenobarbital, St. John's wort); Galactose intolerance, severe lactase deficiency, or glucose-galactose malabsorption (capsules contain lactose); OB: Pregnancy (may cause fetal harm); Lactation: Lactation.
Use Cautiously in: Concurrent use of proton pump inhibitors (may ↓ bioavailability of nilotinib); Electrolyte abnormalities; correct prior to administration to ↓ risk of arrhythmias; Hepatic impairment (↓ dose required for Grade 3 elevated bilirubin, transaminases or lipase); Total gastrectomy (may need to ↑ dose or use alterative therapy); History of pancreatitis; Rep: Women of reproductive potential; Pedi: May affect growth and development; safety and effectiveness not established in children <1 yr.

Adverse Reactions/Side Effects

CNS: fatigue, headache, dizziness. **CV:** MI, STROKE, TORSADES DE POINTES, hypertension, palpitations, pericardial effusion, peripheral arterial disease, QT interval prolongation. **Derm:** pruritus, rash, alopecia, flushing. **EENT:** vertigo. **F and E:** hyperkalemia, hypocalcemia, hypokalemia, hyponatremia, hypophosphatemia. **GI:** HEPATOTOXICITY, ↑ lipase, constipation, diarrhea, nausea, vomiting, abdominal discomfort, anorexia, ascites, dyspepsia, flatulence. **Hemat:** BLEEDING, MYELOSUPRESSION. **Metab:** hyperglycemia. **MS:** ↓ growth, musculoskeletal pain. **Neuro:** paresthesia. **Resp:** pleural effusion, pulmonary edema. **Misc:** fever, hepatitis B virus reactivation, night sweats, tumor lysis syndrome.

Interactions

Drug-Drug: Strong **CYP3A4 inhibitors** including **ketoconazole, itraconazole, voriconazole, clarithromycin, atazanavir, indinavir, nelfinavir, ritonavir, saquinavir**, and **nefazodone** may result in ↑ blood levels and toxicity and should be avoided if possible; if concurrent use is necessary, ↓ nilotinib dose. Strong **CYP3A4 inducers** including **carbamazepine, dexamethasone, phenobarbital, phenytoin, rifabutin, rifampin**, and **rifapentin** may ↓ blood levels and effectiveness and should be avoided. May ↑ levels of **CYP3A4 substrates**, including **alfentanil, cyclosporine, dihydroergotamine, ergotamine, fentanyl, midazolam, sirolimus**, and **tacrolimus**. May ↑ levels of **CYP3A4 substrates**, including **alfentanil, atorvastatin, cyclosporine, dihydroergotamine, ergotamine, fentanyl, lovastatin, midazolam, simvastatin, sirolimus**, and **tacrolimus**. Concurrent use of other **drugs that prolong QT interval**; may ↑ risk of serious arrhythmias; avoid concomitant use. **Proton pump inhibitors, H_2 receptor antagonists**, and **antacids** may ↓ the bioavailability of nilotinib; avoid concurrent use of proton pump inhibitors; doses of H_2 receptor antagonists may be administered 10 hr before or 2 hr after nilotinib; doses of antacids may be administered 2 hr before or after nilotinib.
Drug-Natural Products: St. John's wort may ↓ levels and effectiveness; avoid concurrent use.
Drug-Food: Grapefruit juice may ↑ blood levels and toxicity and should be avoided.

Route/Dosage

Newly Diagnosed Chronic Phase Ph+ CML

PO (Adults): 300 mg twice daily; treatment discontinuation may be considered in patients who have received nilotinib for ≥3 yr and achieved a sustained molecular response; if patients lose molecular response after discontinuing therapy, restart nilotinib within 4 wk at the dose level prior to discontinuation; *Concurrent use of strong CYP3A4 inhibitor (ketoconazole, itraconazole, clarithromycin, atazanavir, indinavir, nefazodone, nelfinavir, ritonavir, saquinavir, voriconazole)*—200 mg once daily.
PO (Children ≥1 yr): 230 mg/m² twice daily (max single dose = 400 mg) until disease progression or unacceptable toxicity; treatment discontinuation may be considered in patients who have received nilotinib for ≥3 yr and achieved a sustained molecular response; if patients lose molecular response after discontinuing therapy, restart nilotinib within 4 wk at the dose level prior to discontinuation; *Concurrent use of strong CYP3A4 inhibitor (ketoconazole, itraconazole, clarithromycin, atazanavir, indinavir, nefazodone, nelfinavir, ritonavir, saquinavir, voriconazole)*—200 mg once daily.

Hepatic Impairment

PO (Adults and Children ≥1 yr): *Mild, moderate or severe hepatic impairment*—200 mg twice daily; may ↑ to 300 mg twice daily if tolerates.

Resistant or Intolerant Chronic Phase Ph+ CML

PO (Adults): 400 mg twice daily; treatment discontinuation may be considered in patients who have received nilotinib for ≥3 yr and achieved a sustained molecular response; if patients lose molecular response after discontinuing therapy, restart nilotinib within 4 wk at the dose level prior to discontinuation; *Concurrent use of strong CYP3A4 inhibitor (ketoconazole, itraconazole, clarithromycin, atazanavir, indinavir, nefazodone, nelfinavir, ritonavir, saquinavir, voriconazole)*—300 mg once daily.

PO (Children ≥1 yr): 230 mg/m^2 twice daily (max single dose = 400 mg) until disease progression or unacceptable toxicity; treatment discontinuation may be considered in patients who have received nilotinib for ≥3 yr and achieved a sustained molecular response; if patients lose molecular response after discontinuing therapy, restart nilotinib within 4 wk at the dose level prior to discontinuation; *Concurrent use of strong CYP3A4 inhibitor (ketoconazole, itraconazole, clarithromycin, atazanavir, indinavir, nefazodone, nelfinavir, ritonavir, saquinavir, voriconazole)*—200 mg once daily.

Hepatic Impairment

PO (Adults and Children ≥1 yr): *Mild or moderate hepatic impairment*—300 mg twice daily; may ↑ to 400 mg twice daily if tolerates; *Severe hepatic impairment*—200 mg twice daily; may ↑ to 300 mg twice daily, and eventually to 400 mg twice daily if tolerates.

Resistant or Intolerant Accelerated Phase Ph+ CML

PO (Adults): 400 mg twice daily; treatment discontinuation may be considered in patients who have received nilotinib for ≥3 yr and achieved a sustained molecular response; if patients lose molecular response after discontinuing therapy, restart nilotinib within 4 wk at the dose level prior to discontinuation; *Concurrent use of strong CYP3A4 inhibitor (ketoconazole, itraconazole, clarithromycin, atazanavir, indinavir, nefazodone, nelfinavir, ritonavir, saquinavir, voriconazole)*—300 mg once daily.

Hepatic Impairment

PO (Adults): *Mild or moderate hepatic impairment*—300 mg twice daily; may ↑ to 400 mg twice daily if tolerates; *Severe hepatic impairment*—200 mg twice daily; may ↑ to 300 mg twice daily, and eventually to 400 mg twice daily if tolerates.

Availability

Capsules: 150 mg, 200 mg.

NURSING IMPLICATIONS

Assessment

- Monitor ECG to assess the QTc interval at baseline, 7 days after initiation of therapy, after any dose adjustment, and periodically thereafter. For ECGs with QTc >480 msec, withhold nilotinib and check serum potassium and magnesium. If below lower limit of normal, correct to normal with supplements. Review concomitant medications for effects on electrolytes. If QTc returns to <450 msec and within 20 msec of baseline within 2 wk, return to prior dose. If QTc is <480 msec and >450 msec after 2 wk, reduce nilotinib dose to 400 mg once daily. Following dose reduction to 400 mg once daily, if QTc return to >480 msec, discontinue nilotinib. Repeat ECG approximately 7 days after any dose adjustment.
- Monitor for myelosuppression. Assess for bleeding (bleeding gums, bruising, petechiae, blood in stools, urine, emesis) and avoid IM injections and taking rectal temperatures if platelet count is low. Apply pressure to venipuncture sites for at least 10 min. Assess for signs of infection during neutropenia. Anemia may occur. Monitor for fatigue, dyspnea, and orthostatic hypotension.
- Monitor for tumor lysis syndrome (malignant disease progression, high WBC counts, hyperuricemia, hyperkalemia, hyperphosphatemia, hypocalcemia, and/or dehydration). Prevent by maintain adequate hydration and correcting uric acid levels prior to starting nilotinib.
- Monitor for signs of severe fluid retention (unexpected rapid weight gain or swelling) and for symptoms of respiratory or cardiac compromise (shortness of breath) periodically during therapy; evaluate cause and treat patients as needed.
- Monitor growth and development in pediatric patients receiving nilotinib.
- ***Lab Test Considerations:*** Obtain negative pregnancy test before starting therapy.
- Monitor serum electrolytes prior to and periodically during therapy. May cause hypokalemia, hypomagnesemia, hypophosphatemia, hyperkalemia, hypocalcemia, hyperglycemia, and hyponatremia.
- Monitor CBC every 2 wk for first 2 mo and monthly thereafter or as indicated. May cause Grade 3/4 thrombocytopenia, neutropenia, and anemia. If ANC is $<1.0 \times 10^9$/L and/or platelet counts $<50 \times 10^9$/L, stop nilotinib and monitor blood counts. Resume within 2 wk at prior dose if ANC $>1.0 \times 10^9$/L and platelets $>50 \times 10^9$/L. If blood counts remain low for >2 wk, reduce dose to 400 mg once daily. Myelosuppression is generally reversible.
- May cause ↑ serum lipase or amylase. If ↑ to ≥Grade 3, withhold nilotinib and monitor serum levels. Resume treatment at 400 mg once daily if serum lipase or amylase return to ≤Grade 1.

N

- May cause ↑ serum bilirubin. If ↑ to ≥Grade 3, withhold nilotinib and monitor bilirubin. Resume treatment at 400 mg once daily if serum lipase or amylase return to ≤Grade 1.
- May cause ↑ serum hepatic transaminases. If ↑ to ≥Grade 3, withhold nilotinib and monitor serum ALT, AST, and alkaline phosphatase. Resume treatment at 400 mg once daily if serum lipase or amylase return to ≤Grade 1.
- Monitor lipid panel and glucose prior to and periodically during first yr of therapy, and then yearly during chronic therapy.
- Upon discontinuation, monitor BCR-ABL transcript levels and CBC with differential monthly for 1 yr, then every 6 wk for 2nd yr, and every 12 wk thereafter.

Implementation

- Do not confuse nilotinib with neratinib or niraparib.
- Correct hypokalemia and hypomagnesemia prior to beginning therapy.
- **PO:** Administer twice daily at 12-hr intervals on an empty stomach, at least 1 hr before and 2 hr after food. Capsule should be swallowed whole with water; do not open capsule.
- Patients unable to swallow capsule may open capsule and sprinkle contents of each capsule in 1 teaspoon of applesauce. Swallow mixture within 15 min. Do not use more than 1 teaspoon of applesauce and use only applesauce.
- Avoid antacids less than 2 hr before or after and H_2 antagonists less than 10 hr before or less than 2 hr after administration.

Patient/Family Teaching

- Instruct patient to take nilotinib as directed, approximately 12 hr apart. If a dose is missed, skip dose and resume taking next prescribed dose. Nilotinib is a long-term treatment; do not stop medication or change dose without consulting health care professional. Advise patient to read the *Medication Guide* before starting and with each Rx refill, in case of changes.
- Advise patient to avoid grapefruit, grapefruit juice or products with grapefruit extract during therapy; may cause toxicity.
- May cause dizziness. Caution patient to avoid driving or other activities requiring alertness until response to medication is known.
- Advise patient to notify health care professional of all Rx or OTC medications, vitamins, or herbal products being taken and to consult with health care professional before taking other medications, especially St. John's wort, during therapy.
- Instruct patient to notify health care professional promptly if fever; chills; cough; hoarseness; sore throat; signs of infection; lower back or side pain; painful or difficulty urination; bleeding gums; bruising; petechiae; blood in stools, urine, or emesis; increased fatigue; dyspnea; signs of fluid retention, or orthostatic hypotension occurs. Caution patient to avoid crowds and persons with known infections. Instruct patients to use a soft toothbrush and electric razor and to avoid falls. Caution patient not to drink alcoholic beverages or take medication containing aspirin or NSAIDs; may precipitate bleeding.
- Instruct patient not to receive any vaccinations without advice of health care professional.
- Discuss the possibility of hair loss with patient. Explore methods of coping. Regrowth usually occurs 2–3 mo after discontinuation of therapy.
- Rep: Advise women of reproductive potential to use highly effective contraception during therapy and for at least 14 days following last dose and to avoid breast feeding for at least 14 days following last dose.

Evaluation/Desired Outcomes

- Decrease in production of leukemic cells.

niMODipine (nye-moe-di-peen)

Nimotop, Nymalize

Classification

Therapeutic: subarachnoid hemorrhage therapy agents

Pharmacologic: calcium channel blockers

Indications

Management of subarachnoid hemorrhage.

Action

Inhibits the transport of calcium into vascular smooth muscle cells, resulting in inhibition of excitation-contraction coupling and subsequent contraction. Potent peripheral vasodilator. **Therapeutic Effects:** Prevention of vascular spasm after subarachnoid hemorrhage, resulting in decreased neurologic impairment.

Pharmacokinetics

Absorption: Well absorbed following oral administration but extensively metabolized, resulting in ↓ bioavailability.

Distribution: Crosses the blood-brain barrier; remainder of distribution unknown.

Protein Binding: >95%.

Metabolism and Excretion: Mostly metabolized by the liver; ≤10% excreted unchanged by kidneys.

Half-life: 1–2 hr.

TIME/ACTION PROFILE (vasodilation)

ROUTE	ONSET	PEAK	DURATION
PO	unknown	1 hr	4 hr

Contraindications/Precautions

Contraindicated in: Hypersensitivity; Systolic BP <90 mm Hg; Concurrent use of strong CYP3A4 inhibitors (↑ risk of hypotension); Concurrent use of strong CYP3A4 inducers (↓ efficacy).

Use Cautiously in: Severe hepatic impairment (dose ↓ recommended); Severe renal impairment; History of serious ventricular arrhythmias or HF; OB, Lactation, Pedi: Safety not established; Geri: Dose ↓ recommended due to↑ risk of hypotension.

Adverse Reactions/Side Effects

CNS: abnormal dreams, anxiety, confusion, dizziness, drowsiness, headache, nervousness, psychiatric disturbances, weakness. **EENT:** blurred vision, disturbed equilibrium, epistaxis, tinnitus. **Resp:** cough, dyspnea. **CV:** ARRHYTHMIAS, HF, chest pain, hypotension, palpitations, peripheral edema, syncope, tachycardia. **GI:** ↑ liver enzymes, anorexia, constipation, diarrhea, dry mouth, dysgeusia, dyspepsia, nausea, vomiting. **GU:** dysuria, nocturia, polyuria, sexual dysfunction, urinary frequency. **Derm:** dermatitis, erythema multiforme, flushing, ↑ sweating, photosensitivity, pruritus/urticaria, rash. **Endo:** gynecomastia, hyperglycemia. **Hemat:** anemia, leukopenia, thrombocytopenia. **Metab:** weight gain. **MS:** joint stiffness, muscle cramps. **Neuro:** paresthesia, tremor. **Misc:** STEVENS-JOHNSON SYNDROME, gingival hyperplasia.

Interactions

Drug-Drug: **Strong CYP3A4 inhibitors**, including **clarithromycin**, **indinavir**, **nelfinavir**, **ritonavir**, **saquinavir**, **ketoconazole**, **itraconazole**, **posaconazole**, **voriconazole**, **conivaptan**, and **nefazodone** may ↑ levels and the risk of hypotension; avoid concurrent use. **Strong CYP3A4 inducers**, including **carbamazepine**, **phenobarbital**, **phenytoin**, and **rifampin** may ↓ levels and effects; avoid concurrent use. Additive hypotension may occur when used concurrently with **fentanyl**, other **antihypertensives**, **nitrates**, acute ingestion of **alcohol**, or **quinidine**.
Drug-Natural Products: **St. John's wort** may ↓ levels and effect; avoid concurrent use.
Drug-Food: **Grapefruit** and **grapefruit juice** ↑ levels and effect; avoid concurrent use.

Route/Dosage

PO (Adults): 60 mg every 4 hr for 21 days; therapy should be started within 96 hr of subarachnoid hemorrhage.

Hepatic Impairment

PO (Adults): 30 mg every 4 hr for 21 days; therapy should be started within 96 hr of subarachnoid hemorrhage.

Availability (generic available)

Capsules: 30 mg. **Oral solution:** 3 mg/mL.

NURSING IMPLICATIONS

Assessment

- Assess patient's neurologic status (level of consciousness, movement) prior to and periodically following administration.
- Monitor BP and pulse prior to therapy and periodically during therapy.
- Monitor intake and output ratios and daily weight. Assess for signs of HF (peripheral edema, rales/crackles, dyspnea, weight gain, jugular venous distention).
- Assess for rash periodically during therapy. May cause Stevens-Johnson syndrome. Discontinue therapy if severe or if accompanied with fever, general malaise, fatigue, muscle or joint aches, blisters, oral lesions, conjunctivitis, hepatitis, and/or eosinophilia.
- ***Lab Test Considerations:*** Total serum calcium concentrations are not affected by calcium channel blockers.
- Monitor serum potassium periodically. Hypokalemia ↑ risk of arrhythmias; should be corrected.
- Monitor renal and hepatic functions periodically. Several days of therapy may cause ↑ hepatic enzymes, which return to normal upon discontinuation of therapy.
- May occasionally cause ↓ platelet count.

Implementation

- Do not confuse nimodipine with nicardipine or nifedipine.
- Begin administration within 96 hr of subarachnoid hemorrhage and continue every 4 hr for 21 consecutive days.
- Administer by PO route ONLY; when administered IV or parenterally, may cause serious adverse events, including death.
- **PO:** If patient is unable to swallow capsule, make a hole in both ends of the capsule with a sterile 18-gauge needle and extract the contents into a syringe. Empty contents into water or nasogastric tube and flush with 30 mL normal saline.
- Administer oral solution 1 hr before or 2 hr after meals. For administration via NG or gastric tube, administer via syringe included, then refill syringe with 20 mL of 0.9% saline water solution; flush remaining contents from NG or gastric tube into stomach.

Patient/Family Teaching

- Advise patient to take medication as directed, even if feeling well. Take missed doses as soon as possible unless almost time for next dose; do not double doses. May need to be discontinued gradually.
- Advise patient to avoid grapefruit or grapefruit juice during therapy.
- Caution patient to change positions slowly to minimize orthostatic hypotension.
- May cause drowsiness or dizziness. Advise patient to avoid driving or other activities requiring alertness until response to the medication is known.
- Instruct patient to notify health care professional of all Rx or OTC medications, vitamins, or herbal products being taken and to avoid concurrent use of al-

N

cohol or OTC medications and herbal products, especially cold preparations, without consulting health care professional.

- Advise patient to notify health care professional if rash, irregular heartbeats, dyspnea, swelling of hands and feet, pronounced dizziness, nausea, constipation, or hypotension occurs or if headache is severe or persistent.
- Caution patient to wear protective clothing and use sunscreen to prevent photosensitivity reactions.
- Advise female patient to notify health care professional if pregnancy is planned or suspected or if breast feeding.

Evaluation/Desired Outcomes

- Improvement in neurologic deficits due to vasospasm following subarachnoid hemorrhage.

niraparib (nye-rap-a-rib)

Zejula

Classification

Therapeutic: antineoplastics

Pharmacologic: enzyme inhibitors

Indications

Maintenance treatment of recurrent epithelial ovarian, fallopian tube, or primary peritoneal cancer in patients who are in a complete or partial response to platinum-based chemotherapy.

Action

Acts as a poly (ADP-ribose) polymerase (PARP-1 and PARP-2) inhibitor; results in DNA damage, apoptosis, and cell death. **Therapeutic Effects:** Decreased progression of ovarian, fallopian tube, or primary peritoneal cancer and improved survival.

Pharmacokinetics

Absorption: 73% absorbed following oral administration.

Distribution: Extensively distributed to tissues.

Metabolism and Excretion: Primarily metabolized by carboxylesterases to an inactive metabolite; 48% excreted in urine (11% as unchanged drug), 39% in feces (19% as unchanged drug).

Half-life: 36 hr.

TIME/ACTION PROFILE (blood levels)

ROUTE	ONSET	PEAK	DURATION
PO	unknown	3 hr	24 hr

Contraindications/Precautions

Contraindicated in: OB: Pregnancy (may cause fetal harm); Lactation: Lactation.

Use Cautiously in: Ischemic heart disease, arrhythmias, or hypertension; Severe renal impairment (CCr <30 mL/min); Moderate or severe hepatic impairment; Rep: Women of reproductive potential; Pedi: Safety and effectiveness not established.

Adverse Reactions/Side Effects

CNS: anxiety, dizziness, fatigue, headache, insomnia. **CV:** palpitations, hypertension. **Derm:** rash. **GI:** abdominal pain/distention, constipation, ↓ appetite, diarrhea, dry mouth, dysgeusia, dyspepsia, ↑ liver enzymes, nausea, stomatitis, vomiting. **GU:** urinary tract infection, ↓ fertility (males). **Hemat:** MYELODYSPLASTIC SYNDROME/ACUTE MYELOID LEUKEMIA, NEUTROPENIA, anemia, leukopenia, thrombocytopenia. **MS:** arthralgia, myalgia. **Resp:** cough, dyspnea.

Interactions

Drug-Drug: None reported.

Route/Dosage

PO (Adults): 300 mg once daily. Continue until disease progression or unacceptable toxicity.

Availability

Capsules: 100 mg.

NURSING IMPLICATIONS

Assessment

- Monitor for signs and symptoms of myelodysplastic syndrome (MDS) or acute myeloid leukemia (AML) (weakness, feeling tired, fever, weight loss, frequent infections, bruising, bleeding easily, breathlessness, blood in urine or stool, and/or low blood cell counts, or need for blood transfusions) periodically during therapy.
- Monitor BP and HR weekly for first 2 mo, then monthly for first year and periodically during therapy. Closely monitor patients with cardiovascular disorders, especially coronary insufficiency, cardiac arrhythmias, and hypertension. Manage hypertension with antihypertensive medications and adjustment of nirapanib dose, if necessary.
- ***Lab Test Considerations:*** Verify negative pregnancy test before starting therapy.
- Monitor CBC weekly for first mo, monthly for next 11 mo, and periodically during therapy. Do not start niraparib until recovery of hematological toxicity from previous chemotherapy has recovered. **If platelet count <100,000 mm³/L:** *First occurrence:* Hold niraparib for a maximum of 28 days and monitor blood counts weekly until platelet counts return to ≥100,000 mm³/L. Resume at same or reduced dose. If platelet count is <75,000 mm³/L, resume at a reduced dose. *Second occurrence:* Hold niraparib for a maximum of 28 days and monitor blood counts weekly until platelet counts return to ≥100,000 μL. Resume at a reduced dose. Discontinue niraparib if platelet count has not returned to acceptable levels within 28 days of the dose interruption period, or if dose already reduced to 100 mg once daily. *For platelet count ≤10,000/mm³/L,* consider platelet transfusion. If other risk factors such as co-administration of anticoagulation or antiplatelet drugs exist, consider interrupting these

drugs and/or transfusion. Resume therapy at a reduced dose.

- *If neutrophil <1,000/µL or Hemoglobin <8 g/dL:* Hold niraparib for a maximum of 28 days and monitor blood counts weekly until neutrophil counts return to ≥1,500/µL or hemoglobin returns to ≥9 g/dL. Resume at a reduced dose. Discontinue therapy if neutrophils and/or hemoglobin have not returned to acceptable levels within 28 days of dose interruption, or if dose already reduced to 100 mg once daily.
- May cause anemia.
- May cause ↑ AST and ALT.

Implementation

- Do not confuse niraparib with neratinib or nilotinib.
- **PO:** Administer once daily, at the same time each day, without regard to food. Nausea may be minimized by administering at bedtime. Swallow capsules whole; do not open, crush, or chew.

Patient/Family Teaching

- Instruct patient to take niraparib as directed at the same time each day. Do not stop therapy without consulting health care professional. If dose missed or patient vomits after dose, omit and take next dose at scheduled time; do not double doses. Advise patient to read *Patient Information* before starting therapy and with each Rx refill in case of changes.
- Advise patient to notify health care professional if symptoms of MDS or AML (weakness, fever, feeling tired, weight loss, shortness of breath, blood in urine or stool, frequent infections, unusual bruising or bleeding) occur.
- Advise patient to notify health care professional of all Rx or OTC medications, vitamins, or herbal products being taken and consult health care professional before taking any new medications.
- Rep: May be teratogenic. Advise patient to use effective contraception during and for 6 mo after last dose and to avoid breast feeding during and for 1 mo after last dose of therapy. Inform male patients niraparib may impair fertility.

Evaluation/Desired Outcomes

- Decreased progression of ovarian, fallopian tube, or primary peritoneal cancer and improved survival.

BEERS

nitrofurantoin

(nye-troe-fyoor-**an**-toyn)

Furadantin, Furantoin, Macrobid, Macrodantin

Classification

Therapeutic: anti-infectives

Indications

Prevention and treatment of urinary tract infections caused by susceptible organisms; not effective in systemic bacterial infections.

Action

Interferes with bacterial enzymes. **Therapeutic Effects:** Bactericidal or bacteriostatic action against susceptible organisms. **Spectrum:** Many gram-negative and some gram-positive organisms, specifically: *Citrobacter, Corynebacterium, Enterobacter, Escherichia coli, Klebsiella, Neisseria, Salmonella, Shigella, Staphylococcus aureus, Staphylococcus epidermidis, Enterococcus.*

Pharmacokinetics

Absorption: Readily absorbed after oral administration. Absorption is slower but more complete with macrocrystals (Macrodantin).

Distribution: Crosses placenta; enters breast milk.

Protein Binding: 40%.

Metabolism and Excretion: Partially metabolized by the liver; 30–50% excreted unchanged by the kidneys.

Half-life: 20 min (↑ in renal impairment).

TIME/ACTION PROFILE (urine levels)

ROUTE	ONSET	PEAK	DURATION
PO	unknown	30 min	6–12 hr

Contraindications/Precautions

Contraindicated in: Hypersensitivity; Hypersensitivity to parabens (suspension); Oliguria, anuria, or significant renal impairment (CCr <60 mL/min); History of cholestatic jaundice or hepatic impairment with previous use of nitrofurantoin; Pregnancy near term and infants <1 mo (↑ risk of hemolytic anemia).

Use Cautiously in: Glucose-6-phosphate dehydrogenase (G6PD) deficiency (↑ risk of hemolytic anemia, especially in Blacks and Mediterranean and Near-Eastern ethnic groups); Patients with diabetes or debilitated patients (neuropathy may be more common); OB: Safety not established but has been used safely in pregnant women. Lactation: May cause hemolysis in infants with G6PD deficiency who are breast fed; Geri: Appears on Beers list; ↑ risk for renal, hepatic, and pulmonary reactions.

Adverse Reactions/Side Effects

CNS: dizziness, drowsiness, headache. **EENT:** nystagmus. **Resp:** PNEUMONITIS, PULMONARY FIBROSIS. **CV:** chest pain. **GI:** HEPATOTOXICITY, CLOSTRIDIUM DIFFICILE-ASSOCIATED DIARRHEA (CDAD), <u>anorexia</u>, <u>nausea</u>, <u>vomiting</u>, abdominal pain, diarrhea. **GU:** rust/brown discoloration of urine. **Derm:** photosensitivity. **Hemat:** blood dyscrasias, hemolytic anemia. **Neuro:** peripheral neuropathy. **Misc:** <u>hypersensitivity reactions</u>.

Interactions

Drug-Drug: Probenecid prevents high urinary concentrations; may ↓ effectiveness. **Antacids** may ↓ absorption. ↑ risk of neurotoxicity with **neurotoxic drugs**. ↑ risk of hepatotoxicity with **hepatotoxic drugs**. ↑ risk of pneumonitis with **drugs having pulmonary toxicity**.

Route/Dosage

PO (Adults): *Treatment of active infection*—50–100 mg every 6–8 hr *or* 100 mg every 12 hr as extended-release product. *Chronic suppression*—50–100 mg single evening dose.

PO (Children >1 mo): *Treatment of active infection*—5–7 mg/kg/day divided every 6 hr; maximum dose: 400 mg/day. *Chronic suppression*—1–2 mg/kg/day as a single dose at bedtime; maximum dose: 100 mg/day (unlabeled).

Availability (generic available)

Oral suspension: 25 mg/5 mL. **Cost:** *Generic*—$608.68/230 mL. **Capsules:** 25 mg, 50 mg, 100 mg. **Cost:** *Generic*—50 mg $199.00/100, 100 mg $338.00/100. **Extended-release capsules:** 100 mg. **Cost:** *Generic*—$320.92/100.

NURSING IMPLICATIONS

Assessment

- Assess for signs and symptoms of urinary tract infection (frequency, urgency, pain, and burning on urination; fever; cloudy or foul-smelling urine) before and periodically during therapy.
- Obtain specimens for culture and sensitivity before and during drug administration.
- Monitor intake and output ratios. Report significant discrepancies in totals.
- Monitor bowel function. Diarrhea, abdominal cramping, fever, and bloody stools should be reported to health care professional promptly as a sign of Clostridium difficile-associated diarrhea (CDAD). May begin up to several wk following cessation of therapy.
- Assess for signs and symptoms of pulmonary reactions periodically during therapy. Acute reactions (fever, chills, cough, chest pain, dyspnea, pulmonary infiltration with consolidation or pleural effusion on x-ray, eosinophilia) usually occur within first wk of treatment and resolve when therapy is discontinued. Chronic reactions (malaise, dyspnea on exertion, cough, altered pulmonary function) may indicate pneumonitis or pulmonary fibrosis and are more common in patients taking nitrofurantoin for 6 mo or longer.
- ***Lab Test Considerations:*** Monitor CBC routinely with patients on prolonged therapy.
- Monitor liver function tests periodically during therapy. May cause ↑ serum glucose, bilirubin, alkaline phosphatase, BUN, and creatinine. If hepatotoxicity occurs, discontinue therapy.
- Monitor renal function periodically during therapy.

Implementation

- **PO:** Administer with food or milk to minimize GI irritation, to delay and increase absorption, to increase peak concentration, and to prolong duration of therapeutic concentration in the urine.
- Do not crush tablets or open capsules.
- Administer liquid preparations with calibrated measuring device. Shake well before administration. Oral suspension may be mixed with water, milk, fruit juices, or infant formula. Rinse mouth with water after administration of oral suspension to avoid staining teeth.

Patient/Family Teaching

- Instruct patient to take medication around the clock, as directed. Take missed doses as soon as remembered and space next dose 2–4 hr apart. Do not skip or double up on missed doses.
- May cause dizziness or drowsiness. Caution patient to avoid driving or other activities requiring alertness until response to medication is known.
- Inform patient that medication may cause a rust-yellow to brown discoloration of urine, which is not significant.
- Advise patient to notify health care professional if fever, chills, cough, chest pain, dyspnea, skin rash, numbness or tingling of the fingers or toes, or intolerable GI upset occurs. Signs of superinfection (milky, foul-smelling urine; perineal irritation; dysuria) should also be reported.
- Instruct patient to notify health care professional if fever and diarrhea develop, especially if stool contains blood, pus, or mucus. Advise patient not to treat diarrhea without consulting health care professional.
- Instruct patient to consult health care professional if no improvement is seen within a few days after initiation of therapy.

Evaluation/Desired Outcomes

- Resolution of the signs and symptoms of infection. Therapy should be continued for a minimum of 7 days and for at least 3 days after the urine has become sterile.
- Decrease in the frequency of infections in chronic suppressive therapy.

NITROGLYCERIN

(nye-tro-**gli**-ser-in)

nitroglycerin extended-release capsules
Nitro-Time, ✤Nitrogard SR

nitroglycerin intravenous
~~Nitro-Bid IV~~, ✤Nitroject, ~~Tridil~~

nitroglycerin sublingual powder
GoNitro

nitroglycerin sublingual tablets
Nitrostat

nitroglycerin transdermal ointment
Nitro-Bid, ✱Nitrol

nitroglycerin transdermal patch
Minitran, Nitro-Dur, ✱Trinipatch

nitroglycerin translingual spray
Nitrolingual, Nitromist, ✱Rho-Nitro

Classification
Therapeutic: antianginals
Pharmacologic: nitrates

Indications

Acute (**translingual, SL, ointment**) and long-term prophylatic (**oral, transdermal**) management of angina pectoris. **PO:** Adjunct treatment of HF. **IV:** Adjunct treatment of acute MI. Production of controlled hypotension during surgical procedures. Treatment of HF.

Action

Increases coronary blood flow by dilating coronary arteries and improving collateral flow to ischemic regions. Produces vasodilation (venous greater than arterial). Decreases left ventricular end-diastolic pressure and left ventricular end-diastolic volume (preload). Reduces myocardial oxygen consumption. **Therapeutic Effects:** Relief or prevention of anginal attacks. Increased cardiac output. Reduction of BP.

Pharmacokinetics

Absorption: Well absorbed after oral, buccal, and sublingual administration. Also absorbed through skin. Orally administered nitroglycerin is rapidly metabolized, leading to ↓ bioavailability.
Distribution: Unknown.
Metabolism and Excretion: Undergoes rapid and almost complete metabolism by the liver; also metabolized by enzymes in bloodstream.
Half-life: 1–4 min.

TIME/ACTION PROFILE (cardiovascular effects)

ROUTE	ONSET	PEAK	DURATION
SL/Translingual	1–3 min	unknown	30–60 min
PO-ER	40–60 min	unknown	8–12 hr
Oint	20–60 min	unknown	4–8 hr
Patch	40–60 min	unknown	8–24 hr
IV	immediate	unknown	several min

Contraindications/Precautions

Contraindicated in: Hypersensitivity; ↑ intracranial pressure; Severe anemia; Pericardial tamponade; Constrictive pericarditis; Uncorrected hypovolemia; Alcohol intolerance (large IV doses only); Concurrent use of PDE-5 inhibitor (avanafil, sildenafil, tadalafil, vardenafil) or riociguat.
Use Cautiously in: Head trauma or cerebral hemorrhage; Glaucoma; Hypertrophic cardiomyopathy; Severe liver impairment; Malabsorption or hypermotility (PO); Cardioversion (remove transdermal patch before procedure); OB: May compromise maternal/fetal circulation; Lactation, Pedi: Safety not established.

Adverse Reactions/Side Effects

CNS: dizziness, headache, apprehension, restlessness, weakness. **EENT:** blurred vision. **CV:** hypotension, tachycardia, syncope. **GI:** abdominal pain, nausea, vomiting. **Derm:** contact dermatitis (transdermal). **Misc:** alcohol intoxication (large IV doses only), cross-tolerance, flushing, tolerance.

Interactions

Drug-Drug: Concurrent use of **avanafil**, **sildenafil**, **tadalafil**, or **vardenafil** may result in severe hypotension (do not use within 24 hr of isosorbide dinitrate or mononitrate); concurrent use contraindicated. Concurrent use of **riociguat** may result in severe hypotension; concurrent use contraindicated. Additive hypotension with **antihypertensives**, acute ingestion of **alcohol**, **beta blockers**, **calcium channel blockers**, **haloperidol**, or **phenothiazines**. Agents having anticholinergic properties (**tricyclic antidepressants**, **antihistamines**, **phenothiazines**) may ↓ absorption of translingual or sublingual nitroglycerin.

Route/Dosage

SL (Adults): *Tablets*—0.3–0.6 mg; may repeat every 5 min for 2 additional doses for acute attack; may also be used prophylactically 5–10 min before activities that may precipitate an acute attack. *Powder*—1–2 packets (400–800 mcg); may then administer 1 packet every 5 min (not to exceed 3 packets within 15–min period); may also be used prophylactically 5–10 min before activities that may precipitate an acute attack.
Translingual Spray (Adults): 1–2 sprays; may be repeated every 5 min for 2 additional doses for acute attack; may also be used prophylactically 5–10 min before activities that may precipitate an acute attack.
PO (Adults): 2.5–9 mg every 8–12 hr.
IV (Adults): 5 mcg/min; ↑ by 5 mcg/min every 3–5 min to 20 mcg/min; if no response, ↑ by 10–20 mcg/min every 3–5 min (dosing determined by hemodynamic parameters; max: 200 mcg/min).
Transdermal (Adults): *Ointment*—1–2 in. every 6–8 hr. *Transdermal patch*—0.2–0.4 mg/hr initially; may titrate up to 0.4–0.8 mg/hr. Patch should be worn 12–14 hr/day and then taken off for 10–12 hr/day.

Availability (generic available)

Extended-release capsules: 2.5 mg, 6.5 mg, 9 mg. **Sublingual powder:** 400 mcg/pkt. **Sublingual tab-**

N

lets: 0.3 mg, 0.4 mg, 0.6 mg. **Translingual spray:** 400 mcg/spray in 4.9–g bottle (60 doses) or 14.6-g bottle (200 doses) (Nitrolingual), 400 mcg/spray in 8.5–g bottle (230 doses) (Nitromist). **Transdermal patch:** 0.1 mg/hr, 0.2 mg/hr, 0.3 mg/hr, 0.4 mg/hr, 0.6 mg/hr, 0.8 mg/hr. **Transdermal ointment:** 2%. **Solution for injection:** 5 mg/mL. **Premixed solution (in D5W):** 25 mg/250 mL, 50 mg/250 mL, 100 mg/250 mL.

NURSING IMPLICATIONS

Assessment

- Assess location, duration, intensity, and precipitating factors of patient's anginal pain.
- Monitor BP and pulse before and after administration. Patients receiving IV nitroglycerin require continuous ECG and BP monitoring. Additional hemodynamic parameters may be monitored.
- ***Lab Test Considerations:*** May cause ↑ urine catecholamine and urine vanillylmandelic acid concentrations.
- Excessive doses may cause ↑ methemoglobin concentrations.
- May cause falsely ↑ serum cholesterol levels.

Implementation

- **PO:** Administer dose 1 hr before or 2 hr after meals with a full glass of water for faster absorption. Sustained-release preparations should be swallowed whole; do not break, crush, or chew.
- **SL:** Tablet should be held under tongue until dissolved. Avoid eating, drinking, or smoking until tablet is dissolved.
- **SL Powder:** Administer 1–2 packets under tongue at onset of attack. Empty contents of packet under tongue; close mouth and breathe normally. Allow powder to dissolve without swallowing. Do not rinse mouth or spit for 5 min after dosing.
- **Translingual spray:** Spray *Nitrolingual* under tongue. Spray *Nitromist* on or under tongue.

IV Administration

- **IV:** Doses must be diluted and administered as an infusion. Standard infusion sets made of polyvinyl chloride (PVC) plastic may absorb up to 80% of the nitroglycerin in solution. Use glass bottles only and special tubing provided by manufacturer.
- **Continuous Infusion:** ***Diluent:*** Vials must be diluted in D5W or 0.9% NaCl. Premixed infusions already diluted in D5W and are ready to be administered (no further dilution needed). Admixed solutions stable for 48 hr at room temperature or 7 days if refrigerated. Stability of premixed solutions based on manufacturer's expiration date. ***Concentration:*** Should not exceed 400 mcg/mL. ***Rate:*** See Route/Dosage section. Administer via infusion pump to ensure accurate rate. Titrate rate according to patient response.
- **Y-Site Compatibility:** acyclovir, alemtuzumab, alfentanil, amikacin, aminocaproic acid, aminophylline, amiodarone, amphotericin B deoxycholate, amphotericin B lipid complex, amphotericin B liposome, ampicillin, ampicillin/sulbactam, anidulafungin, argatroban, ascorbic acid, atracurium, atropine, azithromycin, aztreonam, benztropine, bivalirudin, bleomycin, bumetanide, buprenorphine, butorphanol, calcium chloride, calcium gluconate, cangrelor, carboplatin, carmustine, caspofungin, cefazolin, cefotaxime, cefotetan, cefoxitin, ceftazidime, ceftriaxone, cefuroxime, chloramphenicol, chlorpromazine, cisatracurium, cisplatin, clindamycin, cyanocobalamin, cyclophosphamide, cyclosporine, cytarabine, dactinomycin, dexamethasone, dexmedetomidine, dexrazoxane, digoxin, diltiazem, diphenhydramine, dobutamine, docetaxel, dopamine, doxorubicin hydrochloride, doxorubicin liposomal, doxycycline, enalaprilat, ephedrine, epinephrine, epirubicin, epoetin alfa, eptifibatide, ertapenem, erythromycin, esmolol, etoposide, etoposide phosphate, famotidine, fenoldopam, fentanyl, fluconazole, fludarabine, fluorouracil, folic acid, foscarnet, fosphenytoin, ganciclovir, gemcitabine, gentamicin, glycopyrrolate, granisetron, heparin, hydrocortisone, hydromorphone, idarubicin, ifosfamide, imipenem-cilastatin, indomethacin, insulin, irinotecan, isoproterenol, ketorolac, labetalol, leucovorin, lidocaine, linezolid, lorazepam, magnesium sulfate, mannitol, meperidine, mesna, methotrexate, methyldopate, methylprednisolone, metoclopramide, metronidazole, metoprolol, metronidazole, micafungin, midazolam, milrinone, minocycline, mitoxantrone, morphine, moxifloxacin, multivitamins, mycophenolate, nafcillin, nalbuphine, naloxone, nicardipine, nitroprusside, norepinephrine, octreotide, ondansetron, oxacillin, oxaliplatin, oxytocin, paclitaxel, palonosetron, pamidronate, pancuronium, pantoprazole, papaverine, pemetrexed, penicillin G, pentamidine, pentobarbital, phenobarbital, phenylephrine, phytonadione, piperacillin/tazobactam, potassium acetate, potassium chloride, procainamide, prochlorperazine, promethazine, propofol, propranolol, protamine, pyridoxine, quinupristin-dalfopristin, ranitidine, remifentanil, rocuronium, sodium bicarbonate, streptokinase, succinylcholine, sufentanil, tacrolimus, theophylline, thiamine, thiopental, thiotepa, tigecycline, tirofiban, tobramycin, topotecan, vancomycin, vasopressin, vecuronium, verapamil, vincristine, vinorelbine, voriconazole, warfarin, zoledronic acid.
- **Y-Site Incompatibility:** alteplase, dantrolene, daptomycin, diazepam, hydroxycobalamin, levofloxacin, phenytoin, trimethoprim/sulfamethoxazole.
- **Additive Incompatibility:** Manufacturer recommends that nitroglycerin not be admixed with other medications.
- **Topical:** Sites of topical application should be rotated to prevent skin irritation. Remove patch or ointment from previous site before application.
- Doses may be increased to the highest dose that does not cause symptomatic hypotension.

- Apply ointment by using dose-measuring application papers supplied with ointment. Squeeze ointment onto measuring scale printed on paper. Use paper to spread ointment onto nonhairy area of skin (chest, abdomen, thighs; avoid distal extremities) in a thin, even layer, covering a 2–3-in. area. Do not allow ointment to come in contact with hands. Do not massage or rub in ointment; this will increase absorption and interfere with sustained action. Apply occlusive dressing if ordered.
- Transdermal patches may be applied to any hairless site (avoid distal extremities or areas with cuts or calluses). Apply firm pressure over patch to ensure contact with skin, especially around edges. Apply a new dose unit if the first one becomes loose or falls off. Units are waterproof and not affected by showering or bathing. Do not cut or trim system to adjust dosage. Do not alternate between brands of transdermal products; dose may not be equivalent. Remove patches before MRI, cardioversion or defibrillation to prevent patient burns. Patch may be worn for 12–14 hr and removed for 10–12 hr at night to prevent development of tolerance.

Patient/Family Teaching

- Instruct patient to take medication as directed, even if feeling better. Take missed doses as soon as remembered unless next dose is scheduled within 2 hr (6 hr with extended-release preparations). Do not double doses. Do not discontinue abruptly; gradual dose reduction may be necessary to prevent rebound angina.
- Caution patient to change positions slowly to minimize orthostatic hypotension. First dose should be taken while in a sitting or reclining position, especially in geriatric patients.
- Advise patient to avoid concurrent use of alcohol with this medication. Patient should also consult health care professional before taking OTC medications while taking nitroglycerin.
- Inform patient that headache is a common side effect that should decrease with continuing therapy. Aspirin or acetaminophen may be ordered to treat headache. Notify health care professional if headache is persistent or severe.
- Advise patient to notify health care professional if dry mouth or blurred vision occurs.
- **Acute Anginal Attacks:** Advise patient to sit down and use medication at first sign of attack. Relief usually occurs within 5 min. Dose may be repeated if pain is not relieved in 5–10 min. Call health care professional or go to nearest emergency room if anginal pain is not relieved by 3 tablets in 15 min.
- **SL:** Inform patient that tablets should be kept in original glass container or in specially made metal containers, with cotton removed to prevent absorption. Tablets lose potency in containers made of plastic or cardboard or when mixed with other capsules or tablets. Exposure to air, heat, and moisture also causes loss of potency. Instruct patient not to open bottle frequently, handle tablets, or keep bottle of tablets next to body (i.e., shirt pocket) or in automobile glove compartment. Advise patient that tablets should be replaced 6 mo after opening to maintain potency.
- **Lingual Spray:** Instruct patient to lift tongue and spray dose under tongue (*Nitrolingual, NitroMist*) or on tongue (*NitroMist*).

Evaluation/Desired Outcomes

- Decrease in frequency and severity of anginal attacks.
- Increase in activity tolerance. During long-term therapy, tolerance may be minimized by intermittent administration in 12–14 hr or 10–12 hr off intervals.
- Controlled hypotension during surgical procedures.
- Treatment of HF associated with acute MI.

HIGH ALERT

N

nitroprusside

(nye-troe-**pruss**-ide)

✱Nipride, Nipride RTU, Nitropress

Classification

Therapeutic: antihypertensives

Pharmacologic: vasodilators

Indications

Hypertensive crises. Controlled hypotension during anesthesia. Cardiac pump failure or cardiogenic shock (alone or with dopamine).

Action

Produces peripheral vasodilation by a direct action on venous and arteriolar smooth muscle. **Therapeutic Effects:** Rapid lowering of BP. Decreased cardiac preload and afterload.

Pharmacokinetics

Absorption: IV administration results in complete bioavailability.

Distribution: Unknown.

Metabolism and Excretion: Rapidly metabolized in RBCs and tissues to cyanide and subsequently by the liver to thiocyanate.

Half-life: 2 min.

TIME/ACTION PROFILE (hypotensive effect)

ROUTE	ONSET	PEAK	DURATION
IV	immediate	rapid	1–10 min

Contraindications/Precautions

Contraindicated in: Hypersensitivity; ↓ cerebral perfusion.

Use Cautiously in: Renal disease (↑ risk of thiocyanate accumulation); Hepatic disease (↑ risk of cyanide accumulation); Hypothyroidism; Hyponatremia; Vitamin B deficiency; OB, Lactation: Safety not established; Geri: May have ↑ sensitivity to drug effects.

Adverse Reactions/Side Effects

CNS: dizziness, headache, restlessness. **CV:** dyspnea, hypotension, palpitations. **EENT:** blurred vision, tinnitus. **F and E:** acidosis. **GI:** abdominal pain, nausea, vomiting. **Local:** phlebitis at IV site. **Misc:** CYANIDE TOXICITY, thiocyanate toxicity.

Interactions

Drug-Drug: ↑ hypotensive effect with **ganglionic blocking agents**, **general anesthetics**, and other **antihypertensives**. **Estrogens** and **sympathomimetics** may ↓ the response to nitroprusside.

Route/Dosage

IV (Adults and Children): 0.3 mcg/kg/min initially; may be ↑ as needed up to 10 mcg/kg/min (usual dose is 3 mcg/kg/min; not to exceed 10 min of therapy at 10 mcg/kg/min infusion rate).

Availability (generic available)

Premixed infusion: 10 mg/50 mL 0.9% NaCl, 20 mg/100 mL 0.9% NaCl, 50 mg/100 mL 0.9% NaCl. **Solution for injection (requires dilution):** 25 mg/mL.

NURSING IMPLICATIONS

Assessment

- Monitor BP, heart rate, and ECG frequently throughout therapy; continuous monitoring is preferred. Consult physician for parameters. Monitor for rebound hypertension following discontinuation of nitroprusside.
- Pulmonary capillary wedge pressure (PCWP) may be monitored in patients with MI or HF.
- ***Lab Test Considerations:*** May cause ↓ bicarbonate concentrations, Pco_2, and pH.
- May cause ↑ lactate concentrations.
- May cause ↑ serum cyanide and thiocyanate concentrations.
- Monitor serum methemoglobin concentrations in patients receiving >10 mg/kg and exhibiting signs of impaired oxygen delivery despite adequate cardiac output and arterial Pco_2 (blood is chocolate brown without change on exposure to air). Treatment of methemoglobinemia is 1–2 mg/kg of methylene blue IV administered over several min.
- ***Toxicity and Overdose:*** If severe hypotension occurs, drug effects are quickly reversed, within 1–10 min, by decreasing rate or temporarily discontinuing infusion. May place patient in Trendelenburg position to maximize venous return.
- Monitor plasma thiocyanate levels daily in patients receiving prolonged infusions at a rate >3 mcg/kg/min or 1 mcg/kg/min in patients with anuria. Thiocyanate levels should not exceed 1 mmol/L.
- Signs and symptoms of thiocyanate toxicity include tinnitus, toxic psychoses, hyperreflexia, confusion, weakness, seizures, and coma.
- Cyanide toxicity may manifest as lactic acidosis, hypoxemia, tachycardia, altered consciousness, seizures, and characteristic breath odor similar to almonds.
- Acute treatment of cyanide toxicity includes 4–6 mg/kg of *sodium nitrite* (as a 3% solution) over 2–4 min. This acts as a buffer for cyanide by converting 10% of hemoglobin to methemoglobin. If administration of sodium nitrite is delayed, inhalation of crushed ampule (vaporole, aspirole) of *amyl nitrite* for 15–30 sec of every min should be started until sodium nitrite is running. Following completion of sodium nitrite infusion, administer *sodium thiosulfate* 150–200 mcg/kg (available as 25% and 50% solutions). This will convert cyanide to thiocyanate, which may then be eliminated. If required, entire regimen may be repeated in 2 hr at 50% of the initial doses.

Implementation

- If infusion of 10 mcg/kg/min for 10 min does not produce adequate reduction in BP, manufacturer recommends nitroprusside be discontinued.
- May be administered in left ventricular HF concurrently with an inotropic agent (dopamine, dobutamine) when effective doses of nitroprusside restore pump function and cause excessive hypotension.

IV Administration

- **Continuous Infusion:** ***Diluent:*** Dilute 50 mg of nitroprusside in 250–1000 mL of D5W. Wrap infusion in aluminum foil to protect from light; administration set tubing need not be covered. Amber plastic bags do not offer sufficient protection from light; wrap must be opaque. Freshly prepared solution has a slight brownish tint; discard if solution is dark brown, orange, blue, green, or dark red. Solution must be used within 24 hr of preparation. ***Concentration:*** 50–200 mcg/mL. ***Rate:*** Based on patient's weight (see Route/Dosage section). Administer via infusion pump to ensure accurate dosage rate.
- **Y-Site Compatibility:** alemtuzumab, alfentanil, alprostidil, amikacin, aminocaproic acid, aminophylline, amphotericin B lipid complex, amphotericin B liposome, argatroban, atropine, azithromycin, aztreonam, benztropine, bivalirudin, bleomycin, bumetanide, buprenorphine, butorphanol, calcium chloride, calcium gluconate, cangrelor, carboplatin, carmustine, cefazolin, cefotaxime, cefoxitin, ceftriaxone, cefuroxime, chloramphenicol, cisplatin, clindamycin, cyclophosphamide, cyclosporine, cytarabine, dacarbazine, daptomycin, dexamethasone, dexmedetomidine, dexrazoxane, digoxin, diltiazem, docetaxel, dopamine, doxorubicin, doxorubicin liposomal, doxycycline, enalaprilat, epinephrine, epirubicin, epoetin alfa, eptifibatide, ertapenem, esmolol, etoposide, etoposide phosphate, famotidine,

fenoldopam, fentanyl, fluconazole, fludarabine, fluorouracil, folic acid, foscarnet, fosphenytoin, furosemide, ganciclovir, gemcitabine, gentamicin, glycopyrrolate, granisetron, heparin, hetastarch, hydrocortisone, hydromorphone, idarubicin, ifosfamide, insulin, regular, isoproterenol, ketorolac, labetalol, leucovorin calcium, lidocaine, linezolid, lorazepam, magnesium sulfate, mannitol, meperidine, metaraminol, methyldopate, methylprednisolone, metoclopramide, metoprolol, metronidazole, micafungin, midazolam, milrinone, morphine, multivitamins, nafcillin, nalbuphine, naloxone, nicardipine, nitroglycerin, norepinephrine, octreotide, ondansetron, oxacillin, oxaliplatin, oxytocin, paclitaxel, palonosetron, pamidronate, pancuronium, pantoprazole, penicillin G, pentamidine, pentobarbital, phenobarbital, phentolamine, phenylephrine, phytonadione, piperacillin/tazobactam, potassium acetate, potassium chloride, potassium phosphate, procainamide, propofol, propranolol, protamine, pyridoxime, ranitidine, rocuronium, sodium acetate, sodium bicarbonate, streptokinase, succinylcholine, sufentanil, tacrolimus, theophylline, thiamine, tigecycline, tirofiban, tobramycin, tolazoline, topotecan, vancomycin, vasopressin, vecuronium, verapamil, vinblastine, vincristine, zoledronic acid.

- **Y-Site Incompatibility:** acyclovir, ascorbic acid, azathioprine, caspofungin, ceftazidime, chlorpromazine, dantrolene, daunorubicin hydrochloride, diazepam, diphenhydramine, erythromycin, hydralazine, irinotecan, levofloxacin, mesna, mitomycin, mitoxantrone, moxifloxacin, mycophentolate, papaverine, pemetrexed, phenytoin, prochlorperazine, promethazine, quinupristin/dalfopristin, thiptepa, trimethoprim/sulfamethoxazole, vinorelbine, voriconazole.

Patient/Family Teaching

- Advise patient to report the onset of tinnitus, dyspnea, dizziness, headache, or blurred vision immediately.

Evaluation/Desired Outcomes

- Decrease in BP without the appearance of side effects.
- Treatment of cardiac pump failure or cardiogenic shock.

nivolumab (nye-vol-ue-mab)

Opdivo

Classification

Therapeutic: antineoplastics

Pharmacologic: antibodies, programmed death-1 inhibitors

Indications

Unresectable/metastatic melanoma (as monotherapy or in combination with ipilimumab). Adjuvant treatment of melanoma in patients that have involvement of lymph nodes or metastatic disease and have undergone complete resection. Metastatic non-small cell lung cancer (NSCLC) with progression on or after platinum-based chemotherapy. Patients with epidermal growth factor receptor (EGFR) or anaplastic lymphoma kinase (ALK) genomic tumor aberrations should have disease progression on FDA-approved therapy for these aberrations prior to receiving nivolumab. Metastatic small cell lung cancer (SCLC) with progression after platinum-based chemotherapy and ≥1 other line of therapy. Advanced renal cell carcinoma (RCC) in patients who have previously received anti-angiogenic therapy (as monotherapy). Immediate or poor risk, previously untreated advanced RCC (in combination with ipilimumab). Classic Hodgkin's lymphoma that has relapsed or progressed after either autologous hematopoietic stem cell transplantation (HSCT) and brentuximab or ≥3 lines of systemic therapy that includes autologous HSCT. Recurrent or metastatic squamous cell carcinoma of the head and neck with progression on or after platinum-based therapy. Locally advanced or metastatic urothelial carcinoma in patients who either have progression during or following platinum-based therapy or progression within 12 mo of neoadjuvant or adjuvant treatment with platinum-based therapy. Microsatellite instability-high (MSI-H) or mismatch repair deficient (dMMR) metastatic colorectal cancer (CRC) that has progressed following treatment with a fluoropyrimidine, oxaliplatin, and irinotecan (as monotherapy or in combination with ipilimumab). Hepatocellular carcinoma (HCC) previously treated with sorafenib.

Action

Programmed death receptor-1 (PD-1) blocking antibody (an IgG4 kappa immunoglobulin) that binds to PD-1 and blocks its interaction with its ligands, PD-L1 and PD-L2, resulting in activation of the immune system and decreased tumor growth. **Therapeutic Effects:** Decreased progression of melanoma, Hodgkin's lymphoma, urothelial carcinoma, colorectal cancer, SCLC, and HCC. Decreased progression of and improved survival with NSCLC and advanced RCC. Improved survival with squamous cell carcinoma of head and neck.

Pharmacokinetics

Absorption: IV administration results in complete bioavailability.

Distribution: Unknown.

Metabolism and Excretion: Unknown.

Half-life: 26.7 days.

TIME/ACTION PROFILE

ROUTE	ONSET	PEAK	DURATION
IV	unknown	unknown	unknown

Contraindications/Precautions

Contraindicated in: OB: Pregnancy (may cause fetal harm); Lactation: Discontinue breast feeding.

Use Cautiously in: Patients undergoing allogenic HSCT before or after nivolumab therapy (↑ risk of complications); Patients with multiple myeloma receiving a thalidomide analogue and dexamethasone (↑ risk of mortality); Rep: Women of reproductive potential; Pedi: Children <12 yr (safety and effectiveness not established for MSI-H dMMR CRC); Children <18 yr (safety and effectiveness not established for all other indications).

Adverse Reactions/Side Effects

CNS: IMMUNE-MEDIATED ENCEPHALITIS. **CV:** peripheral edema. **Derm:** STEVENS-JOHNSON SYNDROME, TOXIC EPIDERMAL NECROLYSIS, rash. **Endo:** ADRENAL INSUFFICIENCY, IMMUNE-MEDIATED HYPOPHYSITIS, hypothyroidism, hyperglycemia, hyperthyroidism. **F and E:** hyperkalemia. **GI:** IMMUNE-MEDIATED COLITIS, IMMUNE-MEDIATED HEPATITIS. **GU:** immune-mediated nephritis/renal dysfunction. **Resp:** IMMUNE-MEDIATED PNEUMONITIS, cough. **Misc:** INFUSION-RELATED REACTIONS.

Interactions

Drug-Drug: None noted.

Route/Dosage

Melanoma

IV (Adults): *As monotherapy*— 240 mg every 2 wk *or* 480 mg every 4 wk until disease progression or unacceptable toxicity; *With ipilimumab*— 1 mg/kg followed by ipilimumab on the same day every 3 wk for 4 doses, then 240 mg as monotherapy every 2 wk *or* 480 mg every 4 wk until disease progression or unacceptable toxicity.

Adjuvant Treatment of Melanoma

IV (Adults): 240 mg every 2 wk *or* 480 mg every 4 wk until disease progression or unacceptable toxicity for up to 1 yr.

NSCLC, Classical Hodgkin's Lymphoma, Urothelial Carcinoma, Squamous Cell Carcinoma of Head and Neck, and HCC

IV (Adults): 240 mg every 2 wk *or* 480 mg every 4 wk until disease progression or unacceptable toxicity.

SCLC

IV (Adults): 240 mg every 2 wk until disease progression or unacceptable toxicity.

Advanced RCC

IV (Adults): *As monotherapy*— 240 mg every 2 wk *or* 480 mg every 4 wk until disease progression or unacceptable toxicity; *With ipilimumab*— 3 mg/kg followed by ipilimumab on the same day every 3 wk for 4 doses, then 240 mg as monotherapy every 2 wk *or* 480 mg every 4 wk until disease progression or unacceptable toxicity.

MSI-H dMMR CRC

IV (Adults and Children ≥12 yr and ≥40 kg): *As monotherapy*— 240 mg every 2 wk *or* 480 mg every 4 wk until disease progression or unacceptable toxicity; *With ipilimumab*— 3 mg/kg followed by ipilimumab on the same day every 3 wk for 4 doses, then 240 mg as monotherapy every 2 wk or 480 mg as monotherapy every 4 wk until disease progression or unacceptable toxicity.

IV (Children ≥12 yr and <40 kg): *As monotherapy*— 3 mg/kg every 2 wk until disease progression or unacceptable toxicity; *With ipilimumab*— 3 mg/kg followed by ipilimumab on the same day every 3 wk for 4 doses, then 3 mg/kg as monotherapy every 2 wk until disease progression or unacceptable toxicity.

Availability

Solution for injection: 10 mg/mL.

NURSING IMPLICATIONS

Assessment

- Monitor for signs and symptoms of immune-mediated pneumonitis (shortness of breath, chest pain, new or worse cough) periodically during therapy. Treat with corticosteroids 1–2 mg/kg/day prednisone equivalents for ≥Grade 2 pneumonitis followed by corticosteroid taper. Withhold nivolumab and monitor symptoms for moderate (Grade 2) pneumonitis; resume therapy when recovery to Grade 0 to 1. Permanently discontinue for severe (Grade 3) or life-threatening (Grade 4) pneumonitis.
- Assess for signs and symptoms of infusion reactions (chills or shaking, itching or rash, flushing, difficulty breathing, dizziness, fever, feeling faint) periodically during therapy. Withhold or slow infusion for mild to moderate reactions. Discontinue therapy for severe or life-threatening reactions.
- Monitor for signs and symptoms of immune-mediated colitis (diarrhea, abdominal pain, mucus or blood in stool, with or without fever). Treat with corticosteroids at doses of 1–2 mg/kg/day of prednisone or equivalents followed by corticosteroid taper for severe (Grade 3) or life-threatening (Grade 4) colitis. Treat with corticosteroids at a dose of 0.5 mg/kg/day of prednisone or equivalent followed by corticosteroid taper for moderate (Grade 2) colitis or >5 days; if worsening or no improvement despite corticosteroids increase dose to 1–2 mg/kg/day prednisone equivalents. Withhold nivolumab for Grade 2 or 3 colitis; permanently discontinue nivolumab for Grade 4 colitis or for recurrent colitis upon restarting nivolumab. *If administered with ipilimumab,* withhold for Grad 2 colitis. For moder-

ate or severe (Grade 3 or 4) or recurrent colitis, permanently discontinue nivolumb and ipilimumab.

- Monitor for signs and symptoms of hepatitis (yellowing of skin or whites of eyes, severe nausea or vomiting, right-sided abdominal pain, drowsiness, dark urine, unusual bleeding or bruising, anorexia) periodically during therapy.
- Assess for rash periodically during therapy. May cause Stevens-Johnson syndrome (SJS) and toxic epidermal necrolysis (TEN). If rash, itching, blistering, or ulcers in mouth or other mucous membranes occur, withhold dose and refer for assessment and treatment. If SJS or TEN occur, permanently discontinue therapy. Discontinue therapy if severe or if accompanied with fever, general malaise, fatigue, muscle or joint aches, blisters, oral lesions, conjunctivitis, hepatitis and/or eosinophilia. For immune-mediated rash, administer corticosteroids at doses of 1–2 mg/kg/day of prednisone or equivalents followed by corticosteroid taper for severe (Grade 3) or life-threatening (Grade 4) rash. Withhold for severe rash; permanently discontinue for life threatening rash.
- Monitor for signs and symptoms of hypophysitis (headaches, extreme tiredness, weight gain or loss, dizziness or fainting, mood changes, hair loss, feeling cold, constipation, deepening voice, excessive thirst and urination) periodically during therapy. Administer hormone replacement and corticosteroids at a dose of 1 mg/kg/day prednisone equivalents followed by corticosteroid taper for moderate or severe hypophysitis. Withhold therapy for moderate or severe hypophysitis. Discontinue for life threatening Grade 4.
- Monitor for signs and symptoms of adrenal insufficiency. Administer corticosteroids at a dose of 1–2 mg/kg/day prednisone equivalents followed by corticosteroid taper for severe (Grade 3) or life threatening (Grade 4) symptoms. Withhold for moderate (Grade 2) and permanently discontinue therapy for severe or life-threatening adrenal insufficiency.
- Monitor for signs and symptoms of encephalitis (headache, fever, tiredness or weakness, confusion, memory problems, sleepiness, hallucinations, seizures, stiff neck) periodically during therapy. Withhold therapy for patients with new-onset moderate to severe neurologic symptoms during diagnosis. Permanently discontinue nivolumab and administer corticosteroids at dose of 1–2 mg/kg/day prednisone equivalents for immune-mediated encephalitis, followed by corticosteroid taper.
- Monitor for signs and symptoms of kidney dysfunction (decrease in amount of urine, blood in urine, swelling in ankles, anorexia) periodically during therapy.
- ***Lab Test Considerations:*** Monitor for abnormal liver tests prior to and periodically during therapy. Administer corticosteroids at dose of 1–2 mg/kg/day prednisone equivalents for ≥Grade 2 transaminase ↑, with or without ↑ in total bilirubin. Withhold for moderate (Grade 2) and permanently discontinue for severe (Grade 3) or life-threatening (Grade 4) immune-mediated hepatitis.
- Monitor for ↑ serum creatinine prior to and periodically during therapy. Administer corticosteroids at a dose of 1–2 mg/kg/day prednisone equivalents followed by corticosteroid taper for life-threatening (Grade 4) ↑ serum creatinine and permanently discontinue nivolumab. Withhold nivolumab for severe (Grade 3) or moderate (Grade 2) ↑ serum creatinine and administer corticosteroids at a dose of 0.5–1 mg/kg/day prednisone equivalents followed by corticosteroid taper. If worsening or no improvement occurs, increase dose of corticosteroids to 1–2 mg/kg/day prednisolone equivalents and permanently discontinue nivolumab.
- Monitor thyroid function prior to and periodically during therapy. Treat hypothyroidism with replacement therapy. Use medical management for hyperthyroidism. Immune-mediated thyroid dysfunction does not require dose modification of nivolumab.
- Monitor for hyperglycemia. If severe, withhold therapy until metabolic control achieved. If life-threatening, permanently discontinue nivolumab.

Implementation

IV Administration

- **Intermittent Infusion: *Diluent:*** 0.9% NaCl or D5W. ***Concentration:*** 1 mg/mL to 10 mg/mL. Mix by gentle inversion; do not shake. Solution is clear to slightly opalescent, colorless to slightly yellow; do not administer solution if discolored or contains particulate matter other than translucent to white proteinaceous particles. Solution is stable at room temperature for up to 8 hr and 24 hr if refrigerated. ***Rate:*** Infuse through a sterile, non-pyrogenic, low-protein binding 0.2 micrometer to 1.2 micrometer in-line filter over 30 min. Flush line at end of infusion.
- **Y-Site Incompatibility:** Do not administer other drugs through same infusion line.

Patient/Family Teaching

- Explain purpose of nivolumab to patient.
- Advise patient to notify health care professional immediately if signs and symptoms of pneumonitis, colitis, hepatitis (jaundice, severe nausea or vomiting, pain on right side of abdomen, lethargy, easy bruising or bleeding), kidney problems (decreased urine output, blood in urine, swollen ankles, loss of appetite), hormone gland problems (rapid heart beat, weight loss, increased sweating, weight gain, hair loss, feeling cold, constipation, deepening of voice,

muscle aches, dizziness or fainting, persistent or unusual headache) occur.

- Instruct patient to notify health care professional of all Rx or OTC medications, vitamins, or herbal products being taken and to consult with health care professional before taking other medications.
- Rep: Advise females of reproductive potential to use highly effective contraception during and for 5 mo after last dose; may cause fetal harm. Avoid breast feeding during therapy.
- Emphasize importance of keeping scheduled appointments for blood work or other laboratory tests.

Evaluation/Desired Outcomes

- ↓ spread of melanoma.
- ↓ spread of NSCLC.

nizatidine, **See HISTAMINE H_2 ANTAGONISTS.**

HIGH ALERT

norepinephrine

(**nor**-ep-i-nef-rin)

Levophed

Classification

Therapeutic: vasopressors

Indications

Produces vasoconstriction and myocardial stimulation, which may be required after adequate fluid replacement in the treatment of severe hypotension and shock.

Action

Stimulates alpha-adrenergic receptors located mainly in blood vessels, causing constriction of both capacitance and resistance vessels. Also has minor beta-adrenergic activity (myocardial stimulation). **Therapeutic Effects:** Increased BP. Increased cardiac output.

Pharmacokinetics

Absorption: IV administration results in complete bioavailability.
Distribution: Concentrates in sympathetic nervous tissue. Does not cross the blood-brain barrier but readily crosses the placenta.
Metabolism and Excretion: Taken up and metabolized rapidly by sympathetic nerve endings.
Half-life: Unknown.

TIME/ACTION PROFILE (effects on BP)

ROUTE	ONSET	PEAK	DURATION
IV	immediate	rapid	1–2 min

Contraindications/Precautions

Contraindicated in: Vascular, mesenteric, or peripheral thrombosis; OB: ↓ uterine blood flow; Hypoxia; Hypercarbia; Hypotension secondary to hypovolemia (without appropriate volume replacement); Hypersensitivity to bisulfites.
Use Cautiously in: Hypertension; Concurrent use of MAO inhibitors, tricyclic antidepressants, or cyclopropane or halothane anesthetics; Hyperthyroidism; Cardiovascular disease; Lactation: Safety not established.

Adverse Reactions/Side Effects

CNS: anxiety, dizziness, headache, insomnia, restlessness, tremor, weakness. **Resp:** dyspnea. **CV:** arrhythmias, bradycardia, chest pain, hypertension. **GU:** ↓ urine output, renal failure. **Endo:** hyperglycemia. **F and E:** metabolic acidosis. **Local:** phlebitis at IV site. **Misc:** fever.

Interactions

Drug-Drug: Use with **cyclopropane** or **halothane anesthesia**, **cardiac glycosides**, **doxapram**, or local use of **cocaine** may result in ↑ myocardial irritability. Use with **MAO inhibitors**, **methyldopa**, **doxapram**, or **tricyclic antidepressants** may result in severe hypertension. **Alpha-adrenergic blockers** can prevent pressor response. **Beta blockers** may exaggerate hypertension or block cardiac stimulation. Concurrent use with **ergot alkaloids** (**ergotamine**, **methylergonovine**, or **oxytocin** may result in enhanced vasoconstriction and hypertension.

Route/Dosage

IV (Adults): 0.5–1 mcg/min initially, followed by maintenance infusion of 2–12 mcg/min titrated by BP response (average rate 2–4 mcg/min, up to 30 mcg/min for refractory shock have been used).
IV (Children): 0.1 mcg/kg/min initially; may be followed by infusion titrated to BP response, up to 1 mcg/kg/min.

Availability (generic available)

Injection: 1 mg/mL.

NURSING IMPLICATIONS

Assessment

- Monitor BP every 2–3 min until stabilized and every 5 min thereafter. Systolic BP is usually maintained at 80–100 mm Hg or 30–40 mm Hg below the previously existing systolic pressure in previously hypertensive patients. Consult physician for parameters. Continue to monitor BP frequently for hypotension following discontinuation of norepinephrine.
- ECG should be monitored continuously. CVP, intra-arterial pressure, pulmonary artery diastolic pressure, pulmonary capillary wedge pressure (PCWP), and cardiac output may also be monitored.
- Monitor urine output and notify health care professional if it decreases to <30 mL/hr.
- Assess IV site frequently throughout infusion. A large vein should be used to minimize risk of extravasation, which may cause tissue necrosis. If prolonged therapy is required or if blanching along the course

of the vein occurs, change injection sites to provide relief from vasoconstriction.

- ***Toxicity and Overdose:*** If overdose occurs, discontinue norepinephrine and administer fluid and electrolyte replacement therapy. An alpha-adrenergic blocking agent may be administered intravenously to treat hypertension.

Implementation

- ***High Alert:*** Vasoactive medications are inherently dangerous. Have second practitioner independently check original order, dose calculations, and infusion pump programming. Establish maximum dose limits. Norepinephrine overdose can result in severe peripheral vasoconstriction with resultant ischemia and necrosis of peripheral tissue. Assess peripheral circulation frequently.
- Volume depletion should be corrected, if possible, prior to initiation of norepinephrine.
- Heparin may be added to each 500 mL of solution to prevent thrombosis in the infused vein, perivenous reactions, and necrosis in patients with severe hypotension following MI.
- Norepinephrine may deplete plasma volume and cause ischemia of vital organs, resulting in hypotension when discontinued, if used for prolonged periods. Prolonged or large doses may also decrease cardiac output.
- Infusion should be discontinued gradually, upon adequate tissue perfusion and maintenance of BP, to prevent hypotension. Do not resume therapy unless BP falls to 70–80 mm Hg.

IV Administration

- **Continuous Infusion:** ***Diluent:*** Dilute 4 mg in 1000 mL of D5W or D5/0.9% NaCl. Do not dilute in 0.9% NaCl without dextrose. ***Concentration:*** 4 mcg/mL. Do not use discolored solutions (pink, yellow, brown) or those containing a precipitate. ***Rate:*** Titrate infusion rate according to patient response, using slowest possible rate to correct hypotension. Administer via infusion pump to ensure accurate dosage.
- **Y-Site Compatibility:** alemtuzumab, alfentanil, amikacin, anidulafungin, argatroban, ascorbic acid, atracurium, atropine, aztreonam, benztropine, bivalirudin, bleomycin, bumetanide, buprenorphine, butorphanol, calcium chloride, calcium gluconate, carboplatin, carmustine, caspofungin, cefazolin, cefotaxime, cefotetan, cefoxitin, ceftaroline, ceftazidime, ceftriaxone, cefuroxime, chloramphenicol, chlorpromazine, cisatracurium, cisplatin, clindamycin, cyanocobalamin, cyclophosphamide, cyclosporine, cytarabine, dactinomycin, daptomycin, dexamethasone, dexrazoxane, digoxin, diltiazem, diphenhydramine, dobutamine, docetaxel, dopamine, doxycycline, doxorubicin liposomal, enalaprilat, ephedrine, epinephrine, epirubicin, epoetin alfa, ertapenem, erythromycin, esmolol, etoposide, etoposide phosphate, famotidine, fenoldopam, fentanyl, fluconazole, fludarabine, gemcitabine, gentamicin, glycopyrrolate, granisetron, heparin, hetastarch, hydrocortisone sodium succinate, hydromorphone, idarubicin, ifosfamide, imipenem/cilastatin, irinotecan, isoproterenol, ketorolac, labetalol, leucovorin calcium, lidocaine, linezolid, lorazepam, magnesium sulfate, mannitol, meperidine, meropenem, metaraminol, methotrexate, methoxamine, methyldopate, methylprednisolone, metoclopramide, metoprolol, metronidazole, micafungin, midazolam, milrinone, mitoxantrone, morphine, moxifloxacin, multivitamins, mycophenolate, nafcillin, nalbuphine, naloxone, nicardipine, nitroglycerin, nitroprusside, octreotide, ondansetron, oxacillin, oxaliplatin, oxytocin, paclitaxel, palonosetron, pamidronate, pancuronium, papaverine, pemetrexed, penicillin G, pentamidine, phenylephrine, phytonadione, piperacillin/tazobactam, potassium acetate, potassium chloride, procainamide, prochlorperazine, promethazine, propofol, propranolol, protamine, pyridoxime, ranitidine, remifentanil, streptokinase, succinylcholine, sufentanil, tacrolimus, telavancin, theophylline, thiamine, thiotepa, tigecycline, tirofiban, tobramycin, tolazoline, vancomycin, vasopressin, vecuronium, verapamil, vinblastine, vincristine, vinorelbine, vitamin B complex with C, voriconazole, zoledronic acid.
- **Y-Site Incompatibility:** aminophylline, amphotericin B deoxycholate, amphotericin B lipid complex, azathioprine, dantrolene, diazepam, diazoxide, folic acid, foscarnet, ganciclovir, indomethacin, pentobarbital, phenobarbital, phenytoin, sodium bicarbonate, thiopental, trimethoprim/sulfamethoxazole.

Patient/Family Teaching

- Instruct patient to report headache, dizziness, dyspnea, chest pain, or pain at infusion site promptly.

Evaluation/Desired Outcomes

- Increase in BP to normal range.
- Increased tissue perfusion.

norethindrone, See CONTRACEPTIVES, HORMONAL.

BEERS

nortriptyline (nor-trip-ti-leen)

Aventyl, Pamelor

Classification

Therapeutic: antidepressants
Pharmacologic: tricyclic antidepressants

N

Indications

Various forms of depression. **Unlabeled Use:** Management of chronic neurogenic pain.

Action

Potentiates the effect of serotonin and norepinephrine. Has significant anticholinergic properties. **Therapeutic Effects:** Antidepressant action that develops slowly over several wk.

Pharmacokinetics

Absorption: Well absorbed after oral administration.
Distribution: Widely distributed. Enters breast milk in small amounts; probably crosses the placenta.
Protein Binding: 92%.
Metabolism and Excretion: Mostly metabolized by the liver (CYP2D6 isoenzyme); the CYP2D6 enzyme system exhibits genetic polymorphism; ~7% of population may be poor metabolizers (PMs) and may have significantly ↑ nortriptyline concentrations and an ↑ risk of adverse effects.
Half-life: 18–28 hr.

TIME/ACTION PROFILE (antidepressant effect)

ROUTE	ONSET	PEAK	DURATION
PO	2–3 wk	6 wk	unknown

Contraindications/Precautions

Contraindicated in: Hypersensitivity; Angle-closure glaucoma; Alcohol intolerance (solution only); Brugada syndrome; Concurrent use of MAO inhibitors or MAO-like drugs (linezolid or methylene blue).
Use Cautiously in: Pre-existing cardiovascular disease; History of seizures; Asthma; May ↑ risk of suicide attempt/ideation especially during early treatment or dose adjustment; OB: Use only if clearly needed and maternal benefits outweigh risk to fetus; Lactation: May result in sedation in infant; discontinue drug or bottle-feed; Pedi: Suicide risk may be greater in children or adolescents. Safety not established in children; Geri: More susceptible to adverse reactions; dose ↓ recommended. Geriatric men with prostatic hyperplasia may be more susceptible to urinary retention.

Adverse Reactions/Side Effects

CNS: SUICIDAL THOUGHTS, drowsiness, fatigue, lethargy, agitation, confusion, extrapyramidal reactions, hallucinations, headache, insomnia. **CV:** ARRHYTHMIAS, hypotension, ECG changes. **Derm:** photosensitivity. **EENT:** blurred vision, dry eyes, dry mouth. **Endo:** gynecomastia. **GI:** constipation, nausea, paralytic ileus, unpleasant taste, weight gain. **GU:** urinary retention. **Hemat:** blood dyscrasias.

Interactions

Drug-Drug: Concurrent use with **MAO inhibitors** may result in serious potentially fatal reactions (MAO inhibitors should be stopped at least 14 days before nortriptyline therapy. Nortriptyline should be stopped at least 14 days before MAO inhibitor therapy). Concurrent use with **MAO-inhibitor like drugs**, such as **linezolid** or **methylene blue** may ↑ risk of serotonin syndrome; concurrent use contraindicated; do not start therapy in patients receiving **linezolid** or **methylene blue**; if **linezolid** or **methylene blue** need to be started in a patient receiving nortriptyline, immediately discontinue nortriptyline and monitor for signs/symptoms of serotonin syndrome for 2 wk or until 24 hr after last dose of linezolid or methylene blue, whichever comes first (may resume nortriptyline therapy 24 hr after last dose of linezolid or methylene blue). May prevent the therapeutic response to most **antihypertensives**. Hypertensive crisis may occur with **clonidine**. ↑ CNS depression with other **CNS depressants**, including **alcohol**, **antihistamines**, **opioids**, and **sedative/hypnotics**. Adrenergic effects may be ↑ with other **adrenergic agents**, including **vasoconstrictors** and **decongestants**. ↑ anticholinergic effects with other **drugs possessing anticholinergic properties**, including **antihistamines**, **antidepressants**, **atropine**, **haloperidol**, **phenothiazines**, **quinidine**, and **disopyramide**. **Cimetidine**, **fluoxetine**, or **hormonal contraceptives** ↑ blood levels and risk of toxicity. ↑ risk of agranulocytosis with **antithyroid agents**. Drugs that affect serotonergic neurotransmitter systems, including **SSRIs**, **SNRIs**, **fentanyl**, **buspirone**, **tramadol**, and **triptans** ↑ risk of serotonin syndrome.
Drug-Natural Products: Concomitant use of **kava-kava**, **valerian**, or **chamomile** can ↑ CNS depression. Use with **St. John's wort** ↑ of serotonin syndrome. ↑ anticholinergic effects with **jimson weed** and **scopolia**.

Route/Dosage

PO (Adults): 25 mg 3–4 times daily, up to 150 mg/day.
PO (Geriatric Patients or Adolescents): 30–50 mg/day in divided doses or as a single dose.

Availability (generic available)

Capsules: 10 mg, 25 mg, 50 mg, 75 mg. **Cost:** *Generic*—10 mg $40.50/100, 25 mg $80.31/100, 50 mg $145.55/100, 75 mg $221.95/100. **Oral solution:** 10 mg/5 mL. **Cost:** *Generic*—$182.95/473 mL.

NURSING IMPLICATIONS

Assessment

- Monitor mental status (orientation, mood, behavior).
- Assess weight and BMI initially and throughout treatment. For overweight/obese individuals, monitor fasting blood glucose and cholesterol levels.
- Monitor BP and pulse rate before and during initial therapy. Report significant decreases in BP or a sudden increase in pulse rate.
- Monitor baseline and periodic ECGs in geriatric patients or patients with heart disease. May cause prolonged PR and QT intervals and may flatten T waves.
- Assess for suicidal tendencies, especially during early therapy. Restrict amount of drug available to

patient. Risk may be increased in children, adolescents, and adults ≤24 yrs. After starting therapy, children, adolescents, and young adults should be seen by health care professional at least weekly for 4 wk, every 3 wk for next 4 wk, and on advice of health care professional thereafter.

- **Pain:** Assess type, location, and severity of pain before and periodically during therapy. Use pain scale to monitor effectiveness of medication.
- ***Lab Test Considerations:*** Assess leukocyte and differential blood counts, liver function, and serum glucose periodically. May cause ↑ serum bilirubin and alkaline phosphatase. May cause bone marrow depression. Serum glucose may be ↑ or ↓.
- Serum levels may be monitored in patients who fail to respond to usual therapeutic dose. Therapeutic plasma concentration range is 50–150 ng/mL.
- May cause alterations in blood glucose levels.
- ***Toxicity and Overdose:*** Symptoms of acute overdose include disturbed concentration, confusion, restlessness, agitation, seizures, drowsiness, mydriasis, arrhythmias, fever, hallucinations, vomiting, and dyspnea.
- Treatment of overdose includes gastric lavage, activated charcoal, and a stimulant cathartic. Maintain respiratory and cardiac function (monitor ECG for at least 5 days) and temperature. Medications may include digoxin for HF, antiarrhythmics, and anticonvulsants.

Implementation

- Do not confuse Pamelor (nortriptyline) with Tambocor (flecainide).
- Taper to avoid withdrawal effects. Reduce dose 50% for 3 days, then by 50% for 3 more days, then discontinue.
- **PO:** Administer medication with meals to minimize gastric irritation.
- May be given as a single dose at bedtime to minimize sedation during the day. Dose increases should be made at bedtime because of sedation.

Patient/Family Teaching

- Instruct patient to take medication as directed. Take missed doses as soon as possible unless almost time for next dose; if regimen is a single dose at bedtime, do not take in the morning because of side effects. Advise patient that drug effects may not be noticed for at least 2 wk. Abrupt discontinuation may cause nausea, vomiting, diarrhea, headache, trouble sleeping with vivid dreams, and irritability.
- May cause drowsiness and blurred vision. Caution patient to avoid driving and other activities requiring alertness until response to drug is known.
- Instruct patient to notify health care professional if visual changes occur. Inform patient that periodic glaucoma testing may be required during long-term therapy.
- Caution patient to make position changes slowly to minimize orthostatic hypotension. (This side effect is less pronounced with this medication than with other tricyclic antidepressants.).
- Advise patient, family, and caregivers to look for suicidality, especially during early therapy or dose changes. Notify health care professional immediately if thoughts about suicide or dying, attempts to commit suicide, new or worse depression or anxiety, agitation or restlessness, panic attacks, insomnia, new or worse irritability, aggressiveness, acting on dangerous impulses, mania, or other changes in mood or behavior or if symptoms of serotonin syndrome occur.
- Advise patient to avoid alcohol or other CNS depressant drugs during therapy and for at least 3–7 days after therapy has been discontinued.
- Instruct patient to notify health care professional if urinary retention occurs or if dry mouth or constipation persists. Sugarless candy or gum may diminish dry mouth, and an increase in fluid intake or bulk may prevent constipation. If symptoms persist, dose reduction or discontinuation may be necessary. Consult health care professional if dry mouth persists for more than 2 wk.
- Caution patient to use sunscreen and protective clothing to prevent photosensitivity reactions.
- Alert patient that urine may turn blue-green in color.
- Inform patient of need to monitor dietary intake. Increase in appetite may lead to undesired weight gain. Refer as appropriate for nutritional, weight, or medical management.
- Advise patient to notify health care professional of medication regimen before treatment or surgery.
- Rep: May have teratogenic effects. Advise females of reproductive potential to use effective contraception during and for at least 5 mo after last dose and to avoid breast feeding during therapy. Advise patient to notify health care professional immediately if pregnancy is planned or suspected.
- Therapy for depression is usually prolonged. Emphasize the importance of follow-up exams.

Evaluation/Desired Outcomes

- Increased sense of well-being.
- Renewed interest in surroundings.
- Increased appetite.
- Improved energy level.
- Improved sleep.
- Decrease in severity of chronic neurogenic pain. Patients may require 2–6 wk of therapy before full therapeutic effects of medication are seen.

NPH/regular insulin mixtures, See INSULIN (mixtures).

nystatin (nye-stat-in)

Mycostatin, ✤Nadostine, Nilstat, ✤PMS-Nystatin

Classification

Therapeutic: antifungals (topical/local)

For other nystatin dosage forms, see antifungals (topical) and antifungals (vaginal)

Indications

Lozenges, oral suspension: Local treatment of oropharyngeal candidiasis. Treatment of intestinal candidiasis.

Action

Binds to fungal cell membrane, allowing leakage of cellular contents. **Therapeutic Effects:** Fungistatic or fungicidal action. **Spectrum:** Active against most pathogenic *Candida* species, including *C. albicans*.

Pharmacokinetics

Absorption: Poorly absorbed; action is primarily local.
Distribution: Unknown.
Metabolism and Excretion: Excreted unchanged in the feces after oral administration.
Half-life: Unknown.

TIME/ACTION PROFILE (antifungal effects)

ROUTE	ONSET	PEAK	DURATION
Top	rapid	unknown	2 hr†

†Maintenance of saliva levels required to inhibit growth of Candida species after oral dissolution of 2 lozenges.

Contraindications/Precautions

Contraindicated in: Hypersensitivity; Some products may contain ethyl alcohol or benzyl alcohol—avoid use in patients who may be hypersensitive to or intolerant of these additives.
Use Cautiously in: Denture wearers (dentures require soaking in nystatin suspension); Pedi: Lozenges, pastilles, or troches may pose a choking risk for children <5 yr .

Adverse Reactions/Side Effects

GI: diarrhea, nausea, stomach pain (large doses), vomiting. **Derm:** contact dermatitis, Stevens-Johnson syndrome.

Interactions

Drug-Drug: None significant.

Route/Dosage

PO (Adults and Children): 400,000–600,000 units 4 times daily as oral suspension or 200,000–400,000 units 4–5 times daily as pastilles (lozenges).
PO (Infants): 200,000 units 4 times daily or 100,000 units to each side of the mouth 4 times daily.
PO (Neonates, Premature, and Low Birth Weight): 100,000 units 4 times daily or 50,000 units to each side of the mouth 4 times a day.

Availability (generic available)

Oral suspension: 100,000 units/mL. **Oral pastilles (lozenges, troches):** 200,000 units/troche. **Powder for oral suspension:** 1/8 tsp = 500,000 units. **Oral tablets:** 500,000 units.

NURSING IMPLICATIONS

Assessment

- Inspect oral mucous membranes before and frequently throughout therapy. Increased irritation of mucous membranes may indicate need to discontinue medication.

Implementation

- **PO:** Suspension should be administered by placing ½ of dose in each side of mouth. Patient should hold suspension in mouth or swish throughout mouth for several min before swallowing, then gargle and swallow. Use calibrated measuring device for liquid doses. Shake well before administration. Pedi: For neonates and infants, paint suspension into recesses of the mouth.
- To prepare oral solution from powder, add ⅛ tsp (approximately 500,000 units) to 120 mL of water and stir well. Prepare immediately before use; contains no preservatives.
- Lozenges (pastilles) should be allowed to dissolve slowly and completely in mouth; do not chew or swallow whole. Nystatin vaginal tablets can be administered orally for treatment of oral candidiasis.

Patient/Family Teaching

- Instruct patient to take medication as directed. If a dose is missed, take as soon as remembered but not if almost time for next dose. Do not double doses. Therapy should be continued for at least 2 days after symptoms subside.
- Pedi: Instruct parents or caregivers of infants and children on correct dose and administration. Remind them to use only the measuring device dispensed with the product.
- Advise patient to report increased irritation of mucous membranes or lack of therapeutic response to health care professional.

Evaluation/Desired Outcomes

- Decrease in stomatitis.
- To prevent relapse after oral therapy, therapy should be continued for 48 hr after symptoms have disappeared and cultures are negative.
- Therapy for a period of 2 wk is usually sufficient, but more prolonged therapy may be necessary.

nystatin, See ANTIFUNGALS (TOPICAL).

ocrelizumab (ok-re-liz-ue-mab)

Ocrevus

Classification

Therapeutic: anti-multiple sclerosis agents
Pharmacologic: monoclonal antibodies

Indications

Relapsing forms of multiple sclerosis (MS), including clinically isolated syndrome, relapsing-remitting disease, and active secondary progressive disease. Primary progressive MS.

Action

Binds to the CD20 antigen on pre-B and mature B lymphocytes, which results in antibody-dependent and complement-mediated cell lysis. **Therapeutic Effects:** Reduction in relapse rate and decreased progression toward disability.

Pharmacokinetics

Absorption: IV administration results in complete bioavailability.
Distribution: Binds specifically to CD20 binding sites on B lymphocytes.
Metabolism and Excretion: Unknown.
Half-life: 26 days.

TIME/ACTION PROFILE

ROUTE	ONSET	PEAK	DURATION
IV	unknown	unknown	unknown

Contraindications/Precautions

Contraindicated in: Active hepatitis B virus infection (may reactivate infection during and for several mo after treatment); History of life-threatening infusion reaction to ocrelizumab.

Use Cautiously in: Patients who are immunocompromised or receiving other immunosuppressants; OB: Can pass placental barrier potentially causing fetal B-cell depletion. Give only if clearly needed; Lactation: Weigh benefits of breast feeding against possible adverse effects; Rep: Women of reproductive potential; Pedi: Safety and effectiveness not established.

Adverse Reactions/Side Effects

CNS: PROGRESSIVE MULTIFOCAL LEUKOENCEPHALOPATHY (PML), depression. **CV:** peripheral edema. **GI:** diarrhea. **MS:** back pain. **Hemat:** neutropenia. **Resp:** cough. **Misc:** INFECTION, INFUSION REACTIONS, MALIGNANCY (primarily breast cancer).

Interactions

Drug-Drug: Concurrent use with **immunosuppressive therapies** may ↑ risk of immunosuppression. May ↓ antibody response to or ↑ risk of adverse reactions to **non-live vaccines** and **live vaccines**.

Route/Dosage

IV (Adults): 300 mg initially, then 300 mg in 2 wk, then 600 mg every 6 mo.

Availability

Solution for injection: 30 mg/mL.

NURSING IMPLICATIONS

Assessment

- Assess for active infection prior to each infusion. Delay infusion until infection resolves.
- Monitor for signs and symptoms of infusion reaction (pruritus, rash, urticaria, erythema, bronchospasm, throat irritation, oropharyngeal pain, dyspnea, pharyngeal or laryngeal edema, flushing, hypotension, pyrexia, fatigue, headache, dizziness, nausea, tachycardia) during and for at least 1 hr after completion of infusion. *If mild to moderate infusion reaction occurs,* reduce infusion rate by half at onset of reaction and for at least 30 min. If rate tolerated, increase rate (see Rate below). Will increase duration of infusion, but not total dose. *If severe reaction occurs,* immediately stop infusion and administer supportive treatment. Restart infusion only after all symptoms resolved. Restart at half rate at time of onset of reaction. If tolerated, increase (see Rate below). Will increase duration of infusion, but not total dose. *If life-threatening infusion reaction occurs,* immediately stop infusion and permanently discontinue ocrelizumab. Provide supportive treatment.
- Assess for signs and symptoms of progressive multifocal leukoencephalopathy (PML) (progressive weakness on one side of body or clumsiness of limbs, disturbance of vision, and changes in thinking, memory, and orientation leading to confusion and personality changes) periodically during therapy. Symptoms are diverse and progress over days to wk. At first sign of PML, suspend ocrelizumab and perform diagnostic evaluation. MRI findings may be apparent before clinical signs or symptoms.
- ***Lab Test Considerations:*** Determine current or prior HBV infection by measuring hepatitis B surface antigen (HBsAg) and hepatitis B core antibody (anti-HBc) before initiating therapy. Do not administer to patients with active HBV infection.

Implementation

- Administer all necessary immunizations at least 6 wk before starting therapy. Avoid immunizations during therapy and after discontinuation until B-cell repletion.
- Premedicate to reduce frequency and severity of infusion reactions with methylprednisolone 100 mg IV or equivalent 30 min and an antihistamine, diphenhydramine, 30–60 min before each infusion before each infusion. May add an antipyretic, acetaminophen.

O

- **Intermittent Infusion:** ***Diluent:*** Dilute each dose with 250 mL or 500 mL 0.9% NaCl. Do not use other diluents. Do not shake. Allow infusion bag to come to room temperature before infusion. ***Concentration:*** 1.2 mg/mL. Solution is clear or slightly opalescent, and colorless to pale brown; do not administer solutions that are discolored or contain particulate matter. Solution is stable for 24 hr if refrigerated or up to 8 hrs (including infusion time) at room temperature. ***Rate:*** Administer using a dedicated line with a 0.2 or 0.22 micron in-line filter. *For first 2 infusions (300 mg in 250 mL),* begin at 30 mL/hr. Increase by 30 mL/hr every 30 min to 180 mL/hr. over 2.5 hrs or longer. *For subsequent infusions (600 mg in 500 mL),* begin at 40 mL/hr. Increase by 40 mL/hr every 30 min to 200 mL/hr over 3.5 hrs or longer.

Patient/Family Teaching

- Explain purpose of infusions and importance of maintaining schedule to patient. If infusion is missed, administer as soon as possible; do not wait for next scheduled dose. Reset schedule for 6 mo after missed dose is given. Separate doses by at least 5 mo. Advise patient to read *Medication Guide* before starting therapy and with each dose in case of changes.
- Inform patient that infusion reactions may occur up to 24 hr after infusion. Advise patient to notify health care professional immediately if infusion reaction symptoms occur.
- Advise patient to notify health care professional if signs and symptoms of infection (fever, chills, constant cough, cold sore, shingles, genital sores) or PML (problems with thinking, balance, eyesight, weakness on 1 side of body, strength, using arms or legs) occur.
- Instruct patient to notify health care professional of all Rx or OTC medications, vitamins, or herbal products being taken and to consult health care professional before taking other Rx, OTC, or herbal products.
- Instruct patient to avoid live vaccines during therapy. Administer any live or live-attenuated vaccines ≥4 wk prior to start of therapy and administer any non-live vaccines ≥2 wk prior to start of therapy. Do not administer live or live-attenuated vaccines to infants born to mothers taking ocrelizumab until recovery of B-cell counts confirmed; may administer non-live vaccines to these infants, but should consider assessing vaccine immune responses to determine whether protective immune response mounted.
- Inform patient of increased risk of malignancy. Advise patient to receive regular breast cancer screening.
- Rep: Advise female patient of reproductive potential to use effective contraception during and for 6 mo after last infusion and to notify health care professional if breast feeding.

Evaluation/Desired Outcomes

- Reduction in relapse rate and decreased progression toward disability in patients with multiple sclerosis.

octreotide (ok-tree-oh-tide)

SandoSTATIN, SandoSTATIN LAR, SandoSTATIN LAR Depot

Classification

Therapeutic: antidiarrheals, hormones

Indications

Severe diarrhea and flushing episodes in patients with GI endocrine tumors, including metastatic carcinoid tumors and vasoactive intestinal peptide tumors (VIPomas). Acromegaly. **Unlabeled Use:** Management of diarrhea associated with, chemotherapy, or graft-versus-host disease. Gastroesophageal variceal hemorrhage.

Action

Suppresses secretion of serotonin and gastroenterohepatic peptides. Increases absorption of fluid and electrolytes from the GI tract and increases transit time. Decreases levels of serotonin metabolites. Also suppresses growth hormone, insulin, and glucagon. **Therapeutic Effects:** Normalization of growth hormone and insulin-like growth factor 1 levels. Control of severe flushing and diarrhea associated with GI endocrine tumors.

Pharmacokinetics

Absorption: Well absorbed following subcut administration and IM administration of depot form.

Distribution: Unknown.

Protein Binding: 65%.

Metabolism and Excretion: Extensive hepatic metabolism; 32% excreted unchanged in urine.

Half-life: 1.5 hr.

TIME/ACTION PROFILE (control of symptoms)

ROUTE	ONSET	PEAK	DURATION
Subcut, IV	unknown	unknown	up to 12 hr
IM (LAR depot)	unknown	2 wk	up to 4 wk

Contraindications/Precautions

Contraindicated in: Hypersensitivity.

Use Cautiously in: Gallbladder disease (↑ risk of stone formation); Renal impairment (dose ↓ may be necessary); Hyperglycemia or hypoglycemia (changes in blood glucose may occur); Fat malabsorption (may be aggravated); OB: Safety not established; Lactation: Use while breast feeding only if benefit to patient outweighs potential risk to infant; Pedi: Safety and effectiveness of depot injection not established in children.

Adverse Reactions/Side Effects

CNS: dizziness, drowsiness, fatigue, headache, weakness. **CV:** bradycardia, edema, orthostatic hypotension, palpitations. **Derm:** flushing. **EENT:** visual disturbances. **Endo:** hyperglycemia, hypoglycemia, hypothyroidism. **GI:** ILEUS, PANCREATITIS, cholelithiasis, abdominal pain, cholecystitis, diarrhea, fat malabsorption, nausea, vomiting. **Local:** injection-site pain.

Interactions

Drug-Drug: May alter requirements for **insulin** or **oral hypoglycemic agents**. May ↓ blood levels of **cyclosporine**. May ↑ levels of QTc-prolonging agents.

Route/Dosage

Carcinoid Tumors

Subcut, IV (Adults): 100–600 mcg/day in 2–4 divided doses during first 2 wk of therapy (range 50–1500 mcg/day).
IM (Adults): *Sandostatin LAR*—20 mg every 4 wk for 2 mo; dose may be further adjusted.

VIPomas

Subcut, IV (Adults): 200–300 mcg/day in 2–4 divided doses during first 2 wk of therapy (range 150–750 mcg/day).
IM (Adults): *Sanostatin LAR*—20 mg every 2 wk for 2 mo; dose may be further adjusted.

Acromegaly

Subcut, IV (Adults): 50–100 mcg 3 times daily; titrate to achieve growth hormone levels <5 ng/mL or IGF-I levels <1.9 units/mL (males) or <2.2 units/mL (females) (usual effective dose = 100–200 mcg 3 times daily).
IM (Adults): *Sandostatin LAR*—20 mg every 4 wk for 3 mo, then adjusted on the basis of growth hormone levels.

Diarrhea Associated with Chemotherapy (off-label)

Subcut, IV (Adults): 100–150 mcg subcut every 8 hr; may ↑ to 500–1500 mcg subcut or IV every 8 hr for severe diarrhea.
Subcut (Children): 1–10 mcg/kg every 8–12 hr.

Diarrhea Associated with Graft-Versus-Host Disease (off-label)

IV (Adults): 500 mcg every 8 hr; do not continue for longer than 7 days (discontinue within 24 hr of diarrhea resolution).
Subcut (Children): 1–10 mcg/kg every 8–12 hr.

Gastroesophageal Variceal Hemorrhage (off-label)

IV (Adults): 25–100 mcg bolus (may repeat in 1st hr if hemorrhage uncontrolled), followed by continuous infusion of 25–50 mcg/hr for 2–5 days.
IV (Children): 1–2 mcg/kg bolus, followed by continuous infusion of 1–2 mcg/kg/hr; taper dose by 50% every 12 hr when no active bleeding for 24 hr; discontinue when dose is 25% of initial dose.

Availability (generic available)

Solution for injection: 50 mcg/mL, 100 mcg/mL, 200 mcg/mL, 500 mcg/mL, 1000 mcg/mL. **Suspension for injection (depot):** 10 mg/6 mL, 20 mg/6 mL, 30 mg/6 mL.

NURSING IMPLICATIONS

Assessment

- Assess frequency and consistency of stools and bowel sounds throughout therapy.
- Monitor pulse and BP prior to and periodically during therapy.
- Assess patient's fluid and electrolyte balance and skin turgor for dehydration.
- Monitor diabetic patients for signs of hypoglycemia. May require reduction in requirements for insulin and sulfonylureas and treatment with diazoxide.
- Assess for gallbladder disease; assess for pain and monitor ultrasound examinations of gallbladder and bile ducts prior to and periodically during prolonged therapy.
- ***Lab Test Considerations:*** Monitor growth hormone, IGF-1 (somatomedin C) in patients with acromegaly, 5-HIAA (urinary 5-hydroxyindoleacetic acid), plasma serotonin, and plasma substance P in patients with carcinoid; plasma vasoactive intestinal peptide (VIP) in patients with VIPoma; and free T_4 and serum glucose concentrations prior to and periodically during therapy in all patients taking octreotide.
- Monitor quantitative 72-hr fecal fat and serum carotene determinations periodically for possible drug-induced aggravations of fat malabsorption.
- May cause a slight ↑ in liver enzymes.
- May cause ↓ serum thyroxine (T_4) concentrations.

Implementation

- Do not confuse Sandostatin (octreotide) with Sandimmune (cyclosporine).
- Do not use solution that is discolored or contains particulate matter. Ampules should be refrigerated but may be stored at room temperature for the days they will be used. Discard unused solution.
- **Subcut:** Administer the smallest volume needed to achieve required dose to prevent pain at injection site. Rotate injection sites; avoid multiple injections

O

in same site within short periods of time. Preferred injection sites are the hip, thigh, or abdomen.

- Administer injections between meals and at bedtime to avoid GI side effects.
- Allow medication to reach room temperature prior to injection to minimize local reactions at injection site.
- **IM:** Mix IM solution by adding diluent included in kit. Administer immediately after mixing into the gluteal muscle. Avoid using deltoid site due to pain of injection.
- Patients with carcinoid tumors and VIPomas should continue to receive subcut dose for 2 wk following switch to IM depot form to maintain therapeutic level.

IV Administration

- **IV Push:** ***Diluent:*** May be administered undiluted. ***Rate:*** Administer over 3 min.
- **Intermittent Infusion:** ***Diluent:*** Dilute in 50–200 mL of 0.9% NaCl or D5W. ***Concentration:*** 1.5–250 mcg/mL. ***Rate:*** Infuse over 15–30 min.
- **Y-Site Compatibility:** acyclovir, alfentanyl, allopurinol, amifostine, amikacin, aminocaproic acid, aminophylline, amiodarone, amphotericin B lipid complex, amphotericin B liposome, ampicillin, ampicillin/sulbactam, anidulafungin, argatroban, atracurium, azithromycin, aztreonam, bivalirudin, bleomycin, bumetanide, buprenorphine, busulfan, butorphanol, calcium chloride, calcium gluconate, capreomycin, carboplatin, carmustine, caspofungin, cefazolin, cefepime, cefotaxime, cefotetan, cefoxitin, ceftazidime, ceftriaxone, cefuroxime, chloramphenicol, chlorpromazine, ciprofloxacin, cisatracurium, cisplatin, clindamycin, cyclosporine, cytarabine, dacarbazine, dactinomycin, daptomycin, daunorubicin hydrochloride, daunorubicin liposome, dexamethasone sodium phosphate, dexmedetomidine, dexrazoxane, digoxin, diltiazem, diphenhydramine, dobutamine, docetaxel, dolasetron, dopamine, doxorubicin hydrochloride, doxorubicin liposome, doxycycline, droperidol, enalaprilat, ephedrine, epinephrine, epirubicin, eptifibitide, ertapenem, erythromycin, esmolol, etoposide, etoposide phosphate, famotidine, fenoldopam, fentanyl, fluconazole, fludarabine, fluorouracil, foscarnet, fosphenytoin, furosemide, ganciclovir, gemcitabine, gentamicin, glycopyrrolate, granisetron, haloperidol, heparin, hydralazine, hydrocortisone, hydromorphone, idarubicin, ifosfamide, imipenem/cilastatin, insulin, regular, irinotecan, isoproterenol, ketorolac, labetalol, leucovorin calcium, levofloxacin, lidocaine, linezolid, lorazepam, magnesium hydroxide, mannitol, melphalan, meperidine, meropenem, mesna, methohexital, methotrexate, methylprednisolone, methyldopate, metoclopramide, metoprolol, metronidazole, midazolam, milrinone, minocycline, mitomycin, mitoxantrone, morphine, mycophenolate, nafcillin, nalbuphine, naloxone, nicardipine, nitroglycerin, nitroprusside, norepinephrine, ondansetron, oxaliplatin, paclitaxel, palonosetron, pamidronate, pancuronium, pemetrexed, pentamidine, pentobarbital, phenobarbital, phentolamine, phenylephrine, piperacillin/tazobactam, potassium acetate, potassium chloride, potassium phosphates, procainamide, prochlorperazine, promethazine, propranolol, quinapristin/dalfopristin, ranitidine, remifentanyl, rocuronium, sodium acetate, sodium bicarbonate, sodium phosphates, streptozocin, succinylcholine, sufentanil, tacrolimus, thiopental, thiotepa, tigecycline, tirofiban, tobramycin, topotecan, trimethoprim/sulfamethoxazole, vancomycin, vasopressin, vecuronium, verapamil, vinblastine, vincristine, vinorelbine, voriconazole, zidovudine, zoledronic acid.
- **Y-Site Incompatibility:** dantrolene, diazepam, micafungin, phenytoin.

Patient/Family Teaching

- May cause dizziness, drowsiness, or visual disturbances. Caution patient to avoid driving or other activities requiring alertness until response to medication is known.
- Advise patient to change positions slowly to minimize orthostatic hypotension.
- Rep: Inform females of reproductive potential that therapy with octreotide may result in improved fertility. Caution patient to use contraception to prevent unintended pregnancy.
- **Home Care Issues:** Instruct patients administering octreotide at home on correct technique for injection, storage, and disposal of equipment.
- Instruct patient to administer octreotide exactly as directed. If a dose is missed, administer as soon as possible, then return to regular schedule. Do not double doses.

Evaluation/Desired Outcomes

- Decrease in severity of diarrhea and improvement of electrolyte imbalances in patients with carcinoid or VIP-secreting tumors.
- Relief of symptoms and suppressed tumor growth in patients with pituitary tumors associated with acromegaly.
- Management of diarrhea in patients with AIDS.

BEERS REMS

OLANZapine (oh-lan-za-peen)

ZyPREXA, ZyPREXA Relprevv, ZyPREXA Zydis

Classification

Therapeutic: antipsychotics, mood stabilizers

Pharmacologic: thienobenzodiazepines

Indications

Schizophrenia. Acute therapy of manic or mixed episodes associated with bipolar I disorder (as monother-

apy [adults and adolescents] or with lithium or valproate [adults only]). Maintenance therapy of bipolar I disorder. Acute agitation due to schizophrenia or bipolar I mania (IM). Depressive episodes associated with bipolar I disorder (when used with fluoxetine). Treatment-resistant depression (when used with fluoxetine).
Unlabeled Use: Management of anorexia nervosa. Treatment of nausea and vomiting related to highly emetogenic chemotherapy.

Action

Antagonizes dopamine and serotonin type 2 in the CNS. Also has anticholinergic, antihistaminic, and anti–alpha$_1$-adrenergic effects. **Therapeutic Effects:** Decreased manifestations of psychoses.

Pharmacokinetics

Absorption: Well absorbed but rapidly metabolized by first-pass effect, resulting in 60% bioavailability. Conventional tablets and orally disintegrating tablets (Zydis) are bioequivalent. IM administration results in significantly higher blood levels (5 times that of oral).
Distribution: Extensively distributed.
Protein Binding: 93%.
Metabolism and Excretion: Highly metabolized (mostly by the hepatic P450 CYP 1A2 system); 7% excreted unchanged in urine.
Half-life: 21–54 hr.

TIME/ACTION PROFILE (antipsychotic effects)

ROUTE	ONSET	PEAK*	DURATION
PO	unknown	6 hr	unknown
IM	rapid	15–45 min	2–4 hr

*Blood levels.

Contraindications/Precautions

Contraindicated in: Hypersensitivity; Phenylketonuria (orally disintegrating tablets contain aspartame); Lactation: Lactation.
Use Cautiously in: Hepatic impairment; Patients at risk for aspiration or falls; Cardiovascular or cerebrovascular disease; History of seizures; History of attempted suicide; Diabetes or risk factors for diabetes (may worsen glucose control); Prostatic hyperplasia; Angle-closure glaucoma; History of paralytic ileus; Dysphagia and aspiration have been associated with antipsychotic drug use; use with caution in patients at risk for aspiration; OB: Use only if potential maternal benefit justifies potential fetal risk; neonates at ↑ risk for extrapyramidal symptoms and withdrawal after delivery when exposed during the 3rd trimester; Pedi: Children <13 yr (safety and effectiveness not established); adolescents at ↑ risk for weight gain and hyperlipidemia; Geri: May require ↓ doses; ↑ risk of mortality in elderly patients treated for dementia-related psychosis.

Adverse Reactions/Side Effects

CNS: NEUROLEPTIC MALIGNANT SYNDROME, SEIZURES, SUICIDAL THOUGHTS, agitation, delirium, dizziness, headache, restlessness, sedation, weakness, dystonia, insomnia, mood changes, personality disorder, speech impairment, tardive dyskinesia. **CV:** orthostatic hypotension, bradycardia, chest pain, tachycardia. **Derm:** DRUG REACTION WITH EOSINOPHILIA AND SYSTEMIC SYMPTOMS (DRESS), photosensitivity. **EENT:** amblyopia, rhinitis, ↑ salivation, pharyngitis. **Endo:** amenorrhea, galactorrhea, goiter, gynecomastia, hyperglycemia. **GI:** constipation, dry mouth, ↑ liver enzymes, weight loss or gain, abdominal pain, ↑ appetite, nausea, ↑ thirst. **GU:** impotence, ↓ libido, urinary incontinence. **Hemat:** AGRANULOCYTOSIS, leukopenia, neutropenia. **Metab:** dyslipidemia. **MS:** hypertonia, joint pain. **Neuro:** tremor. **Resp:** cough, dyspnea. **Misc:** fever, flu-like syndrome.

Interactions

Drug-Drug: Effects may be ↓ by concurrent **carbamazepine**, **omeprazole**, or **rifampin**. ↑ hypotension may occur with **antihypertensives**. ↑ CNS depression may occur with concurrent use of **alcohol** or other **CNS depressants**; concurrent use of IM olanzapine and parenteral benzodiazepines should be avoided. May antagonize the effects of **levodopa** or other **dopamine agonists**. **Fluvoxamine** may ↑ levels. **Nicotine** can ↓ olanzapine levels.

Route/Dosage

Schizophrenia

PO (Adults —Most Patients): 5–10 mg/day initially; may ↑ at weekly intervals by 5 mg/day (target dose = 10 mg/day; not to exceed 20 mg/day).
PO (Adults —Debilitated or Nonsmoking Female Patients ≥65 yr): Initiate therapy at 5 mg/day.
PO (Children 13–17 yr): 2.5–5 mg/day initially; may ↑ at weekly intervals by 2.5–5 mg/day (target dose = 10 mg/day; not to exceed 20 mg/day).
IM (Adults): *Oral olanzapine dose = 10 mg/day*—210 mg every 2 wk or 410 mg every 4 wk for the first 8 wk, then 150 mg every 2 wk or 300 mg every 4 wk as maintenance therapy; *Oral olanzapine dose = 15 mg/day*—300 mg every 2 wk for the first 8 wk, then 210 mg every 2 wk or 405 mg every 4 wk as maintenance therapy; *Oral olanzapine dose = 20 mg/day*—300 mg every 2 wk for the first 8 wk, then 300 mg every 2 wk as maintenance therapy.
IM (Adults —Debilitated or Nonsmoking Female Patients ≥65 yr): Initiate therapy at 150 mg every 4 wk.

Acute Manic or Mixed Episodes Associated with Bipolar I Disorder

PO (Adults): 10–15 mg/day initially (use 10 mg/day when used with lithium or valproate); may ↑ every 24 hr by 5 mg/day (not to exceed 20 mg/day).
PO (Children 13–17 yr): 2.5–5 mg/day initially; may ↑ by 2.5–5 mg/day (target dose = 10 mg/day; not to exceed 20 mg/day).

Maintenance Treatment of Bipolar I Disorder

PO (Adults): Continue at the dose required to maintain symptom remission (usual dose: 5–20 mg/day).
PO (Children 13–17 yr): Continue at the lowest dose required to maintain symptom remission.

Acute Agitation due to Schizophrenia or Bipolar I Mania

IM (Adults): 10 mg, may repeat in 2 hr, then 4 hr later.
IM (Adults >65 yr): Initiate therapy with 5 mg.

Depressive Episodes Associated with Bipolar I Disorder

PO (Adults): 5 mg/day with fluoxetine 20 mg/day (both given in evening); may ↑ fluoxetine dose up to 50 mg/day and olanzapine dose up to 12.5 mg/day.
PO (Children 10–17 yr): 20 mg/day with olanzapine 2.5 mg/day (both given in evening); may ↑ fluoxetine dose up to 50 mg/day and olanzapine dose up to 12 mg/day.

Treatment-Resistant Depression

PO (Adults): 5 mg/day with fluoxetine 20 mg/day (both given in evening); may ↑ fluoxetine dose up to 50 mg/day and olanzapine dose up to 20 mg/day.

Availability (generic available)

Extended-release powder for suspension for intramuscular injection (requires reconstitution) (Zyprexa Relprevv): 210 mg/vial, 300 mg/vial, 405 mg/vial. **Orally disintegrating tablets (Zydis):** 5 mg, 10 mg, 15 mg, 20 mg. **Cost:** 5 mg $1,298.66/90, 15 mg $2,880.85/90. **Powder for intramuscular injection (requires reconstitution):** 10 mg/vial. **Tablets:** 2.5 mg, 5 mg, 7.5 mg, 10 mg, 15 mg, 20 mg. **Cost:** *Generic*—2.5 mg $31.23/90, 5 mg $24.47/90, 7.5 mg $30.83/90, 10 mg $37.19/90, 15 mg $53.38/90, 20 mg $71.55/90. ***In combination with:*** fluoxetine (Symbyax; see Appendix B).

NURSING IMPLICATIONS

Assessment

- Assess mental status (orientation, mood, behavior) before and periodically during therapy. Monitor closely for notable changes in behavior that could indicate the emergence or worsening of suicidal thoughts or behavior or depression.
- Monitor BP (sitting, standing, lying), ECG, pulse, and respiratory rate before and frequently during dose adjustment.
- Assess weight and BMI initially and throughout therapy.
- Observe patient carefully when administering medication to ensure that medication is taken and not hoarded or cheeked.
- Assess fluid intake and bowel function. Increased bulk and fluids in the diet may help minimize constipation.
- Monitor patient for onset of akathisia (restlessness or desire to keep moving) and extrapyramidal side effects (*parkinsonian*—difficulty speaking or swallowing, loss of balance control, pill rolling of hands, mask-like face, shuffling gait, rigidity, tremors; and *dystonic*—muscle spasms, twisting motions, twitching, inability to move eyes, weakness of arms or legs) every 2 mo during therapy and 8–12 wk after therapy has been discontinued. Report these symptoms if they occur, as reduction in dose or discontinuation of medication may be necessary. Trihexyphenidyl or benztropine may be used to control symptoms.
- Monitor for tardive dyskinesia (uncontrolled rhythmic movement of mouth, face, and extremities; lip smacking or puckering; puffing of cheeks; uncontrolled chewing; rapid or worm-like movements of tongue, excessive blinking of eyes). Discontinue olanzapine and report immediately; may be irreversible.
- Monitor for development of neuroleptic malignant syndrome (fever, respiratory distress, tachycardia, seizures, diaphoresis, hypertension or hypotension, pallor, tiredness, severe muscle stiffness, loss of bladder control). Notify health care professional immediately if these symptoms occur.
- Monitor for symptoms related to hyperprolactinemia (menstrual abnormalities, galactorrhea, sexual dysfunction).
- Assess for falls risk. Drowsiness, orthostatic hypotension, and motor and sensory instability increase risk. Institute prevention if indicated.
- Monitor for signs and symptoms of DRESS (fever, rash, lymphadenopathy, and/or facial swelling), associated with involvement of other organ systems (hepatitis, nephritis, hematologic abnormalities, myocarditis, myositis) during therapy. May resemble an acute viral infection. Eosinophilia is often present. Discontinue therapy if signs occur.
- *Zyprexa Relprevv*: Observe for signs and symptoms of Post-injection Delirium/Sedation Syndrome (dizziness, confusion, disorientation, slurred speech, altered gait, difficulty ambulating, weakness, agitation, extrapyramidal symptoms, hypertension, convulsion, reduced level of consciousness ranging from mild sedation to coma) for at least 3 hr after injection.
- ***Lab Test Considerations:*** Evaluate CBC, liver function tests, and ocular examinations periodically

during therapy. May cause ↓ platelets. May cause ↑ bilirubin, AST, ALT, GGT, CPK, and alkaline phosphatase.
- Monitor blood glucose prior to and periodically during therapy.
- Monitor serum prolactin prior to and periodically during therapy. May cause ↑ serum prolactin levels.
- Monitor CBC frequently during initial mo of therapy in patients with pre-existing or history of low WBC. May cause leukopenia, neutropenia, or agranulocytosis. Discontinue therapy if this occurs.
- May cause hyperlipidemia; monitor serum lipids prior to and periodically during therapy.

Implementation

- Do not confuse Zyprexa (olanzapine) with Celexa (citalopram), Zyrtec (cetirizine), Reprexain (hydrocodone/ibuprofen), Zestril (lisinopril), or Zelapar (selegiline). Do not confuse olanzapine with quetiapine.
- *Zyprexa Relprevv* is only prescribed through the *Zyprexa Relprevv Patient Care Program*. Prescribers, pharmacies, and patients must be educated about the program and must comply with the program requirements.
- **PO:** May be administered without regard to meals.
- For orally disintegrating tablets, peel back foil on blister, do not push tablet through foil. Using dry hands, remove from foil and place entire tablet in mouth. Tablet will disintegrate with or without liquid.
- **IM:** Reconstitute with 2.1 mL of sterile water for injection for a concentration of 5 mg/mL. Solution should be clear and yellow; do not administer solutions that are discolored or contain particulate matter. Inject slowly, deep into muscle. Do not administer IV or subcutaneously. Administer within 1 hr of reconstitution. Discard unused solution.
- For *Zyprexa Relprevv*: Use gloves when preparing; solution may be irritating to skin. Use only diluent provided by manufacturer. Dilute 150 mg or 210 mg dose with 1.3 mL, 300 mg with 1.8 mL, and 405 mg with 2.3 mL of diluent. Loosen powder by tapping vial; inject diluent into powder. Remove needle from vial holding vial upright to prevent loss of solution. Engage needle safety device as explained by manufacturer. Pad a hard surface and tap vial repeatedly until no powder or yellow, dry clumps are visible. Shake vial vigorously until suspension appears smooth and consistent in color and texture. Solution will be yellow and opaque. Allow foam to dissipate. Suspension is stable for 24 hr at room temperature; if not used immediately, shake to resuspend. ***Concentration:*** 150 mg/mL. Replace needle with 19 gauge, 1.5 inch or 2 inch for obese patients. Slowly withdraw desired amount from vial; 150 mg = 1 mL, 210 mg = 1.4 mL, 300 mg = 2 mL, 405 mg = 2.7 mL. Administer immediately deep IM gluteal after withdrawing. Do not massage injection site. Patient must be observed for at least 3 hr after injection for Post-Injection Delirium/Sedation Syndrome.

Patient/Family Teaching

- Advise patient to take medication as directed and not to skip doses or double up on missed doses. May need to discontinue gradually. Advise patient to read the *Medication Guide* prior to starting therapy and with each Rx refill in case of changes. Explain the *Zyprexa Relprevv Patient Care Program* to patient and encourage patient to enroll in the *Zyprexa Relprevv Patient Care Program* registry.
- Inform patient of possibility of extrapyramidal symptoms and tardive dyskinesia. Instruct patient to report these symptoms immediately to health care professional.
- Advise patient to change positions slowly to minimize orthostatic hypotension. Protect from falls.
- Medication may cause drowsiness. Caution patient to avoid driving or other activities requiring alertness until response to the medication is known. Patients receiving *Zyprexa Relprevv* should not drive for 24 hr following injection.
- Advise patient and family to notify health care professional if thoughts about suicide or dying, attempts to commit suicide; new or worse depression; new or worse anxiety; feeling very agitated or restless; panic attacks; trouble sleeping; new or worse irritability; acting aggressive; being angry or violent; acting on dangerous impulses; an extreme increase in activity and talking, other unusual changes in behavior or mood occur.
- Advise patient to notify health care professional of all Rx or OTC medications, vitamins, or herbal products being taken and to consult with health care professional before taking other medications and alcohol.
- Advise patient to use sunscreen and protective clothing when exposed to the sun. Extremes of temperature (exercise, hot weather, hot baths, or showers) should also be avoided; this drug impairs body temperature regulation.
- Instruct patient to use saliva substitute, frequent mouth rinses, good oral hygiene, and sugarless gum or candy to minimize dry mouth. Consult dentist if dry mouth continues for >2 wk.
- Advise patient to notify health care professional of medication regimen before treatment or surgery.
- Instruct patient to notify health care professional promptly if sore throat, fever, unusual bleeding or bruising, rash, symptoms of Post-Injection Delirium/Sedation Syndrome, or weakness, tremors, visual disturbances, dark-colored urine, clay-colored stools, menstrual abnormalities, galactorrhea, or sexual dysfunction occur.

- Rep: Advise females of reproductive potential to notify health care professional if pregnancy is planned or suspected, and to avoid breast feeding. Encourage women who become pregnant while taking olanzapine to enroll in the National Pregnancy Registry for Atypical Antipsychotics at 1-866-961-2388 or visit http://womensmentalhealth.org/clinical-and-research-programs/pregnancyregistry/. Monitor neonates for extrapyramidal and/or withdrawal symptoms and manage symptoms appropriately.
- Emphasize the importance of routine follow-up exams and continued participation in psychotherapy.

Evaluation/Desired Outcomes

- Decrease in excitable, manic behavior.
- Decrease in positive symptoms (delusions, hallucinations) of schizophrenia.
- Decrease in negative symptoms (social withdrawal, flat, blunted affect) of schizophrenia.
- Increased sense of well-being.
- Decreased agitation.

olaparib (oh-lap-a-rib)

Lynparza

Classification

Therapeutic: antineoplastics

Pharmacologic: enzyme inhibitors

Indications

Treatment of deleterious/suspected deleterious germline *BRCA*-mutated advanced ovarian cancer following ≥3 previous lines of chemotherapy. Maintenance treatment of recurrent epithelial ovarian, fallopian tube, or primary peritoneal cancer in patients who are in a complete or partial response to platinum-based chemotherapy. Maintenance treatment of deleterious/suspected deleterious germline or somatic *BRCA*-mutated advanced epithelial ovarian, fallopian tube, or primary peritoneal cancer in patients who are in a complete or partial response to first-line platinum-based chemotherapy. Treatment of deleterious/suspected deleterious germline *BRCA*-mutated HER2–negative metastatic breast cancer in patients who have been treated with chemotherapy in the neoadjuvant, adjuvant, or metastatic setting (should have been previously treated with or considered intolerant to an endocrine therapy).

Action

Acts as a poly (ADP-ribose) polymerase (PARP) inhibitor; disrupts DNA transcription, cell cycle regulation, and DNA repair. **Therapeutic Effects:** Decreased growth and spread of ovarian cancer, fallopian tube, primary peritoneal cancer, or breast cancer.

Pharmacokinetics

Absorption: Well absorbed following oral administration.

Distribution: Unknown.

Metabolism and Excretion: Extensively metabolized (mostly by CYP3A enzyme system); 15% excreted unchanged in urine, 6% in feces.

Half-life: 14.9 hr.

TIME/ACTION PROFILE (blood levels)

ROUTE	ONSET	PEAK	DURATION
PO	unknown	1–3 hr	12 hr

Contraindications/Precautions

Contraindicated in: OB: Pregnancy (may cause fetal harm); Lactation: Lactation.

Use Cautiously in: Concurrent use of strong/moderate CYP3A inhibitors (avoid if possible, if concurrent use is necessary ↓ olaparib dose); Concurrent use of strong/moderate CYP3A inducers (avoid if possible, if concurrent use is necessary effectiveness of olaparib may be ↓); Moderate or severe hepatic impairment; Moderate or severe renal impairment (CCr <50 mL/min) (dose ↓ may be needed); Rep: Women of reproductive potential and men with female partners of reproductive potential; Pedi: Safety and effectiveness not established.

Adverse Reactions/Side Effects

CNS: fatigue, headache, weakness. **Derm:** dermatitis/rash. **GI:** abdominal pain, ↓ appetite, diarrhea, dyspepsia, nausea, vomiting, dysgeusia. **Hemat:** MYELODYSPLASTIC SYNDROME/ACUTE MYELOID LEUKEMIA, anemia, lymphopenia, neutropenia, thrombocytopenia. **MS:** arthralgia, back pain, musculoskeletal pain, myalgia. **Resp:** PNEUMONITIS, cough.

Interactions

Drug-Drug: ↑ risk of prolonged myelosuppression with other **antineoplastics**. Concurrent use with **strong CYP3A4 inhibitors**, including **clarithromycin, indinavir, itraconazole, ketoconazole, lopinavir/ritonavir, nefazodone, nelfinavir, posaconazole, ritonavir, saquinavir**, or **voriconazole** ↑ levels and risk of toxicity; avoid concurrent use if possible but if necessary, ↓ olaparib dose. Concurrent use with **moderate CYP3A4 inhibitors**, including **aprepitant, atazanavir, ciprofloxacin, crizotinib, darunavir/ritonavir, diltiazem, erythromycin, fluconazole, fosamprenavir, imatinib**, or **verapamil** ↑ levels and risk of toxicity; avoid concurrent use if possible but if necessary, ↓ olaparib dose. Concurrent use with **strong CYP3A inducers** including **carbamazepine, phenytoin**, and **rifampin** ↓ blood levels and effectiveness and should be avoided. Concurrent use with **moderate CYP3A inducers** including **bosentan, efavirenz, etravirine, modafinil**, and **nafcillin** ↓ blood levels and effectiveness; avoid if possible.

Drug-Natural Products: St. John's wort may ↓ blood levels and effectiveness and should be avoided.

Drug-Food: Concurrent ingestion of **grapefruit** and **Seville oranges** may ↑ blood levels and the risk of toxicity and should be avoided.

Route/Dosage

First-Line Maintenance Treatment of *BRCA*-Mutated Advanced Ovarian Cancer

PO (Adults): 300 mg twice daily until disease progression, unacceptable toxicity, or completion of 2 yr of treatment. If complete response achieved after 2 yr of treatment (i.e. no radiological evidence of disease), can stop therapy. If evidence of disease at 2 yr, may continue therapy. *Concurrent use of strong CYP3A4 inhibitor*—100 mg twice daily until disease progression, unacceptable toxicity, or completion of 2 yr of treatment. If complete response achieved after 2 yr of treatment (i.e. no radiological evidence of disease), can stop therapy. If evidence of disease at 2 yr, may continue therapy. *Concurrent use of moderate CYP3A4 inhibitor*—150 mg twice daily until disease progression, unacceptable toxicity, or completion of 2 yr of treatment. If complete response achieved after 2 yr of treatment (i.e. no radiological evidence of disease), can stop therapy. If evidence of disease at 2 yr, may continue therapy.

Renal Impairment

PO (Adults): *CCr 31–50 mL/min*—200 mg twice daily until disease progression, unacceptable toxicity, or completion of 2 yr of treatment. If complete response achieved after 2 yr of treatment (i.e. no radiological evidence of disease), can stop therapy. If evidence of disease at 2 yr, may continue therapy.

Maintenance Treatment of Recurrent Ovarian Cancer, Advanced *gBRCA*-Mutated Ovarian Cancer, or Germline *BRCA*-Mutated HER2–Negative Metastatic Breast Cancer

PO (Adults): 300 mg twice daily until disease progression or unacceptable toxicity. *Concurrent use of strong CYP3A4 inhibitor*—100 mg twice daily until disease progression or unacceptable toxicity. *Concurrent use of moderate CYP3A4 inhibitor*—150 mg twice daily until disease progression or unacceptable toxicity.

Renal Impairment

PO (Adults): *CCr 31–50 mL/min*—200 mg twice daily until disease progression or unacceptable toxicity.

Availability

Tablets: 100 mg, 150 mg.

NURSING IMPLICATIONS

Assessment

- Monitor for signs and symptoms of pneumonitis (new or worsening respiratory symptoms, dyspnea, fever, cough, wheezing, radiological abnormality) during therapy. Interrupt therapy; if pneumonitis confirmed, discontinue therapy.
- ***Lab Test Considerations:*** Use an FDA-approved test to detect deleterious or suspected deleterious germline BRCA-mutations before starting therapy.
- Obtain a negative pregnancy test prior to starting therapy.
- Monitor CBC at baseline and monthly during therapy. Do not start olaparib until patient has recovered from hematological toxicities from previous chemotherapy (≤CTCAE Grade 1). For prolonged hematological toxicities, interrupt olaparib and monitor CBC weekly until recovery. If levels have not recovered to Grade ≤1 after 4 wk, refer to hematologist. Discontinue olaparib if myelodysplastic syndrome or acute myeloid leukemia is confirmed.
- May cause ↓ hemoglobin, neutrophils, platelets, and lymphocytes. May cause ↑ mean corpuscular volume and serum creatinine.

Implementation

- **PO:** Take eight 50 mg capsules twice daily (800 mg/day) without regard to food. Swallow capsules whole; do not open, chew, or dissolve capsule; do not take capsules that are deformed or leak.
- If dose reduction is needed, reduce dose to 200 mg (four 50 mg capsules) twice daily or 400 mg/day. If further final dose reduction is needed, reduce to 100 mg (two 50 mg capsules) twice daily or 200 mg.

Patient/Family Teaching

- Instruct patient to take olaparib as directed. If a dose is missed, do not take another to make up; omit dose and take next scheduled dose.
- Inform patient that mild to moderate nausea and/or vomiting is common when taking olaparib. Notify health care professional for antiemetic options if this is problematic.
- Advise patient to avoid grapefruit or Seville oranges during therapy.
- Advise patient to notify health care professional if signs and symptoms of pneumonitis or hematological toxicity (weakness, feeling tired, fever, weight loss, frequent infections, bruising, bleeding easily, shortness of breath, blood in urine or stool, low blood cell counts on laboratory findings, need for blood transfusions). May also be myelodysplastic syndrome (MDS) or acute myeloid leukemia (AML).
- Instruct patient to notify health care professional of all Rx or OTC medications, vitamins, or herbal products being taken and to consult with health care professional before taking other medications.
- Rep: Inform female patient that olaparib is teratogenic. Advise females of reproductive potential to use effective contraception during and for at least 6 mo after last dose and to avoid breast feeding for 1 mo after last dose. Advise patient to notify health care professional if pregnancy is planned or sus-

O

pected. Advise males with female partners of reproductive potential to use effective contraception during and for 3 mo after last dose. Advise male patients not to donate sperm during therapy and for 3 mo following the last dose.

- Emphasize importance of lab test to monitor for side effects.

Evaluation/Desired Outcomes

- Decreased growth and spread of ovarian cancer, fallopian tube, primary peritoneal cancer, or breast cancer.

olmesartan, See ANGIOTENSIN II RECEPTOR ANTAGONISTS.

olodaterol (oh-loh-**dat**-er-ole)

Striverdi Respimat

Classification

Therapeutic: bronchodilators

Pharmacologic: beta-adrenergic agonists

Indications

Maintenance treatment of airflow obstruction in patients with COPD, including chronic bronchitis and emphysema.

Action

A long-acting beta$_2$-adrenergic agonist (LABA) that stimulates adenyl cyclase, resulting in accumulation of cyclic adenosine monophosphate (cAMP) at beta$_2$-adrenergic receptors resulting in bronchodilation. **Therapeutic Effects:** Bronchodilation with decreased airflow obstruction.

Pharmacokinetics

Absorption: 30% absorbed following oral inhalation (from lung surface); swallowed drug is minimally absorbed.

Distribution: Extensive tissue distribution; probably enters breast milk.

Metabolism and Excretion: Extensively metabolized (some by CYP 3A4), only one metabolite binds to B$_2$ adrenergic receptors. Following inhalation, 5–7% excreted unchanged in urine, remainder in feces as drug and metabolites (84%).

Half-life: 45 hr (following inhalation).

TIME/ACTION PROFILE (improvement in FEV$_1$)

ROUTE	ONSET	PEAK	DURATION
inhaln	within 1 hr	1–5 hr	24 hr

Contraindications/Precautions

Contraindicated in: Acutely deteriorating COPD or acute respiratory symptoms; Asthma.

Use Cautiously in: History of seizures; Thyrotoxicosis; History of cardiovascular disorders (coronary insufficiency, arrhythmias, hypertension); Sensitivity to sympathomimetics (adrenergics); Severe hepatic impairment; OB: Use only if potential maternal benefit justifies potential fetal risk; may interfere with uterine contractility during labor; Lactation: Use while breast feeding only if potential maternal benefit justifies potential risk to infant; Pedi: Safety and effectiveness not established.

Exercise Extreme Caution in: Concurrent use with MAOIs, tricyclic antidepressants, or drugs that prolong QTc (↑ risk of adverse cardiovascular reactions).

Adverse Reactions/Side Effects

CNS: dizziness . **CV:** ↑ BP, ECG changes, tachycardia. **EENT:** nasopharyngitis. **Endo:** hyperglycemia. **F and E:** hypokalemia. **GI:** diarrhea. **MS:** arthralgia, back pain. **Resp:** PARADOXICAL BRONCHOSPASM, cough. **Misc:** HYPERSENSITIVITY REACTIONS (including angioedema).

Interactions

Drug-Drug: Concurrent use with **MAOIs, tricyclic antidepressants**, or **drugs that prolong QTc** ↑ risk of adverse cardiovascular reactions (use with extreme caution). Concurrent use of other **adrenergics** ↑ risk of adverse adrenergic adverse reactions (tachycardia, ↑ BP). Concurrent use with **corticosteroids, non-potassium sparing diuretics**, or **xanthine derivatives** (including **theophylline**) may ↑ risk of hypokalemia and adverse cardiovascular reactions (use cautiously). Concurrent use with **beta blockers** may ↓ effectiveness and cause severe bronchospasm (use cautiously). Should not be used concurrently with any other **long-acting beta$_2$-adrenergic blockers** (LABAs). Blood levels may be ↑ by ketoconazole.

Route/Dosage

Inhaln (Adults): 2 inhalations once daily.

Availability

Inhalation spray: 2.7 mcg (delivers 2.5 mcg) per actuation in cartridges containing 14 doses/cartridge (one actuation lost in priming) for use with Respimat inhaler. ***In combination with:*** tiotropium (Stiolto Respimat). See Appendix B.

NURSING IMPLICATIONS

Assessment

- Assess respiratory status (rate, breath sounds, degree of dyspnea, pulse) before administration and at peak of medication. Consult health care professional about alternative medication if severe bronchospasm is present; onset of action is too slow for patients in acute distress. If paradoxical bronchospasm (wheezing) occurs, withhold medication and notify health care professional immediately.
- Monitor for signs and symptoms of allergic reactions (difficulties in breathing or swallowing, swelling of

tongue, lips and face, urticaria, skin rash). Discontinue therapy if symptoms occur.

- ***Lab Test Considerations:*** May cause transient hypokalemia and hyperglycemia.

Implementation

- **Inhaln:** Prior to first use, prime the inhaler by actuating toward ground until aerosol cloud is visible, then repeat procedure 3 more times. If not used for 3 days, actuate inhaler once to prepare for use. *Striverdi Respimat* has a slow-moving mist to assist with inhalation. Use once (2 puffs), at the same time daily.
- A rescue inhaler of short-acting $beta_2$-agonists should always be available to treat sudden bronchospasm.

Patient/Family Teaching

- Instruct patient in the correct use of *Striverdi Respimat*. Take missed doses as soon as remembered. Do not take more than 1 dose (2 puffs) in 24 hr. Advise patient not to discontinue without consulting health care professional; symptoms may recur.
- Inform patient that olodaterol is a long-acting bronchodilator and should not be used for treating sudden breathing problems of COPD or asthma.
- Advise patient to notify health care professional if signs and symptoms of allergic reaction, worsening symptoms; decreasing effectiveness of inhaled, short-acting $beta_2$–agonists; need for more inhalations than usual of inhaled, short-acting $beta_2$-agonists; or significant decrease in lung function occur.
- Instruct patient to notify health care professional of all Rx or OTC medications, vitamins, or herbal products being taken and to avoid concurrent use of Rx, OTC, and herbal products without consulting health care professional.
- Advise female patient to notify health care professional if pregnancy is planned or suspected, or if breast feeding.

Evaluation/Desired Outcomes

- Bronchodilation with decreased airflow obstruction.

olsalazine (ole-**sal**-a-zeen)

Dipentum

Classification

Therapeutic: gastrointestinal anti-inflammatories

Indications

Ulcerative colitis (when patients cannot tolerate sulfasalazine).

Action

Locally acting anti-inflammatory action in the colon, where activity is probably due to inhibition of prostaglandin synthesis. **Therapeutic Effects:** Reduction in the symptoms of inflammatory bowel disease.

Pharmacokinetics

Absorption: Acts locally in colon, where 98–99% is converted to mesalamine (5-aminosalicylic acid).

Distribution: Action is primarily local and remains in the colon.

Metabolism and Excretion: 2% absorbed into systemic circulation is rapidly metabolized; mostly eliminated as mesalamine in the feces.

Half-life: 0.9 hr.

TIME/ACTION PROFILE (levels)

ROUTE	ONSET	PEAK	DURATION
PO	unknown	1 hr; 4–8 hr	12 hr

Contraindications/Precautions

Contraindicated in: Hypersensitivity reactions to salicylates; Cross-sensitivity with furosemide, sulfonylurea hypoglycemic agents, or carbonic anhydrase inhibitors may exist; Glucose-6–phosphate dehydrogenase (G6PD) deficiency; Urinary tract or intestinal obstruction; Porphyria; Lactation: Lactation; Pedi: Children <2 yr (safety not established).

Use Cautiously in: Severe hepatic or renal impairment; Renal impairment (↑ risk of renal tubular damage); OB: Pregnancy; Geri: Consider ↓ body mass, hepatic/renal/cardiac function, intercurrent illness and drug therapies.

Adverse Reactions/Side Effects

CNS: ataxia, confusion, dizziness, drowsiness, headache, mental depression, psychosis, restlessness. **GI:** diarrhea, abdominal pain, anorexia, exacerbation of colitis, drug-induced hepatitis, nausea, vomiting. **Derm:** itching, rash. **Hemat:** blood dyscrasias.

Interactions

Drug-Drug: ↑ risk of bleeding after neuraxial anesthesia with **low molecular weight heparins** and **heparinoids**; discontinue olsalazine before initiation of therapy or monitor closely if discontinuation not possible. May ↓ metabolism, and ↑ effects/toxicity of **mercaptopurine** or **thioguanine** with and ↑ risk of myelosuppression (use lowest possible dose and monitor closely). ↑ risk of developing Reye's syndrome; avoid olsalazine during 6 wk after **varicella vaccine**.

Route/Dosage

PO (Adults): 500 mg twice daily.

Availability

Capsules: 250 mg.

NURSING IMPLICATIONS

Assessment

- Assess patient for allergy to sulfonamides and salicylates. Patients allergic to sulfasalazine may take mesalamine or olsalazine without difficulty, but therapy should be discontinued if rash or fever occur.
- Monitor intake and output ratios. Fluid intake should be sufficient to maintain a urine output of at least 1200–1500 mL daily to prevent crystalluria and stone formation.
- **Inflammatory Bowel Disease:** Assess abdominal pain and frequency, quantity, and consistency of stools at the beginning of and throughout therapy.
- ***Lab Test Considerations:*** Monitor urinalysis, BUN, and serum creatinine prior to and periodically during therapy.
- Olsalazine may cause ↑ AST and ALT levels.
- Monitor CBC prior to and every 3–6 mo during prolonged therapy. Discontinue olsalazine if blood dyscrasias occur.

Implementation

- **PO:** Administer with food in evenly divided doses every 12 hr.

Patient/Family Teaching

- Instruct patient to take medication as directed, even if feeling better. Take missed doses as soon as remembered unless almost time for next dose.
- May cause dizziness. Caution patient to avoid driving or other activities that require alertness until response to medication is known.
- Advise patient to notify health care professional if skin rash, sore throat, fever, mouth sores, unusual bleeding or bruising, wheezing, fever, or hives occurs.
- Instruct patient to notify health care professional if symptoms do not improve after 1–2 mo of therapy.
- Instruct patient to notify health care professional if symptoms worsen or do not improve. If symptoms of acute intolerance (cramping, acute abdominal pain, bloody diarrhea, fever, headache, rash) occur, discontinue therapy and notify health care professional immediately.
- Inform patient that proctoscopy and sigmoidoscopy may be required periodically during treatment to determine response.

Evaluation/Desired Outcomes

- Decrease in diarrhea and abdominal pain.
- Return to normal bowel pattern in patients with inflammatory bowel disease. Effects may be seen within 3–21 days. The usual course of therapy is 3–6 wk.
- Maintenance of remission in patients with inflammatory bowel disease.
- Decrease in pain and inflammation, and increase in mobility in patients with rheumatoid arthritis.

omadacycline
(oh-**mad**-a-**sye**-kleen)
Nuzyra

Classification
Therapeutic: anti-infectives
Pharmacologic: tetracyclines

Indications

Community-acquired bacterial pneumonia (CABP). Acute bacterial skin and skin structure infections (ABSSSI).

Action

Inhibits bacterial protein synthesis by binding to the 30S bacterial ribosome. **Therapeutic Effects:** Bacteriostatic action against susceptible bacteria. **Spectrum:** Includes activity against some gram-positive pathogens: *Enterococcus faecalis*, *Staphylococcus aureus* (including methicillin-sensitive and methicillin-resistant strains), *Staphylococcus lugdunensis*, *Streptococcus anginosus*, *Streptococcus constellatus*, *Streptococcus intermedius*, *Streptococcus pneumoniae*, *Streptococcus pyogenes*. Active against some gram-negative pathogens: *Enterobacter cloacae*, *Haemophilus influenzae*, *Haemophilus parainfluenzae*, *Klebsiella pneumoniae*. Also active against several other pathogens, including: *Chlamydophila pneumoniae*, *Legionella pneumophila*, *Mycoplasma pneumoniae*.

Pharmacokinetics

Absorption: 35% absorbed following oral administration (high-fat meal ↓ rate and extent of absorption); IV administration results in complete bioavailability.
Distribution: Extensively distributed to tissues.
Metabolism and Excretion: Does not undergo metabolism in the liver. Primarily excreted in feces (78–84%), with 14% excreted in urine (27% as unchanged drug).
Half-life: 15–16 hr.

TIME/ACTION PROFILE (plasma concentrations)

ROUTE	ONSET	PEAK	DURATION
IV	unknown	0.5 hr	24 hr
PO	unknown	2.5 hr	24 hr

Contraindications/Precautions

Contraindicated in: Hypersensitivity to omadacycline or other tetracycline derivatives; OB: Pregnancy (may lead to permanent staining of teeth and inhibition of bone growth in fetus if used during 2nd or 3rd trimester); Lactation: Lactation; Pedi: Children <8 yr (may lead to permanent staining of teeth and ↓ growth).
Use Cautiously in: Rep: Women of reproductive potential; Pedi: Safety and effectiveness not established;

Geri: ↑ risk of mortality, especially those with multiple comorbidities.

Adverse Reactions/Side Effects

CNS: headache, insomnia, intracranial hypertension. **Derm:** photosensitivity. **CV:** hypertension. **GI:** CLOSTRIDIUM DIFFICILE-ASSOCIATED DIARRHEA (CDAD), nausea, vomiting, constipation, diarrhea, ↑ liver enzymes. **GU:** ↓ fertility. **Local:** injection site reactions. **Misc:** HYPERSENSITIVITY REACTIONS (including anaphylaxis).

Interactions

Drug-Drug: May ↑ effect of **warfarin**. Medications containing **aluminum**, **calcium**, or **magnesium** may ↓ absorption of oral tablets; separate administration by ≥4 hr.

Drug-Food: Dairy products may ↓ absorption of oral tablets; separate administration by ≥4 hr.

Route/Dosage

Community-Acquired Bacterial Pneumonia

IV, PO (Adults): *Loading dose*—200 mg IV as single dose on Day 1 *or* 100 mg IV twice daily on Day 1. *Maintenance dose*—100 mg IV once daily for additional 6–13 days *or* 300 mg orally once daily for additional 6–13 days.

Acute Bacterial Skin and Skin Structure Infections

IV, PO (Adults): *Loading dose*—200 mg IV as single dose on Day 1 *or* 100 mg IV twice daily on Day 1 *or* 450 mg orally once daily on Days 1 and 2. *Maintenance dose*—100 mg IV once daily for additional 6–13 days *or* 300 mg orally once daily for additional 6–13 days.

Availability

Lyophilized powder for injection (requires reconstitution and dilution): 100 mg/vial. **Tablets:** 150 mg.

NURSING IMPLICATIONS

Assessment

- Assess for infection (vital signs; appearance of wound, sputum, urine, and stool; WBC) at beginning of and during therapy, especially in geriatric patients.
- Obtain specimens for culture and sensitivity before initiating therapy. First dose may be given before receiving results.
- Monitor bowel function. Diarrhea, abdominal cramping, fever, and bloody stools should be reported to health care professional promptly as a sign of Clostridium difficile-associated diarrhea (CDAD). May begin up to several wk following cessation of therapy.
- Monitor for signs and symptoms of hypersensitivity reactions (rash, hives, swelling of face or throat) during therapy.

Implementation

- May cause yellow-brown discoloration and softening of teeth and bones if administered prenatally or during early childhood. Not recommended for children under 8 yr of age or during pregnancy or lactation.
- **PO:** Fast for at least 4 hrs and then take with water. After oral dosing, consume no food or drink (except water) for 2 hr and no dairy products, antacids, or multivitamins for 4 hr.

IV Administration

- **Intermittent Infusion:** Reconstitute each 100 mg vial with 5 mL of sterile water for injection, 0.9% NaCl, or D5W. Gently swirl and let vial stand until cake has completely dissolved and any foam disperses. Do not shake. Solution is yellow to dark orange; do not administer solutions that are discolored or contain particulate matter. ***Diluent:*** Within 1 hr, withdraw 5–10 ml of reconstituted solution and further dilute in 100 mL 0.9% NaCl or D5W. ***Concentration:*** 1 mg/mL or 2 mg/mL. Discard unused solution. Solution is stable for 12 hr at room temperature or 7 days if refrigerated. Allow solution to reach room temperature before administration. ***Rate:*** Infuse through a dedicated line or a Y-site over 60 min for 200-mg dose, or 30 min for a 100-mg dose. If line used for other infusions, flush with 0,9% NaCl or D5W before and after infusion.
- **Y-Site Incompatibility:** Solutions containing calcium and magnesium.

Patient/Family Teaching

- Instruct patient to take medication and to finish the drug completely as directed, even if feeling better. Instruct patient to fast 4 hr before and 2 hr after taking omadacycline and not to consume dairy products, antacids, or multivitamins for 4 hr after taking dose.
- Instruct patient to notify health care professional immediately if rash, diarrhea, abdominal cramping, fever, or bloody stools occur and not to treat with antidiarrheals without consulting health care professionals.
- Caution patient to use sunscreen and protective clothing to prevent photosensitivity reactions.
- Advise patient to report the signs of superinfection (black, furry overgrowth on the tongue, vaginal itching or discharge, loose or foul-smelling stools) to health care professional.
- Advise patient to notify health care professional of all Rx or OTC medications, vitamins, or herbal products being taken and to consult with health care professional before taking other medications.

- Rep: Advise females of reproductive potential to use a nonhormonal method of contraception while taking omadacycline and until next menstrual period and to avoid breast feeding during and for 4 days after last dose.

Evaluation/Desired Outcomes

- Resolution of the signs and symptoms of infection. Length of time for complete resolution depends on the organism and site of infection.

ombitasvir/paritaprevir/ritonavir/dasabuvir

(om-**bit**-as-vir/par-i-**ta**-pre-vir/ri-**toe**-na-vir/da-**sa**-bue-vir)

Holkira Pak, Viekira Pak

Classification

Therapeutic: antivirals

Pharmacologic: NS5 inhibitors, protease inhibitors, enzyme inhibitors, non-nucleoside NS5B palm polymerase inhibitors

Indications

Treatment of (with or without ribavirin) genotype 1 chronic hepatitis C infection (HCV) including those with compensated cirrhosis.

Action

Ombitasvir—is an inhibitor of HCV NS5A which is necessary for RNA replication and virion assembly. *Paritaprevir*—is an inhibitor of NS3/4A protease an enzyme necessary for viral replication. *Ritonavir* is not active against HCV, but inhibits CYP3A resulting in ↑ blood levels and effectiveness of paritaprevir. *Dasabuvir*—inhibits RNA-dependent RNA polymerase necessary for viral genome replication. **Therapeutic Effects:** Decreased levels of HCV with sustained virologic response and lessened sequelae of chronic HCV infection.

Pharmacokinetics

Absorption: Well absorbed following oral administration: *ombitasvir*—48%, *paritaprevir*—53%, *dasabuvir*—70%.

Distribution: *Ritonavir*—poor CNS penetration.

Protein Binding: *Ombitasvir*—99.9%, *paritaprevir*—97–98.6%, *ritonavir*—>99%, *dasabuvir*—>99.5%.

Metabolism and Excretion: *Ombitasvir*—metabolized by amide hydrolysis and then oxidative metabolism, excreted mainly in feces mostly as unchanged drug, minimal urinary excretion; *paritaprevir*—primarily metabolized by CYP3A, 88% excreted in feces mostly as metabolites; negligible urinary excretion; *ritonavir*—highly metabolized by CYP3A and CYP2D6, 86% excreted in feces (mostly as metabolites), 11.8% excreted in urine, *dasabuvir*—mostly metabolized by CYP2C8 and smaller amounts by CYP3A, 95% excreted in feces (26% as unchanged drug), minimal urinary excretion.

Half-life: *Ombitasvir*—21–25 hr, *paritaprevir*—5.5 hr, *ritonavir*—4 hr, *dasabuvir*—5.5–6 hr.

TIME/ACTION PROFILE (blood levels)

ROUTE	ONSET	PEAK	DURATION
ombitasvir PO	unknown	4–5 hr	24 hr
paritaprevir PO	unknown	4–5 hr	24 hr
ritonavir PO	rapid	4 hr	24 hr
dasabuvir PO	unknown	4–5 hr†	12 hr

†Peak is 8 hr for dasabuvir in ER formulation.

Contraindications/Precautions

Contraindicated in: Hypersensitivity to any components including previous history of Stevens-Johnson syndrome or toxic epidermal necrolysis from ritonavir; Concurrent use of medications that are metabolized by CYP3A4, strong/moderate inducers of CYP3A4, or strong inducers/inhibitors of CYP2C8; Moderate-to-severe hepatic impairment; OB: When used with ribavirin should not be used in pregnant patients or male patients whose partners are pregnant.

Use Cautiously in: Diabetes mellitus; Hemophilia (↑ risk of bleeding); Structural heart disease, conduction abnormalities, ischemic heart disease, or heart failure (↑ risk of heart block); Concurrent HIV infection (additional HIV-suppressive regimen required); Receiving immunosuppressant or chemotherapy medications (↑ risk of hepatitis B virus reactivation); OB: If used without ribavirin consider maternal benefits and possible adverse effects on the fetus; Lactation: Consider maternal benefits and possible adverse effects on infants; breast feeding not recommended in concurrently HIV-infected patients; Rep: Women of reproductive potential; Pedi: Safety and effectiveness not established.

Adverse Reactions/Side Effects

CNS: fatigue, insomnia (↑ with ribavirin), weakness (↑ with ribavirin). **Derm:** ERYTHEMA MULTIFORME, STEVENS-JOHNSON SYNDROME, TOXIC EPIDERMAL NECROLYSIS, pruritus, rash. **GI:** HEPATOTOXICITY, nausea (↑ with ribavirin), ↑ liver enzymes. **Misc:** HYPERSENSITIVITY REACTIONS (including anaphylaxis and angioedema), hepatitis B virus reactivation.

Interactions

Drug-Drug: ↑ levels and risk of serious adverse reactions with **alfuzosin** (hypotension); **dihydroergotamine**, **ergotamine**, or **methylergonovine** (ergot toxicity); **dronedarone** (arrhythmias); **atorvastatin**, **lovastatin** or **simvastatin** (myopathy/rhabdomyolysis); **pimozide** (arrhythmias); **efavirenz** (↑ liver enzymes); **ranolazine** (serious or life-threatening reactions); **sildenafil** (when used for pulmonary hypertension ↑ risk of visual disturbances/hypotension/priapism/syncope), **triazolam** (↑ sedation/respiratory depression); **ethinyl estradiol** containing preparations including oral hormonal contraceptives (↑ liver enzymes); **colchicine** (serious or life-threatening reactions in patients with renal or hepatic impairment); **everolimus**, **sirolimus**, or **tacrolimus** (serious or life-threatening immunosuppressant adverse reactions); **lurasidone** (serious or life-threatening reactions); and **gemfibrozil** (QT interval prolongation); concurrent use contraindicated. Levels and antiviral effectiveness are ↓ by **carbamazepine**, **phenobarbital**, **phenytoin**, and **rifampin**; concurrent use contraindicated. ↑ levels and risk of **digoxin** toxicity; ↓ digoxin dose by 30–50%, monitor carefully. ↑ levels and risk of adverse cardiovascular reactions with **amiodarone**, **disopyramide**, **flecainide**, **lidocaine**, **mexiletine**, **propafenone**, and **quinidine**; careful monitoring recommended. ↑ levels and risk of adverse reactions with **ketoconazole** (daily dose of ketoconazole should not exceed 200 mg). ↓ levels and effectiveness of **voriconazole**; concurrent use is not recommended. ↑ levels and risk of adverse reactions with **quetiapine**; ↓ quetiapine dose to 1/6th and monitor carefully, consider alternative anti-HCV treatments). ↑ levels and risk of hypotension with **amlodipine**, **nifedipine**, **diltiazem**, and **verapamil**; ↓ dose of amlodipine by ≥50%. ↑ levels and effects of **furosemide**; monitor and adjust dose. Concurrent use with **atazanavir**, **atazanavir/ritonavir**, or **lopinavir/ritonavir** ↑ levels of paritaprevir; concurrent use is not recommended. ↓ levels and may ↓ effectiveness of **darunavir**; darunavir (800 mg once daily) without ritonavir should be taken at the same time as ombitasvir/paritaprevir/ritonavir. ↑ levels and risk of adverse cardiovascular reactions with **rilpivirine**; concurrent use is not recommended. ↑ levels and risk of adverse muscular reactions with **pravastatin**; pravastatin dose should not exceed 40 mg/day. ↑ levels and risk of adverse reactions with **cyclosporine**; ↓ cyclosporine dose to 1/5th, monitor and readjust carefully. ↑ levels and risk of adverse cardiovascular reactions with **salmeterol**; Concurrent use is not recommended. ↑ levels of **buprenorphine**; monitor for sedation/cognitive impairment. ↑ levels of **hydrocodone**; ↓ hydrocodone dose by 50% and monitor for sedation and respiratory depression. ↑ levels of **fentanyl**; monitor for sedation and respiratory depression. ↓ levels and effectiveness of **omeprazole**; ↑ dose of omeprazole if necessary, but should not exceed 40 mg/day. ↑ levels and effects of **alprazolam**; monitor for sedation/cognitive impairment and adjust dose. ↓ levels and effectiveness of **diazepam**; ↑ dose of diazepam, if necessary. May ↑ levels of **valsartan**, **losartan**, and **candesartan**; ↓ dose of angiotensin II receptor blocker and monitor for hypotension and renal impairment. ↑ risk of lactic acidosis with **metformin**; concomitant use in patients with renal or hepatic impairment not recommended. May ↓ levels and effectiveness of **carisoprodol** or **cyclobenzaprine**; ↑ dose of carisoprodol or cyclobenzaprine, if necessary. May cause fluctuations in INR when used with **warfarin**; closely monitor INR.

Drug-Natural Products: Levels and antiviral effectiveness are ↓ by **St. John's wort**; concurrent use contraindicated.

Route/Dosage

Viekira Pak

PO (Adults): *Genotype 1a without cirrhosis*—Two tablets (each tablet containing ombitasvir 12.5 mg/paritaprevir 75 mg/ritonavir 50 mg) once daily with dasabuvir 250 mg twice daily with ribavirin for 12 wk; *Genotype 1a with compensated cirrhosis*—Two tablets (each tablet containing ombitasvir 12.5 mg/paritaprevir 75 mg/ritonavir 50 mg) once daily with dasabuvir 250 mg twice daily with ribavirin for 24 wk (some patients may respond to 12 wk); *Genotype 1b with or without compensated cirrhosis*—Two tablets (each tablet containing ombitasvir 12.5 mg/paritaprevir 75 mg/ritonavir 50 mg) once daily with dasabuvir 250 mg twice daily for 12 wk; *Liver transplant patients*—Two tablets (each tablet containing ombitasvir 12.5 mg/paritaprevir 75 mg/ritonavir 50 mg) once daily with dasabuvir 250 mg twice daily with ribavirin for 24 wk.

Availability

Tablets (Viekira Pak): ombitasvir 12.5 mg/paritaprevir 75 mg/ritonavir 50 mg (copackaged with dasabuvir 250 mg in a 28–day convenience pak separated into weekly amounts).

NURSING IMPLICATIONS

Assessment

- Monitor signs of hepatitis (jaundice, fatigue, anorexia, pruritus) during therapy.
- Assess for rash periodically during therapy. May cause Stevens-Johnson syndrome or Toxic Epidermal Necrolysis. Discontinue therapy if severe or if accompanied with fever, general malaise, fatigue, muscle or joint aches, blisters, oral lesions, conjunctivitis, hepatitis, and/or eosinophilia.
- Monitor for signs and symptoms of worsening liver disease (ascites, hepatic encephalopathy, variceal hemorrhage, increases in direct serum bilirubin).
- Monitor for signs and symptoms of hepatitis B reactivation (jaundice, dark urine, light colored stools, fatigue, weakness, loss of appetite, nausea, vomiting, stomach pain) during therapy.
- ***Lab Test Considerations:*** Determine current or prior HBV infection by measuring hepatitis B surface antigen (HBsAg) and hepatitis B core antibody (anti-HBc) before initiating HCV therapy. *In patients with HBV infection*, monitor for clinical and laboratory signs of hepatitis flare or HBV reactivation (rapid ↑

O

in serum HBV DNA level) during HCV therapy and during post-therapy follow-up.

- *For patients with compensated cirrhosis:* Monitor liver function tests including direct bilirubin levels at baseline and during first 4 wk of therapy and as clinically indicated. Signs of hepatic decompensation usually include ↑ bilirubin without ↑ ALT, and ascites, hepatic encephalopathy, variceal hemorrhage. Discontinue therapy if signs of hepatic decompensation occur.
- Monitor liver function tests prior to and during first 4 wk of therapy. If ALT is ↑, repeat test and monitor closely. Discontinue therapy if ALT levels are persistently ↑ >10 × upper limit of normal or if accompanied by signs of liver inflammation or ↑ direct bilirubin, alkaline phosphatase, or INR.
- May cause ↑ serum bilirubin; peaks by wk 1 of therapy and not associated with ↑ ALT.
- May cause ↓ hemoglobin requiring dose reduction.

Implementation

- **PO:** Administer 2 ombitasvir/paritaprevir/ritonavir 12.5/75/50 mg tablets once daily (in the morning) and 1 dasabuvir 250 mg tablet twice daily (morning and evening) with a meal without regard to fat or calorie content. Usually given in combination with ribavirin.

Patient/Family Teaching

- Instruct patient to take *Viekira Pak* as directed. Take missed doses of ombitasvir/paritaprevir/ritonavir within 12 hrs or of dasabuvir within 6 hrs; if more than 12 hrs or 6 hrs, respectively, since missed dose, skip dose and take next dose at scheduled time; do not double doses. Advise patient to read *Medication Guide* before starting therapy and with each Rx refill in case of changes.
- Advise patient to notify health care professional promptly if signs and symptoms of liver dysfunction (fatigue, weakness, lack of appetite, nausea and vomiting, jaundice, discolored feces) occur.
- Instruct patient to notify health care professional of all Rx or OTC medications, vitamins, or herbal products being taken and to consult health care professional before taking other Rx, OTC, or herbal products, especially St. John's wort. Medications containing ethinyl estradiol must be stopped; if taking for birth control, another method must be used.
- Rep: Inform patient about teratogenic effects of *Viekira Pak* and ribavirin. Instruct women of reproductive potential, and men, to use 2 forms of effective non-hormonal contraception (ethinyl estradiol-containing medications including oral hormonal contraceptives are contraindicated due to ↑ risk of liver impairment; effective alternative contraception is recommended) during and for at least 6 mo following conclusion of therapy. Men must use a condom. Avoid breast feeding during use. Advise patient to notify health care professional if pregnancy occurs.

Evaluation/Desired Outcomes

- Protection from liver damage caused by chronic hepatitis C infection; decreases viral load.

omega-3-acid ethyl esters

(oh-**me**-ga three **as**-id **eth**-il **es**-ters)

Lovaza

Classification

Therapeutic: lipid-lowering agents

Pharmacologic: fatty acids

Indications

Hypertriglyceridemia (triglycerides ≥500 mg/dL) in adults; used with specific diet.

Action

Inhibits synthesis of triglycerides. **Therapeutic Effects:** Lowering of triglycerides.

Pharmacokinetics

Absorption: Well absorbed.

Distribution: Unknown.

Metabolism and Excretion: Incorporated into phospholipids.

Half-life: Unknown.

TIME/ACTION PROFILE (lowering of triglycerides)

ROUTE	ONSET	PEAK	DURATION
PO	unknown	2 mo	unknown

Contraindications/Precautions

Contraindicated in: Hypersensitivity.

Use Cautiously in: Allergy/hypersensitivity to fish; OB, Lactation: Pregnancy or lactation; Pedi: Safety not established.

Adverse Reactions/Side Effects

Derm: rash. **GI:** altered taste, eructation, ↑ liver enzymes.

Interactions

Drug-Drug: May ↑ risk of bleeding with **aspirin** or **warfarin**.

Route/Dosage

PO (Adults): 4 g/day; may be given as a single dose or 2 g twice daily.

Availability (generic available)

Gelatin capsules (oil-filled) (Lovaza): 1 g. **Cost:** $196.69/100.

NURSING IMPLICATIONS

Assessment

- Obtain a diet history, especially with regard to fat consumption.

- ***Lab Test Considerations:*** Monitor serum triglyceride levels prior to and periodically during therapy.
- Monitor serum ALT periodically during therapy. May cause ↑ serum ALT without concurrent ↑ in AST levels.
- Monitor serum LDL cholesterol levels periodically during therapy. May cause ↑ in serum LDL levels.

Implementation

- Do not confuse Lovaza (omega-3–acid ethyl esters) with lorazepam.
- An appropriate lipid-lowering diet should be followed before therapy and should continue during therapy.
- **PO:** May be taken as a single 4-g dose or as 2 g twice daily. May be administered with meals. Swallow capsules whole; do not break, dissolve, or chew.

Patient/Family Teaching

- Instruct patient to take medication as directed, not to skip doses or double up on missed doses. Take missed doses as soon as remembered, but if a day is missed, do not double doses the next day. Medication helps control but does not cure elevated serum triglyceride levels.
- Advise patient that this medication should be used in conjunction with diet restrictions (fat, cholesterol, carbohydrates, alcohol), exercise, weight loss in overweight patients, and control of medical problems (such as diabetes mellitus and hypothyroidism) that may contribute to hypertriglyceridemia.
- Advise females of reproductive potential to notify health care professional if pregnancy is planned or suspected, or if breast feeding.
- Emphasize the importance of follow-up exams to determine effectiveness.

Evaluation/Desired Outcomes

- Lowering of serum triglyceride levels. Patients who do not have an adequate response after 2 mo of treatment should be withdrawn from therapy.

BEERS

omeprazole (o-mep-ra-zole)

Losec, PriLOSEC, PriLOSEC OTC

Classification
Therapeutic: antiulcer agents
Pharmacologic: proton-pump inhibitors

Indications

GERD/maintenance of healing in erosive esophagitis. Duodenal ulcers (with or without anti-infectives for *Helicobacter pylori*). Short-term treatment of active benign gastric ulcer. Pathologic hypersecretory conditions, including Zollinger-Ellison syndrome. Reduction of risk of GI bleeding in critically ill patients. **OTC:** Heartburn occurring ≥twice/wk.

Action

Binds to an enzyme on gastric parietal cells in the presence of acidic gastric pH, preventing the final transport of hydrogen ions into the gastric lumen. **Therapeutic Effects:** Diminished accumulation of acid in the gastric lumen with lessened gastroesophageal reflux. Healing of duodenal ulcers.

Pharmacokinetics

Absorption: Rapidly absorbed following oral administration; immediate release formulation contains bicarbonate to prevent acid degradation.
Distribution: Good distribution into gastric parietal cells.
Protein Binding: 95%.
Metabolism and Excretion: Mostly metabolized by the liver via the cytochrome P450 (CYP) system (primarily CYP2C19 isoenzyme, but also the CYP3A4 isoenzyme) (the CYP2C19 enzyme system exhibits genetic polymorphism; 15–20% of Asian patients and 3–5% of Caucasian and Black patients may be poor metabolizers and may have significantly ↑ omeprazole concentrations and an ↑ risk of adverse effects); inactive metabolites are excreted in urine (77%) and feces.
Half-life: 0.5–1 hr (↑ in liver disease to 3 hr).

TIME/ACTION PROFILE (antisecretory effects)

ROUTE	ONSET	PEAK	DURATION
PO-delayed release	within 1 hr	within 2 hr	72–96 hr

Contraindications/Precautions

Contraindicated in: Hypersensitivity to omeprazole or related drugs (benzimidazoles); Concurrent use of rilpivirine.
Use Cautiously in: Hepatic impairment (dose ↓ may be necessary); Patients using high-doses for >1 yr (↑ risk of hip, wrist, or spine fractures and fundic gland polyps); Patients using therapy for >3 yr (↑ risk of vitamin B_{12} deficiency); OB, Lactation: Use only if potential benefit outweighs potential risk; Pedi: Children <1 mo (safety and effectiveness not established).

Adverse Reactions/Side Effects

CNS: dizziness, drowsiness, fatigue, headache, weakness. **CV:** chest pain. **Derm:** cutaneous lupus erythematosus, itching, rash. **F and E:** hypomagnesemia (especially if treatment duration ≥3 mo). **GI:** CLOSTRIDIUM DIFFICILE-ASSOCIATED DIARRHEA (CDAD), abdominal pain, acid regurgitation, constipation, diarrhea, flatulence, fundic gland polyps, nausea, vomiting. **GU:** acute interstitial nephritis. **Hemat:** vitamin B_{12} deficiency. **MS:** bone fracture. **Misc:** allergic reactions, systemic lupus erythematosus.

Interactions

Drug-Drug: Omeprazole is metabolized by the CYP450 enzyme system and may compete with other agents metabolized by this system. May ↑ levels and risk of toxicity of **antifungal agents**, **cilostazol**, **citalopram**, **diazepam**, **flurazepam**, **triazolam**, **cyclosporine**, **phenytoin**, **saquinavir**, **tacrolimus**, and **warfarin**; consider ↓ dose of cilostazol from 100 mg twice daily to 50 mg twice daily. May ↓ absorption of drugs requiring acid pH, including **ketoconazole**, **itraconazole**, **iron salts**, **dasatinib**, **erlotinib**, **nilotinib**, **atazanavir**, **nelfinavir**, **rilpivirine**, and **mycophenolate mofetil**; concurrent use with **rilpivirine** contraindicated; avoid concurrent use with **atazanavir** and **nelfinavir**. Has been used safely with **antacids**. May ↑ levels of **digoxin** and **methotrexate**. **Voriconazole** may ↑ levels. May ↓ the antiplatelet effects of **clopidogrel**; avoid concurrent use. **Rifampin** may ↓ levels and may ↓ response; avoid concurrent use. Hypomagnesemia ↑ risk of **digoxin** toxicity.
Drug-Natural Products: St. John's wort may ↓ levels and may ↓ response; avoid concurrent use.

Route/Dosage

PO (Adults): *GERD/erosive esophagitis and maintenance of healing of erosive esophagitis*—20 mg once daily. *Duodenal ulcers associated with H. pylori*—40 mg once daily in the morning with clarithromycin for 2 wk, then 20 mg once daily for 2 wk *or* 20 mg twice daily with clarithromycin 500 mg twice daily and amoxicillin 1000 mg twice daily for 10 days (if ulcer is present at beginning of therapy, continue omeprazole 20 mg daily for 18 more days); has also been used with clarithromycin and metronidazole. *Gastric ulcer*—40 mg once daily for 4–6 wk. *Reduction of the risk of GI bleeding in critically ill patients*—40 mg initially, then another 40 mg 6–8 hr later, followed by 40 mg once daily for up to 14 days. *Gastric hypersecretory conditions*—60 mg once daily initially; may be increased up to 120 mg 3 times daily (doses >80 mg/day should be given in divided doses); *OTC*—20 mg once daily for up to 14 days.
PO (Children 1–16 yr and ≥20 kg): *GERD/erosive esophagitis*—20 mg once daily for 4–8 wk.
PO (Children 1–16 yr and 10–19 kg): *GERD/erosive esophagitis*—10 mg once daily for 4–8 wk.
PO (Children 1–16 yr and 5–9 kg): *GERD/erosive esophagitis*—5 mg once daily for 4–8 wk.
PO (Children 1 mo–<1 yr and ≥10 kg): *Erosive esophagitis*—10 mg once daily for up to 6 wk.
PO (Children 1 mo–<1 yr and 5–9 kg): *Erosive esophagitis*—5 mg once daily for up to 6 wk.
PO (Children 1 mo–<1 yr and 3–4 kg): *Erosive esophagitis*—2.5 mg once daily for up to 6 wk.

Availability (generic available)

Delayed-release capsules: 10 mg, 20 mg, 40 mg. **Delayed-release powder for oral suspension (peach-mint flavor):** 2.5 mg/packet, 10 mg/packet. **Delayed-release tablets:** 🍁 10 mg, 20 mg^{OTC}. ***In combination with:*** metronidazole and clarithromycin in a compliance package (Losec 1-2-3 M); amoxicillin and clarithromycin in a compliance package (Losec 1-2-3-A) (both in Canada only); sodium bicarbonate (Zegerid [OTC]). See Appendix B.

NURSING IMPLICATIONS

Assessment

- Assess patient routinely for epigastric or abdominal pain and frank or occult blood in the stool, emesis, or gastric aspirate.
- Monitor bowel function. Diarrhea, abdominal cramping, fever, and bloody stools should be reported to health care professional promptly as a sign of Clostridium difficile-associated diarrhea (CDAD). May begin up to several wk following cessation of therapy.
- ***Lab Test Considerations:*** Monitor CBC with differential periodically during therapy.
- May cause ↑ AST, ALT, alkaline phosphatase, and bilirubin.
- May cause serum gastrin concentrations to ↑ during first 1–2 wk of therapy. Levels return to normal after discontinuation of omeprazole.
- Monitor INR and prothrombin time in patients taking warfarin.
- May cause hypomagnesemia. Monitor serum magnesium prior to and periodically during therapy.
- May cause false positive results in diagnostic investigations for neuroendocrine tumors due to ↑ serum chromogranin A (CgA) levels secondary to drug-induced ↓ gastric acidity. Temporarily stop esomeprazole at least 14 days before assessing CgA levels and consider repeating test if initial CgA levels are high.

Implementation

- Do not confuse Prilosec (omeprazole) with Prozac (fluoxetine) or Pristiq (desvenlafaxine). Do not confuse omeprazole with fomepizole.
- **PO:** Administer doses before meals, preferably in the morning. Capsules and tablets should be swallowed whole; do not crush or chew. Capsules may be opened and sprinkled on cool applesauce, entire mixture should be ingested immediately and followed by a drink of water. Do not store for future use.
- *Powder for oral suspension:* Administer on empty stomach, as least 1 hr before a meal. Empty contents of 2.5 mg packet into 5 mL of water or contents of 10 mg packet into 15 mL of water. Stir. Leave 2–3 min to thicken. Stir and drink within 30 min. If material remains after drinking, add more water, stir and drink immediately. For patients with nasogastric or enteral feeding, suspend feeding for 3 hr before and 1 hr after administration. Empty packet contents into a small cup containing 5 mL of water for 2.5 mg dose or 15 mL water for 10 mg dose using a catheter tipped syringe. **Do not use other liquids or**

foods. Immediately shake syringe and leave 2–3 min to thicken. Administer within 30 min. Refill the syringe with an equal amount of water. Shake and flush remaining contents from nasogastric or gastric tube into stomach.
- May be administered concurrently with antacids.

Patient/Family Teaching
- Instruct patient to take medication as directed for the full course of therapy, even if feeling better. Take missed doses as soon as remembered but not if almost time for next dose. Do not double doses.
- May cause occasional drowsiness or dizziness. Caution patient to avoid driving or other activities requiring alertness until response to medication is known.
- Instruct patient to notify health care professional of all Rx or OTC medications, vitamins, or herbal products being taken and consult health care professional before taking any new medications, especially St. John's wort.
- Advise patient to avoid alcohol, products containing aspirin or NSAIDs, and foods that may cause an increase in GI irritation.
- Advise patient to report onset of black, tarry stools; diarrhea; abdominal pain; or persistent headache to health care professional promptly.
- Instruct patient to notify health care professional of onset of black, tarry stools; diarrhea; abdominal pain; or persistent headache or if fever and diarrhea develop, especially if stool contains blood, pus, or mucus. Advise patient not to treat diarrhea without consulting health care professional.
- Advise female patient to notify health care professional if pregnancy is planned or suspected, or if breast feeding.

Evaluation/Desired Outcomes
- Decrease in abdominal pain or prevention of gastric irritation and bleeding. Healing of duodenal ulcers can be seen on x-ray examination or endoscopy.
- Decrease in symptoms of GERD and erosive esophagitis. Therapy is continued for 4–8 wk after initial episode.

ondansetron (on-dan-se-tron)
✱Ondissolve ODF, Zofran, Zofran ODT, Zuplenz

Classification
Therapeutic: antiemetics
Pharmacologic: 5-HT$_3$ antagonists

Indications
Prevention of nausea and vomiting associated with highly or moderately emetogenic chemotherapy. **PO:** Prevention of nausea and vomiting associated with radiation therapy. Prevention and treatment of postoperative nausea and vomiting.

Action
Blocks the effects of serotonin at 5-HT$_3$ receptor sites (selective antagonist) located in vagal nerve terminals and the chemoreceptor trigger zone in the CNS. **Therapeutic Effects:** Decreased incidence and severity of nausea and vomiting following chemotherapy or surgery.

Pharmacokinetics
Absorption: IV administration results in complete bioavailability; 100% absorbed following oral administration.
Distribution: Unknown.
Metabolism and Excretion: Extensively metabolized by the liver (primarily by CYP3A4); 5% excreted unchanged by the kidneys.
Half-life: *Adults*—3.5–5.5 hr; *Children 5 mo–12 yr*—2.9 hr.

TIME/ACTION PROFILE (antiemetic effect)

ROUTE	ONSET	PEAK	DURATION
PO, IV	rapid	15–30 min	4–8 hr
IM	rapid	40 min	unknown

Contraindications/Precautions
Contraindicated in: Hypersensitivity; Orally disintegrating tablets contain aspartame and should not be used in patients with phenylketonuria; Congenital long QT syndrome; Concurrent use of apomorphine.
Use Cautiously in: Hepatic impairment (daily dose not to exceed 8 mg); Abdominal surgery (may mask ileus); Phenylketonuria (orally disintegrating tablets contain phenylalanine); OB, Lactation, Pedi: Pregnancy, lactation, or children ≤3 yr (PO) or <1 mo (parenteral) (safety not established).

Adverse Reactions/Side Effects
CNS: SEROTONIN SYNDROME, headache, dizziness, drowsiness, fatigue, weakness. **CV:** TORSADE DE POINTES, QT interval prolongation. **GI:** constipation, diarrhea, abdominal pain, dry mouth, ↑ liver enzymes. **Neuro:** extrapyramidal reactions. **Derm:** STEVENS-JOHNSON SYNDROME, TOXIC EPIDERMAL NECROLYSIS.

Interactions
Drug-Drug: Use with **apomorphine** ↑ risk of severe hypotension and loss of consciousness; concurrent use contraindicated. **Carbamazepine**, **phenytoin**, and **rifampin** may ↓ levels. Drugs that affect serotonergic neurotransmitter systems, including **SSRIs**, **SNRIs**, **tricyclic antidepressants**, **MAOIs**, **fentanyl**, **lithium**, **buspirone**, **tramadol**, **methylene blue**, and **triptans** ↑ risk of serotonin syndrome.

O

Route/Dosage

PO (Adults): *Prevention of nausea/vomiting associated with highly-emetogenic chemotherapy*—24 mg 30 min prior to chemotherapy.

PO (Adults and Children >11 yr): *Prevention of nausea/vomiting associated with moderately emetogenic chemotherapy*—8 mg 30 min prior to chemotherapy and repeated 8 hr later; 8 mg every 12 hr may be given for 1–2 days following chemotherapy. *Prevention of radiation-induced nausea/vomiting*—8 mg 1–2 hr prior to radiation; may be repeated every 8 hr, depending on type, location, and extent of radiation. *Prevention of postoperative nausea/vomiting*—16 mg 1 hr before induction of anesthesia.

PO (Children 4–11 yr): *Prevention of nausea/vomiting associated with moderately emetogenic chemotherapy*—4 mg 30 min prior to chemotherapy and repeated 4 and 8 hr later; 4 mg every 8 hr may be given for 1–2 days following chemotherapy.

IV (Adults): *Prevention of chemotherapy-induced nausea/vomiting*—0.15 mg/kg (max dose = 16 mg) 30 min prior to chemotherapy, repeated 4 and 8 hr later.

IM, IV (Adults): *Prevention of postoperative nausea/vomiting*—4 mg before induction of anesthesia or postoperatively.

IV (Children 6 mo–18 yr): *Prevention of chemotherapy-induced nausea/vomiting*—0.15 mg/kg (max dose = 16 mg) 30 min prior to chemotherapy, repeated 4 and 8 hr later.

IV (Children 1 mo–12 yr and >40 k g): *Prevention of postoperative nausea/vomiting*—4 mg.

IV (Children 1 mo–12 yr and ≤40 kg): *Prevention of postoperative nausea/vomiting*—0.1 mg/kg.

Hepatic Impairment

PO, IM, IV (Adults): *Severe hepatic impairment*—Not to exceed 8 mg/day.

Availability (generic available)

Orally disintegrating tablets (contain aspartame) (strawberry flavor): 4 mg, 8 mg. **Cost:** *Generic*—4 mg $668.78/30, 8 mg $1,113.95/30. **Oral soluble film (Zuplenz):** 4 mg, 8 mg. **Cost:** All strengths $16.50/1. **Tablets:** 4 mg, 8 mg, 24 mg. **Cost:** *Generic*—4 mg $735.05/30, 8 mg $1,217.42/30, 24 mg $105.50/1. **Oral solution (strawberry flavor):** 4 mg/5 mL. **Cost:** $269.74/50 mL. **Solution for injection:** 2 mg/mL.

NURSING IMPLICATIONS

Assessment

- Assess patient for nausea, vomiting, abdominal distention, and bowel sounds prior to and following administration.
- Assess patient for extrapyramidal effects (involuntary movements, facial grimacing, rigidity, shuffling walk, trembling of hands) periodically during therapy.
- Monitor ECG in patients with hypokalemia, hypomagnesemia, HF, bradyarrhythmias, or patients taking concomitant medications that prolong the QT interval.
- Monitor for signs and symptoms of serotonin syndrome (mental status changes [agitation, hallucinations, delirium, coma], autonomic instability [tachycardia, labile BP, dizziness, diaphoresis, flushing, hyperthermia], neuromuscular symptoms [tremor, rigidity, myoclonus, hyperreflexia, incoordination], seizures, gastrointestinal symptoms [nausea, vomiting, diarrhea]). If symptoms occur, discontinue therapy.
- Assess for rash periodically during therapy. May cause Stevens-Johnson syndrome or toxic epidermal necrolysis. Discontinue therapy if severe or if accompanied with fever, general malaise, fatigue, muscle or joint aches, blisters, oral lesions, conjunctivitis, hepatitis, and/or eosinophilia.
- ***Lab Test Considerations:*** May cause transient ↑ in serum bilirubin, AST, and ALT levels.

Implementation

- First dose is administered prior to emetogenic event.
- **PO:** For orally disintegrating tablets, do not attempt to push through foil backing; with dry hands, peel back backing and remove tablet. Immediately place tablet on tongue; tablet will dissolve in sec, then swallow with saliva. Administration of liquid is not necessary.

IV Administration

- **IV Push:** Administer undiluted (2 mg/mL) immediately before induction of anesthesia or postoperatively if nausea and vomiting occur shortly after surgery. ***Rate:*** Administer over at least 30 sec and preferably over 2–5 min.
- **Intermittent Infusion:** ***Diluent:*** Dilute doses for prevention of nausea and vomiting associated with chemotherapy in 50 mL of D5W, 0.9% NaCl, D5/0.9% NaCl, D5/0.45% NaCl. Solution is clear and colorless. Stable for 7 days at room temperature following dilution. ***Concentration:*** 1 mg/mL. ***Rate:*** Administer each dose over 15 min.
- **Y-Site Compatibility:** acetaminophen, aldesleukin, alemtuzumab, alfentanil, amifostine, amikacin, aminocaproic acid, anakinra, anidulafungin, argatroban, ascorbic acid, atropine, azithromycin, aztreonam, benztropine, bivalirudin, bleomycin, bumetanide, buprenorphine, busulfan, butorphanol, calcium chloride, calcium gluconate, carboplatin, carmustine, caspofungin, cefazolin, cefotaxime, cefoxitin, ceftaroline, ceftazidime, cefuroxime, chlorpromazine, ciprofloxacin, cisatracurium, cisplatin, cladribine, clindamycin, cyanocobalamin, cyclophosphamide, cyclosporine, cytarabine, dacarbazine, dactinomycin, daunorubicin hydrochloride, dexamethasone, dexmedetomidine, dexrazoxane, digoxin, diltiazem, diphenhydramine, dobutamine, docetaxel, dopamine, doxorubicin hydrochloride, doxorubicin liposomal, doxycycline, droperidol,

enalaprilat, ephedrine, epinephrine, epirubicin, epoetin alfa, eptifibatide, erythromycin, esmolol, etoposide, etoposide phosphate, famotidine, fenoldopam, fentanyl, filgrastim, floxuridine, fluconazole, fludarabine, folic acid, fosaprepritant, fosphenytoin, gemcitabine, gentamicin, glycopyrrolate, heparin, hetastarch, hydrocortisone, hydromorphone, idarubicin, ifosfamide, imipenem/cilastatin, irinotecan, isoproterenol, ketorolac, labetalol, levofloxacin, lidocaine, linezolid, magnesium sulfate, mannitol, melphalan, meperidine, mesna, methotrexate, methyldopate, metoclopramide, metoprolol, metronidazole, midazolam, mitomycin, mitoxantrone, morphine, moxifloxacin, multivitamins, mycophenolate, nafcillin, nalbuphine, naloxone, nitroglycerin, nitroprusside, norepinephrine, octreotide, oxacillin, oxaliplatin, oxytocin, paclitaxel, pamidronate, pancuronium, papaverine, penicillin G, pentamidine, pentostatin, phentolamine, phenylephrine, phytonadione, piperacillin/tazobactam, potassium acetate, potassium chloride, potassium phosphates, procainamide, prochlorperazine, promethazine, propranolol, protamine, pyridoxine, ranitidine, remifentanil, rocuronium, sodium acetate, sodium phosphates, streptokinase, streptozocin, succinylcholine, sufentanil, tacrolimus, telavancin, theophylline, thiotepa, tigecycline, tirofiban, tobramycin, topotecan, vancomycin, vasopressin, vecuronium, verapamil, vinblastine, vincristine, vinorelbine, voriconazole, zidovudine, zoledronic acid.

- **Y-Site Incompatibility:** acyclovir, allopurinol, aminophylline, amphotericin B deoxycholate, amphotericin B lipid complex, amphotericin B liposome, ampicillin, ampicillin/sulbactam, amsacrine, cefepime, chloramphenicol, dantrolene, ertapenem, foscarnet, furosemide, ganciclovir, indomethacin, lorazepam, micafungin, milrinone, pantoprazole, pemetrexed, pentobarbital, phenobarbital, phenytoin, rituximab, sargramostim, sodium bicarbonate, thiopental, trastuzumab, trimethoprim/sulfamethoxazole.

Patient/Family Teaching

- Instruct patient to take ondansetron as directed.
- Advise patient to notify health care professional immediately if symptoms of irregular heart beat, serotonin syndrome, or involuntary movement of eyes, face, or limbs occur.

Evaluation/Desired Outcomes

- Prevention of nausea and vomiting associated with emetogenic cancer chemotherapy.
- Prevention of postoperative nausea and vomiting.
- Prevention of nausea and vomiting due to radiation therapy.

oritavancin (oh-rit-a-**van**-sin)

Orbactiv

Classification

Therapeutic: anti-infectives

Pharmacologic: lipoglycopeptides

Indications

Treatment of acute bacterial skin and skin structure infections caused by or suspected to be caused by susceptible designated Gram-positive bacteria.

Action

Binds to bacterial cell wall resulting in cell death. **Therapeutic Effects:** Bactericidal action against susceptible bacteria with resolution of infection. **Spectrum:** Active against *Staphylococcus aureus* (including methicillin-susceptible and resistant strains), *Streptococcus pyogenes*, *Streptococcus agalactiae*, *Streptococcus dysgalactiae*, *Streptococcus anginosus* (including *S. anginosus*, *S. intermidius*, and *S. constellatus*) and *Enterococcus faecalis* (vancomycin-susceptible strains only).

Pharmacokinetics

Absorption: IV administration results in complete bioavailability.

Distribution: Penetrates skin/skin structures.

Metabolism and Excretion: Slowly excreted unchanged in urine (5% in two wk) and feces (1% in two wk).

Half-life: 245 hr (terminal).

TIME/ACTION PROFILE (blood levels)

ROUTE	ONSET	PEAK	DURATION
IV	rapid	end of infusion	at least 2 wk

Contraindications/Precautions

Contraindicated in: Hypersensitivity (cross-sensitivity with other glycopeptides may occur); Heparin use for 120 hr (5 days) following administration of oritavancin (causes false ↑ aPTT); Concurrent warfarin (↑ risk of bleeding, use only if benefit outweighs bleeding risk); Confirmed/suspected osteomyelitis (alternate treatment required).

Use Cautiously in: Concurrent use of drugs with narrow therapeutic indices that are metabolized by the CYP450 enzyme system (effects may be altered); Severe hepatic/renal impairment; Geri: Elderly patients may be ↑ sensitive to drug effects; OB: Use during pregnancy only if potential benefit justifies fetal risk; Lactation: Use cautiously if breast feeding; Pedi: Safety and effectiveness not established.

O

Adverse Reactions/Side Effects

CNS: headache. **CV:** tachycardia. **GI:** diarrhea including CLOSTRIDIUM DIFFICILE, ↑ liver enzymes, nausea, vomiting. **Local:** infusion site reactions. **Misc:** hypersensitivity reactions including ANAPHYLAXIS, infusion reactions including "Red-Man Syndrome," limb/subcutaneous abscess formation.

Interactions

Drug-Drug: ↑ risk of bleeding with **warfarin** (avoid if possible). Affects the activities of several CYP450 enzymes (careful monitoring of other **drugs metabolized by the CYP450 system** that have narrow therapeutic indices to assess for toxicity or ineffectiveness is recommended).

Route/Dosage

IV (Adults >18 yr): 1200 mg single dose.

Availability

Lyophylized powder for injection: 400 mg/vial.

NURSING IMPLICATIONS

Assessment

- Assess for infection (vital signs; appearance of wound, sputum, urine, and stool; WBC) at beginning of and during therapy.
- Obtain specimens for culture and sensitivity prior to therapy. First dose may be given before receiving results.
- Monitor bowel function. Diarrhea, abdominal cramping, fever, and bloody stools should be reported to health care professional promptly as a sign of Clostridium difficile-associated diarrhea (CDAD). May begin up to 2 mo following cessation of therapy.
- Monitor for infusion reactions (Red-man syndrome—flushing of upper body, urticaria, pruritus, rash). May resolve with stopping or slowing infusion.
- ***Lab Test Considerations:*** Monitor hepatic function tests. May cause ↑ ALT, AST, and bilirubin.
- May cause hyperuricemia and hypoglycemia.
- Causes falsely ↑ aPTT for 120 hrs after infusion. Avoid heparin administration during this time. Use a non-phospholipid dependent coagulation test such as Factor Xa assay if needed.
- Artificially prolongs PT and INR for up to 12 hr. May increase risk of bleeding with warfarin.

Implementation

- Using three 400 mg vials, add 40 mL of sterile water for injection to each vial for a 10 mg/mL solution/vial. Swirl gently to avoid foaming and ensure powder is completely reconstituted. Solution is clear and colorless to pale yellow; do not administer solutions that are discolored or contain particulate matter. ***Diluent:*** Withdraw and discard 120 mL from 1000 mL bag of D5W. Withdraw 40 mL from each vial and add to D5W bag. Do not use 0.9% NaCl; may cause precipitation. ***Concentration:*** 1.2 mg/mL. Use within 6 hr at room temperature or 12 hr if refrigerated, including 3 hr infusion. ***Rate:*** Infuse over 3 hr.
- **Y-Site Incompatibility:** Do not mix with other solutions or medications. Flush line before and after infusion.

Patient/Family Teaching

- Instruct patient to notify health care professional if signs and symptoms of hypersensitivity reactions (rash, hives, dyspnea, facial swelling) occur.
- Instruct patient to notify health care professional immediately if diarrhea, abdominal cramping, fever, or bloody stools occur and not to treat with antidiarrheals without consulting health care professionals.
- Advise patient to notify health care professional of all Rx or OTC medications, vitamins, or herbal products being taken and to consult with health care professional before taking other medications.
- Advise female patients to notify health care professional if pregnancy is planned or suspected or if breast feeding.
- Instruct the patient to notify health care professional if symptoms do not improve.

Evaluation/Desired Outcomes

- Resolution of the signs and symptoms of infection. Length of time for complete resolution depends on the organism and site of infection.

oseltamivir (o-sel-**tam**-i-vir)

Tamiflu

Classification
Therapeutic: antivirals
Pharmacologic: neuraminidase inhibitors

Indications

Treatment of uncomplicated acute illness due to influenza infection in adults and children ≥2 wk who have had symptoms for ≤2 days. Prevention of influenza in patients ≥1 yr.

Action

Inhibits the enzyme neuraminidase, which may alter virus particle aggregation and release. **Therapeutic Effects:** Reduced duration or prevention of flu-related symptoms.

Pharmacokinetics

Absorption: Rapidly absorbed from the GI tract and converted by the liver to the active form, oseltamivir carboxylate. 75% reaches systemic circulation as the active drug.
Distribution: Unknown.
Protein Binding: oseltamivir phosphate: 42%; oseltamivir carboxylate: 3%.
Metabolism and Excretion: Rapidly metabolized by the liver to oseltamivir carboxylate, the active drug. >99% excreted unchanged in urine.

Half-life: *Oseltamivir carboxylate*—6–10 hr.

TIME/ACTION PROFILE (blood levels)

ROUTE	ONSET	PEAK	DURATION
PO	unknown	unknown	12 hr

Contraindications/Precautions

Contraindicated in: Hypersensitivity; End stage renal disease and not receiving dialysis.

Use Cautiously in: Renal impairment (↓ dose if CCr ≤60 mL/min); Hereditary fructose intolerance (75 mg of oral suspension contains 2 g of sorbitol); OB: Use during pregnancy only if benefit to patient outweighs potential fetal risk; Lactation: Use during breast feeding only if benefit to patient outweighs potential risk to infant; Pedi: Children <2 wk (safety and efficacy not established for treatment); children <1 yr (safety and efficacy not established for prevention). Oral suspension contains sodium benzoate, avoid use in neonates.

Adverse Reactions/Side Effects

CNS: SEIZURES, abnormal behavior, agitation, confusion, delirium, hallucinations, insomnia, nightmares, vertigo. **GI:** nausea, vomiting. **Resp:** bronchitis.

Interactions

Drug-Drug: May ↓ the therapeutic effect of **influenza virus vaccine** avoid use 2 days prior to and 2 wk after vaccine administration.

Route/Dosage

Treatment of Influenza

PO (Adults and Children ≥13 yr): 75 mg twice daily for 5 days.
PO (Children 1–12 yr and >40 kg): 75 mg twice daily for 5 days.
PO (Children 1–12 yr and 23.1–40 kg): 60 mg twice daily for 5 days.
PO (Children 1–12 yr and 15.1–23 kg): 45 mg twice daily for 5 days.
PO (Children 1–12 yr and ≤15 kg): 30 mg twice daily for 5 days.
PO (Infants 2 wk–<1 yr): 3 mg/kg/dose twice daily for 5 days.

Renal Impairment

PO (Adults): *CCr 30–60 mL/min*—30 mg twice daily for 5 days; *CCr 10–30 mL/min*—30 mg once daily for 5 days; *CCr ≥10 mL/min and on HD*—30 mg after each HD session (not to exceed 5 days); *CCr ≥10 mL/min and on PD*—30 mg single dose immediately after a dialysis exchange; *CCr <10 mL/min and not on dialysis*—Not recommended.

Influenza Prevention

PO (Adults and Children ≥13 yr): 75 mg once daily for ≥10 days.
PO (Children 1–12 yr and >40 k g): 75 mg once daily for 10 days.
PO (Children 1–12 yr and 23.1–40 kg): 60 mg once daily for 10 days.
PO (Children 1–12 yr and 15.1–23 kg): 45 mg once daily for 10 days.
PO (Children 1–12 yr and ≤15 kg): 30 mg once daily for 10 days.

Renal Impairment

PO (Adults): *CCr 30–60 mL/min*—30 mg once daily for ≥10 days; *CCr 10–30 mL/min*—30 mg every other day for ≥10 days; *CCr ≥10 mL/min and on HD*—30 mg after alternate HD sessions (treatment duration ≥10 days); *CCr ≥10 mL/min and on PD*—30 mg once weekly immediately after a dialysis exchange (treatment duration ≥10 days); *CCr <10 mL/min and not on dialysis*—Not recommended.

Availability (generic available)

Capsules: 30 mg, 45 mg, 75 mg. **Oral suspension (tutti-frutti flavor):** 6 mg/mL.

O

NURSING IMPLICATIONS

Assessment

- Monitor influenza symptoms (sudden onset of fever, cough, headache, fatigue, muscular weakness, sore throat). Additional supportive treatment may be indicated to treat symptoms.

Implementation

- Treatment with oseltamivir should be started as soon as possible from the first sign of flu symptoms within 2 days of exposure.
- Consider available information on influenza drug susceptibility patterns and treatment effects before using oseltamivir for prophylaxis.
- **PO:** May be administered with food or milk to minimize GI irritation.
- Use correct oral dosing device for measuring oral solution. Dosing errors have occurred due to oseltamivir dosing in mg and solution in mL. Make sure units of measure on prescription instructions match dosing device provided with the drug.
- If oral suspension is not available, capsules can be opened and mixed with flavored foods (regular or sugar-free chocolate syrup, corn syrup, caramel topping, light brown sugar dissolved in water). If correct dose and oral suspension are not available, pharmacist may compound emergency supply of oral suspension from 75 mg capsules.

Patient/Family Teaching

- Instruct patient to take oseltamivir as soon as influenza symptoms appear and to continue to take it as directed, for the full course of therapy, even if feeling better. Take missed doses as soon as remembered

unless within 2 hr of next dose. Do not double doses.
- Caution patient that oseltamivir should not be shared with anyone, even if they have the same symptoms.
- Advise patient that oseltamivir is not a substitute for a flu shot. Patients should receive annual flu shot according to immunization guidelines.
- Advise patients to report behavioral changes (hallucinations, delirium, and abnormal behavior) to health care professional immediately.
- Advise patient to notify health care professional of all Rx or OTC medications, vitamins, or herbal products being taken and to consult with health care professional before taking other medications.
- Advise females of reproductive potential to notify health care professional if pregnancy is planned or suspected, or if breast feeding.

Evaluation/Desired Outcomes

- Reduced duration or prevention of flu-related symptoms.

osimertinib (oh-si-mer-ti-nib)

Tagrisso

Classification

Therapeutic: antineoplastics

Pharmacologic: epidermal growth factor receptor (EGFR) inhibitors

Indications

Treatment of metastatic epidermal growth factor receptor (EGFR) T790M mutation-positive non–small-cell lung cancer (NSCLC) in patients who have progressed on or after EGFR tyrosine kinase inhibitor therapy. First-line treatment of metastatic NSCLC in patients whose tumors have EGFR exon 19 deletions or exon 21 L858R mutations.

Action

Irreversibly binds to select mutant forms of EGFR (including T790M), resulting in inactivation of kinases that regulate proliferation and transformation; the T790M mutation is the most common mechanism of resistance to EGFR tyrosine kinase inhibitors. **Therapeutic Effects:** Decreased spread of NSCLC.

Pharmacokinetics

Absorption: Well absorbed following oral administration.

Distribution: Extensively distributed to tissues.

Protein Binding: 95%.

Metabolism and Excretion: Mostly metabolized by the liver (CYP3A4 enzyme system) to 2 active metabolites; 68% excreted in feces (2% as unchanged drug); 14% excreted in urine (2% as unchanged drug).

Half-life: 48 hr.

TIME/ACTION PROFILE (blood levels)

ROUTE	ONSET	PEAK	DURATION
Oral	unknown	6 hr	24 hr

Contraindications/Precautions

Contraindicated in: Concurrent use of strong CYP3A4 inhibitors or inducers; OB: Pregnancy (may cause fetal harm); Lactation: Breast feeding should be avoided during treatment and for 2 wk after therapy.

Use Cautiously in: Congenital long QT syndrome, HF, electrolyte abnormalities, or taking QT interval prolonging medications; End-stage renal disease (CCr <15 mL/min); Severe hepatic impairment; Rep: Women of reproductive potential and men with female partners of reproductive potential; Pedi: Safety and effectiveness not established.

Adverse Reactions/Side Effects

CNS: STROKE, fatigue, headache. **CV:** CARDIOMYOPATHY, QT INTERVAL PROLONGATION, VENOUS THROMBOEMBOLISM. **Derm:** dry skin, nail disorders, pruritus, rash. **EENT:** blepharitis, blurred vision, cataracts, dry eye, eye pain, ↑ lacrimation, keratitis. **F and E:** hypermagnesemia, hyponatremia. **GI:** constipation, ↓ appetite, diarrhea, nausea, stomatitis. **Hemat:** NEUTROPENIA, THROMBOCYTOPENIA, anemia, lymphopenia. **MS:** back pain. **Resp:** INTERSTITIAL LUNG DISEASE, cough.

Interactions

Drug-Drug: Strong CYP3A4 inhibitors, including **itraconazole**, **nefazodone**, and **ritonavir** may ↑ levels and the risk of toxicity; avoid concurrent use. **Strong CYP3A4 inducers**, including **carbamazepine**, **rifampin**, and **phenytoin** may ↓ levels and its effectiveness; avoid concurrent use. May ↑ or ↓ **carbamazepine**, **cyclosporine**, **ergot derivatives**, **fentanyl**, **phenytoin**, or **quinidine**; avoid concurrent use. **QT interval prolonging drugs** may ↑ risk of torsade de pointes; avoid concurrent use. May ↑ levels of **P-gp substrates**, including **fexofenadine**. May ↑ levels of **breast cancer resistant protein (BCRP) substrates**, including **rosuvastatin**.

Drug-Natural Products: St. John's wort may ↓ levels and its effectiveness; avoid concurrent use.

Route/Dosage

PO (Adults): 80 mg once daily until disease progression or unacceptable toxicity.

Availability

Tablets: 40 mg, 80 mg.

NURSING IMPLICATIONS

Assessment

- Assess for worsening respiratory symptoms (dyspnea, coughing, fever) during therapy; may indicate interstitial lung disease or pneumonitis. If signs and symptoms occur, permanently discontinue osimertinib.

- Monitor cardiac status (ECG, electrolytes) periodically during therapy, especially in patients with congenital long QTc syndrome, HF, electrolyte abnormalities, or taking medications that prolong QTc interval. *If QTc interval >500 msec on at least 2 separate ECGs,* withhold therapy until QTc interval is <481 msec or recovery to baseline if baseline is ≥481 msec, resume at 40 mg dose. *If QTc interval prolongation occurs with signs and symptoms of life threatening arrhythmia,* permanently discontinue therapy.
- Assess for signs and symptoms of cardiomyopathy (cardiac failure, pulmonary edema, ejection fraction decreased, stress cardiomyopathy) by echo cardiogram, multigated acquisition (MUGA) scan prior to starting therapy and every 3 mo during therapy. *If asymptomatic and absolute decrease in LVEF of 10% from baseline and below 50%,* withhold therapy for up to 4 wk. If improved to baseline, resume. If not improved to baseline, permanently discontinue. *If symptomatic HF develops,* permanently discontinue therapy.
- ***Lab Test Considerations:*** Obtain a negative pregnancy test before starting therapy.
- Monitor CBC with differential periodically during therapy. May cause lymphopenia, thrombocytopenia, anemia, and neutropenia. *If ≥Grade 3 reaction occurs,* withhold osimertinib for up to 3 wk. *If improved to Grade 0–2,* resume at 80 mg or 40 mg daily. *If no improvement in 3 wk,* permanently discontinue osimertinib.
- May cause hyponatremia and hypermagnesemia.

Implementation

- **PO:** Administer once daily without regard to food.
- For patients with difficulty swallowing, disperse tablet in 4 tbsp (50 mL) of only non-carbonated water. Stir until tablet is completely dispersed and swallow or administer through NG tube immediately; do not crush, heat, or ultrasonicate during preparation. Rinse container with 4–8 oz of water and drink or administer through NG tube immediately.

Patient/Family Teaching

- Instruct patient to take osimertinib as directed. If dose missed, omit and take next dose as scheduled. Advise patient to read *Patient Information* prior to starting therapy and with each Rx dose refill in case of changes.
- Advise patient to notify health care professional if signs and symptoms of lung problems (worsening lung symptoms, trouble breathing, shortness of breath, cough, fever) or heart problems (pounding or racing heart, shortness of breath, swollen ankles or feet, lightheadedness) occur.
- Instruct patient to notify health care professional of all Rx or OTC medications, vitamins, or herbal products being taken and consult health care professional before taking any new medications.
- Rep: May be teratogenic and may impair fertility in males and females. Caution women of reproductive potential to use effective contraception during and for at least 6 wk after final dose. Advise males with female partners of reproductive potential to use effective contraception during and for at least 4 mo after final dose. Advise females patient to avoid breast feeding during and for at least 2 wk after final dose.

Evaluation/Desired Outcomes

- Decreased spread of NSCLC.

ospemifene (os-pem-i-feen)

Osphena

Classification

Therapeutic: hormones

Pharmacologic: estrogen agonists/antagonists

Indications

Moderate to severe dyspareunia due to menopausal vulvar/vaginal atrophy. Moderate to severe vaginal dryness due to menopausal vulvar/vaginal atrophy.

Action

Has agonist (estrogen-like) effects on the endometrium of the uterus; effects are tissue-specific. **Therapeutic Effects:** Decreased dyspareunuia. Decreased vaginal dryness.

Pharmacokinetics

Absorption: Well absorbed following oral administration; food enhances absorption 2–3 fold.

Distribution: Unknown.

Protein Binding: >99%.

Metabolism and Excretion: Mostly metabolized by the liver (CYP3A4 and CYP2C9 enzyme systems); 75% excreted in feces, 7% in urine as metabolites; minimal amounts excreted unchanged in urine.

Half-life: 26 hr.

TIME/ACTION PROFILE (improvement in symptoms)

ROUTE	ONSET	PEAK	DURATION
PO	within 12 wk	unknown	unknown

Contraindications/Precautions

Contraindicated in: Hypersensitivity; Undiagnosed abnormal genital bleeding; History/ suspicion of estrogen-dependent cancer; History of/current thromboembolic disorder, including DVT, PE, MI, or stroke; Concurrent use of estrogens, estrogen agonists/antagonists, fluconazole, or rifampin; Severe hepatic impairment;

O

OB: Known/suspected pregnancy (may cause fetal harm); Lactation: Breast feeding should be avoided.

Use Cautiously in: Patients with risk factors for cardiovascular disease, arterial vascular disease, or venous thromboembolism (including hypertension, obesity, family history, tobacco use, diabetes mellitus, history of DVT/PE, or systemic lupus erythematosus); Women with a uterus (estrogen use without a progestin ↑ risk of endometrial cancer); Known or suspected breast cancer.

Adverse Reactions/Side Effects

CV: DEEP VEIN THROMBOSIS/PE, MI, STROKE. **Derm:** hot flush, hyperhydrosis. **GU:** ENDOMETRIAL CANCER, genital/vaginal discharge. **MS:** muscle spasms. **Misc:** HYPERSENSITIVITY REACTIONS (including angioedema).

Interactions

Drug-Drug: Fluconazole may ↑ levels and risk of toxicity; avoid concurrent use. **Ketoconazole** or other **CYP3A4 or CYP2C9 inhibitors** may ↑ levels and risk of toxicity. **Rifampin** may ↓ levels and effectiveness; avoid concurrent use. Avoid concurrent use of other **estrogens** or **estrogen agonist/antagonists** due to ↑ estrogen effects. May displace or be displaced by other **drugs that are highly protein bound**.

Route/Dosage

PO (Adults): 60 mg once daily.

Availability

Tablets: 60 mg.

NURSING IMPLICATIONS

Assessment

- Assess amount of pain during intercourse and vaginal dryness prior to and periodically during therapy.
- Determine methods previously use to treat dyspareunia.
- Assess BP before and periodically during therapy.
- Monitor for hypersensitivity reactions (angioedema, urticaria, rash, pruritus). If symptoms occur discontinue ospemifene and treat symptomatically.

Implementation

- **PO:** Administer once daily with food.

Patient/Family Teaching

- Instruct patient to take ospemifene as directed. Advise patient to read *Patient Information* sheet before starting therapy and with each Rx refill in case of changes.
- Advise patient to report signs and symptoms of unusual vaginal bleeding, changes in vision or speech, sudden new severe headaches, severe pains in chest or legs with or without shortness of breath, weakness, or fatigue promptly to health care professional immediately.
- Inform patient that ospemifene may cause hot flashes, vaginal discharge, muscle spasm, and increased sweating.
- Patients who still have a uterus should discuss addition of progestin with health care professional.
- Instruct patient to notify health care professional of all Rx or OTC medications, vitamins, or herbal products being taken and consult health care professional before taking any new medications.
- Advise patient to notify health care professional of medication regimen before treatment or surgery.
- Advise women to follow yearly exams (pelvic exam, breast exam, mammogram) to monitor for breast and uterine cancer.
- Caution patient that cigarette smoking, high BP, high cholesterol, diabetes, and being overweight during estrogen therapy may increase risk of heart disease.
- Ospemifene should not be taken during pregnancy or breast feeding. Instruct patient to notify health care professional immediately if pregnancy is planned or suspected or if breast feeding.
- Advise patient to discuss dose and need for ospemifene every 3–6 mo.

Evaluation/Desired Outcomes

- Decrease in pain during intercourse.
- Decreased vaginal dryness.

oxacillin, See PENICILLINS, PENICILLINASE RESISTANT.

oxaliplatin (ox-a-li-pla-tin)

Eloxatin

Classification

Therapeutic: antineoplastics

Pharmacologic: alkylating agents

Indications

Adjuvant treatment of stage III colon cancer in patients who have undergone complete resection of the primary tumor (in combination with 5–fluorouracil and leucovorin). Treatment of advanced colorectal cancer (in combination with 5–fluorouracil and leucovorin). **Unlabeled Use:** Treatment of ovarian cancer that has progressed despite treatment with other agents.

Action

Inhibits DNA replication and transcription by incorporating platinum into normal cross-linking (cell-cycle nonspecific). **Therapeutic Effects:** Death of rapidly replicating cells, particularly malignant ones.

Pharmacokinetics

Absorption: IV administration results in complete bioavailability.

Distribution: Extensive tissue distribution.

Protein Binding: >90% (platinum).

Metabolism and Excretion: Undergoes rapid and extensive nonenzymatic biotransformation; excreted mostly by the kidneys.

Half-life: 391 hrs.

TIME/ACTION PROFILE

ROUTE	ONSET	PEAK	DURATION
IV	unknown	unknown	unknown

Contraindications/Precautions

Contraindicated in: Hypersensitivity; Hypersensitivity to other platinum compounds; OB, Lactation: Pregnancy or lactation (may cause fetal harm).

Use Cautiously in: Renal impairment; HF, bradycardia, concomitant use of QT interval prolonging medications, hypokalemia, and hypomagnesemia; Geri: ↑ risk of adverse reactions; Pedi: Safety not established.

Adverse Reactions/Side Effects

Adverse reactions are noted for the combination of oxaliplatin, 5–fluorouracil and leucovorin.

CNS: REVERSIBLE POSTERIOR LEUKOENCEPHALOPATHY SYNDROME, fatigue. **CV:** QT INTERVAL PROLONGATION, TORSADE DE POINTES, chest pain, edema, thromboembolism. **EENT:** visual abnormalities. **Resp:** PULMONARY FIBROSIS, cough, dyspnea. **GI:** diarrhea, nausea, vomiting, abdominal pain, anorexia, gastroesophageal reflux, stomatitis. **F and E:** dehydration, hypokalemia. **Hemat:** leukopenia, NEUTROPENIA, THROMBOCYTOPENIA, anemia. **Local:** injection site reactions. **MS:** RHABDOMYOLYSIS, back pain. **Neuro:** neurotoxicity. **Misc:** ANAPHYLAXIS/ANAPHYLACTOID REACTIONS, fever.

Interactions

Drug-Drug: Concurrent use of **nephrotoxic agents** may ↑ toxicity. Concurrent use of QT interval prolonging medications, including **Class Ia antiarrhythmics** and **Class III antiarrhythimics** may ↑ risk of torsade de pointes.

Route/Dosage

IV (Adults): *Day 1*—85 mg/m² with leucovorin 200 mg/m² at the same time over 2 hr, followed by 5–fluorouracil 400 mg/m² bolus over 2–4 min, then 5–fluorouracil 600 mg/m² as a 22 hr infusion. *Day 2*—leucovorin 200 mg/m² over 2 hr, followed by 5–fluorouracil 400 mg/m² bolus over 2–4 min, then 5–fluorouracil 600 mg/m² as a 22 hr infusion. Cycle is repeated every 2 wk. Dosage reduction/alteration may be required for neurotoxicity or other serious adverse effects.

Renal Impairment

IV (Adults): *CCr <30 mL/min*—↓ dose on Day 1 to 65 mg/m².

Availability (generic available)

Solution for injection: 5 mg/mL.

NURSING IMPLICATIONS

Assessment

- Assess for peripheral sensory neuropathy. *Acute onset* occurs within hr to 1–2 days of dosing, resolves within 14 days, and frequently recurs with further dosing (transient paresthesia, dysesthesia, and hypothesia of hands, feet, perioral area, or throat). Symptoms may be precipitated or exacerbated by exposure to cold or cold objects; avoid ice during symptoms. May also cause jaw spasm, abnormal tongue sensation, dysarthria, eye pain, and a feeling of chest pressure. *Persistent* (>14 days) causes paresthesias, dysethesias, and hypoesthesias, but may also include deficits in proprioception that may interfere with daily activities (walking, writing, swallowing). Persistent neuropathy may occur without prior acute neuropathy and may improve upon discontinuation of oxaliplatin. **Adjuvant Therapy in Patients with Stage III Colon Cancer:** *For persistent Grade 2 neurosensory events that do not resolve,* reduce dose of oxaliplatin to 75 mg/m². *For patients with persistent Grade 3 neurosensory events,* consider discontinuing therapy. Do not alter infusional 5-fluorouracil/leucovorin regimen. **Therapy in Previously Untreated and Previously Treated Patients with Advanced Colorectal Cancer:** *For persistent Grade 2 neurosensory events that do not resolve, reduce dose to 65 mg/m². For patients with persistent Grade 3 neurosensory events,* consider discontinuing therapy. Do not alter infusional 5-fluorouracil/leucovorin regimen.
- Assess for signs of pulmonary fibrosis (non-productive cough, dyspnea, crackles, radiological; infiltrates). May be fatal. Discontinue oxaliplatin if pulmonary fibrosis occurs.
- Monitor for signs of anaphylaxis (rash, hives, swelling of lips or tongue, sudden cough). Epinephrine, corticosteroids, and antihistamines should be readily available.
- Monitor for signs and symptoms of reversible posterior leukoencephalopathy syndrome (headache, altered mental functioning, seizures, abnormal vision from blurriness to blindness, associated or not with hypertension).
- ***Lab Test Considerations:*** Monitor WBC with differential, hemoglobin, platelet count, and blood chemistries (ALT, AST, bilirubin, and creatinine) before each oxaliplatin cycle. **Adjuvant Therapy in Patients with Stage III Colon Cancer:** *For Grade 4 neutropenia, or febrile neutropenia, or Grade 3/4 thrombocytopenia,* reduce dose of oxaliplatin to 75 mg/m² and infusional 5-fluorouracil to 300 mg/m² bolus and 500 mg/m² 22 hr infusion. Delay next dose until neutrophils ≥1.5 x 10^9/L and platelets ≥75 x 10^9/L. **Therapy in Previously Un-**

O

treated and Previously Treated Patients with Advanced Colorectal Cancer: *After recovery from grade 3/4 gastrointestinal (despite prophylactic treatment), or grade 4 neutropenia, or febrile neutropenia, or grade 3/4 thrombocytopenia:* reduce dose of oxaliplatin to 65 mg/m^2 and 5-fluorouracil by 20% (300 mg/m^2 bolus and 500 mg/m^2 22-hr infusion). Delay next dose until neutrophils $\geq$1.5 x 10^9/L and platelets $\geq$75 x 10^9/L.

Implementation

- Extravasation may result in local pain and inflammation that may be severe and lead to necrosis.
- Premedicate patient with antiemetics with or without dexamethasone. Prehydration is not required.

IV Administration

- **Intermittent Infusion:** Protect concentrated solution from light; do not freeze. ***Diluent:*** Must be further diluted with 250–500 mL of D5W. **Do not use 0.9% NaCl or any other chloride-containing solution for final solution.** Do not use aluminum needles or administration sets containing aluminum parts; aluminum may cause degradation of platinum compounds. May be stored in refrigerator for 24 hr or 6 hr at room temperature. Diluted solution is not light-sensitive. Do not administer solutions that are discolored or contain particulate matter. ***Concentration:*** 0.2–0.6 mg/mL. ***Rate:*** Administer oxaliplatin simultaneously with leucovorin in separate bags via Y-line over 120 min. Prolonging infusion time to 6 hr may decrease acute toxicities. Infusion times for fluorouracil and leucovorin do not need to change.
- **Y-Site Compatibility:** alemtuzumab, alfentanil, amifostine, amikacin, aminocaproic acid, amiodarone, amphotericin B deoxycholate, amphotericin B lipid complex, amphotericin B liposome, ampicillin, ampicillin/sulbactam, anidulafungin, argatroban, atracurium, azithromycin, aztreonam, bivalirudin, bleomycin, bumetanide, buprenorphine, butorphanol, calcium gluconate, carboplatin, caspofungin, cefotetan, cefoxitin, ceftazidime, ceftriaxone, cefuroxime, chloramphenicol, ciprofloxacin, cisatracurium, cisplatin, clindamycin, cyclophosphamide, cyclosporine, cytarabine, dacarbazine, dactinomycin, daptomycin, daunorubicin hydrochloride, dexamethasone, dexmedetomidine, dexrazoxane, digoxin, diltiazem, diphenhydramine, dobutamine, docetaxel, dopamine, doxacurium, doxorubicin, doxorubicin liposomal, doxycycline, droperidol, enalaprilat, ephedrine, epinephrine, epirubicin, ertapenem, erythromycin, esmolol, etoposide, etoposide phosphate, famotidine, fenoldopam, fentanyl, fluconazole, fludarabine, foscarnet, fosphenytoin, furosemide, gemcitabine, gentamicin, glycopyrrolate, granisetron, haloperidol, heparin, hetastarch, hydralazine, hydrocortisone, hydromorphone, idarubicin, ifosfamide, imipenem/cilastatin, insulin, irinotecan, isoproterenol, ketorolac, labetalol, leucovorin calcium, levofloxacin, leucovorin calcium, levorphanol, lidocaine, linezolid, lorazepam, magnesium sulfate, mannitol, meperidine, meropenem, mesna, metaraminol, methyldopate, methylprednisolone sodium succinate, metoclopramide, metoprolol, metronidazole, midazolam, milrinone, mitoxantrone, morphine, moxifloxacin, nafcillin, nalbuphine, naloxone, nicardipine, nitroglycerin, nitroprusside, norepinephrine, octreotide, ondansetron, paclitaxel, palonosetron, pancuronium, pemetrexed, pentamidine, phentolamine, phenylephrine, potassium acetate, potassium chloride, potassium phosphates, procainamide, prochlorperazine, promethazine, propranolol, quinupristin/dalfopristin, ranitidine, rocuronium, sodium acetate, sodium phosphates, succinylcholine, sufentanil, tacrolimus, theophylline, thiotepa, tigecycline, tirofiban, tobramycin, tolazoline, topotecan, trimethoprim/sulfamethoxazole, vancomycin, vasopressin, vecuronium, verapamil, vinblastine, vincristine, vinorelbine, voriconazole, zidovudine, zoledronic acid.
- **Y-Site Incompatibility:** calcium chloride, cefepime, dantrolene, diazepam.Alkaline solutions, chloride-containing solutions. Infusion line should be flushed with D5W prior to administration of other solutions or medications.

Patient/Family Teaching

- Inform patients and caregivers of potential for peripheral neuropathy and potentiation by exposure to cold or cold objects. Advise patient to avoid cold drinks, use of ice in drinks or as ice packs, and to cover exposed skin prior to exposure to cold temperature or cold objects. Caution patients to cover themselves with a blanket during infusion, do not breathe deeply when exposed to cold air, wear warm clothing, and cover mouth and nose with a scarf or pull-down ski cap to warm the air that goes to their lungs, do not take things from the freezer or refrigerator without wearing gloves, drink fluids warm or at room temperature, always drink through a straw, do not use ice chips for nausea, be aware that most metals (car doors, mailbox) are cold; wear gloves to touch, do not run air conditioning at high levels in house or car, if hands get cold wash them with warm water. Advise health care professional of how you did since last treatment before next infusion.
- Instruct patient to notify health care professional immediately if signs of reversible posterior leukoencephalopathy syndrome, low blood cell counts (fever, persistent diarrhea, infection) or if persistent vomiting, signs of dehydration, cough or breathing difficulty, thirst, dry mouth, dizziness, decreased urination, signs of infection (fever, temperature of $\geq$100.5° F, cough that brings up mucus, chills or shivering, burning or pain on urination, pain on swallowing, sore throat, redness or swelling at intravenous site) or signs of allergic reactions occur.

- Advise female patient to use effective contraception during therapy and to avoid breasfeeeding; oxaliplatin is teratogenic.

Evaluation/Desired Outcomes

- Decrease in size and spread of malignancies.

BEERS

oxazepam (ox-az-e-pam)

Novoxapam, Oxpam, Serax

Classification
Therapeutic: antianxiety agents, sedative/hypnotics
Pharmacologic: benzodiazepines

Schedule IV

Indications

Management of anxiety, anxiety associated with depression. Symptomatic treatment of alcohol withdrawal.

Action

Depresses the CNS, probably by potentiating GABA, an inhibitory neurotransmitter. **Therapeutic Effects:** Decreased anxiety. Diminished symptoms of alcohol withdrawal.

Pharmacokinetics

Absorption: Well absorbed following oral administration. Absorption is slower than with other benzodiazepines.
Distribution: Widely distributed. Crosses the blood-brain barrier. May cross the placenta and enter breast milk.
Metabolism and Excretion: Metabolized by the liver to inactive compounds.
Protein Binding: 97%.
Half-life: 5–15 hr.

TIME/ACTION PROFILE (sedation)

ROUTE	ONSET	PEAK	DURATION
PO	45–90 min	unknown	6–12 hr

Contraindications/Precautions

Contraindicated in: Hypersensitivity; Cross-sensitivity with other benzodiazepines may exist; Comatose patients or those with pre-existing CNS depression; Uncontrolled severe pain; Angle-closure glaucoma; Some products contain tartrazine and should be avoided in patients with known intolerance; OB, Lactation: Pregnancy or lactation.
Use Cautiously in: Hepatic dysfunction (may be preferred over some benzodiazepines due to short half-life); History of suicide attempt or substance use disorder; Debilitated patients (initial dosage ↓ recommended); Severe chronic obstructive pulmonary disease; Myasthenia gravis; Pedi: Children <6 yr (safety not established); Geri: Appears on Beers list (associated with ↑ risk of falls; ↓ dose required); ↑ sensitivity to benzodiazepines.

Adverse Reactions/Side Effects

CNS: <u>dizziness</u>, <u>drowsiness</u>, confusion, hangover, headache, impaired memory, mental depression, paradoxical excitation, slurred speech. **EENT:** blurred vision. **Resp:** respiratory depression. **CV:** tachycardia. **GI:** constipation, diarrhea, drug-induced hepatitis, nausea, vomiting, weight gain (unusual). **GU:** urinary problems. **Derm:** rashes. **Hemat:** leukopenia. **Misc:** physical dependence, psychological dependence, tolerance.

Interactions

Drug-Drug: Additive CNS depression with other **CNS depressants**, including **alcohol**, **antihistamines**, **antidepressants**, **opioid analgesics**, and other **sedative/hypnotics** (including other **benzodiazepines**). May ↓ the therapeutic effectiveness of **levodopa**. **Hormonal contraceptives** or **phenytoin** may ↓ effectiveness. **Theophylline** may ↓ sedative effects.
Drug-Natural Products: Concomitant use of **kava-kava**, **valerian**, **skullcap**, **chamomile**, or **hops** can ↑ CNS depression.

Route/Dosage

PO (Adults): *Antianxiety agent*—10–30 mg 3–4 times daily. *Sedative/hypnotic/management of alcohol withdrawal*—15–30 mg 3–4 times daily.
PO (Geriatric Patients): 5 mg 1–2 times daily initially or 10 mg 3 times daily; may be ↑ as needed.

Availability (generic available)

Capsules: 10 mg, 15 mg, 30 mg. **Tablets:** 10 mg, 15 mg, 30 mg.

NURSING IMPLICATIONS

Assessment

- Assess patient for anxiety and orientation, mood and behavior.
- Assess level of sedation (ataxia, dizziness, slurred speech) periodically throughout therapy.
- Assess regularly for continued need for treatment.
- Prolonged high-dose therapy may lead to psychological or physical dependence. Restrict the amount of drug available to patient.
- Geri: Assess CNS effects and risk of falls. Institute falls prevention strategies.
- ***Lab Test Considerations:*** Monitor CBC and liver function tests periodically during prolonged therapy.
- May cause decreased thyroidal uptake of ^{123}I and ^{131}I.

Implementation

- Medication should be tapered at the completion of therapy (taper by 0.5 mg every 3 days). Sudden cessation of medication may lead to withdrawal (insomnia, irritability, nervousness, tremors).

- **PO:** Administer with food if GI irritation becomes a problem.

Patient/Family Teaching

- Instruct patient to take oxazepam exactly as directed. Missed doses should be taken within 1 hr; if remembered later, omit and return to regular dosing schedule. Do not double or increase doses. If dose is less effective after a few wk, notify health care professional.
- Inform patient that oxazepam is usually prescribed for short-term use.
- Encourage patient to participate in psychotherapy to address source of anxiety and improve coping skills.
- Teach other methods to decrease anxiety, such as increased exercise, support group, relaxation techniques.
- May cause drowsiness or dizziness. Caution patient to avoid driving or other activities requiring alertness until response to medication is known.
- Advise patient to avoid the use of alcohol and to consult health care professional prior to the use of OTC preparations that contain antihistamines or alcohol.
- Advise patient to notify health care professional of medication regimen prior to treatment or surgery.
- Advise patient to inform health care professional if pregnancy is planned or suspected.
- Emphasize the importance of follow-up exams to monitor effectiveness of medication.
- Geri: Instruct patient and family how to reduce falls risk at home.

Evaluation/Desired Outcomes

- Decreased sense of anxiety.
- Increased ability to cope.
- Prevention or relief of acute agitation, tremor, and hallucinations during alcohol withdrawal.

OXcarbazepine

(ox-kar-**baz**-e-peen)

Oxtellar XR, Trileptal

Classification

Therapeutic: anticonvulsants

Pharmacologic: carbamazepine analogues

Indications

Monotherapy or adjunctive therapy of partial seizures. **Unlabeled Use:** Management of trigeminal neuralgia.

Action

Blocks sodium channels in neural membranes, stabilizing hyperexcitable states, inhibiting repetitive neuronal firing, and decreasing propagation of synaptic impulses. **Therapeutic Effects:** Decreased incidence of seizures.

Pharmacokinetics

Absorption: Rapidly absorbed after oral administration and rapidly converted to the active 10-hydroxy metabolite (MHD).

Distribution: Enters breast milk in significant amounts.

Metabolism and Excretion: Extensively converted to MHD, which is then primarily excreted by the kidneys.

Half-life: *Oxcarbazepine*—2 hr; *MHD*—9 hr.

TIME/ACTION PROFILE (blood levels)

ROUTE	ONSET	PEAK	DURATION
PO 12 hr	PO	rapid	4.5 hr†

†Steady-state levels of MHD are reached after 2–3 days during twice-daily dosing.

Contraindications/Precautions

Contraindicated in: Hypersensitivity to oxcarbazepine, carbamazepine, or eslicarbazepine.

Use Cautiously in: All patients (may ↑ risk of suicidal thoughts/behaviors); Renal impairment (dose ↓ recommended if CCr <30 mL/min); Severe hepatic impairment; OB: May be teratogenic (associated with oral clefts and cardiac abnormalities); levels of active metabolites may gradually ↓ during pregnancy which may ↑ seizure risk; use during pregnancy only if maternal benefit outweighs potential risk to fetus; Lactation: Use while breast feeding only if maternal benefit outweighs potential risk to infant; Rep: Women of reproductive potential; Pedi: Children <2 yr (immediate-release) and <6 yr (extended-release) (safety not established).

Exercise Extreme Caution in: Patients positive for HLA-B*1502 alleles (unless benefits clearly outweigh the risks) (↑ risk of serious skin reactions).

Adverse Reactions/Side Effects

CNS: SEIZURES, SUICIDAL THOUGHTS, dizziness/vertigo, drowsiness/fatigue, headache, cognitive symptoms. **Derm:** DRUG REACTION WITH EOSINOPHILIA AND SYSTEMIC SYMPTOMS (DRESS), STEVENS-JOHNSON SYNDROME, TOXIC EPIDERMAL NECROLYSIS, acne, rash, urticaria. **EENT:** abnormal vision, diplopia, nystagmus. **Endo:** hypothyroidism. **F and E:** hyponatremia. **GI:** abdominal pain, dyspepsia, nausea, vomiting, thirst. **Neuro:** ataxia, gait disturbances, tremor. **Misc:** hypersensitivity reactions, lymphadenopathy.

Interactions

Drug-Drug: May ↑ levels and risk of toxicity of **CYP2C19 substrates**, including **phenytoin** when used at doses greater than 1200 mg/day; may need to ↓ dose of phenytoin. May ↓ levels and effectiveness of **CYP3A4 substrates**, including **hormonal contraceptives**. **Carbamazepine, phenobarbital, phenytoin**, and **rifampin** may ↓ levels; monitor MHD levels during titration period; may need to adjust dose of oxcarbazepine.

Route/Dosage

(Immediate-release tablets and oral suspension can be interchanged at equal doses.).

PO (Adults): *Adjunctive therapy (immediate–release)*—300 mg twice daily, may ↑ by up to 600 mg/day at weekly intervals up to 1200 mg/day (up to 2400 mg/day may be needed); *Conversion to monotherapy (immediate–release)*—300 mg twice daily; may ↑ by 600 mg/day at weekly intervals, while other antiepileptic drugs are tapered over 3–6 wk; dose of oxcarbazepine should be ↑ up to 2400 mg/day over a period of 2–4 wk; *Initiation of monotherapy (immediate–release)*—300 mg twice daily, ↑ by 300 mg/day every 3rd day, up to 1200 mg/day. Maximum maintenance dose should be achieved over 2–4 wk; *Adjunctive therapy or monotherapy (extended–release)*—600 mg once daily for 1 wk; may ↑ by 600 mg/day at weekly intervals up to 1200–2400 mg once daily; *Concurrent use of strong CYP3A4 inducer (carbamazepine, phenobarbital, phenytoin, rifampin) (extended–release)*—consider initiating therapy with 900 mg once daily.

PO (Children 2–16 yr): *Adjunctive therapy (immediate release)*—4–5 mg/kg twice daily (up to 600 mg/day), ↑ over 2 wk to achieve 900 mg/day in patients 20–29 kg, 1200 mg/day in patients 29.1–39 kg and 1800 mg/day in patients >39 kg (range 6–51 mg/kg/day). In patients <20 kg, initial dose of 16–20 mg/kg/day may be used not to exceed 60 mg/kg/day. *Conversion to monotherapy (immediate release)*—8–10 mg/kg/day given twice daily; may ↑ by 10 mg/kg/day at weekly intervals, whereas other antiepileptic drugs are tapered over 3–6 wk; dose of oxcarbazepine should be ↑ up to 600–900 mg/day in patients ≤20 kg, 900–1200 mg/day in patients 25–30 kg, 900–1500 mg/day in patients 35–40 kg. 1200–1500 mg/day in patients 45 kg, 1200–1800 mg/day in patients 50–55 kg, 1200–2100 mg/day in patients 60–65 kg, and 1500–2100 mg/day in patients 70 kg. Maximum maintenance dose should be achieved over 2–4 wk.

PO (Children 6–17 yr): *Adjunctive therapy or monotherapy (extended-release)*—8–10 mg/kg once daily (up to 600 mg/day) for 1 wk; may ↑ by 8–10 mg/kg/day at weekly intervals over 2–3 wk to achieve 900 mg/day in patients 20–29 kg, 1200 mg/day in patients 29.1–39 kg and 1800 mg/day in patients >39 kg; *Concurrent use of strong CYP3A4 inducer (carbamazepine, phenobarbital, phenytoin, rifampin) (extended–release)*—consider initiating therapy with 12–15 mg/kg (max dose = 900 mg) once daily.

Renal Impairment

PO (Adults): *CCr<30 mL/min (immediate and extended–release)*. Initiate therapy at 300 mg/day and ↑ slowly to achieve desired response.

Availability (generic available)

Extended-release tablets: 150 mg, 300 mg, 600 mg. **Cost:** 150 mg $357.60/100, 300 mg $496.80/100, 600 mg $909.60/100. **Oral suspension (lemon-flavor):** 300 mg/5 mL. **Cost:** *Generic*—$206.80/250 mL. **Tablets:** 150 mg, 300 mg, 600 mg. **Cost:** *Generic*—150 mg $145.36/100, 300 mg $264.46/100, 600 mg $487.92/100.

NURSING IMPLICATIONS

Assessment

- Monitor closely for notable changes in behavior that could indicate the emergence or worsening of suicidal thoughts or behavior or depression.
- **Seizures:** Assess frequency, location, duration, and characteristics of seizure activity. Hyponatremia may increase frequency and severity of seizures.
- Monitor patient for CNS changes. May manifest as cognitive symptoms (psychomotor slowing, difficulty with concentration, speech or language problems), somnolence or fatigue, or coordination abnormalities (ataxia, gait disturbances).
- Monitor for skin reactions (rash, erythema, urticaria, pruritus, fever, blistering). Patients with HLA-B*1502 alleles are at increased risk for Stevens Johnson syndrome and toxic epidermal necrolysis. Discontinue oxcarbazepine if symptoms occur.
- Monitor for signs and symptoms of DRESS (fever, rash, lymphadenopathy, and/or facial swelling), associated with involvement of other organ systems (hepatitis, nephritis, hematologic abnormalities, myocarditis, myositis) during therapy. May resemble an acute viral infection. Eosinophilia is often present. Discontinue therapy if signs occur.
- ***Lab Test Considerations:*** Monitor ECG and serum electrolytes before and periodically during therapy. May cause hyponatremia. Usually occurs during the first 3 mo of therapy. May require dose reduction, fluid restriction, or discontinuation of therapy. Sodium levels return to normal within a few days of discontinuation.

Implementation

- Do not confuse oxcarbazepine with carbamazepine or oxaprozin.
- Implement seizure precautions as indicated.
- **PO:** Administer twice daily with or without food.
- Administer extended-release tablets on an empty stomach, at least 1 hr before or 2 hr after meals; giving with food increases risks of adverse effects. Swallow extended-release tablets whole, do not crush, break, or chew.
- Shake oral suspension well and prepare dose immediately after. Withdraw using oral dosing syringe supplied by manufacturer. May be mixed in a small

O

glass of water just prior to administration or swallowed directly from syringe. Rinse syringe with warm water and allow to dry.

Patient/Family Teaching

- Instruct patient to take oxcarbazepine in equally spaced doses, as directed. Take missed doses as soon as possible but not just before next dose; do not double dose. Notify health care professional if more than 1 dose is missed. Medication should be gradually discontinued to prevent seizures. Instruct patient to read the *Medication Guide* before starting and with each Rx refill, changes may occur.
- May cause dizziness, drowsiness, or CNS changes. Advise patients to avoid driving or other activities requiring alertness until response to medication is known. Do not resume driving until physician gives clearance based on control of seizure disorder.
- Instruct patient to notify health care professional of all Rx or OTC medications, vitamins, or herbal products being taken and to consult with health care professional before taking other medications. Advise patient not to take alcohol or other CNS depressants concurrently with this medication.
- Advise patient and family to notify health care professional if thoughts about suicide or dying, attempts to commit suicide; new or worse depression; new or worse anxiety; feeling very agitated or restless; panic attacks; trouble sleeping; new or worse irritability; acting aggressive; being angry or violent; acting on dangerous impulses; an extreme increase in activity and talking, other unusual changes in behavior or mood occur.
- Instruct patient to notify health care professional of medication regimen before treatment or surgery. Rep: Advise females of reproductive potential to use an additional nonhormonal method of contraception during therapy and until next menstrual period. Instruct patient to notify health care professional if pregnancy is planned or suspected. Encourage patients who become pregnant to enroll in the North American Antiepileptic Drug (NAAED) Pregnancy Registry by calling 1-888-233-2334 or on the web at www.aedpregnancyregistry.org. Enrollment must be done by patients themselves.
- Advise patients to carry identification describing disease and medication regimen at all times.

Evaluation/Desired Outcomes

- Absence or reduction of seizure activity.

oxiconazole, **See ANTIFUNGALS (TOPICAL).**

OXYBUTYNIN (ox-i-**byoo**-ti-nin)

oxybutynin (oral)
~~Ditropan~~, Ditropan XL
oxybutynin (gel)
Gelnique
oxybutynin (transdermal system)
Oxytrol, Oxytrol for Women

Classification
Therapeutic: urinary tract antispasmodics
Pharmacologic: anticholinergics

Indications

Urinary symptoms that may be associated with neurogenic bladder including: Frequent urination, Urgency, Nocturia, Urge incontinence. Overactive bladder with symptoms of urge incontinence, urgency, and frequency.

Action

Inhibits the action of acetylcholine at postganglionic receptors. Has direct spasmolytic action on smooth muscle, including smooth muscle lining the GU tract, without affecting vascular smooth muscle. **Therapeutic Effects:** Increased bladder capacity. Delayed desire to void. Decreased urge incontinence, urinary urgency, and frequency and decreased number of urinary accidents associated with overactive bladder.

Pharmacokinetics

Absorption: Rapidly absorbed following oral administration, but undergoes extensive first-pass metabolism; XL tablets provide extended release. Transdermal absorption occurs by passive diffusion through intact skin and bypasses the first-pass effect.
Distribution: Highly bound (>99%) to plasma proteins. Widely distributed.
Metabolism and Excretion: Extensively metabolized by the liver (CYP3A4 enzyme system); 1 metabolite is pharmacologically active; metabolites are renally excreted with negligible (<0.1%) excretion of unchanged drug.
Half-life: 7–8 hr (oral and patch); 30–64 hr (gel).

TIME/ACTION PROFILE (urinary spasmolytic effect)

ROUTE	ONSET	PEAK	DURATION
PO	30–60 min	3–6 hr	6–10 hr (up to 24 hr with XL tablet)
TD-patch	within 24 hr	36 hr	3–4 days
TD-gel	unknown	unknown	24 hr

Contraindications/Precautions

Contraindicated in: Hypersensitivity; Uncontrolled angle-closure glaucoma; Intestinal obstruction or atony; Urinary retention.

Use Cautiously in: Hepatic/renal impairment; Bladder outflow obstruction; Ulcerative colitis; Benign prostatic hyperplasia; Cardiovascular disease; Reflux esophagitis or gastrointestinal obstructive disorders; Patients with dementia receiving acetylcholinesterase inhibitors; Myasthenia gravis; Parkinson's disease (may worsen symptoms); Autonomic neuropathy (may worsen ↓ GI motility); OB, Lactation: Pregnancy or lactation; Pedi: Oral: Safety not established in children <5 yr; Patch and gel: Safety not established in children <18 yr; Geri: Appears on Beers list. Poorly tolerated due to anticholinergic effects. Initiate treatment at lower doses.

Adverse Reactions/Side Effects

CNS: dizziness, drowsiness, agitation, confusion, hallucinations, headache. **CV:** chest pain, edema, tachycardia. **Derm:** ↓ sweating, hot flushes, *transdermal only:* application site reactions, pruritus. **EENT:** blurred vision, hoarseness. **GI:** constipation, dry mouth, nausea, abdominal pain, anorexia, diarrhea, dysphagia. **GU:** ↑ thirst, urinary retention. **Metab:** hyperthermia. **Misc:** HYPERSENSITIVITY REACTIONS (including anaphylaxis and angioedema).

Interactions

Drug-Drug: ↑ anticholinergic effects with other **agents having anticholinergic properties**, including **amantadine**, **antidepressants**, **phenothiazines**, **disopyramide**, and **haloperidol**. Additive CNS depression with other **CNS depressants**, including **alcohol**, **antihistamines**, **antidepressants**, **opioids**, and **sedative/hypnotics**. **Ketoconazole**, **itraconazole**, **erythromycin**, and **clarithromycin** may ↑ effects. May ↓ the GI promotility effects of **metoclopramide**.

Route/Dosage

PO (Adults): *Immediate-release tablets*—5 mg 2–3 times daily (not to exceed 5 mg 4 times daily) (may start with 2.5 mg 2–3 times daily in elderly). *Extended-release tablets*—5–10 mg once daily; may ↑, as needed (in 5-mg increments) up to maximum dose of 30 mg/day.

PO (Children >5 yr): *Immediate-release tablets*—5 mg 2–3 times daily (not to exceed 15 mg/day). *Extended-release tablets (children ≥6 yr)*—5 mg once daily; may ↑, as needed, (in 5-mg increments) up to maximum dose of 20 mg/day.

PO (Children 1–5 yr): 0.2 mg/kg/dose 2–3 times daily.

Transdermal (Adults): *Patch*—Apply one 3.9 mg system twice weekly (every 3–4 days); *Gel*—Apply contents of one sachet once daily.

Availability (generic available)

Extended-release tablets: 5 mg, 10 mg, 15 mg. **Cost:** *Generic*—5 mg $105.23/100, 10 mg $106.08/100, 15 mg $117.04/100. **Immediate-release tablets:** 5 mg. **Cost:** *Generic*—$52.94/100. **Syrup:** 5 mg/5 mL. **Cost:** *Generic*—$38.95/473 mL. **Topical gel:** 10%. **Cost:** $30.12/3 g. **Transdermal patch:** 3.9 mg/24 hr[OTC].

NURSING IMPLICATIONS

Assessment

- Monitor voiding pattern and intake and output ratios, and assess abdomen for bladder distention prior to and periodically during therapy. Catheterization may be used to assess postvoid residual. Cystometry is usually performed to diagnose type of bladder dysfunction prior to prescription of oxybutynin.
- Geri: Assess geriatric patients for anticholinergic effects (sedation and weakness).

Implementation

- Do not confuse Ditropan XL (oxybutynin) with Diprivan (propofol). Do not confuse oxybutynin with oxycodone.
- **PO:** Immediate release tabs should be administered on an empty stomach; XL tablets may be given with or without food. XL tablets should be swallowed whole; do not break, crush, or chew.
- **Transdermal patch:** Apply patch on same two days each wk (Sunday/Wednesday, Monday/Thursday) to hip, abdomen, or buttock in an area that is clean, dry, and without irritation. Patch should be worn continuously.
- **Transdermal gel:** Apply clear, colorless gel once daily to intact skin on abdomen (avoid area around navel), upper arms/shoulders, or thighs until dry. Rotate sites; do not use same site on consecutive days.

Patient/Family Teaching

- Instruct patient to take oxybutinin as directed. Take missed doses as soon as remembered unless almost time for next dose. Advise patient to read *Information for the Patient* prior to beginning therapy and with each Rx refill in case of new information.
- May cause drowsiness or blurred vision. Advise patient to avoid driving and other activities requiring alertness until response to medication is known.
- Advise patient to avoid concurrent use of alcohol and other CNS depressants while taking this medication.
- Instruct patient that frequent rinsing of mouth, good oral hygiene, and sugarless gum or candy may decrease dry mouth. Health care professional should be notified if mouth dryness persists >2 wk.
- Advise patient to stop taking oxybutinin and notify health care professional immediately if signs of angioedema and/or anaphylaxis (swelling of face, tongue, or throat; rash; dyspnea).

O

- Inform patient that oxybutynin decreases the body's ability to perspire. Avoid strenuous activity in a warm environment because overheating may occur.
- Advise patient to notify health care professional if urinary retention occurs or if constipation persists. Discuss methods of preventing constipation, such as increasing dietary bulk, increasing fluid intake, and increasing mobility.
- Advise patient to notify health care professional of all Rx or OTC medications, vitamins, or herbal products being taken and to consult with health care professional before taking other medications.
- Advise patient to notify health care professional if pregnancy is planned or suspected or if breast feeding.
- Discuss need for continued medical follow-up. Periodic cystometry may be used to evaluate effectiveness. Ophthalmic exams should be performed periodically to detect glaucoma, especially in patients over 40 yr of age.
- **Transdermal patch:** Instruct patient on correct application and disposal of patch. Open pouch by tearing along arrows; apply immediately. Apply ½ patch to skin by removing ½ protective cover and applying firmly to skin. Apply 2nd half by bending in half and rolling patch onto skin while removing protective liner. Press patch firmly in place.
- Remove slowly; fold in half, sticky sides together, and discard. Wash site with mild soap and water or a small amount of baby oil.
- Advise patient referred for MRI to remove patch prior to test and give directions for replacing patch.
- **Transdermal gel:** Instruct patient on correct application of oxybutynin gel. Do not apply to recently shaved skin, skin with rashes, or areas treated with lotions, oils, or powders; may be used with sunscreen. Wash area with mild soap and water and dry completely before applying. Tear packet open just before use and squeeze entire contents into hand or directly onto application site of abdomen, arms/shoulders, or thighs. Amount of gel will be size of a nickel on the skin. Gently rub into skin until dry. Wash hands immediately following application. Avoid application near open fire or when smoking; medication is flammable. Do not shower, bathe, swim, exercise, or immerse the application site in water within 1 hr after application. Cover application site with clothing if close skin-to-skin contact at application site is anticipated.

Evaluation/Desired Outcomes

- Relief of bladder spasm and associated symptoms (frequency, urgency, nocturia, and incontinence) in patients with a neurogenic or overactive bladder.

REMS HIGH ALERT

oxyCODONE (ox-i-koe-done)

Oxaydo, OxyCONTIN, ✱Oxy IR, ✱OxyNEO, Roxicodone, Xtampza ER, ✱Supeudol

Classification

Therapeutic: opioid analgesics

Pharmacologic: opioid agonists, opioid agonists/nonopioid analgesic combinations

Schedule II

Indications

Moderate to severe pain. Pain severe enough to require daily, around-the-clock long-term opioid treatment and for which alternative treatment options are inadequate (extended-release) (children ≥11 yr should be tolerating a minimum opioid dose of ≥20 mg of oxycodone or equivalent for ≥5 days before initiating extended-release oxycodone therapy).

Action

Binds to opiate receptors in the CNS. Alters the perception of and response to painful stimuli, while producing generalized CNS depression. **Therapeutic Effects:** Decreased pain.

Pharmacokinetics

Absorption: Well absorbed from the GI tract.
Distribution: Widely distributed. Crosses the placenta; enters breast milk.
Protein Binding: 38–45%.
Metabolism and Excretion: Mostly metabolized by the liver by the CYP3A4 isoenzyme; also metabolized by the CYP2D6 to a minor extent.
Half-life: 2–3 hr.

TIME/ACTION PROFILE (analgesic effects)

ROUTE	ONSET	PEAK	DURATION
PO	10–15 min	60–90 min	3–6 hr
PO-ER†	10–15 min	3 hr	12 hr

†Extended-release.

Contraindications/Precautions

Contraindicated in: Hypersensitivity; Some products contain alcohol or bisulfites and should be avoided in patients with known intolerance or hypersensitivity; Significant respiratory depression; Paralytic ileus; Acute or severe bronchial asthma; Acute, mild, intermittent, or postoperative pain (extended-release).
Use Cautiously in: Head trauma; ↑ intracranial pressure; Severe renal or hepatic disease; Hypothyroidism; Adrenal insufficiency; Alcoholism; Seizure disorders; Undiagnosed abdominal pain; Prostatic hyperplasia; Difficulty swallowing or GI disorders that may predispose patient to obstruction (↑ risk for GI obstruction); OB, Lactation: Avoid chronic use; prolonged use of opioids during pregnancy can result in neonatal

opioid withdrawal syndrome; Geri: Elderly or debilitated patients (↑ risk of respiratory depression; initial dose ↓ recommended); Pedi: Children <11 yr (safety and effectiveness of extended-release products not established).

Adverse Reactions/Side Effects

CNS: confusion, sedation, dizziness, dysphoria, euphoria, floating feeling, hallucinations, headache, unusual dreams. **CV:** orthostatic hypotension. **Derm:** flushing, sweating. **EENT:** blurred vision, diplopia, miosis. **Endo:** adrenal insufficiency. **GI:** constipation, dry mouth, choking, GI obstruction, nausea, vomiting. **GU:** urinary retention. **Resp:** RESPIRATORY DEPRESSION. **Misc:** physical dependence, psychological dependence, tolerance.

Interactions

Drug-Drug: Use with caution in patients receiving **MAO inhibitors** (may result in unpredictable reactions—↓ initial dose of oxycodone to 25% of usual dose). Additive CNS depression with **alcohol**, **antihistamines**, and **sedative/hypnotics**. Administration of **partial-antagonist opioid analgesics** may precipitate withdrawal in physically dependent patients. **Nalbuphine** or **buprenorphine** may ↓ analgesia. Concurrent use of **CYP3A4 inhibitors** including **ritonavir**, **ketoconazole**, **itraconazole**, **fluconazole**, **clarithromycin**, **erythromycin**, **nefazodone**, **diltiazem**, **verapamil**, **nelfinavir**, and **fosamprenavir** ↑ levels and risk of opioid toxicity; careful monitoring during initiation, dose changes, or discontinuation of the inhibitor is recommended. Concurrent use with **CYP3A4 inducers** including **barbiturates**, **carbamazepine**, **efavirenz**, **corticosteroids**, **modafinil**, **nevirapine**, **oxcarbazepine**, **phenobarbital**, **phenytoin**, **rifabutin**, or **rifampin** may ↓ fentanyl levels and analgesia; if inducers are discontinued or dosage ↓, patients should be monitored for signs of opioid toxicity and necessary dose adjustments should be made. **CYP2D6 inhibitors** may ↑ levels. Use with **benzodiazepines** or other **CNS depressants** including other **opioids**, **non-benzodiazepine sedative/hypnotics**, **anxiolytics**, **general anesthetics**, **muscle relaxants**, **antipsychotics**, and **alcohol** may cause profound sedation, respiratory depression, coma, and death; reserve concurrent use for when alternative treatment options are inadequate. Drugs that affect serotonergic neurotransmitter systems, including **tricyclic antidepressants**, **SSRIs**, **SNRIs**, **MAO inhibitors**, **TCAs**, **tramadol**, **trazodone**, **mirtazapine**, **$5-HT_3$ receptor antagonists**, **linezolid**, **methylene blue**, and **triptans** ↑ risk of serotonin syndrome.

Route/Dosage

Larger doses may be required during chronic therapy. ER capsules are NOT bioequivalent to ER tablets.

PO (Adults ≥50 kg): *Opioid-naive patients*—5–10 mg every 3–4 hr initially, as needed. Once optimal analgesia is obtained, patients with chronic pain may be converted to an equivalent 24-hr dose given in 2 divided doses as extended-release tablets every 12 hr.
PO (Adults <50 kg): *Opioid-naive patients*—0.2 mg/kg every 3–4 hr initially, as needed. Once optimal analgesia is obtained, patients with chronic pain may be converted to an equivalent 24-hr dose given in 2 divided doses as extended-release tablets every 12 hr.
PO (Children ≥11 yr): 0.05–0.15 mg/kg every 4–6 hr as needed, as immediate-release product. Once optimal analgesia is obtained, patients with chronic pain may be converted to an equivalent 24-hr dose given in 2 divided doses as extended-release tablets every 12 hr.
Rect (Adults): 10–40 mg 3–4 times daily initially, as needed.

Hepatic Impairment

PO (Adults): ↓ initial dose by 50–66%.

Availability (generic available)

Capsules: 5 mg. **Cost:** *Generic*—$79.59/100. **Extended-release capsules (abuse deterrent) (Xtampza ER):** 9 mg, 13.5 mg, 18 mg, 27 mg, 36 mg. **Extended-release tablets (abuse-deterrent) (Oxycontin):** 10 mg, 15 mg, 20 mg, 30 mg, 40 mg, 60 mg, 80 mg. **Cost:** 10 mg $52.54/20, 15 mg $78.60/20, 20 mg $100.42/20, 30 mg $142.16/20, 40 mg $178.10/20, 60 mg $259.32/20, 80 mg $335.08/20. **Oral solution:** 5 mg/5 mL, 100 mg/5 mL (concentrated). **Cost:** *Generic*—$142.50/500 mL. **Rectal suppositories:** 🍁 10 mg, 🍁 20 mg. **Tablets (Roxicodone):** 5 mg, 10 mg, 15 mg, 20 mg, 30 mg. **Cost:** *Generic*—5 mg $47.99/100, 10 mg $62.50/100, 15 mg $75.90/100, 20 mg $110.30/100, 30 mg $145.47/100. **Tablets (abuse-deterrent) (Oxaydo):** 5 mg, 7.5 mg. ***In combination with:*** aspirin (Endodan, Percodan), acetaminophen (Endocet, Magnacet, Oxycet, Percocet, Roxicet, Xartemis XR); see Appendix B.

NURSING IMPLICATIONS

Assessment

- Assess type, location, and intensity of pain prior to and 1 hr (peak) after administration. When titrating opioid doses, increases of 25–50% should be administered until there is either a 50% reduction in the patient's pain rating on a numerical or visual analog scale or the patient reports satisfactory pain relief. A repeat dose can be safely administered at the time of the peak if previous dose is ineffective and side effects are minimal.
- Patients taking extended-release tablets may also be given supplemental short-acting opioid doses for breakthrough pain.

- An equianalgesic chart (see Appendix J) should be used when changing routes or when changing from one opioid to another.
- Assess BP, pulse, and respirations before and periodically during administration. If respiratory rate is <10/min, assess level of sedation. Physical stimulation may be sufficient to prevent significant hypoventilation. Dose may need to be decreased by 25–50%. Initial drowsiness will diminish with continued use.
- Prolonged use may lead to physical and psychological dependence and tolerance. This should not prevent patient from receiving adequate analgesia. Patients who receive oxycodone for pain rarely develop psychological dependence. Progressively higher doses may be required to relieve pain with long-term therapy.
- Assess bowel function routinely. Prevention of constipation should be instituted with increased intake of fluids and bulk, and laxatives to minimize constipating effects. Stimulant laxatives should be administered routinely if opioid use exceeds 2–3 days, unless contraindicated. Consider drugs for opioid induced constipation.
- Assess risk for opioid addiction, abuse, or misuse prior to administration. Abuse or misuse of extended-release preparations by crushing, chewing, snorting, or injecting dissolved product will result in uncontrolled delivery of oxycodone and can result in overdose and death.
- ***Lab Test Considerations:*** May ↑ plasma amylase and lipase levels.
- ***Toxicity and Overdose:*** If an opioid antagonist is required to reverse respiratory depression or coma, naloxone is the antidote. Dilute the 0.4-mg ampule of naloxone in 10 mL of 0.9% NaCl and administer 0.5 mL (0.02 mg) by IV push every 2 min. For children and patients weighing <40 kg, dilute 0.1 mg of naloxone in 10 mL of 0.9% NaCl for a concentration of 10 mcg/mL and administer 0.5 mcg/kg every 2 min. Titrate dose to avoid withdrawal, seizures, and severe pain.

Implementation

- ***High Alert:*** Accidental overdose of opioid analgesics has resulted in fatalities. Before administering, clarify all ambiguous orders; have second practitioner independently check original order and dose calculations.
- Do not confuse short-acting oxycodone with long-acting Oxycontin. Do not confuse oxycodone with hydrocodone, oxybutynin, or oxymorphone. Do not confuse Oxycontin with MS Contin or oxymorphone.
- Explain therapeutic value of medication prior to administration to enhance the analgesic effect. Abuse deterrent: *Oxaydo*, *Xtampza ER*, and *Oxycontin* are abuse deterrent formulations that are difficult to crush, and if crushed result in a gel.
- Regularly administered doses may be more effective than prn administration. Analgesic is more effective if given before pain becomes severe.
- Coadministration with nonopioid analgesics may have additive analgesic effects and may permit lower doses.
- Oxycodone should be discontinued gradually after long-term use to prevent withdrawal symptoms. For patients on long-acting agents who are physically opioid-dependent, initiate the taper by a small enough increment (no greater than 10%–25% of total daily dose) to avoid withdrawal symptoms, and proceed with dose-lowering at an interval of every 2–4 wk. Patients who have been taking opioids for briefer periods of time may tolerate a more rapid taper.
- **PO:** May be administered with food or milk to minimize GI irritation.
- Administer solution with properly calibrated measuring device.
- **Extended-Release:** Take 1 tablet at a time. Swallow extended-release tablet whole; do not crush, break, or chew. Taking broken, chewed, crushed, or dissolved extended-release tablets may lead to rapid release and absorption of a potentially fatal dose of oxycodone. Advise patients not to pre-soak, lick, or wet controlled-release tablets prior to placing in the mouth. Take each tablet with enough water to ensure complete swallowing immediately after placing in mouth. Dose should be based on 24-hr opioid requirement determined with short-acting opioids then converted to extended-release form.
- Do not use *Oxaydo* for administration via nasogastric, gastric, or other feeding tubes as it may cause obstruction of feeding tubes.
- FDA strongly encourages health care professionals to complete a REMS-compliant education program that includes all the elements of the FDA Education *Blueprint for Health Care Providers Involved in the Management or Support of Patients with Pain,* available at www.fda.gov/OpioidAnalgesicREMSBlueprint. Information on programs can be found at 1-800-503-0784 or www.opioidanalgesicrems.com.

Patient/Family Teaching

- Instruct patient on how and when to ask for and take pain medication. Do not stop taking without discussing with health care professional; may cause withdrawal symptoms if discontinued abruptly after prolonged use. Discuss safe use, risks, and proper storage and disposal of opioid analgesics with patients and caregivers with each Rx. The Patient Counseling Guide (PCG) is available at www.fda.gov/OpioidAnalgesicREMSPCG.
- Advise patient that oxycodone is a drug with known abuse potential. Protect it from theft, and never give to anyone other than the individual for whom it was prescribed. Store out of sight and reach of children, and in a location not accessible by others.

- Medication may cause drowsiness or dizziness. Advise patient to call for assistance when ambulating or smoking. Caution patient to avoid driving and other activities requiring alertness until response to medication is known.
- Advise patients taking *Oxycontin* tablets that empty matrix tablets may appear in stool.
- Advise patient to make position changes slowly to minimize orthostatic hypotension.
- Advise patient to avoid concurrent use of alcohol or other CNS depressants with this medication.
- Instruct patient to notify health care professional of all Rx or OTC medications, vitamins, or herbal products being taken and consult health care professional before taking any new medications.
- Encourage patient to turn, cough, and breathe deeply every 2 hr to prevent atelectasis.
- Rep: Advise patient to notify health care professional if pregnancy is planned or suspected, or if breast feeding. Inform patient of potential for neonatal opioid withdrawal syndrome with prolonged use during pregnancy. Monitor neonate for signs and symptoms of withdrawal symptoms (irritability, hyperactivity and abnormal sleep pattern, high pitched cry, tremor, vomiting, diarrhea, and/or failure to gain weight); usually occur the first days after birth.

Evaluation/Desired Outcomes

- Decrease in severity of pain without a significant alteration in level of consciousness or respiratory status.

HIGH ALERT

oxytocin (ox-i-**toe**-sin)

Pitocin

Classification

Therapeutic: hormones

Pharmacologic: oxytocics

Indications

IV: Induction of labor at term. **IV:** Facilitation of threatened abortion. **IV, IM:** Postpartum control of bleeding after expulsion of the placenta.

Action

Stimulates uterine smooth muscle, producing uterine contractions similar to those in spontaneous labor. Has vasopressor and antidiuretic effects. **Therapeutic Effects:** Induction of labor. Control of postpartum bleeding.

Pharmacokinetics

Absorption: IV administration results in 100% bioavailability.

Distribution: Widely distributed in extracellular fluid. Small amounts reach fetal circulation.

Metabolism and Excretion: Rapidly metabolized by liver and kidneys.

Half-life: 3–9 min.

TIME/ACTION PROFILE (reduction in uterine contractions)

ROUTE	ONSET	PEAK	DURATION
IV	immediate	unknown	1 hr
IM	3–5 min	unknown	30–60 min

Contraindications/Precautions

Contraindicated in: Hypersensitivity; Anticipated nonvaginal delivery.

Use Cautiously in: OB: 1st and 2nd stages of labor; slow infusion over 24 hr has caused water intoxication with seizure and coma or maternal death due to oxytocin's antidiuretic effect.

Adverse Reactions/Side Effects

Maternal adverse reactions are noted for IV use only.

CNS: *maternal*—COMA, SEIZURES; *fetal*—INTRACRANIAL HEMORRHAGE. **Resp:** *fetal*—ASPHYXIA, hypoxia. **CV:** *maternal*—hypotension; *fetal*—arrhythmias. **F and E:** *maternal*—hypochloremia, hyponatremia, water intoxication. **Misc:** *maternal*—↑ uterine motility, painful contractions, abruptio placentae, ↓ uterine blood flow, hypersensitivity.

Interactions

Drug-Drug: Severe hypertension may occur if oxytocin follows administration of **vasopressors**.

Route/Dosage

Induction/Stimulation of Labor

IV (Adults): 0.5–1 mU/min; ↑ by 1–2 mU/min every 30–60 min until desired contraction pattern established; dose may be ↓ after desired frequency of contractions is reached and labor has progressed to 5–6 cm dilation.

Postpartum Hemorrhage

IV (Adults): 10 units infused at 20–40 mU/min.

IM (Adults): 10 units after delivery of placenta.

Incomplete/Inevitable Abortion

IV (Adults): 10 units at a rate of 20–40 mU/min.

Availability (generic available)

Solution for injection: 10 units/mL.

NURSING IMPLICATIONS

Assessment

- Fetal maturity, presentation, and pelvic adequacy should be assessed prior to administration of oxytocin for induction of labor.
- Assess character, frequency, and duration of uterine contractions; resting uterine tone; and fetal heart

O

rate frequently throughout administration. If contractions occur <2 min apart and are >50–65 mm Hg on monitor, if they last 60–90 sec or longer, or if a significant change in fetal heart rate develops, stop infusion and turn patient on her left side to prevent fetal anoxia. Notify health care professional immediately.

- Monitor maternal BP and pulse frequently and fetal heart rate continuously throughout administration.
- This drug occasionally causes water intoxication. Monitor patient for signs and symptoms (drowsiness, listlessness, confusion, headache, anuria) and notify physician or other health care professional if they occur.
- ***Lab Test Considerations:*** Monitor maternal electrolytes. Water retention may result in hypochloremia or hyponatremia.

Implementation

- Do not administer oxytocin simultaneously by more than one route.

IV Administration

- **Continuous Infusion:** Rotate infusion container to ensure thorough mixing. Store solution in refrigerator, but do not freeze.
- Infuse via infusion pump for accurate dose. Oxytocin should be connected via Y-site injection to an IV of 0.9% NaCl for use during adverse reactions.
- Magnesium sulfate should be available if needed for relaxation of myometrium.
- **Induction of Labor:** ***Diluent:*** Dilute 1 mL (10 units) in 1 L of compatible infusion fluid (0.9% NaCl, D5W, or LR). ***Concentration:*** 10 mU/mL. ***Rate:*** Begin infusion at 0.5–2 mU/min (0.05–0.2 mL); increase in increments of 1–2 mU/min at 15–30-min intervals until contractions simulate normal labor.
- **Postpartum Bleeding:** ***Diluent:*** For control of postpartum bleeding, dilute 1–4 mL (10–40 units) in 1 L of compatible infusion fluid. ***Concentration:*** 10–40 mU/mL. ***Rate:*** Begin infusion at a rate of 20–40 mU/min to control uterine atony. Adjust rate as indicated.
- **Incomplete or Inevitable Abortion:** ***Diluent:*** For incomplete or inevitable abortion, dilute 1 mL (10 units) in 500 mL of 0.9% NaCl or D5W. ***Concentration:*** 20 mU/mL. ***Rate:*** Infuse at a rate of 20–40 mU/min.
- **Y-Site Compatibility:** acyclovir, alfentanil, allopurinol, amikacin, aminocaproic acid, aminophylline, amphotericin B liposome, anidulafungin, argatroban, ascorbic acid, atropine, azathioprine, azithromycin, aztreonam, benztropine, bivalirudin, bumetanide, buprenorphine, butorphanol, calcium chloride, calcium gluconate, capreomycin, caspofungin, cefazolin, cefepime, cefotaxime, cefotetan, cefoxitin, ceftazidime, ceftriaxone, cefuroxime, chloramphenicol, ciprofloxacin, cisatracurium, clindamycin, cyanocobalamin, cyclosporine, daptomycin, dexamethasone, dexmedetomidine, digoxin, digoxin, diphenhydramine, dobutamine, dolasetron, dopamine, doxycycline, droperidol, enalaprilat, ephedrine, epinephrine, epoetin alfa, eptifibatide, ertapenem, erythromycin, esmolol, famotidine, fenoldopam, fentanyl, fluconazole, folic acid, foscarnet, fosphenytoin, furosemide, ganciclovir, gentamicin, glycopyrrolate, granisetron, heparin, hydrocortisone sodium succinate, hydromorphone, imipenem/cilastatin, isoproterenol, ketamine, ketorolac, labetalol, leucovorin calcium, levofloxacin, lidocaine, linezolid, lorazepam, magnesium sulfate, mannitol, meperidine, meropenem, metaraminol, methyldopate, methylprednisolone, metoclopramide, metoprolol, metronidazole, midazolam, milrinone, morphine, moxifloxacin, multivitamins, mycophenolate, nafcillin, nalbuphine, naloxone, nicardipine, nitroglycerin, nitroprusside, norepinephrine, ondansetron, oxacillin, palonosetron, pamidronate, papaverine, penicillin G, pentamidine, pentobarbital, phenobarbital, phentolamine, phenylephrine, phytonadione, piperacillin/tazobactam, potassium acetate, potassium chloride, potassium phosphates, procainamide, prochlorperazine, promethazine, propranolol, protamine, pyridoxime, quinupristin/dalfopristin, ranitidine, sodium acetate, sodium bicarbonate, sodium phosphates, streptokinase, succinylcholine, sufentanil, tacrolimus, theophylline, thiamine, tigecycline, tirofiban, tobramycin, tolazoline, vancomycin, vasopressin, verapamil, vitamin B complex with C, voriconazole, warfarin, zidovudine, zoledronic acid.
- **Y-Site Incompatibility:** dantrolene, diazepam, diazoxide, indomethacin, methohexital, phenytoin, remifentanil, trimethoprim/sulfamethoxazole.
- **Solution Compatibility:** dextrose/Ringer's or lactated Ringer's combinations, dextrose/saline combinations, Ringer's or lactated Ringer's injection, D5W, D10W, 0.45% NaCl, 0.9% NaCl.

Patient/Family Teaching

- Advise patient to expect contractions similar to menstrual cramps after administration has started.

Evaluation/Desired Outcomes

- Onset of effective contractions.
- Increase in uterine tone.
- Reduction in postpartum bleeding.

PACLitaxel (pak-li-tax-el)

~~Taxol~~

PACLitaxel protein-bound particles (albumin-bound)

Abraxane

Classification

Therapeutic: antineoplastics

Pharmacologic: taxoids

Indications

Paclitaxel: Advanced ovarian cancer (with cisplatin). Non-small cell lung cancer (NSCLC) when potentially curative surgery and/or radiation therapy is not an option. Metastatic breast cancer unresponsive to other therapy. Node-positive breast cancer when administered sequentially to standard combination chemotherapy that includes doxorubicin. Treatment of AIDS-related Kaposi's sarcoma. **Paclitaxel (albumin-bound):** Metastatic breast cancer after treatment failure or relapse where therapy included an anthracycline. Locally advanced or metastatic NSCLC when potentially curative surgery or radiation therapy is not an option (with carboplatin). Metastatic pancreatic adenocarcinoma (with gemcitabine).

Action

Interferes with the normal cellular microtubule function that is required for interphase and mitosis. **Therapeutic Effects:** Death of rapidly replicating cells, particularly malignant ones.

Pharmacokinetics

Absorption: IV administration results in complete bioavailability.

Distribution: Cross the placenta.

Protein Binding: 89–98%.

Metabolism and Excretion: Highly metabolized by the liver (primarily by CYP2C8 and CYP3A4), <10% excreted unchanged in urine.

Half-life: *Paclitaxel*—13–52 hr; *Paclitaxel protein-bound particles (albumin-bound)*—27 hr.

TIME/ACTION PROFILE (effect on WBCs)

ROUTE	ONSET	PEAK	DURATION
IV	unknown	11 days	3 wk

Contraindications/Precautions

Contraindicated in: Hypersensitivity to paclitaxel, other taxanes, or to castor oil (non-protein-bound vehicle contains polyoxyethylated castor oil); AST >10 × ULN or total bilirubin >5 × ULN (paclitaxel protein-bound particles); Moderate or severe hepatic impairment (pancreatic adenocarcinoma only for paclitaxel protein-bound particles); Known alcohol intolerance; ANC ≤1500/mm^3 in patients with ovarian, lung, breast, or pancreatic cancer; ANC ≤1000/mm^3 in patients with AIDS-related Kaposi's sarcoma; OB: Pregnancy (may cause fetal harm).

Use Cautiously in: Moderate or severe hepatic impairment (↓ dose); Active infection; ↓ bone marrow reserve; Geri: ↑ risk of adverse reactions; Rep: Women of reproductive potential and men with female partners of reproductive potential; Pedi: Safety and effectiveness not established.

Adverse Reactions/Side Effects

CNS: dizziness, headache, seizures. **CV:** ECG changes, edema, hypotension, bradycardia. **Derm:** STEVENS-JOHNSON SYNDROME, TOXIC EPIDERMAL NECROLYSIS, alopecia. **GI:** diarrhea, ↑ liver enzymes, mucositis, nausea, vomiting, pancreatitis. **Hemat:** anemia, neutropenia, thrombocytopenia. **Local:** injection site reactions. **MS:** arthralgia, myalgia. **GU:** renal failure. **Neuro:** peripheral neuropathy. **Resp:** PULMONARY EMBOLISM, PULMONARY FIBROSIS, cough, dyspnea, interstitial pneumonia. **Misc:** HYPERSENSITIVITY REACTIONS (including anaphylaxis), SEPSIS.

Interactions

Drug-Drug: CYP3A4 inhibitors including **atazanavir**, **clarithromycin**, **indinavir**, **itraconazole**, **ketoconazole**, **nefazodone**, **nelfinavir**, **ritonavir**, and **saquinavir** may ↑ levels and risk of toxicity; concurrent use should be undertaken with caution. **CYP3A4 inducers** including **carbamazepine**, **rifampin**, and **phenytoin** may ↓ levels and ↑ risk of treatment failure; concurrent use should be undertaken with caution. **Gemfibrozil** may ↑ levels and risk of toxicity; concurrent use should be undertaken with caution. ↑ risk of myelosuppression with other **antineoplastics** or **radiation therapy**. Myelosuppression ↑ when given after **cisplatin**. May ↑ levels and toxicity of **doxorubicin**. May ↓ antibody response to and ↑ risk of adverse reactions from **live-virus vaccines**.

Route/Dosage

Many other regimens are used.

Paclitaxel

Ovarian Cancer

IV (Adults): *Previously untreated patients*—175 mg/m^2 over 3 hr every 3 wk, or 135 mg/m^2 over 24 hr every 3 wk, followed by cisplatin; *Previously treated patients*—135 mg/m^2 or 175 mg/m^2 over 3 hr every 3 wk.

Breast Cancer

IV (Adults): *Adjuvant treatment of node-positive breast cancer*—175 mg/m^2 over 3 hr every 3 wk for 4 courses administered sequentially to doxorubicin-containing combination chemotherapy; *Failure of initial therapy for metastatic disease or relapse within 6 mo of adjuvant therapy*—175 mg/m^2 over 3 hr every 3 wk.

P

NSCLC

IV (Adults): 135 mg/m² over 24 hr every 3 wk, followed by cisplatin.

AIDS-Related Kaposi's Sarcoma

IV (Adults): 135 mg/m² over 3 hr every 3 wk or 100 mg/m² over 3 hr every 2 wk (dose ↓/adjustment may be necessary in patients with advanced HIV infection).

Paclitaxel Protein-Bound Particles (albumin-bound)

Breast Cancer

IV (Adults): 260 mg/m² over 30 min every 3 wk.

Hepatic Impairment

IV (Adults): *Moderate hepatic impairment (AST levels <10 × ULN and bilirubin levels 1.51–3 × ULN)*—200 mg/m² over 30 min every 3 wk; dose may be ↑ to 260 mg/m² for the 3rd course based on individual tolerance; *Severe hepatic impairment (AST levels <10 × ULN and bilirubin levels 3.01–5× ULN)*—200 mg/m² over 30 min every 3 wk; dose may be ↑ to 260 mg/m² for the 3rd course based on individual tolerance; *Severe hepatic impairment (AST levels >10 × ULN or bilirubin levels >5 × ULN)*—Avoid use.

NSCLC

IV (Adults): 100 mg/m² over 30 min on Days 1, 8, and 15 of each 21-day cycle.

Hepatic Impairment

IV (Adults): *Moderate hepatic impairment (AST levels <10 × ULN and bilirubin levels 1.51–3 × ULN)*—80 mg/m² over 30 min on Days 1, 8, and 15 of each 21–day cycle; dose may be ↑ to 100 mg/m² for the 3rd course based on individual tolerance; *Severe hepatic impairment (AST levels <10 × ULN and bilirubin levels 3.01–5 × ULN)*—80 mg/m² over 30 min on Days 1, 8, and 15 of each 21–day cycle; dose may be ↑ to 100 mg/m² for the 3rd course based on individual tolerance; *Severe hepatic impairment (AST levels >10 × ULN or bilirubin levels >5 × ULN)*—Avoid use.

Pancreatic Adenocarcinoma

IV (Adults): 125 mg/m² over 30–40 min on Days 1, 8, and 15 of each 28–day cycle.

Hepatic Impairment

IV (Adults): *Moderate or severe hepatic impairment*—Avoid use.

Availability

Paclitaxel (generic available)

Solution for injection (requires dilution): 6 mg/mL.

Paclitaxel Protein-Bound Particles (albumin-bound)

Lyophilized powder for injection (requires reconstitution): 100 mg/vial.

NURSING IMPLICATIONS

Assessment

- Monitor vital signs frequently, especially during first hr of the infusion.
- Monitor cardiovascular status especially during first 3 hr of infusion. Hypotension and bradycardia are common but usually do not require treatment. Continuous ECG monitoring is recommended only for patients with serious underlying conduction abnormalities or those concurrently taking doxorubicin.
- Monitor for bone marrow depression. Assess for bleeding (bleeding gums, bruising, petechiae, guaiac stools, urine, and emesis) and avoid IM injections and taking rectal temperatures if platelet count is low. Apply pressure to venipuncture sites for 10 min. Assess for signs of infection during neutropenia. Anemia may occur. Monitor for dyspnea and orthostatic hypotension. Granulocyte-colony stimulating factor (G-CSF) may be used if necessary.
- Assess for development of peripheral neuropathy. If severe symptoms occur, subsequent dose should be reduced by 20%.
- Monitor intake and output, appetite, and nutritional intake. Paclitaxel causes nausea and vomiting in 50% of patients. Prophylactic antiemetics may be used. Adjust diet as tolerated to help maintain fluid and electrolyte balance and nutritional status.
- Assess patient for arthralgia and myalgia, which usually begin 2–3 days after therapy and resolve within 5 days. Pain is usually relieved by nonopioid analgesics but may be severe enough to require treatment with opioid analgesics.
- Assess for rash periodically during therapy. May cause Stevens-Johnson syndrome and toxic epidermal necrolysis. Discontinue therapy if severe or if accompanied with fever, general malaise, fatigue, muscle or joint aches, blisters, oral lesions, conjunctivitis, hepatitis, and/or eosinophilia.
- **Paclitaxel:** Monitor for hypersensitivity reactions continuously during the first 30 min and frequently thereafter. These occur frequently (19%), usually during the first 10 min of paclitaxel infusion, after the 1st or 2nd dose. Pretreatment is recommended for **all** patients and should include dexamethasone 20 mg PO (10 mg for patients with advanced HIV disease) 12 and 6 hr prior to paclitaxel, diphenhydramine 50 mg IV 30–60 min prior to paclitaxel, and ranitidine 50 mg IV 30–60 min prior to paclitaxel. Most common manifestations are dyspnea, flushing, tachycardia, rash, hypotension, and chest pain. If these occur, stop infusion and notify health care professional. Treatment may include bronchodilators, epinephrine, antihistamines, and corticosteroids. Keep these agents and resuscitative equipment close by in the event of an anaphylactic reaction. Other manifestations of hypersensitivity reactions include flushing and rash.
- No premedication for hypersensitivity is required for *paclitaxel protein-bound (albumin-bound)*.

- ***Lab Test Considerations:*** Obtain a negative pregnancy test before starting therapy.
- **Paclitaxel: :** Monitor CBC and differential prior to and periodically during therapy. The nadir of leukopenia occurs in 11 days, with recovery by days 15–21. Notify health care professional if the leukocyte count is $<1500/mm^3$ ($1000/mm^3$ in AIDS-related Kaposi's sarcoma) or if the platelet count is $<100,000/mm^3$. Subsequent doses are usually held until leukocyte count is $>1500/mm^3$ ($1000/mm^3$ in AIDS-related Kaposi's sarcoma) and platelet count is $>100,000/mm^3$.
- **Paclitaxel Protein-Bound Particles (albumin-bound):** Monitor CBC and differential prior to therapy and prior to dosing on Days 1, 8, and 15. Do not administer if neutrophil count is $<1500/mm^3$. If severe neutropenia (neutrophils <500 cells/mm^3 for seven days or more), reduce dose in subsequent courses. Monitor liver function studies (AST, ALT, LDH, bilirubin) prior to and periodically during therapy to detect hepatotoxicity.

Implementation

- Do not confuse paclitaxel with docetaxel or paclitaxel protein-bound particles.

Paclitaxel

IV Administration

- **Continuous Infusion:** Paclitaxel must be diluted prior to injection. ***Diluent:*** Dilute contents of 5-mL (30-mg) vials with the following diluents: 0.9% NaCl, D5W, D5/0.9% NaCl, or dextrose in Ringer's solution. ***Concentration:*** 0.3–1.2 mg/mL. Although haziness in solution is normal, inspect for particulate matter or discoloration before use. Use an in-line filter of not >0.22-micron pore size. Solutions are stable for 27 hr at room temperature and lighting. Do not use PVC containers or administration sets. ***Rate:*** Dose for *breast cancer or AIDS-related Kaposi's sarcoma* is administered over 3 hr. Dose for *ovarian cancer* is administered as a 24-hr infusion.
- **Y-Site Compatibility:** acyclovir, alemtuzumab, alfentanil, allopurinol, amifostine, amikacin, aminophylline, amphotericin B lipid complex, ampicillin, ampicillin/sulbactam, anidulafungin, argatroban, azithromycin, aztreonam, bivalirudin, bleomycin, bumetanide, buprenorphine, busulfan, butorphanol, calcium chloride, calcium gluconate, carboplatin, carmustine, caspofungin, cefazolin, cefepime, cefotaxime, cefotetan, cefoxitin, ceftazidime, ceftriaxone, cefuroxime, chloramphenicol, ciprofloxacin, cisatracurium, cisplatin, cladribine, clindamycin, cyclophosphamide, cyclosporine, cytarabine, dacarbazine, dactinomycin, dantrolene, daptomycin, daunorubicin hydrochloride, dexamethasone, dexmedetomidine, dexrazoxane, diltiazem, diphenhydramine, dobutamine, dolasetron, dopamine, doxorubicin hydrochloride, doxycycline, droperidol, enalaprilat, ephedrine, epinephrine, epirubicin, ertapenem, erythromycin, esmolol, etoposide, etoposide phosphate, famotidine, fenoldopam, fentanyl, floxuridine, fluconazole, fludarabine, fluorouracil, foscarnet, fosphenytoin, furosemide, ganciclovir, gemcitabine, gentamicin, glycopyrrolate, granisetron, haloperidol, heparin, hetastarch, hydralazine, hydrocortisone, hydromorphone, ifosfamide, imipenem/cilastatin, insulin, regular, irinotecan, isoproterenol, ketorolac, leucovorin calcium, levofloxacin, levorphanol, lidocaine, linezolid, lorazepam, magnesium sulfate, mannitol, meperidine, meropenem, mesna, methotrexate, methyldopate, metoclopramide, metoprolol, metronidazole, midazolam, milrinone, mitomycin, morphine, moxifloxacin, nafcillin, nalbuphine, naloxone, nicardipine, nitroglycerin, nitroprusside, norepinephrine, octreotide, ondansetron, oxaliplatin, palonosetron, pamidronate, pancuronium, pantoprazole, pemetrexed, pentamidine, pentobarbital, pentostatin, phenobarbital, phenylephrine, piperacillin/tazobactam, potassium acetate, potassium chloride, potassium phosphates, procainamide, prochlorperazine, promethazine, propofol, quinupristin/dalfopristin, ranitidine, remifentanil, rituximab, sodium acetate, sodium bicarbonate, sodium phosphates, streptozocin, succinylcholine, sufentanil, tacrolimus, theophylline, thiopental, thiotepa, tigecycline, tirofiban, tobramycin, topotecan, trastuzumab, trimethoprim/sulfamethoxazole, vancomycin, vasopressin, vecuronium, verapamil, vinblastine, vincristine, vinorelbine, voriconazole, zidovudine, zoledronic acid.
- **Y-Site Incompatibility:** amiodarone, amphotericin B cholesteryl, amphotericin B colloidal, amphotericin B liposome, chlorpromazine, diazepam, digoxin, doxorubicin liposomal, hydroxyzine, idarubicin, indomethacin, labetalol, methylprednisolone, mitoxantrone, phenytoin, propranolol.

Paclitaxel Protein-Bound Particles (albumin-bound)

IV Administration

- **Intermittent Infusion:** Reconstitute by slowly adding 20 mL to each vial over at least 1 min for a concentration of 5 mg/mL. Direct solution to inside wall of vial to prevent foaming. Allow vial to sit for at least 5 min to ensure proper wetting of cake/powder. Gently swirl or invert vial for at least 2 min until powder is completely dissolved; avoid foaming. If foaming or clumping occurs, allow vial to stand for 15 min until foaming dissolves. Solution should be milky and homogenous without visible particles. If particles or settling are visible, gently invert vial to resuspend. Inject appropriate amount into sterile PVC IV bag. Do not use an in-line filter during administration. Do not administer solutions that are discolored or contain particulate matter. Reconstituted solution should be administered immediately but is stable for 8 hr if refrigerated. Discard unused portion. ***Rate:*** Administer over 30–40 min. Monitor infusion site closely for infiltration.

Patient/Family Teaching

- Explain purpose of paclitaxel to patient.
- Advise patient to notify health care professional immediately of rash, difficulty breathing, or symptoms of hypersensitivity reaction occurs.
- Instruct patient to notify health care professional promptly if fever; chills; cough; hoarseness; sore throat; signs of infection; lower back or side pain; painful or difficult urination; bleeding gums; bruising; petechiae; blood in stools, urine, or emesis; dyspnea; or orthostatic hypotension occurs. Caution patient to avoid crowds and persons with known infections. Instruct patient to use soft toothbrush and electric razor and to avoid falls. Caution patient not to drink alcoholic beverages or to take medication containing aspirin or NSAIDs; may precipitate gastric bleeding.
- May cause dizziness. Caution patient to avoid driving or other activities requiring alertness until response to medication is known.
- Instruct patient to notify health care professional if abdominal pain, yellow skin, weakness, paresthesia, gait disturbances, or joint or muscle aches occur.
- Instruct patient to inspect oral mucosa for redness and ulceration. If mouth sores occur, advise patient to use sponge brush and rinse mouth with water after eating and drinking. Stomatitis usually resolves in 5–7 days.
- Discuss with patient the possibility of hair loss. Complete hair loss usually occurs between days 14 and 21 and is reversible after discontinuation of therapy. Explore coping strategies.
- Instruct patient not to receive any vaccinations without advice of health care professional.
- Rep: Advise females of reproductive potential to use a nonhormonal method of contraception during and for at least 6 mo after last dose of therapy and to avoid breast feeding during and for 2 wk after last dose. Advise male patients with female partners of reproductive potential to use effective contraception during and for at least 3 mo after last dose. May impair fertility in females and males.
- Emphasize the need for periodic lab tests to monitor for side effects.

Evaluation/Desired Outcomes

- Decrease in size or spread of malignancy.

palbociclib (pal-**bo**-si-klib)
Ibrance

Classification
Therapeutic: antineoplastics
Pharmacologic: kinase inhibitors

Indications

Advanced or metastatic hormone receptor (HR)-positive, human epidermal growth factor 2 (HER2)-negative breast cancer in post-menopausal women or in men as initial endocrine-based therapy (in combination with an aromatase inhibitor). Advanced or metastatic HR-positive, HER2-negative breast cancer in women or men with disease progression following endocrine therapy (in combination with fulvestrant).

Action

Inhibits kinases (cyclin-dependent kinases 4 and 6) that are part of the signaling pathway for cell proliferation. **Therapeutic Effects:** Improved survival and decreased spread of breast cancer.

Pharmacokinetics

Absorption: 46% absorbed following oral administration.
Distribution: Unknown.
Metabolism and Excretion: Mostly metabolized (by CYP3A and sulfontransferase [SULT]); also acts as an inhibitor of CYP3A; 6.9% excreted unchanged in urine, 2.3% in feces.
Half-life: 29 hr.

TIME/ACTION PROFILE (improvement in progression-free survival)

ROUTE	ONSET	PEAK	DURATION
PO	within 4 mo	unknown	maintained throughout treatment

Contraindications/Precautions

Contraindicated in: Concurrent use of strong/moderate CYP3A inhibitors; Concurrent use of CYP3A inducers; OB: Pregnancy (may cause fetal harm); Lactation: Discontinue palbociclib or discontinue breast feeding.
Use Cautiously in: Concurrent use of sensitive CYP3A substrates (narrow therapeutic indices); Severe renal impairment; Severe hepatic impairment; Rep: Women of reproductive potential and men with female partners of reproductive potential; Pedi: Safety and effectiveness not established.

Adverse Reactions/Side Effects

CNS: weakness. **Derm:** alopecia. **EENT:** epistaxis. **GI:** ↓ appetite, diarrhea, nausea, stomatitis, vomiting. **GU:** ↓ fertility. **Hemat:** NEUTROPENIA, anemia, leukopenia, thrombocytopenia. **Neuro:** peripheral neuropathy. **Resp:** INTERSTITIAL LUNG DISEASE.

Interactions

Drug-Drug: Concurrent use with **CYP3A inhibitors** including **clarithromycin**, **indinavir**, **itraconazole**, **ketoconazole**, **lopinavir/ritonavir**, **nefazodone**, **nelfinavir**, **posaconazole**, **ritonavir**, **saquinavir**, **verapamil**, and **voriconazole** ↑ levels and the risk of toxicity; avoid, if possible (if unavoidable, ↓ dose of palbociclib [resume original dose after 3–5 half-lives of offending drug have passed following discontinuation]). **Strong CYP3A inducers** including **carbamazepine**, **phenytoin**, **rifampin** can ↓ levels and effectiveness; concurrent use should be avoided. Moderate CYP inducers including **bosentan**, **efavirenz**, **etravirine**, **modafinil**, and **nafcillin** may also ↓ levels and effectiveness; avoid concurrent use. ↑ levels and effects/toxicity of **alfentanil**, **cyclosporine**, **dihydroergotamine**, **ergotamine**, **everolimus**, **fentanyl**, **midazolam**, **pimozide**, **quinidine**, **sirolimus**, and **tacrolimus**; if concurrent use is required dose ↓ may be necessary.

Drug-Natural Products: St. John's wort may ↓ levels and effectiveness; avoid concurrent use.

Drug-Food: Grapefruit/grapefruit juice ↑ levels and the risk of toxicity, avoid ingestion.

Route/Dosage

PO (Adults): 125 mg once daily for 21 days, followed by 7 days off; *Concurrent use of strong CYP3A4 inhibitor*—75 mg once daily for 21 days, followed by 7 days off.

Hepatic Impairment

PO (Adults): *Severe hepatic impairment (Child-Pugh C)*—75 mg once daily for 21 days, followed by 7 days off.

Availability

Capsules: 75 mg, 100 mg, 125 mg.

NURSING IMPLICATIONS

Assessment

- Monitor for signs and symptoms of infection (fever, chills, dizziness, shortness of breath, weakness, increased bleeding or bruising) during therapy. Treat as medically appropriate. No dose adjustment is needed for Grade 1 or 2 non-hematologic toxicities. *For Grade ≥3 (if persisting despite medical treatment)*, withhold palbociclib until symptoms resolve to: Grade ≤1; Grade ≤2 (if not considered a safety risk for patient). Resume at next lower dose.
- Monitor for signs and symptoms of interstitial lung disease or pneumonitis (hypoxia, cough, dyspnea) during therapy. If symptoms are severe, permanently discontinue therapy.
- ***Lab Test Considerations:*** Obtain a negative pregnancy test before starting therapy.
- Monitor CBC prior to and at beginning of each cycle, on Day 15 of first 2 cycles, and as clinically indicated. May cause ↓ neutrophil counts; median time to first episode is 15 days (13–117 days) and median duration of Grade ≥3 neutropenia was 7 days. May cause febrile neutropenia.
- No dose adjustment is needed for Grade 1 or 2 hematologic toxicities. *For Grade 3 Day 1 of cycle:* withhold palbociclib, repeat CBC monitoring within 1 wk. When recovered to Grade ≤2, start next cycle at same dose. *For Grade 3 Day 15 of first 2 cycles:* If Grade 3 on Day 15, continue palbociclib at current dose to complete cycle and repeat CBC on Day 22. *If Grade 4 on Day 22,* withhold palbociclib until recovery to Grade ≤2. Resume at next lower dose. Consider dose reduction in cases of prolonged (>1 wk) recovery from Grade 3 neutropenia or recurrent Grade 3 neutropenia on Day 1 of subsequent cycles. *For Grade 3 ANC (500–<1000/mm^3) plus fever ≥38.5°C and/or infection,* withhold palbociclib until recovery to Grade ≤2. Resume at next lower dose. *For Grade 4,* withhold palbociclib until recovery to Grade ≤2. Resume at next lower dose.
- May cause ↓ WBC, lymphocytes, hemoglobin, and platelets.

Implementation

- **PO:** Administer once daily at the same time each day, for 21 consecutive days followed by 7 days off treatment, with food in combination with letrozole once daily given throughout 28 day cycle. Swallow capsules whole; do not open, crush, or chew; do not swallow capsules that are broken, cracked, or not intact.
- If dose reduction needed for adverse reactions starting dose is 125 mg/day. 1st dose reduction is to 100 mg/day, 2nd dose reduction is to 75 mg/day; if further dose reduction needed, discontinue therapy.

Patient/Family Teaching

- Instruct patient to take palbociclib as directed. If a dose is vomited or missed, omit dose and take next dose at usual time; do not take an additional dose that day. Do not change dose or stop taking without consulting health care professional. Advise patient to read *Patient Information* before starting therapy and with each Rx refill in case of changes.
- Advise patient to avoid grapefruit or grapefruit products during therapy; may increase amount of palbociclib in blood.
- Advise patient to notify health care professional if signs and symptoms of infection occur.
- Instruct patient to notify health care professional of all Rx or OTC medications, vitamins, or herbal products being taken and to consult with health care professional before taking other medications, especially St. John's wort.
- Rep: Advise females of reproductive potential to use effective contraception and avoid breast feeding dur-

ing and for at least 3 wk after last dose. Advise patient to notify health care professional if pregnancy is planned or suspected. Advise males with female partners of reproductive potential to use effective contraception during and for at least 3 wk after last dose. Inform male patient that palbociclib may impair fertility.

Evaluation/Desired Outcomes

- Decrease in the spread of breast cancer.

palifermin (pa-liff-er-min)

Kepivance

Classification

Therapeutic: cytoprotective agents
Pharmacologic: keratinocyte growth factors (rDNA)

Indications

To decrease incidence/duration of severe oral mucositis (≥WHO grade 3) associated with myelotoxic therapy in patients requiring autologous hematopoietic stem cell support for hematologic malignancies.

Action

Enhances proliferation of epithelial cells. **Therapeutic Effects:** Decreased incidence/duration of mucositis.

Pharmacokinetics

Absorption: IV administration results in complete bioavailability.
Distribution: Distributes into extravascular space.
Metabolism and Excretion: Unknown.
Half-life: 4.5 hr.

TIME/ACTION PROFILE (levels)

ROUTE	ONSET	PEAK	DURATION
IV	unknown	end of dose	unknown

Contraindications/Precautions

Contraindicated in: Hypersensitivity to palifermin or other *E. coli*-derived proteins.
Use Cautiously in: Allogeneic hematopoietic stem cell support (↑ risk of exacerbated mucositis); OB: Use only if maternal benefit outweighs fetal risk; Lactation, Pedi: Safety not established.

Adverse Reactions/Side Effects

Derm: erythema, pruritus, rash. **GI:** taste disturbance, tongue thickening/discoloration. **Metab:** ↑ amylase, ↑ lipase. **MS:** arthralgia. **Neuro:** dysesthesia.

Interactions

Drug-Drug: Unfractionated heparin and **low-molecular weight heparin** ↑ levels (flush tubing with saline between use). Administration within 24 hr after **myelotoxic therapy (chemotherapy/radiation)** ↑ severity and duration of mucositis.

Route/Dosage

IV (Adults): 60 mcg/kg/day for 3 days before and 3 days after myelotoxic therapy.

Availability

Powder for injection: 6.25 mg/vial.

NURSING IMPLICATIONS

Assessment

- Assess level of oral mucositis prior to and periodically during therapy.
- ***Lab Test Considerations:*** May cause ↑ serum lipase and amylase; usually reversible.
- May cause proteinuria.

Implementation

- Do not administer palifermin within 24 hr before, during infusion, or 24 hr after infusion of myelotoxic chemotherapy.
- Administer doses for 3 consecutive days before (3rd dose 24–48 hr prior to chemotherapy) and 3 consecutive days after myelotoxic chemotherapy (4th dose on same day as hematopoietic stem cells infusion after infusion is completed and at least 4 days after most recent palifermin administration) for a total of 7 doses.

IV Administration

- **IV Push:** ***Diluent:*** Reconstitute palifermin powder by slowly injecting 1.2 mL of sterile water for injection aseptically. ***Concentration:*** 5 mg/mL. Swirl gently; do not shake or vigorously agitate. Solution should be clear and colorless; do not administer solution that is discolored or contains particulate matter. Dissolution usually takes less than 3 min. Administer immediately after reconstitution or refrigerate and administer within 24 hr. Do not freeze. Allow to reach room temperature for up to 1 hr. Protect from light. Discard palifermin after expiration date or if left at room temperature for more than 1 hr. ***Rate:*** Administer via bolus injection. Do not use a filter.
- **Y-Site Incompatibility:** heparin. If heparin solution is used to maintain IV line, flush with 0.9% NaCl prior to and after use of palifermin.

Patient/Family Teaching

- Explain the purpose of palifermin to patient.
- Inform patient of evidence of tumor growth and stimulation in cell culture and animal models.
- Advise patient to notify health care professional if rash, erythema, edema, pruritus, oral/perioral dysesthesia (tongue discoloration, tongue thickening, alteration of taste) occur.
- Advise female patient to notify health care professional if pregnancy is planned or suspected and to avoid breast feeding during therapy.

Evaluation/Desired Outcomes

- Decrease in incidence and duration of oral mucositis in patients receiving myelotoxic therapy requiring hematopoietic stem cell support.

BEERS

paliperidone (pa-li-per-i-done)

Invega, Invega Sustenna, Invega Trinza

Classification
Therapeutic: antipsychotics
Pharmacologic: benzisoxazoles

Indications

PO, IM: Acute and maintenance treatment of schizophrenia (Invega and Invega Sustenna). **IM:** Maintenance treatment of schizophrenia after patients have been adequately treated with Invega Sustenna for at least 4 mo (Invega Trinza). **PO, IM:** Acute treatment of schizoaffective disorder (as monotherapy or as adjunct to mood stabilizers and/or antidepressants) (Invega and Invega Sustenna).

Action

May act by antagonizing dopamine and serotonin in the CNS. Paliperidone is the active metabolite of risperidone. **Therapeutic Effects:** Decreased manifestations of schizophrenia. Decreased manifestations of schizoaffective disorder.

Pharmacokinetics

Absorption: 28% absorbed following oral administration, food ↑ absorption; slowly absorbed after IM administration (concentrations higher and more rapidly achieved with administration into deltoid muscle).

Distribution: Unknown.

Metabolism and Excretion: 59% excreted unchanged in urine; 32% excreted in urine as metabolites.

Half-life: 23 hr (PO); 25–49 days (IM —Sustenna); 84–139 days (IM —Trinza).

TIME/ACTION PROFILE (blood levels)

ROUTE	ONSET	PEAK	DURATION
PO	unknown	24 hr	24 hr
IM —Sustenna	unknown	13 days	1 mo
IM —Trinza	unknown	30–33 days	3 mo

Contraindications/Precautions

Contraindicated in: Hypersensitivity to paliperidone or risperidone; Concurrent use of drugs known to cause QTc prolongation (including quinidine, procainamide, sotalol, amiodarone, chlorpromazine, thioridazine, moxifloxacin); History of congenital QTc prolongation or other cardiac arrhythmias; Bradycardia, hypokalemia, hypomagnesemia (↑ risk of QTc prolongation); Pre-existing severe GI narrowing (due to nature of tablet formulation); CCr <50 mL/min (for IM).

Use Cautiously in: Patients with Parkinson's disease or dementia with Lewy Bodies (↑ sensitivity to effects of antipsychotics); History of suicide attempt; History of HF, MI, conduction abnormalities, stroke, TIA (↑ risk of orthostatic hypotension and syncope); Patients at risk for aspiration pneumonia or falls; History of seizures; Conditions which may ↑ body temperature (strenuous exercise, exposure to extreme heat, concurrent anticholinergics or risk of dehydration); ↓ GI transit time (may ↑ blood levels); May mask symptoms of some drug overdoses, intestinal obstruction, Reye's Syndrome, or brain tumor (due to antiemetic effect); Diabetes mellitus; Severe hepatic impairment; Renal impairment (dose ↓ recommended if CCr <80 mL/min); OB: Neonates at ↑ risk for extrapyramidal symptoms and withdrawal after delivery when exposed during the 3rd trimester; use only if maternal benefit outweighs fetal risk; Lactation: Use while breast feeding only if maternal benefit outweighs potential risk to infant; Pedi: Children <12 yr (safety and effectiveness not established); Geri: ↑ risk of mortality and stroke/TIA in elderly patients treated for dementia-related psychosis; consider age-related ↓ in renal function.

Adverse Reactions/Side Effects

CNS: NEUROLEPTIC MALIGNANT SYNDROME, SEIZURES, drowsiness, extrapyramidal disorders (dose related), headache, insomnia, anxiety, confusion, dizziness, dysarthria, fatigue, syncope, tardive dyskinesia, weakness. **CV:** QT INTERVAL PROLONGATION, palpitations, tachycardia (dose related), bradycardia, orthostatic hypotension. **EENT:** blurred vision. **Endo:** amenorrhea, dyslipidemia, galactorrhea, gynecomastia, hyperglycemia, weight gain. **GI:** abdominal pain, dry mouth, dyspepsia, nausea, swollen tongue. **GU:** ↓ fertility (females), impotence, priapism. **Hemat:** AGRANULOCYTOSIS, leukopenia, neutropenia. **MS:** back pain, dystonia (dose related). **Neuro:** akathisia, tardive dyskinesia, tremor (dose related). **Resp:** dyspnea, cough. **Misc:** HYPERSENSITIVITY REACTIONS (including anaphylaxis and angioedema), fever.

Interactions

Drug-Drug: ↑ risk of CNS depression with other **CNS depressants** including **alcohol**, **antihistamines**, **sedative/hypnotics**, or **opioid analgesics**. May antagonize the effects of **levodopa** or other **dopamine agonists**. ↑ risk of orthostatic hypotension with **antihypertensives**, **nitrates**, or other **agents that lower BP**. **Strong CYP3A4 inducers** or **strong P-glycoprotein inducers**, including **carbamazepine** or **rifampin** may ↓ levels/effects; avoid concurrent use with Invega Sustenna (if use of strong CYP3A4 or P-glycoprotein inducer necessary, consider using paliperidone ER tablets). **Valproic acid** may ↑ levels (may need to ↓ dose of paliperidone).

Drug-Natural Products: **St. John's wort** may ↓ levels/effects; avoid concurrent use with Invega Sustenna.

P

Route/Dosage

Schizophrenia

PO (Adults): 6 mg once daily; may titrate by 3 mg/day at intervals of at least 5 days (range 3–12 mg/day).
PO (Children 12–17 yr): 3 mg once daily; may titrate by 3 mg/day at intervals of at least 5 days (not to exceed 6 mg if <51 kg or 12 mg if ≥51 kg).
IM (Adults): *Invega Sustenna*—234 mg initially, then 156 mg one wk later; continue with monthly maintenance dose of 117 mg (range of 39–234 mg based on efficacy and/or tolerability); *Invega Trinza*—Dose should be based on dose of previous 1–mo injection dose of Invega Sustenna. If last dose of Invega Sustenna was 78 mg, administer 273 mg of Invega Trinza; if last dose of Invega Sustenna was 117 mg, administer 410 mg of Invega Trinza; if last dose of Invega Sustenna was 156 mg, administer 546 mg of Invega Trinza; if last dose of Invega Sustenna was 234 mg, administer 819 mg of Invega Trinza. Administer dose every 3 mo; may adjust dose based on efficacy and/or tolerability (range: 273–819 mg).

Renal Impairment

PO (Adults): *CCr 50–79 mL/min*—3 mg/day initially; dose may be ↑ to maximum of 6 mg/day; *CCr 10–<50 mL/min*—1.5 mg/day initially; dose may be ↑ to maximum of 3 mg/day.

Renal Impairment

IM (Adults): *CCr 50–79 mL/min*—Invega Sustenna: 156 mg initially, then 117 mg one wk later; continue with monthly maintenance dose of 78 mg; Invega Trinza: once stabilized on Invega Sustenna, can then transition to appropriate dose of Invega Trinza (see above) *CCr <50 mL/min*—Contraindicated.

Schizoaffective Disorder

PO (Adults): 6 mg/day; may titrate by 3 mg/day at intervals of at least 4 days (range 3–12 mg/day).

Renal Impairment

PO (Adults): *CCr 50–79 mL/min*—3 mg/day initially; dose may be ↑ to maximum of 6 mg/day; *CCr 10–<50 mL/min*—1.5 mg/day initially; dose may be ↑ to maximum of 3 mg/day.

Availability (generic available)

Extended-release tablets (Invega): 1.5 mg, 3 mg, 6 mg, 9 mg. **Extended-release intramuscular injection (Invega Sustenna):** 39 mg/0.25 mL, ✱ 50 mg/0.5 mL, ✱ 75 mg/0.75 mL, 78 mg/0.5 mL, ✱ 100 mg/mL, 117 mg/0.75 mL, ✱ 150 mg/1.5 mL, 156 mg/mL, 234 mg/1.5 mL. **Extended-release intramuscular injection (Invega Trinza):** ✱ 175 mg/0.875 mL, ✱ 263 mg/1.315 mL, 273 mg/0.875 mL, ✱ 350 mg/1.75 mL, 410 mg/1.315 mL, ✱ 525 mg/2.625 mL, 546 mg/1.75 mL, 819 mg/2.625 mL.

NURSING IMPLICATIONS

Assessment

- Monitor patient's mental status (orientation, mood, behavior) before and periodically during therapy. Monitor closely for notable changes in behavior that could indicate the emergence or worsening of suicidal thoughts or behavior or depression, especially during early therapy. Restrict amount of drug available to patient.
- Assess weight and BMI initially and throughout therapy.
- Monitor BP (sitting, standing, lying down) and pulse before and periodically during therapy. May cause prolonged QT interval, tachycardia, and orthostatic hypotension.
- Observe patient when administering medication to ensure that medication is actually swallowed and not hoarded or cheeked.
- Monitor patient for onset of extrapyramidal side effects (*akathisia*—restlessness; *dystonia*—muscle spasms and twisting motions; or *pseudoparkinsonism*—mask-like face, rigidity, tremors, drooling, shuffling gait, dysphagia). Report these symptoms; reduction of dose or discontinuation of medication may be necessary.
- Monitor for tardive dyskinesia (involuntary rhythmic movement of mouth, face, and extremities). Report immediately; may be irreversible.
- Monitor for development of neuroleptic malignant syndrome (fever, respiratory distress, tachycardia, seizures, diaphoresis, hypertension or hypotension, pallor, tiredness). Discontinue paliperidone and notify health care professional immediately if these symptoms occur.
- Monitor for symptoms related to hyperprolactinemia (menstrual abnormalities, galactorrhea, sexual dysfunction).
- Assess for falls risk. Drowsiness, orthostatic hypotension, and motor and sensory instability increase risk. Institute prevention if indicated.
- ***Lab Test Considerations:*** Monitor fasting blood glucose and cholesterol levels before and periodically during therapy.
- Monitor serum prolactin prior to and periodically during therapy. May cause ↑ serum prolactin levels.
- Monitor CBC frequently during initial mo of therapy in patients with pre-existing or history of low WBC. May cause leukopenia, neutropenia, or agranulocytosis. Discontinue therapy if this occurs.

Implementation

- ***High Alert:*** Do not confuse *Invega Sustenna* with *Invega Trinza*.
- **PO:** Administer once daily in the morning without regard to food. Tablets should be swallowed whole; do not crush, break or chew.
- **IM:** *Invega Sustenna:* Administer initial and 2nd doses in deltoid using a 1 ½-inch, 22 gauge needle for patients ≥90 kg (≥200 lb) or 1-inch 23 gauge

needle for patients <90 kg (<200 lb). Monthly maintenance doses can be administered in either deltoid or gluteal sites. For gluteal injection, use 1 ½-inch, 22 gauge needle regardless of patient weight. To avoid missed dose, may give 2nd dose 4 days before or after the 1-wk timepoint. Monthly doses may be given up to 7 days before or after the monthly timepoint. *After 1st mo, if missed dose is within 4 wk of scheduled dose*, administer 2nd dose of 156 mg as soon as possible. Give 3rd dose of 117 mg in either deltoid or gluteal muscle 5 wk after 1st injection (regardless of timing of 2nd injection). Then return to normal monthly injections in either deltoid or gluteal muscle. *If >4 wk and <7 wk since 1st injection,* resume by administering 156 mg dose in deltoid as soon as possible, a 2nd 156 mg dose in deltoid in 1 wk, followed by monthly doses in deltoid or gluteal sites. *If >7 mo since scheduled dose,* administer using initial dosing schedule. During regular monthly dose schedule, *if <6 wk since last injection*, administer previously stabilized dose as soon as possible, then monthly. *If >6 wk since last injection*, resume dose previously stabilized on, unless stabilized on 234 mg (then 1st two injections should be 156 mg). Administer 1 dose in deltoid as soon as possible, then another deltoid injection of same dose 1 wk later, then resume regular monthly schedule. *If >6 mo since last injection*, administer using initial dosing schedule.

- **IM:** *Invega Trinza:* Use only after at least 4 mo of monthly *Invega Sustenna* therapy. Prior to administration, shake the prefilled syringe vigorously for at least 15 sec within 5 min prior to administration to ensure a homogeneous suspension. *Deltoid injection:* For patients weighing <90 kg, use the 1-inch 22 gauge thin wall needle. For patients weighing ≥90 kg, use the 1½-inch 22 gauge thin wall needle. *Gluteal injection:* Regardless of patient weight, use 1½-inch 22 gauge thin wall needle. Initiate *Invega Trinza* when next 1-mo paliperidone dose is scheduled. *Avoid missed doses;* dose may be given 2 wk before or after 3 mo scheduled dose. *If more than 3½ mo (up to but <4 mo) since last dose,* administer previously administered dose as soon as possible, then continue with 3-mo injections. *If 4 mo up to and including 9 mo since last dose,* do NOT administer next dose. *If last dose was 273 mg,* administer 2 doses of 78 mg of *Invega Sustenna* one wk apart into deltoid muscle, then one dose of *Invega Trinza* 273 mg one mo after 2nd dose of *Invega Sustenna. If last dose was 410 mg,* administer 2 doses of 117 mg of *Invega Sustenna* one wk apart into deltoid muscle, then one dose of *Invega Trinza* 410 mg one mo after 2nd dose of *Invega Sustenna. If last dose was 819 mg,* administer 2 doses of 156 mg of *Invega Sustenna* one wk apart into deltoid muscle, then one dose of *Invega Trinza* 819 mg one mo after 2nd dose of *Invega Sustenna*. If >9 mo have elapsed since last injection of *Invega Trinza*, re-initiate treatment with *Invega Sustenna*. Then resume *Invega Trinza* after at least 4 mo of *Invega Sustenna*.

Patient/Family Teaching

- Instruct patient to take medication as directed. Advise patient that appearance of tablets in stool is normal and not of concern.
- Inform patient of the possibility of extrapyramidal symptoms. Instruct patient to report these symptoms immediately to health care professional.
- Advise patient to change positions slowly to minimize orthostatic hypotension. Protect from falls.
- May cause drowsiness. Caution patient to avoid driving or other activities requiring alertness until response to medication is known.
- Advise patient and family to notify health care professional if thoughts about suicide or dying, attempts to commit suicide; new or worse depression; new or worse anxiety; feeling very agitated or restless; panic attacks; trouble sleeping; new or worse irritability; acting aggressive; being angry or violent; acting on dangerous impulses; an extreme increase in activity and talking, other unusual changes in behavior or mood occur.
- Advise patient that extremes in temperature should also be avoided; this drug impairs body temperature regulation.
- Advise patient to notify health care professional of all Rx or OTC medications, vitamins, or herbal products being taken and to consult with health care professional before taking other medications, especially St. John's wort and alcohol.
- Advise patient to seek nutritional, weight, or medical management as needed for weight gain or cholesterol elevation.
- Instruct patient to notify health care professional promptly if sore throat, fever, unusual bleeding or bruising, rash, tremors, menstrual abnormalities, galactorrhea, or sexual dysfunction occur.
- Advise patient to notify health care professional of medication regimen before treatment or surgery.
- Rep: Advise female patients to notify health care professional if pregnancy is planned or suspected, and to avoid breast feeding. Encourage women who become pregnant while taking paloperidone to enroll in the National Pregnancy Registry for Atypical Antipsychotics at 1-866-961-2388 or visit http://womensmentalhealth.org/clinical-and-research-programs/pregnancyregistry/. Monitor neonates for extrapyramidal and/or withdrawal symptoms and manage symptoms appropriately. May temporarily cause female infertility.

P

- Emphasize the importance of routine follow-up exams to monitor side effects and continued participation in psychotherapy to improve coping skills.

Evaluation/Desired Outcomes

- Decrease in excited, manic behavior.
- Decrease in positive symptoms (delusions, hallucinations) of schizophrenia.
- Decrease in negative symptoms (social withdrawal, flat, blunted affect) of schizophrenia.

palonosetron

(pa-lone-**o**-se-tron)

Aloxi

Classification

Therapeutic: antiemetics

Pharmacologic: 5-HT_3 antagonists

Indications

Prevention of acute and delayed nausea and vomiting caused by initial or repeat courses of moderately or highly emetogenic chemotherapy (moderately emetogenic chemotherapy for adults only). Prevention of postoperative nausea and vomiting (PONV) for up to 24 hr after surgery.

Action

Blocks the effects of serotonin at receptor sites (selective antagonist) located in vagal nerve terminals and in the chemoreceptor trigger zones in the CNS. **Therapeutic Effects:** Decreased incidence and severity of nausea and vomiting following emetogenic chemotherapy or surgery.

Pharmacokinetics

Absorption: IV administration results in complete bioavailability.

Distribution: Unknown.

Metabolism and Excretion: 50% metabolized; 40% excreted unchanged in urine.

Half-life: 40 hr.

TIME/ACTION PROFILE

ROUTE	ONSET	PEAK	DURATION
IV	within 30 min	unknown	7 days

Contraindications/Precautions

Contraindicated in: Hypersensitivity; cross sensitivity with other 5-HT_3 antagonists may occur; Lactation: Lactation.

Use Cautiously in: OB: Safety not established; Pedi: Neonates <1 mo (safety not established).

Adverse Reactions/Side Effects

CNS: dizziness, headache. **GI:** constipation, diarrhea. **Misc:** SEROTONIN SYNDROME.

Interactions

Drug-Drug: Drugs that affect serotonergic neurotransmitter systems, including **SSRIs**, **SNRIs**, **tricyclic antidepressants**, **MAOIs**, **fentanyl**, **lithium**, **buspirone**, **tramadol**, **methylene blue**, and **triptans** ↑ risk of serotonin syndrome.

Route/Dosage

Prevention of Chemotherapy-Induced Nausea/Vomiting

IV (Adults): 0.25 mg given 30 min before start of chemotherapy.

IV (Children 1 mo–<17 yr): 20 mcg/kg (max = 1.5 mg) given 30 min before start of chemotherapy.

Prevention of PONV

IV (Adults): 0.075 mg given immediately before induction of anesthesia.

Availability (generic available)

Solution for injection: 0.05 mg/mL.

NURSING IMPLICATIONS

Assessment

- Assess patient for nausea, vomiting, abdominal distention, and bowel sounds prior to and following administration.
- ***Lab Test Considerations:*** May cause transient ↑ in serum bilirubin, AST, and ALT levels.

Implementation

- 1st dose is administered prior to emetogenic event.
- Repeated dose within a 7-day period is not recommended.

IV Administration

- **IV Push:** Administer dose undiluted 30 min prior to chemotherapy or immediately prior to the induction of anesthesia. Flush line prior to and after administration with 0.9% NaCl. Do not administer solutions that are discolored or contain particulate matter.
- ***Concentration:*** 0.05 mg/mL. ***Rate:*** Administer over 30 sec in adults and 15 sec in children 30 min before starting chemotherapy and over 10 sec for postoperative nausea and vomiting.
- **Y-Site Compatibility:** alemtuzumab, alfentanil, amifostine, amikacin, aminocaproic acid, aminophylline, amiodarone, amphotericin B liposome, ampicillin, ampicillin/sulbactam, anidulafungin, argatroban, atropine, azithromycin, aztreonam, bivalirudin, bleomycin, bumetanide, buprenorphine, busulfan, butorphanol, calcium acetate, calcium chloride, calcium gluconate, carboplatin, carmustine, caspofungin, cefazolin, cefepime, cefotaxime, cefotetan, cefoxitin, ceftazidime, ceftriaxone, cefuroxime, chloramphenicol, chlorpromazine, ciprofloxacin, cisatracurium, cisplatin, clindamycin, cyclophosphamide, cyclosporine, cytarabine, dacarbazine, dactinomycin, dantrolene, daptomycin, daunorubicin hydrochloride, dexamethasone, dexmedetomidine, dexrazoxane, digoxin, diltiazem, diphenhydramine, dobutamine, docetaxel, dopamine, doxorubicin hydrochloride, droperidol, enalaprilat,

ephedrine, epinephrine, epirubicin, eptifibitide, erythromycin, esmolol, etoposide, etoposide phosphate, famotidine, fenoldopam, fentanyl, fluconazole, fludarabine, fluorouracil, foscarnet, fosphenytoin, furosemide, gemcitabine, gentamicin, glycopyrrolate, haloperidol, heparin, hydralazine, hydrocortisone, hydromorphone, idarubicin, ifosfamide, insulin, irinotecan, isoproterenol, ketorolac, labetalol, leucovorin, levofloxacin, lidocaine, linezolid, lorazepam, magnesium sulfate, mannitol, melphalan, meperidine, meropenem, mesna, methotrexate, methyldopate, metoclopramide, metoprolol, metronidazole, midazolam, milrinone, mitomycin, mitoxantrone, morphine, moxifloxacin, nalbuphine, naloxone, neostigmine, nicardipine, nitroglycerin, nitroprusside, norepinephrine, octreotide, oxaliplatin, oxytocin, paclitaxel, pamidronate, pancuronium, phenobarbital, phenylephrine, piperacillin/tazobactam, potassium acetate, potassium chloride, potassium phosphates, procainamide, prochlorperazine, promethazine, propranolol, quinupristin/dalfopristin, ranitidine, remifentanil, rocuronium, sodium acetate, sodium bicarbonate, sodium phosphates, streptozocin, succinylcholine, sufentanil, tacrolimus, theophylline, thiotepa, tigecycline, tirofiban, tobramycin, topotecan, trimethoprim/sulfamethoxazole, vancomycin, vasopressin, vecuronium, verapamil, vinblastine, vincristine, vinorelbine, zidovudine.

- **Y-Site Incompatibility:** acyclovir, allopurinol, amphotericin B deoxycholate, diazepam, doxycycline, ganciclovir, imipenem/cilastatin, methylprednisolone, minocycline, nafcillin, pantoprazole, pentamidine, pentobarbital, phenytoin, thiopental.

Patient/Family Teaching
- Inform patient of purpose of medication.
- Advise patient to notify health care professional if nausea or vomiting occur.

Evaluation/Desired Outcomes
- Prevention of nausea and vomiting associated with initial and repeat courses of emetogenic cancer chemotherapy or surgery.

pamidronate (pa-mid-roe-nate)
Aredia

Classification
Therapeutic: bone resorption inhibitors
Pharmacologic: biphosphonates, hypocalcemics

Indications
Moderate to severe hypercalcemia associated with malignancy. Osteolytic bone lesions associated with multiple myeloma or breast cancer. Moderate to severe Paget's disease.

Action
Inhibits resorption of bone. **Therapeutic Effects:** Decreased serum calcium. Decreased skeletal destruction in multiple myeloma or breast cancer. Decreased skeletal complications in Paget's disease.

Pharmacokinetics
Absorption: IV administration results in complete bioavailability.
Distribution: Rapidly absorbed by bone. Reaches high concentrations in bone, liver, spleen, teeth, and tracheal cartilage. Approximately 50% of a dose is retained by bone and then slowly released.
Metabolism and Excretion: 50% is excreted unchanged in the urine.
Half-life: Elimination half-life from plasma is biphasic—1st phase 1.6 hr, 2nd phase 27.2 hr. Elimination half-life from bone is 300 days.

TIME/ACTION PROFILE (effect on serum calcium)

ROUTE	ONSET	PEAK	DURATION
IV	24 hr	7 days	unknown

Contraindications/Precautions
Contraindicated in: Hypersensitivity to pamidronate, other biphosphonates, or mannitol; OB, Lactation: Pregnancy or lactation.
Use Cautiously in: Underlying cardiovascular disease, especially HF (initiate saline hydration cautiously); Invasive dental procedures, cancer, receiving chemotherapy or corticosteroids, poor oral hygiene, periodontal disease, dental disease, anemia, coagulopathy, infection, or poorly-fitting dentures (may ↑ risk of jaw osteonecrosis); History of thyroid surgery (may be at ↑ risk for hypocalcemia); Renal impairment (dose ↓ recommended); Pedi: Safety not established.

Adverse Reactions/Side Effects
CNS: fatigue. **EENT:** conjunctivitis, blurred vision, eye pain/inflammation, rhinitis. **Resp:** rales. **CV:** arrhythmias, hypertension, syncope, tachycardia. **GI:** nausea, abdominal pain, anorexia, constipation, vomiting. **F and E:** hypocalcemia, hypokalemia, hypomagnesemia, hypophosphatemia, fluid overload. **GU:** nephrotoxicity. **Hemat:** leukopenia, anemia. **Local:** phlebitis at injection site. **Metab:** hypothyroidism. **MS:** muscle stiffness, musculoskeletal pain, femur fractures, osteonecrosis (primarily of jaw). **Misc:** fever, generalized pain.

Interactions
Drug-Drug: Hypokalemia and hypomagnesemia may ↑ risk of **digoxin** toxicity. **Calcium** and **vitamin D** will antagonize the beneficial effects of pamidronate. Concurrent use of **thalidomide** may ↑ risk of renal dysfunction.

Route/Dosage

Single doses should not exceed 90 mg.

Hypercalcemia of Malignancy

IV (Adults): *Moderate hypercalcemia*—30–90 mg; may be repeated after 7 days.

Osteolytic Lesions from Multiple Myeloma

IV (Adults): 90 mg monthly.

Osteolytic Lesions from Metastatic Breast Cancer

IV (Adults): 90 mg q 3–4 wk.

Paget's Disease

IV (Adults): 90–180 mg/treatment; may be given as 30 mg daily for 3 days up to 30 mg/wk for 6 wk. Single doses of 60–90 mg may also be effective.

Availability (generic available)

Powder for injection: 30 mg/vial, 90 mg/vial.

NURSING IMPLICATIONS

Assessment

- Monitor intake/output ratios and BP frequently during therapy. Assess for signs of fluid overload (edema, rales/crackles).
- Monitor symptoms of hypercalcemia (nausea, vomiting, anorexia, weakness, constipation, thirst, and cardiac arrhythmias).
- Observe for evidence of hypocalcemia (paresthesia, muscle twitching, laryngospasm, and Chvostek's or Trousseau's sign). Protect symptomatic patients by elevating and padding side rails; keep bed in low position.
- Monitor IV site for phlebitis (pain, redness, swelling). Symptomatic treatment should be used if this occurs.
- Assess for bone pain. Treatment with nonopioid or opioid analgesics may be necessary.
- ***Lab Test Considerations:*** Assess serum creatinine prior to each treatment. Withhold dose if renal function has deteriorated in patients treated for bone metastases.
- Monitor serum electrolytes (including calcium, phosphate, potassium, and magnesium), hemoglobin, and creatinine closely. Monitor CBC and platelet count during the first 2 wk of therapy. May cause hyperkalemia or hypokalemia, hypernatremia, and hematuria.
- Monitor renal function periodically during therapy.

Implementation

- Initiate a vigorous saline hydration, maintaining a urine output of 2000 mL/24 hr, concurrently with pamidronate therapy. Patients should be adequately hydrated, but avoid overhydration. Use caution in patients with underlying cardiovascular disease, especially HF. Do not use diuretics prior to treatment of hypovolemia.
- Patients with severe hypercalcemia should be started at the 90-mg dose.
- **IV:** Reconstitute by adding 10 mL of sterile water for injection to each vial. ***Concentration:*** 30 mg/10 mL or 90 mg/10 mL. Allow drug to dissolve before withdrawing. Solution is stable for 24 hr if refrigerated.
- **Hypercalcemia:** ***Diluent:*** Dilute further in 1000 mL of 0.45% NaCl, 0.9% NaCl, or D5W. Solution is stable for 24 hr at room temperature. ***Rate:*** Administer 60-mg infusion over at least 4 hr and 90-mg infusion over 24 hr.
- **Multiple Myeloma:** ***Diluent:*** Dilute reconstituted solution in 500 mL of 0.45% NaCl, 0.9% NaCl, or D5W. ***Rate:*** Administer over 4 hr.
- **Paget's Disease:** Dilute reconstituted solution in 500 mL of 0.45% NaCl, 0.9% NaCl, or D5W.
- ***Rate:*** Administer over 4 hr.
- **Y-Site Compatibility:** acyclovir alemtuzumab, alfentanil, allopurinol, amifostine, amikacin, aminophylline, amphotericin B lipid complex, amphotericin B liposome, ampillicin, ampicillin/sulbactam, anidulafungin, argatroban, atracurium, azithromycin, aztreonam, bivalirudin, bleomycin, bumetanide, buprenorphine, butorphanol, carboplatin, carmustine, cefazolin, cefepime, cefotaxime, cefotetan, cefoxitin, ceftazidime, ceftriaxone, cefuroxime, chloramphenicol, chlorpromazine, ciprofloxacin, cisatracurium, cisplatin, clindamycin, cyclophosphamide, cyclosporine, cytarabine, dacarbazine, daptomycin, dexamethasone, dexmedetomidine, dexrazoxane, digoxin, diltiazem, diphenhydramine, dobutamine, docetaxel, dolasetron, dopamine, doxacurium, doxorubicin, doxorubicin liposomal, doxycycline, droperidol, enalaprilat, ephedrine, epinephrine, epirubicin, ertapenem, erythromycin, esmolol, etoposide, etoposide phosphate, famotidine, fenoldopam, fentanyl, fluconazole, fludarabine, fluorouracil, foscarnet, fosphenytoin, furosemide, ganciclovir, gemcitabine, gentamicin, glycopyrrolate, granisetron, haloperidol, heparin, hydralazine, hydrocortisone, hydromorphone, ifosfamide, imipenem/cilastatin, insulin, isoproterenol, ketorolac, labetalol, levofloxacin, levorphanol, lidocaine, linezolid, lorazepam, magnesium sulfate, mannitol, melphalan, meperidine, meropenem, mesna, metaraminol, methotrexate, methyldopate, methylprednisolone, metoclopramide, metoprolol, metronidazole, midazolam, milrinone, mitoxantrone, morphine, moxifloxacin, mycophenolate, nafcillin, nalbuphine, naloxone, nicardipine, nitroglycerin, nitroprusside, norepinephrine, octreotide, ondansetron, oxytocin, paclitaxel, palonosetron, pancuronium, pemetrexed, pentamidine, pentobarbital, phenobarbital, phentolamine, phenylephrine, piperacillin/tazobactam, potassium acetate, potassium chloride, potassium phosphates, procainamide, prochlorperazine, promethazine, propranolol, quinupristin/dalfopristin, ranitidine, remifentanil, rocuronium, sodium ac-

etate, sodium bicarbonate, sodium phosphates, succinylcholine, sufentanil, tacrolimus, theophylline, thiopental, thiotepa, tigecycline, tirofiban, tobramycin, tolazoline, topotecan, trimethoprim/sulfamethoxazole, vancomycin, vasopressin, vecuronium, verapamil, vinblastine, vincristine, vinorelbine, voriconazole, zidovudine.

- **Y-Site Incompatibility:** amphotericin B deoxycholate, caspofungin, dantrolene, diazepam, leucovorin, phenytoin.
- **Additive Incompatibility:** Calcium-containing solutions, such as Ringer's solution.

Patient/Family Teaching

- Advise patient to report signs of hypercalcemic relapse (bone pain, anorexia, nausea, vomiting, thirst, lethargy) or eye problems (pain, inflammation, blurred vision, conjunctivitis) to health care professional promptly.
- Advise patient to notify nurse of pain at the infusion site.
- Encourage patient to comply with dietary recommendations. Diet should contain adequate amounts of calcium and vitamin D.
- Advise patient to notify health care professional if bone pain is severe or persistent.
- Advise patient to maintain good oral hygiene and have regular dental examinations. Instruct patient to inform health care professional of pamidronate therapy prior to dental surgery.
- Emphasize the need for keeping follow-up exams to monitor progress, even after medication is discontinued, to detect relapse.

Evaluation/Desired Outcomes

- Lowered serum calcium levels.
- Decreased pain from lytic lesions.

pancrelipase (pan-kre-li-pase)

✱Cotazym, Creon, ✱Pancrease MT, Pancreaze, Pertyze, Ultresa, Viokace, Zenpep

Classification
Therapeutic: digestive agent
Pharmacologic: pancreatic enzymes

Indications

Pancreatic insufficiency associated with: Chronic pancreatitis, Pancreatectomy, Cystic fibrosis, GI bypass surgery, Ductal obstruction secondary to tumor.

Action

Contains lipolytic, amylolytic, and proteolytic activity.
Therapeutic Effects: Increased digestion of fats, carbohydrates, and proteins in the GI tract.

Pharmacokinetics

Absorption: Unknown.
Distribution: Unknown.
Metabolism and Excretion: Unknown.
Half-life: Unknown.

TIME/ACTION PROFILE (digestant effects)

ROUTE	ONSET	PEAK	DURATION
PO	rapid	unknown	unknown

Contraindications/Precautions

Contraindicated in: Hypersensitivity to hog proteins.
Use Cautiously in: Gout, renal impairment, or hyperuricemia (may ↑ uric acid levels); OB, Lactation: Safety not established.

Adverse Reactions/Side Effects

EENT: nasal stuffiness. **Resp:** dyspnea, shortness of breath, wheezing. **GI:** FIBROSING COLONOPATHY (high doses only), abdominal pain (high doses only), diarrhea, nausea, stomach cramps, oral irritation. **GU:** hematuria. **Derm:** hives, rash. **Metab:** hyperuricemia. **Misc:** allergic reactions.

Interactions

Drug-Drug: Antacids (**calcium carbonate** or **magnesium hydroxide**) may ↓ effectiveness of pancrelipase. May ↓ the absorption of concurrently administered **iron supplements**.
Drug-Food: **Alkaline foods** destroy coating on enteric-coated products.

Route/Dosage

PO (Adults and Children ≥4 yr): Initiate with 500 lipase units/kg/meal; dose should be adjusted based on weight, clinical symptoms, and stool fat content; maximum dose = 2500 lipase units/kg/meal (or 10,000 lipase units/kg/day).
PO (Children >1 yr and <4 yr): Initiate with 1000 lipase units/kg/meal; dose should be adjusted based on weight, clinical symptoms, and stool fat content; maximum dose = 2500 lipase units/kg/meal (or 10,000 lipase units/kg/day).
PO (Children ≤1 yr): 2000–4000 lipase units per 120 mL of formula or breast milk.

Availability (generic available)

Delayed-release capsules: 2600 units lipase/6200 units protease/10,850 units amylase, 3000 units lipase/9500 units protease/15,000 units amylase, 3000 units lipase/10,000 units protease/16,000 units amylase, 4000 units lipase/14,375 units protease/15,125 units amylase, 4200 units lipase/14,200 units protease/24,600 units amylase, 5000 units lipase/17,000 units protease/27,000 units amylase, 6000 units lipase/19,000 units protease/30,000 units amylase, 8000 units lipase/28,750 units protease/30,250 units amylase, 🍁 8000 units lipase/30,000 units protease/30,000 units amylase, 10,000 units lipase/34,000 units protease/55,000 units amylase, 10,500 units lipase/35,500 units protease/61,500 units amylase, 12,000 units lipase/38,000 units protease/60,000 units amylase, 13,800 units lipase/27,600 units protease/27,600 units amylase, 15,000 units lipase/51,000 units protease/82,000 units amylase, 16,000 units lipase/57,500 units protease/60,500 units amylase, 16,800 units lipase/56,800 units protease/98,400 units amylase, 🍁 20,000 units lipase/55,000 units protease/55,000 units amylase, 20,000 units lipase/68,000 units protease/109,000 units amylase, 20,700 units lipase/41,400 units protease/41,400 units amylase, 21,000 units lipase/54,700 units protease/83,900 units amylase, 23,000 units lipase/46,000 units protease/46,000 units amylase, 24,000 units lipase/76,000 units protease/120,000 units amylase, 25,000 units lipase/85,000 units protease/136,000 units amylase, 36,000 units lipase/114,000 units protease/180,000 units amylase, 40,000 units lipase/136,000 units protease/218,000 units amylase. **Tablets:** 10,440 units lipase/39,150 units protease/39,150 units amylase, 20,880 units lipase/78,300 units protease/78,300 units amylase.

NURSING IMPLICATIONS

Assessment

- Assess patient's nutritional status (height, weight, skin-fold thickness, arm muscle circumference, and lab values) prior to and periodically throughout therapy.
- Monitor stools for high fat content (steatorrhea). Stools will be foul-smelling and frothy.
- Assess patient for allergy to pork; sensitivity to pancrelipase may exist.
- ***Lab Test Considerations:*** May cause ↑ serum and urine uric acid concentrations.

Implementation

Pancreaze is not interchangerable with any other pancrelipase product.

- **PO:** Administer immediately before or with meals and snacks.
- Swallow tablets whole; do not crush, break, or chew.
- Swallow capsules whole. If unable to swallow, capsules may be opened and sprinkled on foods. Delayed-release capsules filled should not be chewed (sprinkle on soft, acidic foods that can be swallowed without chewing, such as applesauce or Jell-O) and followed immediately by water or juice to ensure complete ingestion. These medications should not be chewed or mixed with alkaline foods prior to ingestion or coating will be destroyed.
- Half of the prescribed *Pancreaze* and *Pertyze* dose for an individualized full meal should be given with each snack. The total daily dose should reflect approximately three meals plus two or three snacks per day.
- Do not mix contents of *Pancreaze*, *Pertyze*, or *Creon* capsules directly into breast milk or formula. Capsule contents may be sprinkled on small amounts of acidic soft food with a pH of 4.5 or less (applesauce) and given to the infant within 15 min. Contents of the capsule may also be administered directly to the mouth. Follow administration with breast milk or formula. Applesauce mixture of *Pertyze* can also be administered via G tube.
- Do not mix *Zenpep* capsule contents directly into formula or breast milk prior to administration. Administer with applesauce, bananas, or pears (commercially prepared) and follow with breast milk or formula.
- Do not chew or retain *Ultressa* capsule in mouth.

Patient/Family Teaching

- Encourage patients to comply with diet recommendations of health care professional (generally high-calorie, high-protein, low-fat). Dose should be adjusted for fat content of diet. Usually 300 mg of pancrelipase is necessary to digest every 17 g of dietary fat. If a dose is missed, it should be omitted and next dose taken with next snack, as directed. Do not increase dose without consulting health care professional. Several days may be required to determine correct dose. Advise patient to read *Medication Guide* before starting therapy and with each Rx refill; information may be updated.
- Instruct patient not to chew tablets and to swallow them quickly with plenty of liquid to prevent mouth and throat irritation. Sit upright to enhance swallowing. Eating immediately after taking medication helps further ensure that the medication is swallowed and does not remain in contact with mouth and esophagus for a prolonged period. Patient should avoid sniffing powdered contents of capsules, as sensitization of nose and throat may occur (nasal stuffiness or respiratory distress).
- Advise patients and caregivers to notify health care professional if symptoms of fibrosing colonopathy (abdominal pain, distention, vomiting, constipation) occur. Occur more frequently with doses exceeding 6000 lipase units/kg of body weight per meal (10,000 lipase units/kg of body weight/day) and have been associated with colonic strictures in children below the age of 12 yr.
- Instruct patient to notify health care professional if joint pain, swelling of legs, gastric distress, or rash occurs.
- Advise female patients to notify health care professional if pregnancy is planned or suspected, or if breast feeding.

Evaluation/Desired Outcomes

- Improved nutritional status in patients with pancreatic insufficiency.
- Normalization of stools in patients with steatorrhea.

HIGH ALERT

pancuronium
(pan-cure-**oh**-nee-yum)
~~Pavulon~~

Classification
Therapeutic: neuromuscular blocking agents—nondepolarizing

Indications
Induction of skeletal muscle paralysis and facilitation of intubation after induction of anesthesia in surgical procedures. Facilitation of compliance during mechanical ventilation.

Action
Prevents neuromuscular transmission by blocking the effect of acetylcholine at the myoneural junction. Has no analgesic or anxiolytic properties. **Therapeutic Effects:** Skeletal muscle paralysis.

Pharmacokinetics
Absorption: Following IV administration, absorption is essentially complete.
Distribution: Rapidly distributes into extracellular fluid; small amounts cross the placenta.
Metabolism and Excretion: Excreted mostly unchanged by the kidneys; small amounts are eliminated in bile.
Half-life: 2 hr.

TIME/ACTION PROFILE (neuromuscular blockade)

ROUTE	ONSET	PEAK	DURATION
IV	30–45 sec	3–4.5 min	40–60 min

Contraindications/Precautions
Contraindicated in: Hypersensitivity; Hypersensitivity to bromides; Pedi: Products containing benzyl alcohol should be avoided in neonates.
Use Cautiously in: Underlying cardiovascular disease (↑ risk of arrhythmias); Dehydration or electrolyte abnormalities (should be corrected); Situations in which histamine release would be problematic; Fractures or muscle spasm; Renal impairment (↓ elimination); Hyperthermia (↑ duration/intensity of paralysis); Hepatic impairment (altered response); Shock; Extensive burns (may be more resistant to effects); Low plasma pseudocholinesterase levels (may be seen in association with anemia, dehydration, cholinesterase inhibitors/insecticides, severe liver disease, pregnancy, or hereditary predisposition); Obese patients; OB, Lactation: Safety not established; may be used during caesarian section; Pedi: Contains benzyl alcohol which can cause potentially fatal gasping syndrome in neonates; Geri: Age-related ↓ in renal function may result in prolonged effects.
Exercise Extreme Caution in: Patients with neuromuscular diseases such as myasthenia gravis (small test dose may be used to assess response).

Adverse Reactions/Side Effects
Resp: bronchospasm. **CV:** hypertension, tachycardia. **GI:** excessive salivation. **Derm:** rash. **Misc:** allergic reactions including ANAPHYLAXIS.

Interactions
Drug-Drug: Intensity and duration of paralysis may be prolonged by pretreatment with **succinylcholine**, **general anesthesia** (inhalation), **aminoglycosides**, **vancomycin**, **tetracyclines**, **polymyxin B**, **colistin**, **cyclosporine**, **calcium channel blockers**, **clindamycin**, **lidocaine**, and other **local anesthetics**, **lithium**, **quinidine**, **procainamide**, **beta blockers**, **potassium-losing diuretics**, or **magnesium**. **Inhalation anesthetics** including **enflurane**, **isoflurane**, **halothane**, **desflurane**, **sevoflurane** may enhance effects. Higher infusion rates may be required and duration of action may be shortened in patients receiving long-term **carbamazepine**, **steroids (chronic)**, **azathioprine**, or **phenytoin**.

Route/Dosage
IV (Adults and Children >1 mo): *Initial intubating dose*—0.06–0.1 mg/kg initially; additional doses of 0.01 mg/kg may be given every 25–60 min to maintain paralysis. *Continuous infusion*—1–2 mcg/kg/min.

Availability (generic available)
Injection: 1 mg/mL.

NURSING IMPLICATIONS
Assessment
- Assess respiratory status continuously throughout therapy with neuromuscular blocking agents. These medications should be used only to facilitate intubation or in patients already intubated.
- Neuromuscular response should be monitored with a peripheral nerve stimulator intraoperatively. Paralysis is initially selective and usually occurs sequentially in the following muscles: levator muscles of eyelids, muscles of mastication, limb muscles, abdominal muscles, muscles of the glottis, intercostal muscles, and the diaphragm. Recovery of muscle function usually occurs in reverse order.
- Monitor ECG, heart rate, and BP throughout administration.
- Observe the patient for residual muscle weakness and respiratory distress during the recovery period.
- Monitor infusion site frequently. If signs of tissue irritation or extravasation occur, discontinue and restart in another vein.

P

- ***Toxicity and Overdose:*** If overdose occurs, use peripheral nerve stimulator to determine the degree of neuromuscular blockade. Maintain airway patency and ventilation until recovery of normal respirations occurs.
- Administration of anticholinesterase agents (neostigmine, pyridostigmine) may be used to antagonize the action of neuromuscular blocking agents once the patient has demonstrated some spontaneous recovery from neuromuscular block. Atropine is usually administered prior to or concurrently with anticholinesterase agents to counteract the muscarinic effects.
- Administration of fluids and vasopressors may be necessary to treat severe hypotension or shock.

Implementation

- ***High Alert:*** Unintended administration of a neuromuscular blocking agent instead of administration of the intended medication or administration of a neuromuscular blocking agent in the absence of ventilatory support has resulted in serious harm or death. Confusing similarities in packaging and insufficiently controlled access to these medications are often implicated in these medication errors. Store these products in a separate, locked container.
- Dose is titrated to patient response.
- Neuromuscular blocking agents have *no* effect on consciousness or pain threshold. Adequate anesthesia/analgesia should *always* be used when neuromuscular blocking agents are used as an adjunct to surgical procedures or when painful procedures are performed. Benzodiazepines and/or analgesics should be administered concurrently when prolonged neuromuscular blocker therapy is used for ventilator patients, because patient is awake and able to feel all sensations.
- If eyes remain open throughout prolonged administration, protect corneas with artificial tears.
- Store pancuronium in refrigerator. To prevent absorption by plastic, pancuronium should not be stored in plastic syringes. May be administered in plastic syringes.
- Most neuromuscular blocking agents are incompatible with barbiturates and sodium bicarbonate. Do not admix.

IV Administration

- **IV Push:** ***Diluent:*** May be administered undiluted. ***Concentration:*** 1 mg/mL (10-mL vial); 2 mg/mL (2-mL or 5-mL vial). ***Rate:*** Administer over 1–2 min.
- **Intermittent Infusion:** ***Diluent:*** Add 100 mg of pancuroniuum to 250 mL of D5W, 0.9% NaCl, D5/0.9% NaCl, or LR. ***Concentration:*** 0.4 mg/mL. ***Rate:*** Based on patient's weight (see Route/Dosage section).
- **Y-Site Compatibility:** acyclovir, alemtuzumab, alfentanil, amifostine, amikacin, aminocaproic acid, aminophylline, amphotericin B liposome, ampicillin, ampicillin/sulbactam, anidulafungin, argatroban, azithromycin, aztreonam, bivalirudin, bleomycin, bumetanide, buprenorphine, busulfan, butorphanol, calcium chloride, calcium gluconate, carboplatin, carmustine, cefazolin, cefepime, cefotaxime, cefotetan, cefoxitin, ceftazidime, ceftriaxone, cefuroxime, chloramphenicol, chlorpromazine, ciprofloxacin, cisplatin, clindamycin, cyclophosphamide, cyclosporine, cytarabine, dactinomycin, daptomycin, dexamethasone, dexmedetomidine, dexrazoxane, diltiazem, diphenhydramine, dobutamine, docetaxel, dolasetron, dopamine, doxorubicin, doxorubicin liposomal, doxycycline, droperidol, enalaprilat, ephedrine, epinephrine, epirubicin, eptifibatide, ertapenem, erythromycin, esmolol, etomidate, etoposide, etoposide phosphate, famotidine, fenoldopam, fentanyl, fluconazole, fludarabine, fluorouracil, foscarnet, ganciclovir, gemcitabine, gentamicin, glycopyrrolate, granisetron, haloperidol, heparin, hydralazine, hydrocortisone sodium succinate, hydromorphone, idarubicin, ifosfamide, imipenem-cilastatin, insulin, irinotecan, isoproterenol, ketamine, ketorolac, labetalol, leucovorin calcium, levofloxacin, lidocaine, linezolid, lorazepam, magnesium sulfate, mannitol, melphalan, meperidine, meropenem, methohexital, methotrexate, methyldopate, methylprednisolone, metoclopramide, metoprolol, metronidazole, midazolam, milrinone, mitoxantrone, morphine, moxifloxacin, mycophenolate, nafcillin, nalbuphine, naloxone, nitroglycerin, nitroprusside, norepinephrine, octreotide, ondansetron, oxaliplatin, paclitaxel, palonosetron, pamidronate, pemetrexed, pentamidine, pentobarbital, phenobarbital, phenylephrine, piperacillin/tazobactam, potassium acetate, potassium chloride, potassium phosphates, procainamide, prochlorperazine, promethazine, propranolol, quinupristin/dalfopristin, ranitidine, remifentanil, sodium acetate, sodium bicarbonate, sodium phosphates, streptozocin, sufentanil, tacrolimus, theophylline, thiotepa, tigecycline, tirofiban, tobramycin, trimethoprim/sulfamethoxazole, vancomycin, verapamil, vinblastine, vincristine, vinorelbine, voriconazole, zidovudine, zoledronic acid.
- **Y-Site Incompatibility:** allopurinol, amphotericin B deoxycholate, amphotericin B lipid complex, caspofungin, dantrolene, diazepam, furosemide, pantoprazole, phenytoin, thiopental.

Patient/Family Teaching

- Explain all procedures to patient receiving neuromuscular blocker therapy without general anesthesia, because consciousness is not affected by neuromuscular blocking agents alone.
- Reassure patient that communication abilities will return as the medication wears off.

Evaluation/Desired Outcomes

- Adequate suppression of the twitch response when tested with peripheral nerve stimulation and subsequent muscle paralysis.
- Improved compliance during mechanical ventilation.

panitumumab

(pan-i-**tu**-mu-mab)

Vectibix

Classification

Therapeutic: antineoplastics

Pharmacologic: kinase inhibitors

Indications

Treatment of wild-type *RAS* (wild type in *KRAS* and *NRAS*) metastatic colorectal cancer that has failed fluoropyrimidine-, oxaliplatin-, and irinotecan-containing chemotherapy (to be used as monotherapy). Treatment of wild-type *RAS* (wild type in *KRAS* and *NRAS*) metastatic colorectal cancer (as first-line therapy with FOLFOX).

Action

Binds to EGFR resulting in inactivation of kinases that regulate proliferation and transformation. **Therapeutic Effects:** Decreased progression of colorectal cancer.

Pharmacokinetics

Absorption: IV administration results in complete bioavailability.

Distribution: Monoclonal antibodies cross the placenta and enter breast milk.

Metabolism and Excretion: Unknown.

Half-life: 7.5 days.

TIME/ACTION PROFILE

ROUTE	ONSET	PEAK	DURATION
IV	unknown	end of infusion	unknown

Contraindications/Precautions

Contraindicated in: Concurrent leucovorin; *RAS*—mutant metastatic colorectal cancer or unknown *RAS* mutation status (↑ mortality and tumor progression); OB: May cause fetal harm; Lactation: Avoid breast feeding.

Use Cautiously in: Rep: Women of reproductive potential; Pedi: Safety not established.

Adverse Reactions/Side Effects

CNS: fatigue. **Derm:** NECROTIZING FASCIITIS, acneiform dermatitis, dry skin, erythema, paronychia, pruritus, rash, skin exfoliation, skin fissures, abscesses, photosensitivity. **EENT:** OCULAR TOXICITY, eyelash growth. **F and E:** edema, hypocalcemia, hypomagnesemia. **GI:** abdominal pain, constipation, diarrhea, nausea, vomiting, stomatitis. **GU:** acute renal failure. **Resp:** INTERSTITIAL LUNG DISEASE, PULMONARY FIBROSIS, cough. **Misc:** INFUSION REACTIONS, SEPSIS.

Interactions

Drug-Drug: None noted.

Route/Dosage

IV (Adults): 6 mg/kg every 14 days.

Availability

Solution for injection (requires dilution): 20 mg/mL.

NURSING IMPLICATIONS

Assessment

- Assess for dermatologic toxicity (dermatitis acneiform, pruritus, erythema, rash, skin exfoliation, paronychia, dry skin, skin fissures). If severe, may lead to infection (sepsis, septic death, abscesses requiring incision and drainage). With severe reactions, hold panitumumab and monitor for inflammatory or infectious sequelae. *If severe dermatologic toxicities (Grade 3 or higher) or those considered intolerable occur,* hold panitumumab. *Upon 1st occurrence of a grade 3 dermatologic toxicity,* hold 1–2 doses; if skin improves to <Grade 3, reinitiate at original dose. *For 2nd occurrence of a grade 3 dermatologic toxicity,* hold 1–2 doses; if skin improves to <Grade 3, reinitiate at 80% of original dose. *For 3rd occurrence of a grade 3 dermatologic toxicity,* hold 1–2 doses; if skin improves to <Grade 3, reinitiate at 60% of original dose. *For 4th occurrence of a grade 3 dermatologic toxicity,* permanently discontinue panitumumab.
- Monitor for severe infusion reactions (anaphylactic reaction, bronchospasm, fever, chills, hypotension). If severe reaction occurs, stop panitumumab; may require permanent discontinuation.
- Assess for pulmonary fibrosis (cough, wheezing, exertional dyspnea, interstitial lung disease, pneumonitis, lung infiltrates). Permanently discontinue panitumumab if these signs occur.
- Monitor for diarrhea and dehydration during therapy.
- Monitor for signs and symptoms of interstitial lung disease (persistent or recurrent coughing, wheezing, dyspnea) during therapy; discontinue panitumumab if symptoms occur.
- ***Lab Test Considerations:*** Monitor electrolyte levels periodically during and for 8 wk after completion of therapy. May cause hypomagnesemia, hypocalcemia, and hypokalemia. Replace electrolytes as needed.

P

Implementation

- Prior to administration, assess RAS mutational status in colorectal tumors and confirm the absence of a RAS mutation.
- **Intermittent Infusion:** ***Diluent:*** Withdraw necessary amount of panitumumab. Dilute to a volume of 100 mL with 0.9% NaCl; dilute doses >1000 mg with 150 mL. ***Concentration:*** 10 mg/mL. Mix by inverting gently; do not shake. Administer via infusion pump using a low-protein binding 0.2 mcg or 0.22 mcg in-line filter. Solution is colorless and may contain a small amount of visible translucent to white, amorphous, proteinaceous particles. Do not administer solutions that are discolored or contain particulate matter. Store in refrigerator; do not freeze. Use diluted solution within 6 hr of preparation if stored at room temperature or within 24 hr if refrigerated. ***Rate:*** Administer over 60 min every 14 days. If 1st infusion is tolerated, subsequent infusions may be infused over 30–60 min. Administer doses >1000 mg over 90 min.
- *If mild to moderate infusion reaction (Grade 1 or 2) occurs,* decrease infusion rate by 50%. *If severe reaction (Grade 3 or 4) occurs,* immediately and permanently discontinue panitumumab.
- **Y-Site Incompatibility:** Flush line before and after administration with 0.9% NaCl. Do not mix with other medications or solutions.

Patient/Family Teaching

- Explain purpose of panitumumab to patient.
- May cause photosensitivity. Caution patient to wear sunscreen and hats and to limit sun exposure.
- Advise patient to notify health care professional if signs and symptoms of dermatologic toxicity, infusion reactions, pulmonary fibrosis, or ocular changes occur.
- Rep: Advise patient that panitumumab may cause fertility impairment and may have teratogenic effects. Caution women of reproductive potential to use contraception and avoid breast feeding during and for at least 2 mo after last dose.
- Emphasize the need for periodic blood tests to monitor electrolyte levels.

Evaluation/Desired Outcomes

- Decreased progression of colorectal cancer.

BEERS

pantoprazole

(pan-**toe**-pra-zole)

Pantoloc, Protonix, Protonix IV, Tecta

Classification

Therapeutic: antiulcer agents

Pharmacologic: proton-pump inhibitors

Indications

Erosive esophagitis associated with GERD. Maintenance of healing of erosive esophagitis. Pathologic gastric hypersecretory conditions. **Unlabeled Use:** Adjunctive treatment of duodenal ulcers associated with *Helicobacter pylori*.

Action

Binds to an enzyme in the presence of acidic gastric pH, preventing the final transport of hydrogen ions into the gastric lumen. **Therapeutic Effects:** Diminished accumulation of acid in the gastric lumen, with lessened acid reflux. Healing of duodenal ulcers and esophagitis. Decreased acid secretion in hypersecretory conditions.

Pharmacokinetics

Absorption: Tablet is enteric-coated; absorption occurs only after tablet leaves the stomach.

Distribution: Unknown.

Protein Binding: 98%.

Metabolism and Excretion: Primarily metabolized by the CYP2C19 and CYP3A4 isoenzymes in the liver; the CYP2C19 enzyme system exhibits genetic polymorphism; 15–20% of Asian patients and 3–5% of Caucasian and Black patients may be poor metabolizers and may have significantly ↑ pantoprazole concentrations and an ↑ risk of adverse effects); inactive metabolites are excreted in urine (71%) and feces (18%).

Half-life: 1 hr.

TIME/ACTION PROFILE (effect on acid secretion)

ROUTE	ONSET†	PEAK	DURATION†
PO	2.5 hr	unknown	1 wk
IV	15–30 min	2 hr	unknown

†Onset = 51% inhibition; duration = return to normal following discontinuation.

Contraindications/Precautions

Contraindicated in: Hypersensitivity to rabeprazole or related drugs (benzimidazoles).

Use Cautiously in: Patients using high-doses for >1 yr (↑ risk of hip, wrist, or spine fractures and fundic gland polyps); Patients using therapy for >3 yr (↑ risk of vitamin B_{12} deficiency); OB: Use only if potential maternal benefit justifies potential fetal risk; Lactation: Use while breast feeding only if potential maternal benefit justifies potential risk to infant; Pedi: Safety and effectiveness not established.

Adverse Reactions/Side Effects

CNS: headache. **Derm:** cutaneous lupus erythematosus. **Endo:** hyperglycemia. **F and E:** hypomagnesemia (especially if treatment duration ≥3 mo). **GI:** CLOSTRIDIUM DIFFICILE-ASSOCIATED DIARRHEA (CDAD), abdominal pain, diarrhea, eructation, flatulence, fundic gland polyps. **GU:** acute interstitial nephritis. **Hemat:** vitamin B_{12} deficiency. **MS:** bone fracture. **Misc:** systemic lupus erythematosis.

Interactions

Drug-Drug: May ↓ levels of **atazanavir** and **nelfinavir**; avoid concurrent use with either of these antiretrovirals. May ↓ absorption of drugs requiring acid pH, including **ketoconazole**, **itraconazole**, **ampicillin esters**, **iron salts**, **erlotinib**, and **mycophenolate mofetil**; concomitant use with **atazanavir** not recommended. May ↑ risk of bleeding with **warfarin** (monitor INR/PT). Hypomagnesemia ↑ risk of **digoxin** toxicity. May ↑ **methotrexate** levels.

Route/Dosage

GERD

PO (Adults): *Short-term treatment of erosive esophagitis associated with GERD*—40 mg once daily for up to 8 wk; *Maintenance of healing of erosive esophagitis*—40 mg once daily.
PO (Children ≥5 yr): *15–39 kg*—20 mg once daily for up to 8 wk; *≥40 kg*—40 mg once daily for up to 8 wk.
IV (Adults): 40 mg once daily for 7–10 days.

Gastric Hypersecretory Conditions

PO (Adults): 40 mg twice daily, up to 120 mg twice daily.
IV (Adults): 80 mg every 12 hr (up to 240 mg/day).

Availability (generic available)

Delayed-release tablets: 20 mg, 40 mg. **Cost:** *Generic*—All strengths $368.22/90. **Powder for injection:** 40 mg/vial. **Delayed-release oral suspension:** 40 mg/packet. **Cost:** $7.60/1 pkt.

NURSING IMPLICATIONS

Assessment

- Assess patient routinely for epigastric or abdominal pain and for frank or occult blood in stool, emesis, or gastric aspirate.
- ***Lab Test Considerations:*** May cause abnormal liver function tests, including ↑ AST, ALT, alkaline phosphatase, and bilirubin.
- May cause hypomagnesemia. Monitor serum magnesium prior to and periodically during therapy.

Implementation

- Do not confuse Protonix (pantoprazole) with Lotronex (alosetron) or protamine.
- Patients receiving pantoprazole IV should be converted to PO dosing as soon as possible.
- Monitor bowel function. Diarrhea, abdominal cramping, fever, and bloody stools should be reported to health care professional promptly as a sign of Clostridium difficile-associated diarrhea (CDAD). May begin up to several wk following cessation of therapy.
- **PO:** May be administered with or without food. Do not break, crush, or chew tablets.
- Antacids may be used concurrently.

IV Administration

- **IV:** Reconstitute each vial with 10 mL of 0.9% NaCl. Reconstituted solution is stable for 6 hr at room temperature.
- **IV Push:** ***Diluent:*** Administer undiluted. ***Concentration:*** 4 mg/mL. ***Rate:*** Administer over at least 2 min.
- **Intermittent Infusion:** ***Diluent:*** Dilute further with D5W, 0.9% NaCl, or LR. ***Concentration:*** 0.4–0.8 mg/mL. Diluted solution is stable for 24 hr at room temperature. ***Rate:*** Administer over 15 min at a rate of <3 mg/min.
- **Y-Site Compatibility:** allopurinol, alprostadil, amifostine, aminocaproic acid, amikacin, aminophylline, amphotericin B lipid complex, amphotericin B liposome, ampicillin, ampicillin/sulbactam, anidulafungin, argatroban, azithromycin, bleomycin, bumetanide, cangrelor, carboplatin, carmustine, ceftaroline, ceftriaxone, cyclophosphamide, cytarabine, docetaxel, doxorubicin liposomal, doxycycline, ertapenem, fluorouracil, foscarnet, fosphenytoin, ganciclovir, granisetron, imipenem/cilastatin, irinotecan, mesna, paclitaxel, penicillin G sodium, pentobarbital, phenobarbital, phenylephrine, potassium chloride, procainamide, rifampin, succinylcholine, sufentanil, telavancin, theophylline, tigecycline, tirofiban, vasopressin, zidovudine, zoledronic acid.
- **Y-Site Incompatibility:** alemtuzumab, alfentanil, atropine, aztreonam, buprenorphine, butorphanol, calcium acetate, calcium chloride, cefepime, cefotaxime, cefotetan, chloramphenicol, chlorpromazine, ciprofloxacin, cisatracurium, cisplatin, dacarbazine, dactinomycin, dantrolene, daptomycin, daunorubicin hydrochloride, dexamethasone, dexmedetomidine, dexrazoxane, diazepam, diltiazem, diphenhydramine, dobutamine, doxorubicin hydrochloride, droperidol, ephedrine, epirubicin, esmolol, etoposide, etoposide phosphate, famotidine, fenoldopam, fentanyl, fluconazole, fludarabine, furosemide, gemcitabine, glycopyrrolate, haloperidol, hydralazine, hydromorphone, hydroxyzine, idarubicin, ifosfamide, insulin, regular, ketorolac, labetalol, leucovorin, levofloxacin, lidocaine, linezolid, lorazepam, melphalan, meperidine, meropenem, methotrexate, methylprednisolone, metoprolol, metronidazole, midazolam, milrinone, mitomycin, mitoxantrone, moxifloxacin, multivitamins, mycophenolate, nalbuphine, naloxone, nicardipine, norepinephrine, ondansetron, palonosetron, pancuronium, pemetrexed, pentamidine, phenytoin, potassium acetate, potassium phosphates, prochlorperazine, promethazine, propranolol, quinupristin/dalfopristin, ranitidine, remifentanil, rocuronium,

P

sodium acetate, sodium phosphates, streptozocin, thiotepa, topotecan, vecuronium, verapamil, vinblastine, vincristine, vinorelbine, voriconazole, solutions containing zinc.

Patient/Family Teaching

- Instruct patient to take medication as directed for the full course of therapy, even if feeling better. Advise patient to read *Medication Guide* before starting therapy and with each Rx refill in case of changes.
- Advise patient to avoid alcohol, products containing aspirin or NSAIDs, and foods that may cause an increase in GI irritation.
- Advise patient to report onset of black, tarry stools; diarrhea; or abdominal pain to health care professional promptly. Instruct patient to notify health care professional immediately if rash, diarrhea, abdominal cramping, fever, or bloody stools occur and not to treat with antidiarrheals without consulting health care professional.
- Instruct patient to notify health care professional of all Rx or OTC medications, vitamins, or herbal products being taken and consult health care professional before taking any new medications.
- Advise females of reproductive potential to notify health care professional if pregnancy is planned or suspected, or if breast feeding.

Evaluation/Desired Outcomes

- Decrease in abdominal pain, heartburn, gastric irritation, and bleeding in patients with GERD; may require up to 4 wk of therapy.
- Healing in patients with erosive esophagitis. Therapy is continued for up to 8 wk.

paricalcitol, **See VITAMIN D COMPOUNDS.**

BEERS

PARoxetine

PARoxetine hydrochloride

(par-**ox**-e-teen)

Paxil, Paxil CR

PARoxetine mesylate

Brisdelle, Pexeva

Classification

Therapeutic: antianxiety agents, antidepressants

Pharmacologic: selective serotonin reuptake inhibitors (SSRIs)

Indications

Paxil, Paxil CR, Pexeva: Major depressive disorder, panic disorder. **Paxil, Pexeva**: Obsessive compulsive disorder (OCD), generalized anxiety disorder (GAD). **Paxil, Paxil CR**: Social anxiety disorder. **Paxil**: Posttraumatic stress disorder (PTSD). **Paxil CR**: Premenstrual dysphoric disorder (PMDD). **Brisdelle**: Moderate to severe vasomotor symptoms associated with menopause.

Action

Inhibits neuronal reuptake of serotonin in the CNS, thus potentiating the activity of serotonin; has little effect on norepinephrine or dopamine; mechanism for benefit in treating vasomotor symptoms unknown. **Therapeutic Effects:** Antidepressant action. Decreased frequency of panic attacks, OCD, or anxiety. Improvement in manifestations of post-traumatic stress disorder. Decreased dysphoria prior to menses. Decreased vasomotor symptoms in postmenopausal women.

Pharmacokinetics

Absorption: Completely absorbed following oral administration. Controlled-release tablets are enteric-coated and control medication release over 4–5 hr.

Distribution: Widely distributed throughout body fluids and tissues, including the CNS; cross the placenta and enter breast milk.

Protein Binding: 95%.

Metabolism and Excretion: Highly metabolized by the liver (partly by P450 2D6 enzyme system); the CYP2D6 enzyme system exhibits genetic polymorphism; ~7% of population may be poor metabolizers (PMs) and may have significantly ↑ paroxetine concentrations and an ↑ risk of adverse effects. 2% excreted unchanged in urine.

Half-life: 21 hr.

TIME/ACTION PROFILE (antidepressant action)

ROUTE	ONSET	PEAK	DURATION
PO	1–4 wk	unknown	unknown

Contraindications/Precautions

Contraindicated in: Hypersensitivity; Concurrent use of MAO inhibitors or MAO-like drugs (linezolid or methylene blue); Concurrent use of thioridazine or pimozide; Lactation: Lactation.

Use Cautiously in: Risk of suicide (may ↑ risk of suicide attempt/ideation especially during early treatment or dose adjustment); History of mania; History of seizures; History of bipolar disorder; Angle-closure glaucoma; Severe renal/hepatic impairment; OB: Use during the 1st trimester may be associated with an ↑ risk of cardiac malformations—consider fetal risk/maternal benefit; use during 3rd trimester may result in neonatal serotonin syndrome requiring prolonged hospitalization, respiratory and nutritional support; Pedi: May ↑ risk of suicide attempt/ideation especially during early treatment or dose adjustment; may be greater in children and adolescents (safety and effectiveness in children/adolescents not established); Geri:

↑ risk of hyponatremia; daily dose should not exceed 40 mg.

Adverse Reactions/Side Effects

CNS: NEUROLEPTIC MALIGNANT SYNDROME, SUICIDAL THOUGHTS, anxiety, dizziness, drowsiness, headache, insomnia, weakness, agitation, amnesia, confusion, emotional lability, hangover, impaired concentration, malaise, mental depression, syncope. **CV:** chest pain, edema, hypertension, palpitations, postural hypotension, tachycardia, vasodilation. **Derm:** STEVENS-JOHNSON SYNDROME, sweating, photosensitivity, pruritus, rash. **EENT:** blurred vision, rhinitis. **F and E:** hyponatremia. **GI:** constipation, diarrhea, dry mouth, nausea, abdominal pain, ↓/↑ appetite, dyspepsia, flatulence, taste disturbances, vomiting. **GU:** ejaculatory disturbance, ↓ libido, genital disorders, infertility, urinary disorders, urinary frequency. **Metab:** weight gain/loss. **MS:** back pain, bone fracture, myalgia, myopathy. **Neuro:** paresthesia, tremor. **Resp:** cough, pharyngitis, respiratory disorders, yawning. **Misc:** SEROTONIN SYNDROME, chills, fever.

Interactions

Drug-Drug: Concurrent use with **MAO inhibitors** may result in serious, potentially fatal reactions (wait at least 2 wk after stopping MAO inhibitor before initiating paroxetine; wait at least 2 wk after stopping paroxetine before starting MAO inhibitors). Concurrent use with **MAO-inhibitor like drugs**, such as **linezolid** or **methylene blue** may ↑ risk of serotonin syndrome; concurrent use contraindicated; do not start therapy in patients receiving **linezolid** or **methylene blue**; if **linezolid** or **methylene blue** need to be started in a patient receiving paroxetine, immediately discontinue paroxetine and monitor for signs/symptoms of serotonin syndrome for 2 wk or until 24 hr after last dose of linezolid or methylene blue, whichever comes first (may resume paroxetine therapy 24 hr after last dose of linezolid or methylene blue). Concurrent use with **pimozide** or **thioridazine** may ↑ risk of QT interval prolongation and torsades de pointes; concurrent use contraindicated. May ↓ metabolism and ↑ effects of certain **drugs that are metabolized by the liver**, including other **antidepressants**, **phenothiazines**, **class IC antiarrhythmics**, **risperidone**, **atomoxetine**, **theophylline**, and **quinidine**. Concurrent use should be undertaken with caution. **Cimetidine** ↑ blood levels. **Phenobarbital** and **phenytoin** may ↓ effectiveness. Concurrent use with **alcohol** is not recommended. May ↓ the effectiveness of **digoxin** and **tamoxifen**. May ↑ risk of bleeding with **warfarin**, **aspirin**, or **NSAIDS**. Drugs that affect serotonergic neurotransmitter systems, including **tricyclic antidepressants**, **SNRIs**, **fentanyl**, **buspirone**, **tramadol**, **amphetamines**, and **triptans** ↑ risk of serotonin syndrome.

Drug-Natural Products: ↑ risk of serotonergic side effects including serotonin syndrome with **St. John's wort**, **SAMe**, and **tryptophan**.

Route/Dosage

Depression

PO (Adults): 20 mg as a single dose in the morning; may ↑ by 10 mg/day at weekly intervals (not to exceed 50 mg/day). *Controlled-release tablets*—25 mg once daily initially. May ↑ at weekly intervals by 12.5 mg (not to exceed 62.5 mg/day).

PO (Geriatric Patients or Debilitated Patients): 10 mg/day initially; may be slowly ↑ (not to exceed 40 mg/day). *Controlled-release tablets*—12.5 mg once daily initially; may be slowly ↑ (not to exceed 50 mg/day).

Obsessive-Compulsive Disorder

PO (Adults): 20 mg/day initially; ↑ by 10 mg/day at weekly intervals up to 40 mg (not to exceed 60 mg/day).

Panic Disorder

PO (Adults): 10 mg/day initially; ↑ by 10 mg/day at weekly intervals up to 40 mg (not to exceed 60 mg/day). *Controlled-release tablets*—12.5 mg/day initially; ↑ by 12.5 mg/day at weekly intervals (not to exceed 75 mg/day).

Social Anxiety Disorder

PO (Adults): 20 mg/day. *Controlled-release tablets*—12.5 mg/day initially; may ↑ by 12.5 mg/day weekly intervals (not to exceed 37.5 mg/day).

Generalized Anxiety Disorder

PO (Adults): 20 mg once daily initially; ↑ by 10 mg/day at weekly intervals (not to exceed 50 mg/day).

Post-Traumatic Stress Disorder

PO (Adults): 20 mg/day initially; may ↑ by 10 mg/day at weekly intervals (not to exceed 50 mg/day).

Premenstrual Dysphoric Disorder

PO (Adults): *Controlled-release tablets*—12.5 mg once daily throughout menstrual cycle or during luteal phase of menstrual cycle only; may ↑ to 25 mg/day after one wk.

Menopausal Vasomotor Symptoms

PO (Adults): 7.5 mg once daily at bedtime.

Hepatic Impairment

PO (Adults): Paxil, Paxil CR, or Pexeva: *Severe hepatic impairment*—10 mg/day initially; may slowly ↑ (not to exceed 40 mg/day). *Controlled-release tablets*—12.5 mg once daily initially; may slowly ↑ (not to exceed 50 mg/day).

P

Renal Impairment

PO (Adults): Paxil, Paxil CR, or Pexeva: *Severe renal impairment*—10 mg/day initially; may slowly ↑ (not to exceed 40 mg/day). *Controlled-release tablets*—12.5 mg once daily initially; may slowly ↑ (not to exceed 50 mg/day).

Availability (generic available)

Paroxetine hydrochloride tablets: 10 mg, 20 mg, 30 mg, 40 mg. **Cost:** *Generic*—10 mg $9.93/90, 20 mg $9.93/90, 30 mg $18.82/90, 40 mg $14.88/90. **Paroxetine hydrochloride controlled-release tablets:** 12.5 mg, 25 mg, 37.5 mg. **Cost:** *Generic*—12.5 mg $263.62/90, 25 mg $254.13/90, 37.5 mg $270.06/90. **Paroxetine hydrochloride oral suspension (orange flavor):** 10 mg/5 mL. **Cost:** $268.35/250 mL. **Paroxetine mesylate tablets (Pexeva):** 10 mg, 20 mg, 30 mg, 40 mg. **Cost:** 10 mg $235.38/30, 20 mg $244.69/30, 30 mg $253.99/30, 40 mg $263.33/30. **Paroxetine mesylate capsules (Brisdelle):** 7.5 mg. **Cost:** $161.64/30.

NURSING IMPLICATIONS

Assessment

- Monitor appetite and nutritional intake. Weigh weekly. Notify health care professional of continued weight loss. Adjust diet as tolerated to support nutritional status.
- **Depression:** Monitor mental status (orientation, mood, behavior). Inform health care professional if patient demonstrates significant increase in anxiety, nervousness, or insomnia.
- Assess for suicidal tendencies, especially during early therapy. Restrict amount of drug available to patient. Risk may be increased in children, adolescents, and adults ≤24 yr.
- Assess for serotonin syndrome (mental changes [agitation, hallucinations, coma], autonomic instability [tachycardia, labile BP, hyperthermia], neuromuscular aberations [hyper reflexia, incoordination], and/or GI symptoms [nausea, vomiting, diarrhea]), especially in patients taking other serotonergic drugs (SSRIs, SNRIs, triptans).
- Monitor for development of neuroleptic malignant syndrome (fever, respiratory distress, tachycardia, seizures, diaphoresis, hypertension or hypotension, pallor, tiredness). Discontinue paroxetine and notify health care professional immediately if these symptoms occur.
- Assess for rash periodically during therapy. May cause Stevens-Johnson syndrome. Discontinue therapy if severe or if accompanied with fever, general malaise, fatigue, muscle or joint aches, blisters, oral lesions, conjunctivitis, hepatitis, and/or eosinophilia.
- **OCD:** Assess patient for frequency of obsessive-compulsive behaviors. Note degree to which these thoughts and behaviors interfere with daily functioning.
- **Panic Attacks:** Assess frequency and severity of panic attacks.
- **Social Anxiety Disorder:** Assess frequency and severity of episodes of anxiety.
- **Post-traumatic Stress Disorder:** Assess manifestations of post-traumatic stress disorder periodically during therapy.
- **Premenstrual Dysphoria:** Assess symptoms of premenstrual distress prior to and during therapy.
- ***Lab Test Considerations:*** Monitor CBC and differential periodically during therapy. Report leukopenia or anemia.

Implementation

- Do not confuse paroxetine with fluoxetine, duloxetine, or piroxicam. Do not confuse Paxil (paroxetine) with Doxil (doxorubicin liposomal) or Plavix (clopidogrel). Do not confuse Pexeva (paroxetine mesylate) with Lexiva (fosamprenavir).
- Paroxetine mesylate (Pexeva) cannot be substituted with paroxetine (Paxil or Paxil CR) or generic paroxetine.
- Periodically reassess dose and continued need for therapy.
- **PO:** Administer as a single dose in the morning. May administer with food to minimize GI irritation.
- Swallow tablets whole. Do not crush, break, or chew. Shake suspension before administering.
- Taper to avoid potential withdrawal reactions.

Patient/Family Teaching

- Instruct patient to take paroxetine as directed. Take missed doses as soon as possible and return to regular dosing schedule. Do not double doses. Caution patient to consult health care professional before discontinuing paroxetine. Daily doses should be decreased slowly. Abrupt withdrawal may cause dizziness, sensory disturbances, agitation, anxiety, nausea, and sweating. Advise patient to read *Medication Guide* before starting and with each Rx refill in case of changes.
- May cause drowsiness or dizziness. Caution patient to avoid driving and other activities requiring alertness until response to the drug is known.
- Advise patient, family, and caregivers to look for suicidality, especially during early therapy or dose changes. Notify health care professional immediately if thoughts about suicide or dying, attempts to commit suicide, new or worse depression or anxiety, agitation or restlessness, panic attacks, insomnia, new or worse irritability, aggressiveness, acting on dangerous impulses, mania, or other changes in mood or behavior, or if symptoms of serotonin syndrome or neuroleptic malignant syndrome occur.
- Instruct patient to notify health care professional of all Rx or OTC medications, vitamins, or herbal products being taken and consult health care professional before taking any new medications and to avoid alcohol or other CNS-depressant drugs during therapy.

- Inform patient that frequent mouth rinses, good oral hygiene, and sugarless gum or candy may minimize dry mouth. Saliva substitute may be used. Consult dentist if dry mouth persists for more than 2 wk.
- Advise patient to notify health care professional if headache, weakness, nausea, anorexia, anxiety, or insomnia persists.
- Advise females of reproductive potential to notify health care professional if pregnancy is planned or suspected, or if breast feeding.
- Emphasize the importance of follow-up exams to monitor progress. Encourage patient participation in psychotherapy to improve coping skills.

Evaluation/Desired Outcomes

- Increased sense of well-being.
- Renewed interest in surroundings. May require 1–4 wk of therapy to obtain antidepressant effects.
- Decrease in obsessive-compulsive behaviors.
- Decrease in frequency and severity of panic attacks.
- Decrease in frequency and severity of episodes of anxiety.
- Improvement in manifestations of post-traumatic stress disorder.
- Decreased dysphoria prior to menses.

patiromer (pa-tir-oh-mer)

Veltassa

Classification

Therapeutic: electrolyte modifiers, hypokalemic

Pharmacologic: cationic exchange resins

Indications

Mild to moderate hyperkalemia (if severe, more immediate measures such as calcium IV or insulin/glucose IV should be instituted).

Action

Contains calcium-sorbitol counterion and ↑ fecal potassium excretion through binding of potassium in the lumen of the GI tract. **Therapeutic Effects:** Reduced serum potassium concentrations.

Pharmacokinetics

Absorption: Not systemically absorbed.

Distribution: Not distributed.

Metabolism and Excretion: Eliminated in the feces.

Half-life: Unknown.

TIME/ACTION PROFILE (↓ in serum potassium concentrations)

ROUTE	ONSET	PEAK	DURATION
PO	7–12 hr	unknown	24 hr

Contraindications/Precautions

Contraindicated in: Hypersensitivity; History of bowel impaction, bowel obstruction, or severe constipation (may be ineffective and worsen condition).

Use Cautiously in: Pedi: Safety and effectiveness not established.

Adverse Reactions/Side Effects

F and E: hypokalemia, hypomagnesemia. **GI:** constipation, diarrhea, flatulence, nausea.

Interactions

Drug-Drug: May ↓ absorption of any other orally administered medication; administer other oral medications ≥6 hr before or after patiromer.

Route/Dosage

PO (Adults): 8.4 g once daily; titrate dose at ≥1 wk intervals by 8.4 g once daily as needed to achieve desired serum potassium concentration (max = 25.2 g once daily).

Availability

Powder for oral suspension: 8.4 g/pkt, 16.8 g/pkt, 25.2 g/pkt.

P

NURSING IMPLICATIONS

Assessment

- Monitor for bowel sounds and frequency and consistency of stools periodically during therapy. May cause constipation.
- ***Lab Test Considerations:*** Monitor serum potassium and magnesium periodically during therapy. May cause hypokalemia and hypomagnesemia. Consider magnesium supplements if hypomagnesemia occurs.

Implementation

- Due to delayed action, do not use patiromer as an emergency treatment of life-threatening hyperkalemia.
- **PO:** Prepare dose by measuring 1/3 cup of water, add half of water into glass, then add patiromer and stir. Add remaining water and stir thoroughly. Powder will not dissolve, mixture will look cloudy; add more water to mixture for desired consistency. Administer immediately at least 3 hr before or 3 hr after other PO medications. If powder remains in glass after drinking, add more water, stir and drink immediately. Repeat as necessary for entire dose. Do not heat (microwave) or add to heated foods or liquids. Do not take in dry form. Stable for 3 mo at room temperature or until the package expiration date if refrigerated.

Patient/Family Teaching

- Instruct patient to take patiromer as directed and adhere to prescribed diet.

- Advise patient to take patiromer ≥3 hrs before or 3 hrs after other medications.

Evaluation/Desired Outcomes

- Reduced serum potassium concentrations.

PAZOPanib (pah-zoe-puh-nib)

Votrient

Classification

Therapeutic: antineoplastics

Pharmacologic: kinase inhibitors

Indications

Advanced renal cell carcinoma. Advanced soft tissue sarcoma in patients who have previously received chemotherapy.

Action

Acts as a tyrosine kinase inhibitor of several vascular endothelial growth factor (VEGF) receptors, platelet-derived growth factor receptor, fibroblast growth factor receptor, cytokine receptor, interleukin-2 receptor inducible T-cell kinase, leukocyte-specific protein tyrosine kinase, and transmembrane glycoprotein receptor tyrosine kinase. Overall effect is decreased angiogenesis in tumors. **Therapeutic Effects:** Decreased growth and spread of renal cell carcinoma. Improvement in progression-free survival.

Pharmacokinetics

Absorption: Well absorbed following oral administration; crushing tablet and ingesting food ↑ absorption.

Distribution: unknown.

Protein Binding: >99%.

Metabolism and Excretion: Mostly metabolized by the liver (primarily by the CYP3A4 enzyme system, minor amounts by CYP1A2 and CYP2C8) followed by elimination in feces; <4% excreted by the kidneys.

Half-life: 30.9 hr.

TIME/ACTION PROFILE (blood levels)

ROUTE	ONSET	PEAK	DURATION
PO	PO	2–4 hr	24 hr

Contraindications/Precautions

Contraindicated in: Severe hepatic impairment; History of hemoptysis, cerebral or GI bleeding in preceding 6 mo; Risk/history of arterial thrombotic events, including MI, angina or ischemic stroke within preceding 6 mo; Concurrent use of strong CYP3A4 inhibitors (if concurrent use is necessary, ↓ dose of pazopanib); Concurrent use of strong CYP3A4 inducers (may ↓ effectiveness); Concurrent use of drugs that have narrow therapeutic windows and that are metabolized by CYP3A4, CYP2D6, or CYP2C8 enzyme systems; OB: May cause fetal harm, avoid use during pregnancy; Lactation: Avoid use during breast feeding.

Use Cautiously in: Congenital prolonged QTc interval or concurrent medications/diseases that prolong QTc (may ↑ risk of torsades de pointes); Electrolyte abnormalities (correct prior to use; may ↑ risk of potentially serious arrhythmia); Patients at risk for gastrointestinal perforation/fistula; Surgery; interruption of therapy recommended; Hypertension; control before therapy is initiated; Hypothyroidism (may worsen condition); Concurrent use of inducers of the CYP3A4 enzyme system; consider alternate concurrent medication with little or no enzyme induction potential or avoid pazopanib; Moderate hepatic impairment (dose ↓ recommended); Patients of East-Asian descent (↑ risk of neutropenia, thrombocytopenia, and palmar-plantar erythrodysesthesia); Geri: May be more sensitive to drug effects, consider age-related ↓ in cardiac, renal, and hepatic function, concurrent disease states and drug therapy; ↑ risk of hepatotoxicity; Rep: Women of reproductive potential; Pedi: Safety and effectiveness not established.

Adverse Reactions/Side Effects

CNS: POSTERIOR REVERSIBLE ENCEPHALOPATHY SYNDROME (PRES), STROKE, fatigue, weakness. **CV:** HF, MYOCARDIAL INFARCTION, QT INTERVAL PROLONGATION, DEEP VEIN THROMBOSIS, bradycardia, hypertension, altered taste, chest pain, dyspepsia, heart failure. **GI:** GI PERFORATION/FISTULA, HEPATOTOXICITY, PANCREATITIS, abdominal pain, anorexia, diarrhea, nausea, vomiting. **GU:** HEMOLYTIC UREMIC SYNDROME, ↓ fertility, proteinuria. **Derm:** alopecia, facial edema, palmar-plantar erythrodysesthesia (hand-foot syndrome), rash, skin depigmentation. **Endo:** hypothyroidism. **Hemat:** BLEEDING, THROMBOEMBOLIC EVENTS, THROMBOTIC THROMBOCYTOPENIC PURPURA, neutropenia, thrombocytopenia. **Metab:** ↑ lipase, weight loss. **MS:** arthralgia, muscle spasms. **Resp:** INTERSTITIAL LUNG DISEASE, PULMONARY EMBOLISM. **Misc:** hair color changes (depigmentation).

Interactions

Drug-Drug: Concurrent use of **strong CYP3A4 inhibitors**, including **ketoconazole**, **ritonavir**, and **clarithromycin** may ↑ levels and should be avoided; if required, dose of pazopanib should be ↓ to 400 mg daily or more if necessary. Concurrent use of **strong CYP3A4 inducers**, including **rifampin**, may ↓ levels and effectiveness and should be avoided. Concurrent use with **drugs with narrow therapeutic windows that are metabolized by CYP3A4, CYP2D6, or CYP2C8** may ↑ levels of such drugs and the risk of toxicity/adverse reactions is not recommended. ↑ risk of hepatotoxicity with **simvastatin**. **Drugs that ↑ the pH**, including **proton pump inhibitors** and **H_2 receptor antagonists** may ↓ levels; avoid concurrent use; use short-acting antacid instead. **Antacids** may ↓ levels; separate doses by several hrs.

Drug-Food: **Grapefruit juice** may ↑ levels; avoid concurrent use.

Route/Dosage

PO (Adults): 800 mg once daily; *Concurrent use of strong CYP3A4 inhibitors*—400 mg once daily, further reductions may be necessary.

Hepatic Impairment

PO (Adults): *Moderate hepatic impairment*—200 mg once daily.

Availability

Tablets: 200 mg.

NURSING IMPLICATIONS

Assessment

- Monitor BP during frequent therapy; may cause hypertension. BP should be well-controlled prior to initiating therapy. If persistent hypertension occurs despite antihypertensive therapy, reduce dose. If hypertension persists and is severe, discontinue therapy. Baseline and periodic evaluation of LVEF is recommended in patients at risk of cardiac dysfunction.
- Obtain baseline ECG and monitor periodically during therapy. Maintain serum calcium, magnesium, and potassium within normal range during therapy.
- Monitor for signs and symptoms of GI perforation and fistula (abdominal pain; swelling in stomach area; vomiting blood; black sticky stools; GI bleeding) during therapy.
- ***Lab Test Considerations:*** Verify negative pregnancy status prior to starting therapy.
- Monitor serum liver tests before initiation and wks 3, 5, 7, and 9, then at mo 3 and mo 4 if symptoms occur. Monitor periodically after mo 4. *If isolated ALT ↑ between 3 and 8 times the upper limit of normal,* therapy may continue with weekly monitoring of liver function until ALT returns to Grade 1 or baseline. *If isolated ALT ↑ >8 times the upper limit of normal,* stop therapy until ALT returns to Grade 1 or baseline. If benefit outweighs risk, may reintroduce at reduced dose of 400 mg/day with weekly serum liver tests for 8 wk. Following reintroduction, if ALT ↑ >3 times the upper limit of normal recurs, permanently discontinue pazopanib. *If ALT ↑ occurs concurrently with ↑ serum bilirubin >2 times the upper limit of normal,* discontinue pazopanib permanently. Monitor liver function tests until return to baseline. *Patients with only mild indirect hyperbilirubinemia (Gilbert's syndrome) and ↑ ALT >3 times the upper limit of normal* should be managed as per recommendations for ↑ ALT.
- Monitor thyroid function periodically during therapy. May cause hypothyroidism.
- Obtain baseline urinalysis and monitor periodically. May cause proteinuria. Discontinue therapy if Grade 4 proteinuria develops.
- May cause leukopenia, neútropenia, thrombocytopenia, and lymphocytopenia.
- May cause ↑ AST and ↓ serum phosphorous, sodium, and magnesium. May cause ↑ or ↓ serum glucose.

Implementation

- Do not confuse pazopanib with ponatinib.
- **PO:** Administer at least 1 hr before or 2 hr after a meal. Swallow tablets whole; do not crush tablets.

Patient/Family Teaching

- Instruct patient to take pazopanib on an empty stomach as directed. Take missed doses as soon as remembered; if less than 12 hr before next dose, omit dose. Advise patient to read the *Medication Guide* prior to taking pazopanib and with each Rx refill; new information may be available.
- Advise patient to avoid drinking grapefruit juice or eating grapefruit during therapy; may increase amounts of pazopanib absorbed.
- Advise patient to notify health care professional immediately if signs and symptoms of liver problems (yellowing of skin or whites of eyes, unusual darkening of urine, unusual tiredness, pain in the right upper stomach area), heart failure (shortness of breath), heart attack or stroke (chest pain or pressure; pain in arms, back, neck or jaw; shortness of breath; numbness or weakness on one side of body; trouble talking; headache; dizziness), blood clots (new chest pain, trouble breathing or shortness of breath that starts suddenly; leg pain; swelling of arms and hands, or legs and feet; cool or pale arm or leg), bleeding problems (unusual bleeding, bruising, wounds that do not heal), GI perforation or fistula, reversible posterior leukoencephalopathy syndrome (headaches, seizures, lack of energy, confusion, high BP, loss of speech, blindness or changes in vision, and problems thinking), severe increase in BP (severe chest pain, severe head ache, blurred vision, confusion, nausea and vomiting, severe anxiety, shortness of breath, seizures, unconsciousness), interstitial lung disease (persistent cough, shortness of breath), or severe infections (fever; cold symptoms such as runny nose or sore throat that do not go away; flu symptoms such as cough, tiredness, and body aches; pain when urinating; cuts, scrapes or wounds that are red, warm, swollen or painful) occur.
- Inform patient that diarrhea frequently occurs. Instruct patient on ways to manage diarrhea and to notify health care professional if moderate to severe diarrhea occurs.
- Inform patient that loss of color (depigmentation) of skin or hair may occur during therapy. Explore methods of coping.

P

- Instruct patient to notify health care professional of all Rx or OTC medications, vitamins, or herbal products being taken and consult health care professional before taking any new medications.
- Advise patient to notify health care professional of any impending surgery. Pazopanib must be stopped for at least 7 days prior to surgery due to the effects on healing.
- Rep: Advise female patients and male patients with partners of reproductive potential to use effective contraception during therapy and for at least 2 wk after discontinuing therapy, and to notify health care professional immediately if pregnancy is suspected. Advise patient to avoid breast feeding during therapy. Inform patients that pazopanib may impair fertility for both men and women during therapy.

Evaluation/Desired Outcomes

- Decreased growth and spread of renal cell carcinoma.
- Improvement in spread of sarcoma.

pegaspargase

(peg-ass-**par**-jase)

Oncaspar

Classification

Therapeutic: antineoplastics

Pharmacologic: enzymes

Indications

First-line treatment of acute lymphoblastic leukemia (ALL) (in combination with other chemotherapy agents). Treatment of ALL in patients who have had a previous hypersensitivity reaction to native L-asparaginase (in combination with other chemotherapy agents).

Action

Consists of L-asparaginase bound to polyethylene glycol (PEG). This compound depletes asparagine, which leukemic cells cannot synthesize. Normal cells are able to produce their own asparagine and are less susceptible to the effects of asparaginase. Binding to PEG renders asparaginase less antigenic and therefore less likely to induce hypersensitivity reactions. **Therapeutic Effects:** Death of leukemic cells.

Pharmacokinetics

Absorption: IV administration results in complete bioavailability.

Distribution: Unknown.

Metabolism and Excretion: Metabolized by serum proteases and in the reticuloendothelial system.

Half-life: 5.7 days (less in patients with previous hypersensitivity to native L-asparaginase).

TIME/ACTION PROFILE (hematologic effects)

ROUTE	ONSET	PEAK	DURATION
IV	rapid	unknown	14 days

Contraindications/Precautions

Contraindicated in: Hypersensitivity to pegaspargase; History of serious thrombosis with previous L-asparaginase therapy; History of pancreatitis, including pancreatitis association with previous L-asparaginase therapy; History of serious hemorrhagic events to previous L-asparaginase therapy; Severe hepatic impairment; OB: Pregnancy (may cause fetal harm); Lactation: Lactation.

Use Cautiously in: History of previous hypersensitivity reaction to L-asparaginase (↑ risk of hypersensitivity reaction); Rep: Women of reproductive potential.

Adverse Reactions/Side Effects

CNS: SEIZURES, headache, malaise. **Endo:** hypercholesterolemia, hyperglycemia, hypertriglyceridemia. **CV:** peripheral edema. **GI:** HEPATOTOXICITY, PANCREATITIS, abdominal pain, anorexia, diarrhea, nausea, vomiting. **Hemat:** HEMORRHAGE, THROMBOSIS, neutropenia. **Local:** injection site reactions. **MS:** arthralgia, myalgia. **Neuro:** paresthesia. **Misc:** HYPERSENSITIVITY REACTIONS (including anaphylaxis and angioedema), chills, night sweats.

Interactions

Drug-Drug: May alter response to **anticoagulants** or **antiplatelet agents**.

Route/Dosage

IM, IV (Adults >21 yr): 2500 units/m^2 no more frequently than every 14 days.

IM, IV (Adults and Children ≤21 yr): 2000 units/m^2 no more frequently than every 14 days.

Availability

Solution for injection: 750 units/mL.

NURSING IMPLICATIONS

Assessment

- Assess patient for previous hypersensitivity reactions to native L-asparaginase. Monitor for infusion and hypersensitivity reaction (urticaria, diaphoresis, facial swelling, joint pain, hypotension, bronchospasm) for at least 1 hr following administration. *If Grade 1 reaction occurs,* reduce infusion rate by 50%. *If Grade 2 reaction occurs,* hold infusion and treat symptoms. When symptoms resolve, resume infusion and reduce infusion rate by 50%. *If Grade 3 to 4 reaction occurs,* permanently discontinue infusion. Epinephrine and resuscitation equipment should be readily available. Reaction may occur up to 2 hr after administration.
- Monitor for development of bone marrow depression. Assess for fever, sore throat, and signs of infection. Monitor platelet count throughout therapy. Assess for bleeding (bleeding gums, bruising, petechiae, guaiac test stools, urine, and emesis). Avoid giving IM injections and taking rectal temperatures. Apply pressure to venipuncture sites for 10 min. *If Grade 3 to 4 hemorrhage occurs,* hold infusion. Evaluate for coagulop-

athy and consider clotting factor replacement as needed. Resume pegaspargase with next scheduled dose if bleeding is controlled. Anemia may occur. Monitor for increased fatigue, dyspnea, and orthostatic hypotension.

- Monitor patient frequently for signs of pancreatitis (nausea, vomiting, abdominal pain). *If Grade 3 to 4 pancreatitis occurs,* hold pegaspargase for elevations in lipase or amylase >3 x upper limit of normal (ULN) until enzyme levels stabilize or are declining, Discontinue pegaspargase permanently if pancreatitis is confirmed.
- Monitor for signs and symptoms of thromboembolism (headache, arm or leg swelling, shortness of breath, chest pain) during therapy. *If uncomplicated deep vein thrombosis occurs,* hold infusion and treat with antithrombotic therapy. Upon resolution of symptoms consider resuming pegaspargase, while continuing antithrombotic therapy. *If severe or life-threatening thrombosis occurs,* discontinue pegaspargase permanently. Treat with antithrombotic therapy.
- Assess nausea, vomiting, and appetite. Weigh patient weekly. Prophylactic antiemetics may be used prior to administration.
- ***Lab Test Considerations:*** Obtain negative pregnancy test before starting therapy.
- Monitor CBC prior to and periodically throughout therapy. May alter coagulation studies. Fibrinogen may be decreased; PT and partial thromboplastin time (PTT) may be ↑.
- Monitor serum amylase frequently to detect pancreatitis.
- Monitor blood glucose; may cause hyperglycemia.
- May cause elevated BUN and serum creatinine.
- Hepatotoxicity may be manifested by increased AST, ALT, alkaline phosphatase, or bilirubin. Liver function tests usually return to normal after therapy. *If total bilirubin >3 times to <10 times UNL,* hold infusion until total bilirubin is ≤1.5 times ULN. *If total bilirubin >10 times ULN,* discontinue pegaspargase and do not make up for missed doses.
- May cause ↓ serum calcium.
- May cause elevated serum and urine uric acid and hyponatremia.
- May cause hypercholesterolemia and hypertriglyceridemia.

Implementation

- IM is the preferred route because of a lower incidence of adverse reactions.
- Solutions should be prepared in a biologic cabinet. Wear gloves, gown, and mask while handling medication. Discard equipment in specially designated containers.
- **IM:** Limit single injection volume to 2 mL. If volume of injection is >2 mL, use multiple injection sites.

IV Administration

- **Intermittent Infusion:** ***Diluent:*** Dilute each dose in 100 mL of 0.9% NaCl or D5W. Do not shake or agitate. Do not use if solution is cloudy or has formed a precipitate.
- Use only 1 dose per vial; do not re-enter the vial. Discard unused portions.
- Keep refrigerated but do not freeze. Freezing destroys activity but does not change the appearance of pegaspargase. ***Rate:*** Administer over 1–2 hr via Y-site through an infusion that is already running.
- **Additive Incompatibility:** Information unavailable. Do not admix with other medications or solutions.

Patient/Family Teaching

- Inform patient of the possibility of hypersensitivity reactions, including anaphylaxis.
- Advise patient that concurrent use of other medications may increase the risk of bleeding and the toxicity of pegaspargase. Consult health care professional before taking any other medications, including OTC drugs.
- Instruct patient to notify health care professional if abdominal pain, severe nausea and vomiting, jaundice, fever, chills, sore throat, bleeding or bruising, excess thirst or urination, or mouth sores occur. Caution patient to avoid crowds and persons with known infections. Instruct patient to use soft toothbrush, electric razor, and to be especially careful to avoid falls. Patients should also be cautioned not to drink alcoholic beverages or take medications containing aspirin or NSAIDs because these may precipitate gastric bleeding.
- Instruct patient not to receive any vaccinations without advice of health care professional. Advise parents that this may alter child's immunization schedule.
- Rep: Advise females of reproductive potential to use 2 methods of effective contraception, including a barrier method, and avoid breast feeding during therapy and for at least 3 mo after last dose. Pegaspargase may decrease effectiveness of oral contraceptives, oral contraceptives are not recommended.
- Emphasize the need for periodic lab tests to monitor for side effects.

Evaluation/Desired Outcomes

- Improvement of hematologic status in patients with leukemia.

P

pegfilgrastim (peg-fil-**gra**-stim)

Fulphila, ✦Lapelga, Neulasta, Neulasta Onpro, Udenyca

Classification

Therapeutic: colony-stimulating factors

Indications

To decrease the incidence of infection (febrile neutropenia) in patients with nonmyeloid malignancies receiving myelosuppressive antineoplastics associated with a high risk of febrile neutropenia.

Action

Filgrastim is a glycoprotein that binds to and stimulates neutrophils to divide and differentiate. Also activates mature neutrophils. Binding to a polyethylene glycol molecule prolongs its effects. **Therapeutic Effects:** Decreased incidence of infection in patients who are neutropenic from chemotherapy.

Pharmacokinetics

Absorption: Well absorbed following subcut administration.
Distribution: Unknown.
Metabolism and Excretion: Unknown.
Half-life: 15–80 hr.

TIME/ACTION PROFILE

ROUTE	ONSET	PEAK	DURATION
Subcut	unknown	unknown	unknown

Contraindications/Precautions

Contraindicated in: Hypersensitivity to filgrastim or *Escherichia coli*-derived proteins.
Use Cautiously in: Patients with sickle cell disease (↑ risk of sickle cell crisis); Concurrent use of lithium; Malignancy with myeloid characteristics; OB, Lactation: Pregnancy or lactation.

Adverse Reactions/Side Effects

CV: aortitis. **GI:** SPLENIC RUPTURE. **GU:** glomerulonephritis. **Hemat:** SICKLE CELL CRISIS, leukocytosis. **MS:** medullary bone pain. **Resp:** ADULT RESPIRATORY DISTRESS SYNDROME (ARDS). **Misc:** CAPILLARY LEAK SYNDROME, HYPERSENSITIVITY REACTIONS (including anaphylaxis).

Interactions

Drug-Drug: Simultaneous use with **antineoplastics** may have adverse effects on rapidly proliferating neutrophils; avoid use for 24 hr before and 24 hr following chemotherapy. **Lithium** may potentiate the release of neutrophils; concurrent use should be undertaken cautiously.

Route/Dosage

Subcut (Adults and Children ≥45 kg): 6 mg per chemotherapy cycle.
Subcut (Children 31–44 kg): 4 mg per chemotherapy cycle.
Subcut (Children 21–30 kg): 2.5 mg per chemotherapy cycle.
Subcut (Children 10–20 kg): 1.5 mg per chemotherapy cycle.
Subcut (Children <10 kg): 0.1 mg/kg per chemotherapy cycle.

Availability

Solution for injection (prefilled syringes): 6 mg/0.6 mL.

NURSING IMPLICATIONS

Assessment

- Assess patient for bone pain throughout therapy. Pain is usually mild to moderate and usually controllable with nonopioid analgesics, but may require opioid analgesics.
- Assess patient periodically for signs of ARDS (fever, lung infiltration, respiratory distress). If ARDS occurs, treat condition and discontinue pegfilgrastim and/or withhold until symptoms resolve.
- Monitor for signs and symptoms of capillary leak syndrome (hypotension, hypoalbuminemia, edema, hemoconcentration). Treat symptomatically.
- Assess for signs and symptoms of aortitis (fever, abdominal pain, malaise, back pain, increased inflammatory markers [c-reactive protein, white blood cell count]). Discontinue pegfilgrastim if aortitis is suspected.
- May cause transient positive nuclear bone imaging changes.
- ***Lab Test Considerations:*** Obtain CBC and platelet count before chemotherapy. Monitor hematocrit, WBC, and platelet count regularly.
- May cause elevated LDH, alkaline phosphatase, and uric acid.

Implementation

- Do not confuse Neulasta (pegfilgrastim) with Lunesta (eszopiclone) or Neumega (oprelvekin).
- Pegfilgrastim should not be administered between 14 days before and 24 hrs after administration of cytotoxic chemotherapy.
- Keep patients with sickle cell disease receiving pegfilgrastim well hydrated and monitor for sickle cell crisis.
- **Subcut:** Administer subcut once per chemotherapy cycle. Do not administer solutions that are discolored or contain particulate matter. Do not shake. Store refrigerated; may be allowed to reach room temperature for a at least 30 min and maximum of 48 hr, but protect from light.
- Supplied in prefilled syringes. Following administration, activate UltraSafe Needle Guard to prevent needle sticks by placing hands behind needle, grasping guard with one hand, and sliding guard forward until needle is completely covered and guard clicks into place. If audible click is not heard, guard may not be completely activated. Dispose of by placing entire prefilled syringe with guard activated into puncture-proof container.
- **On-body Injector**: Small, one-time use, lightweight, battery-powered, and waterproof up to 8

feet for 1 hr. Fill by health care professional with a prefilled syringe before application. The prefilled syringe with *Neulasta* and the *On-body Injector* are part of *Neulasta Onpro kit*. The *On-body Injector* is applied directly to skin using a self-adhesive backing. The *On-body Injector* uses sounds and lights to informs its status. The prefilled syringe gray needle cap contains dry natural rubber, a derived from latex; do not use if allergic to latex. Apply to intact, non-irritated skin on abdomen or back of arm. Back of arm may only be used if there is a caregiver available to monitor the status of the *On-body Injector*. Approximately 27 hrs after the *On-body Injector* is applied, *Neulasta* will be delivered over approximately 45 min. Follow manufacturer's instructions for monitoring and removal. Instruct patients using the *On-body Injector*to notify health care professional immediately if they suspect the device may not have performed as intended in order to determine need for a replacement dose.

Patient/Family Teaching

- Advise patient to notify health care professional immediately if signs of allergic reaction (shortness of breath, hives, rash, pruritus, laryngeal edema) or signs of splenic rupture (left upper abdominal or shoulder tip pain) occur.
- Advise females of reproductive potential to notify health care professional if pregnancy is planned or suspected, or if breast feeding.
- Emphasize the importance of adherence with therapy and regular monitoring of blood counts.
- **Home Care Issues:** Instruct patient on correct disposal technique for home administration. Caution patient not to reuse needle, syringe, or drug product. Provide patient with a puncture-proof container for disposal of prefilled syringe.

Evaluation/Desired Outcomes

- Decreased incidence of infection in patients who receive bone marrow–depressing antineoplastics.

peginterferon alpha-2a, See INTERFERONS, ALPHA.

peginterferon beta-1a

(peg-in-ter-**feer**-on **bay**-ta)

Plegridy

Classification

Therapeutic: immune modifiers

Pharmacologic: interferons

Indications

Relapsing forms of multiple sclerosis, including clinically isolated syndrome, relapsing-remitting disease, and active secondary progressive disease.

Action

Antiviral and immunoregulatory properties produced by interacting with specific receptor sites on cell surfaces may explain beneficial effects. Produced by recombinant DNA technology. Pegylation prolongs duration of action. **Therapeutic Effects:** Reduced incidence of relapse (neurologic dysfunction) and slowed physical disability.

Pharmacokinetics

Absorption: Absorption follows subcutaneous administration.

Distribution: Unknown.

Metabolism and Excretion: Undergoes catabolism; excretion is mainly renal.

Half-life: 78 hr.

TIME/ACTION PROFILE (reduction in relapse rate)

ROUTE	ONSET	PEAK	DURATION
subcutaneous	within one mo	24–36 wk	unknown

Contraindications/Precautions

Contraindicated in: Hypersensitivity to natural or recombinant interferon beta or peginterferon.

Use Cautiously in: History of depression or suicidal ideation; History of seizures; Renal impairment (risk of adverse reactions may be ↑); OB: Use during pregnancy only if potential maternal benefit justifies potential fetal risk; Lactation: Use cautiously if breast feeding; Pedi: Safety and effectiveness not established; Geri: Safety and effectiveness not established.

Adverse Reactions/Side Effects

CNS: SEIZURES, SUICIDAL IDEATION, headache, depression, weakness. **CV:** HF. **Derm:** pruritus. **GI:** HEPATOTOXICITY, nausea, vomiting. **Hemat:** THROMBOTIC THROMBOCYTOPENIC PURPURA, HEMOLYTIC UREMIC SYNDROME, ↓ peripheral blood counts. **Local:** injection site pain/pruritus/reactions. **MS:** arthralgia, myalgia. **Misc:** AUTOIMMUNE DISORDERS, HYPERSENSITIVITY REACTIONS (including anaphylaxis), chills, fever, flu-like symptoms.

Interactions

Drug-Drug: ↑ myelosuppression may occur with other **myelosuppressives** including **antineoplastics**. Concurrent use of **hepatotoxic agents** may ↑ the risk of hepatotoxicity (↑ liver enzymes).

Drug-Natural Products: Avoid concommitant use with **immunomodulating natural products** such as **astragalus**, **echinacea**, and **melatonin**.

Route/Dosage

Subcut (Adults): 63 mcg initially, followed by 94 mcg on day 15, then 125 mcg every 14 days.

Availability

Solution for injection (prefilled pens and prefilled syringes): 63 mcg/0.5 mL, 94 mcg/0.5 mL, 125 mcg/0.5 mL.

NURSING IMPLICATIONS

Assessment

- Assess frequency of exacerbations of symptoms of multiple sclerosis periodically during therapy.
- Monitor patient for signs of depression during therapy. If depression occurs, notify health care professional immediately.
- Monitor for injection site reactions (erythema, pain, pruritus, edema, bruising, drainage, necrosis). Avoid injecting near area of reaction.
- Monitor patient with significant cardiac disease for worsening symptoms during initiation and periodically during therapy.
- ***Lab Test Considerations:*** Monitor serum AST, ALT and bilirubin periodically during therapy.
- Monitor CBC with differential and platelet counts periodically during therapy. May cause anemia, ↓ lymphocyte, ↓ neutrophil, and ↓ platelet counts.

Implementation

- Administer prophylactic analgesics and/or antipyretics to prevent or minimize flu-like symptoms.
- **Subcut:** Inject subcut in abdomen, back of upper arm, and thigh every 14 days; rotate sites. Prefilled pens are for single dose; discard after use.

Patient/Family Teaching

- Instruct patient in correct technique for injection and care and disposal of equipment. Avoid injecting into areas of skin irritation, redness, bruising, infection, or scarring. Check injection site 2 hr after injection for redness, swelling, and tenderness. Notify health care professional if skin reaction does not clear in a few days. Caution patient not to reuse needles or syringes and provide patient with a puncture-resistant container for disposal.
- Instruct patient to take medication as directed; do not change dose or schedule without consulting health care professional. Advise patient to read *Medication Guide* prior to starting therapy and with each Rx refill in case of changes.
- Inform patient that flu-like symptoms (headache, fever, chills, myalgia, sweating, malaise, tiredness) may occur during therapy. Acetaminophen may be used for relief of fever and myalgias. Flu-like symptoms are not contagious.
- Advise patient to notify health care professional immediately if signs and symptoms of liver disease (yellowing of skin or whites of eyes, nausea, loss of appetite, tiredness, bleeding easily, confusion, sleepiness, dark colored urine, pale stools), depression, suicidal thoughts, seizures, allergic reactions (itching; swelling of face, eyes, lips, tongue, throat; trouble breathing; feeling faint; anxiousness; rash; hives) or autoimmune diseases (easy bleeding or bruising, thyroid gland problems, autoimmune hepatitis) occur.
- Instruct patient to notify health care professional of all Rx or OTC medications, vitamins, or herbal products being taken and to consult with health care professional before taking other medications.
- Rep: Advise patient to notify health care professional if pregnancy is planned or suspected or if breast feeding. Encourage patients to enroll in Pregnancy Registery by calling 1-866-810-1462 or visiting https://www.plegridypregnancyregistry.com/.

Evaluation/Desired Outcomes

- Decrease in the frequency of relapse (neurologic dysfunction) in patients with relapsing-remitting multiple sclerosis.

pegloticase (peg-**loe**-ti-kase)

Krystexxa

Classification

Therapeutic: antigout agents

Pharmacologic: enzymes

Indications

Treatment of chronic gout in adults who have not responded to/cannot tolerate xanthine oxidase inhibitors, including allopurinol.

Action

Consists of recombinant uricase covalently bonded to monomethoxypoly(ethylene glycol) [mPEG] uricase catalyzes the oxidation of uric acid to allantoin, a water soluble byproduct that is readily excreted in urine. **Therapeutic Effects:** ↓ serum uric acid levels with resultant ↓ in attacks of gout and its sequelae.

Pharmacokinetics

Absorption: IV administration results in complete bioavailability.

Distribution: Unknown.

Metabolism and Excretion: Unknown.

Half-life: Unknown.

TIME/ACTION PROFILE (effects on serum uric acid)

ROUTE	ONSET	PEAK	DURATION
IV	rapid	within 24 hr	>300 hr

Contraindications/Precautions

Contraindicated in: Glucose-6–phosphate dehydrogenase (G6–PD) deficiency (↑ risk of hemolysis and methemoglobinemia); Lactation: Breast feeding is not recommended.

Use Cautiously in: HF (may ↑ risk of exacerbation); Retreatment after a drug-free interval (↑ risk of allergic reactions, monitor carefully); Geri: May be more sensitive to drug effects; OB: Use during pregnancy only if clearly needed; Pedi: Safety and effectiveness not established.

Adverse Reactions/Side Effects

CV: chest pain. **EENT:** nasopharyngitis. **GI:** nausea, constipation, vomiting. **Derm:** contusion/ecchymoses. **Hemat:** HEMOLYSIS, METHEMOGLOBINEMIA. **Metab:** gout flare. **Misc:** allergic reactions including ANAPHYLAXIS, INFUSION REACTIONS.

Interactions

Drug-Drug: May interfere with the action of other **PEG-containing therapies**.

Route/Dosage

IV (Adults): 8 mg every 2 wk.

Availability

Solution for injection: 8 mg/mL.

NURSING IMPLICATIONS

Assessment

- Monitor for joint pain and swelling. Gout flares frequently occur upon initiation of therapy, but do not require discontinuation. Administer prophylactic doses of colchicine or an NSAID at least 1 wk before and concurrently during the first 6 mo of therapy.
- Monitor for signs and symptoms of anaphylaxis (wheezing, peri-oral or lingual edema, hemodynamic instability, rash, urticaria) during and following infusion. May occur with any infusion, including initial infusion; usually occurs with 2 hr of infusion. Delayed reactions have also been reported. Risk is higher in patients with uric acid level >6 m g/dL.
- Monitor for infusion reactions (rash, redness of skin, dyspnea, flushing, chest discomfort, chest pain) during and periodically after infusion. If infusion reaction occurs, slow or stop infusion; restart at slower rate. If severe reaction occurs, discontinue infusion and treat as needed. Risk is greater in patients who have lost therapeutic response. Monitor patient for at least 1 hr following infusion.
- ***Lab Test Considerations:*** Screen patients at risk for G6PD deficiency prior to starting therapy. Patients of African, Mediterranean (including Southern European and Middle Eastern), and Southern Asian ancestry are at increased risk for G6PD deficiency. Do not administer pegloticase to patients with G6PD deficiency.
- Monitor serum uric acid levels prior to infusion. Consider discontinuing therapy if levels ↑ to >6 mg/dL, especially if 2 consecutive levels are >6 mg/dL.

Implementation

- Premedicate patient with antihistamines and corticosteroids prior to infusion to minimize risk of anaphylaxis and infusion reaction. Administer in a setting with professionals prepared to manage anaphylaxis and infusion reactions.
- Discontinue all oral urate-lowering medications prior to and during therapy.

IV Administration

- **Intermittent Infusion:** Withdraw 1 mL of pegloticase from vial and inject into 250 mL bag of NaCl; discard unused portion. Invert bag several times to mix; do not shake. Solution is clear and colorless; do not administer solutions that are discolored or contain a precipitate. Solution is stable for 4 hr if refrigerated or at room temperature. Store in refrigerator and protect from light; do not freeze. Allow solution to reach room temperature before administering; do not use artificial heating. ***Rate:*** Infuse over 120 min. Do not administer via IV push or bolus.
- **Additive Incompatibility:** Do not mix with other medications.

Patient/Family Teaching

- Explain purpose of pegloticase to patient. Instruct patient to read *Medication Guide* before starting therapy before each infusion.
- Advise patient to notify health care professional immediately if signs of anaphylaxis or infusion reaction occur.
- Advise patient not to take pegloticase if they have G6PD deficiency.
- Inform patient that gout flares may initially ↑ at the start of pegloticase. Advise patient to not to stop therapy but to take medication (colchicine, NSAID) to reduce flares regularly for the first few mo of pegloticase therapy.
- Instruct patient to not to take oral urate-lowering medications before or during therapy.
- Advise female patient to notify health care professional if pregnancy is planned or suspected or if breast feeding.

Evaluation/Desired Outcomes

- ↓ in uric acid levels with resultant improvement in gout symptoms in patients with chronic gout.

pembrolizumab

(pem-broe-li-zoo-mab)

Keytruda

Classification

Therapeutic: antineoplastics

Pharmacologic: monoclonal antibodies, programmed death-1 inhibitors

Indications

Unresectable or metastatic melanoma. Adjuvant treatment of melanoma with involvement of lymph node(s)

following complete resection. First-line treatment of patients with stage III non-small cell lung cancer (NSCLC), who are not candidates for surgical resection or definitive chemoradiation, or metastatic NSCLC and whose tumors express PD-L1 (tumor proportion score [TPS] ≥1%) and have no epidermal growth factor receptor (EGFR) or anaplastic lymphoma kinase (ALK) genomic tumor aberrations (as monotherapy). Metastatic NSCLC expressing PD-L1 (TPS ≥1%) that has progressed on or after platinum-containing chemotherapy (as monotherapy). Patients with EGFR or ALK genomic tumor aberrations should have disease progression on FDA-approved therapy for these aberrations prior to receiving pembrolizumab. First-line treatment of metastatic non-squamous NSCLC with no EGFR or ALK genomic tumor aberrations (in combination with pemetrexed and platinum chemotherapy). Metastatic small-cell lung cancer (SCLC) that has progressed on or after platinum-containing chemotherapy and ≥1 other previous line of therapy. First-line treatment of metastatic non-squamous NSCLC (in combination with carboplatin and either paclitaxel or nab-paclitaxel [albumin-bound]). Recurrent or metastatic head and neck squamous cell carcinoma (HNSCC) that has progressed on or after platinum-containing chemotherapy. First-line treatment of metastatic or unresectable, recurrent HNSCC (in combination with platinum and fluorouracil). First-line treatment of metastatic or unresectable, recurrent HNSCC expressing PD-L1 (combined positve score [CPS] ≥1). Refractory classical Hodgkin lymphoma (cHL) in patients who have relapsed after ≥3 prior lines of therapy. Locally advanced or metastatic urothelial carcinoma in patients whose tumors express PD-L1 (CPS ≥10) and who are not eligible for cisplatin-containing chemotherapy or in patients who are not eligible for any platinum-containing chemotherapy regardless of PD-L1 status. Locally advanced or metastatic urothelial carcinoma in patients who have disease progression during or following platinum-containing chemotherapy or within 12 mo of neoadjuvant or adjuvant treatment with platinum-containing chemotherapy. Unresectable or metastatic, microsatellite instability-high (MSI-H) or mismatch repair deficient (dMMR) solid tumors that have progressed following prior treatment and have no satisfactory alternative treatment options. Unresectable or metastatic, MSI-H, or mismatch repair deficient colorectal cancer that has progressed following treatment with a fluoropyrimidine, oxaliplatin, and irinotecan. Recurrent locally advanced or metastatic gastric or gastroesophageal junction adenocarcinoma expressing PD-L1 (CPS ≥1) that has progressed on or after ≥2 prior lines of therapy including fluoropyrimidine- and platinum-containing chemotherapy and if appropriate, HER2/neu-targeted therapy. Recurrent or metastatic cervical cancer expressing PD-L1 (CPS ≥1) that has progressed on or after chemotherapy. Refractory primary mediastinal large B-cell lymphoma in patients who have relapsed after ≥2 prior lines of therapy (should not be used in patients who require urgent cytoreductive therapy). Hepatocellular carcinoma (HCC) in patients previously treated with sorafenib. Recurrent locally advanced or metastatic Merkel cell carcinoma (MCC). First-line treatment of advanced renal cell carcinoma (RCC) (in combination with axitinib). Recurrent locally advanced or metastatic squamous cell carcinoma of the esophagus expressing PD-L1 (CPS ≥10) that has progressed after ≥1 prior lines of systemic therapy. Advanced endometrial carcinoma that is not MSI-H or dMMR in patients who have disease progression following prior systemic therapy and are not candidates for curative surgery or radiation (in combination with lenvatinib).

Action

Programmed death (PD) receptor-1–blocking antibody (an IgG4 kappa immunoglobulin) that blocks the interaction between PD-1 and its ligands PD-L1 and PD-L2 resulting in inhibition of T-cell proliferation and decreased cytokine production. **Therapeutic Effects:** Decreased spread of melanoma, NSCLC, SCLC, HNSCC, cHL, urothelial carcinoma, MSI-H, gastric tumors, cervical cancer, endometrial cancer, esophageal cancer, primary mediastinal large B-cell lymphoma, HCC, MCC, and RCC.

Pharmacokinetics

Absorption: IV administration results in complete bioavailability.
Distribution: Unknown.
Metabolism and Excretion: Unknown.
Half-life: 26 days.

TIME/ACTION PROFILE (response)

ROUTE	ONSET	PEAK	DURATION
IV	within 3 mo	unknown	may persist for >8.8 mo

Contraindications/Precautions

Contraindicated in: OB: Pregnancy (may cause fetal harm); Lactation: Discontinue pembrolizumab or discontinue breast feeding.
Use Cautiously in: Moderate to severe hepatic impairment; Solid organ transplant recipients (may ↑ risk of rejection); Rep: Women of reproductive potential; Pedi: Children <2 yr (safety and effectiveness not established for cHL, MSI-H cancer, primary mediastinal large B-Cell lymphoma, or MCC); Children <18 yr (safety and effectiveness not established for all other indications); Pedi: Safety and effectiveness not established.

Adverse Reactions/Side Effects

CNS: dizziness, fatigue, headache, insomnia. **Derm:** BULLOUS PEMPHIGOID, EXFOLIATIVE DERMATITIS, STEVENS-JOHNSON SYNDROME, TOXIC EPIDERMAL NECROLYSIS, pruritus, rash, immune-mediated dermatitis, vitiligo. **EENT:** immune-mediated optic neuritis. **Endo:** IMMUNE-MEDIATED HYPOPHYSITIS, immune-mediated hypothyroidism, immune-mediated hyperthyroidism, immune-mediated type 1 diabetes. **GI:** IMMUNE-MEDIATED COLITIS, IMMUNE-MEDIATED HEPATITIS, ↓ appetite, constipation, diarrhea, nausea. **GU:** IMMUNE-MEDIATED NEPHRITIS. **Hemat:** anemia. **MS:** IMMUNE-MEDIATED RHABDOMYOLYSIS, arthralgia, back pain, extremity pain, myalgia, immune-mediated myasthenic syndrome. **Resp:** IMMUNE-MEDIATED PNEUMONITIS. **Misc:** INFUSION-RELATED REACTIONS, SEPSIS.

Interactions

Drug-Drug: None noted.

Route/Dosage

Melanoma

IV (Adults): 200 mg every 3 wk until disease progression or unacceptable toxicity; *Adjuvant treatment*—200 mg every 3 wk until disease recurrence, unacceptable toxicity, or up to 12 mo in patients without disease recurrence.

NSCLC or HNSCC

IV (Adults): 200 mg every 3 wk until disease progression, unacceptable toxicity, or up to 24 mo in patients without disease progression. If being administered in combination with chemotherapy, should be administered prior to chemotherapy when given on the same day.

SCLC, Urothelial Carcinoma, Gastric Cancer, Cervical Cancer, Endometrial Carcinoma, Esophageal Cancer, HCC, or RCC

IV (Adults): 200 mg every 3 wk until disease progression, unacceptable toxicity, or up to 24 mo in patients without disease progression.

cHL, MSI-H Cancer, Primary Mediastinal Large B-Cell Lymphoma, or MCC

IV (Adults): 200 mg every 3 wk until disease progression, unacceptable toxicity, or up to 24 mo in patients without disease progression.

IV (Children ≥2 yr): 2 mg/kg (max = 200 mg) every 3 wk until disease progression, unacceptable toxicity, or up to 24 mo in patients without disease progression.

Availability

Lyophilized powder for injection (requires reconstitution and dilution): 50 mg/vial. **Solution for injection:** 25 mg/mL.

NURSING IMPLICATIONS

Assessment

- Monitor for signs and symptoms of immune-mediated pneumonitis (shortness of breath, chest pain, new or worse cough) periodically during therapy. Evaluate with x-ray. Treat with corticosteroids for ≥Grade 2 pneumonitis. *If Grade 2 immune-mediated pneumonitis occurs,* hold pembrolizumab. Resume therapy in patients with complete or partial resolution (Grades 0 to 1) after corticosteroid taper. *If Grades 3 or 4 or recurrent Grade 2 occur,* permanently discontinue therapy.
- Monitor for signs and symptoms of colitis (diarrhea, abdominal pain, mucus or blood in stool, with or without fever). *If Grades 2 or 3 immune-mediated colitis occur,* hold dose. Resume therapy in patients with complete or partial resolution (Grades 0 to 1) after corticosteroid taper. *If Grade 4 occurs,* permanently discontinue pembrolizumab.
- Assess for signs and symptoms of immune-mediated hepatitis (yellowing of skin or whites of eyes, unusual darkening of urine, unusual tiredness, pain in right upper stomach) before each dose. *If AST or ALT ≥5 times upper limit of normal (ULN) if baseline <2 times ULN; AST or ALT >3 times baseline if baseline ≥2 times ULN; total bilirubin >2.0 mg/dL if baseline <1.5 mg/dL; or total bilirubin >3.0 mg/dL, regardless of baseline levels occur in patients with hepatocellular carcinoma,* hold dose. Resume therapy in patients with complete or partial resolution (Grades 0 to 1) after corticosteroid taper. *If ALT or AST >10 times ULN; or Child-Pugh score greater ≥9 points; gastrointestinal bleeding suggestive of portal hypertension; or new onset of clinically detectable ascites; or encephalopathy occur in patients with hepatocellular carcinoma,* permanently discontinue pembrolizumab. *If AST or ALT >3 but ≤5 times ULN or total bilirubin >1.5 but ≤3 times ULN in patients without hepatocellular carcinoma occurs,* hold dose. Resume therapy in patients with complete or partial resolution (Grades 0 to 1) after corticosteroid taper. *If in patients without liver metastases, AST or ALT >5 times ULN or total bilirubin >3 times ULN or in patients with liver metastasis and Grade 2 AST or ALT at baseline, with an increase in AST or ALT of 50% or more relative to baseline that persists for at least 1 wk occurs,* permanently discontinue pembrolizumab.
- Monitor for signs and symptoms of infusion-related reactions (rigors, chills, wheezing, pruritus, flushing, rash, hypotension, hypoxemia, fever). *If Grades 1 or 2 infusion-related reactions occur,* hold or slow rate of infusion. *If Grades 3 or 4 reactions occur,* stop infusion and permanently discontinue therapy.
- Monitor for clinical signs and symptoms of hypophysitis (persistent or unusual headache, extreme weakness, dizziness or fainting, vision changes) during therapy. *If Grade 3 or 4 immune-mediated endocrinopathies occur,* hold dose until clinically stable.

- Assess for rash periodically during therapy. May cause Stevens-Johnson syndrome or toxic epidermal necrolysis. If Grade 3 or suspected Stevens-Johnson Syndrome (SJS) or toxic epidermal necrolysis (TEN) occurs, hold dose. If Grade 4 or confirmed SJS or TEN occur, permanently discontinue therapy.
- ***Lab Test Considerations:*** Obtain a negative pregnancy test prior to starting therapy.
- Monitor for changes in renal function. Treat with corticosteroids for ≥Grade 2 nephritis. If Grade 2 nephritis occurs, hold dose. Resume therapy in patients with complete or partial resolution (Grades 0 to 1) after corticosteroid taper. If Grade 3 or 4 nephritis occurs, permanently discontinue therapy.
- Monitor for changes in thyroid function at start of and periodically during therapy, and as indicated based on clinical evaluation. Administer corticosteroids for ≥Grade 3 hyperthyroidism, withhold pembrolizumab for severe (Grade 3) hyperthyroidism and resume therapy when recovery to Grade 0 to 1. Permanently discontinue for life-threatening (Grade 4) hyperthyroidism. Manage hypothyroidism with thyroid replacement without interruption of therapy or corticosteroids.
- Monitor serum blood glucose. May cause hyperglycemia or other signs and symptoms of diabetes.

Implementation

IV Administration

- **Intermittent Infusion:** Reconstitute by injecting 2.3 mL of sterile water for injection along vial walls; swirl slowly, do not shake. Allow up to 5 min for bubbles to clear. Solution is clear to slightly opalescent, colorless to slightly yellow; do not administer solution if discolored or contains particulate matter other than translucent to white proteinaceous particles. Solution is stable at room temperature for up to 4 hr and 24 hr if refrigerated. ***Diluent:*** 0.9% NaCl. Mix using gently inversion. ***Concentration:*** 1 mg/mL to 10 mg/mL. ***Rate:*** Infuse through a sterile, non-pyrogenic, low-protein binding 0.2 micron to 0.5 micron in-line or add-on filter over 30 min.
- **Y-Site Incompatibility:** Do not administer other drugs through same infusion line.

Patient/Family Teaching

- Explain purpose of pembrolizumab to patient.
- Advise patient to notify health care professional immediately if signs and symptoms of pneumonitis, colitis, hepatitis, kidney problems (change in amount or color of urine), hormone gland problems (rapid heart beat, weight loss, increased sweating, weight gain, hair loss, feeling cold, constipation, deepening of voice, muscle aches, dizziness or fainting, persistent or unusual headache) occur.
- Instruct patient to notify health care professional of all Rx or OTC medications, vitamins, or herbal products being taken and to consult with health care professional before taking other medications.
- Rep: Advise female patient of reproductive potential to use highly effective contraception and avoid breast feeding during and for ≥4 mo after last dose; may cause fetal harm.
- Emphasize importance of keeping scheduled appointments for blood work or other laboratory tests.

Evaluation/Desired Outcomes

- Decreased spread of melanoma, NSCLC, SCLC, HNSCC, cHL, urothelial carcinoma, MSI-H, gastric tumors, cervical cancer, endometrial cancer, esophageal cancer, primary mediastinal large B-cell lymphoma, HCC, MCC, and RCC.

PEMEtrexed (pe-me-**trex**-ed)

Alimta

Classification

Therapeutic: antineoplastics

Pharmacologic: antimetabolites, folate antagonists

Indications

Malignant pleural mesothelioma as initial therapy when tumor is unresectable or patient is not a candidate for surgery (in combination with cisplatin). Metastatic non-squamous non-small cell lung cancer (NSCLC) as initial therapy in patients without EGFR or ALK genomic tumor aberrations (in combination with platinum—based therapy and pembrolizumab). Locally advanced or metastatic non-squamous NSCLC as initial therapy (in combination with cisplatin). Locally advanced or metastatic non-squamous NSCLC as maintenance treatment in patients whose disease has not progressed after four cycles of platinum-based first-line chemotherapy (as monotherapy). Recurrent, metastatic non-squamous NSCLC after previous chemotherapy (as monotherapy).

Action

Disrupts folate dependent metabolic processes involved in thymidine and purine synthesis. Converted intracellularly to polyglutamate form which increases duration of action. **Therapeutic Effects:** Decreases growth and spread of mesothelioma. Improved survival in patients with non-squamous NSCLC.

Pharmacokinetics

Absorption: IV administration results in complete bioavailability.

Distribution: Unknown.

Metabolism and Excretion: Minimal metabolism; 70–90% excreted unchanged in urine.

Half-life: 3.5 hr (normal renal function).

TIME/ACTION PROFILE (hematologic effects)

ROUTE	ONSET	PEAK	DURATION
IV	unknown	8–15 days	21 days

Contraindications/Precautions

Contraindicated in: Hypersensitivity; CCr <45 mL/min; OB: Pregnancy (may cause fetal harm); Lactation: Lactation.

Use Cautiously in: Concurrent use of NSAIDs in patients with CCr 45–79 mL/min (avoid those with short half-lives); 3rd space fluid accumulation (ascites, pleural effusions); consider drainage prior to therapy; Hepatic impairment (dose alteration recommended); Rep: Women of reproductive potential and men with female sexual partners of reproductive potential; Pedi: Safety and effectiveness not established.

Adverse Reactions/Side Effects

CV: chest pain. **Derm:** STEVENS-JOHNSON SYNDROME, TOXIC EPIDERMAL NECROLYSIS, desquamation, rash, radiation recall. **GI:** constipation, nausea, stomatitis, vomiting, anorexia, diarrhea, esophagitis, mouth pain. **GU:** ↓ fertility (men). **Hemat:** anemia, hemolytic anemia, leukopenia, thrombocytopenia. **Neuro:** neuropathy. **Resp:** INTERSTITIAL PNEUMONITIS, pharyngitis. **Misc:** fever, infection.

Interactions

Drug-Drug: **NSAIDs**, especially those with short half-lives, ↑ levels and risk of toxicity; avoid for 2 days before, day of, and 2 days after treatment. **Probenecid** ↑ levels. Concurrent use of **nephrotoxic agents** ↑ risk of nephrotoxicity.

Route/Dosage

Non-Squamous NSCLC

IV (Adults): *Initial therapy (with cisplatin)*—500 mg/m² on Day 1 of each 21-day cycle for up to 6 cycles (administer before cisplatin); *Initial therapy (with platinum-based therapy and pembrolizumab)*—500 mg/m² on Day 1 of each 21-day cycle for 4 cycles (administer before carboplatin or cisplatin and after pembrolizumab). Following completion of platinum-based therapy, pemetrexed may be administered as monotherapy or with pembrolizumab as maintenance therapy until disease progression or unacceptable toxicity; *Maintenance treatment (as monotherapy) or disease recurrence (as monotherapy)*—500 mg/m² on Day 1 of each 21-day cycle until disease progression or unacceptable toxicity.

Mesothelioma

IV (Adults): 500 mg/m² on Day 1 of each 21-day cycle until disease progression or unacceptable toxicity.

Availability

Lyophilized powder for injection (requires reconstitution and dilution): 100 mg/vial, 500 mg/vial.

NURSING IMPLICATIONS

Assessment

- Monitor for rash during therapy. Pretreatment with dexamethasone 4 mg orally twice daily the day before, the day of, and the day after administration reduces incidence and severity or reaction.
- Monitor for hematologic and GI (mucositis, diarrhea) toxicities. *If any Grade 3 or 4 toxicities, except mucositis or diarrhea, requiring hospitalization occur,* decrease doses of pemetrexed and cisplatin by 75%. *If Grade 3 or 4 mucositis occurs,* decrease pemetrexed dose by 50% and cisplatin by 100% of previous dose.
- Monitor for bone marrow depression. Assess for bleeding (bleeding gums, bruising, petechiae, guaiac stools, urine, and emesis) and avoid IM injections and taking rectal temperatures if platelet count is low. Apply pressure to venipuncture sites for 10 min. Assess for signs of infection during neutropenia. Anemia may occur; monitor for increased fatigue, dyspnea, and orthostatic hypotension.
- Assess for neurotoxicity during therapy. *If Grade 0–1 neurotoxicity occurs,* decrease pemetrexed and cisplatin doses by 100% of previous dose. *If Grade 2 neurotoxicity occurs,* decrease pemetrexed dose by 100% and cisplatin dose by 50% of previous dose. *If Grade 3 or 4 neurotoxicity occurs,* discontinue therapy.
- ***Lab Test Considerations:*** Monitor CBC and platelet counts for nadir and recovery and renal function, before each dose and on days 8 and 15 of each cycle and chemistry for renal and liver functions periodically. May cause neutropenia, thrombocytopenia, leukopenia, and anemia. A new cycle should not be started unless the ANC is at least 1500 cells/mm³, platelet count is at least 100,000 cells/mm³, and creatinine clearance is at least 45 mL/min. *If nadir of ANC is <500/mm³ and nadir of platelets are at least 50,000/mm³,* decrease doses of pemetrexed and cisplatin by 75%. *If nadir of platelets is <50,000/mm³ regardless of ANC nadir,* decrease pemetrexed and cisplatin doses by 50%.

Implementation

- Do not confuse pemetrexed with pralatrexate.
- Pemetrexed should be administered under supervision of a physician experienced in the use of chemotherapeutic agents.
- To reduce toxicity, 0.4–1 mg of folic acid must be taken daily for 7 days preceding 1st dose of pemetrexed and should continue during and for 21 days after last dose. Patients must also receive an injection of vitamin B_{12} 1 mg IM during the wk preceding 1st dose of pemetrexed and every 3 cycles thereafter. Subsequent doses of vitamin B_{12} may be given on same day as pemetrexed. Also administer dexame-

P

thasone 4 mg twice daily the day before, the day of, and the day after pemetrexed administration.

IV Administration

- Prepare solution in a biologic cabinet. Wear gloves, gown, and mask while handling medication. Discard equipment in designated containers.
- **Intermittent Infusion:** Calculate number of pemetrexed 500-mg vials needed; vials contain excess to facilitate delivery. Reconstitute 500 mg with 20 mL of preservative–free 0.9% NaCl. ***Concentration:*** 25 mg/mL. Swirl gently until powder is completely dissolved. Solution is clear and colorless to yellow or green-yellow. Do not administer if discolored or containing particulate matter. ***Diluent:*** Dilute further to 100 mL with preservative–free 0.9% NaCl. Solution is stable at room temperature or if refrigerated for up to 24 hr. ***Rate:*** Administer over 10 min.
- **Y-Site Compatibility:** acyclovir, alfentanil, allopurinol, amifostine, amikacin, aminocaproic acid, aminophylline, amiodarone, amphotericin B lipid complex, amphotericin B liposome, ampicillin, ampicillin/sulbactam, atracurium, azithromycin, aztreonam, bivalirudin, bleomycin, bumetanide, buprenorphine, butorphanol, carboplatin, carmustine, ceftriaxone, cefuroxime, cisatracurium, cisplatin, clindamycin, cyclophosphamide, cyclosporine, cytarabine, dactinomycin, daptomycin, dexamethasone sodium phosphate, dexmedetomidine, dexrazoxane, digoxin, diltiazem, diphenhydramine, docetaxel, dolasetron, dopamine, doxacurium, doxorubicin liposome, enalaprilat, ephedrine, epinephrine, eptifibitide, ertapenem, esmolol, etoposide, etoposide phosphate, famotidine, fenoldopam, fentanyl, fluconazole, fludarabine, fluorouracil, foscarnet, fosphenytoin, furosemide, ganciclovir, glycopyrrolate, granisetron, haloperidol, heparin, hydrocortisone sodium succinate, hydromorphone, ifosfamide, imipenem/cilastatin, insulin, regular, isoproterenol, ketorolac, labetalol, leucovorin calcium, levofloxacin, lidocaine, linezolid, lorazepam, magnesium sulfate, mannitol, meperidine, meropenem, mesna, methyldopate, methylprednisolone sodium succinate, metoclopramide, metoprolol, midazolam, milrinone, mitomycin, morphine, moxifloxacin, nafcillin, naloxone, nitroglycerin, norepinephrine, octreotide, oxaliplatin, paclitaxel, pamidronate, pancuronium, pentobarbital, phenobarbital, phentolamine, piperacillin/tazobactam, potassium acetate, potassium chloride, potassium phosphates, procainamide, promethazine, propranolol, ranitidine, remifentanil, rocuronium, sodium acetate, sodium bicarbonate, sodium phosphates, succinylcholine, sufentanil, tacrolimus, theophylline, thiopental, thiotepa, tigecycline, tirofiban, trimethoprim/sulfamethoxazole, vancomycin, vecuronium, verapamil, vinblastine, vincristine, vinorelbine, zidovudine, zoledronic acid.
- **Y-Site Incompatibility:** anidulafungin, calcium acetate, calcium chloride, calcium gluconate, caspofungin, cefazolin, cefepime, cefotaxime, cefotetan, cefoxitin, ceftazidime, chloramphenicol, chlorpromazine, ciprofloxacin, dacarbazine, dantrolene, daunorubicin hydrochloride, diazepam, dobutamine, doxorubicin, doxycycline, droperidol, epirubicin, erythromycin, gemcitabine, gentamicin, hydralazine, idarubicin, irinotecan, metronidazole, mitoxantrone, nalbuphine, nicardipine, nitroprusside, ondansetron, pantoprazole, pentamidine, phenytoin, prochlorperazine, quinupristin/dalfopristin, tobramycin, topotecan, vasopressin.
- **Additive Incompatibility:** Solutions containing calcium, including Lactated Ringer's and Ringer's solution.

Patient/Family Teaching

- Emphasize the importance of taking prophylactic folic acid and vitamin B_{12} to reduce treatment-related hematologic and GI toxicity.
- Advise patient to notify health care professional immediately if signs and symptoms of infection (fever, sore throat), anemia, or neurotoxicity occur.
- Instruct patients to notify health care professional if persistent vomiting, diarrhea, or signs of dehydration appear.
- Instruct patient to notify health care professional of all Rx or OTC medications, vitamins, or herbal products being taken and consult health care professional before taking any new medications, especially NSAIDs, and to avoid alcohol during therapy.
- Rep: Advise females of reproductive potential to use effective contraception during and for at least 6 mo after last dose of pemetrexed and to avoid breast feeding for at least 1 wk after last dose. Advise males with female partners of reproductive potential to use effective contraception during and for at least 3 mo after last dose. If pregnancy is planned or suspected, notify health care professional promptly. May impair fertility in males.

Evaluation/Desired Outcomes

- Decreased growth and spread of mesothelioma or non–small cell lung cancer.

PENICILLINS (pen-i-sill-ins)

penicillin G
Crystapen, Pfizerpen

penicillin G benzathine
Bicillin L-A

penicillin G procaine
~~Wycillin~~

penicillin V
Pen-VK

Classification
Therapeutic: anti-infectives
Pharmacologic: penicillins

Indications

Treatment of a wide variety of infections including: Pneumococcal pneumonia, Streptococcal pharyngitis, Syphilis, Gonorrhea strains. Treatment of enterococcal infections (requires the addition of an aminoglycoside). Prevention of rheumatic fever. Should not be used as a single agent to treat anthrax. **Unlabeled Use:** Treatment of Lyme disease. Prevention of recurrent *Streptococcal pneumoniae* septicemia in children with sickle-cell disease.

Action

Bind to bacterial cell wall, resulting in cell death. **Therapeutic Effects:** Bactericidal action against susceptible bacteria. **Spectrum:** Active against: Most gram-positive organisms, including many streptococci (*Streptococcus pneumoniae*, group A beta-hemolytic streptococci), staphylococci (non–penicillinase-producing strains), and *Bacillus anthracis*; Some gram-negative organisms, such as *Neisseria meningitidis* and *Neisseria gonorrhoeae* (only penicillin susceptible strains); Some anaerobic bacteria and spirochetes including *Borellia burgdorferi*.

Pharmacokinetics

Absorption: Variably absorbed from the GI tract. *Penicillin V*—resists acid degradation in the GI tract. *Procaine and benzathine penicillin*—IM absorption is delayed and prolonged and results in sustained therapeutic blood levels.
Distribution: Widely distributed, although CNS penetration is poor in the presence of uninflamed meninges. Crosses the placenta and enters breast milk.
Metabolism and Excretion: Minimally metabolized by the liver, excreted mainly unchanged by the kidneys.
Half-life: 30–60 min.

TIME/ACTION PROFILE (blood levels)

ROUTE	ONSET	PEAK	DURATION
Penicillin V PO	rapid	0.5–1 hr	4–6 hr
Penicillin G IM	rapid	0.25–0.5 hr	4–6 hr
Penicillin G IV	rapid	end of infusion	4–6 hr
Benzathine penicillin IM	delayed	12–24 hr	3 wk
Procaine penicillin IM	delayed	1–4 hr	12 hr

Contraindications/Precautions

Contraindicated in: Previous hypersensitivity to penicillins (cross-sensitivity may exist with cephalosporins and other beta-lactams); Hypersensitivity to procaine or benzathine (procaine and benzathine preparations only); Some products may contain tartrazine and should be avoided in patients with known hypersensitivity.
Use Cautiously in: Severe renal impairment (dose ↓ recommended); OB: Although safety not established, has been used safely; Lactation: Safety not established; Geri: Consider ↓ body mass, age-related ↓ in renal, hepatic, and cardiac function, comorbidities, and concurrent drug therapy when prescribing and dosing.

Adverse Reactions/Side Effects

CNS: SEIZURES. **Derm:** rash, urticaria. **GI:** CLOSTRIDIUM DIFFICILE-ASSOCIATED DIARRHEA (CDAD), diarrhea, epigastric distress, nausea, vomiting. **GU:** interstitial nephritis. **Hemat:** eosinophilia, hemolytic anemia, leukopenia. **Local:** pain at IM site, phlebitis at IV site. **Misc:** HYPERSENSITIVITY REACTIONS (including anaphylaxis and serum sickness), superinfection.

Interactions

Drug-Drug: May ↓ effectiveness of oral contraceptive agents. **Probenecid** ↓ renal excretion and ↑ blood levels of penicillin (therapy may be combined for this purpose). **Neomycin** may ↓ absorption of penicillin V. ↓ elimination of **methotrexate** and ↑ risk of serious toxicity.

Route/Dosage

Penicillin G

IM, IV (Adults): *Most infections*—1–5 million units every 4–6 hr.
IM, IV (Children): 8333–16,667 units/kg every 4 hr; 12,550–25,000 units/kg every 6 hr; up to 250,000 units/kg/day in divided doses, some infections may require up to 300,000 units/kg/day.
IV (Infants >7 days): 25,000 units/kg every 8 hr; *Meningitis*—50,000–75,000 units/kg every 6 hr.
IV (Infants <7 days): 25,000 units/kg every 12 hr; *Streptococcus B meningitis*—100,000–150,000 units/kg/day in divided doses.

Penicillin G Benzathine

IM (Adults): *Streptococcal infections/erysipeloid*—1.2 million units single dose. *Primary, secondary, and early latent syphilis*—2.4 million units single dose. *Tertiary and late latent syphilis (not neurosyphilis)*—2.4 million units once weekly for 3 wk. *Prevention of rheumatic fever*—1.2 million units every 3–4 wk.
IM (Children >27 kg): *Streptococcal infections/erysipeloid*—900,000–1.2 million units (single dose). *Primary, secondary, and early latent syphilis*—up to 2.4 million units single dose. *Late latent or latent syphilis of undetermined duration*—50,000 units/kg weekly for 3 wk. *Prevention of rheumatic fever*—1.2 million units every 2–3 wk.
IM (Children <27 kg): *Streptococcal infections/erysipeloid*—300,000–600,000 units single dose. *Primary, secondary, and early latent syphilis*—up to

2.4 million units single dose. *Late latent or latent syphilis of undetermined duration*—50,000 units/kg weekly for 3 wk. *Prevention of rheumatic fever*—1.2 million units every 2–3 wk.

Penicillin G Procaine

IM (Adults): *Moderate or severe infections*—600,000–1.2 million units/day as a single dose or in 2 divided doses. *Neurosyphilis*—2.4 million units/day with 500 mg probenecid PO 4 times daily for 10–14 days.
IM (Children): *Congenital syphilis*—50,000 units/kg/day for 10–14 days.

Penicillin V

PO (Adults and Children ≥12 yr): *Most infections*—125–500 mg every 6–8 hr. *Rheumatic fever prevention*—125–250 mg every 12 hr.
PO (Children <12 yr): *Lyme disease*—12.5 mg/kg every 6 hr (unlabeled); prevention of *Streptococcus pneumoniae* sepsis in children with sickle cell disease—125 mg twice daily.

Availability

Penicillin G Potassium (generic available)

Powder for injection (requires reconstitution and dilution): 1 million units/vial, 5 million units/vial, 20 million units/vial. **Premixed solution for injection:** 1 million units/50 mL, 2 million units/50 mL, 3 million units/50 mL.

Penicillin G Sodium (generic available)

Powder for injection (requires reconstitution and dilution): 5 million units/vial.

Penicillin G Benzathine

Suspension for IM injection: 600,000 units/mL.

Penicillin G Procaine (generic available)

Suspension for IM injection: 300,000 units/mL, 600,000 units/mL.

Penicillin V Potassium (generic available)

Oral solution: 125 mg/5 mL, 250 mg/5 mL. **Cost:** *Generic*—125 mg/5 mL $3.84/100 mL, 250 mg/5 mL $4.31/100 mL. **Tablets:** 250 mg, 500 mg. **Cost:** *Generic*—250 mg $45.75/100, 500 mg $77.77/100.

NURSING IMPLICATIONS

Assessment

- Assess for infection (vital signs; appearance of wound, sputum, urine, and stool; WBC) at beginning of and during therapy.
- Obtain a history to determine previous use of and reactions to penicillins, cephalosporins, or other beta-lactam antibiotics. Persons with a negative history of penicillin sensitivity may still have an allergic response.
- Obtain specimens for culture and sensitivity before initiating therapy. 1st dose may be given before receiving results.
- Observe patient for signs and symptoms of anaphylaxis (rash, pruritus, laryngeal edema, wheezing). Discontinue drug and notify health care professional immediately if these symptoms occur. Keep epinephrine, an antihistamine, and resuscitation equipment close by in case of an anaphylactic reaction.
- Monitor bowel function. Diarrhea, abdominal cramping, fever, and bloody stools should be reported to health care professional promptly as a sign of Clostridium difficile-associated diarrhea (CDAD). May begin up to several wk following cessation of therapy.
- ***Lab Test Considerations:*** May cause positive direct Coombs' test results. Hyperkalemia may develop after large doses of penicillin G potassium. Monitor serum sodium concentrations in patient with hypertension or HF. Hypernatremia may develop after large doses of penicillin sodium. May cause ↑ AST, ALT, LDH, and serum alkaline phosphatase concentrations. May cause leukopenia and neutropenia, especially with prolonged therapy or hepatic impairment.

Implementation

- Do not confuse penicillin with penicillamine. Do not confuse penicillin G aqueous (potassium or sodium salt) with penicillin G procaine.
- **PO:** Administer around the clock. Penicillin V may be administered without regard for meals.
- Use calibrated measuring device for liquid preparations. Solution is stable for 14 days if refrigerated.
- **IM:** Reconstitute according to manufacturer's directions with sterile water for injection, D5W, or 0.9% NaCl.
- **IM:** Shake medication well before injection. Inject penicillin deep into a well-developed muscle mass at a slow, consistent rate to prevent blockage of the needle. Massage well. Accidental injury near or into a nerve can result in severe pain and dysfunction.
- Penicillin G potassium or sodium may be diluted with lidocaine (without epinephrine) 1% or 2% to minimize pain from IM injection.
- Never give penicillin G benzathine or penicillin G procaine suspensions IV. May cause embolism or toxic reactions.

IV Administration

- **IV:** Change IV sites every 48 hr to prevent phlebitis.
- Administer slowly and observe patient closely for signs of hypersensitivity.
- **Intermittent Infusion:** ***Diluent:*** Doses of 3 million units or less should be diluted in at least 50 mL of D5W or 0.9% NaCl; doses of more than 3 million units should be diluted with 100 mL. ***Concentration:*** 100,000–500,000 units/mL (50,000 units/mL in neonates). ***Rate:*** Infuse over 1–2 hr in adults or 15–30 min in children.
- **Continuous Infusion:** Doses of 10 million units or more may be diluted in 1 or 2 L.
- ***Rate:*** Infuse over 24 hr.

Penicillin G Potassium

- **Y-Site Compatibility:** acyclovir, amiodarone, ascorbic acid, atropine, aztreonam, benztropine, bumetanide, buprenorphine, butorphanol, calcium chloride, calcium gluconate, cefazolin, cefotaxime, ceftazidime, ceftriaxone, cefuroxime, chloramphenicol, chlorpromazine, clindamycin, cyanocobalamin, cyclophosphamide, cyclosporine, dexamethasone, digoxin, diltiazem, diphenhydramine, dopamine, enalaprilat, ephedrine, epinephrine, epoetin alfa, esmolol, famotidine, fentanyl, fluconazole, folic acid, foscarnet, furosemide, glycopyrrolate, heparin, hydrocortisone, hydromorphone, imipenem/cilastatin, indomethacin, insulin, regular, isoproterenol, ketamine, ketorolac, lidocaine, magnesium sulfate, mannitol, meperidine, methyldopate, methylprednisolone, metoclopramide, metoprolol, midazolam, morphine, nafcillin, nalbuphine, naloxone, nicardipine, nitroglycerin, nitroprusside, norepinephrine, ondansetron, oxacillin, oxytocin, penicillin G sodium, phenylephrine, phytonadione, potassium chloride, procainamide, prochlorperazine, propranolol, pyridoixine, ranitidine, sodium bicarbonate, streptokinase, succinylcholine, tacrolimus, theophylline, thiamine, tobramycin, vancomycin, vasopressin, verapamil, vitamin B complex with C.
- **Y-Site Incompatibility:** If aminoglycosides and penicillins must be administered concurrently, administer in separate sites at least 1 hr apart, aminophylline, ampicillin, dantrolene, diazepam, dobutamine, doxycycline, erythromycin, ganciclovir, haloperidol, papaverine, pentamidine, pentobarbital, phenobarbital, phentolamine, phenytoin, promethazine, protamine, tranexamic acid, trimethoprim/sulfamethoxazole.

Penicillin G Sodium

- **Y-Site Compatibility:** alfentanil, ascorbic acid, atropine, aztreonam, benztropine, bumetanide, buprenorphine, butorphanol, calcium chloride, calcium gluconate, chloramphenicol, clindamycin, cyanocobalamin, cyclosporine, dexamethasone, digoxin, diphenhydramine, dopamine, enalaprilat, ephedrine, epinephrine, epoetin alfa, esmolol, famotidine, fentanyl, fluconazole, folic acid, furosemide, glycopyrrolate, heparin, hydrocortisone, imipenem/cilastatin, indomethacin, insulin, regular, isoproterenol, ketamine, ketorolac, levofloxacin, lidocaine, magnesium sulfate, mannitol, meperidine, methyldopate, methylprednisolone, metoclopramide, metoprolol, morphine, multivitamins, nafcillin, naloxone, nitroglycerin, nitroprusside, norepinephrine, ondansetron, oxacillin, oxytocin, penicillin G potassium, phenylephrine, phytonadione, potassium chloride, procainamide, prochlorperazine, propranolol, pyridoxine, ranitidine, sodium bicarbonate, streptokinase, sufentanil, theophylline, thiamine, vancomycin, vasopressin, verapamil.
- **Y-Site Incompatibility:** If aminoglycosides and penicillins must be administered concurrently, administer in separate sites at least 1 hr apart, aminophylline, amphotericin B colloidal, dantrolene, diazepam, dobutamine, doxycycline, erythromycin, ganciclovir, haloperidol, labetalol, papaverine, pentamidine, pentobarbital, phenobarbital, phenytoin, promethazine, protamine, succinylcholine, tranexamic acid, trimethoprim/sulfamethoxazole.
- **Additive Incompatibility:** Incompatible with aminoglycosides; do not admix.

Patient/Family Teaching

- Instruct patient to take medication around the clock and to finish drug completely as directed, even if feeling better. Advise patient that sharing this medication may be dangerous.
- Advise patient to report signs of superinfection (black, furry overgrowth on tongue; vaginal itching or discharge; loose or foul-smelling stools) and allergy.
- Instruct patient to notify health care professional if fever and diarrhea develop, especially if stool contains blood, pus, or mucus. Advise patient not to treat diarrhea without consulting health care professional.
- Instruct patient to notify health care professional if symptoms do not improve.
- Advise patient taking oral contraceptives to use an additional nonhormonal method of contraception during therapy with penicillin and until next menstrual period.
- Patient with an allergy to penicillin should be instructed to always carry an identification card with this information.

Evaluation/Desired Outcomes

- Resolution of signs and symptoms of infection. Length of time for complete resolution depends on the organism and site of infection.

PENICILLINS, PENICILLINASE RESISTANT

dicloxacillin (dye-klox-a-**sill**-in)

nafcillin (naf-**sill**-in)

oxacillin (ox-a-**sill**-in)

Classification

Therapeutic: anti-infectives

Pharmacologic: penicillinase resistant penicillins

P

Indications
Treatment of the following infections due to penicillinase-producing staphylococci: Respiratory tract infections, Sinusitis, Skin and skin structure infections. **Dicloxacillin:** Osteomyelitis. **Nafcillin, oxacillin:** Are also used to treat: Bone and joint infections, Urinary tract infections, Endocarditis, Septicemia, Meningitis.

Action
Bind to bacterial cell wall, leading to cell death. Not inactivated by penicillinase enzymes. **Therapeutic Effects:** Bactericidal action. **Spectrum:** Active against most gram-positive aerobic cocci but less so than penicillin. Spectrum is notable for activity against: Penicillinase-producing strains of *Staphylococcus aureus*, *Staphylococcus epidermidis*. Not active against methicillin-resistant staphylococci.

Pharmacokinetics
Absorption: *Dicloxacillin*—Rapidly but incompletely (35–76%) absorbed from the GI tract. *Nafcillin and oxacillin*—Completely absorbed following IV administration; well absorbed from IM sites.
Distribution: Widely distributed; penetration into CSF is minimal, but sufficient in the presence of inflamed meninges; cross the placenta and enter breast milk.
Metabolism and Excretion: *Dicloxacillin*—Some metabolism by the liver (6–10%) and some renal excretion of unchanged drug (60%); small amounts eliminated in the feces via the bile. *Nafcillin, oxacillin*—Partially metabolized by the liver (nafcillin 60%, oxacillin 49%), partially excreted unchanged by the kidneys.
Half-life: *Dicloxacillin*—0.5–1.1 hr (↑ in severe hepatic and renal dysfunction); *Nafcillin*—Neonates: 1–5 hr; Children 1 mo – 14 yr: 0.75–1.9 hr; Adults: 0.5–1.5 hr (↑ in renal impairment); *Oxacillin*—Neonates: 1.6 hr; Children up to 2 yr: 0.9–1.8 hr; Adults: 0.3–0.8 hr (↑ in severe hepatic impairment).

TIME/ACTION PROFILE (blood levels)

ROUTE	ONSET	PEAK	DURATION
Dicloxacillin	30 min	30–120 min	6 hr
Nafcillin IM	30 min	60–120 min	4–6 hr
Nafcillin IV	rapid	end of infusion	4–6 hr
Oxacillin IM	rapid	30 min	4–6 hr
Oxacillin IV	rapid	end of infusion	4–6 hr

Contraindications/Precautions
Contraindicated in: Hypersensitivity to penicillins (cross-sensitivity with cephalosporins may exist).
Use Cautiously in: Severe renal or hepatic impairment; OB, Lactation: Safety not established.

Adverse Reactions/Side Effects
CNS: SEIZURES (high doses). **Derm:** rash, urticaria. **GI:** CLOSTRIDIUM DIFFICILE-ASSOCIATED DIARRHEA (CDAD), diarrhea, nausea, vomiting, ↑ liver enzymes. **GU:** acute kidney injury, hematuria, interstitial nephritis, proteinuria. **Hemat:** eosinophilia, leukopenia. **Local:** pain at IM sites, phlebitis at IV sites. **Misc:** HYPERSENSITIVITY REACTIONS (including anaphylaxis and serum sickness), superinfection.

Interactions
Drug-Drug: Probenecid ↓ renal excretion and ↑ blood levels (treatment may be combined for this purpose). May ↓ effectiveness of **oral contraceptive agents.** May ↓ elimination of **methotrexate** and ↑ risk of serious toxicity.

Route/Dosage
Dicloxacillin
PO (Adults and Children ≥40 kg): 125–250 mg every 6 hr (max dose = 2 g/day).
PO (Children <40 kg): 6.25–12.5 mg/kg every 6 hr; (up to 12.25 mg/kg every 6 hr has been used for osteomyelitis) (max dose = 2 g/day).

Nafcillin
IV (Adults): 500–2000 mg every 4–6 hr.
IM (Adults): 500 mg every 4–6 hr.
IM, IV (Children and Infants): 50–200 mg/kg/day divided every 4–6 hr (max dose = 12 g/day).
IM, IV (Neonates >2 kg): 25 mg/kg every 8 hr for the 1st 7 days of life, then 25 mg/kg every 6 hr.
IM, IV (Neonates 1.2–2 kg): 25 mg/kg every 12 hr for the 1st 7 days of life, then 25 mg/kg every 8 hr.
IM, IV (Neonates 0–4 wk, <1.2 kg): 25 mg/kg every 12 hr.

Oxacillin
IM, IV (Adults and Children ≥40 kg): 250–2000 mg every 4–6 hr (max dose = 12 g/day).
IM, IV (Children <40 kg): 100–200 mg/kg/day divided every 4–6 hr (max dose = 12 g/day).
IM, IV (Neonates ≥2 kg): 25 mg/kg every 8 hr for the 1st 7 days of life, then 25 mg/kg every 6 hr.
IM, IV (Neonates 1.2–2 kg): 25 mg/kg every 12 hr for the 1st 7 days of life, then 25 mg/kg every 8 hr.
IM, IV (Neonates <1.2 kg): 25 mg/kg every 12 hr.

Availability
Dicloxacillin (generic available)
Capsules: 250 mg, 500 mg.

Nafcillin (generic available)
Powder for injection (requires reconstitution and dilution): 1 g/vial, 2 g/vial, 10 g/vial. **Premixed infusion:** 1 g/50 mL D5W, 2 g/100 mL D5W.

Oxacillin (generic available)
Powder for injection (requires reconstitution and dilution): 1 g/vial, 2 g/vial, 10 g/vial. **Premixed infusion:** 1 g/50 mL D5W, 2 g/50 mL D5W.

NURSING IMPLICATIONS

Assessment

- Assess patient for infection (vital signs; appearance of wound, sputum, urine, and stool; WBC) at beginning of and throughout therapy.
- Obtain a history before initiating therapy to determine previous use of and reactions to penicillins, cephalosporins, or other beta-lactam antibiotics. Persons with a negative history of penicillin sensitivity may still have an allergic response.
- Obtain specimens for culture and sensitivity prior to initiating therapy. 1st dose may be given before receiving results.
- Observe patient for signs and symptoms of anaphylaxis (rash, pruritus, laryngeal edema, wheezing, abdominal pain). Discontinue the drug and notify health care professional immediately if these occur. Keep epinephrine, an antihistamine, and resuscitation equipment close by in the event of an anaphylactic reaction.
- Assess vein for signs of irritation and phlebitis. Change IV site every 48 hr to prevent phlebitis.
- ***Lab Test Considerations:*** May cause leukopenia and neutropenia, especially with prolonged therapy or hepatic impairment.
- May cause positive direct Coombs' test result.
- May cause ↑ AST, ALT, LDH, and serum alkaline phosphatase concentrations.

Implementation

- **PO:** Administer around the clock on an empty stomach at least 1 hr before or 2 hr after meals. Take with a full glass of water; acidic juices may decrease absorption of penicillins.
- Use calibrated measuring device for liquid preparations. Shake well. Solution is stable for 14 days if refrigerated.

Nafcillin

IV Administration

- **IV, IM:** To reconstitute, add 3.4 mL to each 1-g vial or 6.8 mL to each 2-g vial, for a concentration of 250 mg/mL. Stable for 2–7 days if refrigerated.
- **IV Push:** ***Diluent:*** Dilute reconstituted solution with 15–30 mL of sterile water, 0.45% NaCl, or 0.9% NaCl for injection. ***Concentration:*** 100 mg/mL. ***Rate:*** Administer over 5–10 min.
- **Intermittent Infusion:** ***Diluent:*** Dilute with sterile water for injection, 0.9% NaCl, D5W, D10W, D5/0.25% NaCl, D5/0.45% NaCl, D5/0.9% NaCl, D5/LR, Ringer's or LR. Stable for 24 hr at room temperature, 96 hr if refrigerated. ***Concentration:*** 2–40 mg/mL. ***Rate:*** Infuse over at least 30–60 min to avoid vein irritation.
- **Y-Site Compatibility:** acyclovir, alfentanil, aminophylline, amphotericin B lipid complex, anidulafungin, argatroban, ascorbic acid, atracurium, atropine, aztreonam, benztropine, bivalirudin, bleomycin, bumetanide, buprenorphine, butorphanol, calcium chloride, calcium gluconate, carboplatin, carmustine, chlorpromazine, cisplatin, clindamycin, cyanocobalamin, cyclophosphamide, dactinomycin, daptomycin, dexamethasone, digoxin, dobutamine, docetaxel, dopamine, enalaprilat, ephedrine, epinephrine, epoetin alfa, erythromycin, etoposide, etoposide phosphate, famotidine, fenoldopam, fentanyl, fluconazole, fludarabine, foscarnet, furosemide, ganciclovir, glycopyrrolate, granisetron, heparin, hetastarch, hydrocortisone, hydromorphone, imipenem/cilastatin, indomethacin, isoproterenol, ketorolac, lidocaine, linezolid, lorazepam, magnesium sulfate, mannitol, methoxamine, methyldopate, methylprednisolone, metoclopramide, metoprolol, metronidazole, milrinone, morphine, multivitamins, naloxone, nicardipine, nitroglycerin, nitroprusside, norepinephrine, octreotide, ondansetron, oxacillin, oxytocin, paclitaxel, pamidronate, pnacuronium, pantoprazole, pemetrexed, penicillin G, pentobarbital, perphenazine, phenobarbital, phentolamine, phenylephrine, phytonadione, potassium acetate, potassium chloride, procainamide, prochlorperazine, propofol, propranolol, ranitidine, sodium bicarbonate, streptokinase, sufentanil, tacrolimus, theophylline, thiamine, thiotepa, tigecycline, tirofiban, tolazoline, trimetaphan, vasopressin, voriconazole, zidovudine, zoledronic acid.
- **Y-Site Incompatibility:** alemtuzumab, ampicillin, azathioprine, caspofungin, chloramphenicol, dantrolene, diazoxide, doxycycline, droperidol, epirubicin, folic acid, gemcitabine, haloperidol, hydralazine, hydroxyzine, idarubicin, irinotecan, meperidine, metaraminol, mitoxantrone, mycophenolate, palonosetron, pentamidine, phenytoin, promethazine, protamine, pyridoxime, succinylcholine, trimethoprim/sulfamethoxazole, vecuronium, vincristine, vinrelbine. If penicillins and aminoglycosides must be administered concurrently, administer at separate sites.

Oxacillin

IV Administration

- **IV, IM:** To reconstitute for IM or IV use, add 1.4 mL of sterile water for injection to each 250-mg vial, 2.7 mL to each 500-mg vial, 5.7 mL to each 1-g vial, 11.5 mL to each 2-g vial, and 23 mL to each 4-g vial, for a concentration of 250 mg/1.5 mL. Stable for 3 days at room temperature or 7 days if refrigerated.
- **IV Push:** ***Diluent:*** Further dilute each reconstituted 250-mg or 500-mg vial with 5 mL of sterile water or 0.9% NaCl for injection, 10 mL for each 1-g vial, 20 mL for each 2-g vial, and 40 mL for each 4-g vial. ***Concentration:*** 100 mg/mL. ***Rate:*** Administer slowly over 10 min.

P

- **Intermittent Infusion:** ***Diluent:*** Dilute with 0.9% NaCl, D5W, D5/0.9% NaCl, or LR. ***Concentration:*** 0.5–40 mg/mL. ***Rate:*** May be infused for up to 6 hr.
- **Y-Site Compatibility:** acyclovir, alfentanil, aminophylline, ascorbic acid, atracurium, atropine, aztreonam, benztropine, bumetanide, buprenorphine, butorphanol, chloramphenicol, chlorpromazine, clindamycin, cyanocobalamin, cyclophosphamide, cyclosporine, dexamethasone, digoxin, diltiazem, dopamine, doxapram, enalaprilat, ephedrine, epinephrine, epoetin alfa, erythromycin, famotidine, fentanil, fluconazole, folic acid, foscarnet, furosemide, glycopyrrolate, heparin, hydrocortisone sodium succinate, hydromorphone, imipenem/cilastatin, insulin, regular, isoproterenol, ketorolac, labetalol, levofloxacin, lidocaine, mannitol, methotrexate, methoxamine, methyldopate, metoclopramide, metoprolol, midazolam, milrinone, morphine, multivitamins, nafcillin, naloxone, nitroglycerin, nitroprusside, norepinephrine, ondansetron, oxytocin, papaverine, penicillin G, pentobarbital, perphenazine, phenobarbital, phenylephrine, phytonadione, potassium chloride, procainamide, prochlorperazine, propranolol, ranitidine, streptokinase, sufentanil, tacrolimus, theophylline, thiamine, tolazoline, trimetaphan, vancomycin, vasopressin, vitamin B complex with C, zidovudine.
- **Y-Site Incompatibility:** calcium chloride, calcium gluconate, dantrolene, diazepam, diazoxide, dobutamine, doxycycline, esmolol, haloperidol, hydralazine, metaraminol, pentamidine, phenytoin, promethazine, pyridoxime, succinylcholine, trimethoprim/sulfamethoazole. If penicillins and aminoglycosides must be administered concurrently, administer at separate sites.

Patient/Family Teaching

- Instruct patient to take medication around the clock and to finish the drug completely as directed, even if feeling better. Missed doses should be taken as soon as remembered. Advise patient that sharing of this medication may be dangerous.
- Advise patient to report signs of superinfection (black, furry overgrowth on the tongue; vaginal itching or discharge; loose or foul-smelling stools) and allergy.
- Instruct patient to notify health care professional if fever and diarrhea develop, especially if stool contains blood, pus, or mucus. Advise patient not to treat diarrhea without consulting health care professional.
- Instruct patient to notify health care professional if symptoms do not improve.

Evaluation/Desired Outcomes

- Resolution of the signs and symptoms of infection. Length of time for complete resolution depends on the organism and site of infection.

pentosan (pen-toe-san)

Elmiron

Classification

Therapeutic: interstitial cystitis agents

Pharmacologic: heparin-like compounds

Indications

Management symptoms (bladder pain/discomfort) of chronic interstitial cystitis (IC).

Action

Adheres to uroepithelium, providing a protective barrier against irritating solutes in urine. Has anticoagulant and fibrinolytic properties. **Therapeutic Effects:** ↓ pain and discomfort in chronic IC.

Pharmacokinetics

Absorption: 6% absorbed following oral administrations.

Distribution: Distributes into uroepithelium of the genitourinary tract with less found in liver, spleen, lung, skin, perisoteum, and bone marrow.

Metabolism and Excretion: Metabolized by saturable enzyme systems in liver, spleen and kidney. Majority (58–84%) excreted in feces as unchanged (unabsorbed drug). Metabolites of absorbed drug are renally excreted; minimal renal excretion of unchanged drug.

Half-life: 27 hr.

TIME/ACTION PROFILE (↓ symptoms)

ROUTE	ONSET	PEAK	DURATION
PO	within 4 wk-6 mos	unknown	unknown

Contraindications/Precautions

Contraindicated in: Hypersensitivity.

Use Cautiously in: Underlying coagulopathy, concurrent medications that ↑ bleeding risk, history of aneurysms. thrombocytopenia, hemophilia, GI ulceration/bleeding, polyps, diverticula; History of heparin-induced thrombocytopenia; risk of bleeding may be ↑ Hepatic insufficiency; OB: Use in pregnancy only if clearly needed; Lactation: Use cautiously in breast-feeding women; Pedi: Safe and effective use in children <16 yr has not been established.

Adverse Reactions/Side Effects

CNS: dizziness, headache. **EENT:** epistaxis. **GI:** abdominal pain, diarrhea, dyspepsia, gum bleeding, ↑ liver enzymes, nausea, rectal bleeding. **Derm:** alopecia, ecchymosis, rash. **Hemat:** bleeding, ↑ bleeding time.

Interactions

Drug-Drug: Concurrent use of **coumarin anticoagulants**, **heparins**, **t-PA**, **streptokinase**, high dose **aspirin**, or **NSAIDs** may ↑ risk of bleeding.

Route/Dosage

PO (Adults): 100 mg three times daily.

Availability

Capsules: 100 mg.

NURSING IMPLICATIONS

Assessment

- Assess pain intensity, frequency, and duration in patient with interstitial cystitis.
- ***Lab Test Considerations:*** Doses of <1200 mg/day are unlikely to affect PT or PTT.
- May cause liver function abnormalities.
- May rarely cause anemia, ↑ PT, ↑ PTT, leukopenia, and thrombocytopenia.

Implementation

- **PO:** Administer on an empty stomach 3 times daily, at least 1 hr before or 2 hr after meals.

Patient/Family Teaching

- Instruct patient to take pentosan as directed, taking no more or no more frequently than prescribed.
- Advise patient to notify health care professional if surgery, anticoagulant therapy (warfarin, heparin), or therapy with high doses of aspirin or NSAIDs is planned.
- Advise patient to notify health care professional if pregnancy is planned or suspected or if breast feeding.

Evaluation/Desired Outcomes

- ↓ in pain and discomfort of interstitial cystitis. Reassess after 3 mo of therapy. If no improvement but no limiting adverse events are present, may be continued for 3 more mo.

perampanel (per-am-pa-nel)

Fycompa

Classification

Therapeutic: anticonvulsants

Pharmacologic: glutamate receptor antagonists

Schedule III

Indications

Treatment (with or without other anti-epileptic drugs [AEDs]) of partial-onset seizures with or without secondarily generalized seizures. Adjunctive treatment (with other AEDs) of primary generalized tonic-clonic seizures.

Action

Acts as a non-competitive α-amino-3–hydroxy-5–methyl-4–isoxazolepropionic acid (AMPA) antagonist on post-synaptic neuronal glutamate (excitatory) receptors. **Therapeutic Effects:** Decreased incidence and severity of partial-onset seizures and primary generalized tonic-clonic seizures.

Pharmacokinetics

Absorption: Rapidly and completely absorbed following oral administration.

Distribution: Unknown.

Protein Binding: 95–96%.

Metabolism and Excretion: Extensively metabolized by CYP3A4/5 enzyme systems; excreted in urine and feces primarily as metabolites.

Half-life: 105 hr.

TIME/ACTION PROFILE

ROUTE	ONSET	PEAK	DURATION†
PO	unknown	unknown	2 wk

†Duration of effects following cessation.

Contraindications/Precautions

Contraindicated in: Concurrent use of strong CYP450 inducers (other than AEDs); Severe hepatic impairment.

Use Cautiously in: History of homicidal/suicidal ideation or other psychiatric/behavioral issues; OB: Use in pregnancy only when potential benefits outweigh potential fetal risks; Lactation: Use cautiously; Pedi: Children <4 yr (safety and effectiveness not established); Geri: ↑ risk of adverse reactions; slower titration recommended.

Adverse Reactions/Side Effects

CNS: dizziness, drowsiness, headache, aggression, anger, fatigue, psychiatric/behavioral problems, hostility, irritability, suicidal ideation, vertigo. **Derm:** DRUG REACTION WITH EOSINOPHILIA AND SYSTEMIC SYMPTOMS (DRESS). **Metab:** weight gain. **Neuro:** ataxia, balance disorder, gait disturbance. **Misc:** falls.

Interactions

Drug-Drug: Doses >12 mg/day may ↓ effectiveness of **levonorgestrel-containing hormonal contraceptives**. **CYP450 inducers** including **carbamazepine**, **oxcarbazepine**, **phenobarbital**, **phenytoin**, **primidone**, and **topiramate** can ↓ levels and effectiveness; careful monitoring is required especially during initiation and withdrawal. Dosage adjustments may be required. ↑ risk of CNS depression with other **CNS depressants** including **alcohol**, sedating **antihistamines**, **barbiturates**, **benzodiazepines**, **opioids**, and **sedative/hypnotics**.

Drug-Natural Products: Levels and effectiveness may be ↓ by **St. John's wort**; concurrent use should be avoided.

Route/Dosage

Partial-Onset Seizures

PO (Adults and Children ≥4 yr): 2 mg once daily at bedtime initially; may ↑ by 2 mg/day at weekly intervals (usual dosage range = 4–12 mg once daily); *Concurrent use of moderate or strong CYP3A4 enzyme-inducers (e.g. phenytoin, carbamazepine, oxcarbazepine)*—4 mg once daily at bedtime initially; may ↑ by 2 mg/day at weekly intervals (maximum dose = 12 mg once daily).

PO (Geriatric Patients): 2 mg once daily at bedtime initially; may ↑ by 2 mg/day every 2 wk (usual dosage range = 4–12 mg once daily); *Concurrent use of moderate or strong CYP3A4 enzyme-inducers (e.g. phenytoin, carbamazepine, oxcarbazepine)*—4 mg once daily at bedtime initially; may ↑ by 2 mg/day every 2 wk (maximum dose = 12 mg once daily).

Hepatic Impairment

PO (Adults and Children ≥4 yr): *Mild hepatic impairment*—2 mg once daily at bedtime initially; may ↑ by 2 mg/day every 2 wk (maximum dose = 6 mg once daily); *Moderate hepatic impairment*—2 mg once daily at bedtime initially; may ↑ by 2 mg/day after 2 wk up to 4 mg once daily.

Primary Generalized Tonic-Clonic Seizures

PO (Adults and Children ≥12 yr): 2 mg once daily at bedtime initially; may ↑ by 2 mg/day at weekly intervals (usual dosage range = 8–12 mg once daily); *Concurrent use of moderate or strong CYP3A4 enzyme-inducers (e.g. phenytoin, carbamazepine, oxcarbazepine)*—4 mg once daily at bedtime initially; may ↑ by 2 mg/day at weekly intervals (maximum dose = 12 mg once daily).

PO (Geriatric Patients): 2 mg once daily at bedtime initially; may ↑ by 2 mg/day every 2 wk (usual dosage range = 4–12 mg once daily); *Concurrent use of moderate or strong CYP3A4 enzyme-inducers (e.g. phenytoin, carbamazepine, oxcarbazepine)*—4 mg once daily at bedtime initially; may ↑ by 2 mg/day every 2 wk (maximum dose = 12 mg once daily).

Hepatic Impairment

PO (Adults and Children ≥12 yr): *Mild hepatic impairment*—2 mg once daily at bedtime initially; may ↑ by 2 mg/day every 2 wk (maximum dose = 6 mg once daily); *Moderate hepatic impairment*—2 mg once daily at bedtime initially; may ↑ by 2 mg/day after 2 wk up to 4 mg once daily.

Availability

Oral suspension: 0.5 mg/mL. **Tablets:** 2 mg, 4 mg, 6 mg, 8 mg, 10 mg, 12 mg.

NURSING IMPLICATIONS

Assessment

- Assess location, duration, and characteristics of seizure activity. Institute seizure precautions. Assess response to and continued need for perampanel periodically during therapy.
- Monitor closely for notable changes in behavior that could indicate the emergence or worsening of suicidal thoughts or behavior, new or worse aggressive behavior, or depression.
- Monitor for signs and symptoms of neurologic effects (dizziness, gait disturbance, somnolence, fatigue) during therapy. More common during titration phase and with geriatric patients.
- Monitor for signs and symptoms of DRESS (fever, rash, lymphadenopathy, and/or facial swelling, associated with involvement of other organ systems (hepatitis, nephritis, hematologic abnormalities, myocarditis, myositis) during therapy. May resemble an acute viral infection. Eosinophilia is often present. Discontinue therapy if signs occur.

Implementation

- **PO:** Administer once daily at bedtime.
- Shake oral solution well prior to use. Use provided adaptor and graduated oral dosing syringe for accurate dosing.

Patient/Family Teaching

- Instruct patient to take perampanel as directed. Missed doses should be omitted and dosing resumed the following day. Notify health care professional if more than 1 day of dosing is missed. Medication should be gradually discontinued, do not stop abruptly, to prevent seizures. Advise patient to read the *Medication Guide* prior to starting perampanel and with each Rx refill in case of changes.
- May cause dizziness, sleepiness, fatigue, and gait disturbance, increasing risk of falls. Caution patient to avoid driving or other activities requiring alertness until response to medication is known.
- Inform patients and families of risk of suicidal thoughts and behavior (behavioral changes, emerging or worsening signs and symptoms of depression, unusual changes in mood, or emergence of suicidal thoughts, behavior, or thoughts of self-harm) and aggressive behavior (hostility, anger, anxiety, irritability, being suspicious or distrustful, believing things that are not true). Advise that these should be reported to health care professional immediately.
- Instruct patient to notify health care professional of all Rx or OTC medications, vitamins, or herbal products being taken and consult health care professional before taking any new medications, especially carbamazepine, phenytoin, oxcarbazepine, rifampin, and St. John's wort. Advise patient to avoid taking other CNS depressants or alcohol.
- Rep: Perampanel decreases efficacy of levonorgestrel; advise patients to use a non-hormonal form of birth control during therapy. Advise female patients to notify health care professional if pregnancy is planned or suspected or if breast feeding. Encourage pregnant patients to enroll in the North American Antiepileptic Drug (NAAED) Pregnancy Registry

by calling 1-888-233-2334; information is available at www.aedpregnancyregistry.org.

Evaluation/Desired Outcomes

- Decreased seizure activity.

perindopril, See ANGIOTENSIN-CONVERTING ENZYME (ACE) INHIBITORS.

pertuzumab

(per-**tue**-zue-mab)

Perjeta

Classification

Therapeutic: antineoplastics

Pharmacologic: HER2/neu receptor antagonists, monoclonal antibodies

Indications

HER2-positive metastatic breast cancer in patients who have not yet been treated with anti-HER2 agents or chemotherapy (in combination with docetaxel and trastuzumab). Neoadjuvant treatment of HER2-positive locally advanced, inflammatory, or early stage breast cancer (either >2 cm in diameter or node-positive) (in combination with trastuzumab and chemotherapy). Adjuvant treatment of HER2–positive early breast cancer at high risk of recurrence (in combination with trastuzumab and chemotherapy).

Action

A monoclonal antibody that attaches to and blocks the human epidermal growth factor receptor 2 protein (HER2), resulting in cell growth arrest and apoptosis. **Therapeutic Effects:** Decreased spread of breast cancer.

Pharmacokinetics

Absorption: IV administration results in complete bioavailability.

Distribution: Unknown.

Metabolism and Excretion: Unknown.

Half-life: 18 days.

TIME/ACTION PROFILE

ROUTE	ONSET	PEAK	DURATION
IV	unknown	unknown	20 mo†

†Median duration of response.

Contraindications/Precautions

Contraindicated in: Hypersensitivity; OB: Pregnancy (may cause fetal harm).

Use Cautiously in: HER2 testing is required prior to treatment; Asian patients (↑ incidence of febrile neutropenia); Lactation: Use while breast feeding only if potential maternal benefit justifies potential risk to infant; Rep: Women of reproductive potential; Pedi: Safety and effectiveness not established.

Adverse Reactions/Side Effects

May reflect combination treatment with docetaxel and trastuzumab.

CNS: dizziness, fatigue, headache, insomnia, weakness. **CV:** HF, peripheral edema. **Derm:** alopecia, rash, dry skin, itching, nail disorder. **EENT:** ↑ lacrimation. **GI:** ↓ appetite, diarrhea, dysgeusia, nausea, vomiting. **Hemat:** ANEMIA, LEUKOPENIA, NEUTROPENIA. **MS:** athralgia, myalgia. **Neuro:** peripheral neuropathy. **Resp:** dyspnea. **Misc:** HYPERSENSITIVITY REACTIONS (including anaphylaxis and angioedema), chills, infusion reactions, fever.

Interactions

Drug-Drug: ↑ risk of bone marrow depression/immunosuppression with other **bone marrow depressants/immunosuppressants** or **radiation therapy**.

Route/Dosage

Metastatic Breast Cancer

IV (Adults): 840 mg initially, then 420 mg every 3 wk.

Neoadjuvant Treatment of Breast Cancer

IV (Adults): 840 mg initially, then 420 mg every 3 wk for 3–6 cycles given preoperatively. Following surgery, administer 420 mg every 3 wk to complete 1 yr of treatment (up to 18 cycles).

Adjuvant Treatment of Breast Cancer

IV (Adults): 840 mg initially, then 420 mg every 3 wk for 1 yr (up to 18 cycles) or until disease recurrence or unacceptable toxicity.

Availability

Solution for injection: 30 mg/mL.

NURSING IMPLICATIONS

Assessment

- Metastatic Breast Cancer: *If pretreatment left ventricular ejection fraction (LVEF) ≥50%,* monitor prior to and about every 12 wk. *If LVEF ↓ to <40% or 40%-45% with a fall of ≥10%-points below pretreatment value,* hold pertuzumab and trastuzumab for at least 3 wk. *If after 3 wk LVEF recovered to >45% or 40%-45% with a fall of <10%-points below pretreatment value,* resume pertuzumab and trastuumab. Early Breast Cancer: *If pretreatment left ventricular ejection fraction (LVEF) ≥55%,* monitor prior to and about every 12 wk or once neoadjuvant therapy. *If LVEF ↓ to <50% with a fall of ≥10%-points below pretreatment value,* hold pertuzumab and trastuzumab for at least

P

3 wk. *If after 3 wk LVEF recovered to >50% with a fall of <10%-points below pretreatment value,* resume pertuzumab and trastuumab. For patients receiving anthracycline-based chemotherapy, a LVEF of ≥ 50% is required after completion of anthracyclines, before starting pertuzumab and trastuzumab.

- If trastuzumab is withheld or discontinued, withhold or discontinue pertuzumab. If docetaxel is discontinued, pertuzumab and trastuzumab therapy may continue. Dose reductions are not recommended for pertuzumab.
- Assess patient closely for 60 min after initial infusion and 30 min after subsequent infusions for signs and symptoms of infusion-associated reactions (pyrexia, chills, fatigue, headache, asthenia, hypersensitivity, vomiting). If a significant infusion-associated reaction occurs, slow or interrupt infusion and administer appropriate medical therapies. Monitor until complete resolution of signs and symptoms. If severe infusion reactions occur, consider discontinuation of pertuzumab.
- Monitor patient for signs and symptoms of hypersensitivity reactions (rash, hives, itching, dyspnea, swelling of throat, lips, tongue) occurs.
- ***Lab Test Considerations:*** Obtain a negative preganacy status before starting therapy.
- Determine HER protein overexpression prior to therapy.
- Verify pregnancy status prior to initiation of pertuzumab.
- Monitor CBC with differential periodically during therapy.

Implementation

IV Administration

- When administered with pertuzumab, initial dose of trastuzumab is 8 mg/kg infused over 90 min, followed every 3 wk by 6 mg/kg infused over 30–90 min.
- When administered with pertuzumab, initial dose of docetaxel is 75 mg/m^2 as an IV infusion. Dose of docetaxel may be ↑ to 100 mg/m^2 every 3 wk if initial dose is tolerated.
- Administer pertuzumab, trastuzumab, and docetaxel. Administer pertuzumab and trastuzumab in any order. Administer docetaxel after pertuzumab and trastuzumab. Observe patient for 30 to 60 min after pertuzumab infusion and before any subsequent infusion of trastuzumab or docetaxel.
- **Intermittent Infusion: *Diluent:*** 0.9% NaCl; do not use D5W. Withdraw appropriate volume of pertuzumab and dilute in 250 mL using a PVC or non-PVC polyolefin infusion bag. Gently invert to mix; do not shake. If not administered immediately, may be refrigerated for 24 hr; do not freeze. ***Rate:*** Infuse initial 840 mg over 60 min, followed every 3 wk by 420 mg over 30–60 min.
- For delayed or missed doses, if time between 2 sequential infusions is <6 wk, administer 420 mg dose of pertuzumab; do not wait until next planned dose. If time between 2 sequential infusions ≥6 wk, re-administer initial 840 mg dose over 60 min, followed every 3 wk by 420 mg dose over 30–60 min.

Patient/Family Teaching

- Explain purpose of medication to patient.
- Advise patient to report signs and symptoms of infusion-associated reactions immediately.
- Advise patient to notify health care professional immediately if signs and symptoms of left ventricular dysfunction (new onset or worsening shortness of breath, cough, swelling of the ankles/legs, swelling of the face, palpitations, weight gain of more than 5 pounds in 24 hrs, dizziness or loss of consciousness) occur.
- Instruct patient to notify health care professional promptly if fever; chills; cough; hoarseness; sore throat; signs of infection; lower back or side pain; painful or difficult urination; bleeding gums; bruising; petechiae; blood in stools, urine, or emesis; increased fatigue; dyspnea. Caution patient to avoid crowds and persons with known infections. Instruct patient to use soft toothbrush and electric razor and to avoid falls. Caution patient not to drink alcoholic beverages or take medication containing aspirin or NSAIDs; may precipitate gastric bleeding.
- Instruct patient to notify health care professional of all Rx or OTC medications, vitamins, or herbal products being taken and consult health care professional before taking any new medications.
- Rep: Advise females of reproductive potential that pertuzumab is teratogenic and to notify health care professional immediately if pregnancy is planned or suspected or if breast feeding. Caution patient to use effective contraception during and for 7 mo following the last dose. Women who are breast feeding should be advised to discontinue nursing or discontinue pertuzumab. Encourage women who may be exposed during pregnancy to report exposure to the Genentech Adverse Event Line at 1-888-835-2555. Monitor patients who become pregnant for oligohydramnios.

Evaluation/Desired Outcomes

- Decreased spread of metastatic breast cancer.

phenazopyridine

(fen-az-oh-**peer**-i-deen)

Baridium, Phenazo, Pyridium, Pyridium Plus

Classification

Therapeutic: nonopioid analgesics

Pharmacologic: urinary tract analgesics

Indications

Provides relief from the following urinary tract symptoms, which may occur in association with infection or following urologic procedures: Pain, Itching, Burning, Urgency, Frequency.

Action

Acts locally on the urinary tract mucosa to produce analgesic or local anesthetic effects. Has no antimicrobial activity. **Therapeutic Effects:** Diminished urinary tract discomfort.

Pharmacokinetics

Absorption: Appears to be well absorbed following oral administration.
Distribution: Unknown. Small amounts cross the placenta.
Metabolism and Excretion: Rapidly excreted unchanged in the urine.
Half-life: Unknown.

TIME/ACTION PROFILE (urinary analgesia)

ROUTE	ONSET	PEAK	DURATION
PO	unknown	5–6 hr	6–8 hr

Contraindications/Precautions

Contraindicated in: Hypersensitivity; Glomerulonephritis; Severe hepatitis, uremia, or renal failure; Renal insufficiency; Glucose-6–phosphate dehydrogenase (G6PD) deficiency.
Use Cautiously in: Hepatitis; OB, Lactation: Safety not established.

Adverse Reactions/Side Effects

CNS: headache, vertigo. **GI:** hepatotoxicity, nausea. **GU:** bright-orange urine, renal failure. **Derm:** rash. **Hemat:** hemolytic anemia, methemoglobinemia.

Interactions

Drug-Drug: None significant.

Route/Dosage

PO (Adults): 200 mg 3 times daily for 2 days.
PO (Children): 4 mg/kg 3 times daily for 2 days.

Availability (generic available)

Tablets: 95 mg^{OTC}, 100 mg, ✱100 mg^{OTC}, ✱200 mg^{OTC}, 200 mg.

NURSING IMPLICATIONS

Assessment

- Assess patient for urgency, frequency, and pain on urination prior to and throughout therapy.
- ***Lab Test Considerations:*** Renal function should be monitored periodically during course of therapy.
- Interferes with urine tests based on color reactions (glucose, ketones, bilirubin, steroids, protein).

Implementation

- ***High Alert:*** Do not confuse Pyridium (phenazopyridine) with pyridoxine.
- Medication should be discontinued after pain or discomfort is relieved (usually 2 days for treatment of urinary tract infection). Concurrent antibiotic therapy should continue for full prescribed duration.
- **PO:** Administer medication with or following meals to decrease GI irritation. Do not crush, break, or chew tablet.

Patient/Family Teaching

- Instruct patient to take medication exactly as directed. If a dose is missed, take as soon as remembered unless almost time for next dose.
- Advise patient that while phenazopyridine administration is stopped once pain or discomfort is relieved, concurrent antibiotic therapy must be continued for full duration of therapy. Do not save unused portion of phenazopyridine without consulting health care professional.
- Inform patient that drug causes reddish-orange discoloration of urine that may stain clothing or bedding. Sanitary napkin may be worn to avoid clothing stains. May also cause staining of soft contact lenses.
- Instruct patient to notify health care professional if rash, skin discoloration, or unusual tiredness occurs.

Evaluation/Desired Outcomes

- Decrease in pain and burning on urination.

BEERS

PHENobarbital

(fee-noe-**bar**-bi-tal)
✱Ancalixir, ~~Luminal~~

Classification
Therapeutic: anticonvulsants, sedative/hypnotics
Pharmacologic: barbiturates

Schedule IV

Indications

Anticonvulsant in tonic-clonic (grand mal), partial, and febrile seizures in children. Preoperative sedative and in other situations in which sedation may be required. Hypnotic (short-term). **Unlabeled Use:** Prevention/treatment of hyperbilirubinemia in neonates.

Action

Produces all levels of CNS depression. Depresses the sensory cortex, decreases motor activity, and alters cerebellar function. Inhibits transmission in the nervous system and raises the seizure threshold. Capable of inducing (speeding up) enzymes in the liver that metabolize drugs, bilirubin, and other compounds. **Therapeutic Effects:** Anticonvulsant activity. Sedation.

Pharmacokinetics

Absorption: Absorption is slow but relatively complete (70–90%).

Distribution: Unknown.
Metabolism and Excretion: 75% metabolized by the liver, 25% excreted unchanged by the kidneys.
Half-life: Neonates: 1.8–8.3 days; Infants: 0.8–5.5 days; Children: 1.5–3 days; Adults: 2–6 days.

TIME/ACTION PROFILE (sedation†)

ROUTE	ONSET	PEAK	DURATION
PO	30–60 min	unknown	>6 hr
IM, subcut	10–30 min	unknown	4–6 hr
IV	5 min	30 min	4–6 hr

†Full anticonvulsant effects occur after 2–3 wk of chronic dosing unless a loading dose has been used.

Contraindications/Precautions

Contraindicated in: Hypersensitivity; Comatose patients or those with pre-existing CNS depression; Severe respiratory disease with dyspnea or obstruction; Uncontrolled severe pain; Known alcohol intolerance (elixir only); Lactation: Discontinue drug or bottle feed.
Use Cautiously in: Hepatic dysfunction; Severe renal impairment; History of suicide attempt or drug abuse; Hypnotic use should be short-term. Chronic use may lead to dependence; OB: Chronic use during pregnancy results in drug dependency in the infant; may result in coagulation defects and fetal malformation; acute use at term may result in respiratory depression in the newborn; Geri: Initial dose ↓ recommended.

Adverse Reactions/Side Effects

CNS: hangover, delirium, depression, drowsiness, excitation, lethargy, vertigo. **Resp:** respiratory depression; *IV*, LARYNGOSPASM, bronchospasm. **CV:** *IV*—hypotension. **GI:** constipation, diarrhea, nausea, vomiting. **Derm:** photosensitivity, rashes, urticaria. **Local:** phlebitis at IV site. **MS:** arthralgia, myalgia, neuralgia. **Misc:** hypersensitivity reactions including ANGIOEDEMA and SERUM SICKNESS, physical dependence, psychological dependence.

Interactions

Drug-Drug: Additive CNS depression with other **CNS depressants**, including **alcohol**, **antihistamines**, **opioid analgesics**, and other **sedative/hypnotics**. May induce hepatic enzymes that metabolize other drugs, ↓ their effectiveness, including **hormonal contraceptives**, **warfarin**, **chloramphenicol**, **cyclosporine**, **dacarbazine**, **corticosteroids**, **tricyclic antidepressants**, **felodipine**, **clonazepam**, **carbamazepine**, **verapamil**, **theophylline**, **metronidazole**, and **quinidine**. May ↑ risk of hepatic toxicity of **acetaminophen**. **MAO inhibitors**, **valproic acid**, or **divalproex** may ↓ metabolism of phenobarbital, ↑ sedation. **Rifampin** may ↑ metabolism of and ↓ effects of phenobarbital. May ↑ risk of hematologic toxicity with **cyclophosphamide**.
Drug-Natural Products: Concomitant use of **kava-kava**, **valerian**, **chamomile**, or **hops** can ↑ CNS depression. **St. John's wort** may ↓ effects.

Route/Dosage

Status Epilepticus

IV (Adults and Children >1 mo): 15–18 mg/kg in a single or divided dose, maximum loading dose 20 mg/kg.
IV (Neonates): 15–20 mg/kg in a single or divided dose.

Maintenance Anticonvulsant

IV, PO (Adults and Children >12 yr): 1–3 mg/kg/day as a single dose or 2 divided doses.
IV, PO (Children 5–12 yr): 4–6 mg/kg/day in 1–2 divided doses.
IV, PO (Children 1–5 yr): 6–8 mg/kg/day in 1–2 divided doses.
IV, PO (Infants): 5–6 mg/kg/day in 1–2 divided doses.
IV, PO (Neonates): 3–4 mg/kg/day once daily, may need to increase up to 5 mg/kg/day by 2nd wk of therapy.

Sedation

PO, IM (Adults): 30–120 mg/day in 2–3 divided doses. *Preoperative sedation*—100–200 mg IM 1–1.5 hrs before the procedure.
PO (Children): 2 mg/kg 3 times daily. *Preoperative sedation*—1–3 mg/kg PO/IM/IV 1–1.5 hrs before the procedure.

Hypnotic

PO, Subcut, IV, IM (Adults): 100–320 mg at bedtime.
IV, IM, Subcut (Children): 3–5 mg/kg at bedtime.

Hyperbilirubinemia

PO (Adults): 90–180 mg/day in 2–3 divided doses.
PO (Children <12 yr): 3–8 mg/kg/day in 2–3 divided doses, doses up to 12 mg/kg/day have been used.

Availability (generic available)

Tablets: 15 mg, 30 mg, 60 mg, 100 mg. **Elixir:** 20 mg/5 mL. **Injection:** 65 mg/mL, 130 mg/mL.

NURSING IMPLICATIONS

Assessment

- Monitor respiratory status, pulse, and BP, and signs and symptoms of angioedema (swelling of lips, face, throat, dyspnea) frequently in patients receiving phenobarbital IV. Equipment for resuscitation and artificial ventilation should be readily available. Respiratory depression is dose-dependent.
- Prolonged therapy may lead to psychological or physical dependence. Restrict amount of drug available to patient, especially if depressed, suicidal, or with a history of addiction.
- Geri: Elderly patients may react to phenobarbital with marked excitement, depression, and confusion. Monitor for these adverse reactions.
- **Seizures:** Assess location, duration, and characteristics of seizure activity.
- **Sedation:** Assess level of consciousness and anxiety when used as a preoperative sedative.

- Assess postoperative patients for pain with a pain scale. Phenobarbital may increase sensitivity to painful stimuli.
- ***Lab Test Considerations:*** Patients on prolonged therapy should have hepatic and renal function and CBC evaluated periodically.
- Monitor serum folate concentrations periodically during therapy because of increased folate requirements of patients on long-term anticonvulsant therapy with phenobarbital.
- May cause ↓ serum bilirubin concentrations in neonates, in patients with congenital nonhemolytic unconjugated hyperbilirubinemia, and in epileptics.
- ***Toxicity and Overdose:*** Serum phenobarbital levels may be monitored when used as an anticonvulsant. Therapeutic blood levels are 10–40 mcg/mL. Symptoms of toxicity include confusion, drowsiness, dyspnea, slurred speech, and staggering.

Implementation

- Do not confuse phenobarbital with pentobarbital.
- Supervise ambulation and transfer of patients following administration. Two side rails should be raised and call bell within reach at all times. Keep bed in low position. Institute seizure and fall precautions.
- When changing from phenobarbital to another anticonvulsant, gradually decrease phenobarbital dose while concurrently increasing dose of replacement medication to maintain anticonvulsant effects.
- **PO:** Tablets may be crushed and mixed with food or fluids (do not administer dry) for patients with difficulty swallowing. Oral solution may be taken undiluted or mixed with water, milk, or fruit juice. Use calibrated measuring device for accurate measurement of liquid doses.
- **IM:** Injections should be given deep into the gluteal muscle to minimize tissue irritation. Do not inject >5 mL into any one site, because of tissue irritation.

IV Administration

- **IV:** Doses may require 15–30 min to reach peak concentrations in the brain. Administer minimal dose and wait for effectiveness before administering 2nd dose to prevent cumulative barbiturate-induced depression.
- **IV Push:** ***Diluent:*** Reconstitute sterile powder for IV dose with a minimum of 3 mL of sterile water for injection. Dilute further with 10 mL of sterile water. Do not use solution that is not absolutely clear within 5 min after reconstitution or that contains a precipitate. Discard powder or solution that has been exposed to air for longer than 30 min.
- Solution is highly alkaline; avoid extravasation, which may cause tissue damage and necrosis. If extravasation occurs, injection of 5% procaine solution into affected area and application of moist heat may be ordered.
- ***Concentration:*** 130 mg/mL (undiluted). ***Rate:*** Do not inject IV faster than 1 mg/kg/min with a maximum of 30 mg over 1 min in infants and children and 60 mg over 1 min in adults. Titrate slowly for desired response. Rapid administration may result in respiratory depression.
- **Y-Site Compatibility:** acyclovir, alfentanil, amikacin, aminocaproic acid, aminophylline, amphotericin B lipid complex, amphotericin B liposome, anidulafungin, argatroban, ascorbic acid, atropine, azathioprine, aztreonam, benztropine, bivalirudin, bleomycin, bumetanide, butorphanol, calcium chloride, calcium gluconate, carboplatin, cefazolin, ceftazidime, ceftriaxone, chloramphenicol, cisplatin, clindamycin, cyanocobalamin, cyclophosphamide, cytarabine, dactinomycin, daptomycin, dexamethasone, dexmedetomidine, digoxin, docetaxel, dopamine, doxacurium, doxapram, enalaprilat, ephedrine, epoetin alfa, eptifibatide, ertapenem, etoposide, etoposide phosphate, famotidine, fenoldopam, fentanyl, fluconazole, fludarabine, fluorouracil, folic acid, fosphenytoin, furosemide, ganciclovir, gemcitabine, gentamicin, glycopyrrolate, granisetron, heparin, hetastarch, hydrocortisone, ifosfamide, indomethacin, insulin, irinotecan, ketorolac, labetalol, linezolid, lorazepam, magnesium sulfate, mannitol, meropenem, metaraminol, methadone, methotrexate, methoxamine, methylprednisolone, metoclopramide, metoprolol, metronidazole, milrinone, mitoxantrone, morphine, multivitamins, nafcillin, naloxone, nitroglycerin, nitroprusside, octreotide, oxacillin, oxytocin, paclitaxel, palonosetron, pamidronate, pancuronium, pantoprazole, pemetrexed, pentobarbital, phenylephrine, phytonadione, piperacillin/tazobactam, potassium acetate, potassium chloride, procainamide, propofol, propranolol, ranitidine, rocuronium, sodium acetate, sodium bicarbonate, streptokinase, sufentanil, theophylline, thiotepa, tigecycline, tirofiban, tobramycin, tolazoline, trimetaphan, vancomycin, vasopressin, vecuronium, vincristine, voriconazole, zoledronic acid.
- **Y-Site Incompatibility:** alemtuzumab, amphotericin B cholesteryl, ampicillin, atracurium, buprenorphine, carmustine, caspofungin, cefotaxime, cefotetan, cefoxitin, cefuroxime, chlorpromazine, cyclophosphamide, dantrolene, diazepam, diazoxide, diltiazem, diphenhydramine, dobutamine, doxorubicin, doxycycline, epinephrine, erythromycin, esmolol, haloperidol, hydroxyzine, idarubicin, isoproterenol, lidocaine, meperidine, methyldopate, midazolam, mycophenolate, nalbuphine, norepinephrine, ondansetron, papaverine, penicillin G, pentamidine, phenytoin, prochlorperazine, promethazine, protamine, pyridoxime, quinupristin/dalfo-

P

pristin, succinylcholine, thiamine, trimethoprim/sulfamethoxazole, verapamil, vinorelbine.

Patient/Family Teaching

- Advise patient to take medication as directed. Take missed doses as soon as remembered if not almost time for next dose; do not double doses.
- Advise patients on prolonged therapy not to discontinue medication without consulting health care professional. Abrupt withdrawal may precipitate seizures or status epilepticus.
- Medication may cause daytime drowsiness. Caution patient to avoid driving and other activities requiring alertness until response to medication is known. Do not resume driving until physician gives clearance based on control of seizure disorder.
- Caution patient to avoid taking alcohol or other CNS depressants concurrently with this medication.
- Advise patient to notify health care professional if signs and symptoms of angioedema, fever, sore throat, mouth sores, unusual bleeding or bruising, nosebleeds, or petechiae occur.
- Teach sleep hygiene techniques (dark room, quiet, bedtime ritual, limit daytime napping, avoid nicotine and caffeine).
- Advise female patients using oral contraceptives to use an additional nonhormonal contraceptive during therapy and until next menstrual period. Instruct patient to contact health care professional immediately if pregnancy is planned or suspected.
- Pedi: Advise parents or caregivers that child may experience irritability, hyperactivity, and/or sleep disturbances, which may diminish in a few days to a few wk or may persist until drug is stopped. An alternative medication can be considered. Instruct parents to monitor for skin rash occurring 7–20 days after treatment begins and to contact a health care provider if rash occurs. Teach family about symptoms of toxicity (staggering, drowsiness, slurred speech).

Evaluation/Desired Outcomes

- Decrease or cessation of seizure activity without excessive sedation. Several wk may be required to achieve maximum anticonvulsant effects.
- Preoperative sedation.
- Improvement in sleep patterns.
- Decrease in serum bilirubin levels.

REMS

phentermine/topiramate

(**fen**-ter-meen/toe-**pyre**-a-mate)

Qsymia

Classification

Therapeutic: weight control agents

Pharmacologic: appetite suppressants

Schedule IV

Indications

Weight management as part of a program including caloric restriction and increased exercise in patients with an initial body mass index (BMI) of ≥30 kg/m² or a BMI of ≥27 kg/m² with at least one other risk factor (hypertension, type 2 diabetes mellitus, or dyslipidemia).

Action

Phentermine—↓ appetite and food consumption; *Topiramate*—↓ appetite and enhances satiety. **Therapeutic Effects:** Weight loss.

Pharmacokinetics

Absorption: *Phentermine*—Unknown; *Topiramate*—80% absorbed following oral administration.

Distribution: *Phentermine*—Unknown; *Topiramate*—Unknown.

Metabolism and Excretion: *Phentermine*—metabolized by the liver; *Topiramate*—70% excreted unchanged in urine.

Half-life: *Phentermine*—19–24 hr; *Topiramate*—21 hr.

TIME/ACTION PROFILE (phentermine—appetite suppression, topiramate—blood levels)

ROUTE	ONSET	PEAK	DURATION
PO (weight loss)	within 8 wk	16–32 wk	unknown

Contraindications/Precautions

Contraindicated in: Hypersensitivity/idiosyncracy to sympathomimetics; OB: May cause fetal harm; Lactation: Avoid breast feeding; Glaucoma; Hyperthyroidism; During/within 14 days of MAO inhibitors; Severe renal impairment (CCr <30 mL/min); Severe hepatic impairment; History of suicidal thought/active suicidal ideation.

Use Cautiously in: Diabetes (weight loss may ↑ risk of hypoglycemia); History of substance abuse; Rep: Women of reproductive potential; Geri: ↑ risk of adverse effects, consider age-related ↓ in cardiac, renal, and hepatic function, concurrent chronic disease states and medications; Pedi: Safety and effectiveness not established.

Adverse Reactions/Side Effects

CNS: SEIZURES (FOLLOWING ABRUPT DISCONTINUATION), headache, insomnia, cognitive impairment, dizziness, mood disorders, suicidal ideation. **CV:** tachycardia, hypotension, palpitations. **Derm:** ERYTHEMA MULTIFORME, STEVENS-JOHNSON SYNDROME, TOXIC EPIDERMAL NECROLYSIS, alopecia, oligohydrosis (↓ sweating). **EENT:** acute myopia, blurred vision, eye pain, secondary angle closure glaucoma. **Endo:** hypoglycemia. **F and E:** metabolic acidosis, hypokalemia. **GI:** HEPATOTOXICITY, altered taste, constipation, dry mouth. **GU:** ↑ serum creatinine, kidney stones. **Neuro:** paraesthesia. **Misc:** hyperthermia.

Interactions

Drug-Drug: ↑ risk of hypokalemia with **non-potassium sparing diuretics**. ↑ risk of CNS depression with **other CNS depressants** including **alcohol**, some **antihistamines**, **sedative/hypnotics**, **antipsychotics**, and **opioid analgesics**; avoid concurrent use of alcohol. Altered exposure to **oral contraceptives** may ↑ risk of irregular bleeding. Blood levels of topiramate may be ↓ by **carbamazepine** or **phenytoin**. Concurrent use of topiramate with **valproic acid** may ↑ risk of hyperammonemia. Concurrent use of topiramate with **carbonic anhydrase inhibitors** may ↑ risk of metabolic acidosis and kidney stones. ↑ risk of hypotension with **antihypertensive** and **diuretics**. May ↓ **pioglitazone** levels.

Route/Dosage

PO (Adults): *Initial dose*—one phentermine 3.75 mg/topiramate 23 mg capsule once daily for 14 days, then ↑ to one phentermine 7.5 mg/topiramate 46 mg capsule once daily for 12 wk, then assess weight loss. If weight loss has not exeeded 3% of baseline, discontinue or ↑ dose to one phentermine 11.25 mg/topiramate 69 mg capsule once daily for 14 days, then one phentermine 15 mg/topiramate 92 mg capsule once daily for 12 wk, if weight loss has not exceeded 5% of baseline, discontinue as success is unlikely. Discontinuation should proceed by taking the phentermine 15 mg/topiramate 92 mg capsule every other day for 1 wk.

Renal Impairment

PO (Adults): *CCr ≥30 mL/min–<50 mL/min*—daily dose should not exceed one phentermine 7.5 mg/topiramate 46 mg capsule once daily.

Hepatic Impairment

PO (Adults): *Child-Pugh score 7–9*—daily dose should not exceed one phentermine 7.5 mg/topiramate 46 mg capsule once daily.

Availability

Capsules (contain tartrazine): phentermine 3.75 mg (immediate-release)/topiramate 23 mg (extended-release) (for titration only), phentermine 7.5 mg (immediate-release)/topiramate 46 mg (extended-release), phentermine 11.25 mg (immediate-release)/topiramate 69 mg (extended-release) (for titration only), phentermine 15 mg (immediate-release)/topiramate 92 mg (extended-release). **Cost:** 3.75 mg/23 mg $163.24/30, 7.5 mg/46 mg $184.49/30, 11.25 mg/69 mg $221.38/30, 15 mg/92 mg $239.40/30.

NURSING IMPLICATIONS

Assessment

- Monitor patients for weight loss and adjust concurrent medications (antihypertensives, antidiabetics, lipid-lowering agents) as needed. Evaluate weight loss after each 12 wk of therapy.
- Monitor closely for notable changes in behavior that could indicate the emergence or worsening of suicidal thoughts or behavior or depression. Discontinue phentermine/topiramate if these occur.
- Monitor BP and heart rate periodically during therapy; may cause increase in resting heart rate. May cause hypotension in patients treated with antihypertensives.
- ***Lab Test Considerations:*** Obtain a negative pregnancy test prior to starting therapy and monthly during therapy.
- May cause hypoglycemia; monitor blood glucose closely in diabetic patients.
- May cause metabolic acidosis; monitor serum bicarbonate, prior to starting and periodically during therapy.
- May cause ↑ serum creatinine; peak increases observed after 4–8 wk of therapy. Monitor serum creatinine prior to and periodically during therapy; if persistent elevations occur, decrease dose or discontinue therapy.
- May cause hypokalemia; monitor serum potassium periodically during therapy.

Implementation

- Qsymia is only available through certified pharmacies that are enrolled in the Qsymia certified pharmacy network. Information can be obtained at www.QsymiaREMS.com or by calling 1-888-998-4887.
- **PO:** Administer once daily in the morning without regard to food. Avoid dosing in the evening; may cause insomnia.

Patient/Family Teaching

- Instruct patient to take phentermine/topiramate as directed. Do not stop taking without consulting health care professional. Discontinue gradually taking 1 dose every other day for at least 1 wk to prevent seizures.
- Advise patient to notify health care professional if sustained periods of heart pounding or racing while at rest; severe and persistent eye pain or significant changes in vision; changes in attention, concentration, memory, and/or difficulty finding words; factors that can increase risk of acidosis (prolonged diarrhea, surgery, high protein/low carbohydrate diet, and/or concomitant medications).
- Inform patients and families of risk of suicidal thoughts and behavior (behavioral changes, emerging or worsening signs and symptoms of depression, unusual changes in mood, or emergence of suicidal thoughts, behavior, or thoughts of self-harm). Advise that these should be reported to health care professional immediately.
- May cause changes in mental performance, motor performance, and/or vision. Caution patients to

P

avoid driving and other activities requiring alertness until response to medication is known.

- Instruct patient to increase fluid intake to increase urinary output and decrease risk of kidney stones.
- Advise patient to monitor for decreased sweating and increased body temperature during physical activity, especially in hot weather.
- Instruct patient to notify health care professional of all Rx or OTC medications, vitamins, or herbal products being taken and consult health care professional before taking any new medications. Advise patient to avoid taking other CNS depressants or alcohol.
- Phentermine/topiramate is teratogenic. Advise females of reproductive potential to use effective contraception and avoid breast feeding during therapy. Advise female patients to notify health care professional if pregnancy is planned or suspected. Encourage patients who become pregnant during therapy to enroll in the pregnancy registry to monitor maternal fetal outcomes by calling 1-888-998-4887.

Evaluation/Desired Outcomes

- Decrease in weight and BMI. If 3% of baseline body weight is not lost by Week 12, increase dose or discontinue phentermine/topiramate. Evaluate after second 12 wk of therapy. If 5% of baseline body weight is not lost by second 12 wk of therapy, as it is unlikely patient will achieve and sustain clinically meaningful weight loss with continued treatment.

HIGH ALERT

phenylephrine (fen-il-eff-rin)

Neo-Synephrine, Vazculep

Classification

Therapeutic: vasopressors

Pharmacologic: adrenergics, alpha adrenergic agonists, vasopressors

For ophthalmic use see Appendix C

Indications

Management of hypotension associated with shock that may persist after adequate fluid replacement. Management of hypotension associated with anesthesia. **Anesthesia adjunct:** Prolongation of the duration of spinal anesthesia. Localization of the effect of regional anesthesia.

Action

Constricts blood vessels by stimulating alpha-adrenergic receptors. **Therapeutic Effects:** Increased BP.

Pharmacokinetics

Absorption: Well absorbed from IM sites. IV administration results in complete bioavailability.

Distribution: Highly distributed into organs and tissues.

Metabolism and Excretion: Metabolized by the liver into inactive metabolites.

Half-life: 2.5 hr.

TIME/ACTION PROFILE (vasopressor effects)

ROUTE	ONSET	PEAK	DURATION
IV	immediate	unknown	15–20 min
IM	10–15 min	unknown	0.5–2 hr
Subcut	10–15 min	unknown	50–60 min

Contraindications/Precautions

Contraindicated in: Hypersensitivity to bisulfites.

Use Cautiously in: HF, coronary artery disease, or peripheral arterial disease; OB, Lactation: Safety not established.

Adverse Reactions/Side Effects

CNS: blurred vision, headache, insomnia, nervousness, tremor. **Resp:** dyspnea. **CV:** ARRHYTHMIAS, bradycardia, chest pain, hypertension, ischemia, tachycardia. **Derm:** pruritis. **GI:** epigastric pain, nausea, vomiting. **Local:** phlebitis, sloughing at IV sites.

Interactions

Drug-Drug: Use with **general anesthetics** may result in myocardial irritability; use with extreme caution. Use with **MAO inhibitors**, **ergot alkaloids (methylergonovine)**, **oxytocics**, **tricyclic antidepressants**, **atropine**, **corticosteroids**, or **atomoxetine** results in severe hypertension. **Alpha-adrenergic blockers**, **phosphodiesterase-5 inhibitors**, **calcium channel blockers**, **benzodiazepines**, **ACE inhibitors**, or **guanfacine** may antagonize vasopressor effects.

Route/Dosage

Hypotension

Subcut, IM (Adults): 2–5 mg.

Subcut, IM (Children): 0.1 mg/kg/dose every 1–2 hr as needed, maximum dose 5 mg.

IV (Adults): 0.2 mg (range 0.1–0.5 mg), may be repeated every 10–15 min *or* as an infusion at 100–180 mcg/min initially, 40–60 mcg/min maintenance.

IV (Children): 5–20 mcg/kg/dose every 10–15 min as needed or 0.1–0.5 mcg/kg/min infusion, titrate to effect.

Hypotension during Anesthesia

Subcut, IM (Adults): 2–3 mg has been used 3–4 min before spinal anesthesia to prevent hypotension.

IM, Subcut (Children): —0.5–1 mg/25 lb body weight.

IV (Adults): 40–100 mcg; may repeat every 1–2 min as needed (not to exceed total dose of 200 mcg); if BP remains low, initiate continuous infusion at 10–35 mcg/min (not to exceed 200 mcg/min).

Vasoconstrictor for Regional Anesthesia

Local (Adults): Add 1 mg to every 20 mL of local anesthetic (yields a 1:20,000 solution).

Prolongation of Spinal Anesthesia

Spinal (Adults): 2–5 mg added to anesthetic solution.

Availability (generic available)

Injection: 10 mg/mL.

NURSING IMPLICATIONS

Assessment

- Monitor BP every 2–3 min until stabilized and every 5 min thereafter during IV administration.
- Monitor ECG continuously for arrhythmias during IV administration.
- Assess IV site frequently throughout infusion. Antecubital or other large vein should be used to minimize risk of extravasation, which may cause tissue necrosis.

Implementation

- ***High Alert:*** Patient harm and fatalities have occurred from medication errors with phenylephrine. Prior to administration, have second practitioner independently check original order, dose calculations, concentration, route of administration and infusion pump settings.

IV Administration

- **IV:** Blood volume depletion should be corrected, if possible, before initiation of IV phenylephrine.
- **IV Push: *Diluent:*** Dilute each 1 mg with 9 mL of sterile water for injection or D5W. ***Rate:*** Administer each single dose over 1 min.
- **Continuous Infusion: *Diluent:*** Dilute 10 mg in 250 or 500 mL of D5W or 0.9% NaCl. ***Concentration:*** 125,000 or 150,000 solution, respectively. ***Rate:*** Titrate rate according to patient response. Infuse via infusion pump to ensure accurate dose rate.
- **Y-Site Compatibility:** alemtuzumab, alfentanil, amikacin, aminophylline, amiodarone, amphotericin B liposome, anidulafungin, argatroban, ascorbic acid, asparaginase, atracurium, atropine, aztreonam, benztropine, bivalirudin, bleomycin, bumetanide, buprenorphine, butorphanol, calcium chloride, calcium gluconate, cangrelor, carboplatin, carmustine, caspofungin, cefazolin, cefotaxime, cefotetan, cefoxitin, ceftazidime, ceftriaxone, chloramphenicol, cisatracurium, cisplatin, clindamycin, cyanocobalamin, cyclophosphamide, cyclosporine, cytarabine, dactinomycin, daptomycin, daunorubicin, dexamethasone, dexmedetomidine, dexrazoxane, digoxin, diltiazem, diphenhydramine, dobutamine, docetaxel, dolasetron, dopamine, doxacurium, doxorubicin hydrochloride, doxycycline, enalaprilat, ephedrine, epinephrine, epirubicin, epoetin alfa, eptifibatide, ertapenem, erythromycin, esmolol, etomidate, etoposide, etoposide phosphate, famotidine, fenoldopam, fentanyl, fluconazole, fludarabine, fluorouracil, folic acid, foscarnet, fosphenytoin, gentamicin, glycopyrrolate, granisetron, heparin, hetastarch, hydrocortisone, hydromorphone, idarubicin, ifosfamide, imipenem/cilastatin, irinotecan, isoproterenol, ketorolac, labetalol, leucovorin calcium, levofloxacin, lidocaine, linezolid, lorazepam, magnesium sulfate, mannitol, meperidine, mesna, metaraminol, methotrexate, methylprednisolone, metoclopramide, metoprolol, metronidazole, micafungin, midazolam, milrinone, mitoxantrone, morphine, multivitamins, mycophenolate, nafcillin, nalbuphine, naloxone, nicardipine, nitroglycerin, nitroprusside, norepinephrine, octreotide, ondansetron, oxacillin, oxaliplatin, oxytocin, paclitaxel, palonosetron, pamidronate, pancuronium, pantoprazole, penicillin G, pentobarbital, phenobarbital, phytonadione, piperacillin/tazobactam, potassium acetate, potassium chloride, procainamide, prochlorperazine, promethazine, propranolol, protamine, pyridoxime, quinupristin/dalfopristin, ranitidine, remifentanil, rocuronium, sodium acetate, sodium bicarbonate, streptokinase, succinylcholine, sufentanil, tacrolimus, telavancin, theophylline, thiamine, thiotepa, tigecycline, tirofiban, tobramycin, tolazoline, topotecan, vancomycin, vasopressin, vecuronium, verapamil, vinblastine, vincristine, vinorelbine, voriconazole, zidovudine, zoledronic acid.
- **Y-Site Incompatibility:** acyclovir, amphotericin B deoxycholate, amphotericin B lipid complex, azathioprine, dantrolene, diazepam, diazoxide, ganciclovir, indomethacin, insulin, mitomycin, pentamidine, phenytoin, trimethoprim/sulfamethoxazole, thiopental.
- **Anesthesia:** Phenylephrine 2–5 mg may be added to spinal anesthetic solution to prolong anesthesia.
- Phenylephrine 1 mg may be added to each 20 mL of local anesthetic to produce vasoconstriction.

Patient/Family Teaching

- **IV:** Instruct patient to report headache, dizziness, dyspnea, or pain at IV infusion site promptly.

Evaluation/Desired Outcomes

- Increase in BP to normal range.
- Prolonged duration of spinal anesthesia.
- Localization of regional anesthesia.

♒ phenytoin (fen-i-toyn)

Dilantin, Phenytek, ✱Tremytoine

Classification

Therapeutic: antiarrhythmics (group IB), anticonvulsants

Pharmacologic: hydantoins

Indications

Treatment/prevention of tonic-clonic (grand mal) seizures and complex partial seizures. **Unlabeled Use:** As an antiarrhythmic, particularly for ventricular arrhythmias associated with digoxin toxicity, prolonged QT interval, and surgical repair of congenital heart diseases in children. Management of neuropathic pain, including trigeminal neuralgia.

P

Action

Limits seizure propagation by altering ion transport. May also decrease synaptic transmission. Antiarrhythmic properties as a result of shortening the action potential and decreasing automaticity. **Therapeutic Effects:** Diminished seizure activity. Termination of ventricular arrhythmias.

Pharmacokinetics

Absorption: Absorbed slowly from the GI tract. Bioavailability differs among products; the Dilantin and Phenytek preparations are considered to be "extended" products. Other products are considered to be prompt release.

Distribution: Distributes into CSF and other body tissues and fluids. Enters breast milk; crosses the placenta, achieving similar maternal/fetal levels. Preferentially distributes into fatty tissue.

Protein Binding: Adults 90–95%; ↓ protein binding in neonates (up to 20% free fraction available), infants (up to 15% free), and patients with hyperbilirubinemia, hypoalbuminemia, severe renal dysfunction or uremia.

Metabolism and Excretion: Mostly metabolized by the liver; minimal amounts excreted in the urine.

Half-life: 22 hr (range 7–42 hr).

TIME/ACTION PROFILE (anticonvulsant effect)

ROUTE	ONSET	PEAK	DURATION
PO	2–24 hr (1 wk)*	1.5–3 hr	6–12 hr
PO-ER	2–24 hr (1 wk)	4–12 hr	12–36 hr
IV	0.5–1 hr (1 wk)	rapid	12–24 hr

*() = time required for onset of action without a loading dose.

Contraindications/Precautions

Contraindicated in: Hypersensitivity; Hypersensitivity to propylene glycol (phenytoin injection only); History of hepatotoxicity related to phenytoin; Alcohol intolerance (phenytoin injection and liquid only); Sinus bradycardia, sinoatrial block, 2nd- or 3rd-degree heart block, or Stokes-Adams syndrome (phenytoin injection only); Concurrent use of delavirdine; OB: May cause fetal harm (↑ risk of congenital anomalies; ↑ risk of hemorrhage in newborn if used at term).

Use Cautiously in: All patients (may ↑ risk of suicidal thoughts/behaviors); Hepatic or renal disease (↑ risk of adverse reactions; dose reduction recommended for hepatic impairment); Severe cardiac or respiratory disease (use of IV phenytoin may result in an ↑ risk of serious adverse reactions); Cardiac disease (↑ risk of cardiac arrest or bradycardia); Lactation: Present in breast milk; should weigh risk of potential adverse effects on infant versus potential benefit to mother; Pedi: Suspension contains sodium benzoate, a metabolite of benzyl alcohol that can cause potentially fatal gasping syndrome in neonates; Geri: Use of IV phenytoin may result in an ↑ risk of serious adverse reactions.

Exercise Extreme Caution in: Patients positive for HLA-B*1502 allele (unless exceptional circumstances exist where benefits clearly outweigh the risks).

Adverse Reactions/Side Effects

Most listed are for chronic use of phenytoin.

CNS: SUICIDAL THOUGHTS, ataxia, agitation, confusion, dizziness, drowsiness, dysarthria, dyskinesia, extrapyramidal syndrome, headache, insomnia, vertigo, weakness. **CV:** CARDIAC ARREST, hypotension (↑ with IV phenytoin), bradycardia, tachycardia. **Derm:** ACUTE GENERALIZED EXANTHEMATOUS PUSTULOSIS, DRUG REACTION WITH EOSINOPHILIA AND SYSTEMIC SYMPTOMS (DRESS), STEVENS-JOHNSON SYNDROME, TOXIC EPIDERMAL NECROLYSIS, hypertrichosis, rash, exfoliative dermatitis, pruritus, purple glove syndrome. **EENT:** diplopia, nystagmus. **GI:** ACUTE HEPATIC FAILURE, gingival hyperplasia, nausea, constipation, drug-induced hepatitis, vomiting. **Hemat:** AGRANULOCYTOSIS, APLASTIC ANEMIA, leukopenia, megaloblastic anemia, thrombocytopenia. **MS:** osteomalacia, osteoporosis. **Misc:** ANGIOEDEMA, fever, lymphadenopathy.

Interactions

Drug-Drug: May ↓ the effects of **delavirdine**, resulting in loss of virologic response and potential resistant (concurrent use contraindicated). Acute ingestion of **alcohol**, **amiodarone**, **benzodiazepines**, **capecitabine**, **chloramphenicol**, **chlordiazepoxide**, **cimetidine**, **disulfiram**, **estrogens**, **ethosuximide**, **felbamate**, **fluconazole**, **fluorouracil**, **fluoxetine**, **fluvastatin**, **fluvoxamine**, **halothane**, **isoniazid**, **itraconazole**, **ketoconazole**, **methylphenidate**, **miconazole**, **oxcarbazepine**, **omeprazole**, **phenothiazines**, **salicylates**, **sertraline**, **succinamides**, **sulfonamides**, **tolbutamide**, **trazodone**, **voriconazole**, and **warfarin** may ↑ levels. Chronic ingestion of **alcohol**, **barbiturates**, **carbamazepine**, **diazepam**, **diazoxide**, **fosamprenavir**, **nelfinavir**, **rifampin**, **ritonavir**, **sucralfate**, **theophylline**, and **vigabatrin** may ↓ levels. May ↓ the effects of **albendazole**, **amiodarone**, **atorvastatin**, **benzodiazepines**, **carbamazepine**, **clozapine**, **cyclosporine**, **digoxin**, **efavirenz**, **estrogens**, **felbamate**, **fluvastatin**, **indinavir**, **lamotrigine**, **lopinavir/ritonavir**, **methadone**, **mexiletine**, **nelfinavir**, **nifedipine**, **nimodipine**, **nisoldipine**, **oxcarbazepine**, **oral contraceptives**, **quetiapine**, **quinidine**, **rifampin**, **ritonavir**, **saquinavir**, **simvastatin**, **tacrolimus**, **theophylline**, **topiramate**, **verapamil**, and **warfarin**. IV phenytoin and **dopamine** may cause additive hypotension. Additive CNS depression with other **CNS depressants**, including **alcohol**, **antihistamines**, **antidepressants**, **opioids**, and **sedative/hypnotics**. **Antacids** may ↓ absorption of orally administered phenytoin. ↑ systemic clearance of antileukemic drug **methotrexate** which

has been associated with a worse event free survival, phenytoin use is not recommended in children undergoing chemotherapy for acute lymphocytic leukemia.
Drug-Natural Products: St. John's wort may ↓ levels.
Drug-Food: Phenytoin may ↓ absorption of **folic acid**. Concurrent administration of **enteral tube feedings** may ↓ phenytoin absorption. **Folic acid** may ↓ levels.

Route/Dosage

IM administration is not recommended due to erratic absorption and pain on injection. Oral route should be used whenever possible.

Anticonvulsant

PO (Adults): Loading dose of 15–20 mg/kg as extended capsules in 3 divided doses given every 2–4 hr; maintenance dose 5–6 mg/kg/day given in 1–3 divided doses; usual dosing range = 200–1200 mg/day.
PO (Children 10–16 yr): 6–7 mg/kg/day in 2–3 divided doses.
PO (Children 7–9 yr): 7–8 mg/kg/day in 2–3 divided doses.
PO (Children 4–6 yr): 7.5–9 mg/kg/day in 2–3 divided doses.
PO (Children 0.5–3 yr): 8–10 mg/kg/day in 2–3 divided doses.
PO (Neonates up to 6 mo): 5–8 mg/kg/day in 2 divided doses, may require every 8 hr dosing.
IV (Adults): *Status epilepticus loading dose*—15–20 mg/kg. Rate not to exceed 25–50 mg/min. *Maintenance dose*—same as PO dosing above.
IV (Children): *Status epilepticus loading dose*—15–20 mg/kg at 1–3 mg/kg/min. *Maintenance dose*—same as PO dosing above.

Antiarrhythmic

IV (Adults): 50–100 mg every 10–15 min until arrhythmia is abolished, or a total of 15 mg/kg has been given, or toxicity occurs.
PO (Adults): Loading dose: 250 mg 4 times daily for 1 day, then 250 mg twice daily for 2 days, then maintenance at 300–400 mg/day in divided doses 1–4 times/day.
IV (Children): 1.25 mg/kg every 5 min, may repeat up to total loading dose of 15 mg/kg. *Maintenance dose*—5–10 mg/kg/day in 2–3 divided doses IV or PO.

Availability (generic available)

Chewable tablets: 50 mg. **Cost:** *Generic*—$52.63/100. **Extended-release capsules:** 30 mg, 100 mg, 200 mg, 300 mg. **Cost:** *Generic*—100 mg $33.90/100, 200 mg $24.00/30, 300 mg $34.94/30. **Oral suspension:** 🍁 30 mg/5 mL, 125 mg/5 mL. **Cost:** $36.97/237 mL. **Solution for injection:** 50 mg/mL.

NURSING IMPLICATIONS

Assessment

- Monitor closely for notable changes in behavior that could indicate the emergence or worsening of suicidal thoughts or behavior or depression.
- Assess oral hygiene. Vigorous cleaning beginning within 10 days of initiation of phenytoin therapy may help control gingival hyperplasia.
- Assess patient for phenytoin hypersensitivity syndrome (fever, skin rash, lymphadenopathy). Rash usually occurs within the first 2 wk of therapy. Hypersensitivity syndrome usually occurs at 3–8 wk but may occur up to 12 wk after initiation of therapy. May lead to renal failure, rhabdomyolysis, or hepatic necrosis; may be fatal.
- Observe patient for development of rash. Discontinue phenytoin at the first sign of skin reactions. Serious adverse reactions such as exfoliative, purpuric, or bullous rashes or the development of lupus erythematosus, Stevens-Johnson syndrome, or toxic epidermal necrolysis preclude further use of phenytoin or fosphenytoin. 🧬 Stevens-Johnson syndrome and toxic epidermal necrolysis are significantly more common in patients with a particular human leukocyte antigen (HLA) allele, HLA-B*1502 (occurs almost exclusively in patients with Asian ancestry, including Han Chinese, Filipinos, Malaysians, South Asian Indians, and Thais). Avoid using phenytoin or fosphenytoin as alternatives to carbamazepine for patients who test positive. If less serious skin eruptions (measles-like or scarlatiniform) occur, phenytoin may be resumed after complete clearing of the rash. If rash reappears, further use of fosphenytoin or phenytoin should be avoided.
- Assess mental status (orientation, mood, behavior) before and periodically during therapy. Monitor closely for notable changes in behavior that could indicate the emergence or worsening of suicidal thoughts or behavior or depression.
- Monitor for signs and symptoms of DRESS (fever, rash, lymphadenopathy, and/or facial swelling), associated with involvement of other organ systems (hepatitis, nephritis, hematologic abnormalities, myocarditis, myositis) during therapy. May resemble an acute viral infection. Eosinophilia is often present. Discontinue therapy if signs occur.
- **Seizures:** Assess location, duration, frequency, and characteristics of seizure activity. EEG may be monitored periodically throughout therapy.
- Monitor BP, ECG, and respiratory function continuously during administration of IV phenytoin and throughout period when peak serum phenytoin levels occur (15–30 min after administration).
- **Arrhythmias:** Monitor ECG continuously during treatment of arrhythmias.

- ***Lab Test Considerations:*** Monitor CBC, serum calcium, albumin, and hepatic function tests prior to and monthly for the first several mo, then periodically during therapy.
- May cause ↑ serum alkaline phosphatase, GGT, and glucose levels.
- Monitor serum folate concentrations periodically during prolonged therapy.
- ***Toxicity and Overdose:*** Monitor serum phenytoin levels routinely. Therapeutic blood levels are 10–20 mcg/mL (8–15 mcg/mL in neonates) in patients with normal serum albumin and renal function. In patients with altered protein binding (neonates, patients with renal failure, hypoalbuminemia, acute trauma), free phenytoin serum concentrations should be monitored. Therapeutic serum free phenytoin levels are 1–2 mcg/mL.
- Progressive signs and symptoms of phenytoin toxicity include nystagmus, ataxia, confusion, nausea, slurred speech, and dizziness.

Implementation

- Implement seizure precautions.
- When transferring from phenytoin to another anticonvulsant, dosage adjustments are made gradually over several wk.
- When substituting *fosphenytoin* for oral *phenytoin* therapy, the same total daily dose may be given as a single dose. Unlike parenteral phenytoin, fosphenytoin may be given safely by the IM route.
- Administer vitamin K just before delivery to women taking phenytoin during pregnancy to prevent potentially life-threatening bleeding disorder related to decreased levels of vitamin K-dependent clotting factors which may occur in newborns exposed to phenytoin in utero.
- **PO:** Administer with or immediately after meals to minimize GI irritation. Shake liquid preparations well before pouring. Use a calibrated measuring device for accurate dose. Chewable tablets must be crushed or chewed well before swallowing. Capsules may be opened and mixed with food or fluids for patients with difficulty swallowing. To prevent direct contact of alkaline drug with mucosa, have patient swallow a liquid first, follow with mixture of medication, then follow with a full glass of water or milk or with food.
- If patient is receiving enteral tube feedings, 2 hr should elapse between feeding and phenytoin administration. If phenytoin is administered via nasogastric tube, flush tube with 2–4 oz water before and after administration.
- Do not interchange chewable phenytoin tablets with phenytoin sodium capsules, because they are not bioequivalent.
- Capsules labeled "extended" may be used for once-a-day dose; those labeled "prompt" may result in toxic serum levels if used for once-a-day dose.

IV Administration

- **IV:** Slight yellow color will not alter solution potency. If refrigerated, may form precipitate, which dissolves after warming to room temperature. Discard solution that is not clear.
- To prevent precipitation and minimize local venous irritation, follow infusion with 0.9% NaCl through the same needle or catheter. Avoid extravasation; phenytoin is caustic to tissues; may lead to purple glove syndrome. Monitor infusion site closely.
- **IV Push:** Administer undiluted. ***Rate:*** Administer at a rate not to exceed 50 mg over 1 min in adults or 1–3 mg/kg/min in neonates. Rapid administration may result in severe hypotension, cardiovascular collapse, or CNS depression.
- **Intermittent Infusion:** ***Diluent:*** Administer by mixing with no more than 50 mL of 0.9% NaCl. ***Concentration:*** 1–10 mg/mL. Administer immediately following admixture. Use tubing with a 0.45- to 0.22-micron in-line filter. ***Rate:*** Complete infusion within 1 hr at a rate not to exceed 50 mg/min. In patients who may develop hypotension, patients with cardiovascular disease, or geriatric patients maximum rate of 25 mg/min [may be as low as 5–10 mg/min]. Maximum rate in neonates is 1–3 mg/kg/min. Monitor cardiac function and BP throughout infusion.
- **Y-Site Compatibility:** cisplatin.
- **Y-Site Incompatibility:** acyclovir, alemtuzumab, alfentanil, amikacin, aminocaproic acid, aminophylline, amphotericin B lipid complex, amphotericin B liposome, ampicillin, ampicillin/sulbactam, anidulafungin, argatroban, ascorbic acid, atropine, aztreonam, benztropine, bivalirudin, bumetanide, buprenorphine, butorphanol, calcium chloride, calcium gluconate, carboplatin, carmustine, caspofungin, cefazolin, cefepime, cefotaxime, cefotetan, cefoxitin, ceftazidime, ceftriaxone, cefuroxime, chloramphenicol, chlorpromazine, ciprofloxacin, clindamycin, cyanocobalamin, cyclophosphamide, cyclosporine, cytarabine, dactinomycin, dantrolene, daptomycin, dexamethasone, dexmedetomidine, dexrazoxane, diltiazem, digoxin, diltiazem, diphenhydramine, dobutamine, docetaxel, dopamine, doxorubicin hydrochloride, doxorubicin liposomal, doxycycline, enalaprilat, ephedrine, epinephrine, epirubicin, epoetin alfa, eptifibatide, ertapenem, erythromycin, etoposide, etoposide phosphate, fenoldopam, fentanyl, fludarabine, fluorouracil, folic acid, furosemide, ganciclovir, gemcitabine, gentamicin, glycopyrrolate, granisetron, haloperidol, heparin, hetastarch, hydralazine, hydrocortisone, hydromorphone, hydroxyzine, idarubicin, ifosfamide, imipenem/cilastatin, indomethacin, insulin, regular, irinotecan, isoproterenol, ketamine, ketorolac, labetalol, levofloxacin, lidocaine, linezolid, lorazepam, magnesium sulfate, mannitol, meperidine, mesna, methadone, methotrexate, methylprednisolone, metoclopramide, micafungin, midazolam, milrinone, mitoxantrone, morphine, moxifloxacin, multivitamin

infusion, mycophenolate, nafcillin, nalbuphine, naloxone, nicardipine, nitroglycerin, nitroprusside, norepinephrine, octreotide, ondansetron, oxacillin, oxytocin, paclitaxel, palonosetron, pamidronate, pantoprazole, papaverine, pemetrexed, penicillin G, pentamidine, pentobarbital, phenobarbital, phenylephrine, phytonadione, piperacillin/tazobactam, potassium acetate, potassium chloride, procainamide, prochlorperazine, promethazine, propofol, propranolol, protamine, pyridoxine, quinupristin/dalfopristin, ranitidine, rocuronium, sodium acetate, sodium bicarbonate, streptokinase, succinylcholine, sufentanil, tacrolimus, theophylline, thiamine, thiotepa, tigecycline, tirofiban, tobramycin, trimethoprim/sulfamethoxazole, vancomycin, vasopressin, vecuronium, verapamil, vinblastine, vincristine, vinorelbine, vitamin B complex with C, voriconazole, zoledronic acid.

- **Additive Incompatibility:** Do not admix with other solutions or medications, especially dextrose, because precipitation will occur.

Patient/Family Teaching

- Instruct patient to take medication as directed, at the same time each day. If a dose is missed from a once-a-day schedule, take as soon as possible and return to regular dosing schedule. If taking several doses a day, take missed dose as soon as possible within 4 hr of next scheduled dose; do not double doses. Consult health care professional if doses are missed for 2 consecutive days. Abrupt withdrawal may lead to status epilepticus.
- May cause drowsiness or dizziness. Caution patient to avoid driving or other activities requiring alertness until response to medication is known. Do not resume driving until physician gives clearance based on control of seizure disorder.
- Caution patient to avoid alcohol and CNS depressants. Advise patient to notify health care professional of all Rx or OTC medications, vitamins, or herbal products being taken and to consult with health care professional before taking other medications and alcohol.
- Instruct patient on importance of maintaining good dental hygiene and seeing dentist frequently for teeth cleaning to prevent tenderness, bleeding, and gingival hyperplasia. Institution of oral hygiene program within 10 days of initiation of phenytoin therapy may minimize growth rate and severity of gingival enlargement. Patients under 23 yr of age and those taking doses >500 mg/day are at increased risk for gingival hyperplasia.
- Advise patient that brands of phenytoin may not be equivalent. Check with health care professional if brand or dose form is changed.
- Advise diabetic patients to monitor blood glucose carefully and to notify health care professional of significant changes.
- Instruct patient to notify health care professional of medication regimen prior to treatment or surgery.
- Advise patient not to take phenytoin within 2–3 hr of antacids.
- Advise patient to carry identification describing disease process and medication regimen at all times.
- Instruct patients that behavioral changes, skin rash, fever, sore throat, mouth ulcers, easy bruising, petechiae, unusual bleeding, abdominal pain, chills, pale stools, dark urine, jaundice, severe nausea or vomiting, drowsiness, slurred speech, unsteady gait, swollen glands, or persistent headache should be reported to health care professional immediately. Advise patient and family to notify health care professional if thoughts about suicide or dying, attempts to commit suicide; new or worse depression; new or worse anxiety; feeling very agitated or restless; panic attacks; trouble sleeping; new or worse irritability; acting aggressive; being angry or violent; acting on dangerous impulses; an extreme increase in activity and talking, other unusual changes in behavior or mood occur.
- Rep: Advise female patients to use an additional nonhormonal method of contraception during therapy and until next menstrual period. Instruct patient to notify health care professional if pregnancy is planned or suspected. Encourage patients who become pregnant to enroll in the North American Antiepileptic Drug (NAAED) Pregnancy Registry by calling 1-888-233-2334 or on the web at www.aedpregnancyregistry.org. Enrollment must be done by patients themselves.
- Emphasize the importance of routine exams to monitor progress. Patient should have routine physical exams, especially monitoring skin and lymph nodes, and EEG testing.

Evaluation/Desired Outcomes

- Decrease or cessation of seizures without excessive sedation.
- Suppression of arrhythmias.
- Relief of neuropathic pain.

phosphate/biphosphate
(**foss**-fate/bye-**foss** -fate)
Fleet Enema, OsmoPrep

Classification
Therapeutic: laxatives (saline)

Indications
Intermittent treatment of chronic constipation. **OsmoPrep:** Cleansing of the bowel as a preparation for colonoscopy.

Action
Osmotically active in the lumen of the GI tract. Produces laxative effect by causing water retention and stimulation of peristalsis. Stimulates motility and inhibits fluid and electrolyte absorption from the small intestine. **Therapeutic Effects:** Relief of constipation. Emptying of the bowel.

Pharmacokinetics
Absorption: 1–20% of rectally administered sodium and phosphate may be absorbed; some absorption follows oral administration.
Distribution: Unknown.
Metabolism and Excretion: Excreted by the kidneys.
Half-life: Unknown.

TIME/ACTION PROFILE (laxative effect)

ROUTE	ONSET	PEAK	DURATION
PO	0.5–3 hr	unknown	unknown
Rect	2–5 min	unknown	unknown

Contraindications/Precautions
Contraindicated in: Hypersensitivity; Abdominal pain, nausea, or vomiting, especially when associated with fever or other signs of an acute abdomen; Severe renal or cardiovascular disease; Intestinal obstruction; OB: Not recommended for use at term; *OsmoPrep*—HF, ascites, unstable angina, acute colitis, toxic megacolon, or hypomotility syndrome; Pedi: Children <2 yr.
Use Cautiously in: Excessive or chronic use (may lead to dependence); Renal or cardiovascular disease, dehydration or concurrent use of diuretics or other drugs known to alter electrolytes (correct abnormalities prior to administration); Dehydration, renal dysfunction, bowel obstruction, active colitis, or concurrent use of diuretics, ACE inhibitors, ARBs, or NSAIDs (↑ risk of acute phosphate nephropathy); OB: May cause sodium retention and edema; Geri: May be more sensitive to effects.

Adverse Reactions/Side Effects
CNS: *Visicol*—dizziness, headache. **CV:** ARRHYTHMIAS. **GI:** cramping, nausea, colonic aphtous ulcerations, ischemic colitis; *OsmoPrep*, abdominal bloating, abdominal pain, vomiting. **F and E:** hyperphosphatemia, hypocalcemia, hypokalemia, sodium retention. **GU:** renal dysfunction.

Interactions
Drug-Drug: *OsmoPrep*—Concurrently administered oral medications may not be absorbed due to rapid peristalsis and diarrhea.

Route/Dosage
Each Fleet Enema contains 4.4 g sodium/118 mL.

Bowel Cleansing
PO (Adults): *OsmoPrep*—evening before colonoscopy: 4 tablets every 15 min (with at least 8 oz of water) for a total of 20 tablets; on morning of colonoscopy starting 3–5 hr before procedure, 4 tablets every 15 min (with at least 8 oz of clear liquids), for a total of 12 tablets; should not be repeated in less than 7 days.

Constipation
PO (Adults): 15 mL as single dose.
PO (Children 5–9 yr): 7.5 mL as single dose.
Rect (Adults and Children >12 yr): 118 mL Fleet Enema.
Rect (Children >2 yr): ½ of the adult dose.

Availability (generic available)
Oral solution: 0.9 g dibasic sodium phosphate and 2.4 g monobasic sodium biphosphate/5 mL. **Enema:** 7 g dibasic sodium phosphate and 19 g monobasic sodium biphosphate/118 mL. **Tablets (OsmoPrep):** 1.5 g.

NURSING IMPLICATIONS

Assessment
- Assess patient for fever, abdominal distention, presence of bowel sounds, and usual pattern of bowel function.
- Assess color, consistency, and amount of stool produced.
- May rarely cause arrhythmias. Monitor patients with underlying cardiovascular disease, renal disease, bowel perforation, misuse or overdose.
- ***Lab Test Considerations:*** May cause ↑ serum sodium and phosphorus levels, ↓ serum calcium and potassium levels, and acidosis. Electrolyte changes are transient, self-limiting, do not require treatment, and are not usually associated with adverse clinical events.

Implementation
- Do not administer at bedtime or late in the day.
- **PO:** Administer on an empty stomach for more rapid results. Mix dose in at least ½ glass cold water. May be followed by carbonated beverage or fruit juice to improve flavor.
- See Route and Dosage section for dosing of *OsmoPrep*.
- *Osmoprep:* Do not drink any red—or purple-colored liquids.
- **Rect:** Position patient on left side with knee slightly flexed. Insert prelubricated tip about 2 inches into rectum, aiming toward the umbilicus. Gently squeeze bottle until empty. Discontinue if resistance is met, because perforation may occur if contents are forced into rectum.

Patient/Family Teaching
- Advise patient that laxatives should be used only for short-term therapy. Avoid using more than 1 dose of OTC laxatives/day. Long-term therapy may cause electrolyte imbalance and dependence.

- Caution patient on sodium restriction that this product has a high sodium content.
- Advise patient not to take oral form of this medication within 2 hr of other medications.
- Encourage patient to use other forms of bowel regulation, such as increasing bulk in the diet, fluid intake, and mobility. Normal bowel habits may vary from 3 times/day to 3 times/wk.
- Advise patient to notify health care professional if unrelieved constipation, rectal bleeding, or symptoms of electrolyte imbalance (muscle cramps or pain, weakness, dizziness, and so forth) occur.

Evaluation/Desired Outcomes

- Soft, formed bowel movement.
- Evacuation of the bowel.

phytonadione

(fye-toe-na-**dye**-one)

Mephyton, vitamin K

Classification

Therapeutic: antidotes, vitamins

Pharmacologic: fat-soluble vitamins

Indications

Prevention and treatment of hypoprothrombinemia, which may be associated with: Excessive doses of oral anticoagulants, Salicylates, Certain anti-infective agents, Nutritional deficiencies, Prolonged total parenteral nutrition. Prevention and treatment of vitamin K-deficiency bleeding in neonates.

Action

Required for hepatic synthesis of blood coagulation factors II (prothrombin), VII, IX, and X. **Therapeutic Effects:** Prevention of bleeding due to hypoprothrombinemia.

Pharmacokinetics

Absorption: Well absorbed following oral or subcut administration. Oral absorption requires presence of bile salts. Some vitamin K is produced by bacteria in the GI tract.
Distribution: Crosses the placenta; does not enter breast milk.
Metabolism and Excretion: Rapidly metabolized by the liver.
Half-life: Unknown.

TIME/ACTION PROFILE

ROUTE	ONSET	PEAK†	DURATION‡
PO	6–12 hr	unknown	unknown
Subcut	1–2 hr	3–6 hr	12–14 hr
IV	1–2 hr	3–6 hr	12 hr

†Control of hemorrhage.
‡Normal PT achieved.

Contraindications/Precautions

Contraindicated in: Hypersensitivity; Hypersensitivity or intolerance to benzyl alcohol (injection only).
Use Cautiously in: Hepatic impairment; Pedi: Use of injection formulations containing benzyl alcohol may lead to "gasping syndrome" in neonates and infants.
Exercise Extreme Caution in: Severe life-threatening reactions have occurred following IV administration, use other routes unless risk is justified.

Adverse Reactions/Side Effects

GI: gastric upset, unusual taste. **Derm:** eczematous reactions, flushing, kernicterus, rash, scleroderma-like lesions, urticaria. **GI:** hyperbilirubinemia (large doses in very premature infants). **Hemat:** hemolytic anemia. **Local:** erythema, pain at injection site, swelling. **Misc:** HYPERSENSITIVITY REACTIONS.

Interactions

Drug-Drug: Large doses will counteract the effect of **warfarin**. Large doses of **salicylates** or broad-spectrum **anti-infectives** may ↑ vitamin K requirements. **Bile acid sequestrants**, **mineral oil**, and **sucralfate** may ↓ vitamin K absorption from the GI tract.

P

Route/Dosage

IV use of phytonadione should be reserved for patients with serious or life-threatening bleeding and elevated INR. Oral route is preferred in patients with elevated INRs and no serious or life-threatening bleeding. IM route should generally be avoided because of risk of hematoma formation.

Treatment of Hypoprothrombinemia due to Vitamin K Deficiency (from factors other than warfarin)

Subcut, IV (Adults): 10 mg.
PO (Adults): 2.5–25 mg/day.
Subcut, IV (Children >1 mo): 1–2 mg single dose.
PO (Children >1 mo): 2.5–5 mg/day.

Vitamin K Deficiency (Supratherapeutic INR) Secondary to Warfarin

PO (Adults): *INR ≥5 and <9 (no significant bleeding)*—Hold warfarin and give 1–2.5 mg vitamin K; if more rapid reversal required, given ≤5 mg vitamin K; *INR >9 (no significant bleeding)*—Hold warfarin and give 2.5–5 mg vitamin K.
IV (Adults): *Elevated INR with serious or life-threatening bleeding*—10 mg slow infusion.

Prevention of Hypoprothrombinemia during Total Parenteral Nutrition

IV (Adults): 5–10 mg once weekly.
IV (Children): 2–5 mg once weekly.

Prevention of Vitamin K-Deficiency Bleeding in Neonates

IM (Neonates): 0.5–1 mg, within 1 hr of birth, may repeat in 6–8 hr if needed. May be repeated in 2–3 wk if mother received previous anticonvulsant/anticoagulant/anti-infective/antitubercular therapy. 1–5 mg may be given IM to mother 12–24 hr before delivery.

Treatment of Vitamin K-Deficiency Bleeding in Neonates

IM, Subcut (Neonates): 1–2 mg/day.

Availability (generic available)

Tablets: 5 mg. **Solution for injection:** 1 mg/0.5 mL, 10 mg/mL.

NURSING IMPLICATIONS

Assessment

- Monitor for frank and occult bleeding (guaiac stools, Hematest urine, and emesis). Monitor pulse and BP frequently; notify health care professional immediately if symptoms of internal bleeding or hypovolemic shock develop. Inform all personnel of patient's bleeding tendency to prevent further trauma. Apply pressure to all venipuncture sites for at least 5 min; avoid unnecessary IM injections.
- Pedi: Monitor for side effects and adverse reactions. Children may be especially sensitive to the effects and side effects of vitamin K. Neonates, especially premature neonates, may be more sensitive than older children.
- ***Lab Test Considerations:*** Monitor INR prior to and throughout vitamin K therapy to determine response to and need for further therapy.

Implementation

- Do not confuse Mephyton (phytonadione) with methadone.
- The parenteral route is preferred for phytonadione therapy but, because of severe, potentially fatal hypersensitivity reactions, IV vitamin K is not recommended.
- Administration of whole blood or plasma may also be required in severe bleeding because of the delayed onset of this medication.
- Phytonadione is an antidote for warfarin overdose but does not counteract the anticoagulant activity of heparin.

IV Administration

- **Intermittent Infusion:** ***Diluent:*** Dilute in 0.9% NaCl, D5W, or D5/0.9% NaCl. ***Rate:*** Administer over 30–60 min. Rate should not exceed 1 mg/min.
- **Y-Site Compatibility:** alfentanil, amikacin, aminophylline, ascorbic acid, atracurium, atropine, azathioprine, aztreonam, benztropine, bumetanide, buprenorphine, butorphanol, calcium chloride, calcium gluconate, cefazolin, cefotaxime, cefotetan, cefoxitin, ceftazidime, ceftriaxone, cefuroxime, chloramphenicol, chlorpromazine, clindamycin, cyanocobalamin, cyclosporine, dexamethasone sodium phosphate, digoxin, diphenhydramine, dopamine, doxycycline, enalaprilat, ephedrine, epinephrine, epoetin alfa, erythromycin, esmolol, famotidine, fentanyl, fluconazole, folic acid, furosemide, ganciclovir, gentamicin, glycopyrrolate, heparin, hydrocortisone sodium succinate, imipenem/cilastatin, indomethacin, insulin, isoproterenol, ketorolac, labetalol, lidocaine, mannitol, meperidine, methyldopate, metoclopramide, metoprolol, metronidazole, midazolam, morphine, multivitamins, nafcillin, nalbuphine, naloxone, nitroglycerin, nitroprusside, norepinephrine, ondansetron, oxacillin, oxytocin, papaverine, penicillin G, pentamidine, pentobarbital, phenobarbital, phentolamine, phenylephrine, potassium chloride, procainamide, prochlorperazine, propranolol, pyridoxine, ranitidine, sodium bicarbonate, streptokinase, succinylcholine, sufentanil, theophylline, thiamine, tobramycin, vancomycin, vasopressin, verapamil, vitamin B complex with C.
- **Y-Site Incompatibility:** dantrolene, diazepam, diazoxide, magnesium sulfate, phenytoin, trimethoprim/sulfamethoxazole.

Patient/Family Teaching

- Instruct patient to take phytonadione as directed. Take missed doses as soon as remembered unless almost time for next dose. Notify health care professional of missed doses.
- Cooking does not destroy substantial amounts of vitamin K. Patient should not drastically alter diet while taking vitamin K. See Appendix K for foods high in vitamin K.
- Caution patient to avoid IM injections and activities leading to injury. Use a soft toothbrush, do not floss, and shave with an electric razor until coagulation defect is corrected.
- Advise patient to report any symptoms of unusual bleeding or bruising (bleeding gums; nosebleed; black, tarry stools; hematuria; excessive menstrual flow).
- Advise patient to notify health care professional of all Rx or OTC medications, vitamins, or herbal products being taken and to consult with health care professional before taking other medications and alcohol.
- Advise patient to inform health care professional of medication regimen prior to treatment or surgery.
- Advise patient to carry identification at all times describing disease process.
- Emphasize the importance of frequent lab tests to monitor coagulation factors.

Evaluation/Desired Outcomes

- Prevention of spontaneous bleeding or cessation of bleeding in patients with hypoprothrombinemia secondary to impaired intestinal absorption or oral anticoagulant, salicylate, or anti-infective therapy.
- Prevention of hemorrhagic disease in the newborn.

pimavanserin
(pim-a-**van**-ser-in)
Nuplazid

Classification
Therapeutic: antipsychotics

Indications
Hallucinations and delusions associated with Parkinson's disease psychosis.

Action
Exact mechanism is unknown. May work by acting as an inverse agonist and antagonist primarily at 5-HT[2A] receptors and less at 5–HT[2C] receptors. **Therapeutic Effects:** Reduced frequency and/or severity of hallucinations and delusions in patients with Parkinson's disease psychosis.

Pharmacokinetics
Absorption: Unknown.
Distribution: Extensively distributed to tissues.
Protein Binding: 95%.
Metabolism and Excretion: Mostly metabolized by the liver (CYP3A4 and CYP3A5 isoenzymes) to an active metabolite. Primarily excreted in feces.
Half-life: 57 hr (pimavanserin); 200 hr (active metabolite).

TIME/ACTION PROFILE (blood levels)

ROUTE	ONSET	PEAK	DURATION
PO	unknown	6 hr	unknown

Contraindications/Precautions
Contraindicated in: Hypersensitivity; QT interval prolongation; Concurrent use of agents that prolong the QT interval, including sotalol, quinidine, disopyramide, procainamide, amiodarone, thioridazine, chlorpromazine, moxifloxacin, and ziprasidone (↑ risk of serious arrhythmias); History of arrhythmias, including bradycardia; Hypokalemia or hypomagnesemia (↑ risk of serious arrhythmias); Congenital long QT syndrome (↑ risk of serious arrhythmias); Severe renal impairment (CCr <30 mL/min).
Use Cautiously in: OB, Lactation: Safety not established; Pedi: Safety and effectiveness not established; Geri: ↑ risk of mortality in elderly patients treated for psychosis related to dementia/neurocognitive disorders.

Adverse Reactions/Side Effects
CNS: confusion, hallucinations. **CV:** TORSADES DE POINTES, peripheral edema, QT interval prolongation. **GI:** constipation, nausea. **Neuro:** gait disturbance. **Misc:** HYPERSENSITIVITY REACTIONS (including angioedema).

Interactions
Drug-Drug: Concurrent use of **amiodarone, sotalol, quinidine, disopyramide, procainamide, thioridazine, chlorpromazine, moxifloxacin,** and **ziprasidone** ↑ the risk of serious ventricular arrhythmias and should be avoided. **Strong CYP3A4 inhibitors,** including **clarithromycin, indinavir, itraconazole,** and **ketoconazole,** may ↑ levels; ↓ dose of pimavanserin. **Strong CYP3A4 inducers,** including **carbamazepine, phenytoin,** and **rifampin** as well as **moderate CYP3A4 inducers,**including **efavirenz, modafinil, nafcillin,** and **thioridazine** may ↓ levels; avoid concurrent use.
Drug-Natural Products: St. John's wort may ↓ levels; avoid concurrent use.

Route/Dosage
PO (Adults): 34 mg once daily. *Concurrent use of strong CYP3A4 inhibitors*— 10 mg once daily.

Availability
Capsules: 34 mg. **Tablets:** 10 mg.

NURSING IMPLICATIONS
Assessment
- Assess mental status (orientation, mood, behavior) before and periodically during therapy.

Implementation
- **PO:** Administer 2 tablets once daily without regard to food.

Patient/Family Teaching
- Instruct patient to take pimavanserin as directed.
- Instruct patient to notify health care professional of all Rx or OTC medications, vitamins, or herbal products being taken and consult health care professional before taking any new medications, especially St. John's wort.
- Advise female patient to notify health care professional if pregnancy is planned or suspected or if breast feeding.

Evaluation/Desired Outcomes
- Reduced frequency and/or severity of hallucinations and delusions in patients with Parkinson's disease psychosis.

pimecrolimus
(pi-me-**cro**-li-mus)
Elidel

Classification
Therapeutic: immunosuppressants (topical)

P

Indications

Short-term and intermittent long-term management of mild to moderate atopic dermatitis unresponsive to or in patients intolerant of conventional treatment.

Action

Inhibits T-cell and mast cell activation by interfering with production of inflammatory cytokines. **Therapeutic Effects:** Decreased severity of atopic dermatatis.

Pharmacokinetics

Absorption: Minimally absorbed through intact skin.
Distribution: Local distribution after topical administration.
Metabolism and Excretion: Systemic metabolism and excretion is negligible with local application.
Half-life: Not applicable.

TIME/ACTION PROFILE (improvement in symptoms)

ROUTE	ONSET	PEAK	DURATION
topical	within 6 days	unknown	unknown

Contraindications/Precautions

Contraindicated in: Hypersensitivity; Should not be applied to areas of active cutaneous viral infections (↑ risk of dissemination); Concurrent use of occlusive dressings; Netherton's syndrome (↑ absorption of pimecrolimus); Lactation: Discontinue breast feeding.
Use Cautiously in: Possible risk of cancer. Do not use as first-line therapy; Clinical infection at treatment site (infection should be treated/cleared prior to use); Skin papillomas (warts); allow treatment/resolution prior to use; Natural/artificial sunlight (minimize exposure); OB: Use only if maternal benefit outweighs potential risk to fetus; Pedi: Children <2 yr (safety not established); use only if other treatments have failed.

Adverse Reactions/Side Effects

Local: burning. **Misc:** ↑ risk of lymphoma/skin cancer.

Interactions

Drug-Drug: None significant as systemic absorption is negligible.

Route/Dosage

Topical (Adults and Children ≥2 yr): Apply thin film twice daily; rub in gently and completely.

Availability (generic available)

Cream: 1%.

NURSING IMPLICATIONS

Assessment

- Assess skin lesions prior to and periodically during therapy. Discontinue therapy after signs and symptoms of atopic dermatitis have resolved. Resume treatment at the first signs and symptoms of recurrence.

Implementation

- **Topical:** Apply a thin layer to affected area twice daily and rub in gently and completely. May be used on all skin areas including head, neck, and intertriginous areas. Do not use with occlusive dressings.

Patient/Family Teaching

- Instruct patient on correct technique for application. Apply only as directed to external areas. Wash hands following application, unless hands are areas of application. Advise patient to read *Medication Guide* before starting and with each Rx refill in case of changes.
- Caution patient to avoid exposure to natural or artificial sunlight, including tanning beds, while using cream.
- Advise patient that pimecrolimus may cause skin burning. This occurs most commonly during 1st few days of application, is of mild to moderate severity, and improves within 5 days or as atopic dermatitis resolves.
- Advise patient to notify health care professional if pregnancy is planned or suspected, or if breast feeding.
- Advise patient to notify health care provider if no improvement is seen following 6 wk of treatment or at any time if condition worsens.

Evaluation/Desired Outcomes

- Resolution of signs and symptoms of atopic dermatitis.

pioglitazone (pi-o-**glit**-a-zone)

Actos

Classification
Therapeutic: antidiabetics (oral)
Pharmacologic: thiazolidinediones

Indications

Type 2 diabetes mellitus (with diet and exercise); may be used with metformin, sulfonylureas, or insulin.

Action

Improves sensitivity to insulin by acting as an agonist at receptor sites involved in insulin responsiveness and subsequent glucose production and utilization. Requires insulin for activity. **Therapeutic Effects:** Decreased insulin resistance, resulting in glycemic control without hypoglycemia.

Pharmacokinetics

Absorption: Well absorbed following oral administration.
Distribution: Unknown.
Protein Binding: >99% bound to plasma proteins. Active metabolites are also highly (>99%) bound.
Metabolism and Excretion: Extensively metabolized by the liver (primarily by CYP2C8); at least two metabolites have pharmacologic activity. Minimal renal excretion of unchanged drug.

Half-life: *Pioglitazone*—3–7 hr; *total pioglitazone (pioglitazone plus metabolites)*—16–24 hr.

TIME/ACTION PROFILE (effects on blood glucose)

ROUTE	ONSET	PEAK	DURATION
PO	30 min	2–4 hr	24 hr

Contraindications/Precautions

Contraindicated in: Hypersensitivity; Type 1 diabetes; Diabetic ketoacidosis; Clinical evidence of active liver disease or ↑ ALT (>2.5 times upper limit of normal); Active bladder cancer; OB, Lactation: Insulin should be used to control blood glucose levels; Pedi: Children.

Use Cautiously in: Edema; HF (avoid use in moderate to severe HF); Hepatic impairment; History of bladder cancer; Women (may ↑ distal upper and lower limb fractures); Women with childbearing potential (may restore ovulation and ↑ risk of pregnancy).

Adverse Reactions/Side Effects

CV: HF, edema. **EENT:** macular edema. **GI:** LIVER FAILURE, ↑ liver enzymes. **GU:** BLADDER CANCER. **Hemat:** anemia. **MS:** RHABDOMYOLYSIS. **Misc:** fractures (arm, hand, foot) in female patients.

Interactions

Drug-Drug: May ↓ efficacy of **hormonal contraceptives**. Strong **CYP2C8 inhibitors**, including **gemfibrozil** may ↑ levels. **Ketoconazole** may ↑ levels. Concurrent use with **insulin** may ↑ risk of fluid retention and worsening HF. **Topiramate** may ↓ levels.

Drug-Natural Products: **Glucosamine** may worsen blood glucose control. **Chromium** and **coenzyme Q-10** may produce ↑ hypoglycemic effects.

Route/Dosage

PO (Adults): *No heart failure*—15–30 mg once daily, may be ↑ in increments of 15 mg/day to 45 mg/day if needed; *NYHA class I-II heart failure*—15 mg once daily; may be ↑ in increments of 15 mg/day to 45 mg/day if needed; *Concurrent use of gemfibrozil*—do not exceed 15 mg once daily.

Availability (generic available)

Tablets: 15 mg, 30 mg, 45 mg. **Cost:** *Generic*—15 mg $25.49/90, 30 mg $22.75/90, 45 mg $38.12/90. ***In combination with:*** metformin (Actoplus Met, Actoplus Met XR), glimepiride (Duetact), alogliptin (Oseni); see Appendix B.

NURSING IMPLICATIONS

Assessment

- Observe patient taking concurrent insulin for signs and symptoms of hypoglycemic reactions (sweating, hunger, weakness, dizziness, tremor, tachycardia, anxiety).
- Assess for signs and symptoms of heart failure (edema, dyspnea, rapid weight gain, unusual tiredness) after initiation and with dose increases.
- ***Lab Test Considerations:*** Monitor serum glucose and HbA_{1c} periodically during therapy to evaluate effectiveness.
- Monitor CBC with differential periodically during therapy. May cause ↓ in hemoglobin and hematocrit, usually during the first 4–12 wk of therapy; then levels stabilize.
- Monitor serum AST, ALT, alkaline phosphatase, and total bilirubin levels before starting therapy and periodically thereafter or if jaundice or symptoms of hepatic dysfunction occur. Pioglitazone should not be started in patients with active liver disease or ALT levels >2.5 times the upper limit of normal. Patients with mild ALT ↑ should have more frequent monitoring. If ALT ↑ to >3 times the upper limit of normal, recheck ALT promptly. Discontinue pioglitazone if ALT remains >3 times normal.
- May cause transient ↑ in CPK levels.

Implementation

- Do not confuse Actos (pioglitazone) with Actonel (risedronate).
- Patients stabilized on a diabetic regimen who are exposed to stress, fever, trauma, infection, or surgery may require administration of insulin.
- **PO:** May be administered with or without meals.

Patient/Family Teaching

- Instruct patient to take medication as directed. If dose for 1 day is missed, do not double dose the next day.
- Explain to patient that this medication controls hyperglycemia but does not cure diabetes. Therapy is long-term.
- Review signs of hypoglycemia and hyperglycemia with patient. If hypoglycemia occurs, advise patient to take a glass of orange juice or 2–3 tsp of sugar, honey, or corn syrup dissolved in water and notify health care professional.
- Encourage patient to follow prescribed diet, medication, and exercise regimen to prevent hypoglycemic or hyperglycemic episodes.
- Instruct patient in proper testing of serum glucose and ketones. These tests should be closely monitored during periods of stress or illness, and health care professional should be notified if significant changes occur.
- Advise patient to notify health care professional immediately if signs of hepatic dysfunction (nausea, vomiting, upper right abdominal pain, fatigue, anorexia, dark urine, jaundice), bladder cancer (hematuria, dysuria, urinary urgency), or HF (edema, shortness of breath, rapid weight gain, tiredness) occur.
- Advise patient to inform health care professional of medication regimen before treatment or surgery.

P

- Insulin is the preferred method of controlling blood glucose during pregnancy. Counsel female patients that higher doses of oral contraceptives or a form of contraception other than oral contraceptives may be required and to notify health care professional promptly if pregnancy is planned or suspected.
- Advise patient to carry a form of sugar (sugar packets, candy) and identification describing disease process and medication regimen at all times.
- Emphasize the importance of routine follow-up exams.

Evaluation/Desired Outcomes

- Control of blood glucose levels.

piperacillin/tazobactam

(pi-**per**-a-sill-in/tay-zoe-**bak**-tam)

Tazocin, Zosyn

Classification

Therapeutic: anti-infectives

Pharmacologic: extended spectrum penicillins

Indications

Appendicitis and peritonitis. Skin and skin structure infections. Gynecologic infections. Community-acquired and nosocomial pneumonia caused by piperacillin-resistant, beta-lactamase–producing bacteria.

Action

Piperacillin: Binds to bacterial cell wall membrane, causing cell death. Spectrum is extended compared with other penicillins. **Tazobactam:** Inhibits beta-lactamase, an enzyme that can destroy penicillins. **Therapeutic Effects:** Death of susceptible bacteria. **Spectrum:** Active against piperacillin-resistant, beta-lactamase–producing: *Bacteroides fragilis*, *E. coli*, *Acinetobacter baumanii*, *Klebsiella pneumoniae*, *Pseudomonas aeruginosa*, *Staphylococcus aureus*, *Haemophilus influenzae*.

Pharmacokinetics

Absorption: Piperacillin is well absorbed (80%) from IM sites.

Distribution: Widely distributed. Enters CSF well only when meninges are inflamed. Crosses the placenta and enters breast milk in low concentrations.

Metabolism and Excretion: Piperacillin (68%) and tazobactam (80%) are mostly excreted unchanged by the kidneys.

Half-life: Adults: 0.7–1.2 hr; Children 6 mo–12 yr: 0.7–0.9 hr; Infants 2–5 mo: 1.4 hr.

TIME/ACTION PROFILE (piperacillin blood levels)

ROUTE	ONSET	PEAK	DURATION
IV	rapid	end of infusion	4–6 hr

Contraindications/Precautions

Contraindicated in: Hypersensitivity to penicillins, beta-lactams, cephalosporins, or tazobactam (cross-sensitivity may occur).

Use Cautiously in: Renal impairment (dosage reduction or increased interval recommended if CCr <40 mL/min); Sodium restriction; Critically ill patients (↑ risk of renal failure; use alternative antibiotic, if possible); OB, Lactation: Safety not established.

Adverse Reactions/Side Effects

CNS: SEIZURES (higher doses), confusion, dizziness, headache, insomnia, lethargy. **GI:** CLOSTRIDIUM DIFFICILE-ASSOCIATED DIARRHEA (CDAD), diarrhea, constipation, drug-induced hepatitis, nausea, vomiting. **GU:** interstitial nephritis, renal failure. **Derm:** ACUTE GENERALIZED EXANTHEMATOUS PUSTULOSIS, DRUG REACTION WITH EOSINOPHILIA AND SYSTEMIC SYMPTOMS (DRESS), STEVENS-JOHNSON SYNDROME, TOXIC EPIDERMAL NECROLYSIS, rashes (↑ in cystic fibrosis patients), urticaria. **Hemat:** bleeding, leukopenia, neutropenia, thrombocytopenia. **Local:** pain, phlebitis at IV site. **Misc:** hypersensitivity reactions, including ANAPHYLAXIS and SERUM SICKNESS, fever (↑ in cystic fibrosis patients), superinfection.

Interactions

Drug-Drug: Probenecid ↓ renal excretion and ↑ blood levels. May alter excretion of **lithium**. **Potassium-losing diuretics**, **corticosteroids**, or **amphotericin B** may ↑ risk of hypokalemia. ↑ risk of hepatotoxicity with other **hepatotoxic agents**. May ↓ levels/effects of **aminoglycosides** in patients with renal impairment. May ↑ levels and risk of toxicity from **methotrexate**. ↑ risk of acute kidney injury when concomitantly administered with **vancomycin**.

Route/Dosage

Contains 2.84 mEq (65 mg) sodium/g of piperacillin; adult doses below expressed as combined piperacillin/tazobactam content.

IV (Adults): *Most infections*—3.375 g every 6 hr. *Nosocomial pneumonia*—4.5 g every 6 hr.

IV (Adults): *Nosocomial pneumonia*—4.5 g every 6 hr.

IV (Adults and Children >40 kg): *Appendicitis and/or peritonitis*—3.375 g every 6 hr.

IV (Children ≥9 mo and ≤40 kg): *Appendicitis and/or peritonitis*—300 mg piperacillin component/kg/day divided every 8 hr.

IV (Infants 2–9 mo): *Appendicitis and/or peritonitis*—240 mg piperacillin component/kg/day divided every 8 hr.

IV (Infants and Children ≥6 mo): 240–400 mg/piperacillin component/kg/day divided every 6–8 hr (higher end of dosing range for serious pseudomonal infections); Max dose: 16 g piperacillin/day.

IV (Infants <6 mo): 150–300 mg/piperacillin component/kg/day divided every 6–8 hr.

Renal Impairment

IV (Adults): *CCr 20–40 mL/min*—2.25 g every 6 hr (3.375 g every 6 hr for nosocomial pneumonia); *CCr <20 mL/min*—2.25 g every 8 hr (2.25 g every 6 hr for nosocomial pneumonia); *Hemodialysis*—2.25 g every 12 h (2.25 g every 8 hr for nosocomial pneumonia).

Availability (generic available)

Powder for injection: 2-g piperacillin/0.25-g tazobactam vials and 50-mL premixed frozen containers, 3-g piperacillin/0.375-g tazobactam vials and 50-mL premixed frozen containers, 4-g piperacillin/0.5-g tazobactam vials and 100-mL premixed frozen containers, 36-g piperacillin/4.5-g tazobactam bulk vials.

NURSING IMPLICATIONS

Assessment

- Assess patient for infection (vital signs; appearance of wound, sputum, urine, and stool; WBC) at beginning of and during therapy.
- Obtain a history before initiating therapy to determine previous use of and reactions to penicillins or cephalosporins. Persons with a negative history of penicillin sensitivity may still have an allergic response.
- Obtain specimens for culture and sensitivity prior to initiating therapy. 1st dose may be given before receiving results.
- Observe patient for signs and symptoms of anaphylaxis (rash, pruritus, laryngeal edema, wheezing). Discontinue the drug and notify health care professional immediately if these occur. Keep epinephrine, an antihistamine, and resuscitation equipment close by in the event of an anaphylactic reaction.
- Monitor bowel function. Diarrhea, abdominal cramping, fever, and bloody stools should be reported to health care professional promptly as a sign of Clostridium difficile-associated diarrhea (CDAD). May begin up to several wk following cessation of therapy.
- Assess for skin reactions (rash, fever, edema, mucosal erosions or ulcerations, red or inflamed eyes). Monitor patient with mild to moderate rash for progression. If rash becomes severe or systemic symptoms occur, discontinue piperacillin/tazobactam.
- Monitor for signs and symptoms of DRESS (fever, rash, lymphadenopathy, and/or facial swelling), associated with involvement of other organ systems (hepatitis, nephritis, hematologic abnormalities, myocarditis, myositis) during therapy. May resemble an acute viral infection. Eosinophilia is often present. Discontinue therapy if signs occur.
- ***Lab Test Considerations:*** Evaluate renal and hepatic function, CBC, serum potassium, and bleeding times prior to and routinely during therapy.
- May cause positive direct Coombs' test result.
- May cause ↑ BUN, creatinine, AST, ALT, serum bilirubin, alkaline phosphatase, and LDH.
- May cause leukopenia and neutropenia, especially with prolonged therapy or hepatic impairment.
- May cause prolonged prothrombin and partial thromboplastin time.
- May cause ↓ hemoglobin and hematocrit and thrombocytopenia, eosinophilia, leukopenia, and neutropenia. It also may cause proteinuria; hematuria; pyuria; hyperglycemia; ↓ total protein or albumin; and abnormalities in sodium, potassium, and calcium levels.

Implementation

IV Administration

- **Intermittent Infusion:** Reconstitute each 1 g of piperacillin with at least 5 mL of 0.9% NaCl, sterile water for injection, or D5W. ***Diluent:*** Dilute further in 50–100 mL of 0.9% NaCl, D5W, D5/0.9% NaCl, or LR. Reconstituted vials stable for 24 hr at room temperature or 48 hr if refrigerated. Infusion stable for 24 hr at room temperature or 7 days if refrigerated. ***Rate:*** Infuse over 30 min.
- **Y-Site Compatibility:** alfentanil, allopurinol, amifostine, aminocaproic acid, aminophylline, amphotericin B lipid complex, amphotericin B liposome, anidulafungin, argatroban, aztreonam, bivalirudin, bleomycin, bumetanide, buprenorphine, busulfan, butorphanol, calcium acetate, calcium chloride, calcium gluconate, carboplatin, carmustine, cefepime, chloramphenicol, clindamycin, cyclophosphamide, cyclosporine, cytarabine, dactinomycin, daptomycin, dexamethasone, dexmedetomidine, dexrazoxane, diazepam, digoxin, diphenhydramine, docetaxel, dopamine, doxacurium, enalaprilat, ephedrine, epinephrine, eptifibatide, erythromycin, esmolol, etoposide, etoposide phosphate, fenoldopam, fentanyl, floxuridine, fluconazole, fludarabine, fluorouracil, foscarnet, fosphenytoin, furosemide, granisetron, heparin, hetastarch, hydrocortisone, hydromorphone, ifosfamide, isoproterenol, ketamine, ketorolac, leucovorin calcium, lidocaine, linezolid, lorazepam, magnesium sulfate, mannitol, melphalan, meperidine, mesna, metaraminol, methotrexate, methylprednisolone, metoclopramide, metoprolol, metronidazole, milrinone, morphine, naloxone, nitroglycerin, nitroprusside, norepinephrine, octreotide, ondansetron, oxytocin, paclitaxel, palonosetron, pancuronium, pantoprazole, pemetrexed, pentobarbital, phenobarbital, phentolamine, phenylephrine, potassium acetate, potassium chloride, potassium phosphates, procainamide, ranitidine, remifentanil, rituximab, sargramostim, sodium acetate, sodium bicarbonate, sodium phosphates, succinylcholine, sufentanil, tacrolimus, telavancin, theophylline, thiotepa, tigecycline, tirofiban, trimeth-

P

oprim/sulfamethoxazole, vasopressin, vinblastine, vincristine, voriconazole, zidovudine, zoledronic acid.

- **Y-Site Incompatibility:** acyclovir, alemtuzumab, amiodarone, amphotericin B deoxycholate, azithromycin, caspofungin, chlorpromazine, ciprofloxacin, cisplatin, dacarbazine, dantrolene, daunorubicin hydrocloride, diltiazem, dobutamine, doxorubicin, doxorubicin liposome, doxycycline, droperidol, epirubicin, famotidine, ganciclovir, gemcitabine, glycopyrrolate, haloperidol, hydralazine, hydroxyzine, idarubicin, insulin, irinotecan, labetalol, levofloxacin, methyldopate, midazolam, mitomycin, mitoxantrone, nalbuphine, nicardipine, pentamidine, phenytoin, prochlorperazine, promethazine, propranolol, quinupristin/dalfopristin, rocuronium, streptozocin, thiopental, tobramycin, tranexamic acid, trastuzumab, vecuronium, verapamil, vinorelbine.

Patient/Family Teaching

- Advise patient to report rash and signs of superinfection (black furry overgrowth on tongue, vaginal itching or discharge, loose or foul-smelling stools) and allergy.
- Caution patient to notify health care professional if fever and diarrhea occur, especially if stool contains blood, pus, or mucus. Advise patient not to treat diarrhea without consulting health care professional. May occur up to several wk after discontinuation of medication.

Evaluation/Desired Outcomes

- Resolution of the signs and symptoms of infection. Length of time for complete resolution depends on the organism and site of infection.

pitavastatin, See HMG-CoA REDUCTASE INHIBITORS (statins).

plecanatide (ple-**kan**-a-tide)

Trulance

Classification

Therapeutic: laxatives

Pharmacologic: guanylate cyclase-C agonists

Indications

Chronic idiopathic constipation (CIC). Irritable bowel syndrome with constipation (IBS-C).

Action

Locally ↑ cyclic guanosine monophosphate (cGMP) concentrations which ↑ intestinal fluid and accelerates transit time. **Therapeutic Effects:** Increased frequency of complete spontaneous bowel movements.

Pharmacokinetics

Absorption: Minimally absorbed, action is primarily local.

Distribution: Stays within the GI tract with minimal distribution.

Metabolism and Excretion: Converted to its principal active metabolite within the GI tract. Plecanatide and active metabolite then degraded in intestinal lumen to smaller peptides and amino acids. Excretion information unknown.

Half-life: Unknown.

TIME/ACTION PROFILE (improvement in CIC symptoms)

ROUTE	ONSET	PEAK	DURATION
PO	1 wk	2–12 wk	2 wk†

†Following discontinuation.

Contraindications/Precautions

Contraindicated in: Known/suspected mechanical GI obstruction; Pedi: Children <6 yr (↑ risk of dehydration) and 6–18 yr (safety and effectiveness not established in).

Use Cautiously in: OB, Lactation: Fetal exposure unlikely; safety not established.

Adverse Reactions/Side Effects

GI: abdominal distention, diarrhea, flatulence, ↑ liver enzymes.

Interactions

Drug-Drug: None known.

Route/Dosage

PO (Adults): 3 mg once daily.

Availability

Tablets: 3 mg.

NURSING IMPLICATIONS

Assessment

- Monitor bowel function (frequency, consistency) periodically during therapy. If severe diarrhea occurs, withhold plecanatide and rehydrate patient.
- ***Lab Test Considerations:*** May cause ↑ ALT, and AST.

Implementation

- **PO:** Administer once daily without regard to food. Swallow tablet whole. Tablets can be crushed and mixed in applesauce or water and administered orally or with water in a nasogastric or gastric feeding tube. Do not mix with other foods or liquids.

Patient/Family Teaching

- Instruct patient to take plecanatide as directed. If a dose is missed, omit and take next dose at regular time; do not double doses.
- Instruct patient to notify health care professional of all Rx or OTC medications, vitamins, or herbal prod-

ucts being taken and consult health care professional before taking any new medications.

- Advise female patient to notify health care professional if pregnancy is planned or suspected or if breast feeding.

Evaluation/Desired Outcomes

- Increased frequency of complete spontaneous bowel movements.

polyethylene glycol 3350

(po-lee-**eth**-e-leen **glye**-kole)

🍁 ClearLax, GlycoLax, 🍁 Lax-a-Day, MiraLax, 🍁 PegaLax, 🍁 PolyLax, 🍁 Relaxa, 🍁 RestoraLax

Classification

Therapeutic: laxatives

Pharmacologic: osmotics

Indications

Treatment of occasional constipation.

Action

Polyethylene glycol (PEG) in solution acts as an osmotic agent, drawing water into the lumen of the GI tract. **Therapeutic Effects:** Evacuation of the GI tract without water or electrolyte imbalance.

Pharmacokinetics

Absorption: Nonabsorbable.

Distribution: Unknown.

Metabolism and Excretion: Excreted in fecal contents.

Half-life: Unknown.

TIME/ACTION PROFILE (bowel movement)

ROUTE	ONSET	PEAK	DURATION
PO	unknown	1–3 days	unknown

Contraindications/Precautions

Contraindicated in: GI obstruction; Gastric retention; Toxic colitis; Megacolon; Bowel perforation.

Use Cautiously in: Abdominal pain of uncertain cause, particularly if accompanied by fever; OB, Pedi: Safety not established.

Adverse Reactions/Side Effects

Derm: urticaria. **GI:** abdominal bloating, cramping, flatulence, nausea.

Interactions

Drug-Drug: None significant.

Route/Dosage

PO (Adults): 17 g (heaping tablespoon) in 8 oz of water once daily; may be used for up to 2 wk.

PO (Children >6 mo): 0.5–1.5 g/kg daily, titrate to effect (maximum: 17 g/day).

Availability (generic available)

Powder: 14-oz, 24-oz, and 26-oz containers.

NURSING IMPLICATIONS

Assessment

- Assess patient for abdominal distention, presence of bowel sounds, and usual pattern of bowel function.
- Assess color, consistency, and amount of stool produced.

Implementation

- Do not confuse Miralax (polyethylene glycol) with Mirapex (pramipexole). Do not confuse polyethylene glycol with propylene glycol.
- **PO:** Dissolve powder in 8 oz of water prior to administration.

Patient/Family Teaching

- Inform patient that 2–4 days may be required to produce a bowel movement. PEG should not be used for more than 2 wk. Prolonged, frequent, or excessive use may result in electrolyte imbalance and laxative dependence.
- Advise patient to notify health care professional if unusual cramps, bloating, or diarrhea occurs.

Evaluation/Desired Outcomes

- A soft, formed bowel movement.

posaconazole

(po-sa-**kon**-a-zole)

Noxafil, 🍁 Posanol

Classification

Therapeutic: antifungals

Pharmacologic: triazoles

Indications

Prevention of invasive aspergillus and candida infections in severely immunocompromised patients. Treatment of oropharyngeal candidiasis (including candidiasis unresponsive to itraconazole or fluconazole).

Action

Blocks ergosterol synthesis, a major component of fungal plasma membrane. **Therapeutic Effects:** Fungistatic/fungicidal action against susceptible fungi.

Pharmacokinetics

Absorption: Well absorbed following oral administration; absorption is optimized by food; IV administration results in complete bioavailability.

Distribution: Extensive extravascular distribution and penetration into body tissues.

Protein Binding: >98%.

P

Metabolism and Excretion: Some metabolism via UDP glucuronidation; 66% eliminated unchanged in feces, 13% in urine (mostly as metabolites).
Half-life: 35 hr.

TIME/ACTION PROFILE (blood levels)

ROUTE	ONSET	PEAK	DURATION
PO (suspension)	unknown	3–5 hr	8 hr
PO-ER	unknown	4–5 hr	24 hr
IV	unknown	2 hr	24 hr

Contraindications/Precautions

Contraindicated in: Hypersensitivity to posaconazole or other azole antifungals; Concurrent use of pimozide, quinidine, ergot alkaloids, sirolimus, simvastatin, atorvastatin, or lovastatin.
Use Cautiously in: History of/predisposition to QTc prolongation including congenital QTc prolongation, concurrent medications that prolong QTc, or electrolyte abnormalities (hypokalemia, hypomagnesemia); correct pre-existing abnormalities prior to administration; Moderate-severe renal impairment (CCr <50 mL/min); use only if justified by risk/benefit assessment (IV form should be avoided, use oral form only); Severe diarrhea, vomiting, or renal impairment (monitor for breakthrough fungal infections); OB: May cause fetal harm (based on animal data); use only if potential maternal benefit outweighs potential fetal risk; Lactation: Use while breast feeding only if potential maternal benefit outweighs potential risk to infant; Pedi: Children <18 yr (IV) or <13 yr (oral) (safety and effectiveness not established).

Adverse Reactions/Side Effects

CNS: headache. **CV:** TORSADES DE POINTES, QT interval prolongation. **Endo:** adrenal insufficiency. **F and E:** hypokalemia, hypomagnesemia, hypocalcemia. **GI:** HEPATOCELLULAR DAMAGE, PANCREATITIS, diarrhea, nausea, vomiting. **Resp:** cough. **Misc:** HYPERSENSITIVITY REACTIONS, fever.

Interactions

Drug-Drug: Posaconazole inhibits the CYP3A4 enzyme systems and should be expected to interact with other drugs affected by this system. ↑ **cyclosporine**, **sirolimus**, and **tacrolimus** levels and risk of toxicity; use with sirolimus contraindicated; for cyclosporine and tacrolimus, ↓ dose initially and monitor levels frequently. May ↑ **quinidine** and **pimozide** levels and the risk for arrhythmias; concurrent use contraindicated. May ↑ levels and risk of toxicity from **ergot alkaloids**, including **ergotamine** and **dihydroergotamine**; concurrent use contraindicated. May ↑ levels of **simvastatin**, **atorvastatin**, or **lovastatin** and the risk for rhabdomyolysis; concurrent use contraindicated. **Rifabutin**, **phenytoin**, **cimetidine**, and **efavirenz** ↓ levels and may ↓ antifungal effectiveness; avoid concurrent use. **Esomeprazole** and **metoclopramide** may ↓ levels and may ↓ antifungal effectiveness. ↑ **rifabutin** levels; avoid concurrent use. **QT interval prolonging drugs** may ↑ risk for QT interval prolongation and torsades de pointes; avoid concurrent use. May ↑ **digoxin** levels; monitor levels frequently. ↑ **phenytoin**, **midazolam**, **ritonavir**, and **atazanavir** levels; monitor for excess clinical effect. May ↑ levels of and risk of neurotoxicity, SIADH, and paralytic ileus with concurrent use of **vinca alkaloids**, including **vincristine** and **vinblastine**; consider using an alternative non-azole antifungal. ↑ levels and risk of toxicity of **HMG CoA reductase inhibitors (statins)**; consider ↓ statin dose. May ↑ levels and risk of adverse cardiovascular reactions to **calcium channel blockers**; consider dosage reduction.

Route/Dosage

The delayed-release tablets and oral suspension are NOT interchangeable.

Prophylaxis of Invasive Fungal Infections

IV (Adults): 300 mg twice daily on day 1, then 300 mg once daily starting on day 2.
PO (Adults and Children ≥13 yr): *Delayed-release tablets*—300 mg twice daily on day 1, then 300 mg once daily starting on day 2; *Oral suspension*—200 mg 3 times daily.

Oropharyngeal Candidiasis

PO (Adults and Children ≥13 yr): *Oral suspension*—100 mg twice daily on day 1, then 100 mg once daily for the next 13 days; for refractory oropharyngeal candidiasis, give 400 mg twice daily.

Availability (generic available)

Delayed-release tablets: 100 mg. **Oral suspension (cherry-flavor):** 40 mg/mL. **Solution for injection:** 18 mg/mL.

NURSING IMPLICATIONS

Assessment

- Assess for signs and symptoms of fungal infection.
- ***Lab Test Considerations:*** Monitor liver function tests prior to and periodically during therapy. May cause ↑ ALT, ↑ AST, ↑ alkaline phosphatase and ↑ total bilirubin levels; generally reversible on discontinuation. Discontinue posaconazole if clinical signs and symptoms of liver disease develop.
- Monitor electrolyte levels (potassium, magnesium, calcium) before starting and during therapy. Correct as necessary before and during therapy.

Implementation

- Delayed-release tablet and oral suspension are not interchangeable. Tablets are the preferred oral formulation for prophylaxis because they achieve higher plasma concentrations of drug.
- **PO:** Shake suspension well before use. Administer with a full meal, liquid nutritional supplement or an acidic carbonated beverage (ginger ale) to enhance

absorption. Rinse spoon for administration with water after each use. Alternative therapy or close monitoring for breakthrough fungal infections should be considered for patients unable to eat a full meal or tolerate a nutritional supplement.

- Administer delayed-release tablets with food. Swallow tablets whole; do not divide, crush, or chew.

IV Administration

- **Intermittent Infusion:** Allow solution to reach room temperature before administering. ***Diluent:*** Dilute in D5W, D5/0.45% NaCl, D5/0.9% NaCl, D5/20 mEq potassium, 0.45% NaCl or 0.9% NaCl. ***Concentration:*** 1–2 mg/mL. Do not dilute with other solutions. Use immediately; stable for 24 hrs if refrigerated. Discard unused solution. Solution is clear, colorless to yellow; do not administer solutions that are discolored or contain particulate matter. Administer through a 0.22 micron polyethersulfone (PES) or polyvinylidene difluoride (PVDF) filter via central venous line, including a central venous catheter or peripherally inserted central catheter (PICC) line. If no central catheter available, may be administered through a peripheral venous catheter by slow intravenous infusion over 30 min only as a single dose in advance of central venous line placement or to bridge the period during which a central venous line is replaced or is in use for other intravenous treatment. ***Rate:*** Infuse slowly over 90 min. Do not give as a bolus.
- **Y-Site Compatibility:** amikacin, caspofungin, ciprofloxacin, daptomycin, dobutamine, famotidine, filgrastim, gentamicin, hydromorphone, levofloxacin, lorazepam, meropenem, micafungin, morphine, norepinephrine, potassium chloride, vancomycin.

Patient/Family Teaching

- Instruct patient to take posaconazole during or immediately (within 20 min) following a full meal or liquid nutritional supplement in order to enhance absorption. Take missed doses as soon as remembered. Instruct patient to read the *Patient Information* before taking posaconazole and with each Rx refill; may be new information.
- Advise patient to notify health care professional if severe diarrhea or vomiting occur; may decrease posaconazole blood levels and allow breakthrough fungal infections or if signs and symptoms of liver injury (itching, yellow eyes or skin, fatigue, flu-like symptoms) or change in heart rate or rhythm occur.
- Instruct patient to notify health care professional of all Rx or OTC medications, vitamins, or herbal products being taken and consult health care professional before taking any new medications.
- Advise patient to notify health care professional if pregnancy is planned or suspected and to avoid breast feeding during therapy.

Evaluation/Desired Outcomes

- Resolution of clinical and laboratory indications of fungal infections. Duration of therapy is based on recovery from infection or neutropenia or immunosuppression.

potassium and sodium phosphates

(po-**tas**-e-um/**soe**-dee-um **foss**-fates)

K-Phos M.F, K-Phos Neutral, K-Phos No. 2, Neutra-Phos, Uro-KP Neutral

Classification

Therapeutic: antiurolithics, mineral and electrolyte replacements/supplements

Indications

Treatment and prevention of phosphate depletion in patients who are unable to ingest adequate dietary phosphate. Adjunct therapy of urinary tract infections with methenamine hippurate or mandelate. Prevention of calcium urinary stones. Phosphate salts of potassium may be used in hypokalemic patients with metabolic acidosis or coexisting phosphorus deficiency.

Action

Phosphate is present in bone and is involved in energy transfer and carbohydrate metabolism. Serves as a buffer for the excretion of hydrogen ions by the kidneys. Dibasic potassium phosphate is converted in renal tubule to monobasic salt, resulting in urinary acidification, which is required for methenamine hippurate or mandelate to be active as urinary anti-infectives. Acidification of urine increases solubility of calcium, decreasing calcium stone formation. **Therapeutic Effects:** Replacement of phosphorus in deficiency states. Urinary acidification. Increased efficacy of methenamine. Decreased formation of calcium urinary tract stones.

Pharmacokinetics

Absorption: Well absorbed following oral administration. Vitamin D promotes GI absorption of phosphates.

Distribution: Phosphates enter extracellular fluids and are then actively transported to sites of action.

Metabolism and Excretion: Excreted mainly (>90%) by the kidneys.

Half-life: Unknown.

TIME/ACTION PROFILE (effects on serum phosphate levels)

ROUTE	ONSET	PEAK	DURATION
PO	unknown	unknown	unknown

P

Contraindications/Precautions

Contraindicated in: Hyperkalemia (potassium salts); Hyperphosphatemia; Hypocalcemia; Severe renal impairment; Untreated Addison's disease (potassium salts).

Use Cautiously in: Hyperparathyroidism; Cardiac disease; Hypernatremia (sodium phosphate only); Hypertension (sodium phosphate only); Renal impairment.

Adverse Reactions/Side Effects

Related to hyperphosphatemia, unless otherwise indicated.

CNS: confusion, dizziness, headache, weakness. **CV:** ARRHYTHMIAS, CARDIAC ARREST, bradycardia, ECG changes (absent P waves, widening of the QRS complex with biphasic curve, peaked T waves), edema. **GI:** diarrhea, abdominal pain, nausea, vomiting. **F and E:** hyperkalemia, hypernatremia, hyperphosphatemia, hypocalcemia, hypomagnesemia. **MS:** *hypocalcemia, hyperkalemia*—muscle cramps. **Neuro:** flaccid paralysis, heaviness of legs, paresthesias, tremors.

Interactions

Drug-Drug: Concurrent use of **potassium-sparing diuretics**, **ACE inhibitors**, or **angiotensin II receptor blockers** with potassium phosphates may result in hyperkalemia. Concurrent use of **corticosteroids** with sodium phosphate may result in hypernatremia. Concurrent administration of **calcium-**, **magnesium-**, or **aluminum-containing compounds** ↓ absorption of phosphates by formation of insoluble complexes. **Vitamin D** enhances the absorption of phosphates.

Drug-Food: Oxalates (in spinach and rhubarb) and **phytates** (in bran and whole grains) may ↓ absorption of phosphates by binding them in the GI tract.

Route/Dosage

Phosphorous Supplementation

PO (Adults and Children >4 yr): 250–500 mg (8–16 mmol) phosphorus (1–2 packets) 4 times daily.

PO (Children <4 yr): 250 mg (8 mmol) phosphorus (1 packet) 4 times daily.

Urinary Acidification

PO (Adults): 2 tablets 4 times/day.

Maintenance Phosphorus

PO (Adults): 50–150 mmol/day in divided doses.

PO (Children): 2–3 mmol/kg/day in divided doses.

Availability

Potassium and Sodium Phosphates

Tablets (K-Phos MF): elemental phosphorus 125.6 mg (4 mmol), sodium 67 mg (2.9 mEq), and potassium 44.5 mg (1.1 mEq). **Tablets (K-Phos Neutral):** elemental phosphorus 250 mg (8 mmol), sodium 298 mg (13 mEq), and potassium 45 mg (1.1 mEq). **Tablets (K-Phos No.2):** elemental phosphorus 250 mg (8 mmol), sodium 134 mg (5.8 mEq), and potassium 88 mg (2.3 mEq). **Tablets (Uro-KP Neutral):** elemental phosphorus 258 mg, sodium 262.4 mg (10.8 mEq), and potassium 49.4 mg (1.3 mEq). **Powder for oral solution (Neutra-Phos):** elemental phosphorus 250 mg (8 mmol), sodium 164 mg (7.1 mEq), and potassium 278 mg (7.1 mEq)/packet.

NURSING IMPLICATIONS

Assessment

- Assess patient for signs and symptoms of hypokalemia (weakness, fatigue, arrhythmias, presence of U waves on ECG, polyuria, polydipsia) and hypophosphatemia (anorexia, weakness, decreased reflexes, bone pain, confusion, blood dyscrasias) throughout therapy.
- Monitor intake and output ratios and daily weight. Report significant discrepancies.
- ***Lab Test Considerations:*** Monitor serum phosphate, potassium, sodium, and calcium levels prior to and periodically throughout therapy. Increased phosphate may cause hypocalcemia.
- Monitor renal function studies prior to and periodically throughout therapy.
- Monitor urinary pH in patients receiving potassium and sodium phosphate as a urinary acidifier.

Implementation

- **PO:** Tablets should be dissolved in a full glass of water. Allow mixture to stand for 2–5 min to ensure it is fully dissolved. Solutions prepared by pharmacy should not be further diluted.
- Medication should be administered after meals to minimize gastric irritation and laxative effect.
- Do not administer simultaneously with antacids containing aluminum, magnesium, or calcium.

Patient/Family Teaching

- Explain to the patient the purpose of the medication and the need to take as directed. Take missed doses as soon as remembered unless within 1 or 2 hr of the next dose. Explain that the tablets should not be swallowed whole. Tablets should be dissolved in water.
- Instruct patients in low-sodium diet (see Appendix K).
- Advise patient of the importance of maintaining a high fluid intake (drinking at least one 8-oz glass of water each hr) to prevent kidney stones.
- Instruct the patient to promptly report diarrhea, weakness, fatigue, muscle cramps, unexplained weight gain, swelling of lower extremities, shortness of breath, unusual thirst, or tremors.

Evaluation/Desired Outcomes

- Prevention and correction of serum phosphate and potassium deficiencies.
- Maintenance of acid urine.
- Decreased urine calcium, which prevents formation of renal calculi.

potassium iodide, See **IODINE, IODIDE.**

HIGH ALERT

POTASSIUM SUPPLEMENTS
(poe-**tass**-ee-um)

potassium acetate

potassium bicarbonate/potassium chloride

potassium bicarbonate/potassium citrate
Effer-K, K-Lyte DS

potassium chloride
Klor-Con, Klor-Con M10, Klor-Con M15, Klor-Con M20, K-Tab, Micro-K, Micro-K 10

potassium gluconate

Classification
Therapeutic: mineral and electrolyte replacements/supplements

Indications
PO, IV: Treatment/prevention of potassium depletion. **IV:** Arrhythmias due to digoxin toxicity.

Action
Maintain acid-base balance, isotonicity, and electrophysiologic balance of the cell. Activator in many enzymatic reactions; essential to transmission of nerve impulses; contraction of cardiac, skeletal, and smooth muscle; gastric secretion; renal function; tissue synthesis; and carbohydrate metabolism. **Therapeutic Effects:** Replacement. Prevention of deficiency.

Pharmacokinetics
Absorption: Well absorbed following oral administration.
Distribution: Enters extracellular fluid; then actively transported into cells.
Metabolism and Excretion: Excreted by the kidneys.
Half-life: Unknown.

TIME/ACTION PROFILE (↑ in serum potassium levels)

ROUTE	ONSET	PEAK	DURATION
PO	unknown	1–2 hr	unknown
IV	rapid	end of infusion	unknown

Contraindications/Precautions
Contraindicated in: Hyperkalemia; Severe renal impairment; Untreated Addison's disease; Severe tissue trauma; Hyperkalemic familial periodic paralysis; Some products may contain tartrazine (FDC yellow dye #5) or alcohol; avoid using in patients with known hypersensitivity or intolerance; Potassium acetate injection contains aluminum, which may become toxic with prolonged use to high risk groups (renal impairment, premature neonates).
Use Cautiously in: Cardiac disease; Renal impairment; Diabetes mellitus (liquids may contain sugar); Hypomagnesemia (may make correction of hypokalemia more difficult); GI hypomotility including dysphagia or esophageal compression from left atrial enlargement (tablets, capsules); Patients receiving potassium-sparing drugs.

Adverse Reactions/Side Effects
CNS: confusion, restlessness, weakness. **CV:** ARRHYTHMIAS, ECG changes. **GI:** abdominal pain, diarrhea, flatulence, nausea, vomiting; *tablets, capsules only*, GI ulceration, stenotic lesions. **Local:** irritation at IV site. **Neuro:** paralysis, paresthesia.

Interactions
Drug-Drug: Use with **potassium-sparing diuretics** or **ACE inhibitors** or **angiotensin II receptor antagonists** may lead to hyperkalemia. **Anticholinergics** may ↑ GI mucosal lesions in patients taking wax-matrix potassium chloride preparations.

Route/Dosage
Expressed as mEq of potassium. Potassium acetate contains 10.2 mEq/g; potassium bicarbonate contains 10 mEq potassium/g; potassium chloride contains 13.4 mEq potassium/g; potassium gluconate contains 4.3 mEq/g.

Normal Daily Requirements
PO, IV (Adults): 40–80 mEq/day.
PO, IV (Children): 2–3 mEq/kg/day.
PO, IV (Neonates): 2–6 mEq/kg/day.

Prevention of Hypokalemia during Diuretic Therapy
PO (Adults): 20–40 mEq/day in 1–2 divided doses; single dose should not exceed 20 mEq.
PO (Neonates, Infants, and Children): 1–2 mEq/kg/day in 1–2 divided doses.

Treatment of Hypokalemia
PO (Adults): 40–100 mEq/day in divided doses.
PO (Neonates, Infants, and Children): 2–5 mEq/kg/day in divided doses.
IV (Adults): *Serum potassium >2.5 mEq/L*—Up to 20 mEq/day as an infusion (not to exceed 10 mEq/hr) or a concentration of 40 mEq/L via peripheral line (up

P

to 100 mEq/L have been used via central line [unlabeled]). *Serum potassium <2 mEq/L with symptoms*—Up to 40 mEq/day as an infusion (rate should generally not exceed 20 mEq/hr).
IV (Neonates, Infants, and Children): 0.5–1 mEq/kg/dose (maximum 30 mEq/dose) as an infusion to infuse at 0.3–0.5 mEq/kg/hr (maximum infusion rate 1 mEq/kg/hr).

Availability

Potassium Acetate (generic available)

Concentrate for injection (contains aluminum): 2 mEq/mL, 4 mEq/mL.

Potassium Bicarbonate/Potassium Chloride (generic available)

Tablets for effervescent oral solution: 🍁 12 mEq, 25 mEq.

Potassium Bicarbonate/Potassium Citrate (generic available)

Tablets for effervescent oral solution: 10 mEq, 20 mEq, 25 mEq, 50 mEq.

Potassium Chloride (generic available)

Extended-release tablets: 8 mEq, 10 mEq, 15 mEq, 20 mEq. **Cost:** *Generic*—8 mEq $53.64/100, 10 mEq $45.97/100, 20 mEq $45.97/100. **Extended-release capsules:** 8 mEq, 10 mEq. **Cost:** *Generic*—8 mEq $70.40/100, 10 mEq $72.62/100. **Oral solution:** 20 mEq/15 mL, 40 mEq/15 mL. **Cost:** *Generic*—20 mEq/15 mL $14.51/473 mL, 40 mEq/15 mL $27.11/473 mL. **Powder/packets for oral solution:** 20-mEq/packet, 25-mEq/packet. **Cost:** 20 mEq $58.21/30 pkts, 25 mEq $69.20/30 pkts. **Concentrate for injection:** 0.1 mEq/mL in 10-mEq ampules and vials, 0.2 mEq/mL in 10- and 20-mEq ampules and vials, 0.3 mEq/mL in 30-mEq ampules and vials, 0.4 mEq/mL in 20- and 40-mEq ampules and vials, 1.5 mEq/mL, 2 mEq/mL, 3 mEq/mL. **Solution for IV infusion:** 10 mEq/L in various dextrose and saline solutions in 250-, 500-, and 100-mL containers, 20 mEq/L in dextrose/saline/LRs in 250-, 500-, and 100-mL containers, 30 mEq/L in various dextrose and saline solutions in 250-, 500-, and 100-mL containers, 40 mEq/L in various dextrose and saline solutions in 250-, 500-, and 100-mL containers.

Potassium Gluconate (generic available)

Tablets: 2 mEq, 5 mEq. **Elixir:** 20 mEq/15 mL.

NURSING IMPLICATIONS

Assessment

- Assess for signs and symptoms of hypokalemia (weakness, fatigue, U wave on ECG, arrhythmias, polyuria, polydipsia) and hyperkalemia (see Toxicity and Overdose).
- Monitor pulse, BP, and ECG periodically during IV therapy.
- ***Lab Test Considerations:*** Monitor serum potassium before and periodically during therapy. Monitor renal function, serum bicarbonate, and pH. Determine serum magnesium level if patient has refractory hypokalemia; hypomagnesemia should be corrected to facilitate effectiveness of potassium replacement. Monitor serum chloride because hypochloremia may occur if replacing potassium without concurrent chloride.
- ***Toxicity and Overdose:*** Symptoms of toxicity are those of hyperkalemia (slow, irregular heartbeat; fatigue; muscle weakness; paresthesia; confusion; dyspnea; peaked T waves; depressed ST segments; prolonged QT segments; widened QRS complexes; loss of P waves; and cardiac arrhythmias).
- Treatment includes discontinuation of potassium, administration of sodium bicarbonate to correct acidosis, dextrose and insulin to facilitate passage of potassium into cells, calcium salts to reverse ECG effects (in patients who are not receiving digoxin), sodium polystyrene used as an exchange resin, and/or dialysis for patient with impaired renal function.

Implementation

- ***High Alert:*** Medication errors involving too rapid infusion or bolus IV administration of potassium chloride have resulted in fatalities. See IV administration guidelines below.
- For most purposes, potassium chloride should be used, except for renal tubular acidoses (hyperchloremic acidosis), in which other salts are more appropriate (potassium bicarbonate, potassium citrate, or potassium gluconate).
- If hypokalemia is secondary to diuretic therapy, consideration should be given to decreasing the dose of diuretic, unless there is a history of significant arrhythmias or concurrent digitalis glycoside therapy.
- **PO:** Administer with or after meals to decrease GI irritation.
- Use of tablets and capsules should be reserved for patients who cannot tolerate liquid preparations.
- Dissolve effervescent tablets in 3–8 oz of cold water. Ensure that effervescent tablet is fully dissolved. Powders and solutions should be diluted in 3–8 oz of cold water or juice (do not use tomato juice if patient is on sodium restriction). Instruct patient to drink slowly over 5–10 min.
- Tablets and capsules should be taken with a meal and full glass of water. Do not chew or crush enteric-coated or extended-release tablets or capsules. Micro-K ExtenCaps capsules can be opened and sprinkled on soft food (pudding, applesauce) and swallowed immediately with a glass of cool water or juice.
- **IV:** Assess for extravasation; severe pain and tissue necrosis may occur. ***High Alert:*** Never administer potassium IV push or bolus.

Potassium Acetate

- **Continuous Infusion:** ***High Alert:*** Do not administer undiluted. Each single dose *must* be diluted and thoroughly mixed in 100–1000 mL of dextrose, saline, Ringer's or LR, dextrose/saline, dextrose/Ringer's, or LR combinations. Usually limited to 80 mEq/L via peripheral line (200 mEq/L via central line).

- ***Rate: High Alert:*** Infuse slowly, at a rate up to 10 mEq/hr in adults or 0.5 mEq/kg/hr in children on general care areas. Check hospital policy for maximum infusion rates (maximum rate in monitored setting 40 mEq/hr in adults or 1 mEq/kg/hr in children).
- **Y-Site Compatibility:** ciprofloxacin.

Potassium Chloride

- **Continuous Infusion:** ***High Alert:*** Do not administer concentrations of ≥1.5 mEq/mL undiluted; fatalities have occurred. Concentrated products have black caps on vials or black stripes above constriction on ampules and are labeled with a warning about dilution requirement. Each single dose must be diluted and thoroughly mixed in 100–1000 mL of IV solution. Usually limited to 80 mEq/L via peripheral line (200 mEq/L via central line).
- Concentrations of 0.1 and 0.4 mEq/mL are intended for administration via calibrated infusion device and do not require dilution.
- ***Rate: High Alert:*** Infuse slowly, at a rate up to 10 mEq/hr in adults or 0.5 mEq/kg/hr in children in general care areas. Check hospital policy for maximum infusion rates (maximum rate in monitored setting 40 mEq/hr in adults or 1 mEq/kg/hr in children). Use an infusion pump.
- **Solution Compatibility:** May be diluted in dextrose, saline, Ringer's solution, LR, dextrose/saline, dextrose/Ringer's solution, and dextrose/LR combinations. Commercially available premixed with many of the above IV solutions.
- **Y-Site Compatibility:** acyclovir, alemtuzumab, alfentanil, allopurinol, alprostadil, amifostine, amikacin, aminophylline, amiodarone, amphotericin B liposome, anidulafungin, argatroban, ascorbic acid, atropine, aztreonam, benztropine, betamethasone, bivalirudin, bleomycin, bumetanide, buprenorphine, butorphanol, calcium chloride, calcium gluconate, carboplatin, carmustine, caspofungin, cefazolin, cefotaxime, cefotetan, cefoxitin, ceftaroline, ceftazidime, ceftriaxone, cefuroxime, chloramphenicol, chlorpromazine, ciprofloxacin, cisatracurium, cisplatin, cladribine, clindamycin, cyanocobalamin, cyclophosphamide, cyclosporine, cytarabine, dactinomycin, daptomycin, dexamethasone sodium phosphate, dexmedetomidine, digoxin, diltiazem, diphenhydramine, dobutamine, docetaxel, dopamine, doxorubicin hydrochloride, doxorubicin liposome, doxycycline, droperidol, enalaprilat, ephedrine, epinephrine, epirubicin, epoetin alfa, eptifibatide, ertapenem, esmolol, conjugated estrogens, etoposide, etoposide phosphate, famotidine, fenoldopam, fentanyl, filgrastim, fluconazole, fludarabine, fluorouracil, folic acid, furosemide, ganciclovir, gemcitabine, gentamicin, granisetron, heparin, hydrocortisone, hydromorphone, idarubicin, ifosfamide, imipenem/cilastatin, indomethacin, insulin, irinotecan, isoproterenol, ketamine, ketorolac, labetalol, levofloxacin, lidocaine, linezolid, lorazepam, magnesium sulfate, mannitol, melphalan, meperidine, meropenem, methotrexate, methoxamine, methyldopate, methylergonovine, meticlopramide, metoprolol, metronidazole, micafungin, midazolam, milrinone, mitoxantrone, morphine, multivitamins, mycophenolate, nafcillin, nalbuphine, naloxone, neostigmine, nicardipine, nitroglycerin, nitroprusside, norepinephrine, octreotide, ondansetron, oxacillin, oxaliplatin, oxytocin, paclitaxel, palonosetron, pamidronate, pancuronium, pantoprazole, papaverine, pemetrexed, penicillin G, pentobarbital, phenobarbital, phentolamine, phenylephrine, phytonadione, piperacillin/tazobactam, procainamide, prochlorperazine, propofol, propranolol, protamine, pyridostigmine, pyridoxime, quinupristin/dalfopristin, ranitidine, remifentanil, rituximab, rocuronium, sargramostim, scopolamine, sodium acetate, sodium bicarbonate, streptokinase, succinylcholine, tacrolimus, telavancin, theophylline, thiamine, thiotepa, tirofiban, tobramycin, tolazoline, trastuzumab, trimetaphan, vancomycin, vasopressin, verapamil, vincristine, vinorelbine, voriconazole, warfarin, zidovudine, zoledronic acid.
- **Y-Site Incompatibility:** amphotericin B cholesteryl, amphotericin B deoxycholate, azithromycin, dantrolene, diazepam, diazoxide, haloperidol, hydralazine, pentamidine, phenytoin, trimethoprim/sulfamethoxazole.

P

Patient/Family Teaching

- Explain to patient purpose of the medication and the need to take as directed, especially when concurrent digoxin or diuretics are taken. Take missed doses as soon as remembered within 2 hr; if not, return to regular dose schedule. Do not double dose.
- Emphasize correct method of administration. GI irritation or ulceration may result from chewing enteric-coated tablets or insufficient dilution of liquid or powder forms.
- Some extended-release tablets are contained in a wax matrix that may be expelled in the stool. This occurrence is not significant.
- Instruct patient to avoid salt substitutes or low-salt milk or food unless approved by health care professional. Patient should be advised to read all labels to prevent excess potassium intake.
- Advise patient regarding sources of dietary potassium (see Appendix K). Encourage compliance with recommended diet.

- Instruct patient to report dark, tarry, or bloody stools; weakness; unusual fatigue; or tingling of extremities. Notify health care professional if nausea, vomiting, diarrhea, or stomach discomfort persists. Dosage may require adjustment.
- Emphasize the importance of regular follow-up exams to monitor serum levels and progress.

Evaluation/Desired Outcomes
- Prevention and correction of serum potassium depletion.
- Cessation of arrhythmias caused by digoxin toxicity.

pramipexole (pra-mi-**pex**-ole)
Mirapex, Mirapex ER

Classification
Therapeutic: antiparkinson agents
Pharmacologic: dopamine agonists

Indications
Management of Parkinson's disease. Restless leg syndrome (immediate-release only).

Action
Stimulates dopamine receptors in the striatum of the brain. **Therapeutic Effects:** Decreased tremor and rigidity in Parkinson's disease. Decreased leg restlessness.

Pharmacokinetics
Absorption: >90% absorbed following oral administration.
Distribution: Widely distributed.
Metabolism and Excretion: 90% excreted unchanged in urine.
Half-life: 8 hr (↑ in geriatric patients and patients with renal impairment).

TIME/ACTION PROFILE (blood levels)

ROUTE	ONSET	PEAK	DURATION
PO	unknown	2 hr	8 hr
PO-ER	unknown	6 hr	24 hr

Contraindications/Precautions
Contraindicated in: Hypersensitivity; Major psychotic disorder.
Use Cautiously in: Renal impairment (↑ dosing interval recommended if CCr <60 mL/min [immediate-release] or CCr <50 mL/min [extended-release]); OB, Lactation, Pedi: Safety not established; Geri: ↑ risk of hallucinations.

Adverse Reactions/Side Effects
CNS: SLEEP ATTACKS, amnesia, dizziness, drowsiness, hallucinations, weakness, abnormal dreams, aggressive behavior, agitation, confusion, delirium, delusions, disorientation, dyskinesia, extrapyramidal syndrome, headache, insomnia, paranoid ideation, psychotic-like behavior, urges (gambling, sexual). **CV:** orthostatic hypotension. **Derm:** pruritis. **Endo:** SIADH. **GI:** constipation, dry mouth, dyspepsia, nausea, tooth disease. **GU:** urinary frequency. **MS:** RHABDOMYOLYSIS, leg cramps, muscle pain, postural deformities. **Neuro:** hypertonia, unsteadiness/falling.

Interactions
Drug-Drug: Concurrent **levodopa** ↑ risk of hallucinations and dyskinesia. **Cimetidine**, **ranitidine**, **diltiazem**, **triamterene**, **verapamil**, **quinidine**, **quinine**, and **cisplatin** may ↑ levels. Effectiveness may be ↓ by **dopamine antagonists**, including **butyrophenones**, **metoclopramide**, **phenothiazines**, or **thioxanthenes**.

Route/Dosage
When switching from immediate-release to extended-release product, the same total daily dose can be used.

Parkinson's Disease
PO (Adults): *Immediate-release*—0.125 mg 3 times daily initially; may be ↑ every 5–7 days (range 1.5–4.5 mg/day in 3 divided doses); *Extended-release*—0.375 mg once daily; may be ↑ to 0.75 mg once daily in 5–7 days, and then ↑ every 5–7 days by 0.75 mg/day (max dose = 4.5 mg/day).

Renal Impairment
PO (Adults Immediate-release): *CCr 35–59 mL/min*—0.125 mg twice daily initially, may be ↑ every 5–7 days up to 1.5 mg twice daily; *CCr 15–34 mL/min*—0.125 mg daily initially, may be ↑ every 5–7 days up to 1.5 mg daily.

Renal Impairment
PO (Adults Extended-release): *CCr 30–50 mL/min*—0.375 mg every other day; may consider ↑ dose to 0.375 mg once daily after 1 wk based on response and tolerability; may ↑ in 0.375 mg increments after 1 wk (max dose = 2.25 mg/day).

Restless Leg Syndrome
PO (Adults): 0.125 mg daily 1–3 hr before bedtime. May be ↑ at 4–7 day intervals to 0.25 mg daily, then up to 0.5 mg daily.

Renal Impairment
PO (Adults Immediate-release): *CCr 20–60 mL/min*—0.125 mg daily 1–3 hr before bedtime. May be ↑ at 14-day intervals to 0.25 mg daily, then up to 0.5 mg daily.

Availability (generic available)
Extended-release tablets: 0.375 mg, 0.75 mg, 1.5 mg, 2.25 mg, 3 mg, 3.75 mg, 4.5 mg. **Cost:** 0.375 mg $103.92/7, 0.75 mg $103.92/7, 1.5 mg $103.92/7, 2.25 mg $445.40/30, 3 mg $445.40/30, 3.75 mg $445.40/30, 4.5 mg $445.40/30. **Tablets:** 0.125 mg, 0.25 mg, 0.5 mg, 0.75 mg, 1 mg, 1.5 mg. **Cost:** *Generic*—0.125 mg $265.47/90, 0.25 mg $277.55/90, 0.5 mg $265.47/90, 0.75 mg $265.47/90, 1 mg $277.55/90, 1.5 mg $277.55/90.

NURSING IMPLICATIONS

Assessment

- Assess patient for signs and symptoms of psychotic-like behavior (confusion, paranoid ideation, delusions, hallucinations, psychotic-like behavior, disorientation, aggressive behavior, agitation, delirium, hallucinations). Risk of symptoms increases with age. Notify health care professional if these occur.
- Monitor ECG and BP frequently during dose adjustment and periodically throughout therapy.
- Assess patient for drowsiness and sleep attacks. Drowsiness is a common side effect of pramipexole, but sleep attacks or episodes of falling asleep during activities that require active participation may occur without warning. Assess patient for concomitant medications that have sedating effects or may increase serum pramipexole levels (see Interactions). May require discontinuation of therapy.
- **Parkinson's Disease:** Assess patient for signs and symptoms of Parkinson's disease (tremor, muscle weakness and rigidity, ataxia) before and throughout therapy.
- **Restless Leg Syndrome:** Assess sleep patterns and frequency of restless leg disturbances.

Implementation

- Do not confuse Mirapex (pramipexole) with Miralax (polyethylene glycol).
- An attempt to reduce the dose of levodopa/carbidopa may be made cautiously during pramipexole therapy.
- **PO:** Administer with meals to minimize nausea; usually resolves with continued therapy. Swallow extended-release tablets whole; do not crush, break, or chew.

Patient/Family Teaching

- Instruct patient to take medication as directed. Take missed doses or immediate-release product as soon as remembered if it is not almost time for next dose. If extended release tablets are missed, skip dose and take next regular dose. Do not double doses. Consult health care professional before reducing dose or discontinuing medication; may cause fever, confusion, or severe muscle stiffness. Advise patient to read the *Patient Information* sheet before taking and with each Rx refill, changes may occur.
- May cause drowsiness and unexpected episodes of falling asleep. Caution patient to avoid driving or other activities requiring alertness until response to medication is known. Advise patient to notify health care professional if episodes of falling asleep occur.
- Advise patient to change position slowly to minimize orthostatic hypotension. May occur more frequently during initial therapy.
- Instruct patient to notify health care professional of all Rx or OTC medications, vitamins, or herbal products being taken and consult health care professional before taking any new medications.
- Advise patient to have periodic skin exams to check for lesions that may be melanoma.
- Advise patient to notify health care professional if new or increased gambling, sexual, or other intense urges or psychotic-like behaviors occur.
- Advise patient to notify health care professional if pregnancy is planned or suspected or if breast feeding.

Evaluation/Desired Outcomes

- Decreased tremor and rigidity in Parkinson's disease.
- Decrease in restless legs and improved sleep.

prasterone (pras-ter-one)
Intrarosa

Classification
Therapeutic: none assigned
Pharmacologic: steroids

Indications
Moderate to severe dyspareunia.

Action
Inactive steroid that is converted into active androgens and/or estrogens. Exact mechanism in treatment of vulvar and vaginal atrophy in menopausal women not fully established. **Therapeutic Effects:** Reduced severity of dyspareunia.

Pharmacokinetics
Absorption: Unknown.
Distribution: Unknown.
Metabolism and Excretion: Metabolized via dehydrogenase, reductase, and aromatase to estradiol and testosterone.
Half-life: Unknown.

TIME/ACTION PROFILE (improvement in dyspareunia severity)

ROUTE	ONSET	PEAK	DURATION
Vag	unknown	12 wk	unknown

Contraindications/Precautions
Contraindicated in: Undiagnosed abnormal genital bleeding; Current or history of breast cancer; OB, Lactation, Pedi: Only indicated in postmenopausal women.
Use Cautiously in: None noted.

Adverse Reactions/Side Effects
GU: vaginal discharge.

Interactions
Drug-Drug: None noted.

Route/Dosage

Vag (Adults): Insert one vaginal insert at bedtime.

Availability

Vaginal insert: 6.5 mg.

NURSING IMPLICATIONS

Assessment

- Assess for pain during intercourse periodically during therapy.

Implementation

- **Vag:** Insert vaginal insert at bedtime using applicator provided. Vaginal inserts can be stored at room temperature or refrigerated.

Patient/Family Teaching

- Explain purpose of prasterone to patient. Instruct patient to read *Instructions for Use* before inserting prasterone.
- Inform patient that vaginal discharge and abnormal PAP smear findings may occur with prasterone.
- Advise patient to notify health care professional of all Rx or OTC medications, vitamins, or herbal products being taken and to consult with health care professional before taking other medications during therapy.

Evaluation/Desired Outcomes

- Decreased pain during intercourse.

prasugrel (pra-soo-grel)

Effient

Classification

Therapeutic: antiplatelet agents

Pharmacologic: thienopyridines

Indications

Reduction of thrombotic cardiovascular events (including stent thrombosis) in patients with acute coronary syndrome who will be managed with percutaneous coronary intervention (PCI) including patients with unstable angina or non-ST-elevation myocardial infarction (NSTEMI). Reduction of thrombotic cardiovascular events (including stent thrombosis) in patients with ST-elevation myocardial infarction (STEMI) when managed with either primary/delayed PCI.

Action

Acts by irreversibly binding its active metabolite to the $P2Y_{12}$ class of ADP receptors on platelets; inhibiting platelet activation and aggregation. **Therapeutic Effects:** Decreased thrombotic events including cardiovascular death, nonfatal myocardial infarction (MI), and nonfatal stroke.

Pharmacokinetics

Absorption: Well absorbed following oral administration (79%), then rapidly converted to an active metabolite.

Distribution: Unknown.

Protein Binding: *Active metabolite*—98%.

Metabolism and Excretion: Active metabolite is metabolized to two inactive compounds; 68% excreted in the urine and 27% in feces as inactive metabolites.

Half-life: *Active metabolite*—7 hr (range 2–15 hr).

TIME/ACTION PROFILE (effect on platelet function)

ROUTE	ONSET	PEAK	DURATION
PO	within 1 hr	2 hr	5–9 days†

†Following discontinuation.

Contraindications/Precautions

Contraindicated in: Hypersensitivity; Active pathological bleeding; History of transient ischemic attack or stroke.

Use Cautiously in: Patients about to undergo coronary artery bypass grafting (CABG) (↑ risk of bleeding; discontinue at least 7 days prior to surgery); Premature discontinuation (↑ risk of stent thrombosis, MI, and death); Body weight <60 kg, propensity to bleed, severe hepatic impairment, concurrent use of medications that ↑ the risk of bleeding (↑ risk of bleeding); Hypotension in the setting of recent coronary angiography, PCI, CABG, or other surgical procedure (suspect bleeding but do not discontinue prasugrel); Geri: Use in patients ≥75 yr of age generally not recommended (↑ risk of fatal/intracranial bleeding and questionable benefit, except in high-risk patients such as diabetes or prior MI); OB: Use only if potential benefit to mother justifies potential risk to fetus; Lactation: Use only if potential benefit to the mother justifies potential risk to nursing infant; Pedi: Safety and effectiveness not established.

Adverse Reactions/Side Effects

CNS: dizziness, fatigue, headache. **Resp:** cough, dyspnea. **CV:** atrial fibrillation, bradycardia, hypertension, hypotension, peripheral edema. **GI:** diarrhea, nausea. **Derm:** rash. **Hemat:** BLEEDING, THROMBOTIC THROMBOCYTOPENIC PURPURA, leukopenia. **Metab:** hyperlipidemia. **MS:** back pain, extremity pain. **Misc:** allergic reactions including ANGIOEDEMA, fever, non-cardiac chest pain.

Interactions

Drug-Drug: ↑ risk of bleeding with **warfarin** and **NSAIDs. Opioids** may ↓ absorption of active metabolite and ↓ antiplatelet effects; consider using parenteral antiplatelet in patients with acute coronary syndrome if concurrent use of opioids needed.

Route/Dosage

Aspirin 75–325 mg/daily should be taken concurrently.

PO (Adults ≥60 kg): 60 mg initially as a loading dose, then 10 mg once daily.

PO (Adults <60 kg): Consider maintenance dose of 5 mg once daily.

Availability (generic available)

Tablets: 5 mg, 10 mg.

NURSING IMPLICATIONS

Assessment

- Assess patient for symptoms of stroke, peripheral vascular disease, or MI periodically during therapy.
- Monitor patient for signs of thrombotic thrombocytopenic purpura (thrombocytopenia, microangiopathic hemolytic anemia, neurologic findings, renal dysfunction, fever). May rarely occur, even after short exposure (<2 wk). Requires prompt treatment.
- ***Lab Test Considerations:*** Monitor bleeding time during therapy. Prolonged bleeding time, which is time- and dose-dependent, is expected.
- Monitor CBC with differential and platelet count periodically during therapy. Thrombocytopenia and anemia may rarely occur.

Implementation

- Discontinue prasugrel 7 days before planned surgical procedures.
- Patients should take aspirin 75–325 mg daily with prasugrel.
- *In patients with unstable angina (UA) or NSTEMI,* dose is usually administered at time of diagnosis or at time of PCI.
- *In patients with STEMI* presenting within 12 hrs of symptom onset, loading dose is usually administered at time of diagnosis or at time of PCI.
- **PO:** Administer once daily without regard to food. Swallow tablets whole; do not break.

Patient/Family Teaching

- Instruct patient to take medication as directed. Take missed doses as soon as possible unless almost time for next dose; do not double doses. Do not discontinue without consulting health care professional. Advise patient to read *Medication Guide* before taking and with each Rx refill; in case of changes. Instruct patient to keep prasugrel in original container with dessicant, and keep tightly capped to protect from moisture.
- Advise patient to notify health care professional promptly if fever, weakness, skin paleness, purple skin patches, yellowing of skin or eyes, chills, sore throat, neurological changes, or unusual bleeding or bruising, swelling of lips, difficulty breathing, rash, or hives occurs.
- Advise patient to notify health care professional of medication regimen prior to treatment or surgery.
- Instruct patient to notify health care professional of all Rx or OTC medications, vitamins, or herbal products being taken and consult health care professional before taking any new medications, especially NSAIDs.
- Advise female patient to notify health care professional if pregnancy is planned or suspected and to avoid breast feeding during therapy.

Evaluation/Desired Outcomes

- Prevention of stroke, MI, and vascular death in patients at risk.

pravastatin, See HMG-CoA REDUCTASE INHIBITORS (statins).

BEERS

prazosin (pra-zoe-sin)

Minipress

Classification
Therapeutic: antihypertensives
Pharmacologic: peripherally acting antiadrenergics

Indications

Mild to moderate hypertension. **Unlabeled Use:** Management of urinary outflow obstruction in patients with benign prostatic hyperplasia.

Action

Dilates both arteries and veins by blocking postsynaptic $alpha_1$-adrenergic receptors. Decreases contractions in smooth muscle of prostatic capsule. **Therapeutic Effects:** Lowering of BP. Decreased cardiac preload and afterload. Decreased symptoms of prostatic hyperplasia (urinary urgency, urinary hesitancy, nocturia).

Pharmacokinetics

Absorption: 60% absorbed following oral administration.
Distribution: Widely distributed.
Protein Binding: 97%.
Metabolism and Excretion: Extensively metabolized by the liver. Minimal (5–10%) renal excretion of unchanged drug.
Half-life: 2–3 hr.

TIME/ACTION PROFILE (antihypertensive effects)

ROUTE	ONSET	PEAK	DURATION
PO	2 hr	2–4 hr†	10 hr

†Following single dose; maximal antihypertensive effects occur after 3–4 wk of chronic dosing.

Contraindications/Precautions

Contraindicated in: Hypersensitivity.
Use Cautiously in: Renal insufficiency (↑ sensitivity to effects; dose ↓ may be required); OB, Lactation,

P

Pedi: Safety not established; Angina pectoris; When adding diuretics (↓ dose of prazosin); Patients undergoing cataract surgery (↑ risk of intraoperative floppy iris syndrome).

Adverse Reactions/Side Effects

CNS: dizziness, headache, weakness, drowsiness, mental depression, syncope. **EENT:** blurred vision, intraoperative floppy iris syndrome. **CV:** first-dose orthostatic hypotension, palpitations, angina, edema. **GI:** abdominal cramps, diarrhea, dry mouth, nausea, vomiting. **GU:** erectile dysfunction, priapism.

Interactions

Drug-Drug: Additive hypotension with acute ingestion of **alcohol**, other **antihypertensives**, or **nitrates**. Antihypertensive effects may be ↓ by **NSAIDs**.

Route/Dosage

Hypertension

PO (Adults): 1 mg 2–3 times daily (give 1st dose at bedtime) for initial 3 days of therapy, then ↑ gradually to maintenance dose of 6–15 mg/day in 2–3 divided doses (not to exceed 20–40 mg/day).

PO (Children): 50–400 mcg (0.05–0.4 mg)/kg/day in 2–3 divided doses (not to exceed 7 mg/dose or 15 mg/day).

Benign Prostatic Hyperplasia

PO (Adults): 1–5 mg twice daily.

Availability (generic available)

Capsules: 1 mg, 2 mg, 5 mg. **Tablets:** 🍁 1 mg, 🍁 2 mg, 🍁 5 mg.

NURSING IMPLICATIONS

Assessment

- Assess for first-dose orthostatic reaction (dizziness, weakness) and syncope. May occur 30 min–2 hr after initial dose and occasionally thereafter. Incidence may be dose related. Volume-depleted or sodium-restricted patients may be more sensitive. Observe patient closely during this period; take precautions to prevent injury. 1st dose may be given at bedtime to minimize this reaction.
- Monitor intake and output ratios and daily weight; assess for edema daily, especially at beginning of therapy.
- **Hypertension:** Monitor BP and pulse frequently during initial dosage adjustment and periodically throughout therapy. Report significant changes.
- Monitor frequency of prescription refills to determine adherence.
- **Benign Prostatic Hyperplasia:** Assess patient for symptoms of prostatic hyperplasia (urinary hesitancy, feeling of incomplete bladder emptying, interruption of urinary stream, impairment of size and force of urinary stream, terminal urinary dribbling, straining to start flow, dysuria, urgency) before and periodically during therapy.
- Rule out prostatic carcinoma before therapy; symptoms are similar.

Implementation

- May be used in combination with diuretics or beta blockers to minimize sodium and water retention. If these are added to prazosin therapy, reduce dose of prazosin initially and titrate to effect.
- **PO:** Administer daily dose at bedtime. If necessary, dose may be increased to twice daily.

Patient/Family Teaching

- Instruct patient to take medication at the same time each day. Take missed doses as soon as remembered. If not remembered until next day, omit; do not double doses.
- Advise patient to weigh self twice weekly and assess feet and ankles for fluid retention.
- May cause dizziness or drowsiness. Advise patient to avoid driving or other activities requiring alertness until response to the medication is known.
- Caution patient to avoid sudden changes in position to decrease orthostatic hypotension. Alcohol, CNS depressants, standing for long periods, hot showers, and exercising in hot weather should be avoided because of enhanced orthostatic effects.
- Advise patient to notify health care professional of all Rx or OTC medications, vitamins, or herbal products being taken and to consult with health care professional before taking other medications, especially NSAIDs and cough, cold, or allergy remedies.
- Instruct patient to notify health care professional of medication regimen before any surgery.
- Advise patient to notify health care professional immediately if erection last for 4 hr or longer or if frequent dizziness, fainting, or swelling of feet or lower legs occurs.
- Advise female patient to notify health care professional if pregnancy is planned or suspected or if breast feeding.
- Emphasize the importance of follow-up exams to evaluate effectiveness of medication.
- **Hypertension:** Emphasize the importance of continuing to take this medication as directed, even if feeling well. Medication controls but does not cure hypertension.
- Encourage patient to comply with additional interventions for hypertension (weight reduction, low-sodium diet, smoking cessation, moderation of alcohol consumption, regular exercise, and stress management).
- Instruct patient and family on proper technique for BP monitoring. Advise them to check BP at least weekly and to report significant changes.

Evaluation/Desired Outcomes

- Decrease in BP without appearance of side effects.
- Decrease in symptoms of prostatic hyperplasia.

prednicarbate, See CORTICOSTEROIDS (TOPICAL/LOCAL).

prednisoLONE, See CORTICOSTEROIDS (SYSTEMIC).

predniSONE, See CORTICOSTEROIDS (SYSTEMIC).

pregabalin (pre-gab-a-lin)

Lyrica, Lyrica CR

Classification

Therapeutic: analgesics, anticonvulsants

Pharmacologic: gamma aminobutyric acid (GABA) analogues, nonopioid analgesics

Schedule V

Indications

Immediate-release and extended-release: Treatment of the following conditions: Neuropathic pain associated with diabetic peripheral neuropathy, Postherpetic neuralgia. **Immediate-release:** Treatment of the following conditions: Fibromyalgia, Neuropathic pain associated with spinal cord injury, Partial-onset seizures (adjunctive therapy).

Action

Binds to calcium channels in CNS tissues which regulate neurotransmitter release. Does not bind to opioid receptors. **Therapeutic Effects:** Decreased neuropathic or post-herpetic pain. Decreased partial-onset seizures.

Pharmacokinetics

Absorption: Well absorbed (>90%) following oral administration.

Distribution: Probably crosses the blood-brain barrier.

Metabolism and Excretion: Minimally metabolized; 90% excreted unchanged in urine.

Half-life: 6 hr.

TIME/ACTION PROFILE (↓ post–herpetic pain)

ROUTE	ONSET	PEAK	DURATION
PO	unknown	2–4 wk	unknown

Contraindications/Precautions

Contraindicated in: Hypersensitivity; Myopathy (known/suspected); Severe renal impairment (CCr <30 mL/min) (extended-release only); Lactation: Lactation.

Use Cautiously in: All patients (may ↑ risk of suicidal thoughts/behaviors); Renal impairment (dose alteration recommended for CCr <60 mL/min); HF; History of drug dependence/drug-seeking behavior; OB: Use only if maternal benefit outweighs fetal risk; may ↑ risk of male-mediated teratogenicity; Pedi: Children <1 mo (safety and effectiveness not established); Geri: Consider age-related ↓ in renal function when determining dose.

Adverse Reactions/Side Effects

CNS: SUICIDAL THOUGHTS/BEHAVIORS, dizziness, drowsiness, headache, impaired attention/concentration/thinking. **CV:** peripheral edema, PR interval prolongation. **EENT:** blurred vision, double vision, vertigo. **GI:** dry mouth, abdominal pain, constipation, diarrhea, ↑ appetite, nausea, vomiting. **Hemat:** thrombocytopenia. **Metab:** weight gain. **MS:** ↑ creatine kinase. **Misc:** HYPERSENSITIVITY REACTIONS (including angioedema), fever.

Interactions

Drug-Drug: Concurrent use with **thiazolidinediones (pioglitazone, rosiglitazone)** may ↑ risk of fluid retention. ↑ risk of CNS depression with other **CNS depressants** including **opioids**, **alcohol**, **benzodiazepines**, or other **sedatives/hypnotics**.

Route/Dosage

Diabetic Neuropathic Pain

PO (Adults): *Immediate-release*—50 mg 3 times daily, ↑ over 7 days up to 100 mg 3 times daily. *Extended-release*—165 mg once daily after an evening meal; ↑ to 330 mg once daily after an evening meal within 1 wk.

Renal Impairment

PO (Adults): *CCr 30–60 mL/min*—Immediate–release: 75–300 mg/day in 2–3 divided doses; Extended-release: 82.5–330 mg once daily after an evening meal; *CCr 15–30 mL/min*—Immediate–release: 25–150 mg/day in 1–2 divided doses; *CCr <15 mL/min*—Immediate–release: 25–75 mg/day as a single daily dose.

Postherpetic Neuralgia

PO (Adults): *Immediate-release*—75 mg twice daily or 50 mg 3 times daily initially, may ↑ over 7 days to 300 mg/day in 2–3 divided doses; after 2–4 wk may ↑ to 600 mg/day in 2–3 divided doses. *Extended-release*—165 mg once daily after an evening meal; ↑ to 330 mg once daily after an evening meal within 1 wk; if pain is persistent after 2–4 wk, may then ↑ dose of up to 660 mg once daily after an evening meal.

Renal Impairment

PO (Adults): *CCr 30–60 mL/min*—Immediate-release: 75–300 mg/day in 2–3 divided doses; Extended-release: 82.5–330 mg once daily after an evening meal; *CCr 15–30 mL/min*—Immediate-release: 25–150 mg/day in 1–2 divided doses; *CCr <15 mL/min*—Immediate-release: 25–75 mg/day as a single daily dose.

Fibromyalgia

PO (Adults): *Immediate-release*—75 mg twice daily initially, may ↑ to 150 mg twice daily within 1 wk based on efficacy and tolerability. May ↑ to 225 twice daily.

Renal Impairment

PO (Adults): *CCr 30–60 mL/min*—Immediate-release: 75–300 mg/day in 2–3 divided doses *CCr 15–30 mL/min*—Immediate-release: 25–150 mg/day in 1–2 divided doses; *CCr <15 mL/min*—Immediate-release: 25–75 mg/day as a single daily dose.

Spinal Cord Injury Neuropathic Pain

PO (Adults): *Immediate-release*—75 mg twice daily initially, may be ↑ to 150 mg twice daily within 1 wk based on efficacy and tolerability; if insufficient pain relief after 2–3 wk, may ↑ to 300 twice daily.

Renal Impairment

PO (Adults): *CCr 30–60 mL/min*—Immediate-release: 75–300 mg/day in 2–3 divided doses; *CCr 15–30 mL/min*—Immediate-release: 25–150 mg/day in 1–2 divided doses; *CCr <15 mL/min*—Immediate-release: 25–75 mg/day as a single daily dose.

Partial Onset Seizures

PO (Adults): *Immediate-release*—75 mg twice daily or 50 mg 3 times daily initially; may gradually ↑ on a weekly basis up to a max dose of 600 mg/day (in 2–3 divided doses).

PO (Children ≥1 mo and ≥30 kg): *Immediate-release*—2.5 mg/kg/day in 2–3 divided doses; may gradually ↑ on a weekly basis up to a max dose of 10 mg/kg/day in 2–3 divided doses (max = 600 mg/day).

PO (Children ≥1 mo and <30 kg): *Immediate-release*—3.5 mg/kg/day in 2–3 divided doses for patients ≥4 yr old or in 3 divided doses for patients 1 mo–<4 yr old; may gradually ↑ on a weekly basis up to a max dose of 14 mg/kg/day in 2–3 divided doses for patients ≥4 yr old or in 3 divided doses for patients 1 mo–<4 yr old.

Renal Impairment

PO (Adults): *CCr 30–60 mL/min*—Immediate-release: 75–300 mg/day in 2–3 divided doses; *CCr 15–30 mL/min*—Immediate-release: 25–150 mg/day in 1–2 divided doses; *CCr <15 mL/min*—Immediate-release: 25–75 mg/day as a single daily dose.

Availability (generic available)

Extended-release tablets: 82.5 mg, 165 mg, 330 mg. **Immediate-release capsules:** 25 mg, 50 mg, 75 mg, 100 mg, 150 mg, 200 mg, 225 mg, 300 mg. **Cost:** 25 mg $411.71/100, 50 mg $409.80/100, 75 mg $409.80/100, 100 mg $409.80/100, 150 mg $409.80/100, 200 mg $411.71/100, 225 mg $411.71/100. **Oral solution:** 20 mg/mL. **Cost:** $553.82/473 mL.

NURSING IMPLICATIONS

Assessment

- Monitor closely for notable changes in behavior that could indicate the emergence or worsening of suicidal thoughts or behavior, or depression.
- **Diabetic Peripheral Neuropathy, Postherpetic Neuralgia, Fibromyalgia, and Spinal Cord Injury Pain:** Assess location, characteristics, and intensity of pain periodically during therapy.
- **Seizures:** Assess location, duration, and characteristics of seizure activity.
- ***Lab Test Considerations:*** May cause ↑ creatine kinase levels.
- May cause ↓ platelet count.

Implementation

- Do not confuse Lyrica (pregabalin) with Lopressor (metoprolol). Do not confuse Lyrica with Hydrea (hydroxyurea).
- Pregabalin should be discontinued gradually over at least 1 wk. Abrupt discontinuation may cause insomnia, nausea, headache, anxiety, sweating, and diarrhea when used for pain and may cause increase in seizure frequency when treating seizures.
- **PO:** May be administered without regard to meals. Oral solution may be stored at room temperature.

Patient/Family Teaching

- Instruct patient to take medication as directed. Take missed doses as soon as remembered unless almost time for next dose; do not double doses. Do not discontinue abruptly. Advise patient to read the *Patient Information Leaflet* prior to taking pregabalin and with each Rx refill in case of changes.
- May cause dizziness, drowsiness, and blurred vision. Caution patient to avoid driving or activities requiring alertness until response to medication is known. Advise patient to notify health care professional if changes in vision occur. Patients with seizures should not resume driving until health care professional gives clearance based on control of seizure disorder.
- Instruct patient to promptly report unexplained muscle pain, tenderness, or weakness, especially if accompanied by malaise or fever. Discontinue therapy if myopathy is diagnosed or suspected or if markedly elevated creatine kinase levels occur.
- Advise patient and family to notify health care professional if thoughts about suicide or dying, attempts to commit suicide; new or worse depression; new or worse anxiety; feeling very agitated or restless; panic attacks; trouble sleeping; new or worse irritability; acting aggressive; being angry or violent; acting on

dangerous impulses; an extreme increase in activity and talking, other unusual changes in behavior or mood occur.

- Inform patient that pregabalin may cause edema and weight gain.
- Advise patient to notify health care professional of all Rx or OTC medications, vitamins, or herbal products being taken and to consult with health care professional before taking other medications.
- Caution patient to avoid alcohol or other CNS depressants with pregabalin.
- Instruct patient to notify health care professional of medication regimen before treatment or surgery.
- Rep: Advise female patient to notify health care professional if pregnancy is planned or suspected or if breast feeding. Inform male patients who plan to father a child of the potential risk of male-mediated teratogenicity. Encourage patients who become pregnant to enroll in the NAAED Pregnancy Registry by calling 1-800-233-2334.
- Advise patient to carry identification describing disease process and medication regimen at all times.

Evaluation/Desired Outcomes

- Decrease in intensity of chronic pain.
- Decrease in the frequency or cessation of seizures.

procaine penicillin G, See PENICILLINS.

BEERS

prochlorperazine

(proe-klor-**pair**-a-zeen)

~~Compazine~~, Compro, Prochlorazine

Classification
Therapeutic: antiemetics, antipsychotics
Pharmacologic: phenothiazines

Indications

Management of nausea and vomiting. Treatment of psychoses. Treatment of anxiety.

Action

Alters the effects of dopamine in the CNS. Possesses significant anticholinergic and alpha-adrenergic blocking activity. Depresses the chemoreceptor trigger zone (CTZ) in the CNS. **Therapeutic Effects:** Diminished nausea and vomiting. Diminished signs and symptoms of psychoses or anxiety.

Pharmacokinetics

Absorption: Absorption from tablet is variable; may be better with oral liquid formulations. Well absorbed after IM administration.

Distribution: Widely distributed, high concentrations in the CNS. Crosses the placenta and probably enters breast milk.

Protein Binding: ≥90%.

Metabolism and Excretion: Highly metabolized by the liver and GI mucosa. Converted to some compounds with antipsychotic activity.

Half-life: Unknown.

TIME/ACTION PROFILE (antiemetic effect)

ROUTE	ONSET	PEAK	DURATION
PO	30–40 min	unknown	3–4 hr
Rect	60 min	unknown	3–4 hr
IM	10–20 min	10–30 min	3–4 hr
IV	rapid (min)	10–30 min	3–4 hr

Contraindications/Precautions

Contraindicated in: Hypersensitivity; Cross-sensitivity with other phenothiazines may exist; Angle-closure glaucoma; Bone marrow depression; Severe liver or cardiovascular disease; Hypersensitivity to bisulfites or benzyl alcohol (some parenteral products); Pedi: Children <2 yr or <9.1 kg.

Use Cautiously in: Diabetes mellitus; Respiratory disease; Prostatic hypertrophy; CNS tumors; Epilepsy; Intestinal obstruction; Patients at risk for falls; OB, Lactation: Safety not established; Geri: Dose ↓ recommended; ↑ risk of mortality in elderly patients treated for dementia-related psychosis.

Adverse Reactions/Side Effects

CNS: NEUROLEPTIC MALIGNANT SYNDROME, extrapyramidal reactions, sedation, tardive dyskinesia. **EENT:** blurred vision, dry eyes, lens opacities. **CV:** ECG changes, hypotension, tachycardia. **GI:** constipation, dry mouth, anorexia, drug-induced hepatitis, ileus. **GU:** pink or reddish-brown discoloration of urine, urinary retention. **Derm:** photosensitivity, pigment changes, rashes. **Endo:** galactorrhea. **Hemat:** AGRANULOCYTOSIS, leukopenia. **Metab:** hyperthermia. **Misc:** allergic reactions.

Interactions

Drug-Drug: Additive hypotension with **antihypertensives**, **nitrates**, or acute ingestion of **alcohol**. Additive CNS depression with other **CNS depressants**, including **alcohol**, **antidepressants**, **antihistamines**, **opioid analgesics**, **sedative/hypnotics**, or **general anesthetics**. Additive anticholinergic effects with other **drugs possessing anticholinergic properties**, including **antihistamines**, some **antidepressants**, **atropine**, **haloperidol**, and other **phenothiazines**. **Lithium** ↑ risk of extrapyramidal reactions. May mask early signs of **lithium** toxicity. ↑ risk of agranulocytosis with **antithyroid agents**. ↓ beneficial effects of **levodopa**. **Antacids** may ↓ absorption.

P

Drug-Natural Products: Concomitant use of **kava-kava**, **valerian**, **chamomile**, or **hops** can ↑ CNS depression. ↑ anticholinergic effects with **angel's trumpet**, **jimson weed**, and **scopolia**.

Route/Dosage

Pediatric dose should not exceed 10 mg on the 1st day and then should not exceed 20 mg/day in children 2–5 yr or 25 mg/day in children 6–12 yr.

Antiemetic

PO (Adults and Children ≥12 yr): 5–10 mg 3–4 times daily (not to exceed 40 mg/day).
PO (Children 18–39 kg): 2.5 mg 3 times daily *or* 5 mg twice daily (not to exceed 15 mg/day).
PO (Children 14–17 kg): 2.5 mg 2–3 times daily (not to exceed 10 mg/day).
PO (Children 9–13 kg): 2.5 mg 1–2 times daily (not to exceed 7.5 mg/day).
IM (Adults and Children ≥12 yr): 5–10 mg every 3–4 hr as needed. *Nausea/vomiting associated with surgery*—5–10 mg; may be repeated once.
IM (Children 2–12 yr): 132 mcg (0.132 mg)/kg; usually only 1 dose is required.
IV (Adults and Children ≥12 yr): 2.5–10 mg (not to exceed 40 mg/day). *Nausea/vomiting associated with surgery*—5–10 mg; may be repeated once.
Rect (Adults): 25 mg twice daily.
Rect (Children 18–39 kg): 2.5 mg 3 times daily or 5 mg twice daily (not to exceed 15 mg/day).
Rect (Children 14–17 kg): 2.5 mg 2–3 times daily (not to exceed 10 mg/day).
Rect (Children 9–13 kg): 2.5 mg 1–2 times daily (not to exceed 7.5 mg/day).

Antipsychotic

PO (Adults and Children ≥12 yr): 5–10 mg 3–4 times daily; may be ↑ every 2–3 days (up to 150 mg/day).
PO (Children 2–12 yr): 2.5 mg 2–3 times daily.
IM (Adults): 10–20 mg every 2–4 hr for up to 4 doses, then 10–20 mg every 4–6 hr (up to 200 mg/day).
IM (Children 2–12 yr): 132 mcg (0.132 mg)/kg (not to exceed 10 mg/dose).
IV (Adults and Children ≥12 yr): 2.5–10 mg (up to 40 mg/day).
Rect (Adults): 10 mg 3–4 times daily; may be ↑ by 5–10 mg every 2–3 days as needed.

Antianxiety

PO (Adults and Children ≥12 yr): 5 mg 3–4 times daily (not to exceed 20 mg/day or longer than 12 wk).
IM (Adults and Children ≥12 yr): 5–10 mg every 3–4 hr as needed (up to 40 mg/day).
IM (Children 2–12 yr): 132 mcg (0.132 mg)/kg.
IV (Adults): 2.5–10 mg (up to 40 mg/day).

Availability (generic available)

Tablets: 5 mg, 10 mg. **Cost:** *Generic*—5 mg $59.35/100, 10 mg $89.25/100. **Solution for injection:** 5 mg/mL (edisylate), 🍁 5 mg/mL (mesylate). **Suppositories:** 🍁 10 mg, 25 mg. **Cost:** *Generic*—$160.77/12.

NURSING IMPLICATIONS

Assessment

- Monitor BP (sitting, standing, lying down), ECG, pulse, and respiratory rate before and frequently during the period of dosage adjustment. May cause Q-wave and T-wave changes in ECG.
- Assess patient for level of sedation after administration.
- Monitor patient for onset of akathisia (restlessness or desire to keep moving) and extrapyramidal side effects (*parkinsonian*—difficulty speaking or swallowing, loss of balance control, pill rolling, mask-like face, shuffling gait, rigidity, tremors; and *dystonic*—muscle spasms, twisting motions, twitching, inability to move eyes, weakness of arms or legs) every 2 mo during therapy and 8–12 wk after therapy has been discontinued. Report these symptoms; reduction in dose or discontinuation may be necessary. Trihexyphenidyl or diphenhydramine may be used to control these symptoms.
- Monitor for tardive dyskinesia (uncontrolled rhythmic movement of mouth, face, and extremities; lip smacking or puckering; puffing of cheeks; uncontrolled chewing; rapid or worm-like movements of tongue). Report immediately; may be irreversible.
- Monitor for development of neuroleptic malignant syndrome (fever, respiratory distress, tachycardia, seizures, diaphoresis, hypertension or hypotension, pallor, tiredness, severe muscle stiffness, loss of bladder control). Notify health care professional immediately if these symptoms occur.
- Assess for falls risk. Drowsiness, orthostatic hypotension, and motor and sensory instability increase risk. Institute prevention if indicated.
- **Antiemetic:** Assess patient for nausea and vomiting before and 30–60 min after administration.
- **Antipsychotic:** Monitor patient's mental status (orientation to reality and behavior) before and periodically during therapy.
- Observe patient carefully when administering oral medication to ensure that medication is actually taken and not hoarded.
- Assess fluid intake and bowel function. Increased bulk and fluids in the diet may help minimize constipation.
- **Anxiety:** Assess degree and manifestations of anxiety and mental status before and periodically during therapy.
- ***Lab Test Considerations:*** CBC and liver function tests should be evaluated periodically during therapy. May cause blood dyscrasias, especially between wk 4 and 10 of therapy. Hepatotoxicity is more likely to occur between wk 2 and 4 of therapy. May recur if medication is restarted. Liver function abnormalities may require discontinuation of therapy.

- May cause false-positive or false-negative pregnancy test results and false-positive urine bilirubin test results.
- May cause ↑ serum prolactin levels.

Implementation

- To prevent contact dermatitis, avoid getting solution on hands.
- Phenothiazines should be discontinued 48 hr before and not resumed for 24 hr after myelography; they lower seizure threshold.
- **PO:** Administer with food, milk, or a full glass of water to minimize gastric irritation.
- **IM:** Do not inject subcut. Inject slowly, deep into well-developed muscle. Keep patient recumbent for at least 30 min after injection to minimize hypotensive effects. Slight yellow color will not alter potency. Do not administer solution that is markedly discolored or that contains a precipitate.

IV Administration

- **IV Push:** ***Concentration:*** Dilute to a concentration of 1 mg/mL. ***Rate:*** Administer at a rate of 1 mg/min; not to exceed 5 mg/min.
- **Intermittent Infusion:** ***Diluent:*** Dilute 20 mg in up to 1 L dextrose, saline, Ringer's or LR, dextrose/saline, dextrose/Ringer's, or lactated Ringer's combinations.
- **Continuous Infusion:** Has been used as infusion with 20 mg/L of compatible solution.
- **Y-Site Compatibility:** acetaminophen, alemtuzumab, alfentanil, amikacin, amsacrine, anidulafungin, argatroban, ascorbic acid, atracurium, atropine, benztropine, bleomycin, bumetanide, buprenorphine, butorphanol, carboplatin, carmustine, caspofungin, chlorpromazine, cisatracurium, cisplatin, cladribine, cyanocobalamin, cyclophosphamide, cyclosporine, cytarabine, dactinomycin, daptomycin, dexmedetomidine, dexrazoxane, digoxin, diltiazem, diphenhydramine, dobutamine, docetaxel, dolasetron, dopamine, doxacurium, doxorubicin hydrochloride, doxorubicin liposome, doxycycline, enalaprilat, ephedrine, epinephrine, epirubicin, eptifibatide, erythromycin, esmolol, etoposide, famotidine, fentanyl, fluconazole, gentamicin, glycopyrrolate, granisetron, hetastarch, hydrocortisone sodium succinate, hydromorphone, idarubicin, ifosfamide, irinotecan, isoproterenol, labetalol, leucovorin calcium, lidocaine, linezolid, magnesium sulfate, mannitol, melphalan, meperidine, methotrexate, methyldopate, methylprednisolone, metoclopramide, metoprolol, metronidazole, milrinone, morphine, moxifloxacin, multivitamins, mycophenolate, nafcillin, nalbuphine, naloxone, nicardipine, nitroglycerin, norepinephrine, octreotide, ondansetron, oxacillin, oxaliplatin, oxytocin, paclitaxel, palonosetron, pamidronate, pancuronium, papaverine, penicillin G, phentolamine, phenylephrine, phytonadione, potassium acetate, potassium chloride, procainamide, promethazine, propofol, propranolol, protamine, pyridoxime, quinupristin/dalfopristin, ranitidine, remifentanil, rituximab, rocuronium, sargramostim, sodium acetate, succinylcholine, sufentanil, tacrolimus, theophylline, thiamine, thiotepa, tigecycline, tirofiban, tobramycin, tolazoline, topotecan, trastuzumab, vancomycin, vasopressin, vecuronium, verapamil, vinblastine, vincristine, vinorelbine, vitamin B complex with C, zoledronic acid.
- **Y-Site Incompatibility:** acyclovir, aldesleukin, allopurinol, amifostine, aminophylline, amphotericin B deoxycholate, amphotericin B lipid complex, amphotericin B liposome, ampicillin, ampicillin/sulbactam, azathioprine, aztreonam, bivalirudin, calcium chloride, cefazolin, cefepime, cefotaxime, cefotetan, cefoxitin, ceftazidime, ceftriaxone, cefuroxime, chloramphenicol, clindamycin, dantrolene, dexamethasone, diazoxide, epoetin alfa, ertapenem, etoposide phosphate, fenoldopam, filgrastim, fludarabine, fluorouracil, folic acid, foscarnet, furosemide, ganciclovir, gemcitabine, imipenem/cilastatin, indomethacin, insulin, ketorolac, levofloxacin, midazolam, nitroprusside, pantoprazole, pemetrexed, pentamidine, pentobarbital, phenobarbital, phenytoin, piperacillin/tazobactam, sodium bicarbonate, streptokinase, trimethoprim/sulfamethoxazole.

Patient/Family Teaching

- Instruct patient to take medication as directed, not to skip doses or double up on missed doses. Take missed doses as soon as remembered unless almost time for next dose. If more than 2 doses are scheduled each day, missed dose should be taken within about 1 hr of the ordered time. Abrupt withdrawal may lead to gastritis, nausea, vomiting, dizziness, headache, tachycardia, and insomnia.
- Inform patient of possibility of extrapyramidal symptoms and tardive dyskinesia. Instruct patient to report these symptoms immediately to health care professional.
- Advise patient to change positions slowly to minimize orthostatic hypotension. Protect from falls.
- May cause drowsiness. Caution patient to avoid driving or other activities requiring alertness until response to medication is known.
- Caution patient to avoid alcohol and CNS depressants. Advise patient to notify health care professional of all Rx or OTC medications, vitamins, or herbal products being taken and to consult with health care professional before taking other medications and alcohol.
- Advise patient to use sunscreen and protective clothing when exposed to the sun to prevent photosensi-

P

tivity reactions. Extremes in temperature should also be avoided, because this drug impairs body temperature regulation.

- Instruct patient to use frequent mouth rinses, good oral hygiene, and sugarless gum or candy to minimize dry mouth. Consult health care professional if dry mouth continues for >2 wk.
- Advise patient not to take prochlorperazine within 2 hr of antacids or antidiarrheal medication.
- Advise patient that increasing bulk and fluids in the diet and exercise may help minimize the constipating effects of this medication.
- Inform patient that this medication may turn urine pink to reddish-brown.
- Advise patient to notify health care professional of medication regimen before treatment or surgery.
- Instruct patient to notify health care professional promptly if sore throat, fever, unusual bleeding or bruising, skin rashes, weakness, tremors, visual disturbances, dark-colored urine, or clay-colored stools are noted.
- Advise female patients to notify health care professional if pregnancy is planned or suspected or if breast feeding.
- Emphasize the importance of routine follow-up exams to monitor response to medication and detect side effects. Periodic ocular exams are indicated. Encourage continued participation in psychotherapy as ordered by health care professional.

Evaluation/Desired Outcomes

- Relief of nausea and vomiting.
- Decrease in excitable, paranoic, or withdrawn behavior when used as an antipsychotic.
- Decrease in feelings of anxiety.

progesterone
(proe-**jess**-te-rone)
Crinone, Endometrin, Prometrium, ✱Utrogestan

Classification
Therapeutic: hormones
Pharmacologic: progestins

Indications
Secondary amenorrhea and abnormal uterine bleeding due to hormonal imbalance. **Prometrium:** Prevention of cell overgrowth in the uterine lining in postmenopausal women who have not had a hysterectomy (with estrogen). Part of assisted reproductive technology (ART) in the management of infertility (4% and 8% vaginal gel). **Endometrin:** Support of embryo implantation and early pregnancy. **Unlabeled Use:** Corpus luteum dysfunction.

Action
Produces: Secretory changes in the endometrium, Increase in basal body temperature, Histologic changes in vaginal epithelium, Relaxation of uterine smooth muscle, Mammary alveolar tissue growth, Pituitary inhibition, Withdrawal bleeding in the presence of estrogen. **Therapeutic Effects:** Restoration of hormonal balance with control of uterine bleeding. Successful outcome in assisted reproduction.

Pharmacokinetics
Absorption: Micronization increases oral and vaginal absorption.
Distribution: Enters breast milk.
Protein Binding: ≥90%.
Metabolism and Excretion: Metabolized by the liver; 50–60% eliminated by kidneys; 10% eliminated in feces.
Half-life: Several min.

TIME/ACTION PROFILE (blood levels)

ROUTE	ONSET	PEAK	DURATION
PO	unknown	2–4 hr	unknown
Vaginal	unknown	34.8–55 hr	unknown
IM	unknown	19.6–28 hr	unknown

Contraindications/Precautions
Contraindicated in: Hypersensitivity; Hypersensitivity to parabens or sesame oil/seeds (IM suspension only); Hypersensitivity to peanuts (Prometrium only); Thromboembolic disease; Cerebrovascular disease; Severe liver disease; Breast or genital cancer; Porphyria; Missed abortion; OB: Contraindicated except in corpus luteum dysfunction.
Use Cautiously in: History of liver disease; Renal disease; Cardiovascular disease; Seizure disorders; Mental depression.

Adverse Reactions/Side Effects
CNS: depression. **CV:** PULMONARY EMBOLISM, THROMBOEMBOLISM, thrombophlebitis. **Derm:** chloasma, melasma, rashes. **EENT:** retinal thrombosis. **Endo:** amenorrhea, breakthrough bleeding, breast tenderness, changes in menstrual flow, galactorrhea, spotting. **F and E:** edema. **GI:** gingival bleeding, hepatitis. **GU:** cervical erosions. **Local:** irritation or pain at IM injection site. **Metab:** weight gain, weight loss. **Misc:** HYPERSENSITIVITY REACTIONS (including anaphylaxis and angioedema).

Interactions
Drug-Drug: May ↓ effectiveness of **bromocriptine** when used concurrently for galactorrhea and amenorrhea.

Route/Dosage
PO (Adults): *Secondary amenorrhea*—400 mg once daily in the evening for 10 days; *prevention of postmenopausal estrogen-induced endometrial hyperplasia*—200 mg once daily at bedtime for 14 days on days 8–21 of a 28-day cycle or on days 12–25 of a 30-day cycle; if patient currently receives ≥1.25 mg/day of estrogen, then a daily of dose of 300 mg of progester-

one as 100 mg 2 hr after breakfast and 200 mg at bedtime is used; further adjustments may be required.
Vag (Adults): *Secondary amenorrhea*—45 mg (1 applicatorful of 4% gel) once every other day for up to 6 doses, may be ↑ to 90 mg (1 applicatorful of 8% gel) once every other day for up to 6 doses; *Corpus luteum insufficiency or assisted reproduction technology*—For luteal phase support: 90 mg (1 applicatorful of 8% gel) once daily; for *in vitro* fertilization: 90 mg (1 applicatorful of 8% gel) once daily beginning within 24 hr of embryo transfer and continued through day 30 post-transfer (if pregnancy occurs, treatment may be continued for up to 10–12 wk); *partial or complete ovarian failure*—90 mg (1 applicatorful of 8% gel) twice daily while undergoing donor oocyte transfer (if pregnancy occurs, treatment may be continued for up to 10–12 wk); *Support of embryo implantation and early pregnancy (Endometrin)*—100 mg insert 2 or 3 times daily for up to 10 wk; *Luteal phase support during in vitro fertilization cycles (Utrogestan)*—600 mg/day in divided doses, from the day of embryo transfer until at least the 7th wk of pregnancy and not later than the 12th wk of pregnancy.
IM (Adults): *Secondary amenorrhea*—100–150 mg (single dose) or 5–10 mg daily for 6–8 days given 8–10 days before expected menstrual period. *Dysfunctional uterine bleeding*—5–10 mg daily for 6 days. *Corpus luteum insufficiency*—12.5 mg/day at onset of ovulation for 2 wk; may continue until 11th wk of gestation (unlabeled).

Availability (generic available)
Capsules (Prometrium): 100 mg, 200 mg. **Oil for injection:** 50 mg/mL. **Vaginal capsules (Utrogestan):** 🍁 200 mg. **Vaginal gel (Crinone):** 4%, 8%. **Vaginal inserts (Endometrin):** 100 mg. ***In combination with:*** estradiol (Bijuva). See Appendix B.

NURSING IMPLICATIONS
Assessment
- Monitor BP periodically during therapy.
- Monitor intake and output ratios and weekly weight. Report significant discrepancies or steady weight gain.
- **Amenorrhea:** Assess patient's usual menstrual history. Administration of drug usually begins 8–10 days before anticipated menstruation. Withdrawal bleeding usually occurs 48–72 hr after course of therapy. Therapy should be discontinued if menses occur during injection series.
- **Dysfunctional Bleeding:** Monitor pattern and amount of vaginal bleeding (pad count). Bleeding should end by 6th day of therapy. Therapy should be discontinued if menses occur during injection series.
- ***Lab Test Considerations:*** Monitor hepatic function before and periodically during therapy.
- May cause ↑ plasma amino acid and alkaline phosphatase levels.
- May ↓ pregnanediol excretion concentrations.
- May cause ↑ serum concentrations of LDL and ↓ concentrations of HDL.
- High doses may ↑ sodium and chloride excretion.
- May alter thyroid function test results.

Implementation
- **IM:** Shake vial before preparing IM dose. Administer deep IM. Rotate sites.
- **Vag:** Vaginal gel and insert are administered with disposable applicator provided by manufacturer.
- If dose increase is required from 4% gel to 8% gel, doubling the volume of the 4% gel will not accomplish dose increase; changing to 8% gel is required.

Patient/Family Teaching
- Advise patient to report signs and symptoms of fluid retention (swelling of ankles and feet, weight gain), thromboembolic disorders (pain, swelling, tenderness in extremities, headache, chest pain, blurred vision), mental depression, or hepatic dysfunction (yellowed skin or eyes, pruritus, dark urine, light-colored stools) to health care professional.
- Instruct patient to notify health care professional if change in vaginal bleeding pattern or spotting occurs.
- Caution patient to use sunscreen and protective clothing to prevent photosensitivity reactions.
- Advise patient to notify health care professional of medication regimen before treatment or surgery.
- Advise patient notify health care professional immediately if pregnancy is planned or suspected, or if breast feeding.
- Emphasize the importance of routine follow-up physical exams, including BP; breast, abdomen, and pelvic examinations; and Pap smears.
- **Vag:** Instruct patient not to use vaginal gel concurrently with other vaginal agents. If these agents must be used concurrently, administer at least 6 hr before or after vaginal gel. Small, white globules may appear as a vaginal discharge possibly due to gel accumulation, even several days after use.

Evaluation/Desired Outcomes
- Development of normal cyclic menses.
- Successful outcome in assisted reproduction.

HIGH ALERT

propofol (proe-poe-fol)
Diprivan

Classification
Therapeutic: general anesthetics

P

Indications

Induction of general anesthesia in children >3 yr and adults. Maintenance of balanced anesthesia when used with other agents in children >2 mo and adults. Initiation and maintenance of monitored anesthesia care (MAC). Sedation of intubated, mechanically ventilated patients in intensive care units (ICUs).

Action

Short-acting hypnotic. Mechanism of action is unknown. Produces amnesia. Has no analgesic properties. **Therapeutic Effects:** Induction and maintenance of anesthesia.

Pharmacokinetics

Absorption: Administered IV only, resulting in complete absorption.
Distribution: Rapidly and widely distributed. Crosses the blood-brain barrier well; rapidly redistributed to other tissues. Crosses the placenta and enters breast milk.
Protein Binding: 95–99%.
Metabolism and Excretion: Rapidly metabolized by the liver.
Half-life: 3–12 hr (blood-brain equilibration half-life 2.9 min).

TIME/ACTION PROFILE (loss of consciousness)

ROUTE	ONSET	PEAK	DURATION†
IV	40 sec	unknown	3–5 min

†Time to recovery is 8 min (up to 19 min if opioid analgesics have been used).

Contraindications/Precautions

Contraindicated in: Hypersensitivity to propofol, soybean oil, egg lecithin, or glycerol; OB: Crosses placenta; may cause neonatal depression; may affect child's brain development when used during 3rd trimester; Lactation: Enters breast milk; effects on newborn unknown.
Use Cautiously in: Cardiovascular disease; Lipid disorders (emulsion may have detrimental effect); ↑ intracranial pressure; Cerebrovascular disorders; Hypovolemic patients (lower induction and maintenance dosage ↓ recommended); Pedi: Not recommended for induction of anesthesia in children <3 yr, or for maintenance of anesthesia in infants <2 mo; not for ICU or pre-procedure sedation; may affect brain development in children <3 yr; Geri: Lower induction and maintenance dose ↓ recommended.

Adverse Reactions/Side Effects

CNS: dizziness, headache. **Resp:** APNEA, cough. **CV:** bradycardia, hypotension, hypertension. **GI:** abdominal cramping, hiccups, nausea, vomiting. **Derm:** flushing. **Local:** burning, pain, stinging, coldness, numbness, tingling at IV site. **MS:** involuntary muscle movements, perioperative myoclonia. **GU:** discoloration of urine (green). **Misc:** PROPOFOL INFUSION SYNDROME, fever.

Interactions

Drug-Drug: Additive CNS and respiratory depression with **alcohol, antihistamines, opioid analgesics**, and **sedative/hypnotics** (dose ↓ may be required). **Theophylline** may antagonize the CNS effects of propofol. Propofol may ↑ levels of **alfentanil**. Cardiorespiratory instability can occur when used with **acetazolamide**. Serious bradycardia can occur with concurrent use of **fentanyl** in children. ↑ risk of hypertriglyceridemia with **intravenous fat emulsion**.

Route/Dosage

General Anesthesia

IV (Adults <55 yr): *Induction*—40 mg every 10 sec until induction achieved (2–2.5 mg/kg total). *Maintenance*—100–200 mcg/kg/min. Rates of 150–200 mcg/kg/min are usually required during first 10–15 min after induction, then ↓ by 30–50% during first 30 min of maintenance. Rates of 50–100 mcg/kg/min are associated with optimal recovery time. May also be given intermittently in increments of 25–50 mg.
IV (Geriatric Patients, Cardiac patients, Debilitated Patients, or Hypovolemic Patients): *Induction*—20 mg every 10 sec until induction achieved (1–1.5 mg/kg total). *Maintenance*—50–100 mcg/kg/min (dose in cardiac anesthesia ranges from 50–150 mcg/kg/min depending on concurrent use of opioid).
IV (Adults Undergoing Neurosurgical Procedures): *Induction*—20 mg every 10 sec until induction achieved (1–2 mg/kg total). *Maintenance*—100–200 mcg/kg/min.
IV (Children ≥3 yr–16 yr): *Induction*—2.5–3.5 mg/kg, use lower dose for children ASA III or IV.
IV (Children 2 mo–16 yr): *Maintenance*—125–300 mcg/kg/min (following first 30 min of maintenance, rate should be ↓ if possible), younger children may require larger infusion rates compared to older children.

Monitored Anesthesia Care (MAC) Sedation

IV (Adults <55 yr): *Initiation*—100–150 mcg/kg/min infusion *or* 0.5 mg/kg as slow injection. *Maintenance*—25–75 mcg/kg/min infusion or incremental boluses of 10–20 mg.
IV (Geriatric Patients , Debilitated Patients, or ASA III/IV Patients): *Initiation*—Use slower infusion or injection rates. *Maintenance*—20% less than the usual adult infusion dose; rapid/repeated bolus dosing should be avoided.

ICU Sedation

IV (Adults): 5 mcg/kg/min for a minimum of 5 min. Additional increments of 5–10 mcg/kg/min over 5–10 min may be given until desired response is obtained. (Range 5–50 mcg/kg/min.) Dose should be reassessed every 24 hr.

Availability (generic available)

Solution for injection: 10 mg/mL.

NURSING IMPLICATIONS

Assessment

- Assess respiratory status, pulse, and BP continuously throughout propofol therapy. Frequently causes apnea lasting ≥60 sec. Maintain patent airway and adequate ventilation. Propofol should be used only by individuals experienced in endotracheal intubation, and equipment for this procedure should be readily available.
- Assess level of sedation and level of consciousness throughout and following administration.
- When using for ICU sedation, wake-up and assessment of CNS function should be done daily during maintenance to determine minimum dose required for sedation. Maintain a light level of sedation during these assessments; do not discontinue. Abrupt discontinuation may cause rapid awakening with anxiety, agitation, and resistance to mechanical ventilation.
- Monitor for propofol infusion syndrome (severe metabolic acidosis, hyperkalemia, lipemia, rhabdomyolysis, hepatomegaly, cardiac and renal failure). Most frequent with prolonged, high-dose infusions (>5 mg/kg/hr for >48 hr) but has also been reported following large-dose, short-term infusions during surgical anesthesia. If prolonged sedation or increasing dose is required, or metabolic acidosis occurs, consider alternative means of sedation.
- ***Toxicity and Overdose:*** If overdose occurs, monitor pulse, respiration, and BP continuously. Maintain patent airway and assist ventilation as needed. If hypotension occurs, treatment includes IV fluids, repositioning, and vasopressors.

Implementation

- Do not confuse Diprivan (propofol) with Diflucan (fluconazole) or Ditropan (oxybutynin).
- Dose is titrated to patient response.
- Propofol has no effect on the pain threshold. Adequate analgesia should *always* be used when propofol is used as an adjunct to surgical procedures.

IV Administration

- **IV Push:** ***Diluent:*** Usually administered undiluted. If dilution is necessary, use only D5W. Shake well before use. Solution is opaque, making detection of contaminants difficult. Do not use if separation of the emulsion is evident. Contains no preservatives; maintain sterile technique and administer immediately after preparation. ***Concentration:*** Undiluted: 10 mg/mL. If dilution is necessary, dilute to concentration ≥2 mg/mL.
- Discard unused portions and IV lines at the end of anesthetic procedure or within 6 hr. For ICU sedation, discard after 12 hr if administered directly from vial or after 6 hr if transferred to a syringe or other container. Do not administer via filter <5-micron pore size.
- Aseptic technique is essential. Solution is capable of rapid growth of bacterial contaminants. Infections and subsequent deaths have been reported. ***Rate:*** Administer over 3–5 min. Titrate to desired level of sedation. Frequently causes pain, burning, and stinging at injection site; use larger veins of the forearm, antecubital fossa, or a dedicated IV catheter. Lidocaine 10–20 mg IV may be administered prior to injection to minimize pain. Pedi: Induction doses may be administered over 20–30 sec.
- **Intermittent/Continuous Infusion:** ***Diluent:*** Administer undiluted. Allow 3 to 5 min between dose adjustments to allow for and assess the clinical effects. ***Concentration:*** 10 mg/mL. ***Rate:*** Based on patient's weight (see Route/Dosage section).
- **Solution Compatibility:** D5W, LR, D5/LR, D5/0.45% NaCl, D5/0.2% NaCl.
- **Y-Site Compatibility:** acyclovir, alfentanil, aminophylline, ampicillin, aztreonam, bumetanide, buprenorphine, butorphanol, calcium gluconate, carboplatin, cefazolin, cefepime, cefotaxime, cefoxitin, ceftriaxone, cefuroxime, chlorpromazine, cisplatin, clindamycin, cyclophosphamide, cyclosporine, cytarabine, dexamethasone, dexmedetomidine, diphenhydramine, dobutamine, dopamine, doxycycline, droperidol, enalaprilat, epinephrine, esmolol, famotidine, fenoldopam, fentanyl, fluconazole, fluorouracil, furosemide, ganciclovir, glycopyrrolate, granisetron, haloperidol, heparin, hydrocortisone sodium succinate, hydromorphone, ifosfamide, imipenem/cilastatin, insulin, isoproterenol, ketamine, labetalol, levorphanol, lidocaine, lorazepam, magnesium sulfate, mannitol, meperidine, milrinone, nafcillin, nalbuphine, naloxone, nitroglycerin, nitroprusside, norepinephrine, paclitaxel, pentobarbital, phenobarbital, potassium chloride, prochlorperazine, propranolol, ranitidine, scopolamine, sodium bicarbonate, succinylcholine, sufentanil, thiopental, vecuronium.
- **Y-Site Incompatibility:** amikacin, amphotericin B deoxycholate, calcium chloride, ciprofloxacin, diazepam, digoxin, doxorubicin, gentamicin, levofloxacin, methotrexate, methylpredisolone sodium succinate, metoclopramide, mitoxantrone, phenytoin, tobramycin, verapamil.

Patient/Family Teaching

- Inform patient that this medication will decrease mental recall of the procedure.
- May cause drowsiness or dizziness. Advise patient to request assistance prior to ambulation and transfer and to avoid driving or other activities requiring alertness for 24 hr following administration.

P

- Advise patient to avoid alcohol or other CNS depressants without the advice of a health care professional for 24 hr following administration.

Evaluation/Desired Outcomes

- Induction and maintenance of anesthesia.
- Amnesia.
- Sedation in mechanically ventilated patients in an intensive care setting.

HIGH ALERT

propranolol

(proe-**pran**-oh-lole)

Hemangeol, ~~Inderal~~, Inderal LA, InnoPran XL

Classification

Therapeutic: antianginals, antiarrhythmics (Class II), antihypertensives, vascular headache suppressants

Pharmacologic: beta blockers

Indications

Management of hypertension, angina, arrhythmias, hypertrophic cardiomyopathy, thyrotoxicosis, essential tremors, pheochromocytoma (all but Hemangeol). Also used in the prevention and management of MI, and the prevention of vascular headaches (all but Hemangeol). Proliferating infantile hemangioma requiring systemic therapy (Hemangeol only). **Unlabeled Use:** Also used to manage alcohol withdrawal, aggressive behavior, antipsychotic-associated akathisia, situational anxiety, and esophageal varices. Post-traumatic stress disorder (PTSD) (ongoing clinical trials at National Institute for Mental Health [NIMH]).

Action

Blocks stimulation of beta$_1$ (myocardial) and beta$_2$ (pulmonary, vascular, and uterine)-adrenergic receptor sites; its mechanism for the treatment of infantile hemangiomas is unknown. **Therapeutic Effects:** Decreased heart rate and BP. Suppression of arrhythmias. Prevention of MI. Hemangioma resolution.

Pharmacokinetics

Absorption: Well absorbed but undergoes extensive first-pass hepatic metabolism.

Distribution: Moderate CNS penetration. Crosses the placenta; enters breast milk.

Protein Binding: 93%.

Metabolism and Excretion: Almost completely metabolized by the liver (primarily for CYP2D6 isoenzyme) (the CYP2D6 enzyme system exhibits genetic polymorphism; ~7% of population may be poor metabolizers and may have significantly ↑ propranolol concentrations and an ↑ risk of adverse effects).

Half-life: 3.4–6 hr.

TIME/ACTION PROFILE (cardiovascular effects)

ROUTE	ONSET	PEAK	DURATION
PO	30 min	60–90 min†	6–12 hr
PO–ER	unknown	6 hr	24 hr
IV	immediate	1 min	4–6 hr

†Following single dose, full effect not seen until several wk of therapy.

Contraindications/Precautions

Contraindicated in: Hypersensitivity; Uncompensated HF; Pulmonary edema; Cardiogenic shock; Bradycardia, sick sinus syndrome, or heart block (unless pacemaker present); Premature infants with corrected age <5 wk (Hemangeol only); Infants <2 kg (Hemangeol only); Asthma or history of bronchospasm (Hemangeol only); BP <50/30 mmHg (Hemageol only); Pheochromocytoma (Hemangeol only).

Use Cautiously in: Renal or hepatic impairment; Pulmonary disease (including asthma); Diabetes mellitus (may mask signs of hypoglycemia); Thyrotoxicosis (may mask symptoms); History of severe allergic reactions (may ↑ intensity of response); Skeletal muscle disease (may exacerbate myopathy); OB: Crosses the placenta and may cause fetal/neonatal bradycardia, hypotension, hypoglycemia, or respiratory depression. May also ↓ blood supply to the placenta, ↑ the risk for premature birth or fetal death, and cause intrauterine growth retardation. May ↑ risk of cardiac and pulmonary complications in the infant during the neonatal time frame. Lactation: Appears in breast milk; use formula if propranolol must be taken; Pedi: ↑ risk of hypoglycemia, especially during periods of fasting such as before surgery, during prolonged exertion, or with coexisting renal insufficiency; Geri: ↑ sensitivity to all beta blockers; initial dose reduction and careful titration recommended.

Adverse Reactions/Side Effects

CNS: fatigue, weakness, anxiety, dizziness, drowsiness, insomnia, memory loss, mental depression, mental status changes, nervousness, nightmares. **EENT:** blurred vision, dry eyes, nasal stuffiness. **Resp:** bronchospasm, wheezing. **CV:** ARRHYTHMIAS, BRADYCARDIA, HF, PULMONARY EDEMA, orthostatic hypotension, peripheral vasoconstriction. **GI:** constipation, diarrhea, nausea. **GU:** erectile dysfunction, ↓ libido. **Derm:** ERYTHEMA MULTIFORME, EXFOLIATIVE DERMATITIS, STEVENS-JOHNSON SYNDROME, TOXIC EPIDERMAL NECROLYSIS, itching, rash. **Endo:** hyperglycemia, hypoglycemia (↑ in children). **MS:** arthralgia, back pain, muscle cramps, myopathy. **Neuro:** paresthesia. **Misc:** ANAPHYLAXIS, drug-induced lupus syndrome.

Interactions

Drug-Drug: General anesthesia, **IV phenytoin**, and **verapamil** may cause additive myocardial depression. Additive bradycardia may occur with **digoxin**. Additive hypotension may occur with other **anti-**

hypertensives, acute ingestion of **alcohol**, or **nitrates**. Levels may be ↓ with chronic **alcohol** use. Concurrent use with **amphetamines**, **cocaine**, **ephedrine**, **epinephrine**, **norepinephrine**, **phenylephrine**, or **pseudoephedrine** may result in unopposed alpha-adrenergic stimulation (excessive hypertension, bradycardia). Concurrent **thyroid** administration may ↓ effectiveness. May alter the effectiveness of **insulin** or **oral hypoglycemics** (dose adjustments may be necessary). May ↓ effectiveness of **beta-adrenergic bronchodilators** and **theophylline**. May ↓ beneficial beta cardiovascular effects of **dopamine** or **dobutamine**. Use cautiously within 14 days of **MAO inhibitor** therapy (may result in hypertension). **Cimetidine** may ↑ blood levels and toxicity. Concurrent **NSAIDs** may ↓ antihypertensive action. **Smoking** ↑ metabolism and ↓ effects; smoking cessation may ↑ effects. May ↑ levels of **lidocaine** and **bupivacaine**.

Route/Dosage

PO (Adults): *Antianginal*—80–320 mg/day in 2–4 divided doses or once daily as extended/sustained-release capsules. *Antihypertensive*—40 mg twice daily initially; may be ↑ as needed (usual range 120–240 mg/day; doses up to 1 g/day have been used); *or* 80 mg once daily as extended/sustained-release capsules, ↑ as needed up to 120 mg. *InnoPran XL* dosing form is designed to be given once daily at bedtime. *Antiarrhythmic*—10–30 mg 3–4 times daily. *Prevention of MI*—180–240 mg/day in divided doses. *Hypertrophic cardiomyopathy*—20–40 mg 3–4 times daily. *Adjunct therapy of pheochromocytoma*—20 mg 3 times daily to 40 mg 3–4 times daily concurrently with alpha-blocking therapy, started 3 days before surgery is planned. *Vascular headache prevention*—20 mg 4 times daily *or* 80 mg/day as extended/sustained-release capsules; may be ↑ as needed up to 240 mg/day. *Management of tremor*—40 mg twice daily; may be ↑ up to 120 mg/day (up to 320 mg have been used).

PO (Children): *Antihypertensive/antiarrhythmic*—0.5–1 mg/kg/day in 2–4 divided doses; may be ↑ as needed (usual range for maintenance dose is 2–4 mg/kg/day in 2 divided doses).

PO (Children 5 wk–5 mo): *Infantile hemangioma*—0.6 mg/kg twice daily (at least 9 hr apart); after 1 wk, ↑ to 1.1 mg/kg twice daily; after another wk, ↑ to 1.7 mg/kg twice daily and maintain for 6 mo.

IV (Adults): *Antiarrhythmic*—1–3 mg; may be repeated after 2 min and again in 4 hr if needed.

IV (Children): *Antiarrhythmic*—10–100 mcg (0.01–0.1 mg)/kg (up to 1 mg/dose); may be repeated every 6–8 hr if needed.

Availability (generic available)

Oral solution: 20 mg/5 mL, 40 mg/5 mL. **Oral solution (Hemangeol):** 4.28 mg/mL. **Tablets:** 10 mg, 20 mg, 40 mg, 60 mg, 80 mg. **Extended-release capsules:** 60 mg, 80 mg, 120 mg, 160 mg. **Solution for injection:** 1 mg/mL. ***In combination with:*** hydrochlorothiazide (generic only).

NURSING IMPLICATIONS

Assessment

- Monitor BP and pulse frequently during dose adjustment period and periodically during therapy.
- Abrupt withdrawal of propranolol may precipitate life-threatening arrhythmias, hypertension, or myocardial ischemia. Drug should be tapered over a 2-wk period before discontinuation. Assess patient carefully during tapering and after medication is discontinued. Consider that patients taking propranolol for non-cardiac indications may have undiagnosed cardiac disease. Abrupt discontinuation or withdrawal over too-short a period of time (less than 9 days) should be avoided.
- Pedi: Assess pediatric patients for signs and symptoms of hypoglycemia, particularly when oral foods and fluids are restricted.
- Patients receiving **propranolol IV** must have continuous ECG monitoring and may have pulmonary capillary wedge pressure (PCWP) or central venous pressure (CVP) monitoring during and for several hrs after administration.
- Assess for orthostatic hypotension when assisting patient up from supine position.
- Monitor intake and output ratios and daily weight. Assess patient routinely for evidence of fluid overload (peripheral edema, dyspnea, rales/crackles, fatigue, weight gain, jugular venous distention).
- Assess for rash periodically during therapy. May cause Stevens-Johnson syndrome. Discontinue therapy if severe or if accompanied with fever, general malaise, fatigue, muscle or joint aches, blisters, oral lesions, conjunctivitis, hepatitis and/or eosinophilia.
- **Angina:** Assess frequency and characteristics of anginal attacks periodically during therapy.
- **Vascular Headache Prophylaxis:** Assess frequency, severity, characteristics, and location of vascular headaches periodically during therapy.
- **PTSD:** Assess frequency of symptoms (flashbacks, nightmares, efforts to avoid thoughts or activities that may trigger memories of the trauma, and hypervigilance) periodically throughout therapy.
- **Infantile Hemangioma:** Monitor heart rate and BP for 2 hrs after propranolol initiation or dose increases. May worsen bradycardia or hypotension. Discontinue if severe (<80 beats per min) or symptomatic bradycardia or hypotension (systolic BP <50 mmHg) occurs.
- ***Lab Test Considerations:*** May cause ↑ BUN, serum lipoprotein, potassium, triglyceride, and uric acid levels.
- May cause ↑ ANA titers.

P

- May cause ↓ or ↑ in blood glucose levels. In labile diabetic patients, hypoglycemia may be accompanied by precipitous ↑ of BP.
- ***Toxicity and Overdose:*** Monitor patients receiving beta blockers for signs of overdose (bradycardia, severe dizziness or fainting, severe drowsiness, dyspnea, bluish fingernails or palms, seizures). Notify health care professional immediately if these signs occur.
- Hypotension may be treated with modified Trendelenburg position and IV fluids unless contraindicated. Vasopressors (epinephrine, norepinephrine, dopamine, dobutamine) may also be used. Hypotension does not respond to beta agonists.
- Glucagon has been used to treat bradycardia and hypotension.

Implementation

- ***High Alert:*** IV vasoactive medications are inherently dangerous. Before administering intravenously, have second practitioner independently check the original order, dose calculations, and infusion pump settings. Also, patient harm or fatalities have occurred when switching from oral to IV *propranolol*; oral and parenteral doses are not interchangeable. IV dose is 1/10 of the oral dose. Change to oral therapy as soon as possible.
- ***High Alert:*** Do not confuse propranolol with Pravachol. Do not confuse Inderal (propranolol) with Adderall (an amphetamine/dextroamphetamine combination drug).
- **PO:** Take apical pulse prior to administering. If <50 bpm or if arrhythmia occurs, withhold medication and notify physician or other health care professional.
- Administer with meals or directly after eating to enhance absorption.
- Swallow extended release tablets whole; do not crush, break, or chew. *Propranolol tablets* may be crushed and mixed with food.
- Mix propranolol oral solution with liquid or semisolid food (water, juices, applesauce, puddings). To ensure entire dose is taken, rinse glass with more liquid or have patient consume all of the applesauce or pudding. Do not store after mixing.
- Administer *Hemangeol* during or right after a feeding to prevent hypoglycemia. Skip dose if child is not eating or vomiting. Administer using oral syringe provided; if necessary may be diluted in small amount of milk or fruit juice and given in baby's bottle.

IV Administration

- **IV Push:** ***Diluent:*** Administer undiluted or dilute each 1 mg in 10 mL of D5W for injection. ***Concentration:*** Undiluted: 1 mg/mL. Diluted in 10 mL of D5W: 0.1 mg/mL. ***Rate:*** Administer at 0.5 mg/ min for adults to avoid hypotension and cardiac arrest; do not exceed 1 mg/min. Pedi: Administer over 10 min.
- **Intermittent Infusion:** ***Diluent:*** May be diluted in 50 mL of 0.9% NaCl, D5W, D5/0.45% NaCl, D5/0.9% NaCl, or lactated Ringer's injection. ***Concentration:*** Depends on dose. ***Rate:*** Infuse over 10–15 min.
- **Y-Site Compatibility:** acyclovir, alemtuzumab, alfentanil, alteplase, amikacin, aminocaproic acid, aminophylline, amiodarone, anidulafungin, argatroban, ascorbic acid, atropine, azathioprine, aztreonam, benztropine, bivalirudin, bleomycin, bumetanide, buprenorphine, butorphanol, calcium chloride, calcium gluconate, carboplatin, carmustine, caspofungin, cefazolin, cefotetan, ceftazidime, ceftriaxone, cefuroxime, chloramphenicol, chlorpromazine, cisplatin, clindamycin, cyanocobalamin, cyclophosphamide, cyclosporine, cytarabine, dactinomycin, daptomycin, daptomycin, daunorubicin hydrochloride, dexamethasone, dexmedetomidine, dexrazoxane, digoxin, diltiazem, diphenhydramine, dobutamine, docetaxel, dopamine, doxorubicin, doxorubicin liposomal, doxycycline, enalaprilat, ephedrine, epinephrine, epirubicin, epoetin alfa, eptifibatide, ertapenem, erythromycin, esmolol, etoposide, etoposide phosphate, famotidine, fenoldopam, fentanyl, fluconazole, fludarabine, fluorouracil, folic acid, foscarnet, fosphenytoin, furosemide, ganciclovir, gemcitabine, gentamicin, glycopyrrolate, granisetron, heparin, hydrocortisone, hydromorphone, idarubicin, ifosfamide, imipenem/cilastatin, isoproterenol, ketorolac, labetalol, leucovorin, levofloxacin, lidocaine, linezolid, lorazepam, magnesium sulfate, mannitol, meperidine, mesna, methotrexate, methylprednisolone, metoclopramide, metoprolol, metronidazole, midazolam, milrinone, mitoxantrone, morphine, moxifloxacin, multivitamins, mycophenolate, nafcillin, nalbuphine, naloxone, nicardipine, nitroglycerin, nitroprusside, norepinephrine, octreotide, ondansetron, oxacillin, oxaliplatin, oxytocin, palonosetron, pamidronate, pancuronium, papaverine, pemetrexed, penicillin G, pentamidine, pentobarbital, phenobarbital, phenylephrine, phytonadione, potassium acetate, potassium chloride, procainamide, prochlorperazine, promazine, promethazine, propofol, protamine, pyridoxine, quinupristin/dalfopristin, ranitidine, rocuronium, sodium acetate, sodium bicarbonate, streptokinase, succinylcholine, sufentanil, tacrolimus, theophylline, thiamine, thiotepa, tigecycline, tirofiban, tobramycin, topotecan, vancomycin, vasopressin, vecuronium, verapamil, vinblastine, vincristine, vinorelbine, vitamin B complex with C, voriconazole, zoledronic acid.
- **Y-Site Incompatibility:** amphotericin B deoxycholate, amphotericin B lipid complex, amphotericin B liposome, dantrolene, diazepam, diazoxide, indomethacin, insulin, mitomycin, paclitaxel, pantoprazole, phenytoin, piperacillin/tazobactam, trimethoprim/sulfamethoxazole.

Patient/Family Teaching

- Instruct patient to take medication as directed, at the same time each day, even if feeling well; do not skip or double up on missed doses. Take missed doses as soon as possible up to 4 hr before next dose (8 hr with extended-release propranolol). Inform patient that abrupt withdrawal can cause life-threatening arrhythmias, hypertension, or myocardial ischemia. Advise parent to read medication guide prior to starting and with each Rx refill in case of changes in *Hemangeol*.
- Advise patient to make sure enough medication is available for weekends, holidays, and vacations. A written prescription may be kept in wallet in case of emergency.
- Teach patient and family how to check pulse daily and BP biweekly. Advise patient to hold dose and contact health care professional if pulse is <50 bpm or BP changes significantly.
- May cause drowsiness or dizziness. Caution patients to avoid driving or other activities that require alertness until response to the drug is known.
- Advise patients to change positions slowly to minimize orthostatic hypotension, especially during initiation of therapy or when dose is increased.
- Caution patient that this medication may increase sensitivity to cold.
- Instruct patient to notify health care professional of all Rx or OTC medications, vitamins, or herbal products being taken and to consult health care professional before taking other Rx, OTC, or herbal products, especially NSAIDs and cold preparations, concurrently with this medication.
- Advise diabetic patients to closely monitor blood sugar, especially if weakness, malaise, irritability, or fatigue occurs. Medication may mask some signs of hypoglycemia, but dizziness and sweating may still occur. Acute hypertension may occur following insulin-induced hypoglycemia in patients receiving propranolol. Instruct parents/caregivers of children receiving *Hemangeol* how to recognize signs of hypoglycemia, and to notify health care professional and take child to nearest emergency department if hypoglycemia is suspected.
- Advise patient to notify health care professional if slow pulse, difficulty breathing, wheezing, cold hands and feet, dizziness, light-headedness, confusion, depression, rash, fever, sore throat, unusual bleeding, or bruising occurs.
- Instruct patient to inform health care professional of medication regimen prior to treatment or surgery.
- Advise patient to carry identification describing disease process and medication regimen at all times.
- **Hypertension:** Reinforce the need to continue additional therapies for hypertension (weight loss, sodium restriction, stress reduction, regular exercise, moderation of alcohol consumption, and smoking cessation). Medication controls but does not cure hypertension.
- **Angina:** Caution patient to avoid overexertion with decrease in chest pain.
- **Vascular Headache Prophylaxis:** Caution patient that sharing this medication may be dangerous.
- **PTSD:** Advise patient that medication may relieve distressing symptoms but that psychotherapy is the primary treatment for the disorder. Refer patient and family to a PTSD support group.

Evaluation/Desired Outcomes

- Decrease in BP.
- Control of arrhythmias without appearance of detrimental side effects.
- Reduction in frequency of anginal attacks.
- Increase in activity tolerance.
- Prevention of MI.
- Prevention of vascular headaches.
- Management of thyrotoxicosis.
- Management of pheochromocytoma.
- Decrease in tremors.
- Management of hypertrophic cardiomyopathy.
- Decrease in symptoms associated with PTSD.
- Resolution of Infantile hemangioma (propranolol only).

P

propylthiouracil

(proe-pill-thye-oh-**yoor**-a-sill)

✱Propyl-Thyracil

Classification

Therapeutic: antithyroid agents

Pharmacologic: thioamides

Indications

Patients with Graves' disease with hyperthyroidism or toxic multinodular goiter who are intolerant to methimazole and for whom surgery or radioactive iodine therapy is not appropriate. Adjunct in the control of hyperthyroidism in preparation for thyroidectomy or radioactive iodine therapy in patients who are intolerant to methimazole.

Action

Inhibits the synthesis of thyroid hormones. **Therapeutic Effects:** Decreased signs and symptoms of hyperthyroidism.

Pharmacokinetics

Absorption: Rapidly absorbed from the GI tract.

Distribution: Concentrates in the thyroid gland; crosses the placenta and enters breast milk in low concentrations.

Metabolism and Excretion: Metabolized by the liver.

Half-life: 1–2 hr.

TIME/ACTION PROFILE (effects on clinical thyroid status)

ROUTE	ONSET	PEAK	DURATION
PO	10–21 days†	6–10 wk	wk

†Effects on serum thyroid hormone concentration may occur within 60 min of a single dose.

Contraindications/Precautions

Contraindicated in: Hypersensitivity.

Use Cautiously in: ↓ bone marrow reserve; OB: May be used during 1st trimester (consider using methimazole during 2nd and 3rd trimesters); however, fetus may develop thyroid problems; mother and fetus may be at ↑ risk for hepatotoxicity; Lactation: Enters breast milk (safety not established); Geri: May have ↑ sensitivity; should initiate therapy with lowest dose; Pedi: Children <6 yr (safety not established); not recommended unless methimazole not tolerated and surgery or radioactive iodine therapy not appropriate.

Adverse Reactions/Side Effects

CNS: drowsiness, headache, paresthesia, vertigo. **CV:** edema, vasculitis. **GI:** HEPATOTOXICITY, nausea, vomiting, diarrhea, loss of taste. **Derm:** STEVENS-JOHNSON SYNDROME, TOXIC EPIDERMAL NECROLYSIS, rash, exfoliative dermatitis, hair loss, skin discoloration, urticaria. **Endo:** hypothyroidism. **GU:** glomerulonephritis. **Hemat:** AGRANULOCYTOSIS, APLASTIC ANEMIA, BLEEDING, leukopenia, thrombocytopenia. **MS:** arthralgia, myalgia. **Resp:** interstitial pneumonitis. **Misc:** fever, lymphadenopathy, parotitis, splenomegaly.

Interactions

Drug-Drug: Additive bone marrow depression with **antineoplastics** or **radiation therapy**. Additive antithyroid effects with **lithium**, or **potassium iodide**. ↑ risk of agranulocytosis with **phenothiazines**.

Route/Dosage

PO (Adults): 100 mg every 8 hr; may be ↑ to 400 mg/day (occasional patient may require 600–900 mg/day); usual maintenance dose = 100–150 mg/day.

PO (Children >10 yr): 50–300 mg/day given once daily or in 2–4 divided doses.

PO (Children 6–10 yr): 50–150 mg/day given once daily or in 2–4 divided doses.

Availability (generic available)

Tablets: 50 mg, 🍁100 mg.

NURSING IMPLICATIONS

Assessment

- Monitor response of symptoms of hyperthyroidism or thyrotoxicosis (tachycardia, palpitations, nervousness, insomnia, fever, diaphoresis, heat intolerance, tremors, weight loss, diarrhea).
- Assess patient for development of hypothyroidism (intolerance to cold, constipation, dry skin, headache, listlessness, tiredness, or weakness). Dose adjustment may be required.
- Assess patient for skin rash or swelling of cervical lymph nodes. Treatment may be discontinued if this occurs.
- ***Lab Test Considerations:*** Thyroid function studies should be monitored prior to therapy, monthly during initial therapy, and every 2–3 mo throughout therapy.
- WBC and differential counts should be monitored periodically throughout therapy. Agranulocytosis may develop rapidly and usually occurs during first 2 mo. This necessitates discontinuation of therapy.
- May cause increased AST, ALT, LDH, alkaline phosphatase, serum bilirubin, and prothrombin time.

Implementation

- Do not confuse propylthiouracil with Purinethol (mercaptopurine).
- Can be compounded by pharmacist into enema or suppository.
- **PO:** Administer at same time in relation to meals every day. Food may either increase or decrease absorption.

Patient/Family Teaching

- Instruct patient to take medication exactly as directed, around the clock. If a dose is missed, take as soon as remembered; take both doses together if almost time for next dose; check with health care professional if more than 1 dose is missed. Consult health care professional prior to discontinuing medication.
- Instruct patient to monitor weight 2–3 times weekly. Report significant changes.
- May cause drowsiness. Caution patient to avoid driving or other activities requiring alertness until response to medication is known.
- Advise patient to consult health care professional regarding dietary sources of iodine (iodized salt, shellfish).
- Advise patient to report sore throat, fever, chills, headache, malaise, weakness, yellowing of eyes or skin, unusual bleeding or bruising, symptoms of hyperthyroidism or hypothyroidism, or rash to health care professional promptly.
- Advise patient to notify health care professional of all Rx or OTC medications, vitamins, or herbal products being taken and to consult with health care professional before taking other medications.
- Advise patient to carry identification describing medication regimen at all times and to notify health care professional of medication regimen prior to treatment or surgery.
- Advise female patient to notify health care professional if pregnancy is planned or suspected or if breast feeding.
- Emphasize the importance of routine exams to monitor progress and to check for side effects.

Evaluation/Desired Outcomes

- Decrease in severity of symptoms of hyperthyroidism (lowered pulse rate and weight gain).
- Return of thyroid function studies to normal.
- May be used as short-term adjunctive therapy to prepare patient for thyroidectomy or radiation therapy or may be used in treatment of hyperthyroidism. Treatment of 6 mo to several yr may be necessary, usually averaging 1 yr.

protamine sulfate
(proe-ta-meen)

Classification
Therapeutic: antidotes
Pharmacologic: antiheparins

Indications

Acute management of severe heparin overdosage. Used to neutralize heparin received during dialysis, cardiopulmonary bypass, and other procedures. **Unlabeled Use:** Management of overdose of heparin-like compounds.

Action

A strong base that forms a complex with heparin (an acid). **Therapeutic Effects:** Inactivation of heparin.

Pharmacokinetics

Absorption: Administered IV only, resulting in complete bioavailability.
Distribution: Unknown.
Metabolism and Excretion: Metabolic fate not known. Protamine-heparin complex eventually degrades.
Half-life: Unknown.

TIME/ACTION PROFILE (reversal of heparin effect)

ROUTE	ONSET	PEAK	DURATION
IV	30 sec–1 min	unknown	2 hr†

†Depends on body temperature.

Contraindications/Precautions

Contraindicated in: Hypersensitivity to protamine or fish.
Use Cautiously in: Patients who have received previous protamine-containing insulin or vasectomized men (↑ risk of hypersensitivity reactions); OB, Lactation, Pedi: Safety not established.

Adverse Reactions/Side Effects

Resp: dyspnea. **CV:** bradycardia, hypertension, hypotension, pulmonary hypertension. **GI:** nausea, vomiting. **Derm:** flushing, warmth. **Hemat:** bleeding. **MS:** back pain. **Misc:** hypersensitivity reactions, including ANAPHYLAXIS, ANGIOEDEMA, and PULMONARY EDEMA.

Interactions

Drug-Drug: None significant.

Route/Dosage

IV (Adults and Children): *Heparin overdose*—1 mg/100 units of heparin. If given >30 min after heparin, give 0.5 mg/100 units of heparin (not to exceed 100 mg/2 hr). Further doses should be determined by coagulation tests. If heparin was administered subcutaneously, use 1–1.5 mg protamine per 100 units of heparin, give 25–50 mg of the protamine dose slowly followed by a continuous infusion over 8–16 hr. *Enoxaparin overdose*—1 mg/each mg of enoxaparin to be neutralized (unlabeled). *Dalteparin overdose*—1 mg/100 anti-Xa IU of dalteparin. If required, a 2nd dose of 0.5 mg/100 anti-Xa IU of dalteparin may be given 2–4 hr later if laboratory assessment indicates need (unlabeled).

Availability (generic available)

Injection: 10 mg/mL.

NURSING IMPLICATIONS

Assessment

- Assess for bleeding and hemorrhage throughout therapy. Hemorrhage may recur 8–9 hr after therapy because of rebound effects of heparin. Rebound may occur as late as 18 hr after therapy in patients heparinized for cardiopulmonary bypass.
- Assess for allergy to fish (salmon), previous reaction to or use of protamine insulin or protamine sulfate. Vasectomized and infertile men also have higher risk of hypersensitivity reaction.
- Observe patient for signs and symptoms of hypersensitivity reaction (hives, edema, coughing, wheezing). Keep epinephrine, an antihistamine, and resuscitative equipment close by in the event of anaphylaxis.
- Assess for hypovolemia before initiation of therapy. Failure to correct hypovolemia may result in cardiovascular collapse from peripheral vasodilating effects of protamine sulfate.
- ***Lab Test Considerations:*** Monitor clotting factors, activated clotting time (ACT), activated partial thromboplastin time (aPTT), and thrombin time (TT) 5–15 min after therapy and again as necessary.

Implementation

- Do not confuse protamine with Protonix (pantoprazole).
- Discontinue heparin infusion. In milder cases, overdosage may be treated by heparin withdrawal alone.
- In severe cases, fresh frozen plasma or whole blood may also be required to control bleeding.
- Dose varies with type of heparin, route of heparin therapy, and amount of time elapsed since discontinuation of heparin.

- Do not administer >100 mg in 2 hr without rechecking clotting studies, as protamine sulfate has its own anticoagulant properties.

IV Administration

- **IV Push:** ***Diluent:*** May be administered undiluted. If further dilution is desired, D5W or 0.9% NaCl may be used. ***Concentration:*** 10 mg/mL. ***Rate:*** Administer by slow IV push over 1–3 min. Rapid infusion rate may result in hypotension, bradycardia, flushing, or feeling of warmth. If these symptoms occur, stop infusion and notify physician. No more than 50 mg should be administered within a 10-min period.
- **Y-Site Compatibility:** alfentanil, amikacin, aminophylline, ascorbic acid, atropine, azathioprine, aztreonam, benztropine, bumetanide, buprenorphine, butorphanol, calcium chloride, calcium gluconate, ceftazidime, chlorpromazine, clindamycin, cyanocobalamin, cyclosporine, digoxin, diphenhydramine, dobutamine, dopamine, doxycycline, enalaprilat, ephedrine, epinephrine, epoetin alfa, erythromycin, esmolol, famotidine, fentanyl, fluconazole, ganciclovir, gentamicin, glycopyrrolate, imipenem/cilastatin, isoproterenol, labetalol, lidocaine, magnesium sulfate, mannitol, meperidine, metaraminol, methoxamine, methyldopate, metoclopramide, metoprolol, midazolam, morphine, multivitamins, nalbuphine, naloxone, nitroglycerin, nitroprusside, norepinephrine, ondansetron, oxytocin, papaverine, phentolamine, phenylephrine, potassium chloride, procainamide, prochlorperazine, promethazine, propranolol, pyridoxime, ranitidine, sodium bicarbonate, succinylcholine, sufentanil, tobramycin, tolazoline, trimetaphan, vancomycin, vasopressin, verapamil.
- **Y-Site Incompatibility:** amphotericin B deoxycholate, ampicillin, ampicillin/sulbactam, cefazolin, cefotaxime, cefoxitin, ceftazidime, cefuroxime, chloramphenicol, dantrolene, dexamethasone sodium phosphate, diazepam, diazoxide, folic acid, furosemide, heparin, hydrocortisone sodium succinate, indomethacin, insulin, ketorolac, methylprednisolone sodium succinate, nafcillin, oxacillin, penicillin G, pentamidine, pentobarbital, phenobarbital, phenytoin, trimethoprim/sulfamethoxazole.

Patient/Family Teaching

- Explain purpose of the medication to patient. Instruct patient to report recurrent bleeding immediately.
- Advise patient to avoid activities that may result in bleeding (shaving, brushing teeth, receiving injections or rectal temperatures, or ambulating) until risk of hemorrhage has passed.

Evaluation/Desired Outcomes

- Control of bleeding.
- Normalization of clotting factors in heparinized patients.

prucalopride
(proo-**kal**-oh-pride)
Motegrity

Classification
Therapeutic: prokinetic agents
Pharmacologic: 5-HT_4 agonists

Indications

Treatment of chronic idiopathic constipation (CIC).

Action

Acts as a selective serotonin type 4 (5-HT_4) receptor agonist, which stimulates colonic peristalsis and leads to increased bowel motility. **Therapeutic Effects:** Increased frequency of complete spontaneous bowel movements.

Pharmacokinetics

Absorption: >90% absorbed following oral administration.
Distribution: Extensively distributed to tissues.
Metabolism and Excretion: Primarily excreted by the kidneys, with 60–65% being excreted unchanged in the urine, and 5% in feces.
Half-life: 24 hr.

TIME/ACTION PROFILE (plasma concentrations)

ROUTE	ONSET	PEAK	DURATION
PO	unknown	2–3 hr	24 hr

Contraindications/Precautions

Contraindicated in: Hypersensitivity; Intestinal perforation or obstruction, obstructive ileus, Crohn's disease, ulcerative colitis, or toxic megacolon/megarectum; End-stage renal disease requiring dialysis.
Use Cautiously in: Depression; Severe renal impairment (CCr <30 mL/min) (↓ dose); OB: Use only if potential maternal benefit justifies potential fetal risk; Lactation: Use while breast feeding only if potential maternal benefit justifies potential risk to infant; Pedi: Safety and effectiveness not established; Geri: May need to ↓ dose due to age-related ↓ in renal function.

Adverse Reactions/Side Effects

CNS: SUICIDAL THOUGHTS/BEHAVIOR, headache, dizziness, fatigue. **GI:** abdominal pain, diarrhea, nausea, abdominal distension, flatulence, vomiting.

Interactions

Drug-Drug: None reported.

Route/Dosage

PO (Adults): 2 mg once daily.

Renal Impairment

PO (Adults): *CCr <30 mL/min*—1 mg once daily.

Availability

Tablets: 1 mg, 2 mg.

NURSING IMPLICATIONS

Assessment

- Assess bowel sounds and frequency, quantity, and consistency of stools periodically during therapy.
- Monitor for signs and symptoms of persistent worsening of depression or the emergence of suicidal thoughts and behaviors.

Implementation

- **PO:** Administer once daily without regard to food.

Patient/Family Teaching

- Instruct patient to take prucalopride as directed. Advise patient to read *Patient Information* before starting therapy and with each Rx refill in case of changes.
- Advise patient and family members to discontinue prucalopride and notify health care professional immediately if suicidal ideation and behavior (unusual changes in mood or behavior, persistent worsening of depression, feeling sad or hopeless, thoughts or attempts at self harm, emergence of suicidal thoughts or behavior) occur.
- Instruct patient to notify health care professional of all Rx or OTC medications, vitamins, or herbal products being taken and consult health care professional before taking any new medications.
- Advise females of reproductive potential to notify health care professional if pregnancy is planned or suspected, or if breast feeding.

Evaluation/Desired Outcomes

- Increased frequency of complete spontaneous bowel movements.

pseudoephedrine

(soo-doe-e-**fed**-rin)

Silfedrine Children's, Sudafed 12 Hour, Sudafed 24 Hour, Sudafed Children's, SudoGest, SudoGest 12 Hour

Classification

Therapeutic: allergy, cold, and cough remedies, nasal drying agents/decongestants

Pharmacologic: adrenergics, alpha adrenergic agonists

Indications

Symptomatic management of nasal congestion associated with acute viral upper respiratory tract infections. Used in combination with antihistamines in the management of allergic conditions. Used to open obstructed eustachian tubes in chronic otic inflammation or infection.

Action

Stimulates alpha- and beta-adrenergic receptors. Produces vasoconstriction in the respiratory tract mucosa (alpha-adrenergic stimulation) and possibly bronchodilation ($beta_2$-adrenergic stimulation). **Therapeutic Effects:** Reduction of nasal congestion, hyperemia, and swelling in nasal passages.

Pharmacokinetics

Absorption: Well absorbed after oral administration.
Distribution: Appears to enter the CSF; probably crosses the placenta and enters breast milk.
Metabolism and Excretion: Partially metabolized by the liver. 55–75% excreted unchanged by the kidneys (depends on urine pH).
Half-life: Children: 3.1 hr; Adults: 9–16 hr (depends on urine pH).

TIME/ACTION PROFILE (decongestant effects)

ROUTE	ONSET	PEAK	DURATION
PO	15–30 min	unknown	4–6 hr
PO-ER	60 min	unknown	12 hr

Contraindications/Precautions

Contraindicated in: Hypersensitivity to sympathomimetic amines; Hypertension, severe coronary artery disease; Concurrent MAO inhibitor therapy; Known alcohol intolerance (some liquid products).
Use Cautiously in: Hyperthyroidism; Diabetes mellitus; Prostatic hyperplasia; Ischemic heart disease; Glaucoma; OB, Lactation: Safety not established; Pedi: Avoid OTC cough and cold products containing this medication in children <4 yr.

Adverse Reactions/Side Effects

CNS: SEIZURES, anxiety, nervousness, dizziness, drowsiness, excitability, fear, hallucinations, headache, insomnia, restlessness, weakness. **Resp:** respiratory difficulty. **CV:** CARDIOVASCULAR COLLAPSE, palpitations, hypertension, tachycardia. **GI:** anorexia, dry mouth. **GU:** dysuria. **Misc:** diaphoresis.

Interactions

Drug-Drug: Concurrent use with **MAO inhibitors** may cause hypertensive crisis. Additive adrenergic effects with other **adrenergics**. Concurrent use with **beta blockers** may result in hypertension or bradycardia. **Drugs that acidify the urine** may ↓ effectiveness. **Phenothiazines** and **tricyclic antidepressants** potentiate pressor effects. **Drugs that alkalinize the urine (sodium bicarbonate, high-dose antacid therapy)** may intensify effectiveness.
Drug-Food: **Foods that acidify the urine** may ↓ effectiveness. **Foods that alkalinize the urine** may intensify effectiveness (see lists in Appendix K).

Route/Dosage

PO (Adults and Children >12 yr): 60 mg every 6 hr as needed (not to exceed 240 mg/day) *or* 120 mg

P

extended-release preparation every 12 hr *or* 240 mg extended-release preparation every 24 hr.
PO (Children 6–12 yr): 30 mg every 6 hr as needed (not to exceed 120 mg/day).
PO (Children 4–5 yr): 15 mg every 6 hr (not to exceed 60 mg/day).

Availability (generic available)

Tablets: 30 mg^OTC, 60 mg^OTC. **Extended-release tablets:** 120 mg^OTC, 240 mg^OTC. **Capsules:** ✱ 60 mg^OTC **Extended-release capsules:** ✱ 240 mg^OTC. **Liquid (grape and others):** 15 mg/5 mL^OTC, 30 mg/5 mL^OTC. ***In combination with:*** antihistamines, acetaminophen, cough suppressants, and expectorants^OTC. See Appendix B.

NURSING IMPLICATIONS

Assessment

- Assess congestion (nasal, sinus, eustachian tube) before and periodically during therapy.
- Monitor pulse and BP before beginning therapy and periodically during therapy.
- Assess lung sounds and character of bronchial secretions. Maintain fluid intake of 1500–2000 mL/day to decrease viscosity of secretions.

Implementation

- Do not confuse Sudafed with sotalol or Sudafed PE. Do not confuse Sudafed 12 Hour with Sudafed 12 Hour Pressure + Pain.
- Administer pseudoephedrine at least 2 hr before bedtime to minimize insomnia.
- **PO:** Extended-release tablets and capsules should be swallowed whole; do not crush, break, or chew. Contents of the capsule can be mixed with jam or jelly and swallowed without chewing for patients with difficulty swallowing.

Patient/Family Teaching

- Instruct patient to take medication as directed and not to take more than recommended. Take missed doses within 1 hr; if remembered later, omit. Do not double doses. Caution parents to avoid OTC cough and cold products while breast feeding or to children <4 yr.
- Instruct patient to notify health care professional if nervousness, slow or fast heart rate, breathing difficulties, hallucinations, or seizures occur, because these symptoms may indicate overdose.
- Instruct patient to contact health care professional if symptoms do not improve within 7 days or if fever is present.

Evaluation/Desired Outcomes

- Decreased nasal, sinus, or eustachian tube congestion.

pyrazinamide

(peer-a-**zin**-a-mide)
✱ Tebrazid

Classification
Therapeutic: antituberculars

Indications

Used in combination with other agents in the treatment of active tuberculosis.

Action

Converted to pyrazinoic acid in susceptible strains of Mycobacterium which lowers the pH of the environment. **Therapeutic Effects:** Bacteriostatic action against susceptible mycobacteria. **Spectrum:** Active against mycobacteria only.

Pharmacokinetics

Absorption: Well absorbed after oral administration.
Distribution: Widely distributed. Reaches high concentrations in the CNS (same as plasma). Excreted in breast milk.
Protein Binding: 50%.
Metabolism and Excretion: Mostly metabolized by the liver. Metabolite (pyrazinoic acid) has antimycobacterial activity; 3–4% excreted unchanged by the kidneys.
Half-life: *Pyrazinamide*—9.5 hr. *Pyrazinoic acid*—12 hr. Both are ↑ in renal impairment.

TIME/ACTION PROFILE (blood levels)

ROUTE	ONSET	PEAK	DURATION
PO	unknown	1–2 hr (4–5 hr†)	24 hr

†For pyrazinoic acid.

Contraindications/Precautions

Contraindicated in: Hypersensitivity; Cross-sensitivity with ethionamide, isoniazid, niacin, or nicotinic acid may exist; Severe liver impairment.
Use Cautiously in: Gout; Renal failure; Diabetes mellitus; Acute intermittent porphyria; OB: Safety not established.

Adverse Reactions/Side Effects

GI: HEPATOTOXICITY, anorexia, diarrhea, nausea, vomiting. **GU:** dysuria. **Derm:** acne, itching, photosensitivity, rash. **Hemat:** anemia, thrombocytopenia. **Metab:** hyperuricemia. **MS:** arthralgia, gouty arthritis.

Interactions

Drug-Drug: Concurrent use with **rifampin** may result in life-threatening hepatoxicity and should be avoided. May ↓ blood levels and effectiveness of **cyclosporine**. May ↓ effectiveness of **antigout agents**.

Route/Dosage

PO (Adults and Children): 15–30 mg/kg/day as a single dose. Up to 60 mg/kg/day has been used in isoniazid-resistant tuberculosis (not to exceed 2 g/day as a single dose or 3 g/day in divided doses). May also be given as 50–70 mg/kg 2–3 times weekly (not to exceed 2 g/dose on daily regimen, 3 g/dose for 3-times-weekly regimen, or 4 g/dose for twice-weekly regimen). *Patients with HIV*—20–40 mg/kg/day for first 2 mo of therapy (maximum: 2 g/day); further dosing depends on regimen employed.

Availability (generic available)

Tablets: 500 mg. ***In combination with:*** rifampin and isoniazid (Rifater). See Appendix B.

NURSING IMPLICATIONS

Assessment

- Perform mycobacterial studies and susceptibility tests before and periodically during therapy to detect possible resistance.
- ***Lab Test Considerations:*** Evaluate hepatic function before and every 2–4 wk during therapy. Increased AST and ALT may not be predictive of clinical hepatitis and may return to normal levels during treatment. Patients with impaired liver function should receive pyrazinamide therapy only if crucial to treatment.
- Monitor serum uric acid concentrations during therapy. May cause ↑ resulting in precipitation of acute gout.
- May interfere with urine ketone determinations.

Implementation

- **PO:** May be given concurrently with isoniazid.

Patient/Family Teaching

- Advise patient to take medication as directed and not to skip doses or double up on missed doses. Take missed doses as soon as remembered unless almost time for next dose. Emphasize the importance of continuing therapy even after symptoms have subsided. Length of therapy depends on regimen being used and underlying disease states.
- Inform diabetic patients that pyrazinamide may interfere with urine ketone measurements.
- Advise patients to notify health care professional if no improvement is noticed after 2–3 wk of therapy or if fever, anorexia, malaise, nausea, vomiting, darkened urine, yellowish discoloration of the skin and eyes, pain, or swelling of the joints occurs.
- Advise patients to use sunscreen and protective clothing to prevent photosensitivity reactions.
- Advise female patient to notify health care professional if pregnancy is planned or suspected or if breast feeding.
- Emphasize the importance of regular follow-up exams to monitor progress and check for side effects.

Evaluation/Desired Outcomes

- Resolution of signs and symptoms of tuberculosis.
- Negative sputum cultures.

pyridoxine (peer-i-**dox**-een)

Neuro-K–250 TD, Neuro-K-250 Vitamin B6, Neuro-K-50, Neuro-K-500, Pyri 500, vitamin B_6

Classification

Therapeutic: vitamins

Pharmacologic: water soluble vitamins

Indications

Treatment and prevention of pyridoxine deficiency (may be associated with poor nutritional status or chronic debilitating illnesses). Treatment of pyridoxine-dependent seizures in infants. Treatment and prevention of neuropathy, which may develop from isoniazid, penicillamine, or hydralazine therapy. Management of isoniazid overdose >10 g.

Action

Required for amino acid, carbohydrate, and lipid metabolism. Used in the transport of amino acids, formation of neurotransmitters, and synthesis of heme. **Therapeutic Effects:** Prevention of pyridoxine deficiency. Prevention or reversal of neuropathy associated with hydralazine, penicillamine, or isoniazid therapy.

Pharmacokinetics

Absorption: Well absorbed from the GI tract.
Distribution: Stored in liver, muscle, and brain. Crosses the placenta and enters breast milk.
Metabolism and Excretion: Converted in RBCs to pyridoxal phosphate and another active metabolite. Amounts in excess of requirements are excreted unchanged by the kidneys.
Half-life: 15–20 days.

TIME/ACTION PROFILE

ROUTE	ONSET	PEAK	DURATION
PO, IM, IV	unknown	unknown	unknown

Contraindications/Precautions

Contraindicated in: Hypersensitivity to pyridoxine or any component.
Use Cautiously in: Parkinson's disease (treatment with levodopa only); OB: Chronic ingestion of large doses may produce pyridoxine-dependency syndrome in newborn.

Adverse Reactions/Side Effects

Adverse reactions listed are seen with excessive doses only.
Neuro: sensory neuropathy, paresthesia. **Misc:** pyridoxine-dependency syndrome.

P

Interactions

Drug-Drug: Interferes with the therapeutic response to **levodopa** when used without carbidopa. Requirements are increased by **isoniazid**, **hydralazine**, **chloramphenicol**, **penicillamine**, **estrogens**, and **immunosuppressants**. Decreases serum levels of **phenobarbital** and **phenytoin**.

Route/Dosage

Prevention of Deficiency (Recommended Daily Allowance)

PO (Adults and Children >14 yr): 1.2–1.7 mg/day (larger doses required with cycloserine, ethionamide, hydralazine, immunosuppressants, isoniazid, penicillamine, and estrogen-containing oral contraceptives).
PO (Children 9–13 yr): 1 mg/day (larger doses required with cycloserine, ethionamide, hydralazine, immunosuppressants, isoniazid, and penicillamine).
PO (Children 1–8 yr): 0.5–0.6 mg/day (larger doses required with cycloserine, ethionamide, hydralazine, immunosuppressants, isoniazid, and penicillamine).
PO (Infants 6–12 mo): 0.3 mg/day.
PO (Infants <6 mo): 0.1 mg/day.

Treatment of Deficiency

PO (Adults): 2.5–10 mg/day until clinical signs are corrected, then 2–5 mg/day.
PO (Children): 5–25 mg/day for 3 wk, then 1.5–2.5 mg/day.

Pyridoxine-Dependent Seizures

PO, IM, IV (Neonates and Infants): 10–100 mg initially then 50–100 mg/day orally.

Drug-Induced Neuritis

PO (Adults): Treatment—100–300 mg/day; Prophylaxis—25–100 mg/day.
PO (Children): Treatment—10–50 mg/day; Prophylaxis—1–2 mg/kg/day.

Isoniazid Overdose (>10 g)

IM, IV (Adults and Children): Amount in mg equal to amount of isoniazid ingested given as 1–4 g IV, then 1 g IM every 30 min.

Availability (generic available)

Capsules: 250 mg^OTC^. **Tablets:** 25 mg^OTC^, 50 mg^OTC^, 100 mg^OTC^, 250 mg^OTC^, 500 mg^OTC^. **Extended-release tablets:** 200 mg^OTC^, 500 mg^OTC^. **Injection:** 100 mg/mL. ***In combination with:*** vitamins, minerals, and trace elements in a variety of multivitamin preparations^OTC^.

NURSING IMPLICATIONS

Assessment

- Assess patient for signs of vitamin B_6 deficiency (anemia, dermatitis, cheilosis, irritability, seizures, nausea, and vomiting) before and periodically throughout therapy. Institute seizure precautions in pyridoxine-dependent infants.
- ***Lab Test Considerations:*** May cause false elevations in urobilinogen concentrations.

Implementation

- ***High Alert:*** Do not confuse pyridoxine with Pyridium (phenazopyridine).
- Because of infrequency of single B-vitamin deficiencies, combinations are commonly administered.
- Administration of parenteral vitamin B_6 is limited to patients who are NPO or who have nausea and vomiting or malabsorption syndromes.
- Protect parenteral solution from light; decomposition will occur.
- **PO:** Extended-release capsules and tablets should be swallowed whole, without crushing, breaking, or chewing. For patients unable to swallow capsule, contents of capsules may be mixed with jam or jelly.
- **IM:** Rotate sites; burning or stinging at site may occur.
- **IV:** May be administered slowly by IV push or as infusion in standard IV solutions. Monitor respiratory rate, heart rate, and BP when administering large IV doses.
- Pyridoxine-dependent seizures should cease within 2–3 min of IV administration.
- ***Rate:*** Infusion rates of 15–30 min and up to 3 hr have been used.
- **Additive Incompatibility:** alkaline solutions, riboflavin.

Patient/Family Teaching

- Instruct patient to take medication as directed. If a dose is missed, it may be omitted because an extended period of time is required to become deficient in vitamin B_6.
- Encourage patient to comply with diet recommended by health care professional. Explain that the best source of vitamins is a well-balanced diet with foods from the four basic food groups. Foods high in vitamin B_6 include bananas, whole-grain cereals, potatoes, lima beans, and meats.
- Patients self-medicating with vitamin supplements should be cautioned not to exceed RDA. The effectiveness of megadoses for treatment of various medical conditions is unproved and may cause side effects, such as unsteady gait, numbness in feet, and difficulty with hand coordination.
- Advise female patient to notify health care professional if pregnancy is planned or suspected or if breast feeding.
- Emphasize the importance of follow-up exams to evaluate progress.

Evaluation/Desired Outcomes

- Decrease in the symptoms of vitamin B_6 deficiency.

BEERS

QUEtiapine (kwet-eye-a-peen)

SEROquel, SEROquel XR

Classification

Therapeutic: antipsychotics, mood stabilizers

Indications

Schizophrenia. Depressive episodes with bipolar disorder. Acute manic episodes associated with bipolar I disorder (as monotherapy [for adults or adolescents] or with lithium or divalproex [adults only]). Maintenance treatment of bipolar I disorder (with lithium or divalproex). Adjunctive treatment of depression.

Action

Probably acts by serving as an antagonist of dopamine and serotonin. Also antagonizes histamine H_1 receptors and $alpha_1$-adrenergic receptors. **Therapeutic Effects:** Decreased manifestations of psychoses, depression, or acute mania.

Pharmacokinetics

Absorption: Well absorbed after oral administration.
Distribution: Widely distributed.
Metabolism and Excretion: Extensively metabolized by the liver (mostly by P450 CYP3A4 enyzme system); <1% excreted unchanged in the urine.
Half-life: 6 hr.

TIME/ACTION PROFILE (antipsychotic effects)

ROUTE	ONSET	PEAK	DURATION
PO	unknown	unknown	8–12 hr
PO-XR	unknown	unknown	unknown

Contraindications/Precautions

Contraindicated in: Hypersensitivity; Concurrent use of agents that prolong the QT interval, including dofetilide, sotalol, quinidine, disopyramide, amiodarone, dronedarone, thioridazine, chlorpromazine, droperidol, moxifloxacin, mefloquine, pentamidine, arsenic trioxide, dolasetron, tacrolimus, ziprasidone, erythromycin, citalopram, escitalopram, and clarithromycin (↑ risk of serious arrhythmias); History of arrhythmias, including bradycardia; Hypokalemia or hypomagnesemia (↑ risk of serious arrhythmias); Congenital long QT syndrome (↑ risk of serious arrhythmias).
Use Cautiously in: Cardiovascular disease, cerebrovascular disease, dehydration or hypovolemia (↑ risk of hypotension); History of seizures or Alzheimer's dementia; Diabetes (may ↑ risk of hyperglycemia); Patients at risk for aspiration pneumonia or falls; Hepatic impairment (dose ↓ may be necessary); Hypothyroidism (may be exacerbated); History of suicide attempt; Low white blood cell count or history of drug-induced leukopenia/neutropenia (↑ risk of leukopenia/neutropenia); Urinary retention, prostatic hypertrophy, constipation, or ↑ intraocular pressure; OB: Neonates at ↑ risk for extrapyramidal symptoms and withdrawal after delivery when exposed during the 3rd trimester; use only if potential maternal benefit justifies potential fetal risk; Lactation: Use while breast feeding only if potential maternal benefit justifies potential risk to infant; Pedi: May ↑ risk of suicide attempt/ideation especially during early treatment or dose adjustment; risk may be greater in children or adolescents; Geri: May require ↓ doses; ↑ risk of mortality and stroke in elderly patients treated for dementia-related psychosis.

Adverse Reactions/Side Effects

CNS: NEUROLEPTIC MALIGNANT SYNDROME, SEIZURES, dizziness, cognitive impairment, extrapyramidal symptoms, sedation, tardive dyskinesia. **CV:** ↑ BP (children), palpitations, peripheral edema, postural hypotension. **Derm:** DRUG REACTION WITH EOSINOPHILIA AND SYSTEMIC SYMPTOMS (DRESS), STEVENS-JOHNSON SYNDROME, sweating. **EENT:** ear pain, rhinitis, pharyngitis. **Endo:** weight gain, hyperglycemia, hyperlipidemia, hyperprolactinemia, hypertriglyceridemia, hypothyroidism. **GI:** GI OBSTRUCTION, PANCREATITIS, anorexia, constipation, dry mouth, dyspepsia. **GU:** ↓ fertility (females). **Hemat:** AGRANULOCYTOSIS, ↓ hemoglobin, leukopenia, neutropenia. **MS:** rhabdomyolysis. **Resp:** cough, dyspnea. **Misc:** flu-like syndrome.

Q

Interactions

Drug-Drug: Concurrent use of **macrolide anti-infectives (erythromycin, clarithromycin), dofetilide, sotalol, quinidine, disopyramide, procainamide, thioridazine, chlorpromazine, droperidol, gemifloxacin, moxifloxacin, mefloquine, pentamidine, arsenic trioxide, dolasetron, citalopram, escitalopram, tacrolimus,** and **ziprasidone** ↑ the risk of serious ventricular arrhythmias and should be avoided. ↑ CNS depression may occur with **alcohol, antihistamines, opioid analgesics,** and **sedative/hypnotics**. ↑ risk of hypotension with acute ingestion of **alcohol** or **antihypertensives**. **Phenytoin** and **thioridazine** ↑ clearance and ↓ effectiveness of quetiapine (dose change may be necessary); similar effects may occur with **carbamazepine, barbiturates, rifampin,** or **corticosteroids**. Effects may be ↑ by **ketoconazole, itraconazole, fluconazole, protease inhibitors,** or **erythromycin**, as well as by other **agents that inhibit the cytochrome P450 CYP3A4 enzyme**. Concurrent use of **anticholinergic medications** may ↑ risk of anticholinergic adverse reactions.

Route/Dosage

Schizophrenia

PO (Adults): *Immediate-release*—25 mg twice daily on Day 1, ↑ by 25–50 mg 2–3 times daily on Days 2 and 3, up to 300–400 mg/day in 2–3 divided doses by Day 4 (not to exceed 800 mg/day); *Extended-release*—300 mg once daily, ↑ by 300 mg/day (not to exceed 800 mg/day); elderly patients or patients with hepatic impairment should be started on immediate-release product and converted to extended-release product once effective dose is reached.

PO (Children 13–17 yr): *Immediate-release*—25 mg twice daily on Day 1, ↑ to 50 mg twice daily on Day 2, then ↑ to 100 mg twice daily on Day 3, then ↑ to 150 mg twice daily on Day 4, then ↑ to 200 mg twice daily on Day 5; may then ↑ by no more than 100 mg/day (not to exceed 800 mg/day).

Acute Manic Episodes Associated with Bipolar I Disorder

PO (Adults): *Immediate-release*—50 mg twice daily on Day 1, then ↑ to 100 mg twice daily on Day 2, then ↑ to 150 mg twice daily on Day 3, then ↑ to 200 mg twice daily on Day 4; may then ↑ by no more than 200 mg/day up to 400 mg twice daily on Day 6 if needed; *Extended-release*—300 mg once daily on Day 1, then 600 mg once daily on Day 2, then 400–800 mg once daily starting on Day 3.

PO (Children 10–17 yr): *Immediate-release*—25 mg twice daily on Day 1, then ↑ to 50 mg twice daily on Day 2, then ↑ to 100 mg twice daily on Day 3, then ↑ to 150 mg twice daily on Day 4, then ↑ to 200 mg twice daily on Day 5; may then ↑ by no more than 100 mg/day (not to exceed 600 mg/day).

Acute Depressive Episodes Associated with Bipolar Disorder

PO (Adults): *Immediate-release or extended-release*—50 mg once daily at bedtime on Day 1, then ↑ to 100 mg daily at bedtime on Day 2, then ↑ to 200 mg daily at bedtime on Day 3, then ↑ to 300 mg daily at bedtime thereafter.

Maintenance Treatment of Bipolar I Disorder

PO (Adults): Continue at the dose required to maintain symptom remission (usual dosage: 400–800 mg/day given as once daily dose [extended-release] or in two divided doses [immediate-release]).

PO (Children 10–17 yr): Continue at the lowest dose required to maintain symptom remission.

Depression

PO (Adults): *Extended-release*—50 mg once daily on Days 1 and 2, then ↑ to 150 mg once daily starting on Day 3 (not to exceed 300 mg/day).

Availability (generic available)

Extended-release tablets: 50 mg, 150 mg, 200 mg, 300 mg, 400 mg. **Cost:** 50 mg $460.84/60, 150 mg $827.50/60, 200 mg $910.78/60, 300 mg $1,194.14/60, 400 mg $1,403.42/60. **Tablets:** 25 mg, 50 mg, 100 mg, 200 mg, 300 mg, 400 mg. **Cost:** *Generic*—25 mg $17.59/100, 100 mg $26.94/100, 200 mg $39.30/100.

NURSING IMPLICATIONS

Assessment

- Monitor mental status (mood, orientation, behavior) before and periodically during therapy.
- Assess for suicidal tendencies, especially during early therapy. Restrict amount of drug available to patient. Risk may be increased in children, adolescents, and adults ≤24 yr.
- Assess weight and BMI initially and during therapy.
- Monitor BP (sitting, standing, lying) and pulse before and frequently during initial dose titration. If hypotension occurs during dose titration, return to the previous dose.
- Observe patient carefully to ensure medication is swallowed and not hoarded or cheeked.
- Monitor for onset of extrapyramidal side effects (*akathisia*—restlessness; *dystonia*—muscle spasms and twisting motions; or *pseudoparkinsonism*—mask-like faces, rigidity, tremors, drooling, shuffling gait, dysphagia). Report these symptoms; reduction of dose or discontinuation may be necessary. Trihexyphenidyl or benztropine may be used to control these symptoms.
- Monitor for tardive dyskinesia (involuntary rhythmic movement of mouth, face, and extremities). Report immediately; may be irreversible.
- Monitor for development of neuroleptic malignant syndrome (fever, respiratory distress, tachycardia, seizures, diaphoresis, hypertension or hypotension, pallor, tiredness). Notify health care professional immediately if these symptoms occur.
- Assess for rash periodically during therapy. May cause Stevens-Johnson syndrome. Discontinue therapy if severe or if accompanied with fever, general malaise, fatigue, muscle or joint aches, blisters, oral lesions, conjunctivitis, hepatitis, and/or eosinophilia.
- Monitor for signs of pancreatitis (nausea, vomiting, anorexia, persistent severe abdominal pain, sometimes radiating to the back) during therapy.
- Monitor for symptoms related to hyperprolactinemia (menstrual abnormalities, galactorrhea, sexual dysfunction).
- Assess for falls risk. Drowsiness, orthostatic hypotension, and motor and sensory instability increase risk. Institute prevention if indicated.
- Monitor for signs and symptoms of DRESS (fever, rash, lymphadenopathy, and/or facial swelling), associated with involvement of other organ systems (hepatitis, nephritis, hematologic abnormalities, myocarditis, myositis) during therapy. May resemble an acute viral infection. Eosinophilia is often present. Discontinue therapy if signs occur.
- ***Lab Test Considerations:*** May cause asymptomatic ↑ in AST and ALT.

- May also cause anemia, thrombocytopenia, leukocytosis, and leukopenia.
- May cause ↑ total cholesterol and triglycerides.
- Obtain fasting blood glucose and cholesterol levels initially and throughout therapy.
- Monitor serum prolactin prior to and periodically during therapy. May cause ↑ serum prolactin levels.

Implementation

- Do not confuse quetiapine with olanzapine. Do not confuse Seroquel with Seroquel XR, Serzone (nefazodone), or Sinequan (doxepin).
- If therapy is reinstituted after an interval of ≥1 wk off, follow initial titration schedule.
- **PO:** May be administered without regard to food. Extended-release tablets should be swallowed whole, do not break, crush, or chew.

Patient/Family Teaching

- Instruct patient to take medication as directed. Take missed doses as soon as remembered unless almost time for next dose; do not double doses. Consult health care professional prior to stopping quetiapine; should be discontinued gradually. Stopping abruptly may cause insomnia, nausea, and vomiting.
- Advise patient and caregiver that quetiapine should not be given to elderly patients with dementia-related psychosis; may ↑ risk of death.
- Inform patient of the possibility of extrapyramidal symptoms. Instruct patient to report symptoms immediately to health care professional.
- Advise patient to change positions slowly to minimize orthostatic hypotension. Protect from falls.
- May cause drowsiness. Caution patient to avoid driving or other activities requiring alertness until response to medication is known.
- Advise patient to avoid extremes in temperature; this drug impairs body temperature regulation.
- Advise patient to notify health care professional of all Rx or OTC medications, vitamins, or herbal products being taken and to consult with health care professional before taking other medications and alcohol, especially other CNS depressants.
- Advise patient and family to notify health care professional if thoughts about suicide or dying, attempts to commit suicide; new or worse depression; new or worse anxiety; feeling very agitated or restless; panic attacks; trouble sleeping; new or worse irritability; acting aggressive; being angry or violent; acting on dangerous impulses; an extreme increase in activity and talking; other unusual changes in behavior or mood occur.
- Refer patient for nutritional, weight, or medical management of dyslipidemia as indicated.
- Advise patient to notify health care professional of medication regimen before treatment or surgery.
- Instruct patient to notify health care professional promptly of sore throat, fever, unusual bleeding or bruising, or rash.
- Rep: Advise female patients to notify health care professional if pregnancy is planned or suspected, and to avoid breast feeding. Encourage women who become pregnant while taking quitiapine to enroll in the National Pregnancy Registry for Atypical Antipsychotics at 1-866-961-2388 or visit http://womensmentalhealth.org/clinical-and-research-programs/pregnancyregistry/. Monitor neonates for extrapyramidal and/or withdrawal symptoms and manage symptoms appropriately. May lead to temporary, reversible infertility for females.
- Emphasize importance of routine follow-up exams to monitor side effects and continued participation in psychotherapy as indicated to improve coping skills. Ophthalmologic exams should be performed before and every 6 mo during therapy.

Evaluation/Desired Outcomes

- Decrease in excited, manic, behavior.
- Decrease in signs of depression in patients with bipolar disorder.
- Decrease in manic episodes in patients with bipolar I disorder.
- Decrease in positive symptoms (delusions, hallucinations) of schizophrenia.
- Decrease in negative symptoms (social withdrawal, flat, blunt affect) of schizophrenia.

quinapril, **See ANGIOTENSIN-CONVERTING ENZYME (ACE) INHIBITORS.**

Q

BEERS

RABEprazole (ra-bep-ra-zole)

Aciphex, Aciphex Sprinkle, Pariet

Classification
Therapeutic: antiulcer agents
Pharmacologic: proton-pump inhibitors

Indications

Gastroesophageal reflux disease (GERD). Duodenal ulcers (including combination therapy with clarithromycin and amoxicillin to eradicate *Helicobacter pylori* and prevent recurrence). Pathological hypersecretory conditions, including Zollinger-Ellison syndrome.

Action

Binds to an enzyme in the presence of acidic gastric pH, preventing the final transport of hydrogen ions into the gastric lumen. **Therapeutic Effects:** Diminished accumulation of acid in the gastric lumen, with lessened acid reflux. Healing of duodenal ulcers and esophagitis. Decreased acid secretion in hypersecretory conditions.

Pharmacokinetics

Absorption: Delayed-release tablet is designed to allow rabeprazole, which is not stable in gastric acid, to pass through the stomach intact. Subsequently 52% is absorbed after oral administration.
Distribution: Unknown.
Protein Binding: 96.3%.
Metabolism and Excretion: Mostly metabolized by the CYP3A4 and CYP2C19 isoenzymes in the liver; (the CYP2C19 enzyme system exhibits genetic polymorphism; 15–20% of Asian patients and 3–5% of Caucasian and Black patients may be poor metabolizers and may have significantly ↑ rabeprazole concentrations and an ↑ risk of adverse effects); 10% excreted in feces; remainder excreted in urine as inactive metabolites.
Half-life: 1–2 hr.

TIME/ACTION PROFILE (acid suppression)

ROUTE	ONSET	PEAK	DURATION
PO	within 1 hr	unknown	24 hr†

†Suppression continues to increase over the first wk of therapy.

Contraindications/Precautions

Contraindicated in: Hypersensitivity to rabeprazole or related drugs (benzimidazoles); Concurrent use of rilpivirine; Lactation: Discontinue breast feeding or discontinue the drug.
Use Cautiously in: Severe hepatic impairment (dose reduction may be necessary); Patients using high-doses for >1 yr (↑ risk of hip, wrist, or spine fractures and fundic gland polyps); Patients using therapy for >3 yr (↑ risk of vitamin B_{12} deficiency; OB: Use only if benefit outweighs potential risk to fetus; Pedi: Children <12 yr (safety not established).

Adverse Reactions/Side Effects

CNS: dizziness, headache, malaise. **Derm:** cutaneous lupus erythematosus, photosensitivity, rash. **F and E:** hypomagnesemia (especially if treatment duration ≥3 mo). **GI:** CLOSTRIDIUM DIFFICILE-ASSOCIATED DIARRHEA (CDAD), abdominal pain, constipation, diarrhea, fundic gland polyps, nausea. **GU:** acute interstitial nephritis. **Hemat:** vitamin B_{12} deficiency. **MS:** bone fracture, neck pain. **Misc:** HYPERSENSITIVITY REACTIONS (including anaphylaxis, angioedema, bronchospasm, or urticaria), chills, fever, systemic lupus erythematosus.

Interactions

Drug-Drug: Rabeprazole is metabolized by the CYP450 enzyme system and may interact with other drugs metabolized by this system. May ↓ absorption of drugs requiring acid pH, including **ketoconazole**, **itraconazole**, **atazanavir**, **iron salts**, **erlotinib**, **dasatinib**, **nelfinavir**, **nilotinib**, **rilpivirine**, and **mycophenolate mofetil**; concurrent use with **rilpivirine** contraindicated; avoid concurrent use with **nelfinavir**. May ↑ levels of **digoxin**, **methotrexate**, **saquinavir**, and **tacrolimus**. Hypomagnesemia ↑ risk of **digoxin** toxicity. May ↑ the risk of bleeding with **warfarin** (monitor INR/PT).

R

Route/Dosage

Gastroesophageal Reflux Disease

PO (Adults): *Healing of erosive or ulcerative GERD*—20 mg once daily for 4–8 wk; *Maintenance of healing of erosive or ulcerative GERD*—20 mg once daily; *Symptomatic GERD*—20 mg once daily for 4 wk (additional 4 wk may be considered for nonresponders).
PO (Children ≥12 yr): *Short-term treatment of symptomatic GERD*—20 mg once daily for up to 8 wk.
PO (Children 1–11 yr): *≥15 kg*—10 mg once daily for up to 12 wk (given as sprinkle); *<15 kg*—5 mg once daily for up to 12 wk (given as sprinkle); may ↑ up to 10 mg once daily if inadequate response.

Duodenal Ulcers

PO (Adults): *Healing of duodenal ulcers*—20 mg once daily for up to 4 wk.

H. pylori Eradication to Reduce the Risk of Duodenal Ulcer Recurrence (Triple Therapy)

PO (Adults): 20 mg twice daily for 7 days, with amoxicillin 1000 mg twice daily for 7 days and clarithromycin 500 mg twice daily for 7 days.

Pathological Hypersecretory Conditions Including Zollinger-Ellison Syndrome

PO (Adults): 60 mg once daily initially, may be adjusted as needed and continued as necessary; doses up to 100 mg daily or 60 mg twice daily have been used.

Availability (generic available)

Delayed-release capsules (Sprinkle): 5 mg, 10 mg.
Delayed-release tablets: 🍁 10 mg, 20 mg.

NURSING IMPLICATIONS

Assessment

- Assess routinely for epigastric or abdominal pain and frank or occult blood in the stool, emesis, or gastric aspirate.
- Monitor bowel function. Diarrhea, abdominal cramping, fever, and bloody stools should be reported to health care professional promptly as a sign of Clostridium difficile-associated diarrhea (CDAD). May begin up to several wk following cessation of therapy.
- ***Lab Test Considerations:*** Monitor CBC with differential periodically during therapy.
- May cause hypomagnesemia. Monitor serum magnesium prior to and periodically during therapy.

Implementation

- ***High Alert:*** Do not confuse rabeprazole with aripiprazole. Do not confuse Aciphex with Accupril or Aricept.
- **PO:** Administer doses before meals, preferably in the morning. Tablets should be swallowed whole; do not break, crush, or chew.
- *Aciphex Sprinkle:* open capsule and sprinkle granule contents on a small amount of soft food (apple sauce, fruit, or vegetable-based baby food, yogurt) or empty contents into small amount of liquid (infant formula, apple juice, pediatric electrolyte solution). Food or liquid should be at or below room temperature. Whole dose should be taken within 15 min of being sprinkled. Granules should not be chewed or crushed. Dose should be taken 30 min before a meal. Do not store mixture for future use.

Patient/Family Teaching

- Instruct patient to take medication as directed for the full course of therapy, even if feeling better. Take missed doses as soon as remembered but not if almost time for next dose. Do not double doses.
- May cause occasional drowsiness or dizziness. Caution patient to avoid driving or other activities requiring alertness until response to medication is known.
- Advise patient to avoid alcohol, products containing aspirin or NSAIDs, and foods that may cause an increase in GI irritation.
- Caution patients to wear sunscreen and protective clothing to prevent photosensitivity reactions.
- Advise patient to report onset of black, tarry stools; diarrhea; abdominal pain; or persistent headache to health care professional promptly.
- Instruct patient to notify health care professional of all Rx or OTC medications, vitamins, or herbal products being taken and consult health care professional before taking any new medications.
- Instruct patient to notify health care professional of onset of black, tarry stools; diarrhea; abdominal pain; or persistent headache or if fever and diarrhea develop, especially if stool contains blood, pus, or mucus. Advise patient not to treat diarrhea without consulting health care professional.
- Advise female patients to notify health care professional if pregnancy is planned or suspected or if breast feeding.

Evaluation/Desired Outcomes

- Decrease in abdominal pain or prevention of gastric irritation and bleeding. Healing of duodenal ulcers can be seen on x-ray examination or endoscopy.
- Decrease in symptoms of GERD. Therapy is continued for 4–8 wk after initial episode.

raloxifene (ra-lox-i-feen)

Evista

Classification
Therapeutic: bone resorption inhibitors
Pharmacologic: selective estrogen receptor modulators

Indications

Treatment and prevention of osteoporosis in postmenopausal women. Reduction of the risk of breast cancer in postmenopausal women with osteoporosis and those at high risk for invasive breast cancer.

Action

Binds to estrogen receptors, producing estrogen-like effects on bone, resulting in reduced resorption of bone and decreased bone turnover. **Therapeutic Effects:** Prevention of osteoporosis in patients at risk. Decreased risk of breast cancer.

Pharmacokinetics

Absorption: Although well absorbed (>60%), after oral administration, extensive first-pass metabolism results in 2% bioavailability.
Distribution: Highly bound to plasma proteins; remainder of distribution unknown.
Protein Binding: Highly bound to plasma proteins.
Metabolism and Excretion: Extensively metabolized by the liver; undergoes enterohepatic cycling; excreted primarily in feces.
Half-life: 27.7 hr.

TIME/ACTION PROFILE (effects on bone turnover)

ROUTE	ONSET	PEAK	DURATION
PO	unknown	3 mo	unknown

Contraindications/Precautions

Contraindicated in: Hypersensitivity; History of thromboembolic events; OB: May cause fetal harm (not indicated for women of reproductive potential; avoid use in pregnancy); Lactation: Not indicated for women of reproductive potential (avoid use during breast feeding); Pedi: Safety not established.

Use Cautiously in: Potential immobilization (↑ risk of thromboembolic events); History of stroke or transient ischemic attack; Atrial fibrillation; Hypertension; Cigarette smoking.

Adverse Reactions/Side Effects

CNS: STROKE. **CV:** THROMBOEMBOLISM. **EENT:** retinal vein thrombosis. **MS:** leg cramps. **Misc:** hot flashes.

Interactions

Drug-Drug: Cholestyramine ↓ absorption (avoid concurrent use). May alter effects of **warfarin** and other **highly protein-bound drugs**. Concurrent systemic **estrogen** therapy is not recommended.

Route/Dosage

PO (Adults): 60 mg once daily.

Availability (generic available)

Tablets: 60 mg. **Cost:** $630.76/100.

NURSING IMPLICATIONS

Assessment

- Assess patient for bone mineral density with x-ray, serum, and urine bone turnover markers (bone-specific alkaline phosphatase, osteocalcin, and collagen breakdown products) before and periodically during therapy.
- ***Lab Test Considerations:*** May cause ↑ apolipoprotein A-I and reduced serum total cholesterol, LDL cholesterol, fibrinogen, apolipoprotein B, and lipoprotein.
- May cause ↑ hormone-binding globulin (sex steroid-binding globulin, thyroxine-binding globulin, corticosteroid-binding globulin) with ↑ total hormone concentrations.
- May cause small ↓ in serum total calcium, inorganic phosphate, total protein, and albumin.
- May also cause slight decrease in platelet count.

Implementation

- **PO:** May be administered without regard to meals.
- Calcium supplementation should be added to diet if daily intake is inadequate.

Patient/Family Teaching

- Instruct patient to take raloxifene as directed. Discuss the importance of adequate calcium and vitamin D intake or supplementation. Instruct patient to read the *Medication Guide* when initiating therapy and again with each prescription refill in case of changes.
- Advise patient to discontinue smoking and alcohol consumption.
- Emphasize the importance of regular weight-bearing exercise. Advise patient that raloxifene should be discontinued at least 72 hr before and during prolonged immobilization (recovery from surgery, prolonged bedrest). Instruct patient to avoid prolonged restrictions of movement during travel because of the increased risk of venous thrombosis.
- Advise patient that raloxifene will not reduce hot flashes or flushes associated with estrogen deficiency and may cause hot flashes.
- Instruct patient to notify health care professional immediately if leg pain or a feeling of warmth in the lower leg (calf); swelling of the legs, hands, or feet; sudden chest pain; shortness of breath or coughing up blood; or sudden change in vision, such as loss of vision or blurred vision occur. Being still for a long time (sitting still during a long car or airplane trip, being in bed after surgery) can increase risk of blood clots.
- Advise patient that raloxifene may have teratogenic effects. Instruct patient to notify health care provider immediately if pregnancy is planned or suspected or if breast feeding.

Evaluation/Desired Outcomes

- Prevention of osteoporosis in postmenopausal women.
- Reduced risk of breast cancer in postmenopausal women with osteoporosis and those at high risk for invasive breast cancer.

raltegravir (ral-teg-ra-veer)

Isentress, Isentress HD

Classification

Therapeutic: antiretrovirals

Pharmacologic: integrase strand transfer inhibitors (INSTIs)

Indications

HIV-1 infection (with other antiretrovirals).

Action

Inhibits HIV-1 integrase, which is required for viral replication. **Therapeutic Effects:** Evidence of decreased viral replication and reduced viral load with slowed progression of HIV and its sequelae.

R

Pharmacokinetics

Absorption: Well absorbed following oral administration.

Distribution: Unknown.

Metabolism and Excretion: Mostly metabolized by the uridine diphosphate glucuronosyltransferase (UGT) A1A enzyme system; 23% excreted in urine as parent drug and metabolite.

Half-life: 9 hr.

TIME/ACTION PROFILE (blood levels)

ROUTE	ONSET	PEAK	DURATION
PO	unknown	3 hr	12 hr

Contraindications/Precautions

Contraindicated in: Lactation: Breast feeding not recommended in HIV-infected patients.

Use Cautiously in: Concurrent use of medications associated with rhabdomyolysis/myopathy (may ↑ risk); Phenylketonuria (chewable tablets contain phenylalanine); Geri: Choose dose carefully, considering concurrent disease states, drug therapy, and age-related ↓ in hepatic and renal function; OB: Use in pregnancy only if maternal benefit outweighs fetal risk; Pedi: Pre-term neonates (safety and effectiveness not established).

Adverse Reactions/Side Effects

CNS: SUICIDAL THOUGHTS, headache, depression, dizziness, fatigue, insomnia, weakness. **CV:** MYOCARDIAL INFARCTION. **GI:** diarrhea, abdominal pain, gastritis, hepatitis, nausea, vomiting. **GU:** renal failure/impairment. **Hemat:** anemia, neutropenia. **Metab:** lipodystrophy. **Derm:** STEVENS JOHNSON SYNDROME, TOXIC EPIDERMAL NECROLYSIS, rash. **MS:** RHABDOMYOLYSIS, ↑ creatine kinase, myopathy. **Misc:** hypersensitivity reactions, immune reconstitution syndrome, fever.

Interactions

Drug-Drug: Concurrent use with **strong inducers of the UGT A1A enzyme system** including **rifampin** may ↓ blood levels and effectiveness. Concurrent use with **strong inhibitors of the UGT A1A enzyme system** including **atazanavir** may ↑ blood levels. ↑ risk of rhabomyolysis/myopathy **HMG-CoA reductase inhibitors**. **Proton pump inhibitors** may ↑ levels. **Efavirenz**, **etravirine**, and **tipranavir/ritonavir** may ↓ levels. Administration with **antacids**, containing **magnesium** or **aluminum** ↓ absorption of raltegravir; separate administration of raltegravir and magnesium- or aluminum-containing antacids by ≥6 hr.

Route/Dosage

Do not substitute the chewable tablets or oral suspension for the film-coated tablets.

PO (Adults): *Treatment-naïve patients or patients who are virologically suppressed on an initial regimen of raltegravir 400 mg twice daily*—Two 600-mg tablets (1200 mg) once daily or 400 mg twice daily; *Treatment-experienced patients*—400 mg twice daily; *Concurrent use of rifampin (either treatment-naïve or treatment-experienced patients)*—800 mg twice daily.

PO (Children ≥40 kg and either treatment-naïve or virologically suppressed on an initial regimen of raltegravir 400 mg twice daily): *Tablet*—Two 600-mg tablets (1200 mg) once daily or 400 mg twice daily; *Chewable tablets*—300 mg twice daily.

PO (Children ≥25 kg): *Tablet*—400 mg twice daily; *Chewable tablets (if unable to swallow tablet)*—25–28 kg: 150 mg twice daily; 28–39.9 kg: 200 mg twice daily; ≥40 kg: 300 mg twice daily.

PO (Children ≥4 wk and 20–<25 kg): *Chewable tablets*—150 mg twice daily.

PO (Children ≥4 wk and 14–<20 kg): *Oral suspension*—100 mg twice daily; *Chewable tablets*—100 mg twice daily.

PO (Children ≥4 wk and 11–<14 kg): *Oral suspension*—80 mg twice daily; *Chewable tablets*—75 mg twice daily.

PO (Children ≥4 wk and 8–<11 kg): *Oral suspension*—60 mg twice daily.

PO (Children ≥4 wk and 6–<8 kg): *Oral suspension*—40 mg twice daily.

PO (Children ≥4 wk and 4–<6 kg): *Oral suspension*—30 mg twice daily.

PO (Children ≥4 wk and 3–<4 kg): *Oral suspension*—25 mg twice daily.

PO (Neonates 1–4 wk and 4–<5 kg): *Oral suspension*—15 mg twice daily.

PO (Neonates 1–4 wk and 3–<4 kg): *Oral suspension*—10 mg twice daily.

PO (Neonates 1–4 wk and 2–<3 kg): *Oral suspension*—8 mg twice daily.

PO (Neonates 0–1 wk and 4–<5 kg): *Oral suspension*—7 mg once daily.

PO (Neonates 0–1 wk and 3–<4 kg): *Oral suspension*—5 mg once daily.

PO (Neonates 0–1 wk and 2–<3 kg): *Oral suspension*—4 mg once daily.

Availability

Tablets: 400 mg, 600 mg. **Chewable tablets (orange-banana):** 25 mg, 100 mg. **Packet for oral suspension (banana-flavor):** 100 mg/pkt.

NURSING IMPLICATIONS

Assessment

- Assess patient for change in severity of HIV symptoms and for symptoms of opportunistic infections during therapy.
- Monitor for anxiety, depression (especially in patients with a history of psychiatric illness), suicidal ideation, and paranoia during therapy.
- Assess for rash periodically during therapy. May cause Stevens-Johnson syndrome. Discontinue ther-

apy if severe or if accompanied with fever, general malaise, fatigue, muscle or joint aches, blisters, oral lesions, conjunctivitis, hepatitis, and/or eosinophilia.

- ***Lab Test Considerations:*** Monitor viral load and CD4 counts regularly during therapy.
- May cause ↓ ANC, hemoglobin, and platelet counts.
- May cause ↑ serum glucose, AST, ALT, GGT, total bilirubin, alkaline phosphatase, pancreatic amylase, serum lipase, and creatinine kinase concentrations.

Implementation

- Tablets are not interchangeable with chewable tablets or packets for oral suspension.
- **PO:** May be administered without regard to meals.
- Swallow tablets whole; do not break, crush, or chew.
- Chewable tablets may be chewed or swallowed.
- *Oral suspension:* Pour packet for oral solution into 10 mL of water and mix in provided mixing cup. Gently swirl for 45 sec until mix is uniform; do not shake. Once mixed, administer with syringe orally within 30 min of mixing. Discard unused solution.

Patient/Family Teaching

- Emphasize the importance of taking raltegravir as directed, at evenly spaced times throughout day. Do not take more than prescribed amount and do not stop taking without consulting health care professional. Take missed doses as soon as remembered unless almost time for next dose. Do not double doses. Advise patient to read *Patient Information* sheet before starting therapy and with each Rx renewal in case of changes.
- Instruct patient that raltegravir should not be shared with others.
- Instruct patient to notify health care professional of all Rx or OTC medications, vitamins, or herbal products being taken and consult health care professional before taking any new medications.
- Inform patient that raltegravir does not cure AIDS or prevent associated or opportunistic infections. Raltegravir does not reduce the risk of transmission of HIV to others through sexual contact or blood contamination. Caution patient to use a condom during sexual contact and to avoid sharing needles or donating blood to prevent spreading the AIDS virus to others. Advise patient that the long-term effects of raltegravir are unknown at this time.
- Advise patient to notify health care professional if they develop any unusual symptoms, if any known symptom persists or worsen, or if signs and symptoms of rhabdomyolysis (unexplained muscle pain, tenderness, weakness), rash, or depression or suicidal thoughts occur.
- Immune reconstitution syndrome may trigger opportunistic infections or autoimmune disorders. Notify health care professional if symptoms occur.
- Rep: Advise patient to notify health care professional if pregnancy is planned or suspected. Encourage pregnant women to enroll in the Antiretroviral Pregnancy Registry by calling 1-800-258-4263. Advise female patient to avoid breast feeding during therapy.
- Emphasize the importance of regular follow-up exams and blood counts to determine progress and monitor for side effects.

Evaluation/Desired Outcomes

- Delayed progression of AIDS and decreased opportunistic infections in patients with HIV.
- Decrease in viral load and improvement in CD4 cell counts.

ramipril, See ANGIOTENSIN-CONVERTING ENZYME (ACE) INHIBITORS.

ramucirumab

(ra-mue-**sir**-ue-mab)

Cyramza

Classification

Therapeutic: antineoplastics

Pharmacologic: vascular endothelial growth factor antagonists

R

Indications

Advanced gastric cancer or gastro-esophageal junction adenocarcinoma following unsuccessful combination treatment that included a fluoropyrimidine or platinum compound (as monotherapy or in combination with paclitaxel). Metastatic non-small cell lung cancer (NSCLC) with disease progression on or after platinum-based chemotherapy (in combination with docetaxel). Metastatic colorectal cancer (CRC) with disease progression on or after treatment with bevacizumab, oxaliplatin, and a fluoropyrimidine (in combination with irinotecan, folinic acid, and 5–fluorouracil [FOLFIRI]). Hepatocellular carcinoma (HCC) in patients with an alpha fetoprotein of ≥400 ng/mL who have been previously treated with sorafenib.

Action

A monoclonal antibody that binds to vascular endothelial growth factor receptor 2 (VEGFR 2), antagonizing its effects, resulting in decreased angiogenesis. **Therapeutic Effects:** Decreased growth and spread of gastric cancer, gastro-esophageal junction adenocarcinoma, NSCLC, CRC, and HCC.

Pharmacokinetics

Absorption: IV administration results in complete bioavailability.

Distribution: Unknown.
Metabolism and Excretion: Unknown.
Half-life: Unknown.

TIME/ACTION PROFILE (improved survival)

ROUTE	ONSET	PEAK	DURATION
IV	within 1 mo	7–8 mos	24 mos

Contraindications/Precautions

Contraindicated in: OB: Pregnancy (may cause fetal harm); Lactation: Lactation.
Use Cautiously in: Child-Pugh Class B or C cirrhosis (use only if benefits outweigh risk of further deterioration); Surgery (discontinue prior to surgery, reinstate when healing is complete); Serious or non-healing wounds; Hypertension (must be controlled prior to treatment); Rep: Women of reproductive potential; Pedi: Safety and effectiveness not established.

Adverse Reactions/Side Effects

CNS: REVERSIBLE POSTERIOR LEUKOENCEPHALOPATHY SYNDROME, encephalopathy, headache. **CV:** ARTERIAL THROMBOTIC EVENTS, hypertension. **Endo:** hypothyroidism. **F and E:** hyponatremia. **GI:** GASTROINTESTINAL OBSTRUCTION/PERFORATION, diarrhea, worsened cirrhosis/hepatorenal syndrome, diarrhea. **GU:** impaired female fertility, nephrotic syndrome, proteinuria. **Hemat:** BLEEDING, neutropenia. **Misc:** INFUSION-RELATED REACTIONS, impaired wound healing.

Interactions

Drug-Drug: ↑ risk of bleeding with **anticoagulants, antiplatelet agents** and **NSAIDs**.

Route/Dosage

Gastric Cancer or HCC

IV (Adults): 8 mg/kg every 2 wk continued until disease progression or unacceptable toxicity.

NSCLC

IV (Adults): 10 mg/kg on Day 1 of a 21-day cycle prior to docetaxel; continued until disease progression or unacceptable toxicity.

CRC

IV (Adults): 8 mg/kg every 2 wk prior to FOLFIRI administration; continued until disease progression or unacceptable toxicity.

Availability

Solution for injection (requires dilution): 10 mg/mL.

NURSING IMPLICATIONS

Assessment

- Monitor for infusion-related reactions (rigors/tremors, back pain/spasms, chest pain and/or tightness, chills, flushing, dyspnea, wheezing, hypoxia, paresthesia, bronchospasm, supraventricular tachycardia, hypotension) during infusion. Reduce infusion rate by 50% for Grade 1 or 2 reactions, and immediately and permanently discontinue ramucirumab if Grade 3 or 4 reactions occur.
- Monitor BP prior to and at least every 2 wk during therapy. Hold therapy for severe hypertension until BP is under control. Permanently discontinue if unable to control hypertension.
- Avoid administration for at least 28 days prior to and 28 days after surgery or until wound is healed.
- If arterial thromboembolic events (myocardial infarction, cardiac arrest, cerebrovascular accident, cerebral ischemia), permanently discontinue.
- Monitor for signs and symptoms of bleeding (bleeding, lightheadedness) during therapy. *If Grade 3 or 4 bleeding occur,* permanently discontinue medication.
- Monitor for signs and symptoms of gastrointestinal perforation (severe diarrhea, vomiting, severe abdominal pain) during therapy. Discontinue medication permanently if perforation occurs.
- ***Lab Test Considerations:*** Obtain a negative pregnancy test before starting therapy.
- Monitor urinary protein periodically during therapy. Hold ramucirumab for urine protein ≥2 g/24 hr. Reinitiate therapy at reduced dose (Reduce 8 mg dose to 6 mg/kg and 10 mg to 8 mg) every 2 wk once urinary protein levels <2 g/24 hr. If protein level returns to ≥2 g/24 hr hold therapy until urine protein <2 g per 24 hrs and reduce dose (Reduce 6 mg to 5 mg/kg and 8 mg to 6 mg) every 2 wk once urinary protein levels return to <2 g/24 hr. Discontinue therapy permanently if urine protein level >3 g/24 hr or if nephrotic syndrome occurs.

Implementation

- Prior to each dose, premedicate all patients with IV histamine H_1 antagonist (diphenhydramine). Premedicate patients who have experienced a Grade 1 or 2 infusion reaction with dexamethasone and acetaminophen prior to each infusion.

IV Administration

- **Intermittent Infusion:** Withdraw required volume from vial. ***Diluent:*** Dilute with 0.9% NaCl for a final volume of 250 mL. Do not use dextrose-containing solutions. Gently invert to ensure adequate mixing. Solution is clear to slightly opalescent and colorless to slightly yellow; do not administer solutions that are discolored or contain particulate material. Solution is stable for 24 hr if refrigerated or 4 hr at room temperature. Discard unused solution. ***Rate:*** Infuse over 60 min via infusion pump through a separate infusion line using a 0.22 micron filter; do not administer as IV push or bolus. Flush line with 0.9% NaCl at end of infusion. If 1st infusion is tolerated, administer all subsequent infusions over 30 min.
- **Y-Site Incompatibility:** Do not dilute with other solutions or infuse with other electrolyte solutions or medications.

Patient/Family Teaching

- Explain purpose of ramucirumab to patient.
- Advise patient to notify health care professional if bleeding or lightheadedness occur.
- Instruct patient in self BP monitoring and advise patient to notify health care professional if signs and symptoms of hypertension (elevated BP, severe headache, lightheadedness, neurologic symptoms) or if severe diarrhea, vomiting, or severe abdominal pain occur.
- Advise to notify health care professional of medication regimen prior to surgery; may impair wound healing.
- Advise females of reproductive potential to use effective contraception during and for at least 3 mo after last dose and avoid breast feeding for 2 mo after last dose. Notify health care professional if pregnancy is suspected. and avoid breast feeding during therapy. Advise patient that ramucirumab may impair fertility in females.

Evaluation/Desired Outcomes

- Decreased growth and spread of cancer.

raNITIdine, See HISTAMINE H_2 ANTAGONISTS.

ranolazine (ra-nole-a-zeen)

Ranexa

Classification

Therapeutic: antianginals

Indications

Chronic angina pectoris.

Action

Does not ↓ BP or heart rate; remainder of mechanism is not known. **Therapeutic Effects:** Decreased frequency of angina.

Pharmacokinetics

Absorption: Highly variable.

Distribution: Unknown.

Metabolism and Excretion: Metabolized in the gut (P-glycoprotein) and by the liver (primarily CYP3A and less by CYP2D6); <5% excreted unchanged in urine and feces.

Half-life: 7 hr.

TIME/ACTION PROFILE (blood levels)

ROUTE	ONSET	PEAK	DURATION
PO	unknown	2–5 hr	12 hr

Contraindications/Precautions

Contraindicated in: Hypersensitivity; Concurrent use of potent inhibitors of CYP3A; Concurrent use of inducers of CYP3A; Hepatic impairment; Lactation: Lactation.

Use Cautiously in: Renal impairment; OB: Use only when potential benefit outweighs risk to fetus; Pedi: Safety and effectiveness not established; Geri: ↑ risk of adverse reactions in patients >75 yr.

Adverse Reactions/Side Effects

CNS: dizziness, headache. **CV:** TORSADES DE POINTES, palpitations, QTc prolongation. **EENT:** tinnitus. **GI:** abdominal pain, constipation, dry mouth, nausea, vomiting. **GU:** acute renal failure.

Interactions

Drug-Drug: **Ketoconazole, itraconazole, clarithromycin, nefazodone, nelfinavir, ritonavir, indinavir,** and **saquinavir** significantly ↑ levels; concurrent use contraindicated. **Rifampin, rifabutin, rifapentin, phenobarbital, phenytoin,** and **carbamazepine** significantly ↓ levels; concurrent use contraindicated. **Verapamil, diltiazem, aprepitant, erythromycin,** and **fluconazole** ↑ levels (do not exceed ranolazine dose of 500 mg twice daily). **Cyclosporine** may ↑ levels. **Paroxetine** may ↑ levels. May ↑ levels of **simvastatin.** May ↓ metabolism and ↑ effects of **metoprolol, tricyclic antidepressants,** and **antipsychotics**; dosage adjustments may be necessary. May ↑ **digoxin** levels; dose adjustment may be required.

Drug-Natural Products: St. John's wort significantly ↓ levels (contraindicated).

Drug-Food: Grapefruit juice↑ levels (do not exceed ranolazine dose of 500 mg twice daily).

Route/Dosage

PO (Adults): 500 mg twice daily initially, may be ↑ to 1000 mg twice daily.

Availability (generic available)

Extended-release tablets: 500 mg, 1000 mg.

NURSING IMPLICATIONS

Assessment

- Assess location, duration, intensity, and precipitating factors of anginal pain.
- Monitor ECG at baseline and periodically during therapy to evaluate effects on QT interval.
- ***Lab Test Considerations:*** Monitor renal function after starting and periodically during therapy in patients with moderate to severe renal impairment (CCr <60 mL/min) for ↑ serum creatinine accompanied by ↑ BUN. Usually has a rapid onset, but does not progress during therapy and is reversible with discontinuation of ranolazine. If acute renal failure develops, discontinue ranolazine.

R

- May cause transient eosinophilia.
- May cause small mean ↓ in hematocrit.

Implementation

- Ranolazine should be used in combination with amlodipine, beta blockers, or nitrates.
- Do not administer with grapefruit juice or grapefruit products.
- **PO:** May be administered without regard to food. Tablets should be swallowed whole; do not break, crush, or chew.

Patient/Family Teaching

- Instruct patient to take ranolazine as directed. If a dose is missed, take the usual dose at the next scheduled time; do not double doses. Explain to patient that ranolazine is used for chronic therapy and will not help an acute angina episode.
- Advise patient to avoid grapefruit juice and grapefruit products when taking ranolazine.
- May cause dizziness and light-headedness. Caution patient to avoid driving and other activities requiring alertness until response to medication is known.
- Advise patient to notify health care professional if fainting occurs.
- Inform patient that ranolazine may cause changes in the ECG. Patient should inform health care professional if they have a personal or family history of QTc prolongation, congenital long QT syndrome, or proarrhythmic conditions such as hypokalemia.
- Instruct patient to notify health care professional of all Rx or OTC medications, vitamins, or herbal products being taken and consult health care professional before taking any new medications.
- Advise patient to notify health care professional if pregnancy if planned or suspected, or if breast feeding.

Evaluation/Desired Outcomes

- Decrease in frequency of angina attacks.

rasagiline (ra-za-ji-leen)

Azilect

Classification

Therapeutic: antiparkinson agents

Pharmacologic: monoamine oxidase type B inhibitors

Indications

Parkinson's disease.

Action

Irreversibly inactivates monoamine oxidase (MAO) by binding to it at type B (brain sites); inactivation of MAO leads to increased amounts of dopamine available in the CNS. Differs from selegiline by its nonamphetamine characteristics. **Therapeutic Effects:** Improvement in symptoms of Parkinson's disease, allowing increase in function.

Pharmacokinetics

Absorption: 36% absorbed following oral administration.

Distribution: Readily crosses the blood-brain barrier.

Metabolism and Excretion: Extensively metabolized by the liver (CYP1A2 enzyme) to an inactive metabolite; less than 1% excreted in urine.

Half-life: 1.3 hr; does not correlate with duration of MAO-B inhibition.

TIME/ACTION PROFILE

ROUTE	ONSET	PEAK	DURATION
PO	rapid	1 hr	40 days*

*Recovery of MAO-B function.

Contraindications/Precautions

Contraindicated in: Hypersensitivity; Concurrent meperidine, tramadol, methadone, sympathomimetic amines, dextromethorphan, mirtazapine, cyclobenzaprine, cocaine, St. John's wort, or another MAO inhibitor; Moderate to severe hepatic impairment; Elective surgery requiring general anesthesia; allow 14 days after discontinuation; Pheochromocytoma; Psychotic disorder.

Use Cautiously in: Mild hepatic impairment (↑ blood levels); OB: Safety not established; Lactation: Use during breast feeding only if benefit to patient outweighs potential risk to infant; Pedi: Safety and effectiveness not established.

Adverse Reactions/Side Effects

CNS: depression, dizziness, drowsiness, hallucinations, impulse control disorders (gambling, sexual), malaise, sleep driving, vertigo. **CV:** orthostatic hypotension (may ↑ levodopa-induced hypotension), ↑ BP, chest pain, syncope. **Derm:** alopecia, ecchymosis, ↑ melanoma risk, rash. **EENT:** conjunctivitis, rhinitis. **Endo:** weight loss. **GI:** anorexia, dizziness, dyspepsia, gastroenteritis, vomiting. **GU:** albuminuria, ↓ libido. **Hemat:** leukopenia. **MS:** arthralgia, arthritis, neck pain. **Neuro:** dyskinesia (may ↑ levodopa-induced dyskinesia), paresthesia. **Resp:** asthma. **Misc:** fever, flu-like syndrome, ↑ fall risk.

Interactions

Drug-Drug: Concurrent use of **meperidine, tramadol, methadone**, or other **MAO inhibitors** may ↑ risk of serotonin syndrome; concurrent use contraindicated. **Ciprofloxacin** and other **inhibitors of the CYP1A2 enzyme** ↑ rasagiline levels; dose adjustment is recommended. Concurrent use with **dextromethorphan** may result in psychosis/bizarre behavior and should be avoided. ↑ risk of adverse reactions with **mirtazapine** and **cyclobenzapine**; concurrent use should be avoided. Hypertensive crisis may occur with **sympathomimetic amines** including **amphetamines**, **cold products**, and some **weight loss products** containing **vasoconstrictors** such as **pseudoephedrine**, **phenylephrine**, or **ephedrine**; avoid concurrent use. ↑ risk of serotonin syndrome with **tricyclic antidepressants**, **SSRIs**, and **SNRIs**; rasagiline should be discontinued ≥14 days prior to initiation of antidepressants (**fluoxetine** should be discontinued ≥5 wk prior to rasagiline therapy).

Drug-Natural Products: Risk of toxicity is ↑ with **St. John's wort**.

Drug-Food: Ingestion of foods containing high amounts of **tyramine** (>150 mg) (e.g., cheese) may result in life-threatening hypertensive crisis.

Route/Dosage

PO (Adults): *Monotherapy or as adjunct therapy in patients not taking levodopa*—1 mg once daily; *Concurrent levodopa therapy*—0.5 mg once daily, may ↑ to 1 mg once daily; *Concurrent ciprofloxacin or other CYP1A2 inhibitors*—0.5 mg once daily.

Hepatic Impairment

PO (Adults): *Mild hepatic impairment*—0.5 mg once daily.

Availability (generic available)

Tablets: 0.5 mg, 1 mg.

NURSING IMPLICATIONS

Assessment

- Assess signs and symptoms of Parkinson's disease (tremor, muscle weakness and rigidity, ataxic gait) prior to and during therapy.
- Monitor BP periodically during therapy.
- Assess skin for melanomas periodically during therapy.
- Assess for serotonin syndrome (mental changes [agitation, hallucinations, coma], autonomic instability [tachycardia, labile BP, hyperthermia], neuromuscular aberrations [hyperreflexia, incoordination], and/or GI symptoms [nausea, vomiting, diarrhea]), especially in patients taking other serotonergic drugs (SSRIs, SNRIs, triptans).
- ***Lab Test Considerations:*** May cause albuminuria, leukopenia, and abnormal liver function tests.
- ***Toxicity and Overdose:*** Concurrent ingestion of tyramine-rich foods and many medications may result in a life-threatening hypertensive crisis. Signs and symptoms of hypertensive crisis include chest pain, tachycardia or bradycardia, severe headache, neck stiffness or soreness, nausea and vomiting, sweating, photosensitivity, and enlarged pupils.

Implementation

- Do not confuse Azilect (rasagiline) with Aricept (donepezil).
- If used in combination with levodopa, a reduction in levodopa dose may be considered based on individual results.
- **PO:** Administer once daily.

Patient/Family Teaching

- Instruct patient to take rasagiline as directed. Missed doses should be omitted and next dose taken at usual time the following day. Do not double doses. Do not discontinue abruptly; may cause elevated temperature, muscular rigidity, altered consciousness, and autonomic instability.
- Caution patient to avoid alcohol, CNS depressants, and foods or beverages containing tyramine (see Appendix K) during and for at least 2 wk after therapy has been discontinued; they may precipitate a hypertensive crisis. Contact health care professional immediately if symptoms of hypertensive crisis or serotonin syndrome develop.
- Instruct patient to notify health care professional of all Rx or OTC medications, vitamins, or herbal products being taken and consult health care professional before taking any new medications. Caution patient to avoid use of St. John's wort and analgesics meperidine, tramadol, or methadone during therapy.
- Caution patient to avoid elective surgery requiring general anesthesia, cocaine, or local anesthesia containing sympathomimetic vasoconstrictors within 14 days of discontinuing rasagiline. If surgery is necessary sooner, benzodiazepines, rapacuronium, fentanyl, morphine, and codeine may be used cautiously.
- May cause dizziness or drowsiness. Caution patient to avoid driving and other activities requiring alertness until response to medication is known.
- Caution patient to change positions slowly to minimize orthostatic hypotension. Geriatric patients are at increased risk for this side effect.
- Advise patient to monitor for melanomas frequently and on a regular basis.
- Caution patient to notify health care professional if new skin lesions, agitation, aggression, delirium, hallucinations, sleep driving or new or increased gambling, sexual, or other intense urges occur.
- Advise patient to notify health care professional immediately if severe headache, neck stiffness, heart racing, or palpitations, occur.
- Advise female patients to notify health care professionals if pregnancy is planned or suspected, or if breast feeding.

Evaluation/Desired Outcomes

- Improvement in symptoms of Parkinson's disease, allowing increase in function.

R

rasburicase

(ras-**byoor**-i-case)

Elitek, Fasturtec

Classification

Therapeutic: antigout agents, antihyperuricemics

Pharmacologic: enzymes

Indications

Initial management of increased uric acid levels in patients with leukemia, lymphoma, or other malignancies who are being treated with antineoplastics, which are expected to produce hyperuricemia.

Action

An enzyme that promotes the conversion of uric acid to allantoin, an inactive, water-soluble compound. Produced by recombinant DNA technology. **Therapeutic Effects:** Decreased sequelae of hyperuricemia (nephropathy, arthropathy).

Pharmacokinetics

Absorption: IV administration results in complete bioavailability.
Distribution: Unknown.
Metabolism and Excretion: Unknown.
Half-life: 18 hr.

TIME/ACTION PROFILE (↓ in uric acid)

ROUTE	ONSET	PEAK	DURATION
IV	rapid	unknown	4–24 hr

Contraindications/Precautions

Contraindicated in: G6PD deficiency (↑ risk of severe hemolysis); Previous allergic reaction, hemolysis, or methemoglobinemia from rasburicase; Lactation: Lactation.
Use Cautiously in: OB: Pregnancy (use only if clearly needed).

Adverse Reactions/Side Effects

CNS: headache. **Resp:** respiratory distress. **GI:** abdominal pain, constipation, diarrhea, nausea, vomiting, mucositis. **Derm:** rash. **Hemat:** HEMOLYSIS, METHEMOGLOBINEMIA, neutropenia. **Misc:** hypersensitivity reactions including ANAPHYLAXIS, fever, sepsis.

Interactions

Drug-Drug: None known.

Route/Dosage

IV (Adults and Children): 0.2 mg/kg daily as a single dose for 5 days.

Availability

Lyophilized powder for injection: 1.5 mg/vial, 7.5 mg/vial.

NURSING IMPLICATIONS

Assessment

- Monitor patients for signs of allergic reactions and anaphylaxis (chest pain, dyspnea, hypotension, urticaria). If these signs occur, rasburicase should be immediately and permanently discontinued.
- ***Lab Test Considerations:*** Monitor patients for hemolysis. Screen patients at higher risk for G6PD deficiency (patients of African American or Mediterranean ancestry) prior to therapy. If hemolysis occurs, discontinue and do not restart rasburicase.
- Monitor patients for methemoglobinemia. Discontinue rasburicase and do not restart in patients who develop methemoglobinemia.
- May cause spuriously low uric acid levels in blood samples left at room temperature. Collect blood for uric acid levels in pre-chilled tubes containing heparin and immediately immerse and maintain in an ice water bath. Uric acid must be analyzed in plasma. Plasma samples must be assayed within 4 hr of collection.

Implementation

- Chemotherapy is initiated 4–24 hr after 1st dose of rasburicase.

IV Administration

- **Intermittent Infusion:** Determine number of vials of rasburicase needed based on patient's weight and dose/kg. Reconstitute in diluent provided. Add 1 mL of diluent provided to each vial and mix by swirling very gently. Do not shake or vortex. Solution should be clear and colorless. Do not use solutions that are discolored or contain particulate matter. ***Diluent:*** Remove dose from reconstituted vials and inject into infusion bag of 0.9% NaCl for a final total volume of 50 mL. Administer within 24 hr of reconstitution. Store reconstituted or diluted solution in refrigerator for up to 24 hr. ***Rate:*** Administer over 30 min. Do not administer as a bolus.
- **Y-Site Incompatibility:** Infuse through a separate line. Do not use a filter with infusion. If separate line is not possible, flush line with at least 15 mL of 0.9% NaCl prior to rasburicase infusion.

Patient/Family Teaching

- Inform patient and family of purpose of rasburicase infusion.

Evaluation/Desired Outcomes

- Decrease in plasma uric acid levels in pediatric patients receiving antineoplastics expected to result in tumor lysis and subsequent elevation of plasma uric acid levels. More than 1 course of therapy or administration beyond 5 days is not recommended.

regorafenib (re-goe-**raf**-e-nib)

Stivarga

Classification
Therapeutic: antineoplastics
Pharmacologic: kinase inhibitors

Indications

Metastatic colorectal cancer (CRC) that has failed previous treatment that included a fluoropyrimidine, oxaliplatin, irinotecan, an anti-VEGF therapy, and additional anti-EGFR therapy if tumor is of the RAS wild type. Locally advanced, unresectable, or metastatic gastrointestinal stromal tumor (GIST) in patients who have previously been treated with imatinib and sunitinib.

Hepatocellular carcinoma (HCC) in patients who have previously been treated with sorafenib.

Action

Inhibits kinases, which are responsible for many phases of cell function and proliferation. **Therapeutic Effects:** Decreased progression of HCC and metastatic CRC with improved survival. Decreased progression of GIST.

Pharmacokinetics

Absorption: Well absorbed following oral administration (69–83%).
Distribution: Unknown.
Protein Binding: *Regorafenib*—>99.5%, *M-2 metabolite*—99.8%, *M-5 metabolite*—99.95%.
Metabolism and Excretion: Highly metabolized (by CYP3A4 and UGT1A9), 2 metabolites (M-2 and M-5) have antineoplastic activity. Undergoes enterohepatic circulation.
Half-life: *Regorafenib*—28 hr (range 14–58 hr), *M-2 metabolite*—25 hr (range 14–32 hr), *M-5 metabolite*—51 hr (range 32–70 hr). 47% excreted in feces as parent compound, 24% as metabolites; 19% excreted in urine (mostly as inactive metabolites).

TIME/ACTION PROFILE (improved survival)

ROUTE	ONSET	PEAK	DURATION
PO	3 mo	3 mo	up to 10 mo

Contraindications/Precautions

Contraindicated in: Avoid strong inducers/inhibitors of CYP3A4; OB: May cause fetal harm; Lactation: Breast feeding should be avoided; Severe hepatic impairment (Child-Pugh Class C).
Use Cautiously in: History of hypertension/cardiovascular disease (BP should be controlled prior to treatment); Elective surgical procedures (discontinue 2 wk prior to surgery); Asian patients (↑ risk of palmar-plantar erythrodysesthesia); Rep: Women of reproductive potential and men with female partners of reproductive potential; Pedi: Safety and effectiveness not established.

Adverse Reactions/Side Effects

CNS: REVERSIBLE POSTERIOR LEUKOENCEPHALOPATHY, fatigue, headache. **EENT:** dysphonia. **CV:** HYPERTENSION, MYOCARDIAL ISCHEMIA/INFARCTION. **GI:** GASTROINTESTINAL FISTULA/PERFORATION, HEPATOTOXICITY, ↓ appetite, diarrhea, mucositis, altered taste, dry mouth, gastrointestinal reflux, ↑ transaminases. **Derm:** ERYTHEMA MULTIFORME, PALMAR-PLANTAR ERYTHRODYSESTHESIA, STEVENS-JOHNSON SYNDROME, TOXIC EPIDERMAL NECROLYSIS, alopecia, impaired wound healing, rash. **Endo:** hypothyroidism. **F and E:** hypocalcemia, hypokalemia, hypophosphatemia, hyponatremia. **GU:** proteinuria, ↓ fertility. **Hemat:** BLEEDING, THROMBOCYTOPENIA, anemia, lymphopenia. **Metab:** weight loss, ↑ lipase, ↑ amylase. **MS:** pain, musculoskeletal stiffness. **Neuro:** tremor. **Misc:** HYPERSENSITIVITY REACTIONS, INFECTION, fever.

Interactions

Drug-Drug: Strong inhibitors of CYP3A4 including **clarithromycin, itraconazole, ketoconazole, posaconazole**, and **voriconazole** ↑ levels and the risk of toxicity, avoid concurrent use. **Strong inducers of CYP3A4** including **carbamazepine, phenobarbital, phenytoin**, and **rifampin** ↓ levels and effectiveness, avoid concurrent use. May ↑ risk of bleeding with **warfarin**. May ↑ levels and risk of toxicity of **breast cancer resistance protein (BCRP) substrates**, including **methotrexate, fluvastatin**, or **atorvastatin**.
Drug-Natural Products: St. John's wort ↓ blood levels and effectiveness, avoid concurrent use.
Drug-Food: Grapefruit juice ↑ blood levels and the risk of toxicity, avoid concurrent use.

Route/Dosage

PO (Adults): 160 mg daily on days 1–21 of a 28-day cycle. Continue treatment until disease progression or unacceptable toxicity.

Availability

Tablets: 40 mg.

NURSING IMPLICATIONS

Assessment

- Monitor BP prior to and weekly during the first 6 wk, then every cycle of therapy. Do not initiate regorafenib until BP is well controlled.
- Assess for cardiac ischemia or infarction during therapy.
- Assess for bleeding during therapy. Interrupt therapy if severe hemorrhage occurs.
- Assess for rash periodically during therapy. May cause Stevens-Johnson syndrome or Toxic Epidermal Necrolysis. Discontinue therapy if severe or if accompanied with fever, general malaise, fatigue, muscle or joint aches, blisters, oral lesions, conjunctivitis, hepatitis and/or eosinophilia.
- ***Lab Test Considerations:*** Obtain liver function test (ALT, AST, bilirubin) before starting, at least every 2 wk during first 2 mo of therapy, and monthly thereafter. Monitor liver function tests weekly in patients with ↑ liver function tests until improvement to $<3 \times$ the upper limit of normal or baseline.
- May cause anemia, thrombocytopenia, neutropenia, and lymphopenia.
- May cause hypocalcemia, hypokalemia, hyponatremia, and hypophosphatemia.
- May cause proteinuria, ↑ serum lipase, and ↑ serum amylase.

R

- May cause ↑ INR. Monitor INR levels more frequently in patients receiving warfarin.

Implementation

- ***High Alert:*** Fatalities have occurred with incorrect administration of chemotherapeutic agents. Before administering, clarify all ambiguous orders; double check single, daily, and course-of-therapy dose limits; have second practitioner independently double check original order and dose calculations. Therapy should be initiated by physician experienced in the treatment of patients with colorectal cancer.
- **PO:** Administer four 40 mg tablets once daily at same time of day with a whole glass of water for the first 21 days of each 28-day cycle. Swallow tablets whole with a low-fat meal that contains <30% fat and <600 calories.
- **Dose modifications:** *Interrupt therapy for* Grade 2 hand-foot skin reaction (HFSR) that is recurrent or does not improve in 7 days despite dose reduction; interrupt therapy for a minimum of 7 days for Grade 3 (HFSR), symptomatic Grade 2 hypertension, any Grade 3 or 4 adverse reactions.
- *Reduce dose to 120 mg daily for* 1st occurrence of Grade 2 HFSR of any duration, after 1st recovery of any Grade 3 or 4 adverse reaction, for Grade 3 ↑ AST or ALT; only resume if potential benefit outweighs risk of hepatotoxicity.
- *Reduce dose to 80 mg daily for* re-occurrence of Grade 2 HFSR at 120 mg dose, after recovery of any Grade 3 or 4 adverse reaction at 120 mg dose (except hepatotoxicity).
- *Discontinue regorafenib permanently for* failure to tolerate 80 mg dose, any occurrence of ↑ AST or ALT >20 × upper limit of normal, any occurrence of ↑ AST or ALT >3 × upper limit of normal with concurrent bilirubin >2 × upper limit of normal, re-occurrence of ↑ AST or ALT >5 × upper limit of normal despite reduction to 120 mg dose, any Grade 4 adverse reaction; only resume if the potential benefits outweigh the risks.

Patient/Family Teaching

- Instruct patient to take tablets at the same time each day with a low-fat meal. Take missed doses on the same day as soon as remembered; do not take 2 doses on the same day to make up for a missed dose. Store medicine in original container; do not place in daily or weekly pill boxes. Discard remaining tablets 28 days after opening bottle. Tightly close bottle after each opening and keep desiccant in bottle.
- Advise patient to avoid drinking grapefruit juice or eating grapefruit during regorafenib therapy.
- Advise patient to notify health care professional immediately if signs and symptoms of liver problems (yellowing of skin or white part of eyes, nausea, vomiting, dark tea-colored urine, change in sleep pattern), bleeding, skin changes (redness, pain, blisters, bleeding, swelling), hypertension (severe headache, lightheadedness, neurologic symptoms), myocardial ischemia or infarction (chest pain, shortness of breath, dizziness, fainting), or GI perforation or fistula (severe abdominal pain, persistent swelling of abdomen, high fever, chills, nausea, vomiting, severe diarrhea, dehydration) occur.
- Advise patient to notify health care provider of therapy prior to surgery or if had recent surgery.
- Advise patient to maintain adequate hydration to minimize risk and to notify health care professional promptly if signs and symptoms of reversible posterior leukoencephalopathy syndrome (RPLS) (headache, seizures, weakness, confusion, high BP, blindness or change in vision, problems thinking) occur.
- Instruct patient to notify health care professional of all Rx or OTC medications, vitamins, or herbal products being taken and consult health care professional before taking any new medications, especially St. John's wort.
- Rep: Inform female patient that regorafenib can cause fetal harm. Advise women with reproductive potential and men of the need for effective contraception during and for at least 2 mo after completion of therapy. Notify health care provider immediately if pregnancy is planned or suspected and to avoid breast feeding during and for at least 2 wk after final dose.
- Emphasize importance of monitoring lab values to monitor for adverse reactions.

Evaluation/Desired Outcomes

- Decreased progression of HCC and metastatic CRC.
- Decreased progression of GIST.

reteplase, See THROMBOLYTIC AGENTS.

revefenacin (rev-e-fen-a-sin)

Yupelri

Classification

Therapeutic: bronchodilators

Pharmacologic: anticholinergics

Indications

Maintenance treatment of COPD (not for acute [rescue] use).

Action

Acts as an anticholinergic by inhibiting the M_3 receptor in bronchial smooth muscle, which leads to bronchodilation. **Therapeutic Effects:** Bronchodilation with lessened symptoms of COPD.

Pharmacokinetics

Absorption: 3% systemically absorbed following oral inhalation.

Distribution: Extensively distributed to tissues.

Metabolism and Excretion: Rapidly hydrolyzed to an active metabolite. Primarily eliminated in feces (88%) with less than 5% excreted in urine.
Half-life: 22–70 hr.

TIME/ACTION PROFILE (plasma concentrations)

ROUTE	ONSET	PEAK	DURATION
Nebulization	rapid	14–41 min	24 hr

Contraindications/Precautions
Contraindicated in: Hypersensitivity; Hepatic impairment.
Use Cautiously in: Narrow-angle glaucoma; Prostatic hyperplasia or bladder neck obstruction; OB: Safety not established; Lactation: Use while breast feeding only if potential maternal benefit justifies potential risk to infant; Pedi: Safety and effectiveness not established.

Adverse Reactions/Side Effects
CNS: headache. **Resp:** cough, paradoxical bronchospasm. **Misc:** HYPERSENSITIVITY REACTIONS (including anaphylaxis and angioedema).

Interactions
Drug-Drug: May ↑ risk of anticholinergic effects with other **anticholingerics**. **Rifampin** or **cyclosporine** may ↑ levels of active metabolite; concurrent use not recommended.

Route/Dosage
Inhaln (Adults): 175 mcg via nebulization once daily.

Availability
Inhalation solution: 175 mcg/3 mL.

NURSING IMPLICATIONS
Assessment
- Assess lung sounds, pulse, and BP before administration and during peak of medication. Note amount, color, and character of sputum produced. Closely monitor patients on higher dose for adverse effects.
- Monitor pulmonary function tests before initiating and periodically during therapy to determine effectiveness.
- Observe for paradoxical bronchospasm (wheezing, dyspnea, tightness in chest) during therapy. If condition occurs, hold medication and notify health care professional immediately.
- Monitor patient for signs of hypersensitivity reactions (rash, hives, severe itching, swelling of face, mouth, and tongue, difficulty breathing or swallowing) during therapy. Discontinue therapy and consider alternative if reaction occurs.

Implementation
- **Inhaln:** Administer once daily by oral inhalation via a standard jet nebulizer connected to an air compressor.

Patient/Family Teaching
- Instruct patient to use medication as directed. Do not discontinue therapy without discussing with health care professional, even if feeling better. Use a rapid-acting bronchodilator if symptoms occur before next dose is due. Caution patient not to use more than once a day; may cause adverse effects, paradoxical bronchospasm, or loss of effectiveness of medication. Instruct patient to review *Patient Information* before starting therapy and with each Rx refill in case of changes.
- Caution patient not to use medication to treat acute symptoms. Use a rapid-acting inhaled beta-adrenergic bronchodilator for relief of acute asthma attacks. Notify health care professional immediately if symptoms get worse or more inhalations than usual are needed from rescue inhaler.
- Instruct patient to contact health care professional immediately if shortness of breath is not relieved by medication or nausea, vomiting, shakiness, headache, fast or irregular heartbeat, sleeplessness, or signs and symptoms of narrow angle glaucoma (eye pain or discomfort, blurred vision, visual halos or colored images, red eyes) or urinary retention (difficulty passing urine, painful urination) occur.
- Advise patient to consult health care professional before taking any Rx, OTC, or herbal products or alcohol concurrently with this therapy. Caution patient also to avoid smoking and other respiratory irritants.
- Advise patient to notify health care professional if pregnancy is planned or suspected, or if breast feeding.

Evaluation/Desired Outcomes
- Bronchodilation with decreased airflow obstruction.

Rh_0(D) IMMUNE GLOBULIN
(arr aych oh dee im-**yoon glob**-yoo-lin)

Rh_0(D) immune globulin standard dose IM
HyperRHO S/D Full Dose, RhoGAM

Rh_0(D) immune globulin microdose IM
HyperRHO S/D Mini-Dose, MICRhoGAM, Mini-Gamulin R

Rh_0(D) immune globulin IV
WinRho SDF

R

Rh_0(D) immune globulin microdose IM, IV
Rhophylac

Classification
Therapeutic: vaccines/immunizing agents
Pharmacologic: immune globulins

Indications
IM, IV: Administered to Rh_0(D)-negative patients who have been exposed to Rh_0(D)-positive blood by: Pregnancy or delivery of a Rh_0(D)-positive infant, Abortion of a Rh_0(D)-positive fetus, Fetal-maternal hemorrhage due to amniocentesis, other obstetrical manipulative procedure, or intra-abdominal trauma while carrying a Rh_0(D)-positive fetus, Transfusion of Rh_0(D)-positive blood or blood products to a Rh_0(D)-negative patient. **IV:** Management of immune thrombocytopenic purpura (ITP).

Action
Prevent production of anti-Rh_0(D) antibodies in Rh_0(D)-negative patients who were exposed to Rh_0(D)-positive blood. Increase platelet counts in patients with ITP. **Therapeutic Effects:** Prevention of antibody response and hemolytic disease of the newborn (erythroblastosis fetalis) in future pregnancies of women who have conceived a Rh_0(D)-positive fetus. Prevention of Rh_0(D) sensitization following transfusion accident. Decreased bleeding in patients with ITP.

Pharmacokinetics
Absorption: Completely absorbed with IV administration. Well absorbed from IM sites.
Distribution: Unknown.
Metabolism and Excretion: Unknown.
Half-life: approximately 25–30 days.

TIME/ACTION PROFILE (blood levels)

ROUTE	ONSET	PEAK	DURATION
IM	rapid	5–10 days	unknown
IV†	unknown	2 hr	unknown

†When given for ITP, platelet counts start to rise in 1–2 days, peak after 5–7 days, and last for 30 days.

Contraindications/Precautions
Contraindicated in: Prior hypersensitivity reaction to human immune globulin; Rh_0(D)- or Du-positive patients.
Use Cautiously in: ITP patients with pre-existing anemia (decrease dose if Hgb <10 g/dL). May also cause disseminated intravascular coagulation in ITP patients.

Adverse Reactions/Side Effects
CNS: dizziness, headache. **CV:** hypertension, hypotension. **Derm:** rash. **GI:** diarrhea, nausea, vomiting. **GU:** acute renal failure. **Hemat:** *ITP*—DISSEMINATED INTRAVASCULAR COAGULATION, INTRAVASCULAR HEMOLYSIS, anemia. **MS:** arthralgia, myalgia. **Local:** pain at injection site. **Misc:** fever.

Interactions
Drug-Drug: May ↓ antibody response to some **live-virus vaccines (measles, mumps, rubella)**.

Route/Dosage
Rh_0(D) Immune Globulin (for IM use only)
Following Delivery
IM (Adults): *HyperRHO S/D Full Dose, RhoGAM*—1 vial standard dose (300 mcg) within 72 hr of delivery.

Before Delivery
IM (Adults): *HyperRHO S/D Full Dose, RhoGAM*—1 vial standard dose (300 mcg) at 26–28 wk.

Termination of Pregnancy (<13 wk Gestation)
IM (Adults): *HyperRHO S/D Mini-Dose, MICRhoGAM*—1 vial of microdose (50 mcg) within 72 hr.

Termination of Pregnancy (>13 wk Gestation)
IM (Adults): *RhoGAM*—1 vial standard dose (300 mcg) within 72 hr.

Large Fetal-Maternal Hemorrhage (>15 mL)
IM (Adults): *RhoGAM*—20 mcg/mL of Rh_0(D)-positive fetal RBCs.

Transfusion Accident
IM (Adults): *HyperRHO S/D Full Dose, RhoGAM*—(Volume of Rh-positive blood administered × Hct of donor blood)/15 = number of vials of standard dose (300 mcg) preparation (round to next whole number of vials).

Rh_0(D) Immune Globulin IV (for IM or IV Use)
Following Delivery
IM, IV (Adults): *WinRho SDF*—600 IU (120 mcg) within 72 hr of delivery. *Rhophylac*—1500 IU (300 mcg) within 72 hr of delivery.

Prior to Delivery
IM, IV (Adults): *WinRho SDF, Rhophylac*—1500 IU (300 mcg) at 28 wk; if initiated earlier in pregnancy, repeat every 12 wk.

Following Amniocentesis or Chorionic Villus Sampling
IM, IV (Adults): *WinRho SDF (before 34 wk gestation)*—1500 IU (300 mcg) immediately; repeat every 12 wk during pregnancy. *Rhophylac*—1500 IU (300 mcg) within 72 hr of procedure.

Termination of Pregnancy, Amniocentesis, or Any Other Manipulation

IM, IV (Adults): *WinRho SDF*—600 IU (120 mcg) within 72 hr after event.

Large Fetal-Maternal Hemorrhage/Transfusion Accident

IM (Adults): *WinRho SDF*—6000 IU (1200 mcg) every 12 hr until total dose is given (total dose determined by amount of blood loss/hemorrhage).

IV (Adults): 3000 IU (600 mcg) every 8 hr until total dose is given (total dose determined by amount of blood loss/hemorrhage).

Immune Thrombocytopenic Purpura

IV (Adults and Children): *WinRho SDF, Rhophylac*—50 mcg (250 IU)/kg initially (if Hgb <10 g/dL, ↓ dose to 25–40 mcg [125–200 IU]/kg); further dosing/frequency determined by clinical response (range 25–60 mcg [125–300 IU]/kg). Each dose may be given as a single dose or in 2 divided doses on separate days.

Availability

Rh_o(D) Immune Globulin (for IM Use)

Injection: 50 mcg/vial (microdose—MICRhoGAM, HyperRHO S/D Mini-Dose), 300 mcg/vial (standard dose—RhoGAM, HyperRHO S/D Full Dose).

Rh_o(D) Immune Globulin Intravenous (for IM or IV Use)

Injection: 600 IU (120 mcg)/vial, 1500 IU (300 mcg)/vial, 2500 IU (500 mcg)/vial, 5000 IU (1000 mcg)/vial, 15,000 IU (3000 mcg)/vial. **Prefilled syringes:** 1500 IU (300 mcg/2 mL).

NURSING IMPLICATIONS

Assessment

- **IV:** Assess vital signs periodically during therapy in patients receiving IV Rh_o(D) immune globulin.
- **ITP:** Monitor patient for signs and symptoms of intravascular hemolysis (IVH) (back pain, shaking chills, fever, hemoglobinuria), anemia, and renal insufficiency. If transfusions are required, use Rh_o(D)-negative packed red blood cells to prevent exacerbation of IVH.
- ***Lab Test Considerations:*** *Pregnancy:* Type and crossmatch of mother and newborn's cord blood must be performed to determine need for medication. Mother must be Rh_o(D)-negative and Du-negative. Infant must be Rh_o(D)-positive. If there is doubt regarding infant's blood type or if father is Rh_o(D)-positive, medication should be given.
- An infant born to a woman treated with Rh_o(D) immune globulin antepartum may have a weakly positive direct Coombs' test result on cord or infant blood.
- *ITP:* Monitor platelet counts, RBC counts, hemoglobin, and reticulocyte levels to determine effectiveness of therapy.

Implementation

- Do not give to infant, to Rh_o(D)-positive individual, or to Rh_o(D)-negative individual previously sensitized to the Rh_o(D) antigen. However, there is no more risk than when given to a woman who is not sensitized. When in doubt, administer Rh_o(D) immune globulin.
- Do not confuse IM and IV formulations. Rh immune globulin for IV administration is labeled "Rh Immune Globulin Intravenous." Rh Immune Globulin Intravenous may be given IM; however, Rh Immune Globulin (microdose and standard dose) is for IM use only and cannot be given IV.
- When using prefilled syringes, allow solution to reach room temperature before administration.
- **IM:** Reconstitute Rh_o(D) immune globulin IV for IM use immediately before use with 1.25 mL of 0.9% NaCl. Inject diluent onto inside wall of vial and wet pellet by gently swirling until dissolved. Do not shake.
- Administer into the deltoid muscle. Dose should be given within 3 hr but may be given up to 72 hr after delivery, miscarriage, abortion, or transfusion.

IV Administration

- **IV Push:** Reconstitute Rh_o(D) immune globulin IV for IV administration immediately before use with 2.5 mL of 0.9% NaCl. Inject diluent onto inside wall of vial and wet pellet by gently swirling until dissolved. Do not shake. ***Rate:*** Administer over 3–5 min.

Patient/Family Teaching

- **Pregnancy:** Explain to patient that the purpose of this medication is to protect future Rh_o(D)-positive infants.
- **ITP:** Explain purpose of medication to patient.

Evaluation/Desired Outcomes

- Prevention of erythroblastosis fetalis in future Rh_o(D)-positive infants.
- Prevention of Rh_o(D) sensitization following incompatible transfusion.
- Decreased bleeding episodes in patients with ITP.

ribociclib (rye-boe-**sye**-klib)

Kisqali

Classification

Therapeutic: antineoplastics

Pharmacologic: kinase inhibitors

Indications

In combination with an aromatase inhibitor for the treatment of advanced or metastatic hormone receptor (HR)-positive, human epidermal growth factor 2 (HER2)-negative breast cancer in pre-/perimenopausal or postmenopausal women (as initial endocrine-based therapy). In combination with fulvestrant for the treatment of advanced or metastatic hormone receptor (HR)-positive, human epidermal growth factor 2 (HER2)-negative breast cancer in postmenopausal women (as initial endocrine-based therapy or following disease progression on endocrine therapy).

Action

Inhibits kinases (cyclin-dependent kinases 4 and 6) that are part of the signaling pathway for cell proliferation. **Therapeutic Effects:** Improved survival and decreased spread of breast cancer.

Pharmacokinetics

Absorption: Unknown.

Distribution: Extensively distributed to the tissues.

Metabolism and Excretion: Mostly metabolized by CYP3A4; 17% excreted unchanged in feces, 12% in urine.

Half-life: 32 hr.

TIME/ACTION PROFILE (plasma levels)

ROUTE	ONSET	PEAK	DURATION
PO	unknown	1–4 hr	unknown

Contraindications/Precautions

Contraindicated in: QT interval prolongation (QT interval ≥450 msec); Uncorrected hypokalemia or hypomagnesemia; Recent MI, HF, unstable angina, or bradycardia; Concurrent use of QT interval prolonging medications or strong CYP3A4 inhibitors; CYP3A inducers (may ↓ effectiveness); OB: May cause fetal harm; Lactation: Avoid breast feeding.

Use Cautiously in: Concurrent use of sensitive CYP3A substrates (narrow therapeutic indices), dose of substrate may need to be ↓; Severe renal impairment (↓ dose); Moderate or severe hepatic impairment (↓ dose); Rep: Women of reproductive potential; Pedi: Safety and effectiveness not established.

Adverse Reactions/Side Effects

CNS: fatigue, headache, insomnia. **CV:** TORSADES DE POINTES, peripheral edema, QT interval prolongation, syncope. **Derm:** alopecia, pruritis, rash. **F and E:** hypokalemia, hypophosphatemia. **GI:** abdominal pain, constipation, ↓ appetite, diarrhea, nausea, ↑ liver enzymes, stomatitis, vomiting, hyperbilirubinemia. **GU:** ↑ creatinine, ↓ fertility (males). **Hemat:** NEUTROPENIA, THROMBOCYTOPENIA, anemia. **MS:** back pain. **Resp:** INTERSTITIAL LUNG DISEASE, dyspnea. **Misc:** fever.

Interactions

Drug-Drug: Strong CYP3A4 inhibitors, including **clarithromycin**, **conivaptan**, **indinavir**, **itraconazole**, **ketoconazole**, **lopinavir/ritonavir**, **nefazodone**, **nelfinavir**, **posaconazole**, **ritonavir**, **saquinavir**, or **voriconazole** may ↑ levels and the risk of toxicity; avoid concurrent use, if possible (if unavoidable, ↓ dose of ribociclib). **Strong CYP3A4 inducers**, including **carbamazepine**, **phenytoin**, or **rifampin** can ↓ levels and effectiveness; avoid concurrent use. May ↑ levels and effects/toxicity of **alfentanil**, **cyclosporine**, **dihydroergotamine**, **ergotamine**, **everolimus**, **fentanyl**, **midazolam**, **pimozide**, **quinidine**, **sirolimus** and **tacrolimus**; if concurrent use is required dose ↓ may be necessary. **QT-interval-prolonging medications**, including **amiodarone**, **chloroquine**, **clarithromycin**, **disopyramide**, **haloperidol**, **methadone**, **moxifloxacin**, **ondansetron**, **pimozide**, **procainamide**, **quinidine**, **sotalol**, and **tamoxifen** may ↑ risk of QT interval prolongation; avoid concurrent use.

Drug-Natural Products: St. John's wort may ↓ levels and effectiveness; avoid concurrent use.

Drug-Food: Grapefruit/grapefruit juice or **pomegranate/pomegranate juice** may ↑ levels and the risk of toxicity; avoid ingestion.

Route/Dosage

PO (Adults): 600 mg once daily for 21 days, followed by 7 days off to complete a 28-day treatment cycle; continue treatment cycles until disease progression or unacceptable toxicity. *Concurrent use of strong CYP3A4 inhibitor*—400 mg once daily for 21 days, followed by 7 days off to complete a 28-day treatment cycle; continue treatment cycles until disease progression or unacceptable toxicity.

Renal Impairment

PO (Adults): *Severe renal impairment*—200 mg once daily for 21 days, followed by 7 days off to complete a 28-day treatment cycle; continue treatment cycles until disease progression or unacceptable toxicity.

Hepatic Impairment

PO (Adults): *Moderate or severe hepatic impairment*—400 mg once daily for 21 days, followed by 7 days off to complete a 28-day treatment cycle; continue treatment cycles until disease progression or unacceptable toxicity.

Availability

Tablets: 200 mg.

NURSING IMPLICATIONS

Assessment

- Monitor ECG prior to starting therapy. Avoid administering ribociclib to patient with QT interval >450 msec. Repeat ECG on Day 14 of first cycle, beginning of 2nd cycle, and as indicated. *If QT interval >480 msec,* suspend therapy. *If QT interval prolongation resolves to <481 msec,* resume therapy at same dose level. *If QT ≥481 msec recurs,* interrupt dose until QT interval resolves to <481 msec;

then resume ribociclib at next lower dose level. *If QT interval >500 msec,* withhold therapy if >500 msec on at least 2 separate ECGs (within same visit). *If QT interval prolongation resolves to <481 msec,* resume therapy at next lower dose. *If QT interval prolongation is either >500 msec or >60 msec change from baseline AND associated with any of the following: Torsades de Pointes, polymorphic ventricular tachycardia, unexplained syncope, or signs and symptoms of serious arrhythmia,* permanently discontinue ribociclib.

- Monitor for signs and symptoms of ILD/pneumonitis (hypoxia, cough, dyspnea) during therapy. If Grade 1 symptoms (asymptomatic) occur, continue dose and treat symptoms. If Grade 2 symptoms (symptomatic) occur, hold therapy until ≤Grade 1. Resume at next lower dose. If Grade 2 recurs, discontinue ribiciclib permanently. If Grade 3 (severe symptomatic) or 4 symptoms (life-threatening) occur, permanently discontinue therapy.
- ***Lab Test Considerations:*** Obtain a negative pregnancy test prior to starting therapy.
- Monitor serum electrolytes (potassium, calcium, phosphorous, magnesium) prior to starting therapy, at beginning of first 6 cycles, and as indicated. Correct abnormalities before starting therapy.
- Monitor liver function before starting therapy, every 2 wk for first 2 cycles, at beginning of each subsequent 4 cycles, and as indicated. **For AST and/or ALT ↑ from baseline, WITHOUT ↑ total bilirubin >2 × upper limit of normal (ULN):** *Grade 1 (>ULN to 3 × ULN),* No dose adjustment. *Grade 2 (>3 to 5 × ULN),* Baseline at <Grade 2: Hold dose until recovery to ≤baseline grade, then resume at same dose. *If Grade 2 recurs,* resume ribociclib at next lower dose. Do not interrupt dose for Grade 2 at baseline. *Grade 3 (>5 to 20 × ULN),* withhold dose until recovery to ≤baseline grade, then resume at next lower dose. *If Grade 3 recurs,* discontinue ricociclib. *Grade 4 (>20 × ULN),* discontinue ribociclib. **Combined ↑ in AST and/or ALT WITH total bilirubin ↑, in absence of cholistasis:** *If ALT and/or AST >3 × ULN along with total bilirubin >2 × ULN irrespective of baseline grade,* discontinue ribociclib.
- Monitor CBC before starting therapy, every 2 wk for first 2 cycles, at beginning of each subsequent 4 cycles, and as indicated. *If Grade 1 or 2 (ANC 1000/mm^3 to <lower limit of normal [LLN]) occurs,* no dose adjustment required. *If Grade 3 (ANC 500–1000/mm^3) occurs,* interrupt dose until recovery to Grade ≤2. Resume therapy at same dose. *If toxicity recurs at Grade 3,* hold dose until recovery, then resume ribociclib at next lower dose. *If Grade 3 fibrile neutropenia occurs,* suspend therapy until recovery of neutropenia to Grade ≤2. Resume therapy at next lower dose. *If Grade 4 (ANC <500/mm^3 occurs,* withhold therapy until recovery to Grade ≤2. Resume ribociclib at next lower dose.

Implementation

- **PO:** Administer once daily, at the same time each day, preferably in the morning, without regard to food. Swallow tablets whole; do not crush, break or chew. Do not administer tablets that are broken, cracked, or not intact.
- Pre/perimenopausal women taking ribociclib and an aromatase inhibitor or fulvestrant should also be treated with a luteinizing hormone-releasing hormone (LHRH) agonist.

Patient/Family Teaching

- Instruct patient to take ribociclib as directed. If patient vomits after taking dose or misses dose, do not take more that day. Take next dose next day at usual time. Advise patient to read *Patient Information* prior to starting and with each Rx refill in case of changes.
- Advise patient to avoid eating pomegranate or grapefruit and to avoid drinking pomegranate or grapefruit juice during therapy.
- Advise patient to notify health care professional if signs and symptoms of heart rhythm problems (change in heartbeat [fast or irregular], dizziness, feeling faint), low white blood cell counts (fever and chills), or liver problems (yellowing of skin or whites of eyes, jaundice, dark or brown, tea-colored urine, feeling very tired, loss of appetite, pain on upper right side of abdomen, unusual bleeding or bruising) occur.
- Instruct patient to notify health care professional of all Rx or OTC medications, vitamins, or herbal products being taken and to consult with health care professional before taking other medications.
- Rep: May be teratogenic. Advise female patient of reproductive potential to use effective contraception to avoid breast feeding during and for at least 3 wk after last dose of therapy. Inform male patients that ribociclib may impair fertility.

Evaluation/Desired Outcomes

- Improved survival and decreased spread of breast cancer.

rifabutin (riff-a-**byoo**-tin)

Mycobutin

Classification

Therapeutic: agents for atypical mycobacterium

R

Indications

Prevention of disseminated *Mycobacterium avium* complex (MAC) disease in patients with advanced HIV infection.

Action

Appears to inhibit DNA-dependent RNA polymerase in susceptible organisms. **Therapeutic Effects:** Antimycobacterial action against susceptible organisms. **Spectrum:** Active against *M. avium* and most strains of *M. tuberculosis*.

Pharmacokinetics

Absorption: Well absorbed following oral administration (50–85%). Absorption ↓ in HIV-positive patients (20%).
Distribution: Widely distributed to body tissues and fluids.
Metabolism and Excretion: Mostly metabolized by the liver; <5% excreted unchanged by the kidneys.
Half-life: 45 hr.

TIME/ACTION PROFILE (blood levels)

ROUTE	ONSET	PEAK	DURATION
PO	rapid	2–4 hr	24 hr

Contraindications/Precautions

Contraindicated in: Hypersensitivity. Cross-sensitivity with other rifamycins (rifampin) may occur; Active tuberculosis; Concurrent use of ritonavir or delavirdine.
Use Cautiously in: OB, Lactation, Pedi: Safety not established. Use in pregnancy only if potential benefit justifies potential risk to fetus.

Adverse Reactions/Side Effects

CV: chest pain, chest pressure. **Derm:** rash, skin discoloration. **EENT:** ocular disturbances. **GI:** CLOSTRIDIUM DIFFICILE-ASSOCIATED DIARRHEA (CDAD), altered taste, drug-induced hepatitis. **Hemat:** hemolysis, neutropenia, thrombocytopenia. **MS:** arthralgia, myositis. **Resp:** dyspnea. **Misc:** brown-orange discoloration of body fluids (urine, tears, saliva), flu-like syndrome.

Interactions

Drug-Drug: May ↓ levels and effectiveness of **efavirenz**, **indinavir**, **nelfinavir**, **nevirapine**, **saquinavir** (dosage adjustment may be necessary), **delavirdine** (concurrent use should be avoided), **corticosteroids**, **disopyramide**, **quinidine**, **opioid analgesics**, **oral hypoglycemic agents**, **warfarin**, **estrogens**, **estrogen-containing contraceptives**, **phenytoin**, **verapamil**, **fluconazole**, **quinidine**, **theophylline**, **zidovudine**, and **chloramphenicol**. **Ritonavir** ↑ levels; (concurrent use contraindicated), similar effects occur with **efavirenz** and **nevirapine**.

Route/Dosage

PO (Adults): 300 mg once daily. If GI upset occurs, may give as 150 mg twice daily with food.

Availability (generic available)

Capsules: 150 mg.

NURSING IMPLICATIONS

Assessment

- Monitor patient for signs of active tuberculosis (purified protein derivative [PPD], chest x-ray, sputum culture, blood culture, urine culture, biopsy of suspicious lymph nodes) prior to and throughout therapy. Rifabutin must not be administered to patients with active tuberculosis.
- Monitor bowel function. Diarrhea, abdominal cramping, fever, and bloody stools should be reported to health care professional promptly as a sign of Clostridium difficile-associated diarrhea (CDAD). May begin up to several wk following cessation of therapy.
- ***Lab Test Considerations:*** Monitor CBC periodically during therapy. May cause neutropenia and thrombocytopenia.

Implementation

- Do not confuse rifabutin with rifapentine.
- **PO:** May be administered without regard to meals. High-fat meals slow rate but not extent of absorption. May be mixed with foods such as applesauce. If GI upset occurs, administer with food.

Patient/Family Teaching

- Advise patient to take medication as directed. Do not skip doses or double up on missed doses. Emphasize the importance of continuing therapy even if asymptomatic.
- Advise patient to notify health care professional promptly if signs and symptoms of neutropenia (sore throat, fever, signs of infection), thrombocytopenia (unusual bleeding or bruising), or hepatitis (yellow eyes and skin, nausea, vomiting, anorexia, unusual tiredness, weakness) occur.
- Caution patient to avoid the use of alcohol during this therapy, because this may increase the risk of hepatotoxicity.
- Instruct patient to notify health care professional immediately if diarrhea, abdominal cramping, fever, or bloody stools occur and not to treat with antidiarrheals without consulting health care professionals.
- Instruct patient to report symptoms of myositis (myalgia, arthralgia) or uveitis (intraocular inflammation) to health care professional promptly.
- Inform patient that skin, saliva, sputum, sweat, tears, urine, and feces may become brown-orange and that soft contact lenses may become permanently discolored.
- Rep: Advise patient that this medication has teratogenic properties and may decrease the effectiveness of oral contraceptives. Counsel patient to use a nonhormonal form of contraception during therapy.

- Emphasize the importance of regular follow-up exams to monitor progress and to check for side effects.

Evaluation/Desired Outcomes

- Prevention of disseminated MAC in patients with advanced HIV infection.

rifAMPin (rif-am-pin)

Rifadin, Rimactane, Rofact

Classification

Therapeutic: antituberculars
Pharmacologic: rifamycins

Indications

Active tuberculosis (with other agents). Elimination of meningococcal carriers. **Unlabeled Use:** Prevention of disease caused by *Haemophilus influenzae* type B in close contacts. Synergy with other antimicrobial agents for *S. aureus* infections.

Action

Inhibits RNA synthesis by blocking RNA transcription in susceptible organisms. **Therapeutic Effects:** Bactericidal action against susceptible organisms. **Spectrum:** Broad spectrum notable for activity against: *Mycobacterium* spp., *Staphylococcus aureus*, *H. influenzae*, *Legionella pneumophila*, *Neisseria meningitidis*.

Pharmacokinetics

Absorption: Well absorbed following oral administration.
Distribution: Widely distributed; enters CSF. Crosses placenta; enters breast milk.
Protein Binding: 80%.
Metabolism and Excretion: Mostly metabolized by the liver; 60% eliminated in feces via biliary elimination.
Half-life: 3 hr.

TIME/ACTION PROFILE (blood levels)

ROUTE	ONSET	PEAK	DURATION
PO	rapid	2–4 hr	12–24 hr
IV	rapid	end of infusion	12–24 hr

Contraindications/Precautions

Contraindicated in: Hypersensitivity; Concurrent use of atazanavir, darunavir, fosamprenavir, praziquantel, saquinavir, tipranavir, or ritonavir-boosted saquinavir.
Use Cautiously in: History of liver disease (↑ risk of hepatotoxicity); Chronic liver disease, poor nutritional status, or prolonged use of antibacterial drugs or anticoagulants (↑ risk of vitamin K deficiency and subsequent coagulation disorders); Diabetes; Concurrent use of other hepatotoxic agents; OB, Lactation: Pregnancy or lactation.

Adverse Reactions/Side Effects

CNS: ataxia, confusion, drowsiness, fatigue, headache, weakness. **Derm:** ACUTE GENERALIZED EXANTHEMATOUS PUSTULOSIS, DRUG REACTION WITH EOSINOPHILIA AND SYSTEMIC SYMPTOMS (DRESS), STEVENS-JOHNSON SYNDROME, TOXIC EPIDERMAL NECROLYSIS, rash, pruritus. **EENT:** red discoloration of tears. **GI:** HEPATOTOXICITY, abdominal pain, diarrhea, flatulence, heartburn, nausea, vomiting, red discoloration of saliva and teeth. **GU:** red discoloration of urine. **Hemat:** bleeding, hemolytic anemia, thrombocytopenia. **MS:** arthralgia, muscle weakness, myalgia. **Misc:** HYPERSENSITIVITY REACTIONS (including angioedema), flu-like syndrome.

Interactions

Drug-Drug: ↑ risk of hepatotoxicity with ritonavir-boosted **saquinavir**; concurrent use contraindicated. Significantly ↓ blood levels of **atazanavir**, **darunavir**, **fosamprenavir**, **praziquantel**, **saquinavir**, and **tipranavir**; concurrent use contraindicated. ↑ risk of hepatotoxicity with other **hepatotoxic agents**, including **alcohol**, **ketoconazole**, **isoniazid**, **pyrazinamide** (concurrent use with **pyrazinamide** may result in potentially fatal hepatotoxicity and should be avoided). Significantly ↓ blood levels of **delavirdine**, **indinavir**, and **nelfinavir**. Stimulates liver enzymes, which may ↑ metabolism and ↓ effectiveness of other drugs, including **ritonavir**, **nevirapine**, and **efavirenz** (dose adjustment may be necessary), **ciprofloxacin**, **clarithromycin**, **corticosteroids**, **cyclosporine**, **diazepam**, **diltiazem**, **disopyramide**, **doxycycline**, **levothyroxine**, **methadone**, **nifedipine**, **quinidine**, **opioid analgesics**, **oral hypoglycemic agents**, **warfarin**, **estrogens**, **phenytoin**, **phenobarbital**, **tacrolimus**, **verapamil**, **fluconazole**, **ketoconazole**, **itraconazole**, **quinidine**, **theophylline**, **zidovudine**, **chloramphenicol**, and **hormonal contraceptive agents**. **Cefazolin** may ↑ risk of vitamin K-dependent coagulation disorders; avoid concurrent use in patients at ↑ risk for bleeding.

Route/Dosage

Tuberculosis

PO, IV (Adults): 600 mg/day or 10 mg/kg/day (up to 600 mg/day) single dose; may also be given twice weekly.
PO, IV (Children and Infants): 10–20 mg/kg/day single dose or divided every 12 hr (not to exceed 600 mg/day); may also be given twice weekly.

Asymptomatic Carriers of Meningococcus

PO, IV (Adults): 600 mg every 12 hr for 2 days.
PO, IV (Children ≥1 mo): 10 mg/kg every 12 hr for 2 days (max: 600 mg/dose).
PO (Infants <1 mo): 5 mg/kg every 12 hr for 2 days.

H. influenzae Prophylaxis

PO (Adults): 600 mg/day for 4 days.
PO (Children): 20 mg/kg/day for 4 days (max: 600 mg/dose).
PO (Neonates): 10 mg/kg/day for 4 days.

Synergy for *S. aureus* infections

PO (Adults): 300–600 mg twice daily.
PO (Children and Neonates): 5–20 mg/kg/day divided every 12 hr (max: 600 mg/dose).

Availability (generic available)

Capsules: 150 mg, 300 mg. **Powder for injection (requires reconstitution and dilution):** 600 mg/vial. ***In combination with:*** isoniazid (IsonaRif, Rifamate); isoniazid and pyrazinamide (Rifater). See Appendix B.

NURSING IMPLICATIONS

Assessment

- Perform mycobacterial studies and susceptibility tests prior to and periodically during therapy to detect possible resistance.
- Assess lung sounds and character and amount of sputum periodically during therapy.
- Monitor for signs and symptoms of DRESS (fever, rash, lymphadenopathy, and/or facial swelling), associated with involvement of other organ systems (hepatitis, nephritis, hematologic abnormalities, myocarditis, myositis) during therapy. May resemble an acute viral infection. Eosinophilia is often present. Discontinue therapy if signs occur.
- ***Lab Test Considerations:*** Evaluate renal function, CBC, and urinalysis periodically and during therapy.
- Monitor hepatic function at least monthly during therapy. May cause ↑ BUN, AST, ALT, and serum alkaline phosphatase, bilirubin, and uric acid concentrations.
- May cause false-positive direct Coombs' test results. May interfere with folic acid and vitamin B assays.
- May interfere with dexamethasone suppression test results; discontinue rifampin 15 days prior to test.
- May interfere with methods for determining serum folate and vitamin B levels and with urine tests based on color reaction.
- Monitor coagulation tests (PT, INR, aPTT) during therapy in patients at risk for vitamin K deficiency.

Implementation

- Do not confuse rifampin with rifaximin or Rifamate (isoniazid/rifampin).
- May use vitamin K supplementation in patients at risk for vitamin K deficiency.
- **PO:** Administer medication on an empty stomach at least 1 hr before or 2 hr after meals with a full glass (240 mL) of water. If GI irritation becomes a problem, may be administered with food. Antacids may also be taken 1 hr prior to administration. Capsules may be opened and contents mixed with applesauce or jelly for patients with difficulty swallowing.
- Pharmacist can compound a syrup for patients unable to swallow solids.

IV Administration

- **Intermittent Infusion:** Reconstitute each 600-mg vial with 10 mL of sterile water for injection for a concentration of 60 mg/mL. ***Diluent:*** Dilute further in 100 mL or 500 mL of D5W or 0.9% NaCl. Reconstituted vials are stable for 24 hr at room temperature. Infusion is stable at room temperature for 4 hr (in D5W) or 24 hr (in 0.9% NaCl). ***Concentration:*** Not to exceed 6 mg/mL. ***Rate:*** Administer solutions diluted in 100 mL over 30 min and solutions diluted in 500 mL over 3 hr.
- **Y-Site Compatibility:** amiodarone, bumetanide, ciprofloxacin, daptomycin, midazolam, pantoprazole, tigecycline, vancomycin.
- **Y-Site Incompatibility:** diltiazem.

Patient/Family Teaching

- Advise patient to take medication once daily (unless biweekly regimens are used), as directed, and not to skip doses or double up on missed doses. Emphasize the importance of continuing therapy even after symptoms have subsided. Length of therapy for tuberculosis depends on regimen being used and underlying disease states. Patients on short-term prophylactic therapy should also be advised of the importance of compliance with therapy.
- Advise patient to notify health care professional promptly if signs and symptoms of hepatitis (yellow eyes and skin, nausea, vomiting, anorexia, unusual tiredness, weakness) or of thrombocytopenia (unusual bleeding or bruising) occur.
- Caution patient to avoid the use of alcohol during this therapy, because this may increase the risk of hepatotoxicity.
- Instruct patient to report the occurrence of flu-like symptoms (fever, chills, myalgia, headache) promptly.
- Rifampin may occasionally cause drowsiness. Caution patient to avoid driving or other activities requiring alertness until response to medication is known.
- Inform patient that saliva, sputum, teeth, sweat, tears, urine, and feces may become red-orange to red-brown and that soft contact lenses may become permanently discolored.
- Advise patient that this medication has teratogenic properties and may decrease the effectiveness of oral contraceptives. Counsel females of reproductive po-

tential to use a nonhormonal form of contraception throughout therapy.
- Emphasize the importance of regular follow-up exams to monitor progress and to check for side effects.

Evaluation/Desired Outcomes
- Decreased fever and night sweats.
- Diminished cough and sputum production.
- Negative sputum cultures.
- Increased appetite.
- Weight gain.
- Reduced fatigue.
- Sense of well-being in patients with tuberculosis.
- Prevention of meningococcal meningitis.
- Prevention of *H. influenzae* type B infection. Prophylactic course is usually short term.

rifAXIMin (ri-fax-i-min)
Xifaxan, ✤Zaxine

Classification
Therapeutic: anti-infectives
Pharmacologic: rifamycins

Indications
Travelers' diarrhea due to noninvasive strains of *Escherichia coli*. Reduction in risk of overt hepatic encephalopathy recurrence. Treatment of irritable bowel syndrome (IBS) with diarrhea.

Action
Inhibits bacterial RNA synthesis by binding to bacterial DNA-dependent RNA polymerase. **Therapeutic Effects:** Decreased severity of travelers' diarrhea. Decreased episodes of overt hepatic encephalopathy. Decreased signs/symptoms of IBS. **Spectrum:** *Escherichia coli* (enterotoxigenic and enteroaggregative strains).

Pharmacokinetics
Absorption: Poorly absorbed (<0.4%), action is primarily in GI tract.
Distribution: 80–90% concentrated in gut.
Metabolism and Excretion: Almost exclusively excreted unchanged in feces.
Half-life: 6 hr.

TIME/ACTION PROFILE

ROUTE	ONSET	PEAK	DURATION
PO	unknown	unknown	unknown

Contraindications/Precautions
Contraindicated in: Hypersensitivity to rifaximin or other rifamycins; Diarrhea with fever or bloody stools; Diarrhea caused by other infectious agents; Lactation: Potential for adverse effects in the infant. Switch to formula for duration of treatment.
Use Cautiously in: OB: Use only if benefit to mother outweighs risk to fetus; Pedi: Safety not established in children <18 yr (hepatic encephalopathy) or <12 yr (travelers' diarrhea).

Adverse Reactions/Side Effects
CNS: dizziness. **CV:** peripheral edema. **GI:** CLOSTRIDIUM DIFFICILE-ASSOCIATED DIARRHEA (CDAD).

Interactions
Drug-Drug: P-glycoprotein inhibitors, including **cyclosporine**, may ↑ levels. May cause fluctuations in INR when used with **warfarin**; closely monitor INR.

Route/Dosage
Travelers' Diarrhea
PO (Adults and Children ≥12 yr): 200 mg 3 times daily for 3 days.

Hepatic Encephalopathy
PO (Adults): 550 mg twice daily.

IBS with Diarrhea
PO (Adults): 550 mg 3 times daily for 14 days; if recurrence of symptoms, may treat up to an additional 2 times.

Availability
Tablets: 200 mg, 550 mg.

NURSING IMPLICATIONS
Assessment
- **Traveler's Diarrhea:** Assess frequency and consistency of stools and bowel sounds prior to and during therapy.
- Assess fluid and electrolyte balance and skin turgor for dehydration.
- **Hepatic Encephalopathy:** Assess mental status periodically during therapy.
- **IBS with Diarrhea:** Assess frequency and consistency of stools and other IBS symptoms (bloating, cramping) daily.
- Monitor bowel function. Diarrhea, abdominal cramping, fever, and bloody stools should be reported to health care professional promptly as a sign of Clostridium difficile-associated diarrhea (CDAD). May begin up to several wk following cessation of therapy.
- ***Lab Test Considerations:*** May cause lymphocytosis, monocytosis, and neutropenia.

Implementation
- Do not confuse rifaximin with rifampin.
- **PO:** Administer with or without food.

R

Patient/Family Teaching

- Instruct patient to take rifaximin as directed and to complete therapy, even if feeling better. Caution patient to stop taking rifaximin if diarrhea symptoms get worse, persist more than 24–48 hr, or are accompanied by fever or blood in the stool. Consult health care professional if these occur. Advise patient not to treat diarrhea without consulting health care professional. May occur up to several wk after discontinuation of medication.
- May cause dizziness. Caution patient to avoid driving and other activities requiring alertness until response to medication is known.
- Advise female patients to notify health care professional if pregnant or if pregnancy is suspected, or if breast feeding.

Evaluation/Desired Outcomes

- Decreased severity of travelers' diarrhea.
- Reduction in risk of overt hepatic encephalopathy recurrence.
- Reduction in symptoms of IBS with diarrhea.

rilpivirine (ril-pi-vir-een)

Edurant

Classification

Therapeutic: antiretrovirals

Pharmacologic: non-nucleoside reverse transcriptase inhibitors

Indications

Treatment-naïve adult patients with HIV infection with HIV-1 RNA ≤100,000 copies/mL at start of therapy.

Action

Inhibits HIV-replication by non-competitively inhibiting HIV reverse transcriptase. **Therapeutic Effects:** Slowed progression of HIV infection and decreased occurrence of sequelae. Increases CD4 cell counts and decreases viral load.

Pharmacokinetics

Absorption: Well absorbed following oral administration.

Distribution: Unknown.

Protein Binding: 99.7%.

Metabolism and Excretion: Mostly metabolized by the liver (CYP3A enzyme system); 25% excreted in feces unchanged, <1% excreted unchanged in urine.

Half-life: 50 hr.

TIME/ACTION PROFILE (blood levels)

ROUTE	ONSET	PEAK	DURATION
PO	unknown	4–5 hr	24 hr

Contraindications/Precautions

Contraindicated in: Concurrent use of drugs that induce the CYP3A enzyme system or ↑ gastric pH (↓ blood levels and effectiveness, ↑ resistance); Lactation: Avoid breast feeding due to possible transmission of virus in breast milk.

Use Cautiously in: Concurrent use of drugs that ↑ risk of torsades de pointes (may ↑ risk of arrhythmias); History of depression or suicide attempt; Hepatitis B or C; Concurrent use of antacids or H_2 antagonists (↓ levels and effectiveness); Geri: Consider ↓ hepatic/renal/cardiac function, concurrent diseases, and drug therapy; OB: Has been used safely during pregnancy; Pedi: Children <12 yr (safety and effectiveness not established).

Adverse Reactions/Side Effects

CNS: <u>depression (↑ in children)</u>, dizziness, headache, insomnia. **Derm:** DRUG REACTION WITH EOSINOPHILIA AND SYSTEMIC SYMPTOMS (DRESS), rash. **Endo:** fat redistribution, Grave's disease. **GI:** autoimmune hepatitis, hepatotoxicity. **MS:** polymyositis. **Neuro:** Guillain-Barré syndrome. **Misc:** immune reconstitution syndrome.

Interactions

Drug-Drug: **Drugs that induce the CYP3A enzyme system** including **carbamazepine**, **dexamethasone** (more than a single dose), **oxcarbazepine**, **phenobarbital**, **phenytoin**, **rifampin**, or **rifapentine** ↓ levels and effectiveness and promote virologic resistance; concurrent use contraindicated. **Proton pump inhibitors** including **esomeprazole**, **lansoprazole**, **omeprazole**, **pantoprazole**, and **rabeprazole** ↓ levels and effectiveness and may ↑ resistance; concurrent use contraindicated. Concurrent use with **antacids** may ↓ levels and effectiveness; use with caution, administer at least 2 hr before or 4 hr after rilpivirine. Concurrent use with **H_2 antagonists** may ↓ levels and effectiveness; use with caution, administer at least 12 hr before or 4 hr after rilpivirine. **Rifabutin** may ↓ levels; ↑ rilpivirine dose during concurrent use. **Delavirdine** may ↑ levels; avoid concurrent use. **Efavirenz**, **etravirine**, and **nevirapine** may ↓ levels; avoid concurrent use. **Darunavir/ritonavir**, **lopinavir/ritonavir**, **atazanavir/ritonavir**, **fosamprenavir/ritonavir**, **saquinavir/ritonavir**, **tipranavir/ritonavir**, **atazanavir**, **fosamprenavir**, **indinavir**, and **nelfinavir** may ↑ levels. **Clarithromyin**, **erythromycin**, or **troleandomycin** may ↑ levels; consider azithromycin. **Fluconazole**, **itraconazole**, **ketoconazole**, **posaconazole**, and **voriconazole** may ↑ levels; rilpivirine may ↓ **ketoconazole** levels. Concurrent use with **drugs that ↑ risk of torsades de pointes** may ↑ risk of serious arrhythmias. May ↓ levels of **methadone**; monitor clinical effects.

Drug-Natural Products: Concurrent use of **St. John's wort** ↓ blood levels and effectiveness and promote virologic resistance; concurrent use contraindicated.

Route/Dosage

PO (Adults and Children ≥12 yr and ≥35 kg): 25 mg once daily; *Pregnant patients on stable rilpivirine regimen prior to pregnancy and virologically suppressed (HIV RNA <50 copies/mL)*—25 mg once daily; *Concurrent rifabutin therapy*—50 mg once daily (↓ dose to 25 mg once daily when rifabutin discontinued).

Availability

Tablets: 25 mg. ***In combination with:*** dolutegravir (Juluca); emtricitabine and tenofovir (Complera). See Appendix B.

NURSING IMPLICATIONS

Assessment

- Assess for change in severity of HIV symptoms and for symptoms of opportunistic infections during therapy.
- Monitor closely for notable changes in behavior that could indicate the emergence or worsening of suicidal thoughts or behavior or depression.
- Assess for rash periodically during therapy. May cause Stevens-Johnson syndrome. Discontinue therapy if severe or if accompanied with fever, general malaise, fatigue, muscle or joint aches, blisters, oral lesions, conjunctivitis, hepatitis, and/or eosinophilia.
- ***Lab Test Considerations:*** Monitor viral load and CD4 cell count regularly during therapy.
- Monitor liver function tests before and periodically during therapy in patients with underlying liver disease, hepatitis B or C, or marked ↑ transaminase. May cause ↑ serum creatinine, AST, ALT, total bilirubin, total cholesterol, LDL, and triglycerides.

Implementation

- **PO:** Administer once daily with a meal.

Patient/Family Teaching

- Emphasize the importance of taking rilpivirine as directed, at the same time each day. It must always be used in combination with other antiretroviral drugs. Do not take more than prescribed amount and do not stop taking without consulting health care professional. Take missed doses with a meal if remembered <12 hr of the time it is usually taken, then return to regular schedule. If more than 12 hr from time dose is usually taken, omit dose and resume dosing schedule; do not double doses. Advise patient to read *Patient Information* prior to starting therapy and with each Rx refill in case of changes.
- Advise patient to take antacids 2 hr before or 4 hr after and H_2 antagonists 12 hr before or 4 hr after rilpivirine.
- Instruct patient that rilpivirine should not be shared with others.
- Inform patient that rilpivirine does not cure AIDS or prevent associated or opportunistic infections. Rilpivirine does not reduce the risk of transmission of HIV to others through sexual contact or blood contamination. Caution patient to use a condom and to avoid sharing needles or donating blood to prevent spreading the AIDS virus to others. Advise patient that the long-term effects of rilpivirine are unknown at this time.
- Inform patients and families of risk of suicidal thoughts and behavior and advise that behavioral changes, emergency or worsening signs and symptoms of depression, unusual changes in mood, or emergence of suicidal thoughts, behavior, or thoughts of self-harm should be reported to health care professional immediately.
- Immune reconstitution syndrome may trigger opportunistic infections or autoimmune disorders. Notify health care professional if symptoms or rash occur.
- May cause dizziness. Caution patient to avoid driving or other activities requiring alertness until response to medication is known.
- Advise patient to notify health care professional of all Rx or OTC medications, vitamins, or herbal products being taken and to consult with health care professional before taking other medications, especially St. John's wort.
- Inform patient that changes in body fat (increased fat in upper back and neck, breast, and around back, chest, and stomach area; loss of fats from legs, arms, and face) may occur.
- Rep: Advise patient taking oral contraceptives to use a nonhormonal method of birth control during rilpivirine therapy. If pregnancy is suspected notify health care professional promptly. Encourage pregnant women to enroll in the Antiretroviral Pregnancy Registry by calling 1-800-258-4263. Advise female patient to avoid breast feeding during therapy.
- Emphasize the importance of regular follow-up exams and blood counts to determine progress and monitor for side effects.

Evaluation/Desired Outcomes

- Delayed progression of AIDS and decreased opportunistic infections in patients with HIV.
- Decrease in viral load and increase in CD4 cell counts.

risedronate (riss-ed-roe-nate)

Actonel, Actonel DR, Atelvia

Classification
Therapeutic: bone resorption inhibitors
Pharmacologic: biphosphonates

Indications

Prevention and treatment of postmenopausal and corticosteroid-induced osteoporosis. Treatment of Paget's

R

disease in men and women. Treatment of osteoporosis in men.

Action

Inhibits bone resorption by binding to bone hydroxyapatite, which inhibits osteoclast activity. **Therapeutic Effects:** Reversal of the progression of osteoporosis with decreased fractures and other sequelae. Reduced bone turnover and resorption; normalization of serum alkaline phosphatase with reduced complications of Paget's disease.

Pharmacokinetics

Absorption: Rapidly but poorly absorbed following oral administration (0.63% bioavailability).

Distribution: 60% of absorbed dose distributes to bone.

Metabolism and Excretion: 40% of absorbed dose is excreted unchanged by kidneys; unabsorbed drug is excreted in feces.

Half-life: *Initial*—1.5 hr; *terminal*—220 hr (reflects dissociation from bone).

TIME/ACTION PROFILE (effects on serum alkaline phosphatase)

ROUTE	ONSET	PEAK	DURATION
PO	within days	30 days	up to 16 mo

Contraindications/Precautions

Contraindicated in: Hypersensitivity; Hypocalcemia; Abnormalities of the esophagus, which delay esophageal emptying (i.e., strictures, achalasia); Inability to stand/sit upright for at least 30 min; Lactation: Lactation; Severe renal impairment (CCr <30 mL/min).

Use Cautiously in: History of upper GI disorders; Other disturbances of bone or mineral metabolism (correct abnormalities before initiating therapy); Dietary deficiencies (supplemental vitamin D and calcium may be required); Invasive dental procedures, cancer, receiving chemotherapy, corticosteroids, or angiogenesis inhibitors, poor oral hygeine, periodontal disease, dental disease, anemia, coagulopathy, infection, or poorly fitting dentures (may ↑ risk of jaw osteonecrosis); OB, Pedi: Safety not established; use in pregnancy only if potential benefit justifies potential risks.

Adverse Reactions/Side Effects

CNS: weakness. **EENT:** amblyopia, conjunctivitis, dry eyes, eye pain/inflammation, tinnitus. **CV:** chest pain, edema. **GI:** abdominal pain, diarrhea, belching, colitis, constipation, dysphagia, esophagitis, esophageal cancer, esophageal ulcer, gastric ulcer, nausea. **Derm:** STEVENS-JOHNSON SYNDROME, TOXIC EPIDERMAL NECROLYSIS, rash. **MS:** arthralgia, musculoskeletal pain, femur fractures, osteonecrosis (primarily of jaw). **Resp:** asthma exacerbation. **Misc:** flu-like syndrome.

Interactions

Drug-Drug: Concurrent use with **NSAIDs** or **aspirin** ↑ risk of GI irritation. Absorption is ↓ by **calcium supplements** or **antacids**. **Proton pump inhibitors** and **H2 antagonists** may cause a faster release of drug from the delayed-release product that can ↑ drug levels; concurrent use not recommended.

Drug-Food: Food ↓ absorption (administer at least 30 min before breakfast).

Route/Dosage

PO (Adults): *Postmenopausal osteoporosis*—5 mg daily; *or* 35 mg once weekly (immediate- or delayed-release); *or* 75 mg taken on 2 consecutive days for a total of 2 tablets each mo; *or* 150 mg once monthly. *Osteoporosis in men*—35 mg once weekly (immediate-release); *Glucocorticoid-induced osteoporosis*—5 mg daily; *Paget's disease*—30 mg daily for 2 mo; retreatment may be considered after 2 mo off therapy.

Availability (generic available)

Tablets: 5 mg, 30 mg, 35 mg, 150 mg. **Delayed-release tablets (Atelvia):** 35 mg.

NURSING IMPLICATIONS

Assessment

- Perform a routine oral exam prior to initiation of therapy. Dental exam with appropriate preventative dentistry should be considered prior to therapy. Patients with history of tooth extraction, poor oral hygiene, gingival infections, diabetes, or use of a dental appliance or those taking immunosuppressive therapy, angiogenesis inhibitors, or systemic corticosteroids are at greater risk for osteonecrosis of the jaw.
- **Osteoporosis:** Assess patients via bone density study for low bone mass before and periodically during therapy.
- **Paget's disease:** Assess for symptoms of Paget's disease (bone pain, headache, decreased visual and auditory acuity, increased skull size).
- ***Lab Test Considerations:*** *Osteoporosis:* Assess serum calcium before and periodically during therapy. Hypocalcemia and vitamin D deficiency should be treated before initiating alendronate therapy. May cause mild, transient ↑ of calcium and phosphate.
- *Paget's disease:* Monitor alkaline phosphatase prior to and periodically during therapy to monitor effectiveness of therapy.

Implementation

- Do not confuse Actonel (risedronate) with Actos (pioglitazone).
- **PO:** Administer *Actonel* first thing in the morning with 6–8 oz of water, 30 min prior to other medications, beverages, or food. Waiting longer than 30 min will improve absorption. Administer *Atelvia* right after breakfast with 4 oz of water. Tablet should be swallowed whole; do not crush, break, or chew.
- Calcium-, magnesium-, or aluminum-containing agents may interfere with absorption of risedronate

and should be taken at a different time of day with food.

- Avoid administering delayed-release product with proton pump inhibitors or H_2 antagonists; may allow a faster release and increased drug level.

Patient/Family Teaching

- Instruct patient on the importance of taking as directed. Risedronate should be taken with 6–8 oz of water (mineral water, orange juice, coffee, and other beverages decrease absorption). *If a dose of Actonel 35 is missed,* take 1 tablet the morning remembered, then return to the 1 tablet/wk on the originally scheduled day; do not take 2 pills at once. *If 1 or both tablets of Actonel 75 are missed and the next month's scheduled doses are more than 7 days away:* if both Actonel 75 are missed take 1 the morning remembered and 1 the next morning. If only 1 Actonel 75 tablet is missed: take the missed tablet on the morning of the day after you remember, then return to original schedule. Do not take more than two 75 mg tablets within 7 days. *If 1 or both tablets of Actonel 75 are missed and the next month's scheduled doses are within 7 days,* omit and return to schedule next mo. *If 1 or both tablets of Actonel 150 are missed and the next month's scheduled doses are more than 7 days away,* take the missed tablet on the morning of the day after you remember, then return to original schedule. Do not take more than two 150-mg tablets within 7 days. *If 1 or both tablets of Actonel 75 are missed and the next month's scheduled doses are within 7 days,* omit and return to schedule next mo. Encourage patient to read the *Medication Guide* before starting therapy and with each Rx refill in case of changes.
- Caution patients to remain upright for 30 min following dose to facilitate passage to stomach and minimize risk of esophageal irritation.
- Advise patient to eat a balanced diet and consult health care professional about the need for supplemental calcium and vitamin D (see Appendix K).
- Inform patient that severe musculoskeletal pain may occur within days, mo, or yr after starting risendronate. Symptoms my resolve completely after discontinuation or slow or incomplete resolution may occur. Notify health care professional if severe pain occurs.
- Encourage patient to participate in regular exercise and to modify behaviors that increase the risk of osteoporosis (stop smoking, reduce alcohol consumption).
- Advise patient to inform health care professional of risedronate therapy prior to dental surgery.
- Advise female patients to notify health care professional if pregnancy is planned or suspected or if breast feeding.

Evaluation/Desired Outcomes

- Reversal of the progression of osteoporosis with decreased fractures and other sequelae. For patients at low risk of fracture, discontinue after 3 to 5 yr of use.
- Decrease in serum alkaline phosphatase and the progression of Paget's disease.

BEERS

risperiDONE (riss-**per**-i-done)

Perseris, RisperDAL, RisperDAL Consta, RisperDAL M-TAB

Classification

Therapeutic: antipsychotics, mood stabilizers

Pharmacologic: benzisoxazoles

Indications

Schizophrenia. Short-term treatment of acute manic or mixed episodes associated with Bipolar I Disorder (oral only) and maintenance treatment of Bipolar I Disorder (IM only); can be used with lithium or valproate (adults only). Irritability associated with autistic disorder (oral only).

Action

May act by antagonizing dopamine and serotonin in the CNS. **Therapeutic Effects:** Decreased symptoms of psychoses, bipolar mania, or autism.

Pharmacokinetics

Absorption: 70% after administration of tablets, solution, or orally disintegrating tablets. Following IM administration, small initial release of drug, followed by 3-wk lag; the rest of release starts at 3 wk and lasts 4–6 wk. Following subcutaneous administration, initial release of drug occurs at 4–6 hr, with the rest of release occurring at 10–14 days after administration.

Distribution: Unknown.

Metabolism and Excretion: Extensively metabolized by the liver. Metabolism is genetically determined; extensive metabolizers (most patients) convert risperidone to 9-hydroxyrisperidone rapidly. Poor metabolizers (6–8% of Whites) convert it more slowly. The 9-hydroxyrisperidone is an antipsychotic compound. Risperidone and its active metabolite are renally eliminated.

Half-life: *Extensive metabolizers*—3 hr for risperidone, 21 hr for 9-hydroxyrisperidone. *Poor metabolizers*—20 hr for risperidone and 30 hr for 9-hydroxyrisperidone; *Subcutaneous*—9–11 days.

R

TIME/ACTION PROFILE (clinical effects)

ROUTE	ONSET	PEAK	DURATION
PO	1–2 wk	unknown	up to 6 wk†
IM	3 wk	4–6 wk	up to 6 wk†
Subcut	2 wk	6–8 wk	unknown

†After discontinuation.

Contraindications/Precautions

Contraindicated in: Hypersensitivity to risperidone or paliperidone; Lactation: Discontinue drug or bottle feed.

Use Cautiously in: Debilitated patients, patients with renal or hepatic impairment (initial dose reduction recommended); Underlying cardiovascular disease (↑ risk of arrhythmias and hypotension); History of seizures; History of drug abuse; Diabetes or risk factors for diabetes (may worsen glucose control); Patients at risk for aspiration or falls; Renal or hepatic impairment; OB, Pedi: Safety not established; Geri: Initial dose ↓ recommended. ↑ risk of mortality and cerebrovascular events in elderly patients treated for dementia-related psychosis.

Adverse Reactions/Side Effects

CNS: NEUROLEPTIC MALIGNANT SYNDROME, SEIZURES, aggressive behavior, dizziness, extrapyramidal reactions, headache, ↑ dreams, ↑ sleep duration, insomnia, sedation, fatigue, impaired temperature regulation, nervousness, tardive dyskinesia. **CV:** arrhythmias, orthostatic hypotension, tachycardia. **Derm:** itching/skin rash, dry skin, ↑ pigmentation, sweating, photosensitivity, seborrhea. **EENT:** pharyngitis, rhinitis, visual disturbances. **Endo:** dyslipidemia, galactorrhea, hyperglycemia. **GI:** constipation, diarrhea, dry mouth, nausea, abdominal pain, anorexia, dyspepsia, dysphagia, polydipsia, ↑ salivation, vomiting. **GU:** ↓ libido, dysmenorrhea/menorrhagia, amenorrhea, difficulty urinating, gynecomastia, impotence, polyuria, priapism. **Hemat:** AGRANULOCYTOSIS, leukopenia, neutropenia. **Metab:** weight gain, weight loss. **MS:** arthralgia, back pain. **Resp:** cough, dyspnea. **Misc:** HYPERSENSITIVITY REACTIONS (including anaphylaxis and angioedema).

Interactions

Drug-Drug: May ↓ the antiparkinsonian effects of **levodopa** or other **dopamine agonists**. **Strong CYP3A4 inducers**, including **carbamazepine**, **phenytoin**, **rifampin**, and **phenobarbital** may ↑ metabolism and may ↓ effectiveness; dose adjustments may be necessary. **Fluoxetine** and **paroxetine** ↑ blood levels and may ↑ effects; dose adjustments may be necessary. **Clozapine** ↓ metabolism and may ↑ effects of risperidone. ↑ CNS depression may occur with other **CNS depressants**, including **alcohol**, **antihistamines**, **sedative/hypnotics**, or **opioid analgesics**.

Drug-Natural Products: Kava, valerian, or chamomile can ↑ CNS depression.

Route/Dosage

Schizophrenia

PO (Adults): 1 mg twice daily, ↑ by 1–2 mg/day no more frequently than every 24 hr to 4–8 mg daily.

PO (Children 13–17 yr): 0.5 mg once daily, ↑ by 0.5–1.0 mg no more frequently than every 24 hr to 3 mg daily. May administer half the daily dose twice daily if drowsiness persists.

IM (Adults): 25 mg every 2 wk; some patients may benefit from a higher dose of 37.5 or 50 mg every 2 wk.

Subcut (Adults): *Currently taking 3 mg/day of oral risperidone*—90 mg once monthly; *Currently taking 4 mg/day of oral risperidone*—120 mg once monthly; *Planned therapy with fluoxetine or paroxetine*—Initiate 90 mg once monthly 2–4 wk before starting fluoxetine or paroxetine therapy; *Concurrent use of strong CYP3A4 inducer*—If receiving 90 mg once monthly regimen, consider ↑ dose to 120 mg once monthly; if receiving 120 mg once monthly regimen, consider using additional oral risperidone.

Hepatic/Renal Impairment

PO (Adults): *Severe renal impairment (CCr <30 mL/min) or severe hepatic impairment*—Start with 0.5 mg twice daily; ↑ by 0.5 mg twice daily, up to 1.5 mg twice daily; then ↑ at weekly intervals if necessary.

Hepatic/Renal Impairment

Subcut (Adults): Titrate patients up to at least 3 mg/day of oral risperidone before initiating subcutaneous risperidone. If patient tolerates this dose of oral risperidone, consider subcutaneous dose of 90 mg once monthly.

Acute Manic or Mixed Episodes Associated with Bipolar I Disorder

PO (Adults): 2–3 mg/day as a single daily dose, dose may be ↑ at 24-hr intervals by 1 mg (range 1–5 mg/day).

PO (Children 13–17 yr): 0.5 mg once daily, ↑ by 0.5–1 mg no more frequently than every 24 hr to 2.5 mg daily. May administer half the daily dose twice daily if drowsiness persists.

PO (Geriatric Patients or Debilitated Patients): Start with 0.5 mg twice daily; ↑ by 0.5 mg twice daily, up to 1.5 mg twice daily; then ↑ at weekly intervals if necessary. May also be given as a single daily dose after initial titration.

Hepatic/Renal Impairment

PO (Adults): *Severe renal impairment (CCr <30 mL/min) or severe hepatic impairment*—Start with 0.5 mg twice daily; ↑ by 0.5 mg twice daily, up to 1.5 mg twice daily; then ↑ at weekly intervals if necessary.

Maintenance Treatment of Bipolar I Disorder

IM (Adults): 25 mg every 2 wk; some patients may benefit from a higher dose of 37.5 or 50 mg every 2 wk.

Irritability Associated with Autistic Disorder

PO (Children 5–16 yr weighing <20 kg): 0.25 mg/day initially. After at least 4 days of therapy, may ↑ to 0.5 mg/day. Dose ↑ in increments of 0.25 mg/day may be considered at 2 wk or longer intervals. May be given as a single or divided dose.

PO (Children 5–16 yr weighing >20 kg): 0.5 mg/day initially. After at least 4 days of therapy, may ↑ to 1 mg/day. Dose ↑ in increments of 0.5 mg/day may be considered at 2 wk or longer intervals. May be given as a single or divided dose.

Hepatic/Renal Impairment

PO (Adults): *Severe renal impairment (CCr <30 mL/min) or severe hepatic impairment*—Start with 0.5 mg twice daily; ↑ by 0.5 mg twice daily, up to 1.5 mg twice daily; then ↑ at weekly intervals if necessary.

Availability (generic available)

Extended-release microspheres for IM injection (Risperdal Consta) (requires reconstitution): 12.5 mg/vial kit, 25 mg/vial kit, 37.5 mg/vial kit, 50 mg/vial kit. **Extended-release suspension for subcut injection (Perseris):** 90 mg/vial kit, 120 mg/vial kit. **Oral solution:** 1 mg/mL. **Cost:** *Generic*—$152.56/30 mL. **Orally disintegrating tablets (Risperdal M-Tabs):** 0.25 mg, 0.5 mg, 1 mg, 2 mg, 3 mg, 4 mg. **Cost:** *Generic*—0.5 mg $131.86/28, 1 mg $154.07/28, 2 mg $250.49/28, 3 mg $316.12/28, 4 mg $424.45/28. **Tablets:** 0.25 mg, 0.5 mg, 1 mg, 2 mg, 3 mg, 4 mg. **Cost:** *Generic*—0.25 mg $18.40/180, 0.5 mg $22.58/180, 1 mg $24.13/180, 2 mg $28.94/180, 3 mg $34.94/180, 4 mg $38.30/180.

NURSING IMPLICATIONS

Assessment

- Monitor patient's mental status (orientation, mood, behavior) and mood before and periodically during therapy. Monitor closely for notable changes in behavior that could indicate the emergence or worsening of suicidal thoughts or behavior or depression, especially during early therapy. Restrict amount of drug available to patient.
- Assess weight and BMI initially and throughout therapy. Monitor for symptoms of hyperglycemia polydipsia, polyuria, polyphagia,weakness) periodically during therapy.
- Monitor BP (sitting, standing, lying down) and pulse before and frequently during initial dose titration. May cause prolonged QT interval, tachycardia, and orthostatic hypotension. If hypotension occurs, dose may need to be decreased.
- Observe patient when administering medication to ensure medication is swallowed and not hoarded or cheeked.
- Monitor patient for onset of extrapyramidal side effects (*akathisia*—restlessness; *dystonia*—muscle spasms and twisting motions; or *pseudoparkinsonism*—mask-like face, rigidity, tremors, drooling, shuffling gait, dysphagia). Report these symptoms; reduction of dose or discontinuation may be necessary. Trihexyphenidyl or benztropine may be used to control symptoms.
- Monitor for tardive dyskinesia (involuntary rhythmic movement of mouth, face, and extremities). Report immediately; may be irreversible.
- Monitor for development of neuroleptic malignant syndrome (fever, respiratory distress, tachycardia, seizures, diaphoresis, hypertension or hypotension, pallor, tiredness). Notify health care professional immediately if these symptoms occur.
- Monitor for symptoms related to hyperprolactinemia (menstrual abnormalities, galactorrhea, sexual dysfunction).
- Assess for falls risk. Drowsiness, orthostatic hypotension, and motor and sensory instability increase risk. Institute prevention if indicated.
- ***Lab Test Considerations:*** May cause ↑ serum prolactin levels.
- May cause ↑ AST and ALT.
- May also cause anemia, thrombocytopenia, leukocytosis, and leukopenia.
- Obtain fasting blood glucose and cholesterol levels initially and periodically during therapy.
- Monitor CBC frequently during initial mo of therapy in patients with pre-existing or history of low WBC. May cause leukopenia, neutropenia, or agranulocytosis. Discontinue therapy if this occurs.
- Monitor serum prolactin prior to and periodically during therapy. May cause ↑ serum prolactin levels.

Implementation

- Do not confuse risperidone with ropinirole. Do not confuse Risperdal with Restoril (temazepam) or ropinirole.
- When switching from other antipsychotics, discontinue previous agents when starting risperidone and minimize the period of overlapping antipsychotic agents.
- If therapy is reinstituted after an interval off risperidone, follow initial titration schedule.
- For IM use, establish tolerance with oral dosing before IM use and continue oral dosing for 3 wk following initial IM injection. Do not increase dose more frequently than every 4 wk.
- **PO:** Daily doses can be taken in the morning or evening.

- For orally disintegrating tablets, open blister pack by pealing back foil to expose tablet; do not try to push tablet through foil. Use dry hands to remove tablet from blister and immediately place entire tablet on tongue. Tablets disintegrate in mouth within sec and can be swallowed with or without liquid. Do not attempt to split or chew tablet. Do not try to store tablets once removed from blister.
- Oral solution can be mixed with water, coffee, orange juice, or low-fat milk; do not mix with cola or tea.
- **Subcut:** Mix *Perseris* according to manufacturer's instructions. With patient in supine position, inject into abdomen; avoid areas with nodules, lesions, excessive pigment, irritation, redness, bruising, infection or scarring. Hold syringe upright for several sec to allow air bubbles to rise; depress the plunger to expel excess air. Pinch skin to avoid IM injection. Do not rub site after injection. Advise patient that they may have a lump for several wk; will decrease in size over time. Instruct patient not to rub or massage injection site and avoid constriction by belts or clothing waistbands.
- **IM:** Reconstitute with 2 mL of diluent provided by manufacturer. Administer via deep deltoid (1-in. needle) or gluteal (2-in. needle) injection using enclosed safety needle; alternate arms or buttocks with each injection. Allow solution to warm to room temperature prior to injection. Administer immediately after mixed with diluent; shake well to mix suspension. Must be administered within 6 hr of reconstitution. Store dose pack in refrigerator.
- Do not combine dose strengths in a single injection.

Patient/Family Teaching

- Instruct patient to take medication as directed.
- Inform patient of the possibility of extrapyramidal symptoms. Instruct patient to report these symptoms immediately to health care professional.
- Advise patient to change positions slowly to minimize orthostatic hypotension. Protect from falls.
- May cause drowsiness. Caution patient to avoid driving or other activities requiring alertness until response to medication is known.
- Advise patient and family to notify health care professional if thoughts about suicide or dying, attempts to commit suicide; new or worse depression; new or worse anxiety; feeling very agitated or restless; panic attacks; trouble sleeping; new or worse irritability; acting aggressive; being angry or violent; acting on dangerous impulses; an extreme increase in activity and talking; other unusual changes in behavior or mood occur.
- Advise patient to use sunscreen and protective clothing when exposed to the sun to prevent photosensitivity reactions. Extremes in temperature should also be avoided; this drug impairs body temperature regulation.
- Instruct patient to notify health care professional of all Rx or OTC medications, vitamins, or herbal products being taken and consult health care professional before taking any new medications. Caution patient to avoid concurrent use of alcohol and other CNS depressants.
- Advise patient to notify health care professional of medication regimen before treatment or surgery.
- Instruct patient to notify health care professional promptly if sore throat, fever, unusual bleeding or bruising, rash, tremors, or symptoms of hyperglycemia occur.
- Rep: Advise female patients to notify health care professional if pregnancy is planned or suspected, and to avoid breast feeding. Encourage women who become pregnant while taking iloperidone to enroll in the National Pregnancy Registry for Atypical Antipsychotics at 1-866-961-2388 or visit http://womensmentalhealth.org/clinical-and-research-programs/pregnancyregistry/. Monitor neonates for extrapyramidal and/or withdrawal symptoms and manage symptoms appropriately. May impair fertility in females, usually reversible.
- Emphasize the importance of routine follow-up exams to monitor side effects and continued participation in psychotherapy to improve coping skills.

Evaluation/Desired Outcomes

- Decrease in excited, manic behavior.
- Decrease in positive symptoms (delusions, hallucinations) of schizophrenia.
- Decreased aggression toward others, deliberate self-injury, temper tantrums, and mood changes in children with autism.
- Decrease in negative symptoms (social withdrawal, flat, blunted affects) of schizophrenia.
- Decrease in autism symptoms.

ritonavir (ri-toe-na-veer)

Norvir

Classification
Therapeutic: antiretrovirals
Pharmacologic: protease inhibitors

Indications

HIV infection (with other antiretrovirals).

Action

Inhibits the action of HIV protease and prevents the cleavage of viral polyproteins. **Therapeutic Effects:** Increased CD4 cell counts and decreased viral load with subsequent slowed progression of HIV infection and its sequelae.

Pharmacokinetics

Absorption: Appears to be well absorbed after oral administration.
Distribution: Poor CNS penetration.
Protein Binding: 98–99%.
Metabolism and Excretion: Primarily metabolized by the CYP3A4 and CYP2D6 isoenzymes in the

liver; one metabolite has antiretroviral activity; 3.5% excreted unchanged in urine.

Half-life: 3–5 hr.

TIME/ACTION PROFILE (blood levels)

ROUTE	ONSET	PEAK	DURATION
PO	rapid	4 hr*	12 hr

*Nonfasting.

Contraindications/Precautions

Contraindicated in: Hypersensitivity; Concurrent use of alfuzosin, amiodarone, colchicine, dihydroergotamine, dronedarone, ergotamine, flecainide, fluticasone, lomitapide, lovastatin, lurasidone, meperidine, methylergonovine, midazolam (PO), pimozide, propafenone, quinidine, ranolazine, simvastatin, sildenafil (Revatio), St. John's wort, triazolam, or voriconazole; Hypersensitivity or intolerance to alcohol or castor oil (present in liquid); OB: Avoid oral solution during pregnancy (because of alcohol content); Lactation: Breast feeding not recommended in HIV-infected patients.

Use Cautiously in: Impaired hepatic function, history of hepatitis; Diabetes mellitus; Hemophilia (↑ risk of bleeding); Structural heart disease, conduction abnormalities, ischemic heart disease, or heart failure (↑ risk of heart block); OB, Pedi: Pregnancy or children <1 mo (safety not established).

Adverse Reactions/Side Effects

CNS: SEIZURES, abnormal thinking, weakness, dizziness, headache, malaise, somnolence, syncope. **CV:** heart block, orthostatic hypotension, PR interval prolongation, vasodilation. **Derm:** STEVENS-JOHNSON SYNDROME, TOXIC EPIDERMAL NECROLYSIS, rash, skin eruptions, sweating, urticaria. **EENT:** pharyngitis, throat irritation. **Endo:** hyperglycemia. **F and E:** dehydration. **GI:** abdominal pain, altered taste, anorexia, diarrhea, nausea, vomiting, constipation, dyspepsia, flatulence. **GU:** renal insufficiency. **Metab:** hyperlipidemia. **MS:** ↑ creatine kinase, myalgia. **Neuro:** circumoral paresthesia, peripheral paresthesia. **Resp:** bronchospasm. **Misc:** HYPERSENSITIVITY REACTIONS (including anaphylaxis and angioedema), fat redistribution, fever, immune reconstitution syndrome.

Interactions

Drug-Drug: ↑ levels and risk of toxicity from some **antiarrhythmics (amiodarone, dronedarone, flecainide, pimozide, propafenone, quinidine)**, **ergot derivatives (dihydroergotamine, ergotamine, methylergonovine)**, **fluticasone (inhalation)**, **lomitapide**, **lurasidone**, **meperidine**, **ranolazine**, **sildenafil (Revatio)**, **alfuzosin**, **lovastatin**, **simvastatin**, **voriconazole**, **midazolam (oral)**, and **triazolam**; concurrent use contraindicated. May ↑ **colchicine** levels; concurrent use in patients with renal or hepatic impairment contraindicated; ↓ dose of colchicine in patients without renal or hepatic impairment. ↑ levels of **maraviroc**; ↓ maraviroc dose to 150 mg twice daily. ↑ levels of **clarithromycin**; ↓ clarithromycin dose if CCr <60 mL/min. ↑ levels of **rifabutin**; ↓ rifabutin dose to 150 mg every other day or 3 times weekly. May also ↑ levels and effects of some **opioid analgesics (alfentanil, fentanyl, hydrocodone, oxycodone)**, **tramadol**; some **NSAIDs (diclofenac, ibuprofen, indomethacin)**; some **antiarrhythmics (disopyramide, lidocaine, mexiletine)**; many **antidepressants (amitriptyline, clomipramine, desipramine, imipramine, nortriptyline, nefazodone, sertraline, trazodone, fluoxetine, paroxetine, venlafaxine)**; some **antiemetics (dronabinol, ondansetron)**; some **beta blockers (metoprolol, pindolol, propranolol, timolol)**; many **calcium channel blockers (amlodipine, diltiazem, felodipine, isradipine, nicardipine, nifedipine, nimodipine, nisoldipine, verapamil)**; some **immunosuppressants (cyclosporine, tacrolimus)**; some **antipsychotics (chlorpromazine, haloperidol, perphenazine, risperidone, thioridazine)**; and also **atazanavir**, **darunavir**, **fosamprenavir**, **quinidine**, **saquinavir**, **tipranavir**, **bedaquiline**, **methamphetamine**, and **warfarin**; dosage ↓ may be necessary. May ↑ **vincristine** and **vinblastine** levels; consider holding or switching to another antiretroviral regimen that does not contain a CYP3A or P-glycoprotein inhibitor. May ↑ **dasatinib** and **nilotinib** levels; may need to ↓ doses of dasatinib and nilotinib. May ↑ **venetoclax** and **ibrutinib** levels and ↑ risk of tumor lysis syndrome; avoid concurrent use. May ↑ **abemaciclib** and **neratinib** levels and risk of toxicity; avoid concurrent use. May ↑ levels and risk of toxicity of **glecaprevir/pibrentasvir** and **sofosbuvir/velpatasvir/voxilaprevir**, **ombitasvir**, and **paritaprevir**; avoid concurrent use. May ↑ levels of systemic, inhaled, nasal, or ophthalmic **corticosteroids (betamethasone, budesonide, ciclesonide, dexamethasone, fluticasone, methylprednisolone, mometasone, prednisone**, or **triamcinolone**; consider alternative corticosteroid such as beclomethasone or prednisolone. ↓ levels and effects of **hormonal contraceptives**, **zidovudine**, **bupropion**, and **theophylline**; dose alteration or alternative therapy may be necessary. Levels may be ↑ by **clarithromycin** or **fluoxetine**. ↑ risk of heart block with **beta blockers**, **verapamil**, **diltiazem**, **digoxin**, or **atazanavir**. May ↑ concentrations of phosphodiesterase type 5 inhibitors (PDE5) causing hypotension, visual changes, priapism; ↓ starting doses not to exceed 25 mg within 48 hr for **sildenafil** (Viagra), 2.5 mg every 72 hr for **vardenafil** and 10 mg every 72 hr for **tadalafil**. May ↑ risk of adverse effects with **salmeterol**; concurrent use not recom-

R

mended. ↑ risk of myopathy with **atorvastatin** or **rosuvastatin**; use lowest possible dose of statin. May ↑ **bosentan** levels; initiate bosentan at 62.5 mg once daily or every other day; if patient already receiving bosentan, discontinue bosentan at least 36 hr before initiation of ritonavir and then restart bosentan at least 10 days later at 62.5 mg once daily or every other day. May ↑ **tadalafil (Adcirca)** levels; initiate tadalafil (Adcirca) at 20 mg once daily; if patient already receiving tadalafil (Adcirca), discontinue tadalafil (Adcirca) at least 24 hr before initiation of ritonavir and then restart tadalafil (Adcirca) at least 7 days later at 20 mg once daily. May ↑ **colchicine** levels; ↓ dose of colchicine; do not administer colchicine if patients have renal or hepatic impairment. May ↑ **quetiapine** levels; ↓ quetiapine dose to ⅙ of current dose. **Dexamethasone** may ↓ levels/effects; consider use of alternative corticosteroid, such as beclomethasone or prednisolone.

Drug-Natural Products: St. John's wort ↓ levels and may promote resistance; avoid concomitant use.

Drug-Food: Food ↑ absorption.

Route/Dosage

PO (Adults): 300 mg twice daily for 2–3 days, then 400 mg twice daily for 2–3 days, then 500 mg twice daily for 2–3 days, then 600 mg twice daily as maintenance.

PO (Children >1 mo): 250 mg/m^2 twice daily initially; ↑ by 50 mg/m^2 twice daily every 2–3 days up to 400 mg/m^2 twice daily (if unable to get up to 400 mg/m^2 twice daily, consider alternative antiretroviral therapy).

Availability (generic available)

Oral powder: 100 mg/pkt. **Oral solution (contains alcohol):** 80 mg/mL. **Tablets:** 100 mg.

NURSING IMPLICATIONS

Assessment

- Assess patient for change in severity of HIV symptoms and for symptoms of opportunistic infections during therapy.
- Assess patient for rash (mild to moderate rash usually occurs in the 2nd wk of therapy and resolves within 1–2 wk of continued therapy). If rash is severe (extensive erythematous or maculopapular rash with moist desquamation or angioedema) or accompanied by systemic symptoms (serum sickness-like reaction, Stevens-Johnson syndrome, toxic epidermal necrolysis), therapy must be discontinued immediately.
- ***Lab Test Considerations:*** Monitor viral load and CD4 counts regularly during therapy.
- Monitor for hyperglycemia, new onset diabetes mellitus, or an exacerbation of diabetes mellitus. May cause hyperglycemia.
- Monitor serum triglycerides and total cholesterol prior to and periodically during therapy. May cause ↑ serum AST, ALT, GGT, total bilirubin, CK, triglycerides, and uric acid concentrations.

Implementation

- Do not confuse ritonavir with Retrovir (zidovudine).
- **PO:** Administer with a meal or light snack.
- Oral powder may be mixed with apple sauce, vanilla pudding, water, chocolate milk, or infant formula. Oral solution may be mixed with chocolate milk, *Ensure*, or *Advera* within 1 hr of dosing to improve taste. Use calibrated oral dosing syringe for oral solution. Oral solution does not require refrigeration if used within 30 days and stored below 77°F in the original container. Keep cap tightly closed. Tablets should be swallowed whole; do not crush, break, or chew. Store tablets at room temperature.
- May be administered via feeding tubes compatible with ethanol and propylene glycol, such as silicone and polyvinyl chloride (PVC); do not use with polyurethane feeding tubes due to potential incompatibility.
- If nausea occurs on dose of 600 mg twice daily, may titrate by 300 mg twice daily for 1 day, then 400 mg twice daily for 2 days, then 500 mg twice daily for 1 day, then 600 mg twice daily thereafter.
- Patients initiating concurrent therapy with nucleoside analogues may have less GI intolerance by initiating ritonavir for 2 wk and then adding the nucleoside analogue.

Patient/Family Teaching

- Emphasize the importance of taking ritonavir as directed, at evenly spaced times throughout day. Do not take more than prescribed amount and do not stop taking without consulting health care professional. Take missed doses as soon as remembered; do not double doses.
- Instruct patient that ritonavir should not be shared with others.
- Advise patient to notify health care professional of all Rx or OTC medications, vitamins, or herbal products being taken and consult health care professional before taking any new medications, especially St. John's wort.
- Inform patient that ritonavir does not cure AIDS or prevent associated or opportunistic infections. Ritonavir does not reduce the risk of transmission of HIV to others through sexual contact or blood contamination. Caution patient to use a condom during sexual contact and to avoid sharing needles or donating blood to prevent spreading the AIDS virus to others. Advise patient that the long-term effects of ritonavir are unknown at this time.
- Inform patient that ritonavir may cause hyperglycemia. Advise patient to notify health care professional if increased thirst or hunger; unexplained weight loss; increased urination; fatigue; or dry, itchy skin occurs.
- Instruct patient to notify health care professional immediately if rash occurs.
- Inform patient that redistribution and accumulation of body fat may occur, causing central obesity, dor-

socervical fat enlargement (buffalo hump), peripheral wasting, breast enlargement, and cushingoid appearance. The cause and long-term effects are not known.

- Rep: Advise patient taking oral contraceptives to use a nonhormonal method of birth control during ritonavir therapy. If pregnancy is suspected notify health care professional promptly. Encourage pregnant women to enroll in the Antiretroviral Pregnancy Registry by calling 1-800-258-4263. Advise female patient to avoid breast feeding during therapy.
- Emphasize the importance of regular follow-up exams and blood counts to determine progress and monitor for side effects.

Evaluation/Desired Outcomes

- Delayed progression of AIDS and decreased opportunistic infections in patients with HIV.
- Decrease in viral load and improvement in CD4 cell counts.

riTUXimab (ri-tux-i-mab)

Rituxan, Ruxience, Truxima

Classification

Therapeutic: antineoplastics

Pharmacologic: monoclonal antibodies

Indications

Rituxan, Ruxience, and Truxima: Treatment of the following conditions: Relapsed or refractory, low-grade or follicular, CD20-positive, B-cell non-Hodgkin's lymphoma (NHL) (as monotherapy). Previously untreated follicular, CD20-positive, B-cell NHL in combination with first-line chemotherapy and, in patients achieving a complete or partial response to rituximab in combination with chemotherapy, as single-agent maintenance therapy. Non-progressing, low-grade, CD20-positive, B-cell NHL following treatment with cyclophosphamide, vincristine, and prednisone (as monotherapy). Previously untreated diffuse large B-cell, CD20–positive, NHL (in combination with CHOP or another anthracycline-based chemotherapy regimen). CD-20 positive chronic lymphocytic leukemia (CLL) (in combination with fludarabine and cyclophosphamide. **Rituxan and Ruxience:** Treatment of the following condition: Granulomatosis with polyangiitis (GPA) (Wegener's granulomatosis) and microscopic polyangiitis (MPA) (in combination with glucocorticoids). **Rituxan only:** Treatment of the following conditions: Moderately-to-severely active rheumatoid arthritis in patients who have had an inadequate response to ≥1 TNF antagonist therapies (with methotrexate), Moderate to severe pemphigus vulgaris.

Action

Binds to the CD20 antigen on the surface of lymphoma cells, preventing the activation process for cell cycle initiation and differentiation. **Therapeutic Effects:** Death of lymphoma cells. Prolonged progression-free survival in CLL. Reduced signs and symptoms of rheumatoid arthritis. Achievement of complete remission in GPA, MPA, and pemphigus vulgaris.

Pharmacokinetics

Absorption: IV administration results in complete bioavailability.

Distribution: Binds specifically to CD20 binding sites on lymphoma cells.

Metabolism and Excretion: Unknown.

Half-life: 59.8–174 hr (depending on tumor burden).

TIME/ACTION PROFILE (B-cell depletion)

ROUTE	ONSET	PEAK	DURATION
IV	within 14 days	3–4 wk	6–9 mo†

†Duration of depletion after 4 wk of treatment.

Contraindications/Precautions

Contraindicated in: Hypersensitivity to murine (mouse) proteins; OB: Can pass placental barrier potentially causing fetal B-cell depletion. Give only if clearly needed; Lactation: Potential for immunosuppression in infant. Discontinue nursing.

Use Cautiously in: Pre-existing bone marrow depression; Hepatitis B infection (may reactivate infection during and for several mo after treatment); Systemic lupus erythematosus (may cause fatal progressive multifocal leukoencephalopathy); HIV infection (may increase risk of HIV-associated lymphoma); Rep: Women of reproductive potential; Pedi: Safety and effectiveness only established for children ≥2 yr with GPA or MPA.

Adverse Reactions/Side Effects

CNS: PROGRESSIVE MULTIFOCAL LEUKOENCEPHALOPATHY, headache. **CV:** ARRHYTHMIAS, hypotension, peripheral edema. **Derm:** MUCOCUTANEOUS SKIN REACTIONS, flushing, urticaria. **Endo:** hyperglycemia. **F and E:** hypocalcemia. **GI:** HEPATITIS B REACTIVATION, abdominal pain, altered taste, dyspepsia. **GU:** renal failure. **Hemat:** ANEMIA, NEUTROPENIA, THROMBOCYTOPENIA. **MS:** arthralgia, back pain. **Resp:** bronchospasm, cough, dyspnea. **Misc:** HYPERSENSITIVITY REACTIONS (including anaphylaxis and angioedema), INFUSION REACTIONS, TUMOR LYSIS SYNDROME, fever/chills/rigors (infusion related), infection.

Interactions

Drug-Drug: May ↓ antibody response to or ↑ risk of adverse reactions to **live vaccines**; avoid use during treatment; inactive vaccines should be administered ≥4 wk prior to start of therapy.

Route/Dosage

Relapsed or Refractory, Low-Grade or Follicular, CD20-Positive, B-Cell NHL

IV (Adults): 375 mg/m² once weekly for 4 or 8 doses; may retreat with 375 mg/m² once weekly for 4 doses.

Previously Untreated Follicular, CD20–Positive, B-Cell NHL

IV (Adults): 375 mg/m² given on Day 1 of each cycle of CVP for up to 8 doses; if patients experience complete or partial response, give 375 mg/m² (as monotherapy) every 8 wk for 12 doses (initiate this maintenance therapy 8 wk after completion of rituximab + CVP regimen).

Non-Progressing Low-Grade, CD20-Positive, B-Cell NHL

IV (Adults): For patients who have not progressed following 6–8 cycles of CVP chemotherapy, 375 mg/m² given once weekly for 4 doses given every 6 mo for up to 16 doses.

Diffuse Large B-Cell NHL

IV (Adults): 375 mg/m² given on Day 1 of each cycle of chemotherapy for up to 8 infusions.

CLL

IV (Adults): 375 mg/m² given on the day before initiating FC chemotherapy, then 500 mg/m² on Day 1 of cycles 2–6 (every 28 days).

Rheumatoid Arthritis

IV (Adults): 1000 mg every 2 wk for 2 doses; subsequent courses should be administered every 24 wk (not sooner than every 16 wk).

GPA and MPA

IV (Adults): *Induction treatment*—375 mg/m² once weekly for 4 wk; *Follow-up treatment in patients who have achieved disease control with induction treatment*—500 mg every 2 wk for 2 doses (should be started 16–24 wk after last rituximab induction dose; if achieved disease control with another agent, start follow-up treatment within 4 wk after last induction dose of that agent), then 500 mg every 6 mo thereafter.
IV (Children ≥2 yr): *Induction treatment*—375 mg/m² once weekly for 4 wk; *Follow-up treatment in patients who have achieved disease control with induction treatment*—250 mg/m² every 2 wk for 2 doses (should be started 16–24 wk after last rituximab induction dose; if achieved disease control with another agent, start follow-up treatment within 4 wk after last induction dose of that agent), then 250 mg/m² every 6 mo thereafter.

Pemphigus Vulgaris

IV (Adults): 1000 mg every 2 wk for 2 doses, then maintenance dose of 500 mg infusion at month 12 and then every 6 mo thereafter. Upon relapse, administer 1000 mg.

Availability

Solution for injection (requires dilution): 10 mg/mL.

NURSING IMPLICATIONS

Assessment

- Monitor patient for fever, chills/rigors, nausea, urticaria, fatigue, headache, pruritus, bronchospasm, dyspnea, sensation of tongue or throat swelling, rhinitis, vomiting, hypotension, flushing, and pain at disease sites. Infusion-related events occur frequently within 30 min–2 hr of beginning 1st infusion and may resolve with slowing or discontinuing infusion and treatment with IV saline, diphenhydramine, and acetaminophen. Patients with increased risk (females, patients with pulmonary infiltrates, chronic lymphocytic leukemia, or mantle cell leukemia) may have more severe reactions, which may be fatal. Signs of severe reactions include hypotension, angioedema, hypoxia, or bronchospasm and may require interruption of infusion. May result in pulmonary infiltrates, adult respiratory distress syndrome, MI, ventricular fibrillation, and cardiogenic shock. Monitor closely. Incidence decreases with subsequent infusions.
- Monitor patient for tumor lysis syndrome due to rapid reduction in tumor volume (acute renal failure, hyperkalemia, hypocalcemia, hyperuricemia, or hypophosphatemia) usually occurring 12–24 hr after 1st infusion. Risks are higher in patients with greater tumor burden; may be fatal. Correct electrolyte abnormalities, monitor renal function and fluid balance, and administer supportive care, including dialysis, as indicated.
- Assess patient for hypersensitivity reactions (hypotension, bronchospasm, angioedema) during administration. May respond to decrease in infusion rate. Premedication with diphenhydramine and acetaminophen is recommended. Treatment includes diphenhydramine, acetaminophen, bronchodilators, or IV saline as indicated. Epinephrine, antihistamines, and corticosteroids should be readily available in the event of a severe reaction. If severe reactions occur, discontinue infusion; may be resumed at 50% of the rate when symptoms have resolved completely.
- Monitor ECG during and immediately after infusion in patients with pre-existing cardiac conditions (arrhythmias, angina) or patients who have developed arrhythmias during previous infusions of rituximab. Life-threatening arrhythmias may occur.
- Assess for signs of progressive multifocal leukoencephalopathy (hemiparesis, apathy, confusion, cognitive deficiencies, and ataxia) periodically during therapy.
- Assess for infection during and for 1 yr after therapy. Bacterial, fungal, and new or reactivated viral infections may occur. Screen patient for hepatitis B infec-

tion prior to therapy. Discontinue rituximab and any concomitant chemotherapy in patients who develop viral hepatitis or other serious infections, and institute appropriate treatment.

- Assess for mucocutaneous reactions periodically during therapy. May cause Stevens-Johnson syndrome and toxic epidermal necrolysis. Discontinue therapy if severe or if accompanied with fever, general malaise, fatigue, muscle or joint aches, blisters, oral lesions, conjunctivitis, hepatitis, and/or eosinophilia.
- ***Lab Test Considerations:*** Monitor CBC and platelet count regularly during therapy and frequently in patients with blood dyscrasias. May cause anemia, thrombocytopenia, or neutropenia.
- Frequently causes B-cell depletion with an associated ↓ in serum immunoglobulins in a minority of patients; does not appear to cause an increased incidence of infection.
- Obtain HBsAg and anti-HBc to screen patient for HBV infection before initiating therapy. May cause reactivation of hepatitis B up to 24 mo after therapy.

Implementation

- Do not confuse rituximab with infliximab.
- Transient hypotension may occur during infusion; antihypertensive medications may be held for 12 hr before infusion.
- **Rheumatoid Arthritis:** Administer 100 mg methylprednisolone IV or equivalent 30 min prior to each infusion to minimize infusion reactions.
- **GPA and MPA:** Administer methylprednisolone 1000 mg IV per day for 1 to 3 days followed by oral prednisone 1 mg/kg/day (not to exceed 80 mg/day and tapered per clinical need) to treat severe vasculitis symptoms. Begin regimen within 14 days prior to or with the initiation of rituximab and may continue during and after the 4 wk course of rituximab treatment.
- Prophylaxis against *Pneumocystis jiroveci* pneumonia and herpes virus recommended during treatment and for up to 12 mo following treatment as appropriate for patients with CLL, and during and for at least 6 mo following last rituximab infusion for patients with WG and MPA.

IV Administration

- **Intermittent Infusion:** ***Diluent:*** Dilute with 0.9% NaCl or D5W. ***Concentration:*** 1–4 mg/mL. Gently invert bag to mix. Solution is clear and colorless; do not administer solutions that are discolored or contain particulate matter. Discard unused portion remaining in vial. Solution is stable for 12 hr at room temperature and for 24 hr if refrigerated. ***Rate:*** Do not administer as an IV push or bolus.
- *First infusion:* Administer at an initial rate of 50 mg/hr. If hypersensitivity or infusion-related events do not occur, rate may be escalated in 50-mg/hr increments every 30 min to a maximum of 400 mg/hr.
- *Subsequent infusions:* May be administered at an initial rate of 100 mg/hr and increased by 100-mg/hr increments at 30-min intervals to a maximum of 400 mg/hr.
- For previously untreated non-Hodgkins lymphoma and B-cell non-Hodgkin's lymphoma, if no Grade 3 or 4 infusion-related reactions occurred in Cycle 1, may administer via 90-min infusion using glucocorticoids. Begin at rate of 20% of dose over 30 min, with remaining 80% dose over 60 min. If tolerated, then can be used for remainder of therapy.
- **Y-Site Compatibility:** acyclovir, amifostine, amikacin, aminophylline, ampicillin, ampicillin/sulbactam, aztreonam, bleomycin, bumetanide, buprenorphine, busulfan, butorphanol, calcium gluconate, carboplatin, carmustine, cefazolin, cefotaxime, cefotetan, cefoxitin, ceftazidime, ceftriaxone, cefuroxime, chlorpromazine, cisplatin, clindamycin, cyclophosphamide, cytarabine, dactinomycin, daunorubicin hydrochloride, dexamethasone sodium phosphate, dexrazoxane, digoxin, diphenhydramine, dobutamine, docetaxel, dopamine, doxorubicin liposome, doxycycline, droperidol, enalaprilat, etoposide phosphate, famotidine, fentanyl, filgrastim, floxuridine, fluconazole, fludarabine, fluorouracil, ganciclovir, gemcitabine, gentamicin, granisetron, haloperidol, heparin, hydrocortisone, hydromorphone, idarubicin, ifosfamide, imipenem/cilastatin, irinotecan, leucovorin calcium, levorphanol, lorazepam, magnesium sulfate, mannitol, meperidine, mesna, methotrexate, methylprednisolone, metoclopramide, metronidazole, mitomycin, mitoxantrone, morphine, nalbuphine, paclitaxel, pentamidine, piperacillin/tazobactam, potassium chloride, prochlorperazine, promethazine, ranitidine, sargramostim, streptozocin, theophylline, thiotepa, tobramycin, trimethoprim/sulfamethoxazole, vinblastine, vincristine, vinorelbine, zidovudine.
- **Y-Site Incompatibility:** aldesleukin, amphotericin B deoxycholate, ciprofloxacin, cyclosporine, doxorubicin hydrochloride, furosemide, levofloxacin, minocycline, ondansetron, quinapristin/dalfopristin, sodium bicarbonate, topotecan, vancomycin.
- **Additive Incompatibility:** Do not admix with other medications.

Patient/Family Teaching

- Inform patient of the purpose of the medication. Advise patient to read the *Medication Guide* prior to starting therapy and before each infusion in case of changes.
- Advise patient to report infusion-related events or symptoms of hypersensitivity reactions immediately.
- Instruct patient to notify health care professional promptly if fever; chills; cough; hoarseness; sore

R

throat; signs of infection; lower back or side pain; painful or difficult urination; bleeding gums; bruising; petechiae; blood in stools, urine, or emesis; increased fatigue; dyspnea; orthostatic hypotension; or painful ulcers or sores on your skin, lips, or in mouth, blisters, peeling skin, rash, pustule occurs. Caution patient to avoid crowds and persons with known infections. Instruct patient to use soft toothbrush and electric razor and to avoid falls. Caution patient not to drink alcoholic beverages or take medication containing aspirin or NSAIDs; may precipitate gastric bleeding.

- Advise patient to consult health care professional prior to receiving any vaccinations.
- Rep: Advise females of reproductive potential to use effective contraception during therapy and for 12 mo following therapy, and to avoid breast feeding during and for at least 6 mo after last dose. Observe newborns and infants of women taking rituximab during pregnancy for signs of infection.

Evaluation/Desired Outcomes

- Decrease in spread of malignancy.
- Reduced signs and symptoms of rheumatoid arthritis.
- Achievement of complete remission in GPA and MPA.

rivaroxaban (ri-va-**rox**-a-ban)

Xarelto

Classification

Therapeutic: anticoagulants

Pharmacologic: antithrombotics, factor Xa inhibitors

Indications

Prevention of deep vein thrombosis that may lead to pulmonary embolism (PE) following knee or hip replacement surgery. Reduction in risk of stroke/systemic embolism in patients with nonvalvular atrial fibrillation (AF). Treatment of deep vein thrombosis (DVT) or PE. Reduction in risk of recurrence of DVT and/or PE in patients at continued risk for recurrent DVT or PE after completion of initial treatment for at least 6 mo. Reduction in risk of major cardiovascular events (cardiovascular death, MI, and stroke) in patients with chronic coronary artery disease or peripheral arterial disease (in combination with aspirin).

Action

Acts as selective factor X inhibitor that blocks the active site of factor Xa, inactivating the cascade of coagulation. **Therapeutic Effects:** Treatment and prevention of thromboembolic events and major cardiovascular events.

Pharmacokinetics

Absorption: Well absorbed (80%) following oral administration; absorption occurs in the stomach and ↓ as it enters the small intestine.

Distribution: Unknown.

Metabolism and Excretion: 51% metabolized by the liver; 36% excreted unchanged in urine. Metabolites do not have anticoagulant activity.

Half-life: 5–9 hr.

TIME/ACTION PROFILE (anticoagulant effect)

ROUTE	ONSET	PEAK	DURATION
PO	unknown	2–4 hr†	24 hr

†Blood levels.

Contraindications/Precautions

Contraindicated in: Hypersensitivity; Active major bleeding; Severe renal impairment (CCr <30 mL/min [DVT/PE treatment or prevention]) Prosthetic heart valves; Moderate to severe hepatic impairment (Child-Pugh B or C) or any liver pathology resulting in altered coagulation; PE with hemodynamic instability or requiring thrombolysis or pulmonary embolectomy; Concurrent use of drugs that are combined P-gp inducers/strong CYP3A4 inducers or combined P-gp inhibitors/strong CYP3A4 inhibitors; Antiphospholipid syndrome; Lactation: Avoid breast feeding.

Use Cautiously in: Neuroaxial spinal anesthesia or spinal puncture, especially if concurrent with an indwelling epidural catheter, drugs affecting hemostasis, history of traumatic/repeated spinal puncture or spinal deformity (↑ risk of spinal hematoma); Use of feeding tube (proper placement of tube must be documented to ensure absorption); OB: Use only if potential benefit outweighs potential risk.

Adverse Reactions/Side Effects

CNS: syncope. **Derm:** blister, pruritus. **Hemat:** BLEEDING. **Local:** wound secretion. **MS:** extremity pain, muscle spasm.

Interactions

Drug-Drug: Rivaroxaban acts as a substrate of these subsets of the CYP450 enzyme system: CYP3A4/5, CYP2J2, and ATP-binding cassette G2 (ABCG2). Drugs that inhibit or induce these systems may alter effectiveness. Concurrent use of drugs that are combined P-gp inhibitors/strong CYP3A4 inhibitors, including **ketoconazole**, **itraconazole**, **lopinavir/ritonavir**, **ritonavir**, **indinavir**, and **conivaptan** may ↑ levels; avoid concomitant use. Concurrent use of drugs that are combined P-gp inducers/strong CYP3A4 inducers, including **carbamazepine**, **phenytoin**, or **rifampin** may ↓ levels; avoid concomitant use. Concurrent use of drugs that are combined P-gp inhibitors/moderate CYP3A4 inhibitors, including **erythromycin** in patients with renal impairment (CCr 15–79 mL/min) may ↑ levels; avoid concomitant use. ↑ risk of bleeding with other **anticoagulants**, **aspirin**, **clopidogrel**, **tica-**

grelor, prasugrel, fibrinolytics, NSAIDs, SNRIs, or SSRIs.

Drug-Natural Products: **St. John's wort** may ↓ levels; avoid concomitant use.

Route/Dosage

Prevention of Deep Vein Thrombosis Following Knee or Hip Replacement Surgery

PO (Adults): 10 mg once daily, initiated 6–10 hr postoperatively (when hemostasis is achieved) continued for 35 days after hip replacement or 12 days after knee replacement.

Reduction in Risk of Stroke/Systemic Embolism in Nonvalvular Atrial Fibrillation

PO (Adults): 20 mg once daily with evening meal.

Renal Impairment

PO (Adults): *CCr ≤50 mL/min*—15 mg once daily with evening meal.

Treatment of Deep Vein Thrombosis or Pulmonary Embolism

PO (Adults): 15 mg twice daily for 21 days, then 20 mg once daily for remainder of treatment period.

Reduction in Risk of Recurrent Deep Vein Thrombosis and/or Pulmonary Embolism in Patients at Continued Risk for Recurrent Deep Vein Thrombosis and/or Pulmonary Embolism

PO (Adults): 10 mg once daily to be initiated after ≥6 mo of standard anticoagulant treatment.

Reduction in Risk of Major Cardiovascular Events in Patients with Chronic Coronary Artery Disease or Peripheral Arterial Disease

PO (Adults): 2.5 mg twice daily.

Availability

Tablets: 2.5 mg, 10 mg, 15 mg, 20 mg.

NURSING IMPLICATIONS

Assessment

- Assess for signs of bleeding and hemorrhage (bleeding gums; nosebleed; unusual bruising; black, tarry stools; hematuria; fall in hematocrit or BP; guaiac-positive stools); bleeding from surgical site. Notify health care professional if these occur. May use prothrombin concentrate complex, activated prothrombin complex concentrate or recombinant factor VIIa attempt to reverse life-threatening bleeding; efficacy and safety studies have not been done.
- Monitor patients with epidural catheters frequently for signs and symptoms of neurologic impairment (midline back pain, sensory and motor deficits [numbness, tingling, weakness in lower limbs], bowel and/or bladder dysfunction). Epidural catheter should not be removed earlier than 18 hr in young patients aged 20–45 yrs and 26 hrs in elderly patients aged 60–76 yrs after last administration of rivaroxaban; next dose should be at least 6 hr after catheter removal.
- ***Lab Test Considerations:*** May cause ↑ serum AST, ALT, total bilirubin, and GGT levels.
- Monitor renal function periodically during therapy.
- ***Toxicity and Overdose:*** Antidote is andexanet alfa; effects persist for at least 24 hr after last dose. Other agents and hemodialysis do not have a significant effect. Consider using prothrombin complex concentrate (PCC) or Factor VIIa.

Implementation

- *When switching from warfarin to rivaroxaban,* discontinue warfarin and start rivaroxaban as soon as INR <3.0 to avoid periods of inadequate anticoagulation. *When switching from anticoagulants other than warfarin to rivaroxaban,* start rivaroxaban 0–2 hr prior to next scheduled evening dose and omit dose of other anticoagulant. For continuous heparin, discontinue heparin and administer rivaroxaban at same time. *When switching from rivaroxaban to warfarin or other anticoagulants,* no data is available. May discontinue rivaroxaban and begin both parenteral anticoagulant and warfarin at time of next rivaroxaban dose.
- Discontinue at least 24 hr prior to surgery and other interventions. Restart as soon as hemostasis has been re-established.
- If rivaroxaban must be discontinued for other than bleeding, consider replacing with another anticoagulant; discontinuation increases risk of thrombotic events.
- **PO:** *Prophylaxis of DVT following surgery:* Administer 1st dose 6–10 hr after surgery, once hemostasis has been established. 10-mg tablet may be administered without regard to food; 15-mg and 20-mg tablet should be taken with food.
- If unable to swallow tablet, 15-mg and 20-mg tablets may be crushed, mixed with applesauce, and administered immediately after mixing. Follow dose immediately with food. Tablets are stable in applesauce for up to 4 hr.
- If administering crushed tablet via GI feeding tube, check placement of tube. Rivaroxaban is absorbed from the GI tract, not the small intestine. Suspend crushed tablet in 50 mL water and administer. Follow administration of 15-mg or 20-mg tablet immediately with food.
- Crushed tablets are stable in water or applesauce for up to 4 hr.
- *Reduction in Risk of Stroke in Nonvalvular Atrial Fibrillation:* Administer with evening meal.

R

- *Treatment of DVT and/or PE:* Administer with food, at the same time each day.
- *Reduction in the Risk of Recurrence of DVT and/ or PE in patients at continued risk for DVT and/or PE, Prophylaxis of VTE in Acutely Ill Medical Patients at Risk for Thromboembolic Complications Not at High Risk of Bleeding, or Reduction of Risk of Major Cardiovascular Events (CV Death, MI, and Stroke) in Chronic CAD or PAD:* Administer without regard for food.

Patient/Family Teaching

- Instruct patient to take medication as directed. Take missed doses as soon as remembered that day. If taking 2.5 mg twice daily, take a single 2.5 mg dose at next scheduled dose. If taking 15 mg twice daily, may take two 15-mg tablets to achieve 30 mg daily dose, then return to regular schedule. If taking 10 mg, 15 mg, or 20 mg once daily, take missed dose immediately; do not double dose. Inform health care professional of missed doses at time of checkup or lab tests. Inform patients that anticoagulant effect may persist for 2–5 days following discontinuation. Advise patient to read the *Medication Guide* before starting therapy and with each Rx refill in case of changes. Caution patients not to discontinue medication early without consulting health care professional.
- Advise patient to report any symptoms of unusual bleeding or bruising (bleeding gums; nosebleed; black, tarry stools; hematuria; excessive menstrual flow) and symptoms of spinal or epidural hematoma (tingling; numbness, especially in lower extremities; muscular weakness) to health care professional immediately.
- Instruct patient not to drink alcohol or take other Rx, OTC, or herbal products, especially those containing aspirin, NSAIDs, or St. John's wort, or to start or stop any new medications during rivaroxaban therapy without advice of health care professional.
- Advise females of reproductive potential to notify health care professional if pregnancy is planned or suspected, or if breast feeding. Monitor for bleed in fetus and/or neonate of women taking rivaroxaban during pregnancy.

Evaluation/Desired Outcomes

- Prevention of blood clots and subsequent pulmonary emboli following knee/hip replacement surgery. Duration of treatment is 35 days for patients with hip replacement and 12 days for patients with knee replacement surgery.

rivastigmine (rye-va-**stig**-meen)

Exelon

Classification

Therapeutic: anti-Alzheimer's agents
Pharmacologic: cholinergics (cholinesterase inhibitors)

Indications

PO: Mild to moderate dementia associated with Alzheimer's disease. **Transdermal:** Treatment of mild, moderate, or severe dementia associated with Alzheimer's disease and mild to moderate dementia associated with Parkinson's disease.

Action

Enhances cholinergic function by reversible inhibition of cholinesterase. Does not cure the disease. **Therapeutic Effects:** Decreased dementia (temporary) associated with Alzheimer's disease and Parkinson's disease. Enhanced cognitive ability.

Pharmacokinetics

Absorption: Well absorbed following oral administration. Transdermal patch is slowly absorbed over 8 hr.

Distribution: Widely distributed.

Metabolism and Excretion: Rapidly and extensively metabolized by the liver; metabolites are excreted by the kidneys.

Half-life: *PO*—1.5 hr; *Transdermal*—24 hr.

TIME/ACTION PROFILE (improvement in dementia)

ROUTE	ONSET	PEAK	DURATION
PO	within 2 wk	up to 12 wk	unknown
Transdermal	unknown	unknown	unknown

Contraindications/Precautions

Contraindicated in: Hypersensitivity to rivastigmine or other carbamates; History of application site reactions with transdermal product suggestive of allergic contact dermatitis.

Use Cautiously in: History of asthma or obstructive pulmonary disease; History of GI bleeding; Sick sinus syndrome or other supraventricular cardiac conduction abnormalities; Moderate or severe renal impairment (dose ↓ may be needed); Mild or moderate hepatic impairment (dose ↓ may be needed); Patients weighing <50 kg; at risk for ↑ adverse reactions (dose ↓ may be needed); OB: Safety not established; Lactation: Use during breast feeding only if benefit to patient outweighs potential risk to infant; Pedi: Safety and effectiveness not established.

Adverse Reactions/Side Effects

CNS: weakness, dizziness, drowsiness, headache, sedation (unusual). **CV:** edema, heart failure, hypotension. **Derm:** allergic dermatitis. **GI:** anorexia, dyspepsia, nausea, vomiting, abdominal pain, diarrhea, flatulence. **Local:** application reactions (for transdermal patch only). **Metab:** weight gain (unusual), weight loss. **Neuro:** tremor. **Misc:** fever.

Interactions

Drug-Drug: Nicotine may ↑ metabolism and ↓ levels.

Route/Dosage

PO (Adults): 1.5 mg twice daily initially; after at least 2 wk, dose may be ↑ to 3 mg twice daily. Further increments may be made at 2-wk intervals up to 6 mg twice daily.

Transdermal (Adults): *Initial Dose*—4.6 mg/24-hr transdermal patch intially; ↑ to 9.5 mg/24-hr transdermal patch after at least 4 wk; may ↑ to 13.3 mg/24-hr transdermal patch if needed (is recommended effective dose for patients with severe Alzheimer's disease).

Hepatic Impairment

Transdermal (Adults): *Mild-moderate hepatic impairment*—Do not exceed dose of 4.6 mg/24 hr.

Availability (generic available)

Capsules: 1.5 mg, 3 mg, 4.5 mg, 6 mg. **Transdermal patch:** 4.6 mg/24 hr, 9.5 mg/24 hr, 13.3 mg/24 hr.

NURSING IMPLICATIONS

Assessment

- Assess cognitive function (memory, attention, reasoning, language, ability to perform simple tasks) periodically throughout therapy.
- Monitor patient for nausea, vomiting, anorexia, and weight loss. Notify health care professional if these side effects occur.
- Monitor for hypersensitivity skin reactions; may occur after oral or transdermal administration. If allergic contact dermatitis is suspected after transdermal use, may switch to oral rivastigmine after negative allergy testing. If disseminated hypersensitivity reaction of the skin occurs, discontinue therapy.

Implementation

- Patients switching from oral doses of <6 mg to transdermal doses should use 4.6 mg/24 hr patch. Patients taking oral doses of 6–12 mg may be converted directly to 9.5 mg/24 hr patch. Apply patch on the day following the last oral dose.
- **PO:** Administer in the morning and evening with food.
- **Transdermal:** Apply patch to clean, dry, hairless area that will not be rubbed by tight clothing. Upper or lower back is recommended, may also use upper arm or chest. Do not apply to red, irritated, or cut skin. Rotate sites to prevent irritation, do not use same site within 14 days. Remove adhesive liner and apply by pressing patch firmly until edges stick well. May be worn during bathing and hot weather. Each 24 hr, remove old patch and discard by folding in half and apply new patch to a new area.

Patient/Family Teaching

- **PO:** Emphasize the importance of taking rivastigmine at regular intervals as directed.
- Caution patient and caregiver that rivastigmine may cause dizziness. Caution patient to avoid driving or other activities requiring alertness until response to medication is known.
- Advise patient and caregiver to notify health care professional if nausea, vomiting, anorexia, or weight loss occur. If adverse effects become intolerable during treatment with *transdermal patch,* instruct patient to discontinue patches for several days and then restart at same or next lower dose level. If treatment is interrupted for more than several days, lowest dose level should be used when restarting and titrate according to Route and Dosage section.
- Advise patient and caregiver to notify health care professional of medication regimen prior to treatment or surgery.
- Inform patient and caregiver that improvement in cognitive functioning may take wk to mo and that the degenerative process is not reversed.
- Advise patient to notify health care professional if pregnancy is planned or suspected, or if breast feeding.
- **Transdermal:** Instruct patient and caregiver on the correct application, rotation, and discarding of patch. Patch should be folded in half and discarded out of reach of children and pets; medication remains in discarded patch. Replace missed doses immediately and apply next patch at usual time. Advise patient and caregiver to avoid contact with eyes and to wash hands after applying patch. Avoid exposure to heat sources (excessive sunlight, saunas, heating pads) for long periods.
- Advise patient and caregiver to notify health care professional if skin reactions occur.
- Advise patient referred for MRI test to discuss patch with referring health care professional and MRI facility to determine if removal of patch is necessary prior to test and for directions for replacing patch.

Evaluation/Desired Outcomes

- Temporary improvement in cognitive function (memory, attention, reasoning, language, ability to perform simple tasks) in patients with Alzheimer's disease.
- Improvement in cognitive function and overall functioning in patients with Parkinson's disease.

R

rizatriptan (riz-a-**trip**-tan)

Maxalt, Maxalt-MLT

Classification

Therapeutic: vascular headache suppressants

Pharmacologic: 5-HT_1 agonists

Indications

Acute treatment of migraine with or without aura.

Action

Acts as an agonist at specific 5-HT_1 receptor sites in intracranial blood vessels and sensory trigeminal nerves.

Therapeutic Effects: Cranial vessel vasoconstriction with associated decrease in release of neuropeptides and resultant decrease in migraine headache.

Pharmacokinetics

Absorption: Completely absorbed after oral administration, but first-pass metabolism results in 45% bioavailability.

Distribution: Unknown.

Metabolism and Excretion: Primarily metabolized by monoamine oxidase-A (MAO-A); minor conversion to an active compound; 14% excreted unchanged in urine.

Half-life: 2–3 hr.

TIME/ACTION PROFILE (blood levels)

ROUTE	ONSET	PEAK	DURATION
PO	30 min	1–1.5 hr	unknown

Contraindications/Precautions

Contraindicated in: Hypersensitivity; Ischemic or vasospastic cardiovascular, cerebrovascular, or peripheral vascular syndromes; History of significant cardiovascular disease; Uncontrolled hypertension; Should not be used within 24 hr of other 5-HT_1 agonists or ergot-type compounds (dihydroergotamine); Basilar or hemiplegic migraine; Concurrent MAO-A inhibitor therapy or within 2 wk of discontinuing MAO-A inhibitor therapy; Phenylketonuria (orally disintegrating tablet contains aspartame).

Use Cautiously in: Severe renal impairment, especially in patients on dialysis; Moderate hepatic impairment; OB, Lactation, Pedi: Pregnancy, lactation, or children <6 yr (safety not established).

Exercise Extreme Caution in: Cardiovascular risk factors (hypertension, hypercholesterolemia, cigarette smoking, obesity, diabetes, strong family history, menopausal women or men >40 yr); use only if cardiovascular status has been evaluated and determined to be safe and 1st dose is administered under supervision.

Adverse Reactions/Side Effects

CNS: dizziness, drowsiness, weakness. **CV:** CORONARY ARTERY VASOSPASM, MI, VENTRICULAR ARRHYTHMIAS, chest pain, myocardial ischemia. **GI:** dry mouth, nausea. **Misc:** hypersensitivity reactions including ANGIOEDEMA, toxic epidermal necrolysis, pain.

Interactions

Drug-Drug: Concurrent use with **MAO-A inhibitors** ↑ levels and adverse reactions (concurrent use or use within 2 wk of MAO inhibitor is contraindicated). Concurrent use with other **5-HT agonists** or **ergot-type compounds (dihydroergotamine)** may result in ↑ vasoactive properties (avoid use within 24 hr of each other). **Propranolol** ↑ levels and risk of adverse reactions (↓ dose of rizatriptan; rizatriptan not recommended in children <40 kg). ↑ risk of serotonin syndrome when used with **SSRI or SNRI antidepressants**.

Drug-Natural Products: ↑ risk of serotinergic side effects including serotonin syndrome with **St. John's wort** and **SAMe**.

Route/Dosage

PO (Adults): 5–10 mg (use 5-mg dose in patients receiving propranolol); may be repeated in 2 hr; not to exceed 3 doses/24 hr.

PO (Children 6–17 yr): *≥40 kg*—10 mg single dose (use 5-mg dose in patients receiving propranolol); *<40 kg*—5 mg single dose (do NOT use in patients receiving propranolol).

Availability (generic available)

Tablets: 5 mg, 10 mg. **Orally disintegrating tablets (Maxalt-MLT) (peppermint flavor):** 5 mg, 10 mg.

NURSING IMPLICATIONS

Assessment

- Assess pain location, character, intensity, and duration and associated symptoms (photophobia, phonophobia, nausea, vomiting) during migraine attack.
- Assess for serotonin syndrome (mental changes [agitation, hallucinations, coma], autonomic instability [tachycardia, labile BP, hyperthermia], neuromuscular aberations [hyper reflexia, incoordination], and/or GI symptoms [nausea, vomiting, diarrhea]), especially in patients taking other serotonergic drugs (SSRIs, SNRIs).

Implementation

- **PO:** Tablets should be swallowed whole with liquid.
- Orally disintegrating tablets should be left in the package until use. Remove from the blister pouch. Do not push tablet through the blister; peel open the blister pack with dry hands and place tablet on tongue. Tablet will dissolve rapidly and be swallowed with saliva. No liquid is needed to take the orally disintegrating tablet.

Patient/Family Teaching

- Inform patient that rizatriptan should be used only during a migraine attack. It is meant to be used for relief of migraine attacks but not to prevent or reduce the number of attacks.
- Instruct patient to administer rizatriptan as soon as symptoms of a migraine attack appear, but it may be administered at any time during an attack. If migraine symptoms return, a 2nd dose may be used. Allow at least 2 hr between doses, and do not use more than 30 mg in any 24-hr period.
- If 1st dose does not relieve headache, additional rizatriptan doses are not likely to be effective; notify health care professional.
- Caution patient not to take rizatriptan within 24 hr of other vascular headache suppressants.

- Advise patient that lying down in a darkened room after rizatriptan administration may further help relieve headache.
- Advise patient that overuse (use more than 10 days/mo) may lead to exacerbation of headache (migraine-like daily headaches, or as a marked increase in frequency of migraine attacks). May require gradual withdrawal of rizatriptan and treatment of symptoms (transient worsening of headache).
- Advise patient to notify health care professional before next dose of rizatriptan if pain or tightness in the chest occurs during use. If pain is severe or does not subside, notify health care professional immediately. If feelings of tingling, heat, flushing, heaviness, pressure, drowsiness, dizziness, tiredness, or sickness develop, discuss with health care professional at next visit.
- May cause dizziness or drowsiness. Caution patient to avoid driving or other activities requiring alertness until response to medication is known.
- Advise patient to avoid alcohol, which aggravates headaches, during rizatriptan use.
- Advise patient to notify health care professional immediately if signs or symptoms of serotonin syndrome occur.
- Caution female patient to avoid rizatriptan if pregnant or breast feeding, or if pregnancy is suspected or planned. Adequate contraception should be used during therapy.

Evaluation/Desired Outcomes

- Relief of migraine attack.

rolapitant (rol-ap-i-tant)

Varubi

Classification

Therapeutic: antiemetics

Pharmacologic: neurokinin antagonists

Indications

To prevent delayed nausea and vomiting associated with initial/repeat courses of emetogenic cancer chemotherapy (to be used with dexamethasone and a 5–HT_3 antagonist).

Action

Acts as a selective antagonist at substance P/neurokinin 1 (NK_1) receptors in the brain. **Therapeutic Effects:** Decreased nausea and vomiting associated with chemotherapy. Augments the antiemetic effects of dexamethasone and 5-HT_3 antagonists.

Pharmacokinetics

Absorption: Well absorbed following oral administration.

Distribution: Extensively distributed to tissues.

Protein Binding: 99.8%.

Metabolism and Excretion: Mostly metabolized, primarily by CYP3A4; one metabolite, C4–pyrrolidine-hydroxylated rolapitant (M19) has antiemetic activity. Excretion is mainly via hepato/biliary elimination. 14% excreted in urine (8% as metabolites), 73% in feces (38% as unchanged drug).

Half-life: *Rolapitant*—7 days; *M19*—7 days.

TIME/ACTION PROFILE (blood levels)

ROUTE	ONSET	PEAK	DURATION
PO	within 30 min	4 hr	unknown

Contraindications/Precautions

Contraindicated in: Concurrent use of CYP2D6 substrates with a narrow therapeutic index.

Use Cautiously in: Concurrent use of other CYP2D6 substrates; Severe hepatic impairment (avoid if possible; if unavoidable, monitor carefully); OB: Safety not established; Lactation: Weigh maternal benefits against risks to the infant; Pedi: Safety and effectiveness not established; Geri: May be more sensitive to drug effects.

Adverse Reactions/Side Effects

CV: dizziness. **GI:** abdominal pain, ↓ appetite, dyspepsia, hiccups, stomatitis. **GU:** ↓ fertility (females). **Hemat:** anemia, neutropenia. **Misc:** infusion reactions.

Interactions

Drug-Drug: ↑ levels and risk of serious cardiac toxicity with **CYP2D6 substrates** with a narrow therapeutic index, including **thioridazine** and **pimozide**; concurrent use contraindicated. May ↑ levels and risk of toxicity of other **CYP2D6 substrates** for an extended period of time (≥28 days). May ↑ levels and risk of toxicity of **Breast-Cancer-Resistance Protein (BCRP) substrates**, including **irinotecan**, **methotrexate**, **rosuvastatin** and **topotecan**; dose reduction may be necessary. May ↑ levels and risk of toxicity of **P-glycoprotein substrates**, including **digoxin**; avoid concurrent use with P-gp substrates with a narrow therapeutic index. **Strong CYP3A4 inducers**, including **rifampin**, ↓ levels and effectiveness; avoid concurrent use.

Route/Dosage

PO (Adults): 180 mg within 2 hr prior to start of chemotherapy.

Availability

Tablets: 90 mg.

NURSING IMPLICATIONS

Assessment

- Assess nausea, vomiting, appetite, bowel sounds, and abdominal pain prior to and following administration.
- ***Lab Test Considerations:*** May cause ↓ WBC.

R

Implementation

- **PO:** Administer 2 hr before starting chemotherapy without regard to food. Due to long action, administer no more frequently than once every 14 days. Given with dexamethasone and a 5-HT_3 antagonist.
- **Intermittent Infusion:** Administer 2 hr before starting chemotherapy. Solution is translucent white and does not need to be shaken; do not inject solutions that are discolored or contain particulate matter. Insert a vented IV set through septum of vial and use immediately; do not dilute. Infuse through a Y-site of 0.9% NaCl. D5W, D5/LR, or LR. ***Rate:*** Infuse over 30 min.

Patient/Family Teaching

- Instruct patient to take rolapitant as directed. Direct patient to read the *Patient Package Insert* before starting therapy and each time Rx renewed in case of changes.
- Instruct patient to notify health care professional of all Rx or OTC medications, vitamins, or herbal products being taken and consult health care professional before taking any new medications.
- Advise patient and family to use general measures to decrease nausea (begin with sips of liquids and small, nongreasy meals; provide oral hygiene; remove noxious stimuli from environment).
- Advise patient to notify health care professional if pregnancy is planned or suspected, or if breast feeding.

Evaluation/Desired Outcomes

- Decreased delayed nausea and vomiting associated with emetogenic chemotherapy.

rOPINIRole (roe-pin-i-role)

Requip, ~~Requip XL~~

Classification

Therapeutic: antiparkinson agents

Pharmacologic: dopamine agonists

Indications

Management of signs and symptoms of idiopathic Parkinson's disease. Restless leg syndrome (immediate-release only).

Action

Stimulates dopamine receptors in the brain. **Therapeutic Effects:** Decreased tremor and rigidity in Parkinson's disease. Decreased leg restlessness.

Pharmacokinetics

Absorption: 55% absorbed following oral administration.

Distribution: Widely distributed.

Metabolism and Excretion: Extensively metabolized by the liver (by cytochrome P450 CYP1A2 enzyme system); <10% excreted unchanged in urine.

Half-life: 6 hr.

TIME/ACTION PROFILE

ROUTE	ONSET	PEAK	DURATION
PO	unknown	unknown	8 hr

Contraindications/Precautions

Contraindicated in: Hypersensitivity.

Use Cautiously in: Hepatic impairment (slower titration may be required); Severe cardiovascular disease; Geri: ↑ risk of hallucinations; OB: Safety not established; Lactation: Safety not established; may inhibit lactation; Pedi: Safety and effectiveness not established.

Adverse Reactions/Side Effects

CNS: SLEEP ATTACKS, dizziness, syncope, agitation, aggression, confusion, delirium, delusions, disorientation, drowsiness, dyskinesia, fatigue, hallucinations, headache, impulse control disorders (gambling, sexual), paranoid ideation, psychosis, somnolence, weakness. **CV:** orthostatic hypotension, hypertension, peripheral edema, syncope. **EENT:** abnormal vision. **GI:** constipation, dry mouth, dyspepsia, nausea, vomiting. **Derm:** MELANOMA, sweating.

Interactions

Drug-Drug: Drugs that alter the activity of cytochrome P450 CYP1A2 enzyme system may affect the activity of ropinirole. Effects may be ↑ by **estrogens**. Effects may be ↓ by **phenothiazines**, **butyrophenones**, **thioxanthenes**, or **metoclopramide**. May ↑ effects of **levodopa** (may allow dose ↓ of levodopa).

Route/Dosage

Parkinson's Disease

PO (Adults): *Immediate-release*—0.25 mg 3 times daily for 1 wk, then 0.5 mg 3 times daily for 1 wk, then 0.75 mg 3 times daily for 1 wk, then 1 mg 3 times daily for 1 wk; then may ↑ by 1.5 mg/day every wk up to 9 mg/day; then may ↑ by up to 3 mg/day every wk up to 24 mg/day; *Extended-release*—2 mg once daily for 1–2 wk; may ↑ by 2 mg/day; do not exceed 8 mg/day in patients with advanced Parkinson's disease or 12 mg/day in patients with early Parkinson's disease.

Renal Impairment

PO (Adults): *Hemodialysis*—0.25 mg 3 times daily; may ↑ dose as needed based on response and tolerability (not to exceed 18 mg/day).

Restless Leg Syndrome

PO (Adults): *Immediate-release*—0.25 mg once daily initially, 1–3 hr before bedtime. After 2 days, ↑ to 0.5 mg once daily and to 1 mg once daily by the end of first wk of dosing, then ↑ by 0.5 mg weekly, up to 4 mg/day as needed/tolerated.

Renal Impairment

PO (Adults): *Hemodialysis*—0.25 mg once daily; may ↑ dose as needed based on response and tolerability (not to exceed 3 mg/day).

Availability (generic available)

Extended-release tablets: 2 mg, 4 mg, 6 mg, 8 mg, 12 mg. **Cost:** *Generic*—2 mg $82.05/30, 4 mg $164.10/30, 6 mg $246.16/30, 8 mg $246.16/30, 12 mg $410.47/30. **Tablets:** 0.25 mg, 0.5 mg, 1 mg, 2 mg, 3 mg, 4 mg, 5 mg. **Cost:** *Generic*—0.25 mg $250.21/100, 0.5 mg $250.21/100, 1 mg $250.21/100, 2 mg $250.21/100, 3 mg $259.54/100, 4 mg $259.85/100, 5 mg $259.85/100.

NURSING IMPLICATIONS

Assessment

- Assess BP periodically during therapy.
- Assess patient for drowsiness and sleep attacks. Drowsiness is a common side effect of ropinirole, but sleep attacks or episodes of falling asleep during activities that require active participation may occur without warning. Assess patient for concomitant medications that have sedating effects or may increase serum ropinirole levels (see Interactions). May require discontinuation of therapy.
- Assess patient for signs and symptoms of psychotic-like behavior (confusion, paranoid ideation, delusions, hallucinations, psychotic-like behavior, disorientation, aggressive behavior, agitation, delirium, hallucinations). Risk of symptoms increases with age. Notify health care professional if these occur.
- **Parkinson's Disease:** Assess patient for signs and symptoms of Parkinson's disease (tremor, muscle weakness and rigidity, ataxic gait) prior to and during therapy.
- **Restless Leg Syndrome:** Assess sleep patterns and frequency of restless leg disturbances.
- Monitor for *augmentation* (earlier onset of symptoms in the evening or afternoon), increase in symptoms, and spread of symptoms to involve other extremities and *rebound* (new onset of symptoms in the early morning hrs). If symptoms occur, consider dose adjustment or discontinuation of therapy.
- ***Lab Test Considerations:*** May cause ↑ BUN.

Implementation

- Do not confuse ropinirole with Risperdal (risperidone) or risperidone.
- **PO:** May be administered with or without food. Administration with food may decrease nausea. Extended-release tablets should be swallowed whole; do not break, crush, or chew.

Patient/Family Teaching

- Instruct patient to take medication exactly as directed. Missed doses should be taken as soon as possible, but not if almost time for next dose. Do not double doses. Do not stop abruptly; may cause hyperpyrexia and confusion. Taper doses gradually.
- Caution patient to change positions slowly to minimize orthostatic hypotension.
- May cause drowsiness and unexpected episodes of falling asleep. Caution patient to avoid driving or other activities requiring alertness until response to medication is known. Advise patient to notify health care professional if episodes of falling asleep occur.
- Advise patient to avoid alcohol and other CNS depressants concurrently with ropinirole.
- Advise patient that increasing fluids, sugarless gum or candy, ice, or saliva substitutes may help minimize dry mouth. Consult health care professional if dry mouth continues for >2 wk.
- Advise patient to have periodic skin exams to check for lesions that may be melanoma.
- Advise patient to notify health care professional if new or increased gambling, sexual, or other impulse control disorders or psychotic-like behaviors occur.
- Advise patient to notify health care professional if pregnancy is planned or suspected, or if breast feeding. Advise patients that ropinerole could inhibit lactation because ropinirole inhibits prolactin secretion.

Evaluation/Desired Outcomes

- Decreased tremor and rigidity in Parkinson's disease.
- Decrease in restless legs and improved sleep.

R

ropivacaine, See EPIDURAL LOCAL ANESTHETICS.

rosuvastatin, See HMG-CoA REDUCTASE INHIBITORS (statins).

rucaparib (roo-kap-a-rib)

Rubraca

Classification
Therapeutic: antineoplastics
Pharmacologic: enzyme inhibitors

Indications

Deleterious BRCA mutation-associated epithelial ovarian, fallopian tube, or primary peritoneal cancer in patients who have been treated with ≥2 chemotherapies. Maintenance treatment of recurrent epithelial ovarian, fallopian tube, or primary peritoneal cancer in patients who have experienced a complete or partial response to platinum-based chemotherapy.

Action

Acts as a poly (ADP-ribose) polymerase (PARP) inhibitor, thereby disrupting DNA transcription, cell cycle regulation and DNA repair. **Therapeutic Effects:**

Decreased growth and spread of epithelial ovarian, fallopian tube, or primary peritoneal cancer.

Pharmacokinetics

Absorption: 30–45% absorbed following oral administration; bioavailability increased but delayed with high-fat meal.
Distribution: Extensively distributed to tissues.
Metabolism and Excretion: Extensively metabolized (mostly by CYP2D6; minor pathways include CYP1A2 and CYP3A4); information regarding mode of elimination unknown.
Half-life: 17–19 hr.

TIME/ACTION PROFILE (blood levels)

ROUTE	ONSET	PEAK	DURATION
PO	unknown	2 hr	unknown

Contraindications/Precautions

Contraindicated in: OB: May cause fetal harm; Lactation: Breast feeding should be avoided during treatment and for 2 wk after therapy.
Use Cautiously in: Rep: Women of reproductive potential; Pedi: Safety and effectiveness not established.

Adverse Reactions/Side Effects

CNS: dizziness. **Derm:** photosensitivity, rash, palmar-plantar erythrodysaesthesia syndrome, pruritus. **Endo:** hypercholesterolemia. **GI:** abdominal pain, constipation, ↓ appetite, diarrhea, dysgeusia, ↑ liver function tests, nausea, vomiting. **GU:** ↑ serum creatinine. **Hemat:** MYELODYSPLASTIC SYNDROME/ACUTE MYELOID LEUKEMIA, anemia, lymphocytopenia, neutropenia, thrombocytopenia. **Neuro:** fatigue. **Resp:** dyspnea. **Misc:** fever.

Interactions

Drug-Drug: None known.

Route/Dosage

PO (Adults): 600 mg twice daily until disease progression or unacceptable toxicity.

Availability

Tablets: 200 mg, 250 mg, 300 mg.

NURSING IMPLICATIONS

Assessment

- Monitor for signs and symptoms of myelodysplastic syndrome/acute myeloid leukemia during therapy. May require discontinuation of therapy.
- ***Lab Test Considerations:*** For patient selection for BRCA-mutated ovarian cancer, information on the FDA-approved test for the detection of a tumor BRCA mutation in patients with ovarian cancer is available at: http://www.fda.gov/CompanionDiagnostics.
- Obtain a negative pregnancy test prior to starting therapy.
- Monitor CBC prior to and monthly during therapy. Do not start rucaparib until hematologic toxicity from previous chemotherapy has recovered to ≤Grade 1. For prolonged hematologic toxicities, interrupt rucaparib and monitor CBC weekly until recovery. If levels have not recovered to ≤Grade 1 after 4 wk, refer patient to hematologist for further investigations, including bone marrow analysis and blood sample for cytogenetics. If myelodysplastic syndrome/acute myeloid leukemia is confirmed, discontinue rucaparib.
- May cause anemia, thrombocytopenia, lymphocytopenia, and neutropenia.
- May cause ↑ serum creatinine, ALT, AST, and cholesterol.

Implementation

- **PO:** Administer 2 tablets twice daily approximately 12 hr apart, without regard to food.

Patient/Family Teaching

- Instruct patient to take rucaparib as directed. If a dose is missed, omit and take next dose at scheduled time. Do not replace vomited doses.
- Advise patient to notify health care professional if signs and symptoms of myelodysplastic syndrome/acute myeloid leukemia (weakness, feeling tired, fever, weight loss, frequent infections, bruising, bleeding easily, breathlessness, blood in urine or stool) occur.
- Advise patient to wear protective clothing and sunscreen to prevent photosensitivity reactions.
- Instruct patient to notify health care professional of all Rx or OTC medications, vitamins, or herbal products being taken and consult health care professional before taking any new medications.
- Rep: Caution patient rucaparib is teratogenic. Advise females of of reproductive potential to use effective contraception during and for 6 mo following last dose of rucaparib and to avoid breast feeding during and for 2 wk after last dose.

Evaluation/Desired Outcomes

- Decrease in growth and spread of ovarian cancer.

sacubitril/valsartan

(sa-**ku**-bi-tril/val-**sar**-tan)

Entresto

Classification

Therapeutic: vasodilators, antihypertensives

Pharmacologic: angiotensin II receptor antagonists, neprilysin inhibitors

Indications

To ↓ risk of cardiovascular death and hospitalization for chronic heart failure patients (NYHA Class II-IV and ↓ ejection fraction).

Action

sacubitril—a pro-drug converted to LBQ657, its active moeity. LBQ657 inhibits the enzyme neprilysin. Neprilysin degrades vasoactive peptides, including natriuretic peptides, bradykinin, and adrenomedullin resulting in ↑ levels of these peptides, causing vasodilation and ↓ ECF volume via sodium excretion. *Valsartan*—Blocks vasoconstrictor and aldosterone-producing effects of angiotensin II at receptor sites, including vascular smooth muscle and the adrenal glands. **Therapeutic Effects:** Reduced cardiovascular death and hospitalizations due to HF.

Pharmacokinetics

Absorption: *Sacubitril*—≥60% absorbed following oral administration; rapidly converted to LBQ657, its active form. *valsartan*—Absorption in combinations with sacubitril is greater than 10–35% absorbed following oral administration of single-entity formulation.

Distribution: *Sacubitril*—small amounts cross the blood-brain barrier. *valsartan*—crosses the placenta.

Protein Binding: *Sacubitril, valsartan*—94–97%.

Metabolism and Excretion: *Sacubitril*—following conversion to LBQ657 metabolism is minimal; 52–68% excreted in urine. *valsartan*—Minor metabolism by the liver; 13% excreted in urine, 83% in feces.

Half-life: *Sacubitril*—1.4 hr. *LBQ657*—11.5 hr. *valsartan*—9.9 hr.

TIME/ACTION PROFILE (blood levels)

ROUTE	ONSET	PEAK	DURATION
sacubitril	unknown	0.5 hr	12 hr
LBQ657	unknown	2 hr	12 hr
Valsartan	unknown	1.5 hr	12 hr

Contraindications/Precautions

Contraindicated in: Hypersensitivity, hereditary angioedema, or history of angioedema from previous ACE inhibitors or ARBs; Concurrent use of ACE inhibitors during or for 36 hr before or after; Concurrent use with aliskiren in patients with diabetes or moderate-to-severe renal impairment (CCr <60 mL/min); Severe hepatic impairment; OB: Can cause injury or death of fetus—if pregnancy occurs, discontinue immediately; Lactation: Discontinue drug or use formula.

Use Cautiously in: HF (may result in azotemia, oliguria, acute renal failure and/or death); Volume- or salt-depleted patients or patients receiving high doses of diuretics (correct deficits before initiating therapy or initiate at lower doses); Black patients (may not be effective); Impaired renal function due to primary renal disease or HF (may worsen renal function); Rep: Women of reproductive potential; Pedi: Safety and effectiveness not established.

Adverse Reactions/Side Effects

CNS: dizziness. **CV:** hypotension. **F and E:** hyperkalemia. **Resp:** cough. **Misc:** ANGIOEDEMA.

Interactions

Drug-Drug: NSAIDs and selective **COX-2 inhibitors** may ↑ the risk of renal dysfunction. ↑ risk of hypotension with other **antihypertensives** and **diuretics**. Concurrent use of **potassium-sparing diuretics**, **potassium-containing salt substitutes** or **potassium supplements** may ↑ risk of hyperkalemia. ↑ risk of hyperkalemia, renal dysfunction, hypotension, and syncope with concurrent use of **ACE inhibitors** or **aliskiren**; avoid concurrent use with aliskiren in patients with diabetes or CCr <60 mL/min; avoid concurrent use with ACE inhibitors. May ↑ **lithium** levels.

Route/Dosage

PO (Adults): Sacubitril 49 mg/valsartan 51 mg twice daily initially; may double dose every 2–4 wk to target dose of sacubitril 97 mg/valsartan 103 mg as tolerated. *Patients not currently receiving angiotensin-converting enzyme inhibitors or angiotensin receptor blockers or receiving low doses*—Sacubitril 24 mg/valsartan 26 mg twice daily initially; may double dose every 2–4 wk to target dose of sacubitril 97 mg/valsartan 103 mg as tolerated.

Hepatic/Renal Impairment

PO (Adults): *Severe renal impairment (CCr <30 mL/min/1.73 m² or moderate hepatic impairment (Child-Pugh class B)*—Sacubitril 24 mg/valsartan 26 mg twice daily initially; may double dose every 2–4 wk to target dose of sacubitril 97 mg/valsartan 103 mg as tolerated.

Availability

Tablets: sacubitril 24 mg/valsartan 26 mg, sacubitril 49 mg/valsartan 51 mg, sacubitril 97 mg/valsartan 103 mg.

NURSING IMPLICATIONS

Assessment

- Assess BP (lying, sitting, standing) and pulse frequently during initial dose adjustment and periodically throughout therapy. Correct volume or salt depletion prior to administration of therapy. If hypotension occurs, consider reducing dose of diuretics, concomitant antihypertensive agents, and treatment of other causes of hypotension (hypovolemia). If hypotension persist, reduce the dose or temporarily discontinue therapy. Permanent discontinuation of therapy is usually not required.
- Monitor daily weight and assess patient routinely for resolution of fluid overload (peripheral edema, rales/crackles, dyspnea, weight gain, jugular venous distention).
- Monitor frequency of prescription refills to determine compliance.
- Assess patients for signs of angioedema (dyspnea, orofacial swelling); may occur more frequently in Black patients. If signs occur, discontinue therapy, provide supportive therapy, and monitor for airway compromise.
- ***Lab Test Considerations:*** Monitor renal function. May cause increase in BUN and serum creatinine. May require ↓ dose.
- May cause hyperkalemia. May require ↓ dose.
- May cause ↓ in hemoglobin and hematocrit.

Implementation

- **PO:** Administer twice daily.
- If switching from an ACE inhibitor to *Entresto*, allow 36 hrs between last ACE inhibitor dose and starting *Entresto*. For patients unable to swallow pills a suspension can be made by a pharmacist.

Patient/Family Teaching

- Instruct patient to take *Entresto* as directed, at the same time each day, even if feeling well. Take missed doses as soon as remembered if not almost time for next dose; do not double doses. Warn patient not to discontinue therapy unless directed by health care professional. Advise patient to read *Patient Information* before starting therapy and with each Rx refill in case of changes.
- Caution patient to avoid salt substitutes containing potassium or foods containing high levels of potassium or sodium unless directed by health care professional. See Appendix K.
- Instruct patient to notify health care professional if swelling of face, eyes, lips, or tongue or if difficulty swallowing or breathing occur.
- May cause dizziness. Caution patient to avoid driving or other activities requiring alertness until response to medication is known.
- Instruct patient to notify health care professional of all Rx or OTC medications, vitamins, or herbal products being taken and to avoid concurrent use of Rx, OTC, and herbal products, especially NSAIDs, potassium supplements or salt substitute, ACE inhibitors, ARBs, lithium or aliskiren, without consulting health care professional.
- Instruct patient to notify health care professional of medication regimen before treatment or surgery.
- Rep: May be teratogenic. Advise females of reproductive potential to use contraception and avoid breast feeding during therapy. Notify health care professional if pregnancy is planned or suspected. *Entresto* should be discontinued as soon as possible when pregnancy is detected.
- Emphasize the importance of follow-up exams to evaluate effectiveness of medication.

Evaluation/Desired Outcomes

- Decreased heart-failure-related hospitalizations in patients with heart failure.

safinamide (sa-fin-a-mide)

Xadago

Classification

Therapeutic: antiparkinson agents

Pharmacologic: monoamine oxidase type B inhibitors

Indications

Adjunctive treatment to levodopa/carbidopa in patients with Parkinson's disease (PD) who are experiencing "off" episodes.

Action

Irreversibly inhibits monoamine oxidase (MAO) B which leads to ↑ dopamine levels in the CNS. **Therapeutic Effects:** Increased amount of "on" time without dyskinesia or with non-troublesome dyskinesia.

Pharmacokinetics

Absorption: 95% absorbed following oral administration.

Distribution: Extensively distributed to the tissues; readily crosses the blood-brain barrier.

Metabolism and Excretion: Extensively metabolized by hydrolytic oxidation or oxidative cleavage to inactive metabolites; 76% excreted in urine (primarily as inactive metabolites).

Half-life: 20–26 hr.

TIME/ACTION PROFILE (blood levels)

ROUTE	ONSET	PEAK	DURATION
PO	unknown	2–3 hr	24 hr

Contraindications/Precautions

Contraindicated in: Hypersensitivity; Concurrent use of other MAO inhibitors; Concurrent use of opioids, SNRIs, TCAs, cyclobenzaprine, methylphenidate, amphetamine, or St. John's wort; Concurrent use of dextromethorphan; Severe hepatic impairment (Child-Pugh C); Psychotic disorder; Lactation: Discontinue breast feeding or discontinue the safinamide.

Use Cautiously in: Retinal disease; Moderate hepatic impairment (Child-Pugh B) (do not exceed maximum recommended dose); OB: Use only if maternal benefit outweighs fetal risk; Pedi: Safety and effectiveness not established.

Adverse Reactions/Side Effects

CNS: anxiety, drowsiness, hallucinations, impulse control disorders (gambling, sexual, binge eating), ↑ fall risk, insomnia, psychosis, sleep attacks, sleep driving. **CV:** hypertension, orthostatic hypotension. **EENT:** visual changes. **GI:** ↑ liver enzymes, nausea. **Neuro:** dyskinesia, paresthesia. **Resp:** cough. **Misc:** hypersensitivity reactions.

Interactions

Drug-Drug: Concurrent use of other **MAO inhibitors**, including **linezolid** and **isoniazid** may ↑ risk of hypertensive crises and is contraindicated; separate administration by ≥14 days. Concurrent use of **meperidine, methadone, tramadol, SNRIs, TCAs, cyclobenzaprine, methylphenidate**, or **amphetamine** may ↑ risk of serotonin syndrome and is contraindicated; separate administration by ≥14 days; SSRIs may be used at the lowest dose possible. Concurrent use with **dextromethorphan** may result in psychosis/bizarre behavior and is contraindicated. Hypertensive crisis may occur with cough and cold products containing **sympathomimetic amines** including **pseudoephedrine** and **phenylephrine**; monitor patient's BP closely. May ↑ levels/toxicity of **imatinib**, **irinotecan**, **lapatinib**, **methotrexate**, **mitoxantrone**, **rosuvastatin**, **sulfasalazine**, and **topotecan**; monitor closely for adverse effects. **Dopamine antagonists**, including **antipsychotics** and **metoclopramide** may ↓ effectiveness of safinamide.

Drug-Natural Products: Concurrent use with **St. John's wort** may ↑ risk of serotonin syndrome; concurrent use contraindicated.

Drug-Food: Ingestion of foods containing high amounts of **tyramine** (>150 mg) (e.g., cheese) may result in hypertensive crisis.

Route/Dosage

PO (Adults): 50 mg once daily; after 2 wk, may ↑ dose to 100 mg once daily.

Hepatic Impairment

PO (Adults): *Moderate hepatic impairment (Child-Pugh B)*—Do not exceed 50 mg/day; *Severe hepatic impairment (Child-Pugh C)*—Contraindicated.

Availability

Tablets: 50 mg, 100 mg.

NURSING IMPLICATIONS

Assessment

- Assess signs and symptoms of Parkinson's disease (tremor, muscle weakness and rigidity, ataxic gait) prior to and during therapy.
- Monitor for new onset hypertension or hypertension not adequately controlled after starting safinamide. Sustained BP elevation may require dose reduction.
- Assess for serotonin syndrome (mental changes [agitation, hallucinations, coma], autonomic instability [tachycardia, labile BP, hyperthermia], neuromuscular aberrations [hyperreflexia, incoordination], and/or GI symptoms [nausea, vomiting, diarrhea]), especially in patients taking other serotonergic drugs (SSRIs, SNRIs, triptans).
- ***Toxicity and Overdose:*** Concurrent ingestion of tyramine-rich foods and many medications may result in a life-threatening hypertensive crisis. Signs and symptoms of hypertensive crisis include chest pain, tachycardia or bradycardia, severe headache, neck stiffness or soreness, nausea and vomiting, sweating, photosensitivity, and enlarged pupils.

Implementation

- **PO:** Administer once daily, at the same time each day, without regard to food.

Patient/Family Teaching

- Instruct patient to take safinamide as directed. Missed doses should be omitted and next dose taken at usual time the following day. Do not double doses. Do not discontinue abruptly; may cause elevated temperature, muscular rigidity, altered consciousness, and autonomic instability. Advise patient to read *Patient Information* before starting therapy and with each Rx refill in case of changes.
- Caution patient to avoid alcohol, CNS depressants, and foods or beverages containing tyramine (see Appendix K) during and for at least 2 wk after therapy has been discontinued; they may precipitate a hypertensive crisis. Contact health care professional immediately if symptoms of hypertensive crisis or serotonin syndrome develop.
- Instruct patient to notify health care professional of all Rx or OTC medications, vitamins, or herbal products being taken and consult health care professional before taking any new medications. Caution patient to avoid use of St. John's wort, cough or cold products containing dextromethorphan, and analgesics meperidine, tramadol, or methadone during therapy.
- May cause drowsiness and unexpected episodes of falling asleep. Caution patient to avoid driving or other activities requiring alertness until response to medication is known. Advise patient to notify health care professional if episodes of falling asleep occur.

S

- Advise patient to notify health care professional if new or increased gambling, sexual, or other impulse control disorders or psychotic-like behaviors occur.
- Advise female patients to notify health care professionals if pregnancy is planned or suspected or if breast feeding.

Evaluation/Desired Outcomes

- Improvement in symptoms of Parkinson's disease, allowing increase in function.

salmeterol (sal-me-te-role)

Serevent Diskus

Classification

Therapeutic: bronchodilators

Pharmacologic: adrenergics

Indications

As concomitant therapy for the treatment of asthma and the prevention of bronchospasm in patients who are currently taking but are inadequately controlled on a long-term asthma-control medication (e.g., inhaled corticosteroid). Prevention of exercise-induced bronchospasm. Maintenance treatment to prevent bronchospasm in chronic obstructive pulmonary disease (COPD) including chronic bronchitis and emphysema.

Action

Produces accumulation of cyclic adenosine monophosphate (cAMP) at beta$_2$-adrenergic receptors. Relatively specific for beta (pulmonary) receptors. **Therapeutic Effects:** Bronchodilation.

Pharmacokinetics

Absorption: Minimal systemic absorption follows inhalation.

Distribution: Action is primarily local.

Metabolism and Excretion: Unknown.

Half-life: 3–4 hr.

TIME/ACTION PROFILE (bronchodilation)

ROUTE	ONSET	PEAK	DURATION
Inhaln	10–25 min	3–4 hr	12 hr†

†9 hr in adolescents.

Contraindications/Precautions

Contraindicated in: Hypersensitivity to salmeterol or milk proteins; Acute attack of asthma (onset of action is delayed); Patients not receiving a long-term asthma-control medication (e.g., inhaled corticosteroid) (↑ risk of asthma-related death); Patients whose asthma is currently controlled on low- or medium-dose inhaled corticosteroid therapy.

Use Cautiously in: Cardiovascular disease (including angina and hypertension); Seizure disorders; Diabetes; Glaucoma; Hyperthyroidism; Pheochromocytoma; Excessive use (may lead to tolerance and paradoxical bronchospasm); OB: Use only if potential maternal benefit justifies potential fetal risk; may inhibit contractions during labor; Lactation: Use while breast feeding only if potential maternal benefit justifies potential risk to infant; Pedi: Children <4 yr (safety not established); a fixed-dose combination product containing salmeterol and an inhaled corticosteroid should be strongly considered to ensure adherence.

Adverse Reactions/Side Effects

CNS: <u>headache</u>, nervousness. **CV:** palpitations, tachycardia. **GI:** abdominal pain, diarrhea, nausea. **MS:** muscle cramps/soreness. **Neuro:** trembling. **Resp:** paradoxical bronchospasm, cough.

Interactions

Drug-Drug: Beta blockers may ↓ therapeutic effects. **MAO inhibitors** and **tricyclic antidepressants** potentiate cardiovascular effects. ↑ levels and ↑ risk of cardiovascular effects when used with potent CYP3A4 inhibitors (e.g., **ketoconazole**, **itraconazole**, **ritonavir**, **atazanavir**, **clarithromycin**, **indinavir**, **nefazodone**, **nelfinavir**, or **saquinavir**); concurrent use is not recommended.

Drug-Natural Products: Use with caffeine-containing herbs (**cola nut**, **guarana**, **mate**, **tea**, **coffee**) ↑ stimulant effect.

Route/Dosage

Asthma

Inhaln (Adults and Children ≥4 yr): 50 mcg (1 inhalation) twice daily (approximately 12 hr apart).

Prevention of Exercise-Induced Bronchospasm

Inhaln (Adults and Children ≥4 yr): 50 mcg (1 inhalation) ≥30 min before exercise; additional doses should not be used for ≥12 hr.

COPD

Inhaln (Adults): 50 mcg (1 inhalation) twice daily (approximately 12 hr apart).

Availability

Powder for oral inhalation (Serevent Diskus): 50 mcg/blister. ***In combination with:*** fluticasone (Advair Diskus, Advair HFA, AirDuo RespiClick, Wixhela Inhub). See Appendix B.

NURSING IMPLICATIONS

Assessment

- Assess lung sounds, pulse, and BP before administration and periodically during therapy.
- Monitor pulmonary function tests before initiating therapy and periodically during therapy.
- Observe for paradoxical bronchospasm (wheezing, dyspnea, tightness in chest) and hypersensitivity reaction (rash; urticaria; swelling of the face, lips, or eyelids). Frequently occurs with first use of new canister or vial. If condition occurs, withhold medication and notify physician or other health care professional immediately.

- ***Lab Test Considerations:*** May cause ↑ serum glucose concentrations; occurs rarely with recommended doses and is more pronounced with frequent use of high doses.
- May cause ↓ serum potassium concentrations, which are usually transient and dose related; rarely occurs at recommended doses and is more pronounced with frequent use of high doses.
- ***Toxicity and Overdose:*** Symptoms of overdose include persistent agitation, chest pain or discomfort, decreased BP, dizziness, hyperglycemia, hypokalemia, seizures, tachyarrhythmias, persistent trembling, and vomiting.
- Treatment includes discontinuing salmeterol and other beta-adrenergic agonists and providing symptomatic, supportive therapy. Cardioselective beta blockers are used cautiously because they may induce bronchospasm.

Implementation

- Salmeterol should be used along with an inhaled corticosteroid, not as monotherapy. Patients taking salmeterol twice daily should not use additional doses for exercise-induced bronchospasm.
- **Inhaln:** *Serevent Diskus:* Once removed from foil overwrap, discard diskus when every blister has been used or 6 wk have passed, whichever comes first.

Patient/Family Teaching

- Advise patient to take salmeterol as directed. Do not use more than the prescribed dose. If a regularly scheduled dose is missed, use as soon as possible and resume regular schedule. Do not double doses. If symptoms occur before next dose is due, use a rapid-acting inhaled bronchodilator.
- Instruct patient using *powder for inhalation* never to exhale into diskus device and always to hold device in a level horizontal position. Mouthpiece should be kept dry; never wash.
- Caution patient not to use salmeterol to treat acute symptoms. A rapid-acting inhaled beta-adrenergic bronchodilator should be used for relief of acute asthma attacks.
- Advise patients on chronic therapy not to use additional salmeterol to prevent exercise-induced bronchospasm. Patients using salmeterol for prevention of exercise-induced bronchospasm should not use additional doses of salmeterol for 12 hr after prophylactic administration.
- Advise patient to notify health care professional immediately if difficulty in breathing persists after use of salmeterol, if condition worsens, if more inhalations of rapid-acting bronchodilator than usual are needed to relieve an acute attack, or if using 4 or more inhalations of a rapid-acting bronchodilator for 2 or more consecutive days or more than 1 canister in an 8-wk period.
- Salmeterol is often used with inhaled corticosteroids and is not a substitute for corticosteroids or adrenergic bronchodilators. Advise patients using inhalation or systemic corticosteroids to consult health care professional before stopping or reducing therapy.
- Advise patient to notify health care professional if pregnancy is planned or suspected, or if breast feeding.
- Emphasize the importance of regular follow-up exams to determine progress during therapy.

Evaluation/Desired Outcomes

- Prevention of bronchospasm or reduction of frequency of acute asthma attacks in patients with chronic asthma. Improvement in asthma control can occur within 15 min of starting therapy, but full benefit may take 1 wk or longer. Time to onset and degree of symptom relief will vary with individual.
- Prevention of exercise-induced asthma.

sarilumab (sar-il-ue-mab)

Kevzara

Classification

Therapeutic: antirheumatics, immunosuppressants

Pharmacologic: interleukin antagonists

Indications

Moderately- to severely-active rheumatoid arthritis in patients who have not responded to ≥1 disease-modifying antirheumatic drugs [DMARDs]) (as monotherapy or in combination with methotrexate or other non-biologic DMARDs).

Action

Acts as an inhibitor of interleukin-6 (IL-6) receptors by binding to them. IL-6 is a mediator of various inflammatory processes. **Therapeutic Effects:** Slowed progression of rheumatoid arthritis.

Pharmacokinetics

Absorption: Well absorbed via subcutaneous injection.

Distribution: Well distributed.

Metabolism and Excretion: Metabolic pathway has not been defined. Elimination is predominantly through the linear, non-saturable proteolytic pathway at high concentrations; at lower concentrations, elimination is predominately through non-linear saturable target-mediated pathway.

Half-life: *200 mg every 2 wk dose*—up to 10 days; *150 mg every 2 wk dose*—up to 8 days.

S

TIME/ACTION PROFILE (blood levels)

ROUTE	ONSET	PEAK	DURATION
Subcut		2–4 days	28–43 days

Contraindications/Precautions

Contraindicated in: Hypersensitivity; Active infection; Active hepatic disease/impairment; Absolute neutrophil count (ANC) <2000/mm^3 (<500/mm^3 while on therapy) or platelet count <150,000/mm^3 (<50,000/mm^3 while on therapy); Concurrent use with biological DMARDs.

Use Cautiously in: Chronic or recurrent infection; History of serious or opportunistic infection; Exposure to tuberculosis; Lived in or traveled to areas of endemic tuberculosis or endemic mycoses; Diverticulitis or concomitant use of NSAIDs or corticosteroids (↑ risk for GI perforation); Severe renal impairment; Geri: ↑ risk of infections; OB: Use only if potential benefit justifies potential risk to fetus; Lactation: Use only if potential benefit justifies potential risk to infant; Pedi: Safety and effectiveness not established.

Adverse Reactions/Side Effects

GI: GASTROINTESTINAL PERFORATION, ↑ liver enzymes. **Hemat:** NEUTROPENIA, THROMBOCYTOPENIA. **Metab:** dyslipidemia. **Misc:** INFECTIONS (including tuberculosis, disseminated fungal infections, and infections with opportunistic pathogens), MALIGNANCY, hypersensitivity reactions (including rash and urticaria), injection site reactions.

Interactions

Drug-Drug: May alter the activity of CYP450 enzymes; the effects of the following drugs should be monitored: **cyclosporine**, **theophylline**, **warfarin**, **hormonal contraceptives**, **atorvastatin**, and **lovastatin**. Other drugs which are substrates for this system should also be monitored; effect may persist for several wk after discontinuation. May ↓ antibody response to and ↑ risk of adverse reactions to **live virus vaccines**; do not administer concurrently.

Route/Dosage

Subcut (Adults): 200 mg every 2 wk.

Availability

Solution for subcutaneous injection (prefilled syringes and prefilled pens): 150 mg/1.14 mL, 200 mg/1.14 mL.

NURSING IMPLICATIONS

Assessment

- Assess for signs of infection (fever, dyspnea, flu-like symptoms, frequent or painful urination, redness or swelling at the site of a wound), including tuberculosis, prior to injection. Sarilumab is contraindicated in patients with active infection. Monitor new infections closely; most common are upper respiratory tract infections, bronchitis, and urinary tract infections. Signs and symptoms of inflammation may be lessened due to suppression from sarilumab. Infections may be fatal, especially in patients taking immunosuppressive therapy. If patient develops a serious infection, discontinue sarilumab until infection is controlled.
- Monitor for signs and symptoms of viral reactivation: herpes zoster (rash, blisters), hepatitis B (jaundice, dark urine, light colored stools, fatigue, weakness, loss of appetite, nausea, vomiting, stomach pain) during therapy.
- ***Lab Test Considerations:*** Monitor neutrophil count prior to, and 4 and 8 wk after starting, and every 3 mo during therapy. Base dose modifications on measures from end of dosing interval. *If ANC >1000 cells/mm^3,* maintain current dose of sarilumab. *If ANC 500–1000 cells/mm^3,* withhold therapy until ANC >1000. Resume at 150 mg every 2 wk and ↑ to 200 mg every 2 wk as appropriate. If ANC <500 cells/mm^3, discontinue sarilumab.
- Monitor platelet count prior to, and 4 and 8 wk after starting, and every 3 mo during therapy. *If platelet count 50,000–100,000 cells/mm^3,* suspend therapy until platelets >100,000. Resume at 150 mg every 2 wk and ↑ to 200 mg every 2 wk as appropriate.
- Monitor serum AST and ALT prior to, and 4 and 8 wk after starting, and every 3 mo during therapy. *If ALT >upper limits of normal (ULN) to 3 × ULN or less,* consider modifying dose of concomitant DMARDs as clinically appropriate. *If ALT >3 × ULN to 5 × ULN or less,* hold therapy until ALT <3 × ULN. Resume at 150 mg every 2 wk and ↑ to 200 mg every 2 wk as appropriate. *If ALT >5 × ULN,* discontinue sarilumab.
- Monitor serum lipid levels 4–8 wk following start of therapy, then at 6 mo intervals. Manage with clinical guidelines for hyperlipidemia.

Implementation

- Administer a tuberculin skin test prior to administration of sarilumab. Patients with latent TB should be treated for TB prior to therapy.
- Other DMARDs should be continued during sarilumab therapy.
- **Subcut:** Refrigerate in original carton to protect from light. Do not freeze or shake. May be stored for up to 14 days in original carton at room temperature. Inject full amount in syringe. Rotate injection sites; avoid areas where skin is tender, damaged, or has bruises or scars. Solution is clear and colorless to pale yellow; do not administer solutions that are discolored or contain particulate matter.

Patient/Family Teaching

- Instruct patient on the purpose for sarilumab. If a dose is missed, contact health care professional to schedule next infusion. Instruct patient and caregiver in correct technique for subcut injections and care and disposal of equipment. Advise patient to read the *Medication Guide* before starting and with each Rx refill in case of changes.

- Caution patient to notify health care professional immediately if signs of infection (fever, sweating, chills, muscle aches, cough, shortness of breath, blood in phlegm, weight loss, warm, red or painful skin or sores, diarrhea or stomach pain, burning on urination, urinary frequency, feeling tired), fever and stomach-area pain that does not go away, change in bowel habits, severe rash, swollen face, or difficulty breathing occurs while taking. If signs and symptoms of anaphylaxis occur, discontinue injections and notify health care professional immediately.
- Advise patient to avoid receiving live vaccines during therapy.
- Instruct patient to notify health care professional of all Rx or OTC medications, vitamins, or herbal products being taken and consult health care professional before taking any new medications.
- Instruct patient to notify health care professional of medication regimen prior to treatment or surgery.
- Rep: Advise female patients to notify health care professional if pregnancy is planned or suspected, or if breast feeding, Encourage women who become pregnant while taking sarilumab to participate in the pregnancy registry by calling 1-877-311-8972.

Evaluation/Desired Outcomes

- Slowed progression of rheumatoid arthritis.

SAXagliptin (sax-a-**glip**-tin)

Onglyza

Classification

Therapeutic: antidiabetics

Pharmacologic: dipeptidyl peptidase-4 (DDP-4) inhibitors

Indications

Adjunct with diet and exercise to improve glycemic control in adults with type 2 diabetes mellitus.

Action

Acts as a competitive inhibitor of dipeptidyl peptidase-4 (DPP4), which slows inactivation of incretin hormones, thereby increasing their concentrations and reducing fasting and postprandial glucose concentrations.
Therapeutic Effects: Improved control of blood glucose.

Pharmacokinetics

Absorption: Well absorbed following oral administration.
Distribution: Unknown.
Metabolism and Excretion: Metabolized by the liver via the P450 3A4/5 (CYP3A4/5) enzyme system, with conversion to 5–hydroxysaxagliptin, a pharmacologically active metabolite; 24% of saxagliptin is excreted unchanged in urine, 36% of hydroxysaxagliptin is excreted unchanged in urine, 22% is eliminated in feces as unabsorbed drug/metabolites excreted in bile.
Half-life: *Saxagliptin*—2.5 hr; *5–hydroxysaxagliptin*—3.1 hr.

TIME/ACTION PROFILE (DDP-4 inhibition)

ROUTE	ONSET	PEAK	DURATION
PO	unknown	2 hr (4 hr for 5–hydroxysaxagliptin)†	24 hr

†Blood levels.

Contraindications/Precautions

Contraindicated in: Type 1 diabetes; Diabetic ketoacidosis; History of hypersensitivity reaction.
Use Cautiously in: HF or renal impairment (↑ risk of worsening HF); Moderate or severe renal impairment (CCr ≤45 mL/min) (↓ dose required); OB: Use only if potential maternal benefit justifies potential fetal risk; Lactation: Use while breast feeding only if potential maternal benefit outweighs potential risk to infant; Pedi: Safety and effectiveness not established; Geri: May be more sensitive to effects; consider age-related ↓ in renal function.

Adverse Reactions/Side Effects

CNS: headache. **CV:** HF, peripheral edema (↑ with thiazolidinediones). **Derm:** bullous pemphigoid. **Endo:** hypoglycemia (↑ with sulfonylureas). **GI:** PANCREATITIS, abdominal pain, vomiting. **Hemat:** ↓ lymphocyte count. **MS:** RHABDOMYOLYSIS, arthralgia. **Misc:** HYPERSENSITIVITY REACTIONS (including anaphylaxis and angioedema).

Interactions

Drug-Drug: Strong **CYP3A4/5 inhibitors**, including **ketoconazole**, **atazanavir**, **clarithromycin**, **indinavir**, **itraconazole**, **nefazodone**, **nelfinavir**, **ritonavir**, and **saquinavir** ↑ blood levels; daily dose should not exceed 2.5 mg. ↑ risk of hypoglycemia with **sulfonylureas** or **insulin**; may need to ↓ dose of sulfonylureas or insulin.

Route/Dosage

PO (Adults): 2.5–5 mg once daily; *Concurrent use of strong CYP3A4/5 inhibitors*—2.5 mg once daily.

Renal Impairment

PO (Adults): *CCr ≤45 mL/min (including patients undergoing hemodialysis)*—2.5 mg once daily; in patients undergoing hemodialysis, administer after hemodialysis.

Availability

Tablets: 2.5 mg, 5 mg. ***In combination with:*** dapagliflozin (Qtern); dapagliflozin and metformin XR

(Qternmet XR); metformin XR (Kombiglyze XR). See Appendix B.

NURSING IMPLICATIONS

Assessment

- Observe patient for signs and symptoms of hypoglycemic reactions (abdominal pain, sweating, hunger, weakness, dizziness, headache, tremor, tachycardia, anxiety).
- Monitor for signs of pancreatitis (nausea, vomiting, anorexia, persistent severe abdominal pain, sometimes radiating to the back) during therapy. If pancreatitis occurs, discontinue saxagliptin and monitor serum and urine amylase, amylase/creatinine clearance ratio, electrolytes, serum calcium, glucose, and lipase.
- ***Lab Test Considerations:*** Monitor hemoglobin A1C prior to and periodically during therapy.
- Monitor renal function prior to and periodically during therapy.
- May cause ↓ absolute lymphocyte count.

Implementation

- Do not confuse saxagliptin with sitagliptin.
- Patients stabilized on a diabetic regimen who are exposed to stress, fever, trauma, infection, or surgery may require administration of insulin.
- **PO:** May be administered without regard to food. Swallow tablet whole, do not cut or split.

Patient/Family Teaching

- Instruct patient to take saxagliptin as directed. If a dose is missed, take the next dose as prescribed; do not double doses. Advise patient to read the *Patient Package Insert* before starting and with each Rx refill; new information may be available.
- Explain to patient that saxagliptin helps control hyperglycemia but does not cure diabetes. Therapy is usually long term.
- Instruct patient not to share this medication with others, even if they have the same symptoms; it may harm them.
- Encourage patient to follow prescribed diet, medication, and exercise regimen to prevent hyperglycemic or hypoglycemic episodes.
- Review signs of hypoglycemia and hyperglycemia with patient. If hypoglycemia occurs, advise patient to take a glass of orange juice or 2–3 tsp of sugar, honey, or corn syrup dissolved in water, and notify health care professional.
- Instruct patient in proper testing of blood glucose and urine ketones. These tests should be monitored closely during periods of stress or illness and health care professional notified if significant changes occur.
- Advise patient to notify health care professional promptly if swelling of hands, feet, or ankles; rash; hives; or swelling of face, lips, or throat occur.
- Instruct patient to notify health care professional of all Rx or OTC medications, vitamins, or herbal products being taken and consult health care professional before taking any new medications.
- Advise patient to notify health care professional if pregnancy is planned or suspected, or if breast feeding.

Evaluation/Desired Outcomes

- Improved hemoglobin A1C, fasting plasma glucose, and 2-hr post-prandial glucose levels.

BEERS

scopolamine (scoe-pol-a-meen)

Transderm-Scop

Classification

Therapeutic: antiemetics

Pharmacologic: anticholinergics

Indications

Prevention of motion sickness. Prevention of postoperative nausea and vomiting.

Action

Inhibits the muscarinic activity of acetylcholine. Corrects the imbalance of acetylcholine and norepinephrine in the CNS, which may be responsible for motion sickness. **Therapeutic Effects:** Reduction of postoperative nausea and vomiting. Reduction of spasms.

Pharmacokinetics

Absorption: Well absorbed following transdermal administration.

Distribution: Crosses the placenta and blood-brain barrier.

Metabolism and Excretion: Mostly metabolized by the liver.

Half-life: 8 hr.

TIME/ACTION PROFILE (antiemetic, sedative properties)

ROUTE	ONSET	PEAK	DURATION
Transdermal	4 hr	unknown	72 hr

Contraindications/Precautions

Contraindicated in: Hypersensitivity; Angle-closure glaucoma; Acute hemorrhage; Tachycardia secondary to cardiac insufficiency or thyrotoxicosis.

Use Cautiously in: Possible intestinal obstruction; Prostatic hyperplasia; Chronic renal, hepatic, pulmonary, or cardiac disease; OB: Avoid use in pregnant women with severe pre-eclampsia (may cause seizures); otherwise, use only if potential maternal benefit justifies potential fetal risk; Lactation: Use while breast feeding only if potential maternal benefit justifies potential risk to infant; Pedi, Geri: ↑ risk of adverse reactions.

Adverse Reactions/Side Effects

CNS: drowsiness, confusion. **CV:** tachycardia, palpitations. **Derm:** ↓ sweating. **EENT:** blurred vision, mydriasis, photophobia. **GI:** dry mouth, constipation. **GU:** urinary hesitancy, urinary retention.

Interactions

Drug-Drug: ↑ anticholinergic effects with **antihistamines, antidepressants, quinidine**, or **disopyramide**. ↑ CNS depression with **alcohol, antidepressants, antihistamines, opioid analgesics**, or **sedative/hypnotics**. May alter the absorption of other **orally administered drugs** by slowing motility of the GI tract. May ↑ GI mucosal lesions in patients taking oral **wax-matrix potassium chloride preparations**.

Drug-Natural Products: ↑ anticholinergic effects with **jimson weed** and **scopolia**.

Route/Dosage

Transdermal (Adults): *Motion sickness*—Apply 1 patch 4 hr prior to travel and then every 3 days (as needed); *Preoperative*—Apply 1 patch the evening before surgery (remove 24 hr after surgery).

Availability (generic available)

Transdermal system: Transderm-Scop—1.5 mg scopolamine/patch releases 0.5 mg scopolamine over 3 days.

NURSING IMPLICATIONS

Assessment

- Assess patient for signs of urinary retention periodically during therapy.

Implementation

- **Transdermal:** Apply at least 4 hr (US product) before exposure to travel to prevent motion sickness.

Patient/Family Teaching

- **Transdermal:** Instruct patient on application of transdermal patches. Apply at least 4 hr (US product) before exposure to travel to prevent motion sickness. Wash hands and dry thoroughly before and after application. Apply to hairless, clean, dry area behind ear; avoid areas with cuts or irritation. Apply pressure over system to ensure contact with skin. System is effective for 3 days. If system becomes dislodged, replace with a new system on another site behind the ear. System is waterproof and not affected by bathing or showering.
- Instruct patient to remove patch and notify health care professional immediately if symptoms of acute angle-closure glaucoma (pain or reddening of the eyes with pupil dilation) occur.
- Caution patients engaging in underwater sports of potentially distorting effects of scopolamine.
- Advise patient referred for MRI test to discuss patch with referring health care professional and MRI facility to determine if removal of patch is necessary prior to test and for directions for replacing patch.
- Instruct patient to take medication as directed. Take missed doses as soon as remembered. Do not double doses.
- May cause drowsiness or blurred vision. Caution patient to avoid driving or other activities requiring alertness until response to medication is known.
- Advise patient to use caution when exercising and in hot weather; overheating may result in heatstroke.
- Advise patient to avoid concurrent use of alcohol and other CNS depressants with this medication.
- Inform patient that frequent mouth rinses, good oral hygiene, and sugarless gum or candy may minimize dry mouth.
- Advise patient to notify health care professional if pregnancy is planned or suspected, or if breast feeding.

Evaluation/Desired Outcomes

- Prevention of motion sickness.
- Prevention of postoperative nausea and vomiting.

secnidazole (sek-nid-a-zole)

Solosec

Classification

Therapeutic: anti-infectives

Pharmacologic: imidazoles

Indications

Bacterial vaginosis.

Action

Disrupts DNA synthesis in susceptible organisms. **Therapeutic Effects:** Resolution of bacterial vaginosis. **Spectrum:** Active against *Bacteroides spp.*, *Gardnerella vaginalis*, *Prevotella spp.*, and *Mobiluncus spp.*

Pharmacokinetics

Absorption: Rapidly and completely absorbed following oral administration.

Distribution: Extensively distributed to tissues.

Metabolism and Excretion: Primarily metabolized by CYP450 system in liver; 15% excreted unchanged in urine.

Half-life: 17 hr.

TIME/ACTION PROFILE (plasma concentrations)

ROUTE	ONSET	PEAK	DURATION
PO	rapid	4 hr	unknown

Contraindications/Precautions

Contraindicated in: Hypersensitivity; cross sensitivity with other imidazoles may occur; Lactation: Avoid breast feeding.

S

Use Cautiously in: OB: Safety not established in pregnancy; Pedi: Safety and effectiveness not established.

Adverse Reactions/Side Effects

CNS: headache. **GI:** abdominal pain, diarrhea, metallic taste, nausea, vomiting. **GU:** vulvovaginal candidiasis, vulvovaginal pruritus.

Interactions

Drug-Drug: None known.

Route/Dosage

PO (Adults): 2-g single dose.

Availability

Oral granules: 2 g/pkt.

NURSING IMPLICATIONS

Assessment

- Assess for symptoms of bacterial vaginosis before and periodically following secnidazole.
- ***Lab Test Considerations:*** Obtain specimen for culture and sensitivity before starting therapy.

Implementation

- **PO:** Administer packet once without regard to meals. Open packet and sprinkle entire contents onto applesauce, yogurt, or pudding. Granules will not dissolve. Consume all of the mixture within 30 min without chewing or crunching granules. May be followed with a glass of water to aid in swallowing. Granules are not intended to be dissolved in any liquid.

Patient/Family Teaching

- Instruct patient in correct technique for taking secnidazole. Advise patient to read *Patient Information* before taking secnidazole.
- Advise patient to notify health care professional if signs and symptoms of vulvovaginal candidiasis (vaginal itching, white or yellowish discharge [discharge may be lumpy or look like cottage cheese]) occur. May require treatment with antifungal agents.
- Advise patient to notify health care professional of all Rx or OTC medications, vitamins, or herbal products being taken and to consult with health care professional before taking other medications during therapy.
- Advise patient to notify health care professional if pregnancy is planned or suspected. Advise female patient to avoid breast feeding for at least 96 hrs (4 days) following secnidazole dose.

Evaluation/Desired Outcomes

- Resolution of bacterial vaginosis.

selegiline (se-le-ji-leen)

Eldepryl, Zelapar

Classification

Therapeutic: antiparkinson agents
Pharmacologic: monoamine oxidase type B inhibitors

Indications

Management of Parkinson's disease (with levodopa or levodopa/carbidopa) in patients who fail to respond to levodopa/carbidopa alone.

Action

Following conversion by MAO to its active form, selegiline inactivates MAO by irreversibly binding to it at type B (brain) sites. Inactivation of MAO leads to increased amounts of dopamine available in the CNS. **Therapeutic Effects:** Increased response to levodopa/dopamine therapy in Parkinson's disease.

Pharmacokinetics

Absorption: Appears to be well absorbed following oral administration.

Distribution: Widely distributed.

Metabolism and Excretion: Metabolism involves some conversion to amphetamine and methamphetamine. 45% excreted in urine as metabolites.

Half-life: Unknown; orally disintegrating tablets 1.3 hr.

TIME/ACTION PROFILE (onset of beneficial effects in Parkinson's disease)

ROUTE	ONSET	PEAK	DURATION
PO	2–3 days	40–90 min	unknown
Orally disintegrating	5 min	10–15 min	unknown

Contraindications/Precautions

Contraindicated in: Hypersensitivity; Concurrent meperidine or opioid analgesic therapy (possible fatal reactions); Concurrent use of SSRIs or tricyclic antidepressants.

Use Cautiously in: Doses >10 mg/day (↑ risk of hypertensive reactions with tyramine-containing foods and some medications); History of peptic ulcer disease; Geri: ↑ risk of sedation.

Adverse Reactions/Side Effects

CNS: SEROTONIN SYNDROME, confusion, dizziness, fainting, hallucinations, insomnia, sedation, urges (gambling, sexual), vivid dreams. **Derm:** melanoma. **GI:** nausea, abdominal pain, dry mouth.

Interactions

Drug-Drug: Concurrent use with **meperidine** or other **opioid analgesics** may possibly result in a potentially fatal reaction (excitation, sweating, rigidity, and hypertension; or hypotension and coma). Serotonin syndrome (confusion, agitation, hyperpyrexia, hypertension, seizures) may occur with concurrent use of **nefazodone** or **SSRI antidepressants** (fluoxetine should be discontinued 5 wk prior to selegiline, **venlafaxine** should be discontinued 7 days before selegiline, other agents should be discontinued 2 wk before selegiline). Selegiline should be discontinued 2 wk before **SSRIs** are initiated. Concurrent use with **tricyclic antidepressants** may result in asystole, diaphoresis, hypertension, syncope, behavioral changes, altered consciousness, hyperpyrexia, tremors, muscle rigidity, and seizures (avoid concurrent use; discontinue selegiline 2 wk before initiating tricyclic antidepressant therapy). May initially ↑ risk of side effects of **levodopa/carbidopa** (dose of levodopa/carbidopa may need to be ↓ by 10–30%).

Drug-Food: Doses >10 mg/day may produce hypertensive reactions with **tyramine-containing foods** (see Appendix K).

Route/Dosage

PO (Adults): 5 mg twice daily, with breakfast and lunch (some patients may require further dividing of doses—2.5 mg 4 times daily).

PO (Adults): *Orally disintegrating tablets*—1.25 mg once daily for at least 6 wk. After 6 wk, may increase to 2.5 mg if effect not achieved and patient is tolerating medication.

Availability (generic available)

Capsules: 5 mg. **Tablets:** 5 mg. **Orally disintegrating tablets:** 1.25 mg.

NURSING IMPLICATIONS

Assessment

- Assess patient for signs and symptoms of Parkinson's disease (tremor, muscle weakness and rigidity, ataxic gait) prior to and during therapy.
- Assess BP periodically during therapy.

Implementation

- Do not confuse selegiline with Salagen (pilocarpine). Do not confuse Zelapar (selegiline) with Zyprexa (olanzapine).
- An attempt to reduce the dose of levodopa/carbidopa by 10–30% may be made after 2–3 days of selegiline therapy.
- **PO:** Administer 5-mg tablet with breakfast and lunch.
- Administer *orally disintegrating tablets* in the morning, before breakfast and without liquid. Remove tablet gently from blister pack with clean, dry hands immediately before administering. Do not attempt to push tablet through backing. Tablet will disintegrate within sec when placed on tongue. Avoid food or liquid within 5 min of administering orally disintegrating tablets.

Patient/Family Teaching

- Instruct patient to take medication as directed. Take missed doses as soon as possible, but not if late afternoon or evening or almost time for next dose. Do not double doses. Caution patient that taking more than the prescribed dose may increase side effects and place patient at risk for hypertensive crisis if foods containing tyramine are consumed (see Appendix K).
- Advise patients taking selegiline ≥20 mg/day to avoid large amounts of tyramine-containing foods (see Appendix K), alcoholic beverages, large quantities of caffeine-containing beverages, or OTC or herbal cough or cold medications.
- Caution patient and caregiver that selegiline may cause drowsiness and dizziness. Monitor and assist with ambulation and caution patient to avoid driving and other activities requiring alertness until response to medication is known.
- Inform patient and family of the signs and symptoms of MAO inhibitor–induced hypertensive crisis (severe headache, chest pain, nausea, vomiting, photosensitivity, enlarged pupils). Advise patient to notify health care professional immediately if severe headache or any other unusual symptoms occur.
- Caution patient to change positions slowly to minimize orthostatic hypotension.
- Advise patient to notify health care professional of signs and symptoms of serotonin syndrome (mental status changes [agitation, hallucinations, delirium, and coma], autonomic instability [tachycardia, labile BP, dizziness, diaphoresis, flushing, hyperthermia], neuromuscular changes [tremor, rigidity, myoclonus, hyperreflexia, incoordination], seizures, and/or gastrointestinal symptoms [nausea, vomiting, diarrhea]).
- Instruct patient to notify health care professional of all Rx or OTC medications, vitamins, or herbal products being taken and to consult with health care professional before taking other medications.
- Advise patient to have periodic skin exams to check for lesions that may be melanoma.
- Advise patient to notify health care professional if agitation, aggression, delirium, hallucinations, new or increased gambling, sexual, or other intense urges occur.
- Advise patient that increasing fluids, sugarless gum or candy, ice, or saliva substitutes may help minimize dry mouth. Consult health care professional if dry mouth continues for >2 wk.

Evaluation/Desired Outcomes

- Improved response to levodopa/carbidopa in patients with Parkinson's disease.

selegiline transdermal

(se-**le**-ji-leen)

Emsam

Classification

Therapeutic: antidepressants

Pharmacologic: monoamine oxidase type B inhibitors

Indications

Major depressive disorder.

S

Action

Following conversion by MAO to its active form, selegiline inactivates MAO by irreversibly binding to it at type B (brain) sites; this results in higher levels of monoamine neurotransmitters in the brain (dopamine, serotonin, norepinephrine). **Therapeutic Effects:** Decreased symptoms of depression.

Pharmacokinetics

Absorption: 25–30% of patch content is transdermally absorbed, blood levels are higher than those following oral administration because there is less first-pass hepatic metabolism.

Distribution: Rapidly distributes to all body tissues; crosses the blood-brain barrier.

Metabolism and Excretion: Mostly metabolized by the liver, primarily by the CYP2A6, CYP2C9, and CYP3A4/5 enzyme systems. 10% excreted in urine as metabolites, 2% in feces; negligible renal excretion of unchanged drug.

Half-life: 18–25 hr.

TIME/ACTION PROFILE

ROUTE	ONSET	PEAK	DURATION
transdermal	unknown	2 or more wk	2 wk (after discontinuation)

Contraindications/Precautions

Contraindicated in: Hypersensitivity; Pheochromocytoma; Concurrent selective serotonin reuptake inhibitors (fluoxetine, paroxetine, citalopram, escitalopram, and others), nonselective serotonin re-uptake inhibitors (venlafaxine, duloxetine), tricyclic antidepressants (amitriptyline, imipramine, and others), carbamazepine, oxcarbazepine, amphetamines, vasoconstrictors (ephedrine, pseudoephedrine), bupropion, meperidine, tramadol, methadone, dextromethorphan, mirtazapine cyclobenzaprine, other MAO inhibitors (isocarboxazid, phenelzine, tranylcypromine), oral selegiline, sympathomimetic amines, amphetamines, cocaine, local anesthetics with vasoconstrictors, or St. John's wort; Alcohol; Pedi: Children <12 yr (↑ risk of hypertensive crises).

Use Cautiously in: Elective surgery within 10 days; benzodiazepines, rapacuronium, fentanyl, morphine, and codeine may be used cautiously; May ↑ risk of suicide attempt/ideation especially during early treatment or dose adjustment; risk may be greater in children or adolescents (safe use in children <12 yr not established); History of mania; Dosing at 9 mg/24 hr or 12 mg/24 hr requires dietary modification (avoid foods containing large amounts of tyramine); Geri: May be more susceptible to orthostatic hypotension; OB: Use only if benefit outweighs risk to the fetus; Lactation: Safety not established; Pedi: May ↑ risk of suicide attempt/ideation especially during early treatment or dose adjustment; risk may be greater in children or adolescents; Pedi: Children 12–17 yr (safety and effectiveness not established).

Adverse Reactions/Side Effects

CNS: SEROTONIN SYNDROME, insomnia, abnormal thinking, agitation, amnesia, worsening of mania/hypomania. **CV:** HYPERTENSIVE CRISIS, chest pain, orthostatic hypotension, peripheral edema. **Derm:** application site reactions, acne, ecchymoses, pruritus, sweating. **EENT:** tinnitus. **GI:** diarrhea, altered taste, anorexia, constipation, flatulence, gastroenteritis, vomiting. **GU:** dysmenorrhea, metrorrhagia, urinary frequency. **MS:** mylagia, neck pain, pathologic fracture. **Neuro:** paresthesia. **Resp:** cough.

Interactions

Drug-Drug: Concurrent **selective serotonin reuptake inhibitors (fluoxetine, paroxetine, citalopram, escitalopram**, and others), **nonselective serotonin re-uptake inhibitors (venlafaxine, duloxetine), tricyclic antidepressants (amitriptyline, imipramine**, and others), **carbamazepine, oxcarbazepine, amphetamines, vasoconstrictors (ephedrine, pseudoephedrine, phenylpropanolamine), bupropion, meperidine, tramadol, methadone, dextromethorphan, mirtazapine, cyclobenzaprine**, other MAO inhibitors (**isocarboxazid, phenelzine, tranylcypromine**), oral **selegiline, sympathomimetic amines, amphetamines, cocaine**, or **local anesthetics with vasoconstrictors**; these may all ↑ risk of hypertensive crisis. (**Fluoxetine** should not be used within 2 wk of initiating therapy.).

Drug-Natural Products: St. John's wort may ↑ risk of hypertensive crisis.

Route/Dosage

Transdermal (Adults): Apply 6 mg/24 hr patch once daily initially; if necessary, may be ↑ at 2-wk intervals in increments of 3 mg/24 hr patch (max dose = 12 mg/24 hr).

Availability

Transdermal patch : 6 mg/24 hr, 9 mg/24 hr, 12 mg/24 hr.

NURSING IMPLICATIONS

Assessment

- Assess mental status, mood changes, and anxiety level frequently. Assess for suicidal tendencies, agitation, irritability, and unusual changes in behavior especially during early therapy. Assess for any personal or family history of bipolar disorder, mania, or hypomania before starting therapy. Monitor pediatric patients face-to-face weekly during first 4 wk, every other wk for 4 wk, at 12 wk, and as clinically indicated during therapy. Restrict amount of drug available to patient.
- Monitor BP and pulse rate before and frequently during therapy. Report significant changes promptly.

- ***Toxicity and Overdose:*** Concurrent ingestion of tyramine-rich foods and many medications may result in a life-threatening hypertensive crisis. Signs and symptoms of hypertensive crisis include chest pain, tachycardia or bradycardia, severe headache, neck stiffness or soreness, nausea and vomiting, sweating, photosensitivity, and enlarged pupils. If hypertensive crisis occurs, discontinue selegiline transdermal and administer labetalol 20 mg slowly IV to control hypertension. Manage fever with external cooling. Monitor patient closely until symptoms have stabilized.

Implementation

- **Transdermal:** Apply system to dry, intact skin on the upper torso such as chest, back, upper thigh, or outer surface of the upper arm once every 24 hr at the same time each day. Avoid areas that are hairy, oily, irritated, broken, scarred, or calloused. Wash area gently with soap and warm water, rinse thoroughly. Allow skin to dry completely before application. Apply immediately after removing from package. Do not alter the system (i.e., cut) in any way before application. Remove liner from adhesive layer and press firmly in place with palm of hand for 30 sec, especially around the edges, to make sure contact is complete. Remove used system and fold so that adhesive edges are together. Only 1 selegiline patch should be worn at a time. Dispose away from children and pets. Apply new system to a different site. Wash hands thoroughly with soap and water to remove any medicine that may have gotten on them.

Patient/Family Teaching

- Instruct patient to apply patch as directed. Advise patients and caregivers to read the *Medication Guide about Using Antidepressants in Children and Teenagers*. Inform patient that improvement may be noticed after 1 to several wk of therapy. Advise patient not to discontinue therapy without consulting health care professional.
- Caution patient to avoid alcohol and CNS depressants during and for at least 2 wk after therapy has been discontinued; they may precipitate a hypertensive crisis. Contact health care professional immediately if symptoms of hypertensive crisis develop. Patients taking 9 mg/24 hr or 12 mg/24 hr must avoid foods or beverages containing tyramine (see Appendix K) from the 1st day of the increased dose through 2 wk after discontinuation of selegiline transdermal therapy.
- Advise patient to avoid exposing application site to external sources of direct heat such as heating pads, electric blankets, heat lamps, saunas, hot tubs, heated water beds, and prolonged direct sunlight.
- May cause dizziness or drowsiness. Caution patient to avoid driving and other activities requiring alertness until response to medication is known.
- Caution patient to change positions slowly to minimize orthostatic hypotension. Geriatric patients are at increased risk for this side effect.
- Advise patient to notify health care professional of signs and symptoms of serotonin syndrome (mental status changes [agitation, hallucinations, delirium, and coma], autonomic instability [tachycardia, labile BP, dizziness, diaphoresis, flushing, hyperthermia], neuromuscular changes [tremor, rigidity, myoclonus, hyperreflexia, incoordination], seizures, and/or gastrointestinal symptoms [nausea, vomiting, diarrhea]).
- Advise patient referred for MRI test to discuss patch with referring health care professional and MRI facility to determine if removal of patch is necessary prior to test and for directions for replacing patch.
- Advise patients and caregivers to notify health care professional if severe headache, neck stiffness, heart racing or palpitations, anxiety, agitation, panic attacks, insomnia, irritability, hostility, aggressiveness, impulsivity, akathisia, hypomania, mania, change in behavior, worsening of depression, or suicidal ideation occur, especially during initial therapy or during changes in dose.
- Instruct patient to consult health care professional before taking any Rx, OTC, or herbal products. Caution patient to avoid use of St. John's wort and the analgesics meperidine, tramadol, or methadone during therapy.
- Advise patient to notify health care professional of medication regimen before treatment or surgery. If possible, therapy should be discontinued at least 2 wk before surgery.
- Advise patient to notify health care professional if pregnancy is planned or suspected or if breast feeding.

Evaluation/Desired Outcomes

- Improved mood in depressed patients.
- Decreased anxiety.
- Increased appetite.
- Improved energy level.
- Improved sleep. Evaluate effectiveness of therapy periodically.

semaglutide (sem-a-gloo-tide)

Ozempic, Rybelsus

Classification

Therapeutic: antidiabetics

Pharmacologic: glucagon-like peptide-1 (GLP-1) receptor agonists

S

Indications

Adjunct treatment to diet and exercise in the management of adults with type 2 diabetes mellitus (not recommended as first-line therapy).

Action

Stimulates the glucagon-like peptide-1 (GLP-1, an incretin) receptor which leads to a reduction in blood glucose by stimulating insulin release and lowering glucagon secretion (both effects subside as blood glucose decreases toward normal). Also lowers blood glucose by delaying gastric emptying. **Therapeutic Effects:** Improved glycemic control.

Pharmacokinetics

Absorption: 89% absorbed following subcutaneous injection; 0.4–1% absorbed following oral administration.

Distribution: Minimally distributed to tissues.

Protein Binding: >99%.

Metabolism and Excretion: Endogenously metabolized; eliminated in the urine (3% as unchanged drug) and feces.

Half-life: 1 wk.

TIME/ACTION PROFILE (plasma concentrations)

ROUTE	ONSET	PEAK	DURATION
Subcut	unknown	1–3 days	unknown
PO	unknown	1 hr	unknown

Contraindications/Precautions

Contraindicated in: Hypersensitivity; Personal or family history of medullary thyroid carcinoma; Multiple Endocrine Neoplasia syndrome type 2; Type 1 diabetes; Diabetic ketoacidosis.

Use Cautiously in: History of pancreatitis; Diabetic retinopathy (↑ risk of complications); History of angioedema or anaphylaxis to another GLP-1 receptor agonist; History of diabetic retinopathy; OB: Use only if potential maternal benefit justifies potential fetal risk; Lactation: Safety not established in breast feeding; Rep: Women of reproductive potential; Pedi: Safety and effectiveness not established.

Adverse Reactions/Side Effects

EENT: retinopathy complications. **Endo:** THYROID C-CELL TUMORS, hypoglycemia. **GI:** PANCREATITIS, abdominal pain, diarrhea, nausea, cholelithiasis, constipation, ↓ appetite, dyspepsia, flatulence, ↑ amylase, ↑ lipase, vomiting. **GU:** acute kidney injury. **Local:** injection site reactions. **Misc:** HYPERSENSITIVITY REACTIONS (including anaphylaxis and angioedema).

Interactions

Drug-Drug: Concurrent use with **agents that increase insulin secretion**, including **sulfonylureas** or **insulin**, may ↑ the risk of serious hypoglycemia; use cautiously and consider dose ↓ of agent increasing insulin secretion. May alter absorption of concomitantly administered **oral medications** due to delayed gastric emptying.

Route/Dosage

PO (Adults): 3 mg once daily for 30 days, then 7 mg once daily; after 30 days, may ↑ to 14 mg once daily if additional glycemic control needed.

Subcut (Adults): 0.25 mg once weekly initially for 4 wk, then 0.5 mg once weekly for 1 wk; may then ↑ dose after 4 wk, if needed, up to 1 mg once weekly.

Availability

Solution for injection (prefilled pen): 2 mg/1.5 mL (delivers doses of 0.25 mg, 0.5 mg, or 1 mg), 4 mg/3 mL (delivers dose of 1 mg). **Tablets:** 3 mg, 7 mg, 14 mg.

NURSING IMPLICATIONS

Assessment

- Observe patient taking concurrent insulin for signs and symptoms of hypoglycemic reactions (sweating, hunger, weakness, dizziness, tremor, tachycardia, anxiety, headache, blurred vision, slurred speech, irritability).
- Monitor for pancreatitis (persistent severe abdominal pain, sometimes radiating to the back, with or without vomiting). If pancreatitis is suspected, discontinue semaglutide; if confirmed, do not restart semaglutide.
- ***Lab Test Considerations:*** Monitor serum HbA_{1c} periodically during therapy to evaluate effectiveness.
- May ↑ lipase and pancreatic amylase.

Implementation

- Patients stabilized on a diabetic regimen who are exposed to stress, fever, trauma, infection, or surgery may require administration of insulin.
- **Subcut:** Administer once weekly on same day each wk, any time of day without regard to meals. May change day of injection as long as time between doses is >48 hrs. Inject into abdomen, thigh, or upper arm, rotating sites each wk. Solution is clear and colorless; do not administer solutions that are discolored or contain particulate matter.

Patient/Family Teaching

- Instruct patient in correct technique for injection and disposal of materials. Follow manufacturer's instructions for pen use. Pen should never be shared between patients, even if needle is changed. Administer missed doses as soon as remembered within 5 days of missed dose; if >5 days, skip dose and administer next dose on regular scheduled day. Advise patient to read the *Medication Guide* before starting therapy and with each Rx refill in case of changes.
- Advise patient taking insulin and semaglutide to never mix insulin and semaglutide together. Give as

2 separate injections. Both injections may be given in the same body area, but should not be given right next to each other.

- Explain to patient that this medication controls hyperglycemia but does not cure diabetes. Therapy is long-term.
- Review signs of hypoglycemia and hyperglycemia with patient. If hypoglycemia occurs, advise patient to take a glass of orange juice or 2–3 tsp of sugar, honey, or corn syrup dissolved in water and notify health care professional.
- Encourage patient to follow prescribed diet, medication, and exercise regimen to prevent hypoglycemic or hyperglycemic episodes.
- Instruct patient in proper testing of serum glucose and ketones. These tests should be closely monitored during periods of stress or illness, and health care professional should be notified if significant changes occur.
- Advise patient to notify health care professional of all Rx or OTC medications, vitamins, or herbal products being taken and consult health care professional before taking any new medications.
- Advise patient to notify health care professional and discontinue semaglutide immediately if signs of pancreatitis (nausea, vomiting, abdominal pain radiating to back) or hypersensitivity (swelling of face, lips, tongue or throat, problems breathing or swallowing, severe rash or itching, fainting or feeling dizzy, very rapid heartbeat) occur.
- Inform patient of risk of benign and malignant thyroid C-cell tumors. Advise patient to notify health care professional if symptoms of thyroid tumors (lump in neck, hoarseness, trouble swallowing, shortness of breath) occur.
- Advise patient to inform health care professional of medication regimen before treatment or surgery.
- Advise patient to carry a form of sugar (sugar packets, candy) and identification describing disease process and medication regimen at all times.
- Rep: Insulin is the preferred method of controlling blood glucose during pregnancy. Advise female and male patient of reproductive potential to discontinue semaglutide in women at least 2 mo before a planned pregnancy to allow for long washout period of semaglutide. Counsel female patients to notify health care professional if pregnancy is planned or suspected or if breast feeding.
- Emphasize the importance of routine follow-up exams.

Evaluation/Desired Outcomes

- Improved glycemic control.

sennosides (sen-oh-sides)

Black-Draught, Ex-Lax, Ex-Lax Chocolated, Fletchers' Castoria, Maximum Relief Ex-Lax, Sena-Gen, Senexon, Senokot, SenokotXTRA

Classification
Therapeutic: laxatives
Pharmacologic: stimulant laxatives

Indications

Treatment of constipation, particularly when associated with: Slow transit time, Constipating drugs, Irritable or spastic bowel syndrome, Neurologic constipation.

Action

Active components of senna (sennosides) alter water and electrolyte transport in the large intestine, resulting in accumulation of water and increased peristalsis.
Therapeutic Effects: Laxative action.

Pharmacokinetics

Absorption: Minimally absorbed following oral administration.
Distribution: Unknown.
Metabolism and Excretion: Unknown.
Half-life: Unknown.

TIME/ACTION PROFILE (laxative effect)

ROUTE	ONSET	PEAK	DURATION
PO	6–12 hr†	unknown	3–4 days

†May take as long as 24 hr.

Contraindications/Precautions

Contraindicated in: Hypersensitivity; Abdominal pain of unknown cause, especially if associated with fever; Rectal fissures; Ulcerated hemorrhoids; Known alcohol intolerance (some liquid products).
Use Cautiously in: Chronic use (may lead to laxative dependence); Possible intestinal obstruction; OB, Lactation: Safety not established.

Adverse Reactions/Side Effects

GI: cramping, diarrhea, nausea. **GU:** pink-red or brown-black discoloration of urine. **F and E:** electrolyte abnormalities (chronic use or dependence).
Misc: laxative dependence.

Interactions

Drug-Drug: May ↓ absorption of other **orally administered drugs** because of ↓ transit time.

Route/Dosage

Larger doses have been used to treat/prevent opioid-induced constipation. Consult labeling of individual OTC products for more specific dosing information.

PO (Adults and Children >12 yr): 12–50 mg 1–2 times daily.
PO (Children 6–12 yr): 6–25 mg 1–2 times daily.
PO (Children 2–6 yr): 3–12.5 mg 1–2 times daily.

Availability (generic available)

Noted as sennoside content

Tablets: 6 mg[OTC], 8.6 mg[OTC], 15 mg [OTC], 17 mg[OTC], 25 mg[OTC]. **Granules:** 15 mg/5 mL[OTC], 20 mg/5 mL[OTC]. **Syrup:** 8.8 mg/5 mL[OTC]. **Liquid:** 25 mg/15 mL[OTC], 33.3 mg/mL senna concentrate[OTC]. ***In combination with:*** psyllium and docusate[OTC]. See Appendix B.

NURSING IMPLICATIONS

Assessment

- Assess patient for abdominal distention, presence of bowel sounds, and usual pattern of bowel function.
- Assess color, consistency, and amount of stool produced.

Implementation

- **PO:** Take with a full glass of water. Administer at bedtime for evacuation 6–12 hr later. Administer on an empty stomach for more rapid results.
- Shake oral solution well before administering.
- Granules should be dissolved or mixed in water or other liquid before administration.

Patient/Family Teaching

- Advise patient that laxatives should be used only for short-term therapy. Long-term therapy may cause electrolyte imbalance and dependence.
- Encourage patient to use other forms of bowel regulation, such as increasing bulk in the diet, increasing fluid intake, and increasing mobility. Normal bowel habits are individualized and may vary from 3 times/day to 3 times/wk.
- Inform patient that this medication may cause a change in urine color to pink, red, violet, yellow, or brown.
- Instruct patients with cardiac disease to avoid straining during bowel movements (Valsalva maneuver).
- Advise patient not to use laxatives when abdominal pain, nausea, vomiting, or fever is present.

Evaluation/Desired Outcomes

- A soft, formed bowel movement.

sertraline (ser-tra-leen)

Zoloft

Classification
Therapeutic: antidepressants
Pharmacologic: selective serotonin reuptake inhibitors (SSRIs)

Indications

Major depressive disorder. Panic disorder. Obsessive-compulsive disorder (OCD). Post-traumatic stress disorder (PTSD). Social anxiety disorder (social phobia). Premenstrual dysphoric disorder (PMDD). **Unlabeled Use:** Generalized anxiety disorder (GAD).

Action

Inhibits neuronal uptake of serotonin in the CNS, thus potentiating the activity of serotonin. Has little effect on norepinephrine or dopamine. **Therapeutic Effects:** Antidepressant action. Decreased incidence of panic attacks. Decreased obsessive and compulsive behavior. Decreased feelings of intense fear, helplessness, or horror. Decreased social anxiety. Decrease in premenstrual dysphoria.

Pharmacokinetics

Absorption: Appears to be well absorbed after oral administration.
Distribution: Extensively distributed throughout body tissues.
Protein Binding: 98%.
Metabolism and Excretion: Extensively metabolized by the liver; 1 metabolite has some antidepressant activity; 14% excreted unchanged in feces.
Half-life: 24 hr.

TIME/ACTION PROFILE (antidepressant effect)

ROUTE	ONSET	PEAK	DURATION
PO	within 2–4 wk	unknown	unknown

Contraindications/Precautions

Contraindicated in: Hypersensitivity; Concurrent use of MAO inhibitors or MAO-like drugs (linezolid or methylene blue); Concurrent use of pimozide; Oral concentrate contains alcohol; avoid in patients with known intolerance.
Use Cautiously in: Severe hepatic or renal impairment; Patients with a history of mania; History of suicide attempt; Angle-closure glaucoma; OB: Use during 3rd trimester may result in neonatal serotonin syndrome requiring prolonged hospitalization, respiratory and nutritional support. Use only if potential benefit justifies potential risk to fetus; Lactation: May cause sedation in infant; discontinue drug or bottle-feed; Pedi: May ↑ risk of suicide attempt/ideation especially during early treatment or dose adjustment; risk may be greater in children or adolescents.

Adverse Reactions/Side Effects

CNS: SUICIDAL THOUGHTS, dizziness, drowsiness, fatigue, headache, insomnia, agitation, anxiety, confusion, emotional lability, impaired concentration, manic reaction, nervousness, weakness, yawning. **CV:** TORSADES DE POINTES, chest pain, palpitations, QT interval prolongation. **Derm:** ↑ sweating, hot flashes, rash. **EENT:** pharyngitis, rhinitis, tinnitus, visual abnormalities. **Endo:** diabetes. **F and E:** hyponatremia. **GI:** diarrhea, dry mouth, nausea, abdominal pain, altered taste, anorexia, constipation, dyspepsia, flatulence, ↑ appetite, vomiting. **GU:** sexual dysfunction, menstrual disorders, urinary disorders, urinary frequency. **MS:** back pain, myalgia. **Neuro:** tremor, hypertonia, hypoesthesia, paresthesia, twitching. **Misc:** SEROTONIN SYNDROME, fever, ↑ thirst.

Interactions

Drug-Drug: Serious, potentially fatal reactions (hyperthermia, rigidity, myoclonus, autonomic instability, with fluctuating vital signs and extreme agitation, which may proceed to delirium and coma) may occur with concurrent **MAO inhibitors**. MAO inhibitors should be stopped at least 14 days before sertraline therapy. Sertraline should be stopped at least 14 days before MAO inhibitor therapy. Concurrent use with **MAO-inhibitor–like drugs**, such as **linezolid** or **methylene blue** may ↑ risk of serotonin syndrome; concurrent use contraindicated; do not start therapy in patients receiving **linezolid** or **methylene blue**; if **linezolid** or **methylene blue** need to be started in a patient receiving sertraline, immediately discontinue sertraline and monitor for signs/symptoms of serotonin syndrome for 2 wk or until 24 hr after last dose of linezolid or methylene blue, whichever comes first (may resume sertraline therapy 24 hr after last dose of linezolid or methylene blue). May ↑ **pimozide** levels and the risk of QT interval prolongation and ventricular arrhythmias; concurrent use contraindicated. Drugs that affect serotonergic neurotransmitter systems, including **tricyclic antidepressants**, **SNRIs**, **fentanyl**, **buspirone**, **tramadol**, **amphetamines**, and **triptans** ↑ risk of serotonin syndrome. May ↑ sensitivity to **adrenergics** and ↑ the risk of serotonin syndrome. Concurrent use with **alcohol** is not recommended. May ↑ levels/effects of **warfarin**, **phenytoin**, **tricyclic antidepressants**, some **benzodiazepines (alprazolam)**, **cloazapine**, or **tolbutamide**. ↑ risk of bleeding with **NSAIDS**, **aspirin**, **clopidogrel**, or **warfarin**. **Cimetidine** ↑ blood levels and effects. Concurrent use of **QT interval prolonging medications** may ↑ risk of QT interval prolongation and torsade de pointes; avoid concurrent use.

Drug-Natural Products: ↑ risk of serotonergic side effects including serotonin syndrome with **St. John's wort** and **SAMe**.

Route/Dosage

Depression/OCD

PO (Adults): 50 mg once daily in the morning or evening initially; after several wk may be ↑ at weekly intervals up to 200 mg/day, depending on response.

PO (Children 13–17 yr): *OCD*—50 mg once daily.

PO (Children 6–12 yr): *OCD*—25 mg once daily.

Panic Disorder

PO (Adults): 25 mg once daily initially, may ↑ after 1 wk to 50 mg once daily.

PTSD

PO (Adults): 25 mg once daily for 7 days, then ↑ to 50 mg once daily; may then be ↑ if needed at intervals of at least 7 days (range 50–200 mg once daily).

Social Anxiety Disorder

PO (Adults): 25 mg once daily initially, then 50 mg once daily; may be ↑ at weekly intervals up to 200 mg/day.

PMDD

PO (Adults): 50 mg/day initially either daily or daily during luteal phase of cycle. Daily dosing may be titrated upward in 50-mg increments at the beginning of a cycle. In luteal phase–only dosing a 50 mg/day titration step for 3 days at the beginning of each luteal phase dosing period should be used (range 50–150 mg/day).

Availability (generic available)

Capsules: 🍁25 mg, 🍁50 mg, 🍁100 mg. **Oral solution (concentrated) (contains 12% alcohol):** 20 mg/mL. **Cost:** *Generic*—$64.28/60 mL. **Tablets:** 25 mg, 50 mg, 100 mg. **Cost:** *Generic*—25 mg $17.68/90, 50 mg $22.22/90, 100 mg $19.73/90.

NURSING IMPLICATIONS

Assessment

- Assess for suicidal tendencies, especially during early therapy. Restrict amount of drug available to patient. Risk may be increased in children, adolescents, and adults ≤24 yr. After starting therapy, children, adolescents, and young adults should be seen by health care professional at least weekly for 4 wk, every 3 wk for next 4 wk, and on advice of health care professional thereafter.
- Monitor appetite and nutritional intake. Weigh weekly. Notify health care professional of continued weight loss. Adjust diet as tolerated to support nutritional status.
- Assess for serotonin syndrome (mental changes [agitation, hallucinations, coma], autonomic instability [tachycardia, labile BP, hyperthermia], neuromuscular aberrations [hyper-reflexia, incoordination], and/or GI symptoms [nausea, vomiting, diarrhea]), especially in patients taking other serotonergic drugs (SSRIs, SNRIs, triptans).
- **Depression:** Monitor mood changes. Inform health care professional if patient demonstrates significant increase in anxiety, nervousness, or insomnia.
- Assess for suicidal tendencies, especially during early therapy. Restrict amount of drug available to patient.
- **OCD:** Assess patient for frequency of obsessive-compulsive behaviors. Note degree to which these thoughts and behaviors interfere with daily functioning.

S

- **Panic Attacks:** Assess frequency and severity of panic attacks.
- **PTSD:** Assess patient for feelings of fear, helplessness, and horror. Determine effect on social and occupational functioning.
- **Social Anxiety Disorder:** Assess patient for symptoms of social anxiety disorder (blushing, sweating, trembling, tachycardia during interactions with new people, people in authority, or groups) periodically during therapy.
- **Premenstrual Dysphoric Disorder:** Assess patient for symptoms of premenstrual dysphoric disorder (feeling angry, tense, or tired; crying easily, feeling sad or hopeless; arguing with family or friends for no reason; difficulty sleeping or paying attention; feeling out of control or unable to cope; having cramping, bloating, food craving, or breast tenderness) periodically during therapy.
- ***Lab Test Considerations:*** May cause false-positive urine screening tests for benzodiazepines.
- May cause hyperglycemia and diabetes mellitus; monitor serum glucose if clinical symptoms occur.

Implementation

- Do not confuse sertraline with cetirizine or Soriatane (acitretin).
- Periodically reassess dose and continued need for therapy.
- **PO:** Administer as a single dose in the morning or evening.
- For oral concentrate, use dropper provided to remove oral concentrate and mix with 4 oz (1/2 cup) of water, ginger ale, lemon/lime soda, lemonade or orange juice ONLY. Do not mix with other liquids. Take immediately after mixing. Do not mix in advance. Slight haze may appear after mixing; this is normal. Dropper dispenser contains dry natural rubber, advise patient with latex allergy.

Patient/Family Teaching

- Instruct patient to take sertraline as directed. Take missed doses as soon as possible and return to regular dosing schedule. Do not double doses. Do not stop abruptly; may cause dysphoric mood, irritability, agitation, dizziness, sensory disturbances (paresthesias such as electric shock sensations), anxiety, confusion, headache, lethargy, emotional lability, insomnia, and hypomania.
- May cause drowsiness or dizziness. Caution patient to avoid driving and other activities requiring alertness until response to the drug is known.
- Advise patient, family, and caregivers to look for suicidality, especially during early therapy or dose changes. Notify health care professional immediately if thoughts about suicide or dying, attempts to commit suicide; new or worse depression or anxiety; agitation or restlessness; panic attacks; insomnia; new or worse irritability, aggressiveness, acting on dangerous impulses, mania, or other changes in mood or behavior or if symptoms of serotonin syndrome occur.
- Advise patient to avoid alcohol or other CNS depressant drugs during therapy and to consult with health care professional before taking other medications and to avoid alcohol or other CNS depressant drugs during therapy.
- Instruct patient to notify health care professional of all Rx or OTC medications, vitamins, or herbal products being taken and consult health care professional before taking any new medications, especially St. John's wort or SAMe.
- Inform patient that frequent mouth rinses, good oral hygiene, and sugarless gum or candy may minimize dry mouth. If dry mouth persists for more than 2 wk, consult health care professional regarding use of saliva substitute.
- Advise patient to wear sunscreen and protective clothing to prevent photosensitivity reactions.
- Advise patient to notify health care professional if headache, weakness, nausea, anorexia, anxiety, or insomnia persists.
- Instruct female patient to inform health care professional if pregnancy is planned or suspected, or if breast feeding.
- Emphasize the importance of follow-up exams to monitor progress. Encourage patient participation in psychotherapy to improve coping skills.

Evaluation/Desired Outcomes

- Increased sense of well-being.
- Renewed interest in surroundings. May require 1–4 wk of therapy to obtain antidepressant effects.
- Decrease in obsessive-compulsive behaviors.
- Decrease in frequency and severity of panic attacks.
- Decrease in symptoms of PTSD.
- Decrease in social anxiety disorder.
- Decrease in symptoms of premenstrual dysphoric disorder.

sevelamer (se-**vel**-a-mer)

Renagel, Renvela

Classification

Therapeutic: electrolyte modifiers

Pharmacologic: phosphate binders

Indications

Reduction of serum phosphate levels in patients with hyperphosphatemia associated with end-stage renal disease.

Action

A polymer that binds phosphate in the GI tract, preventing its absorption. **Therapeutic Effects:** Decreased serum phosphate levels and reduction in the consequences of hyperphosphatemia (ectopic calcification, secondary hyperparathyroidism with osteitis fibrosa).

Pharmacokinetics

Absorption: Not absorbed; action is local (in GI tract).
Distribution: Unknown.
Metabolism and Excretion: Eliminated in feces.
Half-life: Unknown.

TIME/ACTION PROFILE (↓ in serum phosphate levels)

ROUTE	ONSET	PEAK	DURATION
PO	5 days	2 wk	unknown

Contraindications/Precautions

Contraindicated in: Hypersensitivity; Hypophosphatemia; Bowel obstruction.
Use Cautiously in: Dysphagia, swallowing disorders, severe GI motility disorders, or major GI tract surgery; OB: Not systemically absorbed; no fetal exposure expected. May ↓ levels of folate and fat-soluble minerals; consider supplementation during pregnancy; Lactation: Not systemically absorbed; no expected presence in breast milk. May ↓ levels of folate and fat-soluble minerals; consider supplementation while breast feeding; OB, Lactation, Pedi: Children <18 yr (Renagel) and <6 yr (Renvela) (safety and effectiveness not established).

Adverse Reactions/Side Effects

GI: BOWEL OBSTRUCTION/PERFORATION, ESOPHAGEAL OBSTRUCTION (tablet), diarrhea, dyspepsia, vomiting, choking (tablet), constipation, dysphagia (tablet), flatulence, nausea. **Misc:** hypersensitivity reactions.

Interactions

Drug-Drug: May ↓ absorption of other drugs and ↓ effectiveness, especially **drugs whose efficacy is dependent on tightly controlled blood levels**. ↓ absorption of **ciprofloxacin**.

Route/Dosage

PO (Adults): 800–1600 mg 3 times daily with meals; may titrate by 800 mg every 2 wk to achieve target serum phosphorus levels.
PO (Children ≥6 yr and BSA ≥1.2 m^2): *Renvela*—1600 mg 3 times daily with meals; may titrate by 800 mg every 2 wk to achieve target serum phosphorus levels.
PO (Children ≥6 yr and BSA 0.75–<1.2 m^2): *Renvela*—800 mg 3 times daily with meals; may titrate by 400 mg every 2 wk to achieve target serum phosphorus levels.

Availability (generic available)

Powder for oral suspension: 800 mg/pkt, 2400 mg/pkt. **Tablets:** 400 mg, 800 mg.

NURSING IMPLICATIONS

Assessment

- Assess patient for GI side effects periodically during therapy.
- ***Lab Test Considerations:*** Monitor serum phosphorous, calcium, bicarbonate, and chloride levels periodically during therapy.

Implementation

- Do not confuse Renagel with Renvela.
- Doses of concurrent medications, especially antiarrhythmics, should be spaced at least 1 hr before or 3 hr after sevelamer.
- **PO:** Administer with meals. Do not break, chew, or crush tablets; contents expand in water.
- Place contents of powder packet in a cup and mix thoroughly with at least 1 oz of water for the 0.8-g dose or 2 oz of water for the 2.4-g dose packet. Stir mixture vigorously (it does not dissolve) and drink entire preparation within 30 min or resuspend the preparation right before drinking.

Patient/Family Teaching

- Instruct patient to take sevelamer with meals as directed and to adhere to prescribed diet.
- Caution patient to space concurrent medications at least 1 hr before or 3 hr after sevelamer.
- Advise patient to notify health care professional if GI effects are severe or prolonged.
- Rep: Advise patient to notify health care professional if pregnancy is planned or suspected, or if breast feeding. Sevelamer is not systemically absorbed, but may decrease serum levels of fat soluble vitamins and folic acid in pregnant women. May consider supplementation.

Evaluation/Desired Outcomes

- Decrease in serum phosphorous concentration to ≤6 mg/dL. Dose adjustment is based on serum phosphorous concentrations.

S

sildenafil (sil-den-a-fil)

Revatio, Viagra

Classification
Therapeutic: erectile dysfunction agents, vasodilators
Pharmacologic: phosphodiesterase type 5 inhibitors

Indications

Viagra: Erectile dysfunction. *Revatio:* Pulmonary arterial hypertension (WHO Group I).

Action

Viagra: Enhances effects of nitric oxide released during sexual stimulation. Nitric oxide activates guanylate cyclase, which produces increased levels of cyclic guanosine monophosphate (cGMP). cGMP produces smooth muscle relaxation of the corpus cavernosum, which promotes increased blood flow and subsequent erection. cGMP also leads to vasodilation of the pulmonary vasculature. Sildenafil inhibits the enzyme phosphodiesterase type 5 (PDE5), PDE5 inactivates cGMP. *Revatio:* Produces vasodilation of the pulmonary vascular bed. **Therapeutic Effects:** *Viagra:* Enhanced blood flow to the corpus cavernosum and erection sufficient to allow sexual intercourse. Requires sexual stimulation. *Revatio:* Improved exercise tolerance and delay worsening of disease.

Pharmacokinetics

Absorption: Rapidly absorbed (41%) after oral administration; IV administration results in complete bioavailability.

Distribution: Widely distributed to tissues; negligible amount in semen.

Protein Binding: 96%.

Metabolism and Excretion: Mostly metabolized by the liver (by P450 3A4 enzyme system); 1 metabolite is active and accounts for 20% or more of drug effect. Metabolites excreted mostly (80%) in feces; 13% excreted in urine.

Half-life: 4 hr (for sildenafil and active metabolite).

TIME/ACTION PROFILE (vasodilation, ability to produce erection)

ROUTE	ONSET	PEAK	DURATION
PO	within 1 hr	30–120 min	up to 4 hr

Contraindications/Precautions

Contraindicated in: Hypersensitivity; Concurrent use of nitrates or riociguat; Pulmonary veno-occlusive disease; Pedi: *Revatio*—Chronic use not recommended for pulmonary hypertension due to lack of efficacy and ↑ risk of death.

Use Cautiously in: Serious underlying cardiovascular disease (including history of MI, stroke, or serious arrhythmia within 6 mo), cardiac failure, or coronary artery disease with unstable angina; History of HF, coronary artery disease, uncontrolled hypertension (BP >170/110 mm Hg) or hypotension (BP <90/50 mm Hg), dehydration, autonomic dysfunction, or severe left ventricular outflow obstruction; Pulmonary hypertension secondary to sickle cell anemia (may ↑ risk of vaso-occlusive crises); Concurrent treatment with antihypertensives or glipizide; Renal impairment (CCr <30 mL/min, hepatic impairment; all result in ↑ blood levels; ↓ dose required with Viagra); Anatomic penile deformity (angulation, cavernosal fibrosis, Peyronie disease); Conditions associated with priapism (sickle cell anemia, multiple myeloma, leukemia); Bleeding disorders or active peptic ulceration; History of sudden severe vision loss or at risk for non-arteritic ischemic optic neuropathy (NAION) (low cup to disc ratio in eye, age >50 yr, diabetes, hypertension, coronary artery disease, hyperlipidemia, and smoking); may ↑ risk of recurrence; Retinitis pigmentosa; Alpha adrenergic blockers (patients should be on stable dose of alpha blockers before starting sildenafil); OB: *Revatio*—Use during pregnancy only if maternal benefit outweighs potential risk to fetus; Lactation: Safety not established; Geri: ↑ blood levels and may require lower doses; consider age-related decrease in cardiac, hepatic, and renal function as well as concurrent drug therapy and chronic disease states.

Adverse Reactions/Side Effects

CNS: headache, dizziness, insomnia. **CV:** MYOCARDIAL INFARCTION, SUDDEN DEATH, hypotension, vaso-occlusive crises. **Derm:** flushing, rash. **EENT:** epistaxis, hearing loss, nasal congestion, vision loss. **GI:** dyspepsia, diarrhea. **GU:** priapism, urinary tract infection. **MS:** mylagia. **Neuro:** paresthesias.

Interactions

Drug-Drug: Concurrent use of **nitrates** may cause serious, life-threatening hypotension and is contraindicated. Concurrent use of **riociguat** may result in severe hypotension; concurrent use contraindicated. Blood levels and effects, including the risk of hypotension, may be ↑ by **CYP3A4 inhibitors** including **cimetidine**, **erythromycin**, **tacrolimus**, **ketoconazole**, **itraconazole**, and **protease inhibitor antiretrovirals** including **nelfinavir**, **indinavir**, **ritonavir**, and **saquinavir** (initial dose of sildenafil for erectile dysfunction should be ↓ to 25 mg) (concurrent use of potent CYP3A inhibitors not recommended with oral Revatio). ↑ risk of hypotension with **alpha adrenergic blockers** and acute ingestion of **alcohol**. **CYP3A4 inducers**, including **rifampin**, **bosentan**, **barbiturates**, **carbamazepine**, **phenytoin**, **efavirenz**, **nevirapine**, **rifampin**, or **rifabutin** may ↓ blood levels and effects; dose adjustments may be necessary in the treatment of pulmonary arterial hypertension. ↑ levels of **bosentan**. Use cautiously with **glipizide**. May ↑ risk of bleeding with **warfarin**.

Route/Dosage

Viagra (for erectile dysfunction)

PO (Adults): 50 mg taken 1 hr before sexual activity (range 25–100 mg taken 30 min–4 hr before sexual activity); not more than once daily; *Concurrent use with alpha-blocker antihypertensives*—do not use 50–100 mg dose within 4 hr of alpha blocker, 25-mg dose may be taken anytime.

PO (Geriatric Patients ≥65 yr or with concurrent enzyme inhibitors): 25 mg taken 1 hr before sexual activity (range 25–100 mg taken 30 min–4 hr before sexual activity); not more than once daily.

Hepatic/Renal Impairment

PO (Adults): 25 mg taken 1 hr before sexual activity (range 25–100 mg taken 30 min–4 hr before sexual activity); not more than once daily.

Revatio (for pulmonary arterial hypertension)

IV therapy is indicated for patients unable to take PO therapy

PO (Adults): 5 mg or 20 mg 3 times daily; dose adjustments may be necessary for concurrent bosentan, barbiturates, carbamazepine, phenytoin, efavirenz, nevirapine, rifampin, or rifabutin.
IV (Adults): 2.5 mg or 10 mg 3 times daily.

Availability (generic available)

Powder for oral suspension (requires reconstitution) (Revatio) (grape flavor): 10 mg/mL. **Solution for injection (Revatio):** 0.8 mg/mL. **Tablets (Revatio):** 20 mg. **Tablets (Viagra):** 25 mg, 50 mg, 100 mg.

NURSING IMPLICATIONS

Assessment

- **Viagra:** Determine erectile dysfunction before administration. Sildenafil has no effect in the absence of sexual stimulation.
- **Revatio:** Monitor hemodynamic parameters and exercise tolerance prior to and periodically during therapy.

Implementation

- Do not confuse Viagra (sildenafil) with Allegra (fexofenadine).
- **PO:** Dose for *erectile dysfunction* is usually administered 1 hr before sexual activity. May be administered 30 min–4 hr before sexual activity.
- Dose for *pulmonary arterial hypertension* is administered 3 times daily without regard to food. Doses should be spaced 4–6 hr apart.
- Use syringe provided for accurate dosing of oral suspension. Shake well before using. Solution is stable for 60 days from date of reconstitution.

IV Administration

- **IV Push:** Administer undiluted. Solution is clear and colorless; do not administer solutions that are discolored or contain a precipitate. ***Rate:*** Administer as a bolus three times daily.

Patient/Family Teaching

- Instruct patient to take sildenafil as directed. For *erectile dysfunction,* take approximately 1 hr before sexual activity and not more than once per day. If taking sildenafil for *pulmonary arterial hypertension*, take missed doses as soon as remembered unless almost time for next dose; do not double doses.
- Advise patient that *Viagra* is not indicated for use in women.
- Caution patient not to take sildenafil concurrently with alpha-adrenergic blockers (unless on a stable dose) of nitrates. If chest pain occurs after taking sildenafil, instruct patient to seek immediate medical attention. Advise patient taking sildenafil for *pulmonary arterial hypertension* to notify health care professional of all Rx or OTC medications, vitamins, or herbal products being taken and to consult with health care professional before taking other medications.
- Instruct patient to notify health care professional promptly if erection lasts longer than 4 hr or if experience sudden or decreased vision loss in 1 or both eyes or loss or decrease in hearing, ringing in the ears, or dizziness.
- Inform patient that sildenafil offers no protection against sexually transmitted diseases. Counsel patient that protection against sexually transmitted diseases and HIV infection should be considered.

Evaluation/Desired Outcomes

- Male erection sufficient to allow intercourse.
- Increased exercise tolerance.

silodosin (si-lo-do-sin)

Rapaflo

Classification
Therapeutic: benign prostatic hyperplasia (BPH) agents
Pharmacologic: alpha-adrenergic blockers

Indications

Treatment of the signs/symptoms of benign prostatic hyperplasia (BPH).

Action

Blocks post synaptic $alpha_1$-adrenergic receptors. Decreases contractions in the smooth muscle of the prostatic capsule. **Therapeutic Effects:** Decreased signs and symptoms of BPH (urinary urgency, hesitancy, nocturia).

Pharmacokinetics

Absorption: 32% absorbed following oral administration.
Distribution: Unknown.
Protein Binding: 97%.
Metabolism and Excretion: Extensively metabolized (CYP3A4, UGT2B7, and other metabolic pathways involved); 33.5% excreted in urine and 54.9% in feces.
Half-life: 13.3 hr.

TIME/ACTION PROFILE (effect on symptoms of BPH)

ROUTE	ONSET	PEAK	DURATION
PO	rapid	24 hr	24 hr*

*Following discontinuation.

Contraindications/Precautions

Contraindicated in: Hypersensitivity; Not indicated for use in women or children; Severe renal impairment (CrCl less than 30 mL/min); Severe hepatic impairment (Child-Pugh score of ≥10); Concurrent use of strong CYP3A4 inhibitors or P-gp inhibitors.

Use Cautiously in: Moderate inhibitors of the CYP3A4 enzyme system; Cataract surgery (may cause intraoperative floppy iris syndrome); Moderate renal impairment (lower dose recommended); Geri: ↑ risk of orthostatic hypotention; Pedi: Safety and effectiveness have not been established.

Adverse Reactions/Side Effects

CNS: dizziness, headache. **CV:** orthostatic hypotension. **GI:** diarrhea. **GU:** retrograde ejaculation. **Derm:** pruritis, rash, urticaria. **Misc:** allergic reactions.

Interactions

Drug-Drug: Strong inhibitors of CYP3A4 (including **ketoconazole**, **clarithromycin**, **itraconazole**, and **ritonavir**) ↓ metabolism, ↑ blood levels and risk of toxicity; concurrent use is contraindicated. Concurrent use with **moderate CYP3A4 inhibitors** (including **diltiazem**, **erythromycin**, and **verapamil**) may ↑ levels; use cautiously. Concurrent use with **antihypertensives** (including **calcium channel blockers** and **thiazides**), other **alpha blockers** and **phosphodiesterase type 5 inhibitors** (including **sildenafil**, **tadalafil**, and **vardenafil**) ↑ the risk of dizziness and orthostatic hypotension. **P-glycoprotein (P-gp) inhibitors** including **cyclosporine**) may ↑ levels; concurrent use not recommended.

Route/Dosage

PO (Adults): 8 mg once daily.

Renal Impairment

PO (Adults): *CCr 30–50 mL/min*—4 mg once daily.

Availability (generic available)

Capsules: 4 mg, 8 mg.

NURSING IMPLICATIONS

Assessment

- Assess patient for symptoms of benign prostatic hyperplasia (urinary hesitancy, feeling of incomplete bladder emptying, interruption of urinary stream, impairment of size and force of urinary stream, terminal urinary dribbling, straining to start flow, frequency, dysuria, nocturia, urgency) before and periodically during therapy.
- Assess patient for orthostatic reaction and syncope. Monitor BP (lying and standing) and during initial therapy and periodically thereafter.
- Rule out prostatic carcinoma before therapy; symptoms are similar.

Implementation

- ***High Alert:*** Do not confuse Rapaflo with Rapamune (sirolimus). Do not confuse silodosin with sirolimus.
- **PO:** Administer with food at the same meal each day.
- If unable to swallow capsule, may open capsule and sprinkle powder inside on a tablespoonful of applesauce. Swallow immediately, within 5 min, without chewing; follow with 8 oz of cool water to ensure complete dose is swallowed. Use cool applesauce, soft enough to be swallowed without chewing. Do not store for future use or subdivide capsule contents.

Patient/Family Teaching

- Instruct patient to take medication with the same meal each day.
- May cause dizziness. Caution patient to avoid driving or other activities requiring alertness until response to the medication is known.
- Caution patient to avoid sudden changes in position to decrease orthostatic hypotension, especially patients with low BP or concurrently taking antihypertensives. Geri: Assess risk for falls; instruct patient and family in preventing falls at home.
- Instruct patient to notify health care professional of all Rx or OTC medications, vitamins, or herbal products being taken and consult health care professional before taking any new medications, especially cough, cold, or allergy remedies.
- Instruct patient to notify health care professional of medication regimen before any surgery. Patients planning cataract surgery should notify ophthalmologist of silodosin therapy prior to surgery.
- Inform patient that silodosin may cause retrograde ejaculation (orgasm with reduced or no semen). This does not pose a safety concern and is reversible with discontinuation.
- Emphasize the importance of follow-up exams to evaluate effectiveness of medication.

Evaluation/Desired Outcomes

- Decreased symptoms of benign prostatic hyperplasia.

simvastatin, See HMG-CoA REDUCTASE INHIBITORS (statins).

sirolimus (sir-oh-li-mus)

Rapamune

Classification

Therapeutic: immunosuppressants

Indications

Prevention of organ rejection in allogenic kidney transplantation (with corticosteroids and cyclosporine). Treatment of lymphangioleiomyomatosis (LAM).

Action

Inhibits T-lymphocyte activation/proliferation, which occurs as a response to antigenic and cytokine stimulation; antibody production is also inhibited. **Therapeutic Effects:** Decreased incidence and severity of organ rejection. Improvement in pulmonary function.

Pharmacokinetics

Absorption: Rapidly absorbed following oral administration (14% bioavailability).

Distribution: Concentrates in erythrocytes; distributes to heart, intestines, kidneys, liver, lungs, muscle, spleen, and testes in high concentrations.

Protein Binding: 92%.

Metabolism and Excretion: Extensively metabolized (some metabolism by P450 3A4 system); 91% excreted in feces.

Half-life: 62 hr.

TIME/ACTION PROFILE (blood levels)

ROUTE	ONSET	PEAK	DURATION
PO	rapid	1–2 hr	24 hr

Contraindications/Precautions

Contraindicated in: Hypersensitivity; Alcohol intolerance/sensitivity (solution contains ethanol); Concurrent ketoconazole, voriconazole, itraconazole, erythromycin, clarithromycin, rifampin, rifabutin, or grapefruit juice; Severe hepatic impairment; OB: Pregnancy (may cause fetal harm).

Use Cautiously in: Mild to moderate hepatic impairment; Lactation: Use while breast feeding only if potential maternal benefit justifies potential risk to infant; Rep: Women of reproductive potential; Pedi: Children <13 yr (safety and effectiveness not established).

Adverse Reactions/Side Effects

Reflects combined therapy with corticosteroids and cyclosporine.

CNS: PROGRESSIVE MULTIFOCAL LEUKOENCEPHALOPATHY (PML), insomnia. **CV:** edema, hypotension, pericardial effusion. **Derm:** acne, rash, thrombocytopenic purpura. **F and E:** hypokalemia. **Endo:** hyperglycemia. **GI:** ascites, hepatotoxicity. **GU:** amenorrhea, infertility (males), menorrhagia, ovarian cysts, renal impairment. **Hemat:** leukopenia, thrombocytopenia, anemia. **Metab:** hypercholesterolemia, hypertriglyceridemia. **MS:** arthralgias. **Neuro:** tremor. **Resp:** INTERSTITIAL LUNG DISEASE, PULMONARY HYPERTENSION. **Misc:** ANGIOEDEMA, INFECTION (including activation of latent viral infections such as BK virus-associated nephropathy and *Clostridium difficile*-associated diarrhea [CDAD]), ↓ wound healing, lymphocele, lymphoma.

Interactions

Drug-Drug: Cyclosporine (modified) greatly ↑ blood levels (administer sirolimus 4 hr after cyclosporine). Drugs that inhibit the CYP3A4 enzyme system may be expected to ↑ blood levels and the risk of adverse reactions. **Ketoconazole**, **voriconazole**, **itraconazole**, **clarithromycin**, and **erythromycin** significantly ↑ blood levels (concurrent use is contraindicated). Blood levels are also ↑ by **diltiazem** and **verapamil** (monitor sirolimus levels and adjust dose as necessary) and may be ↑ by **nicardipine**, **verapamil**, **clotrimazole**, **fluconazole**, **metoclopramide**, **cimetidine**, **danazol**, and **protease inhibitors**. **Rifampin** and **rifabutin** ↑ metabolism by stimulating the CYP3A4 enzyme system and significantly ↓ blood levels. Blood levels may also be ↓ by **carbamazepine**, **phenobarbital**, **phenytoin**, and **rifapentine**. Risk of renal impairment may be ↑ by concurrent use of other **nephrotoxic agents**. Concurrent use with **tacrolimus** and **corticosteroids** in lung transplantation may ↑ risk of anastomotic dehiscence; fatalites have been reported (not approved for this use). Concurrent use with **tacrolimus** and **corticosteroids** in liver transplantation may ↑ risk of hepatic artery thrombosis; fatalites have been reported (not approved for this use). Concurrent use with **ACE inhibitors** may ↑ risk of angioedema. May ↓ antibody response to and ↑ risk of adverse reactions to **live-virus vaccines**; avoid vaccination. May ↑ **verapamil** levels.

Drug-Natural Products: Concomitant use with **echinacea** and **melatonin** may interfere with immunosuppression. **St. John's wort** may ↑ blood levels and the risk of toxicity.

Drug-Food: Grapefruit juice ↓ CYP3A4 metabolism and ↑ levels; do not use as a diluent and avoid concurrent ingestion.

Route/Dosage

Kidney Transplantation

PO (Adults and Children ≥13 yr): 6-mg loading dose, followed by 2 mg/day maintenance dose. *Dosing following cyclosporine withdrawal*—Patients at low to moderate risk for rejection after transplantation may be withdrawn from cyclosporine over 4–8 wk beginning 2–4 mo after transplant. Thereafter, sirolimus dose should be titrated upward to maintain a whole blood trough level of 12–14 ng/mL. Clinical assessment should also be used to gauge dose. Dose changes can be made at 7–14 day intervals. The following formula may also be used: sirolimus maintenance dose = current dose × (target concentration/current concentration). If a large ↑ is needed, a loading dose may be given and blood levels reassessed 3–4 days later. Loading dose may be calculated by the following formula: sirolimus loading dose = 3 × (new maintenance dose-current maintenance dose). Loading doses >40 mg should be spread over 2 days.

PO (Adults and Children ≥13 yr and <40 kg): 3 mg/m^2 loading dose, followed by 1 mg/m^2/day mainte-

S

nance dose. *See adjustments above for doses following cyclosporine withdrawal.*

Hepatic Impairment

PO (Adults and Children): *Mild or moderate hepatic impairment*—↓ maintenance dose by 33%; loading dose is unchanged; *Severe hepatic impairment*—↓ maintenance dose by 50%; loading dose is unchanged.

Lymphangioleiomyomatosis

PO (Adults): 2 mg once daily. Monitor whole blood trough level in 10–20 days and titrate dose to maintain level of 5–15 ng/mL. The following formula may also be used to adjust dose: sirolimus maintenance dose = current dose × (target concentration/current concentration). Further dose changes can be made at 7–14 day intervals. Once stable dose achieved, should monitor whole blood trough levels at least every 3 mo.

Hepatic Impairment

(Adults): *Mild or moderate hepatic impairment*—↓ dose by 33%; *Severe hepatic impairment*—↓ dose by 50%.

Availability (generic available)

Oral solution (contains alcohol): 1 mg/mL. **Tablet:** 0.5 mg, 1 mg, 2 mg.

NURSING IMPLICATIONS

Assessment

- Monitor BP closely during therapy. Hypertension is a common complication of sirolimus therapy and should be treated.
- Assess for any new signs or symptoms that may be suggestive of PML, an opportunistic infection of the brain that leads to death or severe disability; withhold dose and notify health care professional promptly. Symptoms of PML may include hemiparesis, apathy, confusion, cognitive deficiencies, and ataxia. Consider decreasing the amount of immunosuppression in these patients.
- **Lymphangioleiomyomatosis:** Monitor for signs and symptoms of LAM (wheezing; cough, which may be bloody; shortness of breath; chest pain; pneumothorax) periodically during therapy.
- ***Lab Test Considerations:*** Monitor sirolimus blood levels when dose forms are changed and in patients likely to have altered drug metabolism, patients ≥13 yr who weigh <40 kg, patients with hepatic impairment, and during concurrent administration of drugs that may interact with sirolimus. Trough concentrations of ≥15 ng/mL are associated with an ↑ in adverse effects.
- Monitor patients for hyperlipidemia. May require additional interventions to treat hyperlipidemia.
- May cause anemia, leukopenia, thrombocytopenia, and hypokalemia.
- May cause ↑ AST, ↑ ALT, hypophosphatemia, and hyperglycemia.

Implementation

- Therapy with sirolimus should be started as soon as possible post-transplant. Concurrent therapy with cyclosporine and corticosteroids is recommended. Sirolimus should be taken 4 hr after cyclosporine (MODIFIED, Neoral).
- Sirolimus should be ordered only by physicians skilled in immunosuppressive therapy, with the staff and facilities to manage renal transplant patients.
- Antimicrobial prophylaxis for *Pneumocystis jirovecii* pneumonia for 1 yr and for cytomegalovirus protection for 3 mo post-transplant are recommended.
- **PO:** Administer consistently with or without food. Swallow tablet whole; do not crush, break, or chew. Do not administer with or mix with grapefruit juice.
- To dilute from bottle, use amber oral dose syringe to withdraw prescribed amount. Empty sirolimus from syringe into a glass or plastic container holding at least 2 oz (60 mL) of water or orange juice; do not use other liquids. Stir vigorously and drink at once. Refill container with at least 4 oz of additional liquid, stir vigorously, and drink at once.
- If using the pouch, empty entire contents of pouch into at least 2 oz of water or orange juice; do not use other liquids. Stir vigorously and drink at once. Refill container with at least 4 oz of additional liquid, stir vigorously, and drink at once.
- Store bottles and pouches in refrigerator. Protect from light. Solution may develop a slight haze when refrigerated; allow to stand at room temperature and shake gently until haze disappears. Sirolimus may remain in syringe at room temperature or refrigerated for up to 24 hr. Discard syringe after 1 use. Oral solution must be used within 1 mo of opening bottle.

Patient/Family Teaching

- Instruct patient to take sirolimus at the same time each day, as directed. Advise patient to avoid taking with or diluting with grapefruit juice. Do not skip or double up on missed doses. Do not discontinue medication without advice of health care professional.
- Advise patient to avoid grapefruit and grapefruit juice during therapy.
- Reinforce the need for lifelong therapy to prevent transplant rejection. Review symptoms of rejection for transplanted organ and stress need to notify health care professional immediately if they occur.
- Advise patient to notify health care professional if swelling of your face, eyes, or mouth; trouble breathing or wheezing; throat tightness; chest pain or tightness; feeling dizzy or faint; rash or peeling of skin; swelling of hands or feet; or symptoms of PML occur.
- Advise patient to wear sunscreen and protective clothing and limit time in sunlight and UV light due to increased risk of skin cancer.
- Caution patient to notify health care professional if signs of infection occur.

- Advise patient to avoid vaccinations with a live virus during therapy; sirolimus may decrease vaccine effectiveness.
- Rep: Advise patient of the risk of taking sirolimus during pregnancy. Caution women of reproductive potential to use effective contraception prior to, during, and for 12 wk following therapy. May cause male infertility.
- Emphasize the importance of repeated lab tests during sirolimus therapy.

Evaluation/Desired Outcomes

- Prevention of transplanted kidney rejection.
- Reduction in symptoms of lymphangioleiomyomatosis (LAM).

SITagliptin (sit-a-glip-tin)

Januvia

Classification

Therapeutic: antidiabetics

Pharmacologic: enzyme inhibitors

Indications

Adjunct to diet and exercise to improve glycemic control in patients with type 2 diabetes mellitus; may be used as monotherapy or combination therapy with metformin, a thiazolidinedione, a sulfonylurea, or insulin.

Action

Inhibits the enzyme dipeptidyl peptidase-4 (DPP-4), which slows the inactivation of incretin hormones, resulting in increased levels of active incretin hormones. These hormones are released by the intestine throughout the day and are involved in regulation of glucose homeostasis. Increased/prolonged incretin levels result in an increase in insulin release and decrease in glucagon levels. **Therapeutic Effects:** Improved control of blood glucose.

Pharmacokinetics

Absorption: 87% absorbed following oral administration.

Distribution: Unknown.

Metabolism and Excretion: 79% excreted unchanged in urine, minor metabolism.

Half-life: 12.4 hr.

TIME/ACTION PROFILE

ROUTE	ONSET	PEAK	DURATION
PO	rapid	1–4 hr	24 hr

Contraindications/Precautions

Contraindicated in: Type 1 diabetes mellitus; Diabetic ketoacidosis; Hypersensitivity.

Use Cautiously in: Renal impairment (dose ↓ required for CCr <50 mL/min); History of pancreatitis; History of angioedema to another DPP-4 inhibitor; History of HF or renal impairment (↑ risk of HF); OB: Use only if clearly needed; Lactation: Excretion into breast milk unknown; Pedi: Safety not established; Geri: Consider age-related ↓ in renal function when determining dose.

Adverse Reactions/Side Effects

CNS: headache. **CV:** HF. **Derm:** STEVENS-JOHNSON SYNDROME, bullous pemphigoid, rash, urticaria. **GI:** PANCREATITIS, nausea, diarrhea. **GU:** acute renal failure. **Resp:** upper respiratory tract infection, nasopharyngitis. **MS:** RHABDOMYOLYSIS, arthralgia, back pain, myalgia. **Misc:** HYPERSENSITIVITY REACTIONS (including anaphylaxis and angioedema).

Interactions

Drug-Drug: May slightly ↑ serum digoxin levels; monitoring recommended. ↑ risk of hypoglycemia when used with **insulin**, **glyburide**, **glipizide**, or **glimepiride** (may need to ↓ dose of insulin or sulfonylurea).

Route/Dosage

PO (Adults): 100 mg once daily.

Renal Impairment

PO (Adults): *CCr 30–<45 mL/min*—50 mg once daily; *CCr <30 mL/min, hemodialysis, or peritoneal dialysis*—25 mg once daily.

Availability

Tables: 25 mg, 50 mg, 100 mg. **Cost:** 25 mg $801.18/90, 50 mg $816.93/90, 100 mg $816.93/90. ***In combination with:*** ertugliflozin (Steglujan); metformin (Janumet); metformin XR (Janumet XR). See Appendix B.

NURSING IMPLICATIONS

Assessment

- Observe patient for signs and symptoms of hypoglycemic reactions (abdominal pain, sweating, hunger, weakness, dizziness, headache, tremor, tachycardia, anxiety).
- Monitor for signs of pancreatitis (nausea, vomiting, anorexia, persistent severe abdominal pain, sometimes radiating to the back) during therapy. If pancreatitis occurs, discontinue sitagliptin and monitor serum and urine amylase, amylase/creatinine clearance ratio, electrolytes, serum calcium, glucose, and lipase.
- Assess for rash periodically during therapy. May cause Stevens-Johnson syndrome. Discontinue therapy if severe or if accompanied with fever, general malaise, fatigue, muscle or joint aches, blisters, oral lesions, conjunctivitis, hepatitis, and/or eosinophilia.

- ***Lab Test Considerations:*** Monitor hemoglobin A1C prior to and periodically during therapy.
- Monitor renal function prior to and periodically during therapy.

Implementation

- Do not confuse sitagliptin with saxagliptin or sumatriptan. Do not confuse Januvia (sitagliptin) with Enjuvia (estrogens, conjugated B), Jantoven (warfarin), or Janumet (sitagliptin/metformin).
- Patients stabilized on a diabetic regimen who are exposed to stress, fever, trauma, infection, or surgery may require administration of insulin.
- **PO:** May be administered without regard to food.

Patient/Family Teaching

- Instruct patient to take sitagliptin as directed. Take missed doses as soon as remembered, unless it is almost time for next dose; do not double doses. Advise patient to read the *Medication Guide* before starting and with each Rx refill in case of changes.
- Explain to patient that sitagliptin helps control hyperglycemia but does not cure diabetes. Therapy is usually long term.
- Instruct patient not to share this medication with others, even if they have the same symptoms; it may harm them.
- Encourage patient to follow prescribed diet, medication, and exercise regimen to prevent hyperglycemic or hypoglycemic episodes.
- Review signs of hypoglycemia and hyperglycemia with patient. If hypoglycemia occurs, advise patient to take a glass of orange juice or 2–3 tsp of sugar, honey, or corn syrup dissolved in water, and notify health care professional.
- Instruct patient in proper testing of blood glucose and urine ketones. These tests should be monitored closely during periods of stress or illness and health care professional notified if significant changes occur.
- Advise patient to stop taking sitagliptin and notify health care professional promptly if symptoms of hypersensitivity reactions (rash; hives; swelling of face, lips, tongue, and throat; difficulty in breathing or swallowing) or pancreatitis occur.
- Advise patient to notify health care professional of all Rx or OTC medications, vitamins, or herbal products being taken and to consult with health care professional before taking other medications.
- Rep: Advise patient to notify health care professional if pregnancy is planned or suspected, or if breast feeding. Encourage patients who become pregnant while taking sitagliptin to join the pregnancy registry by calling 1-800-986-8999 to collect information about pregnancy outcomes.

Evaluation/Desired Outcomes

- Improved hemoglobin A1C, fasting plasma glucose and 2-hr post-prandial glucose levels.

sodium bicarbonate

(**soe**-dee-um bye-**kar**-boe-nate)

Baking Soda, Bell-Ans, Citrocarbonate, Neut, Soda Mint

Classification

Therapeutic: antiulcer agents

Pharmacologic: alkalinizing agents

Indications

PO, IV: Management of metabolic acidosis. **PO, IV:** Used to alkalinize urine and promote excretion of certain drugs in overdosage situations (phenobarbital, aspirin). **PO:** Antacid. **Unlabeled Use:** Stabilization of acid-base status in cardiac arrest and treatment of life-threatening hyperkalemia.

Action

Acts as an alkalinizing agent by releasing bicarbonate ions. Following oral administration, releases bicarbonate, which is capable of neutralizing gastric acid. **Therapeutic Effects:** Alkalinization. Neutralization of gastric acid.

Pharmacokinetics

Absorption: Following oral administration, excess bicarbonate is absorbed and results in metabolic alkalosis and alkaline urine.

Distribution: Widely distributed into extracellular fluid.

Metabolism and Excretion: Sodium and bicarbonate are excreted by the kidneys.

Half-life: Unknown.

TIME/ACTION PROFILE (PO = antacid effect; IV = alkalinization)

ROUTE	ONSET	PEAK	DURATION
PO	immediate	30 min	1–3 hr
IV	immediate	rapid	unknown

Contraindications/Precautions

Contraindicated in: Metabolic or respiratory alkalosis; Hypocalcemia; Hypernatremia; Excessive chloride loss; As an antidote following ingestion of strong mineral acids; Patients on sodium-restricted diets (oral use as an antacid only); Renal failure (oral use as an antacid only); Severe abdominal pain of unknown cause, especially if associated with fever (oral use as an antacid only).

Use Cautiously in: HF; Renal insufficiency; Concurrent corticosteroid therapy; Chronic use as an antacid (may cause metabolic alkalosis and possible sodium overload); Pedi: May ↑ risk of cerebral edema in children with diabetic ketoacidosis.

Adverse Reactions/Side Effects

CV: edema. **GI:** *PO*—flatulence, gastric distention. **F and E:** metabolic alkalosis, hypernatremia, hypocalcemia, hypokalemia, sodium and water retention. **Local:** irritation at IV site. **Neuro:** tetany, cerebral hemorrhage (with rapid injection in infants).

Interactions

Drug-Drug: Following oral administration, may ↓ absorption of **ketoconazole**. Concurrent use with **calcium-containing antacids** may lead to milk-alkali syndrome. Urinary alkalinization may result in ↓ **salicylate** or **barbiturate** blood levels; ↑ blood levels of **quinidine**, **mexiletine**, **flecainide**, or **amphetamines**; ↑ risk of crystalluria from **fluoroquinolones**; ↓ effectiveness of **methenamine**. May negate the protective effects of **enteric-coated products** (do not administer within 1–2 hr of each other).

Route/Dosage

Contains 12 mEq of sodium/g.

Alkalinization of Urine

PO (Adults): 48 mEq (4 g) initially. Then 12–24 mEq (1–2 g) every 4 hr (up to 48 mEq every 4 hr) or 1 tsp of powder every 4 hr as needed.
PO (Children): 1–10 mEq/kg (84–840 mg/kg) per day in divided doses.
IV (Adults and Children): 2–5 mEq/kg as a 4–8 hr infusion.

Antacid

PO (Adults): *Tablets/powder*—325 mg–2 g 1–4 times daily or ½ tsp every 2 hr as needed. *Effervescent powder*—3.9–10 g in water after meals; patients >60 yr should receive 1.9–3.9 g after meals.

Systemic Alkalinization/Cardiac Arrest

IV (Adults and Children and Infants): *Cardiac arrest/urgent situations*—1 mEq/kg; may repeat 0.5 mEq/kg every 10 min. *Less urgent situations*—2–5 mEq/kg as a 4–8 hr infusion.

Renal Tubular Acidosis

PO (Adults): 0.5–2 mEq/kg/day in 4–5 divided doses.
PO (Children): 2–3 mEq/kg/day in 3–4 divided doses.

Availability (generic available)

Oral powder: (20.9 mEq Na/½ tsp) in 120-, 240-, 480-, and 2400-g containers^OTC. **Tablets:** 325 mg (3.9 mEq Na/tablet)^OTC, 🍁500 mg (6.0 mEq Na/tablet^OTC, 520 mg (6.2 mEq Na/tablet)^OTC, 650 mg (7.7 mEq Na/tablet)^OTC. **Solution for injection:** 4.2% (0.5 mEq/mL) in 2.5-, 5-, and 10-mL prefilled syringes, 5% (0.6 mEq/mL) in 500-mL containers, 7.5% (0.9 mEq/mL) in 50-mL vials and prefilled syringes and 200-mL vials, 8.4% (1 mEq/mL) in 10- and 50-mL vials and prefilled syringes. **Neutralizing additive solution for injection:** 4% (0.48 mEq/mL) in 5-mL vials, 4.2% (0.5 mEq/mL) in 6-mL vials.

NURSING IMPLICATIONS

Assessment

- **IV:** Assess fluid balance (intake and output, daily weight, edema, lung sounds) throughout therapy. Report symptoms of fluid overload (hypertension, edema, dyspnea, rales/crackles, frothy sputum) if they occur.
- Assess patient for signs of acidosis (disorientation, headache, weakness, dyspnea, hyperventilation), alkalosis (confusion, irritability, paresthesia, tetany, altered breathing pattern), hypernatremia (edema, weight gain, hypertension, tachycardia, fever, flushed skin, mental irritability), or hypokalemia (weakness, fatigue, U wave on ECG, arrhythmias, polyuria, polydipsia) throughout therapy.
- Observe IV site closely. Avoid extravasation, as tissue irritation or cellulitis may occur. If infiltration occurs, confer with physician or other health care professional regarding warm compresses and infiltration of site with lidocaine or hyaluronidase.
- **Antacid:** Assess patient for epigastric or abdominal pain and frank or occult blood in the stool, emesis, or gastric aspirate.
- ***Lab Test Considerations:*** Monitor serum sodium, potassium, calcium, bicarbonate concentrations, serum osmolarity, acid-base balance, and renal function prior to and periodically throughout therapy.
- Obtain arterial blood gases (ABGs) frequently in emergency situations and during parenteral therapy.
- Monitor urine pH frequently when used for urinary alkalinization.
- Antagonizes effects of pentagastrin and histamine during gastric acid secretion test. Avoid administration during the 24 hr preceding the test.

Implementation

- This medication may cause premature dissolution of enteric-coated tablets in the stomach.
- **PO:** Tablets must be taken with a full glass of water.
- When used in treatment of peptic ulcers, may be administered 1 and 3 hr after meals and at bedtime.

IV Administration

- **IV Push:** Used in cardiac arrest or urgent situations. ***Diluent:*** Use premeasured ampules or prefilled syringes to ensure accurate dose. ***Rate:*** Administer by rapid bolus. Flush IV line before and after administration to prevent incompatible medications used in arrest management from precipitating.
- **Continuous Infusion:** ***Diluent:*** May be diluted in dextrose, saline, and dextrose/saline combinations. Premixed infusions are already diluted and ready to use. ***Rate:*** May be administered over 4–8 hr.
- **Y-Site Compatibility:** acyclovir, amifostine, amikacin, aminophylline, asparaginase, atropine, aztreonam, bivalirudin, bumetanide, cefazolin, cefe-

pime, ceftazidime, ceftriaxone, chloramphenicol, cimetidine, cladribine, clindamycin, cyclophosphamide, cyclosporine, cytarabine, daptomycin, daunorubicin, dexamethasone sodium phosphate, dexmedetomidine, digoxin, docetaxel, doxorubicin, enalaprilat, ertapenem, erythromycin, esmolol, etoposide, etoposide phosphate, famotidine, fentanyl, filgrastim, fluconazole, fludarabine, furosemide, gemcitabine, gentamicin, granisetron, heparin, hydrocortisone sodium succinate, ifosfamide, indomethacin, insulin, ketorolac, labetalol, levofloxacin, lidocaine, linezolid, lorazepam, magnesium sulfate, melphalan, mesna, methylprednisolone sodium succinate, metoclopramide, metoprolol, metronidazole, milrinone, morphine, nafcillin, nitroglycerin, nitroprusside, paclitaxel, palonosetron, pantoprazole, pemetrexed, penicillin G potassium, phenylephrine, phytonadione, piperacillin/tazobactam, potassium chloride, procainamide, propranolol, propofol, protamine, ranitidine, remifentanil, tacrolimus, thiotepa, tirofiban, tobramycin, tolazoline, vasopressin, vitamin B complex with C, voriconazole.

- **Y-Site Incompatibility:** allopurinol, amiodarone, amphotericin B, amphotericin B cholesteryl sulfate complex, ampicillin, anidulafungin, calcium chloride, calcium gluconate, caspofungin, cefotaxime, cefoxitin, cefuroxime, diazepam, diphenhydramine, dobutamine, doxorubicin liposome, doxycycline, epinephrine, fenoldopam, ganciclovir, haloperidol, hydroxyzine, idarubicin, imipenem/cilastatin, isoproterenol, lansoprazole, leucovorin, meperidine, midazolam, nalbuphine, norepinephrine, ondansetron, phenytoin, prochlorperazine, promethazine, quinupristin/dalfopristin, sargramostim, trimethoprim/sulfamethoxazole, verapamil, vincristine, vinorelbine.
- **Solution Incompatibility:** Do not add to Ringer's solution, LR, or Ionosol products, as compatibility varies with concentration.

Patient/Family Teaching

- Instruct patient to take medication as directed. Take missed doses as soon as remembered unless almost time for next dose.
- Review symptoms of electrolyte imbalance with patients on chronic therapy; instruct patient to notify health care professional if these symptoms occur.
- Advise patient not to take milk products concurrently with this medication. Renal calculi or hypercalcemia (milk-alkali syndrome) may result.
- Emphasize the importance of regular follow-up examinations to monitor serum electrolyte levels and acid-base balance and to monitor progress.
- **Antacid:** Advise patient to avoid routine use of sodium bicarbonate for indigestion. Dyspepsia that persists >2 wk should be evaluated by a health care professional.
- Advise patient on sodium-restricted diet to avoid use of baking soda as a home remedy for indigestion.
- Instruct patient to notify health care professional if indigestion is accompanied by chest pain, difficulty breathing, or diaphoresis or if stools become dark and tarry.

Evaluation/Desired Outcomes

- Increase in urinary pH.
- Clinical improvement of acidosis.
- Enhanced excretion of selected overdoses and poisonings.
- Decreased gastric discomfort.

sodium citrate and citric acid

(**soe**-dee-um **sye**-trate and **sit**-rik **as**-id)

~~Bicitra~~, Oracit, Shohl's Solution modified

Classification

Therapeutic: antiurolithics, mineral and electrolyte replacements/supplements

Pharmacologic: alkalinizing agents

Indications

Management of chronic metabolic acidosis associated with chronic renal insufficiency or renal tubular acidosis. Alkalinization of urine. Prevention of cystine and urate urinary calculi. Prevention of aspiration pneumonitis during surgical procedures. Used as a neutralizing buffer.

Action

Converted to bicarbonate in the body, resulting in increased blood pH. As bicarbonate is renally excreted, urine is also alkalinized, increasing the solubility of cystine and uric acid. Neutralizes gastric acid. **Therapeutic Effects:** Provision of bicarbonate in metabolic acidosis. Alkalinization of the urine. Prevention of cystine and urate urinary calculi. Prevention of aspiration pneumonitis.

Pharmacokinetics

Absorption: Well absorbed following oral administration.

Distribution: Rapidly and widely distributed.

Metabolism and Excretion: Rapidly oxidized to bicarbonate, which is excreted primarily by the kidneys. Small amounts (<5%) excreted unchanged by the lungs.

Half-life: Unknown.

TIME/ACTION PROFILE (effects on serum pH)

ROUTE	ONSET	PEAK	DURATION
PO	rapid (min–hr)	unknown	4–6 hr

Contraindications/Precautions

Contraindicated in: Severe renal impairment; Severe sodium restriction; HF, untreated hypertension, edema, or toxemia of pregnancy.

Use Cautiously in: OB, Lactation: Safety not established.

Adverse Reactions/Side Effects

F and E: fluid overload, hypernatremia (severe renal impairment), hypocalcemia, metabolic alkalosis (large doses only). **GI:** diarrhea. **MS:** tetany.

Interactions

Drug-Drug: May partially antagonize the effects of **antihypertensives**. Urinary alkalinization may result in ↓ **salicylate** or **barbiturate** levels or ↑ levels of **quinidine**, **flecainide**, or **amphetamines**.

Route/Dosage

Adjust dosage according to urine pH. Contains 1 mEq sodium and 1 mEq bicarbonate/mL solution.

Alkalinizer

PO (Adults): 10–30 mL solution diluted in water 4 times daily.

PO (Children): 5–15 mL solution diluted in water 4 times daily.

Antiurolithic

PO (Adults): 10–30 mL solution diluted in water 4 times daily.

Neutralizing Buffer

PO (Adults): 15–30 mL solution diluted in 15–30 mL of water.

Availability

Oral solution: sodium citrate 490 mg and citric acid 640 mg/5 mL, sodium citrate 500 mg and citric acid 300 mg/5 mL, sodium citrate 500 mg and citric acid 334 mg/5 mL.

NURSING IMPLICATIONS

Assessment

- Assess patient for signs of alkalosis (confusion, irritability, paresthesia, tetany, altered breathing pattern) or hypernatremia (edema, weight gain, hypertension, tachycardia, fever, flushed skin, mental irritability) throughout therapy.
- Monitor patients with renal dysfunction for fluid overload (discrepancy in intake and output, weight gain, edema, rales/crackles, and hypertension).
- ***Lab Test Considerations:*** Prior to and every 4 mo during chronic therapy, monitor hematocrit, hemoglobin, electrolytes, pH, creatinine, urinalysis, and 24-hr urine for citrate.
- Monitor urine pH if used to alkalinize urine.

Implementation

- **PO:** Solution is more palatable if chilled. Administer with 30–90 mL of chilled water. Administer 30 min after meals or as bedtime snack to minimize saline laxative effect.
- When used as preanesthetic, administer 15–30 mL of sodium citrate with 15–30 mL of chilled water.

Patient/Family Teaching

- Instruct patient to take as directed. Missed doses should be taken within 2 hr. Do not double doses.
- Instruct patients receiving chronic sodium citrate on correct method of monitoring urine pH, maintenance of alkaline urine, and the need to increase fluid intake to 3000 mL/day. When treatment is discontinued, pH begins to fall toward pretreatment levels.
- Advise patients receiving long-term therapy on need to avoid salty foods.

Evaluation/Desired Outcomes

- Correction of metabolic acidosis.
- Maintenance of alkaline urine with resulting decreased stone formation.
- Buffering the pH of gastric secretions, thereby preventing aspiration pneumonitis associated with intubation and anesthesia.

sodium ferric gluconate complex, See IRON SUPPLEMENTS.

S

sodium polystyrene sulfonate

(**soe**-dee-um po-lee-**stye**-reen **sul**-fon-ate)

Kalexate, 🍁Kayexalate, Kionex, 🍁Solystat, SPS

Classification

Therapeutic: hypokalemic, electrolyte modifiers

Pharmacologic: cationic exchange resins

Indications

Mild to moderate hyperkalemia (if severe, more immediate measures such as sodium bicarbonate IV, calcium, or glucose/insulin infusion should be instituted).

Action

Exchanges sodium ions for potassium ions in the intestine (each 1 g is exchanged for 1 mEq potassium).

Therapeutic Effects: Reduction of serum potassium levels.

Pharmacokinetics

Absorption: Distributed throughout the intestine but is nonabsorbable.

Distribution: Not distributed.

Metabolism and Excretion: Eliminated in the feces.

Half-life: Unknown.

TIME/ACTION PROFILE (decrease in serum potassium)

ROUTE	ONSET	PEAK	DURATION
PO	2–12 hr	unknown	6–24 hr
Rectal	2–12 hr	unknown	4–6 hr

Contraindications/Precautions

Contraindicated in: Life-threatening hyperkalemia (other, more immediate measures should be instituted); Hypersensitivity to saccharin or parabens (some products); Ileus; Abnormal bowel function (↑ risk for intestinal necrosis); Postoperative patients with no bowel movement (↑ risk for intestinal necrosis); History of impaction, chronic constipation, inflammatory bowel disease, ischemic colitis, vascular intestinal atherosclerosis, previous bowel resection, or bowel obstruction (↑ risk for intestinal necrosis); Known alcohol intolerance (suspension only).

Use Cautiously in: Geri: Geriatric patients; Heart failure; Hypertension; Edema; Sodium restriction; Constipation.

Adverse Reactions/Side Effects

F and E: hypocalcemia, hypokalemia, sodium retention, hypomagnesemia. **GI:** INTESTINAL NECROSIS, constipation, fecal impaction, anorexia, gastric irritation, ischemic colitis, nausea, vomiting.

Interactions

Drug-Drug: May ↓ absorption of any other orally administered medication; administer sodium polystyrene sulfonate ≥3 hr before or after other oral medications (≥6 hr for patients with gastroparesis). Administration with **calcium** or **magnesium-containing antacids** may ↓ resin-exchanging ability and ↑ risk of systemic alkalosis. Hypokalemia may enhance **digoxin** toxicity. Use with **sorbitol** may ↑ risk of colonic necrosis (concomitant use not recommended).

Route/Dosage

4 level tsp = 15 g (4.1 mEq sodium/g).

PO (Adults): 15 g 1–4 times daily in water (up to 40 g 4 times daily).

Rect (Adults): 30–50 g as a retention enema; repeat as needed every 6 hr.

PO, Rect (Children): 1 g/kg/dose every 6 hr.

Availability (generic available)

Oral suspension: 15 g sodium polystyrene sulfonate with 20 g sorbitol/60 mL, 15 g sodium polystyrene sulfonate with 14.1 g sorbitol/60 mL. **Powder for suspension (requires reconstitution):** 454 g/bottle. **Rectal suspension:** 30 g/120 mL, 50 g/200 mL.

NURSING IMPLICATIONS

Assessment

- Monitor response of symptoms of hyperkalemia (fatigue, muscle weakness, paresthesia, confusion, dyspnea, peaked T waves, depressed ST segments, prolonged QT segments, widened QRS complexes, loss of P waves, and cardiac arrhythmias). Assess for development of hypokalemia (weakness, fatigue, arrhythmias, flat or inverted T waves, prominent U waves).
- Monitor intake and output ratios and daily weight. Assess for symptoms of fluid overload (dyspnea, rales/crackles, jugular venous distention, peripheral edema). Concurrent low-sodium diet may be ordered for patients with HF (see Appendix K).
- In patients receiving concurrent digoxin, assess for symptoms of digoxin toxicity (anorexia, nausea, vomiting, visual disturbances, arrhythmias).
- Assess abdomen and note character and frequency of stools. Discontinue sodium polystyrene sulfonate if patient becomes constipated. Concurrent sorbitol or laxatives may be ordered to prevent constipation or impaction. Some products contain sorbitol to prevent constipation. Patient should ideally have 1–2 watery stools each day during therapy. Monitor for intestinal necrosis if sorbitol is added.
- ***Lab Test Considerations:*** Monitor serum potassium daily during therapy. Notify health care professional when potassium ↓ to 4–5 mEq/L.
- Monitor renal function and electrolytes (especially sodium, calcium, bicarbonate, and magnesium) prior to and periodically throughout therapy.

Implementation

- Solution is stable for 24 hr when refrigerated.
- Consult health care professional regarding discontinuation of medications that may increase serum potassium (angiotensin-converting enzyme inhibitors, potassium-sparing diuretics, potassium supplements, salt substitutes).
- An osmotic laxative (sorbitol) is usually administered concurrently to prevent constipation.
- **PO:** For oral administration, shake commercially available suspension well before use. When using powder, add prescribed amount to 3–4 mL water/g of powder. Shake well. Syrup may be ordered to improve palatability. Resin cookie or candy recipes are available; discuss with pharmacist or dietitian.
- **Retention Enema:** Precede retention enema with cleansing enema. Administer solution via rectal tube or 28-French Foley catheter with 30-mL balloon. Insert tube at least 20 cm and tape in place.
- For retention enema, add powder to 100 mL of prescribed solution (usually sorbitol or 20% dextrose in water). Shake well to dissolve powder thoroughly; should be of liquid consistency. Position patient on left side and elevate hips on pillow if solution begins to leak. Follow administration of medication with additional 50–100 mL of diluent to ensure administra-

tion of complete dose. Encourage patient to retain enema as long as possible, at least 30–60 min.
- After retention period, irrigate colon with 1–2 L of non–sodium-containing solution. Y-connector with tubing may be attached to Foley or rectal tube; cleansing solution is administered through 1 port of the Y and allowed to drain by gravity through the other port.

Patient/Family Teaching
- Explain purpose and method of administration of medication to patient.
- Advise patient to avoid taking antacids or laxatives during therapy, unless approved by health care professional; may cause systemic alkalosis.
- Advise female patient to notify health care professional if pregnant or breast feeding.
- Inform patient of need for frequent lab tests to monitor effectiveness.

Evaluation/Desired Outcomes
- Normalization of serum potassium levels.

⧚ sofosbuvir/velpatasvir
(soe-**fos**-bue-vir/vel-**pat**-as-vir)
Epclusa

Classification
Therapeutic: antivirals
Pharmacologic: NS5B inhibitors, NS5A inhibitors

Indications
⧚ Chronic hepatitis C virus (HCV) genotype 1, 2, 3, 4, 5, or 6 infection in patients: Without cirrhosis or with compensated cirrhosis; With decompensated cirrhosis (with ribavirin).

Action
Sofosbuvir—inhibits the HCV NS5B RNA-dependent RNA polymerase, resulting in inhibition of viral replication. *Velpatasvir*—inhibits the HCV NS5A protein, resulting in inhibition of viral replication. **Therapeutic Effects:** Decreased levels of HCV with sustained virologic response and lessened sequelae of chronic HCV infection.

Pharmacokinetics
Sofosbuvir

Absorption: Rapidly metabolized following absorption (extensive first-pass effect).
Distribution: Unknown.
Metabolism and Excretion: Extensively metabolized primarily to GS-461203, an active antiviral moiety, then converted to GS-331007, which does not have antiviral activity. 80% excreted in urine mostly as GS-331007 (3.5% as unchanged drug), 14% excreted in feces, 2.5% excreted in expired air.
Half-life: *Sofosbuvir*—0.4 hr; *GS-331007*—25 hr.

Velpatasvir

Absorption: Well absorbed following oral administration.
Distribution: Unknown.
Protein Binding: >99.5%.
Metabolism and Excretion: Metabolized primarily via CYP2B6, CYP2C8, and CYP3A4. Primarily undergoes biliary excretion, with 94% excreted in feces and 0.4% eliminated in urine.
Half-life: 47 hr.

TIME/ACTION PROFILE (blood levels)

ROUTE	ONSET	PEAK	DURATION
sofosbuvir (PO)	unknown	0.5–1 hr	24 hr
velpatasvir (PO)	unknown	3 hr	24 hr

Contraindications/Precautions
Contraindicated in: Situations when ribavirin is contraindicated (when ribavirin required); Should not be used with other drugs/regimens containing sofosbuvir; Severe renal impairment (eGFR <30 mL/min/1.73 m²) or end-stage renal disease requiring hemodialysis (no dose recommendation); Receiving immunosuppressant or chemotherapy medications (↑ risk of hepatitis B virus reactivation); OB: Pregnant women or men whose partners are pregnant (when ribavirin is required; ribavirin may cause fetal harm); Lactation: Discontinue sofosbuvir/velpatasvir or discontinue breast feeding (when ribavirin required).
Use Cautiously in: OB: Safety not established (when ribavirin not required); Lactation: Weigh benefits of breast feeding against possible adverse effects (when ribavirin not required); Geri: May be more sensitive to drug effects; Pedi: Safety and effectiveness not established.

Adverse Reactions/Side Effects
Without ribavirin
CNS: headache, insomnia, irritability. **Derm:** rash.
GI: hepatitis B virus reactivation, ↑ lipase, nausea.
Misc: fatigue.

With ribavirin
CNS: headache, insomnia. **Derm:** rash. **GI:** diarrhea, nausea, hepatitis B virus reactivation, ↑ lipase. **Hemat:** anemia. **Misc:** fatigue.

Interactions
Drug-Drug: Concurrent use of **P-gp inducers** may ↓ levels/effectiveness of sofosbuvir and velpatasvir; concurrent use not recommended. Concurrent use of **moderate-to-strong inducers of CYP2B6, CYP2C8, or CYP3A4** may ↓ levels/effectiveness of vel-

S

patasvir; concurrent use not recommended. **Amiodarone** may ↑ risk of symptomatic bradycardia when used with sofosbuvir-containing regimens; concurrent use not recommended; if amiodarone necessary, monitor patients in inpatient setting for first 48 hr of concomitant use and then monitor heart rate on outpatient basis for at least the first 2 wk of treatment; follow same monitoring procedure if discontinuing amiodarone immediately before initiation of sofosbuvir/velpatasvir. **Acid-reducing agents** may ↓ levels of velpatasvir; separate administration from **antacids**, including **magnesium hydroxide** and **aluminum hydroxide** by 4 hr; administer **H_2-receptor antagonists** simultaneously or 12 hr apart from sofosbuvir/velpatasvir (dose of H_2 antagonist should not exceed famotidine 40 mg twice daily or equivalent); concurrent use with **proton-pump inhibitors** not recommended (if proton pump inhibitor necessary, administer sofosbuvir/velpatasvir with food and take 4 hr before **omeprazole** 20 mg; use with other proton pump inhibitors not studied). May ↑ levels/toxicity of **digoxin**; therapeutic monitoring of serum digoxin concentrations recommended. May ↑ levels/toxicity of **topotecan**; concurrent use not recommended. **Carbamazepine**, **phenytoin**, **phenobarbital**, and **oxcarbazepine** may ↓ levels/effectiveness of sofosbuvir and velpatasvir; concurrent use not recommended. **Rifabutin**, **rifampin**, and **rifapentine** may ↓ levels/effectiveness of sofosbuvir and velpatasvir; concurrent use not recommended. **Efavirenz** may ↓ levels/effectiveness of velpatasvir; concurrent use not recommended. May ↑ levels/toxicity of **tenofovir disoproxil fumarate** and **tenofovir disoproxil fumarate-containing combinations**; monitor closely. **Tipranavir/ritonavir** may ↓ levels/effectiveness of sofosbuvir and velpatasvir; concurrent use not recommended. May ↑ levels/toxicity of **rosuvastatin** and **atorvastatin**; rosuvastatin dose should not exceed 10 mg/day; monitor closely for atorvastatin-induced myopathy or rhabdomyolysis. May cause fluctuations in INR when used with **warfarin**; closely monitor INR. May ↑ risk of hypoglycemia when used with certain **antidiabetic agents**.

Drug-Natural Products: St. John's wort may ↓ levels/effectiveness of sofosbuvir and velpatasvir; concurrent use not recommended.

Route/Dosage

Dosing recommendations below may also be followed for patients coinfected with HIV.

PO (Adults): *Patients without cirrhosis or with compensated cirrhosis (Child–Pugh A)*—1 tablet once daily for 12 wk; *Patients with decompensated cirrhosis (Child–Pugh B or C)*—1 tablet once daily for 12 wk in combination with ribavirin.

Availability

Tablets: sofosbuvir 400 mg/velpatasvir 100 mg.

NURSING IMPLICATIONS

Assessment

- Monitor for signs and symptoms of hepatitis B reactivation (jaundice, dark urine, light colored stools, fatigue, weakness, loss of appetite, nausea, vomiting, stomach pain) during therapy.
- ***Lab Test Considerations:*** Measure hepatitis B surface antigen (HBsAg) and hepatitis core antibody (anti-HBc) in all patients before starting hepatitis C virus therapy. May cause hepatitis B virus reactivation. Monitor for clinical and laboratory signs of hepatitis flare (↑ AST, ALT, bilirubin, liver failure, death) or HBV reactivation (rapid ↑ in serum HBV DNA level) during HCV treatment and post-treatment follow-up.
- May cause ↑ serum lipase and amylase levels.
- May cause ↑ creatine kinase and indirect bilirubin levels.

Implementation

- **PO:** Administer one tablet daily without regard to food for 12 wk.
- Administer antacids 4 hrs apart from sofosbuvir/velpatsvir. May administer simultaneously or 12 hr apart with H_2–receptor antagonists at doses not to exceed famotidine 40 mg twice daily. Avoid administration with proton pump inhibitors; if medically necessary, administer sofosbuvir/velpatasvir with food and 4 hr before omeprazole 20 mg.

Patient/Family Teaching

- Instruct patient to take *Epclusa*™ as directed. Do not skip or miss doses or stop medication without consulting health care professional. Advise patient to read *Patient Information* before starting and with each Rx refill in case of changes.
- Advise patient to notify health care professional if they have a history of HBV. May cause reactivation.
- Instruct patient to notify health care professional of all Rx or OTC medications, vitamins, or herbal products being taken and consult health care professional before taking any new medications, especially St. John's wort.
- Rep: Advise patients to notify health care professional if pregnancy is planned or suspected, or if breast feeding. Advise females of reproductive potential who take *Epclusa*™ with ribavirin to use effective contraception during and for 6 mo after therapy is completed. Notify health care professional immediately if pregnancy is suspected.

Evaluation/Desired Outcomes

- Decreased levels of HCV with sustained virologic response and lessened sequelae of chronic HCV infection.

sofosbuvir/velpatasvir/voxilaprevir

(soe-**fos**-bue-vir/vel-**pat**-as-vir/vox-i-**la**-pre-vir)

Vosevi

Classification

Therapeutic: antivirals

Pharmacologic: NS5B inhibitors, NS5A inhibitors, protease inhibitors

Indications

Chronic hepatitis C virus (HCV) genotype 1, 2, 3, 4, 5, or 6 infection in patients without cirrhosis or with compensated cirrhosis (Child-Pugh A) who have previously been treated with an HCV regimen containing an NS5A inhibitor. Chronic HCV genotype 1a or 3 infection in patients without cirrhosis or with compensated cirrhosis (Child-Pugh A) who have previously been treated with an HCV regimen containing sofosbuvir without an NS5A inhibitor.

Action

Sofosbuvir—inhibits the HCV NS5B RNA-dependent RNA polymerase, resulting in inhibition of viral replication. *Velpatasvir*—inhibits the HCV NS5A protein, resulting in inhibition of viral replication. *Voxilaprevir*—inhibitor of NS3/4A protease, an enzyme necessary for viral replication. **Therapeutic Effects:** Decreased levels of HCV with sustained virologic response and lessened sequelae of chronic HCV infection.

Pharmacokinetics

Sofosbuvir

Absorption: Prodrug that is rapidly metabolized to its active form (GS-461203) following absorption.

Distribution: Unknown.

Metabolism and Excretion: Extensively metabolized primarily to GS-461203, an active antiviral moiety, then converted to GS-331007, which does not have antiviral activity. 80% excreted in urine mostly as GS-331007, 14% excreted in feces.

Half-life: *Sofosbuvir*—0.5 hr; *GS-331007*—29 hr.

Velpatasvir

Absorption: Well absorbed following oral administration.

Distribution: Unknown.

Protein Binding: >99%.

Metabolism and Excretion: Metabolized in the liver primarily via CYP2B6, CYP2C8, and CYP3A4. Primarily undergoes biliary excretion, with 94% excreted in feces (77% as unchanged drug) and 0.4% eliminated in urine.

Half-life: 17 hr.

Voxilaprevir

Absorption: Well absorbed following oral administration.

Distribution: Unknown.

Protein Binding: >99%.

Metabolism and Excretion: Metabolized in the liver primarily via CYP3A4. Primarily undergoes biliary excretion, with 94% excreted in feces (40% as unchanged drug) and 0% eliminated in urine.

Half-life: 33 hr.

TIME/ACTION PROFILE (blood levels)

ROUTE	ONSET	PEAK	DURATION
sofosbuvir (PO)	unknown	2 hr	24 hr
velpatasvir (PO)	unknown	4 hr	24 hr
voxilaprevir (PO)	unknown	4 hr	24 hr

Contraindications/Precautions

Contraindicated in: Concurrent use of rifampin; Concurrent use of P-glycoprotein inducers as well as moderate or strong inducers of CYP2B6, CYP2C8, or CYP3A4; Moderate or severe hepatic impairment (Child-Pugh B or C).

Use Cautiously in: Receiving immunosuppressant or chemotherapy medications (↑ risk of HBV reactivation); Severe renal impairment (eGFR <30 mL/min) or end-stage renal disease requiring hemodialysis (no dose recommendation); OB: Safety not established; Lactation: Weigh benefits of breast feeding against possible adverse effects; Geri: May be more sensitive to drug effects; Pedi: Safety and effectiveness not established.

Adverse Reactions/Side Effects

CNS: fatigue, headache, insomnia. **GI:** diarrhea, nausea, hepatitis B virus reactivation, hyperbilirubinemia.

Interactions

Drug-Drug: **Rifampin** may ↓ levels/effectiveness of sofosbuvir, velpatasvir, and voxilaprevir; concurrent use contraindicated. **Amiodarone** may ↑ risk of symptomatic bradycardia when used with sofosbuvir-containing regimens; concurrent use not recommended; if amiodarone necessary, monitor patients in inpatient setting for first 48 hr of concomitant use and then monitor heart rate on outpatient basis for at least the first 2 wk of treatment; follow same monitoring procedure if discontinuing amiodarone immediately before initiation of sofosbuvir/velpatasvir/voxilaprevir. **Acid-reducing agents** may ↓ levels of velpatasvir; separate administration from **antacids**, including **magnesium hydroxide** and **aluminum hydroxide** by 4 hr; administer **H_2-receptor antagonists** simultaneously or 12 hr apart

S

from sofosbuvir/velpatasvir/voxilaprevir (dose of H_2 antagonist should not exceed famotidine 40 mg twice daily or equivalent); may use with **omeprazole** 20 mg (use with other **proton-pump inhibitors** not studied). May ↑ levels/toxicity of **digoxin**; therapeutic monitoring of serum digoxin concentrations recommended. May ↑ levels/risk of bleeding of **dabigatran**; may need to ↓ dose of dabigatran. **Carbamazepine**, **oxcarbazepine**, **phenytoin**, **phenobarbital**, **rifabutin**, and **rifapentine** may ↓ levels/effectiveness of sofosbuvir, velpatasvir, and voxilaprevir; concurrent use not recommended. **Atazanavir** or **lopinavir** may ↑ levels/toxicity of voxilaprevir; concurrent use not recommended. **Tipranavir/ritonavir** may ↓ levels/effectiveness of sofosbuvir and velpatasvir; concurrent use not recommended. **Efavirenz** may ↓ levels/effectiveness of velpatasvir and voxilaprevir; concurrent use not recommended. May ↑ levels/toxicity of **tenofovir disoproxil fumarate**; monitor closely. May ↑ levels/toxicity of **pravastatin**; do not exceed pravastatin dose of 40 mg/day. May ↑ levels/toxicity of **atorvastatin**, **fluvastatin**, **lovastatin**, **pitavastatin**, **pravastatin**, **rosuvastatin**, and **simvastatin**; do not exceed pravastatin dose of 40 mg/day; concurrent use with pitavastatin or rosuvastatin not recommended; use the lowest possible dose of atorvastatin, fluvastatin, lovastatin, and simvastatin. **Cyclosporine** may ↑ levels/toxicity of voxilaprevir; concurrent use not recommended. May ↑ levels/toxicity of **imatinib**, **irinotecan**, **lapatinib**, **methotrexate**, **mitoxantrone**, **sulfasalazine**, or **topotecan**; concurrent use not recommended. May cause fluctuations in INR when used with **warfarin**; closely monitor INR. May ↑ risk of hypoglycemia when used with certain **antidiabetic agents**.

Drug-Natural Products: St. John's wort may ↓ levels/effectiveness of sofosbuvir, velpatasvir, and voxilaprevir; concurrent use not recommended.

Route/Dosage

PO (Adults): 1 tablet once daily for 12 wk.

Availability

Tablets: sofosbuvir 400 mg/velpatasvir 100 mg/voxilaprevir 100 mg.

NURSING IMPLICATIONS

Assessment

- Monitor for signs and symptoms of hepatitis B reactivation (jaundice, dark urine, light colored stools, fatigue, weakness, loss of appetite, nausea, vomiting, stomach pain) during therapy.
- ***Lab Test Considerations:*** Measure hepatitis B surface antigen (HBsAg) and hepatitis core antibody (anti-HBc) in all patients before starting hepatitis C virus therapy. May cause hepatitis B virus reactivation. Monitor for clinical and laboratory signs of hepatitis flare (↑ AST, ALT, bilirubin, liver failure, death) or HBV reactivation (rapid ↑ in serum HBV DNA level) during HCV treatment and post-treatment follow-up.
- Test patient with HCV genotype 1a infection for presence of virus with NS5A resistance-associated polymorphisms prior to starting therapy with Vosevi™ to determine dose regimen and duration.

Implementation

- **PO:** Administer once daily with food.

Patient/Family Teaching

- Instruct patient to take medication as directed. Do not skip or miss doses. Do not stop medication without consulting health care professional. Advise patient to read *Patient Information* before starting therapy and with each Rx refill in case of changes.
- Advise patient to notify health care professional if signs and symptoms of bradycardia (near-fainting or fainting, dizziness or lightheadedness, malaise, weakness, excessive tiredness, shortness of breath, chest pains, confusion, memory problems) occur.
- Advise patient to notify health care professional if they have a history of HBV. May cause reactivation.
- Instruct patient to notify health care professional of all Rx or OTC medications, vitamins, or herbal products being taken and consult health care professional before taking any new medications, especially St. John's wort.
- Advise patient to notify health care professional if pregnancy is planned or suspected, or if breast feeding.

Evaluation/Desired Outcomes

- Decreased levels of HCV with sustained virologic response and lessened sequelae of chronic HCV infection.

solifenacin (so-li-**fen**-a-sin)

VESIcare

Classification

Therapeutic: urinary tract antispasmodics

Pharmacologic: anticholinergics

Indications

Overactive bladder with symptoms (urge incontinence, urgency, frequency).

Action

Acts as a muscarinic (cholinergic) receptor antagonist; antagonizes bladder smooth muscle contraction.

Therapeutic Effects: Decreased symptoms of overactive bladder.

Pharmacokinetics

Absorption: Well absorbed (90%).

Distribution: Unknown.

Protein Binding: 98%.

Metabolism and Excretion: Extensively metabolized by the CYP3A4 enzyme system. 69% excreted in urine as metabolites, 22% in feces.

Half-life: 45–68 hr.

TIME/ACTION PROFILE

ROUTE	ONSET	PEAK	DURATION
Oral	unknown	3–8 hr	24 hr

Contraindications/Precautions

Contraindicated in: Hypersensitivity; Urinary retention; Gastric retention; Uncontrolled angle-closure glaucoma; Severe hepatic impairment; Lactation: Lactation.

Use Cautiously in: Concurrent use of CYP3A4 inhibitors (use lower dose/clinical monitoring may be necessary); Moderate hepatic impairment (lower dose recommended); Renal impairment; Bladder outflow obstruction; GI obstructive disorders, severe constipation, or ulcerative colitis; Myasthenia gravis; Angle-closure glaucoma; OB: Use only if potential maternal benefit justifies potential fetal risk; Pedi: Safety and effectiveness not established.

Adverse Reactions/Side Effects

CNS: confusion, drowsiness, hallucinations, headache. **CV:** palpitations, tachycardia. **EENT:** blurred vision. **GI:** constipation, dry mouth, dyspepsia, nausea. **MS:** muscle weakness. **Misc:** ANGIOEDEMA.

Interactions

Drug-Drug: Drugs that induce or inhibit the CYP3A4 enzyme system may significantly alter levels; **ketoconazole** ↑ levels and risk of toxicity (do not exceed 5 mg/day).

Route/Dosage

PO (Adults): 5 mg once daily, may ↑ to 10 mg once daily; *Concurrent use of ketoconazole or other potent CYP3A4 inhibitors*—Not to exceed 5 mg/day.

Renal Impairment

(Adults): *CCr <30 mL/min*—Not to exceed 5 mg/day.

Hepatic Impairment

(Adults): *Moderate hepatic impairment*—Not to exceed 5 mg/day.

Availability (generic available)

Tablets: 5 mg, 10 mg. **Cost:** All strengths $703.66/90.

NURSING IMPLICATIONS

Assessment

- Monitor voiding pattern and assess symptoms of overactive bladder (urinary urgency, urinary incontinence, urinary frequency) to and periodically during therapy.

Implementation

- **PO:** Administer once daily without regard to food. Tablets must be swallowed whole; do not break, crush, or chew.

Patient/Family Teaching

- Instruct patient to take solifenacin as directed. Advise patient to read the *Patient Information* before starting therapy and with each prescription refill. If a dose is missed, skip dose and take next day; do not take 2 doses in same day.
- Do not share solifenacin with others; may be dangerous.
- May cause dizziness and blurred vision. Caution patient to avoid driving and other activities that require alertness until response to medication is known.
- Advise patient to notify health care professional immediately if hives; rash; swelling or lips, face, tongue, or throat; trouble breathing occurs.
- Inform patient of potential anticholinergic side effects (constipation, urinary retention, blurred vision, heat prostration in a hot environment).
- Instruct patient to notify health care professional of all Rx or OTC medications, vitamins, or herbal products being taken and consult health care professional before taking any new medications.

Evaluation/Desired Outcomes

- Decrease in symptoms of overactive bladder (urge urinary incontinence, urgency, frequency).

sotalol (soe-ta-lole)

Betapace, Betapace AF, ✱Rylosol, Sorine, Sotylize

Classification

Therapeutic: antiarrhythmics (class III)

S

Indications

Management of life-threatening ventricular arrhythmias. **Betapace AF and Sotylize:** Maintenance of normal sinus rhythm in patients with highly symptomatic atrial fibrillation/atrial flutter (AF/AFL) who are currently in sinus rhythm.

Action

Blocks stimulation of $beta_1$ (myocardial) and $beta_2$ (pulmonary, vascular, and uterine) adrenergic receptor sites. **Therapeutic Effects:** Suppression of arrhythmias.

Pharmacokinetics

Absorption: Well absorbed following oral administration (bioavailability 90–100%).

Distribution: Crosses the placenta; enters breast milk.

Metabolism and Excretion: Elimination is mostly renal.

Half-life: 12 hr (↑ in renal impairment).

TIME/ACTION PROFILE (antiarrhythmic effects)

ROUTE	ONSET	PEAK	DURATION
PO	hr	2–3 days	8–12 hr

Contraindications/Precautions

Contraindicated in: Hypersensitivity; Uncompensated HF; Pulmonary edema; Asthma; Cardiogenic shock; Congenital or acquired long QT syndromes; Sinus bradycardia, 2nd- and 3rd-degree AV block (unless a functioning pacemaker is present); CCr <40 mL/min in patients who are being treated with Betapace AF or Sotylize.

Use Cautiously in: Renal impairment (↑ dosing interval recommended if CCr ≤60 mL/min for patients with ventricular arrhythmias); Hepatic impairment; Hypokalemia (↑ risk of arrhythmias); Geri: ↑ sensitivity to beta blockers; Diabetes mellitus (may mask signs of hypoglycemia); Thyrotoxicosis (may mask symptoms); Patients with a history of severe allergic reactions (intensity of reactions may be increased); OB, Lactation, Pedi: Safety not established; may cause fetal/neonatal bradycardia, hypotension, hypoglycemia, or respiratory depression.

Adverse Reactions/Side Effects

CNS: fatigue, weakness, anxiety, dizziness, drowsiness, insomnia, memory loss, mental depression, mental status changes, nervousness, nightmares. **EENT:** blurred vision, dry eyes, nasal stuffiness. **Resp:** bronchospasm, wheezing. **CV:** ARRHYTHMIAS, BRADYCARDIA, HF, PULMONARY EDEMA, orthostatic hypotension, peripheral vasoconstriction. **GI:** constipation, diarrhea, nausea. **GU:** erectile dysfunction, ↓ libido. **Derm:** itching, rash. **Endo:** hyperglycemia, hypoglycemia. **MS:** arthralgia, back pain, muscle cramps. **Neuro:** paresthesia. **Misc:** drug-induced lupus syndrome.

Interactions

Drug-Drug: Concurrent use with other **class 1A antiarrhythmics** is not recommended due to ↑ risk of arrhythmias. **General anesthesia**, **IV phenytoin**, and **verapamil** may cause additive myocardial depression. Additive bradycardia may occur with **digoxin**, **beta-blockers**, **verapamil**, and **diltiazem**. Additive hypotension may occur with other **antihypertensives**, acute ingestion of **alcohol**, or **nitrates**. Concurrent use with **amphetamines**, **cocaine**, **ephedrine**, **epinephrine**, **norepinephrine**, **phenylephrine**, or **pseudoephedrine** may result in unopposed alpha-adrenergic stimulation (excessive hypertension, bradycardia). Concurrent **thyroid hormone** administration may ↓ effectiveness. May alter the effectiveness of **insulin** or **oral hypoglycemic agents** (dose adjustments may be necessary). May ↓ the effectiveness of **beta-adrenergic bronchodilators** and **theophylline**. May ↓ the beneficial $beta_1$ cardiovascular effects of **dopamine** or **dobutamine**. Discontinuation of **clonidine** in patients receiving sotalol may result in excessive rebound hypertension. Use cautiously within 14 days of **MAO inhibitors** (may result in hypertension).

Route/Dosage

Ventricular Arrhythmias

PO (Adults): 80 mg twice daily; may be gradually ↑ (usual maintenance dose is 160–320 mg/day in 2–3 divided doses; some patients may require up to 480–640 mg/day).

Renal Impairment

PO (Adults): *CCr 30–59 mL/min*—initial dose of 80 mg, with subsequent doses given every 24 hr; *CCr 10–29 mL/min*—initial dose of 80 mg, with subsequent doses given every 36–48 hr.

Atrial Fibrillation/Atrial Flutter

PO (Adults): 80 mg twice daily, may be ↑ during careful monitoring to 120 mg twice daily if necessary.

Renal Impairment

PO (Adults): *CCr 40–60 mL/min*—Administer every 24 hr.

Availability (generic available)

Tablets: 80 mg, 120 mg, 160 mg, 240 mg. **Tablets (Betapace AF):** 80 mg, 120 mg, 160 mg. **Oral solution (Sotylize) (grape flavor):** 5 mg/mL.

NURSING IMPLICATIONS

Assessment

- Monitor ECG prior to and periodically during therapy. May cause life-threatening ventricular tachycardia associated with QT interval prolongation. Do not initiate sotalol therapy if baseline QTc is longer than 450 ms. If QT interval becomes ≥500 ms, reduce dose, prolong duration of infusion, or discontinue therapy.
- Monitor BP and pulse frequently during dose adjustment period and periodically during therapy. Assess for orthostatic hypotension when assisting patient up from supine position.
- Monitor intake and output ratios and daily weight. Assess patient routinely for evidence of fluid overload (peripheral edema, dyspnea, rales/crackles, fatigue, weight gain, jugular venous distention).
- ***Lab Test Considerations:*** Calculate creatinine clearance prior to dosing.
- May cause ↑ BUN, serum lipoprotein, potassium, triglyceride, and uric acid levels.
- May cause increased ANA titers.
- May cause increase in blood glucose levels.
- ***Toxicity and Overdose:*** Monitor patients receiving beta blockers for signs of overdose (bradycardia, severe dizziness or fainting, severe drowsiness, dyspnea, bluish fingernails or palms, seizures). Notify health care professional immediately if these signs occur.
- Glucagon has been used to treat bradycardia and hypotension.

Implementation

- Do not confuse sotalol with Sudafed (pseudoephedrine).
- Patients should be hospitalized and monitored for arrhythmias for at least 3 days during initiation of therapy and dose increases.
- Do not substitute Betapace for Betapace AF. Make sure patients transferred from Betapace to Betapace AF have enough Betapace AF upon leaving the hospital to allow for uninterrupted therapy until Betapace AF prescription can be filled.
- **PO:** Take apical pulse prior to administering. If <50 bpm or if arrhythmia occurs, withhold medication and notify health care professional.
- Administer on an empty stomach, 1 hr before or 2 hr after meals. Administration with food, especially milk or milk products, reduces absorption by approximately 20%.
- Avoid administering antacids containing aluminum or magnesium within 2 hr before administration of sotalol.
- For patients unable to swallow pills, pharmacist can convert tablets to a solution.

Patient/Family Teaching

- Instruct patient to take medication as directed, at the same time each day, even if feeling well; do not skip or double up on missed doses. Take missed doses as soon as possible up to 8 hr before next dose. Abrupt withdrawal may precipitate life-threatening arrhythmias, hypertension, or myocardial ischemia. Advise patients taking *Betapace AF* to read the *Medication Guide* before starting and with each Rx refill in case of changes.
- Advise patient to make sure enough medication is available for weekends, holidays, and vacations. A written prescription may be kept in wallet in case of emergency.
- Teach patient and family how to check pulse and BP. Instruct them to check pulse daily and BP biweekly. Advise patient to hold dose and contact physician or other health care professional if pulse is <50 bpm or if BP changes significantly.
- May cause drowsiness or dizziness. Caution patients to avoid driving or other activities that require alertness until response to the drug is known.
- Advise patients to change positions slowly to minimize orthostatic hypotension, especially during initiation of therapy or when dose is increased.
- Caution patient that this medication may increase sensitivity to cold.
- Advise patient to notify health care professional of all Rx or OTC medications, vitamins, or herbal products being taken and to consult with health care professional before taking other medications, especially cold preparations.
- Diabetic patients should closely monitor blood glucose, especially if weakness, malaise, irritability, or fatigue occurs. Medication may mask tachycardia and increased BP as signs of hypoglycemia, but dizziness and sweating may still occur.
- Advise patient to notify health care professional immediately if new fast heartbeats with lightheadedness and fainting occurs, or if slow pulse, difficulty breathing, wheezing, cold hands and feet, dizziness, confusion, depression, rash, fever, sore throat, unusual bleeding, bruising, or if pain or swelling at the infusion site occurs.
- Instruct patient to inform health care professional of medication regimen prior to treatment or surgery.
- Advise patient to carry identification describing disease process and medication regimen at all times.

Evaluation/Desired Outcomes

- Control of arrhythmias without appearance of detrimental side effects.

spironolactone, See DIURETICS (POTASSIUM-SPARING).

streptokinase, See THROMBOLYTIC AGENTS.

streptomycin, See AMINOGLYCOSIDES.

strong iodine solution, See IODINE, IODIDE.

sucralfate (soo-**kral**-fate)

Carafate, ✱Sulcrate, ✱Sulcrate Plus

Classification

Therapeutic: antiulcer agents
Pharmacologic: GI protectants

Indications

Short-term management of duodenal ulcers. Maintenance (preventive) therapy of duodenal ulcers. **Unlabeled Use:** Management of gastric ulcer or gastroesophageal reflux. Prevention of gastric mucosal injury caused by high-dose aspirin or other NSAIDs in patients with rheumatoid arthritis or in high-stress situations (e.g., intensive care unit). **Suspension:** Mucositis/stomatitis/rectal or oral ulcerations from various etiologies.

S

Action

Aluminum salt of sulfated sucrose reacts with gastric acid to form a thick paste, which selectively adheres to the ulcer surface. **Therapeutic Effects:** Protection of ulcers, with subsequent healing.

Pharmacokinetics

Absorption: Systemic absorption is minimal (<5%).
Distribution: Unknown.
Metabolism and Excretion: >90% is eliminated in the feces.
Half-life: 6–20 hr.

TIME/ACTION PROFILE (mucosal protectant effect)

ROUTE	ONSET	PEAK	DURATION
PO	1–2 hr	unknown	6 hr

Contraindications/Precautions

Contraindicated in: Hypersensitivity.
Use Cautiously in: Renal failure (accumulation of aluminum can occur); Diabetes (↑ risk of hyperglycemia with suspension); Impaired swallowing (↑ risk of tablet aspiration).

Adverse Reactions/Side Effects

CNS: dizziness, drowsiness. **Derm:** pruritus, rashes. **Endo:** hyperglycemia (with suspension). **GI:** constipation, diarrhea, dry mouth, gastric discomfort, indigestion, nausea. **Misc:** HYPERSENSITIVITY REACTIONS (including anaphylaxis and angioedema).

Interactions

Drug-Drug: May ↓ absorption of **phenytoin**, **fat-soluble vitamins**, or **tetracycline**. ↓ effectiveness when used with **antacids**, **cimetidine**, or **ranitidine**. ↓ absorption of **fluoroquinolones** (separate administration by 2 hr).

Route/Dosage

Treatment of Ulcers

PO (Adults): 1 g 4 times daily, given 1 hr before meals and at bedtime; or 2 g twice daily, on waking and at bedtime.

Prevention of Ulcers

PO (Adults): 1 g twice daily, given 1 hr before a meal.

Gastroesophageal Reflux

PO (Adults): 1 g 4 times daily, given 1 hr before meals and at bedtime.
PO (Children): 40–80 mg/kg/day divided every 6 hr, given 1 hr before meals and at bedtime.

Stomatitis

PO (Adults and Children): 5–10 mL of suspension, swish and spit or swish and swallow 4 times daily.

Proctitis

Rect (Adults): 2 g of suspension given as an enema once or twice daily.

Availability (generic available)

Oral suspension (cherry flavor): 1 g/10 mL, ✱ 200 mg/mL. **Cost:** $122.42/420 mL. **Tablets:** 1 g. **Cost:** *Generic*—$23.86/100.

NURSING IMPLICATIONS

Assessment

- Assess patient routinely for abdominal pain and frank or occult blood in the stool.

Implementation

- **PO:** Administer on an empty stomach, 1 hr before meals and at bedtime. Tablet may be broken or dissolved in water before ingestion. Shake suspension well before administration.
- Oral suspension is only for oral use; do not administer IV. Shake well before use. Store at room temperature, do not freeze.
- If antacids are also required for pain, administer 30 min before or after sucralfate dose.

Patient/Family Teaching

- Advise patient to continue with course of therapy for 4–8 wk, even if feeling better, to ensure ulcer healing. If a dose is missed, take as soon as remembered unless almost time for next dose; do not double doses.
- Advise patient that increase in fluid intake, dietary bulk, and exercise may prevent drug-induced constipation.
- Emphasize the importance of routine examinations to monitor progress.

Evaluation/Desired Outcomes

- Decrease in abdominal pain.
- Prevention and healing of duodenal ulcers, seen by x-ray examination and endoscopy.

sulconazole, See ANTIFUNGALS (TOPICAL).

sulfaSALAzine

(sul-fa-**sal**-a-zeen)
Azulfidine, Azulfidine EN-tabs, ✱ Salazopyrin

Classification
Therapeutic: antirheumatics (DMARD), gastrointestinal anti-inflammatories

Indications

Mild-to-moderate ulcerative colitis or as adjunctive therapy in severe ulcerative colitis. Rheumatoid arthritis unresponsive or intolerant to salicylates and/or NSAIDs.

Action

Locally acting anti-inflammatory action in the colon, where activity is probably a result of inhibition of prostaglandin synthesis. **Therapeutic Effects:** Reduction in the symptoms of ulcerative colitis or rheumatoid arthritis.

Pharmacokinetics

Absorption: 10–15% absorbed after oral administration.
Distribution: Widely distributed; crosses the placenta and enters breast milk.
Protein Binding: 99%.
Metabolism and Excretion: Split by intestinal bacteria into sulfapyridine and 5-aminosalicylic acid. Some absorbed sulfasalazine is excreted by bile back into intestines; 15% excreted unchanged by the kidneys. Sulfapyridine also excreted mostly by the kidneys.
Half-life: 6 hr.

TIME/ACTION PROFILE (blood levels)

ROUTE	ONSET	PEAK	DURATION
PO	1 hr	1.5–6 hr	6–12 hr

Contraindications/Precautions

Contraindicated in: Hypersensitivity reactions to sulfonamides, salicylates, or sulfasalazine; Cross-sensitivity with furosemide, sulfonylurea hypoglycemic agents, or carbonic anhydrase inhibitors may exist; Glucose-6–phosphate dehydrogenase (G6PD) deficiency; Hypersensitivity to bisulfites (mesalamine enema only); Urinary tract or intestinal obstruction; Porphyria.
Use Cautiously in: Severe hepatic or renal impairment; History of porphyria; Blood dyscrasias; OB: Neural tube defects have been reported; Lactation: Safety not established; may compete with bilirubin for binding sites on plasma proteins in the newborn and cause kernicterus; bloody stools or diarrhea reported in breast-fed infants; Pedi: Children <2 yr (safety not established).

Adverse Reactions/Side Effects

CNS: headache. **Derm:** EXFOLIATIVE DERMATITIS, STEVENS-JOHNSON SYNDROME, TOXIC EPIDERMAL NECROLYSIS, rash, photosensitivity, yellow discoloration. **GI:** anorexia, diarrhea, nausea, vomiting, drug-induced hepatitis. **GU:** crystalluria, infertility, oligospermia, orange-yellow discoloration of urine. **Hemat:** AGRANULOCYTOSIS, APLASTIC ANEMIA, blood dyscrasias, eosinophilia, hemolytic anemia, megaloblastic anemia, thrombocytopenia. **Neuro:** peripheral neuropathy. **Resp:** pneumonitis. **Misc:** HYPERSENSITIVITY REACTIONS (including anaphylaxis and angioedema), fever.

Interactions

Drug-Drug: May ↑ action/risk of toxicity from **oral hypoglycemic agents**, **phenytoin**, **methotrexate**, **zidovudine**, or **warfarin**. ↑ risk of drug-induced hepatitis with other **hepatotoxic agents**. ↑ risk of crystalluria with **methenamine**. May ↓ metabolism and ↑ effects/toxicity of **mercaptopurine** or **thioguanine**.
Drug-Food: May ↓ **iron** and **folic acid** absorption.

Route/Dosage

Ulcerative Colitis

PO (Adults): 1 g every 6–8 hr (may start with 500 mg every 6–12 hr), followed by maintenance dose of 500 mg every 6 hr.
PO (Children >2 yr): *Initial*—6.7–10 mg/kg every 4 hr *or* 10–15 mg/kg every 6 hr *or* 13.3–20 mg/kg every 8 hr. *Maintenance*—7.5 mg/kg every 6 hr (not to exceed 2 g/day).

Rheumatoid arthritis

PO (Adults): 500 mg–1 g/day (as delayed-release tablets) for 1 wk, then ↑ by 500 mg/day every wk up to 2 g/day in 2 divided doses; if no benefit seen after 12 wk, ↑ to 3 g/day in 2 divided doses.
PO (Children ≥6 yr): 30–50 mg/kg/day in 2 divided doses (as delayed-release tablets); initiate therapy at ¼–⅓ of planned maintenance dose and ↑ every 7 days until maintenance dose is reached (not to exceed 2 g/day).

Availability (generic available)

Tablets: 500 mg. **Delayed-release (enteric-coated) tablets (Azulfidine EN-tabs):** 500 mg.

NURSING IMPLICATIONS

S

Assessment

- Assess patient for allergy to sulfonamides and salicylates. Therapy should be discontinued if rash, difficulty breathing, swelling of face or lips, or fever occur.
- Monitor intake and output ratios. Fluid intake should be sufficient to maintain a urine output of at least 1200–1500 mL daily to prevent crystalluria and stone formation.
- Assess for rash periodically during therapy. May cause Stevens-Johnson syndrome. Discontinue therapy if severe or if accompanied with fever, general malaise, fatigue, muscle or joint aches, blisters, oral lesions, conjunctivitis, hepatitis, and/or eosinophilia.
- **Ulcerative Colitis:** Assess abdominal pain and frequency, quantity, and consistency of stools at the beginning of and during therapy.
- **Rheumatoid Arthritis:** Assess range of motion and degree of swelling and pain in affected joints before and periodically during therapy.
- ***Lab Test Considerations:*** Monitor urinalysis, BUN, and serum creatinine before and periodically during therapy. May cause crystalluria and urinary cell calculi formation.
- Monitor CBC with differential and liver function tests before and every 2nd wk during first 3 mo of ther-

apy, monthly during the 2nd 3 mo, and every 3 mo thereafter or as clinically indicated. Discontinue sulfasalazine if blood dyscrasias occur.

- Serum sulfapyridine levels may be monitored; concentrations >50 μg/mL may be associated with increased incidence of adverse reactions.

Implementation

- Do not confuse sulfasalazine with cefuroxime or sulfadiazine.
- Varying dosing regimens of sulfasalazine may be used to minimize GI side effects.
- **PO:** Administer after meals or with food to minimize GI irritation, with a full glass of water. Do not crush or chew enteric-coated tablets.

Patient/Family Teaching

- Instruct patient on the correct method of administration. Advise patient to take medication as directed, even if feeling better. Take missed doses as soon as remembered unless almost time for next dose.
- May cause dizziness. Caution patient to avoid driving or other activities that require alertness until response to medication is known.
- Advise patient to notify health care professional if skin rash, sore throat, fever, mouth sores, unusual bleeding or bruising, wheezing, fever, or hives occur.
- Caution patient to use sunscreen and protective clothing to prevent photosensitivity reactions.
- Inform patient that this medication may cause orange-yellow discoloration of urine and skin, which is not significant. May permanently stain contact lenses yellow.
- Instruct patient to notify health care professional if symptoms worsen or do not improve. If symptoms of acute intolerance (cramping, acute abdominal pain, bloody diarrhea, fever, headache, rash) occur, discontinue therapy and notify health care professional immediately.
- Advise patient to notify health care professional if pregnancy is planned or suspected, and to avoid breast feeding. Monitor newborn for kernicterus if mother taking sulfasalazine; monitor breast-fed infants for bloody stool or diarrhea. Inform male patient that sulfasalazine may cause infertility; usually reversible.
- Instruct patient to notify health care professional if symptoms do not improve after 1–2 mo of therapy.

Evaluation/Desired Outcomes

- Decrease in diarrhea and abdominal pain.
- Return to normal bowel pattern in patients with ulcerative colitis. Effects may be seen within 3–21 days. The usual course of therapy is 3–6 wk.
- Maintenance of remission in patients with ulcerative colitis.
- Decrease in pain and inflammation and increase in mobility in patients with rheumatoid arthritis.

HIGH ALERT

SULFONYLUREAS

glimepiride (glye-**me**-pye-ride)
Amaryl

glipiZIDE (**glip**-i-zide)
Glucotrol, Glucotrol XL

glyBURIDE (**glye**-byoo-ride)
DiaBeta, ✱Euglucon, Glynase

Classification
Therapeutic: antidiabetics
Pharmacologic: sulfonylureas

Indications

Control of blood glucose in type 2 diabetes mellitus when diet therapy fails. Require some pancreatic function.

Action

Lower blood glucose by stimulating the release of insulin from the pancreas and increasing the sensitivity to insulin at receptor sites. May also decrease hepatic glucose production. **Therapeutic Effects:** Lowering of blood glucose in diabetic patients.

Pharmacokinetics

Absorption: All agents are well absorbed after oral administration.

Distribution: *Glyburide*—reaches high concentrations in bile and crosses the placenta.

Protein Binding: *Glimepiride*—99.5%, *glipizide*—99%, *glyburide*—99%.

Metabolism and Excretion: All agents are mostly metabolized by the liver. *Glimepiride*—converted to a metabolite with some hypoglycemic activity; *Glyburide*—Primarily metabolized by CYP2C9.

Half-life: *Glimepiride*—5–9.2; *glipizide*—2.1–2.6 hr; *glyburide*—10 hr.

TIME/ACTION PROFILE (hypoglycemic activity)

ROUTE	ONSET	PEAK	DURATION
Glimepiride	unknown	2–3 hr	24 hr
Glipizide	15–30 min	1–2 hr	up to 24 hr
Glyburide	45–60 min	1.5–3 hr	24 hr

Contraindications/Precautions

Contraindicated in: Hypersensitivity; Hypersensitivity with sulfonamides (cross-sensitivity may occur); Type 1 diabetes; Diabetic coma or ketoacidosis; Concurrent use of bosentan (glyburide only).

Use Cautiously in: Glucose 6-phosphate dehydrogenase deficiency (↑ risk of hemolytic anemia); Renal or hepatic dysfunction (↑ risk of hypoglycemia); Infection, trauma, or surgery (may alter requirements for control of blood glucose); Impaired pituitary or adrenal function; Prolonged nausea or vomiting; Debilitated or malnourished patients (↑ risk of hypoglycemia); OB: Cross the placenta and ↑ risk of neonatal hypoglycemia; should be discontinued ≥2 wk before delivery; insulin recommended during pregnancy; Lactation: May ↑ risk of hypoglycemia in infant; use while breast feeding only if benefit to patient outweighs potential risk to infant; Pedi: Safety and effectiveness not established; Geri: ↑ sensitivity; dose reduction may be required.

Adverse Reactions/Side Effects

CNS: dizziness, drowsiness, headache, weakness. **Derm:** ERYTHEMA MULTIFORME, photosensitivity, exfoliative dermatitis, rash. **Endo:** hypoglycemia. **F and E:** hyponatremia. **GI:** constipation, cramps, diarrhea, drug-induced hepatitis, heartburn, ↑ appetite, nausea, vomiting. **Hemat:** APLASTIC ANEMIA, agranulocytosis, hemolytic anemia, leukopenia, pancytopenia, thrombocytopenia. **Metab:** ↑ weight.

Interactions

Drug-Drug: ↑ risk of elevated liver enzymes when **bosentan** used with glyburide (avoid concurrent use). Effectiveness may be ↓ by concurrent use of **diuretics, corticosteroids, atypical antipsychotics, danazol, phenothiazines, oral contraceptives, estrogens, progestins, glucagon, protease inhibitors, somatropin, thyroid preparations, phenytoin, niacin, sympathomimetics, calcium channel blockers** and **isoniazid. Alcohol, ACE inhibitors, angiotensin II receptor blockers, chloramphenicol, fibric acid derivatives, fluoxetine, disopyramide, fluoroquinolones, MAO inhibitors, NSAIDs** (except diclofenac), **pentoxifylline, probenecid, salicylates, voriconazole, H_2 receptor antagonists, sulfonamides,** and **warfarin** may ↑ risk of hypoglycemia. Concurrent use with **warfarin** may alter the response to both agents (↑ effects of both initially, then ↓ activity); close monitoring recommended during any changes in dose. **Beta blockers** may mask the signs and symptoms of hypoglycemia. May ↑ **cyclosporine** levels. **Colesevelam** may ↓ effects; administer glyburide, glipizide, and glimepiride ≥4 hr before colesevelam. **Topiramate** may ↓ levels and ↓ effects of glyburide.

Route/Dosage

Glimepiride

PO (Adults): 1–2 mg once daily initially; may ↑ every 1–2 wk up to 8 mg/day (usual range 1–4 mg/day).

PO (Geriatric Patients): 1 mg once daily initially.

Glipizide

PO (Adults): 5 mg once daily initially, may ↑ by 2.5–5 mg/day at weekly intervals as needed (max dose = 40 mg/day immediate-release; 20 mg/day extended-release). Extended-release tablets are given once daily. Doses >15 mg/day of immediate-release tablets should be given as 2 divided doses.

PO (Geriatric Patients): 2.5 mg once daily initially.

Glyburide

The nonmicronized formulation (Diabeta) cannot be used interchangeably with the micronized formulation (Glynase PresTab)

PO (Adults): *DiaBeta (nonmicronized)*—2.5–5 mg once daily initially; may ↑ by 2.5–5 mg/day at weekly intervals (range 1.25–20 mg/day). *Glynase PresTab (micronized)*—1.5–3 mg/day initially; may ↑ by 1.5 mg/day at weekly intervals (range 0.75–12 mg/day; doses >6 mg/day should be given as divided doses).

PO (Geriatric Patients): *DiaBeta (nonmicronized)*—1.25 mg once daily initially; may ↑ by 2.5 mg/day at weekly intervals. *Glynase PresTab (micronized)*—0.75 mg once daily /day; may ↑ by 1.5 mg/day at weekly intervals.

Availability

Glimepiride (generic available)

Tablets: 1 mg, 2 mg, 4 mg. **Cost:** *Generic*—1 mg $9.83/100, 2 mg $10.83/100, 4 mg $10.83/100. ***In combination with:*** pioglitazone (Duetact); rosiglitazone (Avandaryl); see Appendix B.

Glipizide (generic available)

Extended-release tablets: 2.5 mg, 5 mg, 10 mg. **Cost:** *Generic*—2.5 mg $23.76/90, 5 mg $22.86/90. **Tablets:** 5 mg, 10 mg. **Cost:** *Generic*—5 mg $10.83/100, 10 mg $7.18/100. ***In combination with:*** Metformin (Metaglip); see Appendix B.

Glyburide (generic available)

Micronized tablets: 1.5 mg, 3 mg, 6 mg. **Cost:** *Generic*—1.5 mg $37.50/100, 3 mg $60.50/100, 6 mg $107.32/100. **Tablets:** 1.25 mg, 2.5 mg, 5 mg. **Cost:** *Generic*—All strengths $10.83/100. ***In combination with:*** metformin (Glucovance); see Appendix B.

NURSING IMPLICATIONS

Assessment

- Observe for signs and symptoms of hypoglycemic reactions (sweating, hunger, weakness, dizziness, tremor, tachycardia, anxiety).
- Assess patient for allergy to sulfonamides.
- Patients on concurrent beta blocker therapy may have very subtle signs of hypoglycemia.
- ***Lab Test Considerations:*** Monitor serum glucose and glycosylated hemoglobin (HbA1C) periodically during therapy to evaluate effectiveness of treatment.
- Monitor CBC periodically during therapy. Report ↓ in blood counts promptly.

S

- May cause an ↑ in AST, LDH, BUN, and serum creatinine.
- ***Toxicity and Overdose:*** Overdose is manifested by symptoms of hypoglycemia. Mild hypoglycemia may be treated with administration of oral glucose. Severe hypoglycemia should be treated with IV D50W followed by continuous IV infusion of more dilute dextrose solution at a rate sufficient to keep serum glucose at approximately 100 mg/dL.

Implementation

- ***High Alert:*** Accidental administration of oral hypoglycemic agents to non-diabetic adults and children has resulted in serious harm or death. Before administering, confirm that patient has type 2 diabetes.
- ***High Alert:*** Do not confuse Diabeta (glyburide) with Zebeta (bisoprolol).
- Patients stabilized on a diabetic regimen who are exposed to stress, fever, trauma, infection, or surgery may require administration of insulin.
- To convert from other oral hypoglycemic agents, gradual conversion is not required. For insulin dose of less than 20 units/day, change to oral hypoglycemic agents can be made without gradual dose adjustment. Patients taking 20 or more units/day should convert gradually by receiving oral agent and a 25–30% reduction in insulin dose every day or every 2nd day with gradual insulin dose reduction as tolerated. Monitor serum or urine glucose and ketones at least 3 times/day during conversion.
- **PO:** May be administered once in the morning with breakfast or divided into 2 doses.
- Administer *glipizide* 30 min before a meal.
- Do not administer *nonmicronized glyburide* with a meal high in fat. *Micronized glyburide* cannot be substituted for *nonmicronized glyburide*. These preparations are not equivalent.

Patient/Family Teaching

- Instruct patient to take medication at same time each day. Take missed doses as soon as remembered unless almost time for next dose. Do not take if unable to eat.
- Explain to patient that this medication controls hyperglycemia but does not cure diabetes. Therapy is long term.
- Review signs of hypoglycemia and hyperglycemia with patient. If hypoglycemia occurs, advise patient to take a glass of orange juice or 2–3 tsp of sugar, honey, or corn syrup dissolved in water or an appropriate number of glucose tablets and notify health care professional.
- Encourage patient to follow prescribed diet, medication, and exercise regimen to prevent hypoglycemic or hyperglycemic episodes.
- Instruct patient in proper testing of serum glucose and ketones. These tests should be closely monitored during periods of stress or illness and health care professional notified if significant changes occur.
- Concurrent use of alcohol may cause a disulfiram-like reaction (abdominal cramps, nausea, flushing, headaches, and hypoglycemia).
- May occasionally cause dizziness or drowsiness. Caution patient to avoid driving or other activities requiring alertness until response to medication is known.
- Caution patient to avoid other medications, especially alcohol, while on this therapy without consulting health care professional.
- Caution patient to use sunscreen and protective clothing to prevent photosensitivity reactions.
- Advise patient to inform health care professional of medication regimen before treatment or surgery.
- Advise patient to carry a form of sugar (sugar packets, candy) and identification describing disease process and medication regimen at all times.
- Advise patient to notify health care professional promptly if unusual weight gain, swelling of ankles, drowsiness, shortness of breath, muscle cramps, weakness, sore throat, rash, or unusual bleeding or bruising occurs.
- Insulin is the recommended method of controlling blood glucose during pregnancy. Counsel females of reproductive potential to use a form of contraception other than oral contraceptives and to notify health care professional promptly if pregnancy is planned or suspected and to avoid breast feeding. If therapy continued during breast feeding monitor infant for hypoglycemia.
- Emphasize the importance of routine follow-up exams.

Evaluation/Desired Outcomes

- Control of blood glucose levels without the appearance of hypoglycemic or hyperglycemic episodes.

SUMAtriptan (soo-ma-**trip**-tan)

Imitrex, ✱Imitrex DF, Imitrex STATdose, Onzetra Xsail, Tosymra, Zembrace SymTouch

Classification

Therapeutic: vascular headache suppressants

Pharmacologic: 5-HT_1 agonists

Indications

Subcut, PO, Intranasal: Acute treatment of migraine attacks. **Subcut:** Acute treatment of cluster headache episodes.

Action

Acts as a selective agonist of 5-HT_1 at specific vascular serotonin receptor sites, causing vasoconstriction in large intracranial arteries. **Therapeutic Effects:** Relief of acute attacks of migraine.

Pharmacokinetics

Absorption: Well absorbed (97%) after subcut administration. Absorption after oral administration is incomplete and significant amounts undergo substantial hepatic metabolism, resulting in poor bioavailability (14%). Well absorbed after intranasal administration.
Distribution: Does not cross the blood-brain barrier. Remainder of distribution not known.
Metabolism and Excretion: Mostly metabolized (80%) by the liver.
Half-life: 2 hr.

TIME/ACTION PROFILE (relief of migraine)

ROUTE	ONSET	PEAK	DURATION
PO	within 30 min	2–4 hr	up to 24 hr
Subcut	30 min	up to 2 hr	up to 24 hr
Nasal	within 60 min	2 hr	unknown

Contraindications/Precautions

Contraindicated in: Hypersensitivity to sumatriptan or latex (needle shield of prefilled syringe contains rubber [latex derivative]); Ischemic heart disease or signs and symptoms of ischemic heart disease, Prinzmetal's angina, or uncontrolled hypertension; Stroke or transient ischemic attack; Peripheral vascular disease (including, but not limited to, ischemic bowel disease); Concurrent MAO inhibitor therapy; Hemiplegic or basilar migraine; Concurrent use of (within 24 hr) ergotamine-containing or ergot-type drugs or other $5HT_1$ agonists; Severe hepatic impairment; Geri: Excessive risk of cardiovascular complications.
Use Cautiously in: OB: Use during pregnancy only if maternal benefit outweighs potential fetal risk; Lactation: Use while breast feeding only if maternal benefit outweighs potential risk to infant; Rep: Women of reproductive potential; Pedi: Safety and effectiveness not established.
Exercise Extreme Caution in: Cardiovascular risk factors (hypertension, hypercholesterolemia, smoking, obesity, diabetes, family history, menopausal women or men >40 yr); use only if cardiovascular status has been evaluated and determined to be safe and 1st dose is administered under supervision.

Adverse Reactions/Side Effects

All adverse reactions are less common after oral administration.
CNS: dizziness, vertigo, anxiety, drowsiness, fatigue, feeling of heaviness, feeling of tightness, headache, malaise, strange feeling, tight feeling in head, weakness. **CV:** MI, angina, chest pressure, chest tightness, coronary vasospasm, ECG changes, transient hypertension. **Derm:** tingling, warm sensation, burning sensation, cool sensation, flushing. **EENT:** alterations in vision, nasal sinus discomfort, throat discomfort. **GI:** abdominal discomfort, dysphagia. **Local:** injection site reaction. **MS:** jaw discomfort, muscle cramps, myalgia, neck pain, neck stiffness. **Neuro:** numbness. **Misc:** HYPERSENSITIVITY REACTIONS (including anaphylaxis and angioedema).

Interactions

Drug-Drug: The risk of vasospastic reactions may be ↑ by concurrent use of **ergotamine** or **dihydroergotamine** (avoid within 24 hr of each other). Avoid concurrent use with other **$5HT_1$ agonists**. **MAO inhibitors** may ↑ levels (do not use within 2 wk of discontinuing MAO inhibitor). ↑ risk of serotonin syndrome with **SSRIs**, **SNRIs**, **TCAs**, **triptans**, **meperidine**, **bupropion**, or **buspirone**; avoid concurrent use.
Drug-Natural Products: ↑ risk of serotonergic side effects including serotonin syndrome with **St. John's wort** and **SAMe**.

Route/Dosage

PO (Adults): 25 mg initially; if response is inadequate at 2 hr, up to 100 mg may be given (initial doses of 25–50 mg may be more effective than 25 mg). If headache recurs, doses may be repeated every 2 hr (not to exceed 300 mg/day). If PO therapy is to follow subcut injection, additional PO sumatriptan may be taken every 2 hr (not to exceed 200 mg/day).
Subcut (Adults): 6 mg; may repeat after 1 hr (not to exceed 12 mg in 24 hr); *Zembrace SymTouch*—3 mg; may repeat after 1 hr (not to exceed 12 mg/24 hr).
Intranasal (Adults): *Nasal spray (Imitrex)*—Single dose of 5, 10, or 20 mg in 1 nostril; may be repeated in 2 hr (not to exceed 40 mg/24 hr or treatment of >5 episodes/mo); *Nasal spray (Tosymra)*—Single dose of 10 mg in 1 nostril; may be repeated in 1 hr (not to exceed 30 mg/24 hr); *Nasal powder*—11 mg in each nostril; may be repeated in 2 hr (not to exceed 44 mg/24 hr or treatment of >4 episodes/mo).

Hepatic Impairment

PO (Adults): 25 mg initially; if response is inadequate at 2 hr, up to 50 mg may be given (initial doses of 25–50 mg may be more effective than 25 mg). If headache recurs, doses may be repeated every 2 hr (not to exceed 300 mg/day). If PO therapy is to follow subcut injection, additional PO sumatriptan may be taken every 2 hr (not to exceed 200 mg/day); no single oral dose should exceed 50 mg.

Availability (generic available)

Nasal powder capsules: 11 mg. **Nasal spray:** 5 mg/spray, 10 mg/spray, 20 mg/spray. **Cost:** *Generic*—All strengths $49.26/device. **Solution for injection:** 3 mg/0.5-mL (autoinjectors), 4 mg/0.5-mL (prefilled syringes), 6 mg/0.5-mL (prefilled syringes or vials). **Cost:** *Generic*—4 mg/0.5 mL $60.56/0.5 mL, 6 mg/0.5 mL $31.20/0.5 mL. **Tablets:** 25 mg, 50 mg, 100 mg. **Cost:** *Generic*—25 mg $243.47/9, 50 mg

S

$226.26/9, 100 mg $226.26/9. ***In combination with:*** naproxen (Treximet); see Appendix B.

NURSING IMPLICATIONS

Assessment

- Assess pain location, intensity, duration, and associated symptoms (photophobia, phonophobia, nausea, vomiting) during migraine attack.
- Give initial subcut dose under observation to patients with potential for coronary artery disease including postmenopausal women, men >40 yr, patients with risk factors for coronary artery disease such as hypertension, hypercholesterolemia, obesity, diabetes, smoking, or family history. Monitor BP before and for 1 hr after initial injection. If angina occurs, monitor ECG for ischemic changes.
- Monitor for serotonin syndrome in patients taking SSRIs or SNRIs concurrently with sumatriptan.

Implementation

- Do not confuse sumatriptan with sitagliptin or zolmitriptan.
- **PO:** Tablets should be swallowed whole; do not crush, break, or chew. Tablets are film-coated to prevent contact with tablet contents, which have an unpleasant taste and may cause nausea and vomiting.
- **Subcut:** Administer as a single injection. Solution is clear and colorless or pale yellow; do not use if dark-colored or cloudy or if beyond expiration date.
- **Intranasal:** 10-mg dose may be administered as 2 sprays of 5 mg in 1 nostril or 1 spray in each nostril.
- **Nasal Powder**: Remove clear device cap from the reusable delivery device, then remove a disposable nosepiece from foil pouch and click nosepiece into device body. Press fully and promptly release white piercing button on device body to pierce capsule inside nosepiece. White piercing button should only be pressed once and released prior to administration to each nostril. Insert nosepiece into nostril making a tight seal. Rotate device to place mouthpiece into the mouth. Patient blows forcefully through mouthpiece to deliver the sumatriptan powder into nasal cavity. Vibration (e.g., a rattling noise) may occur, and indicates that patient is blowing forcefully, as directed. Once medication in the first nosepiece has been administered, remove and discard nosepiece.

Patient/Family Teaching

- Inform patient that sumatriptan should be used only *during* a migraine attack. It is meant to be used for relief of migraine attacks but not to prevent or reduce the number of attacks.
- Instruct patient to administer sumatriptan as soon as symptoms of a migraine attack appear, but it may be administered at any time during an attack. If migraine symptoms return, a 2nd injection may be used. Allow at least 1 hr between doses, and do not use more than 2 injections in any 24-hr period. Additional sumatriptan doses are not likely to be effective, and alternative medications may be used. If no relief from 1st dose, unlikely 2nd dose will provide relief. Advise patient to read *Patient Information* prior to using and with each Rx refill; new information may be available.
- Advise patient that lying down in a darkened room after sumatriptan administration may further help relieve headache.
- Advise patient that overuse (use more than 10 days/mo) may lead to exacerbation of headache (migraine-like daily headaches, or as a marked increase in frequency of migraine attacks). May require gradual withdrawal of sumatriptan and treatment of symptoms (transient worsening of headache).
- Advise patient to notify health care professional before next dose of sumatriptan if pain or tightness in chest occurs during use. If pain is severe or does not subside, notify health care professional immediately. If wheezing; heart throbbing; swelling of eyelids, face, or lips; skin rash; skin lumps; or hives occur, notify health care professional immediately, and do not take more sumatriptan without approval of health care professional. If usual dose fails to relieve 3 consecutive headaches, or if frequency and/or severity increases, notify health care professional. If feelings of tingling, heat, flushing, heaviness, pressure, drowsiness, dizziness, tiredness, or sickness develop, discuss with health care professional at next visit.
- Sumatriptan may cause dizziness or drowsiness. Caution patient to avoid driving or other activities requiring alertness until response to medication is known.
- Advise patient to avoid alcohol, which aggravates headaches, during sumatriptan use.
- Instruct patient to notify health care professional of all Rx or OTC medications, vitamins, or herbal products being taken and consult health care professional before taking any new medications. Patients concurrently taking SSRI or SNRI antidepressants should notify health care professional promptly if signs of serotonin syndrome (mental status changes: agitation, hallucinations, coma; autonomic instability: tachycardia, labile BP, hyperthermia; neuromuscular aberrations: hyper-reflexia, incoordination; and/or gastrointestinal symptoms: nausea, vomiting, diarrhea) occur.
- Caution patient not to use sumatriptan if pregnancy is planned or suspected or if breast feeding. Adequate contraception should be used during therapy.
- **Subcut:** Instruct patient on the proper technique for loading, administering, and discarding the *Imitrex STATdose pen* autoinjector. Patient information pamphlet is provided. Instructional video is available from the manufacturer.
- Inform patient that pain or redness at the injection site usually lasts less than 1 hr.

- **Intranasal:** Instruct patient in proper technique for intranasal administration. Usual dose is a single spray in 1 nostril. If headache returns, a 2nd dose may be administered in ≥2 hr. Do not administer 2nd dose if no relief was provided by 1st dose without consulting health care professional.

Evaluation/Desired Outcomes

- Relief of migraine attack.

SUNItinib (su-ni-ti-nib)

Sutent

Classification

Therapeutic: antineoplastics

Pharmacologic: kinase inhibitors

Indications

Gastrointestinal stromal tumor (GIST) that has progressed or intolerance to imatinib. Advanced renal cell carcinoma (RCC). Adjuvant treatment of patients at high risk of recurrent RCC following nephrectomy. Advanced pancreatic neuroendocrine tumors (pNET).

Action

Inhibits multiple receptor tyrosine kinases, which are enzymes implicated in tumor growth, abnormal vascular growth, and tumor metastases. **Therapeutic Effects:** Decreased tumor spread.

Pharmacokinetics

Absorption: Well absorbed following oral administration.

Distribution: Unknown.

Protein Binding: *Sunitinib*—95%; *primary active metabolite*—90%.

Metabolism and Excretion: Metabolized by the CYP3A4 enzyme system to its primary active metabolite. This metabolite is further metabolized by CYP3A4. Excretion is primarily fecal.

Half-life: *Sunitinib*—40–60 hr; *primary active metabolite*—80–110 hr.

TIME/ACTION PROFILE (blood levels)

ROUTE	ONSET	PEAK	DURATION
PO	unknown	6–12 hr	24 hr

Contraindications/Precautions

Contraindicated in: Hypersensitivity; NYHA class II-IV HF; OB: May cause fetal harm; Lactation: Avoid breast feeding; Concurrent use of ketoconazole or St. John's wort.

Use Cautiously in: Hepatic/renal impairment; Concurrent use of bisphosphonates or a history of dental disease (may ↑ risk of jaw osteonecrosis); History of myocardial ischemia or MI; LVEF <50% and >20% below baseline with no signs/symptoms of HF (need to interrupt therapy or ↓ dose); Diabetes (↑ risk of hypoglycemia); History of QT interval prolongation, use of antiarrhythmics, cardiac disease, bradycardia, or electrolyte disturbances; Rep: Women of reproductive potential and men with female partners of reproductive potential; Pedi: Safety and effectiveness not established.

Adverse Reactions/Side Effects

CNS: POSTERIOR REVERSIBLE ENCEPHALOPATHY SYNDROME (PRES), fatigue, dizziness, headache. **CV:** HF, MI, TORSADES DE POINTES, hypertension, peripheral edema, QT interval prolongation, thromboembolic events. **Derm:** ERYTHEMA MULTIFORME, NECROTIZING FASCIITIS, STEVENS-JOHNSON SYNDROME, TOXIC EPIDERMAL NECROLYSIS, alopecia, hand-foot syndrome, hair color change, impaired wound healing, rash, skin discoloration. **EENT:** epistaxis. **Endo:** hypoglycemia, hypothyroidism, adrenal insufficiency, hyperthyroidism. **F and E:** dehydration, hypophosphatemia. **GI:** HEPATOTOXICITY, diarrhea, dyspepsia, nausea, stomatitis, vomiting, altered taste, anorexia, cholecystitis, constipation, esophagitis, ↑ lipase/amylase, ↑ liver enzymes, oral pain. **GU:** HEMOLYTIC UREMIC SYNDROME, ↓ fertility, nephrotic syndrome, proteinuria, renal failure. **Hemat:** HEMORRHAGE, THROMBOTIC THROMBOCYTOPENIC PURPURA, anemia, lymphopenia, neutropenia, thrombocytopenia. **Metab:** hyperuricemia. **MS:** arthralgia, back pain, limb pain, myalgia, osteonecrosis (primarily of jaw). **Misc:** TUMOR LYSIS SYNDROME, fever.

Interactions

Drug-Drug: Strong CYP3A4 inhibitors, such as **ketoconazole** may ↑ levels and the risk of toxicity; avoid concurrent use, if possible. If strong inhibitor must be used, ↓ sunitinib dose. **Strong CYP3A4 inducers**, such as **rifampin** may ↓ levels and effectiveness; avoid concurrent use, if possible. If strong inducer must be used, ↑ sunitinib dose. Concurrent use with **alendronate**, **etidronate**, **ibandronate**, **pamidronate**, **risedronate**, **tiludronate**, or **zoledronic acid** may ↑ risk of jaw osteonecrosis. ↑ risk of microangiopathic hemolytic anemia when used with **bevacizumab** (concurrent use not recommended). Concurrent use of other **QT-interval prolonging medications** may ↑ risk of torsade de pointes.

Drug-Natural Products: St. John's wort may ↓ levels and effectiveness; avoid concurrent use.

Drug-Food: Blood levels and effects are ↑ by **grapefruit juice**; concurrent use should be avoided.

Route/Dosage

GIST and RCC

PO (Adults): 50 mg once daily for 4 wk, followed by 2 wk off. *Concurrent use of strong CYP3A4 inhibitor*—37.5 mg once daily for 4 wk, followed by 2 wk off. *Con-*

current use of strong CYP3A4 inducer—87.5 mg once daily for 4 wk, followed by 2 wk off.

Renal Impairment

PO (Adults): *End-stage renal disease (on hemodialysis)*—No initial adjustment required; subsequent dosage ↑ (up to 2-fold) may be required due to reduced exposure.

Adjuvant Treatment of RCC

PO (Adults): 50 mg once daily for 4 wk, followed by 2 wk off for a total of nine 6-wk cycles. *Concurrent use of strong CYP3A4 inhibitor*—37.5 mg once daily for 4 wk, followed by 2 wk off for a total of nine 6-wk cycles. *Concurrent use of strong CYP3A4 inducer*—87.5 mg once daily for 4 wk, followed by 2 wk off for a total of nine 6-wk cycles.

Renal Impairment

PO (Adults): *End-stage renal disease (on hemodialysis)*—No initial adjustment required; subsequent dosage ↑ (up to 2-fold) may be required due to reduced exposure.

pNET

PO (Adults): 37.5 mg once daily. *Concurrent use of strong CYP3A4 inhibitor*—25 mg once daily. *Concurrent use of strong CYP3A4 inducer*—62.5 mg once daily.

Renal Impairment

PO (Adults): *End-stage renal disease (on hemodialysis)*—No initial adjustment required; subsequent dosage ↑ (up to 2-fold) may be required due to reduced exposure.

Availability (generic available)

Capsules: 12.5 mg, 25 mg, 37.5 mg, 50 mg.

NURSING IMPLICATIONS

Assessment

- Monitor for signs of HF (dyspnea, edema, jugular venous distention) during therapy. Assess left ventricular ejection fraction (LVEF) at baseline and periodically during therapy in patients with cardiac events in the previous 12 mo and a baseline ejection fraction in patients without cardiovascular risk factors. Discontinue sunitinib if signs of HF occur.
- Monitor for hypertension and treat with standard antihypertensive therapy. If severe hypertension occurs, may discontinue sunitinib until controlled.
- Monitor ECG and electrolytes periodically during therapy; may cause QT prolongation and torsades de pointes.
- Monitor for rash. If progressive skin rash with blisters or mucosal lesions occurs discontinue and do not restart sunitinib.
- ***Lab Test Considerations:*** Monitor CBC with platelet count and serum chemistries including phosphate at the beginning of each treatment cycle. May cause neutropenia, lymphopenia, anemia, and thrombocytopenia. May cause ↑ creatinine, hypokalemia, hyperuricemia, and ↑ uric acid.
- Monitor ALT, AST, and bilirubin before starting therapy, during each cycle of treatment, and as clinically indicated. Stop therapy if Grade 3 or 4 drug-related hepatic adverse events occur and discontinue if there is no resolution. Do not restart sunitinib if patients subsequently experience severe changes in liver function tests or have other signs and symptoms of liver failure. May cause ↑ AST, ALT, alkaline phosphatase, total and indirect bilirubin, amylase, and lipase.
- Monitor thyroid function at baseline and in patients with symptoms of hypothyroidism or hyperthyroidism. May be treated with standard medical practice.
- Monitor urinalysis for urine protein at baseline and periodically during therapy. Follow up with 24-hr urine protein as clinically indicated. Interrupt sunitinib and reduce dose if 24-hr urine protein ≥3 grams. Discontinue for patients with nephrotic syndrome or repeat episodes of urine protein ≥3 grams despite dose reductions.
- Monitor blood glucose levels periodically during and after therapy. Assess if antidiabetic drug dose needs to be adjusted to minimize the risk of hypoglycemia.

Implementation

- Do not confuse sunitinib with sorafenib.
- **PO:** Administer once daily with or without food.

Patient/Family Teaching

- Instruct patient to take sunitinib as directed. Take missed doses as soon as remembered, but not just before next dose. Take next dose at regular time. Do not take more than 1 dose at a time. Tell your health care professional about the missed dose.
- Advise patient to avoid grapefruit juice and grapefruit products during therapy.
- Instruct patient to notify health care professional promptly if signs of liver failure (itching, yellow eyes or skin, dark urine, pain or discomfort in the right upper stomach area), rash, or tumor lysis syndrome (nausea, shortness of breath, irregular heartbeat, clouding of urine, tiredness) occur.
- Advise patient that GI disorders (diarrhea, nausea, stomatitis, dyspepsia, vomiting) are common and may require antiemetic and antidiarrheal medications.
- Inform patient that sunitinib may cause discoloration (yellow) of skin and depigmentation of hair or skin.
- Instruct patient to notify health care professional of all Rx or OTC medications, vitamins, or herbal products being taken and consult health care professional before taking any new medications, especially St. John's wort.
- Advise patient to notify health care professional if bleeding or swelling occur.

- Advise females of reproductive potential to use effective contraception during and after therapy and to avoid breast feeding during and for 4 wk after last dose.

Evaluation/Desired Outcomes

- Decrease in tumor spread.

suvorexant (soo-voe-**rex**-ant)

Belsomra

Classification

Therapeutic: sedative/hypnotics

Pharmacologic: orexin receptor antagonists

Schedule IV

Indications

Treatment of insomnia associated with difficulty in sleep onset and/or maintenance.

Action

Antagonizes the effects of orexins A and B, naturally occurring neuropeptides that promote wakefulness, by binding to their receptors. **Therapeutic Effects:** Improved sleep.

Pharmacokinetics

Absorption: 82% absorbed following oral administration; a high fat meal will delay absorption and sleep onset. ↑ absorption in obese females.

Distribution: Does not distribute into RBCs.

Protein Binding: >99%.

Metabolism and Excretion: Extensively metabolized by CYP3A (minor metabolism by CYP2C19; metabolites are not active). 66% excreted in feces, 23% in urine, mostly as metabolites.

Half-life: 12 hr (↑ in hepatic impairment).

TIME/ACTION PROFILE (sleep)

ROUTE	ONSET	PEAK	DURATION
PO	30 min (delayed by food)	unknown	7 hr†

†Excess sedation may persist for several days after discontinuation.

Contraindications/Precautions

Contraindicated in: Narcolepsy; Concurrent use of strong inhibitors of CYP3A; Severe hepatic impairment.

Use Cautiously in: History of substance abuse or drug dependence; Concurrent use of moderate inhibitors of CYP3A (dose ↓ recommended); Obese patients (↑ levels, especially in women, dose ↓ may be warranted); History of or concurrent psychiatric diagnoses; Underlying pulmonary disease; OB: Use during pregnancy only if potential benefit justifies potential fetal risk; Lactation: Use cautiously if breast feeding; Pedi: Safe and effective use in children has not been established.

Adverse Reactions/Side Effects

Adverse reactions, especially related to CNS depression are dose-related, especially at the 20 mg dose.

CNS: drowsiness, cataplexy, daytime drowsiness, hallucinations (during sleep), worsening of depression/suicidal ideation, sleep driving, sleep paralysis.

Interactions

Drug-Drug: Concurrent use of **strong inhibitors of CYP3A** including **clarithromycin**, **conivaptan**, **indinavir**, **itraconazole**, **ketoconazole**, **nefazodone**, **nelfinavir**, **posaconazole**, **ritonavir**, and **saquinavir** ↑ risk of excessive sedation and should be avoided. Concurrent use of **moderate inhibitors of CYP3A** including **aprepitant**, **atazanavir**, **ciprofloxacin**, **diltiazem**, **erythromycin**, **fluconazole**, **fosamprenavir**, **imatinib**, and **verapamil** may result in ↑ sedation (↓ dose recommended). Risk of CNS depression, next-day impairment, "sleep-driving" and other complex behaviors while not fully awake ↑ with other **CNS depressants** including **alcohol**, some **antihistamines**, **opioids**, other **sedative/hypnotics** (including **benzodiazepines**) and **tricyclic antidepressants**; dose adjustments may be necessary. Concurrent use of **CYP3A inducers** including **carbamazepine**, **phenytoin**, and **rifampin** may ↓ effectiveness. May alter **digoxin** levels (blood level monitoring recommended).

Drug-Food: Grapefruit juice may result in ↑ blood levels and excess sedation (↓ dose recommended).

Route/Dosage

PO (Adults): 10 mg within 30 min of going to bed, if well tolerated but not optimally effective, dose may be increased next night, not to exceed 20 mg (dose may not be repeated on a single night and should be when at least 7 hr of sleep time is anticipated before planned awakening). *Concurrent use of moderate inhibitors of CYP3A* —5 mg initially, dose may be ↑ to 10 mg if lower dose is tolerated but not optimally effective. Lowest effective dose should be used.

Availability

Tablets: 5 mg, 10 mg, 15 mg, 20 mg.

NURSING IMPLICATIONS

Assessment

- Assess mental status, sleep patterns, and potential for abuse prior to administration. Prolonged use of >7–10 days may lead to physical and psychological dependence. Limit amount of drug available to the patient.
- Assess alertness at time of peak effect. Notify health care professional if desired sedation does not occur.

S

Implementation

- Before administering, reduce external stimuli and provide comfort measures to increase effectiveness of medication.
- Protect patient from injury. Raise bed side rails. Assist with ambulation. Remove patient's cigarettes.
- Use lowest effective dose.
- **PO:** Tablets should be swallowed whole with full glass of water. Take no more than once/night and within 30 min of going to bed. Take only if at least 7 hr remaining before awaking. For faster onset of sleep, do not administer with or immediately after a meal.

Patient/Family Teaching

- Instruct patient to take suvorexant as directed. Advise patient not to take suvorexant unless able to stay in bed a full night (7 hr) before being active again. Do not take more than the amount prescribed because of the habit-forming potential. Not recommended for use longer than 7–10 days. Instruct patient to read the *Medication Guide* for correct product before taking and with each Rx refill, changes may occur.
- Because of rapid onset, advise patient to go to bed immediately after taking suvorexant.
- May cause daytime drowsiness or dizziness. Advise patient to avoid driving or other activities requiring alertness until response to this medication is known.
- Caution patient that complex sleep-related behaviors (sleep-driving) may occur while asleep. Inform families and advise to notify health care professional if these behaviors occur.
- Instruct patient to notify health care professional of all Rx or OTC medications, vitamins, or herbal products being taken and to avoid concurrent use of Rx, OTC, and herbal products without consulting health care professional.
- Caution patient to avoid concurrent use of alcohol or other CNS depressants.
- Advise patient to notify health care professional if depression worsens or suicidal thoughts occur.
- Advise patient to notify health care professional immediately if signs of anaphylaxis (swelling of the tongue or throat, trouble breathing, and nausea and vomiting) occur.
- Advise female patient to notify health care professional if pregnancy is planned or suspected or if breast feeding.

Evaluation/Desired Outcomes

- Relief of insomnia.

TACROLIMUS

tacrolimus (oral, IV)
(ta-**kroe**-li-mus)
Advagraf, Astagraf XL,
Envarsus PA, Envarsus XR, Prograf

tacrolimus (topical)
Protopic

Classification
Therapeutic: immunosuppressants

Indications

PO, IV: Prevention of organ rejection in patients who have undergone allogenic liver, kidney, or heart transplantation (used concurrently with corticosteroids) (used concurrently with azathioprine or mycophenolate mofetil in kidney or heart transplants) (extended-release only indicated for kidney transplant). **Topical:** Moderate to severe atopic dermatitis in patients who do not respond to or cannot tolerate alternative, conventional therapies.

Action

Inhibit T-lymphocyte activation. **Therapeutic Effects:** Prevention of transplanted organ rejection. Improvement in signs/symptoms of atopic dermatitis.

Pharmacokinetics

Absorption: Absorption following oral administration is erratic and incomplete (bioavailability ranges 5–67%); minimal amounts absorbed following topical use.
Distribution: Crosses the placenta and enters breast milk.
Protein Binding: 99%.
Metabolism and Excretion: 99% metabolized by the liver; <1% excreted unchanged in the urine.
Half-life: *Liver transplant patients*—11.7 hr; *healthy volunteers*—21.2 hr.

TIME/ACTION PROFILE (immunosuppression)

ROUTE	ONSET	PEAK	DURATION
PO	rapid	1.3–3.2 hr*	12 hr
PO-ER	unknown	unknown	24 hr
IV	rapid	unknown	8–12 hr
Topical†	unknown	1–2 wk	unknown

*Blood level.
†Improvement in atopic dermatitis.

Contraindications/Precautions

Contraindicated in: Hypersensitivity to tacrolimus or to castor oil (a component in the injection); Concurrent use with cyclosporine or sirolimus should be avoided; Congenital long QT syndrome; Weakened/compromised immune system; Malignant or premalignant skin condition; Lactation: Avoid breast feeding.

Use Cautiously in: Heart failure, bradycardia, or electrolyte disorders (hypokalemia, hypomagnesemia, hypocalcemia); Concurrent use of other drugs known to prolong the QT interval; Renal or hepatic impairment (dose ↓ may be required; if oliguria occurs, wait 48 hr before initiating tacrolimus); Exposure to sunlight/UV light (may ↑ risk of malignant skin changes); Superficial skin infections; OB: Hyperkalemia and renal impairment may occur in the newborn; use only if benefit to mother justifies risk to the fetus; Rep: Women and men of reproductive potential; Pedi: Higher end of dosing range required to maintain adequate blood levels.

Adverse Reactions/Side Effects

Noted primarily for PO and IV use.
CNS: POSTERIOR REVERSIBLE ENCEPHALOPATHY SYNDROME (PRES), SEIZURES, dizziness, headache, insomnia, tremor, abnormal dreams, agitation, anxiety, confusion, depression, emotional lability, hallucinations, psychoses, somnolence. **CV:** hypertension, peripheral edema, QTc interval prolongation. **Derm:** pruritus, rash, alopecia, herpes simplex, hirsutism, photosensitivity, sweating. **EENT:** abnormal vision, amblyopia, sinusitis, tinnitus. **Endo:** hyperglycemia, hyperlipidemia. **F and E:** hyperkalemia, hypomagnesemia, hyperphosphatemia, hypocalcemia, hyponatremia, hypophosphatemia, metabolic acidosis, metabolic alkalosis. **GI:** GI BLEEDING, GI PERFORATION, abdominal pain, anorexia, ascites, constipation, diarrhea, dyspepsia, ↑ liver enzymes, nausea, vomiting, cholangitis, cholestatic jaundice, dysphagia, flatulence, ↑ appetite, oral thrush, peritonitis. **GU:** nephrotoxicity, urinary tract infection, ↓ fertility. **Hemat:** anemia, leukocytosis, leukopenia, thrombocytopenia, coagulation defects, pure red cell aplasia. **Local:** *topical*—burning, stinging. **MS:** arthralgia, hypertonia, leg cramps, muscle spasm, myalgia, myasthenia, osteoporosis. **Neuro:** paresthesia, neuropathy. **Resp:** cough, pleural effusion, asthma, bronchitis, pharyngitis, pneumonia, pulmonary edema. **Misc:** HYPERSENSITIVITY REACTIONS (including anaphylaxis, INFECTION (including activation of latent viral infections such as BK virus-associated nephropathy), MALIGNANCY (including lymphoma and skin cancer), generalized pain, abnormal healing, chills, fever.

Interactions

Noted primarily for PO and IV use, but should be considered for topical use.
Drug-Drug: Risk of nephrotoxicity is ↑ by concurrent use of **aminoglycosides**, **amphotericin B**, **cisplatin**, or **cyclosporine** (allow 24 hr to pass after stopping cyclosporine before starting tacrolimus). Concurrent use of **potassium-sparing diuretics**, **ACE inhibitors**, or **angiotensin II receptor blockers** ↑ risk of hyperkalemia. **Strong CYP3A4 inhibitors**, including **clarithromycin**, **itraconazole**, **ketocona-**

T

zole, **letermovir**, **nefazodone**, **posaconazole**, **protease inhibitors**, and **voriconazole**, may significantly ↑ levels; ↓ tacrolimus dose by ⅔ when used with voriconazole or posaconazole; closely monitor tacrolimus whole blood trough concentrations. **Bromocriptine**, **calcium channel blockers**, **chloramphenicol**, **cimetidine**, **lansoprazole**, **cyclosporine**, **amiodarone**, **danazol**, **ethinyl estradiol**, **erythromycin**, **magnesium/aluminum hydroxide methylprednisolone**, **omeprazole**, **nefazodone**, and **metoclopramide**. Concurrent use with **CYP3A4 substrates** or **CYP3A4 inhibitors** that also prolong the QT interval may ↑ the risk of QT interval prolongation. **Strong CYP3A4 inducers**, including **rifampin** and **rifabutin** may significantly ↓ levels; closely monitor tacrolimus whole blood trough concentrations. **Phenobarbital**, **phenytoin**, **caspofungin**, **sirolimus** and **carbamazepine** may ↓ levels; closely monitor tacrolimus whole blood trough concentrations. **Vaccinations** may be less effective if given concurrently with tacrolimus (avoid use of live-virus vaccines). May ↑ levels of **mycophenolate mofetil** or **mycophenolic acid**.

Drug-Natural Products: Concomitant use with **astragalus**, **echinacea**, and **melatonin** may interfere with immunosuppression. **St. John's wort** may ↓ tacrolimus blood levels. **Schisandra sphenanthera** may significantly ↑ levels; closely monitor tacrolimus whole blood trough concentrations.

Drug-Food: Food ↓ the rate and extent of GI absorption. **Grapefruit juice** ↑ levels; avoid concurrent use.

Route/Dosage

Because of the potential risk for anaphylaxis, the IV route of administration should be reserved for those patients unable to take the drug orally. Extended-release capsules are not interchangeable with immediate-release capsules/granules or other extended-release products. When converting between immediate-release capsules and granules, the total daily dose should remain the same. African-American patients may require a higher dose to achieve desired tacrolimus trough concentrations.

Kidney Transplantation

PO (Adults): *Initial dose of immediate-release capsules (with azathioprine)*—0.1 mg/kg every 12 hr; titrate to achieve recommended whole blood trough concentration; *Initial dose of immediate-release capsules (with mycophenolate mofetil and IL-2 antagonist)*—0.05 mg/kg every 12 hr; titrate to achieve recommended whole blood trough concentration; *Extended-release capsules (Astagraf XL) (with basiliximab induction)*—0.15–0.2 mg/kg once daily (to be started prior to reperfusion or within 48 hr of completion of transplant); *Extended-release capsules (Astagraf XL) (without basiliximab induction)*—0.1 mg/kg given as single dose preoperatively within 12 hr prior to reperfusion, followed by 0.2 mg/kg once daily started postoperatively at least 4 hr after preoperative dose and within 12 hr after reperfusion; *Conversion from immediate-release capsules to extended-release capsules (Envarsus XR)*—Initiate extended-release treatment with a once daily dose that is 80% of the total daily dose of the immediate-release product (also appropriate for African-American patients); *Initial dose of extended—release capsules as initial therapy (Envarsus XR)*—0.14 mg/kg once daily; titrate to achieve recommended whole blood trough concentration.

PO (Children): *Immediate-release capsules or granules*—0.15 mg/kg every 12 hr; titrate to achieve recommended whole blood trough concentration; *Extended-release capsules (Astagraf XL) (with basiliximab induction)*—0.3 mg/kg once daily (to be started within 24 hr following reperfusion).

IV (Adults): *Initial dose*—0.03–0.1 mg/kg/day as a continuous infusion; titrate to achieve recommended whole blood trough concentration.

IV (Children): 0.03–0.15 mg/kg/day.

Liver Transplantation

PO (Adults): *Initial dose of immediate–release capsules*—0.1–0.15 mg/kg/day in two divided doses; titrate to achieve recommended whole blood trough concentration.

PO (Children): *Initial dose of immediate–release capsules*—0.075–0.1 mg/kg every 12 hr; titrate to achieve recommended whole blood trough concentration; *Initial dose of immediate–release capsules or granules*—0.1 mg/kg every 12 hr; titrate to achieve recommended whole blood trough concentration.

IV (Adults and Children): Same as for kidney transplant.

Heart Transplantation

PO (Adults): *Initial dose of immediate-release capsules*—0.075 mg/kg/day in two divided doses; titrate to achieve recommended whole blood trough concentration.

PO (Children): *Initial dose of immediate–release capsules*—0.075–0.1 mg/kg every 12 hr; titrate to achieve recommended whole blood trough concentration.

IV (Adults): *Initial dose*—0.01 mg/kg/day as a continuous infusion; titrate to achieve recommended whole blood trough concentration.

Atopic Dermatitis

Topical (Adults): Apply 0.03% or 0.1% ointment twice daily. Discontinue when signs/symptoms of atopic dermatitis resolve.

Topical (Children ≥2–15 yr): Apply 0.03% ointment twice daily. Discontinue when signs/symptoms of atopic dermatitis resolve.

Availability (generic available)

Capsules: 0.5 mg, 1 mg, 5 mg. **Extended-release capsules (Astragraf XL):** 0.5 mg, 1 mg, 3 mg, 5 mg. **Extended-release tablets (Envarsus XR):** 0.75 mg, 1 mg, 4 mg. **Granules for oral suspension:** 0.2 mg/pkt, 1 mg/pkt. **Solution for injection (requires dilution):** 5 mg/mL. **Topical ointment:** 0.03%, 0.1%.

NURSING IMPLICATIONS

Assessment

- Assess for symptoms of PRES (headache, altered mental status, seizures, visual disturbances, hypertension) periodically during therapy. Confirm diagnosis by radiologic procedure. If PRES is suspected or diagnosed, maintain BP control and immediately reduce immunosuppression. Symptoms are usually reversed on reduction or discontinuation of immunosuppression.
- **Prevention of Organ Rejection:** Monitor BP closely during therapy. Hypertension is a common complication of tacrolimus therapy and should be treated.
- Observe patients receiving IV tacrolimus for the development of anaphylaxis (rash, pruritus, laryngeal edema, wheezing) for at least 30 min and frequently thereafter. If signs develop, stop infusion and initiate treatment.
- **Atopic Dermatitis:** Assess skin lesions prior to and periodically during therapy.
- Use only for short time, not continuously, and in the minimum dose possible to decrease risk of developing skin cancer.
- ***Lab Test Considerations:*** Tacrolimus blood level monitoring may be helpful in the evaluation of rejection and toxicity, dose adjustments, and assessment of compliance. *For kidney transplantation*, during the first 3 mo, most patients maintained tacrolimus whole blood concentrations between 7–20 ng/mL and then between 5–15 ng/mL through 1 yr. *For de novo kidney transplantation*, during the first mo, most patients maintained tacrolimus whole blood concentrations between 6–11 ng/mL and then between 4–11 ng/mL through month 1. *For heart transplantation*, from wk 1 to 3 mo, most patients maintained tacrolimus trough whole blood concentrations between 8–20 ng/mL and then between 6–18 ng/mL from 3–18 mo post-transplant.
- Monitor serum creatinine, potassium, and glucose closely. ↑ serum creatinine and ↓ urine output may indicate nephrotoxicity. May also cause insulin-dependent post-transplant diabetes mellitus (🧬 incidence is higher in African American and Hispanic patients).
- May also cause hyperuricemia, hypokalemia, hyperkalemia, hypomagnesemia, metabolic acidosis, metabolic alkalosis, hyperlipidemia, hyperphosphatemia, hypophosphatemia, hypocalcemia, and hyponatremia.
- Monitor CBC. May cause anemia, leukocytosis, and thrombocytopenia.

Implementation

- Do not confuse Prograf (tacrolimus) with Prozac (fluoxetine).
- Do not confuse immediate-release tacrolimus with extended-release tacrolimus.
- Should only be prescribed by health care professionals experienced with immunosuppressive therapy and organ transplant patients.
- Begin therapy with tacrolimus no sooner than 6 hr post-transplantation. Concurrent therapy with corticosteroids is recommended in the early postoperative period.
- Tacrolimus should not be used concomitantly with cyclosporine. Tacrolimus or cyclosporine should be discontinued at least 24 hr before starting the other.
- Oral therapy is preferred because of the risk of anaphylactic reactions with IV tacrolimus. IV therapy should be replaced with oral therapy as soon as possible.
- Adults should be started at the lower end of the dose range; children require a higher doses to maintain blood trough concentrations similar to adults.
- Immediate and extended-release capsules are not interchangeable.
- **PO:** Oral doses can be initiated 8–12 hr after discontinuation of IV doses. May be taken without regard to food, but should be consistent, with or without food and at same time each day.
- Take extended-release capsules at the same time each day, preferably in the morning, on an empty stomach at least 1 hr before or 2 hrs after breakfast. Swallow capsules whole; do not chew, divide, or crush.
- **Topical:** Do not use continuously for a long time.
- **Topical:** Wash hands before applying. Apply a thin layer of ointment twice daily to affected skin. Use smallest amount of ointment needed to control signs and symptoms of eczema. Do not cover treated area with bandages, dressings or wraps. If not treating areas on hands, wash hands with soap and water after applying to remove any ointment on hands.

IV Administration

- **Continuous Infusion:** ***Diluent:*** Dilute in 0.9% NaCl or D5W. ***Concentration:*** 0.004–0.02 mg/mL. May be stored in polyethylene or glass containers for 24 hr following dilution. Do not store in PVC containers. Do not administer solutions that are discolored or contain particulate matter. ***Rate:*** Administer daily dose as a continuous infusion over 24 hr.
- **Y-Site Compatibility:** alemtuzumab, alfentanil, amifostine, amikacin, aminocaproic acid, aminophylline, amiodarone, amphotericin B lipid complex, amphotericin B liposome, anidulafungin, argatroban, azithromycin, aztreonam, benztropine, bivalirudin, bleomycin, bumetanide, buprenorphine, busulfan, butorphanol, calcium acetate, calcium

T

chloride, calcium gluconate, carboplatin, carmustine, caspofungin, cefazolin, cefotaxime, cefotetan, cefoxitin, ceftazidime, ceftriaxone, cefuroxime, chloramphenicol, chlorpromazine, ciprofloxacin, cisatracurium, cisplatin, clindamycin, cyclophosphamide, cyclosporine, cytarabine, dacarbazine, dactinomycin, daptomycin, daunorubicin hydrochloride, dexamethasone, dexmedetomidine, dexrazoxane, digoxin, diltiazem, diphenhydramine, dobutamine, docetaxel, dopamine, doxorubicin hydrochloride, doxorubicin liposomal, doxycycline, droperidol, enalaprilat, ephedrine, epinephrine, epirubicin, ertapenem, erythromycin, esmolol, etoposide, etoposide phosphate, famotidine, fenoldopam, fentanyl, fluconazole, fludarabine, foscarnet, fosphenytoin, gemcitabine, gentamicin, glycopyrrolate, granisetron, haloperidol, heparin, hetastarch, hydralazine, hydrocortisone, hydromorphone, idarubicin, ifosfamide, imipenem/cilastatin, insulin, regular, irinotecan, isoproterenol, ketorolac, labetalol, leucovorin calcium, levofloxacin, levorphanol, lidocaine, linezolid, lorazepam, magnesium sulfate, mannitol, meperidine, meropenem, mesna, methotrexate, methyldopate, methylprednisolone, metoclopramide, metoprolol, metronidazole, micafungin, midazolam, milrinone, mitomycin, mitoxantrone, morphine, moxifloxacin, multivitamins, mycophenolate, nafcillin, nalbuphine, naloxone, nicardipine, nitroglycerin, nitroprusside, norepinephrine, octreotide, ondansetron, oxacillin, oxaliplatin, oxytocin, paclitaxel, palonosetron, pamidronate, pancuronium, pemetrexed, penicillin G potassium, pentamidine, phentolamine, phenylephrine, piperacillin/tazobactam, potassium acetate, potassium chloride, potassium phosphates, procainamide, prochlorperazine, promethazine, propranolol, quinupristin/dalfopristin, ranitidine, remifentanil, rocuronium, sodium acetate, sodium bicarbonate, sodium phosphates, streptozocin, succinylcholine, sufentanil, theophylline, thiotepa, tigecycline, tirofiban, tobramycin, topotecan, vancomycin, vasopressin, vecuronium, verapamil, vinblastine, vincristine, vinorelbine, voriconazole, zidovudine, zoledronic acid.

- **Y-Site Incompatibility:** acyclovir, allopurinol, azathioprine, cefepime, dantrolene, diazepam, esomeprazole, folic acid, ganciclovir, iron sucrose, levothyroxine, phenytoin, thiopental.

Patient/Family Teaching

- Instruct patient to take tacrolimus at the same time each day, with or without food, as directed. Do not skip or double up on missed doses. Do not discontinue medication without advice of health care professional. Take missed doses of extended-release capsule as soon as remembered unless more than 14 hr after scheduled dose; do not double doses. Advise patient to read the *Patient Information* before starting tacrolimus and with each refill in case of changes. Instruct patient to inspect capsules with each new Rx, before taking. Contact health care professional if appearance of capsules or dose has changed.
- Advise patient to avoid grapefruit and grapefruit juice and alcohol during therapy.
- Reinforce the need for lifelong therapy to prevent transplant rejection. Review symptoms of rejection for transplanted organ and stress need to notify health care professional immediately if they occur.
- Advise patient to avoid eating raw oysters or other shellfish; make sure they are fully cooked before eating.
- Instruct patient to notify health care professional if signs of diabetes mellitus (frequent urination, increased thirst or hunger), infection (fever, sweats, chills, cough or flu-like symptoms, muscle aches, warm, red, painful areas on skin), neurotoxicity (vision changes, deliriums, or tremors), or PRES occur.
- Advise patient to wear protective clothing and sunscreen to avoid photosensitivity reactions.
- Instruct patient to avoid exposure to chicken pox, measles, mumps, and rubella. If exposed, see health care professional for prophylactic therapy.
- Instruct patient to notify health care professional of all Rx or OTC medications, vitamins, or herbal products being taken and consult health care professional before taking any new medications.
- Inform patient of the risk of lymphoma or skin cancer with tacrolimus therapy.
- Advise patient of the risk of taking tacrolimus during pregnancy or breast feeding. Caution females of reproductive potential and males with female partners of reproductive potential to use effective contraception before and during therapy. If breast feeding or planning to breast feed discuss with health care professional. Encourage females who become pregnant and males who have fathered a pregnancy during treatment with tacrolimus to enroll in the pregnancy registry to collect information about birth outcomes by calling 1-877- 955-6877.
- Emphasize the importance of repeated lab tests during tacrolimus therapy.
- **Topical:** Instruct apply ointment as directed. Advise patient to read the *Medication Guide* prior to starting and with each Rx renewal; new information may be available.
- Advise patient not to bathe, shower, or swim right after applying; may wash off ointment. May use moisturizers with ointment. Instruct patient to check with health care professional first about products to use. If moisturizers are used, apply them after application of ointment.
- Advise patients to contact health care professional if their symptoms do not improve after 6 wk of therapy, if their symptoms worsen, or they develop a skin infection.
- Instruct patient to use ointment only on areas of skin with atopic dermatitis.

- Advise patient to stop using the ointment when the signs/symptoms of atopic dermatitis go away.
- Advise patient to limit sun exposure during treatment.
- Advise patient of the risk of using topical tacrolimus during pregnancy.
- Inform patient of the risk of lymphoma or skin cancer with topical tacrolimus therapy.

Evaluation/Desired Outcomes

- Prevention of transplanted organ rejection.
- Management of atopic dermatitis.

tadalafil (ta-da-la-fil)

Adcirca, Alyq, Cialis

Classification

Therapeutic: erectile dysfunction agents, vasodilators

Pharmacologic: phosphodiesterase type 5 inhibitors

Indications

Cialis: Treatment of: Erectile dysfunction (ED), Benign prostatic hyperplasia (BPH), ED and BPH. *Adcirca and Alyq:* Pulmonary arterial hypertension.

Action

Increases cyclic guanosine monophosphate (cGMP) levels by inhibiting phosphodiesterase type 5 (PDE5) an enzyme responsible for the breakdown of cGMP. cGMP produces smooth muscle relaxation of the corpus cavernosum, which in turn promotes increased blood flow and subsequent erection. cGMP also leads to vasodilation of the pulmonary vasculature. **Therapeutic Effects:** *Cialis:* Enhanced blood flow to the corpus cavernosum and erection sufficient to allow sexual intercourse. Improved signs and symptoms of BPH. *Adcirca and Alyq:* Improved exercise tolerance.

Pharmacokinetics

Absorption: Well absorbed following oral administration.

Distribution: Extensive tissue distribution; penetrates semen.

Protein Binding: 94%.

Metabolism and Excretion: Mostly metabolized by the liver (mainly CYP3A4 enzyme system); metabolites are excreted in feces (61%) and urine (36%).

Half-life: 17.5 hr.

TIME/ACTION PROFILE (vasodilation, improved erectile function)

ROUTE	ONSET	PEAK	DURATION
PO	rapid	0.5–6 hr	36

Contraindications/Precautions

Contraindicated in: Hypersensitivity; Concurrent use of nitrates or riociguat; Unstable angina, recent history of stroke, life-threatening heart failure within 6 mo, uncontrolled hypertension, arrhythmias, stroke within 6 mo or MI within 90 days; Any other cardiovascular pathology precluding sexual activity; Known hereditary degenerative retinal disorders; Severe hepatic impairment; Severe renal impairment (Adcirca and Alyq); Severe renal impairment (CCr <30 mL/min) (Cialis once daily dosing); Congenital or acquired QT interval prolongation or concurrent use of Class IA or III antiarrhythmics; Concurrent use of ketoconazole, itraconazole, or rifampin (Adcirca and Alyq); Alpha adrenergic blockers (when tadalafil used for BPH); Women; Pedi: Children or newborns.

Use Cautiously in: Left ventricular outflow obstruction; Penile deformity; Renal impairment; Underlying conditions predisposing to priapism including sickle cell anemia, multiple myeloma, or leukemia; Bleeding disorders or active peptic ulcer disease; Strong inhibitors of the CYP3A4 enzyme system; Alpha adrenergic blockers (patients should be on stable dose of alpha blockers before starting tadalafil for ED); History of sudden severe vision loss or non arteritic ischemic optic neuropathy (NAION); may ↑ risk of recurrence; Low cup to disk ratio, age >50 yr, diabetes, hypertension, coronary artery disease, hyperlipidemia, or smoking (↑ risk of NAION); Geri: ↑ risk of diarrhea.

Adverse Reactions/Side Effects

CNS: <u>headache</u>. **CV:** hypotension, peripheral edema. **Derm:** <u>flushing</u>. **EENT:** hearing loss, nasal congestion, vision loss. **GI:** diarrhea, dyspepsia. **GU:** ↓ fertility, priapism. **MS:** back pain, limb pain, myalgia.

Interactions

Drug-Drug: Concurrent use of **nitrates** may cause serious, life threatening hypotension and is contraindicated. Concurrent use of **riociguat** may result in severe hypotension; concurrent use contraindicated. ↑ risk of hypotension with **alpha adrenergic blockers** and acute ingestion of **alcohol**; discontinue alpha-adrenergic blocker therapy ≥1 day before starting Cialis for BPH. Strong inhibitors of CYP3A4 including **ritonavir**, **ketoconazole**, **itraconazole** ↑ effects and the risk of adverse reactions (dose adjustments recommended; ketoconazole and itraconazole contraindicated with Adcirca and Alyq). Similar effects may be expected of other **inhibitors of CY3A4**. **CYP3A4 inducers** may ↓ effects (**rifampin** contraindicated with Adcirca or Alyq).

Route/Dosage

Cialis (for ED)

PO (Adults): 10 mg prior to sexual activity (range 5–20 mg; not to exceed one dose/24 hr) *or* 2.5 mg once daily (max: 5 mg/day); *Concurrent use of CYP3A4 inhibitors including itraconazole, ketoconazole and ritonavir*—single dose should not exceed 10 mg in any 72 hr period; for once daily dose regimen, should not exceed 2.5 mg/day.

Renal Impairment

PO (Adults): *CCr 30–50 mL/min (as needed dosing)*—Initial dose should not exceed 5 mg/day; maximum dose should not exceed 10 mg in 48 hr; *CCr <30 mL/min (as needed dosing)*—Maximum dose should not exceed 5 mg in 72 hr; *CCr <30 mL/min (once daily dosing)*—Not recommended for use.

Hepatic Impairment

PO (Adults): *Mild or moderate hepatic impairment (Child–Pugh class A or B)*—Daily dose should not exceed 10 mg (once daily dose regimen not recommended) *Severe hepatic impairment (Child–Pugh class C)*—Not recommended for use.

Cialis (for BPH or ED/BPH)

PO (Adults): 5 mg once daily; *Concurrent use of CYP3A4 inhibitors including itraconazole, ketoconazole and ritonavir*—Should not exceed 2.5 mg/day.

Renal Impairment

PO (Adults): *CCr 30–50 mL/min*—Initial dose should not exceed 2.5 mg/day; maximum dose should not exceed 5 mg/day; *CCr <30 mL/min*—Not recommended for use.

Hepatic Impairment

PO (Adults): Not recommended for use.

Adcirca and Alyq (for pulmonary arterial hypertension)

PO (Adults): 40 mg once daily; *If receiving ritonavir for ≥1 wk*—start 20 mg once daily; may then ↑ to 40 mg once daily based on tolerability; *If initiating ritonavir while on Adcirca or Alyq*—stop Adcirca or Alyq ≥24 hr before starting ritonavir; may reinitiate Adcirca or Alyq at 20 mg once daily after ≥1 wk of therapy with ritonavir; may then ↑ to 40 mg once daily based on tolerability.

Renal Impairment

(Adults): *CCr 31–80 mL/min*—Start 20 mg once daily; may then ↑ to 40 mg once daily based on tolerability.

Hepatic Impairment

PO (Adults): *Mild or moderate hepatic impairment (Child–Pugh class A or B)*—Start with 20 mg once daily.

Availability (generic available)

Tablets (Cialis): 2.5 mg, 5 mg, 10 mg, 20 mg. **Tablets (Adcirca or Alyq):** 20 mg.

NURSING IMPLICATIONS

Assessment

- *Cialis: for ED* : Determine ED before administration. Tadalafil has no effect in the absence of sexual stimulation.
- *Cialis for BPH*: Assess for symptoms of prostatic hyperplasia (urinary hesitancy, feeling of incomplete bladder emptying, interruption of urinary stream, impairment of size and force of urinary stream, terminal urinary dribbling, straining to start flow, dysuria, urgency) before and periodically during therapy.
- Digital rectal examinations should be performed before and periodically during therapy for BPH.
- *Adcirca*: Monitor hemodynamic parameters and exercise tolerance prior to and periodically during therapy.

Implementation

- **PO:** Administer dose *as needed for ED* at least 30 min prior to sexual activity; effectiveness may continue for 36 hr.
- Administer dose for *pulmonary hypertension, BPH, ED/BPH, or daily for ED* once daily at the same time each day.
- May be administered without regard to food. Swallow tablets whole; do not crush, break, or chew.

Patient/Family Teaching

- Instruct patient to take tadalafil as needed for ED at least 30 min before sexual activity and not more than once per day. Inform patient that sexual stimulation is required for an erection to occur after taking tadalafil.
- Advise patient that tadalafil is not indicated for use in women.
- Caution patient not to take tadalafil concurrently with alpha adrenergic blockers (unless on a stable dose) or nitrates. If chest pain occurs after taking tadalafil, instruct patient to seek immediate medical attention.
- Advise patient to avoid excess alcohol intake (≥5 units) in combination with tadalafil; may increase risk of orthostatic hypotension, increased heart rate, decreased standing BP, dizziness, headache.
- Instruct patient to notify health care professional promptly if erection lasts longer than 4 hr, if they are not satisfied with their sexual performance or develop unwanted side effects or if they experience sudden or decreased vision loss in one or both eyes or loss or decrease in hearing, ringing in the ears, or dizziness.
- Advise patient to notify health care professional of all Rx or OTC medications, vitamins, or herbal products being taken and to consult with health care professional before taking other medications.
- Inform patient that tadalafil offers no protection against sexually transmitted diseases. Counsel patient that protection against sexually transmitted diseases and HIV infection should be considered.

Evaluation/Desired Outcomes

- Male erection sufficient to allow intercourse.
- Decrease in urinary symptoms of benign prostatic hyperplasia.
- Increased exercise tolerance.

tamoxifen (ta-mox-i-fen)

~~Nolvadex~~, ✱Nolvadex-D, Soltamox

Classification
Therapeutic: antineoplastics
Pharmacologic: antiestrogens

Indications

Estrogen-receptor positive metastatic breast cancer. Adjuvant treatment of early-stage estrogen-receptor positive breast cancer. To reduce the occurrence of contralateral breast cancer when used as adjuvant therapy for breast cancer. Prevention of breast cancer in high-risk patients. Treatment of ductal carcinoma *in situ* following breast surgery and radiation.

Action

Competes with estrogen for binding sites in breast and other tissues. Reduces DNA synthesis and estrogen response. **Therapeutic Effects:** Suppression of tumor growth. Reduced incidence of breast cancer in high-risk patients.

Pharmacokinetics

Absorption: Absorbed after oral administration.
Distribution: Widely distributed.
Metabolism and Excretion: Mostly metabolized by the liver. Slowly eliminated in the feces. Minimal amounts excreted in the urine.
Half-life: 7 days.

TIME/ACTION PROFILE (tumor response)

ROUTE	ONSET	PEAK	DURATION
PO	4–10 wk	several mo	several wk

Contraindications/Precautions

Contraindicated in: Hypersensitivity; Concurrent warfarin therapy with history of deep vein thrombosis (patients at high risk for breast cancer only); OB: May cause fetal harm (avoid use during pregnancy); Lactation: Avoid use during breast feeding.
Use Cautiously in: ↓ bone marrow reserve; Rep: Women of reproductive potential.

Adverse Reactions/Side Effects

CNS: STROKE, confusion, depression, headache, weakness. **CV:** THROMBOEMBOLISM, edema. **EENT:** blurred vision. **F and E:** hypercalcemia. **GI:** nausea, vomiting. **GU:** UTERINE MALIGNANCIES, vaginal bleeding. **Hemat:** leukopenia, thrombocytopenia. **Metab:** hot flashes. **MS:** bone pain. **Misc:** tumor flare.

Interactions

Drug-Drug: Estrogens may ↓ effectiveness of concurrently administered tamoxifen. Blood levels are ↑ by **bromocriptine**. May ↑ the anticoagulant effect of **warfarin**. Risk of thromboembolic events is ↑ by concurrent use of other **antineoplastics**.

Route/Dosage

Metastatic Breast Cancer

PO (Adults): 20 mg once daily *or* 20 mg twice daily.

Adjuvant Treatment of Breast Cancer

PO (Adults): 20 mg once daily for 5–10 yrs.

Prevention of Breast Cancer in High-Risk Women or Ductal Carcinoma *in Situ*

PO (Adults): 20 mg once daily for 5 yrs.

Availability (generic available)

Oral solution (licorice aniseed-flavor): 10 mg/5 mL. **Tablets:** 10 mg, 20 mg.

NURSING IMPLICATIONS

Assessment

- Assess for an increase in bone or tumor pain. Confer with health care professional regarding analgesics. This transient pain usually resolves despite continued therapy.
- ***Lab Test Considerations:*** Obtain a negative pregnancy test before starting therapy.
- Monitor CBC, platelets, and calcium levels before and during therapy. May cause transient hypercalcemia in patients with metastases to the bone. An estrogen receptor assay should be assessed before initiation of therapy.
- Monitor serum cholesterol and triglyceride concentrations in patients with pre-existing hyperlipidemia. May cause ↑ concentrations.
- Monitor hepatic function tests and thyroxine (T_4) periodically during therapy. May cause ↑ serum hepatic enzyme and thyroxine concentrations.
- Gynecologic examinations should be performed regularly; may cause variations in Papanicolaou and vaginal smears.

Implementation

- **PO:** Administer with food or fluids if GI irritation becomes a problem. Consult health care professional if patient vomits shortly after administration of medication to determine need for repeat dose.
- Do not crush, break, chew, or administer an antacid within 1–2 hr of enteric-coated tablet.

Patient/Family Teaching

- Instruct patient to take medication as directed. If a dose is missed, it should be omitted.
- If skin lesions are present, inform patient that lesions may temporarily increase in size and number and may have increased erythema.
- Advise patient to report bone pain to health care professional promptly. This pain may be severe. Analgesics should be ordered to control pain. Inform patient that this may be an indication of the drug's effectiveness and will resolve over time.

T

- Instruct patient to monitor weight weekly. Weight gain or peripheral edema should be reported to health care professional.
- Advise patient that medication may cause hot flashes. Notify health care professional if these become bothersome.
- Instruct patient to notify health care professional promptly if pain or swelling of legs, shortness of breath, weakness, sleepiness, confusion, nausea, vomiting, weight gain, dizziness, headache, loss of appetite, or blurred vision occurs. Patient should also report menstrual irregularities, vaginal bleeding, pelvic pain or pressure.
- This medication may induce ovulation and may have teratogenic properties. Advise females of reproductive potential to use a nonhormonal method of contraception during and for 2 mo after last dose of tamoxifen and to avoid breast feeding for 3 mo after last dose. May sometimes cause female infertility.

Evaluation/Desired Outcomes

- Decrease in the size or spread of breast cancer. Observable effects of therapy may not be seen for 4–10 wk after initiation.

tamsulosin (tam-**soo**-loe-sin)

Flomax

Classification
Therapeutic: none assigned
Pharmacologic: peripherally acting antiadrenergics

Indications

Management of signs/symptoms of benign prostatic hyperplasia (BPH).

Action

Decreases contractions in smooth muscle of the prostatic capsule by preferentially binding to $alpha_1$-adrenergic receptors. **Therapeutic Effects:** Decreased symptoms of prostatic hyperplasia (urinary urgency, hesitancy, nocturia).

Pharmacokinetics

Absorption: Slowly absorbed after oral administration.
Distribution: Widely distributed.
Protein Binding: 94–99%.
Metabolism and Excretion: Extensively metabolized by the liver; <10% excreted unchanged in urine.
Half-life: 14 hr.

TIME/ACTION PROFILE (↑ in urine flow)

ROUTE	ONSET	PEAK	DURATION
PO	unknown	2 wk	unknown

Contraindications/Precautions

Contraindicated in: Hypersensitivity.
Use Cautiously in: Patients at risk for prostate carcinoma (symptoms may be similar); Patients undergoing cataract surgery (↑ risk of intraoperative floppy iris syndrome); Sulfa allergy.

Adverse Reactions/Side Effects

CNS: dizziness, headache. **CV:** orthostatic hypotension. **EENT:** intraoperative floppy iris syndrome, rhinitis. **GU:** priapism, retrograde/diminished ejaculation.

Interactions

Drug-Drug: Cimetidine may ↑ levels and the risk of toxicity. ↑ risk of hypotension with other peripherally acting anti-adrenergics (**doxazosin, prazosin, terazosin**); concurrent use should be avoided. ↑ risk of hypotension with **sildenafil, tadalafil,** and **vardenafil**. Strong **CYP3A4 inhibitors** and **CYP2D6 inhibitors** may ↑ levels (concurrent use should be avoided).

Route/Dosage

PO (Adults): 0.4 mg once daily after a meal; may ↑ after 2–4 wk to 0.8 mg/day.

Availability (generic available)

Capsules: 0.4 mg. **Cost:** *Generic*—$26.89/100. ***In combination with:*** dutasteride (Jalyn); see Appendix B.

NURSING IMPLICATIONS

Assessment

- Assess patient for symptoms of BPH (urinary hesitancy, feeling of incomplete bladder emptying, interruption of urinary stream, impairment of size and force of urinary stream, terminal urinary dribbling, straining to start flow, dysuria, urgency) before and periodically during therapy.
- Assess patient for first-dose orthostatic hypotension and syncope. Incidence may be dose related. Observe patient closely during this period and take precautions to prevent injury.
- Monitor intake and output ratios and daily weight, and assess for edema daily, especially at beginning of therapy. Report weight gain or edema.
- Rectal exams prior to and periodically throughout therapy to assess prostate size are recommended.

Implementation

- Do not confuse tamsulosin with tacrolimus.
- **PO:** Administer daily dose 30 min after the same meal each day. Swallow capsules whole; do not open, crush, or chew.
- If dose is interrupted for several days at either the 0.4-mg or 0.8-mg dose, restart therapy with the 0.4-mg/day dose.

Patient/Family Teaching

- Emphasize the importance of continuing to take this medication, even if feeling well. Instruct patient to take medication at the same time each day. If a dose is missed, take as soon as remembered unless almost time for next dose. Do not double doses.
- May cause dizziness. Advise patient to avoid driving or other activities requiring alertness until response to medication is known.

- Caution patient to change positions slowly to minimize orthostatic hypotension.
- Instruct patient to notify health care professional of all Rx or OTC medications, vitamins, or herbal products being taken and consult health care professional before taking any new medications, especially cough, cold, or allergy remedies.
- Emphasize the importance of follow-up visits to determine effectiveness of therapy.

Evaluation/Desired Outcomes

- Decrease in urinary symptoms of BPH.

REMS

tapentadol (ta-pen-ta-dol)

Nucynta, Nucynta IR, Nucynta ER

Classification

Therapeutic: analgesics (centrally acting), opioid analgesics

Pharmacologic: opioid agonists

Schedule II

Indications

Management of acute pain that is severe enough to require an opioid analgesic and for which alternative treatments are inadequate. Moderate to severe chronic pain in opioid-tolerant patients requiring use of daily, around-the-clock long-term opioid treatment and for which alternative treatment options are inadequate (extended-release only). Diabetic pain associated with diabetic peripheral neuropathy in patients requiring around-the-clock opioid analgesia for an extended time (extended-release only).

Action

Acts as μ-opioid receptor agonist. Also inhibits the reuptake of norepinephrine. **Therapeutic Effects:** Decrease in pain severity.

Pharmacokinetics

Absorption: 32% absorbed following oral administration.

Distribution: Widely distributed.

Metabolism and Excretion: Undergoes extensive first-pass hepatic metabolism (97%); metabolites have no analgesic activity; metabolized drug is 99% renally excreted.

Half-life: 4 hr.

TIME/ACTION PROFILE (analgesic effect)

ROUTE	ONSET	PEAK	DURATION
PO	unknown	1 hr	4–6 hr

Contraindications/Precautions

Contraindicated in: Hypersensitivity; Significant respiratory depression in unmonitored settings or where resuscitative equipment is not readily available; Paralytic ileus; Severe hepatic or renal impairment; Concurrent MAO inhibitors or use of MAO inhibitors in the preceding 2 wk; Acute or severe bronchial asthma; Acute, mild, intermittent, or postoperative pain (extended-release only).

Use Cautiously in: Conditions associated with hypoxia, hypercapnea, or ↓ respiratory reserve including asthma, chronic obstructive pulmonary disease, cor pulmonale, extreme obesity, sleep apnea syndrome, myxedema, kyphoscoliosis, CNS depression, use of other CNS depressants or coma (↑ risk of further respiratory depression); use smallest effective dose; History of substance abuse or addiction disorder; Seizure disorders; Moderate hepatic impairment; OB: Labor or delivery; OB, Lactation: Avoid chronic use; prolonged use of opioids during pregnancy can result in neonatal opioid withdrawal syndrome; Geri: Geriatric or debilitated patients (↑ risk of respiratory depression; dose ↓ suggested); Pedi: Safety and effectiveness not established.

Adverse Reactions/Side Effects

CNS: SEIZURES, dizziness, headache, somnolence. **CV:** hypotension. **Endo:** adrenal insufficiency. **GI:** diarrhea, nausea, vomiting. **GU:** ↓ fertility. **Resp:** RESPIRATORY DEPRESSION. **Misc:** HYPERSENSITIVITY REACTIONS (including anaphylaxis and angioedema).

Interactions

Drug-Drug: Concurrent **MAO inhibitors** or use of MAO inhibitors in the preceding 2 wk can result in potentially life-threatening adverse cardiovascular reactions due to additive effects on norepinephrine levels. Use with **benzodiazepines** or other **CNS depressants** including other **opioids**, **non-benzodiazepine sedative/hypnotics**, **anxiolytics**, **general anesthetics**, **muscle relaxants**, **antipsychotics**, and **alcohol** may cause profound sedation, respiratory depression, coma, and death; reserve concurrent use for when alternative treatment options are inadequate. **Alcohol** may ↑ levels and ↑ the risk of toxicity. Drugs that affect serotonergic neurotransmitter systems, including **tricyclic antidepressants**, **SSRIs**, **SNRIs**, **MAO inhibitors**, **TCAs**, **tramadol**, **trazodone**, **mirtazapine**, **5-HT$_3$ receptor antagonists**, **linezolid**, **methylene blue**, and **triptans** ↑ risk of serotonin syndrome.

Route/Dosage

When switching from immediate-release to extended-release product, the same total daily dose can be used.

PO (Adults): *Immediate-release*—50 mg, 75 mg, or 100 mg initially, then every 4–6 hr as needed and tolerated. If pain control is not achieved within first hr of first dose, additional dose may be given. Doses should not exceed 700 mg on the first day or 600 mg/day-

T

thereafter; *Extended-release*— 50 twice daily; titrate dose up to 100–250 mg twice daily (not to exceed dose of 500 mg/day).

Hepatic Impairment

PO (Adults): *Moderate hepatic impairment*—Immediate release: 50 mg every 8 hr initially, then titrate to maintain analgesia without intolerable side effects; Extended-release: 50 mg once daily; may titrate up to maximum dose of 100 mg once daily, if needed.

Availability

Tablets: 50 mg, 75 mg, 100 mg. **Extended-release tablets:** 50 mg, 100 mg, 150 mg, 200 mg, 250 mg.

NURSING IMPLICATIONS

Assessment

- Assess type, location, and intensity of pain before and 1 hr (peak) after administration.
- Assess BP and respiratory rate before and periodically during administration. Monitor for respiratory depression especially during initial dosing and with patients at increased risk.
- Assess bowel function routinely. Prevention of constipation should be instituted with increased intake of fluids and bulk and with laxatives to minimize constipating effects. Administer stimulant laxatives routinely if opioid use exceeds 2–3 days, unless contraindicated. Consider drugs for opioid induced constipation.
- Prolonged use may lead to physical and psychological dependence and tolerance, although these may be milder than with opioids. This should not prevent patient from receiving adequate analgesia. Patients who receive tapentadol for pain rarely develop psychological dependence.
- Monitor patient for seizures. May occur within recommended dose range. Risk is increased in patients with a history of seizures and in patients taking antidepressants (SSRIs, SNRIs, tricyclics) or other drugs that decrease the seizure threshold.
- Monitor for serotonin syndrome (mental-status changes [agitation, hallucinations, coma]), autonomic instability [tachycardia, labile BP, hyperthermia], neuromuscular aberrations [hyperreflexia, incoordination] and/or gastrointestinal symptoms [nausea, vomiting, diarrhea] in patients taking SSRIs, SNRIs, triptans, tricyclic antidepressants, or MAO inhibitors concurrently with tapentadol.
- Assess risk for opioid addiction, abuse, or misuse prior to administration. Abuse or misuse of extended-release preparations by crushing, chewing, snorting, or injecting dissolved product will result in uncontrolled delivery of tapentatol and can result in overdose and death.
- ***Toxicity and Overdose:*** Overdose may cause respiratory depression. Naloxone (Narcan) may reverse some, but not all, of the symptoms of overdose. Treatment should be symptomatic and supportive. Maintain adequate respiratory exchange.

Implementation

- Initial immediate-release dose of 50 mg, 75 mg, or 100 mg is individualized based on pain severity, previous experience with similar drugs, and ability to monitor patient. 2nd dose may be administered as soon as 1 hr after first dose if adequate pain relief is not obtained with first dose.
- Medication should be discontinued gradually after long-term use to prevent withdrawal symptoms. For patients on long-acting agents who are physically opioid-dependent, initiate the taper by a small enough increment (e.g., no greater than 10% to 25% of total daily dose) to avoid withdrawal symptoms, and proceed with dose-lowering at an interval of every 2 to 4 wk. Patients who have been taking opioids for briefer periods of time may tolerate a more rapid taper.
- **PO:** Tapentadol may be administered without regard to meals.
- Swallow extended-release tablets whole; do not crush, break or chew.
- Use calibrated syringe to administer correct dose of oral solution.
- FDA strongly encourages health care professionals to complete a REMS-compliant education program that includes all the elements of the FDA Education *Blueprint for Health Care Providers Involved in the Management or Support of Patients with Pain,* available at www.fda.gov/OpioidAnalgesicREMSBlueprint. Information on programs can be found at 1-800-503-0784 or www.opioidanalgesicrems.com.

Patient/Family Teaching

- Instruct patient on how and when to ask for and take pain medication and to take tapentadol as directed; do not adjust dose without consulting health care professional. Report breakthrough pain and adverse reactions to health care professional. Do not take tapentadol if pain is mild or can be controlled with other pain medications such as NSAIDs or acetaminophen. Do not stop abruptly; may cause withdrawal symptoms (anxiety, sweating, insomina, rigors, pain, nausea, tremors, diarrhea, upper respiratory symptoms, hallucinations). Decrease dose gradually. Advise patient to read the *Medication Guide* prior to taking tapentadol and with each Rx refill, in case of changes. Discuss safe use, risks, and proper storage and disposal of opioid analgesics with patients and caregivers with each Rx. The Patient Counseling Guide (PCG) is available at www.fda.gov/OpioidAnalgesicREMSPCG.
- Advise patient that tapentadol is a drug with known abuse potential. Protect it from theft, and never give to anyone other than the individual for whom it was prescribed; may be dangerous. Store out of sight and reach of children, and in a location not accessible by others.

- May cause dizziness and drowsiness. Caution patient to avoid driving or other activities requiring alertness until response to medication is known.
- Inform patient that tapentadol may cause seizures. Stop taking tapentadol and notify health care professional immediately if seizures occur.
- Advise patient to change positions slowly to minimize orthostatic hypotension.
- Caution patient to avoid concurrent use of alcohol or other CNS depressants with this medication.
- Instruct patient to notify health care professional of all Rx or OTC medications, vitamins, or herbal products being taken and consult health care professional before taking any new medications.
- Advise patient to notify health care professional if signs of serotonin syndrome occur.
- Encourage patient to turn, cough, and breathe deeply every 2 hr to prevent atelectasis.
- Rep: Advise patient to notify health care professional if pregnancy is planned or suspected, or if breast feeding. Inform patient of potential for neonatal opioid withdrawal syndrome with prolonged use during pregnancy. Monitor neonate for signs and symptoms of withdrawal symptoms (irritability, hyperactivity and abnormal sleep pattern, high pitched cry, tremor, vomiting, diarrhea, and/or failure to gain weight); usually occur the first days after birth.

Evaluation/Desired Outcomes

- Decrease in severity of pain without a significant alteration in level of consciousness or respiratory status.

tedizolid (ted-eye-**zoe**-lid)

Sivextro

Classification

Therapeutic: anti-infectives

Pharmacologic: oxazolidinones

Indications

Treatment of acute bacterial skin and skin structure infections (ABSSSI).

Action

Inhibits bacterial protein synthesis at the level of the 23S ribosome of the 50S subunit. **Therapeutic Effects:** Bacteriostatic action against enterococci, staphylococci and streptococci, resulting is resolution of infection. **Spectrum:** Active against *Staphylococcus aureus* including methicillin-resistant strains (MRSA), *Streptococcus pyogens*, *Streptococcus agalactiae*, *Streptococcus anginosus* Group (including *Streptococcus anginosus*, *Streptococcus intermedius*, *Streptococcus constellatus*) and *Enterococcus faecalis*.

Pharmacokinetics

Absorption: IV administration results in complete bioavailability; well absorbed (91%) following oral administration, rapidly converted by phosphatases to its active form.

Distribution: Penetrates interstitial fluid space of adipose and skeletal muscle resulting in similar levels to plasma.

Metabolism and Excretion: Eliminated via liver with inactive metabolites excreted in feces (82%) and urine (18%); <3% excreted unchanged in urine or feces.

Half-life: 12 hr.

TIME/ACTION PROFILE (blood levels)

ROUTE	ONSET	PEAK	DURATION
PO	unknown	2.5 hr	24 hr
IV	rapid	end of infusion	24 hr

Contraindications/Precautions

Contraindicated in: Uncontrolled HTN, pheochromocytoma, thyrotoxicosis, or concurrent use of sympathomimetic agents, vasopressors, or dopaminergic agents (↑ risk of hypertensive response); Concurrent or recent (<2 wk) use of monoamine oxidase (MAO) inhibitors (↑ risk of hypertensive response); Carcinoid syndrome or concurrent use of SSRIs, TCAs, triptans, meperidine, or buspirone (↑ risk of serotonin syndrome).

Use Cautiously in: Neutropenia (safety and efficacy not established if WBC <1000 cells/mm³); OB: Use in pregnancy only if potential maternal benefit justifies potential fetal risk; Lactation: Use cautiously if breast feeding; Pedi: Safety and effectiveness not established.

Adverse Reactions/Side Effects

CNS: dizziness, headache. **GI:** CLOSTRIDIUM DIFFICILE-ASSOCIATED DIARRHEA (CDAD), nausea, diarrhea, vomiting. **Misc:** infusion reactions.

Interactions

Drug-Drug: ↑ risk of hypertensive response with **MAO inhibitors**, **sympathomimetics** (e.g., **pseudoephedrine**), **vasopressors** (e.g., **epinephrine**, **norepinephrine**), and **dopaminergic agents** (e.g., **dopamine**, **dobutamine**); concurrent or recent use should be avoided. ↑ risk of serotonin syndrome with **SSRIs**, **TCAs**, **triptans**, **meperidine**, **bupropion**, or **buspirone**; avoid concurrent use. May ↑ levels of **methotrexate**, **topotecan**, or **rosuvastatin**; discontinue these medications temporarily during tedizolid treatment.

Route/Dosage

PO, IV (Adults): 200 mg once daily for 6 days.

Availability

Lyophilized powder for injection (requires reconstitution and dilution): 200 mg/vial. **Tablets:** 200 mg.

T

NURSING IMPLICATIONS

Assessment

- Assess for infection (vital signs; appearance of wound, sputum, urine, and stool; WBC) at beginning of and during therapy.
- Obtain specimens for culture and sensitivity prior to initiating therapy. First dose may be given before receiving.
- Monitor bowel function. Diarrhea, abdominal cramping, fever, and bloody stools should be reported to health care professional promptly as a sign of Clostridium difficile-associated diarrhea (CDAD). May begin up to several mo following cessation of therapy.
- ***Lab Test Considerations:*** Consider alternate therapies in patients with neutrophil counts <1000 cells/mm^3.
- May cause anemia.

Implementation

- Dose adjustment is not necessary when switching from IV to oral dose.
- **PO:** May be administered with or without food.

IV Administration

- **Intermittent Infusion:** Reconstitute each vial with 4 mL of sterile water for injection. Gently swirl and let vial stand until completely dissolved; avoid shaking. ***Diluent:*** Dilute further with 250 mL of 0.9% NaCl by slowing injecting reconstituted solution into 250 mL bag. Gently invert bag to mix; avoid shaking to minimize foaming. Solution is clear and colorless to pale yellow; do not administer solutions that are discolored or contain particulate material. Must be used within 24 hrs of reconstitution at room temperature or under refrigeration. ***Rate:*** Infuse over 1 hr.
- **Y-Site Incompatibility:** solutions containing calcium or magnesium, Lactated Ringer's, Hartmann's solution.

Patient/Family Teaching

- Advise patients taking oral tedizolid to take as directed, for full course of therapy, even if feeling better. Take missed doses as soon as remembered up to 8 hrs before next dose; if less than 8 hrs before next dose, wait until next scheduled dose. Do not double dose.
- Advise patient to notify health care professional of all Rx or OTC medications, vitamins, or herbal products being taken and to consult with health care professional before taking other medications.
- Instruct patient to notify health care professional if changes in vision occur or immediately if diarrhea, abdominal cramping, fever, or bloody stools occur and not to treat with antidiarrheals without consulting health care professionals.
- Advise female patient to notify health care professional if pregnancy is planned or suspected, or if breast feeding.
- Advise patient to notify health care professional if no improvement is seen in a few days.

Evaluation/Desired Outcomes

- Resolution of signs and symptoms of infection. Length of time for complete resolution depends on organism and site of infection.

telavancin (tel-a-van-sin)

Vibativ

Classification

Therapeutic: anti-infectives

Pharmacologic: lipoglycopeptides

Indications

Treatment of complicated skin/skin structure infections caused by susceptible bacteria. Hospital-acquired and ventilator-associated bacterial pneumonia caused by *Staphylococcus aureus*.

Action

Inhibits bacterial cell wall synthesis by interfering with the polymerization and cross-linking of peptidoglycan. **Therapeutic Effects:** Bactericidal action against susceptible organisms. **Spectrum:** Active against *Staphylococcus aureus* (including methicillin-susceptible and -resistant strains), *Streptococcus pyogenes*, *Streptococcus agalactiae*, *Streptococcus anginosus* (including *S. anginosus*, *S. intermedius*, and *S. constellatus*), and *Enterococcus faecalis* (vancomycin-susceptible strains only).

Pharmacokinetics

Absorption: IV administration results in complete bioavailability.

Distribution: Penetrates blister fluid.

Metabolism and Excretion: Metabolism is not known; 76% excreted unchanged in urine <1% in feces.

Half-life: 8 hr.

TIME/ACTION PROFILE

ROUTE	ONSET	PEAK	DURATION
IV	unknown	end of infusion	24 hr

Contraindications/Precautions

Contraindicated in: Hypersensitivity; Congenital long QT syndrome, known prolongation of the QT interval, uncompensated HF, or severe left ventricular hypertrophy (risk of fatal arrhythmias); Concurrent use of unfractionated heparin (aPTT may be falsely ↑ for up to 18 hr after telavancin therapy); OB: Do not use unless potential maternal benefit outweighs potential risk to fetus.

Use Cautiously in: Renal impairment (efficacy may be ↓ dose ↓ recommended for CCr ≤50 mL/min) (↑ risk of mortality in patients with CCr ≤50 mL/min; use only if benefit outweighs risk) (↑ risk of renal impairment); Diabetes, HF, hypertension (↑ risk of renal impairment); Geri: Consider age-related ↓ in renal function, adjust dose accordingly (↑ risk of adverse renal reactions); Lactation: Use cautiously; Pedi: Safety and effectiveness not established.

Adverse Reactions/Side Effects

CNS: dizziness. **CV:** QT interval prolongation. **GI:** CLOSTRIDIUM DIFFICILE-ASSOCIATED DIARRHEA (CDAD), taste disturbance, nausea, vomiting, abdominal pain. **GU:** foamy urine, nephrotoxicity. **Misc:** ANAPHYLAXIS, infusion reactions.

Interactions

Drug-Drug: Concurrent use of other **medications known to prolong QT interval** may ↑ risk of arrhythmias. Concurrent use of **NSAIDs, ACE inhibitors**, and **loop diuretics** may ↑ risk of adverse renal effects.

Route/Dosage

Complicated Skin/Skin Structure Infections

IV (Adults): 10 mg/kg ever 24 hr for 7–14 days.

Hospital-Acquired/Ventilator-Associated Bacterial Pneumonia

IV (Adults): 10 mg/kg ever 24 hr for 7–21 days.

Renal Impairment

IV (Adults): *CCr 30–50 mL/min*—7.5 mg/kg every 24 hr; *CCr 10–≤30 mL/min*—10 mg/kg every 48 hr.

Availability

Lyophilized powder for injection: 750 mg/vial.

NURSING IMPLICATIONS

Assessment

- Assess for infection (vital signs; appearance of wound, sputum, urine, and stool; WBC) at beginning of and throughout therapy.
- Obtain specimens for culture and sensitivity prior to therapy. First dose may be given before receiving results.
- Rep: Assess women of child bearing age for pregnancy. Women should have a negative serum pregnancy test before starting telavancin.
- Monitor bowel function. Diarrhea, abdominal cramping, fever, and bloody stools should be reported to health care professional promptly as a sign of Clostridium difficile-associated diarrhea (CDAD). May begin up to several wk following cessation of therapy.
- Monitor for infusion reactions (Red-man syndrome—flushing of upper body, urticaria, pruritus, rash). May resolve with stopping or slowing infusion.
- Observe patient for signs and symptoms of anaphylaxis (rash, pruritus, laryngeal edema, wheezing). Discontinue drug and notify health care professional immediately if symptoms occur. Keep epinephrine, an antihistamine, and resuscitation equipment close by in case of anaphylactic reaction.
- ***Lab Test Considerations:*** Monitor renal function (serum creatinine, creatinine clearance) prior to, every 48–72 hrs during, and at the end of therapy. May cause nephrotoxicity. If renal function decreases, reassess need for telavancin.
- May interfere with prothrombin time, INR, aPTT, activated clotting time, and coagulation based factor Xa tests. Collect blood samples for theses tests as close to next dose of telavancin as possible.
- Interferes with urine qualitative dipstick protein assays and quantitative dye methods; may use microalbumin assays.

Implementation

IV Administration

- **Intermittent Infusion:** Reconstitute the 750 mg vial with 45 mL of D5W, sterile water for injection, or 0.9% NaCl for concentrations of 15 mg/mL. Reconstitution time is usually under 2 min but may require up to 20 min. Mix thoroughly with contents dissolved completely. Do not administer solution that is discolored or contains particulate matter. Discard vial if vacuum did not pull diluent into vial. Time in vial plus time in bag should not exceed 4 hr at room temperature or 72 hr if refrigerated. ***Diluent:*** For doses of 150–800 mg dilute further with 100–250 mL of D5W, 0.9% NaCl, or LR. ***Concentration:*** For doses <150 mg or >800 mg dilute for a final concentration of 0.6–8 mg/mL. ***Rate:*** Administer over at least 60 min to minimize infusion reactions. Flush line with D5W, 0.9% NaCl, or LR before and after administration.
- **Y-Site Compatibility:** amphotericin B lipid complex, ampicillin/sulbactam, azithromycin, calcium gluconate, caspofungin, cefepime, ceftazidime, ceftriaxone, ciprofloxacin, dexamethasone, diltiazem, dobutamine, dopamine, doxycycline, ertapenem, famotidine, fluconazole, gentamicin, hydrocortisone, labetalol, magnesium sulfate, mannitol, meropenem, metoclopramide, milrinone, norepinephrine, ondansetron, pantoprazole, phenylephrine, piperacillin/tazobactam, potassium chloride, potassium phosphates, ranitidine, sodium bicarbonate, sodium phosphates, tigecycline, tobramycin, vasopressin.
- **Y-Site Incompatibility:** amphotericin B deoxycholate, amphotericin B liposome, digoxin, esomeprazole, furosemide, levofloxacin, micafungin.

Patient/Family Teaching

- Instruct patient to notify health care professional immediately if diarrhea, abdominal cramping, fever, or bloody stools occur and not to treat with antidiarrheals without consulting health care professionals.
- Inform patient that common side effects include taste disturbance, nausea, vomiting, headache and

T

foamy urine. Notify health care professional if signs of infusion reaction occur.

- Instruct patient to notify health care professional of all Rx or OTC medications, vitamins, or herbal products being taken and consult health care professional before taking any new medications.
- Rep: Advise female patients to use effective contraception during therapy and to notify health care professional if pregnancy is suspected. Encourage pregnant patients to enroll in the VIBATIV pregnancy registry by calling 1-855-633-8479.
- Instruct the patient to notify health care professional if symptoms do not improve.

Evaluation/Desired Outcomes

- Resolution of the signs and symptoms of infection. Length of time for complete resolution depends on the organism and site of infection.

telmisartan, See ANGIOTENSIN II RECEPTOR ANTAGONISTS.

tenecteplase, See THROMBOLYTIC AGENTS.

tenofovir alafenamide

(te-**noe**-fo-veer al-a-**fen**-a-mide)
Vemlidy

Classification
Therapeutic: antiretrovirals
Pharmacologic: nucleoside reverse transcriptase inhibitors

Indications

Chronic hepatitis B virus (HBV) infection in patients with compensated liver disease.

Action

Converted by hydrolysis to tenofovir and subsequently phosphorylated to the active metabolite, tenofovir diphosphate, which inhibits replication of HBV through incorporation into viral DNA by the HBV reverse transcriptase resulting in disruption of DNA synthesis.
Therapeutic Effects: Decreased progression/sequelae of chronic hepatitis B infection.

Pharmacokinetics

Absorption: Tenofovir alafenamide is a prodrug, which is hydrolyzed into tenofovir; absorption enhanced by high-fat meals.
Distribution: Unknown.
Metabolism and Excretion: Tenofovir is phosphorylated to tenofovir diphosphate (active metabolite); 32% excreted in feces, <1% in urine.
Half-life: 0.51 hr.

TIME/ACTION PROFILE (blood levels)

ROUTE	ONSET	PEAK	DURATION
PO	unknown	0.5 hr	24 hr

Contraindications/Precautions

Contraindicated in: End-stage renal disease (CCr <15 mL/min); Decompensated hepatic impairment (Child-Pugh B or C).
Use Cautiously in: Co-infection with HIV and chronic hepatitis B; Renal impairment or receiving nephrotoxic medications (↑ risk of renal impairment); OB: Safety not established; Lactation: Consider benefits of breast feeding against possible risk to infant; Pedi: Safety and effectiveness not established.

Adverse Reactions/Side Effects

CNS: fatigue, headache. **GI:** LACTIC ACIDOSIS/HEPATOMEGALY WITH STEATOSIS, abdominal pain, ↑ amylase, ↑ liver enzymes, nausea. **GU:** glycosuria, renal impairment. **Metab:** hyperlipidemia. **MS:** back pain, ↑ creatine kinase. **Resp:** cough.

Interactions

Drug-Drug: Nephrotoxic agents, including **NSAIDs** ↑ risk of nephrotoxicity; avoid concurrent use. Medications that compete for active tubular secretion, including **acyclovir**, **cidofovir**, **ganciclovir**, **valacyclovir**, **valganciclovir**, or **aminoglycosides** may ↑ tenofovir levels and toxicity; avoid if possible. **Carbamazepine**, **oxcarbazepine**, **phenobarbital**, **phenytoin**, **rifabutin**, **rifampin**, or **rifapentine** may ↓ tenofovir levels and its effectiveness; concurrent use with oxcarbazepine, phenobarbital, phenytoin, rifabutin, rifampin, or rifapentine not recommended; ↑ tenofovir alafenamide dose to 50 mg once daily when used with carbamazepine.
Drug-Natural Products: **St. John's wort** may ↓ tenofovir levels and its effectiveness; concurrent use not recommended.

Route/Dosage

PO (Adults): 25 mg once daily.

Availability

Tablets: 25 mg. ***In combination with:*** bictegravir and emtricitabine (Biktarvy); darunavir, cobicistat, and emtricitabine (Symtuza); elvitegravir, cobicistat, and emtricitabine (Genvoya); emtricitabine (Descovy); emtricitabine and rilpivirine (Odefsey). See Appendix B.

NURSING IMPLICATIONS

Assessment

- Monitor signs of hepatitis (jaundice, fatigue, anorexia, pruritus) during therapy. Upon discontinuation of therapy, monitor for exacerbations of hepatitis B for at least several mos after stopping therapy.
- ***Lab Test Considerations:*** Monitor liver function tests and hepatitis B virus levels throughout and following therapy. If therapy is discontinued, may cause severe exacerbation of hepatitis B. May cause ↑ AST,

ALT, alkaline phosphatase, creatine kinase, amylase, and triglyceride concentrations. Lactic acidosis may occur with hepatic toxicity causing hepatic steatosis; may be fatal, especially in women. May cause renal impairment. Monitor serum creatinine, estimated creatinine clearance, urine glucose, and urine protein before starting and periodically during therapy. Also assess serum phosphorous in patients with chronic kidney disease. Discontinue medication in patients who develop clinically significant ↓ in renal function or evidence of Fanconi syndrome. May cause ↑ ALT, AST, serum creatine kinase, serum amylase, LDL cholesterol, and glycosuria.

Implementation

- **PO:** Administer once daily with food.

Patient/Family Teaching

- Instruct patient to take medication as directed. Avoid missing doses. Advise patient to read *Patient Information* before starting and with each Rx refill in case of changes.
- Advise patient to notify health care professional immediately if symptoms of lactic acidosis (feel very weak or tired, have unusual (not normal) muscle pain, have trouble breathing, have stomach pain with nausea or vomiting, feel cold, especially in your arms and legs, feel dizzy or lightheaded, have a fast or irregular heartbeat) or severe liver problems (yellow skin or whites eyes, dark "tea-colored" urine, light-colored bowel stools, loss of appetite, nausea, pain, aching, or tenderness in right side of abdomen) occur.
- Instruct patient to notify health care professional of all Rx or OTC medications, vitamins, or herbal products being taken and consult health care professional before taking any new medications.
- Rep: Advise patient to notify health care professional if pregnancy is planned or suspected or if breast feeding. Advise patient taking oral contraceptives to use a nonhormonal method of birth control during therapy. Encourage pregnant women to enroll in the Antiretroviral Pregnancy Registry by calling 1-800-258-4263.

Evaluation/Desired Outcomes

- Decreased progression/sequelae of chronic hepatitis B infection.

BEERS

terazosin (ter-**ay**-zoe-sin)

Hytrin, ~~Hytrin~~

Classification

Therapeutic: antihypertensives

Pharmacologic: peripherally acting antiadrenergics

Indications

Mild to moderate hypertension (alone or with other agents). Treatment of signs/symptoms of benign prostatic hyperplasia (BPH).

Action

Dilates both arteries and veins by blocking postsynaptic alpha$_1$-adrenergic receptors. Decreases contractions in smooth muscle of the prostatic capsule. **Therapeutic Effects:** Lowering of BP. Decreased symptoms of prostatic hyperplasia (urinary urgency, hesitancy, nocturia).

Pharmacokinetics

Absorption: Well absorbed after oral administration.
Distribution: Unknown.
Metabolism and Excretion: 50% metabolized by the liver. 10% excreted unchanged by the kidneys. 20% excreted unchanged in feces. 40% eliminated in bile.
Half-life: 12 hr.

TIME/ACTION PROFILE

ROUTE	ONSET†	PEAK‡	DURATION†
PO-hypertension	15 min	6–8 wk	24 hr
PO-BPH	2–6 wk	unknown	unknown

†After single dose.
‡After multiple oral dosing.

Contraindications/Precautions

Contraindicated in: Hypersensitivity.
Use Cautiously in: Deyhdration, volume or sodium depletion (↑ risk of hypotension); Patients undergoing cataract surgery (↑ risk of intraoperative floppy iris syndrome); OB, Lactation, Pedi: Safety not established.

Adverse Reactions/Side Effects

CNS: dizziness, headache, weakness, drowsiness, nervousness. **EENT:** nasal congestion, blurred vision, conjunctivitis, intraoperative floppy iris syndrome, sinusitis. **Resp:** dyspnea. **CV:** first-dose orthostatic hypotension, arrhythmias, chest pain, palpitations, peripheral edema, tachycardia. **GI:** nausea, abdominal pain, diarrhea, dry mouth, vomiting. **GU:** erectile dysfunction, urinary frequency. **Derm:** pruritus. **Metab:** weight gain. **MS:** arthralgia, back pain, extremity pain. **Neuro:** paresthesia. **Misc:** fever.

Interactions

Drug-Drug: ↑ risk of hypotension with **sildenafil**, **tadalafil**, **vardenafil**, other **antihypertensives**, **nitrates**, or acute ingestion of **alcohol**. **NSAIDs**, **sympathomimetics**, or **estrogens** may ↓ effects of antihypertensive therapy.

Route/Dosage

The first dose should be taken at bedtime.

Hypertension

PO (Adults): 1 mg initially, then slowly ↑ up to 5 mg/day (usual range 1–5 mg/day); may be given as single dose or in 2 divided doses (not to exceed 20 mg/day).

Benign Prostatic Hyperplasia

PO (Adults): 1 mg at bedtime; gradually may be ↑ up to 5–10 mg/day.

Availability (generic available)

Capsules: 1 mg, 2 mg, 5 mg, 10 mg. **Tablets:** 1 mg, 2 mg, 5 mg, 10 mg. **Cost:** *Generic*—All strengths $160.38/100.

NURSING IMPLICATIONS

Assessment

- Assess for first-dose orthostatic reaction (dizziness, weakness) and syncope. May occur 30 min–2 hr after initial dose and occasionally thereafter. Incidence may be dose related. Volume-depleted or sodium-restricted patients may be more sensitive. Observe patient closely during this period; take precautions to prevent injury. First dose may be given at bedtime to minimize this reaction.
- Monitor intake and output ratios and daily weight; assess for edema daily, especially at beginning of therapy.
- **Hypertension:** Monitor BP and pulse frequently during initial dosage adjustment and periodically throughout therapy. Report significant changes.
- Monitor frequency of prescription refills to determine adherence.
- **BPH:** Assess patient for symptoms of BPH (urinary hesitancy, feeling of incomplete bladder emptying, interruption of urinary stream, impairment of size and force of urinary stream, terminal urinary dribbling, straining to start flow, dysuria, urgency) before and periodically during therapy.
- Rule out prostatic carcinoma before therapy; symptoms are similar.

Implementation

- May be used in combination with diuretics or beta blockers to minimize sodium and water retention. If these are added to terazosin therapy, reduce dose of terazosin initially and titrate to effect.
- **PO:** Administer daily dose at bedtime. If necessary, dose may be increased to twice daily.

Patient/Family Teaching

- Instruct patient to take medication at the same time each day. Take missed doses as soon as remembered. If not remembered until next day, omit; do not double doses.
- Advise patient to weigh self twice weekly and assess feet and ankles for fluid retention.
- May cause dizziness or drowsiness. Advise patient to avoid driving or other activities requiring alertness until response to the medication is known.
- Caution patient to avoid sudden changes in position to decrease orthostatic hypotension. Alcohol, CNS depressants, standing for long periods, hot showers, and exercising in hot weather should be avoided because of enhanced orthostatic effects.
- Advise patient to notify health care professional of all Rx or OTC medications, vitamins, or herbal products being taken and to consult with health care professional before taking other medications, especially NSAIDs, cough, cold, or allergy remedies.
- Instruct patient to notify health care professional of medication regimen before any surgery.
- Advise patient to notify health care professional if frequent dizziness, fainting, or swelling of feet or lower legs occurs.
- Emphasize the importance of follow-up exams to evaluate effectiveness of medication.
- **Hypertension:** Emphasize the importance of continuing to take this medication as directed, even if feeling well. Medication controls but does not cure hypertension.
- Encourage patient to comply with additional interventions for hypertension (weight reduction, low-sodium diet, smoking cessation, moderation of alcohol consumption, regular exercise, and stress management).
- Instruct patient and family on proper technique for BP monitoring. Advise them to check BP at least weekly and to report significant changes.

Evaluation/Desired Outcomes

- Decrease in BP without appearance of side effects.
- Decreased symptoms of BPH. May require 2–6 wk of therapy before effects are noticeable.

terbinafine, See ANTIFUNGALS (TOPICAL).

terbutaline (ter-**byoo**-ta-leen)

~~Bricanyl~~

Classification

Therapeutic: bronchodilators
Pharmacologic: adrenergics

Indications

Management of reversible airway disease due to asthma or COPD; inhalation and subcut used for short-term control and oral agent as long-term control. **Unlabeled Use:** Management of preterm labor (tocolytic) (the FDA has recommended that injectable terbutaline should not be used in pregnancy for the prevention or prolonged treatment [>48–72 hr] of preterm labor in either the inpatient or outpatient settings because of the potential for serious maternal heart problems and death; oral terbutaline should not be used for the prevention or any treatment of preterm labor because of a lack of efficacy and the potential for serious material heart problems and death).

Action

Results in the accumulation of cyclic adenosine monophosphate (cAMP) at beta-adrenergic receptors. Produces bronchodilation. Inhibits the release of mediators of immediate hypersensitivity reactions from mast cells. Relatively selective for $beta_2$ (pulmonary)-adrenergic receptor sites, with less effect on $beta_1$ (cardiac)-adrenergic receptors. **Therapeutic Effects:** Bronchodilation.

Pharmacokinetics

Absorption: 35–50% absorbed following oral administration but rapidly undergoes first-pass metabolism. Well absorbed following subcut administration.
Distribution: Enters breast milk.
Metabolism and Excretion: Partially metabolized by the liver; 60% excreted unchanged by the kidneys following subcut administration.
Half-life: Unknown.

TIME/ACTION PROFILE (bronchodilation)

ROUTE	ONSET	PEAK	DURATION
PO	within 60–120 min	within 2–3 hr	4–8 hr
Subcut	within 15 min	within 0.5–1 hr	1.5–4 hr

Contraindications/Precautions

Contraindicated in: Hypersensitivity to adrenergic amines.
Use Cautiously in: Cardiac disease; Hypertension; Hyperthyroidism; Diabetes; Glaucoma; Geri: More susceptible to adverse reactions; may require dose ↓; Excessive use may lead to tolerance and paradoxical bronchospasm (inhaler); OB, Lactation: Pregnancy (near term) and lactation.

Adverse Reactions/Side Effects

CNS: nervousness, restlessness, tremor, headache, insomnia. **Resp:** pulmonary edema. **CV:** angina, arrhythmias, hypertension, myocardial ischemia, tachycardia. **GI:** nausea, vomiting. **Endo:** hyperglycemia. **F and E:** hypokalemia.

Interactions

Drug-Drug: Concurrent use with other **adrenergics** (sympathomimetic) will have additive adrenergic side effects. Use with **MAO inhibitors** may lead to hypertensive crisis. **Beta blockers** may negate therapeutic effect.
Drug-Natural Products: Use with caffeine-containing herbs (**cola nut, guarana, mate, tea, coffee**) ↑ stimulant effect.

Route/Dosage

PO (Adults and Children >15 yr): *Bronchodilation*—2.5–5 mg 3 times daily, given every 6 hr (not to exceed 15 mg/24 hr).
PO (Children 12–15 yr): *Bronchodilation*—2.5 mg 3 times daily (given every 6 hr) (not to exceed 7.5 mg/24 hr).
PO (Children <12 yr): *Bronchodilation*—0.05 mg/kg 3 times daily; may ↑ gradually (not to exceed 0.15 mg/kg 3–4 times daily or 5 mg/24 hr).
Subcut (Adults and Children ≥12 yr): *Bronchodilation*—250 mcg; may repeat in 15–30 min (not to exceed 500 mcg/4 hr).
Subcut (Children <12 yr): *Bronchodilation*—0.005–0.01 mg/kg; may repeat in 15–20 min.
IV (Adults): *Tocolysis*—2.5–10 mcg/min infusion; ↑ by 5 mcg/min every 10 min until contractions stop (not to exceed 30 mcg/min). After contractions have stopped for 30 min, ↓ infusion rate to lowest effective amount and maintain for 4–8 hr (unlabeled).

Availability (generic available)

Tablets: 2.5 mg, 5 mg. **Solution for injection:** 1 mg/mL.

NURSING IMPLICATIONS

Assessment

- **Bronchodilator:** Assess lung sounds, respiratory pattern, pulse, and BP before administration and during peak of medication. Note amount, color, and character of sputum produced, and notify health care professional of abnormal findings.
- Monitor pulmonary function tests before initiating therapy and periodically throughout therapy to determine effectiveness of medication.
- **Preterm Labor:** Monitor maternal pulse and BP, frequency and duration of contractions, and fetal heart rate. Notify health care professional if contractions persist or increase in frequency or duration or if symptoms of maternal or fetal distress occur. Maternal side effects include tachycardia, palpitations, tremor, anxiety, and headache.
- Assess maternal respiratory status for symptoms of pulmonary edema (increased rate, dyspnea, rales/crackles, frothy sputum).
- Monitor mother and neonate for symptoms of hypoglycemia (anxiety; chills; cold sweats; confusion; cool, pale skin; difficulty in concentration; drowsiness; excessive hunger; headache; irritability; nausea; nervousness; rapid pulse; shakiness; unusual tiredness; or weakness) and mother for hypokalemia (weakness, fatigue, U wave on ECG, arrhythmias).
- ***Lab Test Considerations:*** May cause transient ↓ in serum potassium concentrations with higher than recommended doses.
- Monitor maternal serum glucose and electrolytes. May cause hypokalemia and hypoglycemia. Monitor neonate's serum glucose, because hypoglycemia may also occur in neonates.

T

- ***Toxicity and Overdose:*** Symptoms of overdose include persistent agitation, chest pain or discomfort, decreased BP, dizziness, hyperglycemia, hypokalemia, seizures, tachyarrhythmias, persistent trembling, and vomiting.
- Treatment includes discontinuing beta-adrenergic agonists and symptomatic, supportive therapy. Cardioselective beta blockers are used cautiously, because they may induce bronchospasm.

Implementation

- **PO:** Administer with meals to minimize gastric irritation.
- Tablet may be crushed and mixed with food or fluids for patients with difficulty swallowing.
- **Subcut:** Administer subcut injections in lateral deltoid area. Do not use solution if discolored.

IV Administration

- **Continuous Infusion:** ***Diluent:*** May be diluted in D5W, 0.9% NaCl, or 0.45% NaCl. ***Concentration:*** 1 mg/mL (undiluted). ***Rate:*** Use infusion pump to ensure accurate dose. Begin infusion at 10 mcg/min. Increase dosage by 5 mcg every 10 min until contractions cease. Maximum dose is 80 mcg/min. Begin to taper dose in 5-mcg decrements after a 30–60 min contraction-free period is attained. Switch to oral dose form after patient is contraction-free 4–8 hr on the lowest effective dose.
- **Y-Site Compatibility:** insulin.

Patient/Family Teaching

- Instruct patient to take medication as directed. If on a scheduled dosing regimen, take a missed dose as soon as possible; space remaining doses at regular intervals. Do not double doses. Caution patient not to exceed recommended dose; may cause adverse effects, paradoxical bronchospasm, or loss of effectiveness of medication.
- Instruct patient to contact health care professional immediately if shortness of breath is not relieved by medication or is accompanied by diaphoresis, dizziness, palpitations, or chest pain.
- Advise patient to consult health care professional before taking any OTC medications or alcoholic beverages concurrently with this therapy. Caution patient also to avoid smoking and other respiratory irritants.
- **Preterm Labor:** Notify health care professional immediately if labor resumes or if significant side effects occur.

Evaluation/Desired Outcomes

- Prevention or relief of bronchospasm.
- Increase in ease of breathing.
- Control of preterm labor in a fetus of 20–36 wk gestational age.

terconazole, See ANTIFUNGALS (VAGINAL).

teriflunomide

(ter-i-**floo**-noe-mide)

Aubagio

Classification

Therapeutic: anti-multiple sclerosis agents

Pharmacologic: immune response modifiers, pyrimidine synthesis inhibitors

Indications

Relapsing forms of multiple sclerosis (MS), including clinically isolated syndrome, relapsing-remitting disease, and active secondary progressive disease.

Action

Inhibits an enzyme required for pyrimidine synthesis; has antiproliferative and anti-inflammatory effects.

Therapeutic Effects: ↓ incidence and severity of relapses in MS, with a decrease in disability progression.

Pharmacokinetics

Absorption: Well absorbed following oral administration.

Distribution: Unknown.

Protein Binding: >99%.

Metabolism and Excretion: Eliminated via biliary excretion of unchanged drug with renal excretion of metabolites (37.5 in feces and 22.6% in urine), some metabolism occurs.

Half-life: 18–19 days.

TIME/ACTION PROFILE (decrease in disability progression)

ROUTE	ONSET	PEAK	DURATION
PO	3–6 mo	unknown	unknown

Contraindications/Precautions

Contraindicated in: Hypersensitivity to teriflunomide or leflunomide; Severe hepatic impairment; Concurrent leflunomide treatment; Live virus vaccinations; Active acute or chronic infection; Severe immunodeficiency, bone marrow disease or severe uncontrolled infection; Lactation: Discontinue teriflunomide or discontinue breast feeding; OB: Pregnancy (may cause fetal harm); Rep: Women of reproductive potential not using effective contraception.

Use Cautiously in: Pre-existing liver disease; Severe immunodeficiency, bone marrow disease or severe uncontrolled infection; Concurrent use of neurotoxic medications or diabetes mellitus (↑ risk of peripheral neuropathy); Hypertension (treat appropriately prior); Rep: Women of reproductive potential and men with female partners of reproductive potential; Pedi: Safety and effectiveness not established; Geri: ↑ risk of peripheral neuropathy.

Adverse Reactions/Side Effects

CV: hypertension. **Derm:** STEVENS-JOHNSON SYNDROME, TOXIC EPIDERMAL NECROLYSIS, alopecia. **F and E:** hyperkalemia, hypophosphatemia. **GI:** HEPATOTOXICITY, diarrhea, ↑ transaminases, nausea. **GU:** acute renal failure (urate nephropathy). **Hemat:** leukopenia, neutropenia, thrombocytopenia. **Neuro:** paresthesia, peripheral neuropathy. **Resp:** INTERSTITIAL LUNG DISEASE (rare). **Misc:** HYPERSENSITIVITY REACTIONS (including anaphylaxis, angioedema, and urticaria), INFECTION (including latent TB and viral infections).

Interactions

Drug-Drug: May ↑ levels and effects of **drugs metabolized by the CYP2C8 enzyme system** including **paclitaxel**, **pioglitazone**, **repaglinide**, and **rosiglitazone**. May ↓ levels and effectiveness of **drugs metabolized by the CYP1A2 enzyme system** including **alosetron**, **duloxetine**, **thoephylline**, and **tizanidine**. May ↓ response to and ↑ risk of adverse reactions from **live vaccines** (avoid live vaccinations and consider long half-life of teriflunomide before administering). May ↑ levels and effects of **ethinylestradiol** and **levonorgestrel**. May ↑ risk of bleeding with **warfarin**. ↑ risk of additive immunosuppression with other **immunosuppressants** or **antineoplastics** (consider long half-life of teriflunomide). Levels and effects may be ↑ by breast cancer resistant protein (BCRP) inhibitors including **cyclosporine**, **eltrombopag**, and **gefitinib**. May alter response to **warfarin**. May ↑ risk of adverse reactions and ↓ antibody response to **live virus vaccines**.

Route/Dosage

PO (Adults): 7 mg or 14 mg once daily.

Availability (generic available)

Film-coated tablets: 7 mg, 14 mg.

NURSING IMPLICATIONS

Assessment

- Assess BP before starting and periodically during therapy. Treat hypertension as needed.
- Assess for rash periodically during therapy. May cause Stevens-Johnson syndrome or Toxic Epidermal Necrolysis. Discontinue therapy if severe or if accompanied with fever, general malaise, fatigue, muscle or joint aches, blisters, oral lesions, conjunctivitis, hepatitis and/or eosinophilia.
- ***Lab Test Considerations:*** Monitor liver function tests (transaminases, bilirubin) within 6 mo of starting therapy and monthly after teriflunomide therapy begins. Do not administer if ALT >2 × upper limit of normal. Consider discontinuing therapy if serum transaminase ↑ >3 × upper limit of normal is confirmed. Monitor serum transaminase and bilirubin in patients with symptoms of liver dysfunction. If liver injury is suspected, discontinue teriflunomide, begin accelerated elimination procedure, and monitor liver function tests weekly until normal.
- Obtain a pregnancy test from female patients of reproductive potential prior to beginning therapy.
- Monitor CBC with platelet count within 6 mo prior to starting and periodically during therapy based on signs and symptoms of infection. Mean decrease in WBC occurs during first 6 wk and remains low during therapy.
- Monitor INR closely in patients taking warfarin, a decrease in warfarin peak may occur.

Implementation

- Administer a tuberculin skin test prior to administration of teriflunomide. Patients with active latent TB should be treated for TB prior to therapy.
- **PO:** Administer once daily without regard to food.
- **Drug Elimination Procedure:** Females of reproductive potential who wish to become pregnant, females who become pregnant during therapy and males who want to father a child must continue teriflunomide and go through one of the drug elimination procedures. Either of the following procedures is recommended to achieve nondetectable plasma levels <0.02 mg/L after stopping treatment with teriflunomide. 1) Administer cholestyramine 8 g 3 times daily (every 8 hrs) for 11 days. If cholestyramine 8 g is not well tolerated, cholestyramine 4 g 3 times/day can be used. *or* 2) Administration of 50 g oral activated charcoal powder every 12 hr for 11 days. (Days do not need to be consecutive unless rapid lowering of levels is desired.) Verify plasma levels <0.02 mg/L by 2 separate tests at least 14 days apart. Plasma levels may take up to 2 yr to reach nondetectable levels without drug elimination procedure.

Patient/Family Teaching

- Instruct patient to take teriflunomide as directed. Advise patient to read *Medication Guide* before starting therapy and with each Rx refill in case of changes.
- Advise patient to notify health care professional promptly if symptoms of liver problems (nausea, vomiting, stomach pain, loss of appetite, tiredness, skin or whites of eyes yellowing, dark urine), serious skin problems (redness or peeling), infection (fever, tiredness, body aches, chills, nausea, vomiting), or interstitial lung disease (cough, dyspnea, with or without fever) occur.
- Instruct patient to notify health care professional if symptoms of peripheral neuropathy (numbness and tingling in hands and feet different from symptoms of MS), kidney problems (flank pain), high potassium level (nausea or racing heartbeat), or high BP occur.
- Instruct patient to notify health care professional of all Rx or OTC medications, vitamins, or herbal products being taken and consult health care professional before taking any new medications.

- Instruct patient to avoid vaccinations with live vaccines during and following therapy without consulting health care professional.
- Discuss the possibility of hair loss with patient. Explore methods of coping.
- Rep: Advise patient that teriflunomide is teratogenic. Effective birth control should be used during therapy and until blood levels of teriflunomide are low enough. If pregnancy is planned or suspected, or if breast feeding notify health care professional immediately, accelerated eliminated procedure may be used to decrease blood levels more rapidly. Male patients with female partner of reproductive potential who plans to become pregnant may also use this method. If female partner does not plan to become pregnant, use effective birth control until blood levels are low enough; may require 2 yr. Females of childbearing potential are recommended to undergo accelerated elimination procedure upon discontinuation of teriflunomide. Patients who become pregnant should be encouraged to enroll in the Aubagio Pregnancy Registry at 1-800-745-4447 to collect information about mother and baby's health.

Evaluation/Desired Outcomes

- Decrease in the number of MS flares (relapses) and slowing of physical problems caused by MS.

tesamorelin (tess-a-**moe**-rel-in)

Egrifta, Egrifta SV

Classification

Therapeutic: none assigned

Pharmacologic: growth hormone-releasing factor analogues

Indications

Reduction of excess abdominal fat (lipodystrophy) seen in HIV-infected patients.

Action

Acts as an analog of human growth hormone-releasing factor (GRF, GHRH), resulting in endogenous production of growth hormone (GH), which has anabolic and lipolytic properties. **Therapeutic Effects:** Reduction of abdominal adipose tissue in HIV-infected patients.

Pharmacokinetics

Absorption: <4% absorbed following subcutaneous administration.

Distribution: Unknown.

Metabolism and Excretion: Unknown.

Half-life: 26–38 min.

TIME/ACTION PROFILE (effect on visceral adipose tissue)

ROUTE	ONSET	PEAK	DURATION
Subcut	within 3 mos	10–12 mos	3 mos†

†Following discontinuation.

Contraindications/Precautions

Contraindicated in: Hypersensitivity to tesamorelin or mannitol; Any pathology that alters the hypothalamic-pituitary axis, including hypophysectomy, hypopituitarism, pituitary surgery/tumor, cranial irradiation/trauma; OB: Pregnancy (may cause fetal harm); Lactation: Breast feeding should be avoided in patients with HIV.

Use Cautiously in: Acute critical illness (may ↑ risk of serious complications; consider discontinuation); Pre-existing malignancy (disease should be inactive or treatment completed); Non-malignant neoplasms (carefully consider benefit); Persistently elevated insulin-like growth factor (IGF-1; may require discontinuation); Diabetes mellitus (may cause glucose intolerance); Pedi: Safety and effectiveness not established.

Adverse Reactions/Side Effects

CV: peripheral edema. **Endo:** glucose intolerance. **Local:** erythema, hemorrhage, irritation, pain, pruritus. **MS:** arthralgia, carpal tunnel syndrome, extremity pain, myalgia. **Misc:** hypersensitivity reactions.

Interactions

Drug-Drug: May alter the clearance and actions of drugs known to be metabolized by the CYPP450 enzyme system including **corticosteroids**, **androgens**, **estrogens** and **progestins** (including **hormonal contraceptives**), **anticonvulsants**, and **cyclosporine**, careful monitoring for efficacy and/or toxicity recommended. Inhibits the conversion of **cortisone acetate** and **prednisone** to active forms; patients on replacement therapy may need ↑ maintenance/stress doses.

Route/Dosage

Subcut (Adults): *Egrifta*—2 mg once daily; *Egrifta SV*—1.4 mg once daily.

Availability

Lyophilized powder for injection (requires reconstitution) (Egrifta): 1 mg/vial. **Lyophilized powder for injection (requires reconstitution) (Egrifta SV):** 2 mg/vial.

NURSING IMPLICATIONS

Assessment

- Assess for fluid retention which manifests as ↑ tissue turgor and musculoskeletal discomfort (edema, arthralgia, extremity pain, carpal tunnel syndrome). May be transient or resolve with discontinuation of treatment.
- ***Lab Test Considerations:*** Monitor serum IGF-I closely during therapy; tesamorelin stimulates growth hormone production and the effect on progression of malignancies is unknown. Consider discontinuing tesamorelin in patients with persistent elevations of IGF-I levels, especially if efficacy response is not strong.
- May cause glucose intolerance and ↑ risk of developing diabetes. Monitor serum glucose prior to

starting and periodically during therapy. Monitor diabetic patients closely for worsening of retinopathy.

Implementation

- **Subcut:** Sterile water for injection 10 mL diluent is provided. *For 1–mg vial,* two vials must be reconstituted for dose. Inject 2.2 mL of sterile water for injection into first 1–mg tesamorelin, angled so that water goes down inside wall to prevent foaming. Roll vial gently between hands for 30 sec to mix; do not shake. Change needle. Withdraw solution and inject into 2nd 1–mg tesamorelin vial with solution against wall of vial. Mix between hands for 30 sec. Withdraw all solution. *For 2–mg vial,* reconstitute 1 vial with 0.5 mL of diluent (2 mg per 0.5 mL). Mix by rolling the vial gently in your hands for 30 sec. Do not shake. Administer 0.35 mL of immediately following reconstitution and throw away any unused solution and diluent. Solution is clear and colorless; do not administer solution that is discolored or contains particulate matter. Use solution immediately upon reconstitution or discard; do not refrigerate or freeze. Change needle to ½ inch 27 gauge needle. Pinch skin and inject at right angle into abdomen below navel; rotate sites. Remove hand from pinched area and inject slowly. Do not inject into scar, bruises, or the navel. Prior to reconstitution, vials must be refrigerated and protected from light.

Patient/Family Teaching

- Instruct patient on correct technique for administration of tesamorelin. Caution patient never to share needles with others.
- Inform patient that tesamorelin may cause symptoms of fluid retention (edema, arthralgia, carpal tunnel syndrome); usually transient or resolve with discontinuation of therapy.
- Advise patient to discontinue tesamorelin and notify health care professional promptly if signs and symptoms of hypersensitivity (rash, urticaria, hives, swelling of face or throat, shortness of breath, fast heartbeat, fainting) occur.
- Advise female patients to notify health care professional if pregnancy is planned or suspected and to avoid breast feeding.

Evaluation/Desired Outcomes

- Reduction of excess abdominal fat in HIV-infected patients with lipodystrophy.

BEERS REMS

TESTOSTERONE
(tess-**toss**-te-rone)

testosterone cypionate
Depo-Testosterone

testosterone enanthate
~~Delatestryl~~, Xyosted

testosterone nasal gel
Natesto

testosterone pellets
Testopel

testosterone topical gel
Androgel, Fortesta, Testim, Vogelxo

testosterone topical solution
~~Axiron~~

testosterone transdermal
Androderm

testosterone undecanoate
Aveed, Jatenzo

Classification
Therapeutic: hormones
Pharmacologic: androgens

Schedule III

Indications

Hypogonadism in men with low testosterone serum concentrations. Delayed puberty in men (enanthate and pellets). Androgen-responsive breast cancer in postmenopausal women (palliative) (enanthate).

Action

Responsible for the normal growth and development of male sex organs. Maintenance of male secondary sex characteristics: Growth and maturation of the prostate, seminal vesicles, penis, scrotum, Development of male hair distribution, Vocal cord thickening, Alterations in body musculature and fat distribution. **Therapeutic Effects:** Correction of hormone deficiency in male hypogonadism: Initiation of male puberty. Suppression of tumor growth in some forms of breast cancer.

Pharmacokinetics

Absorption: Well absorbed from IM or subcut sites, through skin, or through nasal mucosa. Cypionate, enanthate, and undecanoate salts are absorbed slowly. Skin serves as reservoir for sustained release of testosterone into systemic circulation; 10% absorbed into systemic circulation during 24–hr period.
Distribution: Crosses the placenta.
Protein Binding: 98%.
Metabolism and Excretion: Metabolized by the liver. 90% eliminated in urine as metabolites.
Half-life: *Enanthate (IM), nasal gel, pellets, topical gel, topical solution, undecanoate*—10–100 min; *transdermal*—70 min; *cypionate*—8 days; *enanthate (subcut)*—Unknown.

TIME/ACTION PROFILE (androgenic effects†)

ROUTE	ONSET	PEAK	DURATION
IM—cypionate, enanthate	unknown	unknown	2–4 wk
IM—undecanoate	unknown	unknown	10 wk
Subcut —enanthate	unknown	unknown	unknown
Nasal gel	unknown	unknown	3 mo
Oral	unknown	unknown	unknown
Pellets	unknown	unknown	3–6 mo
Topical solution	unknown	14 days	7–10 days
Transdermal (gel)	30 min	unknown	24 hr
Transdermal (patch)	unknown	6–8 hr‡	24 hr§

†Response is highly variable among individuals; may take mo.

‡Plasma testosterone levels following applications of patch.

§Following patch removal.

Contraindications/Precautions

Contraindicated in: Hypersensitivity; Men with breast or prostate cancer; Age-related hypogonadism (undecanoate [PO]); Some products contain benzyl alcohol and should be avoided in patients with known hypersensitivity; Women (pellets, nasal gel, patch, tablets, topical gel, topical solution); OB: Avoid use during pregnancy (may cause fetal virilization); Lactation: Avoid use during breast feeding.

Use Cautiously in: Diabetes mellitus; Established cardiovascular disease or risk factors for cardiovascular disease; Hypertension; Renal or hepatic impairment; Benign prostatic hyperplasia; Hypercalcemia; Obesity or chronic lung disease (↑ risk of sleep apnea); Polycythemia; Nasal disorders, nasal/sinus surgery, nasal fracture in previous 6 mo, nasal fracture that caused deviated anterior nasal septum, mucosal inflammatory disorders (e.g. Sjogren's syndrome), or sinus disorders (nasal gel); Pedi: Prepubertal males exposed to testosterone may experience premature development of secondary sexual characteristics, aggression, and other side effects; Geri: ↑ risk of prostatic hyperplasia/carcinoma.

Adverse Reactions/Side Effects

CNS: SUICIDAL THOUGHTS/BEHAVIOR, anxiety, confusion, depression, fatigue, headache, vertigo. **CV:** MI, STROKE, VENOUS THROMBOEMBOLISM, edema, ↑ blood pressure. **Derm:** male pattern baldness. **EENT:** deepening of voice; *nasal gel*, epistaxis, nasal scabbing, nasopharyngitis, rhinorrhea. **Endo:** *women*—change in libido, clitoral enlargement, ↓ breast size; *men*—, acne, facial hair, gynecomastia, erectile dysfunction, oligospermia, priapism. **F and E:** hypercalcemia, hyperkalemia, hyperphosphatemia. **GI:** HEPATOTOXICITY, abdominal cramps, changes in appetite, nausea, vomiting; *buccal*—, bitter taste, ginigivitis, gum edema, gum tenderness. **GU:** ↓ fertility, ↓ sperm count, menstrual irregularities, nocturia, priapism, prostatic enlargement, urinary hesitancy, urinary incontinence. **Hemat:** ↑ hematocrit. **Local:** ANAPHYLAXIS, chronic skin irritation (transdermal), pain at injection/implantation site, pulmonary oil microembolism reactions (IM). **Metab:** hyperlipidemia. **Resp:** sleep apnea.

Interactions

Drug-Drug: May ↑ action of **warfarin**, **oral hypoglycemic agents**, and **insulin**. Concurrent use with **corticosteroids** may ↑ risk of edema formation.

Route/Dosage

Replacement Therapy

IM (Adults): 50–400 mg every 2–4 wk (enanthate or cypionate); 750 mg initially, then at wk 4, then every 10 wk (undecanoate).

Subcut (Adults): 75 mg once weekly (enanthate).

Intranasal (Adults): 1 actuation (5.5 mg) in each nostril 3 times daily.

PO (Adults): 158 mg twice daily; may titrate up to 396 mg twice daily based on serum testosterone concentrations.

Transdermal(patch) (Adults): One 4–mg/day system applied every 24 hr in the evening; adjust dose based on serum testosterone concentrations (dosing range = 2–6 mg/day).

Transdermal (Adults): *Androgel 1% or Testim*—5 g (contains 50 mg of testosterone; 5 mg systemically absorbed) applied once daily (morning preferable), if needed may be ↑ to maximum of 10 g (contains 100 mg of testosterone; 10 mg systemically absorbed); *Androgel 1.62%*—40.5 mg of testosterone (2 pump actuations) applied once daily (morning preferable); dose may be adjusted down to a minimum of 20.25 mg or up to a maximum of 81 mg of testosterone, if needed (dose based on serum testosterone levels) *Fortesta*—40 mg of testosterone (4 pump actuations) applied once daily (morning preferable); dose may be adjusted down to a minimum of 10 mg or up to a maximum of 70 mg of testosterone, if needed (dose based on serum testosterone levels); *Vogelxo*—50 mg of testosterone (1 tube, 1 packet, or 4 pump actuations) applied once daily; dose may be adjusted up to a maximum of 100 mg of testosterone, if needed (dose based on serum testosterone levels).

Subcut(for subcutaneous implantation) (pellets) (Adults): 150–450 mg every 3–6 mo.

Topical (Adults): 60 mg (2 pump actuations) applied once daily; may be ↑ up to 120 mg (4 pump actuations) based on serum testosterone concentrations.

Delayed Male Puberty

IM (Children): 50–200 mg every 2–4 wk for up to 6 mo (enanthate).

Subcut(for subcutaneous implantation) (pellets) (Children): 150–450 mg every 3–6 mo.

Palliative Management of Breast Cancer

IM (Adults): 200–400 mg every 2–4 wk (enanthate).

Availability (generic available)

Capsules (Jatenzo): 158 mg, 198 mg, 237 mg. **Nasal gel:** 5.5 mg/pump actuation. **Pellets:** 75 mg. **Solution for intramuscular injection (cypionate) (in oil):** 100 mg/mL, 200 mg/mL. **Solution for intramuscular injection (enanthate) (in oil):** 200 mg/mL. **Solution for intramuscular injection (undecanoate) (in oil):** 250 mg/mL. **Solution for subcutaneous injection (enanthate) (autoinjector) (Xyosted):** 50 mg/0.5 mL, 75 mg/0.5 mL, 100 mg/0.5 mL. **Topical gel (Androgel):** 20.25 mg/packet (1.62%), 25 mg/packet (1%), 40.5 mg/packet (1.62%), 50 mg/packet (1%), 75–g metered dose pump (each pump dispenses 60 metered 12.5–mg doses [1%]), 88–g metered dose pump (each pump dispenses 60 metered 20.25–mg doses [1.62%]). **Topical gel (Fortesta):** 60–g metered dose pump (each pump dispenses 120 metered 10–mg doses [2%]). **Topical gel (Testim):** 50 mg/unit–dose tube (1%). **Topical gel (Vogelxo):** 50 mg/packet or unit–dose tube (1%), 75–g metered dose pump (each pump dispenses 60 metered 12.5–mg doses [1%]). **Topical solution:** 30 mg/pump actuation. **Transdermal patch:** 2 mg/24 hr, 4 mg/24 hr.

NURSING IMPLICATIONS

Assessment

- Monitor intake and output ratios, weigh patient twice weekly, and assess patient for edema. Report significant changes indicative of fluid retention.
- Assess for abuse using higher doses than prescribed and usually in conjunction with other anabolic androgenic steroids. May result in heart attack, heart failure, stroke, depression, hostility, aggression, liver toxicity, and infertility. Measure serum testosterone if abuse is suspected.
- **Men:** Monitor for precocious puberty in boys (acne, darkening of skin, development of male secondary sex characteristics—increase in penis size, frequent erections, growth of body hair). Bone age determinations should be measured every 6 mo to determine rate of bone maturation and effects on epiphyseal closure.
- Monitor for breast enlargement, persistent erections, and increased urge to urinate in men. Monitor for difficulty urinating in elderly men, because prostate enlargement may occur.
- **Women:** Assess for virilism (deepening of voice, unusual hair growth or loss, clitoral enlargement, acne, menstrual irregularity).
- In women with metastatic breast cancer, monitor for symptoms of hypercalcemia (nausea, vomiting, constipation, lethargy, loss of muscle tone, thirst, polyuria).
- ***Lab Test Considerations:*** Prior to therapy, measure serum testosterone in the morning on at least two separate days. Normal range (300 to 1050 ng/dL). Monitor serum testosterone concentrations 4–12 wk after starting therapy. Discontinue therapy is concentrations are consistently outside of normal range.
- Monitor hemoglobin and hematocrit periodically during therapy; may cause polycythemia.
- Monitor hepatic function tests, prostate specific antigen and serum cholesterol levels periodically during therapy. May cause ↑ serum AST, ALT, and bilirubin, ↑ cholesterol levels, and suppress clotting factors II, V, VII, and X.
- Monitor serum and urine calcium levels and serum alkaline phosphatase concentrations in women with metastatic breast cancer.
- Monitor serum sodium, chloride, potassium, and phosphate concentrations (may be ↑).
- Monitor blood glucose closely in patients with diabetes who are receiving oral hypoglycemic agents or insulin.
- *Transdermal:* Monitor serum testosterone concentrations 2 wk after starting therapy; these concentrations should be obtained in the morning (following application of patch during the previous evening). Serum testosterone concentrations measured in the early morning outside range of 400 – 930 ng/dL require increasing daily dose to 6 mg (one 4 mg/day and one 2 mg/day system) or decreasing daily dose to 2 mg (one 2 mg/day system), maintaining nightly application.
- *Topical Solution:* Measure serum testosterone concentrations after initiation of therapy to ensure desired concentrations (300 ng/dL–1050 ng/dL) are achieved. Adjust dose based on serum testosterone concentration from a single blood draw 2–8 hrs after applying and at least 14 days after starting treatment or following dose adjustment. If concentration is below 300 ng/dL, daily dose may be increased from 60 mg (2 pump actuations) to 90 mg (3 pump actuations) or from 90 mg to 120 mg (4 pump actuations). If concentration exceeds 1050 ng/dL, the daily testosterone dose should be decreased from 60 mg (2 pump actuations) to 30 mg (1 pump actuation) as instructed by health care professional. If concentration consistently exceeds 1050 ng/dL at lowest daily dose of 30 mg (1 pump actuation), discontinue therapy.
- *Nasal gel:* Monitor serum testosterone concentrations after 1 mo and periodically during therapy. If total testosterone concentrations consistently exceed 1050 ng/dL, discontinue therapy. If total testosterone concentrations are consistently below 300 ng/dL, consider alternative therapy.

Implementation

- Range-of-motion exercises should be done with all bedridden patients to prevent mobilization of calcium from the bone.
- **IM:** Administer IM deep into gluteal muscle. Crystals may form when vials are stored at low temperatures;

T

warming and shaking vial will redissolve crystals. Use of a wet syringe or needle may cause solution to become cloudy but will not affect its potency.

- **Subcut:** Pellets are to be implanted subcutaneously by a health care professional.
- **Transdermal:** Apply patch to clean, dry, hairless skin on the back, abdomen, upper arms, or thighs. Do not apply to the scrotum. Avoid application over bony prominences or a part of the body that may be subject to prolonged pressure during sleep or sitting. The patch does not need to be removed while swimming or taking a shower or bath.
- The sites of application should be rotated; once a patch is removed, the same site should not be used again for at least 1 wk.
- If skin irritation occurs, apply a small amount of OTC topical hydrocortisone cream after system removal or a small amount of 0.1% triamcinolone cream may be applied to the skin under the central drug reservoir of the *Androderm* system without affecting the absorption of testosterone. Ointment formulations should not be used for pretreatment because they may significantly reduce testosterone absorption.
- Patch should be removed if undergoing a magnetic resonance imaging (MRI) scan. The system contains aluminum and may predispose the patient to skin burns during the test.
- **Topical: Solution:** Apply to axilla using applicator at the same time each morning, to clean, dry, intact skin. Do not apply to other parts of the body including to the scrotum, penis, abdomen, shoulders or upper arms. Prime pump when using for first time by depressing pump 3 times, discard any product dispensed directly into a basin, sink, or toilet and then wash liquid away thoroughly. Prime only prior to first use of each pump. After priming, completely depress pump once with nozzle over applicator cup to dispense 30 mg of testosterone. Apply in 30 mg (1 pump actuation) increments. Place actuator into the axilla and wipe steadily down and up into the axilla. If solution drips or runs, wipe back up with applicator cup. Do not rub into skin with fingers or hand. Repeat process for each 30 mg dose needed. When repeat application to same axilla, allow axilla to dry completely before more is applied. Rinse applicator under room temperature, running water and pat dry with a tissue. Allow axilla to dry completely prior to dressing. Solution has an alcohol based and is flammable until dry. Apply deodorant prior to application of testosterone solution. Avoid swimming or washing for 2 hrs after application. Wash hands immediately with soap and water after application.
- **Topical: Gel:** Apply gel once daily, preferably in the morning, to clean dry intact skin of shoulders and upper arms (*Androgel*, *Testim*, and *Vogelxo*) or abdomen (Androgel only) or front or inner thighs (Fortesta). Gel should not be applied to scrotum (5–30 x more permeable than other sites). Refer to the chart on the pump label to determine how many full pump depressions are required for the daily prescribed dose.
- The dose of Fortesta should be titrated based on the serum testosterone concentration from a single blood draw 2 hrs after applying Fortesta and at approximately 14 days and 35 days after starting treatment or following dose adjustment.
- **Intranasal:** Prime pump by inverting, depressing pump 10 times, and discarding any amount dispensed directly into a sink and washing gel away thoroughly with warm water. Wipe tip with a clean, dry tissue. If gel gets on hands, wash hands with warm water and soap. Priming should be done only prior to first use of each dispenser. Blow nose. Place right index finger on pump of actuator and while in front of a mirror, slowly advance tip of actuator into left nostril upwards until finger on the pump reaches the base of the nose. Tilt the actuator so that the opening on the tip of the actuator is in contact with the lateral wall of the nostril to ensure that the gel is applied to the nasal wall. Slowly depress the pump until it stops. Remove the actuator from the nose while wiping the tip along the inside of the lateral nostril wall to fully transfer the gel. Repeat with right nostril. Press on the nostrils at a point just below bridge of the nose and lightly massage. Refrain from blowing nose or sniffing for 1 hr after administration.

Patient/Family Teaching

- Advise patient to report the following signs and symptoms promptly: *in male patients,* priapism (sustained and often painful erections) difficulty urinating, or gynecomastia; *in female patients,* virilism (which may be reversible if medication is stopped as soon as changes are noticed), or hypercalcemia (nausea, vomiting, constipation, and weakness); *in male or female patients,* edema (unexpected weight gain, swelling of feet), hepatitis (yellowing of skin or eyes and abdominal pain), or unusual bleeding or bruising.
- Instruct patient to use testosterone as directed. Do not use higher than prescribed doses. Explain rationale for prohibiting use of testosterone for increasing athletic performance. Testosterone is neither safe nor effective for this use and has a potential risk of serious side effects.
- Advise diabetic patients to monitor blood closely for alterations in blood glucose concentrations.
- Emphasize the importance of regular follow-up physical exams, lab tests, and x-ray exams to monitor progress.
- Radiologic bone age determinations should be evaluated every 6 mo in prepubertal children to determine rate of bone maturation and effects on epiphyseal centers.
- Instruct females to notify health care professional immediately if pregnancy is planned or suspected or if breast feeding.

- **Transdermal:** Advise patient to notify health care professional if their female sexual partner develops signs/symptoms of virilization (e.g. change in body hair distribution, significant increase in acne, deepening of voice, menstrual irregularities).
- Instruct patient that the protective plastic liner must be removed before applying the patch.
- Instruct patient to apply patch to a clean, dry area of skin on back, abdomen, upper arms, or thighs. The patch should not be applied to their genitals or over bony areas (e.g., upper shoulders or upper hip).
- Instruct patient to rotate the sites of application. Once a patch is removed, the site should not be used again for at least 1 wk.
- Advise patient that the patch does not need to be removed while showering, bathing, or swimming.
- Avoid contact of patch with women and children.
- Advise patient that the patch should be removed prior to undergoing an MRI scan.
- If a patch falls off before noon, advise patient to replace it with a fresh patch which should be worn until a new patch is applied in the evening. If a patch falls off after noon, advise patient that it does not need to be replaced until a fresh patch is applied in the evening.
- **Topical:** Explain application to patient.
- Advise patient that women and children should avoid contact with unclothed or unwashed application site. Patients should cover the application site(s) with clothing (T-shirt) after solution has dried. For direct skin-to-skin contact, patient should wash application site thoroughly with soap and water to remove any testosterone residue. If unwashed or unclothed skin with testosterone solution comes in direct contact with skin of another person, wash area of contact with soap and water as soon as possible.
- **Intranasal:** Advise patient to notify health care professional if nasal signs or symptoms (nasopharyngitis, rhinorrhea, epistaxis, nasal discomfort, nasal scabbing) occur.

Evaluation/Desired Outcomes

- Resolution of the signs of androgen deficiency without side effects. Therapy is usually limited to 3–6 mo followed by bone growth or maturation determinations.
- Decrease in the size and spread of breast malignancy in postmenopausal women. In antineoplastic therapy, response may require 3 mo of therapy; if signs of disease progression appear, therapy should be discontinued.

TETRACYCLINES

doxycycline (dox-i-**sye**-kleen)
Acticlate, Apprilon, Atridox, Doryx, Doxy, Doxycin, Doxytab, Monodox, Oracea, Periostat, Vibramycin

minocycline (min-oh-**sye**-kleen)
Dynacin, Minocin, Minolira, Solodyn, Ximino

tetracycline (te-tra-**sye**-kleen)
~~Sumycin~~

Classification
Therapeutic: anti-infectives
Pharmacologic: tetracyclines

Indications

Treatment of various infections caused by unusual organisms, including: *Mycoplasma*, *Chlamydia*, *Rickettsia*, *Borellia burgdorferi*. Treatment of gonorrhea and syphilis in penicillin-allergic patients. Prevention of exacerbations of chronic bronchitis. Treatment of inhalational anthrax (postexposure) and cutaneous anthrax (doxycycline only). Treatment of acne. Malaria prophylaxis (doxycycline only). Inflammatory lesions of nonnodular acne vulgaris (Solodyn and Ximino).

Action

Inhibits bacterial protein synthesis at the level of the 30S bacterial ribosome. **Therapeutic Effects:** Bacteriostatic action against susceptible bacteria. **Spectrum:** Includes activity against some gram-positive pathogens: *Bacillus anthracis*, *Clostridium perfringens*, *Clostridium tetani*, *Listeria monocytogenes*, *Nocardia*, *Propionibacterium acnes*, *Actinomyces israelii*. Active against some gram-negative pathogens: *Haemophilus influenzae*, *Legionella pneumophila*, *Yersinia enterocolitica*, *Yersinia pestis*, *Neisseria gonorrhoeae*, *Neisseria meningitidis*. Also active against several other pathogens, including: *Mycoplasma*, *Treponema pallidum*, *Chlamydia*, *Rickettsia*, *B. burgdorferi*.

Pharmacokinetics

Absorption: *Tetracycline*—60–80% absorbed following oral administration. *Doxycycline, minocycline*—well absorbed from the GI tract.
Distribution: Widely distributed, some penetration into CSF; crosses the placenta and enters breast milk.
Metabolism and Excretion: *Doxycycline*—20–40% excreted unchanged by the urine; some inactivation in the intestine and some enterohepatic circulation with excretion in bile and feces. *Minocycline*—5–20% excreted unchanged by the urine; some metabolism by the liver with enterohepatic circulation and excretion in bile and feces. *Tetracycline*—Excreted mostly unchanged by the kidneys.
Half-life: *Doxycycline*—14–17 hr (↑ in severe renal impairment). *Minocycline*—11–26 hr. *Tetracycline*—6–12 hr.

T

TIME/ACTION PROFILE (blood levels)

ROUTE	ONSET	PEAK	DURATION
Doxycycline-PO	1–2 hr	1.5–4 hr	12 hr
Doxycycline-IV	rapid	end of infusion	12 hr
Minocycline-PO	rapid	2–3 hr	6–12 hr
Minocycline-PO—ER	unknown	3.5–4 hr	24 hr
Tetracycline-PO	1–2 hr	2–4 hr	6–12 hr

Contraindications/Precautions

Contraindicated in: Hypersensitivity; Some products contain alcohol or bisulfites; avoid in patients with known hypersensitivity or intolerance; OB: Risk of permanent staining of teeth in infant if used during last half of pregnancy (doxycycline may be used to treat anthrax in pregnant women due to the seriousness of the disease); Lactation: Lactation; Pedi: Children <8 yr (permanent staining of teeth) (unless used for anthrax; doxycycline may be used to treat anthrax in children due to the seriousness of the disease).

Use Cautiously in: Renal impairment; Hepatic impairment (minocycline); Nephrogenic diabetes insipidus; OB: Women of childbearing age.

Adverse Reactions/Side Effects

CNS: intracranial hypertension; *minocycline*, dizziness. **Derm:** DRUG RASH WITH EOSINOPHILIA AND SYSTEMIC SYMPTOMS (DRESS), ERYTHEMA MULTIFORME, EXFOLIATIVE DERMATITIS, STEVENS-JOHNSON SYNDROME, TOXIC EPIDERMAL NECROLYSIS, photosensitivity, rashes; *minocycline*, pigmentation of skin and mucous membranes. **EENT:** *minocycline*, vestibular reactions. **Endo:** *minocycline*—thyroid disorders. **GI:** CLOSTRIDIUM DIFFICILE-ASSOCIATED DIARRHEA (CDAD), HEPATOTOXICITY, PANCREATITIS, diarrhea, nausea, vomiting, dysphagia, esophagitis, glossitis. **Hemat:** blood dyscrasias. **MS:** *minocycline*—lupus-like syndrome. **Local:** *doxycycline, minocycline*—phlebitis at IV site. **Misc:** HYPERSENSITIVITY REACTIONS (including anaphylaxis and angioedema), superinfection.

Interactions

Drug-Drug: May ↑ effect of **warfarin**. May ↓ effectiveness of **estrogen-containing hormonal contraceptives**. **Antacids**, **calcium**, **iron**, **zinc**, **aluminum**, and **magnesium** form insoluble compounds (chelates) and ↓absorption of tetracyclines. **Sucralfate** may bind to tetracycline and ↓ its absorption from the GI tract. **Cholestyramine** or **colestipol** ↓ oral absorption of tetracyclines. **Adsorbent antidiarrheals** may ↓ absorption of tetracyclines. **Barbiturates**, **carbamazepine**, or **phenytoin** may ↓ activity of doxycycline. **Isotretinoin** may ↑ risk of intracranial hypertension with doxycycline; avoid concomitant use.

Drug-Food: Calcium in foods or **dairy products** ↓ absorption by forming insoluble compounds (chelates).

Route/Dosage

Doxycycline

PO (Adults and Children >8 yr and >45 kg): *Most infections*—100 mg every 12 hr on the 1st day, then 100–200 mg once daily or 50–100 mg every 12 hr; *Gonorrhea*—100 mg every 12 hr for 7 days or 200 mg once daily for 7 days (delayed-release tablets) or 300 mg followed 1 hr later by another 300-mg dose; *Uncomplicated urethral, endocervical, or rectal infection caused by Chlamydia trachomatis*—100 mg every 12 hr for 7 days; *Syphilis (early)*—100 mg every 12 hr for 14 days; *Syphilis (>1 yr duration)*—100 mg every 12 hr for 4 wk; *Malaria prophylaxis*—100 mg once daily; *Lyme disease*—100 mg twice daily; *Periodontitis*—20 mg twice daily; *Rosacea*—40 mg once daily in morning.

PO (Children >8 yr and ≤45 kg): *Most infections*—2.2 mg/kg every 12 hr on the 1st day, then 2.2–4.4 mg/kg once daily or 1.1–2.2 mg/kg every 12 hr; *Malaria prophylaxis*—2 mg/kg once daily.

PO, IV (Adults and Children >45 kg): *Inhalational anthrax (post–exposure)*—100 mg IV every 12 hr; change to 100 mg PO every 12 hr when clinically appropriate for a total of 60 days; one or two other anti-infectives may be added initially, depending on clinical situation; *Cutaneous anthrax*—100 mg PO every 12 hr for 60 days; some patients may require IV therapy initially depending on clinical situation.

PO, IV (Children ≤45 kg): *Inhalational anthrax (post–exposure)*—2.2 mg/kg IV every 12 hr; change to 2.2 mg/kg PO every 12 hr when clinically appropriate for a total of 60 days; one or two other anti-infectives may be added initially, depending on clinical situation; *Cutaneous anthrax*—2.2 mg/kg every 12 hr for 60 days; some patients may require IV therapy initially depending on clinical situation.

Minocycline

PO (Adults): 100–200 mg initially, then 100 mg every 12 hr or 50 mg every 6 hr.

PO, IV (Children ≥8 yr): 4 mg/kg initially, then 2 mg/kg every 12 hr.

PO (Adults and Children ≥12 yrs [Solodyn and Ximino]): *126–136 kg*—135 mg once daily for 12 wk; *111–125 kg*—115 mg once daily for 12 wk; *97–110 kg*—105 mg once daily for 12 wk; *85–96 kg*—90 mg once daily for 12 wk; *72–84 kg*—80 mg once daily for 12 wk; *60–71 kg*—65 mg once daily for 12 wk; *50–59 kg*—55 mg once daily for 12 wk; *45–49 kg*—45 mg once daily for 12 wk.

IV (Adults): 200 mg initially, then 100 mg every 12 hr (max dose = 400 mg/day).

Tetracycline

PO (Adults): 250–500 mg every 6 hr or 500 mg–1 g every 12 hr. *Chronic treatment of acne*—500 mg–2 g/day for 3 wk, then ↓ to 125 mg–1 g/day.

PO (Children ≥8 yr): 6.25–12.5 mg/kg every 6 hr or 12.5–25 mg/kg every 12 hr.

Availability

Doxycycline (generic available)

Capsules: 50 mg, 75 mg, 100 mg, 150 mg. **Cost:** *Generic*—50 mg $118.74/100, 75 mg $1,639.77/100, 100 mg $96.92/50, 150 mg $1,479.01/60. **Delayed-release capsules:** 40 mg. **Cost:** $501.12/30. **Delayed-release tablets:** 50 mg, 75 mg, 100 mg, 120 mg, 150 mg, 200 mg. **Cost:** *Generic*—75 mg $613.45/60, 100 mg $1,314.83/100, 150 mg $1,759.94/100. **Oral suspension (raspberry flavor):** 25 mg/5 mL. **Cost:** *Generic*—$22.77/60 mL. **Powder for injection (requires reconstitution and dilution):** 100 mg/vial, 200 mg/vial. **Syrup (apple-raspberry flavor):** 50 mg/5 mL. **Cost:** $339.47/473 mL. **Tablets:** 20 mg, 50 mg, 75 mg, 100 mg, 150 mg. **Cost:** *Generic*—20 mg $118.90/100, 50 mg $335.71/100, 75 mg $498.35/100, 100 mg $246.02/50, 150 mg $274.17/30.

Minocycline (generic available)

Capsules: 50 mg, 75 mg, 100 mg. **Cost:** *Generic*—50 mg $169.87/100, 75 mg $197.96/100, 100 mg $169.87/50. **Extended-release capsules:** 90 mg, 135 mg. **Extended-release tablets:** 45 mg, 55 mg, 65 mg, 80 mg, 90 mg, 105 mg, 115 mg, 135 mg. **Cost:** *Generic*—45 mg $605.01/30, 90 mg $605.01/30, 135 mg $605.01/30; *Solodyn*—55 mg $1,044.22/30, 65 mg $1,044.22/30, 80 mg $1,044.22/30, 105 mg $1,044.22/30, 115 mg $1,044.22/30. **Lyophilized powder for injection (requires reconstitution):** 100 mg/vial. **Tablets:** 50 mg, 75 mg, 100 mg. **Cost:** *Generic*—50 mg $343.47/100, 75 mg $504.25/100, 100 mg $300.98/50.

Tetracycline (generic available)

Capsules: 250 mg, 500 mg. **Cost:** *Generic*—250 mg $6.88/100, 500 mg $11.80/100.

NURSING IMPLICATIONS

Assessment

- Assess for infection (vital signs; appearance of wound, sputum, urine, and stool; WBC) at beginning of and throughout therapy.
- Obtain specimens for culture and sensitivity before initiating therapy. First dose may be given before receiving results.
- Monitor bowel function. Diarrhea, abdominal cramping, fever, and bloody stools should be reported to health care professional promptly as a sign of Clostridium difficile-associated diarrhea (CDAD). May begin up to several wk following cessation of therapy.
- Assess for rash periodically during therapy. May cause Stevens-Johnson syndrome or toxic epidermal necrolysis. Discontinue therapy if severe or if accompanied with fever, general malaise, fatigue, muscle or joint aches, blisters, oral lesions, conjunctivitis, hepatitis and/or eosinophilia.
- Monitor for signs and symptoms of DRESS (fever, rash, lymphadenopathy, and/or facial swelling), associated with involvement of other organ systems (hepatitis, nephritis, hematologic abnormalities, myocarditis, myositis) during therapy. May resemble an acute viral infection. Eosinophilia is often present. Discontinue therapy if signs occur.
- **IV:** Assess IV site frequently; may cause thrombophlebitis.
- ***Lab Test Considerations:*** Monitor renal and hepatic function and CBC periodically during long-term therapy.
- May cause ↑ AST, ALT, serum alkaline phosphatase, bilirubin, and amylase concentrations. Tetracyclines, except doxycycline, may cause ↑ serum BUN.

Implementation

- Do not confuse Oracea with Orencia (abatacept). Do not confuse Dynacin with Dynacirc (isradipine).
- May cause yellow-brown discoloration and softening of teeth and bones if administered prenatally or during early childhood. Not recommended for children under 8 yr of age or during pregnancy or lactation unless used for the treatment of anthrax.
- **PO:** Administer around the clock. Administer at least 1 hr before or 2 hr after meals. *Doxycycline and minocycline* may be taken with food or milk if GI irritation occurs. Administer with a full glass of liquid and at least 1 hr before going to bed to avoid esophageal ulceration. Use calibrated measuring device for liquid preparations. Shake liquid preparations well. Do not administer within 1–3 hr of other medications.
- Do not open, break, crush or chew extended release capsules and tablets.
- Avoid administration of calcium, zinc, antacids, magnesium- or aluminum-containing medications, sodium bicarbonate, or iron supplements within 1–3 hr of oral tetracyclines.

Doxycycline

- The *Oracea* product is only indicated for rosacea, not for infections.
- **PO: Public Health Emergency —Exposure to Anthrax:** To prepare doses for infants and children exposed to anthrax, place one 100 mg tablet in a small bowl and crush to a fine powder with a metal spoon, leaving no large pieces. Add 4 level teaspoons of lowfat milk, lowfat chocolate milk, regular chocolate milk, chocolate pudding, or apple juice. Mix food or drink and doxycycline powder until powder dissolves. Mixture is stable in a covered container for 24 hr if refrigerated (if made with milk or pudding) or at room temperature (if made with juice). Number of teaspoons to administer/dose is

T

based on child's weight (0–12.5 lb—1/2 tsp; 12.5–25 lb—1 tsp; 25–37.5 lb—1 1/2 tsp; 37.5–50 lb—2 tsp; 50–62.5 lb—2 1/2 tsp; 62.5–75 lb—3 tsp; 75–87.5 lb—3 1/2 tsp; 87.5–100 lb—4 tsp).

- Capsules may also be administered by carefully opening and sprinkling capsule contents on a spoonful of applesauce. The applesauce should be swallowed immediately without chewing and followed with a cool 8 oz glass of water to ensure complete swallowing of the capsule contents. The applesauce should not be hot, and it should be soft enough to be swallowed without chewing. If mixture cannot be taken immediately, discard; do not store for later use.

IV Administration

- **Intermittent Infusion:** Reconstitute each 100 mg with 10 mL of sterile water or 0.9% NaCl for injection. ***Diluent:*** Dilute further in 100–1000 mL of 0.9% NaCl, D5W, D5/LR, Ringer's, or lactated Ringer's solution. Solution is stable for 12 hr at room temperature and 72 hr if refrigerated. If diluted with D5/LR or lactated Ringer's solution, administer within 6 hr. Protect solution from direct sunlight. ***Concentration:*** Concentrations of less than 1 mcg/mL or greater than 1 mg/mL are not recommended. ***Rate:*** Administer over a minimum of 1–4 hr. Avoid rapid administration. Avoid extravasation.
- **Y-Site Compatibility:** acyclovir, alemtuzumab, alfentanyl, amifostine, amikacin, aminophylline, amiodarone, anidulafungin, argatroban, ascorbic acid, atropine, azithromycin, aztreonam, benztropine, bivalirudin, bleomycin, bumetanide, buprenorphine, butorphanol, calcium chloride, calcium gluconate, cangrelor, carboplatin, carmustine, caspofungin, cefotaxime, ceftriaxone, chlorpromazine, cisatracurium, cisplatin, clindamycin, cyanocobalamin, cyclophosphamide, cyclosporine, cytarabine, dacarbazine, dactinomycin, daptomycin, daunorubicin hydrochloride, dexmedetomidine, dexrazoxane, digoxin, diltiazem, diphenhydramine, dobutamine, docetaxel, dopamine, doxorubicin hydrochloride, enalaprilat, ephedrine, epinephrine, epirubicin, epoetin alfa, eptifibatide, ertapenem, esmolol, etoposide, etoposide phosphate, famotidine, fenoldopam, fentanyl, filgrastim, fluconazole, fludarabine, fosphenytoin, gemcitabine, gentamicin, glycopyrrolate, granisetron, hetastarch, hydromorphone, idarubicin, ifosfamide, imipenem/cilastatin, insulin, regular, irinotecan, isoproterenol, labetalol, leucovorin calcium, levofloxacin, lidocaine, linezolid, lorazepam, magnesium sulfate, mannitol, melphalan, meperidine, mesna, methyldopate, metoclopramide, metoprolol, metronidazole, midazolam, milrinone, mitoxantrone, morphine, multivitamins, mycophenolate, nalbuphine, naloxone, nicardipine, nitroglycerin, nitroprusside, norepinephrine, octreotide, ondansetron, oxaliplatin, oxytocin, paclitaxel, pamidronate, pancuronium, pantoprazole, papaverine, pentamidine, phentolamine, phenylephrine, phytonadione, potassium chloride, procainamide, prochlorperazine, promethazine, propofol, propranolol, protamine, pyridoxine, quinupristin/dalfopristin, ranitidine, remifentanil, rituximab, rocuronium, sargramostim, sodium acetate, streptokinase, succinylcholine, sufentanil, tacrolimus, telavancin, theophylline, thiamine, thiotepa, tirofiban, tobramycin, topotecan, trastuzumab, vancomycin, vasopressin, vecuronium, verapamil, vinblastine, vincristine, vinorelbine, voriconazole, zoledronic acid.
- **Y-Site Incompatibility:** allopurinol, aminocaproic acid, amphotericin B lipid complex, amphotericin B liposome, ampicillin, ampicillin/sulbactam, cefazolin, cefotetan, cefoxitin, ceftazidime, cefuroxime, chloramphenicol, dantrolene, dexamethasone, diazepam, erythromycin, fluorouracil, folic acid, furosemide, ganciclovir, heparin, hydrocortisone, indomethacin, ketorolac, methotrexate, methylprednisolone, nafcillin, oxacillin, palonosetron, pemetrexed, penicillin G, pentobarbital, phenobarbital, phenytoin, piperacillin/tazobactam, potassium acetate, sodium bicarbonate, trimethoprim/sulfamethoxazole.

Minocycline

IV Administration

- IV doses are indicated only when oral therapy is not adequate or tolerated. Resume oral doses as soon as possible.
- **Intermittent Infusion:** Reconstitute vial with 5 mL of sterile water for injection. ***Diluent:*** 100 mL–1,000 mL 0.9% NaCl, D5W, or D5/0.9% NaCl, or in 250 mL–1000 mL LR, but not with other solutions containing calcium; precipitate may form especially in neutral and alkaline solutions. Solutions are stable for 4 hr at room temperature or 24 hr if refrigerated. ***Rate:*** Infuse over 60 min. Do not infuse rapidly.
- **Y-Site Incompatibility:** Do not administer with other medications or solutions. Flush line between doses.

Patient/Family Teaching

- Instruct patient to take medication around the clock and to finish the drug completely as directed, even if feeling better. Take missed doses as soon as possible unless it is almost time for next dose; do not double doses. Advise patient that sharing of this medication may be dangerous.
- Advise patient to avoid taking milk or other dairy products concurrently with oral tetracyclines. Also avoid taking antacids, zinc, calcium, magnesium- or aluminum-containing medications, sodium bicarbonate, and iron supplements within 1–3 hr of oral tetracyclines.
- Instruct patient to notify health care professional immediately if rash, diarrhea, abdominal cramping, fe-

ver, or bloody stools occur and not to treat with antidiarrheals without consulting health care professionals.

- *Minocycline* commonly causes dizziness or unsteadiness. Caution patient to avoid driving or other activities requiring alertness until response to medication is known. Notify health care professional if these symptoms occur.
- Caution patient to use sunscreen and protective clothing to prevent photosensitivity reactions.
- Advise patient to report the signs of superinfection (black, furry overgrowth on the tongue; vaginal itching or discharge; loose or foul-smelling stools) or intracranial hypertension (headache, blurred vision, diplopia, vision loss). Women who are overweight, of childbearing age or have a history of IH are at greater risk for developing tetracyclines—associated IH. Skin rash, pruritus, and urticaria should also be reported.
- Advise patient to notify health care professional of all Rx or OTC medications, vitamins, or herbal products being taken and to consult with health care professional before taking other medications.
- Instruct patient to notify health care professional of medication regimen before treatment or surgery.
- Rep: Advise females of reproductive potential to use a nonhormonal method of contraception while taking tetracyclines and until next menstrual period. Men attempting to father a child should not take minocycline.
- Instruct patient to notify health care professional if symptoms do not improve within a few days for systemic preparations.
- Caution patient to discard outdated or decomposed tetracyclines; they may be toxic.
- **Malaria Prophylaxis:** Advise patient to avoid being bitten by mosquitoes by using protective measures, especially from dusk to dawn (e.g., staying in well-screened areas, using mosquito nets, covering the body with clothing, and using an effective insect repellant). Doxycycline prophylaxis should begin 1–2 days before travel to the malarious area, continued daily while in the malarious area and after leaving the malarious area, should be continued for 4 more wk to avoid development of malaria. Do not exceed 4 mo.

Evaluation/Desired Outcomes

- Resolution of the signs and symptoms of infection. Length of time for complete resolution depends on the organism and site of infection.
- Decrease in acne lesions.
- Treatment of inhalation anthrax (post exposure) or treatment of cutaneous anthrax (doxycycline).
- Prevention of malaria.
- Reduction in inflammatory lesions associated with rosacea.

REMS

thalidomide (tha-**lid**-oh-mide)

Thalomid

Classification

Therapeutic: immunosuppressants

Indications

Cutaneous manifestations of moderate to severe erythema nodosum leprosum (ENL). Prevention (maintenance) and suppression of recurrent ENL. Newly diagnosed multiple myeloma (with dexamethasone). **Unlabeled Use:** Bechet's syndrome. HIV-associated wasting syndrome. Aphthous stomatitis (including HIV associated). Crohn's disease.

Action

May suppress excess levels of tumor necrosis factor-alpha (TNF-alpha) in patients with ENL and alter leukocyte migration by altering characteristics of cell surfaces. **Therapeutic Effects:** Decreased skin lesions in ENL and prevention of recurrence.

Pharmacokinetics

Absorption: 67–93% absorbed following oral administration.
Distribution: Crosses the placenta; highly protein bound.
Protein Binding: Highly bound.
Metabolism and Excretion: Hydrolyzed in plasma to multiple metabolites.
Half-life: 5–7 hr.

TIME/ACTION PROFILE (dermatologic effects)

ROUTE	ONSET	PEAK	DURATION
PO	48 hr	1–2 mo	unknown

Contraindications/Precautions

Contraindicated in: Hypersensitivity; Seizure disorders; Concurrent use of pembrolizumab in patients with multiple myeloma (↑ risk of mortality); OB: May cause fetal harm; Lactation: Avoid breast feeding (potential for serious adverse reactions in the infant).
Use Cautiously in: Rep: Women of childbearing potential and men with female sexual partners of childbearing potential; Pedi: Children <12 yr (safety not established).

Adverse Reactions/Side Effects

CNS: SEIZURES, dizziness, drowsiness. **CV:** bradycardia, edema, orthostatic hypotension, thromboembolic events (↑ risk with dexamethasone in multiple myeloma). **Derm:** DRUG REACTION WITH EOSINOPHILIA AND SYSTEMIC SYMPTOMS (DRESS), STEVENS-JOHNSON SYNDROME, TOXIC EPIDERMAL NECROLYSIS, rash, photosensitivity. **GI:** constipation. **Hemat:** neutropenia, throm-

T

bocytopenia. **Neuro:** peripheral neuropathy. **Misc:** HYPERSENSITIVITY REACTIONS (including anaphylaxis and angioedema), SEVERE BIRTH DEFECTS, TUMOR LYSIS SYNDROME, ↑ HIV viral load.

Interactions

Drug-Drug: ↑ CNS depression with concurrent use of **barbiturates**, **sedative/hypnotics**, **alcohol**, **chlorpromazine**, or other **CNS depressants**. Concurrent use of **agents that may cause peripheral neuropathy** ↑ risk of peripheral neuropathy.

Drug-Natural Products: Concommitant use with **echinacea**, and **melatonin** may interfere with immunosuppression.

Route/Dosage

ENL

PO (Adults ≥50 kg): 100–300 mg once daily initially; up to 400 mg/day has been used, depending on previous response. Every 3–6 mo, attempts should be made to taper and discontinue in decrements of 50 mg every 2–4 wk.

PO (Adults <50 kg): 100 mg once daily initially; up to 400 mg/day has been used, depending on previous response. Every 3–6 mo, attempts should be made to taper and discontinue in decrements of 50 mg every 2–4 wk.

Multiple Myeloma

PO (Adults): 200 mg once daily in 28-day treatment cycles.

Availability

Capsules: 50 mg, 100 mg, 150 mg, 200 mg.

NURSING IMPLICATIONS

Assessment

- Assess monthly for initial 3 mo and periodically during therapy to detect early signs of peripheral neuropathy (numbness, tingling, or pain in hands and feet). Commonly occurs with prolonged therapy, but has occurred following short-term use or following completion of therapy. May be severe and irreversible. Electrophysiologic testing may be done at baseline and every 6 mo to detect asymptomatic peripheral neuropathy. If symptoms occur, discontinue thalidomide immediately to limit further damage. Reinstate therapy only if neuropathy returns to baseline.
- Monitor for signs of hypersensitivity reaction (erythematous macular rash, fever, tachycardia, hypotension). May require discontinuation of therapy if severe. If reaction recurs when dosing is resumed, discontinue thalidomide.
- Monitor for signs and symptoms of bleeding (petechiae, epistaxis, gastrointestinal bleeding) during therapy. May require dose interruption, reduction, or discontinuation.
- Monitor for side effects (constipation, oversedation, peripheral neuropathy); may require discontinuation or dose reduction until side effects resolve.
- **Multiple Myeloma:** Assess for venous thromboembolism (dyspnea, chest pain, arm or leg swelling) periodically during therapy, especially in patients concurrently taking dexamethasone. Consider prophylaxis depending on patient risk factors.
- ***Lab Test Considerations:*** Assess pregnancy status prior to starting therapy. Pregnancy tests with a sensitivity of at least 50 mIU/mL must be done within 10–14 days and within 24 hrs of starting therapy. Once treatment has started pregnancy tests should occur weekly during first 4 wk of use, then every 4 wk in females with a regular menstrual cycle and every 2 wk in females with an irregular cycle.
- Monitor WBC with differential and platelet count during therapy. May cause ↓ WBC. Do not initiate therapy with an ANC ≤750/mm³. If ANC ↓ to ≤750/mm³ during therapy, re-evaluate medication regimen; if neutropenia persists, consider discontinuing therapy. May cause thrombocytopenia.
- May cause ↑ viral load levels in patients with HIV.

Implementation

- Do not confuse Thalomid (thalidomide) with thiamine.
- Rep: Due to teratogenic effects, thalidomide may be prescribed only by prescribers registered in the *System for Thalidomide Education and Prescribing Safety (STEPS)* program. Thalidomide is started within 24 hr of a negative pregnancy test with a sensitivity of at least 50 mIU/mL. Pregnancy testing must occur weekly during first mo of therapy, then monthly thereafter in women with a regular menstrual cycle. For women with irregular menses, pregnancy testing should occur every 2 wk. If pregnancy occurs, thalidomide should be discontinued immediately. Any suspected fetal exposure must be reported to the FDA and the manufacturer, and patient should be referred to an obstetrician/gynecologist experienced in reproductive toxicity.
- If health care professionals or other caregivers are exposed to body fluids from patients receiving thalidomide, use appropriate precautions, such as wearing gloves to prevent the potential cutaneous exposure to thalidomide or washing the exposed area with soap and water.
- Corticosteroids may be used concurrently with thalidomide for patients with moderate to severe neuritis associated with a severe ENL reaction. Use of corticosteroids can be tapered and discontinued when neuritis resolves.
- **PO:** Administer once daily with water, preferably at bedtime and at least 1 hr after the evening meal. If divided doses are used, administer at least 1 hr after meals.

Patient/Family Teaching

- Instruct patient to take thalidomide as directed. Do not discontinue without notifying health care professional; dose should be tapered gradually. Explain *STEPS* program to patient.

- Advise patient that thalidomide should not be shared with others.
- Frequently causes drowsiness or dizziness. Caution patient to avoid driving or other activities requiring alertness until response to medication is known.
- Advise patient to change positions slowly to minimize orthostatic hypotension.
- Caution patient to use sunscreen and protective clothing to prevent photosensitivity reactions.
- Instruct patient not to donate blood and male patients not to donate sperm while taking thalidomide and for 1 mo following discontinuation.
- Advise patient to notify health care professional immediately if pain, numbness, tingling, or burning in hands or feet or shortness of breath, chest pain, swelling of arms or legs occur.
- Rep: Inform female patients of reproductive potential that they must use one highly effective method (IUD, hormonal contraceptive, tubal ligation, partner's vasectomy) and one additional method (latex condom, diaphragm, cervical cap) AT THE SAME TIME for at least 4 wk before, during therapy and interruptions of therapy, and for 4 wk following discontinuation of therapy, even with a history of infertility, unless due to a hysterectomy or patient has been postmenopausal naturally for 24 consecutive mo. Advise female patients to avoid breast feeding during therapy. Males with female partners of reproductive potential receiving thalidomide must always use a latex condom during and for up to 4 wk following discontinuation, even if they have undergone a successful vasectomy. Thalidomide must be discontinued if pregnancy is suspected or confirmed. Suspected fetal exposure must be reported to FDA via MedWatch at 1-800-FDA-1088 and to manufacturer at 1-888-668-2528. Inform females there is a Pregnancy Exposure Registry that monitors pregnancy outcomes in females exposed to thalidomide during pregnancy and that they can contact the Pregnancy Exposure Registry by calling 1-888-423-5436.
- Advise patient to notify health care professional of all Rx or OTC medications, vitamins, or herbal products being taken and to consult with health care professional before taking other medications. Concomitant use of HIV-protease inhibitors, modafinil, penicillins, rifampin, rifabutin, phenytoin, carbamazepine, or certain herbal supplements such as St. John's wort with hormonal contraceptive agents may reduce the effectiveness of contraception during and for up to one mo after discontinuation of these concomitant therapies. Therefore, women requiring treatment with one or more of these drugs must use two other effective or highly effective methods of contraception or abstain from heterosexual sexual contact while taking thalidomide.

Evaluation/Desired Outcomes

- Resolution of the signs and symptoms of active ENL reaction. Usually requires at least 2 wk of therapy; then taper medication in 50 mg decrements every 2–4 wk.
- Prevention of recurrent ENL. Tapering off medication should be attempted every 3–6 mo in decrements of 50 mg every 2–4 wk.
- Decrease in serum and urine paraprotein measurements in patients with multiple myeloma.

thiamine (thye-a-min)

🍁Betaxin, vitamin B1

Classification
Therapeutic: vitamins
Pharmacologic: water soluble vitamins

Indications

Treatment of thiamine deficiencies (beriberi). Prevention of Wernicke's encephalopathy. Dietary supplement in patients with GI disease, alcoholism, or cirrhosis.

Action

Required for carbohydrate metabolism. **Therapeutic Effects:** Replacement in deficiency states.

Pharmacokinetics

Absorption: Well absorbed from the GI tract by an active process. Excessive amounts are not absorbed completely. Also well absorbed from IM sites.
Distribution: Widely distributed. Enters breast milk.
Metabolism and Excretion: Metabolized by the liver. Excess amounts are excreted unchanged by the kidneys.
Half-life: Unknown.

TIME/ACTION PROFILE (time for symptoms of deficiency—edema and heart failure—to resolve†)

ROUTE	ONSET	PEAK	DURATION
PO, IM, IV	hr	days	days–wk

†Confusion and psychosis take longer to respond.

Contraindications/Precautions

Contraindicated in: Hypersensitivity; Known alcohol intolerance or bisulfite hypersensitivity (elixir only).
Use Cautiously in: Wernicke's encephalopathy (condition may be worsened unless thiamine is administered before glucose).

Adverse Reactions/Side Effects

Adverse reactions and side effects are extremely rare and are usually associated with IV administration or extremely large doses.
CNS: restlessness, weakness. **EENT:** tightness of the throat. **Resp:** pulmonary edema, respiratory distress.

T

CV: VASCULAR COLLAPSE, hypotension, vasodilation. **GI:** GI bleeding, nausea. **Derm:** cyanosis, pruritus, sweating, tingling, urticaria, warmth. **Misc:** ANGIOEDEMA.

Interactions

Drug-Drug: None significant.

Route/Dosage

Thiamine Deficiency (Beriberi)

PO (Adults): 5–10 mg 3 times daily.
PO (Children): 10–50 mg/day in divided doses.
IM, IV (Adults): 5–100 mg 3 times daily.
IM, IV (Children): 10–25 mg/day.

Dietary Supplement

PO (Adults): 1–1.6 mg/day.
PO (Children 4–10 yr): 0.9–1 mg/day.
PO (Children birth–3 yr): 0.3–0.7 mg/day.

Availability (generic available)

Tablets: 5 mg[OTC], 10 mg[OTC], 25 mg[OTC], 50 mg[OTC], 100 mg[OTC], 250 mg[OTC], 500 mg[OTC]. **Injection:** 100 mg/mL. ***In combination with:*** other vitamins, minerals, and trace elements in multi-vitamin preparations[OTC].

NURSING IMPLICATIONS

Assessment

- Assess for signs and symptoms of thiamine deficiency (anorexia, GI distress, irritability, palpitations, tachycardia, edema, paresthesia, muscle weakness and pain, depression, memory loss, confusion, psychosis, visual disturbances, elevated serum pyruvic acid levels).
- Assess patient's nutritional status (diet, weight) prior to and throughout therapy.
- Monitor patients receiving IV thiamine for anaphylaxis (wheezing, urticaria, edema).
- ***Lab Test Considerations:*** May interfere with certain methods of testing serum theophylline, uric acid, and urobilinogen concentrations.

Implementation

- Do not confuse thiamine with Thalomid (thalidomide).
- Because of infrequency of single B-vitamin deficiencies, combinations are commonly administered.
- **IM, IV:** Parenteral administration is reserved for patients in whom oral administration is not feasible.
- **IM:** Administration may cause tenderness and induration at injection site. Cool compresses may decrease discomfort.

IV Administration

- **IV:** Sensitivity reactions and death have occurred from IV administration. An intradermal test dose is recommended in patients with suspected sensitivity. Monitor site for erythema and induration.
- **IV Push:** ***Concentration:*** Administer undiluted at 100 mg/mL. ***Rate:*** Administer at a rate of 100 mg over 5 min.
- **Continuous Infusion:** ***Diluent:*** May be diluted in dextrose/Ringer's or LR combinations, dextrose/saline combinations, D5W, D10W, Ringer's and LR injection, 0.9% NaCl, or 0.45% NaCl. Usually administered with other vitamins.
- **Y-Site Compatibility:** alfentanil, amikacin, ascorbic acid, atracurium, atropine, aztreonam, benztropine, bumetanide, buprenorphine, butorphanol, calcium chloride, calcium gluconate, cefazolin, cefonocid, cefotaxime, cefotetan, cefoxitin, ceftriaxone, cefuroxime, chlorpromazine, clindamycin, cyanocobalamin, cyclosporine, dexamethasone, digoxin, diphenhydramine, dobutamine, dopamine, doxycycline, enalaprilat, ephedrine, epinephrine, erythromycin, esmolol, famotidine, fentanyl, gentamicin, glycopyrrolate, heparin, insulin, isoproterenol, labetalol, lidocaine, magnesium sulfate, mannitol, meperidine, metaraminol, methoxamine, methyldopate, metoclopramide, metoprolol, morphine, multivitamins, nafcillin, nalbuphine, naloxone, nitroglycerin, nitroprusside, norepinephrine, oxacillin, oxytocin, papaverine, penicillin G, pentamidine, phentolamine, phenylephrine, phytonadione, potassium chloride, procainamide, prochlorperazine, promethazine, propranolol, protamine, pyridoxime, ranitidine, streptokinase, succinylcholine, sufentanil, theophylline, tobramycin, tolazoline, trimetaphan, vancomycin, vasopressin, verapamil.
- **Y-Site Incompatibility:** aminophylline, amphotericin B deoxycholate, azathioprine, ceftazidime, chloramphenicol, dantrolene, diazepam, diazoxide, folic acid, furosemide, ganciclovir, hydrocortisone, imipenem/cilastatin, indomethacin, methylprednisolone, pentobarbital, phenobarbital, phenytoin, sodium bicarbonate, trimethoprim/sulfamethoxazole.
- **Additive Incompatibility:** Solutions with neutral or alkaline pH, such as carbonates, bicarbonates, citrates, and acetates.

Patient/Family Teaching

- Encourage patient to comply with dietary recommendations of health care professional. Explain that the best source of vitamins is a well-balanced diet with foods from the four basic food groups.
- Teach patient that foods high in thiamine include cereals (whole grain and enriched), meats (especially pork), and fresh vegetables; loss is variable during cooking.
- Caution patients self-medicating with vitamin supplements not to exceed RDA. The effectiveness of megadoses of vitamins for treatment of various medical conditions is unproved and may cause side effects.

Evaluation/Desired Outcomes

- Prevention of or decrease in the signs and symptoms of vitamin B deficiency.
- Decrease in the symptoms of neuritis, ocular signs, ataxia, edema, and heart failure may be seen within hrs of administration and may disappear within a few days.
- Confusion and psychosis may take longer to respond and may persist if nerve damage has occurred.

HIGH ALERT

THROMBOLYTIC AGENTS

alteplase (**al**-te-plase)
Activase, ✱Activase rt-PA, Cathflo Activase, tissue plasminogen activator, t-PA

reteplase (**re**-te-plase)
Retavase

streptokinase (strep-toe-**kye**-nase)
Streptase

tenecteplase (te-**nek**-te-plase)
TNKase

Classification
Therapeutic: thrombolytics
Pharmacologic: plasminogen activators

Indications
Alteplase, reteplase, streptokinase, tenecteplase: Acute myocardial infarction (MI). **Alteplase, streptokinase:** Acute massive pulmonary emboli. **Alteplase:** Acute ischemic stroke. **Streptokinase:** Acute deep vein thrombosis. **Streptokinase:** Acute arterial thrombi. **Streptokinase:** Occluded arteriovenous cannulae. **Alteplase:** Occluded central venous access devices.

Action
Convert plasminogen to plasmin, which is then able to degrade fibrin present in clots. Alteplase, reteplase, and tenecteplase directly activate plasminogen. Streptokinase combines with plasminogen to form activator complexes, which then converts plasminogen to plasmin. **Therapeutic Effects:** Lysis of thrombi in coronary arteries, with preservation of ventricular function or improvement of ventricular function (and ↓ risk of HF or death). Lysis of pulmonary emboli or deep vein thrombosis. Lysis of thrombi causing ischemic stroke, reducing risk of neurologic sequelae. Restoration of cannula or catheter patency and function.

Pharmacokinetics
Absorption: Complete after IV administration. Intracoronary administration or administration into occluded catheters or cannulae has a more localized effect.
Distribution: Streptokinase appears to cross the placenta minimally, if at all. Remainder of distribution for streptokinase or other agents is not known.
Metabolism and Excretion: *Alteplase, tenecteplase*—Rapidly metabolized by the liver. *Reteplase*—Cleared primarily by the liver and kidneys. *Streptokinase*—Rapidly cleared from circulation by antibodies and other unknown mechanism.
Half-life: *Alteplase*—35 min; *reteplase*—13–16 min; *streptokinase*—initially 18 min (due to clearance by antibodies), then 83 min; *Tenecteplase*—20–24 min (initial phase), 90–130 min (terminal phase).

TIME/ACTION PROFILE (fibrinolysis)

ROUTE	ONSET	PEAK	DURATION
Alteplase IV	30 min	60 min	unknown
Reteplase IV	30 min	30–90 min	48 hr
Streptokinase IV	immediate	rapid	4 hr (up to 12 hr)
Tenecteplase IV	rapid	unknown	unknown

Contraindications/Precautions
Contraindicated in: Active internal bleeding; History of cerebrovascular accident; Recent (within 2 mo) intracranial or intraspinal injury or trauma; Intracranial neoplasm, AV malformation, or aneurysm; Severe uncontrolled hypertension; Known bleeding tendencies; Hypersensitivity; cross-sensitivity with other thrombolytics may occur.
Use Cautiously in: Recent (within 10 days) major surgery, trauma, GI, or GU bleeding; Left heart thrombus; Severe hepatic or renal disease; Hemorrhagic ophthalmic conditions; Septic phlebitis; Previous puncture of a noncompressible vessel; Subacute bacterial endocarditis or acute pericarditis; Recent streptococcal infection or previous therapy with streptokinase (from 5 days–6 mo); may produce resistance because of antibody formation; ↑ dosage requirements may be encountered (streptokinase only); Geri: >75 yr; ↑ risk of intracranial bleeding; OB, Lactation, Pedi: Safety not established.
Exercise Extreme Caution in: Patients receiving concurrent anticoagulant therapy (↑ risk of intracranial bleeding).

Adverse Reactions/Side Effects
CNS: INTRACRANIAL HEMORRHAGE. **EENT:** epistaxis, gingival bleeding. **Resp:** bronchospasm, hemoptysis. **CV:** hypotension, reperfusion arrhythmias. **GI:** GI BLEEDING, RETROPERITONEAL BLEEDING, nausea, vomiting. **GU:** GU TRACT BLEEDING. **Derm:** ecchymoses, flushing, urticaria. **Hemat:** BLEEDING. **Local:** hemorrhage at injection sites, phlebitis at IV site. **MS:** musculoskeletal pain. **Misc:** allergic reactions including ANAPHYLAXIS, fever.

Interactions
Drug-Drug: Concurrent use of **aspirin**, other **NSAIDs**, **warfarin**, **heparin**, **low-molecular-weight heparins**, **direct thrombin inhibitors**, **eptifibatide**, **tirofiban**, **clopidogrel**, or **dipyridamole** may ↑ risk of bleeding, although these agents are frequently used together or in sequence. Effects may be ↓ by **anti-**

T

fibrinolytic agents, including **aminocaproic acid** or **tranexamic acid**.
Drug-Natural Products: ↑ anticoagulant effect and bleeding risk with **anise**, **arnica**, **chamomile**, **clove**, **dong quai**, **fenugreek**, **feverfew**, **garlic**, **ginger**, **ginkgo**, **Panax ginseng**, **licorice**, and others.

Route/Dosage

Alteplase

Myocardial Infarction (Accelerated or Front-Loading Infusion)

IV (Adults): 15 mg bolus, then 0.75 mg/kg (up to 50 mg) over 30 min, then 0.5 mg/kg (up to 35 mg) over next 60 min; usually accompanied by heparin therapy.

Myocardial Infarction (3-Hr Infusion)

IV (Adults >65 kg): 60 mg over 1st hr (6–10 mg given as a bolus over first 1–2 min), 20 mg over the 2nd hr, and 20 mg over the 3rd hr for a total dose of 100 mg.
IV (Adults <65 kg): 0.75 mg/kg over 1st hr (0.075–0.125 mg/kg given as a bolus over first 1–2 min), 0.25 mg/kg over the 2nd hr, and 0.25 mg/kg over the 3rd hr for a total dose of 1.25 mg/kg (not to exceed 100 mg total).

Pulmonary Embolism

IV (Adults): 100 mg over 2 hr; follow with heparin.

Acute Ischemic Stroke

IV (Adults): 0.9 mg/kg (not to exceed 90 mg), given as an infusion over 1 hr, with 10% of the dose given as a bolus over the 1st min.

Occluded Venous Access Devices

IV (Adults and Children >30 kg): 2 mg/2 mL instilled into occluded catheter; if unsuccessful, may repeat once after 2 hr.
IV (Adults and Children <30 kg): 110% of the lumen volume (not to exceed 2 mg in 2 mL) instilled into occluded catheter; if unsuccessful, may repeat once after 2 hr.

Reteplase

IV (Adults): 10 units, followed 30 min later by an additional 10 units.

Streptokinase

Myocardial Infarction

IV (Adults): 1.5 million units given as a continuous infusion over up to 60 min.
Intracoronary (Adults): 20,000 unit bolus followed by 2000–4000 units/min infusion for 30–90 min.

Deep Vein Thrombosis, Pulmonary Emboli, Arterial Emboli, or Arterial Thromboses

IV (Adults): 250,000 unit loading dose over 30 min, followed by 100,000 unit/hr for 24 hr for pulmonary emboli or arterial thrombosis/embolism, 72 hr for deep vein thrombosis.

Tenecteplase

IV (Adults <60 kg): 30 mg.
IV (Adults ≥60 kg and <70 kg): 35 mg.
IV (Adults ≥70 kg and <80 kg): 40 mg.
IV (Adults ≥80 kg and <90 kg): 45 mg.
IV (Adults ≥90 kg): 50 mg.

Availability

Alteplase

Powder for injection: 2 mg/vial, 50 mg/vial, 100 mg/vial.

Reteplase

Powder for injection: 10.8 units/vial.

Streptokinase

Powder for injection: 250,000 units/vial, 750,000 units/vial, 1,500,000 units/vial.

Tenecteplase

Powder for injection: 50 mg/vial.

NURSING IMPLICATIONS

Assessment

- Begin therapy as soon as possible after the onset of symptoms.
- Monitor vital signs, including temperature, continuously for coronary thrombosis and at least every 4 hr during therapy for other indications. Do not use lower extremities to monitor BP. Notify health care professional if systolic BP >180 mm Hg or diastolic BP >110 mm Hg. Should not be given if hypertension is uncontrolled. Inform health care professional if hypotension occurs. Hypotension may result from the drug, hemorrhage, or cardiogenic shock.
- Assess patient carefully for bleeding every 15 min during the 1st hr of therapy, every 15–30 min during the next 8 hr, and at least every 4 hr for the duration of therapy. Frank bleeding may occur from sites of invasive procedures or from body orifices. Internal bleeding may also occur (decreased neurologic status; abdominal pain with coffee-grounds emesis or black, tarry stools; hematuria; joint pain). If uncontrolled bleeding occurs, stop medication and notify health care professional immediately.
- Inquire about previous reaction to streptokinase therapy. Assess patient for hypersensitivity reaction (rash, dyspnea, fever, changes in facial color, swelling around the eyes, wheezing). If these occur, inform health care professional promptly. Keep epinephrine, an antihistamine, and resuscitation equipment close by in the event of an anaphylactic reaction.
- Inquire about recent streptococcal infection. *Streptokinase* may be less effective if administered between 5 days and 6 mo of a streptococcal infection.
- Assess neurologic status throughout therapy. Altered sensorium or neurologic changes may be indicative of intracranial bleeding.
- **Myocardial Infarction:** Monitor ECG continuously. Notify health care professional if significant arrhyth-

mias occur. Monitor cardiac enzymes. Radionuclide myocardial scanning and/or coronary angiography may be ordered 7–10 days after therapy to monitor effectiveness of therapy.

- Assess intensity, character, location, and radiation of chest pain. Note presence of associated symptoms (nausea, vomiting, diaphoresis). Notify health care professional if chest pain is unrelieved or recurs.
- Monitor heart sounds and breath sounds frequently. Inform health care professional if signs of HF occur (rales/crackles, dyspnea, S_3 heart sound, jugular venous distention).
- **Acute Ischemic Stroke:** Assess neurologic status. Determine time of onset of stroke symptoms. Alteplase must be administered within 3–4.5 hr of onset (within 3 hr in patients older than 80 yr, those taking oral anticoagulants, those with a baseline National Institutes of Health Stroke Scale score 25, or those with both a history of stroke and diabetes).
- **Pulmonary Embolism:** Monitor pulse, BP, hemodynamics, and respiratory status (rate, degree of dyspnea, ABGs).
- **Deep Vein Thrombosis/Acute Arterial Thrombosis:** Observe extremities and palpate pulses of affected extremities every hr. Notify health care professional immediately if circulatory impairment occurs. Computerized tomography, impedance plethysmography, quantitative Doppler effect determination, and/or angiography or venography may be used to determine restoration of blood flow and duration of therapy; however, repeated venograms are not recommended.
- **Cannula/Catheter Occlusion:** Monitor ability to aspirate blood as indicator of patency. Ensure that patient exhales and holds breath when connecting and disconnecting IV syringe to prevent air embolism.
- ***Lab Test Considerations:*** Hematocrit, hemoglobin, platelet count, fibrin/fibrin degradation product (FDP) titer, fibrinogen concentration, prothrombin time, thrombin time, and activated partial thromboplastin time (aPTT) may be evaluated before and frequently during therapy. Bleeding time may be assessed before therapy if patient has received platelet inhibitors.
- Obtain type and crossmatch and have blood available at all times in case of hemorrhage.
- Stools should be tested for occult blood loss and urine for hematuria periodically during therapy.
- ***Toxicity and Overdose: High Alert:*** If local bleeding occurs, apply pressure to site. If severe or internal bleeding occurs, discontinue infusion. Clotting factors and/or blood volume may be restored through infusions of whole blood, packed RBCs, fresh frozen plasma, or cryoprecipitate. Do not administer dextran; it has antiplatelet activity. Aminocaproic acid (Amicar) may be used as an antidote.

Implementation

- ***High Alert:*** Overdose and underdose of thrombolytic medications have resulted in patient harm or death. Have second practitioner independently check original order, dosage calculations, and infusion pump settings. Do not confuse the abbreviation *t-PA* for alteplase (Activase) with the abbreviation *TNK t-PA* for tenecteplase (TNKase) and *r-PA* for reteplase (Retavase). Clarify orders that contain either of these abbreviations.
- Thrombolytic agents should be used only in settings in which hematologic function and clinical response can be adequately monitored.
- Starting two IV lines before therapy is recommended: one for the thrombolytic agent, the other for any additional infusions.
- Avoid invasive procedures, such as IM injections or arterial punctures, with this therapy. If such procedures must be performed, apply pressure to all arterial and venous puncture sites for at least 30 min. Avoid venipunctures at noncompressible sites (jugular vein, subclavian site).
- Acetaminophen may be ordered to control fever.

Alteplase

IV Administration

- **Intermittent Infusion:** Vials are packaged with sterile water for injection (without preservatives) to be used as diluent. Do not use bacteriostatic water for injection. Reconstitute 20-mg vials with 20-mL and 50-mg vials with 50 mL using an 18-gauge needle. Avoid excess agitation during dilution; swirl or invert gently to mix. Solution may foam upon reconstitution. Bubbles will resolve upon standing a few min. Solution will be clear to pale yellow. Stable for 8 hr at room temperature. ***Concentration:*** May be administered as reconstituted (1 mg/mL). ***Diluent:*** May be further diluted immediately before use in an equal amount of 0.9% NaCl or D5W. ***Rate:*** Flush line with 20–30 mL of saline at completion of infusion to ensure entire dose is received. See Route and Dosage section for specific rates.
- **Y-Site Compatibility:** eptifibatide, lidocaine, metoprolol, propranolol.
- **Y-Site Incompatibility:** bivalirudin, dobutamine, dopamine, heparin, nitroglycerin.
- **Cathflo Activase:** Reconstitute by withdrawing 2.2 mL of sterile water (provided) and injecting into Cathflo Activase vial, directing diluent into powder for a concentration of 1 mg/mL. Allow slight foaming to dissipate by letting vial stand undisturbed. Do not use bacteriostatic water. Mix by gently swirling to dissolve; complete dissolution should occur within 3 min. Do not shake. Solution should be colorless to pale yellow. Use solution within 8 hr.

T

- Withdraw 2.0 mL of reconstituted solution and instill into occluded catheter. After 30 min dwell time, attempt to aspirate blood. If catheter remains occluded, allow 120 min dwell time. If catheter function is not restored after one dose, 2nd dose may be instilled. If catheter function is restored, aspirate 4–5 mL of blood to remove Cathflo Activase and residual clot. Gently irrigate catheter with 0.9% NaCl.

Reteplase

IV Administration

- **IV Push:** Reconstitute using diluent, needle, syringe, and dispensing pin provided. Reconstitute only with sterile water for injection without preservatives. Solution is colorless. Do not administer solutions that are discolored or contain a precipitate. Slight foaming may occur; allow vial to stand undisturbed for several min to dissipate bubbles. Reconstitute immediately before use. Stable for 4 hr at room temperature. ***Concentration:*** Administer undiluted. ***Rate:*** Administer each bolus over 2 min into an IV line containing D5W; flush line before and after bolus.
- **Y-Site Incompatibility:** bivalirudin, heparin. No other medication should be infused or injected into line used for reteplase.

Streptokinase

IV Administration

- **Intracoronary:** Dilute 250,000 IU vial to a total volume of 125 mL with 0.9% NaCl or D5W. Administer 20,000 IU (10 mL) via bolus injection.
- ***Rate:*** Intracoronary bolus is administered over 15 sec–2 min.
- **Intermittent Infusion:** Reconstitute with 5 mL of 0.9% NaCl or D5W (direct to sides of vial) and swirl gently; do not shake. ***Diluent:*** Dilute further with 0.9% NaCl for a total volume of 45–500 mL (45 mL for MI, 90 mL for deep vein thrombosis or pulmonary embolism). Solution is slightly yellow in color. Administer through 0.8-micron pore–size filter. Use reconstituted solution within 24 hr. ***Rate:*** Administer dose for MI within 60 min.
- Intracoronary bolus should be followed by an intracoronary maintenance infusion of 2000 IU/min for 60 min.
- Loading dose for *deep vein thrombosis* or *pulmonary embolism* is administered over 30 min, followed by an infusion of 100,000 IU/hr.
- Use infusion pump to ensure accurate dose.
- **Y-Site Compatibility:** alfentanil, amikacin, aminophylline, ascorbic acid, atracurium, atropine, aztreonam, benztropine, bumetanide, buprenorphine, butorphanol, calcium chloride, calcium gluconate, cefazolin, cefonocid, cefotaxime, cefotetan, cefoxitin, ceftazidime, ceftriaxone, cefuroxime, chloramphenicol, clindamycin, cyanocobalamin, cyclosporine, dexamethasone, digoxin, diphenhydramine, dobutamine, dopamine, doxycycline, enalaprilat, ephedrine, epinephrine, epoetin alfa, erythromycin, esmolol, famotidine, fentanyl, fluconazole, folic acid, furosemide, gentamicin, glycopyrrolate, heparin, hydrocortisone, imipenem/cilastatin, indomethacin, insulin, isoproterenol, ketorolac, labetalol, lidocaine, magnesium sulfate, mannitol, meperidine, methoxamine, methyldopate, methylprednisolone, metoclopramide, metoprolol, midazolam, morphine, multivitamins, nafcillin, naloxone, nitroglycerin, nitroprusside, norepinephrine, ondansetron, oxacillin, oxytocin, penicillin G, pentobarbital, phenobarbital, phentolamine, phenylephrine, phytonadione, potassium chloride, procainamide, propranolol, pyridoxime, ranitidine, sodium bicarbonate, succinylcholine, sufentanil, theophylline, thiamine, tobramycin, trimetaphan, verapamil.
- **Y-Site Incompatibility:** azathioprine, bivalirudin, chlorpromazine, dantrolene, diazepam, diazoxide, ganciclovir, hydroxyzine, nalbuphine, pentamidine, phenytoin, prochlorperazine, promethazine, trimethoprim/sulfamethoxazole, vancomycin.
- **Additive Incompatibility:** Do not admix with any other medication.
- **Cannula/Catheter Clearance:** Dilute 250,000 IU in 2 mL of 0.9% NaCl or D5W.
- ***Rate:*** Administer slowly, over 25–35 min, into each occluded limb of cannula, and then clamp for at least 2 hr. Aspirate contents carefully and flush lines with 0.9% NaCl.

Tenecteplase

IV Administration

- **Intermittent Infusion:** Vials are packaged with sterile water for injection (without preservatives) to be used as diluent. Do not use bacteriostatic water for injection. Do not discard shield assembly. To reconstitute aseptically withdraw 10 mL of diluent and inject into the tenectplase vial, directing the stream into the powder. Slight foaming may occur; large bubbles will dissipate if left standing undisturbed for several min. Swirl gently until contents are completely dissolved; do not shake. ***Concentration:*** Solution containing 5 mg/mL is clear and colorless to pale yellow. Withdraw dose from reconstituted vial with the syringe and discard unused portion. Once dose is in syringe, stand the shield vertically on a flat surface (with green side down) and passively recap the red hub cannula. Remove the entire shield assembly, including the red hub cannula, by twisting counter clockwise. Shield assembly also contains the clear-ended blunt plastic cannula; retain for split septum IV access. Reconstitute immediately before use. May be refrigerated and administered within 8 hr. ***Rate:*** Administer as a single IV bolus over 5 sec.
- **Y-Site Incompatibility:** Precipate forms in line when administered with dextrose-containing solutions. Flush line with saline-containing solution prior to and following administration of tenecteplase.
- **Additive Incompatibility:** Do not admix.

Patient/Family Teaching

- Explain purpose of medication and the need for close monitoring to patient and family. Instruct patient to report hypersensitivity reactions (rash, dyspnea) and bleeding or bruising.
- Explain need for bedrest and minimal handling during therapy to avoid injury. Avoid all unnecessary procedures such as shaving and vigorous tooth brushing.

Evaluation/Desired Outcomes

- Lysis of thrombi and restoration of blood flow.
- Prevention of neurologic sequelae in acute ischemic stroke.
- Cannula or catheter patency.

ticagrelor (tye-ka-grel-or)

Brilinta

Classification

Therapeutic: antiplatelet agents

Pharmacologic: platelet aggregation inhibitors

Indications

To decrease the incidence of thrombotic cardiovascular events associated with acute coronary syndrome (ACS). Also reduces the incidence of stent thrombosis in patients who have received an intracoronary stent for ACS.

Action

Both parent drug and its active metabolite inhibit platelet aggregation by reversibly interacting with platelet $P2Y_{12}$ADP-receptors, preventing signal transduction and platelet activation. **Therapeutic Effects:** Reduced sequelae of ACS including cardiovascular death, MI and stroke. Reduction in stent thrombosis.

Pharmacokinetics

Absorption: 36% absorbed following oral administration.

Distribution: Unknown.

Protein Binding: 99% for ticagrelor and its active metabolite.

Metabolism and Excretion: Mostly metabolized in the liver (CYP3A4 enzyme system, some metabolism by CYP3A5) with conversion to an active metabolite (AR-C124910XX); excretion primarily via biliary secretion; <1% excreted unchanged or as active metabolite in urine.

Half-life: *Ticagrelor*—7 hr; *Active metabolite*—9 hr.

TIME/ACTION PROFILE (inhibition of platelet aggregation)

ROUTE	ONSET	PEAK	DURATION
PO	within 30 min	4 hr	5 days†

† Following discontinuation.

Contraindications/Precautions

Contraindicated in: Hypersensitivity; Active bleeding; History of intracranial bleeding; Severe hepatic impairment (↑ risk of bleeding); Impending coronary artery bypass graft (CABG) surgery or other surgery (discontinue 5 days prior); Strong inhibitors/inducers of CYP3A enzyme system (avoid concurrent use if possible); Lactation: Avoid breast feeding.

Use Cautiously in: Moderate hepatic impairment; History of sick sinus syndrome, 2nd or 3rd degree heart block, or bradycardia-related syncope in the absence of a pacemaker; Hypotension following recent CABG or percutaneous coronary intervention (PCI) in patients receiving ticagrelor (consider bleeding as a cause); OB: Use during pregnancy only if potential maternal benefit justifies potential risk to fetus; Pedi: Safety and effectiveness not established; Geri: Some elderly patients may be more sensitive to effects.

Adverse Reactions/Side Effects

CV: bradycardia, heart block. **Endo:** gynecomastia. **Hemat:** BLEEDING. **Resp:** dyspnea. **Misc:** HYPERSENSITIVITY REACTIONS (including angioedema).

Interactions

Drug-Drug: Strong inhibitors of CYP3A4/5 including **atazanavir**, **clarithromycin**, **indinavir**, **itraconazole**, **ketoconazole**, **nefazodone**, **nelfinavir**, **ritonavir**, **saquinavir**, and **voriconazole** ↑ levels and the risk of bleeding and should be avoided. **Potent inducers of CYP3A** including **carbamazepine**, **dexamethasone**, **phenobarbital**, **phenytoin**, **rifampin** may ↓ levels and effectiveness and should be avoided. **P-glycoprotein inhibitors** including **cyclosporine** may ↑ levels and the risk of bleeding. Concurrent use of **lovastatin** or **simvastatin** in doses >40 mg/day ↑ risk of statin-related adverse reactions. Effectiveness is ↓ by **aspirin** >100 mg/day (maintain aspirin at 75–100 mg/day). May alter **digoxin** levels (monitoring recommended). Risk of bleeding ↑ by **anticoagulants**, **fibrinolytics** and chronic **NSAIDs**. **Opioids** may ↓ absorption of ticagrelor and its active metabolite and ↓ antiplatelet effects; consider using parenteral antiplatelet in patients with acute coronary syndrome if concurrent use of opioids needed.

Route/Dosage

PO (Adults): *Loading dose*—180 mg; followed by *maintenance dose*—90 mg twice daily for 1 yr, then 60 mg twice daily.

Availability (generic available)

Tablets: 60 mg, 90 mg.

NURSING IMPLICATIONS

Assessment

- Assess patient for symptoms of stroke, peripheral vascular disease, or MI periodically during therapy.

T

- Observe patient for signs and symptoms of hypersensitivity reactions (rash, facial swelling, pruritus, laryngeal edema, wheezing). Discontinue drug and notify health care professional immediately if symptoms occur. Keep epinephrine, an antihistamine, and resuscitation equipment close by in case of anaphylactic reaction.
- ***Lab Test Considerations:*** May cause ↑ serum uric acid and ↑ serum creatinine.

Implementation

- **PO:** Administer ticagrelor 180 mg (two 90 mg tablets) as a loading dose, followed by 90 mg twice daily for 1 yr, then 60 mg twice daily. After initial 325 mg loading dose of aspirin, administer maintenance dose of 75–100 mg daily. Administer without regard for food.
- For patients unable to swallow, tablets can be crushed and mixed with water. Mixture can also be administered via a nasogastric tube.
- Patients who have received a loading dose of clopidogrel may be started on ticagrelor.
- Discontinue ticagrelor 5 days before planned surgical procedures. If ticagrelor must be temporarily discontinued, restart as soon as possible. Premature discontinuation of therapy may increase risk of myocardial infarction, stent thrombosis, and death.

Patient/Family Teaching

- Instruct patient to take ticagrelor exactly as directed. Take missed doses as soon as possible unless almost time for next dose; do not double doses. Do not discontinue ticagrelor without consulting health care professional; may increase risk of cardiovascular events. Advise patient to read the *Medication Guide* before starting therapy and with each Rx refill in case of changes.
- Advise patient that daily aspirin should not exceed 100 mg and to avoid taking other medications that contain aspirin.
- Inform patient that they will bleed and bruise more easily and it will take longer to stop bleeding. Advise patient to notify health care professional promptly if unusual, prolonged, or excessive bleeding or blood in stool or urine occurs.
- Inform patient that ticagrelor may cause shortness of breath which usually resolved during therapy. Advise patient to notify health care professional if unexpected or severe shortness of breath or symptoms of hypersensitivity reactions occur.
- Advise patient to notify health care professional of medication regimen prior to treatment or surgery or dental procedure. Prescriber should be consulted before stopping ticagrelor.
- Instruct patient to notify health care professional of all Rx or OTC medications, vitamins, or herbal products being taken and consult health care professional before taking any new medications, especially aspirin or NSAIDs.
- Advise patient to notify health care professional if pregnancy is planned or suspected or if breast feeding.

Evaluation/Desired Outcomes

- Decreased thrombotic cardiovascular events in patients with ACS.

tigecycline (tye-gi-**sye**-kleen)

Tygacil

Classification

Therapeutic: anti-infectives

Pharmacologic: glycylcyclines

Indications

Complicated skin/skin structure infections, complicated intra-abdominal infections, or community-acquired bacterial pneumonia caused by susceptible bacteria (Should only be used when alternative treatments are not suitable; should NOT be used for diabetic foot infections).

Action

Inhibits bacterial protein synthesis by binding to the 30S ribosomal subunit. **Therapeutic Effects:** Resolution of infection. **Spectrum:** Active against the following Gram-positive bacteria: *Enterococcus faecalis* (vancomycin-susceptible strains only), *Staphylococcus aureus* (methicillin-sensitive and methicillin-resistant strains), *Streptococcus agalactiae*, *Streptococcus anginosus*, *Streptococcus pneumoniae* (penicillin-susceptible isolates), and *Streptococcus pyogenes*. Also active against these Gram-negative organisms: *Citrobacter freundii*, *Enterobacter cloacae*, *Escherichia coli*, *Haemophilus influenzae*, *Legionella pneumophila*, *Klebsiella oxytoca*, and *Klebsiella pneumoniae*. Additionally active against the following anaerobes: *Bacteroides fragilis*, *Bacteroides thetaiotaomicron*, *Bacteroides uniformis*, *Bacteroides vulgatus*, *Clostridium perfringens*, and *Peptostreptococcus micros*.

Pharmacokinetics

Absorption: IV administration results in complete bioavailability.

Distribution: Widely distributed with good penetration into gall bladder, lung, and colon; crosses the placenta.

Metabolism and Excretion: Minimal metabolism; primary route of elimination is biliary/fecal excretion of unchanged drug and metabolites (59%), 33% renal (22% unchanged).

Half-life: 27.1 hr (after 1 dose); 42.4 hr after multiple doses.

TIME/ACTION PROFILE (blood levels)

ROUTE	ONSET	PEAK	DURATION
IV	rapid	end of infusion	12 hr

Contraindications/Precautions

Contraindicated in: Hypersensitivity; Diabetic foot infections; Hospital-acquired or ventilator-associated pneumonia; Pedi: Children.

Use Cautiously in: Complicated intra-abdominal infections due to perforation; Severe hepatic impairment (↓ maintenance dose recommended); Geri: May be more sensitive to adverse effects; OB, Lactation: Use in pregnancy only when potential maternal benefit outweighs fetal risk; use cautiously during lactation.

Adverse Reactions/Side Effects

CNS: somnolence. **Derm:** STEVENS-JOHNSON SYNDROME. **GI:** PANCREATITIS, CLOSTRIDIUM DIFFICILE-ASSOCIATED DIARRHEA (CDAD), nausea, vomiting, altered taste, anorexia, dry mouth, hepatotoxicity, jaundice. **GU:** ↑ serum creatinine. **Endo:** hyperglycemia, hypoglycemia. **F and E:** hypocalcemia, hyponatremia. **Resp:** pneumonia. **Local:** injection site reactions. **Misc:** DEATH, allergic reactions.

Interactions

Drug-Drug: May ↓ the effectiveness of **hormonal contraceptives**. Effects on **warfarin** are unknown (monitoring recommended).

Route/Dosage

IV (Adults >18 yr): 100 mg initially, then 50 mg every 12 hr for 5–14 days (skin/skin structure infections and intra-abdominal infections) or 7–14 days (pneumonia).

Hepatic Impairment

IV (Adults >18 yr): *Child-Pugh C*— 100 mg initially, then 25 mg every 12 hr.

Availability (generic available)

Lyophilized powder for injection: 50 mg/vial.

NURSING IMPLICATIONS

Assessment

- Assess for infection (vital signs; appearance of wound, sputum, urine, and stool; WBC) at beginning of and throughout therapy.
- Obtain specimens for culture and sensitivity before initiating therapy. 1st dose may be given before receiving results.
- Before initiating therapy, obtain a history of tetracycline hypersensitivity; may also have an allergic response to tigecycline.
- Monitor bowel function. Diarrhea, abdominal cramping, fever, and bloody stools should be reported to health care professional promptly as a sign of Clostridium difficile-associated diarrhea (CDAD). May begin up to several wk following cessation of therapy.
- Assess patient for signs of pancreatitis (nausea, vomiting, abdominal pain, increased serum lipase or amylase) periodically during therapy. May require discontinuation of therapy.
- Assess for rash periodically during therapy. May cause Stevens-Johnson syndrome. Discontinue therapy if severe or if accompanied with fever, general malaise, fatigue, muscle or joint aches, blisters, oral lesions, conjunctivitis, hepatitis and/or eosinophilia.
- ***Lab Test Considerations:*** May cause anemia, leukocytosis, and thrombocythemia.
- May cause ↑ serum alkaline phosphatase, amylase, bilirubin, LDH, AST, and ALT.
- May cause hyperglycemia, hypokalemia, hypoproteinemia, hypocalcemia, hyponatremia, and ↑ BUN level.

Implementation

- May cause yellow-brown discoloration and softening of teeth and bones if administered prenatally or during early childhood. Not recommended for children under 8 yr of age or during pregnancy or lactation unless used for the treatment of anthrax.

IV Administration

- **Intermittent Infusion:** Reconstitute each vial with 5.3 mL of 0.9% NaCl or D5W to achieve a concentration of 10 mg/mL. ***Diluent:*** Dilute further in 100 mL of D5W, LR, or 0.9% NaCl. Reconstituted solution should be yellow to orange in color. Do not administer solutions that are discolored or contain particulate matter. Infusion is stable for up to 24 hr at room temperature or for up to 48 hr if refrigerated. ***Concentration:*** Final concentration of infusion should be ≤1 mg/mL. ***Rate:*** Infuse over 30–60 min. Flush line before and after infusion with 0.9% NaCl or D5W.
- **Y-Site Compatibility:** acetaminophen, acyclovir, alfentanil, allopurinol, amifostine, amikacin, aminocaproic acid, aminophylline, amphotericin B liposome, ampicillin, ampicillin/sulbactam, argatroban, azithromycin, aztreonam, bivalirudin, bumetanide, buprenorphine, busulfan, butorphanol, calcium chloride, calcium gluconate, carboplatin, carmustine, caspofungin, cefazolin, cefepime, cefotaxime, cefotetan, cefoxitin, ceftazidime, ceftriaxone, cefuroxime, ciprofloxacin, cisatracurium, cisplatin, clindamycin, cyclophosphamide, cyclosporine, cytarabine, dacarbazine, dactinomycin, daptomycin, daunorubicin hydrochloride, dexamethasone, dexmedetomidine, dexrazoxane, digoxin, diltiazem, diphenhydramine, dobutamine, docetaxel, dopamine, doxorubicin hydrochloride, doxorubicin liposome, droperidol, enalaprilat, epinephrine, eptifibatide, ertapenem, erythromycin, esmolol, etoposide, etoposide phosphate, famotidine, fenoldopam, fentanyl, fluconazole, fludarabine, fluorouracil, foscarnet, fosphenytoin, furosemide, ganciclovir, gemcitabine, gentamicin, glycopyrrolate, granisetron, haloperidol, heparin, hydrocortisone, hydromorphone, ifosfamide, imipenem/cilastatin, insulin, irinotecan, isoproterenol, ketorolac, labetalol, lansoprazole, leucovorin, levofloxa-

T

cin, lidocaine, linezolid, lorazepam, magnesium sulfate, mannitol, melphalan, meperidine, meropenem, mesna, methohexital, methotrexate, methyldopate, metoclopramide, metoprolol, metronidazole, midazolam, milrinone, mitomycin, mitoxantrone, morphine, moxifloxacin, mycophenolate, nafcillin, nalbuphine, naloxone, nitroglycerin, nitroprusside, norepinephrine, octreotide, ondansetron, oxaliplatin, oxytocin, paclitaxel, palonosetron, pamidronate, pancuronium, pantoprazole, pemetrexed, pemtamidine, pentobarbital, phenobarbital, phenylephrine, piperacillin/tazobactam, potassium acetate, potassium chloride, potassium phosphates, procainamide, prochlorperazine, promethazine, propofol, propranolol, ranitidine, remifentanil, rocuronium, sodium acetate, sodium bicarbonate, sodium phosphates, streptozocin, succinylcholine, sufentanil, tacrolimus, telavancin, theophylline, thiopental, thiotepa, tirofiban, tobramycin, topotecan, trimethoprim/sulfamethoxazole, vancomycin, vasopressin, vecuronium, vinblastine, vincristine, vinorelbine, zidovudine, zoledronic acid.

- **Y-Site Incompatibility:** amiodarone, amphotericin B deoxycholate, amphotericin B lipid complex, bleomycin, chloramphenicol, chlorpromazine, dantrolene, diazepam, epirubicin, esomeprazole, hydralazine, idarubicin, nicardipine, phenytoin, quinupristin/dalfopristin, verapamil.

Patient/Family Teaching

- Advise patient that full course of therapy should be completed, even if feeling better. Skipping doses or not completing full course of therapy may result in decreased effectiveness and increased risk of bacterial resistance.
- Instruct patient to notify health care professional if fever and diarrhea develop, especially if stool contains blood, pus, or mucus. Advise patient not to treat diarrhea without consulting health care professional.
- Advise patient to report the signs of superinfection (black, furry overgrowth on the tongue, vaginal itching or discharge, loose or foul-smelling stools). Skin rash, pruritus, and urticaria should also be reported.
- Instruct female patient to use a nonhormonal method of contraception while taking tigecycline and until next menstrual period. Advise patient to notify health care professional if pregnancy is planned or suspected or if breast feeding.

Evaluation/Desired Outcomes

- Resolution of signs and symptoms of infection.

tildrakizumab

(til-dra-**kiz**-ue-mab)

Ilumya

Classification

Therapeutic: antipsoriatics

Pharmacologic: interleukin antagonists, monoclonal antibodies

Indications

Moderate-to-severe plaque psoriasis in patients who are candidates for phototherapy or systemic therapy.

Action

Binds to the p19 protein subunit of the interleukin (IL)-23 cytokine to prevent its interaction with the IL-23 receptor. This cytokine is normally involved in inflammatory and immune responses. Binding to interleukins antagonizes their effects, inhibiting the release of proinflammatory cytokines and chemokines. **Therapeutic Effects:** Decrease in area and severity of psoriatic lesions.

Pharmacokinetics

Absorption: 73–80% absorbed following subcutaneous administration.

Distribution: Well distributed to tissues.

Metabolism and Excretion: Broken down by catabolic processes into peptides and amino acids.

Half-life: 23 days.

TIME/ACTION PROFILE (plasma concentrations)

ROUTE	ONSET	PEAK	DURATION
Subcut	unknown	6 days	12 wk

Contraindications/Precautions

Contraindicated in: Hypersensitivity; Active, untreated infection.

Use Cautiously in: History of tuberculosis (possibility of reactivation); OB: Use only if potential maternal benefit justifies potential risk to fetus; Lactation: Use only if potential maternal benefit justifies potential risk to fetus; Pedi: Safety and effectiveness not established.

Exercise Extreme Caution in: Chronic infection or history of recurrent infection.

Adverse Reactions/Side Effects

GI: diarrhea. **Local:** injection site reactions. **Misc:** HYPERSENSITIVITY REACTIONS (angioedema, urticaria), infection.

Interactions

Drug-Drug: May ↓ antibody response to and ↑ risk of adverse reactions from **live vaccines**; avoid use during therapy.

Route/Dosage

Subcut (Adults): 100 mg initially and 4 wk later, then 100 mg every 12 wk.

Availability

Solution for subcutaneous injection: 100 mg/mL in prefilled syringes.

NURSING IMPLICATIONS

Assessment

- Assess affected area(s) prior to and periodically during therapy.

- Assess patient for latent tuberculosis with a tuberculin skin test prior to initiation of therapy. Treatment of latent tuberculosis should be started before therapy with tildrakizumab. Monitor patients for signs and symptoms of active TB during and after therapy.
- Assess for signs of infection (fever, dyspnea, flu-like symptoms, frequent or painful urination, redness or swelling at the site of a wound), including tuberculosis, prior to injection. Monitor new infections closely; most common are upper respiratory tract infections, bronchitis, and urinary tract infections.

Implementation

- Injection should be administered by a health care professional.
- Update immunizations to current prior to initiating therapy.
- **Subcut:** Allow prefilled syringe to sit in carton at room temperature for 30 min prior to injection. Solution is clear to slightly opalescent, colorless to slightly yellow solution; do not administer solutions that are cloudy, discolored or contain particulate matter. Air bubbles in solution do not need removal; do not shake. Inject into abdomen, thigh, or upper arm. Do not inject within 2 inches of umbilicus, or into skin that is tender, bruised, erythematous, indurated, affected by psoriasis or into scars, stretch marks, or blood vessels. Follow manufacturer's directions for retractable needle syringe. Store in refrigerator in original carton until time of use; do not freeze. May be stored at room temperature in original carton for up to 30 days.

Patient/Family Teaching

- Explain purpose of tildrakizumab to patient. If a dose is missed, administer as soon as possible. Resume dosing at regularly scheduled interval. Advise patient and caregiver to read the *Medication Guide* before starting therapy and with each Rx refill in case of changes.
- Advise patient to notify health care professional if signs and symptoms of hypersensitivity reaction (feel faint, swelling of face, eyelids, lips, mouth, tongue or throat, skin rash, trouble breathing or throat tightness, chest tightness and infection (fever; sweats; chills; sore throat; cough; shortness of breath); blood in phlegm (mucus); muscle aches; warm, red, or painful skin or sores different from psoriasis; weight loss; diarrhea or stomach pain; burning during urination or urinating more often than normal) occur.
- Instruct patient to avoid receiving live vaccines during therapy.
- Instruct patient to notify health care professional of all Rx or OTC medications, vitamins, or herbal products being taken and consult health care professional before taking any new medications.
- Advise female patient to notify health care professional if pregnancy is planned or suspected or if breast feeding.

Evaluation/Desired Outcomes

- Decrease in extent and severity of psoriatic lesions.

tioconazole, See ANTIFUNGALS (VAGINAL).

tiotropium (tye-o-**trope**-ee-yum)

Spiriva, Spiriva Handihaler, Spiriva Respimat

Classification

Therapeutic: bronchodilators

Pharmacologic: anticholinergics

Indications

Long-term maintenance treatment of bronchospasm due to COPD. Reduce exacerbations in patients with COPD. Long-term maintenance treatment of asthma.

Action

Acts as anticholinergic by selectively and reversibly inhibiting M_3 receptors in smooth muscle of airways. **Therapeutic Effects:** Decreased incidence and severity of bronchospasm in COPD and asthma.

Pharmacokinetics

Absorption: *Handihaler*—19% absorbed following inhalation; *Respimat*—33% absorbed following inhalation.

Distribution: Extensive tissue distribution; due to route of administration ↑ concentrations occur in lung.

Metabolism and Excretion: 74% excreted unchanged in urine; 25% of absorbed drug is metabolized.

Half-life: 5–6 days.

TIME/ACTION PROFILE (bronchodilation)

ROUTE	ONSET	PEAK	DURATION
inhaln	rapid	5 min	24 hr

Contraindications/Precautions

Contraindicated in: Hypersensitivity to tiotropium or ipratropium; Concurrent ipratropium.

Use Cautiously in: Hypersensitivity to atropine or milk proteins; Narrow-angle glaucoma, prostatic hyperplasia, bladder neck obstruction (may worsen condition); CCr ≤60 mL/min (monitor closely); OB, Lactation: Safety not established; Pedi: Children <6 yr (safety and effectiveness not established).

Adverse Reactions/Side Effects

CV: tachycardia. **Derm:** rash. **EENT:** glaucoma. **GI:** dry mouth, constipation. **GU:** urinary difficulty, urinary

T

retention. **Resp:** paradoxical bronchospasm. **Misc:** HYPERSENSITIVITY REACTIONS (including angioedema).

Interactions

Drug-Drug: Should not be used concurrently with **ipratropium** due to risk of additive anticholinergic effects.

Route/Dosage

Inhaln (Adults): *Handihaler*—18 mcg once daily; *Respimat*—2 inhalations of 2.5 mcg once daily.
Inhaln (Adults and Children ≥6 yr): *Respimat*—2 inhalations of 1.25 mcg once daily.

Availability

Dry powder capsules for inhalation (Handihaler): 18 mcg. **Cost:** $317.33/30 capsules. **Inhalation solution (Respimat):** 1.25 mcg/inhalation in cartridge (delivers 28 or 60 metered inhalations), 2.5 mcg/inhalation in cartridge (delivers 28 or 60 metered inhalations).

NURSING IMPLICATIONS

Assessment

- **Inhaln:** Assess respiratory status (rate, breath sounds, degree of dyspnea, pulse) before administration and at peak of medication. Consult health care professional about alternative medication if severe bronchospasm is present; onset of action is too slow for patients in acute distress. If paradoxical bronchospasm (wheezing) occurs, withhold medication and notify health care professional immediately.

Implementation

- Do not confuse Spiriva (tiotropium) with Apidra (insulin glulisine) or Inspra (eplerenone).
- **Inhaln:** See Appendix D for administration of inhalation medications.

Patient/Family Teaching

- Instruct patient to take medication as directed. Capsules are for inhalation only and must not be swallowed. Take missed doses as soon as remembered unless almost time for the next dose; space remaining doses evenly during day. Do not double doses.
- Advise patient that tiotropium is not to be used for acute bronchospasm attacks, but may be continued during an acute exacerbation.
- Advise patient to notify health care professional immediately if signs and symptoms of angioedema (swelling of the lips, tongue, or throat, itching, rash) or signs of glaucoma (eye pain or discomfort, blurred vision, visual halos or colored images in association with red eyes from conjunctival congestion and corneal edema) occur.
- Caution patient to avoid spraying medication in eyes; may cause blurring of vision and pupil dilation.
- Advise patient that rinsing mouth after using inhaler, good oral hygiene, and sugarless gum or candy may minimize dry mouth; usually resolves with continued treatment.
- Instruct patient to notify health care professional of all Rx or OTC medications, vitamins, or herbal products being taken and consult health care professional before taking any new medications, including eye drops.
- Advise patient to inform health care professional if pregnancy is planned or suspected or if breast feeding.
- **Handihaler:** Instruct patient in proper use and cleaning of the Handihaler inhaler. Review the *Patient's Instructions for Use* guide with patient. Capsules should be stored in sealed blisters; remove immediately before use or effectiveness of capsules is reduced. Tear blister strip carefully to expose only one capsule at a time. Discard capsules that are inadvertently exposed to air. *Spiriva* should be administered only via the Handihaler and the Handihaler should not be used with other medications. When disposing of capsule, tiny amount of powder left in capsule is normal.
- **Respimat:** Advise patient to prime inhaler by actuating inhaler toward the ground until an aerosol cloud is visible, then repeat process 3 more times. If not used for >3 days, actuate inhaler once to prepare inhaler for use. If not used for >21 days, actuate inhaler until an aerosol cloud is visible, then repeat 3 more times to prepare inhaler for use. Discard 3 mo from 1st use.

Evaluation/Desired Outcomes

- Decreased dyspnea.
- Improved breath sounds.
- Fewer exacerbations in patients with COPD and asthma.

HIGH ALERT

tirofiban (tye-roe-**fye**-ban)

Aggrastat

Classification
Therapeutic: antiplatelet agents
Pharmacologic: glycoprotein IIb/IIIa inhibitors

Indications

To reduce the incidence of thrombotic cardiovascular events (death, MI, or refractory ischemia/repeat cardiac procedure in patients with non-ST elevation acute coronary syndrome [unstable angina/non–Q-wave MI]).

Action

Decreases platelet aggregation by reversibly antagonizing the binding of fibrinogen to the glycoprotein IIb/IIIa binding site on platelet surfaces. **Therapeutic Effects:** Inhibition of platelet aggregation resulting in decreased incidence of new MI, death, or refractory ischemia with the need for repeat cardiac procedures.

Pharmacokinetics

Absorption: IV administration results in complete bioavailability.
Distribution: Unknown.

Metabolism and Excretion: Excreted mostly unchanged by the kidneys (65%); 25% excreted unchanged in feces.
Half-life: 2 hr.

TIME/ACTION PROFILE (effects on platelet function)

ROUTE	ONSET	PEAK	DURATION
IV	rapid	30 min†	brief‡

†>90% inhibition of platelet aggregation at end of initial 30-min infusion.
‡Inhibition is reversible following cessation of infusion.

Contraindications/Precautions

Contraindicated in: Hypersensitivity; Active internal bleeding or history of bleeding within previous 30 days; History of intracranial hemorrhage, intracranial neoplasm, arteriovenous malformation or aneurysm; History of thrombocytopenia during previous tirofiban therapy; History of hemorrhagic stroke or other stroke within 30 days; Major surgical procedure or severe physical trauma within 30 days; History, symptoms, or other findings associated with aortic aneurysm; Severe hypertension (systolic BP >180 mm Hg and/or diastolic BP >110 mm Hg); Concurrent use of other glycoprotein IIb/IIIa receptor antagonists; Acute pericarditis; Lactation: Lactation.
Use Cautiously in: Platelet count <150,000/mm^3; Hemorrhagic retinopathy; Females (↑ risk of bleeding); Severe renal impairment (↓ rate of infusion if CCr ≤60 mL/min); OB: Use only if potential maternal benefit justifies potential fetal risk; Lactation: Use while breast feeding only if potential maternal benefit justifies potential risk to infant; Pedi: Safety and effectiveness not established; Geri: ↑ risk of bleeding.

Adverse Reactions/Side Effects

Noted for patients receiving heparin and aspirin in addition to tirofiban.
CNS: headache, dizziness. **CV:** bradycardia, coronary dissection, edema, vasovagal reaction. **Derm:** hives, rash, sweating. **GI:** nausea. **Hemat:** bleeding, thrombocytopenia. **MS:** leg pain. **Misc:** HYPERSENSITIVITY REACTIONS (including anaphylaxis), fever, pelvic pain.

Interactions

Drug-Drug: Concurrent use of **aspirin**, **NSAIDs**, **warfarin**, **heparin**, **heparin-like agents**, **eptifibatide**, **clopidogrel**, or **dipyridamole** may ↑ risk of bleeding, although these agents are frequently used together or in sequence. Risk of bleeding may be ↑ by concurrent use of **cefotetan valproic acid**.
Drug-Natural Products: ↑ anticoagulant effect and bleeding risk with **anise**, **arnica**, **chamomile**, **clove**, **dong quai**, **fenugreek**, **feverfew**, **garlic**, **ginger**, **ginkgo**, **Panax ginseng**, **licorice**, and others.

Route/Dosage

IV (Adults): 25 mcg/kg within 5 min, then 0.15 mcg/kg/min for up to 18 hr.

Renal Impairment

IV (Adults): *CCr ≤60 mL/min*—25 mcg/kg within 5 min then 0.075 mcg/kg/min for up to 18 hr.

Availability

Premixed infusion: 5 mg/100 mL 0.9% NaCl, 12.5 mg/250 mL 0.9% NaCl. **Solution for injection:** 250 mcg/mL.

NURSING IMPLICATIONS

Assessment

- Assess for bleeding. Most common is oozing from the arterial access site for cardiac catheterization. Arterial and venous punctures, IM injections, and use of urinary catheters, nasotracheal intubation, and nasogastric tubes should be minimized. Noncompressible sites for IV access should be avoided. If bleeding cannot be controlled with pressure, discontinue tirofiban and heparin immediately.
- During vascular access, avoid puncturing posterior wall of femoral artery. Maintain bedrest with head of bed elevated 30° and affected limb restrained in a straight position while the vascular sheath is in place. Heparin should be discontinued for 3–4 hr and activated clotting time (ACT) <180 sec or activated partial thromboplastin time (aPTT) <45 sec prior to pulling the sheath. Use compressive techniques to obtain hemostasis and monitor closely. Sheath hemostasis should be maintained for >4 hr before discharge from the hospital.
- Monitor for signs of thrombocytopenia (chills, low-grade fever) during therapy.
- ***Lab Test Considerations:*** Assess hemoglobin, hematocrit, and platelet count prior to tirofiban therapy, within 6 hr following loading infusion, and at least daily during therapy (more frequently if evidence of significant decline). May cause ↓ hemoglobin and hematocrit.
- If platelet count ↓ to <90,000/mm^3, perform additional platelet counts to rule out pseudothrombocytopenia. If thrombocytopenia is confirmed, tirofiban and heparin should be discontinued and condition monitored and treated.
- To monitor unfractionated heparin, assess aPTT 6 hr after the start of heparin infusion. Adjust heparin to maintain aPTT at approximately 2 times control.
- May cause presence of urine and fecal occult blood.

Implementation

- Do not confuse Aggrastat (tirofiban) with argatroban.
- ***High Alert:*** Use of antiplatelet medications has resulted in patient harm and/or death from internal

T

hemorrhage or intracranial bleeding. Have second practitioner independently check original order, dosage calculations, and infusion pump settings.

- Most patients receive heparin and aspirin concurrently with tirofiban.
- Do not administer solutions that are discolored or contain particulate matter. Discard unused portion.

IV Administration

- **IV Push:** Withdraw bolus dose from 15 mL premixed bolus vial into a syringe; may also be administered from the 100 mL premixed vial or from the 250 mL premixed bag. Do not dilute. Administer within 5 min via syringe or IV pump. Immediately following bolus dose, administer maintenance infusion from the 100 mL premixed vial or 250 mL premixed bag via an IV pump. Discard any unused portion left in the vial or bag.
- **Intermittent Infusion:** ***Diluent:*** Tirofiban injection premix is ready for administration and dose not require any further dilution. ***Concentration:*** 50 mcg/mL. ***Rate:*** Based on patient's weight (see Route/Dosage section).
- **Y-Site Compatibility:** acyclovir, alfentanil, allopurinol, amifostine, amikacin, aminocaproic acid, aminophylline, amiodarone, ampicillin, ampicillin/sulbactam, anidulafungin, argatroban, arsenic trioxide, atropine, azithromycin, aztreonam, bivalirudin, bleomycin, bumetanide, buprenorphine, busulfan, butorphanol, calcium chloride, calcium gluconate, cangrelor, capreomycin, carboplatin, carmustine, caspofungin, cefazolin, cefepime, cefotaxime, cefotetan, cefoxitin, ceftazidime, ceftriaxone, cefuroxime, chloramphenicol, chlorpromazine, ciprofloxacin, cisatracurium, cisplatin, clindamycin, cyclophosphamide, cyclosporine, cytarabine, dacarbazine, dactinomycin, daptomycin, dexamethasone, dexmedetomidine, dexrazoxane, digoxin, diltiazem, diphenhydramine, dobutamine, docetaxel, dopamine, doxorubicin hydrochloride, doxorubicin liposomal, doxycycline, droperidol, enalaprilat, ephedrine, epinephrine, epirubicin, ertapenem, erythromycin, esmolol, etoposide, etoposide phosphate, famotidine, fenoldopam, fentanyl, fluconazole, fludarabine, fluorouracil, foscarnet, fosphenytoin, furosemide, ganciclovir, gemcitabine, gentamicin, glycopyrrolate, granisetron, haloperidol, heparin, hydralazine, hydrocortisone, hydromorphone, idarubicin, ifosfamide, imipenem/cilastatin, insulin, regular, irinotecan, isoproterenol, ketorolac, labetalol, leucovorin calcium, levofloxacin, lidocaine, linezolid, lorazepam, magnesium sulfate, mannitol, melphalan, meperidine, meropenem, mesna, methotrexate, methyldopate, methylprednisolone, metoclopramide, metoprolol, metronidazole, midazolam, milrinone, mitomycin, mitoxantrone, morphine, moxifloxacin, mycophenolate, nafcillin, nalbuphine, naloxone, nicardipine, nitroglycerin, nitroprusside, norepinephrine, octreotide, ondansetron, oxaliplatin, oxytocin, paclitaxel, palonosetron, pamidronate, pancuronium, pantoprazole, pemetrexed, pentobarbital, phenobarbital, phenylephrine, piperacillin/tazobactam, potassium acetate, potassium chloride, potassium phosphates, procainamide, prochlorperazine, promethazine, propranolol, quinupristin/dalfopristin, ranitidine, remifentanil, rocuronium, sodium acetate, sodium bicarbonate, sodium phosphates, streptozocin, succinylcholine, sufentanil, tacrolimus, theophylline, thiopental, thiotepa, tigecycline, tobramycin, topotecan, vancomycin, vasopressin, vecuronium, verapamil, vinblastine, vincristine, vinorelbine, voriconazole, zidovudine, zoledronic acid.
- **Y-Site Incompatibility:** amphotericin B lipid complex, dantrolene, diazepam, phenytoin.

Patient/Family Teaching

- Inform patient of the purpose of tirofiban.
- Instruct patient to notify health care professional immediately if any bleeding is noted.
- Instruct patient to notify health care professional of all Rx or OTC medications, vitamins, or herbal products being taken and consult health care professional before taking any new medications.
- Advise females of reproductive potential to notify health care professional if pregnancy is planned or suspected, or if breast feeding.

Evaluation/Desired Outcomes

- Inhibition of platelet aggregation resulting in decreased incidence of new MI, death, or refractory ischemia with the need for repeat cardiac procedures.

tobramycin, See AMINOGLYCOSIDES.

tocilizumab (toe-si-**liz**-oo-mab)

Actemra

Classification

Therapeutic: antirheumatics, immunosuppressants

Pharmacologic: interleukin antagonists

Indications

Treatment of adults with moderately- to severely-active rheumatoid arthritis who have not responded to one or more disease-modifying antirheumatic drugs [DMARDs] (as monotherapy or with methotrexate or other non-biologic DMARDs). Active systemic juvenile idiopathic arthritis (as monotherapy or with methotrexate). Active polyarticular juvenile idiopathic arthritis (as monotherapy or with methotrexate). Giant cell arteritis. Chimeric antigen receptor (CAR) T cell-induced severe or life-threatening cytokine release syndrome.

Action

Acts as in inhibitor of interleukin-6 (IL-6) receptors by binding to them. IL-6 is a mediator of various inflammatory processes. **Therapeutic Effects:** Slowed progression of rheumatoid arthritis, systemic/polyarticular juvenile idiopathic arthritis, giant cell arteritis. Resolution of cytokine release syndrome.

Pharmacokinetics

Absorption: IV administration results in complete bioavailability; 80% absorbed following subcut administration.
Distribution: Unknown.
Metabolism and Excretion: Unknown.
Half-life: *4 mg/kg dose*—up to 11 days; *8 mg/kg*—up to 13 days.

TIME/ACTION PROFILE (improvement)

ROUTE	ONSET	PEAK	DURATION
IV	within 1 mo	4 mo	unknown
Subcut	unknown	unknown	unknown

Contraindications/Precautions

Contraindicated in: Hypersensitivity; Serious infections; Active hepatic disease/impairment; Absolute neutrophil count (ANC) <2000/mm³ (<500/mm³ while on therapy) or platelet count below 100,000/mm³ (<50,000/mm³ while on therapy); Lactation: Not recommended.
Use Cautiously in: Patients at risk for GI perforation, including patients with diverticulitis; Renal or hepatic impairment; Concurrent use of other hepatotoxic medications (↑ risk of hepatotoxicity); Patients with tuberculosis risk factors; Geri: ↑ risk of adverse reactions; OB: Use only if potential benefit justifies potential risk to fetus; Pedi: Children <2 yr (safety not established).

Adverse Reactions/Side Effects

CNS: headache, dizziness. **CV:** hypertension. **Derm:** STEVENS-JOHNSON SYNDROME, rash. **EENT:** nasopharyngitis. **GI:** GASTROINTESTINAL PERFORATION, HEPATOTOXICITY, ↑ liver enzymes. **Hemat:** NEUTROPENIA, THROMBOCYTOPENIA. **Metab:** ↑ lipids. **Resp:** upper respiratory tract infections. **Misc:** HYPERSENSITIVITY REACTIONS (including anaphylaxis), INFECTION (including tuberculosis, disseminated fungal infections and infections with opportunistic pathogens), infusion reactions.

Interactions

Drug-Drug: May alter the activity of CYP450 enzymes; the effects of the following drugs should be monitored: **cyclosporine**, **theophylline**, **warfarin**, **hormonal contraceptives**, **atorvastatin** and **lovastatin**. Other drugs which are substrates for this system should also be monitored; effect may persist for several wk after discontinuation. Concurrent use of other hepatotoxic medications, including **methotrexate**, may ↑ risk of hepatotoxicity. May ↓ antibody response to and ↑ risk of adverse reactions to **live virus vaccines**; do not administer concurrently.

Route/Dosage

Rheumatoid Arthritis

IV (Adults): 4 mg/kg every 4 wk; may ↑ to 8 mg/kg every 4 wk based on clinical response.
Subcut (Adults ≥100 kg): 162 mg once weekly.
Subcut (Adults <100 kg): 162 mg every 2 wk, may ↑ to every wk based on clinical response.

Systemic Juvenile Idiopathic Arthritis

IV (Children ≥2 yr and ≥30 kg): 8 mg/kg every 2 wk.
IV (Children ≥2 yr and <30 kg): 12 mg/kg every 2 wk.
Subcut (Children ≥2 yr and ≥30 kg): 162 mg once weekly.
Subcut (Children ≥2 yr and <30 kg): 162 mg every 2 wk.

Polyarticular Juvenile Idiopathic Arthritis

IV (Children ≥2 yr and ≥30 kg): 8 mg/kg every 4 wk.
IV (Children ≥2 yr and <30 kg): 10 mg/kg every 4 wk.
Subcut (Children ≥2 yr and ≥30 kg): 162 mg every 2 wk.
Subcut (Children ≥2 yr and <30 kg): 162 mg every 3 wk.

Giant Cell Arteritis

Subcut (Adults): 162 mg once weekly (with a tapering course of corticosteroids); may also consider giving 162 mg every 2 wk (with a tapering course of corticosteroids) based on clinical response.

Cytokine Release Syndrome

IV (Adults and Children ≥2 yr and ≥30 kg): 8 mg/kg (max = 800 mg/dose) initially; if patient does not clinically improve after initial dose, up to 3 additional doses may be administered every 8 hr.
IV (Adults and Children ≥2 yr and <30 kg): 12 mg/kg initially; if patient does not clinically improve after initial dose, up to 3 additional doses may be administered every 8 hr.

Availability

Solution for intravenous injection: 20 mg/mL. **Solution for subcutaneous injection (autoinjectors or prefilled syringes):** 162 mg/0.9 mL.

NURSING IMPLICATIONS

Assessment

- Assess pain and range of motion before and periodically during therapy.
- Assess for signs of infection (fever, dyspnea, flu-like symptoms, frequent or painful urination, redness or swelling at the site of a wound), including tuberculo-

T

sis, prior to injection. Tocilizumab is contraindicated in patients with active infection. Monitor new infections closely; most common are upper respiratory tract infections, bronchitis, and urinary tract infections. Signs and symptoms of inflammation may be lessened due to suppression from tocilizumab. Infections may be fatal, especially in patients taking immunosuppressive therapy. If patient develops a serious infection, discontinue tocilizumab until infection is controlled.

- Monitor for injection site reactions (redness and/or itching, rash, hemorrhage, bruising, pain, or swelling). Rash will usually disappear within a few days. Application of a towel soaked in cold water may relieve pain or swelling.
- Monitor patient for signs of anaphylaxis (urticaria, dyspnea, facial edema) following injection. Medications (antihistamines, corticosteroids, epinephrine) and equipment should be readily available in the event of a severe reaction. Discontinue tocilizumab immediately if anaphylaxis or other severe allergic reaction occurs.
- Assess patient for latent tuberculosis with a tuberculin skin test prior to initiation of therapy. Treatment of latent tuberculosis should be started before therapy with tocilizumab.
- Assess for signs and symptoms of systemic fungal infections (fever, malaise, weight loss, sweats, cough, dypsnea, pulmonary infiltrates, serious systemic illness with or without concomitant shock). Ascertain if patient lives in or has traveled to areas of endemic mycoses. Consider empiric antifungal treatment for patients at risk of histoplasmosis and other invasive fungal infections until the pathogens are identified. Consult with an infectious diseases specialist. Consider stopping tocilizumab until the infection has been diagnosed and adequately treated.
- ***Lab Test Considerations:*** Assess CBC with platelet count prior to initiating therapy and after 4–8 wk, then every 3 mo during therapy. Do not administer tocilizumab to patients with an ANC <2000/mm^3, platelet count <100,000/mm^3, or ALT or AST above 1.5 times the upper limit of normal (ULN).
- *If ANC >1000/mm^3*, maintain dose. *If ANC 500–1000/mm^3*, interrupt IV tocilizumab until ANC >1000/mm^3, then resume at 4 mg/kg and ↑ to 8 mg/kg as clinically appropriate or reduce subcut tocilizumab to every other wk and increase frequency to every wk as clinically appropriate. *If ANC <500/mm^3*, discontinue tocilizumab.
- *If platelet count 50,000–100,000/mm^3*, interrupt dosing until platelet count is >100,000/mm^3 then resume IV dosing at 4 mg/kg and ↑ to 8 mg/kg as clinically appropriate or reduce subcut tocilizumab to every other wk and increase frequency to every wk as clinically appropriate. *If platelet count is <50,000/mm^3*, discontinue tocilizumab.
- **For rheumatoid arthritis and giant cell arteritis,** obtain liver test panel (serum alanine aminotransferase [ALT], aspartate aminotransferase [AST], alkaline phosphatase, and total bilirubin before starting therapy, every 4–8 wk after start of therapy for first 6 mo and every 3 mo thereafter. *If liver enzymes persistently* ↑ *>1–3 × ULN,* reduce IV tocilizumab dose to 4 mg/kg and reduce subcut injection to every other wk or interrupt until AST/ALT have normalized. *If >3–5 × ULN* (confirmed by repeat testing), interrupt tocilizumab until <3 × ULN and follow recommendations for ↑ >1–3 × ULN. *If persistent* ↑ *>1–3 × ULN or >5 × ULN*, discontinue tocilizumab. **For Systemic Juvenile Idiopathic Arthritis (SJIA) and Polyarticular Juvenile Idiopathic Arthritis (PJIA),** Monitor liver test panel at the time of the 2nd administration and thereafter every 4–8 wk for PJIA and every 2 to 4 wk for SJIA.
- Monitor lipid levels after 4–8 wk of therapy, then follow clinical guidelines for management of hyperlipidemia. May cause ↑ total cholesterol, triglycerides, LDL cholesterol, and/or HDL cholesterol.

Implementation

- Administer a tuberculin skin test prior to administration of tocilizumab. Patients with latent TB should be treated for TB prior to therapy.
- Immunizations should be current prior to initiating therapy. Patients on tocilizumab may receive concurrent vaccinations, except for live vaccines.
- Do not administer solutions that are discolored or contain particulate matter. Discard unused solution.
- Other DMARDs should be continued during tocilizumab therapy.
- **Children:** Do not change dose based on single visit weight; weight fluctuates.
- To switch from IV to Subcut, administer next dose Subcut instead of IV.
- **Subcut:** Only for adult patients with RA. Solution is clear and colorless to pale yellow; do not administer solutions that are discolored or contain particulate matter. Rotate injection sites; avoid sites with moles, scars, areas where skin is tender, bruised, red, hard, or not intact.

IV Administration

- **Intermittent Infusion: *Diluent:*** Withdraw volume of 0.9% NaCl or 0.45% NaCl from a 100 mL bag (50 mL bag for children <30 kg) equal to volume of solution required for patient's dose. Slowly add tocilizumab from each vial to infusion bag. Invert slowly to mix; avoid foaming. Do not infuse solutions that are discolored or contain particulate matter. Diluted solution is stable for 24 hr if refrigerated or at room temperature; protect from light. Allow solution to reach room temperature before infusing. ***Rate:*** Infuse over 60 min. Do not administer via IV push or bolus.
- **Y-Site Incompatibility:** Do not infuse concomitantly in the same line with other drugs.

Patient/Family Teaching

- Instruct patient on the purpose for tocilizumab. If a dose is missed, contact health care professional to schedule next infusion. Instruct patient and caregiver in correct technique for subcut injections and care and disposal of equipment.

- Caution patient to notify health care professional immediately if signs of infection (fever, sweating, chills, muscle aches, cough, shortness of breath, blood in phlegm, weight loss, warm, red or painful skin or sores, diarrhea or stomach pain, burning on urination, urinary frequency, feeling tired), fever and stomach-area pain that does not go away, change bowel habits, severe rash, swollen face, or difficulty breathing occurs while taking. If signs and symptoms of anaphylaxis occur, discontinue injections and notify health care professional immediately.
- Instruct patient to notify health care professional of all Rx or OTC medications, vitamins, or herbal products being taken and consult health care professional before taking any new medications.
- Instruct patient to notify health care professional of medication regimen prior to treatment or surgery.
- Rep: Advise female patients to notify health care professional if pregnancy is planned or suspected, or if breast feeding. Pregnant women should be encouraged to participate in the pregnancy registry to monitor pregnancy outcomes by calling 1-877-311-8972.

Evaluation/Desired Outcomes

- Decreased pain and swelling with decreased rate of joint destruction in patients with rheumatoid arthritis, systemic idiopathic juvenile arthritis, polyarticular juvenile idiopathic arthritis, or giant cell arteritis.

ⵗ **tofacitinib** (toe-fa-**sye**-ti-nib)

Xeljanz, Xeljanz XR

Classification

Therapeutic: antirheumatics

Pharmacologic: kinase inhibitors

Indications

Moderately to severely active rheumatoid arthritis (RA) in patients who have had an inadequate response/intolerance to methotrexate (as monotherapy or in combination with methotrexate or other nonbiologic disease-modifying antirheumatic drugs [DMARDs]) (not to be used with biologic DMARDs or potent immunosuppressants including azathioprine and cyclosporine) (immediate-release and extended-release). Active psoriatic arthritis in patients who have had an inadequate response/intolerance to methotrexate or other DMARDs (in combination with other nonbiologic DMARDs) (not to be used with biologic DMARDs or potent immunosuppressants including azathioprine and cyclosporine) (immediate-release and extended-release). Moderately-to-severely active ulcerative colitis in patients who have had an inadequate response/intolerance to tumor necrosis factor inhibitors (not to be used with biologic therapies or potent immunosuppressants including azathioprine and cyclosporine) (immediate-release only).

Action

Acts as a Janus kinase (JAK) inhibitor. Some results of inhibition include decreased hematopoiesis and immune cell function. Decreases circulating killer cells, increases in B cell count and decreases serum C-reactive protein (CRP). **Therapeutic Effects:** Improvement in clinical and symptomatic parameters of RA, psoriatic arthritis, and ulcerative colitis.

Pharmacokinetics

Absorption: Well absorbed following oral administration (74%).

Distribution: Distributes equally between red blood cells and plasma.

Metabolism and Excretion: 70% metabolized by the liver (primarily CYP3A4 with some contribution from CYP2C19). 30% renal excretion of the parent drug.

Half-life: 3 hr.

TIME/ACTION PROFILE (clinical improvement)

ROUTE	ONSET	PEAK	DURATION
PO	within 2 wk	3 mo	unknown
PO-ER	unknown	unknown	unknown

Contraindications/Precautions

Contraindicated in: Active infection; Administration of live vaccines; Severe hepatic impairment; Increased risk for thrombosis; Lymphocyte count <500 cells/mm^3, absolute neutrophil count (ANC) <1000 cells/mm^3, or hemoglobin levels <9 g/dL; Lactation: Lactation.

Use Cautiously in: Patients with RA who are >50 yr old and have ≥1 cardiovascular risk factor (↑ risk of mortality and thrombosis with use of higher than recommended doses for RA); Risk of GI perforation; Chronic lung disease (↑ risk of infection); ⵗ Japanese patients (↑ risk of herpes zoster); Geri: Infection risk may be ↑ OB: Use during pregnancy only if potential benefit justifies potential fetal risk; Pedi: Safety and effectiveness not established.

Adverse Reactions/Side Effects

CNS: fatigue, headache, insomnia. **CV:** ARTERIAL THROMBOSIS, DEEP VEIN THROMBOSIS, peripheral edema. **Derm:** erythema, pruritus, rash. **F and E:** dehydration. **GI:** GI PERFORATION, abdominal pain, diarrhea, dyspepsia, gastritis, ↑ liver enzymes, vomiting. **GU:** ↑ serum creatinine. **Hemat:** anemia, neutropenia. **Metab:** ↑ lipids. **MS:** arthralgia, joint swelling, musculoskeletal pain, tendonitis. **Neuro:** paresthesia. **Resp:** PULMONARY EMBOLISM. **Misc:** DEATH, HYPERSENSITIVITY REACTIONS (including angioedema and urticaria), INFECTION (including tuberculosis, bacterial, invasive fungal infections, viral, and other infections due to opportunistic pathogens), MALIGNANCY, fever.

Interactions

Drug-Drug: May ↑ risk of adverse reactions and ↓ antibody response to **live vaccines**; avoid concurrent use. Blood levels and effects may be ↑ by **strong CYP3A4 inhibitors** including **ketoconazole** or **moderate CYP3A4 inhibitors/strong CYP2C19 inhibitors** including **fluconazole**; dose ↓ recommended. Blood levels and effectiveness may be ↓ **strong CYP3A4 inducers** including **rifampin**; avoid concurrent use. ↑ risk of immunosuppression when used concurrently with other potent **immunosuppressants** including **azathioprine**, **cyclosporine**, **tacrolimus**, **antineoplastics**, or **radiation therapy**.

Route/Dosage

RA and Psoriatic Arthritis

PO (Adults): *Immediate-release*—5 mg twice daily; *Extended-release*—11 mg once daily; *Concurrent use of strong CYP3A4 inhibitors or concurrent use of moderate CYP3A4 inhibitor with a strong CYP2C19 inhibitor*—5 mg once daily (immediate-release); if previously taking extended-release tofacitinib, then switch to immediate-release tofacitinib 5 mg once daily.

Renal Impairment

PO (Adults): *Moderate or severe renal impairment*—5 mg once daily (immediate-release); if previously taking extended-release tofacitinib, then switch to immediate-release tofacitinib 5 mg once daily; for patients undergoing hemodialysis administer dose after dialysis session.

Hepatic Impairment

PO (Adults): *Moderate hepatic impairment*—5 mg once daily (immediate-release); if previously taking extended-release tofacitinib, then switch to immediate-release tofacitinib 5 mg once daily.

Ulcerative Colitis

PO (Adults): *Immediate-release*—Induction: 10 mg twice daily for 8 wk; based on therapeutic response, may transition to maintenance dose or continue 10 mg twice daily for an additional 8 wk. Discontinue therapy if inadequate response achieved after 16 wk using 10 mg twice daily. Maintenance: 5 mg twice daily; if patient experiences loss of response on 5 mg twice daily, then use 10 mg twice daily after assessing the benefits and risks and use for the shortest duration; use lowest effective dose to maintain response; *Concurrent use of strong CYP3A4 inhibitors or concurrent use of moderate CYP3A4 inhibitor with a strong CYP2C19 inhibitor*—if taking 10 mg twice daily, ↓ to 5 mg twice daily (immediate-release); if taking 5 mg twice daily, ↓ to 5 mg once daily (immediate-release).

Renal Impairment

PO (Adults): *Moderate or severe renal impairment*—if taking 10 mg twice daily, ↓ to 5 mg twice daily (immediate-release); if taking 5 mg twice daily, ↓ to 5 mg once daily (immediate-release).

Hepatic Impairment

PO (Adults): *Moderate hepatic impairment*—if taking 10 mg twice daily, ↓ to 5 mg twice daily (immediate-release); if taking 5 mg twice daily, ↓ to 5 mg once daily (immediate-release).

Availability

Extended-release tablets: 11 mg. **Tablets:** 5 mg, 10 mg.

NURSING IMPLICATIONS

Assessment

- Assess pain and range of motion before and periodically during therapy.
- Assess for signs of infection (fever, dyspnea, flu-like symptoms, frequent or painful urination, redness or swelling at the site of a wound), including tuberculosis, prior to and periodically during therapy. Tofacitinib is contraindicated in patients with active infection. New infections should be monitored closely; most common are pneumonia, cellulitis, herpes zoster, urinary tract infection, diverticulitis, and appendicitis. Infections may be fatal, especially in patients taking immunosuppressive therapy.
- Assess for signs and symptoms of systemic fungal infections (fever, malaise, weight loss, sweats, cough, dypsnea, pulmonary infiltrates, serious systemic illness with or without concomitant shock). Ascertain if patient lives in or has traveled to areas of endemic mycoses. Consider empiric antifungal treatment for patients at risk of histoplasmosis and other invasive fungal infections until the pathogens are identified. Consult with an infectious diseases specialist. Consider stopping tofacitinib until the infection has been diagnosed and adequately treated.
- Assess patient for latent tuberculosis with a tuberculin skin test prior to initiation of therapy. Treatment of latent tuberculosis should be started before therapy with tofacitinib.
- ***Lab Test Considerations:*** Monitor CBC prior to and periodically during therapy. Do not initiate tofacitinib in patients with lymphocyte count <500 cells/mm³, an ANC <1000 cells/mm³, or who have hemoglobin level <9 g/dL.
- Monitor lymphocyte count at baseline and every 3 mo thereafter. *If lymphocyte count ≥500 cells/mm³* maintain dose. *If lymphocyte count <500 cells/mm³ and confirmed by repeat testing,* discontinue tofacitinib.
- Monitor neutrophil count at baseline, after 4–8 wk of therapy, and every 3 mo thereafter. *If ANC >1000 cells/mm³*, maintain dose. *If ANC 500–1000 cells/mm³*, for persistent decreases in this range, interrupt dosing until ANC is >1000 cells/mm³. *If ANC <500 cells/mm³ and confirmed by repeat testing,* discontinue tofacitinib.

- Monitor hemoglobin at baseline, after 4–8 wk of therapy, and every 3 mo thereafter. *If hemoglobin ≤2 g/dL decrease and ≥9.0 g/dL and confirmed by repeat testing*, maintain dose. *If hemoglobin >2 dL decrease and <8.0 g/dL*, interrupt administration of tofacitinib until hemoglobin values have normalized.
- Monitor liver enzymes prior to and periodically during therapy.
- Monitor total cholesterol, LDL cholesterol, HDL cholesterol 4–8 wk following initiation of therapy.

Implementation

- Administer a tuberculin skin test prior to administration of tofacitinib. Patients with active latent TB should be treated for TB prior to therapy.
- Immunizations should be current prior to initiating therapy. Patients on tofacitinib should not receive live vaccines.
- Screen patient for viral hepatitis before starting therapy.
- *To switch from immediate release to extended release,* patients treated with *Xeljanz* 5 mg twice daily may be switched to *Xeljanz XR* 11 mg once daily the day following the last dose of *Xeljanz* 5 mg.
- **PO:** Administer twice daily without regard to food. Swallow extended release tablets whole; do not crush, break, or chew.

Patient/Family Teaching

- Instruct patient to take tofacitinib as directed. Advise patient to read Medication Guide before starting and with each Rx refill in case of changes.
- Caution patient to notify health care professional immediately if signs of infection (fever, sweating, chills, muscle aches, cough, shortness of breath, blood in phlegm, weight loss, warm, red, or painful skin or sores, diarrhea or stomach pain, burning on urination or urinating more often than normal, feeling very tired) or stomach or intestinal perforation (fever, stomach-area pain that does not go away, change in bowel habits) occur.
- Advise patient to notify health care professional of all Rx or OTC medications, vitamins, or herbal products being taken and to consult with health care professional before taking other medications.
- Instruct patient to notify health care professional of medication regimen prior to treatment or surgery.
- Inform patient of increased risk of lymphoma and other cancers. Advise patient to have periodic skin exams for new lesions of skin cancer.
- Rep: Advise female patients to notify health care professional if pregnancy is planned or suspected and to avoid breast feeding during therapy. Encourage patients who become pregnant during therapy to enroll in the pregnancy registry to monitor pregnancy outcomes by calling 1-877-311-8972.
- Emphasize the importance of follow-up lab tests to monitor for adverse reactions.

Evaluation/Desired Outcomes

- Decreased pain and swelling with improved physical functioning and decreased rate of joint destruction in patients with rheumatoid arthritis.

tolcapone (tole-ka-pone)

Tasmar

Classification
Therapeutic: antiparkinson agents
Pharmacologic: catechol-*O*-methyltransferase inhibitors

Indications

Management of Parkinson's disease with carbidopa/levodopa in patients without severe movement abnormalities who do not respond to other treatment.

Action

Acts as a selective and reversible inhibitor of the enzyme catechol-*O*-methyltransferase. Inhibition of this enzyme prevents the breakdown of levodopa, greatly increasing its availability to the CNS. **Therapeutic Effects:** Prolongs duration of response to levodopa without end-of-dose motor fluctuations. Decreased signs and symptoms of Parkinson's disease.

Pharmacokinetics

Absorption: Rapidly absorbed following oral administration with 65% bioavailability.
Distribution: Unknown.
Protein Binding: >99% bound to plasma proteins.
Metabolism and Excretion: Mostly metabolized by the liver; <0.5% excreted unchanged in urine.
Half-life: 2–3 hr.

TIME/ACTION PROFILE (blood levels)

ROUTE	ONSET	PEAK	DURATION
PO	unknown	1.7 hr	8 hr

Contraindications/Precautions

Contraindicated in: Hypersensitivity; Concurrent MAO inhibitor therapy; Clinical evidence of liver disease.
Use Cautiously in: Severe renal impairment (safety not established if CCr <25 mL/min); OB: Lactation: Safety not established.

Adverse Reactions/Side Effects

CNS: headache, sleep disorder, hallucinations, syncope, urges (gambling, sexual). **CV:** orthostatic hypotension. **GI:** HEPATOTOXICITY, constipation, diarrhea, anorexia, ↑ liver enzymes, nausea, vomiting. **GU:** hematuria, yellow discoloration of urine. **Derm:** ↑ sweating, melanoma. **Neuro:** dyskinesia, dystonia.

Interactions

Drug-Drug: Concurrent use with **MAO inhibitors** is not recommended; both agents inhibit the metabolic pathways of catecholamines. May ↑ the effects of **methyldopa**, **apomorphine**, **dobutamine**, or **isoproterenol**; dose reduction may be necessary. ↑ the bioavailability of **levodopa** by two-fold; this is a desired effect.

Route/Dosage

PO (Adults): 100 mg 3 times daily; may cautiously ↑ to 200 mg 3 times daily if benefit is justified.

Availability (generic available)

Tablets: 100 mg.

NURSING IMPLICATIONS

Assessment

- Assess patient for signs and symptoms of Parkinson's disease (tremor, muscle weakness and rigidity, ataxic gait) prior to and throughout therapy.
- Assess BP periodically during therapy.
- Monitor for signs and symptoms of liver dysfunction (persistent nausea, fatigue, lethargy, anorexia, jaundice, dark urine, pruritus, right upper quadrant tenderness) periodically during therapy.
- ***Lab Test Considerations:*** Monitor liver function tests before every 2–4 wk for the first 6 mo following initiation or dose increase and periodically thereafter. Discontinue tolcapone if liver function tests reach two times the upper limit of normal or if jaundice occurs; do not reinstate.

Implementation

- **PO:** Administer 1st dose of the day of tolcapone together with carbidopa/levodopa. Administer subsequent doses 6 and 12 hr later.
- May be administered without regard to food.

Patient/Family Teaching

- Instruct patient to take medication as directed. Caution patient not to discontinue tolcapone without consulting health care professional. Abrupt discontinuation or rapid dose reduction may result in neuroleptic malignant syndrome (↑ temperature, muscular rigidity, altered consciousness).
- Caution patient to make position changes slowly to minimize orthostatic hypotension, especially at the beginning of therapy.
- May affect mental and/or motor performance. Caution patient to avoid driving or other activities requiring alertness until response to medication is known.
- Advise patient to avoid taking alcohol or other CNS depressants concurrently with tolcapone.
- Inform patient and caregiver that hallucinations, nausea, dyskinesia, or dystonia may occur during tolcapone therapy.
- Instruct patient to notify health care professional if persistent diarrhea occurs.
- Advise patient to notify health care professional if symptoms of liver failure (clay-colored stools, jaundice, fatigue, loss of appetite, lethargy), suspicious or unusual skin changes, hallucinations, or new or increased gambling, sexual, or other intense urges occur.
- Advise patient to notify health care professional if pregnancy is planned or suspected.
- Emphasize the importance of routine follow-up exams.

Evaluation/Desired Outcomes

- Decrease in signs and symptoms of Parkinson's disease.

tolnaftate, See ANTIFUNGALS (TOPICAL).

tolterodine (tol-ter-oh-deen)

Detrol, Detrol LA

Classification

Therapeutic: urinary tract antispasmodics

Pharmacologic: anticholinergics

Indications

Treatment of overactive bladder function that results in urinary frequency, urgency, or urge incontinence.

Action

Acts as a competitive muscarinic receptor antagonist resulting in inhibition of cholinergically mediated bladder contraction. **Therapeutic Effects:** Decreased urinary frequency, urgency, and urge incontinence.

Pharmacokinetics

Absorption: Well absorbed (77%) following oral administration.

Distribution: Unknown.

Protein Binding: 96.3%.

Metabolism and Excretion: Extensively metabolized by the liver (primarily by CYP2D6 isoenzyme) (the CYP2D6 enzyme system exhibits genetic polymorphism; ~7% of population may be poor metabolizers and may have significantly ↑ tolterodine concentrations and an ↑ risk of adverse effects); one metabolite (5-hydroxymethyltolterodine) is active; other metabolites are excreted in urine.

Half-life: *Tolterodine*—1.9–3.7 hr; *5-hydroxymethyltolterodine*—2.9–3.1 hr.

TIME/ACTION PROFILE (effects on bladder function)

ROUTE	ONSET	PEAK	DURATION
PO	unknown	unknown	12 hr

Contraindications/Precautions

Contraindicated in: Hypersensitivty to tolterodine or fesoterodine; Urinary retention; Gastric retention;

Severe hepatic impairment; End-stage renal disease (CCr <10 mL/min); Uncontrolled angle-closure glaucoma; Lactation: Lactation.

Use Cautiously in: GI obstructive disorders, including pyloric stenosis (↑ risk of gastric retention); Significant bladder outflow obstruction (↑ risk of urinary retention); Controlled angle-closure glaucoma; Myasthenia gravis; Mild-to-moderate hepatic impairment (↓ dose); Severe renal impairment (CCr 10–30 mL/min) (↓ dose); OB: Use only if potential maternal benefit justifies potential fetal risk; Pedi: Safety and effectiveness not established.

Adverse Reactions/Side Effects

CNS: headache, dizziness, sedation. **Derm:** STEVENS-JOHNSON SYNDROME. **EENT:** blurred vision, dry eyes. **GI:** dry mouth, constipation, dyspepsia. **Misc:** HYPERSENSITIVITY REACTIONS (including anaphylaxis and angioedema).

Interactions

Drug-Drug: Strong CYP3A4 inhibitors, including **Erythromycin**, **clarithromycin**, **cyclosporine**, **itraconazole**, **ketoconazole**, and **vinblastine** may ↑ levels and risk of toxicity.

Route/Dosage

Immediate-Release Tablets

PO (Adults): 2 mg twice daily; may be lowered depending on response; *Concurrent use of strong CYP3A4 inhibitors*—1 mg twice daily.

Hepatic/Renal Impairment

PO (Adults): *Mild-to-moderate hepatic impairment (Child-Pugh Class A or B) or severe renal impairment (CCr 10–30 mL/min)*—1 mg twice daily.

Extended-Release Capsules

PO (Adults): 4 mg once daily; may be lowered depending on response; *Concurrent use of strong CYP3A4 inhibitors*—2 mg once daily.

Hepatic/Renal Impairment

PO (Adults): *Mild-to-moderate hepatic impairment (Child-Pugh Class A or B) or severe renal impairment (CCr 10–30 mL/min)*—2 mg once daily.

Availability (generic available)

Extended-release capsules: 2 mg, 4 mg. **Cost:** 2 mg $458.03/60, 4 mg $447.85/60. **Tablets:** 1 mg, 2 mg. **Cost:** *Generic*—1 mg $198.55/60, 2 mg $203.79/60.

NURSING IMPLICATIONS

Assessment

- Assess patient for urinary urgency, frequency, and urge incontinence periodically during therapy.
- Monitor for signs and symptoms of anaphylaxis and angioedema (difficulty breathing, upper airway obstruction, fall in BP, rash, swelling of face or neck). Have emergency equipment readily available.
- Assess for rash periodically during therapy. May cause Stevens-Johnson syndrome or toxic epidermal necrolysis. Discontinue therapy if severe or if accompanied with fever, general malaise, fatigue, muscle or joint aches, blisters, oral lesions, conjunctivitis, hepatitis and/or eosinophilia.

Implementation

- **PO:** Administer without regard to food.
- Extended-release capsules should be swallowed whole; do not open, crush, dissolve, or chew.

Patient/Family Teaching

- Instruct patient to take tolterodine as directed.
- May cause dizziness and blurred vision. Caution patient to avoid driving or other activities requiring alertness until response to medication is known.
- Instruct patient to notify health care professional immediately if rash or signs and symptoms of anaphylaxis or angioedema occur.
- Advise patient to notify health care professional if pregnancy is planned or suspected, or if breast feeding.

Evaluation/Desired Outcomes

- Decreased urinary frequency, urgency, and urge incontinence.

REMS

tolvaptan (tol-vap-tan)

✱ Jinarc, Jynarque, Samsca

Classification

Therapeutic: electrolyte modifiers
Pharmacologic: vasopressin antagonists

Indications

Samsca: Treatment of significant hypervolemic and euvolemic hyponatremia (serum sodium <125 mEq/L or less marked symptomatic hyponatremia that has resisted correction by fluid restriction), including patients with heart failure and syndrome of inappropriate antidiuretic hormone (SIADH). **Jynarque:** Patients at risk of rapidly progressing autosomal dominant polycystic kidney disease (ADPKD).

Action

Acts as a selective vasopressin V2-receptor antagonist, resulting in increased renal water excretion and increased serum sodium. **Therapeutic Effects:** Correction of hyponatremia (Samsca). Slow deterioration of renal function (Jynarque).

Pharmacokinetics

Absorption: 40% absorbed following oral administration.

T

Distribution: >99%.

Metabolism and Excretion: Extensively metabolized primarily by the CYP3A4 enzyme system; no renal elimination.

Half-life: 12 hr.

TIME/ACTION PROFILE

ROUTE	ONSET	PEAK	DURATION
PO	within 8 hr	2–4 hr†	7 days

† Blood level.

Contraindications/Precautions

Contraindicated in: Hypersensitivity; Liver disease; Urgent need to acutely raise serum sodium (Samsca); Patients who cannot appropriately sense/respond to thirst; Hypovolemia; Uncorrected abnormal serum sodium concentrations (Jynarque); Concurrent use of strong or moderate CYP3A inhibitors (Samsca); Concurrent use of strong CYP3A inhibitors (Jynarque); Anuria; Uncorrect urinary outflow obstruction (Jynarque); Lactation: Avoid use.

Use Cautiously in: Severe malnutrition, alcoholism or advanced liver disease (↑ risk of osmotic demyelination; correct electrolyte abnormalities at a slower rates); Cirrhosis (↑ risk of GI bleeding, use only when the need to treat outweighs risk); Concurrent use of moderate CYP3A inhibitors (↓ dose) (Jynarque); Geri: May have ↑ sensitivity to effects; OB: Use only if the potential benefit justifies the potential risk to the fetus; Pedi: Safety and effectiveness not established.

Adverse Reactions/Side Effects

CNS: dizziness, weakness. **CV:** palpitations. **Derm:** dry skin, rash. **Endo:** hyperglycemia, hyperuricemia. **F and E:** thirst, hypernatremia, hypovolemia. **GI:** HEPATOTOXICITY, constipation, diarrhea, dry mouth, ↓ appetite, dyspepsia. **GU:** polyuria. **Neuro:** osmotic demyelination. **Misc:** HYPERSENSITIVITY REACTIONS (including anaphylaxis).

Interactions

Drug-Drug: **Strong CYP3A inhibitors**, including **ketoconazole**, **clarithromycin**, **itraconazole**, **saquinavir**, **nelfinavir**, **ritonavir**, and **nefazodone** as well as **moderate CYP3A inhibitors**, including **erythromycin**, **fluconazole**, **aprepitant**, **diltiazem**, and **verapamil** may ↑ levels and risk of toxicity; avoid concurrent use. **CYP3A inducers**, including **rifampin**, may ↓ levels and effectiveness; avoid concurrent use with Jynarque; dosage adjustments may be necessary with Samsca. **P-gp inhibitors**, including **cyclosporine** may ↑ levels and risk of toxicity; dosage adjustments may be necessary. Jynarque may ↑ levels of **statins**, **bosentan**, **glyburide**, **nateglinide**, **repaglinide**, **methotrexate**, and **furosemide**; avoid concurrent use. May ↑ **digoxin** levels; monitor carefully. May ↑ risk of hyperkalemia with **angiotensin receptor blockers**, **ACE inhibitors**, and **potassium-sparing diuretics**. **Diuretics** may ↑ risk of too rapid correction of sodium. May inhibit effects of **desmopressin**; avoid concurrent use.

Drug-Food: **Grapefruit juice** ↑ levels and the risk of toxicity; avoid concurrent use.

Route/Dosage

Samsca and Jynarque should not be used interchangeably.

Hyponatremia (Samsca)

PO (Adults): 15 mg once daily initially; may ↑ at intervals of ≥1 day to 30 mg once daily, up to a maximum of 60 mg once daily. Do not use for longer than 30 days.

Autosomal Dominant Polycystic Kidney Disease (Jynarque and Jinarc)

PO (Adults): 60 mg/day initially (taken as 45 mg upon wakening and then 15 mg 8 hr later); may be ↑ after at least 1 wk to 90 mg/day (taken as 60 mg upon wakening and then 30 mg 8 hr later); may then be ↑ after at least 1 wk to 120 mg/day (taken as 90 mg upon wakening and then 30 mg 8 hr later); *Concurrent use of moderate CYP3A inhibitors*—30 mg/day initially (taken as 15 mg upon wakening and then 15 mg 8 hr later); may be ↑ after at least 1 wk to 45 mg/day (taken as 30 mg upon wakening and then 15 mg 8 hr later); may then be ↑ after at least 1 wk to 60 mg/day (taken as 45 mg upon wakening and then 15 mg 8 hr later).

Availability

Tablets (Jynarque and Jinarc): 15 mg, 30 mg, 45 mg, 60 mg, 90 mg. **Tablets (Samsca):** 15 mg, 30 mg.

NURSING IMPLICATIONS

Assessment

- Monitor neurologic status and assess for signs and symptoms of osmotic demyelination syndrome (trouble speaking, dysphagia, drowsiness, confusion, mood changes, involuntary movements, weakness, seizures), especially during initiation and after titration. If a rapid ↑ in sodium or symptoms occur, discontinue tolvaptan and consider administration of hypotonic fluid.
- Monitor fluid balance. If hypovolemia occurs interrupt or discontinue tolvaptan and provide supportive care (monitor vital signs, balance fluid and electrolytes).
- Monitor for signs and symptoms of liver injury (fatigue, anorexia, right upper abdominal discomfort, dark urine, jaundice) periodically during therapy. If symptoms occur, discontinue therapy.
- ***Lab Test Considerations:*** Monitor serum sodium levels frequently during initiation and dose titration and periodically during therapy. Too rapid correction of hyponatremia (>12 mEq/L/24 hr) can cause osmotic demyelination syndrome.
- Monitor serum potassium in patients with serum potassium >5 mEq/L or taking medication known to ↑ potassium.

- Monitor ALT, AST and bilirubin 2 wk and 4 wk after starting therapy, then monthly for first 18 mo and every 3 mo thereafter. If ALT, AST, or bilirubin increase to >2 × ULN, immediately discontinue *Jynarque;* repeat tests as soon as possible (within 48-72 hrs). If levels stabilize or resolve, *Jynarque* may be reinitiated with increased frequency of monitoring as long as ALT and AST remain below 3 times ULN. Do not restart in patients with signs or symptoms of hepatic injury or whose ALT or AST ever exceeds 3 times ULN during therapy with tolvaptan, unless another explanation for liver injury exists and the injury has resolved. In patients with a stable, low baseline AST or ALT, an increase >2 times baseline, even if <2 times ULN, may indicate early liver injury. Suspend and promptly (48-72 hrs) reevaluate liver levels before reinitiating therapy with more frequent monitoring.

Implementation

- Initiate and re-initiate therapy in a hospital.
- REMS requirements are for *Jynaque* product.
- Avoid fluid restriction during first 24 hr of therapy.
- **PO:** Administer once daily without regard to meals.

Patient/Family Teaching

- Instruct patient to take tolvaptan as directed. Avoid drinking grapefruit juice during therapy; may cause ↑ levels. Take missed doses as soon as remembered, but not if just before next dose; do not double doses. Do not stop and restart therapy. Restarting therapy may require hospitalization.
- Explain requirements of Jynarque REMS program (patient must enroll, comply with ongoing monitoring requirements, must get Jynarque from pharmacies participating in REMS program).
- Inform patients they can continue fluid ingestion in response to thirst during therapy and should have water available to drink at all times during therapy. Following discontinuation of therapy, resume fluid restriction.
- Advise patient to notify health care professional immediately if signs and symptoms of hepatotoxicity (feeling tired, fever, loss of appetite, rash, nausea, itching, right upper abdomen pain or tenderness, yellowing of skin and white part of eye, vomiting, dark urine) occur.
- Advise patient to notify health care professional of all Rx or OTC medications, vitamins, or herbal products being taken and to consult with health care professional before taking other medications.
- Advise patient to notify health care professional if signs of dehydration (vomiting, diarrhea, inability to drink normally, dizziness, feeling faint) or bleeding (vomiting bright red blood, dark blood clots, or coffee-ground-like material; black, tarry stools; bloody stools).
- Advise female patients to notify health care professional if pregnancy is planned or suspected, and to avoid breast feeding.

Evaluation/Desired Outcomes

- Normalization of serum sodium levels. Therapy should be limited to 30 days.

topiramate (toe-**peer**-i-mate)

Qudexy XR, Topamax, Topamax Sprinkle, Trokendi XR

Classification

Therapeutic: anticonvulsants, mood stabilizers

Indications

Seizures including: partial-onset, primary generalized tonic-clonic, seizures due to Lennox-Gastaut syndrome. Prevention of migraine headache. **Unlabeled Use:** Adjunct in treatment of bipolar disorder. Infantile spasms.

Action

Action may be due to: Blockade of sodium channels in neurons, Enhancement of gamma-aminobutyrate (GABA), an inhibitory neurotransmitter, Prevention of activation of excitatory receptors. **Therapeutic Effects:** Decreased incidence of seizures. Decreased incidence/severity of migraine headache.

Pharmacokinetics

Absorption: Well absorbed (80%) after oral administration.

Distribution: Unknown.

Metabolism and Excretion: 70% excreted unchanged in urine.

Half-life: 21 hr; *Extended-release*—31 hr.

TIME/ACTION PROFILE (blood levels†)

ROUTE	ONSET	PEAK	DURATION
PO	unknown	2 hr	12 hr
PO-ER	unknown	24 hr	unknown

†After single dose.

Contraindications/Precautions

Contraindicated in: Hypersensitivity; Recent alcohol use (within 6 hr before and after use of extended-release product); Metabolic acidosis (on metformin) (with extended-release product only).

Use Cautiously in: All patients (may ↑ risk of suicidal thoughts/behaviors); Renal impairment (dose ↓ recommended if CCr <70 mL/min/1.73 m^2); Hepatic impairment; Dehydration; Patients predisposed to metabolic acidosis; Sulfa allergy; OB: May ↑ risk for cleft palate and/or cleft lip, and being small for gesta-

T

tional age in infants exposed during pregnancy; use only if maternal benefit outweighs fetal risk; Lactation: Use while breast feeding only if maternal benefit outweighs potential risk to infant; Rep: Women of reproductive potential; Pedi: Children <2 yr (immediate-release) and <6 yr (extended-release) (safety and effectiveness not established); children are more prone to oligohydrosis and hyperthermia; Geri: Consider age-related ↓ in renal/hepatic impairment, concurrent disease states and drug therapy.

Adverse Reactions/Side Effects

CNS: SEIZURES, SUICIDAL THOUGHTS, cognitive disorders, dizziness, drowsiness, fatigue, impaired concentration/memory, nervousness, psychomotor slowing, speech problems, sedation, aggressive reaction, agitation, anxiety, confusion, depression, malaise, mood problems. **Derm:** oligohydrosis (↑ in children). **EENT:** abnormal vision, diplopia, nystagmus, acute myopia/secondary angle closure glaucoma, visual field defects. **F and E:** hyperchloremic metabolic acidosis. **GI:** nausea, abdominal pain, anorexia, constipation, dry mouth, encephalopathy, hyperammonemia. **GU:** kidney stones. **Hemat:** BLEEDING, leukopenia. **Metab:** weight loss, hyperthermia (↑ in children). **Neuro:** ataxia, paresthesia, tremor. **Misc:** fever.

Interactions

Drug-Drug: **Alcohol** use within 6 hr before or after use of Trokendi XR may significantly alter topiramate levels; use during this time frame contraindicated. Levels and effects may be ↓ by **phenytoin**, **carbamazepine**, or **valproic acid**. May ↑ levels and effects of **phenytoin**, **amitriptyline**, or **lithium**. May ↓ levels and effects of **hormonal contraceptives**, **risperidone**, or **valproic acid**. ↑ risk of CNS depression with **alcohol** or other **CNS depressants**. **Carbonic anhydrase inhibitors** (e.g. **acetazolamide** or **zonisamide**) may ↑ risk of metabolic acidosis and kidney stones. Concurrent use with **valproic acid** may ↑ risk of hyperammonemia, encephalopathy, and hypothermia. ↑ risk of bleeding with **aspirin**, **clopidogrel**, **ticagrelor**, **prasugrel**, **warfarin**, **dabigatran**, **rivaroxaban**, **apixaban**, **edoxaban**, **NSAIDs**, or **SSRIs**.

Route/Dosage

Epilepsy (monotherapy)

PO (Adults and Children ≥10 yr): *Immediate-release*—25 mg twice daily initially, gradually ↑ at weekly intervals to 200 mg twice daily over a 6–wk period; *Extended-release (Qudexy XR or Trokendi XR)*—50 mg once daily initially, gradually ↑ at weekly intervals to 400 mg once daily over a 6–wk period.

PO (Children 2–<10 yr [6–<10 yr for Trokendi XR] and >38 kg): *Immediate-release*—25 mg once daily in the evening initially, gradually ↑ at weekly intervals to 125 mg twice daily over a 5–7-wk period; if needed may continue to titrate dose on a weekly basis up to 200 mg twice daily; *Extended-release (Qudexy XR or Trokendi XR)*—25 mg once daily for 1 wk, then ↑ to 50 mg once daily for 1 wk, then ↑ by 25–50 mg/day at weekly intervals over a 5–7-wk period to target dose of 250–400 mg once daily.

PO (Children 2–<10 yr [6–<10 yr for Trokendi XR] and 32–38 kg): *Immediate-release*—25 mg once daily in the evening initially, gradually ↑ at weekly intervals to 125 mg twice daily over a 5–7-wk period; if needed may continue to titrate dose on a weekly basis up to 175 mg twice daily; *Extended-release (Qudexy XR or Trokendi XR)*—25 mg once daily for 1 wk, then ↑ to 50 mg once daily for 1 wk, then ↑ by 25–50 mg/day at weekly intervals over a 5–7-wk period to target dose of 250–350 mg once daily.

PO (Children 2–<10 yr [6–<10 yr for Trokendi XR] and 23–31 kg): *Immediate-release*—25 mg once daily in the evening initially, gradually ↑ at weekly intervals to 100 mg twice daily over a 5–7-wk period; if needed may continue to titrate dose on a weekly basis up to 175 mg twice daily; *Extended-release (Qudexy XR or Trokendi XR)*—25 mg once daily for 1 wk, then ↑ to 50 mg once daily for 1 wk, then ↑ by 25–50 mg/day at weekly intervals over a 5–7-wk period to target dose of 200–350 mg once daily.

PO (Children 2–<10 yr [6–<10 yr for Trokendi XR] and 12–22 kg): *Immediate-release*—25 mg once daily in the evening initially, gradually ↑ at weekly intervals to 100 mg twice daily over a 5–7-wk period; if needed may continue to titrate dose on a weekly basis up to 150 mg twice daily; *Extended-release (Qudexy XR or Trokendi XR)*—25 mg once daily for 1 wk, then ↑ to 50 mg once daily for 1 wk, then ↑ by 25–50 mg/day at weekly intervals over a 5–7-wk period to target dose of 200–300 mg once daily.

PO (Children 2–<10 yr [6–<10 yr for Trokendi XR] and ≤11 kg): *Immediate-release*—25 mg once daily in the evening initially, gradually ↑ at weekly intervals to 75 mg twice daily over a 5–7-wk period; if needed may continue to titrate dose on a weekly basis up to 125 mg twice daily; *Extended-release (Qudexy XR or Trokendi XR)*—25 mg once daily for 1 wk, then ↑ to 50 mg once daily for 1 wk, then ↑ by 25–50 mg/day at weekly intervals over a 5–7-wk period to target dose of 150–250 mg once daily.

Renal Impairment

PO (Adults): *CCr <70 mL/min*—↓ dose by 50%.

Epilepsy (adjunctive therapy)

PO (Adults and Children ≥17 yr): *Immediate-release*—25–50 mg/day initially, ↑ by 25–50 mg/day at weekly intervals up to 200–400 mg/day in 2 divided doses (200–400 mg/day in 2 divided doses for partial seizures or Lennox-Gastaut syndrome and 400 mg/day in 2 divided doses for primary generalized tonic-clonic seizures); *Extended-release (Qudexy XR or Trokendi XR)*—25–50 mg once daily initially, ↑ by 25–50 mg/day at weekly intervals up to 200–400 mg once daily (for partial seizures or Lennox-Gastaut syndrome) and

400 mg once daily (for primary generalized tonic-clonic seizures).
PO (Children 2–16 yr): *Immediate-release and extended-release (Qudexy XR)*—25 mg once daily at night initially for first wk, ↑ at 1–2 wk intervals by 1–3 mg/kg/day up to 5–9 mg/kg/day in 2 divided doses.
PO (Children 6–16 yr): *Extended-release (Trokendi XR)*—25 mg once daily at night initially for first wk, ↑ at 1–2 wk intervals by 1–3 mg/kg/day up to 5–9 mg/kg/day given once daily at night.

Renal Impairment
PO (Adults): *CCr <70 mL/min*—↓ dose by 50%.

Migraine Prevention
PO (Adults and Children ≥12 yr): *Immediate-release*—25 mg at night initially, ↑ by 25 mg/day at weekly intervals up to target dose of 100 mg/day in 2 divided doses; *Extended-release (Qudexy XR)*—25 mg once daily initially, ↑ by 25 mg/day at weekly intervals up to target dose of 100 mg once daily.

Renal Impairment
PO (Adults): *CCr <70 mL/min*—↓ dose by 50%.

Availability (generic available)
Extended-release capsules (Qudexy XR): 25 mg, 50 mg, 100 mg, 150 mg, 200 mg. **Extended-release capsules (Trokendi XR):** 25 mg, 50 mg, 100 mg, 200 mg. **Sprinkle capsules:** 15 mg, 25 mg. **Cost:** *Generic*—15 mg $144.97/60, 25 mg $175.26/60. **Tablets:** 25 mg, 50 mg, 100 mg, 200 mg. **Cost:** *Generic*—25 mg $21.85/180, 50 mg $33.03/180, 100 mg $41.48/180, 200 mg $54.38/180. ***In combination with:*** phentermine (Qsymia). See Appendix B.

NURSING IMPLICATIONS
Assessment
- Monitor closely for notable changes in behavior that could indicate the emergence or worsening of suicidal thoughts or behavior or depression.
- **Seizures:** Assess location, duration, and characteristics of seizure activity.
- **Migraines:** Assess pain location, intensity, duration, and associated symptoms (photophobia, phonophobia, nausea, vomiting) during migraine attack. Monitor frequency and intensity of pain on pain scale.
- **Bipolar Disorder:** Assess mental status (mood, orientation, behavior) and cognitive abilities before and periodically during therapy.
- ***Lab Test Considerations:*** Monitor CBC with differential and platelet count before therapy to determine baseline levels and periodically during therapy. Frequently causes anemia.
- Hepatic function should be monitored periodically throughout therapy. May cause ↑ AST and ALT levels.
- Evaluate serum bicarbonate prior to and periodically during therapy. Monitor for signs and symptoms of metabolic acidosis (hyperventilation, fatigue, anorexia, cardiac arrhythmias, stupor). If metabolic acidosis occurs, dosing taper or discontinuation may be necessary.

Implementation
- Implement seizure precautions.
- Do not confuse Topamax (topiramate) with Toprol XL (metoprolol).
- **PO:** May be administered without regard to meals.
- Do not break/crush tablets because of bitter taste.
- Contents of the sprinkle capsules can be sprinkled on a small amount (teaspoon) of soft food, such as applesauce, custard, ice cream, oatmeal, pudding, or yogurt. To open, hold the capsule upright so that you can read the word "TOP." Carefully twist off the clear portion of the capsule. It may be best to do this over the small portion of the food onto which you will be pouring the sprinkles. Sprinkle the entire contents of the capsule onto the food. Be sure the patient swallows the entire spoonful of the sprinkle/food mixture immediately without chewing. Follow with fluids immediately to make sure all of the mixture is swallowed. Never store a sprinkle/food mixture for use at another time.
- A 6 mg/mL oral suspension may be compounded by pharmacy for pediatric patients.
- Swallow extended-release capsules *(Trokendi XR)* whole; do not sprinkle on food, or break, crush, dissolve, or chew.
- Swallow extended-release capsules *(Qudexy XR)* whole; may be opened and sprinkled on soft food; do not crush or chew. Swallow immediately, do not save for later.

Patient/Family Teaching
- Instruct patient to take topiramate exactly as directed. Take missed doses as soon as possible but not just before next dose; do not double doses. Notify health care professional if more than 1 dose is missed. Medication should be gradually discontinued to prevent seizures and status epilepticus. Instruct patient to read the *Medication Guide* before starting and with each Rx refill in case of changes.
- May cause decreased sweating and increased body temperature. Advise patients, especially parents of pediatric patients, to provide adequate hydration and monitoring, especially during hot weather.
- May cause dizziness, drowsiness, confusion, and difficulty concentrating. Caution patients to avoid driving or other activities requiring alertness until response to medication is known.
- Advise patient to maintain a fluid intake of 2000–3000 mL of fluid/day to prevent the formation of kidney stones.

T

- Instruct patient to notify health care professional immediately if periorbital pain or blurred vision occur. Medication should be discontinued if ocular symptoms occur. May lead to permanent loss of vision.
- Advise patient and family to notify health care professional if thoughts about suicide or dying, attempts to commit suicide; new or worse depression; new or worse anxiety; feeling very agitated or restless; panic attacks; trouble sleeping; new or worse irritability; acting aggressive; being angry or violent; acting on dangerous impulses; an extreme increase in activity and talking, other unusual changes in behavior or mood occur.
- Inform patients that topiramate may cause encephalopathy. If signs and symptoms (unexplained lethargy, vomiting, changes in mental status) occur, notify health care professional.
- Caution patient to make position changes slowly to minimize orthostatic hypotension.
- Instruct patient to notify health care professional of all Rx or OTC medications, vitamins, or herbal products being taken and consult health care professional before taking any new medications.
- Advise patient not to take alcohol or other CNS depressants concurrently with this medication. Avoid alcohol 6 hrs before and 6 hrs after taking *Trokendi XR*.
- Instruct patient to notify health care professional of medication regimen before treatment or surgery.
- Advise patient to use sunscreen and wear protective clothing to prevent photosensitivity reactions.
- Rep: Advise patient to use a nonhormonal form of contraception while taking topiramate; may make hormonal contraceptives less effective. Notify health care professional if pregnancy is planned or suspected or if breast feeding. If pregnancy occurs, encourage patient to enroll in the North American Drug Pregnancy Registry by calling 1-888-233-2334 or online at http://www.aedpregnancyregistry.org/.
- Advise patient to carry identification describing disease and medication regimen at all times.

Evaluation/Desired Outcomes

- Absence or reduction of seizure activity.
- Decrease in incidence and severity of migraine headaches.
- Remission of manic symptoms.

HIGH ALERT

topotecan (toe-poe-**tee**-kan)

Hycamtin

Classification

Therapeutic: antineoplastics

Pharmacologic: enzyme inhibitors

Indications

IV: Metastatic ovarian cancer that has not responded to previous chemotherapy. Small cell lung cancer unresponsive to first line therapy. Stage IV-B persistent or recurrent cervical cancer not amenable to treatment with surgery or radiation (with cisplatin). **PO:** Relapsed small cell lung cancer in patients with a complete or partial prior response and who are at least 45 days from the end of first-line chemotherapy.

Action

Interferes with DNA synthesis by inhibiting the enzyme topoisomerase. **Therapeutic Effects:** Death of rapidly replicating cells, particularly malignant ones.

Pharmacokinetics

Absorption: IV administration results in complete bioavailability.

Distribution: Unknown.

Metabolism and Excretion: 30% excreted in urine; small amounts metabolized by the liver.

Half-life: *PO*—3–6 hr; *IV*—2–3 hr.

TIME/ACTION PROFILE (effects on WBCs)

ROUTE	ONSET	PEAK	DURATION
PO	unknown	1–2 hr	24 hr
IV	within days	11 days	7 days

Contraindications/Precautions

Contraindicated in: Hypersensitivity; OB, Lactation: Pregnancy or lactation.

Use Cautiously in: Impaired renal function (↓ dose if CCr <40 mL/min); Platelet count <25,000 cells/mm³ (↓ dose); History of interstitial lung disease, pulmonary fibrosis, lung cancer, thoracic radiation, or use of pneumotoxic drugs or colony stimulating factors; Rep: Patients with childbearing potential; Geri: May require dose ↓ due to age-related ↓ in renal function.

Adverse Reactions/Side Effects

CNS: headache, fatigue, weakness. **Resp:** INTERSTITIAL LUNG DISEASE, dyspnea. **GI:** abdominal pain, diarrhea, nausea, vomiting, anorexia, constipation, ↑ liver enzymes, stomatitis. **Derm:** alopecia. **Hemat:** anemia, leukopenia, thrombocytopenia. **MS:** arthralgia.

Interactions

Drug-Drug: P-glycoprotein inhibitors, including **amiodarone, azithromycin, captopril, carvedilol, clarithromycin, conivaptan, cyclosporine, diltiazem, dronedarone, erythromycin, felodipine, itraconazole, ketoconazole, lopinavir, ritonavir, quinidine, ranolazine, ticagrelort**, or **verapamil** may ↑ levels; avoid concurrent use. Neutropenia is prolonged by concurrent use of **filgrastim** (do not use until day 6; 24 hr following completion of topotecan). ↑ myelosuppression with other **antineoplastics** (especially **cisplatin**) or **radiation therapy**. May ↓ antibody response to and ↑ risk of adverse reactions from **live virus vaccines**.

Route/Dosage

PO (Adults): 2.3 mg/m²/day for 5 days starting on day 1 of a 21–day course (round calculated oral dose to nearest 0.25 mg and prescribe the minimum number of

1 mg and 0.25 mg capsules with the same number of capsules prescribed for each of the 5 days).

IV (Adults): *Ovarian and Small Cell Lung Cancer*—1.5 mg/m²/day for 5 days starting on day 1 of a 21-day course; *Cervical Cancer*—75 mg/m² on Days 1, 2, and 3 followed by cisplatin on Day 1 and repeated every 21 days.

Renal Impairment

PO (Adults): *CCr 30–49 mL/min*—1.5 mg/m²/day for 5 days starting on day 1 of a 21-day course; dose may be ↑after first course by 0.4 mg/m²/day if no severe hematologic or GI toxicities occur; *CCr <30 mL/min*—0.6 mg/m²/day for 5 days starting on day 1 of a 21-day course; dose may be ↑after first course by 0.4 mg/m²/day if no severe hematologic or GI toxicities occur.

Renal Impairment

IV (Adults): *CCr 20–39 mL/min*—0.75 mg/m²/day for 5 days starting on day 1 of a 21-day course. *Cervical Cancer*—Administer at standard doses only if serum creatinine is ≤1.5 mg/dL. Do not administer if serum creatinine >1.5 m g/dL.

Availability (generic available)

Capsules: 0.25 mg, 1 mg. **Powder for injection:** 4 mg/vial. **Solution for injection:** 1 mg/mL.

NURSING IMPLICATIONS

Assessment

- Monitor vital signs frequently during administration.
- Monitor for bone marrow depression. Assess for bleeding (bleeding gums, bruising, petechiae; guaiac stools, urine, and emesis) and avoid IM injections and taking rectal temperatures if platelet count is low. Apply pressure to venipuncture sites for 10 min. Assess for signs of infection during neutropenia. Anemia may occur. Monitor for increased fatigue, dyspnea, and orthostatic hypotension.
- Nausea and vomiting are common. Pretreatment with antiemetics should be considered.
- Assess IV site frequently for extravasation, which causes mild local erythema and bruising.
- Monitor for signs and symptoms of interstitial lung disease (cough, fever, dyspnea, hypoxia). Discontinue topotecan if interstitial lung disease is confirmed.
- ***Lab Test Considerations:*** Monitor CBC with differential and platelet count prior to administration and frequently during therapy. Baseline neutrophil count of ≥1500 cells/mm³ and platelet count of ≥100,000 cells/mm³ are required before first dose. The nadir of neutropenia occurs in 11 days, with a duration of 7 days. The nadir of thrombocytopenia occurs in 15 days, with a duration of 5 days. The nadir of anemia occurs in 15 days. Subsequent doses should not be administered until neutrophils recover to >1000 cells/mm³, platelets recover to >100,000 cells/mm³, and hemoglobin levels recover to 9.0 mg/dL. **When topotecan used as a single-agent,** ↓ dose to 1.25 mg/m² if *neutrophil <500 cells/mm³*, or administer granulocyte-colony stimulating factor (G-CSF) starting no sooner than 24 hrs following the last dose or *platelet counts less than 25,000 cells/mm³* during previous cycle. **When topotecan used with cisplatin,** ↓ dose to 0.60 mg/m² (and to 0.45 mg/m² if necessary) for febrile neutropenia (*neutrophil counts <1,000 cells/mm³ with temperature of ≥38.0°C (100.4°F)*), or administer G-CSF starting no sooner than 24 hrs following the last dose or *platelet counts less than 25,000 cells/mm³* during previous cycle.
- Monitor liver function. May cause transient ↑ in AST, ALT, and bilirubin concentrations.

Implementation

- ***High Alert:*** Fatalities have occurred with chemotherapeutic agents. Before administering, clarify all ambiguous orders; double check single, daily, and course-of-therapy dose limits; have second practitioner independently double check original order, dose calculations and infusion pump settings.
- **PO:** May be taken without regard to food. Capsules must be swallowed whole; do not open, crush, or chew. If patient vomits after taking dose, do not replace dose.
- Do not administer capsules to patients with Grade 3 or 4 diarrhea. When recovered to ≤Grade 1, resume with dose decreased by 0.4 mg/m²/day for subsequent courses.

IV Administration

- Solution should be prepared in a biologic cabinet. Wear gloves, gown, and mask while handling IV medication. Discard IV equipment in specially designated containers.
- **Intermittent Infusion:** Reconstitute each vial with 4 mL of sterile water for injection. ***Diluent:*** Dilute further in D5W or 0.9% NaCl. Infusion is stable for 24 hr at room temperature or up to 7 days if refrigerated. Solution is yellow to yellow-green. ***Concentration:*** 10–50 mcg/mL. ***Rate:*** Infuse over 30 min.
- **Y-Site Compatibility:** alemtuzumab, alfentanil, amikacin, amiodarone, anidulafungin, argatroban, aztreonam, bivalirudin, buprenorphine, butorphanol, calcium chloride, carboplatin, caspofungin, cefazolin, cefotaxime, cefotetan, cefoxitin, ceftriaxone, cefuroxime, chloramphenicol, chlorpromazine, ciprofloxacin, cisatracurium, cisplatin, cyclophosphamide, cyclosporine, dacarbazine, dactinomycin, daptomycin, daunorubicin hydrochloride, dexmedetomidine, dexrazoxane, diltiazem, diphenhydramine, dobutamine, docetaxel, dopamine, doxorubicin hy-

T

drochloride, doxorubicin liposomal, doxycycline, droperidol, enalaprilat, ephedrine, epinephrine, erythromycin, esmolol, etoposide, etoposide phosphate, famotidine, fenoldopam, fentanyl, fluconazole, fludarabine, furosemide, gemcitabine, gentamicin, glycopyrrolate, granisetron, haloperidol, heparin, hetastarch, hydralazine, hydrocortisone, hydromorphone, idarubicin, ifosfamide, insulin, isoproterenol, labetalol, leucovorin, levofloxacin, lidocaine, linezolid, lorazepam, magnesium sulfate, mannitol, meperidine, methyldopate, methylprednisolone, metoclopramide, metoprolol, metronidazole, midazolam, milrinone, mitoxantrone, morphine, moxifloxacin, nalbuphine, naloxone, nitroglycerin, nitroprusside, norepinephrine, octreotide, ondansetron, oxaliplatin, paclitaxel, palonosetron, pamidronate, pancuronium, pentamidine, phenylephrine, potassium chloride, procainamide, prochlorperazine, promethazine, propranolol, ranitidine, remifentanil, succinylcholine, sufentanil, tacrolimus, theophylline, thiotepa, tigecycline, tirofiban, tobramycin, vancomycin, vasopressin, vecuronium, verapamil, vinblastine, vincristine, vinorelbine, voriconazole, zidovudine, zoledronic acid.

- **Y-Site Incompatibility:** acyclovir, allopurinol, amifostine, aminophylline, amphotericin B deoxycholate, amphotericin B lipid complex, ampicillin, ampicillin/sulbactam, bumetanide, calcium gluconate, cefepime, ceftazidime, clindamycin, dantrolene, dexamethasone, diazepam, digoxin, ertapenem, fluorouracil, foscarnet, fosphenytoin, ganciclovir, hydrocortisone, imipenem/cilastatin, ketorolac, meropenem, mitomycin, nafcillin, pantoprazole, pemetrexed, pentobarbital, phenobarbital, phenytoin, piperacillin/tazobactam, potassium acetate, potassium phosphates, rituximab, sodium bicarbonate, sodium phosphates, thiopental, trastuzumab, trimethoprim/sulfamethoxazole.

Patient/Family Teaching

- Instruct patient to take as directed. If patient vomits after taking, do not replace dose; notify health care professional. Do not take missed doses; take next scheduled dose and notify health care professional. If any capsules are broken or leaking, do not touch with bare hands; dispose of capsules and wash hands with soap and water. Patient should be instructed to read the *Patient Information* guide prior to first dose and with each Rx refill in case of changes.
- May cause drowsiness or sleepiness during and for several days after therapy. Caution patient to avoid driving and other activities requiring alertness until response to medication is known.
- Instruct patient to notify health care professional if fever; chills; sore throat; signs of infection; bleeding gums; bruising; petechiae; blood in urine, stool, emesis or signs and symptoms of interstitial lung disease occur. Caution patient to avoid crowds and persons with known infections. Instruct patient to use soft toothbrush and electric razor. Patient should be cautioned not to drink alcoholic beverages or take products containing aspirin or NSAIDs.
- May cause diarrhea. Advise patient to notify health care professional if diarrhea with fever or stomach pain or cramps or diarrhea that occurs more than 3 times/day.
- Advise patient to notify health care professional of all Rx or OTC medications, vitamins, or herbal products being taken and to consult with health care professional before taking other medications.
- Discuss with patient the possibility of hair loss. Explore methods of coping.
- Instruct patient not to receive any vaccinations without advice of health care professional.
- Rep: Advise male and female patient that topotecan may cause infertility and may have teratogenic effects. Contraception should be used during therapy and for at least 1 mo after last dose; and breast feeding avoided.
- Emphasize the need for periodic lab tests to monitor for side effects.

Evaluation/Desired Outcomes

- Decrease in size and spread of malignancy.

torsemide (tore-se-mide)

Demadex

Classification

Therapeutic: antihypertensives
Pharmacologic: loop diuretics

Indications

Edema due to: HF, Hepatic or renal disease. Hypertension.

Action

Inhibits the reabsorption of sodium and chloride from the loop of Henle and distal renal tubule. Increases renal excretion of water, sodium, chloride, magnesium, hydrogen, and calcium. Effectiveness persists in impaired renal function. **Therapeutic Effects:** Diuresis and subsequent mobilization of excess fluid (edema, pleural effusions). Decreased BP.

Pharmacokinetics

Absorption: 80% absorbed after oral administration.

Distribution: Widely distributed.

Protein Binding: ≥99%.

Metabolism and Excretion: 80% metabolized by liver, 20% excreted in urine.

Half-life: 3.5 hr.

TIME/ACTION PROFILE (diuretic effect)

ROUTE	ONSET	PEAK	DURATION
PO	within 60 min	60–120 min	6–8 hr

Contraindications/Precautions

Contraindicated in: Hypersensitivity; Cross-sensitivity with thiazides and sulfonamides may occur; Hepatic coma or anuria.

Use Cautiously in: Severe liver disease (may precipitate hepatic coma; concurrent use with potassium-sparing diuretics may be necessary); Electrolyte depletion; Diabetes mellitus; Increasing azotemia; Geri: May have ↑ risk of side effects, especially hypotension and electrolyte imbalance, at usual doses; OB, Lactation, Pedi: Safety not established.

Adverse Reactions/Side Effects

CNS: dizziness, headache, nervousness. **EENT:** hearing loss, tinnitus. **CV:** hypotension. **GI:** constipation, diarrhea, dry mouth, dyspepsia, nausea, vomiting. **GU:** ↑ BUN, excessive urination. **Derm:** STEVENS-JOHNSON SYNDROME, TOXIC EPIDERMAL NECROLYSIS, photosensitivity, rash. **Endo:** hyperglycemia, hyperuricemia. **F and E:** dehydration, hypocalcemia, hypochloremia, hypokalemia, hypomagnesemia, hyponatremia, hypovolemia, metabolic alkalosis. **MS:** arthralgia, muscle cramps, myalgia.

Interactions

Drug-Drug: ↑ hypotension with **antihypertensives**, **nitrates**, or acute ingestion of **alcohol**. ↑ risk of hypokalemia with other **diuretics**, **amphotericin B**, **stimulant laxatives**, and **corticosteroids**. Hypokalemia may ↑ risk of **digoxin** toxicity and ↑ risk of arrhythmia in patients taking drugs that prolong the QT interval. May ↑ risk of **lithium** toxicity. ↑ risk of ototoxicity with **aminoglycosides**. **NSAIDS** may ↓ effects. ↑ risk of **salicylate** toxicity (with use of high-dose **salicylate** therapy). **Cholestyramine** may ↓ absorption.

Route/Dosage

HF

PO (Adults): 10–20 mg once daily; dose may be doubled until desired effect is obtained (maximum daily dose = 200 mg).

Chronic Renal Failure

PO (Adults): 20 mg once daily; dose may be doubled until desired effect is obtained (maximum daily dose = 200 mg).

Hepatic Cirrhosis

PO (Adults): 5–10 mg once daily (with aldosterone antagonist or potassium-sparing diuretic); dose may be doubled until desired effect is obtained (maximum daily dose = 40 mg).

Hypertension

PO (Adults): 2.5–5 mg once daily, may be ↑ to 10 mg once daily after 4–6 wk (if still not effective, add another agent).

Availability (generic available)

Tablets: 5 mg, 10 mg, 20 mg, 100 mg. **Cost:** *Generic*—5 mg $63.42/100, 10 mg $70.27/100, 20 mg $82.08/100, 100 mg $304.00/100.

NURSING IMPLICATIONS

Assessment

- Assess fluid status during therapy. Monitor daily weight, intake and output ratios, amount and location of edema, lung sounds, skin turgor, and mucous membranes. Notify health care provider if thirst, dry mouth, lethargy, weakness, hypotension, or oliguria occurs.
- Monitor BP and pulse before and during administration. Monitor frequency of prescription refills to determine adherence in patients treated for hypertension.
- Assess patients receiving digoxin for anorexia, nausea, vomiting, muscle cramps, paresthesia, and confusion. Patients taking digoxin are at increased risk of digoxin toxicity due to potassium-depleting effect of the diuretic. Potassium supplements or potassium-sparing diuretics may be used concurrently to prevent hypokalemia.
- Assess patient for tinnitus and hearing loss. Audiometry is recommended for patients receiving prolonged high-dose IV therapy. Hearing loss is most common following rapid or high-dose IV administration in patients with decreased renal function or those taking other ototoxic drugs.
- Assess for allergy to sulfonamides.
- Assess patient for skin rash frequently during therapy. Discontinue torsemide at first sign of rash; may be life-threatening. Stevens-Johnson syndrome or toxic epidermal necrolysis may develop. Treat symptomatically; may recur once treatment is stopped.
- Geri: Diuretic use is associated with increased risk for falls in older adults. Assess falls risk and implement fall prevention strategies.
- ***Lab Test Considerations:*** Monitor electrolytes, renal and hepatic function, serum glucose, and uric acid levels before and periodically during therapy. May cause ↓ serum sodium, potassium, calcium, and magnesium concentrations. May also cause ↑ BUN, serum glucose, creatinine, and uric acid levels.

Implementation

- Administer medication in the morning to prevent disruption of sleep cycle.
- **PO:** May be taken with food or milk to minimize gastric irritation.

Patient/Family Teaching

- Instruct patient to take torsemide as directed. Take missed doses as soon as possible; do not double doses.
- Caution patient to change positions slowly to minimize orthostatic hypotension. Caution patient that

T

the use of alcohol, exercise during hot weather, or standing for long periods during therapy may enhance orthostatic hypotension.

- Instruct patient to consult health care professional regarding a diet high in potassium (see Appendix K).
- Advise patient to contact health care professional if they gain more than 2–3 lb/day.
- Instruct patient to notify health care professional of all Rx or OTC medications, vitamins, or herbal products being taken and to consult health care professional before taking any OTC medications concurrently with this therapy.
- Instruct patient to notify health care professional of medication regimen prior to treatment or surgery.
- Caution patient to use sunscreen and protective clothing to prevent photosensitivity reactions.
- Advise patient to contact health care professional immediately if rash muscle weakness, cramps, nausea, dizziness, numbness, or tingling of extremities occurs.
- Advise diabetic patients to monitor blood glucose closely; may cause increased blood glucose levels.
- Emphasize the importance of routine follow-up examinations.
- **Hypertension:** Advise patients on antihypertensive regimen to continue taking medication even if feeling better. Torsemide controls but does not cure hypertension.
- Reinforce the need to continue additional therapies for hypertension (weight loss, exercise, restricted sodium intake, stress reduction, regular exercise, moderation of alcohol consumption, cessation of smoking).

Evaluation/Desired Outcomes

- Decrease in edema.
- Decrease in abdominal girth and weight.
- Increase in urinary output.
- Decrease in BP.

REMS

traMADol (tra-ma-dol)

ConZip, Durela, Ralivia, Tridural, Ultram, ~~Ultram ER~~, Zytram XL

Classification

Therapeutic: analgesics (centrally acting)

Schedule IV

Indications

Moderate to moderately severe pain (extended-release formulations indicated for patients who require around-the-clock pain management).

Action

Binds to μ-opioid receptors. Inhibits reuptake of serotonin and norepinephrine in the CNS. **Therapeutic Effects:** Decreased pain.

Pharmacokinetics

Absorption: *Immediate-release*—75% absorbed after oral administration; *Extended-release (Ultram)*—85–90% (compared with immediate-release).

Distribution: Crosses the placenta; enters breast milk.

Metabolism and Excretion: Mostly metabolized by the liver (primarily by CYP2D6 and CYP3A4); primarily metabolized by CYP2D6 to active metabolite with analgesic activity (M1); CYP2D6 enzyme system exhibits genetic polymorphism; ~7% of population may be poor metabolizers and may have significantly ↑ concentrations of tramadol and ↓ concentrations of M1 metabolite. 1–10% of Whites, 3–4% of Blacks, and 1–2% of East Asians may be ultra–rapid metabolizers of CYP2D6 and have significantly ↑ concentrations of M1 metabolite. 30% eliminated unchanged in the urine.

Half-life: *Tramadol*—6–8 hr, *ER*—7.9 hr; *active metabolite*—7–9 hr; both are ↑ in renal or hepatic impairment.

TIME/ACTION PROFILE (analgesia)

ROUTE	ONSET	PEAK	DURATION
PO	1 hr	2–3 hr	4–6 hr
ER	unknown	12 hr	24 hr

Contraindications/Precautions

Contraindicated in: Hypersensitivity; Cross-sensitivity with opioids may occur; Significant respiratory depression; Acute or severe bronchial asthma (in unmonitored setting or in absence of resuscitative equipment); Known or suspected GI obstruction (including paralytic ileus); Concurrent use of MAO inhibitors (or use within the past 14 days); Patients who are acutely intoxicated with alcohol, sedatives/hypnotics, centrally acting analgesics, opioid analgesics, or psychotropic agents; Patients who are physically dependent on opioid analgesics (may precipitate withdrawal); Ultra-rapid metabolizers of CYP2D6 (↑ risk of respiratory depression and death); *ER only*—CCr <30 mL/min or hepatic impairment; Lactation: Avoid use in breast feeding (↑ risk of drowsiness and respiratory depression in infant); Pedi: Children <12 yr, children <18 yr following tonsillectomy and/or adenoidectomy, and children 12–18 yr who are postoperative, have obstructive sleep apnea, obesity, or severe pulmonary disease, neuromuscular disease; or are taking other medications that cause respiratory depression (↑ risk of respiratory depression and death).

Use Cautiously in: Patients with a history of epilepsy or risk factors for seizures; Renal impairment (↑ dosing interval recommended if CCr <30 mL/min); Hepatic impairment (↑ dosing interval recommended in patients with cirrhosis); Patients receiving neuroleptics, SSRIs, or TCAs, or other CNS depressants; Patients who are suicidal or prone to addiction (↑ risk of suicide); Excessive use of alcohol (↑ risk of suicide); ↑ intracranial pressure or head trauma; Patients with a history of opioid dependence or who have recently received large doses of opioids; Geri: *Immediate-release*—Not to exceed 300 mg/day in patients >75 yr; *ER*—Use with extreme caution in patients >75 yr; OB: Prolonged use during pregnancy can result in neonatal opioid withdrawal syndrome.

Adverse Reactions/Side Effects

CNS: SEIZURES, dizziness, headache, somnolence, anxiety, confusion, coordination disturbance, euphoria, malaise, nervousness, sleep disorder, stimulation, weakness. **CV:** vasodilation. **Derm:** pruritus, sweating. **EENT:** visual disturbances. **GI:** constipation, nausea, abdominal pain, anorexia, diarrhea, dry mouth, dyspepsia, flatulence, vomiting. **GU:** ↓ fertility, menopausal symptoms, urinary retention/frequency. **Neuro:** hypertonia. **Misc:** SEROTONIN SYNDROME, physical dependence, psychological dependence, tolerance.

Interactions

Drug-Drug: **MAO inhibitors** ↑ risk of adverse reactions; concurrent use or use within previous 14 days contraindicated. ↑ risk of CNS depression when used concurrently with other **CNS depressants**, including **alcohol**, **antihistamines**, **sedative/hypnotics**, **opioid analgesics**, **anesthetics**, or **psychotropic agents**. ↑ risk of seizures with high doses of **penicillins**, **cephalosporins**, **phenothiazines**, **opioid analgesics**, or **antidepressants**. **Carbamazepine** ↑ metabolism and ↓ effectiveness of tramadol (increased doses may be required). **CYP2D6 inhibitors**, including**quinidine**, **fluoxetine**, **paroxetine**, and **bupropion**, may ↓ levels of active metabolite (M1) and lead to ↓ analgesic effects. **CYP3A4 inhibitors**, including **erythromycin**, **clarithromycin**, **ketoconazole**, **itraconazole**, and **protease inhibitors** may allow for a greater degree of metabolism via CYP2D6 and ↑ levels of the active metabolite (M1) leading to respiratory depression. **CYP3A4 inducers** may ↓ levels. ↑ risk of serotonin syndrome when used with **SSRI and SNRI antidepressants**, **TCAs**, **MAO inhibitors**, **$5HT_1$ agonists**, **CYP2D6 inhibitors**, and **CYP3A4 inhibitors**.

Drug-Natural Products: Concomitant use of **kava-kava**, **valerian**, or **chamomile** can ↑ CNS depression. ↑ risk of serotonin syndrome when used with **St. John's wort**.

Route/Dosage

Immediate-release

PO (Adults ≥18 yr): *Rapid titration*—50–100 mg every 4–6 hr (not to exceed 400 mg/day [300 mg in patients >75 yr]). *Gradual titration*—25 mg/day initially, ↑ by 25 mg/day every 3 days to reach dose of 25 mg 4 times daily, then ↑ by 50 mg/day every 3 days to reach dose of 50 mg 4 times daily; may then use 50–100 mg every 4–6 hr (maximum dose = 400 mg/day).

Renal Impairment

PO (Adults): *CCr <30 mL/min*—↑ dosing interval to every 12 hr (not to exceed 200 mg/day).

Hepatic Impairment

PO (Adults): 50 mg every 12 hr.

Extended-release

PO (Adults): *Not currently receiving immediate-release*—100 mg once daily initially, may then titrate every 5 days up to 300 mg/day; *Currently receiving immediate-release*—calculate 24-hr total dose of immediate-release product and give same dose (rounded down to next lowest 100-mg increment) of ER once daily (maximum dose = 300 mg/day).

Availability (generic available)

Extended-release capsules (Conzip): 100 mg, 150 mg, 200 mg, 300 mg. **Cost:** 100 mg $232.19/30, 200 mg $289.79/30, 300 mg $365.98/30. **Extended-release tablets:** 🍁 75 mg, 100 mg, 🍁 150 mg, 200 mg, 300 mg, 🍁 400 mg. **Cost:** *Generic*—100 mg $126.95/30, 200 mg $209.95/30, 300 mg $292.93/30. **Tablets:** 50 mg. **Cost:** *Generic*—$83.40/100. ***In combination with:*** acetaminophen (Ultracet). See Appendix B.

NURSING IMPLICATIONS

Assessment

- Assess type, location, and intensity of pain before and 2–3 hr (peak) after administration.
- Assess BP and respiratory rate before and periodically during administration. Respiratory depression has not occurred with recommended doses.
- Assess bowel function routinely. Prevention of constipation should be instituted with increased intake of fluids and bulk and with laxatives to minimize constipating effects.
- Prolonged use may lead to physical and psychological dependence and tolerance, although these may be milder than with opioids. This should not prevent patient from receiving adequate analgesia. Patients who receive tramadol for pain rarely develop psychological dependence. If tolerance develops, changing to an opioid agonist may be required to relieve pain.
- Monitor patient for seizures. May occur within recommended dose range. Risk is increased with higher doses and in patients taking antidepressants (SSRIs, SNRIs, tricyclics, or MAO inhibitors), opioid analgesics, or other drugs that decrease the seizure threshold. Also monitor for serotonin syndrome (mental-status changes (e.g., agitation, hallucinations, coma), autonomic instability (e.g., tachycardia, labile BP, hyperthermia), neuromuscular aberrations (e.g., hyperreflexia, incoordination) and/or gastrointestinal symptoms (e.g., nausea, vomiting,

T

diarrhea) in patients taking these drugs concurrently).

- Assess risk for opioid addiction, abuse, or misuse prior to administration. Abuse or misuse of extended-release preparations by crushing, chewing, snorting, or injecting dissolved product will result in uncontrolled delivery of tramadol and can result in overdose and death.
- ***Lab Test Considerations:*** May cause ↑ serum creatinine, ↑ liver enzymes, ↓ hemoglobin, and proteinuria.
- ***Toxicity and Overdose:*** Overdose may cause respiratory depression and seizures. Naloxone may reverse some, but not all, of the symptoms of overdose. Treatment should be symptomatic and supportive. Maintain adequate respiratory exchange. Hemodialysis is not helpful because it removes only a small portion of administered dose. Seizures may be managed with barbiturates or benzodiazepines; naloxone increases risk of seizures.

Implementation

- ***High Alert:*** Do not confuse tramadol with trazodone. Do not confuse Ultram with lithium.
- Tramadol is considered to provide more analgesia than codeine 60 mg but less than combined aspirin 650 mg/codeine 60 mg for acute postoperative pain.
- For chronic pain, daily doses of 250 mg of tramadol provide pain relief similar to that of 5 doses/day of acetaminophen 300 mg/codeine 30 mg, 5 doses/day of aspirin 325 mg/codeine 30 mg, or 2–3 doses/day of acetaminophen 500 mg/oxycodone 5 mg.
- Explain therapeutic value of medication before administration to enhance the analgesic effect.
- Regularly administered doses may be more effective than prn administration. Analgesic is more effective if given before pain becomes severe.
- Tramadol should be discontinued gradually after long-term use to prevent withdrawal symptoms. For patients on long-acting agents who are physically opioid-dependent, initiate the taper by a small enough increment (no greater than 10%–25% of total daily dose) to avoid withdrawal symptoms, and proceed with dose-lowering at an interval of every 2–4 wk. Patients who have been taking opioids for briefer periods of time may tolerate a more rapid taper.
- **PO:** Tramadol may be administered without regard to meals. Swallow extended-release tablets and capsules whole; do not crush, break, dissolve, or chew.
- FDA strongly encourages health care professionals to complete a REMS-compliant education program that includes all the elements of the FDA Education *Blueprint for Health Care Providers Involved in the Management or Support of Patients with Pain,* available at www.fda.gov/OpioidAnalgesicREMSBlueprint. Information on programs can be found at 1-800-503-0784 or www.opioidanalgesicrems.com.

Patient/Family Teaching

- Instruct patient on how and when to ask for pain medication. Do not stop taking without discussing with health care professional; may cause withdrawal symptoms if discontinued abruptly after prolonged use. Discuss safe use, risks, and proper storage and disposal of opioid analgesics with patients and caregivers with each Rx. The Patient Counseling Guide (PCG) is available at www.fda.gov/OpioidAnalgesicREMSPCG.
- May cause dizziness and drowsiness. Caution patient to avoid driving or other activities requiring alertness until response to medication is known.
- Advise patient that tramadol is a drug with known abuse potential. Protect it from theft, and never give to anyone other than the individual for whom it was prescribed. Store out of sight and reach of children, and in a location not accessible by others.
- Advise patient to change positions slowly to minimize orthostatic hypotension.
- Caution patient to avoid concurrent use of alcohol or other CNS depressants with this medication. Advise patient to notify health care professional before taking other RX, OTC, or herbal products concurrently.
- Advise patient to notify health care professional if seizures or if symptoms of serotonin syndrome occur.
- Encourage patient to turn, cough, and breathe deeply every 2 hr to prevent atelectasis.
- Advise females of reproductive potential to notify health care professional if pregnancy is planned or suspected, and to avoid breast feeding.

Evaluation/Desired Outcomes

- Decrease in severity of pain without a significant alteration in level of consciousness or respiratory status.

---

trandolapril, See ANGIOTENSIN-CONVERTING ENZYME (ACE) INHIBITORS.

HIGH ALERT

trastuzumab
(traz-**too**-zoo-mab)

Herceptin, Herzuma, Kanjinti, Ogivri, Ontruzant, Trazimera

Classification
Therapeutic: antineoplastics
Pharmacologic: monoclonal antibodies

Indications

HER2–overexpressing metastatic gastric or gastroesophageal adenocarcinoma in patients who have not received prior treatment for metastatic disease (in combination with cisplatin and capecitabine or 5–fluorouracil). HER2–overexpressing node positive or node negative breast cancer (as part of one of the following regimens: doxorubicin, cyclophosphamide, and either paclitaxel or docetaxel; or docetaxel and carboplatin) (as adjuvant therapy). HER2–overexpressing node positive or node negative breast cancer (to be used alone after multi-modality anthracycline-based therapy) (as adjuvant therapy). Metastatic breast cancer that displays overexpression of the human epidermal growth factor receptor 2 (HER2) protein (as first-line therapy) (in combination with paclitaxel). HER2–overexpressing metastatic breast cancer in patients who have already received ≥1 other chemotherapy regimens for metastatic disease (as monotherapy).

Action

A monoclonal antibody that binds to HER2 sites in breast cancer tissue and inhibits proliferation of cells that overexpress HER2 protein. **Therapeutic Effects:** Regression of breast, gastric, or gastroesophageal cancer and metastases.

Pharmacokinetics

Absorption: IV administration results in complete bioavailability.

Distribution: Binds to HER2 proteins.

Metabolism and Excretion: Unknown.

Half-life: 10-mg dose—1.7 days; 500-mg dose—12 days.

TIME/ACTION PROFILE (blood levels)

ROUTE	ONSET	PEAK	DURATION
IV	unknown	unknown	unknown

Contraindications/Precautions

Contraindicated in: OB: Pregnancy (may cause fetal harm); Lactation: Lactation (may cause harm to infant).

Use Cautiously in: Pre-existing pulmonary conditions; Hypersensitivity to trastuzumab, Chinese hamster ovary cell proteins, or other components of the product; Hypersensitivity to benzyl alcohol (use sterile water for injection instead of bacteriostatic water, which accompanies the vial); Rep: Women of reproductive potential; Pedi: Safety not established; Geri: May have ↑ risk of cardiac dysfunction.

Exercise Extreme Caution in: Patients with preexisting cardiac dysfunction.

Adverse Reactions/Side Effects

CNS: dizziness, headache, insomnia, weakness, depression. **CV:** ARRHYTHMIAS, HF, hypertension, tachycardia. **Derm:** rash, acne, herpes simplex. **F and E:** edema. **GI:** abdominal pain, anorexia, diarrhea, nausea, vomiting. **Hemat:** anemia, leukopenia. **MS:** back pain, arthralgia, bone pain. **Neuro:** neuropathy, paresthesia, peripheral neuritis. **Resp:** INTERSTITIAL PNEUMONITIS, PULMONARY EDEMA, PULMONARY FIBROSIS, dyspnea, increased cough, pharyngitis, rhinitis, sinusitis. **Misc:** HYPERSENSITIVITY REACTIONS (including anaphylaxis and angioedema), INFECTION, chills, fever, pain, flu-like syndrome.

Interactions

Drug-Drug: Concurrent **anthracycline** (**daunorubicin**, **doxorubicin**, or **idarubicin**) therapy may ↑ risk of cardiotoxicity. Blood levels are ↑ by concurrent **paclitaxel**.

Route/Dosage

Adjuvant Treatment of Breast Cancer

IV (Adults): *During and following paclitaxel, docetaxel, or docetaxel/carboplatin*—4 mg/kg initially, then 2 mg/kg once weekly during chemotherapy for the first 12 wk (paclitaxel or docetaxel) or 18 wk (docetaxel/carboplatin); one wk after the last weekly dose, give 6 mg/kg every 3 wk. Do not exceed treatment duration of 1 yr; *As single agent within 3 wk following completion of multi-modality, anthracycline-based chemotherapy regimens*—8 mg/kg initially, then 6 mg/kg every 3 wk. Do not exceed treatment duration of 1 yr.

Metastatic Breast Cancer

IV (Adults): 4 mg/kg initially, then 2 mg/kg once weekly until disease progression.

Metastatic Gastric Cancer

IV (Adults): 8 mg/kg initially, then 6 mg/kg every 3 wk until disease progressiones.

Availability

Lyophilized powder for injection (requires reconstitution and dilution): 150 mg/vial (single-dose vial), 420 mg/vial (multidose vial).

NURSING IMPLICATIONS

Assessment

- Assess for infusion-related symptoms (chills, fever, nausea, vomiting, pain [in some cases at tumor sites], headache, dizziness, dyspnea, hypotension, rash, and asthenia) following initial infusion. Severe reactions (bronchospasm, anaphylaxis, angioedema, hypoxia, severe hypotension) may occur during or immediately following the initial infusion. May be treated with epinephrine, corticosteroids, diphenhydramine, bronchodilators, and oxygen. Discontinue if dyspnea or severe hypotension occurs and discontinue permanently if severe reaction occurs.
- Assess for signs and symptoms of HF (dyspnea, increased cough, paroxysmal nocturnal dyspnea, peripheral edema, S_3 gallop, reduced ejection fraction) prior to and frequently during therapy.

T

Baseline cardiac assessment of history, physical exam, and left ventricular ejection fraction (LVEF) with ECG or multiple gated acquisition (MUGA) scan. Monitor LVEF every 3 mo and at completion of therapy, every 6 mo for 2 yr. Withhold trastuzumab for ≥16% absolute decrease in LVEF from pre-treatment values or an LVEF value below institutional limits of normal and ≥10% absolute decrease in LVEF from pretreatment values. Repeat LVEF measures every 4 wk if dose is withheld. HF associated with trastuzumab may be severe, resulting in cardiac failure, death, and stroke. Trastuzumab should be discontinued upon the development of significant HF.

- Monitor patient for signs of pulmonary hypersensitivity reactions (dyspnea, pulmonary infiltrates, pleural effusion, noncardiogenic pulmonary edema, pulmonary insufficiency, hypoxia, acute respiratory distress syndrome). Patients with symptomatic pulmonary disease or extensive lung tumor involvement are at increased risk. Infusion should be discontinued if severe symptoms occur.
- ***Lab Test Considerations:*** Obtain a negative pregnancy test before starting therapy.
- HER2 protein overexpression is used to determine whether treatment with trastuzumab is indicated. HER2 protein overexpression is detected by HercepTest (IHC assay) and PathVysion (FISH assay).
- Verify negative pregnancy status before starting therapy.
- May cause anemia and leukopenia.

Implementation

- ***High Alert:*** Do not confuse trastuzumab (Herceptin) with ado-trastuzumab (Kadcyla).
- ***High Alert:*** Fatalities have occurred with chemotherapeutic agents. Before administering, clarify all ambiguous orders; double check single, daily, and course-of-therapy dose limits; have second practitioner independently double check original order, dose calculations and infusion pump settings.
- May be administered in the outpatient setting.
- *If a dose is missed by ≤1 wk,* administer usual maintenance dose as soon as possible. Do not wait until next planned cycle. Administer subsequent maintenance doses 7 days or 21 days later according to the weekly or three-weekly schedules, respectively. *If a dose is missed by >1 wk,* administer a re-loading dose as soon as possible. Administer subsequent maintenance doses 7 days or 21 days later according to weekly or three-weekly schedules, respectively.

IV Administration

- **Intermittent Infusion:** Reconstitute each vial with 20 mL of bacteriostatic water for injection, directing the stream of diluent into lyophilized cake of trastuzumab. ***Concentration:*** 21 mg/mL. Swirl the vial gently; do not shake. May foam slightly; allow the vial to stand undisturbed for 5 min. Solution should be clear to slightly opalescent and colorless to pale yellow, without particulate matter. Label vial immediately in the area marked "Do not use after" with the date 28 days from the date of reconstitution. Stable for 24 hr at room temperature or 28 days if refrigerated. If patient is allergic to benzyl alcohol, use sterile water for injection for reconstitution. Use immediately and discard any unused portion. ***Diluent:*** Calculate to volume required for the desired dose, withdraw, and add it to an infusion containing 250 mL of 0.9% NaCl. Invert bag gently to mix. ***Rate:*** Infuse the 4 mg/kg loading dose over 90 min and the weekly 2 mg/kg dose over 30 min or 6 mg/kg dose over 30–90 min every 3 wk, or 8 mg/kg dose over 90 min if the loading dose was well tolerated. Do not administer as an IV push or bolus.
- **Y-Site Compatibility:** acyclovir, amifostine, aminophylline, ampicillin, ampicillin/sulbactam, bleomycin, bumetanide, buprenorphine, busulfan, butorphanol, calcium gluconate, carboplatin, carmustine, cefazolin, ceftazidime, ceftriaxone, cefuroxime, ciprofloxacin, cisplatin, cyclophosphamide, cytarabine, dactinomycin, daunorubicin hydrochloride, dexamethasone, digoxin, diphenhydramine, dobutamine, docetaxel, dopamine, doxorubicin hydrochloride, doxorubicin liposomal, doxycycline, droperidol, enalaprilat, etoposide phosphate, famotidine, fentanyl, filgrastim, fluconazole, fluorouracil, ganciclovir, gemcitabine, gentamicin, granisetron, haloperidol, heparin, hydrocortisone, hydromorphone, ifosfamide, imipenem/cilastatin, leucovorin calcium, lorazepam, magnesium sulfate, mannitol, meperidine, mesna, methotrexate, methylprednisolone, metoclopramide, metronidazole, mitomycin, mitoxantrone, paclitaxel, pentamidine, potassium chloride, prochlorperazine, promethazine, ranitidine, remifentanil, sargramostim, sodium bicarbonate, theophylline, thiotepa, tobramycin, trimethoprim/sulfamethoxazole, vancomycin, vinblastine, vincristine, vinorelbine, zidovudine.
- **Y-Site Incompatibility:** aldesleukin, amikacin, aztreonam, cefotaxime, cefotetan, cefoxitin, chlorpromazine, clindamycin, cyclosporine, fludarabine, furosemide, idarubicin, irinotecan, levofloxacin, levorphanol, morphine, nalbuphine, ondansetron, piperacillin/tazobactam, streptozocin, topotecan.
- **Additive Incompatibility:** Do not dilute trastuzumab with or add to solutions containing dextrose. Do not mix or dilute with other drugs.

Patient/Family Teaching

- Instruct patient to notify health care professional promptly if new onset or worsening shortness of breath, cough, swelling of the ankles/legs, swelling of the face, palpitations, weight gain of more than 5 pounds in 24 hrs, dizziness or loss of consciousness occur. Caution patient to avoid crowds and persons with known infections.
- Advise patient not to receive any vaccinations without advice of health care professional.

- Rep: Advise female patient that trastuzumab is teratogenic and to notify health care professional immediately if pregnancy is planned or suspected or if breast feeding. Caution patient to use effective contraception during and for 7 mo following last dose. Advise women who are breast feeding to discontinue nursing or discontinue trastuzumab. Encourage women who may be exposed during pregnancy to report exposure to the Genentech Adverse Event Line at 1-888-835-2555. Monitor patients who become pregnant for oligohydramnios.

Evaluation/Desired Outcomes

- Regression of breast, gastric, or gastroesophageal cancer and metastases.

traZODone (traz-oh-done)

~~Desyrel~~, ✱Oleptro, ✱Trazorel

Classification

Therapeutic: antidepressants

Indications

Major depression. **Unlabeled Use:** Insomnia, chronic pain syndromes, including diabetic neuropathy, and anxiety.

Action

Alters the effects of serotonin in the CNS. **Therapeutic Effects:** Antidepressant action, which may develop only over several wk.

Pharmacokinetics

Absorption: Well absorbed after oral administration.

Distribution: Widely distributed.

Protein Binding: 89–95%.

Metabolism and Excretion: Extensively metabolized by the liver (CYP3A4 enzyme system); minimal excretion of unchanged drug by the kidneys.

Half-life: 5–9 hr (immediate-release).

TIME/ACTION PROFILE (antidepressant effect)

ROUTE	ONSET	PEAK	DURATION
PO	1–2 wk	2–4 wk	wks

Contraindications/Precautions

Contraindicated in: Hypersensitivity; Recovery period after MI; Concurrent electroconvulsive therapy; Concurrent use of MAO inhibitors or MAO-like drugs (linezolid or methylene blue); Angle-closure glaucoma.

Use Cautiously in: Cardiovascular disease; Suicidal behavior; May ↑ risk of suicide attempt/ideation especially during early treatment or dose adjustment; Severe hepatic or renal disease (dose ↓ recommended); Lactation: Discontinue drug or bottle feed; Pedi: Suicide risk may be greater in children and adolescents; safety not established; Geri: Initial dose ↓ recommended.

Adverse Reactions/Side Effects

CNS: SUICIDAL THOUGHTS, drowsiness, confusion, dizziness, fatigue, hallucinations, headache, insomnia, nightmares, slurred speech, syncope, weakness. **EENT:** blurred vision, tinnitus. **CV:** hypotension, arrhythmias, chest pain, hypertension, palpitations, QT interval prolongation, tachycardia. **GI:** dry mouth, altered taste, constipation, diarrhea, excess salivation, flatulence, nausea, vomiting. **GU:** hematuria, erectile dysfunction, priapism, urinary frequency. **Derm:** rash. **Hemat:** anemia, leukopenia. **MS:** myalgia. **Neuro:** tremor.

Interactions

Drug-Drug: Serious, potentially fatal reactions (hyperthermia, rigidity, myoclonus, autonomic instability, with fluctuating vital signs and extreme agitation, which may proceed to delirium and coma) may occur with concurrent **MAO inhibitors**. MAO inhibitors should be stopped at least 14 days before trazodone therapy. Trazodone should be stopped at least 14 days before MAO inhibitor therapy. Concurrent use with **MAO-inhibitor like drugs**, such as **linezolid** or **methylene blue** may ↑ risk of serotonin syndrome; concurrent use contraindicated; do not start therapy in patients receiving **linezolid** or **methylene blue**; if **linezolid** or **methylene blue** need to be started in a patient receiving trazodone, immediately discontinue trazodone and monitor for signs/symptoms of serotonin syndrome for 2 wk or until 24 hr after last dose of linezolid or methylene blue, whichever comes first (may resume trazodone therapy 24 hr after last dose of linezolid or methylene blue). May ↑ **digoxin** or **phenytoin** serum levels. ↑ CNS depression with other **CNS depressants**, including **alcohol**, **opioid analgesics**, and **sedative/hypnotics**. ↑ hypotension with **antihypertensives**, acute ingestion of **alcohol**, or **nitrates**. Concurrent use with **fluoxetine** ↑ levels and risk of toxicity from trazodone. **Drugs that inhibit the CYP3A4 enzyme system**, including **ritonavir indinavir** and **ketoconazole**↑ levels and the risk of toxicity. **Drugs that induce the CYP3A4 enzyme system**, including **carbamazepine** ↓ levels and may decrease effectiveness. Drugs that affect serotonergic neurotransmitter systems, including **tricyclic antidepressants**, **fentanyl**, **buspirone**, **tramadol** and **triptans** ↑ risk of serotonin syndrome. ↑ risk of bleeding with **NSAIDS**, **aspirin**, **clopidogrel**, or **warfarin**.

Drug-Natural Products: Concomitant use of **kava-kava**, **valerian**, or **chamomile** can ↑ CNS depression. ↑ risk of serotinergic side effects including serotonin syndrome with **St. John's wort** and **SAMe**.

T

Route/Dosage

Depression

PO (Adults): 150 mg/day in 3 divided doses; ↑ by 50 mg/day every 3–4 days until desired response (not to exceed 400 mg/day in outpatients or 600 mg/day in hospitalized patients).

PO (Geriatric Patients): 75 mg/day in divided doses initially; may be ↑ every 3–4 days.

Insomnia

PO (Adults): 25–100 mg at bedtime.

Availability (generic available)

Tablets (immediate-release): 50 mg, 100 mg, 150 mg, 300 mg. **Cost:** *Generic*—All strengths $10.83/100. **Tablets (extended-release) (Oleptro):** 🍁150 mg, 🍁300 mg.

NURSING IMPLICATIONS

Assessment

- Monitor BP and pulse rate before and during initial therapy. Monitor ECGs in patients with pre-existing cardiac disease before and periodically during therapy to detect arrhythmias.
- Assess for possible sexual dysfunction.
- Assess for serotonin syndrome (mental changes [agitation, hallucinations, coma], autonomic instability [tachycardia, labile BP, hyperthermia], neuromuscular aberrations [hyper-reflexia, incoordination], and/or GI symptoms [nausea, vomiting, diarrhea]), especially in patients taking other serotonergic drugs (SSRIs, SNRIs, triptans).
- **Depression:** Assess mental status (orientation, mood, and behavior) frequently.
- Assess for suicidal tendencies, especially during early therapy. Restrict amount of drug available to patient. Risk may be increased in children, adolescents, and adults ≤24 yr. After starting therapy, children, adolescents, and young adults should be seen by health care professional at least weekly for 4 wk, every 3 wk for next 4 wk, and on advice of health care professional thereafter.
- **Pain:** Assess location, duration, intensity, and characteristics of pain before and periodically during therapy. Use pain scale to assess effectiveness of medicine.
- ***Lab Test Considerations:*** Assess CBC and renal and hepatic function before and periodically during therapy. Slight, clinically insignificant ↓ in leukocyte and neutrophil counts may occur.

Implementation

- Do not confuse trazodone with tramadol.
- **PO:** Administer with or immediately after meals to minimize side effects (nausea, dizziness) and allow maximum absorption of trazodone. A larger portion of the total daily dose may be given at bedtime to decrease daytime drowsiness and dizziness.

Patient/Family Teaching

- Instruct patient to take medication as directed. If a dose is missed, take as soon as remembered. Do not take if within 4 hr of next scheduled dose; do not double doses. Consult health care professional before discontinuing medication; gradual dose reduction is necessary to prevent aggravation of condition. Advise patient to read *Medication Guide* prior starting therapy and with each Rx refill in case of changes.
- May cause drowsiness and blurred vision. Caution patient to avoid driving and other activities requiring alertness until response to drug is known.
- Caution patient to change positions slowly to minimize orthostatic hypotension.
- Advise patient to avoid concurrent use of alcohol or other CNS depressant drugs.
- Advise patient, family, and caregivers to look for suicidality, especially during early therapy or dose changes. Notify health care professional immediately if thoughts about suicide or dying, attempts to commit suicide, new or worse depression or anxiety, agitation or restlessness, panic attacks, insomnia, new or worse irritability, aggressiveness, acting on dangerous impulses, mania, or other changes in mood or behavior or if symptoms of serotonin syndrome occur.
- Advise patient to notify health care professional of all Rx or OTC medications, vitamins, or herbal products being taken and to consult with health care professional before taking other medications, especially aspirin and NSAIDs.
- Inform patient that frequent rinses, good oral hygiene, and sugarless candy or gum may diminish dry mouth. Health care professional should be notified if this persists >2 wk. An increase in fluid intake, fiber, and exercise may prevent constipation.
- Advise patient to notify health care professional of medication regimen before treatment or surgery.
- Instruct patient to notify health care professional if priapism, irregular heartbeat, fainting, confusion, skin rash, or tremors occur or if dry mouth, nausea and vomiting, dizziness, headache, muscle aches, constipation, or diarrhea becomes pronounced.
- Instruct patient to notify health care professional if signs of serotonin syndrome (mental status changes: agitation, hallucinations, coma; autonomic instability: tachycardia, labile BP, hyperthermia; neuromuscular aberrations: hyperreflexia, incoordination; and/or gastrointestinal symptoms: nausea, vomiting, diarrhea) occur.
- Advise female patients to notify health care professional if pregnancy is planned or suspected or if breast feeding.
- Emphasize the importance of follow-up exams to evaluate progress.

Evaluation/Desired Outcomes

- Resolution of depression.
- Increased sense of well-being.

- Renewed interest in surroundings.
- Increased appetite.
- Improved energy level.
- Improved sleep.
- Decrease in severity of pain in chronic pain syndromes. Therapeutic effects are usually seen within 1 wk, although 4 wk may be required to obtain significant therapeutic results.

triamcinolone, See CORTICOSTEROIDS (NASAL), CORTICOSTEROIDS (SYSTEMIC), and CORTICOSTEROIDS (TOPICAL/LOCAL).

triamterene, See DIURETICS (POTASSIUM-SPARING).

tricalcium phosphate (39% Ca or 19.5 mEq/g), See CALCIUM SALTS.

trifluridine/tipiracil

(tri-**floo**-ri-deen/ti-**peer**-a-sil)
Lonsurf

Classification
Therapeutic: antineoplastics
Pharmacologic: nucleoside metabolic inhibitors, thymidine phosphorylase inhibitors

Indications

Metastatic colorectal cancer in patients previously treated with fluoropyrmidine-, oxalplatin- or irinotecan-based chemotherapies, an anti-VEGF based biological and an anti-EGFR agent (if RAS wild-type positive). Metastatic gastric or gastroesophageal junction adenocarcinoma previously treated with ≥2 lines of chemotherapy including a fluoropyrimidine, a platinum, either a taxane or irinotecan, and if appropriate, a HER2/neu-targeted therapy.

Action

Trifluridine—following uptake into cells, interferes with DNA synthesis, inhibiting cell proliferation. *tipiracil*—increases trifluridine levels by inhibiting thymidine phosphorylase, the enzyme that metabolizes it.
Therapeutic Effects: Decreases spread of metastatic colorectal cancer.

Pharmacokinetics

Absorption: Well absorbed following oral administration.
Distribution: Unknown.
Protein Binding: *Trifluridine*—>96%.
Metabolism and Excretion: Trifluridine is metabolized by thymidine phosphorylase to an inactive metabolite. *Trifluridine*—1.5% excreted unchanged in urine; *tipiracil*—29.3% excreted unchanged in urine.
Half-life: *Trifluridine*—2.1 hr; *tipiracil*—2.4 hr.

TIME/ACTION PROFILE (improved survival)

ROUTE	ONSET	PEAK	DURATION
PO	1–2 mo	unknown	unknown

Contraindications/Precautions

Contraindicated in: Initial ANC <1500/mm³ or platelets <75,000/mm³, resolution of grade 3 or 4 nonhematologic toxicity to grade 0 or 1; During treatment ANC<500 mm³ or febrile neutropenia, platelets <50,000/mm³ or grade 3 or 4 non-hematologic toxicity; Moderate to severe hepatic impairment; OB: Pregnancy (may cause fetal harm); Lactation: Avoid breast feeding.
Use Cautiously in: Severe renal impairment (effects of drug are not known); Moderate renal impairment (↑ risk of toxicity, dose alteration may be required; Rep: Women of reproductive potential or men with female partners of reproductive potential (use effective contraception); Geri: ↑ risk and severity of myelosuppression in patients ≥65 yr.

Adverse Reactions/Side Effects

CNS: asthenia. **Derm:** alopecia. **GI:** abdominal pain, ↓ appetite, diarrhea, nausea, vomiting, stomatitis. **Hemat:** ANEMIA, NEUTROPENIA, THROMBOCYTOPENIA. **Misc:** fever.

Interactions

Drug-Drug: None noted.

Route/Dosage

PO (Adults): 35 mg/m²/dose (max dose = 80 mg) (based on trifluridine content rounded to the nearest 5 mg) twice daily on days 1–5 and 8–12 of each 28-day cycle; continue until disease progression or unacceptable toxicity.

Availability

Tablets: trifluridine 15 mg/tipiracil 6.14 mg, trifluridine 20 mg/tipiracil 8.19 mg.

NURSING IMPLICATIONS

Assessment

- Monitor for signs and symptoms of infection (fever, chills, body aches) periodically during therapy.
- ***Lab Test Considerations:*** Obtain a negative pregnancy test before starting therapy.
- Obtain CBC prior to and on Day 15 of each cycle and as clinically indicated. *Do not administer un-*

til: absolute neutrophil count (ANC) ≥1500/mm³ or febrile neutropenia resolved, platelet count ≥75,000/mm³, and Grade 3 or 4 non-hematologic adverse reactions are resolved to Grade 0–1. *During treatment cycle, withhold trifluridine/tipiracil if:* ANC <500/mm³ or febrile neutropenia, platelets <50,000/mm³, or Grade 3 or 4 non-hematologic adverse reactions occur. *After recovery, reduce dose by 5 mg/m²/dose from previous dose level if:* febrile neutropenia —uncomplicated Grade 4 neutropenia recovered to ≥1500/mm³ or thrombocytopenia —recovered to ≥75,000/mm³ resulting in >1 wk delay in start of next cycle or nonhematologic Grade 3 or 4 adverse reaction except for Grade 3 nausea and/or vomiting controlled by antiemetic therapy or Grade 3 diarrhea responsive to antidiarrheal medication occur. No more than 3 dose reductions to a minimum dose of 20 mg/m² twice daily are permitted. Do not escalate dose after reductions.

Implementation

- **PO:** Administer twice daily within 1 hr of completion of morning and evening meals on Days 1–5 and Days 8–12 of each 28 day cycle. Swallow tablets whole; do not crush, break, or chew.

Patient/Family Teaching

- Instruct patient to take medication as directed. If dose missed or vomited, omit and take next dose at scheduled time; do not double doses. Inform patient that medication comes in two strengths; both strengths may be required for prescribed dose. Advise patient to read *Patient Information* before starting and with each Rx refill in case of changes.
- Advise patient that anyone who handles medication should wear gloves. Wash hands after handling medication.
- Advise patient to notify health care professional if signs and symptoms of infection, or persistent nausea, vomiting, or diarrhea occur.
- Instruct patient to notify health care professional of all Rx or OTC medications, vitamins, or herbal products being taken and consult health care professional before taking any new medications.
- Rep: Caution patient that medication is teratogenic. Advise females of reproductive potential to use effective contraception during therapy and for 6 mo after last dose, and to notify health care professional if pregnancy is planned or suspected. Advise female patient to avoid breast feeding during and for at least 1 day after last dose of therapy. Advise male patients with female partners of reproductive potential to wear condoms during and for at least 3 mo after last dose of therapy.

Evaluation/Desired Outcomes

- Decreases spread of metastatic colorectal cancer.

trimethoprim/sulfamethoxazole

(trye-**meth**-oh-prim/sul-fa-meth-**ox**-a-zole)

Bactrim, Bactrim DS, Septra, Septra DS, ✱Sulfatrim, ✱Sulfatrim DS, Sulfatrim Pediatric

Classification

Therapeutic: anti-infectives, antiprotozoals

Pharmacologic: folate antagonists, sulfonamides

Indications

Treatment of: Bronchitis, *Shigella* enteritis, Otitis media, *Pneumocystis jirovecii* pneumonia (PCP), Urinary tract infections, Traveler's diarrhea. Prevention of PCP in HIV-positive patients. **Unlabeled Use:** Biliary tract infections, osteomyelitis, burn and wound infections, chlamydial infections, endocarditis, gonorrhea, intra-abdominal infections, nocardiosis, rheumatic fever prophylaxis, sinusitis, eradication of meningococcal carriers, prophylaxis of urinary tract infections, and an alternative agent in the treatment of chancroid. Prevention of bacterial infections in immunosuppressed patients.

Action

Combination inhibits the metabolism of folic acid in bacteria at two different points. **Therapeutic Effects:** Bactericidal action against susceptible bacteria. **Spectrum:** Active against many strains of gram-positive aerobic pathogens including: *Streptococcus pneumoniae*, *Staphylococcus aureus*, Group A beta-hemolytic streptococci, *Nocardia*, *Enterococcus*. Has activity against many aerobic gram-negative pathogens, such as: *Acinetobacter*, *Enterobacter*, *Klebsiella pneumoniae*, *Escherichia coli*, *Proteus mirabilis*, *Shigella*, *Xanthomonas maltophilia*, *Haemophilus influenzae*, including ampicillin-resistant strains. *P. jirovecii*. Not active against *Pseudomonas aeruginosa*.

Pharmacokinetics

Absorption: Well absorbed from the GI tract.

Distribution: Widely distributed. Crosses the blood-brain barrier and placenta and enters breast milk.

Protein Binding: *Trimethoprim*—45%; *Sulfamethoxazole*—68%.

Metabolism and Excretion: Some metabolism by the liver (20%); remainder excreted unchanged by the kidneys.

Half-life: *Trimethoprim*—6–11 hr; *sulfamethoxazole*—9–12 hr, both prolonged in renal failure.

TIME/ACTION PROFILE (blood levels)

ROUTE	ONSET	PEAK	DURATION
PO	rapid	2–4 hr	6–12 hr
IV	rapid	end of infusion	6–12 hr

Contraindications/Precautions

Contraindicated in: Hypersensitivity to sulfonamides or trimethoprim; History of drug-induced immune thrombocytopenia due to sulfonamides or trimethoprim; Megaloblastic anemia secondary to folate deficiency; Severe hepatic or renal impairment; OB, Lactation, Pedi: Pregnancy, lactation, or children <2 mo (can cause kernicterus in neonates). Exception: neonates born to HIV-infected mothers (prophylaxis should be initiated at 4–6 wk of age).

Use Cautiously in: Mild to moderate hepatic or renal impairment (dose ↓ required if CCr <30 mL/min); Glucose–6–phosphate dehydrogenase deficiency (↑ risk hemolysis); HIV-positive patients (↑ incidence of adverse reactions); Concurrent use with other products containing propylene glycol (IV only) (↑ risk of lactic acidosis).

Adverse Reactions/Side Effects

CNS: fatigue, hallucinations, headache, insomnia, mental depression, kernicterus in neonates. **CV:** hypotension. **Derm:** ERYTHEMA MULTIFORME, STEVENS-JOHNSON SYNDROME, TOXIC EPIDERMAL NECROLYSIS, rash, photosensitivity. **Endo:** hypoglycemia. **F and E:** hyperkalemia, hyponatremia. **GI:** CLOSTRIDIUM DIFFICILE-ASSOCIATED DIARRHEA (CDAD), HEPATIC NECROSIS, nausea, vomiting, diarrhea, stomatitis, hepatitis, cholestatic jaundice, pancreatitis. **GU:** crystalluria. **Hemat:** AGRANULOCYTOSIS, APLASTIC ANEMIA, hemolytic anemia, leukopenia, megaloblastic anemia, thrombocytopenia. **Local:** phlebitis at IV site. **Misc:** fever.

Interactions

Drug-Drug: May ↑ half-life, ↓ clearance, and exaggerate folic acid deficiency caused by **phenytoin**. May ↑ effects of **sulfonylureas**, **pioglitazone**, **rosiglitazone**, **repaglinide**, **phenytoin**, **digoxin**, and **warfarin**. May ↑ toxicity of **methotrexate**. ↑ risk of thrombocytopenia from **thiazide diuretics** (↑ in geriatric patients). ↓ levels of and ↑ risk of nephrotoxicity with **cyclosporine**. Concurrent use with **ACE inhibitors** may ↑ risk of hyperkalemia. May ↓ the effects of **tricyclic antidepressants**. Concurrent use with **leucovorin** may result in treatment failure and ↑ risk of death (avoid concurrent use).

Route/Dosage

(TMP = trimethoprim; SMX = sulfamethoxazole). Dosing based on TMP content.

Bacterial Infections

PO, IV (Adults and Children >2 mo): *Mild-moderate infections*—6–12 mg TMP/kg/day divided every 12 hr; *Serious infection/Pneumocystis*—15–20 mg TMP/kg /day divided every 6–8 hr.

PO (Adults): *Urinary tract infection/chronic bronchitis*—1 double-strength tablet (160 mg TMP/800 mg SMX) every 12 hr for 10–14 days.

Urinary Tract Infection Prophylaxis

PO, IV (Adults and Children >2 mo): 2 mg TMP/kg/dose once daily or 5 mg TMP/kg/dose twice weekly.

P. jirovecii Pneumonia (Prevention)

PO (Adults): 1 double-strength tablet (160 mg TMP/800 mg SMX) once daily (may also be given 3 times weekly).

PO (Children >1 mo): 150 mg TMP/m^2/day divided every 12 hr or given as a single dose on 3 consecutive days/wk (not to exceed 320 mg TMP/1600 mg SMX per day).

Availability (generic available)

Oral suspension (cherry, grape flavors): 40 mg TMP/200 mg SMX per 5 mL. **Cost:** *Generic*—$58.10/473 mL. **Solution for injection (requires dilution):** 16 mg TMP/80 mg SMX per mL (contains 40% propylene glycol). **Tablets:** 🍁 20 mg TMP/100 mg SMX, 80 mg TMP/400 mg SMX, 160 mg TMP/800 mg SMX (double-strength). **Cost:** *Generic*—80 mg TMP/400 mg SMX $6.99/30, 160 mg TMP/800 mg SMX $6.70/30.

NURSING IMPLICATIONS

Assessment

- Assess for infection (vital signs; appearance of wound, sputum, urine, and stool; WBC) at beginning of and during therapy.
- Obtain specimens for culture and sensitivity before initiating therapy. First dose may be given before receiving results.
- Inspect IV site frequently. Phlebitis is common.
- Assess patient for allergy to sulfonamides.
- Monitor intake and output ratios. Fluid intake should be sufficient to maintain a urine output of at least 1200–1500 mL daily to prevent crystalluria and stone formation.
- Monitor bowel function. Diarrhea, abdominal cramping, fever, and bloody stools should be reported to health care professional promptly as a sign of Clostridium difficile-associated diarrhea (CDAD). May begin up to several wk following cessation of therapy.
- Assess for rash periodically during therapy. May cause Stevens-Johnson syndrome. Discontinue therapy if severe or if accompanied with fever, general malaise, fatigue, muscle or joint aches, blisters, oral lesions, conjunctivitis, hepatitis and/or eosinophilia.
- ***Lab Test Considerations:*** Monitor CBC and urinalysis periodically during therapy.
- May produce ↑ serum bilirubin, ↑ potassium, creatinine, and alkaline phosphatase.
- May cause hypoglycemia.

T

Implementation

- Do not confuse DS (double-strength) formulations with single-strength formulations.
- Do not administer medication IM.
- **PO:** Administer around the clock with a full glass of water. Use calibrated measuring device for liquid preparations.

IV Administration

- **Intermittent Infusion:** ***Diluent:*** Dilute each 5 mL of trimethoprim/sulfamethoxazole with 125 mL of D5W (stable for 24 hr at room temperature). May also dilute each 5 mL of drug with 75 mL of D5W if fluid restriction is required (stable for 6 hr at room temperature). Do not refrigerate. ***Concentration:*** Should not exceed 1.06 mg/mL. ***Rate:*** Infuse over 60–90 min.
- **Y-Site Compatibility:** acyclovir, aldesleukin, alemtuzumab, allopurinol, amifostine, aminocaproic acid, amphotericin B liposome, anidulafungin, argatroban, azithromycin, bivalirudin, bleomycin, carboplatin, carmustine, cefepime, ceftaroline, cisplatin, cyclophosphamide, cytarabine, dactinomycin, daptomycin, dexmedetomidine, diltiazem, docetaxel, doxorubicin liposome, eptifibatide, ertapenem, etoposide, etoposide phosphate, fenoldopam, filgrastim, fludarabine, fluorouracil, gemcitabine, granisetron, hetastarch, hydromorphone, ifosfamide, irinotecan, levofloxacin, linezolid, lorazepam, melphalan, methotrexate, metronidazole, milrinone, mitoxantrone, nicardipine, octreotide, oxaliplatin, paclitaxel, palonosetron, pamidronate, pancuronium, pantoprazole, pemetrexed, perphenazine, piperacillin/tazobactam, potassium acetate, remifentanil, rituximab, sargramostim, sodium acetate, thiotepa, tigecycline, tirofiban, trastuzumab, vecuronium, vinblastine, vincristine, voriconazole, zidovudine, zoledronic acid.
- **Y-Site Incompatibility:** alfentanil, amikacin, aminophylline, amphotericin B lipid complex, ampicillin, ampicillin/sulbactam, ascorbic acid, atropine, azathioprine, benztropine, bumetanide, buprenorphine, butorphanol, calcium chloride, calcium gluconate, caspofungin, cefazolin, cefotaxime, cefoxitin, ceftazidime, ceftriaxone, cefuroxime, chloramphenicol, chlorpromazine, clindamycin, cyanocobalamin, cyclosporine, dantrolene, dexamethasone, dexrazoxane, diazepam, diazoxide, digoxin, diphenhydramine, dobutamine, dopamine, doxorubicin, doxycycline, ephedrine, epinephrine, epirubicin, epoetin alfa, erythromycin, famotidine, fentanyl, fluconazole, folic acid, furosemide, ganciclovir, gentamicin, glycopyrrolate, haloperidol, heparin, hydralazine, hydrocortisone, hydroxyzine, idarubicin, imipenem/cilastatin, indomethacin, insulin, regular, isoproterenol, ketamine, ketorolac, lidocaine, mannitol, metaraminol, methyldopate, methylprednisolone, metoclopramide, metoprolol, midazolam, multivitamins, mycophenolate, nafcillin, nalbuphine, naloxone, nitroglycerin, nitroprusside, norepinephrine, ondansetron, oxacillin, oxytocin, papaverine, penicillin G, pentamidine, pentobarbital, phenobarbital, phentolamine, phenylephrine, phenytoin, phytonadione, potassium chloride, procainamide, prochlorperazine, promethazine, propranolol, protamine, pyridoxime, quinupristin/dalfopristin, ranitidine, sodium bicarbonate, streptokinase, succinylcholine, sufentanil, theophylline, thiamine, tobramycin, tolazoline, vancomycin, verapamil, vinorelbine.

Patient/Family Teaching

- Instruct patient to take medication around the clock and to finish drug completely as directed, even if feeling well. Take missed doses as soon as remembered unless almost time for next dose. Advise patient that sharing of this medication may be dangerous.
- Instruct patient to notify health care professional if rash, or fever and diarrhea develop, especially if diarrhea contains blood, mucus, or pus. Advise patient not to treat diarrhea without consulting health care professional.
- Caution patient to use sunscreen and protective clothing to prevent photosensitivity reactions.
- Advise patient to notify health care professional if skin rash, sore throat, fever, mouth sores, or unusual bleeding or bruising occurs.
- Instruct patient to notify health care professional if symptoms do not improve within a few days.
- Advise females of reproductive potential to notify health care professional if pregnancy is planned or suspected, or if breast feeding.
- Emphasize importance of regular follow-up exams to monitor blood counts in patients on prolonged therapy.
- **Home Care Issues:** Instruct family or caregiver on dilution, rate, and administration of drug and proper care of IV equipment.

Evaluation/Desired Outcomes

- Resolution of the signs and symptoms of infection. Length of time for complete resolution depends on organism and site of infection.
- Resolution of symptoms of traveler's diarrhea.
- Prevention of *Pneumocystis jirovecii* pneumonia in patients with HIV.

ulipristal, See CONTRACEPTIVES, HORMONAL.

umeclidinium

(ue-mek-li-**din**-ee-um)
Incruse Ellipta

Classification
Therapeutic: bronchodilators
Pharmacologic: anticholinergics

Indications

Maintenance treatment of COPD.

Action

Acts as an anticholinergic by inhibiting M3 muscarinic receptors in bronchial smooth muscle resulting in bronchodilation. **Therapeutic Effects:** Bronchodilation with decreased airflow obstruction.

Pharmacokinetics

Absorption: Minimal oral absorption; remainder of absorption occurs in lungs.
Distribution: Unknown.
Metabolism and Excretion: Primarily metabolized by CYP2D6, metabolites do not contribute to bronchodilation.
Half-life: 11 hr.

TIME/ACTION PROFILE (bronchodilation)

ROUTE	ONSET	PEAK	DURATION
inhaln	1 hr	2–12 hr	24 hr

Contraindications/Precautions

Contraindicated in: Severe/acute symptoms of airflow obstruction; Severe hypersensitivity to milk proteins or other ingredients; Concurrent use with other anticholinergics.
Use Cautiously in: Narrow-angle glaucoma (may cause acute angle closure); Urinary retention, prostatic hyperplasia, bladder-neck obstruction; Severe hepatic impairment; OB: Safety not established; Lactation: Use while breast feeding only if maternal benefit outweighs potential risk to infant; Pedi: Safety and effectiveness not established; Geri: May be more sensitive to drug effects.

Adverse Reactions/Side Effects

CV: chest pain. **EENT:** acute narrow-angle glaucoma, cough, nasopharyngitis. **GU:** urinary retention. **MS:** arthralgia. **Resp:** PARADOXICAL BRONCHOSPASM. **Misc:** HYPERSENSITIVITY REACTIONS (including anaphylaxis and angioedema).

Interactions

Drug-Drug: ↑ risk of adverse anticholinergic adverse reactions when used concurrently with other **anticholinergics** (avoid concurrent use).

Route/Dosage

Inhaln (Adults): One inhalation (62.5 mcg) once daily.

Availability

Powder for inhalation in blister strips (contains lactose): 62.5 mcg/blister. ***In combination with:*** vilanterol (Anoro Ellipta), fluticasone and vilanterol (Trelegy Ellipta). See Appendix B.

NURSING IMPLICATIONS

Assessment

- Assess respiratory status (rate, breath sounds, degree of dyspnea, pulse) before administration and at peak of medication. Consult health care professional about alternative medication if severe bronchospasm is present; onset of action is too slow for patients in acute distress. If paradoxical bronchospasm (wheezing) occurs, withhold medication and notify health care professional immediately.

Implementation

- **Inhaln:** Follow manufacturer's instructions for use of inhaler. Breathe out; do not blow into mouthpiece. Close lips around mouthpiece. Breathe in a long, steady deep breath. Continue to hold breath as long as possible while removing inhaler from mouth. Slide cover over mouthpiece.

Patient/Family Teaching

- Instruct patient in the correct use of inhaler. Advise patient not to discontinue without consulting health care professional; symptoms may recur.
- Inform patient that umeclidinium should not be used for treating sudden breathing problems.
- Advise patient to notify health care professional if worsening symptoms; decreasing effectiveness of inhaled, short-acting beta$_2$–agonists; need for more inhalations than usual of inhaled, short-acting beta$_2$–agonists; or significant decrease in lung function occur.
- Instruct patient to notify health care professional of all Rx or OTC medications, vitamins, or herbal products being taken and to avoid concurrent use of Rx, OTC, and herbal products without consulting health care professional.
- Advise patient to notify health care professional if signs and symptoms of worsening narrow-angle glaucoma (eye pain or discomfort, blurred vision, visual halos, colored images associated with red dyes from conjunctival congestion, corneal edema) or worsening urinary retention (difficulty passing urine, painful urination) occur.
- Advise female patient to notify health care professional if pregnancy is planned or suspected or if breast feeding.

Evaluation/Desired Outcomes

- Decrease in the number of flare-ups or the worsening of COPD symptoms (exacerbations).

U

valACYclovir

(val-ay-**sye**-kloe-veer)
Valtrex

Classification
Therapeutic: antivirals

Indications

Treatment of herpes zoster (shingles). Treatment/suppression of genital herpes. Reduction of transmission of genital herpes. Treatment of chickenpox. Treatment of herpes labialis (cold sores).

Action

Rapidly converted to acyclovir. Acyclovir interferes with viral DNA synthesis. **Therapeutic Effects:** Inhibited viral replication, decreased viral shedding, reduced time to healing of lesions. Reduced transmission of genital herpes.

Pharmacokinetics

Absorption: 54% bioavailable as acyclovir after oral administration of valacyclovir.
Distribution: CSF concentrations of acyclovir are 50% of plasma concentrations. Acyclovir crosses placenta; enters breast milk.
Metabolism and Excretion: Rapidly converted to acyclovir via intestinal/hepatic metabolism.
Half-life: 2.5–3.3 hr; up to 14 hr in renal impairment (acyclovir).

TIME/ACTION PROFILE (blood levels†)

ROUTE	ONSET	PEAK	DURATION
PO	unknown	1.5–2.5 hr	8–24 hr

†Acyclovir.

Contraindications/Precautions

Contraindicated in: Hypersensitivity to valacyclovir or acyclovir.
Use Cautiously in: Renal impairment (↓ dose/↑ dosing interval recommended if CCr <50 mL/min); OB, Lactation, Pedi: Pregnancy, lactation, or children <2 yr (safety not established); Geri: Dose ↓ may be necessary due to ↑ risk of acute renal failure and CNS side effects.

Adverse Reactions/Side Effects

CNS: headache, agitation, confusion, delirium, dizziness, encephalopathy, hallucinations, seizures, weakness. **GI:** nausea, abdominal pain, anorexia, constipation, diarrhea. **GU:** RENAL FAILURE, crystalluria.
Hemat: THROMBOTIC THROMBOCYTOPENIC PURPURA/HEMOLYTIC UREMIC SYNDROME (very high doses in immunosuppressed patients).

Interactions

Drug-Drug: Probenecid and **cimetidine** ↑ blood levels; significant only in renal impairment. Concurrent use of other **nephrotoxic drugs** ↑ risk of adverse renal effects.

Route/Dosage

Herpes Zoster

PO (Adults): 1 g 3 times daily for 7 days.

Genital Herpes

PO (Adults): *Initial treatment*—1 g twice daily for 10 days. *Recurrence*—500 mg twice daily for 3 days. *Suppression of recurrence*—1 g once daily or 500 mg once daily in patients experiencing <10 recurrences/yr. *Suppression of recurrence in HIV-infected patients*—500 mg every 12 hr. *Reduction of transmission*—500 mg once daily for source partner.

Herpes Labialis

PO (Adults and Children ≥12 yr): 2 g then 2 g 12 hr later.

Chickenpox

PO (Children ≥2 yr): 20 mg/kg 3 times daily for 5 days (not to exceed 1 g 3 times daily).

Renal Impairment

PO (Adults): *CCr 30–49 mL/min*—1 g every 12 hr for herpes zoster treatment, no ↓ required for treatment of genital herpes; 1 g then 1 g 12 hr later for herpes labialis. *CCr 10–29 mL/min*—1 g every 24 hr for initial treatment of genital herpes, 500 mg every 24 hr for treatment of recurrent episodes of genital herpes, 500 mg every 48 hr for suppression of genital herpes in patients with 9 or fewer recurrences/yr, 500 mg every 24 hr for suppression of genital herpes in patients with ≥10 recurrences/yr or HIV-infected patients, 1 g every 24 hr for treatment of herpes zoster; 500 mg then 500 mg 12 hr later for herpes labialis. *CCr <10 mL/min*—500 mg every 24 hr for initial treatment of genital herpes, 500 mg every 24 hr for treatment of recurrent episodes of genital herpes, 500 mg every 48 hr for suppression of genital herpes in patients with 9 or fewer recurrences/yr, 500 mg every 24 hr for suppression of genital herpes in patients with ≥10 recurrences/yr or HIV-infected patients, 500 mg every 24 hr for treatment of herpes zoster; single 500 mg dose for herpes labialis.

Availability (generic available)

Tablets: 500 mg, 1 g. **Cost:** *Generic*—500 mg $31.44/30, 1 g $53.34/30.

NURSING IMPLICATIONS

Assessment

- Assess lesions before and daily during therapy.
- Monitor patient for signs of thrombotic thrombocytic purpura/hemolytic uremic syndrome (thrombocytopenia, microangiopathic hemolytic anemia, neurologic findings, renal dysfunction, fever). Requires prompt treatment; may be fatal.

Implementation

- ***High Alert:*** Do not confuse valacyclovir with valganciclovir. Do not confuse Valtrex (valacyclovir) with Valcyte (valganciclovir).
- **PO:** May be administered without regard to meals.
- **Herpes Zoster:** Implement valacyclovir therapy as soon as possible after the onset of signs or symptoms of herpes zoster; most effective if started within 48 hr of the onset of zoster rash. Efficacy of treatment started >72 hr after rash onset is unknown.
- **Genital Herpes and Herpes Labialis:** Implement treatment for genital herpes as soon as possible after onset of symptoms (tingling, itching, burning).
- **Chicken Pox:** Initiate therapy at the earliest sign or symptom; preferably within 24 hr of onset of rash.

Patient/Family Teaching

- Instruct patient to take valacyclovir exactly as directed for the full course of therapy. Take missed doses as soon as remembered if not just before next dose; do not double doses. Advise patient to read the *Patient Information* before starting therapy.
- Advise patient to maintain adequate hydration during therapy.
- Advise patient to notify health care professional promptly if nervous system symptoms (aggressive behavior, unsteady movement, shaky movements, confusion, speech problems, hallucinations, seizures, coma) occur.
- Instruct patient to notify health care professional of all Rx or OTC medications, vitamins, or herbal products being taken and consult health care professional before taking any new medications.
- Instruct female patients to notify health care professional if pregnancy is planned or suspected, or if breast feeding.
- **Herpes Zoster:** Inform patient that valacyclovir does not prevent the spread of infection to others. Precautions should be taken around others who have not had chickenpox or varicella vaccine, or are immunosuppressed, until all lesions have crusted.
- **Genital Herpes and Herpes Labialis:** Inform patient that valacyclovir does not prevent the spread of herpes labialis to others. Advise patient to avoid contact with lesions while lesions or symptoms are present. Valacyclovir reduces transmission of genital herpes to others. Advise patient to practice safe sex (avoid sexual intercourse when lesions are present and wear a condom made of latex or polyurethane during sexual contact).

Evaluation/Desired Outcomes

- Decrease in time to full crusting, loss of vesicles, loss of ulcers, and development of crusts in patients with acute herpes zoster (shingles).
- Decrease in time to full crusting, loss of vesicles, loss of ulcers, and development of crusts in patients with genital herpes.
- Decrease in frequency of outbreaks in patients with genital herpes.
- Decrease in time to full crusting, loss of vesicles, loss of ulcers, and development of crusts in patients with herpes labialis. Decrease in transmission of genital herpes.
- Treatment of chickenpox.

valbenazine (val-**ben**-a-zeen)

Ingrezza

Classification
Therapeutic: none assigned
Pharmacologic: reversible monoamine depleters

Indications

Tardive dyskinesia.

Action

Acts as a reversible inhibitor of the vesicular monoamine transporter 2 (VMAT2), which inhibits the reuptake of serotonin, norepinephrine and dopamine into vesicles in presynaptic neurons. **Therapeutic Effects:** Reduced severity of tardive dyskinesia.

Pharmacokinetics

Absorption: 49% absorbed following oral administration.
Distribution: Well distributed.
Protein Binding: >99%.
Metabolism and Excretion: Rapidly and extensively metabolized by the liver via hydrolysis to the active metabolite, α-dihydrotetrabenazine (α-HTBZ); also metabolized via CYP3A4 to form other minor metabolites. α-HTBZ is further metabolized, in part, via CYP2D6. The CYP2D6 enzyme system exhibits genetic polymorphism; 7% of population may be poor metabolizers and may have significantly ↑ concentrations and an ↑ risk of adverse effects. 60% eliminated in urine (<2% as unchanged drug) and 30% eliminated in feces (<2% as unchanged drug).
Half-life: 15–22 hr (valbenazine and α-HTBZ).

TIME/ACTION PROFILE (blood levels)

ROUTE	ONSET	PEAK	DURATION
PO	unknown	0.5–1 hr	unknown

Contraindications/Precautions

Contraindicated in: Hypersensitivity; Congenital long QT syndrome or history of torsades de pointes; Concurrent use of MAO inhibitors or strong CYP3A4 inducers; Severe renal impairment (CCr <30 mL/min); Lactation: Lactation.
Use Cautiously in: Poor CYP2D6 metabolizers or taking strong CYP2D6 inhibitor (may need to ↓ valbenazine dose); Concurrent use of strong CYP3A4 inhibitor (↓ dose of valbenazine); Moderate or severe hepatic impairment (↓ dose); OB: Safety not established; Pedi: Safety and effectiveness not established.

Adverse Reactions/Side Effects

CNS: fatigue, sedation/somnolence, dizziness, headache. **EENT:** blurred vision. **GI:** constipation, nausea, vomiting, xerostomia. **GU:** urinary retention. **MS:** arthralgia, bradykinesia. **Neuro:** akathisia, balance difficulty, gait disturbances, parkinsonism, restlessness, tremor, unsteady gait. **Misc:** HYPERSENSITIVITY REACTIONS (including angioedema).

Interactions

Drug-Drug: MAO inhibitors may ↑ risk of serotonin syndrome and/or ↓ effect of valbenazine; avoid concurrent use. **Strong CYP3A4 inhibitors**, including **itraconazole**, **ketoconazole**, or **clarithromycin** may ↑ levels of valbenazine and its active metabolite (α-HTBZ); ↓ valbenazine dose. **Strong CYP2D6 inhibitors**, including **fluoxetine**, **paroxetine**, or **quinidine** may ↑ levels of the active metabolite (α-HTBZ); may need to ↓ valbenazine dose. **Strong CYP3A4 inducers**, including **rifampin**, **carbamazepine**, or **phenytoin** may ↓ levels and effect of valbenazine; concurrent use not recommended. May ↑ **digoxin** levels.
Drug-Natural Products: St. John's wort may ↓ levels and effect of valbenazine; concurrent use not recommended.

Route/Dosage

PO (Adults): 40 mg once daily; after 1 wk, ↑ to 80 mg once daily. *Concurrent use of strong CYP3A4 inhibitors*—40 mg once daily (with no additional titration).

Hepatic Impairment

PO (Adults): *Moderate or severe hepatic impairment*—40 mg once daily (with no additional titration).

Availability

Capsules: 40 mg, 80 mg.

NURSING IMPLICATIONS

Assessment

- Monitor for changes in signs and symptoms of tardive dyskinesia (uncontrolled rhythmic movement of mouth, face, and extremities; lip smacking or puckering; puffing of cheeks; uncontrolled chewing; rapid or worm-like movements of tongue, excessive eye blinking) periodically during therapy.

Implementation

- **PO:** Administer once daily without regard to food.

Patient/Family Teaching

- Instruct patient to take valbenazine as directed. Do not stop taking valbenazine without consulting health care professional. Advise patient to read *Patient Information* before starting and with each Rx refill in case of changes.
- May cause drowsiness. Caution patient to avoid driving and other activities requiring alertness until response to medication is known.
- Advise patient to notify health care professional if symptoms of heart rhythm problems (fast, slow, or irregular heartbeat, shortness of breath, dizziness, fainting) or if a fast or irregular heartbeat occurs.
- Instruct patient to notify health care professional of all Rx or OTC medications, vitamins, or herbal products being taken and consult health care professional before taking any new medications.
- Advise patient to notify health care professional if pregnancy is planned or suspected and to avoid breast feeding during and for 5 days after last dose of therapy.

Evaluation/Desired Outcomes

- Decrease in severity of uncontrolled movements.

valGANciclovir

(val-gan-**sye**-kloe-veer)
Valcyte

Classification
Therapeutic: antivirals

Indications

Treatment of cytomegalovirus (CMV) retinitis in patients with AIDS. Prevention of CMV disease in kidney, kidney/pancreas and heart transplant patients at risk.

Action

Valganciclovir is a prodrug which is rapidly converted to ganciclovir by intestinal and hepatic enzymes. CMV virus converts ganciclovir to its active form (ganciclovir phosphate) inside host cell, where it inhibits viral DNA polymerase. **Therapeutic Effects:** Antiviral effect directed preferentially against CMV-infected cells.

Pharmacokinetics

Absorption: 59.4% absorbed following oral administration, rapidly converted to ganciclovir.
Distribution: Unknown.
Metabolism and Excretion: Rapidly converted to ganciclovir; ganciclovir is mostly excreted by the kidneys.
Half-life: 4.1 hr (intracellular half-life of ganciclovir phosphate is 18 hr).

TIME/ACTION PROFILE (ganciclovir blood levels)

ROUTE	ONSET	PEAK	DURATION
PO	rapid	2 hr	12–24 hr

Contraindications/Precautions

Contraindicated in: Hypersensitivity to valganciclovir or ganciclovir; Hemodialysis; Patients undergoing liver transplantation; OB: Pregnancy or planned pregnancy; Lactation: Lactation.
Use Cautiously in: Renal impairment (dosage ↓ recommended if CCr <60 mL/min); Pre-existing bone

V

marrow depression; Previous or concurrent myelosuppressive drug therapy or radiation therapy; Geri: Age-related ↓ in renal function requires dosage reduction; Pedi: Children <4 mo (safety not established).

Adverse Reactions/Side Effects

CNS: SEIZURES, headache, insomnia, agitation, confusion, dizziness, hallucinations, psychosis, sedation. **GI:** abdominal pain, diarrhea, nausea, vomiting. **GU:** ↓ fertility, renal impairment. **Hemat:** NEUTROPENIA, THROMBOCYTOPENIA, anemia, aplastic anemia, bone marrow depression, pancytopenia. **Neuro:** ataxia, paresthesia, peripheral neuropathy. **Misc:** HYPERSENSITIVITY REACTIONS (including anaphylaxis), INFECTION, fever.

Interactions

Drug-Drug: ↑ risk of hematologic toxicity with **zidovudine**. Blood levels and effects may be ↑ by **probenecid**. Patients with renal impairment may experience accumulation of metabolites of **mycophenolate** and valganciclovir. ↑ blood levels and risk of toxicity from **didanosine**.

Drug-Food: Food ↑ absorption.

Route/Dosage

Treatment of CMV Disease

PO (Adults): *Induction*—900 mg twice daily for 21 days; *Maintenance treatment or patients with inactive CMV retinitis*—900 mg once daily.

Renal Impairment

CCr 40–59 mL/min (Adults): *Induction*—450 mg twice daily for 21 days; *Maintenance treatment or patients with inactive CMV retinitis*—450 mg once daily.

Renal Impairment

CCr 25–39 mL/min (Adults): *Induction*—450 mg once daily for 21 days; *Maintenance treatment or patients with inactive CMV retinitis*—450 mg every 2 days.

Renal Impairment

CCr 10–24 mL/min (Adults): *Induction*—450 mg every 2 days for 21 days; *Maintenance treatment or patients with inactive CMV retinitis*—450 mg twice weekly.

Prevention of CMV Disease in Transplant Patients

PO (Adults): *Kidney/pancreas, or heart transplant*—900 mg once daily, starting 10 days prior to transplant and continued for 100 days after; *Kidney transplant*—900 mg once daily, starting 10 days prior to transplant and continued for 200 days after.

Renal Impairment

PO (Adults): *CCr 40–59 mL/min*—450 mg once daily; *CCr 25–39 mL/min*—450 mg every 2 days; *CCr 12–24 mL/min*—450 mg twice weekly.

PO (Children 4 mo-16 yr): *Kidney transplant*—Dose is based on body surface area (BSA) and CCr. Dose = 7 × BSA × CCr (see prescribing information for equations used for BSA and CCr); all calculated doses should be rounded to nearest 10 mg (max = 900 mg) and administered as oral solution; should be started 10 days prior to transplant and continued for 200 days after.

PO (Children 4 mo-16 yr): *Heart transplant*—Dose is based on BSA and CCr. Dose = 7 × BSA × CCr (see prescribing information for equations used for BSA and CCr); all calculated doses should be rounded to nearest 10 mg (max = 900 mg) and administered as oral solution; should be started 10 days prior to transplant and continued for 100 days after.

Renal Impairment

PO (Adults): *CCr 40–59 mL/min*—450 mg once daily; *CCr 25–39 mL/min*—450 mg every 2 days; *CCr 12–24 mL/min*—450 mg twice weekly.

Availability (generic available)

Oral solution (tutti-frutti flavor): 50 mg/mL. **Tablets:** 450 mg.

NURSING IMPLICATIONS

Assessment

- Diagnosis of CMV retinitis should be determined by ophthalmoscopy prior to treatment with valganciclovir.
- Culture for CMV (urine, blood, throat) may be taken prior to administration. However, a negative CMV culture does not rule out CMV retinitis. If symptoms do not respond after several wk, resistance to valganciclovir may have occurred. Ophthalmologic exams should be performed weekly during induction and every 2 wk during maintenance or more frequently if the macula or optic nerve is threatened. Progression of CMV retinitis may occur during or following ganciclovir treatment.
- Assess for signs of infection (fever, chills, cough, hoarseness, lower back or side pain, sore throat, difficult or painful urination). Notify health care professional if these symptoms occur.
- Assess for bleeding (bleeding gums, bruising, petechiae, or guaiac stools, urine, and emesis). Avoid IM injections and taking rectal temperatures. Apply pressure to venipuncture sites for 10 min.
- ***Lab Test Considerations:*** Obtain a negative pregnancy test before starting therapy.
- May cause granulocytopenia, anemia, and thrombocytopenia. Monitor neutrophil and platelet count closely throughout therapy. Do not administer if ANC <500/mm^3, platelet count <25,000/mm^3, or hemoglobin <8 g/dL. Recovery begins within 3–7 days of discontinuation of therapy.
- Monitor BUN and serum creatinine at least once every 2 wk throughout therapy. May cause ↑ in serum creatinine.

Implementation

- Do not confuse valganciclovir with valacyclovir. Do not confuse Valcyte (valganciclovir) with Valtrex (valacyclovir).
- **PO:** Administer tablets and oral solution with food. Adults should take tablets, not oral solution. Handle valganciclovir tablets carefully. Do not break or crush. May be potentially teratogenic; avoid direct contact with broken or crushed tablets. If contact with the skin or mucous membranes occurs, wash thoroughly with soap and water and rinse eyes thoroughly with plain water.
- Oral solution (50 mg/mL) must be prepared by the pharmacist prior to dispensing to the patient. Shake well prior to use. Use oral dispenser provided for accurate dose. Store oral solution in refrigerator for no longer than 49 days.

Patient/Family Teaching

- Instruct patient to take valganciclovir with food, as directed. Take missed doses as soon as remembered, unless almost time for next dose; do not double doses. Advise patient to read *Patient Information* before starting therapy and with each Rx refill in case of changes.
- Inform patient that valganciclovir is not a cure for CMV retinitis. Progression of retinitis may continue in immunocompromised patients during and following therapy. Advise patients to have regular ophthalmic exams at least every 4–6 wk. Duration of therapy for CMV prevention is based on the duration and degree of immunosuppression.
- May cause seizures, sedation, dizziness, ataxia, and/or confusion. Caution patient not to drive or do other activities requiring alertness until response to medication is known.
- Advise patient to notify health care professional if fever; chills; sore throat; other signs of infection; bleeding gums; bruising; petechiae; or blood in urine, stool, or emesis occurs. Caution patient to avoid crowds and persons with known infections. Instruct patient to use soft toothbrush and electric razor. Patient should be cautioned not to drink alcoholic beverages or take products containing aspirin or NSAIDs.
- Caution patient to use sunscreen and protective clothing to prevent photosensitivity reactions.
- Advise patient that valganciclovir may have teratogenic effects. Advise females of reproductive potential to use effective contraception during and for at least 30 days following therapy and to avoid breast feeding. Advise males with female partners of reproductive potential to use a barrier method of contraception during and for at least 90 days following therapy. May cause temporary or permanent infertility.
- Emphasize the importance of frequent follow-up exams to monitor blood counts.

Evaluation/Desired Outcomes

- Management of the symptoms of CMV retinitis in patients with AIDS.
- Prevention of CMV disease in kidney, kidney/pancreas and heart transplant patients at risk.

VALPROATES

divalproex sodium
(dye-val-**proe**-ex **soe**-dee-um)
Depakote, Depakote ER, Depakote Sprinkle, Epival

valproate sodium
(val-**proe**-ate **soe**-dee-um)
~~Depacon~~

valproic acid (val-**proe**-ik **as**-id)
~~Depakene~~

Classification
Therapeutic: anticonvulsants, vascular headache suppressants

Indications

Monotherapy and adjunctive therapy for simple and complex absence seizures. Monotherapy and adjunctive therapy for complex partial seizures. Adjunctive therapy for patients with multiple seizure types, including absence seizures. **Divalproex sodium only.** Manic episodes associated with bipolar disorder. Prevention of migraine headache.

Action

Increase levels of GABA, an inhibitory neurotransmitter in the CNS. **Therapeutic Effects:** Suppression of seizure activity. Decreased manic episodes. Decreased frequency of migraine headaches.

Pharmacokinetics

Absorption: Well absorbed following oral administration; divalproex is enteric-coated, and absorption is delayed. ER form produces lower blood levels. IV administration results in complete bioavailability.

Distribution: Rapidly distributed into plasma and extracellular water. Cross blood-brain barrier and placenta; enters breast milk.

Protein Binding: 80–90%, decreased in neonates, elderly, renal impairment, or chronic hepatic disease.

Metabolism and Excretion: Mostly metabolized by the liver; minimal amounts excreted unchanged in urine.

Half-life: Adults: 9–16 hr.

V

TIME/ACTION PROFILE (onset = anticonvulsant effect; peak = blood levels)

ROUTE	ONSET	PEAK	DURATION
PO—liquid	2–4 days	15–120 min	6–24 hr
PO—capsules	2–4 days	1–4 hr	6–24 hr
PO—delayed-release products	2–4 days	3–5 hr	12–24 hr
PO—extended-release products	2–4 days	7–14 hr	24 hr
IV	2–4 days	end of infusion	6–24 hr

Contraindications/Precautions

Contraindicated in: Hypersensitivity; Hepatic impairment; Known/suspected urea cycle disorders (may result in fatal hyperammonemic encephalopathy); Mitochondrial disorders caused by mutations in mitochondrial DNA polymerase gamma (↑ risk for potentially fatal hepatotoxicity); OB: Pregnancy (may cause fetal harm including ↓ IQ, neurodevelopmental disorders, neural tube defects, and other major congenital malformations; contraindicated for migraine prophylaxis only); Rep: Women of reproductive potential not using effective contraception (contraindicated for migraine prophylaxis only); Pedi: Children <2 yr with suspected mitochondrial disorder caused by mutations in mitochondrial DNA polymerase gamma (↑ risk for potentially fatal hepatotoxicity).

Use Cautiously in: All patients (may ↑ risk of suicidal thoughts/behaviors); Bleeding disorders; History of liver disease; Organic brain disease; Bone marrow depression; Renal impairment; Geri: ↑ risk of adverse effects; OB: Pregnancy (may cause fetal harm including ↓ IQ, neurodevelopmental disorders, neural tube defects, and other major congenital malformations; use for seizure disorders or bipolar disorders only if other medications are ineffective, poorly tolerated, or inappropriate); Lactation: Passes into breast milk. Consider discontinuing nursing when valproates are administered to the nursing mother; Rep: Women of reproductive potential (use for seizure disorders or bipolar disorders only if other medications are ineffective, poorly tolerated, or inappropriate).

Adverse Reactions/Side Effects

CNS: SUICIDAL THOUGHTS agitation, dizziness, headache, insomnia, sedation, confusion, depression. **CV:** peripheral edema. **Derm:** DRUG REACTION WITH EOSINOPHILIA AND SYSTEMIC SYMPTOMS (DRESS), alopecia, rashes. **EENT:** visual disturbances. **GI:** HEPATOTOXICITY, PANCREATITIS, abdominal pain, anorexia, diarrhea, indigestion, nausea, vomiting, constipation, ↑ appetite. **Hemat:** thrombocytopenia, leukopenia. **Metab:** HYPERAMMONEMIA, weight gain. **Neuro:** HYPOTHERMIA, tremor, ataxia.

Interactions

Drug-Drug: ↑ risk of bleeding with **warfarin**. Blood levels and toxicity may be ↑ by **aspirin**, **carbamazepine**, **chlorpromazine**, **cimetidine**, **erythromycin**, or **felbamate**. ↑ CNS depression with other **CNS depressants**, including **alcohol**, **antihistamines**, **antidepressants**, **opioid analgesics**, **MAO inhibitors**, and **sedative/hypnotics**. **MAO inhibitors** and other **antidepressants** may ↓ seizure threshold and ↓ effectiveness of valproate. **Carbamazepine**, **meropenem**, **phenobarbital**, **phenytoin**, **estrogen-containing contraceptives**, or **rifampin** may ↓ valproate levels. May ↑ levels of **carbamazepine**, **diazepam**, **amitriptyline**, **nortriptyline**, **ethosuximide**, **lamotrigine**, **phenobarbital**, **phenytoin**, **rufinamide**, **topiramate**, or **zidovudine**; dosage adjustments of these medications may be necessary. May ↑ levels of **propofol**; ↓ dose of propofol. Concurrent use with **topiramate** may ↑ risk of hypothermia and hyperammonemia with or without encephalopathy. **Ertapenem**, **imipenem**, or **meropenem** may ↓ valproate levels. **Cholestyramine** may ↓ valproate levels; separate administration by 3 hr.

Route/Dosage

Regular-release and delayed-release formulations usually given in 2–4 divided doses daily; extended-release formulation (Depakote ER) usually given once daily.

Anticonvulsant

PO (Adults and Children >10 yr): *Single-agent therapy (complex partial seizures)*—Initial dose of 10–15 mg/kg/day in 1–4 divided doses; ↑ by 5–10 mg/kg/day weekly until therapeutic response achieved (not to exceed 60 mg/kg/day); when daily dose exceeds 250 mg, give in divided doses. *Polytherapy (complex partial seizures)*—Initial dose of 10–15 mg/kg/day; ↑ by 5–10 mg/kg/day weekly until therapeutic response achieved (not to exceed 60 mg/kg/day); when daily dosage exceeds 250 mg, give in divided doses.

PO (Adults and Children >2 yr [>10 yr for Depakote ER]): *Simple and complex absence seizures*—Initial dose of 15 mg/kg/day in 1–4 divided doses; ↑ by 5–10 mg/kg/day weekly until therapeutic response achieved (not to exceed 60 mg/kg/day); when daily dose exceeds 250 mg, give in divided doses.

IV (Adults and Children): Give same daily dose and at same frequency as was given orally; switch to oral formulation as soon as possible.

Rect (Adults and Children): Dilute syrup 1:1 with water for use as a retention enema. Give 17–20 mg/kg load, maintenance 10–15 mg/kg/dose every 8 hr.

Mood Stabilizer

PO (Adults): *Depakote*—Initial dose of 750 mg/day in divided doses initially, titrated rapidly to desired clinical effect or trough plasma levels of 50–125 mcg/mL (not to exceed 60 mg/kg/day). *Depakote ER*—Initial dose of 25 mg/kg once daily; titrated rapidly to desired clinical effect of trough plasma levels of 85–125 mcg/mL (not to exceed 60 mg/kg/day).

Migraine Prevention

PO (Adults and Children ≥16 yr): *Depakote*—250 mg twice daily (up to 1000 mg/day). *Depakote ER*—500 mg once daily for 1 wk, then ↑ to 1000 mg once daily.

Availability

Valproic Acid (generic available)

Capsules: 250 mg, 🍁 500 mg. **Cost:** *Generic*—$37.90/100. **Syrup:** 250 mg/5 mL.

Valproate Sodium (generic available)

Solution for injection: 100 mg/mL.

Divalproex Sodium (generic available)

Delayed-release tablets (Depakote): 125 mg, 250 mg, 500 mg. **Cost:** 125 mg $89.72/100, 250 mg $176.23/100, 500 mg $324.97/100. **Extended-release tablets (Depakote ER):** 250 mg, 500 mg. **Cost:** 250 mg $167.91/100, 500 mg $295.36/100. **Sprinkle capsules:** 125 mg. **Cost:** $137.53/100.

NURSING IMPLICATIONS

Assessment

- **Seizures:** Assess location, duration, and characteristics of seizure activity. Institute seizure precautions.
- **Bipolar Disorder:** Assess mood, ideation, and behavior frequently.
- **Migraine Prophylaxis:** Monitor frequency and intensity of migraine headaches.
- Geri: Assess geriatric patients for excessive somnolence.
- Assess for suicidal tendencies, especially during early therapy. Restrict amount of drug available to patient. Risk may be increased in children, adolescents, and adults ≤24 yr.
- Monitor for signs and symptoms of pancreatitis (abdominal pain, nausea, vomiting, anorexia). If pancreatitis occurs, valproates should be discontinued and alternate therapy initiated.
- Monitor for signs and symptoms of DRESS (fever, rash, lymphadenopathy, hepatitis, nephritis, hematological abnormalities, myocarditis, myositis, eosinophilia). If symptoms occur and DRESS is confirmed, discontinue valproate and do not restart.
- ***Lab Test Considerations:*** Monitor CBC, platelet count, and bleeding time prior to and periodically during therapy. May cause leukopenia and thrombocytopenia.
- Monitor hepatic function (LDH, AST, ALT, and bilirubin) and serum ammonia concentrations prior to and periodically during therapy. May cause hepatotoxicity; monitor closely, especially during initial 6 mo of therapy; fatalities have occurred. Therapy should be discontinued if hyperammonemia occurs.
- May interfere with accuracy of thyroid function tests.
- May cause false-positive results in urine ketone tests.
- ***Toxicity and Overdose:*** Therapeutic serum levels range from 50–100 mcg/mL (50–125 mcg/mL for mania). Doses are gradually ↑ until a pre-dose serum concentration of at least 50 mcg/mL is reached. However, a good correlation among daily dose, serum level, and therapeutic effects has not been established. Monitor patients receiving near the maximum recommended 60 mg/kg/day for toxicity.

Implementation

- Do not confuse *Depakote ER* and regular dose forms. *Depakote ER* produces lower blood levels than *Depakote* dosing forms. If switching from *Depakote* to *Depakote ER*, increase dose by 8-20%.
- Single daily doses are usually administered at bedtime because of sedation.
- **PO:** Administer with or immediately after meals to minimize GI irritation. Extended-release and delayed-release tablets and capsules should be swallowed whole, do not open, break, or chew; will cause mouth or throat irritation and destroy extended release mechanism. Do not administer tablets with milk or carbonated beverages (may cause premature dissolution). Delayed-release divalproex sodium may cause less GI irritation than valproic acid capsules.
- Shake liquid preparations well before pouring. Use calibrated measuring device to ensure accurate dose. Syrup may be mixed with food or other liquids to improve taste.
- Sprinkle capsules may be swallowed whole or opened and entire capsule contents sprinkled on a teaspoonful of soft, cool food (applesauce, pudding). Do not chew mixture. Administer immediately; do not store for future use.
- To convert from valproic acid to divalproex sodium, initiate divalproex sodium at same total daily dose and dosing schedule as valproic acid. Once patient is stabilized on divalproex sodium, attempt administration 2–3 times daily.
- **Rect:** Dilute syrup 1:1 with water for use as a retention enema.

IV Administration

- **Intermittent Infusion:** ***Diluent:*** May be diluted in at least 50 mL of D5W, 0.9% NaCl, or LR. Solution is stable for 24 hr at room temperature. ***Concentration:*** 2 mg/mL. ***Rate:*** Infuse over 60 min (≤20 mg/min). Rapid infusion may cause increased side effects. Has been given as a one-time infusion of 1000 mg over 5–10 min @ 3 mg/kg/min up to 15 mg/kg in patients with no detectable valproate levels.
- **Y-Site Compatibility:** cefepime, ceftazidime, naloxone.
- **Y-Site Incompatibility:** vancomycin.

Patient/Family Teaching

- Instruct patient to take medication as directed. If a dose is missed on a once-a-day schedule, take as soon as remembered that day. If on a multiple-dose schedule, take it within 6 hr of the scheduled time, then space remaining doses throughout the remainder of the day. Abrupt withdrawal may lead to status epilepticus. Advise patient to read the *Medication*

V

Guide before starting therapy and with each Rx refill in case of changes.

- May cause drowsiness or dizziness. Caution patient to avoid driving or other activities requiring alertness until effects of medication are known. Tell patient not to resume driving until physician gives clearance based on control of seizure disorder.
- Instruct patient to notify health care professional of all Rx or OTC medications, vitamins, or herbal products being taken and consult health care professional before taking any new medications, especially CNS depressants. Caution patient to avoid alcohol during therapy.
- Advise patient and family to notify health care professional if thoughts about suicide or dying, attempts to commit suicide; new or worse depression; new or worse anxiety; feeling very agitated or restless; panic attacks; trouble sleeping; new or worse irritability; acting aggressive; being angry or violent; acting on dangerous impulses; an extreme increase in activity and talking, other unusual changes in behavior or mood occur.
- Instruct patient to notify health care professional of medication regimen prior to treatment or surgery.
- Advise patient to notify health care professional if anorexia, abdominal pain, severe nausea and vomiting, yellow skin or eyes, fever, sore throat, malaise, weakness, facial edema, lethargy, unusual bleeding or bruising, pregnancy, or loss of seizure control occurs. Children <2 yr of age are especially at risk for fatal hepatotoxicity.
- Rep: May cause teratogenic effects. Advise females of reproductive potential to use effective contraception during therapy and to notify health care professional immediately if pregnancy is planned or suspected, or if breast feeding. Advise pregnant patients taking valproates to enroll in the NAAED Pregnancy Registry to monitor pregnancy outcomes by calling 1-888-233-2334; call must be made by patient. Registry website is www.aedpregnancyregistry.org. May cause male infertility. Monitor breast-fed infant for signs of liver damage including jaundice and unusual bruising or bleeding.
- Advise patient to carry identification at all times describing medication regimen.
- Emphasize the importance of routine exams to monitor progress.

Evaluation/Desired Outcomes

- Decreased seizure activity.
- Decreased incidence of manic episodes in patients with bipolar disorders.
- Decreased frequency of migraine headaches.

valsartan, See ANGIOTENSIN II RECEPTOR ANTAGONISTS.

vancomycin (van-koe-mye-sin)

Firvanq, Vancocin

Classification
Therapeutic: anti-infectives

Indications

IV: Treatment of potentially life-threatening infections when less toxic anti-infectives are contraindicated. Particularly useful in staphylococcal infections, including: Endocarditis, Meningitis, Osteomyelitis, Pneumonia, Septicemia, Soft-tissue infections in patients who have allergies to penicillin or its derivatives or when sensitivity testing demonstrates resistance to methicillin. **PO:** Treatment of staphylococcal enterocolitis or diarrhea due to *Clostridium difficile*. **IV:** Part of endocarditis prophylaxis in high-risk patients who are allergic to penicillin.

Action

Binds to bacterial cell wall, resulting in cell death. **Therapeutic Effects:** Bactericidal action against susceptible organisms. **Spectrum:** Active against gram-positive pathogens, including: Staphylococci (including methicillin-resistant strains of *Staphylococcus aureus*), Group A beta-hemolytic streptococci, *Streptococcus pneumoniae*, *Corynebacterium*, *Clostridium difficile*, *Enterococcus faecalis*, *Enterococcus faecium*.

Pharmacokinetics

Absorption: Poorly absorbed from the GI tract.
Distribution: Widely distributed. Some penetration (20–30%) of CSF; crosses placenta.
Metabolism and Excretion: Oral doses excreted primarily in the feces; IV vancomycin eliminated almost entirely by the kidneys.
Half-life: Neonates: 6–10 hr; Children 3 mo–3 yr: 4 hr; Children >3 yr: 2–2.3 hr; Adults: 5–8 hr (↑ in renal impairment).

TIME/ACTION PROFILE (blood levels)

ROUTE	ONSET	PEAK	DURATION
IV	rapid	end of infusion	12–24 hr

Contraindications/Precautions

Contraindicated in: Hypersensitivity.
Use Cautiously in: Renal impairment (dosage reduction required if CCr ≤80 mL/min); Hearing impairment; Intestinal obstruction or inflammation (↑ systemic absorption when given orally); OB, Lactation: Safety not established.

Adverse Reactions/Side Effects

CV: hypotension. **Derm:** rash. **EENT:** ototoxicity. **GI:** nausea, vomiting. **GU:** nephrotoxicity. **Hemat:** eosinophilia, leukopenia. **Local:** phlebitis. **MS:** back and neck pain. **Misc:** HYPERSENSITIVITY REACTIONS (including anaphylaxis), chills, fever, "red man" syndrome (with rapid infusion), superinfection.

Interactions

Drug-Drug: May cause additive ototoxicity and nephrotoxicity with other **ototoxic** and **nephrotoxic drugs** (**aspirin**, **aminoglycosides**, **cyclosporine**, **cisplatin**, **loop diuretics**). May enhance neuromuscular blockade from **nondepolarizing neuromuscular blocking agents**. ↑ risk of histamine flush when used with **general anesthetics** in children.

Route/Dosage

Serious Systemic Infections

IV (Adults): 500 mg every 6 hr *or* 1 g every 12 hr (up to 4 g/day).

IV (Children >1 mo): 40 mg/kg/day divided every 6–8 hr *Staphylococcal CNS infection*—60 mg/kg/day divided every 6 hr, maximum dose: 1 g/dose.

IV (Neonates 1 wk–1 mo): <1200 g: 15 mg/kg every 24 hr. 1200–2000 g: 10–15 mg/kg every 8–12 hr. >2000 g: 15–20 mg/kg every 8 hr.

IV (Neonates <1 wk): <1200 g: 15 mg/kg every 24 hr. 1200–2000 g: 10–15 mg/kg every 12–18 hr. >2000 g: 10–15 mg/kg every 8–12 hr.

IT (Adults): 20 mg/day.

IT (Children): 5–20 mg/day.

IT (Neonates): 5–10 mg/day.

Endocarditis Prophylaxis in Penicillin-Allergic Patients

IV (Adults and Adolescents): 1 g single dose 1 hr preprocedure.

IV (Children): 20 mg/kg single dose 1 hr preprocedure.

Diarrhea Due to *C. difficile*

PO (Adults): 125 mg every 6 hr for 10 days.

PO (Children): 40 mg/kg/day divided into 3 or 4 doses for 7–10 days (not to exceed 2 g/day).

Staphylococcal Enterocolitis

PO (Adults): 500–2000 mg/day in 3–4 divided doses for 7–10 days.

PO (Children): 40 mg/kg/day in 3–4 divided doses for 7–10 days (not to exceed 2 g/day).

Renal Impairment

IV (Adults): An initial loading dose of 750 mg–1 g (not less than 15 mg/kg); serum level monitoring is optimal for choosing maintenance dose in patients with renal impairment; these guidelines may be helpful. *CCr 50–80 mL/min*—1 g every 1–3 days; *CCr 10–50 mL/min*—1 g every 3–7 days; *CCr <10 mL/min*—1 g every 7–14 days.

Availability (generic available)

Capsules: 125 mg, 250 mg. **Powder for oral solution (requires reconstitution) (grape-flavor):** 3.75 g/bottle, 7.5 g/bottle, 10.5 g/bottle, 15 g/bottle. **Premixed infusion:** 500 mg/100 mL D5W, 1000 mg/200 mL D5W or 0.9% NaCl, 2000 mg/400 mL. **Solution for injection (requires reconstitution and dilution):** 250 mg/vial, 500 mg/vial, 750 mg/vial, 1 g/vial, 1.5 g/vial, 5 g/vial, 10 g/vial, 100 g/vial.

NURSING IMPLICATIONS

Assessment

- Assess patient for infection (vital signs; appearance of wound, sputum, urine, and stool; WBC) at beginning of and throughout therapy.
- Obtain specimens for culture and sensitivity prior to initiating therapy. First dose may be given before receiving results.
- Monitor IV site closely. Vancomycin is irritating to tissues and causes necrosis and severe pain with extravasation. Rotate infusion site.
- Monitor BP throughout IV infusion.
- Evaluate eighth cranial nerve function by audiometry and serum vancomycin levels prior to and throughout therapy in patients with borderline renal function or those >60 yr of age. Prompt recognition and intervention are essential in preventing permanent damage.
- Monitor intake and output ratios and daily weight. Cloudy or pink urine may be a sign of nephrotoxicity.
- Assess patient for signs of superinfection (black, furry overgrowth on tongue; vaginal itching or discharge; loose or foul-smelling stools). Report occurrence.
- Observe patient for signs and symptoms of anaphylaxis (rash, pruritus, laryngeal edema, wheezing). Discontinue drug and notify health care professional immediately if these problems occur. Keep epinephrine, an antihistamine, and resuscitation equipment close by in case of an anaphylactic reaction.
- **Pseudomembranous Colitis:** Assess bowel status (bowel sounds, frequency and consistency of stools, presence of blood in stools) throughout therapy.
- ***Lab Test Considerations:*** Monitor for casts, albumin, or cells in the urine or decreased specific gravity, CBC, and renal function periodically during therapy.
- May cause increased BUN levels.
- ***Toxicity and Overdose:*** Trough concentrations should not exceed 10 mcg/mL (mild-moderate infections) or 15–20 mcg/mL (for severe infections).

Implementation

- Vancomycin must be given orally for treatment of staphylococcal enterocolitis and *C. difficile*-associated diarrhea. Orally administered vancomycin is not effective for other types of infections.
- **PO:** Use calibrated measuring device for liquid preparations. Oral solution is stable for 14 days if refrigerated.

V

IV Administration

- **Intermittent Infusion:** ***Diluent:*** To reconstitute, add 10 mL of sterile water for injection to 500-mg vial or 20 mL of sterile water for injection to 1-g vial for a concentration of 50 mg/mL. Dilute further with at least 100 mL of 0.9% NaCl, D5W, D5/0.9% NaCl, or LR for every 500 mg of vancomycin being administered. Reconstituted vials stable for 14 days if refrigerated. Infusion is stable for 96 hr if refrigerated. ***Concentration:*** ≤5 mg/mL. ***Rate:*** Infuse over at least 60 min (90 min for doses >1 g). Do not administer rapidly or as a bolus, to minimize risk of thrombophlebitis, hypotension, and "red-man (neck)" syndrome (sudden, severe hypotension; flushing and/or maculopapular rash of face, neck, chest, and upper extremities). May need to slow infusion further to 1.5–2 hr if red-man syndrome occurs.
- **IT:** ***Diluent:*** Dilute with preservative-free NS. ***Concentration:*** 1–5 mg/mL. ***Rate:*** Directly instill into ventricular cerebrospinal fluid.
- **Y-Site Compatibility:** acetylcysteine, acyclovir, aldesleukin, alemtuzumab, alfentanil, allopurinol, alprostadil, amifostine, amikacin, amiodarone, amsacrine, anidulafungin, argatroban, ascorbic acid, atracurium, atropine, azithromycin, benztropine, bleomycin, bumetanide, buprenorphine, butorphanol, calcium chloride, calcium gluconate, carboplatin, carmustine, caspofungin, chlorpromazine, ciprofloxacin, cisatracurium, cisplatin, clindamycin, cyanocobalamin, cyclophosphamide, cyclosporine, cytarabine, dactinomycin, dexamethasone, dexmedetomidine, dexrazoxane, digoxin, diltiazem, diphenhydramine, dobutamine, docetaxel, dolasetron, dopamine, doxacurium, doxapram, doxorubicin hydrochloride, doxorubicin liposome, doxycycline, enalaprilat, ephedrine, epinephrine, epirubicin, eptifibatide, ertapenem, erythromycin, esmolol, etoposide, etoposide phosphate, famotidine, fenoldopam, fentanyl, filgrastim, fluconazole, fludarabine, folic acid, gemcitabine, gentamicin, glycopyrrolate, granisetron, hetastarch, hydromorphone, ifosfamide, insulin regular, irinotecan, isoproterenol, ketamine, labetalol, levofloxacin, lidocaine, linezolid, lorazepam, magnesium sulfate, mannitol, melphalan, meperidine, meropenem, metaraminol, methyldopate, metoclopramide, metoprolol, metronidazole, midazolam, milrinone, mitoxantrone, morphine, multivitamins, mycophenolate, nalbuphine, naloxone, nicardipine, nitroglycerin, nitroprusside, norepinephrine, octreotide, ondansetron, oxacillin, oxaliplatin, oxytocin, paclitaxel, palonosetron, pamidronate, pancuronium, papaverine, pemetrexed, penicillin G, pentamidine, pentobarbital, perphenazine, phenobarbital, phentolamine, phenylephrine, phytonadione, potassium acetate, potassium chloride, procainamide, prochlorperazine, promethazine, propranolol, protamine, pyridoxime, ranitidine, remifentanil, rifampin, sodium acetate, sodium bicarbonate, sodium citrate, succinylcholine, sufentanil, tacrolimus, thiamine, thiotepa, tigecycline, tirofiban, tobramycin, tolazoline, trastuzumab, vasopressin, vecuronium, verapamil, vinblastine, vincristine, vinorelbine, voriconazole, zidovudine, zoledronic acid.
- **Y-Site Incompatibility:** albumin, aminophylline, amphotericin B deoxycholate, amphotericin lipid complex, amphotericin B liposome, azathioprine, bivalirudin, chloramphenicol, dantrolene, daptomycin, diazepam, diazoxide, epoetin alfa, fluorouracil, furosemide, ganciclovir, heparin, ibuprofen, idarubicin, indomethacin, ketorolac, leucovorin calcium, methylprednisolone, mitomycin, moxifloxacin, phenytoin, rituximab, streptokinase, trimethoprim/sulfamethoxazole, valproate sodium.

Patient/Family Teaching

- Advise patients on oral vancomycin to take as directed. Take missed doses as soon as remembered unless almost time for next dose; do not double dose.
- Instruct patient to report signs of hypersensitivity, tinnitus, vertigo, or hearing loss.
- Advise patient to notify health care professional if no improvement is seen in a few days.
- Patients with a history of rheumatic heart disease or valve replacement need to be taught importance of using antimicrobial prophylaxis prior to invasive dental or medical procedures.
- Advise female patient to notify health care professional if pregnancy is planned or suspected or if breast feeding.

Evaluation/Desired Outcomes

- Resolution of signs and symptoms of infection. Length of time for complete resolution depends on organism and site of infection.
- Endocarditis prophylaxis.

REMS

vandetanib (van-det-a-nib)

Caprelsa

Classification

Therapeutic: antineoplastics

Pharmacologic: kinase inhibitors

Indications

Treatment of symptomatic/progressive medullary thyroid cancer in patients with unresectable, locally advanced, or metastatic disease.

Action

Inhibits tyrosine kinase; results in inhibited action of epidermal growth factor (EGFR), vascular endothelial cell growth factor (VEGF) and other kinase based actions. Inhibits endothelial cell migration/proliferation/survival and new blood vessel formation. Also inhibits EGFR-dependent cell survival. **Therapeutic Effects:** Decreased spread of thyroid cancer.

Pharmacokinetics

Absorption: Well absorbed following oral administration.

Distribution: Unknown.

Metabolism and Excretion: Mostly metabolized by the liver; 44% excreted in feces, 25% in urine.

Half-life: 19 days.

TIME/ACTION PROFILE (blood levels)

ROUTE	ONSET	PEAK	DURATION
PO	unknown	4–10 hr	24 hr

Contraindications/Precautions

Contraindicated in: Congenital long QT syndrome or QTcF interval >450 msec; Hypocalcemia (serum calcium should be within normal range), hypokalemia (serum potassium should >4.0 mEq/L and within normal range), or hypomagnesemia (serum magnesium should be within normal range); Concurrent use of strong inducers of the CYP3A4 enzyme system; OB: Can cause fetal harm; Lactation: Avoid breast feeding.

Use Cautiously in: Diarrhea (↑ risk of electrolyte abnormalities and risk of arrhythmias); Renal impairment (dose ↓ recommended for CCr <50 mL/min with close monitoring of QT interval); Moderate to severe hepatic impairment (Child-Pugh Class B or C; safety and effectiveness not established); Rep: Women of reproductive potential; Pedi: Safety and effectiveness not established.

Exercise Extreme Caution in: Concurrent use of other drugs know to prolong QT interval (avoid if possible; if medically necessary, monitoring is required).

Adverse Reactions/Side Effects

CNS: REVERSIBLE POSTERIOR LEUKOENCEPHALOPATHY SYNDROME, fatigue, headache, depression, insomnia, reversible posterior leukoencephalopathy. **Resp:** INTERSTITIAL LUNG DISEASE, upper respiratory tract infection. **CV:** HEART FAILURE, ISCHEMIC CEREBROVASCULAR EVENTS, TORSADE DE POINTES, hypertension, QT interval prolongation. **GI:** abdominal pain, ↓ appetite, diarrhea, nausea, dyspepsia, intestinal perforation, vomiting. **GU:** proteinuria. **Derm:** STEVENS-JOHNSON SYNDROME, TOXIC EPIDERMAL NECROLYSIS, acne, photosensitivity reaction, rash, skin reactions, pruritus. **Endo:** hypothyroidism. **F and E:** hypocalcemia. **Hemat:** BLEEDING.

Interactions

Drug-Drug: Strong CYP3A4 inducers including **carbamazepine**, **dexamethasone**, **phenobarbital**, **phenytoin**, **rifabutin**, **rifampin**, **rifapentine**, and **phenobartital**; may ↓ levels and effectiveness; concurrent use should be avoided. Concurrent use with other drugs that prolong the QT interval should be including some **antiarrhythmics** (**amiodarone**, **disopyramide**, **procainamide**, **sotalol**, **dofetilide**), **chloroquine**, **clarithromycin**, **dolasetreon**, **granisetron**, **haloperidol**, **methadone**, **moxifloxacin**, and **pimozide**. May ↑ **metformin** and **digoxin** levels.

Drug-Natural Products: St. John's wort may ↓ levels and effectiveness and should be avoided.

Route/Dosage

PO (Adults): 300 mg once daily.

Renal Impairment

PO (Adults): *CCr <50 mL/min*—200 mg once daily.

Availability

Tablets: 100 mg, 300 mg.

NURSING IMPLICATIONS

Assessment

- May prolong QT intervals. Obtain ECG at baseline, at 2–4 wk, at 8–12 wk after starting therapy and every 3 mo there after. Use these parameters to assess QT interval following dose reduction for QT prolongation or dose interruption >2 wk. May require more frequent monitoring if diarrhea occurs.
- Assess patient for rash periodically during therapy. Mild to moderate skin reactions may include rash, acne, dry skin, dermatitis, and pruritus and may be treated with topical or systemic corticosteroids, oral antihistamines, and topical and systemic antibiotics. Treatment of severe rash (Grade 3 or greater) may include systemic corticosteroids and discontinuation of treatment until improved. Upon improvement, may be restarted at a reduced dose.
- Assess for signs and symptoms of interstitial lung disease (hypoxia, pleural effusion, cough, dyspnea). If radiological changes occur with few or no symptoms, therapy may continue. If symptoms are moderate, consider interrupting therapy until symptoms improve. If symptoms are severe, discontinue therapy; permanent discontinuation should be considered. Treat with antibiotics and corticosteroids.
- Assess for signs and symptoms of heart failure (intake and output rations, daily weight, peripheral edema, rales and crackles upon lung auscultation, dyspnea) periodically during therapy.
- Monitor BP during therapy. Control hypertension during therapy.
- Monitor for diarrhea. If severe diarrhea develops, hold therapy until resolved.
- Monitor for signs and symptoms of reversible posterior leukoencephalopathy syndrome (seizures, headache, visual disturbances, confusion, altered mental status); may require discontinuation of therapy.
- ***Lab Test Considerations:*** Monitor serum calcium, potassium, and magnesium periodically during therapy. Maintain serum potassium at ≥4 mEq/L. Maintain serum calcium and magnesium within normal limits. May require more frequent monitoring if diarrhea occurs.

- Monitor TSH at baseline, at 2–4 wk, at 8–12 wk, and every 3 mo thereafter in patients with thyroidectomy. If symptoms of hypothyroidism occur, check TSH levels and adjust thyroid replacement.
- May cause ↓ serum glucose, WBC, hemoglobin, neutrophils, and platelets.
- May cause ↑ serum ALT, creatinine, bilirubin, and glucose.

Implementation

- Only prescribers and pharmacies certified with the Caprelsa REMS program are able to prescribe and dispense vandetanib.
- Correct hypocalcemia, hypokalemia, and hypomagnesemia prior to therapy.
- **PO:** May be administered daily without regard to food. Swallow tablets whole, do not crush, break or chew. If unable to swallow tablet, tablet may be dispersed in a class containing 2 oz of non-carbonated water and stirred for approximately 10 min until tablet is dispersed (will not completely dissolve). No other liquids should be used. Swallow dispersion immediately, then mix any residue with 4 oz of non-carbonated water and swallow. Dispersion may also be administered through nasogastric or gastrostomy tubes. Avoid direct contact with crushed tablets with skin or mucous membranes. Wash thoroughly to avoid exposure.

Patient/Family Teaching

- Instruct patient to take vandetanib as directed. Take missed doses as soon as remembered unless within 12 hrs of next dose. Instruct patient to read *Medication Guide* prior to starting therapy and with each Rx refill in case of changes.
- Advise patients to notify health care professional if rash or signs and symptoms of interstitial lung disease or reversible posterior leukoencephalopathy syndrome. If diarrhea occurs, instruct patient to treat with antidiarrheal medications and notify health care professional if diarrhea becomes severe or persistent.
- May cause tiredness, weakness, or blurred vision. Caution patients to avoid driving or other activities requiring alertness until response to medication is known.
- Caution patient to wear sunscreen and protective clothing during and for 4 mo after therapy is discontinued to prevent photosensitivity reactions.
- Advise patient to notify health care professional of all Rx or OTC medications, vitamins, or herbal products being taken and to consult with health care professional before taking other medications, especially St. John's wort.
- Rep: Advise female patients to use effective contraception during and for 4 mo after therapy and to avoid breast feeding.
- Emphasize the importance of regular follow-up exams, ECGs, and blood counts to determine progress and monitor for side effects.

Evaluation/Desired Outcomes

- Decreased spread of thyroid cancer.

vardenafil (var-den-a-fil)

Levitra, Staxyn

Classification

Therapeutic: erectile dysfunction agents

Pharmacologic: phosphodiesterase type 5 inhibitors

Indications

Erectile dysfunction.

Action

Increases cyclic guanosine monophosphate (cGMP) levels by inhibiting phosphodiesterase type 5 (PDE5) an enzyme responsible for the breakdown of cGMP. cGMP produces smooth muscle relaxation of the corpus cavernosum, which in turn promotes increased blood flow and subsequent erection. **Therapeutic Effects:** Enhanced blood flow to the corpus cavernosum and erection sufficient to allow sexual intercourse. Requires sexual stimulation.

Pharmacokinetics

Absorption: 15% absorbed following oral administration; absorption is rapid.

Distribution: Extensive tissue distribution; penetrates semen.

Protein Binding: 95%.

Metabolism and Excretion: Mostly metabolized by the liver (mainly CYP3A4 enzyme system, minor metabolism by CYP2C). M1 metabolite has anti-erectile dysfunction activity. Parent drug and metabolites are mostly excreted in feces. 2–6% renally eliminated.

Half-life: 4–6 hr.

TIME/ACTION PROFILE

ROUTE	ONSET	PEAK	DURATION
PO	rapid	0.5–2 hr	4 hr

Contraindications/Precautions

Contraindicated in: Hypersensitivity; Concurrent use of nitrates or riociguat; Unstable angina, recent history of stroke, life-threatening arrhythmias, HF or MI within 6 mo; End-stage renal disease requiring dialysis; Known hereditary degenerative retinal disorders; Moderate hepatic impairment (Child-Pugh B) (Staxyn only); Severe hepatic impairment (Child-Pugh C); Congenital or acquired QT prolongation or concurrent use of Class IA or III antiarrhythmics; Moderate or potent inhibitors of the CYP3A4 enzyme system (e.g. ketoconazole, itraconazole, ritonavir, indinavir, saquinavir, atazanavir, clarithromycin erythromycin) (Staxyn only); Pedi: Women, children or newborns.

Use Cautiously in: Other serious underlying cardiovascular disease or left ventricular outflow obstruction; Penile deformity; Underlying conditions predisposing to priapism including sickle cell anemia, multiple myeloma or leukemia; Bleeding disorders or active peptic ulcer diseases; History of sudden severe vision loss or non arteritic ischemic optic neuropathy (NAION); may ↑ risk of recurrence; Low cup to disk ratio, age >50 yr, diabetes, hypertension, coronary artery disease, hyperlipidemia, or smoking (↑ risk of NAION); Moderate or potent inhibitors of the CYP3A4 enzyme system (ketoconazole, itraconazole, ritonavir, indinavir, saquinavir, atazanavir, clarithromycin, erythromycin); need to ↓ dose of Levitra; Alpha adrenergic blockers (patients should be on stable dose of alpha blockers before starting vardenafil; should start therapy with tablets (Staxyn should not be used)); Geri: Have ↑ blood levels; ↓ dose required.

Adverse Reactions/Side Effects

CNS: headache, amnesia, dizziness. **EENT:** HEARING LOSS, VISION LOSS, rhinitis, sinusitis. **GI:** dyspepsia, nausea. **GU:** priapism. **Derm:** flushing. **Misc:** flu syndrome.

Interactions

Drug-Drug: Concurrent use of **nitrates** may cause serious, life-threatening hypotension and is contraindicated. Concurrent use of **riociguat** may result in severe hypotension; concurrent use contraindicated. Concurrent use of Class IA antiarrhythmics (such as **quindine** or **procainamide**) or **Class III antiarrhythmics** (such as **amiodarone** or **sotalol**) ↑ risk of serious arrhythmias and should be avoided. Concurrent use of alpha-adrenergic blockers may cause serious hypotension, lowest doses of each should be used initially. Strong inhibitors of CYP3A4 including **ritonavir**, **saquinavir**, **indinavir**, **atazanavir**, **ketoconazole**, **itraconazole**, and **clarithromycin** ↑ levels and the risk of adverse reactions; concurrent use of moderate inhibitors of CYP3A4 including **erythromycin** may also ↑ effects; concurrent use of any of these drugs is contraindicated with Staxyn; dose of Levitra must be ↓. ↑ risk of hypotension with **alpha adrenergic blockers** and acute ingestion of **alcohol**.

Route/Dosage

The tablets and orally disintegrating tablets are not interchangeable; the orally disintegrating tablets provide a higher level of systemic exposure compared to the tablets.

Levitra

PO (Adults): 10 mg taken 1 hr prior to sexual activity (range 5–20 mg; not to exceed one dose/24 hr); *Concurrent use of ritonavir*—single dose should not exceed 2.5 mg in any 72-hr period; *Concurrent use of indinavir, saquinavir, atazanavir, clarithromycin, ketoconazole 400 mg daily, or itraconazole 400 mg daily*—single dose should not exceed 2.5 mg/24 hr; *Concurrent use of ketoconazole 200 mg daily, itraconazole 200 mg daily, or erythromycin*—single dose should not exceed 5 mg/24 hr; *Concurrent use of stable alpha-blocker therapy (not on potent CYP3A4 inhibitor)*—5 mg initial dose; titrate as tolerated; *Concurrent use of stable alpha-blocker and potent CYP3A4 inhibitor therapy*—2.5 mg initial dose; titrate as tolerated.
PO (Geriatric Patients ≥65 yr): 5 mg initial dose; titrate as tolerated.

Hepatic Impairment

PO (Adults): *Moderate hepatic impairment (Child-Pugh B)*—May start with 5 mg dose (not to exceed 10 mg).

Staxyn

PO (Adults): 10 mg taken 1 hr prior to sexual activity (not to exceed one dose/24 hr).

Availability (generic available)

Tablets (Levitra): 2.5 mg, 5 mg, 10 mg, 20 mg. **Orally disintegrating tablets (Staxyn) (peppermint-flavor):** 10 mg.

NURSING IMPLICATIONS

Assessment

- Determine erectile dysfunction before administration. Vardenafil has no effect in the absence of sexual stimulation.

Implementation

- *Levitra* and *Staxyn* are not interchangeable.
- **PO:** *Levitra* is usually administered 1 hr before sexual activity. May be administered 30 min to 4 hr before sexual activity.
- Administer *Staxyn* 1 hr before sexual activity. Orally disintegrating tablets should be left in the package until use. Remove from the blister pouch. Do not push tablet through the blister; peel open the blister pack with dry hands and place tablet on tongue. Tablet will dissolve rapidly and be swallowed with saliva. No liquid is needed to take the orally disintegrating tablet.
- May be administered without regard to food.

Patient/Family Teaching

- Instruct patient to take vardenafil approximately 30 min–1 hr before sexual activity and not more than once per day. Inform patient that sexual stimulation is required for an erection to occur after taking vardenafil.
- Advise patient that vardenafil is not indicated for use in women.
- Caution patient not to take vardenafil concurrently with alpha adrenergic blockers (unless on a stable dose) or nitrates. If chest pain occurs after taking vardenafil, instruct patient to seek immediate medical attention.
- Instruct patient to notify health care professional promptly if erection lasts longer than 4 hr or if sudden or decreased vision loss in one or both eyes, or loss or decrease in hearing, ringing in the ears, or dizziness occurs.

V

- Instruct patient to notify health care professional of all Rx or OTC medications, vitamins, or herbal products being taken and consult health care professional before taking any new medications.
- Inform patient that vardenafil offers no protection against sexually transmitted diseases. Counsel patient that protection against sexually transmitted diseases and HIV infection should be considered.

Evaluation/Desired Outcomes

- Male erection sufficient to allow intercourse.

varenicline (ver-en-i-cline)

Champix, Chantix

Classification

Therapeutic: smoking deterrents

Pharmacologic: nicotine agonists

Indications

Treatment of smoking cessation; in conjunction with nonpharmacologic support (educational materials/counseling).

Action

Selectively binds to alpha$_4$, beta$_2$ nicotinic acetylcholine receptors, acting as a nicotine agonist; prevents the binding of nicotine to receptors. **Therapeutic Effects:** Decreased desire to smoke.

Pharmacokinetics

Absorption: 100% absorbed following oral administration.

Distribution: 24 hr.

Metabolism and Excretion: Minimally metabolized; 92% excreted in urine unchanged.

Half-life: 24 hr.

TIME/ACTION PROFILE

ROUTE	ONSET	PEAK	DURATION
PO	unknown	3–4 hr	24 hr

Contraindications/Precautions

Contraindicated in: Hypersensitivity; Lactation: Lactation; Pedi: Safety not established.

Use Cautiously in: Severe renal impairment (↓ dose recommended if CCr <30 mL/min); Stable cardiovascular disease (may ↑ risk of cardiovascular events); Psychiatric illness; Seizure disorders; Geri: Consider age-related ↓ in renal function; OB: Use only if maternal benefit outweighs fetal risk.

Adverse Reactions/Side Effects

CNS: HOMICIDAL THOUGHTS/BEHAVIOR, SEIZURES, STROKE, SUICIDAL THOUGHTS/BEHAVIOR, ↓ attention span, anxiety, depression, insomnia, irritability, dizziness, restlessness, abnormal dreams, agitation, aggression, amnesia, anxiety, delusions, disorientation, dissociation, hallucinations, hostility, mania, mood changes, migraine, panic, paranoia, psychosis, sleepwalking. **EENT:** blurred vision, visual disturbances. **CV:** MYOCARDIAL INFARCTION, syncope. **GI:** diarrhea, gingivitis, nausea, ↑ appetite, constipation, dyspepsia, dysphagia, enterocolitis, eructation, flatulence, gallbladder disorder, GI bleeding, ↑ liver enzymes, vomiting. **Derm:** STEVENS-JOHNSON SYNDROME, flushing, hyperhydrosis, acne, dermatitis, dry skin. **Hemat:** anemia. **MS:** arthralgia, back pain, musculoskeletal pain, muscle cramps, myalgia, restless legs. **Misc:** ANGIOEDEMA, accidental injury, chills, fever, hypersensitivity, mild physical dependence.

Interactions

Drug-Drug: Smoking cessation may ↓ metabolism of **theophylline**, **warfarin**, and **insulin** resulting in ↑ effects; careful monitoring is recommended. Risk of adverse reactions (nausea, vomiting, dizziness, fatigue, headache) may be ↑ with **nicotine** replacement therapy (nicotine transdermal patches). Concomitant use with **alcohol** may ↑ risk of worsening neuropsychiatric events.

Route/Dosage

PO (Adults): Treatment is started one wk prior to planned smoking cessation (may also begin dosing and then quit smoking between days 8 and 35 of treatment); 0.5 mg once daily on the first three days, then 0.5 mg twice daily for the next 4 days, then 1 mg twice daily.

Renal Impairment

PO (Adults): *CCr <30 mL/min*—0.5 mg daily, may ↑ to 0.5 mg twice daily.

Availability

Tablets: 0.5 mg, 1 mg. **Cost:** All strengths $237.71/56.

NURSING IMPLICATIONS

Assessment

- Assess for desire to stop smoking.
- Assess for nausea. Usually dose-dependent. May require dose reduction.
- Assess mental status and mood changes, especially during initial few mo of therapy and during dose changes. Risk may be increased in children, adolescents, and adults ≤24 yr. Inform health care professional if patient demonstrates significant increase in signs of depression (depressed mood, loss of interest in usual activities, significant change in weight and/or appetite, insomnia or hypersomnia, psychomotor agitation or retardation, increased fatigue, feelings of guilt or worthlessness, slowed thinking or impaired concentration, suicide attempt or suicidal or homicidal ideation). Restrict amount of drug available to patient.
- Assess for rash periodically during therapy. May cause Stevens-Johnson syndrome. Discontinue therapy if severe or if accompanied with fever, general malaise, fatigue, muscle or joint aches, blisters, oral lesions, conjunctivitis, hepatitis and/or eosinophilia.
- ***Lab Test Considerations:*** May cause anemia.

Implementation

- **PO:** Administer after eating with a full glass of water.

Patient/Family Teaching

- Instruct patient to take varenicline as directed. Set a date to stop smoking. Start taking varenicline 1 wk before quit date. Patient may also begin varenicline and then quit smoking between days 8 and 35 of therapy. Begin with 0.5 mg/day for the first 3 days, then for the next 4 days take one 0.5 mg tablet in the morning and in the evening. After first 7 days, increase to 1 mg tablet in the morning and evening. Advise patient to read *Medication Guide* before starting therapy.
- Encourage patient to attempt to quit, even if they had early lapses after quit day.
- Advise patient to stop taking varenicline and contact health care professional promptly if agitation, depressed mood, any changes in behavior that are not typical of nicotine withdrawal, or if suicidal thoughts or behavior; rash with mucosal lesions or skin reaction, or chest pain, pressure, or dyspnea occur. Encourage patient to reduce amount of alcohol consumed until effects of medication are known.
- Provide patient with educational materials and counseling to support attempts to quit smoking.
- Caution patient not to share varenicline with others. May be harmful.
- May cause blurred vision, dizziness, and disturbance in attention. Caution patient to avoid driving and other activities requiring alertness until response to medication is known.
- Inform patient that nausea, insomnia, and vivid, unusual, or strange dreams may occur and are usually transient. Advise patient to notify health care professional if these symptoms are persistent and bothersome; dose reduction may be considered.
- Instruct patient to notify health care professional of all Rx or OTC medications, vitamins, or herbal products being taken and consult health care professional before taking any new medications. Inform patient that some medications may require dose adjustments after quitting smoking.
- Advise patient to notify health care professional if pregnancy is planned or suspected or if breast feeding.

Evaluation/Desired Outcomes

- Smoking cessation. Patients who have successfully stopped smoking at the end of 12 wk, should take an additional 12 wk course to increase the likelihood of long-term abstinence. Patients who do not succeed in stopping smoking during 12 wk of initial therapy or who relapse after treatment, should be encouraged to make another attempt once factors contributing to the failed attempt have been identified and addressed.

vasopressin (vay-soe-press-in)

~~Pitressin~~, Vasostrict

Classification
Therapeutic: hormones
Pharmacologic: antidiuretic hormones, vasopressors

Indications

Central diabetes insipidus due to deficient antidiuretic hormone. Vasodilatory shock. **Unlabeled Use:** Gastrointestinal hemorrhage.

Action

Alters the permeability of the renal collecting ducts, allowing reabsorption of water. Directly stimulates musculature of GI tract. In high doses acts as a nonadrenergic peripheral vasoconstrictor. **Therapeutic Effects:** Decreased urine output and increased urine osmolality in diabetes insipidus. Increased BP.

Pharmacokinetics

Absorption: IM absorption may be unpredictable.
Distribution: Widely distributed throughout extracellular fluid.
Metabolism and Excretion: Rapidly degraded by the liver and kidneys; <5% excreted unchanged by the kidneys.
Half-life: <10 min.

TIME/ACTION PROFILE (antidiuretic effect)

ROUTE	ONSET	PEAK	DURATION
IM, subcut	unknown	unknown	2–8 hr
IV	unknown	unknown	30–60 min

V

Contraindications/Precautions

Contraindicated in: Chronic renal failure with ↑ BUN; Hypersensitivity to 8-L arginine vasopressin or chlorobutanol (only in multidose vial).
Use Cautiously in: Perioperative polyuria (↑ sensitivity to vasopressin effects); Comatose patients; Seizures; Migraine headaches; Asthma; Heart failure; Cardiovascular disease; Renal impairment; OB: Higher doses (0.07 units/min) for vasodilatory shock may be needed in 2nd and 3rd trimesters; Geri: ↑ sensitivity to vasopressin effects.

Adverse Reactions/Side Effects

CNS: dizziness, "pounding" sensation in head. **CV:** MI, angina, chest pain. **Derm:** paleness, perioral blanching, sweating. **GI:** abdominal cramps, belching, diarrhea, flatulence, heartburn, nausea, vomiting. **Neuro:** trembling. **Misc:** allergic reactions, fever, water intoxication (higher doses).

Interactions

Drug-Drug: Antidiuretic effect may be ↓ by concurrent administration of **clozapine**, **lithium**, **demeclo-**

cycline, **foscarnet**. Antidiuretic effect may be ↑ by concurrent administration of **cyclophosphamide**, **enalapril**, **felbamate**, **haloperidol**, **ifosfamide**, **methyldopa**, **pentamidine**, **tricyclic antidepressants**, **SSRIs**, or **vincristine**. Vasopressor effect may be ↑ by concurrent administration of **ganglionic blocking agents**, **indomethacin**, or **catecholamines**. **Furosemide** ↑ urine flow.

Route/Dosage

Diabetes Insipidus

IM, Subcut (Adults): 5–10 units 2–4 times daily.
IM, Subcut (Children): 2.5–10 units 2–4 times daily.
IV (Adults and Children): 0.0005 units/kg/hr, double dose every 30 min as needed to a maximum of 0.01 units/kg/hr.

Vasodilatory Shock

IV (Adults): 0.01 units/min, titrate by 0.005 units/min every 10–15 min until target BP achieved; (max dose = 0.07 units/min).
IV (Infants and Children): 0.0003–0.002 units/kg/min, titrate to effect.

GI Hemorrhage

IV (Adults): 0.2–0.4 units/min then titrate to maximum dose of 0.9 units/min; if bleeding stops continue same dose for 12 hr then taper off over 24–48 hr.
IV (Children): 0.002–0.005 units/kg/min then titrate to maximum dose of 0.01 units/kg/min; if bleeding stops continue same dose for 12 hr then taper off over 24–48 hr.

Availability (generic available)

Solution for injection (requires dilution): 20 units/mL.

NURSING IMPLICATIONS

Assessment

- Monitor BP, HR, and ECG periodically throughout therapy and continuously throughout cardiopulmonary resuscitation.
- **Diabetes Insipidus:** Monitor urine osmolality and urine volume frequently to determine effects of medication. Assess patient for symptoms of dehydration (excessive thirst, dry skin and mucous membranes, tachycardia, poor skin turgor). Weigh patient daily, monitor intake and output, and assess for edema.
- ***Lab Test Considerations:*** Monitor urine specific gravity throughout therapy.
- Monitor serum electrolyte concentrations periodically during therapy.
- ***Toxicity and Overdose:*** Signs and symptoms of water intoxication include confusion, drowsiness, headache, weight gain, difficulty urinating, seizures, and coma.
- Treatment of overdose includes water restriction and temporary discontinuation of vasopressin until polyuria occurs. If symptoms are severe, administration of mannitol, hypertonic dextrose, urea, and/or furosemide may be used.

Implementation

- Aqueous vasopressin injection may be administered subcut or IM for diabetes insipidus.
- Administer 1–2 glasses of water at the time of administration to minimize side effects (blanching of skin, abdominal cramps, nausea).

IV Administration

- **Continuous Infusion:** ***Diluent:*** Dilute 2.5 mg or 5 mg of vasopresssin in 500 mL or 100 mL respectively of 0.9% NaCl or D5W. ***Concentration:*** 0.1 units/mL or 1 unit/mL. Solution is stable for 18 hrs at room temperature or 24 hr if refrigerated. ***Rate:*** See Route/Dosage section.
- **Y-Site Compatibility:** acyclovir, alemtuzumab, alfentanil, allopurinol, amifostine, amikacin, aminocaproic acid, aminophylline, amiodarone, amphotericin B liposome, anidulafungin, argatroban, ascorbic acid, asparaginase, atracurium, atropine, azathioprine, azithromycin, aztreonam, benztropine, bivalirudin, bleomycin, bumetanide, buprenorphine, busulfan, butorphanol, calcium chloride, calcium gluconate, carboplatin, carmustine, caspofungin, cefazolin, cefepime, cefotaxime, cefotetan, cefoxitin, ceftaroline, ceftazidime, ceftriaxone, cefuroxime, chloramphenicol, chlorpromazine, ciprofloxacin, cisatracurium, cisplatin, clindamycin, cyanocobalamin, cyclophosphamide, cyclosporine, cytarabine, dacarbazine, dactinomycin, daptomycin, dexamethasone, dexmedetomidine, dexrazoxane, digoxin, diltiazem, diphenhydramine, dobutamine, docetaxel, dopamine, doxorubicin hydrochloride, doxycycline, droperidol, enalaprilat, ephedrine, epinephrine, epirubicin, epoetin alfa, ertapenem, erythromycin, esmolol, etoposide, etoposide phosphate, famotidine, fenoldopam, fentanyl, fluconazole, fludarabine, fluorouracil, folic acid, foscarnet, fosphenytoin, ganciclovir, gemcitabine, gentamicin, glycopyrrolate, granisetron, heparin, hetastarch, hydrocortisone, hydromorphone, idarubicin, ifosfamide, imipenem/cilastatin, irinotecan, isoproterenol, ketorolac, labetalol, levofloxacin, lidocaine, linezolid, lorazepam, magnesium sulfate, mannitol, melphalan, meperidine, meropenem, mesna, metaraminol, methohexital, methotrexate, methylprednisolone, metoclopramide, metoprolol, metronidazole, micafungin, midazolam, milrinone, mitomycin, mitoxantrone, morphine, moxifloxacin, multivitamins, mycophenolate, nafcillin, nalbuphine, naloxone, nicardipine, nitroglycerin, nitroprusside, norepinephrine, octreotide, ondansetron, oxacillin, oxaliplatin, oxytocin, paclitaxel, palonosetron, pamidronate, pantoprazole, papaverine, penicillin G, pentamidine, phenobarbital, phentolamine, phenylephrine, phytonadione, piperacillin/tazobactam, potassium acetate, potassium chloride, potassium phosphates, procainamide, prochlorperazine, promethazine, propranolol, protamine, pyridoxime, quinupristin/dalfopristin, ranitidine, remifentanil, rocuronium, sodium acetate, sodium bicarbonate, so-

dium phosphates, streptozocin, succinylcholine, sufentanil, tacrolimus, telavancin, theophylline, thiamine, thiopental, thiotepa, tigecycline, tirofiban, tobramycin, tolazoline, topotecan, vancomycin, vecuronium, verapamil, vinblastine, vincristine, vinorelbine, voriconazole, zidovudine, zoledronic acid.

- **Y-Site Incompatibility:** amphotericin B lipid complex, dantrolene, diazepam, diazoxide, indomethacin, pemetrexed, phenytoin.

Patient/Family Teaching

- Instruct patient to take medication as directed. Caution patient not to use more than prescribed amount. Take missed doses as soon as remembered, unless almost time for next dose.
- Advise patient to drink 1–2 glasses of water at time of administration to minimize side effects (blanching of skin, abdominal cramps, nausea). Inform patient that these side effects are not serious and usually disappear in a few min.
- Caution patient to avoid concurrent use of alcohol while taking vasopressin.
- Advise patient to notify health care professional if pregnancy is planned or suspected, or if breast feeding.
- Patients with diabetes insipidus should carry identification at all times describing disease process and medication regimen.

Evaluation/Desired Outcomes

- Decrease in urine volume.
- Relief of polydipsia.
- Increased urine osmolality in patients with central diabetes insipidus.
- Increase in BP.

vedolizumab
(ve-doe-**liz**-yoo-mab)
Entyvio

Classification
Therapeutic: gastrointestinal anti-inflammatories
Pharmacologic: monoclonal antibodies, integrin receptor antagonists

Indications

Moderately to severely active ulcerative colitis or Crohn's disease that has not responded adequately to/lost response to/become intolerant to tumor necrosis factor (TNF) blockers or immunomodulators; or has become intolerant to/dependant on corticosteroids and failed to induce/maintain beneficial response/remission, improved endoscopic appearance (ulcerative colitis) or achieved corticosteroid-free remission.

Action

A monoclonal antibody that binds to certain integrins, blocking their interaction with substances involved in mucosal cell adhesion, also inhibits migration of memory T-lymphocytes across endothelium into inflamed GI tissue. **Therapeutic Effects:** Decreased chronic GI inflammation and symptomatology associated with ulcerative colitis and Crohn's disease.

Pharmacokinetics

Absorption: IV administration results in complete bioavailability.
Distribution: Unknown.
Metabolism and Excretion: Unknown.
Half-life: 25 days.

TIME/ACTION PROFILE (clinical improvement)

ROUTE	ONSET	PEAK	DURATION
IV	within 6 wk	unknown	up to 8 wk

Contraindications/Precautions

Contraindicated in: Hypersensitivity; Active severe infection; Live-virus vaccinations; Concurrent use of natalizumab; Concurrent use of TNF blockers.
Use Cautiously in: OB: Use during pregnancy if maternal benefits outweigh risk to the unborn child; Lactation: Use cautiously if breast feeding; Pedi: Safe and effective use in children has not been established.

Adverse Reactions/Side Effects

CNS: headache, fatigue. **Derm:** pruritus, rash. **GI:** ↑ liver enzymes, oropharyngeal pain. **MS:** arthralgia, back pain, extremity pain. **Resp:** cough. **Misc:** fever, HYPERSENSITIVITY REACTIONS (including anaphylaxis), INFECTION.

Interactions

Drug-Drug: May ↓ antibody response to and ↑ risk of adverse reactions from **live-virus vaccines** (complete immunizations prior to treatment). Concurrent use with **natalizumab** may ↑ risk of infections and Progressive Multifocal Leukoencephalopathy and should be avoided. Concurrent use with **TNF blockers** may ↑ risk of infections and should be avoided.

Route/Dosage

IV (Adults): 300 mg initially, then 2 and 6 wk later, then every 8 wk; treatment may be continued if beneficial response is obtained by wk 14.

Availability

Lyophilized powder for injection (requires reconstitution and dilution): 300 mg/vial.

NURSING IMPLICATIONS

Assessment

- Assess abdominal pain and frequency, quantity, and consistency of stools at beginning and during therapy.
- Assess for signs of hypersensitivity or infusion-related reactions (dyspnea, bronchospasm, urticaria,

V

flushing, rash, swelling of lips, tongue, throat, or face, wheezing, hypertension, tachycardia). If anaphylaxis or serious allergic reactions occur, discontinue vedolizumab and treat symptoms.

- Assess for new signs or symptoms suggestive of progressive multifocal leukoencephalopathy (PML), an opportunistic infection of the brain caused by the JC virus, leading to death or severe disability; withhold dose and notify health care professional promptly. Monitor during therapy and for at least 6 mo following discontinuation. PML symptoms may begin gradually but usually over days to wk and leads to death or severe disability over wk to mo. Symptoms include progressive weakness on one side of body or clumsiness of limbs, disturbance of vision, changes in thinking, memory and orientation leading to confusion and personality changes. Diagnosis is usually made via gadolinium-enhanced MRI and CSF analysis. Withhold vedolizumab at first sign of PML.
- ***Lab Test Considerations:*** May cause ↑ AST, ALT, and serum bilirubin. Discontinue in patients with jaundice or other evidence of liver injury.

Implementation

- Perform test for latent TB. If positive, begin treatment for TB prior to starting vedolizumab therapy. Monitor for TB throughout therapy, even if latent TB test is negative.

IV Administration

- **Intermittent Infusion:** Reconstitute with 4.8 mL sterile water for injection using 21- to 25-gauge needle. Direct stream to wall of vial to prevent excessive foaming. Gently swirl vial for at least 15 sec to dissolve; do not invert of shake vigorously. Allow to sit for up to 20 min at room temperature for reconstitution and settling of foam. If not fully dissolved after 20 min, allow another 10 min. Do not use vial if not dissolved within 30 min. Solution is clear or opalescent, colorless to light brownish yellow; do not administer solutions that are discolored or contain particulate matter. Swirl gently and invert vial 3 times prior to withdrawing. Withdraw 5 mL (300 mg) using 21- to 25-gauge needle. Discard unused portion. ***Diluent:*** 250 mL 0.9% NaCl or LR. Gently mix bag. Use as soon as possible. Stable up to 4 hrs if refrigerated; do not freeze. ***Rate:*** Infuse over 30 min; do not administer as IV push or bolus. Flush line with 30 mL of 0.9% NaCl or LR after infusion.
- **Y-Site Incompatibility:** Do not administer with other solutions or medications.

Patient/Family Teaching

- Explain purpose of vedolizumab to patient. Advise patient to read *Medication Guide* prior to therapy.
- Instruct patient to report symptoms of PML (progressive weakness on one side of the body or clumsiness of limbs; disturbance of vision; changes in thinking, memory, and orientation leading to confusion and personality changes), hypersensitivity reactions, hepatotoxicity (yellowing of the skin and eyes, unusual darkening of the urine, anorexia, nausea, feeling tired or weak, vomiting, right upper abdominal pain), or worsening of symptoms (new or sudden change in your thinking, eyesight, balance, or strength or other problems) that persist over several days to health care professional immediately.
- Inform patient of risk of infection. Advise patient to notify health care professional if symptoms of infection (fever, chills, muscle aches, shortness of breath, runny nose, cough, sore throat, red or painful skin or open cuts or sores, tiredness, pain during urination) occur.
- Advise patient to notify health care professional of all Rx or OTC medications, vitamins, or herbal products being taken and to consult with health care professional before taking other medications.
- Advise females of reproductive potential to notify health care professional if pregnancy is planned or suspected, or if breast feeding. Encourage pregnant women to join Entyvio Pregnancy Registry by calling 1-877-825-3327. Registry monitors pregnancy outcomes in women exposed to vedolizumab during pregnancy.

Evaluation/Desired Outcomes

- Decreased chronic GI inflammation and symptomatology associated with ulcerative colitis and Crohn's disease. Discontinue therapy if no improvement by Week 14.

vemurafenib

(vem-u-**raf**-e-nib)

Zelboraf

Classification

Therapeutic: antineoplastics

Pharmacologic: kinase inhibitors

Indications

Treatment of unresectable or metastatic melanoma with BRAF ^{V600E} mutation. Treatment of Erdheim-Chester Disease (ECD) with BRAF ^{V600E} mutation.

Action

Inhibits mutated forms of the enzyme kinase. Inhibits proliferation that occurs in conjunction with activated BRAF proteins. **Therapeutic Effects:** Decreased spread of melanoma and ECD.

Pharmacokinetics

Absorption: Some absorption follows oral administration, bioavailability is not known.

Distribution: Unknown.

Protein Binding: >99%.

Metabolism and Excretion: Mostly metabolized by the liver (mostly by the CYP3A4 enzyme system), 1% eliminated in urine.

Half-life: 57 hr (range 30–120 hr).

TIME/ACTION PROFILE (blood levels)

ROUTE	ONSET	PEAK	DURATION
PO	unknown	3 hr	12 hr

Contraindications/Precautions

Contraindicated in: Underlying electrolyte abnormalities (↑ risk of serious arrhythmias; correct prior to administration); Congenital or acquired prolonged QT syndromes; Baseline QTc interval >500 msec; Concurrent use of QT-interval prolonging drugs; OB: May cause fetal harm; Lactation: Avoid breast feeding during therapy.

Use Cautiously in: Pre-existing severe hepatic or renal impairment; Concurrent use of strong CYP3A4 inducers/inhibitors or drugs that are substrates of CYP3A4, CYP1A2 or CYP2D6 enzyme systems; monitoring of effects and necessary dose adjustments may be necessary; Receiving radiation therapy prior to, during, or after therapy (↑ risk of radiation sensitization/recall); Geri: ↑ risk of cutaneous squamous cell carcinoma, nausea, ↓ appetite, peripheral edema, keratoacanthoma and atrial fibrillation; Rep: Women of reproductive potential; Pedi: Safety and effectiveness not established.

Adverse Reactions/Side Effects

CNS: fatigue, weakness, headache. **CV:** TORSADES DE POINTES, peripheral edema, QT interval prolongation. **Derm:** DRUG REACTION WITH EOSINOPHILIA AND SYSTEMIC SYMPTOMS (DRESS), SKIN CANCER, STEVENS-JOHNSON SYNDROME, TOXIC EPIDERMAL NECROLYSIS, alopecia, dry skin, rash (↑ in females), pruritus, rash, photosensitivity (↑ in females), skin papilloma, keratocanthoma (↑ in males). **EENT:** iritis, retinal vein occlusion, uveitis. **GI:** HEPATOTOXICITY, ↓ appetite, dysgeusia, nausea. **GU:** acute interstitial nephritis, acute tubular necrosis, ↑ creatinine (↑ in females). **MS:** arthralgia (↑ in females), myalgia, back pain, Dupuytren's contracture, musculoskeletal pain, plantar fascial fibromatosis. **Resp:** cough. **Misc:** HYPERSENSITIVITY REACTIONS (including anaphylaxis), fever, radiation sensitization/recall.

Interactions

Drug-Drug: **QT interval prolonging drugs** may ↑ the risk of QT interval prolongation with arrhythmias; concurrent use contraindicated. Concurrent use with **agents with narrow therapeutic indices that are metabolized by the CYP1A2 enzyme systems** not recommended. Consider dose ↓ of substrates. Strong CYP3A inhibitors, including **atazanavir**, **clarithromycin**, **indinavir**, **itraconazole**, **ketoconazole**, **nefazodone**, **nelfinavir**, **ritonavir**, **saquinavir**, and **voriconazole** may ↑ levels and effects; avoid concurrent use. Strong inducers of CYP3A4 including **carbamazepine**, **phenobarbital**, **phenytoin**, **rifabutin**, **rifampin**, **rifapentine** may ↓ levels and effectiveness; avoid concurrent use. May ↑ risk of bleeding with **warfarin**. Concurrent use with **ipilimumab** may ↑ risk of hepatotoxicity. May ↑ **digoxin** levels and lead to toxicity. May ↑ **tizanidine** levels.

Route/Dosage

PO (Adults): 960 mg (4 tablets) twice daily until disease progression or unacceptable toxicity; *Concurrent use of strong CYP3A4 inducers*—1200 mg (5 tablets) twice daily until disease progression or unacceptable toxicity.

Availability

Tablets: 240 mg.

NURSING IMPLICATIONS

Assessment

- Perform dermatologic evaluation prior to initiation and every 2 mo during therapy. Excise any suspicious lesions, send for dermapathologic evaluation, and treat with standard care. Continue monitoring for 6 mo following discontinuation of therapy.
- Monitor ECG 15 days after initiation of therapy, monthly during first 3 mo, every 3 mo thereafter, and more often if clinically indicated.
- Monitor for hypersensitivity reactions (rash, erythema, hypotension). Permanently discontinue therapy if severe reaction occurs.
- Monitor for signs and symptoms of uveitis periodically during therapy. May require treatment with steroid and mydriatic ophthalmic drops.
- Assess patient for rash (mild to moderate rash usually occurs in the 2nd wk of therapy and resolves within 1–2 wk of continued therapy). If rash is severe (extensive erythematous or maculopapular rash with moist desquamation or angioedema) or accompanied by systemic symptoms (serum sickness-like reaction, Stevens-Johnson syndrome, toxic epidermal necrolysis), therapy must be discontinued immediately.
- ***Lab Test Considerations:*** Information on FDA-approved tests for the detection of BRAF V600 mutations in melanoma is available at www.fda.gov/CompanionDiagnostics.
- Monitor serum potassium, magnesium, and calcium before starting therapy and after dose modification.
- Monitor AST, ALT, alkaline phosphatase, and bilirubin before starting therapy, monthly during therapy, and as clinically indicated. May require dose reduction, treatment interruption or discontinuation.
- Monitor serum creatinine before starting and periodically during therapy.

Implementation

- **PO:** Administer (four 240 mg tablets) twice daily, without regard to food. Take first dose in the morning with 2nd dose about 12 hrs later. Swallow tablets whole, do not crush or chew.

- Adverse reactions or QTc prolongation may occur requiring dose modification. *If Grade 1 or 2 (tolerable) occur,* maintain dose at 960 mg twice daily. *If Grade 2 (Intolerable) or Grade 3, 1st appearance occurs,* interrupt therapy until Grade 0–1. Resume dosing at 720 mg twice daily. *If 2nd appearance,* interrupt therapy until Grade 0–1. Resume dosing at 480 mg twice daily. *If 3rd appearance,* discontinue permanently. *If Grade 4, 1st appearance occurs,* discontinue permanently or interrupt therapy until Grade 0–1. Resume dosing at 480 twice daily. *If 2nd appearance,* discontinue permanently. Doses below 480 mg twice daily are not recommended.

Patient/Family Teaching

- Instruct patient to take venurafenib as directed. If vomiting occurs, do not an additional dose, take next dose as scheduled. Take missed doses as soon as remembered up to 4 hrs before next dose; do not double dose.
- Inform patient that assessment of BRAF mutation is required for selection of patients.
- Instruct patient to stop taking vemurafenib and notify health care professional immediately if signs and symptoms of allergic reaction (rash or redness all over body; feeling faint; difficulty breathing or swallowing; throat tightness or hoarseness; fast heartbeat; swelling of face, lips, or tongue) or severe skin reactions (blisters on skin; blisters or sores in mouth; peeling of skin, fever, redness or swelling of face, hands, or soles of feet) occur.
- Advise patient to wear broad spectrum UVA/UVB sunscreen, lip balm (SPF ≥30) and protective clothing, and to avoid sun exposure to prevent photosensitivity reactions. Severe photosensitivity reactions may require dose modifications.
- Advise patient to notify health care professional if signs and symptoms of liver dysfunction (yellow skin or whites of eyes; feeling tired; urine turns dark or brown; nausea or vomiting; loss of appetite; pain on right side of stomach) or eye problems (eye pain, swelling, or redness; blurred vision; vision changes) occur.
- Instruct patient to notify health care professional of all Rx or OTC medications, vitamins, or herbal products being taken and consult health care professional before taking any new medications.
- Inform patient that regular assessments of skin and assessments for signs and symptoms of other malignancies must be done during and for up to 6 mo after therapy. Advise patient to notify health care professional immediately if any changes in skin occur.
- Rep: Advise women of reproductive potential to use effective contraception during and for at least 2 wk after last dose of vemurafenib, and to avoid breast feeding during and for 2 wk after last dose.

Evaluation/Desired Outcomes

- Decreased spread of melanoma.

venetoclax (ven-**et**-oh-klax)

Venclexta

Classification

Therapeutic: antineoplastics

Pharmacologic: BCL-2 inhibitors

Indications

Chronic lymphocytic leukemia (CLL) or small lymphocytic leukemia (SLL) (as monotherapy or in combination with obinutuzumab or rituximab). Newly diagnosed acute myeloid leukemia (AML) in patients who are ≥75 yr old or who have comorbidities that prevent the use of intensive induction chemotherapy (in combination with azacitidine or decitabine or low-dose cytarabine).

Action

Inhibits BCL-2 which is overexpressed on CLL, SLL, and AML cells, thereby inducing apoptosis. **Therapeutic Effects:** Reduced disease progression.

Pharmacokinetics

Absorption: Well absorbed with food following oral administration; bioavailability ↑ by high-fat foods.

Distribution: Extensively distributed to tissues.

Protein Binding: 99%.

Metabolism and Excretion: Primarily metabolized by CYP3A4/5. 99% excreted in feces (21% as unchanged drug).

Half-life: 26 hr.

TIME/ACTION PROFILE (blood levels)

ROUTE	ONSET	PEAK	DURATION
PO	unknown	5–8 hr	unknown

Contraindications/Precautions

Contraindicated in: Concurrent use with strong CYP3A inhibitors during initiation and ramp-up phases; Concurrent use with moderate CYP3A inhibitors or P-gp inhibitors; Concurrent use with strong or moderate CYP3A inducers; OB: Pregnancy (may cause fetal harm); Lactation: Lactation.

Use Cautiously in: High tumor burden (↑ risk of tumor lysis syndrome); Renal impairment (CCr <80 mL/min) (↑ risk of tumor lysis syndrome); Severe hepatic impairment (↓ dose); Rep: Women of reproductive potential; Pedi: Safety and effectiveness not established.

Adverse Reactions/Side Effects

CNS: headache. **CV:** peripheral edema. **F and E:** hyperkalemia, hyperphosphatemia, hypokalemia, hyperuricemia, hypocalcemia. **GI:** constipation, diarrhea, nausea, vomiting. **GU:** ↓ fertility (males). **Hemat:** anemia, neutropenia, thrombocytopenia. **MS:** back pain. **Resp:** cough. **Misc:** INFECTION, TUMOR LYSIS SYNDROME, fatigue, fever.

Interactions

Drug-Drug: Strong CYP3A inhibitors, including **itraconazole**, **conivaptan**, **clarithromycin**, **indina-**

vir, **lopinavir**, **ritonavir**, **posaconazole**, and **voriconazole** may ↑ levels; concurrent use during initiation and ramp-up phase contraindicated; ↓ venetoclax dose by ≥75% after ramp-up phase if concurrent use necessary. **Moderate CYP3A4 inhibitors**, including **erythromycin**, **ciprofloxacin**, **diltiazem**, **dronedarone**, **fluconazole**, or **verapamil** or **P-gp inhibitors**, including **amiodarone**, **azithromycin**, **captopril**, **carvedilol**, **cyclosporine**, **felodipine**, **quinidine**, **ranolazine**, or **ticagrelor** may ↑ levels; avoid concurrent use; ↓ venetoclax dose by ≥50% if concurrent use necessary. **Strong CYP3A4 inducers**, including **carbamazepine**, **phenytoin**, or **rifampin** or **moderate CYP3A inducers**, including **bosentan**, **efavirenz**, **etravirine**, **modafinil**, or **nafcillin** may ↓ levels; avoid concurrent use. May ↑ levels of **P-gp substrates** with a narrow therapeutic index, including **digoxin**, **sirolimus**, and **everolimus**; if concurrent therapy necessary, give P-gp substrate ≥6 hr before venetoclax. May ↑ levels of **warfarin**. May ↓ antibody response to **live-virus vaccine** and ↑ risk of adverse reactions; do not administer concurrently.

Drug-Natural Products: St. John's wort may ↓ levels; avoid concurrent use.

Drug-Food: Grapefruit products, **Seville oranges**, and **starfruit** may ↑ levels; avoid concurrent use.

Route/Dosage

CLL/SLL

PO (Adults): *Monotherapy*—Start with the following 5–wk venetoclax ramp-up phase: 20 mg once daily during Wk 1, then 50 mg once daily during Wk 2, then 100 mg once daily during Wk 3, then 200 mg once daily during Wk 4, then 400 mg once daily during Wk 5. After completion of ramp-up phase, continue venetoclax therapy at 400 mg once daily until disease progression or unacceptable toxicity. *In combination with rituximab*—Start with the following 5–wk venetoclax ramp-up phase: 20 mg once daily during Wk 1, then 50 mg once daily during Wk 2, then 100 mg once daily during Wk 3, then 200 mg once daily during Wk 4, then 400 mg once daily during Wk 5. After completion of ramp-up phase, start rituximab which will be administered on Day 1 of each 28–day cycle for a total of 6 cycles. Continue venetoclax therapy at 400 mg once daily starting on Day 1 of Cycle 1 and continue for 24 mo (from Day 1 of Cycle 1). *In combination with obinutuzumab*—Start with obinutuzumab on Days 1, 2, 8, and 15 of Cycle 1 and then on Day 1 of each subsequent 28–day cycle for a total of 6 cycles. On Day 22 of Cycle 1, start 5–wk venetoclax ramp-up phase: 20 mg once daily during Wk 1, then 50 mg once daily during Wk 2, then 100 mg once daily during Wk 3, then 200 mg once daily during Wk 4, then 400 mg once daily during Wk 5. After completion of ramp-up phase on Day 28 of Cycle 2, continue venetoclax therapy at 400 mg once daily from Day 1 of Cycle 3 until Day 28 of Cycle 12. *Concurrent use of strong CYP3A inhibitors (including posaconazole) (during ramp–up phase)*—Contraindicated; *Concurrent use of posaconazole (after ramp–up phase)*—↓ venetoclax dose to 70 mg once daily. *Concurrent use of strong CYP3A inhibitors other than posaconazole (after ramp–up phase)*—↓ venetoclax dose to 100 mg once daily. *Concurrent use of moderate CYP3A inhibitors or P-gp inhibitors (during or after ramp–up phase)*—↓ venetoclax dose by ≥50%.

Hepatic Impairment

PO (Adults): *Severe hepatic impairment*—↓ dose by 50%.

AML

PO (Adults): *In combination with azacitidine or decitabine*—Start with the following venetoclax ramp-up phase: 100 mg once daily on Day 1, then 200 mg once daily on Day 2, then 400 mg once daily on Day 3, then 400 mg once daily on Day 4. After completion of ramp-up phase, continue venetoclax therapy at 400 mg once daily until disease progression or unacceptable toxicity. Start azacitidine or decitabine on Day 1. *In combination with low-dose cytarabine*—Start with the following venetoclax ramp-up phase: 100 mg once daily on Day 1, then 200 mg once daily on Day 2, then 400 mg once daily on Day 3, then 600 mg once daily on Day 4. After completion of ramp-up phase, continue venetoclax therapy at 600 mg once daily until disease progression or unacceptable toxicity. Start low-dose cytarabine on Day 1. *Concurrent use of posaconazole*—↓ venetoclax dose during ramp-up phase to 10 mg once daily on Day 1, then 20 mg once daily on Day 2, then 50 mg once daily on Day 3, then 70 mg once daily on Day 4. After completion of ramp-up phase, ↓ venetoclax dose to 70 mg once daily. *Concurrent use of strong CYP3A inhibitors other than posaconazole*—↓ venetoclax dose during ramp-up phase to 10 mg once daily on Day 1, then 20 mg once daily on Day 2, then 50 mg once daily on Day 3, then 100 mg once daily on Day 4. After completion of ramp-up phase, ↓ venetoclax dose to 100 mg once daily. *Concurrent use of moderate CYP3A inhibitors or P-gp inhibitors*—↓ venetoclax dose by ≥50% during or after completion of ramp-up phase.

Hepatic Impairment

PO (Adults): *Severe hepatic impairment*—↓ dose by 50%.

Availability

Tablets: 10 mg, 50 mg, 100 mg.

NURSING IMPLICATIONS

Assessment

- Assess for risk of tumor lysis syndrome and provide prophylactic hydration and anti-hyperuricemis agents prior to 1st dose to reduce tumor lysis syndrome.

V

Prophylaxis for patients with a low tumor burden (All lymph node (LN) <5 cm AND absolute lymphocyte count (ALC) <25 x 10^9/L) includes allopurinol with oral hydration of 1.5–2 L. Monitor blood chemistries (potassium, uric acid, phosphorous, calcium creatinine) on an outpatient basis at pre-dose, 6–8 hrs, 24 hrs at 1st dose of 20 mg and 50 mg and Pre-dose at subsequent ramp-up doses. *Prophylaxis for patients with a medium tumor burden* (Any LN 5 cm-<10 cm OR ALC ≥25 x 10^9/L) includes allopurinol and oral hydration of 1.5–2 L and consider additional IV hydration. Monitor blood chemistries on an outpatient basis at pre-dose, 6–8 hrs, 24 hrs at 1st dose of 20 mg and 50 mg and Pre-dose at subsequent ramp-up doses. Consider hospitalization for patients with creatinine clearance <80 mL/min at 1st dose of 20 mg and 50 mg. *Prophylaxis for patients with a high tumor burden* (Any LN ≥10 cm OR ALC ≥25 x 10^9/L AND any LN ≥5 cm) includes allopurinol; consider rasburicase if baseline uric acid ↑, and oral hydration of 1.5–2 L and IV 150–200 mL/hr as tolerated. Monitor blood chemistries in hospital at 1st dose of 20 mg and 50 mg, pre-dose, 4, 8, 12, and 24 hrs; outpatient at subsequent ramp-up doses, pre-dose, 6–8 hrs, and 24 hrs. Administer IV hydration for patients who cannot tolerate oral hydration. Start allopurinol or xanthine oxidase inhibitor 2–3 days prior to starting venetoclax.

- Monitor for signs and symptoms of infection (fever, chills, dyspnea). Treat infections promptly.
- Monitor for non-hematologic toxicities (pneumonia, fever, diarrhea, nausea, upper respiratory infection, fatigue) during therapy. *For 1st occurrence of Grade 3 or 4 non-hematologic toxicities,* interrupt venetoclax. Once toxicity resolved to Grade 1 or baseline, may resume at same dose. *For 2nd and subsequent occurrences,* interrupt venetoclax. After resolution, resume at decreased dose: if 400 mg resume at 300 mg, if 300 mg resume at 200 mg, if 200 mg resume at 100 mg, if 100 mg resume at 50 mg, if 50 mg resume at 20 mg, if 20 mg resume at 10 mg.
- ***Lab Test Considerations:*** Obtain a negative pregnancy test before starting therapy.
- Assess blood chemistry (serum potassium, uric acid, phosphorous, calcium, creatinine) and correct pre-existing abnormalities prior to starting therapy. *For blood chemistry changes or symptoms of tumor lysis syndrome,* withhold next day's dose. If resolved within 24–48 hrs of last dose, resume at same dose. If >48 hrs to resolve, resume at reduced dose. *If clinical tumor lysis syndrome (renal failure, cardiac arrhythmias, sudden death, seizures) occurs,* resume at reduced dose after resolution.
- Monitor CBC periodically during therapy. May cause neutropenia, anemia, thrombocytopenia, and febrile neutropenia. If 1st occurrence of Grade 3 or 4 neutropenia with infection or fever; or Grade 4 hematologic toxicities (except lymphoma), interrupt venetoclax. May administer granulocyte-colony stimulating factor (G-CSF) to reduce risks of infection. Once toxicity resolved to Grade 1 or baseline, may resume venetoclax at same dose. For 2nd and subsequent occurrences, interrupt venetoclax. Consider using G-CSF as clinically indicated. Resume therapy at reduced dose. If patient required dose reductions to <100 mg for >2 wk, consider discontinuing venetoclax.

Implementation

- Obtain negative pregnancy test prior to starting therapy with venetoclax.
- **PO:** Administer with a meal and water at same time each day. Swallow tablets whole; do not break, crush, or chew.

Patient/Family Teaching

- Instruct patient to take venetoclax as directed; do not change dose or stop taking venetoclax without consulting health care professional. Keep in original packaging for first 4 wk of therapy; do not transfer to another container. Take missed doses as soon as possible within 8 hrs of usual dose time. If missed by >8 hrs, omit and resume next day. If patient vomits do not replace dose.
- Advise patient to avoid grapefruit products, Seville oranges, or starfruit during therapy.
- Advise patient to avoid live vaccines prior to, during, or after treatment until B-cell recovery occurs.
- Advise patient to notify health care professional immediately if signs and symptoms of neutropenia (fever, signs of infection) or tumor lysis syndrome (fever, chills, nausea, vomiting, confusion, shortness of breath, seizure, irregular heartbeat, dark or cloudy urine, unusual tiredness, muscle pain, joint discomfort) occur. Advise patient to hydrate with 6–8 glasses of water/day starting 2 days before and on day of 1st dose and every dose increase to reduce risk of tumor lysis syndrome.
- Instruct patient to notify health care professional of all Rx or OTC medications, vitamins, or herbal products being taken and consult health care professional before taking any new medications.
- Emphasize importance of regular blood work and laboratory tests.
- Rep: Advise patient venetoclax is teratogenic. Use effective contraception during and for at least 30 days after last dose and avoid breast feeding during therapy. May cause male infertility; consider sperm banking for males of reproductive potential.

Evaluation/Desired Outcomes

- Reduced disease progression.

venlafaxine (ven-la-**fax**-een)

~~Effexor~~, Effexor XR

Classification

Therapeutic: antidepressants, antianxiety agents

Pharmacologic: selective serotonin/norepinephrine reuptake inhibitors

Indications

Major depressive disorder. Generalized anxiety disorder (Effexor XR only). Social anxiety disorder (Effexor XR only). Panic disorder (Effexor XR only). **Unlabeled Use:** Premenstrual dysphoric disorder.

Action

Inhibits serotonin and norepinephrine reuptake in the CNS. **Therapeutic Effects:** Decrease in depressive symptomatology, with fewer relapses/recurrences. Decreased anxiety. Decrease in panic attacks.

Pharmacokinetics

Absorption: 92–100% absorbed after oral administration.

Distribution: Extensive distribution into body tissues.

Metabolism and Excretion: Extensively metabolized on first pass through the liver (primarily through CYP2D6 enzyme pathway). A small percentage of the population are poor metabolizers and will have higher blood levels with ↑ effects. One metabolite, O-desmethylvenlafaxine (ODV), has antidepressant activity; 5% of venlafaxine is excreted unchanged in urine; 30% of the active metabolite is excreted in urine.

Half-life: *Venlafaxine*—3–5 hr; *ODV*—9–11 hr (both are ↑ in hepatic/renal impairment).

TIME/ACTION PROFILE (antidepressant action)

ROUTE	ONSET	PEAK	DURATION
PO	within 2 wk	2–4 wk	unknown

Contraindications/Precautions

Contraindicated in: Hypersensitivity; Concurrent use of MAO inhibitors or MAO-like drugs (linezolid or methylene blue); Lactation: Lactation.

Use Cautiously in: Cardiovascular disease, including hypertension; Hepatic or renal impairment (↓ dose recommended); History of seizures or neurologic impairment; History of mania; History of drug abuse; Angle-closure glaucoma; OB: Use only if potential maternal benefit justifies potential fetal risk (potential for discontinuation syndrome or toxicity in the neonate when venlafaxine is taken during the 3rd trimester); Pedi: ↑ risk of suicidal thinking and behavior (suicidality) in children and adolescents with major depressive disorder and other psychiatric disorders. Observe closely for suicidality and behavior changes.

Adverse Reactions/Side Effects

CNS: NEUROLEPTIC MALIGNANT SYNDROME, SEIZURES, SUICIDAL THOUGHTS, abnormal dreams, anxiety, dizziness, headache, insomnia, nervousness, weakness, abnormal thinking, agitation, confusion, depersonalization, drowsiness, emotional lability, worsening depression. **CV:** chest pain, hypertension, palpitations, tachycardia. **Derm:** ecchymoses, itching, photosensitivity, skin rash. **EENT:** rhinitis, visual disturbances, epistaxis, tinnitus. **GI:** abdominal pain, altered taste, anorexia, constipation, diarrhea, dry mouth, dyspepsia, nausea, vomiting, weight loss. **GU:** sexual dysfunction, urinary frequency, urinary retention. **Hemat:** bleeding. **Neuro:** paresthesia, twitching. **Misc:** SEROTONIN SYNDROME, chills, yawning.

Interactions

Drug-Drug: Concurrent use with **MAO inhibitors** may result in serious, potentially fatal reactions (wait at least 2 wk after stopping MAO inhibitor before initiating venlafaxine; wait at least 1 wk after stopping venlafaxine before starting MAO inhibitors). Concurrent use with **MAO-inhibitor like drugs**, such as **linezolid** or **methylene blue** may ↑ risk of serotonin syndrome; concurrent use contraindicated; do not start therapy in patients receiving **linezolid** or **methylene blue**; if **linezolid** or **methylene blue** need to be started in a patient receiving venlafaxine, immediately discontinue venlafaxine and monitor for signs/symptoms of serotonin syndrome for 2 wk or until 24 hr after last dose of linezolid or methylene blue, whichever comes first (may resume venlafaxine therapy 24 hr after last dose of linezolid or methylene blue). Concurrent use with **alcohol** or other **CNS depressants**, including **sedatives/hypnotics**, **antihistamines**, and **opioid analgesics** in depressed patients is not recommended. Drugs that affect serotonergic neurotransmitter systems, including **tricyclic antidepressants**, **SNRIs**, **fentanyl**, **buspirone**, **tramadol**, **amphetamines**, and **triptans** ↑ risk of serotonin syndrome. **Lithium** may have ↑ serotonergic effects with venlafaxine; use cautiously in patients receiving venlafaxine. ↑ blood levels and may ↑ effects of **desipramine** and **haloperidol**. **Cimetidine** may ↑ the effects of venlafaxine (may be more pronounced in geriatric patients, those with hepatic or renal impairment, or those with pre-existing hypertension). **Ketoconazole** may ↑ the effects of venlafaxine. ↑ risk of bleeding with **NSAIDS**, **aspirin**, **clopidogrel**, or **warfarin**.

Drug-Natural Products: Concomitant use of **kava-kava**, **valerian**, **chamomile**, or **hops** can ↑ CNS depression. ↑ risk of serotinergic side effects including serotonin syndrome with **St. John's wort** and **SAMe**.

Route/Dosage

Major Depressive Disorder

PO (Adults): *Tablets*—75 mg/day in 2–3 divided doses; may ↑ by up to 75 mg/day every 4 days, up to 225 mg/day (not to exceed 375 mg/day in 3 divided doses); *Extended-release (XR) capsules*—75 mg once daily (some patients may be started at 37.5 mg once daily) for 4–7 days; may ↑ by up to 75 mg/day at intervals of not less than 4 days (not to exceed 225 mg/day).

V

General Anxiety Disorder

PO (Adults): *Extended-release (XR) capsules*—75 mg once daily (some patients may be started at 37.5 mg once daily) for 4–7 days; may ↑ by up to 75 mg/day at intervals of not less than 4 days (not to exceed 225 mg/day).

Social Anxiety Disorder

PO (Adults): *Extended-release (XR) capsules*—75 mg once daily.

Panic Disorder

PO (Adults): *Extended-release (XR) capsules*—37.5 mg once daily for 7 days; may then ↑ to 75 mg once daily; may then ↑ by 75 mg/day every 7 days (not to exceed 225 mg/day).

Hepatic Impairment

PO (Adults): ↓ daily dose by 50% in patients with mild-to-moderate hepatic impairment.

Renal Impairment

PO (Adults): *CCr 10–70 mL/min*—↓ daily dose by 25–50%; *Hemodialysis*—↓ daily dose by 50%.

Availability (generic available)

Immediate-release tablets: 25 mg, 37.5 mg, 50 mg, 75 mg, 100 mg. **Cost:** *Generic*—25 mg $32.24/100, 37.5 mg $39.41/100, 75 mg $38.00/100. **Extended-release capsules:** 37.5 mg, 75 mg, 150 mg. **Cost:** *Generic*—37.5 mg $32.14/90, 75 mg $271.37/100, 150 mg $29.94/100. **Extended-release tablets:** 37.5 mg, 75 mg, 150 mg, 225 mg. **Cost:** *Generic*—37.5 mg $32.14/90, 75 mg $271.37/100, 150 mg $29.94/100.

NURSING IMPLICATIONS

Assessment

- Assess mental status and mood changes. Inform health care professional if patient demonstrates significant increase in anxiety, nervousness, or insomnia.
- Assess suicidal tendencies, especially in early therapy. Restrict amount of drug available to patient. Risk may be increased in children, adolescents, and adults ≤24 yr.
- Monitor BP before and periodically during therapy. Sustained hypertension may be dose-related; decrease dose or discontinue therapy if this occurs.
- Monitor appetite and nutritional intake. Weigh weekly. Report continued weight loss. Adjust diet as tolerated to support nutritional status.
- Assess for serotonin syndrome (mental changes [agitation, hallucinations, coma], autonomic instability [tachycardia, labile BP, hyperthermia], neuromuscular aberrations [hyper-reflexia, incoordination], and/or GI symptoms [nausea, vomiting, diarrhea]), especially in patients taking other serotonergic drugs (SSRIs, SNRIs, triptans).
- ***Lab Test Considerations:*** Monitor CBC with differential and platelet count periodically during therapy. May cause anemia, leukocytosis, leukopenia, thrombocytopenia, basophilia, and eosinophilia.
- May cause an ↑ in serum alkaline phosphatase, bilirubin, AST, ALT, BUN, and creatinine.
- May also cause ↑ serum cholesterol.
- May cause electrolyte abnormalities (hyperglycemia or hypoglycemia, hyperkalemia or hypokalemia, hyperuricemia, hyperphosphatemia or hypophosphatemia, and hyponatremia).
- May cause false-positive immunoassay screening tests for phencyclidine (PCP) and amphetamine.

Implementation

- Do not confuse Effexor XR (venlafaxine) with Enablex (darifenacin).
- **PO:** Administer venlafaxine with food.
- Swallow extended-release capsules and tablets whole; do not crush, break, or chew.
- Extended-release capsules may be opened and contents sprinkled on a spoonful of applesauce. Take immediately and follow with a glass of water. Do not store mixture for later use.

Patient/Family Teaching

- Instruct patient to take venlafaxine as directed at the same time each day. Take missed doses as soon as possible unless almost time for next dose. Do not double doses or discontinue abruptly. Patients taking venlafaxine for >6 wk should have dose gradually decreased before discontinuation.
- Advise patient, family, and caregivers to look for suicidality, especially during early therapy or dose changes. Notify health care professional immediately if thoughts about suicide or dying, attempts to commit suicide; new or worse depression or anxiety; agitation or restlessness; panic attacks; insomnia; new or worse irritability; aggressiveness; acting on dangerous impulses, mania, or other changes in mood or behavior or if symptoms of serotonin syndrome occur.
- May cause drowsiness or dizziness. Caution patient to avoid driving or other activities requiring alertness until response to the drug is known.
- Instruct patient to notify health care professional of all Rx or OTC medications, vitamins, or herbal products being taken and consult health care professional before taking any new medications. Caution patient to avoid taking alcohol or other CNS-depressant drugs during therapy.
- Instruct patient to notify health care professional if signs of allergy (rash, hives) occur.
- Instruct females of reproductive potential to inform health care professional if pregnancy is planned or suspected, and to avoid breast feeding during therapy.
- Emphasize the importance of follow-up exams to monitor progress. Encourage patient participation in psychotherapy.

Evaluation/Desired Outcomes

- Increased sense of well-being.
- Renewed interest in surroundings. Need for therapy should be periodically reassessed. Therapy is usually continued for several mo.
- Decreased anxiety.

verapamil (ver-ap-a-mil)

Calan, Calan SR, ✱Isoptin SR, Verelan, Verelan PM

Classification

Therapeutic: antianginals, antiarrhythmics (class IV), antihypertensives, vascular headache suppressants

Pharmacologic: calcium channel blockers

Indications

Management of hypertension, angina pectoris, and/or vasospastic (Prinzmetal's) angina. Management of supraventricular arrhythmias and rapid ventricular rates in atrial flutter or fibrillation. **Unlabeled Use:** Prevention of migraine headache.

Action

Inhibits the transport of calcium into myocardial and vascular smooth muscle cells, resulting in inhibition of excitation-contraction coupling and subsequent contraction. Decreases SA and AV conduction and prolongs AV node refractory period in conduction tissue. **Therapeutic Effects:** Systemic vasodilation resulting in decreased BP. Coronary vasodilation resulting in decreased frequency and severity of attacks of angina. Reduction of ventricular rate during atrial fibrillation or flutter.

Pharmacokinetics

Absorption: 90% absorbed after oral administration, but much is rapidly metabolized, resulting in bioavailability of 20–25%.

Distribution: Small amounts enter breast milk.

Protein Binding: 90%.

Metabolism and Excretion: Mostly metabolized by the liver (primarily by CYP3A4).

Half-life: 4.5–12 hr.

TIME/ACTION PROFILE (cardiovascular effects)

ROUTE	ONSET	PEAK	DURATION
PO	1–2 hr	30–90 min†	3–7 hr
PO-ER	unknown	5–7 hr	24 hr
IV	1–5 min‡	3–5 min	2 hr‡

†Single dose; effects from multiple doses may not be evident for 24–48 hr.

‡Antiarrhythmic effects; hemodynamic effects begin 3–5 min after injection and persist for 10–20 min.

Contraindications/Precautions

Contraindicated in: Hypersensitivity; Sick sinus syndrome; 2nd- or 3rd-degree AV block (unless an artificial pacemaker is in place); Systolic BP <90 mm Hg; HF, severe ventricular dysfunction, or cardiogenic shock, unless associated with supraventricular tachyarrhythmias; Concurrent IV beta blocker therapy.

Use Cautiously in: Severe hepatic impairment (dose ↓ recommended); History of serious ventricular arrhythmias or HF; Geri: Dose ↓/slower IV infusion rates recommended (↑ risk of hypotension); OB, Lactation: Safety not established.

Adverse Reactions/Side Effects

CNS: abnormal dreams, anxiety, confusion, dizziness/lightheadedness, drowsiness, extrapyramidal reactions, headache, jitteriness, nervousness, psychiatric disturbances, weakness. **CV:** ARRHYTHMIAS, HF, bradycardia, chest pain, hypotension, palpitations, peripheral edema, syncope, tachycardia. **Derm:** STEVENS-JOHNSON SYNDROME, dermatitis, erythema multiforme, flushing, photosensitivity, pruritus/urticaria, rash, sweating. **EENT:** blurred vision, disturbed equilibrium, epistaxis, tinnitus. **Endo:** gynecomastia, hyperglycemia. **GI:** ↑ liver enzymes, anorexia, constipation, diarrhea, dry mouth, dysgeusia, dyspepsia, nausea, vomiting. **GU:** dysuria, nocturia, polyuria, sexual dysfunction, urinary frequency. **Hemat:** anemia, leukopenia, thrombocytopenia. **Metab:** weight gain. **MS:** joint stiffness, muscle cramps. **Neuro:** paresthesia, tremor. **Resp:** cough, dyspnea. **Misc:** gingival hyperplasia.

Interactions

Drug-Drug: Additive hypotension may occur when used concurrently with **fentanyl**, other **antihypertensives**, **nitrates**, acute ingestion of **alcohol**, or **quinidine**. Antihypertensive effects may be ↓ by concurrent use of **NSAIDs**. May ↑ **digoxin** levels. Concurrent use with **beta blockers**, **digoxin**, **clonidine**, or **ivabradine** may result in bradycardia or conduction defects; avoid concurrent use with ivabradine. ↑ risk of hypotension and bradycardia with **erythromycin**, **clarithromycin**, or **ritonavir**. May ↓ metabolism of and ↑ risk of toxicity from **cyclosporine**, **quinidine**, **theophylline**, or **carbamazepine**. **Rifampin** and **phenobarbital** may ↓ levels. ↑ the muscle-paralyzing effects of **nondepolarizing neuromuscular-blocking agents**. May alter **lithium** levels. May ↑ risk of bleeding with **aspirin**. Concurrent use with **sirolimus**, **temsirolimus**, or **everolimus** may result in ↑ levels of sirolimus, temsirolimus, everolimus, and verapamil; consider ↓ dose of sirolimus, temsirolimus, everolimus, and verapamil. ↑ risk of myopathy with **simvastatin** and **lovastatin**; do not exceed 10 mg/day of simvastatin and 20 mg/day of lovastatin.

Drug-Natural Products: ↑ **caffeine** levels with caffeine-containing herbs (**cola nut**, **guarana**, **mate**, **tea**, **coffee**).

Drug-Food: **Grapefruit juice** ↑ levels and effect.

Route/Dosage

PO (Adults): 80–120 mg 3 times daily, ↑ as needed. *Patients with hepatic impairment or geriatric patients*—40 mg 3 times daily initially. *Extended-re-*

V

lease preparations—120–240 mg/day as a single dose; may be ↑ as needed (range 240–480 mg/day).
PO (Children up to 15 yr): 4–8 mg/kg/day in divided doses.
IV (Adults): 5–10 mg (75–150 mcg/kg); may repeat with 10 mg (150 mcg/kg) after 15–30 min.
IV (Children 1–15 yr): 2–5 mg (100–300 mcg/kg); may repeat after 30 min (initial dose not to exceed 5 mg; repeat dose not to exceed 10 mg).
IV (Children <1 yr): 0.75–2 mg (100–200 mcg/kg); may repeat after 30 min.

Availability (generic available)

Extended-release capsules (Verelan): 120 mg, 180 mg, 240 mg, 360 mg. **Cost:** *Generic*—120 mg $130.25/100, 180 mg $135.16/100, 240 mg $152.54/100, 360 mg $209.94/100. **Extended-release capsules (Verelan PM):** 100 mg, 200 mg, 300 mg. **Cost:** *Generic*—100 mg $195.84/100, 200 mg $252.23/100, 300 mg $366.98/100. **Extended-release tablets:** 120 mg, 180 mg, 240 mg. **Cost:** *Generic*—120 mg $31.44/100, 180 mg $35.98/100, 240 mg $27.80/100. **Solution for injection:** 2.5 mg/mL. **Tablets:** 40 mg, 80 mg, 120 mg. **Cost:** *Generic*—40 mg $21.85/100, 80 mg $10.83/100. ***In combination with:*** trandolapril (Tarka); see Appendix B.

NURSING IMPLICATIONS

Assessment

- Monitor BP and pulse before therapy, during dosage titration, and periodically throughout therapy. Monitor ECG periodically during prolonged therapy. Verapamil may cause prolonged PR interval.
- Monitor intake and output ratios and daily weight. Assess for signs of HF (peripheral edema, rales/crackles, dyspnea, weight gain, jugular venous distention).
- Patients receiving digoxin concurrently with calcium channel blockers should have routine serum digoxin levels and be monitored for signs and symptoms of digoxin toxicity.
- Assess for rash periodically during therapy. May cause Stevens-Johnson syndrome. Discontinue therapy if severe or if accompanied with fever, general malaise, fatigue, muscle or joint aches, blisters, oral lesions, conjunctivitis, hepatitis and/or eosinophilia.
- **Angina:** Assess location, duration, intensity, and precipitating factors of patient's anginal pain.
- **Arrhythmias:** Monitor ECG continuously during administration. Notify health care professional promptly if bradycardia or prolonged hypotension occurs. Emergency equipment and medication should be available. Monitor BP and pulse before and frequently during administration.
- ***Lab Test Considerations:*** Total serum calcium concentrations are not affected by calcium channel blockers.
- Monitor serum potassium periodically. Hypokalemia ↑ risk of arrhythmias and should be corrected.
- Monitor renal and hepatic functions periodically during long-term therapy. May cause ↑ hepatic enzymes after several days of therapy, which return to normal on discontinuation of therapy.

Implementation

- **PO:** Administer verapamil with meals or milk to minimize gastric irritation.
- Do not open, crush, break, or chew sustained-release capsules or tablets. Empty tablets that appear in stool are not significant.

IV Administration

- **IV:** Patients should remain recumbent for at least 1 hr after IV administration to minimize hypotensive effects.
- **IV Push:** ***Diluent:*** Administer undiluted. ***Concentration:*** 2.5 mg/mL. ***Rate:*** Administer over 2 min. Geri: Administer over 3 min.
- **Y-Site Compatibility:** alemtuzumab, alfentanil, amikacin, aminocaproic acid, amphotericin B lipid complex, anidulafungin, argatroban, ascorbic acid, atracurium, atropine, azithromycin, aztreonam, benztropine, bivalirudin, bleomycin, bumetanide, buprenorphine, butorphanol, calcium chloride, calcium gluconate, cangrelor, carboplatin, carmustine, caspofungin, cefazolin, cefotaxime, cefotetan, cefoxitin, ceftriaxone, cefuroxime, chlorpromazine, ciprofloxacin, cisplatin, clindamycin, cyanocobalamin, cyclophosphamide, cyclosporine, cytarabine, dacarbazine, dactinomycin, daptomycin, dexamethasone, dexmedetomidine, dexrazoxane, digoxin, diltiazem, diphenhydramine, dobutamine, docetaxel, dopamine, doxorubicin hydrochloride, doxorubicin liposomal, doxycycline, enalaprilat, ephedrine, epinephrine, epirubicin, epotein alfa, eptifibatide, erythromycin, esmolol, etoposide, etoposide phosphate, famotidine, fenoldopam, fentanyl, fluconazole, fludarabine, gemcitabine, gentamicin, glycopyrrolate, granisetron, heparin, hydrocortisone, hydromorphone, idarubicin, ifosfamide, imipenem/cilastatin, insulin, regular, irinotecan, isoproterenol, ketorolac, labetalol, leucovorin calcium, levofloxacin, lidocaine, linezolid, lorazepam, magnesium sulfate, mannitol, meperidine, mesna, metaraminol, methotrexate, methyldopate, methylprednisolone sodium succinate, metoclopramide, metoprolol, metronidazole, midazolam, milrinone, mitoxantrone, morphine, moxifloxacin, multivitamins, mycophenolate, nalbuphine, naloxone, nitroglycerin, nitroprusside, norepinephrine, octreotide, ondansetron, oxaliplatin, oxytocin, paclitaxel, palonosetron, pamidronate, pancuronium, papaverine, pemetrexed, penicillin G, pentamidine, phentolamine, phenylephrine, phytonadione, potassium acetate, potassium chloride, procainamide, prochlorperazine, promethazine, propranolol, protamine, pyridoxime, quinupristin/dalfopristin, ranitidine, rocuronium, sodium acetate, streptokinase, succinylcholine, sufentanil, tacrolimus, theophylline, thiamine, tirofiban, tobramycin, tolazoline, topotecan, vancomycin, vasopressin, vecuronium, vinblastine, vincristine, vinorelbine, voriconazole, zoledronic acid.

- **Y-Site Incompatibility:** acyclovir, albumin, aminophylline, amphotericin B liposome, ampicillin, ampicillin/sulbactam, azathioprine, ceftazidime, chloramphenicol, dantrolene, diazepam, diazoxide, ertapenem, fluorouracil, folic acid, foscarnet, fosphenytoin, furosemide, ganciclovir, indomethacin, pantoprazole, pentobarbital, phenobarbital, phenytoin, piperacillin/tazobactam, propofol, sodium bicarbonate, thiotepa, tigecycline, trimethoprim/sulfamethoxazole.

Patient/Family Teaching

- Advise patient to take medication as directed, even if feeling well. Take missed doses as soon as possible unless almost time for next dose; do not double doses. May need to be discontinued gradually.
- Advise patient to avoid large amounts (6–8 glasses of grapefruit juice/day) during therapy.
- Instruct patient on correct technique for monitoring pulse. Instruct patient to contact health care professional if heart rate is <50 bpm.
- Caution patient to change positions slowly to minimize orthostatic hypotension.
- May cause drowsiness or dizziness. Advise patient to avoid driving or other activities requiring alertness until response to the medication is known.
- Instruct patient on importance of maintaining good dental hygiene and seeing dentist frequently for teeth cleaning to prevent tenderness, bleeding, and gingival hyperplasia (gum enlargement).
- Instruct patient to notify health care professional of all Rx or OTC medications, vitamins, or herbal products being taken and consult health care professional before taking any new medications, especially cold preparations.
- Advise patient to notify health care professional if irregular heartbeats, rash, dyspnea, swelling of hands and feet, pronounced dizziness, nausea, constipation, or hypotension occurs or if headache is severe or persistent.
- Caution patient to wear protective clothing and use sunscreen to prevent photosensitivity reactions.
- **Angina:** Instruct patient on concurrent nitrate or beta-blocker therapy to continue taking both medications as directed and use SL nitroglycerin as needed for anginal attacks.
- Advise patient to contact health care professional if chest pain does not improve, worsens after therapy, or occurs with diaphoresis; if shortness of breath occurs; or if severe, persistent headache occurs.
- Caution patient to discuss exercise restrictions with health care professional before exertion.
- Advise patient to notify health care professional if pregnancy is planned or suspected, and to avoid breast feeding during therapy.
- **Hypertension:** Encourage patient to comply with other interventions for hypertension (weight reduction, low-sodium diet, smoking cessation, moderation of alcohol consumption, regular exercise, and stress management). Medication controls but does not cure hypertension.
- Instruct patient and family in proper technique for monitoring BP. Advise patient to take BP weekly and to report significant changes to health care professional.

Evaluation/Desired Outcomes

- Decrease in BP.
- Decrease in frequency and severity of anginal attacks.
- Decrease in need for nitrate therapy.
- Increase in activity tolerance and sense of well-being.
- Suppression and prevention of atrial tachyarrhythmias.

vilazodone (vil-az-oh-done)

Viibryd

Classification

Therapeutic: antidepressants

Pharmacologic: selective serotonin reuptake inhibitors (SSRIs), benzofurans

Indications

Treatment of major depressive disorder.

Action

Increases serotonin activity in the CNS by inhibiting serotonin reuptake. Also binds selectively with high affinity to $5\text{-}HT_{1A}$ receptors and is a $5\text{-}HT_{1A}$ receptor partial agonist. **Therapeutic Effects:** Improvement in symptoms of depression.

Pharmacokinetics

Absorption: 72% absorbed following oral administration with food.

Distribution: Unknown.

Protein Binding: 96–99%.

Metabolism and Excretion: Mostly metabolized by the liver, primarily by the CYP3A4 enzyme system; 1% excreted unchanged in urine.

Half-life: 25 hr.

TIME/ACTION PROFILE (blood levels)

ROUTE	ONSET	PEAK	DURATION
PO	unknown	4–5 hr	unknown

Contraindications/Precautions

Contraindicated in: Concurrent use of MAO inhibitors or MAO-like drugs (linezolid or methylene blue).

Use Cautiously in: History of seizure disorder; History of suicide attempt/suicidal ideation; Bipolar disorder; may ↑ risk of mania/hypomania; Angle-closure glaucoma; OB: Use only if potential maternal benefit justifies potential fetal risk; use during third trimester

V

may result in need for prolonged hospitalization, respiratory support and tube feeding; Lactation: Use while breast feeding only if potential maternal benefit justifies potential risk to infant; Pedi: Safety and effectiveness not established; ↑ risk of suicidal thinking/behavior in children, adolescents and young adults.

Adverse Reactions/Side Effects

CNS: NEUROLEPTIC MALIGNANT-LIKE SYNDROME, SEIZURES, SUICIDAL THOUGHTS, insomnia, abnormal dreams, dizziness, sleep paralysis. **Endo:** ↓ libido, sexual dysfunction, syndrome of inappropriate antidiuretic hormone (SIADH). **F and E:** hyponatremia. **GI:** PANCREATITIS, diarrhea, nausea, dry mouth, restlessness, vomiting. **Hemat:** bleeding. **Misc:** SEROTONIN SYNDROME.

Interactions

Drug-Drug: Concurrent use with, or use within 14 days of starting or stopping **MAOIs** may ↑ risk of neuroleptic malignant syndrome or serotonin syndrome and should be avoided. Concurrent use with **MAO-inhibitor like drugs**, such as **linezolid** or **methylene blue** may ↑ risk of serotonin syndrome; concurrent use contraindicated; do not start therapy in patients receiving **linezolid** or **methylene blue**; if **linezolid** or **methylene blue** need to be started in a patient receiving vilazodone, immediately discontinue vilazodone and monitor for signs/symptoms of serotonin syndrome for 2 wk or until 24 hr after last dose of linezolid or methylene blue, whichever comes first (may resume vilazodone therapy 24 hr after last dose of linezolid or methylene blue). Drugs that affect serotonergic neurotransmitter systems, including **tricyclic antidepressants**, **SNRIs**, **fentanyl**, **buspirone**, **tramadol**, **amphetamines**, and **triptans** ↑ risk of serotonin syndrome. Concurrent use with **NSAIDs**, **aspirin**, **antiplatelet drugs**, or other **drugs that affect coagulation** may ↑ risk of bleeding. Concurrent use of **strong inhibitors of CYP3A4**, including **ketoconazole** ↑ blood levels and the risk of adverse reactions/toxicity; daily dose should not exceed 20 mg. Concurrent use of **moderate inhibitors of CYP3A4**, including **erythromycin** may require dose ↓ to 20 mg daily if adverse reactions/toxicity occurs. Concurrent use of **strong inducers of CYP3A4**, including **carbamazepine** for >14 days may require ↑ dose up to 2–fold (do not exceed dose of 80 mg/day). Use cautiously with other **CNS-active drugs**.

Drug-Natural Products: ↑ risk of serotonin syndrome with **St. John's wort**.

Route/Dosage

PO (Adults): 10 mg once daily for one wk, then 20 mg once daily for one wk; dose may be ↑ to 40 mg once daily (recommended dose = 20–40 mg/day). *Concurrent use of strong inhibitors of CYP3A4*—not to exceed 20 mg/day; *Concurrent use of strong inducers of CYP3A4 (if used for >14 days)*—may need to ↑ dose up to 2–fold (daily dose should not exceed 80 mg).

Availability (generic available)

Tablets: 10 mg, 20 mg, 40 mg.

NURSING IMPLICATIONS

Assessment

- Assess mental status and mood changes. Inform health care professional if patient demonstrates significant ↑ in anxiety, nervousness, or insomnia.
- Prior to starting therapy, screen patient for bipolar disorder (detailed psychiatric history, including family/personal history of suicide, bipolar disorder, depression). Use cautiously in patients with a positive history.
- Assess suicidal tendencies, especially in early therapy. Restrict amount of drug available to patient. Risk may be ↑ in children, adolescents, and adults ≤24 yr.
- Assess for signs and symptoms of hyponatremia (headache, difficulty concentrating, memory impairment, confusion, weakness, unsteadiness). May require discontinuation of therapy.
- Assess for serotonin syndrome (mental changes [agitation, hallucinations, coma], autonomic instability [tachycardia, labile BP, hyperthermia], neuromuscular aberrations [hyper-reflexia, incoordination], and/or GI symptoms [nausea, vomiting, diarrhea]), especially in patients taking other serotonergic drugs (SSRIs, SNRIs, triptans).
- Monitor for development of neuroleptic malignant syndrome (fever, muscle rigidity, altered mental status, respiratory distress, tachycardia, seizures, diaphoresis, hypertension or hypotension, pallor, tiredness, loss of bladder control). Discontinue vilazodone and notify health care professional immediately if these symptoms occur.
- ***Lab Test Considerations:*** Monitor serum sodium concentrations periodically during therapy. May cause hyponatremia potentially as a result of syndrome of inappropriate antidiuretic hormone secretion (SIADH).
- May cause altered anticoagulant effects. Monitor patients receiving warfarin, NSAIDs, or aspirin concurrently.

Implementation

- **PO:** Administer vilazodone with food; administration without food can result in inadequate drug concentrations and may ↓ effectiveness.
- When discontinuing therapy, decrease dose gradually; 40 mg once daily to 20 mg once daily for 4 days, followed by 10 mg once daily for 3 days. Taper patients taking 20 mg once daily dose to 10 mg once daily for 7 days. Stopping abruptly may cause flu-like symptoms (headache, sweating, and nausea), anxiety, high or low mood, irritability, feeling restless or sleepy, dizziness, electric shock-like sensations, tremor, and confusion.

Patient/Family Teaching

- Instruct patient to take vilazodone as directed at the same time each day. Take missed doses as soon as possible unless almost time for next dose. Do not double doses or discontinue abruptly. Gradually ↓

dose before discontinuation. Advise patient to read *Medication Guide* before starting therapy and with each Rx refill; new information may be available.

- Advise patient, family, and caregivers to look for activation of maina/hypomania and suicidality, especially during early therapy or dose changes. Notify health care professional immediately if thoughts about suicide or dying, attempts to commit suicide; new or worse depression or anxiety; agitation or restlessness; panic attacks; insomnia; new or worse irritability; aggressiveness; acting on dangerous impulses, mania, or other changes in mood or behavior or if symptoms of serotonin syndrome occur.
- Caution patient of the risk of serotonin syndrome and neuroleptic malignant syndrome, especially when taking triptans, tramadol, tryptophan supplements and other serotonergic or antipsychotic agents.
- May cause dizziness. Caution patient to avoid driving or other activities requiring alertness until response to the drug is known.
- Instruct patient to notify health care professional of all Rx or OTC medications, vitamins, or herbal products being taken and to avoid concurrent use of Rx, OTC, and herbal products, especially NSAIDs, aspirin, and warfarin, without consulting health care professional.
- Caution patient to avoid taking alcohol or other CNS-depressant drugs during therapy.
- Instruct female patients to inform health care professional if pregnancy is planned or suspected or if breast feeding.
- Emphasize the importance of follow-up exams to monitor progress. Encourage patient participation in psychotherapy.

Evaluation/Desired Outcomes

- ↑ sense of well-being.
- Renewed interest in surroundings. Need for therapy should be periodically reassessed. Therapy is usually continued for several mo.
- ↓ anxiety.

HIGH ALERT

vinBLAStine (vin-**blass**-teen)

Classification
Therapeutic: antineoplastics
Pharmacologic: vinca alkaloids

Indications

Combination chemotherapy of: Lymphomas, Nonseminomatous testicular carcinoma, Advanced breast cancer, Other tumors.

Action

Binds to proteins of mitotic spindle, causing metaphase arrest. Cell replication is stopped as a result (cell cycle–specific for M phase). **Therapeutic Effects:** Death of rapidly replicating cells, particularly malignant ones. Has immunosuppressive properties.

Pharmacokinetics

Absorption: Administered IV only, resulting in complete bioavailability.
Distribution: Does not cross the blood-brain barrier well.
Metabolism and Excretion: Converted by the liver to an active antineoplastic compound; excreted in the feces via biliary excretion, some renal elimination.
Half-life: 24 hr.

TIME/ACTION PROFILE (effects on white blood cell counts)

ROUTE	ONSET	PEAK	DURATION
IV	5–7 days	10 days	7–14 days

Contraindications/Precautions

Contraindicated in: Hypersensitivity; OB, Lactation: Pregnancy or lactation.
Use Cautiously in: Infection; ↓ bone marrow reserve; Patients with impaired hepatic function (↓ dose by 50% if serum bilirubin >3 m g/dL); Rep: Women with childbearing potential.

Adverse Reactions/Side Effects

CNS: SEIZURES, mental depression, neurotoxicity, weakness. **Resp:** BRONCHOSPASM. **GI:** nausea, vomiting, anorexia, constipation, diarrhea, stomatitis. **GU:** gonadal suppression. **Derm:** alopecia, dermatitis, vesiculation. **Endo:** syndrome of inappropriate antidiuretic hormone (SIADH). **Hemat:** anemia, leukopenia, thrombocytopenia. **Local:** phlebitis at IV site. **Metab:** hyperuricemia. **Neuro:** neuritis, paresthesia, peripheral neuropathy.

Interactions

Drug-Drug: Additive bone marrow depression with other **antineoplastics** or **radiation therapy**. Bronchospasm may occur in patients who have been previously treated with **mitomycin**. May ↓ antibody response to **live-virus vaccines** and ↑ risk of adverse reactions. May ↓ **phenytoin** levels.

Route/Dosage

Doses may vary greatly, depending on tumor, schedule, condition of patient, and blood counts.
IV (Adults): *Initial*— 3.7 mg/m² (100 mcg/kg), single dose; ↑ weekly as tolerated by 1.8 mg/m² (50 mcg/kg) to maximum of 18.5 mg/m² (usual dose is 5.5–7.4 mg/m²). *Maintenance*— 10 mg 1–2 times/mo or one increment less than last dose every 7–14 days.
IV (Children): *Initial*— 2.5 mg/m², single dose; ↑ weekly as tolerated by 1.25 mg/m² to maximum of 7.5 mg/m². *Maintenance*— one increment less than last dose every 7 days.

V

Availability (generic available)

Solution for injection: 1 mg/mL. **Powder for injection (requires reconstitution):** 10 mg/vial.

NURSING IMPLICATIONS

Assessment

- Monitor BP, pulse, and respiratory rate during therapy. Bronchospasm can be life-threatening and may occur at time of infusion or several hrs to wk later.
- Monitor for bone marrow depression. Assess for bleeding (bleeding gums, bruising, petechiae, guaiac stools, urine, and emesis) and avoid IM injections and taking rectal temperatures if platelet count is low. Apply pressure to venipuncture sites for 10 min. Assess for signs of infection during neutropenia. Anemia may occur. Monitor for increased fatigue, dyspnea, and orthostatic hypotension.
- May cause nausea and vomiting. Monitor intake and output, appetite, and nutritional intake. Prophylactic antiemetics may be used. Adjust diet as tolerated.
- Assess injection site frequently for redness, irritation, or inflammation. If extravasation occurs, infusion must be stopped and restarted elsewhere to avoid damage to subcut tissue. Standard treatment includes infiltration with hyaluronidase and application of heat.
- Monitor for symptoms of gout (increased uric acid, joint pain, edema). Encourage patient to drink at least 2 L of fluid per day. Allopurinol or alkalinization of urine may be used to decrease uric acid levels.
- ***Lab Test Considerations:*** Monitor CBC prior to and routinely throughout therapy. If WBC <2000, subsequent doses are usually withheld until WBC is ≥4000. The nadir of leukopenia occurs in 5–10 days and recovery usually occurs 7–14 days later. Thrombocytopenia may also occur in patients who have received radiation or other chemotherapy agents.
- Monitor liver function studies (AST, ALT, LDH, bilirubin) and renal function studies (BUN, creatinine) prior to and periodically throughout therapy.
- May cause ↑ uric acid. Monitor periodically during therapy.

Implementation

- ***High Alert:*** Fatalities have occurred with chemotherapeutic agents. Before administering, clarify all ambiguous orders; double check single, daily, and course-of-therapy dose limits; have second practitioner independently double check original order, dose calculations, and infusion pump settings. Do not administer subcut, IM, or intrathecally (IT). IT administration is fatal. Vinblastine must be dispensed in an overwrap stating, "For IV use only." Overwrap should remain in place until immediately before administration.
- ***High Alert:*** Do not confuse vinblastine with vincristine.
- Solution should be prepared in a biologic cabinet. Wear gloves, gown, and mask while handling medication. Discard IV equipment in specially designated containers.
- Do not inject into extremities with impaired circulation; may cause thrombophlebitis.

IV Administration

- **IV Push:** ***Diluent:*** Dilute each 10 mg with 10 mL of 0.9% NaCl for injection with phenol or benzyl alcohol. Solution is clear. Reconstituted medication is stable for 28 days if refrigerated. ***Concentration:*** 1 mg/mL. ***Rate:*** Administer each single dose over 1 min through Y-site injection of a free-flowing infusion of 0.9% NaCl or D5W.
- **Intermittent Infusion:** Dilution in large volumes (100–250 mL) or prolonged infusion (≥30 min) increases chance of vein irritation and extravasation.
- **Y-Site Compatibility:** acyclovir, alemtuzumab, alfentanil, allopurinol, amifostine, amikacin, aminophylline, amiodarone, amphotericin B lipid complex, ampicillin, ampicillin/sulbactam, anidulafungin, argatroban, aztreonam, bivalirudin, bleomycin, bumetanide, buprenorphine, busulfan, butorphanol, calcium chloride, calcium gluconate, carboplatin, carmustine, caspofungin, cefazolin, cefotaxime, cefotetan, cefoxitin, ceftazidime, ceftriaxone, cefuroxime, chloramphenicol, chlorpromazine, ciprofloxacin, cisatracurium, cisplatin, clindamycin, cyclophosphamide, cyclosporine, dacarbazine, dactinomycin, daptomycin, daunorubicin hydrochloride, dexamethasone, dexmedetomidine, dexrazoxane, digoxin, diltiazem, diphenhydramine, dobutamine, docetaxel, dolasetron, dopamine, doxorubicin hydrochloride, doxorubicin liposomal, doxycycline, droperidol, enalaprilat, ephedrine, epinephrine, epirubicin, ertapenem, erythromycin, esmolol, etoposide, etoposide phosphate, famotidine, fenoldopam, fentanyl, filgrastim, fluconazole, fludarabine, fluorouracil, foscarnet, fosphenytoin, ganciclovir, gemcitabine, gentamicin, glycopyrrolate, granisetron, haloperidol, heparin, hetastarch, hydralazine, hydrocortisone, hydromorphone, idarubicin, ifosfamide, imipenem/cilastatin, insulin, irinotecan, isoproterenol, ketorolac, labetalol, leucovorin calcium, levofloxacin, lidocaine, linezolid, lorazepam, magnesium sulfate, mannitol, melphalan, meperidine, meropenem, mesna, methotrexate, methyldopate, metoclopramide, metoprolol, metronidazole, midazolam, milrinone, mitomycin, mitoxantrone, morphine, moxifloxacin, nafcillin, nalbuphine, naloxone, nitroglycerin, nitroprusside, norepinephrine, octreotide, ondansetron, oxaliplatin, paclitaxel, palonosetron, pamidronate, pancuronium, pemetrexed, pentamidine, pentobarbital, phenobarbital, phenylephrine, piperacillin/tazobactam, potassium chloride, potassium phosphates, procainamide, prochlorperazine, promethazine, propranolol, quinupristin/dalfopristin, ranitidine, remifentanil, rituximab, sargramostim, sodium acetate, sodium bicarbonate, sodium phosphates, succinylcholine, sufentanil, tacrolimus, theophylline, thiopental, thiotepa, tigecycline, tirofiban, tobramycin, topotecan, trastuzumab, trimethoprim/sulfamethoxazole, vancomycin, vasopres-

sin, vecuronium, verapamil, vincristine, vinorelbine, voriconazole, zidovudine, zoledronic acid.

- **Y-Site Incompatibility:** amphotericin B deoxycholate, amphotericin B liposome, cefepime, dantrolene, diazepam, furosemide, pantoprazole, phenytoin.

Patient/Family Teaching

- Advise patient to notify health care professional if fever; chills; sore throat; signs of infection; bleeding gums; bruising; petechiae; or blood in urine, stool, or emesis occurs. Caution patient to avoid crowds and persons with known infections. Instruct patient to use soft toothbrush and electric razor. Caution patient not to drink alcoholic beverages or take products containing aspirin or NSAIDs.
- Instruct patient to inspect oral mucosa for redness and ulceration. Advise patient that, if ulceration occurs, to avoid spicy foods, use sponge brush, and rinse mouth with water after eating and drinking. Topical agents may be used if mouth pain interferes with eating. Stomatitis pain may require treatment with opioid analgesics.
- Instruct patient to report symptoms of neurotoxicity (paresthesia, pain, difficulty walking, persistent constipation).
- Advise patient that jaw pain, pain in organs containing tumor tissue, nausea, and vomiting may occur. Avoid constipation and report other adverse reactions.
- Discuss with patient the possibility of hair loss. Explore coping strategies.
- Instruct patient not to receive any vaccinations without advice of health care professional.
- Rep: Advise patient that this medication may have teratogenic effects. Contraception should be used during and for at least 2 mo after therapy is concluded.
- Emphasize need for periodic lab tests to monitor for side effects.

Evaluation/Desired Outcomes

- Regression of malignancy without the appearance of detrimental side effects.

HIGH ALERT

vinCRIStine (vin-**kriss**-teen)

~~Vincasar PFS~~

Classification

Therapeutic: antineoplastics

Pharmacologic: vinca alkaloids

Indications

Used alone and in combination with other treatment modalities (antineoplastics, surgery, or radiation therapy) in treatment of: Hodgkin's disease, Leukemias, Neuroblastoma, Malignant lymphomas, Rhabdomyosarcoma, Wilms' tumor, Other tumors.

Action

Binds to proteins of mitotic spindle, causing metaphase arrest. Cell replication is stopped as a result (cell cycle–specific for M phase). Has little or no effect on bone marrow. **Therapeutic Effects:** Death of rapidly replicating cells, particularly malignant ones. Has immunosuppressive properties.

Pharmacokinetics

Absorption: Administered IV only, resulting in complete bioavailability.

Distribution: Rapidly and widely distributed; extensively bound to tissues.

Metabolism and Excretion: Metabolized by the liver and eliminated in the feces via biliary excretion.

Half-life: 10.5–37.5 hr.

TIME/ACTION PROFILE (effects on blood counts†)

ROUTE	ONSET	PEAK	DURATION
IV	unknown	4 days	7 days

†Usually mild.

Contraindications/Precautions

Contraindicated in: Hypersensitivity; OB, Lactation: Pregnancy or lactation.

Use Cautiously in: Infection; ↓ bone marrow reserve; Hepatic impairment (50% dose ↓ recommended if serum bilirubin >3 m g/dL); Rep: Women with childbearing potential.

Adverse Reactions/Side Effects

CNS: agitation, insomnia, mental depression, mental status changes. **EENT:** cortical blindness, diplopia. **Resp:** bronchospasm. **GI:** <u>nausea</u>, <u>vomiting</u>, abdominal cramps, anorexia, constipation, ileus, stomatitis. **GU:** gonadal suppression, nocturia, oliguria, urinary retention. **Derm:** <u>alopecia</u>. **Endo:** syndrome of inappropriate antidiuretic hormone (SIADH). **Hemat:** anemia, leukopenia, thrombocytopenia (mild and brief). **Local:** <u>phlebitis at IV site, tissue necrosis (from extravasation)</u>. **Metab:** hyperuricemia. **Neuro:** <u>ascending peripheral neuropathy</u>.

Interactions

Drug-Drug: Bronchospasm may occur in patients who have been previously treated with **mitomycin**. **L-asparaginase** may ↓ hepatic metabolism of vincristine (give vincristine 12–24 hr prior to asparaginase). May ↓ antibody response to **live-virus vaccines** and ↑ risk of adverse reactions.

Route/Dosage

Many other protocols are used.

IV (Adults): 10–30 mcg/kg (0.4–1.4 mg/m²); may repeat weekly (not to exceed 2 mg/dose).

IV (Children >10 kg): 1.5–2 mg/m² single dose; may repeat weekly.
IV (Children <10 kg): 50 mcg/kg single dose; may repeat weekly.

Availability (generic available)

Solution for injection: 1 mg/mL.

NURSING IMPLICATIONS

Assessment

- Monitor BP, pulse, and respiratory rate during therapy. Report significant changes.
- Monitor neurologic status. Assess for paresthesia (numbness, tingling, pain), loss of deep tendon reflexes (Achilles reflex is usually first involved), weakness (wrist drop or footdrop, gait disturbances), cranial nerve palsies (jaw pain, hoarseness, ptosis, visual changes), autonomic dysfunction (ileus, difficulty voiding, orthostatic hypotension, impaired sweating), and CNS dysfunction (decreased level of consciousness, agitation, hallucinations). Notify physician if these symptoms develop, as they may persist for mo.
- Monitor intake and output ratios and daily weight; report significant discrepancies. Decreased urine output with concurrent hyponatremia may indicate SIADH, which usually responds to fluid restriction.
- Assess infusion site frequently for redness, irritation, or inflammation. If extravasation occurs, infusion must be stopped and restarted elsewhere to avoid damage to subcut tissue. Cellulitis and discomfort may be minimized by infiltration with hyaluronidase and application of moderate heat or by application of cold compresses.
- Assess nutritional status. An antiemetic may be used to minimize nausea and vomiting.
- Monitor for symptoms of gout (increased uric acid, joint pain, edema). Encourage patient to drink at least 2 liters of fluid per day. Allopurinol or alkalinization of urine may be used to decrease uric acid levels.
- ***Lab Test Considerations:*** Monitor CBC prior to and periodically throughout therapy. May cause slight leukopenia 4 days after therapy, which resolves within 7 days. Platelet count may ↑ or ↓.
- Monitor liver function studies (AST, ALT, LDH, bilirubin) and renal function studies (BUN, creatinine) prior to and periodically throughout therapy.
- May cause ↑ uric acid. Monitor periodically during therapy.

Implementation

- ***High Alert:*** Fatalities have occurred with chemotherapeutic agents. Before administering, clarify all ambiguous orders; double check single, daily, and course-of-therapy dose limits; have second practitioner independently double check original order, dose calculations, and infusion pump settings. Do not administer subcut, IM, or intrathecally (IT). IT administration is fatal. Vincristine must be dispensed in an overwrap stating "For IV use only." Overwrap should remain in place until immediately before administration.
- ***High Alert:*** Do not confuse vincristine with vinblastine.
- Solution should be prepared in a biologic cabinet. Wear gloves, gown, and mask while handling medication. Discard IV equipment in specially designated containers.

IV Administration

- **IV Push:** ***Diluent:*** Does not need to be reconstituted. ***Concentration:*** Administer undiluted at 1 mg/mL. ***Rate:*** Administer each dose IV push over 1 min through Y-site injection of a free-flowing infusion of 0.9% NaCl or D5W.
- **Y-Site Compatibility:** acyclovir, alemtuzumab, alfentanil, allopurinol, amifostine, amikacin, aminophylline, amiodarone, amphotericin B lipid complex, amphotericin B liposome, ampicillin, ampicillin/sulbactam, anidulafungin, argatroban, azithromycin, aztreonam, bivalirudin, bleomycin, bumetanide, buprenorphine, butorphanol, calcium chloride, calcium gluconate, carboplatin, carmustine, caspofungin, cefazolin, cefotetan, cefoxitin, ceftazidime, ceftriaxone, cefuroxime, chlorpromazine, ciprofloxacin, cisatracurium, cladribine, cisplatin, cladribine, clindamycin, cyclophosphamide, cyclosporine, cytarabine, dactinomycin, daptomycin, daunorubicin hydrochloride, dexamethasone, dexmedetomidine, dexrazoxane, digoxin, diltiazem, diphenhydramine, dobutamine, docetaxel, dolasetron, dopamine, doxorubicin hydrochloride, doxorubicin liposomal, doxycycline, droperidol, enalaprilat, ephedrine, epinephrine, epirubicin, ertapenem, erythromycin, esmolol, etoposide, etoposide phosphate, famotidine, fenoldopam, fentanyl, filgrastim, fluconazole, fludarabine, fluorouracil, foscarnet, fosphenytoin, fosphenytoin, ganciclovir, gemcitabine, gentamicin, granisetron, haloperidol, heparin, hetastarch, hydrocortisone, hydromorphone, ifosfamide, imipenem/cilastatin, insulin, isoproterenol, ketorolac, labetalol, leucovorin calcium, levofloxacin, levorphanol, lidocaine, linezolid, lorazepam, magnesium sulfate, mannitol, melphalan, meperidine, meropenem, mesna, methotrexate, methoprednisolone, metoclopramide, metoprolol, metronidazole, midazolam, milrinone, mitomycin, mitoxantrone, morphine, moxifloxacin, nalbuphine, naloxone, nicardipine, nitroglycerin, nitroprusside, norepinephrine, octreotide, ondansetron, oxaliplatin, paclitaxel, palonosetron, pancuronium, pemetrexed, pentamidine, pentobarbital, phenobarbital, phenylephrine, piperacillin/tazobactam, potassium acetate, potassium chloride, potassium phosphates, procainamide, prochlorperazine, promethazine, propranolol, quinupristin/dalfopristin, ranitidine, remifentanil, rituximab, rocuronium, sargramostim,

sodium acetate, sodium phosphates, succinylcholine, sufentanil, tacrolimus, theophylline, thiopental, thiotepa, tigecycline, tirofiban, tobramycin, topotecan, trastuzumab, trimethoprim/sulfamethoxazole, vancomycin, vasopressin, vecuronium, verapamil, vinblastine, vinorelbine, voriconazole, zidovudine, zoledronic acid.

- **Y-Site Incompatibility:** amphotericin B deoxycholate, cefepime, diazepam, idarubicin, nafcillin, pantoprazole, phenytoin.

Patient/Family Teaching

- Instruct patient to notify health care professional immediately if redness, swelling, or pain at injection site occurs.
- Instruct patient to report symptoms of neurotoxicity (paresthesia, pain, difficulty walking, persistent constipation). Inform patient that increased fluid intake, dietary fiber, and exercise may minimize constipation. Stool softeners or laxatives may be used. Patient should inform health care professional if severe constipation or abdominal discomfort occurs, as this may be a sign of neuropathy.
- Advise patient to notify health care professional if fever; chills; sore throat; signs of infection; bleeding gums; bruising; petechiae; blood in urine, stool, or emesis; or mouth sores occur. Caution patient to avoid crowds and persons with known infections.
- Discuss with patient the possibility of hair loss. Explore coping strategies.
- Instruct patient not to receive any vaccinations without advice of health care professional.
- Rep: Advise patient that this medication may have teratogenic effects. Contraception should be used during and for at least 2 mo after therapy is concluded.
- Emphasize need for periodic lab tests to monitor for side effects.

Evaluation/Desired Outcomes

- Regression of malignancy without the appearance of detrimental side effects.

HIGH ALERT

vinorelbine (vine-oh-**rel**-been)

~~Navelbine~~

Classification

Therapeutic: antineoplastics

Pharmacologic: vinca alkaloids

Indications

Inoperable non–small-cell cancer of the lung in ambulatory patients (alone or with cisplatin).

Action

Binds to a protein (tubulin) of cellular microtubules, where it interferes with microtubule assembly. Cell replication is stopped as a result (cell cycle–specific for M phase). **Therapeutic Effects:** Death of rapidly replicating cells, particularly malignant ones.

Pharmacokinetics

Absorption: IV administration results in complete bioavailability.

Distribution: Highly bound to platelets and lymphocytes.

Metabolism and Excretion: Mostly metabolized by the liver. At least one metabolite is active. Large amounts eliminated in feces; 11% excreted unchanged by the kidneys.

Half-life: 28–44 hr.

TIME/ACTION PROFILE (effect on WBCs)

ROUTE	ONSET	PEAK	DURATION
IV	unknown	7–10 days	7–15 days

Contraindications/Precautions

Contraindicated in: Hypersensitivity; Active infection; ↓ bone marrow reserve; OB: Pregnancy (may cause fetal harm); Lactation: Lactation.

Use Cautiously in: Hepatic impairment (dose ↓ recommended if total bilirubin >2 m g/dL); Debilitated patients (↑ risk of hyponatremia); Granulocytopenic patients (temporarily discontinue or reduce dose); Pedi: Safety not established; Rep: Women of reproductive potential.

Adverse Reactions/Side Effects

CNS: <u>fatigue</u>. **CV:** chest pain. **Derm:** <u>alopecia</u>, rash. **F and E:** hyponatremia. **GI:** <u>constipation</u>, <u>nausea</u>, abdominal pain, anorexia, diarrhea, transient ↑ in liver enzymes, vomiting. **Hemat:** <u>anemia</u>, <u>neutropenia</u>, thrombocytopenia. **Local:** <u>irritation</u> at IV site, skin reactions, phlebitis. **MS:** arthralgia, back pain, jaw pain, myalgia. **Neuro:** <u>neurotoxicity</u>. **Resp:** shortness of breath. **Misc:** pain in tumor-containing tissue.

Interactions

Drug-Drug: ↑ bone marrow depression with other **antineoplastics** or **radiation therapy**. Concurrent use with **cisplatin** ↑ risk and severity of bone marrow depression. Concurrent use with **mitomycin** or **chest radiation** ↑ risk of pulmonary reactions.

Route/Dosage

IV (Adults): 30 mg/m² once weekly.

Hepatic Impairment

IV (Adults): *Total bilirubin 2.1–3 mg/dL*—15 mg/m² once weekly; *total bilirubin ≥3 mg/dL*—7.5 mg/m² once weekly.

Availability (generic available)

Solution for injection (requires dilution): 10 mg/mL.

NURSING IMPLICATIONS

Assessment

- Monitor BP, pulse, and respiratory rate during therapy. Note significant changes. Acute shortness of breath and severe bronchospasm may occur infrequently shortly after administration. Treatment with corticosteroids, bronchodilators, and supplemental oxygen may be required, especially in patients with a history of pulmonary disease.
- Assess frequently for signs of infection (sore throat, temperature, cough, mental status changes), especially when nadir of granulocytopenia is expected.
- Monitor neurologic status. Assess for paresthesia (numbness, tingling, pain), loss of deep tendon reflexes (Achilles reflex is usually first involved), weakness (wrist drop or footdrop, gait disturbances), cranial nerve palsies (jaw pain, hoarseness, ptosis, visual changes), autonomic dysfunction (constipation, ileus, difficulty voiding, orthostatic hypotension, impaired sweating), and CNS dysfunction (decreased level of consciousness, agitation, hallucinations). These symptoms may persist for mo. The incidence of neurotoxicity associated with vinorelbine is less than that of other vinca alkaloids.
- Monitor intake and output and daily weight for significant discrepancies.
- Assess nutritional status. Mild to moderate nausea is common. An antiemetic may be used to minimize nausea and vomiting.
- Monitor for symptoms of gout (increased uric acid, joint pain, edema). Encourage patient to drink at least 2 L of fluid/day. Allopurinol and alkalinization of urine may decrease uric acid levels.
- ***Lab Test Considerations:*** Monitor CBC prior to each dose and routinely during therapy. The nadir of granulocytopenia usually occurs 7–10 days after vinorelbine administration and recovery usually follows within 7–15 days. If granulocyte count is <1500/mm^3, dose reduction or temporary interruption of vinorelbine may be warranted. If repeated episodes of fever and/or sepsis occur during granulocytopenia, future dose of vinorelbine should be modified. May also cause mild to moderate anemia. Thrombocytopenia rarely occurs.
- Monitor liver function studies (AST, ALT, LDH, bilirubin) and renal function studies (BUN, creatinine) prior to and periodically during therapy. May cause ↑ uric acid; monitor periodically during therapy.

Implementation

- ***High Alert:*** Fatalities have occurred with chemotherapeutic agents. Before administering, clarify all ambiguous orders; double check single, daily, and course-of-therapy dose limits; have second practitioner independently double check original order, dose calculations, and infusion pump settings.
- Solution should be prepared in a biologic cabinet. Wear gloves, gown, and mask while handling medication. Discard IV equipment in specially designated containers.
- Assess infusion site frequently for redness, irritation, or inflammation. Vinorelbine is a vesicant. If extravasation occurs, infusion must be stopped and restarted elsewhere to avoid damage to subcut tissue. Treatment of extravasation includes application of warm compresses applied over the area immediately for 30–60 min, then alternating on/off every 15 min for 1 day to increase systemic absorption of the drug. Hyaluronidase 150 units diluted in 1–2 mL of 0.9% NaCl, 1 mL for each mL extravasated, should be injected through existing IV cannula or subcut if the needle has been removed to enhance absorption and dispersion of the extravasated drug.

IV Administration

- **IV Push: *Diluent:*** Dilute vinorelbine with 0.9% NaCl or D5W. ***Concentration:*** 1.5–3 mg/mL. ***Rate:*** Infuse over 6–10 min into Y-site closest to bag of a free-flowing IV or into a central line.
- Flush vein with at least 75–125 mL of 0.9% NaCl or D5W administered over 10 min or more following administration of vinorelbine.
- **Intermittent Infusion: *Diluent:*** Dilute vinorelbine with 0.9% NaCl, D5W, 0.45% NaCl, D5/0.45% NaCl, Ringer's or lactated Ringer's injection. Solution should be colorless to pale yellow. Do not administer solutions that are discolored or contain particulate matter. Diluted solution is stable for 24 hr at room temperature. ***Concentration:*** 0.5–2 mg/mL. ***Rate:*** Infuse over 6–10 min (up to 30 min) into Y-site closest to bag of a free-flowing IV or into a central line.
- Flush vein with at least 75–125 mL of 0.9% NaCl or D5W administered over 10 min or more following administration of vinorelbine.
- **Y-Site Compatibility:** amikacin, aztreonam, bleomycin, bumetanide, buprenorphine, butorphanol, calcium gluconate, carboplatin, carmustine, cefotaxime, ceftazidime, chlorpromazine, cimetidine, cisplatin, clindamycin, cyclophosphamide, cytarabine, dacarbazine, dactinomycin, daunorubicin, dexamethasone sodium phosphate, diphenhydramine, doxorubicin, doxorubicin liposome, doxycycline, droperidol, enalaprilat, etoposide, famotidine, filgrastim, floxuridine, fluconazole, fludarabine, gemcitabine, gentamicin, granisetron, haloperidol, hydrocortisone, hydromorphone, idarubicin, ifosfamide, imipenem/cilastatin, lorazepam, mannitol, melphalan, meperidine, mesna, methotrexate, metoclopramide, metronidazole, mitoxantrone, morphine, nalbuphine, ondansetron, oxaliplatin, potassium chloride, prochlorperazine, promethazine, ranitidine, streptozocin, tobramycin, vancomycin, vinblastine, vincristine, zidovudine.
- **Y-Site Incompatibility:** acyclovir, allopurinol, aminophylline, amphotericin B deoxycholate, ampicillin, cefazolin, ceftriaxone, cefuroxime, fluoroura-

cil, furosemide, ganciclovir, lansoprazole, methylprednisolone, mitomycin, sodium bicarbonate, thiotepa, trimethoprim/sulfamethoxazole.

Patient/Family Teaching

- Instruct patient to report symptoms of neurotoxicity (paresthesia, pain, difficulty walking, persistent constipation).
- Inform patient that increased fluid intake, dietary fiber, and exercise may minimize constipation. Stool softeners or laxatives may be necessary. Patient should be advised to report severe constipation or abdominal discomfort, as this may be a sign of ileus, which may occur as a consequence of neuropathy.
- Advise patient to notify health care professional if fever; chills; sore throat; signs of infection; bleeding gums; bruising; petechiae; blood in urine, stool, or emesis; or mouth sores occur.
- Caution patient to avoid crowds and persons with known infections.
- Advise patient that this medication may have teratogenic effects. Advise females of reproductive potential to use effective contraception during and for at least 2 mo after last dose of vinorelbine and to avoid breast feeding during and for 9 days after last dose.
- Discuss with patient the possibility of hair loss and explore coping strategies.
- Instruct patient not to receive any vaccinations without advice of health care professional.
- Emphasize the need for periodic lab tests to monitor for side effects.

Evaluation/Desired Outcomes

- Decrease in the size or spread of malignancy without detrimental side effects.

VITAMIN B_{12} PREPARATIONS

cyanocobalamin
(sye-an-oh-koe-**bal**-a-min)
Nascobal

hydroxocobalamin
(hye-drox-oh-koe-**bal**-a-min)
Cyanokit

Classification
Therapeutic: antianemics, vitamins
Pharmacologic: water soluble vitamins

Indications

Vitamin B_{12} deficiency (parenteral product or nasal spray should be used when deficiency is due to malabsorption). Pernicious anemia (only parenteral products should be used for initial therapy; nasal or oral products are not indicated until patients have achieved hematologic remission following parenteral therapy and have no signs of CNS involvement). Part of the Schilling test (vitamin B_{12} absorption test) (diagnostic). Cyanide poisoning (Cyanokit only).

Action

Necessary coenzyme for metabolic processes, including fat and carbohydrate metabolism and protein synthesis. Required for cell production and hematopoiesis.
Therapeutic Effects: Corrects manifestations of pernicious anemia (megaloblastic indices, GI lesions, and neurologic damage). Corrects vitamin B_{12} deficiency. Reverses symptoms of cyanide toxicity (Cyanokit only).

Pharmacokinetics

Absorption: Oral absorption in GI tract requires intrinsic factor and calcium; well absorbed after IM, subcut and nasal administration.
Distribution: Stored in the liver and bone marrow; crosses placenta, enters breast milk.
Metabolism and Excretion: Primarily excreted unchanged in urine.
Half-life: *Cyanocobalamin*—6 days (400 days in liver); *Hydroxocobalamin*—26–31 hr.

TIME/ACTION PROFILE (reticulocytosis)

ROUTE	ONSET	PEAK	DURATION
Cyanocobalamin IM, subcut, nasal	unknown	3–10 days	unknown
Hydroxocobalamin IM	unknown	unknown	unknown

Contraindications/Precautions

Contraindicated in: Hypersensitivity; Lactation: *Cyanokit*—Breast feeding not recommended; Pedi: Avoid using preparations containing benzyl alcohol in premature infants (associated with fatal "gasping syndrome").
Use Cautiously in: Hereditary optic nerve atrophy (accelerates nerve damage); Uremia, folic acid deficiency, concurrent infection, iron deficiency (response to B_{12} will be impaired); Renal dysfunction (when using aluminum-containing products); Pedi: *Cyanokit*—Safety and effectiveness not established; OB: *Cyanokit*—Use during pregnancy only if maternal benefit outweighs potential risk to fetus.

Adverse Reactions/Side Effects

CNS: headache; *Cyanokit*, dizziness, memory impairment, restlessness. **CV:** heart failure; *Cyanokit*, hypertension, chest pain, tachycardia. **Derm:** itching; *Cyanokit*, erythema, rash. **EENT:** *Cyanokit*—dry throat, eye redness, eye swelling. **GI:** diarrhea; *Cyanokit*, abdominal discomfort, dyspepsia, dysphagia,

V

hematochezia, nausea, vomiting. **F and E:** hypokalemia. **GU:** *Cyanokit*—red urine, acute renal failure. **Hemat:** thrombocytosis. **Local:** pain at IM site. **Resp:** pulmonary edema; *Cyanokit*, dyspnea. **Misc:** HYPERSENSITIVITY REACTIONS (including anaphylaxis).

Interactions

Drug-Drug: **Chloramphenicol** and **antineoplastics** may ↓ hematologic response to vitamin B_{12}. **Colchicine**, **aminosalicylic acid**, **cimetidine**, and excess intake of **alcohol**, or **vitamin C** may ↓ oral absorption/effectiveness of vitamin B_{12}.

Route/Dosage

Cyanocobalamin (oral products are usually not recommended due to poor absorption and should be used only if patient refuses the IM, deep subcutaneous, or intranasal route of administration)

PO (Adults and Children): *Vitamin B_{12} deficiency*—amount depends on deficiency (up to 1000 mcg/day have been used).

PO (Adults): *Pernicious anemia (for hematologic remission only)*—1000–2000 mcg once daily.

IM, Subcut (Adults): *Vitamin B_{12} deficiency*—30 mcg once daily for 5–10 days, then 100–200 mcg once monthly. *Pernicious anemia*—100 mcg once daily for 6–7 days; if improvement, give same dose every other day for 7 doses, then every 3–4 days for 2–3 wk; once hematologic values return to normal (remission), can give maintenance dose of 100 mcg once monthly (doses up to 1000 mcg have been used for maintenance) (could alternatively use oral or intranasal formulations below for maintenance at specified doses). *Schilling test*—Flushing dose is 1000 mcg.

IM, Subcut (Children): *Vitamin B_{12} deficiency*—0.2 mcg/kg once daily for 2 days, then 1000 mcg once daily for 2–7 days, then 100 mcg once weekly for 1 mo. *Pernicious anemia*—30–50 mcg once daily for ≥2 wk (to a total dose of 1000–5000 mcg), then give maintenance dose of 100 mcg once monthly (doses up to 1000 mcg have been used for maintenance).

Intranasal (Adults): *Vitamin B_{12} deficiency*—500 mcg (one spray) in one nostril once weekly. *Pernicious anemia (for hematologic remission only)*—500 mcg (one spray) in one nostril once weekly.

Hydroxocobalamin

IM (Adults): *Vitamin B_{12} deficiency*—30 mcg once daily for 5–10 days, then 100–200 mcg once monthly. *Pernicious anemia*—100 mcg once daily for 6–7 days; if improvement, give same dose every other day for 7 doses, then every 3–4 days for 2–3 wk; once hematologic values return to normal (remission), give maintenance dose of 100 mcg once monthly. *Schilling test*—Flushing dose is 1000 mcg.

IM (Children): *Vitamin B_{12} deficiency*—100 mcg once daily for ≥2 wk (to achieve total dose of 1000–5000 mcg), then 30–50 mcg once monthly. *Pernicious anemia*—30–50 mcg once daily for ≥2 wk (to achieve total dose of 1000–5000 mcg), then 100 mcg once monthly.

IV (Adults): *Cyanide poisoning (Cyanokit only)*—5 g over 15 min; another 5 g dose may be infused over 15–120 min depending upon severity of poisoning (maximum cumulative dose = 10 g).

Availability

Cyanocobalamin (generic available)

Extended-release tablets: 1000 mcg^{OTC}. **Lozenges:** 50 mcg ^{OTC}, 100 mcg^{OTC}, 250 mcg^{OTC}, 500 mcg^{OTC}. **Nasal spray:** 500 mcg/0.1 mL actuation (8 sprays/bottle). **Solution for injection:** 1000 mcg/mL. **Sublingual tablets:** 2500 mcg^{OTC}. **Tablets:** 100 mcg^{OTC}, 250 mcg^{OTC}, 500 mcg^{OTC}, 1000 mcg^{OTC}.

Hydroxocobalamin (generic available)

Solution for intramuscular injection: 1000 mcg/mL. **Powder for intravenous injection (requires reconstitution) (Cyanokit):** 5 g/vial.

NURSING IMPLICATIONS

Assessment

- Assess patient for signs of vitamin B_{12} deficiency (pallor; neuropathy; psychosis; red, inflamed tongue) before and periodically during therapy.
- ***Lab Test Considerations:*** Monitor plasma folic acid, vitamin B_{12}, and iron levels, hemoglobin, hematocrit, and reticulocyte count before treatment, 1 mo after the start of therapy, and then every 3–6 mo. Evaluate serum potassium level in patients receiving vitamin B_{12} for pernicious anemia for hypokalemia during the first 48 hr of treatment. Serum potassium and platelet counts should be monitored routinely during the course of therapy.
- **Cyanokit: :** Management of cyanide poisoning should also include establishment of airway, ensuring adequate oxygenation and hydration, cardiovascular support, and seizure management. Monitor BP and heart rate continuously during and after infusion and immediately report significant changes. The maximal ↑ in BP usually occurs toward the end of the infusion. BP usually returns to baseline within 4 hr of drug administration.

Implementation

- Usually administered in combination with other vitamins; solitary vitamin B_{12} deficiencies are rare.
- Administration of vitamin B_{12} by the oral route is useful only for nutritional deficiencies. Patients with small-bowel disease, malabsorption syndrome, or gastric or ileal resections require parenteral administration.
- **PO:** Administer with meals to increase absorption.
- May be mixed with fruit juices. Administer immediately after mixing; ascorbic acid alters stability.
- **Intranasal:** Dose should not be administered within 1 hr of hot food or liquids (these substances may re-

sult in the formation of nasal secretions which may result in ↓ effectiveness of nasal spray).

- **IM, Subcut:** Vials should be protected from light.
- If subcutaneous route used, deep subcutaneous administration is preferred.

IV Administration

- **IV:** IV route should only be used with Cyanokit.
- **Intermittent Infusion:** ***Diluent:*** Dilute each Cyanokit vial with 200 mL of 0.9% NaCl, D5W, or LR. Gently invert the vial for at least 60 sec prior to infusion. Reconstituted vial can be hung for infusion and is stable for 6 hr at room temperature. Discard any unused solution after 6 hr. ***Rate:*** Administer initial 5-g dose over 15 min. Administer additional 5-g dose over 15–120 min.
- **Y-Site Incompatibility:** ascorbic acid, blood products, diazepam, dobutamine, dopamine, fentanyl, nitroglycerin, pentobarbital, propofol, sodium thiosulfate, thiopental.

Patient/Family Teaching

- Encourage patient to comply with diet recommendations of health care professional. Explain that the best source of vitamins is a well-balanced diet with foods from the four basic food groups.
- Foods high in vitamin B_{12} include meats, seafood, egg yolk, and fermented cheeses; few vitamins are lost with ordinary cooking.
- Patients self-medicating with vitamin supplements should be cautioned not to exceed RDA. Effectiveness of megadoses for treatment of various medical conditions is unproved and may cause side effects.
- Inform patients with pernicious anemia of the lifelong need for vitamin B_{12} replacement.
- Emphasize the importance of follow-up exams to evaluate progress.
- **Intranasal:** Instruct patient in proper administration technique. Review *Patient Information Sheet* and demonstrate use of actuator. Unit must be primed with 3 strokes upon using for the first time. Unit must be primed with 1 stroke before each of the remaining doses. Advise patient to clear nose, then place tip approximately 1 inch into nostril and press pump once, firmly and quickly. After dose, remove unit from nose and massage dosed nostril gently for a few sec. Vial delivers 8 doses. Unit should be stored at room temperature and protected from light.
- **Intermittent Infusion:** Advise patient that skin redness may last up to 2 wk and that their urine may remain red for up to 5 wk after drug administration. Instruct patient to avoid sun exposure while their skin is red. Advise patient to contact health care professional if skin or urine redness persist after these time periods. Advise patient that a rash may develop from 7–28 days after drug administration. It will usually resolve without treatment within a few wk. Advise patient to contact health care professional if rash persists after this time period.

Evaluation/Desired Outcomes

- Resolution of the symptoms of vitamin B_{12} deficiency.
- Increase in reticulocyte count.
- Improvement in manifestations of pernicious anemia.
- Resolution of symptoms of cyanide poisoning.

VITAMIN D COMPOUNDS

calcitriol (kal-si-**trye**-ole)
~~Calcijex~~, Rocaltrol

cholecalciferol
(kol-e-kal-**sif**-e-role)
Delta-D3, ✦Euro D

doxercalciferol
(**dox**-er-kal-**sif**-e-role)
Hectorol

ergocalciferol
(**er**-goe-kal-**sif**-e-role)
Drisdol

paricalcitol (par-i-**kal**-si-tole)
Zemplar

Classification
Therapeutic: vitamins
Pharmacologic: fat-soluble vitamins

Indications

Calcitriol: Management of hypocalcemia in chronic renal dialysis (IV and PO). Treatment of hypocalcemia in patients with hypoparathyroidism or pseudohypoparathyroidism (PO only). Management of secondary hyperparathyroidism and resulting metabolic bone disease in predialysis patients with moderate to severe renal insufficiency (CCr 15–55 mL/min) (PO only). **Cholecalciferol:** Treatment or prevention of vitamin D deficiency. **Doxercalciferol:** Treatment of secondary hyperparathyroidism in patients undergoing chronic renal dialysis (IV and PO). Treatment of secondary hyperparathyroidism in patients with Stage 3 or 4 chronic kidney disease (PO only). **Ergocalciferol:** Treatment of familial hypophosphatemia. Treatment of hypoparathyroidism. Treatment of vitamin D-resistant rickets. **Paricalcitol:** Prevention and treatment of secondary hyperparathyroidism in patients with Stage 3 or 4 (PO) or Stage 5 (PO and IV) chronic kidney disease.

Action

Cholecalciferol requires activation in the liver and kidneys to create the active form of vitamin D_3 (calcitriol).

V

Doxercalciferol and ergocalciferol require activation in the liver to create the active form of vitamin D_2. Paricalcitol is a synthetic analogue of calcitriol. Vitamin D: Promotes the absorption of calcium and ↓ parathyroid hormone concentration. **Therapeutic Effects:** Treatment and prevention of deficiency states, particularly bone manifestations. Improved calcium and phosphorous homeostasis in patients with chronic kidney disease.

Pharmacokinetics

Absorption: *Calcitriol, doxercalciferol, ergocalciferol, paricalcitol*—Well absorbed following oral administration. *Calcitriol, doxercalciferol, paricalcitol*—IV administration results in complete bioavailability.

Distribution: Calcitriol and paricalcitol cross the placenta; calcitriol also enters breast milk.

Protein Binding: *Calcitriol and paricalcitol*—99.9%.

Metabolism and Excretion: *Calcitriol*—Undergoes enterohepatic recycling and is excreted mostly in bile. *Cholecalciferol*—Converted by the liver and kidneys to calcitriol (active form of vitamin D_3). *Ergocalciferol*—Converted to active form of vitamin D_2 by sunlight, the liver, and the kidneys. *Doxercalciferol*—Converted by the liver to the active form of vitamin D_2. *Paricalcitol*—mostly metabolized by the liver and excreted via hepatobiliary elimination.

Half-life: *Calcitriol*—5–8 hr. *Cholecalciferol*—14 hr. *Doxercalciferol*—32–37 hr (up to 96 hr). *Paricalcitol*—14–20 hr.

TIME/ACTION PROFILE (effects on serum calcium)

ROUTE	ONSET	PEAK	DURATION
Calcitriol-PO	2–6 hr	2–6 hr	3–5 days
Calcitriol-IV	unknown	unknown	unknown
Cholecalciferol-PO	unknown	unknown	unknown
Doxercalciferol PO	unknown	8 wk	1 wk
Doxercalciferol-IV	unknown	8 wk	1 wk
Ergocalciferol-PO	12–24 hr	unknown	up to 6 mo
Paricalcitol-PO	unknown	2–4 wk	unknown
Paricalitol IV	unknown	up to 2 wk	unknown

Contraindications/Precautions

Contraindicated in: Hypersensitivity; Hypercalcemia; Vitamin D toxicity; Concurrent use of magnesium-containing antacids or other vitamin D supplements; **Ergocalciferol**: Known intolerance to tartrazine; **Cholecalciferol and ergocalciferol**: Malabsorption problems.

Use Cautiously in: Calcitriol, doxercalciferol, paricalcitol: Patients receiving digoxin; OB: Safety not established; Lactation: Use during breast feeding only if potential maternal benefit outweighs risk to infant (infant should be monitored for hypercalcemia).

Adverse Reactions/Side Effects

Seen primarily as manifestations of toxicity (hypercalcemia).

CNS: headache, somnolence, weakness; *doxercalciferol*, dizziness, malaise. **CV:** arrhythmias, edema, hypertension; *doxercalciferol*, bradycardia; *paricalcitol*, palpitations. **Derm:** pruritus. **EENT:** conjunctivitis, photophobia, rhinorrhea. **F and E:** hypercalcemia. **GI:** PANCREATITIS, abdominal pain, anorexia, constipation, dry mouth, ↑ liver enzymes, metallic taste, nausea, polydipsia, vomiting, weight loss. **GU:** albuminuria, azotemia, ↓ libido, nocturia, polyuria. **Local:** pain at injection site. **Metab:** hyperthermia. **MS:** bone pain, muscle pain; *doxercalciferol*, arthralgia; *paricalcitol*, metastatic calcification. **Resp:** *doxercalciferol and ergocalciferol*—dyspnea. **Misc:** *calcitriol*—allergic reactions, chills, fever; *doxercalciferol*, HYPERSENSITIVITY REACTIONS (including anaphylaxis, angioedema, hypotension, dyspnea, and cardiac arrest).

Interactions

Drug-Drug: Cholestyramine, **colestipol**, or **mineral oil** ↓ absorption of vitamin D analogues. Use with **thiazide diuretics** may result in hypercalcemia. **Corticosteroids** ↓ effectiveness of vitamin D analogues. Using calcitriol, doxercalciferol, or paricalcitol with **digoxin** may ↑ risk of arrhythmias. Vitamin D requirements ↓ by **phenytoin** and other **hydantoin anticonvulsants**, **sucralfate**, **barbiturates**, and **primidone**. Concurrent use with **magnesium-containing drugs** may lead to hypermagnesemia. Concurrent use of **calcium-containing drugs** may ↑ risk of hypercalcemia. Concurrent use of other **vitamin D supplements** may ↑ risk of hypercalcemia. **Agents that induce liver enzymes (phenobarbital, rifampin)** and **agents that inhibit liver enzymes (atazanavir, clarithromycin, erythromycin, indinavir, itraconazole, ketoconazole, nefazodone, nelfinavir, ritonavir, saquinavir, verapamil, voriconazole)** may alter requirements for doxercalciferol and paricalcitol (monitoring of calcium and phosphorus recommended).

Drug-Food: Ingestion of **foods high in calcium content** (see Appendix K) may lead to hypercalcemia.

Route/Dosage

Calcitriol

PO (Adults): *Hypocalcemia during dialysis*—0.25 mcg once daily or every other day; if needed, may ↑ by 0.25 mcg/day at 4–8 wk intervals (typical dosage = 0.5–1 mcg/day). *Hypoparathyroidism*—0.25 mcg once daily initially; if needed, may ↑ dose by 0.25 mcg/day at 2–4 wk intervals (typical dosage = 0.5–2 mcg/day). *Predialysis patients*—0.25 mcg once daily (up to 0.5 mcg/day).

PO (Children): *Hypocalcemia during dialysis*—0.25–2 mcg once daily. *Hypoparathyroidism (chil-*

dren ≥6 yr)—0.25 mcg once daily initially; if needed, may ↑ dose by 0.25 mcg/day at 2–4 wk intervals (typical dosage = 0.5–2 mcg/day). *Hypoparathyroidism (children 1–5 yr)*—0.25–0.75 mcg once daily. *Hypoparathyroidism (children <1 yr)*—0.04–0.08 mcg/kg/day. *Predialysis patients (children ≥3 yr)*—0.25 mcg once daily (up to 0.5 mcg/day). *Predialysis patients (children <3 yr)*—10–15 ng/kg/day.
IV (Adults): *Hypocalcemia during dialysis*—0.5 mcg (0.01 mcg/kg) 3 times weekly. May be ↑ by 0.25–0.5 mcg/dose at 2–4 wk intervals (typical maintenance dose = 0.5–3.0 mcg 3 times weekly [0.01–0.05 mcg/kg 3 times weekly]).
IV (Children): *Hypocalcemia during dialysis*—0.01–0.05 mcg/kg 3 times weekly.

Cholecalciferol

PO (Adults): 400–1000 units once daily.
PO (Infants): *Exclusively or partially breast fed*—400 units once daily.

Doxercalciferol

PO (Adults): *Dialysis patients*—10 mcg 3 times weekly (at dialysis); dose may be adjusted by 2.5 mcg at 8-wk intervals based on intact PTH concentrations (maximum dose = 20 mcg 3 times weekly). *Non-dialysis patients*—1 mcg once daily; dose may be adjusted by 0.5 mcg at 2 wk intervals based on intact PTH concentrations (maximum dose = 3.5 mcg/day).
IV (Adults): 4 mcg 3 times weekly at the end of dialysis; dose may be adjusted by 1–2 mcg at 8-wk intervals based on intact PTH concentrations (maximum dose = 6 mcg 3 times weekly).

Ergocalciferol

PO (Adults): *Vitamin D–resistant rickets*—12,000–500,000 units/day (to be used with phosphate supplement). *Familial hypophosphatemia*—10,000–80,000 units/day (with phosphorus 1–2 g/day). *Hypoparathyroidism*—50,000–200,000 units/day (to be used with calcium supplement).
PO (Children): *Vitamin D–resistant rickets*—40,000–80,000 units/day (to be used with phosphate supplement). *Familial hypophosphatemia*—10,000–80,000 units/day (with phosphorus 1–2 g/day). *Hypoparathyroidism*—50,000–200,000 units/day (to be used with calcium supplement).
PO (Infants): *Exclusively or partially breast fed*—400 units once daily.

Paricalcitol

Stage 3 or 4 Chronic Kidney Disease

PO (Adults): *Baseline intact PTH concentration ≤500 pg/mL*—Initiate with 1 mcg once daily or 2 mcg 3 times weekly; dose can be adjusted at 2–4 wk intervals based on intact PTH, calcium, and phosphate concentrations. *Baseline intact PTH concentration >500 pg/mL*—Initiate with 2 mcg once daily or 4 mcg 3 times weekly; dose can be adjusted at 2–4 wk intervals based on intact PTH, calcium, and phosphate concentrations.

Stage 5 Chronic Kidney Disease

PO (Adults): Initial dose (in mcg) is based on following equation: baseline intact PTH concentration (pg/mL)/80; dose should be given 3 times weekly; dose can be adjusted at 2–4 wk intervals based on intact PTH, calcium, and phosphate concentrations.
IV (Adults and Children ≥5 yr): 0.04–0.1 mcg/kg 3 times weekly during dialysis; dose can be adjusted by 2–4 mcg at 2–4 wk intervals based on intact PTH, calcium, and phosphate concentrations (doses up to 0.24 mcg/kg have been used).

Availability

Calcitriol (generic available)

Capsules: 0.25 mcg, 0.5 mcg. **Oral solution:** 1 mcg/mL. **Solution for injection:** 1 mcg/mL.

Cholecalciferol

Capsules: 1,000 units OTC, 2,000 units OTC, 5,000 units OTC, 10,000 units OTC, 25,000 units OTC, 50,000 units OTC. **Chewable tablets:** 400 units OTC. **Oral solution:** 400 units/mL OTC, 5,000 units/mL OTC. **Tablets:** 400 units OTC, 1,000 units OTC, 2,000 units OTC, 3,000 units OTC, 5,000 units OTC, 50,000 units OTC. ***In combination with:*** alendronate (Fosamax Plus D), see Appendix B.

Doxercalciferol (generic available)

Capsules: 0.5 mcg, 1 mcg, 2.5 mcg. **Solution for injection:** 2 mcg/mL.

Ergocalciferol (generic available)

Capsules: 50,000 units. **Oral solution:** 8000 units/mL Rx, OTC. **Tablets:** 400 units, 2,000 units.

Paricalcitol (generic available)

Capsules: 1 mcg, 2 mcg, 4 mcg. **Solution for injection:** 2 mcg/mL, 5 mcg/mL.

NURSING IMPLICATIONS

Assessment

- Assess for symptoms of vitamin deficiency prior to and periodically during therapy.
- Assess patient for bone pain and weakness prior to and during therapy.
- Observe patient carefully for evidence of hypocalcemia (paresthesia, muscle twitching, laryngospasm, colic, cardiac arrhythmias, and Chvostek's or Trousseau's sign). Protect symptomatic patient by raising and padding side rails; keep bed in low position.
- Pedi: Monitor height and weight; growth arrest may occur in prolonged high-dose therapy.
- **Rickets/Osteomalacia:** Assess patient for bone pain and weakness prior to and during therapy.

- ***Lab Test Considerations:*** During *calcitriol* therapy, serum calcium and phosphate concentrations should be drawn twice weekly initially. Serum calcium, magnesium, alkaline phosphatase, and intact PTH should then be monitored at least monthly. During *cholecalciferol* therapy, serum calcium, phosphate, and alkaline phosphatase concentrations should be monitored periodically. During *doxercalciferol* therapy, serum ionized calcium, phosphate, and intact PTH concentrations should be monitored prior to initiation of therapy, and then weekly during the first 12 wk of therapy, then periodically. Alkaline phosphatase should be monitored periodically. During *ergocalciferol* therapy, serum calcium and phosphate concentrations should be monitored every 2 wk. During oral *paricalcitol* therapy, serum calcium, phosphate, and intact PTH concentrations should be monitored at least every 2 wk for the first 3 mo of therapy or after any dosage adjustment, then monthly for 3 mo, then every 3 mo. During IV *paricalcitol* therapy, serum calcium and phosphate concentrations should be monitored twice weekly initially until dosage stabilized, and then at least monthly. Serum intact PTH concentrations should be monitored every 3 mo.
- The serum calcium × phosphate product (Ca × P) should not exceed 70 mg^2/dL^2 (55 mg^2/dL^2 for doxercalciferol) (patients may be at ↑ risk of calcification).
- Calcitriol may cause false ↑ cholesterol levels.
- ***Toxicity and Overdose:*** Toxicity is manifested as hypercalcemia, hypercalciuria, and hyperphosphatemia. Assess patient for appearance of nausea, vomiting, anorexia, weakness, constipation, headache, bone pain, and metallic taste. Later symptoms include polyuria, polydipsia, photophobia, rhinorrhea, pruritus, and cardiac arrhythmias. Notify health care professional immediately if these signs of hypervitaminosis D occur. Treatment usually consists of discontinuation of calcitriol, a low-calcium diet, use of low-calcium dialysate in peritoneal dialysis patients, and administration of a laxative. IV hydration and loop diuretics may be ordered to increase urinary excretion of calcium. Hemodialysis may also be used.

Implementation

- **PO:** May be administered without regard to meals. Measure solution accurately with calibrated dropper provided by manufacturer. May be mixed with juice, cereal, or food, or dropped directly into mouth. Calcitriol capsules or solution should be protected from light.

IV Administration

- **IV Push:** Administer *calcitriol, doxercalciferol, and paracalcitol* undiluted by rapid injection through the catheter at the end of a hemodialysis period.

Patient/Family Teaching

- Advise patient to take medication as directed. Take missed doses as soon as remembered that day, unless almost time for next dose; do not double up on doses.
- Review diet modifications with patient. See Appendix K for foods high in calcium and vitamin D. Renal patients must still consider renal failure diet in food selection. Health care professional may order concurrent calcium supplement.
- Encourage patient to comply with dietary recommendations of health care professional. Explain that the best source of vitamins is a well-balanced diet with foods from the 4 basic food groups and the importance of sunlight exposure. See Appendix K for foods high in vitamin D.
- Patients self-medicating with vitamin supplements should be cautioned not to exceed RDA. The effectiveness of megadoses for treatment of various medical conditions is unproved and may cause side effects.
- Advise patient to avoid concurrent use of antacids containing magnesium.
- Review symptoms of overdose and instruct patient to report these promptly to health care professional.
- Emphasize the importance of follow-up exams to evaluate progress.

Evaluation/Desired Outcomes

- Normalization of serum calcium and parathyroid hormone levels.
- Resolution or prevention of vitamin D deficiency.
- Improvement in symptoms of vitamin D–resistant rickets.

voriconazole

(vor-i-**kon**-a-zole)

Vfend

Classification

Therapeutic: antifungals

Indications

Invasive aspergillosis. Candidemia (in patients without neutropenia) and serious *Candida* infections in skin, bladder, abdomen, kidney, and wounds. Esophageal candidiasis. Scedosporiosis and fusariosis in patients intolerant of or refractory to other therapies.

Action

Inhibits fungal ergosterol synthesis leading to production of abnormal fungal plasma membrane. **Therapeutic Effects:** Antifungal activity. **Spectrum:** Spectrum is notable for activity against: *Aspergillus* spp., *Candida* spp., *Scedosporium apiospermum*, *Fusarium* spp.

Pharmacokinetics

Absorption: Well absorbed following oral administration (96%); IV administration results in complete bioavailability.

Distribution: Extensive tissue distribution.

Protein Binding: 58%.

Metabolism and Excretion: Highly metabolized by the hepatic P450 enzymes (CYP2C19, CYP2C9,

CYP3A4); <2% excreted unchanged in urine. Much individual variation in metabolism; metabolites are inactive. 🧬 The CYP2C19 enzyme system exhibits genetic polymorphism; 15–20% of Asian patients and 3–5% of Caucasian and Black patients may be poor metabolizers and may have significantly ↑ voriconazole concentrations and an ↑ risk of adverse effects.

Half-life: Dose-dependent (adults 6–9 hrs); ↑ in hepatic impairment.

TIME/ACTION PROFILE (blood levels)

ROUTE	ONSET	PEAK	DURATION
PO	rapid	1–2 hr	12 hr
IV	rapid	end of infusion	12 hr

Contraindications/Precautions

Contraindicated in: Concurrent use of high-dose ritonavir (400 mg every 12 hr), rifampin, rifabutin, St. John's wort, carbamazepine, and phenobarbital (↓ antifungal activity); Concurrent use of sirolimus, pimozide, quinidine, ergotamine, and dihydroergotamine (↑ risk of toxicity of these agents); Concurrent use of efavirenz at doses ≥400 mg/day (↓ antifungal activity); Tablets contain lactose and should be avoided in patients with galactose intolerance, Lapp lactase deficiency, or glucose-galactose malabsorption; Severe hepatic impairment.

Use Cautiously in: Mild to moderate hepatic impairment (↓ IV and PO maintenance doses); Renal impairment (CCr <50 mL/min) (Vehicle in IV formulation can accumulate resulting in toxicity; avoid use of IV unless potential benefit greatly outweighs potential risk, use oral form only); Congenital/acquired QT interval prolongation, HF, sinus bradycardia, hypokalemia, hypomagnesemia, or symptomatic arrhythmias; Concurrent use of drugs that prolong the QTc interval; Hematologic malignancy (↑ risk of hepatotoxicity); OB, Lactation: Use only if benefits justify risk; Rep: Women of reproductive potential; Pedi: Children <2 yr (safety and effectiveness not established); suspension contains benzyl alcohol which may cause potentially fatal "gasping syndrome" in neonates; ↑ risk of photosensitivity reactions.

Adverse Reactions/Side Effects

CNS: dizziness, hallucinations, headache. **CV:** changes in BP, peripheral edema, QT interval prolongation, tachycardia. **Derm:** MELANOMA, SQUAMOUS CELL CARCINOMA, STEVENS-JOHNSON SYNDROME, photosensitivity, rash. **EENT:** visual disturbances, eye hemorrhage. **F and E:** hypokalemia, hypomagnesemia, hyperglycemia. **GI:** HEPATOTOXICITY, abdominal pain, diarrhea, nausea, pancreatitis, vomiting. **MS:** fluorosis, periostitis. **Misc:** chills, fever, infusion reactions.

Interactions

Drug-Drug: Voriconazole is a substrate and inhibitor of the **CYP3A4**, **CYP2C9**, and **CYP2C19** enzyme systems. **Carbamazepine**, **ritonavir** (at a dose of 400 mg every 12 hr), **phenobarbital**, **St. John's wort**, **rifabutin**, and **rifampin** may ↓ levels and effectiveness; concurrent use contraindicated. May ↑ levels of **dihydroergotamine**, **ergotamine**, **pimozide**, **quinidine**, **rifabutin**, and **sirolimus**; concurrent use contraindicated. Concurrent use with **efavirenz** at doses of ≥400 mg every 24 hr is contraindicated since it may ↑ efavirenz levels and ↓ voriconazole levels; if used together, ↑ oral maintenance dose of voriconazole to 400 mg every 12 hr and ↓ dose of efavirenz to 300 mg daily. **Fluconazole** may ↑ levels of voriconazole; avoid concurrent use. May ↑ levels of **cyclosporine**; ↓ cyclosporine dose by 50%. May ↑ levels of **tacrolimus**; ↓ tacrolimus dose to ⅓ of the starting dose. May ↑ levels of **HMG-CoA reductase inhibitors**, some **benzodiazepines (alprazolam, midazolam, triazolam)**, **fentanyl**, **oxycodone**, **NSAIDs (ibuprofen, diclofenac)**, some **calcium channel blockers**, **sulfonylureas (glipizide, glyburide)**, **phenytoin**, **alfentanil**, **warfarin**, and **vinca alkaloids (vincristine, vinblastine)**; dose ↓ may be needed and careful monitoring required during concurrent use. May ↑ **methadone** levels and ↑ risk of QT interval prolongation. Concurrent use with **hormonal contraceptives** containing **ethinyl estadiol** and **norethindone** may ↑ voriconazole, ethinyl estradiol and norethindrone levels. May ↑ levels of **everolimus**; concurrent use not recommended. ↑ blood levels of **omeprazole**; if patient receiving ≥40 mg/day of omeprazole, ↓ omeprazole dose by 50%. Similar effects may occur with other **proton-pump inhibitors**. May ↓ metabolism and ↑ blood levels and effects of **protease-inhibitor antiretrovirals** and **non-nucleoside reverse transcriptase inhibitor antiretrovirals**; frequent monitoring recommended. **Non-nucleoside reverse transcriptase inhibitor antiretrovirals**; may induce or inhibit the metabolism of voriconazole; frequent monitoring recommended.

Drug-Natural Products: **St. John's wort** ↑ metabolism and may ↓ effectiveness; concurrent use contraindicated.

Route/Dosage

Invasive Aspergillosis, Scedosporiosis, or Fusariosis

IV, PO (Adults ≥40 kg): *Loading dose (IV)*—6 mg/kg IV every 12 hr for 2 doses, followed by *maintenance dose (IV)* of 4 mg/kg IV every 12 hr (use 5 mg/kg IV every 12 hr if concurrently using with phenytoin). Continue IV therapy for ≥7 days, then switch to oral maintenance dose once patient has clinically improved

V

and can tolerate oral medications. *Maintenance dose (PO)*—200 mg PO every 12 hr (use 400 mg PO every 12 hr if concurrently using with phenytoin or efavirenz); if response inadequate, may ↑ to 300 mg every 12 hr. Total duration of therapy: ≥6–12 wk.

IV, PO (Adults <40 kg): *Loading dose (IV)*—6 mg/kg IV every 12 hr for 2 doses, followed by *maintenance dose (IV)* of 4 mg/kg IV every 12 hr (use 5 mg/kg IV every 12 hr if concurrently using with phenytoin). Continue IV therapy for ≥7 days, then switch to oral maintenance dose once patient has clinically improved and can tolerate oral medications. *Maintenance dose (PO)*—100 mg PO every 12 hr (use 200 mg PO every 12 hr if concurrently using with phenytoin; use 400 mg PO every 12 hr if concurrently using with efavirenz); if response inadequate, may ↑ to 150 mg every 12 hr. Total duration of therapy: ≥6–12 wk.

IV, PO (Children ≥15 yr): *Loading dose (IV)*—6 mg/kg IV every 12 hr for 2 doses, followed by *maintenance dose (IV)* of 4 mg/kg IV every 12 hr. Continue IV therapy for ≥7 days, then switch to oral maintenance dose once patient has clinically improved and can tolerate oral medications. *Maintenance dose (PO)*—200 mg every 12 hr; if response inadequate, may ↑ to 300 mg every 12 hr. Total duration of therapy: ≥6–12 wk.

IV, PO (Children 12–14 yr and ≥50 kg): *Loading dose (IV)*—6 mg/kg IV every 12 hr for 2 doses, followed by *maintenance dose (IV)* of 4 mg/kg IV every 12 hr. Continue IV therapy for ≥7 days, then switch to oral maintenance dose once patient has clinically improved and can tolerate oral medications. *Maintenance dose (PO)*—200 mg every 12 hr; if response inadequate, may ↑ to 300 mg every 12 hr. Total duration of therapy: ≥6–12 wk.

IV, PO (Children 12–14 yr and <50 kg): *Loading dose (IV)*—9 mg/kg IV every 12 hr for 2 doses, followed by *maintenance dose (IV)* of 8 mg/kg IV every 12 hr; if response inadequate, may ↑ maintenance dose by 1 mg/kg. Continue IV therapy for ≥7 days, then switch to oral maintenance dose once patient has clinically improved and can tolerate oral medications. *Maintenance dose (PO)*—9 mg/kg every 12 hr (not to exceed 350 mg every 12 hr); if response inadequate, may ↑ by 1 mg/kg or 50 mg (not to exceed 350 mg every 12 hr). Total duration of therapy: ≥6–12 wk.

IV, PO (Children 2–11 yr): *Loading dose (IV)*—9 mg/kg IV every 12 hr for 2 doses, followed by *maintenance dose (IV)* of 8 mg/kg IV every 12 hr; if response inadequate, may ↑ maintenance dose by 1 mg/kg. Continue IV therapy for ≥7 days, then switch to oral maintenance dose once patient has clinically improved and can tolerate oral medications. *Maintenance dose (PO)*—9 mg/kg every 12 hr (not to exceed 350 mg every 12 hr); if response inadequate, may ↑ by 1 mg/kg or 50 mg (not to exceed 350 mg every 12 hr). Total duration of therapy: ≥6–12 wk.

Hepatic Impairment

IV, PO (Adults): *Child-Pugh Class A and B*—Use standard IV loading dose, ↓ maintenance doses (IV or PO) by 50%; *Child-Pugh Class C*—Not recommended.

Candidemia in Non-Neutropenic Patients or Other Deep Tissue *Candida* Infections

IV, PO (Adults ≥40 kg): *Loading dose (IV)*—6 mg/kg IV every 12 hr for 2 doses, followed by *maintenance dose (IV)* of 3–4 mg/kg IV every 12 hr (use 5 mg/kg IV every 12 hr if concurrently using with phenytoin). Switch to oral dosing once patient has clinically improved and can tolerate oral medications. *Maintenance dose (PO)*—200 mg PO every 12 hr (use 400 mg PO every 12 hr if concurrently using with phenytoin or efavirenz); if response inadequate, may ↑ to 300 mg every 12 hr. Total duration of therapy: ≥14 days following resolution of symptoms or following last positive culture, whichever is longer.

IV, PO (Adults <40 kg): *Loading dose (IV)*—6 mg/kg IV every 12 hr for 2 doses, followed by *maintenance dose (IV)* of 3–4 mg/kg IV every 12 hr (use 5 mg/kg IV every 12 hr if concurrently using with phenytoin). Switch to oral dosing once patient has clinically improved and can tolerate oral medications. *Maintenance dose (PO)*—100 mg PO every 12 hr (use 200 mg PO every 12 hr if concurrently using with phenytoin; use 400 mg PO every 12 hr if using concurrently with efavirenz); if response inadequate, may ↑ to 150 mg every 12 hr. Total duration of therapy: ≥14 days following resolution of symptoms or following last positive culture, whichever is longer.

IV, PO (Children ≥15 yr): *Loading dose (IV)*—6 mg/kg IV every 12 hr for 2 doses, followed by *maintenance dose (IV)* of 3–4 mg/kg IV every 12 hr. Switch to oral dosing once patient has clinically improved and can tolerate oral medications. *Maintenance dose (PO)*—200 mg every 12 hr; if response inadequate, may ↑ to 300 mg every 12 hr. Total duration of therapy: ≥14 days following resolution of symptoms or following last positive culture, whichever is longer.

IV, PO (Children 12–14 yr and ≥50 kg): *Loading dose (IV)*—6 mg/kg IV every 12 hr for 2 doses, followed by *maintenance dose (IV)* of 3–4 mg/kg IV every 12 hr. Switch to oral dosing once patient has clinically improved and can tolerate oral medications. *Maintenance dose (PO)*—200 mg every 12 hr; if response inadequate, may ↑ to 300 mg every 12 hr. Total duration of therapy: ≥14 days following resolution of symptoms or following last positive culture, whichever is longer.

IV, PO (Children 12–14 yr and <50 kg): *Loading dose (IV)*—9 mg/kg IV every 12 hr for 2 doses, followed by *maintenance dose (IV)* of 8 mg/kg IV every 12 hr; if response inadequate, may ↑ maintenance dose by 1 mg/kg. Switch to oral dosing once patient has clinically improved and can tolerate oral medications. *Maintenance dose (PO)*—9 mg/kg every 12 hr (not to exceed 350 mg every 12 hr); if response inadequate,

may ↑ by 1 mg/kg or 50 mg (not to exceed 350 mg every 12 hr). Total duration of therapy: ≥14 days following resolution of symptoms or following last positive culture, whichever is longer.
IV, PO (Children 2–11 yr): *Loading dose (IV)*—9 mg/kg IV every 12 hr for 2 doses, followed by *maintenance dose (IV)* of 8 mg/kg IV every 12 hr; if response inadequate, may ↑ maintenance dose by 1 mg/kg. Switch to oral dosing once patient has clinically improved and can tolerate oral medications. *Maintenance dose (PO)*—9 mg/kg every 12 hr (not to exceed 350 mg every 12 hr); if response inadequate, may ↑ by 1 mg/kg or 50 mg (not to exceed 350 mg every 12 hr). Total duration of therapy: ≥14 days following resolution of symptoms or following last positive culture, whichever is longer.

Hepatic Impairment

IV, PO (Adults): *Child-Pugh Class A and B*—Use standard IV loading dose, ↓ maintenance doses (IV or PO) by 50%; *Child-Pugh Class C*—Not recommended.

Esophageal Candidiasis

PO (Adults ≥40 kg): 200 mg every 12 hr (use 400 mg every 12 hr if concurrently using with phenytoin or efavirenz); if response inadequate, may ↑ to 300 mg every 12 hr. Duration of therapy: ≥14 days and for ≥7 days following resolution of symptoms.
PO (Adults <40 kg): 100 mg every 12 hr (use 200 mg every 12 hr if concurrently using with phenytoin; use 400 mg every 12 hr if using concurrently with efavirenz); if response inadequate, may ↑ to 150 mg every 12 hr. Duration of therapy: ≥14 days and for ≥7 days following resolution of symptoms.
PO (Children ≥15 yr): 200 mg every 12 hr; if response inadequate, may ↑ to 300 mg every 12 hr. Duration of therapy: ≥14 days and for ≥7 days following resolution of symptoms.
PO (Children 12–14 yr and ≥50 kg): 200 mg every 12 hr; if response inadequate, may ↑ to 300 mg every 12 hr. Duration of therapy: ≥14 days and for ≥7 days following resolution of symptoms.
IV, PO (Children 12–14 yr and <50 kg): Initiate therapy with *maintenance dose (IV)* of 4 mg/kg IV every 12 hr; if response inadequate, may ↑ maintenance dose by 1 mg/kg. Switch to oral dosing once patient has clinically improved and can tolerate oral medications. *Maintenance dose (PO)*—9 mg/kg every 12 hr (not to exceed 350 mg every 12 hr); if response inadequate, may ↑ by 1 mg/kg or 50 mg (not to exceed 350 mg every 12 hr). Total duration of therapy: ≥14 days and for ≥7 days following resolution of symptoms.
IV, PO (Children 2–11 yr): Initiate therapy with *maintenance dose (IV)* of 4 mg/kg IV every 12 hr; if response inadequate, may ↑ maintenance dose by 1 mg/kg. Switch to oral dosing once patient has clinically improved and can tolerate oral medications. *Maintenance dose (PO)*—9 mg/kg every 12 hr (not to exceed 350 mg every 12 hr); if response inadequate, may ↑ by 1 mg/kg or 50 mg (not to exceed 350 mg every 12 hr). Total duration of therapy: ≥14 days and for ≥7 days following resolution of symptoms.

Hepatic Impairment

IV, PO (Adults): *Child-Pugh Class A and B*—Use standard IV loading dose, ↓ maintenance doses (IV or PO) by 50%; *Child-Pugh Class C*—Not recommended.

Availability (generic available)

Oral suspension (orange-flavor): 40 mg/mL. **Powder for injection (requires reconstitution and dilution):** 200 mg/vial. **Tablets:** 50 mg, 200 mg.

NURSING IMPLICATIONS

Assessment

- Monitor for signs and symptoms of fungal infections prior to and during therapy.
- Obtain specimens for culture and histopathology prior to therapy to isolate and identify organism. Therapy may be started before results are received.
- Monitor visual function including visual acuity, visual field, and color perception in patients receiving more than 28 days of therapy. Vision usually returns to normal within 14 days after discontinuation of therapy.
- Monitor for allergic reactions during infusion of voriconazole (flushing, fever, sweating, tachycardia, chest tightness, dyspnea, faintness, nausea, pruritus, rash). Symptoms occur immediately upon start of infusion. May require discontinuation.
- Monitor patients with risk factors for acute pancreatitis (recent chemotherapy, hematopoietic stem cell transplantation [HSCT]) for the signs of pancreatitis (abdominal pain, ↑ serum amylase and lipase).
- Assess for rash periodically during therapy. May cause Stevens-Johnson syndrome. Discontinue therapy if severe or if accompanied with fever, general malaise, fatigue, muscle or joint aches, blisters, oral lesions, conjunctivitis, hepatitis and/or eosinophilia.
- ***Lab Test Considerations:*** Monitor liver function tests (AST, ALT, and bilirubin) prior to, weekly during first mo and monthly during therapy. If abnormal liver function tests occur, monitor for development of severe hepatic injury. Discontinue therapy if markedly ↑ or clinical signs and symptoms of liver disease develop.
- Monitor renal function (serum creatinine) during therapy.

Implementation

- Once patient can tolerate oral medication, PO voriconazole may be used.
- Correct electrolyte disturbances (hypokalemia, hypomagnesemia, hypocalcemia) prior to initiation and during therapy.

V

- **PO:** Administer at least 1 hr before or 1 hr after a meal.
- Shake suspension well (approximately 10 sec) before measuring suspension. Do not mix suspension with other medicine, flavored liquid, or syrup. Store suspension at room temperature up to 14 days, then discard.

IV Administration

- Do not administer voriconazole with blood products or concentrated electrolytes, even in separate lines. Non-concentrated electrolytes can be infused at same time, but separate lines must be used. TPN can be administered simultaneously but must be via separate line or via a different port in a multi-lumen catheter.
- **Intermittent Infusion:** Reconstitute each 200-mg vial with 19 mL of sterile water for injection to achieve concentration of 10 mg/mL. Calculate volume of 10 mg/mL solution required for patient dose. ***Diluent:*** Withdraw and discard equal volume of diluent from infusion bag or bottle to be used. Withdraw required volume of voriconazole solution from vial(s) and add to appropriate volume of 0.9% NaCl, LR, D5/LR, D5/0.45% NaCl, D5W, 0.45% NaCl, or D5/0.9% NaCl. Reconstituted solution stable for 24 hr if refrigerated. Discard partially used vials. ***Concentration:*** Final concentration of infusion should be 0.5–5 mg/mL. ***Rate:*** Infuse over 1–2 hr at a rate not to exceed 3 mg/kg/hr.
- **Y-Site Compatibility:** acyclovir, alemtuzumab, alfentanil, allopurinol, amifostine, amikacin, aminophylline, amiodarone, amphotericin B liposome, ampicillin, ampicillin/sulbactam, anidulafungin, argatroban, azithromycin, aztreonam, bivalirudin, bleomycin, buprenorphine, butorphanol, bumetanide, buprenorphine, butorphanol, calcium acetate, calcium chloride, calcium gluconate, cangrelor, carboplatin, carmustine, caspofungin, cefazolin, cefotaxime, cefotetan, cefoxitin, ceftaroline, ceftazidime, ceftriaxone, chloramphenicol, chlorpromazine, ciprofloxacin, cisatracurium, cisplatin, clindamycin, cyclophosphamide, cytarabine, dacarbazine, dactinomycin, daptomycin, daunorubicin hydrochloride, dexamethasone, dexmedetomidine, dexrazoxane, digoxin, diltiazem, diphenhydramine, dobutamine, docetaxel, dolasetron, dopamine, doxycycline, droperidol, enalaprilat, ephedrine, epinephrine, epirubicin, ertapenem, erythromycin, esmolol, etoposide, etoposide phosphate, famotidine, fenoldopam, fentanyl, fluconazole, fludarabine, fluorouracil, foscarnet, fosphenytoin, furosemide, ganciclovir, gemcitabine, gentamicin, glycopyrrolate, granisetron, haloperidol, heparin, hydralazine, hydrocortisone, ifosfamide, imipenem/cilastatin, insulin, regular, irinotecan, isoproterenol, ketorolac, labetalol, leucovorin calcium, levofloxacin, lidocaine, linezolid, lorazepam, magnesium sulfate, mannitol, melphalan, meperidine, meropenem, mesna, methohexital, methotrexate, methyldopate, methylprednisolone, metoclopramide, metoprolol, metronidazole, midazolam, milrinone, mitomycin, morphine, mycophenolate, nafcillin, nalbuphine, naloxone, nicardipine, nitroglycerin, norepinephrine, octreotide, ondansetron, oxaliplatin, oxytocin, paclitaxel, pamidronate, pancuronium, pentamidine, pentobarbital, phenobarbital, phenylephrine, piperacillin/tazobactam, potassium acetate, potassium chloride, potassium phosphates, procainamide, promethazine, propranolol, quinupristin/dalfopristin, remifentanil, rocuronium, sodium acetate, sodium bicarbonate, sodium phosphates, streptozocin, succinylcholine, sufentanil, tacrolimus, theophylline, thiotepa, tirofiban, tobramycin, topotecan, trimethoprim/sulfamethoxazole, vancomycin, vasopressin, vecuronium, verapamil, vinblastine, vincristine, vinorelbine, zidovudine, zoledronic acid.
- **Y-Site Incompatibility:** amphotericin B lipid complex, busulfan, cefepime, cyclosporine, dantrolene, diazepam, doxorubicin hydrochloride, idarubicin, mitoxantrone, moxifloxacin, nitroprusside, pantoprazole, phenytoin, thiopental.

Patient/Family Teaching

- Advise patient to take voriconazole as directed, on an empty stomach.
- May cause blurred vision, photophobia, and dizziness. Caution patient to avoid driving and other activities requiring alertness until response to medication is known. Also advise patient to avoid driving at night during voriconazole therapy.
- Advise patient to avoid direct sunlight, sunlamps and tanning beds during voriconazole therapy. Use sunscreen and protective clothing to prevent severe sunburn. Advise patient to have dermatologic evaluation regular basis to allow early detection and management of premalignant lesions; squamous cell carcinoma of the skin and melanoma have been reported during long-term therapy.
- Instruct patient to notify health care professional of all Rx or OTC medications, vitamins, or herbal products being taken and consult health care professional before taking any new medications.
- Advise patient to notify health care professional if rash or signs and symptoms of allergic reaction occur.
- Rep: Advise females of reproductive potential to use effective contraception and notify health care professional if pregnancy is planned or suspected, or if breast feeding. If pregnancy is detected, discontinue medication as soon as possible.

Evaluation/Desired Outcomes

- Resolution of fungal infections.

HIGH ALERT

warfarin (war-fa-rin)

Coumadin, Jantoven

Classification
Therapeutic: anticoagulants
Pharmacologic: coumarins

Indications

Prophylaxis and treatment of: Venous thrombosis, Pulmonary embolism, Atrial fibrillation with embolization. Management of myocardial infarction: Decreases risk of death, Decreases risk of subsequent MI, Decreases risk of future thromboembolic events. Prevention of thrombus formation and embolization after prosthetic valve placement.

Action

Interferes with hepatic synthesis of vitamin K-dependent clotting factors (II, VII, IX, and X). **Therapeutic Effects:** Prevention of thromboembolic events.

Pharmacokinetics

Absorption: Well absorbed from the GI tract after oral administration.

Distribution: Crosses the placenta but does not enter breast milk.

Protein Binding: 99%.

Metabolism and Excretion: Metabolized by the liver.

Half-life: 42 hr.

TIME/ACTION PROFILE (effects on coagulation tests)

ROUTE	ONSET	PEAK	DURATION
PO	36–72 hr	5–7 days†	2–5 days‡

†At a constant dose
‡After discontinuation

Contraindications/Precautions

Contraindicated in: Uncontrolled bleeding; Open wounds; Active ulcer disease; Recent brain, eye, or spinal cord injury or surgery; Severe liver or kidney disease; Uncontrolled hypertension; OB: Crosses placenta and may cause fatal hemorrhage in the fetus. May also cause congenital malformation.

Use Cautiously in: Malignancy; Patients with history of ulcer, liver disease, or acute kidney injury; History of poor compliance; Asian patients or those who carry the CYP2C9*2 allele and/or the CYP2C9*3 allele, or with the VKORC1 AA genotype (↑ risk of bleeding with standard dosing; lower initial doses should be considered); Geri: Due to greater than expected anticoagulant response, initiate and maintain at lower doses; Rep: Women of reproductive potential; Pedi: Has been used safely but may require more frequent PT/INR assessments.

Adverse Reactions/Side Effects

Derm: dermal necrosis. **GI:** cramps, nausea. **GU:** CALCIPHYLAXIS. **Hemat:** BLEEDING. **Misc:** fever.

Interactions

Drug-Drug: Androgens, capecitabine, cefotetan, chloramphenicol, clopidogrel, disulfiram, fluconazole, fluoroquinolones, itraconazole, metronidazole (including vaginal use), **thrombolytics, eptifibatide, tirofiban, sulfonamides, quinidine, quinine, NSAIDs, valproates,** and **aspirin** may ↑ the response to warfarin and ↑ the risk of bleeding. Chronic use of **acetaminophen** may ↑ the risk of bleeding. Chronic **alcohol** ingestion may ↓ action of warfarin; if chronic **alcohol** abuse results in significant liver damage, action of warfarin may be ↑ due to ↓ production of clotting factor. Acute **alcohol** ingestion may ↑ action of warfarin. **Barbiturates, carbamazepine, rifampin,** and **hormonal contraceptives containing estrogen** may ↓ the anticoagulant response to warfarin. **Many other drugs** may affect the activity of warfarin.

Drug-Natural Products: St. John's wort ↓ effect. ↑ bleeding risk with **anise, arnica, chamomile, clove, dong quai, fenugreek, feverfew, garlic, ginger, ginkgo, Panax ginseng, licorice,** and others.

Drug-Food: Ingestion of large quantities of **foods high in vitamin K content** (see list in Appendix K) may antagonize the anticoagulant effect of warfarin.

Route/Dosage

PO (Adults): 2–5 mg/day for 2–4 days; then adjust daily dose by results of INR. Initiate therapy with lower doses in geriatric or debilitated patients or in Asian patients or those with CYP2C9*2 and/or CYP2C9*3 alleles or VKORC1 AA genotype.

PO (Children >1 mo): *Initial loading dose*—0.2 mg/kg (maximum dose: 10 mg) for 2–4 days then adjust daily dose by results of INR, use 0.1 mg/kg if liver dysfunction is present. *Maintenance dose range*—0.05–0.34 mg/kg/day.

Availability (generic available)

Tablets: 1 mg, 2 mg, 2.5 mg, 3 mg, 4 mg, 5 mg, 6 mg, 7.5 mg, 10 mg. **Cost:** *Generic*—1 mg $10.83/100, 2 mg $10.83/100, 2.5 mg $10.83/100, 3 mg $10.83/100, 4 mg $10.83/100, 5 mg $8.52/100, 6 mg $10.64/100, 7.5 mg $10.83/100, 10 mg $10.83/100.

NURSING IMPLICATIONS

Assessment

- Assess for signs of bleeding and hemorrhage (bleeding gums; nosebleed; unusual bruising; tarry, black stools; hematuria; fall in hematocrit or BP; guaiac-positive stools, urine, or nasogastric aspirate).

W

- Assess for evidence of additional or increased thrombosis. Symptoms depend on area of involvement.
- ***Lab Test Considerations:*** Monitor PT, INR and other clotting factors frequently during therapy; monitor more frequently in patients with renal impairment. Therapeutic PT ranges 1.3–1.5 times greater than control; however, the INR, a standardized system that provides a common basis for communicating and interpreting PT results, is usually referenced. Normal INR (not on anticoagulants) is 0.8–1.2. An INR of 2.5–3.5 is recommended for patients at very high risk of embolization (for example, patients with mitral valve replacement and ventricular hypertrophy). Lower levels are acceptable when risk is lower. Heparin may affect the PT/INR; draw blood for PT/INR in patients receiving both heparin and warfarin at least 5 hr after the IV bolus dose, 4 hr after cessation of IV infusion, or 24 hr after subcut heparin injection. Asian patients and those who carry the CYP2C9*2 allele and/or the CYP2C9*3 allele, or those with VKORC1 AA genotype may require more frequent monitoring and lower doses.
- Geri: Patients over 60 yr exhibit greater than expected PT/INR response. Monitor for side effects at lower therapeutic ranges.
- Pedi: Achieving and maintaining therapeutic PT/INR ranges may be more difficult in pediatric patients. Assess PT/INR levels more frequently.
- Monitor hepatic function and CBC before and periodically throughout therapy.
- Monitor stool and urine for occult blood before and periodically during therapy.
- ***Toxicity and Overdose:*** Withholding 1 or more doses of warfarin is usually sufficient if INR is excessively elevated or if minor bleeding occurs. If overdose occurs or anticoagulation needs to be immediately reversed, the antidote is vitamin K (phytonadione, Aquamephyton). Administration of whole blood or plasma also may be required in severe bleeding because of the delayed onset of vitamin K.

Implementation

- ***High Alert:*** Do not confuse Coumadin (warfarin) with Avandia (rosiglitazone) or Cardura (doxazosin). Do not confuse Jantoven (warfarin) with Janumet (sitagliptin/metformin) or Januvia (sitagliptin).
- Because of the large number of medications capable of significantly altering warfarin's effects, careful monitoring is recommended when new agents are started or other agents are discontinued. Interactive potential should be evaluated for all new medications (Rx, OTC, and herbal products).
- **PO:** Administer medication at same time each day. Medication requires 3–5 days to reach effective levels; usually begun while patient is still on heparin.
- Do not interchange brands; potencies may not be equivalent.

Patient/Family Teaching

- Instruct patient to take medication as directed. Take missed doses as soon as remembered that day; do not double doses. Inform health care professional of missed doses at time of checkup or lab tests. Inform patients that anticoagulant effect may persist for 2–5 days following discontinuation. Advise patient to read *Medication Guide* before starting therapy and with each Rx refill in case of changes.
- Review foods high in vitamin K (see Appendix K). Patient should have consistent limited intake of these foods, as vitamin K is the antidote for warfarin, and alternating intake of these foods will cause PT levels to fluctuate. Advise patient to avoid cranberry juice or products during therapy.
- Caution patient to avoid IM injections and activities leading to injury. Instruct patient to use a soft toothbrush, not to floss, and to shave with an electric razor during warfarin therapy. Advise patient that venipunctures and injection sites require application of pressure to prevent bleeding or hematoma formation.
- Advise patient to report any symptoms of unusual bleeding or bruising (bleeding gums; nosebleed; black, tarry stools; hematuria; excessive menstrual flow) and pain, color, or temperature change to any area of your body to health care professional immediately. Patients with a deficiency in protein C and/or S mediated anticoagulant response may be at greater risk for tissue necrosis.
- Instruct patient not to drink alcohol or take other Rx, OTC, or herbal products, especially those containing aspirin or NSAIDs, or to start or stop any new medications during warfarin therapy without advice of health care professional.
- Advise patient to notify health care professional if pregnancy is planned or suspected or if breast feeding.
- Instruct patient to carry identification describing medication regimen at all times and to inform all health care personnel caring for patient on anticoagulant therapy before lab tests, treatment, or surgery.
- Emphasize the importance of frequent lab tests to monitor coagulation factors.

Evaluation/Desired Outcomes

- Prolonged PT (1.3–2.0 times the control; may vary with indication) or INR of 2–4.5 without signs of hemorrhage.

BEERS

zaleplon (za-lep-lon)

Sonata

Classification

Therapeutic: sedative/hypnotics

Schedule IV

Indications

Short-term management of insomnia in patients unable to get at least 4 hr of sleep; especially useful in sleep initiation disorders.

Action

Produces CNS depression by binding to GABA receptors in the CNS. Has no analgesic properties. **Therapeutic Effects:** Induction of sleep.

Pharmacokinetics

Absorption: Rapidly absorbed following oral administration.

Distribution: Enters breast milk.

Metabolism and Excretion: Extensively metabolized in the liver (mostly by aldehyde oxidase and some by CYP 450 3A4 enzymes).

Half-life: Unknown.

TIME/ACTION PROFILE

ROUTE	ONSET	PEAK	DURATION
PO	within min	unknown	3–4 hr

Contraindications/Precautions

Contraindicated in: Hypersensitivity; History of experiencing complex sleep behaviors with zaleplon; Severe hepatic impairment; OB, Lactation: Pregnancy or lactation.

Use Cautiously in: Mild to moderate hepatic impairment, weight ≤50 kg, or concurrent cimetidine therapy (initiate therapy at lowest dose); Impaired respiratory function; History of suicide attempt; Pedi: Safety not established; Geri: ↑ risk of cognitive impairment and falls. Initial dose ↓ recommended.

Adverse Reactions/Side Effects

CNS: COMPLEX SLEEP BEHAVIORS (including sleep driving, sleep walking, or engaging in other activities while sleeping), abnormal thinking, amnesia, anxiety, behavior changes, depersonalization, dizziness, drowsiness, hallucinations, headache, impaired memory (briefly following dose), impaired psychomotor function (briefly following dose), malaise, nightmares, vertigo, weakness. **CV:** peripheral edema. **Derm:** photosensitivity. **EENT:** abnormal vision, ear pain, epistaxis, hearing sensitivity, ocular pain, altered sense of smell. **GI:** abdominal pain, anorexia, colitis, dyspepsia, nausea. **GU:** dysmenorrhea. **Neuro:** hyperesthesia, paresthesia, tremor. **Misc:** fever.

Interactions

Drug-Drug: Cimetidine ↓ metabolism and ↑ effects (initiate therapy at a lower dose). Additive CNS depression with other **CNS depressants** including **alcohol**, **antihistamines**, **opioid analgesics**, other **sedative/hypnotics**, **phenothiazines**, and **tricyclic antidepressants**. Effects may be ↓ by drugs that induce the CYP 450 3A4 enzyme system including **rifampin**, **phenytoin**, **carbamazepine**, and **phenobarbital**.

Drug-Natural Products: Concomitant use of **kava-kava**, **valerian**, **chamomile**, or **hops** can ↑ CNS depression.

Drug-Food: Concurrent ingestion of a **high-fat meal** slows the rate of absorption.

Route/Dosage

PO (Adults <65 yr): 10 mg (range 5–20 mg) at bedtime.

PO (Geriatric Patients or Patients <50 kg): Initiate therapy at 5 mg at bedtime (not to exceed 10 mg at bedtime).

Hepatic Impairment

PO (Adults): Initiate therapy at 5 mg at bedtime (not to exceed 10 mg at bedtime).

Availability (generic available)

Capsules: 5 mg, 10 mg.

NURSING IMPLICATIONS

Assessment

- Assess mental status, sleep patterns, and potential for abuse prior to administering this medication. Zaleplon is used to treat short-term difficulty in falling asleep; decreases time to sleep onset. May not increase total sleep time or decrease number of wakenings after falling asleep. Prolonged use of >7–10 days may lead to physical and psychological dependence. Limit amount of drug available to the patient.
- Assess alertness at time of peak effect. Notify health care professional if desired sedation does not occur.
- Assess patient for pain. Medicate as needed. Untreated pain decreases sedative effects.

Implementation

- Do not confuse Sonata with Soriatane.
- Before administering, reduce external stimuli and provide comfort measures to increase effectiveness of medication.
- Protect patient from injury. Supervise ambulation and transfer of patients after administration. Remove cigarettes. Side rails should be raised and call bell within reach at all times.
- **PO:** Tablets should be swallowed whole with full glass of water immediately before bedtime or after

Z

going to bed and experiencing difficulty falling asleep. Do not administer with or immediately after a high-fat or heavy meal.

Patient/Family Teaching

- Instruct patient to take zaleplon as directed. Do not take more than the amount prescribed because of the habit-forming potential. Not recommended for use longer than 7–10 days. Rebound insomnia (1–2 nights) may occur when stopped. If used for 2 wk or longer, abrupt withdrawal may result in dysphoria, insomnia, abdominal or muscle cramps, vomiting, sweating, tremors, and seizures.
- Because of rapid onset, advise patient to go to bed immediately after taking zaleplon.
- May cause daytime drowsiness or dizziness. Advise patient to avoid driving or other activities requiring alertness until response to this medication is known.
- Inform patient that amnesia may occur, but can be avoided if zaleplon is only taken when patient is able to get >4 hr sleep.
- Caution patient that complex sleep-related behaviors (sleep-driving, making phone calls, preparing and eating food, having sex, sleep walking) may occur while asleep. Inform patient to notify health care professional if sleep-related behaviors, (may include sleep-driving—driving while not fully awake after ingestion of a sedative-hypnotic product, with no memory of the event) occur.
- Caution patient to avoid concurrent use of alcohol or other CNS depressants.
- Advise females of reproductive potential to notify health care professional if pregnancy is planned or suspected, or if breast feeding.

Evaluation/Desired Outcomes

- Improved ability to fall asleep; decreased time to sleep onset.

zidovudine (zye-**doe**-vue-deen)

Retrovir

Classification

Therapeutic: antiretrovirals

Pharmacologic: nucleoside reverse transcriptase inhibitors

Indications

HIV infection (with other antiretrovirals). Reduction of maternal/fetal transmission of HIV. **Unlabeled Use:** Chemoprophylaxis after occupational exposure to HIV.

Action

Following intracellular conversion to its active form, inhibits viral RNA synthesis by inhibiting the enzyme DNA polymerase (reverse transcriptase). Prevents viral replication. **Therapeutic Effects:** Virustatic action against selected retroviruses. Slowed progression and decreased sequelae of HIV infection. Decreased viral load and improved CD4 cell counts. Decreased transmission of HIV to infants born to HIV-infected mothers.

Pharmacokinetics

Absorption: Well absorbed following oral administration.

Distribution: Widely distributed; enters the CNS. Crosses the placenta.

Metabolism and Excretion: Mostly (75%) metabolized by the liver; 15–20% excreted unchanged by the kidneys.

Half-life: 1 hr.

TIME/ACTION PROFILE (blood levels)

ROUTE	ONSET	PEAK	DURATION
PO	unknown	0.5–1.5 hr	4 hr
IV	rapid	end of infusion	4 hr

Contraindications/Precautions

Contraindicated in: Hypersensitivity; Lactation: Breast feeding not recommended in women with HIV.

Use Cautiously in: ↓ bone marrow reserve (dose ↓ required for anemia or granulocytopenia); Women and obese patients (↑ risk of lactic acidosis and severe hepatomegaly); Severe hepatic or renal disease (dose modification may be required); Latex allergy (IV only); Geri: Select dose carefully due to potential for age-related ↓ in hepatic, renal, or cardiac function.

Adverse Reactions/Side Effects

CNS: SEIZURES, headache, weakness, anxiety, confusion, ↓ mental acuity, dizziness, insomnia, mental depression, restlessness, syncope. **Derm:** nail pigmentation. **Endo:** gynecomastia, lipoatrophy. **F and E:** LACTIC ACIDOSIS. **GI:** HEPATOMEGALY (with steatosis), PANCREATITIS, abdominal pain, diarrhea, nausea, anorexia, dyspepsia, oral mucosa pigmentation, vomiting. **Hemat:** anemia, granulocytopenia, pure red-cell aplasia, thrombocytosis. **MS:** back pain, myopathy. **Neuro:** tremor. **Misc:** immune reconstitution syndrome.

Interactions

Drug-Drug: ↑ bone marrow depression with other **agents having bone marrow–depressing properties, antineoplastics, radiation therapy**, or **ganciclovir**. ↑ neurotoxicity may occur with **acyclovir**. Toxicity may be ↑ by concurrent administration of **probenecid** or **fluconazole**. Levels are ↓ by **clarithromycin**.

Route/Dosage

Management of HIV Infection

PO (Adults): 100 mg every 4 hr while awake or 200 mg 3 times daily or 300 mg twice daily (depends on combination and clinical situation).

PO (Children 4 wk–<18 yr): *4–8.9 kg*—12 mg/kg twice daily or 8 mg/kg 3 times daily; *9–29.9 kg*—9

mg/kg twice daily or 6 mg/kg 3 times daily; ≥*30 kg*—300 mg twice daily or 200 mg 3 times daily.
IV (Adults and Children >12 yr): 1 mg/kg every 4 hr. Change to oral therapy as soon as possible.
IV (Children): 120 mg/m² every 6 hr (not to exceed 160 mg/dose) or 20 mg/m²/hr as a continuous infusion.

Prevention of Maternal/Fetal Transmission of HIV Infection

PO (Adults >14 wk Pregnant): 100 mg 5 times daily until onset of labor.
IV (Adults during Labor and Delivery): 2 mg/kg over 1 hr, then continuous infusion of 1 mg/kg/hr until umbilical cord is clamped.
PO (Neonates): 2 mg/kg every 6 hr until 6 wk of agee.
IV (Neonates): 1.5 mg/kg every 6 hr until 6 wk of age.

Availability (generic available)

Capsules: 100 mg. **Oral syrup:** 50 mg/5 mL. **Solution for injection (requires dilution):** 10 mg/mL. **Tablets:** 300 mg. ***In combination with:*** lamivudine (Combivir); abacavir and lamivudine (Trizivir); see Appendix B.

NURSING IMPLICATIONS

Assessment

- Assess patient for change in severity of symptoms of HIV and for symptoms of opportunistic infections during therapy.
- ***Lab Test Considerations:*** Monitor viral load and CD4 counts prior to and periodically during therapy.
- Monitor CBC every 2 wk during the first 8 wk of therapy in patients with advanced HIV disease, and decrease to every 4 wk after the first 2 mo if zidovudine is well tolerated or monthly during the first 3 mo and every 3 mo thereafter unless indicated in patients who are asymptomatic or have early symptoms. Commonly causes granulocytopenia and anemia. Anemia may occur 2–4 wk after initiation of therapy. Anemia may respond to epoetin administration (see epoetin monograph). Granulocytopenia usually occurs after 6–8 wk of therapy. Consider dose reduction, discontinuation of therapy, or blood transfusions if hemoglobin is <7.5 g/dL or reduction of >25% from baseline and/or granulocyte count is <750/mm³ or reduction of >50% from baseline. Therapy may be gradually resumed when bone marrow recovery is evident.
- May cause ↑ serum AST, ALT, and alkaline phosphatase levels. Lactic acidosis may occur with hepatic toxicity, causing hepatic steatosis; may be fatal, especially in women.
- Monitor serum amylase, lipase, and triglycerides periodically during therapy. Elevated serum levels may indicate pancreatitis and require discontinuation.

Implementation

- Do not confuse Retrovir (zidovudine) with ritonavir.
- **PO:** Administer doses around the clock.
- For neonates, use a syringe with 0.1-mL graduations to ensure accurate dosing of the syrup.
- **IV:** Patient should receive the IV infusion only until oral therapy can be administered.

IV Administration

- **Intermittent Infusion:** *Retrovir* vial stoppers contain latex; may cause allergic reactions in latex-sensitive individuals. ***Diluent:*** Remove calculated dose from the vial and dilute with D5W or 0.9% NaCl. Do not use solutions that are discolored. Stable for 8 hr at room temperature or 24 hr if refrigerated. ***Concentration:*** Not to exceed 4 mg/mL. ***Rate:*** Infuse at a constant rate over 1 hr or over 30 min in neonates. Avoid rapid infusion or bolus injection.
- **Continuous Infusion:** Has also been administered via continuous infusion.
- **Y-Site Compatibility:** acyclovir, alemtuzumab, allopurinol, amifostine, amikacin, aminocaproic acid, amiodarone, amphotericin B lipid complex, amphotericin B liposome, anidulafungin, argatroban, azithromycin, aztreonam, bivalirudin, bleomycin, carboplatin, carmustine, caspofungin, cefepime, ceftazidime, ceftriaxone, cisatracurium, cisplatin, clindamycin, cyclophosphamide, cytarabine, dactinomycin, daptomycin, daunorubicin hydrochloride, dexamethasone, dexmedetomidine, diltiazem, dobutamine, docetaxel, dopamine, doxacurium, doxorubicin hydrochloride, doxorubicin liposome, epirubicin, eptifibatide, ertapenem, erythromycin lactobionate, etoposide, etoposide phosphate, fenoldopam, filgrastim, fluconazole, fludarabine, fluorouracil, foscarnet, fosphenytoin, gemcitabine, gentamicin, granisetron, heparin, hydromorphone, idarubicin, ifosfamide, imipenem/cilastatin, irinotecan, leucovorin calcium, levofloxacin, linezolid, lorazepam, melphalan, meperidine, meropenem, mesna, methotrexate, metoclopramide, metronidazole, milrinone, mitoxantrone, morphine, mycophenolate, nafcillin, nicardipine, octreotide, ondansetron, oxacillin, oxaliplatin, oxytocin, paclitaxel, palonosetron, pamidronate, pancuronium, pantoprazole, pemetrexed, pentamidine, phenylephrine, piperacillin/tazobactam, potassium acetate, potassium chloride, quinapristin/dalfopristin, ranitidine, remifentanil, rituxumab, rocuronium, sargramostim, sodium acetate, tacrolimus, thiotepa, tigecycline, tirofiban, tobramycin, topotecan, trastuzumab, trimethoprim/sulfamethoxazole, vancomycin, vasopressin, vecuronium, vinblastine, vincristine, vinorelbine, voriconazole, zoledronic acid.
- **Y-Site Incompatibility:** dexrazoxane.
- **Additive Incompatibility:** blood products or protein solutions, dexrazoxane.

Z

Patient/Family Teaching

- Instruct patient to take zidovudine as directed, around the clock, even if sleep is interrupted. Emphasize the importance of compliance with therapy, not taking more than prescribed amount, and not discontinuing without consulting health care professional. Take missed doses as soon as remembered unless almost time for next dose; do not double doses. Inform patient that long-term effects of zidovudine are unknown at this time.
- Instruct patient that zidovudine should not be shared with others.
- Zidovudine may cause dizziness or fainting. Caution patient to avoid driving or other activities requiring alertness until response to medication is known.
- Inform patient that zidovudine does not cure HIV and does not reduce the risk of transmission of HIV to others through sexual contact or blood contamination. Caution patient to use a condom during sexual contact and avoid sharing needles or donating blood to prevent spreading the AIDS virus to others.
- Instruct patient to notify health care professional promptly if fever, sore throat, signs of infection, muscle weakness, or shortness of breath occurs. Caution patient to avoid crowds and persons with known infections. Instruct patient to use soft toothbrush, to use caution when using toothpicks or dental floss, and to have dental work done prior to therapy or deferred until blood counts return to normal. Patient should also notify health care professional immediately if shortness of breath, muscle weakness, muscle aches, symptoms of hepatitis or pancreatitis, or other unexpected reactions occur.
- Advise patient to notify health care professional of all Rx or OTC medications, vitamins, or herbal products being taken and to consult with health care professional before taking other medications.
- Inform patient that redistribution and accumulation of body fat may occur, causing central obesity, dorsocervical fat enlargement (buffalo hump), peripheral wasting, breast enlargement, and cushingoid appearance. The cause and long-term effects are not known.
- Rep: Advise patient to notify health care professional if pregnancy is planned or suspected or if breast feeding. Advise patient taking oral contraceptives to use a nonhormonal method of birth control during therapy. Encourage pregnant women to enroll in the Antiretroviral Pregnancy Registry by calling 1-800-258-4263.
- Emphasize the importance of regular follow-up exams and blood counts to determine progress and monitor for side effects.

Evaluation/Desired Outcomes

- Decrease in viral load and increase in CD4 counts in patients with HIV.
- Delayed progression of AIDS and decreased opportunistic infections in patients with HIV.
- Reduction of maternal/fetal transmission of HIV.

BEERS

ziprasidone (zi-pra-si-done)

Geodon, Zeldox

Classification
Therapeutic: antipsychotics, mood stabilizers
Pharmacologic: piperazine derivatives

Indications

Schizophrenia; IM form is reserved for control of acutely agitated patients. Treatment of acute manic or mixed episodes associated with Bipolar I Disorder (oral only). Maintenance treatment of Bipolar I Disorder (as adjunct to lithium or valproate) (oral only).

Action

Effects probably mediated by antagonism of dopamine type 2 (D2) and serotonin type 2 (5-HT_2). Also antagonizes α_2 adrenergic receptors. **Therapeutic Effects:** Diminished schizophrenic behavior.

Pharmacokinetics

Absorption: 60% absorbed following oral administration; 100% absorbed from IM sites.
Distribution: Unknown.
Protein Binding: 99%; potential for drug interactions due to drug displacement is minimal.
Metabolism and Excretion: 99% metabolized by the liver; <1% excreted unchanged in urine.
Half-life: *PO*—7 hr; *IM*—2–5 hr.

TIME/ACTION PROFILE (blood levels)

ROUTE	ONSET	PEAK	DURATION
PO	within hrs	1–3 days†	unknown
IM	rapid	60 min	unknown

†Steady state achieved following continuous use.

Contraindications/Precautions

Contraindicated in: Hypersensitivity; History of QT prolongation (persistent QTc measurements >500 msec), arrhythmias, recent MI or uncompensated heart failure; Concurrent use of other drugs known to prolong the QT interval including quinidine, dofetilide, sotalol, other class Ia and III antiarrhythmics, pimozide, sotalol, thioridazine, chlorpromazine, pentamidine, arsenic trioxide, mefloquine, dolasetron, tacrolimus, droperidol, and moxifloxacin; Hypokalemia or hypomagnesemia; Lactation: Discontinue drug or bottle feed.
Use Cautiously in: Concurrent diuretic therapy or diarrhea (may ↑ the risk of hypotension, hypokalemia, or hypomagnesemia); Significant hepatic impairment; History of cardiovascular or cerebrovascular disease; Hypotension, concurrent antihypertensive therapy, dehydration, or hypovolemia (may ↑ risk of orthostatic hypotension); Patients at risk for aspiration pneumonia or falls; History of suicide attempt; OB: Neonates at ↑ risk for extrapyramidal symptoms and withdrawal after

delivery when exposed during the 3rd trimester; use only if maternal benefit outweighs risk to fetus; Pedi: Safety not established; Geri: Alzheimer's dementia or age >65 yr (may ↑ risk of seizures). Geriatric patients (may require ↓ doses; ↑ risk of mortality, stroke, and transient ischemic attack in elderly patients treated for dementia-related psychosis).

Adverse Reactions/Side Effects

CNS: NEUROLEPTIC MALIGNANT SYNDROME, seizures, dizziness, drowsiness, restlessness, extrapyramidal reactions, syncope, tardive dyskinesia. **CV:** QT INTERVAL PROLONGATION, orthostatic hypotension. **Derm:** DRUG REACTION WITH EOSINOPHILIA AND SYSTEMIC SYMPTOMS (DRESS), STEVENS-JOHNSON SYNDROME, rash, urticaria. **Endo:** galactorrhea, hyperglycemia, hyperlipidemia, weight gain. **GI:** constipation, diarrhea, nausea, dysphagia. **GU:** amenorrhea, impotence. **Hemat:** AGRANULOCYTOSIS, leukopenia, neutropenia. **Resp:** cough, rhinorrhea.

Interactions

Drug-Drug: Concurrent use of **quinidine, dofetilide, other class Ia and III antiarrhythmics, pimozide, sotalol, thioridazine, chlorpromazine, pentamidine, arsenic trioxide, mefloquine, dolasetron, tacrolimus, droperidol, moxifloxacin,** or other agents that prolong the QT interval may result in potentially life-threatening adverse drug reactions (concurrent use contraindicated). Additive CNS depression may occur with **alcohol, antidepressants, antihistamines, opioid analgesics,** or **sedative/hypnotics**. Blood levels and effectiveness may be ↓ by **carbamazepine**. Blood levels and effects may be ↑ by **ketoconazole**.

Route/Dosage

Schizophrenia

PO (Adults): 20 mg twice daily initially; dose increments may be made at 2-day intervals up to 80 mg twice daily.

IM (Adults): 10–20 mg as needed up to 40 mg/day; may be given as 10 mg every 2 hr or 20 mg every 4 hr.

Acute Manic or Mixed Episodes Associated with Bipolar I Disorder

PO (Adults): 40 mg twice on first day, then 60 or 80 mg twice daily on 2nd day, then 40–80 mg twice daily.

Maintenance Treatment of Bipolar I Disorder (as adjunct to lithium or valproate)

PO (Adults): Continue same dose on which patient was initially stabilized (range: 40–80 mg twice daily).

Availability (generic available)

Capsules: 20 mg, 40 mg, 60 mg, 80 mg. **Cost:** *Generic*—20 mg $380.02/180, 40 mg $544.16/180, 60 mg $451.99/180, 80 mg $451.99/180. **Lyophilized powder for injection (requires reconstitution):** 20 mg/vial.

NURSING IMPLICATIONS

Assessment

- Monitor patient's mental status (orientation, mood, behavior) prior to and periodically during therapy.
- Assess weight and BMI initially and periodically during therapy.
- Monitor BP (sitting, standing, lying) and pulse rate prior to and frequently during initial dose titration. Patients found to have persistent QTc measurements of >500 msec should have ziprasidone discontinued. Patients who experience dizziness, palpitations, or syncope may require further evaluation (i.e., Holter monitoring).
- Assess for rash during therapy. May be treated with antihistamines or corticosteroids. Usually resolves upon discontinuation of ziprasidone. Medication should be discontinued if no alternative etiology for rash is found. May cause Stevens-Johnson syndrome or DRESS. Discontinue therapy if severe or if accompanied with fever, general malaise, fatigue, muscle or joint aches, blisters, oral lesions, conjunctivitis, hepatitis and/or eosinophilia.
- Observe carefully when administering medication to ensure medication is actually taken and not hoarded or cheeked.
- Monitor for onset of akathisia (restlessness or desire to keep moving) and extrapyramidal side effects (*parkinsonian*—difficulty speaking or swallowing, loss of balance control, pill rolling of hands, mask-like face, shuffling gait, rigidity, tremors and dystonic muscle spasms, twisting motions, twitching, inability to move eyes, weakness of arms or legs) every 2 mo during therapy and 8–12 wk after therapy has been discontinued. Notify health care professional if these symptoms occur, as reduction in dose or discontinuation of medication may be necessary. Trihexyphenidyl or benztropine may be used to control these symptoms.
- Although not yet reported for ziprasidone, monitor for possible tardive dyskinesia (uncontrolled rhythmic movement of mouth, face, and extremities, lip smacking or puckering, puffing of cheeks, uncontrolled chewing, rapid or worm-like movements of tongue). Report these symptoms immediately; may be irreversible.
- Monitor frequency and consistency of bowel movements. Increasing bulk and fluids in the diet may help to minimize constipation.
- Ziprasidone lowers the seizure threshold. Institute seizure precautions for patients with history of seizure disorder.

Z

- Monitor for development of neuroleptic malignant syndrome (fever, respiratory distress, tachycardia, seizures, diaphoresis, hypertension or hypotension, pallor, tiredness). Notify health care professional immediately if these symptoms occur.
- Monitor for symptoms related to hyperprolactinemia (menstrual abnormalities, galactorrhea, sexual dysfunction).
- Assess for falls risk. Drowsiness, orthostatic hypotension, and motor and sensory instability increase risk. Institute prevention if indicated.
- ***Lab Test Considerations:*** Monitor serum potassium and magnesium prior to and periodically during therapy. Patients with low potassium or magnesium should have levels treated and checked prior to resuming therapy. Obtain fasting blood glucose and cholesterol levels initially and periodically during therapy.
- Monitor CBC frequently during initial mo of therapy in patients with pre-existing or history of low WBC. May cause leukopenia, neutropenia, or agranulocytosis. Discontinue therapy if this occurs.
- Monitor serum prolactin prior to and periodically during therapy. May cause ↑ serum prolactin levels.

Implementation

- Dose adjustments should be made at intervals of no less than 2 days. Usually patients should be observed for several wk before dose titration.
- Patients on parenteral therapy should be converted to oral doses as soon as possible.
- **PO:** Administer capsules with food or milk to decrease gastric irritation. Swallow capsules whole; do not open.
- **IM:** Add 1.2 mL of sterile water for injection to the vial; shake vigorously until all drug is dissolved for a concentration of 20 mg/mL. Discard unused portion. Do not mix with other products or solutions. Do not administer solutions that are discolored or contain particulate matter.

Patient/Family Teaching

- Instruct patient to take medication as directed, at the same time each day. Do not discontinue medication without discussing with health care professional, even if feeling well. Patients on long-term therapy may need to discontinue gradually.
- Inform patient of possibility of extrapyramidal symptoms. Instruct patient to report these symptoms immediately.
- Advise patient to change positions slowly to minimize orthostatic hypotension. Protect from falls.
- May cause seizures and drowsiness. Caution patient to avoid driving or other activities requiring alertness until response to medication is known.
- Advise patient to notify health care professional of all Rx or OTC medications, vitamins, or herbal products being taken and to consult with health care professional before taking other medications. Caution patient to avoid concurrent use of alcohol and other CNS depressants.
- Advise patient to notify health care professional of medication regimen prior to treatment or surgery.
- Instruct patient to notify health care professional promptly if dizziness, loss of consciousness, palpitations, menstrual abnormalities, galactorrhea or sexual dysfunction occur.
- Advise females of reproductive potential to notify health care professional if pregnancy is planned or suspected, and to avoid breast feeding during therapy.
- Advise patient of need for continued medical follow-up for psychotherapy, eye exams, and laboratory tests.

Evaluation/Desired Outcomes

- Decrease in acute excited, manic behavior.
- Decrease in positive (delusions, hallucinations) and negative symptoms (social withdrawal, flat, blunted affect) of schizophrenia.
- Management of signs and symptoms of Bipolar I Disorder.

zoledronic acid

(zoe-led-**dron**-ic **as**-id)

✱ Aclasta, Reclast, Zometa

Classification

Therapeutic: bone resorption inhibitors, electrolyte modifiers, hypocalcemics

Pharmacologic: biphosphonates

Indications

Hypercalcemia of malignancy (Zometa only). Multiple myeloma and metastatic bone lesions from solid tumors (Zometa only). Paget's disease (Reclast only). Treatment of osteoporosis in men (Reclast only). Treatment and prevention of osteoporosis in postmenopausal women (Reclast only). Treatment and prevention of glucocorticoid-induced osteoporosis in patients expected to be on glucocorticoids for at least 12 mo (Reclast only).

Action

Inhibits bone resorption. Inhibits increased osteoclast activity and skeletal calcium release induced by tumors. **Therapeutic Effects:** Decreased serum calcium. Decreased serum alkaline phosphatase. Decreased fractures, radiation/surgery to bone, or spinal cord compression in patients with multiple myeloma or metastatic bone lesions. Decreased hip, vertebral, or non-vertebral osteoporosis-related fractures in postmenopausal women. Increased bone mass in men, postmenopausal women, and patients on prolonged corticosteroid therapy.

Pharmacokinetics

Absorption: IV administration results in complete bioavailability.

Distribution: Unknown.
Metabolism and Excretion: Mostly excreted unchanged by the kidneys.
Half-life: 167 hr.

TIME/ACTION PROFILE (effect on serum calcium)

ROUTE	ONSET	PEAK	DURATION
IV	within 4 days	4–7 days	30 days

Contraindications/Precautions

Contraindicated in: Hypersensitivity to zoledronic acid or other bisphosphonates; Severe renal impairment (CCr <35 mL/min) or acute renal failure; Hypocalcemia (correct before administering); adequate supplemental calcium and vitamin D required; OB: Pregnancy (may cause fetal harm); Lactation: Lactation (may cause harm to infant).
Use Cautiously in: History of aspirin-induced asthma; Chronic renal impairment; Chronic renal impairment, concurrent use of diuretics or nephrotoxic drugs, or dehydration (↑ risk of renal impairment; correct deficits prior to use); Concurrent use of nephrotoxic drugs; Invasive dental procedures, cancer, receiving chemotherapy, corticosteroids, or angiogenesis inhibitors, undergoing radiation, poor oral hygiene, periodontal disease, dental disease, anemia, coagulopathy, infection, or poorly-fitting dentures (may ↑ risk of jaw osteonecrosis); Rep: Women of reproductive potential; Pedi: Potential for long-term retention in bone in children; use only if potential benefit outweighs potential risk; Geri: ↑ risk of renal impairment.

Adverse Reactions/Side Effects

CNS: agitation, anxiety, confusion, insomnia. **CV:** hypotension, chest pain, leg edema. **Derm:** STEVENS-JOHNSON SYNDROME, TOXIC EPIDERMAL NECROLYSIS, pruritus, rash. **EENT:** conjunctivitis. **F and E:** hypophosphatemia, hypocalcemia, hypokalemia, hypomagnesemia. **GI:** abdominal pain, constipation, diarrhea, nausea, vomiting, dysphagia. **GU:** ↓ fertility (females), renal impairment/failure. **Hemat:** anemia. **MS:** musculoskeletal pain, femur fractures, osteonecrosis (primarily of jaw). **Resp:** asthma exacerbation. **Misc:** fever, flu-like syndrome.

Interactions

Drug-Drug: Concurrent use of **loop diuretics, calcitonin,** or **aminoglycosides** ↑ risk of hypocalcemia. Concurrent use of **NSAIDs** may ↑ risk of nephrotoxicity.

Route/Dosage

Reclast

IV (Adults): *Paget's disease*—5 mg as a single dose (information regarding retreatment unknown); *Treatment of osteoporosis in men or postmenopausal women, treatment/prevention of glucocorticoid-induced osteoporosis*—5 mg once yearly; *Prevention of osteoporosis in postmenopausal women*—5 mg every 2 yr.

Zometa

IV (Adults): *Hypercalcemia of malignancy*—4 mg; may be repeated after 7 days; *Multiple myeloma and bone metastases from solid tumors*—4 mg every 3–4 wk (has been used for up to 15 mo).

Availability (generic available)

Premixed infusion (Reclast): 5 mg/100 mL. **Premixed infusion (Zometa):** 4 mg/100 mL. **Solution for injection (Zometa):** 0.8 mg/mL.

NURSING IMPLICATIONS

Assessment

- Monitor intake and output ratios. Initiate a vigorous saline hydration promptly and maintain a urine output of 2 L/day during therapy. Patients should be adequately hydrated, but avoid overhydration. Do not use diuretics prior to treatment of hypovolemia.
- Assess for acute-phase reaction (fever, mylagia, flu-like symptoms, headache, arthralgia). Usually occur within 3 days of dose and resolve within 3 days of onset, but may take 7–14 days to resolve; incidence decreases with repeat dosing.
- Perform a routine oral exam prior to initiation of therapy. Dental exam with appropriate preventative dentistry should be considered prior to therapy. Patients with history of tooth extraction, poor oral hygiene, gingival infections, diabetes, cancer, receiving radiation, anemia, coagulopathy, or use of a dental appliance or those taking immunosuppressive therapy, angiogenesis inhibitors, or systemic corticosteroids are at greater risk for osteonecrosis of the jaw.
- **Hypercalcemia:** Monitor symptoms of hypercalcemia (nausea, vomiting, anorexia, weakness, constipation, thirst, cardiac arrhythmias).
- Observe for evidence of hypocalcemia (paresthesia, muscle twitching, laryngospasm, Chvostek's or Trousseau's sign).
- **Paget's Disease:** Assess for symptoms of Paget's disease (bone pain, headache, decreased visual and auditory acuity, increased skull size) periodically during therapy.
- **Osteoporosis:** Assess patients via bone density study for low bone mass before and periodically during therapy.
- ***Lab Test Considerations:*** Obtain a negative pregnancy test before starting therapy.
- Monitor serum creatinine, calculated based on actual body weight using the Cockcroft-Gault formula, prior to each treatment. Patients with a normal serum creatinine prior to treatment, who develop an

Z

increase of 0.5 mg/dL within 2 wk of next dose should have next dose withheld until serum creatinine is within 10% of baseline value. Patients with an abnormal serum creatinine prior to treatment who have an increase of 1.0 mg/dL within 2 wk of next dose should have next dose withheld until serum creatinine is within 10% of baseline value.

- Assess serum calcium, phosphate, and magnesium before and periodically during therapy. If hypocalcemia, hypophosphatemia, or hypomagnesemia occur, temporary supplementation may be required. Hypocalcemia and vitamin D deficiency should be treated before initiating zoledronic acid therapy.
- Monitor CBC with differential and hemoglobin and hematocrit closely during therapy.
- *Paget's Disease:* Monitor serum alkaline phosphatase prior to and periodically during therapy to monitor effectiveness.

Implementation

- Vigorous saline hydration alone may be sufficient to treat mild, asymptomatic hypercalcemia. Adequate rehydration is required prior to administration.
- Patients on long-term therapy should have 1200 mg of oral calcium and 800–1000 units of Vitamin D each day.
- Patients treated for *Paget's disease* should receive 1500 mg elemental calcium and 800 IU of vitamin D daily, particularly during the 2 wk after dosing. Patients with osteoporosis should take 1200 mg of calcium and 800–1000 IU of Vitamin D daily. Patients with multiple myeloma and bone metastasis of solid tumors take an oral calcium supplement of 500 mg and a multiple vitamin containing 400 international units of vitamin D daily.
- Administration of acetaminophen or ibuprofen following administration may reduce the incidence of acute-phase reaction symptoms.

IV Administration

- **Intermittent Infusion:** ***Diluent:*** Reconstitute *Zometa* by adding 5 mL of sterile water for injection to each vial for a solution containing 4 mg of zoledronic acid. Medication must be completely dissolved prior to withdrawal of solution. Dilute 4-mg dose further with 100 mL of 0.9% NaCl or D5W. If not used immediately, may be refrigerated for up to 24 hr. *Reclast* comes ready to use 5 mg in 100-mL solution. If refrigerated, allow solution to reach room temperature prior to administration. Do not administer solution that is discolored or contains particulate matter. ***Rate:*** Administer as a single infusion over at least 15 min. Rapid infusions increase risk of renal deterioration and renal failure.
- **Y-Site Compatibility:** acyclovir, alfentanil, allopurinol, amifostine, amikacin, aminophylline, amiodarone, amphotericin B lipid complex, amphotericin B liposome, ampicillin, ampicillin/sulbactam, anidulafungin, argatroban, azithromycin, aztreonam, bivalirudin, bleomycin, bumetanide, buprenorphine, busulfan, butorphanol, carboplatin, carmustine, caspofungin, cefazolin, cefepime, cefotaxime, cefotetan, cefoxitin, ceftazidime, ceftriaxone, cefuroxime, chloramphenicol, chlorpromazine, ciprofloxacin, cisatracurium, cisplatin, clindamycin, cyclophosphamide, cyclosporine, cytarabine, dacarbazine, dactinomycin, daptomycin, daunorubicin hydrochloride, dexamethasone, dexmedetomidine, dexrazoxane, digoxin, diltiazem, diphenhydramine, dobutamine, docetaxel, dolasetron, dopamine, doxorubicin hydrochloride, doxorubicin liposomal, doxycycline, droperidol, enalaprilat, ephedrine, epinephrine, epirubicin, eptifibatide, ertapenem, erythromycin, esmolol, etoposide, etoposide phosphate, famotidine, fenoldopam, fentanyl, fluconazole, fludarabine, fluorouracil, foscarnet, fosphenytoin, furosemide, ganciclovir, gemcitabine, gentamicin, glycopyrrolate, granisetron, haloperidol, heparin, hydralazine, hydrocortisone, hydromorphone, idarubicin, ifosfamide, imipenem/cilastatin, insulin, regular, irinotecan, isoproterenol, ketorolac, labetalol, levofloxacin, lidocaine, linezolid, lorazepam, magnesium sulfate, mannitol, melphalan, meperidine, meropenem, mesna, methotrexate, methyldopate, methylprednisolone, metoclopramide, metoprolol, metronidazole, midazolam, milrinone, mitomycin, mitoxantrone, morphine, moxifloxacin, mycophenolate, nafcillin, nalbuphine, naloxone, nicardipine, nitroglycerin, nitroprusside, norepinephrine, octreotide, ondansetron, oxaliplatin, oxytocin, paclitaxel, pancuronium, pantoprazole, pemetrexed, pentamidine, pentobarbital, phenobarbital, phenylephrine, piperacillin/tazobactam, potassium acetate, potassium chloride, potassium phosphates, procainamide, prochlorperazine, promethazine, propranolol, quinupristin/dalfopristin, ranitidine, remifentanil, rocuronium, sodium acetate, sodium bicarbonate, sodium phosphates, streptozocin, succinylcholine, sufentanil, tacrolimus, theophylline, thiopental, thiotepa, tigecycline, tirofiban, tobramycin, topotecan, trimethoprim/sulfamethoxazole, vancomycin, vecuronium, verapamil, vinblastine, vincristine, vinorelbine, voriconazole, zidovudine.
- **Y-Site Incompatibility:** alemtuzumab, calcium-containing solutions, dantrolene, diazepam, phenytoin. Manufacturer recommends administration as a single infusion in a line separate from all other drugs.
- **Additive Incompatibility:** Do not mix with solutions containing calcium, such as Lactated Ringer's solution.

Patient/Family Teaching

- Explain the purpose of zoledronic acid to patient. Advise patient to read *Medication Guide* prior to each administration in case of changes.
- Advise patients of the importance of adequate hydration. Patient should be instructed to drink at least two glasses of water prior to receiving dose.

- Advise patient to notify health care professional of all Rx or OTC medications, vitamins, or herbal products being taken and to consult with health care professional before taking other medications.
- Advise patient to eat a balanced diet and consult health care professional about the need for supplemental calcium and vitamin D.
- Inform patient that severe musculoskeletal pain may occur within days, mo, or yr after starting zoledronic acid. Symptoms may resolve completely after discontinuation or slow or incomplete resolution may occur. Notify health care professional if severe pain occurs.
- Encourage patient to participate in regular exercise and to modify behaviors that increase the risk of osteoporosis (stop smoking, reduce alcohol consumption).
- Advise patient to notify health care professional if signs and symptoms if osteonecrosis of the jaw (pain, numbness, swelling of or drainage from the jaw, mouth, or teeth) or hypocalcemia (spasms, twitches, or cramps in muscles; numbness or tingling in fingers, toes, or around mouth) or thigh, hip, or groin pain occur.
- Advise patient to inform health care professional of zoledronic acid therapy prior to dental surgery.
- Rep: Advise females of reproductive potential use effective contraception and avoid breast feeding during and after therapy. May impair fertility in females.
- Emphasize the importance of lab tests to monitor progress.

Evaluation/Desired Outcomes

- Decrease in serum calcium.
- Decrease in serum alkaline phosphatase and the progression of Paget's disease.
- Reversal of the progression of osteoporosis with decreased fractures and other sequelae. Discontinuation after 3–5 yr should be considered for postmenopausal women with low risk for fractures.

ZOLMitriptan (zole-mi-**trip**-tan)

Zomig, Zomig-ZMT

Classification

Therapeutic: vascular headache suppressants

Pharmacologic: 5-HT_1 agonists

Indications

Acute treatment of migraine headache.

Action

Acts as an agonist at specific 5-HT_1 receptor sites in intracranial blood vessels and sensory trigeminal nerves. **Therapeutic Effects:** Cranial vessel vasoconstriction with resultant decrease in migraine headache.

Pharmacokinetics

Absorption: Well absorbed (40%) following oral and intranasal administration.

Distribution: Unknown.

Metabolism and Excretion: Mostly metabolized by the liver; some conversion to metabolites that are more active than zolmitriptan. 8% excreted unchanged in urine.

Half-life: 3 hr (for zolmitriptan and active metabolite).

TIME/ACTION PROFILE (relief of headache)

ROUTE	ONSET	PEAK	DURATION
PO	unknown	1.5 hr*	unknown
Intranasal	unknown	3 hr	unknown

*3 hr for orally disintegrating tablets.

Contraindications/Precautions

Contraindicated in: Hypersensitivity; Significant underlying heart disease (including ischemic heart disease, history of MI, coronary artery vasospasm, uncontrolled hypertension); Stroke or transient ischemic attack; Peripheral vascular disease (including, but not limited to ischemic bowel disease); Concurrent (or within 24 hr) use of other 5-HT agonists, ergotamine, or ergot-type medications; Concurrent (or within 2 wk) use of MAO inhibitors; Hemiplegic or basilar migraine; Symptomatic Wolff-Parkinson-White syndrome or other arrhythmias; Moderate-severe hepatic impairment (nasal spray only).

Use Cautiously in: Cardiovascular risk factors (hypertension, hypercholesterolemia, cigarette smoking, obesity, diabetes, strong family history, menopausal females or males >40 yr [use only if cardiovascular status has been evaluated and determined to be safe and 1st dose is administered under supervision]); Hepatic impairment (use lower doses of oral); OB: Safety not established; Lactation: Use while breast feeding only if benefit to patient outweighs potential risk to infant; Pedi: Children <18 yr (safety and effectiveness not established for PO); children <12 yr (safety and effectiveness not established for intranasal).

Adverse Reactions/Side Effects

CNS: dizziness, drowsiness, vertigo, weakness. **CV:** MI, angina, chest pain/pressure/tightness/heaviness, hypertension, palpitations. **Derm:** sweating, warm/cold sensation. **EENT:** throat pain/tightness/pressure. **GI:** dry mouth, dyspepsia, dysphagia, nausea. **MS:** myalgia, myasthenia. **Neuro:** hypesthesia, paresthesia. **Misc:** pain.

Interactions

Drug-Drug: Because of ↑ risk of cerebral vasospasm, avoid concurrent use of other **5-HT agonists (naratriptan, sumatriptan, rizatriptan)** and/or er-

Z

got-type preparations (dihydroergotamine). Concurrent use of **MAO inhibitors** ↑ blood levels and risk of toxicity (avoid use within 2 wk of MAO inhibitors). Blood levels may be ↑ by **hormonal contraceptives**. **Cimetidine** ↑ half-life of zolmitriptan and its active metabolite. ↑ risk of serotonin syndrome with **SSRIs**, **SNRIs**, **TCAs**, **triptans**, **meperidine**, **bupropion**, or **buspirone**; avoid concurrent use.

Drug-Natural Products: ↑ risk of serotinergic side effects including serotonin syndrome with **St. John's wort** and **SAMe**.

Route/Dosage

PO (Adults): 1.25–2.5 mg initially; if headache returns, dose may be repeated after 2 hr (not to exceed 10 mg/24 hr); *Concurrent cimetidine therapy*—Single dose not to exceed 2.5 mg (not to exceed 5 mg/24 hr).

Hepatic Impairment

PO (Adults): *Moderate-severe hepatic impairment (oral tablets only)*—1.25 mg initially; if headache returns, dose may be repeated after 2 hr (not to exceed 5 mg/24 hr).

Intranasal (Adults and Children ≥12 yr): Single 2.5 mg initially (maximum single dose = 5 mg); may be repeated after 2 hr (not to exceed 10 mg/24 hr); *Concurrent cimetidine therapy*—Single dose not to exceed 2.5 mg (not to exceed 5 mg/24 hr).

Availability (generic available)

Orally disintegrating tablets: 2.5 mg, 5 mg. **Nasal spray:** 2.5 mg/100 mcL unit-dose spray device (package of 6), 5 mg/100 mcL unit-dose spray device (package of 6). **Tablets:** 2.5 mg, 5 mg.

NURSING IMPLICATIONS

Assessment

- Assess pain location, intensity, duration, and associated symptoms (photophobia, phonophobia, nausea, vomiting) during migraine attack.
- Monitor for serotonin syndrome in patients taking SSRIs or SNRIs concurrently with zolmitriptan.

Implementation

- Do not confuse zolmitriptan with sumatriptan.
- **PO:** Initial dose is 2.5 mg. Lower doses can be achieved by breaking 2.5-mg tablet.
- Orally disintegrating tablets should be left in the package until use. Remove from the blister pouch. Do not push tablet through the blister; peel open the blister pack with dry hands and place tablet on tongue. Do not break orally disintegrating tablet. Tablet will dissolve rapidly and be swallowed with saliva. No liquid is needed to take the orally disintegrating tablet.
- **Intranasal:** Remove cap from nasal spray. Hold upright and block one nostril. Tilt head slightly back, insert device into opposite nostril, and depress plunger. May repeat in 2 hr.

Patient/Family Teaching

- Inform patient that zolmitriptan should be used only during a migraine attack. It is meant to be used to relieve migraine attack but not to prevent or reduce the number of attacks.
- Instruct patient to administer zolmitriptan as soon as symptoms appear, but it may be administered any time during an attack. If migraine symptoms return, a 2nd dose may be used. Allow at least 2 hr between doses, and do not use more than 10 mg in any 24-hr period.
- If dose does not relieve headache, additional zolmitriptan doses are not likely to be effective; notify health care professional.
- Advise patient that lying down in a darkened room following zolmitriptan administration may further help relieve headache.
- May cause dizziness or drowsiness. Caution patient to avoid driving or other activities requiring alertness until response to medication is known.
- Advise patient to notify health care professional prior to next dose of zolmitriptan if pain or tightness in the chest occurs during use. If pain is severe or does not subside, notify health care professional immediately. If wheezing; heart throbbing; swelling of eyelids, face, or lips; skin rash; skin lumps; or hives occur, notify health care professional immediately and do not take more zolmitriptan without approval of health care professional. If feelings of tingling, heat, flushing, heaviness, pressure, drowsiness, dizziness, tiredness, or sickness develop, discuss with health care professional at next visit.
- Advise patient to avoid alcohol, which aggravates headaches, during zolmitriptan use.
- Advise patient that overuse (use more than 10 days/mo) may lead to exacerbation of headache (migraine-like daily headaches, or as a marked increase in frequency of migraine attacks). May require gradual withdrawal of zolmitriptan and treatment of symptoms (transient worsening of headache).
- Advise patient to notify health care professional of all Rx or OTC medications, vitamins, or herbal products being taken and to consult with health care professional before taking other medications. Patients concurrently taking SSRI or SNRI antidepressants should notify health care professional promptly if signs of serotonin syndrome (mental status changes: agitation, hallucinations, coma; autonomic instability: tachycardia, labile BP, hyperthermia; neuromuscular aberrations: hyper-reflexia, incoordination; and/or gastrointestinal symptoms: nausea, vomiting, diarrhea) occur.
- Advise females of reproductive potential to notify health care professional if pregnancy is planned or suspected, or if breast feeding.

Evaluation/Desired Outcomes

- Relief of migraine attack.

BEERS

zolpidem (zole-pi-dem)

Ambien, Ambien CR, Edluar, Intermezzo, ♣Sublinox, Zolpimist

Classification

Therapeutic: sedative/hypnotics

Schedule IV

Indications

Insomnia with difficulties in sleep initiation (Intermezzo is indicated for insomnia when a middle-of-the-night awakening is followed by difficulty returning to sleep).

Action

Produces CNS depression by binding to GABA receptors. Has no analgesic properties. **Therapeutic Effects:** Sedation and induction of sleep.

Pharmacokinetics

Absorption: Rapidly absorbed following oral administration. Controlled-release formulation releases 10 mg immediately, then another 2.5 mg later.

Distribution: Minimal amounts enter breast milk; remainder of distribution not known.

Metabolism and Excretion: Converted to inactive metabolites, which are excreted by the kidneys; clearance of Intermezzo lower in women than in men.

Half-life: 2.5–3 hr (↑ in geriatric patients and patients with hepatic impairment).

TIME/ACTION PROFILE (sedation)

ROUTE	ONSET	PEAK*	DURATION
PO	rapid	30 min–2 hr	6–8 hr
PO-ER	rapid	2–4 hr	6–8 hr
PO-Spray	rapid	unknown	unknown
SL	rapid	unknown	unknown

*Food delays peak levels and effects.

Contraindications/Precautions

Contraindicated in: Hypersensitivity; History of experiencing complex sleep behaviors with zolpidem; Sleep apnea; Severe hepatic impairment (↑ risk of hepatic encephalopathy).

Use Cautiously in: History of previous psychiatric illness, suicide attempt, drug or alcohol abuse; Mild or moderate hepatic impairment (↑ risk of hepatic encephalopathy; initial dose ↓ recommended); Pulmonary disease; Sleep apnea; Myasthenia gravis; OB: May ↑ risk of respiratory depression in neonates after birth; Lactation, Pedi: Safety not established; Geri: Initial dose ↓ recommended; at ↑ risk for falls.

Adverse Reactions/Side Effects

CNS: COMPLEX SLEEP BEHAVIORS (including sleep driving, sleep walking, or engaging in other activities while sleeping), <u>daytime drowsiness</u>, <u>dizziness</u>, abnormal thinking, agitation, amnesia, behavior changes, hallucinations, prolonged reaction time. **EENT:** blurred vision, double vision. **GI:** diarrhea, nausea, vomiting. **Misc:** HYPERSENSITIVITY REACTIONS (including anaphylaxis), physical dependence, psychological dependence, tolerance.

Interactions

Drug-Drug: CNS depression may ↑ with **sedatives/hypnotics**, **alcohol**, **phenothiazines**, **tricyclic antidepressants**, **opioid analgesics**, or **antihistamines**. Concurrent use of **CYP3A4 inducers**, including **rifampin**, may ↓ levels. Concurrent use of **CYP3A4 inhibitors**, including **ketoconazole**, may ↑ levels; consider ↓ zolpidem dose.

Drug-Natural Products: Concomitant use of **kava-kava**, **valerian**, or **chamomile** can ↑ CNS depression. **St. John's wort** may ↓ levels; avoid concurrent use.

Drug-Food: Food ↓ and delays absorption.

Route/Dosage

PO, SL (Adults): *Tablets, spray, or SL tablets (Edluar)*—5 mg (for women) and 5–10 mg (for men) at bedtime; may ↑ to 10 mg at bedtime if 5–mg dose not effective; *SL tablets (Intermezzo)*—1.75 mg (for women) or 3.5 mg (for men) once upon awakening in the middle-of-the-night; *Extended-release tablets*—6.25 mg (for women) and 6.25–12.5 mg (for men) at bedtime; may ↑ to 12.5 mg at bedtime if 6.25–mg dose not effective.

PO, SL (Geriatric Patients , Debilitated Patients, or Patients with Mild/Moderate Hepatic Impairment): *Tablets, spray or SL tablets (Edluar)*—Do not exceed dose of 5 mg at bedtime; *Extended-release tablets*—Do not exceed dose of 6.25 mg at bedtime.

SL (Geriatric Patients , Patients taking concomitant CNS depressants, or Patients with Mild/Moderate Hepatic Impairment): *SL tablets (Intermezzo)*—Do not exceed dose of 1.75 mg at bedtime (in either men or women).

Availability (generic available)

Extended-release tablets: 6.25 mg, 12.5 mg. **Cost:** *Generic*—6.25 mg $42.14/30, 12.5 mg $37.39/30. **Oral spray (Zolpimist) (cherry-flavor):** 5 mg/spray (60 sprays/container). **Cost:** $79.20/7.7 mL. **Sublingual tablets (Edluar):** 5 mg, 10 mg. **Cost:** All strengths $235.19/30. **Sublingual tablets (Intermezzo):** 1.75 mg, 3.5 mg. **Cost:** All strengths $248.46/30. **Tablets:** 5 mg, 10 mg. **Cost:** *Generic*—5 mg $7.81/30.

Z

NURSING IMPLICATIONS

Assessment

- Assess mental status, sleep patterns, and potential for abuse prior to administration. Prolonged use of >7–10 days may lead to physical and psychological dependence. Limit amount of drug available to the patient.
- Assess alertness at time of peak effect. Notify health care professional if desired sedation does not occur.
- Assess patient for pain. Medicate as needed. Untreated pain decreases sedative effects.

Implementation

- ***High Alert:*** Do not confuse zolpidem with Zyloprim (allopurinol).
- Before administering, reduce external stimuli and provide comfort measures to increase effectiveness of medication.
- Protect patient from injury. Raise bed side rails. Assist with ambulation. Remove patient's cigarettes.
- Use lowest effective dose.
- **PO:** Swallow tablets whole with full glass of water. For faster onset of sleep, do not administer with or immediately after a meal.
- Swallow extended-release tablets whole; do not crush, break, or chew.
- **SL:** To open the blister pack, separate the individual blisters at the perforations. Peel off top layer of paper and push tablet through foil. Place the tablet under the tongue, allow to disintegrate; do not swallow or take with water.
- *Intermezzo*—Only take if at least 4 hr left prior to time to awakening.
- **Oral Spray:** Do not take with or immediately after a meal; may slow effect. Spray is a clear, colorless, and cherry-flavor solution.

Patient/Family Teaching

- Instruct patient to take zolpidem as directed. Take as a single dose and do not readminister during the same night. Advise patient not to take zolpidem unless able to stay in bed a full night (7–8 hr) before being active again. Do not take more than the amount prescribed because of the habit-forming potential. Not recommended for use longer than 7–10 days. If used for 2 wk or longer, abrupt withdrawal may result in fatigue, nausea, flushing, light-headedness, uncontrolled crying, vomiting, GI upset, panic attack, or nervousness. Instruct patient to read *Patient Information* for correct product before taking and with each Rx refill in case of changes.
- Because of rapid onset, advise patient to go to bed immediately after taking zolpidem.
- May cause daytime drowsiness or dizziness. Advise patient to avoid driving or other activities requiring alertness until response to this medication is known.
- Caution patient that complex sleep-related behaviors (sleep-driving) may occur while asleep.
- Advise patient to notify health care professional immediately if signs of anaphylaxis (swelling of the tongue or throat, trouble breathing, and nausea and vomiting) occur.
- Caution patient to avoid concurrent use of alcohol or other CNS depressants.
- Rep: Advise females of reproductive potential to notify health care professional if pregnancy is planned or suspected or if breast feeding. Monitor neonates exposed to zolpidem during pregnancy and labor for signs of excess sedation, hypotonia, and respiratory depression.
- **Oral Spray:** To prime, patients should be told to point the black spray opening away from their face and other people and spray 5 times. For administration, hold container upright with the black spray opening pointed directly into the mouth. Press down fully on pump to make sure a full dose (5 mg) is sprayed directly into mouth over tongue. For 10-mg dose, a 2nd spray should be administered. If not used for 14 days, re-prime with 1 spray.

Evaluation/Desired Outcomes

- Relief of insomnia.
- Re-evaluate insomnia after 7–10 days of *Intermezzo*.

Drugs Approved in Canada

These monographs describe medications approved for use in Canada by the Therapeutic Products Directorate, a division of Health Canada's Health Products and Food Branch. The medications are not approved by the United States Food and Drug Administration; however, similar formulations carrying different generic or brand names might be available in the US.

alfacalcidol (al-fa-kal-si-dol)

One-Alpha

Classification
Therapeutic: vitamins
Pharmacologic: vitamin D analogues

Indications
Management of hypocalcemia, secondary hyperparathyroidism and osteodystrophy associated with chronic renal failure.

Action
Stimulates intestinal absorption of calcium and phosphorus, reabsorption of calcium from bone and renal reabsorption of calcium. Does not require renal activation. **Therapeutic Effects:** Improved calcium and phosphorus homeostasis in patients with chronic kidney disease.

Pharmacokinetics
Absorption: Completely absorbed following oral administration.
Distribution: Unknown.
Protein Binding: Extensively protein bound.
Metabolism and Excretion: Following absorption, 50 % is rapidly converted by liver to active metabolite (1.25–$(OH)_2D$; 13% renally excreted.
Half-life: 3 hr.

TIME/ACTION PROFILE (levels of active metabolite)

ROUTE	ONSET†	PEAK	DURATION‡
PO	6 hr	12 hr	few days–1 wk
IV	unknown	4 hr	few days–1 wk

†Effect on intestinal calcium absorption, bone pain and muscle weakness improve within 2 wk–3 mo.
‡Effect on serum calcium levels following discontinuation.

Contraindications/Precautions
Contraindicated in: Concurrent use of other vitamin D analogs or magnesium-containing antacids; Lactation: Avoid breast feeding.
Use Cautiously in: OB: Potential benefits should be weighed against hazards to fetus and mother; Pedi: Safety and effectiveness not been established.

Adverse Reactions/Side Effects
CNS: headache, drowsiness, weakness. **CV:** ARRHYTHMIAS, hypertension. **EENT:** conjunctivitis, photophobia. **GI:** constipation, nausea, anorexia, dry mouth, metallic taste, pancreatitis, polydipsia, vomiting. **Derm:** pruritus. **F and E:** HYPERCALCEMIA, hyperphosphatemia, hyperthermia, ↑ thirst. **GU:** albuminuria, hypercalcuria, ↓ libido, nocturia, polyuria. **Metab:** ectopic calcification, hypercholesterolemia, hyperthermia. **MS:** bone pain, muscle pain.

Interactions
Drug-Drug: Hypercalcemia ↑ risk of toxicity from **digoxin**. ↑ risk of toxicity and adverse reactions with concurrent use of other **vitamin D analogs**. Concurrent use of **bile acid sequestrants**, including **cholestyramine**, or **mineral oil** ↓ absorption and effectiveness. Concurrent use of **barbiturates** and other **anticonvulsants** may ↓ effectiveness; larger doses of alfacalcidol may be required.

Route/Dosage
PO (Adults): *Pre-dialysis patients*—0.25 mcg/day for 2 mo initially, if necessary dose increments of 0.25 mg/day may be made at 2 mo intervals (usual range 0.5–1.0 mcg/day); *dialysis patients* —1 mcg/day, if necessary dose increments of 0.5 mcg/day may be made at 2–4 wk intervals (usual range 1–2 mcg/day, up to 3 mcg/day). When normalization occurs, dose should be ↓ to minimum amount required to maintain normal serum calcium levels.
IV (Adults): *Dialysis patients*—1 mcg during each dialysis session (2–3 times weekly), if necessary dose may be ↑ weekly by 1 mcg per dialysis session up to 12 mcg/wk (range 1.5–12 mcg/wk). When normalization occurs, dose should be ↓ to minimum amount required to maintain normal serum calcium levels.

Availability
Soft gel capsules: 0.25 mcg, 1 mcg; Oral drops: 2 mcg/mL; Solution for injection (contains ethanol and propylene glycol): 2 mcg/mL.

NURSING IMPLICATIONS

Assessment
- Assess for signs of vitamin D deficiency prior to and during treatment.
- Assess for bone pain and weakness during therapy; usually decreases within 2 wk to 3 mo.
- ***Lab Test Considerations:*** *For pre-dialysis patients:* Monitor serum calcium and phosphate levels monthly and electrolytes periodically during treatment. *For dialysis patients:* Monitor serum calcium at least twice weekly during dose titration.

If hypercalcemia occurs decrease dose of alfacalcidol by 50% and stop all calcium supplements until calcium levels return to normal. May cause ↑ plasma phosphorous levels. Maintain serum phosphate levels <2.0 mmol/L. Monitor inorganic phosphorus, magnesium, alkaline phosphatase, creatinine, BUN, 24-hr urinary calcium and protein as needed.

- ***Toxicity and Overdose:*** Toxicity is manifested as hypercalcemia, hypercalciuria, and hyperphosphatemia. Assess for appearance of nausea, vomiting, anorexia, weakness, constipation, headache, bone pain, and metallic taste. Later symptoms include polyuria, polydipsia, photophobia, rhinorrhea, pruritus, and cardiac arrhythmias. Notify health care professional immediately if these signs of hypervitaminosis D occur. Treatment usually consists of discontinuation of alfacalcidol, a low-calcium diet, stopping calcium supplements. Persistent or markedly elevated serum calcium levels in hemodialysis patients may be corrected by dialysis against a calcium-free dialysate.

Implementation

- **PO:** Administer with food. Use calibrated dropper with oral for accurate dose. Oral solution may be mixed with water or milk.
- **IV:** Administer IV during hemodialysis. Shake well before use. Keep refrigerated. Single use vials; discard unused portion.

Patient/Family Teaching

- Advise patient to take medication as directed. Do not stop taking without consulting with health care professional.
- Advise patient and family to notify health care professional if signs and symptoms of hypercalcemia occur.
- Review diet modifications with patient. See Appendix K for foods high in calcium and vitamin D. Renal patients must still consider renal failure diet in food selection. Health care professional may order concurrent calcium supplement.
- Encourage patient to comply with dietary recommendations. Explain that best source of vitamins is a well-balanced diet with foods from all 4 basic food groups, and sunlight exposure for Vitamin D.
- Advise patient to avoid concurrent use of antacids containing magnesium during therapy.
- Instruct patient to notify health care professional of all Rx or OTC medications, vitamins, or herbal products being taken and to consult health care professional before taking any other Rx, OTC, or herbal products.
- Advise female patient to notify health care professional if pregnancy is planned or suspected or if breast feeding.
- Emphasize the importance of follow-up exams to evaluate progress.

Evaluation

- Improved levels of calcium and phosphorous in patients with kidney disease.

bezafibrate (bezz-uh-fibe-rate)

Bezalip SR

Classification
Therapeutic: lipid-lowering agents
Pharmacologic: fibric acid derivatives

Indications

Use in conjunction with diet and other modalities in the treatment of hypercholesterolemia (Type IIa and IIb mixed hyperlipidemia, to decrease serum TG, LDL cholesterol and apolipoprotein B and increase HDL cholesterol and apolipoprotein A). Treatment of adults with hypertriglyceridemia (Type IV and V hyperlipidemias) at risk pancreatitis and other sequelae.

Action

Inhibits triglyceride synthesis. **Therapeutic Effects:** Lowered cholesterol and triglycerides, increased HDL, with decreased risk of pancreatitis and other sequelae.

Pharmacokinetics

Absorption: Well absorbed (100%) following oral adminiinistration.

Distribution: Unknown.

Metabolism and Excretion: 50% metabolized, 50% excreted unchanged in urine, remainder as metabolites. 3% excreted in feces.

Half-life: 1–2 hr.

TIME/ACTION PROFILE (blood levels)

ROUTE	ONSET	PEAK	DURATION
PO	unknown	3–4 hr	24 hr

Contraindications/Precautions

Contraindicated in: Hypersensitivity/photosensitivity to bezafibrate or other fibric acid or fibrate derivatives; Severe hepatic or renal impairment (CCr <60 mL/min), primary biliary cirrhosis, gallstone or gallbladder disease or hypoalbuminemia; OB: Avoid use during pregnancy (discontinue several mo prior to conception); Lactation: Discontinue breast feeding.

Use Cautiously in: History of liver disease; Doses >400 mg/day in conjuction with HMG CoA reductase inhibitors (statins) with any risk factors (renal impairment, infection, trauma, surgery, hormonal or electrolyte imbalance) ↑ risk for rhabdomyolysis; Geri: Consider age-related ↓ in renal function; avoid in patients >70 yr; Pedi: Limited experience in children at a dose of 10–20 mg/kg/day.

Adverse Reactions/Side Effects

CNS: dizziness, headache. **GI:** dyspepsia, flatulence, gastritis, abdominal distension, abdominal pain, ↓ appetite, cholestasis, constipation, diarrhea, nausea. **GU:** erectile dysfunction, renal failure. **Derm:** alopecia, pruritus, urticaria, photosensitivity reaction, alopecia, rash. **MS:** RHABDOMYOLYSIS, muscle cramps, muscular weakness, myalgia. **Misc:** hypersensitivity reactions including ANAPHYLAXIS.

Interactions

Drug-Drug: ↑ risk of bleeding with **oral anticoagulants**; ↓ dose of anticoagulant by 50% with frequent monitoring. **Cyclosporine** ↑ risk of severe myositis/rhabdomyolysis; risk of combined therapy should be undertaken with caution. Concurrent use of **immunosuppressants** may ↑ risk of reversible renal impairment. ↑ risk of myopathy with **HMG CoA reductase inhibitors (statins)**; combination therapy should be undertaken with extreme caution and must be discontinued at the first signs of myopathy and should not be undertaken in the presence of predisposing factors including impaired renal function, severe infection, trauma, surgery, hormonal /electrolyte imbalance or ↑ alcohol intake. ↑ risk of serious hypoglycemia with **insulin** or **sulfonylureas**. Concurrent use with **MAO inhibitors** may ↑ risk of hepatotoxicity. **Cholestyramine** and other **bile-acid sequestrants** may ↓ absorption, separate administration by ≥2 hr. Effectiveness may be ↓ by concurrent **estrogen**.

Route/Dosage

PO (Adults): 400 mg once daily.

Availability

Sustained-release tablet: 400 mg.

NURSING IMPLICATIONS

Assessment

- Obtain a diet history with regard to fat consumption. Before starting benzafibrate, every attempt should be made to obtain a normal triglyceride level with diet, exercise and weight loss.
- Assess for cholelithiasis. If gallbladder studies are indicated, and gallstones are found, discontinue therapy.
- ***Lab Test Considerations:*** Monitor serum lipids prior to and periodically during therapy.
- ***Lab Test Considerations:*** Monitor AST and ALT serums periodically during therapy to assess for ↑ levels. Discontinue therapy if levels rise >3 times normal value.
- ***Lab Test Considerations:*** If patient develops muscle tenderness during therapy, monitor CPK levels. If CPK levels are markedly ↑ or myopathy occurs, discontinue therapy.

Implementation

- **PO:** Administer without regards to meals. Swallow sustained-release tablets whole; do not crush, break, or chew.

Patient/Family Teaching

- Instruct the patient to take the medication as directed, and to not share medication. Missed doses should be taken as soon as remembered; do not double dose. Medication helps control but does not cure elevated serum triglyceride levels.
- Advise patient that medication should be taken in conjunction with diet restrictions of fat, cholesterol, carbohydrates, and alcohol, as well as an exercise regimen, and cessation of smoking.
- Instruct patient to notify health care professional of unexplained muscle pain or weakness, tiredness, fever, nausea, vomiting, abdominal pain.
- Instruct patient to notify health care professional of all Rx or OTC medications, vitamins, or herbal products being taken and to consult health care professional before taking any other Rx, OTC, or herbal products.
- Instruct female patients to immediately notify health care professional if pregnancy is planned or suspected.
- Emphasize importance of follow-up appointments, and lab tests to evaluate effectiveness.

Evaluation

- A decrease in serum triglyceride and LDL cholesterol levels.
- An increase in HDL levels.

buserelin (bue-se-**rel**-in)

🍁Suprefact

Classification

Therapeutic: antineoplastics, hormones

Pharmacologic: luteinizing hormone-releasing hormone (LHRH) analogues

Indications

Subcutaneous injection—Initial and maintenance palliative treatment of advanced hormone-dependent prostate cancer (usually given with an anti-androgen). *Nasal solution*—Maintenance palliative treatment of advanced hormone-dependent prostate cancer (usually given with an anti-androgen). *Nasal solution*—Non-surgical treatment of endometriosis (course of treatment 6–9 mo).

Action

Acts as a synthetic analog of endogenous gonadotropin-releasing hormone (GnRH/LHRH). Chronic use results in inhibited secretion of gonadotropin release and gonadal steroid production. The overall effect is due to down-regulation of pituitary LHRH receptors. In males, testosterone synthesis and release is decreased. In females, secretion of estrogen in decreased. **Therapeutic Effects:** Decreased spread of advanced prostate cancer. Decreased sequelae of endometriosis (pain, dysmenorrhea).

Pharmacokinetics

Absorption: *Subcut*—70%; *intranasal*—1–3%; *implant*—drug is slowly absorbed over 2–3 mo.
Distribution: Accumulates in liver, kidneys and anterior pituitary lobe; enters breast milk in small amounts.
Metabolism and Excretion: Metabolized in liver, kidneys and by enzymes on membranes in the pituitary gland.
Half-life: *Subcut*—80 min; *intranasal*—1–2 hr; *implant*—20–30 days.

TIME/ACTION PROFILE

ROUTE	ONSET	PEAK	DURATION
prostate cancer †	7 days	4 mo	until discontinuation
endometriosis ‡(intranasal)	unknown	unknown	duration of treatment

†↓ in testosterone levels.
‡Symptom improvement.

Contraindications/Precautions

Contraindicated in: Hypersensitivity; Non-hormonal-dependent prostate cancer or previous orchiectomy; Females with undiagnosed vaginal bleeding; OB: Pregnancy (avoid use); Lactation: Avoid breast feeding (small amounts enter breast milk; injection contains benzyl alcohol).

Use Cautiously in: Prostate cancer with urinary tract obstruction or spinal lesions; Pedi: Safety and effectiveness not established (injection contains benzyl alcohol).

Adverse Reactions/Side Effects

CNS: depression, dizziness. **CV:** hypertension. **Endo:** glucose intolerance. **Hemat:** anemia. **Local:** injection site reactions. **MS:** osteoporosis (long-term use).
Misc: transient exacerbation of metastatic prostate cancer or endometriosis.

Prostate cancer

CNS: headache (nasal solution). **EENT:** nasal irritation (nasal spray). **GU:** ↓ libido, impotence. **Derm:** hot flushes. **Endo:** gynecomastia, testosterone flair. **MS:** bone pain.

Endometriosis

CNS: headache, weakness, insomnia. **CV:** edema. **GI:** constipation, gastrointestinal disorders, nausea. **GU:** ↓ libido, vaginal dryness, menorrhagia. **Derm:** hot flushes, acne. **Endo:** supression of ovulation. **MS:** back pain.

Interactions

Drug-Drug: Risk of serious arrhythmias may be ↑ by concurrent **amiodarone**, **disopyramide**, **dofetilide**, **flecainide ibutilide**, **propafenone quinidine**, **sotalol**, **antipsychotics** (including **chlorpromazine**) **antidepressants** (including **amitrypline** and **nortriptyline**), **opioids** (including **methadone**), **macrolide anti-infectives** (including **azithromycin**, **erythromycin** and **clarithromycin**), **fluoroquinolones** (including **moxifloxacin**), **azole antifungals**, **5-HT3 antagonists** (including **ondansetron**), **beta-2 receptor agonists** (including **salbutamol**), **pentamidine**, and **quinine**.

Route/Dosage

Prostate cancer

Subcut (Adults): *Initial treatment*—500 mcg every 8 hr for 7 days, *Maintenance treatment*—200 mcg daily.
Intranasal (Adults): *Maintenance treatment*—400 mcg (200 mcg in each nostril) 3 times daily.
Subcut implant (Adults): 6.3 mg every 2 mo or 9.45 mg every 3 mo.

Endometriosis

Intranasal (Adults): 400 mcg (200 mcg in each nostril) 3 times daily. Treatment is usually continued for 6 mo; not to exceed 9 mo.

Availability

Solution for subcutaneous injection (contains benzyl alcohol): 1000 mcg/mL; Intranasal Solution: 1000 mcg/mL (delivers 100 mcg per actuation); Subcutaneous implant (depot): 6.3 mg (2–mo implant), 9.45 mg (3–mo implant).

NURSING IMPLICATIONS

Assessment

- **Cancer:** Monitor patients with vertebral metastases for increased back pain and decreased sensory/motor function.
- Monitor intake and output ratios and assess for bladder distention in patients with urinary tract obstruction during initiation of therapy.
- **Endometriosis:** Assess for signs and symptoms of endometriosis before and periodically during therapy. Amenorrhea usually occurs within 8 wk of initial administration and menses usually resume 8 wk after completion.
- ***Lab Test Considerations:*** Monitor serum testosterone levels every 3 mo during treatment with male patients. When treatment begins, testosterone levels can temporarily markedly ↑ and patients may need another medication to ↓ levels.
- Monitor blood glucose in patients with diabetes frequently; may affect blood glucose levels.
- Verify negative pregnancy test before starting therapy for women.

Implementation

Prostate Cancer

- **Subcut:** Only use syringes that come with kit for accurate dose. Inject into fatty tissue of abdomen, arm, or leg 3 times/day for 7 days; then daily during maintenance.
- **Intranasal:** When used as maintenance, begin nasal spray in each nostril 3 times daily. If patient also receives decongestant nasal spray, wait 30 min to give buserelin spray before or after the decongestant.
- **Implant:** Implant is inserted in subcut tissue of upper abdominal wall every 28 days. Local anesthesia may be used before injection.
- If the implant needs to be removed for any reason, it can be located by ultrasound.

Endometriosis

- **Intranasal:** One spray in each nostril 3 times daily for 6–9 mo.

Patient/Family Teaching

- Inform male patients that they may experience breast swelling and tenderness, decreased libido, hot flashes and sweats, impotence and weight gain. Notify health care professional if these symptoms occur.
- Inform female patients that they may experience decreased libido, constipation, painful sexual intercourse, menopausal symptoms, changes in hair

growth. Notify health care professional if these symptoms occur.

- Caution both male and female patients to use contraception while taking this drug. Advise female patient to inform health care professional if pregnancy is suspected. Buserelin can be harmful to a fetus.
- **Subcut:** Instruct patient in proper technique for self-injection, care and disposal of equipment. Use only syringes included in kit. Instruct patients that syringes may only be used once, and then discarded.
- **Intranasal:** Instruct patient on proper nasal spray technique. Prime pump before use.
- Advise patients that the nasal spray can cause nose bleeds, and may change smell and taste senses.

Evaluation

- Decrease in the spread of prostate cancer.
- Decrease in lesions and pain in endometriosis.

cannabidiol (ka-na-bi-dye-ole)

delta-9-tetrahydrocannabinol (THC)

(**del**-ta nine tet-re-hye-dro-ka-**na**-bi-nole)

✱Sativex

Classification

Therapeutic: analgesic adjuncts, therapeutic antispasticity agents

Pharmacologic: cannabinoids

Indications

Adjunct treatment of spasticity in adults with multiple sclerosis (MS) who have not responded to other therapies. Analgesic adjunct in the management of neuropathic pain in patients with MS or advanced cancer who have not responded to opioids or other analgesics for severe pain.

Action

Acts on cannabinoid receptors located in pain pathways in the brain, spinal cord and peripheral nerve terminals. Has analgesic and muscle relaxant properties. **Therapeutic Effects:** Decreased pain and spasticity.

Pharmacokinetics

Absorption: Buccal absorption is slower than inhalation.

Distribution: Highly lipid soluble, distributes and accumulates in fatty tissues. Cannabinoids enter breast milk in considerable amounts.

Metabolism and Excretion: Some first-pass hepatic metabolism occurs; highly metabolized by the CYP450 enzyme system. Metabolites can be stored in fatty tissues and re-released over time (up to weeks); one metabolite of THC is pharmacologically active (11-hydroxy-THC). Further metabolism occurs in renal and biliary systems.

Half-life: Bi-exponential half-lives with short initial phases of *Cannabidiol*—1.4–1.8 hr; *THC*—1.3–1.7 hr *11-hydroxy-THC*—1.9–2.1 hr; terminal elimination half-life of *cannabinoids*—24–26 hr or more.

TIME/ACTION PROFILE (analgesic and antispasticity effects)

ROUTE	ONSET	PEAK†	DURATION
cannabidiol	unknown	1.6–2.8 hr	up to 12 hr
THC	unknown	1.6–2.4 hr	up to 12 hr

†Blood levels peak more quickly when administered under the tongue.

Contraindications/Precautions

Contraindicated in: Allergy/hypersensitivity to cannabinoids, propylene glycol or peppermint oil; Serious cardiovascular disease, including ischemic heart disease, arrhythmias, poorly controlled hypertension or severe heart failure; History of schizophrenia/psychoses; Patients with childbearing potential who are not using reliable contraception; Sore/inflamed mucosa (may alter absorption); OB: Pregnancy (avoid use); Lactation: Avoid breast feeding (cannabinoids enter breast milk in considerable amounts); Pedi: Safety and effectiveness not established.

Use Cautiously in: Epilepsy/recurrent seizures; Substance abuse; Perioperative state (consider possible changes in cardiovascular status); History of depression/suicide attempt or ideation; Significant hepatic/renal impairment; Women of reproductive potential (reliable contraception must be ensured); Cancer patients with urinary tract pathology (↑ risk of urinary tract adverse reactions); Geri: Use cautiously.

Adverse Reactions/Side Effects

CNS: dizziness, fatigue, confusion, depression, disorientation, drowsiness, euphoria, hallucinations, psychotic reactions, suicidal ideation, weakness. **CV:** hypertension, palpitations, tachycardia, postural hypotension. **GI:** appetite change, constipation, dry mouth, dysgeusia, mucosal/teeth discoloration, nausea (↑ in cancer patients), stomatitis. **GU:** urinary retention (↑ in cancer patients). **Local:** application site irritation. **Misc:** physical dependence, psychological dependence.

Interactions

Drug-Drug: ↑ risk of CNS depression with other **CNS depressants** including **alcohol**, some **antidepressants**, some **antihistamines**, **benzodiazepines**, **GABA inhibitors**, **sedative/hypnotics**, **opioids**, and **psychotropics/antipsychotics**. Cannabidiol inhibits the CYP450 enzyme system; may ↑ effects of **amitriptyline**, **alfentanil**, **fentanyl** and **sufentanil**.

Drug-Natural Products: ↑ risk of intoxication with other forms of **cannibis**.

Route/Dosage

Buccal (Adults): *Day 1*—One spray in the morning and one in the evening; may ↑ by 1 spray/day on subsequent days. If unacceptable effects occur, temporarily discontinue and restart at a lower # of sprays/day or use longer intervals between sprays. Titrate to optimal maintenance dose (usual range 4–8 sprays/day, usually not more than 12 sprays/day; higher doses have been used/tolerated). Adjust dose to changes in patient condition.

Availability

Buccal spray contains ethanol (50% v/v), propylene glycol and peppermint oil: Each ml contains *Cannabidiol*—25 mg and *THC*—27 mg/ml. Delivers 100 microliter/spray, each spray provides cannabidiol 2.5 mg and THC 2.7 mg.

NURSING IMPLICATIONS

Assessment

- Assess patient's pain level before and after cannabidiol.

Implementation

- Prime pump before first use. Shake vial gently and remove protective cap. Hold vial in an upright position and press firmly and quickly on the actuator 2 or 3 times, until a fine spray appears. Point spray into a tissue, away from patient.
- Administer one spray 2 times/day, in morning and in evening, on first day. Administer under tongue or in buccal area. Rotate sites in mouth to avoid irritation. Effects should be noticed in about 30 min. Do not spray the back of throat or into nose. After first day, increase dose by 1 spray every 24 hr, spacing doses evenly. No more than 12 doses should be used over a 24 hr period. Space each spray by at least 15 min.

Patient/Family Teaching

- Caution patient to use medication as directed.
- Instruct patient on correct spray technique. Instruct patient to rotate sites in the mouth between under the tongue and buccal locations.
- Instruct patient to store unopened bottles in refrigerator. Do not freeze. Keep away from sources of heat such as direct sunlight or flames (product is flammable). Opened bottles may be stored at room temperature. Keep out of reach of children.
- Inform patient that any unused contents should be discarded after 28 days. Do not dispose of medications in wastewater (e.g. down the sink or in the toilet) or in household garbage. Consult pharmacist how to dispose of expired or unneeded medication.
- Caution patient to avoid alcohol while taking cannabidiol.
- Advise patient to notify health care professional if pregnancy is planned or suspected or if breast feeding.

Evaluation

- Decrease in pain.
- Decrease in muscle spasticity.

cilazapril (sye-**lay**-za-pril)

Inhibace

Classification

Therapeutic: antihypertensives

Pharmacologic: ACE inhibitors

Indications

Alone or with other agents in the management of hypertension. HF.

Action

ACE inhibitors block the conversion of angiotensin I to the vasoconstrictor angiotensin II. ACE inhibitors also prevent the degradation of bradykinin and other vasodilatory prostaglandins. ACE inhibitors also ↑ plasma renin levels and ↓ aldosterone levels. Net result is systemic vasodilation. **Therapeutic Effects:** Lowering of BP in hypertensive patients. Improved symptoms in patients with HF.

Pharmacokinetics

Absorption: Well absorbed following oral administration, rapidly converted to active metabolite, cilazaprilat (57% bioavailability for cilazaprilat).

Distribution: Enters breast milk.

Metabolism and Excretion: Cilazaprilat is eliminated unchanged by the kidneys (91%).

Half-life: *Early elimination phase*—0.9 hr; *terminal elimination phase (enzyme–bound cilazaprilat)* 36–49 hr.

TIME/ACTION PROFILE (effects on hemodynamics)

ROUTE	ONSET	PEAK	DURATION
PO (hypertension)	within 1 hr	3–7 hr	12–24 hr
PO (heart failure)	1–2 hr	2–4 hr	24 hr

Contraindications/Precautions

Contraindicated in: Hypersensitivity; History of angioedema with previous use of ACE inhibitors; Concurrent use with aliskiren in patients with diabetes or moderate-to-severe renal impairment (CCr <60 mL/min); OB: Can cause injury or death of fetus—if pregnancy occurs, discontinue immediately; Lactation: Discontinue drug or use formula.

Use Cautiously in: Renal impairment, hepatic impairment, hypovolemia, hyponatremia, concurrent diuretic therapy; Black patients with hypertension (monotherapy less effective, may require additional therapy; ↑ risk of angioedema); Women of reproductive potential; Surgery/anesthesia (hypotension may be exaggerated); Geri: Initial dose ↓ recommended for most agents due to age-related ↓ in renal function; Pedi: Safety and effectiveness not established.

Exercise Extreme Caution in: Family history of angioedema.

Adverse Reactions/Side Effects

CNS: dizziness, drowsiness, fatigue, headache, insomnia, vertigo, weakness. **Resp:** cough, dyspnea. **CV:** hypotension, chest pain, edema, tachycardia. **Endo:** hyperuricemia. **GI:** taste disturbances, abdominal pain, anorexia, constipation, diarrhea, nausea, vomiting. **GU:** erectile dysfunction, proteinuria, renal dysfunction, renal failure. **Derm:** flushing, pruritis, rashes. **F and E:** hyperkalemia. **Hemat:** AGRANULOCYTOSIS. **MS:** back pain, muscle cramps, myalgia. **Misc:** ANGIOEDEMA, fever.

Interactions

Drug-Drug: Excessive hypotension may occur with concurrent use of **diuretics** or other **antihypertensives** or **alcohol**. ↑ risk of hyperkalemia with concurrent use of **potassium supplements**, **potassium-sparing diuretics**, or **potassium-containing salt substitutes**. ↑ risk of hyperkalemia, renal impairment, hypotension, and syncope with concurrent use of **angiotensin II receptor antagonists** or **aliskiren**; avoid concurrent use with aliskiren in patients with diabetes or CCr <60 mL/min. **NSAIDs** and selective **COX-2 inhibitors** may blunt the antihypertensive effect and ↑ the risk of renal dysfunction. ↑ levels and may ↑ risk of **lithium** toxicity.

Route/Dosage

Hypertension

PO (Adults ≤65 yr): *As monotherapy*—2.5 mg once daily initially, may be increased every 2 wk by 2.5 mg/day; usual dose 2.5–5 mg once daily, not to exceed 10 mg/day. Twice daily administration may be necessary in some patients; *With diuretics*—0.5 mg once daily initially, titrate carefully.

PO (Adults >65 yr): *As monotherapy*—1.25 mg once daily initially, titrate carefully.

Renal Impairment

PO (Adults): *CCr >40 mL/min*—1 mg once daily initially, titrate carefully, not to exceed 5 mg once daily; *CCr 10–40 mL/min*—0.5 mg once daily initially, titrate carefully, not to exceed 2.5 mg once daily; *CCr <10 mL/min*—0.25–0.5 mg once or twice weekly depending on blood pressure response.

Hepatic Impairment

PO (Adults): 0.5 mg once daily or less.

Heart Failure

PO (Adults): After considering concurrent diuretic therapy/salt/volume depletion, *Initial dose*—0.5 mg/day with careful monitoring, after 5 days dose may be ↑ to 1 mg/day, dose may then be carefully titrated as needed/tolerated up to 2.5 mg/day, rarely patients may require 5 mg/day.

Renal Impairment/hyponatremia

PO (Adults): *CCr 10–40 mL/min*—0.25–0.5 mg once daily; *CCr <10 mL/min*—0.25–0.5 mg once or twice weekly depending on response.

Availability

Tablets: 1 mg, 2.5 mg, 5 mg. ***In combination with:*** hydrochlorothiazide 12.5 mg (Inhibace Plus).

NURSING IMPLICATIONS

Assessment

- Assess patient for signs of angioedema; dyspnea and facial swelling.
- **Hypertension:** Monitor BP and pulse frequently during initial dose adjustment and periodically during therapy. Notify health care professional of significant changes.
- **Heart Failure:** Monitor daily weight and assess frequently for fluid overload (dyspnea, rales/crackles, weight gain, jugular venous distention).
- ***Lab Test Considerations:*** Monitor BUN, creatinine, and serum electrolyte levels periodically during therapy.
- Monitor CBC periodically. May cause agranulocytosis.
- May cause ↑ AST, ALT, alkaline phosphatase, serum bilirubin, uric acid, and glucose.

Implementation

- **PO:** Tablets may be taken before or after meals.

Patient/Family Teaching

- Instruct patient to take cilazapril as directed. Take missed dose as soon as remembered. If not until the following day, skip missed dose. Do not double doses.
- Caution patient to change positions slowly to minimize hypotension. Use of alcohol, standing for long periods, exercising, and hot weather may ↑ orthostatic hypotension.
- May cause dizziness. Caution patient to avoid driving and other activities requiring alertness until response to medication is known.
- Instruct patient on proper technique for monitoring blood pressure. Advise patient to check BP and weight weekly and record and report results to health care professional.
- Provide patient with additional interventions for hypertension control (weight reduction, low sodium diet, cessation of smoking, exercise regimen, stress management, and moderation of alcohol consumption). Medication controls but does not cure hypertension.
- Instruct patient to notify health care professional of all Rx or OTC medications, vitamins, or herbal products being taken and consult health care professional before taking any new medications, especially cough, cold, or allergy remedies.
- Advise women of childbearing potential to use contraception and to notify health care professional if planning or suspecting pregnancy. Discontinue medication immediately if pregnancy is confirmed.

Evaluation

- Decrease in blood pressure.
- Decrease in signs and symptoms of heart failure.

cloxacillin (klox-a-**sill**-in)

Classification
Therapeutic: anti-infectives
Pharmacologic: penicillinase resistant penicillins

Indications

Treatment of the following infections due to penicillinase-producing staphylococci: respiratory tract infections, sinusitis, septicemia, endocarditis, osteomyelitis, skin and skin structure infections.

Action

Bind to bacterial cell wall, leading to cell death. Not inactivated by penicillinase enzymes. **Therapeutic Effects:** Bactericidal action. **Spectrum:** Active against most gram-positive aerobic cocci. Spectrum is notable for activity against: Penicillinase-producing strains of *Staphylococcus aureus Staphylococcus epidermidis*. Not active against methicillin-resistant bacteria (MRSA).

Pharmacokinetics

Absorption: IV administration results in complete bioavailability. Moderately absorbed (50%) following oral administration.
Distribution: Widely distributed; penetration into CSF is minimal but sufficient in the presence of inflamed meninges; crosses the placenta and enters breast milk.
Metabolism and Excretion: Some metabolism by the liver (9–22%) and some renal excretion of unchanged drug (20 %).
Half-life: 0.5–1.1 hr (↑ in severe hepatic impairment, renal impairment, and in neonates).

TIME/ACTION PROFILE

ROUTE	ONSET	PEAK	DURATION
PO	30 min	30–120 min	6 hr
IM	unknown	unknown	6 hr
IV	rapid	end of injection/infusion	6 hr

Contraindications/Precautions

Contraindicated in: Previous hypersensitivity to penicillins (cross-sensitivity exists with cephalosporins and other beta-lactam antibiotics).
Use Cautiously in: Severe renal or hepatic impairment; OB: Safety not established; Pedi: Safety in premature and newborn infants not established.

Adverse Reactions/Side Effects

CNS: SEIZURES. **GI:** CLOSTRIDIUM DIFFICILE-ASSOCIATED DIARRHEA (CDAD), diarrhea, epigastric distress, nausea, vomiting. **GU:** interstitial nephritis. **Derm:** rash, urticaria. **Hemat:** eosinophilia, leukopenia. **Misc:** allergic reactions including ANAPHYLAXIS and SERUM SICKNESS, superinfection.

Interactions

Drug-Drug: May ↓ effectiveness of **oral contraceptive agents**. **Probenecid** ↓ renal excretion and ↑ levels (therapy may be combined for this purpose). **Neomycin** may ↓ absorption. Concurrent use with **methotrexate** ↓ methotrexate elimination and ↑ risk of serious toxicity.
Drug-Food: Food ↓ oral absorption by 50%.

Route/Dosage

PO (Adults): 250–500 mg every 6 hr.
PO (Children >1 mo): 50–100 mg/kg/day divided every 6 hr up to a maximum of 4 g/day.
IM, IV (Adults): 250–500 mg every 6 hr, maximum dose 6 g/day.
IM, IV (Children up to 20 kg): 25–50 mg/kg/day in 4 equally divided doses every 6 hr.

Availability

Capsules: 🍁 250 mg, 🍁 500 mg; Oral solution: 🍁 125 mg/5 mL; Powder for injection (requires reconstitution/ dilution: 🍁 250 mg/vial, 🍁 500 mg/vial, 🍁 1 g/vial, 🍁 2 g/vial.

NURSING IMPLICATIONS

Assessment

- Assess for infection (vital signs; appearance of wound, sputum, urine, and stool; WBC) at beginning of and throughout therapy.
- Obtain a history before initiating therapy to determine previous use of and reactions to cephalosporins or other beta-lactam antibiotics. Persons with no history of penicillin sensitivity may still have an allergic response.
- Obtain specimens for culture and sensitivity prior to initiating therapy. First dose may be given before receiving results.
- Observe patient for signs and symptoms of anaphylaxis (rash, pruritus, laryngeal edema, wheezing, abdominal pain). Discontinue drug and notify health care professional immediately if these occur. Keep epinephrine, an antihistamine, and resuscitation equipment close by in event of an anaphylactic reaction.
- Monitor bowel function. Diarrhea, abdominal cramping, fever, and bloody stools should be reported to health care professional promptly as a sign of Clostridium difficile-associated diarrhea (CDAD). May begin up to several wk following cessation of therapy.
- ***Lab Test Considerations:*** May cause leukopenia and neutropenia, especially with prolonged therapy or hepatic impairment.
- May cause positive direct Coombs' test result.
- May cause ↑ AST, ALT, LDH, and serum alkaline phosphatase concentrations.

Implementation

- **PO:** Administer around the clock on an empty stomach at least 1 hr before or 2 hr after meals. Take with a full glass of water; acidic juices may decrease absorption of penicillins. Swallow capsules whole; do not crush, chew, or open capsules.
- Use calibrated measuring device for liquid preparations. Shake well. Solution is stable for 14 days if refrigerated.
- **IM:** Reconstitute by adding 1.9 mL and 1.7 mL sterile water to 250 mg and 500 mg respectively, for concentrations of 125 mg/mL and 250 mg/mL. Shake well to dissolve. Stable for 24 hr at room temperature or 48 hr if refrigerated.
- **IV:** For IV use, reconstitute 250 mg vial with 4.9 mL, 500 mg vial with 4.8 mL, and 1000 mg vial with 9.6 mL sterile water for concentrations of 50 mg/mL, 100 mg/mL, and 100 mg/mL respectively. Shake well. Use reconstituted solution immediately. Infuse over 2–4 min.
- **IV:** Reconstitute for infusion with sterile water for injection using 3.4 mL for 1000 mg, 6.8 mL for 2000 mg, and 34 mL for 10,000 mg, resulting in 250 mg/

mL. Add to an appropriate infusion fluid in amount calculated to give desired dose. Shake well to dissolve. Use solution immediately. Infuse over 30-40 min.
- **Y-Site Compatibility:** epinephrine, ketamine.
- **Y-Site Incompatibility:** pantoprazole, rocuronium.

Patient/Family Teaching
- Instruct patient to take medication around the clock and to finish the drug completely as directed, even if feeling better. Missed doses should be taken as soon as remembered. Advise patient that sharing of this medication may be dangerous.
- Advise patient to report signs of superinfection (black, furry overgrowth on the tongue; vaginal itching or discharge; loose or foul-smelling stools) and allergy.
- Instruct patient to notify health care professional if fever and diarrhea develop, especially if stool contains blood, pus, or mucus. Advise patient not to treat diarrhea without consulting health care professional.
- Instruct patient to notify health care professional if symptoms do not improve.

Evaluation
- Resolution of the signs and symptoms of infection. Length of time for complete resolution depends on the organism and site of infection.

cyproterone (sy-**proe**-te-rone)
Androcur

Classification
Therapeutic: antineoplastics, hormones
Pharmacologic: antiandrogens

Indications
Palliative treatment of advanced prostate cancer.

Action
Has antiandrogenic and progestogenic/antigonadotropic properties, resulting in blocked binding of the active metabolite of testosterone on the surface of prostatic cancer cells and decreased production of testicular testosterone. **Therapeutic Effects:** Decreased spread of prostate cancer.

Pharmacokinetics
Absorption: Completely absorbed following oral administration. Absorption after IM depot injection is delayed and prolonged.
Distribution: Unknown.
Metabolism and Excretion: Metabolized by the CYP3A enzyme system; excreted in feces (60%) and urine (33%), as unchanged drug and metabolites.
Half-life: *PO*—38 hr; *IM*—4 days.

TIME/ACTION PROFILE (blood levels)

ROUTE	ONSET	PEAK	DURATION
PO	unknown	3–4 hr	8–12 hr
IM (depot)	unknown	3.4 days	1–2 wk

Contraindications/Precautions
Contraindicated in: Hypersensitivity; Liver disease/hepatic impairment/liver tumors (not due to prostate cancer); Dubin Johnson syndrome; Rotor syndrome; History of meningioma; Wasting diseases (not related to prostate cancer); Severe depression; Thromboembolism; OB: Not indicated for use in women; Pedi: Not recommended for use in children <18 yr.
Use Cautiously in: History of cardiovascular disease; Renal impairment.

Adverse Reactions/Side Effects
CNS: MENINGIOMAS, fatigue, weakness, depression. **Resp:** cough, dyspnea, pulmonary microembolism. **CV:** THROMBOEMBOLISM, edema, heart failure, myocardial infarction, hypotension, syncope, tachycardia, vasovagal reactions. **GI:** HEPATOTOXICITY, LIVER TUMORS, anorexia, constipation, diarrhea, nausea, vomiting. **Derm:** dry skin, hot flashes, ↑ sweating, patchy hair loss. **Endo:** adrenal suppression, antiandrogen withdrawal syndrome, gynecomastia. **F and E:** hypercalcemia. **GU:** infertility, impotence. **Hemat:** anemia, thrombocytopenia. **Metab:** glucose intolerance, hyperlipidemia. **MS:** osteoporosis (long term use). **Misc:** allergic reactions.

Interactions
Drug-Drug: Antiandrogenic effect may be ↓ by **alcohol**. Effectiveness/long-term survival may be ↓ by concurrent **GnRH agonist** treatment. ↑ risk of myopathy with **HMG CoA reductase inhibitors (statins)**. Blood levels and effects may be ↑ by **strong inhibitors of CYP3A4** including **clotrimazole**, **itraconazole**, **ketoconazole** and **ritonavir**. Blood levels and effectiveness may be ↓ by **inducers of CYP3A4** including **phenytoin** and **rifampicin**. Use cautiously with other **drugs that are substrates of the P450 enzymes**.
Drug-Natural Products: Blood levels and effectiveness may be ↓ by **St. John's wort**.

Route/Dosage
PO (Adults): 200–300 mg/day in 2–3 divided doses, not to exceed 300 mg/day; *After orchiectomy*—100–200 mg/day.
IM (Adults): 300 mg once weekly; *After orchiectomy*—300 mg every 2 wk.

Availability
Tablets: 50 mg; Depot injection: 100 mg/mL in 3–mL. ***In combination with:*** Ethinyl estradiol (Diane-35, Cyestra-35, Cleo-35).

NURSING IMPLICATIONS
Assessment
- Assess for signs and symptoms of thromboembolism (chest pain, dyspnea, vital signs, level of consciousness). Discontinue therapy if symptoms occur.
- Monitor mood changes, especially during first 6–8 wk. Note degree to which these thoughts and behaviors interfere with daily functioning. Inform health

= Canadian drug name. = Genetic implication. ~~Strikethrough~~ = Discontinued.
*CAPITALS indicates life-threatening; underlines indicate most frequent.

care professional if patient demonstrates significant increase in anxiety, nervousness, or insomnia.

- ***Lab Test Considerations:*** Monitor PSA during therapy. May cause increase in PSA. If PSA increase occurs discontinue therapy and monitor for 6–8 wk for withdrawal response prior to any decision to proceed with other prostate cancer therapy.
- ***Lab Test Considerations:*** May impair carbohydrate metabolism. Monitor fasting blood glucose and glucose tolerance tests periodically during therapy, especially in patients with diabetes. May require dose changes in insulin or oral antidiabetic agents.
- ***Lab Test Considerations:*** Monitor CBC and platelet count periodically during therapy.
- ***Lab Test Considerations:*** Monitor liver function tests prior to and periodically during therapy and if symptoms of hepatotoxicity occur. May develop several wk to mo after therapy starts. Discontinue therapy if hepatotoxicity occurs.
- ***Lab Test Considerations:*** Monitor adrenocortical function tests by serum cortisol assay periodically during therapy.

Implementation

- **PO:** Take by mouth two or three times a day with or just after meals as directed. Dose is usually lower after orchiectomy.

Patient/Family Teaching

- Instruct patient to take cyproterone as directed. Take missed doses as soon as remembered, unless almost time for next dose, then skip missed dose and resume usual dosing schedule. Do not double dose.
- Inform patient that benign breast lumps may occur; they generally subside 1–3 mo after discontinuation of therapy and/or after dose reduction. Dose reduction should be weighed against the risk of inadequate tumor control.
- Advise patient to avoid alcohol during therapy.
- May cause fatigue and lassitude during first few wk of therapy; then diminishes. Caution patient to avoid driving and other activities requiring alertness until response to medication is known.
- Inform patient that sperm count and volume of ejaculate decrease with therapy. Infertility is common but is reversible when therapy is discontinued.
- Discuss with patient potential for patchy hair loss. Explore methods of coping.
- Instruct patient to notify health care professional of all Rx or OTC medications, vitamins, or herbal products being taken and consult health care professional before taking any new medications, especially St. John's wort.
- Advise patient to notify health care professional if pregnancy is planned or suspected or if breast feeding.
- Emphasize the importance of follow-up appointments and blood tests to monitor progression of treatment.

Evaluation

- Decreased spread of prostate cancer.

danaparoid (da-nap-a-roid)

Orgaran

Classification

Therapeutic: anticoagulants

Pharmacologic: heparins (low molecular weight)

Indications

Prevention of thromboembolic phenomena including deep vein thrombosis and pulmonary emboli after surgical procedures known to increase the risk of such complications (knee/hip replacement, abdominal surgery). Management of non-hemorrhagic stroke. Treatment/prevention of thromboembolic phenomena in patients with a history of heparin-induced thrombocytopenia (HIT).

Action

Potentiates the inhibitory effect of antithrombin on factor Xa and thrombin. Danaparoid is a heparinoid. **Therapeutic Effects:** Prevention of thrombus formation.

Pharmacokinetics

Absorption: 100% absorbed after subcut administration; IV administration results in complete bioavailability.

Distribution: Unknown.

Metabolism and Excretion: Excreted mostly by the kidneys.

Half-life: 24 hr.

TIME/ACTION PROFILE (anticoagulant effect)

ROUTE	ONSET	PEAK	DURATION
Subcut	unknown	2–5 hr	12 hr

Contraindications/Precautions

Contraindicated in: Hypersensitivity to danaparoid, pork products, or sulfites; Uncontrolled bleeding; Imminent/threatened abortion; Lactation: Avoid breast feeding.

Use Cautiously in: Severe hepatic or renal impairment (dosage ↓ may be necessary in severe renal impairment); Retinopathy (hypertensive or diabetic); Untreated hypertension; Recent history of ulcer disease; Spinal/epidural anesthesia; History of congenital or acquired bleeding disorder; Malignancy; History of thrombocytopenia related to heparin (HIT), has been used successfully; OB: Safe use in pregnancy has not been established; Geri: Dosage ↓ may be necessary in severe renal impairment; Pedi: Safety not established.

Exercise Extreme Caution in: Severe uncontrolled hypertension; Bacterial endocarditis, bleeding disorders; GI bleeding/ulceration/pathology; Hemorrhagic stroke; Recent CNS or ophthalmologic surgery; Active GI bleeding/ulceration.

Adverse Reactions/Side Effects

CNS: dizziness, headache, insomnia. **CV:** edema. **GI:** constipation, nausea, reversible increase in liver enzymes, vomiting. **GU:** urinary retention. **Derm:** ecchymoses, pruritus, rash, urticaria. **Hemat:** BLEEDING, anemia, thrombocytopenia. **Local:** erythema at injection site, hematoma, irritation, pain. **Misc:** fever.

Interactions

Drug-Drug: Risk of bleeding may be ↑ by concurrent use of other **anticoagulants** including **warfarin** or **drugs that affect platelet function**, including **aspirin**, **NSAIDs**, **dipyridamole**, some **penicillins**, **clopidogrel**, **ticlopidine**, and **dextran**.

Route/Dosage

Prophylaxis of DVT (non HIT patients)

Subcut (Adults): 750 anti-factor Xa IU every 12 hr starting 1–4 hr preop and at least 2 hr postop for 7–10 days or until ambulatory (up to 14 days). *Prophylaxis of DVT following Orthopedic, Major Abdominal Surgery and Thoracic Surgery*—750 anti-factor Xa units, twice daily up to 14 days, initiate 1–4 hr preop.

IV, Subcut (Adults): *Prophylaxis of Deep Vein Thrombosis in Non-hemorrhagic Stroke Patients*—up to 1000 anti-Xa units IV, followed by 750 anti-Xa units subcutaneously, twice daily for 7–14 days.

HIT

IV, Subcut (Adults): *DVT prophylaxis, current HIT, ≤90 kg*—750 anti-Xa units SC two or three times daily for 7–10 days (initial bolus of 1250 anti-Xa units IV may be used); *DVT prophylaxis, current HIT, >90 kg*—1250 anti-Xa units SC two or three times daily for 7–10 days (initial bolus of 1250 anti-Xa units IV may be used); *DVT prophylaxis, past (>3 mos) HIT, ≤90 kg*—750 anti-Xa units SC two or three times daily for 7–10 days; *DVT prophylaxis, past (>3 mos) HIT, >90 kg*—750 anti-Xa units SC three times daily or 1250 anti-Xa units SC twice daily for 7–10 days; *Established pulmonary embolism or DVT, thrombus <5 days, >90 kg*—3750 anti-Xa units IV bolus, then 400 anti-Xa units/hr for 4 hr, then 300 anti-Xa units/hr for 4 hr, then 150–200 anti-Xa units/hr for 5–7 days or 1750 anti-Xa units SC twice daily for 4–7 days; *Established pulmonary embolism or DVT, thrombus <5 days, 55–90 kg*—2250–2500 anti-Xa units IV bolus, then 400 anti-Xa units/hr for 4 hr, then 300 anti-Xa units/hr for 4 hr, then 150–200 anti-Xa units/hr for 5–7 days or 2000 anti-Xa units SC twice daily for 4–7 days; *Established pulmonary embolism or DVT, thrombus <5 days, <55 kg*—1250–1500 anti-Xa units IV bolus, then 400 anti-Xa units/hr for 4 hr, then 300 anti-Xa units/hr for 4 hr, then 150–200 anti-Xa units/hr for 5–7 days or 1500 anti-Xa units SC twice daily for 4–7 days; *Established pulmonary embolism or DVT, thrombus ≥5 days, >90 kg*—1250 anti-Xa units IV bolus, then 750 anti-Xa units SC three times daily or 1250 anti-Xa units twice daily; *Established pulmonary embolism or DVT, thrombus ≥5 days, ≤90 kg*—1250 anti-Xa units IV bolus, then 750 anti-Xa units SC 2–3 times daily; *Surgical prophylaxis, nonvascular surgery, >90 kg*—750 anti-Xa units SC, repeat ≥6 hr after procedure, then 1250 anti-Xa units SC twice daily for 7–10 days; *Surgical prophylaxis, nonvascular surgery, ≤90 kg*—750 anti-Xa units SC, repeat ≥6 hr after procedure, then 750 anti-Xa units SC twice daily for 7–10 days; *Surgical prophylaxis, embolectomy, >90 kg*—2250–2500 anti-Xa units IV bolus before procedure, then 150–200 anti-Xa units/hr IVstarting ≥6 hr after procedure for 5–7 days or 750 anti-Xa units 2–3 times daily or change to oral anticoagulants after several days; *Surgical prophylaxis, embolectomy, 55–90 kg*—2250–2500 anti-Xa units IV bolus before procedure, then 1250 anti-Xa units SC twice daily starting ≥6 hr after procedure, then 750 anti-Xa units 2–3 times daily or change to oral anticoagulants after several days; *Cardiac catheterization >90 k g*—3750 anti-Xa units IV bolus prior to procedure; *Cardiac catheterization <90 kg*—2500 anti-Xa units IV bolus prior to procedure; *Percutaneous transluminal coronary angioplasty*—2500 anti-Xa units IV prior to procedure, then 150–200 anti-Xa units/hr IV for 1–2 days after procedure, may be followed by 750 anti-Xa units SC for several several days; *Intra-aortic balloon pump catherization, >90 kg*—3750 anti-Xa units IV bolus before procedure, then 150–200 anti-Xa units/hr IV or a 2nd bolus of 1250 anti-Xa units IV or 750 anti-Xa units SC two or three times daily or 1250 anti-Xa units SC twice daily; *Intra-aortic balloon pump catherization, <90 kg*—2500 anti-Xa units IV bolus before procedure, then 150–200 anti-Xa units/hr IV of a 2nd bolus of 1250 anti-Xa units IV or 750 anti-Xa units SC two or three times daily or 1250 anti-Xa units SC twice daily; *Peripheral vascular bypass*—2250–2500 anti-Xa units IV bolus before procedure, then 150–200 anti-Xa units/hr IV started ≥6 hr after procedure for 5–7 days or 750 anti-Xa units SC two or three times daily or change to oral anticoagulants.

Availability

Solution for injection (contains sulfites): 750 anti-factor Xa units/0.6 mL ampule.

NURSING IMPLICATIONS

Assessment

- Assess for signs of bleeding and hemorrhage (bleeding gums; nosebleed; unusual bruising; black, tarry stools; hematuria; fall in hematocrit or BP; guaiac-positive stools); bleeding from surgical site. Notify health care professional if these occur.
- Assess for evidence of additional or increased thrombosis. Symptoms will depend on area of involvement. Monitor neurological status frequently for signs of neurological impairment. May require urgent treatment.
- Monitor patient for hypersensitivity reactions (chills, fever, urticaria).
- Monitor patients with epidural catheters frequently for signs and symptoms of neurologic impairment.
- **Subcut:** Observe injection sites for hematomas, ecchymosis, or inflammation.
- ***Lab Test Considerations:*** Monitor CBC, and stools for occult blood periodically during therapy.

Monitor platelet count every other day for first wk, twice weekly for next 2 wk, and weekly thereafter. If thrombocytopenia occurs, monitor closely. If hematocrit decreases unexpectedly, assess patient for potential bleeding sites.

- Special monitoring of clotting times (aPTT) is not necessary.
- May cause ↑ in AST, ALT, and alkaline phosphatase levels.
- ***Toxicity and Overdose:*** Danaparoid is not reversed with protamine sulfate. If overdose occurs, discontinue danaparoid. Transfusion with fresh frozen plasma and plasmapheresis has been used if bleeding is uncontrollable.

Implementation

- Cannot be used interchangeably (unit for unit) with unfractionated heparin or other low-molecular-weight heparins.
- Conversion to oral anticogulant therapy (unless it is contraindicated) should not be started until adequate anti-thrombotic control with parenteral danaparoid has been achieved; conversion may take up to 5 days.
- **Subcut:** Administer deep into subcut tissue. Alternate injection sites daily between the left and right anterolateral and left and right posterolateral abdominal wall. Inject entire length of needle at a 45° or 90° angle into a skin fold held between thumb and forefinger; hold skin fold throughout injection. Do not aspirate or massage. Rotate sites frequently. Do not administer IM because of danger of hematoma formation. Solution should be clear; do not inject solution containing particulate matter.
- If excessive bruising occurs, ice cube massage of site before injection may lessen bruising.

IV Administration

- **IV Push:** Subcut is preferred route. ***Diluent:*** If administered IV, give as a bolus. May dilute with 0.9% NaCl, D5/0.9% NaCl, Ringer's, LR, and mannitol. Stable for up to 48 hr at room temperature.
- **Y-Site Incompatibility:** Administer separately; do not mix with other drugs.

Patient/Family Teaching

- Instruct patient in correct technique for self injection, care and disposal of equipment.
- Advise patient to report any symptoms of unusual bleeding or bruising, dizziness, itching, rash, fever, swelling, or difficulty breathing to health care professional immediately.
- Instruct patient not to take aspirin, naproxen, or ibuprofen without consulting health care professional while on danaparoid therapy.
- Advise female patient to notify health care professional if pregnancy is planned or suspected or if breast feeding.

Evaluation

- Prevention of deep vein thrombosis and pulmonary emboli.

domperidone (dom-per-i-done)

Classification
Therapeutic: gastric stimulant
Pharmacologic: butyrophenones dopamine antagonists

Indications

Management of symptoms associated with GI motility disorders including subacute/chronic gastritis and diabetic gastroparesis. Treatment of nausea/vomiting associated with dopamine agonist antiparkinson therapy. **Unlabeled Use:** To stimulate lactation.

Action

Acts as a peripheral dopamine receptor blocker. Increases GI motility, peristalsis and lower esophageal sphincter pressure. Facilitates gastric emptying and decreases small bowel transit time. Also increases prolactin levels. **Therapeutic Effects:** Improved GI motility. Decreased nausea/vomiting associated with dopamine agonist antiparkinson therapy.

Pharmacokinetics

Absorption: Well absorbed following oral administration.
Distribution: Does not cross the blood-brain barrier; enters breast milk in low concentrations.
Metabolism and Excretion: Undergoes extensive first-pass hepatic metabolism; much via the CYP3A4 enzyme system. 31% excreted in urine, 66% in feces.
Half-life: 7 hr.

TIME/ACTION PROFILE

ROUTE	ONSET	PEAK	DURATION
PO	unknown	30 min (blood levels)	6–8 hr

Contraindications/Precautions

Contraindicated in: Known hypersensitivity/intolerance; Concurrent use of ketoconazole; Prolactinoma; Conditions where GI stimulation is dangerous including GI hemorrhage/mechanical obstruction/perforation; Lactation: Breast feeding is not recommended unless potential benefits outweigh potential risks.
Use Cautiously in: History of breast cancer; Hepatic impairment; Severe renal impairment (dose adjustment may be necessary during chronic therapy); OB: Use only if expected benefit outweighs potential hazard; Pedi: Safety and effectiveness not established.

Adverse Reactions/Side Effects

CNS: headache, insomnia. **GI:** dry mouth. **GU:** amenorrhea, impotence. **Derm:** hot flushes, rash. **Endo:** galactorrhea, gynecomastia, hyperprolactinemia.

Interactions

Drug-Drug: Ketoconazole↑ levels and the risk of cardiovascular toxicity; concurrent use contraindicated; other **azole antifungals**, **macrolide anti-infectives** and **protease inhibitors** may have similar effects. Risk of adverse cardiovascular reactions may be ↑ by concurrent use of **drugs known to ↑ QT interval** including

antiarrhythmics, some **fluoroquinolones**, **antipsychotics**, **beta-2 adrenergic agonists**, **antimalarials**, **SSRIs**, **tri/tetracyclic antidepressants** and **nefazodone** and should be undertaken cautiously, especially if other risk factors for *torsade de pointes* exists. Effectiveness may be ↓ by concurrent use of **anticholinergics**. Due to effects on gastric motility, absorption of drugs from the small intestine may be accelerated, while absorption of drugs from the stomach may be slowed, especially **sustained-release** or **enteric-coated** formulations. Concurrent use with **MAOIs** should be undertaken with caution.
Drug-Food: Grapefruit juice may ↑ levels.

Route/Dosage
PO (Adults): *Upper GI motility disorders*—10 mg 3–4 times daily; may be ↑ to 20 mg 3–4 times daily; *Nausea/vomiting due to dopamine agonist antiparkinson agents*—20 mg 3–4 times daily, higher doses may be required during dose titration.

Renal Impairment
PO (Adults): Depending on degree of impairment, dosing during chronic therapy should be reduced to once or twice daily.

Availability
Tablets: 10 mg.

NURSING IMPLICATIONS

Assessment
- Assess for nausea, vomiting, abdominal distention, and bowel sounds before and after administration.
- Monitor BP (sitting, standing, lying down) and pulse before and periodically during therapy. May cause prolonged QT interval, tachycardia, and orthostatic hypotension, especially in patients older than 60 yrs or taking >30 mg/day.
- Monitor for symptoms related to hyperprolactinemia (menstrual abnormalities, galactorrhea, sexual dysfunction).
- ***Lab Test Considerations:*** May cause ↑ serum ALT, AST, and cholesterol.
- Monitor serum prolactin prior to and periodically during therapy. May cause ↑ serum prolactin levels.

Implementation
- Use lowest effective dose.
- Administer 3–4 times daily, 15–30 min before meals and at bedtime.

Patient/Family Teaching
- Instruct patient to take as directed. Advise patient to avoid grapefruit juice during therapy.
- Advise patient to notify health care professional if galactorrhea (excessive or spontaneous flow of breast milk), gynecomastia (excessive development of male mammary gland), menstrual irregularities (spotting or delayed periods), palpitations, irregular heart beat (arrhythmia), dizziness, or fainting occur.
- Advise female patient to notify health care professional if pregnancy is planned or suspected or if breast feeding.

Evaluation
- Prevention or relief of nausea and vomiting.
- Decreased symptoms of gastric stasis.

flupentixol (floo-pen-tiks-ol)
Fluanxol

Classification
Therapeutic: antipsychotics
Pharmacologic: thioxanthenes

Indications
Maintenance treatment of schizophrenia in patients whose symptomatology does not include excitement, agitation or hyperactivity. Not indicated for the treatment of dementia in the elderly.

Action
Alters the effects of dopamine in the CNS. Has some anticholinergic and alpha-adrenergic blocking activity.
Therapeutic Effects: Diminished signs and symptoms of schizophrenia.

Pharmacokinetics
Absorption: *Flupentixol dihydrochloride*—40% absorbed following oral administration; *Flupentixol decanoate*—slowly released from IM injection sites.
Distribution: Distributes to lungs, liver and spleen, enter CNS; extensive tissue distribution.
Protein Binding: 99%.
Metabolism and Excretion: Mostly metabolized, metabolites do not have antipsychotic activity. Most metabolites are excreted in feces, some renal elimination.
Half-life: *Flupentixol dihydrochloride*—35 hr; *Flupentixol decanoate*—3 wk.

TIME/ACTION PROFILE (antipsychotic effect)

ROUTE	ONSET	PEAK	DURATION
PO	within 2–3 days	3–8 hr (blood level)	8 hr
IM (depot)	24–72 hr	4–7 days (blood level)	2–4 wk

Contraindications/Precautions
Contraindicated in: Hypersensitivity to flupentixol or other thioxanthines (cross sensitivity with phenothiazines may occur); CNS depression due to any cause, including comatose states, cortical brain damage (known or suspected), or circulatory collapse; Opiate, alcohol or barbiturate intoxication; Hepatic impairment, cerebrovascular insufficiency or severe cardiovascular pathology; Concurrent use of other drugs known to prolong QT interval; Pedi: Safety and effectiveness not established; not recommended.

Use Cautiously in: Brain tumors or intestinal obstruction (may mask symptoms); Patients exposed to extreme heat or organophosphorous insecticides; Risk factors for/history of stroke; Any risk factors for QT prolongation including hypokalmia, hypomagnesemia, genetic predisposition, cardiovascular disease history (including bradycardia), recent MI, HF or arrhythmias; Known/suspected glaucoma; History of seizures (may ↓ seizure threshold); Parkinson's disease (may worsen symptoms); Geri: Consider age-related ↓ in renal, cardiac and hepatic function; OB: Use only if expected benefit outweighs potential risks to infant; Lactation: Safe use not established; low levels in breast milk are not expected to affect infant if therapeutic doses are used.

Adverse Reactions/Side Effects

CNS: NEUROLEPTIC MALIGNANT SYNDROME dizziness. **EENT:** blurred vision. **CV:** QT INTERVAL PROLONGATION, THROMBOEMBOLISM, extrapyramidal symptoms, tachycardia, hypotension, sedation, tardive dyskinesia. **GI:** constipation, dry mouth, excess salivation, hepatotoxicity. **GU:** ↓ libido, urinary retention. **Derm:** photosensitivity reactions, rash, sweating. **Endo:** glucose intolerance, hyperprolactinemia, menstrual irregularity. **Hemat:** agranulocytosis, granulocytopenia, neutropenia. **Metab:** weight change. **MS:** osteoporosis (long term use).

Interactions

Drug-Drug: ↑ CNS depression with other **CNS depressants** including **alcohol**, some **antidepressants**, some **antihistamines**, **anxiolytics**, **benzodiazepines** and **sedative/hypnotics**. ↑ risk of QT prolongation and serious arrhythmias with **Class Ia and III antiarrhythmics** (including **quinidine**, **amiodarone** and **sotalol**), some **antipsychotics** (including **thioridazine**), some **macrolides** (including **erythromycin**) and some **fluoroquinolones** (including **moxifloxacin**); concurrent use should be avoided. Concurrent use of **diuretics** and other **drugs affecting electrolytes** may ↑ risk of QT interval prolongation and serious arrhythmias. ↑ risk of anticholinergic adverse reactions, including paralytic ileus when used concurrently with other **anticholinergics** or **drugs with anticholinergic side effects**. May ↓ metabolism and ↑ effects of **tricyclic antidepressants**. ↑ risk of extrapyramidal symptoms with **metoclopramide**. May ↓ effectiveness of **levodopa** and **dopamine agonists**.

Route/Dosage

PO (Adults): 1 mg 3 times daily initially; ↑ by 1 mg every 2–3 days until desired response, usual effective dose is 3–6 mg/day in divided doses (up to 12 mg/day has been used); if insomnia occurs, evening dose may be ↓.

IM (Adults): Initiate with a 5–20 mg test dose (use 5 mg dose in elderly/frail/cachectic patients) as the 2% injection. Patients previously treated with long-acting neuroleptic injections may tolerate initial doses of 20 mg. A 2nd 20 mg dose may be given 4–10 days later and then 20–40 mg every 2–3 wk depending on response. Oral flupentixol should be continued, but gradually decreased in the first wk following depot injection. Guidelines for conversion from PO to depot IM injection: daily oral dose (mg) × 4 = dose of depot injection (mg) given every 2 wk *or* daily oral dose (mg) × 8 = depot injection (mg) given every 4 wk.

Availability

Tablets (flupentixol dihydrochloride): 0.5 mg, 3 mg, 5 mg; Depot injection (flupentixol decanoate—contains medium-chain triglycerides [coconut oil]): 20 mg/mL (2%), 100 mg/mL (10%).

NURSING IMPLICATIONS

Assessment

- Assess mental status (orientation, mood, behavior) before and periodically during therapy.
- Monitor BP (sitting, standing, lying), ECG, pulse, and respiratory rate before and frequently during the period of dose adjustment. May cause Q-T prolongation.
- Observe carefully when administering oral medication to ensure that medication is actually taken and not hoarded.
- Assess weight and BMI initially and throughout therapy.
- Assess fluid intake and bowel function. Increased bulk and fluids in the diet help minimize constipation.
- Monitor for onset of akathisia (restlessness or desire to keep moving) and extrapyramidal side effects (*parkinsonian*—difficulty speaking or swallowing, loss of balance control, pill rolling, mask-like face, shuffling gait, rigidity, tremors; *dystonic*—muscle spasms, twisting motions, twitching, inability to move eyes, weakness of arms or legs) every 2 mo during therapy and 8–12 wk after therapy has been discontinued. Reduction in dose or discontinuation of medication may be necessary. Benztropine or diphenhydramine may be used to control these symptoms.
- Monitor for tardive dyskinesia (uncontrolled rhythmic movement of mouth, face, and extremities; lip smacking or puckering; puffing of cheeks; uncontrolled chewing; rapid or worm-like movements of tongue). Report immediately; may be irreversible.
- Monitor for development of neuroleptic malignant syndrome (fever, respiratory distress, tachycardia, seizures, diaphoresis, arrhythmias, hypertension or hypotension, pallor, tiredness, severe muscle stiffness, loss of bladder control). Report immediately.
- Monitor for symptoms related to hyperprolactinemia (menstrual abnormalities, galactorrhea, sexual dysfunction).
- ***Lab Test Considerations:*** Monitor CBC and liver function tests periodically during treatment. May cause ↑ AST, ALT, and alkaline phosphatase.
- Monitor blood glucose prior to and periodically during therapy. May cause hyperglycemia.
- Monitor serum prolactin prior to and periodically during therapy. May cause ↑ serum prolactin levels.
- May cause false-positive pregnancy tests.

Implementation

- **PO:** Initially, take tablets 3 times daily, without regard to food. Dose will increase for first few days until desired results. Maintenance dose is usually taken in morning.
- When converting to IM doses, PO dose is usually continued in decreasing doses for first wk.
- **IM:** Inject deep IM preferably into gluteus maximus. Solution is a yellow viscous oil, aspirate prior to injection to ensure dose is not injected IV. Do not administer solutions that are discolored, hazy, or contain particulate matter.
- For large doses or pain with large volume, flupentizol decanoate BP 10% (100 mg/mL) may be used instead of flupentixol decanoate BP 2% (20 mg/mL).

Patient/Family Teaching

- Instruct patient to take as directed. If a dose is missed, omit and take next dose as scheduled. Discontinuation should be gradual; abrupt discontinuation may cause withdrawal symptoms (nausea, vomiting, anorexia, diarrhoea, rhinorrhoea, sweating, myalgias, paraesthesias, insomnia, restlessness, anxiety, agitation, vertigo, feelings of warmth and coldness, tremor). Symptoms begin within 1 to 4 days of withdrawal and abate within 7 to 14 days. Advise patient to read *Patient Information* leaflet prior to starting therapy and with each Rx refill in case of changes.
- Inform patient of possibility of extrapyramidal symptoms and tardive dyskinesia. Caution patient to report these symptoms immediately to health care professional.
- Advise patient to change positions slowly to minimize orthostatic hypotension.
- Medication may cause drowsiness. Caution patient to avoid driving or other activities requiring alertness until response to medication is known.
- Advise patient to notify health care professional of all Rx or OTC medications, vitamins, or herbal products being taken and to consult with health care professional before taking other medications.
- Caution patient to avoid concurrent use of alcohol and other CNS depressants.
- Instruct patient to notify health care professional promptly if sore throat, fever, unusual bleeding or bruising, rash, weakness, tremors, visual disturbances, dark-colored urine, or clay-colored stools occur.
- Instruct patient to avoid sun exposure and to wear protective clothing and sunscreen when outdoors.
- Advise patient to notify health care professional of medication regimen before treatment or surgery.
- Advise female patients to notify health care professional if pregnancy is planned or suspected or if breast feeding.

Evaluation

- Decreased symptoms of schizophrenia (delusions, hallucinations, social withdrawal, flat, blunt affect).

fusidic acid (fyoo-**sid**-ik **as**-id)

🍁Fucidin, 🍁Fucithalmic

Classification

Therapeutic: anti-infectives

Indications

Topical: Local treatment of primary and secondary bacterial skin infections including impetigo contagiosa, erythrasma and secondary skin infections such as infected wounds/burns. **Ophth:** Treatment of superficial eye infections.

Action

Inhibits bacterial protein synthesis. **Therapeutic Effects:** Resolution of localized bacterial infections. Not active against Gram-negative organisms; active against Staphylococci, Streptococci and Corynebacterium.

Pharmacokinetics

Absorption: Unknown.

Distribution: Systemically absorbed drug crosses the placenta and enters breast milk.

Metabolism and Excretion: Absorbed drug is extensively metabolized.

Half-life: 5–6 hr.

TIME/ACTION PROFILE

ROUTE	ONSET	PEAK	DURATION
Top	unknown	unknown	6–8 hr
Ophth	unknown	unknown	12 hr

Contraindications/Precautions

Contraindicated in: Hypersensitivity to fusidic acid or other components of the formulation (topical ointment contains lanolin).

Use Cautiously in: OB: Potential benefits should be weighed against the possible hazards to the fetus (crosses the placenta); Lactation: Safe use during breast feeding has not been established (enters breast milk).

Adverse Reactions/Side Effects

Derm: mild local irritation.

Interactions

Drug-Drug: None noted.

Route/Dosage

Topical (Adults and Children): Apply to affected area 3–4 times daily.

Ophth (Adults and Children): One drop into conjunctival sac of both eyes every 12 hr for 7 days.

Availability

Topical cream: 2% (20 mg/g); Topical ointment (contains lanolin): 2% (20 mg/g); Ophthalmic viscous drops (microcrystalline suspension): 1%. ***In combination with:*** hydrocortisone (Fucidin H).

NURSING IMPLICATIONS

Assessment

- Inspect involved areas of skin and mucous membranes before and frequently during therapy. Increased skin irritation may indicate need to discontinue medication.

Implementation

- Do not confuse topical product with ophthalmic product.
- **Topical:** Consult health care professional for proper cleansing technique before applying medication. Apply small amount to cover affected area completely. Avoid the use of occlusive wrappings or dressings unless directed by health care professional.
- **Ophth:** Administer 1 drop into conjunctival sac of both eyes every 12 hr for 7 days. See Appendix D for instructions.

Patient/Family Teaching

- Instruct patient to apply medication as directed for full course of therapy, even if feeling better. Emphasize the importance of avoiding the eyes.
- Advise patient to report increased skin irritation or lack of response to therapy to health care professional.

Evaluation

- Resolution of skin or eye infection.

gliclazide (glik-la-zide)

Diamicron MR

Classification

Therapeutic: antidiabetics

Pharmacologic: sulfonylureas

Indications

Control of blood sugar in type 2 diabetes mellitus when control of diet and exercise fails or when insulin is not an option. Requires some pancreatic function.

Action

Lowers blood glucose by stimulating the release of insulin from the pancreas and increasing sensitivity to insulin at receptor sites. **Therapeutic Effects:** Lowering of blood glucose in diabetic patients.

Pharmacokinetics

Absorption: Well absorbed following oral administration (97%).

Distribution: Unknown.

Protein Binding: 95%.

Metabolism and Excretion: Extensively metabolized, metabolites are mostly eliminated (60–70%) in urine, 10–20% in feces; <1% excreted unchanged in urine.

Half-life: *Tablets*—10.4 hr; *modified-release tablets*—16 hr.

TIME/ACTION PROFILE (effect on blood sugar)

ROUTE	ONSET	PEAK	DURATION
PO	unknown	4–6 hr (blood levels)	12–24 hr

Contraindications/Precautions

Contraindicated in: Hypersensitivity; cross sensitivity with other sulfonylureas may occur; Unstable diabetes, type 1 diabetes mellitus, diabetic ketoacidosis, diabetic coma or pre-coma; Severe hepatic or renal impairment; Concurrent use of oral/oromucosal miconazole, alcohol or alcohol-containing medications, or systemic phenylbutazone; OB: Should not be used during pregnancy, insulin is preferred; Lactation: Should not be used during lactation, insulin is perferred.

Use Cautiously in: Glucose 6-phosphate dehydrogenase deficiency (↑ risk of hemolytic anemia); Infection, stress, or changes in diet may alter requirements for control of blood sugar or require use of insulin; Impaired thyroid, pituitary, or adrenal function; Malnutrition, high fever, prolonged nausea, or vomiting; Pedi: Safety and effectiveness not established.

Adverse Reactions/Side Effects

Endo: hypoglycemia. **GI:** abdominal pain, diarrhea, dyspepsia, ↑ liver enzymes, nausea, vomiting. **Derm:** photosensitivity, rash.

Interactions

Drug-Drug: Concurrent use of **alcohol**, **angiotensin converting-enzyme inhibitors**, **antituberculars**, **azole antifungals**, **beta-blockers**, **clarithromycin**, **clofibrate**, **disopyramide**, **H2–receptor antagonists**, **MAO inhibitors**, **NSAIDs**, **phenylbutazone**, **salicylates**, long-acting **sulfonamides**, **warfarin**, may ↑ risk of hypoglycemia. ↑ risk of hypoglycemia with other **antidiabetic agents** including **alpha glucosidase inhibitors**, **biguanides**, and **insulin**. Concurrent use of **chlorpromazine**, **corticosteroids**, **danazol**, **diuretics**, (including **thiazides**, and **furosemide**), **hormonal contraceptives** (**estrogen** and **progestogen**), **nicotinic acid** (pharmacologic doses), **ritodrine**, **salbutamol**, **terbutaline**, or **tetracosactrin** may ↑ risk of hyperglycemia and lead to loss of diabetic control. May ↑ risk of bleeding with **warfarin**. Concurrent use with **alcohol** may result in a disulfiram-like reaction and should be avoided. **Beta-blockers** may ↓ some symptoms of hyperglycemia.

Route/Dosage

PO (Adults): *Tablets*—80–320 mg/day, doses >160 mg/day should be divided and given twice daily; *modified-release tablets*—30 mg daily, may be ↑ in 30–mg increments every 2 wk until blood sugar is controlled up to 120 mg/day.

Availability

Tablets (contain lactose): 80 mg; Modified-release tablets: 30 mg, 60 mg.

NURSING IMPLICATIONS

Assessment

- Observe for signs and symptoms of hypoglycemia (hunger, weakness, sweating, dizziness, tachycardia, anxiety).
- Assess patient for allergy to sulfonyureas.
- ***Lab Test Considerations:*** Monitor serum glucose and glycosylated hemoglobin periodically during therapy to evaluate effectiveness of treatment.

- Monitor liver function periodically in patients with mild to moderate liver dysfunction. May cause ↑ AST, ALT, alkaline phosphatase and LDH.
- Monitor renal function periodically in patients with mild to moderate renal dysfunction. May cause ↑ creatinine and hyponatremia.
- ***Toxicity and Overdose:*** Overdose is manifested by symptoms of hypoglycemia. Mild hypoglycemia may be treated with administration of oral glucose. Treat severe hypoglycemia with IV D50W followed by continuous IV infusion of more dilute dextrose solution at a rate sufficient to keep serum glucose at approximately 100 mg/dL.

Implementation

- Patients on a diabetic regimen exposed to stress, fever, infection, trauma, or surgery may require administration of insulin.
- **PO:** Administer with meals at the same time every day.

Patient/Family Teaching

- Instruct patient to take gliclazides as directed at the same time every day.
- Explain to patient that this medication does not cure diabetes and must be used in conjunction with a prescribed diet, exercise regimen, to prevent hypoglycemic and hyperglycemic events.
- Instruct patient on proper technique for home glucose monitoring. Monitor closely during periods of stress or illness and health care professional notified if significant changes occur.
- Review signs of hypoglycemia and hyperglycemia with patient. If hypoglycemia occurs, advise patient to drink a glass of orange juice or ingest 2–3 tsp of sugar, honey, or corn syrup dissolved in water or an appropriate number of glucose tablets and notify health care professional.
- Encourage patient to follow prescribed diet, medication, and exercise regimen to prevent hypoglycemic or hyperglycemic episodes.
- Concurrent use of alcohol may cause a disulfiram-like reaction (abdominal cramps, nausea, flushing, headaches, and hypoglycemia).
- Instruct patient to avoid sun exposure and to wear protective clothing and sunscreen when outdoors.
- Caution patient to avoid other medications, especially aspirin and alcohol, while on this therapy without consulting health care professional.
- Advise patient to notify health care professional promptly if unusual weight gain, swelling of ankles, drowsiness, shortness of breath, muscle cramps, weakness, sore throat, rash, or unusual bleeding or bruising occurs.
- Advise patient to inform health care professional of medication regimen prior to treatment or surgery.
- Advise patient to carry sugar packets or candy, and identification describing diabetes diagnosis and medication regimen.
- Insulin is the recommended method of controlling blood sugar during pregnancy. Counsel female patients to use a form of contraception other than oral contraceptives and to notify health care professional promptly if pregnancy is planned or suspected.
- Emphasize the importance of routine follow-up exams.

Evaluation

- Control of blood glucose levels to avoid episodes of hypoglycemia and hyperglycemia.

methotrimeprazine

(meth-oh-try-**mep**-ra-zeen)

🍁Methoprazine, 🍁 Nozinan

Classification

Therapeutic: antipsychotics, nonopioid analgesics

Pharmacologic: phenothiazines

Indications

Management of psychotic disturbances. Management of conditions associated with anxiety/tension. As an analgesic and adjunct in pain due to cancer, zona, trigeminal neuralgia, intercostal neuralgia, phantom limb pain, and muscular discomforts. Used as a preoperative sedative. As an antiemetic. As a sedative in the treatment of insomnia.

Action

Sedation. **Therapeutic Effects:** Reduction in severity of pain.

Pharmacokinetics

Absorption: Well absorbed after PO/IM administration. IV administration results in complete bioavailability.

Distribution: Enters CSF and crosses the placenta. Minimal amounts enter breast milk.

Metabolism and Excretion: Mostly metabolized by the liver. Some metabolites are active; 1% excreted unchanged by the kidneys.

Half-life: *PO*—10.3–10.8 hr; *IM*—15–30 hr.

TIME/ACTION PROFILE

ROUTE	ONSET	PEAK	DURATION
PO (blood levels)	unknown	2.7–2.9 hr	8–12 hr
IM (analgesia)	unknown	20–40 min	8 hr (up to 24 hr in children)

Contraindications/Precautions

Contraindicated in: Blood dyscrasias; Hepatic impairment; Hypersensitivity to methotrimeprazine, phenothiazines or sulfites; Comatose patients or those who have overdosed on CNS depressants including alcohol, analgesics, opioids or sedative/hypnotics; OB: Third-trimester use may result in agitation, hypotonia, tremor,

somnolence, respiratory distress and feeding disturbances in newborn and should be avoided.
Use Cautiously in: History of seizures; History of glaucoma or prostatic hypertrophy (↑ risk of anticholinergic adverse reactions); Bradycardia, electrolyte abnormalities, congenital/acquired prolonged QT interval or concurrent use of drugs that may prolong QT interval (↑ risk of serious arrhythmias); Underlying cardiovascular disease including stroke, arteriosclerosis, or thromboembolism (↑ risk of adverse cardiovascular effects); Geri: Initial dosage ↓ recommended, ↑ risk of death in elderly patients with dementia; Lactation: Safety not established; Pedi: Safety not established.

Adverse Reactions/Side Effects

CNS: NEUROLEPTIC MALIGNANT SYNDROME, SEIZURES, amnesia, drowsiness, excess sedation, disorientation, euphoria, extrapyramidal reactions, headache, slurred speech, tardive dyskinesia, weakness. **EENT:** nasal congestion. **CV:** orthostatic hypotension, bradycardia, palpitations, tachycardia. **GI:** constipation, abdominal discomfort, dry mouth, nausea, vomiting. **GU:** difficulty in urination. **Endo:** hyperglycemia, hyperprolactinemia. **Hemat:** blood dyscrasias. **Local:** pain at injection site. **Misc:** chills.

Interactions

Drug-Drug: ↑ CNS depression with other **CNS depressants**, including **alcohol**, **antihistamines**, **antidepressants**, **opioids**, or **sedative/hypnotics**; ↓ dose of these agents by 50% initially. ↑ anticholinergic effects with **antihistamines**, **antidepressants**, **phenothiazines**, **quinidine**, **disopyramide**, **atropine**, or **scopolamine**; ↓ doses of concurrent atropine or scopolamine. Reverses vasopressor effects of **epinephrine**; avoid concurrent use—if vasopressor required, use phenylephrine or norepinephrine. ↑ risk of hypotension with acute ingestion of **alcohol**, **nitrates**, **MAO inhibitors**, or **antihypertensives**. Concurrent use with **succinylcholine** may result in tachycardia, hypotension, CNS stimulation, delirium, and ↑ extrapyramidal symptoms.
Drug-Natural Products: Concomitant use of **kava**, **valerian**, **skullcap**, **chamomile**, or **hops** ↑ risk of CNS depression.

Route/Dosage

PO (Adults): *Minor conditions*—6–25 mg/day in 3 divided doses (if sedation occurs, use smaller daytime doses and a larger dose at bedtime); *Night time sedative*—10–25 mg as a single bedtime dose; *Psychoses/intense pain*—50–75 mg/day in 2–3 divided doses, dose may be titrated upward to desired effect (doses of 1 g/day have been used, if daily dose exceeds 100–200 mg, administer in divided doses and keep patient at bed-rest).
PO (Children): 0.25 mg/kg/day in 2–3 divided doses (not to exceed 40 mg/day in children <12 yr).
IM (Adults): *Post-operative analgesic adjunct*—10–25 mg every 8 hr, if given with opioids, ↓ opioid dose by 50%.
IM (Children): *Analgesia*—62.5–125 mcg (0.0625–0.125 mg)/kg/day single dose or divided doses, change to oral medication as soon as possible.
IV (Children): *Palliative care setting*—62.5 mcg (0.0625 mg)/kg/day in 250 mL of 5% dextrose solution as a slow infusion (20–40 drops/min).

Availability

Tablets: 2 mg, 5 mg, 25 mg, 50 mg; Solution for injection: 25 mg/mL.

NURSING IMPLICATIONS

Assessment

- Assess type, location, and intensity of pain before and 30 min after administration.
- Monitor BP frequently after injection. Orthostatic hypotension, fainting, syncope, and weakness frequently occur from 10 min to 12 hr after administration. Patient should remain supine for 6–12 hr after injection.
- Assess weight and BMI initially and throughout therapy.
- Observe patient carefully for extrapyramidal side effects (*parkinsonian*—difficulty speaking or swallowing, loss of balance control, pill rolling, mask-like face, shuffling gait, rigidity, tremors; *dystonic*—muscle spasms, twisting motions, twitching, inability to move eyes, weakness of arms or legs). Usually occur only after prolonged or high-dose therapy. Usually resolve with dose decrease or administration of antiparkinsonian agent.
- Monitor for tardive dyskinesia (involuntary rhythmic movement of mouth, face, and extremities). Report immediately and discontinue therapy; may be irreversible.
- Monitor for development of neuroleptic malignant syndrome (fever, respiratory distress, tachycardia, seizures, diaphoresis, hypertension or hypotension, pallor, tiredness). Discontinue methotrimeprazine and notify health care professional immediately if these symptoms occur.
- Methotrimeprazine potentiates the action of other CNS depressants but can be given in conjunction with modified doses of opioid analgesics for management of severe pain. This medication does not significantly depress respiratory status and can be useful where pulmonary reserve is low.
- Monitor for symptoms related to hyperprolactinemia (menstrual abnormalities, galactorrhea, sexual dysfunction).
- ***Lab Test Considerations:*** Monitor CBC prior to and periodically during therapy and liver function tests should be evaluated periodically throughout long-term (>30 days) therapy.
- Monitor blood glucose prior to and periodically during therapy may therapy. May cause hyperglycemia.
- Monitor serum prolactin prior to and periodically during therapy. May cause ↑ serum prolactin levels.

Implementation

- **PO:** May be administered during day or only at night depending on indication.
- **IM:** Do not inject subcut. Inject slowly into deep, well-developed muscle. Rotate injection sites.

- **Intermittent Infusion:** For patients in palliative care, may be infused as 0.0625 mg/kg/day in 250 mL of D5W. ***Rate:*** Infuse slowly 20–40 drops per min.
- **Y-Site Compatibility:** fentanyl hydromorphone, methadone, morphine, sufentanil.
- **Y-Site Incompatibility:** heparin.

Patient/Family Teaching

- Instruct patient on how and when to ask for pain medication.
- Instruct patient to take medication as directed. Take missed doses as soon as remembered unless almost time for next dose; do not double dose. Advise patient to read *Patient Information* leaflet prior to starting therapy and with each Rx refill in case of changes.
- Advise patients to make position changes slowly and to remain recumbent for 6–12 hr after administration to minimize orthostatic hypotension.
- May cause drowsiness. Caution patient to request assistance with ambulation and transfer and to avoid driving or other activities requiring alertness until response to the medication is known.
- Advise patient to notify health care professional of all Rx or OTC medications, vitamins, or herbal products being taken and to consult with health care professional before taking other medications.
- Caution patient to avoid taking alcohol or other CNS depressants concurrently with this medication.
- Advise patient to use sunscreen and protective clothing when exposed to the sun. Extremes of temperature should also be avoided because this drug impairs body temperature regulation.
- Instruct patient to use frequent mouth rinses, good oral hygiene, and sugarless gum or candy to minimize dry mouth.
- Instruct patient to notify health care professional promptly if sore throat, fever, unusual bleeding or bruising, rash, weakness, tremors, dark-colored urine, or clay-colored stools or signs of blood clots (swelling, pain and redness in an arm or leg that can be warm to touch, sudden chest pain, difficulty breathing, heart palpitations) occur.

Evaluation

- Decrease in severity of pain.
- Sedation.

moclobemide

(moe-**kloe**-be-mide)

Manerix

Classification

Therapeutic: antidepressants

Pharmacologic: monamine oxidase (MAO) inhibitors, benzamides

Indications

Treatment of depression.

Action

Short-acting, reversible inhibitor of monoamine oxidase type A. Increases concentrations of serotonin, norepinephrine, and dopamine. **Therapeutic Effects:** Decreased symptoms of depression, with improved mood and quality of life.

Pharmacokinetics

Absorption: 98% absorbed following oral administration, but undergoes first-pass hepatic metabolism resulting in 90% bioavailability.

Distribution: Unknown.

Metabolism and Excretion: Extensively metabolized (partially by CYP2C19 and CYP2D6), very small amounts are pharmacologically active, less than 1% excreted unchanged in urine.

Half-life: 1.5 hr (↑ with dose).

TIME/ACTION PROFILE

ROUTE	ONSET	PEAK	DURATION
PO	days–several wk (antidepressant effect)	0.5–3.5 hr (blood levels)	24 hr (MAO-A inhibition)

Contraindications/Precautions

Contraindicated in: Known hypersensitivity; Acute confusional states; Concurrent use of tricyclic antidepressants; Concurrent use of SSRIs or other MAO inhibitors; Concurrent use of dextromethorphan, meperidine, selegiline or thioridazine; Pedi: Safety not established, use is not recommended.

Use Cautiously in: History of suicide attempt or ideation; History of thyrotoxicosis or pheochromocytoma (possible risk of hypertensive reaction); Severe hepatic impairment (↓ dose required); Renal impairment; OB: Should not be used unless anticipated benefits justify potential harm to fetus; Lactation: Not recommended unless anticipated benefits justify potential harm to infant.

Adverse Reactions/Side Effects

CNS: SUICIDAL IDEATION, agitation, insomnia, restlessness, tremor. **CV:** hypotension.

Interactions

Drug-Drug: ↑ levels and risk of QT prolongation with **thioridazine**, avoid concurrent use. Concurrent use with **selegiline** greatly ↑ sensitivity to tyramine and is contraindicated. Concurrent use with **tricyclic antidepressants** may result in severe adverse reactions and is contraindicated. Should not be used with **SSRIs** or other **MAO inhibitors**; when making a switch allow 4–5 half-lives of previous drug; for **fluoxetine** wait at least 5 wk. Exessive **alcohol** should be avoided. **Cimetidine** ↓ metabolism and ↑ blood levels, ↓ moclobemide dose by 50%. Because of the potential for interactions with **anesthetics**, especially local anesthetics containing **epinephrine**, moclo-

bemide should be discontinued at least 2 days prior to procedures. Concurrent use with **opioids** should be avoided; dosage adjustments may be necessary. Concurrent use of **sympathomimetics** including **ephedrine** and **amphetamines** may ↑ blood pressure and should be avoided. Concurrent use with **dextromethorphan** may result in vertigo, tremor, nausea and vomiting and should be avoided. Concurrent use with **antihypertensives** should be carefully monitored.
Drug-Food: Ingestion of large amounts of **tyramine-containing foods** including some cheeses and **Marmite yeast extract** may result in hypertension and arrhythmias and should be undertaken with caution.

Route/Dosage

PO (Adults): 150 mg twice daily initially; may be ↑ gradually after one wk as needed/tolerated up to 600 mg/day.

Hepatic Impairment

PO (Adults): *Severe hepatic impairment or concurrent enzyme inhibitor (cimetidine)*—↓ daily dose to ⅓ to ½ of standard dose.

Availability

Tablets: 100 mg, 150 mg, 300 mg.

NURSING IMPLICATIONS

Assessment

- Assess mental status for orientation, mood, behavior and anxiety. Assess for suicidal tendencies. Restrict amount of drug available to patient.
- Monitor BP and pulse before and frequently during therapy. Report significant changes promptly.
- Monitor mood changes. Assess for suicidal tendencies, especially during early therapy. Restrict amount of drug available to patient.
- Monitor intake and output ratios and daily weight. Assess patient for peripheral edema and urinary retention.
- ***Lab Test Considerations:*** Monitor liver and kidney function periodically during treatment.
- Monitor serum glucose closely in diabetic patients; hypoglycemia may occur.
- ***Toxicity and Overdose:*** Concurrent ingestion of tyramine-rich foods and many medications may result in a life-threatening hypertensive crisis. Signs and symptoms of hypertensive crisis include chest pain, tachycardia, severe headache, nausea and vomiting, photosensitivity, and enlarged pupils. Treatment includes IV phentolamine.
- Symptoms of overdose include anxiety, irritability, tachycardia, hypertension or hypotension, respiratory distress, dizziness, drowsiness, hallucinations, confusion, seizures, fever, and diaphoresis. Treatment includes induction of vomiting or gastric lavage and supportive therapy as symptoms arise.

Implementation

- Administer after meals. Swallow tablet whole; do not crush, break, or chew. Dose may be adjusted gradually during the first wk of therapy.

Patient/Family Teaching

- Instruct patient to take medication as directed. Take missed doses if remembered unless almost time for next dose; do not double doses. Do not discontinue abruptly; withdrawal symptoms (nausea, vomiting, malaise, nightmares, agitation, psychosis, seizures) may occur. Advise patient to read *Patient Information* leaflet prior to starting and with each Rx refill in case of changes.
- Caution patient to avoid alcohol, CNS depressants, OTC drugs, and foods or beverages containing tyramine (see Appendix K) during and for at least 2 wk after therapy has been discontinued; they may precipitate a hypertensive crisis. Contact health care professional immediately if symptoms of hypertensive crisis develop.
- Caution patient to notify health care professional if neck stiffness, changes in vision, diarrhea, constipation, rapid/pounding heart beat, sudden and severe headache, stiff neck, confusion, disorientation, slurred speech, behavioral changes, seizures.
- Advise patient and family to notify health care professional if thoughts about suicide or dying, attempts to commit suicide; new or worse depression; new or worse anxiety; feeling very agitated or restless; panic attacks; trouble sleeping; new or worse irritability; acting aggressive; being angry or violent; acting on dangerous impulses; an extreme increase in activity and talking; other unusual changes in behavior or mood occur.
- Instruct patient to carry identification describing medication regimen.
- Advise female patients to notify health care professional if pregnancy is planned or suspected or if breast feeding.
- Encourage patient to participate in psychotherapy in conjunction with taking medication.

Evaluation

- Improved mood in depressed patients.
- Decreased anxiety.

pinaverium

(pin-ah-**veer**-ee-um)
Dicetel

Classification
Therapeutic: anti-irritable bowel syndrome agents
Pharmacologic: calcium channel blockers

Indications

Management of symptoms of irritable bowel syndrome (IBS) including abdominal pain, bowel disturbances and discomfort. Treatment of symptoms related to biliary tract disorders.

Action

Acts as a calcium channel blocker with specific selectivity for intestinal smooth muscle. Relaxes gastrointestinal (mainly colon) and biliary tracts, inhibits colonic motor response to food/pharmacologic stimulation. **Therapeutic Effects:** Decreased symptoms of IBS.

Pharmacokinetics

Absorption: Poorly absorbed (1–10%).
Distribution: Distributes selectively to digestive tract.
Protein Binding: 97%.
Metabolism and Excretion: Minimal enterohepatic cycling, eliminated almost entirely in feces. Some metabolism.
Half-life: 1.5 hr.

TIME/ACTION PROFILE (blood levels)

ROUTE	ONSET	PEAK	DURATION
PO	unknown	1 hr	unknown

Contraindications/Precautions

Contraindicated in: Known hypersensitivity; Galactose intolerance/Lapp lactase deficiency/glucose-galactose malabsorption (tablets contain lactose); Lactation: Avoid use if breast-feeding; Pedi: Safety and effectiveness not established, use is not recommended.
Use Cautiously in: Pre-existing eosphageal lesions/hiatal hernia (glass of water and snack should be taken with each dose); OB: Should be used only if essential to welfare of patient.

Adverse Reactions/Side Effects

All less than 1%. **CNS:** drowsiness headache, vertigo. **GI:** constipation, diarrhea, distention, dry mouth, epigastric pain/fullness, esophageal irritation, nausea. **Derm:** rash.

Interactions

Drug-Drug: Concurrent use of **anticholinergics** may ↑ spasmolytic effects.

Route/Dosage

PO (Adults): 50 mg 3 times daily; may be ↑ as needed/tolerated up to 100 mg 3 times daily.

Availability

Tablets (contain lactose): 50 mg, 100 mg.

NURSING IMPLICATIONS

Assessment

- Assess for symptoms of IBS (abdominal pain or discomfort, bloating, constipation).
- Assess for lactose intolerance; product contains lactose.

Implementation

- **PO:** Administer tablet with a glass of water and food. Swallow tablet whole, do not crush, chew or suck. If >3 tablets/day prescribed, take additional tablets with glass of water and a snack. May be irritating to esophagus. Do not take the tablet while lying down or just before bedtime.

Patient/Family Teaching

- Instruct patient to take pinaverium as directed. Take missed doses as soon as remembered unless almost time for next dose; do not double doses.
- Caution patient to inform health care professional if the following side effects persist or worsen; stomach pain or fullness, nausea, constipation or diarrhea, heartburn, headache, dry mouth, dizziness, skin rash.
- Instruct patient to avoid alcohol intake while taking this medication.
- Advise female patient to inform health care professional if pregnancy is planned or suspected or if breast feeding.

Evaluation

- A decrease in symptoms of irritable bowel syndrome. The length of treatment depends on the condition being treated.

prucalopride

(proo-**kal**-o-pride)

Resotran

Classification
Therapeutic: prokinetic agents
Pharmacologic: dihydrobenzofurancarboxamides

Indications

Treatment of chronic idiopathic constipation in adult females who do not respond to laxatives.

Action

Acts as a serotonin (5–HT_4) receptor agonist with prokinetic properties. Enhances peristalsis and gastrointestinal propulsion. **Therapeutic Effects:** Laxative effect.

Pharmacokinetics

Absorption: Rapidly absorbed (90%) following oral administration.
Distribution: Rapidly and extensively distributed, enters breast milk.
Metabolism and Excretion: 60% excreted unchanged in urine, 3–8% unchanged in feces, minor amounts are extensively metabolized.
Half-life: 24 hr.

TIME/ACTION PROFILE (normalization of bowel movements)

ROUTE	ONSET	PEAK	DURATION
PO	3–4 days	1–4 wk	unknown

Contraindications/Precautions

Contraindicated in: Hypersensitivity; Renal impairment requiring dialysis; Intestinal obstruction/perforation (structural or function), obstructive ileus, severe gastrointestinal inflammatory disease, including Crohn's disease, ulcerative colitis, toxic megacolon/megarectum; Galactose intolerance, Lapp lactase deficiency or glucose/galactose malabsorption (tablets contain lactose); OB: Not recommended for use during pregnancy; Lactation: Not recommended for use while breast feeding;

Pedi: Safety and effectiveness not established; not recommended for use.

Use Cautiously in: Severe/clinically stable concurrent chronic diseases including liver, cardiovascular or lung disease, neurological or psychiatric disorders, cancer, AIDS or other disorders or insulin-dependent diabetes mellitus; History of arrhythmias or cardiovascular disease, ischemic heart disease, pre-excitation syndromes (including Wolff-Parkinson-White syndrome, Lown-Ganong-Levine syndrome or AV nodal disorders (↑ risk of arrhythmias); Severe renal impairment (↓ dose recommended); Geri: Due to age-related ↓ in renal function, ↓ dose is recommended.

Adverse Reactions/Side Effects

CNS: headache, dizziness, fatigue. **CV:** palpitations, ↓ PR interval, tachycardia. **GI:** abdominal pain, diarrhea, nausea, vomiting.

Interactions

Drug-Drug: Severe diarrhea may ↓ effectiveness of **oral hormonal contraceptives**; additional method of contraception recommended. Blood levels and effects are ↑ by concurrent CYP3A4 and P-gp inhibitors including **ketoconazole**, **verapamil**, **cyclosporine** and **quinidine**. Beneficial effects may be ↓ by concurrent use of **anticholinergics**.

Route/Dosage

PO (Adults): 2 mg once daily. If no bowel movement occurs in 3–4 days, add-on laxatives should be considered. If benefit is not obtained after 4 wk, prucalopride should be discontinued.

PO (Adults >65 yr): 1 mg once daily.

Renal Impairment

PO (Adults): *GFR <30 mL/min/1.73m²*—1 mg once daily.

Availability

Tablets (contain lactose): 1 mg, 2 mg.

NURSING IMPLICATIONS

Assessment

- Assess for symptoms of chronic constipation (abdominal pain or discomfort, bloating, constipation).

Implementation

- **PO:** Medication should be taken with food or on an empty stomach at the same time each day.

Patient/Family Teaching

- Instruct patient to take prucalopride as directed.
- Caution the patient to discontinue the medication and notify health care professional with occurrence of severe diarrhea, signs of heart attack, black tarry stools, vomiting of blood or material that looks like coffee grounds.
- Advise patient on a nutritional regimen and hydration, and exercise to decrease constipation.
- Inform patient that if no bowel movement within 3 days of treatment, a "rescue" laxative may be added occasionally while taking prucalopride.
- Advise women of childbearing age who are taking prucalopride to use an effective method of birth control during treatment. If pregnant occurs while taking this medication, contact health care professional immediately.

Evaluation

- A soft formed bowel movement.

trimebutine (try-meh-boo-teen)

🍁Modulon

Classification

Therapeutic: lower gastrointestinal tract motility regulators, spasmolytics

Indications

Symptomatic treatment of irritable bowel syndrome (IBS). Treatment of postoperative paralytic ileus.

Action

Acts as a spasmolytic. **Therapeutic Effects:** ↓ symptoms of IBS. Resumption of intestinal transit following abdominal surgical procedures.

Pharmacokinetics

Absorption: Rapidly absorbed following oral administration.

Distribution: Unknown.

Metabolism and Excretion: Extensively metabolized, <2.4% excreted unchanged in urine.

Half-life: 2.7–3.1 hr.

TIME/ACTION PROFILE (symptom relief)

ROUTE	ONSET	PEAK	DURATION
PO	within 3 days–2 wk	1 hr (blood level)	>1 wk (following discontinuation)

Contraindications/Precautions

Contraindicated in: Hypersensitivity.

Use Cautiously in: OB: Not recommended for use; Pedi: Children <12 yr (safety and effectiveness not established).

Adverse Reactions/Side Effects

CNS: dizziness, drowsiness, fatigue, headache. **GI:** diarrhea, dry mouth, dysguesia, dyspepsia, epigastric pain, nausea. **Derm:** hot/cold sensation, rash.

Interactions

Drug-Drug: None known.

Route/Dosage

PO (Adults): 200 mg 3 times daily.

Availability

Tablets: 100 mg, 200 mg.

NURSING IMPLICATIONS

Assessment

- Assess for symptoms of irritable bowel syndrome (cramping, constipation and diarrhea, mucus in stools).
- Assess for abdominal distention and assess bowel sounds.
- Monitor intake and output and record.

Implementation
- **PO:** Administer three times daily before meals.

Patient/Family Teaching
- Instruct patient to take trimebutine as directed.
- Advise female patient to inform health care professional if pregnancy is planned or suspected or if breast feeding.

Evaluation
- Decrease signs and symptoms of irritable bowel disease.

zopiclone (zoe-pi-clone)
Imovane

Classification
Therapeutic: sedative/hypnotics
Pharmacologic: cyclopyrrolones

Indications
Short-term treatment of insomnia characterized by difficulty falling asleep and frequent/early awakenings.

Action
Interacts with GABA-receptor complexes; not a benzodiazepine. **Therapeutic Effects:** Improved sleep with decrease latency and increased maintenance of sleep.

Pharmacokinetics
Absorption: Rapidly absorbed (75%) following oral administration.
Distribution: Rapidly distributed from extravascular compartment. Enters breast milk in concentrations that are 50% of plasma levels.
Metabolism and Excretion: Extensively metabolized (mostly by the CYP3A4 enzyme system), metabolites have minimal sedative/hypnotic activity; 4–5% excreted unchanged in urine.
Half-life: 5 hr.

TIME/ACTION PROFILE

ROUTE	ONSET	PEAK	DURATION
PO	rapid	2 hr	6 hr

Contraindications/Precautions
Contraindicated in: Hypersensitivity; Myasthenia gravis; Severe hepatic impairment; Severe respiratory impairment (including sleep apnea); Galactose intolerance (5 mg tablet contains lactose); OB: May cause fetal harm, neonatal CNS depression or withdrawal; Lactation: Breast feeding not recommended.
Use Cautiously in: Renal, hepatic or pulmonary impairment (dosage ↓ may be recommended); Past history of paradoxical reactions to sedative/hypnotics or alcohol or violent behavior; History of depression or suicidal ideation; Geri: ↑ sensitivity may ↑ the risk of falls, confusion or anterograde amnesia (use lowest effective dose); Pedi: Safety and effectiveness not established.
Exercise Extreme Caution in: History of substance/alcohol abuse.

Adverse Reactions/Side Effects
CV: abnormal thinking, behavioral changes, sleep-driving. **GI:** bitter taste, anorexia, constipation, dry mouth, dyspepsia. **Misc:** allergic reactions including ANAPHYLAXIS, ANAPHYLACTOID REACTIONS and ANGIOEDEMA.

Interactions
Drug-Drug: ↑ risk of CNS depression with other **CNS depressants** including **antihistamines, antidepressants, opioids, sedative/hypnotics,** and **antipsychotics.** ↑ levels and risk of CNS depression with **drugs that inhibit the CYP3A4 enzyme system,** including **erythromycin ketoconazole, itraconazole, clarithromycin, nefazodone, ritonavir,** and **nelfinavir;** ↓ dose may be necessary. Levels and effectiveness may be ↓ by **drugs that induce the CYP3A4 enzyme system,** including **carbamazepine, phenobarbital, phenytoin, rifampicin,** and **rifampin;** dose ↑ may be necessary.

Route/Dosage
PO (Adults): 5–7.5 mg taken immediately before bedtime; not to exceed 7.5 mg or 7–10 days use. Geri: 3.75 mg initially taken immediately before bedtime; may be ↑ up to 7.5 mg if needed.

Hepatic/Renal Impairment
PO (Adults): 3.75 mg initially taken immediately before bedtime; may be ↑ up to 7.5 mg if needed.

Availability
Tablets: 5 mg, 7.5 mg.

NURSING IMPLICATIONS

Assessment
- Assess mental status, sleep patterns, and previous use of sedative/hypnotics. Prolonged use of >7–10 days may lead to physical and psychological dependence.
- Assess alertness at time of peak of drug. Notify health care professional if desired sedation does not occur.
- Assess patient for pain. Medicate as needed. Untreated pain decreases sedative effects.

Implementation
- Before administering, reduce external stimuli and provide comfort measures to increase effectiveness of medication.
- Protect patient from injury. Raise bed side rails. Assist with ambulation. Remove patient's cigarettes.
- Use lowest effective dose.
- **PO:** Tablets should be swallowed with full glass of water. For faster onset of sleep, do not administer with or immediately after a meal.

Patient/Family Teaching
- Instruct patient to take zopiclone as directed. Advise patient not to take zopiclone unless able to stay in bed a full night (7–8 hr) before being active again. Do not take more than the amount prescribed

DRUGS APPROVED IN CANADA

because of the habit-forming potential. Not recommended for use longer than 7–10 days. If used for 2 wk or longer, abrupt withdrawal may result in fatigue, nausea, flushing, light-headedness, uncontrolled crying, vomiting, GI upset, panic attack, or nervousness. Instruct patient to read *Patient Information* for correct product before taking and with each Rx refill, changes may occur.

- Because of rapid onset, advise patient to go to bed immediately after taking zopiclone.
- May cause daytime drowsiness or dizziness. Advise patient to avoid driving or other activities requiring alertness until response to this medication is known.
- Caution patient that complex sleep-related behaviors (sleep-driving) may occur while asleep.
- Advise patient to notify health care professional immediately if signs of anaphylaxis (swelling of the tongue or throat, trouble breathing, and nausea and vomiting) occur.
- Caution patient to avoid concurrent use of alcohol or other CNS depressants.

Evaluation

- Relief of insomnia by improved falling asleep and decreased frequency of nocturnal and early morning awakenings.

zuclopenthixol

(zoo-kloe-pen-**thix**-ole)

Clopixol, Clopixol-Acuphase, Clopixol Depot

Classification
Therapeutic: antipsychotics
Pharmacologic: thioxanthenes

Indications

Management of schizophrenia; *oral*—initial and maintenance management; *IM (acuphase)*—initial treatment of acute psychotic episodes or exacerbation of psychosis due to schizophrenia; *IM (depot)*—maintenance management of schizophrenia.

Action

Has high affinity for dopamine D_1 and D_2 receptors, α_1–adrenergic and 5–HT_2 receptors. Dopaminergic blockade produces neuroleptic activity. **Therapeutic Effects:** Decreases psychoses due to schizophrenia.

Pharmacokinetics

Absorption: *PO*—well absorbed following oral administration; *IM (depot and acuphase)*—slowly absorbed from IM sites.
Distribution: Enters breast milk.
Metabolism and Excretion: Mostly metabolized (partially by the CYP2D6 enzyme system), metabolites do not have antipsychotic activity; minimal amounts excreted unchanged in urine.
Half-life: *PO*—20 hr.

TIME/ACTION PROFILE (antipsychotic effect)

ROUTE	ONSET	PEAK	DURATION
PO	within hrs	4 hr (blood level)	8–24 hr
IM (acetate [Acuphase])	2–4 hr	8 hr (sedation)	2–3 days
IM (decanoate [Depot])	within 3 days	3–7 days (blood level)	2–4 wk

Contraindications/Precautions

Contraindicated in: Treatment of dementia; Narrow angle glaucoma; Pedi: Safety and effectiveness not established, use not recommended.
Use Cautiously in: Hepatic or renal impairment; Electrolyte abnormalities, including hypokalemia, hypomagnesemia, concurrent diuretic therapy or drugs affecting QT interval or cardiovascular disease/history (↑ risk of serious arrhythmias); Intestinal pathology or brain lesions (anti-emetic effect may mask symptoms); History of seizures (may ↓ threshold); Parkinson's disease (may cause deterioration); Risk factors/history of stroke; Abrupt discontinuation (should be tapered); Geri: Consider age-related ↓ in renal, hepatic and cardiovascular function, concurrent disease states and drug therapies; OB: Infants exposed in the third trimester may exhibit extrapyramidal and withdrawal reactions including agitation, hyertonia, hypotonia, tremor, somnolence, respiratory distress and feeding disorders, do not use in pregnancy unless expected benefit to the mother outweighs potential fetal risks; Lactation: Enters breast milk; safety not established.

Adverse Reactions/Side Effects

CNS: NEUROLEPTIC MALIGNANT SYNDROME, dizziness, extrapyramidal symptoms, fatigue, sedation, tardive dyskinesia, weakness, syncope. **EENT:** abnormal vision accommodation. **CV:** THROMBOEMBOLISM, arrhythmias, hypotension, tachycardia. **GI:** constipation, dry mouth, diarrhea, thirst, vomiting. **Derm:** photosensitivity reactions, ↑ sweating. **Endo:** hyperprolactinemia, hyperglycemia. **GU:** ↓ libido, abnormal urination. **Hemat:** anemia, granulocytopenia. **Metab:** weight change. **MS:** myalgia.

Interactions

Drug-Drug: ↑ risk of CNS depression with other **CNS depressants** including **alcohol**, some **antihistamines**, some **antidepressants**, **anxiolytics**, **barbiturates**, **benzodiazepines**, and **sedative/hypnotics**. ↑ levels and risk of toxicity with **CYP2D6 inhibitors**. Concurrent use of **diuretics**, **lithium**, **Class Ia and III antiarrhythmics** including **amiodarone**, **sotalol**, and **quinidine**; some **antipsychotics** including **thioridazine**, some **macrolides** including **erythromycin**; and some **fluoroquinolones** including **moxifloxacin** ↑ risk of QT interval prolongation and serious arrhythmias; concurrent use should be avoided. ↑ risk of anticholinergic adverse reactions with other **anticholinergic drugs**. ↑ risk of hypotension with **antihypertensives** and **diuretics**. Concurrent use with **tricyclic antidepressants** may result in altered metabolism and effects of both. ↑ risk of extrapyramidal symptoms with **metoclopramide**. May ↓ beneficial effects of **levodopa** and **dopamine agonists**.

Route/Dosage

PO (Adults): *Acute psychoses*— 10–50 mg/day in 2–3 divided doses initially; may be ↑ by 10–20 mg/day every 2–3 days, titrate according to response. Usual dose range is 20–60 mg/day; doses >100 mg/day are not recommended. Dose should be ↓ to lowest dose needed to control symptoms (usual range 20–40 mg/day). Once maintenance dose is established, may be given as a single daily dose.
IM (Adults): *Zuclopenthixol acetate [Acuphase]*— 50–150 mg, may be repeated every 2–3 days if necessary, some patients may need an additional dose 1–2 days after first injection only; care must be taken to avoid over-medicating due to delay in absorption and antipsychotic effects. Maximum cumulative dose should not exceed 400 mg or four injections. *Zuclopenthixol acetate (Acuphase)* dose form is not meant for long-term use, duration should not exceed 2 wk. If injection volume exceeds 2 mL, dose should be divided and given in two sites. If oral maintenance is to be used, treatment with tablets should be initiated 2–3 days following the last dose of the *Zuclopenthixol acetate (Acuphase)* dose form; if *Zucopenthixol decanoate (Depot)* dose form is to be used for maintenance, may be given concurrently with the last injection of *Zuclopenthixol acetate (Acuphase)* dose form. *Suggested transfer regimen to oral dosing*—If *Zuclopenthixol acetate (Acuphase)* dose was 50 mg, then daily oral dose could be 20 mg; if *Zuclopenthixol acetate (Acuphase)* dose was 100 mg, then daily oral dose could be 40 mg; if *Zuclopenthixol acetate (Acuphase)* dose was 150 mg, then daily oral dose could be 60 mg. *Suggested transfer regimen to Zuclopenthixol decanoate (Depot) dosing*—If *Zuclopenthixol acetate (Acuphase)* dose was 50 mg, then IM dose of *Zuclopenthixol decanoate (Depot)* could be 100 mg every 2 wk; if *Zuclopenthixol acetate (Acuphase)* dose was 100 mg, then IM dose of *Zuclopenthixol decanoate (Depot)* could be 200 mg every 2 wk; if *Zuclopenthixol acetate (Acuphase)* dose was 150 mg, then IM dose of *Zuclopenthixol decanoate (Depot)* could be 300 mg every 2 wk.
IM (Adults): *Zuclopenthixol decanoate [depot]*— Usual maintenance dose is 150–300 mg every 2–4 wk, regimens should be individualized according to response, care must be taken not to over-medicate due to delayed/prolonged absorption and effects. If injection volume exceeds 2 mL, dose should be divided and given in two sites.

Availability

Zuclopenthixol hydrochloride tablets —contain castor oil: 10 mg, 25 mg; Zuclopenthixol acetate injection (Acuphase)—contains medium-chain triglycerides: 50 mg/mL; Zuclopenthixol decanoate injection (Depot) —contains medium-chain triglycerides: 200 mg/mL.

NURSING IMPLICATIONS

Assessment

- Assess mental status (orientation, mood, behavior) before and periodically during therapy.
- Observe carefully when administering oral medication to ensure that medication is actually taken and not hoarded.
- Assess weight and BMI initially and throughout therapy.
- Assess fluid intake and bowel function. Increased bulk and fluids in the diet help minimize constipation.
- Monitor for onset of akathisia (restlessness or desire to keep moving) and extrapyramidal side effects (*parkinsonian*—difficulty speaking or swallowing, loss of balance control, pill rolling, mask-like face, shuffling gait, rigidity, tremors; *dystonic*—muscle spasms, twisting motions, twitching, inability to move eyes, weakness of arms or legs) every 2 mo during therapy and 8–12 wk after therapy has been discontinued. Reduction in dose or discontinuation of medication may be necessary. Benztropine or diphenhydramine may be used to control these symptoms.
- Monitor for tardive dyskinesia (uncontrolled rhythmic movement of mouth, face, and extremities; lip smacking or puckering; puffing of cheeks; uncontrolled chewing; rapid or worm-like movements of tongue). Report immediately; may be irreversible.
- Monitor for development of neuroleptic malignant syndrome (fever, respiratory distress, tachycardia, seizures, diaphoresis, arrhythmias, hypertension or hypotension, pallor, tiredness, severe muscle stiffness, loss of bladder control). Report immediately.
- Monitor for symptoms related to hyperprolactinemia (menstrual abnormalities, galactorrhea, sexual dysfunction).
- ***Lab Test Considerations:*** Monitor CBC and liver function tests every 6 mo and periodically as needed during treatment. May cause ↑ AST, ALT, and alkaline phosphatase.
- Monitor blood glucose prior to and periodically during therapy. May cause hyperglycemia.
- Monitor serum prolactin prior to and periodically during therapy. May cause ↑ serum prolactin levels.

Implementation

- **PO:** Administer tablets before or after meals.
- **IM:** Administer deep in large muscle. A test dose may be ordered for first administration.

Patient/Family Teaching

- Instruct patient to take as directed. If a dose is missed, omit and take next dose as scheduled. Discontinuation should be gradual.
- Inform patient of possibility of extrapyramidal symptoms and tardive dyskinesia. Caution patient to report these symptoms immediately to health care professional.
- Advise patient to change positions slowly to minimize orthostatic hypotension.

- Medication may cause drowsiness. Caution patient to avoid driving or other activities requiring alertness until response to medication is known.
- Advise patient to notify health care professional of all Rx or OTC medications, vitamins, or herbal products being taken and to consult with health care professional before taking other medications.
- Instruct patient to notify health care professional promptly if sore throat, fever, unusual bleeding or bruising, rash, weakness, tremors, visual disturbances, dark-colored urine, or clay-colored stools occur.
- Instruct patient to avoid sun exposure and to wear protective clothing and sunscreen when outdoors.
- Advise patient to notify health care professional of medication regimen before treatment or surgery.
- Advise female patients to notify health care professional if pregnancy is planned or suspected or if breast feeding or planning to breast feed.

Evaluation

- Decreased symptoms of schizophrenia (delusions, hallucinations, social withdrawal, flat, blunt affect).

Natural/Herbal Products

The following monographs introduce some commonly used natural products. Because the amounts of active ingredients in these agents are not standardized or currently subject to FDA guidelines for medicines, *Davis's Drug Guide for Nurses*, although respectful of patients' right to choose from a variety of therapeutic options, does not endorse their routine use unless supervised by a knowledgeable health care professional. Users should take into account the possibility of adverse reactions and interactions and consider the relative lack of data supporting widespread use of these products. Doses are poorly standardized, and individuals are advised to read package labels carefully to ensure safe and efficacious use.

aloe (al-oh)

Other Name(s):
Aloe vera, Cape aloe, Aloe latex, Burn plant, Curacao aloe

Classification
Therapeutic: laxatives, wound/ulcer/decubiti healing agent

Common Uses
PO: Cathartic laxative. **Topical:** Use on burns/sunburns, wounds, irritated skin, psoriasis; topical anti-infective.

Action
PO: Exerts a laxative effect bycausing increased mucous secretion and peristalsis. The cathartic effects occur within 10 hr. Water and electrolyte reabsorption are inhibited. **Topical:** May help accelerate wound healing through inhibition of thromboxane A2 and increased microcirculation preventing ischemia in wounds, although the evidence is inconsistent. May have some activity against gram-positive, gram-negative bacteria and yeast. **Therapeutic Effects:** Relief of constipation. Improved wound healing.

Pharmacokinetics
Absorption: Unknown.
Distribution: Unknown.
Metabolism and Excretion: Unknown.
Half-life: Unknown.

TIME/ACTION PROFILE

ROUTE	ONSET	PEAK	DURATION
PO, Topical	unknown	unknown	unknown

Contraindications/Precautions
Contraindicated in: Intestinal obstruction; Inflammatory intestinal diseases (including Crohn's disease); Appendicitis and abdominal pain of unknown origin; OB: Safety not established; Pedi: Oral aloe not appropriate for children <12 yr. Topically applied aloe gel-containing formulations have been safely used in clinical trials.
Use Cautiously in: Renal disease; Fluid or electrolyte abnormalities; Diabetes; Alcohol containing products should be used cautiously in patients with known intolerance or liver disease; Pedi: Cautious use in children >12 yr.

Adverse Reactions/Side Effects
Derm: Contact dermatitis, skin irritation. **Endo:** hypoglycemia. **F and E:** HYPOKALEMIA, dehydration. **GI:** Cramping, diarrhea, laxative dependence (chronic use). **GU:** hematuria.

Interactions
Natural Product-Drug: Combining oral aloe with potassium-wasting drugs (e.g., **diuretics**, other **laxatives**, **corticosteroids**, **cisplatin**, **amphotericin B**) may worsen hypokalemia. Hypokalemia may ↑ risk of toxicity from **digoxin** and some **antiarrhythmics**. May have additive effects with **antidiabetic** agents. May ↑ bleeding risk with **warfarin**. **Alcohol**-containing preparations may interact with **disulfiram** and **metronidazole**.
Natural-Natural: ↑ hypokalemia risk with **licorice** and **horsetail**. Additive effects with stimulant laxative herbs and herbs with hypoglycemic potential. ↑ bleeding risk with antiplatelet herbs.

Route/Commonly Used Doses
PO (Adults): *Constipation*—100–200 mg aloe or 50 mg of aloe extract taken in the evening. Do not use for >1–2 wk without medical advice; *Juice*—1 teaspoonful tid after meals.
Topical (Adults): Aloe gel can be applied liberally to affected areas 2–3 times daily.

Availability
Alone or in combination with other herbal medicinals^OTC; Capsules^OTC; Juice^OTC; Tincture (1:10 in 50% alcohol)^OTC; Topical or gel or applied directly from cut plant.

NATURAL/HERBAL PRODUCTS

NURSING IMPLICATIONS

Assessment

- **Constipation:** Assess for abdominal distention, presence of bowel sounds, and usual pattern of elimination.
- Assess color, consistency, and amount of stool produced.
- **Topical:** Perform baseline skin assessment prior to applying aloe to minor wounds, burns, and abrasions. Observe the size, character, and location of the affected area prior to the application of aloe.
- Note topical response assessing for increased inflammation, drainage, pain, warmth, and/or pruritus.
- ***Lab Test Considerations:*** Monitor serum potassium in patients with chronic use and CBC in patients who self-medicate and experience bloody diarrhea or have ulcerative colitis or Crohn's disease.

Implementation

- **PO:** Administer laxative at bedtime to induce a bowel movement in the morning.
- **Topical:** Wash hands and then apply liberally to affected area of skin. Cover broken areas of skin with a light non-adhering dressing (e.g., band-aid dressing with *Telfa* lining) to facilitate keeping area clean. Do not apply an occlusive dressing over site of application.

Patient/Family Teaching

- **Constipation:** Instruct patients with pre-existing intestinal disorders (e.g., ulcerative colitis, Crohn's disease, irritable bowel syndrome) not to take aloe juice without the advice of a health care professional.
- Counsel patients that the oral juice should not be taken if they are experiencing abdominal pain, nausea, vomiting, or fever.
- Inform patients that occasional constipation may not be an issue but persistent constipation may represent a more serious health problem and to consult their health care professional.
- Advise patients to expect laxative response to the oral juice in 8–12 hr.
- Caution patients that the laxative effects may be dramatic and that accompanying dehydration and electrolyte imbalances may occur. If severe diarrhea occurs or persists, seek out treatment from their health care professional.
- Advise patients other than those with spinal cord injury that laxatives should only be used for short-term therapy. Although this is considered by some to be a natural way of correcting constipation it still carries the risk of electrolyte imbalance and dependency with chronic use.
- Encourage patients to use other forms of bowel regulation: increasing bulk in the diet, increasing fluid intake, and increasing mobility, as appropriate. Normal bowel habits are individualized and may vary from 3 times/day to 3 times/wk.
- Advise patients to consume 1500–2000 mL/day of fluids during therapy to prevent dehydration.
- Caution patients with a known cardiac history not to take this herbal supplement without the advice of their health care professional because of the risk of hypokalemia worsening arrhythmias.
- Caution patients with cardiac history to avoid straining during bowel movements (Valsalva maneuver).
- **Topical:** Advise patients that topical applications should only be used for minor burns, abrasions, or wounds. Wounds of larger size or more serious burns should be treated by a health care professional.
- Instruct patients using topical application on a non-intact skin surface about signs and symptoms of infection (milky or discolored drainage, redness, warmth, swelling, pain) and to promptly seek out treatment of a health care professional if this occurs.
- Counsel patients that if improvement in the wound is not occurring or it worsens, stop treatment with aloe vera and seek the advice of a health care professional.
- Warn patients with risk factors for delayed wound healing (e.g., diabetic patients, vascular disease) not to self-medicate with aloe vera without the approval of their health care professional.

Evaluation

- A soft, formed bowel movement.
- Evacuation of the colon.
- Relief of sunburn pain.
- Wound healing in small localized burns or abrasions.

arnica (ar-ni-cuh)

Other Name(s):
Arnica montana, leopard's bane, mountain tobacco, mountain snuff, wolf's bane

Classification
Therapeutic: anti-inflammatories, immune stimulants

Common Uses
Topical treatment of insect bites, bruises, acne, boils, sprains, muscle, and joint pain.

Action
Polysaccharides in arnica may produce a slight anti-inflammatory and analgesic effect. Some antibacterial effects are seen, in addition to a counterirritant effect, which may aid in wound healing. **Therapeutic Effects:** Decreased inflammation. Pain relief.

Pharmacokinetics
Absorption: Systemic absorption may occur following topical application to broken skin.
Distribution: Unknown.
Metabolism and Excretion: Unknown.
Half-life: Unknown.

TIME/ACTION PROFILE

ROUTE	ONSET	PEAK	DURATION
Topical	unknown	unknown	unknown

Contraindications/Precautions
Contraindicated in: Not for oral use (except in highly diluted homeopathic preparations); Arnica allergy; Avoid use on broken skin; Infectious or inflammatory GI conditions; OB: Pregnancy and lactation.
Use Cautiously in: Infectious or inflammatory GI conditions; Surgery (discontinue use 2 wk prior to procedure due to antiplatelet effects).

Adverse Reactions/Side Effects
GI: abdominal pain, vomiting, diarrhea (if taken orally). **Derm:** edematous dermatitis with pustules (chronic treatment of damaged skin), eczema (prolonged use). **Misc:** local allergic reactions.

Interactions
Natural Product-Drug: Alcohol-containing preparations may interact with **disulfiram** and **metronidazole**. May potentiate the effects of **anticoagulants** and **antiplatelet agents**, increasing the risk of bleeding.
Natural-Natural: May increase risk of bleeding with **clove**, **garlic**, **ginger**, **ginkgo**, and **ginseng**.

Route/Commonly Used Doses
Topical (Adults): *Topical*— rub or massage arnica tincture, cream, or gel onto injured area 2–3 times a day. Do not apply to broken skin; *Compress*— dilute 1 tablespoon of arnica tincture in ½ L water. Wet a gauze pad with solution and apply to affected area for 15 min. For use in poultices, dilute tincture 3–10 times with water.

Availability
Cream, tincture, salve, ointment, gel, and oil^OTC; Topical (preparations should contain not more than 20–25% arnica tincture or 15% arnica oil)^OTC; Homeopathic preparations^OTC.

NURSING IMPLICATIONS

Assessment
- Inspect skin for breaks prior to application to ensure arnica is applied only to an intact surface. Note the size, character, and location of affected area prior to application of arnica.
- After application, monitor affected area for signs of allergic response.
- ***Toxicity and Overdose:*** Systemic absorption may result in nausea, vomiting, organ damage, hypertension, cardiotoxicity, arrhythmias, muscular weakness, collapse, vertigo, renal dysfunction, coma, and death. If ingested orally, induce emesis and gastric lavage to remove undigested contents. Supportive care may be necessary. Do not take orally or apply to non-intact skin to avoid systemic absorption.

Implementation
- Clean skin with a non-alcohol containing cleanser prior to applying arnica. Apply topically to affected area, or site of injury, ensuring skin is intact.
- Do not take orally or apply to an open wound because of potential for systemic absorption with toxicity.

Patient/Family Teaching
- Teach patients to inspect the affected area for breaks in the skin and not to apply arnica to any areas where the skin is broken.
- Warn patients that use on non-intact skin and oral ingestion may cause life-threatening toxicity.
- Advise patients that arnica should only be used for short period of time in the treatment of minor aches and pains associated with local muscle, joint, or skin pain. Prolonged use may cause allergic/hypersensitivity reactions to develop.
- Instruct patients taking antihypertensive agents to avoid concurrent use of arnica.
- Advise females of reproductive potential to notify health care professional if pregnancy is planned or suspected. Arnica should be avoided during pregnancy.

Evaluation
- Relief of, or improvement in, minor aches and pains associated with muscle or joint overuse, or sprains and/or local skin irritation from insect bites, bruises, boils, or acne.

NATURAL/HERBAL PRODUCTS

bilberry (bill-beh-ree)

Other Name(s):
Vaccinium myrtillus, Tegens

Classification
Therapeutic: ocular agents, vascular agents

Common Uses
Visual acuity improvement, atherosclerosis, venous insufficiency, varicose veins, diabetes mellitus, diarrhea, hemorrhoids, peptic ulcer disease, osteoarthritis, and chronic fatigue syndrome.

Action
Anthocyanidins in bilberry have a variety of effects including increased glycosaminoglycans synthesis, decreasing vascular permeability, reducing membrane thickness, redistribution of microvascular blood flow, and formation of interstitial fluid. **Therapeutic Effects:** Decreased inflammation. Decreased edema. Decreased blood glucose. Improved circulation.

Pharmacokinetics
Absorption: Unknown.
Distribution: Unknown.
Metabolism and Excretion: Eliminated by the kidneys.
Half-life: Unknown.

TIME/ACTION PROFILE

ROUTE	ONSET	PEAK	DURATION
PO	Unknown	Unknown	Unknown

Contraindications/Precautions
Contraindicated in: Hypersensitivity or allergy to bilberry; Leaves are potentially toxic with chronic use of 1.5 g/kg/day.
Use Cautiously in: Diabetic patients; Patients at risk for bleeding; OB: Avoid use in pregnancy due to lack of safety data.

Adverse Reactions/Side Effects
Endo: low blood sugar. **GI:** diarrhea, upset stomach. **Hemat:** bleeding, bruising.

Interactions
Natural Product-Drug: May ↑ effects of **anticoagulants and antiplatelet drugs** and ↓ platelet activity. May ↑ effects of **antidiabetic agents** and cause hypoglycemia.
Natural-Natural: Avoid use with chromium-containing herbs and supplements (bilberry contains chromium). Avoid use with herbs with hypoglycemic properties.

Route/Commonly Used Doses
PO (Adults): *General use*—80–160 mg of aqueous extract three times daily. *Retinopathy*—160 mg of bilberry extract (Tegens®) has been taken twice daily for one mo. *Chronic venous insufficiency*—A bilberry extract equivalent to 173 mg of anthocyanins has been taken daily for 30 days.

Availability
Liquid extract; Tablets; Softgel capsules 160 mg.

NURSING IMPLICATIONS

Assessment
- Monitor BP periodically during therapy, coagulation panel, blood glucose.
- ***Lab Test Considerations:*** Monitor coagulation studies in patients on anticoagulants and antiplatelet agents.
- Monitor blood glucose periodically during therapy. May cause hypoglycemia.

Implementation
- Administer without regard to food.

Patient/Family Teaching
- Instruct patient to take bilberry as directed.

Evaluation
- Improvement in vascular insufficiency.
- Decrease in diarrhea.

black cohosh (blak coe-hosh)
Remifemin

Other Name(s):
baneberry black snakeroot, bugbane, phytoestrogen, rattle root, rattleweed, rattle top, squaw root

Classification
Therapeutic: menopausal agents

Do not confuse black cohosh with blue or white cohosh

Common Uses
Management of menopausal symptoms. Premenstrual discomfort. Dysmenorrhea. Mild sedative. Rheumatism.

Action
Therapeutic effects are produced by glycosides isolated from the fresh or dried rhizome with attached roots. Mechanism of action is unclear. **Therapeutic Effects:** May decrease symptoms of menopause, including hot flashes, sweating, sleep disturbance, and anxiety. Has no effect on vaginal epithelium.

Pharmacokinetics
Absorption: Unknown.
Distribution: Unknown.

Metabolism and Excretion: Unknown.
Half-life: Unknown.

TIME/ACTION PROFILE

ROUTE	ONSET	PEAK	DURATION
PO	unknown	unknown	unknown

Contraindications/Precautions

Contraindicated in: OB: Pregnancy and lactation.
Use Cautiously in: Breast cancer (may increase risk of metastasis); Hormone-sensitive cancers; Protein S deficiency (increased risk for thrombosis); Liver disease.

Adverse Reactions/Side Effects

Neuro: SEIZURES (in combination with evening primrose and chasteberry), headache, dizziness. **GI:** GI upset, hepatotoxicity. **Derm:** rash. **Misc:** weight gain, cramping, breast tenderness, vaginal spotting/bleeding.

Interactions

Natural Product-Drug: Unknown effects when combined with hormone replacement therapy and **antiestrogens** (e.g., **tamoxifen**). Concurrent use with **hepatotoxic drugs** may ↑ risk of liver damage. **Alcohol-containing preparations** may interact with **disulfiram** and **metronidazole**. May ↓ cytotoxic effects of **cisplatin**. May precipitate hypotension when used in combination with **antihypertensives**.
Natural-Natural: May ↑ risk of hepatotoxicity when used with **chaparral**, **comfrey**, **kava-kava**, and **niacin**.

Route/Commonly Used Doses

PO (Adults): *Tablets (Remifemin)*—20 mg twice daily. *Liquid extract*—0.3–2 mL 2–3 times daily. *Tincture*—2–4 mL 2–3 times daily. *Dried rhizome*—0.3–2 g 3 times daily. Do not use for more than 6 mo.

Availability

Alone or in combination with other herbal medicinals^OTC; Tablets (Remifemin 20 mg [best studied black cohosh product])^OTC; Liquid extract (1:1 in 90% alcohol)^OTC; Tincture (1:10 in 60% alcohol)^OTC; Dried rhizome.

NURSING IMPLICATIONS

Assessment

- Assess frequency and severity of menopausal symptoms.
- Monitor BP for patients on antihypertensive drugs; may increase effects and cause hypotension.
- Assess for history of seizures or liver disease.

Implementation

- Administration with food may help to minimize nausea.

Patient/Family Teaching

- Advise patients with seizures, liver dysfunction, excessive alcohol intake, cancer, or other medical problems to consult their health care professional prior to initiating self-therapy with this herb.
- Advise patient to consult health care professional before taking with other estrogen replacements.
- Advise patient to notify health care professional if pregnancy is planned or suspected. Avoid use during pregnancy; may induce a miscarriage.

Evaluation

- Resolution of menopausal vasomotor symptoms.

chondroitin (konn-**droy**-tinn)

Other Name(s):
chondroitin polysulfate, CPS, CDS

Classification
Therapeutic: nonopioid analgesics

Common Uses

Osteoarthritis. Ischemic heart disease. Hyperlipidemia. Osteoporosis. **Ophth:** In combination with sodium hyaluronate, for use as a surgical aid in cataract extraction or lens implantation, and as a lubricant.

Action

May serve as a building block of articular cartilage. May protect cartilage against degradation. May have antiatherogenic properties. **Therapeutic Effects:** Improvement in osteoarthritis symptoms.

Pharmacokinetics

Absorption: 8–18% is absorbed orally.
Distribution: Unknown.
Metabolism and Excretion: Unknown.
Half-life: Unknown.

TIME/ACTION PROFILE

ROUTE	ONSET	PEAK	DURATION
PO	unknown	unknown	unknown

Contraindications/Precautions

Contraindicated in: OB: Pregnancy and lactation.
Use Cautiously in: Asthma (may exacerbate symptoms); Clotting disorders (may ↑ risk of bleeding); Prostate cancer (may ↑ risk of metastasis or recurrence).

Adverse Reactions/Side Effects

GI: heartburn, nausea, diarrhea. **Hemat:** bleeding (antiplatelet effect). **Misc:** allergic reactions, edema, hair loss.

Interactions

Natural Product-Drug: Use of chondroitin with **anticoagulant** and **antiplatelet** drugs, **thrombolytics, NSAIDs**, some **cephalosporins**, and **valproates** may ↑ risk of bleeding.
Natural-Natural: Herbs with anticoagulant or antiplatelet properties may ↑ bleeding risk when combined with chondroitin, including: **anise**, **arnica**, **chamomile**, **clove**, **dong quai**, **fenugreek**, **feverfew**, **ginger**, **ginkgo**, **Panax ginseng**, **licorice**, and others.

Route/Commonly Used Doses

PO (Adults): *Osteoarthritis*—800–2000 mg daily, as a single dose or in 2–3 divided doses. *Prevention of recurrent myocardial infarction*—10 g daily in 3 divided doses for 3 mo followed by 1.5 g daily in 3 divided doses as maintenance therapy.
IM (Adults): *Osteoarthritis*—50 mg twice weekly for 8 wk every 4 mo.

Availability

TabletsOTC; **Capsules**OTC; **Injection (not available in US)**; Ophthalmic Drops Rx in combination with sodium hyaluronate (Viscoat).

NURSING IMPLICATIONS

Assessment

- Evaluate drug profile before starting therapy with this herbal supplement. If the patient is taking anticoagulants or antiplatelet drugs, avoid use of this herb.
- Monitor pain (type, location, and intensity) and range of motion on an ongoing basis as an indicator of drug efficacy.
- Assess for gastric discomfort and instruct patient to seek out the advice of a health care professional if persistent gastric discomfort occurs.
- Assess for signs of bleeding and discontinue herbal supplement promptly and seek out health care professional for follow-up.

Implementation

- **PO:** Administer with food.

Patient/Family Teaching

- Advise patients that this herbal supplement is usually taken with glucosamine.
- Caution patients who take aspirin or NSAIDs or other non-prescription medications not to take this herbal supplement without conferring with their health care professional.
- Instruct patients that this medication works by building up cartilage and that this requires that the medication be taken consistently over a period of time. It is not recommended as a supplemental pain medication.
- Advise female patients to notify health care professional if pregnancy is planned or suspected or if breast feeding; avoid use.

Evaluation

- Improvement in pain and range of motion.
- Reduced need for supplemental or breakthrough pain medication.

dong quai (don kwi)

Other Name(s):
Angelica sinensis, Chinese Angelica, Dang Gui, Danggui, Don Quai, Ligustilides, Phytoestrogen, *Radix angelicae gigantis*, Tang Kuei, Tan Kue Bai Zhi

Classification
Therapeutic: none assigned

Common Uses

Premenstrual syndrome. Various uses as a blood purifier. Topically in combination with other ingredients for premature ejaculation.

Action

May have vasodilating and antispasmodic properties. Binds to estrogen receptors. **Therapeutic Effects:** Improved ejaculatory latency.

Pharmacokinetics

Absorption: Unknown.
Distribution: Unknown.
Metabolism and Excretion: Unknown.
Half-life: Unknown.

TIME/ACTION PROFILE

ROUTE	ONSET	PEAK	DURATION
PO	unknown	unknown	unknown

Contraindications/Precautions

Contraindicated in: Allergy to carrot, celery, mugwort, or other members of the Apiaceae family; OB: Pregnancy and lactation.
Use Cautiously in: Hormone sensitive cancers and conditions (may exacerbate effects or stimulate growth of cancer cells); Protein S deficiency (↑ risk for thrombosis); Surgery (discontinue 2 wk prior to procedure).

Adverse Reactions/Side Effects

Derm: photosensitivity. **GI:** diarrhea. **Misc:** Some constituents are carcinogenic and mutagenic.

Interactions

Natural Product-Drug: Alcohol-containing preparations may interact with **disulfiram** and **metro-**

nidazole. Use of dong quai with **anticoagulant** and **antiplatelet** drugs, **thrombolytics**, **NSAIDs**, some **cephalosporins**, and **valproates** may increase risk of bleeding.
Natural-Natural: Herbs with antiplatelet or anticoagulant properties may increase bleeding risk when combined with dong quai including: **angelica**, **clove**, **danshen**, **garlic**, **ginger**, **ginkgo**, ***Panax ginseng***, and **willow**.

Route/Commonly Used Doses

PO (Adults): *Bulk herb*—3–4.5 g per day in divided doses with meals; *Extract*—1 mL (20–40 drops) three times daily.

Availability

Bulk herb[OTC]; **Extract**[OTC].

NURSING IMPLICATIONS

Assessment

- Assess pain and menstrual patterns prior to and following menstrual cycle to determine effectiveness of this herbal supplement.
- Assess for pregnancy prior to recommending use of the herbal supplement.
- Assess for history of hormone sensitive cancers or conditions and warn against use.
- Assess medication profile including prescription and over-the-counter use of products such as aspirin- and ibuprofen-based products to treat menstrual pain.

Implementation

- **PO:** Take with meals.

Patient/Family Teaching

- Caution patients to avoid use of aspirin or other NSAIDs concurrently because of the risk of bleeding.
- Notify patients that there are no studies supporting the use of this herbal supplement for treatment of menopausal symptoms.
- Advise patients to consult their health care professional if taking prescription medications before taking dong quai.
- Discontinue the herbal supplement if diarrhea or excessive bleeding occurs and contact a health care provider if symptoms do not resolve.
- Inform patients that photosensitivity may occur and to wear sunscreen and protective clothing if sun exposure is anticipated.
- Advise females of reproductive potential to avoid use if pregnancy is planned or suspected.

Evaluation

- Reduction in menstrual pain and cramping and regular periods with normal flow.

echinacea (*Echinacea purpurea*) (ek-i-nay-sha)

Other Name(s):
American coneflower, black sampson, black susan, *brauneria angustifolia*, kansas snakeroot, purple coneflower, red sunflower, *rudbeckia*, sampson root, scurvy root

Classification
Therapeutic: immune stimulants

Common Uses

Bacterial and viral infections. Prevention and treatment of colds, coughs, flu, and bronchitis. Fevers. Wounds and burns. Inflammation of the mouth and pharynx. Urinary tract infections. Vaginal candidiasis.

Action

Medicinal parts derived from the roots, leaves, or whole plant of perennial herb (Echinacea). *Echinacea purpurea herba* has been reported to promote wound healing, which may be due to an increase in white blood cells, spleen cells, and increased activity of granulocytes, as well as an increase in helper T cells and cytokines. *E. purpurea radix* has been shown to have antibacterial, antiviral, anti-inflammatory, and immune-modulating effects. **Therapeutic Effects:** Resolution of respiratory and urinary tract infections. Decreased duration and intensity of common cold. Improved wound healing. Stimulates phagocytosis; inhibits action of hyaluronidase (secreted by bacteria), which helps bacteria gain access to healthy cells. Externally, has antifungal and bacteriostatic properties.

Pharmacokinetics

Absorption: Unknown.
Distribution: Unknown.
Metabolism and Excretion: Unknown.
Half-life: Unknown.

TIME/ACTION PROFILE

ROUTE	ONSET	PEAK	DURATION
PO	unknown	unknown	unknown

Contraindications/Precautions

Contraindicated in: Multiple sclerosis, leukosis, collagenoses, AIDS, tuberculosis, autoimmune diseases; Hypersensitivity and cross-sensitivity in patients allergic to plants in *Asteraceae/Compositae* plant family (daisies, chrysanthemums, marigolds, etc.); OB: Pregnancy and lactation.
Use Cautiously in: Diabetes; Pedi: May increase risk of rash in children; Tinctures should be used

cautiously in alcoholics or patients with liver disease; Do not take longer than 8 wk—may suppress immune function.

Adverse Reactions/Side Effects

CNS: dizziness, fatigue, headache, somnolence. **EENT:** tingling sensation on tongue, sore throat. **GI:** nausea, vomiting, heartburn, constipation, abdominal pain, diarrhea. **Derm:** allergic reaction, rash (more common in children). **Misc:** fever.

Interactions

Natural Product-Drug: May possibly interfere with **immunosuppressants** because of its immunostimulant activity. May ↑ risk for hepaotoxicity from **anabolic steroids**, **methotrexate**, or **ketoconazole** when taken with echinacea. May ↑ **midazolam** availability.
Natural-Natural: May ↑ risk for hepatotoxicity when taken with **kava**.

Route/Commonly Used Doses

PO (Adults): *Tablets*—6.78 mg tablets, take 2 tabs 3 times daily. *Capsules*—500–1000 mg 3 times a day for 5–7 days. *Fluid extract*—1–2 mL tid; solid form (6.5:1)—150–300 mg tid. Should not be used for more than 8 wk at a time. *Tea*—½ tsp comminuted drug, steeped and strained after 10 min, 1 cup 5–6 times daily on the first day, titrating down to 1 cup daily over the next 5 days. *Echinacea purpuren herb juice*—6–9 mL/day. *Liquid*—20 drops every 2 hr for the first day of symptoms, then 3 times daily for up to 10 days.
Topical (Adults): *Ointment, lotion, tincture used externally*—1.5–7.5 mL tincture, 2–5 g dried root.

Availability

Capsules^{OTC}**; Tablets** ; Dried Root^{OTC}; **The dried root can be steeped and strained in boiling water and taken as a tea**^{OTC}**; Liquid extract**^{OTC}**; 1:1 in 45% alcohol**^{OTC}**; Tincture**^{OTC}**; 1:5 in 45% alcohol**^{OTC}**; Blended teas**^{OTC}**; *Echinacea purpuren* herb juice**^{OTC}.

NURSING IMPLICATIONS

Assessment

- Assess wound for size, appearance, and drainage prior to the start of and periodically during therapy.
- Assess frequency of common mild illnesses (such as a cold) in response to use.

Implementation

- Tinctures may contain significant concentrations of alcohol and may not be suitable for children, alcoholics, patients with liver disease, or those taking disulfiram, metronidazole, some cephalosporins, or sulfonylurea oral antidiabetic agents.
- Prolonged use of this agent may cause overstimulation of the immune system, and use beyond 8 wk is not recommended. Therapy of 10–14 days is usually considered sufficient.
- May be taken without regard to food.

Patient/Family Teaching

- Herb is more effective for treatment than prevention of colds. Take at first sign of symptoms.
- Advise patient to seek immediate treatment for an illness that does not improve after taking this herb.
- Instruct patient that the usual course of therapy is 10–14 days and 8 wk is the maximum.
- Inform patient that use of this herb is not recommended in severe illnesses (e.g., AIDS, tuberculosis) or autoimmune diseases (e.g., multiple sclerosis, collagen diseases, etc.).
- Caution patient that prolonged use of this herb may result in overstimulation of the immune system, possibly with subsequent immunosuppression.
- Instruct patient to consult health care professional before taking any prescription or OTC medications concurrently with echinacea.
- Keep tincture in a dark bottle away from sunlight. Should be taken several times a day.
- Store herb in airtight container away from sunlight.
- Advise females of reproductive potential to avoid pregnancy or breast feeding during use.

Evaluation

- Improved wound healing.
- Infrequent common illnesses.
- Illnesses of shorter duration and less severity.

feverfew (fee-vurr-fyoo)

Other Name(s):

Altamisa, Bachelor's Buttons, *Chrysanthemum parethenium*, Featerfoiul, Featherfew, Featherfoil, Flirtwort Midsummer Daisy, *Pyrethrum parthenium*, Santa Maria, *Tanaceti parthenii*, Wild chamomile, Wild quinine

Classification

Therapeutic: vascular headache suppressants

Common Uses
PO: Migraine headache prophylaxis. **Topical:** Toothaches and as an antiseptic.

Action
The sesquiterpene lactone, parthenolide, may provide feverfew's migraine prophylaxis effects. Feverfew may also have antiplatelet and vasodilatory effects and block prostaglandin synthesis.
Therapeutic Effects: May reduce the symptoms and frequency of migraine headaches.

Pharmacokinetics
Absorption: Unknown.
Distribution: Unknown.
Metabolism and Excretion: Unknown.
Half-life: Unknown.

TIME/ACTION PROFILE

ROUTE	ONSET	PEAK	DURATION
PO	2–4 mo	unknown	unknown

Contraindications/Precautions
Contraindicated in: OB: Pregnancy and lactation; Feverfew hypersensitivity or allergy to *Asteraceae/Compositae* family plants, including ragweed, chrysanthemums, daisies, and marigolds.
Use Cautiously in: Use >4 mo (safety and efficacy not established).

Adverse Reactions/Side Effects
CNS: "Post-Feverfew Syndrome" (anxiety, headache, insomnia, muscle and joint aches). **CV:** *with long-term use*—tachycardia. **GI:** nausea, vomiting, diarrhea, heartburn, mouth ulceration and soreness (from chewing fresh leaves). **Derm:** contact dermatitis (when used topically).

Interactions
Natural Product-Drug: Use of feverfew with **anticoagulant** and **antiplatelet** drugs, **thrombolytics**, **NSAIDs**, some **cephalosporins**, and **valproates** may increase risk of bleeding. Concomitant use with **NSAIDs** may also reduce feverfew effectiveness.
Natural-Natural: Use with **anise**, **arnica**, **chamomile**, **clove**, **dong quai**, **fenugreek**, **garlic**, **ginger**, **gingko**, **licorice**, and ***Panax ginseng*** may increase anticoagulant potential of feverfew.

Route/Commonly Used Doses
PO (Adults): 50–100 mg feverfew extract daily (standardized to 0.2–0.35% parthenolide) or 50–125 mg freeze-dried leaf daily with or after food.

Availability
Feverfew extract standardized to 0.2-0.35% parthenolide[OTC]; **Fresh leaf**[OTC]; **Freeze-dried leaf**[OTC].

NURSING IMPLICATIONS

Assessment
- Monitor frequency, intensity, and duration of migraine headaches prior to and during ongoing therapy.
- Assess for mouth ulcers or skin ulcerations during therapy.

Implementation
- Take with food or on a full stomach.

Patient/Family Teaching
- Instruct patients to take this medication on a consistent basis to prevent migraine headaches. This herbal supplement is not for treatment of migraines.
- Warn patients about mouth ulcers and sores and that if this occurs to seek the advice of a health care professional. Encourage proper oral hygiene.
- Advise patients not to abruptly stop this product because of the possibility of post- feverfew syndrome. Inform patients that anxiety, headache, insomnia, and muscle aches may indicate withdrawal. Feverfew should be gradually tapered.
- Review dietary and medication profile of patient to identify potential interactions. Instruct patient about other herbs that may interact with feverfew.
- Counsel patients on anticoagulants not to take feverfew except as directed by their health care provider.
- Advise patients to avoid using NSAIDs as this may reduce the effectiveness of feverfew.
- Instruct patients to look for signs of bleeding such as unusual bruising or inability to clot after a cut and to seek the advice of a health care professional if this occurs.
- Inform patients that feverfew should reduce the number of migraines and severity of symptoms but that duration of the migraine may not be affected.

Evaluation
- Reduction in the frequency and severity of migraine headaches.

garlic (gar-lik)

Other Name(s):
Alli sativa bulbus, *Allium sativum*

Classification
Therapeutic: lipid-lowering agents

Common Uses
PO: Hypertension, hyperlipidemia, cardiovascular disease prevention, colorectal and gastric cancer

prevention. **Topical:** Dermal fungal infections including tinea corporis, cruris, and pedis.

Action

May have HMG-CoA inhibitor properties in lowering cholesterol, but less effectively than statin drugs; vasodilatory and antiplatelet properties. **Therapeutic Effects:** Decreased cholesterol levels. Decreased platelet aggregation.

Pharmacokinetics

Absorption: Garlic oil is well absorbed.
Distribution: Unknown.
Metabolism and Excretion: Kidney and lungs.
Half-life: Unknown.

TIME/ACTION PROFILE

ROUTE	ONSET	PEAK	DURATION
PO	4–25 wk	unknown	unknown

Contraindications/Precautions

Contraindicated in: Bleeding disorders. Discontinue use 1–2 wk prior to surgery.
Use Cautiously in: Diabetes, gastrointestinal infection or inflammation.

Adverse Reactions/Side Effects

CNS: dizziness. **GI:** Irritation of the mouth, esophagus, and stomach, nausea, bad breath, vomiting, flatulence, diarrhea. **Derm:** Contact dermatitis and other allergic reactions (asthma, rash, anaphylaxis [rare]), Diaphoresis. **Hemat:** Chronic use or excessive dose may lead to ↓ hemoglobin production and lysis of RBCs, platelet dysfunction, prolonged bleeding time. **Misc:** body odor.

Interactions

Natural Product-Drug: Use of garlic with **anticoagulants**, **antiplatelet agents**, and **thrombolytics** may ↑ risk of bleeding. May ↓ the effectiveness of **contraceptive drugs** and **cyclosporine**. May ↓ plasma concentrations of **saquinavir**, **nevirapine**, **delavirdine**, and **efavirenz**. May ↓ **isoniazid** levels by 65%.
Natural-Natural: Herbs with anticoagulant or antiplatelet properties may increase bleeding risk when combined with garlic, including: **angelica**, **anise**, **asafoetida**, **bogbean**, **boldo**, **capsicum**, **celery**, **chamomile**, **clove**, **danshen**, **dong quai**, **fenugreek**, **feverfew**, **ginger**, **ginkgo**, ***Panax ginseng***, **horse chestnut**, **horseradish**, **licorice**, **meadowsweet**, **prickly ash**, **onion**, **papain**, **passionflower**, **poplar**, **quassia**, **red clover**, **turmeric**, **wild carrot**, **wild lettuce**, **willow**, and others.

Route/Commonly Used Doses

PO (Adults): 200–400 mg tid of standardized garlic powder extract with 1.3% allin. *Fresh garlic*—1–7 cloves per day. One clove contains approximately 4 g of garlic.
Topical (Adults): *Tinea infections*—0.4% cream, 0.6% gel, or 1% gel applied bid x 7 days.

Availability

CapsulesOTC; **Tablets**OTC; **Topical cream**; Topical gel; Fresh garlicOTC.

NURSING IMPLICATIONS

Assessment

- Obtain usual dietary intake from patient, especially in regard to fat consumption.
- Assess patient's reason for using this herbal remedy and knowledge about hyperlipidemia.
- Ascertain the amount of garlic the patient consumes on a regular basis.

Implementation

- Take orally as fresh clove, capsule, or tablet.
- Do not exceed recommended dose.

Patient/Family Teaching

- Instruct patients about the need to follow a healthy diet (low in fat and high in vegetables and fruits) in conjunction with garlic. Other lipid-reducing strategies, such as exercise and smoking cessation, should also be employed.
- Inform patients that there are other more effective agents for lipid reduction available.
- Caution patients about the potential for bleeding and not to take this herbal remedy without notifying their health care provider if they are taking other medications. Instruct patients undergoing elective surgery to stop using garlic 2 wk prior to surgery and to notify the surgeon that they are taking garlic in the event of emergent surgery.
- Notify patients that allergies may occur and to discontinue use if symptoms develop.
- Emphasize the need for follow-up exams with a healthcare professional to assess effectiveness of the regimen.

Evaluation

- Normalization of lipid profile.
- Prevention of cardiac disease.

ginger (*Zingiber officinale*) (jin-jer)

Other Name(s):
Calicut, cochin, gengibre, ginger root, imber, ingwerwurzel, ingwer, Jamaica ginger, jenjibre, kankyo, jiang, zingiber

Classification
Therapeutic: antianemics

Common Uses
Prevention and treatment of nausea and vomiting associated with motion sickness, loss of appetite, pregnancy, surgery, and chemotherapy. Prevention of postoperative nausea and vomiting. May be used for dyspepsia, flatulence, relief of joint pain in rheumatoid arthritis, cramping, and diarrhea. Migraine headache. Tonic (toning/strengthening agent) in gout, gas, respiratory infections, anti-inflammatory, stimulant (tones the gut, increases saliva and gastric juices, acts as anticoagulant, decreases blood cholesterol).

Action
Antiemetic effect due to increasing GI motility and transport; may act on serotonin receptors. Shown to be hypoglycemic, hypotensive, or hypertensive, and positive inotropic agent. Inhibits prostaglandins and platelets, lowers cholesterol, and improves appetite and digestion. **Therapeutic Effects:** ↓ nausea and vomiting due to motion sickness, surgery, and chemotherapy. ↓ joint pain and improvement of joint motion in rheumatoid arthritis. Antioxidant.

Pharmacokinetics
Absorption: Unknown.
Distribution: Unknown.
Metabolism and Excretion: Unknown.
Half-life: Unknown.

TIME/ACTION PROFILE

ROUTE	ONSET	PEAK	DURATION
PO	unknown	unknown	unknown

Contraindications/Precautions
Contraindicated in: Lactation (if using large amounts); Gallstones.
Use Cautiously in: Pregnancy (preliminary evidence that ginger might affect fetal sex hormones); Patients with ↑ risk of bleeding; Diabetes; Anticoagulant therapy; Cardiovascular disease.

Adverse Reactions/Side Effects
GI: minor heartburn. **Derm:** dermatitis (when used topically).

Interactions
Natural Product-Drug: May ↑ risk of bleeding when used with **anticoagulants**, **antiplatelet agents**, and **thrombolytics**. May have additive effects with **antidiabetic agents** (causing hypoglycemia) and **calcium channel blockers** (causing hypotension).
Natural-Natural: May theoretically ↑ risk of bleeding when used with other **herbs** that have anticoagulant or antiplatelet activities.

Route/Commonly Used Doses
PO (Adults): *Motion sickness*— 1000 mg dried ginger root taken 30 min–4 hr before travel or 250 mg qid. *Postoperative nausea prevention*— 1000 mg ginger taken 1 hr before induction or anesthesia. *Chemotherapy–induced nausea*— 2–4 g/day. Up to 2 g freshly powdered drug has been used as an antiemetic (not to exceed 4 g/day). *Migraine headache*— 500 mg at onset then 500 mg every 4 hrs up to 1.5–2 g/day for 3–4 days. *Osteoarthritis*— 170 mg tid or 255 mg bid of ginger extract. *Whole root rhizome*— 0.25–1 g for other illnesses. *Tea*— pour 150 mL boiling water over 0.5–1 g of ginger and strain after 5 min. *Tinture*— 0.25–3 mL.

Availability
Alone or in combination with other herbal medicinals^OTC^; Dried powdered root^OTC^; Syrup^OTC^; Tincture^OTC^; Tablets^OTC^; Capsules (≥550 mg)^OTC^; Spice^OTC^; Tea^OTC^.

NURSING IMPLICATIONS

Assessment
- Assess patient for nausea, vomiting, abdominal distention, and pain prior to and after administration of the herb when used as an antiemetic agent.
- Assess pain location, duration, intensity, and associated symptoms (photophobia, phonophobia, nausea, vomiting) during migraine attack.
- Assess pain, swelling, and range of motion in affected joints prior to and after administration when used in the treatment of arthritis.
- Assess patient for epigastric pain prior to and after administration when used as a gastroprotective agent.
- Monitor BP and heart rate in patients with cardiovascular disease including hypertension.
- ***Lab Test Considerations:*** Monitor blood glucose and coagulation panels periodically during therapy.

Implementation
- Administer ginger prior to situations where nausea or vomiting is anticipated (e.g., motion sickness).
- Dose form and strengths vary with each disease state. Ensure that proper formulation and dose are administered for the indicated use.

Patient/Family Teaching
- Instruct patients receiving anticoagulants not to take this herb without the advice of health care professional (increased risk of bleeding).

- Advise patient to stop the herb immediately if palpitations occur and notify health care professional.
- Advise patient to observe for easy bruising or other signs of bleeding. If they occur, stop the herb immediately and notify health care professional.
- Counsel patients with a history of gallbladder disease to use this herb only under the supervision of health care professional.
- Instruct patient to consult health care professional before taking any Rx, OTC, or other herbal products concurrently with ginger.
- Herb is meant to be used as a tonic, not for long-term use.

Evaluation

- Prevention of nausea and vomiting.
- Relief of epigastric pain.
- Improved joint mobility and relief of pain.
- Relief of migraine headache.

ginkgo (ging-ko)

Other Name(s):
Bai guo ye, fossil tree, ginkgo folium, Japanese silver apricot, kew tree, maidenhair-tree, *salisburia adiantifolia*, yinhsing

Classification
Therapeutic: antiplatelet agents, central nervous system stimulants

Common Uses

Symptomatic relief of organic brain dysfunction (dementia syndromes, short-term memory deficits, inability to concentrate, depression). Intermittent claudication. Vertigo and tinnitus of vascular origin. Improvement of peripheral circulation. Premenstrual syndrome.

Action

Improves tolerance to hypoxemia, especially in cerebral tissue. Inhibits development of cerebral edema and accelerates its regression. Improves memory, blood flow (microcirculation), compensation of disequilibrium, and rheological properties of blood. Inactivates toxic oxygen radicals. Antagonizes platelet-activating factor. Interferes with bronchoconstriction and phagocyte chemotaxis. **Therapeutic Effects:** Symptomatic relief of dementia syndromes. Inhibits arterial spasm, decreases capillary fragility and blood viscosity. Improves venous tone, relaxes vascular smooth muscle.

Pharmacokinetics

Absorption: 70–100% absorption.
Distribution: Unknown.
Metabolism and Excretion: Unknown.
Half-life: Unknown.

TIME/ACTION PROFILE

ROUTE	ONSET	PEAK	DURATION
PO	unknown	unknown	unknown

Contraindications/Precautions

Contraindicated in: Hypersensitivity; Pregnancy and lactation.
Use Cautiously in: Bleeding disorders; Children (fresh seeds have caused seizures and death); Diabetes; Epilepsy; Surgery (discontinue use 2 wk prior).

Adverse Reactions/Side Effects

CNS: CEREBRAL BLEEDING, dizziness, headache, vertigo, seizure. **CV:** palpitations. **GI:** flatulence, stomach upset. **Derm:** allergic skin reaction. **Hemat:** bleeding. **Misc:** hypersensitivity reactions.

Interactions

Natural Product-Drug: Theoretically may potentiate effects of **anticoagulants**, **thrombolytics**, **antiplatelet agents**, and **MAO inhibitors**. May also ↑ risk of bleeding with some **cephalosporins**, **valproic acid**, and **NSAIDs**. May ↓ effectiveness of **anticonvulsants**. May alter **insulin** metabolism requiring dose adjustments of antidiabetic drugs.
Natural-Natural: May ↑ risk of bleeding when used with other **herbs** with antiplatelet effects (including **angelica**, **arnica**, **chamomile**, **feverfew**, **garlic**, **ginger**, and **licorice**).

Route/Commonly Used Doses

Organic Brain Syndromes

PO (Adults): 120–240 mg ginkgo leaf extract daily in 2 or 3 doses.

Intermittent Claudication

PO (Adults): 120–240 mg ginkgo leaf extract daily in 2 or 3 doses.

Vertigo and Tinnitus

PO (Adults): 120–160 mg ginkgo leaf extract daily in 2 or 3 doses.

Cognitive Function Improvement

PO (Adults): 120–600 mg per day.

Premenstrual Syndrome

PO (Adults): 80 mg BID starting on the 16th day of the menstrual cycle until the 5th day of the next cycle.

NATURAL/HERBAL PRODUCTS

Availability

Ginkgo leaf extract (acetone/water) 22–27% flavonoid glycosides, 5–7% terpene lactones, 2.6–3.2% bilobalide, <5 ppm of ginkgolic acids.

NURSING IMPLICATIONS

Assessment

- Assess cognitive function (memory, attention, reasoning, language, ability to perform simple tasks) prior to and periodically during therapy. Exclude other treatable causes of dementia prior to instituting treatment with ginkgo.
- Assess frequency, duration, and severity of muscle cramps (claudication) experienced by the patient prior to and periodically throughout therapy.
- Assess for headache and neurologic changes (thromboembolism).

Implementation

- **PO:** Start dose at 120 mg per day and increase as needed to minimize side effects.
- May be administered without regard to food. Administer at same time each day.
- Use of dried leaf preparations in the form of a tea is not recommended because of insufficient quantity of active ingredients.
- Advise patients to avoid crude ginkgo plant parts which can cause severe allergic reactions.

Patient/Family Teaching

- Advise patient to observe for easy bruising and other signs of bleeding and report to health care professional if they occur.
- Caution patient to keep this herb out of the reach of children; may cause seizures.
- Caution patient to avoid handling the pulp or seed coats because of the risk of contact dermatitis. Wash skin under free-flowing water promptly if contact does occur.
- Instruct patient not to exceed recommended doses; large doses may result in toxicity (restlessness, diarrhea, nausea and vomiting, headache).
- Notify patients receiving anticoagulant or antiplatelet therapy not to take this medication without approval of health care professional and frequent monitoring.
- Instruct patient to consult health care professional before taking any prescription or OTC medications concurrently with ginkgo.

Evaluation

- Improvement in walking distances pain-free.
- Improvement in tinnitus and vertigo.
- Improvement in short-term memory, attention span, and ability to perform simple tasks.
- Improvement in sexual function.
- Decreased symptoms of premenstrual syndrome.
- Administration for a minimum of 6–8 wk of 80 mg (tid) (not <6 wk) is required to determine response.

ginseng (*Panax ginseng*)
(jin-seng)

Other Name(s):
Asian ginseng, Chinese ginseng, hong shen, Japanese ginseng, Korean ginseng, red ginseng, renshen, white ginseng

Classification
Therapeutic: none assigned

Common Uses

Improving physical and mental stamina. General tonic to energize during times of fatigue and inability to concentrate. Sedative, sleep aid, antidepressant. Diabetes. Enhanced sexual performance/aphrodisiac. Increased longevity. Adjunctive treatment of cancer. Increased immune response. Increased appetite.

Action

Main active ingredient is ginsenoside from the dried root. Serves as CNS stimulant and depressant. Enhances immune function. Interferes with platelet aggregation and coagulation. Has analgesic, anti-inflammatory, and estrogen-like effects. **Therapeutic Effects:** Improves mental and physical ability. May improve appetite, memory, sleep pattern. May reduce fasting blood glucose level in diabetic patients.

Pharmacokinetics

Absorption: Unknown.
Distribution: Unknown.
Metabolism and Excretion: Unknown.
Half-life: Unknown.

TIME/ACTION PROFILE

ROUTE	ONSET	PEAK	DURATION
PO	unknown	unknown	unknown

Contraindications/Precautions

Contraindicated in: Pregnancy (androgenization of fetus); Lactation; Children; Manic-depressive disorders and psychosis; Hypertension; Asthma; Infection; Organ transplant recipients (can interfere with immunosuppressive therapy); Hormone-sensitive cancers.
Use Cautiously in: Autoimmune diseases; Cardiovascular disease; Diabetics (may have hypoglycemic

effects); Patients receiving anticoagulants; Bleeding disorders; Schizophrenia (may cause agitation).

Adverse Reactions/Side Effects

CNS: agitation, depression, dizziness, euphoria, headaches, insomnia, nervousness. **CV:** hypertension, tachycardia. **GI:** diarrhea. **GU:** amenorrhea, vaginal bleeding. **Derm:** skin eruptions. **Endo:** estrogen-like effects. **Misc:** fever, mastalgia, STEVENS-JOHNSON SYNDROME.

Interactions

Natural Product-Drug: May ↓ anticoagulant activity of **warfarin**. May interfere with **MAO inhibitors** treatment and cause headache, tremulousness, and manic episodes. May enhance blood glucose lowering effects of **oral hypoglycemics** and **insulin**. May interfere with **immunosuppressant** therapy. Use with caution when taking **estrogens**.
Natural-Natural: May ↑ risk of bleeding when used with **herbs** that have antiplatelet or anticoagulant activities. May prolong the QT interval when used with **bitter orange**, **country mallow**, and **ephedra** and ↑ risk of life-threatening arrhythmias. May ↑ risk of hypoglycemia when used with herbs with hypoglycemic potential.
Natural-Food: May potentiate effects of **caffeine** in **coffee** or **tea** and CNS stimulant effects of **mate**.

Route/Commonly Used Doses

PO (Adults): *Capsule*— 200–600 mg/day; *extract*— 100–300 mg 3 times daily; *crude root*— 1–2g/day; *infusion*—*tea*— 1–2 g root daily (½ tbsp/cup water) up to 3 times daily (*P. ginseng* tea bag usually contains 1500 mg of ginseng root). Do not use for longer than 3 mo. *Cold/flu prevention*— 100 mg daily 4 wk prior to influenza vaccination and continued for 8 wk; *Chronic bronchitis*— 100 mg BID for 9 days combined with antibiotic therapy; *Erectile dysfunction*— 900 mg TID; *Type 2 diabetes*— 200 mg daily.

Availability (generic available)

Root powder[OTC]**; Extract in alcohol**[OTC]**; Capsules**[OTC]**; Tea bags**[OTC]**.**

NURSING IMPLICATIONS

Assessment

- Assess level of energy, attention span, and fatigue person is experiencing prior to initiating and periodically during therapy.
- Assess appetite; sleep duration; and perceived quality, emotional lability, and work efficiency prior to and during therapy.
- Patients with chronic medical problems should not use this herb without the advice of health care professional.
- Assess for ginseng toxicity (nervousness, insomnia, palpitations, and diarrhea).
- Monitor patients with diabetes more frequently for hypoglycemia until response to the agent is ascertained.
- Assess for the development of ginseng abuse syndrome (occurs when large doses of the herb are taken concomitantly with other psychomotor stimulants such as coffee and tea. May present as diarrhea, hypertension, restlessness, insomnia, skin eruptions, depression, appetite suppression, euphoria, and edema).

Implementation

- May be taken without regard to food.
- Take at the same time daily and do not increase dose above the recommended amount because of potential toxic effects.

Patient/Family Teaching

- Caution patients with cardiovascular disease, hypertension or hypotension, or on steroid therapy to avoid the use of this herb.
- Instruct patient in the symptoms of ginseng toxicity and to reduce dose or stop use of the herb if they occur.
- Advise patient to limit the amount of caffeine consumed.
- Advise patients with diabetes to monitor blood sugar levels until response to this agent is known.
- Teach patient about the signs and symptoms of hepatitis (yellow skin or whites of eyes, dark urine, light-colored stools, lack of appetite for several days or longer, nausea, abdominal pain) and to stop use of the herb and promptly contact health care professional if they occur. (This herb is hepatoprotectant at low doses, but hepatodestructive at high doses.).
- Caution patient not to exceed recommended doses because of potential side effects and toxicity.
- Instruct patient to discontinue ginseng if diarrhea develops.
- Instruct patient to consult health care professional before taking any Rx or OTC medications concurrently with ginseng.
- Advise females of reproductive potential to avoid use of ginseng if pregnancy is planned or suspected or if breast feeding.

Evaluation

- Improved energy level and sense of well-being.
- Improved quality of sleep.
- Improved concentration and work efficiency.
- Improved appetite.

*CAPITALS indicates life-threatening; underlines indicate most frequent.

- May need to take for several wk before seeing results.
- Recommended course of therapy is 3 wk. A repeated course is feasible. Do not use for longer than 3 mo.

glucosamine
(glew-**kos**-ah-meen)

Other Name(s):
2-amino-2-deoxyglucose sulfate, chitosamine

Classification
Therapeutic: antirheumatics

Common Uses
Osteoarthritis. Temporomandibular joint (TMJ) arthritis. Glaucoma.

Action
May stop or slow osteoarthritis progression by stimulating cartilage and synovial tissue metabolism.
Therapeutic Effects: Decreased pain and improved joint function.

Pharmacokinetics
Absorption: 0.9% absorbed.
Distribution: Unknown.
Metabolism and Excretion: 74% eliminated via first-pass metabolism.
Half-life: Unknown.

TIME/ACTION PROFILE

ROUTE	ONSET	PEAK	DURATION
PO	unknown	unknown	unknown

Contraindications/Precautions
Contraindicated in: Shellfish allergy (glucosamine is often derived from marine exoskeletons); Pregnancy and lactation.
Use Cautiously in: Diabetes (may worsen glycemic control); Asthma (may exacerbate symptoms); Surgery (may affect blood glucose levels, discontinue glucosamine 2 wk before elective procedures).

Adverse Reactions/Side Effects
GI: nausea, heartburn, diarrhea, constipation. **CNS:** headache, drowsiness. **Derm:** skin reactions. **Endo:** hyperglycemia.

Interactions
Natural Product-Drug: May antagonize the effects of **antidiabetics**. May induce resistance to some chemotherapy drugs such as **etoposide**, **teniposide**, and **doxorubicin**. May increase anticoagulant effects of **warfarin**.
Natural-Natural: None known.

Route/Commonly Used Doses
PO (Adults): 500 mg three times daily.
Topical (Adults): use cream as needed for up to 8 wk.

Availability
Tablets500 mg^{OTC}; **Capsules**500 mg^{OTC}; **Topical cream**30 mg/g in combination with other ingredients^{OTC}.

NURSING IMPLICATIONS

Assessment
- Assess for shellfish allergy prior to initiating therapy.
- Monitor pain (type, location, and intensity) and range of motion periodically during therapy.
- Assess bowel function periodically during therapy. Constipation may be reduced by increased fluid intake and bulk in diet; bulk laxatives may be added if necessary.
- ***Lab Test Considerations:*** Monitor serum glucose levels periodically during therapy for patients with diabetes.

Implementation
- Administer prior to meals.

Patient/Family Teaching
- Instruct patients that effects of this drug come from stimulating cartilage and synovial tissue metabolism and that the supplement must be taken on a regular basis to achieve benefit. Do not use as an intermittent pain medication.
- Caution patients with a shellfish allergy that this herbal supplement should not be used.
- Advise patient to notify health care professional if gastric discomfort develops and persists.
- Advise diabetic patients to monitor glucose values closely during initial therapy.

Evaluation
- Improvement in pain and range of motion.

grape seed extract
(grayp seed **ex**-trakt)

Other Name(s):
Vitis vinifera, *Vitis coignetiae*, Oligomeric Proanthocyanidins (OPCs)

Classification
Therapeutic: cardioprotective agents

Common Uses
Chronic venous insufficiency, edema, diabetic retinopathy, varicose veins, cancer prevention, atherosclerosis, cirrhosis, prevention of collagen break-

NATURAL/HERBAL PRODUCTS

down, vision problems, constipation, antioxidant, wound healing.

Action

Grape flavonoids have a wide range of effects including antioxidant, vasodilatory, antiplatelet, decreased superoxide production, free-radical removal, and inhibition of collagenase. **Therapeutic Effects:** Reduced risk of coronary disease. Decreased skin and vasculature breakdown.

Pharmacokinetics

Absorption: unknown.
Distribution: unknown.
Metabolism and Excretion: unknown.
Half-life: unknown.

TIME/ACTION PROFILE

	ONSET	PEAK	DURATION
PO	Unknown	Unknown	Unknown

Contraindications/Precautions

Contraindicated in: Hypersensitivity or allergy to grape seed extract; Patients with bleeding disorders or receiving anticoagulant therapy.
Use Cautiously in: OB: Avoid use in pregnancy due to lack of safety data.

Adverse Reactions/Side Effects

CV: hypertension. **CNS:** dizziness, headache. **Derm:** dry skin. **EENT:** sore throat, cough. **GI:** nausea, diarrhea. **Hemat:** ↑ risk of bleeding.

Interactions

Natural Product-Drug: May ↑ anticoagulant effects of **warfarin**. May ↓ plasma levels of CYP1A2 substrates.
Natural-Natural: May inhibit the growth of **lactobacillus acidophilus**. May ↑ BP in hypertensive patients also taking **vitamin c**.

Route/Commonly Used Doses

PO (Adults): 75–300 mg daily.

Availability

Tablets; Capsules.

NURSING IMPLICATIONS

Assessment

- Monitor BP periodically during therapy.
- ***Lab Test Considerations:*** Monitor serum cholesterol levels periodically during therapy.

Implementation

- Administer as directed. Doses may vary.

Patient/Family Teaching

- Advise patient not to take grape seed extract with vitamin C; may cause increase in BP.
- Advise females of reproductive potential to notify health care professional if pregnancy is planned or suspected.

Evaluation

- Decrease in cholesterol.
- Decrease in BP.

green tea (green tee)

Other Name(s):
Camellia sinensis

Classification
Therapeutic: central nervous system stimulants

Common Uses

Bladder, esophageal, ovarian, and pancreatic cancer risk reduction, mental alertness, hypotension, cervical dysplasia associated with human papillomavirus infection, hyperlipidemia, weight loss, protection of the skin from sun damage, genital warts, dental caries, Parkinson's disease.

Action

Caffeine in green tea stimulates the CNS and cardiovascular system through adenosine receptor blockade and phosphodiesterase inhibition. **Therapeutic Effects:** Improved cognitive performance and mental alertness.

Pharmacokinetics

Absorption: Unknown.
Distribution: Unknown.
Metabolism and Excretion: Unknown.
Half-life: Unknown.

TIME/ACTION PROFILE

ROUTE	ONSET	PEAK	DURATION
PO	Unknown	Unknown	Unknown

Contraindications/Precautions

Contraindicated in: Allergy/hypersensitivity; Pregnancy and lactation (doses >200 mg/day due to caffeine content).
Use Cautiously in: Patients with caffeine sensitivity. Long-term use of doses >250 mg/day may produce tolerance, psychological dependence, tachyarrhythmias, and sleep disturbances; Iron deficiency anemia (may worsen); Diabetes (may impair glucose control); Cardiac conditions (may induce arrhythmias in sensitive individuals); Bleeding disorders.

Adverse Reactions/Side Effects

CV: arrhythmia, tachycardia. **CNS:** agitation, dizziness, excitement, insomnia, tremors. **GI:** nausea, vomiting, diarrhea, hepatotoxicity, abdominal pain. **F and E:** hypokalemia. **Endo:** hyperglycemia. **Hemat:** prolonged bleeding time.

Interactions

Natural Product-Drug: Green tea may ↓ effects of **adenosine**. ↑ risk of bleeding with **anticoagu-**

lants or **antiplatelet** agents. ↑ effects of **CNS stimulants**. May impair glucose control from **antidiabetic** agents. Abrupt withdrawal can ↑ **lithium** levels. May ↓ **dipyridamole**—induced vasodilation. **Verapamil** can ↑ caffeine concentrations by 25%. Additive effects with **methylxanthines**.
Natural-Natural: ↑ risk of adverse cardiovascular effects with **bitter orange**. ↑ risk of hepatotoxicity with hepatotoxic herbs or supplements. ↑ risk of seizures, hypertension, or stroke with **ephedra** and **creatine**.

Route/Commonly Used Doses

PO (Adults): Range: 1–10 cups/day. One cup provides approximately 60 mg of caffeine.

Availability

Tea leaves.

NURSING IMPLICATIONS

Assessment

- Monitor BP and heart rate periodically during therapy.
- ***Lab Test Considerations:*** Monitor serum glucose, homocysteine, and uric acid levels periodically during therapy.
- Monitor liver and kidney function periodically during therapy.

Implementation

- May be taken as tea or as an extract in capsules.

Patient/Family Teaching

- Advise females of reproductive potential to limit green tea due to the caffeine content.

Evaluation

- Improvement in memory.

hawthorn (Crataegus Species) (haw-thorn)

Other Name(s):
aubepine crataegi folium, cum flore, hagedorn, maybush, whitehorn

Classification
Therapeutic: antihypertensives, inotropics

Common Uses

Hypertension. Mild to moderate HF. Angina. Spasmolytic. Sedative.

Action

Active compounds in hawthorn include flavonoids and procyanidins. Increase coronary blood flow. Positive inotropic and chronotropic effects because of increased permeability to calcium and inhibition of phosphodiesterase. **Therapeutic Effects:** Increased cardiac output. Decreased BP, myocardial workload, and oxygen consumption.

Pharmacokinetics

Absorption: Unknown.
Distribution: Unknown.
Metabolism and Excretion: Unknown.
Half-life: Unknown.

TIME/ACTION PROFILE

ROUTE	ONSET	PEAK	DURATION
PO	unknown	6–8 wk	unknown

Contraindications/Precautions

Contraindicated in: Pregnancy (potential uterine activity); Lactation.
Use Cautiously in: Concurrent use with ACE inhibitors and digoxin; Do not discontinue use abruptly.

Adverse Reactions/Side Effects

CNS: agitation, dizziness, fatigue, vertigo, headache, sedation (high dose), sleeplessness, sweating. **CV:** hypotension (high dose), palpitations. **Derm:** rash. **GI:** nausea.

Interactions

Natural Product-Drug: May potentiate effects of **digoxin, calcium channel blockers**, and **beta blockers**. Concurrent use with **phosphodiesterase-5 inhibitors (sildenafil, tadalafil, vardenafil)** and **nitrates** may potentiate vasodilatory effects. May cause additive CNS depression when used with other **CNS depressants**.
Natural-Natural: Additive effect with other cardiac glycoside–containing **herbs (digitalis leaf, black hellebore, oleander leaf**, and others). Additive hypotensive effects with herbs than lower BP such as **ginger, *Panax ginseng*, coenzyme Q-10** and **valerian**. Additive effect with other cardioactive herbs (**devil's claw, fenugreek**, and others).

Route/Commonly Used Doses

PO (Adults): *Heart failure*—160–1800 mg standardized hawthorn leaf with flower extract in 2–3 divided doses daily. *Hawthorn fluid extract (1:1 in 25% alcohol)*—0.5–1 mL tid; *hawthorn fruit tincture (1:5 in 45% alcohol)*—1–2 mL tid; *dried hawthorn berries*—300–1000 mg tid.

Availability (generic available)

Dried fruit^OTC; Liquid extract of the fruit or leaf^OTC; Tincture of the fruit or leaf^OTC.

NURSING IMPLICATIONS

Assessment

- Monitor intake and output rations and daily weight. Assess for peripheral edema, auscul-

NATURAL/HERBAL PRODUCTS

tate lungs for rales and crackles during therapy.

- Assess BP and pulse periodically during therapy.

Implementation

- Administered as 2–3 divided doses daily at the same time.
- May be taken without regard to food.

Patient/Family Teaching

- Advise patients that there are other proven therapies available for treatment of heart failure. These therapies should be employed prior to initiating treatment with hawthorn.
- Tell patient not to take hawthorn without the advice of health care professional.
- Instruct patients in the symptoms of a heart attack (pain in the region of the heart, jaw, arm, or upper abdomen; sweating; chest tightness) and heart failure (shortness of breath, chest tightness, dizziness, sweating) and to promptly notify health care professional and obtain emergency services if they occur.
- Advise patient to report weight gain or persistent swelling of the feet to health care professional.
- May cause dizziness and fatigue. Patients should avoid driving or other activities that require mental alertness until response to herb is known.
- Avoid alcohol and other CNS depressants while taking hawthorn without consulting health care professional.
- Profuse sweating and dehydration under extreme heat may increase the BP-lowering properties of hawthorn, leading to severe hypotension. Caution patients to avoid exertion in hot weather to minimize the risk of side effects.
- Instruct patients that hawthorn helps control the symptoms of heart failure but does not cure the disease. Lifestyle changes (salt restriction, weight management, exercise as tolerated, adherence to medication regimens) still need to be followed.
- Instruct patient to consult health care professional before taking Rx, OTC, or other herbal products concurrently with hawthorn.
- Advise females of reproductive potential to use effective contraception during therapy and to notify health care professional if pregnancy is planned or suspected or if breast feeding.

Evaluation

- Decrease in symptoms of HF. Effects may not be seen for 6 wks.
- Improved cardiac output as evidenced by improved activity tolerance.

kava-kava (Piper Methysticum) (ka-va ka-va)

Other Name(s):
Ava pepper, intoxicating pepper, kao, kew, tonga, wurzelstock, yagona

Classification
Therapeutic: antianxiety agents, sedative/hypnotics

Common Uses

Anxiety, stress, restlessness, insomnia, benzodiazepine withdrawal. Mild muscle aches and pains. Menstrual cramps and PMS.

Action

Alters the limbic system modulation of emotional processes. Shown to have centrally-acting skeletal muscle relaxant properties activated. **Therapeutic Effects:** Relief of anxiety. Sedation.

Pharmacokinetics

Absorption: Peak plasma level occurs about 1.8 hr after an oral dose.
Distribution: Enters breast milk.
Metabolism and Excretion: Elimination occurs primarily by renal excretion (both unchanged and metabolites) and in the feces. Metabolized by the liver (reduction or demethylation).
Half-life: Approximately 9 hr.

TIME/ACTION PROFILE

ROUTE	ONSET	PEAK	DURATION
PO	1.8 hr	unknown	8 hr

Contraindications/Precautions

Contraindicated in: OB, Lactation: Pregnancy (may affect uterine tone) and lactation; Patients with endogenous depression (may ↑ risk of suicide); Children <12 yr; Hepatitis or other liver disease.
Use Cautiously in: Concurrent use of other hepatotoxic agents; Depression and Parkinson's disease (may worsen symptoms); Should not be used for >3 mo to prevent psychological dependence.

Adverse Reactions/Side Effects

CNS: dizziness, headache, drowsiness, sensory disturbances, extrapyramidal effects. **EENT:** Pupil dilation, red eyes, visual accommodation disorders. **GI:** HEPATOTOXICITY, gastrointestinal complaints. **Derm:** allergic skin reactions, yellow discoloration of skin, pellagroid dermopathy. **Hemat:** ↓ lymphocytes, decreased platelets. **Metab:** weight loss (long term, high dose). **Neuro:** ataxia, muscle weakness.

Interactions

Natural Product-Drug: Additive effect when used with **alprazolam**. Potentiates effect of **CNS de-**

pressants (ethanol, barbiturates, benzodiazepines, opioid analgesics). Has ↓ effectiveness of **levodopa** in few cases. May have additive effects with **antiplatelet agents**. May ↑ risk of liver damage with other **hepatotoxic agents**.
Natural-Natural: Concurrent use with other hepatotoxic products such as **DHEA**, **coenzyme Q-10** (high doses), and **niacin** can ↑ risk of liver damage. May have additive sedative effects when used with other **herbs** with sedative properties.

Route/Commonly Used Doses

PO (Adults): *Antianxiety*— 50–100 mg (70 mg kavalactones) 3 times daily; *Benzodiazepine withdrawal*— 50–300 mg/day over one wk while tapering benzodiazepine over 2 wk (use 70% kavalactone extract). *Insomnia*— 180–210 mg kavalactones. Typically taken as a tea by simmering the root in boiling water and then straining.

Availability (generic available)

Dried root extracts (alcohol or acetone based) containing 30–70% kavapyrones.

NURSING IMPLICATIONS

Assessment

- Assess muscle spasm, associated pain, and limitations of movement prior to and periodically during therapy.
- Assess degree of anxiety and level of sedation (visual disturbances and changes in motor reflexes are side effects) prior to and periodically during therapy.
- Assess sleep patterns and level of sedation upon arising.
- Prolonged use may lead to ↓ of platelet and lymphocyte counts and ↑ liver function tests.

Implementation

- Prepared as a drink from pulverized roots, tablets, capsules, or extract.

Patient/Family Teaching

- Inform patient that significant, serious side effects may occur with prolonged use. Use for longer than 1 mo is not recommended without supervision of health care professional.
- Caution patient to avoid alcohol or other CNS depressants while taking this herb; may increase sedative effect.
- May cause drowsiness. Caution patient to avoid driving or other activities requiring alertness until response to herb is known.
- Caution patients to stop use of the herb immediately and notify health care professional if shortness of breath or signs of liver disease (yellowing of the skin or whites of the eyes, brown urine, nausea, vomiting, light-colored stools, unusual tiredness, weakness, stomach or abdominal pain, loss of appetite) occur.
- Instruct patients with liver disease, or taking drug products that can affect the liver, to consult health care professional before using kava-containing supplements.
- Inform patient that although there is no evidence of physiological dependence, the risk of psychological dependence still exists.
- Instruct patient to consult health care professional before taking any Rx, OTC, or other herbal products concurrently with kava-kava.
- Advise females of reproductive potential to use effective contraception during therapy and to notify health care professional immediately if pregnancy is planned or suspected or if breast feeding.
- **Kava has been banned in other countries due to hepatotoxicity.**

Evaluation

- Decrease in anxiety level.
- Decrease in muscle spasms.
- Relief of insomnia.

milk thistle (milk this-ul)

Other Name(s):
Holy thistle, Lady's thistle, Mary Thistle, Silybin, Silymarin

Classification
Therapeutic: antidotes

Common Uses

Cirrhosis, chronic hepatitis, gallstones, psoriasis, liver cleansing and detoxification, treatment of liver toxicity due to Amanita mushroom poisoning (European IV formulation), and chemicals. Dyspepsia (in combination with other herbs). Diabetes.

Action

The active component, silymarin, has antioxidant and hepatoprotectant actions. Silymarin helps prevent toxin penetration and stimulates hepatocyte regeneration. **Therapeutic Effects:** Liver detoxification. Improved dyspepsia symptoms. Decreased fasting blood glucose.

Pharmacokinetics

Absorption: 23–47% absorbed after oral administration.
Distribution: Unknown.
Metabolism and Excretion: Hepatic metabolism by cytochrome P450 3A4.
Half-life: 6 hr.

TIME/ACTION PROFILE

ROUTE	ONSET	PEAK	DURATION
PO	5–30 days or more	unknown	unknown

Contraindications/Precautions

Contraindicated in: Pregnancy and lactation (insufficient information available); Allergy to chamomile, ragweed, asters, chrysanthemums, and other members of the family *Asteraceae/Compositae*.
Use Cautiously in: Hormone sensitive cancers/conditions (milk thistle plant parts may have estrogenic effects).

Adverse Reactions/Side Effects

GI: Laxative effect, nausea, bloating, anorexia. **Misc:** Allergic reactions.

Interactions

Natural Product-Drug: In vitro, milk thistle extract inhibited the drug-metabolizing enzyme **cytochrome P450 3A4**. Interactions have not been reported in humans, but milk thistle should be used cautiously with other drugs metabolized by 3A4, such as **cyclosporine**, **carbamazepine**, **HMG-CoA inhibitors**, **ketoconazole**, and **alprazolam**.
Natural-Natural: Herbs with hypoglycemic potential may have additive hypoglycemic effects.

Route/Commonly Used Doses

PO (Adults): *Hepatic cirrhosis*—420 mg/day of extract containing 70–80% silymarin; *Chronic active hepatitis*—140 mg tid of silymarin; 240 mg bid of silibinin; *Diabetes*—200 mg tid of silymarin; *Tea*—3–4 times daily 30 min before meals. Tea is not recommended as silymarin is not sufficiently water soluble.
IV (Adults): 20–50 mg/kg over 24 hr, 48 hr post mushroom ingestion (IV formulation not available in US).

Availability

Capsules^OTC^**; Tablets**^OTC^**; Crude drug**^OTC^**; Tea**^OTC^**; Extract**^OTC^.

NURSING IMPLICATIONS

Assessment

- Assess patients for signs of liver failure (jaundice, mental status changes, abdominal distention, ascites, generalized edema).
- Evaluate consistency and frequency of bowel movements.
- ***Lab Test Considerations:*** Monitor liver function, lipid profile, and blood glucose periodically during therapy.

Implementation

- **PO:** Orally as an extract, capsule, tablets, or as a dried fruit as a single daily dose or divided into three doses.
- Tea is not recommended as milk thistle is not water-soluble.

Patient/Family Teaching

- Inform patient of symptoms of liver failure; advise patient to report worsening symptomatology promptly to health care professional.
- Advise patients to avoid alcohol and follow diet for liver or gall bladder disease being treated.
- Emphasize the need for blood tests to monitor liver function tests.

Evaluation

- Normalization of liver function tests.
- Reduction in jaundice, abdominal distention, fatigue and other symptoms associated with liver disease.

SAMe (sam-ee)

Other Name(s):
Ademetionine, S-adenosylmethionine

Classification
Therapeutic: antidepressants

Common Uses

Treatment of depression. Has also been used to manage: osteoarthritis, fibromyalgia, liver disease, migraine headaches.

Action

May aid in the production, activation, and metabolism of various amines, phospholipids, hormones, and neurotransmitters. May stimulate articular cartilage growth and repair. **Therapeutic Effects:** Decreased depression. Anti-inflammatory and analgesic effects improve symptoms of osteoarthritis.

Pharmacokinetics

Absorption: Rapidly and extensively metabolized following oral administration.
Distribution: Unknown.
Metabolism and Excretion: Actively metabolized by the liver.
Half-life: 100 min.

TIME/ACTION PROFILE (antidepressant action)

ROUTE	ONSET	PEAK	DURATION
PO (depression)	1–2 wk	unknown	unknown
PO (osteoarthritis)	30 days	unknown	unknown

Contraindications/Precautions
Contraindicated in: Hypersensitivity; Bipolar disorder; Lactation.
Use Cautiously in: Pregnancy or children (safety not established); Bipolar disorder (can induce mania); Parkinson's disease (may worsen symptoms); Surgery (discontinue 2 wk prior to elective procedures).

Adverse Reactions/Side Effects
CNS: agitation, dizziness, mild insomnia, manic reactions (in patients with bipolar disorder). **GI:** vomiting, diarrhea, flatulence.

Interactions
Natural Product-Drug: Avoid use with **antidepressants, meperidine, pentazocine, tramadol**, and **dextromethorphan** (additive serotonergic effects may occur). May ↓ effectiveness of **levodopa** and worsen Parkinsonian symptoms. Should not be used concurrently with **MAO inhibitors**. Avoid use of SAMe within 2 wk of using a **MAO inhibitor**.
Natural-Natural: Avoid use with natural products that increase serotonin levels such as **l-tryptophan** and **St. John's wort**.

Route/Commonly Used Doses
PO (Adults): *Depression*—200 mg once or twice daily, adjusted upward over 2 wk (range 400–1600 mg/day); *Liver disorders*—1200–1600 mg/day; *Osteoarthritis*—200–400 mg three times daily; *Fibromyalgia*—800 mg/day.

Availability
Tablets 100 mg, 200 mg, 400 mg[OTC].

NURSING IMPLICATIONS

Assessment
- Assess mental status for symptoms of depression prior to and periodically during therapy; advise patients with depression to be evaluated by a health care professional.
- Assess symptoms of pain and fatigue prior to and periodically during therapy.

Implementation
- **PO:** Administer on an empty stomach. Initial dose should be 200 mg once or twice daily to minimize GI disturbances. Dose may be adjusted upward over 1–2 wk depending on response and tolerance.

Patient/Family Teaching
- Instruct patient to take SAMe as directed.
- Advise patients to discontinue 2 wk prior to elective surgical procedures.
- Advise females of reproductive potential to consult health care professional if pregnancy is planned or suspected or if breast feeding.

Evaluation
- Decrease in symptoms of depression.
- Improvement in osteoarthritis symptoms.

saw palmetto
(saw pal-**met**-toe)

Other Name(s):
American Dwarf Palm Tree, Cabbage Palm, Ju-Zhong, Palmier Nain, Sabal, Sabal Fructus, Saw Palmetto Berry, *Serenoa repens*

Classification
Therapeutic: benign prostatic hyperplasia (BPH) agents

Common Uses
Benign prostatic hyperplasia.

Action
Exerts antiandrogenic, anti-inflammatory, and antiproliferative properties in prostate tissue resulting in improvement in BPH symptoms such as frequent urination, hesitancy, urgency, and nocturia. Comparable in efficacy to finasteride but may be less effective than prazosin. **Therapeutic Effects:** Decreased urinary symptoms of BPH.

Pharmacokinetics
Absorption: Unknown.
Distribution: Unknown.
Metabolism and Excretion: Unknown.
Half-life: Unknown.

TIME/ACTION PROFILE

ROUTE	ONSET	PEAK	DURATION
PO	1–2 mo	unknown	48 wk (longest studied treatment duration)

Contraindications/Precautions
Contraindicated in: Pregnancy and lactation.
Use Cautiously in: Prior to surgery (discontinue 2 wk before to prevent bleeding).

Adverse Reactions/Side Effects
CNS: dizziness, headache. **GI:** nausea, vomiting, constipation, and diarrhea.

Interactions
Natural Product-Drug: Hormonal action may interfere with other hormonal therapies (**testosterone, hormonal contraceptives**). Avoid use with **antiplatelet** or **anticoagulant drugs** (may ↑ bleeding risk).

NATURAL/HERBAL PRODUCTS

Natural-Natural: Concomitant use with herbs that affect platelet aggregation such as **ginger**, **garlic**, **gingko**, and **ginseng** may ↑ bleeding risk.

Route/Commonly Used Doses

PO (Adults): *Lipophilic extract (80–90% fatty acids)*—160 mg twice daily or 320 mg once daily. *Whole berries*—1–2 g daily. *Liquid extract from berry pulp*—1–2 mL three times daily. *Tea (efficacy is questionable due to lipophilicity of active constituents)*—1 cup three times daily. Tea is prepared by steeping 0.5–1 g dried berry in 150 mL boiling water for 5–10 min.

Availability

Lipophilic extract (80-90% fatty acids)[OTC]; **Whole berries**[OTC]; **Liquid extract**[OTC].

NURSING IMPLICATIONS

Assessment

- Assess patient for symptoms of benign prostatic hypertrophy (BPH) (urinary hesitancy, feeling of incomplete bladder emptying, interruption in urinary stream, impairment in size and force of urinary stream, terminal urinary dribbling, straining to start flow, dysuria, urgency) before and periodically during therapy.
- Perform rectal exams prior to and periodically during therapy to assess prostate size are recommended.

Implementation

- Take on a full stomach to minimize GI effects.

Patient/Family Teaching

- Advise patients to start therapy with saw palmetto only after evaluation by a health care professional who will provide continued follow-up care.
- Inform patients that saw palmetto does not alter the size of the prostate but still should relieve the symptoms associated with BPH.
- Advise patient that taking saw palmetto with food may reduce GI effects and improve tolerability.

Evaluation

- Decrease in urinary symptoms of BPH.

St. John's wort (*Hypericum perforatum*)

(saynt **jonz** wort)

Other Name(s):
Amber, Demon chaser, Goatweed, Hardhay, Klamath weed, Rosin rose, Tipton weed

Classification
Therapeutic: antidepressants

Common Uses

PO: Management of mild to moderate depression and obsessive compulsive disorder (OCD). (Not effective for major depression.). **Topical:** Inflammation of the skin, blunt injury, wounds, and burns. Other uses are for capillary strengthening, decreasing uterine bleeding, and reducing tumor size.

Action

Derived from *Hypericum perforatum*; the active component is *hypericin*. **PO:** Antidepressant action may be due to ability to inhibit reuptake of serotonin and other neurotransmitters. **Topical:** Anti-inflammatory, antifungal, antiviral, and antibacterial properties. **Therapeutic Effects: PO:** Decreased signs and symptoms of depression. **Topical:** Decreased inflammation of burns or other wounds.

Pharmacokinetics

Absorption: Unknown.
Distribution: Unknown.
Metabolism and Excretion: Unknown.
Half-life: *Hypericum constituents*—24.8–26.5 hr.

TIME/ACTION PROFILE

ROUTE	ONSET	PEAK	DURATION
PO	10–14 days	within 4–6 wk	unknown

Contraindications/Precautions

Contraindicated in: Pregnancy and lactation.
Use Cautiously in: Children 6–17 years: use orally no longer than 8 wk; History of phototoxicity; Surgery (discontinue 2 wk prior to surgical procedures); Alzheimer's disease (may induce psychosis); Patients undergoing general anesthesia (may cause cardiovascular collapse); History of suicide attempt, severe depression, schizophrenia, or bipolar disorder (can induce hypomania or psychosis).

Adverse Reactions/Side Effects

CNS: dizziness, restlessness, sleep disturbances. **CV:** hypertension. **GI:** abdominal pain, bloating, diarrhea, dry mouth, feeling of fullness, flatulence, nausea, vomiting. **Neuro:** neuropathy. **Derm:** allergic skin reactions (hives, itching, skin rash), phototoxicity. **Misc:** serotonin syndrome.

Interactions

Natural Product-Drug: Concurrent use with **alcohol** or other **antidepressants** (including **SSRIs** and **MAO inhibitors**) may ↑ risk of adverse CNS reactions. May ↓ the effectiveness and serum concentrations of **digoxin**, **alprazolam**, **amitriptyline**, **imatinib**, **irinotecan**, **warfarin**, and **protease inhibitors**. Use with **MAO Inhibitors**,

NATURAL/HERBAL PRODUCTS

tramadol, **pentazocine**, and **selective serotonin agonists** could result in serotonin syndrome. May ↓ effectiveness of **oral contraceptives**. May ↓ plasma **cyclosporine** and **tacrolimus** levels by 30–70% and cause acute transplant rejection. May ↑ metabolism of **phenytoin** and **phenobarbital** and cause loss of seizure control. Avoid use of St. John's wort and **MAO Inhibitors** within 2 wk of each other.
Natural-Natural: May ↑ risk of serotonin syndrome when taken with **tryptophan** and **SAM-e**.

Route/Commonly Used Doses

PO (Adults): *Mild Depression*—300 mg of St. John's wort (standardized to 0.3% hypericin) 3 times daily or 250 mg twice daily of 0.2% hypericin extract. *OCD*-450 mg twice daily of extended release preparation.
Topical (Adults): 0.2–1 mg total hypericin daily.

Availability

Preparations for Oral Use
Dried herb[OTC]; **Dried (hydroalcoholic) extract**[OTC]; **Oil**[OTC]; **Tincture**[OTC].
Preparations for Topical Application
Liquid[OTC]; **Semisolid**[OTC].

NURSING IMPLICATIONS

Assessment

- **Depression:** Assess for depression periodically during therapy.
- **Inflammation:** Assess skin or skin lesions periodically during therapy.

Implementation

- **PO:** Tea can be prepared by mixing 2–4 dried herbs in 150 mL of boiling water and steeping for 10 min.

Patient/Family Teaching

- Instruct patient to take St. John's wort as directed.
- Patients with depression should be evaluated by health care professional. Standard therapy may be of greater benefit for moderate to severe depression.
- Instruct patient to consult health care professional before taking other Rx, OTC, or herbal products concurrently with St. John's wort. May reduce the therapeutic effectiveness of other drugs. May potentiate effect of sedatives and side effects of other antidepressants. Do not take within 2 wk of MAO inhibitor therapy.
- Caution patients to avoid sun exposure and use protective sunscreen to reduce the risk of photosensitivity reactions.
- Inform patient to purchase herbs from a reputable source and that products and their contents vary among different manufacturers.
- Caution patient not to use alcohol while taking St. John's wort.
- Advise patient to notify health care professional of medication regimen prior to treatment or surgery.
- Inform patient that St. John's wort is usually taken for a period of 4–6 wk. If no improvement is seen, another therapy should be considered.

Evaluation

- Decrease in signs and symptoms of depression or anxiety.
- Improvement in skin inflammation.

valerian (vuh-lare-ee-en)

Other Name(s):
Amantilla, All-Heal, Baldrian, Baldrianwurzel, Belgium Valerian, Common Valerian, Fragrant Valerian, Garden Heliotrope, Garden Valerian, Indian Valerian, Mexican Valerian, Pacific Valerian, Tagara, Valeriana, *Valeriana officinalis*, *Valerianae radix*, Valeriana rhizome, Valeriane

Classification
Therapeutic: antianxiety agents, sedative/hypnotics

Common Uses

Insomnia. Anxiety.

Action

May increase concentrations of the inhibitory CNS transmitter GABA. **Therapeutic Effects:** Improvement in sleep quality.

Pharmacokinetics

Absorption: Unknown.
Distribution: Unknown.
Metabolism and Excretion: Unknown.
Half-life: Unknown.

TIME/ACTION PROFILE

ROUTE	ONSET	PEAK	DURATION
PO	30–60 min	2 hr	unknown

Contraindications/Precautions

Contraindicated in: Pregnancy and lactation.
Use Cautiously in: Alcohol use (may have additive sedative effects); Surgery (discontinue use 2 wk prior to elective procedures); Children (do not use longer than 8 wk).

Adverse Reactions/Side Effects

CNS: drowsiness, headache. **GI:** dry mouth. **Misc:** Benzodiazepine-like withdrawal symptoms with discontinuation after long-term use.

Interactions

Natural Product-Drug: Additive CNS depression with **alcohol**, **antihistamines**, **anesthetic agents**, **sedative hypnotics**, and other **CNS depressants**. Alcohol-containing preparations may interact with **disulfiram** and **metronidazole**.
Natural-Natural: Additive sedative effects can occur when used with herbal supplements with sedative properties such as **kava**, **l-tryptophan**, **melatonin**, **SAMe**, and **St. John's wort**.

Route/Commonly Used Doses

PO (Adults): *Tea*—1 cup tea 1–5 times daily. Tea is made by steeping 2–3 g root in 150 mL boiling water for 5–10 min then straining. *Tincture*—1–3 mL 1–5 times daily. *Extract*—400–900 mg up to 2 hr before bedtime or 300–450 mg divided tid.

Availability

Capsules^{OTC}; **Extract**^{OTC}; **Tea**^{OTC}; **Tincture**^{OTC}.

NURSING IMPLICATIONS

Assessment

- Assess degree of anxiety and level of sedation prior to and periodically throughout therapy.
- Assess sleep patterns.
- Assess response in the elderly population where drowsiness and loss of balance may pose a significant risk for injury.

Implementation

- Take 1–2 hr before bedtime if used for nighttime hypnotic.
- Administer orally three to five times daily to control anxiety.

Patient/Family Teaching

- Encourage patients to avoid stimulants such as caffeine and to provide an environment that promotes restful sleep.
- May cause drowsiness. Caution patient to avoid driving or other activities requiring alertness until response to drug is known.
- Caution patient to avoid use of alcohol and other medications or herbals that have a sedative effect; may increase drowsiness.
- Advise patients to discontinue 2 wk prior to elective surgical procedures.
- Inform patients that dependence with withdrawal symptoms may develop with prolonged use.
- Advise females of reproductive potential to avoid valerian if pregnancy is planned or suspected or breast-feeding.

Evaluation

- Decreased anxiety level.
- Improvement in sleep with a feeling of restfulness without drowsiness upon awakening.

PEDIATRIC INTRAVENOUS MEDICATION QUICK REFERENCE CHART

Risk of fluid overload in infants and children is always a consideration when administering IV medications. The following table provides maximum concentrations—the smallest amount of fluid necessary for diluting specific medications—and the maximum rate at which the medications be given.

Drug	Maximum Concentration	Maximum Rate
acetaminophen	10 mg/mL	Give over 15 min
acetazolamide	100 mg/mL	500 mg/min²
acyclovir	7 mg/mL	Give over 1 hr
adenosine	3 mg/mL	Give over 1–2 sec
allopurinol	6 mg/mL	Give over 30 min
amikacin	10 mg/mL	Give over 30–60 min
aminocaproic acid	20 mg/mL	Give over 1 hr
aminophylline	25 mg/mL	25 mg/min
amphotericin B deoxycholate (conventional)	0.1 mg/mL (peripherally) 0.5 mg/mL (centrally)	Give over 2–6 hr Give over 2–6 hr
amphotericin B lipid complex	2 mg/mL	Give over 2 hr
amphotericin B liposomal	2 mg/mL	Give over 2 hr
ampicillin	100 mg/mL	100 mg/min
ampicillin/sulbactam	30 mg/mL (ampicillin)	Give over 15–30 min
anidulafungin	0.77 mg/mL	1.1 mg/min
atropine	1 mg/mL	Give over 1 min
azithromycin	2 mg/mL	Give over 1 hr
aztreonam	20 mg/mL	Give over 20–60 min
bumetanide	0.25 mg/mL	Give over 1–2 min
caffeine citrate	20 mg/mL	Give over 10–20 min
calcitriol	2 mcg/mL	Give over 15 sec
calcium chloride	100 mg/mL	100 mg/min
calcium gluconate	100 mg/mL	100 mg/min
caspofungin	0.5 mg/mL	Give over 1 hr
cefazolin	138 mg/mL (IVP) 20 mg/mL (intermittent infusion)	Give over 3–5 min Give over 10–60 min
cefepime	160 mg/mL	Give over 30 min
cefotaxime	200 mg/mL (IVP) 60 mg/mL (intermittent infusion)	Give over 3–5 min Give over 10–30 min
cefoxitin	200 mg/mL (IVP) 40 mg/mL (intermittent infusion)	Give over 3–5 min Give over 10–60 min
ceftazidime	180 mg/mL (IVP) 40 mg/mL (intermittent infusion)	Give over 3–5 min Give over 10–30 min
ceftriaxone	40 mg/mL	Give over 10–30 min
cefuroxime	100 mg/mL (IVP) 137 mg/mL (intermittent infusion)	Give over 3–5 min Give over 15–30 min
chlorothiazide	28 mg/mL	Give over 3–5 min
chlorpromazine	1 mg/mL	0.5 mg/min
ciprofloxacin	2 mg/mL	Give over 60 min
clindamycin	18 mg/mL	30 mg/min
cyclosporine	2.5 mg/mL	Give over 2–6 hr
dexamethasone	10 mg/mL	Doses ≤10 mg: Give over 1–4 min Doses >10 mg: Give over 15–30 min
dexmedetomidine	4 mcg/mL	Give bolus over 5–10 min
diazepam	5 mg/mL	2 mg/min
digoxin	100 mcg/mL	Give over 5 min
diphenhydramine	25 mg/mL	25 mg/min
doxycycline	1 mg/mL	Give over 1 hr
enalaprilat	1.25 mg/mL	Give over 5 min
erythromycin	5 mg/mL	Give over 20–120 min
esomeprazole	8 mg/mL	Give over 10–30 min
ethacrynic acid	2 mg/mL	Give over 5–30 min
famotidine	4 mg/mL (IVP) 0.2 mg/mL (intermittent infusion)	10 mg/min Give over 15–30 min
fentanyl	50 mcg/mL	Give over 1–3 min
fluconazole	2 mg/mL	Give over 1–2 hr
flumazenil	0.1 mg/mL	0.2 mg/min
foscarnet	12 mg/mL (peripherally) 24 mg/mL (centrally)	60 mg/kg/hr
fosphenytoin	25 mg/mL	3 mg/kg/min
furosemide	10 mg/mL	0.5 mg/kg/min
ganciclovir	10 mg/mL	Give over 1 hr
gentamicin	10 mg/mL	Give over 30 min
glycopyrrolate	0.2 mg/mL	20 mcg/min
granisetron	1 mg/mL (IVP) 50 mcg/mL (intermittent infusion)	Give over 30 sec Give over 30–60 min

PEDIATRIC INTRAVENOUS MEDICATION QUICK REFERENCE CHART

Drug	Maximum Concentration	Maximum Rate
hydralazine	20 mg/mL	0.2 mg/kg/min
hydrocortisone sodium succinate	50 mg/mL (IVP) 5 mg/mL (intermittent infusion)	Give over 30 sec Give over 10–30 min
ibuprofen	10 mg/mL	Give over 15 min
imipenem/cilastatin	7 mg/mL	Give over 15–60 min
indomethacin	1 mg/mL	Give over 20–30 min
ketamine	50 mg/mL (IVP) 2 mg/mL (intermittent infusion)	0.5 mg/kg/min 0.5 mg/kg/min
ketorolac	30 mg/mL	Give over 1–5 min
labetalol	5 mg/mL (IVP)	2 mg/min
lacosamide	10 mg/mL	Give over 30–60 min
levetiracetam	15 mg/mL	Give over 5–15 min
levocarnitine	200 mg/mL	Give over 2–3 min
levothyroxine	100 mcg/mL	Give over 2–3 min
linezolid	2 mg/mL	Give over 30–120 min
lorazepam	4 mg/mL	2 mg/min or 0.05 mg/kg over 2–5 min
magnesium sulfate	200 mg/mL	Give over 10–20 min
meperidine	10 mg/mL	Give over 5 min
meropenem	50 mg/mL (IVP) 20 mg/mL (intermittent infusion)	Give over 3–5 min Give over 15–30 min
methylprednisolone	125 mg/mL (IVP) 2.5 mg/mL (intermittent infusion)	Give over 1–30 min Give over 20–60 min
metoclopramide	5 mg/mL	5 mg/min
metronidazole	8 mg/mL	Give over 1 hr
micafungin	1.5 mg/mL	Give over 1 hr
midazolam	5 mg/mL	Give over 20–30 sec (5 min in neonates)
milrinone	800 mcg/mL	Give over 10 min (loading dose)
morphine	5 mg/mL	Give over 5–30 min
nafcillin	125 mg/mL	Give over 15–60 min
naloxone	1 mg/mL	Give over 30 sec
ondansetron	2 mg/mL	Give over 2–15 min
oxacillin	100 mg/mL (IVP) 40 mg/mL (intermittent infusion)	Give over 10 min Give over 15–30 min
pancuronium	2 mg/mL (IVP)	Give over 3–5 sec
pantoprazole	4 mg/mL	Give over 2–15 min
penicillin G	100,000 units/mL	Give over 15–30 min
pentamidine	6 mg/mL	Give over 1–2 hr
pentobarbital	50 mg/mL	50 mg/min
phenobarbital	130 mg/mL	30 mg/min
phenytoin	10 mg/mL	1 mg/kg/min (neonates) 3 mg/kg/min (children)
phytonadione	10 mg/mL	1 mg/min
piperacillin/tazobactam	200 mg/mL	Give over 30 min
potassium chloride	80 mEq/L (peripherally) 200 mEq/L (centrally)	1 mEq/kg/hr
promethazine	25 mg/mL	25 mg/min
propranolol	1 mg/mL	1 mg/min
protamine	10 mg/mL	5 mg/min
ranitidine	2.5 mg/mL	10 mg/min
rifampin	6 mg/mL	Give over 30 min
tacrolimus	0.02 mg/mL	Give over 4–24 hr
terbutaline	1 mg/mL	Give over 5–10 min
tobramycin	10 mg/mL	Give over 30 min
trimethoprim/sulfamethoxazole	1 mL drug per 10 mL diluent	Give over 1–1.5 hr
valproate sodium	50 mg/mL	3 mg/kg/min
vancomycin	5 mg/mL	Give over 60 min
vasopressin	1 unit/mL	Give over 5–30 min
verapamil	2.5 mg/mL (IVP)	Give over 2–3 min
voriconazole	5 mg/mL	3 mg/kg/hr
zidovudine	4 mg/mL	Give over 60 min

1. Phelps SJ, Hagemann TM, Lee KR, Thompson AJ: Pediatric Injectable Drugs, 11th Edition. American Society of Health-System Pharmacists, Bethesda, MD 2018.
2. Taketomo CK, Hodding JH, Kraus DM: Pediatric and Neonatal Dosage Handbook, 25th Edition, Lexi-Comp, Hudson, OH 2018.

BEERS CRITERIA

The Beers criteria for potentially inappropriate medication use in adults 65 and older in the United States is a compilation of drugs and drug classes found to increase the risk of adverse events in older adults. Frequently, older adults are more sensitive to the medications or their side effects. These adverse events have significant economic and quality of life costs for society and individuals and can result in more frequent hospitalizations, permanent injury, or death. Often, the potential for adverse events can be minimized by prescribing safer alternatives or prescribing at the lowest effective dose. The list of medications below represents an update to the list previously published in 2015.

- alprazolam (Xanax, Xanax XR)
- amiodarone (avoid using as first-line therapy for atrial fibrillation unless heart failure or significant left ventricular hypertrophy present) (Pacerone)
- amitriptyline
- amobarbital (Amytal Sodium)
- amoxapine
- aripiprazole (avoid use, except in schizophrenia or bipolar disorder) (Abilify, Abilify Maintena)
- asenapine (avoid use, except in schizophrenia or bipolar disorder) (Saphris)
- aspirin (avoid using dosage >325 mg/day)
- atropine (does not apply to ophthalmic formulations) (Atropen)
- belladonna alkaloids (Donnatal)
- benztropine (oral only) (Cogentin)
- brexpiprazole (avoid use, except in schizophrenia) (Rexulti)
- brompheniramine
- butabarbital (Butisol Sodium)
- butalbital
- carbinoxamine (Karbinal ER)
- cariprazine (avoid use, except in schizophrenia or bipolar disorder) (Vraylar)
- carisoprodol (Soma)
- chlordiazepoxide (Librium)
- chlordiazepoxide-amitriptyline
- chlorpheniramine (Chlor-Trimeton)
- chlorpromazine (avoid use, except in schizophrenia or bipolar disorder or for short-term use as antiemetic during chemotherapy)
- chlorzoxazone
- clemastine (Dayhist Allergy)
- clidinium-chlordiazepoxide (Librax)
- clomipramine (Anafranil)
- clonazepam (Klonopin)
- clonidine (avoid use for first-line treatment of hypertension) (Catapres, Duraclon, Kapvay)
- clorazepate (Tranxene)
- clozapine (avoid use, except in schizophrenia or bipolar disorder) (Clozaril, Versacloz)
- cyclobenzaprine (Amrix, Fexmid)
- cyproheptadine
- desipramine (Norpramin)
- desmopressin (avoid use for treatment of nocturia or nocturnal polyuria) (DDAVP, Nocdurna, Noctiva, Stimate)
- dessicated thyroid (Armour Thyroid)
- dexbrompheniramine
- dexchlorpheniramine
- dexlansoprazole (avoid scheduled use for >8 wk unless for high-risk patients or patients with erosive esophagitis, Barrett esophagitis, or pathological hypersecretory condition) (Dexilant)
- diazepam (Valium)
- diclofenac (Cambia, Zipsor, Zorvolex)
- dicyclomine (Bentyl)
- diflunisal
- digoxin (avoid using for first-line treatment of atrial fibrillation or heart failure; avoid using dosage >0.125 mg/day) (Lanoxin)
- dimenhydrinate (Dramamine)
- diphenhydramine (Benadryl)
- dipyridamole (short-acting)
- disopyramide (Norpace, Norpace CR)
- doxazosin (avoid using for treatment of hypertension) (Cardura)
- doxepin (avoid using dosage >6 mg/day) (Silenor)
- doxylamine
- dronedarone (avoid use in permanent atrial fibrillation or in patients with severe or recently decompensated heart failure) (Multaq)
- ergoloid mesylates
- esomeprazole (avoid scheduled use for >8 wk unless for high-risk patients or patients with erosive esophagitis, Barrett esophagitis, or pathological hypersecretory condition) (Nexium, Nexium 24HR)
- estazolam
- estrogens (with or without progestins) (avoid systemic estrogens; intravaginal formulations acceptable to use)
- eszopiclone (Lunesta)
- etodolac
- fenoprofen (Nalfon)
- fluphenazine (avoid use, except in schizophrenia)
- flurazepam
- glimepiride (Amaryl)
- glyburide (Diabeta, Glynase)
- growth hormone (avoid unless used for confirmed growth hormone deficiency)
- guanfacine (Intuniv)
- haloperidol (avoid use, except in schizophrenia or bipolar disorder or for short-term use as antiemetic during chemotherapy) (Haldol)
- hydroxyzine (Vistaril)
- hyoscyamine (Anaspaz, Levsin)
- ibuprofen (Advil, Motrin)
- iloperidone (avoid use, except in schizophrenia) (Fanapt)
- imipramine (Tofranil)
- indomethacin (Indocin, Tivorbex)
- insulin (avoid use of regimens containing only short- or rapid-acting insulin without concurrent use of basal or long-acting insulin)
- isoxsuprine
- ketoprofen
- ketorolac
- lansoprazole (avoid scheduled use for >8 wk unless for high-risk patients or patients with erosive esophagitis, Barrett esophagitis, or pathological hypersecretory condition) (Prevacid, Prevacid 24HR, Prevacid SoluTab)
- lorazepam (Ativan)
- loxapine (avoid use, except in schizophrenia or bipolar disorder) (Adasuve)
- lurasidone (avoid use, except in schizophrenia or bipolar disorder) (Latuda)
- meclizine
- meclofenamate
- mefenamic acid (Ponstel)
- megestrol (Megace ES)
- meloxicam (Mobic, Qmiiz ODT, Vivlodex)
- meperidine (Demerol)
- meprobamate
- metaxalone (Skelaxin)

BEERS CRITERIA

methocarbamol (Robaxin)	pimozide
methscopolamine	piroxicam (Feldene)
methyldopa	prazosin (avoid using for treatment of hypertension) (Minipress)
methyltestosterone (avoid unless used for confirmed hypogonadism) (Android, Testred)	prochlorperazine (avoid use, except for short-term use as antiemetic during chemotherapy) (Compro)
metoclopramide (avoid use, except in gastroparesis [use should generally not exceed 12 wk]) (Reglan)	promethazine
mineral oil (oral)	propantheline
nabumetone	protriptyline
naproxen (Aleve, Anaprox, Naprelan, Naprosyn)	pyrilamine
nifedipine (immediate-release) (Procardia)	quazepam (Doral)
nitrofurantoin (avoid using if CCr <30 mL/min or for long-term suppression of urinary tract infections) (Furadantin, Macrobid, Microdantin)	quetiapine (avoid use, except in schizophrenia or bipolar disorder) (Seroquel, Seroquel XR)
nortriptyline (Pamelor)	rabeprazole (avoid scheduled use for >8 wk unless for high-risk patients or patients with erosive esophagitis, Barrett esophagitis, or pathological hypersecretory condition) (Aciphex, Aciphex Sprinkle)
olanzapine (avoid use, except in schizophrenia or bipolar disorder or for short-term use as antiemetic during chemotherapy) (Zyprexa, Zyprexa Relprevv, Zyprexa Zydis)	risperidone (avoid use, except in schizophrenia or bipolar disorder) (Perseris Kit, Risperdal, Risperdal Consta)
olanzapine-fluoxetine (avoid use, except in bipolar disorder) (Symbyax)	scopolamine (Transderm-Scop)
omeprazole (avoid scheduled use for >8 wk unless for high-risk patients or patients with erosive esophagitis, Barrett esophagitis, or pathological hypersecretory condition) (Prilosec, Prilosec OTC)	secobarbital (Seconal)
orphenadrine	sulindac
oxaprozin (Daypro)	temazepam (Restoril)
oxazepam	terazosin (avoid using for treatment of hypertension)
paliperidone (avoid use, except in schizophrenia or bipolar disorder) (Invega, Invega Sustenna, Invega Trinza)	testosterone (avoid unless used for confirmed hypogonadism) (Androderm, Androgel, Aveed, Fortesta, Natesto, Striant, Testim, Vogelxo, Xyosted)
pantoprazole (avoid scheduled use for >8 wk unless for high-risk patients or patients with erosive esophagitis, Barrett esophagitis, or pathological hypersecretory condition) (Protonix)	thioridazine (avoid use, except in schizophrenia)
paroxetine (Brisdelle, Paxil, Paxil CR, Pexeva)	thiothixene (avoid use, except in schizophrenia)
pentobarbital (Nembutal)	tolmetin
perphenazine (avoid use, except in schizophrenia or for short-term use as antiemetic during chemotherapy)	triazolam (Halcion)
perphenazine-amitriptyline (avoid use, except in schizophrenia)	trifluoperazine (avoid use, except in schizophrenia)
phenobarbital	trihexyphenidyl
	trimipramine
	triprolidine
	zaleplon (Sonata)
	ziprasidone (avoid use, except in schizophrenia or bipolar disorder) (Geodon)
	zolpidem (Ambien, Ambien CR, Edluar, Intermezzo, Zolpimist)

The 2019 American Geriatrics Society Beers Criteria Update Expert Panel. American Geriatrics Society 2019 updated AGS Beers Criteria for potentially inappropriate medication use in older adults. *J Am Geriatr Soc.* 2019;67:674–694.

DRUGS ASSOCIATED WITH INCREASED RISK OF FALLS IN THE ELDERLY

Many factors are associated with falls in the elderly, including frailty, disease, vision, polypharmacy, and certain medications. Below is a list of drugs associated with falls. Assess geriatric patients on these medications for fall risk and implement fall reduction strategies.

ACE Inhibitors

- benazepril (Lotensin)
- captopril
- enalapril (Vasotec)
- fosinopril
- lisinopril (Prinivil, Zestril)
- moexipril
- perindopril
- quinapril (Accupril)
- ramipril (Altace)
- trandolapril

Angiotensin II Receptor Antagonists

- azilsartan (Edarbi)
- candesartan (Atacand)
- eprosartan
- irbesartan (Avapro)
- losartan (Cozaar)
- olmesartan (Benicar)
- telmisartan (Micardis)
- valsartan (Diovan)

Antiarrhythmics

- digoxin (Lanoxin)
- disopyramide (Norpace)

Anticonvulsants

- carbamazepine (Carbatrol, Epitol, Equetro, Tegretol)
- ethosuximide (Zarontin)
- felbamate (Felbatol)
- gabapentin (Gralise, Neurontin)
- lamotrigine (Lamictal)
- levetiracetam (Keppra, Spritam)
- methsuximide (Celontin)
- phenobarbital
- phenytoin (Dilantin, Phenytek)
- pregabalin (Lyrica)
- primidone (Mysoline)
- tiagabine (Gabatril)
- topiramate (Qudexy XR, Topamax, Trokendi XR)
- valproate (Depakote)
- zonisamide (Zonegran)

Antidepressants

- amitriptyline
- amoxapine
- bupropion (Aplenzin, Forfivo XL, Wellbutrin XL)
- citalopram (Celexa)
- clomipramine (Anafranil)
- desipramine (Norpramin)
- doxepin (Silenor)
- duloxetine (Cymbalta, Drizalma Sprinkle)
- escitalopram (Lexapro)
- fluoxetine (Prozac)
- fluvoxamine
- imipramine (Tofranil)
- isocarboxazid (Marplan)
- maprotiline
- mirtazapine (Remeron)
- nefazodone
- paroxetine (Paxil, Pexeva)
- phenelzine (Nardil)
- protriptyline (Vivactil)
- sertraline (Zoloft)
- tranylcypromine (Parnate)
- trazodone
- trimipramine
- venlafaxine (Effexor XR)

Antihistamines/Antinauseants

- dimenhydrinate (Dramamine)
- diphenhydramine (Benadryl)
- hydroxyzine (Vistaril)
- meclizine (Bonine)
- metoclopramide (Reglan)
- prochlorperazine (Compro)
- promethazine
- scopolamine patch (Transderm Scop)

Antiparkinsonian Agents

- amantadine (Gocovri, Osmolex ER)
- bromocriptine (Parlodel)
- entacapone (Comtan)
- levodopa/carbidopa (Duopa, Rytary, Sinemet, Sinemet CR)
- pramipexole (Mirapex, Mirapex ER)
- selegiline (Zelapar)

Antipsychotics (Atypical)

- aripiprazole (Abilify, Abilify Maintena, Aristada, Aristada Initio)
- clozapine (Clozaril, Versacloz)
- olanzapine (Zyprexa, Zyprexa Relprevv, Zyprexa Zydis)
- paliperidone (Invega, Invega Sustenna, Invega Trinza)
- quetiapine (Seroquel, Seroquel XR)
- risperidone (Perseris, Risperdal, Risperdal Consta)
- ziprasidone (Geodon)

Antipsychotics (Typical)

- chlorpromazine
- fluphenazine
- haloperidol (Haldol)
- loxapine (Adasuve)
- perphenazine
- pimozide
- thioridazine
- thiothixine
- trifluoperazine

Anxiolytics

- buspirone
- meprobamate

Benzodiazepines (Long-Acting)

- chlordiazepoxide (Librium)
- clonazepam (Klonopin)
- clorazepate (Tranxene)
- diazepam (Valium)
- flurazepam

Benzodiazepines (Intermediate-Acting)

- alprazolam (Xanax, Xanax XR)
- estazolam
- lorazepam (Ativan)
- oxazepam
- temazepam (Restoril)

Benzodiazepines (Short-Acting)

- triazolam (Halcion)

Beta Blockers

- acebutolol
- atenolol (Tenormin)
- bisoprolol
- carvedilol (Coreg, Coreg CR)
- labetalol (Trandate)
- metoprolol (Kaspargo Sprinkle, Lopressor, Toprol XL)
- propranolol (Inderal LA, InnoPran XL)
- timolol

Calcium Channel Blockers

- amlodipine (Katerzia, Norvasc)
- diltiazem (Cardizem, Cardizem CD, Cardizem LA, Cartia XT, Taztia XT, Tiazac)
- felodipine
- isradipine
- nicardipine (Cardene)
- nifedipine (Adalat CC, Procardia XL)
- nisoldipine (Sular)
- verapamil (Calan SR, Verelan, Verelan PM)

Diuretics

- amiloride/hydrochlorothiazide
- bumetanide (Bumex)
- furosemide (Lasix)
- hydrochlorothiazide (Microzide)
- triamterene/hydrochlorothiazide (Dyazide, Maxzide)

Opioid Analgesics

- codeine
- fentanyl (Abstral, Actiq, Duragesic, Fentora, Ionsys, Lazanda, Sublimaze, Subsys)
- hydrocodone (Hysingla ER, Zohydro ER)
- hydromorphone (Dilaudid)
- levorphanol
- meperidine (Demerol)
- methadone (Dolophine, Methadose)
- morphine (Duramorph, Infumorph, Kadian, Mitigo, Morphabond ER, MS Contin)
- oxycodone (Oxaydo, OxyContin, Roxicodone, Xtampza ER)
- oxymorphone (Opana)

Skeletal Muscle Relaxants

- baclofen (Gablofen, Lioresal, Ozobax)

Vasodilators

- doxazosin (Cardura, Cardura XL)
- hydralazine
- isosorbide dinitrate/mononitrate (Dilatrate SR, Isordil, Monoket)
- nitroglycerin (GoNitro, Minitran, Nitro-Dur, Nitrolingual, Nitromist, Nitrostat)
- prazosin (Minipress)
- terazosin

American Geriatrics Society, British Geriatrics Society, and American Academy of Orthopedic Surgeons Panel on Falls Prevention. Guideline for the prevention of falls in older persons. J Am Geriatr Soc. 49:664–672, 2001.
Keys PA. Preventing falls in the elderly: the role of the pharmacist. J Pharm Pract. 17(2):149–152, 2004.
Cooper JW, Burfield AH. Medication interventions for fall prevention in the older adult. J Am Pharm Assoc. 49:e70-84, 2009.

LIST OF CONFUSED DRUG NAMES

Drug Name	Confused Drug Name
Abelcet	amphotericin B
Accupril	Aciphex
acetaminophen	aceta**ZOLAMIDE**
aceta**ZOLAMIDE**	acetaminophen
acetic acid for irrigation	glacial acetic acid
Aciphex	Accupril
Aciphex	Aricept
Activase	Cathflo Activase
Activase	TNKase
Actonel	Actos
Actos	Actonel
Adacel (Tdap)	Daptacel (DTaP)
ado-trastuzumab emtansine	trastuzumab
Aggrastat	argatroban
Aldara	Alora
Alkeran	Leukeran
Alkeran	Myleran
Allegra	Allegra Anti-Itch Cream (diphenhydramine/ allantoin)
Allegra	Viagra
Allegra Anti-Itch Cream (diphenhydramine/ allantoin)	Allegra
Alora	Aldara
ALPRAZolam	clonaze**PAM**
ALPRAZolam	**LOR**azepam
amantadine	amiodarone
Ambisome	amphotericin B
a**MIL**oride	am**LODIP**ine
amiodarone	amantadine
am**LODIP**ine	a**MIL**oride
amphotericin B	Abelcet
amphotericin B	Ambisome
amphotericin B	amphotericin B liposomal
amphotericin B liposomal	amphotericin B
antacid	Atacand
anticoagulant citrate dextrose solution formula A	anticoagulant sodium citrate solution
anticoagulant sodium citrate solution	anticoagulant citrate dextrose solution formula A
Apidra	Spiriva
argatroban	Aggrastat
Aricept	Aciphex
Aricept	Azilect
ARIPiprazole	proton pump inhibitors
ARIPiprazole	**RABE**prazole
Arista AH (absorbable hemostatic agent)	Arixtra
Arixtra	Arista AH (absorbable hemostatic agent)
Asacol	Os-Cal
Atacand	antacid
atomoxetine	atorvastatin
atorvastatin	atomoxetine
Avandia	Coumadin
aza**CITID**ine	aza**THIO**prine

Drug Name	Confused Drug Name
aza**THIO**prine	aza**CITID**ine
Azilect	Aricept
B & O (belladonna and opium)	Beano
BabyBIG	HBIG (hepatitis B immune globulin)
Beano	B & O (belladonna and opium)
Benadryl	benazepril
benazepril	Benadryl
Betadine (with povidone-iodine)	Betadine (without povidone-iodine)
Betadine (without povidone-iodine)	Betadine (with povidone-iodine)
betaine (anhydrous form)	betaine HCl
betaine HCl	betaine (anhydrous form)
Bicillin C-R	Bicillin L-A
Bicillin L-A	Bicillin C-R
Bidex	Videx
Brevibloc	Brevital
Brevital	Brevibloc
buprenorphine	**HYDRO**morphone
bu**PROP**ion	bus**PIR**one
bus**PIR**one	bu**PROP**ion
captopril	carvedilol
car**BAM**azepine	**OX**carbazepine
CARBOplatin	**CIS**platin
Cardene	Cardizem
Cardizem	Cardene
Cardura	Coumadin
carvedilol	captopril
Cathflo Activase	Activase
ce**FAZ**olin	cef**TRIAX**one
cef**TRIAX**one	ce**FAZ**olin
cefuroxime	sulfa**SALA**zine
Cele**BREX**	Cele**XA**
Cele**BREX**	Cerebyx
Cele**XA**	Cele**BREX**
Cele**XA**	Cerebyx
Cele**XA**	Zy**PREXA**
Cerebyx	Cele**BREX**
Cerebyx	Cele**XA**
cetirizine	sertraline
cetirizine	stavudine
chlordiaze**POXIDE**	chlorpro**MAZINE**
chlorpro**MAZINE**	chlordiaze**POXIDE**
CISplatin	**CARBO**platin
Claritin (loratadine)	Claritin Eye (ketotifen fumarate)
Claritin-D	Claritin-D 24
Claritin-D 24	Claritin-D
Claritin Eye (ketotifen fumarate)	Claritin (loratadine)
Clindesse	Clindets
Clindets	Clindesse
clo**BAZ**am	clonaze**PAM**
clomi**PHENE**	clomi**PRAMINE**
clomi**PRAMINE**	clomi**PHENE**

Brand names always start with an upper case letter. Some brand names incorporate tall man letters in initial characters and may not be readily recognized as brand names. Brand name products appear in black; generic/other products appear in red.

LIST OF CONFUSED DRUG NAMES continued

Drug Name	Confused Drug Name
clonazePAM	ALPRAZolam
clonazePAM	cloBAZam
clonazePAM	cloNIDine
clonazePAM	cloZAPine
clonazePAM	LORazepam
cloNIDine	clonazePAM
cloNIDine	cloZAPine
cloNIDine	KlonoPIN
cloZAPine	clonazePAM
cloZAPine	cloNIDine
Clozaril	Colazal
coagulation factor IX (recombinant)	factor IX complex, vapor heated
Colace	Cozaar
Colazal	Clozaril
colchicine	Cortrosyn
Cortrosyn	colchicine
Coumadin	Avandia
Coumadin	Cardura
Cozaar	Colace
Cozaar	Zocor
Cubicin	Cubicin RF
Cubicin RF	Cubicin
cyclophosphamide	cycloSPORINE
cycloSERINE	cycloSPORINE
cycloSPORINE	cyclophosphamide
cycloSPORINE	cycloSERINE
Cymbalta	Symbyax
dabigatran	vigabatrin
DACTINomycin	DAPTOmycin
Daptacel (DTaP)	Adacel (Tdap)
DAPTOmycin	DACTINomycin
DAUNOrubicin	DOXOrubicin
DAUNOrubicin	IDArubicin
Denavir	indinavir
Depakote	Depakote ER
Depakote ER	Depakote
DEPO-Medrol	SOLU—Medrol
Depo-Provera	Depo-subQ provera 104
Depo-subQ provera 104	Depo-Provera
desipramine	disopyramide
desmopressin	vasopressin
dexamethasone	dexmedetomidine
Dexilant	DULoxetine
dexmedetomidine	dexamethasone
dexmethylphenidate	methadone
diazePAM	dilTIAZem
Diflucan	Diprivan
dilTIAZem	diazePAM
dimenhyDRINATE	diphenhydrAMINE
diphenhydrAMINE	dimenhyDRINATE
Diprivan	Diflucan
Diprivan	Ditropan
disopyramide	desipramine
Ditropan	Diprivan
DOBUTamine	DOPamine
DOCEtaxel	PACLitaxel

Drug Name	Confused Drug Name
DOPamine	DOBUTamine
Doxil	Paxil
DOXOrubicin	DAUNOrubicin
DOXOrubicin	DOXOrubicin liposomal
DOXOrubicin	IDArubicin
DOXOrubicin liposomal	DOXOrubicin
Dramamine (dimenhyDRINATE)	Dramamine (ginger root)
Dramamine (dimenhyDRINATE)	Dramamine (meclizine)
Dramamine (ginger root)	Dramamine (dimenhyDRINATE)
Dramamine (ginger root)	Dramamine (meclizine)
Dramamine (meclizine)	Dramamine (dimenhyDRINATE)
Dramamine (meclizine)	Dramamine (ginger root)
Dulcolax (bisacodyl)	Dulcolax (docusate sodium)
Dulcolax (docusate sodium)	Dulcolax (bisacodyl)
DULoxetine	Dexilant
DULoxetine	FLUoxetine
DULoxetine	PARoxetine
Effexor XR	Enablex
elvitegravir, cobicistat, emtricitabine, and tenofovir alafenamide	elvitegravir, cobicistat, emtricitabine, and tenofovir disoproxil fumarate
elvitegravir, cobicistat, emtricitabine, and tenofovir disoproxil fumarate	elvitegravir, cobicistat, emtricitabine, and tenofovir alafenamide
Enablex	Effexor XR
Enbrel	Levbid
Engerix-B adult	Engerix-B pediatric/adolescent
Engerix-B pediatric/adolescent	Engerix-B adult
ePHEDrine	EPINEPHrine
EPINEPHrine	ePHEDrine
epiRUBicin	eriBULin
eriBULin	epiRUBicin
factor IX complex, vapor heated	coagulation factor IX (recombinant)
Fanapt	Xanax
Farxiga	Fetzima
Femara	Femhrt
Femhrt	Femara
fentaNYL	SUFentanil
Fetzima	Farxiga
Fioricet	Fiorinal
Fiorinal	Fioricet
flavoxATE	fluvoxaMINE
Flonase	Flovent
Floranex	Florinef
Florastor	Florinef
Florinef	Floranex
Florinef	Florastor
Flovent	Flonase

Brand names always start with an upper case letter. Some brand names incorporate tall man letters in initial characters and may not be readily recognized as brand names. Brand name products appear in black; generic/other products appear in red.

LIST OF CONFUSED DRUG NAMES continued

Drug Name	Confused Drug Name
flumazenil	influenza virus vaccine
FLUoxetine	DULoxetine
FLUoxetine	PARoxetine
fluPHENAZine	fluvoxaMINE
fluvoxaMINE	flavoxATE
fluvoxaMINE	fluPHENAZine
fomepizole	omeprazole
gabapentin	gemfibrozil
gemfibrozil	gabapentin
gentamicin	gentian violet
gentian violet	gentamicin
glacial acetic acid	acetic acid for irrigation
glipiZIDE	glyBURIDE
glyBURIDE	glipiZIDE
guaiFENesin	guanFACINE
guanFACINE	guaiFENesin
HBIG (hepatitis B immune globulin)	BabyBIG
Healon	Hyalgan
heparin	Hespan
Hespan	heparin
HMG-CoA reductase inhibitors ("statins")	nystatin
HumaLOG	HumuLIN
HumaLOG	NovoLOG
HumaLOG Mix 75/25	HumuLIN 70/30
HumuLIN	HumaLOG
HumuLIN	NovoLIN
HumuLIN 70/30	HumaLOG Mix 75/25
HumuLIN R U-100	HumuLIN R U-500
HumuLIN R U-500	HumuLIN R U-100
Hyalgan	Healon
hydrALAZINE	hydroCHLOROthiazide
hydrALAZINE	hydrOXYzine
Hydrea	Lyrica
hydroCHLOROthiazide	hydrALAZINE
hydroCHLOROthiazide	hydrOXYzine
HYDROcodone	oxyCODONE
HYDROmorphone	buprenorphine
HYDROmorphone	morphine
HYDROmorphone	oxyMORphone
hydroxychloroquine	hydroxyurea
HYDROXYprogesterone	medroxyPROGESTERone
hydroxyurea	hydroxychloroquine
hydroxyurea	hydrOXYzine
hydrOXYzine	hydrALAZINE
hydrOXYzine	hydroCHLOROthiazide
hydrOXYzine	hydroxyurea
IDArubicin	DAUNOrubicin
IDArubicin	DOXOrubicin
IDArubicin	idaruCIZUmab
idaruCIZUmab	IDArubicin
indinavir	Denavir
inFLIXimab	riTUXimab
influenza virus vaccine	flumazenil
influenza virus vaccine	perflutren lipid microspheres

Drug Name	Confused Drug Name
influenza virus vaccine	tuberculin purified protein derivative (PPD)
Inspra	Spiriva
Intuniv	Invega
Invega	Intuniv
ISOtretinoin	tretinoin
Jantoven	Janumet
Jantoven	Januvia
Janumet	Jantoven
Janumet	Januvia
Janumet	Sinemet
Januvia	Jantoven
Januvia	Janumet
K-Phos Neutral	Neutra-Phos-K
Kaletra	Keppra
Keflex	Keppra
Keppra	Kaletra
Keppra	Keflex
Ketalar	ketorolac
ketorolac	Ketalar
ketorolac	methadone
KlonoPIN	cloNIDine
labetalol	LaMICtal
labetalol	lamoTRIgine
LaMICtal	labetalol
LaMICtal	LamISIL
LamISIL	LaMICtal
lamiVUDine	lamoTRIgine
lamoTRIgine	labetalol
lamoTRIgine	lamiVUDine
lamoTRIgine	levETIRAcetam
lamoTRIgine	levothyroxine
Lanoxin	levothyroxine
Lanoxin	naloxone
lanthanum carbonate	lithium carbonate
Lantus	Latuda
Lantus	Lente
Lasix	Luvox
Latuda	Lantus
leucovorin calcium	Leukeran
leucovorin calcium	LEVOleucovorin
Leukeran	Alkeran
Leukeran	leucovorin calcium
Leukeran	Myleran
Levbid	Enbrel
Levemir	Lovenox
levETIRAcetam	lamoTRIgine
levETIRAcetam	levOCARNitine
levETIRAcetam	levoFLOXacin
levOCARNitine	levETIRAcetam
levoFLOXacin	levETIRAcetam
LEVOleucovorin	leucovorin calcium
levothyroxine	lamoTRIgine
levothyroxine	Lanoxin
levothyroxine	liothyronine
Lexiva	Pexeva

Brand names always start with an upper case letter. Some brand names incorporate tall man letters in initial characters and may not be readily recognized as brand names. Brand name products appear in black; generic/other products appear in red.

LIST OF CONFUSED DRUG NAMES continued

Drug Name	Confused Drug Name
linaCLOtide	linaGLIPtin
linaGLIPtin	linaCLOtide
liothyronine	levothyroxine
Lipitor	ZyrTEC
lithium	Ultram
lithium carbonate	lanthanum carbonate
Lopressor	Lyrica
LORazepam	ALPRAZolam
LORazepam	clonazePAM
LORazepam	Lovaza
Lotronex	Protonix
Lovaza	LORazepam
Lovenox	Levemir
Lunesta	Neulasta
Lupron Depot-3 Month	Lupron Depot-Ped
Lupron Depot-Ped	Lupron Depot-3 Month
Luvox	Lasix
Lyrica	Hydrea
Lyrica	Lopressor
Malarone	mefloquine
Maxzide	Microzide
medroxyPROGESTERone	HYDROXYprogesterone
medroxyPROGESTERone	methylPREDNISolone
medroxyPROGESTERone	methylTESTOSTERone
mefloquine	Malarone
memantine	methadone
Mephyton	methadone
Metadate	methadone
metFORMIN	metroNIDAZOLE
methadone	dexmethylphenidate
methadone	ketorolac
methadone	memantine
methadone	Mephyton
methadone	Metadate
methadone	methylphenidate
methadone	metOLazone
methazolAMIDE	methIMAzole
methazolAMIDE	metOLazone
methIMAzole	methazolAMIDE
methIMAzole	metOLazone
methotrexate	metOLazone
methylene blue	VisionBlue
methylphenidate	methadone
methylPREDNISolone	medroxyPROGESTERone
methylPREDNISolone	methylTESTOSTERone
methylTESTOSTERone	medroxyPROGESTERone
methylTESTOSTERone	methylPREDNISolone
metOLazone	methadone
metOLazone	methazolAMIDE
metOLazone	methIMAzole
metoprolol succinate	metoprolol tartrate
metoprolol tartrate	metoprolol succinate
metroNIDAZOLE	metFORMIN
metyraPONE	metyroSINE
metyroSINE	metyraPONE
Microzide	Maxzide

Drug Name	Confused Drug Name
miFEPRIStone	miSOPROStol
Miralax	Mirapex
Mirapex	Miralax
miSOPROStol	miFEPRIStone
mitoMYcin	mitoXANTRONE
mitoXANTRONE	mitoMYcin
morphine	HYDROmorphone
morphine - non-concentrated oral liquid	morphine - oral liquid concentrate
morphine - oral liquid concentrate	morphine - non-concentrated oral liquid
Motrin	Neurontin
MS Contin	OxyCONTIN
Mucinex D	Mucinex DM
Mucinex DM	Mucinex D
Myleran	Alkeran
Myleran	Leukeran
nalbuphine	naloxone
naloxone	Lanoxin
naloxone	nalbuphine
Neo-Synephrine (oxymetazoline)	Neo-Synephrine (phenylephrine)
Neo-Synephrine (phenylephrine)	Neo-Synephrine (oxymetazoline)
neratinib	nilotinib
neratinib	niraparib
Neulasta	Lunesta
Neulasta	Nuedexta
Neurontin	Motrin
Neutra-Phos-K	K-Phos Neutral
NexAVAR	NexIUM
NexIUM	NexAVAR
niCARdipine	NIFEdipine
niCARdipine+	niMODipine
NIFEdipine	niCARdipine
NIFEdipine	niMODipine
nilotinib	neratinib
nilotinib	niraparib
niMODipine	niCARdipine
niMODipine	NIFEdipine
niraparib	neratinib
niraparib	nilotinib
NovoLIN	HumuLIN
NovoLIN	NovoLOG
NovoLIN 70/30	NovoLOG Mix 70/30
NovoLOG	HumaLOG
NovoLOG	NovoLIN
NovoLOG FLEXPEN	NovoLOG Mix 70/30 FLEXPEN
NovoLOG Mix 70/30	NovoLIN 70/30
NovoLOG Mix 70/30 FLEXPEN	NovoLOG FLEXPEN
Nuedexta	Neulasta
nystatin	HMG-CoA reductase inhibitors ("statins")
OLANZapine	QUEtiapine
omeprazole	fomepizole

Brand names always start with an upper case letter. Some brand names incorporate tall man letters in initial characters and may not be readily recognized as brand names. Brand name products appear in black; generic/other products appear in red.

LIST OF CONFUSED DRUG NAMES continued

Drug Name	Confused Drug Name
Oracea	Orencia
Orencia	Oracea
OrthoTri-Cyclen	Ortho Tri-Cyclen LO
Ortho Tri-Cyclen LO	OrthoTri-Cyclen
Os-Cal	Asacol
oxaprozin	OXcarbazepine
OXcarbazepine	carBAMazepine
OXcarebazepine	oxaprozin
oxybutynin	oxyCODONE
oxyCODONE	HYDROcodone
oxyCODONE	oxybutynin
oxyCODONE	OxyCONTIN
oxyCODONE	oxyMORphone
OxyCONTIN	MS Contin
OxyCONTIN	oxyCODONE
OxyCONTIN	oxyMORphone
oxyMORphone	HYDROmorphone
oxyMORphone	oxyCODONE
oxyMORphone	OxyCONTIN
PACLitaxel	DOCEtaxel
PACLitaxel	PACLitaxel protein-bound particles
PACLitaxel protein-bound particles	PACLitaxel
Pamelor	Tambocor
PARoxetine	DULoxetine
PARoxetine	FLUoxetine
PARoxetine	piroxicam
Paxil	Doxil
Paxil	Plavix
PAZOPanib	PONATinib
PEMEtrexed	PRALAtrexate
penicillAMINE	penicillin
penicillin	penicillAMINE
perflutren lipid microspheres	influenza virus vaccine
PENTobarbital	PHENobarbital
Pexeva	Lexiva
PHENobarbital	PENTobarbital
piroxicam	PARoxetine
Plavix	Paxil
Plavix	Pradaxa
polyethylene glycol	propylene glycol
PONATinib	PAZOPanib
potassium acetate	sodium acetate
Pradaxa	Plavix
PRALAtrexate	PEMEtrexed
prednisoLONE	predniSONE
predniSONE	prednisoLONE
Prenexa	Ranexa
PriLOSEC	Pristiq
PriLOSEC	PROzac
Pristiq	PriLOSEC
Prograf	Proscar
Prograf	PROzac
propylene glycol	polyethylene glycol
propylthiouracil	Purinethol

Drug Name	Confused Drug Name
Proscar	Prograf
Proscar	Provera
protamine	Protonix
proton pump inhibitors	ARIPiprazole
Protonix	Lotronex
Protonix	protamine
Provera	Proscar
Provera	PROzac
PROzac	PriLOSEC
PROzac	Prograf
PROzac	Provera
Purinethol	propylthiouracil
Pyridium	pyridoxine
pyridoxine	Pyridium
QUEtiapine	OLANZapine
quiNIDine	quiNINE
quiNINE	quiNIDine
RABEprazole	ARIPiprazole
Ranexa	Prenexa
raNITIdine	riMANTAdine
Rapaflo	Rapamune
Rapamune	Rapaflo
Razadyne	Rozerem
Renagel	Renvela
Renvela	Renagel
repaglinide	rasagiline
Restoril	RisperDAL
Retrovir	ritonavir
ribavirin	riboflavin
riboflavin	ribavirin
rifabutin	rifapentine
Rifadin	Rifater
Rifamate	rifampin
rifAMPin	Rifamate
rifAMPin	rifAXIMin
rifapentine	rifabutin
Rifater	Rifadin
rifAXIMin	rifAMPin
riMANTAdine	raNITIdine
RisperDAL	Restoril
RisperDAL	rOPINIRole
risperiDONE	rOPINIRole
ritonavir	Retrovir
Rituxan	Rituxan Hycela
Rituxan Hycela	Rituxan
riTUXimab	inFLIXimab
romiDEPsin	romiPLOStim
romiPLOStim	romiDEPsin
rOPINIRole	RisperDAL
rOPINIRole	risperiDONE
Rozerem	Razadyne
Salagen	selegiline
SandIMMUNE	SandoSTATIN
SandoSTATIN	SandIMMUNE
sAXagliptin	SITagliptin
selegiline	Salagen

Brand names always start with an upper case letter. Some brand names incorporate tall man letters in initial characters and may not be readily recognized as brand names. Brand name products appear in black; generic/other products appear in red.

LIST OF CONFUSED DRUG NAMES continued

Drug Name	Confused Drug Name
SEROquel	SEROquel XR
SEROquel XR	SEROquel
sertraline	cetirizine
sertraline	Soriatane
silodosin	sirolimus
Sinemet	Janumet
sirolimus	silodosin
SITagliptin	sAXagliptin
SITagliptin	SUMAtriptan
sodium acetate	potassium acetate
Solu-CORTEF	SOLU-Medrol
SOLU-Medrol	DEPO-Medrol
SOLU-Medrol	Solu-CORTEF
Sonata	Soriatane
SORAfenib	SUNItinib
Soriatane	sertraline
Soriatane	Sonata
sotalol	Sudafed
Spiriva	Apidra
Spiriva	Inspra
stavudine	cetirizine
Sudafed	sotalol
Sudafed	Sudafed PE
Sudafed 12 Hour	Sudafed 12 Hour Pressure + Pain
Sudafed 12 Hour Pressure + Pain	Sudafed 12 Hour
Sudafed PE	Sudafed
SUFentanil	fentaNYL
sulfADIAZINE	sulfaSALAzine
sulfaSALAzine	cefuroxime
sulfaSALAzine	sulfADIAZINE
SUMAtriptan	SITagliptin
SUMAtriptan	ZOLMitriptan
SUNItinib	SORAfenib
Symbyax	Cymbalta
tacrolimus	tamsulosin
Tambocor	Pamelor
Tarceva	Tresiba
Taxol	Paxil
Taxol	Taxotere
Taxotere	Taxol
TEGretol	TEGretol XR
TEGretol XR	TEGretol
tetanus diphtheria toxoid (Td)	tuberculin purified protein derivative (PPD)
Thalomid	thiamine
thiamine	Thalomid
tiaGABine	tiZANidine
Tiazac	Ziac
tiZANidine	tiaGABine
TNKase	Activase
TNKase	t-PA
Tobradex	Tobrex
Tobrex	Tobradex
Topamax	Toprol-XL
Toprol-XL	Topamax

Drug Name	Confused Drug Name
Toujeo	Tradjenta
Toujeo	Tresiba
Toujeo	Trulicity
t-PA	TNKase
Tracleer	Tricor
Tradjenta	Toujeo
Tradjenta	Tresiba
Tradjenta	Trulicity
traMADol	traZODone
trastuzumab	ado-trastuzumab emtansine
traZODone	traMADol
Tresiba	Tarceva
Tresiba	Toujeo
Tresiba	Tradjenta
Tresiba	Trulicity
tretinoin	ISOtretinoin
Tricor	Tracleer
Trulicity	Toujeo
Trulicity	Tradjenta
Trulicity	Tresiba
tuberculin purified protein derivative (PPD)	influenza virus vaccine
tuberculin purified protein derivative (PPD)	tetanus diphtheria toxoid (Td)
Tylenol	Tylenol PM
Tylenol PM	Tylenol
Ultram	lithium
valACYclovir	valGANciclovir
Valcyte	Valtrex
valGANciclovir	valACYclovir
Valtrex	Valcyte
Varivax	VZIG (varicella-zoster immune globulin)
vasopressin	desmopressin
Venofer	Vfend
Venofer	Vimpat
Vfend	Venofer
Vfend	Vimpat
Viagra	Allegra
Videx	Bidex
vigabatrin	dabigatran
Vimpat	Venofer
Vimpat	Vfend
vinBLAStine	vinCRIStine
vinCRIStine	vinBLAStine
Viracept	Viramune
Viramune	Viracept
VisionBlue	methylene blue
VZIG (varicella-zoster immune globulin)	Varivax
Wellbutrin SR	Wellbutrin XL
Wellbutrin XL	Wellbutrin SR
Xanax	Fanapt
Xanax	Tenex
Xanax	Zantac
Xeloda	Xenical

Brand names always start with an upper case letter. Some brand names incorporate tall man letters in initial characters and may not be readily recognized as brand names. Brand name products appear in black; generic/other products appear in red.

LIST OF CONFUSED DRUG NAMES continued

Drug Name	Confused Drug Name
Xenical	Xeloda
Yasmin	Yaz
Yaz	Yasmin
Zantac	Xanax
Zantac	ZyrTEC
Zegerid	Zestril
Zelapar	ZyPREXAZydis
Zerit	ZyrTEC
Zestril	Zegerid
Zestril	Zetia
Zestril	ZyPREXA
Zetia	Zestril
Ziac	Tiazac
Zocor	Cozaar
Zocor	ZyrTEC
ZOLMitriptan	SUMAtriptan
zolpidem	Zyloprim
Zostrix	Zovirax
Zovirax	Zostrix

Drug Name	Confused Drug Name
Zovirax	Zyvox
Zyloprim	zolpidem
ZyPREXA	CeleXA
ZyPREXA	Zestril
ZyPREXA	ZyrTEC
ZyPREXA Zydis	Zelapar
ZyrTEC	Lipitor
ZyrTEC	Zantac
ZyrTEC	Zerit
ZyrTEC	Zocor
ZyrTEC	ZyPREXA
ZyrTEC	ZyrTEC-D
ZyrTEC (cetirizine)	ZyrTEC Itchy Eye Drops (ketotifen fumarate)
ZyrTEC-D	ZyrTEC
ZyrTEC Itchy Eye Drops (ketotifen fumarate)	ZyrTEC (cetirizine)
Zyvox	Zovirax

Brand names always start with an upper case letter. Some brand names incorporate tall man letters in initial characters and may not be readily recognized as brand names. Brand name products appear in black; generic/other products appear in red.

DO NOT CRUSH!

Do not crush any oral medication that is labeled as:

Antineoplastic **(AN)**
Buccal **(BU)**
Delayed Release **(DR)**
Enteric-Coated **(EC)**
Extended Release **(ER)**
Effervescent Tablet **(EVT)**
Mucous Membrane Irritant **(MMI)**
Orally Disintegrating Tablets **(ODT)**
Sustained-Release **(SR)**
Sublingual **(SL)**

Do not crush any oral medication that ends in the following letters:

CD CR ER LA SR XL XR XT

MEDICATIONS THAT SHOULD NOT BE CRUSHED:

Absorica Capsule **(MMI)**
Aciphex Tablet **(SR)**
Aciphex Sprinkle **(SR)**—see code "C"
Acticlate Tablet **(film-coated)**—see code "B"
Actiq Lozenge **(SR) (chewing or swallowing may ↓ bioavailability)**
Actonel Tablet **(MMI)**
Adalat CC Tablet **(SR)**
Adderall XR Capsule **(SR)**—see code "C"
Adzenys XR-ODT Tablet **(ODT, SR)**—see code "E"
Afeditab CR Tablet **(SR)**
Afinitor Tablet **(MMI)**
Aggrenox Capsule **(SR)**
Alecensa Capsule **(AN)**
Altoprev Tablet **(SR)**
Alunbrig Tablet **(AN)**
Ambien CR Tablet **(SR)**
Amitiza Capsule **(SR)**
Amnesteem Capsule **(MMI)**
Ampyra Tablet **(SR)**
Amrix Capsule **(SR)**—see code "C"
Aplenzin Tablet **(SR)**
Apriso Capsule **(SR)**—see code "C"
Aptensio XR Capsule **(SR)**—see code "C"
Aptivus Capsule **(oil emulsion within spheres)**—taste issue—see code "A"
Aricept 23-mg Tablet **(crushing may ↑ rate of absorption)**
Arthrotec Tablet **(EC)**
Asacol HD Tablet **(SR)**
Aspirin Caplet or Tablet **(EC, SR)**
Astagraf XL Capsule **(SR)**
Atelvia Tablet **(SR, MMI)**
Augmentin XR Tablet **(SR)**—see codes "A," "B"
Austedo Tablet
Avodart Capsule **(MMI)**—see code "F"
Azulfidine EN-Tablet **(SR)**
Bayer Low-Dose Aspirin Tablet **(EC)**
Belbuca Buccal Film **(BU, film-coated) (chewing or swallowing may ↓ bioavailability)**—see code "E"
Biaxin-XL Tablet **(SR)**
Biltricide Tablet **(crushing, breaking or chewing can leave bitter taste)**—see code "B"
Binosto Tablet **(EVT)**—see code "G"
Bisac-Evac Tablet **(EC)**—see code "D"
Bisacodyl Tablet **(EC)**—see code "D"
Boniva Tablet **(MMI)**
Bonjesta Tablet **(SR)**
Bosulif Tablet **(AN)**
Briviact Tablet **(film-coated)**—see code "A"
Bunavail Buccal Film **(BU, EC) (chewing or swallowing may ↓ bioavailability)**
Bupropion ER Tablet **(SR)**
Cabometyx Tablet **(film-coated)**
Caprelsa Tablet **(MMI)**
Carbaglu Tablet **(tablets should be completely dispersed in water)**
Carbatrol Capsule **(SR)**—see code "C"
Cardizem Tablet
Cardizem CD Capsule **(SR)**
Cardizem LA Tablet **(SR)**
Cardura XL Tablet **(SR)**
Cartia XT Capsule **(SR)**
Cefaclor ER Tablet **(SR)**—see code "A"
Cefuroxime Tablet **(may cause unpleasant taste)**—see code "A"
CellCept Capsule, Tablet—see codes "A," "H"
Cerdelga Capsule **(preferably taken with water)**
Cholbam Capsule —see code "C"
Cipro XR Tablet **(SR)**—see code "A"
Claravis Capsule **(MMI)**
Colace Capsule **(crushing, breaking, or chewing can leave bitter taste)**
Colestid Tablet **(SR)**
Cometriq Capsule **(AN)**
Concerta Tablet **(SR)**
Contrave Tablet **(SR)**
Conzip Capsule **(SR) (crushing, chewing or dissolving may ↑ risk of fatal overdose)**
Coreg CR Capsule **(SR)**—see code "C"
Cotempla XR-ODT Tablet **(ODT, SR)**—see code "E"
Creon Capsule **(SR)**—see code "C"
Cresemba Capsule
Crixivan Capsule **(crushing, breaking, or chewing can leave bitter taste)**—see code "C"
Cyclophosphamide Tablet **(may be crushed; however, injection preferred)**
Cymbalta Capsule **(SR)**
Delzicol Capsule **(SR)**—see code "C"
Depakote Tablet **(SR)**
Depakote ER Tablet **(SR)**
Detrol LA Capsule **(SR)**
Dexilant Capsule **(SR)**—see code "C"
Diclegis Tablet **(SR)**
Dilatrate-SR Capsule **(SR)**
Ditropan XL Tablet **(SR)**
Doryx Tablet **(SR)**
Doryx MPC Tablet **(SR)**
Drisdol Capsule **(filled with liquid)**
Droxia Capsule **(wear gloves to administer)**
Duavee Tablet
Duexis Tablet
Dulcolax Tablet, Capsule **(EC)**—see code "D"
EC-Naprosyn Tablet **(SR, EC)**—see code "A"
Ecotrin Tablet **(EC)**
Edluar Sublingual Tablet **(SL)**—see code "E"
Effer-K Tablet **(EVT)**—see code "G"
Effexor XR Capsule **(SR)**—see code "C"
Enablex Tablet **(SR)**
Entocort EC Capsule **(EC)**—see code "C"
Envarsus XR Tablet **(SR)**
Equetro Capsule **(SR)**—see code "C"
Ergomar Sublingual Tablet **(SL)**—see code "E"
Erivedge Capsule—see code "F"
Ery-Tab Tablet **(SR, EC)**
Erythromycin Base Tablet **(EC)**
Erythromycin Delayed-Release Capsule **(SR) (contains pellets)**—see code "C"
Evista Tablet—see code "F"
Exjade Tablet **(tablets must be dispersed in liquid)**
Farydak Capsule **(MMI)**
Feldene Capsule **(MMI)**
Felodipine Tablet **(SR)**
Fentanyl Lozenge **(SR)**
Fentora Buccal Tablet **(BU) (crushing could ↓ effectiveness)**
Fetzima Capsule **(SR)**
Fibricor Tablet
Fleet Laxative Tablet **(EC)**—see code "D"
Flomax Capsule **(SR)**
Fluvoxamine ER Capsule **(SR)**
Focalin XR Capsule **(SR)**—see code "C"
Forfivo XL Tablet **(SR)**
Fortamet Tablet **(SR)**
Fosamax Tablet **(MMI)**
Fosamax Plus D Tablet **(MMI)**
Gleevec Tablet **(MMI) (may be dissolved in water or apple juice)**
Glucophage XR Tablet **(SR)**
Glucotrol XL Tablet **(SR)**
Glumetza Tablet **(SR)**
Gralise Tablet **(SR)**—see code "A"
Halfprin Tablet **(EC)**
Hetlioz Capsule
Horizant Tablet **(SR)**—see code "A"
Hydrea Capsule **(wear gloves to administer)**
Hydromorphone ER Tablet **(SR) (crushing, chewing or dissolving may ↑ risk of fatal overdose)**
Hysingla ER Tablet **(SR) (crushing, chewing or dissolving may ↑ risk of fatal overdose)**
Ibrance Capsule **(AN)**
Iclusig Tablet **(AN)**
Idhifa Tablet **(AN)**
Imbruvica Capsule **(AN)**
Impavido Capsule
Inderal LA Capsule **(SR)**
Inlyta **(AN)**
Indomethacin SR Capsule **(SR)**—see codes "A," "C"
InnoPran XL Capsule **(SR)**
Intelence Tablet **(may disperse in water)**
Intermezzo Sublingual Tablet **(SL)**—see code "E"
Intuniv Tablet **(SR)**
Invega Tablet **(SR)**
Invokamet XR Tablet **(SR)**
Iressa Tablet **(may dissolve in water)**
Isosorbide Dinitrate ER Capsule, Tablet **(SR)**
Isosorbide Mononitrate ER Tablet **(SR)**—see code "B"
Jakafi Tablet **(may disperse in water)**
Jalyn Capsule **(MMI)**—see codes "F," "H"

DO NOT CRUSH!

MEDICATIONS THAT SHOULD NOT BE CRUSHED:

Janumet XR Tablet **(SR)**
Jentadueto XR Tablet **(SR)**
Juxtapid Capsule
Kadian Capsule **(SR) (do not give via NG tube; crushing, chewing or dissolving may ↑ risk of fatal overdose)**—see code "C"
Kaletra Tablet **(film-coated)**—see code "A"
Kapvay Tablet **(SR)**
Kazano Tablet
Keppra Tablet **(crushing, breaking or chewing can leave bitter taste)**—see code "A"
Keppra XR Tablet **(SR)**—see code "A"
Kisqali Tablet **(AN)**
Klor-Con Tablet **(SR)**—see code "A"
Klor-Con M Tablet **(SR)**—see codes "A," "B"
Kombiglyze XR Tablet **(SR)**
Korlym Tablet
K-Tab Tablet **(SR)**—see code "A"
Lamictal XR Tablet **(SR)**
Lenvima Capsule **(may dissolve in water or apple juice)**
Lescol XL Tablet **(SR)**
Letairis Tablet
Levbid Tablet **(SR)**—see code "B"
Lialda Tablet **(SR)**
Linzess Capsule—see code "C"
Lithobid Tablet **(SR)**
Lovaza Capsule **(do not put contents in styrofoam or plastic container)**
Lynparza Capsule **(AN)**
Mestinon ER Tablet **(SR)**—see code "A"
Metadate CD Capsule **(SR)**—see code "C"
Metadate ER Tablet **(SR)**
Methylin ER Tablet **(SR)**
Metoprolol Succinate Tablet **(SR)**
Micro-K Capsule **(SR)** see codes "A," "C"
Minocin Capsule **(MMI)**
Minolira Tablet **(SR)**—see code "B"
Mirapex ER Tablet **(SR)**
Morphabond ER Tablet **(SR) (crushing, chewing or dissolving may ↑ risk of fatal overdose)**—see code "A"
Motrin Tablet **(crushing, breaking or chewing can leave bitter taste)**—see code "A"
MS Contin Tablet **(SR) (crushing, chewing or dissolving may ↑ risk of fatal overdose)**—see code "A"
Mucinex Tablet **(SR)**
Mucinex DM Tablet **(SR)**
Mydayis Capsule **(SR)**—see code "C"
Myfortic Tablet **(SR)**
Myorisan Capsule **(MMI)**
Myrbetriq Tablet **(SR)**
Mytesi Tablet **(SR)**
Namenda XR Capsule **(SR)**—see codes "A," "C"
Namzaric Capsule **(SR)**—see code "C"
Naprelan Tablet **(SR)**
Nerlynx Tablet **(AN)**
Neurontin Capsule, Tablet—see codes "A," "B"
Nexium Capsule **(SR)**—see code "C"
Nexium 24HR Capsule, Tablet **(SR)**
Niaspan Tablet **(SR)**
Ninlaro Capsule **(AN)**
Nitrostat Sublingual Tablet **(SL)**—see code "E"
Norpace CR Capsule **(SR)**
Northera Capsule
Norvir Tablet **(crushing may ↓ bioavailability)**—see code "A"
Noxafil Tablet **(SR)**—see code "A"
Nucynta ER Tablet **(SR) (crushing, chewing or dissolving may ↑ risk of fatal overdose)**
Ofev Capsule **(crushing or chewing can leave bitter taste)**
Omeprazole Capsule **(SR)**—see codes "A," "C"
Opsumit Tablet
Oravig Buccal Tablet **(BU)**
Orenitram Tablet **(SR)**
Orphenadrine Citrate ER Tablet **(SR)**
Oseni Tablet
Otezla Tablet **(film-coated)**
Oxaydo Tablet **(may obstruct feeding tubes if crushed)**—see code "A"
Oxtellar XR Tablet **(SR)**
OxyContin Tablet **(SR) (crushing, chewing or dissolving may ↑ risk of fatal overdose)**
Pancreaze Capsule **(EC, SR)**—see code "C"
Paxil Tablet **(film-coated)**—see code "A"
Paxil CR Tablet **(SR)**
Pentasa Capsule **(SR)**—see code "C"
Pentoxifylline ER Tablet **(SR)**
Pertyze Capsule **(SR)**—see code "C"
Pexeva Tablet **(film-coated)**—see code "A"
Pomalyst Capsule **(AN)**
Pradaxa Capsule **(breaking, chewing, or emptying may ↑ bioavailability)**
Prevacid 24HR Capsule **(SR)**
Prevacid Capsule **(SR)**—see code "C"
Prevacid SoluTab Tablet **(ODT) (may dissolve in water to administer via NG tube)**
Prilosec OTC Tablet **(SR)**
Pristiq Tablet **(SR)**
Procardia XL Tablet **(SR)**
Procysbi Capsule **(SR)**—see code "C"
Propecia Tablet—see code "F"
Proscar Tablet—see code "F"
Protonix Tablet **(SR)**—see code "A"
Prozac Weekly Capsule **(EC)**
Pylera Capsule **(MMI)**
Qtern Tablet
Qudexy XR Capsule **(SR)**—see code "C"
Ranexa Tablet **(SR)**
Rapamune Tablet—see code "A"
Rayaldee Capsule **(SR)**
Rayos Tablet **(SR)**—see code "A"
Razadyne ER Capsule **(SR)**
Renagel Tablet **(expands in liquid when crushed or broken)**—see code "A"
Renvela Tablet **(expands in liquid when crushed or broken)**—see code "A"
Requip XL Tablet **(SR)**
Revlimid Capsule—see code "F"
Reyataz Capsule **(oral powder available)**
Ritalin LA Capsule **(SR)**—see code "C"
Roweepra Tablet **(crushing or chewing can leave bitter taste)**—see code "A"
Roweepra ER Tablet **(SR)**—see code "A"
Rydapt Capsule **(AN)**
Rytary Capsule **(SR)**—see code "C"
Rythmol SR Capsule **(SR)**
Sensipar Tablet **(cutting tablets may cause variable dosing accuracy)**
Seroquel XR Tablet **(SR)**
Sinemet CR Tablet **(SR)**—see code "B"
Sirturo Tablet
Sitavig Buccal Tablet **(BU)**
Solodyn Tablet **(SR)**
Sprycel Tablet **(film-coated)**—see code "F"
Stalevo Tablet **(combining portions of tablets may lead to overdose of entacapone)**
Staxyn Sublingual Tablet **(SL)**—see code "E"
Stivarga Tablet **(SR)**
Straterra Capsule **(contents can cause ocular irritation)**
Suboxone Sublingual Film **(SL)**—see code "E"
Sular Tablet **(SR)**
Symax Duotab Tablet **(SR)**
Symax SR Tablet **(SR)**
Synjardy XR Tablet **(SR)**
Tafinlar Capsule **(AN)**
Tagrisso Tablet **(may be dissolved in water)**
Tasigna Capsule —see code "C"
Taztia XT Capsule **(SR)**—see code "C"
Tecfidera Capsule **(SR)**
Tegretol-XR Tablet **(SR)**
Temodar Capsule **(SR, MMI)**—see code "H"
Tessalon Perles Capsule **(chewing or crushing may cause local anesthesia of mucous membranes which could lead to choking)**
Theo-24 Capsule **(SR)**
Theochron Tablet **(SR)**
Tiazac Capsule **(SR)**—see code "C"
Topamax Tablet, Capsule **(crushing, breaking or chewing can leave bitter taste)**—see code "C"
Toprol XL Tablet **(SR)**—see code "B"
Toviaz Tablet **(SR)**
Traceleer Tablet—see code "F"
Treximet Tablet **(chewing, crushing, or breaking may cause rapid absorption)**
Trilipix Capsule **(SR)**
Trokendi XR Capsule **(SR)**
Uceris Tablet **(SR)**
Ultresa Capsule **(SR)**—see code "C"
Uptravi Tablet **(film-coated)**
Urocit-K Tablet **(SR)**
Uroxatral Tablet **(SR)**
Valcyte Tablet—see codes "A," "F"
Valproic Acid Capsule **(SR, MMI)**—see code "A"
Vascepa Capsule
Venclexta Tablet **(AN, film-coated)**
Verelan Capsule **(SR)**—see code "C"
Verelan PM Capsule **(SR)**—see code "C"
Vesicare Tablet **(crushing, breaking or chewing can leave bitter taste)**
Videx EC Capsule **(EC, SR)**

DO NOT CRUSH!

MEDICATIONS THAT SHOULD NOT BE CRUSHED:		
Viekira XR Tablet **(SR)** Vimovo Tablet **(SR)** Viokace Tablet **(MMI)** Viramune XR Tablet **(SR)**—see code **"A"** VoSpire ER Tablet **(SR)** Votrient Tablet **(crushing may ↑ bioavailability)** Wellbutrin SR, XL Tablet **(SR)** Xalkori Capsule **(AN)** Xanax XR Tablet **(SR)**	Xarelto Tablet **(crushed tablet must be given within 4 hr)** Xeljanz XR Tablet **(SR)** Xigduo XR Tablet **(SR)** Ximino Capsule **(SR)** Xtampza ER Tablet **(SR)**—see code **"A"** Xtandi Capsule **(AN)** Yosprala Tablet **(SR)** Zegerid OTC Capsule **(SR)**—see code **"A"** Zejula Capsule **(AN)** Zelboraf Tablet **(AN)** Zenatane Capsule **(MMI)**	Zenpep Capsule **(SR)**—see code **"C"** Zohydro ER Capsule **(SR) (crushing, chewing or dissolving may ↑ risk of fatal overdose)** Zolinza Capsule **(MMI)** Zortress Tablet **(MMI)** Zubsolv Sublingual Tablet **(SL)**—see code **"E"** Zuplenz Oral Film—see code **"E"** Zydelig Tablet **(AN, film-coated)** Zyflo CR Tablet **(SR)** Zytiga Tablet **(AN)**

CODES:		
A: Liquid forms are available **B:** Tablets that are scored may be broken in half **C:** Capsule can be opened—contents may be used/sprinkled on certain foods or liquids as recommended by the manufacturer	**D:** Do not take with antacids or milk products **E:** Disintegrates on or under the tongue—do not chew **F:** Women who are of childbearing age should not handle crushed or broken tablets or the contents of opened capsules	**G:** Effervescent tablets must be dissolved in the volume of diluent recommended by the manufacturer **H:** Avoid direct contact with skin as may enhance tumor development

FDA-APPROVED LIST OF GENERIC DRUG NAMES WITH TALL MAN LETTERS

Drug Name with Tall Man Letters	Confused with
buPROPion	busPIRone
busPIRone	buPROPion
clomiPHENE	clomiPRAMINE
clomiPRAMINE	clomiPHENE
cycloSERINE	cycloSPORINE
cycloSPORINE	cycloSERINE
DAUNOrubicin	DOXOrubicin
dimenhyDRINATE	diphenhydrAMINE
diphenhydrAMINE	dimenhyDRINATE
DOBUTamine	DOPamine
DOPamine	DOBUTamine
DOXOrubicin	DAUNOrubicin
glipiZIDE	glyBURIDE
glyBURIDE	glipiZIDE
hydrALAZINE	hydrOXYzine—HYDROmorphone
HYDROmorphone	hydrOXYzine—hydrALAZINE

Drug Name with Tall Man Letters	Confused with
hydrOXYzine	hydrALAZINE—HYDROmorphone
medroxyPROGESTERone	methylPREDNISolone—methylTESTOSTERone
methylPREDNISolone	medroxyPROGESTERone—methylTESTOSTERone
methylTESTOSTERone	medroxyPROGESTERone—methylPREDNISolone
mitoXANTRONE	Not specified
niCARdipine	NIFEdipine
NIFEdipine	niCARdipine
predniSOLONE	predniSONE
predniSONE	predniSOLONE
risperiDONE	rOPINIRole
rOPINIRole	risperiDONE
vinBLAStine	vinCRIStine
vinCRIStine	vinBLAStine

ISMP LIST OF ADDITIONAL DRUG NAMES WITH TALL MAN LETTERS

Drug Name with Tall Man Letters	Confused with
ALPRAZolam	LORazepam—clonazePAM
aMILoride	amLODIPine
amLODIPine	aMILoride
ARIPiprazole	RABEprazole
azaCITIDine	azaTHIOprine
azaTHIOprine	azaCITIDine
carBAMazepine	OXcarbazepine
CARBOplatin	CISplatin
ceFAZolin	cefoTEtan—cefOXitin—cefTAZidime—cefTRIAXone
cefoTEtan	ceFAZolin—cefOXitin—cefTAZidime—cefTRIAXone
cefOXitin	ceFAZolin—cefoTEtan—cefTAZidime—cefTRIAXone
cefTAZidime	ceFAZolin—cefoTEtan—cefOXitin—cefTRIAXone
cefTRIAXone	ceFAZolin—cefoTEtan—cefOXitin—cefTAZidime
CeleBREX*	CeleXA*
CeleXA*	CeleBREX*
chlordiazePOXIDE	chlorproMAZINE
chlorproMAZINE	chlordiazePOXIDE
CISplatin	CARBOplatin
cloBAZam	clonazePAM
clonazePAM	cloNIDine—cloZAPine—cloBAZam—LORazepam
cloNIDine	clonazePAM—cloZAPine—KlonoPIN*

Drug Name with Tall Man Letters	Confused with
cloZAPine	clonazePAM —cloNIDine
DACTINomycin	DAPTOmycin
DAPTOmycin	DACTINomycin
DEPO-Medrol*	SOLU-Medrol*
diazePAM	dilTIAZem
dilTIAZem	diazePAM
DOCEtaxel	PACLitaxel
DOXOrubicin	IDArubicin
DULoxetine	FLUoxetine—PARoxetine
ePHEDrine	EPINEPHrine
EPINEPHrine	ePHEDrine
epiRUBicin	eriBULin
eriBULin	epiRUBicin
fentaNYL	SUFentanil
flavoxATE	fluvoxaMINE
FLUoxetine	DULoxetine—PARoxetine
fluPHENAZine	fluvoxaMINE
fluvoxaMINE	fluPHENAZine—flavoxATE
guaiFENesin	guanFACINE
guanFACINE	guaiFENesin
HumaLOG*	HumuLIN*
HumuLIN*	HumaLOG*
hydrALAZINE	hydroCHLOROthiazide—hydrOXYzine
hydroCHLOROthiazide	hydrOXYzine—hydrALAZINE

*Brand names always start with an upper case letter. Some brand names incorporate tall man letters in initial characters and may not be readily recognized as brand names. An asterisk follows all brand names in IMSP List of Additional Drug Names with Tall Man Letters.

 Report actual and potential medication errors to the Medication Errors Reporting Program (MERP) via the Web at www.ismp.org or by calling 1-800-FAIL-SAF(E).

ISMP LIST OF ADDITIONAL DRUG NAMES WITH TALL MAN LETTERS

Drug Name with Tall Man Letters	Confused with
HYDROcodone	oxyCODONE
HYDROmorphone	morphine—oxyMORphone
HYDROXYprogesterone	medroxyPROGESTERone
hydrOXYzine	hydrALAZINE—hydroCHLOROthiazide
IDArubicin	DOXOrubicin—idaruCIZUmab
idaruCIZUmab	IDArubicin
inFLIXimab	riTUXimab
ISOtretinoin	tretinoin
KlonoPIN*	cloNIDine
LaMICtal*	LamISIL*
LamISIL*	LaMICtal*
lamiVUDine	lamoTRIgine
lamoTRIgine	lamiVUDine
levETIRAcetam	levOCARNitine—levoFLOXacin
levOCARNitine	levETIRAcetam
levoFLOXacin	levETIRAcetam
LEVOleucovorin	leucovorin
LORazepam	ALPRAZolam—clonazePAM
medroxyPROGESTERone	HYDROXYprogesterone
metFORMIN	metroNIDAZOLE
methazolAMIDE	methiMAZOLE—metOLazone
methiMAZOLE	metOLazone—methazolAMIDE
metOLazone	methiMAZOLE—methazolAMIDE
metroNIDAZOLE	metFORMIN
metyraPONE	metyroSINE
metyroSINE	metyraPONE
miFEPRIStone	miSOPROStol
miSOPROStol	miFEPRIStone
mitoMYcin	mitoXANTRONE
mitoXANTRONE	mitoMYcin
NexAVAR*	NexIUM*
NexIUM*	NexAVAR*
niCARdipine	niMODipine—NIFEdipine
NIFEdipine	niMODipine—niCARdipine
niMODipine	NIFEdipine—niCARdipine
NovoLIN*	NovoLOG*
NovoLOG*	NovoLIN*
OLANZapine	QUEtiapine
OXcarbazepine	carBAMazepine
oxyCODONE	HYDROcodone—OxyCONTIN*—oxyMORphone
OxyCONTIN*	oxyCODONE—oxyMORphone
oxyMORphone	HYDROmorphone—oxyCODONE—OxyCONTIN*

Drug Name with Tall Man Letters	Confused with
PACLItaxel	DOCEtaxel
PARoxetine	FLUoxetine—DULoxetine
PAZOPanib	PONATinib
PEMEtrexed	PRALAtrexate
penicillAMINE	penicillin
PENTobarbital	PHENobarbital
PHENobarbital	PENTobarbital
PONATinib	PAZOPanib
PRALAtrexate	PEMEtrexed
PriLOSEC*	PROzac*
PROzac*	PriLOSEC*
QUEtiapine	OLANZapine
quiNIDine	quiNINE
quiNINE	quiNIDine
RABEprazole	ARIPiprazole
raNITIdine	riMANTAdine
rifAMPin	rifAXIMin
rifAXIMin	rifAMPin
riMANTAdine	raNITIdine
RisperDAL*	rOPINIRole
risperiDONE	rOPINIRole
riTUXimab	inFLIXimab
romiDEPsin	romiPLOStim
romiPLOStim	romiDEPsin
rOPINIRole	RisperDAL*—risperiDONE
SandIMMUNE*	SandoSTATIN*
SandoSTATIN*	SandIMMUNE*
SAXagliptin	SITagliptin
SEROquel*	SINEquan*
SINEquan*	SEROquel*
SITagliptin	SAXagliptin—SUMAtriptan
Solu—CORTEF*	SOLU—Medrol*
SOLU—Medrol*	Solu—CORTEF*—DEPO Medrol*
SORAfenib	SUNItinib
SUFentanil	fentaNYL
sulfADIAZINE	sulfaSALAzine
sulfaSALAzine	sulfADIAZINE
SUMAtriptan	SITagliptin—ZOLMitriptan
SUNItinib	SORAfenib
tiaGABine	tiZANidine
tiZANidine	tiaGABine
traMADol	traZODone
traZODone	traMADol
valACYclovir	valGANciclovir
valGANciclovir	valACYclovir
ZOLMitriptan	SUMAtriptan
ZyPREXA*	ZyrTEC*
ZyrTEC*	ZyPREXA*

*Brand names always start with an upper case letter. Some brand names incorporate tall man letters in initial characters and may not be readily recognized as brand names. An asterisk follows all brand names in IMSP List of Additional Drug Names with Tall Man Letters.

APPENDICES

APPENDIX A

Recent Drug Approvals

To view full-text monographs of drugs that have been recently released from the FDA or to learn about changes to dosage forms, please visit www.DrugGuide.com.

acalabrutinib

(a-**kal**-a-broo-ti-nib)
Calquence

Classification
Therapeutic: antineoplastics
Pharmacologic: kinase inhibitors

Indications

Mantle cell lymphoma (MCL) in patients who have not responded to ≥1 previous therapy.

Contraindications/Precautions

Contraindicated in: Concurrent use of strong CYP3A4 inducers/inhibitors; OB: May cause fetal harm; avoid pregnancy; Lactation: Avoid breast feeding.

Use Cautiously in: Concurrent use of moderate inhibitors of CYP3A4 (↓ dose of acalabrutinib); Concurrent use of antiplatelet agents/anticoagulants (↑ risk of bleeding); Surgical procedures (if possible withhold for 3–7 days pre- and post-operatively); Pedi: Safety and effectiveness in children not established.

Adverse Reactions/Side Effects

CNS: PROGRESSIVE MULTIFOCAL LEUKOENCEPHALOPATHY (PML), headache. **CV:** atrial fibrillation/flutter. **Derm:** rash. **GI:** abdominal pain, constipation, diarrhea, nausea, vomiting. **GU:** ↑ serum creatinine. **Hemat:** HEMORRHAGE, anemia, neutropenia, thrombocytopenia. **MS:** myalgia. **Misc:** INFECTION, SECOND MALIGNANCIES, fatigue.

Route/Dosage

PO (Adults): 100 mg twice daily until disease progression or unacceptable toxicity. *Concurrent use of moderate CYP3A inhibitors*—100 mg once daily until disease progression or unacceptable toxicity; *Concurrent use of strong CYP3A inducers*—200 mg twice daily until disease progression or unacceptable toxicity.

adapalene (a-**dap**-a-leen)

Differin

Classification
Therapeutic: antiacne agents
Pharmacologic: retinoids

Indications

Management of acne vulgaris.

Contraindications/Precautions

Contraindicated in: Hypersensitivity.

Use Cautiously in: OB: Use during pregnancy only if potential benefit justifies the potential risk to the fetus; Lactation: Safety not established; Pedi: Children <12 yr (safety and effectiveness not established).

Adverse Reactions/Side Effects

Derm: burning, dryness, erythema, pruritus, scaling, photosensitivity.

Route/Dosage

Topical (Adults and Children ≥12 yr): Apply once daily at bedtime.

angiotensin II

(an-jee-oh-**ten**-sin too)
Giapreza

Classification
Therapeutic: vasopressors
Pharmacologic: vasopressors

Indications

Increases blood pressure in septic or other distributive shock.

Contraindications/Precautions

Contraindicated in: None.

Use Cautiously in: OB: Use only if potential maternal benefit outweighs potential fetal risk; Lactation: Safety not established; Pedi: Safety and effectiveness in children not established.

Adverse Reactions/Side Effects

CNS: delirium. **CV:** THROMBOEMBOLIC EVENTS, peripheral ischemia, tachycardia. **Endo:** hyperglycemia. **Hemat:** thrombocytopenia. **Misc:** fungal infection.

Route/Dosage

IV (Adults): 20 ng/kg/min continuous infusion; may be titrated every 5 min of up to 15 ng/kg/min to achieve or maintain target mean arterial pressure. Do not exceed dose of 80 ng/kg/min during first 3 hr.

During maintenance therapy, do not exceed dose of 40 ng/kg/min. Once shock has adequately improved, titrate down by 15 ng/kg/min every 5–15 min based on mean arterial pressure.

apalutamide
(a-pa-**loo**-ta-mide)
Erleada

Classification
Therapeutic: antineoplastics
Pharmacologic: androgen receptor inhibitors

Indications
Non-metastatic castration-resistant prostate cancer. Metastatic castration-sensitive prostate cancer.

Contraindications/Precautions
Contraindicated in: OB: Pregnancy (may cause fetal harm).
Use Cautiously in: History of seizures, underlying brain pathology, cerebrovascular accident, transient ischemic attack, brain metastases or brain arteriovenous malformation (may ↑ risk of seizures); Ischemic heart disease or HF; Rep: Men with female partners of reproductive potential; Pedi: Safety and effectiveness not established.

Adverse Reactions/Side Effects
CNS: SEIZURES, falls, fatigue. **CV:** MI, hypertension, peripheral edema, unstable angina. **Derm:** hot flush, rash, pruritus. **Endo:** hyperglycemia, hypothyroidism. **F and E:** hyperkalemia. **GI:** ↓ appetite, diarrhea, nausea. **GU:** ↓ fertility (males). **Hemat:** anemia, leukopenia, lymphopenia. **Metab:** ↓ weight, hypercholesterolemia, hypertriglyceridemia. **MS:** arthralgia, fracture.

Route/Dosage
PO (Adults): 240 mg once daily.

avatrombopag
(a-va-**trom**-boe-**pag**)
Doptelet

Classification
Therapeutic: antithrombocytopenics
Pharmacologic: thrombopoietin receptor agonists

Indications
Treatment of thrombocytopenia in patients with chronic liver disease who are scheduled to undergo a medical or dental procedure. Treatment of thrombocytopenia in patients with chronic immune thrombocytopenia who have had insufficient response to a previous treatment.

Contraindications/Precautions
Contraindicated in: OB: Pregnancy (may cause fetal harm); Lactation: Avoid breast feeding.
Use Cautiously in: Factor V Leiden, prothrombin 20210A, antithrombin deficiency or protein C or S deficiency (↑ risk for thromboembolism); Pedi: Safety and effectiveness not established.

Adverse Reactions/Side Effects
CNS: fatigue, headache. **CV:** THROMBOEMBOLISM, peripheral edema. **F and E:** hyponatremia. **GI:** abdominal pain, nausea. **Hemat:** anemia. **MS:** myalgia. **Misc:** fever.

Route/Dosage

Patients with Chronic Liver Disease
PO (Adults): *Platelet count <40 × 10^9/L*—60 mg once daily for 5 days (should be initiated 10–13 days prior to scheduled procedure; procedure should be performed 5–8 days after last dose); *Platelet count 40–<50 × 10^9/L*—40 mg once daily for 5 days (should be initiated 10–13 days prior to scheduled procedure; procedure should be performed 5–8 days after last dose).

Patients with Chronic Immune Thrombocytopenia
PO (Adults): Dose levels recommended for titration of therapy based on platelet counts: *Dose Level 1*—20 mg once weekly; *Dose Level 2*—20 mg twice weekly *OR* 40 mg once weekly; *Dose Level 3*—20 mg 3 times weekly; *Dose Level 4*—20 mg once daily; *Dose Level 5*—40 mg 3 times weekly *AND* 20 mg the remaining 4 days of the wk; *Dose Level 6*—40 mg once daily; Initiate therapy at Dose Level 4 (20 mg once daily); if platelet count <50 × 10^9/L after 2 wk of therapy, ↑ one Dose Level; if platelet count 50–200 × 10^9/L after 2 wk of therapy, continue current Dose Level; if platelet count 200–400 × 10^9/L after 2 wk of therapy, ↓ one Dose Level; if platelet count >400 × 10^9/L, discontinue avatrombopag and restart therapy (↓ one Dose Level) once platelet count <150 × 10^9/L. *Concurrent use of moderate or strong dual inhibitors of CYP3A4 and CYP2C9*—Initiate therapy at Dose Level 3 (20 mg 3 times weekly). *Concurrent use of moderate or strong dual inducers of CYP3A4 and CYP2C9*—Initiate therapy at Dose Level 6 (40 mg once daily).

avelumab (a-vel-ue-mab)
Bavencio

Classification
Therapeutic: antineoplastics
Pharmacologic: programmed death ligand 1 (PD-L1) inhibitors

Indications
Metastatic Merkel cell carcinoma (MCC). Locally advanced or metastatic urothelial carcinoma in patients who have disease progression during or following platinum-containing chemotherapy or have disease progression within 12 mo of neoadjuvant or adjuvant treatment with platinum-containing chemotherapy. Advanced renal cell carcinoma (RCC) as first-line therapy (in combination with axitinib).

Contraindications/Precautions
Contraindicated in: OB: May cause fetal harm in pregnancy; Lactation: Avoid breast feeding.
Use Cautiously in: Diabetes, hypertension, and/or dyslipidemia; Rep: Women of reproductive potential; Pedi: Children <12 yr (safety and effectiveness not established).

Adverse Reactions/Side Effects
CNS: dizziness, headache. **CV:** HF, MI, hypertension, peripheral edema. **Derm:** pruritus, rash. **Endo:** adrenal insufficiency, hyperglycemia, hyperthyroidism, hypothyroidism, type 1 diabetes mellitus. **F and E:** hyponatremia, hyperkalemia. **GI:** COLITIS, HEPATITIS, abdominal pain, constipation, ↓ appetite, diarrhea, ↑ lipase, ↑ liver enzymes, nausea, vomiting, ↑ amylase. **GU:** renal impairment, urinary tract infection. **Hemat:** anemia, lymphopenia, thrombocytopenia, neutropenia. **Metab:** ↓ weight. **MS:** pain. **Resp:** PNEUMONITIS, cough, dyspnea, fever. **Misc:** INFUSION-RELATED REACTIONS, fatigue.

Route/Dosage

MCC
IV (Adults and Children ≥12 yr): 800 mg every 2 wk until disease progression or unacceptable toxicity.

Urothelial Carcinoma and RCC
IV (Adults): 800 mg every 2 wk until disease progression or unacceptable toxicity.

defibrotide (de-fib-ro-tide)
Defitelio

Classification
Therapeutic: anticoagulants
Pharmacologic: fibrinolysis inhibitors

Indications
Treatment of hepatic veno-occlusive disease (VOD), also known as sinusoidal obstruction syndrome (SOS), with renal or pulmonary impairment following hematopoietic stem-cell transplantation (HSCT).

Contraindications/Precautions
Contraindicated in: Hypersensitivity; Concurrent use with systemic anticoagulants or fibrinolytics; Active bleeding; Lactation: Avoid breast feeding.
Use Cautiously in: OB: Safety not established in pregnancy.

Adverse Reactions/Side Effects
CV: hypotension. **Endo:** hyperuricemia. **GI:** diarrhea, nausea, vomiting. **Hemat:** BLEEDING. **Misc:** HYPERSENSITIVITY REACTIONS (including anaphylaxis and angioedema), graft versus host disease, infection.

Route/Dosage
IV (Adults and Children): 6.25 mg/kg every 6 hr for at least 21 days; may continue for up to 60 days if signs/symptoms of VOD persist after 21 days.

deflazacort (de-flaze-a-kort)
Emflaza

Classification
Therapeutic: anti-inflammatories, immunosuppressants, none assigned
Pharmacologic: corticosteroids

Indications
Duchenne muscular dystrophy (DMD).

Contraindications/Precautions
Contraindicated in: Hypersensitivity; Active untreated infections.
Use Cautiously in: Hypopituitarism, primary adrenal insufficiency, congenital adrenal hyperplasia, thyroid dysfunction, or pheochromocytoma (↑ risk of endocrine abnormalities); HF, hypertension, recent MI, or renal impairment; Peptic ulcer disease, diverticulitis, recent intestinal anastomoses, or ulcerative colitis (↑ risk of GI perforation); Myasthenia gravis (↑ risk of

myopathy); OB: Use only if potential maternal benefit justifies potential fetal risk; Lactation: Use only if potential maternal benefit justifies potential risks to infant; Pedi: Children <2 yr (safety and effectiveness not established); oral suspension contains benzyl alcohol which can cause gasping syndrome in premature neonates and low birth weight infants.

Adverse Reactions/Side Effects

CNS: headache, depression, euphoria, insomnia, irritability, mood swings. **CV:** THROMBOEMBOLIC EVENTS, hypertension, peripheral edema. **Derm:** TOXIC EPIDERMAL NECROLYSIS, acne, hirsutism, erythema, rash, skin striae. **EENT:** cataracts, epistaxis, glaucoma, rhinorrhea. **Endo:** Cushingoid appearance, adrenal suppression, ↓ bone density, ↓ growth (children), hyperglycemia. **GI:** PEPTIC ULCERATION, abdominal pain, constipation, ↑ appetite, nausea. **Metab:** ↑ weight. **MS:** avascular necrosis of joints, back pain, myopathy. **Resp:** cough. **Misc:** HYPERSENSITIVITY REACTIONS (including anaphylaxis), INFECTION, KAPOSI'S SARCOMA, fever.

Route/Dosage

PO (Adults and Children ≥2 yr): 0.9 mg/kg once daily. *Concurrent use of moderate or strong CYP3A4 inhibitors*—Give ⅓ the recommended dose.

deutetrabenazine
(du-tet-ra-**ben**-a-zeen)
Austedo

Classification
Therapeutic: antichoreas
Pharmacologic: reversible monoamine depleters

Indications

Chorea due to Huntington's Disease. Tardive dyskinesia.

Contraindications/Precautions

Contraindicated in: Hepatic impairment; Concurrent use of reserpine, MAO inhibitors, tetrabenazine, or valbenazine; Patients who are suicidal or have untreated or inadequately treated depression; Congenital long QT syndrome or cardiac arrhythmias.
Use Cautiously in: History of/propensity for depression or history of psychiatric illness; history of suicidality; Poor CYP2D6 metabolizers; initial dose ↓ required; Concurrent use of strong CYP2D6 inhibitors; initial dose ↓ required; Bradycardia, hypokalemia, hypomagnesemia, or concurrent use of QT-interval prolonging drugs; History of breast cancer; OB: Use only when potential maternal benefit justifies potential fetal risk; Lactation: Use while breast feeding only when potential maternal benefit justifies potential risk to infant; Pedi: Safety and effectiveness not established.

Adverse Reactions/Side Effects

CNS: NEUROLEPTIC MALIGNANT SYNDROME, SUICIDAL THOUGHTS/IDEATION, sedation/somnolence, agitation, anxiety, depression, dizziness, fatigue, insomnia. **Endo:** hyperprolactinemia. **CV:** QTc interval prolongation. **GI:** constipation, diarrhea, dry mouth. **GU:** urinary tract infection. **MS:** bradykinesia. **Neuro:** akathisia, gait disturbances, parkinsonism, restlessness, tremor.

Route/Dosage

Huntington's Disease

PO (Adults): 6 mg once daily; may ↑ dose by 6 mg/day at weekly intervals (max dose = 48 mg/day). Daily doses exceeding 12 mg should be administered in 2 divided doses. *Concurrent use of strong CYP2D6 inhibitors or poor CYP2D6 metabolizers*—Do not exceed dose of 36 mg/day.

Tardive Dyskinesia

PO (Adults): 6 mg twice daily; may ↑ dose by 6 mg/day at weekly intervals (max dose = 48 mg/day). Daily doses exceeding 12 mg should be administered in 2 divided doses. *Concurrent use of strong CYP2D6 inhibitors or poor CYP2D6 metabolizers*—Do not exceed dose of 36 mg/day.

doravirine (dor-a-**vir**-een)
Pifeltro

Classification
Therapeutic: antiretrovirals
Pharmacologic: non-nucleoside reverse transcriptase inhibitors

Indications

HIV-1 infection in patients with no prior antiretroviral treatment history (in combination with other antiretrovirals). To replace the current antiretroviral regimen in patients with HIV-1 infection who are virologically suppressed (HIV-1 RNA <50 copies/mL), receiving a stable antiretroviral regimen with no history of treatment failure, and have no known substitutions associated with resistance to doravirine (in combination with other antiretrovirals).

Contraindications/Precautions

Contraindicated in: Concurrent use of carbamazepine, enzalutamide, mitotane, oxcarbazepine, phenobarbital, phenytoin, rifampin, rifapentine, and St. John's wort; Lactation: Breast feeding not recommended in women infected with HIV.

Use Cautiously in: End-stage renal disease; Severe hepatic impairment (Child-Pugh Class C); OB: Safety not established; Pedi: Safety and effectiveness not established; Geri: Consider age-related ↓ in organ function and body mass, concurrent disease states and medications.

Adverse Reactions/Side Effects

CNS: abnormal dreams, dizziness, fatigue, headache, insomnia, sedation. **Derm:** rash. **Endo:** Graves' disease. **GI:** diarrhea, abdominal pain, autoimmune hepatitis, hyperbilirubinemia, ↑ lipase, ↑ liver enzymes, nausea. **GU:** ↑ serum creatinine. **MS:** ↑ creatine kinase, polymyositis. **Neuro:** Guillan-Barré syndrome. **Misc:** immune reconstitution syndrome.

Route/Dosage

PO (Adults): 100 mg once daily.

durvalumab (dur-val-ue-mab)

Imfinzi

Classification

Therapeutic: antineoplastics

Pharmacologic: monoclonal antibodies, programmed death ligand 1 (PD-L1) inhibitors

Indications

Locally advanced or metastatic urothelial carcinoma in patients who have disease progression during or following platinum-containing chemotherapy or have disease progression within 12 mo of neoadjuvant or adjuvant treatment with platinum-containing chemotherapy. Unresectable, stage III non-small cell lung cancer (NSCLC) in patients whose disease has not progressed with concurrent platinum-containing chemotherapy and radiation.

Contraindications/Precautions

Contraindicated in: OB: May cause fetal harm; avoid pregnancy; Lactation: Avoid breast feeding.

Use Cautiously in: Rep: Woman of reproductive potential; Pedi: Safety and effectiveness not established.

Adverse Reactions/Side Effects

CV: peripheral edema. **Derm:** STEVENS-JOHNSON SYNDROME, TOXIC EPIDERMAL NECROLYSIS, pruritus, rash, bullous dermatitis. **Endo:** hyperglycemia, hypothyroidism, adrenal insufficiency, hyperthyroidism, hypophysitis, type 1 diabetes mellitus. **F and E:** hyperkalemia, hypocalcemia, hyponatremia, hypercalcemia, hypermagnesemia, hypokalemia. **GI:** COLITIS/DIARRHEA, HEPATITIS, abdominal pain, constipation, ↓ appetite, nausea, ↑ liver enzymes. **GU:** acute kidney injury, glomerulonephritis, ↑ serum creatinine, renal failure. **Hemat:** NEUTROPENIA, lymphopenia, anemia. **Metab:** hypoalbuminemia. **MS:** pain. **Resp:** PNEUMONITIS, cough, dyspnea. **Misc:** INFECTION, INFUSION-RELATED REACTIONS, fatigue, fever.

Route/Dosage

Urothelial Carcinoma

IV (Adults): 10 mg/kg every 2 wk until disease progression or unacceptable toxicity.

NSCLC

IV (Adults): 10 mg/kg every 2 wk until disease progression, unacceptable toxicity, or a maximum of 12 mo.

ertugliflozin (er-too-gli-floe-zin)

Steglatro

Classification

Therapeutic: antidiabetics

Pharmacologic: sodium-glucose co-transporter 2 (SGLT2) inhibitors

Indications

Adjunct to diet and exercise in the management of type 2 diabetes mellitus.

Contraindications/Precautions

Contraindicated in: Hypersensitivity; Severe renal impairment (eGFR <30 mL/min/1.73 m^2), end-stage renal disease or on dialysis; Type 1 diabetes; Diabetic ketoacidosis; Severe hepatic impairment; OB: Avoid use during 2nd and 3rd trimesters (↑ risk of renal impairment in fetus); Lactation: Avoid use during breast feeding.

Use Cautiously in: Moderate renal impairment (eGFR 30–59 mL/min/1.73 m^2) (↑ risk of adverse reactions related to ↓ intravascular volume) (use not recommended); Renal impairment (eGFR <60 mL/min/1.73 m^2), age ≥65 yr, low systolic BP, or concurrent use of diuretics (↑ risk of hypotension); Acute febrile illness, reduced caloric intake due to illness or surgery, history of pancreatitis or pancreatic surgery, or alcohol abuse (↑ risk of ketoacidosis); Hypovolemia, chronic kidney disease, HF, or concurrent use of diuretics, NSAIDs, ACE inhibitors, or ARBs (↑ risk of acute kidney injury); Previous amputation, peripheral vascular disease, neuropathy, or diabetic foot infection

(↑ risk of lower limb amputation); History of genital mycotic infections or uncircumcised (↑ risk of genital mycotic infections); Geri: ↑ risk of adverse reactions related to ↓ intravascular volume; OB: Use during first trimester only if potential maternal benefit justifies potential fetal risk; Pedi: Safety and effectiveness not established.

Adverse Reactions/Side Effects

CNS: dizziness, headache, syncope. **CV:** hypotension. **Endo:** hypoglycemia (↑ with other medications). **F and E:** KETOACIDOSIS, dehydration, polydipsia. **GU:** NECROTIZING FASCIITIS OF PERINEUM (FOURNIER'S GANGRENE), UROSEPSIS, genital mycotic infection, acute kidney injury, polyuria, urinary tract infection (including pyelonephritis), vaginal pruritus. **Metab:** ↓ weight, hyperlipidemia. **MS:** back pain, lower limb amputation (primarily toe).

Route/Dosage

PO (Adults): *eGFR* $\geq$ *60 mL/min/1.73 m²*—5 mg once daily initially; may ↑ to 15 mg once daily if needed.

eteplirsen (e-**tep**-lir-sen)

Exondys 51

Classification
Therapeutic: none assigned
Pharmacologic: antisense oligonucleotides

Indications

Treatment of Duchenne muscular dystrophy (DMD) in patients who have a confirmed mutation of the DMD gene that is amenable to exon 51 skipping.

Contraindications/Precautions

Contraindicated in: None.
Use Cautiously in: OB, Lactation: Safety and effectiveness not established.

Adverse Reactions/Side Effects

Derm: rash. **GI:** vomiting. **Neuro:** balance disorder. **MS:** arthralgia. **Resp:** upper respiratory tract infection. **Misc:** HYPERSENSITIVITY REACTIONS (including rash, urticaria, pyrexia, flushing, dyspnea, bronchospasm, and hypotension).

Route/Dosage

IV (Children): 30 mg/kg once weekly.

glycopyrrolate, oral inhalation

(glye-koe-**pye**-roe-late)
Lonhala Magnair, Seebri Neohaler

Classification
Therapeutic: bronchodilators
Pharmacologic: anticholinergics

Indications

Maintenance treatment of COPD.

Contraindications/Precautions

Contraindicated in: Hypersensitivity to any components or severe hypersensitivity to milk proteins; Acute attack of COPD (onset of action is delayed).
Use Cautiously in: Narrow-angle glaucoma; Urinary retention, prostatic hyperplasia, bladder-neck obstruction; OB, Lactation: Safety not established; Pedi: Safety and effectiveness not established.

Adverse Reactions/Side Effects

CNS: fatigue. **EENT:** nasopharyngitis, rhinitis, sinusitis. **GI:** diarrhea, nausea. **MS:** arthralgia. **Resp:** dyspnea, paradoxical bronchospasm, upper respiratory tract infection. **Misc:** HYPERSENSITIVITY REACTIONS (including angioedema, urticaria, or rash).

Route/Dosage

Inhaln (Adults): *Lonhala Magnair*—1 vial (25 mcg) twice daily; *Seebri Neohaler*—1 capsule (15.6 mcg) twice daily.

imipenem/cilastatin/relebactam

(i-me-**pen**-em/sye-la-**stat**-in/**rel**-e-**bak**-tam)
Recarbrio

Classification
Therapeutic: anti-infectives
Pharmacologic: carbapenems, beta lactamase inhibitors

Indications

Complicated urinary tract infections (cUTI), including pyelonephritis (for patients with limited or no alternative treatment options). Complicated intra-abdominal infections (for patients with limited or no alternative treatment options).

Contraindications/Precautions

Contraindicated in: Hypersensitivity (cross-sensitivity may occur with penicillins and cephalosporins).

Use Cautiously in: Seizure disorders; Renal impairment (dose ↓ required if CCr <90 mL/min); OB: Use only if potential maternal benefit justifies potential fetal risk; Lactation: Use while breast feeding only if potential maternal benefit justifies potential risk to infant; Pedi: Safety and effectiveness not established; Geri: May be at ↑ risk for adverse reactions due to age-related renal impairment.

Adverse Reactions/Side Effects

CNS: SEIZURES, headache. **CV:** hypertension. **GI:** CLOSTRIDIUM DIFFICILE-ASSOCIATED DIARRHEA (CDAD), diarrhea, ↑ lipase, ↑ liver enzymes, nausea, vomiting. **Hemat:** anemia. **Local:** phlebitis. **Misc:** HYPERSENSITIVITY REACTIONS (including anaphylaxis), fever.

Route/Dosage

IV (Adults): 1.25 g every 6 hr.

Renal Impairment

IV (Adults): *CCr 60–89 mL/min*— 1 g every 6 hr; *CCr 30–59 mL/min*— 750 mg every 6 hr; *CCr 15–29 mL/min*— 500 mg every 6 hr; *CCr <15 mL/min on hemodialysis*— 500 mg every 6 hr (on dialysis days, administer doses after hemodialysis).

indacaterol/glycopyrrolate

(in-da-**kat**-e-role/glye-koe-**pye**-roe-late)

❖Ultibrol Breezhaler, Utibron Neohaler

Classification

Therapeutic: bronchodilators

Pharmacologic: anticholinergics, long-acting beta$_2$-adrenergic agonists (LABAs)

Indications

Maintenance treatment of airflow obstruction in patients with COPD.

Contraindications/Precautions

Contraindicated in: Hypersensitivity to any component; Acutely deteriorating COPD or acute respiratory symptoms; Asthma; Lactation: Discontinue drug or discontinue breast feeding.

Use Cautiously in: History of cardiovascular disorders (coronary insufficiency, arrhythmias, hypertension); History of seizures; Thyrotoxicosis; Narrow-angle glaucoma; Urinary retention, prostatic hyperplasia, bladder-neck obstruction; Severe hepatic impairment; OB: Use only if potential maternal benefit justifies potential fetal risk; indacaterol may interfere with uterine contractility during labor; Pedi: Safety and effectiveness not established.

Exercise Extreme Caution in: Concurrent use of MAO inhibitors, tricyclic antidepressants or drugs that prolong the QTc interval.

Adverse Reactions/Side Effects

Combination. **CNS:** headache **CV:** hypertension, tachycardia. **EENT:** nasopharyngitis, rhinitis. **F and E:** hypokalemia. **GI:** diarrhea. **Metab:** hyperglycemia. **Resp:** paradoxical bronchospasm, respiratory tract infection. **Misc:** HYPERSENSITIVITY REACTIONS (including angioedema, urticaria, or rash).

Route/Dosage

Inhaln (Adults): 1 capsule (indacaterol 27.5 mcg/glycopyrrolate 15.6 mcg) twice daily.

letermovir (le-**term**-oh-vir)

Prevymis

Classification

Therapeutic: antivirals

Indications

Prevention of cytomegalovirus (CMV) infection and disease in adult CMV-seropositive recipients of an allogeneic hematopoietic stem cell transplant (HSCT).

Contraindications/Precautions

Contraindicated in: Concurrent use of pimozide or ergot alkaloids; Concurrent use of pitavastatin and simvastatin when administered with cyclosporine; Severe hepatic impairment.

Use Cautiously in: Renal impairment (CCr <50 mL/min; accumulation of IV vehicle may occur [closely monitor serum creatinine]); OB, Lactation: Safety not established; Pedi: Safety and effectiveness not established.

Adverse Reactions/Side Effects

CNS: headache. **CV:** peripheral edema, atrial fibrillation, tachycardia. **GI:** abdominal pain, diarrhea, nausea, vomiting. **GU:** ↑ serum creatinine. **Hemat:** anemia, neutropenia, thrombocytopenia. **Resp:** cough. **Misc:** fatigue.

Route/Dosage

IV therapy should only be used when patients are unable to take oral therapy.

IV, PO (Adults): 480 mg once daily started between Day 0 and Day 28 post-transplantation and continued through Day 100 post-transplantation. *Concurrent* *use with cyclosporine*—240 mg once daily started between Day 0 and Day 28 post-transplantation and continued through Day 100 post-transplantation.

obeticholic acid
(oh-bet-i-**koe**-lik **as**-id)
Ocaliva

Classification
Therapeutic: none assigned
Pharmacologic: farnesoid X receptor agonists

Indications
Treatment of primary biliary cholangitis (PBC) in patients with an inadequate response to ursodeoxycholic acid (UDCA) (in combination with UDCA) or unable to tolerate UDCA (as monotherapy).

Contraindications/Precautions
Contraindicated in: Complete biliary obstruction.
Use Cautiously in: Decompensated cirrhosis or Child-Pugh Class B or C hepatic impairment; OB, Lactation: Safety not established; Pedi: Safety and effectiveness not established.

Adverse Reactions/Side Effects
CNS: HEPATIC ENCEPHALOPATHY, dizziness. **CV:** palpitations, peripheral edema. **Derm:** pruritus, eczema, rash. **EENT:** oropharyngeal pain. **Endo:** ↓ high-density lipoprotein cholesterol, hypothyroidism. **GI:** VARICEAL BLEEDING, abdominal pain, ascites (worsening), constipation, ↑ liver enzymes, jaundice. **MS:** arthralgia. **Misc:** fatigue, fever.

Route/Dosage
PO (Adults): *Non-cirrhotic or compensated Child-Pugh Class A*—5 mg once daily for 3 mo; if adequate reduction in alkaline phosphatase and/or total bilirubin not achieved and tolerating medication, ↑ dose to 10 mg once daily; *Child-Pugh Class B or C or prior hepatic decompensation event*—5 mg once weekly for 3 mo; if adequate reduction in alkaline phosphatase and/or total bilirubin not achieved and tolerating medication, ↑ dose to 5 mg twice weekly (with doses given ≥3 days apart); may further titrate to 10 mg twice weekly (with doses given ≥3 days apart) based on clinical response and tolerability.

ozenoxacin (oz-en-**ox**-a-sin)
Xepi

Classification
Therapeutic: anti-infectives
Pharmacologic: fluoroquinolones

Indications
Impetigo.

Contraindications/Precautions
Contraindicated in: None.
Use Cautiously in: OB, Lactation: Safety not established; fetal exposure not expected due to minimal systemic absorption; Pedi: Children <2 mo (safety and effectiveness not established).

Adverse Reactions/Side Effects
Derm: rosacea, seborrheic dermatitis.

Route/Dosage
Topical (Adults and Children ≥2 mo): Apply to affected area twice daily for 5 days.

sodium zirconium cyclosilicate
(**soe**-dee-um zir-**koe**-nee-um **sye**-kloe-**sil**-i-kate)
Lokelma

Classification
Therapeutic: hypokalemic, electrolyte modifiers
Pharmacologic: cationic exchange resins

Indications
Hyperkalemia.

Contraindications/Precautions
Contraindicated in: Severe constipation, bowel obstruction/impaction, post-operative motility disorders (ineffective and may worsen condition).
Use Cautiously in: Heart failure or renal impairment (sodium content may cause edema); Pedi: Safety and effectiveness not established.

Adverse Reactions/Side Effects
CV: edema. **F and E:** hypokalemia.

Route/Dosage
PO (Adults): 10 g 3 times daily in water for up to 48 hr, then 10 g once daily (if treatment continued beyond 48 hr); may titrate chronic therapy in increments of 5 g at 1–wk intervals (recommended maintenance dose range = 5–15 g once daily).

NEW DOSAGE FORMS

Generic Name (Brand Name)	New Dosage Form
abiraterone (Yonsa)	Oral tablet
amantadine (Osmolex ER)	Extended-release oral tablet
amikacin (Arikayce)	Liposomal suspension for oral inhalation
amlodipine (Katerzia)	Oral suspension
amphetamine (Evekeo ODT)	Orally disintegrating tablet
aripiprazole lauroxil (Aristada Initio)	Extended-release suspension for IM injection
baclofen (Ozobax)	Oral solution
bendamustine (Belrapzo)	Solution for IV injection
cladribine (Mavenclad)	Oral tablet
clobazam (Sympazan)	Oral film
colchicine (Gloperba)	Oral solution
colesevelam (Welchol)	Chewable bar
cyclosporine (Cequa)	Ophthalmic solution
desmopressin (Nocdurna)	Sublingual tablet
duloxetine (Drizalma Sprinkle)	Delayed-release capsule
efavirenz/lamivudine/tenofovir disoproxil fumarate (Symfi Lo)	Oral tablet
estradiol (Imvexxy)	Vaginal insert
gemcitabine (Infugem)	Solution for IV injection
glucagon (Baqsimi)	Nasal powder
glucagon (Gvoke)	Solution for subcutaneous injection
glycopyrrolate (Glyrx-PF)	Solution for IV/IM injection
glycopyrronium (Qbrexza)	Topical cloth
halobetasol (Bryhali)	Topical lotion for plaque psoriasis
halobetasol (Lexette)	Topical foam for plaque psoriasis
ibrutinib (Imbruvica)	Oral tablet
ivabradine (Corlanor)	Oral solution
latanoprost (Xelpros)	Ophthalmic emulsion
ledipasvir/sofosbuvir (Harvoni)	Oral pellets
levodopa (Inbrija)	Capsule for oral inhalation
lidocaine (ZTlido)	Transdermal patch
loteprednol (Inveltys)	Ophthlalmic suspension
lumacaftor/ivacaftor (Orkambi)	Oral granules
meloxicam (Qmiiz ODT)	Orally disintegrating tablet
metformin (Riomet ER)	Extended-release oral suspension
methylphenidate (Jornay PM)	Extended-release oral capsule
metoprolol succinate (Kaspargo Sprinkle)	Extended-release oral capsule
midazolam (Nayzilam)	Nasal spray

NEW DOSAGE FORMS (continued)

Generic Name (Brand Name)	New Dosage Form
pimavanserin (Nuplazid)	Oral capsule
riluzole (Tiglutek)	Oral suspension
risperidone (Perseris)	Extended-release suspension for subcutaneous injection
rosuvastatin (Ezallor)	Oral capsule
semaglutide (Rybelsus)	Oral tablet
sofosbuvir (Sovaldi)	Oral pellets
stiripentol (Diacomit)	Powder for oral suspension
sufentanil (Dsuvia)	Sublingual tablet
tacrolimus (Prograf)	Granules for oral suspension
testosterone enanthate (Xyosted)	Solution for subcutaneous injection
testosterone undecanoate (Jatenzo)	Oral capsule
tretinoin (Altreno)	Topical lotion
vancomycin (Firvanq)	Powder for oral solution

DISCONTINUED DRUGS

Generic Name (Brand Name)	Reason for Discontinuation
abciximab (Reopro)	Discontinued by manufacturer
daclatasvir (Daklinza)	Discontinued by manufacturer
interferon alfa-2b (Intron A)	Discontinued by manufacturer
lesinurad (Zurampic)	Discontinued by manufacturer
liotrix (Thyrolar)	Discontinued by manufacturer
nesiritide (Natrecor)	Discontinued by manufacturer
olaratumab (Lartruvo)	Discontinued by manufacturer
ombitasvir/paritaprevir/ritonavir (Technivie)	Discontinued by manufacturer
peginterferon alfa-2b (Pegintron, Sylatron)	Discontinued by manufacturer

APPENDIX B

Combination Drugs

Note: The drugs listed in this section are in alphabetical order according to trade names. If the trade name does not specify dose form, the dose form is either a tablet or capsule. Following each trade name are the generic names and doses of the active ingredients contained in each preparation. For information on these drugs, look up each generic name in the combination. For inert ingredients, see drug label. **(OTC)** signifies "over-the-counter" or nonprescription medication.

Acanya Topical Gel—1.2% clindamycin + 2.5% benzoyl peroxide
Accuretic 10/12.5—quinapril 10 mg + hydrochlorothiazide 12.5 mg
Accuretic 20/12.5—quinapril 20 mg + hydrochlorothiazide 12.5 mg
Accuretic 20/25—quinapril 20 mg + hydrochlorothiazide 25 mg
Activella 0.5/0.1—estradiol 0.5 mg + norethindrone 0.1 mg
Activella 1/0.5—estradiol 1 mg + norethindrone 0.5 mg
Actoplus Met 15/500—pioglitazone 15 mg + metformin 500 mg
Actoplus Met 15/850—pioglitazone 15 mg + metformin 850 mg
Advair Diskus 100—(per actuation) fluticasone 100 mcg + salmeterol 50 mcg
Advair Diskus 250—(per actuation) fluticasone 250 mcg + salmeterol 50 mcg
Advair Diskus 500—(per actuation) fluticasone 500 mcg + salmeterol 50 mcg
Advair HFA 45—(per actuation) fluticasone 45 mcg + salmeterol 21 mcg
Advair HFA 115—(per actuation) fluticasone 115 mcg + salmeterol 21 mcg
Advair HFA 230—(per actuation) fluticasone 230 mcg + salmeterol 21 mcg
Advil Allergy & Congestion Relief—phenylephrine 10 mg + ibuprofen 200 mg + chlorpheniramine 4 mg **(OTC)**
Advil Allergy Sinus—pseudoephedrine 30 mg + ibuprofen 200 mg + chlorpheniramine 2 mg **(OTC)**
Advil Cold & Sinus—pseudoephedrine 30 mg + ibuprofen 200 mg **(OTC)**
Advil PM—diphenhydramine citrate 38 mg + ibuprofen 200 mg **(OTC)**
Advil PM Liquigels—diphenhydramine 25 mg + ibuprofen 200 mg **(OTC)**
Advil Sinus Congestion & Pain—phenylephrine 10 mg + ibuprofen 200 mg **(OTC)**
Aggrenox—aspirin 25 mg + extended-release dipyridamole 200 mg
Airduo RespiClick 55—(per actuation) fluticasone 55 mcg + salmeterol 14 mcg
Airduo RespiClick 113—(per actuation) fluticasone 113 mcg + salmeterol 14 mcg
Airduo Respiclick 232—(per actuation) fluticasone 232 mcg + salmeterol 14 mcg
Alavert Allergy and Sinus D-12—loratadine 5 mg + pseudoephedrine 120 mg **(OTC)**
Aldactazide 25/25—hydrochlorothiazide 25 mg + spironolactone 25 mg
Aldactazide 50/50—hydrochlorothiazide 50 mg + spironolactone 50 mg
Aleve-D Sinus & Cold—naproxen 220 mg + extended-release pseudoephedrine 120 mg **(OTC)**
Aleve-D Sinus & Headache—naproxen 220 mg + extended-release pseudoephedrine 120 mg **(OTC)**
Aleve PM—naproxen 220 mg + diphenhydramine 25 mg **(OTC)**
Alka-Seltzer Effervescent, Extra-Strength—citric acid 1000 mg + sodium bicarbonate 1985 mg + aspirin 500 mg **(OTC)**
Alka-Seltzer Effervescent, Original—citric acid 1000 mg + sodium bicarbonate 1916 mg + aspirin 325 mg **(OTC)**
Alka-Seltzer Plus Cold & Cough Effervescent Tablets—dextromethorphan 10 mg + phenylephrine 7.8 mg + chlorpheniramine 2 mg + aspirin 325 mg **(OTC)**
Alka-Seltzer Plus Cold Effervescent Tablets—phenylephrine 7.8 mg + chlorpheniramine 2 mg + aspirin 325 mg **(OTC)**

Alka-Seltzer Plus Cold Night Effervescent Tablets—dextromethorphan 10 mg + phenylephrine 7.8 mg + doxylamine 6.25 mg + aspirin 500 mg **(OTC)**
Alka-Seltzer Plus Day Severe Cold & Flu—(per packet) dextromethorphan 20 mg + phenylephrine 10 mg + acetaminophen 500 mg + guaifenesin 400 mg **(OTC)**
Alka-Seltzer Plus Maximum-Strength Cold & Cough Liquid Gels—dextromethorphan 10 mg + phenylephrine 5 mg + chlorpheniramine 2 mg + acetaminophen 325 mg **(OTC)**
Alka-Seltzer Plus Maximum-Strength Day Cold & Flu Liquid Gels—dextromethorphan 10 mg + phenylephrine 5 mg + acetaminophen 325 mg **(OTC)**
Alka-Seltzer Plus Maximum-Strength Night Cold & Flu Liquid Gels—acetaminophen 325 mg + doxylamine 6.25 mg + dextromethorphan 10 mg + phenylephrine 5 mg **(OTC)**
Alka-Seltzer Plus Maximum-Strength Severe Sinus, Allergy, & Cough Liquid Gels—acetaminophen 325 mg + doxylamine 6.25 mg + dextromethorphan 10 mg + phenylephrine 5 mg **(OTC)**
Alka-Seltzer Plus Severe Cold & Flu Formula Effervescent Tablets—dextromethorphan 10 mg + phenylephrine 5 mg + chlorpheniramine 2 mg + acetaminophen 250 mg **(OTC)**
Alka-Seltzer Plus Severe Cough, Mucus, & Congestion Liquid Gels—dextromethorphan 10 mg + phenylephrine 5 mg + acetaminophen 250 mg + guaifenesin 200 mg **(OTC)**
Alka-Seltzer Plus Severe Sinus Cold & Cough Liquid Gels—dextromethorphan 10 mg + phenylephrine 5 mg + acetaminophen 250 mg + guaifenesin 200 mg **(OTC)**
Allegra-D 12 Hour—fexofenadine 60 mg + extended-release pseudoephedrine 120 mg
Allegra-D 24 Hour—fexofenadine 180 mg + extended-release pseudoephedrine 240 mg
Allzital—acetaminophen 325 mg + butalbital 25 mg
Altavera—levonorgestrel 0.15 mg + ethinyl estradiol 30 mcg
Alyacen 1/35—norethindrone 1 mg + ethinyl estradiol 35 mcg
Alyacen 7/7/7
  Phase I—norethindrone 0.5 mg + ethinyl estradiol 35 mcg
  Phase II—norethindrone 0.75 mg + ethinyl estradiol 35 mcg
  Phase III—norethindrone 1 mg + ethinyl estradiol 35 mcg
Amabelz 0.5/0.1—estradiol 0.5 mg + norethindrone 0.1 mg
Amabelz 1/0.5—estradiol 1 mg + norethindrone 0.5 mg
Amethia—levonorgestrel 0.15 mg + ethinyl estradiol 30 mcg
Amethia Lo—levonorgestrel 0.1 mg + ethinyl estradiol 20 mcg
Amethyst—levonorgestrel 0.09 mg + ethinyl estradiol 20 mcg
Anacin—aspirin 400 mg + caffeine 32 mg **(OTC)**
Anexsia 5/325—hydrocodone 5 mg + acetaminophen 325 mg
Anexsia 7.5/325—hydrocodone 7.5 mg + acetaminophen 325 mg
Angeliq 0.25/0.5—drospirenone 0.25 mg + estradiol 0.5 mg
Angeliq 0.5/1—drospirenone 0.5 mg + estradiol 1 mg
Anoro Ellipta—(per actuation) umeclidinium 62.5 mcg + vilanterol 25 mcg
Apri-28—desogestrel 0.15 mg + ethinyl estradiol 30 mcg
Aranelle
  Phase I—norethindrone 0.5 mg + ethinyl estradiol 35 mcg
  Phase II—norethindrone 1 mg + ethinyl estradiol 35 mcg
  Phase III—norethindrone 0.5 mg + ethinyl estradiol 35 mcg
Arthrotec 50/200—diclofenac 50 mg + misoprostol 200 mcg
Arthrotec 75/200—diclofenac 75 mg + misoprostol 200 mcg
Ashlyna—levonorgestrel 0.15 mg + ethinyl estradiol 30 mcg/10 mcg
Atacand HCT 16/12.5—candesartan 16 mg + hydrochlorothiazide 12.5 mg
Atacand HCT 32/12.5—candesartan 32 mg + hydrochlorothiazide 12.5 mg
Atacand HCT 32/25—candesartan 32 mg + hydrochlorothiazide 25 mg
🍁 **Atacand Plus 16/12.5**—candesartan 16 mg + hydrochlorothiazide 12.5 mg
🍁 **Atacand Plus 32/12.5**—candesartan 32 mg + hydrochlorothiazide 12.5 mg
🍁 **Atacand Plus 32/25**—candesartan 32 mg + hydrochlorothiazide 25 mg
Atripla—efavirenz 600 mg + emtricitabine 200 mg + tenofovir disoproxil fumarate 300 mg
Aubra—levonorgestrel 0.1 mg + ethinyl estradiol 20 mcg

Avalide 150/12.5—irbesartan 150 mg + hydrochlorothiazide 12.5 mg
Avalide 300/12.5—irbesartan 300 mg + hydrochlorothiazide 12.5 mg
Aviane-28—levonorgestrel 0.1 mg + ethinyl estradiol 20 mcg
Azor 5/20—amlodipine 5 mg + olmesartan 20 mg
Azor 5/40—amlodipine 5 mg + olmesartan 40 mg
Azor 10/20—amlodipine 10 mg + olmesartan 20 mg
Azor 10/40—amlodipine 10 mg + olmesartan 40 mg
Azurette—desogestrel 0.15 mg + ethinyl estradiol 20 mcg/10 mcg
Balziva-28—norethindrone 0.4 mg + ethinyl estradiol 35 mcg
Bekyree—desogestrel 0.15 mg + ethinyl estradiol 20 mcg/10 mcg
Benicar HCT 20/12.5—olmesartan 20 mg + hydrochlorothiazide 12.5 mg
Benicar HCT 40/12.5—olmesartan 40 mg + hydrochlorothiazide 12.5 mg
Benicar HCT 40/25—olmesartan 40 mg + hydrochlorothiazide 25 mg
BenzaClin Topical Gel—1% clindamycin + 5% benzoyl peroxide
Benzamycin Topical Gel—5% benzoyl peroxide + 3% erythromycin
Bevespi Aerosphere—(per actuation) glycopyrrolate 9 mcg + formoterol 4.8 mcg
Beyaz
Phase I—drospirenone 3 mg + ethinyl estradiol 20 mcg + levomefolate 0.451 mg
Phase II—levomefolate 0.451 mg
Bicitra Solution—(per 5 ml) sodium citrate 500 mg + citric acid 334 mg
Bidil—isosorbide dinitrate 20 mg + hydralazine 37.5 mg
Bijuva—estradiol 1 mg + progesterone 100 mg
Biktarvy—bictegravir 50 mg + emtricitabine 200 mg + tenofovir alafenamide 25 mg
Blephamide Ophthalmic Suspension/Ointment—0.2% prednisolone + 10% sodium sulfacetamide
Breo Ellipta 100/25—(per blister for inhalation) fluticasone 100 mcg + vilanterol 25 mcg
Breo Ellipta 200/25—(per blister for inhalation) fluticasone 200 mcg + vilanterol 25 mcg
Brevicon-28—norethindrone 0.5 mg + ethinyl estradiol 35 mcg
Briellyn—norethindrone 0.4 mg + ethinyl estradiol 35 mcg
Bromfed DM Liquid—(per 5 mL) brompheniramine 2 mg + dextromethorphan 10 mg + pseudoephedrine 30 mg
Bronkaid Dual Action—ephedrine 25 mg + guaifenesin 400 mg **(OTC)**
Bufferin—aspirin 325 mg + calcium carbonate 158 mg + magnesium oxide 63 mg + magnesium carbonate 34 mg **(OTC)**
Bunavail 2.1/0.3—buprenorphine 2.1 mg + naloxone 0.3 mg
Bunavail 4.2/0.7—buprenorphine 4.2 mg + naloxone 0.7 mg
Bunavail 6.3/1—buprenorphine 6.3 mg + naloxone 1 mg
Caduet 2.5/10—amlodipine 2.5 mg + atorvastatin 10 mg
Caduet 2.5/20—amlodipine 2.5 mg + atorvastatin 20 mg
Caduet 2.5/40—amlodipine 2.5 mg + atorvastatin 40 mg
Caduet 5/10—amlodipine 5 mg + atorvastatin 10 mg
Caduet 5/20—amlodipine 5 mg + atorvastatin 20 mg
Caduet 5/40—amlodipine 5 mg + atorvastatin 40 mg
Caduet 5/80—amlodipine 5 mg + atorvastatin 80 mg
Caduet 10/10—amlodipine 10 mg + atorvastatin 10 mg
Caduet 10/20—amlodipine 10 mg + atorvastatin 20 mg
Caduet 10/40—amlodipine 10 mg + atorvastatin 40 mg
Caduet 10/80—amlodipine 10 mg + atorvastatin 80 mg
Cafergot—ergotamine 1 mg + caffeine 100 mg
Caltrate 600+D$_3$—vitamin D 800 IU + calcium 600 mg **(OTC)**
Caziant
Phase I—desogestrel 0.1 mg + ethinyl estradiol 25 mcg
Phase II—desogestrel 0.125 mg + ethinyl estradiol 25 mcg
Phase III—desogestrel 0.15 mg + ethinyl estradiol 25 mcg
Cetacaine Topical Spray—14% benzocaine + 2% tetracaine + 2% butamben + 0.005% cetyl dimethyl ethyl ammonium bromide

Chateal—levonorgestrel 0.15 mg + ethinyl estradiol 30 mcg

Children's Tylenol Cold + Cough + Runny Nose Suspension—(per 5 mL) acetaminophen 160 mg + dextromethorphan 5 mg + chlorpheniramine 1 mg **(OTC)**

Children's Tylenol Cold + Cough + Sore Throat Suspension—(per 5 mL) acetaminophen 160 mg + dextromethorphan 5 mg **(OTC)**

Children's Tylenol Cold + Flu Suspension—(per 5 mL) acetaminophen 160 mg + dextromethorphan 5 mg + chlorpheniramine 1 mg + phenylephrine 2.5 mg **(OTC)**

Cimduo—lamivudine 300 mg + tenofovir disoproxil fumarate 300 mg

Cipro HC Otic Suspension—0.2% ciprofloxacin + 1% hydrocortisone

Ciprodex Otic Suspension—0.3% ciprofloxacin + 0.1% dexamethasone

Clarinex-D 12 Hour—desloratadine 2.5 mg + pseudoephedrine 120 mg

Clarinex-D 24 Hour—desloratadine 5 mg + pseudoephedrine 240 mg

Claritin-D 12 Hour—loratadine 5 mg + pseudoephedrine 120 mg **(OTC)**

Claritin-D 24-Hour—loratadine 10 mg + pseudoephedrine 240 mg **(OTC)**

Climara Pro Transdermal Patch (release per day)—estradiol 0.045 mg + levonorgestrel 0.015 mg

Col-Probenecid—probenecid 500 mg + colchicine 0.5 mg

Coly-Mycin S Otic Suspension—1% hydrocortisone + 0.33% neomycin base + 0.3% colistin + 0.05% thonzonium bromide

Colyte—PEG 3350 240 g + sodium sulfate 22.72 g + sodium bicarbonate 6.72 g + sodium chloride 5.84 g + potassium chloride 2.98 g

Combigan Ophthalmic Solution—0.2% brimonidine + 0.5% timolol

CombiPatch 0.05/0.14—estradiol 0.05 mg/day + norethindrone 0.14 mg/day

CombiPatch 0.05/0.25—estradiol 0.05 mg/day + norethindrone 0.25 mg/day

Combivent Respimat—(per actuation) ipratropium bromide 20 mcg + albuterol 100 mcg

Combivir—lamivudine 150 mg + zidovudine 300 mg

Complera—emtricitabine 200 mg + rilpivirine 25 mg + tenofovir disoproxil fumarate 300 mg

Consensi 2.5/200—amlodipine 2.5 mg + celecoxib 200 mg

Consensi 5/200—amlodipine 5 mg + celecoxib 200 mg

Consensi 10/200—amlodipine 10 mg + celecoxib 200 mg

Contac Cold & Flu Day Maximum Strength Caplets—phenylephrine 5 mg + acetaminophen 500 mg **(OTC)**

Contac Cold & Flu Night Cooling Relief Liquid—(per 15 mL) doxylamine 6.25 mg + dextromethorphan 15 mg + acetaminophen 500 mg **(OTC)**

Contac Cold & Flu Night Maximum Strength Caplets—chlorpheniramine 2 mg + phenylephrine 5 mg + acetaminophen 500 mg **(OTC)**

Coricidin HBP Chest Congestion & Cough Liquid Gels—dextromethorphan 10 mg + guaifenesin 200 mg **(OTC)**

Coricidin HBP Cold & Flu Tablets—acetaminophen 325 mg + chlorpheniramine 2 mg **(OTC)**

Coricidin HBP Cough & Cold Tablets—chlorpheniramine 4 mg + dextromethorphan 30 mg **(OTC)**

Coricidin HBP Maximum Strength Flu Tablets—acetaminophen 325 mg + chlorpheniramine 2 mg + dextromethorphan 15 mg **(OTC)**

Coricidin HBP Nighttime Multi-Symptom Cold Liquid—(per 15 mL) acetaminophen 325 mg + doxylamine 6.25 mg + dextromethorphan 15 mg **(OTC)**

Cortisporin Topical Cream—(per g) neomycin 3.5 mg + polymyxin B 10,000 units + 0.5% hydrocortisone

Corzide 40/5—nadolol 40 mg + bendroflumethiazide 5 mg

Corzide 80/5—nadolol 80 mg + bendroflumethiazide 5 mg

Cosopt Ophthalmic Solution—2% dorzolamide + 0.5% timolol

Coversyl Plus—perindopril 4 mg + indapamide 1.25 mg

Coversyl Plus HD—perindopril 8 mg + indapamide 2.5 mg

Coversyl Plus LD—perindopril 2 mg + indapamide 0.625 mg

Creon—lipase 3000 units + amylase 15,000 units + protease 9,500 units

Creon—lipase 6000 units + amylase 30,000 units + protease 19,000 units

Creon—lipase 12,000 units + amylase 60,000 units + protease 38,000 units
Creon—lipase 24,000 units + amylase 120,00 units + protease 76,000 units
Creon—lipase 36,000 units + amylase 180,000 units + protease 114,000 units
Cryselle—norgestrel 0.3 mg + ethinyl estradiol 30 mcg
Cyclafem 1/35—norethindrone 1 mg + ethinyl estradiol 35 mcg
Cyclafem 7/7/7
  Phase I—norethindrone 0.5 mg + ethinyl estradiol 35 mcg
  Phase II—norethindrone 0.75 mg + ethinyl estradiol 35 mcg
  Phase III—norethindrone 1 mg + ethinyl estradiol 35 mcg
Cyclessa
  Phase I—desogestrel 0.1 mg + ethinyl estradiol 25 mcg
  Phase II—desogestrel 0.125 mg + ethinyl estradiol 25 mcg
  Phase III—desogestrel 0.15 mg + ethinyl estradiol 25 mcg
Cyclomydril Ophthalmic Solution—0.2% cyclopentolate + 1% phenylephrine
Dasetta 1/35—norethindrone 1 mg + ethinyl estradiol 35 mcg
Dasetta 7/7/7
  Phase I—norethindrone 0.5 mg + ethinyl estradiol 35 mcg
  Phase II—norethindrone 0.75 mg + ethinyl estradiol 35 mcg
  Phase III—norethindrone 1 mg + ethinyl estradiol 35 mcg
Dayquil Cold & Flu Relief LiquiCaps—acetaminophen 325 mg + dextromethorphan 10 mg + phenylephrine 5 mg **(OTC)**
Dayquil Cold & Flu Relief Liquid—(per 15 mL) acetaminophen 325 mg + dextromethorphan 10 mg + phenylephrine 5 mg **(OTC)**
Dayquil Cough & Congestion Liquid—(per 15 mL) dextromethorphan 10 mg + guaifenesin 200 mg **(OTC)**
Dayquil HBP Cold & Flu LiquiCaps—acetaminophen 325 mg + dextromethorphan 10 mg + **(OTC)**
Dayquil Severe Cold & Flu Relief Caplets/LiquiCaps—acetaminophen 325 mg + dextromethorphan 10 mg + guaifenesin 200 mg + phenylephrine 5 mg **(OTC)**
Dayquil Severe Cold & Flu Relief Liquid—(per 15 mL) acetaminophen 325 mg + dextromethorphan 10 mg + guaifenesin 200 mg + phenylephrine 5 mg **(OTC)**
Daysee—levonorgestrel 0.15 mg + ethinyl estradiol 30 mcg/10 mcg
Delstrigo—doravirine 100 mg + lamivudine 300 mg + tenofovir disoproxil fumarate 300 mg
Descovy—emtricitabine 200 mg + tenofovir alafenamide 25 mg
Diclegis—doxylamine 10 mg + pyridoxine 10 mg
Dimetapp Cold & Allergy Syrup—(per 10 mL) phenylephrine 5 mg + brompheniramine 2 mg **(OTC)**
Dimetapp Cold & Cough Syrup—(per 10 mL) phenylephrine 5 mg + brompheniramine 2 mg + dextromethorphan 10 mg **(OTC)**
Dimetapp Multi-Symptom Cold & Flu Syrup—(per 10 mL) acetaminophen 320 mg + diphenhydramine 12.5 mg + phenylephrine 5 mg **(OTC)**
Dimetapp Nighttime Cold & Congestion Syrup—(per 10 mL) diphenhydramine 12.5 mg + phenylephrine 5 mg **(OTC)**
Diovan HCT 80/12.5—valsartan 80 mg + hydrochlorothiazide 12.5 mg
Diovan HCT 160/12.5—valsartan 160 mg + hydrochlorothiazide 12.5 mg
Diovan HCT 160/25—valsartan 160 mg + hydrochlorothiazide 25 mg
Diovan HCT 320/12.5—valsartan 320 mg + hydrochlorothiazide 12.5 mg
Diovan HCT 320/25—valsartan 320 mg + hydrochlorothiazide 25 mg
Donnatal Elixir—(per 5 mL) phenobarbital 16.2 mg + hyoscyamine 0.1037 mg + atropine 0.0194 mg + scopolamine 0.0065 mg + 23% alcohol
Donnatal Tablets—phenobarbital 16.2 mg + hyoscyamine 0.1037 mg + atropine 0.0194 mg + scopolamine 0.0065 mg
Dovato—dolutegravir 50 mg + lamivudine 300 mg
Duac Topical Gel—1.2% clindamycin + 5% benzoyl peroxide
Duaklir Pressair—(per actuation) aclidinium 400 mcg + formoterol 12 mcg
Duavee—conjugated estrogens 0.45 mg + bazedoxifene 20 mg
Duetact 2/30—glimepiride 2 mg + pioglitazone 30 mg

Duetact 4/30—glimepiride 4 mg + pioglitazone 30 mg
Duexis—ibuprofen 800 mg + famotidine 26.6 mg
Dulera 100/5—(per actuation) mometasone 100 mcg + formoterol 5 mcg
Dulera 200/5—(per actuation) mometasone 200 mcg + formoterol 5 mcg
Duobrii Topical Lotion—0.01% halobetasol + 0.04% tazarotene
Dutoprol 12.5/25—hydrochlorothiazide 12.5 mg + metoprolol succinate 25 mg
Dutoprol 12.5/50—hydrochlorothiazide 12.5 mg + metoprolol succinate 50 mg
Dutoprol 12.5/100—hydrochlorothiazide 12.5 mg + metoprolol succinate 100 mg
Dyazide—hydrochlorothiazide 25 mg + triamterene 37.5 mg
Dymista—(per actuation) azelastine 137 mcg + fluticasone 50 mcg
Edarbyclor 40/12.5—azilsartan 40 mg + chlorthalidone 12.5 mg
Edarbyclor 40/25—azilsartan 40 mg + chlorthalidone 25 mg
Elinest—norgestrel 0.3 mg + ethinyl estradiol 30 mcg
Eluryng—etonogestrel 0.12 mg/day + ethinyl estradiol 15 mcg/day
Embeda 20/0.8—morphine sulfate 20 mg + naltrexone 0.8 mg
Embeda 30/1.2—morphine sulfate 30 mg + naltrexone 1.2 mg
Embeda 50/2—morphine sulfate 50 mg + naltrexone 2 mg
Embeda 60/2.4—morphine sulfate 60 mg + naltrexone 2.4 mg
Embeda 80/3.2—morphine sulfate 80 mg + naltrexone 3.2 mg
Embeda 100/4—morphine sulfate 100 mg + naltrexone 4 mg
EMLA Topical Cream—2.5% lidocaine + 2.5% prilocaine
Emoquette—ethinyl estradiol 30 mcg + desogestrel 0.15 mg
Endocet 2.5/325—oxycodone 2.5 mg + acetaminophen 325 mg
Endocet 5/325—oxycodone 5 mg + acetaminophen 325 mg
Endocet 7.5/325—oxycodone 7.5 mg + acetaminophen 325 mg
Endocet 10/325—oxycodone 10 mg + acetaminophen 325 mg
Enpresse-28
  Phase I—levonorgestrel 0.05 mg + ethinyl estradiol 30 mcg
  Phase II—levonorgestrel 0.075 mg + ethinyl estradiol 40 mcg
  Phase III—levonorgestrel 0.125 mg + ethinyl estradiol 30 mcg
Enskyce—desogestrel 0.15 mg + ethinyl estradiol 30 mcg
Enstilar Topical Foam—0.005% calcipotriene + 0.064% betamethasone
Entresto 24/26—sacubitril 24 mg + valsartan 26 mg
Entresto 49/51—sacubitril 49 mg + valsartan 51 mg
Entresto 97/103—sacubitril 97 mg + valsartan 103 mg
Epiduo Forte Topical Gel—0.3% adapalene + 2.5% benzoyl peroxide
Epiduo Topical Gel—0.1% adapalene + 2.5% benzoyl peroxide
Epifoam Aerosol Foam—1% hydrocortisone + 1% pramoxine
Epzicom—abacavir 600 mg + lamivudine 300 mg
Estarylla—norgestimate 0.25 mg + ethinyl estradiol 35 mcg
Estrostep Fe
  Phase I—norethindrone 1 mg + ethinyl estradiol 20 mcg
  Phase II—norethindrone 1 mg + ethinyl estradiol 30 mcg
  Phase III—norethindrone 1 mg + ethinyl estradiol 35 mcg
  Phase IV—ferrous fumarate 75 mg
Evotaz—atazanavir 300 mg + cobicstat 150 mg
Excedrin Extra Strength Caplets—acetaminophen 250 mg + aspirin 250 mg + caffeine 65 mg **(OTC)**
Excedrin Migraine Caplets—aspirin 250 mg + acetaminophen 250 mg + caffeine 65 mg **(OTC)**
Excedrin P.M. Headache Caplets—acetaminophen 250 mg + aspirin 250 mg + diphenhydramine citrate 38 mg **(OTC)**
Excedrin Tension Headache Caplets—acetaminophen 500 mg + caffeine 65 mg **(OTC)**
Exforge 5/160—amlodipine 5 mg + valsartan 160 mg
Exforge 5/320—amlodipine 5 mg + valsartan 320 mg
Exforge 10/160—amlodipine 10 mg + valsartan 160 mg
Exforge 10/320—amlodipine 10 mg + valsartan 320 mg

Exforge HCT 5/160/12.5—amlodipine 5 mg + valsartan 160 mg + hydrochlorothiazide 12.5 mg
Exforge HCT 5/160/25—amlodipine 5 mg + valsartan 160 mg + hydrochlorothiazide 25 mg
Exforge HCT 10/160/12.5—amlodipine 10 mg + valsartan 160 mg + hydrochlorothiazide 12.5 mg
Exforge HCT 10/160/25—amlodipine 10 mg + valsartan 160 mg + hydrochlorothiazide 25 mg
Exforge HCT 10/320/25—amlodipine 10 mg + valsartan 320 mg + hydrochlorothiazide 25 mg
Falmina—levonorgestrel 0.1 mg + ethinyl estradiol 20 mcg
Femhrt 0.5/2.5—norethindrone 0.5 mg + ethinyl estradiol 2.5 mcg
Femhrt 1/5—norethindrone 1 mg + ethinyl estradiol 5 mcg
Fioricet—acetaminophen 300 mg + caffeine 40 mg + butalbital 50 mg
Fioricet with Codeine—acetaminophen 300 mg + caffeine 40 mg + butalbital 50 mg + codeine 30 mg
Fiorinal—aspirin 325 mg + caffeine 40 mg + butalbital 50 mg
Fiorinal with Codeine—aspirin 325 mg + caffeine 40 mg + butalbital 50 mg + codeine 30 mg
Fosamax Plus D 70/2800—alendronate 70 mg + cholecalciferol 2800 IU
Fosamax Plus D 70/5600—alendronate 70 mg + cholecalciferol 5600 IU
Gaviscon Extra Strength Liquid—(per 5 mL) aluminum hydroxide 254 mg + magnesium carbonate 237.5 mg **(OTC)**
Gaviscon Extra Strength Tablets—magnesium carbonate 105 mg + aluminum hydroxide 160 mg **(OTC)**
Gaviscon Regular Strength Liquid—(per 15 mL) aluminum hydroxide 95 mg + magnesium carbonate 358 mg **(OTC)**
Gaviscon Regular Strength Tablets—magnesium trisilicate 14.2 mg + aluminum hydroxide 80 mg **(OTC)**
Gelusil—aluminum hydroxide 200 mg + magnesium hydroxide 200 mg + simethicone 25 mg **(OTC)**
Generess Fe—norethindrone 0.8 mg + ethinyl estradiol 25 mcg + ferrous fumarate 75 mg
Genvoya—elvitegravir 150 mg + cobicistat 150 mg + emtricitabine 200 mg + tenofovir alafenamide 10 mg
Gianvi—drospirenone 3 mg + ethinyl estradiol 20 mcg
Gildagia—norethindrone 0.4 mg + ethinyl estradiol 35 mcg
Gildess 1/20—norethindrone 1 mg + ethinyl estradiol 20 mcg
Gildess Fe 1/20—norethindrone 1 mg + ethinyl estradiol 20 mcg + ferrous fumarate 75 mg
Gildess 1.5/30—norethindrone 1.5 mg + ethinyl estradiol 30 mcg
Gildess Fe 1.5/30—norethindrone 1.5 mg + ethinyl estradiol 30 mcg + ferrous fumarate 75 mg
Glyxambi 10/5—empagliflozin 10 mg + linagliptin 5 mg
Glyxambi 25/5—empagliflozin 25 mg + linagliptin 5 mg
Golytely—PEG 3350 236 g + sodium sulfate 22.74 g + sodium bicarbonate 6.74 g + sodium chloride 5.86 g + potassium chloride 2.97 g
Golytely Packets—PEG 3350 227.1 g + sodium sulfate 21.5 g + sodium bicarbonate 6.36 g + sodium chloride 5.53 g + potassium chloride 2.82 g
Hyzaar 50/12.5—losartan 50 mg + hydrochlorothiazide 12.5 mg
Hyzaar 100/12.5—losartan 100 mg + hydrochlorothiazide 12.5 mg
Hyzaar 100/25—losartan 100 mg + hydrochlorothiazide 25 mg
Imodium Multi-Symptom Relief—loperamide 2 mg + simethicone 125 mg **(OTC)**
Introvale—levonorgestrel 0.15 mg + ethinyl estradiol 30 mcg
Invokamet 50/500—canagliflozin 50 mg + metformin 500 mg
Invokamet 50/1000—canagliflozin 50 mg + metformin 1000 mg
Invokamet 150/500—canagliflozin 150 mg + metformin 500 mg
Invokamet 150/1000—canagliflozin 150 mg + metformin 1000 mg
Invokamet XR 50/500—canagliflozin 50 mg + metformin extended-release 500 mg
Invokamet XR 50/1000—canagliflozin 50 mg + metformin extended-release 1000 mg
Invokamet XR 150/500—canagliflozin 150 mg + metformin extended-release 500 mg
Invokamet XR 150/1000—canagliflozin 150 mg + metformin extended-release 1000 mg
Isibloom—desogestrel 0.15 mg + ethinyl estradiol 30 mcg
IsonaRif—isoniazid 150 mg + rifampin 300 mg
Jalyn—dutasteride 0.5 mg + tamsulosin 0.4 mg

Janumet 50/500—sitagliptin 50 mg + metformin 500 mg
Janumet 50/1000—sitagliptin 50 mg + metformin 1000 mg
Janumet XR 50/500—sitagliptin 50 mg + metformin extended-release 500 mg
Janumet XR 50/1000—sitagliptin 50 mg + metformin extended-release 1000 mg
Janumet XR 100/1000—sitagliptin 100 mg + metformin extended-release 500 mg
Jentadueto 2.5/500—linagliptin 2.5 mg + metformin 500 mg
Jentadueto 2.5/850—linagliptin 2.5 mg + metformin 850 mg
Jentadueto 2.5/1000—linagliptin 2.5 mg + metformin 1000 mg
Jentadueto XR 2.5/1000—linagliptin 2.5 mg + metformin extended-release 1000 mg
Jentadueto XR 5/1000—linagliptin 5 mg + metformin extended-release 1000 mg
Jinteli—norethindrone 1 mg + ethinyl estradiol 5 mcg
Jolessa—levonorgestrel 0.15 mg + ethinyl estradiol 30 mcg
Juluca—dolutegravir 50 mg + rilpivirine 25 mg
Junel 1/20—norethindrone 1 mg + ethinyl estradiol 20 mcg
Junel 1.5/30—norethindrone 1.5 mg + ethinyl estradiol 30 mcg
Junel Fe 1/20—norethindrone 1 mg + ethinyl estradiol 20 mcg + ferrous fumarate 75 mg
Junel Fe 1.5/30—norethindrone 1.5 mg + ethinyl estradiol 30 mcg + ferrous fumarate 75 mg
Kariva—desogestrel 0.15 mg + ethinyl estradiol 20 mcg/10 mcg
Kazano 12.5/500—alogliptin 12.5 mg + metformin 500 mg
Kazano 12.5/1000—alogliptin 12.5 mg + metformin 1000 mg
Kelnor 1/35—ethynodiol 1 mg + ethinyl estradiol 35 mcg
Kelnor 1/50—ethynodiol 1 mg + ethinyl estradiol 50 mcg
Kimidess—desogestrel 0.15 mg + ethinyl estradiol 20 mcg/10 mcg
Kombiglyze XR 2.5/1000—saxagliptin 2.5 mg + metformin extended-release 1000 mg
Kombiglyze XR 5/500—saxagliptin 5 mg + metformin extended-release 500 mg
Kombiglyze XR 5/1000—saxagliptin 5 mg + metformin extended-release 1000 mg
Kurvelo—levonorgestrel 0.15 mg + ethinyl estradiol 30 mcg
Lactinex—mixed culture of *Lactobacillus acidophilus* and *L. bulgaricus* **(OTC)**
Larin 1/20—norethindrone 1 mg + ethinyl estradiol 20 mcg
Larin 1.5/30—norethindrone 1.5 mg + ethinyl estradiol 30 mcg
Larin Fe 1/20—norethindrone 1 mg + ethinyl estradiol 20 mcg + ferrous fumarate 75 mg
Larin Fe 1.5/30—norethindrone 1.5 mg + ethinyl estradiol 30 mcg + ferrous fumarate 75 mg
Leena
  Phase I—norethindrone 0.5 mg + ethinyl estradiol 35 mcg
  Phase II—norethindrone 1 mg + ethinyl estradiol 35 mcg
  Phase III—norethindrone 0.5 mg + ethinyl estradiol 35 mcg
Lessina-28—levonorgestrel 0.1 mg + ethinyl estradiol 20 mcg
Levonest
  Phase I—levonorgestrel 0.05 mg + ethinyl estradiol 30 mcg
  Phase II—levonorgestrel 0.075 mg + ethinyl estradiol 40 mcg
  Phase III—levonorgestrel 0.125 mg + ethinyl estradiol 30 mcg
Levora-28—levonorgestrel 0.15 mg + ethinyl estradiol 30 mcg
Librax—clidinium 2.5 mg + chlordiazepoxide 5 mg
Loestrin 21 1/20—norethindrone 1 mg + ethinyl estradiol 20 mcg
Loestrin 21 1.5/30—norethindrone 1.5 mg + ethinyl estradiol 30 mcg
Loestrin Fe 1/20—norethindrone 1 mg + ethinyl estradiol 20 mcg with 7 tablets of ferrous fumarate 75 mg per container
Loestrin Fe 1.5/30—norethindrone 1.5 mg + ethinyl estradiol 30 mcg with 7 tablets of ferrous fumarate 75 mg per container
Lo Loestrin Fe
  Phase I—norethindrone 1 mg + ethinyl estradiol 10 mcg
  Phase II—ethinyl estradiol 10 mcg
  Phase III—ferrous fumarate 75 mg
Lopressor HCT 50/25—metoprolol tartrate 50 mg + hydrochlorothiazide 25 mg
Lopressor HCT 100/25—metoprolol tartrate 100 mg + hydrochlorothiazide 25 mg

Lorcet—hydrocodone 5 mg + acetaminophen 325 mg
Lorcet HD—hydrocodone 10 mg + acetaminophen 325 mg
Lorcet Plus—hydrocodone 7.5 mg + acetaminophen 325 mg
Loryna—drospirenone 3 mg + ethinyl estradiol 20 mcg
LoSeasonique—levonorgestrel 0.1 mg + ethinyl estradiol 20 mcg
Lotensin HCT 10/12.5—benazepril 10 mg + hydrochlorothiazide 12.5 mg
Lotensin HCT 20/12.5—benazepril 20 mg + hydrochlorothiazide 12.5 mg
Lotensin HCT 20/25—benazepril 20 mg + hydrochlorothiazide 25 mg
Lotrel 2.5/10—amlodipine 2.5 mg + benazepril 10 mg
Lotrel 5/10—amlodipine 5 mg + benazepril 10 mg
Lotrel 5/20—amlodipine 5 mg + benazepril 20 mg
Lotrel 5/40—amlodipine 5 mg + benazepril 40 mg
Lotrel 10/20—amlodipine 10 mg + benazepril 20 mg
Lotrel 10/40—amlodipine 10 mg + benazepril 40 mg
Lotrisone Topical Cream/Lotion—0.05% betamethasone + 1% clotrimazole
Low-Ogestrel-28—norgestrel 0.3 mg + ethinyl estradiol 30 mcg
Lutera—levonorgestrel 0.1 mg + ethinyl estradiol 20 mcg
Malarone—atovaquone 250 mg + proguanil 100 mg
Malarone Pediatric—atovaquone 62.5 mg + proguanil 25 mg
Marlissa—levonorgestrel 0.15 mg + ethinyl estradiol 30 mcg
Maxitrol Ophthalmic Suspension/Ointment—(per g) neomycin 3.5 mg + 0.1% dexamethasone + polymyxin B 10,000 units
Maxzide—hydrochlorothiazide 50 mg + triamterene 75 mg
Maxzide-25—hydrochlorothiazide 25 mg + triamterene 37.5 mg
Micardis HCT 40/12.5—telmisartan 40 mg + hydrochlorothiazide 12.5 mg
Micardis HCT 80/12.5—telmisartan 80 mg + hydrochlorothiazide 12.5 mg
Micardis HCT 80/25—telmisartan 80 mg + hydrochlorothiazide 25 mg
Microgestin 1/20—norethindrone 1 mg + ethinyl estradiol 20 mcg
Microgestin 1.5/30—norethindrone 1.5 mg + ethinyl estradiol 30 mcg
Microgestin Fe 1/20—norethindrone 1 mg + ethinyl estradiol 20 mcg + ferrous fumarate 75 mg
Microgestin Fe 1.5/30—norethindrone 1.5 mg + ethinyl estradiol 30 mcg + ferrous fumarate 75 mg
Midol Caplets—acetaminophen 500 mg + pamabrom 25 mg **(OTC)**
Midol Complete Caplets—acetaminophen 500 mg + caffeine 60 mg + pyrilamine 15 mg **(OTC)**
Migergot Suppositories—ergotamine 2 mg + caffeine 100 mg
Minastrin 24 Fe—norethindrone 1 mg + ethinyl estradiol 20 mcg + ferrous fumarate 75 mg
Mono-Linyah—norgestimate 0.25 mg + ethinyl estradiol 35 mcg
Mononessa—norgestimate 0.25 mg + ethinyl estradiol 35 mcg
Motrin PM—ibuprofen 200 mg + diphenhydramine 38 mg **(OTC)**
Moviprep—PEG 3350 100 g + sodium sulfate 7.5 g + sodium chloride 2.69 g + potassium chloride 1.02 g
Mucinex Cold, Cough, & Sore Throat Liquid for Children—(per 10 mL) acetaminophen 325 mg + guaifenesin 200 mg + dextromethorphan 10 mg + phenylephrine 5 mg **(OTC)**
Mucinex Congestion & Cough Liquid for Children—(per 5 mL) guaifenesin 100 mg + dextromethorphan 5 mg + phenylephrine 2.5 mg **(OTC)**
Mucinex Cough Liquid for Children—(per 5 mL) guaifenesin 100 mg + dextromethorphan 5 mg **(OTC)**
Mucinex Cough Mini-Melts—guaifenesin 100 mg + dextromethorphan 5 mg **(OTC)**
Mucinex D Maximum Strength Tablets—guaifenesin 1200 mg + pseudoephedrine 120 mg **(OTC)**
Mucinex D Tablets—guaifenesin 600 mg + pseudoephedrine 60 mg **(OTC)**
Mucinex DM Maximum Strength Tablets—guaifenesin 1200 mg + dextromethorphan 60 mg **(OTC)**
Mucinex DM Tablets—guaifenesin 600 mg + dextromethorphan 30 mg **(OTC)**
Mucinex Maximum Strength Fast-Max Cold, Flu, & Sore Throat Caplets/Liquid Gels—acetaminophen 325 mg + guaifenesin 200 mg + dextromethorphan 10 mg + phenylephrine 5 mg **(OTC)**

Mucinex Maximum Strength Fast-Max Cold, Flu, & Sore Throat Liquid—(per 20 mL) acetaminophen 650 mg + guaifenesin 400 mg + dextromethorphan 20 mg + phenylephrine 10 mg **(OTC)**
Mucinex Maximum Strength Fast-Max Congestion & Headache Caplets/Liquid Gels—acetaminophen 325 mg + guaifenesin 200 mg + phenylephrine 5 mg **(OTC)**
Mucinex Maximum Strength Fast-Max Congestion & Headache Liquid—(per 20 mL) acetaminophen 325 mg + guaifenesin 200 mg + phenylephrine 5 mg **(OTC)**
Mucinex Maximum Strength Fast-Max DM Max Liquid—(per 20 mL) guaifenesin 400 mg + dextromethorphan 20 mg **(OTC)**
Mucinex Maximum Strength Fast-Max Night Time Cold & Flu Caplets—acetaminophen 325 mg + diphenhydramine 25 mg + phenylephrine 5 mg **(OTC)**
Mucinex Maximum Strength Fast-Max Night Time Cold & Flu Liquid—(per 20 mL) acetaminophen 650 mg + diphenhydramine 25 mg + phenylephrine 10 mg **(OTC)**
Mucinex Maximum Strength Fast-Max Severe Congestion & Cough Caplets—guaifenesin 200 mg + dextromethorphan 10 mg + phenylephrine 5 mg **(OTC)**
Mucinex Maximum Strength Fast-Max Severe Congestion & Cough Liquid—(per 20 mL) guaifenesin 400 mg + dextromethorphan 20 mg + phenylephrine 10 mg **(OTC)**
Mucinex Maximum Strength Sinus-Max Night Time Congestion & Cough Liquid—(per 20 mL) acetaminophen 650 mg + diphenhydramine 25 mg + phenylephrine 10 mg **(OTC)**
Mucinex Maximum Strength Sinus-Max Pressure & Pain Caplets—acetaminophen 325 mg + guaifenesin 200 mg + phenylephrine 5 mg **(OTC)**
Mucinex Maximum Strength Sinus-Max Severe Congestion Relief Caplets/Liquid Gels—acetaminophen 325 mg + guaifenesin 200 mg + phenylephrine 5 mg **(OTC)**
Mucinex Maximum Strength Sinus-Max Severe Congestion Relief Liquid—(per 20 mL) acetaminophen 650 mg + guaifenesin 400 mg + phenylephrine 10 mg **(OTC)**
Mucinex Multi-Symptom Cold & Fever Liquid for Children—(per 10 mL) acetaminophen 325 mg + guaifenesin 200 mg + dextromethorphan 10 mg + phenylephrine 5 mg **(OTC)**
Mucinex Multi-Symptom Cold Liquid for Children—(per 5 mL) guaifenesin 100 mg + dextromethorphan 5 mg + phenylephrine 2.5 mg **(OTC)**
Mucinex Night Time Multi-Symptom Cold Liquid for Children—(per 10 mL) acetaminophen 325 mg + diphenhydramine 12.5 mg + phenylephrine 5 mg **(OTC)**
Mucinex Stuffy Nose & Cold Liquid for Children—(per 5 mL) guaifenesin 100 mg + phenylephrine 2.5 mg **(OTC)**
Myzilra
  Phase I—levonorgestrel 0.05 mg + ethinyl estradiol 30 mcg
  Phase II—levonorgestrel 0.075 mg + ethinyl estradiol 40 mcg
  Phase III—levonorgestrel 0.125 mg + ethinyl estradiol 30 mcg
Namzaric 7/10—memantine extended-release 7 mg + donepezil 10 mg
Namzaric 14/10—memantine extended-release 14 mg + donepezil 10 mg
Namzaric 21/10—memantine extended-release 21 mg + donepezil 10 mg
Namzaric 28/10—memantine extended-release 28 mg + donepezil 10 mg
Natazia
  Phase I—estradiol valerate 3 mg
  Phase II—estradiol valerate 2 mg + dienogest 2 mg
  Phase III—estradiol valerate 2 mg + dienogest 3 mg
  Phase IV—estradiol valerate 1 mg
Necon 0.5/35—norethindrone 0.5 mg + ethinyl estradiol 35 mcg
Necon 1/35—norethindrone 1 mg + ethinyl estradiol 35 mcg
Necon 7/7/7
  Phase I—norethindrone 0.5 mg + ethinyl estradiol 35 mcg
  Phase II—norethindrone 0.75 mg + ethinyl estradiol 35 mcg
  Phase III—norethindrone 1 mg + ethinyl estradiol 35 mcg
Neo-Synalar Topical Cream—0.35% neomycin + 0.025% fluocinolone
Neosporin Antibiotic Topical Ointment—(per g) neomycin 3.5 mg + bacitracin 400 units + polymyxin B 5000 units **(OTC)**
Neosporin G.U. Irrigant—(per mL) neomycin 40 mg + polymyxin B 200,000 units

Neosporin + Pain Relief Antibiotic Topical Cream—(per g) neomycin 3.5 mg + polymyxin B 10,000 units + pramoxine 10 mg **(OTC)**
Neosporin + Pain Relief Antibiotic Topical Ointment—(per g) neomycin 3.5 mg + polymyxin B 10,000 units + bacitracin 500 units + pramoxine 10 mg **(OTC)**
Nikki—drospirenone 3 mg + ethinyl estradiol 20 mcg
Norco 5/325—hydrocodone 5 mg + acetaminophen 325 mg
Norco 7.5/325—hydrocodone 7.5 mg + acetaminophen 325 mg
Norco 10/325—hydrocodone 10 mg + acetaminophen 325 mg
Norinyl 1/35—norethindrone 1 mg + ethinyl estradiol 35 mcg
Nortrel 0.5/35—norethindrone 0.5 mg + ethinyl estradiol 35 mcg
Nortrel 1/35—norethindrone 1 mg + ethinyl estradiol 35 mcg
Nortrel 7/7/7
Phase I—norethindrone 0.5 mg + ethinyl estradiol 35 mcg
Phase II—norethindrone 0.75 mg + ethinyl estradiol 35 mcg
Phase III—norethindrone 1 mg + ethinyl estradiol 35 mcg
Nuedexta—dextromethorphan 20 mg + quinidine sulfate 10 mg
NuLytely—PEG 3350 420 g + sodium bicarbonate 5.72 g + sodium chloride 11.2 g + potassium chloride 1.48 g
Nuvaring—etonogestrel 0.12 mg/day + ethinyl estradiol 15 mcg/day
Nyquil Cold & Flu Nighttime Relief Liquicaps—acetaminophen 325 mg + dextromethorphan 15 mg + doxylamine 6.25 mg **(OTC)**
Nyquil Cold & Flu Nighttime Relief Liquid—(per 30 mL) acetaminophen 650 mg + dextromethorphan 30 mg + doxylamine 12.5 mg **(OTC)**
Nyquil Cough Suppressant Liquid—(per 30 mL) dextromethorphan 30 mg + doxylamine 12.5 mg **(OTC)**
Nyquil HBP Cold & Flu Liquid—(per 30 mL) acetaminophen 650 mg + dextromethorphan 30 mg + doxylamine 12.5 mg **(OTC)**
Nyquil Severe Cold & Flu Nighttime Relief Liquicaps— acetaminophen 325 mg + dextromethorphan 10 mg + doxylamine 6.25 mg + phenylephrine 5 mg **(OTC)**
Nyquil Severe Cold & Flu Nighttime Relief Liquid—(per 30 mL) acetaminophen 650 mg + dextromethorphan 20 mg + doxylamine 12.5 mg + phenylephrine 10 mg **(OTC)**
Nyquil Severe Vapocool Nighttime Cough, Cold, & Flu Relief Caplets—acetaminophen 325 mg + dextromethorphan 10 mg + doxylamine 6.25 mg + phenylephrine 5 mg **(OTC)**
Nyquil Severe Vapocool Nighttime Cough, Cold, & Flu Relief Liquid—(per 30 mL) acetaminophen 650 mg + dextromethorphan 20 mg + doxylamine 12.5 mg + phenylephrine 10 mg **(OTC)**
Ocella—drospirenone 3 mg + ethinyl estradiol 30 mcg
Odefsey—emtricitabine 200 mg + rilpivirine 25 mg + tenofovir alafenamide 25 mg
Ogestrel-28—norgestrel 0.5 mg + ethinyl estradiol 50 mcg
Onexton Topical Gel—1.2% clindamycin + 3.75% benzoyl peroxide
Opcon-A Ophthalmic Solution—0.027% naphazoline + 0.3% pheniramine **(OTC)**
Oraqix Periodontal Gel—2.5% lidocaine + 2.5% prilocaine
Orsythia—levonorgestrel 0.1 mg + ethinyl estradiol 20 mcg
Ortho-Novum 1/35—norethindrone 1 mg + ethinyl estradiol 35 mcg
Ortho-Novum 7/7/7
Phase I—norethindrone 0.5 mg + ethinyl estradiol 35 mcg
Phase II—norethindrone 0.75 mg + ethinyl estradiol 35 mcg
Phase III—norethindrone 1 mg + ethinyl estradiol 35 mcg
Ortho Tri-Cyclen-28
Phase I—norgestimate 0.18 mg + ethinyl estradiol 35 mcg
Phase II—norgestimate 0.215 mg + ethinyl estradiol 35 mcg
Phase III—norgestimate 0.25 mg + ethinyl estradiol 35 mcg
Ortho Tri-Cyclen Lo
Phase I—norgestimate 0.18 mg + ethinyl estradiol 25 mcg
Phase II—norgestimate 0.215 mg + ethinyl estradiol 25 mcg
Phase III—norgestimate 0.25 mg + ethinyl estradiol 25 mcg

Oseni 12.5/15—alogliptin 12.5 mg + pioglitazone 15 mg
Oseni 12.5/30—alogliptin 12.5 mg + pioglitazone 30 mg
Oseni 12.5/45—alogliptin 12.5 mg + pioglitazone 45 mg
Oseni 25/15—alogliptin 25 mg + pioglitazone 15 mg
Oseni 25/30—alogliptin 25 mg + pioglitazone 30 mg
Oseni 25/45—alogliptin 25 mg + pioglitazone 45 mg
Otovel Otic Solution—0.3% ciprofloxacin + 0.025% fluocinolone
Oxycet—oxycodone 5 mg + acetaminophen 325 mg
Pamprin Maximum Strength Max—acetaminophen 250 mg + aspirin 250 mg + caffeine 65 mg **(OTC)**
Pamprin Maximum Strength Multi-Symptom—acetaminophen 500 mg + pamabrom 25 mg + pyrilamine 15 mg **(OTC)**
Pancreaze—lipase 2600 units + amylase 10,850 units + protease 6200 units
Pancreaze—lipase 4200 units + amylase 24,600 units + protease 14,200 units
Pancreaze—lipase 10,500 units + amylase 61,500 units + protease 35,500 units
Pancreaze—lipase 16,800 units + amylase 98,400 units + protease 56,800 units
Pancreaze—lipase 21,000 units + amylase 54,700 units + protease 83,900 units
Pediacare Children's Cough & Congestion Liquid—(per 5 mL) dextromethorphan 5 mg + guaifenesin 100 mg **(OTC)**
Pediacare Children's Cough & Runny Nose Liquid—(per 5 mL) acetaminophen 160 mg + chlorpheniramine 1 mg + dextromethorphan 5 mg **(OTC)**
Pediacare Children's Multi-Symptom Cold Liquid—(per 5 mL) acetaminophen 160 mg + chlorpheniramine 1 mg + phenylephrine 2.5 mg + dextromethorphan 5 mg **(OTC)**
Pepcid Complete—calcium carbonate 800 mg + magnesium hydroxide 165 mg + famotidine 10 mg **(OTC)**
Percocet 2.5/325—oxycodone 2.5 mg + acetaminophen 325 mg
Percocet 5/325—oxycodone 5 mg + acetaminophen 325 mg
Percocet 7.5/325—oxycodone 7.5 mg + acetaminophen 325 mg
Percocet 10/325—oxycodone 10 mg + acetaminophen 325 mg
Percodan—oxycodone 4.84 mg + aspirin 325 mg
Peri-Colace—docusate sodium 50 mg + sennosides 8.6 mg **(OTC)**
Pertyze—lipase 4000 units + amylase 15,125 units +protease 14,375 units
Pertyze—lipase 8000 units + amylase 30,250 units +protease 28,750 units
Pertyze—lipase 16,000 units + amylase 60,500 units +protease 57,500 units
Pertyze—lipase 24,000 units + amylase 90,750 units +protease 86,250 units
Philith—norethindrone 0.4 mg + ethinyl estradiol 35 mcg
Pimtrea—desogestrel 0.15 mg + ethinyl estradiol 20 mcg/10 mcg
Pirmella 1/35—norethindrone 1 mg + ethinyl estradiol 35 mcg
Pirmella 7/7/7
- **Phase I**—norethindrone 0.5 mg + ethinyl estradiol 35 mcg
- **Phase II**—norethindrone 0.75 mg + ethinyl estradiol 35 mcg
- **Phase III**—norethindrone 1 mg + ethinyl estradiol 35 mcg

Pliaglis Topical Cream—7% lidocaine + 7% tetracaine
Polysporin Topical Ointment—(per g) polymyxin B 10,000 units + bacitracin 500 units **(OTC)**
Polytrim Ophthalmic Solution—(per mL) polymyxin B 10,000 units + trimethoprim 1 mg
Portia-28—levonorgestrel 0.15 mg + ethinyl estradiol 30 mcg
Pramosone Topical Cream 1/0.5—1% pramoxine + 0.5% hydrocortisone
Pramosone Topical Cream/Lotion 1/1—1% pramoxine + 1% hydrocortisone
Pramosone Topical Cream/Lotion 1/2.5—1% pramoxine + 2.5% hydrocortisone
PrandiMet 1/500—repaglinide 1 mg + metformin 500 mg
PrandiMet 2/500—repaglinide 2 mg + metformin 500 mg
Pred G Ophthalmic Ointment—0.6% prednisolone + 0.3% gentamicin
Pred G Ophthalmic Suspension—1% prednisolone + 0.3% gentamicin
Premphase—conjugated estrogens 0.625 mg + medroxyprogesterone 5 mg (14 tablets) plus conjugated estrogens 0.625 mg (14 tablets) in a compliance package

Prempro 0.3/1.5—conjugated estrogens 0.3 mg + medroxyprogesterone 1.5 mg
Prempro 0.45/1.5—conjugated estrogens 0.45 mg + medroxyprogesterone 1.5 mg
Prempro 0.625/2.5—conjugated estrogens 0.625 mg + medroxyprogesterone 2.5 mg
Prempro 0.625/5—conjugated estrogens 0.625 mg + medroxyprogesterone 5 mg
Prestalia 3.5/2.5—perindopril 3.5 mg + amlodipine 2.5 mg
Prestalia 7/5—perindopril 7 mg + amlodipine 5 mg
Prestalia 14/10—perindopril 14 mg + amlodipine 10 mg
Previfem—norgestimate 0.25 mg + ethinyl estradiol 35 mcg
Prevpac—amoxicillin 500-mg capsules + clarithromycin 500-mg tablets + lansoprazole 30-mg capsules in a compliance package
Prezcobix—darunavir 800 mg + cobicistat 150 mg
Primatene—ephedrine 12.5 mg + guaifenesin 200 mg **(OTC)**
Primlev 5/300—oxycodone 5 mg + acetaminophen 300 mg
Primlev 7.5/300—oxycodone 7.5 mg + acetaminophen 300 mg
Primlev 10/300—oxycodone 10 mg + acetaminophen 300 mg
Proctofoam-HC Rectal Foam—1% hydrocortisone + 1% pramoxine
Pylera—bismuth subcitrate potassium 140 mg + metronidazole 125 mg + tetracycline 125 mg
Qsymia 3.75/23—phentermine 3.75 mg + extended-release topiramate 23 mg
Qsymia 7.5/46—phentermine 7.5 mg + extended-release topiramate 46 mg
Qsymia 11.25/69—phentermine 11.25 mg + extended-release topiramate 69 mg
Qsymia 15/92—phentermine 15 mg + extended-release topiramate 92 mg
Qtern 5/5—dapagliflozin 5 mg + saxagliptin 5 mg
Qtern 10/5—dapagliflozin 10 mg + saxagliptin 5 mg
Qternmet XR 2.5/1000/2.5—dapagliflozin 2.5 mg + metformin extended-release 1000 mg + saxagliptin 2.5 mg
Qternmet XR 5/1000/2.5—dapagliflozin 5 mg + metformin extended-release 1000 mg + saxagliptin 2.5 mg
Qternmet XR 5/1000/5—dapagliflozin 5 mg + metformin extended-release 1000 mg + saxagliptin 5 mg
Qternmet XR 10/1000/5—dapagliflozin 10 mg + metformin extended-release 1000 mg + saxagliptin 5 mg
Quartette
  Phase I—levonorgestrel 0.15 mg + ethinyl estradiol 20 mcg
  Phase II—levonorgestrel 0.15 mg + ethinyl estradiol 25 mcg
  Phase III—levonorgestrel 0.15 mg + ethinyl estradiol 30 mcg
  Phase IV—ethinyl estradiol 10 mcg
Quasense—levonorgestrel 0.15 mg + ethinyl estradiol 30 mcg
Quinaretic 10/12.5—quinapril 10 mg + hydrochlorothiazide 12.5 mg
Quinaretic 20/12.5—quinapril 20 mg + hydrochlorothiazide 12.5 mg
Quinaretic 20/25—quinapril 20 mg + hydrochlorothiazide 25 mg
Reclipsen—desogestrel 0.15 mg + ethinyl estradiol 30 mcg
Reprexain 2.5/200—hydrocodone 2.5 mg + ibuprofen 200 mg
Reprexain 10/200—hydrocodone 10 mg + ibuprofen 200 mg
RID Lice Killing Shampoo—0.33% pyrethrins + 4% piperonyl butoxide **(OTC)**
Rifamate—isoniazid 150 mg + rifampin 300 mg
Rifater—rifampin 120 mg + isoniazid 50 mg + pyrazinamide 300 mg
🍁 **Robaxacet**—methocarbamol 400 mg + acetaminophen 325 mg **(OTC)**
🍁 **Robaxacet Extra Strength**—methocarbamol 400 mg + acetaminophen 500 mg **(OTC)**
Robitussin Children's Cough & Chest Congestion DM Liquid—(per 5 mL) guaifenesin 100 mg + dextromethorphan 5 mg **(OTC)**
Robitussin Children's Cough & Cold CF Liquid—(per 10 mL) guaifenesin 100 mg + phenylephrine 5 mg + dextromethorphan 10 mg **(OTC)**
Robitussin Children's Cough & Cold Long-Acting Liquid—(per 10 mL) chlorpheniramine 2 mg + dextromethorphan 15 mg **(OTC)**

Robitussin Children's Nighttime Cough Long-Acting DM Liquid—(per 10 mL) chlorpheniramine 2 mg + dextromethorphan 15 mg **(OTC)**
Robitussin Cough + Chest Congestion DM Liquid—(per 20 mL) guaifenesin 200 mg + dextromethorphan 20 mg **(OTC)**
Robitussin Maximum Strength 12–Hour Cough + Mucus Extended-Release Tablets—guaifenesin 1200 mg + dextromethorphan 60 mg **(OTC)**
Robitussin Maximum Strength Cough + Chest Congestion DM Capsules—guaifenesin 200 mg + dextromethorphan 10 mg **(OTC)**
Robitussin Maximum Strength Cough + Chest Congestion DM Liquid—(per 10 mL) guaifenesin 400 mg + dextromethorphan 20 mg **(OTC)**
Robitussin Maximum Strength Nighttime Cough DM Liquid—(per 10 mL) dextromethorphan 30 mg + doxylamine 12.5 mg **(OTC)**
Robitussin Maximum Strength Severe Cough + Sore Throat Liquid—(per 20 mL) acetaminophen 650 mg + dextromethorphan 20 mg **(OTC)**
Robitussin Maximum Strength Severe Multi-Symptom Cough, Cold & Flu Liquid—(per 20 mL) acetaminophen 650 mg + guaifenesin 400 mg + phenylephrine 10 mg + dextromethorphan 20 mg **(OTC)**
Robitussin Maximum Strength Severe Multi-Symptom Cough, Cold & Flu Nighttime Liquid—(per 20 mL) acetaminophen 650 mg + phenylephrine 10 mg + diphenhydramine 25 mg **(OTC)**
Robitussin Peak Cold Multi-Symptom Cold Liquid—(per 10 mL) guaifenesin 200 mg + phenylephrine 10 mg + dextromethorphan 20 mg **(OTC)**
Rolaids Advanced Tablets—calcium carbonate 1000 mg + magnesium hydroxide 200 mg + simethicone 40 mg **(OTC)**
Rolaids Extra Strength Tablets—calcium carbonate 675 mg + magnesium hydroxide 135 mg **(OTC)**
Rolaids Regular Strength Tablets—calcium carbonate 550 mg + magnesium hydroxide 110 mg **(OTC)**
Rolaids Ultra Strength Tablets—calcium carbonate 1000 mg + magnesium hydroxide 200 mg **(OTC)**
Roxicet 5/325—oxycodone 5 mg + acetaminophen 325 mg
Safyral
  Phase I—drospirenone 3 mg + ethinyl estradiol 30 mcg + levomefolate 0.451 mg
  Phase II—levomefolate 0.451 mg
Scot-Tussin DM Maximum Strength Cough Suppressant & Cold Relief Liquid—(per 5 mL) chlorpheniramine 2 mg + dextromethorphan 15 mg **(OTC)**
Scot-Tussin Senior Maximum Strength Cough Suppressant & Expectorant Liquid—(per 5 mL) guaifenesin 200 mg + dextromethorphan 15 mg **(OTC)**
Seasonale—levonorgestrel 0.15 mg + ethinyl estradiol 30 mcg
Seasonique—levonorgestrel 0.15 mg + ethinyl estradiol 30 mcg/10 mcg
Segluromet 2.5/500—ertugliflozin 2.5 mg + metformin 500 mg
Segluromet 2.5/1000—ertugliflozin 2.5 mg + metformin 1000 mg
Segluromet 7.5/500—ertugliflozin 7.5 mg + metformin 500 mg
Segluromet 7.5/1000—ertugliflozin 7.5 mg + metformin 1000 mg
Semprex-D—acrivastine 8 mg + pseudoephedrine 60 mg
Senokot-S—sennosides 8.6 mg + docusate sodium 50 mg **(OTC)**
Setlakin—levonorgestrel 0.15 mg + ethinyl estradiol 30 mcg
Simbrinza Ophthalmic Suspension—0.2% brimonidine + 1% brinzolamide
Soliqua—(per mL) insulin glargine 100 units + lixisenatide 33 mcg
Sprintec—norgestimate 0.25 mg + ethinyl estradiol 35 mcg
Sronyx—levonorgestrel 0.1 mg + ethinyl estradiol 20 mcg
Stalevo 50—carbidopa 12.5 mg + entacapone 200 mg + levodopa 50 mg
Stalevo 75—carbidopa 18.75 mg + entacapone 200 mg + levodopa 75 mg
Stalevo 100—carbidopa 25 mg + entacapone 200 mg + levodopa 100 mg
Stalevo 125—carbidopa 31.25 mg + entacapone 200 mg + levodopa 125 mg

Stalevo 150—carbidopa 37.5 mg + entacapone 200 mg + levodopa 150 mg
Stalevo 200—carbidopa 50 mg + entacapone 200 mg + levodopa 200 mg
Steglujan 5/100—ertugliflozin 5 mg + sitagliptin 100 mg
Steglujan 15/100—ertugliflozin 15 mg + sitagliptin 100 mg
Stiolto Respimat—(per actuation) tiotropium 2.5 mcg + olodaterol 2.5 mcg
Suboxone 2/0.5—buprenorphine 2 mg + naloxone 0.5 mg
Suboxone 4/1—buprenorphine 4 mg + naloxone 1 mg
Suboxone 8/2—buprenorphine 8 mg + naloxone 2 mg
Suboxone 12/3—buprenorphine 12 mg + naloxone 3 mg
Sudafed PE Cough + Cold Children's Liquid—(per 5 mL)phenylephrine 2.5 mg + dextromethorphan 5 mg **(OTC)**
Sudafed PE Head Congestion + Flu Severe Caplets—acetaminophen 325 mg + phenylephrine 5 mg + guaifenesin 100 mg + dextromethorphan 10 mg **(OTC)**
Sudafed PE Head Congestion + Mucus Caplets—phenylephrine 5 mg + guaifenesin 200 mg + acetaminophen 325 mg **(OTC)**
Sudafed PE Head Congestion + Pain Caplets—phenylephrine 10 mg + ibuprofen 200 mg **(OTC)**
Sudafed PE Pressure + Pain + Cough Liquid—(per 15 mL) phenylephrine 5 mg + dextromethorphan 10 mg + acetaminophen 325 mg **(OTC)**
Sudafed PE Sinus Pressure + Pain Caplets—acetaminophen 325 mg + phenylephrine 5 mg **(OTC)**
Sudafed Sinus 12-Hour Pressure + Pain Caplets—naproxen 220 mg + extended-release pseudoephedrine 120 mg **(OTC)**
Syeda—drospirenone 3 mg + ethinyl estradiol 30 mcg
Symbicort 80/4.5—(per actuation) budesonide 80 mcg + formoterol 4.5 mcg
Symbicort 160/4.5—(per actuation) budesonide 160 mcg + formoterol 4.5 mcg
Symbyax 3/25—olanzapine 3 mg + fluoxetine 25 mg
Symbyax 6/25—olanzapine 6 mg + fluoxetine 25 mg
Symbyax 6/50—olanzapine 6 mg + fluoxetine 50 mg
Symbyax 12/25—olanzapine 12 mg + fluoxetine 25 mg
Symbyax 12/50—olanzapine 12 mg + fluoxetine 50 mg
Symfi—efavirenz 600 mg + lamivudine 300 mg + tenofovir disoproxil fumarate 300 mg
Symfi Lo—efavirenz 400 mg + lamivudine 300 mg + tenofovir disoproxil fumarate 300 mg
Symtuza—darunavir 800 mg + cobicistat 150 mg + emtricitabine 200 mg + tenofovir alafenamide 10 mg
Synera Transdermal Patch—lidocaine 70 mg + tetracaine 70 mg
Synjardy 5/500—empagliflozin 5 mg + metformin 500 mg
Synjardy 5/1000—empagliflozin 5 mg + metformin 1000 mg
Synjardy 12.5/500—empagliflozin 12.5 mg + metformin 500 mg
Synjardy 12.5/1000—empagliflozin 12.5 mg + metformin 1000 mg
Synjardy XR 5/1000—empagliflozin 5 mg + metformin extended-release 1000 mg
Synjardy XR 10/1000—empagliflozin 10 mg + metformin extended-release 1000 mg
Synjardy XR 12.5/1000—empagliflozin 12.5 mg + metformin extended-release 1000 mg
Synjardy XR 25/1000—empagliflozin 25 mg + metformin extended-release 1000 mg
Taclonex Topical Ointment/Suspension—0.005% calcipotriene + 0.064% betamethasone
Tarka 1/240—trandolapril 1 mg + sustained-release verapamil 240 mg
Tarka 2/180—trandolapril 2 mg + sustained-release verapamil 180 mg
Tarka 2/240—trandolapril 2 mg + sustained-release verapamil 240 mg
Tarka 4/240—trandolapril 4 mg + sustained-release verapamil 240 mg
Tekturna HCT 150/12.5—aliskiren 150 mg + hydrochlorothiazide 12.5 mg
Tekturna HCT 150/25—aliskiren 150 mg + hydrochlorothiazide 25 mg
Tekturna HCT 300/12.5—aliskiren 300 mg + hydrochlorothiazide 12.5 mg
Tekturna HCT 300/25—aliskiren 300 mg + hydrochlorothiazide 25 mg
Temixys—lamivudine 300 mg + tenofovir disoproxil fumarate 300 mg
Tenoretic 50/25—atenolol 50 mg + chlorthalidone 25 mg

Tenoretic 100/25—atenolol 100 mg + chlorthalidone 25 mg
TheraFlu Cough Relief Hot Liquid Powder—(per packet) guaifenesin 400 mg + dextromethorphan 20 mg **(OTC)**
TheraFlu Daytime Severe Cold & Cough Hot Liquid Powder—(per packet) acetaminophen 650 mg + phenylephrine 10 mg + dextromethorphan 20 mg **(OTC)**
TheraFlu Expressmax Daytime Severe Cold & Cough Caplets—acetaminophen 325 mg + phenylephrine 5 mg + dextromethorphan 10 mg **(OTC)**
TheraFlu Expressmax Daytime Severe Cold & Cough Liquid—(per 30 mL) acetaminophen 650 mg + phenylephrine 10 mg + dextromethorphan 20 mg **(OTC)**
TheraFlu Expressmax Flu, Cough & Sore Throat Liquid—(per 30 mL) acetaminophen 650 mg + phenylephrine 10 mg + diphenhydramine 25 mg **(OTC)**
TheraFlu Expressmax Nighttime Severe Cold & Cough Caplets—acetaminophen 325 mg + phenylephrine 5 mg + diphenhydramine 12.5 mg **(OTC)**
TheraFlu Expressmax Nighttime Severe Cold & Cough Liquid—(per 30 mL) acetaminophen 650 mg + phenylephrine 10 mg + diphenhydramine 25 mg **(OTC)**
TheraFlu Expressmax Severe Cold & Flu Caplets—acetaminophen 325 mg + phenylephrine 5 mg + dextromethorphan 10 mg + guaifenesin 200 mg **(OTC)**
TheraFlu Expressmax Severe Cold & Flu Liquid—(per 30 mL) acetaminophen 650 mg + phenylephrine 10 mg + dextromethorphan 20 mg + guaifenesin 400 mg **(OTC)**
TheraFlu Flu & Sore Throat Hot Liquid Powder—(per packet) acetaminophen 650 mg + phenylephrine 10 mg + pheniramine 20 mg **(OTC)**
TheraFlu Multi-Symptom Severe Cold Hot Liquid Powder—(per packet) acetaminophen 500 mg + phenylephrine 10 mg + dextromethorphan 20 mg **(OTC)**
TheraFlu Nighttime Multi-Symptom Severe Cold Hot Liquid Powder—(per packet) acetaminophen 500 mg + phenylephrine 10 mg + diphenhydramine 25 mg **(OTC)**
TheraFlu Nighttime Severe Cold & Cough Hot Liquid Powder—(per packet) acetaminophen 650 mg + phenylephrine 10 mg + diphenhydramine 25 mg **(OTC)**
Tilia Fe
Phase I—norethindrone 1 mg + ethinyl estradiol 20 mcg
Phase II—norethindrone 1 mg + ethinyl estradiol 30 mcg
Phase III—norethindrone 1 mg + ethinyl estradiol 35 mcg
Phase IV—ferrous fumarate 75 mg
TobraDex Ophthalmic Suspension/Ointment—0.1% dexamethasone + 0.3% tobramycin
TobraDex ST Ophthalmic Suspension—0.05% dexamethasone + 0.3% tobramycin
Trelegy Ellipta—(per inhalation) fluticasone 100 mcg + umeclidinium 62.5 mcg + vilanterol 25 mcg
Treximet 10/60—sumatriptan 10 mg + naproxen 60 mg
Treximet 85/500—sumatriptan 85 mg + naproxen 500 mg
Tri–Estarylla
Phase I—norgestimate 0.18 mg + ethinyl estradiol 35 mcg
Phase II—norgestimate 0.215 mg + ethinyl estradiol 35 mcg
Phase III—norgestimate 0.25 mg + ethinyl estradiol 35 mcg
Tri–Legest–21
Phase I—norethindrone 1 mg + ethinyl estradiol 20 mcg
Phase II—norethindrone 1 mg + ethinyl estradiol 30 mcg
Phase III—norethindrone 1 mg + ethinyl estradiol 35 mcg
Tri–Legest Fe
Phase I—norethindrone 1 mg + ethinyl estradiol 20 mcg
Phase II—norethindrone 1 mg + ethinyl estradiol 30 mcg
Phase III—norethindrone 1 mg + ethinyl estradiol 35 mcg
Phase IV—ferrous fumarate 75 mg
Tri–Linyah
Phase I—norgestimate 0.18 mg + ethinyl estradiol 35 mcg
Phase II—norgestimate 0.215 mg + ethinyl estradiol 35 mcg
Phase III—norgestimate 0.25 mg + ethinyl estradiol 35 mcg

Tri-Lo-Estarylla

Phase I—norgestimate 0.18 mg + ethinyl estradiol 25 mcg
Phase II—norgestimate 0.215 mg + ethinyl estradiol 25 mcg
Phase III—norgestimate 0.25 mg + ethinyl estradiol 25 mcg

Tri-Luma Topical Cream—0.01% fluocinolone + 4% hydroquinone + 0.05% tretinoin

Tri-Norinyl

Phase I—norethindrone 0.5 mg + ethinyl estradiol 35 mcg
Phase II—norethindrone 1 mg + ethinyl estradiol 35 mcg
Phase III—norethindrone 0.5 mg + ethinyl estradiol 35 mcg

Tri-Previfem

Phase I—norgestimate 0.18 mg + ethinyl estradiol 35 mcg
Phase II—norgestimate 0.215 mg + ethinyl estradiol 35 mcg
Phase III—norgestimate 0.25 mg + ethinyl estradiol 35 mcg

Tri-Sprintec

Phase I—norgestimate 0.18 mg + ethinyl estradiol 35 mcg
Phase II—norgestimate 0.215 mg + ethinyl estradiol 35 mcg
Phase III—norgestimate 0.25 mg + ethinyl estradiol 35 mcg

Triacin-C Cough Syrup—(per 5 mL) codeine 10 mg + pseudoephedrine 30 mg + triprolidine 1.25 mg

Triaminic Cough & Congestion Liquid—(per 5 mL) guaifenesin 100 mg + dextromethorphan 5 mg **(OTC)**

Triaminic Cough & Sore Throat Liquid—(per 5 mL) acetaminophen 160 mg + dextromethorphan 5 mg **(OTC)**

Triaminic Day Time Cold & Cough Liquid—(per 5 mL) phenylephrine 2.5 mg + dextromethorphan 5 mg **(OTC)**

Triaminic Multi-Symptom Fever & Cold Liquid—(per 5 mL) acetaminophen 160 mg + dextromethorphan 5 mg + chlorpheniramine 1 mg + phenylephrine 2.5 mg **(OTC)**

Triaminic Night Time Cold & Cough Liquid—(per 5 mL) phenylephrine 2.5 mg + diphenhydramine 6.25 mg **(OTC)**

Tribenzor 20/5/12.5—olmesartan 20 mg + amlodipine 5 mg + hydrochlorothiazide 12.5 mg

Tribenzor 40/5/12.5—olmesartan 40 mg + amlodipine 5 mg + hydrochlorothiazide 12.5 mg

Tribenzor 40/5/25—olmesartan 40 mg + amlodipine 5 mg + hydrochlorothiazide 25 mg

Tribenzor 40/10/12.5—olmesartan 40 mg + amlodipine 10 mg + hydrochlorothiazide 12.5 mg

Tribenzor 40/10/25—olmesartan 40 mg + amlodipine 10 mg + hydrochlorothiazide 25 mg

TriLyte—PEG 3350 420 g + sodium bicarbonate 5.72 g + sodium chloride 11.2 g + potassium chloride 1.48 g

TriNessa

Phase I—norgestimate 0.18 mg + ethinyl estradiol 35 mcg
Phase II—norgestimate 0.215 mg + ethinyl estradiol 35 mcg
Phase III—norgestimate 0.25 mg + ethinyl estradiol 35 mcg

Triumeq—abacavir 600 mg + dolutegravir 50 mg + lamivudine 150 mg

Trivora-28

Phase I—levonorgestrel 0.05 mg + ethinyl estradiol 30 mcg
Phase II—levonorgestrel 0.075 mg + ethinyl estradiol 40 mcg
Phase III—levonorgestrel 0.125 mg + ethinyl estradiol 30 mcg

Trizivir—abacavir 300 mg + lamivudine 150 mg + zidovudine 300 mg

Truvada 100/150—emtricitabine 100 mg + tenofovir disoproxil fumarate 150 mg

Truvada 133/200—emtricitabine 133 mg + tenofovir disoproxil fumarate 200 mg

Truvada 167/250—emtricitabine 167 mg + tenofovir disoproxil fumarate 250 mg

Truvada 200/300—emtricitabine 200 mg + tenofovir disoproxil fumarate 300 mg

TussiCaps 5/4—hydrocodone 5 mg + chlorpheniramine 4 mg

TussiCaps 10/8—hydrocodone 10 mg + chlorpheniramine 8 mg

Tussigon—hydrocodone 5 mg + homatropine 1.5 mg

Tuzistra XR—(per 5 mL) chlorpheniramine polistirex 2.8 mg + codeine polistirex 14.7 mg

Twynsta 40/5—telmisartan 40 mg + amlodipine 5 mg
Twynsta 40/10—telmisartan 40 mg + amlodipine 10 mg
Twynsta 80/5—telmisartan 80 mg + amlodipine 5 mg
Twynsta 80/10—telmisartan 80 mg + amlodipine 10 mg
Tylenol Cold & Flu & Cough Nighttime Liquid—(per 15 mL) acetaminophen 325 mg + phenylephrine 5 mg + dextromethorphan 10 mg + doxylamine 6.25 mg **(OTC)**
Tylenol Cold & Flu Severe Caplets—acetaminophen 325 mg + phenylephrine 5 mg + dextromethorphan 10 mg + guaifenesin 200 mg **(OTC)**
Tylenol Cold & Flu Severe Warming Liquid—(per 15 mL) acetaminophen 325 mg + phenylephrine 5 mg + dextromethorphan 10 mg + guaifenesin 200 mg **(OTC)**
Tylenol Cold & Head Congestion Severe Caplets—acetaminophen 325 mg + phenylephrine 5 mg + guaifenesin 200 mg **(OTC)**
Tylenol Cold Max Daytime Caplets—acetaminophen 325 mg + phenylephrine 5 mg + dextromethorphan 10 mg **(OTC)**
Tylenol Cold Max Daytime Liquid—(per 15 mL) acetaminophen 325 mg + phenylephrine 5 mg + dextromethorphan 10 mg **(OTC)**
Tylenol Cold & Mucus Severe Liquid—(per 15 mL) acetaminophen 325 mg + guaifenesin 200 mg + phenylephrine 5 mg + dextromethorphan 10 mg **(OTC)**
Tylenol PM Caplets—acetaminophen 500 mg + diphenhydramine 25 mg **(OTC)**
Tylenol PM Liquid—(per 30 mL) acetaminophen 1000 mg + diphenhydramine 50 mg **(OTC)**
Tylenol Sinus & Headache Daytime Caplets—acetaminophen 325 mg + phenylephrine 5 mg **(OTC)**
Tylenol Sinus Severe Daytime Caplets—acetaminophen 325 mg + phenylephrine 5 mg + guaifenesin 200 mg **(OTC)**
Tylenol with Codeine No. 3—acetaminophen 300 mg + codeine 30 mg
Tylenol with Codeine No. 4—acetaminophen 300 mg + codeine 60 mg
Ultracet—tramadol 37.5 mg + acetaminophen 325 mg
Ultresa—lipase 13,800 units + amylase 27,600 units + protease 27,600 units
Ultresa—lipase 20,700 units + amylase 41,400 units + protease 41,400 units
Ultresa—lipase 23,000 units + amylase 46,000 units + protease 46,000 units
Utibron Neohaler—(per inhalation capsule) indacaterol 27.5 mcg + glycopyrrolate 15.6 mcg
Vaseretic 5/12.5—enalapril 5 mg + hydrochlorothiazide 12.5 mg
Vaseretic 10/25—enalapril 10 mg + hydrochlorothiazide 25 mg
Velivet
Phase I—desogestrel 0.1 mg + ethinyl estradiol 25 mcg
Phase II—desogestrel 0.125 mg + ethinyl estradiol 25 mcg
Phase III—desogestrel 0.15 mg + ethinyl estradiol 25 mcg
Veltin Topical Gel—1.2% clindamycin + 0.025% tretinoin
Vienva—levonorgestrel 0.1 mg + ethinyl estradiol 20 mcg
Vimovo 375/20—naproxen delayed-release 375 mg + esomeprazole 20 mg
Vimovo 500/20—naproxen delayed-release 500 mg + esomeprazole 20 mg
Viokace—lipase 10,440 units + amylase 39,150 units + protease 39,150 units
Viokace—lipase 20,880 units + amylase 78,300 units + protease 78,300 units
Viorele—desogestrel 0.15 mg + ethinyl estradiol 20 mcg/10 mcg
Visine Allergy Eye Relief Multi-Action Ophthalmic Solution—0.025% naphazoline + 0.3% pheniramine **(OTC)**
Vusion Topical Ointment—0.25% miconazole + 15% zinc oxide
Vyfemla—norethindrone 0.4 mg + ethinyl estradiol 35 mcg
Vytorin 10/10—ezetimibe 10 mg + simvastatin 10 mg
Vytorin 10/20—ezetimibe 10 mg + simvastatin 20 mg
Vytorin 10/40—ezetimibe 10 mg + simvastatin 40 mg
Vytorin 10/80—ezetimibe 10 mg + simvastatin 80 mg
Vyxeos—daunorubicin 44 mg + cytarabine 100 mg
Wera—norethindrone 0.5 mg + ethinyl estradiol 35 mcg

Wymzya Fe—norethindrone 0.4 mg + ethinyl estradiol 35 mcg + ferrous fumarate 75 mg
Xartemis XR—oxycodone 7.5 mg + acetaminophen 325 mg
Xerese Topical Cream—5% acyclovir + 1% hydrocortisone
Xigduo XR 2.5/1000—dapagliflozin 2.5 mg + metformin extended-release 1000 mg
Xigduo XR 5/500—dapagliflozin 5 mg + metformin extended-release 500 mg
Xigduo XR 5/1000—dapagliflozin 5 mg + metformin extended-release 1000 mg
Xigduo XR 10/500—dapagliflozin 10 mg + metformin extended-release 500 mg
Xigduo XR 10/1000—dapagliflozin 10 mg + metformin extended-release 1000 mg
Xulane—norelgestromin 150 mcg/day + ethinyl estradiol 35 mcg/day
Xultophy—(per mL) insulin degludec 100 units + liraglutide 3.6 mg
Xylocaine with Epinephrine Injection 0.5/0.0005—0.5% lidocaine + 0.0005% epinephrine
Xylocaine with Epinephrine Injection 1/0.001—1% lidocaine + 0.001% epinephrine
Xylocaine with Epinephrine Injection 2/0.001—2% lidocaine + 0.001% epinephrine
Yaela—drospirenone 3 mg + ethinyl estradiol 30 mcg
Yasmin—drospirenone 3 mg + ethinyl estradiol 30 mcg
Yaz—drospirenone 3 mg + ethinyl estradiol 20 mcg
Yosprala 81/40—aspirin 81 mg + omeprazole 40 mg
Yosprala 325/40—aspirin 325 mg + omeprazole 40 mg
Zarah—drospirenone 3 mg + ethinyl estradiol 30 mcg
Zegerid Capsules 20/1100—omeprazole 20 mg + sodium bicarbonate 1100 mg
Zegerid Capsules 40/1100—omeprazole 40 mg + sodium bicarbonate 1100 mg
Zegerid OTC Capsules—omeprazole 20 mg + sodium bicarbonate 1100 mg **(OTC)**
Zegerid Powder for Oral Suspension 20/1680—(per pkt) omeprazole 20 mg + sodium bicarbonate 1680 mg **(OTC)**
Zegerid Powder for Oral Suspension 40/1680—(per pkt) omeprazole 40 mg + sodium bicarbonate 1680 mg
Zenchent—norethindrone 0.4 mg + ethinyl estradiol 35 mcg
Zenchent Fe—norethindrone 0.4 mg + ethinyl estradiol 35 mcg + ferrous fumarate 75 mg
Zenpep—lipase 3000 units + amylase 14,000 units + protease 10,000 units
Zenpep—lipase 5000 units + amylase 24,000 units + protease 17,000 units
Zenpep—lipase 10,000 units + amylase 42,000 units + protease 32,000 units
Zenpep—lipase 15,000 units + amylase 63,000 units + protease 47,000 units
Zenpep—lipase 20,000 units + amylase 84,000 units + protease 63,000 units
Zenpep—lipase 25,000 units + amylase 105,000 units + protease 79,000 units
Zenpep—lipase 40,000 units + amylase 168,000 units + protease 126,000 units
Zestoretic 10/12.5—lisinopril 10 mg + hydrochlorothiazide 12.5 mg
Zestoretic 20/12.5—lisinopril 20 mg + hydrochlorothiazide 12.5 mg
Zestoretic 20/25—lisinopril 20 mg + hydrochlorothiazide 25 mg
Ziac 2.5/6.25—bisoprolol 2.5 mg + hydrochlorothiazide 6.25 mg
Ziac 5/6.25—bisoprolol 5 mg + hydrochlorothiazide 6.25 mg
Ziac 10/6.25—bisoprolol 10 mg + hydrochlorothiazide 6.25 mg
Ziana Topical Gel—1.2% clindamycin + 0.025% tretinoin
Zovia 1/35—ethynodiol 1 mg + ethinyl estradiol 35 mcg
Zovia 1/50—ethynodiol 1 mg + ethinyl estradiol 50 mcg
Zubsolv 0.7/0.18—buprenorphine 0.7 mg + naloxone 0.18 mg
Zubsolv 1.4/0.36—buprenorphine 1.4 mg + naloxone 0.36 mg
Zubsolv 2.9/0.71—buprenorphine 2.9 mg + naloxone 0.71 mg
Zubsolv 5.7/1.4—buprenorphine 5.7 mg + naloxone 1.4 mg
Zubsolv 8.6/2.1—buprenorphine 8.6 mg + naloxone 2.1 mg
Zubsolv 11.4/2.9—buprenorphine 11.4 mg + naloxone 2.9 mg
Zylet Ophthalmic Suspension—0.5% loteprednol + 0.3% tobramycin
Zyrtec-D Allergy & Congestion—cetirizine 5 mg + pseudoephedrine 120 mg **(OTC)**

APPENDIX C

Ophthalmic Medications

General Info: See Appendix D for administration techniques for ophthalmic agents.
Consult health care professional regarding:
Concurrent use of contact lenses (medication or additives may be absorbed by the lens).
Concurrent administration of other ophthalmic agents (order and spacing may be important).
ADRs = adverse reactions.

DRUG NAME	DOSE	NOTES
Anesthetics		
Uses: Provide brief local anesthesia to allow measurement of intraocular pressure, removal of foreign bodies, or other superficial procedures. **CAUTIONS:** Repeated use may result in ↑ risk of CNS and cardiovascular toxicity; cross-sensitivity with some local anesthetics may occur.		
lidocaine (Akten)	**Adults and children:** 2 drops of 3.5% gel (single dose).	• Does not interact with ophthalmic cholinesterase inhibitors • ADRs: ophthalmic—irritation; systemic—irregular heartbeat, CNS depression
proparacaine (Alcaine)	**Adults and children:** 1–2 drops of 0.5% solution (single dose).	• Does not interact with ophthalmic cholinesterase inhibitors • ADRs: ophthalmic—irritation; systemic—irregular heartbeat, CNS depression
tetracaine (Altacaine, Tetcaine)	**Adults:** 1–2 drops of 0.5% solution (single dose).	• May interact with ophthalmic cholinesterase inhibitors, resulting in ↑ duration of action and risk of toxicity • ADRs: ophthalmic—irritation; systemic—irregular heartbeat, CNS depression
Antihistamines		
Uses: Various forms of allergic conjunctivitis.		
alcaftadine (Lastacaft)	**Adults and children ≥2 yr:** 1 drop of 0.25% solution once daily.	• ADRs: transient burning/stinging, headache
azelastine	**Adults and children ≥3 yr:** 1 drop of 0.05% solution twice daily.	• ADRs: transient burning/stinging, headache, bitter taste
bepotastine (Bepreve)	**Adults and children ≥2 yr:** 1 drop of 1.5% solution twice daily.	• ADRs: taste disturbance, headache, local irritation
epinastine (Elestat)	**Adults and children ≥2 yr:** 1 drop of 0.05% solution twice daily.	• ADRs: headache, local irritation
ketotifen (Alaway, Claritin Eye, Zaditor)	**Adults and children ≥3 yr:** 1 drop of 0.025% solution twice daily (given 8–12 hr apart).	• OTC • ADRs: local irritation
olopatadine (Pataday, Patanol, Pazeo)	**Adults and children ≥2 yr (Pataday, Pazeo); ≥3 yr (Patanol):** *Patanol*—1 drop of 0.1% solution twice daily (given 6–8 hr apart); *Pataday*—1 drop of 0.2% solution once daily; *Pazeo*—1 drop of 0.7% solution once daily.	• Small amounts are absorbed; excreted in urine • ADRs: headache, conjunctival irritation
Antibacterials/Antifungals/Antivirals		
Uses: Localized superficial ophthalmic infections (e.g., bacterial conjunctivitis). **CAUTIONS:** Small amounts may be absorbed and result in hypersensitivity reactions.		
azithromycin (AzaSite)	**Adults and children ≥1 yr:** 1 drop of 1% solution twice daily (given 8–12 hr apart) for 2 days, then once daily for 5 more days.	• When used to treat ocular chlamydial infections, concurrent systemic therapy is required • ADRs: eye irritation

DRUG NAME	DOSE	NOTES
bacitracin	**Adults and children:** ¼–½-in. ointment strip every 3–4 hr for acute infections or 2–3 times daily for mild-moderate infections.	• ADRs: eye irritation
besifloxacin (Besivance)	**Adults and children ≥1 yr:** 1 drop of 0.6% suspension 3 times daily (given 4–12 hr apart) for 7 days.	• ADRs: headache, eye irritation
ciprofloxacin (Ciloxan)	**Adults and children of all ages (solution) or ≥2 yr (ointment):** *Bacterial conjunctivitis*—Solution: 1–2 drops of 0.3% solution every 2 hr while awake for 2 days, then every 4 hr while awake for 5 more days; Ointment: ½-in. strip 3 times daily for 2 days, then twice daily for 5 more days; *Corneal ulcers*—Solution: 2 drops of 0.3% solution every 15 min for 6 hr, then every 30 min while awake for rest of day, then every hr while awake for next 24 hr, then every 4 hr while awake for next 12 days or longer if re-epithelialization does not occur.	• May cause harmless white crystalline precipitate that resolves over time • ADRs: altered taste, systemic allergic reactions, photophobia, discomfort
erythromycin	**Adults and children:** *Treatment of infections*—½-in. ointment strip 2–6 times daily. **Infants:** *Prophylaxis of ophthalmia neonatorum*—½-in. ointment strip in each eye as a single dose.	• ADRs: irritation
fusidic acid (🍁 Fucithalmic)	**Adults and children ≥2 yr:** 1 drop of 1% suspension twice daily for 7 days.	• ADRs: irritation
gatifloxacin (🍁 Zymar, Zymaxid)	**Adults and children of all ages (Zymar) or ≥1 yr (Zymaxid):** *Zymaxid*—1 drop of 0.5% solution every 2 hr while awake (up to 8 times/day) for 1 day, then 2–4 times daily while awake for 6 more days; *Zymar*—1 drop of 0.3% solution every 2 hr while awake (up to 8 times/day) for 2 days, then 4 times daily while awake for 5 more days.	• ADRs: irritation, headache, ↓ visual acuity, taste disturbance
gentamicin (Genoptic, Gentak)	**Adults and children:** *Solution*—1–2 drops of 0.3% solution every 2–4 hr; *Ointment*—½-in. strip every 8–12 hr.	• ADRs: irritation, burning, stinging, blurred vision (ointment)
levofloxacin	**Adults and children ≥6 yr:** 1–2 drops of 0.5% solution every 2 hr while awake for 2 days (up to 8 times/day); then every 4 hr while awake for 5 more days (up to 4 times/day).	• ADRs: altered taste, systemic allergic reactions, photophobia
moxifloxacin (Moxeza, Vigamox)	**Adults and children ≥4 mo (Moxeza) or of all ages (Vigamox):** *Moxeza*—1 drop of 0.5% solution twice daily for 7 days; *Vigamox*—1 drop of 0.5% solution 3 times daily for 7 days.	• ADRs: irritation, ↓ visual acuity

DRUG NAME	DOSE	NOTES
ofloxacin (Ocuflox)	**Adults and children ≥1 yr:** *Bacterial conjunctivitis*—1–2 drops of 0.3% solution every 2–4 hr while awake for 2 days, then 4 times daily for 5 more days; *Corneal ulcer*—1–2 drops of 0.3% solution every 30 min while awake and every 4–6 hr while sleeping for 2 days, then every hr while awake for 4–6 more days, then 4 times daily until cured.	• ADRs: altered taste, systemic allergic reactions, photophobia
sulfacetamide (Bleph-10)	**Adults and children ≥2 mo:** *Solution*—1–2 drops of 10% solution every 2–3 hr while awake (less frequently at night) for 7–10 days; *Ointment*—½-in. strip every 3–4 hr and at bedtime for 7–10 days.	• Cross-sensitivity with other sulfonamides (including thiazides) may occur • ADRs: local irritation
tobramycin (AK-Tob, Tobrex)	**Adults and children ≥2 mo:** *Solution*—1–2 drops of 0.3% solution every 2–4 hr depending on severity of infection; *Ointment*—½-in. strip every 8–12 hr.	• Ointment may retard corneal wound healing • ADRs: irritation, burning, stinging, blurred vision (ointment)
Antifungal		
natamycin (Natacyn)	**Adults:** *Fungal keratitis*—1 drop of 5% suspension every 1–2 hr for 3–4 days, then 6–8 times/day for 2–3 wk; *Fungal blepharitis or conjunctivitis*—1 drop of 5% suspension every 4–6 hr for 2–3 wk.	• ADRs: irritation, swelling
Antivirals		
ganciclovir (Zirgan)	**Adults and children ≥2 yr:** 1 drop of 0.15% gel 5 times daily (every 3 hr while awake) until corneal ulcer heals, then 3 times daily for 7 days.	• ADRs: blurred vision, irritation, keratopathy
trifluridine (Viroptic)	**Adults and children ≥6 yr:** 1 drop of 1% solution every 2 hr while awake (up to 9 drops/day) until re-epithelialization occurs, then every 4 hr while awake for 7 more days (not to exceed 21 days).	• ADRs: burning, stinging, keratopathy
Artificial Tears/Ocular Lubricants (sterile buffered isotonic solutions/ointments)		
Uses: Artificial tears—keep the eyes moist with isotonic solutions and wetting agents in the management of dry eyes due to lack of tears; also provide lubrication for artificial eyes. Ocular lubricants—provide lubrication and protection in a variety of conditions including exposure keratitis, ↓ corneal sensitivity, corneal erosions, keratitis sicca, during/following ocular surgery or removal of a foreign body.		
Artificial tears (Bion Tears, Genteal Tears, HypoTears, LiquiTears, Murine Tears, Nature's Tears, Soothe, Systane, 🍁 Teardrops, Tears Naturale, Viva-Drops)	**Adults and children:** *Artificial tears*—Solution: 1–2 drops 3–4 times daily; Insert: 1 insert 1–2 times daily; *Ocular lubricants*—small amount instilled into conjunctiva several times daily.	• May alter effects of other concurrently administered ophthalmic medications • ADRs: photophobia, lid edema stinging (insert only), transient blurred vision, eye discomfort

Beta Blockers

Uses: Treatment of open-angle glaucoma and other forms of ocular hypertension (↓ formation of aqueous humor).
CAUTIONS: Systemic absorption is minimal but may occur. Systemic absorption may result in additive adverse cardiovascular effects (bradycardia, hypotension), especially when used with other cardiovascular agents (antihypertensives, antiarrhythmics). Other systemic adverse reactions may occur, including bronchospasm or delirium (geriatric patients). Concurrent use with ophthalmic epinephrine may ↓ effectiveness.

DRUG NAME	DOSE	NOTES
betaxolol (Betoptic, Betoptic S)	**Adults:** *Betoptic*—1–2 drops of 0.5% solution twice daily; *Betoptic S*—1 drop of 0.25% suspension twice daily. **Children:** *Betoptic S*—1 drop of 0.25% suspension twice daily.	• ADRs: conjunctivitis, ↓ visual acuity, ocular burning, rash (may be less likely than others to cause bronchospasm if systemically absorbed)
carteolol	**Adults:** 1 drop of 1% solution twice daily.	• ADRs: ocular burning, ↓ visual acuity
levobunolol (AKBeta, Betagan)	**Adults:** 1–2 drops of 0.25% solution twice daily or 1–2 drops of 0.5% solution once daily.	• ADRs: conjunctivitis, ↓ visual acuity, ocular burning, rash
timolol (Betimol, Istalol, Timoptic, Timoptic-XE)	**Adults:** *Solution*—1 drop of 0.25–0.5% solution 1–2 times daily; *Gel-forming solution*—1 drop of 0.25–0.5% solution once daily. **Children:** *Solution*—1 drop of 0.25–0.5% solution twice daily; *Gel-forming solution*—1 drop of 0.25–0.5% solution once daily.	• Lasts up to 24 hr • ADRs: conjunctivitis, ↓ visual acuity, ocular burning, rash

Carbonic Anhydrase Inhibitors

Uses: Treatment of open-angle glaucoma and other forms of ocular hypertension (↓ formation of aqueous humor).
CAUTIONS: May exacerbate kidney stones; should not be used in patients with CCr <30 mL/min; may have cross-sensitivity with sulfonamides.

DRUG NAME	DOSE	NOTES
brinzolamide (Azopt)	**Adults:** 1 drop of 1% suspension 3 times daily.	• ADRs: burning, stinging, unusual taste
dorzolamide (Trusopt)	**Adults and children:** 1 drop of 2% solution 3 times daily.	• ADRs: bitter taste, ocular irritation, or allergy

Cholinergics (direct-acting)

Uses: Treatment of open-angle glaucoma (facilitates the outflow of aqueous humor); also used to facilitate miosis after ophthalmic surgery or before examination (to counteract mydriatics).
CAUTIONS: Conditions in which pupillary constriction occurs should be avoided. If significant systemic absorption occurs, bronchospasm, sweating, and ↑ urination and salivation may occur.

DRUG NAME	DOSE	NOTES
acetylcholine (Miochol-E)	**Adults:** 0.5–2 mL instilled into anterior chamber before or after securing one or more sutures.	• ADRs: corneal edema, corneal clouding
carbachol (Miostat)	**Adults:** *Glaucoma*—1–2 drops of 0.01 solution 1–3 times daily; *To facilitate miosis*—0.5 mL instilled into anterior chamber before or after securing sutures.	• ADRs: blurred vision, altered vision, stinging, eye pain
pilocarpine (Isopto Carpine)	**Adults and children ≥2 yr:** *Glaucoma*—1–2 drops of 0.5–4% solution up to 6 times daily; *Counteracting mydriatic sympathomimetics*—1 drop of 1–2% solution (may be repeated prior to surgery). **Children <2 yr:** *Glaucoma*—1 drop of 1% solution 3 times daily.	• ADRs: blurred vision, altered vision, stinging, eye pain, headache

Cholinergics (cholinesterase inhibitors)

Uses: Treatment of open-angle glaucoma not controlled with short-acting miotics or other agents; also used in varying doses for accommodative esotropia (diagnosis and treatment).
CAUTIONS: Enhance neuromuscular blockade from succinylcholine; intensify the actions of cocaine and some other local anesthetics; additive toxicity with antimyasthenics, anticholinergics, and cholinesterase inhibitors (including some pesticides). Use cautiously in patients with history or risk of retinal detachment.

DRUG NAME	DOSE	NOTES
echothiophate (Phospholine Iodide)	**Adults:** 1 drop of 0.125% solution 1–2 times daily.	• Irreversible cholinesterase inhibitor • May cause hyperactivity in patients with Down syndrome • ADRs: blurred vision, change in vision, brow ache, miosis, eyelid twitching, watering eyes

DRUG NAME	DOSE	NOTES
Corticosteroids		
Uses: Management of inflammatory eye conditions including allergic conjunctivitis, nonspecific superficial keratitis, anterior endogenous uveitis; infectious conjunctivitis (with anti-infectives); management of corneal injury; suppression of graft rejection following keratoplasty; prevention of postoperative inflammation. **CAUTIONS:** Use cautiously in patients with infectious ocular processes (avoid in herpes simplex keratitis), especially fungal and viral ocular infections (may mask symptoms); diabetes, glaucoma, or epithelial compromise.		
dexamethasone (Maxidex)	**Adults and children:** *Solution*—1–2 drops of 0.1% solution every hr during the day and every 2 hr during the night, gradually ↓ the dose to 1 drop every 4 hr, then to 3–4 times daily; *Suspension*—1–2 drops of 0.1% suspension up to 4–6 times daily.	• As condition improves, ↓ frequency of administration • ADRs: corneal thinning, ↑ intraocular pressure, irritation
difluprednate (Durezol)	**Adults and children:** *Postoperative inflammation*—1 drop of 0.05% emulsion 4 times daily beginning 24 hr after surgery and continued for 2 wk, then 2 times daily for 1 wk, then taper; *Uveitis*—1 drop of 0.05% emulsion 4 times daily for 14 days, then taper.	• As condition improves, ↓ frequency of administration • ADRs: blepharitis, photophobia, ↓ visual acuity
fluorometholone (Flarex, FML, FML Forte)	**Adults and children ≥2 yr:** *Suspension*—1–2 drops of 0.1% suspension 4 times daily (up to 2 drops every 2 hr during initial 24–48 hr) or 1 drop of 0.25% suspension 2–4 times daily (up to 1 drop every 4 hr during initial 24–48 hr); *Ointment*—½-in. strip 1–3 times daily (up to every 4 hr during initial 24–48 hr).	• As condition improves, ↓ frequency of administration • ADRs: blurred vision (ointment), corneal thinning, ↑ intraocular pressure, irritation
loteprednol (Alrex, Inveltys, Lotemax, Lotemax SM)	**Adults:** *Allergic conjunctivitis*—Alrex: 1 drop of 0.2% suspension 4 times daily; *Inflammatory conditions*—Lotemax: 1–2 drops of 0.5% suspension 4 times daily (up to 1 drop every hr may be used in first wk); *Postoperative inflammation/pain*—Lotemax gel/suspension: 1–2 drops of 0.5% gel/suspension 4 times daily beginning 24 hr after surgery and continued for 2 wk or 1 drop of 0.38% gel 3 times daily beginning 24 hr after surgery and continued for 2 wk; Lotemax ointment: ½-in. strip 4 times daily beginning 24 hr after surgery and continued for 2 wk; Inveltys suspension: 1–2 drops of 1% suspension 2 times daily beginning 24 hr after surgery and continued for 2 wk. **Children:** *Postoperative inflammation/pain*—Lotemax gel: 1–2 drops of 0.5% gel 4 times daily beginning 24 hr after surgery and continued for 2 wk.	• ADRs: corneal thinning, ↑ intraocular pressure, irritation
prednisolone (Omnipred, Pred Forte, Pred Mild)	**Adults and children:** 1–2 drops of 0.12–1% solution/suspension 2–4 times daily.	• As condition improves, ↓ frequency of administration • ADRs: corneal thinning, ↑ intraocular pressure, irritation
Cycloplegic Mydriatics		
Uses: Preparation for cycloplegic refraction; induction of mydriasis; management of uveitis (not tropicamide). **CAUTIONS:** Use cautiously in patients with a history of glaucoma; systemic absorption may cause anticholinergic effects such as confusion, unusual behavior, flushing, hallucinations, slurred speech, drowsiness, swollen stomach (infants), tachycardia, or dry mouth.		

DRUG NAME	DOSE	NOTES
atropine (Isopto Atropine)	**Adults and children ≥3 mo:** *Cycloplegia/mydriasis*—Solution: 1–2 drops of 1% solution 40 min before procedure; Ointment: 0.3–0.5 cm strip 1–2 times daily.	• Effects on accommodation may last 6 days; mydriasis may last 12 days • ADRs: irritation, blurred vision, photophobia
cyclopentolate (Cyclogyl)	**Adults:** 1–2 drops of 0.5–2% solution; may repeat in 5–10 min. **Children:** 1 drop of 0.5–2% solution; may be followed 5–10 min later by 1 drop of 0.5–1% solution.	• Peak of cycloplegia is within 25–75 min and lasts 6–24 hr • Peak of mydriasis is within 30–60 min and may last several days • 2% solution used for heavily pigmented iris • ADRs: irritation, blurred vision, photophobia
homatropine	**Adults:** *Cycloplegic refraction*—1–2 drops of 2–5% solution, may repeat in 5–10 min for 2 more doses; *Uveitis*—1–2 drops of 2–5% solution 2–3 times daily (up to every 4 hr). **Children ≥3 mo:** *Cycloplegic refraction*—1–2 drops of 2% solution, may repeat in 10–15 min if needed; *Uveitis*—1–2 drops of 2% solution 2–3 times daily (up to every 4 hr).	• Cycloplegia and mydriasis may last for 24–72 hr • ADRs: irritation, blurred vision, photophobia
tropicamide (Mydriacyl, Tropicacyl)	**Adults and children:** 1–2 drops of 0.5–1% solution.	• Stronger solution/repeated dosing may be required in patients with dark irides • Peak effect occurs in 20–40 min • Cycloplegia lasts 2–6 hr; mydriasis lasts up to 7 hr • ADRs: irritation, blurred vision, photophobia

Immunomodulators

Uses: ↑ tear production when the cause of dry eye is inflammation secondary to keratoconjunctivitis sicca.
CAUTIONS: Tear production is not ↑ during concurrent use of ophthalmic NSAIDs or punctal plugs.

cyclosporine (Cequa, Restasis)	**Adults and children ≥16 yr:** Restasis: 1 drop of 0.05% emulsion every 12 hr. **Adults:** Cequa: 1 drop of 0.09% solution every 12 hr.	• Emulsion should be inverted to obtain uniform opaque appearance prior to use. • ADRs: irritation, blurred vision, conjunctival hyperemia
lifitegrast (Xiidra)	**Adults:** 1 drop of 5% solution every 12 hr.	• Emulsion should be inverted to obtain uniform opaque appearance prior to use. • ADRs: headache, irritation, blurred vision, metallic taste

Mast Cell Stabilizers

Uses: Vernal keratoconjunctivitis.
CAUTIONS: Require several days of treatment before effects are seen.

cromolyn	**Adults and children ≥4 yr:** 1–2 drops of 4% solution 4–6 times daily.	• ADRs: irritation
lodoxamide (Alomide)	**Adults and children ≥2 yr:** 1–2 drops of 0.1% solution 4 times daily for up to 3 mo.	• ADRs: blurred vision, foreign body sensation, irritation
nedocromil (Alocril)	**Adults and children ≥3 yr:** 1–2 drops of 2% solution twice daily throughout period of exposure to allergen.	• ADRs: headache, ocular burning, unpleasant taste, nasal congestion

Nonsteroidal Anti-inflammatory Drugs

Uses: Management of pain/inflammation following surgery (bromfenac, diclofenac, ketorolac, nepafenac), allergic conjunctivitis (ketorolac), inhibition of perioperative miosis (flurbiprofen).
CAUTIONS: Cross-sensitivity with systemic NSAIDs may occur; concurrent use of anticoagulants, other NSAIDs, thrombolytics, some cephalosporins, and valproates may ↑ the risk of bleeding. May slow/delay healing. Avoid contact lens use.

DRUG NAME	DOSE	NOTES
bromfenac (Bromsite, Prolensa)	**Adults:** *Generic*—1 drop of 0.09% solution once daily starting 1 day before surgery and continued on day of surgery and for 2 wk after surgery; *Bromsite*—1 drop of 0.075% solution once daily starting 1 day before surgery and continued on day of surgery and for 2 wk after surgery; *Prolensa*—1 drop of 0.07% solution once daily starting 1 day before surgery and continued on day of surgery and for 2 wk after surgery.	• Contains sulfites • ADRs: irritation, headache
diclofenac (Voltaren)	**Adults:** *Cataract surgery*—1 drop of 0.1% solution 4 times daily starting 24 hr after surgery and for 2 wk after surgery; *Corneal refractive surgery*—1–2 drops of 0.1% solution within hr before surgery, within 15 min after surgery, then continue 4 times daily for up to 3 days.	• ADRs: irritation, allergic reactions
flurbiprofen (Ocufen)	**Adults:** 1 drop of 0.03% solution every 30 min, beginning 2 hr prior to surgery (4 drops total in each eye).	• ADRs: irritation, allergic reactions
ketorolac (Acular, Acular LS, Acuvail)	**Adults and children ≥2 yr:** *Allergic conjunctivitis*—Acular: 1 drop of 0.5% solution 4 times daily; *Postoperative pain/inflammation*—Acular: 1 drop of 0.5% solution 4 times daily starting 24 hr after cataract surgery and for 2 wk after surgery; Acular LS: 1 drop of 0.4% solution 4 times daily for up to 4 days after corneal refractive surgery; Acuvail: 1 drop of 0.45% solution twice daily starting 1 day before cataract surgery and continued for 2 wk after surgery.	• ADRs: irritation, allergic reactions
nepafenac (Ilevro, Nevanac)	**Adults and children ≥10 yr:** *Ilevro*—1 drop of 0.3% suspension once daily starting one day before cataract surgery and continued for 2 wk after surgery; instill 1 additional drop 30–120 min before surgery; *Nevanac*—1 drop of 0.1% suspension 3 times daily starting one day before cataract surgery and continued for 2 wk after surgery.	• ADRs: irritation, photophobia, headache, hypertension, nausea/vomiting

Ocular Decongestants/Vasoconstrictors

Uses: ↓ ocular congestion due to irritation by vasoconstricting conjunctival blood vessels; stronger solutions have mydriatic effects.
CAUTIONS: Systemic absorption may result in adverse cardiovascular effects; excessive/prolonged use may produce rebound hyperemia; use caution in patients at risk for acute angle-closure glaucoma; cardiovascular effects may be exaggerated by MAO inhibitors and dose adjustment may be required within 21 days of MAO inhibitors; ↑ risk of arrhythmias with inhalation anesthetics.

DRUG NAME	DOSE	NOTES
naphazoline (🍁 Albalon, Clear Eyes Redness Relief, 🍁 Diopticon, 🍁 Naphcon Forte)	**Adults:** 1–2 drops of 0.012–0.025% solution up to 4 times daily (for up to 3 days) or 1–2 drops of 0.1% solution every 3–4 hr as needed.	• ADRs: ophthalmic-rebound hyperemia; systemic-dizziness, headache, nausea, sweating, weakness
oxymetazoline (Visine LR)	**Adults and children ≥6 yr:** 1–2 drops of 0.025% solution every 6 hr as needed (for up to 3 days).	• ADRs: ophthalmic-rebound hyperemia; systemic-headache, insomnia, nervousness, tachycardia

DRUG NAME	DOSE	NOTES
phenylephrine (🍁 Mydfrin)	**Adults:** *Decongestant*—1–2 drops of 0.12% solution up to 4 times daily as needed (for up to 3 days); *Mydriasis*—1 drop of 2.5–10% solution, may repeat in 10–60 min as needed. **Children ≥1 yr:** *Mydriasis*—1 drop of 2.5–10% solution, may repeat in 10–60 min as needed.	• ADRs: ophthalmic-blurred vision, irritation; systemic-dizziness, tachycardia, hypertension, paleness, sweating, trembling
tetrahydrozoline (Visine)	**Adults:** 1–2 drops of 0.05% solution 2–4 times daily.	• ADRs: ophthalmic—irritation; systemic—tachycardia, hypertension

Prostaglandin Agonists

Uses: Treatment of open-angle glaucoma (↑ outflow of aqueous humor).
CAUTIONS: May change eye color to brown; will form precipitate with thimerosal-containing products; can be used with other agents to ↓ intraocular pressure.

DRUG NAME	DOSE	NOTES
bimatoprost (Lumigan, 🍁 Vistitan)	**Adults and children ≥16 yr:** 1 drop of 0.01–0.03% solution once daily in the evening.	• ADRs: local irritation, foreign body sensation, ↑ eyelash growth, ↑ brown pigmentation in iris
latanoprost (Xalatan, Xelpros)	**Adults:** 1 drop of 0.005% solution/emulsion once daily in the evening.	• ADRs: local irritation, foreign body sensation, ↑ eyelash growth, ↑ brown pigmentation in iris
latanoprostene (Vyzulta)	**Adults:** 1 drop of 0.024% solution once daily in the evening.	• ADRs: conjunctival hyperemia, local irritation, eye pain, ↑ eyelash growth, ↑ brown pigmentation in iris
tafluprost (Zioptan)	**Adults:** 1 drop of 0.0015% solution once daily in the evening.	• ADRs: local irritation, foreign body sensation, ↑ eyelash growth, ↑ brown pigmentation in iris
travoprost (Travatan Z)	**Adults and children ≥16 yr:** 1 drop of 0.004% solution once daily in the evening.	• ADRs: local irritation, foreign body sensation, ↑ eyelash growth, ↑ brown pigmentation in iris

Rho Kinase Inhibitor

Uses: Treatment of open-angle glaucoma or ocular hypertension (↑ outflow of aqueous humor).
CAUTIONS: Can be used with other agents to ↓ intraocular pressure.

DRUG NAME	DOSE	NOTES
netarsudil (Rhopressa)	**Adults:** 1 drop of 0.02% solution once daily in the evening.	• ADRs: conjunctival hyperemia, corneal verticillata, conjunctival hemorrhage eye pain

Sympathomimetics

Uses: Treatment of open-angle glaucoma and other forms of intraocular hypertension (↓ formation of aqueous humor); brimonidine also available as over-the-counter product to ↓ ocular redness.
CAUTIONS: Systemic absorption may result in adverse cardiovascular and CNS reactions (especially in patients with cardiovascular disease); avoid use in patients predisposed to acute angle-closure glaucoma.

DRUG NAME	DOSE	NOTES
apraclonidine (Iopidine)	**Adults:** *Postoperative reduction of intraocular pressure*—1–2 drops of 0.5% solution 3 times daily or 1 drop of 1% solution 1 hr before surgery and upon completion of surgery.	• Used to ↓ intraocular pressure after surgery • A selective alpha-adrenergic agonist • Monitor pulse and blood pressure • Avoid concurrent use with MAO inhibitors • ADRs: ophthalmic-irritation, mydriasis; systemic-allergic reactions, arrhythmias, bradycardia, drowsiness, dry nose, fainting, headache, nervousness, weakness
brimonidine (Alphagan P, Lumify [OTC])	**Adults and children ≥2 yr:** *Glaucoma*—1 drop of 0.1–0.2% solution 3 times daily (8 hr apart). **Adults and children ≥5 yr:** *Ocular redness*—1 drop of 0.025% solution every 6–8 hr as needed (up to 4 times daily).	• A selective alpha-adrenergic agonist • Avoid concurrent use with MAO inhibitors • Tricyclic antidepressants may ↓ effectiveness; additive CNS depression may occur with other CNS depressants, additive adverse cardiovascular effects with other cardiovascular agents • ADRs: ophthalmic—irritation; systemic—drowsiness, dizziness, dry mouth, headache, weakness, muscular pain

APPENDIX D

Medication Administration Techniques

Subcutaneous Injection Sites

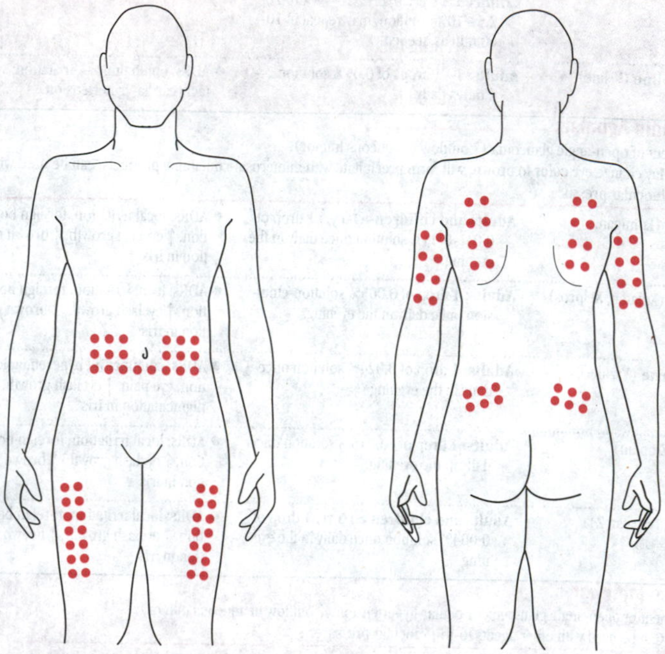

Administration of Ophthalmic Medications

For instillation of ophthalmic solutions, instruct patient to lie down or tilt head back and look at ceiling. Pull down on lower lid, creating a small pocket, and instill solution into pocket. With systemically acting drugs, apply pressure to the inner canthus for 1–2 min to minimize systemic absorption. Instruct patient to gently close eye. Wait 5 min before instilling second drop or any other ophthalmic solutions.

For instillation of ophthalmic ointment, instruct patient to hold tube in hand for several minutes to warm. Squeeze a small amount of ointment (¼–½ in.) inside lower lid. Instruct patient to close eye gently and roll eyeball around in all directions with eye closed. Wait 10 min before instilling any other ophthalmic ointments.

Do not touch cap or tip of container to eye, fingers, or any surface.

Administration of Medications with Metered-Dose Inhalers

Instruct patient on the proper use of the metered-dose inhaler. There are 3 methods of using a metered-dose inhaler. Shake inhaler well. (1) Take a drink of water to moisten the throat; place the inhaler mouthpiece 2 finger-widths away from mouth; tilt head back slightly. While activating the inhaler, take a slow, deep breath for 3–5 sec; hold the breath for 10 sec; and breathe out slowly. (2) Exhale and close lips firmly around mouthpiece. Administer during second half of inhalation, and hold breath for as long as possible to ensure deep instillation of medication. (3) Use of spacer. Consult health care professional to determine method desired prior to instruction. Allow 1–2 min between inhalations. Rinse mouth with water or mouthwash after each use to minimize dry mouth and hoarseness. Wash inhalation assembly at least daily in warm running water.

For use of dry powder inhalers, turn head away from inhaler and exhale (do not blow into inhaler). Do not shake. Close mouth tightly around the mouthpiece of the inhaler and inhale rapidly.

Steps for Using Your Inhaler*

1. Remove the cap and hold inhaler upright.
2. Shake the inhaler.
3. Tilt your head back slightly and breathe out slowly.
4. Position the inhaler in one of the following ways (A or B is optimal, but C is acceptable for those who have difficulty with A or B. C is required for breath-activated inhalers):

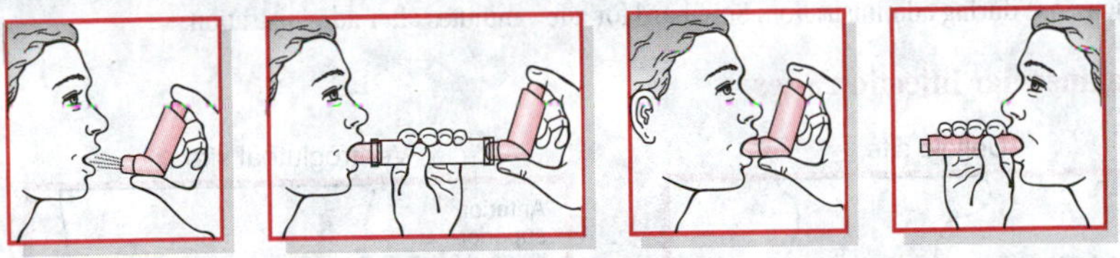

A. Open mouth with inhaler 1 to 2 inches away.

B. Use space/holding chamber (this is recommended especially for young children and for people using corticosteroids).

C. In the mouth. Do not use for corticosteroids.

D. NOTE: Inhaled dry powder capsules require a different inhalation technique. To use a dry powder inhaler, it is important to close the mouth tightly around the mouthpiece of the inhaler and to inhale rapidly.

5. Press down on the inhaler to release medication as you start to breathe in slowly.
6. Breathe in slowly (3–5 sec).
7. Hold your breath for 10 sec to allow the medicine to reach deeply into your lungs.
8. Repeat puff as directed. Waiting 1 min between puffs may permit second puff to penetrate your lungs better.
9. Spacers/holding chambers are useful for all patients. They are particularly recommended for young children and older adults and for use with **inhaled corticosteroids**.

Avoid common inhaler mistakes. Follow these inhaler tips:

- Breathe out before pressing your inhaler.
- Inhale slowly.
- Breathe in through your mouth, not your nose.
- Press down on your inhaler at the start of inhalation (or within the first sec of inhalation).
- Keep inhaling as you press down on inhaler.
- Press your inhaler only once while you are inhaling (one breath for each puff).
- Make sure you breathe in evenly and deeply.
- If you are using a short-acting bronchodilator inhaler and a corticosteroid inhaler, use the bronchodilator first, and allow 5 min to elapse before using the corticosteroid.

Other inhalers have become available in addition to the one illustrated here. Different types of inhalers may require different techniques.

Administration of Medications by Nebulizer

Administer in a location where patient can sit comfortably for 10–15 min. Plug in compressor. Mix medication as directed, or empty unit-dose vials into nebulizer. Do not mix different types of medications

*Source: Expert Panel Report 2: Guidelines for the Diagnosis and Management of Asthma. National Asthma Education and Prevention Program, National Heart, Lung, and Blood Institute, 1997.

without checking with health care professional. Assemble mask or mouthpiece and connect tubing to port on compressor. Have patient sit in a comfortable upright position. Make sure that mask fits properly over nose and mouth and that mist does not flow into eyes, or put mouthpiece into mouth. Turn on compressor. Instruct patient to take slow deep breaths. If possible, patient should hold breath for 10 sec before slowly exhaling. Continue this process until medication chamber is empty. Wash mask in hot soapy water; rinse well and allow to air dry before next use.

Administration of Nasal Sprays

Clear nasal passages of secretions prior to use. If nasal passages are blocked, use a decongestant immediately prior to use to ensure adequate penetration of the spray. Keep head upright. Breathe in through nose during administration. Sniff hard for a few minutes after administration.

Intramuscular Injection Sites

Deltoid site

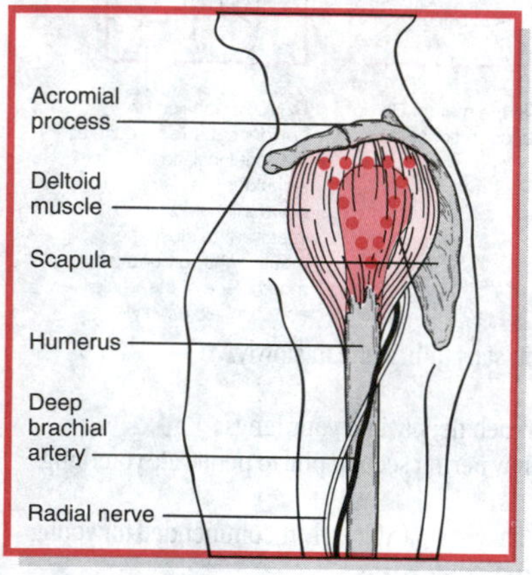

Ventrogluteal site

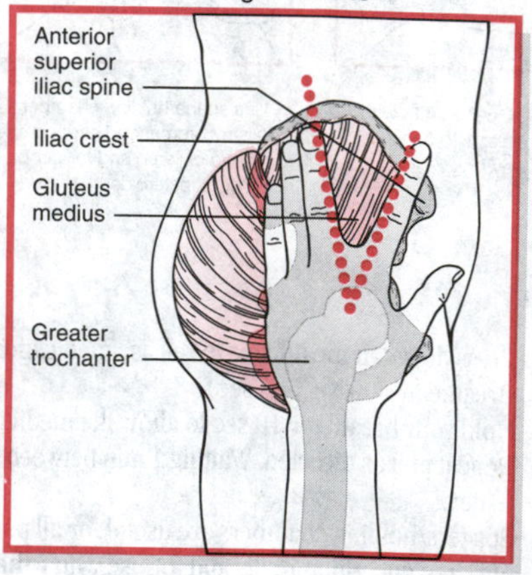

Vastus lateralis site

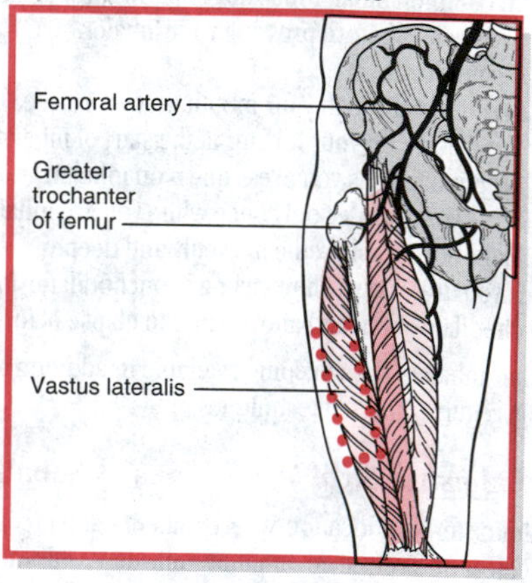

The deltoid and ventrogluteal sites are the preferred sites for adults; the vastus lateralis site is preferred in children under 2 yr of age.

APPENDIX E

Administering Medications to Children

General Guidelines

Medication administration to a pediatric patient can be challenging. Prescribers should order dosage forms that are age appropriate for their patients. If a child is unable to take a particular dosage form, ask the pharmacist if another form is available or for other options.

Oral Liquids

Pediatric liquid medicines may be given with plastic medicine cups, oral syringes, oral droppers, or cylindrical dosing spoons. Parents should be taught to use these calibrated devices rather than using household utensils. If a medicine comes with a particular measuring device, do not use it with another product. For young children, it is best to squirt a little of the dose at a time into the side of the cheek away from the bitter taste buds at the back of the tongue.

Eye Drops/Ointments

Tilt the child's head back and gently press the skin under the lower eyelid and pull the lower lid away slightly until a small pouch is visible. Insert the ointment or drop (1 at a time) and close the eye for a few minutes to keep the medicine in the eye.

Ear Drops

Shake otic suspensions well before administration. For children <3 yr, pull the outer ear outward and downward before instilling drops. For children ≥3 yr, pull the outer ear outward and upward. Keep child on side for 2 min and instill a cotton plug into ear.

Nose Drops

Clear nose of secretions prior to use. A nasal aspirator (bulb syringe) or a cotton swab may be used in infants and young children. Ask older children to blow their nose. Tilt child's head back over a pillow and squeeze dropper without touching the nostril. Keep child's head back for 2 min.

Suppositories

Keep refrigerated for easier administration. Wearing gloves, moisten the rounded end with water or petroleum jelly prior to insertion. Using your pinky finger for children <3 yr and your index finger for those ≥3 yr, insert the suppository into the rectum about ½ to 1 inch beyond the sphincter. If the suppository slides out, insert it a little farther than before. Hold the buttocks together for a few minutes and have the child hold their position for about 20 min, if possible.

Topicals

Clean affected area and dry well prior to application. Apply a thin layer to the skin and rub in gently. Do not apply coverings over the area unless instructed to do so by the prescriber.

Metered-Dose Inhalers

Generally the same principles apply in children as in adults, except the use of spacers is recommended for young children (see Appendix D).

APPENDIX F

Formulas Helpful for Calculating Doses

Ratio and Proportion

A ratio is the same as a fraction and can be expressed as a fraction (½) or in the algebraic form (1:2). This relationship is stated as *one is to two*.

A proportion is an equation of equal fractions or ratios.

$$\frac{1}{2} = \frac{4}{8}$$

To calculate doses, begin each proportion with the two known values, for example 15 grains = 1 gram (known equivalent) or 10 milligrams = 2 milliliters (dosage available) on one side of the equation. Next, make certain that the units of measure on the opposite side of the equation are the same as the units of the known values and are placed on the same level of the equation.

Problem A: $$\frac{15 \text{ gr}}{1 \text{ g}} = \frac{10 \text{ gr}}{x \text{ g}}$$

Problem B: $$\frac{10 \text{ mg}}{2 \text{ mL}} = \frac{5 \text{ mg}}{x \text{ mL}}$$

Once the proportion is set up correctly, cross-multiply the opposing values of the proportion.

Problem A: $$\frac{15 \text{ gr}}{1 \text{ g}} \times \frac{10 \text{ gr}}{x \text{ g}}$$

$$15x = 10$$

Problem B: $$\frac{10 \text{ mg}}{2 \text{ mL}} \times \frac{5 \text{ mg}}{x \text{ mL}}$$

$$10x = 10$$

Next, divide each side of the equation by the number with the x to determine the answer. Then, add the unit of measure corresponding to x in the original equation.

Problem A: $$\frac{15x}{15} = \frac{10}{15}$$

$$x = \frac{2}{3} \text{ or } 0.6 \text{ g}$$

Problem B: $$\frac{10x}{10} = \frac{10}{10}$$

$$x = 1 \text{ mL}$$

Calculation of IV Drip Rate

To calculate the drip rate for an intravenous infusion, 3 values are needed:

I. The amount of solution and corresponding time for infusion. May be ordered as:

1000 mL over 8 hr

or

125 mL/hr

II. The equivalent in time to convert hr to min.

$$1 \text{ hr} = 60 \text{ min}$$

III. The drop factor or number of drops that equal 1 mL of fluid. (This information can be found on the IV tubing box.)

$$10 \text{ gtt} = 1 \text{ mL}$$

Set up the problem by placing each of the 3 values in a proportion.

$$\frac{125 \text{ mL}}{1 \text{ hr}} \times \frac{1 \text{ hr}}{60 \text{ min}} \times \frac{10 \text{ gtt}}{1 \text{ mL}}$$

Units of measure can be canceled out from the upper and lower levels of the equation. The units cancel, leaving:

$$\frac{125}{1} \times \frac{1}{60 \text{ min}} \times \frac{10 \text{ gtt}}{1}$$

Next, multiply each level across and divide the numerator by the denominator for the answer.

$$\frac{125}{1} \times \frac{1}{6 \text{ min}} \times \frac{1 \text{ gtt}}{1}$$

$$125/6 = 20.8 \text{ or } 21 \text{ gtt/min}$$

Calculation of Creatinine Clearance (CCr) in Adults from Serum Creatinine

$$\text{Men: CCr} = \frac{\text{ideal body weight (kg)} \times (140 - \text{age})}{72 \times \text{serum creatinine (mg/dL)}}$$

$$\text{Women: CCr} = 0.85 \times \text{calculation for men}$$

Calculation of Body Surface Area (BSA) in Adults and Children

Dubois method:

$$\text{SA (cm}^2) = \text{wt (kg)}^{0.425} \times 71.84$$

$$\text{SA (m}^2) \; K \times \sqrt[3]{\text{wt}^2 \text{ (kg)}}$$ (common K value 0.1 for toddlers, 0.103 for neonates)

Simplified method:

$$\text{BSA (m}^2) = \sqrt{\frac{\text{ht (cm)} \times \text{wt (kg)}}{3600}}$$

Body Mass Index

$$\text{BMI} = \text{wt (kg)/ht (m}^2)$$

APPENDIX G

Pediatric Dosage Calculations

Most drugs in children are dosed according to body weight (mg/kg) or body surface area (BSA) (mg/m^2). Care must be taken to properly convert body weight from pounds to kilograms (1 kg= 2.2 lb) before calculating doses based on body weight. Doses are often expressed as mg/kg/day or mg/kg/dose, therefore orders written "mg/kg/d," which is confusing, *require further clarification from the prescriber.*

Chemotherapeutic drugs are commonly dosed according to body surface area, which requires an extra verification step (BSA calculation) prior to dosing. Medications are available in multiple concentrations, therefore *orders written in "mL" rather than "mg" are not acceptable and require further clarification.*

Dosing also varies by indication, therefore diagnostic information is helpful when calculating doses. The following examples are typically encountered when dosing medication in children.

Example 1.

Calculate the dose of amoxicillin suspension in mLs for otitis media for a 1-yr-old child weighing 22 lb. The dose required is 40 mg/kg/day divided BID and the suspension comes in a concentration of 400 mg/5 mL.

Step 1. Convert pounds to kg:	22 lb × 1 kg/2.2 lb = 10 kg
Step 2. Calculate the dose in mg:	10 kg × 40 mg/kg/day = 400 mg/day
Step 3. Divide the dose by the frequency:	400 mg/day ÷ 2 (BID) = 200 mg/dose BID
Step 4. Convert the mg dose to mL:	200 mg/dose ÷ 400 mg/5 mL = **2.5 mL BID**

Example 2.

Calculate the dose of ceftriaxone in mLs for meningitis for a 5-yr-old weighing 18 kg. The dose required is 100 mg/kg/day given IV once daily and the drug comes prediluted in a concentration of 40 mg/mL.

Step 1. Calculate the dose in mg:	18 kg × 100 mg/kg/day = 1800 mg/day
Step 2. Divide the dose by the frequency:	1800 mg/day ÷ 1 (daily) = 1800 mg/dose
Step 3. Convert the mg dose to mL:	1800 mg/dose ÷ 40 mg/mL = **45 mL once daily**

Example 3.

Calculate the dose of vincristine in mLs for a 4-yr-old with leukemia weighing 37 lb and is 97 cm tall. The dose required in 2 mg/m^2 and the drug comes in 1 mg/mL concentration.

Step 1. Convert pounds to kg:	37 lb × 1 kg/2.2 lb = 16.8 kg
Step 2. Calculate BSA:	$\sqrt{16.8 \text{ kg} \times 97 \text{ cm}/3600} = 0.67 \text{ m}^2$
Step 3. Calculate the dose in mg:	2 mg/m^2 × 0.67 m^2 = 1.34 mg
Step 4. Calculate the dose in mL:	1.34 mg ÷ 1 mg/mL = **1.34 mL**

APPENDIX H

Normal Values of Common Laboratory Tests

SERUM TESTS

HEMATOLOGIC	MEN	WOMEN
Hemoglobin	13.5–18 g/dL	12–16 g/dL
Hematocrit	40–54%	38–47%
Red blood cells (RBC)	4.6–6.2 million/mm^3	4.2–5.4 million/mm^3
Mean corpuscular volume (MCV)	76–100 (micrometer)^3	76–100 (micrometer)^3
Mean corpuscular hemoglobin (MCH)	27–33 picogram	27–33 picogram
Mean corpuscular hemoglobin concentration (MCHC)	33–37 g/dL	33–37 g/dL
Erythrocyte sedimentation rate (ESR)	≤20 mm/hr	≤30 mm/hr
Leukocytes (WBC)	5000–10,000/mm^3	5000–10,000/mm^3
Neutrophils	54–75% (3000–7500/mm^3)	54–75% (3000–7500/mm^3)
Bands	3–8% (150–700/mm^3)	3–8% (150–700/mm^3)
Eosinophils	1–4% (50–400/mm^3)	1–4% (50–400/mm^3)
Basophils	0–1% (25–100/mm^3)	0–1% (25–100/mm^3)
Monocytes	2–8% (100–500/mm^3)	2–8% (100–500/mm^3)
Lymphocytes	25–40% (1500–4500/mm^3)	25–40% (1500–4500/mm^3)
T lymphocytes	60–80% of lymphocytes	60–80% of lymphocytes
B lymphocytes	10–20% of lymphocytes	10–20% of lymphocytes
Platelets	150,000–450,000/mm^3	150,000–450,000/mm^3
Prothrombin time (PT)	9.6–11.8 sec	9.5–11.3 sec
Partial thromboplastin time (PTT)	30–45 sec	30–45 sec
Bleeding time (duke)	1–3 min	1–3 min
(ivy)	3–6 min	3–6 min
(template)	3–6 min	3–6 min

CHEMISTRY	MEN	WOMEN
Sodium	135–145 mEq/L	135–145 mEq/L
Potassium	3.5–5.0 mEq/L	3.5–5.0 mEq/L
Chloride	95–105 mEq/L	95–105 mEq/L
Bicarbonate (HCO_3)	19–25 mEq/L	19–25 mEq/L
Total calcium	9–11 mg/dL or 4.5–5.5 mEq/L	9–11 mg/dL or 4.5–5.5 mEq/L
Ionized calcium	4.2–5.4 mg/dL or 2.1–2.6 mEq/L	4.2–5.4 mg/dL or 2.1–2.6 mEq/L
Phosphorus/phosphate	2.4–4.7 mg/dL	2.4–4.7 mg/dL
Magnesium	1.8–3.0 mg/dL or 1.5–2.5 mEq/L	1.8–3.0 mg/dL or 1.5–2.5 mEq/L
Glucose	65–99 mg/dL	65–99 mg/dL
Osmolality	285–310 mOsm/kg	285–310 mOsm/kg
Ammonia (NH_3)	10–80 mcg/dL	10–80 mcg/dL
Amylase	≤130 U/L	≤130 U/L
Creatine phosphokinase total (CK, CPK)	<150 U/L	<150 U/L
Creatine kinase isoenzymes, MB fraction	>5% in MI	>5% in MI
Lactic dehydrogenase (LDH)	50–150 U/L	50–150 U/L
Protein, total	6–8 g/d	6–8 g/d
Albumin	4–6 g/dL	4–6 g/dL

HEPATIC	MEN	WOMEN
AST	8–46 U/L	7–34 U/L
ALT	10–30 IU/mL	10–30 IU/mL
Total bilirubin	0.3–1.2 mg/dL	0.3–1.2 mg/dL
Conjugated bilirubin	0.0–0.2 mg/dL	0.0–0.2 mg/dL
Unconjugated (indirect) bilirubin	0.2–0.8 mg/dL	0.2–0.8 mg/dL
Alkaline phosphatase	20–90 U/L	20–90 U/L

RENAL	MEN	WOMEN
BUN	6–20 mg/dL	6–20 mg/dL
Creatinine	0.6–1.3 mg/dL	0.5–1.0 mg/dL
Uric acid	4.0–8.5 mg/dL	2.7–7.3 mg/dL

ARTERIAL BLOOD GASES	MEN	WOMEN
pH	7.35–7.45	7.35–7.45
Po_2	80–100 mm Hg	80–100 mm Hg
Pco_2	35–45 mm Hg	35–45 mm Hg
O_2 saturation	95–97%	95–97%
Base excess	+2–(−2)	+2–(−2)
Bicarbonate (HCO_3^-)	22–26 mEq/L	22–26 mEq/L

URINE TESTS

URINE	MEN	WOMEN
pH	4.5–8.0	4.5–8.0
Specific gravity	1.010–1.025	1.010–1.025

APPENDIX I

Controlled Substances Schedules

General

A controlled substance is any type of drug that the federal government has categorized as having significant potential for abuse or addiction. While controlled substances are regulated in both the United States (U.S.) and Canada, differences exist between the two countries with respect to scheduling and enforcement.

IN THE UNITED STATES:

The Drug Enforcement Agency (DEA), an arm of the United States Justice Department, classifies controlled substances according to five schedules, based on the potential for abuse and dependence liability (physical and psychological) of the medication. Some states may have stricter prescription regulations. Physicians, dentists, podiatrists, and veterinarians may prescribe controlled substances. Nurse practitioners and physician assistants may also prescribe controlled substances with limitations that vary from state to state.

Schedule I (C-I)

Potential for abuse is so high as to be unacceptable. May be used for research with appropriate limitations. Examples are LSD and heroin.

Schedule II (C-II)

High potential for abuse and extreme liability for physical and psychological dependence (amphetamines, opioid analgesics, dronabinol, certain barbiturates). Outpatient prescriptions must be in writing. In emergencies, telephone orders may be acceptable if a written prescription is provided within 72 hr. No refills are allowed.

Schedule III (C-III)

Intermediate potential for abuse (less than C-II) and intermediate liability for physical and psychological dependence (certain nonbarbiturate sedatives, certain nonamphetamine CNS stimulants, and certain opioid analgesics). Outpatient prescriptions can be refilled 5 times within 6 mo from date of issue if authorized by prescriber. Telephone orders are acceptable.

Schedule IV (C-IV)

Less abuse potential than Schedule III with minimal liability for physical or psychological dependence (certain sedative/hypnotics, certain antianxiety agents, some barbiturates, benzodiazepines, chloral hydrate, pentazocine, and propoxyphene). Outpatient prescriptions can be refilled 6 times within 6 mo from date of issue if authorized by prescriber. Telephone orders are acceptable.

Schedule V (C-V)

Minimal abuse potential. Number of outpatient refills determined by prescriber. Some products (cough suppressants with small amounts of codeine, antidiarrheals containing paregoric) may be available without prescription to patients >18 yr of age.

IN CANADA:

The federal *Controlled Drugs and Substances Act (CDSA)* along with the *Narcotic Control Regulations*, Part G of the *Food and Drug Regulations*, and the *Benzodiazepines and Other Targeted Substances Regulations* regulate narcotics, controlled drugs, and targeted substances.

The CDSA classifies controlled substances according to eight schedules and three classes of precursors. While a few examples are listed below, a complete list of drugs scheduled in Canada's Controlled Drugs and Substances act can be accessed at: http://laws-lois.justice.gc.ca/eng/acts/C%2D38.8/

Schedule I
—opioids and derivatives and related drugs (e.g., morphine, oxycodone, heroin)

Schedule II
—cannabis (marihuana) and derivatives

Schedule III
—amphetamines and related drugs and substances (e.g., methylphenidate, LSD)

Schedule IV
—barbiturates and derivatives, anabolic steroids and related drugs, and benzodiazepines (e.g., diazepam)

Schedule V
—propylhexedrine

Schedule VI
—precursors Class A (e.g., pseudoephedrine and salts)
—precursors Class B (e.g., acetone, toluene)
—precursors Class C mixtures of the above

Schedules VII & VIII
—cannabis and its resins in varying amounts
(Note: In Canada marihuana may be used for medical purposes. It is regulated by the Access to Cannabis for Medical Purposes Regulations, which can be accessed at: http://www.laws-lois.justice.gc.ca/eng/regulations/SOR-2016-230/page-1.html)

The CDSA federally regulates conditions of sale, distribution, and accountability relating to controlled substances. Provincial legislation compliments how patients access controlled substances from regulated health professionals. As such, it is imperative for an individual to become familiar with legislation pertaining to the specific province he/she is working in. Some federal regulations are as follows:

Narcotic drug—Two subcategories of prescription narcotics—"Straight" Narcotics and Verbal Prescription Narcotics
(e.g., codeine, morphine, fentanyl, oxycodone)

Straight Narcotics
- All single active ingredient products containing a narcotic, along with all narcotics for parenteral use and narcotic compounds containing more than one narcotic entity or less than two non-narcotic ingredients.
- Prescription can be written, faxed, or generated electronically in an authorized provincial electronic health record and must be signed and dated by prescriber.
- Refills are not permitted, but a prescription may be dispensed in divided portions. Prescription transfers from one pharmacist to another are not permitted.

Verbal Prescription Narcotic

(e.g., Tylenol No.2 and Tylenol No.3)

- Refers to oral combination products containing only one narcotic and two or more non-narcotic ingredients in a therapeutic dose. (Excluding diacetylmorphine, oxycodone, hydrocodone, methadone, or pentazocine. This means that an oral combination product that contains these drugs cannot be classified as a Verbal Prescription Narcotic.)
- Similar rules as above but prescriptions may also be verbal.

Exempted Codeine Preparations

(e.g., Tylenol No.1)

- Under federal regulations, products containing codeine (meaning codeine phosphate or its equivalent) may be purchased over the counter, without a prescription, provided they have two other medicinal ingredients and a **maximum** of 8 mg of codeine per solid oral dosage unit or 20 mg per 30 mL of liquid.
- The product may not be supplied if there are reasonable grounds to suspect the product will be used for other than recognized medical or dental purposes.

Controlled Drugs—Part 1

(e.g., Dexedrine, Ritalin, pentobarbital, secobarbital)

- Refers to drugs listed in Part I of the Schedule to Part G of the Food and Drug Regulations.
- Prescription may be written or verbal; no refills allowed if prescription is verbal.
- Refills are permitted if the number of repeats and the frequency or interval between refills is specified. Prescription transfers are not permitted.

Controlled Drugs—Parts 2 and 3

(e.g., other barbiturates and anabolic steroids)

- Refers to drugs listed in Parts II and III of the Schedule to Part G of the Food and Drug Regulations.
- Prescription may be written or verbal.
- Refills are permitted if prescribed in writing or verbally and the number of repeats and frequency or interval between refills is specified. Prescription transfers are not permitted.

Benzodiazepines and Other Targeted Substances

(e.g., lorazepam, diazepam)

- Refers to all benzodiazepines except flunitrazepam, which is listed in Schedule III of the Act as an illicit substance.
- Prescriptions may be written or verbal. Refills are permitted if the prescription is less than 1 year old and the prescriber specifies the number of times it can be refilled. If the prescriber indicated the interval between refills, the pharmacist cannot refill the prescription if that interval has expired. Prescription transfers are permitted, but only once.

References:

New Classes of Practitioners Regulations. http://laws-lois.justice.gc.ca/eng/regulations/SOR-2012-230/page-1.html (accessed 7 September 2017).

Controlled Drugs and Substances Act (S.C. 1996, c. 19). Available at http://laws-lois.justice.gc.ca/eng/acts/C-38.8/index.html (accessed 7 September 2017).

National Association of Pharmacy Regulatory Authorities (www.napra.org)

APPENDIX J

Equianalgesic Dosing Guidelines

OPIOID ANALGESICS STARTING ORAL DOSE COMMONLY USED FOR SEVERE PAIN

	EQUIANALGESIC DOSE		STARTING ORAL DOSE			
NAME	ORAL*	PARENTERAL†	ADULTS	CHILDREN	COMMENTS	PRECAUTIONS AND CONTRAINDICATIONS
Morphine-like agonists (mu agonists)						
morphine	30 mg	10 mg	15–30 mg	0.3 mg/kg	Standard of comparison for opioid analgesics. Sustained release preparations (MS Contin) release over 8–12 hr. Other formulations (Kadian, Morphabond ER, MS Contin) last 12–24 hr. Generic sustained release morphine preparations are now available.	For all opioids, caution in patients with impaired ventilation, bronchial asthma, ↑ intracranial pressure, liver failure.
hydromorphone (Dilaudid)	7.5 mg	1.5 mg	Opioid naïve: 4–8 mg	0.06 mg/kg	Slightly shorter duration than morphine. Sustained release preparations release over 24 hr.	
fentanyl	—	0.1 mg	—	—		
oxycodone	20 mg	—	10–20 mg	0.2 mg/kg		
methadone	10 mg	5 mg	5–10 mg	0.2 mg/kg	Good oral potency, long plasma half-life (24–36 hr).	Accumulates with repeated dosing, requiring decreases in dose size and frequency, especially on days 2–5. Use with caution in older adults.
levorphanol	2 mg (acute), 1 mg (chronic)	—	2–4 mg	0.04 mg/kg	Long plasma half-life (12–16 hr, but may be as long as 90–120 hr after one wk of dosing).	Accumulates on days 2 and 3. Use with caution in older adults.
oxymorphone (Opana)	10 mg	—	—	—	—	

meperidine (Demerol)	300 mg	100 mg	Not Recommended	—	Slightly shorter acting than morphine; accumulates with repetitive dosing causing CNS excitation; avoid in children with impaired renal function or who are receiving monoamine oxidase inhibitors.‡	Use with caution. Normeperidine (toxic metabolite) accumulates with repetitive dosing causing CNS excitation and a high risk of seizure. Avoid in children, renal impairment, and patients on monoamine oxidase inhibitors.‡
Centrally-acting mu agonists						
tramadol (UltramConZip)	120 mg	—	50–100 mg every 4–6 hr	—	Prodrug; significant serotonin reuptake inhibition. Maximum dose: IR 400 mg/day; ER 300 mg/day.	Caution with pre-existing seizure disorder, concurrent use of medications that ↓ seizure threshold, or medications that ↑ risk of serotonin syndrome.
tapentadol (Nucynta)	100 mg	—	50–100 mg every 4–6 hr	—	Sustained release preparation (Nucynta ER) releases over 12 hr. Blocks reuptake of norepinephrine > serotonin.	Caution with pre-existing seizure disorder or concurrent use of medications that ↓ seizure threshold.
Mixed agonists–antagonists (kappa agonists)						
nalbuphine	—	10 mg	10 mg every 3–6 hr	0.1–0.2 mg/kg every 3–4 hr	Not available orally; not scheduled under Controlled Substances Act. Kappa agonist, partial mu antagonist.	Incidence of psychotomimetic effects lower than with pentazocine; may precipitate withdrawal in opioid-dependent patients.
butorphanol	—	2 mg	1–4 mg every 3–4 hr (IM); 0.5–2 mg every 3–4 hr (IV)	—	Kappa agonist, partial mu antagonist. Also available in nasal spray.	Like nalbuphine.
pentazocine (Talwin)	—	30 mg	30–60 mg every 3–4 hr (IM); 30 mg every 3–4 hr (IV)	—	Kappa agonist, partial mu antagonist. Significant psychotomimetic side effects.	
Partial agonist						
buprenorphine (Buprenex)	—	0.4 mg	0.3 mg every 6–8 hr (IM/IV)	2–12 yr: 0.2–0.6 mg every 4–6 hr (IM/IV)	Sublingual tablets now available both plain and with naloxone for opioid-dependent patient management for specially certified physicians. These tablets are not approved as analgesics. Also available as a long-acting transdermal patch (Butrans), buccal film (Belbuca), and subdermal insert (Probuphine).	May precipitate withdrawal in opioid-dependent patients; not readily reversed by naloxone; avoid in labor.

*Starting dose should be lower for older adults.

†These are standard parenteral doses for acute pain in adults and can also be used to convert doses for IV infusions and repeated small IV boluses. For single IV boluses, use half the IM dose. IV doses for children >6 mo. = parenteral equianalgesic dose times weight (kg)/100.

‡Irritating to tissues with repeated IM injections.

Modified from *American Pain Society, Principles of Analgesic Use in the Treatment of Acute Pain and Cancer Pain*, ed.7. American Pain Society, 2016.

GUIDELINES FOR PATIENT-CONTROLLED INTRAVENOUS OPIOID ADMINISTRATION FOR ADULTS WITH ACUTE PAIN

DRUG*	USUAL STARTING DOSE AFTER LOADING	USUAL DOSE RANGE	USUAL LOCKOUT (MIN)	USUAL LOCKOUT RANGE (MIN)
Morphine (1 mg/mL)	1 mg	0.5–2.5 mg	8	5–10
Hydromorphone (0.2 mg/mL)	0.2 mg	0.05–0.4 mg	8	5–10
Fentanyl (50 mcg/mL)	20 mcg	10–50 mcg	6	5–8

*Standard concentrations for most PCA machines are listed in parentheses.
Modified from *American Pain Society, Principles of Analgesic Use in the Treatment of Acute Pain and Cancer Pain*, ed.7. American Pain Society, 2016.

FENTANYL TRANSDERMAL DOSE BASED ON DAILY MORPHINE DOSE*

ORAL 24-HRMORPHINE (mg/day)	TRANSDERMAL FENTANYL (mg/day)	FENTANYL TRANSDERMAL (mcg/hr)
30–90	0.6	25
91–150	1.2	50
151–210	1.8	75
211–270	2.4	100
271–330	3.0	125
331–390	3.6	150
391–450	4.2	175
451–510	4.8	200
511–570	5.4	225
571–630	6.0	250
631–690	6.6	275
691–750	7.2	300
For each additional 60 mg/day	+0.6	+25

*A 10-mg IM or 60-mg oral dose of morphine every 4 hr for 24 hr (total of 60 mg/day IM or 360 mg/day oral) was considered approximately equivalent to fentanyl transdermal 100 mcg/hr.

APPENDIX K

Food Sources for Specific Nutrients

Potassium-Rich Foods

artichoke
avocados
bananas
cantaloupe
cassava
dried fruits
grapefruit
honey dew
jack fruit
kiwi
kohlrabi
lima beans
mango
meats
milk
dried peas and beans
nuts
oranges/orange juice
papaya
peaches
pears
plantains
pomegranate
potatoes (white and sweet)
prunes/prune juice
pumpkin
rhubarb
salt substitute
spinach
sunflower seeds
Swiss chard
tomatoes/tomato juice
vegetable juice
winter squash

Sodium-Rich Foods

baking mixes (pancakes, muffins)
barbecue sauce
buttermilk
butter/margarine
canned chili
canned seafood
canned soups
canned spaghetti sauce
cured meats
dry onion soup mix
"fast" foods
frozen dinners
macaroni and cheese
microwave dinners
Parmesan cheese
pickles
potato salad
pretzels, potato chips
salad dressings (prepared)
salt
sauerkraut
tomato ketchup

Calcium-Rich Foods

almond (milk/nuts)
calcium fortified foods
canned salmon/sardines
cheese
cream soups (with milk)
greens: collard/mustard/turnip
kale
milk
soy (beans/milk)
spinach
tofu
yogurt

Vitamin K-Rich Foods

asparagus
beet greens
broccoli
brussel sprouts
cabbage
collard greens
dandelion leaves
garden cress
green tea leaves
kale
mustard greens
parsley
spinach
swiss chard
turnip greens

Low-Sodium Foods

baked or broiled poultry
canned pumpkin
cooked turnips
egg yolk
fresh vegetables
fruit
grits (not instant)
honey
jams and jellies
lean meats
low-calorie mayonnaise
macaroons
potatoes
puffed wheat and rice
red kidney and lima beans
sherbet
unsalted nuts
whiskey

Foods that Acidify Urine

cheeses
corn
cranberries
eggs
fish
grains (breads and cereals)
lentils
meats
nuts (Brazil, filberts, walnuts)
pasta
plums
poultry
prunes
rice

Foods that Alkalinize Urine

all fruits except cranberries, prunes, plums
all vegetables (except corn)
milk
nuts (almonds, chesnuts)

Foods Containing Tyramine

aged cheeses (blue, Boursault, brick, Brie, Camembert, cheddar, Emmenthaler, Gruyère, mozzarella, Parmesan, Romano, Roquefort, Stilton, Swiss)
American processed cheese
avocados (especially over-ripe)
bananas
bean curd
beer and ale
caffeine-containing beverages (coffee, tea, colas)
caviar
chocolate
distilled spirits
fermented sausage (bologna, salami, pepperoni, summer sausage)
liver
meats prepared with tenderizer
miso soup
over-ripe fruit
peanuts
raisins
raspberries
red wine (especially Chianti)
sauerkraut
sherry
shrimp paste
smoked or pickled fish
soy sauce
vermouth
yeasts
yogurt

Iron-Rich Foods

cereals
clams
dried beans and peas
dried fruit
leafy green vegetables
lean red meats
molasses (blackstrap)
organ meats

Vitamin D-Rich Foods

canned salmon, sardines, tuna
cereals
fish
fish liver oils
fortified milk
nonfat dry milk

Foods that Interact with/Inhibit the CYP3A4 Isoenzyme

grapefruit
grapefruit juice
Seville oranges
tangelos

APPENDIX L

Insulins and Insulin Therapy

The goal of therapy for diabetic patients is to provide insulin coverage that most closely resembles endogenous insulin production and results in the best glycemic control without hypoglycemia. Although daytime control of hyperglycemia may be accomplished with bolus doses of rapid-acting insulin analogs, elevations in fasting glucose may remain a problem. If fasting blood glucose levels remain elevated, the basal insulin dose (intermediate or long-acting) may have to be adjusted.

Most insulins used today are recombinant DNA human insulins. Produced through genetic engineering, synthetic human insulin is "manufactured" by yeast or nonpathogenic *E. coli*. In recent years, pharmaceutical companies have developed several new types and formulations of insulin.

Different insulins are distinguished by how quickly they are absorbed, the time and length of peak activity, and overall duration of action. Onset, peak, and duration of action times are approximate and vary according to individual factors such as injection site, blood supply, concurrent illnesses, lifestyle, and exercise level. These factors can vary from patient to patient and can vary in any patient from day to day.

There are 5 kinds of insulins: rapid-acting, short-acting, intermediate-acting, long-acting, and combination insulins.

Rapid-Acting Insulins

Rapid-acting insulins are analogs of regular insulin. An analog is a chemical structure very similar to another but differing in one component. Admelog/Humalog (lispro), Apidra (glulisine), and Fiasp/Novolog (aspart) are rapid-acting insulin analogs. The amino acid sequences of these analogs are nearly identical to human insulin. They differ in the positioning of certain proteins, which allow them to enter the bloodstream rapidly—within 15 min of subcutaneous injection. This closely mimics the body's own insulin response and allows greater flexibility in eating schedules for diabetic patients. Also, because these insulins leave the bloodstream quickly, the risk of hypoglycemic episodes several hours after the meal is lessened. The peak time for rapid-acting insulins is 1–2 hr and the duration is 3–4 hr. Rapid-acting insulin solutions are clear. Insulin aspart, insulin glulisine, and insulin lispro (100 units/mL only) can be given intravenously in selected situations under medical supervision.

Short-Acting Insulins

Regular insulin is a short-acting insulin and is available commercially as Humulin R or Novolin R. The onset of regular insulin is 0.5–1 hr; its peak activity occurs 2–4 hr after subcutaneous injection and its duration of action is 5–7 hr. This time/action profile makes rigid meal scheduling necessary, as the patient must estimate that a meal will occur within 45 min of injection. Short-acting insulin solutions are clear. Regular insulin (100 units/mL only) can be given intravenously.

Intermediate-Acting Insulins

Intermediate-acting insulin contains protamine, which delays onset, peak, and duration of action to provide basal insulin coverage. Basal insulins are given to control blood glucose levels throughout the day when not eating. Commercially, intermediate-acting insulins are available as Humulin N or Novolin N. (The "N" stands for NPH.) Action starts between 2 and 4 hr after injecting. Peak activity occurs between 4 and 10 hr. Duration of action lasts 10–16 hr. The addition of protamine causes the cloudy appearance of intermediate-acting insulins and results in the formulation being a suspension rather than a solution. This is why these insulins must be gently mixed before administering. Intermediate-acting insulins can be mixed with short- or rapid-acting insulins to provide both basal and bolus coverage.

Long-Acting Insulins

Long-acting insulins have the most delayed onset and the longest duration of all insulins. Products include Basaglar/Lantus/Toujeo (insulin glargine), Levemir (insulin detemir), and Tresiba (insulin degludec). Peaks are not as prominent in long-acting insulins. In fact, insulin glargine has no real peak action because it forms slowly dissolving crystals in the subcutaneous tissue. The onset of action of insulin glargine and insulin detemir is 3–4 hr and for insulin degludec is within 2 hr after subcutaneous injection. Full activity occurs within 4 to 5 hr and remains constant for 24 hr. Even though these insulins are clear solutions, they cannot be diluted or mixed with any other insulin or solution. Mixing these insulins with other insulin products can alter the onset of action and time to peak effect. If bolus insulin is to be given at the same time as insulin glargine, insulin detemir, or insulin degludec, two separate syringes and injection sites must be used.

Combination Insulins

Various combinations of premixed insulins are available, containing fixed proportions of two different insulins, usually a short- and an intermediate-acting insulin. Typically the intermediate-acting insulin makes up 70–75% of the mixture, with rapid- or short-acting insulin making up the remainder. Onset, peak, and duration vary according to each specific product. Brand names of these products include Humulin 70/30 (70% NPH, 30% regular), Humalog Mix 75/25 (75% insulin lispro protamine suspension and 25% insulin lispro), Humalog Mix 50/50 (50% insulin lispro protamine suspension and 50% insulin lispro), and Novolin 70/30 (70% NPH, 30% regular), or Novolog Mix 70/30 (70% insulin aspart protamine suspension and 30% insulin aspart).

BRAND NAME	GENERIC NAME	TYPE OF INSULIN	ONSET/PEAK/DURATION
Humalog Mix 75/25 Humalog Mix 50/50	insulin lispro protamine suspension & insulin lispro injection mixtures	Combination	15–30 min/2.8 hr/24 hr
Novolog Mix 70/30	insulin aspart protamine suspension & insulin aspart injection mixtures	Combination	15 min/1–4 hr/18–24 hr
Humulin 70/30	NPH/regular insulin mixture	Combination	30 min/2–12 hr/24 hr
Novolin 70/30	NPH/regular insulin mixture	Combination	30 min/2–12 hr/24 hr
Apidra	insulin glulisine	Rapid-Acting	Within 15 min/1–2 hr/3–4 hr
Admelog or Humalog	insulin lispro	Rapid-Acting	Within 15 min/1–2 hr/3–4 hr
Fiasp or Novolog	insulin aspart	Rapid-Acting	Within 15 min/1–2 hr/3–4 hr
Humulin R	regular insulin (subcut)	Short-Acting	½–1 hr/2–4 hr/5–7 hr
Novolin R	regular insulin (subcut)	Short-Acting	½–1 hr/2–4 hr/5–7 hr
Humulin R	regular insulin (IV)	Short-Acting	10–30 min/15–30 min/30–60 min
Novolin R	regular insulin (IV)	Short-Acting	10–30 min/15–30 min/30–60 min
Humulin N	NPH	Intermediate-Acting	2–4 hr/4–10 hr/10–16 hr
Novolin N	NPH	Intermediate-Acting	2–4 hr/4–10 hr/10–16 hr
Levemir	insulin detemir	Long-Acting	3–4 hr/3–14 hr/6–24 hr
Basaglar, Lantus, or Toujeo	insulin glargine	Long-Acting	3–4 hr/No Peak/24 hr
Tresiba	insulin degludec	Long-Acting	Within 2 hr/12 hr/up to 42 hr

APPENDIX M

Differences in U.S. and Canadian Pharmaceutical Practices

In the United States (U.S.) and Canada, most drugs are prescribed and used similarly. However, certain processes and actions of the U.S. and Canadian pharmaceutical industries differ in significant ways, affecting both consumers and health care providers. Safety, marketing, and availability are three of these issues.

Safety

Controversy related to the importation of medications from Canada by U.S. consumers has sometimes raised concerns about the safety of these drugs. These fears are unfounded; in fact, the Canadian approval and manufacturing processes are very similar to U.S. processes. Both countries have pharmaceutical-related standards, laws, and policies to ensure that chemical entities marketed for human diseases and conditions are safe and effective. The process of taking a new drug from the laboratory to the pharmacy shelves includes:

Scientific development. The process begins with research. Scientists develop a new molecular entity targeted at a specific disease, symptom, or condition.

Patenting. A manufacturer applies for a patent, which prevents other drug companies from manufacturing a chemically identical drug. Patent protection lasts 17 years in the U.S. and 20 years in Canada. After a patent expires, any manufacturer can make generic versions of the chemical; generic drugs typically cost much less than the brand-name drugs.

Preclinical testing. Before a drug is taken by human subjects, preclinical testing of the chemical is performed first on animals. Testing helps identify drug action, toxicity effects, side effects, adverse reactions, dosage amounts and routes, and administration procedures. This phase can last anywhere from 3–5 years.

Permission to begin clinical testing. Once a drug is found to have demonstrable positive health effects and is safe for animal consumption, a manufacturer seeks permission to begin clinical studies with human subjects. In the U.S., this process is called New Drug Application (NDA) and is administered by the Food and Drug Administration (FDA). In Canada, the process is referred to as a Clinical Trial Application (CTA) and is administered by Health Canada.

Clinical trials. Clinical trials are initiated to establish the potential benefits and risks for humans. Several sub-phases are required in the clinical trials phase whereby increasingly larger sample sizes are necessary.

Phase 0: A new designation for first-in-human trials, which are designed to assess whether the drug affects humans in a manner that is expected.

Phase 1: Between 20 and 80 healthy volunteers are recruited to assess safety, tolerance, dosage ranges, pharmacokinetics, and pharmacodynamics.

Phase 2: Up to 300 patient volunteers with the drug-targeted disease are enrolled to assess efficacy and toxicity. Variables from Phase I trials may also be assessed.

Phase 3: Between 1000 and 3000 patient volunteers are entered into a randomized, double-blinded study designed to confirm drug effectiveness, comparability with existing treatments, and further exploration of potential and real side effects.

Ongoing surveillance of a drug for rare or long-term effects continues after approval is received and marketing begun.

Approval. The results of the clinical studies are reviewed by Health Canada in Canada and by the FDA in the U.S. These regulatory bodies assess all aspects of a drug, including the labeling. The approval process is often deemed excessively long by physicians and patients who are anxious to try new remedies for refractory or terminal diseases. Efforts are ongoing to shorten the process in both countries. For example, Health Canada is collaborating with the FDA to develop a harmonized system for new drug submissions. A jointly planned Common Electronic Submissions Gateway (CESG) has been developed to allow submissions to be sent to both Canada and the U.S. in a common platform, while the review of these submissions continues to be a separate process.[1]

Marketing. Once a drug has been approved, it can be prescribed to consumers or, if it does not require a prescription, purchased by them.

Postmarketing Surveillance. More clinical data become available when a drug is marketed and used by many people for longer periods of time. Pharmacovigilance is the term used to refer to the process of ongoing assessment of a drug's safety and effectiveness during this phase. In Canada, this includes Adverse Drug Reaction reporting by consumers and health professionals as described in "Detecting and Managing Adverse Drug Reactions."

Differences Between Canadian and U.S. Drug Pricing and Marketing

One major difference between Canadian and U.S drug regulatory processes is pricing. In Canada, the Patented Medicine Prices Review Board (PMPRB) regulates the prices that manufacturers can charge for prescription and nonprescription medicines. This is to ensure that prices are not excessive. No such control exists in the U.S., which is why many citizens purchase their medications from Canadian online pharmacies. One study identified that U.S. citizens can save approximately 24% if they buy their medications from Canadian pharmacies rather than from a U.S. chain pharmacies.[2]

Another difference is in advertising. In the U.S., manufacturers can market drugs directly, and forcefully, to consumers, a controversial privilege that has resulted in consumers requesting specific medications despite not necessarily understanding all of the risks and benefits. In Canada, such advertising is limited and subject to the approval of the Advertising Standards Canada (ASC) agency and the Pharmaceutical Advertising Advisory Board (PAAB). To address this issue in the U.S., the Institute of Medicine (IOM) has recommended that the FDA ban direct-to-consumer advertising during the first 2 years after a drug is marketed. Such a delay may help to prevent large numbers of people experiencing side effects not observed in the clinical trials, such as occurred with sildenafil (Viagra) when several patients died or developed vision problems in the first months after marketing began. Despite the differences in regulation of marketing, it is important to note that the overlap of television and print media between the U.S. and Canada leads to significant inadvertent exposure of the marketing techniques to the Canadian population.

Natural Health Products

In Canada, Natural Health Products (NHPs) are regulated by Health Canada under the Natural Health Products Regulations. All NHPs must have a product license, and the Canadian sites that manufacture, package, label, and import these products must have a site license. A Natural Product Number (NPN) or Homeopathic Medicine Number (DIN-HM) is issued for the product only after it has been reviewed by Health Canada for its safety and efficacy. The term "Natural Product" refers to vitamins and mineral supplements, herbal remedies, traditional and homeopathic medicines, probiotics and other products such as amino acids, enzymes, essential fatty acids, protein supplements, or personal care items for consumption that contain natural ingredients.

In the U.S., the FDA classifies natural products as food products under the Dietary Supplements Health Education Act, so claims about the ability of a supplement to diagnose, prevent, treat or cure a disease is prohibited. It is not necessary, however, for natural products to undergo review or approval, or for testing to be done for identity, purity of active ingredients.

Drug Schedule, Availability, and Pregnancy Category Differences

In Canada, drug schedules are used to classify medication according to accessibility. The Canadian drug schedules as defined by NAPRA (the National Pharmacy Regulatory Authorities) are:

- **Schedule I:** Available only by prescription and provided by a pharmacist.
- **Schedule II:** Available only from a pharmacist; does not require a prescription; must be kept in an area with no public access (i.e. behind-the-counter).
- **Schedule III:** Available via open access in a pharmacy only (i.e. over-the-counter) to guarantee access to a pharmacist; does not require a prescription.
- **Unscheduled:** Can be sold in any store without professional supervision.

Each province and territory in Canada decides where to schedule each individual drug (except narcotics and controlled substances), frequently changing schedules as new evidence is obtained. (note: The province of Québec has not adopted this national model.)

The U.S., in contrast, categorizes medications according to two general classes:

- **Prescription Only:** Available only by prescription and provided by a pharmacist.
- **Over-the-Counter (OTC):** Available via open access in the pharmacy.

As a result of these differences in accessibility some potentially dangerous drugs (such as heparin, insulin, and codeine-containing cough medicines) are available only with a prescription in the U.S. and available without a prescription but in consultation with a pharmacist in Canada. Similarly, some Canadian drugs are available in combinations not found in the U.S. (see Appendix B for new Canadian combination drugs). There can also be significant variation within Canada due to each province and territory independently scheduling drugs, with the exception of narcotics and controlled substances. Other differences also exist with respect to drug availability between the two countries.

SOURCES CITED

1. Rawson, Nigel, S.B. "New Drug Approval Times and Safety Warnings in the United States and Canada, 1992-2011." J Popul Ther Clin Pharmacol Vol 20(2):e67-e81; April 22, 2013.
2. Quon B., Firszt R., Eisenberg M. "A Comparison of Brand-Name Drug Prices Between Canadian-Based Internet Pharmacies and Major U.S. Drug Chain Pharmacies. Ann Intern Med. 143(6):397–403, 2005. http://www.annals.org/cgi/content/abstract/143/6/397 (accessed 10 December 2007).

ADDITIONAL REFERENCES

Canadian Pharmacists Association. "From Research Lab to Pharmacy Shelf." http://people.stfx.ca/ksaulnie/DrugApprovalProcess_Mar2007.pdf (accessed 6 September 2017).

Common Electronic Submissions Gateway. https://www.canada.ca/en/health-canada/services/drugs-health-products/drug-products/applications-submissions/guidance-documents/common-electronic-submissions-gateway.html (accessed 6 September 2017).

Health Canada. https://www.canada.ca/en/health-canada.html (accessed 6 September 2017).

Natural and Non-Prescription Health Products. https://www.canada.ca/en/health-canada/services/drugs-health-products/natural-non-prescription/regulation.html (accessed 6 September 2017).

Tomalin A. "Drugs Used in Pregnancy: The Regulatory Process." Can J Clin Pharmacol. 14(1):e5–e9, 2007. http://www.jptcp.com/articles/drugs-used-in-pregnancy-the-regulatory-process.pdf (accessed 6 September 2017).

U.S. Food and Drug Administration. http://www.fda.gov (accessed 15 December 2007).

APPENDIX N

Routine Pediatric and Adult Immunizations

Immunization recommendations change frequently. For the latest recommendations see http://www.cdc.gov/vaccines/schedules/hcp/index.html.
For Canadian recommendations see the Canadian Immunization Guide (Public Health Agency of Canada) http://www.phac-aspc.gc.ca/publicat/cig-gci/index-eng.php

ROUTINE PEDIATRIC IMMUNIZATIONS (0–18 yr)

GENERIC NAME (BRAND NAMES)	ROUTE/DOSAGE	CONTRAINDICATIONS	ADVERSE REACTIONS/ SIDE EFFECTS	NOTES
Diphtheria toxoid, tetanus toxoid, and acellular pertussis vaccine (DTaP, Daptacel, Infanrix)	0.5 mL IM at 2, 4, 6, 15–18 mo and 4–6 yr (1st dose may be given as early as age 6 wk; 4th dose may be given as early as age 12 mo).	Anaphylactic reaction after a previous dose or to vaccine component; encephalopathy within 7 days of administration of previous dose of Tdap, DTP, or DTaP vaccines.	Crying, ↓ appetite, fever, irritability, malaise, redness, tenderness, vomiting.	Individual components may be given as separate injections if unusual reactions occur. The same product should be used for all doses when possible. Do not give to children ≥7 yr.
Haemophilus b conjugate vaccine (Hib, ActHIB, Hiberix, PedvaxHIB)	*ActHIB or Hiberix*—0.5 mL IM at 2, 4, and 6 mo, with a booster at 12–15 mo (1st dose may be given as early as age 6 wk); *PedvaxHIB*—0.5 mL IM at 2 and 4 mo, with a booster dose at 12–15 mo (1st dose may be given as early as age 6 wk).	Anaphylactic reaction after a previous dose or to vaccine component.	Anorexia, crying, diarrhea, fever, irritability, malaise, tenderness, vomiting, weakness.	If different brands of vaccine are used for 1st and 2nd doses, need to administer 3rd dose followed by a booster after 12 mo. Give only one dose to unvaccinated children 5–18 yr who are at ↑ risk for invasive Hib disease (i.e., HIV, splenectomy, chemotherapy/radiation). Give only one dose to unvaccinated children 15–59 mo.
Hepatitis A vaccine (HepA, Havrix, Vaqta)	0.5 mL IM of pediatric formulation initiated at 12–23 mo, followed by 0.5 mL IM of pediatric formulation *Vaqta* 6–18 mo or *Havrix* 6–12 mo later.	Anaphylactic reaction after a previous dose or to vaccine component.	↓ appetite, drowsiness, fever, headache, irritability, pain at injection site, weakness.	Also recommended in children ≥2 yr who live in areas with high rates of hepatitis A or are in other high-risk groups (e.g., chronic liver disease, clotting factor disorders, illicit drug users, adolescent males who have sex with other males, close personal contact within first 60 days of arrival of international adoptee from country where hepatitis A is endemic).

GENERIC NAME (BRAND NAMES)	ROUTE/DOSAGE	CONTRAINDICATIONS	ADVERSE REACTIONS/ SIDE EFFECTS	NOTES
Hepatitis B vaccine (HepB, Engerix-B, Recombivax HB)	0.5 mL IM within 24 hr of birth, and then at 1–2 mo, and then ≥8 wk after 2nd dose or ≥16 wk after 1st dose (but no earlier than age 24 wk); if mother's HBsAg status is unknown, administer hepatitis B vaccine within 12 hr of birth. *Infants born to HBsAg-positive mothers:* Administer 0.5 mL of hepatitis B immune globulin IM and 1st dose of hepatitis B vaccine within 12 hr of birth; give 2nd and 3rd doses of hepatitis B vaccine at 1–2 mo and then ≥8 wk after 2nd dose or ≥16 wk after 1st dose (but no earlier than age 24 wk), respectively.	Anaphylactic reaction after a previous dose or to vaccine component (including yeast).	Injection site reactions.	A 2-dose series (separated by ≥4 mo) of the adult formulation (Recombivax HB) can be used in children 11–15 yr.
Human papillomavirus vaccine, quadrivalent (HPV4, Gardasil)	0.5 mL IM in males and females age ≥11 yr; if initiated before age 15, give 2 doses (1st dose may be given as early as age 9 yr), with 2nd dose being given 6–12 mo after 1st dose. If initiated at ≥15 yr, give 3 doses, with 2nd and 3rd doses being given at 1–2 mo and 6 mo, respectively after 1st dose.	Anaphylactic reaction after a previous dose or to vaccine component (including yeast).	Diarrhea, dizziness, fever, headache, nausea, pain at injection site, syncope.	Used to prevent cervical, vulvar, and vaginal cancer caused by HPV types 16 and 18 in females and to prevent genital warts caused by HPV types 6 and 11 and anal cancer caused by HPV types 16 and 18 in males and females. HPV series should be completed with same product, when possible.
Human papillomavirus vaccine, 9–valent (HPV9, Gardasil 9)	0.5 mL IM in females age 11–26 yr; if initiated before age 15, give 2 doses (1st dose may be given as early as age 9 yr), with 2nd dose being given 6–12 mo after 1st dose. If initiated at ≥15 yr, give 3 doses, with 2nd and 3rd doses being given at 1–2 mo and 6 mo, respectively after 1st dose.	Anaphylactic reaction after a previous dose or to vaccine component (including yeast).	Dizziness, fever, headache, pain at injection site, syncope.	Used to prevent cervical, vulvar, and vaginal cancer caused by HPV types 16, 18, 31, 33, 45, 52, and 58 in females and to prevent genital warts caused by HPV types 6 and 11 and anal cancer caused by HPV types 16, 18, 31, 33, 45, 52, and 58 in males and females. HPV series should be completed with same product, when possible.
Influenza vaccine (Afluria, Afluria Quadrivalent, Fluarix Quadrivalent, Flucelvax Quadrivalent, FluLaval Quadrivalent, Fluvirin, Fluzone Quadrivalent)	For 2019, infants and children 6 mo to <9 years of age who received at least 2 doses of trivalent or quadrivalent influenza vaccine prior to July 1, 2018 need only 1 dose of the 2019–2020 seasonal influenza vaccine. The 2 doses need not have been received during the same season or consecutive seasons. All other children <9 years of age (including those whose vaccination status cannot be determined) should receive 2 doses separated by ≥4 wk in order to achieve satisfactory antibody response. *Age 6–35 mo:* 1–2 doses (see note above) of 0.25 mL (Fluzone Quadrivalent) or 0.5 mL (FluLaval Quadrivalent) IM. *Age 3–8 yr:* 1–2 doses (see above note) of 0.5 mL IM. *Age ≥9 yr:* 0.5 mL IM single dose annually.	Anaphylactic reaction after a previous dose or to vaccine component, including eggs/egg products and thimerosal (injection only). Avoid use in patients with acute neurologic compromise.	Local soreness, fever, myalgia, possible neurologic toxicity.	Afluria and Afluria Quadrivalent should only be used in children ≥5 yr. Fluarix Quadrivalent should only be used in children ≥3 yr. Flucelvax Quadrivalent and Fluvirin should only be used in children ≥4 yr. FluLaval Quadrivalent and Fluzone Quadrivalent should only be used in children ≥6 mo. If patient experiences anaphylactic reaction to eggs or egg-containing foods, inactivated influenza vaccine should be administered by health care professional with experience in recognition and management of severe allergic conditions and patient should be closely monitored for ≥15 min after vaccination.

GENERIC NAME (BRAND NAMES)	ROUTE/DOSAGE	CONTRAINDICATIONS	ADVERSE REACTIONS/ SIDE EFFECTS	NOTES
Measles, mumps, and rubella vaccine (MMR, M-M-R II)	0.5 mL subcut at 12–15 mo and at 4–6 yr (2nd dose may be given earlier if ≥4 wk have elapsed since the 1st dose).	Anaphylactic reaction after a previous dose or to vaccine component (including, eggs, neomycin, or gelatin); severe immunosuppression (in the absence of severe immunosuppression, HIV is not a contraindication); pregnancy.	Arthralgia, encephalitis, fever, pain at injection site.	If unusual reactions occur, individual components may be given as separate injections. Immunosuppression may ↓ antibody response to injection and ↑ the risk of viral transmission.
Meningococcal conjugate vaccine *Serogroups A, C, W, and Y conjugate vaccines:* (Menactra [MCV4 or MenACWY-D], Menveo [MenACWY-CRM]); *Serogroup B vaccines:* (Bexsero [MenB-4C], Trumenbra [MenB-FHbp])	0.5 mL IM single dose of Menactra or Menveo at 11–12 yr with a booster dose at age 16 yr; single dose can be given at age 13–18 yr if not previously vaccinated (if received 1st dose at age 13–15 yr, should receive booster dose at age 16–18 yr [with an interval of ≥8 wk between doses] if received 1st dose at age ≥16 yr, no booster dose needed). Single dose should be given to previously unvaccinated college freshmen (≤21 yr) living in dormitories. Young adults aged 16–23 yr who are not at ↑ risk for meningococcal disease may be given 2 doses of either Bexsero (give doses ≥1 mo apart) or Trumenba (give doses 6 mo apart).	Anaphylactic reaction after a previous dose or to vaccine component.	Anorexia, arthralgia, diarrhea, fatigue, fever, headache, myalgia, nausea, irritability, malaise, pain at injection site, vomiting.	Routine vaccination with meningococcal vaccine also is recommended for certain children (≥2 mo) who are at high risk (anatomic or functional asplenia; HIV; persistent complement component deficiency; travel or reside in areas in which meningococcal disease is epidemic).
Pneumococcal conjugate vaccine, 13–valent (PCV13, Prevnar 13)	0.5 mL IM at 2, 4, 6, and 12–15 mo.	Anaphylactic reaction after a previous dose or to vaccine component (including diphtheria toxoid).	Arthralgia, chills, ↓ appetite, fatigue, fever, headache, insomnia, irritability, myalgia, pain at injection site, rash.	One dose may also be given to previously unvaccinated healthy children age 24–59 mo. For high-risk children (e.g., sickle cell disease; anatomic or functional asplenia; chronic cardiac, pulmonary, or renal disease; diabetes; HIV; immunosuppression; cerebrospinal fluid leaks; cochlear implant) age 2–5 yr, give 2 doses (≥8 wk apart, with 1st dose being given ≥8 wk after most recent dose) if previously unvaccinated or received <3 doses (if previously received 3 doses, give 1 dose ≥8 wk after most recent dose).
Pneumococcal polysaccharide vaccine (PPSV23, Pneumovax 23)	0.5 mL IM or subcut ≥8 wk after final dose of PCV in high-risk children ≥2 yr (see Notes section for pneumococcal conjugate vaccine for definition of high risk).	Anaphylactic reaction after a previous dose or to vaccine component.	Chills, fever, injection site reactions.	A 2nd dose may be given 5 yr later in children with immunosuppression, sickle cell disease, chronic renal failure, or anatomic/functional asplenia.
Polio vaccine, inactivated (IPV, IPOL)	0.5 mL IM or subcut at 2, 4, and 6–18 mo and at 4–6 yr.	Anaphylactic reaction after a previous dose or to vaccine component (including neomycin, streptomycin, or polymyxin B).	Anorexia, fatigue, fever, Irritability, pain at injection site, vomiting.	Oral polio vaccine (OPV) is no longer recommended for use in the United States.

GENERIC NAME (BRAND NAMES)	ROUTE/DOSAGE	CONTRAINDICATIONS	ADVERSE REACTIONS/ SIDE EFFECTS	NOTES
Rotavirus vaccine (RV, Rotarix [RV1], RotaTeq [RV5])	*Rotarix*—1 mL PO at 2 and 4 mo; *RotaTeq*—2 mL PO at 2, 4, and 6 mo. First dose of either product may be given as early as age 6 wk; final dose should be given no later than age 8 mo.	Anaphylactic reaction after a previous dose or to vaccine component (if allergic to latex, do not use Rotarix); history of uncorrected congenital malformation of GI tract (Rotarix only); history of intussusception; severe combined immunodeficiency disease.	Diarrhea, fever, irritability, vomiting.	Series should not be started in infants ≥15 wk. Series should be completed with same product, when possible. If RotaTeq used in any of the doses, a total of 3 doses should be given.
Tetanus toxoid, **reduced** diphtheria toxoid, and acellular pertussis vaccine absorbed (Tdap, Adacel, Boostrix)	0.5 mL IM given at age 11–12 yr if previously completed DTaP series, then followed by booster doses of Td every 10 yr; one-time dose may be given if age ≥7 yr if did not previously complete DTaP series; one-time dose (in place of single Td booster) may be given to all adolescents who have not received previous Tdap at age 11 or 12.	Anaphylactic reaction after a previous dose or to vaccine component; encephalopathy within 7 days of administration of previous dose of Tdap, DTP, or DTaP vaccines.	Abdominal pain, arthralgia, chills, diarrhea, fatigue, headache, myalgia, nausea, pain at injection site, vomiting.	Should also be given to pregnant adolescents during each pregnancy (preferably during 27–36 wk gestation) regardless of interval since prior Td or Tdap.
Varicella vaccine (Var, Varivax)	0.5 mL subcut at 12–15 mo and at 4–6 yr (2nd dose may be given earlier if ≥3 mo have elapsed since the 1st dose); for persons 7–18 yr who do not have evidence of immunity, 2 doses should be given (≥3 mo apart if 7–12 yr or ≥4 wk apart if ≥13 yr).	Anaphylactic reaction after a previous dose or to vaccine component (including gelatin or neomycin); severe immunosuppression (in the absence of severe immunosuppression, HIV is not a contraindication); pregnancy.	Anorexia, chills, diarrhea, fatigue, fever, headache, injection site reaction, irritability, nausea, vomiting.	Immunosuppression may ↓ antibody response to injection and ↑ the risk of viral transmission.

Nursing Implications:

Assessment

Assess previous immunization history and history of hypersensitivity.

Assess for history of latex allergy. Some prefilled syringes may use latex components and should be avoided in those with hypersensitivity.

Implementation

Measles, mumps, and rubella vaccine and diphtheria toxoid, tetanus toxoid, and pertussis vaccine may be given concomitantly.

Administer each immunization by appropriate route:

PO: Rotavirus.

Subcut: measles, mumps, rubella, polio, varicella, pneumococcal polysaccharide.

IM: diphtheria, tetanus toxoid, pertussis, polio, Haemophilus b, hepatitis B, meningococcal conjugate, hepatitis A, pneumococcal conjugate, pneumococcal polysaccharide, influenza injection, human papillomavirus.

Patient/Family Teaching

Inform parent of potential and reportable side effects of immunization. Notify health care professional if patient develops fever higher than 39.4° C (103° F); difficulty breathing; hives; itching; swelling of eyes, face, or inside of nose; sudden, severe tiredness or weakness; or convulsions.

Review next scheduled immunization with parent.

Evaluation

Prevention of diseases through active immunity.

ROUTINE ADULT IMMUNIZATIONS

GENERIC NAME (BRAND NAMES)	INDICATIONS	DOSAGE/ROUTE	CONTRAINDICATIONS	ADVERSE REACTIONS/ SIDE EFFECTS
Hepatitis A vaccine (HepA, Havrix, Vaqta)	High-risk groups (e.g., chronic liver disease, receive clotting factor concentrates, users of injection/non-injection illicit drugs, men who have sex with men, working with infected primates or with hepatitis A virus in a research laboratory setting); travel to endemic areas; unvaccinated individuals who anticipate close personal contact with an international adoptee during the initial 60 days after their arrival in the U.S. from a country with intermediate or high endemicity.	1 mL IM, followed by 1 mL IM 6–12 mo (for Havrix) or 6–18 mo (for Vaqta) later.	Anaphylactic reaction after a previous dose or to vaccine component.	↓ appetite, drowsiness, fever, injection site reactions, irritability, headache.
Hepatitis B vaccine (HepB, Engerix-B, Recombivax HB)	High-risk patients (e.g., household contacts or sex partners of persons with chronic hepatitis B virus infection, injection drug users, sexually active persons not in a long-term monogamous relationship [having >1 sex partner in past 6 mo], men who have sex with men, HIV, STDs, end-stage renal disease, hemodialysis, health care workers, chronic liver disease; clients and staff of institutions for those with developmental disabilities; adults in STD treatment facilities, HIV testing/treatment facilities, drug abuse prevention/treatment facilities, facilities providing services to injection drug users or men who have sex with men, correctional facilities, end-stage renal disease programs, hemodialysis facilities, or facilities for those with developmental disabilities); travel to endemic areas; unvaccinated adults (19–59 yr) with diabetes (may also be administered at prescriber's discretion to adults ≥60 yr with diabetes).	Immunocompetent: 1 mL IM, given at 0, 1 and 6 mo. Immunosuppressed: 1 mL (Recombivax HB) or 2 mL (Engerix-B) IM at 0, 1, and 6 mo.	Anaphylactic reaction after a previous dose or to vaccine component.	Injection site reactions.
Human papillomavirus vaccine, quadrivalent (HPV4, Gardasil)	All previously unvaccinated females (through age 26) and males (through age 21 yr). Males age 22–26 yr may be vaccinated if they have sex with other men or are immunocompromised.	0.5 mL IM, repeat at 1–2 and 6 mo after initial dose.	Anaphylactic reaction after a previous dose or to vaccine component; pregnancy.	Dizziness, fever, headache, injection site reactions, syncope.
Human papillomavirus vaccine, 9–valent (HPV9, Gardasil 9)	All previously unvaccinated females (through age 26) and males (through age 21 yr). Males age 22–26 yr may be vaccinated if they have sex with other men or are immunocompromised.	0.5 mL IM, repeat at 1–2 and 6 mo after initial dose.	Anaphylactic reaction after a previous dose or to vaccine component (including yeast); pregnancy.	Dizziness, fever, headache, pain at injection site, syncope.

GENERIC NAME (BRAND NAMES)	INDICATIONS	DOSAGE/ROUTE	CONTRAINDICATIONS	ADVERSE REACTIONS/ SIDE EFFECTS
Influenza vaccine *Injection (inactivated):* (Afluria, Afluria Quadrivalent, Fluarix Quadrivalent, Flucelvax Quadrivalent, FluLaval Quadrivalent, Fluvirin, Fluzone Quadrivalent)	All adults.	0.5 mL IM annually.	If patient experiences anaphylactic reaction to eggs or egg-containing foods, inactivated influenza vaccine should be administered by health care professional with experience in recognition and management of severe allergic conditions and patient should be closely monitored for ≥15 min after vaccination.	Fever, injection site reactions, myalgia.
Measles, mumps, and rubella vaccine (MMR, M-M-R II)	Adults born in or after 1957 with unreliable documentation of previous vaccination (unless have laboratory evidence of immunity to all 3 diseases); health care workers born before 1957 who do not have laboratory evidence of immunity to measles, mumps, or rubella.	Adults born in or after 1957 with unreliable history: 1 or 2 doses of 0.5 mL subcut (with ≥28 days between doses); high-risk groups should receive a total of 2 doses (with ≥28 days between doses).	Allergy to egg, gelatin, or neomycin; severe immunosuppression (in the absence of severe immunosuppression, HIV is not a contraindication); pregnancy (also avoid becoming pregnant for 4 wk after immunization).	Burning, stinging, pain at injection site; arthritis/arthralgia; fever; encephalitis; allergic reactions. Immunosuppression may ↓ antibody response to injection and ↑ the risk of viral transmission (live vaccine).
Meningococcal conjugate vaccine *Serogroups A, C, W, and Y conjugate vaccines:* (Menactra [MCV4 or MenACWY-D], Menveo [MenACWY-CRM]); *Serogroup B vaccines:* (Bexsero [MenB-4C], Trumenbra [MenB-FHbp])	College freshmen (up to age 21) living in dormitories if they have not previously received a dose on or after their 16th birthday; military recruits; anatomic or functional asplenia; HIV; persistent complement component deficiency; travel or reside in areas in which meningococcal disease is hyperendemic or epidemic; persons at risk during an outbreak due to a vaccine serogroup.	Age ≤55 yr: 0.5 mL IM single dose; Age ≤55 yr with anatomic or functional asplenia, persistent complement component deficiency, or HIV: 0.5 mL IM, repeat at least 2 mo after initial dose. Revaccination with MenACWY every 5 yr is indicated in patients previously vaccinated with MenACWY and who also remain at ↑ risk for infection; patients with functional asplenia or persistent complement component deficiency or those at risk because of a serogroup B meningococcal outbreak should also receive 2 doses of MenB-4C ≥1 mo apart or 3 doses of MenB-FHbp with the 2nd and 3rd doses being given 1–2 mo and 6 mo, respectively, after the 1st dose; MenACWY is preferred for adults ≥56 yr who previously received MenACWY and need to be revaccinated or for whom multiple doses are needed.	Anaphylactic reaction after a previous dose or to vaccine component.	Anorexia, arthralgia, diarrhea, fatigue, fever, headache, myalgia, nausea, irritability, malaise, pain at injection site, vomiting.
Pneumococcal conjugate vaccine, 13–valent (PCV13, Prevnar 13)	All adults ≥65 yr; adults ≤64 yr with chronic renal failure, anatomic or functional asplenia, sickle cell disease, cerebrospinal fluid leaks, cochlear implants, or immunosuppression (including HIV).	Adults ≥65 yr: 0.5 mL IM single dose followed by single dose of PPSV23 ≥1 yr later; if already received PPSV23, give PCV13 single dose (0.5 mL IM) ≥1 yr after dose of PPSV23. Adults ≥19 yr with specified medical conditions (under Indications column): 0.5 mL IM single dose followed by single dose of PPSV23 ≥8 wk later; if already received PPSV23, give PCV13 single dose (0.5 mL IM) ≥1 yr after dose of PPSV23.	Anaphylactic reaction after a previous dose or to vaccine component including diphtheria toxoid.	Arthralgia, chills, ↓ appetite, fatigue, fever, headache, insomnia, irritability, myalgia, pain at injection site, rash.

GENERIC NAME (BRAND NAMES)	INDICATIONS	DOSAGE/ROUTE	CONTRAINDICATIONS	ADVERSE REACTIONS/ SIDE EFFECTS
Pneumococcal polysaccharide vaccine (PPSV23, Pneumovax 23)	All adults ≥65 yr; high-risk adults ≤64 yr (e.g., chronic cardiac [excluding hypertension] or pulmonary disease [including COPD and asthma], chronic liver disease, alcoholism, diabetes, cigarette smoker, anatomic or functional asplenia, sickle cell disease; immunosuppression (including HIV), chronic renal failure, cochlear implants, cerebrospinal fluid leaks).	0.5 mL IM or subcut; one-time revaccination should also be given ≥5 yr after 1st dose to those ≥65 yr (if 1st dose was given ≥5 yr ago and before age 65) and to high-risk patients age 19–64 yr (chronic renal failure, anatomic or functional asplenia, sickle cell disease, immunosuppression) ≥5 yr after 1st dose (if the most recent dose of PPSV23 was administered before age 65 yr, at age ≥65 yr, give another dose of PPSV23 ≥8 wk after PCV13 and ≥5 yr after the most recent dose of PPSV23).	Anaphylactic reaction after a previous dose or to vaccine component.	Chills, fever, injection site reactions.
Tetanus toxoid, **reduced** diphtheria toxoid and acellular pertussis vaccine absorbed (Tdap, Adacel, Boostrix)	Single dose should be given to replace one of the 10-yr Td boosters in all adults who did not previously receive a dose of Tdap or if their vaccine status is unknown. Single dose should also be given as soon as feasible to all pregnant women (preferred during 27–36 wks' gestation), close contacts of infants <12 mo, and health care workers with direct patient contact.	0.5 mL IM single dose.	Anaphylactic reaction after a previous dose or to vaccine component; encephalopathy within 7 days of administration of previous dose of Tdap, DTP, or DTaP vaccines.	Abdominal pain, arthralgia, chills, diarrhea, fatigue, headache, myalgia, nausea, pain at injection site, vomiting.
Tetanus-diphtheria (Td, Tenivac)	All adults who lack written documentation of a primary series consisting of ≥3 doses of tetanus– and diphtheria–toxoid-containing vaccine; booster dose should be given to all adults every 10 yr (see info above regarding use of Tdap to replace one dose of Td in booster series).	*Unimmunized:* 2 doses of 0.5 mL IM ≥4 wk apart, then a 3rd dose 6–12 mo later; *Immunized:* 0.5 mL IM booster every 10 yr.	Anaphylactic reaction after a previous dose or to vaccine component.	Arthralgia, chills, diarrhea, fatigue, headache, myalgia, nausea, pain at injection site.
Varicella vaccine (Var, Varivax)	Any adult without a history of chickenpox or herpes zoster (shingles), without a history of receiving 2 doses of varicella vaccine ≥4 wk apart, or without laboratory evidence of immunity. Health care workers and pregnant women born in U.S. before 1980 who do not meet the above criteria should be tested for immunity.	0.5 mL subcut; repeated 4–8 wk later.	Anaphylactic reaction after a previous dose or to vaccine component (including gelatin or neomycin); severe immunosuppression (in the absence of severe immunosuppression, HIV is not a contraindication); pregnancy (also avoid becoming pregnant for 4 wk after immunization).	Fever, pain at injection site. Immunosuppression may ↓ antibody response to injection and ↑ the risk of viral transmission (live vaccine).
Zoster vaccine (Shingrix, Zos, Zostavax)	All adults ≥50 yr (regardless of previous history of chickenpox or herpes zoster).	(Shingrix 2 doses, 0.5 mL IM each, 2nd dose 2–6 mo after first dose. Zostavax 0.65 mL subcut single dose.)	Anaphylactic reaction after a previous dose or to vaccine component (including gelatin or neomycin); severe immunosuppression (in the absence of severe immunosuppression, HIV is not a contraindication); pregnancy (also avoid becoming pregnant for 4 wk after immunization).	Fever, pain at injection site. Immunosuppression may ↓ antibody response to injection and ↑ the risk of viral transmission (live vaccine).

SOURCE: Adapted from the recommendations of the Department of Health and Human Services, Centers for Disease Control and Prevention: http://www.cdc.gov/vaccines/schedules/hcp/index.html.

BIBLIOGRAPHY

American Pain Society: Principles of Analgesic Use, 7th ed. American Pain Society, Skokie, IL, 2016.

American Society of Health-System Pharmacists: Handbook on Injectable Drugs, 16th ed. American Society of Health-System Pharmacists, Bethesda, MD, 2016.

Blumenthal, M, et al: The Complete German Commission E Monographs: Therapeutic Guide to Herbal Medicines. Integrative Medical Communications, Boston, 1998.

DRUGDEX® System [intranet database]. Version 5.1. Greenwood Village, Colo: Thomson Healthcare.

Facts and Comparisons. Wolters Kluwer Clinical Drug Information, Inc., Hudson, Ohio.

Fetrow, CW, and Avila, JR: Professional's Handbook of Complementary & Alternative Medicines, ed. 3. Lippincott Williams & Wilkins, Philadelphia, PA, 2004.

Kemp, SF, and deShazo, RD: Prevention and treatment of anaphylaxis. Clin Allergy Immunol 2008;21:477–498.

Kuhn, MA, and Winston, D: Herbal Therapy and Supplements: A Scientific and Traditional Approach. 2nd ed. Lippincott Williams & Wilkins, Philadelphia, 2007.

Lexi-Comp, Inc: (Lexi-Drugs [Comp + Specialties]). Lexi-Comp, Inc., Hudson, Ohio.

MICROMEDEX® 2.0 and MICROMEDEX® 1.0 (Healthcare Series).

National Institutes of Health Office of Dietary Supplements. Vitamin and Mineral Fact Sheets, Bethesda, MD. https://ods.od.nih.gov/factsheets/list-VitaminsMinerals.

National Kidney Foundation: A-Z Guide for High Potassium Foods, National Kidney Foundation. https://www.kidney.org/atoz/content/potassium.

PDR for Herbal Medicines, ed 4. Thomson Healthcare, New York, NY, 2011.

Pennington, JAT, and Spungen, J: Bowes and Church's Food Values of Portions Commonly Used, 19th ed. Philadelphia: Lippincott Williams & Wilkins, 2009.

Phelps, SJ, Hagemann, TM, Lee, KR, and Thompson, AJ: Pediatric Injectable Drugs, 10th ed. American Society of Health-System Pharmacists, Bethesda, MD, 2013.

Polovich, M, Olsen, M, and Lefebvre, K: Chemotherapy and Biotherapy Guidelines and Recommendations for Practice, 4th ed. Oncology Nursing Society, Pittsburgh, PA, 2014.

Taketomo, CK, Hodding, JH, and Kraus, DM: Pediatric Dosage Handbook, 21st. Lexi-Comp, Hudson, Ohio, 2014.

Van Leeuwen, AM, and Bladh, ML: Davis's Comprehensive Handbook of Laboratory and Diagnostic Tests with Nursing Implications, 7th ed. FA Davis Company, Philadelphia, PA, 2017.

https://www.fda.gov/drugs.

http://www.accessdata.fda.gov/scripts/cder/drugsatfda/.

COMPREHENSIVE INDEX*

*Entries for **generic** names appear in **boldface type.** Trade names appear in regular type, with Canadian names preceded by a maple leaf icon (🍁). **CLASSIFICATIONS** appear in **BOLDFACE SMALL CAPS.** *Combination Drugs* appear in *italics,* herbal products are preceded by a yin-yang icon (☯), and drugs with genetic implications are preceded by a double-helix icon (🧬).

*Entries for **generic** names appear in **boldface type.** Trade names appear in regular type, with Canadian names preceded by a maple leaf icon (🍁). **CLASSIFICATIONS** appear in **BOLDFACE SMALL CAPS.** *Combination Drugs* appear in *italics,* herbal products are preceded by a yin-yang icon (☯), and drugs with genetic implications are preceded by a double-helix icon (🧬).

*Entries for **generic** names appear in **boldface type**. Trade names appear in regular type, with Canadian names preceded by a maple leaf icon (🍁). CLASSIFICATIONS appear in BOLDFACE SMALL CAPS. *Combination Drugs* appear in *italics*, herbal products are preceded by a yin-yang icon (☯), and drugs with genetic implications are preceded by a double-helix icon (🧬).

COMPREHENSIVE INDEX

*Entries for **generic** names appear in **boldface type.** Trade names appear in regular type, with Canadian names preceded by a maple leaf icon (🍁). **CLASSIFICATIONS** appear in **BOLDFACE SMALL CAPS.** *Combination Drugs* appear in *italics,* herbal products are preceded by a yin-yang icon (☯), and drugs with genetic implications are preceded by a double-helix icon (🧬).

*Entries for **generic** names appear in **boldface type.** Trade names appear in regular type, with Canadian names preceded by a maple leaf icon (🍁). **CLASSIFICATIONS** appear in **BOLDFACE SMALL CAPS.** *Combination Drugs* appear in *italics,* herbal products are preceded by a yin-yang icon (☯), and drugs with genetic implications are preceded by a double-helix icon (🧬).

*Entries for **generic** names appear in **boldface type.** Trade names appear in regular type, with Canadian names preceded by a maple leaf icon (🍁). **CLASSIFICATIONS** appear in **BOLDFACE SMALL CAPS.** *Combination Drugs* appear in *italics,* herbal products are preceded by a yin-yang icon (☯), and drugs with genetic implications are preceded by a double-helix icon (🧬).

*Entries for **generic** names appear in **boldface type.** Trade names appear in regular type, with Canadian names preceded by a maple leaf icon ( ). **CLASSIFICATIONS** appear in **BOLDFACE SMALL CAPS.** *Combination Drugs* appear in *italics,* herbal products are preceded by a yin-yang icon ( ), and drugs with genetic implications are preceded by a double-helix icon ( ).

*Entries for **generic** names appear in **boldface type.** Trade names appear in regular type, with Canadian names preceded by a maple leaf icon (🍁). **CLASSIFICATIONS** appear in **BOLDFACE SMALL CAPS.** *Combination Drugs* appear in *italics,* herbal products are preceded by a yin-yang icon (☯), and drugs with genetic implications are preceded by a double-helix icon (🧬).

E

*Entries for **generic** names appear in **boldface type.** Trade names appear in regular type, with Canadian names preceded by a maple leaf icon (🍁). **CLASSIFICATIONS** appear in **BOLDFACE SMALL CAPS.** *Combination Drugs* appear in *italics,* herbal products are preceded by a yin-yang icon (☯), and drugs with genetic implications are preceded by a double-helix icon (🧬).

F

*Entries for **generic** names appear in **boldface type.** Trade names appear in regular type, with Canadian names preceded by a maple leaf icon. **CLASSIFICATIONS** appear in **BOLDFACE SMALL CAPS.** *Combination Drugs* appear in *italics,* herbal products are preceded by a yin-yang icon, and drugs with genetic implications are preceded by a double-helix icon.

*Entries for **generic** names appear in **boldface type.** Trade names appear in regular type, with Canadian names preceded by a maple leaf icon ( ). **CLASSIFICATIONS** appear in **BOLDFACE SMALL CAPS.** *Combination Drugs* appear in *italics,* herbal products are preceded by a yin-yang icon ( ), and drugs with genetic implications are preceded by a double-helix icon ( ).

*Entries for **generic** names appear in **boldface type.** Trade names appear in regular type, with Canadian names preceded by a maple leaf icon (🍁). CLASSIFICATIONS appear in BOLDFACE SMALL CAPS. *Combination Drugs* appear in *italics,* herbal products are preceded by a yin-yang icon (☯), and drugs with genetic implications are preceded by a double-helix icon (🧬).

*Entries for **generic** names appear in **boldface type.** Trade names appear in regular type, with Canadian names preceded by a maple leaf icon. **CLASSIFICATIONS** appear in **BOLDFACE SMALL CAPS.** *Combination Drugs* appear in *italics*, herbal products are preceded by a yin-yang icon, and drugs with genetic implications are preceded by a double-helix icon.

COMPREHENSIVE INDEX

*Entries for **generic** names appear in **boldface type.** Trade names appear in regular type, with Canadian names preceded by a maple leaf icon (🍁). **CLASSIFICATIONS** appear in **BOLDFACE SMALL CAPS.** *Combination Drugs* appear in *italics,* herbal products are preceded by a yin-yang icon (☯), and drugs with genetic implications are preceded by a double-helix icon (🧬).

COMPREHENSIVE INDEX

*Entries for **generic** names appear in **boldface type.** Trade names appear in regular type, with Canadian names preceded by a maple leaf icon (🍁). **CLASSIFICATIONS** appear in **BOLDFACE SMALL CAPS.** *Combination Drugs* appear in *italics,* herbal products are preceded by a yin-yang icon (☯), and drugs with genetic implications are preceded by a double-helix icon (🧬).

*Entries for **generic** names appear in **boldface type.** Trade names appear in regular type, with Canadian names preceded by a maple leaf icon (🍁). **CLASSIFICATIONS** appear in **BOLDFACE SMALL CAPS.** *Combination Drugs* appear in *italics,* herbal products are preceded by a yin-yang icon (☯), and drugs with genetic implications are preceded by a double-helix icon (🧬).

P

*Entries for **generic** names appear in **boldface type.** Trade names appear in regular type, with Canadian names preceded by a maple leaf icon (). **CLASSIFICATIONS** appear in **BOLDFACE SMALL CAPS.** *Combination Drugs* appear in *italics,* herbal products are preceded by a yin-yang icon (), and drugs with genetic implications are preceded by a double-helix icon ().

*Entries for **generic** names appear in **boldface type.** Trade names appear in regular type, with Canadian names preceded by a maple leaf icon (🍁). **CLASSIFICATIONS** appear in **BOLDFACE SMALL CAPS.** *Combination Drugs* appear in *italics,* herbal products are preceded by a yin-yang icon (☯), and drugs with genetic implications are preceded by a double-helix icon (🧬).

*Entries for **generic** names appear in **boldface type.** Trade names appear in regular type, with Canadian names preceded by a maple leaf icon (🍁). **CLASSIFICATIONS** appear in **BOLDFACE SMALL CAPS.** *Combination Drugs* appear in *italics,* herbal products are preceded by a yin-yang icon (☯), and drugs with genetic implications are preceded by a double-helix icon (🧬).

*Entries for **generic** names appear in **boldface type.** Trade names appear in regular type, with Canadian names preceded by a maple leaf icon (🍁). CLASSIFICATIONS appear in **BOLDFACE SMALL CAPS.** *Combination Drugs* appear in *italics*, herbal products are preceded by a yin-yang icon (☯), and drugs with genetic implications are preceded by a double-helix icon (🧬).

*Entries for **generic** names appear in **boldface type.** Trade names appear in regular type, with Canadian names preceded by a maple leaf icon. **CLASSIFICATIONS** appear in **BOLDFACE SMALL CAPS.** *Combination Drugs* appear in *italics,* herbal products are preceded by a yin-yang icon, and drugs with genetic implications are preceded by a double-helix icon.

*Entries for **generic** names appear in **boldface type.** Trade names appear in regular type, with Canadian names preceded by a maple leaf icon ( ). **CLASSIFICATIONS** appear in **BOLDFACE SMALL CAPS.** *Combination Drugs* appear in *italics,* herbal products are preceded by a yin-yang icon ( ), and drugs with genetic implications are preceded by a double-helix icon ( ).

Measurement Conversion Table

Metric System Equivalents

1 gram (g) = 1000 milligrams (mg)
1000 grams = 1 kilogram (kg)
0.001 milligram = 1 microgram (mcg)
1 liter (L) = 1000 milliliters (ml)
1 milliliter = 1 cubic centimeter (cc)
1 meter = 100 centimeters (cm)
1 meter = 1000 millimeters (mm)

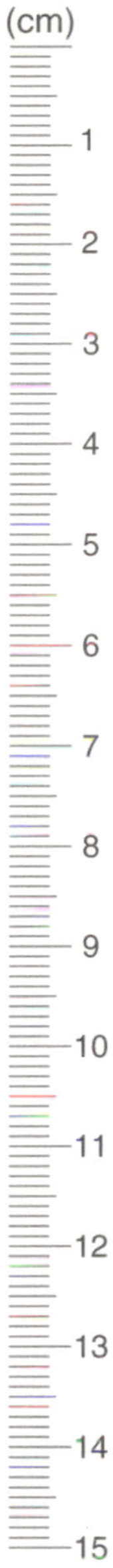

Conversion Equivalents

Volume

1 milliliter = 15 minims (M) = 15 drops (gtt)

5 milliliters = 1 fluidram = 1 teaspoon (tsp)

15 milliliters = 4 fluidrams = 1 tablespoon (T)

30 milliliters = 1 ounce (oz) = 2 tablespoons

480 milliliters = 1 pint (pt)

960 milliliters = 1 quart (qt)

Weight

1 kilogram = 2.2 pounds (lb)
1 gram (g) = 1000 milligrams
0.6 gram = 600 milligrams
0.5 gram = 500 milligrams
0.325 gram = 325 milligrams = 5 grains (gr)
0.065 gram = 65 milligrams = 1 grain

Length

2.5 centimeters = 1 inch

Centigrade/Fahrenheit Conversions

$C = (F - 32) \times {}^{5}/_{9}$
$F = (C \times {}^{9}/_{5}) + 32$

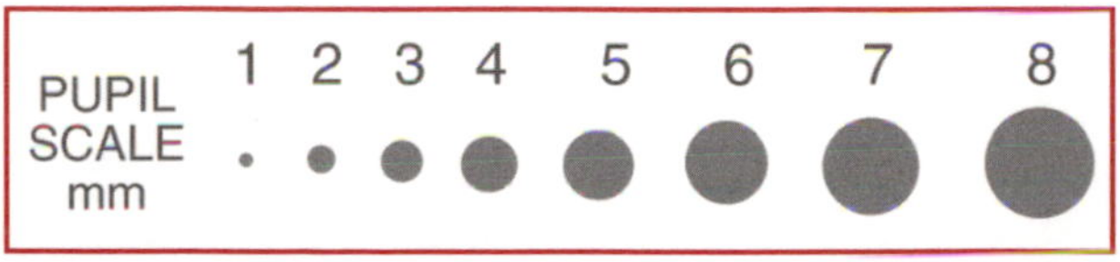